AIDS Therapy

Commissioning Editor: Karen Bowler, Thu Nguyen
Development Editor: Karen Carter
Project Manager: Cheryl Brant, Naughton Project Management
Design: Gene Harris
Illustration Manager: Karen Giacomucci
Illustrator: Beach Studios, Inc.

AIDS Therapy

Third Edition

Raphael Dolin MD

Maxwell Finland Professor of Medicine (Microbiology and Molecular Genetics)
Dean for Academic and Clinical Programs
Harvard Medical School
Boston, Massachusetts, USA

Henry Masur MD

Chief, Critical Care Medicine Department
The NIH Clinical Center
National Institutes of Health
Bethesda, Maryland, USA

Michael Saag MD

Professor of Medicine
Director, Division of Infectious Disease and
The William C Gorgas Center for International Health
Director, Center for AIDS Research
University of Alabama at Birmingham
Birmingham, Alabama, USA

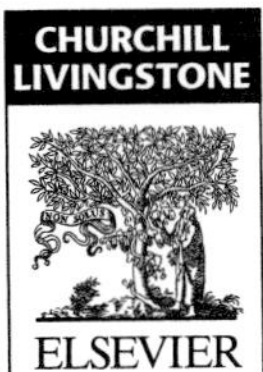

CHURCHILL
LIVINGSTONE
ELSEVIER

CHURCHILL LIVINGSTONE
An imprint of Elsevier Inc

First edition © 1999
Second edition © 2002
Third edition © 2008

ISBN: 978-0-443-06752-5

British Library Cataloguing in Publication Data
A catalogue record for this book is available from the British Library

Library of Congress Cataloging in Publication Data
A catalog record for this book is available from the Library of Congress

Notice
Medical knowledge is constantly changing. Standard safety precautions must be followed, but as new research and clinical experience broaden our knowledge, changes in treatment and drug therapy may become necessary or appropriate. Readers are advised to check the most current product information provided by the manufacturer of each drug to be administered to verify the recommended dose, the method and duration of administration, and contraindications. It is the responsibility of the practitioner, relying on experience and knowledge of the patient, to determine dosages and the best treatment for each individual patient. Neither the Publisher nor the author assume any liability for any injury and/or damage to persons or property arising from this publication.

The Publisher

Printed in Canada
Last digit is the print number: 9 8 7 6 5 4 3 2 1

Contents

Section VIII Approach to Specific Syndromes

Section IX Drug Administration and Interactions

Section X HIV/AIDS-Related Internet Resources

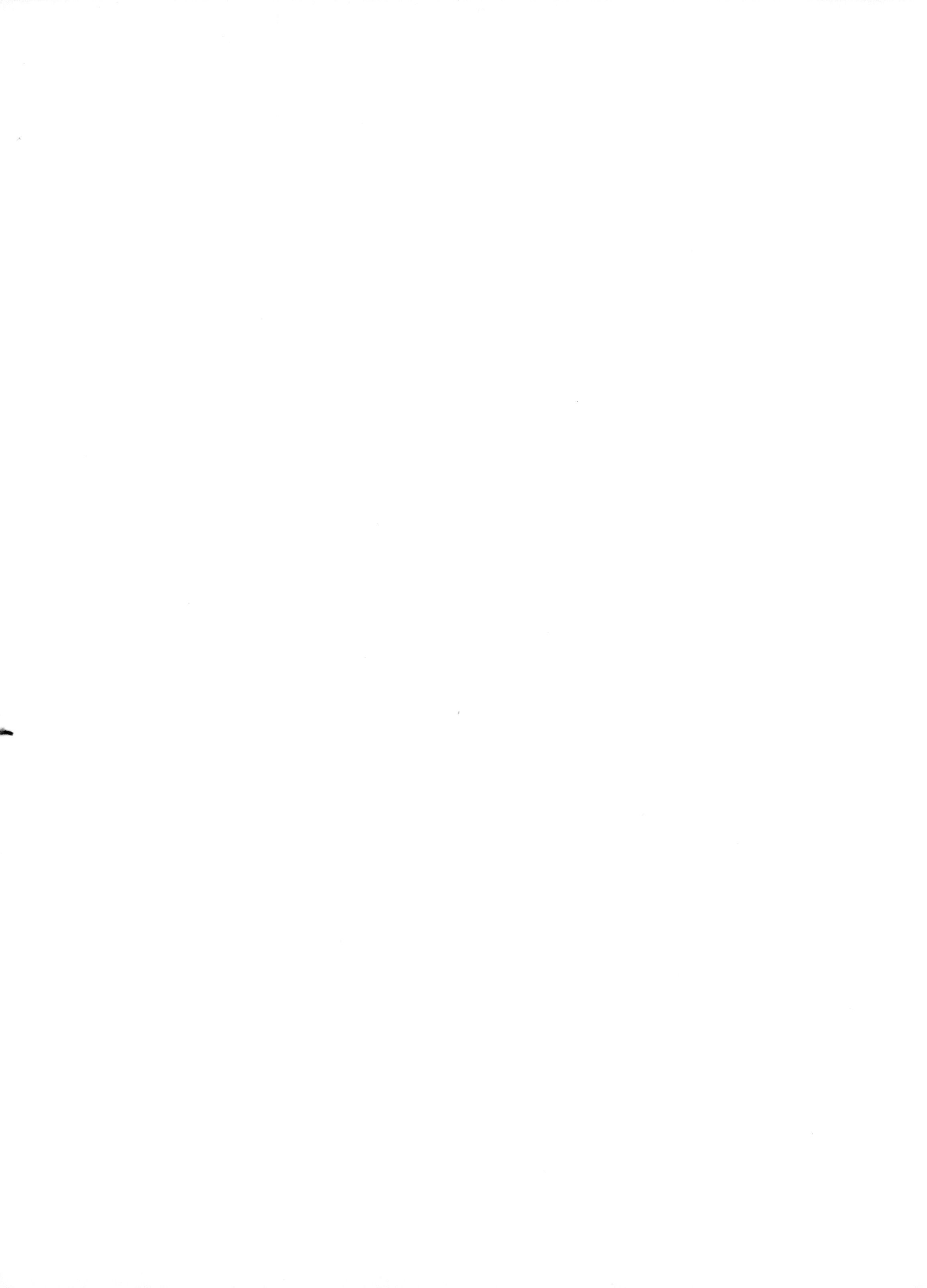

Preface

The first 25 years of the AIDS pandemic have witnessed considerable changes in the management of infected patients. As understanding of pathogenesis has improved, and as new diagnostic, therapeutic, and preventive tools have expanded, the management of patients with HIV infection has become dramatically more successful, but dramatically more complex. There are now over 25 different antiretroviral drugs and countless numbers of potential drug combinations, with even more novel classes of antiretroviral drugs likely to be approved in the near future. How to use these drugs, how to avoid drug–drug interactions, and how to manage their adverse effects requires eminently more knowledge than was necessary a decade ago. Thus, this third edition of *AIDS Therapy* has new chapters dealing with metabolic and cardiovascular issues as well as chapters on drugs that were not available when the second edition was published.

During the past several years it has also become clear that the management of HIV/AIDS differs considerably in different geographical regions of the world. This book is focused primarily on management of patients in North America, Western Europe, Japan, and Australia. Yet, we have included a specific chapter on differences in patient populations in developing countries. Our hope is that by the time the 4th Edition of this book is published, there will be very little distinction between the treatment of patients regardless of what area of the world they reside in.

This book has in depth information about managing patients. While the field of HIV/AIDS changes so rapidly that internet resources are needed to keep current with important developments, we feel strongly that there is a real need for a text book that focuses in depth on important issues about drug efficacy, safety, and about strategies for managing different syndromes. In essence, a 'one-stop' resource for busy clinicians working in busy practice settings.

Writing concise, accurate, and organized chapters is a time consuming undertaking. We thank the international experts who have contributed to this edition, which should continue to expand the impact of this book in North America, Europe, and beyond. We also thank Erin Cromack and Lisa Ruprecht for their assistance in making this edition possible and Karen Carter for producing a well organized and readable product. We also would like to thank our families, in particular our wives Kelly, Grace, and Amy, who put up with our late night reviews of chapters and time away from home as the Third Edition came together. And finally, we would like to acknowledge our colleagues, from whom we derive tremendous stimulation and support, and our patients, who motivate us to strive for excellence and who serve as a constant source of inspiration as they struggle to live full and complete lives while dealing with the horror of this pandemic plague.

List of Contributors

Judith A Aberg MD
Principal Investigator, AIDS Clinical Trials Unit
Director of Virology, Bellevue Hospital Center
Associate Professor of Medicine
New York University School of Medicine
New York, NY, USA

Donald I Abrams MD
Chief, Hematology-Oncology
San Francisco General Hospital
Director of Clinical Programs
UCSF Osher Center for Integrative Medicine
Professor of Clinical Medicine
University of California San Francisco
San Francisco, CA, USA

Val K Amorosa MD
Assistant Professor of Clinical Medicine
Department of Medicine, School of Medicine
University of Pennsylvania
Philadelphia, PA, USA

Neil M Ampel MD
Professor of Medicine
University of Arizona
Staff Physician
Southern Arizona VA Health Care System
Tucson, AZ, USA

Andrew F Angelino MD, DFAPA
Assistant Professor
Department of Psychiatry and Behavioral Sciences
Johns Hopkins University School of Medicine
Clinical Director
Department of Psychiatry
Johns Hopkins Bayview Medical Center
Baltimore, MD, USA

Roberto Badaró MD, PhD
Professor of Infectious Diseases
Federal University of Bahia, Brazil
Visiting Research Professor
Department of Medicine
University of California San Diego
La Jolla, CA, USA

Dan H Barouch MD, PhD
Associate Professor of Medicine
Harvard Medical School
Division of Viral Pathogenesis
Department of Medicine
Beth Israel Deaconess Medical Center
Boston, MA, USA

John A Bartlett MD
Professor of Medicine
Division of Infectious Diseases/Department of Medicine
Duke University Medical Center
Durham, NC, USA
Professor of Medicine
Kilimanjaro Christian Medical Centre
Moshi, Tanzania

Constance A Benson, MD
Professor of Medicine and Infectious Diseases
Division of Infectious Diseases
Director, Antiviral Research Center
University of California, San Diego School of Medicine
La Jolla, CA, USA

Ruth E Berggren MD
Associate Professor of Medicine
Division of Infectious Diseases
University of Texas Health Science Center-San Antonio
San Antonio, TX, USA

William Bonnez MD
Associate Professor of Medicine
University of Rochester School of Medicine
Infectious Disease Unit
Rochester, NY, USA

Charles A B Boucher MD
Professor of Virology
Coordinator Unite More Program
Eijkman-Winkler Institute
University Medical Centre
Utrecht, The Netherlands

Bernard M Branson, MD
Associate Director for Laboratory Diagnostics
Centers for Disease Control and Prevention
National Center for HIV/AIDS, Viral Hepatitis, STD and TB Prevention
Division of HIV/AIDS Prevention
Atlanta, GA, USA

Sunil Chauhan MD, MsPH
Clinical Assistant Professor of Neurology
Department of Neurology
University of Illinois School of Medicine
Peoria, IL, USA

Raymond T Chung MD
Director of Hepatology
Medical Director, Liver Transplant Program
Massachusetts General Hospital
Associate Professor of Medicine
Harvard Medical School
Boston, MA, USA

Connie L Celum MD, MPH
Professor of Global Health and Medicine
Adjunct Professor of Epidemiology
University of Washington
Seattle, WA, USA

Bonaventura Clotet MD, PhD
Director
IrsiCaixa Retrovirology Laboratory
Hospital Germans Trias i Pujol
Universitat Autònoma de Barcelona
Badalona, Catalonia, Spain

Richard A Colvin MD, PhD
Instructor in Medicine
Harvard Medical School
Department of Medicine, Division of Infectious Diseases
Massachusetts General Hospital
Boston, MA, USA

Judith S Currier MD, MSc
Professor of Medicine
Associate Chief, Division of Infectious Diseases
Associate Director, Center for Clinical AIDS Research and Education
David Geffen School of Medicine, UCLA
Los Angeles, CA, USA

Richard T D'Aquila MD
Addison B Scoville Jr Professor of Medicine
Professor of Microbiology and Immunology
Director, Division of Infectious Diseases
Department of Medicine
Vanderbilt AIDS Center
Vanderbilt University School of Medicine
Nashville TN, USA

Sven A Danner MD, PhD
Professor of Medicine
Chief, Department of Internal Medicine
Vrije Universiteit Medical Center
Amsterdam, The Netherlands

Lisa M Demeter MD
Associate Professor
Department of Medicine, Infectious Diseases Division
University of Rochester School of Medicine and Dentistry
Rochester, NY, USA

Thomas E Dobbs MD, MPH
Technical Consultant to Gorgas TB Initiative
University of Alabama at Birmingham
Birmingham, AL, USA

Raphael Dolin MD
Maxwell Finland Professor of Medicine (Microbiology and Molecular Genetics)
Dean for Academic and Clinical Programs
Harvard Medical School
Boston, MA, USA

Joseph J Eron Jr MD
Professor of Medicine
Division of Infectious Diseases
Department of Medicine
University of North Carolina School of Medicine
University of North Carolina at Chapel Hill
Chapel Hill, NC, USA

John JW Fangman MD
Assistant Professor of Medicine
Division of Infectious Diseases
Medical College of Wisconsin
Milwaukee, WI, USA

Carl J Fichtenbaum MD
Associate Professor of Clinical Medicine
Director Residency Research Program
University of Cincinnati College of Medicine
Cincinnati, OH, USA

Margaret A Fischl MD
Professor of Medicine
Director, AIDS Clinical Research Unit
University of Miami Medical School
Miami, FL, USA

Timothy P Flanigan MD
Professor of Medicine
Miriam Hospital
Department of Medicine
Brown University School of Medicine
Providence, RI, USA

Charles Flexner MD
Professor of Medicine
Professor of Pharmacology and Molecular Science
Professor of International Health
Johns Hopkins University
Baltimore, MD, USA

Jose M Gatell MD, PhD
Senior Consultant & Head, Infectious Diseases & AIDS Units
Clinical Institute of Medicine & Dermatology. Hospital Clinic
Professor of Medicine, University of Barcelona
Barcelona, Spain

John W Gnann Jr MD
Professor of Medicine, Pediatrics and Microbiology
Department of Medicine, Division of Infectious Diseases
University of Alabama at Birmingham and Birmingham VA Medical Center
Birmingham, AL, USA

Miguel A Goicoechea MD
Assistant Professor of Medicine
Department of Medicine – Division of Infectious Diseases
University of California, San Diego
La Jolla, CA, USA

John R Graybill MD
Professor Emeritus
The University of Texas Health Science Center
Department of Medicine
San Antonio, TX, USA

Paul D Griffiths MD, DSc
Professor of Virology
Centre for Virology
Royal Free and University College Medical School
London, United Kingdom

Steven Grinspoon MD
Associate Professor of Medicine
Harvard Medical School
Director MGH Program in Nutritional Metabolism
Massachusetts General Hospital
Boston, MA, USA

Lisa A Grohskopf MD, MPH
Medical Officer
Division of HIV/AIDS Prevention
National Center for HIV, STD & TB Prevention
Centers for Disease Control and Prevention
Atlanta, GA, USA

Carl Grunfeld MD, PhD
Professor of Medicine, University of California, San Francisco
Chief, Metabolism and Endocrine Sections, Veterans Affairs Medical Center
San Francisco, CA, USA

Roy M Gulick MD, MPH
Professor of Medicine
Director, Cornell HIV Clinical Trials Unit
Weill Medical College of Cornell University
New York, NY, USA

Colleen Hadigan MD, MPH
Staff Clinician
Laboratory of Immunoregulation
National Institutes of Allergy and Infectious Diseases
National Institutes of Health
Bethesda, MD, USA

Colin D Hall MB ChB
Professor of Neurology
University of North Carolina at Chapel Hill
Depar tment of Neurology
Chapel Hill, NC, USA

Marianne Harris MD, CCFP
Clinical Research Advisor
AIDS Research Program, St Paul's Hospital
Canadian HIV Trials Network
Vancouver, BC, Canada

Richard H Haubrich MD
Professor of Medicine
Division of Infectious Diseases
University of California, San Diego
Antiviral Research Center
San Diego, CA, USA

Jeffery D Hill DMD
Associate Professor and Director
1917 Dental Clinic
University of Alabama at Birmingham
Birmingham, AL, USA

Martin S Hirsch MD
Professor of Medicine
Harvard Medical School
Professor in the Department of Immunology & Infectious Diseases
Harvard School of Public Health
Director, Clinical AIDS Research
Department of Medicine, Infectious Disease Unit
Massachusetts General Hospital
Boston, MA, USA

Craig J Hoesley MD
Associate Professor of Medicine
Division of Infectious Diseases
Department of Medicine
University of Alabama at Birmingham
Birmingham, AL, USA

Robert Hogg PhD
BC Centre for Excellence in HIV/AIDS
Vancouver, BC
and Faculty of Health Sciences
Simon Fraser University
Burnaby, BC, Canada

Laurence Huang MD
Professor of Medicine
University of California
San Francisco General Hospital
AIDS Program
San Francisco, CA, USA

Douglas A Jabs MD MBA
Professor and Chairman
Department of Ophthalmology
The Mount Sinai School of Medicine
New York, NY, USA

Richard A Johnson MD
Instructor in Dermatology
Harvard Medical School
Massachusetts General Hospital
Boston, MA, USA

Steven C Johnson MD
Professor of Medicine
Division of Infectious Diseases
University of Colorado Health Sciences Center
Aurora, CO, USA

Victoria A Johnson MD
Professor of Medicine and Microbiology
Division of Infectious Diseases, Department of Medicine
Senior Scientist, UAB Center for AIDS Research
University of Alabama at Birmingham School of Medicine
Birmingham, AL, USA

Véronique Joly MD
Hospital Bichat-Claude Bernard
Paris, France

Eric C Johannsen MD
Assistant Professor of Medicine
Harvard Medical School
Associate Physician, Division of Infectious Diseases
Brigham & Women's Hospital
Channing Laboratory
Boston, MA, USA

Moses R Kamya MD
CDC Fellow
Centers for Disease Control and Prevention
Atlanta, GA, USA

Jonathan E Kaplan MD
Acting Director
Division of AIDS, STD and TB Laboratory
Centers for Disease Control and Prevention
Atlanta, GA, USA

Christine Katalama MD
Professor of Infectious Diseases
University Paris VI Pierre and Marie Curie Pitié-Salpêtrière
Hospital Department of Infectious Diseases
AIDS Clinical Research Unit
Paris, France

Harold A Kessler MD
Professor of Medicine and Immunology/Microbiology
St Luke's Medical Center
Rush University Medical Center
Chicago, IL, USA

J Michael Kilby MD
Associate Professor of Medicine
Medical Director, UAB 1917 Clinic
University of Alabama at Birmingham
Birmingham, AL, USA

Richard Kim MD
Professor, Clinical Pharmacology
University of Western Ontario
London, ON, Canada

David W Kimberlin MD
Professor of Pediatrics
Division of Pediatric Infectious Diseases
The University of Alabama at Birmingham
Birmingham, AL, USA

Michael E Kimerling MD, MPH
Professor of Medicine
Department of Medicine
University of Alabama at Birmingham
Birmingham, AL, USA

Paul E Klotman MD
Professor & Chair Medicine/Nephrology
Professor of Immunobiology
Professor of Genetics and Cell Biology
Department of Medicine
Mount Sinai Hospital
New York, NY, USA

Jane E Koehler MD
Professor of Medicine
Division of Infectious Diseases
University of California-San Francisco
San Francisco, CA, USA

Jens J Kort MD, PhD
Associate Professor of Clinical Medicine
Keck School of Medicine
University of Southern California
Associate Medical Director
Rand Schrader Health & Research Center
USC & LAC Medical Center
Los Angeles, CA, USA

Joseph A Kovacs MD
Head, AIDS Section
Critical Care Medicine Department
NIH Clinical Center
Bethesda, MD, USA

Susan E Krown MD
Attending Physician and Member
Memorial Sloan-Kettering Cancer Center
New York, NY, USA

Shawn E Kuhmann MD
Instructor
Department of Microbiology and Immunology
Weill Medical College of Cornell University
New York, NY, USA

Daniel R Kuritzkes MD
Director of AIDS Research
Brigham and Women's Hospital
Professor of Medicine
Harvard Medical School
Section of Retroviral Therapeutics
Brigham and Women's Hospital
Cambridge, MA, USA

Matthew B Laurens MD, MPH
Fellow
Center for Vaccine Development
Assistant Professor of Pediatrics
University of Maryland School of Medicine
Baltimore, MD, USA

Miriam K Laufer MD, MPH
Assistant Professor of Pediatrics
Center for Vaccine Development
University of Maryland School of Medicine
Baltimore, MD, USA

Jeffrey L Lennox MD
Professor of Medicine
Director HIV Center
Emory University
Atlanta, GA, USA

Richard F Little MD
Senior Investigator
Head, Hematologic & AIDS-related Malignancies
and Hematopoietic Stem Cell Transplantation
Clinical Investigations Branch
National Cancer Institute
Bethesda, MD, USA

Joan C Lo MD
Physician Scientist
Division of Research
San Francisco General Hospital
San Francisco, CA, USA

Jens D Lundgren MD DMSc
University of Copenhagen & Rigshospitalet
Professor of Viral Diseases
Faculty of Health Sciences & Rigshospitalet
Copenhagen, Denmark

Simon Mallal MD
Adjunct Professor
Centre for Clinical Immunology and Biomedical Statistics
Royal Perth Hospital
Perth, Australia

Christina M Marra MD
Professor, Neurology
Adjunct Professor Medicine (Infectious Diseases)
University of Washington School of Medicine
Seattle, WA, USA

Martin Markowitz MD
Clinical Director
Staff Investigator
The Aaron Diamond AIDS Research Center
New York, NY, USA

Nicole M Martin MD
Clinical Fellow in Medicine
Massachusetts General Hospital
Department of Internal Medicine
Boston, MA, USA

Catia Marzolini PharmD, PhD
Research Fellow
Clinical Pharmacology
Vanderbilt University School of Medicine
Nashville, TN, USA

Henry Masur MD
Chief, Critical Care Medicine Department
The NIH Clinical Center
National Institutes of Health
Bethesda, MD, USA

Kenneth H Mayer MD
Professor of Medicine and Community Health
Director, Brown University AIDS Program
Warren Alpert Medical School of Brown University
Medical Director of Research, Fenway Community Health
The Miriam Hospital – Infectious Diseases Division
Providence, RI, USA

J Steve McDougal MD
Chief, Immunology Branch
Centers for Disease Control and Prevention
Division of HIV/AIDS
Atlanta, GA, USA

James McIntyre MB ChB, FRCOG
Executive Director
Perinatal HIV Research Unit
University of The Witwatersrand
Chris Hani Baragwanath Hospital
Johannesburg, South Africa

Saurabh Mehandru MD
Visiting Scientist
The Aaron Diamond AIDS Research Center
New York, NY, USA

Sanjay Mehta MD
Fellow, Division of Infectious Diseases
University of California, San Diego
La Jolla CA, USA

Jonathan Mermin MD, MPH
Director, CDC Uganda
Centers for Disease Control and Prevention
Atlanta, GA, USA

José M Miró MD, PhD
Senior Consultant, Infectious Diseases Service
Associate Professor of Medicine
Hospital Clinic – IDIBAPS
University of Barcelona
Barcelona, Spain

Julio S G Montaner MD
Professor of Medicine & Chair of AIDS Research
University of British Columbia
Director, AIDS Research Program and Immunodeficiency Clinic
St Paul's Hosptial – University of British Columbia
Vancouver, BC, Canada

John P Moore PhD
Professor of Microbiology and Immunology
Weill Medical College of Cornell University
New York, NY, USA

Richard D Moore MD, MHSc
Professor, Medicine and Epidemiology
Director, Johns Hopkins HIV Clinic
Johns Hopkins University School of Medicine
Baltimore, MD, USA

Graeme Moyle MD
Associate Specialist in HIV Medicine
Associate Director of HIV Research
Honorary Clinical Teacher in Medicine
Chelsea & Westminster Hospital
London, UK

Michael J Mugavero MD, MHS
Assistant Professor of Medicine
Division of Infectious Diseases
University of Alabama at Birmingham
Birmingham, AL, USA

Holly Murphy MD, MPH
Research Assistant Professor
Tulane University School of Medicine
Department of Medicine, Section of Medical Hematology Medical Oncology
New Orleans, LA, USA

Henry W Murray MD
Arthur R Ashe, Jr Professor of Medicine
Associate Chairman, Department of Medicine
Weill Medical College of Cornell University
New York Presbyterian Hospital
New York, NY, USA

David Nolan MD
Senior Clinical Research Fellow
Centre for Clinical Immunology and Biomedical Statistics
Royal Perth Hospital and Murdoch University
Perth, Australia

Adelisa L Panlilio MD, MPH, CAPT, UPHS
Medical Epidemiologist
Division of Healthcare Quality Promotion
Centers for Disease Control and Prevention
Atlanta, GA, USA

Peter G Pappas MD
Professor of Medicine
Department of Infectious Diseases
University of Alabama at Birmingham
Birmingham, Alabama, USA

Roger Paredes MD
Senior Researcher
IrsiCaixa Retrovirology Laboratory
Hospital Germans Trias i Pujol
Universitat Autònoma de Barcelona
Badalona, Catalonia, Spain

Thomas F Patterson MD
Director, San Antonio Center for Medical Mycology
Professor of Medicine
Department of Medicine
The University of Texas Health Science Center
San Antonio, TX, USA

Alice K Pau PharmD
Staff Scientist (Clinical)
Division of Clinical Research
National Institute of Allergy and Infectious Diseases
National Institutes of Health
Bethesda, MD, USA

Andrew T Pavia MD
Professor of Medicine
University of Utah School of Medicine
Division of Pediatric Infectious Diseases
University of Utah Medical Center
Salt Lake City, UT, USA

Paul A Pham PharmD
Research Associate
Division of Infectious Diseases
Johns Hopkins University School of Medicine
Maryland, MD, USA

Stefania Pittaluga MD
Staff Clinician
National Cancer Institutes
Laboratory of Pathology
National Institutes of Health
Bethesda, MD, USA

Richard W Price MD
Professor and Vice Chair of Neurology
University of California San Francisco
San Francisco, CA, USA

Michael A Polis MD, MPH
Chief
Collaborative Clinical Research Branch
Laboratory of Immunoregulation
National Institute for Allergies and Infectious Diseases
National Institutes of Health
Bethesda, MD, USA

William G Powderly MD
Professor of Medicine and Therapeutics
Head, School of Medicine and Medical Science
Medical Professorial Unit
University College Dublin, Mater University Hospital
Dublin, Ireland

Anton Pozniak MD
Consultant Physician and Senior Lecturer
The St Stephens Centre
Chelsea & Westminster Hospital
London, UK

Richard C Reichman MD
Professor of Medicine and of Microbiology and Immunology
University of Rochester School of Medicine and Dentistry
Rochester, NY, USA

Peter Reiss MD, PhD
Associate Professor of Medicine
Academic Medical Center
University of Amsterdam, The Netherlands
Deputy Director of the Dutch National AIDS Therapy Evaluation Center
Amsterdam, The Netherlands

David Reznik, DDS
Chief, Dental Services Director
Oral Health Center Infectious Disease Program
Grady Health System
Atlanta, GA, USA

Sarah Robertson PharmD
Clinical Pharmacology Reviewer
Center for Drug Evaluation and Research
Anti-infective and Ophthalmologic Products
Office of Clinical Pharmacology
Food and Drug Administration
White Oak, MD, USA

Lidia Ruiz PhD
Senior Researcher
IrsiCaixa Retrovirology Laboratory
Hospital Germans Trias i Pujol
Universitat Autònoma de Barcelona
Badalona, Catalonia, Spain

Michael Saag MD
Professor of Medicine
Director, Division of Infectious Disease and The William C Gorgas Center for International Health
Director, Center for AIDS Research
University of Alabama at Birmingham
Birmingham, AL, USA

Arturo Saavedra-Lauzon MD PhD
Instructor in Dermatology
Harvard Medical School
Brigham and Women's Hospital
Boston, MA, USA

Fred R Sattler MD
Chief, Division of Infectious Diseases
Professor of Medicine
Senior Associate Dean for Faculty Affairs
Associate Program Director, USC GCRC
Keck School of Medicine
University of Southern California
Los Angeles, CA, USA

Morris Schambelan MD
Professor of Medicine
Associate Chair, Clinical and Translational Research
Program Director, CTSI Clinical Research Center
University of California, San Francisco
San Francisco, CA, USA

Irini Sereti MD
Clinical and Molecular Retrovirology Section
Laboratory of Immunoregulation
National Institute for Allergy and Infectious Diseases
National Institutes of Health
Bethesda, MD, USA

Kenneth E Sherman MD, PhD
Gould Professor of Medicine
Director, Division of Digestive Diseases
University of Cincinnati College of Medicine
Cincinnati, OH, USA

Kasha P Singh MB, BS, BA, MPH, FRACP
Clinical Research Fellow
Chelsea and Westminster Hospital NHS Foundation Trust
London, UK

Benjamin C Silverman MD
Psychiatry Resident
Massachusetts General Hospital
Boston, MA, USA

Kimberly Y Smith MD, MPH
Associate Professor of Medicine
Section of Infectious Diseases
Rush Presbyterian St Luke's Medical Center
Chicago, IL, USA

Anette Sjøl MD
Head of Department
Department of Internal Medicine
Nordsjællands Hospital
Frederikssund
Capital Region of Denmark
Frederikssund, Dermark

David H Spach MD
Professor of Medicine, Division of Infectious Diseases
University of Washington, School of Medicine
Clinical Director and Medical Educator
Northwest AIDS Education and Training Center
Harborview Medical Center
Seattle, WA, USA

Serena S Spudich MD
Assistant Adjunct Professor
Department of Neurology
University of California, San Francisco
San Francisco, CA, USA

Schlomo Staszewski MD
Senior Physician for Internal Medicine
Director of HIV Outpatient Clinic
Director of Antiretroviral Resarch Unit
Johann Wolfgang Goethe University
Frankfurt, Germany

Lara B Strick MD, MSc
Clinical Instructor in Medicine
University of Washington School of Medicine
Madison Clinic
Harborview Medical Center
Seattle, WA, USA

Mark S Sulkowski MD
Associate Professor of Medicine
Medical Director, Viral Hepatitis Center
Johns Hopkins University School of Medicine
Baltimore, MD, USA

Pablo Tebas MD
Associate Professor of Medicine
Division of Infectious Diseases
Hospital of the University of Pennsylvania
Philadelphia, PA, USA

Amalio Telenti MD, PhD
Professor of Biology and Medicine
University of Lausanne
Lausanne, Switzerland

Alex Thompson MD, MBA
Acting Instructor
Department of Psychiatry and Behavioral Sciences
University of Washington School of Medicine
Seattle, WA, USA

Jennifer E Thorne MD, PhD
Assistant Professor of Ophthalmology
Division of Ocular Immunology
Wilmer Eye Institute
Johns Hopkins School of Medicine
Baltimore, MD, USA

Anna R Thorner MD
Instructor in Medicine
Division of Infectious Diseases
Department of Medicine
Harvard Medical School
Brigham and Women's Hospital
Boston, MA, USA

Jason Tokumoto MD
Assistant Professor of Medicine
University of California, San Francisco
San Francisco, CA, USA

Glenn J Treisman MD, PhD
Associate Professor of Psychiatry
Johns Hopkins University School of Medicine
Director of AIDS Psychiatry
Johns Hopkins Hospital
Baltimore, MD, USA

Marc van der Valk MD, PhD
Department of Internal Medicine
Academic Medical Center
University of Amsterdam
Amsterdam, The Netherlands

Christine A Wanke MD
Professor of Medicine and Community Health
Tufts Sackler School of Biomedical Sciences
Boston, MA, USA

Louis M Weiss MD, MPH
Professor of Medicine & Pathology
Albert Einstein College of Medicine
New York, NY, USA

Melissa F Wellons MD, MHS
Assistant Professor of Medicine
University of Alabama at Birmingham
Birmingham, AL, USA

Lawrence J Wheat MD
President and Director
MiraVista Diagnostics & MiraBella Technologies
Indianapolis, IN, USA

C Mel Wilcox MD
Professor of Medicine
Director, Division of Gastrointestinal Medicine
University of Alabama at Birmingham
Birmingham, AL, USA

James H Willig MD
Senior Clinical Research Fellow
Division of Infectious Diseases
University of Alabama at Birmingham
Alabama, AL, USA

Jonathan A Winston MD
Associate Professor, Medicine/Nephrology
Mount Sinai School of Medicine
New York, NY, USA

Robert Yarchoan MD
Chief, HIV and AIDS Malignancy Branch
Center for Cancer Research
National Cancer Institute
Bethesda, MA, USA

Patrick Yeni MD
Director
Department of Infectious and Tropical Medicine
Hôpital Bichat-Claude Bernard
X Bichat Medical School
Paris, France

Carlos Zala MD
Director, Clinical Research
Foundation Huesped
Beunos Aires, Argentina

Andrew R Zolopa MD
Associate Professor of Medicine
Stanford University School of Medicine
Stanford, CA, USA

Chapter 1

Establishing the Diagnosis of HIV Infection

Bernard M. Branson, MD, J. Steven McDougal, MD

Treatment, especially highly active antiretroviral therapy (HAART), has dramatically improved survival for persons infected with human immunodeficiency virus (HIV).[1] However, because of late diagnosis, many people do not realize the full benefits of therapy. In 2004, 39% were diagnosed with acquired immunodeficiency syndrome (AIDS) within 1 year of their first positive HIV test.[2] Although many with HIV infection visit healthcare settings in the years before their diagnosis, they are often not tested for HIV.[3–5] Moreover, the changing demographics of the HIV/AIDS epidemic in the US have diminished the effectiveness of testing based solely on reported risk behaviors to identify HIV-infected persons.[6] Since the 1980s, increasing proportions of infected persons are found among youth, minority races and ethnicities, persons who reside outside metropolitan areas, and heterosexual men and women.

During its clinical stages, HIV infection produces numerous biologic indicators of virus infection including clinical symptoms, viremia, circulating viral proteins, antibodies against viral proteins, and immunologic markers of infection such as changes in the absolute number of and ratio of CD4 and CD8 lymphocytes (Fig. 1-1). These markers can be detected and in many cases quantified by the correct use of diagnostic tests to substantiate the presence of HIV infection. Selecting the most appropriate test for accurate diagnosis depends upon knowledge of the kinetic characteristics and relationships of the various biologic markers and the performance characteristics (sensitivity and specificity) of the various detection systems. This chapter reviews various techniques currently used in the diagnosis of HIV infection (Table 1-1) and their sequence of reactivity over the course of HIV infection.

THE HIV VIRION

Morphologically, HIV is an enveloped, roughly spherical virus that contains a capsid enclosing two copies of genomic RNA (Fig. 1-2).[7] Replication, via the action of the enzyme reverse

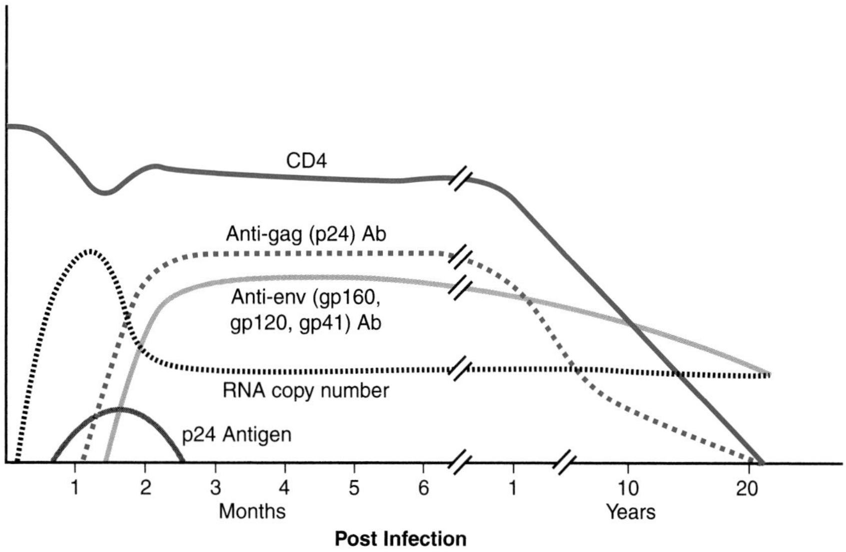

Figure 1-1 ■ Sequence of viral and antiviral responses after HIV infection.

Tests Available for HIV Diagnosis

Table 1-1

Antibody Blood Tests
EIA for antibody to HIV-1, HIV-2, HIV-1/2 (serum/plasma)
Rapid antibody tests for HIV-1, HIV-1/2 (serum/plasma/whole blood)
Indirect IFA for HIV-1 (serum/plasma)
Western blot for HIV-1, HIV-2 (serum/plasma)

Other Blood Tests
HIV-1 p24 antigen EIA (serum/plasma)
Combination HIV-1 p24 antigen–HIV-1/2 antibody assays (serum/plasma)
HIV-1 DNA PCR (PBMCs)
Qualitative HIV-1 RNA RT-PCR assays (plasma)
Qualitative HIV-1 RNA TMA assays (plasma)
Cell culture for HIV-1/2 (plasma/peripheral blood mononuclear cells)

Other Fluid Tests
Oral fluid HIV-1 antibody EIA/Western blot
Oral fluid HIV-1/2 rapid antibody test
Urine HIV-1 antibody EIA/Western blot

Quantitative HIV-1 RNA Viral Load (Plasma)
RT-PCR
Branched bDNA
NASBA

transcriptase, proceeds by the reverse transcription of genomic RNA into a DNA intermediate. The DNA intermediate is integrated into the host cell genome where it is referred to as proviral DNA. Provirus is the template from which progeny RNA and proteins are synthesized using the host cell's synthetic machinery. The viral components subsequently assemble below the host cell membrane and bud from the membrane as mature virions potentially capable of spreading infection to other cells or transmitting infection to other hosts.[8] HIV replicates in an error-prone manner that generates a mutation virtually every time it replicates.[9] Thus, the viruses circulating in the host are not an absolutely homogeneous population; rather, they consist of a swarm of similar yet divergent variants known as quasi-species. This existing variation and ongoing mutation is the substrate upon which selective pressures act to allow the emergence of different variants in the host such as drug resistant strains or immunologic escape-mutants.

The HIV genome consists of three major genes that encode the viral enzymatic and structural proteins: *gag* (group-specific antigens or capsid proteins), *pol* (polymerase, protease, and integrase enzymes), and *env* (envelope glycoproteins).[10]

HIV viruses are classified based on phylogenetic relatedness of nucleotide sequences. The current classification is hierarchical and consists of types, groups, subtypes, sub-subtypes, and recombinant forms (Fig. 1-3).[11] Subtypes are often referred to as clades. The most distantly related HIVs are categorized as types: HIV type 1 and HIV type 2.[12] The HIV-1 type is further characterized into groups: the major (M) group; the more divergent outlier (O) group, and the non-M, non-O (N) group.[9,12] Most HIV infections occur with group M HIV-1 which is differentiated into subtypes (HIV-1 group M subtypes A, B, C, D, F, G, H, J, and K).[9] Subtypes A and F are further classified into sub-subtypes A1, A2, A3, F1, and F2. HIV-2 has two major subtypes, A and B.[12] When

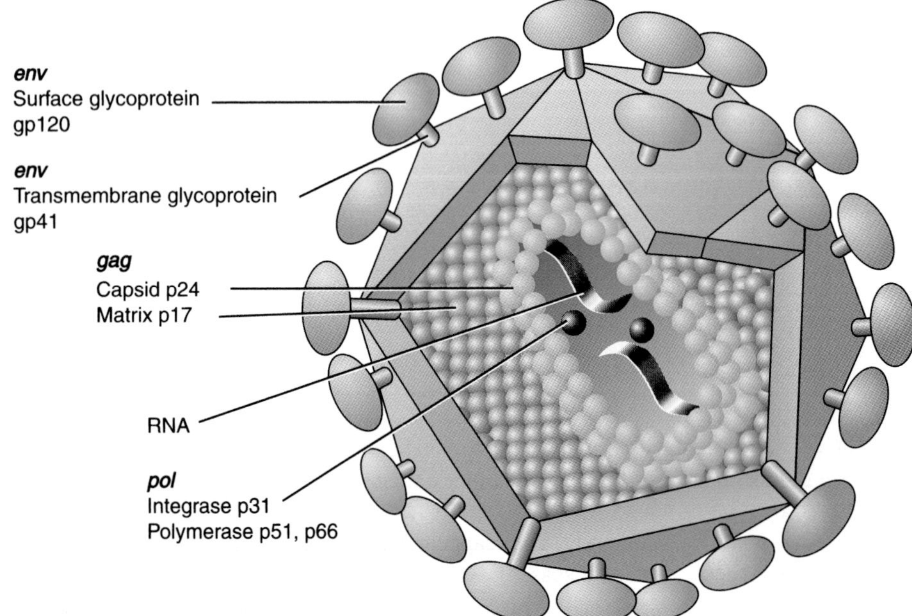

Figure 1-2 ■ Schematic of HIV-1 viral elements useful for establishing a diagnosis of HIV infection.

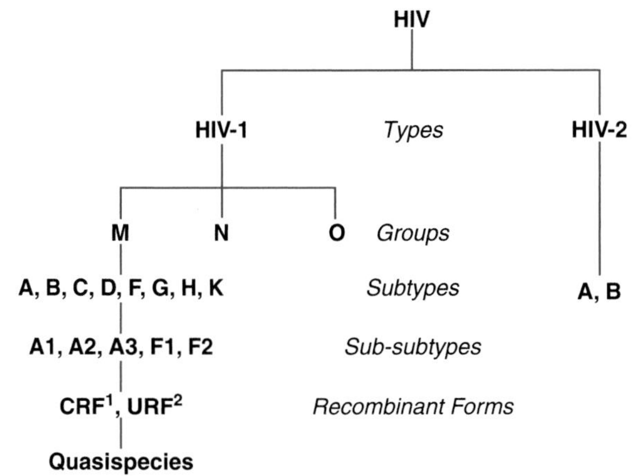

Figure 1-3 ■ Classification of HIV. [1]Circulating recombinant forms. [2]Unique recombinant forms.

Redrawn with permission from Constantine NT, Saville RD, Dax EM. Retroviral Testing and Quality Assurance: Essentials for Laboratory Diagnosis. 2005, p 37.

viruses from two or more HIV-1 lineages infect one individual and exchange their genetic material, they are termed recombinant viruses.[13] If transmission of the recombinant virus has been documented by whole genome sequences to three or more persons, it is referred to as a circulating recombinant form (CRF), and the CRF is given a numeric designation. As of July 2007, CRF01 to CRF34 are recognized. Recombinant viruses that have been identified but are not documented to have been further transmitted are referred to as unique recombinant forms (URF). The variation in nucleotide sequences can have implications for the biology and transmission of the virus, for patient survival, and also helps explain the geographic distribution, and epidemiology of HIV infection.[9,12,13] From the diagnostic perspective, sequence variation can have significant implications for the reactivity and cross-reactivity of diagnostic tests designed to detect specific viral proteins or peptides.

NATURAL HISTORY AND RESPONSE TO HIV INFECTION

HIV is a blood-borne pathogen transmitted by the exchange of blood or bodily fluids through sexual contact, sharing of injection paraphernalia, transfusion of blood products, or from mother to child during pregnancy or through breastfeeding. By virtue of having a receptor for the CD4 molecule and co-receptors that facilitate membrane fusion, HIV targets, infects, and replicates in CD4 T lymphocytes and CD4-positive monocytes and macrophages. CD4 T lymphocytes play a pivotal role in the initial recognition of foreign antigen and in the induction of responses by other cells of the immune system. Their gradual depletion by HIV infection renders the host increasingly susceptible to opportunistic infections and certain malignancies.

Clinically, HIV infection progresses through several stages, each with characteristic laboratory findings. Within weeks of infection, a flu-like syndrome may develop in some 40–90% of patients.[14–16] Symptoms, including fever, malaise, myalgia, lymphadenopathy, and macular rash, lasting from a few days to several weeks, can be sufficiently severe to prompt as many as half of patients to seek medical attention.[16] Primary HIV infection or PHI, as the syndrome is called, lasts a few weeks and is associated with high levels of viremia, a transient depression in CD4 T lymphocytes, elevation of CD8 T lymphocytes, and generally resolves concomitantly with the onset of a cellular and humoral immune response to HIV. Following PHI, most patients then enter an asymptomatic or "latent" phase that has been observed to last from several months to more than 15 years. During this clinically latent phase, HIV replication establishes a steady state where virus levels in plasma reach a "set point" and CD4 T lymphocyte counts slowly decline. Both the viral set point and rate of decline of CD4 T-lymphocyte levels have prognostic value in predicting progression to advanced disease.[17] With continued viral replication and progressive decline in CD4 T lymphocytes, patients may develop constitutional symptoms (fever, malaise, lymphadenopathy) and non-life-threatening diseases related to immunodeficiency such as oral candidiasis, oral hairy leukoplakia, and thrombocytopenia. Finally, and often precipitously, CD4 T-lymphocyte levels decline to less than 200 cells/μL, virus levels climb, the immune system collapses, and patients are prone to life-threatening opportunistic infections and malignancies – the full-fledged AIDS.

There are corresponding phases in reactivity of various laboratory diagnostic tests during clinical stages of HIV infection (Fig. 1-4). Shortly after infection, viral replication reaches levels that can be detected by sensitive molecular assays for viral nucleic acid (nucleic acid amplification tests or NAATs). The duration of time between initial infection and first detection of viral nucleic acid in plasma, the "eclipse period", has not been accurately defined and likely varies with the infection route and inoculum size as well as with the sensitivity of the particular NAAT assay. The eclipse period has been estimated by back regression of the initial slopes of a plot of virus load versus time and by analysis of patients with an accurately known infection event. These types of studies estimate a duration of ~6–12 days for the eclipse period.[18,19] Viral antigens, particularly the most abundant viral protein, the capsid protein p24, are also detectable in the first few weeks after infection. There are ~2000–3000 copies of the p24 molecule in each virion, compared with two RNA molecules. Detection thresholds for p24 assays during acute infection correspond to ~10 000 viral RNA copies per milliliter; p24 antigen can first be detected ~5 days after plasma viral RNA.[18,19] p24 antigen detection is transient and its disappearance usually coincides with the development of anti-p24 antibodies, whereas RNA usually remains detectable throughout infection. The disappearance of p24 antigen with seroconversion may be due in part to blocking of p24 detection by the formation of immune complexes with anti-p24 antibody. The reappearance of detectable p24 antigen in late-stage disease is associated with the reduction in p24 antibody and the increased viral replication that occurs in that phase.

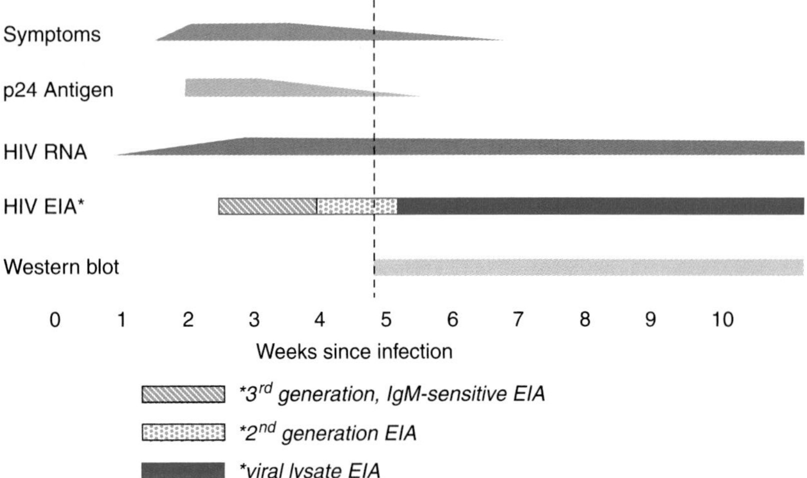

Figure 1-4 ■ Sequence of reactivity of diagnostic tests for HIV in early infection.

Specific anti-HIV antibody signifies past exposure to HIV and current active infection. Patients mount and generally sustain a vigorous humoral immune response to HIV infection. Detection of anti-HIV antibodies is the mainstay of diagnosis for HIV infection in the vast majority of patients. Immunoglobulin M (IgM) antibodies to HIV appear first. They are of low titer, usually transient, but may be detected intermittently throughout infection.[20–23] The IgM response is followed by a long-lived immunoglobulin G (IgG) response. Antibodies to protein products of the *gag* gene (p17, p24, and p55) and *env* gene (gp41, gp120, and gp160) appear first, followed days to weeks later by antibodies to *pol* gene proteins (p31, p51, and p66).[18,19,24] The period of time from infection until antibody seroconversion (known as the preseroconversion window period) varies between different persons and also depends on the assay used to detect antibody (Fig. 1-4). The newer, most sensitive third generation enzyme immunoassays (EIAs) are generally positive 7–14 days after viral RNA is first detected.[18,19] It may take longer (15–30 days) for earlier, less sensitive first generation EIAs to become reactive, or for development of a sufficient number of bands on Western blot to meet diagnostic criteria.[18,19] Almost all patients meet the criteria for serologic diagnosis of HIV infection within 3 months after infection.[18,19,24–27] In cases in which either the EIA or Western blot assays are found to be negative or indeterminate, repeat testing is recommended 8–12 weeks later. In rare cases, infection can be documented by virologic techniques, but seroconversion is delayed or absent.[28–30] Usually, such cases have extremely high levels of viremia and rapid progression of clinical disease. It is not clear why this occurs. Some patients have an underlying, preexistent immunodeficiency such as common variable immunodeficiency, but most do not.[19,25,26,31–34] Perhaps it is due to B-lymphocyte loss or dysfunction, although most of these patients appear to generate antibodies against other pathogens.[30] With advanced disease or with effective antiretroviral therapy in patients with established seropositivity, antibody levels decline, but total loss of seroreactivity is extremely rare.[31,34–37] Early and intensive antiretroviral therapy, initiated before seroconversion, can also blunt or abolish the antibody response to HIV infection.[31,35,38] Spontaneous seroreversion, in the absence of early therapy or advanced disease, is extremely rare and has been difficult to document.[39,40]

METHODOLOGIES

Screening and Confirmatory Tests for Diagnosis of HIV Infection

Detection of antibody to HIV proteins is the most common means to diagnose HIV infection. HIV antibody tests in current use have very high sensitivity and specificity, exceeding 98%. They can be selected for greater relative sensitivity or specificity depending on the intended use of the test results. A highly sensitive test is used for initial screening to detect almost all specimens from infected persons at the expense of incorrectly classifying some specimens from uninfected persons as false positive. Thus, a negative test result engenders great confidence that the patient is uninfected, but some positive test results will be incorrect. Conversely, a highly specific test may sometimes yield a negative test result from an infected person, but a positive result conclusively indicates presence of infection. For diagnostic purposes, a test that is both extremely sensitive and extremely specific would be preferable, but in practice, this is difficult to achieve. Therefore, serologic testing for HIV relies upon a testing algorithm which employs an initial highly sensitive screening test designed to identify all potentially infected patients, followed by a more specific supplemental test for confirmation of the positive screening test result.

A listing of HIV diagnostic tests approved by the US Food and Drug Administration (FDA) is at http://www.FDA.gov/cber/products/testkits.htm. The World Health Organization (WHO) also evaluates HIV tests and maintains a list of HIV tests and results of their evaluation at http://www.who.int/diagnostics_laboratory/publications/evaluations/en/index.html.

EIA for Detection of HIV Antibody

The EIA has been the predominant screening test for laboratory-based HIV testing. HIV EIAs have gone through several iterations since they were first developed in 1985, resulting in continued improvements in technology, sensitivity, specificity, and reproducibility. They are based on techniques that capture serum antibodies against HIV, if present, with viral antigen applied to the solid phase (micro-plate wells, beads, or paper strips) in the test kit. The antigen–antibody complex is then detected using an anti-human IgG antibody conjugated to an enzyme such as alkaline phosphatase or horseradish peroxidase. A substrate is then added from which the bound enzyme generates a colorimetric reaction. Color development is measured by optical density (OD) at an appropriate wave length with a spectrophotometer. OD is proportionate to the amount of bound enzyme conjugate which, in turn, is proportionate to the amount of antibody bound to solid-phase viral antigen. The EIA does not distinguish which specific antibodies are present in the patient's serum; as a qualitative test, it is scored as positive if any antibodies are present.

In the earliest first generation versions of the EIA, antigen in the form of a whole-virus lysate is coated on the surface of microtiter wells as the solid-phase antigen (Fig. 1-5A). The HIV-1 viral lysates contain native antigens from virtually all structural components of the virus, and will generally detect all subtypes of group M, many group O, and cross-react with many HIV-2 viruses. However, they are prone to false-positive results because of cross-reactions with host cell proteins from which the virus is propagated, and they are less sensitive during early seroconversion because they do not detect IgM and because of the large dilutions necessary to attain adequate specificity. The second generation tests replace crude viral lysates with recombinant viral proteins or peptides from conserved immunodominant regions of HIV-1 and HIV-2 (Fig. 1-5A), and many have been modified to detect the outlier (O) group of HIV-1. Not only is the sensitivity for detection of a range of HIV types and subtypes expanded, but the false-positive rate due to reaction with viral lysate contaminants or cross-reactions with viral antigens is lower, resulting in greater specificity. Third generation tests (or immunometric tests) rely on a somewhat different principle (Fig. 1-5B). Like first and second generation tests, viral antigens are in the solid phase. In third generation tests, however, detection is accomplished with enzyme conjugated to HIV antigen (instead of to anti-human IgG). Antibody in patient serum thus binds to HIV antigen in the solid phase and also to the HIV antigen in the enzyme conjugate. This "antigen sandwich" detects any class of antibody, including IgM, and is subject to lower background ODs, which improves analytic sensitivity. As a result, the third generation tests detect seroconversion about a week before second generation tests.[18,19,41,42] Newer third generation assays incorporate antigens from HIV-1 group M subtypes, group O and HIV-2. These combination formats have excellent sensitivity when assessing subjects with established infection and may have lower false-positive rates (i.e., higher specificity) than earlier generation tests.[18,19,41,43–48] Fourth generation EIAs have been developed that combine antibody and p24 antigen detection in the same assay (Fig. 1-5C).[47,49,50] This increases sensitivity during acute infection, because antigen detection has been shown to shorten the preseroconversion window by ~5 days. However, the fourth generation assay requires a more formidable confirmatory procedure to validate reactivity against antibody or antigen. Further, the combination assay may not be as sensitive for antigen detection as separate p24 antigen testing, and the test may not be equally sensitive for all subtypes of HIV-1.[51]

All EIAs are subject to false-positive reactions. These may be due to procedural mistakes, coincidental cross-reactions, or be associated with acute or chronic inflammation, autoimmunity, or hypergammaglobulinemia (Table 1-2).[52–54] False positives related to the latter associations are usually transient or unstable and do not confirm with supplemental tests based on a different principle. HIV vaccine-induced antibodies may also be detected by current tests and may cause false-positive results in vaccine trial participants; true infection status can be difficult to resolve. Persons whose test results are HIV-positive and who are identified as vaccine trial participants should be encouraged to contact or return to their trial site or an associated trial site for confirmatory testing. A referenced list of possible and variably documented associations with false-positive HIV EIA results can be found at http://healtoronto.com/testcross.html.

Western Blot

The HIV Western blot identifies antibodies to individual viral proteins. Because the technique separates and concentrates specific viral proteins for detection and identification of specific anti-HIV antibodies, it is generally considered to be a more specific test than the EIA. The Western blot is widely used to confirm HIV infection in specimens that have screened as positive by EIA. To create the Western blot, HIV proteins from a viral lysate are subjected to gel electrophoresis, separating the component viral proteins based on their molecular weights. Higher molecular weight proteins have slower mobility than lower molecular weight proteins. The individual proteins are then transferred as resolved proteins to nitrocellulose paper. When the strips are reacted with test sera, antibody to the viral proteins binds at the location where the HIV protein is immobilized. Bound antibody is then detected with anti-IgG enzyme conjugated to a colorimetric substrate. This produces a colored band corresponding to the particular viral protein's molecular weight (Fig. 1-6).

The nomenclature of viral proteins indicates either "gp" for glycoprotein or "p" for protein followed by a number indicating its molecular weight in kilodaltons. The glycoprotein bands on Western blot tend to be diffuse because of variable glycosylation, whereas the protein bands are more discreet. The major bands of diagnostic utility for HIV-1 include envelope proteins (gp160, gp120, gp41), the *gag* core gene proteins (p55, p24, p17), and polymerase gene proteins (p66, p51, p31). HIV-2 Western blot bands are similar but differ

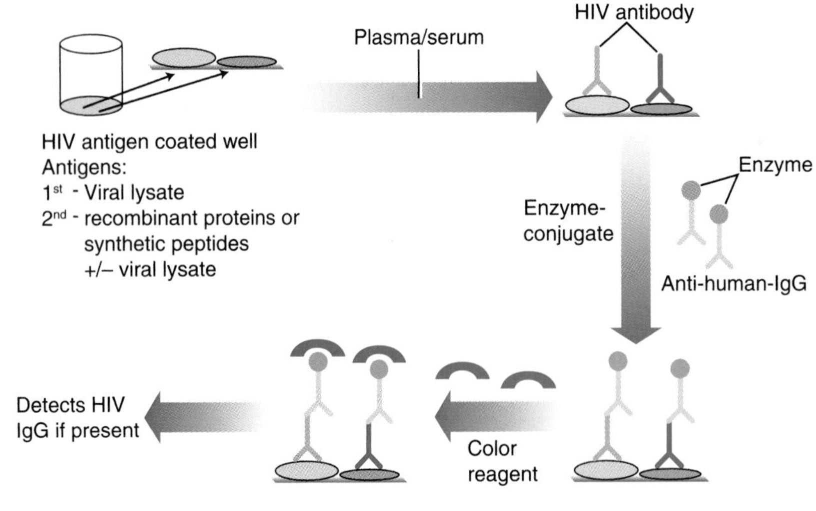

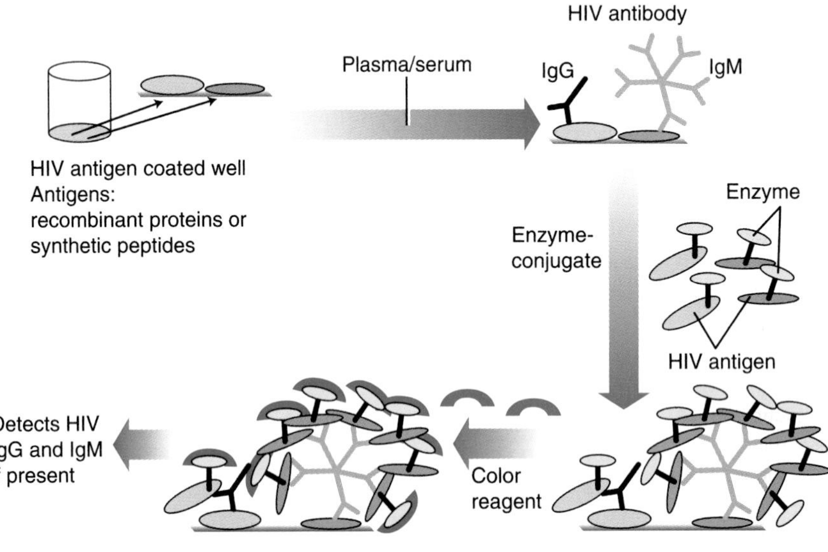

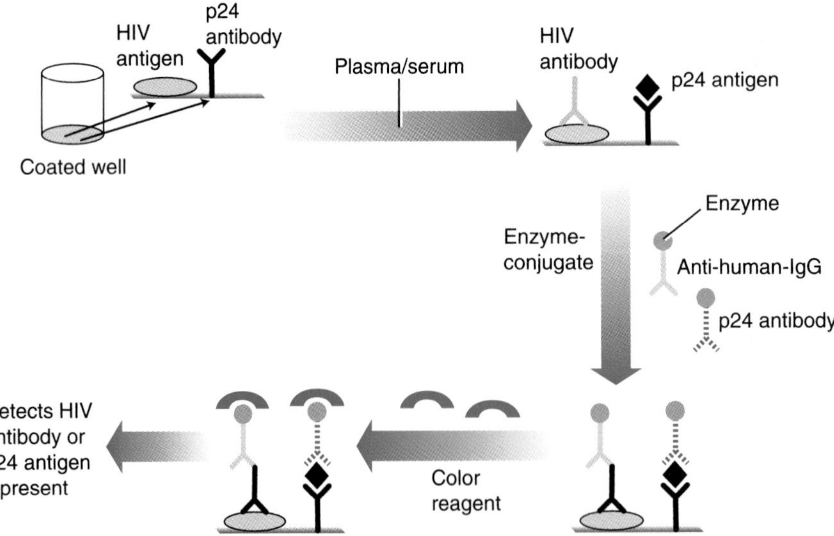

Figure 1-5 ■ Principles of different EIAs. A: 1st and 2nd generation EIAs. B: 3rd generation EIA. C: 4th generation EIA.

Causes of False-Positive or False-Negative HIV EIA Results

Table 1-2

Causes of False-Positive Results for HIV Antibody on EIA
Hematologic malignant disorders
DNA viral infections
Autoimmune disorders
Multiple myeloma
Primary biliary cirrhosis
Alcoholic hepatitis
Influenza vaccination
Hepatitis B vaccination
Rabies vaccination
Passively transferred antibodies
Antibodies to class II leukocytes
Renal transplantation
Chronic renal failure
Stevens–Johnson syndrome
Positive rapid plasma regain test
Malaria
Dengue
Increased parity
Systemic lupus erythematosus
Causes of False-Negative Results for HIV Antibody on EIA
Preseroconversion “window’ period
Immunosuppressive therapy
Replacement transfusion
Malignant disorders
B-lymphocyte dysfunction
Bone marrow transplantation
Starch powder from laboratory gloves

Adapted from Cordes RJ, Ryan ME. Pitfalls in HIV testing: application and limitations of current tests. Postgrad Med 98:177, 1995; Mylonakis E, Paliou M, Lally M, et al. Laboratory testing for infection with the human immunodeficiency virus: established and novel approaches. Am J Med 109:568, 2000. Related article: Daikh BE, Holyst MM. Lupus-specific autoantibodies in concomitant human immunodeficiency virus and systemic lupus erythematosus: case report and literature review. Semin Arthritis Rheum 30:418, 2001.

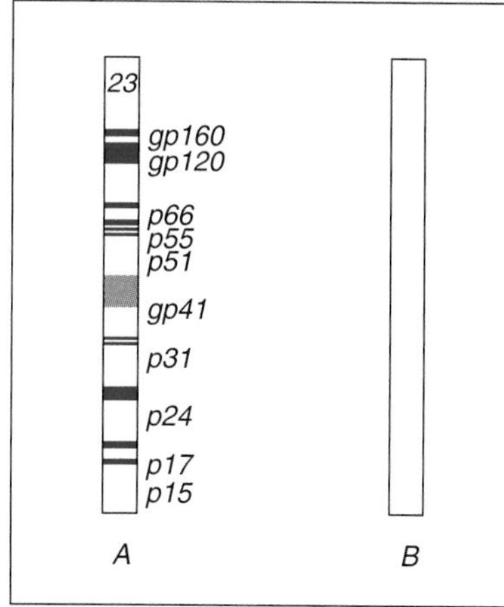

Figure 1-6 ■ Western blot results: (A) positive result (reactive to all antigens); (B) negative result.

Reprinted with permission from Contantine NT, Callahan JD, Watts DM. Retroviral Testing: Essentials of Quality Control and Laboratory Diagnosis. Boca Raton, FL: CRC Press; 1992, p 63.

HIV Proteins Represented on Western Blot Test

Table 1-3

	Viral Protein/Glycoprotein Molecular Weight	
HIV Gene and Products	**HIV-1**	**HIV-2**
env		
Precursor	gp160	gp140
External glycoprotein	gp120	gp105/125
Transmembrane glycoprotein	gp41	gp36
pol		
Reverse transcriptase	p66	p68
Reverse transcriptase	p51	p53
Endonuclease	p31	p31/34
gag		
Precursor	p55	p56
Core	p24	p26
Matrix	p17	p16

somewhat in the molecular weight of the three gene products (Table 1-3). Other bands corresponding to smaller viral proteins may be present but are not part of the diagnostic scoring criteria.[55]

The antigen preparation for Western blot is generally purified extracellular virus representing mature virions. The protein profile of mature virions as detected by Western blot may differ somewhat from that of intracellular replicating virus because not all proteins required for virus replication are packaged with extracellular virus. For example, gp160 is proteolytically cleaved by host cell proteases into gp120 and gp41. Intact gp160 is not efficiently incorporated into viral membranes, and its presence in extracellular virus is somewhat unexpected. Thus, only a small portion of the gp160 band in Western blot is authentic gp160; the majority represents polymerized gp41 (tetramers).[56–59] Immunoblot assays that use purified recombinant proteins as an alternative to viral lysate antigens have also been developed. These perform as well as standard Western blot, though none are approved by FDA.[60,61]

Interpretation of the Western blot is somewhat subjective, and test specimens are compared to a control strip that has been reacted with low-positive serum. If no colored bands are present, the Western blot is interpreted as negative. Interpretive criteria for a positive Western blot place heavy emphasis on the presence of envelope glycoproteins and the core protein p24 because these appear first in serum following seroconversion (Fig. 1-1). Depending on which organization's criteria are used, a blot is interpreted as positive when at least two bands or band clusters (e.g., p24, gp41, gp120/160) are present, or if one band from each of the gene products is present (Table 1-4).[62–64] If bands are present but do not meet interpretive criteria for a positive test, the blot is scored as indeterminate.

Given sufficient time after infection, most subjects develop a full banding pattern, and there is little difference in interpretation by the various scoring criteria.[18,19,52,63,64] An indeterminate result may represent early seroconversion or reflect nonspecific, irrelevant cross-reactivity. In studies of serial specimens from early infection, the Western blot becomes criterion-positive 0–20 days after the EIA is positive (depending on the sensitivity of the EIA) and 10–30 days after tests for viral nucleic acid or antigen are positive.[18,19,25,27,47,41] Viral nucleic acid or antigen testing may be a useful supplementary test for resolving indeterminate Western blot results.[52,65–67] However, the ultimate resolution requires follow-up testing. Specimens from infected persons with an initially indeterminate blot will usually evolve into a pattern indicative of HIV infection within 4 weeks.[18,19,25,27,41,47,67] Nonspecific indeterminate blot patterns generally do not evolve and may recede.[67] The most common cause of an indeterminate Western blot result, which may occur in 10–15% of uninfected persons, is an isolated p24 or p17 band.[47,53,63] In a long-term study of uninfected patients with repeatedly reactive HIV EIAs and indeterminate Western blots, independent risk factors for an indeterminate blot among males were a tetanus booster during the preceding 2 years and sexual contact with a prostitute. For uninfected women, indeterminate Western blots were associated with having given birth to one or more children, and the presence of rheumatoid factor or antinuclear antibodies.[63] Other variably documented associations with nonspecific or indeterminate banding patterns are listed in Table 1-5.[32,52,53]

False-positive Western blots are rare but problematic. Historically, Western blot positivity has become the gold standard for evaluating the sensitivity and specificity of other HIV tests. Discordance between a positive Western blot result and an independent test is generally ascribed to imperfect sensitivity of the independent test rather than to the imperfect specificity of the blot.[52,65,66] Kleinman et al[52] evaluated blot performance in a blood donor population, a low prevalence setting where the proportion of false positives is expected to be magnified. Specimens with criterion-positive blots were subjected to supplemental testing and follow-up to assign true infection status. Of the positive blots, 4.8% were thought to be false positive. A true positive was more likely in first time donors, when a p31 band was present, or when three or more bands were present. The probability that a positive blot is a true positive (positive predictive value, PPV) varies with prevalence. In this study with an HIV prevalence of 0.008%, PPV was 95%. In populations with prevalence above 0.1%, the PPV of a positive blot exceeds 99.9%.

Table 1-4

Interpretive Criteria for a Positive HIV-1 Western Blot Test

Organization	Criteria
APHL/CDC	Any two: p24, gp41, gp120/160
ARC	Three or more bands, one from each gene product group: *gag*, *pol*, *env*
CRSS	Two or more bands: p24 or p31 and gp41 or gp120/160
WHO	Two *env* bands with or without *gag* or *pol*

APHL/CDC, Association of Public Health Laboratories/Centers for Disease Control and Prevention; ARC, American Red Cross; CRSS, Consortium for Retrovirus Serological Standardization; WHO, World Health Organization.

Data from Proffitt MR, Yen-Lieberman B. Laboratory diagnosis of human immunodeficiency virus infection. Infect Dis Clin North Am 7:203, 1993; George JR, Schochetman G. Serologic tests for the detection of human immunodeficiency virus infection. In: George JR, Schochetman G (eds) AIDS Testing: Methodology and Management Issues. New York: Springer; 1992, p 48.

Table 1-5

Causes of False-Positive and Indeterminate Western Blot Results for HIV

- Normal human ribonucleoproteins
- Other human retroviruses
- Antibodies to mitochondrial, nuclear, and T-lymphocyte antigens
- Globulins produced during polyclonal gammopathy
- Proteins on filter paper
- Anticarbohydrate antibodies
- Heat-inactivated serum
- High concentration of bilirubin in serum
- Passively acquired antibodies
- Heterophil antibodies to bovine, ovine, caprine, and murine IgG
- HIV vaccines

From Cordes RI, Ryan ME. Pitfalls in HIV testing: application and limitations of current tests. Postgrad Med 98:177, 1995; Willman JH, Hill HR, Martins TB, et al. Multiplex analysis of heterophile antibodies in patients with indeterminate HIV immunoassay results. Am J Clin Pathol 115:764, 2001.

Indirect Immunofluorescence Assay

The indirect immunofluorescence assay (IFA) is an alternative supplemental test used following a positive EIA result. In the IFA, HIV-infected cells are fixed on a microscope slide. The cell preparations are incubated with patient serum, washed, and further incubated with a fluorescein-labeled anti-human

IgG reagent. Uninfected cells serve as an internal control for nonspecific binding or reaction with cellular antigens. Antibody-positive sera exhibit a characteristic cytoplasmic fluorescence. If both the control cells and virus-infected cells are fluorescent, the IFA is reported as indeterminate. Results are generally concordant with that of the Western blot.[68] The IFA is sometimes used to resolve the infection status of a patient with an indeterminate Western blot. Although turnaround time is similar to that for the Western blot, the IFA is not widely used because it requires more hands-on time and a technician who is skilled at reading the IFA.

Simple, Rapid HIV Antibody Tests

A major advance has been the development of rapid HIV assays that provide results within an hour of sample collection without the need for specialized equipment or sophisticated technical expertise. A number of rapid tests can be performed on whole blood and some on oral fluid, in addition to serum or plasma. These features greatly enhance opportunities for HIV testing in resource-limited and outreach settings. Programmatic studies have indicated that the use of on-site rapid tests significantly increases the number of clients who actually receive their test results compared with conventional EIA testing.[69–73] Rapid HIV tests also have demonstrated value for clinical situations in which decisions regarding antiviral prophylaxis are urgent, such as for pregnant women who present in labor with unknown HIV infection status, and for testing the source patient after occupational exposures to blood or body fluids.[47,74–78] Rapid tests are more expensive than the EIA, but they offer advantages because they can be performed during initial contact with the patient in the field, clinic, or emergency department; do not require laboratory equipment or specialized technicians; and provide test results during the same visit. Negative test results require no further confirmation and can be reported immediately to the patient. As with any HIV screening test, a reactive rapid test result requires confirmation, but the patient can be counseled about a provisionally positive test result while confirmatory testing is in progress. Performing an EIA after a positive rapid HIV test is optional; supplemental testing with Western blot or IFA is required regardless of the EIA result.[79]

Many rapid tests achieve sensitivity and specificity equivalent to that of the EIA and Western blot. Most rapid tests are assembled in kit form, require no additional reagents or equipment, and many can be stored at ambient temperatures.

Three main test formats are used: particle agglutination, immunoconcentration (flow-through), and immunochromatography (lateral flow).[80] In particle agglutination tests, latex particles coated with HIV antigen are mixed with patient serum. If HIV antibodies are present, they cross-link the particles and produce agglutination that can be observed visually. Some test kits enhance agglutination by causing the specimen to pass through narrowed capillary channels. Interpretation is simple in strong agglutination reactions, but weak agglutination can be difficult to detect and accurate interpretation is possible only after much experience and practice.[81] Automated readers have been developed to improve sensitivity, but with added cost and complexity. Flow-through devices consist of a cartridge with one or more HIV antigens immobilized on a porous membrane. Patient specimen is allowed to flow through the membrane (by gravity or wicked by an absorbent pad on the other side of the porous membrane). Antibody binds to the immobilized antigen, and is detected by the subsequent addition of anti-human IgG bound to a reagent that produces a red or blue color. In the presence of antibody, a dot or visible line forms on the membrane at the antigen location. Many flow-through tests also incorporate anti-human IgG immobilized on the membrane to serve as an internal control: appearance of color at the control location demonstrates that specimen has been added and that the test has been performed correctly. Some tests allow differentiation of HIV-1 from HIV-2 by applying different antigens in different locations on the membrane. The flow-through devices require several steps for application of specimen, wash buffer, and the indicator reagent. Most are suitable for serum or plasma, though some are equipped with a filter or hemolyzing reagent to allow their use with whole blood. Lateral flow devices consist of a nitrocellulose strip, often encased in a plastic cartridge, and incorporate both antigen and signal reagent into the nitrocellulose strip. The specimen (usually followed by a buffer) is added to an absorbent pad. Alternatively, the specimen is diluted in a vial of buffer, to which the device is added. The specimen migrates through the nitrocellulose strip and combines with a colored anti-human IgG signal reagent. The complex then continues to migrate along the strip, over lines where HIV antigen has been applied. A positive reaction results in a colored line on the strip where the HIV antibody–anti-IgG conjugate complex is bound to the HIV antigen. A control line, consisting of immobilized anti-IgG, is often applied to the strip distal to the antigen line. Appearance of a colored line at the control location ensures adequate flow of sample and integrity of the reagents. Most lateral flow devices require only a single step and no additional equipment or refrigeration; test results can be obtained in less than 30 min. Many can be used with multiple types of specimen: finger stick or venipuncture whole blood, plasma, serum, or oral fluid.

Six rapid assays were approved by the US FDA as of July 2006, and many more are available internationally. A listing of commercially available rapid HIV tests is available at http://www.rapid-diagnostics.org/rti-hiv-com.htm. Systematic evaluations have established that most rapid tests adequately detect all subtypes of group M, but performance is more variable with group O and HIV-2.[82–92] Limited data from seroconversion panels indicate that analytic sensitivity for early infection is comparable to that of first and second generation EIAs currently licensed by the FDA.[84,88] The WHO maintains results of its periodic rapid HIV test evaluations at http://www.who.int/diagnostics_laboratory/publications/evaluations/en/index.html. Sequential algorithms that use combinations of rapid tests for screening and confirmation are recommended by the WHO (Fig. 1-7) and have been used effectively in international settings for years.[47,71,93–95] Similar

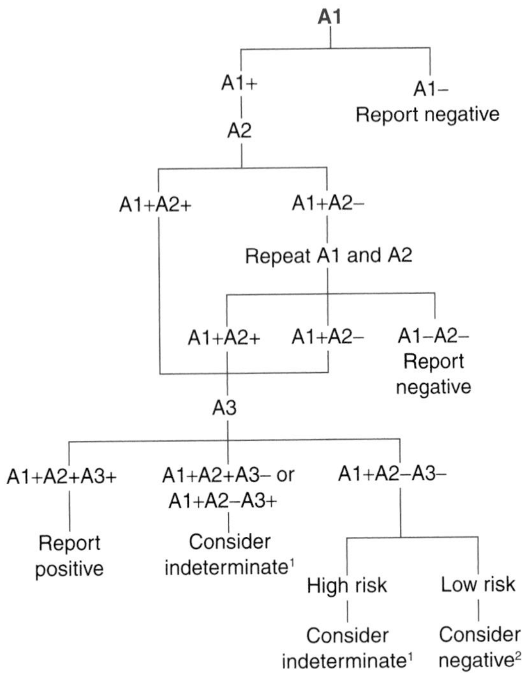

Figure 1-7 ■ Schematic representation of the UNAIDS WHO diagnostic testing algorithm using combinations of screening or rapid tests. A1, A2, and A3 represent 3 different assays. [1] Testing should be repeated on a second sample taken after 14 days. [2] In the absence of any risk for HIV infection.

Redrawn with permission from World Health Organization, Weekly Epidemiologic Record, vol 72, no 12, 1997, p 84.

evaluations are underway in the US, and a same-visit confirmation procedure would be a major advance.

Alternative Specimens: Oral Fluid and Urine

For settings where blood collection is impractical, for the needle-phobic, and for improved compliance, tests have been devised to detect HIV antibody in oral fluid and urine. Initially, these tests were not as sensitive or specific as blood tests, but the current tests perform comparably.[35,86,87,95–99] Many patients find HIV testing with oral fluid and urine to be more acceptable than conventional blood tests.[100,101]

Because antibody levels in whole saliva are low, oral fluid HIV tests are designed for use with oral mucosal transudate, secreted at the crevice between the tooth and the gum. This oral fluid contains a quantity of HIV antibody, predominately of the IgG isotype, that is sufficient for testing. When used with oral fluid obtained from both adults and children, commercial HIV assays show sensitivity and specificity comparable to those of tests performed with serum.[97,102] Two oral fluid tests have been approved for HIV diagnosis by the FDA. The Orasure test (OraSure Technologies, Bethlehem, PA, USA) uses an oral fluid collection device to obtain antibody-rich oral fluid. After collection, the device is inserted into a vial containing an antibacterial preservative and sent to a laboratory for testing with an EIA and Western blot specifically optimized for use with oral fluid. Compared to serum-based testing, the sensitivity and specificity of the Orasure test process approach 100%.[97,98] The Oraquick Advance HIV-1/2 rapid antibody test, from the same manufacturer, is a lateral flow rapid test that is used to both collect and test oral fluid. Test results can be obtained in less than 30 min, but sensitivity and specificity, though greater than 99%, are slightly lower than those obtained when the same device is used with blood or plasma.[99] Relative performance in early seroconversion has not been extensively evaluated.

Several studies have shown that, despite very low IgG levels in urine compared with serum, EIAs can be performed on urine with results that are similar to those with serum.[103–106] Both a urine EIA and Western blot (Calypte Biomedical, Inc., Lake Oswego, OR) are FDA approved for HIV-1 diagnosis. However, because sensitivity and specificity with urine are slightly lower than with parallel serum testing,[107] reactive HIV test results from urine may require confirmation with serum testing.

Tests for p24 Antigen

Tests for p24 antigen were initially pursued to aid HIV diagnosis during the preseroconversion window period and for infants in whom the persistence of passively transferred maternal antibody precluded definitive diagnosis with antibody tests. The HIV-1 p24 core protein is the most abundant viral protein, and can be measured in plasma during early infection before seroconversion. However, p24 antigen disappears with seroconversion and is present only intermittently during the phase of clinical latency. The p24 antigen test has been used to detect PHI before serococonversion, and was formerly used to screen seronegative blood donors for early infection.[108,109] Its use for blood bank purposes has now been supplanted by NAAT testing for viral RNA.[110–114] However, the p24 test is less expensive and technically less complicated than NAAT and may continue to be useful in settings with insufficient resources or inadequate laboratory infrastructure. Currently, p24 antigen detection has found widespread acceptance in international settings as part of fourth generation EIAs that detect both p24 antigen and HIV antibody with a single screening test.[47,49,50]

Commercial assays for p24 detection and quantitation use a sandwich capture EIA format in which anti-p24 antibody, applied to the solid phase, binds p24 antigen from patient serum or plasma. Bound antigen is detected with an enzyme-conjugated anti-p24 antibody, and the subsequent colorimetric reaction is proportionate to the amount of p24 antigen in the specimen. A neutralization test is used to confirm both this assay and fourth generation EIAs. The neutralization test requires demonstration of a loss or reduction in OD when the assay is performed after p24 antigen-negative, antibody-positive serum is mixed with the patient serum to block or compete with the binding of the patient's p24 antigen.

During and after seroconversion, antibodies against p24 result in the formation of immune complexes containing p24 antigen. Conventional assays fail to detect p24 antigen in immune complexes. Procedural modifications have been introduced that involve pretreatment with acid or heat to dissociate the antigen antibody complexes, after which free p24 can then be measured.[115–117] Such "ultrasensitive" techniques may be especially useful as a low-cost method for diagnosis of HIV infection in perinatally exposed infants.[118]

Nucleic Acid Amplification Tests

Both quantitative and qualitative assays for detecting HIV-1 RNA molecules in plasma are commercially available. All of these rely on molecular amplification techniques, that is, multiplication of the RNA molecule or a related signal until the number of molecules produced is sufficient to be detected by diagnostic methods. Quantitative viral load assays are now used routinely for assessing disease prognosis, making decisions regarding the initiation of antiretroviral therapy, and monitoring the response to therapy.[17,119] Qualitative assays are currently used for blood donor screening[112,113,120] and for HIV-1 diagnosis in infants.[121–127] The qualitative assays are optimized for analytic sensitivity at low thresholds, whereas the quantitative assays are optimized to produce reliable, reproducible results over a dynamic range of HIV-1 RNA levels. In practice, the quantitative assays, particularly the "ultrasensitive" versions, have a sufficiently low threshold of detection for diagnostic use.

During clinical latency or late infection, HIV antibody testing should be adequate for diagnosis because RNA testing for primary diagnosis is expensive and unnecessary. However, RNA testing may be of value for diagnosing HIV antibody-negative patients with suspected PHI, and as a supplemental test on specimens with indeterminate Western blot results.[18,19,47,52] The HIV viral load levels during PHI are usually extremely high and are detectable well before seroconversion.[19,45,128–131] Levels may range from 10^4 to 10^7 RNA copies per milliliter, exceeding the threshold for HIV-1 detection of most RNA assays.[17,19,128,132] Several evaluations of the clinical value of screening for PHI by RNA testing in settings other than the blood bank have been published or are underway.[108,128,133–135] Unlike p24 antigen testing, RNA levels are generally measurable throughout the course of infection in the absence of effective ART.[136]

Three quantitative viral load assays were FDA approved as of July 2006 for monitoring HIV-1 infection: Roche Amplicor HIV-1 Monitor Test (Roche Molecular Systems, Inc., Branchburg Township, NJ); NucliSens HIV-1 QT (bioMerieux, Inc., Durham, NC); and Versant HIV-1 RNA 3.0 bDNA (Bayer Corp., Berkeley, CA). None of these has a designation for HIV diagnosis. Three qualitative assays are also FDA approved for screening of pooled specimens from blood donors for HIV-1: UltraQual HIV-1 RT-PCR Assay (National Genetics Institute, Los Angeles, CA); COBAS Ampliscreen HIV-1 Test (Roche Molecular Systems, Inc., Pleasanton, CA); and the multiplex Procleix (Gen-Probe, San Diego, CA), which screens for HIV-1 and hepatitis C virus (HCV). Aptima (Gen Probe, San Diego, CA) is a qualitative RNA assay used to identify the presence of HIV-1, and is FDA approved as an aid to HIV-1 diagnosis. It may be used for screening antibody-negative specimens to detect acute infection. Aptima may also be used as an additional test, when it is reactive, to confirm HIV infection after a reactive HIV antibody test. If the antibody test is reactive and the Aptima test is negative, however, further testing with Western blot or IFA is required for confirmation.

The RNA molecular diagnostic tests in current use in the US employ three different principles for RNA detection and quantitation. The Amplicor viral load test and the qualitative Ampliscreen and UltraQual tests are based on reverse transcriptase polymerase chain reaction (RT-PCR) technology.[137] To perform these tests, RNA is extracted from plasma, from which RNA is reverse transcribed into cDNA. The DNA and a known standard is then amplified by PCR. The HIV-1 *gag* gene product is detected with an enzyme-linked DNA probe, and the subsequent color reaction is proportionate to the amount of input RNA. The known copy-number standard allows conversion of the colorimetric readings into copies of RNA per milliliter of plasma, and also serves as an internal control for the efficiency of RNA extraction. The Nucli-Sens HIV-1 QT viral load test is a nucleic acid sequence-based amplification (NASBA) assay based on a different principle: transcription mediated amplification (TMA).[138] RNA extracted from plasma is subjected to the activity of two enzymes, reverse transcriptase (containing RNAse H activity) and T7 polymerase, in the presence of two primers complementary to a nucleic acid sequence in the *gag* region of HIV-1. The result is a single-strand DNA (cDNA) template for multiple rounds of RNA transcription. Amplification of RNA and internal calibration standards generate a luminescent signal proportional to the input RNA copy number.[138] The qualitative Aptima RNA assay also accomplishes target amplification with TMA; detection is achieved by chemiluminescent nucleic acid probes that hybridize to the amplification products. The Versant uses a signal amplification technique known as branched DNA (bDNA) for RNA quantitation.[139,140] HIV-1 RNA is captured onto a microtiter plate. Multiple DNA probes are hybridized to specific polymerase gene segments. The probes have tandem sequences that allow further hybridization to a branched probe that, in turn, can bind multiple copies of an alkaline phosphatase conjugate. The alkaline phosphatase acts on a substrate to generate a chemiluminescent reaction; the relative light units produced are converted to an RNA copy number by reference to an external standard. Thus, in contrast to the RT-PCR and NASBA techniques, which amplify the actual RNA target, the bDNA amplifies the signal from the RNA–DNA hybridization reaction. In direct comparisons of the three quantitative assays, all show similar lower limits of detection, sensitivity, and specificity.[141–149] Results with the three assays are highly correlated although the absolute RNA value for an individual specimen may differ somewhat.[141–149]

Direct DNA PCR of proviral HIV-1 DNA from peripheral blood mononuclear cells (PBMCs) has also been used for diagnosis. Qualitative DNA PCR has traditionally been used for diagnosis of HIV-1 in infants.[123–125,150] In fact, DNA PCR of PBMC was used in the first demonstrations of the power of NAAT technology for detecting HIV-1 in clinical specimens.[151–153] Roche Molecular Diagnostics markets a commercial DNA-PCR assay that is currently not FDA approved, nor had application for approval been made. There is a theoretical disadvantage related to analytic sensitivity of DNA PCR in terms of the relatively smaller numbers of copies of DNA than of RNA in clinical specimens. Analytic sensitivity could be improved by performing both RT PCR and DNA PCR simultaneously on cellular specimens. The wide availability of RNA tests for monitoring HIV levels and the requirement for an alternative specimen type for DNA extraction (whole blood or cells as opposed to plasma) are practical drawbacks favoring the use of RNA NAAT. Nevertheless, DNA NAAT appears to perform as well as RNA-based assays for detection of HIV in clinical specimens.[151]

Although there may have been problems with detection of nonclade B isolates with earlier versions of the quantitative and qualitative tests, the current versions reliably detect HIV-1 group M subtypes and group O.[46,154] Antiretroviral therapy is the most common cause of undetectable RNA in plasma, but an occasional HIV-1 specimen may not amplify (false negative). This may be due to very low levels of virus, specimen degradation, the presence of an inhibitor such as heparin, or a mismatch of the primer–probe sequence with the target RNA. Mismatch of primer–probe can sometimes be resolved by using an alternate commercial test, by isolation in cell culture, or amplification of other regions of the viral genome.[155] There is also a low rate of false-positive RNA tests.[18,156,157] False positives usually register low levels of RNA (<5000 copies/mL), and they are generally negative on repeat testing. None of the NAAT tests detect HIV-2, and no quantitative RNA assays for HIV-2 are commercially available.

HIV Isolation by Cell Culture

Infectious virus can be isolated from plasma or PBMC by co-culture with susceptible cell lines or activated PBMC from a seronegative donor. Culture supernatants are monitored for viral replication by detecting p24 antigen or reverse transcriptase activity over a period of several weeks. The advantage of virus isolation is that it provides definitive evidence of infection (barring contamination). The disadvantages are that it is relatively insensitive,[158] requires up to 4 weeks to complete, and involves specialized laboratory facilities and expertise. Viral culture is also expensive and not well standardized. Because of these drawbacks, viral culture is not used routinely for diagnostic purposes. It is reserved for resolution and investigation of specimens with unusual or discordant serologic results in which a variant HIV is suspected.

Diagnosis of HIV-2

HIV-2 was first detected in West Africa, and is found infrequently in the rest of the world, except in patients with a direct or indirect connection to West Africa.[159–162] HIV-1 and HIV-2 share cross-reactive epitopes in the *gag* and *pol* region, but envelope cross-reactivity is weak or nonexistent.[159,161,163,164] Thus, an HIV-2 specimen may react in some HIV-1 screening tests, and give a characteristic indeterminate banding pattern (with the absence of envelope bands) in an HIV-1 Western blot. A completely negative HIV-1 Western blot result with HIV-2 serum is very unusual but may occur in patients with advanced HIV-2 disease. Current HIV-1/HIV-2 combination EIAs and rapid tests specifically target HIV-2 by inclusion of a gp36 antigen to increase the yield of HIV-2 detection compared with reliance on cross-reactivity with HIV-1. Thus, in most current testing algorithms, a repeatedly positive HIV-1/HIV-2 EIA or HIV-1 EIA followed by an indeterminate HIV-1 supplemental test is a flag for investigating the possibility of HIV-2 infection. An independent indication for HIV-2 testing relates to clinical suspicion of HIV-2 infection (negative HIV-1 results in a symptomatic patient with links to West Africa). An HIV-2 screening EIA is available commercially (BioRad Laboratories, Hercules, CA). This test is based on an HIV-2 viral lysate that may cross-react with HIV-1 sera. It is FDA-approved for screening but is of limited value in distinguishing HIV-1 from HIV-2. The Multispot HIV-1/2 rapid test from the same manufacturer is FDA-approved for distinguishing HIV-1 from HIV-2. It is a flow-through device with separate antigen spots for recombinant HIV-1 protein and two spots for non-cross-reactive HIV-1 and HIV-2 peptides. The type-specific antigens are derived from the respective transmembrane envelope proteins, gp41 in HIV-1 and gp36 in HIV-2. Western blots for HIV-2 are available, but none is currently licensed by the FDA. An HIV-1/HIV-2 recombinant immunoblot assay (Chiron) that incorporates both HIV-1 and HIV-2 antigens in a single blot and performs equivalently to standard Western blot in HIV diagnosis is also available but not FDA-approved.[60,61] NAAT tests do not detect HIV-2. Gene sequencing to distinguish HIV-1 from HIV-2 is relatively straightforward and may be available by referral to specialized research laboratories.

THE IMPORTANCE OF FOLLOW-UP TESTING

After a positive HIV test, it is clinically prudent to repeat testing on a second specimen to assure that no procedural error or specimen mix-up has occurred. Discordant or indeterminate results (EIA-positive, WB-negative; NAAT-positive, EIA-negative; WB indeterminate) require testing of a follow-up specimen for definitive resolution. If there is some indication of reactivity from initial testing and the patient is infected, follow-up testing at 1 and, if needed, 3 months will usually resolve the issue.[18,19,25,27] After a known exposure to HIV, data from observations after a known infectious exposure such as a needle stick injury are informative. Most who will seroconvert will do so within 3 months of exposure, although rarely, infected persons have remained antibody negative for more than 6 months.[19,25–27,165] Although the documentation of these cases have been called into question,[19,26] there do appear to be some patients who exhibit delayed seroconversion.[19,25,26] In addition, the effect of postexposure prophylaxis on the evolution of seroconversion is unknown. Taken together, there is no entirely secure way of ruling out infection after an exposure other than following for at least 6 months. We generally test at 1, 3, and 6 months and try to communicate the declining risk with successive negative tests without raising undue alarm.

DIAGNOSIS OF HIV INFECTION IN INFANTS

HIV can be transmitted from an infected mother to child during gestation, labor, or through breastfeeding. Most infections occur late in pregnancy or during delivery.[166] Mother-to-child transmission can be reduced to <2% with universal screening of pregnant women in combination with prophylactic administration of antiretroviral drugs, scheduled caesarean delivery, when indicated, and avoidance of breastfeeding.[167,168] The use of intrapartum and postpartum antiretroviral prophylaxis can also reduce transmission substantially.[169,170] Appropriate treatment of HIV-infected infants requires HIV-exposed infants to be identified as soon as possible, which can be best accomplished through the identification of HIV-infected women before or during pregnancy with routine HIV antibody testing. If women are not tested for HIV during pregnancy, a rapid HIV antibody test should be performed during labor, if possible, or during the immediate postnatal period. When maternal HIV status has not been determined during the prenatal or immediate postpartum period, newborns should undergo rapid HIV antibody testing.[171,172] The HIV exposure status of infants should be determined promptly because the neonatal component of the recommended zidovudine prophylaxis regimen should begin as soon as possible after birth, and because prophylaxis against *pneumocystis* pneumonia should be initiated at age 4–6 weeks in all infants born to HIV-infected women.[173]

HIV antibody tests are ineffective for establishing the diagnosis of HIV infection in HIV-exposed infants because maternal IgG antibody crosses the placenta and may cause positive antibody tests in uninfected infants for more than a year after birth.[127,174–178] Maternal antibody levels decline in the infant over 9–12 months, and virtually all uninfected infants are antibody-negative by 18 months of age; infected infants will demonstrate rising titers and persistence of antibody.[127,174–178]

HIV infection can be definitely diagnosed in most infected infants by age 1 month and in virtually all infected infants by age 6 months with the use of virologic tests (NAAT assays or viral culture).[173] HIV-1 NAAT (cellular DNA or plasma RNA assays) are the virologic methods of choice for the diagnosis or exclusion of infection in infants. HIV culture is more complex, less well standardized, and less sensitive than NAAT.[158,179,180] p24 antigen detection is highly specific, but it is less sensitive than NAAT, especially in the presence of antibody, and it is not useful for excluding infection.[115,180–182] The specificity of a standardized NAAT test in experienced hands approaches 100%. Sensitivity varies with the timing of infection but approaches 100% if performed after 4 months of age in infants who were infected pre- or perinatally.[121–127,158] The timing of transmission (intrauterine, peripartum, or through breastfeeding) dictates the amount of time required for viral replication to rise to the threshold of detection by NAAT assays. Intrauterine infection has been operationally defined as having a positive DNA test within 48 h of birth, whereas peripartum infections are negative in the first week of life but become positive within 4–6 weeks.[177,179,183,184] Transmission due to breastfeeding can first be detected at any time during or up to 6 weeks after breastfeeding has stopped.[177,183] Once infected, infants have a rapid rise in plasma virus to high levels that exceed that of adults by several orders of magnitude. These levels are sustained or decline only slightly during the first 18 months of life.[121,123,125–127,177,185,186] Thus, detection of well-established infection poses little problem for most virologic tests.

Diagnostic testing in the infant is recommended within 48h after birth and at 14 days, 1–2 months, and at 3–6 months of age.[171,173] Although the specificity of a single, standardized NAAT test is extremely high, it is prudent to repeat the testing on a positive specimen before concluding that infection is present.[156–158,178,187] HIV infection is diagnosed by two positive HIV virologic tests performed on separate blood samples, regardless of age. Umbilical cord blood should not be used for diagnosis because of the possibility of contamination with maternal blood. In a meta-analysis representing 271 HIV-infected children, the estimated sensitivity of the HIV DNA-PCR assay was 38% at birth, increasing to 93% at 14 days of age, and 96% at 28 days of age.[150] In the absence of antiretroviral prophylaxis, comparisons of DNA versus RNA testing for infant diagnosis have shown little difference[122,124,125] or a small advantage for RNA testing.[121,123,158] Antiretroviral prophylaxis of the infant has been reported to cause little or no delay in the onset of RNA detection.[123,127,158,188] It remains to be determined whether the more intensive combination antiretroviral regimens women may receive during pregnancy for treatment of their own HIV infection will affect the sensitivity of RNA detection in their infants. Because of the easier availability and standardization of RNA tests, RNA testing is likely to be used more often than DNA testing for infant diagnosis.

Excluding HIV infection in an exposed infant is more difficult. HIV-1-exposed infants are generally followed with periodic testing for 18–24 months before concluding that infection is absent. In an unpublished analysis of several large data sets conducted by the CDC, HIV infection could be reasonably excluded in non-breast fed infants with two or more negative NAAT tests performed at age >1 month, with one of those performed at age ≥4 months. Because of the possibility of mutation/recombination involving the target sequences detected by a particular NAAT assay, it is possible that an occasional infection might go undetected. Demonstration of reactivity in a specimen from the mother provides reassurance that the particular test used is appropriate for the infant. However, if suspicion is high and results are negative, it may be prudent to with another assay. Negative HIV antibody test results more than 6 months after birth are clinically useful and reliable for ruling out infection.[174–178] Two or more negative IgG antibody tests performed at age 6 months with an interval of at least 1 month between the tests excludes HIV infection in HIV-exposed infants with no other clinical or laboratory evidence of HIV infection.[173] Serology after 12 months is recommended to confirm that transferred maternal antibodies have disappeared. If the child is still antibody positive at 12 months, then testing should be repeated between 15 and 18 months. Loss of HIV antibody in a child with previously negative HIV NAAT tests definitively confirms that the child is uninfected. The WHO recommends waiting 6 weeks after stopping breastfeeding before conducting tests to exclude infection.[183]

ALGORITHMS FOR HIV TESTING

In practice, HIV diagnostics involves a testing sequence designed to capture all potentially infected persons with an initial screening test followed by a more specific test to confirm infection. The performance and selection of a testing algorithm depends on a number of factors. These include the test sensitivity and specificity relevant to the population being tested, the purpose of testing, cost, testing infrastructure, and turnaround time. No single test is perfect and no single algorithm fits all situations. Optimally designed algorithms leave only a small number of discordant specimens that need further testing or follow-up specimens for resolution of infection status.

Operationally, a negative screening assay is taken as prima facie evidence for the absence of HIV antibody. All screening tests are prone to giving occasional weakly reactive results that most often are not reproducible. Therefore, most laboratories repeat an initially reactive screening EIA result in duplicate before proceeding to confirmatory testing. This avoids a substantial amount of unnecessary confirmatory testing. There is little advantage to doing the initial screen with two different screening assays, other than as a check on procedure. Discordant dual screening test results rarely indicate infection on supplemental testing, and there is almost no gain in sensitivity and considerable increase in cost. Strong reactive results in the current screening assays are the norm for specimens from infected persons, but the degree of reactivity is not a reliable distinction between true positives and false positives. Further testing is required. Supplemental tests should be selected that are not prone to the same false-positive effect that gave rise to false-positive results in the initial screen. False positives can be minimized by selecting assays that contain different HIV antigens (viral lysate, recombinant proteins, or peptides) or that differ in assay format. All algorithms are plagued by occasional discordant or equivocal results. These can sometimes be resolved by additional

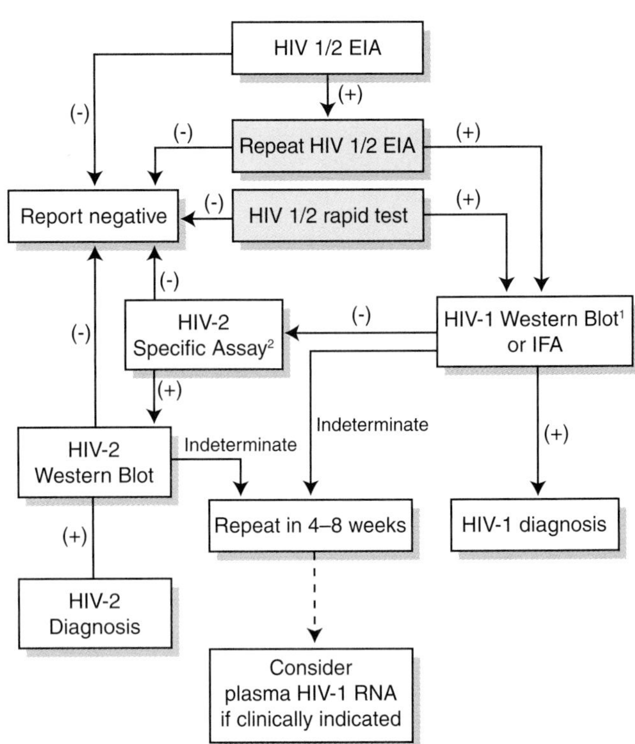

Figure 1-8 ■ US Public Health Service algorithm for serologic diagnosis of HIV-1/HIV-2 infection.

testing. More often, a second specimen drawn weeks to months later is required to determine whether the pattern of reactivity has evolved into a definitive diagnostic category.

Three algorithms are described below. They are representative of varied algorithms for different testing situations, constraints, and intended purpose. A more extensive outline of 12 algorithms, their applicability to the test population, and relative merits can be found in reference.[47]

A typical algorithm consistent with the US Public Health Service recommendations, often referred to as the "classic" algorithm, is shown in Figure 1-8. Specimens are screened with an EIA or rapid test that detects HIV-1 and HIV-2. Negative results are reported as such. Reactive EIAs are repeated; and specimens positive by rapid test or repeatedly reactive by EIA advance to supplemental HIV-1 Western blot or IFA testing. If the Western blot is positive, the specimen is reported as HIV-1 positive. If the Western blot is negative or indeterminate (especially with the unusual indeterminate pattern of *gag* plus *pol* bands in the absence of *env* bands), the specimen is tested specifically for HIV-2, either with an HIV-2 EIA or the Multispot HIV-1/2 rapid test. If negative for HIV-2, an HIV-1 Western blot-negative specimen is reported as HIV-negative. If the HIV-1 Western blot is indeterminate, the specimen is reported as indeterminate and a follow-up specimen is requested.

The US blood banking algorithm incorporates NAAT testing, both for detection of PHI[108,111–114,120,189] and for confirmatory testing. EIA negative specimens are tested in a pooled specimen strategy (see the discussion under

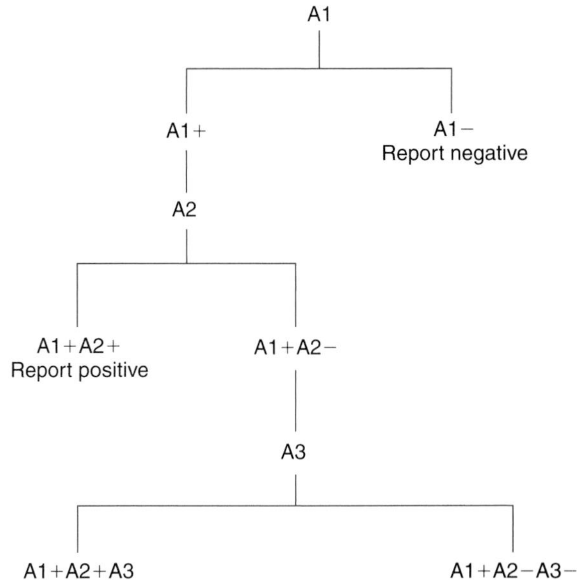

Figure 1-9 ■ Modified algorithm for establishing the diagnosis of HIV infection using combinations of rapid tests. A1, A2 and A3 represent different assays.

Redrawn with permission from World Health Organization and Join United Nations Programme on HIV/AIDS, Guidelines for Using HIV Testing Technologies in Surveillance. 2001, p 23.

"Screening for PHI"). EIA repeatedly reactive specimens are tested with individual NAAT. If positive, the specimen is reported as positive. If negative, Western blot testing is done and the subsequent sequence is the same as in the US Public Health Service algorithm.

The WHO developed a set of three testing strategies designed to be appropriate to the purpose of the testing (blood screening, surveillance or diagnosis) and the expected prevalence of HIV in the population, and to help mitigate the delays and high cost inherent to confirmatory testing with the Western blot.[93] The WHO strategy for diagnosis is based on sequential combinations of EIA or rapid screening tests (Fig. 1-7). An initial negative test result is reported as such. If the initial screen is positive, a second and third test are performed. If all three tests are positive, the result is reported as positive. All other combinations following an initial positive test are reported as indeterminate. Indeterminate results are resolved either by follow-up testing on a second specimen collected after 14 days, or by supplemental tests such as the Western blot. In practice, a modified three-test algorithm is used in many international settings (Fig. 1-9).[71,72,89,94,95] If the first test is positive, a second test is performed. If both tests are positive, the specimen is reported as positive. If the second test is negative, a third test is performed, and the result is reported based on the concordance of two of the three test results.

SCREENING FOR PHI

PHI spans the period after infection and before seroconversion, the so-called window period. During this period and the subsequent 3 months, patients can have extremely high viral loads, are disproportionately contagious relative to persons with longer-term infection, and present an opportunity for early intervention.[18,19,28,128–130,190–194] In order to narrow the diagnostic window that is undetected by antibody assays, HIV antigen or nucleic acid detection may be used.[14,18,19]

Screening seronegatives for p24 antigen, which shortens the window by ~5 days,[18,19] was instituted by US blood banks in the 1990s. In 1999, NAAT screening using qualitative tests was introduced, which shortens the window by ~10–15 days[18,19] and has since replaced p24 screening in blood banks. Highly sensitive and specific, standardized, qualitative NAAT assays are used in a "multiplex" configuration for simultaneous detection of HIV-1 and HCV.[111–114,189] To improve throughput and reduce cost, 16 to 24 seronegative donor specimens are pooled, and the pool is tested. For HIV, virtually all PHI specimens detected by individual NAAT have sufficiently high viral load to register positive in a pool despite the 1:16–24 dilution factor.[14,28,114,131,156,157] Pools with a positive reaction are resolved and confirmed by discriminatory NAAT performed on the individual specimens that constitute the reactive pool.[111–114,189] In the low prevalence US blood donor population, the yield of reactive NAAT tests was low: one infection in three million seronegative donors were detected with NAAT in the initial evaluation of the program.[112,113,120,189] Despite the low yield and high cost, NAAT screening of blood donors is now routine in developed countries in order to optimally protect the blood supply.[109,120,134,195]

The utility of screening for PHI in the diagnostic or public health arena is under evaluation.[14,28,129,131,133,194,196,197] In published studies, the yield of new infections detected as a percent of seronegatives screened ranges from 0.02% to 0.15%.[28,131,197] The incremental yield of HIV-1 infections detected over that of serology alone ranges from 4% to 7%.[28,131,197] Unpublished yields are more extreme. The Maryland State Health Department detected no NAAT-positive specimens among more than 68 000 EIA-negatives. The San Francisco Health Department detected NAAT reactivity in 0.40% of seronegatives, increasing the diagnostic yield of infections detected by 11%. Undoubtedly, the wide range of yields relate to the risk for HIV infection in the populations being screened. It is also notable that newer generation EIAs detect HIV infection earlier than previous tests, further narrowing the window and likely decreasing the yield of a NAAT screening program. Despite the demonstrated ability to accurately detect PHI, the benefits of such a program relative to the intensive resource demands remain to be determined.[134]

WHO SHOULD BE TESTED

Since the introduction of the first EIA for HIV in 1985, recommendations for HIV testing have focused on those persons whose increased risk for HIV characterized the early epidemic: men who have sex with men, injection drug users, hemophiliacs, and persons seeking treatment for sexually transmitted diseases.[198,199] Specific HIV testing sites were established where persons who considered themselves at risk could seek voluntary testing. Since 1993, routine HIV counseling and testing has been recommended for hospital inpatients and outpatients in areas where the prevalence of HIV infection is higher than 1%.[200] Of adults age 18–64 in the US, 38–42% report that they have been tested for HIV, and 16–22 million persons are tested annually; more than 75% report they were tested by private doctors, in health maintenance organizations, hospitals, emergency departments, and community clinics.[201] Despite these efforts, approximately one quarter of the estimated 1–1.2 million HIV-infected persons in the US are unaware of their HIV infection and, therefore, unable to benefit from clinical care to reduce morbidity and mortality.[202] Treatment, especially since HAART was introduced in 1995, has dramatically improved survival rates, but insufficient progress has been made in effecting earlier diagnosis. Nearly half of persons diagnosed with AIDS are first tested for HIV because of illness, late in the course of their disease.[203]

Accumulating evidence demonstrates that risk-based testing fails to identify many HIV-infected persons.[204,205] In 2003, CDC introduced *Advancing HIV Prevention: New Strategies for a Changing Epidemic.* A key strategy is making HIV testing a routine part of medical care on the same voluntary basis as other diagnostic or screening tests.[206] HIV screening is recommended for all pregnant women during each pregnancy, and, based on cost-effectiveness analyses, for all persons ages 13–64 in healthcare settings.[172,207,208] Subsequently, repeat testing is recommended at least annually for all persons known to be at increased risk for HIV. Providers should also encourage HIV screening for patients and their prospective partners before they initiate a new sexual relationship. All patients with signs or symptoms consistent with HIV infection or an opportunistic infection should receive diagnostic testing for HIV, and when PHI is a possibility (patients with a compatible clinical syndrome and a recent high-risk exposure), a plasma RNA test should be used in conjunction with an HIV antibody test to diagnose acute infection.[172]

HIV testing must be voluntary, and confidentiality must be assured. Patients should receive oral or written information about HIV infection and the meanings of positive and negative test results, and have the opportunity to ask questions and to decline testing. HIV screening need not be contingent on assessment of patients' risk behaviors. Prevention counseling is not required as a part of HIV screening programs in healthcare settings, and need not be linked to HIV testing. Assessment of risk for infection with HIV and other STDs and provision of prevention information should be incorporated into routine primary care of all sexually active persons, and prevention counseling is strongly encouraged for persons at high risk for HIV when risk behaviors are routinely assessed, such as when patients seek treatment for STD-related symptoms.

Identifying persons with HIV infection is important from both a clinical and public health standpoint. The US Preventive Services Task Force concluded that there is good evidence that when HIV is diagnosed early, appropriately timed interventions, particularly HAART, lead to improved health outcomes, including slower clinical progression and reduced mortality.[209] Most persons who are aware of their HIV infections substantially reduce sexual behaviors that might transmit HIV after they become aware they are infected. In a meta-analysis of findings from eight studies, the prevalence of unprotected anal or vaginal intercourse with uninfected partners was an average of 68% lower for HIV-infected persons aware of their status than for HIV-infected persons unaware of their status.[210] Because viral load is the chief predictor of HIV transmission,[129] reduction in viral load through timely initiation of HAART may reduce transmission, even for HIV-infected patients who do not change their risk behavior.[208]

HIV infection meets all of the generally accepted criteria that justify routine screening: HIV infection is a serious health disorder that can be diagnosed before symptoms develop; HIV can be detected by reliable, inexpensive, noninvasive screening tests; infected patients have years of life to gain if treatment is initiated early, before symptoms develop; and the costs of screening are reasonable in relation to the anticipated benefits.[211] Prevention strategies that incorporate universal HIV screening have been highly effective. For example, screening blood donors for HIV has virtually eliminated transfusion-associated HIV infection in the US.[110] The incidence of pediatric HIV/AIDS declined substantially since the 1990s, when prevention strategies began to include specific recommendations for routine HIV testing of pregnant women regardless of risk.[212,213] The number of children reported with AIDS attributed to perinatal HIV transmission peaked at 945 in 1992 and declined 95% to 48 in 2004, largely because of the identification of HIV-infected pregnant women and the effectiveness of antiretroviral prophylaxis in reducing mother-to-child transmission of HIV.[2,214] In 2006, the CDC recommended that HIV screening should be a part of routine clinical care in all healthcare settings, preserving the patient's option to decline HIV testing and ensuring a provider-patient relationship conducive to optimal clinical and preventive care.[172]

REFERENCES

1. Palella FJ, Deloria-Knoll M, Chimel JS. Survival benefit of initiating antiretroviral therapy in HIV-infected persons in different CD4+ cell strata. Ann Intern Med 138:620, 2003.
2. Centers for Disease Control and Prevention. HIV/AIDS surveillance report, 2004. 16:1, 2005.
3. Klein D, Hurley LB, Merrill D, Quesenberry CP. Review of medical encounters in the 5 years before a diagnosis of HIV-1 infection: implications for early detection. J Acquir Immune Defic Syndr 32:143, 2003.
4. Liddicoat RV, Horton NJ, Urban R, et al. Assessing missed opportunities for HIV testing in medical settings. J Gen Intern Med 19:349, 2004.
5. Kuo AM, Haukoos JS, Witt MD, et al. Recognition of undiagnosed HIV infection: an evaluation of missed opportunities in a predominantly minority urban population. AIDS Patient Care STDs 19:239, 2005.

6. Institute of Medicine. No Time to Lose: Getting More from HIV Prevention. Washington, DC: National Academy of Sciences Press; 2001.
7. Kieny MP. Structure and regulation of the human AIDS virus. J Acquir Immune Defic Syndr 3:395, 1990.
8. Greene WC. The molecular biology of human immunodeficiency virus type 1 infection. N Engl J Med 324:308, 1991.
9. McCutchan FE. Global epidemiology of HIV. J Med Virol 78(Suppl 1):S7, 2006.
10. Peterlin BM, Luciw PA. Molecular biology of HIV. AIDS 2(Suppl 1):S29, 1988.
11. Gorny MK, Conley AJ, Karwowska S, et al. Neutralization of diverse human immunodeficiency virus type 1 variants by an anti-V3 human monoclonal antibody. J Virol 66:7538, 1992.
12. McCutchan FE. Understanding the genetic diversity of HIV-1. AIDS 14:S31, 2000.
13. Kijak GH, McCutcheon FE. HIV diversity, molecular epidemiology, and the role of recombination. Curr Infect Dis Rep 7:480, 2005.
14. Hecht FM, Busch MP, Rawal B, et al. Use of laboratory tests and clinical symptoms for identification of primary HIV infection. AIDS 16:1119, 2002.
15. Kahn JO, Walker BD. Acute human immunodeficiency virus type 1 infection. N Engl J Med 339:33, 1998.
16. Celum CL, Buchbinder SP, Donnel D. Early human immunodeficiency virus (HIV) infection in the HIV Network for Prevention Trials Vaccine Preparedness cohort: risk behaviors, symptoms, and early plasma and genital tract virus load. J Infect Dis 183:23, 2001.
17. Mellors JW, Munoz A, Giorgi JV, et al. Plasma viral load and CD4+ lymphocytes as prognostic markers of HIV-1 infection. Ann Intern Med 126:946, 1997.
18. Fiebig EW, Wright DJ, Rawal BD, et al. Dynamics of HIV viremia and antibody seroconversion in plasma donors: implications for diagnosis and staging of primary HIV infection. AIDS 17:1871, 2003.
19. Lindback S, Thorstensson R, Karlsson AC, et al. Diagnosis of primary HIV-1 infection and duration of follow-up after HIV exposure. AIDS 14:2333, 2000.
20. McDougal JS, Kennedy MS, Nicholson JK, et al. Antibody response to human immunodeficiency virus in homosexual men. Relation of antibody specificity, titer, and isotype to clinical status, severity of immunodeficiency and disease progression. J Clin Invest 80:316, 1987.
21. Gaines H, von Sydow M, Parry JV, et al. Detection of immunoglobulin M antibody in primary human immunodeficiency virus infection. AIDS 2:11, 1988.
22. Nkengasong J, Van Kerckhoven I, Vercauteren G, et al. Alternative confirmatory strategy for anti-HIV antibody detection. J Virol Methods 36:159, 1992.
23. Cooper DA, Imrie AA, Penney R. Antibody response to human immunodeficiency virus after primary infection. J Infect Dis 155:1113, 1987.
24. Gaines H, von Sydow M, Sonnerborg A, et al. Antibody response in primary human immunodeficiency virus infection. Lancet 1:1249, 1987.
25. Busch MP, Satten GA. Time course of viremia and antibody seroconversion following human immunodeficiency virus exposure. Am J Med 102(5B):117, 1997.
26. Heptonstall J, Gill ON. HIV, occupational exposure, and medical responsibilities. Lancet 346:578, 1995.
27. Busch MP, Lee LL, Satten GA, et al. Time course of detection of viral and serologic markers preceding human immunodeficiency virus type 1 seroconversion: implications for screening of blood and tissue donors. Transfusion 35:91, 1995.
28. Pilcher CD, Fiscus SA, Nguyen TQ, et al. Detection of acute infections during HIV testing in North Carolina. N Engl J Med 352:1873, 2005.
29. Centers for Disease Control and Prevention. Persistent lack of detectable HIV-1 antibody in a person with HIV infection – Utah, 1995. MMWR 25:181, 1996.
30. Ellenberger DL, Sullivan PS, Dorn J. Viral and immunologic examination of human immunodeficiency virus type 1-infected, persistently seronegative persons. J Infect Dis 180:1033, 1999.
31. Hare CB, Pappalardo BL, Busch MP, et al. Seroreversion in subjects receiving antiretroviral therapy during acute/early HIV infection. Clin Infect Dis 42:700, 2006.
32. Willman JH, Hill HR, Martins TB, et al. Multiplex analysis of heterophile antibodies in patients with indeterminate HIV immunoassay results. Immunopathology 115:764, 2001.
33. Padeh YC, Rubinstein A, Shliozberg J. Common variable immunodeficiency and testing for HIV-1. N Engl J Med 353:1074, 2005.
34. Ho DD, Moudgil T, Robin HS, et al. Human immunodeficiency virus type 1 in a seronegative patient with visceral Kaposi's sarcoma and hypogammaglobulinemia. Am J Med 86:349, 1989.
35. O'Connell RJ, Merritt TM, Malia JA, et al. Performance of the OraQuick rapid antibody test for diagnosis of human immunodeficiency virus type 1 infection in patients with various levels of exposure to highly active antiretroviral therapy. J Clin Microbiol 41:2153, 2003.
36. Gutierrez M, Soriano V, Bravo R, et al. Seroreversion in patients with end-stage HIV infection. Vox Sang 67:238, 1994.
37. Pan LZ, Cheng-Mayer C, Levy JA. Patterns of antibody response in individuals infected with the human immunodeficiency virus. J Infect Dis 155:626, 1987.
38. Markowitz M, Vesanen M, Tenner-Racz K, et al. The effect of commencing combination anti-retroviral therapy soon after human immunodeficiency virus type 1 infection on viral replication and antiviral immune responses. J Infect Dis 179:527, 1999.
39. Frenkel LM, Mullins JI, Learn GH, et al. Genetic evaluation of suspected cases of transient HIV-1 infection of infants. Science 280:1073, 1998.
40. Roy MJ, Damato JJ, Burke DS. Absence of true seroreversion of HIV-1 antibody in seroreactive individuals. JAMA 269:2876, 1993.
41. Constantine NT, van der Groen G, Belsey EM, Tamashiro H. Sensitivity of HIV-antibody assays determined by seroconversion panels. AIDS 8:1715, 1994.
42. Weber B, Moshtaghi-Boronjeni M, Brunner M, et al. Evaluation of the reliability of 6 current anti-HIV-1/HIV-2 enzyme immunoassays. J Virol Methods 55:97, 1995.
43. Ghosh K, Javeri KN, Mohanty D, et al. False-positive serologic tests in acute malaria. Brit J Biomed Science 58:20, 2001.
44. Koch WH, Sullivan PS, Roberts C, et al. Evaluation of United States-licensed human immunodeficiency virus immunoassays for detection of group M viral variants. J Clin Microbiol 39:1017, 2001.
45. Kinloch-de Loes S, de Saussure P, Saurat JH, et al. Symptomatic primary infection due to human immunodeficiency virus type 1: review of 31 cases. Clin Infect Dis 17:59, 1993.
46. van Binsberen J, de Rijk D, Peels H, et al. Evaluation of a new third generation anti-HIV-1/anti-HIV2 assay with increased sensitivity for HIV-1 group O. J Virol Methods 60:131, 1996.
47. Constantine NT, Saville RD, Dax EM. Retroviral Testing and Quality Assurance. Halifax: MedMira Laboratories; 2005.
48. Loussert-Ajaka I, Ly TD, Chaix ML, et al. HIV-1/HIV-2 seronegativity in HIV-1 subtype O infected patients. Lancet 343:1393, 1994.
49. Polywka S, Feldner J, Duttmann H, Laufs R. Diagnostic evaluation of a new combined HIV p24 antigen and anti-HIV1/2/O screening assay. Clin Lab 47:351, 2001.

50. Saville RD, Constantine NT, Cleghorn FR, et al. Fourth-generation enzyme-linked immunosorbent assay for the simultaneous detection of human immunodeficiency virus antigen and antibody. J Clin Microbiol 39:2518, 2001.
51. Laperche S, Maniez-Montreuil M, Courouce AM. Screening tests combined with p24 antigen and anti-HIV antibodies in early detection of HIV-1. Transfus Clin Biol 1(Suppl 1):18S, 2000.
52. Kleinman S, Busch MP, Hall L, et al. False-positive HIV-1 test results in a low-risk screening setting of voluntary blood donation. Retrovirus Epidemiology Donor Study. JAMA 280:1080, 1998.
53. Celum CL, Coombs RW, Jones M, et al. Risk factors for repeatedly reactive HIV-1 EIA and indeterminate Western blots. A population-based case-control study. Arch Intern Med 154:1129, 1994.
54. Cordes RJ, Ryan ME. Pitfalls in HIV testing. Application and limitations of current tests. Postgrad Med 98:177, 1995.
55. Reiss P, De Ronde A, Dekker J, et al. Seroconversion to HIV-1 rev- and tat-gene-encoded proteins. AIDS 2:105, 1989.
56. Parekh BS, Pau CP, Granade TC, et al. Oligomeric nature of transmembrane glycoproteins of HIV-2: procedures for their efficient dissociation and preparation of Western blots for diagnosis. AIDS 5:1009, 1991.
57. Pau CP, Granade TC, Parekh B, et al. Misidentification of HIV-2 proteins by Western blots. Lancet 337:616, 1991.
58. Pinter A, Honnen WJ, Tilley SA, et al. Oligomeric structure of gp41, the transmembrane protein of human immunodeficiency virus type 1. J Virol 63:2674, 1989.
59. Zolla-Pazner S, Gorny MK, Honnen WJ, Pinter A. Reinterpretation of human immunodeficiency virus Western blot patterns. N Engl J Med 320:1280, 1989.
60. Zaaijer HL, van Rixel T, van Exel-Ochlers P, et al. New anti-human immunodeficiency virus immunoblot assays resolve nonspecific Western blot results. Transfusion 37:193, 1997.
61. Kline RL, McNairn D, Holodniy M, et al. Evaluation of Chiron HIV-1/HIV-2 recombinant immunoblot assay. J Clin Microbiol 34:2650, 1996.
62. Centers for Disease Control and Prevention. Interpretation and use of the Western blot assay for serodiagnosis of human immunodeficiency virus type 1 infections. MMWR 38(S-7):1, 1989.
63. O'Gorman MR, Weber D, Landis SE, et al. Interpretive criteria of the Western blot assay for serodiagnosis of human immunodeficiency virus type 1 infection. Arch Pathol Lab Med 115:26, 1991.
64. George JR, Schochetman G. Serologic tests for the detection of human immunodeficiency virus infection. In: George JR, Schochetman G (eds) AIDS Testing: Methodology and Management Issues. New York: Springer; 1992, p 48.
65. Pasquier C, Sandres-Saune K, Mansuy J-M, et al. Virologic exploration of individuals with discordant HIV screening tests. J Clin Virol 30:218, 2004.
66. Laperche S, Morel P, Deschaseaux M, et al. HIV antibody screening remains indispensable for ensuring viral safety of blood components despite NAT implementation. Transfusion 43:1428, 2003.
67. Jackson JB, Hanson MR, Johnson GM, et al. Long-term follow-up of blood donors with indeterminate human immunodeficiency virus type 1 results on Western blot. Tranfusion 35:98, 1995.
68. Carlson JR, Yee J, Hinrichs SH, et al. Comparison of indirect immunofluorescence and Western blot for detection of anti-human immunodeficiency virus antibodies. J Clin Microbiol 25:494, 1987.
69. Kane B. Rapid testing for HIV: why so fast. Ann Intern Med 131:481, 1999.
70. Centers for Disease Control and Prevention. Update: HIV counseling and testing using rapid tests – United States, 1995. MMWR 47:211, 1998.
71. Downing R, Otten R, Marum E. Optimizing the delivery of HIV counseling and testing services: the Uganda experience using rapid HIV antibody test algorithms. J Acquir Immune Defic Syndr 18:384, 1998.
72. Kassler W, Alwano-Edyegu M, Marum E. Rapid HIV testing with same-day results: a field trial in Uganda. Int J STD AIDS 9:134, 1998.
73. Kassler W, Dillon B, Haley C. On-site, rapid HIV testing with same-day results and counseling. AIDS 11:1045, 1997.
74. Bulterys M, Jamieson DJ, O'Sullivan MJ, et al. Mother–Infant Rapid Intervention At Delivery (MIRIAD) Study Group. Rapid HIV-1 testing during labor: a multicenter study. JAMA 292:219, 2004.
75. Mrus JM, Tsevat J. Cost-effectiveness of interventions to reduce vertical HIV transmission from pregnant women who have not received prenatal care. Med Decis Making 24:30, 2004.
76. Doyle NM, Levison JE, Gardner MO. Rapid HIV versus enzyme-linked immunosorbent assay screening in a low-risk Mexican American population presenting in labor: a cost-effectiveness analysis. Am J Obstet Gynecol 193:1280, 2005.
77. Puro V, Francisci D, Sighinolfi L, et al. Benefits of a rapid HIV test for evaluation of the source patient after occupational exposure of healthcare workers. J Hosp Infect 57:179, 2005.
78. Landrum ML, Wilson CH, Perri LP, et al. Usefulness of a rapid human immunodeficiency virus-1 antibody test for the management of occupational exposure to blood and body fluid. Infect Control Hosp Epidemiol 26:768, 2005.
79. Centers for Disease Control and Prevention. Protocol for confirmation of rapid HIV tests. MMWR 53:221, 2004.
80. Branson BM. Point of care rapid tests for HIV antibodies. J Lab Med 27:288, 2003.
81. Dax EM, O'Connell R. Standardization of subjectively scored HIV immunoassays: developing a quality assurance program to assist in reproducible interpretation of results using an anti-HIV particle agglutination assay as a model. J Virol Methods 82:113, 1999.
82. Windsor IM, Gomes Dos Santos ML, De La Hunt LI, et al. An evaluation of the Capillus HIV-1/HIV-2 latex agglutination test using serum and whole blood. Int J STD AIDS 8:192, 1997.
83. Ray CS, Mason PR, Smith H, et al. An evaluation of dipstick-dot immunoassay in the detection antibodies to HIV-1 and 2 in Zimbabwe. Trop Med Int Health 2:83, 1997.
84. Kuun E, Brashaw M, Heyns AD. Sensitivity and specificity of standard and rapid HIV-antibody tests evaluated by seroconversion and non-seroconversion low titre panels. Vox Sang 72:11, 1997.
85. Phillips S, Granade TC, Pau C-P, et al. Diagnosis of human immunodeficiency virus type 1 infection with different subtypes using rapid tests. Clin Diagn Lab Immunol 7:698, 2000.
86. Tamashiro H, Constantine NT. Serological diagnosis of HIV infection using oral fluid samples. Bull World Heath Organ 72:135, 1994.
87. Lu XS, Delfraissy JF, Grangeot-Keros L, et al. Rapid and constant detection of HIV antibody response in saliva of HIV-infected patients; selective distribution of anti-HIV activity in the IgG isotype. ResVirol 145:369, 1994.
88. Giles RE, Perry KR, Parry JV. Simple/rapid test devices for anti-HIV screening: do they come up to the mark? J Med Virol 59:104, 1999.
89. Stetler HC, Granade TC, Nunez CA, et al. Field evaluation of rapid HIV serologic tests for screening and confirming HIV-1 infection in Honduras. AIDS 11:369, 1997.

90. Constantine NT, Zeking L, Sangare AK, et al. Diagnostic challenges for rapid human immunodeficiency virus assays: performance using HIV-1 group O, HIV-1 group M, and HIV-2 samples. J Virol Methods 1:45, 1997.
91. Makuwa M, Souquiere S, Niangui MT, et al. Reliability of rapid diagnostic tests for HIV variant infection. J Virol Methods 103:183, 2002.
92. Reynold SJ, Ndongala LM, Luo CC, et al. Evaluation of a rapid test for the detection of antibodies to human immunodeficiency virus type1 and 2 in the setting of multiple transmitted subtypes. Int J STD AIDS 12:171, 2002.
93. Joint United Nations Programme on HIV/AIDS. The importance of simple/rapid assays in HIV testing. Wkly Epidemiol Rec 73:321, 1998.
94. Nkengasong JN, Maurice C, Koblavi S, et al. Evaluation of HIV serial and parallel serologic testing algorithms in Abidjan, Cote d'Ivoire. AIDS 13:109, 1999.
95. Koblavi-Demi S, Maurice C, Yavo D, et al. Sensitivity and specificity of human immunodeficiency virus rapid serologic assays and testing algorithms in an antenatal clinic in Abidjan, Ivory Coast. J Clin Microbiol 39:1808, 2001.
96. Hodinka RL, Nagashunmugam T, Malamud D. Detection of human immunodeficiency virus antibodies in oral fluids. Clin Diag Lab Immunol 5:419, 1998.
97. Gallo D, George JR, Fitchen JH, et al. Evaluation of a system using oral mucosal transudate for HIV-1 antibody screening and confirmatory testing. OraSure HIV Clinical Trial Group. JAMA 277:254, 1997.
98. King SD, Wynter SH, Bain BC, et al. Comparison of testing saliva and serum for detection of antibody to human immunodeficiency virus in Jamaica, West Indies. J Clin Virol 19: 157, 2000.
99. Delaney KP, Branson BM, Uniyal A, et al. Performance of an oral fluid rapid HIV1/2 test: experience from four CDC studies. AIDS 20:1655, 2006.
100. Meehan MP, Sewankambo NK, Wawer MJ, et al. Sensitivity and specificity of HIV-1 testing of urine compared with serum specimens: Rakai, Uganda. The Rakai Project Team. Sex Transm Dis 10:590, 1999.
101. Spielberg F, Branson BM, Goldaum GM, et al. Choosing HIV counseling and testing strategies for outreach settings: a randomized trial. J Acquir Immune Defic Syndr 38:348, 2005.
102. McFarland W, Busch MP, Kellogg TA, et al. Detection of early HIV infection and estimation of incidence using a sensitive/less-sensitive enzyme immunoassay testing strategy at anonymous counseling and testing sites in San Francisco. J Acquir Immune Defic Syndr 22:484, 1999.
103. Sterne JA, Turner AC, Connell JA, et al. Human immunodeficiency virus: GACPAT and GACELISA as diagnostic tests for antibodies in urine. Trans R Soc Trop Med Hyg 87:181, 1993.
104. Hashida S, Hashinaka K, Saitoh A, et al. Diagnosis of HIV-1 infection by detection of antibody IgG to HIV-1 in urine with ultrasensitive enzyme immunoassay (immune complex transfer enzyme immunoassay) using recombinant proteins as antigens. J Clin Lab Anal 8:237, 1994.
105. Constantine NT, Zhang X, Li L, et al. Application of a rapid assay for detection of antibodies to human immunodeficiency virus in urine. Am J Clin Pathol 101:157, 1994.
106. Berrios DC, Avins AL, Haynes-Sanstad K, et al. Screening for human immunodeficiency virus antibody in urine. Arch Pathol Lab Med 119:139, 1995.
107. Urnovitz HB, Sturge JC, Gottfried TD, Murphy WH. Urine antibody tests: new insights into the dynamics of HIV-1 infection. Clin Chem 45:1602, 1999.
108. Gallarda JL, Dragon E. Blood screening by nucleic acid amplification technology: current issues, future challenges. Mol Diagn 5:11, 2000.
109. Schreiber GB, Busch MP, Kleinman SH, Korelitz JJ. The risk of transfusion-transmitted viral infections. The Retrovirus Epidemiology Donor Study. N Engl J Med 334:1685, 1996.
110. Dodd RY, Notari EP, Stramer SL. Current prevalence and incidence of infectious disease markers and estimated window-period risk in the American Red Cross blood donor population. Transfusion 42:975, 2002.
111. Roth WK, Weber M, Seifried E. Feasibility and efficacy of routine PCR screening of blood donations for hepatitis C virus, hepatitis B virus, and HIV-1 in a blood bank setting. Lancet 353:359, 1999.
112. Stramer SL, Caglioti S, Strong DM. NAT of the United States and Canadian blood supply. Transfusion 40:1165, 2000.
113. Stramer SL, Glynn SA, Kleinman SH, et al. Detection of HIV-1 and HCV infections among antibody-negative blood donors by nucleic acid-amplification testing. N Engl J Med 351:760, 2004.
114. Grant PR, Busch MP. Nucleic acid amplification technology methods used in blood donor screening. Transfus Med 12:229, 2002.
115. Schupbach J. Measurement of HIV-1 p24 antigen by signal-amplification-boosted ELISA of heat-denatured plasma is a simple and inexpensive alternative to tests for viral RNA. AIDS Rev 4:83, 2002.
116. Nishanian P, Huskins KR, Stehn S, et al. A simple method for improved assay demonstrates that HIV p24 antigen is present as immune complexes in most sera from HIV-infected individuals. J Infect Dis 162:21, 1990.
117. Bollinger RC, Kline RL, Francis HL, et al. Acid dissociation increases the sensitivity of p24 antigen detection for the evaluation of antiviral therapy and disease progression in asymptomatic human immunodeficiency virus infected persons. J Infect Dis 165:913, 1992.
118. Patton JC, Sherman GG, Coovadia AH, et al. Ultrasensitive human immunodeficiency virus type 1 p24 antigen assay modified for use on dried whole-blood spots as a reliable, affordable test for infant diagnosis. Clin Vaccine Immunol 13:152, 2006.
119. Holodniy M. Viral load monitoring in HIV infection. Curr Infect Dis Rep 1:497, 1999.
120. Busch MP, Kleinman SH, Jackson B, et al. Committee report. Nucleic acid amplification testing of blood donors for transfusion-transmitted infectious diseases: report of the interorganizational task force on nucleic acid amplification testing of blood donors. Transfusion 40:143, 2000.
121. Steketee RW, Abrams EJ, Thea DM, et al. Early detection of perinatal human immunodeficiency virus (HIV) type 1 infection using HIV RNA amplification and detection. New York City Perinatal HIV Transmission Collaborative Study. J Infect Dis 175:707, 1997.
122. Rouet F, Montcho C, Rouzioux C, et al. Early diagnosis of paediatric HIV-1 infection among African breast-fed children using a quantitative plasma HIV RNA assay. AIDS 15:1849, 2001.
123. Young NL, Shaffer N, Chaowanachan T, et al. Early diagnosis of HIV-1-infected infants in Thailand using RNA and DNA PCR assays sensitive to non-B subtypes. J Acquir Immune Defic Syndr 24:401, 2000.
124. Nesheim S, Palumbo P, Sullivan K. Quantitative RNA testing for diagnosis of HIV-infected infants. J Acquir Immune Defic Syndr 32:192, 2003.
125. Cunningham CK, Charbonneau TT, Song K, et al. Comparison of human immunodeficiency virus 1 DNA polymerase chain reaction and qualitative and quantitative RNA polymerase chain reaction in human immunodeficiency virus 1-exposed infants. Ped Infecti Dis J 18:30, 1999.
126. Shearer WT, Quinn TC, LaRussa P, et al. Viral load and disease progression in infants infected with human immunodeficiency

virus type 1. Women and Infants Transmission Study Group. N Engl J Med 336:1337, 1997.
127. Palumbo PE, Kwok S, Waters S, et al. Viral measurement by polymerase chain reaction-based assays in human immunodeficiency virus-infected infants. J Pediatr 126:592, 1995.
128. Brookmeyer R, Gail MH. AIDS Epidemiology: A Quantitative Approach. New York: Oxford University Press; 1994.
129. Daar EC, Little S, Pitt J, et al. Diagnosis of primary HIV-1 infection. Ann Intern Med 134:25, 2001.
130. Niu MT, Bethel J, Holodniy M, et al. Zidovudine treatment in patients with primary (acute) human immunodeficiency virus type 1 infection: a randomized, double-blind, placebo-controlled trial. J Infect Dis 178:80, 1998.
131. Stekler J, Swenson PD, Wood RW, et al. Targeted screening for primary HIV infection through pooled HIV-RNA testing in men who have sex with men. AIDS 19:1323, 2005.
132. Piatak M, Saag MS, Yang LC, et al. High levels of HIV-1 in plasma during all stages of infection determined by competitive PCR. Science 259:1749, 1993.
133. Pilcher CD, McPherson JT, Leone PA, et al. Real-time, universal screening for acute HIV infection in a routine HIV counseling and testing population. JAMA 288:216, 2002.
134. Busch MP, Hecht FR. Nucleic acid amplification testing for diagnosis of acute HIV infection: has the time come? AIDS 19:1317, 2005.
135. Nguyen K-A, Busch MP. Evolving strategies for diagnosing human immunodeficiency virus infection. Am J Med 109:595, 2000.
136. Henrard DR, Phillips JF, Muenz LR, et al. Natural history of HIV-1 cell-free viremia. JAMA 274:554, 1995.
137. Sun R, Ku J, Jayakar H, et al. Ultrasensitive reverse transcription-PCR assay for quantitation of human immunodeficiency virus type 1 RNA in plasma. J Clin Microbiol 36:2964, 1998.
138. Kievits T, van Gemen B, van Strijp D, et al. NASBA isothermal enzymatic in vitro nucleic acid amplification optimized for the diagnosis of HIV-1 infection. J Virol Methods 35:273, 1991.
139. Urdea MS, Wilber JC, Yeghiazarian T, et al. Direct and quantitative detection of HIV-1 RNA in human plasma with a branched DNA signal amplification assay. AIDS 7:S11, 1993.
140. Collins ML, Irvine B, Tyner D, et al. A branched DNA signal amplification assay for quantification of nucleic acid targets below 100 molecules/ml. Nucleic Acids Res 25:2979, 1997.
141. Berndt C, Muller U, Bergmann F, et al. Comparison between a nucleic acid sequence-based amplification and branched DNA test for quantifying HIV RNA load in blood plasma. J Virol Methods 89:177, 2000.
142. Murphy DG, Cote L, Fauvel M, et al. Multicenter comparison of Roche COBAS Amplicor Monitor Version 1.5, Organon Teknika Nuclisens QT with Extractor, and Bayer Quantiplex Version 3.0 for quantitation of human immunodeficiency virus type 1 RNA in plasma. J Clin Microbiol 38:4034, 2000.
143. Lin JH, Pedneault L, Hollinger FB. Intra-assay performance characteristics of five assays for quantification of human immunodeficiency virus type 1 RNA in plasma. J Clin Microbiol 36:835, 1998.
144. Schmitt Y. Performance characteristics of quantification assays for human immunodeficiency virus type 1 RNA. J Clin Virol 20:31, 2001.
145. Anastassopoulou CG, Touloumi G, Katsoulidou A, et al. Comparative evaluation of the Quantiplex HIV-1 RNA 2.0 and 3.0 (bDNA) assays and the Amplicor HIV-1 Monitor v1.5 test for the quantitation of human immunodeficiency virus type 1 RNA in plasma. J Virol Methods 91:67, 2001.
146. Highbarger HC, Alvord WG, Jiang MK, et al. Comparison of the Quantiplex Version 3.0 assay and a sensitized Amplicor Monitor assay for measurement of human immunodeficiency virus type 1 RNA levels in plasma samples. J Clin Microbiol 37:3612, 1999.
147. Elbeik T, Charlebois E, Nassos P, et al. Quantitative and cost comparison of ultrasensitive human immunodeficiency virus type 1 RNA viral load assays: Bayer bDNA Quantiplex Versions 3.0 and 2.0 and Roche PCR Amplicor Monitor Version 1.5. J Clin Microbiol 38:1113, 2000.
148. Coste J, Montes B, Reynes J, et al. Comparative evaluation of three assays for the quantitation of human immunodeficiency virus type 1 RNA in plasma. J Med Virol 50:293, 1996.
149. Schuurman R, Descamps D, Weverling GJ, et al. Multicenter comparison of three commercial methods for quantification of human immunodeficiency virus type 1 RNA in plasma. J Clin Microbiol 34:3016, 1996.
150. Dunn DT, Brandt CD, Krivine A, et al. The sensitivity of HIV-1 DNA polymerase chain reaction in the neonatal period and the relative contributions of intra-uterine and intra-partum transmission. AIDS 9:7, 1995.
151. Owens DK, Holodniy M, Garber AM, et al. Polymerase chain reaction for the diagnosis of HIV infection in adults. A meta-analysis with recommendations for clinical practice and study design. Ann Intern Med 124:803, 1996.
152. Kwok S, Mack DH, Mullis KB, et al. Identification of human immunodeficiency virus sequences by using in vitro enzymatic amplification and oligomer cleavage detection. J Virol 61:1690, 1987.
153. Ou C-Y, Kwok S, Mitchell SW, et al. DNA amplification for direct detection of HIV-1 in DNA of peripheral blood mononuclear cells. Science 239:295, 1988.
154. Respess RA, Butcher A, Wang H, et al. Detection of genetically diverse human immunodeficiency virus type 1 group M and O isolates by PCR. J Clin Microbiol 35:1284, 1997.
155. Yang C, Bipin C, Simon F, et al. Detection of diverse variants of human immunodeficiency virus-1 groups M, N, and O and simian immunodeficiency viruses from chimpanzees by using generic pol and env primer pairs. J Infect Dis 181:1791, 2000.
156. Havlichek DH, Hage-Korban E. False positive HIV diagnosis by HIV-1 plasma viral load testing. Ann Intern Med 130:37, 1999.
157. Rich JD, Merriman NA, Mlonakis E, et al. Misdiagnosis of HIV infection by HIV-1 plasma viral load testing: a case series. Ann Intern Med 130:37, 1999.
158. Lambert JS, Harris DR, Stiehm ER, et al. Performance characteristics of HIV-1 culture and HIV-1 DNA and RNA amplification assays for early diagnosis of perinatal HIV-1 infection. J Acquir Immune Defic Syndr 34:512, 2003.
159. George JR, Ou CY, Parekh B, et al. Prevalence of HIV-1 and HIV-2 mixed infections in Cote d'Ivoire. Lancet 340:337, 1992.
160. Kim SS, Kim EY, Park KY, et al. Introduction of human immunodeficiency virus 2 infection into South Korea. Acta Virol 44:15, 2000.
161. Markovitz DM. Infection with the human immunodeficiency virus type 2. Ann Intern Med 118:211, 1993.
162. O'Brien TR, George JR, Epstein JS, Schochetman G. Testing for antibodies to human immunodeficiency virus type 2 in the United States. MMWR 41(RR12):1, 1992.
163. George JR, Rayfield MA, Phillips S, et al. Efficacies of US Food and Drug Administration-licensed HIV-1-screening enzyme immunoassays for detecting antibodies to HIV-2. AIDS 4:321, 1990.
164. Gottlieb GS, Sow PS, Hawes SE, et al. Molecular epidemiology of dual HIV-1/HIV-2 seropositive adults from Senegal, West Africa. AIDS Res Hum Retroviruses 19:575, 2003.
165. Ciesielski CA, Metler RP. Duration of time between exposure and seroconversion in healthcare workers with occupationally acquired infection with human immunodeficiency virus. Am J Med 102(5B):115, 1997.
166. Kourtis AP, Bulterys M, Nesheim SR, Lee FK. Understanding the timing of HIV transmission from mother to infant. JAMA 285:709, 2002.

167. Cooper ER, Chaurat M, Mofenson L. Combination antiretroviral strategies for the treatment of pregnant HIV-1-infected women and prevention of perinatal HIV-1 transmission. J Acquir Immune Defic Syndr 29:484, 2002.
168. International Perinatal HIV Group. The mode of delivery and the risk of vertical transmission of human immunodeficiency virus type-1: a meta-analysis of 15 prospective cohort studies. N Engl J Med 340:977, 1999.
169. Wade NA, Birkhead GS, Warren BL, et al. Abbreviated regimens of zidovudine prophylaxis and perinatal transmission of the human immunodeficiency virus. N Engl J Med 339:1409, 1998.
170. Shaffer N, Bulterys M, Simonds RJ. Short courses of zidovudine and perinatal transmission of HIV. N Engl J Med 340:1042, 1999.
171. Mofenson L. Technical report: perinatal human immunodeficiency virus testing and prevention of transmission. Committee on Pediatric AIDS. Pediatrics 106:E88, 2000.
172. Centers for Disease Control and Prevention. Revised recommendations for HIV testing of adults, adolescents, and pregnant women in health care settings. MMWR 55(RR-14):1, 2006.
173. US Public Health Service. Guidelines for the use of antiretroviral agents in pediatric HIV infection. Available: http://aidsinfo.nih.gov/ContentFiles/PediatricGuidelines.pdf 2006.
174. Chantry CJ, Cooper ER, Pelton SI, et al. Seroreversion in human immunodeficiency virus-exposed but uninfected infants. Pediatr Infect Dis J 14:382, 1995.
175. Madurai S, Moodley D, Coovadia HM, et al. Use of HIV-1 specific immunoglobulin G3 as a serological marker of vertical transmission. J Trop Pediatr 42:359, 1996.
176. Parekh BS, Shaffer N, Coughlin R, et al. Human immunodeficiency virus 1-specific IgA capture enzyme immunoassay for early diagnosis of human immunodeficiency virus 1 infection in infants. NYC Perinatal HIV Transmission Study Group. Pediatr Infect Dis J 12:908, 1993.
177. Fowler MG, Simonds RJ, Roongpisuthipong A. Update on perinatal HIV transmission. Pediatr Clin North Am 47:21, 2000.
178. Kline MW, Lewis DE, Hollinger FB, et al. A comparative study of human immunodeficiency virus culture, polymerase chain reaction and anti-human immunodeficiency virus immunoglobulin A antibody detection in the diagnosis during early infancy of vertically acquired human immunodeficiency virus infection. Pediatr Infect Dis J 13:90, 1994.
179. Kalish LA, Pitt J, Lew J, et al. Defining the time of fetal or perinatal acquisition of human immunodeficiency virus type 1 infection on the basis of age at first positive culture. Women and Infants Transmission Study (WITS). J Infect Dis 175:712, 1997.
180. Borkowsky W, Krasinsky K, Pollack H, et al. Early diagnosis of human immunodeficiency virus infection in children less than 6 months of age: comparison of polymerase chain reaction, culture, and plasma antigen capture techniques. J Infect Dis 166:616, 1992.
181. Zijenah LS, Tobaiwa O, Rusakaniko S, et al. Signal boosted qualitative ultrasensitive p24 antigen assay for diagnosis of subtype C HIV-1 infection in infants under the age of 2 years. J Acquir Immune Defic Syndr 39:391, 2005.
182. Schupbach J, Boni J, Tomasik Z, et al. Sensitive detection and early prognostic significance of p24 antigen in heat-denatured plasma of human immunodeficiency virus type 1-infected infants. Swiss Neonatal HIV Study Group. J Infect Dis 170:318, 1994.
183. Nduati R, John G, Mbori-Ngacha D, et al. Effect of breastfeeding and formula feeding on transmission of HIV-1: a randomized clinical trial. JAMA 283:1167, 2000.
184. Bryson YJ, Luzuriaga K, Sullivan JL, Wara DW. Proposed definitions for in utero versus intrapartum transmission of HIV-1. N Engl J Med 327:1246, 1992.
185. Hermaszewski RA, Webster ADB. Primary hypogammaglobulinemia: a survey of clinical manifestations and complications. QJM 86:31, 1993.
186. Abrams EJ, Weedon J, Steketee RW, et al. Association of human immunodeficiency virus (HIV) load early in life with disease progression among HIV-infected infants. New York City Perinatal HIV Transmission Collaborative Study Group. J Infect Dis 178:101, 1998.
187. Lujan-Zilbermann J, Bitar W, Knapp K, Flynn P. Human immunodeficiency virus type 1 RNA polymerase chain reaction reasonably excludes infection in exposed infants. Pediatr Infect Dis J 22:97, 2003.
188. Dunn DT, Simonds RJ, Bulterys M, et al. Interventions to prevent vertical transmission of HIV-1: effect on viral detection rate in early infant samples. AIDS 14:1421, 2000.
189. Busch MP, Dodd RY. NAT and blood safety: what is the paradigm? Transfusion 40:1157, 2000.
190. Wawer MJ, Gray RH, Sewankambo NK, et al. Rates of HIV-1 transmission per coital act, by stage of HIV-1 infection, in Rakai, Uganda. J Infect Dis 191:1403, 2005.
191. Koopman JS, Jacquez JA, Welch GW, et al. The role of early infection in the spread of HIV through populations. J Acquir Immune Defic Syndr 14:249, 1997.
192. Pilcher CD, Tien HC, Eron JJ, et al. Brief but efficient: acute HIV infection and the sexual transmission of HIV. J Infect Dis 189:1785, 2004.
193. Jacquez JA, Koopman JS, Simon CP, Longini IM. Role of the primary infection in epidemics of HIV infection in gay cohorts. J Acquir Immune Defic Syndr 7:1169, 1994.
194. Quinn TC, Wawer MJ, Sewankambo N, et al. Viral load and heterosexual transmission of human immunodeficiency virus type 1. Rakai Project Study Group. N Engl J Med 342:921, 2000.
195. Jackson BR, Busch MP, Stramer SL, AuBuchon JP. The cost-effectiveness of NAT for HIV, HCV, and HBV in whole-blood donations. Transfusion 43:721, 2003.
196. Roland ME, Elbeik TA, Kahn JO, et al. HIV RNA testing in the context of nonoccupational postexposure prophylaxis. J Infect Dis 190:598, 2004.
197. Patel P, Klausner JD, Bacon OM, et al. Detection of acute HIV infections in high-risk patients in California. J Acquir Immune Defic Syndr 42:75, 2006.
198. Centers for Disease Control and Prevention. Public Health Service guidelines for counseling and antibody testing to prevent HIV infection and AIDS. MMWR 36:509, 1987.
199. Centers for Disease Control and Prevention. Revised guidelines for HIV counseling, testing, and referral. MMWR 50(RR-19):1, 2001.
200. Centers for Disease Control and Prevention. Recommendations for HIV testing services for inpatients and outpatients in acute-care hospital settings. MMWR 42(RR-2):1, 1993.
201. Centers for Disease Control and Prevention. Number of persons tested for HIV – United States, 2002. MMWR 53:1110, 2004.
202. Glynn M, Rhodes P. Estimated HIV prevalence in the United States at the end of 2003. Abstract from National HIV Prevention Conference, Atlanta, GA, 12–15 June 2005.
203. Centers for Disease Control and Prevention. Late versus early testing of HIV – 16 sites, United States, 2000–2003. MMWR 52:581, 2003.
204. Chen Z, Branson B, Ballenger A, Peterman TA. Risk assessment to improve targeting of HIV counseling and testing services for STD clinic patients. Sex Transm Dis 25:539, 1998.
205. Jenkins TC, Gardner EM, Thrun MW. Risk-based human immunodeficiency virus (HIV) testing fails to detect the majority of HIV-infected persons in medical care settings. Sex Transm Dis 5:329, 2006.

206. Centers for Disease Control and Prevention. Advancing HIV prevention: new strategies for a changing epidemic – United States, 2003. MMWR 52:329, 2003.
207. Patiel AD, Weinstein MC, Kimmel AD, et al. Expanded screening for HIV in the United States – an analysis of cost-effectiveness. N Engl J Med 352:586, 2005.
208. Sanders GD, Bayoumi AM, Sundaram V, et al. Cost effectiveness of screening for HIV in the era of highly active antiretroviral therapy. N Engl J Med 352:570, 2005.
209. US Preventive Services Task Force. Screening for HIV: recommendation statement. Ann Intern Med 143:32, 2005.
210. Marks G, Crepaz N, Senterfitt JW, Janssen RS. Meta-analysis of high-risk sexual behavior in persons aware and unaware they are infected with HIV in the United States: implications for HIV prevention programs. J Acquir Immune Defic Syndr 39:446, 2005.
211. Wilson JM, Jungmer CT. Principles and practice of screening for disease. WHO Public Health Paper 34:1968.
212. Centers for Disease Control and Prevention. HIV/AIDS Surveillance Report, 1999. HIV/AIDS Surveillance Report 11:1, 2000.
213. Centers for Disease Control and Prevention. US Public Health Service recommendations for human immunodeficiency virus counseling and voluntary testing of pregnant women. MMWR 44(RR-7):1, 1995.
214. Lindegren ML, Byers RH, Thomas P. Trends in perinatal transmission of HIV/AIDS in the United States. JAMA 282:531, 1999.

Chapter 2

Primary Care in Developed Countries

David H. Spach, MD, Kenneth H. Mayer, MD

In developed countries, persons infected with human immunodeficiency virus (HIV) have experienced a profound improvement in survival, mainly as a result of the widespread availability and use of highly active antiretroviral therapy (HAART). With this tremendous success and with persons living much longer, the role of long-term primary care of HIV-infected persons has taken on increased importance. In the US and other developed nations, a wide range of medical providers, including infectious diseases specialists, internists, family practitioners, physician assistants, and advanced registered nurse practitioners, now serve in the capacity as HIV primary medical care providers. Excellent primary care for HIV-infected individuals consists of competent management of both HIV-related issues, as well as those general medical issues not directly related to HIV. Fundamental elements of competent HIV-specific primary care consist of identifying HIV-infected persons, recognizing common HIV-related manifestations, performing the initial comprehensive evaluation, providing appropriate vaccinations, prescribing appropriate medications to prevent major opportunistic infections, diagnosing common opportunistic infections, initiating optimal antiretroviral therapy when indicated, and providing counseling for prevention of the transmission of HIV to others. In addition, because of the rapidly changing nature of the field of HIV, those medical providers not considered HIV experts should make every effort to remain current with updated key treatment guidelines and receive consultation advice as needed, particularly for complicated HIV-related issues, such as interpretation of resistance tests and management of serious opportunistic infections. Conversely, many HIV experts may not have expertise in general medical care, and thus should attempt to remain current on the management of common primary care problems, such as hyperlipidemia, hypertension, and diabetes, as well as on the provision of essential preventive medicine services. This chapter will focus on HIV-related clinical issues essential for the primary care management of HIV-infected individuals.

IDENTIFYING HIV-INFECTED PATIENTS

Unfortunately, approximately one-fourth of persons now living with HIV in the US remain unaware of their HIV infections, and many persons who eventually obtain a diagnosis of HIV do not get tested until late in the course of their disease.[1] The rationale for emphasizing early diagnosis of persons with HIV infection is twofold: those individuals identified earlier in the course of their disease are likely to benefit more from antiretroviral therapy and opportunistic infection prophylaxis and, moreover, persons who are aware of their HIV status may be less likely to transmit HIV to others. Four major settings exist in which a medical provider might identify an HIV-infected individual: (1) routine HIV screening of an individual, (2) recognizing acute (primary) HIV infection, (3) recognizing a non-life-threatening HIV-related manifestation, such as oral hairy leukoplakia or oral candidiasis, and (4) diagnosing an AIDS-related complication, such as *Pneumocystis* pneumonia or *Toxoplasma* encephalitis.

During the early years of the HIV epidemic in the US, as well as in other industrialized countries, identification of HIV-infected persons focused on specific populations, particularly men who had sex with men (MSM), injection-drug users, hemophiliacs, and other blood product recipients; and these different populations were often described as 'high-risk groups'.[2,3] This terminology implies that certain individuals have greater susceptibility to HIV infection when compared with others, but as the HIV epidemic progressed, it became clear that HIV could infect persons from any population if they engaged in high-risk behavior. Thus, the HIV epidemic in the US now affects persons from a wide spectrum of socioeconomic and cultural groups. In 2003, the Centers for Disease Control and Prevention (CDC) issued recommendations to test for HIV infection in the following individuals: (1) all patients in all high HIV-prevalence clinical settings (such as a sexually transmitted diseases clinic), (2) those with risks for HIV in low-prevalence clinical settings, and (3) patients admitted to high HIV-prevalence acute care hospitals (HIV seroprevalence exceeds 1% or where the AIDS case rate exceeds 1 per 1000 discharges), and (4) all pregnant women.[4] Despite these recommendations for testing, the number of undiagnosed HIV-infected persons has remained at ~25%. Moreover, despite broad prevention efforts, the number of new HIV infections in the US has remained at ~40 000 new cases per year, and there has been great concern that a disproportionate number of the new cases have resulted from HIV transmission from individuals who do not know they have HIV infection. These factors, when taken together, led the CDC to revamp their strategy for HIV testing and in 2006, the CDC issued sweeping new HIV testing guidelines. These new guidelines have four essential components: (1) routine voluntary HIV screening of all persons in the US aged 13–64 (not based on HIV risk or HIV prevalence), (2) repeat HIV screening at least annually in persons with ongoing risk factors, (3) opt-out testing with an opportunity for the patient to ask questions and to decline, and (4) formal consent and prevention counseling will no longer be required (Table 2-1).[5] Even with the new CDC recommendations for broad HIV testing, a significant proportion of HIV-infected persons will remain undiagnosed, particularly if they do not access a healthcare system or if their medical provider fails to perform HIV testing. Since these undiagnosed individuals may present to medical care with an initial HIV-related complication, medical providers should remain alert to recognition of HIV-related clinical findings.

Diagnosing a patient with acute (primary) HIV has major implications for the long-term health of this person and for their risk of transmitting HIV to others. Overall, ~40–90% of individuals who acquire HIV will have a symptomatic illness associated with this initial infection.[6] Clinical manifestations of acute retroviral illness may appear within days to weeks of exposure to HIV, and most commonly occur between 2 and 6 weeks.[7] The clinical presentation most often consist of a mononucleosis-like illness that includes fever, lethargy, myalgias, headache, pharyngitis, fatigue, lymphadenopathy, and a nonpruritic erythematous maculopapular rash (Table 2-2). The differential diagnosis for patients with acute retroviral syndrome is relatively broad and includes infectious mononucleosis, streptococcal pharyngitis, viral respiratory tract infections, secondary syphilis, acute toxoplasmosis, viral hepatitis, or viral meningitis (Table 2-3). Because of the nonspecific nature of the syndrome, the initial clinical findings and laboratory results can overlap with numerous other diseases; thus, the clinician should obtain relevant medical

Summary of 2006 Revised CDC Recommendations for HIV Screening

Table 2-1

Recommendation
Routine HIV voluntary screening of all persons aged 13–64 in healthcare settings
Screening not based on risk or prevalence
Screening performed as opt-out testing (patient advised to have test and patient can refuse test)
Formal consent no longer required
Prevention counseling in conjunction with HIV screening no longer required
Separate recommendations apply to correctional facilities
Patients with positive HIV test should be provided reliable clinical care or referred to qualified provider

Signs and Symptoms Associated With Acute Retroviral Syndrome

Table 2-2

Clinical Finding	Percent of Patients
Fever	>80
Fatigue	>70
Weight loss	70
Pharyngitis	50–70
Myalgia	50–70
Night sweats	50
Diarrhea	50
Rash	40–80
Lymphadenopathy	40–70
Headache	32–70
Nausea, vomiting	30–60
Aseptic meningitis	24
Oral or genital ulcers	10–20
Thrombocytopenia	45
Leukopenia	40
Elevated liver enzymes	21

Adapted from Kahn JO, Walker BD. Acute human immunodeficiency virus type 1 infection. N Engl J Med 339:33–9 1998, with permission; and Schacker T, Collier AC, Hughes J, et al. Clinical and epidemiologic features of primary HIV infection. Ann Intern Med 125:257–64, 1996. Erratum. Ann Intern Med 126:74, 1997.

Differential Diagnosis of Acute Retroviral Syndrome

Table 2-3

Infectious mononucleosis (Epstein-Barr virus or cytomegalovirus)
Toxoplasmosis
Streptococcal pharyngitis
Rubella
Secondary syphilis
Viral meningitis
Other viral infections (e.g., influenza)
Viral hepatitis
Disseminated gonococcal infection
Drug reaction

history related to a potential HIV exposure during the preceding 6–8 weeks. The diagnosis is confirmed by a positive HIV RNA assay (or p24 antigen test) in conjunction with a negative HIV antibody test (or a positive enzyme immunoassay and an indeterminate Western blot test).[6] Because patients with newly acquired HIV are probably more infectious to others than at any other stage of their HIV disease course, making a diagnosis at this stage provides an opportunity to impact this patient's potential transmission of HIV to others. In addition, if a patient with acute infection does not have a diagnosis made with this initial illness, their infection may remain unrecognized for many years and optimal medical care for their HIV illness will be delayed. A detailed discussion of acute HIV is presented in Chapter 33.

Early manifestations of altered cell-mediated immunity may raise the clinical suspicion of HIV; furthermore, many of these common clinical manifestations require recognition and management in routine care of persons with known HIV infection. Examples of such clinical findings include oral candidiasis, molluscum contagiosum, oral hairy leukoplakia, herpes zoster, generalized lymphadenopathy, unexplained cytopenias, pneumococcal pneumonia, tuberculosis, and specifically in women, refractory vulvovaginal candidiasis, cervical dysplasia, and any stage of cervical carcinoma.[8] Making a diagnosis of HIV at this stage is critical since the patient has already displayed some facet of immunosuppression and likely would need antiretroviral therapy at this stage or in the near future.

Although the number of severe opportunistic infections has dramatically declined among HIV-infected persons as a result of HAART, a significant proportion of HIV-infected individuals remain undiagnosed until they present with a major complication late in the course of their disease. This scenario would most likely take place when a patient presents to an emergency room or in a hospital setting. The most common HIV-related complications related to severe immune suppression that would present in this manner consist of *Pneumocystis* pneumonia, cryptococcal meningitis, *Toxoplasma* encephalitis, esophageal candidiasis, wasting syndrome, and severe dementia. In the initial evaluation of these severe situations, when the diagnosis of HIV is not yet confirmed, it is also important to search for other potential HIV-related manifestations, such as oral candidiasis and oral hairy leukoplakia, since these findings may further point to a diagnosis of HIV infection and prompt early empiric treatment of the severe HIV-related complication while HIV test results are pending. Making a diagnosis of HIV in this setting is obviously important for survival of this potential life-threatening event. In addition, the diagnosis of HIV will enable the administration of antiretroviral therapy in this setting, as well as prophylaxis for other opportunistic infections.

NATURAL HISTORY OF HIV

The clinical course of untreated HIV infection is now well established.[9] In most cases HIV causes progressive loss of T-helper lymphocytes, which eventually renders the patient unable to mount an adequate immune response against a variety of opportunistic pathogens. The time course of this decline varies considerably from patient to patient (Fig. 2-1). Indeed, in some individuals, no apparent loss of immunologic function is detectable as long as 10 years or more after untreated infection (the so-called long-term nonprogressors). Antiretroviral drug therapy is generally not indicated for this subset of patients, as they are apparently able to control HIV replication. Conversely, some patients have very rapid progression of their disease with development of severe immune suppression within 2 years of acquiring HIV infection. In most cases, however, T-helper lymphocyte counts in untreated individuals gradually decline to the point that major HIV-related complications develop ~7–10 years after becoming infected with HIV. The patient's initial baseline plasma HIV RNA level (prior to starting antiretroviral therapy) serves as a powerful predictor of the pace of T-lymphocyte cell decline and subsequent risk of progression to AIDS.[10] The HIV RNA value tends to remain relatively stable after the host controls the acute HIV infection, with the establishment of a type of equilibrium between viral replication on one hand and T-helper lymphocyte generation on the other, which typically occurs ~6 months to a year after the initial infection. The decision to start HAART is based on an assessment of the likelihood of clinical progression and the risk of subsequent development of major HIV-related complications and this issue is discussed in detail in Chapter 4. Since the course of HIV disease is highly variable, individual patients will need close long-term follow-up to optimize the timing of initiation of antiretroviral therapy.

A fairly well-defined correlation exists between a patient's T-helper lymphocyte count and the risk of developing specific infections (Fig. 2-2).[11,12] In general, certain virulent

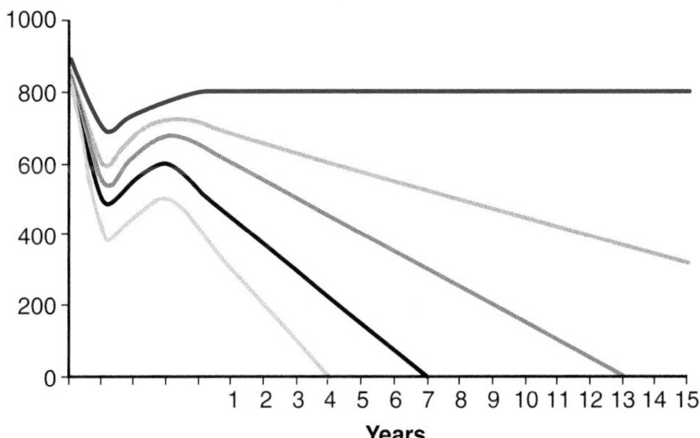

Figure 2-1 ■ Natural history of persons infected with HIV: variable CD4 cell count decline. This schematic drawing shows variable patterns of CD4 cell count decline. The top curve represents a long-term nonprogressor and the bottom curve represents a rapid CD4 decline and rapid progression to AIDS. The middle two curves represent a more typical CD4 cell count decline and progression to AIDS.

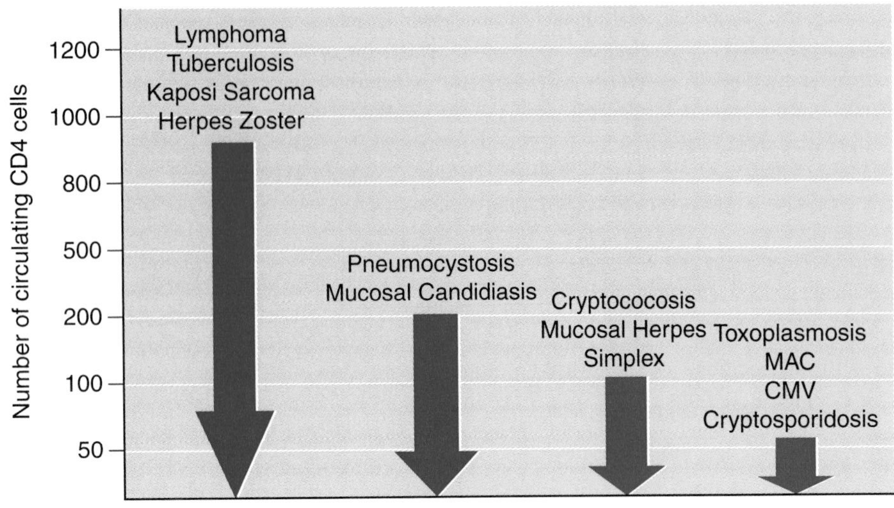

Figure 2-2 ■ Typical relation of clinical manifestations to the CD4+ T-lymphocyte count in HIV-infected patients. Abbreviations: CMV, cytomegalovirus; MAC, *M. avium* complex.

bacterial pathogens, such as *Mycobacterium tuberculosis* and *Streptococcus pneumoniae*, may cause disease in patients with relatively high CD4+ T-helper lymphocyte counts (in excess of 300 cells/μL). Other life-threatening opportunistic pathogens generally pose a threat only at levels below a certain threshold CD4+ T-helper lymphocyte count: *Pneumocystis jiroveci* (below 200 cells/μL), *Toxoplasma gondii* (below 100 cells/μL), disseminated *Mycobacterium avium* complex (below 50 cells/mm^3), and cytomegalovirus (below 50 cells/μL).

INITIAL EVALUATION OF THE HIV-INFECTED PATIENT

During the initial evaluation when an HIV-infected individual establishes a primary care relationship, a crucial interface takes place between the provider and the patient that may set the tone for future long-term care. In this initial encounter, the medical provider should make the most of the opportunity to establish rapport with the patient. For practical purposes, many clinicians have the initial evaluation of an HIV-infected patient include two visits that are spaced ~1–2 weeks apart. The first visit should typically involve three key components: (1) obtaining a detailed medical history relevant to the patient's HIV disease, (2) performing a complete physical examination, and (3) ordering relevant laboratory studies. The second visit should primarily focus on reviewing the patient's laboratory results, estimating the stage of HIV disease based on the CD4+ T-cell count, and, if applicable, providing vaccinations, antiretroviral therapy, and prophylaxis for opportunistic infections. At either of these visits, the patient should have tuberculin skin testing performed. During both of these initial encounters, the medical provider should assess the patient's fundamental understanding of HIV disease and address concerns or questions the patient may have. A typical flow sheet for initial evaluation of the HIV-infected patient is shown in Figure 2-3.

Medical History

As part of the initial clinical management of a patient with HIV infection, the medical provider should review the date of the first positive HIV antibody test result, the last negative HIV antibody test (if available), and any prior CD4+ T-lymphocyte counts, quantitative HIV RNA measurements, and HIV resistance assays that were obtained if the patient was previously in the care of another provider. It is helpful to document clear-cut laboratory evidence of a HIV diagnosis, as there have been cases of factitious HIV infection in which individuals misrepresented themselves as HIV-infected for secondary gain, such as health insurance benefits and housing benefits. It is also helpful to ascertain why the patient was tested for HIV, and what the presumed mode of HIV acquisition was. Occasionally, a patient will not know how they became infected, and this can serve as an opportunity to provide basic information regarding prevention of HIV transmission. When newly HIV-infected patients are identified, it is important to ask if they know or suspect the source of their infection, to ask the patients to notify their contacts, and to refer the contacts for HIV counseling and testing. Although many HIV-infected patients do not know when they acquired HIV, some will recall an acute seroconversion illness; this latter information may prove useful in predicting the overall course of disease progression.

During this initial evaluation, the medical provider should assess the patient's general medical history and perform a complete review of systems, including a review of symptoms associated with earlier stage HIV-related disease, such as fever, night sweats, unanticipated weight loss, generalized lymphadenopathy, herpes zoster, diarrhea, and oral candidiasis (Table 2-4). Questions should also address history of (or active symptoms that would suggest) an AIDS-related complication, including recurrent bacterial pneumonia, *Pneumocystis* pneumonia, tuberculosis (including extrapulmonary disease), *Toxoplasma* encephalitis, cryptococcal meningitis, cytomegalovirus infection, disseminated *M. avium* complex infection,

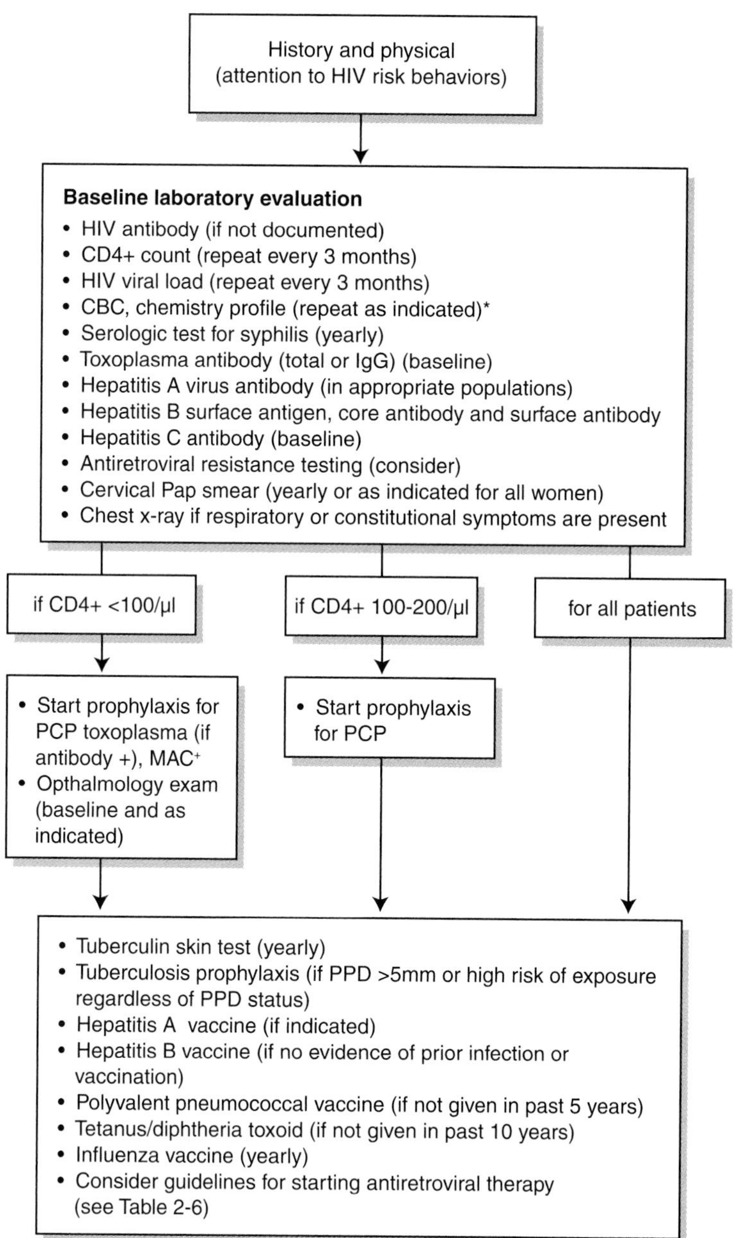

History and physical
(attention to HIV risk behaviors)
Baseline laboratory evaluation
• HIV antibody (if not documented)
• CD4+ count (repeat every 3 months)
• HIV viral load (repeat every 3 months)
• CBC, chemistry profile (repeat as indicated)*
• Serologic test for syphilis (yearly)
• Toxoplasma antibody (total or IgG) (baseline)
• Hepatitis A virus antibody (in appropriate populations)
• Hepatitis B surface antigen, core antibody and surface antibody
• Hepatitis C antibody (baseline)
• Antiretroviral resistance testing (consider)
• Cervical Pap smear (yearly or as indicated for all women)
• Chest x-ray if respiratory or constitutional symptoms are present
if CD4+ <100/µl
if CD4+ 100-200/µl
for all patients
• Start prophylaxis for PCP toxoplasma (if antibody +), MAC+
• Opthalmology exam (baseline and as indicated)
• Start prophylaxis for PCP
• Tuberculin skin test (yearly)
• Tuberculosis prophylaxis (if PPD >5mm or high risk of exposure regardless of PPD status)
• Hepatitis A vaccine (if indicated)
• Hepatitis B vaccine (if no evidence of prior infection or vaccination)
• Polyvalent pneumococcal vaccine (if not given in past 5 years)
• Tetanus/diphtheria toxoid (if not given in past 10 years)
• Influenza vaccine (yearly)
• Consider guidelines for starting antiretroviral therapy (see Table 2-6)

Figure 2-3 ■ Flow chart for initial evaluation of the HIV-infected patient.

Table 2-4 Relevant Clinical History for HIV-Infected Patients

Medical Issues
Prior medical, surgical, or psychiatric conditions
Current medications
Drug allergies
Prior or current infection with tuberculosis, sexually transmitted infections, and/or viral hepatitis (A, B, or C)
Reproductive health history
Travel history
Immunizations

HIV-Specific Issues
Duration of infection
CD4 T-lymphocyte counts
Plasma viral load measurements
History of opportunistic infections or neoplasms
Antiretroviral therapy history
Prophylactic medications
Nutritional history

Behavioral Issues
Prior and current alcohol and other drug use
Cigarette and other nicotine use
Awareness of how HIV infection is transmitted, and current pattern of risk behaviors
Emotional status: presence of depression
Family and other primary support systems
Employment/insurance status
Community involvement

cervical cancer, and Kaposi sarcoma. The provider should also obtain a specific geographic history since patients may have previously become infected with a regionally prevalent fungal organism, and thus have an increased risk of developing a reactivation fungal disease, which can occur with histoplasmosis, blastomycosis, and coccidioidomycosis. Because of the nature of HIV transmission, a detailed sexual and drug history (including use of recreational drugs) should also be included, and any history of specific sexually transmitted diseases or viral hepatitis should be elicited. In addition, providers should also ascertain whether patients have had a prior hepatitis A or B vaccination.

A detailed tuberculosis exposure history should be elicited, which includes known exposure to tuberculosis, the date of their last chest radiograph (if any), the date of the patient's last tuberculin skin test, whether the patient has ever had a positive tuberculin skin test, and, if they have ever received chemoprophylaxis, the details regarding the type and duration of the prophylaxis regimen. If the patient has a prior history of active clinical tuberculosis, it is imperative to document the adequacy of therapy, adherence to a full-course regimen, and resolution of clinical symptoms.

Medication and Drug History

Obtaining an accurate and thorough medication history is essential, especially if antiretroviral therapy is to be initiated. The medical provider should ask the patient about all medications being taken, including over-the-counter drugs, complementary and alternative medications, such as herbal preparations and nutritional supplements. Because many patients tend to consider herbal medications benign and do not mention their use, they should be reminded that any pharmacologically active substance might have unwanted side effects or interactions with other medications. For example, St John's wort, which is sold over-the-counter as an antidepressant, may significantly alter the metabolism of protease inhibitors.[13] Our understanding of the safety and efficacy of many alternative therapeutics remains incomplete, and thus careful monitoring should take place if the patient discloses the use of nonprescription medications. In addition to determining the patient's medication history, the medical provider should, in a nonjudgmental fashion, obtain an accurate and detailed history regarding the use of tobacco, alcohol, and illicit drugs. Information regarding illicit drug use may have particular relevance when considering the timing of initiation of antiretroviral therapy, adherence to antiretroviral medications, and possible transmission of HIV to others.

Physical Examination

A thorough physical examination should be done at the initial visit, focusing on organ systems likely to be affected by opportunistic illnesses. Height and weight should be measured at baseline; in particular, a change in weight can be a sensitive marker of systemic illness. With regard to vital signs, fever suggests infection or an inflammatory process, and hemodynamic instability suggests hypovolemia, a serious infection, or adrenal insufficiency. A thorough skin examination should look for lesions suggestive of Kaposi sarcoma and other opportunistic illnesses. The ocular fundi should be visualized to look for retinal lesions, particularly those associated with cytomegalovirus infection, toxoplasmosis, or HIV-related lesions (*see* Chapter 66). In the oropharynx, candidiasis and oral hairy leukoplakia are sensitive markers of immunosuppression. Kaposi sarcoma can be observed in the mouth or on the skin. An assiduous search should be made for significantly enlarged lymph nodes in all palpable areas. Hepatomegaly or splenomegaly suggests a number of possible systemic infections, ranging from viral hepatitis to disseminated mycobacterial disease. A careful neurologic examination should also be done on all patients at baseline. A detailed anogenital examination is important, since many HIV-infected patients are also at risk for sexually transmitted diseases, including herpes simplex virus and human papilloma virus (HPV) infection. Although some experts have suggested men who engage in anal sex should have anal Pap smears checked yearly, the 2002 US Public Health Service/Infection Disease Society of America (USPHS/IDSA) Guidelines for the Prevention of Opportunistic Infections states that further studies of screening and treatment programs for high-grade squamous intraepithelial lesions need to be performed prior to making a recommendation for routine anal cytology screening.[14]

Laboratory Tests

A baseline laboratory evaluation of a newly diagnosed HIV-infected patient (Fig. 2-3) should include a complete blood count, platelet count, routine serum chemistries, blood urea nitrogen, serum creatinine, total bilirubin, alkaline phosphatase, and hepatic aminotransferase levels. These tests can help identify asymptomatic common co-morbid conditions, such as anemia, thrombocytopenia, HIV-associated nephropathy, and viral hepatitis, as well as to serve as a valuable baseline prior to initiating antiretroviral therapy. In addition, because antiretroviral therapy may cause or contribute to new-onset glucose intolerance or hyperlipidemia,[15] patients should also be screened with fasting blood glucose and lipid determinations to determine an accurate baseline value.

The CD4+ T-lymphocyte count is the most readily available quantitative measure of the status of the cell-mediated immune system, and should be checked at baseline and every 3–4 months thereafter. The CD4+ T-lymphocyte count has a wide dynamic range in HIV-infected and HIV-uninfected persons; normal values typically range from 500 to 1200 cells/μL in noninfected persons. For HIV-infected persons clinical manifestations related to cell-mediated immune dysfunction infrequently occur when CD4+ T-lymphocyte counts are greater than 350 cells/μL; herpes zoster is one major exception since it can occur at relatively high CD4+ T-cell counts. At counts less than 350 cells/μL, oral candidiasis, oral hairy leukoplakia, recurrent dermatoses, and other mucosal infections may begin to manifest and connote impaired immune function. Those patients with counts less than 200 cells/μL have severe immune dysfunction and have a significant increased risk for developing life-threatening opportunistic infections.[12] Thus, in an asymptomatic patient with a stable CD4+ T-lymphocyte count of 500 cells/μL or more, it is not necessary to monitor the CD4+ T-lymphocyte counts more frequently than every 3 months, but in patients whose count are less than 350 cells/μL and show more rapid decline, more frequent monitoring may be warranted.

Similar to the monitoring of CD4+ T-lymphocyte counts, a quantitative plasma HIV RNA assay should be followed on a regular basis, typically every 3–4 months in a patient not receiving antiretroviral therapy. However, if the patient is receiving antiretroviral therapy, monitoring the HIV RNA levels more frequently may be indicated, particularly during the first 4–6 months after initiation of therapy, or when breakthrough viremia has occurred and resistance to antiretroviral medications is suspected. There are three commonly used assays that measure plasma HIV RNA and offer comparable information: polymerase chain reaction (PCR), branched DNA (bDNA), and nucleic acid sequence-based amplification (NASBA) (*see* Chapter 1 for more detail).[16] The HIV RNA level should be measured when a patient is first diagnosed, prior to any planned change in antiretroviral therapy, and at least every 4 weeks after a change until it has reached a stable level.[17] For antiretroviral-naive patients with established HIV infection, baseline HIV genotypic or phenotypic resistance testing should be considered[17] and many experts have increasingly begun performing resistance tests in this setting given the increased transmission of resistant HIV (*see* Chapter 28).[18]

Screening for Concomitant Infections

Newly diagnosed HIV-infected patients should also be tested for concomitant infections that may be transmitted by sexual or parenteral contact, such as hepatitis B virus (HBV), hepatitis C virus (HCV), syphilis, gonorrhea, and *Chlamydia* infection. As a minimum, baseline testing should include serologic screening for prior hepatitis A virus (HAV) infection, prior and active hepatitis B infection (hepatitis B surface antigen and antibody, and core antibody), and for hepatitis C infection. Antibodies against *T. gondii* should also be measured at baseline[14]; this assay simply provides evidence of prior exposure, and indicates latent *T. gondii* infection and a risk for subsequent reactivation. Therefore, a single titer of total or immunoglobulin G (IgG) antibodies is adequate. This contrasts with testing immunocompetent symptomatic patients for acute toxoplasmosis, in whom acute and convalescent antibody levels or immunoglobulin M (IgM) antibodies are measured.

All HIV-infected patients should be tested for syphilis with a nontreponenal assay (rapid plasma regain (RPR) or venereal diseases research laboratory (VDRL)) test and treated if a treponemal-specific confirmatory serologic test (fluorescent treponemal antibody absorbed (FTA-ABS) or *Treponema pallidum* particle agglutination (TP-PA)) is reactive.[19,20] This population is at increased risk of complications from syphilis, including neurosyphilis, rapid progression of disease, and failure of treatment (*see* Chapter 58).[19] For this reason a lumbar puncture should be strongly considered for all HIV-infected patients diagnosed with syphilis of unknown duration. The use of tetracyclines for treating syphilis in HIV-positive patients is discouraged because of the drug's limited ability to cross the blood–brain barrier; instead, penicillin desensitization is preferred in penicillin-allergic individuals, as the spirochete tends to disseminate early to the central nervous system in the setting of HIV infection. Tuberculin skin testing at baseline and annually should also be routine for HIV-infected patients.[21] Any HIV-infected patient with a reactive tuberculin skin test (at least 5 mm in diameter) or a known exposure to a person with active tuberculosis should receive antituberculous prophylaxis for a year if previously untreated (*see* Chapter 40).

Immunizations

There are several immunizations routinely recommended for HIV-infected patients (Table 2-5).[14] Earlier, investigators had shown that plasma HIV RNA measurements obtained immediately after vaccination may transiently increase if the patient was not on effective suppressive antiretroviral therapy.[22] There are, however, no data that suggest such vaccine-related transient 'blips' lead to a sustained rise in viral load or to subsequent development of antiretroviral resistance; thus immunizations now appear to have negligible risks to adversely affect the course of HIV disease.[23] Current recommendations suggest that all HIV-infected patients receive the 23-valent pneumococcal vaccine as soon as possible after their diagnosis of HIV infection.[24] In addition, patients younger than 65 should receive a one-time revaccination after 5 or more years have elapsed from the time of the initial pneumococcal vaccination. For patients with a CD4+ T-lymphocyte count of less than 200 cells/μL, the likelihood of developing an effective humoral response to the pneumococcal vaccination is diminished, but the vaccine is safe and can nevertheless still be given. Some experts, however, would defer vaccinating such severely immunocompromised patients if imminent improvement in immunologic function is expected after starting HAART. Although the benefit of this vaccine is somewhat in question, current Advisory Committee on Immunization Practices (ACIP) and USPHS/IDSA guidelines recommend vaccination based on the theoretical benefit and the safety of the vaccine. Yearly influenza vaccination with inactivated influenza is warranted for all HIV-infected patients, independent of their immune status. The live attenuated nasal influenza vaccine should not be administered to HIV-infected persons. All HIV-infected patients should receive tetanus-diphtheria booster vaccinations every 10 years, in accordance with the recommendation for the general adult population.

The ACIP recommends all HIV-infected patients who do not have evidence of prior HBV infection should receive HBV vaccination.[24] At 1–6 months following completion of the hepatitis B vaccine series, patients be tested for antibody to HBV surface antigen (anti-HBs) to assess whether they have achieved the target protective titer of at least 10 IU/L. Whether patients with 'isolated hepatitis B core antibody'

Immunizations for HIV-Infected Patients

Table 2-5

Vaccine	Status	Dose/Regimen	Comments
Pneumococcal vaccine	Recommended	0.5 mL IM	One time revaccination after 5 years
Hepatitis B vaccine	Recommended for patients who do not have anti-HBcAb	*Engerix*-B 20 μg (give at 0, 1, 6 months) or *Recombivax* HB 10 μg IM (give at 0, 1, 6 months)	Test vaccinated pts for HBsAb after third dose (anti-HBs titer >10 IU/L protective); Nonresponders should receive up to three more doses and have HBsAb checked after last dose
Hepatitis A vaccine	Recommended for at-risk patients	1 mL IM (give at 0 and 6–12 months)	Give to MSM, injection-drug users, persons with clotting factor disorder; those with planned travel to hepatitis A endemic regions, and patients with hepatitis B or C
Combined hepatitis A and B vaccine	Option for patients who require both hepatitis A and B vaccine	*Twinrix* (give at 0, 1, 6 months)	This vaccine requires fewer shots than giving hepatitis A and B vaccines separately
Influenza (inactivated) vaccine	Recommended	0.5 mL IM annually	Live attenuated intranasal vaccine contraindicated, regardless of CD4 cell count
Tetanus toxoid	Recommended	Td 0.5 mL IM	Same as for HIV(−); reboost every 10 years
Haemophilus influenzae vaccine	See comments	0.5 mL IM	No formal recommendation (but no contraindication) for giving to HIV-infected adults
Meningococcal vaccine	Recommended for at-risk patients	1 dose	Conditions or situations for which meningococcal vaccine recommended include asplenia, terminal complement deficiency, first year college students living in a dormitory, US military recruits, travel to region hyperendemic for meningococcal disease; conjugate vaccine preferred for persons under 55 years of age
Polio vaccine	IPV	0.5 mL SC in three doses for primary immunization series over 12 months	Routine immunization not necessary for adults residing in the US IPV indicated for travel to endemic areas. OPV contraindicated

HAV, hepatitis A virus; HBsAb, hepatitis B surface antibody; IM, intramuscular; IPV, enhanced inactivated polio vaccine; MSM, men who have sex with men; OPV, oral polio vaccine; pts, patients; SC, subcutaneous; Td, tetanus-diphtheria toxoid.

(positive anti-HBc, negative anti-HBs, and negative HBsAg) should receive hepatitis B vaccine remains controversial, and the optimal approach to these patients remains unclear. The current ACIP guidelines recommend giving hepatitis A vaccine to HIV-infected persons who have one or more of the following risk factors for acquiring HAV infection: male-to-male sex, use of illegal drugs, travel to an HAV endemic region, chronic liver disease, or a clotting factor disorder.[24] Younger patients are unlikely to have preexisting hepatitis A immunity, so it may be more cost-effective simply to vaccinate against HAV than to test for baseline HAV antibodies. Unfortunately, current data indicate that most HIV-infected patients eligible for hepatitis B and hepatitis A vaccines are not receiving appropriate immunizations.[25]

In general, HIV-infected adults should not receive live virus vaccines, including oral polio vaccine, varicella-zoster vaccine, attenuated intranasal influenza vaccine, smallpox vaccine, and measles, mumps, and rubella vaccine[24]; the exception is that measles, mumps, and rubella vaccine can be given to HIV-infected individuals who have mild to moderate immune suppression (CD4+ T-lymphocyte count greater than 200 cells/μL). Household members of an HIV-infected patient should not receive oral polio vaccine because of the risk of infecting the HIV-infected house member as a result of fecal shedding of live poliovirus. If someone in the patient's household has received oral polio vaccine, the HIV-infected patient should avoid contact with that person for 4 weeks from the time the vaccine was administered.

Prophylaxis for Opportunistic Infections

Providing appropriate prophylaxis against opportunistic infections is a critical component of the primary care of HIV-infected persons in developed countries. The USPHS/IDSA guidelines[14] for prophylaxis to prevent first-episode opportunistic infections in adults and adolescents infected with HIV are presented in Table 2-6 and those to prevent recurrence of opportunistic infections are presented in Table 2-7. Salient features of these recommendations are discussed below.

Table 2-6 Prophylaxis to Prevent First Episode of Opportunistic Disease in Adults and Adolescents Infected with HIV

Pathogen	Indication	Preventive Regimens: First Choice	Preventive Regimens: Alternatives
Strongly Recommended as Standard of Care			
Pneumocystis pneumonia[a]	CD4 T-lymphocyte count <200/μL or oropharyngeal candidiasis	TMP-SMZ 1 DS PO qd (AI); TMP-SMZ 1 SS PO qd (AI)	Dapsone 50 mg PO bid or 100 mg PO qd (BI); dapsone 50 mg PO qd plus pyrimethamine 50 mg PO q week plus leucovorin 25 mg PO q week (BI); dapsone 200 mg PO plus pyrimethamine 75 mg PO plus leucovorin 25 mg PO q week (BI); aerosolized pentamidine 300 mg q month via Respirgard II nebulizer (BI); atovaquone 1500 mg PO qd (BI); TMP-SMZ 1 DS PO three times weekly (BI)
Mycobacterium tuberculosis Isoniazid-sensitive[b]	TST reaction ≥5 mm or prior positive TST result without treatment or contact with case of active tuberculosis, regardless of TST result (BIII)	Isoniazid 300 mg PO qd plus pyridoxine 50 mg PO qd × 9 months (AII) or isoniazid 900 mg PO twice weekly plus pyridoxine 100 mg PO twice weekly × 9 months (BII)	Rifabutin 600 mg PO qd × 4 months (BIII); rifampin 600 mg PO qd × 4 months (BIII)
Isoniazid-resistant	Same as above; increased probability of exposure to isoniazid-resistant tuberculosis	Rifampin 600 mg PO qd × 4 months (AIII) or rifabutin 300 mg PO qd × 4 months (BIII)	Rifabutin 300 mg plus pyrazinamide 15–20 mg/kg; pyrazinamide 15–20 mg/kg body weight PO qd × 2 months plus either rifampin 600 mg PO qd × 2 months (BI) or rifabutin 300 mg PO qd × 2 months (CIII)
Multidrug (isoniazid and rifampin)-resistant	Same as above; increased probability of exposure to multidrug-resistant tuberculosis	Choice of drugs requires consultation with public health authorities; depends on susceptibility of isolate from source patient	
Toxoplasma gondi[c]	IgG antibody to Toxoplasma and CD4 count <100/μL	TMP-SMZ 1 DS PO qd (AII)	TMP-SMZ 1 SS PO qd (BIII); dapsone 50 mg PO qd plus pyrimethamine 50 mg PO q week plus leucovorin 25 mg PO q week (BI); atovaquone 1500 mg PO qd with or without pyrimethamine 25 mg PO qd plus leucovorin 10 mg PO qd if pyrimethamine used (CIII)
Mycobacterium avium complex[d]	CD4 count <50/μL	Azithromycin 1200 mg PO q week (AI) or clarithromycin[e] 500 mg PO bid (AI)	Rifabutin, 300 mg PO qd (BI); azithromycin 1200 mg PO q week plus rifabutin 300 mg PO qd (CI)
Varicella zoster virus (VZV)	Substantial exposure to chickenpox or shingles for patients who have no history of either condition or, if available, negative antibody to VZV	Varicella zoster immune globulin (VZIG), 5 vials (1.25 mL each) IM, administered ≤96 h after exposure, ideally within 48 h (AIII)	

(*Continued*)

Table 2-6

(Continued)

Pathogen	Indication	Preventive Regimens	
		First Choice	**Alternatives**
Generally Recommended			
Streptococcus pneumoniae[f]	*CD4 count* >200/μL	23 Valent polysaccharide vaccine, 0.5 mL IM (BII)	None
Hepatitis B virus[g,h]	All susceptible (anti-HBc-negative) patients	Hepatitis B vaccine: three doses (BII)	None
Influenza virus[g,i]	All patients (annually, before influenza season)	Inactivated trivalent influenza virus vaccine one annual dose (0.5 mL) IM (BIII)	Oseltamivir 75 mg PO qd (influenza A or B) (CIII); rimantadine 100 mg PO bid (CIII) or amantadine 100 mg PO bid (CIII) (influenza A only)
Hepatitis A virus[g]	All susceptible patients (anti-HAV-negative) at risk for hepatitis A infection	Hepatitis patients at increased risk for HAV infection (e.g., illicit drug users, men who have sex with men, hemophiliacs) or with chronic liver disease, including chronic hepatitis B or hepatitis CA vaccine: two doses (BIII)	None
Evidence for Efficacy but not Routinely Indicated			
Bacteria	Neutropenia	G-CSF 5–10 μg/kg SC qd for 2–4 weeks or GM-CSF 250 μg/m^2 SC qd 3 2–4 weeks (CII)	
Cryptococcus neoformans	CD4 count <50/μL	Fluconazole 100–200 mg PO qd (CI)	Itraconazone capsule 200 mg PO qd (CIII)
Histoplasma capsulatum[j]	CD4 count <100/μL, endemic geographic area	Itraconazole capsule 200 mg PO qd (CI)	None
Cytomegalovirus (CMV)[k]	CD4 count <50/μL and CMV antibody positivity	Oral ganciclovir 1 g PO tid (CI)	None

Note: Information included in these guidelines might not represent Food and Drug Administration (FDA) approval or approved labeling for the particular products or indications in question. Specifically, the terms 'safe' and 'effective' might not be synonymous with the FDA-defined legal standards for product approval. The Respirgard II nebulizer is manufactured by Marquest, Englewood, Co. Letters and Roman numerals in parentheses after regimens indicate the strength of the recommendation and the quality of evidence supporting it (see Rating System below. Anti-HBc, antibody to hepatitis B core antigen; DS, double-strength tablet; GM-CSF, granulocyte/macrophage colony-stimulating factor; HAART, highly active antiretroviral therapy; HAV, hepatitis A virus; HIV, human immunodeficiency virus; qd, daily; SS, single-strength tablet; TMP-SMZ, trimethoprim-sulfamethoxazole; TST, tuberculin skin test.

[a]Prophylaxis should also be considered for persons with a CD41 T-lymphocyte percentage of <14%, for persons with a history of an AIDS-defining illness and possibly for those with CD4 T-lymphocyte counts of >200 but <250 cells/μL. TMP-SMZ also reduces the frequency of toxoplasmosis and some bacterial infections. Patients receiving dapsone should be tested for glucose-6-phosphate dehydrogenase deficiency. A dosage of 50 mg qd is probably less effective than 100 mg qd. The efficacy of parenteral pentamidine (e.g., 4 mg kg^{-1} month^{-1}) is uncertain. Fansidar (sulfadoxine–pyrimethamine) is rarely used because of severe hypersensitivity reactions. Patients who are being administered therapy for toxoplasmosis with sulfadiazine–pyrimethamine are protected against *Pneumocystis carinii* pneumonia (PCP) and do not need additional prophylaxis against PCP.

[b]Directly observed therapy is recommended for isoniazid, e.g., 900 mg biw; isoniazid regimens should include pyridoxine to prevent peripheral neuropathy. If rifampin or rifabutin are adminstered concurrently with protease inhibitors or non-nucleoside reverse transcriptase inhibitors, careful consideration should be given to potential pharmacokinetic interactions exposure to multidrug-resistant tuberculosis might require prophylaxis with two drugs; consult public health authorities. Possible regimens include pyrazinamide plus either ethambutol or a fluoroquinolone.

[c]Protection against toxoplasmosis is provided by TMP-SMZ, dapsone plus pyrimethamine, and possibly by atovaquone. Atovaquone may be used with or without pyrimethamine. Pyrimethamine alone probably provides little if any protection.

[d]See 'Disseminated Infection with *M avium* complex' for a discussion of drug interactions.

[e]During pregnancy azithromycin is preferred over clarithromycin because of the teratogenicity of clarithromycin in animals.

[f]Vaccination may be offered to persons who have a CD41 T-lymphocyte count of <200 cells/μL, although the efficacy is likely to be diminished. Revaccination 5 years after the first dose or sooner if the initial immunization was given when the CD41 T-lymphocyte count was <200 cells/μL and has increased to >200 cells/μL on HAART is considered optional. Some authorities are concerned that immunizations might stimulate the replication of HIV.

[g]Data do not conclusively demonstrate a clinical benefit of these vaccines in this population, although it is logical to assume that those patients who develop antibody responses will derive some protection. Some authorities are concerned that immunizations might stimulate HIV replication, although for influenza vaccination a large observational study of HIV-infected persons in clinical care showed no adverse effect of this vaccine, including multiple doses, on patient survival (J Ward, CDC, personal communication). Also this concern may be less relevant in the setting of HAART. However, because of the theoretical concern that increases in HIV plasma RNA following vaccination during pregnancy might increase the risk of perinatal transmission of HIV, providers may wish to defer vaccination for such patients until after HAART is initiated.

[h]Hepatitis B vaccine has been recommended for all children and adolescents and for all adults with risk factors for hepatitis B virus (HBV).

[i]Oseltamivir is appropriate during outbreaks of influenza A or B. Rimantadine and amantadine are appropriate during outbreaks of influenza A (although neither rimantadine nor amantadine is recommended during pregnancy). Dosage reduction for antiviral chemoprophylaxis against influenza might be indicated for decreased renal or hepatic function and for persons with seizure disorders. Physicians should consult the drug package inserts and the annual CDC influenza guidelines for more specific information about adverse effects and dosage adjustments. For additional information regarding vaccination against hepatitis A and B and vaccination and antiviral therapy against influenza see: CDC. Prevention of hepatitis A through active or passive immunization: recommendations of the Advisory Committee on Immunization Practices (ACIP). MMWR 48(RR-12), 1999; CDC. Hepatitis B virus: a comprehensive strategy for eliminating transmission in the United States through universal childhood vaccination: recommendations of the Advisory Committee on Immunization Practices (ACIP). MMWR 40(RR-13), 1991; and CDC. Prevention and control of influenza: recommendations of the Advisory Committee on Immunization Practices (ACIP). For additional information about vaccination and antiviral therapy against influenza, see: CDC. Prevention and control of influenza: recommendations of the Advisory Committee on Immunization Practices (ACIP). MMWR 50(RR-4), 2000.

[j]In a few unusual occupational or other circumstances, prophylaxis should be considered; consult a specialist.

[k]Acyclovir is not protective against CMV. Valacyclovir is not recommended because of an unexplained trend toward increased mortality observed in persons with AIDS who were being administered this drug for prevention of CMV disease.

Adapted and modified from Kaplan JE, Masur H, Holmes KK; USPHS; Infectious Disease Society of America. Guidelines for preventing opportunistic infections among HIV-infected persons–2002. Recommendations of the U.S. Public Health Service and the Infectious Diseases Society of America. MMWR Recomm Rep 51(RR-8):1–52, 2002.

System Used to Rate the Strength of Recommendations and Quality of Supporting Evidence

Rating	Criteria
Strength of the Recommendation	
A	Strong evidence for efficacy and substantial clinical benefit support recommendation for use. Should always be offered.
B	Moderate evidence for efficacy – or strong evidence for efficacy but only limited clinical benefit – supports recommendation for use. Should generally be offered.
C	Evidence for efficacy is insufficient to support a recommendation for or against use, or the evidence might not outweigh adverse consequences (e.g., drug toxicity, drug interactions) or cost of the chemoprophylaxis or alternative approaches. Optional.
D	Moderate evidence for lack of efficacy or for adverse outcome supports a recommendation against use. Should generally not be offered.
E	Good evidence for lack of efficacy or for adverse outcome supports a recommendation against use. Should never be offered.
Quality of Evidence Supporting the Recommendation	
I	Evidence from at least one properly randomized, controlled trial.
II	Evidence from at least one well designed clinical trial without randomization, from cohort or case-controlled analytic studies (preferably from more than one center), or from multiple time series studies; or dramatic results from uncontrolled experiments.
III	Evidence from opinions of respected authorities based on clinical experience, descriptive studies, or reports of expert committees.

Table 2-7

Prophylaxis to Prevent Recurrence of Opportunistic Disease (After Chemotherapy for Acute Disease) in Adults and Adolescents Infected with HIV

Pathogen	Indication	Preventive Regimens: First Choice	Preventive Regimens: Alternatives
Recommended as Standard of Care			
Pneumocystis pneumonia	Prior Pneumocystis pneumonia	TMP-SMZ 1 DS PO qd (AI); TMP-SMZ 1 SS PO qd (AI)	Dapsone 50 mg PO bid or 100 mg PO qd (BI); dapsone 50 mg PO qd plus pyrimethamine 50 mg PO q week plus leucovorin 25 mg PO q week (BI); dapsone 200 mg PO plus pyrimethamine 75 mg PO plus leucovorin 25 mg PO q week (BI); aerosolized pentamidine 300 mg qm via Respirgard II nebulizer (BI); atovaquone 1500 mg PO qd (BI); TMP-SMZ 1 DS PO three times weekly (CI)
Toxoplasma gondii[a]	Prior toxoplasmic encephalitis	Sulfadiazine 500–1000 mg PO qid, plus pyrimethamine 25–50 mg PO qd plus leucovorin 10–25 mg PO qd (AI)	Clindamycin 300–450 mg PO q6-8h plus pyrimethamine 25–50 mg PO qd plus leucovorin 10–25 mg PO qd (BI); atovaquone 750 mg PO q6-12h with or without pyrimethanine 25 mg PO qd plus leucovorin 10 mg PO qd (if pyrimethamine used) (CIII)
Mycobacterium avium complex[b]	Documented disseminated disease	Clarithromycin[c] 500 mg PO bid (AI) plus ethambutol 15 mg/kg PO qd (AII); with or without rifabutin 300 mg PO qd (CI)	Azithromycin 500 mg PO qd (AII) plus ethambutol, 15 mg/kg PO qd (AII); with or without rifabutin, 300 mg PO qd (CI)
Cytomegalovirus	Prior end-organ disease	Ganciclovir 5–6 mg kg^{21} day^{21} IV 5–7 days/week or 1000 mg PO tid (AI); or foscarnet 90–120 mg/kg IV qd (AI); or (for retinitis) ganciclovir sustained-release implant q6-9 months plus ganciclovir 1.0–1.5 g PO tid (AI)	Cidofovir 5 mg/kg IV every other week with probenecid 2 g PO 3 h before the dose followed by 1 g PO 2 h after the dose, and 1 g PO 8 h after the dose (total 4 g) (AI); fomivirsen 1 vial (330 mg) injected into the vitreous, then repeated every 2–4 weeks with ganciclovir 1.0–1.5 g PO tid (AI) or valganciclovir 900 mg PO qd (BI)
Cryptococcus neoformans	Documented disease	Fluconazole 200 mg PO qd (AI)	Amphotericin B 0.6–1.0 mg/kg IV weekly to three times weekly (AI); itraconazole 200 mg PO qd (BI)
Histoplasma capsulatum	Documented disease	Itraconazole capsule 200 mg PO bid (AI)	Amphotericin B 1.0 mg/kg IV q week (AI)

Coccidioides immitis	Documented disease	Fluconazole 400 mg PO qd (AII)	Amphotericin B 1.0 mg/kg IV q week (AI); itraconazole 200 mg capsule PO bid (AII)
Salmonella species, (non-typhi)[d]	Bacteremia	Ciprofloxacin 500 mg PO bid for at least 2 months (BII)	Antibiotic chemoprophylaxis with another active agent (CIII)
Recommended Only if Subsequent Episodes Are Frequent or Severe			
Herpes simplex virus	Frequent/severe recurrences	Acyclovir 200 mg PO tid or 400 mg PO bid (AI); famciclovir 500 mg PO bid (AI)	Valacyclovir 500 mg PO bid (CIII)
Candida (oropharyngeal or vaginal)	Frequent/severe recurrences	Fluconazole 100–200 mg PO qd (CI)	Itraconazole solution 200 mg PO qd (CI)
Candida (esophageal)	Frequent/severe recurrences	Fluconazole 100–200 mg PO qd (BI)	Itraconazole solution 200 mg PO qd (BI)

Note: Information included in these guidelines might not represent Food and Drug Administration (FDA) approval or approved labeling for the particular products or indications in question. Specifically, the terms 'safe' and 'effective' might not be synonymous with the FDA-defined legal standards for product approval. The Respirgard II nebulizer is manufactured by Marquest, Englewood, CO. Letters and Roman numerals in parentheses after regimens indicate the strength of the recommendation and the quality of evidence supporting it (as in Table 2-6).

bid, twice a day; DS, double-strength tablet; qd, daily; SS, single-strength tablet; tid, three times a day; TMP-SMZ, trimethoprim-sulfamethoxazole.

[a]Pyrimethamine–sulfadiazine confers protection against PCP as well as toxoplasmosis; clindamycin–pyrimethamine does not offer protection against PCP.

[b]Many multiple-drug regimens are poorly tolerated. Drug interactions (e.g., those seen with clarithromycin and rifabutin) can be problematic; rifabutin has been associated with uveitis, especially when administered at daily doses of .300 mg or concurrently with fluconazole or clarithromycin.

[c]During pregnancy, azithromycin is recommended instead of clarithromycin because clarithromycin is teratogenic in animals.

[d]Efficacy for eradication of Salmonella has been demonstrated only for ciprofloxacin.

From Kaplan JE, Masur H, Holmes KK; USPHS; Infectious Disease Society of America. Guidelines for preventing opportunistic infections among HIV-infected persons – 2002. Recommendations of the U.S. Public Health Service and the Infectious Diseases Society of America. MMWR Recomm Rep 51(RR-8):1–52, 2002.

P. jiroveci Pneumonia

Chemoprophylaxis against *P. jiroveci* pneumonia is associated with decreased mortality and is indicated in patients with a CD4+ T-lymphocyte count of less than 200 cells/μL, a CD4+ T-lymphocyte percentage less than 14%, oral thrush, or a history of *Pneumocystis* pneumonia.[14] Trimethoprim-sulfamethoxazole is more efficacious than other preventive therapies (dapsone, atovaquone, or inhaled pentamidine) and should be used whenever possible. Trimethoprim-sulfamethoxazole also provides protection against *Toxoplasma* encephalitis, as well as some protection against bacterial pneumonia and sinusitis. Patients who develop a mild nonurticarial skin rash from trimethoprim-sulfamethoxazole can cautiously continue the medication and use antihistamines as needed, as these mild rashes frequently abate. In patients with a history of a mild to moderately severe reaction to sulfonamides, an oral desensitization regimen can be considered. Those with a history of severe reactions, such as Stevens–Johnson syndrome, should not be rechallenged with this medication.

Toxoplasma Encephalitis

Prophylaxis against *Toxoplasma* encephalitis is indicated for HIV-infected patients who have a CD4+ T-lymphocyte count of less than 100 cells/μL and evidence of latent infection (as shown by a positive IgG *Toxoplasma* antibody test).[14] Similar to recommendations for preventing *Pneumocystis* pneumonia, trimethoprim-sulfamethoxazole is the first-line agent. The recommended alternative regimen consists of pyrimethamine plus dapsone. If a patient cannot tolerate either of these options, then atovaquone, with or without pyrimethamine, should be considered, but limited data exist with the use of atovaquone for this purpose. Patients who do not have serologic evidence of prior infection with *T. gondii* should receive instructions to prevent acquisition of *T. gondii*, namely to avoid direct contact with material contaminated with cat feces and not to ingest undercooked or raw red meat.

Disseminated *M. avium* Complex

Use of azithromycin or clarithromycin for primary prophylaxis against disseminated *M. avium* complex disease is recommended for patients with a CD4+ T-lymphocyte count of less than 50 cells/μL.[14] Combining rifabutin with either azithromycin or clarithromycin provides no additional advantage over using either azithromycin or clarithromycin alone, and thus combination of the drugs for prophylaxis is not recommended. Azithromycin or clarithromycin likely also provides some protection against community-acquired pneumonia.

Other Opportunistic Infections

Long-term primary prophylaxis is not recommended for infections caused by cytomegalovirus, *Candida* species, *Cryptococcus neoformans*, or endemic fungal organisms, such as *Histoplasma capsulatum*. In contrast, patients with established clinical disease caused by cytomegalovirus, *C. neoformans*, or *H. capsulatum* should receive secondary prophylaxis to control the disease process. Many experts would now also recommend long-term suppressive therapy in patients with recurrent herpes simplex infections to decrease the frequency of recurrences, as well as to possibly diminish the shedding of HIV.[26]

Discontinuing Opportunistic Infection Prophylaxis

Within 6 months to a year after starting HAART, many patients with advanced immune suppression have major improvements in their immunologic function. Multiple studies have established that patients with such improvement in immunologic function and sustained suppression of HIV are able to eventually discontinue both primary and secondary opportunistic infection prophylaxis for *Pneumocystis* pneumonia, *Toxoplasma* encephalitis, and disseminated *M. avium* complex infection.[14,27–29] Specific thresholds of CD4+ T-lymphocyte counts at which time opportunistic infection prophylaxis can be discontinued are listed in Table 2-8.

MEDICATION ADHERENCE

Antiretroviral therapy and prophylactic medicines to prevent the onset of opportunistic infections cannot be effective if patients do not adhere to the regimen, and suboptimal adherence to antiretroviral therapy has been associated with less durable viral suppression and increased risk of clinical progression.[30] Providers should feel comfortable discussing strategies to optimize adherence with their patients and should take into consideration patient preferences, such as decreased pill burden, less frequent dosing of medications, and greater flexibility related to meals.

PRIMARY CARE FOR HIV-INFECTED WOMEN

Women who are HIV-infected have unique clinical and psychological issues that should be addressed as part of their comprehensive care.[31] They have unrelated rates of recurrent candida vaginitis, bacterial vaginosis, and *Trichomonas*-induced vaginitis. They may also develop complications associated with pelvic inflammatory disease, such as tubo-ovarian abscess, more frequently than HIV-uninfected women and thus they require careful monitoring for this serious condition if pelvic pain, vaginal discharge, or both are present. Overall, comprehensive, accessible gynecologic services play a vital role in the care of HIV-infected women.[32]

Infection with HPV is common among HIV-infected women, putting them at increased risk for cervical neoplasia.[33] Although cervical cancer is more common among HIV-infected women than HIV-uninfected women, routine Pap smear screening can lower morbidity and mortality associated with cervical cancer. The USPHS/IDSA opportunistic infection

Table 2-8

Discontinuing Opportunistic Infection Prophylaxis in Persons with Immune Recovery in Response to Antiretroviral Therapy

Opportunistic Illness	Criteria for Discontinuing Primary Prophylaxis	Criteria for Discontinuing Secondary Prophylaxis
Pneumocystis pneumonia	CD4 count >200 cells/μL for ≥3 months (AI)	CD4 count >200 cells/μL for ≥3 months (BII)
Toxoplasmosis	CD4 count >200 cells/μL for ≥3 months (AI)	CD4 count >200 cells/μL for sustained period (e.g., ≥6 months) and completed initial therapy and asymptomatic for Toxoplasma (CIII)
Disseminated *Mycobacterium avium* complex (MAC)	CD4 count >100 cells/μL for ≥3 months (AI)	CD4 count >100 cells/μL for sustained period (e.g., ≥6 months) and completed 12 months of MAC therapy and asymptomatic for MAC (CIII)
Cryptococcosis	Not applicable	CD4 count >100–200 cells/μL for sustained period (e.g., ≥6 months) and completed initial therapy and asymptomatic for cryptococcosis (CIII)
Histoplasmosis	Not applicable	No criteria recommended for stopping
Coccidioidomycosis	Not applicable	No criteria recommended for stopping
Cytomegalovirus retinitis	Not applicable	CD4 count >100–150 cells/μL for sustained period (e.g., ≥6 months) and completed initial therapy and no evidence of active disease; regular ophthalmic examination (BII)

Adapted from Kaplan JE, Masur H, Holmes KK; USPHS; Infectious Disease Society of America. Guidelines for preventing opportunistic infections among HIV-infected persons – 2002. Recommendations of the U.S. Public Health Service and the Infectious Diseases Society of America. MMWR Recomm Rep 51(RR-8):1–52, 2002.

Table 2-9

Follow-up Recommendations for Abnormal Cervical Cytology

Pap Smear Result	Recommendation
ASCUS (with severe inflammation)	Evaluate for infection; if found, treat and recheck Pap smear in 2–3 months
ASCUS	Follow-up Pap smear every 4–6 months for 2 years (until three consecutive Pap smears are negative) If another ASCUS, consider colposcopy
ASCUS (neoplastic process suspected)	Follow-up Pap smear every 4–6 months; *or* colposcopy and biopsy if LSIL persists; *or* immediate colposcopy
LSIL	Follow-up Pap smear every 4–6 months; *or* colposcopy and biopsy if LSIL persists; *or* immediate colposcopy
HSIL (cervical intraepithelial neoplasia 2 or 3, carcinoma *in situ*) *or* Squamous cell carcinoma	Colposcopy and biopsy of abnormal area

Pap, Papanicolaou test; ASCUS, atypical cells of undetermined significance; LSIL, low-grade squamous intraepithelial lesion; HSIL, high-grade squamous intraepithelial lesion.

From Kaplan JE, Masur H, Holmes KK; USPHS; Infectious Disease Society of America. Guidelines for preventing opportunistic infections among HIV-infected persons – 2002. Recommendations of the U.S. Public Health Service and the Infectious Diseases Society of America. MMWR Recomm Rep 51(RR-8):1–52, 2002.

prevention guidelines recommend HIV-infected women undergo Pap smear screening twice in the first year after a diagnosis of HIV infection and then annually (as long as the Pap smears remain normal). If the woman has an abnormal Pap smear, the follow-up becomes intensified and the specific recommendations depend on whether the abnormal findings consist of atypical squamous cells of undetermined significance (ASCUS), low-grade squamous intraepithelial lesion (LSIL), or more invasive lesions consisting of either high-grade SIL (HSIL) or squamous cell carcinoma (Table 2-9).[14] For those women with ASCUS, the approach varies based on the presence or absence of inflammation and whether the Pap smear suggests the presence of a neoplastic process. Some experts also recommend twice yearly Pap smears in women who have CD4+ T-lymphocyte counts less than 200 cells/μL, even if patients have normal Pap smears. Although women who engage in anal intercourse probably have an increased risk of developing anal HPV and neoplasia, no consensus exists for monitoring these women for anal squamous cell carcinoma.

Although the same general criteria exist for initiating antiretroviral therapy for men and nonpregnant women, unique considerations exist regarding the use of specific antiretroviral medications in women. Several studies have shown that women have a disproportionately higher rate of hepatic-related adverse reactions with nevirapine than do men, and initiating nevirapine is not recommended in women who have a prenevirapine T-lymphocyte count greater than 250 cells/μL, unless the benefit clearly outweighs the risk.[17] In addition, efavirenz should not be used in women who are pregnant or have pregnancy potential (women with child bearing potential implies women who want to conceive or those who are not using effective contraception).[17] Issues related to the management of HIV-infected pregnant women are discussed in Chapter 35.

Women living with HIV often have other unique concerns, such as providing the sole support for a family unit that may include dependent children or elders. Programs that care for these women need to develop social service supports, such as the availability of an on-site case manager, who can assist the women and their families to find stable, safe housing, deal with substance use concerns, and address related issues that may affect a woman's ability to adhere to a complex antiretroviral regimen.

SOCIAL CONCERNS

In recent years, the HIV epidemic in the US has increasingly involved persons who have concomitant problems with homelessness, unemployment, mental health, and substance abuse. Accordingly, integrating social workers and case managers into the clinical team is vital, so that issues related to personal finances, housing, substance use, legal difficulties, and partners or families can be appropriately addressed. In addition, social workers and case managers often can provide critical assistance with issues related to funding for medical care, including drug assistance programs for antiretroviral therapy. The patient's long-term treatment success may depend on the their ability to maintain a stable home and work environment, minimize or abstain from substance abuse, and adequately address any mental disorder. Clearly, more favorable outcomes will occur if the clinic provides a multidisciplinary approach for care and the patient establishes trust with the care team.

SUBSTANCE ABUSE

As the HIV epidemic in the US continues to evolve, substance abuse increasingly plays a significant role in the management of HIV-infected persons. Substance use that involves injection of drugs and potential sharing of blood-borne contaminated needles and syringes can result in the acquisition and subsequent transmission of blood-borne pathogens, most importantly HIV, HCV, and HBV. In addition many patients with substance abuse problems present major challenges for clinicians, particularly through erratic engagement in medical care, difficulties with medication adherence, and increased rates of incarceration. The following discussion will focus on substance use associated with heroin, methamphetamine, cocaine, and recreational 'club' drugs. Other substances, such as alcohol, marijuana, and tobacco, can certainly adversely affect HIV-infected individuals, but these topics will not be addressed here, since most medical providers have significant experience in dealing with abuse of those substances.

Heroin Use and Management

During the US HIV epidemic, heroin-related injection drug use has accounted for a substantial number of new HIV infections. Injection drug use with heroin can directly lead to HIV acquisition or transmission via sharing of contaminated needles or syringes, and indirectly to HIV acquisition or transmission by increasing high-risk sexual behavior. Moreover, ongoing use of heroin can have severe adverse medical and social consequences. The long-term management of HIV-infected heroin addiction is thus extremely important and requires a two-pronged approach consisting of medical therapy and long-term addiction counseling services. Specific medical therapy for heroin addiction now consists of either methadone or buprenorphine. Overall, methadone is generally safe and is associated with good long-term success, especially if given in conjunction with a rigorous counseling program. In the US, only designated methadone maintenance treatment clinics are allowed to administer long-term methadone for heroin addiction. Most patients start on methadone at a dose of 20–30 mg once daily and typically require 50–60 mg once daily as a long-term maintenance dose; however, some patients will require much higher maintenance doses.

More recently, buprenorphine, a partial agonist at the opiate receptor, has received Food and Drug Administration (FDA) approval for the medical management of heroin addiction.[34] When used in clinical practice for long-term management of heroin addiction, buprenorphine is generally combined with naloxone in a fixed dose buprenorphine-naloxone pill and is administered via the sublingual route. The naloxone component does not undergo significant absorption by the sublingual route, but if a patient tries to crush the pill and inject it, the naloxone will immediately generate withdrawal symptoms and thus provide intense negative reinforcement. Buprenorphine-naloxone is typically given at a dose of 8–24 mg once daily (dose based on the buprenorphine component). In the US, buprenorphine and buprenorphine-naloxone can be prescribed in the office setting by physicians who undergo the required training related to the management of opiate-addicted patients; these trainings are organized by the Center for Substance Abuse Treatment

(CSAT) branch of the Substance Abuse and Mental Health Administration (SAMSA) and are offered on-line or as all day conferences. In general, buprenorphine has a relatively low abuse potential for two reasons: the drug has a ceiling effect beyond which increasing the dose will not likely provide substantial differences in effect and the naloxone component deters any use via injection. Nevertheless, overdoses have been reported in situations when buprenorphine was taken without the naloxone component in conjunction with taking benzodiazepines.[35]

Methamphetamine Use

In recent years, methamphetamine use has markedly increased among HIV-infected individuals, and this drug now plays a significant role from multiple standpoints, especially by increasing high-risk behavior associated with transmission of HIV, negatively affecting adherence with antiretroviral medications, and adversely impacting the long-term physical and mental health of HIV-infected individuals. Methamphetamine is an easily synthesized compound that acts as a stimulant, similar to amphetamine. It is most often snorted, inhaled, or injected. The use of methamphetamine has become increasingly popular among HIV-infected persons, especially HIV-infected MSM. Several studies have clearly shown that methamphetamine use is associated with high-risk sexual practices among MSM, including sex with multiple partners, sex with casual or anonymous partners, and unprotected anal sex.[36] Most clinicians have observed the negative impact of methamphetamine use in relation to patient adherence to HAART, mainly by disruptions in sleep patterns caused by methamphetamine, chaotic schedules, missed meals, and mental health disturbances.[37] Indeed, the use of methamphetamine can clearly negatively impact the success of HAART, as shown by one study that documented significantly higher HIV RNA levels among active methamphetamine users taking HAART compared to nonusers taking HAART.[38] In addition, chronic and heavy use of methamphetamine can cause a range of psychiatric disturbances, such as depression, delusions, paranoia, and uncontrolled violent behavior; unfortunately many of these disturbances may not resolve after more than a year of abstinence from methamphetamine use.[39] The long-term treatment of methamphetamine abuse often is very difficult and intensive behavioral therapy remains the mainstay of therapy.

Cocaine Use

Similar to the high-risk behavior associated with methamphetamine use that may increase the risk of HIV transmission, the use of cocaine has clearly been associated with high-risk drug behavior and high-risk sexual behavior, even among those persons known to have HIV infection.[40,41] In particular, multiple studies have shown a high incidence of exchanging sex-for-drugs among African-American women who use 'crack cocaine' (inhaling or smoking cocaine).[42,43] Indeed, this epidemic of crack cocaine use among African-American women is likely playing a pivotal role in the marked increase in heterosexual transmission of HIV in the US, particularly in southeastern states. Along with the multitude of medical problems associated with cocaine use, HIV-infected persons who use cocaine have decreased adherence with antiretroviral medications.[44] Furthermore, one study has suggested that cocaine use increases HIV neuroinvasion via remodeling of brain microvascular endothelial cells, thus possibly augmenting the risk of developing HIV-associated dementia.[45]

Recreational 'Club' Drugs

Among MSM, the use of recreational 'club' drugs, such as methylenedioxybutyrate (ecstasy, MDMA), ketamine, and gamma hydroxybutyrate (GHB), have increased in use in recent years. These drugs cause disinhibition, enhance energy, and augment sexual experiences; their use has become particularly popular at all-night dance parties known as raves.[46] Similar to methamphetamine, the use of these drugs has been associated with unsafe sex behaviors. In addition, the use of methylenedioxybutyrate may be associated with transient decline in immune function. Several reports have documented HIV-infected persons on HAART who developed severe consequences from using club drugs, presumably from an interaction of antiretroviral medication and the club drug.[47,48] Specifically, ritonavir's inhibition of cytochrome CYP450 enzymes is believed to have caused a significant increase in levels of methylenedioxybutyrate, since this drug is also metabolized via the cytochrome CYP450 system.[46]

PREVENTING TRANSMISSION OF HIV

The CDC has estimated that there are 30000–40000 new HIV infections annually in the US.[1] Studies from recent years have shown an increase in STDs among persons known to have HIV infection,[1] thus raising major concerns regarding transmission of HIV. These data, as well as other concerns, led to a publication in 2003 from the CDC, the Health Resources and Services Administration, the National Institutes of Health, and the HIV Medicine Association of the IDSA which focused HIV prevention strategies on individuals already infected with HIV. This document is now commonly referred to as the 'Prevention for Positives' initiative.[1] Medical professionals who provide primary care for HIV-infected patients have a prime opportunity to evaluate and counsel their patients regarding sexual and injection-drug practices. When discussing issues related to potential HIV transmission, it is important to discuss risk behaviors in a frank yet nonjudgmental manner. In addition, the medical provider should clearly address the concept of relative risk: the patient should understand that some behaviors (e.g., unprotected anal or vaginal intercourse, sharing contaminated needles) are associated with a high risk of transmitting infection, others (e.g., fellatio) present intermediate risk, and others (e.g., intercourse with a latex condom) are considered to have a low risk.

Although the actual per-contact rates of HIV transmission are not precisely known, cohort studies suggest that the average per-contact transmission rate varies widely based on the actual sex act, with a general consensus that the highest rates of transmission occur with unprotected receptive anal or unprotected receptive vaginal intercourse.[49] Recent data have shown higher rates of HIV acquisition among uncircumcised men.[50,51] In addition, an earlier study found a circumcised infected man to be four times more likely to transmit HIV to his female partner than vice versa, but uncircumcised men have a risk of HIV acquisition comparable to that of women in serodiscordant couples.[52] Men engaging in receptive anal intercourse are far more likely to acquire HIV from their insertive partner than the reverse. The reasons for the wide variability include the fact that certain tissues (e.g., foreskin, cervix, rectal mucosa) are more susceptible to HIV infection, predominantly due to the presence of numbers and types of cells which can bind or transmit HIV. Other factors that may alter HIV susceptibility or infectiousness, include the presence of concomitant genital tract infections, sexual trauma, the HIV level in the infected partners' genital secretions, and possibly the strain of virus to which one is exposed. One additional factor that can play a role in HIV susceptibility is whether a woman is prepubescent or postmenopausal (estrogen thickens the cervicovaginal epithelium and protects against HIV). Finally, oral exposure to HIV appears to have a markedly lower risk than anal or vaginal intercourse,[53] possibly because of endogenous anti-HIV substances that are present in the oropharynx. Nonetheless, it is important to note that multiple well-documented case reports have described HIV acquisition after oral exposure to ejaculate. Thus, although fellatio does not pose as high a risk as unprotected anal or vaginal intercourse, it is not risk-free.[54] Ultimately, the patient will make their own decision regarding how much risk he or she is willing to accept with partners, and providers should serve as nonjudgmental advisors. Health professionals, however, should remind patients that even if their plasma viral load is undetectable they could still transmit HIV to others.

In addition to the concern of an HIV-infected patient transmitting HIV to others, those HIV-infected patients who engage in unsafe sex or drug practices may place themselves at risk of acquiring resistant strains of HIV. Indeed, several recent reports have documented clear-cut cases of HIV 'superinfection' – a term used to describe acquisition of HIV from two different people at distinct points in time.[55] Several cases of HIV superinfection have involved acquisition of resistant strains of HIV that apparently caused virologic breakthrough and antiretroviral therapy failure.[56] Any attempt by the medical provider to assign a precise risk of HIV superinfection occurring with a single high-risk act is not likely to be helpful; instead, patients should understand the general concept that having unprotected sex with another HIV-infected persons is not risk-free, and if superinfection does occur, it may have a serious impact on the patient's ongoing response to antiretroviral therapy.

Patients at risk for HIV infection may be from relatively stigmatized groups, including injection drug users and the MSM group. Accurate assessment of HIV risk and appropriate counseling for risk reduction depend on complete reporting of all potential risk behaviors. This includes activities that may be socially unacceptable or illegal, or which the clinician may find personally objectionable. In such circumstances, it is essential for the clinician to remain absolutely nonjudgmental while questioning the patient. Such marginalized patients are not likely to be forthcoming with accurate information if they believe their medical provider disapproves of specific behaviors, or is inclined to judge patients differently based on what patients relate about themselves. Conversely, once a bond of trust has been established between the medical provider and the patient, the patient is more likely to discuss high-risk behavior frankly and to accept the medical provider's counseling regarding risk reduction.

CONCLUSIONS

The primary care management of HIV infection has become increasingly complex as people with HIV live longer, treatment options become more extensive, and the epidemic increasingly involves persons with concomitant social, mental health, and drug problems. Unfortunately, ~25% of persons infected with HIV in the US remain undiagnosed. During the current era, it is recommended that all medical care providers involved in HIV care become skilled in recognizing all phases of HIV infection and maintain an up-to-date fund of knowledge related to HIV clinical care. In the US, the medical care of HIV-infected persons is most often performed by an infectious diseases specialist, or a generalist who has devoted significant time and energy to become a highly skilled HIV provider. Since the annual number of new HIV infections in the US far exceeds the number of deaths, the population of HIV-infected individuals is expanding, and continued effort is needed to identify and train medical providers interested in providing excellent HIV clinical care.

REFERENCES

1. Centers for Disease Control and Prevention (CDC); Health Resources and Services Administration; National Institutes of Health; HIV Medicine Association of the Infectious Diseases Society of America. Incorporating HIV prevention into the medical care of persons living with HIV: recommendations of CDC, the Health Resources and Services Administration, the National Institutes of Health and the HIV Medicine Association of the Infectious Diseases Society of America. MMWR Morb Mortal Wkly Rep 52(RR-12):1–24, 2003.
2. Centers for Disease Control and Prevention. Kaposi's sarcoma and Pneumocystis pneumonia among homosexual men – New York City and California. MMWR Morb Mortal Wkly Rep 30:305–8, 1981.
3. Masur H, Michelis MA, Greene JB, et al. An outbreak of community-acquired *Pneumocystis carinii* pneumonia: initial manifestation of cellular immune dysfunction. N Engl J Med 305:1431–8, 1981.
4. Centers for Disease Control and Prevention (CDC). Advancing HIV prevention: new strategies for a changing epidemic –

United States, 2003. MMWR Morb Mortal Wkly Rep 52(15): 329–32, 2003.

5. Centers for Disease Control and Prevention (CDC). Revised recommendations for HIV testing of adults, adolescents, and pregnant women in health-care settings. MMWR Recomm. Rep. Sep 22; 55:(RR1-4):1–17, 2006.
6. Kahn JO, Walker BD. Acute human immunodeficiency virus type 1 infection. N Engl J Med 339:33–9, 1998.
7. Schacker T, Collier AC, Hughes J, et al. Clinical and epidemiologic features of primary HIV infection. Ann Intern Med 125:257–64, 1996. Erratum. Ann Intern Med 126:74, 1997.
8. Orenstein R. Presenting syndromes of human immunodeficiency virus. Mayo Clin Proc 77:1093–102, 2002
9. Phair JP. Determinants of the natural history of human immunodeficiency virus type 1 infection. J Infect Dis 179(Suppl 2): S384–6, 1999.
10. Lyles RH, Munoz A, Yamashita TE, et al. Natural history of human immunodeficiency virus type 1 viremia after seroconversion and proximal to AIDS in a large cohort of homosexual men: Multicenter AIDS Cohort Study. J Infect Dis 181:872–80, 2000.
11. Masur H, Ognibene F, Yarchoan R, et al. CD4 counts as predictors of opportunistic pneumonias in human immunodeficiency virus (HIV) infection. Ann Intern Med 111:223–31, 1989.
12. Crowe SM, Carlin JB, Stewart KI, et al. Predictive value of CD4 lymphocyte numbers for the development of opportunistic infections and malignancies in HIV-infected persons. J Acquir Immune Defic Syndr 4:770–6, 1991.
13. Piscitelli SC, Burstein AH, Chaitt D, et al. Indinavir concentrations and St. John's wort. Lancet 355:547–8, 2000.
14. Kaplan JE, Masur H, Holmes KK; USPHS; Infectious Disease Society of America. Guidelines for preventing opportunistic infections among HIV-infected persons – 2002. Recommendations of the US Public Health Service and the Infectious Diseases Society of America. MMWR Recomm Rep 51(RR-8):1–52, 2002.
15. Hadigan C, Meigs J, Corcoran C, et al. Metabolic abnormalities and cardiovascular disease risk factors in adults with human immunodeficiency virus infection and lipodystrophy. Clin Infect Dis 32:130–9, 2001.
16. Parekh B, Phillips S, Granade T, et al. Impact of HIV type 1 subtype variation on viral RNA quantitation. AIDS Res Hum Retroviruses 15:133–42, 1999.
17. Bartlett JG, Lane HC; The Panel on Clinical Practices for Treatment of HIV Infection. Guidelines for the use of antiretroviral agents in HIV-1-infected adults and adolescents. May 4, 2006. Available: www.aidsinfo.nih.gov/ 15 May 2006.
18. Tang JW, Pillay D. Transmission of HIV-1 drug resistance. J Clin Virol 30:1–10, 2004.
19. Golden MR, Marra CM, Holmes KK. Update on syphilis: resurgence of an old problem. JAMA 290:1510–14, 2003.
20. Centers for Disease Control and Prevention. Sexually transmitted diseases treatment guidelines. MMWR Morb Mortal Wkly Rep 51(RR-6):1–80, 2002.
21. Centers for Disease Control and Prevention. Prevention and treatment of tuberculosis among patients infected with human immunodeficiency virus: principles of therapy and revised recommendations MMWR Morb Mortal Wkly Rep 47:1–58, 1998.
22. Stanley SK, Ostrowski MA, Justement JS, et al. Effect of immunization with a common recall antigen on viral expression in patients infected with human immunodeficiency virus type 1. N Engl J Med 334:1222–30, 1996.
23. Gunthard HF, Wong JK, Spina CA, et al. Effect of influenza vaccination on viral replication and immune response in persons infected with human immunodeficiency virus receiving potent antiretroviral therapy. J Infect Dis 181:522–31, 2000.
24. Centers for Disease Control and Prevention. Recommended adult immunization schedule – United States, October 2004–September 2005. MMWR Morb Mortal Wkly Rep 53:Q1-4, 2004.
25. Tedaldi EM, Baker RK, Moorman AC, et al; HIV Outpatient Study (HOPS) Investigators. Hepatitis A and B vaccination practices for ambulatory patients infected with HIV. Clin Infect Dis 38:1478–84, 2004.
26. Celum CL, Robinson NJ, Cohen MS. Potential effect of HIV type 1 antiretroviral and herpes simplex virus type 2 antiviral therapy on transmission and acquisition of HIV type 1 infection. J Infect Dis 191(Suppl 1):S107–14, 2005.
27. Furrer H, Egger M, Opravil M, et al. Discontinuation of primary prophylaxis against *Pneumocystis carinii* pneumonia in HIV-1-infected adults treated with combination antiretroviral therapy. Swiss HIV Cohort Study. N Engl J Med 340:1301–6, 1999.
28. Mussini C, Pezzotti P, Govoni A, et al. Discontinuation of primary prophylaxis for *Pneumocystis carinii* pneumonia and toxoplasmic encephalitis in human immunodeficiency virus type I-infected patients: the changes in opportunistic prophylaxis study. J Infect Dis 181:1635–42, 2000.
29. Currier JS, Williams PL, Koletar SL, et al. Discontinuation of Mycobacterium avium complex prophylaxis in patients with antiretroviral therapy-induced increases in CD4+ cell count. A randomized, double-blind, placebo-controlled trial. AIDS Clinical Trials Group 362 Study Team. Ann Intern Med 133:493–503, 2000.
30. Paterson DL, Swindells S, Mohr J, et al. Adherence to protease inhibitor therapy and outcomes in patients with HIV infection. Ann Intern Med 133:21–30, 2000.
31. Klirsfeld D. HIV disease and women. Med Clin North Am 82:335–57, 1998.
32. Sobel J. Gynecologic infections in human immunodeficiency virus-infected women. Clin Infect Dis 31:1225–33, 2000.
33. Ellerbrock TV, Chiasson MA, Bush TJ, et al. Incidence of cervical squamous intraepithelial lesions in HIV-infected women. JAMA 283:1031–7, 2000.
34. McCance-Katz EF. Treatment of opioid dependence and coinfection with HIV and hepatitis C virus in opioid-dependent patients: the importance of drug interactions between opioids and antiretroviral agents. Clin Infect Dis 41:S89–95, 2005.
35. Tracqui A, Kintz P, Ludes B. Buprenorphine-related deaths among drug addicts in France: a report on 20 fatalities. J Anal Toxicol 22:430–4, 1998.
36. Semple SJ, Patterson TL, Grant I. Motivations associated with methamphetamine use among HIV+ men who have sex with men. J Subst Abuse Treat 22:149–56, 2002.
37. Reback CJ, Larkins S, Shoptaw S. Methamphetamine abuse as a barrier to HIV medication adherence among gay and bisexual men. AIDS Care 15:775–85, 2003.
38. Ellis RJ, Childers ME, Cherner M, et al; HIV Neurobehavioral Research Center Group. Increased human immunodeficiency virus loads in active methamphetamine users are explained by reduced effectiveness of antiretroviral therapy. J Infect Dis 188:1820–6, 2003.
39. Urbina A, Jones K. Crystal methamphetamine, its analogues, and HIV infection: medical and psychiatric aspects of a new epidemic. Clin Infect Dis 38:890–4, 2004.
40. Buchanan D, Tooze JA, Shaw S, et al. Demographic, HIV risk behavior, and health status characteristics of 'crack' cocaine injectors compared to other injection drug users in three New England cities. Drug Alcohol Depend 81:221–9, 2006.
41. Campsmith ML, Nakashima AK, Jones JL. Association between crack cocaine use and high-risk sexual behaviors after HIV diagnosis. J Acquir Immune Defic Syndr 25:192–8, 2000.
42. Inciardi JA, Surratt HL. Drug use, street crime, and sex-trading among cocaine-dependent women: implications for public health and criminal justice policy. J Psychoactive Drugs 33:379–89, 2001.

43. Feist-Price S, Logan TK, Leukefeld C, et al. Targeting HIV prevention on African American crack and injection drug users. Subst Use Misuse 38:1259–84, 2003.
44. Sharpe TT, Lee LM, Nakashima AK, et al. Crack cocaine use and adherence to antiretroviral treatment among HIV-infected black women. J Community Health 29:117–27, 2004.
45. Fiala M, Eshleman AJ, Cashman J, et al. Cocaine increases human immunodeficiency virus type 1 neuroinvasion through remodeling brain microvascular endothelial cells. J Neurovirol 11:281–91, 2005.
46. Romanelli F, Smith KM, Pomeroy C. Use of club drugs by HIV-seropositive and HIV-seronegative gay and bisexual men. Top HIV Med 11:25–32, 2003.
47. Harrington RD, Woodward JA, Hooton TM, Horn JR. Life-threatening interactions between HIV-1 protease inhibitors and the illicit drugs MDMA and gamma-hydroxybutyrate. Arch Intern Med 159:2221–4, 1999.
48. Henry JA, Hill IR. Fatal interaction between ritonavir and MDMA. Lancet 352:1751–2, 1998.
49. Gray RB, Wawer MJ, Brookmeyer R, et al. The probability of HIV-1 transmission per coital act in monogamous HIV-discordant couples, Rakai, Uganda. Lancet 357:1149–53, 2001.
50. Buchbinder SP, Vittinghoff E, Heagerty PJ, et al. Sexual risk, nitrite inhalant use, and lack of circumcision associated with HIV seroconversion in men who have sex with men in the United States. J Acquir Immune Defic Syndr 39:82–9, 2005.
51. Auvert B, Taljaard D, Lagarde E, et al. Randomized, controlled intervention trial of male circumcision for reduction of HIV infection risk: the ANRS 1265 Trial. PLoS Med 2:e298, 2005.
52. Gray RH, Kiwanuka N, Quinn TC, et al. Male circumcision and HIV acquisition and transmission: cohort studies in Rakai, Uganda: Rakai project team. AIDS 14:2371–81, 2000.
53. Vittinghoff F, Douglas J, Judson F, et al. Per-contact risk of human immunodeficiency virus transmission between male sexual partners. Am J Epidemiol 150:306–11, 1999.
54. Page-Shafer K, Veugelers PJ, Moss AR, et al. Sexual risk behavior and risk factors for HIV-1 seroconversion in homosexual men participating in the Tricontinental Seroconverter Study, 1982–1994. Am J Epidemiol 146:531–42, 1997.
55. Smith DM, Richman DD, Little SJ. HIV superinfection. J Infect Dis 192:438–44, 2005.
56. Smith DM, Wong JK, Hightower GK, et al. HIV drug resistance acquired through superinfection. AIDS 19:1251–6, 2005.

Chapter 3

Antiretroviral Therapy and Comprehensive HIV Care in Resource-Limited Settings

Moses R. Kamya, MD, MPH, Jonathan Mermin, MD, MPH, Jonathan E. Kaplan, MD

INTRODUCTION

In 2006, 39.5 million people worldwide were living with HIV, and over 4 million people were newly infected with the virus in 2006.[1] Combating the AIDS pandemic requires a multi-sectoral, multi-faceted approach with a goal to ensure that countries everywhere come as close as possible to achieving universal access to HIV prevention, antiretroviral therapy (ART), and basic care. In resource-poor settings in Africa and Asia, where 90% of people with HIV/AIDS live, access to ART is limited. Over the past four years, the increasing availability of cheaper generic drug formulations and the launch of initiatives by international agencies, including the Global Fund to Fight AIDS, Tuberculosis, and Malaria and the United States President's Emergency Plan for AIDS Relief (PEPFAR), have permitted expanded HIV-treatment programs to take root in many countries. As of December 2005, an estimated 1.3 million people were receiving ART in low- and middle-income countries. This represented only 20% of the estimated 6.5 million people in urgent need of antiretroviral therapy in those regions.[2]

There is compelling evidence that ART can be feasibly administered in resource-limited settings (RLSs) in both adults and children.[3–5] Virologic and immunologic effectiveness, reduction in morbidity, and increased survival among patients in RLS are similar to those seen in Western countries.[6–11] A review of multiple studies reported a substantial increase in CD4+ T-lymphocyte cell counts, and 73% of patients with an undetectable viral load by a median follow-up of 6 months).[3] Many studies report high levels of treatment adherence that are comparable to or better than those of industrialized countries.[12,13]

Several factors could limit the effectiveness of ART in RLS, including: (1) patients often starting ART with advanced HIV infection, e.g., CD4+ T-lymphocyte cell counts <100 cells/μL)[3]; (2) a high prevalence of co-infections, including tuberculosis (TB) and bacterial diseases[14–16]; (3) Interruptions in treatment due to the high cost of antiretroviral (ARV) drugs or transportation to clinics[17,18] (e.g., the percentage lost to follow-up in RLS ranges from 3.7% to 44%[19]); (4) maintaining an uninterrupted supply of drugs[20,21]; (5) monitoring the efficacy and safety of ARV treatment in countries with limited resources (which is problematic because of the lack of laboratory facilities that can conduct tests indicated for HIV care, such as CD4+ T-lymphocyte cell counts and viral loads, and even where such tests can be performed, most patients with HIV infection do not have access to or cannot afford them[22]); and (6) other challenges of ART, including organizational constraints, inadequate human resources, and limited healthcare infrastructure.

Comprehensive care (ART and non-ART) is important in preserving the health of HIV-infected persons and improving quality of life. Ideally, programs should implement care that includes prevention and treatment of opportunistic and other common illnesses, psychosocial support, and prevention of transmission of HIV. To optimize care and treatment for persons with HIV in Africa a two-pronged approach of ARV therapy and prophylaxis/treatment of opportunistic illness is important. Whereas many of the strategies regarding ART are similar regardless of place, the opportunistic infections (OIs) affecting adults and children with HIV vary depending on climate, environment, local infections, and economic conditions. For example, certain illnesses, such as malaria, are common in sub-Saharan Africa; at the same time, some of the infections discussed in current US-based guidelines,[23] such as *Mycobacterium avium* complex, may be less common in some areas of Africa. Some interventions, such as provision of clean drinking water, are regularly provided by governmental services in the industrialized world, but are less available elsewhere. Because of these differences, it is useful to develop a locally applicable package of standard interventions that can be provided to patients with HIV. Cotrimoxazole (trimethoprim-sulfamethoxazole), which is inexpensive, widely available, and effective in reducing morbidity and mortality, should be the cornerstone of such a preventive care package.[24]

Taking daily prophylaxis and using other preventive interventions has the additional benefit of providing a foundation for ARV implementation, both on an individual basis with regard to adherence and HIV disclosure to family members, and on a health system level in relation to establishing reliable drug and commodity distribution mechanisms.

This chapter considers some issues related to ART and non-ART care in RLS: when ART should begin, which regimens should be used, how to promote adherence to therapy and prevention of development of drug resistance, how treatment should be monitored, with specific reference to ART toxicity and efficacy, and when to change ART. We also address issues of organizing an ART program and ensuring that patients receive a comprehensive care package including a basic preventive care package and treatment of OIs. We do not address other aspects of HIV care, such as psychosocial and spiritual support and end-of-life care.

WHEN AND HOW TO INITIATE ART

When to Start ARV Treatment – WHO Eligibility Criteria

In April 2002, WHO published the first edition of the WHO ARV guidelines, a Public Health Approach, with simplified standardized tools for the delivery of ART. Updates of these guidelines have been published frequently, considering new scientific data and the experiences of increasing ART scale up in many countries.[25] Modified versions of the WHO guidelines are generally implemented in RLS.[3] The 2006 criteria for initiating ART are shown in Table 3-1.

The majority of patients in the developing world who present for ART have CD4+ T-lymphocyte cell counts far below 200 cells/μL. Most of these patients receive a diagnosis of HIV infection only when they present to the hospital with a life-threatening OI.[26] At the Infectious Diseases Institute clinic at Makerere University and Mulago Hospital in Kampala, Uganda, the median CD4+ T-lymphocyte cell count at the start of ART was 97.5 cells/μL for 918 patients who started therapy. There is urgent need to establish and scale up routine HIV testing in clinical and other settings to identify HIV-infected patients earlier in the course of HIV infection and to link them to HIV care programs.[27]

Table 3-1 WHO Clinical and Immunologic Criteria for Initiating ART

Clinical Staging for Initiation of ART

Clinical Stage (see Revised WHO Clinical Staging, Box 3-1)	CD4+ T-lymphocyte Available	CD4+ T-lymphocyte Not Available
I	CD4+ T-lymphocyte guided	Do not treat
II	CD4+ T-lymphocyte guided	TLC guided
III	Consider CD4+ T-lymphocyte	Treat
IV	Treat	Treat

CD4+ T-lymphocyte Count Criteria for Initiation of ART

CD4+ T-Lymphocyte Count (cells/μL)	Actions
<200	Treat irrespective of clinical stage
200–350	Consider treatment, initiate before count drops below 200 cells/μL
>350	Do not initiate treatment

TLC, total lymphocyte count.

Evaluating the level of immune suppression is important for making decisions regarding initiation of ART and is a challenge in RLS. Flow cytometry serves as the gold standard technique to quantify the CD4+ T-lymphocyte cell population; however, other methods are also available. Table 3-2 shows the different methods of CD4+ T-lymphocyte testing (standard flow cytometry vs alternatives), and some of the advantages and disadvantages of each method. FACSCalibur equipment (Becton-Dickinson (BD) Biosciences, San Jose, CA, USA and EPICS XL, Beckman Coulter, Miami, FL, USA) is expensive but has the highest throughput and less cost per test, making it appropriate for central laboratories. The FACSCount System (BD) for measuring CD4+ T-lymphocyte cell counts is simpler to perform but requires more expensive reagents and therefore costs $5–10 US/test. One of the most crucial needs in the developing world is universal access to affordable and locally usable CD4+ T-lymphocyte testing technology. As access to ART increases worldwide, alternative laboratory monitoring methods are being considered for use in RLS. For example, the Guava Easy CD4+ T-lymphocyte assay (Guava Technologies, Hayward, CA, USA) utilizes microcapillary cytometry for CD4+ T-lymphocyte cell enumeration. Due to small reagent amounts and no requirement for sheath fluid, costs can be minimized – about

Laboratory Methods to Monitor CD4+ T-lymphocyte Counts in Resource-limited Settings

Table 3-2

CD4+ T-Lymphocyte Tests	Test Cost	System	Advantages	Disadvantages
FACSCalibur (Becton Dickinson Biosciences) or EPICS XL (Beckman Coulter)	4–8, 5–10 USD (BD TriTest CD45/CD3/CD4, BD MultiTest CD45/CD3/CD8/CD4); 6 USD (Beckman Coulter)	Large flow cytometers	Automated add-on loaders available to increase capacity. Can be used in single or dual platform assays. Dedicated reagents not required, potentially lower reagent costs. Can run older specimens	High initial instrument cost. Requires more technologist training. More expensive maintenance costs
FACSCount (Becton Dickinson Biosciences)	5–10; 4–7 USD CD4 and CD8, CD4 alone	Self-contained machine	Single platform. Ease of operation. Built in software for analysis. Less costly than standard flow cytometers	Must use dedicated reagents (MoAbs and TruCount beads). Expensive reagents. Limited number of specimens that can be run in one day. Accurate pipetting crucial. Does not give CD4+T-lymphocyte percentage
Guava Easy CD4 (Guava Technologies)	1.00–1.50, 1.50–2.00 USD CD4+ count, CD4+ %	Microcapillary flow cytometer	Single platform. Simple platform volumetric. Low reagent cost. Low volume of blood needed (10 μL). Easy to operate. Includes CD4+ T-lymphocyte percentage	Laptop computer for analysis (risk of theft). Instrument cost higher than other dedicated smaller machines
CyFlow Counter or SL (Partec)	1.75, 2.50 Euros CD4 count, CD4 %	Volumetric flow cytometer	Single platform. Built in software for analysis (Counter). Lower cost instrument. Can be powered by a 12 V battery. Mobile laboratory also being marketed	Not well validated. Limited service network. Laptop computer for analysis (risk of theft) for SL model
AuRICA (PointCare Technologies)	8–10 USD	Gold-based reagent	Reagents do not require refrigeration. Little training required for operation. Lower cost instrument. Lower biohazard risk (closed tube sampling and reagent system). Also provides lymphocyte count and percent. No pipetting required	Single sample per run; run time 14 min. Low throughput. Higher reagent cost. Not well validated. Limited service network
Cytospheres CD4 (Coulter)	~8 USD	Manual latex bead assay	Minimal equipment, light microscope. Modest technical skill required	Labor intensive. Tedious to count. Learning curve to distinguish monocytes from lymphocytes

(*Continued*)

(Continued)

Table 3-2

CD4+ T-Lymphocyte Tests	Test Cost	System	Advantages	Disadvantages
				Low throughput. Does not give CD4+ T-lymphocyte percentage. Not compatible with external quality assurance materials
Dynabeads T4-T8 system (Dynal)	~5 USD	Manual magnetic bead assay	Minimal equipment, light microscope. Modest technical skill required	Labor intensive. Tedious to count. Low throughput; Less accurate at CD4+ T-lymphocyte >500. Does not give CD4+ T-lymphocyte percentage. Not compatible with external quality assurance materials
Panleukogating (Beckman Coulter)	3–6 USD	Gating strategy using only two monoclonal antibodies Dual platform assay	Lower reagent costs. Better reproducibility (comparable to other single platform techniques). Older specimens can be tested	Requires standard flow cytometer. Requires white blood cell count from hematology instrument. No automated software. Requires training

Note: The estimated costs in this table represent per test costs, once the test is set up; the purchase of equipment and maintenance availability and cost must be considered in the overall costs of a test but have not been included here. Other factors including manpower availability, ease of training and its cost, space requirements, workflow requirements and age of specimens need to be considered.

$1.25 per test. However, the relatively low throughput of the Guava means that this technology has to be applied in smaller health centers with lower demand for CD4+ T-lymphocyte testing. Josefowicz et al conducted a five-site evaluation in the US and Canada and demonstrated that the Easy CD4+ T-lymphocyte assay is precise and accurate when compared to flow cytometry.[28] Our recent study showed that the CD4+ T-lymphocyte cell count determined by the GuavaTech Easy CD4+ T-lymphocyte was comparable to that determined by flow cytometry, with a sensitivity and specificity for CD4+ T-lymphocyte below 200 cells/μL of 90% and 98%, respectively.[29] Low-cost manual methods for CD4+ T-lymphocyte cell enumeration such as the Dynabeads technique[30–32] now exist. Studies evaluating the performance of the Dynabeads methods for the determination of CD4+ T-lymphocyte cells show high overall correlation coefficients between Dynabeads and FACSCount.[31,33] Since the Dynabeads method is simpler and cheaper than flow cytometry, it provides an alternative option for the enumeration of CD4+ T-lymphocyte cells in laboratories with limited facilities. However, the manual methods (Dynabeads, Cytospheres) are much more labor intensive, and their application in ART scale-up in RLS is less clear. Considerations in making decisions regarding choice of CD4+ T-lymphocyte testing method besides instrument and reagent costs include training requirements, throughput, equipment maintenance, supply chain, compatibility with proficiency testing materials, and technician time.

Studies from Africa show simple markers such as HIV-related symptoms (e.g., WHO clinical stage 4); anemia (e.g., hemoglobin less than 8 g/dL) and total lymphocyte count (TLC) (e.g., less than 1200 cells/μL) are relatively specific for a CD4+ T-lymphocyte cell count <200 cells/μL and can be used to determine initiation of ART; however, they are not sensitive predictors of CD4+ T-lymphocyte cell counts below 200 cells/μL.[34,35] The TLC cutoff point has major impact on the sensitivity and specificity of this marker in predicting CD4+ T-lymphocyte cell counts.[36] A higher cutoff increases sensitivity, reducing the likelihood of failing to identify those patients who might benefit from ART. With a lower cutoff (e.g., 1000–1200 cells/μL), sensitivity is lost, but specificity increases.[35,36] In RLS, a lower TLC cutoff point with maximal specificity may be a more practical and cost-effective public health approach for determining eligibility for initiation of ART in asymptomatic or mildly symptomatic HIV-infected patients where CD4+ T-lymphocyte testing is unavailable.[36] In RLS (as well as in industrialized countries), the clinical advantages of starting treatment at CD4+ T-lymphocyte cell counts above 200 cells/μL are unclear.[37]

Viral load testing is very costly and is not of much benefit for initiating ART, even in industrialized countries. It should not be part of screening algorithms for initiating ART in RLS.[38]

How to Start ART

Confirming HIV Infection

Confirming HIV infection is critical before ART is initiated. Patients may present for ART with false-positive HIV serologic results or with only presumed HIV infection. In case of any doubt, clinicians should perform a repeat HIV test before initiating ART.

Baseline Clinical Assessment

Before any patient is started on ART, he/she should undergo baseline clinical assessment including a medical history, physical examination, laboratory investigations, staging of disease (WHO clinical criteria) and counseling and assessment of patients' readiness to start therapy. The treatment of coexisting infection takes priority over starting ART. ART should not be started in patients with serious co-morbidities or those who are terminally ill. However, in most HIV treatment centers in RLS, the facilities to diagnose OIs are limited. Particularly, in countries with a high burden of TB (which includes most middle- and low-income countries), ART programs are challenged with diagnosing TB. In our

BOX 3-1 Revised WHO Clinical Staging of HIV/AIDS for Adults and Adolescents

Primary HIV Infection

- Asymptomatic
- Acute retroviral syndrome

Clinical Stage I

- Asymptomatic
- Persistent generalized lymphadenopathy (PGL)

Clinical Stage II

- Moderate unexplained weight loss (<10% of presumed or measured body weight)
- Recurrent respiratory tract infections (RTIs, sinusitis, bronchitis, otitis media, pharyngitis)
- Herpes zoster
- Angular cheilitis
- Recurrent oral ulcerations
- Papular pruritic eruptions
- Seborrheic dermatitis
- Fungal nail infections of fingers

Clinical Stage III

Conditions where a presumptive diagnosis can be made on the basis of clinical signs or simple investigations:

- Unexplained severe weight loss (>10% of presumed or measured body weight)
- Unexplained chronic diarrhea for longer than 1 month
- Unexplained persistent fever (intermittent or constant for longer than 1 month)
- Persistent oral candidiasis
- Oral hairy leukoplakia
- Pulmonary TB (current)
- Severe bacterial infections (e.g., pneumonia, empyema, pyomyositis, bone or joint infection, meningitis, bacteremia)
- Acute necrotizing ulcerative stomatitis, gingivitis, or periodontitis

Conditions where confirmatory diagnostic testing is necessary:

Unexplained anemia (<8 g/dL), and/or neutropenia (<500/mm^3), and/or thrombocytopenia (<50 000/mm^3) for more than 1 month

Clinical Stage IV

Conditions where a presumptive diagnosis can be made on the basis of clinical signs or simple investigations:

- HIV wasting syndrome
- Pneumocystis pneumonia
- Recurrent bacterial pneumonia
- Chronic herpes simplex infection (orolabial genital or anorectal of more than 1 month's duration)
- Oesophageal candidiasis
- Extrapulmonary TB
- Kaposi's sarcoma
- Central nervous system (CNS) toxoplasmosis
- HIV encephalopathy

Conditions where confirmatory diagnostic testing is necessary:

- Extrapulmonary cryptococcosis including meningitis
- Disseminated nontuberculous mycobacteria infection
- Progressive multifocal leukoencephalopathy (PML)
- Candida of trachea, bronchi or lungs
- Chronic cryptosporidiosis
- Chronic isosporiasis
- Visceral herpes simplex infection
- Cytomegalovirus (CMV) infection (retinitis or of an organ other than liver, spleen or lymph nodes)
- Any disseminated mycosis (e.g., histoplasmosis, coccidiomycosis, penicilliosis)
- Recurrent nontyphoidal salmonella septicemia
- Lymphoma (cerebral or B cell non-Hodgkin)
- Invasive cervical carcinoma
- Atypical disseminated visceral leishmaniasis
- Symptomatic HIV-associated nephropathy or HIV-associated cardiomyopathy

experience, ART initiation commonly causes the unmasking of occult TB.[39] The rolling out of ART therefore requires that TB diagnostic capacity be strengthened. TB screening protocols should be part of any ART program in endemic areas.

The baseline medical history should include essential demographic characteristics; HIV risk behaviors; the past medical history including major illnesses (particularly TB) and sexually transmitted infections (STIs), hospitalizations and surgeries; the length of time since the diagnosis of HIV infection; symptoms and current medications (including anti-TB drugs, traditional therapies, etc) that could interact with ART or potentially cause additive toxic effect if co-administered with ARV drugs. For women, current or planned pregnancy and the access to contraceptive services should be reviewed.

The physical examination should include vital signs, weight, and detailing of any abnormalities of the skin, eyes (including fundi if possible), oral-pharynx (oropharyngeal thrush generally indicates severe immune suppression), lymph nodes, lungs, heart, abdomen, extremities, nervous system, and genital tract and evidence for symptomatic liver (e.g., jaundice, ascites) or kidney disease (e.g., body swelling).

Laboratory testing involves tests that are helpful before starting ART because they may discourage use of a particular regimen or may be helpful in diagnosing an underlying OI. Absence of laboratory testing should not be a barrier to initiating ART. In almost all cases, if laboratory testing is not available, it is still preferable to begin a clinically eligible patient on ART than to not provide her or him with therapy. If laboratory capacity is available, in addition to assessing the level of immune suppression by CD4+ T-lymphocyte cell testing, a full blood count (or at least a hemoglobin) for patients starting on a zidovudine (ZDV)-containing regimen and a pregnancy test for women of child-bearing potential starting on an efavirenz (EFV)-containing regimen, which is potentially teratogenic, are beneficial before initiating ART. Other baseline tests are important to assess the patient's health and diagnose any preexisting HIV complications. These tests include:

- Chest radiograph for patients with cough.
- A sputum smear for patients who have coughed for more than 2–3 weeks.
- Syphilis screening (15% of an ART cohort in Botswana were RPR positive[26]).
- Symptom-directed laboratory tests needed to diagnose preexisting illnesses.

The cost-effectiveness of performing baseline serum chemistry tests (liver and renal function tests) at baseline in RLSs is not clear, but studies to answer this question are ongoing.[40] In Uganda, 11% of patients beginning ART had a positive serum cryptococcal antigen (CRAG) test at baseline.[41] About two-thirds of patients with a positive CRAG test who did not have a prior history of cryptococcal infection developed cryptococcal meningitis while on ART. However, there are no specific data on the impact of an intervention of routine screening and treatment of CRAG-positive asymptomatic persons on morbidity or mortality. Table 3-3 summarizes a baseline clinical evaluation checklist for patients starting ART.

Treatment Education and Assessment of Readiness to Start

Initiation of ART requires a team effort, involving counselors, nurses, caretakers, doctors, and the patient. The preparation of the patient for ART should start with baseline counseling. Time should be spent with the patient to assess his/her 'readiness' to start ART. The issues discussed should include:

- Basic knowledge about HIV and available treatment options.
- Interest and motivation in taking therapy and understanding of the life-long commitment to ART.
- A review of the expected benefits and potential side effects of the regimen chosen and the need to report any perceived side effects of the medications. In some cases, the latter may be life saving, for example, the recognition of symptoms related to abacavir (ABC) hypersensitivity or nevirapine (NVP)-associated hepatotoxicity.
- A review of possible drug interactions (such as with oral contraceptives) and food restrictions.
- The critical need to maintain safe sex practices to prevent HIV transmission and re-infection.
- Reproductive health and how to access contraceptive services.
- The importance of drug adherence to a successful outcome. The patient must be willing to complete a personal adherence plan with a counselor, including a discussion on fitting drug dosing into the patient's routine. If resources are limited, priority for ART slots should be given to patients most likely to be adherent, such as those who have been faithful to their appointments and have adhered to prophylactic medication.
- The importance of disclosure of HIV status to spouse and other family members to allow for adherence support and family HIV testing. Disclosure may be an important indicator that the patient will be adherent.
- The potential benefits of having a treatment supporter to observe treatment on a daily basis.
- Avoidance of drug sharing and drug shopping.
- Assessment of psychosocial and financial barriers that may interfere with clinic visits.

It is common for one or more orientation meetings to occur between the patient and his/her treatment supporter before ART is begun. Adherence should be emphasized at all visits. Motivation sessions that include presentations by persons living with HIV/AIDS are particularly useful. Patients should be informed about the symptoms of ARV drug toxicities and should be aware of the need to seek care and/or to stop therapy in the interim if the need so arises.

Table 3-3 Baseline Clinical Evaluation Checklist for Patients Starting ART

Assessment
1 History Level of understanding of HIV/AIDS; the length of time since the diagnosis of HIV infection Demographics and lifestyle: whether employed and nature of work History of previous ART, prior use of nevirapine during pregnancy Pregnancy risks: contraception options and choices, current or planned pregnancy, access to contraceptive services Sexual risks and disclosure: willingness to practice safer sex, disclosure of HIV serostatus, use of condoms, HIV counseling and testing of sex partners and children Symptoms of chronic pain and depression History of opportunistic infections and other significant illnesses, e.g., TB and STIs, hospitalizations, and surgeries Current medications (including anti-TB drugs, traditional therapies, etc)
2 Physical Exam Weight Nutritional status Functional capacity and level of disability Examination of vital signs, skin, eyes, oropharynx (presence of thrush), lymph nodes, lungs, heart, abdomen, genital tract (STIs), extremities, nervous system
3 Baseline Laboratory Testing to Assess Immunosuppression and Decide on Regimen Confirming HIV serostatus CD4+ T-lymphocyte testing A full blood count for patients starting on a ZDV-containing regimen A pregnancy test for women of child-bearing potential starting on EFV-containing regimen
4 Baseline Laboratory Testing to Assess General Health and Diagnose any Preexisting HIV Complications A sputum smear for AFB for patients who have coughed for more than 2–3 weeks and a chest radiograph for patients who have unproductive cough or whose AFB smears are negative Syphilis screening Serum chemistries (liver and renal function tests), if available Symptom directed laboratory tests to diagnose preexisting illnesses
5 Staging of Disease Using WHO Clinical Criteria
6 Counseling and Assessment of Patients' Readiness to Start Therapy Including Assessment for Specific Education/Information/Counseling Support Needs

Table 3-4 First- and Second-Line ARV Drug Regimens in Adults and Adolescents (2006) as Recommended by WHO[42]

First-Line Regimens	Second-Line Regimens: RTI Component[a]	Second-Line Regimens: PI Component[b]
(ZDV or d4T) + (3TC or FTC) + (EFV or NVP)	ABC + ddI or ABC + TDF or TDF + 3TC ± ZDV	ATV/r or LPV/r or SQV/r
TDF + (3TC or FTC) + (EFV or NVP)	ABC + ddI or ddI + 3TC ± ZDV	ATV/r or LPV/r or SQV/r
ABC + (3TC or FTC) + (EFV or NVP)	ddI + 3TC ± ZDV or TDF + 3TC ± ZDV	ATV/r or LPV/r or SQV/r
(ZDV or d4T) + (3TC or FTC) + (ABC or TDF)	EFV or NVP ± ddI	

ZDV, zidovudine; d4T, stavudine; 3TC, lamivudine; FTC, emtricitabine; EFV, efavirenz; NVP, nevirapine; ABC, abacavir; ddI, didanosine; TDF, tenofovir; ATV/r, ritonavir-boosted atazanavir; LPV/r, ritonavir-boosted lopinavir; SQV/r, ritonavir-boosted saquinavir.

[a] 3TC can be considered to be maintained in second-line regimens to reduce viral fitness.
[b] Nelfinavir (NFV) or ATV in places without cold chain. TDF cannot be used with unboosted ATV.

CHOICE OF ART REGIMENS IN ADULTS AND ADOLESCENTS

Table 3-4 shows the first- and second-line ARV regimens in adults and adolescents recommended by WHO in 2006.[42] Most countries have their own guidelines that are generally derived from the WHO guidelines.

Choices for First Line

First-line regimens are generally recommended at the national level to cover the majority of patients; the choice of preferred regimens is largely driven by cost and availability.

Rationale for Choice of Initial ART Regimens

Currently the initial treatment regimens that are widely used in RLS are: non-nucleoside reverse transcriptase inhibitor (NNRTI): EFV or NVP plus a nucleoside reverse transcriptase inhibitor (NRTI) backbone: stavudine (d4T) plus lamivudine

(3TC) or ZDV plus 3TC. These first-line regimens prolong life, have a low pill burden, and have the lowest cost at the present time. The current treatment regimens permit rapid scale-up. However, they are also associated with drug toxicities that may be irreversible or lethal.[43] Patients at highest risk of these toxicities are those with advanced disease who are often given the highest priority in ART programs in RLS. Currently the data on the incidence and severity of ARV drug toxicities in African patients are still limited.

Nucleoside Reverse Transcriptase Inhibitors

Concerns are increasingly being voiced about the widespread use of stavudine (d4T), given its propensity to cause a progressive disabling peripheral neuropathy especially among patients with advanced HIV and preexisting peripheral neuropathy[26] and those taking concomitant anti-TB drugs.[44] An ongoing program in rural Uganda is following a cohort of 1029 adult patients on a stavudine-containing regimen. Thirty-six per cent of the patients developed neuropathy (9% severe grade) after 11,268 patient months of observation.[45] Stavudine is also associated with stigmatizing facial lipoatrophy,[46] limb fat loss, and lactic acidosis (rare but potentially fatal). Since stavudine is widely used in first-line regimens, patients on stavudine should be monitored closely for neuropathy and lipoatrophy and should be switched to ZDV in a timely fashion to minimize effects of stavudine cumulative toxicity.

Zidovudine also is not without problems; ZDV is associated with anemia, which may lead to blood transfusions and rarely to death. In the DART trial, 21% of patients on ZDV developed a new episode of anemia following initiation of therapy, and 6.6% developed new grade-4 anemia by week 48.[47]

There are alternative drugs without toxicities of this magnitude, although they are all considerably more expensive. Tenofovir (TDF) is at least as potent as d4T and does not have the toxicity profile of d4T or ZDV. TDF-containing regimens may be considered for alternative first-line therapy for the following reasons:

- Relatively low toxicity profile.
- Can be used in pregnancy, and concurrently with TB medication.
- Gilead has recently reduced prices of TDF and emtricitabine (FTC) for the 97 developing countries served by the Gilead Access Program and the new agreement of Gilead with Aspin to produce a generic version may bring the cost down further.
- Once-daily administration: currently TDF is co-formulated with FTC. A single combination pill of EFV, TDF, and FTC has been developed. This combination allows for the possibility of a 1 pill per day regimen, with the obvious potential for improved adherence.
- Added advantage of TDF for treatment of patients co-infected with hepatitis B. Hepatitis co-infection (hepatitis B surface antigenemia) is present in ~10% of HIV infected patients beginning ART in Botswana.[26] This high prevalence has implications for empirical treatment with drugs that have activity against both HIV and hepatitis B.
- The current 'cost' of toxic first-line drugs that are cheaper to purchase than less toxic alternatives may be underestimated. The cost of the extra clinic visits, treatment switches, and laboratory monitoring of drug toxicity may be more than purchasing less toxic first-line agents.
- If TDF is used in the first-line regimen, this approach reserves the thymidine analogs (d4T and ZDV) and PIs for second-line therapy.
- Use of TDF, FTC, and EFV has superior treatment outcomes compared to ZDV/3TC plus EFV.[48]

The use of ABC is currently limited by cost.

Non-Nucleoside Reverse Transcriptase Inhibitors

The use of an NNRTI as the third drug is preferable to use of a protease inhibitor (PI), since an NNRTI-containing first-line regimen:

- is less expensive;
- provides the option to use a PI at a later date;
- appears to be safe during pregnancy (NVP, not EFV); and
- allows treatment of TB co-infected patients who are on rifampicin (EFV, not NVP).

Using the fixed-dose combination (currently the least expensive regimen) of d4T, 3TC, and NVP poses a complication with regard to starting and stopping treatment. The recommended NVP dosing regimen starts with a lower lead-in dose of 200 mg q.d. for 2 weeks, followed by 200 mg b.i.d. thereafter. This is based on analyses suggesting that this regimen is less frequently associated with rash. Starting a fixed-dose regimen of combination NNRTI–NRTI treatment without the 'lead in' dose of NVP may be associated with increased toxicity. In addition, NVP has a very long pharmacokinetic tail after discontinuation, and a low genetic barrier to resistance. Therefore, stopping use of the fixed-dose combination without continuing the NRTIs for an additional 5 days may lead to NNRTI resistance.[49]

Concern about the use of NNRTIs as first-line ARV treatment is growing because of the increased use of NVP monotherapy to prevent mother-to-child transmission of HIV infection.[50] One dose of NVP during delivery has been shown to cause significant resistance mutations.[51,52] Johnson et al[53] showed that resistance mutations emerge in at least 65% of the women after single dose NVP. In a study in Thailand, women who received intrapartum NVP were less likely to have virologic suppression after 6 months of postpartum treatment with an NVP-containing regimen than those who had not received NVP.[50] The HIV-1 RNA level was less than 50 copies/mL in 49% of the women who had received intrapartum NVP, compared with 68% of the women who had not received intrapartum NVP ($P = 0.03$). More recent data do not support an adverse impact of NVP monotherapy for

PMTCT on subsequent response to NVP-based ART if ART is initiated 6 months or more after receipt of a single, peripartum dose of nevirapine.[54] Further research to determine clinical implications is needed.

Regimens that contain EFV should not be used by women at risk of pregnancy because of the teratogenic potential for the fetus.[55] The potential teratogenicity of EFV means that effective contraception is strongly recommended for women taking this drug. Despite the increasing attention to ART in RLS, support for reproductive choice in HIV-infected individuals has lagged behind.[56] More research is needed to understand reproductive decisions in HIV-infected women and the factors that influence them. Because of drug interactions with rifampin, the use of NVP is generally avoided in patients who require both TB and ART.[57]

PI-Based Regimens

PI-based regimens are an accepted standard of care for initial regimens. However, their high cost relative to NNRTI-based regimens makes their use problematic in RLS seeking to achieve rapid scale-up of therapy. Disadvantages are higher pill counts, food and water requirements in some cases, significant interactions with other drugs that preclude or complicate their use with TB treatment regimens including rifampin, metabolic abnormalities, and the need for a functioning cold chain for ritonavir (RTV)-boosted regimens. In RLS, PIs are generally reserved for second-line therapy.[24]

Triple NRTIs

The triple-nucleoside combination of ABC, ZDV, and 3TC was associated with an inferior virological outcome, compared with a regimen containing EFV and two or three nucleosides.[58] However, emerging data suggest that select triple NRTI regimens are simple to administer, have low pill burden, are associated with acceptable HIV RNA reductions and CD4+ T-lymphocyte cell increases, are relatively safe, have fewer drug–drug interactions and are less likely than NNRTI-containing regimens to cause ARV drug resistance when treatment is interrupted. These regimens are being studied[59] and may be good choices for patients with TB or in whom a preferred or alternative NNRTI- or PI-based regimen may be less desirable due to concerns about toxicity, drug interactions, or regimen complexity. Examples of triple NRTI regimens include: ZDV + 3TC + TDF; ZDV + 3TC + ABC.

MONITORING AND SWITCHING ART

Once patients have been started on ART, they must be monitored for efficacy and toxicity. In developed countries, the efficacy of an ARV treatment regimen is monitored by viral load testing, and decisions to switch therapy are based on increasing viral load, decreasing CD4+ T-lymphocyte cell counts and resistance testing.[60] Western style monitoring is not affordable and is severely limited by laboratory infrastructure in RLS. Unlike the prices for ARV drugs, the prices for laboratory reagents have not decreased significantly in recent years, although there are efforts to find new and less expensive ways to monitor efficacy of treatment.[61,62] The lack of laboratory monitoring should not prevent initiating or continuing ART. In fact, the minimum laboratory testing (in addition to clinical monitoring) that is adequate for monitoring for drug toxicity in RLS is not known. Several studies looking at the effect of different levels of monitoring on patient health outcomes are underway.[40,59] In the meantime, WHO recommends clinical monitoring, with symptom- and ART drug regimen-directed laboratory assessment as needed for monitoring ART.

Clinical Monitoring

Without laboratory support, especially in rural settings, clinicians rely more on clinical monitoring only, using symptoms and signs to indicate treatment failure or drug toxicity. Once therapy has begun, clinical assessment should cover: the patient's perception of how he/she is doing on treatment; changes in body weight over the course of therapy (assuming a reliable food supply); intercurrent symptoms and signs (including changes in the frequency and/or severity of HIV-associated symptoms); signs like fever, diarrhea, thrush; signs of immune reconstitution syndromes; and symptoms and signs of drug toxicities.

Patients must be evaluated for the range of potential adverse events caused by their medications. Patients may complain of minor difficulties in tolerating ARVs, which are often transient and do not necessitate stopping the drug. In contrast, drug toxicities may be severe enough to necessitate change of therapy or temporary discontinuation to assess whether the adverse effect is due to the suspected drug. Major toxicities of commonly used ARV drugs include ZDV-related anemia, EFV-associated CNS symptoms, NVP-associated hepatotoxicity and rash and d4T-related neuropathy, lipoatrophy, and lactic acidosis.

Using clinical symptoms to assess the possibility of treatment failure is a challenge and may be inaccurate, especially during the first 3–6 months of ART. Patients may develop symptoms that are not caused by treatment failure but instead represent the side effects of ARV therapy, an immune reactivation inflammatory syndrome,[63] OIs that continue to appear because the patient is still immunocompromised, or an infection/reinfection by a common endemic pathogen such as TB or malaria. If a patient has been adherent with a good ART regimen and has not had previous ARV exposure, very few treatment failures will occur during the first 6 months.[64] After 6 months to 1 year of ART, clinical manifestations will be more useful for predicting treatment success/failure. This will be particularly so in patients who were symptomatic (WHO clinical stage III and IV) at the start of ART, a group that currently represents the majority of those who start ART in countries with limited resources. Development of a new OI or loss of weight may signal treatment failure. Following the effect of ART on relatively mild HIV-related symptoms and signs such as prurigo may be useful markers of treatment response but remain unproven. Prurigo occurs in at least 10% of African patients with advanced HIV disease.[65] Once prurigo appears, in the absence of ARV treatment the itching and the papular eruption generally persist and symptomatic treatment is ineffective. In a Ugandan study, pruritic papular eruption significantly improved and in some cases disappeared among patients with advanced HIV infection started on ART (Colebunders Robert, Byakwaga Helen, personal observation).

Immunological Monitoring

CD4+ T-lymphocyte cell counts are useful in detecting asymptomatic patients or patients with minor symptoms (WHO stage-II disease) who require ART. A CD4+ T-lymphocyte cell count may also help in deciding when to start or stop prophylaxis for OIs but is of less value as an indirect tool to monitor antiviral efficacy. Indeed, in most instances, once a patient has failed immunologically (or clinically), viral resistance has already evolved. Moreover, the change in CD4+ T-lymphocyte cell count may vary from one patient to another regardless of the virological efficacy of a regimen. A slight increase in CD4+ T-lymphocyte cell count (<50 cells/μL after 1 year of ART) does not necessarily imply treatment failure.[66,67] Conversely, a patient on a virologically failing regimen whose virus is resistant to only one or two drugs of the regimen may have a continued increase in CD4+ T-lymphocyte cell count.[68,69] The criteria proposed by the WHO for immunological treatment failure are (1) a CD4+ T-lymphocyte cell count below 100 cells/mm^3 after six months of therapy; (2) a return to, or a decrease to below the pre-therapy CD4+ T-lymphocyte cell count after six months of therapy; or (3) a 50% decline from the on-treatment peak CD4+ T-lymphocyte cell value (if known).[42] Ideally, CD4+ T-lymphocyte cell count testing should be done when the patient does not have an active OI since intercurrent infections may cause CD4+ T-lymphocyte cell count levels to decline.[70] A problem in resource poor settings is that many OIs are difficult to diagnose. Therefore, in a patient who is not doing well clinically, with a decreasing CD4+ T-lymphocyte cell count, it is often unclear whether this is because of an intercurrent illness, HIV disease progression, or both.

Virological Monitoring

Virological monitoring is considered the ideal method for assessing the efficacy of an ARV regimen since it directly assesses the effect of therapy and typically occurs before immunological or clinical failure. A recent study in Uganda showed that health status and Karnofsky scores were high for all study participants regardless of virologic status.[18] This finding emphasizes that virologic failure occurs in the setting of clinical well-being. Patients with virologic failure may progress to drug resistance prior to the development of illness. Although the combined cost of medications and laboratory-based monitoring may require resources that are not yet available in developing countries, the consequences of continuing to provide a failing regimen must be considered.

HIV RNA viral load testing is costly ($15–150 US per test), and requires both a sophisticated laboratory infrastructure and well-trained personnel. Alternative technologies are being developed as substitutes or surrogates for HIV RNA testing, such as heat-denatured quantitative ultrasensitive (Up24) antigen measurement and real time reverse transcriptase-based assays.[71–75] However, these tests are also expensive (about $3–30 US per test) and have not yet been validated in resource limited settings. In our clinic population of Ugandans infected with HIV-1 non-B subtypes, the Up24 antigen test demonstrated low sensitivity, especially at lower viral loads, when compared with reverse transcriptase polymerase chain reaction (RT-PCR). This may limit the usefulness of the Up24 assay to monitor patients treated with ART in patients infected with non-B subtypes.[76]

WHEN AND HOW TO CHANGE THERAPY

The reason for changing a patient's ART regimen should be clearly defined. Common indications include: adverse drug effects, treatment failure, occurrence of active TB, and/or pregnancy, inconvenient regimens such as dosing/number of pills that may compromise adherence, and economic constraints for those buying their own drugs. When changing therapy for indications other than treatment failure, the provider should substitute for only the offending drug(s).

Diagnosing Drug Toxicity and Switching Therapies

The most common reason for modifying therapy is the development of an adverse drug effect.[77] In the setting of a good therapeutic response, the development of a clearly definable toxicity permits single drug substitutions without compromising the overall regimen. For example, ZDV can be substituted for d4T-induced neuropathy and NVP can be substituted for EFV when EFV-related central nervous system symptoms are unremitting. For other toxicities, for which a specific agent cannot be identified as causal, and/or low-grade but intolerable side effects which frequently compromise adherence, a complete regimen switch to the second-line drugs may be indicated. If an interruption in therapy is indicated to permit resolution of toxicity, the entire regimen should be temporarily interrupted in order to prevent the emergence of drug resistance (NRTIs should be continued for at least 5 days to avoid monotherapy with NNRTIs, due to the long half-life of the NNRTIs). Monitoring for some adverse effects of ARV drugs in RLS is a challenge. For example, because ART centers do not have access to measurement of serum lactate, lactic acidosis may be an underdiagnosed problem and its effect on patient outcomes may be underestimated.

Diagnosing Treatment Failure and Switching Therapies

Physicians in RLS have great difficulties in diagnosing treatment failure. In assessing treatment failure, the following must be reviewed: treatment history, adherence, potential drug interactions, clinical evidence of failure, and available laboratory test results (CD4+ T-lymphocyte, viral load). Treatment failure should be considered only after ascertaining that poor response is not due to nonadherence. According to the WHO HIV treatment guidelines,[42] in settings where viral load testing is unavailable, treatment failure, defined by clinical or CD4+ T-lymphocyte cell count, can include any one of the following: (1) occurrence of new OIs or malignancy signifying clinical disease progression (rule out IRIS), (2) recurrence of previous OIs, (3) onset or recurrence of WHO stage III or IV conditions, (4) return of CD4+ T-lymphocyte cell count to pretherapy baseline or below without concomitant infection to explain transient CD4+ T-lymphocyte cell decrease, or (5) >50% fall from therapy on-treatment CD4+ T-lymphocyte peak level without concomitant infection to explain a transient CD4+ T-lymphocyte cell decrease, or (6) persistent CD4+ levels below 100 cells/mm^3. There are no data currently to support these CD4+ T-lymphocyte cell count criteria. As mentioned before, in a patient who is not doing well clinically, with a decreasing CD4+ T-lymphocyte cell count, it is often unclear whether the latter is due to intercurrent illness, HIV disease progression, or test variation.

The availability of treatment options affects switching decisions. Clinicians are encouraged to make decisions to change therapy on a case-by-case basis and should seek the opinion of colleagues experienced in the management of HIV. This is important because a small number of patients may have poor immunologic response despite good virologic suppression (the disconnect syndromes) and the symptoms of immune reconstitution inflammatory syndrome (IRIS) (see section on IRIS) may be confused with clinical failure. It is important to identify the factors that may have contributed to failure of the initial regimen and address them before the change is made to avoid premature failure of the second-line regimen.

Choices for Second-Line ART

Optimal second-line therapy for HIV is unclear in resource-limited countries. Management of treatment failure and presumed drug resistance is particularly challenging in sub-Saharan Africa, where genotyping and viral load testing, the cornerstones of decision making regarding salvage therapy in the developed countries, remain prohibitively expensive. The current WHO guidelines for management of ART failure recommend discontinuation of all medications in the initial failing regimen and changing to at least three new drugs, usually a PI and two nucleoside analogs.[42] To maximize the possibility of virologic suppression and sustained benefit from the second-line regimen, the WHO recommends that these new drugs should have a low probability of cross-resistance to drugs in the failing regimen. For example, NVP should not be replaced with EFV, and d4T should not be replaced with ZDV.[78] ZDV and d4T share a high rate of cross-resistance and the use of one of these drugs in the first-line regimen generally precludes the use of the other in second-line combinations. However, switching to an entirely new regimen for second-line therapy can be problematic if formularies are restricted by both cost and limited supply. In addition, some of the alternative nucleoside combinations for empiric salvage therapy may incur a worrisome risk of generating the potent K65R mutation, as seen with the combination of TDF/ABC.[79] Mutational interactions such as the resensitization to ZDV that occurs in the presence of the 3TC/FTC M184V resistance mutation could potentiate the antiviral activity of the NRTI component of the second-line regimen.[80] The current WHO guidelines technical advisory group suggest that continuation of 3TC as part of a second-line regimen can be considered to reduce viral fitness. For patients who develop TB and who are receiving second-line RTV-boosted PIs, the choice of another second-line regimen is particularly difficult in RLS where access to rifabutin is limited.

The recommendation of RTV-boosted lopinavir (LPV/r) in the second-line regimen poses a challenge in places without a cold chain. In Uganda, we have recommended that patients who do not have access to a refrigerator should wrap their LPV/r container in a polythene bag and store it in a wet sand-filled clay pot in a cool place. A new formulation of LPV/r (Meltrex, Aluvia) that does not need refrigeration has recently been approved by the Food and Drug Administration (FDA) in the USA and may soon become available. The alternative PIs that do not need refrigeration such as nelfinavir (NFV) and unboosted atazanavir (ATV) are more expensive and less available.

WHAT TO DO AFTER SECOND-LINE TREATMENT FAILURE

Salvage regimens are not currently readily available and no salvage therapy regimens have been recommended by WHO. Decisions to continue a failing second-line regimen should be made on a case-by-case basis and in consultation with experts in ART. Because a failing ARV regimen, containing nucleoside analogs and a PI, may still have a beneficial effect on the immune status of the patient,[81] there is reason to continue a failing ARV regimen if no other treatment option is available and particularly if there is evidence of good clinical response. Stopping may be considered if a patient fails to tolerate available second-line regimen or has fulminant life-threatening and incurable OIs. It is important to carefully evaluate the benefits (reducing viral fitness), adverse effects and cost of continuing ART. Laboratory monitoring needs, pill burden, toxicity/drug interactions and drug costs generally increase progressively when a patient moves from first-line to salvage regimens.

IMMUNE RECONSTITUTION SYNDROMES

Soon after initiating ART some patients may experience symptoms and signs of inflammation due to IRISs. IRIS events may occur very quickly after starting ART (within 2–6 weeks). Less commonly, IRIS may occur after many months of ART. IRIS reactions may fluctuate on and off over time. IRIS, an adverse consequence of restoration of pathogen-specific immune responses is particularly problematic in the context of known or occult TB and cryptococcal infection.[82–84] In settings where HIV/TB endemicity is high and where ART is often initiated in advanced stages of HIV disease, clinicians should be alert to the manifestations of immune reconstitution syndromes. Patients with known co-infections should also be educated regarding this possibility to reassure them of drug efficacy and to encourage continued adherence. Inflammatory reactions occur commonly in co-infected patients receiving both ART and TB treatment,[84,85] and may contribute to the higher mortality in co-infected patients. The incidence of IRIS among patients co-infected with *Cryptococcus neoformans* may also be very common (30% in one study).[63] Studies are urgently needed to determine incidence and to better characterize IRIS resulting from the multiple co-morbidities in patients taking ART in RLS.

It is our experience that undiagnosed TB is being commonly unmasked by ART. The diagnosis of IRIS should be considered by ART providers when a patient who has recently started ART (within 3 months) develops new symptoms when he/she should be getting better. Clinical features typical of TB-related IRIS include rapidly increasing tender lymphadenopathy with abscess formation. Patients may present with painful and swollen lymph nodes, chest symptoms, and unexplained fever, among other symptoms. IRIS events associated with cryptococcal meningitis include increased intracranial pressure and therefore increasing headache and/or vomiting, confusion and fits and visual disturbance. They may cause dangerous clinical deterioration.[63]

The management of IRIS should be based upon appropriate management of the responsible OI. OIs (especially TB) must be excluded before starting ART and ART should be delayed as much as possible in patients receiving OI treatment. If an IRIS event occurs, the ART should be continued. There are very little data to support the use of nonsteroidal antiinflammatory drugs and steroids in IRIS, but it is our experience that they may offer some benefit.

ART FOR TB/HIV CO-INFECTED PATIENTS

With the onset of the HIV epidemic, there has been a fourfold increase in TB in some parts of Africa. One-third of HIV-positive patients are co-infected with TB, and 50–70% of TB cases occur in persons with HIV. In one study,[86] approximately one-quarter of the ART cohort received treatment for TB during a median follow-up of 40 weeks.

According to current WHO guidelines, ART is recommended for all patients with TB who have CD4+ T-lymphocyte cell counts below 200 cells/μL (start ART two to eight weeks after starting TB treatment), and for patients with CD4+ T-lymphocyte counts between 200 and 350 cells/μL (start ART after eight weeks of TB treatment). In the absence of CD4+ T-lymphocyte cell counts, ART is recommended for all patients with TB. In HIV-infected patients with confirmed or presumptive TB disease, initiation of TB treatment is the priority. Despite WHO recommendations, the optimal timing for initiation of ART during TB treatment is not known. The decision on when to start ART after starting TB treatment involves a consideration of pill burden and potential for adherence, potential drug interactions (particularly rifampin drug interactions with NNRTI and PI drugs), overlapping toxicities and possible IRIS versus the risk of further progression of immune suppression with its associated increase in mortality and morbidity. The drug interactions may result in subtherapeutic ARV drug levels, and overlapping toxicity profiles may result in increased risk of toxicity. These interactions can be avoided with rifabutin, but rifampin is the only affordable rifamycin drug in RLS.

In patients with severe immune suppression (WHO stage 4 or very low CD4+ T-lymphocyte cell counts) WHO recommends that ART be started between 2 and 8 weeks after the start of TB therapy, after the patient has stabilized on TB therapy. Patients with higher CD4+ T-lymphocyte counts have a lower short-term risk of HIV disease progression or death, and response to TB therapy can guide the decision regarding the urgency of starting ART (starting during the 2-month induction phase vs starting after the induction phase vs deferral and re-assessing for ART after TB treatment is completed). In patients already receiving ART who are diagnosed with TB, ART should be continued. Patients who develop TB while receiving NNRTI-based regimens, a change to EFV-based regimens instead of NVP-based regimens should be made because of cytochrome p450 interactions. Available and emerging data suggest that select triple NRTI regimens such as ZDV + 3TC + TDF; ZDV + 3TC + ABC, may be good choices for patients with TB. The choice of an ART regimen among patients who have failed NNRTI first-line regimens and are receiving RTV-boosted PIs, is more difficult in RLS where rifabutin is unavailable. Options of dealing with this situation includes stopping ART or using triple nucleosides.

ADHERENCE TO ART AND PREVENTING DRUG RESISTANCE

Encouraging Adherence

A clear association between degree of adherence and treatment outcome has been documented.[86] Recent studies conducted in South Africa, Uganda, and Senegal demonstrate high medication adherence in RLS.[9,13,87] However, with the introduction of free drugs and widespread use of ART, the rates of adherence might potentially decrease. Optimization of adherence has the advantage that one may prevent treatment failure and the development of virological resistance. Sustained viral suppression with ART may also render individuals less infectious and may prevent risk of HIV transmission to others. Quinn et al observed that virologic suppression (<1500 copies/mL) reduced the risk of sexual transmission in discordant couples.[88] It is extremely important that ART programs in RLS invest in strategies to obtain optimal adherence to prevent drug failure and the emergence of HIV drug resistance.

Avoidance of Treatment Interruption

Adherence studies from RLS show that the majority of nonadherence is due to treatment interruption as a result of inadequate supply and financial constraints rather than decisions by patients to otherwise stop taking drugs. Studies conducted in RLS[20,89,90] show that treatment interruption due to unreliable drug supply is a significant challenge. However, financial constraints also pose a significant barrier.[77] At the Infectious Diseases Clinic at Mulago Hospital in Kampala, Uganda, we conducted a cross-sectional study between August and December 2003. The 137 participants were paying for their own drug supply without the additional support of clinical trial infrastructure. The study showed that patients who reported a history of unplanned treatment interruption were five times more likely to have virologic failure compared to patients with no such history.[18] Of 32 patients who interrupted ART, 20 cited financial constraints as the cause of lapse in treatment.

ART interruption is particularly problematic for those treated with NNRTI-based regimens. Due to the long half-life of NNRTIs, patients who interrupt NNRTI-based combination therapy are exposed to monotherapy with NNRTIs due to the comparatively short half-life of NRTIs. Stopping the commonly used fixed-dose combination d4T, 3TC, NVP without continuing the NRTI for at least 5 days may lead to resistance because of the long half-life of NVP[49] and the low genetic barrier of NNRTIs to drug resistance.

Ability to pay for ART during the initial phase of therapy does not mean that households have the ability to pay for extended periods of time. Most of the programs for free ARVs give priority to naive patients with the assumption that if they have not bought ART at all, they are poorer and therefore in greater need of free medication than those who are paying for their drugs. The experienced patients who started ART before the free ART programs are excluded to give priority to poor patients.[91] However, paying for medications may lead to treatment interruption and in some cases, discontinuing therapy[17,18] and less optimal treatment outcomes.[3] A solution would be that the patients who are buying medications should be switched to free programs, when resources permit.[91] Monitoring treatment interruptions is an important part of adherence monitoring.

Loss to follow-up among patients on ART may be high in low-income settings; the proportion of patients lost to follow-up can be as high as 44%.[19] Inadequate clinical and biologic follow-up may lead to high rates of drug resistance.[92,93] Evaluation of small cohorts in Côte d'Ivoire,[92] Zimbabwe,[94] and Uganda[95,96] has demonstrated drug resistance. There is a need to identify methods to sustain provision of long-term care for patients receiving comprehensive HIV care, including consideration of home, community, and decentralized services.

Strategies to Improve Adherence

In some settings, adherence counseling is provided by a specialized ART counselor or adherence nurse. Messages on adherence should be reinforced by the entire ART team – doctors, pharmacists, and nurses – and patients should go through multiple adherence counseling sessions before ART is started. Strategies to improve adherence include: (1) disclosure to spouse, which may improve adherence support from family members and may also result in testing the spouse for HIV and preventing pill sharing; (2) fitting the dosing into a patient's routine. A maximum of twice-daily dosing is desirable; some patients find it difficult to take pills at the work place; (3) using adherence aids such as pill boxes and telephone reminders; and (4) directly observed therapy (DOT). Although DOT may be logistically difficult, there is some evidence that this method is superior to self-administration in RLS[97]; an attempt to replicate the success of DOT TB programs by using a treatment supporter as part of the ART program is done in some ART programs. This person is identified by the patient and helps to motivate and ensure patient compliance with the ART regimen. The supporter is included in training sessions to ensure that a proper and informed orientation to HIV care and treatment issues is completed and that the role of the supporter is well defined. In contrast to many TB programs, this person is often a family member; this model may be more sustainable and less expensive than other DOT models.

Some programs have provided home-based care to enhance adherence. Follow-up of patients in their homes is an attractive model as it enables the provision of home HIV care and family VCT. If an ART program has no home care program, home visiting could be provided to difficult patients or those with adherence problems. Involvement of people living with HIV/AIDS (PLWHAs), and community-based organizations (CBOs) and support groups and community volunteers has been used to support adherence at the community level.

ORGANIZATIONAL ISSUES INVOLVED IN THE SETUP, IMPLEMENTATION, AND MONITORING OF AN ART PROGRAM

With the increased availability of ARV drugs, HIV treatment clinics are being overwhelmed by patients. Routine HIV testing is increasingly offered, and is national policy in Botswana and Uganda. During a 3-month period at Mulago Hospital in Uganda, as part of a routine testing program, 12911 patients without prior HIV testing were tested and over 4000 new HIV-infected patients were identified and linked to care. In this circumstance, new clinics had to be opened to care for the increasing number of newly identified patients. The infrastructure of each new ART center must be assessed and accredited by the national ministry of health to ensure that it has the basic physical infrastructure for clinical care, a minimum number of qualified personnel with training and experience in the management of HIV/AIDS, record keeping, drug procurement, and referral system. A standardized assessment procedure should be in place for this purpose. Facilities and the necessary human resources to deal with large numbers of HIV-infected patients requiring care are currently lacking in most areas.[98] To cope with the increasing demand for outlets for HIV care (including ART), public and private providers must organize themselves to provide quality services. Development of national care guidelines including ART and non-ART care, a national implementation plan and a plan to evaluate/ensure quality of programs are essential. The major issues in setting up an ART program include:

- ensuring that the minimum physical infrastructure is available;
- identifying and training providers;
- establishing or strengthening drug logistics systems: procurement, storage, and distribution of drugs;
- setting up the necessary laboratory services for ARV monitoring (determine laboratory tests that can be done on-site, off-site, and organization of a specimen referral mechanism);
- establishing a system for record keeping; ensuring adequate records/data facilities and personnel to manage records;
- choosing the model of care (home-based care or facility-based care) and establishing referral systems between levels of service delivery (tertiary institution, district/health subdistrict, community, and/or home-based levels) to ensure a comprehensive continuum of care for the patient from the home to the highest level and back to the home;
- ensuring program sustainability and leadership: maintaining sustainable resources, fundraising from national or local government budgets, deciding if cost sharing by patients is an option; and
- developing standard operating procedures for:
  1. ART eligibility, screening and initiation, choice of first-line drug regimens;
  2. diagnosing treatment failure and choice of second-line regimens;
  3. clinical and laboratoy monitoring and management of side effects;
  4. clinic appointments: follow-up mechanism; frequency of appointments and services offered at each patient visit; patient flow patterns and referral mechanisms with regard to asymptomatic patients, symptomatic patients, patients on ARVs, and very sick patients; involvement of nurses in follow-up;
  5. ART counseling including strategies for maximizing and measuring of adherence;
  6. prevention counseling;
  7. tracking of patients on ART; and
  8. TB diagnosis and treatment.

Physical Infrastructure

Before starting an ART program, a basic physical infrastructure should ideally be in place. Space should be identified to accommodate the essential activities of an AIDS clinic including: waiting area, consultation rooms, a private counseling space, a space for drug storage, and a laboratory.

ART Team Training and Community Education

The limited numbers of healthcare workers in RLS – doctors, nurses, dispensers, clinical pharmacists, and counselors – must be organized into effective clinical teams for providing HIV care services. An ART program requires personnel with adequate clinical expertise. This will require major training initiatives, as well as reorganization of health services. Investing in the training program of ART teams including treatment counselors dedicated to carefully following each patient on ART is critical to effective delivery of ART services, optimizing treatment and preventing drug resistance.

The community should be provided with information and education about the ARV service (e.g., who is eligible for ARV and the need for community support of patients on ART).

Drug Logistics/Procurement/Storage

The ART program must ensure an uninterrupted supply of appropriate ARV and OI drugs and other supplies. A decision on the ARV drug regimens and other necessary commodities for the program must be made. Forecasting the quantities needed to treat a specified number of patients and ensuring no 'stock-outs' is essential. There is also need for procurement planning to ensure timely delivery of shipments and clearance of products through customs and quality control checks. ART programs require a strong inventory management and distribution system, which includes all the storage facilities and transport links at the various levels throughout the system.

Referral Systems

The needs of patients with HIV are physical, social, psychological, and spiritual. If these needs are not met, an ART program might be compromised. Therefore, HIV care is a lifetime commitment to providing comprehensive care. The ART program must identify needs manageable within the program, needs that cannot be addressed within the program, and possible referral or networking partners for unaddressed needs (such as family planning services). Patients may be started on ART at a tertiary health center and then referred to a lower level health center for follow-up. The patient may be referred back up to the tertiary center if he/she develops complications or requires second-line regimens. Community-based support groups and networks of PLWHAs are useful for psychosocial support, motivating and educating patients and their families and informing the health center staff about any problems. Private physicians and traditional healers play a significant role in the provision of HIV care in poor countries. National policies that engage those in the private sector in ART are essential in providing continuity of care and supporting treatment.[99]

RECORD KEEPING AND DATA MANAGEMENT

Collecting ART-specific data is critical in monitoring and evaluation of an ART program. As much as possible, collection of data related to ART should be integrated into the existing national Health Management Information System (HMIS) to avoid duplication. However, there is usually a need for a parallel data collection system to collect specific information on ART-related data that are not routinely collected through the HMIS. This includes information such as: WHO stage, Karnofsky score, weight, CD4+ T-lymphocyte cell count, OI prophylaxis, TB status, pregnancy status, prior use of ART, ART eligibility, past and current OIs, ART regimens, reasons for regimen change, toxicity to ART, follow-up status at end of each month, ART source, missed doses, missed refills/appointments. Some countries have introduced Facility HIV Care Registers (pre-ART and ART) to record the minimum information on each patient enrolled into HIV care. These data are used to fill out monthly and quarterly reporting forms.

A patient-held card is recommended. The card contains personal identification details, information on treatment and appointments, and dates of prescription and refills of ARV drugs. The patient and his/her treatment supporter can use the card to monitor medication adherence. It can also contribute to adherence monitoring by the nurse/counselor.

In the absence of sophisticated data management, in order to keep track of patients on ART, box files or shelves are recommended. The box files or shelves should have divisions for each month of the year. If the patient starts ART, the patient's personal file or continuing care card can be put in the month of the section or shelf for the next appointment. If they attend and are resupplied and given an appointment for the following month, then the card is put in the division or shelf for that month. If the patient does not attend, then the card will still be in the section or shelf of the previous month – making it clear that the patient has not attended, and needs to be contacted and encouraged to attend.

LABORATORY SUPPORT

Laboratory support is crucial for initiating and monitoring ARV use. Prior to initiating an ART program, laboratory services should be strengthened to provide adequate support to the ART program. The laboratory at the ART site should be able to carry out the minimum tests including HIV testing and hemoglobin,[25] and possibly malaria and TB microscopy. When laboratory tests cannot be done at the point of collection, arrangements can be made for the collection and referral of samples to the nearest referral laboratory. A clear plan should be in place detailing collection, and transport of samples and communication of results.

COMPREHENSIVE HIV CARE

Basic HIV Preventive Care

In Table 3-5, we have listed some basic interventions for HIV-infected adults and children focusing primarily on those that have been associated with the prevention of illness and mortality or HIV transmission. These can improve the health of patients with minimal cost and infrastructure and are often overlooked by HIV programs. Interventions include cotrimoxazole (trimethoprim-sulfamethoxazole, CTX) prophylaxis, safe drinking water, isoniazid (INH) prophylaxis, insecticide-treated bed nets, micronutrients, and provision of HIV testing and counseling to family members.[24] Additional interventions may be applicable and available in certain settings.[23]

Daily CTX prophylaxis (160 mg trimethoprim/800 mg sulfamethoxazole for adults and equivalent dose per kilogram for children) in HIV-infected people in Africa has been associated with up to 46% reduction in mortality,[100–102] and reductions in malaria, diarrhea, and hospitalization.[100,101,103,104] It is the mainstay of prevention of *Pneumocystis jiroveci* pneumonia. There is evidence of effectiveness even in areas with high bacterial resistance to CTX,[101–103,105,106] and it is recommended for use by persons with AIDS throughout the world.[23,107] Although most commonly used among persons with symptomatic HIV disease or lower CD4+ T-lymphocyte cell counts, e.g., <200 cells/μL, there are indications that CTX prophylaxis might benefit even those persons with high CD4+ T-lymphocyte counts,[101,108,109] and potentially reduce the rate of decline in CD4+ T-lymphocyte count and stabilize viral load.[101] Adverse reactions are rare in Africa.[100,103] Often, primary or secondary CTX prophylaxis is not recommended for persons whose CD4+ T-lymphocyte cell counts have risen above predetermined levels,[23] although it is unclear at what CD4+ T-lymphocyte level discontinuation might be considered for patients living in tropical areas.

In sub-Saharan Africa (SSA), diarrhea is four times more common among children with HIV and seven times more common among adults with HIV than among their HIV-negative household members.[101] Bacterial contamination of drinking water is common in many parts of the world. A randomized controlled trial of the provision of a small-mouthed plastic water vessel with a spigot and a supply of dilute chlorine solution for water purification was associated with a reduction in microbial contamination of household water and less diarrhea and dysentery among persons with HIV.[110] In addition, this type of drinking water intervention was associated with reduced mortality in a population with unknown HIV status in Kenya.[111]

TB is the leading cause of severe morbidity and mortality among persons with HIV in SSA[15] where a substantial proportion of persons have latent TB. It is estimated that 5–10% of persons with HIV and TB co-infection will develop active TB per year.[15] Although the priority for TB programs is to find and treat all cases of TB disease, daily INH prophylaxis for 6–9 months has been associated with a substantial

Table 3-5

Potential Basic Care and Prevention Interventions for Persons With HIV/AIDS in Resource-Limited Settings

Intervention	Impact: Individual with HIV	Impact: Household	Comments
Cotrimoxazole prophylaxis	Reduction in mortality, malaria, diarrhea, clinic visits, hospitalizations[100–103,105,106,108] Possible effect on stabilization of viral load and rate of decline of CD4+ T-lymphocyte cell count[101,103,105,106]	Reduction in diarrhea, malaria, and mortality in children[158]	Reduction in morbidity for wide range of CD4+ T-lymphocyte cell counts[100,108,109] Low rate of adverse events in Africa[100,103,105,106]
Safe drinking water	Reduction in diarrhea[110]	Reduction in diarrhea and mortality[111]	Efficacy data among people with HIV based on home-based disinfection with chlorine and a plastic water vessel with spigot
Isoniazid prophylaxis	Reduction in incidence of TB[112] Possible reduction in mortality[112]	Theoretical benefit of reduced TB transmission	Questionnaire and physical exam may be adequate to screen out persons with active TB[113] Need for diagnosis and treatment for persons with possible active TB
Insecticide-treated bed nets	Reduction in incidence of malaria	Reductions in malaria and all cause mortality among children[116]	Long-lasting insecticide-treated bed nets available that eliminate need for re-treatment
Micronutrients and vitamin A	Reduction in morbidity, mortality, and disease progression in adults[119,120,123] Possible beneficial effect on CD4+ T-lymphocyte cell count and HIV viral load[119,120] Vitamin A reduces morbidity and mortality, and improves growth among children with HIV/AIDS[124]	Micronutrient supplementation for pregnant or lactating women improves infant outcomes and may reduce rate of mother-to-child transmission of HIV [121,122,159]	One study suggests that regimens containing high levels of vitamin A may not be as beneficial for pregnant women as vitamin B complex, vitamin C, and vitamin E alone[119,120,121]
Family HIV counseling and testing	Psychological benefits of HIV-status disclosure[125–127] Reduction in HIV transmission[132–136,139]	High proportion of adults and children in family have undiagnosed HIV and benefit from care and prevention efforts[128,129]	High uptake with home-based VCT[101]

reduction in the incidence of TB, and possible reductions in mortality.[112] The effect has almost exclusively been observed among persons with HIV who have a positive tuberculin skin test.[112] To avoid treating persons who have active TB with monotherapy it is important to screen for symptoms of active disease for which a simple questionnaire and physical exam may be adequate.[113] Screening should be conducted and active TB ruled out before initiating INH prophylaxis. Persons with potential symptoms of active TB (e.g., prolonged cough, fever, night sweats) should be provided with further evaluation and treatment. Persons who report no symptoms and have a normal exam can be given a tuberculin skin test and if positive receive INH prophylaxis. If skin testing is not available in areas where the prevalence of latent TB infection is relatively high, all persons without active TB can be offered prophylaxis, although a greater number of persons need to be treated per case of TB prevented.

Malaria is twice as common, and *Plasmodium falciparum* parasitemia is more frequent and more severe in adults and children with HIV than in persons without HIV.[101,114] Severe complications from malaria, including death, are probably more common among persons with HIV, at least in areas with episodic transmission.[115] Randomized trials of bed nets have shown a 50% reduction in malaria and a 17% reduction in all cause mortality among children,[116] and a similar reduction in malaria has also been demonstrated among HIV-infected adults beyond what is achieved with CTX and ART.[117] Although generally enough bed nets are provided to cover all sleeping areas in a household, benefits also accrue to members of the household who do not sleep under the nets.[118]

Several studies have shown that persons with HIV have micronutrient deficiencies, and a few studies have evaluated the effect of micronutrient supplementation among persons with HIV. In a randomized trial of pregnant women, multivitamins containing vitamins B, C, and E, but not vitamin A, were associated with reduced maternal and infant mortality, lower rates of mother-to-child transmission of HIV, higher birth weight, and short- and long-term beneficial effects on CD4+ T-lymphocyte cell count and viral load.[119–122] One randomized trial among men and women with HIV in Thailand found that a multivitamin and mineral supplement containing vitamin A was associated with reduced mortality.[123] Children with HIV receive substantial morbidity, mortality, and growth benefits from vitamin A supplementation.[124]

Providing HIV counseling and testing to family members of HIV-positive clients can be an effective method for facilitating HIV disclosure among couples and family members, for identifying and preventing new HIV infections within the family, and linking previously undiagnosed family members with care and treatment. HIV disclosure has been shown to increase support to infected persons and to reduce negative psychological outcomes,[125] including depression.[126,127] A substantial proportion of family members, especially spouses and children under 5 years old, of persons with HIV are infected.[128,129] About 2.5 million children in Africa have HIV,[130] and without effective care almost half will die before their third birthday.[131]

Providing couples with HIV testing and counseling decreases high-risk sexual behavior and HIV transmission,[132,133] particularly among HIV-discordant couples.[134–136] Many persons with HIV believe that their partners are already infected and therefore do not avoid high-risk practices; however, more than 30% of HIV-positive patients in Africa have HIV-negative spouses.[129,136–138] Although facility-based prevention of mother-to-child-transmission programs have had limited success with partner testing, generally less than 10%[138]; over 95% of family members of men and women with HIV accepted testing when it was offered in their homes.[101]

Counseling for HIV-infected persons and their partners can include information regarding HIV discordance, abstinence, safer sex, and the consistent use of condoms. The provision of condoms and education has been associated with an 80% reduction in HIV transmission among HIV-discordant couples.[139]

TREATMENT OF OIS

The diagnosis of OIs in RLS is often complicated by limited knowledge of the incidence and prevalence of OI, poorly equipped laboratories, limited availability and/or affordability of diagnostic tests, lack of training of laboratory personnel, and good quality laboratory systems that increase providers' confidence in the accuracy of test results. Proper treatment of OI is limited by availability and affordability of OI drugs and the potential for poor drug quality due to suboptimal drug regulatory mechanisms. However, despite these limitations, numerous studies of the prevalence of AIDS-related conditions among patients presenting for care, primarily in hospital settings, affords some appreciation for the OIs of importance in various regions.[140–150]

Tuberculosis

TB is the most common serious OI in RLS around the world – in sub-Saharan Africa, in Asia, and in many parts of Latin America as well.[140,141,145,146,149,150] TB is thought to account for 11% of AIDS-related deaths worldwide – more than any other infectious disease.[151] In sub-Saharan Africa, depending on the setting in which HIV is diagnosed, as many as 10% of HIV-infected persons will be found to have active TB at the time HIV is diagnosed.[152] Therefore, screening for active TB is critical in all situations in which HIV is diagnosed. Screening should consist of one or more questions designed to elicit symptoms of TB (e.g., cough for 2–3 weeks). Patients who respond positively to one or more screening questions should be evaluated further by at least a physical examination and sputum studies; if nondiagnostic, then chest radiography and other diagnostic procedures should be performed as indicated.

Accurate and reliable examination of sputum smears for AFB is the most important OI diagnostic procedure that should be in place in all settings in which HIV care is provided in RLS. In most RLS, national TB programs oversee a network of laboratories that perform AFB smears, but quality may be variable. Laboratory technicians should be trained in reading AFB smears and should be supervised by personnel from the regional or national TB program on a regular basis. Laboratories should participate in an external quality assurance (EQA) system in which a sample of slides is examined for AFB in a blinded fashion by an expert on a regular basis.

Diagnosis of TB in RLS is generally made on the basis of a positive AFB smear in the setting of compatible symptoms, signs, and when available, chest radiography, since confirmatory culture and identification of *Mycobacterium tuberculosis* are generally unavailable. A diagnosis of smear-negative TB requires clinical judgment, and is usually made in a patient with symptoms and signs compatible with TB and a negative AFB smear, frequently after a brief trial of antibiotics which has not resulted in clinical improvement.

Treatment of TB should be standardized, with the drug regimen specified by the national TB program. Generally, treatment consists of a 2-month course of rifampin, INH and two additional drugs, directly observed on a daily basis, followed by a continuation phase of two drugs for a total of 6–9 months of therapy.[153] The continuation phase of therapy should ideally be observed, and may be administered thrice weekly, but in practice it is frequently self-administered at home. TB drugs, at least for smear-positive TB, are generally provided at no cost by the national TB program.

Treatment of TB is complicated by the existence of drug-resistant TB, including multi-drug-resistant (MDR) TB (defined by resistance to INH and rifampin) and, more recently, extensively drug-resistant (XDR) TB (defined by resistance to INH, rifampin, a fluoroquinolone), and at least one of three injectable second-line drugs (i.e., amikacin, kanamycin, or capreomycin).[154] Since culture and drug susceptibility testing (DST) of *Mycobacterum tuberculosis* are generally unavailable in RLS, diagnosis and management of drugs-resistant TB is problematic; consultation of an expert is advised.

Patients with HIV and active TB are generally also candidates for ART, but the presence of TB complicates ART since treatment of both conditions involves administration of multiple drugs, with increased potential for drug intolerance and/or toxicity and difficulty in determining the identity of the offending drug. Also, significant drug interactions between rifampin and NNRTI and PI ARV drugs do not permit the co-administration of rifampin with any of these drugs except EFV and RTV (the latter only when administered as the sole PI).[153] Treatment of active TB is always the priority and should always be undertaken immediately. For patients with moderately advanced HIV disease (e.g., CD4+ T-lymphocyte cell count >200 cells/μL), most providers would complete the rifampin-containing phase of the TB treatment before starting ARVs. For patients with advanced disease, earlier initiation of ART should be considered, while rifampin is still being administered, provided that EFV can be used as part of the ARV regimen.

Bacterial Diseases

Bacterial pneumonia is common in HIV-infected persons and is most commonly caused by *S. pneumoniae*, *H. influenzae*, *S. aureus*, and various other gram-negative organisms. Accurate identification and drug susceptibility of pathogens in respiratory specimens is generally unavailable, due to the limited availability of microbiology laboratories. If available, gram stain of sputum may provide helpful information. Generally, patients with symptoms and signs suggestive of bacterial pneumonia (acute onset of cough, fever, chest pain, sputum production, and a chest film suggesting bacterial pneumonia) must be treated presumptively, usually with a penicillin derivative (e.g., ampicillin) ± an aminoglycoside. Third generation cephalosporins, e.g., ceftriazidine, are appropriate but may be unavailable or unaffordable. The same is true for fluoroquinolones active against *S. pneumoniae* (e.g., moxifloxacin or gatifloxacin).

Bacteria are generally less frequent than parasites as causes of diarrhea in HIV-infected persons, but bacterial diarrhea can be caused by nontyphoidal *Salmonella*, *Shigella*, or *Campylobacter* species. The limited availability of microbiology facilities generally obviates against specific diagnosis, but a bacterial etiology should be suspected in patients with severe diarrhea, pus or blood in the stool, and fever. A fluoroquinolone, e.g., ciprofloxacin, should be used in such situations.

Fungal Diseases

Oral candidiasis (OC) is likely the most common OI in HIV-infected persons in RLS, where it is usually diagnosed by visual inspection. OC is a marker for advanced immunosuppression; that is, its presence is associated with CD4+ T-lymphocyte cell counts <200 cells/μL and therefore indicates a risk for other, more serious OIs. Patients with OC and odynophagia (painful swallowing) likely have esophageal candidiasis; this diagnosis can be confirmed by esophagoscopy, which ideally should be performed to differentiate this condition from other causes of esophageal pathology (e.g., herpes simplex virus, cytomegalovirus, Kaposi sarcoma). However, this procedure is not generally available in RLS. OC is usually treated topically in RLS using gentian violet or clotrimazole troches for 5–10 days but can be treated with oral fluconazole if the drug is available. Esophageal candidiasis requires treatment with fluconazole for at least 2 weeks; patients who respond should receive chronic maintenance therapy for several weeks after resolution of the acute episode.[153]

Cryptococcosis is the most common serious fungal OI in most RLS and generally presents as meningitis, with severe headache, fever, and increasing levels of mental disturbance. Focal neurological signs are usually absent on physical examination. Diagnosis requires a lumbar puncture (LP), although in the absence of an LP a presumptive diagnosis of cryptococcal meningitis can be made on the basis of a positive serum CRAG test in the setting of compatible signs and symptoms. Performance of an LP may require clinical judgment in RLS, since a space-occupying lesion should ideally be ruled out by an imaging procedure such as computerized tomography (CT) or magnetic resonance imaging (MRI) before an LP is performed; however, these procedures are generally not available. Hence, the clinician frequently must rely on fundoscopic examination, the absence of focal neurological signs on physical examination, and clinical judgment before proceeding with an LP. The cerebrospinal fluid (CSF) is characterized by pleocytosis and elevated protein concentration; the causative organism, *C. neoformans*, may be detected by Indian ink stain or by a positive CSF CRAG test, if available. Opening pressure is frequently elevated. The differential diagnosis usually includes TB meningitis. Treatment of cryptococcal meningitis requires intravenous amphotericin B for at least 2 weeks, followed by oral fluconazole for 6–10 additional weeks.[153] Repeated LPs may be required to reduce intracranial pressure. Chronic maintenance therapy is required after resolution of acute disease.[153]

P. jiroveci pneumonia (PCP) appears to be less common in HIV-infected persons in SSA compared with other areas of the world, although the disease does seem to be common in HIV-infected children in that region.[155,156] It should be suspected in patients with advanced HIV and a subacute onset of cough, fever, shortness of breath, and hypoxemia, the latter out of proportion to chest film abnormalities, particularly if the patient has not responded to treatment with antibiotics for possible bacterial pneumonia. Definitive diagnosis requires bronchoscopy and examination of bronchoalveolar lavage (BAL) fluid by special stains, but neither the procedures nor the stains are commonly available in RLS; hence, diagnosis is usually presumptive. PCP should be treated with CTX; patients generally respond in 4–7 days, and therapy should continue for a total of 21 days.[153] Adjunctive use of corticosteroids has been associated with improved outcome in persons with severe PCP[153] but such treatment should be used cautiously in RLS because of the possibility of TB. After successful therapy for PCP, patients should receive chronic maintenance therapy with CTX.[153]

Parasitic Diseases

Toxoplasmic encephalitis (TE) is probably the most common cause of mass lesions in the brain in HIV-infected persons in RLS and hence should be suspected in any HIV-infected person with advanced immunodeficiency and physical evidence of a focal neurological deficit. TE is characteristically associated with multiple ring-enhancing lesions on CT or MRI scans; however, these procedures are usually unavailable or unaffordable by patients in RLS. Hence, TE is often treated presumptively in such settings. The treatment of choice is pyrimethamine plus sulfadiazine or pyrimethamine plus clindamycin, but pyrimethamine is frequently unavailable. There is some evidence supporting the use of CTX for treatment of TE, and this drug is often used for this purpose. Fansidar, which is a combination of pyrimethamine and sulfadoxine, has also been used, although supportive data are unavailable. Successful treatment of TE should result in clinical improvement within 2 weeks. If successful, therapy should continue for 8 weeks and should be followed by chronic maintenance therapy after resolution of acute disease.[153]

Cryptosporidium parvum is a common cause of chronic diarrhea in patients with advanced HIV. However, diagnosis requires special staining of stool specimens, which is generally unavailable, and no drug has been proven to be effective for cryptosporidiosis. However, most patients with cryptosporidiosis have advanced immunodeficiency and are eligible for ARTs. ART generally results in clinical improvement and possibly eradication of the causative organism[153] and is therefore of high priority in such patients.

Drugs and doses for treatment of selected OIs in RLS in adults are shown in Table 3-6.

Initiation of ART

Patients with severe OI generally have advanced immunodeficiency and are nearly always candidates for ART. There are few data to guide the timing of treatment of OI vs initiation of ART, even in industrialized countries. However, in general, treatment of the OI, if it is available, is of higher priority. Concomitant initiation of ART is complicated by simultaneous introduction of multiple drugs, with the attendant increased probability of drug intolerance or toxicity, and the difficulty in identifying the offending drug. Therefore, most providers would treat the OI first, and initiate ARTs only when the patient is improving and when it is feasible to introduce additional drugs. The introduction of ARTs may be complicated by exacerbation of symptoms of the OI within the first 2–6 weeks of treatment due to immune reconstitution.[153] Such IRISs may be challenging to the healthcare provider. In general, both ART and treatment of the OI should be continued, with the addition of antiinflammatory medication for the IRIS.[153]

Discontinuation of Chronic Maintenance Therapy

In industrialized countries, numerous studies support the discontinuation of chronic maintenance therapy for some OIs when use of ART has resulted in an increase in CD4+ T-lymphocyte cell count and when the patient no longer has signs or symptoms of the OI.[153] However, data to support such a practice in RLS are lacking. Therefore, discontinuation of therapy in RLS cannot be routinely recommended; clinicians must exercise judgment in making such decisions in these settings.

Syndromic Treatment of OI

Because of the lack of diagnostic facilities at most levels of the healthcare system in RLS, particularly in SSA, a syndromic

Table 3-6

Therapy of OIS in HIV-Infected Adults in Resource-Limited Settings

Agent	Clinical Manifestations	Diagnosis	Primary	Comment/Alternative
Bacteria				
M. tuberculosis	Fever, cavitary lung disease, pneumonia, lymphadenopathy, wasting, bone disease	AFB sputum microscopy, culture for Mycobacteria	INH 5 mg/kg orally/day Rifampicin 10 mg/kg orally/day Ethambutol 15–20 mg/kg orally/day Pyrazinamide 20–30 mg/kg orally/day	Treat × 2 months, then continue with two drugs for an additional 4–7 months
M. avium	Fever, lymphadenopathy, hepatosplenomegaly	Mycobacteria culture of blood or bone marrow	Clarithromycin 500 mg, orally twice daily, plus ethambutol 15 mg/kg/day orally; can add rifabutin 300 mg/day orally	Treat for 6–10 weeks. Secondary prophylaxis required
S. pneumoniae	Fever, pneumonia, bacteremia	Sputum Gram stain, culture; blood culture	Amoxicillin 500 mg orally 3 times/day × 7 days	
H. influenzae	Fever, pneumonia, bacteremia	Sputum Gram stain, culture; blood culture	Amoxicillin 500 mg orally 3 times/day × 7 days	
S. aureus	Fever, pneumonia, bacteremia	Sputum Gram stain, culture; blood culture	Dicloxacillin 125–250 mg orally every 6 h × 7–14 days	
K. pneumoniae	Fever, pneumonia, bacteremia	Sputum Gram stain, culture; blood culture	Ciprofloxacin 500–750 mg orally 2 times/day × 7–10 days	
Salmonella sp	Fever, diarrhea, bacteremia	Stool, blood culture	Ciprofloxacin 500–750 mg orally 2 times/day × 10–14 days	
Shigella sp	Fever, diarrhea	Stool culture	Ciprofloxacin 500 mg orally 2 times/day × 5 days	
Campylobacter sp	Fever, diarrhea	Stool culture	Ciprofloxacin 500 mg orally or norfloxacin 400 mg orally 2 times/day × 7 days	Azithromycin 500 mg orally/day × 7 days
T. pallidum	Genital ulcer, skin rash, tertiary manifestations	Darkfield microscopy, RPR/VDRL treponemal antibody test	Benzathine pencillin 2.4 million units IM × 1 (primary or secondary syphilis) or weekly × 3 (late latent or tertiary syphilis)	Neurosyphilis requires treatment with IV penicillin G × 10–14 days
N. gonorrhoeae	Urethral, cervico-vaginal discharge	Gram stain, culture	Ceftriaxone 125 mg IM or cefixime 400 mg orally (one dose only)	Fluoroquinolone resistance is common in Southeast Asia

C. trachomatis	Urethral, cervico-vaginal discharge	Culture	Doxycycline 100 mg twice daily orally × 7 days	Erythromycin 500 mg orally 4 times/day × 7 days or ofloxacin 300 mg orally twice daily × 7 days
H. ducreyi	Genital ulcer	Gram stain, culture	Azithromycin 1 gm orally or ceftriaxone 250 mg IM (one dose only)	Ciprofloxacin 500 mg twice daily orally × 3 days
Fungi				
Candida sp	Thrush, esophagitis	Visual inspection, KOH prep, fungal culture	Clotrimazole troches 10 mg, 5 times/day orally × 14 days	Fluconazole 100 mg/day orally × 7–14 days
C. neoformans	Fever, meningitis, pneumonia, skin lesions	India ink stain (spinal fluid); Wright stain (skin lesion); fungal culture	Amphotericin B 0.7 mg/kg/day IV × 10–14 days then fluconazole 400 mg orally/day × 8 weeks	Fluconazole 400 mg/2 times/day orally × 10–14 days, then 400 mg/day × 10 weeks. Secondary prophylaxis required
H. capsulatum	Fever, weight loss, pneumonia, sepsis, skin lesions	Blood culture; Wright stain (skin lesion); fungal culture	Amphotericin B 0.7 mg/kg/day IV × 10–14 days, then itraconazole 200 mg 3 times/day orally × 3 days, then reduce to 200 mg 2 times/day × 10 weeks.	Itraconazole 200 mg 3 times/day orally × 3 days, then reduce to 200 mg 2 times/day × 12 weeks. Secondary prophylaxis required
P. marneffei	Fever, weight loss, pneumonia, skin lesions	Blood culture; Wright stain (skin lesion); fungal culture	Amphotericin B 0.7–1.0 mg/kg/day IV × 10–14 days, then itraconazole 200 mg 2 times/day orally × 4 weeks, then 200 mg/day × 4 weeks	Itraconazole 200 mg 3 times/day orally × 3 days then 200 mg 2 times/day × 12 weeks. Secondary prophylaxis required
P. jiroveci	Fever, pneumonia	Gomori-methenamine silver, Giemsa, or Wright stain of induced sputum or BAL fluid	Trimethoprim sulfamethoxazole 15–20 mg/kg of trimethoprim component/day orally in 3–4 divided doses, × 21 days	Trimethoprim 15 mg/kg/day orally plus dapsone 100 mg/day orally × 21 days, or pentamidine 4 mg/kg IV per day × 21 days; or clindamycin 600 mg IV every 8 h plus primaquine 15 mg/day orally × 21 days. Secondary prophylaxis required

(*Continued*)

Table 3-6 (Continued)

Agent	Clinical Manifestations	Diagnosis	Primary	Comment/Alternative
Parasites				
C. parvum	Diarrhea	Modified acid-fast stain of stool	Hydration; no antibiotics known to be effective	
Microspordia	Diarrhea	Various (e.g., Chromotrope 2A) stains of stool	Albendazole 400 mg 2 times/day orally × several weeks	Effective against most but not all species of Microsporidia
I. belli	Diarrhea	Stool microscopy	Cotrimoxazole (480mg tab) 2 tab orally 2 times per day × 10 days, then 2 tabs per day x 3 weeks	Pyrimethamine 75 mg/day orally plus folinic acid 5–10 mg/day orally × 4 weeks
T. gondii	Focal neurological disease, brain lesions	CT, MRI scan of brain	Pyrimethamine 50 mg/day plus folinic acid 10–20 mg/day plus sulfadiazine 1 g 4 times/day orally × 8 weeks	Pyrimethamine 50 mg/day plus folinic acid 10–20 mg/day plus clindamycin 600 mg 3–4 times/day orally × 8 weeks or cotrimoxazole (960 mg tab) 2 tabs 2 times/day orally × 8 weeks. Secondary prophylaxis required
T. vaginalis	Vaginal discharge	Wet mount of vaginal discharge	Metronidazole 2 g orally (one dose only)	Metronidazole 0.5 g orally twice daily × 7 days
Viruses				
H. simplex	Genital ulcers	Visual inspection, herpes culture	Acyclovir 400 mg 3 times/day orally × 5 days	
H. zoster	Shingles	Visual inspection, herpes culture	Acyclovir 800 mg orally 5 times/day or famciclovir 500 mg orally 3 times/day or valacyclovir 1 g orally 3 times/day × 7–10 days	
Cytomegalovirus	Retinitis, pneumonia, colitis	Characteristic retinal findings	Ganciclovir 5 mg/kg IV over 1–2 h 2 times/day × 14–21 days, or foscarnet 60 mg/kg by IV infusion every 8 h × 14–21 days	Secondary prophylaxis required
M. contagiosum	Skin lesions	Visual inspection	Surgical removal by scraping or de-coring; or freezing	
Papillomavirus	Venereal warts	Visual inspection	Podophyllin resin 10–25% in tincture of benzoin, applied weekly	

approach to diagnosis and treatment of OIs must be considered. The WHO has developed a module for acute care of HIV-infected persons that addresses this issue[157]; this module has undergone in-country adaptation, and HCWs have been trained in its use in a few countries in SSA (Sandy Gove, personal communication). Such an approach appears promising but will require additional in-country adaptations, training, implementation, and evaluation.

REFERENCES

1. UNAIDS/WHO AIDS Epidemic Update: December 2006. http://www.unaids.org.
2. WHO/UNAIDS. Global access to HIV therapy tripled in past two years, but significant challenges remain. Press release, Geneva, March 28, 2006.
3. Akileswaran C, Lurie MN, Flanigan TP, Mayer KH. Lessons learned from use of highly active antiretroviral therapy in Africa. Clin Infect Dis 41:376–85, 2005.
4. Puthanakit T, Oberdorfer A, Akarathum N, et al. Efficacy of highly active antiretroviral therapy in HIV-infected children participating in Thailand's National Access to Antiretroviral Program. Clin Infect Dis 41:100–7, 2005.
5. Severe P, Leger P, Charles M, et al. Antiretroviral therapy in a thousand patients with AIDS in Haiti. N Engl J Med 353:2325–34, 2005.
6. Gadelha AJ, Accacio N, Costa RL, et al. Morbidity and survival in advanced AIDS in Rio de Janeiro, Brazil. Rev Inst Med Trop Sao Paulo 44:179–86, 2002.
7. Marins JR, Jamal LF, Chen SY, et al. Dramatic improvement in survival among adult Brazilian AIDS patients. AIDS 17:1675–82, 2003.
8. Djomand G, Roels T, Ellerbrock T, Hanson D, et al. Virologic and immunologic outcomes and programmatic challenges of an antiretroviral treatment pilot project in Abidjan, Cote d'Ivoire. AIDS 17(Suppl 3):S5–15, 2003.
9. Laurent C, Diakhate N, Gueye NF, et al. The Senegalese government's highly active antiretroviral therapy initiative: an 18-month follow-up study. AIDS 16:1363–70, 2002.
10. Weidle PJ, Malamba S, Mwebaze R, et al. Assessment of a pilot antiretroviral drug therapy programme in Uganda: patients' response, survival, and drug resistance. Lancet 360:34–40, 2002.
11. Bartlett JA, DeMasi R, Quinn J, et al. Overview of the effectiveness of triple combination therapy in antiretroviral-naive HIV-1 infected adults. AIDS 15:1369–77, 2001.
12. Laniece I, Ciss M, Desclaux A, et al. Adherence to HAART and its principal determinants in a cohort of Senegalese adults. AIDS 17(Suppl 3):S103–8, 2003.
13. Oyugi JH, Byakika-Tusiime J, Charlebois ED, et al. Multiple validated measures of adherence indicate high levels of adherence to generic HIV antiretroviral therapy in a resource-limited setting. J Acquir Immune Defic Syndr 36:1100–2, 2004.
14. Aaron L, Saadoun D, Calatroni I, et al. Tuberculosis in HIV-infected patients: a comprehensive review. Clin Microbiol Infect 10:388–98, 2004.
15. Holmes CB, Losina E, Walensky RP, et al. Review of human immunodeficiency virus type 1-related opportunistic infections in sub-Saharan Africa. Clin Infect Dis 36:652–62, 2003.
16. Attia A, Huet C, Anglaret X, et al. HIV-1-related morbidity in adults, Abidjan, Cote d'Ivoire: a nidus for bacterial diseases 7.
17. Kabugo C, Bahendeka S, Mwebaze R, et al. Long-term experience providing antiretroviral drugs in a fee-for-service HIV clinic in Uganda: evidence of extended virologic and CD4+ cell count responses. J Acquir Immune Defic Syndr 38:578–83, 2005.
18. Spacek LA, Shihab HM, Kamya MR, et al. Response to antiretroviral therapy in HIV-infected patients attending a public, urban clinic in Kampala, Uganda. Clin Infect Dis 42:252–9, 2006.
19. Cohort Profile: antiretroviral therapy in lower income countries (ART-LINC): international collaboration of treatment cohorts. Int J Epidemiol 1–8, 2005.
20. Laurent C, Meilo H, Guiard-Schmid JB, et al. Antiretroviral therapy in public and private routine health care clinics in Cameroon: lessons from the Douala antiretroviral (DARVIR) initiative. Clin Infect Dis 41:108–11, 2005.
21. Colebunders R, Ronald A, Katabira E, Sande M. Rolling out antiretrovirals in Africa: there are still challenges ahead. Clin Infect Dis 41:386–9, 2005.
22. Nkengasong JN, dje-Toure C, Weidle PJ. HIV antiretroviral drug resistance in Africa. AIDS Rev 6:4–12, 2004.
23. Kaplan JE, Masur H, Holmes KK. Centers for disease control and prevention. guidelines for preventing opportunistic infections among HIV-infected persons. Recommendations of the US Public Health Service and the Infectious Diseases Society of America, 2002. MMWR 51(RR-8), PM:12617574, 2002.
24. Mermin J, Bunnell R, Lule J, et al. Developing an evidence-based, preventive care package for persons with HIV in Africa. Trop Med Int Health10:961–70, 2005.
25. World Health Organization. Scaling up Antiretroviral Therapy in Resource Limited Settings: Guidelines for a Public Health Approach. Geneva: WHO; 2003. Available: http://www.who.int/3by5/publications/documents/arv_guidelines/en.
26. Wester CW, Kim S, Bussmann H, et al. Initial response to highly active antiretroviral therapy in HIV-1C-infected adults in a public sector treatment program in Botswana. J Acquir Immune Defic Syndr 40:336–43, 2005.
27. Wanyenze R, Kamya M, Liechty CA, et al. HIV Counseling and Testing Practices at an Urban Hospital in Kampala, Uganda. AIDS Behav 1–7, 2006.
28. Josefowicz S, Louzao R, Lam L, et al. 5-Site evaluation of the Guava EasyCD4 Assay for the enumeration of human CD4+ T Cells. 12th Conference on Retroviruses and Opportunistic Infections, Hynes Convention Center, Boston, MA, USA, 2005.
29. Spacek LA, Shihab HM, Lutwama F, et al. Evaluation of a low-cost method, the Guava EasyCD4 assay, to enumerate CD4-positive lymphocyte counts in HIV-infected patients in the United States and Uganda. J Acquir Immune Defic Syndr 41:607–10, 2006.
30. Pattanapanyasat K, Lerdwana S, Shain H, et al. Low-cost CD4 enumeration in HIV-infected patients in Thailand. Asian Pac J Allergy Immunol 21:105–13, 2003.
31. Diagbouga S, Chazallon C, Kazatchkine MD, et al. Successful implementation of a low-cost method for enumerating CD4+ T lymphocytes in resource-limited settings: the ANRS 12–26 study. AIDS 17:2201–8, 2003.
32. Didier JM, Kazatchkine MD, Demouchy C, et al. Comparative assessment of five alternative methods for CD4+ T-lymphocyte enumeration for implementation in developing countries. J Acquir Immune Defic Syndr 26:193–5, 2001.
33. Lyamuya EF, Kagoma C, Mbena EC, et al. Evaluation of the FACScount, TRAx CD4 and Dynabeads methods for CD4 lymphocyte determination. J Immunol Methods 195:103–12, 1996.
34. Mekonnen Y, Dukers NH, Sanders E, et al. Simple markers for initiating antiretroviral therapy among HIV-infected Ethiopians. AIDS 17:815–19, 2003.
35. Kamya MR, Semitala FC, Quinn TC, et al. Total lymphocyte count of 1200 is not a sensitive predictor of CD4 lymphocyte count among patients with HIV disease in Kampala, Uganda. Afr Health Sci 4:94–101, 2004.

36. Schreibman T, Friedland G. Use of total lymphocyte count for monitoring response to antiretroviral therapy. Clin Infect Dis 38:257–62, 2004.
37. Rabkin M, El Sadr W, Katzenstein DA, et al. Antiretroviral treatment in resource-poor settings: clinical research priorities. Lancet 360:1503–5, 2002.
38. Diomande FV, Bissagnene E, Nkengasong JN, et al. The most efficient use of resources to identify those in need of antiretroviral treatment in Africa: empirical data from Cote d'Ivoire's Drug Access Initiative. AIDS 17(Suppl 3):S87–93, 2003.
39. Baalwa J, Mayanja-Kizza H, Kamya M, et al. *Mycobacterium tuberculosis* immune reconstitution inflammatory syndrome in Uganda. The 36th IUATLD World Conference on Lung Health: Late-Breaker Session, Paris, France.
40. Bunnell R, Ekwaru JP, Solberg P, et al. Changes in sexual behavior and risk of HIV transmission after antiretroviral therapy and prevention interventions in rural Uganda. AIDS 20:85–92, 2006.
41. Kamya MR, Kambugu A, Semitala F, et al. Routine cryptococcal antigen (CRAG) screening in AIDS patients on HAART at the Infectious Diseases Institute, Kampala, Uganda. IDSA 43rd Annual Meeting, San Francisco; 2005.
42. World Health Organization. Antiretroviral therapy for HIV infection in adults and adolescents: Recommendations for a public health approach. Geneva: World Health Organization, 2006 revision.
43. Colebunders R, Kamya MR, Laurence J, et al. First-line antiretroviral therapy in Africa – how evidence-base are our recommendations? AIDS Rev 7:148–54, 2005.
44. Ndiaye IP, Ndiaye MM, Mauferon JB, et al. Etiological aspects of polyneuritis in Senegal. Dakar Med 34:68–71, 1989.
45. Forna F, Liechty C, Solberg P, Asiimwe F, Were W, Mermin J, et al. Clinical toxicity of highly active antiretroviral therapy in a home-based AIDS care program in rural Uganda. J Acquir Immune Defic Syndr 44(4): 456–62, 2007.
46. Treatment with generics: tolerability, safety and resistance. 2004. http://www.i-base info/pub/htb/v5/htb5-3/Treatment.html
47. Ssali F, Stohr W, Munderi P, Reid A, Walker AS, Gibb DM, et al. Prevalence, incidence and predictors of severe anaemia with zidovudine-containing regimens in African adults with HIV infection within the DART trial. Antivir Ther 11(6): 741–9, 2006.
48. Gallant JE, DeJesus E, Arribas JR, et al. Tenofovir DF, emtricitabine, and efavirenz vs. zidovudine, lamivudine, and efavirenz for HIV. N Engl J Med 354:251–60, 2006.
49. Mackie NE, Fidler S, Tamm N, et al. Clinical implications of stopping nevirapine-based antiretroviral therapy: relative pharmacokinetics and avoidance of drug resistance. HIV Med 5:180–4, 2004.
50. Jourdain G, Ngo-Giang-Huong N, Le Coeur S, et al. Intrapartum exposure to nevirapine and subsequent maternal responses to nevirapine-based antiretroviral therapy. N Engl J Med 351:229–40, 2004.
51. Eshleman SH, Guay LA, Mwatha A, et al. Comparison of nevirapine (NVP) resistance in Ugandan women 7 days vs. 6–8 weeks after single-dose nvp prophylaxis: HIVNET 012. AIDS Res Hum Retroviruses 20:595–9, 2004.
52. Eshleman SH, Guay LA, Mwatha A, et al. Characterization of nevirapine resistance mutations in women with subtype A vs. D HIV-1 6–8 weeks after single-dose nevirapine (HIVNET 012). J Acquir Immune Defic Syndr 35:126–30, 2004.
53. Johnson JA, Li JF, Morris L, et al. Emergence of drug-resistant HIV-1 after intrapartum administration of single-dose nevirapine is substantially underestimated. J Infect Dis 192:16–23, 2005.
54. Lockman S, Shapiro RL, Smeaton LM, Wester C, Thior I, Stevens L, et al. Response to antiretroviral therapy after a single, peripartum dose of nevirapine. N Engl J Med 356(2): 135–47, 2007.
55. Taylor GP, Low-Beer N. Antiretroviral therapy in pregnancy: a focus on safety. Drug Saf 24:683–702, 2001.
56. Myer L, Morroni C, El-Sadr WM. Reproductive decisions in HIV-infected individuals. Lancet 366:698–700, 2005.
57. Oliva J, Moreno S, Sanz J, et al. Co-administration of rifampin and nevirapine in HIV-infected patients with tuberculosis. AIDS 17:637–8, 2003.
58. Gulick RM, Ribaudo HJ, Shikuma CM, et al. Triple-nucleoside regimens versus efavirenz-containing regimens for the initial treatment of HIV-1 infection. N Engl J Med 350:1850–61, 2004.
59. Kaleebu P, Pillay D, Walker AS, et al. Virological response to a triple nucleoside/nucleotide analogue regimen over 48 weeks in HIV-1-infected adults in Africa. AIDS 20:1391–9, 2006.
60. Smith CJ, Staszewski S, Sabin CA, et al. Use of viral load measured after 4 weeks of highly active antiretroviral therapy to predict virologic outcome at 24 weeks for HIV-1-positive individuals. J Acquir Immune Defic Syndr 37:1155–9, 2004.
61. Kumarasamy N, Flanigan TP, Mahajan AP, et al. Monitoring HIV treatment in the developing world. Lancet Infect Dis 2:656–7, 2002.
62. Stephenson J. Cheaper HIV drugs for poor nations bring a new challenge: monitoring treatment. JAMA 288:151–3, 2002.
63. Shelburne SA III, Darcourt J, White AC Jr, et al. The role of immune reconstitution inflammatory syndrome in AIDS-related cryptococcus neoformans disease in the era of highly active antiretroviral therapy. Clin Infect Dis 40:1049–52, 2005.
64. van LF, Phanuphak P, Ruxrungtham K, et al. Comparison of first-line antiretroviral therapy with regimens including nevirapine, efavirenz, or both drugs, plus stavudine and lamivudine: a randomised open-label trial, the 2NN Study. Lancet 363:1253–63, 2004.
65. Colebunders R, Mann JM, Francis H, et al. Generalized papular pruritic eruption in African patients with human immunodeficiency virus infection. AIDS 1:117–21, 1987.
66. Florence E, Lundgren J, Dreezen C, et al. Factors associated with a reduced CD4 lymphocyte count response to HAART despite full viral suppression in the EuroSIDA study. HIV Medicine 4:255–62, 2003.
67. Lederman HM, Williams PL, Wu JW, et al. Incomplete immune reconstitution after initiation of highly active antiretroviral therapy in human immunodeficiency virus-infected patients with severe CD4+ cell depletion. J Infect Dis 188:1794–803, 2003.
68. Brigido L, Rodrigues R, Casseb J, et al. CD4+ T-cell recovery and clinical outcome in HIV-1-infected patients exposed to multiple antiretroviral reimens: partial control of viremia is associated with favorable outcome. AIDS Patient Care STDS 18:189–98, 2004.
69. Buckheit RW. Understanding HIV resistance, fitness, replication capacity and compensation: targeting viral fitness as a therapeutic strategy. Opin Investig Drugs 13:933–58, 2004.
70. Wolday D, Hailu B, Girma M, et al. Low CD4+ T-cell count and high HIV viral load precede the development of tuberculosis disease in a cohort of HIV-positive ethiopians. Int J Tuberc Lung Dis 7:110–16, 2003.
71. Pascual A, Cachafeiro A, Funk ML, Fiscus SA. Comparison of an assay using signal amplification of the heat-dissociated p24 antigen with the Roche Monitor human immunodeficiency virus RNA assay. J Clin Microbiol 40:2472–5, 2002.
72. Ledergerber B, Flepp M, Boni J, et al. Human immunodeficiency virus type 1 p24 concentration measured by boosted ELISA of heat-denatured plasma correlates with decline in CD4 cells, progression to AIDS, and survival: comparison with viral RNA measurement. J Infect Dis 181:1280–8, 2000.
73. Braun J, Plantier JC, Hellot MF, et al. A new quantitative HIV load assay based on plasma virion reverse transcriptase activity for the different types, groups and subtypes. AIDS 17:331–6, 2003.

74. Schupbach J, Boni J, Bisset LR, et al. HIV-1 p24 antigen is a significant inverse correlate of CD4 T-cell change in patients with suppressed viremia under long-term antiretroviral therapy. J Acquir Immune Defic Syndr 33:292–9, 2003.
75. Schupbach J, Boni J, Flepp M, et al. Antiretroviral treatment monitoring with an improved HIV-1 p24 antigen test: an inexpensive alternative to tests for viral RNA. J Med Virol 65:225–32, 2001.
76. Lutwama F, Shihab HM, Summerton J, et al. Evaluation of heat-denatured HIV-1 p24 antigen as an inexpensive marker for HIV-1 viral load in non-B subtypes in Kampala, Uganda. IDSA 43rd Annual Meeting, San Francisco, 2005.
77. Kumarasamy N, Vallabhaneni S, Cecelia AJ, et al. Reasons for modification of generic highly active antiretroviral therapeutic regimens among patients in southern India. J Acquir Immune Defic Syndr 41:53–8, 2006.
78. Pollard RB, Tierney C, Havlir D, et al. A phase II randomized study of the virologic and immunologic effect of zidovudine + stavudine versus stavudine alone and zidovudine + lamivudine in patients with >300 CD4 cells who were antiretroviral naive (ACTG 298). AIDS Res Hum Retroviruses 18:699–704, 2002.
79. Stone C. Human immunodeficiency virus type 1 reverse transcriptase mutation selection during in vitro exposure to tenofovir alone or combined with abacavir or lamivudine. Antimicrob Agents Chemother 48:1413–15, 2004.
80. Catucci M, Venturi G, Romano L, et al. Development and significance of the HIV-1 reverse transcriptase M184V mutation during combination therapy with lamivudine, zidovudine, and protease inhibitors. J Acquir Immune Defic Syndr 21:203–8, 1999.
81. Deeks SG, Hoh R, Neilands TB, et al. Interruption of treatment with individual therapeutic drug classes in adults with multi-drug-resistant HIV-1 infection. J Infect Dis 192:1537–44, 2005.
82. Hirsch HH, Kaufmann G, Sendi P, Battegay M. Immune reconstitution in HIV-infected patients. Clin Infect Dis 38:1159–66, 2004.
83. Shelburne SA, Visnegarwala F, Darcourt J, et al. Incidence and risk factors for immune reconstitution inflammatory syndrome during highly active antiretroviral therapy. AIDS 19:399–406, 2005.
84. Kumarasamy N, Chaguturu S, Mayer KH, et al. Incidence of immune reconstitution syndrome in HIV/tuberculosis-coinfected patients after initiation of generic antiretroviral therapy in India. J Acquir Immune Defic Syndr 37:1574–6, 2004.
85. Breton G, Duval X, Estellat C, et al. Determinants of immune reconstitution inflammatory syndrome in HIV type 1-infected patients with tuberculosis after initiation of antiretroviral therapy. Clin Infect Dis 39:1709–12, 2006.
86. Wools-Kaloustian K, Kimaiyo S, Diero L, et al. Viability and effectiveness of large-scale HIV treatment initiatives in sub-Saharan Africa: experience from western Kenya. AIDS 20:41–8, 2006.
87. Orrell C, Bangsberg DR, Badri M, Wood R. Adherence is not a barrier to successful antiretroviral therapy in South Africa. AIDS 17:1369–75, 2003.
88. Quinn TC, Wawer MJ, Sewankambo N, et al. Viral load and heterosexual transmission of human immunodeficiency virus type 1. N Engl J Med 342:921–9, 2000.
89. Livesley N, Morris C. Antiretroviral therapy in a primary care clinic in rural South Africa. AIDS 17:2005–6, 2003.
90. Macharia DK, Chang LW, Lule G, et al. Antiretroviral therapy in the private sector of Nairobi, Kenya: a review of the experience of five physicians. AIDS 17:938–40, 2003.
91. Colebunders R, Kamya M, Semitala F, et al. Free antiretrovirals must not be restricted only to treatment-naive patients. PLoS Med 2:e276, 2005.
92. Adje C, Cheingsong R, Roels TH, et al. High prevalence of genotypic and phenotypic HIV-1 drug-resistant strains among patients receiving antiretroviral therapy in Abidjan, Cote d'Ivoire. J Acquir Immune Defic Syndr 26:501–6, 2001.
93. Vergne L, Malonga-Mouellet G, Mistoul I, et al. Resistance to antiretroviral treatment in Gabon: need for implementation of guidelines on antiretroviral therapy use and HIV-1 drug resistance monitoring in developing countries. J Acquir Immune Defic Syndr Hum Retrovirol 29:165–8, 2002.
94. Kantor R, Zijenah LS, Shafer RW, et al. HIV-1 subtype C reverse transcriptase and protease genotypes in Zimbabwean patients failing antiretroviral therapy. AIDS Res Hum Retroviruses 18:1407–13, 2002.
95. Weidle PJ, Kityo CM, Mugyenyi P, et al. Resistance to antiretroviral therapy among patients in Uganda. JAIDS 26:495–500, 2001.
96. Richard N, Juntilla M, Abraha A, et al. High prevalence of antiretroviral resistance in treated Ugandans infected with non-subtype B human immunodeficiency virus type 1. AIDS Res Hum Retroviruses 20:355–64, 2004.
97. Liechty CA, Bangsberg DR. Doubts about DOT: antiretroviral therapy for resource-poor countries. AIDS 17:1383–7, 2003.
98. Kober K, Van DW. Scaling up access to antiretroviral treatment in southern Africa: who will do the job? Lancet 364:103–7, 2004.
99. Brugha R. Antiretroviral treatment in developing countries: the peril of neglecting private providers. BMJ 326:1382–4, 2003.
100. Wiktor SZ, Sassan MM, Grant AD, et al. Efficacy of trimethoprim-sulphamethoxazole prophylaxis to decrease morbidity and mortality in HIV-1-infected patients with tuberculosis in Abidjan, Cote d'Ivoire: a randomised controlled trial. Lancet 353:1469–75, 1999.
101. Mermin J, Lule J, Ekwaru JP, et al. Effect of cotrimoxazole prophylaxis on morbidity, mortality, CD4 cell count, and HIV viral load among persons with HIV in rural Uganda. Lancet 364:1428–34, 2004.
102. Lowrance D, Makombe S, Clin D, et al. Lower early mortality rates among patients receiving antiretroviral treatment at clinics offering cotrimoxazole prophylaxis in Malawi. J Acquir Defic Syndr Jul 19, 2007. Epub.
103. Zachariah R, Spielmann MP, Harries AD, et al. Cotrimoxazole prophylaxis in HIV-infected individuals after completing anti-tuberculosis treatment in Thyolo, Malawi. Int J Tuberc Lung Dis 6:1046–50, 2002.
104. Zar HJ, Dechaboon A, Hanslo D, et al. *Pneumocystis carinii* pneumonia in South African children infected with human immunodeficiency virus. Pediatr Infect Dis J 19:603–7, 2000.
105. Badri M, Ehrlich R, Wood R, Maartens G. Initiating co-trimoxazole prophylaxis in HIV-infected patients in Africa: an evaluation of the provisional WHO/UNAIDS recommendations. AIDS 15:1143–8, 2001.
106. Castetbon K, Anglaret X, Attia A, et al. Effect of early chemoprophylaxis with co-trimoxazole on nutritional status evolution in HIV-1-infected adults in Abidjan, Cote d'Ivoire. AIDS 15:869–76, 2001.
107. World Health Organization, 2006. Guidelines on co-trimoxazole prophylaxis for HIV-related infections among children, adolescents, and adults. Available at http://www.who.int.
108. Anglaret X, Chêne G, Attia A, et al. Early chemoprophylaxis with trimethoprim-sulphamethoxazole for HIV-1-infected adults in Abidjan, Côte d'Ivoire: a randomised trial. Lancet 353:1463–8, 1999.
109. Mermin J, Lule JR, Ekwaru JP, Pitter C. Should cotrimoxazole prophylaxis be taken by all adults with HIV in Africa? AIDS 19:845–6, 2005.
110. Lule JR, Mermin JH, Malamba S, et al. Effect of safe water and cotrimoxazole on diarrhea among people with HIV and their family. 13th International Conference on AIDS and STIs in Africa (ICASA), Nairobi, abstract no 776099.
111. Crump JA, Otieno PO, Slutsker L, et al. Household based treatment of drinking water with flocculant-disinfectant

for preventing diarrhoea in areas with turbid source water in rural western Kenya: cluster randomised controlled trial. BMJ 2005.

112. Grant AD, Kaplan JE, De Cock KM. Preventing opportunistic infections among human immunodeficiency virus-infected adults in African countries. Am J Trop Med Hyg 65:810–21, 2001.
113. Mosimaneotsile B, Talbot EA, Moeti TL, et al. Value of chest radiography in a tuberculosis prevention programme for HIV-infected people, Botswana. Lancet 362:1551–2, 2003.
114. Whitworth J, Morgan D, Quigley M, et al. Effect of HIV-1 and increasing immunosuppression on malaria parasitaemia and clinical episodes in adults in rural Uganda: a cohort study. Lancet 356:1051–6, 2000.
115. Grimwade K, French N, Mbatha DD, et al. HIV infection as a cofactor for severe falciparum malaria in adults living in a region of unstable malaria transmission in South Africa. AIDS 18:547–54, 2004.
116. Lengeler C. Insecticide-treated bed nets and curtains for preventing malaria. Cochrane Database Syst Rev 2:CD000363, 2004.
117. Mermin J, Ekwaru JP, Liechty CA, et al. Effect of co-trimoxazole, antiretroviral therapy, and insecticide-treated bed-nets on the frequency of malaria in HIV-1-infected adults in Uganda: a prospective cohort study. Lancet 367:1256–61, 2006.
118. Howard SC, Omumbo J, Nevill C, et al. Evidence for a mass community effect of insecticide-treated bednets on the incidence of malaria on the Kenyan coast. Trans R Soc Trop Med Hyg 94:357–60, 2000.
119. Fawzi WW, Msamanga GI, Spiegelman D, et al. A randomized trial of multivitamin supplements and HIV disease progression and mortality. N Engl J Med 351:23–32, 2004.
120. Villamor E, Msamanga G, Spiegelman D, et al. Effect of multivitamin and vitamin A supplements on weight gain during pregnancy among HIV-1-infected women. Am J Clin Nutr 76:1082–90, 2002.
121. Fawzi WW, Msamanga GI, Hunter D, et al. Randomised trial of vitamin supplements in relation to transmission of HIV-1 through breastfeeding and early child mortality. AIDS 16:1935–44, 2002.
122. Coutsoudis A, Pillay K, Spooner E, et al. Randomized trial testing the effect of vitamin A supplementation on pregnancy outcomes and early mother-to-child HIV-1 transmission in Durban, South Africa. South African Vitamin A Study Group. AIDS 13:1517–24, 1999.
123. Jiamton S, Pepin J, Suttent R, et al. A randomized trial of the impact of multiple micronutrient supplementation on mortality among HIV-infected individuals living in Bangkok. AIDS 17:2461–9, 2003.
124. Fawzi WW, Mbise RL, Hertzmark E, et al. A randomized trial of vitamin A supplements in relation to mortality among human immunodeficiency virus-infected and uninfected children in Tanzania. Pediatr Infect Dis J 18:127–33, 1999.
125. Maman S, Mbwambo JK, Hogan NM, et al. High rates and positive outcomes of HIV-serostatus disclosure to sexual partners: reasons for cautious optimism from a voluntary counseling and testing clinic in Dar es Salaam, Tanzania. AIDS Behav 7:373–82, 2003.
126. Armistead L, Morse E, Forehand R, et al. African-American women and self-disclosure of HIV infection: rates, predictors, and relationship to depressive symptomatology. AIDS Behav 3:195–204, 1999.
127. Hays RB, McKusick L, Pollack L, et al. Disclosing HIV seropositivity to significant others. AIDS 7:425–31, 1993.
128. Lurie MN, Williams BG, Zuma K, et al. Who infects whom? HIV-1 concordance and discordance among migrant and non-migrant couples in South Africa. AIDS 17:2245–52, 2003.
129. Kabatesi D, Ransom R, Lule JR, et al. HIV prevalence among household members of persons living with HIV in rural Uganda. XIV International Aids Conference, Barcelona, 2002, abstract TuPeD4910.
130. UNAIDS. Epidemiology of HIV/AIDS among children and adults 2004. Available: http://www.unaids.org/html/pub/Topics/Epidemiology/Slides02/Epicore2003_en_ppt.ppt.
131. Spira R, Lepage P, Msellati P, et al. Natural history of human immunodeficiency virus type 1 infection in children: a five-year prospective study in Rwanda. Mother-to-Child HIV-1 Transmission Study Group. Pediatrics 104:e56, 1999.
132. Allen S, Tice J, van de Perre P, et al. Effect of serotesting with counselling on condom use and seroconversion among HIV discordant couples in Africa. Br Med J 304:1605–9, 1992.
133. The Voluntary HIV-1 Counseling and Testing Efficacy Study Group. Efficacy of voluntary HIV-1 counselling and testing in individual and couples in Kenya, Tanzania, and Trinidad: a randomised trial. Lancet 356:103–12, 2000.
134. Kamenga M, Ryder RW, Jingu M, et al. Evidence of marked sexual behavior change associated with low HIV-1 seroconversion in 149 married couples with discordant HIV-1 serostatus: experience at an HIV counselling center in Zaire. AIDS 5:61–7, 1991.
135. Allen S, Meinzen-Derr J, Kautzman M, et al. Sexual behavior of HIV discordant couples after HIV counseling and testing. AIDS 17:733–40, 2003.
136. Allen S, Serufilira A, Bogaerts J, et al. Confidential HIV testing and condom promotion in Africa. Impact on HIV and gonorrhea rates. JAMA 268:3338–43, 1992.
137. Trask SA, Derdeyn CA, Fideli U, et al. Molecular epidemiology of human immunodeficiency virus type 1 transmission in a heterosexual cohort of discordant couples in Zambia. J Virol 76:397–405, 2002.
138. Kilewo C, Massawe A, Lyamuya EF, et al. HIV counseling and testing of pregnant women in sub-Saharan Africa: experiences from a study on prevention of mother-to-child HIV-1 transmission in Dar es Salaam, Tanzania. J Acquir Immune Defic Syndr Hum Retrovirol 28:458–62, 2001.
139. Weller S, Davis K. Condom effectiveness in reducing heterosexual HIV transmission. Cochrane Database Syst Rev 3: CD003255, 2001.
140. Grant AD, Sidibe K, Domoua K, Bonard D, Sylla-Koko F, Dosso M, et al. Spectrum of disease among HIV-infected adults hospitalised in a respiratory medicine unit in Abidjan, Cote d'Ivoire. Int J Tuberc Lung Dis 2(11):926–34, 1998.
141. Okongo M, Morgan D, Mayanja B, et al. Causes of death in a rural, population-based human immunodeficiency virus type 1 (HIV-1) natural history cohort in Uganda. Int J Epidemiol 27:698–702, 1998.
142. Colvin M, Dawood S, Kleinschmidt I, Mullick S, Lallo U. Prevalence of HIV and HIV-related diseases in the adult medical wards of a tertiary hospital in Durban, South Africa. Int J STD AIDS 12:386–9, 2001.
143. Rana FS, Hawken MP, Mwachari C, et al. Autopsy study of HIV-1-positive and HIV-1-negative adult medical patients in Nairobi, Kenya. J Acquir Immune Defic Syndr 24:23–9, 2000.
144. Ansari NA, Kombe AH, Kenyon TA, et al. Pathology and causes of death in a group of 128 predominantly HIV-positive patients in Botswana, 1997–1998. Int J Tuberc Lung Dis 6:55–63, 2002.
145. Anekthananon T, Ratanasuwan W, Techasathit W, Rongrungruang Y, Suwanagool S. HIV infection/acquired immunodeficiency syndrome at Siriraj Hospital, 2002: time for secondary prevention. J Med Assoc Thai 87:173–9, 2004.
146. Sharma SK, Kadhiravan T, Banga A, Goyal T, Bhatia I, Saha PK. Spectrum of clinical disease in a series of 135 hospitalized HIV-infected patients from north India. BMC Infect Dis 4:52, 2004.

147. Bellamy R, Sangeetha S, Paton NI. AIDS-defining illnesses among patients with HIV in Singapore, 1985 to 2001: results from the Singapore HIV Observational Cohort Study (SHOCS). BMC Infect Dis 4:47, 2004.
148. Nissapatorn V, Lee CK, Rohela M, Anuar AK. Spectrum of opportunistic infections among HIV-infected patients in Malaysia. Southeast Asian J Trop Med Public Health 35(Suppl 2):26–32, 2004.
149. Nobre V, Braga E, Rayes A, et al. Opportunistic infections in patients with AIDS admitted to an university hospital of the Southeast of Brazil. Rev Inst Med Trop Sao Paulo 45:69–74, 2003.
150. Mohar A, Romo J, Salido F, et al. The spectrum of clinical and pathological manifestations of AIDS in a consecutive series of autopsied patients in Mexico. AIDS 6:467–73, 1992.
151. Corbett EL, Watt CJ, Walker N, et al. The growing burden of tuberculosis: global trends and interactions with the HIV epidemic. Arch Intern Med 163:1009–21, 2003.
152. World Health Organization. Interim policy on collaborative TB/HIV activities. 2004. Available: http://whqlibdoc.who.int/hq/2004/WHO_HTM_TB_2004.330.pdf.
153. Benson CA, Kaplan JE, Masur H, et al. Treating opportunistic infections among HIV-infected adults and adolescents. MMWR 53(RR-15):1–112, 2004.
154. Centers for Disease Control and Prevention. Revised definition of extensively drug-resistant tuberculosis (Notice to Readers). MMWR 43:1176, 2006.
155. Lucas SB, Hounnou A, Koffi K, et al. Pathology of paediatric human immunodeficiency virus infections in Cote d'Ivoire. East Afr Med J 73(5 Suppl):S7–8, 1996.
156. Ruffini DD, Madhi SA. The high burden of *Pneumocystis carinii* pneumonia in African HIV-1-infected children hospitalized for severe pneumonia. AIDS 16:105–12, 2002.
157. World Health Organization. Integrated management of adolescent and adult illness (IMAI): acute care. Interim guidelines for first-level facility health workers. 2006. Available: htpp://www.who.int/3by5/publications/briefs/en/IMAI 2006.
158. Mermin J, Lule J, Ekwaru JP, et al. Cotrimoxazole prophylaxis by HIV-infected persons in Uganda reduces morbidity and mortality among HIV-uninfected family members. AIDS 19:1035–42, 2005.
159. Kumwenda N, Miotti PG, Taha TE, et al. Antenatal vitamin A supplementation increases birth weight and decreases anemia among infants born to human immunodeficiency virus-infected women in Malawi. Clin Infect Dis 35:618–24, 2002.

Chapter 4

Strategic Use of Antiretroviral Therapy

Michael S. Saag, MD

Over the last decade, highly active antiretroviral therapy (HAART) has revolutionized the care of human immunodeficiency virus (HIV) infected patients. Advances in the understanding of HIV pathogenesis, the routine use of viral load and resistance testing in clinical practice, and the availability of over 23 Food and Drug Administration (FDA) approved antiretroviral (ARV) agents (Table 4-1) have created the promise for most HIV-infected patients to live, and live well, for decades such that HIV ultimately has little impact on the duration or quality of their life.[1–5] Persistent, high-level viral replication is the driving force of HIV pathogenesis, with up to 10 billion virions produced in an infected individual each day.[6–9] Viral load measurements enable the clinician to determine the degree to which an ARV therapeutic regimen is working and, more importantly, when the regimen is failing.[10–14] This allows therapy to be switched at the time of ARV failure rather than at the time of clinical failure. Once a regimen begins to fail, clinicians can utilize resistance test information to choose from dozens of potential alternative regimens, utilizing both existing approved drugs and experimental therapeutic agents with novel mechanisms of action now in development.[15] Through the contributions of all of these developments,

ARV Drugs Approved for Use in the United States as of 2006

Table 4-1

Year Approved	Agent (Trade Name)
1987	Zidovudine (retrovir)
1991	Didanosine (videx)
1992	Zalcitabine (hivid)
1994	Stavudine (zerit)
1995	Saquinavir (invirase)
	Lamivudine (epivir)
1996	Indinavir (crixivan)
	Ritonavir (norvir)
	Nevirapine (viramune)
1997	Delavirdine (rescriptor)
	Nelfinavir (viracept)
1998	Efavirenz (sustiva)
	Abacavir (ziagen)
1999	Amprenavir (agenerase)
2000	Lopinavir/ritonavir (kaletra)
2001	Tenofovir DF (viread)
2003	Atazanavir (reyataz)
	Emtricitabine (emtriva)
	Enfuvirtide (fusion)
2004	Fos-amprenavir (lexiva)
2005	Tipranavir (aptivus)
2006	Darunavir (prezista)
	Miraviroc
2007 (in expanded access)	Raltegravir
	Etravirine

clinicians have the potential to achieve long-term clinical benefits by keeping the viral load as low as possible for as long as possible.

The use of modern ARV therapies has led to a striking reduction in HIV-associated mortality.[16–18] Despite these advances, newly recognized toxicities of ARV treatment have begun to limit the long-term benefits of chronic therapy.[19–27] Moreover, the durability of the ARV effect is quite variable. Many factors influence the ability to sustain suppression of viral replication, including pharmacokinetic properties of the regimen, tissue penetration, cellular penetration, appropriate intracellular processing, ARV drug history, tolerability of the regimen, adherence, potency of the regimen, and the development of or preexisting presence of resistant virus.[15,28–34] To achieve the most durable effect of ARV therapy (ART), clinicians must develop a strategic approach that maximizes the likelihood of success of each given regimen through a thorough understanding of the biology of HIV disease and the principles of ART.

THE BIOLOGY OF HIV INFECTION

Since HIV was identified in 1983, several landmark discoveries have helped elucidate the mechanisms by which HIV causes the immune system dysfunction associated with AIDS. These discoveries are usually linked to the application of newly developed technology in the laboratory. Soon after discovery of the virus, investigators demonstrated the presence of HIV in virtually all tissues of the body, including the brain.[35,36] Utilizing p24 antigen assays, an association was made between the level of p24 antigen in plasma and the stage of disease, with higher levels of viremia observed during the time of acute seroconversion and again in the later stages of advanced HIV disease.[37–39] Most of the individuals who were asymptomatic with high CD4+ T-lymphocyte counts had no appreciable p24 antigenemia detected. During the late 1980s, utilizing tissue culture techniques investigators were able to titrate the amount of infectious virus in plasma.[37,40,41] Much like p24 antigenemia, higher levels of infectious virus in plasma were noted at the time of acute seroconversion and again in later stages of disease.[38,39,42] Although the plasma culture technique was more sensitive than the p24 antigen technique, substantial numbers of patients with asymptomatic disease, as well as those on ART, had undetectable levels of infectious virus.[37,40,41]

Utilizing this information, a picture of HIV pathogenesis emerged whereby the virus established widespread infection early in the course of disease (at the time of seroconversion), stimulating a potent immune system response. During the period of clinical latency, which typically lasts up to 10–12 years, initial models of pathogenesis suggested that viral replication was under effective control by the immune system, only to reappear as high-level viremia during later stages of disease (Fig. 4-1).[38,39,42] This model, however, could not explain the slow, yet progressive decline in CD4+ T-lymphocyte counts and immune system function that occurs during the period of clinical latency. With the advent of quantitative polymerase chain reaction (PCR) technology during the early 1990s, the association of HIV replication and immune system destruction was more completely described. Piatak and colleagues were the first to describe the presence of detectable virus at all stages of HIV infection, including the period of clinical latency.[12,13] As was demonstrated with p24 antigen and quantitative plasma culture techniques, the highest levels of viral RNA were detected at the time of acute seroconversion and during later stages of disease.[12,43] However, lower levels of virus were detected even at the early, asymptomatic stages of the disease, implying that viral replication is a continuous, ongoing process even during the period of clinical latency.

The application of viral load testing to determine the activity of ARV therapeutic regimens led to the opportunity to define further the nature of HIV replication *in vivo*. Even with the use of relatively weak ARV regimens, such as zidovudine monotherapy, an 80% (0.9 log) reduction in viral load was noted within 1 week of the initiation of therapy, with a relatively symmetrical return to baseline within 1 week after discontinuing treatment.[44] Based on these observations, it

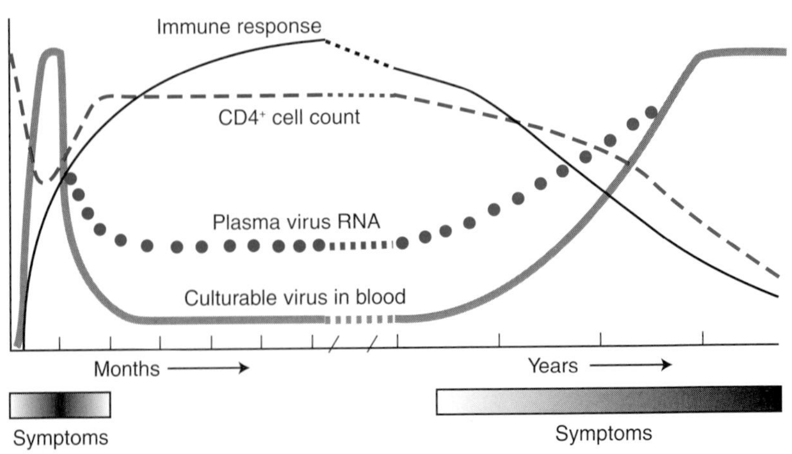

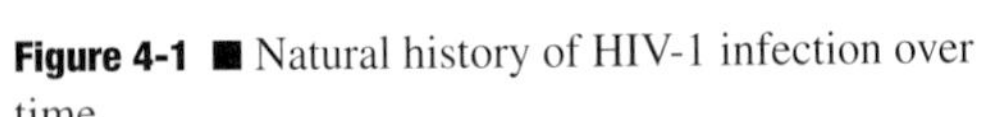
Figure 4-1 ■ Natural history of HIV-1 infection over time.

Modified from Saag MA, Holodniy M, Kuritzkes DR, et al. HIV viral load markers in clinical practice. Nature Med 2:625, 1996. Copyright 1996 Macmillan Magazines Limited.

was apparent that viral replication was not only continuous but also quite rapid.[45] However, it was not until the dramatic responses to HIV protease and non-nucleoside reverse transcriptase (RT) inhibitors were observed that the magnitude of the rate of viral replication *in vivo* was fully appreciated.

In separate reports, Wei et al and Ho et al quantitated the rapid turnover of HIV *in vivo*, demonstrating the production and clearance of up to 10 billion virions each day (~400 million virions per hour).[6,7] The half-life of virions in the circulation is estimated to be 1–2 h or less. When new rounds of viral replication are blocked by ART, the amount of measurable virus drops by more than 99% within 2–7 days of initiating therapy. The estimated life cycle (or generation time) of HIV, which represents the time from release of a virion until it infects another cell resulting in the release of new progeny, is estimated to be 1–2 days (Fig. 4-2).[8,46,47] These data were generated by observing the rapid decay in viral load over the first few weeks of potent therapy and represent the contribution of the acutely infected cells in the host, which have a half-life of 1–2 days. These cells represent more than 99% of the daily virus production. The remaining production of virus comes from a longer-lived population of cells that contribute to the slower, 'second phase' decay of plasma viremia (Fig. 4-3).[47,48] Therefore within 8–12 weeks after initiation of potent therapy, plasma HIV RNA levels generally fall below 400 copies/mL of plasma. It usually takes several weeks longer to reach undetectable levels when utilizing ultrasensitive virologic techniques (limit of detection ~5–50 copies/mL). Most viral replication takes place in lymphoid organs, where most of the CD4+ T lymphocytes reside.[28,49–54] The detection of virus in plasma, as measured for example by the plasma 'viral load', represents spillover of virus from the site of production (lymphatic tissue) into the bloodstream where it can be readily detected. In addition to the gradual reduction in absolute CD4+ T lymphocytes over time, loss of lymphoid architecture within lymph nodes also occurs

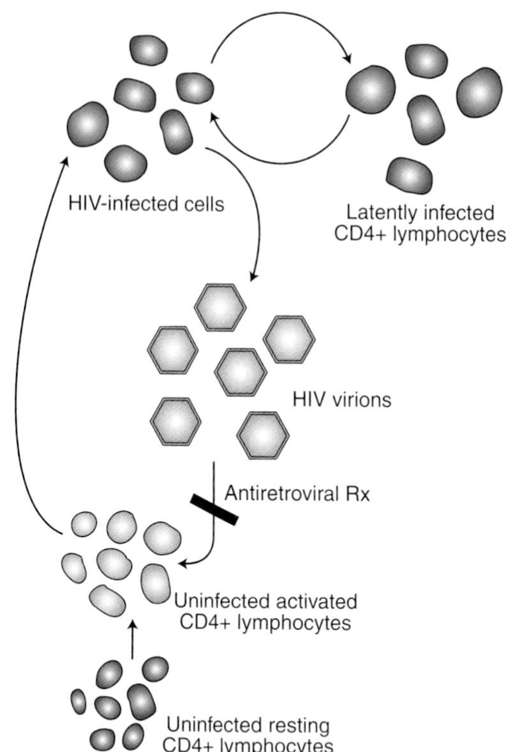

Figure 4-2 ■ HIV-1 replication is rapid *in vivo*. Plasma HIV-1 viremia, depicted here as HIV-1 virions results from spillover of recently produced virus from infected cells in lymphatic tissue. Uninfected, activated CD4+ T lymphocytes are the predominant target of HIV-1 infection. Once infected, these cells produce virus within 1–2 days and continue producing virus for an estimated 1–3 days. More than 99% of the virus detected in the bloodstream comes from recently infected CD4+ T lymphocytes. The remaining less than 1% of virus comes from chronically infected CD4+ T lymphocytes or macrophages, which have life spans ranging from a few days to several years.

Redrawn with modification from Perelson et al. HIV-1 dynamics in vivo: virion clearance rate, infected cell life-span, and viral generation time. Science 271:1582, 1996. Copyright 1996 American Association for the Advancement of Science.

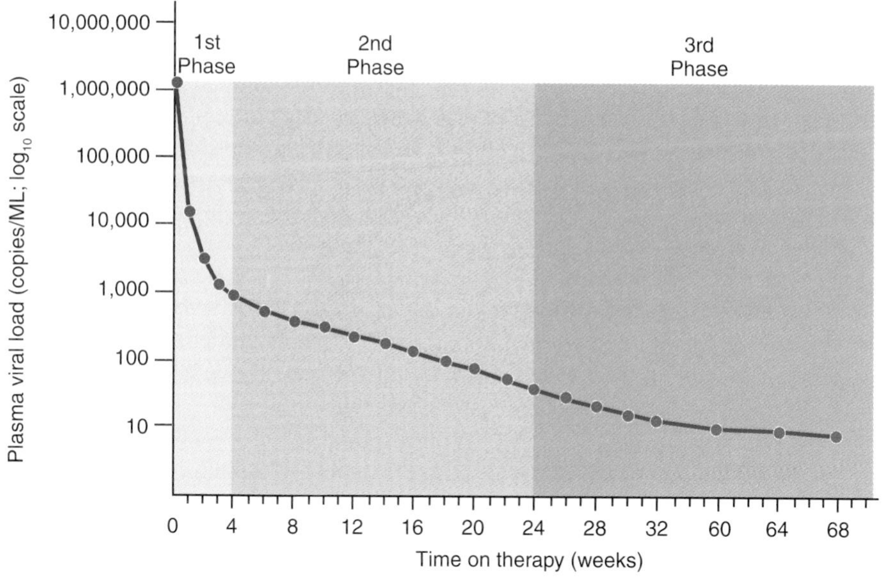

Figure 4-3 ■ Typical plasma HIV RNA response to potent ART. After initiation of treatment, a sharp decrease in viral load is observed over the first 2–4 weeks of therapy. Thereafter a steady, less steep decline in plasma viral load is observed. These differential rates of decline have been arbitrarily divided into 'phases' for purposes of mathematic modeling. In reality, they represent a continuum of viral decay as the life span of productively infected cells is exhausted. If all further new infection is completely blocked for a sufficient period of time (new estimates: many years) to allow all existing infected cells to die, a cure is theoretically possible.

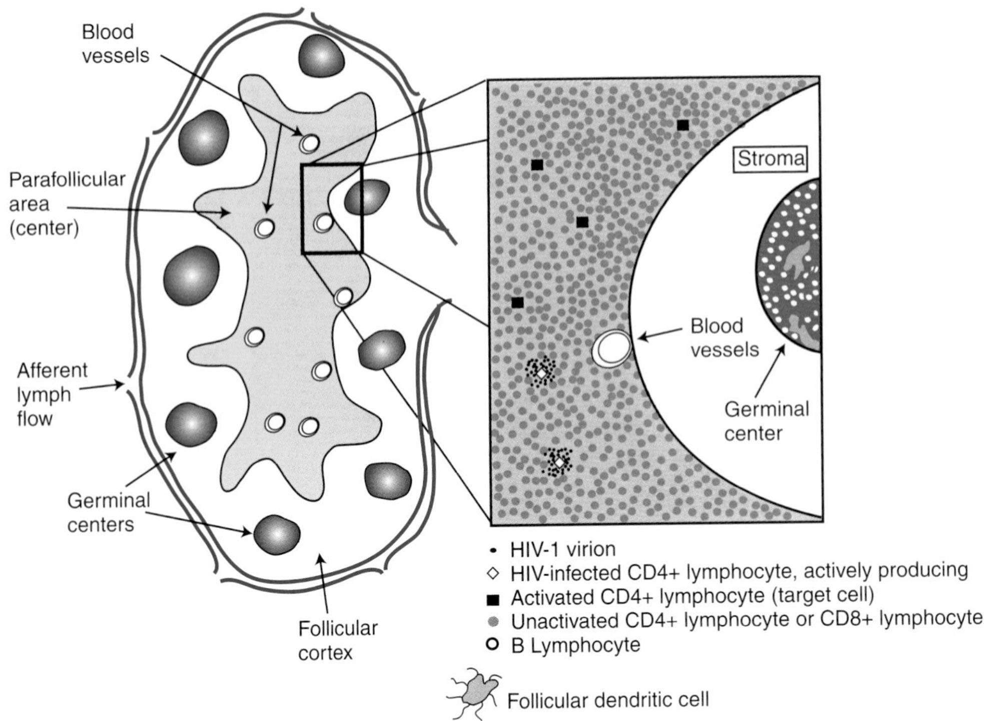

Figure 4-4 ■ Lymph node from a patient with established HIV infection. The actively producing cells (diamonds) excrete high levels of HIV virions (black dots), with an average instantaneous burst size of 4000 copies per cell. These newly produced virions are trapped by follicular dendritic cells (large cells in germinal center), are absorbed onto circulating resting CD4+ T lymphocytes (black closed circles) or activated CD4+ T lymphocytes (black squares) passing by, or spill into the circulation. The actual number of target (activated) cells infected by virus produced by any actively producing cell is small: about one new cell infected over the life span of each actively producing cell at steady state.

and is believed to contribute to the relative lack of immune system efficiency at later stages of the disease.[49,50] Although most newly formed virions do not result in infection of a neighboring cell, on average several million new CD4+ T lymphocytes are infected each day.[7,46] This high-level, continuous production of virus and subsequent infection of new CD4+ T lymphocytes helps explain how the CD4+ cells decline and immune system destruction occur during the time of clinical latency.

Activated CD4+ T lymphocytes are the principal targets of HIV replication. The estimated life span of an infected CD4+ T lymphocyte is 1–2 days.[55] Each infected cell has an instantaneous burst size of ~4000 copies per cell.[28] The calculated burst size per cell is remarkably constant and is independent of stage of disease, plasma viral load, and ARV treatment status.[28] Thus the plasma viral load is a direct reflection of the number of infected cells in the body producing virus at any moment in time.

Whereas the instantaneous burst size, defined as the number of measurable virions produced by an infected cell at any given moment, is ~4000 copies per cell, the effective burst size, defined as the number of viruses produced that result in productive infection of a neighboring cell, at steady state is ~1 virion per cell (Fig. 4-4). At steady state, each patient establishes an equilibrium between the production and destruction of virus producing cells such that as each productive cell is destroyed or stops producing virus it is replaced by another newly infected, productive cell. Clinically, this equilibrium establishes a relatively stable viral load value over time, defined as the viral 'set point'.[8,56] Mellors and colleagues have demonstrated a direct relation between the viral load, or set point, and the rate of CD4+ T-lymphocyte count decline.[57] When viewed in the context of the direct relation between plasma viral load and the number of productively infected cells at any moment in time, these findings are not surprising. Yet, when this concept is applied to individual patients the ability of the plasma viral load to predict the rate of CD4+ T-lymphocyte decline for a specific patient is quite poor, indicating that other factors, as yet unmeasured, are playing a role in causing the loss of T cells in HIV-infected patients.[58]

Much attention has focused on how actively producing cells are eliminated.[59,60] The leading possibilities are the direct cytopathic effect of the virus (or deleterious effects of virions budding from the cell membrane), virus-induced cell apoptosis, or direct destruction via an effective immune system response. Initial experience with tissue culture growth of the virus supported the concept of a direct cytopathic effect.[61] Under the stimulation of phytohemaglutinin and interleukin-2 (IL-2), most virus-infected cells died within several days of becoming infected in tissue culture, often through the development of large syncytia. Syncytia have never been demonstrated *in vivo*, and so the concept of death of cells via this mechanism remains uncertain. Apoptosis, or programmed cell death, is a natural mechanism for eliminating lymphocytes of the immune system. Viral proteins, or cytokines released in response to viral infection, may trigger the apoptotic pathway in actively producing cells, although the degree to which this occurs is not known. What is clear, however, is the tremendous loss of CD+ T lymphocytes in the gut during the first several days to weeks after initial infection.[62–64] Studies in both animals (infected with SIV) and humans with acute HIV infection demonstrate profound loss of immune cells and disruption of normal architecture of the gut in the first several days after infection. These data suggest strong consideration of aggressive use of ART during the period of acute infection.

A large body of evidence supports the role of HIV-specific immune system responses to eliminate virus-producing cells.[65–69] The early and rapid development of the HIV quasi-species is a direct consequence of HIV-specific immunity, both cellular and humoral. Neutralizing antibody studies have demonstrated a very dynamic virologic escape phenomena within the first several weeks of HIV infection, with persistent generation of novel viral variants in response to antibody responses over the life of infection.[70,71] Enhanced HIV-specific immunologic responses were postulated to be responsible for the lower virologic set points observed among seroconverters who were treated within days to a couple of weeks after the onset of symptoms of their initial HIV infection and had therapy periodically withdrawn.[72] High levels of anti-HIV-specific CD4+ T-lymphocyte activity were demonstrated in association with control of replication. This level of CD4+ T-lymphocyte help is typical in 'long-term nonprogressor' patients, who naturally control viral infection and do not suffer CD4+ T lymphopenia despite chronic HIV infection. In contrast, when therapeutic withdrawal of treatment was performed in patients with chronic, well-established HIV infection who were not treated within 12–20 weeks of acute infection, viral load values typically rebound back to high levels.[73,74] These patients have extremely low or absent HIV-specific CD4+ T-helper lymphocyte responses. Longer-term follow-up of the treated acute seroconversion patients revealed a return to higher viral load set points indicating some loss of the initial immunologic priming from therapy. Of more concern, one patient in the initial intermittent therapy study became superinfected with virus from another patient following sexual exposure while off therapy. This story has created a challenge and some controversy for those working on development of a preventative HIV vaccine.

Taken together, HIV pathogenesis is best depicted as a vicious cycle of production of large numbers of HIV virions that infect activated CD4+ target cells, which in turn produce more viruses that infect additional cells (Fig. 4-5).[9] The function of the targeted CD4+ T lymphocytes, ironically, is to create an HIV-specific, coordinated response against the virus that is attacking them. Current thinking supports the concept that cytotoxic CD8+ T lymphocytes, under the support of an HIV-specific CD4+ T-lymphocyte response, are responsible, at least in part, for eliminating the active virus-producing HIV-infected cells.[68–72,75–78] The HIV-specific CD4+ T-helper lymphocyte responses appear to be lost early (within the first few weeks after infection), perhaps never to return. The continuous infection of other activated CD4+ cells is believed to lead to impairment of the immune responses to other antigens/pathogens, thereby creating potential deficits in the immune system's response to opportunistic processes. The goal of effective ART therefore is to block, as completely as possible, the ability of the virus to infect uninfected CD4+ T lymphocytes, thereby inhibiting *de novo* production of virus and, at the same time, preserving immune system competence.[61]

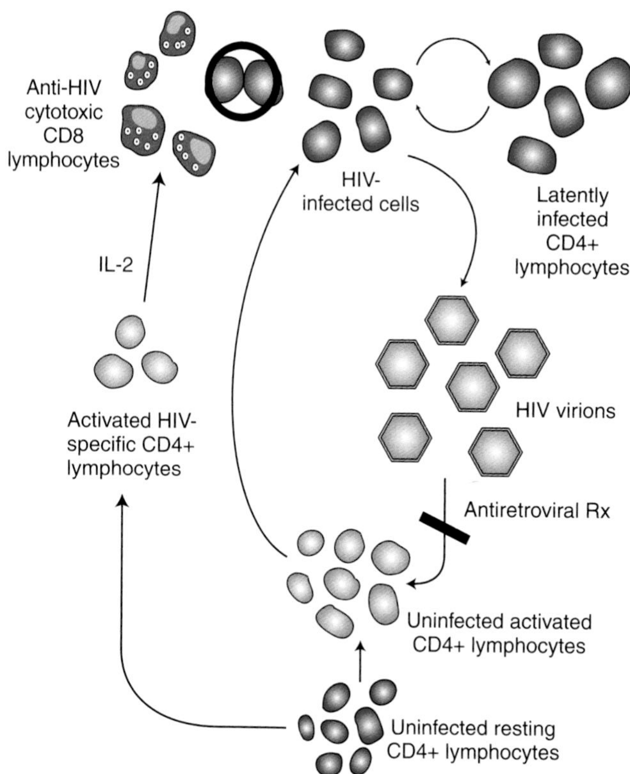

Figure 4-5 ■ More complete picture of HIV pathogenesis. Actively producing CD4+ lymphocytes are killed, at least in part, by HIV-specific CD8+ cytotoxic lymphocytes. These cytotoxic cells are stimulated by cytokines (e.g., IL-2) produced by HIV-specific CD4+ lymphocytes. In the presence of functioning CD4+ T lymphocytes, the inherent anti-HIV immune response is capable of controlling viral replication in an efficient manner. Unfortunately, early during the course of infection (soon after the time of seroconversion), most of the HIV-specific CD4+ activity is lost, and the immune response is much less efficient. Early treatment, prior to the time of seroconversion, helps preserve the HIV-specific immune response, potentially abrogating the need for ART.

STRATEGIC USE OF ART

Simply stated, the goal of ART is to inhibit completely viral replication *in vivo* and sustain the effect for as long as possible.

Theoretically, if complete suppression is sustained for a long enough time to allow the population of chronically infected cells to decay to extinction, eradication of HIV (or a true cure) is possible. Whether a cure is truly achievable is critical to establishing the foundation of an ARV therapeutic strategy. If cure is indeed possible, all patients should be treated with the most potent agents early and aggressively during the course of their infection, much like the treatment of acute lymphocytic leukemia. If a cure with ART alone is not a realistic possibility, other strategic approaches must be considered, more like the treatment of chronic lymphocytic leukemia.

Whether eradication is possible depends in large part on the life span of longer-lived, chronically infected cells and whether complete (or relatively complete) suppression of viral replication is achievable. About 99% of the plasma viremia is generated by actively producing CD4+ T lymphocytes with a relatively short half-life (1–2 days), the remaining 1% or less of plasma viremia is produced by longer-lived cells that previously were predicted to have an estimated average half-life of 14–28 days, although some of the cells could have a life span as short as 2–4 days or as long as more than 400 days (Fig. 4-2).[46,48,79] If the life span of these long-lived cells is 28 days or less and all *de novo* infection is completely blocked, eradication may be achieved as early as 3–5 years after initiation of therapy[46,47]; however, if the life span of the longer-lived chronically infected cells is substantially longer (on the order of 400 days) or if latently infected cells (that contain proviral DNA) are able to circulate, multiply or expand, and express virus at a later time, the time required for complete eradication of HIV could be on the order of decades and may not be achievable, even with complete block of *de novo* rounds of replication sustained over a prolonged period of time.[50,67] Data generated during the latter portion of the 1990s demonstrated that the half-life of the chronically infected population of cells was not 14–28 days as originally assumed but, rather, 6 months at the shortest or over 44 months at the longest.[29,60,80–82] Thus the time to eradication under the assumption of complete arrest of all *de novo* infection now ranges from 12 to well over 60 years of continuous, maximally effective ART.

As indicated above, the concept of eradicating HIV from an infected individual requires chronically infected cells to have a relatively short half-life but also requires complete block of all new rounds of de novo infection and this block must be sustained for a long enough time to allow all chronically infected, productive cells within the body to be destroyed or die off. To achieve eradication, inhibitory levels of ART must be maintained above inhibitory concentrations within all body compartments and within all susceptible target cells, ideally on a continuous basis. Thus a ‘cure’ for HIV infection assumes complete penetration of ARV drugs into the cells in all compartments of the body where the virus is replicating and strict adherence to the regimen for a period long enough to allow the infected cells to die off. An important issue in the discussion of a potential ‘cure’ relates to the relation of ‘undetectable’ levels of plasma virus to complete suppression of viral replication. ‘Undetectable’ levels of HIV in plasma are a function of a laboratory assay; complete suppression is a biologic phenomenon. All too often patients and clinicians assume that achieving an undetectable level of virus is synonymous with complete suppression. Even when plasma viral load values are less than a theoretical 1 $\log_{10}$ copy/mL, an estimated 75 000–150 000 cells are still producing virus in lymphoid tissue (Fig. 4-6).[28] Zhang et al reported evidence of genetic drift in the envelope region in virus isolated from a patient who was treated at the time of seroconversion and sustained levels of less than 50 copies/mL for more than 20 months, supporting the notion of ongoing low-level replication when plasma viral load values are undetectable.[29] Therefore low-level viral replication appears to be ongoing even in the face of potent, yet incomplete viral suppression.[59] This implies that breakthrough viremia may ultimately occur in any given patient with sustained plasma HIV RNA levels below 50 copies/mL, although the likelihood of such breakthrough is a function of the probability of emergent resistant virus in the face of strong selective drug pressure (as discussed in the following section). Inevitably, more sensitive virologic assays will become commercially available and help narrow the gap between ‘undetectable’ and ‘complete suppression’. At the present time, however, it does not appear that currently available ARV agents, even when used in combination, are potent enough to achieve and maintain truly complete suppression. Thus a gap continues to exist between the ideal goal of ART (defined as complete suppression of *de novo* infection) and the achievable goal of ART (defined as

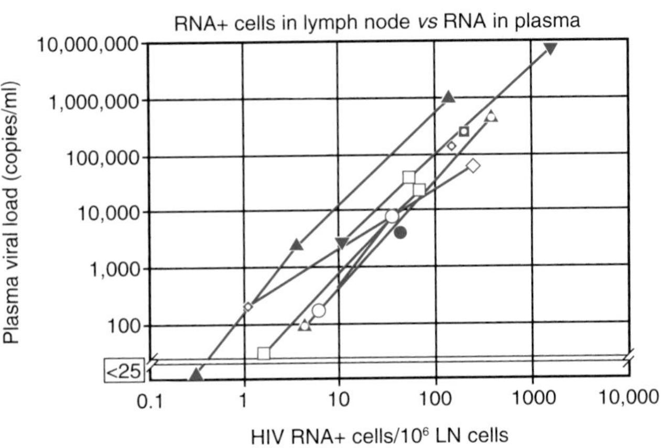

Figure 4-6 ■ A log–log plot of the relation between plasma viral load (copies per milliliter) and the number of cells actively producing virus in lymphatic tissue. Each point represents a separate biopsy time point paired with the plasma viral load obtained at the time of biopsy. The lines connecting points with the same symbol represent values obtained from the same patient before and after initiation of potent ART. The slope of this line is 1.6, and the Pearson correlation coefficient (R) is 0.95, indicating a strong relation between the number of cells producing virus in the body and the plasma viral load.

Modified from Hockett RD, Kilby JM, Derdeyn CA, et al. Constant mean viral copy number per infected cell in tissues regardless of high, low, or undetectable plasma HIV RNA. J Exp Med 189:1545, 1999.

achieving undetectable levels of virus by available viral load techniques). With earlier, less potent regimens, many patients were unable to achieve undetectable levels of virus.[83–85] In such circumstances, the ability to achieve undetectable levels of virus was more difficult among patients with higher baseline viral load levels and heavier treatment experience.[86–92] However, with more potent and tolerable regimens available today, over 80–85% of patients are able to achieve <50 c/mL with their initial regimens and increasingly the <50 c/mL target can be achieved even among very heavily treatment experienced patients.[93–95]

Taken together, evidence of chronically infected cells living for extended periods of time combined with evidence of ongoing, low-level replication in the face of 'undetectable' levels of plasma viremia indicates that eradication of HIV is not likely to occur with potent ART alone. Although eradication of HIV remains the ultimate goal of therapy, a more realistic goal at the present time would be to sustain suppression as completely as possible for as long as possible utilizing existing therapy over time.

Initiation of Therapy

The ultimate success of ART is total eradication, or cure, as discussed above. In the case of healthcare workers who have been exposed to infected blood through percutaneous needlestick exposure, the use of ART appears to help abort early infection and, in this regard, is the best example of eradication occurring as a result of ART.[96,97] Similarly, prevention of perinatal infection through the use of prepartum and peripartum treatment of the mother and postpartum treatment of the neonate is another example where early infection is either prevented or aborted after exposure through the use of ART.[98] Other than these two situations, success with ART in total eradication or cure has not been achieved. Rather, antiretroviral 'success' is defined more as the absence of ARV failure rather than as success *per se*. Therefore, prevention of ARV failure becomes the principal goal of ART.

With the development of a large number of more potent ARV agents, there has been a paradigm shift in the approach to therapy: the focus of therapy has changed from keeping patients alive from this year to the next to keeping patients alive from this decade to the next. The goals of chronic administration of ART can be seen as twofold: to prevent clinical progression and to prevent or delay development of resistance. Over the last decade the guidelines for treatment of HIV infection have vacillated, owing in large part to the emerging realization that a cure was not readily achievable with ART alone.[99] The 'treat early, treat hard' approach to therapy was initially linked with the idea that complete, maintained viral suppression could result in the eradication of HIV from the body within a short time.[61] In addition, confusion regarding the goals of therapy at different stages of disease contributes to the apparent 'change' in guidelines. To prevent the emergence of viral resistance, relatively complete viral suppression is required. Therefore, in all newly treated patients the principal goal of treatment should be to achieve virologic suppression to undetectable levels.[1,100] While clinical benefit can still be realized with less than maximal suppression of viral load,[83,89,101,102] use of more modern drugs has led to the emergence of a new treatment paradigm whereby the target of ARV therapy ideally should be <50 c/mL even in heavily experienced patients.[1,4] Yet, for those patients who cannot achieve this degree of virologic suppression, a reduction in HIV RNA levels of 0.5 $\log_{10}$ copies/mL below baseline is associated with relative maintenance of the CD4+ T-lymphocyte count over time, provided this degree of viral suppression is sustained.[83,89,102] Therefore for patients who have experienced multiple regimens and cannot achieve <50 c/mL, the goal of therapy changes from prevention of further resistance mutations to prevention of clinical progression. In this setting, a reasonable target is to achieve and sustain viral load values at least 0.5 $\log_{10}$ copies/mL, and preferably 1.0 $\log^{10}$ copies/mL below baseline.

The 'treat early, treat hard' approach to therapy was grounded in concepts other than eradication.[61,99] Most clinical trials confirm that the first treatment represents the 'best shot' at achieving profound suppression of viral replication. Based on current knowledge of HIV pathogenesis, early and profound suppression also prevents the development of resistance by limiting replication, preserving immune system integrity (before there is loss of critical clones of responsive cells), and creating a higher virologic hurdle for emergence of viral resistance.[103–105] Although this rationale is clearly sound, the approach rests on assumptions concerning adherence, toxicity, pharmacokinetics/pharmacodynamics, and the absence of meaningful immune system recovery. First, complete adherence to complex ARV regimens is difficult for most patients to maintain.[34,106,107] Multiple studies demonstrate a striking relation between adherence and success of ARV therapeutic regimens. Second, although serious toxicity is relatively uncommon with initial treatment for early disease, prolonged exposure to treatment is associated with a number of metabolic and hepatic complications.[20,21,108–114] Third, drug pharmacokinetics and pharmacodynamics are subject to variability that can reduce the effectiveness of treatment.[31,115] Not all patients are able to achieve and sustain similar levels of intracellular concentrations of drug or are able to metabolize drugs in a predictable fashion.[32,116,117] Fourth, although treatment that is initiated late in the course of disease (e.g., at CD4+ T-lymphocyte counts of less than 100 cells/μL) is associated with a worse outcome, treatment started at moderate CD4+ T-lymphocyte counts (e.g., 350 cells/μL) can be accompanied by preservation of immune competence that does not seem to be clinically distinguishable from that seen when starting therapy at earlier stages (e.g., CD4+ T-lymphocyte count of 600 cells/μL).[87,118,119]

There are additional considerations that argue against universal application of very early treatment.[120] Much of the data on progression of HIV disease from the Multicenter AIDS Cohort Study (MACS), which has been used to support earlier intervention, is derived from untreated individuals (Fig. 4-7A).[56] The use of data from untreated cohorts, although providing information on the natural history of

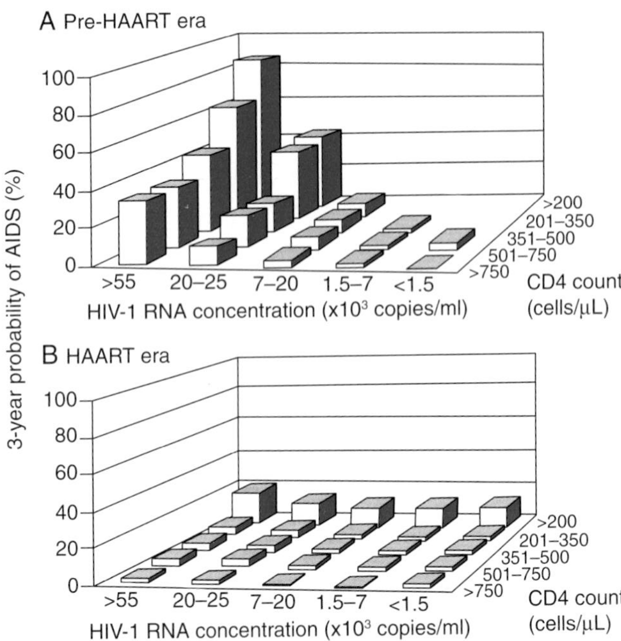

Figure 4-7 ■ Likelihood of progression to AIDS or death in the pretreatment (A) and treatment (B) era.

Used from Egger M, May M, Chene G, et al. Prognosis of HIV-1 infected drug naive patients starting potent antiretroviral therapy: a collaborative analysis of prospective studies. Lancet 360:119–29, 2002, as presented in US Department of Health and Human Services Panel on Clinical Practices for Treatment of HIV Infection. Guidelines for the Use of Antiretroviral Agents in HIV-1 Infected Adults and Adolescents. Washington, DC, DHHS. Available: http://aidsinfo.nih.gov/Guidelines/GuidelinesDetail.aspx?MenuItem=Guidelines&Search=Off&GuidelineID=7&ClassID=1 10 Oct 2006.

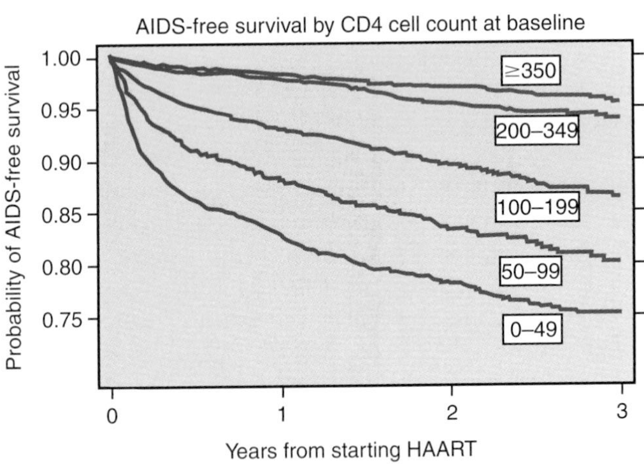

Figure 4-8 ■ Progression of HIV disease to AIDS or death by initial CD4 count.

Used from Egger M, May M, Chene G, et al. Prognosis of HIV-1 infected drug naive patients starting potent antiretroviral therapy: a collaborative analysis of prospective studies. Lancet 360:119–29, 2002.

disease prior to the influence of ART, is anachronistic during the treatment era. Because the impact of treatment on the viral load determinants of progression is immediate, its predictive value is negated once potent treatment is initiated. Moreover, most clinicians do not idly observe progression of disease in their patients without introducing some intervention prior to the onset of profound CD4+ T-lymphocyte depletion or the development of clinical disease. More recent data sets derived from clinical cohorts of treated individuals are more valuable for the 'treatment era' (Figs 4-7B and 4-8).[119] Data from the ART-Cohort Collaborative, a compilation of treatment experience of over 23 000 patients from over 50 clinical sites, demonstrate little short-term disease progression among patients who initiated therapy with more moderate CD4+ T-lymphocyte counts (e.g., 350–500 cells/μL), even if their viral load values at the time of treatment initiation are high (e.g., >100 000 copies/mL).[87,118]

Based on such considerations, along with the increased frequency of long-term adverse events of treatment, a more conservative approach than 'treat early, treat hard' is advocated currently, although as therapies become better tolerated the recommendations continue to be in flux (Table 4-2).[1,4] Among asymptomatic patients, treatment may be initiated relatively early (e.g., at CD4+ T-lymphocyte counts of 350–500 cells/μL; while guidelines suggest consideration of treatment at these CD4+ T-lymphocyte counts, some experts now recommend treatment at this level) rather than very early (e.g., CD4 counts >500 cells/μL) using ARV combinations that are likely to reduce the viral load below 50 copies/mL.[1,4,5] In contrast, all symptomatic patients should have treatment initiated regardless of CD4+ count and viral load. Similarly, all HIV-infected pregnant women should have treatment initiated by the beginning of the second trimester, regardless of viral load or CD4+ count, to eliminate the transmission of HIV to her baby. Once the mother has delivered, therapy can be stopped among those women who had initial CD4+ counts above 350–500 cells/μL and who are not breast-feeding (Table 4-2).[1,4]

Selection of the specific regimen is based on the predicted likelihood of patient tolerance and adherence, with consideration of short- and long-term toxicities. The dramatically improved outcomes of more modern initial regimens, whereby over 85% of patients achieve target values of <50 c/mL at 1 year of treatment, is due in large part to improved tolerability. Simply put, adherence is most directly related to drug tolerance. Medications and regimens that create even low-grade symptoms, such as intermittent nausea, mild headache, or occasional crampy diarrhea, ultimately lead to skipped doses. These skipped doses result in resolution of the offending symptoms, thus reinforcing the nonadherent behavior. Over time, skipped doses become more common, ultimately leading to the emergence of drug-resistant virus and regimen failure.

Drugs cannot work if they are not taken. Creating a regimen that is relatively easy for the patient to take therefore is essential when designing initial treatment (Fig. 4-9A). Moreover, frequently missed doses not only decrease the ability of the drugs to work, it is a recipe for the development of ARV resistance. A study comparing outcomes among prisoners versus patients who participated in clinical trials using the

Table 4-2 Recommendations for Initiating ART in Treatment-Naive Adults[a] with Chronic HIV Infection

Parameter	Recommendation: IAS-USA[1]	Recommendation: HHS[4]
Symptomatic HIV Disease	ART is recommended	ART is recommended
Asymptomatic HIV Disease		
CD4+ ≤200 cells/μL	ART is recommended	ART is recommended
CD4+ <350 cells/μL but >200 cells/μL	ART should be considered[b] and the decision is individualized (see text); monitoring and counseling for HIV transmission prevention should continue if therapy is deferred	Treatment should be offered following discussion of pros and cons of therapy
CD4+ >350 cells/μL but ≤500 cells/μL	ART is generally not recommended[c]; monitoring and counseling for HIV transmission prevention should continue	VL > 100 000 c/mL, most clinicians recommend deferring ART, but some would treat; VL < 100 000 c/mL, defer therapy
CD4+ >500 cells/μL	ART is generally not recommended; monitoring and counseling for HIV transmission prevention should continue	VL > 100 000 c/mL, most clinicians recommend deferring ART, but some would treat; VL < 100 000 c/mL, defer therapy

[a]Nonpregnant adults.
[b]The closer the CD4+ cell count is to 200/μL, the stronger the recommendation, particularly if the plasma viral load is high (>100 000 copies/mL) or if the CD4+ count is declining rapidly (>100 cells μL^{-1} $year^{-1}$).
[c]Consider treatment for patients with high plasma viral load or with rapid decline of CD4+ cell count.

Adapted from IAS-USA Guidelines 2006[1]

identical regimens from the clinical trials, demonstrated that the prisoners, who had drugs administered under conditions of directly observed therapy, had substantially better virologic outcomes (90% vs 75% achieved viral load values of less than 400 copies/mL).[121] These data underscore the importance of drug-taking behavior, commitment to the regimen, simplicity of regimens, and overall adherence to the success of the initial regimen.

Other considerations in the selection of the initial regimen include the availability of the treatments and, indirectly, their costs. In the past, selection of the initial regimen was made with a focus on keeping subsequent treatment options open in the case of failure of the first regimen, which was believed to be inevitable for most patients. However, with more modern regimens that have reduced pill burdens (some requiring only one pill once a day) and markedly improved tolerability, the concept of 'planning for failure' has been replaced with a strategy of 'planning for success', wherein regimens are tailored and adjusted for each patient on an individual basis. Once a regimen is initiated, frequent questioning regarding tolerance, for even mild or intermittent symptoms related to the regimen, should occur at each clinic visit and the regimen should be modified to eliminate the offending ARV agent. Most importantly, to ensure the best chance for success, patients should understand the rationale for treatment prior to treatment initiation and genuinely be 'ready to start' therapy.

The potency of the initial regimen is critical to long-term success. Regimens for initial treatment should be of sufficient potency to ensure a high likelihood of achieving viral load levels below the limit of detection (<50 c/μL). Preexisting drug resistant virus, which has been reported with increased

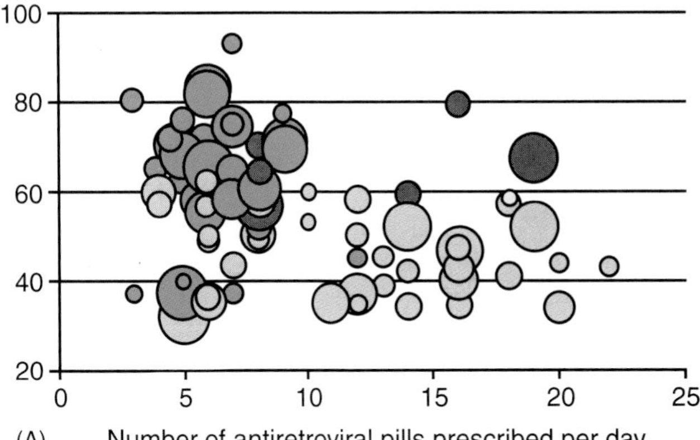

Figure 4-9 ■ Proportion of patients achieving virologic success based on number of pills required per day in the regimen (Pill Burden). These data were derived from a meta-analysis of 53 trials that enrolled 14 264 patients into 90 treatment arms. Each regimen evaluated contained two nucleosides plus either a boosted-BPI (grey), an NNRTI (dark blue), a third nucleoside (blue), or a nonboosted PI (very light blue). Overall 55% of patients had plasma HIV RNA levels <50 copies/mL at week 48. Pill count correlated with the percentage of patients with plasma HIV RNA levels <50 copies/mL at week 48 **(A)**. In this figure, the size of the circles represents the standard error associated with the point estimate. Significantly greater numbers of patients receiving NNRTI (64%) and boosted-PI (BPI; 64%) had RNA <50 copies/mL at 48 weeks compared to those receiving triple nucleoside (54%) or nonboosted PI (43%) regimens. However, when the individual trials are listed, more NNRTI-based treatment regimens are associated with success **(B)**.

Adapted from Bartlett JA, Fath MJ, Demasi R, et al. An updated systematic overview of triple combination therapy in antiretroviral-naive HIV-infected adults. AIDS 20:2051–64, 2006.

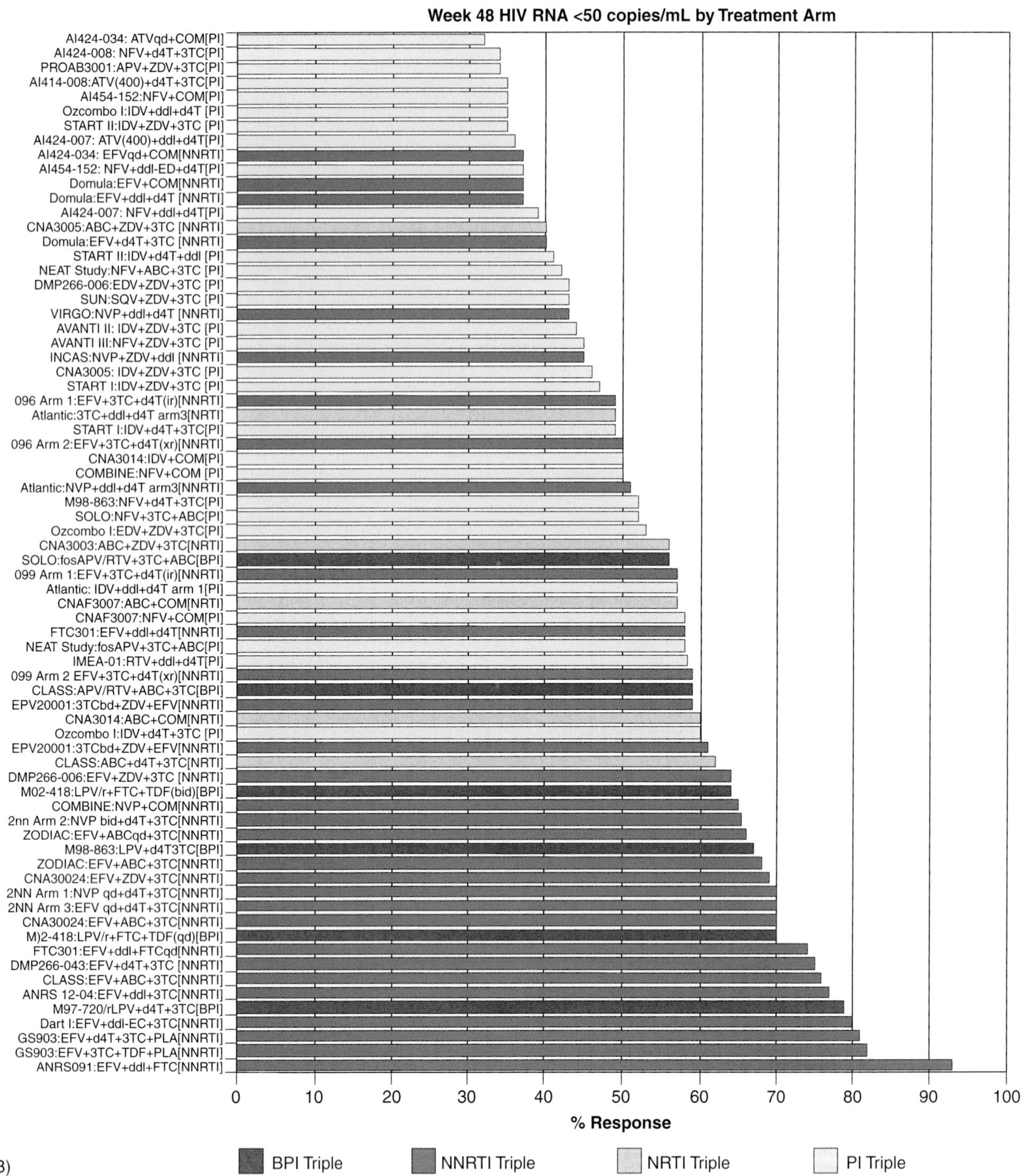

Figure 4-9 ■ Continued

frequency (between <3% and 14%), significantly hampers the potency of the initial regimen. Current guidelines suggest obtaining a pre-ARV treatment genotypic resistance test for any patient living in an area where a high prevalence (>5%) of resistant virus is known to exist, for patients presenting with acute seroconversion syndrome, and for pregnant women in selected cases.

Once a decision has been made to initiate therapy the proper choice of regimen is essential. Meta-analyses have shown that efavirenz plus two nucleoside reverse transcriptase inhibitors (NRTIs) demonstrates ARV effectiveness activity comparable, if not superior, to that of ritonavir boosted protease inhibitor (PI)-containing regimens (Fig. 4-9B).[30,122,127] However, ritonavir-boosted regimens are more likely to be associated with hypertriglyceridemia and possibly insulin resistance and lipodystrophy, reinforcing the trend for use of PI-sparing regimens as initial therapy. Unboosted PI-containing regimens are universally inferior to boosted-PI

Initial Treatment (HHS Guidelines^{+})

Table 4-3

Preferred Option	
NNRTI Option	**NRTI Options**
• Efavirenz*	Tenofovir + emtricitabine**
OR	*OR*
PI Options • Atazanavir + ritonavir • Fosamprenavir + ritonavir (BID) • Lopinavir/ritonavir (BID)	Zidovudine + lamivudine**
Alternative Options	
NNRTI Option	**NRTI Options**
• Nevirapine#	Abacavir + lamivudine
OR	*OR*
PI Options • Atazanavir## • Fosamprenavir • Fosamprenavir + ritonavir (1x/day) • Lopinavir/ritonavir (1x/day)	Didanosine + (emtricitabine or lamivudine)

$^{+}$ As of October 2006; reference 4.
* Avoid in pregnant women and women with significant pregnancy potential.
** Emtricitabine can be used in place of lamivudine and vice versa.
# Nevirapine should not be initiated in women with CD4 counts >250 cells/mm^3 or men with CD4 counts >400 cells/mm^3.
Atazanavir must be boosted with ritonavir if used in combination with tenofovir.

and most non-nucleoside reverse transcriptase inhibitor (NNRTI) containing regimens and should be used only in selected clinical situations, such as in some active intravenous drug users, in those with significant hepatic compromise, or in patients requiring therapy for concomitant diseases where the drugs interact with ritonavir or NNRTI agents. In head-to-head studies, efavirenz has generally been more effective (by intent to treat) than nevirapine, although the outcomes were at the margin of statistical significance. Nevirapine should not be used in patients with higher CD4+ T-lymphocyte counts (>250 cells/μL for women; >350 cells/μL for men) owing to a higher risk of hepatic toxicity.[27] Efavirenz should generally be avoided in pregnant women, especially in the first trimester when the neural tube maturation is occurring. The preferred and alternative regimens according to the HHS guidelines are shown in Table 4-3.

Notwithstanding all of the considerations listed above, the most important issue related to the long-term success of ART is the degree to which the patient desires to start therapy.[128] Patients' 'buy in' is based in large part on their understanding of the rationale of treatment (i.e., why should they start) and the degree to which they believe they have a role to play when selecting of the regimen. The 'best' choice of therapy must encompass not just potency, appropriate pharmacokinetics, minimal toxicity, and relative ease of administration, it must include strong consideration of how the regimen fits into the patients' day-to-day activities and their beliefs regarding the likelihood that the regimen will work. Taken together, the timing of therapy initiation is a complex decision process that requires an understanding of HIV biology, pathogenesis, natural history, pharmacology, toxicology, psychology, and behavior. In this regard, therapy is genuinely 'tailored' for each patient, making guidelines for the initiation of therapy entirely relative rather than absolute.

Management of ARV Failure

ART 'failure' is a relative term that can be defined in terms of both clinical and virologic parameters. Clinical failure is the easiest to define: progression of clinical symptomatology or the development of a new opportunistic infection or death in the face of ART. From a virologic standpoint, ARV failure simply means the loss of control of viral replication; however, this loss of control is often incremental and in most cases is only partially lost. When viral load testing was first used in clinical practice, virologic failure was originally defined as a return toward (within 0.3–0.5 $\log^{10}$ copies/mL) the original baseline viral load.[10] Soon thereafter the definition was more stringently defined as a confirmed return to detectable levels of virus (>200–500 c/mL) or the inability to achieve undetectable HIV RNA after 16–20 weeks of therapy.[129] This definition of failure was deemed most appropriate for a patient's first regimen, with the goal of therapy being driven predominantly by the desire to avoid the development of resistance. For patients who have experienced multiple regimen failures, the new target of therapy is the same as the first regimen. However, not all patients can achieve this level of suppression. Since the development of clinical progression (clinical failure) is infrequent provided the viral load level is maintained below 0.5 $\log^{10}$ copies/mL (threefold) of the original viral load set point,[89,101] the definition of virologic 'failure' becomes dependent on the clinical setting and must be individualized for each patient, taking into account the history of ART, baseline viral load, response to therapy, and availability of options for treatment once 'failure' has occurred. Once the definitions of success and failure have been delineated, the choice of subsequent regimens depends on the prior exposure to ARV agents, previous adverse experiences, potential drug–drug interactions, underlying disease, CD4+ T-lymphocyte count/viral load status, and the perspective of the patient regarding the ability to adhere to a complex drug regimen. Fortunately, with the newer generation of drugs, the ability to achieve <50 c/mL even in experienced patients is easier than in the past.[93–95]

The reasons for ART failure are multifactorial. The four primary reasons for failure include toxicity/intolerance, development of resistance, pharmacodynamics, and nonadherence. Each of these factors is discussed individually below.

Toxicity/Intolerance

Each pharmaceutical agent is associated with a unique set of toxicities. The degree to which a given toxicity is tolerated by the patient depends on a number of factors, including the nature and severity of the toxicity, the degree to which the toxicity interferes with day-to-day living, and the willingness of the patient to live with the toxicity. Generally, a patient who is totally asymptomatic is less willing to tolerate an adverse experience from a medication than a patient who has more advanced, symptomatic disease or has previously experienced disease progression. In addition, the degree to which a patient believes the regimen will provide benefit is proportional to the patient's willingness to tolerate an adverse experience.

With the use of combination therapy, the individual adverse experience profile for a given agent is compounded by drug–drug interactions, altered pharmacokinetic profiles, and synergistic toxicities of the drugs. Some adverse experiences develop soon after initiation of therapy, and the symptoms may wane after several weeks (tachyphylaxis). Depending on the nature of the toxicity, its severity, the tendency of the toxicity to develop tachyphylaxis, and the willingness of the patient to tolerate the toxicity, the decision to discontinue a specific agent (or not) must be individualized. In general, intolerance reported on a patients first regimen is of special concern owing to the association with nonadherence. Dose reduction or withholding a single agent for even a short period of time generally is not an option based on concern of inducing resistant virus to the agent while using a suboptimal dose or exposing the virus to a partially suppressive regimen with inadequate potency from the remaining agents in the regimen.

Development of Resistance

Resistance is a function of two principal conditions: (1) innate susceptibility of the virus (typically expressed in terms of 50% (IC^{50}) or 90% (IC^{90}) inhibitory concentration from an *in vitro* assay); and (2) the achievable level of drug in susceptible target cells, where viral replication takes place. In the case of antibacterial therapy, the difference between the *in vitro* susceptibility and the tissue concentration of drug is often as much as 100–1000-fold; however, in the case of antiviral therapy, the therapeutic window is generally much smaller. The maximum tolerated dose of most ARV agents limits tissue levels of drug to single-digit multiples of the IC_{90} (e.g., three- to sevenfold) at trough levels. Therefore any genetic mutation that reduces the susceptibility of the virus to even a modest degree may have significant clinical implications.

To manage resistance clinically, the biology of how resistance develops should be understood. HIV exists *in vivo* as a quasi-species.[130] After initial infection with a predominant genotype, viral replication ensues at an extraordinary rate, resulting in the production of progenitor viruses that are highly related yet genetically distinct. The major reason for the generation of such enormous diversity is a combination of immune system pressure and the relative infidelity of the RT enzyme. RT is a relatively error-prone enzyme, creating a transcriptional error every 3000–4000 basepairs (bp) transcribed.[131,132] Because HIV is a 9000-bp virus, on average one to two transcriptional errors occur with each replication cycle. With the generation of up to 10 billion virions per day, a wide variety of genetic mutants are theoretically produced on a daily basis. Most of these transcriptional errors are believed to lead to stop codons and defective virions, although critical point mutations that confer resistance to antiviral therapy may be generated. Under the conditions of selective pressure of either the immune system or drug therapy, these mutated viruses become the predominant genotype. Although most of these errors are neutral or lead to stop codons, several mutations may lead to the development of new virions with altered fitness or selective advantage.[133] When the mutation results in reduced fitness, the mutant virus grows less well and becomes a minor component of the quasi-species. However, when the mutant virus is more fit and has a selective growth advantage, it may dominate the quasi-species rapidly (within days).[6] Therefore a major difference between antibacterial susceptibility testing and ARV testing becomes immediately obvious: antibacterial tests are performed against a single clone of bacteria isolated from an infected source, whereas ARV tests are performed on a swarm of viruses that coexist in different frequencies and change in rapid fashion upon challenge with a new selective pressure (e.g., initiation of a new ARV regimen).

The likelihood of the development of resistance mutations *in vivo* is a function of two factors: the relative potency of the ARV regimen and the degree of ongoing replication occurring while the regimen is being administered. A regimen that has relatively poor potency creates little selective pressure on the virus to mutate; in such cases, resistance mutations are unlikely to develop (Fig. 4-10). In contrast, a highly active regimen generates substantial selected pressure for the virus to mutate. The likelihood of resistance development then becomes a function of the degree of replication allowed to occur while the regimen is being administered: the more replication allowed to occur under strong selective pressure, the faster resistance develops. Theoretically, if a regimen is completely suppressive, no resistance develops because no replication is taking place and resistance mutations do not have the chance to develop.

Virally encoded RT and protease enzymes, the two primary targets of most ARTs, are highly plastic molecules. Some of the mutations induced by one agent may lead to reduced susceptibility of the virus to other agents (cross-resistance), especially to agents with the same mechanism of action (e.g., NNRTIs and PIs). Conversely, some mutations that confer high-level resistance to one agent may increase the susceptibility of the virus to another, resulting in a so-called 'hypersusceptable' virus to the other agent.[15] Additionally, many resistance-conferring mutations cause substantially less

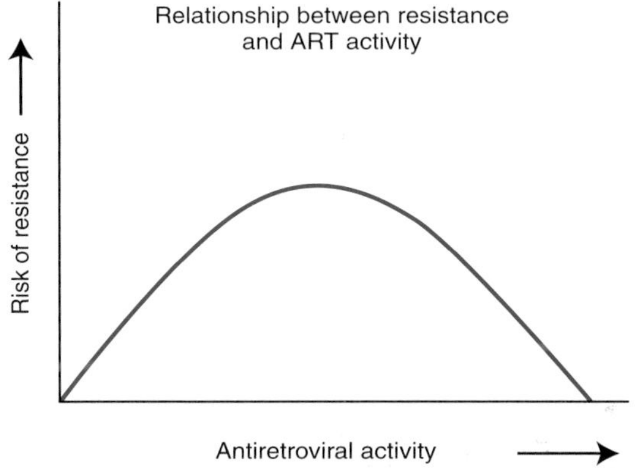

Figure 4-10 ■ Likelihood of developing resistance is directly related to the relative activity of ART. In the absence of meaningful activity (far left-hand side) there is no selective pressure exerted that can lead to resistance. Similarly, in the absence of viral replication (complete suppression of virus; far right-hand side), no resistance can develop because there is no ongoing replication. However, when regimens are only partially suppressive (middle portion of figure), there is ongoing replication in the presence of ample selective pressure, creating a higher likelihood of resistance.

Modified from presentations by Doug Richman and Emilio Emini.

efficient replication capacity than wild-type virus, resulting in a virus that is less 'fit' than wild-type virus.[133]

Common mutations selected by NRTIs, NNRTIs and PIs are shown in Figure 4-11.[134] Although there is general concordance between laboratory-selected mutations induced by serial passage of the virus in the presence of drug and those mutations observed in clinical isolates, some mutations selected *in vitro* have not been identified from clinical specimens among patients receiving drug.[15] In either case, mutations can be viewed as primary or secondary. Primary mutations are defined as those that have a demonstrable effect on the degree of resistance to the given agent. Secondary mutations often have no discernible effect on the susceptibility of the virus to the drug but are likely selected on the basis of their ability to improve the fitness of the virus, usually as a compensatory mutation that allows more effective viral replication or enzyme function (*see* Chapter 28).

Variable degrees of resistance are conferred by single point mutations, depending on the specific agent and the ease of resistance development. For example, a single point mutation at amino acid position 181 of the RT enzyme (e.g., Y181C) can lead to profound reduction in susceptibility to most NNRTIs, whereas single amino acid changes in RT (e.g., M41L or T215Y) may lead to only partial reduction in susceptibility to zidovudine.[135,136] Upon development of subsequent mutations, the degree of resistance increases incrementally, ultimately resulting in high-level resistance when four or five resistance-conferring mutations are present.[137,138] A similar pattern of sequential mutation acquisition within the protease gene product region is required for the development of high-level PI resistance.[139,140] To complicate matters, although the sequential acquisition of mutations may be common among agents within a particular class, the precise mutation responsible for conferring resistance is generally agent-specific with varying degrees of cross-reactivity (depending on the drugs and the mutation in question). As an example, a single point mutation at amino acid position 30 (D30N) of the protease gene product leads to a several-fold reduction in susceptibility of the virus to nelfinavir but not other PIs.[141,142] Subsequent acquisition of other mutations, at amino acid positions 82 or 84 of the protease gene product leads to high-level resistance to nelfinavir and other PIs as well. To complicate matters further, some point mutations create secondary changes in the functional gene product, leading to improved fitness or some degree of reversal of resistance.[133] In the case of lamivudine and entricitabine, an M184V mutation results in substantial reduction of the susceptibility of these drugs while partially reversing zidovudine resistance or delaying the emergence of zidovudine resistance when the two agents are used together in a regimen.[143] Taken together, drug-induced mutations occur under the influence of multiple factors, often resulting in variable phenotypic expression and clinical consequences.

In addition to *de novo* development of resistance, some viral variants with resistance-conferring mutations may preexist as subpopulations within infected T lymphocytes and macrophages.[91,144] Under the conditions of strong selective

A

MUTATIONS IN THE REVERSE TRANSCRIPTASE GENE ASSOCIATED WITH RESISTANCE TO REVERSE TRANSCRIPTASE INHIBITORS

Nucleoside and Nucleotide Reverse Transcriptase Inhibitors (nRTIs)

Multi-nRTI Resistance: 69 Insertion Complex (affects all nRTIs currently approved by the US FDA)

M	A	▼	K	L	T	K
41	**62**	**69**	**70**	**210**	**215**	**219**
L	V	Insert	R	W	Y F	Q E

Multi-nRTI Resistance: 151 Complex (affects all nRTIs currently approved by the US FDA except tenofovir)

A	V	F	F	Q
62	**75**	**77**	**116**	**151**
V	I	L	Y	M

Multi-nRTI Resistance: Thymidine Analogue-associated Mutations (TAMs; affects all nRTIs currently approved by the US FDA)

M	D	K	L	T	K
41	**67**	**70**	**210**	**215**	**219**
L	N	R	W	Y F	Q E

Abacavir	K	L	Y	M
	65	**74**	**115**	**184**
	R	V	F	V

Didanosine	K	L
	65	**74**
	R	V

Emtricitabine	K	M
	65	**184**
	R	V I

Lamivudine	K	M
	65	**184**
	R	V I

Stavudine	M	D	K	L	T	K
	41	**67**	**70**	**210**	**215**	**219**
	L	N	R	W	Y F	Q E

Tenofovir	K	K
	65	**70**
	R	E

Zidovudine	M	D	K	L	T	K
	41	**67**	**70**	**210**	**215**	**219**
	L	N	R	W	Y F	Q E

B

Nonnucleoside Reverse Transcriptase Inhibitors (NNRTIs)

Efavirenz	L	K	V	V	Y	Y	G	P
	100	**103**	**106**	**108**	**181**	**188**	**190**	**225**
	I	N	M	I	C I	L	S A	H

Etravirine (expanded access)	V	A	L	K	V	V	Y	G
	90	**98**	**100**	**101**	**106**	**179**	**181**	**190**
	I	G	I	E P	I	D F	C I V	S A

Nevirapine	L	K	V	V	Y	Y	G
	100	**103**	**106**	**108**	**181**	**188**	**190**
	I	N	A M	I	C I	C L H	A

Figure 4-11 ■ Common point mutations conferred by use of PIs **(A)**, nucleoside RT inhibitors **(B)**, and non-nucleoside RT inhibitors **(C)**, mutations associated with decreased susceptibility to PIs. For each amino acid residue listed, the letter above the listing represents the wild-type virus, and the letter below the listing represents the mutation. Amino acids: A, alanine; C, cysteine; D, aspartate; E, glutamate; F, phenylalanine; G, glycine; H, histidine; I, isoleucine; K, lysine; L, leucine; M, methionine; N, asparagine; P, proline; Q, glutamine; R, arginine; S, serine; T, theronine; V, valine; W, tryptophan; Y, tyrosine. For full details of footnotes refer to chapter.

Reprinted from the International AIDS Society-USA. Johnson VA, Brun-Vezinet F, Clotet B, et al. Update of the drug resistance mutations in HIV-1: fall 2006. Top HIV Med 14:125–30, 2006. Updated information and thorough explanatory notes is available at http://www.iasusa.org.

C **MUTATIONS IN THE PROTEASE GENE ASSOCIATED WITH RESISTANCE TO PROTEASE INHIBITORS**

Atazanavir +/− ritonavir

Amino acid, wild-type	Position	Substitutions
L	10	I F V C
G	16	E
K	20	R M I T V
L	24	I
V	32	I
L	33	I F V
E	34	Q
M	36	I L V
M	46	I L
G	48	V
I	**50**	L
F	53	L Y
I	54	L V M T A
D	60	E
I	62	V
I	64	L M V
A	71	V I T L
G	73	C S T A
V	82	A T F I
I	**84**	V
I	85	V
N	**88**	S
L	90	M
I	93	L M

Fosamprenavir/ritonavir

Amino acid, wild-type	Position	Substitutions
L	10	F I R V
V	32	I
M	46	I L
I	47	V
I	**50**	V
I	54	L V M
G	73	S
L	76	V
V	82	A F S T
I	**84**	V
L	90	M

Darunavir/ritonavir

Amino acid, wild-type	Position	Substitutions
V	11	I
V	32	I
L	33	F
I	47	V
I	**50**	V
I	**54**	M L
G	73	S
L	**76**	V
I	**84**	V
L	89	V

Indinavir/ritonavir

Amino acid, wild-type	Position	Substitutions
L	10	I R V
K	20	M R
L	24	I
V	32	I
M	36	I
M	**46**	I L
I	54	V
A	71	V T
G	73	S A
L	76	V
V	77	I
V	**82**	A F T
I	**84**	V
L	90	M

Lopinavir/ritonavir

Amino acid, wild-type	Position	Substitutions
L	10	F I R V
K	20	M R
L	24	I
V	**32**	I
L	33	F
M	46	I L
I	**47**	V A
I	50	V
F	53	L
I	54	V L A M T S
L	63	P
A	71	V T
G	73	S
L	76	V
V	**82**	A F T S
I	84	V
L	90	M

Nelfinavir

Amino acid, wild-type	Position	Substitutions
L	10	F I
D	**30**	N
M	36	I
M	46	I L
A	71	V T
V	77	I
V	82	A F T S
I	84	V
N	88	D S
L	**90**	M

Saquinavir/ritonavir

Amino acid, wild-type	Position	Substitutions
L	10	I R V
L	24	I
G	**48**	V
I	54	V L
I	62	V
A	71	V T
G	73	S
V	77	I
V	82	A F T S
I	84	V
L	**90**	M

Tipranavir/ritonavir

Amino acid, wild-type	Position	Substitutions
L	10	V
I	13	V
K	20	M R
L	**33**	F
E	35	G
M	36	I
K	43	T
M	46	L
I	47	V
I	54	A M V
Q	58	E
H	69	K
T	74	P
V	**82**	L T
N	83	D
I	**84**	V
L	90	M

MUTATIONS IN THE ENVELOPE GENE ASSOCIATED WITH RESISTANCE TO ENTRY INHIBITORS

Enfuvirtide

Amino acid, wild-type	Position	Substitutions
G	36	D S
I	37	V
V	38	A M E
Q	39	R
Q	40	H
N	42	T
N	43	D

Maraviroc

MUTATIONS IN THE INTEGRASE GENE ASSOCIATED WITH RESISTANCE TO INTEGRASE INHIBITORS

Raltegravir (expanded access)

Amino acid, wild-type	Position	Substitutions
Q	**148**	H K R
N	**155**	H

Amino acid abbreviations: A, alanine; C, cysteine; D, aspartate; E, glutamate; F, phenylalanine; G, glycine; H, histidine; I, isoleucine; K, lysine; L, leucine; M, methionine; N, asparagine; P, proline; Q, glutamine; R, arginine; S, serine; T, threonine; V, valine; W, tryptophan; Y, tyrosine.

D

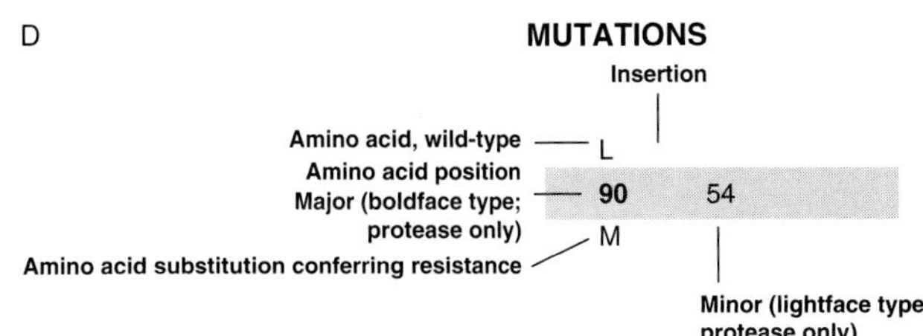

Figure 4-11 ■ Continued

pressure, these preexistent mutants may rapidly become the predominant species expressed *in vivo*. The best example of this phenomenon is the development of rapid resistance observed when NNRTIs are administered as monotherapy.[6,144] Resistant viral variants have been observed as early as 5 days after the initiation of NNRTI monotherapy, with complete conversion of the predominant genotype in plasma from wild-type to resistant within 14–28 days after initiation of therapy.[6] Monotherapy with NRTIs (e.g., lamivudine) typically emerges within 2–4 weeks of therapy and for PIs (e.g., indinavir) within 4–12 weeks of treatment initiation.[6,145]

The concept of preexistent viral mutants plays a critical role in the sequencing of ARV regimens and the ability of a new regimen to succeed after a previous regimen has failed. At the time a regimen fails because of the development of resistance, resistant genotypes predominate in the plasma. As the regimen is changed, if these virions are susceptible to the new regimen, a shift in the population generally occurs, with suppression of the previous resistant viruses (ideally to undetectable levels).[6,144] If the new regimen is not completely suppressive, some degree of replication continues, potentially utilizing the preexisting resistant mutants as substrates for the ongoing production of virus. This may lead to the creation of individual virions with multiple resistance mutations. This scenario is most likely to occur in the context of so-called sequential monotherapy, whereby a single agent is added to an existing failing regimen. A common example of sequential monotherapy is the addition of indinavir to a failing regimen of zidovudine/lamivudine. In this case, resistance mutations to zidovudine and lamivudine already exist at the time indinavir is added. If the new regimen is only partially suppressive, mutations that confer resistance to indinavir begin to appear sequentially on the background of zidovudine and lamivudine resistance mutations, potentially leading to multidrug-resistant virions.[139]

The development of resistance is often an incremental process, perhaps best thought of as a function of chance; that is, the likelihood of resistance development is directly related to the degree of ongoing replication and the chance that a resistance mutant may be precisely the virus that infects a susceptible, activated CD4+ lymphocyte passing by at that moment in time. Even with regimens that are highly potent, yet not completely suppressive, a single point mutation may occur that confers partial reduction in susceptibility.[139,146] This results in a slightly higher degree of viral replication, thereby increasing the likelihood of the development of a second resistance-conferring mutation, leading to even further reduction in susceptibility and increased replication in the face of drug selective pressure. Therefore mutations occurring after the first mutation often appear more rapidly because of the higher degree of replication that occurs after development of the first mutation. The resultant end-product is a highly resistant mutant that has multiple coexisting resistance mutations. From a clinical perspective, the more rapid acquisition of subsequent mutations suggests that regimens should be changed early in the course of virologic failure to avoid the development of higher-level resistance, assuming that viable therapeutic options exist for the patient in question.

Pharmacologic Aspects

For ARV drugs to have activity *in vivo*, the drugs must be absorbed and delivered to the site where viral replication is occurring (e.g., CD4+ T lymphocytes) and be appropriately processed by the target cell into an active moiety (e.g., the triphosphate derivative of nucleosides). The relative amount of drug in plasma may or may not reflect the amount of drug at the active, intracellular site of replication; therefore measuring plasma levels may only partially describe the relative activity of an agent. Just like toxicity profiles and resistance patterns, each drug has its own unique characteristics of absorption, metabolism, tissue penetration (including penetration into various body compartments, such as the central nervous system), intracellular processing, intracellular half-life, and mechanism of elimination (including the first-pass effect; *see* Chapter 79). Not only is the pharmacologic profile unique for each agent, but the absorption and metabolic processing may vary from patient to patient. This interpatient variability, due to weight, volume of distribution, hepatic metabolism, renal function, or genetic polymorphisms influencing drug absorption and clearance, becomes critical when interpreting data from studies that involve large populations of patients receiving combination ARV regimens. Even when patients within a given population adhere completely to the regimen, a fixed-dose regimen of a drug given every 8 h may lead to adequate concentrations at the target site for most individuals but be too low to sustain complete suppression in some or too high in others, resulting in early drug failure or excess toxicity, respectively.[147] Because most ARV agents have narrow therapeutic windows, these issues become critical when trying to implement a strategy of complete suppression of viral replication for all patients. Thus many current studies focus on measuring drug levels as part of a strategy to achieve improved virologic outcome with less toxicity. To date, not enough data have been generated to recommend this approach in clinical practice.

Adherence

To achieve and maintain complete suppression of viral replication as a goal of therapy, patients must take all of the agents comprising a combination regimen at the prescribed time and under the proper conditions. Because of drug–drug interactions and the interference of food with the absorption of some agents, many patients must adhere to complicated regimens that require careful planning of meals, sometimes in conjunction with taking multiple tablets at different times during the day. Even the most dedicated and committed patients find it difficult to remember to take each pill as prescribed every day over several months to years. Based on experience with other chronic diseases, such as hypertension, up to one-third of patients are able to adhere to their regimen 90% of the time, but most patients adhere poorly or intermittently.[148–150] For diseases in which the consequences of nonadherence result in some degree of morbidity, such as the use of insulin in brittle diabetics, the adherence is much better but still not 100%. In most instances, HIV infection is more like hypertension than diabetes; that is, most individuals with HIV infection are relatively asymptomatic and even those with symptoms usually do not experience the consequences of missed doses of their medicines. Because the objective of therapy is to maintain complete suppression and to achieve this objective drug levels must remain above the IC_{90} at the target site throughout the entire viral life cycle, intermittent dosing that allows some degree of replication to occur in the face of high selective pressure becomes a recipe for the development of resistance and ultimate ARV failure.

Several factors may contribute to poor or intermittent adherence. The most common factor is poor instructions given to the patient regarding the regimen and its possible adverse experiences.[150] The development of side effects and their severity have a significant impact on a patient's willingness to take medications as prescribed or to continue a given regimen. The degree to which a patient is willing to tolerate adverse effects of medications is related to several factors, including the nature of the side effect, how much it interferes with the patient's ability to carry on daily activities, the severity of the patient's underlying condition (the more serious the disease, the higher the rate of adherence), and the patient's belief that the regimen is likely to be effective.[151] Even mild or intermittent symptoms, such as low-grade nausea or headache, can lead to skipped doses that result in reinforcement of skipped dose behavior, especially among patients asymptomatic to their HIV infection. Regimens given once or twice daily have a higher degree of adherence, and therefore effectiveness, than three or four time a day regimens or those that require strict timing of drug administration in relation to meals (Fig. 4-9A). Other factors, such as level of education, socioeconomic status, and underlying substance abuse, generally do not predict adherence behavior.[34]

STRATEGIES FOR CHANGING THERAPY

Failure of ART can generally be divided into two categories: failure resulting from toxicity and that resulting from virologic escape. The strategies for managing toxicity and virologic escape are quite different and are discussed separately.

Strategies for Changing Therapy because of Toxicity

Toxicity may be due to a single agent in a regimen or to multiple agents. Adverse events may manifest either through the inherent toxicity of the offending agent(s), through additive toxicity between two or more agents, or through adverse drug–drug interactions. Even though most of the approved agents have been in widespread use for only a few years, the most common adverse experiences are well established and fairly distinctive for each drug. In cases where a side effect occurs that is commonly associated with a particular drug in the regimen, it is relatively easy to ascribe the toxicity to the most likely offending agent and adjust the regimen accordingly. However, in other cases, overlapping toxicities or uncommon side effects occur that are difficult to ascribe to a particular drug. In such cases it is best to stop the entire regimen, wait for the adverse effect to abate or decrease in severity, and reinstate therapy with a new regimen that substitutes one or more new drugs for the most likely offending agent(s).

When adjusting regimens because of toxic effects, several guidelines should be followed. When toxicities are noted within 2–4 weeks after initiating a new regimen, the most likely offending agent can be removed and a new drug without overlapping toxicity added to the remaining drugs in the regimen. For example, the development of rash from nevirapine usually occurs 14–28 days after initiating the regimen, in which case another agent of similar potency can be substituted into the regimen without changing the nucleoside backbone. Similarly, early manifestations of distal symmetric peripheral neuropathy (DSPN) in patients who are taking didanosine or stavudine or anemia among patients taking zidovudine should prompt the substitution of another NRTI for the offending agent. When toxicity to an agent develops weeks to months after the regimen had been initiated and the virologic response has achieved and maintained undetectable levels of virus, substitution of a new drug for the most likely offending agent is still an appropriate approach. In this case it is assumed that the existing regimen has suppressed viral replication sufficiently to prevent the development of resistance-conferring mutations to the drugs remaining in the regimen as the regimen is changed. Perhaps the best example of this is the development of metabolic or lipid abnormalities among patients taking a PI-containing regimen who replace the PI with an NNRTI agent while maintaining the nucleoside backbone (Table 4-4). Multiple small studies have been reported demonstrating successful maintenance of virologic control with improvement in lipid profiles but variable success in correcting insulin resistance or body composition abnormalities. Conversely, when side effects are noted weeks to months after starting a regimen that has not successfully achieved an optimal virologic response, it is best to change at least two, and possibly all, of the agents in the regimen (including the drug most likely responsible for the adverse effect) based on resistance testing results because of concerns regarding rapid development of resistance to a new drug when it is added as 'sequential monotherapy'.

Strategies for Changing Therapy because of Virologic Failure

Virologic failure may result from an inability to achieve the desired level of viral suppression initially or from the return of plasma HIV RNA to unacceptable levels after having achieved and sustained the targeted degree of viral suppression for months or years previously. In either case, the existence of the undesirable plasma HIV RNA value should be confirmed with repeat testing before any change in therapy

Table 4-4

Effects of Switching from Initial Regimens to Alternative Regimens

Study	No.	Follow-Up (week)	TGs	Chol	Glu/IR	Body Change	Comments
2NRTI + PI to 2NRTI + efavirenz[154]	33	40	NC	NC	NC	NC	Subset analysis of a cohort of 624 patients evaluated for body fat, lipid, and glucose abnormalities
2NRTI + PI to 2NRTI + efavirenz[155]	39	24	<↓	NC	NC	NC	Virologic control maintained. Modest increase in HDL-cholesterol
2NRTI + PI to 2NRTI + efavirenz[156]	43	24	<↓	NC	–	NC	Viral load remained <50 copies/mL in all patients. HDL-cholesterol unchanged
2NRTI + PI to 2NRTI + efavirenz[157]	25	24	<↑	NC	–	NC	Randomized to NVP, EFV, or control. Only one patient had rebound VL in NEV group vs 2 EFV vs 1 PI
2NRTI + PI to 2NRTI + efavirenz[158]	25	24	<↓	<↓	↑	<pVAT	All patients remained at <500 copies/mL 2NRTI + efavirenz[143]
2NRTI + PI to 2NRTI + efavirenz[159]	165	24	–	NC	–	–	Improvement in HDL-cholesterol in EFV group
2NRTI + PI to 2NRTI (+ABC) + efavirenz[160]	27	36	<↑	<↑	<↑	NC	Some overall fat loss by BIA (2.5 kg), but no change in symptoms of fat redistribution. Virologic failure in one patient
2NRTI + PI to 2NRTI[161]	56	24	↑	↓HDL	–	NC	No virologic failure. Some increase in lipoatrophy (five patients)
2NRTI + PI to 2NRTI + efavirenz[162]	45	48	↑	<↑	–	–	Virologic failure in two patients
2NRTI + PI to 2NRTI + efavirenz[163]	20	24	NC	NC	NC	NC	No virologic failures. Subjective improvement in morphologic appearance but no change in anthropometric studies
2NRTI + PI to 2NRTI + efavirenz[164]	93	52	↑	NC	↑	↑WHR ↑VAT	Switch (46) vs controls (47) Moderate increase in HDL with EFV; no difference in VL outcome. SQ fat loss no different
2NRTI + PI to 2NRTI + efavirenz[165]	41	52	–	–	NC	–	Patients with lipodystrophy syndrome; only IR and Glu tolerance evaluated
2NRTI + PI to 2NRTI + EFV or NVP[166]	100	52	↑	↑	–	NC	VL suppression maintained in 80%. No difference between EFV and NVP groups

2NRTI + PI to 2NRTI + nevirapine[167]	23	24	↑	↑	↑	↑WHR	Diet not reported
2NRTI + PI to 2NRTI + nevirapine[168]	138	24	<↑	<↑	–	<↑	Rebound in HIV RNA occurred more often in PI group than NVP group (29% vs 11%; $P < 0.5$)
2NRTI + PI to 2NRTI + nevirapine[169]	60	36	↑	↑	NC	NC	Randomized study. Virologic failure: 4 NVP, 3 PI
2NRTI + PI to 2NRTI + NVP + adefovir + OH-urea[170]	80	24	↑	↑	NC	↑VAT	Randomized (2:3) study. No effect on HDL-cholesterol. Virologic failure: 3 (6%) exp, 6 (19%) PI. Intolerance in 15 exp patients
2NRTI + PI to 2NRTI + NVP or 2NRTI + EFV[171]	116	12	<↑	NC	↑	NC	Offered switch to NNRTI due to intolerance of PI; 67% <200 copies/mL at switch. No change in viral load
2NRTI + PI to 2NRTI + nevirapine[172]	40	48	↑	NC	↑	NC	Severe rash in six patients; therapy changed to EFV. One patient with virologic failure
2NRTI + PI to 2NRTI + nevirapine[157]	26	24	↑	↑	–	NC	Randomized to NVP, EFV, or control. Only one patient had rebound VL in NVP group vs 2 EFV and 1 control
2NRTI + PI to 2NRTI + nevirapine[173]	63	60	↑	NC	–	NC	Nonrandomized; 10 patients received EFZ, 63 NVP. Infrequent virologic failure. CD4+ T-lymphocyte count increase of 82 cells/mL
2NRTI + PI to 2NRTI + nevirapine[174]	68	24	<↑	NC	—	—	Virologic failure in four cases.
d4T : ZDV or ABC[175]	59	36	↑	NC	NC	↑SAT VAT NC	Modest CD4+ T-lymphocyte increase Some patients ($n = 18$) on dual NRTI; remainder ($n = 41$) on PI/NRTI. Lactate declined significantly
2NRTI + PI to 2NRTI + ABC[176]	211	24	<↑	↑	↑	–	Randomized to continue PI or not. Failures: ABC (9; 3 virologic); PI (14; 2 virologic)
2NRTI + PI to 2NRTI + ABC[177]	163	52	↑	↑	–	–	Randomized to continue PI or not. Virologic failures: ABC (11), PI (5)
2NRTI + PI to 2NRTI + ABC[178]	105	45	<↑	<↑	–	–	Randomized to continue PI (106) or not (105). Virologic failures: ABC (4) vs PI (2)

ABC, abacavir; BIA, bioelectrical impedence analysis; Chol, cholesterol; d4T, stavudine; EFV, efavirenz; exp, experimental; Glu/IR, glucose/insulin resistance; HDL, high density lipoprotein; NC, no change; NNRTI, non-nucleoside reverse transcriptase inhibitor; NR, not reported; NRTI, nucleoside reverse transcriptase inhibitor; NVP, nevirapine; PI, protease inhibitor; VL, viral load; SAT, subcutaneous adipose tissue; 3TC, lamivudine; TGs, triglycerides; VAT, visceral adipose tissue; WHR, waist hip ratio; ZDV, zidovudine; – not done; ↓ or ↑, significant increase or decrease; <↓ or <↑, nonsignificant trend of increase or decrease.

Comparison of Genotypic and Phenotypic Resistance Assays

Table 4-5

Issues	Genotypic Assays	Phenotypic Assays
Availability	Generally available	Restricted availability
Time to results	Days	Weeks
Technical issues	Straightforward	Demanding
Susceptibility measurement	Indirect	Direct
Sensitivity (minor species)	Poor	Poor
Interpretation	Complex	Straightforward
Cost	Moderately expensive	Expensive
Major limitations	May not correlate with phenotype	Cutoff values poorly defined

is initiated. This point has been emphasized with results from many studies, where solitary increases in viral load ('blips') up to 1000 c/mL were noted among several patients who had otherwise maintained undetectable levels of virus.[152,153] The blips were followed by a second value <50 c/mL and were not associated with an increased risk of long-term virologic failure or with an increased risk of developing resistance. Even patients who experience multiple isolated blips during the course of the therapy experience no apparent long-term adverse consequences.

Once an elevated plasma HIV RNA level has been confirmed, resistance testing can help identify which drugs, if any, may be contributing to the rebounding viral load (Table 4-5) (*see* Chapter 28).[15] The absence of resistance mutations in the face of rising viral load implies problems with adherence or potential pharmacologic difficulties, such as poor absorption, increased metabolism (possibly due to a drug–drug interaction), decreased intracellular processing, or increased extrusion of drug from the intracellular compartment (e.g., as occurs with induction of P-glycopeptide pumps). Additionally, it is vital to confirm that the patient was still on the failing regimen at the time the sample for resistance testing was obtained, otherwise the viral quasispecies may have reverted back to wild-type falsely indicating that resistance mutations were not the cause of the virologic failure. When only one of the drugs in the regimen has induced detectable resistance mutations, changing only the single drug is acceptable; however, some consideration should be given to changing some of the other drugs in the regimen owing to the theoretical presence of low-level resistance to the other agents in the form of subpopulations. The activity of the next regimen should be at least as potent as the original regimen and ideally of more potency. In the absence of resistance testing, failure should be associated with the entire regimen rather than attempting to ascribe the failure to a particular drug in the regimen. In general, intensification with the addition of a single agent added to a failing regimen should be avoided except in circumstances where a substantial reduction in viral load has been achieved but not to undetectable levels within 16–20 weeks of initiating therapy. Even when these conditions are met, great care should be used to ensure that the persistent detectable viral load is not due to problems with adherence, which would be aggravated with the addition of yet another pill to take. The addition of single new drugs, 'sequential monotherapy', is less likely to achieve either the targeted virologic effect or a durable response and is more likely to lead to the development of multidrug-resistant isolates. Conversely, in cases where adherence is judged to be the reason for failure, the substitution of ritonavir-boosted PIs (e.g., low-dose ritonavir added to saquinavir, indinavir, amprenavir, or lopinavir) for single PIs enable the regimen to be given less frequently. Several studies with regimens of boosted PIs given twice daily have reported comparable virologic results, lower total drug costs, greater tolerability, and improved adherence.

Selection of the next regimen must be individualized based, in relatively equal parts, on the last regimen, the resistance test results obtained while the patient is still taking the failing regimen, and prior exposure to other agents, with emphasis on tolerability and potential residual (archived) resistant viruses that are being harbored in latently infected cells. As when selecting the initial regimen, consideration must be given to what the patient is willing to take and likely to tolerate. In situations where options are limited because of previous toxicity or prior failure of available agents, it may be necessary to 'recycle' an ARV drug back into a new regimen. When this is necessary, it is best to use agents that have not been utilized in the last two or three regimens and to avoid recycling two or three agents from a single previous regimen back together. Ideally, the new regimen should consist of two or more agents deemed to be active, preferably with drugs that have not been used together in previous regimens. Most often it is prudent to maintain the presence of either lamivudine or emtricitabine in the next regimen owing to both the observation that these drugs still exert a substantial antiviral effect (0.5–0.8 log reduction in viral load) even it the face of an M184V mutation and the high degree of tolerability of these drugs.[145,179]

Pharmacokinetic enhancement, such as boosting PI levels with low-dose ritonavir, should be exploited whenever possible in the setting of multiple-regimen failure. The use of 'double-boosted PIs' (two PI agents along with low-dose ritonavir) has not been shown to have any benefit over single-boosted PI therapy and is associated with increased toxicity and unpredictable drug–drug interactions.[1] Similarly, the use of multidrug (six or more drugs) rescue therapy has shown variable ARV activity.[180–182] However, this approach often leads to substantial toxicity and problems with adherence, drug–drug interactions, and cost. With newer, more potent drugs available, such as tipranavir, darunavir, and enfuvirtide, multiple drug regimens (so-called 'mega-HAART') is no longer a meaningful consideration.

Except in cases of toxicity, it is preferable to continue even 'failing' drug regimens that maintain selective pressure on the viruses rather than permanently discontinuing all ART, especially in settings in which the CD4+ T-lymphocyte counts are maintained despite a rebound in viral replication.[179] In cases where the regimen is changed, the same concepts of defining the target plasma RNA values that define success and failure of the regimen in the current clinical setting still apply and should be discussed with the patient.

Treatment Interruptions

Use of a 'supervised' treatment interruption (STI) has been postulated to be of clinical benefit among certain patient populations. In the setting of multidrug-resistant virus, STIs have been used in an attempt to exploit the rapid reversion to wild-type viruses.[183–185] Such a strategy should be undertaken with great caution owing to the rapid increase in viral load and marked reduction in CD4+ T-lymphocyte count in association with reversion to wild-type virus around week eight of the STI.[183] Studies of this approach have yielded mixed results, mostly due to differences in the timing of reinitiation of therapy (prior to week 12 of the STI vs at week 16).[186–190] Therefore, if an STI is employed in the setting of multiply resistant virus, frequent assessments should be performed during the STI with early resumption of treatment with any sign of plummeting CD4+ T-lymphocyte count. Of significant concern is the higher incidence of cardiovascular events in studies of planned treatment interruptions.[186] This unexpected safety outcome occurred most commonly among those patients who stopped ART with lower CD4+ counts and those who had a lower CD4 count nadir.

STIs have also been postulated to be a strategy among successfully treated patients in an attempt to reduce drug exposure, long-term toxicities, and costs. Several studies that employed this strategy have demonstrated harm associated with routine use of STIs in this setting.[186] In particular, the SMART study, which randomized patients to standard of care (continuous treatment) versus routine cessation of ARV therapy when their CD4+ count rose above 400 cells/μL and have treatment reinstated when the CD4+ count dropped below 250 cells/μL, demonstrated clear harm associated with the STI strategy. The study was stopped early by a Data Safety and Monitoring Board owing to a significantly higher degree of clinical events, including cardiac events, among the STI managed patients.

Another proposed use of an STI is to enhance and stimulate immunologic responses to HIV with the goal of reducing the need for ARV therapy. The concept is to use periodic treatment interruptions as a natural vaccine using autologous virus as the immunogen.[191,192] The few studies that have been conducted to evaluate this concept have demonstrated some evidence of partial lowering of the viral load set-point, but the magnitude of response is quite meager and this approach cannot be recommended.

The most common and perhaps only appropriate use of an STI is in the management of treatment toxicities as discussed above.

Other ARV Management Issues

On occasion, patients present with a 'discordant' response, whereby the viral load is successfully suppressed but the CD4+ T-lymphocyte count fails to increase. Several options exist for managing a 'discordant' response, but because the reasons for the discordant responses are not well understood there is no clearly defined or optimal approach to management. Drug-related toxic effects, inhibition of *de novo* CD4+ T-lymphocyte synthesis, sequestration of cells within lymphoid tissue, and interference with clonal expansion of memory CD4+ T lymphocytes have been proposed as potential mechanisms. The approach to management depends on the suspected reason for the discordant response. For those patients with viral load values <50 c/mL, it is best to continue the current regimen and evaluate for other causes of bone marrow or cellular toxicity. For example, substituting specific drugs in the regimen, removing potentially cytotoxic drugs, and eliminating hydroxyurea-containing regimens are valid options when bone marrow toxicity is suspected. Alternatively, the use of cytokines, such as IL-2 or granulocyte- and granulocyte/macrophage colony-stimulating factors, are potential approaches to expand the cell populations directly (*see* Chapter 30). However there are not enough data to recommend cytokine therapy at this time. Trials of IL-2 (3.0–4.5 million units twice daily for 5 days every 2 months) are being evaluated among patients with low (SILCAAT) and high (ESPRIT) CD4+ T-lymphocyte counts in an attempt to raise the CD4+ T-lymphocyte cell counts among patients who have achieved successful suppression of HIV but did not have concomitant increases in their CD4+ T-lymphocyte counts. To date, these trials have not yielded definitive recommendations on the use of IL-2; but it is important to note the high degree of toxicity associated with IL-2 treatment and the low degree of observed disease progression among patients with low CD4 T-lymphocyte counts and persistent viral load values <50 c/mL.

The use of therapeutic drug monitoring (TDM) has been proposed as a means of enhancing virologic outcomes and assessing reasons for virologic failure or toxicity (*see* Chapter 79). TDM is a process whereby drug levels are measured at fixed time intervals after a dose of medicine has been ingested. The PK curve of a given drug can be modeled with as few as one or two measurements. Once determined, the peak and trough levels can be estimated and used to assess the likelihood of virologic suppression or development of toxicity. Although the concept is attractive on face value, multiple assumptions limit the usefulness of TDM in practice. For example, to model accurately, the time of dosing must be known precisely. Relying on verbal reports of dosing is inaccurate. Moreover, the modeling assumes that the patient is at steady state, which means that all previous doses were taken correctly and on time, which may not be the case. The modeling is inaccurate if it utilizes levels determined on samples obtained within the first 2 h (absorption/distribution phase) of dosing; therefore, only levels for samples obtained 'postpeak' can be used. Finally, it is unclear which 'level' is the optimal target for best virologic response for each individual drug. Because TDM is based solely on plasma levels, there is no consideration for intracellular drug concentrations or intracellular processing, creating further limitations of the technique. Nonetheless, TDM can be a useful adjunct to therapy when assessing the possibility of nonadherence or poor absorption (e.g., absence of drug in the bloodstream) or in cases of extremely advanced disease where higher doses of drug are being considered to maximize ARV benefit. Outside of these two circumstances, TDM remains a research tool.

REFERENCES

1. Hammer SM, Saag MS, Schechter M, et al. Treatment of adult HIV infection: 2006 recommendations of the International AIDS Society-USA panel. JAMA 296:827–883, 2006.
2. National Institutes of Health Panel to define principles of therapy of HIV infection. Guidelines for the use of antiretroviral agents in HIV-infected adults and adolescents. Ann Intern Med 128:1079–100, 1998.
3. Gazzard B, Moyle G, BHIVA Guidelines Writing Committee. Revision to the British HIV Association guidelines for antiretroviral treatment of HIV seropositive individuals. Lancet 352:314–16, 1998.
4. US Department of Health and Human Services Panel on Clinical Practices for Treatment of HIV Infection. Guidelines for the use of antiretroviral agents in HIV-1 infected adults and adolescents. Washington, DC: DHHS. Available: http://aidsinfo.nih.gov/Guidelines/GuidelineDetail.aspx?MenuItem=Guidelines&Search=Off&GuidelineID=7&ClassID=1 10 Oct 2006.
5. US Department of Health and Human Services Panel on Clinical Practices for Treatment of HIV Infection. Guidelines for the use of antiretroviral agents in HIV-1 infected adults and adolescents. MMWR Morb Mortal Wkly Rep 47(RR-5):1–41, 1998.
6. Wei X, Ghosh SK, Taylor ME, et al. Viral dynamics in HIV-1 infection. Nature 373:117–22, 1995.
7. Ho DD, Neumann AU, Perelson AS, et al. Rapid turnover of plasma virions and CD4+ lymphocytes in HIV-1 infection. Nature 373:123–26, 1995.
8. Coffin JM. HIV population dynamics in vivo: implications for genetic variation, pathogenesis, and therapy. Science 267: 483–9, 1995.
9. Wain-Hobson S. AIDS: virological mayhem. Nature 373:102, 1995.
10. Saag MS, Holodniy M, Kuritzkes DR, et al. HIV viral load markers in clinical practice. Nat Med 2:625–9, 1996.
11. Holodniy M, Katzenstein DA, Sengupta S. Detection and quantification of human immunodeficiency virus RNA in patient serum by use of the polymerase chain reaction. J Infect Dis 163:862–6, 1991.
12. Piatak M, Saag MS, Yang LC, et al. High levels of HIV-1 in plasma during all stages of infection determined by competitive PCR. Science 259:1749–54, 1993.
13. Piatak M Jr, Saag MS, Yang LC, et al. Determination of plasma viral load in HIV-1 infection by quantitative competitive polymerase chain reaction. AIDS 7(Suppl 2):S65–71, 1993.
14. Cao Y, Ho DD, Todd J, et al. Clinical evaluation of branched DNA signal amplification for quantifying HIV type 1 in human plasma. AIDS Res Hum Retroviruses 11:353–61, 1995.
15. Hirsch MS, Brun-Vézinet F, Clotet B, et al. Antiretroviral drug resistance testing in adults infected with human immunodeficiency virus type I: 2003 recommendations of an International AIDS Society-USA panel. Clin Infect Dis 37:113–28, 2003.
16. Hogg RS, Heath KV, Yip B, et al. Improved survival among HIV-infected individuals following initiation of antiretroviral therapy. JAMA 279:450–54, 1998.
17. Palella FJ, Delaney KM, Moorman AC, et al. Declining morbidity and mortality among patients with advanced human immunodeficiency virus infection. N Engl J Med 338:853–60, 1998.
18. Palella F, Moorman A, Chmiel J, et al. Continued low morbidity and mortality among patients with advanced HIV infection and their patterns of highly active antiretroviral therapy (HAART) usage. Presented at the 7th Conference on Retroviruses and Opportunistic Infections, 2000, p 216.
19. Carr A, Samaras K, Burton S, et al. A syndrome of peripheral lipodystrophy, hyperlipidaemia and insulin resistance in patients receiving HIV protease inhibitors. AIDS 12:F51–8, 1998.
20. Carr A, Miller J, Law M, Cooper DA. A syndrome of lipoatrophy, lactic acidaemia and liver dysfunction associated with HIV nucleoside analogue therapy: contribution to protease inhibitor-related lipodystrophy syndrome. AIDS 14:F25–32, 2000.
21. Carr A, Samaras K, Chisholm DJ, Cooper DA. Pathogenesis of HIV-1-protease inhibitor-associated peripheral lipodystrophy, hyperlipidaemia, and insulin resistance. Lancet 351:1881–3, 1998.
22. Yarasheski KE, Tebas P, Sigmund C, et al. Insulin resistance in HIV protease inhibitor-associated diabetes. J Acquir Immune Defic Syndr 21:209–16, 1999.
23. Schambelan M, Benson C, Carpenter CCJ, et al. Metabolic complications guidelines: recommendation of the International AIDS Society-USA panel. JAIDS 31:257–75, 2002.
24. Masur H, Miller KD, Jones EC, et al. High prevalence of avascular necrosis (AVN) of the hip in HIV infection: magnetic resonance imaging of 339 asymptomatic patients. Presented at the 38th Annual Meeting of the Infectious Diseases Society of America, 2000.
25. Gupta SK, Eustace JA, Winston JA, et al. Guidelines for the management of chronic kidney disease in HIV-infected patients: recommendations of the HIV Medicine Association of the Infectious Diseases Society of America. Clin Infect Dis 40:1559–85, 2005.
26. Lo JC, Kazemi MR, Hsue PY, et al. The relationship between nucleoside analogue treatment duration, insulin resistance, and fasting arterialized lactate level in patients with HIV infection. Clin Infect Dis 41:1335–40, 2005.
27. Sanne I, Mommeja-Marin H, Hinkle J, et al. Severe hepatotoxicity associated with nevirapine use in HIV-infected subjects. J Infect Dis 192:545–6, 2005.
28. Hockett RD, Kilby JM, Derdeyn CA, et al. Constant mean viral copy number per infected cell in tissues regardless of high, low, or undetectable plasma HIV RNA. J Exp Med 189:1545–59, 1999.
29. Zhang L, Ramratnam B, Tenner-Racz K, et al. Quantifying residual HIV-1 replication in patients receiving combination antiretroviral therapy. N Engl J Med 340:1605–13, 1999.
30. Acosta EP, Henry K, Baken L, et al. Indinavir concentrations and antiviral effect. Pharmacotherapy 19:708–12, 1999.
31. Acosta EP, Kakuda TN, Brundage RC, et al. Pharmacodynamics of human immunodeficiency virus type 1 protease inhibitors. Clin Infect Dis 30(Suppl 2):S151–9, 2000.
32. Sommadossi JP, Zhou XJ, Moore J, et al. Impairment of stavudine phosphorylation in patients receiving a combination of zidovudine and stavudine. Presented at the 5th Conference on Retroviruses and Opportunistic Infections, 1998.

33. Hsu A, Granneman GR, Bertz RJ. Ritonavir-clinical pharmacokinetics and interactions with other anti-HIV agents. Clin Pharmacokinet 35:275–91, 1998.
34. Chesney MA, Morin M, Sherr L. Adherence to HIV combination therapy. Soc Sci Med 50:1599–605, 2000.
35. Shaw GM, Harper ME, Hahn BH, et al. HTLV-III infection in brains of children and adults with AIDS encephalopathy. Science 227:177–81, 1985.
36. Bagasra O, Lavi E, Bobroski L. Cellular reservoirs of HIV-1 in the central nervous system of infected individuals: identification by the combination of in situ polymerase chain reaction and immunohistochemistry. AIDS 10:573–85, 1996.
37. Coombs RW, Welles SL, Hooper C. Association of plasma human immunodeficiency virus type-1 RNA level with risk of clinical progression in patients with advanced infection. J Infect Dis 174:704–12, 1996.
38. Daar ES, Moudgil T, Meyer RD, Ho DD. Transient high levels of viremia in patients with primary human immunodeficiency virus type 1 infection. N Engl J Med 324:961–4, 1991.
39. Clark SJ, Saag MS, Decker WD, et al. High titers of cytopathic virus in plasma of patients with symptomatic primary HIV-1 infection. N Engl J Med 324:954–60, 1991.
40. Ho DD, Moudgil T, Alam M. Quantitation of human immunodeficiency virus type 1 in the blood of infected persons. N Engl J Med 321:1621–5, 1989.
41. Saag MS, Crain MJ, Decker WD. High-level viremia in adults and children infected with human immunodeficiency virus: relation to disease stage and CD4+ lymphocyte levels. J Infect Dis 164:72–80, 1991.
42. Clark SJ, Shaw GM. Acute retroviral syndrome and the pathogenesis of HIV-1 infection. Semin Immunol 5:149–55, 1993.
43. Schacker T, Hughes JP, Shea T, et al. Biological and virologic characteristics of primary HIV infection. Ann Intern Med 128:613–20, 1998.
44. Kappes JC, Saag MS, Shaw GM, et al. Assessment of antiretroviral therapy by plasma viral load testing: standard and ICD HIV-1 p24 antigen and viral RNA (QC-PCR) assays compared. Acquir Immune Defic Syndr Hum Retrovir 10:139–49, 1995.
45. Saag MS, Emini EA, Laskin OL. Short-term clinical evaluation of L-697,661, a nonnucleoside inhibitor of HIV-1 reverse transcriptase. N Engl J Med 329:1065–72, 1993.
46. Perelson AS, Neumann AU, Markowitz M, et al. HIV-1 dynamics in vivo: virion clearance rate, infected cell life-span, and viral generation time. Science 271:1582–6, 1996.
47. Perelson AS, Essunger P, Cao Y, et al. Decay characteristics of HIV-1 infected compartments during combination therapy. Nature 387:188–91, 1997.
48. Perelson AS, Essunger P, Ho DD. Dynamics of HIV-1 and CD4 lymphocytes in vivo. AIDS 11(Suppl A):517–24, 1997.
49. Fauci AS. Host factors and the pathogenesis of HIV-induced disease. Nature 384:529–34, 1996.
50. Chun TW, Fauci AS. Latent reservoirs of HIV: obstacles to the eradication of virus. Proc Natl Acad Sci USA 96:10958–61, 1999.
51. Wong JK, Gunthard HF, Havlir DV, et al. Reduction of HIV in blood and lymph nodes after potent antiretroviral therapy and the virologic correlates of treatment failure. Proc Natl Acad Sci USA 94:12574–9, 1997.
52. Dybul M, Chun TW, Ward DJ, et al. Evaluation of lymph node virus burden in human immunodeficiency virus-infected patients receiving efavirenz-based protease inhibitor-sparing highly active antiretroviral therapy. J Infect Dis 181:1273–9, 2000.
53. Boucher C, Nijhuis M, Schipper P, et al. Reduction of HIV in blood and lymph nodes after potent antiretroviral therapy. Presented at the 4th Conference on Retroviruses and Opportunistic Infections, 1997.
54. Cavert W, Notermans DW, Staskus K, et al. Kinetics of response in lymphoid tissues to antiretroviral therapy of HIV-1 infection. Science 276:960–4, 1997.
55. Nelson PW, Mittler JE, Perelson A. Effect of drug efficacy and the eclipse phase of the viral life cycle on estimates of HIV viral dynamic parameters. J Acquir Defic Syndr Hum Retrovir 26:405–12, 2001.
56. Mellors JW, Rinaldo CR Jr, Gupta P, et al. Prognosis in HIV-1 infection predicted by the quantity of virus in plasma. Science 272:1167–70, 1996.
57. Mellors JW, Munoz AM, Giorgi JV, et al. Plasma viral load and CD4+ lymphocytes as prognostic markers of HIV-1 infection. Ann Intern Med 126:946–54, 1997.
58. Rodriguez B, Sethi AK, Cheruvu VK, et al. Predictive value of plasma HIV RNA level on rate of CD4 T-cell decline in untreated HIV infection. JAMA 296:1498–506, 2006.
59. Ferguson NM, deWolf F, Ghani AC, et al. Antigen-driven CD4+ T cell and HIV-1 dynamics: residual viral replication under highly active antiretroviral therapy. Proc Natl Acad Sci USA 96:15167–72, 1999.
60. Finzi D, Siliciano RF. Viral dynamics in HIV-1 infection. Cell 93:665–71, 1998.
61. Ho DD. Time to hit HIV, early and hard. N Engl J Med 333:450–1, 1995.
62. Brenchley JM, Price DA, Douek DC. HIV disease: fallout from a mucosal catastrophe? Nat Immunol 7:235–9, 2006.
63. Brenchley JM, Schacker TW, Ruff LE, et al. CD4+ T cell depletion during all stages of HIV disease occurs predominantly in the gastrointestinal tract. J Exp Med 200:749–59, 2004.
64. Mattapallil JJ, Douek DC, Hill B, et al. Massive infection and loss of memory CD4+ T cells in multiple tissues during acute SIV infection. Nature 434:1093–7, 2005.
65. Autran B, Carcelain G, Li TS, et al. Positive effects of combined antiretroviral therapy on CD4+ T cell homeostasis and function in advanced HIV disease. Science 277:112–16, 1997.
66. Bucy RP. Immune clearance of HIV type 1 replication-active cells: a model of two patterns of steady state HIV infection. AIDS Res Hum Retroviruses 15:223–7, 1999.
67. Saag MS, Kilby JM. HIV-1 and HAART: a time to cure, a time to kill. Nat Med 5:609–11, 1999.
68. Rosenberg ES, Billingsley JM, Caliendo AM, et al. Vigorous HIV-1-specific CD4+ T cell responses associated with control of viremia. Science 278:1447–50, 1997.
69. Rosenberg ES, Walker BD. HIV type 1-specific helper T cells: a critical host defense. AIDS Res Hum Retroviruses 14(Suppl 2):S143–7, 1998.
70. Wei X, Decker JM, Wang S, et al. Antibody neutralization and escape by HIV-1. Nature Mar 20; 422:307–12, 2003.
71. Decker JM, Bibollet-Ruche F, Wei X, et al. Antigenic conservation and immunogenicity of the HIV co-receptor binding site. J Exp Med 201:1407–19, 2005.
72. Rosenberg ES, Altfeld M, Poon SH, et al. Immune control of HIV-1 after early treatment of acute infection. Nature 407:523–6, 2000.
73. Davey RT Jr, Bhat N, Yoder C, et al. HIV-1 and T cell dynamics after interruption of highly active antiretroviral therapy (HAART) in patients with a history of sustained viral suppression. Proc Natl Acad Sci USA 96:15109–14, 1999.
74. Ruiz L, Martinez-Picado J, Romeu J, et al. Structured treatment interruption in chronically HIV-1 infected patients after long-term viral suppression. AIDS 14:397–403, 2000.
75. Borrow P, Lewicki H, Wei X, et al. Antiviral pressure exerted by HIV-1-specific cytotoxic T lymphocytes (CTLs) during primary infection demonstrated by rapid selection of CTL escape virus. Nat Med 3:205–11, 1997.

76. Borrow P, Lewicki H, Hahn BH, et al. Virus-specific CD8+ cytotoxic T-lymphocyte activity associated with control of viremia in primary human immunodeficiency virus type 1 infection. J Virol 68:6103–10, 1994.
77. Altfeld M, Rosenberg ES, Mukherjee J, et al. Enhancement of HIV-1 specific CTL responses during structured treatment interuptions (STI) following treated acute HIV-1-infection is associated with control of HIV-1 viremia. Presented at the XIII International AIDS Conference, 2000.
78. Walker CM, Moody DJ, Stites DP, Levy JA. CD8+ lymphocytes can control HIV infection in vitro by suppressing virus replication. Science 234:1563–6, 1986.
79. Mclean AR, Michie CA. In vivo estimates of division and death rates of human T-lymphocytes. Proc Natl Acad Sci USA 92:3707–11, 1995.
80. Chun TW, Carruth L, Finzi D, et al. Quantification of latent tissue reservoirs and total body fat viral load in HIV-1 infection. Nature 387:183–8, 1997.
81. Wong JK, Hezareh M, Gunthard HF, et al. Recovery of replication-competent HIV despite prolonged suppression of plasma viremia. Science 278:1291–5, 1997.
82. Finzi D, Hermankova M, Pierson T, et al. Identification of a reservoir for HIV-1 in patients on highly active antiretroviral therapy. Science 278:1295–300, 1997.
83. Deeks SG, Hecht FM, Swanson M, et al. HIV RNA and CD4 cell count response to protease inhibitor therapy in an urban AIDS clinic: response to both initial and salvage therapy. AIDS 13:F35–43, 1999.
84. Hammer SM, Squires KE, Hughes MD, et al. A controlled trial of two nucleoside analogues plus indinavir in persons with human immunodeficiency virus infection and CD4 cell counts of 200/μl or less. N Engl J Med 337:725–33, 1997.
85. Gulick RM, Mellors JW, Havlir D, et al. Treatment with indinavir, zidovudine, and lamivudine in adults with human immunodeficiency virus infection and prior antiretroviral therapy. N Engl J Med 337:734–9, 1997.
86. Chaisson RE, Keruly JC, Moore RD. Association of initial CD4 cell count and viral load with response to highly active antiretroviral therapy. JAMA 284:3128–9, 2000.
87. Hogg RS, Yip B, Wood E, et al. Diminished effectiveness of antiretroviral therapy among patients initiating therapy with CD4+ cell counts below $200/mm^3$. Presented at the 8th Conference on Retroviruses and Opportunistic Infections, 2001.
88. Moore R, Keruly J, Bartlett J, Chaisson R. Start HAART early (CD4 > 350 cells/μl) or later? Evidence for greater effectiveness if started early. Presented at the 7th Conference on Retroviruses and Opportunistic Infections, 2000, p 174.
89. Marschner IC, Collier AC, Coombs RW, et al. Use of changes in plasma levels of human immunodeficiency virus type 1 RNA to assess clinical benefit to antiretroviral therapy. J Infect Dis 177:40–7, 1998.
90. Yerly S, Kaiser L, Perneger TV, et al. Time of initiation of antiretroviral therapy: impact on HIV-1 viraemia: the Swiss HIV Cohort Study. AIDS 14:243–9, 2000.
91. Chun TW, Davey RT Jr, Ostrowski M, et al. Relationship between pre-existing viral reservoirs and the re-emergence of plasma viremia after discontinuation of highly active anti-retroviral therapy. Nat Med 6:757–61, 2000.
92. Kempf DJ, Rode RA, Xu Y, et al. The duration of viral suppression during protease inhibitor therapy for HIV-1 infection is predicted by plasma HIV-1 RNA at the nadir. AIDS 12:F9–14, 1998.
93. Cahn P. 24-week data from RESIST 2: phase 3 study of the efficacy and safety of either tipranavir/ritonavir (TPV/r) or an optimized ritonavir (RTV)-boosted standard-of-care (SOC) comparator PI (CPI) in a large randomized multicenter trial in treatment-experienced HIV+ patients. 7th International Congress on Drug Therapy in HIV Infection, Glasgow, Scotland, 14–18 Nov 2004, abstract PL14.3.
94. Katlama C, Carvalho MT, Cooper D, et al. TMC114/r outperforms investigator-selected PI(s) in 3-class-experienced patients: week 24 primary analysis of POWER 1 (TMC114-C213). 3rd IAS Conference on HIV Pathogenesis and Treatment, Rio de Janeiro, Brazil, 24–27 Jul 2005, abstract WeOaLB0102.
95. Wilkin T, Haubrich R, Steinhart CR, et al. TMC114/r superior to standard of care in 3-class-experienced patients: 24-wks primary analysis of the Power 2 Study (C202). 45th Interscience Conference on Antimicrobial Agents and Chemotherapy, Washington, DC, 16–19 Dec 2005, abstract H-413.
96. Clerici M, Levin JM, Kessler HA. HIV-specific T-helper activity in seronegative health care workers exposed to contaminated blood. JAMA 271:42–6, 1994.
97. Centers for Disease Control and Prevention. Public health service guidelines for the management of health-care worker exposures to HIV and recommendations for post-exposure prophylaxis. MMWR Morb Mortal Wkly Rep 47(RR-7):1–33, 1998.
98. Connor EM, Sperling RS, Gelber R, et al. Reduction of maternal-infant transmission of human immunodeficiency virus type 1 with zidovudine treatment: pediatric AIDS Clinical Trials Group Protocol 076 Study Group. N Engl J Med 331:1173–80, 1994.
99. Saag MS, Schooley RT. Initiation of antiretroviral therapy: current controversies in when and with what to start. Top HIV Med 8:8–13, 2000.
100. Raboud JM, Rae S, Hogg RS, et al. Suppression of plasma viral load below the detection limit of a human immunodeficiency virus kit is associated with longer virologic response than suppression below the limit of quantitation. J Infect Dis 180: 1347–50, 1999.
101. Deeks S, Barbour J, Martin JN, et al. Sustained CD4+ T cell response after virologic failure of protease inhibitor-based regimens in patients with human immunodeficiency virus infection. J Infect Dis 181:946–53, 2000.
102. Deeks SG, Barbour JD, Martin JN, Grant RM. Delayed immunologic deterioration among patients who virologically fail protease inhibitor-based therapy. Presented at the 7th Conference on Retroviruses and Opportunistic Infections, 2000, p 120.
103. Emini EA, Graham DJ, Gotlib L. HIV and multidrug resistance. Nature 364:679, 1993.
104. Richman DD. Resistance of clinical isolates of human immunodeficiency virus to antiretroviral agents. Antimicrob Agents Chemother 37:1207–13, 1993.
105. Richman DD, Havlir D, Corbeil J, et al. Nevirapine resistance mutations of human immunodeficiency virus type 1 selected during therapy. J Virol 68:1660–6, 1994.
106. Bangsberg DR, Hecht FM, Charlebois ED, et al. Adherence to protease inhibitors, HIV-1 viral load, and development of drug resistance in an indigent population. AIDS 14:357–66, 2000.
107. Arnsten J, Demas P, Gourevitch M, et al. Adherence and viral load in HIV-infected drug users: comparison of self-report and medication event monitors (MEMS). Presented at the 7th Conference on Retroviruses and Opportunistic Infections, 2000, p 88.
108. Carr A, Samaras K, Thorisdottir A, et al. Diagnosis, prediction, and natural course of HIV-1 protease inhibitor-associated lipodystrophy, hyperlipidaemia, and diabetes mellitus: a cohort study. Lancet 353:2093–9, 1999.
109. Hadigan C, Meigs JB, Corcoran C, et al. Metabolic abnormalities and cardiovascular disease risk factors in adults with human immunodeficiency virus infection and lipodystrophy. Clin Infect Dis 32:130–9, 2001.
110. Blacksin MF, Kloser PC, Simon J. Avascular necrosis of bone in human immunodeficiency virus infected patients. Clin Imaging 23:314–18, 1999.

111. Brinkman K, Smeitink JA, Romijn JA, Reiss P. Mitochondrial toxicity induced by nucleoside-analogue reverse-transcriptase inhibitors is a key factor in the pathogenesis of antiretroviral-therapy-related lipodystrophy. Lancet 354:1112–15, 1999.
112. Tebas P, Powderly WG, Claxton S, et al. Accelerated bone mineral loss in HIV-infected patients receiving potent antiretroviral therapy. AIDS 14:F63–7, 2000.
113. Hoy J, Hudson J, Law M, Cooper DA. Osteopenia in a randomized multicenter study of protease inhibitor (PI) substitution in patients with the lipodystrophy syndrome and well-controlled HIV viremia. Presented at the 7th Conference on Retroviruses and Opportunistic Infections, 2000, p 114.
114. Glesby MJ, Hoover PR, Vaamonde CM. Osteonecrosis in patients infected with HIV: a case-control study. J Infect Dis 184:519–23, 2001.
115. Fletcher CV, Anderson PL, Kakuda TN, et al. A novel approach to integrate pharmacologic and virologic characteristics: an in vivo potency (IVP) index for antiretroviral agents. Presented at the 8th Conference on Retroviruses and Opportunistic Infections, 2001.
116. Flexner C, Speck RR. Role of multidrug transporters in HIV pathogenesis. Presented at the 8th Conference on Retroviruses and Opportunistic Infections, 2001, p 281.
117. Haas DW, Ribaudo HJ, Kim RB, et al. Pharmacogenetics of efavirenz and central nervous system side effects: an Adult AIDS Clinical Trials Group study. AIDS 18:2391–400, 2004.
118. Chen R, Westfall A, Cloud G, et al. Long-term survival after initiation of antiretroviral therapy. Presented at the 8th Conference on Retroviruses and Opportunistic Infections, 2001.
119. Egger M, May M, Chene G, et al. Prognosis of HIV-1 infected drug naive patients starting potent antiretroviral therapy: a collaborative analysis of prospective studies. Lancet 360:119–29, 2002.
120. Henry K. The case for more cautious, patient-focused antiretroviral therapy. Ann Intern Med 132:306–22, 2000.
121. Kirkland LR, Fischl MA, Tashira KT, et al. Response to lamivudine-zidovudine plus abacavir twice daily in ART-NAIVE, incarcerated patients with HIV taking directly observed treatment. Clin Infect Dis 34:511–18, 2002.
122. Staszewski S, Morales-Ramirez J, Tashima KT, et al. Efavirenz plus zidovudine and lamivudine, efavirenz plus indinavir, and indinavir plus zidovudine and lamivudine in the treatment of HIV-1 infection in adults: study 006 team. N Engl J Med 341:1865–73, 1999.
123. Acosta EP, Gulick R, Katzenstein D, et al. Pharmacokinetic (PK) evaluation of saquinavir soft gel capsules (SQV)/ritonavir (RTV) or SQV/nelfinavir (NFV) in combination with delavirdine (DLV) and/or adefovir dipivoxil (ADV)-ACTG 359. Presented at the 6th Conference on Retroviruses and Opportunistic Infections, 1999.
124. Andrade A, Flexner C. HIV-related drug metabolism and cytochrome P450 enzymes. AIDS Clin Care 12:91–5, 2000.
125. Benson C, Brun S, King M, et al. Two year follow-up of ABT378/ritonavir (ABT-378/r) in antiretroviral naive HIV + patients. Presented at the 40th Interscience Conference on Antimicrobial Agents and Chemotherapy, 2000, p 282.
126. Cameron DW, Japour AJ, Xu Y, et al. Ritonavir and saquinavir combination therapy for the treatment of HIV infection. AIDS 13:213–24, 1999.
127. Casado JL, Moreno A, Marti-Belda P, et al. Increased indinavir levels using twice daily ritonavir/indinavir at 100/800 mg improves virological response even after multiple failure. Presented at the 40th Interscience Conference on Antimicrobial Agents and Chemotherapy, 2000, p 301.
128. Hammer SM. Clinical practice. Management of newly diagnosed HIV infection. N Engl J Med 353:1702–10, 2005.
129. Carpenter CCJ, Fischl MA, Hammer SM, et al. Antiretroviral therapy for HIV infection in 1998: updated recommendations of the International AIDS Society-USA panel. JAMA 280:78–86, 1998.
130. Saag MS, Hahn BH, Gibbons J, et al. Extensive variation of human immunodeficiency virus type-1 in vivo. Nature 334:440–4, 1988.
131. Drake JW. Rates of spontaneous mutation among RNA viruses. Proc Natl Acad Sci USA 90:4171–5, 1993.
132. Mansky LM, Temin HM. Lower in vivo mutation rate of human immunodeficiency virus type 1 than that predicted from the fidelity of purified reverse transcriptase. J Virol 69:5087–94, 1995.
133. Deeks SG, Wrin T, Duecy E, et al. Decreased HIV-1 fitness after long-term virologic failure of protease inhibitor-based therapy: relationship to immunologic response. Presented at the 7th Conference on Retroviruses and Opportunistic Infections, 2000, p 104.
134. International AIDS Society-USA Resistance Mutations Project Panel. Update on drug resistance mutations in HIV-1. Top HIV Med 14:125–30, 2006.
135. Kuritzkes DR, Bell S, Shugarts D, Abrams D. Development of resistance to lamivudine (3TC) in NUCA 3001, a phase II comparative study of 3TC versus zidovudine versus 3TC plus zidovudine. Presented at the 2nd National Conference on Human Retroviruses and Related Infections, 1995.
136. Saag MS, Emini EA, Laskin OL, et al. A short-term clinical evaluation of L-697,661, a non-nucleoside inhibitor of HIV-1 reverse transcriptase: L-697,661 working group. N Engl J Med 329:1065–72, 1993.
137. Larder BA, Darby G, Richman DD. HIV with reduced sensitivity to zidovudine (AZT) isolated during prolonged therapy. Science 243:1731–4, 1989.
138. Larder BA, Chesebro B, Richman DD. Susceptibilities of zidovudine-susceptible and -resistant human immunodeficiency virus isolates to antiviral agents determined by using a quantitative plaque reduction assay. Antimicrob Agents Chemother 34:436–41, 1990.
139. Condra JH, Schleif WA, Blahy OM. In vivo emergence of HIV-1 variants resistant to multiple protease inhibitors. Nature 374:569–71, 1995.
140. Condra JH, Holder DJ, Schleif WA, et al. Genetic correlates of in vivo viral resistance to indinavir, a human immunodeficiency virus type 1 protease inhibitor. J Virol 70:8270–6, 1996.
141. Patrick A, Mo H, Markowitz M. Antiviral and resistance studies of AG1343, an orally bioavailable inhibitor of human immunodeficiency virus protease. Antimicrob Agents Chemother 40:292–7, 1996.
142. Kravcik S, Farnsworth A, Patick A, et al. Long-term follow-up of combination protease inhibitor therapy with nelfinavir and saquinavir (soft gel) in HIV infection. Presented at the 5th Conference on Retroviruses and Opportunistic Infections, 1998.
143. Larder BA, Kemp SD, Harrigan PR. Antiviral potency of AZT + 3TC combination therapy supports virological observations. Presented at the 2nd National Conference on Human Retroviruses and Related Infections, 1995.
144. Havlir DV, Gamst A, Eastman S, Richman DD. Nevirapine-resistant human immunodeficiency virus: kinetics of replication and estimated prevalence in untreated patients. J Virol 70:7894–9, 1996.
145. Eron JJ, Benoit SL, Jemsek J, et al. Treatment with lamivudine, zidovudine, or both in HIV-positive patients with 200 to 500 CD4+ cells per cubic millimeter. N Engl J Med 333:1662–9, 1995.
146. Larder BA, Kellam P, Kemp SD. Convergent combination therapy can select viable multidrug-resistant HIV-1 in vitro. Nature 365:451–3, 1993.
147. Murphy RL, Sommadossi JP, Lamson M, et al. Antiviral effect and pharmacokinetic interaction between nevirapine and

indinavir in persons infected with human immunodeficiency virus type 1. J Infect Dis 179:1116–23, 1999.
148. Urquhart J. Partial compliance in cardiovascular disease: risk implications. Br J Clin Pract 73(Suppl):2, 1994.
149. Greenberg RN. Overview of patient compliance with medication dosing: a literature review. Clin Ther 65:590, 1984.
150. Wright EC. Non-compliance: or how many aunts has Matilda? Lancet 342:909, 1993.
151. Urquhart J. Patient non-compliance with drug regimens: measurement, clinical correlates, economic impact. Eur Heart J 17(Suppl A):8, 1996.
152. Havlir D, Levitan D, Bassett R, et al. Prevalence and predictive value of intermittent viraemia in patients with viral suppression. Antiviral Ther 5(Suppl 3):89, 2000.
153. Havlir DV, Marschner IC, Hirsch MS, et al. Maintenance antiretroviral therapies in HIV infected patients with undetectable plasma HIV RNA after triple-drug therapy: AIDS Clinical Trials Group Study 343 team. N Engl J Med 339:1261–8, 1998.
154. Gharakhanian S, Salhi Y, Adda N, et al. Identification of fat redistribution/metabolic anomalies in a cohort treated by 2 NRTIs + 1 PI, and absence of significant modification following PI substitution. Presented at the 7th Conference on Retroviruses and Opportunistic Infections, 2000, p 84.
155. Viciana P, Alarcon A, Martin D, et al. Partial improvement of lipodystrophy after switching from HIV-1 protease inhibitors (PI) to efavirenz (EFV). Presented at the 7th Conference on Retroviruses and Opportunistic Infections, 2000, p 84.
156. Bonnet E, Lepec R, Bluteau M, et al. Evolution of lipodystrophy syndrome and lipidic profile in HIV patients after switching from protease inhibitors to efavirenz. Presented at the 7th Conference on Retroviruses and Opportunistic Infections, 2000, p 84.
157. Negredo E, Cruz L, Ruiz L, et al. Impact of switching from protease inhibitors (PI) to nevirapine (NVP) or efavirenz (EFV) in patients with viral suppression. Presented at the 40th Interscience Conference on Antimicrobial Agents and Chemotherapy, 2000, p 277.
158. Moyle GJ, Baldwin C, Dent N, et al. Management of protease inhibitor (PI)-associated lipodystrophy by substitution with efavirenz (EFV) in virologically controlled HIV-infected persons. Presented at the 39th Interscience Conference on Antimicrobial Agents and Chemotherapy, 1999, p 526.
159. Katlama C. Successful substitution of protease inhibitors with Sustiva (efavirenz) in patients with undetectable plasma HIV-1 RNA levels: results of a prospective, randomized, multicenter, open-label study (DMP 266–027). Presented at the XIII International AIDS Conference, 2000.
160. Bickel M, Rickerts V, Klauke S, et al. The Protra study: switch from PI to abacavir (ABC) and efavirenz (EFV) in HIV-1 infected adults previously treated with 2 NRTIs and a PI with undetectable HIV-RNA levels (vRNA). Presented at the 40th Interscience Conference on Antimicrobial Agents and Chemotherapy, 2000, p 324.
161. Knechten H, Sturner KH, Hohn C, Braun P. 24-Week follow-up of patients switching from a protease inhibitor (PI) containing regimen with lamivudine (3TC) and stavudine (d4T) or zidovudine (AZT) to an efavirenz (EFV) based therapy. Presented at the 40th Interscience Conference on Antimicrobial Agents and Chemotherapy, 2000, p 324.
162. Maggiolo F, Migliorino M, Pravettoni G, et al. Management of PI-associated metabolic changes by substitution with efavirenz in virologically controlled HIV + persons. Presented at the 40th Interscience Conference on Antimicrobial Agents and Chemotherapy, 2000, p 325.
163. Lafon E, Bani Sadr F, Chandemerle C, et al. LIPSTOP study: evolution of clinical lipodystrophy (LD), blood lipids, visceral (VAT) and subcutaneous (SAT) adipose tissue after switching from protease inhibitor (PI) to efavirenz (EFV) in HIV-1 infected patients. Presented at the 40th Interscience Conference on Antimicrobial Agents and Chemotherapy, 2000, p 325.
164. Martinez E, Romeu J, Garcia-Viejo MA, et al. An open randomized study on the replacement of HIV-1 protease inhibitors by efavirenz in chronically suppressed HIV-1-infected patients with lipodystrophy. Presented at the 8th Conference on Retroviruses and Opportunistic Infections, 2001.
165. Estrada V, De Villar NGP, Martinez-Larrad T, et al. Switching to efavirenz from protease inhibitor-based therapy does not improve insulin resistance after one year in HIV patients with lipodystrophy syndrome. Presented at the 8th Conference on Retroviruses and Opportunistic Infections, 2001.
166. Casado JL, Arrizabalaga J, Antela A, et al. Long-term efficacy and tolerance of switching the protease inhibitor for nonnucleoside reverse transcriptase inhibitors: a 52-week, multicenter, prospective study. Presented at the 8th Conference on Retroviruses and Opportunistic Infections, 2001.
167. Martinez E, Conget I, Lozano L, et al. Reversion of metabolic abnormalities after switching from HIV-1 protease inhibitors to nevirapine. AIDS 13:805–10, 1999.
168. Barreiro P, Soriano V, Blanco F, et al. Risks and benefits of replacing protease inhibitors by nevirapine in HIV-infected subjects under long-term successful triple combination therapy. AIDS 14:807–12, 2000.
169. Ruiz L, Negredo E, Domingo P, et al. Clinical, virological, and immunological benefit of switching the protease inhibitor (PI) by nevirapine (NVP) in HAART-experienced patients suffering lipodystrophy (LD): 36-week follow-up. Presented at the 7th Conference on Retroviruses and Opportunistic Infections, 2000, p 114.
170. Carr A, Hudson J, Chuah J, et al. HIV protease inhibitor substitution in patients with lipodystrophy: a randomised, multicentre, open-label study. AIDS 15:1811–15, 2001.
171. Munoz V, Casado JL, Moreno A, et al. Persistent viral suppression after switching a protease inhibitor (PI)-containing regimen to a nonnucleoside reverse transcriptase inhibitor (NNRTI)-based therapy (BEGIN study). Presented at the 39th Interscience Conference on Antimicrobial Agents and Chemotherapy, 1999, p 524.
172. Tebas P, Yarasheski K, Powderly WG, et al. A prospective open-label pilot trial of a maintenance nevirapine (NVP)-containing regimen in patients with undetectable viral loads (VL) on protease inhibitor (PI) regimens for at least 6 months. Presented at the 7th Conference on Retroviruses and Opportunistic Infections, 2000, p 83.
173. Raffi F, Esnault JL, Reliquet V, et al. The maintavir study, substitution of a nonnucleoside reverse transcriptase inhibitor (NNRTI) for a protease inhibitor (PI) in patients with undetectable plasma HIV-1 RNA: 18 months follow-up. Presented at the 40th Interscience Conference on Antimicrobial Agents and Chemotherapy, 2000, p 277.
174. Buisson M, Grappin M, Piroth L, et al. Simplified maintenance therapy with NNRTI (nevirapine) in patients with long-term suppression of HIV-1 RNA: first results of a cohort study. Presented at the 40th Interscience Conference on Antimicrobial Agents and Chemotherapy, 2000, p 327.
175. Saint-Marc T, Partisani M, Poizot-Martin I, Touraine JL. Reversibility of peripheral fat wasting (lipoatrophy) on stopping stavudine therapy. Presented at the 7th Conference on Retroviruses and Opportunistic Infections, 2000, p 85.
176. Goebel FD, Walli RK. A novel use of abacavir to simplify therapy in PI-experienced patients successfully treated with HAART: CNA30017. Presented at the 7th Conference on Retroviruses and Opportunistic Infections, 2000, p 84.
177. Opravil M, Hirschel B, Lazzarin A, et al. Simplified maintenance therapy with abacavir + lamivudine + zidovudine in patients with HAART-induced long-term suppression of

HIV-1 RNA: final results. Presented at the 40th Interscience Conference on Antimicrobial Agents and Chemotherapy, 2000, p 278.

178. Montaner JSG. A novel use of abacavir to simplify therapy and reduce toxicity in PI experienced patients successfully treated with HAART: 48-week results (CNA30017). Presented at the 40th Interscience Conference on Antimicrobial Agents and Chemotherapy, 2000, p 278.
179. Deeks SG, Hoh R, Neilands TB, et al. Interruption of treatment with individual therapeutic drug classes in adults with multidrug-resistant HIV-1 infection. J Infect Dis 192:1537–44, 2005.
180. Miller V, Gute P, Carlebach A, et al. Baseline resistance and virological response to mega-HAART salvage therapies. Presented at the 6th Conference on Retroviruses and Opportunistic Infections, 1999.
181. Workman C, Mussen R, Sullivan J. Salvage therapy using six drugs in heavily pretreated patients. Presented at the 5th Conference on Retroviruses and Opportunistic Infections, 1998.
182. Montaner JSG, Harrigan R, Jahnke N, et al. Multi-drug rescue therapy (MDRT) following failure to multiple regimens: preliminary results [abstract 76c]. Antiviral Ther 3(Suppl 2):80, 1998.
183. Deeks SG, Wrin T, Liegler T, et al. Virologic and immunologic consequences of discontinuing combination antiretroviral-drug therapy in HIV-infected patients with detectable viremia. N Engl J Med 344:472–80, 2001.
184. Miller V, Sabin C, Hertogs K, et al. Virological and immunological effects of treatment interruptions in HIV-1 infected patients with treatment failure. AIDS 14:2857–67, 2000.
185. Miller V, Sabin C, Hertogs K, et al. Antiretroviral treatment interruptions in patients with treatment failure: analyses from the Frankfurt HIV cohort [abstract 25]. Antivir Ther 5(Suppl 2):22, 2000.
186. El-Sadr W, Neaton J. Episodic CD4-guided use of ART is inferior to continuous therapy: results of the SMART study. NEJM 355:2283–2296, 2006.
187. Ananworanich J, Gayet-Agernon A, Lebraz M, et al. CD4 guided scheduled treatment interruption compared to continuous therapy: Results of the Staccato Trial. 13th Conference on Retroviruses and Opportunistic Infections, Denver, CO, 5–8 Feb 2006, abstract 102.
188. Marchou B, Tangre P, Charreau I, et al. Structured treatment interruptions in HIV-infected patients with high CD4 cell counts and virologic suppression: results of a prospective, randomized, open-label trial (Window-ANRS 106). 13th Conference on Retroviruses and Opportunistic Infections, Denver, CO, 5–8 Feb 2006, abstract 104.
189. Danel C, Moh R, Sorho S, et al. The CD4-guided strategy arm stopped in a randomized structured treatment interruption trial in West-African adults: ANRS 1269 Trivacan Trial. 13th Conference on Retroviruses and Opportunistic Infections, Denver, CO, 5–8 Feb 2006, abstract 105LB.
190. Palmisano L, Giuliano M, Bucciardini R, et al. Final results of a randomized, controlled trial of structured treatment interruptions vs continuous HAART in chronic HIV-infected subjects with persistent suppression of viral replication. 13th Conference on Retroviruses and Opportunistic Infections, Denver, CO, 5–8 Feb 2006, abstract 103.
191. Jacobson JM, Bucy PR, Spritzler J, et al. Evidence that intermittent structured treatment interruption, but not immunization with ALVAC-HIV vCP1452, promotes host control of HIV replication: the results of AIDS Clinical Trials Group 5068. J Infect Dis 194:623–32, 2006.
192. Kilby JM, Bucy RP, Mildvan D, et al. A randomized, partially blinded phase 2 trial of antiretroviral therapy, HIV-specific immunizations, and interleukin-2 cycles to promote efficient control of viral replication (ACTG A5024). J Infect Dis 194:1672–6, 2006.

Chapter 5

Zidovudine

Jeffrey L. Lennox, MD, Margaret A. Fischl, MD

Zidovudine (3′-azido-3′-deoxythymidine, AZT) (ZDV) is a pyrimidine nucleoside analog of thymidine (Fig. 5-1). ZDV differs from thymidine in that the 3′-hydroxyl group of thymidine has been replaced. ZDV (Retrovir) was first synthesized in 1964.[1] It was the first nucleoside analog available for the treatment of human immunodeficiency virus (HIV) infection. It was approved by the United States Food and Drug Administration in 1987 based on demonstrable survival benefit in patients with acquired immunodeficiency syndrome (AIDS), and clinical benefit in those with symptomatic or asymptomatic HIV disease who had a CD4+ T-lymphocyte count of 500 cells/mm^3 or less.

MECHANISM OF ACTION AND *IN VITRO* ACTIVITIES

In order to inhibit HIV-1 reverse transcriptase (RT) ZDV requires the addition of three phosphate groups by cellular kinases, forming the active agent zidovudine triphosphate (ZDV-TP).[2,3] Once formed, ZDV-TP is then incorporated into the nascent DNA strand by HIV-1 RT. However, the lack of a 3′-hydroxyl group in ZDV leads to termination of the elongating DNA chain. The initial phosphorylation of ZDV is performed by cellular thymidine kinase-1 (TK-1) and results in ZDV monophosphate (ZDV-MP). TK-1 is a cytosolic enzyme that is primarily active in proliferating cells.[4] Cells from patients with HIV-1 infection have been shown to have higher median TK-1 activity levels, and more variability in activity, than cells from healthy matched controls.[5,6] In a cross-sectional study, patients receiving ZDV therapy were found to have lower TK-1 activity levels when compared to treatment naïve patients, whereas TK-1 activity levels from stavudine-treated patients were not similarly reduced.[5] The clinical importance of this finding is questionable since sequential measures of total cellular ZDV phosphates did not show a significant decline after 12 months of therapy.[7] TK-1 mediated phosphorylation is inhibited by both ribavirin and by doxorubicin, reducing intracellular AMP levels.[8,9] However, subsequent phosphorylation steps are not affected, and ribavirin does not reduce the intracellular activity of ZDV.[10]

Following the initial phosphorylation, ZDV-MP accumulates intracellularly since the conversion of ZDV-MP to ZDV-DP and ZDV-TP is less than 1% as efficient as the conversion of thymidine-MP to thymidine-TP.[2] The accumulation of intracellular ZDV-MP may be responsible for some of the toxicity of ZDV.[11] ZDV-MP binds to the ATP-binding site of TK, further

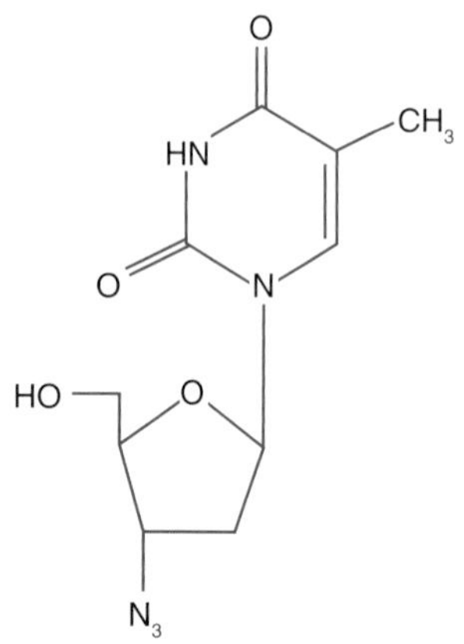

Figure 5-1 ■ Structure of ZDVs.

decreasing its activity. It therefore appears that ZDV works as a chain terminator, also by competitively inhibiting the binding of TTP at the active site in RT, and potentially by depleting intracellular pools of phosphorylated nucleosides. ZDV-TP may also decrease RNAase activity, preventing the degradation of the viral RNA template and inhibiting the formation of the complete viral preintegration complex.[12] The *in vitro* activity of ZDV against HIV-1 is dependent on the activation state of the cell. ZDV has its greatest activity in cells which are metabolically active, such as CD4+ T cells.[13,14] *In vitro*, ZDV has ~100–1000 times more antiviral activity in activated cells versus resting cells. ZDV is much less active in macrophages than is didanosine. ZDV is also less efficiently converted to its active triphosphate form in monocyte-derived dendritic or langerhans cells than is lamivudine or tenofovir.[15] Synergistic activity against HIV-1 has been demonstrated by combinations of ZDV and either abacavir, didanosine, lamivudine, or zalcitabine.[16,17] Since ZDV and stavudine utilize the same phosphorylation pathways, they are antagonistic *in vivo*, although some studies have indicated *in vitro* synergy.[18]

ZDV is active *in vitro* against human immunodeficiency type two (HIV-2) in certain experiments, but not in others.[19] Isolated HIV-2 RT is fourfold less sensitive to ZDV than is HIV-1 RT.[20] Studies from HIV-2 infected patients treated with ZDV have demonstrated the development of ZDV resistance, confirming that ZDV has some activity against this virus.[21] ZDV is also active *in vitro* against human T-cell leukemia/lymphoma virus (HTLV-1). In a single cycle replication assay model for HTLV-1, the 50% inhibitory concentration for ZDV was 0.11 μM/L, versus 22.0 μM/L for lamivudine, 4.6 μM/L for abacavir and 0.005 μM/L for tenofovir.[22] ZDV may also have activity as an antitumor agent for human herpes virus-8 (HHV-8) associated primary effusion lymphoma and for Epstein–Barr virus (EBV) associated Burkett's lymphoma. In a mouse model ZDV was found to induce apoptosis of human-derived EBV-associated primary central nervous system lymphoma cells following induction of EBV-TK expression by ionizing radiation.[23] In cell lines derived from HHV-8 and EBV-associated lymphomas ZDV inhibited the phosphorylation of IκB, reducing the antiapoptotic effects of NFκB and enhancing tumor cell apoptosis.[24] Since interferon alpha (IFN-α) increases tumor cell apoptosis, the combination of IFN-α and ZDV may be a useful treatment for these viral-associated lymphomas.[25,26]

ZDV has activity *in vitro* against certain enteric bacteria, primarily *Salmonella* and Enterobacteriaceae species. The minimal inhibitory concentrations for ZDV against *S. typhimurium* and *E. coli* were 0.5 μg/mL (0.125–4 μg/mL) and 0.125 μg/mL (0.031–1.0 μg/mL) respectively. For the same organisms the inhibitory concentrations for both didanosine and stavudine were approximately 10-fold higher.[27] In a macrophage cell line ZDV had greater inhibitory activity against *S. typhimurium* than did ceftriaxone. ZDV is not inhibitory *in vitro* for *Pseudomonas* sp., gram-positive bacteria, anaerobes, spirochetes, mycobacteria, *Candida* sp., *Mycoplasma* sp., or *Ureaplasma* sp.[28,29] ZDV does not have antiviral activity against hepatitis B virus, hepatitis C virus, herpes simplex virus or cytomegalovirus.

CLINICAL PHARMACOLOGY

ZDV may be administered both orally and intravenously. Following a 2 mg/kg intravenous dose of ZDV plasma levels were found to peak (T_{max}) within 1 h at 1.5–2 μM/L.[30] The T_{max} of ZDV following a 300 mg oral dose is 1.03 h, the C_{max} is 2.59 ± 0.52 μM/L, the AUC_{02-12} hours is 4.59 ± 0.79 μM/L, average bioavailability is 63 ± 13% and the mean volume of distribution is 3.0 + 0.6 L/kg.[31–33] With decreasing CD4+ count levels there is decreasing bioavailability of ZDV in HIV-infected patients.[34] There is conflicting data about the effect of food on ZDV absorption. In patients given a high-fat meal, there was decreased absorption, an increased maximal concentration and an increased half-life of ZDV.[35] However, in another study, patients who were given a standard breakfast had little change in the bioavailability of ZDV.[36] Since ZDV is lipophilic it is likely that its absorption may be influenced by high-fat meals. When ZDV is used as a fixed-dose combination with lamivudine, dose adjustment for meal content would be difficult. ZDV elixir administered rectally produced lower peak plasma levels than was observed when ZDV capsules were administered orally.[37]

ZDV is less than 25% protein bound, primarily to albumin.[38] Intracellularly, the C_{max} of ZDV-TP was 82 FMOL per 10^6 cells following a 300 mg dose.[39] The intracellular half-life of ZDV-TP is ~8–12 h, making ZDV compatible with twice-daily dosing.[32,40] Women may have higher intracellular ZDV-TP levels than men. In AIDS Clinical Trials Group (ACTG) study 161 the AUC of total intracellular phosphorylates of ZDV was significantly higher for women than men.[41] In a separate study, ZDV-TP concentrations were two-fold higher in women than in men, and women had a shorter time to virologic suppression on ZDV therapy.[42]

Approximately 75% of ZDV is metabolized by the enzyme uridine diphosphoglucuronyltransferase to form 5′-glucuronylzidovudine (GZDV).[43] This enzyme has been shown to be induced by both rifampin and rifabutin. Of the remaining 25% of ZDV, 15–20% is excreted as the parent compound in urine, and ~2% is metabolized to 3′-amino-3′-deoxythymidine (AMT).[44,45] In a study of ZDV clearance in children, it was found that those less than 2 weeks of age had impaired glucuronidation.[46] Infants therefore had higher levels of ZDV, and decreased ZDV clearance, compared to older children.

Since ZDV is excreted in the urine, patients with reduced glomerular filtration rates have impaired ZDV clearance. Clearance of ZDV has been shown to be decreased by ~50% in those with severe renal insufficiency.[47] Dose adjustment for ZDV is therefore necessary in patients who have a creatinine clearance of less than 10–20 mL/min. Dialysis has little effect on ZDV levels, since ZDV is highly lipophilic. Probenecid decreases excretion of GZDV.[48] Renal excretion of GZDV is also reduced by the histamine H2 receptor antagonist cimetidine, but not by ranitidine.[49] This effect is not sufficient to be clinically significant. ZDV clearance is also affected by a hepatic disease. In HIV uninfected patients with cirrhosis, the glucuronidation of ZDV has been found to be reduced by approximately threefold.[50] Similar findings have been found in a small study of patients with AIDS and hepatic disease, in which clearance was reduced by 63%.[51] In a study of patients with mild liver disease ZDV clearance was reduced by only 32%.[52] Pregnancy does not appear to affect the pharmacokinetics of ZDV.[53]

As expected of a lipophilic compound, the penetration of ZDV into the central nervous system is relatively high. In several studies, the cerebrospinal fluid (CSF) to plasma ZDV ratio ranged from 0.15 to 1.53.[33,54,55] In adults given ZDV at doses ranging from 600 to 1500 mg/day, the median CSF ZDV concentration equaled 0.153 μM/L (0.056–0.027 μM/L) and the CSF:plasma ratio varied from 0.09 to 1.2.[54] In other studies, sequential sampling of individual patients has shown up to a 200% difference in CSF ZDV concentrations over time.[54] This high degree of variability may be due, in part, to differences in adherence over the interval studied. Intravenous dosing of ZDV eliminates this potential effect. In children given intravenous ZDV, the CSF to plasma ratio was ~0.25 ± 0.09.[56] In adults treated intravenously the CSF to plasma ratio was ~0.75 ± 0.26.[57] Nucleoside analog levels in brain parenchyma may not be accurately predicted by CSF levels since brain endothelial transport proteins actively remove nucleosides from the central nervous system.[57] However, ZDV is less of a substrate for these transporters than is didanosine. ZDV has also been shown to improve cognition in patients with AIDS dementia complex.[58]

ZDV levels in other bodily fluids and compartments have been extensively studied. ZDV levels in salivary fluid have been found to be correlated with those in plasma.[59] ZDV levels in semen have varied, depending on the fraction of the semen studied. In one study, the semen to serum ratio varied from 0.35 to 5.5.[60] It is likely that lipid-rich components of semen, and cells in semen, will have therapeutic levels of ZDV. ZDV treatment in nonpregnant women has been shown to lead to a significantly faster decay in viral RNA levels in cervix and vaginal secretions than that observed for plasma.[61] Approximately 70% of ZDV crosses the placenta.[62] In newborns, umbilical and venous ZDV levels have been found to be approximately equivalent.[53] In aborted fetuses from 26 HIV-infected women given a 200 mg dose of ZDV, the fetal plasma level was 92% of the maternal plasma level.[63] In two studies of a total of 30 lactating women who were receiving treatment with ZDV, drug levels in breast milk were found to exceed those in plasma by 1.48–3.21-fold.[64,65] This result is in agreement with the lipophilic properties of ZDV.

ADVERSE REACTIONS

Common symptoms and laboratory abnormalities reported with ZDV include headache, fatigue, malaise, myalgia, anorexia, nausea, anemia, and neutropenia (Table 5-1).[66–68]

Table 5-1 Side Effects Associated with ZDV

Headache	Vomiting	Myopathy[a]
Fatigue	Anorexia	Fever[b]
Myalgia	Anemia	Rash[b]
Insomnia	Neutropenia	Hepatitis[b]
Nausea	Nail pigmentation[a]	Steatosis/lactic acidosis[b]
	Lipoatrophy[a]	

[a]Associated with long-term use.

[b]Rare events.

Atlas of Infectious Diseases. Philadelphia: Current Medicine, with permission.

Of the symptom side effects, only vomiting was statistically significantly greater with ZDV use in randomized trials comparing ZDV to either stavudine or abacavir.[69,70] Initial symptoms, particularly headache, insomnia, fatigue, and gastrointestinal problems, are mild and can be managed symptomatically. In a small percentage of patients, particularly those receiving three- and four-drug regimens, persistent symptoms may require modification of the dose of ZDV or substitution by another nucleoside analog. Rare cases of rash and fever have been described that necessitated discontinuing ZDV.

Anemia is more prominent in advanced disease than in early disease (7% vs 1%, respectively). Serum folate levels are normal or elevated, and vitamin B_{12} levels are normal or slightly decreased. The reticulocyte count is frequently depressed and may be the first sign of bone marrow toxicity. Bone marrow examinations in cases of severe anemia show a decrease or absence of red blood cell precursors. Erythropoietin levels are commonly elevated and in some cases are quite high (>500 IU/L), suggesting that ZDV-induced erythroid hypoplasia is not due to interference with erythropoietin production but is more likely due to inhibition of cell commitment to the erythroid line or direct toxic effects on committed erythroid stem cells.[71] Anemia can be seen as early as 4–6 weeks after initiation of ZDV. Progressive declines in the hemoglobin concentration should signal the potential for severe anemia, particularly if the hemoglobin concentration declines to 7.5–8.0 g/dL. In cases of severe anemia, ZDV (whenever possible) should be temporarily interrupted until the hemoglobin concentration increases, which typically takes 7–14 days. Recombinant human erythropoietin has been shown to be safe and to decrease blood transfusion requirements in patients without marked elevation in endogenous erythropoietin levels who develop severe anemia while receiving ZDV.[72] Alternatively, the dose of ZDV can be decreased or another antiretroviral agent substituted for ZDV. Abacavir, stavudine, and tenofovir have all been shown to cause less anemia than ZDV in comparative trials.[69,70,73] Macrocytosis with an elevation in the mean corpuscular volume of 25–40 units is common and is typically not associated with anemia. Increases in mean corpuscular volume can occur within 6–8 weeks of starting ZDV and are most prominent after 16–24 weeks.

Neutropenia also occurs more frequently during advanced HIV disease than in the early stages of the disease (37% vs

8%, respectively) and is noted within 12–24 weeks of initiating ZDV. ZDV suppresses the receptor for granulocyte-monocyte colony stimulating factor (GM-CSF) on murine bone marrow cells.[74] It is not known whether ZDV causes neutropenia in humans by a similar mechanism. Mild to moderate neutropenia, manifested by neutrophil counts of 750–1000 cells/mm^3, may be more frequent and does not require any adjustments in the ZDV dose. Declines in the neutrophil count to less than 750 cells/mm^3 suggest a need to decrease the dose of ZDV or temporarily interrupt the drug (when possible) until the neutrophil count increases. If persistent or recurrent neutropenia occurs, another antiretroviral agent can be substituted for ZDV. In an open label trial comparing indinavir plus lamivudine, in combination with either ZDV or stavudine, there was no significant difference in the occurrence of neutropenia between ZDV and stavudine.[70] In two double-blind trials ZDV was shown to cause neutropenia more frequently than does tenofovir, but not more frequently than abacavir.[69,73]

Long-term use of ZDV may be associated with several toxicities, including nail hyperpigmentation, hepatic toxicity, muscle toxicity and lipoatrophy. The nail hyperpigmentation consists of multiple longitudinal streaks and diffuse pigment changes ranging from shades of blue to brown-black.[75] Nails on both the hands and feet can be involved, and pigment changes appear to move distally from the base of the nail. Hyperpigmentation changes in the nail appear to occur more frequently among those of the black African population. Associated skin pigment changes have not been described.

Muscle toxicity manifested by myalgia, progressive muscle wasting, weakness, and elevation of the serum creatine kinase concentration has been described, as well as rare cases of cardiomyopathy. The lower extremities and gluteal muscles appear to be preferentially involved. Muscle biopsy histology is consistent with a destructive mitochondrial myopathy with ragged-red fibers and proliferation of abnormal mitochondria.[76] Reduction of mitochondrial DNA has been noted and is likely due to inhibition of mitochondrial DNA replication by DNA polymerase-γ.[77] Asymptomatic elevations in creatine kinase may also be seen.

Increased liver enzyme levels have been noted with ZDV use, although in a comparative trial stavudine was more likely to cause such abnormalities than was ZDV.[70] In comparative trials ZDV was not more likely to cause liver enzyme elevations than either tenofovir or abacavir.[69,73] In a subset of patients ZDV use may be associated with severe steatosis, lactic acidosis, and death. This syndrome is typically characterized by progressive increases in liver aminotransferase levels and moderate to severe hepatomegaly. Scans and biopsy of the liver are consistent with steatosis. Associated symptoms of tachypnea, dsypnea, and severe acidosis with progressive liver and renal failure and death have been described and are mostly due to dysfunction of hepatic mitochondria. This syndrome has now been described with most nucleoside RT inhibitors (NRTIs). Most of these cases have been in women. Obesity and prolonged administration may be risk factors. In a case series of eight patients, and a review of 50 other reported cases, use of ZDV was associated with higher mortality than that observed with stavudine or lamivudine.[78] However, fatalities associated with ZDV may have been more frequent due to failure to recognize and treat this syndrome in the 1980s and early 1990s. If this syndrome is suspected, antiretroviral therapy should be interrupted. Uridine has shown *in vitro* beneficial effects on reducing the toxic effects of ZDV on hepatocytes.[79] A sugarcane extract, mitocnol, increases uridine levels in humans and is being tested for other nucleoside-associated toxicities.

Changes in body fat composition, particularly lipoatrophy, have been reported in patients receiving ZDV. The incidence of lipoatrophy appears to be less for ZDV-treated patients than for stavudine-treated patients. In two prospective studies that compared stavudine to ZDV, both in combination with lamivudine and a third agent, the incidence of lipoatrophy at 30–36 weeks was 48–57% in the stavudine arm and 19–22% in the ZDV arm.[80,81] The combination of ZDV and lamivudine also appears to produce less lipoatrophy than a stavudine/didanosine combination. In a substudy of ACTG Study 384, in which these two nucleoside combinations were compared in treatment naive patients, 157 patients underwent body fat measurements and dual-energy X-ray absorptiometry (DEXA) scanning at 16 week intervals.[82] After the first 16 weeks of treatment, limb fat increased by 9.4% in the stavudine-containing arm and by 11.6% in the ZDV-containing arm. Limb fat subsequently decreased in both groups after week 16, but to a greater extent in the stavudine-containing arm. By week 64 total limb fat in the ZDV group had decreased nearly to baseline, whereas the stavudine group had a net loss of 16.8% of limb fat compared to baseline. In contrast to stavudine, tenofovir is less likely to result in lipoatrophy than ZDV. In a randomized study comparing tenofovir and ZDV, both in combination with emtricitabine and efavirenz, week-48 total limb fat was significantly less in a subgroup of patients in the ZDV–lamivudine group who underwent DEXA scanning than in a subgroup of patients in the tenofovir–emtricitabine group (mean, 6.9 kg vs 8.9 kg respectively; $P = 0.03$).[73] In a separate study, 12 patients who replaced ZDV with tenofovir had approximately a 4% increase in limb fat over 24 weeks.[83] This result indicates that ZDV-induced lipoatrophy is partially reversible after discontinuation of ZDV.

The mechanisms by which ZDV therapy causes lipoatrophy in humans have not been completely determined. In 20 HIV-uninfected patients who were given either stavudine or ZDV for 2 weeks, and who then had a biopsy of adipose tissue performed, both nucleoside analogs produced a decrease in adipose mitochondrial DNA transcription compared to baseline.[84] Another group compared 12 HIV-uninfected controls to 18 lipoatrophic patients who had been treated with stavudine (12) or ZDV (6) containing regimens for ~30 months.[85] Compared to the controls, the nucleoside-treated patients had no difference in adipose mitochondrial DNA content and no difference in tumor necrosis factor alpha levels in plasma or in adipose tissue. There was a decrease in plasma adiponectin levels of 50% in those receiving ZDV and of 58% in those receiving stavudine. Both groups had equal reductions in mitochondrial respiratory chain enzymes. These results suggest that ZDV may cause dysfunction of adipose mitochondria and of adiponectin production.

CLINICAL EFFICACY

ZDV in combination with other antiretroviral agents is discussed in subsequent chapters of this book. Monotherapy trials and comparative trials of ZDV are detailed in Table 5-2 and discussed below.

ZDV Placebo-Controlled Trials

ZDV was the first antiretroviral agent to indicate that treatment intervention can improve the outcome in HIV disease. For advanced HIV disease, the probability of surviving more than 24 weeks was significantly better for ZDV recipients than for placebo recipients (0.98 vs 0.78; $P < 0.001$).[86] Similarly, the risk of disease progression over 24 weeks was significantly lower for ZDV recipients than for placebo recipients (0.23 vs 0.43; $P < 0.001$). Subsequent placebo-controlled studies showed that the risk of disease progression was decreased more than threefold by 18 months for patients with symptomatic disease (3.23; $P = 0.0002$) and by 12 months for patients with asymptomatic disease (3.1; $P = 0.005$).[67,87] No differences in survival were demonstrable in either study. Early versus delayed use of ZDV therapy has also been evaluated in patients with asymptomatic and with symptomatic HIV infection. The estimated 3-year survival probabilities were 92% for immediate therapy and 94% for delayed therapy for asymptomatic patients. Similar findings were noted for progression to AIDS or death.[88] Another study compared ZDV therapy in symptomatic patients who started treatment at CD4+ counts between 200 and 500/mm^3 versus ZDV begun when the CD4+ counts fell below 200/mm^3.[89] There were 23 deaths in the early-therapy group ($n = 170$) and 20 deaths in the late-therapy group ($n = 168$) ($P = 0.48$). In the early-therapy group fewer patients developed AIDS ($P = 0.02$; relative risk, 1.76); and early therapy prolonged the time to a CD4+ count below 200/mm^3. These data confirmed the benefit of ZDV but pointed out the limited duration of the benefit.

ZDV Perinatal Transmission Trials

ZDV is approved for the prevention of perinatal transmission in pregnant women with HIV infection and newborns of women with HIV infection. In one study the estimated risk of HIV infection in the newborn was 8.3% for ZDV recipients compared to 25.5% for placebo recipients, a 67.5% reduction in the relative risk of HIV transmission.[90] Chemoprophylaxis consisted of three components, including oral ZDV administration to pregnant women during the second and third trimesters, intravenous administration to pregnant women during labor and delivery, and oral administration to infants during the first 6 weeks of life. Short antepartum and intrapartum regimens of ZDV also reduced perinatal transmission by 50%.[91] (For a detailed discussion of the use of zidovudine and other antiretrovirals during pregnancy, *see* Chapter 36.)

ZDV Primary Infection Trials

ZDV has been evaluated for the treatment of primary HIV infection. In one study, disease progression among ZDV recipients (one case) was significantly less than in placebo recipients (seven cases; $P = 0.009$).[92] The relative risk of disease progression for ZDV recipients compared with placebo recipients was 0.008 ($P = 0.03$).

ZDV Comparative Trials

Comparing ZDV and zalcitabine among patients with minimal prior therapy, ZDV proved more effective.[93] In patients with advanced HIV disease who had little or no prior ZDV therapy, ZDV provided a 1.5-fold decrease in disease progression compared with zalcitabine. Estimated 1-year survival rates were 85% for zalcitabine recipients and 92% for ZDV recipients ($P = 0.007$). Comparing ZDV and didanosine among patients with extensive prior ZDV therapy, didanosine provided a threefold decrease in disease progression compared with continuing ZDV (relative risk (RR) 1.39; confidence interval (CI) 1.06–1.82; $P = 0.0015$).[94] However, for patients with advanced HIV disease and no or minimal prior ZDV therapy, ZDV provided a more than twofold decrease in disease progression compared with didanosine (RR 1.43, CI 1.02–2.00).[95]

ZDV Efficacy for Other Conditions

In areas where HTLV-1 is endemic, co-infection with HIV-1 may occur and HTLV-1-associated complications may develop. HIV-uninfected patients with HTLV-1 associated leukemia or lymphoma have shown favorable therapeutic responses to the combination of ZDV and IFN-α. Clinical response rates of 25–58% have been reported from various case series.[96–98] Others have not had similarly favorable results.[99] ZDV has also shown promise in a pilot study of 10 patients with HTLV-1 associated myelopathy.[100] Seven out of 10 had significant improvement in their ability to ambulate. In the developing world ZDV may also be useful for preventing relapses of salmonella bacteremia. In one study, nine of 17 patients who did not receive ZDV had a relapse of bacteremia, versus none of the 15 ZDV treated patients ($p < 0.01$).[101] Another study found that patients taking ZDV were less likely to experience a relapse of *Salmonella* than those taking ampicillin or trimethopim/sulfamethoxazole.[102]

ZDV RESISTANCE

Resistance to ZDV generally requires the accumulation of several mutations in the viral *pol* gene. The rate of change in susceptibility of viral isolates to ZDV is associated with the stage of HIV disease (Fig. 5-2).[103] Recent advances in

Table 5-2

Trials of ZDV Monotherapy

Trial	Design	Dosage	No. of Subjects	Entry Criteria	CD4+/Lymphocytes on Entry (cells/mm^3)
Fischl et al[86] (BWO2)	Placebo controlled, randomized, double blind	ZDV 250 mg q4 h	282	AIDS or ARC; CD4 <100, 101–499	49(p), 54(z) (medians); 128(p), 190(z) (medians)
Fischl et al[87] (ACTG 016)	Placebo controlled, randomized, double blind	ZDV 200 mg q4 h	711	Mildly symptomatic; CD4 >200, <800	225 (median)
Volberding et al[67] (ACTG 019)	Placebo controlled, randomized, double blind	300 mg 5×/day or 100 mg 5×/day	1338	Asymptomatic; CD4 <500	350
Anonymous[88] Concorde	Placebo controlled, randomized, double blind	250 mg bid initially; or deferred until start of symptoms or low CD4 counts[a] (open label ZDV then)	1749	Asymptomatic	42% >500; 52% >201, <500; 6% <200
Hamilton et al[89,140] (V.A. Cooperative Study 298)	Placebo controlled, randomized, double blind	250 mg bid initially; or deferred until CD4 counts less than 200 (open label ZDV then)	338	Symptomatic, CD4 200-500 cells/mm^3	348(p), 359(z) (mean)
Kinloch-De Loes et al[92]	Placebo controlled, randomized, double blind	ZDV 250 mg bid for 6 months	77	Acute retroviral syndrome, p24 antigenemia, and low or negative HIV ab tests	519(p), 477(z) (mean)
Dolin et al[33] (ACTG 116a)	ddI vs ZDV; randomized, double blind	ddI: 500 or 750 mg/day ZDV: 600 mg/day	617	Symptomatic: CD4 <300 or Asymptomatic: CD4 <200; Previous ZDV experience of <16 weeks	130 (median)
Kahn et al[94] (ACTG 116b/117)	ddI vs ZDV; randomized, double blind	ddI: 500 or 750 mg/day ZDV: 600 mg/day	913	As for ACTG 116a above, but >16 weeks of previous ZDV experience	95 (median)
Follansbee et al[93] (ACTG 114/ Ro3300)	ddC vs ZDV; randomized, double blind	ddC: 2.25 mg/day ZDV: 600 mg/day	635	AIDS or ARC, less than 3 months of prior ZDV use	Unknown

CD4+ Lymphocyte Response	Antiviral Response	Clinical Outcome	Comments
Counts increased in ZDV recipients[86]	p24 antigenemia decreased in ZDV recipients	ZDV increased survival and decreased OIs over 24 weeks	Benefits demonstrated for CD4 count[a] <100; study was halted before effect on higher CD4 counts could be fully evaluated.
Counts increased by 44 in pts with entry counts of >200, but <500; no significant changes in counts for those with >500 on entry[87]	Rate of p24 antigenemia decreased by 50% in 65% of ZDV recipients and in 15% of placebo recipients	ZDV decreased progression of disease in pts with CD4 >200, but <500; no effect on survival	Insufficient events occurred to assess effects on pts. With CD4 >500, less toxicity than in pts with more advanced disease (BWO2).
Median increase of[67] 26–39/mm^3	Decrease in rate of p24 antigenemia compared to placebo.	ZDV decreased progression of disease; no effects on survival	ZDV dose of 1500 mg/day was more toxic than 500 mg/day dose.
Increase of 20/mm^3 in immediate ZDV and decrease of 9/mm^3 in deferred ZDV, at 3 months[88]		No difference in clinical outcomes between immediate and deferred ZDV at 3 years; transient delay in disease progression at 1 year with immediate ZDV therapy	Indicated that benefit of monotherapy with ZDV was temporally limited.
ZDV recipients gained 0.3 cells at 12 months; placebo lost 48.7 cells at 12 months[140]	At 16 weeks 15/19 ZDV recipients had negative p24, vs 6/7. Peak ZDV RNA response −0.6 $\log_{10}$	No difference in deaths, placebo group had a 1.75 relative risk of progressing to AIDS	Indicated that ZDV prolonged the time to AIDS if given between 200 and 500 CD4+ cells/mm^3
ZDV recipients gained 8.9 cells/month; placebo lost 12.0 cells/month[92]	No difference in p24 or HIV RNA responses	Disease progression (primarily minor OI) was less frequent in ZDV group; no effect on acute retroviral syndrome	Long-term benefits not assessed. ZDV was relatively well tolerated.

(Continued)

Table 5-2 (Continued)

CD4+ Lymphocyte Response	Antiviral Response	Clinical Outcome			Comments
ddI 500 mg group had slower decline in counts than ddI 750 mg or ZDV group[33]	No difference in p24 declines among three treatment groups	**Group**	**Deaths (No.)**	**AIDS Events or Deaths (/100 pt-year)**	ZDV more effective than 750 ddI in ZDV-naive patients; 500 ddI more effective than ZDV in patients with >8 but <16 weeks ddI. No significant differences in efficacy between 500 and 750 ddI, but 750 ddI was more toxic.
		ZDV naive			
		500 ddI	10	32.3	
		750 ddI	10	36.6	
		ZDV	9	26.6	
		ZDV <8 weeks			
		500 ddI	3	27.8	
		750 ddI	4	25.1	
		ZDV	3	24.1	
		ZDV >8, but <16 weeks			
		500 ddI	4	24.8	
		750 ddI	3	31.5	
		ZDV	3	52.5	
CD4 change/mm^3 at 24 weeks: 500 ddI: −10 750 ddI: −10 ZDV: −23[94]	% of subjects with at least 50% p24 decrease at 24 weeks: 500 ddI: 21 750 ddI: 32 ZDV: 21	**Group**	**Deaths (/100 pt-year)**	**AIDS Events or Deaths(/100 pt-year)**	Dose of 500 ddI more effective than ZDV for reduction of risk of primary endpoints.
		500 ddI	15.5	37.1	
		750 ddI	17.5	42.5	
		ZDV	16.9	52.8	
Not Done[93]	Not Done	ddC-treated group had a 1.76 increase in the relative risk of death compared to the ZDV-treated group.			Indicated that monotherapy with ZDV superior to monotherapy with ddC.

ab, antibody; ARC, AIDS-related complex; ddI, didanosine; OI, opportunistic infection; pt, patient; ZDV, zidovudine.

[a]CD4+ lymphocyte count.

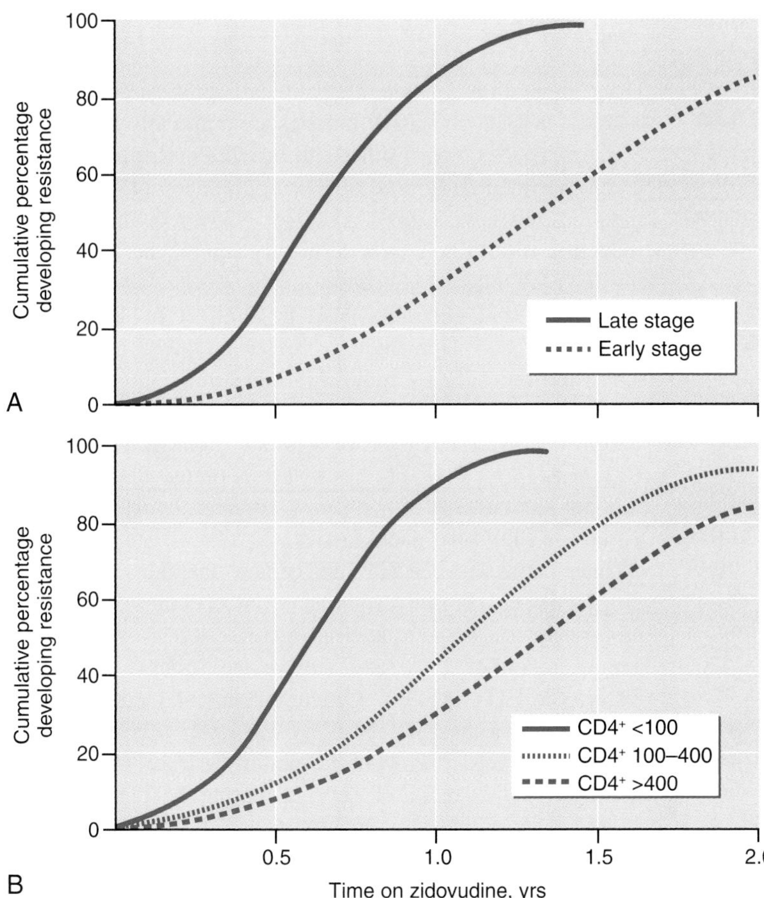

Figure 5-2 ■ Proportion of patients developing viral resistance to ZDV based on stage of disease (**A**) and CD4+ T-lymphocyte count (**B**).

From Fischl MA. Antiviral treatments. In: Mandell GL, Mildvan D (eds) Atlas of Infectious Diseases. Philadelphia: Current Medicine, with permission.

the elucidation of the mechanisms behind the development of resistance to ZDV have provided new insights into the general mechanisms of antiretroviral nucleoside analog resistance. In general, resistance to ZDV can develop through two distinct mechanisms. The most common of these is the excision of ZDV-MP subsequent to its incorporation into the nascent DNA strand, also known as 'primer unblocking'.[104] In the wild-type RT enzyme of HIV-1, the incorporation of ZDV-MP liberates a pyrophosphate group from ZDV-TP. In the subsequent step of the reverse transcription process, the newly incorporated ZDV-MP moves from the N site to the H site of the enzyme. The incoming native nucleotide then binds to the N site, protecting the ZDV-MP from excision. Prior to the binding of the incoming nucleotide, the liberated pyrophosphate from ZDV-TP may bind to the incorporated ZDV-MP, and the RT enzyme can then excise the incorporated analog. This process, which occurs in the wild-type enzyme, is called pyrophosphorolysis. Any process which delays the transition of the ZDV-MP from the N site to the H site, or which allows the entry of a pyrophosphate donor into the active site, enhances the resistance of the HIV-1 to ZDV. For patients who have been treated with ZDV, a group of RT mutants called thymidine analog mutations (TAMS) enhances the excision of ZDV-MP.

The most common TAMS are M41L, D67N, K70R, L210W, T215Y and F, and K219Q and E. Generally, the TAMS develop through two separate pathways and result in a partially overlapping complex of mutations. In one pathway the L210W and T215Y mutations develop, and in the other pathway the K70R and T215F mutations develop. A RT enzyme which contains three to six TAMS confers greater than 500-fold resistance to ZDV. Mechanistic studies have revealed that TAMS confer resistance by facilitating the entry of pyrophosphate and ATP into the RT active site, and by stabilizing the RT structure with ZDV-MP bound in the N site.[105–108] ATP is the most common pyrophosphate donor when TAMS are present. When ATP enters the active site and binds to ZDV-MP, RT-mediated excision removes the ZDV-MP, liberates ZDVppppA, and restores the ability of the viral RNA to be transcribed. Primer unblocking is more complete in viral RT enzymes that possess the 67/70/219Q complex than viral enzymes with 41/210/215Y.[109] TAMS are not the only mutations that result in primer unblocking. A two base insertion at position 69 (69INS) causes broad nucleoside analog cross resistance through ATP-mediated primer unblocking.[110,111]

Mutations in the RNAseH domain of the RT may increase the primer unblocking effect of TAMS. RNAseH is necessary to degrade the viral RNA template following the process of reverse transcription. Theoretically, reductions in RNAseH activity will increase the time available for excision of ZDV-MP from a terminated primer since the viral reverse transcription complex will be stabilized by the continued presence of the RNA template. Evidence supporting this concept comes from experiments in which the introduction of an RNAseH mutation in position 539 in an RT that contains four TAMS increased ZDV resistance ninefold compared to the TAMS alone.[112] Detecting such mutations is difficult outside of a research laboratory since current, commercially available genotype and phenotype assays do not detect mutations in the RNAseH domain.

Other mutations in the viral RT can either slow the development of TAMS, or partially reverse their primer unblocking properties. The M184V mutation, which causes resistance to lamivudine and stavudine, decreases the effect of TAMS on primer unblocking and also delays the development of TAMS.[113,114] A similar effect is observed with the tenofovir-associated K65R mutation.[115] The M184V and the K65R mutations therefore do not reduce the sensitivity of the viral RT to ZDV. The binding of non-nucleoside RT inhibitors (NNRTIs) *in vitro* to wild-type RT changes the structure of the nucleoside binding pocket and reduces the likelihood of pyrophosphorolysis.[116] NNRTI-induced mutations can have a similar effect. The Y181C mutation associated with nevirapine resistance reduces primer unblocking of ZDV-MP.[117,118] Such effects of NNRTI, and the effect of M184V, may partially explain the favorable efficacy of combinations which include ZDV, lamivudine, and an NNRTI.

The alternative method by which RT develops resistance to ZDV is through a reduction of the ability of ZDV to enter the active site and bind to the N domain of RT. The best studied example of this type of resistance is the M184V mutation, which imparts resistance to lamivudine and emtricitabine. This mutation changes the shape of the active site and interferes with binding by lamivudine and emtricitabine through steric interference. For ZDV a similar process has been observed with a complex of mutations which includes Q151M. The Q151M complex may contain Q151M, F116Y, F77L, V75I, and A62V. RT enzymes which possess this complex are sensitive to tenofovir and lamivudine, but are resistant to the remaining nucleoside analogs. The Q151M complex does not create a steric interference preventing ZDV-entry into the active site. However, it does decrease the electrostatic interactions between ZDV-TP and the components of the active site, which allows preferential entry and binding of native nucleotides.[119] This pathway to resistance is particularly important for HIV-2. The RT of HIV-2 is fourfold less sensitive to ZDV *in vitro* than the HIV-1 enzyme. The HIV-1 RT enzyme has been shown to be more efficient at incorporation of ZDV than the HIV-2 RT enzyme. However, the HIV-1 RT is also more efficient at primer unblocking.[20] HIV-2 is therefore more likely to develop resistance through the Q151M pathway. This has been confirmed *in vivo*, where Q151M has been found to be present in over a quarter of HIV-2 infected patients whose viral load is not suppressed on thymidine analog-containing regimens.[21]

The development of resistance to ZDV in bacteria has been associated with either decreased TK activity, or with TK deficient mutants.[120,121]

DRUG INTERACTIONS

Drug interactions of potential clinical significance are summarized in Table 5-3. ZDV kinetics are minimally affected by concurrent use of most other antiretrovirals. Ritonavir, when given in a total daily dose of 600 mg, induces ZDV glucuronidation and lowers ZDV AUC by ~25%.[122] This level of reduction is not likely to be clinically significant. Nevirapine lowers ZDV plasma concentration by ~30%, whereas both delavirdine and efavirenz have little effect on ZDV pharmacokinetics.[123] Tipranavir decreases the AUC of ZDV by 43%, and the C_{max} by 61%.[124] Studies to establish whether this degree of decrease has a clinical effect have not been performed. Atazanavir given without ritonavir reduces the C_{min} of ZDV by 31%, but has no effect on the ZDV AUC.[125] It is not known what effect, if any, ritonavir boosted atazanavir has on ZDV pharmacokinetics.

Interactions between ZDV and certain other nonantiretroviral drugs may be clinically significant. Atovaquone, methadone, probenecid and valproic acid all increase levels of ZDV. Co-administration of ZDV and atovaquone resulted in a 31% increase in ZDV AUC.[126] Concurrent use of methadone and ZDV increased the ZDV AUC by 29–41%, without affecting methadone levels.[127] Probenecid inhibits both the glucuronidation and renal excretion of ZDV, increasing the ZDV AUC by 45%, and causing rash in three-fourths of HIV-infected patients who were given ZDV and probenecid.[48,128] Valproic acid inhibits the glucuronidation of ZDV and increases the ZDV AUC by 80%.[129] This effect may be clinically relevant given the recent interest in using valproic acid to reduce the size of the latently infected cell reservoir. The co-administration of ZDV with a daily dose of 400 mg of fluconazole in 12 HIV-infected patients demonstrated a 74% increase in the AUC of ZDV.[130] In contrast, the same fluconazole dose given to 20 other HIV-infected patients produced no change in ZDV pharmacokinetics.[131] ZDV AUC is decreased 32% by rifabutin and 47% by rifampin.[132,133] For both of these medications no dosing change is recommended for ZDV since the effect on intracellular ZDV-TP levels is unknown. Clarithromycin given simultaneously with ZDV reduced the ZDV C_{max} and AUC, but did not have a similar effect in another study in which clarithromycin was given 2–4 h prior to ZDV.[134,135] Azithromycin did not affect plasma concentrations of ZDV, but did increase the intracellular ZDV-TP concentration significantly.[136] ZDV in combination with ganciclovir, hydroxyurea, IFN-α and bone marrow suppressive agents may result in increased hematological toxicity.

CLINICAL USE

Regimens

ZDV has been used alone and in various combination regimens for the treatment of patients with HIV infection. As a result of improved clinical outcomes with combination regimens and the decreased risk for viral resistance, ZDV monotherapy for the treatment of patients with HIV infection is no

Drug Interactions With ZDV

Table 5-3

Medication	Effect on ZDV	Clinical Recommendations	References
Atazanavir (reyataz)	Inhibits glucuronidation. No change in AUC or C_{max}, but 31% decrease in C_{min}	No dosing change	125
Atovaquone (mepron)	Inhibits glucuronidation. AUC increased 31%	Monitor for toxicity	126
Azithromycin (Zithromax)	Enhances phosphorylation	No dosing change	136
Clarithromycin (biaxin)	Enhances phosphorylation. C_{max} decreased 41% when given simultaneously. C_{max} and AUC unchanged if dosed separately	No dosing change	134, 135
Fluconazole (diflucan)	Possibly inhibits glucuronidation. Inconsistent study results	No dosing change	130, 131
Ganciclovir (cytovene) Valganciclovir (valcyte)	Inhibits phosphorylation, C_{max} increased 62% and AUC decreased 22%	Avoid use due to overlapping toxicities	141
Hydroxyurea	Enhances phosphorylation 2–3 fold	Avoid use due to overlapping toxicities	142
Methadone (dolophine)	Inhibits glucuronidation and renal clearance. AUC increased 29–41%	Monitor for toxicity	127
Nevirapine (viramune)	Induces glucuronidation, C_{max} decreased 30%	No dosing change	123
Probenecid	Decreases renal clearance by 45% and inhibits glucuronidation	Monitor for toxicity	48, 128
Ribavirin (rebetrol, Ribasphere, copegus)	May decrease phosphorylation	Avoid use due to overlapping toxicities	8–10
Rifabutin (mycobutin)	Induces glucuronidation. C_{max} decreased 48%, AUC decreased 32%	No dosing change, effect on intracellular ZDV-TP levels unknown	132
Rifampin	Induces glucuronidation. C_{max} decreased 43%, AUC decreased 47%	No dosing change, effect on intracellular ZDV-TP levels unknown	133
Ritonavir (norvir) (given 300 mg TID)	Mechanism of interaction unknown Decreases C_{max} 27%, decreases AUC 26%	No dosing change	122
Tipranavir (aptivus)	Induces glucuronidation. Decreases C_{max} 39%, decreases AUC 57%	Appropriate dose not established	124
Valproic acid	Inhibits glucuronidation. Increase in AUC 80%	Monitor for toxicity	129, 143

longer recommended. ZDV is currently recommended as the initial treatment of choice for treatment-naive patients in combination with either lamivudine or emtricitabine, and both in combination with either efavirenz or lopinavir/ritonavir fixed-dose combination.[137] The combination of ZDV, lamivudine, and abacavir should not be used as initial therapy when one of the preferred combinations listed above can be used instead.

ZDV has also been used to decrease the risk of HIV transmission when administered to HIV-infected pregnant women or uninfected individuals following an occupational exposure.[90] It has also been used to improve platelet counts in patients with HIV-related thrombocytopenia and to improve cognitive function in patients with AIDS-related dementia.[58]

Dosage and Dose Frequency

ZDV was initially administered as 200 mg every 4 h. This regimen was selected based on a rapid elimination half-life of 1 h and target serum concentration of 1 mM. Subsequent studies of early and advanced HIV disease utilizing lower daily doses (100 mg five or six times daily) demonstrated equivalent efficacy with less toxicity (Fig. 5-3).[66] Based on the estimated intracellular half-life for ZDV 5′-triphosphate of 8–11 h, ZDV dosing was changed to 200 mg three times a day and most recently to 300 mg twice daily. ZDV, given as 100 mg every 4 h or as 300 mg every 12 h for 48 weeks in one study, resulted in no significant differences in adverse experiences.[138] Although

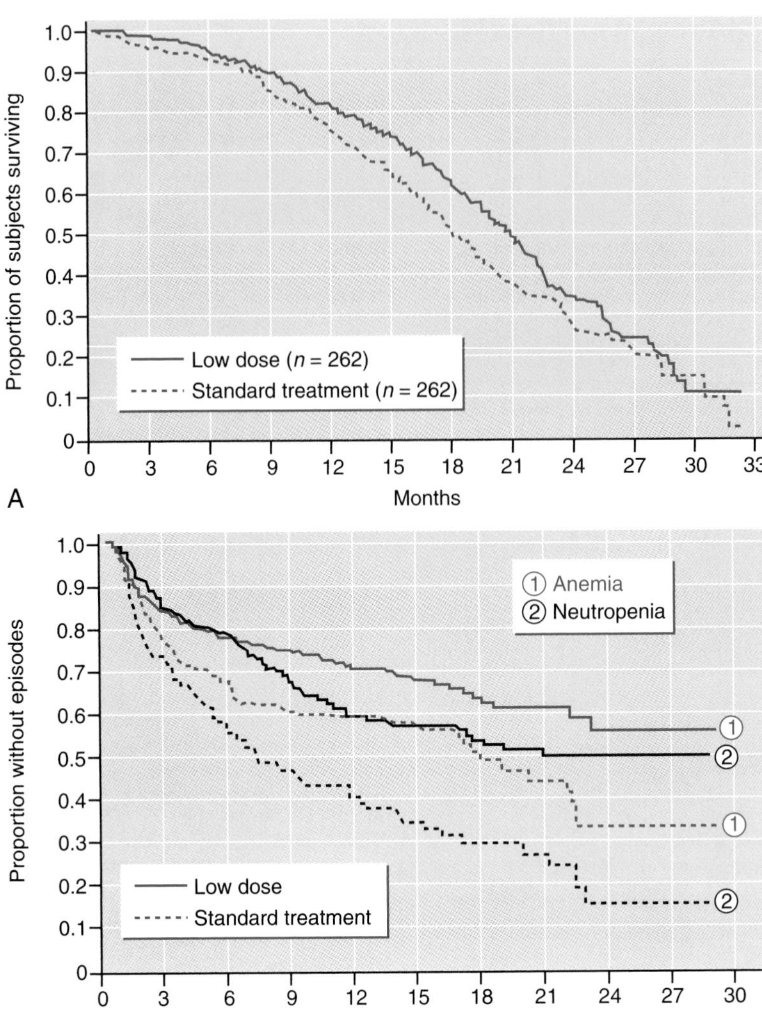

Figure 5-3 ■ Proportion of patients surviving after two doses of ZDV (standard dose 1500 mg/day vs low dose 600 mg/day) **(A)** and the proportion of patients with anemia or neutropenia receiving either the initial standard ZDV dose (1500 mg/day) or the low dose (600 mg/day) **(B)**.

From Fischl MA. Antiviral treatments. In: Mandell GL, Mildvan D (eds) Atlas of Infectious Diseases. Philadelphia: Current Medicine.

the study was not designed as an efficacy study, no differences in clinical events were noted between the two regimens. ZDV given at 600 mg daily has been compared to ZDV given 300 mg twice daily for 13 days in antiretroviral naive patients.[139] At day 14, the once a day dosing group had a lower mean reduction in HIV-1 RNA from baseline (-0.585 $\log_{10}$ copies/mL) compared with the twice a day group (-0.849 $\log_{10}$ copies/mL, $p = 0.056$). Intracellular ZDV-TP were also lower in the once daily group, indicating that ZDV should not be used as a single daily dose.

CONCLUSIONS

ZDV was the first antiretroviral agent approved for use against HIV infection. It continues to be an important component of combination therapy and has been used extensively in regimens with lamivudine, for which a FDC tablet is available. An FDC tablet of ZDV/lamivudine/abacavir is also available. ZDV monotherapy markedly reduces perinatal transmission of HIV and has also provided benefit in the treatment of primary HIV infection. ZDV appears to be additive or synergistic with currently available nucleoside analogs, NNRTIs, and protease inhibitors (PIs). An important exception is stavudine, which is antagonistic *in vivo* with ZDV; the two drugs should not be used in combination.

Toxicities associated with ZDV, particularly anemia and neutropenia, occur more frequently in patients with advanced HIV disease and can generally be managed in those patients. The toxicity of ZDV is leading to its use primarily in antiretroviral-experienced patients, where it's continuing activity in the face of the K65R and M184V mutations in HIV-1 RT make it a useful agent.

REFERENCES

1. Horwitz JP, Noel M. The monomesylates of 1-(2′-deoxy-B-D-lyxofuranosyl)thymine. J Org Chem 29:2076–8, 1964.
2. Furman PA, Fyfe JA, St Clair MH, et al. Phosphorylation of 3′-azido-3′-deoxythymidine and selective interaction of the 5′-triphosphate with human immunodeficiency virus reverse transcriptase. Proc Natl Acad Sci 83:8333–7, 1986.
3. St Clair MH, Richards CA, Spector T, et al. 3′-Azido-3′-deoxythymidine triphosphate as an inhibitor and substrate of

purified human immunodeficiency virus reverse transcriptase. Antimicrob Agents Chemother 31:1972–7, 1987.
4. Balzarini J, Herdewijn P, De Clercq E. Differential patterns of intracellular metabolism of 2′,3′-didehydro-2′,3′-dideoxythymidine and 3′-azido-2′,3′-dideoxythymidine, two potent anti-human immunodeficiency virus compounds. J Biol Chem 264:6127–33, 1989.
5. Turriziani O, Gianotti N, Bambacioni F, et al. Lack of reduction of thymidine kinase activity in stavudine-treated HIV-infected patients. AIDS Res Hum Retroviruses 20:701–3, 2004.
6. Groschel B, Miller V, Doerr HW, Cinatl J Jr. Activity of cellular thymidine kinase 1 in PBMC of HIV-1-infected patients: novel therapy marker. Infection 28:209–13, 2000.
7. Hoggard PG, Lloyd J, Khoo SH, et al. Zidovudine phosphorylation determined sequentially over 12 months in human immunodeficiency virus-infected patients with or without previous exposure to antiretroviral agents. Antimicrob Agents Chemother 45:976–80, 2001.
8. Sim SM, Hoggard PG, Sales SD, et al. Effect of ribavirin on zidovudine efficacy and toxicity in vitro: a concentration-dependent interaction. AIDS Res Hum Retroviruses 14:1661–7, 1998.
9. Vogt MW, Hartshorn KL, Furman PA, et al. Ribavirin antagonizes the effect of azidothymidine on HIV replication. Science 235:1376–9, 1987.
10. Rodriguez-Torres M, Torriani FJ, Soriano V, et al. Effect of ribavirin on intracellular and plasma pharmacokinetics of nucleoside reverse transcriptase inhibitors in patients with human immunodeficiency virus-hepatitis C virus coinfection: results of a randomized clinical study. Antimicrob Agents Chemother 49:3997–4008, 2005.
11. Lavie A, Schlichting I, Vetter IR, et al. The bottleneck in AZT activation [see comment]. Nat Med 3:922–4, 1997.
12. Tan CK, Civil R, Mian AM, et al. Inhibition of the RNase H activity of HIV reverse transcriptase by azidothymidylate. Biochemistry 30:4831–5, 1991.
13. Gao WY, Agbaria R, Driscoll JS, Mitsuya H. Divergent anti-human immunodeficiency virus activity and anabolic phosphorylation of 2′,3′-dideoxynucleoside analogs in resting and activated human cells. J Biol Chem 269:12633–8, 1994.
14. Aquaro S, Perno CF, Balestra E, et al. Inhibition of replication of HIV in primary monocyte/macrophages by different antiviral drugs and comparative efficacy in lymphocytes. J Leukoc Biol 62:138–43, 1997.
15. Balzarini J, Van Herrewege Y, Vanham G. Metabolic activation of nucleoside and nucleotide reverse transcriptase inhibitors in dendritic and Langerhans cells. AIDS 16:2159, 2002.
16. Merrill DP, Moonis M, Chou TC, Hirsch MS. Lamivudine or stavudine in two- and three-drug combinations against human immunodeficiency virus type 1 replication in vitro. J Infect Dis 173:355–64, 1996.
17. Eron JJ Jr, Johnson VA, Merrill DP, et al. Synergistic inhibition of replication of human immunodeficiency virus type 1, including that of a zidovudine-resistant isolate, by zidovudine and 2′,3′-dideoxycytidine in vitro. Antimicrob Agents Chemother 36:1559–62, 1992.
18. Hoggard P, Khoo S, Barry M, Back D. Intracellular metabolism of zidovudine and stavudine in combination. J Infect Dis 174:671–2, 1996.
19. Reid P, MacInnes H, Cong M-E, et al. Natural resistance of human immunodeficiency virus type 2 to zidovudine. Virology 336:251–64, 2005.
20. Boyer PL, Sarafianos SG, Clark PK, et al. Why do HIV-1 and HIV-2 use different pathways to develop AZT resistance? PLoS Pathogens 2:e10, 2006.
21. Descamps D, Damond F, Matheron S, et al. High frequency of selection of K65R and Q151M mutations in HIV-2 infected patients receiving nucleoside reverse transcriptase inhibitors containing regimen. J Med Virol 74:197–201, 2004.
22. Hill SA, Lloyd PA, McDonald S, et al. Susceptibility of human T cell leukemia virus type I to nucleoside reverse transcriptase inhibitors. J Infect Dis 188:424–7, 2003.
23. Roychowdhury S, Peng R, Baiocchi RA, et al. Experimental treatment of Epstein-Barr virus-associated primary central nervous system lymphoma. Cancer Res 63:965–71, 2003.
24. Kurokawa M, Ghosh SK, Ramos JC, et al. Azidothymidine inhibits NF-kappaB and induces Epstein-Barr virus gene expression in Burkitt lymphoma. Blood 106:235–40, 2005.
25. Ghosh SK, Wood C, Boise LH, et al. Potentiation of TRAIL-induced apoptosis in primary effusion lymphoma through azidothymidine-mediated inhibition of NF-kappa B. Blood 101:2321–7, 2003.
26. Sperber SJ, Feibusch EL, Damiani A, Weinstein MP. In vitro activities of nucleoside analog antiviral agents against salmonellae. Antimicrob Agents Chemother 37:106–10, 1993.
27. Herrmann JL, Lagrange PH. Intracellular activity of zidovudine (3′-azido-3′-deoxythymidine, AZT) against Salmonella typhimurium in the macrophage cell line J774-2. Antimicrob Agents Chemother 36:1081–5, 1992.
28. Keen MG, Stamm LV, Bassford PJ. Susceptibility of Treponema pallidum and other selected spirochaetes to zidovudine. J Antimicrob Chemother 29:447–53, 1992.
29. Madoff S, Ferraro MJ, Merrill DP, Hirsch MS. Lack of activity of zidovudine against Ureaplasma urealyticum and Mycoplasma hominis [comment]. Lancet 340:484, 1992.
30. Yarchoan R, Mitsuya H, Myers CE, Broder S. Clinical pharmacology of 3′-azido-2′,3′-dideoxythymidine (zidovudine) and related dideoxynucleosides. N Engl J Med 321:726–38, 1989. Erratum. N Engl J Med 322:280, 1990.
31. Wintergerst U, Rolinski B, Vocks-Hauck M, et al. Pharmacokinetics of orally administered zidovudine in HIV-infected children and adults. Infection 23:344–8, 1995.
32. Barry MG, Khoo SH, Veal GJ, et al. The effect of zidovudine dose on the formation of intracellular phosphorylated metabolites. AIDS 10:1361–7, 1996.
33. Klecker RW Jr, Collins JM, Yarchoan R, et al. Plasma and cerebrospinal fluid pharmacokinetics of 3′-azido-3′-deoxythymidine: a novel pyrimidine analog with potential application for the treatment of patients with AIDS and related diseases. Clin Pharmacol Ther 41:407–12, 1987.
34. Macnab KA, Gill MJ, Sutherland LR, et al. Erratic zidovudine bioavailability in HIV seropositive patients. J Antimicrob Chemother 31:421–8, 1993.
35. Unadkat JD, Collier AC, Crosby SS et al. Pharmacokinetics of oral zidovudine (azidothymidine) in patients with AIDS when administered with and without a high-fat meal [see comment]. AIDS 4:229–32, 1990.
36. Ruhnke M, Bauer FE, Seifert M, et al. Effects of standard breakfast on pharmacokinetics of oral zidovudine in patients with AIDS. Antimicrob Agents Chemother 37:2153–8, 1993.
37. Wintergerst U, Rolinski B, Bogner JR, et al. Pharmacokinetics of zidovudine after rectal administration in human immunodeficiency virus-infected patients. Antimicrob Agents Chemother 41:1143–5, 1997.
38. Luzier A, Morse GD. Intravascular distribution of zidovudine: role of plasma proteins and whole blood components. Antiviral Res 21:267–80, 1993.
39. Slusher JT, Kuwahara SK, Hamzeh FM, et al. Intracellular zidovudine (ZDV) and ZDV phosphates as measured by a validated combined high-pressure liquid chromatography-radioimmunoassay procedure. Antimicrob Agents Chemother 36:2473–7, 1992.
40. Rodriguez JF, Rodriguez JL, Santana J, et al. Simultaneous quantitation of intracellular zidovudine and lamivudine triphosphates in human immunodeficiency virus-infected individuals. Antimicrob Agents Chemother 44:3097–100, 2000.

41. Stretcher BN, Pesce AJ, Frame PT, Stein DS. Pharmacokinetics of zidovudine phosphorylation in peripheral blood mononuclear cells from patients infected with human immunodeficiency virus. Antimicrob Agents Chemother 38:1541–7, 1994.
42. Anderson PL, Kakuda TN, Kawle S, Fletcher CV. Antiviral dynamics and sex differences of zidovudine and lamivudine triphosphate concentrations in HIV-infected individuals. AIDS 17:2159–68, 2003.
43. Good SS, Reynolds DJ, de Miranda P. Simultaneous quantification of zidovudine and its glucuronide in serum by high-performance liquid chromatography. J Chromatogr 431:123–33, 1988.
44. Blum MR, Liao SH, Good SS, de Miranda P. Pharmacokinetics and bioavailability of zidovudine in humans. Am J Med 85:189–94, 1988.
45. Stagg MP, Cretton EM, Kidd L, et al. Clinical pharmacokinetics of 3′-azido-3′-deoxythymidine (zidovudine) and catabolites with formation of a toxic catabolite, 3′-amino-3′-deoxythymidine. Clin Pharmacol Ther 51:668–76, 1992.
46. Boucher FD, Modlin JF, Weller S, et al. Phase I evaluation of zidovudine administered to infants exposed at birth to the human immunodeficiency virus. J Pediatrics 122:137–44, 1993.
47. Singlas E, Pioger JC, Taburet AM, et al. Zidovudine disposition in patients with severe renal impairment: influence of hemodialysis. Clin Pharmacol Ther 46:190–7, 1989.
48. de Miranda P, Good SS, Yarchoan R, et al. Alteration of zidovudine pharmacokinetics by probenecid in patients with AIDS or AIDS-related complex. Clin Pharmacol Ther 46:494–500, 1989.
49. Fletcher CV, Henry WK, Noormohamed SE, et al. The effect of cimetidine and ranitidine administration with zidovudine. Pharmacotherapy 15:701–8, 1995.
50. Taburet AM, Naveau S, Zorza G, et al. Pharmacokinetics of zidovudine in patients with liver cirrhosis. Clin Pharmacol Ther 47:731–9, 1990.
51. Fletcher CV, Rhame FS, Beatty CC, et al. Comparative pharmacokinetics of zidovudine in healthy volunteers and in patients with AIDS with and without hepatic disease. Pharmacotherapy 12:429–34, 1992.
52. Moore KH, Raasch RH, Brouwer KL, et al. Pharmacokinetics and bioavailability of zidovudine and its glucuronidated metabolite in patients with human immunodeficiency virus infection and hepatic disease (AIDS Clinical Trials Group protocol 062). Antimicrob Agents Chemother 39:2732–7, 1995.
53. O'Sullivan MJ, Boyer PJ, Scott GB, et al. The pharmacokinetics and safety of zidovudine in the third trimester of pregnancy for women infected with human immunodeficiency virus and their infants: phase I acquired immunodeficiency syndrome clinical trials group study (protocol 082). Zidovudine Collaborative Working Group. Am J Obstet Gynecol 168:1510–16, 1993.
54. Tartaglione TA, Collier AC, Coombs RW, et al. Acquired immunodeficiency syndrome. Cerebrospinal fluid findings in patients before and during long-term oral zidovudine therapy. Arch Neurol 48:695–9, 1991. Erratum. Arch Neurol 48:1238, 1991.
55. Burger DM, Kraaijeveld CL, Meenhorst PL, et al. Penetration of zidovudine into the cerebrospinal fluid of patients infected with HIV. AIDS 7:1581–7, 1993.
56. Balis FM, Pizzo PA, Murphy RF, et al. The pharmacokinetics of zidovudine administered by continuous infusion in children. Ann Intern Med 110:279–85, 1989.
57. Rolinski B, Bogner JR, Sadri I, et al. Absorption and elimination kinetics of zidovudine in the cerebrospinal fluid in HIV-1-infected patients. J Acquir Immune Defic Syndr 15:192–7, 1997.
58. Sidtis JJ, Gatsonis C, Price RW, et al. Zidovudine treatment of the AIDS dementia complex: results of a placebo-controlled trial. AIDS Clinical Trials Group. Ann Neurol 33:343–9, 1993.
59. Rolinski B, Wintergerst U, Matuschke A, et al. Evaluation of saliva as a specimen for monitoring zidovudine therapy in HIV-infected patients. AIDS 5:885–8, 1991. Erratum. AIDS 5: following 1155, 1991.
60. Henry K, Chinnock BJ, Quinn RP, et al Concurrent zidovudine levels in semen and serum determined by radioimmunoassay in patients with AIDS or AIDS-related complex. JAMA 259:3023–6, 1988.
61. Chuachoowong R, Shaffer N, Siriwasin W, et al. Short-course antenatal zidovudine reduces both cervicovaginal human immunodeficiency virus type 1 RNA levels and risk of perinatal transmission. Bangkok Collaborative Perinatal HIV Transmission Study Group. J Infect Dis 181:99–106, 2000.
62. Bawdon RE, Sobhi S, Dax J. The transfer of anti-human immunodeficiency virus nucleoside compounds by the term human placenta. Am J Obstet Gynecol 167:1570–4, 1992.
63. Siu S-S, Yeung JH-K, Pang M-W, et al. Placental transfer of Zidovudine in first trimester of pregnancy. Obstet Gynecol 106:824–7, 2005.
64. Ruprecht RM, Sharpe AH, Jaenisch R, Trites D. Analysis of 3′-azido-3′-deoxythymidine levels in tissues and milk by isocratic high-performance liquid chromatography. J Chromatogr 528:371–83, 1990.
65. Shapiro RL, Holland DT, Capparelli E, et al. Antiretroviral concentrations in breast-feeding infants of women in Botswana receiving antiretroviral treatment [see comment]. J Infect Dis 192:720–7, 2005.
66. Fischl MA, Parker CB, Pettinelli C, et al. A randomized controlled trial of a reduced daily dose of zidovudine in patients with the acquired immunodeficiency syndrome. The AIDS Clinical Trials Group. N Engl J Med 323:1009–14, 1990.
67. Volberding PA, Lagakos SW, Koch MA, et al. Zidovudine in asymptomatic human immunodeficiency virus infection. A controlled trial in persons with fewer than 500 CD4-positive cells per cubic millimeter. The AIDS Clinical Trials Group of the National Institute of Allergy and Infectious Diseases [see comment]. N Engl J Med 322:941–9, 1990.
68. Richman DD, Fischl MA, Grieco MH, et al. The toxicity of azidothymidine (AZT) in the treatment of patients with AIDS and AIDS-related complex. A double-blind, placebo-controlled trial. N Engl J Med 317:192–7, 1987.
69. DeJesus EHG, Teofilo E, Gerstoft J, et al. Abacavir versus zidovudine combined with lamivudine and efavirenz, for the treatment of antiretroviral-naive HIV-infected adults. Clin Infect Dis 39:1038–46, 2004.
70. Squires KE, Gulick R, Tebas P, et al. A comparison of stavudine plus lamivudine versus zidovudine plus lamivudine in combination with indinavir in antiretroviral naive individuals with HIV infection: selection of thymidine analog regimen therapy (START I). AIDS 14:1591–600, 2000.
71. Walker RE, Parker RI, Kovacs JA, et al. Anemia and erythropoiesis in patients with the acquired immunodeficiency syndrome (AIDS) and Kaposi sarcoma treated with zidovudine. Ann Intern Med 108:372–6, 1988.
72. Fischl M, Galpin JE, Levine JD, et al. Recombinant human erythropoietin for patients with AIDS treated with zidovudine [see comment]. N Engl J Med 322:1488–93, 1990.
73. Gallant JE, DeJesus E, Arribas JR, et al. Tenofovir DF, emtricitabine, and efavirenz vs. zidovudine, lamivudine, and efavirenz for HIV. N Engl J Med 354:251–60, 2006.
74. Chitnis S, Mondal D, Agrawal KC. Zidovudine (AZT) treatment suppresses granulocyte-monocyte colony stimulating factor receptor type alpha (GM-CSFR alpha) gene expression in murine bone marrow cells. Life Sci 71:967–78, 2002.
75. Don PC, Fusco F, Fried P, et al. Nail dyschromia associated with zidovudine. Ann Intern Med 112:145–6, 1990.
76. Dalakas MC, Illa I, Pezeshkpour GH, et al. Mitochondrial myopathy caused by long-term zidovudine therapy [see comment]. N Engl J Med 322:1098–105, 1990.

77. Arnaudo E, Dalakas M, Shanske S, et al. Depletion of muscle mitochondrial DNA in AIDS patients with zidovudine-induced myopathy. Lancet 337:508–10, 1991.
78. Tripuraneni NS, Smith PR, Weedon J, et al. Prognostic factors in lactic acidosis syndrome caused by nucleoside reverse transcriptase inhibitors: report of eight cases and review of the literature. AIDS Patient Care STDs 18:379–84, 2004.
79. Walker UA, Venhoff N. Uridine in the prevention and treatment of NRTI-related mitochondrial toxicity. Antivir Ther 10(Suppl 2):M117–23, 2005.
80. Joly V, Flandre P, Meiffredy V, et al. Increased risk of lipoatrophy under stavudine in HIV-1-infected patients: results of a substudy from a comparative trial. AIDS 16:2447–54, 2002.
81. Amin J, Moore A, Carr A, et al. Combined analysis of two-year follow-up from two open-label randomized trials comparing efficacy of three nucleoside reverse transcriptase inhibitor backbones for previously untreated HIV-1 infection: OzCombo 1 and 2. HIV Clin Trial 4:252–61, 2003.
82. Dube MP, Parker RA, Tebas P, et al. Glucose metabolism, lipid, and body fat changes in antiretroviral-naive subjects randomized to nelfinavir or efavirenz plus dual nucleosides. AIDS 19:1807–18, 2005.
83. Moyle G, Sabin CA, Cartledge J et al. A randomized comparative trial of tenofovir DF or abacavir as replacement for a thymidine analogue in persons with lipoatrophy. AIDS 20: 2043–50, 2006.
84. Mallon PWG, Unemori P, Sedwell R, et al. In vivo, nucleoside reverse-transcriptase inhibitors alter expression of both mitochondrial and lipid metabolism genes in the absence of depletion of mitochondrial DNA. J Infect Dis 191:1686–96, 2005.
85. Jones SP, Qazi N, Morelese J, et al. Assessment of adipokine expression and mitochondrial toxicity in HIV patients with lipoatrophy on stavudine- and zidovudine-containing regimens. J Acquir Immune Defic Syndr 40:565–72, 2005.
86. Fischl MA, Richman DD, Grieco MH, et al. The efficacy of azidothymidine (AZT) in the treatment of patients with AIDS and AIDS-related complex. A double-blind, placebo-controlled trial. N Engl J Med 317:185–91, 1987.
87. Fischl MA, Richman DD, Hansen N, et al. The safety and efficacy of zidovudine (AZT) in the treatment of subjects with mildly symptomatic human immunodeficiency virus type 1 (HIV) infection. A double-blind, placebo-controlled trial. The AIDS Clinical Trials Group. Ann Intern Med 112:727–37, 1990.
88. Anonymous. Concorde: MRC/ANRS randomised double-blind controlled trial of immediate and deferred zidovudine in symptom-free HIV infection. Concorde Coordinating Committee. Lancet 343:871–81, 1994.
89. Hamilton JD, Hartigan PM, Simberkoff MS, et al. A controlled trial of early versus late treatment with zidovudine in symptomatic human immunodeficiency virus infection. Results of the Veterans Affairs Cooperative Study. N Engl J Med 326:437–43, 1992.
90. Connor EM, Sperling RS, Gelber R, et al. Reduction of maternal-infant transmission of human immunodeficiency virus type 1 with zidovudine treatment. Pediatric AIDS Clinical Trials Group Protocol 076 Study Group [see comment]. N Engl J Med 331:1173–80, 1994.
91. Shaffer N, Chuachoowong R, Mock PA, et al. Short-course zidovudine for perinatal HIV-1 transmission in Bangkok, Thailand: a randomised controlled trial. Bangkok Collaborative Perinatal HIV Transmission Study Group. Lancet 353:773–80, 1999.
92. Kinloch-De Loes S, Hirschel BJ, Hoen B, et al. A controlled trial of zidovudine in primary human immunodeficiency virus infection. N Engl J Med 333:408–13, 1995.
93. Follansbee SDL, Olson R, Pollard R, et al. The efficacy of zalcitabine (ddC, HIVID) versus zidovudine (ZDV) as monotherapy in ZDV naive patients with advanced HIV disease: a randomized, double-blind, comparative trial (ACTG 114; N3300). International Conference on AIDS; 1993, abstract no PO-B26-2113.
94. Kahn JO, Lagakos SW, Richman DD, et al. A controlled trial comparing continued zidovudine with didanosine in human immunodeficiency virus infection. The NIAID AIDS Clinical Trials Group. N Engl J Med 327:581–7, 1992.
95. Dolin R, Amato DA, Fischl MA, et al. Zidovudine compared with didanosine in patients with advanced HIV type 1 infection and little or no previous experience with zidovudine. AIDS Clinical Trials Group. Arch Intern Med 155:961–74, 1995.
96. Bazarbachi A, Hermine O. Treatment with a combination of zidovudine and alpha-interferon in naive and pretreated adult T-cell leukemia/lymphoma patients. J Acquir Immune Defic Syndr Hum Retrovirol 13(Suppl 1):S186–90, 1996.
97. Gill PS, Harrington W Jr, Kaplan MH, et al. Treatment of adult T-cell leukemia-lymphoma with a combination of interferon alfa and zidovudine. N Engl J Med 332:1744–8, 1995.
98. Hermine O, Allard I, Levy V, et al. A prospective phase II clinical trial with the use of zidovudine and interferon-alpha in the acute and lymphoma forms of adult T-cell leukemia/lymphoma. Hematol J 3:276–82, 2002.
99. White JD, Wharfe G, Stewart DM, et al. The combination of zidovudine and interferon alpha-2B in the treatment of adult T-cell leukemia/lymphoma. Leuk Lymphoma 40:287–94, 2001.
100. Sheremata WA, Benedict D, Squilacote DC, et al. High-dose zidovudine induction in HTLV-I-associated myelopathy: safety and possible efficacy. Neurology 43:2125–9, 1993.
101. Salmon D, Detruchis P, Leport C, et al. Efficacy of zidovudine in preventing relapses of Salmonella bacteremia in AIDS. J Infect Dis 163:415–16, 1991.
102. Casado JL, Valdezate S, Calderon C, et al. Zidovudine therapy protects against Salmonella bacteremia recurrence in human immunodeficiency virus-infected patients. J Infect Dis 179:1553–6, 1999.
103. Richman DD, Grimes JM, Lagakos SW. Effect of stage of disease and drug dose on zidovudine susceptibilities of isolates of human immunodeficiency virus. J Acquir Immune Defic Syndr 3:743–6, 1990.
104. Meyer PR, Matsuura SE, Mian AM, et al. A mechanism of AZT resistance: an increase in nucleotide-dependent primer unblocking by mutant HIV-1 reverse transcriptase. Mol Cell 4:35–43, 1999.
105. Meyer PR, Matsuura SE, So AG, Scott WA. Unblocking of chain-terminated primer by HIV-1 reverse transcriptase through a nucleotide-dependent mechanism. Proc Natl Acad Sci 95:13471–6, 1998.
106. Arion D, Kaushik N, McCormick S, et al. Phenotypic mechanism of HIV-1 resistance to 3′-azido-3′-deoxythymidine (AZT): increased polymerization processivity and enhanced sensitivity to pyrophosphate of the mutant viral reverse transcriptase. Biochemistry 37:15908–17, 1998.
107. Boyer PL, Sarafianos SG, Arnold E, Hughes SH. Selective excision of AZTMP by drug-resistant human immunodeficiency virus reverse transcriptase. J Virol 75:4832–42, 2001.
108. Ray AS, Murakami E, Basavapathruni A, et al. Probing the molecular mechanisms of AZT drug resistance mediated by HIV-1 reverse transcriptase using a transient kinetic analysis. Biochemistry 42:8831–41, 2003.
109. Miranda LR, Gotte M, Liang F, Kuritzkes DR. The L74V mutation in human immunodeficiency virus type 1 reverse transcriptase counteracts enhanced excision of zidovudine monophosphate associated with thymidine analog resistance mutations. Antimicrob Agent Chemother 49:2648–56, 2005.

110. Boyer PL, Sarafianos SG, Arnold E, Hughes SH. Nucleoside analog resistance caused by insertions in the fingers of human immunodeficiency virus type 1 reverse transcriptase involves ATP-mediated excision. J Virol 76:9143–51, 2002.
111. Meyer PR, Matsuura SE, Zonarich D, et al. Relationship between 3′-azido-3′-deoxythymidine resistance and primer unblocking activity in foscarnet-resistant mutants of human immunodeficiency virus type 1 reverse transcriptase. J Virol 77:6127–37, 2003.
112. Nikolenko GN, Palmer S, Maldarelli F, et al. Mechanism for nucleoside analog-mediated abrogation of HIV-1 replication: balance between RNase H activity and nucleotide excision. Proc Natl Acad Sci 102:2093–8, 2005.
113. Picard V, Angelini E, Maillard A, et al. Comparison of genotypic and phenotypic resistance patterns of human immunodeficiency virus type 1 isolates from patients treated with stavudine and didanosine or zidovudine and lamivudine. J Infect Dis 184:781–4, 2001.
114. Boyer PL, Sarafianos SG, Arnold E, Hughes SH. The M184V mutation reduces the selective excision of zidovudine 5′-monophosphate (AZTMP) by the reverse transcriptase of human immunodeficiency virus type 1. J Virol 76:3248–56, 2002.
115. Sluis-Cremer N, Arion D, Kaushik N, et al. Mutational analysis of Lys65 of HIV-1 reverse transcriptase. Biochem J 348 (Pt 1):77–82, 2000.
116. Temiz NA, Bahar I. Inhibitor binding alters the directions of domain motions in HIV-1 reverse transcriptase. Proteins 49:61–70, 2002.
117. Blanca G, Baldanti F, Paolucci S, et al. Nevirapine resistance mutation at codon 181 of the HIV-1 reverse transcriptase confers stavudine resistance by increasing nucleotide substrate discrimination and phosphorolytic activity. J Biol Chem 278:15469–72, 2003.
118. Selmi B, Deval J, Alvarez K, et al. The Y181C substitution in 3′-azido-3′-deoxythymidine-resistant human immunodeficiency virus, type 1, reverse transcriptase suppresses the ATP-mediated repair of the 3′-azido-3′-deoxythymidine 5′-monophosphate-terminated primer. J Biol Chem 278:40464–72, 2003.
119. Deval J, Selmi B, Boretto J, et al. The molecular mechanism of multidrug resistance by the Q151M human immunodeficiency virus type 1 reverse transcriptase and its suppression using alpha-boranophosphate nucleotide analogues. J Biol Chem 277:42097–104, 2002.
120. Lewin CS, Allen RA, Amyes SG. Mechanisms of zidovudine resistance in bacteria. J Med Micro 33:235–8, 1990.
121. Elwell LP, Ferone R, Freeman GA, et al. Antibacterial activity and mechanism of action of 3′-azido-3′-deoxythymidine (BW A509U). Antimicrob Agent Chemother 31:274–80, 1987.
122. Cato A 3rd, Qian J, Hsu A, et al. Multidose pharmacokinetics of ritonavir and zidovudine in human immunodeficiency virus-infected patients. Antimicrob Agent Chemother 42:1788–93, 1998.
123. Viramune. Data on file Boehringer-Ingleheim Viramune Package Insert: 6, 2005.
124. Tipranavir. Data on file Boehringer-Ingleheim Tipranavir Package Insert: 12, 2006.
125. Atazanavir. Data on file, Bristol Myers Squibb. Atazanavir Package Insert: 4, 2005.
126. Lee BL, Tauber MG, Sadler B, et al. Atovaquone inhibits the glucuronidation and increases the plasma concentrations of zidovudine. Clin Pharmacol Ther 59:14–21, 1996.
127. McCance-Katz EF, Rainey PM, Jatlow P, Friedland G. Methadone effects on zidovudine disposition (AIDS Clinical Trials Group 262). J Acquir Immune Defic Syndr 18:435–43, 1998.
128. Petty BG, Kornhauser DM, Lietman PS. Zidovudine with probenecid: a warning. Lancet 335:1044–5, 1990.
129. Lertora JJ, Rege AB, Greenspan DL, et al. Pharmacokinetic interaction between zidovudine and valproic acid in patients infected with human immunodeficiency virus. Clin Pharmacol Ther 56:272–8, 1994.
130. Sahai J, Gallicano K, Pakuts A, Cameron DW. Effect of fluconazole on zidovudine pharmacokinetics in patients infected with human immunodeficiency virus. J Infect Dis 169:1103–7, 1994.
131. Brockmeyer NH, Tillmann I, Mertins L, et al. Pharmacokinetic interaction of fluconazole and zidovudine in HIV-positive patients. Eur J Med Res 2:377–83, 1997.
132. Blaschke TF, Skinner MH. The clinical pharmacokinetics of rifabutin. Clin Infect Dis 22(Suppl 1):S15–21; discussion S21–2, 1996.
133. Gallicano KD, Sahai J, Shukla VK, et al. Induction of zidovudine glucuronidation and amination pathways by rifampicin in HIV-infected patients. Br J Clin Pharmacol 48:168–79, 1999.
134. Polis MA, Piscitelli SC, Vogel S, et al. Clarithromycin lowers plasma zidovudine levels in persons with human immunodeficiency virus infection. Antimicrob Agent Chemother 41:1709–14, 1997.
135. Vance E, Watson-Bitar M, Gustavson L, Kazanjian P. Pharmacokinetics of clarithromycin and zidovudine in patients with AIDS. Antimicrob Agents Chemother 39:1355–60, 1995.
136. Amsden G, Flaherty J, Luke D. Lack of an effect of azithromycin on the disposition of zidovudine and dideoxyinosine in HIV-infected patients. J Clin Pharmacol 41:210–16, 2001.
137. Anonymous. Department of Health and Human Services (DHHS) panel on antiretroviral guidelines for adults and adolescents: guidelines for the use of antiretroviral agents in HIV-1-infected adults and adolescents. Available: http://AIDSinfo.nih.gov: 1-112, 2006.
138. Shepp DH, Ramirez-Ronda C, Dall L, et al. A comparative trial of zidovudine administered every four versus every twelve hours for the treatment of advanced HIV disease. J Acquir Immune Defic Syndr 15:283–8, 1997.
139. Ruane PJ, Richmond GJ, DeJesus E, Hill-Zabala CE, et al. Pharmacodynamic effects of zidovudine 600 mg once/day versus 300 mg twice/day in therapy-naive patients infected with human immunodeficiency virus. Pharmacotherapy 24:307–12, 2004.
140. O'Brien WA, Hartigan PM, Martin D, et al. Changes in plasma HIV-1 RNA and CD4+ lymphocyte counts and the risk of progression to AIDS. N Engl J Med 334:426–31, 1996.
141. Cimoch PJ, Lavelle J, Pollard R, Griffy KG, et al. Pharmacokinetics of oral ganciclovir alone and in combination with zidovudine, didanosine, and probenecid in HIV-infected subjects. J Acquir Immune Defic Syndr 17:227–34, 1998.
142. Palmer S, Cox S. Increased activation of the combination of 3′-azido-3′-deoxythymidine and 2′-deoxy-3′-thiacytidine in the presence of hydroxyurea. Antimicrob Agent Chemother 41:460–4, 1997.
143. Antoniou T, Gough K, Yoong D, Arbess G. Severe anemia secondary to a probable drug interaction between zidovudine and valproic acid. Clin Infect Dis 38:e38–40, 2004.

Chapter 6

Didanosine

Raphael Dolin, MD

STRUCTURE

Didanosine (2′,3′-dideoxyinosine, ddI, Videx, Videx EC) is a nucleoside analog active against human immunodeficiency virus type 1 (HIV-1), HIV-2, simian immunodeficiency virus, and human T-cell lymphotropic virus-1 (HTLV-1)[1,2] (Fig. 6-1). It is acid-labile and under acidic conditions is hydrolyzed to 2′,3′-dideoxyribose and the base hypoxanthine.[3] Didanosine is also the deamination product *in vivo* of 2′,3′-dideoxyadenosine (ddA) through the action of the ubiquitous enzyme adenosine deaminase.[4] Didanosine was the second antiretroviral drug approved by the US Food and Drug Administration (FDA) in 1991.

MECHANISM OF ACTION

Didanosine exerts its antiviral action through its triphosphorylated metabolite 2′,3′-dideoxyadenosine 5′-triphosphate (ddATP), which competes with the naturally occurring nucleoside 2′-deoxyadenosine 5′-triphosphate (dATP) for binding to HIV-1 reverse transcriptase (RT).[5] In addition, ddATP serves as a chain terminator after incorporation into viral DNA because it lacks the requisite 3′-hydroxyl group for elongation of the DNA nascent chain.[6,7]

Didanosine enters the cell by means of nonfacilitated diffusion through a nucleobase carrier.[8] It is initially phosphorylated to the monophosphate form (ddIMP) by a 5′-nucleotidase and then converted to ddA monophosphate by an adenylosuccinate synthetase and adenylosuccinate lyase.[3] It is subsequently phosphorylated to the diphosphate (ddADP) and finally the triphosphate (ddATP), which is the active antiviral moiety. ddATP has a prolonged intracellular half-life, estimated to be 8–40 h.[9,10] This provides the rationale for the prolonged dosing intervals of once or twice per day for didanosine used in clinical trials.

Didanosine is active against HIV-1 in both lymphocytes and macrophages, with a median inhibitory concentration (IC_{50}) of 0.24–0.6 mg/L in T-cell cultures and 0.002–0.020 mg/L in monocyte/macrophage cultures.[6,11–13] Didanosine appears to have more activity in resting cells than in activated cells, in contrast to zidovudine or stavudine for which the reverse is true.[14,15] The antiviral activity of didanosine also appears to be relatively unaffected by the presence of endogenous nucleosides such as 2′-deoxyadenosine.[3] *In vitro*, didanosine almost completely inhibits HIV replication at concentrations of 4.8 mg/L.[16] Against HIV-1, didanosine demonstrates additive effects or synergy with nucleoside analogs such as zidovudine and stavudine,[17] non-nucleoside reverse transcriptase inhibitors (NNRTIs) such as delavirdine,[18] and protease inhibitors (PIs) such as saquinavir[18] or indinavir.[19] Hydroxyurea demonstrates a synergistic effect against HIV-1 when combined with didanosine through inhibition of the ribonucleotide reductase enzyme.

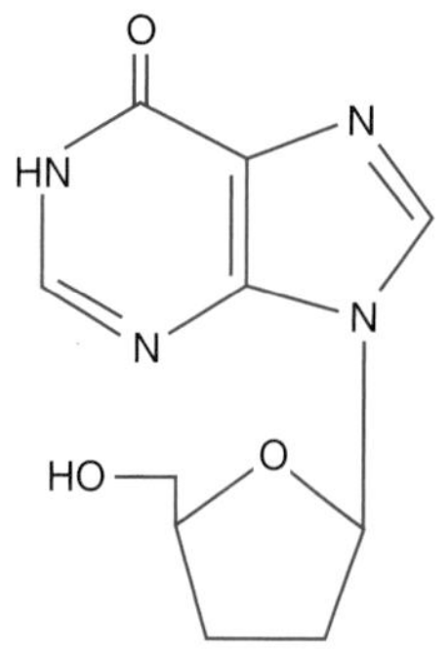

Figure 6-1 ■ Structure of didanosine (2′,3′-dideoxyinosine, ddI, Videx).

Didanosine Dosage in Adults

Table 6-1

Patient Weight	Buffered Tablets[a]	Buffered Powder	Enteric Coated Capsules
Recommended Dosage			
⩾60 kg	200 mg bid	250 mg bid	[b]
<60 kg	125 mg bid	167 mg bid	[b]
Dosage for Patients Whose Management Requires Once-Daily Frequency			
⩾60 kg	400 mg qd	[c]	400 mg qd
<60 kg	250 mg qd	[c]	250 mg qd

[a]The 200 mg strength tablet should only be used as a component of a once-daily regimen.
[b]The enteric coated capsule contains delayed release beadlets and should be administered no more frequently than once daily.
[c]Not suitable for once-daily dosing except for patients with renal impairment.

From Prescribing Information. Videx (Didanosine). Princeton, NJ: Bristol-Myers Squibb, Oct 2005; and Prescribing Information, Videx EC. Princeton, NJ: Bristol-Myers Squibb, Mar 2006.

This results in the decrease of intracellular dATP with which the active metabolite of didanosine (ddATP) competes for binding to RT.[20] Didanosine is approximately 100-fold less toxic than zidovudine against bone marrow progenitor cells,[16] which likely accounts for the lack of hematopoietic toxicity of the drug observed in clinical trials.

PHARMACOKINETICS

The *N*-glycocidic bond of didanosine is highly acid-labile, and significant degradation occurs at the low pH found in gastric fluid.[21] Thus, oral preparations have been formulated with buffers to prevent degradation or as an enteric coated delayed release preparation (Videx EC). The sachet (powder) form contains citrate phosphate buffer, and the chewable/dispersible tablet contains calcium carbonate and magnesium hydroxide as antacids. A pediatric powder formulation of didanosine is also available without buffer and must be reconstituted with water and administered with a concomitant antacid. The nonbuffered, enteric coated, delayed-release formulation consists of a capsule with enteric coated beadlets that contain didanosine (see further ahead).[22]

Oral bioavailability of didanosine has been reported to be somewhat variable and dose dependent.[3,23] The buffered chewable/dispersible tablet is 20–25% more bioavailable than the sachet form, which accounts for the lower recommended daily dose of the tablet (usually 400 mg/day for patients weighing 60 kg or more) compared to the powder (500 mg/day).[4,10] Twice-a-day dosing of the buffered tablet was the regimen initially recommended and studied most extensively. However, once-daily administration of twice the dose given BID results in similar plasma concentration–time curves (area under the curve, or AUC),[24] as does administration of the enteric coated delayed-release formulation, which should be administrated only once a day (Table 6-1).[22] Once-a-day dosing has been approved by the FDA, and is now used most frequently, although the FDA states in the package insert that twice-a-day dosing is preferred because "there is more evidence to support its effects" (see further ahead). The bioavailability of didanosine is decreased up to 50% when administered with food and so should be taken on an empty stomach, either 30 min before or 2 h after a meal.[22,25,26]

Oral absorption of buffered didanosine preparations is generally rapid, and time to peak plasma concentrations (T_{max}) occurs 0.50–1.13 h after oral administration.[3,6,7,27] Peak concentrations range between 5 and 9 μmol/L when currently recommended doses are used.[3] The peak concentration for the EC delayed-release preparation is ~40% lower, and T_{max} is prolonged to 2 h.[22] Approximately 5% of didanosine is bound to protein.[16] The plasma elimination half-life of didanosine after administration is relatively short, ranging from 0.50 to 2.74 h after multiple oral doses.[6,7] Thirty to sixty percent of an oral dose is excreted unchanged by the kidneys via glomerular filtration and tubular secretion.[23,28] Reduction of dosage is recommended for patients with significant renal dysfunction (creatinine clearance is less than 60 mL/min), as shown in Table 6-2.[10,22] Didanosine is partially removed during hemodialysis, with an extraction ratio of 53%.[29] For patients requiring hemodialysis or continuous ambulatory peritoneal dialysis (CAPD), didanosine buffered or EC formulations should be given the dose which is appropriate for those with a creatinine clearance of less than 10 mL/min.[10,22]

As noted above, didanosine is converted to the active moiety ddATP and then further metabolized to hypoxanthine and eventually to uric acid. Didanosine is converted to hypoxanthine by a purine nucleoside phosphorylase (PNP), which is also inhibited by tenofovir (TDF). This apparently accounts for the increased concentrations of ddI when administered with TDF,[30] and was the basis for attempts to use combinations of TDF and ddI to avoid dietary restrictions with the latter.[31,32] However, the ddI–TDF combination has resulted in increased rates of toxicity (see further ahead). The volume of distribution of didanosine is 0.76–1.29 L/kg,[33] which is less than the distribution of zidovudine, likely reflecting the lower lipid solubility of didanosine. Mean cerebrospinal fluid concentrations have been reported to be 21% of serum concentrations (range 12–85%), although the concentrations were more variable in children.[28,33,34]

Didanosine Dosage During Renal Impairment

Table 6-2

Creatinine Clearance (mL/min)	≥60 kg Buffered Tablet[a] (mg)	≥60 kg Buffered Powder[b] (mg)	≥60 kg Enteric Coated Capsule[c] (mg)	<60 kg Buffered Tablet[a] (mg)	<60 kg Buffered Powder[b] (mg)	<60 kg Enteric Coated Capsule[c] (mg)
>60	200 bid[d]	250 bid	400 qd	125 bid[d]	167 bid	250 qd
30–59	200 qd or 100 bid	100 bid	200 qd	150 qd or 75 bid	100 bid	125 qd
10–29	150 qd	167 qd	125 qd	100 qd	100 qd	125 qd
<10	100 qd	100 qd	125 qd	75 qd	100 qd	[e]

[a]Chewable/dispersible buffered tablet. Two tablets must be taken with each dose: different strengths of tablets may be combined to yield the recommended dose.
[b]Buffered powder for oral solution.
[c]Enteric coated capsule containing delayed release beadlets.
[d]400 mg qd (≥60 kg) or 250 mg qd (<60 kg) for patients whose management requires once-daily frequency of administration.
[e]Not suitable for use in patients <60 kg and creatinine clearance <10 mL/min.

From Prescribing Information. Videx (Didanosine). Princeton, NJ: Bristol-Myers Squibb, Oct 2005; and Prescribing Information, Videx EC. Princeton, NJ: Bristol-Myers Squibb, Mar 2006.

Toxicities Associated With Didanosine

Table 6-3

Toxicity	Frequency	Comment	Refs
Peripheral neuropathy	9–15%	ZDV monotherapy in same studies had rates of 7–14%; Increased in combinations with d4T, HU, TDF	42–44, 50, 51, 61
Pancreatitis	4–7%	ZDV monotherapy in same studies had rates of 3–4%; Increased with TDF, d4T	31, 42–44, 60, 61
Diarrhea	16% in expanded access program	Not significantly increased compared to ZDV monotherapy in some studies; possibly less frequent in extended release formulation	42, 43, 62
Elevated serum amylase (>1.4 × normal)	13–20%	ZDV monotherapy in same studies had rates of 3–4%	42, 43, 61
Elevated AST, ALT (>5.1 × normal)	6–9%	Rare fulminant hepatitis has been noted	42, 43, 63, 64
Lactic acidosis and hepatic steatosis	Rare	As with other NRTIs[a]	10, 22, 65–67

ALT, alanine transaminase; AST, aspartate transaminase; NRTIs, nucleoside reverse transcriptase inhibitors; ZDV, zidovudine; d4T, stavudine; HU, hydroxyurea; TDF, tenofovir.

[a]Letter of warning has been issued regarding fatal cases of lactic acidosis that have occurred in pregnant women who were receiving didanosine and stavudine.[67]

Pharmacokinetic measurements in pregnant patients were not significantly different from those obtained in nonpregnant patients.[35] Didanosine was found in placental and fetal circulations at concentrations that were 20–50% of those in the maternal circulation, presumably because of placental metabolism of the drug.[35–37] The pharmacokinetics of didanosine in pediatric patients are similar to those described in adults, although bioavailability was somewhat lower in some studies of children.[38–40] Once-daily dosing of didanosine (180 mg/m^2) in pediatric patients had similar bioavailability (90 mg/m^2) when given twice-daily.[41]

TOXICITY

The currently available formulations of didanosine, including the dispersible buffered tablet and the extended-release capsule, are more palatable than earlier formulations. This, along with once-daily dosing, has improved acceptability of the drug. Overall, didanosine has been a reasonably well tolerated drug as ascertained by large-scale clinical studies of HIV-infected patients at various stages of disease progression.[42–44] However, significant toxicities may be encountered, of which the most common are listed in Table 6-3. The most well-established side effects are peripheral neuropathy and pancreatitis, which have also been the dose-limiting toxicities encountered in phase I dose-escalation studies.[44] Adverse effects occur most frequently in patients with advanced HIV disease and do not appear to differ significantly between once-a-day and twice-a-day regimens of didanosine, except for rates of diarrhea, which may be decreased with the EC formulation.[10,22]

Peripheral neuropathy associated with didanosine is indistinguishable from that seen with other nucleoside analogs such as zalcitabine. It is primarily a sensory polyneuropathy that is usually symmetrical and distal; and it most commonly involves the lower extremities.[45–47] Initial symptoms are often dysesthesias, which are described as aching, burning, tingling or numbness. They can progress to markedly disabling pain on ambulation or even at rest. Phase I studies indicated that the frequency of neuropathy was dose-related and decreased when doses below 12 mg/kg/day were used.[45] In the expanded access program in which patients with advanced HIV disease received didanosine, the reported frequency of peripheral neuropathy was 16%,[10] which undoubtedly includes a background of neuropathy caused by other drugs and by underlying HIV infection. In two large-scale clinical trials that compared didanosine and zidovudine monotherapy (AIDS Clinical Trial Group (ACTG) 116a[42] and ACTG 116b/117[43]), the rates of peripheral neuropathy were not significantly different between the didanosine- and zidovudine-treated groups. Because zidovudine is not known to cause peripheral neuropathy, these studies indicate that peripheral neuropathy caused by didanosine is uncommonly encountered when recommended doses of the drug are employed. Nonetheless, clinicians must be aware of risk factors for the development of neuropathy with didanosine, which include the presence of underlying peripheral neuropathy from other causes, concurrent treatment with other potentially neurotoxic drugs,[48] and low CD4+ T-lymphocyte counts.[49] Rates of peripheral neuropathy appear to be increased when didanosine is combined with hydroxyurea or with stavudine and probably with TDF (see further ahead).[50,51] Peripheral neuropathy associated with didanosine generally resolves over several weeks after discontinuing the drug, although occasionally symptoms worsen for 1–2 weeks after the drug has been stopped. Some patients with didanosine-associated peripheral neuropathy have been able to tolerate reinstitution of the drug at lower doses,[52] but this is rarely necessary in an era when multiple alternative antiretroviral therapies are available. The pathogenesis of nucleoside-induced peripheral neuropathy is not fully understood but appears to be related to inhibition of mitochondrial DNA polymerases in neurons by this class of drugs.[53]

Acute pancreatitis is a dose-related toxic effect of didanosine that is infrequently encountered at currently recommended doses.[54] As is the case with peripheral neuropathy, pancreatitis unrelated to didanosine can develop in HIV-infected patients because of opportunistic infections or neoplasms that involve the pancreas and the use of other pancreatotoxic drugs.[55] Among 7806 patients who participated in the expanded access program for didanosine, pancreatitis was noted in 5% who received the drug for at least 5 months.[10] Acute pancreatitis associated with didanosine can present with variable severity, ranging from mild abdominal pain to life-threatening illness on rare occasions.[54,56] Fatalities associated with pancreatitis occurred in 0.35% of patients in the expanded access program.[10] Asymptomatic elevations in serum amylase and, to a lesser extent, lipase and triglycerides have also been observed.[3,57] In the large-scale studies that compared zidovudine and didanosine monotherapy noted above (ACTG 116a[42] and ACTG 116b/117[43]), an excessive rate of pancreatitis (3–4%) was noted in the didanosine arm (500 mg/day) compared to the zidovudine monotherapy arm. In the ACTG 175 trial, which examined patients with somewhat less advanced HIV disease, the overall frequency of pancreatitis was 0.5% in the entire study population and was not increased in the didanosine-treated groups.[58] Risk factors for the development of pancreatitis include a history of pancreatitis, a history of alcohol or drug abuse, hypertriglyceridemia, and possibly renal dysfunction.[10,59] Co-administration with TDF also increases risk of pancreatitis (see further ahead).[31] Combination of didanosine with stavudine, with or without hydroxyurea, may also increase the risk of pancreatitis.[10,22,60] Clinicians who treat patients with didanosine should be alert to signs and symptoms of pancreatitis, and the drug should be stopped promptly if pancreatitis is suspected. Some patients with risk factors for the development of pancreatitis may benefit from periodic monitoring of amylase, lipase, and triglycerides. If amylase concentrations rise 1.5–2.0 times above the upper limit of normal or if triglycerides rise above 7 g/L, didanosine administration should be stopped.[48] Fractionation of serum amylase into total and salivary components may increase the specificity of such monitoring. Although some patients with didanosine-associated pancreatitis have been able to tolerate lower doses of the drug once the acute episode has resolved,[45,48] didanosine should be avoided in such patients unless there is no other alternative for antiretroviral therapy (ART).

Diarrhea has also been associated with didanosine administration. It has been attributed, at least in part, to the citrate phosphate buffer in the powdered preparation and may be less frequent with the EC formulation.[22] Diarrhea was reported in 16% of patients in the didanosine expanded-access program in which patients had a far advanced HIV disease and were receiving multiple other medications.[61] In studies of monotherapy with didanosine in which the chewable/dispersible tablet was employed, rates of diarrhea were not significantly different from those seen with zidovudine monotherapy arms in some studies. Elevations in aminotransferases (more than five times normal) were seen in 6–9% of subjects who received didanosine monotherapy,[10,42,43] and rare cases of fulminant hepatitis have been reported.[62,63]

As with other nucleoside analogs, life-threatening lactic acidosis and hepatic steatosis may occur with didanosine.[64–66] The FDA and the manufacturers of didanosine issued a letter of warning reporting three fatal cases of lactic acidosis in pregnant women who were receiving didanosine combined with stavudine and recommended that this combination be used in pregnant women only when the 'potential benefit clearly outweighs the risk.'[67] Asymptomatic elevations in uric acid have also been noted, primarily in patients with preexisting hyperuricemia.[61] Rarely, depigmented retinal lesions and optic neuritis have been reported in patients receiving didanosine,[68,69] and consideration of periodic retinal examinations for patients on didanosine have been suggested.[10,22,70]

Of particular note has been the absence of hematopoietic toxicity associated with didanosine administration. In fact, in several studies, improvement in hemoglobin, white blood cells, and platelet counts occurred on didanosine therapy, presumably because of the beneficial effects of the drug in inhibiting replication of HIV.[4,71]

The recommended dosage schedule for didanosine was twice a day for the buffered formulation, but in 1999 the FDA approved once-a-day dosing,[10] as well as the EC delayed-release formulation, which should be administered only once a day.[22] Comparative trials of twice- and once-a-day regimens of didanosine in combination with stavudine have demonstrated equivalent effects on virologic and CD4 cell count parameters,[72,73] and similar findings were noted when twice- and once-a-day regimens of didanosine were used in combination with zidovudine.[74] Once-a-day dosing of didanosine, in combination with stavudine and nelfinavir, had an antiretroviral effect equivalent to that of a combination of zidovudine, lamivudine, and nelfinavir.[10] Buffered didanosine preparations administered on a once-a-day regimen has also been employed in other comparative and noncomparative studies of didanosine in a wide variety of combination trials, including nucleoside reverse transcriptase inhibitors (NRTIs), NNRTIs, and PIs.[7,75–78] The FDA currently points out that for adults, 'the preferred dosing frequency of VIDEX (ddI chewable/dispersible buffered tablets) is twice daily because there is more evidence to support the effectiveness of this dosing regiment.'[10] Once-daily dosing should be considered only for 'adults whose management requires once-daily administration of Videx.'[10] Videx EC (delayed release capsules containing enteric coated beadlets) should be administered once daily.[22]

RESISTANCE

After didanosine monotherapy, five- to 26-fold reduction in didanosine sensitivity has been reported; it is associated with a change in the *pol* gene at codon 74 (Leu:Val), which appears to be the predominant mutation associated with resistance.[13] Isolates from 60% to 65% of patients who have received didanosine therapy for at least 1 year demonstrate this mutation.[79–81] Viruses with the L74V mutation also manifested decreased virus replication ('fitness') *in vitro*.[82] A similar level of resistance with a change at codon 184 (Met: Val) has been reported.[83,84] A mutation at codon 65 (Lys:Arg) has resulted in a three- to fivefold decrease in sensitivity[85]; and mutations at 135 (Ile:Val) and 200 (Thr:Ala), which confer resistance, have also been described.[86]

Mutations at codon 74 are also associated with partial restoration of susceptibility to zidovudine but with an approximately 10-fold reduction in sensitivity to zalcitabine.[12,87] The position K65R mutation is associated with a reduction in sensitivity to both zalcitabine and lamivudine,[88] and appeared to have an added effect on resistance to didanosine when present with the M184V mutation.[89] The development of a mutation at codon 41, 67, 70, 215, or 219 conferred resistance to zidovudine in patients who received prolonged didanosine therapy but apparently had not received zidovudine therapy.[90] This suggests that viruses resistant to both zidovudine and didanosine occasionally emerge in patients on didanosine therapy alone. Resistance mutations at codon 74 have been associated with poorer CD4 responses and higher virus loads in patients receiving didanosine.[81]

Combination therapy with zidovudine and didanosine reduced the rate of emergence of genotypic didanosine resistance to less than 4% compared to patients who received didanosine monotherapy.[79,80,91–93] Combination therapy with didanosine and zidovudine did not decrease the emergence of viruses resistant to zidovudine in studies that examined the sensitivity of isolates to both drugs.[91,94]

Viruses resistant to both didanosine and zidovudine have been detected after prolonged combination therapy with both drugs, with amino acid substitutions at codons 62, 75, 77, 116, and 151.[91,95–97] These viruses are also resistant to zalcitabine and stavudine and are partially resistant to lamivudine. The inclusion of the mutation Glu to Met at codon 151 (Q151M) and three or four other mutations that result in broad NRTI resistance have been associated with loss of favorable effect on CD4+ T-lymphocyte counts.[98–99] A 6-bp insert between codons 69 and 70 that confers broad resistance to NRTIs has also been identified in patients who received didanosine or zalcitabine alone or in combination with zidovudine.[100]

DRUG INTERACTIONS

Drug interactions that occur with the buffered formulations of didanosine are most frequently related to the antacid activity in the tablet or powder or to the divalent calcium and magnesium cations present in the tablet form or in antacids added to the pediatric powder (Table 6-4). These interactions can be minimized by administering other drugs 2 h before or 2–6 h after administration of didanosine. An example of this type of interaction is the reduction in the absorption of drugs such as itraconazole[101,102] or ketoconazole,[103,104] which require gastric acidity for optimal absorption when these drugs are given concomitantly with didanosine. Dapsone also requires low gastric pH for optimal absorption, and there was concern that buffering by didanosine might account for the apparent failure of dapsone prophylaxis for *Pneumocystis jerovici* infection when both drugs were administered to patients.[105] However, pharmacokinetic studies in humans receiving didanosine did not show a reduction of plasma dapsone levels.[10,22,106] Absorption of tetracycline[107] and ciprofloxacin[108] (and possibly other quinolone antibiotics) is decreased by chelation with divalent cations in didanosine tablets. Concurrent administration with ranitidine and presumably other H2-blockers results in a small increase in bioavailability of buffered didanosine preparations by decreasing gastric acidity.[109] Concomitant ganciclovir

Drug Interactions with Didanosine

Table 6-4

Type of Interaction	Drug	Refs
Decreased absorption of drugs requiring gastric acidity for optimal absorption[a]	Itraconazole	101, 102
	Ketoconazole	103, 104
Decreased absorption of drugs by chelation with cations[a]	Tetracycline	107
	Ciprofloxacin	108
Increased absorption of didanosine by block of gastric acid production	Ranitidine	109
Increased plasma concentration of didanosine	Ganciclovir	110–112
Decreased plasma concentration of drug when given at the same time as didanosine[b]	Delavirdine	116, 117
	Indinavir	116, 118
Decreased plasma concentration of didanosine when given with drug	Delavirdine	116, 117
	Methadone	118
Possibly increased rate of peripheral neuropathy when given with didanosine	Isoniazid	48
	Ethambutol	
	Metronidazole	
	Zalcitabine	
	Hydroxyurea	50, 51
	Stavudine	
Possibly increased pancreatic toxicity when given with didanosine	Pentamidine	55
	Azathioprine	
	Ethambutol	
	Zalcitabine	
	Stavudine	60
Increased plasma concentration of didanosine through inhibition of PNP	Allopurinol	10, 30
	Tenofovir	130, 131

[a]Interaction is avoided if a nonbuffered preparation (VIDEX EC) is used.
[b]Interaction is avoided if didanosine is administered 1–2 h before indinavir or 1 h apart from delavirdine.

administration increases plasma didanosine concentrations by 57.7% (C_{max}) and AUC values by 71.5%,[110–112] so clinicians should be alert to the possibility of increased didanosine toxicity when the two drugs are given together. Studies of interactions between didanosine and zidovudine have shown only minor changes in the pharmacokinetics of either drug.[113–115] When delavirdine and didanosine were administered simultaneously, reductions in the concentrations of both delavirdine (32% decrease in AUC) and didanosine (20% decrease in AUC) were noted[116,117]; hence the two drugs should be given at least 1 h apart. Decreased absorption of indinavir has also been noted when the drug is administered simultaneously with didanosine,[116,118] but not if didanosine is taken 1 h before indinavir.[119] Minor interactions, without clinical significance, have been observed between didanosine and ritonavir.[120] Clinically significant pharmacokinetic interactions have not been observed between didanosine and the following drugs: trimethoprim-sulfamethoxazole,[121] rifabutin,[122] isoniazid,[123] foscarnet,[124] stavudine,[125] loperamide,[22] metoclopramide,[22] clarithromycin,[126] nevirapine,[127] and nelfinavir.[128] Administration of allopurinol increases the AUC of didanosine approximately fourfold through inhibition of the enzyme, PNP, so the two drugs should not be administered together.[10,22] Chronic methadone administration reduces the AUC of didanosine by 57% and the C_{max} by 66%.[129]

Administration of TDF may increase the plasma levels of didanosine by 40% or more,[130,131] through inhibition of PNP. This likely accounts for the increased toxicity observed in co-administration of TDF and didanosine, particularly as increased rates of pancreatitis,[132] and possibly peripheral neuropathy as well. An interaction between didanosine and TDF resulting in enhanced mitochondrial toxicity has been suggested as well.[133] Increased rates of hyperglycemia have also been reported in combination therapy with the two drugs.[134] Because of the above toxicities, and apparent decreased efficacies (see further ahead), concomitant use of TDF and didanosine should be avoided if possible. If they need to be used together, the manufacturers suggest that the dosage of didanosine be reduced to 250 mg daily for adults weighing 60 kg or greater, or 200 mg for adults weighing under 60 kg with creatinine clearances of 60 mL/min.[10,22] The EC formulation of didanosine, which does not contain buffer, should not be expected to result in drug interactions that depend on the antacid or cation contents of didanosine tablets. However, drug interactions with didanosine based on other mechanisms, such as those involving allopurinol, ganciclovir, or methadone, would be expected to occur with the EC formulation as well.[22]

As noted in the section on toxicity, clinicians should be alert to the development of didanosine toxicity when drugs that are known to cause or potentiate peripheral neuropathy[49] (e.g., isoniazid, ethambutol, metronidazole, vincristine, hydroxyurea, stavudine and possibly TDF) or pancreatitis[54,60] (pentamidine, azathioprine, TDF, stavudine) are co-administered, and alternative drugs should be considered. Because of the potential for additive toxicities involving peripheral neuropathy and pancreatitis, didanosine and zalcitabine should not be administered concurrently.

EFFICACY

Didanosine Monotherapy or Dual Nucleoside Combination Therapy

Clinical studies of didanosine monotherapy or dual combination therapy were carried out at times when the use of one or two antiretrovirals was the standard of care. The major studies of this type are summarized in Table 6-5. Studies conducted by the ACTG showed that changing to didanosine monotherapy was more effective than continuing zidovudine monotherapy in patients with advanced HIV infection who had previously received at least 8 weeks of zidovudine (ACTG 116a, ACTG 116b/117),[42,43] although zidovudine appeared to be somewhat more effective than didanosine in antiretroviral-naive patients.[42] Studies of patients who received at least 6 months of zidovudine and were either clinically stable[135] or deteriorating[61] also showed benefits after their therapy was changed to didanosine. A meta-analysis of the above studies and ACTG 175 (see further ahead) supported the beneficial effect of switching from zidovudine to didanosine across a broad range of CD4 and HIV disease categories.[136] A comparison of didanosine with zidovudine as initial monotherapy in patients with 'mildly symptomatic disease' and CD4 counts lower than 500/μL showed that the clinical efficacies of the two drugs were similar.[137]

Three large-scale studies have examined the clinical benefit of didanosine as part of dual combination therapy with zidovudine in patients with a broad range of underlying CD4+ T-lymphocyte counts and previous experience with zidovudine (Table 6-5). Two of these studies, ACTG 175[58,138] and Delta,[139] found combination therapy to be superior to zidovudine monotherapy in the study population as a whole, and the third study, CPRA 007,[140] found the combination to be superior in a subgroup of patients with less than 12 months of previous zidovudine experience.

An additional study indicated that combinations of didanosine and zidovudine were superior to zidovudine alone in patients who were largely antiretroviral-naive and had CD4 counts of less than 300/μL.[94] A study of patients who had been receiving zidovudine for a median of 3 years showed a modest survival benefit if didanosine replaced or was added to zidovudine.[141]

The combination of didanosine and stavudine has been investigated in dose-range and comparative trials (Table 6-5). In antiretroviral-naive patients, didanosine (200–400 mg/day) plus stavudine (20 mg/day) resulted in a decrease in RNA levels of 0.9–1.3 $\log_{10}$ after 49 weeks.[141] High-dose and low-dose combinations of didanosine and stavudine reduced the HIV RNA levels by 1.22–2.09 $\log_{10}$ copies/mL in a study in Thailand.[142] The ALBI trial found that 24 weeks of didanosine plus stavudine resulted in a greater drop in HIV RNA (2.26 $\log_{10}$ copies/mL) than either zidovudine plus lamivudine (1.26 $\log_{10}$ copies/mL) or alternating didanosine and stavudine followed by zidovudine plus lamivudine (1.58 $\log_{10}$ copies/mL).[143] Studies of didanosine and stavudine in highly antiretroviral-experienced patients have generally resulted in less profound decreases in HIV RNA levels than those seen in antiretroviral-naive patients.[74,144,145] In antiretroviral-naive patients studied in ACTG 306, didanosine plus lamivudine did not increase antiretroviral effects compared to didanosine monotherapy, whose antiretroviral effects in turn were similar to those of lamivudine plus zidovudine.[146] As noted earlier, concomitant administration of didanosine and d4T has been associated with increased toxicity, and use of the combination must be approached with caution. Studies of combination therapy with didanosine and stavudine, and with didanosine and lamivudine are also reviewed in Chapters 8 and 9, respectively.

Triple Combination Therapy with Didanosine

Dual nucleoside antiretroviral regimens have not been able to achieve the potency and durability of triple antiretroviral combinations, and the latter have generally become the standard of therapy in which didanosine is now used most frequently. Didanosine has been studied as part of triple combination regimens with other nucleoside analogs, NNRTIs, and PIs in both noncomparative and comparative trials as reviewed below.

Didanosine in Primary Infection

A triple combination of zidovudine/didanosine/lamivudine was employed to treat 10 patients with primary HIV-1 infection. This combination reduced plasma HIV RNA below detectable levels in all subjects after 108 ± 32 days of therapy. Infectious HIV could not be detected in lymph nodes from five patients on day 90, and HIV-1 RNA was at extremely low levels in lymph nodes after 1 year.[147]

Triple NRTI

A small study of 20 antiretroviral-naive subjects treated with didanosine and lamivudine and TDF showed poor virologic responses at week 12, as only 25% had a decrease of more than 1 $\log_{10}$ viral copies/mL, and 20% had an increase in viral RNA levels.[148] The poor responses were attributed to the presence of M184V and K65R resistance mutations.[89,149,150]

Didanosine in Regimens with NNRTIs

Triple regimens that include didanosine and NNRTIs have been compared with dual regimens in various stages of HIV infection. The ACTG 241 study evaluated the combination of didanosine/zidovudine/nevirapine versus didanosine/zidovudine in patients who had 350 or fewer CD4+ cells/μL and who had undergone more than 6 months of previous nucleoside therapy (Table 6-6).[151] The triple combination regimen

Table 6-5

Trials of Didanosine Monotherapy and Dual Nucleoside Combination Therapy

Trial	Design	Dosage	No. of Subjects	Entry Criteria	CD4 cells/μL on Entry	CD4 Response	Antiviral Response	Clinical Outcome			Comments
									Death/ 100 pt-year	AIDS event or death/ 100 pt-year	
ACTG 116a (Dolin et al[42])	ddI vs ZDV; randomized, double-blind	ddI: 500 or 750 mg/ day ZDV: 600 mg/ day	617	Symptomatic: c: CD4 <300/μL or Asymptomatic: CD4 <200/μL Previous ZDV experience of <16 weeks	130 (mean)	ddI 500 mg had slower decline in CD4 than ddI 750 mg or ZDV group	No difference in p24 declines among three treatment groups ZDV	500 ddI 750 ddI 11.1	17.7 15.4 30.4	30.0 33.1 500 ddI	ZDV more effective than 750 ddI in ZDV naive patients; more effective than ZDV in patients with >8 weeks <16 weeks ddI
ACTG 116b/117 (Kahn et al[43])	ddI vs ZDV; randomized, double-blind	ddI: 500 or 750 mg/ day ZDV: 600 mg/day	913	AS for ACTG 116a but ≥16 weeks of previous ZDV experience	95 (median)	CD4 change/ mm^3 at 24 weeks ddI 500 mg: −10 ddI 750 ddI 750 mg: −10 ZDV 600 mg: −23	Percent of subjects with ≥50% p24 decrease at 24 weeks: 500 ddI: 21 750 ddI: 32 ZDV: 21	500 ddI 750 ddI ZDV	Death/ 100 pt-year 15.5 17.5 16.9	AIDS event or death/ 100 pt-year 37.1 42.5 52.8	500 mg ddI more effective than ZDV in reducing risk of primary endpoints
BMS 010 (Spruance et al[61])	Switch to ddI or continue ZDV; randomized, double-blind	ddI 600 mg/ day (≥60 kg) 400 mg/day (<60 mg) ZDV: 600 mg/day	312	CD4 ≤300/μL ZDV for at least 6 months Clinical deterioration	70–75 (median)	Less decrease in CD4 in ddI group through week 24 ($P < 0.0001$)	No difference	New AIDS-defining events or death, or ≥50% CD4 decline ddI 53/100 pt-year ZDV 75/100 pt-years ($P = 0.02$)			Switching to ddI superior to continuation of ZDV in patients who are failing on ZDV

CTN 002 (Montaner et al[135])	Switch to ddI or continue ZDV; double-blind, randomized	ddI 400 mg/day (≥60 kg) 200 mg/day (<60 kg) ZDV: 600 mg/day	246	CD4 200–500/μL ZDV for at least 6 months Clinically stable	324	Increase in CD4 in ddI, decrease in ZDV at 48 weeks ($P < 0.01$)		New AIDS-defining events or death (no.) ddI(1); ZDV(8) ($P = 0.02$)	Switching to ddI superior to continuation of ZDV in patients clinically stable on ZDV
ACTG 175 (Hammer et al[58,138])	ddI vs zidovudine (ZDV) vs ddI + ZDV vs ddC + ZDV; randomized, double-blind	ddI: 400 mg/day ZDV: 600 mg/day Same in combination ddC: 2.25 mg/day in combination	2467	CD4 200–500/μL No AIDS-defining illness Antiretroviral naive or experienced	352 (mean)	Significantly better for ddI or combination therapy than for ZDV ($P < 0.006$)	Decrease in HIV RNA copies/mL $\log_{10}$ at 8 weeks: ZDV 0.26 ddI 0.65 ddI + ZDV 0.93 ddI + ddC 0.89	Progression to AIDS-defining events or death or >50% decline in CD4 counts ZDV 32% ddI 22% ddI + ZDV 18% ddC + ZDV 20% ($P < 0.001$ global)	Survival benefit for ddI, ddI + ZDV, and a trend for ddI + ddC ($P = 0.1$) Benefits for both antiretroviral viral naive and experienced, except for naive only for ddC + ZDV
ALBI Trial (Molina et al[143])	1. ddI + d4T 2. ZDV + 3TC or 3. ddI + d4T followed by ZDV + 3TC	ddI: 400 mg/day d4T: 80 mg/day ZDV: 500 mg/day 3TC: 300 mg/day	151	CD4 ≥200/μL Antiretroviral naive	382–384 (median)	Mean increase/μL 1. 124 2. 62 3. 18	Decrease in HIV RNA copies/mL/$\log_{10}$ at 24 weeks 1. 2.26 2. 1.26 3. 1.58		Antiretroviral effects greater with ddI + d4T CD4 greater with both ddI and ddT regimens

ddC, dideoxycytidine; ddI, dideoxyinosine; d4T, stavudine; 3TC, lamivudine.

resulted in higher mean CD4+ T-lymphocyte counts, lower mean infectious HIV-1 titers in peripheral blood mononuclear cells, and lower mean plasma HIV RNA levels than patients who received the double-combination regimen. The risk for disease progression did not differ between the two groups, but the study may have been underpowered to detect clinical differences.[151] In the ISSIS 047[152] and Incas[153] studies, the triple combination of didanosine, zidovudine, and nevirapine was superior in reduction of HIV RNA levels compared to the combination of didanosine plus zidovudine. At weeks 48–52, HIV RNA was undetectable in 38–51% of patients, and CD4+ T-lymphocyte counts had increased by 117 and 139 cells/μL, respectively, which were also significantly better than in recipients of dual therapy (Table 6-6).[152,153] The VIRGO trial also showed marked reductions in HIV RNA levels (−2.5 $\log_{10}$ copies/mL) and increases in CD4+ T-lymphocyte counts (168–139 cells/μL) with a combination of didanosine/zidovudine/nevirapine (NVP) (Table 6-6).[154] ACTG 261 compared a combination of didanosine/zidovudine/delavirdine with dual combinations of its components.[155] At 48 weeks, recipients of triple therapy had a higher rate of undetectable HIV RNA in plasma (26%), although the mean reductions in plasma levels were relatively modest in all the treatment groups (Table 6-6). A small trial in antiretroviral-naive patients showed no differences in virologic or CD4 responses among three aims comparing ddI + d4T + NVP, ZDV + 3TC + NVP or d4T + 3TC + NVP regimens.[156]

A small, single-aim study of didanosine + lamivudine + efavirenz administered once daily showed a reduction of HIV RNA levels to less than 50 copies/mL at 48 weeks.[157] Two studies of once-daily combination of didanosine/efavirenz/emtricitabine in antiretroviral-naive patients also showed potent antiviral and CD4 responses (Table 6-6).[158,159] A comparison of ddI + 3TC + efavirenz (EFV) with ddI + TDF + EFV in antiretroviral-naive patients demonstrated a significantly poorer virologic response in the TDF containing arm at week 12, but no differences in CD4 responses.[160] The patient population under study had median CD4 counts of 158–174 cells/μL and virus loads of 4.9–5.1 $\log_{10}$ copies/mL (Table 6-6). A small study of antiretroviral-naive patients who were treated with ddI + TDF + EFV found virologic failure in 6/14 (43%) which was attributed to the presence of resistance.[161,162]

Didanosine in Regimens with PIs

Didanosine has been studied in combination with many of the available PIs. Combinations of didanosine/stavudine/indinavir were studied in the OZCOMBO 1,[163] START II,[164] and ATLANTIC[165,166] trials in patients who were largely antiretroviral-naive. In OZCOMBO 1, this combination resulted in a decrease in HIV RNA levels of 2.68 $\log_{10}$ copies/mL at week 52 and an increase in CD4 cells of 120/μL[163]; in the START II trial there was a decrease of 2.6 $\log_{10}$ copies/mL and an increase in CD4 cells of 214/μL at 48 weeks (Table 6-7).[164] The ATLANTIC study found similar results for the combination of didanosine/stavudine/indinavir and for didanosine plus stavudine combined with either lamivudine or nevirapine.[165,166] Didanosine/lamivudine/indinavir therapy also demonstrated antiviral effects and improved CD4 counts at 24 weeks in another study of antiretroviral-naive patients among whom 41% were intravenous drug users.[167]

The combination of didanosine/stavudine/nelfinavir decreased the virus load (−1.36 $\log_{10}$ copies/mL) and increased CD4+ T-lymphocyte counts (111/μL) in patients without previous experience with any of the drugs in this regimen (Table 6-7).[128] A study carried out in 16 HIV-infected drug users with partly observed therapy with didanosine/stavudine/nelfinavir also showed either a more than 2 $\log_{10}$ drop in RNA levels or a more than 100/μL in CD4 counts in most of the subjects.[168] Didanosine and stavudine in combination with ritonavir resulted in a 3.1 $\log_{10}$ reduction of RNA copies/mL after 72 weeks, although nearly one-half of the subjects discontinued medication because of adverse side effects (Table 6-7).[169] A study reported that didanosine and 3TC as one of four nucleoside regimens combined with ritonavir/indinavir resulted in potent reductions of viral loads and rises in CD4 counts in antiretroviral-naive patients with high baseline viral loads, although specific results for the didanosine containing arm were not reported.[170] Didanosine combined with atazanavir[171] also showed strong antiretroviral effects.

A CPCRA study compared the combination of didanosine + d4T with abacavir (ABC) + 3TC added to a regimen consisting of either a PI + NRTI, NNRTI + NRTI, or PI + NNRTI + NRTI. At 24 months, a trend was reported for superior responses in the ABC + 3TC regimen with respect to the primary endpoint of virus load of less than 50 copies/mL, CD4 rises, and tolerability[172] (Table 6-6).

ACTG 384 compared the effect of starting treatment with one of four, three drug regimens: (1) ddI + d4T + EFV; (2) ddI + d4T + nelfinavir; (3) ZDV + 3TC + EFV; or (4) ZDV + 3TC + nelfinavir, followed by sequential therapy with the other three drug regimens as needed. Also included were two groups, with a four drug regimen: (5) ddI + d4T + EFV + nelfinavir; and (6) ZDV + 3TC + EFV + nelfinavir.[173,174] Among the three drug regimens, starting with ZDV + 3TC + EFV appeared to be superior to the other regimens (Table 6-7).[173] Results in four drug regimens were not significantly different from three drug regimens.[174] Regimens containing d4T + didanosine appeared to be more toxic than those containing ZDV + 3TC, particularly with respect to peripheral neuropathy and lactic acidosis (Table 6-7).

Combinations of Didanosine and Hydroxyurea

As noted above, hydroxyurea does not inhibit HIV replication directly but, rather, potentiates the effects of didanosine.[20,175,176] Thus administration of hydroxyurea alone did not reduce HIV-1 RNA levels; but when given in combination with didanosine, reductions of HIV RNA of 0.02–2.10 $\log_{10}$ copies/mL were achieved.[177–182] A greater effect on HIV RNA levels was seen when higher doses of hydroxyurea were used (1000 mg/day compared to 500 mg/day).[177] Because hydroxyurea also has antiproliferative cellular

Table 6-6

Triple Combination Therapy with Didanosine and Nonnucleoside Reverse Transcriptase Inhibitors

Trial	Design	Dosage	No. of Subjects	Entry Criteria	CD4 cells/μl; HIV RNA[a] on Entry	CD 4 Response	Antiviral Response[a]	Clinical Outcome	Comments
ACTG 241 (D'Aquila et al[151])	ddI + ZDV vs. ddI + ddI: 400 mg/d ZDV + NVP Double-blind, randomised	ZDV: 600 mg/d NVP: 200 mg/d for 2wk, then 400 mg/d	398	CD4: ≤350; >6 mo of prior nucleoside therapy	135–139 (median)	At 48 wks, triple combination had 18% higher mean CD4 counts	At 48 wks: triple combination had lower mean plasma RNA levels	No difference in disease progression	Severe rashes more common in NVP group
INCAS (Montaner et al[153])	ddI + ZDV + NVP vs. ZDV + NVP vs. ZDV + ddI Double-blind, randomised	As for ACTG 241	153	CD4: 200–600 Antiretroviral-naive	340 (median) 4.25–4.54 (median) RNA	At 52 wks Triple Rx: increase of 139/μl ZDV + ddI: increase of 87/μl ZDV + NVP: decrease of 6/μl	At 52 wks: RNA levels log_{10} Triple Rx: −2.71 to −0.72 ZDV + ddI: −2.11 to −0.01 ZDV + NVP: −0.41 to −0.08	Disease progression or death Triple Rx: 12% ZDV + ddI: 25% ZDV + NVP: 23%	Trend toward improved clinical outcome in triple Rx (P = 0.08)
Virgo I and II (Raffi et al[154])	ddI + d4T + NVP Open label	ddI: 400 mg/d d4T: 80 mg/d NVP: 400 mg/d	100	Antiretroviral-naive	412–414 (mean) 4.59–4.87 (mean)	139–168 increase at wk 24	At wk 52: 67% of pts had <50 copies/ml	–	20% discontinued study because of an adverse event
ACTG 261 (Friedland et al[155])	ddI + ZDV + delavirdine (DLV) vs. ddI + ZDV vs. ddI + DLV vs. ZDV + DLV Double-blind, randomised	ddI: 400 mg/d ZDV: 600 mg/d DLV 1.2 g/d	544	CD4: 100–500; <6 mo of monotherapy	2.95 (median) 4.45 (median)	At 40–48 wks, increase of 65 (mean) for triple Rx	At 40–48 wks: decrease of 0.73 for triple Rx	–	Generally better responses for triple Rx; 30% experienced rash (1 severe)
Molina et al[158]	ddI + EFV + emtricitabine	ddI: 400 mg/d EFV: 600 mg/d Emitricitabine: 200 mg/d	40	Antiretroviral-naive	373 median 4.77 median	159 (median); increase at wk 24	At wk 24: 3.5 Decrease	–	Well tolerated; mild to moderate CNS symptoms in 73%

(Continued)

Table 6-6 **(Continued)**

Inhibitors									
Trial	Design	Dosage	No. of Subjects	Entry Criteria	CD4 cells/μl; HIV RNA[a] on Entry	CD 4 Response	Antiviral Response[a]	Clinical Outcome	Comments
OzCombo 2 (French et al[156])	ZDV + 3TC + NVP or d4T + ddI + NVP or d4T + 3TC + NVP Randomized	ddI: 200 mg/bid ZDV: 250 mg bid d4T: 40 mg bid NVP: 200 mg bid	70	CD4 >50/μl Antiretroviral-naive 4.63 (mean)	399 (mean) 4.63 (mean)	174 (mean)	−1.60 (mean)		No significant difference among treatment arms – low power to detect differences
Maitland et al[160]	ddI + 3TC + EFV or ddI + TDF + EFV Randomized	ddI: 400 mg qd with 3TC: 300 mg qd or TDF: 300 mg qd with ddI: 200–250 mg pd plus EFV: 600 mg qd	76	Antiretroviral-naive	174–158 (median) 5.13–4.99 (mean)	At week 12 3TC group: 117 TDF group: 108	At week 12 3TC: −3.16 TDF: −2.85		TDF/ddI/EFV regimens had poorer virologic sequences than 3TC/ddI/EFV regimens; CD4 responses were similar

DLV, delavirdine; NVP, nevirapine; EFV, efavirenz; 3TC, lamivudine; TDF, tenofovir.

[a] Log_{10} of copies of plasma HIV RNA/mL.

Table 6-7

Triple Combination Therapy with Didanosine and Protease Inhibitors

Trial	Design	Dosage	No. of Subjects	Entry Criteria	CD4 cells/μl; HIV RNA[a] at Entry	CD4 Response	Antiviral Response[a]	Comments
OzCombo1 (Carr et al[163])	ZDV + 3TC + IDV or d4T + 3TC + IDV or d4T + ddI + IDV Randomized	ddI: 400 mg/d d4t: 80 mg/d IDV: 2.4 g/d 3TC: 300 mg/d ZDV: 500 mg/d	109	CD4 < 500/μl or RNA > 30,0000 copies/ml Antiretroviral-naive	267–313 (mean) 5.00–5.21 (mean)	120–159/μl mean increase at wk 52	−2.68 to −3.28 mean decrease at wk 52	DTH responses improved but remained impaired; quality of life improved DdI + d4T + IDV comparable or superior to ZDV + 3TC + IDV Well tolerated; no
START II (Eron et al[164])	ZDV + 3TC + IDV or d4T + ddI + IDV Randomized	As above, except ZDV given 600 mg/d	205	CD4 >200 μl and RNA >10,000 copies/ml, <4 wks of Rx; naïve to 3TC and protease inhibitors	422 (median) 4.5 (median)	214/μl median increase for ddI arm and 142 for ZDV arm at wk 48	−2.6 for both arms at wk 48	ddI + d4T + ZDV comparable or superior to ZDV + 3TC + IDV
Elion et al[128]	d4T + ddI + NFV Open label	ddI: 400 mg/d d4T: 80 mg/d NFV: 2250 mg/d	22	RNA >10,000 copies/ml; naive to d4T, ddI or protease inhibitors	315 (median) 4.8 $\log_{10}$ (median)	+111 mean at wk 12	−1.36 mean at wk 12	Well tolerated; no pharmacokinetic interaction between ddI, d4T, and NFV
Saimot et al[169]	ddI + d4T + ritonavir Open label	ddI: 200 mg bid d4T: 40 mg bid Ritonavir: NR	36	CD4: 5–350 Antiretroviral-naive	252 (mean)	At wk 12, mean CD4 increase of 138 cells/μl	Decrease in plasma RNA levels by 3.1 $\log_{10}$ at wk 72	15/36 patients discontinued assigned dosage because of adverse effects
McArthur et al[172]	ddI + d4T or ABC + 3TC in combination with PI + RTI, NNRTI + NRTI, or PI + NNRTI + NRTI Randomized	–	182	Antiretroviral-naive	212 (mean) 5.1	At 24 months: ABC + 3TC regimen had 35 cells/μl increase more than ddI + d4T regimen $P = 0.6$	At 24 months, >50 copies/ml: ddI + d4T: 79% ABC + 3TC: 73% $P = 0.23$	Author concluded that a trend favors ABC + 3TC regimen over ddI + d4T

(*Continued*)

Table 6-7

(Continued)

Trial	Design	Dosage	No. of Subjects	Entry Criteria	CD4 cells/μl; HIV RNA[a] at Entry	CD4 Response	Antiviral Response[a]	Comments
ACTG 384 (Robbins et al[173,174])	d4T + ddI + EFV; d4T + ddI + Nelfinavir; ZDV + 3TC + EFV; ZDV + 3TC + Nelfinavir; d4T + ddI + EFV + Nelfinaviar; ZDV + 3TC + EFV + Nelfinavir Randomized; double Blind with respect to EFV and Nelfinavir; factorial design	ddI: 400 mg bd d4t: 40 mg bd 3TC: 150 mg bd EFV: 600 mg qd Nelfinvir: 1250 mg bd	980 (620) in sequential three drug regimens	Antiretroviral-naive RNA copies ≥500 ml	278 (median) 4.9 (median)	At 12 months: 285 (median) without difference among groups	In 3 drug regimens, time to 1° endpoint of virologic failure was delayed in ZDV + 3TC and in EFV regimens; Results in 4 drug regimens were not significantly different from 3 drug regimens	Regimens with ZDV + 3TC had delayed onset of toxicity, compared to d4T + ddI, particularly peripheral neuropathy. Lactic acidosis occurred in 9 subjects on ddI + d4T

[a] Log_{10} of plasma HIV RNA copies/ml.

activity, CD4 responses generally have been absent or blunted, which is an important limitation on use of the drug. In a comparative study, combination therapy with didanosine and hydroxyurea was superior to monotherapy with either drug, with zidovudine alone, or with zidovudine along with hydroxyurea.[183] Triple combination therapy with didanosine/stavudine/hydroxyurea was superior to that seen with didanosine/hydroxyurea[184,185] but appeared less effective than that observed with didanosine/stavudine/nelfinavir in another study.[186] Treatment of patients with primary infection with didanosine/indinavir/hydroxyurea resulted in undetectable (fewer than 50 copies/mL) levels of HIV RNA in 11 of 11 patients after 68 weeks.[187] Prolonged suppression of HIV RNA levels with didanosine/hydroxyurea also resulted in improvement of some immune parameters.[188] Triple combination therapy with didanosine/hydroxyurea/PIs has also been shown to suppress HIV RNA levels for up to 21 months.[189]

The combination of didanosine/hydroxyurea has been reported to be well tolerated in general,[50,187,190–192] although significant toxicities have also been encountered, and in one long-term study, most of the patients who had started with a hydroxyurea-containing regimen were no longer taking hydroxyurea at the end of the study.[185] The most commonly encountered toxicity was reversible bone marrow suppression consistent with the drug's antiproliferative effect.[50,193] The addition of hydroxyurea also increased the rate of peripheral neuropathy when combined with either didanosine or stavudine[194] or when added to a combination of the two drugs.[50,185,195] Pancreatitis has also been reported in patients receiving hydroxyurea/didanosine[196,197] and in patients receiving hydoxyurea, stavudine and didanosine.[10,22] A report from the FDA Adverse Event Reporting System suggested that the use of hydroxyurea in combination with an NRTI may enhance the risk of death caused by hepatoxicity, and that this risk may be further enhanced if hydroxyurea were used in combination with didanosine and stavudine. The report stated: 'Interpretations of data from such voluntary reporting systems have limitations; however, clinicians should be particularly aware of this potential toxicity when combinations of these drugs are used.'[198]

STUDIES IN PEDIATRIC PATIENTS

Didanosine buffered formulations are approved for use in pediatric patients, and a powder for oral solutions is available for pediatric use. The recommended dose for pediatric administration for patients between 2 weeks and 8 months of age is 100 mg/m^2 bid and for those over 8 months of age is 120 mg/m^2 bid. Recommendations for children below 2 weeks of age are not available. Studies of the efficacy of once-daily dosing in children have not been reported, and the EC formulation is approved for use in adults only.

Didanosine, alone or in combination with other antiretroviral agents, has been studied in children of various ages and HIV-related disease states; the major studies in this area are summarized in Table 6-8. Initial studies showed that didanosine monotherapy was well tolerated and associated with antiretroviral activity and improved CD4 counts.[199–201] Combination therapy with didanosine and zidovudine also demonstrated beneficial antiretroviral and CD4 count responses[202] and was superior to zidovudine monotherapy in terms of clinical endpoints in the ACTG 152 study.[203] In that study, didanosine/zidovudine combination therapy was not significantly better than didanosine monotherapy.

In the PACTG 300 study zidovudine/didanosine or zidovudine/lamivudine was associated with lower rates of disease progression than didanosine alone.[204] Didanosine/stavudine[205,206] or didanosine/lamivudine[207] also had a beneficial effect on HIV-1 virus markers. Marked decreases in HIV-1 RNA levels have been observed in pediatric studies of didanosine/stavudine as part of triple combinations with saquinavir,[208] indinavir,[209,210] or nelfinavir[211] and with zidovudine/nevirapine.[212]

CLINICAL INDICATIONS AND CONCLUSIONS

Didanosine is a potent antiretroviral agent whose efficacy has been demonstrated in large-scale clinical trials involving adults and children at various stages of HIV disease progression. The initial trials consisted of monotherapy and dual combination therapy, which have now been supplanted by triple combination regimens that have demonstrated potent antiretroviral and CD4 responses. These have included various regimens of didanosine in combination with other NRTIs (zidovudine, lamivudine, emtricitabine, stavudine, TDF), NNRTIs (nevirapine, delavirdine, efavirenz) and PIs (indinavir, nelfinavir, ritonavir, atazanavir). The addition of hydroxyurea potentiated the antiretroviral effect of didanosine, but the resultant CD4 responses were blunted because of the antiproliferative activity of hydroxyurea, and the combination potentiates certain toxicities (see further ahead). As part of combination therapy of antiretroviral-naive patients, some didanosine containing regimens appeared to be less potent than other alternatives. Didanosine tolerability has been significantly improved overall with the use of the currently available buffered tablets (VIDEX) and extended release capsule (VIDEX EC), and their use in once-a-day dosing regimens.

The major toxicities of didanosine to which clinicians should be alert are pancreatitis and peripheral neuropathy which if recognized early are often reversible upon discontinuation of the drug. These toxicities may be potentiated by concurrent administration of didanosine with antiretrovirals such as stavudine, TDF, zalcitabine, or by hydroxyurea, and such combinations should be avoided whenever possible. As with any NRTI, lactic acidosis and hepatic injury can occur with didanosine and may be particularly severe in patients who receive the drug in combination with hydroxyurea or stavudine (or both), and in pregnant patients.

Didanosine Therapy in Children

Table 6-8

Trial	Design	Dosage	No. of Subjects	Entry Criteria
Mueller et al[199]	ddI Dose ranging	20–180 mg/m^2 q8h	103	6 months to 18 years: CD4 <500/μL
Husson et al[202]	ddI + zidovudine (ZDV) Dose ranging	ddI: 90–180 mg/m^2 q12h ZDV: 60 mg/m^2 q6h	54	3 months to 18 years: CD4 <500/μL
ACTG 152 (Englund et al[203])	ZDV vs ddI vs ZDV + ddI Double-blind, randomized	ZDV: 180 mg/m^2 q6h or ddI: 120 mg/m^2 q12h or ZDV: 120 mg/m^2 q6h plus ddI: 90 mg/m^2 q12h	831	3 months to 18 years: CD4 <1000/μL if <15 months; CD4 <500 if >15 months but <18 years
Luzuriaga et al[212]	ddI + ZDV + nevirapine; open-label	ddI: 120 mg/m^2 q12h plus ZDV: 180 mg/m^2 q8h plus Nevirapine: 120 mg/m^2 qd × 28 days, then 200 mg/m^2 q12h	8	2–18 months
PACTG 300[207]	ZDV + 3TC vs ddI vs ddI + ZDV; randomized, double-blind	ZDV: 160 mg/m^2 tid 3TC: 4 mg/kg q12h ddI monotherapy: 120 mg/m^2 q12h ddI combination: 90 mg/m^2 q12h	471	Immunosuppression or symptomatic infection;<56 days of prior Rx; ages 42 days to 15 years
Kline et al[209]	ddI + d4T + IDV; open-label d4T: 1 mg/kg q12h IDV: 500 mg/m^2 q12h	ddI: 90 mg/m^2 q12h	12	Symptomatic infection; >1 year of NRTI therapy; 4.2–13.5 years
Funk et al[211]	ddI + d4T + NFV; open-label d4T: 2 mg/kg bid; NFV: 60–90 mg/kg tid	ddI: 180 mg/m^2 bid	8	CDC category A1, B1, or B3; no prior Rx; 14–132 months

AUC, area under the curve; IDV, indinavir; HYD, hydroxyurea; NFV, nelfinavir; URIs, upper respiratory infections.

[a] Log_{10} of plasma HIV RNA copies/mL.

Drug interactions with didanosine are generally infrequent (Table 6-4), and those related to the antacid and cation content of buffered didanosine formulations can be minimized by appropriately spacing the administration of didanosine and other medications. Such interactions would not be present with the delayed-release EC formulation, which does not contain buffer.

Because of the evidence for decreased potency of certain didanosine containing regimens as initial therapy and because of its toxicity profile, didanosine is no longer recommended as part of dual NRTI components of initial therapy in the 2006 Recommendations of International AIDS Society – USA Panel.[213] The most recent recommendations from the Department of Health and Human Services also do not list didanosine as part of the dual NRTI component of initial therapy, but didanosine in combination with either lamivudine or emtricitabine is listed as an alternative.[214] For antiretroviral experienced patients, didanosine may be a useful component of salvage therapy with appropriate monitoring for virologic resistance and awareness of toxicity profiles.

REFERENCES

1. Hitchcock MJM. In vitro antiviral activity of didanosine compared with that of other dideoxynucleoside analogs against laboratory strains and clinical isolates of human immunodeficiency virus. Clin Infect Dis 16(Suppl 1):S16, 1993.
2. McGowan JJ, Tomaszewski JE, Cradock J, et al. Overview of the preclinical development of an antiretroviral drug, 2′,3′-dideoxyinosine. Rev Infect Dis 12(Suppl 5):S513, 1990.
3. Shelton MJ, O'Donnell AM, Morse GD. Didanosine. Ann Pharmacother 26:660, 1992.
4. Cooney DA, Ahluwalia G, Mitsuay H, et al. Initial studies on the cellular pharmacology of 2′,3′-dideoxyadenosine, an inhibitor of HTLV-III infectivity. Biochem Pharmacol 36:1765, 1987.
5. Reinke CM, Drach JC, Shipman C Jr. Differential inhibition of mammalian DNA polymerases α, β, and γ herpes simplex virus-induced DNA polymerase by the 5′-triphosphates of arabinosyladenine and arabinosylcytosine. In: de The G, Henle W, Rapp F (eds) Oncogenesis and Herpesviruses III. Lyon: IARC Scientific Publications; 1978, p 999.
6. Perry CM, Balfour JA. Didanosine: an update on its antiviral activity, pharmacokinetic properties and therapeutic efficacy in the management of HIV disease. Drugs 52:928, 1996.

CD4 cells/μL on Entry; HIV RNA[a] on Entry	CD4 Response	Antiviral Response[a]	Clinical Outcome	Comments
10–37 (median)	>50 cell/μL increases in 28/87 after 6 months and in 11/27 after 3 years	Decrease in p24 below 50 pg/ml in 17/40 at 6 months and in 57–80% at >60 months	Longer survival with entry CD4 >100/μL	Interpatient variability in AUC
33 (median)	Median increase of 225/μL at 24 weeks	Median decrease of 64 pg/L	84% Gained weight; no overall increase in IQ	ZDV-intolerant patients tolerated lower doses of ZDV in combinations
809 (median)	At 96 weeks, CD4 counts were 86% higher in ddI, and 76% were higher in ddI + ZDV than in ZDV monotherapy	At 48 weeks, p24 levels were 40% lower for both ddI and ddI + ZDV than in ZDV group	Interim analysis for primary endpoint: ZDV: 27% ddI: 19% ddI + ZDV: 18% ($P = 0.007$) Final analysis: no difference between ddI and ddI + ZDV groups	More hematologic toxicity with ZDV + ddI than ddI alone
18–58% of peripheral lymphocytes	Stable or slightly increased CD4 counts	At four weeks decrease of plasma RNA of >1.5 $\log_{10}$ in 7/8; during 6 month treatment, RNA was undetectable in two; 0.5–1.5 $\log_{10}$ decrease in 5/6		Well-tolerated
699 (median); 5.1 (median)	ZDV + 3TC: +73/μL ddI: +4/μL at 36–48 weeks	ZDV + 3TC: −0.80 ddI: −0.28 at week 12		Randomization to ZDV + ddI stopped early because of ACTG152 results; both combination arms had lower rates of disease progression than HIV monotherapy
11–878 (range)	317/μL median increase at week 48	−2.0 decrease at week 48		9/12 completed 48-week course; 6/12 had crystalluria
606 (median); 606 000 RNA copies/mL	183/μL median increase at week 12	−2.4 decrease at week 12	Some improvement in adenopathy, and possibly decreased URIs or otitis media	Generally well-tolerated; mild diarrhea and elevated triglycerides were seen; no difference in results from a comparative group given ZDV + 3TC + NFV

7. Perry CM, Noble S. Didanosine: an updated review of its use in HIV infection. Drugs 58:1099, 1999.
8. Domin BA, Mahoney WB, Zimmerman TP. Membrane permeation mechanisms of 2′,3′-dideoxynucleosides. Biochem Pharmacol 46:725, 1993.
9. St Clair MH, Pennington KN, Rooney J. In vitro comparison of selected triple-drug combinations for suppression of HIV-1 replication: the inter-company collaboration protocol. J Acquir Immune Defic Syndr Hum Retrovirol 10(Suppl 2):83, 1995.
10. Prescribing Information. Videx (Didanosine). Princeton, NJ: Bristol-Meyers Squibb, Oct 2005.
11. Reichman RC, Tejani N, Lambert LJ, et al. Didanosine (ddI) and zidovudine (ZDV) susceptibilities of human immunodeficiency virus (HIV) isolates from long-term recipients of ddI. Antiviral Res 20:267, 1993.
12. McLeod GX, McGrath JM, Ladd EA, et al. Didanosine and zidovudine resistance patterns in clinical isolates of human immunodeficiency virus type 1 as determined by a replication endpoint concentration assay. Antimicrob Agents Chemother 36:920, 1992.
13. St Clair MH, Martin JL, Tudor-Williams G, et al. Resistance to ddI and sensitivity to AZT induced by a mutation in HIV-1 reverse transcriptase. Science 253:1557, 1991.
14. Gao W-Y, Agbaria R, Driscoll JS, et al. Divergent anti-human immunodeficiency virus activity and anabolic phosphorylation of 2′3′-dideoxynucleoside analogs in resting and activated human cells. J Biol Chem 269:12633, 1994.
15. Aquaro S, Perno C-F, Balestra E, et al. Inhibition of replication of HIV in primary monocyte/macrophages by different antiviral drugs and comparative efficacy in lymphocytes. J Leukoc Biol 62:138, 1997.
16. Faulds D, Brodgen RN. Didanosine: a review of its antiviral activity, pharmacokinetic properties and therapeutic potential in human immunodeficiency virus infection. Drugs 44:94, 1992.
17. Merrill DP, Moonis M, Chou TC, et al. Lamivudine or stavudine in two- and three-drug combinations against human immunodeficiency virus type 1 replication in vitro. J Infect Dis 173:355, 1996.
18. Manion DJ, Hirsh MS. Mechanisms underlying combination anti-retroviral therapies. In: Merigan TJ, Bartlett JG, Bolognesi D (eds) Textbook of AIDS Medicine. Baltimore: Williams & Wilkins; 2000, p 886.
19. Hammer SM, Inouye RT. Antiviral agents. In: Richman DD, Whitley RJ, Hayden FG (eds) Clinical Virology. Washington, DC: ASM Press; 2002, p 193.

20. Lori F, Malykh A, Cara A, et al. Hydroxyurea as an inhibitor of human immunodeficiency virus-type 1 replication. Science 266:801, 1994.
21. Burger DM, Meenhorst PL, Beijnen JH. Concise overview of the clinical pharmacokinetics of dideoxynucleoside antiretroviral agents. Pharm World Sci 17:25, 1995.
22. Prescribing Information, Videx EC. Princeton, NJ: Bristol-Myers Squibb, Mar 2006.
23. Knupp CA, Shyu WC, Dolin R, et al. Pharmacokinetics of didanosine in patients with acquired immunodeficiency syndrome or acquired immunodeficiency syndrome complex. Clin Pharmacol Ther 49:523, 1991.
24. Hoetelmans RMW, van Heeswijk RPG, Profijt M, et al. Comparison of the plasma pharmacokinetics and renal clearance of didanosine during once and twice daily dosing in HIV-1 infected individuals. AIDS 12(Suppl 1):F211, 1998.
25. Shyu WC, Knupp CA, Pittman KA, et al. Food-induced reduction in bioavailability of didanosine. Clin Pharmacol Ther 50:503, 1991.
26. Knupp CA, Milbrath R, Barbhaiya RH. Effect of time of food administration on the bioavailability of didanosine from a chewable tablet formulation. J Clin Pharmacol 33:568, 1993.
27. Dudley MN. Clinical pharmacokinetics of nucleoside antiretroviral agents. J Infect Dis 171(Suppl 2):S99, 1995.
28. Hartman NR, Yarchoan R, Pluda JM, et al. Pharmacokinetics of 2′,3′-dideoxyadenosine and 2′,3′-dideoxyinosine in patients with severe human immunodeficiency virus infection. Clin Pharmacol Ther 47:647, 1990.
29. Singlas E, Taburet AM, Borsa Lebas LF, et al. Didanosine pharmacokinetics in patients with normal and impaired renal function: influence of hemodialysis. Antimicrob Agents Chemother 36:1519, 1992.
30. Ray AS, Olson L, Fridland A. Role of purine nucleoside phosphorylase in interactions between 2′,3′-dideoxyinosine and allopurinol, ganciclovir, or tenofovir. Antimicrob Agents Chemother 48:1089, 2004.
31. Waters L, Maitland D, Moyle GJ. Tenofovir and didanosine: a dangerous liaison. AIDS Read 15:403–6, 413, 2005.
32. Tung MY, Mandalia S, Bower M, et al. The durability of virological success of tenofovir and didanosine dosed at either 400 or 250 mg once daily. HIV Med 6:151, 2005.
33. Klecker RW Jr, Collins JM, Yarchoan R, et al. Plasma and cerebrospinal fluid pharmacokinetics of 3′-azido-3′-deoxythimidine: a novel pyrimidine analog with potential application for the treatment of patients with AIDS and related diseases. Clin Pharmacol Ther 41:407, 1987.
34. Burger DM, Kraayeveld CL, Meenhorst PL, et al. Study on didanosine concentrations in cerebrospinal fluid: implications for the treatment and prevention of AIDS dementia complex. Pharm World Sci 17:218, 1995.
35. Wang Y, Livingston E, Patil S, et al. Pharmacokinetics of didanosine in antepartum and postpartum human immunodeficiency virus-infected pregnant women and their neonates: an AIDS clinical trials group study. J Infect Dis 180:1536, 1999.
36. Dancis J, Lee JD, Mendoza S, et al. Transfer and metabolism of dideoxyinosine by the perfused human placenta. J Acquir Immune Defic Syndr 6:2, 1993.
37. Henderson GI, Perez AB, Yang Y, et al. Transfer of dideoxyinosine across the human isolated placenta. Br J Clin Pharmacol 38:237, 1994.
38. Balis FM, Pizzo PA, Butler KM, et al. Clinical pharmacology 2′,3′-dideoxyinosine in human immunodeficiency virus-infected children. J Infect Dis 165:99, 1992.
39. Stevens RC, Rodman JH, Yong FH, et al. Effect of food and pharmacokinetic variability on didanosine systemic exposure in HIV-infected children: pediatric AIDS Clinical Trials Group protocol 144 study team. AIDS Res Hum Retroviruses 16:415, 2000.
40. Marra CM, Booss J. Does brain penetration of anti-HIV drugs matter? Sex Transm Infect 76:1, 2000.
41. Abreu T, Plaisance K, Rexroad V, et al. Bioavailability of once- and twice-daily regimens of didanosine in human immunodeficiency virus-infected children. Antimicrob Agents Chemother 44:1375, 2000.
42. Dolin R, Amato DA, Fischl MA, et al. Zidovudine compared with didanosine in patients with advanced HIV type 1 infection and little or no previous experience with zidovudine. Arch Intern Med 155:961, 1995.
43. Kahn JO, Lagakos SW, Richman DD, et al. A controlled trial comparing continued zidovudine with didanosine in human immunodeficiency virus infection. N Engl J Med 327:581, 1992.
44. Dolin R. Didanosine (dideoxyinosine, ddI). In: Mills J, Corey L (eds) Antiviral Chemotherapy: New Directions for Clinical Application and Research. Englewood Cliffs, NJ: Prentice-Hall; 1993, p 363.
45. Lambert JS, Seidlin M, Reichman RC, et al. 2′,3′-Dideoxyinosine (ddI) in patients with the acquired immunodeficiency syndrome or AIDS-related complex: a phase I trial. N Engl J Med 322:1333, 1990.
46. Styrt BA, Piazza-Hepp TD, Chikami GK. Clinical toxicity of antiretroviral nucleoside analogs. Antivir Res 31:121, 1996.
47. Rozencweig M, McLaren C, Beltangady M, et al. Overview of phase I trials of 2′,3′-dideoxyinosine (ddI) conducted on adult patients. Rev Infect Dis 12(Suppl 5):S570, 1990.
48. Yarchoan R, Mitsuya H, Pluda JM, et al. The National Cancer Institute phase I study of 2′,3′-dideoxyinosine administration in adults with AIDS or AIDS-related complex: analysis of activity and toxicity profiles. Rev Infect Dis 12(Suppl 5):S522, 1990.
49. Kelleher T, Cross A, Dunkle L. Relation of peripheral neuropathy to HIV treatment in four randomized clinical trials including didanosine. Clin Ther 21:118, 1999.
50. Seminari E, Lisziewicz J, Tinelli C, et al. Hydroxyurea toxicity combined with didanosine (ddI) in HIV-1-seropositive asymptomatic individuals. Int J Clin Pharmacol Ther 37:514, 1999.
51. Moore RD, Wong WM, Keruly JC, McArthur JC. Incidence of neuropathy in HIV-infected patients on monotherapy versus those on combination therapy with didanosine, stavudine and hydroxyurea. AIDS 14:273, 2000.
52. Kieburtz KD, Seidlin M, Lambert JS, et al. Extended follow up of peripheral neuropathy in patients with AIDS and AIDS-related complex treated with dideoxyinosine. J Acquir Immune Defic Syndr 5:60, 1992.
53. Chen CH, Cheng YC. Delayed cytotoxicity and selective loss of mitochondrial DNA in cells treated with anti-human immunodeficiency virus compound 2′,3′-dideoxycytidine. J Biol Chem 264:11934, 1989.
54. Grasela TH, Walawander CA, Beltangady M, et al. Analysis of potential risk factors associated with the development of pancreatitis in phase I patients with AIDS or AIDS-related complex receiving didanosine. J Infect Dis 169:1250, 1994.
55. Schwartz MS, Brandt LJ. The spectrum of pancreatic disorders in patients with the acquired immunodeficiency syndrome. Am J Gastroenterol 84:459, 1989.
56. Jablonowski H, Arasteh K, Staszewski S, et al. A dose comparison study of didanosine in patients with very advanced HIV infection who are intolerant to or clinically deteriorate on zidovudine. AIDS 9:463, 1995.
57. Nguyen B-Y, Yarchoan R, Wyvill KM, et al. Five-year follow up of a phase I study of didanosine in patients with advanced human immunodeficiency virus infection. J Infect Dis 171:1180, 1994.
58. Hammer SM, Katzenstein DA, Hughes MD, et al. A trial comparing nucleoside monotherapy with combination therapy in HIV-infected adults with CD4 cell counts from 200 to 500 per cubic millimeter. N Engl J Med 335:1091, 1996.

59. Whitfield RM, Bechtel L, Schroeder G, et al. Pancreatitis in HIV/AIDS patients taking dideoxyinosine or dideoxycytosine who use ethanol, tobacco, or controlled substances [abstract]. Clin Res 42:46A, 1994.
60. Reisler RB, Murphy RL, Redfield RR, Parker RA. Incidence of pancreatitis in HIV-1-infected individuals enrolled in 20 adult AIDS clinical trials group studies: lessons learned. J Acquir Immune Defic Syndr 39:159, 2005.
61. Spruance SL, Pavia AT, Peterson D, et al. Didanosine compared with continuation of zidovudine in HIV-infected patients with signs of clinical deterioration while receiving zidovudine: a randomized, double-blind clinical trial. Ann Intern Med 120:360, 1994.
62. Pike IM, Nicaise C. The didanosine expanded access program: safety analysis. Clin Infect Dis 16(Suppl 1):S63, 1993.
63. Lai KK, Gang DL, Zawacki JK. Fulminant hepatic failure associated with 2′,3′-dideoxyinosine (ddI). Ann Intern Med 115:283, 1991.
64. Ware AJ, Berggren RA, Taylor WE. Didanosine-induced hepatitis. Am J Gastroenterol 95:2141, 2000.
65. Bissuel F, Bruneel F, Habersetzer F, et al. Fulminant hepatitis with severe lactate acidosis in HIV-infected patients on didanosine therapy. J Intern Med 235:367, 1994.
66. Ter Hofstede HJM, de Marie D, Foudraine NA, et al. Clinical features and risk factors of lactic acidosis following long-term antiretroviral therapy: 4 fatal cases. Int J STD AIDS 11:611, 2000.
67. Important Drug Warning [letter]. Princeton, NJ: Bristol-Myers Squibb, 5 Jan 2001.
68. Whitcup SM, Dastgheib K, Nussenblatt RB, et al. A clinicopathologic report of the retinal lesions associated with didanosine. Arch Ophthalmol 112:1594, 1994.
69. Whitcup SM, Butler KM, Pizzo PA. Retinal lesions in children treated with dideoxyinosine. N Engl J Med 326:1226, 1992.
70. Zapor MJ, Cozza KL, Wynn GH, et al. Antiretrovirals. Part II: Focus on non-protease inhibitor antiretrovirals (NRTIs, NNRTIs, and fusion inhibitors). Psychosomatics 45: 524, 2004.
71. Allan JD, Connolly KJ, Fitch H, et al. Long-term follow-up of didanosine administered orally twice daily to patients with advanced human immunodeficiency virus infection and hematologic intolerance of zidovudine. Clin Infect Dis 16(Suppl 1): S46, 1993.
72. Monno L, Cargnel A, Soranzo ML, et al. Comparison of once- and twice-daily dosing of didanosine in combination with stavudine for the treatment of HIV-1 infection. Antivir Ther 4:195, 1999.
73. Mobley JE, Pollard RB, Schrader S, et al. Virological and immunological responses to once-daily dosing of didanosine in combination with stavudine. AIDS 13:F87, 1999.
74. Kazatchkine MD, Van PN, Costagliola D, et al. Didanosine dosed daily is equivalent to twice daily dosing for patients on double or triple combination antiretroviral therapy. J Acquir Immune Defic Syndr 24:418, 2000.
75. Youle M. Didanosine once daily: an overview. Antivir Ther 3(Suppl 4):35, 1998.
76. Pollard RB. Didanosine once-daily: potential for expanded use [review]. AIDS 14:2421, 2000.
77. Van Heeswijk RPG, Veldkamp AI, Mulder JW, et al. Nevirapine plus didanosine: once or twice daily combination? J Acquir Immune Defic Syndr 25:93, 2000.
78. Garcia F, Knobel H, Sambeat MA, et al. Comparison of twice-daily stavudine plus once- or twice-daily didanosine and nevirapine in early stages of HIV infection: the scan study. AIDS 14:2485, 2000.
79. Mayers D, Bethel J, Wainberg MA, et al. Human immunodeficiency virus proviral DNA from peripheral blood and lymph nodes demonstrates concordance resistance mutations to zidovudine (codon 215) and didanosine (codon 74). J Infect Dis 177:1730, 1998.
80. Nielsen C, Bruun L, Mathiesen LR, et al. Development of resistance to zidovudine (ZDV) and didanosine (ddI) in HIV from patients in ZDV, ddI and alternating ZDV/ddI therapy. AIDS 10:625, 1996.
81. Kozal MJ, Kroodsma K, Winters MA, et al. Didanosine resistance in HIV-infected patients switched from zidovudine to didanosine monotherapy. Ann Intern Med 121:263, 1994.
82. Sharma PL, Crumpacker CS. Attenuated replication of human immunodeficiency virus type 1 with a didanosine-selected reverse transcriptase mutation. J Virol 71:8846, 1997.
83. Gu ZX, Gao Q, Li XG, et al. Novel mutation in the human immunodeficiency virus type-1 reverse transcriptase gene that encodes cross-resistance to 2′,3′-dideoxyinosine and 2′,3′-dideoxycytidine. J Virol 66:7128, 1992.
84. Gao Q, Gu Z, Parniak MA, et al. The same mutation that encodes low-level human immunodeficiency virus type 1 resistance to 2′,3′-dideoxyinosine and 2′,3′-dideoxycytidine confers high-level resistance to the (−) enantiomer of 2′,3′-dideoxy-3′-thiacytidine. Antimicrob Agents Chemother 37:1390, 1993.
85. Zhang D, Caliendo AM, Eron JJ, et al. Resistance to 2′,3′-dideoxycytidine conferred by a mutation in codon 65 of the human immunodeficiency virus type 1 reverse transcriptase. Antimicrob Agents Chemother 38:282, 1994.
86. Yerly S, Rakik A, Kaiser L, et al. Analyses of HIV-1 reverse transcriptase genotype in long-term ddI-treated patients. In: Abstracts of the HIV Drug Resistance 4th International Workshop, Sardinia, Italy, 1995, abstract 29.
87. Moyle G. Influence of emergence of viral resistance on HIV treatment choice [letter]. Int J STD AIDS 6:225, 1995.
88. Eron JJ, Chow Y-K, Caliendo AM, et al. Pol mutations conferring zidovudine and didanosine resistance with different effects in vitro yield multiply resistant human immunodeficiency virus type 1 isolates in vivo. Antimicrob Agents Chemother 37:1480, 1993.
89. Saag MS. Initiation of antiretroviral therapy: implications of recent findings. Top HIV Med 12:83, 2004.
90. Demeter LM, Nawaz T, Morse G, et al. Development of zidovudine resistance mutations in patients receiving prolonged didanosine monotherapy. J Infect Dis 172:1480, 1995.
91. Shafer RW, Kozal MJ, Winters MA, et al. Combination therapy with zidovudine and didanosine selects for drug-resistant human immunodeficiency virus type 1 strains with unique patterns of pol gene mutations. J Infect Dis 169:722, 1994.
92. Kojima E, Shirasaka T, Anderson BD, et al. Human immunodeficiency virus type 1 (HIV-1) viremia changes and development of drug-related mutations in patients with symptomatic HIV-1 infection receiving alternating or simultaneous zidovudine and didanosine therapy. J Infect Dis 102(Suppl 5B):70, 1995.
93. Brun-Vezinet F, Boucher C, Loveday C, et al. HIV-1 viral load, phenotype, and resistance in a subset of drug-naive participants from the Delta trial: the National Virology Groups, Delta Virology Working Group and Coordinating Committee. Lancet 350:983, 1997.
94. Schooley RT, Ramirez-Ronda C, Lange JMA, et al. Virologic and immunologic benefits of initial combination therapy with zidovudine and zalcitabine or didanosine compared with zidovudine monotherapy. J Infect Dis 173:1354, 1996.
95. Shafer RW, Iversen AKN, Winters MA, et al. Drug resistance and heterogeneous long-term virologic responses of human immunodeficiency virus type 1-infected subjects to zidovudine and didanosine combination therapy. J Infect Dis 172:70, 1995.
96. Shirasaka T, Kavlick MR, Veno T, et al. Emergence of human immunodeficiency virus type 1 variants with resistance to multiple dideoxynucleosides in patients receiving therapy with dideoxynucleosides. Proc Natl Acad Sci USA 92:2398, 1995.
97. Garcia-Lerma JG, Gerrish PJ, Wright AC, et al. Evidence of a role for the Q151L mutation and the viral background in

development of multiple dideoxynucleoside-resistant human immunodeficiency virus type 1. J Virol 74:9339, 2000.

98. Kavlick MF, Wyvill K, Yarchoan R, et al. Emergence of multi-dideoxynucleoside-resistant human immunodeficiency virus type 1 variants, viral sequence variation, and disease progression in patients receiving antiretroviral chemothapy. J Infect Dis 177:1506, 1998.
99. Shirasaka T, Kavlick MF, Ueno T, et al. Emergence of human immunodeficiency virus type 1 variants with resistance to multiple dideoxynucleosides in patients receiving therapy with dideoxynucleosides. Proc Natl Acad Sci USA 92:2398, 1995.
100. Winters MA, Coolley KL, Girard YA, et al. A 6-basepair insert in the reverse transcriptase gene of human immunodeficiency virus type 1 confers resistance to multiple nucleoside inhibitors. J Clin Invest 37:A61, 1998.
101. Moreno F, Hardin TC, Rinaldi MG, et al. Itraconazole–didanosine excipient interaction [letter]. JAMA 269:1508, 1993.
102. May DB, Drew RH, Yedinak KC, et al. Effect of simultaneous didanosine administration on itraconazole absorption in healthy volunteers. Pharmacotherapy 14:509, 1994.
103. Acosta EP, Fletcher CV. Antiretroviral drug interactions. Int J Antimicrob Agents 5:73, 1995.
104. Knupp CA, Brater DC, Relue J. Pharmacokinetics of didanosine and ketoconazole after coadministration to patients seropositive for the human immunodeficiency virus. J Clin Pharmacol 33:912, 1993.
105. Huengsberg M, Castelino S, Sherrard J, et al. Does drug interaction cause failure of PCP prophylaxis with dapsone? Lancet 341:48, 1993.
106. Sahai J, Garber G, Gallicano K, et al. Effects of the antacids in didanosine tablets on dapsone pharmacokinetics. Ann Intern Med 123:584, 1995.
107. Prescribing Information. Didanosine. American Hospital Formulary Service, Bethesda, MD, 1996.
108. Knupp CA, Barbhaiya RH. A multiple-dose pharmacokinetic interaction study between didanosine (videx) and ciprofloxacin (cipro) in male subjects seropositive for HIV but asymptomatic. Biopharm Drug Dispos 18:65, 1997.
109. Knupp CA, Graziano FM, Dixon RM, et al. Pharmacokinetic-interaction study of didanosine and ranitidine in patients seropositive for human immunodeficiency virus. Antimicrob Agents Chemother 36:2075, 1992.
110. Cimoch PJ, Lavelle J, Pollard R, et al. Pharmacokinetics of oral ganciclovir alone and in combination with zidovudine, didanosine, and probenecid in HIV-infected subjects. J Acquir Immune Defic Syndr Hum Retrovir 17:227, 1998.
111. Jung D, Griffy K, Dorr A, et al. Effect of high-dose oral ganciclovir on didanosine disposition in human immunodeficiency virus (HIV)-positive patients. J Clin Pharmacol 38:1057, 1998.
112. Trapnell CB, Cimoch P, Gaines K, et al. Altered didanosine pharmacokinetics with concomitant oral ganciclovir. In: Abstracts of the 95th Annual Meeting of the American Society of Clinical Pharmacology and Therapeutics, 1994, abstract 193.
113. Collier AC, Coombs RW, Fischl MA, et al. Combination therapy with zidovudine and didanosine compared with zidovudine alone in HIV-1 infection. Ann Intern Med 119:786, 1993.
114. Burger DM, Meenhorst PL, Kroon FP, et al. Pharmacokinetic interaction study of zidovudine and didanosine. J Drug Dev 6:187, 1994.
115. Barry M, Howe JL, Ormesher S, et al. Pharmacokinetics of zidovudine and dideoxyinosine alone and in combination in patients with the acquired immunodeficiency syndrome. Br J Clin Pharmacol 37:421, 1994.
116. Drugs for HIV infection. Med Lett 39:115, 1997.
117. Morse GD, Fischl MA, Shelton MJ, et al. Single-dose pharmacokinetics of delavirdine mesylate and didanosine in patients with human immunodeficiency virus infection. Antimicrob Agents Chemother 41:169, 1997.
118. Mummaneni V, Kaul S, Knupp CA. Single oral dose pharmacokinetic interaction study of didanosine and indinavir sulfate in healthy subjects [abstract]. J Clin Pharmacol 37:865, 1997.
119. Shelton MJ, Mei HJ, Hewitt RG. If taken 1 hour before indinavir (IDV), didanosine does not affect IDV exposure, despite persistent buffering effects. Antimicrob Agents Chemother 45:298, 2001.
120. Cato A, Qian J, Hsu A, et al. Pharmacokinetic interaction between ritonavir and didanosine when administered concurrently to HIV-infected patients. J Acquir Immune Defic Syndr Hum Retrovir 18:466, 1998.
121. Knupp C, Srinivas N, Batteiger B. A pK interaction study of didanosine coadministered with or without TMP and/or SMX in HIV seropositive patients [abstract]. Pharm Res 11(Suppl):399, 1994.
122. Sahai J, Narang PK, Hawley-Foss N, et al. A phase I evaluation of concomitant rifabutin and didanosine in symptomatic HIV-infected patients. J Acquir Immune Defic Syndr Hum Retrovir 9:274, 1995.
123. Gallicano K, Sahai J, Zaror-Behrens G, et al. Effect of antacids in didanosine tablet on bioavailability of isoniazid. Antimicrob Agents Chemother 38:894, 1994.
124. Aweeka FT, Mathur V, Dorsey R, et al. Pharmacokinetics of concomitant foscarnet and didanosine in patients with HIV disease [abstract]. Clin Pharmacol Ther 57:143, 1995.
125. Seifert RD, Stewart MB, Sramek JJ, et al. Pharmacokinetics of co-administered didanosine and stavudine in HIV-seropositive male patients. Br J Clin Pharmacol 38:405, 1994.
126. Gillum JG, Bruzzese VL, Israel DS, et al. Effect of clarithromycin on the pharmacokinetics of 2′,3′-dideoxyinosine in patients who are seropositive for human immunodeficiency virus. Clin Infect Dis 22:716, 1996.
127. MacGregor TR, Lamson MJ, Cort S, et al. Steady state pharmacokinetics of nevirapine, didanosine, zalcitabine, and zidovudine combination therapy in HIV-1 positive patients [abstract]. Pharm Res 12(Suppl):S101, 1995.
128. Elion R, Kaul S, Knupp C, et al. safety profile and antiviral activity of the combination of stavudine, didanosine and nelfinavir in patients with HIV infection. Clin Ther 21:1853, 1999.
129. Rainey PM, Friedland G, McCance-Katz EF, et al. Interaction of methadone with didanosine and stavudine. J Acquir Immune Defic Syndr 24:241, 2000.
130. Cheng AK, Kearney BP, Damle B, et al. Tenofovir DF (TDF) and didanosine EC (ddI EC): investigation of pharmacokinetic (PK) drug–drug and drug–food interactions. Presented at the XIV International AIDS Conference, Barcelona, Spain, 7–12 Jul 2002, abstract LBPE9026.
131. Kearney BP, Isaacson E, Sayre J, et al. Didanosine and tenofovir DF drug-drug interaction: assessment of didanosine dose reduction. Presented at the 10th Conference on Retroviruses and Opportunistic Infections, Boston, 10–14 Feb 2003, abstract 533.
132. Martinez E, Milinkovic A, de Lazzari E, et al. Pancreatic toxic effects associated with co-administration of didanosine and tenofovir in HIV-infected adults. Lancet 364:65, 2004.
133. Lopez S, Negredo E, Garrabou G, et al. Longitudinal study on mitochondrial effects of didanosine–tenofovir combination. AIDS Res Hum Retroviruses 22:33, 2006.
134. Garcia-Benayas T, Rendon AL, Rodriguez-Novoa S, et al. Higher risk of hyperglycemia in HIV-infected patients treated with didanosine plus tenofovir. AIDS Res Hum Retroviruses 22:333, 2006.
135. Montaner JSC, Schechter MT, Rachlis A, et al. Didanosine compared with continuous zidovudine therapy for HIV infected patients, with 200–500 CD4 cells/mm^3. Ann Intern Med 123:561, 1995.

136. Raboud JM, Montaner JSG, Rae S, et al. Meta-analysis of five randomized controlled trials comparing continuation of zidovudine vs. switching to didanosine in HIV infected individuals. Antivir Ther 2:237, 1997.
137. Floridia M, Vella S, Seeber AC, et al. A randomized trial (ISS902) of didanosine versus zidovudine in previously untreated patients with mildly symptomatic human immunodeficiency virus infection. J Infect Dis 175:255, 1997.
138. Katzenstein DA, Hammer SM, Hughes MD, et al. The relation of virologic and immunologic markers to clinical outcomes after nucleoside therapy in HIV-infected adults with 200 to 500 CD4 cells per cubic millimeter. N Engl J Med 335:1091, 1996.
139. Delta Coordinating Committee. Delta: a randomised double-blind controlled trial comparing combinations of zidovudine plus didanosine or zalcitabine with zidovudine alone in HIV-infected individuals. Lancet 348:283, 1996.
140. Saravolatz LD, Winslow DL, Collins G, et al. Zidovudine alone or in combination with didanosine or zalcitabine in HIV-infected patients with the acquired immunodeficiency syndrome or fewer than 200 CD4 cells per cubic millimeter. N Engl J Med 335:1099, 1996.
141. Graham NMH, Hoover DR, Park LP, et al. Survival in HIV infected patients who have received zidovudine: comparison of combination therapy with sequential monotherapy and continued zidovudine monotherapy. Ann Intern Med 124:1031, 1996.
142. Ruxruntham K, Kroon EDMB, Ungsedhapand C, et al. A randomized dose-finding study with didanosine plus stavudine versus didanosine (ddI) stavudine (d4T) in HIV-infected Thais. AIDS 14:1375, 2000.
143. Molina J-M, Chene G, Ferchal F, et al. The ALBI trial: a randomized controlled trial comparing stavudine plus didanosine with zidovudine plus lamivudine and a regimen alternating both combinations in previously untreated patients infected with human immunodeficiency virus. J Infect Dis 180:351, 1999.
144. Raffi F, Reliquet V, Auger S, et al. Efficacy and safety of stavudine and didanosine combination therapy in antiretroviral-experienced patients. AIDS 12:1999, 1998.
145. Henry K, Erice A, Tierney C, et al. A randomized, controlled, double-blind study of d4T + ddI vs. ZDV + ddI as initial treatment HIV-infected subjects with CD4 counts <500 cells/mm^3 [abstract]. Presented at the 37th Interscience Conference on Anti-Microbial Agents and Chemotherapy, Sep 1997, p 266.
146. Kuritzkes DR, Marschner I, Johnson VA, et al. Lamivudine in combination with zidovudine, stavudine, or didanosine in patients with HIV-1 infection: a randomized double-blind, placebo-controlled trial. AIDS 13:685, 1999.
147. Lafeuillade A, Poggi C, Tamalet C, et al. Effects of a combination of zidovudine, didanosine, and lamivudine on primary human immunodeficiency virus type 1 infection. J Infect Dis 175:1051, 1997.
148. Jemsek J, Hutcherson P, Harper E. Poor virologic responses and early emergence of resistance in treatment naïve, HIV-infected patients receiving a once daily triple nucleoside regimen of didanosine, lamivudine, and tenofovir DF. 11th Conference on Retroviruses and Opportunistic Infections, San Francisco, CA, 8–11 Feb 2004, abstract 51.
149. Parikh U, Koontz D, Sluis-Cremer N, et al. K65R: a multinucleoside resistance mutation of increasing prevalence exhibits bi-directional phenotypic antagonism with TAM. 11th Conference on Retroviruses and Opportunistic Infections, San Francisco, CA, 8–11 Feb 2004, abstract 54.
150. White KL, Margot NA, Chen JM, et al. The HIV-1 K65R RT mutant utilizes a combination of decreased incorporation and decreased excision to evade NRTI. 11th Conference on Retroviruses and Opportunistic Infections, San Francisco, CA, 8–11 Feb 2004, abstract 55.
151. D'Aquila RT, Hughes MD, Johnson VA, et al. Nevirapine, zidovudine, and didanosine compared with zidovudine and didanosine in patients with HIV-1 infection. Ann Intern Med 124:1019, 1996.
152. Floridia M, Bucciardini R, Ricciardulle D, et al. A randomized, double-blind trial on the use of a triple combination including nevirapine, a nonnucleoside reverse transcriptase HIV inhibitor, in antiretroviral-naive patients with advanced disease. J Acquir Immune Defic Syndr Hum Retrovir 20:11, 1999.
153. Montaner JS, Reiss P, Cooper D, et al. A randomized, double-blind trial comparing combinations of nevirapine, didanosine, and zidovudine for HIV-infected patients: the INCAS trial: Italy, The Netherlands, Canada and Australian study. JAMA 279:930, 1998.
154. Raffi F, Reliquet V, Ferre V, et al. The VIRGO study: nevirapine, didanosine and stavudine combination therapy in anti-retroviral naive HIV-1 infected adults. Antivir Ther 5:267, 2000.
155. Friedland GH, Pollard R, Griffith B, et al. Efficacy and safety of delavirdine mesylate with zidovudine and didanosine compared with two-drug combinations of these agents in persons with HIV disease with CD4 counts of 100 to 500 cells/mm^3 (ACTG 261). J Acquir Immune Defic Syndr 21:281, 1999.
156. French M, Amin J, Roth N, et al. Randomized, open-label, comparative trial to evaluate the efficacy and safety of three antiretroviral drug combinations including two nucleoside analogues and nevirapine for previously untreated HIV-1 infection: the OzCombo 2 study. HIV Clin Trials 3:177–185, 2002.
157. Maggiolo F, Migliorino M, Maserati R, et al. Virological and immunological responses to a once-a-day antiretroviral regimen with didanosine, lamivudine and efavirenz. Antivir Ther 6:249, 2001.
158. Molina JM, Ferchal F, Rancinan C, et al. Once-daily combination therapy with emtricitabine, didanosine, and efavirenz in human immunodeficiency virus-infected patients. J Infect Dis 182:599, 2000.
159. Saag MS, Cahn P, Raffi F, et al. Efficacy and safety of emtricitabine vs stavudine in combination therapy in antiretroviral-naïve patients: a randomized trial. JAMA 292:180, 2004.
160. Maitland D, Moyle G, Hand J, et al. Early virologic failure in HIV-1 infected subjects on didanosine/tenofovir/efavirenz: 12-week results from a randomized trial. AIDS 19:1183, 2005.
161. Ruane PJ, DeJesus E: New nucleoside/nucleotide backbone options: a review of recent studies. J Acquir Immune Defic Syndr 37(Suppl 1):S21, 2004.
162. Podzamozer D, Ferrer E, Gatell JM, et al. Early virological failure and occurrence of resistance in naïve patients receiving tenofovir, didanosine and efavirenz. Antivir Ther 9:S172 (abstract 156), 2004.
163. Carr A, Chauh J, Hudson J. A randomized, open-label comparison of three highly active antiretroviral therapy regimens including two nucleoside analogues and indinavir for previously untreated HIV-1 infection: the OzCombo 1 study. AIDS 14:1171, 2000.
164. Eron JJ, Murphy RL, Peterson D, et al. A comparison of stavudine, didanosine, and indinavir with zidovudine, lamivudine and indinavir for the initial treatment of HIV-1 infected individuals: selection of thymidine analog regimen therapy (START II). AIDS 14:1601, 2000.
165. Gatell J, Murphy R, Katlama C, et al. The Atlantic study: a randomized open-label study comparing two protease inhibitors (PI)-sparing antiretroviral strategies versus a standard PI-containing regimen. Presented at the 6th Conference on Retroviruses and Opportunistic Infections, Chicago, 1999, abstract 18.
166. Gatell J, Murphy R, Katlama C, et al. The Atlantic study: a randomized open-label study comparing two protease inhibitors

(PI)-sparing antiretroviral strategies versus a standard PI-containing regimen, 48 week data. Presented at the 7th European Conference on Clinical Aspects and Treatment of HIV Infection, Lisbon, 1999, p 14.
167. De Mendoza C, Soriano V, Perez-Olmeda M, et al. Efficacy and safety didanosine and lamivudine both once daily plus indinavir in human immunodeficiency virus-infected patients. J Hum Virol 3:335, 2000.
168. Flepp M, Wang J, Nigg C, et al. Nelfinavir, didanosine, and stavudine in HIV-infected drug users enrolled in opiate substitution programs at four outpatients clinics-the Zurich Prometheus Study [abstract]. AIDS 12(Suppl 4):S41, 1998.
169. Saimot AG, Landman R, Damond F, et al. Stavudine, didanosine and ritonavir as a triple therapy in antiretroviral-naive patients: results at 72 weeks [abstract]. Presented at the 12th World AIDS Conference, Geneva, 1998, p 344.
170. Lichterfeld M, Nischalke HD, Bergmann F, et al. Long-term efficacy and safety of ritonavir/indinavir at 400/400 mg twice a day in combination with two nucleoside reverse transcriptase inhibitors as first line antiretroviral therapy. HIV Med 3:37, 2002.
171. Sanne I, Piliero P, Squires K, et al. Results of a phase 2 clinical trial at 48 weeks (AI424-007): a dose-ranging, safety, and efficacy comparative trial of atazanavir at three doses in combination with didanosine and stavudine in antiretroviral-naive subjects. JAIDS 32:18, 2003.
172. MacArthur RD, Chen L, Peng G, et al. Efficacy and safety of abacavir plus lamivudine versus didanosine plus stavudine when combined with a protease inhibitor, a non-nucleoside reverse transcriptase inhibitor, or both in HIV-1 positive antiretroviral-naïve person. HIV Clin Trials 5:361–370, 2004.
173. Robbins GK, De Gruttola V, Shafer RW, et al. Comparison of sequential three-drug regimens as initial therapy for HIV-1 infection. N Engl J Med 349:2293, 2003.
174. Shafer RW, Smeaton LM, Robbins GK, et al. Comparison of four-drug regimens and pairs of sequential three-drug regimens as initial therapy for HIV-1 infection. N Engl J Med 349:2304, 2003.
175. Luzzati R, Di Perri G, Fendt D, et al. Pharmacokinetics, safety and anti-human immunodeficiency virus (HIV) activity of hydroxyurea in combination with didanosine. J Antimicrob Chemother 42:565, 1998.
176. De BRJ, Boucher CAB, Perelson AS. Target cell availability and the successful suppression of HIV by hydroxyurea and didanosine. AIDS 12:1567, 1998.
177. Montaner JSG, Zala C, Raboud JM, et al. A pilot study of hydroxyurea (HO-urea) as adjuvant therapy among patients with advanced HIV disease receiving didanosine (ddI) therapy: Canadian HIV Trials Network Protocol 080. J Infect Dis 175:801, 1997.
178. Hellinger JA, Iwane MK, Smith JJ, et al. A randomized study of the safety and antiretroviral activity of hydroxyurea combined with didanosine in persons infected with human immunodeficiency virus type 1. American Foundation for AIDS Research Community-Based Clinical Trials Network. J Infect Dis 181:540, 2000.
179. Clotet B, Ruiz L, Cabrerea C, et al. Short-term anti-HIV activity of the combination of didanosine and hydroxyurea. Antivir Ther 1:189, 1996.
180. Biron F, Lucht F, Peyramond D, et al. Pilot clinical trial of the combination of hydroxyurea and didanosine in HIV-1 infected individuals. Antivir Res 29:111, 1996.
181. Foli A, Lori F, Maserati R, et al. Hydroxyurea and didanosine is a more potent combination than hydroxyurea and zidovudine. Antivir Ther 2:31, 1997.
182. Lori F, Jessen H, Foli A, et al. Long-term suppression of HIV-1 by hydroxyurea and didanosine. JAMA 277:1437, 1997.
183. Foli A, Lori F, Maserati R, et al. Hydroxyurea and didanosine is a more potent combination than hydroxyurea and zidovudine. Antivir Ther 2:31, 1997.
184. Rutschmann OT, Opravil M, Iten A. A placebo-controlled trial of didanosine plus stavudine, with and without hydroxyurea, for HIV infection. AIDS 12:F71, 1998.
185. Rutschmann OT, Vernazza PL, Bucher HC, et al. Long-term hydroxyurea in combination with didanosine and stavudine for the treatment of HIV-1 infection. AIDS 14:2145, 2000.
186. Jaegel-Guedes E, Wolf E, Goeppner S, et al. d4T/ddI plus hydroxyurea: an alternative to a PI containing triple regimen in ART-naive HIV$^+$ patients [abstract]. Presented at the 12th World AIDS Conference, Geneva, 1998, p 583.
187. Lisziewicz J, Jessen H, Finzi D, et al. HIV-1 suppression by early treatment with hydroxyurea, didanosine, and a protease inhibitor. Lancet 352:199, 1998.
188. Lori F, Rosenberg E, Lieberman J, et al. Hydroxyurea and didanosine long-term treatment prevents HIV breakthrough and normalizes immune parameters. AIDS Res Hum Retroviruses 15:1333, 1999.
189. Lori F, Jessen H, Foli A. Long-term suppression of HIV replication and cell proliferation leads to minimal levels of proviral DNA and to immune recovery [abstract]. Presented at the 12th World AIDS Conference, Geneva, 1998, p 778.
190. Lori F, Lisziewicz J. Rationale for the use of hydroxyurea as an anti-human immunodeficiency virus drug. Clin Infect Dis 30(Suppl 2):S193, 2000.
191. Zala C, Rouleau D, Montaner JS. Role of hydroxyurea in treatment of disease due to human immunodeficiency virus infection. Clin Infect Dis 30(Suppl 2):S143, 2000.
192. Biron F, Ponceau B, Bouhour D. Long-term safety and antiretroviral activity of hydroxyurea and didanosine in HIV-infected patients. J Acquir Immune Defic Syndr 25:329, 2000.
193. Hydroxyurea in the treatment of HIV-1 infection: toxicity and side effects [review]. J Biol Regul Homeost Agents 13:181, 1999.
194. McCarthy WF, Gable J, Lawrence J, et al. A retrospective study to determine if hydroxyurea augmentation of antiretroviral drug regimens that contain ddI and/or d4T increases the risk of developing peripheral neuropathy in HIV-1 infected individuals. Pharmacoepidemiol Drug Safety 9:49, 2000.
195. Cepeda JA, Wilks D. Excess peripheral neuropathy in patients treated with hydroxyurea plus didanosine and stavudine for HIV infection [letter]. AIDS 14:332, 2000.
196. Longhurst HJ, Pinching AJ. Drug points: pancreatitis associated with hydroxyurea in combination with didanosine. BMJ 322:81, 2001.
197. Havlir DV, Gilbert PB, Bennett K, et al. Effects of treatment intensification with hydroxyurea in HIV-infected patients with virologic suppression. AIDS 15:1379, 2001.
198. Boxwell D, Toerner J. Fatal hepatoxicity associated with combination hydroxyurea and nucleoside reverse transcriptase inhibitors (NRTIs): cases from the FDA adverse event reporting system (AERS). Presented at the 8th Conference on Retroviruses and Opportunistic Infections, Chicago, 2001, abstract 671.
199. Mueller BU, Butler KM, Stocker VL, et al. Clinical and pharmacokinetic evaluation of long-term therapy with didanosine in children with HIV infection. Pediatrics 94:724, 1994.
200. Butler KM, Husson RN, Balis FM, et al. Dideoxyinosine in children with symptomatic human immunodeficiency virus infection. N Engl J Med 324:137, 1991.
201. Blanche S, Calvez T, Rouzioux C, et al. Randomized study of two doses of didanosine in children infected with human immunodeficiency virus. J Pediatr 122:966, 1993.
202. Husson RN, Mueller BU, Farley M, et al. Zidovudine and didanosine combination therapy in children with human immunodeficiency virus infection. Pediatrics 93:316, 1994.

203. Englund JA, Baker CJ, Raskino C, et al. Zidovudine, didanosine, or both as the initial treatment for symptomatic HIV-infected children. N Engl J Med 336:1704, 1997.
204. McKinney RE Jr, Johnson GM, Stanley K, et al. A randomized study of combined zidovudine-naive HIV-1 infection: the pediatric AIDS Clinical Trials Group protocol 300 study team. J Pediatr 133:500, 1998.
205. Kline MW, Fletcher CV, Federici ME, et al. Combination therapy with stavudine and didanosine in children with advanced human immunodeficiency virus infection: pharmacokinetic properties, safety and immunologic and virologic effects. Pediatrics 97:886, 1996.
206. Kline MW, Van Dyke RB, Lindsey JC, et al. Combination therapy with stavudine (d4T) plus didanosine (ddI) in children with human immunodeficiency virus infection: the pediatric AIDS Clinical Trials Group 327 team. Pediatrics 103:e62, 1999.
207. Paediatric European Network for Treatment of AIDS. A randomized double-blind trial of the addition of lamivudine or matching placebo to current nucleoside analogue reverse transcriptase inhibitor therapy in HVI-infected children: the PENTA-4 trial. AIDS 12:F151, 1998.
208. Kline M, Fletcher CV, Brundage RC, et al. Combination therapy with saquinavir soft gelatin capsules plus nucleoside anti-retroviral agents in HIV-infected children [abstract]. Presented at the 12th World AIDS Conference, Geneva, 1998, p 64.
209. Kline MW, Fletcher CV, Harris AT, et al. A pilot study of combination therapy with indinavir, stavudine (d4T), and didanosine (ddI) in children infected with the human immunodeficiency virus. J Pediatr 132:543, 1998.
210. Fletcher CV, Brundage RC, Remmel RP, et al. Pharmacologic characteristics of indinavir, didanosine, and stavudine in human immunodeficiency virus-infected children receiving combination therapy. Antimicrob Agents Chemother 44:1029, 2000.
211. Funk MB, Linde R, Wintergerst U, et al. Preliminary experiences with triple therapy including nelfinavir and two reverse transcriptase inhibitors in previously untreated HIV-infected children. AIDS 13:1653, 1999.
212. Luzuriaga K, Bryson Y, Krogstad P, et al. Combination treatment with zidovudine, didanosine, and nevirapine in infants with human immunodeficiency virus type 1 infection. N Engl J Med 336:1343, 1997.
213. Hammer SM, Saag MS, Schechter M, et al. Treatment for adult HIV infection: 2006 recommendations of the International AIDS Society-USA Panel. JAMA 296:827, 2006.
214. DHHS panel. Guidelines for the use of antiretrovirals in adults and adolescents. Available: http://AIDSinfo.nih.gov 10 Oct 2006.

Chapter 7

Zalcitabine

John A. Bartlett, MD

Zalcitabine (2′,3′-dideoxycytidine, ddC, HIVID) is a pyrimidine analog whose synthesis was originally described by Horwitz et al in 1966.[1] The antiretroviral activity of zalcitabine was first recognized in 1986,[2] and it was approved by the Food and Drug Administration (FDA) in 1992, initially only for use in combination with zidovudine. Historically, zalcitabine was the third antiretroviral drug approved by the FDA and the first agent to receive licensure through the FDA's accelerated approval process.

STRUCTURE

Zalcitabine is derived from cytidine (similar to lamivudine) and lacks the 3′-OH moiety on the ribose sugar (Fig. 7-1). Zalcitabine shares its nucleotide base with lamivudine, but they differ in their sugar moieties and stereochemistry. To become active as an antiretroviral agent, zalcitabine must undergo triphosphorylation to the 5′-triphosphate form.

MECHANISMS OF ACTION AND *IN VITRO* ACTIVITY

Zalcitabine acts as an inhibitor of human immunodeficiency virus type 1 (HIV-1) reverse transcriptase and as a chain terminator.[2] It inhibits HIV-1 replication and protects against cytopathogenicity at concentrations of 0.5 μM.[2–4] Zalcitabine is active against HIV-1 in a variety of cell lines, including peripheral blood lymphocytes and those derived from lymphocytes or monocyte/macrophages, although its inhibitory activity and metabolism may be different across cell lines.[4] Zalcitabine is especially active against macrophage-tropic strains in monocyte/macrophage cell lines, with a median inhibitory concentration (IC_{50}) of 0.002 μM, compared to 0.01 μM for didanosine and 0.20 μM for zidovudine.[5] Zalcitabine is active against zidovudine-resistant HIV-1 isolates,[6–8] HIV-2,[9] and hepatitis B virus[10,11] but not against herpes simplex virus 1 or 2.[12] Zalcitabine has synergy with zidovudine, delavirdine, saquinavir, and interferon-*a*.[13–15] In contrast, zalcitabine has demonstrated antagonism with ribavirin, perhaps through ribavirin's inhibition of zalcitabine's phosphorylation.[16,17] *In vitro* cytotoxicity from zalcitabine has usually been demonstrated at concentrations of 10 μM or higher, although Molt-4 cells have demonstrated an increased doubling time, decreased cellular content of mitochondrial DNA, and decreased rate of glycolysis at 0.5 or 0.2 μM.[18]

The intracellular metabolism of zalcitabine begins with cellular entry through both nucleoside carrier-mediated and non-carrier-mediated mechanisms.[19–21] Zalcitabine then undergoes triphosphorylation by cellular kinases that are also used by 2′-deoxycytidine.[22] The process of triphosphorylation occurs in both HIV-infected and HIV-uninfected cell lines.[19,23,24] Anywhere from 2% to 40% of zalcitabine is converted to its triphosphate form, 2′,3′-dideoxycytidine

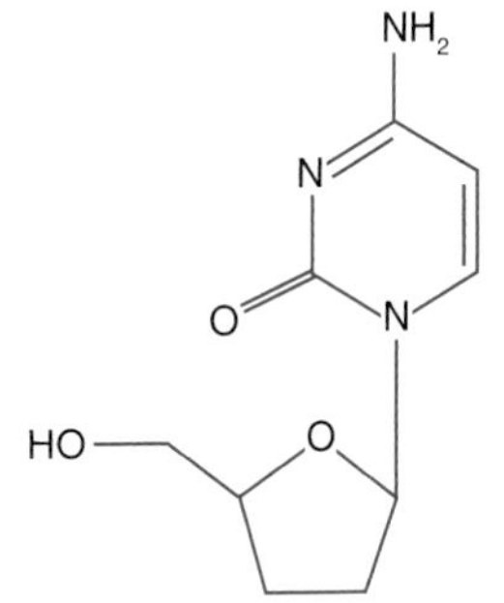

Figure 7-1 ■ Biochemical structure of zalcitabine.

5′-triphosphate (ddCTP), depending on the cell line studied.[19,25,26] Zalcitabine is most efficiently triphosphorylated in resting peripheral blood mononuclear cells, in contrast to zidovudine, which is most efficiently triphosphorylated in activated cells.[27,28] The ddCTP binds to HIV-1 reverse transcriptase with a ^{K}I of 0.2–0.9 μM[29,30]; it does not bind efficiently to host *a* DNA polymerase, but it has been speculated that zalcitabine's neurotoxicity may be related to its inhibition of host β and γ DNA polymerases.[18] The efflux of ddCTP from Molt-4 cells follows a biphasic pattern with an initial retention half-life of 2.6 h.[25]

PHARMACOKINETICS

Zalcitabine has been administered over the dose range of 0.007–0.50 mg/kg, although a clear dose-response relation with peripheral neuropathy at doses of more than 0.01 mg/kg has limited the use of higher doses.[31–34] Zalcitabine has linear pharmacokinetics over the dose range of 0.03–0.5 mg/kg.[32,33] It is ~70–90% bioavailable following oral administration of zalcitabine oral solution or tablets.[32,33] The maximum plasma concentration of zalcitabine after an oral dose of 1.5 mg is 0.12 μM, which occurs 0.8 h after dosing. Administration of zalcitabine with food decreases the maximum plasma concentration by 39%, prolongs the time to achieve maximum concentrations to 1.6 h, and decreases the plasma concentration area under the curve (AUC) by 14%.[9]

Zalcitabine is rapidly eliminated, with a total body clearance of ~250 mL min^{-1} m^{-2} after single and multiple doses. In patients with normal renal function, the plasma elimination half-life is 1–3 h and no significant drug accumulation was noted after 14 days of intravenous dosing.[32,33] As a result, zalcitabine is recommended for every-8-hour oral dosing. Two small studies of zalcitabine dosed twice daily have been published and demonstrated promising activity.[34,35] However, their sample sizes were small (total 41 subjects) and there was no comparisons with zalcitabine dosed every 8 h.

Zalcitabine reaches a steady-state volume of distribution of 0.5–0.6 L/kg in adults, and less than 4% is bound to plasma proteins.[9] Zalcitabine concentrations in cerebrospinal fluid approximate 20% of plasma levels.[31] Zalcitabine does not undergo hepatic metabolism, and ~75% and 62% of intravenous and oral doses, respectively, are recovered unchanged in the urine over 24 h.[32] In seven patients with creatinine clearances of less than 55 mL/min, the plasma half-life of zalcitabine was prolonged to 8.5 h.[9] Similar pharmacokinetics have been observed in HIV-infected children, although zalcitabine bioavailability is more variable in children (29–100%) than in adults.[36]

TOXICITY

The reported toxicities of zalcitabine include peripheral neuropathy, stomatitis, rash, and pancreatitis. The major studies of zalcitabine that describe toxicities are summarized in Table 7-1.

Peripheral Neuropathy

The most common toxicity related to zalcitabine is a peripheral neuropathy.[37–40] The frequency of peripheral neuropathy is clearly dose related and was reported in up to 100% of subjects receiving zalcitabine 0.03 mg/kg q4h.[37] Moderate peripheral neuropathy has been reported in 3–23% of patients taking zalcitabine, and severe peripheral neuropathy has been reported in 0–15%.[40–43] In randomized trials comparing zalcitabine-containing and didanosine-containing regimens, the frequency of zalcitabine-associated severe peripheral neuropathy was higher (5% vs 1%[42] and 15.0% vs 6.6%,[44] respectively). Two small studies observed infrequent peripheral neuropathy in subjects receiving zalcitabine 1.125 mg twice daily for up to 48 weeks (1/41 subjects).[34,35] Baseline characteristics associated with a higher frequency of zalcitabine-associated peripheral neuropathy include a lower absolute CD4+ T-lymphocyte number,[39] diabetes mellitus,[45] lower baseline vitamin B^{12} levels, heavy alcohol consumption, and a history of symptomatic peripheral neuropathy.[46] Symptoms typically begin at a mean of 10–18 weeks after initiating zalcitabine[45–47] and most commonly involve the distal lower extremities.[45,46] The symptoms usually begin in a symmetrical stocking distribution, with numbness, aching, and burning dysesthesias. On examination, patients may have diminished sensation in response to light touch, pinprick, temperature, and vibration; and up to 60% may have absent ankle deep tendon reflexes.[45,48] Nerve conduction studies reveal a sensory axonal neuropathy with decreased to absent sensory nerve action potentials and normal distal latencies and velocities.[48] The symptoms of zalcitabine-associated peripheral neuropathy may worsen for up to 5 weeks following its discontinuation[31,48] but then slowly improve. More severe neuropathic symptoms may not return to baseline. If symptoms resolve, most patients are able to tolerate the careful reintroduction of half-dose zalcitabine.[45] Preexisting zalcitabine-associated peripheral neuropathy may predispose to neuropathic exacerbation on didanosine,[49] so didanosine should be substituted for zalcitabine with caution.

Stomatitis

Stomatitis was reported in eight of 20 patients in the first dose-escalation phase I trial of zalcitabine.[31] The ulcerations most commonly occur on the buccal mucosa, soft palate, tongue, or pharynx. They are usually self-limited and resolve with continued therapy. In large clinical trials utilizing zalcitabine at doses of 0.75 mg q8h, the reported frequency of moderate to severe oral ulcerations is 2–4%.[40–42,50] One case of more severe esophageal ulceration that required discontinuation of zalcitabine has also been reported.[51]

Rash

Rash was reported in 14 of 20 patients in the first dose-escalation phase I trial of zalcitabine.[31] The rash is most commonly an erythematous, maculo-papular eruption over the

Table 7-1 Toxicities Associated with Zalcitabine

Trial	Dose	Entry Criteria	Peripheral Neuropathy	Stomatitis	Pancreatitis	Other Toxicities	Comments
Yarchoan et al[31]	0.03–0.25 mg/kg IV and PO q8h	ARC or AIDS CD4 <350/mm^3	All 10 subjects treated for >6 weeks	8/20	None reported	Rash 14/20	
Merigan et al[37]	0.005–0.06 mg/kg PO q4h	Advanced ARC or AIDS p24 antigen ⩾100 pg/mL	0.005 mg/kg q4h 17% 0.01 mg/kg q4h 80% 0.03 mg/kg q4h 100% 0.06 mg/kg q4h 100%	0.005 mg/kg q4h 7/15 0.01 mg/kg q4h 9/11 0.03 mg/kg q4h 11/15 0.06 mg/kg q4h 16/18	None reported	Rash 39/61	
ACTG 047 (Skowron et al[38])	0.01–0.03 mg/kg PO q4h	ARC or AIDS p24 antigen >70 pg/mL	0.1 mg/kg 15% 0.03 mg/kg 34%* (*$P = 0.04$)	None reported	None reported	Anaphylactoid symptoms (1), fever (1) reversible hearing loss (1)	Dose–response relation with peripheral neuropathy; neuropathic symptoms occurred within first 24 weeks in 68%
ACTG 119 (Fischl et al[39])	0.75 mg PO q8h	Severe ARC or AIDS ⩾48 weeks prior ZDV	Severe peripheral neuropathy in 6/59 (10%) on ddC; 0/52 on ZDV	Mouth ulcers (1) and esophageal ulcers (1) leading to ddC discontinuation	One subject on ddC	Hepatotoxicity (1) leading to ddC discontinuation; (1) leading to ZDV discontinuation	
ACTG 155 (Fischl et al[40])	00.75 mg PO q8h	ARC or AIDS with CD4 <300/mm^3 or asymptomatic with CD4 <200/mm^3 >6 months prior ZDV	Moderate or worse neuropathy ZDV 13% ddC 23% ZDV + ddC 22% ($P = 0.005$)	ddC 4% ddC + ZDV 1% ZDV 1%	ddC 9 (3%) ddC + ZDV 8 (2%) ZDV 4 (1%) One fatal episode of pancreatitis in ZDV + ddC group	None reported	Increased frequency of peripheral neuropathy at lower baseline CD4; one fatal pancreatitis case
			Severe neuropathy ZDV 4% ddC 6% ZDV + ddC 6% ($P = 0.51$)		None reported	Arthralgias (1) Myalgias (1)	
ACTG 106 (Meng et al[41])	0.005–0.01 mg/kg q8h	Advanced ARC or AIDS CD4 <200/mm^3 Treatment naive	1/29 severe neuropathy at 0.005 mg/kg; 1/18 severe neuropathy at 0.01 mg/kg	None reported	None reported	Transaminase elevations ×3 ULN in four subjects	

(Continued)

Table 7-1

(Continued)

Trial	Dose	Entry Criteria	Peripheral Neuropathy	Stomatitis	Pancreatitis	Other Toxicities
ACTG 175 (Hammer et al[42])	0.75 mg q8h	Asymptomatic with CD4 200–500/mm^3	Not reported	Not reported	Not reported	Not reported
Delta Coordinating Committee[43]	0.75 mg PO q8h	CD4 50–350/mm^3	Severe neuropathy ZDV + ddC 5% ZDV + ddC 1% ZDV 2%	Mouth ulcers ZDV + ddC 0.3%	ZDV + ddC 0.5% ZDV + ddI 1%	Transaminase elevations ZDV + ddC 7% ZDV + ddI 5% ZDV 5%
NV14256[46]	0.75 mg PO q8h	CD4 50–350/mm^3, >16 weeks prior ZDV	Treatment-limiting peripheral neuropathy 14% ddC alone arm, 9% ddC+SQV, 3% SQV alone	Mouth ulcers 2.5% ddC alone, 2% ddC + SQV, 0% SQV alone	None reported	Transaminase elevations (>5 × ULN) 2% ddC alone
HIVBID[35]	1.125 mg PO q12h	CD4 >200, RNA >5000 No preexisting PN		None reported	None reported	None reported
Moyle and Gazzard[34]	1.125 mg PO q12h	Previously treated with zalcitabine for a median of 19 months	1/17 (6%)	None reported	None reported	
MIKADO[48]	0.75 mg PO q8h	CD4 ≥250; RNA ≥5000	5/35 (14%) ddC + d4T + SQV	None reported	None reported	
Quattro[47]	0.75 mg PO q8h	CD4 50–350	1/34 (3%) ddC + ZDV+ LMV + loviride	None reported	1/34 (3%)	

ddI, didanosine; SQV, saquinavir; 3TC, lamivudine; ULN, upper limit of normal; ZDV, zidovudine.
CD4 indicates the CD4+ T-lymphocyte count.

trunk and extremities. It usually begins after 10–14 days of zalcitabine therapy and is self-limited. Larger trials have not reported the frequency of zalcitabine-associated rash, presumably because it is mild and self-limited. Skin biopsies of the rash reveal perivascular lymphocytic infiltrates.[52]

Pancreatitis

Pancreatitis has been reported infrequently in zalcitabine-treated patients. Large trials suggest a frequency of 0.5–3.0%.[38,39,41,42] Trials that have randomized subjects to either zalcitabine or didanosine suggest that zalcitabine-associated pancreatitis occurs less commonly (0.5% vs 1%[41] and 0.5% vs 2.2%,[53] respectively). One case of fatal zalcitabine-associated pancreatitis has been reported.[39]

Other Toxicities

Miscellaneous toxicities attributed to zalcitabine include cardiomyopathy,[9] anaphylactoid reactions,[38] fever,[38] reversible hearing loss,[38] arthralgias,[50] and myalgias.[50] Zalcitabine's potential to cause hepatotoxicity remains unclear; transaminase elevations led to drug discontinuation in one subject,[40] and a large randomized trial revealed transaminase elevations in 7.1% of subjects receiving zalcitabine/zidovudine, 5% of subjects receiving didanosine/zidovudine, and 5.1% of subjects receiving zidovudine alone.[42] There are no available data regarding the use of zalcitabine during pregnancy.

EFFICACY

Zalcitabine has been evaluated extensively as monotherapy and two- and three-drug combinations in HIV-infected subjects. The results of major efficacy studies are summarized in Table 7-2.

Zalcitabine Monotherapy

Many early trials evaluated zalcitabine monotherapy in subjects with relatively late-stage HIV infection.[31,37–40,54] The designs of these trials included dose-escalation studies,[31,37] zalcitabine alternating with zidovudine,[38] and comparisons of zalcitabine monotherapy with zidovudine,[39,40,55] didanosine,[56] or saquinavir[54] monotherapies. Increases in absolute CD4+ T-lymphocyte number of zalcitabine-treated subjects were extremely small,[31] if they changed at all from baseline.[37] In patients with severe acquired immunodeficiency syndrome (AIDS)-related complex (ARC) or AIDS and 48 weeks or less of prior zidovudine, subjects randomized to zalcitabine had less decline in absolute CD4+ T lymphocytes than zidovudine-treated subjects at 28 weeks.[39]

In contrast to the modest absolute CD4+ T-lymphocyte response in zalcitabine-treated subjects, serum p24 antigen levels responded more favorably.[31,37,38] In one dose-escalation study, most subjects experienced at least a 50% decline from baseline in serum p24 antigen levels.[37] Similar results were seen in subjects receiving alternating zalcitabine and zidovudine compared to those receiving zidovudine alone. Zidovudine-experienced subjects were less likely to have p24 antigen suppression, and in the ACTG 155 study no significant difference was noted between zalcitabine- and zidovudine-treated subjects.[40]

The clinical outcomes reported in zalcitabine-treated subjects are variable, and their inconsistency probably reflects the inadequacy of antiretroviral monotherapy. The ACTG 114 study, performed in subjects with ARC or AIDS and less than 3 months of prior zidovudine, reported more frequent progression to AIDS or death in zalcitabine-treated subjects compared to those receiving zidovudine.[52] Studies ACTG 119 and 155, both performed in subjects with ARC or AIDS and more zidovudine experience (ACTG 119: =48 weeks; ACTG 155: >6 months), revealed no differences in progression to AIDS or death, or survival, between zalcitabine- and zidovudine-treated subjects.[39,40] The CPCRA 002 study was performed in subjects with absolute CD4+ T-lymphocyte counts of less than 300 cells/mm^3 and either zidovudine intolerance or more than 6 months of prior zidovudine with disease progression. Subjects were randomized to zalcitabine or didanosine monotherapy, and the results suggested a possible survival advantage for zalcitabine over didanosine, with an adjusted relative risk of 0.65 ($P = 0.003$).[56] In the NV 14256 trial subjects were randomized to receive zalcitabine or saquinavir monotherapy, or the combination.[54] There were no significant differences in plasma HIV RNA levels, CD4+ T-lymphocyte numbers and AIDS-defining events or deaths between the zalcitabine or saquinavir monotherapy arms.

Combination Therapy with Zalcitabine

Combination treatment with zalcitabine and zidovudine can clearly increase the absolute CD4+ T-lymphocyte number more than zidovudine monotherapy in treatment-naive subjects.[42,50,53] The magnitude of the absolute CD4+ T-lymphocyte increase in zalcitabine/zidovudine-treated subjects in these trials varied between 40 and 100 cells/mm^3 at 8 weeks. In one trial, the absolute CD4+ T-lymphocyte change from baseline was not significantly different at 72 weeks in subjects treated with zalcitabine/zidovudine or didanosine/zidovudine.[50]

Zidovudine-experienced subjects who add zalcitabine to their treatment may have higher absolute CD4+ T-lymphocyte increases than those who are randomized to continue on zidovudine monotherapy,[40,53] although one trial failed to show this difference.[42] The NUCA 3002 trial compared zalcitabine/zidovudine to lamivudine/zidovudine in experienced subjects. The results showed that adding zalcitabine to zidovudine provided an extremely small increase in absolute CD4+ T-lymphocyte number of short duration, and that the lamivudine/zidovudine group had greater absolute CD4+ T-lymphocyte increases.[57] Cumulatively, these results suggest that adding zalcitabine to zidovudine therapy can increase the absolute CD4+ T-lymphocyte number modestly, but the magnitude of this increase in experienced subjects is lower than in naive subjects and varies between 0 and 30 cells/mm^3 at 8 weeks.

Major Activity and Efficacy Trials Evaluating Zalcitabine Monotherapy and Combination Therapy

Table 7-2

Trial	Design	No. of Dose	Subjects	Entry Criteria	CD4 Response
ACTG 047 (Skowron et al[38])	Alternating ddC + ZDV vs, continuous ZDV	0.01–0.03 mg/kg q4h ddC	131	ARC or AIDS p24 >70 pg/mL	Greatest in alternating limbs
ACTG 114[56]	ddC vs, ZDV	0.75 mg PO q8h ddC	635 CD4 ≤200/mm³ <3 months prior ZDV	ARC or AIDS	
ACTG 155 (Fischl et al[40])	ddC vs, ZDV vs, ZDV + ddC	0.75 mg PO q8h	1001	ARC or AIDS with CD4 <300/mm³ or asymptomatic with CD4 <200/mm³ ZDV >6 months	No significant difference vs, ZDV + ddC
CPCRA 002 (Abrams et al[57])	ddC vs, ddI	0.75 mg PO q8h	467	CD4 <300/mm³ ZDV intolerant or ≥6 months prior ZDV with disease progression	Not included
ACTG 175 (Hammer et al[42]) Overall	ZDV vs, ddI vs, ddI + ZDV vs, ddC + ZDV	0.75 mg PO q8h	2467	Asymptomatic with CD4 200–500/mm³	Not reported
Naive subjects	ZDV vs, ddI vs, ddI + ZDV vs, ddC + ZDV	0.75 mg PO q8h	1067		Week 8 ZDV 114/mm³* ddI + ZDV 163/mm³* ddC + ZDV 141/mm³* (*P <0.05 compared to ZDV)
Experienced subjects	ZDV vs, ddI vs, ddI + ZDV vs, ddC + ZDV	0.75 mg PO q8h	1400		Week 8 ZDV −22/mm³ ddI +34/mm³* ddI + ZDV +40/mm³* ddC + ZDV +13/mm³* (*P >0.05 compared to ZDV)
Delta Coordinating Committee[43] Overall	ZDV vs, ddI + ZDV vs, ddC + ZDV	0.75 mg PO q8h	3207	CD4 50–350/mm³	Not provided
Naive subjects	ZDV vs, ddI + ZDV vs, ddC + ZDV	0.75 mg PO q8h	2124		Week 8 ZDV +30/mm³ ddI + ZDV +80/mm³* ddC + ZDV +67/mm³* (*P < 0.05 compared to ZDV)
Experienced subjects	ZDV vs, ddI + ZDV vs, ddC + ZDV	0.7 mg PO q8h	1083		Week 8 ZDV −12/mm³ ddI + ZDV +20/mm³* ddC + ZDV +3/mm³ (*P < 0.05 compared to ZDV)

(Continued)

(Continued)

Table 7-2

Trial	Design	No. of Dose	Subjects	Entry Criteria	CD4 Response
CPCRA (Saravolatz et al[45])	ZDV vs, ddI + ZDV vs, ddC + ZDV	0.75 mg PO q8h	1102	AIDS or CD4 <200/mm^3	Month 2 ZDV −4/mm^3 ddI + ZDV +19.2/mm^3* ddC + ZDV +12.9/mm^3 (*$P < 0.001$ compared to ZDV)
ACTG 193A (Henry et al[58])	ZDV alternating with ddI vs, ZDV + ddI vs, ZDV + ddI + NVP	0.75 mg PO q8h	1314	CD4 <50/mm^3	Not available
SV 14604[59]	ZDV vs, ZDV + ddC vs, ZDV + SQV vs, ZDV + ddC + SQV	0.75 mg PO q8h	3485	≤16 weeks prior ZDV	Not available
SV14256[46]	ddC vs, SQV vs, ddC +SQV		940	<16 weeks prior ZDV, CD4 50–350	48 weeks ddC −27/mm^3 SQV −22/mm^3 ddC +SQV −21/mm^3
Quattro[47]	ddC + ZDV + LMV+ loviride vs, 8-week cycles of each as monotherapy vs, ZDV + LMV		100	Naive, CD4 50–350	64 weeks 4 drugs + 87/mm^3 cycles + 18/mm^3 2 drugs + 40/mm^3
MIKADO[48]	ddC + d4T + SQV		35	Naive, CD ≥ 250, RNA ≥ 5000	24 weeks significant increase from baseline
Idoka et al[66]	ddC + ZDV + NLV		40	CD4 100–500	24 weeks + 141/mm^3 in the 26 patients still on treatment
HIVBID[35]	ddC bid + ZDV + SQV or NLV vs, LMV + ZDV + SQV or NLV		47	Naive, CD ≥ 200, RNA ≥ 5000	48 weeks ddC + 128/mm^3 LMV + 115/mm^3

Antiviral Response	Clinical Outcome	Comments
p24 Decline greatest in alternating limbs	Not studied	Alternating ddC and ZDV superior to intermittent ddC or ZDV
	Treatment / **AIDS or Death** / **Death** ddC / 41% / 59 ZDV / 30% / 33 P / 0.02 / 0.07	ZDV monotherapy superior to ddC monotherapy

(*Continued*)

(Continued)

Table 7-2

Antiviral Response	Clinical Outcome: Treatment	AIDS or Death	Death	Comments
No significant difference in p24 decline vs, ZDV	ddC ZDV ddC + ZDV *P*	125 11 16 NS	51 43 78 NS	No difference in clinical outcomes in ZDV-experienced subjects
Not included	ddC ddI Adjusted RR *P*	153 157 0.84 0.15	88 100 0.65 0.003	Possible survival advantage for ddC over ddI
Not reported	ddC + ZDV vs, ZDV *P*	0.77 NS	0.71 NS	
Not reported	ddC + ZDV vs, ZDV ($P < 0.05$)	0.49*	0.55 NS	Combination therapy with ddC + ZDV offers improved clinical outcomes over ZDV alone in naive subjects
Not reported	ddC + ZDV vs, ZDV (*$P < 0.05$)	0.91*	0.81 NS	No differences in clinical outcomes in ZDV-experienced subjects
Not provided	ddC + ZDV vs, ZDV ddI + ZDV vs, ddC + ZDV (*$P < 0.05$)	0.86* 0.85*	0.79* 0.85	
Not provided	ddC + ZDV vs, ZDV ddI + ZDV vs, ddC + ZDV (*$P < 0.05$)	0.80* 0.79*	0.68* 0.85	Combination therapy with ddC + ZDV offers improved clinical outcomes compared to ZDV but not ZDV + ddI in naive subjects
Not provided	ddC + ZDV vs, ZDV ddI + ZDV vs, ddC + ZDV	0.95 0.92	0.91 0.84	No differences in clinical outcomes in ZDV-experienced subjects
Not provided	ddC + ZDV vs, ZDV ddI + ZDV vs, ddC + ZDV	0.92 0.93	0.96 0.92	Treatment ddC + ZDV vs, ZDV ddI + ZDV vs, ddC + ZDV
Not available	AIDS or Death ZDV + ddI + NVP vs, ZDV + ddC* ZDV + ddI + NVP vs, ZDV alternating with ddI* (*$P < 0.05$)			Three drugs improve clinical outcomes compared to ZDV + ddC in subjects with CD4 <50/mm^3
Not available	ZDV + ddC ZDV + ddC + SQV (*$P < 0.001$)	142 116*	34 31	Three drugs improve clinical outcomes compared to ZDV + ddC
48 weeks ddC + SQV −0.62 $\log_{10}$	ddC + SQV had fewer AIDS-defining events ($p = 0.0006$) and fewer deaths ($p = 0.0002$) than ddC alone; ddC and SQV monotherapy groups not significantly different			Clear advantage for ddC + SQV
64 weeks 4 drugs −1.25 $\log_{10}$ Cycles −0.41 $\log_{10}$ 2 drugs −0.75 $\log_{10}$	No difference			

(*Continued*)

(Continued)

Table 7-2

Antiviral Response	Clinical Outcome: Treatment	AIDS or Death	Death	Comments
24 weeks 63% <200 copies/mL 34% <20 copies/mL	Not available			
22 patients had baseline and week 24 measures; 17/22 had decreased RNA 2/22 <400 4/22 >2 $\log_{10}$ decrease 6/22 >1 $\log_{10}$ decrease	Not available			Resource-limited setting
48 weeks RNA ddC −2.31 $\log_{10}$ LMV −2.32 $\log_{10}$	Not available			

ddI, didanosine; LMV, lamivudine; NVP, nevirapine; RR, relative risk; SQV, saquinavir; ZDV, zidovudine. CD4 indicates the CD4+ T-lymphocyte count.

Suppression of serum p24 antigen levels was greater in subjects receiving zalcitabine/zidovudine than in those receiving zalcitabine or zidovudine alone.[40] Serum p24 antigen suppression has shown a dose-response relation with zalcitabine and zidovudine doses, and the greatest suppression has been achieved at full doses of both drugs.[41] In more recent trials, plasma HIV RNA levels were monitored in subjects receiving zalcitabine/zidovudine. Treatment-naive subjects receiving both drugs achieved greater suppression of plasma HIV RNA levels than those receiving zidovudine alone.[41] In treatment-naive subjects, the magnitude of the change in plasma HIV RNA levels at 52 weeks was ~0.6 $\log_{10}$ copies /mL in the zalcitabine/zidovudine recipients and was not significantly different from those receiving didanosine/zidovudine.[50] In experienced subjects, no significant difference was seen in plasma HIV RNA suppression over 52 weeks between those receiving zalcitabine/zidovudine or lamivudine/zidovudine.[57] In treatment-experienced subjects receiving zalcitabine/zidovudine, the magnitude of suppression was ~0.4 $\log_{10}$ copies/mL over 52 weeks.

The clinical outcomes associated with zalcitabine/zidovudine have been studied in several large clinical trials. In treatment-naive subjects, progression to AIDS or death was less frequent for zalcitabine/zidovudine recipients compared with those receiving zidovudine alone[42,53] (relative risk 0.49[53] to 0.80[42]). Survival was improved in one trial [42] but did not achieve statistical significance in the other.[53] In one study, didanosine/zidovudine had a lower relative risk of progression to AIDS or death than zalcitabine/zidovudine, but survival was not significantly different.[42] Prolonged follow-up of subjects enrolled in the Delta trial (median 43 months) revealed that the maximum effects on mortality were observed between 2 and 3 years with a 26% decrease in those receiving zalcitabine plus zidovudine, (a 48% decrease was seen in subjects receiving didanosine plus zidovudine[58]). A systematic overview of 6 randomized trials included 7700 subjects receiving zidovudine monotherapy, zalcitabine plus zidovudine, or didanosine plus zidovudine. The combination of zalcitabine + zidovudine provided improved survival (relative risk of death = 0.87 [0.77–0.98]) and less disease progression (RR = 0.86 [0.78–0.94]) compared with zidovudine monotherapy.[59] However, didanosine plus zidovudine was significantly better than zalcitabine plus zidovudine in prolonging survival (RR = 0.86 [0.77–0.96]) and delaying disease progression (RR = 0.87 [0.79–0.96]). Zalcitabine and saquinavir were given as a 2 drug combination in the NV 14256 study, and this combination provided better RNA suppression, increases in CD4+ T-lymphocyte counts, and clinical outcomes compared to either drug alone.[54] Quality of life scores were also higher for subjects receiving zalcitabine plus saquinavir.[60]

In treatment-experienced subjects it has been much more difficult to show improved clinical outcomes for any double nucleoside reverse transcriptase inhibitor (NRTI) combination. The ACTG 155, ACTG 175, CPCRA 007, and Delta 2 studies have all failed to show any improvement regarding progression to AIDS or death, or survival alone, in the recipients of zalcitabine/zidovudine compared to continued zidovudine monotherapy.[40,42,44,53] Only a stratified analysis in ACTG 155 identified improvements in disease progression or death in subjects with baseline absolute CD4+ T-lymphocyte counts higher than 150 cells/mm^3. The CPCRA 007 and Delta 2 studies also showed no difference in clinical outcomes between zalcitabine/zidovudine recipients versus didanosine/zidovudine recipients.[42,44]

Three-drug combinations including zalcitabine have also undergone evaluation.[61–63] In the ACTG 229 study, the magnitude of absolute CD4+ T-lymphocyte increases was greater for the recipients of zalcitabine/zidovudine/saquinavir versus zalcitabine or zidovudine alone.[63] Plasma HIV RNA levels also achieved better suppression with three drugs than with two drugs in the same trial.[63] Clinical outcomes have been studied in two other trials, ACTG 193A and SV 14604. ACTG 193A studied two-drug combinations of didanosine alternating with zidovudine, didanosine/zidovudine, and zalcitabine/zidovudine versus a three-drug combination of didanosine/zidovudine/nevirapine in subjects with absolute CD4+ T-lymphocyte counts of more than 50 cells/mm^3.[61] The three-drug combination offered improved clinical outcomes compared to didanosine alternating with zidovudine or zalcitabine/zidovudine. SV 14604 studied zidovudine alone, zalcitabine/zidovudine, saquinavir/zidovudine, and zalcitabine/zidovudine/saquinavir in 3485 subjects with zidovudine experience of 16 weeks or more,[62] and the three-drug combination resulted in significantly less risk of the occurrence of a primary endpoint (disease progression or death) than zalcitabine/zidovudine but did not significantly affect survival when analyzed separately. Subjects receiving the three-drug combination had stable quality of life scores after 48 weeks, in contrast with decreasing scores among subjects receiving zalcitabine plus zidovudine.[64] The HIVBID study randomized 47 subjects to receive zalcitabine 1.125 mg BID or lamivudine 150 mg BID in combination with zidovudine and either saquinavir or nelfinavir.[61] There were no significant differences in the proportions of subjects with plasma HIV RNA levels <400 or 50 copies/mL, or in the increases in absolute CD4+ T lymphocytes after 48 weeks. Zalcitabine, stavudine and saquinavir were given to 35 subjects in the MIKADO study,[54] and plasma HIV RNA levers were <200 and <20 copies/mL in 63% and 34% of subjects after 24 weeks. Zalcitabine, zidovudine and nelfinavir were given to 40 Nigerian patients, and 31/40 completed 24 weeks of treatment.[65] Although many patients experienced clinical improvements, only two suppressed plasma HIV RNA levels below detectable limits. Finally a four-drug combination of zalcitabine, zidovudine, lamivudine and loviride was given to 34 subjects in the Quattro Study,[66] and their mean decline in plasma HIV RNA levels was -1.25 $\log_{10}$ copies/mL after 64 weeks.

RESISTANCE

Zalcitabine resistance is not easily identified from *in vitro* serial HIV passages or clinical isolates. High-level resistance ($>$100-fold changes in IC_{50}) has not been reported to date from *in vitro* studies or clinical trials.[67] Low-level to moderate-level resistance has been associated with five mutations in the *pol* gene: Lys_{65}:Arg, Thr_{69}:Arg, Leu_{74}:Val, Gln_{151}:Met, and Met_{184}:Val/Ile.[67] All five mutations are within or close to conserved motifs near the catalytic site of reverse transcriptase. All of these mutations may be associated with cross-resistance to didanosine, lamivudine, or zidovudine, except Thr_{69}:Asp.

The results of phenotypic and genotypic assays indicate the infrequent detection of zalcitabine resistance in subjects receiving zalcitabine/zidovudine. In the BW 34, 225-02 trial studying treatment-naive subjects, no change in phenotypic zalcitabine sensitivity was noted in 10 subjects receiving zalcitabine/zidovudine over 48 weeks.[50] However, two of these subjects did have codon 184 mutations when genotypic assays were performed. A subsequent study did not identify any M184V mutations in eight persons with treatment failure receiving zidovudine/zalcitabine.[68] Interestingly, zalcitabine/zidovudine therapy did not delay the onset of phenotypic zidovudine resistance in the BW 34, 225-02 study compared with zidovudine alone. Similar results in the ACTG 106 study documented a lack of zalcitabine resistance in phenotypic assays in 15 treatment-naive subjects receiving zalcitabine/zidovudine for 36 months.[69] In Delta 1 study subjects receiving zalcitabine/zidovudine, no zalcitabine resistance mutations were found in genotypic assays after 112 weeks.[70] Using the sensitive LiPA technique to detect point mutations, no L74V mutations were noted in eight patients who failed a zidovudine/zalcitabine regimen.[68] In the Quattro study, the cycle of zalcitabine monotherapy initially selected M184V variants, but they disappeared with continued therapy.[71] Overall, zalcitabine resistance was rarely identified in this study.

In zidovudine-experienced patients, it is also difficult to detect zalcitabine resistance when zalcitabine is added, although these subjects can have zalcitabine-resistant strains prior to the initiation of zalcitabine therapy as a result of cross-resistance with zidovudine.[72,73] Zalcitabine resistance was not observed at baseline in the NUCA 3002 trial, and none of 14 subjects treated with zalcitabine/zidovudine developed phenotypic zalcitabine resistance after 12 weeks of therapy.[74] In addition, none of these subjects had phenotypic evidence of cross-resistance to lamivudine. In contrast, among subjects treated with lamivudine/zidovudine who developed phenotypic lamivudine resistance at week 12, the median zalcitabine IC_{50} values increased 3.3- to 4.4-fold, suggesting the occurrence of cross-resistance to zalcitabine in lamivudine-treated subjects.[74] Similar observations of decreased zalcitabine susceptibility were made following the development of lamivudine resistance in a second study.[75]

DRUG INTERACTIONS

Zalcitabine has few recognized drug interactions.[76] However, caution should be used when prescribing drugs that may have overlapping toxicities (Table 7-3). For example, other antiretroviral agents with neuropathic toxicities, such as didanosine and stavudine, should not be co-administered with zalcitabine.

Potential Drug Interactions: Overlapping Toxicities With Zalcitabine

Table 7-3

Neuropathy
Didanosine
Stavudine
Dapsone
Disulfiram
Isoniazid
Lithium carbonate
Metronidazole
Pentamidine
Phenytoin
Ribavirin
Vincristine
Pancreatitis
Didanosine
Stavudine
Pentamidine

Other drugs that can cause neuropathy, such as dapsone, disulfiram, isoniazid, lithium carbonate, metronidazole, pentamidine, phenytoin, ribavirin, and vincristine, should be given with caution. Zalcitabine is predominantly eliminated through the kidneys; hence renal function should be monitored to avoid overdosage, especially in patients who may be receiving concurrent nephrotoxic medications.

CONCLUSIONS

Zalcitabine is a nucleoside analog that is rarely used in current antiretroviral regimens because other, less toxic and equally or more potent drugs are available. It has been demonstrated to have antiviral and clinical benefits, particularly in treatment-naive patients. Recipients of zalcitabine should be monitored carefully for peripheral neuropathy, which is the principal toxicity of the drug. Zalcitabine should not be used in combination regimens with didanosine or stavudine because of overlapping toxicities of the drugs. Cross-resistance between other nucleoside analogs and zalcitabine is common, particularly in patients treated with lamivudine.

REFERENCES

1. Horwitz JP, Chua J, DaRooge M, et al. Nucleosides. IX. The formation of 2′,3′-unsaturated pyrimidine nucleosides via a novel β-elimination reaction. J Org Chem 31:205, 1966.
2. Mitsuya H, Broder S. Inhibition of the in vitro infectivity and cytopathic effect of T-lymphotrophic virus type III/lymphadenopathy-associated virus (HTLV III/LAV) by 2′,3′-dideoxynucleosides. Proc Natl Acad Sci USA 82:7096, 1986.
3. Mitsuya H, Broder S. Strategies for antiviral therapy in AIDS. Nature 325:773, 1987.
4. Balzarini J, Pauwels R, Baba M, et al. The in vitro and in vivo anti-retrovirus activity, and intracellular metabolism of 2′,3′-azido-2′,3′-dideoxythymidine and 2′,3′-dideoxcytidine are highly dependent on the cell species. Biochem Pharmacol 37:897, 1988.
5. Perno C-F, Yarchoan R, Cooney D. Replication of human immunodeficiency virus in monocytes: granulocyte/macrophage colony-stimulating factor (GMCSF) potentiates viral production yet enhances the antiviral effect mediated by 3′-azido-2′,3′-dideoxythymidine (AZT) and other dideoxynucleosides. J Exp Med 167:988, 1989.
6. Larder BA, Darby G, Richman D. HIV with reduced sensitivity to zidovudine (AZT) isolated during prolonged therapy. Science 243:1731, 1989.
7. Richman D. Susceptibility to nucleoside analogues of zidovudine-resistant isolates of human immunodeficiency virus. Am J Med 88 (Suppl 5B):85, 1990.
8. Eron J, Johnson V, Merrill D, et al. Synergistic inhibition of replication of human immunodeficiency virus type 1, including that of a zidovudine-resistant isolate, by zidovudine and 2′,3′-dideoxycytidine in-vitro. Antimicrob Agents Chemother 35:394, 1991.
9. Zalcitabine package insert. Nutley, NJ: Roche Laboratories, 1996.
10. Kassianides C, Hoonagle J, Miller R, et al. Inhibition of duck hepatitis B virus replication by 2′,3′-dideoxycytidine. Gastroenterology 97:1276, 1989.
11. Yokota T, Mochizuki S, Kommo K, et al. Inhibitory effects of selected antiviral compounds on human hepatitis B virus DNA synthesis. Antimicrob Agents Chemother 35:394, 1991.
12. Balzarini J, Pauwels R, Herdewijn P, et al. Potent and selective anti-HTLV III/LAV activity of 2′,3′-dideoxycytidine, the 2N,3N-unsaturated derivative of 2′,3′-dideoxycytidine. Biochem Biophys Res Commun 140:735, 1986.
13. Vogt M, Durno A, Chou T-C. Synergistic interaction of 2′,3′-dideoxycytidine and recombinant interferon-alpha on replication of human immunodeficiency virus type 1. J Infect Dis 158:378, 1988.
14. Johnson V, Merrill D, Chou T-C. Human immunodeficiency virus type 1 (HIV-1) inhibitory interactions between protease inhibitor Ro 31-8959 and zidovudine, 2′,3′-dideoxycytidine, or recombinant interferon-alpha against zidovudine-sensitive or resistant HIV-1 in-vitro. J Infect Dis 166:1143, 1992.
15. Chong K-T, Pagano P, Hinshaw R. Bisheteroarylpiperazine reverse transcriptase inhibitor in combination with 3′-azido-3′-deoxythymidine or 2′,3′-dideoxycytidine synergistically inhibits human immunodeficiency virus type 1 replication in vitro. Antimicrob Agents Chemother 38:288, 1994.

16. Vogt M, Hartshorn K, Furman P. Ribavirin antagonizes the effects of azidothymidine on HIV replication. Science 235:1376, 1987.
17. Baba M, Pauwels R, Balzarini J. Ribavirin antagonizes inhibitory effects of pyrimidine 2′,3′-dideoxynucleosides but enhances inhibitory effects of purine 2′,3′-dideoxynucleosides on replication of human immunodeficiency virus in-vitro. Antimicrob Agents Chemother 31:1613, 1987.
18. Chen C-H, Cheng Y-C. Delayed cytotoxicity and selective loss of mitochondrial DNA in cells treated with the anti-human immunodeficiency virus compound 2′,3′-dideoxycytidine. J Biol Chem 264:11934, 1989.
19. Cooney DA, Dala M, Mitsuga H, et al. Initial studies on the cellular pharmacology of 2′,3′-dideoxycytidine, an inhibitor of HTLV III infectivity. Biochem Pharmacol 35:2065, 1986.
20. Ullman B, Coons T, Rockwell S, et al. Genetic analysis of 2′,3′-dideoxycytidine incorporation into cultured human T lymphoblasts. J Biol Chem 263:12391, 1988.
21. Plagemann P, Woffendi C. Dideoxycytidine permeation and salvage by mouse leukemia cells and human erythrocytes. Biochem Pharmacol 38:3469, 1989.
22. Yarchoan R, Mitsuya H, Myers C, et al. Clinical pharmacology of 3′-azido-2′,3′-dideoxythymidine (zidovudine) and related dideoxynucleosides. N Engl J Med 321:726, 1989.
23. Broder S. Pharmacodynamics of 2′,3′-dideoxycytidine: an inhibitor of human immunodeficiency virus infection. Am J Med 88(Suppl 5B):25, 1990.
24. Brandi G, Rossi L, Schiavano G, et al. In vitro toxicity and metabolism of 2′,3′-dideoxycytidine, an inhibitor of human immunodeficiency virus infectivity. Chem Biol Interactions 79:53, 1991.
25. Starnes M, Cheng Y. Cellular metabolism of 2N,3N-dideoxycytidine, a compound active against human immunodeficiency virus in vitro. J. Biol Chem 262:988, 1987.
26. Tornerik Y, Eriksson S. 2′,3′-Dideoxycytidine toxicity in cultured human CEM T lymphoblasts: effects of combination with 3′-azido-3N-deoxythymidine and thymidine. Mol Pharmacol 38:237, 1990.
27. Gao W-Y, Shirasaka T, Johns D. Differential phosphorylation of azidothymidine, dideoxycytidine and dideoxyinosine in resting and activated peripheral blood mononuclear cells. J Clin Invest 91:2326, 1993.
28. Gao W-Y, Agbaria R, Driscoll J. Divergent anti-human immunodeficiency virus activity and anabolic phosphorylation of 2′,3′-dideoxynucleoside analogs in resting and activated human cells. J Biol Chem 269:12633, 1994.
29. Chen M, Oshana S. Inhibition of HIV reverse transcriptase by 2′,3′-dideoxynucleoside triphosphates. Biochem Pharmacol 36:4361, 1987.
30. Hao Z, Cooney D, Hartman N, et al. Factors determining the activity of 2′,3′-dideoxynucleosides in suppressing human immunodeficiency virus in-vitro. Mol Pharmacol 34:431, 1988.
31. Yarchoan R, Devno C, Thomas R, et al. Phase I studies of 2′,3′-dideoxycytidine in severe human immunodeficiency virus infection as a single agent and alternating with zidovudine (AZT). Lancet 1:76, 1988.
32. Klecker R, Collins J, Yarchoan R, et al. Pharmacokinetics of 2′,3′-dideoxycytidine in patients with AIDS and related disorders. J Clin Pharmacol 28:835, 1988.
33. Gustavson L, Fukuda E, Rubio F, et al. A pilot study of the bioavailability and pharmacokinetics of 2′,3′-dideoxycytidine in patients with AIDS or AIDS-related complex. J Acquir Immune Defic Syndr 3:28, 1990.
34. Moyle G, Gazzard B. Finding a role for zalcitabinein the HAART era. Antivir Ther 3:125, 1998.
35. Antunes F, Walker M, Moyle G, on behalf of the HIVBID Study Group. Efficacy and tolerability of zalcitabine twice daily. J Acquir Immune Defic Syndr 35:205, 2004.
36. Pizzo P, Butler K, Balis F, et al. Dideoxycytidine alone and in an alternating schedule with zidovudine in children with symptomatic human immunodeficiency virus infection. J Pediatr 117:799, 1990.
37. Merigan T, Skowron G, Bozzette S, et al; ddC Study Group of the AIDS Clinical Trials Group. Circulating p24 antigen levels and responses to dideoxycytidine in human immunodeficiency virus (HIV) infections. Ann Intern Med 110:189, 1989.
38. Skowron G, Bozzette S, Lim L, et al. Alternating and intermittent regimens of zidovudine and dideoxycytidine in patients with AIDS or AIDS-related complex. Ann Intern Med 118:321, 1993.
39. Fischl M, Olson R, Follansbee S, et al. Zalcitabine compared with zidovudine in patients with advanced HIV-1 infection who received previous zidovudine therapy. Ann Intern Med 118:762, 1993.
40. Fischl M, Stanley K, Collier A, et al. NIAID AIDS Clinical Trials Group. Combination and monotherapy with zidovudine and zalcitabine in patients with advanced HIV disease. Ann Intern Med 122:24, 1995.
41. Meng T-C, Fischl M, Boota A, et al. Combination therapy with zidovudine and dideoxycytidine in patients with advanced human immunodeficiency virus infection. Ann Intern Med 116:13, 1992.
42. Delta Coordinating Committee. Delta: a randomised double-blind controlled trial comparing combinations of zidovudine plus didanosine or zalcitabine with zidovudine alone in HIV-infected individuals. Lancet 348:283, 1996.
43. Katlama C, Pelligrin J-L, Lacoste D, et al. MIKADO: A multicenter, open-label pilot study to evaluate the antiretroviral activity and safety of saquinavir with stavudine and zalcitabine. HIV Medicine 2:20, 2001.
44. Saravolatz L, Winslow D, Collins G, et al; Investigators for the Terry Beirn Community Programs for Clinical Research on AIDS. Zidovudine alone or in combination with didanosine or zalcitabine in HIV-infected patients with the acquired immunodeficiency syndrome or fewer than 200 CD4 cells per cubic millimeter. N Engl J Med 335:1099, 1996.
45. Blum A, Dal Pan G, Feinberg J, et al. Low dose zalcitabine (ddC)-related toxic neuropathy: frequency, natural history, and risk factors. Neurology 46:999, 1996.
46. Fichtenbaum C, Clifford D, Powderly W. Risk factors for dideoxynucleoside-induced toxic neuropathy in patients with human immunodeficiency virus infection. J Acquir Immune Defic Syndr 10:169, 1995.
47. Berger A, Arezzo J, Schaumberg H, et al. 2′,3′-Dideoxycytidine (ddC) toxic neuropathy: a study of 52 patients. Neurology 43:358, 1993.
48. Dubinsky R, Yarchoan R, Dalakas M, et al. Reversible axonal neuropathy from the treatment of AIDS and related disorders with 2′,3′-dideoxycytidine (ddC). Muscle Nerve 12:856, 1989.
49. LeLacheor S, Simon G. Exacerbation of dideoxycytidine-induced neuropathy with dideoxyinosine. J Acquir Immune Defic Syndr 4:538, 1991.
50. Schooley R, Ramirez-Ronda C, Lange J, et al; Wellcome Resistance Study Collaborative Group. Virologic and immunologic benefits of initial combination therapy with zidovudine and zalcitabine or didanosine compared with zidovudine monotherapy. J Infect Dis 173:1354, 1996.
51. Indorf A, Pegram P. Esophageal ulceration due to zalcitabine (ddC). Ann Intern Med 117:133, 1992.
52. McNeely M, Yarchoan R, Broder S, et al. Dermatologic complications associated with administration of 2′,3′-dideoxycytidine in patients with human immunodeficiency virus infection. J Am Acad Dermatol 21:1213, 1989.
53. Hammer S, Katzenstein D, Hughes M, et al; AIDS Clinical Trials Group Study 175 Team. A trial comparing nucleoside monotherapy with combination therapy in HIV-infected adults

with CD4 cell counts from 200 to 500 per cubic millimeter. N Engl J Med 335:1081, 1996.
54. Haubrich R, Lalezari J, Follansbee S, et al. Improved survival and reduced clinical progression in HIV-infected patients with advanced disease treated with saquinavir plus zalcitabine. Antivir Ther 3:33, 1998.
55. Letter to investigators. Nutley, NJ: Hoffman-LaRoche, 1991.
56. Abrams D, Goldman A, Launer C, et al; Terry Beirn Community Programs for Clinical Research on AIDS. A comparative trial of didanosine or zalcitabine after treatment with zidovudine in patients with human immunodeficiency virus infection. N Engl J Med 330:657, 1994.
57. Bartlett J, Benoit S, Johnson V, et al; North American HIV Working Party. Lamivudine plus zidovudine compared with zalcitabine plus zidovudine in patients with HIV infection. Ann Intern Med 125:161, 1996.
58. Delta Coordinating Committee. Evidence for prolonged clinical benefit from initial combination therapy: Delta extended follow-up. HIV Med 2:181, 2001.
59. HIV Trialist's Collaborative Group. Zidovudine, didanosine, and zalcitabine in the treatment of HIV infection: meta-analysis of the randomised evidence. Lancet 353:2014, 1999.
60. Revicki D, Swartz C, Wu A, et al. Quality of life outcomes of saquinavir, zalcitabine, and combination saquinavir plus zalcitabine therapy for adults with advanced HIV infection with CD4 counts between 50 and 300 cells/mm^3. Antivir Ther 4:35, 1999.
61. Henry K, Erice A, Tierney C, et al; ACTG 193A Study Team. A randomized, controlled double-blind study comparing the survival benefit of four different reverse transcriptase inhibitor therapies (three-drug, two-drug, and alternating drug) for the treatment of advanced AIDS. J Acqui Imm Syndr Human Retr 19:339, 1998.
62. Letter to investigators. Nutley, NJ: Roche Laboratories, 1997.
63. Collier A, Coombs R, Schoenfeld D, et al; AIDS Clinical Trials Group. Treatment of human immunodeficiency virus infection with saquinavir, zidovudine and zalcitabine. N Engl J Med 334:1011, 1996.
64. Revicki D, Moyle G, Stellbrink H, Barker C. Quality of life outcomes of combination zalcitabine–zidovudine, saquinavir–zidovudine, and saquinavir–zalcitabine–zidovudine therapy for HIV-infected adults with CD4 cell counts between 50 and 350 per cubic millimeter. AIDS 13: 851, 1999.
65. Idoka J, Akinsete L, Abalaka A, et al. A multicentre study to determine the efficacy and tolerability of a combination of nelfinavir, zalcitabine and zidovudine in treatment of HIV infected Nigerian patients. West Afr J Med 21:83, 2002.
66. Quattro Steering Committee. A randomized trial comparing regimens of four reverse transcriptase inhibitors given together or cyclically in HIV-1 infection – The Quattro Trial. AIDS 13:2209, 1999.
67. Craig C, Moyle G. The development of resistance of HIV-1 to zalcitabine. AIDS 11:271, 1997.
68. Rusconi S, La Seta Catamancio S, Sheridan F, Parker D. A genotypic analysis of patients receiving zidovudine, didanosine or zalcitabine dual therapy using the LiPA point mutations assay to detect genotypic variation at codons 41, 69, 70, 74, 184 and 215. J Clin Virol 3:135, 2000.
69. Richman D, Meng T-C, Spector S, et al. Resistance to AZT and ddC during long-term combination therapy in patients with advanced infection with human immunodeficiency virus. J Acquir Immune Defic Syndr 7:135, 1994.
70. Loveday C; Delta Virology Group. HIV-1 genotypic and phenotypic resistance in Delta patients. In: Abstracts of the XIth International Conference on AIDS, Vancouver, 1996, abstract Th.B 4354.
71. Quattro Steering Committee. Observations of HIV-1 genotypic drug resistance in a trial of four reverse transcriptase inhibitors (Quattro trial). Antivir Ther 7:11, 2002.
72. Cox S, Aperia K, Sandstrom E, et al. Cross-resistance between AZT, ddI and other antiretroviral drugs in primary isolates of HIV-1. Antivir Chem Chemother 5:7, 1994.
73. Mayers D, Japour A, Arduino J-M, et al; RV43 Study Group. Dideoxynucleoside resistance emerges with prolonged zidovudine monotherapy. Antimicrob Agents Chemother 38:307, 1994.
74. Johnson V, Quinn J, Benoit S, et al. Drug resistance and viral load in NUCA 3002: a randomized trial of lamivudine plus zidovudine versus zalcitabine plus zidovudine in zidovudine-experienced HIV-infected subjects. In: Abstracts of the 4th Conference on Retroviruses and Opportunistic Infections, Washington, DC. Alexandria, VA: Westover Management Group; 1997, abstract 580.
75. Schmit J-C, Martinez-Picado J, Ruiz L, et al. Evolution of HIV drug resistance in zidovudine/zalcitabine- and zidovudine/didanosine-experienced patients receiving lamivudine-containing combination therapy. Antivir Ther 3:81, 1998.
76. Shelton M, O'Donnell A, Morse G. Zalcitabine. Ann Pharmacother 27:480, 1993.

Chapter 8

Stavudine

Andrew T. Pavia, MD

STRUCTURE

Stavudine (2′,3′didehydro-2′,3′-didoxythymidine: d4T), like zidovudine, is an analog of thymidine (Fig. 8-1). It differs from thymidine by replacement of the hydroxyl group at the 3′ position by a hydrogen. It is relatively water soluble with solubility of 83 mg/mL in water at 23°C.[1–3]

MECHANISM OF ACTION AND *IN VITRO* ACTIVITY

Like other nucleoside analogs, stavudine is not active as the parent compound, but must be phosphorylated to the active intracellular form, stavudine triphosphate.[1,4] The parent compound enters the cell by passive diffusion.[5] It is phosphorylated by thymidine kinase, thymidylate kinase, and pyrimidine diphosphate kinase.[6] The initial phosphorylation by thymidine kinase appears to be the rate-limiting step in the activation of stavudine.[7] Unlike zidovudine, there is no accumulation of the monophosphate. The mono-, di-, and triphosphate forms of d4T are present in approximately 1:1:1 ratio, and increasing the extracellular concentration of stavudine results in proportional increases in intracellular concentration of the active form.[6–8] The accumulation of zidovudine monophosphate and the difficulty in achieving high levels of the active triphosphate may limit the antiviral activity of zidovudine and contribute to toxicity.[9,10] In contrast to zidovudine, stavudine does not result in depletion of the intracellular pools of thymidine-5′-triphosphate in bone marrow progenitor cells. This was hypothesized to explain the lack of hematologic toxicity,[11] but other studies have suggested that depletion of thymidine-5′-triphosphate does not explain zidovudine's bone marrow toxicity.[12,13]

The triphosphate form of stavudine acts as a competitive inhibitor of reverse transcriptase by competing with the natural substrate, 2′-deoxy-thymidine-5′-triphosphate.[1,6,14,15] The alterations in the ribose ring at the 3′ position prevent formation of a new 3′-5′ phosphodiester bond with the next nucleotide. Therefore, stavudine also acts as an obligate chain terminator.

Stavudine shows antiviral activity *in vitro* against both HIV-1 and HIV-2, but not against hepatitis B, herpes simplex, or CMV.[8,16,17] The 50% inhibitory concentration (IC_{50}) for stavudine against laboratory and clinical isolates ranges from 0.009 to 4.1 μM (0.002–0.9 μg/mL) depending on the cell type and the assay system (Table 8-1). [1,8,11,13] Like zidovudine, stavudine is primarily active in HIV-infected activated cells, such as phytohemagglutinin-stimulated peripheral blood mononuclear cells, probably because thymidine kinase is an S-phase-specific enzyme. [13,18,19] Stavudine exhibits partial cross-resistance with zidovudine; isolates with multiple zidovudine

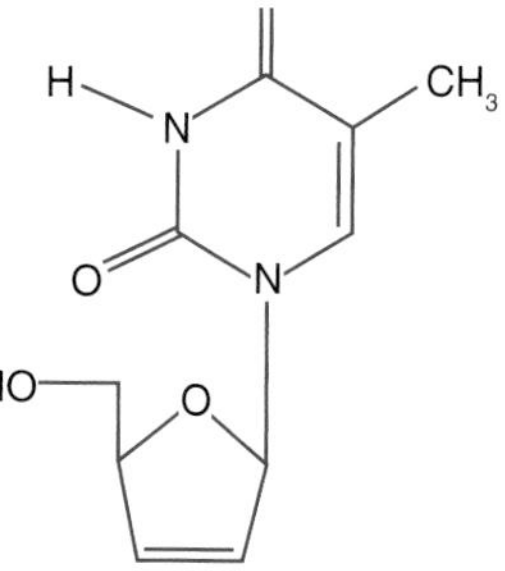

Figure 8-1 ■ Structure of stavudine (2′,3′-didehydro-2′,3′-dideoxythymidine; d4T, Zerit).

Antiviral Activity of Nucleoside Analogs Against HIV in Different Cell Systems

Table 8-1

Cell System (Strain)	EC_{50} (μM)			
	Stavudine	Zidovudine	Zalcitabine	Didanosine
MT-4 ($HTLV-III_B$)	0.01	0.006	0.06	10.0
ATH-8 ($HTLV-III_B$)	4.1	2.4	0.2	7.0
PBMC (LAV-1)	0.04	0.0006	0.011	3.0–5.0
Monocyte/Macrophages ($HTLV-III_B$)	0.3	0.2	0.002	0.01

Adapted from Sommadossi JP. Comparison of metabolism and in vitro antiviral activity of stavudine versus other 2′,3′-dideoxynucleoside analogues. J Infect Dis 171(Suppl 2):S88–92, 1995.

resistance mutations (M41L, D67N, T215Y) have reduced susceptibility.[20–23] Stavudine shows additive or synergistic activity *in vitro* when combined with didanosine, lamivudine, nevirapine, saquinavir, indinavir, and nelfinavir. [24–27] Zidovudine and stavudine compete for activation by thymidine kinase.[28] When they are co-administered *in vivo*, the amounts of stavudine triphosphate are reduced relative to zidovudine triphosphate.[6] As might be predicted, the combination of zidovudine and stavudine shows antagonism *in vitro* against zidovudine resistant strains of HIV.[24]

PHARMACOKINETICS

Stavudine is well absorbed. Initial studies suggested a bioavailablity of 82–86%,[2,29,30] but population pharmacokinetic analysis on 33 patients calculated bioavailability of greater than 99%[31,32], consistent with complete bioavailability observed in mice.[33] The area under the time-concentration curve (AUC) is identical when stavudine is taken while fasting or with a high fat meal, but the maximal concentration (C_{max}) is reduced when given with a meal.[34] Peak plasma concentrations increase in a dose-related manner. After a 0.67 mg/kg dose, the peak serum concentration of 1.2 μg/mL is reached in within 1 h.[29] The estimated volume of distribution is 0.53 L/kg,[29,33] and there is negligible protein binding.

Plasma concentrations of stavudine decline in a biphasic manner, independent of dose. The mean plasma half-life following single oral doses in HIV-infected volunteers was 1.6 ± 0.8 h. The intracellular half-life, however, is between 3 and 4 h.[19] Interpatient variation in the absorption and excretion of stavudine is relatively low.[35] About 40% of stavudine is excreted unchanged in the urine; therefore, dose adjustment is necessary for patients with renal failure (creatinine clearance <50–mL/min – see recommendations for use).[36] Two small studies have examined the clearance of stavudine in patients on hemodialysis (Bristol-Myers Squibb Investigational Drug Service written communication, Nov 1996). C_{max} was unchanged but the terminal half-life was prolonged up to 12 h. The mean hemodialysis clearance value of stavudine was 120 ± 18 mL/min. No dose adjustment is necessary in patients with hepatic impairment.[37]

Based on primate studies, the nonrenal metabolism is thought to involve cleavage of the sugar to yield thymine, which is degraded to beta-aminoisobutyric acid, or used in the pyrimidine salvage pathway.[38]

Stavudine crosses the blood–brain barrier. Levels above the IC_{50} were measured in brain tissue of rats, dogs, and monkeys after a single oral dose of 25 mg/kg.[33] Single-dose studies using a 40 mg oral dose in healthy volunteers demonstrated a mean concentration of 61 ng/mL at 4–5 h, with a mean CSF to plasma ratio of 40% (Bristol-Myers Squibb Investigational Drug Service, written communication, Apr 1997). Foudraine reported CSF concentrations of stavudine at week 12 in 17 HIV-infected patients treated with stavudine and lamivudine. The concentration of stavudine ranged from 0.2 to 0.27 μmol/L and the mean CSF to plasma ratio was 38%.[39] The concentration exceeded the mean IC_{50} for clinical isolates. Foudraine and others[40] also made the important observation that calculation of the CSF to plasma ratio can be misleading, since the ratio is highly dependent of the timing of sampling. This is because the clearance rate from plasma is much faster than from CSF. Absolute concentrations of drug relative to antiviral activity may be more reliable indicators. In HIV-infected children on stable dosing, CSF stavudine concentrations, obtained ~2–3 h after oral doses, ranged from 16% to 97% of simultaneous plasma concentrations.[41] The clinical relevance of stavudine concentrations in the CSF was suggested in Prometheus, a trial that randomized patients to ritonavir and saquinavir with or without stavudine. Twelve of 13 patients on the stavudine arm suppressed CSF HIV RNA to undetectable levels compared to only four of 14 of those not on stavudine.[42]

In pregnant macaques, stavudine reached the fetal circulation with a maternal to fetal ratio of 77–81%.[43] In *ex vivo* studies using human placenta, stavudine crossed the placenta via rapid, nonfacilitated, nonsaturable diffusion, with similar pharmacokinetic properties to zidovudine.[44] Concentrations within placental tissue were approximately twofold lower for stavudine than for zidovudine, however, probably reflecting stavudine's lower lipid solubility.[44]

TOXICITY

Stavudine is generally well tolerated in the short term and side effects are modest. Thus, it was initially thought of as one of the safest nucleosides. However, it required several years of widespread clinical use before the long-term toxicities

Table 8-2

Clinical Toxicities of Stavudine from a Phase III Randomized Clinical Trial of Monotherapy[a]

	Rate per 100 person years	
Adverse Event	**Stavudine (40 mg bid) $n = 417$**	**Zidovudine (200 mg tid) $n = 405$**
Headache	36	38
Chills/fever	34	40
Diarrhea	33	34
Rash	27	27
Nausea and vomiting	26	35
Abdominal pain	23	21
Myalgia	21	27
Insomnia	20	24
Pancreatitis	<1	<1
Neuropathy any grade	11.7	3.9
Neuropathy grade 3–4	2	1
Hyperamylasemia (>1.4 X ULN)	12.6	10.7
Elevated AST any grade	65.6	44
Elevated AST > 5 X ULN	8.6	9.3
Elevated ALT any grade	69.1	41.3
Elevated ALT > 5 X ULN	12.1	9.9
Anemia grade 3–4	0.6	14.2
Neutropenia grade 3–4	3.0	6.4

[a] Events among patients on zidovudine are included for comparison.

From Spruance SL, Pavia AT, Mellors JW, et al. Clinical efficacy of monotherapy with stavudine compared with zidovudine in HIV-infected, zidovudine-experienced patients. A randomized, double-blind, controlled trial. Bristol-Myers Squibb Stavudine/019 Study Group. Ann Intern Med 126:355–63, 1997 and Final Report of Protocol AI455-019.

were better understood. These long-term toxicities are the most clinically important, including mitochondrial toxicity, lipoatrophy, lactic acidemia and lactic acidosis (discussed in more detail in Chapters 73 and 74). These long-term adverse events now limit the long-term use of stavudine to exceptional clinical situations, such as in patients who harbor HIV with a K6 mutation and cannot tolerate zidovudine, and in resource-constrained countries where other nucleoside agents are not available.

Preclinical studies predicted the major clinical toxicities of stavudine. *In vitro*, stavudine is substantially less toxic to bone marrow precursors than zidovudine.[45,46] However, stavudine inhibits outgrowth of neurites in an *in vitro* model of neurotoxicity, with slightly less toxicity than didanosine or zalcitabine, but substantially more than zidovudine.[47,48] The neurotoxicity of these nucleoside analogs was thought by some investigators to be due to inhibition of mitochondrial DNA polymerase-gamma.[49]

Clinical toxicities of stavudine monotherapy from phase III studies are shown in Table 8-2. Stavudine does not cause significant bone marrow suppression.[50–54] Initial phase I and phase II dose-ranging trials demonstrated that peripheral neuropathy, and to a lesser extent, elevations of hepatic transaminases are the major dose-limiting toxicities of stavudine. The maximum tolerated dose of stavudine established in phase I studies was 2 mg kg^{-1} day^{-1}.[50–53]

The risk of peripheral neuropathy is dose related. In an analysis of data from three phase 1 studies and one phase II study, the incidence of neuropathy (of any severity) was 17–21/100 person years in patients receiving doses of 0.5 mg $kg^{-1}day^{-1}$, 21/100 person years at 1.0 mg kg^{-1} day^{-1}, and 41–66/100 person years at 2.0 mg kg^{-1} day^{-1}. Patients receiving 4 mg kg^{-1} day^{-1} for extended periods had a cumulative incidence of peripheral neuropathy of 64–71%.[53] In BMS 019, the phase III efficacy trial among zidovudine-experienced patients (using the currently recommended dose of 40 mg po bid, ~1 mg kg^{-1} day^{-1}), the rate of neuropathy sufficient to require dose modification was 11.7/100 person years among stavudine-treated patients compared to 3.9/100 person years in the zidovudine group.[54] The occurrence of neuropathy was strongly associated with a baseline diagnosis of AIDS, preexisting neuropathy, and with low CD4 counts at study entry.

Neuropathy associated with stavudine is usually reversible when the drug is discontinued or the dose is modified promptly. Among 56 stavudine-treated patients who developed neuropathy in the phase III trial, 63% had complete resolution of neurologic symptoms within a median of 17 days. These patients all tolerated rechallenge at half of the original dose.[54] In pediatric trials, peripheral neuropathy has been rare.[41,55–57] Higher rates of neuropathy have been observed in patients treated with stavudine in combination with didanosine and hydroxyurea.[58]

Modest elevations of hepatic transaminases are common with stavudine therapy, but significant elevations and clinical hepatitis are uncommon. Grade III or IV elevations of hepatic transaminases (greater than five times the upper limit of normal) occurred in 9–13% of patients receiving doses of 2.0 mg kg^{-1} day^{-1} of stavudine in the phase I and II studies.[53,59] Significant elevations were not apparently related to dose, but were significantly associated with abnormal baseline levels. In the phase III study, grade III or IV elevations of alaninine aminotransferase (ALT) or aspartate aminotransferase occurred in similar rates in the stavudine and zidovudine groups (12/100 person years vs 10/100 person years) but milder elevations were common and significantly more frequent in the stavudine group (69 vs 44/100 person years).[54]

Lactic acidemia, lactic acidosis, and hepatic steatosis were recognized early as rare but severe complications of nucleoside analogs, including zidovudine, zalcitabine, didanosine, and stavudine.[60–64] Severity ranges from asymptomatic lactic acidemia to fatal fulminant disease. Symptoms are nonspecific and include fatigue, nausea, vomiting, and abdominal pain. Mitochondrial dysfunction appears to be an underlying defect,[65–70] although other factors, including the rate of lactate clearance, may be critical.[71,72] A number of case reports and case series have implicated stavudine in lactic acidemia and lactic acidosis.[62,70,73–78] However, it has been difficult to determine the risk associated with stavudine relative to other nucleoside analogs, and to determine the role of host factors.[79] However, there appears to be a hierarchy of risk with ddC > didanosine > stavudine > zidovudine >> tenofovir, abacavir, or lamivudine.

A study that involved 18 months of prospective monitoring of 349 patients found lactate levels to rise modestly after the initiation of stavudine- or zidovudine-based HAART.[78] However, the increase was an average 0.23 mmol/L greater in those on stavudine. Severe hyperlactatemia and hepatic steatosis, however, were rare. In Africa, where stavudine-based combination therapy is widely used, symptomatic lactic acidosis is being increasingly recognized, although the incidence and risk factors remain to be defined.[80] The combination of stavudine and didanosine is associated with markedly increased risk of lactic acidosis, and hepatic steatosis.

It has been proposed that stavudine-induced mitochondrial dysfunction plays a role in lipodystrophy, especially lipoatrophy.[81–83] (*See also* Chapters 72 and 73.) Many studies are plagued by the complexity of overlapping syndromes, cross-sectional design, and multiple confounders and interactions, both biologic and statistical. Nucleoside analog use, duration of therapy, age, and gender have been consistent risk factors for lipoatrophy.[84,85] Many studies identified an association between stavudine and lipodystrophy although early studies were not able to adequately control for common prescribing of stavudine or duration of therapy.[82,86] However, prospective cohort studies do show an increased risk of lipodystrophy associated with stavudine use. Among 277 patients participating in the Western Australia cohort, stavudine-containing regimens were associated with an increased relative risk of fat wasting, as were PI use, white race, age, and duration of nucleoside analog therapy.[85] Among 1035 patients participating in the British Columbia drug treatment program, lipodystrophy was diagnosed based on prospectively collected self-report. Lipodystrophy syndrome was independently associated with age, use of PI therapy, being employed, use of alternative therapy and duration of stavudine therapy[87] (*see* Chapter 73).

Perhaps the clearest demonstration of the role of stavudine comes from several trials which examined the effect of stopping stavudine and changing to other nucleoside analogs on lactic acidosis, mitochondrial function and lipoatrophy. In a study of 118 patients with lipoatrophy who were switched to abacavir ($n = 86$) or zidovudine ($n = 32$), lactic acidosis stabilized or improved.[88] Modest improvements in limb fat were measured, but not in facial lipoatrophy.[89] The high prevalence of facial lipoatrophy and the lack of improvement in facial fat after stopping stavudine has led to a significant decrease in the use of this drug in clinical practice. Improvements in the DNA content of adipocyte mitochondria have also been demonstrated after switching.[90]

In contrast to didanosine, stavudine alone is not clearly associated with increased risk of pancreatitis or hyperamylasemia.[54,91,92]

Stavudine is classified as FDA pregnancy category C. Long-term animal carcinogenicity studies are negative.[93] Animal toxicology studies of stavudine in pregnancy show no specific embryopathy. Exposure of early embryos to high levels of stavudine (10 μmol/L) inhibited blastocyst formation.[94] There was no reduction in fertility at doses greater than 200 times the human levels. Teratology studies using 400 times the human serum concentrations in rats and 183 times the human serum concentration in rabbits did not show any increase in birth defects. In rats exposed to the highest doses, there were decreases in sternal bone calcification and mild increases in neonatal mortality. These changes are consistent with nonspecific toxicity.[93,95,96]

EFFICACY

Since 1996, combination therapy has become the standard of care. However, in many trials of combination therapy, it is not possible to discern the individual role of the nucleoside analog component. Therefore, it is useful to review data on monotherapy (Table 8-3) and dual-therapy trials (Table 8-4).

Monotherapy

In a phase II dose-ranging study, beneficial effects on CD4 cell count, p24 antigenemia, cellular viremia, and weight gain were observed at doses of 0.5 mg kg^{-1} day^{-1} or 2.0 mg kg^{-1} day^{-1}.[59] Little or no response was observed at 0.1 mg kg^{-1} day^{-1}. The median CD4 cell increase was 20–30 cells/mm^3; greater responses were observed in zidovudine-naive patients. The greatest antiviral response was seen at 2.0 mg kg^{-1} day^{-1}, with a 77% decrease in the median titer of infected PBMCs. Another small study of 15 patients demonstrated

Table 8-3

Summary of Major Trials Involving Stavudine Monotherapy

Study (Reference)	Design	Arms	No. of Subjects	Patients	CD4/μL at Entry	Antiviral Response	Immunologic and Clinical Response
Phase II dose ranging[59]	3 arm dose escalation	d4T 0.1 mg/kg vs d4T 0.5 mg/kg vs d4T 2.0 mg/kg	152	Treatment naive	250 (median)	Not done	CD4 and virologic response increased with increasing dose. Neuropathy more prominent at 2.0 mg/kg
Stavudine parallel track program[91]	Simple trial; randomized, double blind dose comparison	d4T 20 mg bid vs d4T 40 mg	15 000	ZDV experienced, advanced disease, failing or intolerant to available drugs	41 (median)	Not done	Weight gain, hematologic improvement and hospitalizations favored 40 mg dose. No difference in mortality. Neuropathy requiring dose modification 23% vs 17%
BMS 019[54]	Double blind RCT	d4T 40 mg bid vs ZDV 200 mg tid	822	ZDV experienced >6 months	236 (median)	Not done	Decreased progression to AIDS or death in stavudine group. Improved CD4 count (30–50 cell difference). No difference in mortality
BMS 024[98]	Double blind RCT	d4T 40 mg bid vs d4T 20 mg bid vs placebo	66	Treatment naive; CD4 <350	527 (median)	HIV RNA decrease 0.8 $\log_{10}$ in 40 mg arm, dec 0.4 log in 20 mg arm	CD4 inc 40 cells in 40 mg, 25 cells in 20 mg, dec 50 cells in placebo
ACTG 240[56]	Initially double blind RCT; unblinded early	d4T 1 mg/kg bid vs ZDV 180 mg/m^2 q 6 h	266	Children 3 months to 6 years Treatment naive	965 (median)	No difference in progression to endpoints (but underpowered due to early unblinding)	Clinical endpoints met in 19% on d4T vs 24% on ZDV (ns). Better weight gain and maintenance of CD4 cell count in d4T group

RCT, randomized controlled trial; ZDV, zidovudine.

Table 8-4

Summary of Major Trials Involving Stavudine Dual Therapy

Study (Reference)	Design	Arms	No. of Subjects	Patients	CD4/μL at Entry	Antiviral Response[a]	Immunologic and Clinical Response[b]
ALTIS 1[103]	Open label 24 week	d4T 40 mg + 3TC 150 mg bid	42	Treatment naive; CD4 50–400; RNA > 15 000	258 (median)	HIV RNA decrease 1.66 $\log_{10}$ at week 24; 21% <200 copies;	CD4 increase 108 cells
ALTIS 2[103]	Open label 24 week	d4T 40 mg + 3TC 150 mg bid	41	ZDV, ddI, ddC experienced, median 35 months; CD4, RNA as above	172 (median)	HIV RNA decrease 0.55 $\log_{10}$ at week 24; 5% <200 copies;	CD4 increase 46 cells
ACTG 306[99]	Double blind RCT 48 week	d4T 40 mg bid vs d4T + 3TC 150 mg bid vs ZDV 200 mg tid	146 (d4T limb)	Nucleoside naive; CD4 200–600. Median HIV RNA 10 146 copies	407 (median)	HIV RNA decrease 1.59 $\log_{10}$ at week 20–24 in d4T+3TC group vs 1.05 $\log_{10}$ in ZDV+3TC group vs 0.55 $\log_{10}$ in d4T monotherapy (analysis adjusted for censoring since 35–57% fell below 500 copies). At week 40–48, RNA decrease 1.50 $\log_{10}$ in d4T+3TC group vs 1.50 $\log_{10}$ in ZDV+3TC group vs 0.96 $\log_{10}$ in d4T monotherapy	Mean CD4 increase 80 cells in d4T monotherapy, 118 d4T/3TC, 79 in ZDV/3TC at week 40/48 (ns)
Amsterdam Cohort[104]	Open label RCT	d4T/3TC vs ZDV/3TC	47	Treatment naive	300 (median)	HIV RNA decrease 1.65 $\log_{10}$ at week 12 in d4T+3TC group vs 1.53 $\log_{10}$ in ZDV+3TC group ($P < 0.0001$)	120 cell increase in d4T/3TC at 24 weeks compared to 90 in ZDV/3TC group ($P = 0.002$)
BMS 460[106]	Randomized double blind dose comparison 48 week	d4T 10 + ddI 100 d4T 20 + ddI 100 d4T 20 + ddI 200 d4T 40 + ddI 100 d4T 40 + ddI 400	94	Treatment naive		HIV RNA decrease 1.2 to 1.4 $\log_{10}$ at week 28 across groups.	CD4 increase 42 to 112 cells. Better response with higher dose
Swiss HIV Cohort study[107]	Double blind RCT 48 week	d4T/ddI vs d4T/ddI/hydroxyurea	142	d4T and hydroxyurea naive	370 (mean)	HIV RNA decrease 1.6 $\log_{10}$ in d4T/ddI arm vs 1.9 log in d4T/ddI/HU arm at week 12.	CD4 increase 91 cells in d4T/ddI vs 10 cells in d4T/ddI/HU
ALBI[108]	Open label RCT 24 week	d4T/ddI vs ZDV/3TC vs d4T/ddI followed by ZDV/3TC	153	Treatment naive	385 (median)	HIV RNA decrease 2.3 $\log_{10}$ in d4T + ddI arm vs 1.26 $\log_{10}$ in ZDV/3TC arm vs 1.58 $\log_{10}$ in sequential arm. Proportion less than 500 copies on treatment (bDNA) 91% vs 42% vs 60%	CD4 increase 124 cells in d4T + ddI arm vs 62 ZDV/3TC arm vs 1.58 $\log_{10}$ in sequential vs 118 in sequential arm
PACTG 327[153]	Partially randomized double blind 48 weeks	d4T 1 mg/kg/ddI 90 mg/m² bid vs d4T 1 mg/kg bid	108	d4T or ZDV monotherapy experienced children	730 (median)	HIV RNA decrease 0.51 $\log_{10}$ with d4T+ ddI in ZDV-experienced group, 0.17 $\log_{10}$ with d4T monotherapy in ZDV-experienced ($P - 0.026$) and 0.3 $\log_{10}$ with d4T +ddI in d4T experienced (ns)	No statistical difference in CD4 response
ACTG 290[147]	Partially blinded randomized 4 arm study	d4T vs d4T/ZDV vs ddI vs ddI/ZDV	145	ZDV experienced patients (median 135 weeks)	401 (median)	HIV RNA decrease 0.14 $\log_{10}$ in d4T and d4T/ZDV arm at week 16 vs 0.39 $\log_{10}$ in ddI arm and 0.56 $\log_{10}$ in ddI/ZDV arm	CD4 count decreased 22 cells in d4T/ZDV arm at week 16 compared to 17 cell increase in d4T arm

ddc, zalcitabine; ddI, didanosine; ZDV, zidovudine; d4T, stavudine; 3TC, lamivudine; RCT, randomized clinical trial.

[a]HIV RNA copies/μL.

[b]CD4+ T lymphocyte/μL.

median drops in the infectious titer of 1–2 $\log_{10}$ and a median decrease in viral RNA of 0.5 $\log_{10}$ at 52 weeks.[97] Katlama and colleagues examined short-term antiviral effect of stavudine among 66 treatment-naive subjects randomized to either stavudine at 20 mg bid (~0.5 mg kg^{-1} day^{-1}), stavudine 40 mg bid (1.0 mg kg^{-1} day^{-1}) or placebo.[98] Responses tended to favor the 40 mg bid dose compared to the 20 mg bid dose. The median CD4 increase at week 8 was 63 cells/mm^3 in the 40 mg bid group against 33 cells in the low-dose group and a 50-cell decline in the placebo group. The median decrease in cellular viremia was 1.0 $\log_{10}$ versus 0.7 $\log_{10}$, and the median decrease in plasma HIV RNA at week 12 (measured by NASBA) was 0.8 $\log_{10}$ versus 0.4 $\log_{10}$. In ACTG 306, 34 treatment-naive patients were randomized to stavudine monotherapy at 40 mg bid. At 24 weeks, the mean decrease in viral load was 0.55 $\log_{10}$, or 1.04 after adjustment for censoring.[99] In patients with prolonged zidovudine therapy, the response to stavudine is attenuated. Among patients with very prolonged zidovudine monotherapy (mean 3.6 years) in ACTG trial 175 who were switched to stavudine monotherapy, the virologic response at 48 weeks was modest (mean decrease 0.18 $\log_{10}$).[100]

The only clinical endpoint study of stavudine monotherapy (BMS 019) compared stavudine (40 mg bid) with continued zidovudine in 822 patients with CD4 cell counts of 50–500 at least 6 months of prior zidovudine treatment.[54] Median duration of follow-up was 115 weeks. Patients receiving stavudine reached clinical endpoints (AIDS-defining events or death) at a significantly lower rate than those randomized to continue zidovudine (26/100 person years vs 32/100 person years; relative risk 0.75; $p = 0.03$; Fig. 8-2). This benefit was apparent in all strata of baseline CD4 cell count. Survival was not significantly different, but there was a trend favoring longer survival in the stavudine group (relative risk 0.74; $p = 0.066$). Patients assigned to stavudine remained on initial therapy significantly longer (79 weeks compared to 53 weeks). Quality of life as measured by the MOS SF-36 was significantly better among stavudine-treated patients at week 12, but by week 36 the difference was not significant.[101] Patients in the stavudine group had significantly less anemia and neutropenia, better weight gain. The CD4 count initially increased a median of 20 cells, but then declined. The count remained 30–40 cells/mm^3 higher than the zidovudine group (Fig. 8-2). Viral RNA was not measured in this study.

Stavudine Combined with Lamivudine

Because of the convenient dosing and the favorable side effect profile, the combination of stavudine and lamivudine became popular before clinical trial data were available to demonstrate efficacy.[102] *In vitro*, the combination shows additive to synergistic effects.[24] The combination appears at least as active as zidovudine and lamivudine.

In an open-label prospective study (ALTIS I) among 42 treatment-naive patients,[103] the combination of stavudine and lamivudine resulted in a median decrease in viral RNA of 1.96 $\log_{10}$ at 4 weeks, sustained at -1.66 $\log_{10}$ at 24 weeks with an increase in the CD4 count of 108 cells/mm^3 at 24 weeks. RNA levels were below 500 copies/mL at week 24 in 30%. In a parallel study of 41 antiretroviral-experienced but stavudine- and lamivudine-naive patients (ALTIS II), more modest effects were observed. The median maximum change in HIV RNA was -1.3 $\log_{10}$ at week 4, but only -0.55 $\log_{10}$ at week 24 accompanied by a CD4 increase of 46 cells/mm^3.

Two studies have compared stavudine plus lamivudine with zidovudine plus lamivudine. ACTG 306 was a six-arm study among antiretroviral-naive patients.[99] The stavudine arm compared stavudine monotherapy, stavudine plus lamivudine, and zidovudine plus lamivudine. Adjusted for censoring, the change in viral load at week 20–24 was -0.55 $\log_{10}$

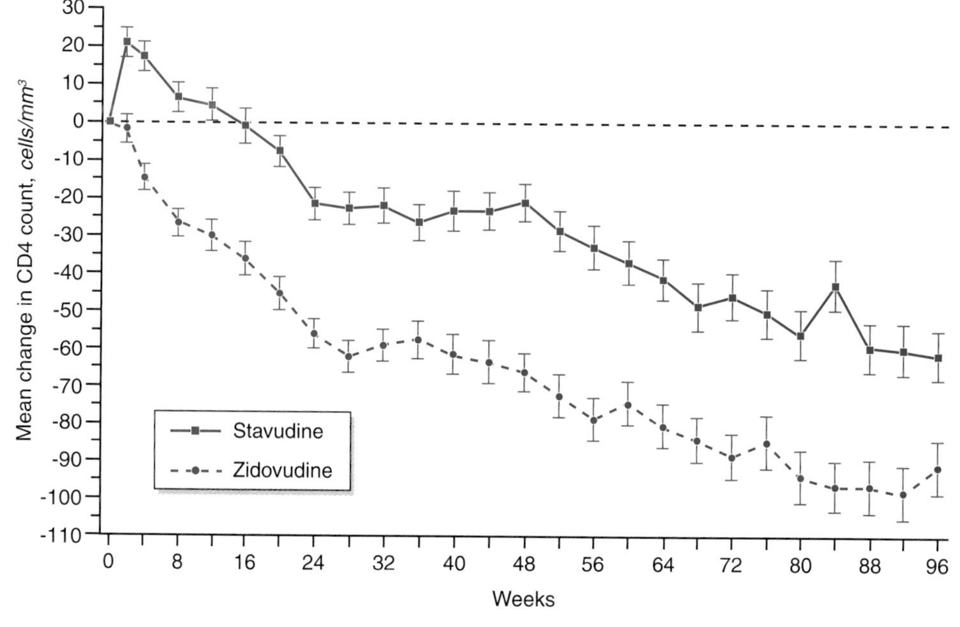

Figure 8-2 ■ Mean change in CD4+ cell count from baseline by treatment group in BMS 019. Bars represent standard error.

From Spruance SL, Pavia AT, Mellors JW, et al. Clinical efficacy of monotherapy with stavudine compared with zidovudine in HIV-infected, zidovudine-experienced patients. A randomized, double-blind, controlled trial. Bristol-Myers Squibb Stavudine/019 Study Group. Ann Intern Med 126:355–63, 1997.

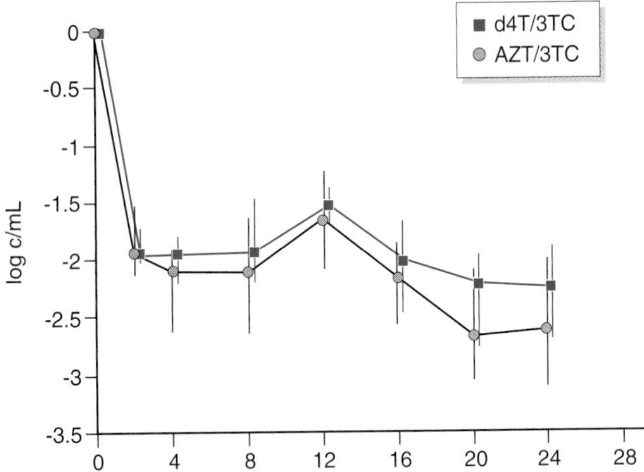

Figure 8-3 ■ Mean change in HIV RNA from baseline in antiretroviral-naive patients on stavudine and lamivudine or zidovudine and lamivudine.

From Foudraine NA, de Jong JJ, Jan Weverling G, et al. An open randomized controlled trial of zidovudine plus lamivudine versus stavudine plus lamivudine. AIDS 12:1513–19, 1998.

in the stavudine monotherapy arm, $-1.59 \log_{10}$ in the stavudine/lamivudine arm, and $-1.05 \log_{10}$ in the zidovudine arm. The difference favoring stavudine/lamivudine over zidovudine was of borderline statistical significance ($p = 0.052$) at week 24, but no difference was seen at week 48. A low baseline viral load complicates the analysis. Using an ultrasensitive assay (lower limit 20 copies/mL), there was no difference between stavudine/lamivudine and zidovudine/lamivudine (-1.64 vs $-1.57 \log_{10}$). In another randomized trial among 47 patients who received stavudine/lamivudine or zidovudine/lamivudine for 12 weeks, the viral load decreased by -1.65 compared to $-1.53 \log_{10}$ (Fig. 8-3). However, all patients had developed lamivudine resistance by 12 weeks.[104] In 28 patients who underwent lumbar puncture before and after therapy, both regimens resulted in CSF HIV RNA becoming undetectable by quantitative PCR in all patients.[39]

Stavudine Combined with Didanosine

Additive to synergistic antiviral effects are seen *in vitro* when stavudine is combined with didanosine.[24,26,27] There is no significant pharmacokinetic interaction.[105] Data from several trials suggested that this combination was clinically effective and well tolerated. A double-blind dose-ranging trial compared five regimens of stavudine plus didanosine among 76 treatment-naive patients with a median CD4 count of 325 cell/μL (stavudine 10 mg and didanosine 100 mg, 20 mg and 100 mg, 40 mg and 100 mg, 20 mg and 200 mg, or 40 mg and 200 mg, all dosed bid).[106] The reduction in plasma viral RNA was $-1.1 \log_{10}$- $-1.8 \log_{10}$ across groups. The reduction was sustained for 52 weeks, and patients receiving the two highest doses (close to full dose of each agent) had somewhat greater responses. CD4 cell counts increased 42–112 cells/μL across the groups. Increases of 80–100 cells/mm^3 were sustained at 52 weeks in the higher-dose regimens. Only one episode of neuropathy occurred (grade 2), despite the concern over potential synergistic toxicity.

A double-blind randomized trial comparing stavudine plus didanosine (at standard doses) with stavudine, didanosine and hydroxyurea (500 mg bid) confirmed the antiviral efficacy of stavudine plus didanosine.[107] The trial enrolled 144 patients, 80% of whom were treatment-naive. In the stavudine plus didanosine arm, the mean reduction in viral RNA was $-1.6 \log_{10}$ at week 12 using the Roche PCR assay with a detection limit of 200 copies. RNA levels were below the limit of detection in 28%. CD4 counts increased by 91 cells/mm^3 at week 12. In an open-label extension, the viral load remained $1.5 \log_{10}$ below baseline at 24 months. In the group that received hydroxyurea, the viral load reduction was slightly greater ($-1.8 \log_{10}$ at week 12, $p = 0.06$), and 54% were below 200 copies/mL, but the change in CD4 count was less substantial (+10 cells at week 12, $p = 0.003$). Toxicity was greater when hydroxyurea was added. In another trial among 151 naive patients, stavudine plus didanosine was compared to zidovudine plus lamivudine or alternating use of the two combinations. Stavudine didanosine resulted in greater reductions of viral load than zidovudine lamivudine ($-2.26 \log_{10}$ vs 1.26; $p < 0.001$; Fig. 8-4).[108]

These data led to a period of enthusiasm for the combination of stavudine with didanosine. However, in ACTG 384, the combination of stavudine and didanosine was clearly associated with shorter time to regimen failure than zidovudine with lamivudine.[109] This was due to more frequent discontinuation. In a substudy, a greater loss of limb fat was seen with stavudine/didanosine. With the advent of other less toxic alternatives, the combination of stavudine with didanosine is no longer recommended.[110]

Stavudine Combined with Protease Inhibitors or Non-nucleoside Reverse Transcriptase Inhibitors

A small number of studies have stavudine plus a protease inhibitor as a two-drug combination, before it became clear that this was inadequate therapy.[111–113]

Stavudine plus lamivudine combination has been used as a backbone in a number of trials with different agents or strategies (Table 8-5).[114–117] Two trials have compared the use of stavudine lamivudine plus indinavir versus zidovudine lamivudine plus indinavir. In START 1, 204 antiretroviral-naive patients were enrolled in a randomized, open-label trial. At 48 weeks, there was no significant difference between the arms in the proportion below 500 copies/mL (62% vs 54%; $p = 0.2$), below 50 copies/mL (49% vs 47%), or in the CD4 response (226 cells vs 198) (Fig. 8-5).[118] The Ozcombo study randomized 109 therapy-naive patients to indinavir with either stavudine lamivudine, stavudine didanosine or zidovudine lamivudine.[119] There were no significant differences in virologic outcome or CD4 response. Fewer patients in the stavudine didanosine group discontinued therapy because of adverse events ($p = 0.06$).

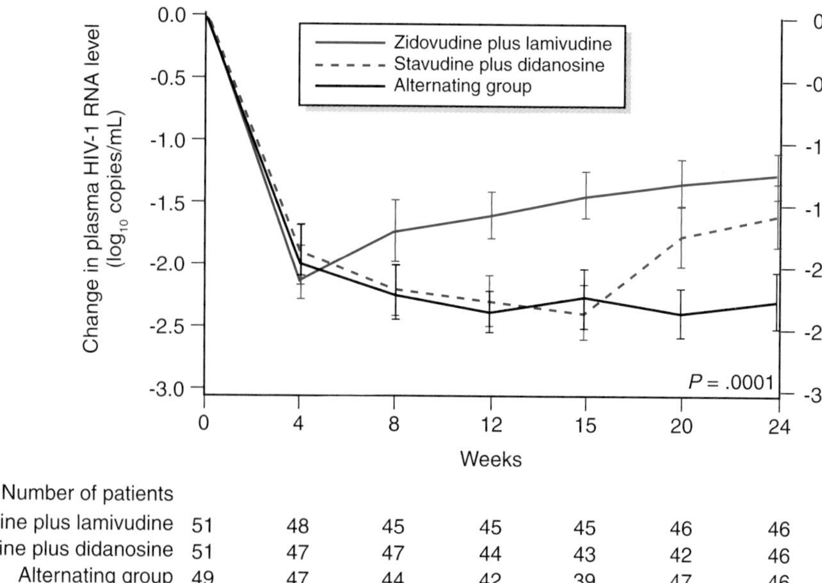

Figure 8-4 ■ Mean change in HIV RNA from baseline in antiretroviral-naive patients on stavudine and didanosine, zidovudine and lamivudine, or stavudine and didanosine followed by zidovudine and lamivudine (alternating group).

From Molina JM, Chene G, Ferchal F, et al. The ALBI trial: a randomized controlled trial comparing stavudine plus didanosine with zidovudine plus lamivudine and a regimen alternating both combinations in previously untreated patients infected with human immunodeficiency virus. J Infect Dis 180:351–8, 1999.

Most comparisons are hampered by limited follow-up. Gilead 903 compared stavudine and lamivudine to tenofovir and emtricitabine, both combined with efavirenz over 3 years, and led to important insights. At 144 weeks, the antiviral efficacy was equivalent and impressive; 69% of those on stavudine lamivudine compared to 73% on tenofovir emtricitabine had viral loads less than 50 copies by intent to treat analysis. However, there were significantly greater increases in triglycerides, total cholesterol, and LDL cholesterol among patients on stavudine lamivudine. Moreover, there was a much higher rate of investigator-defined lipodystrophy and lower limb fat in the stavudine-treated patients.[120]

Stavudine and didanosine combination has also been used as a backbone with protease inhibitors, non-nucleoside reverse transcriptase inhibitors and triple nucleoside regimens. The START II trial compared indinavir with stavudine didanosine or zidovudine lamivudine in a randomized, open-label study of 205 therapy-naive patients (Fig. 8-6).[121] At the 48-week primary endpoint, the viral load reduction and the proportion of patients with less than 500 RNA copies/mL or less than 50 copies/mL were similar. The patients in the stavudine didanosine group had significantly greater increases in CD4 cell count (214 vs 142; $p = 0.026$). The frequency of adverse events was similar. The Atlantic trial compared stavudine and didanosine with indinavir, nevirapine, or lamivudine in 298 antiretroviral-naive patients.[122] At 48 weeks, the three regimens had similar rates of virologic responses of HIV-1 RNA copies of <500/mL (57–58.7%); at 96 weeks the lamivudine arm had lower rates of virologic responses when a criterion of <50 copies/mL was used. Patients in the nevirapine arm had smaller increases in CD4+ T-lymphocytes. There were no significant differences in rates of serious adverse effects among the treatment arms.

The most important evaluation of stavudine and didanosine as a backbone was performed in ACTG 384. Patients were randomized to either stavudine and didanosine or zidovudine and lamivudine, combined with either efavirenz, nelfinavir or both. Patients randomized to zidovudine and lamivudine-containing regimens had significantly longer time to treatment failure or to toxicity than those randomized to stavudine and didanosine-containing regimens.[109] These differences were driven by increased toxicity.

RESISTANCE

Early on, it was noted that stavudine-based regimens lose effectiveness with time,[54] consistent with the evolution of resistance. Full understanding of resistance to stavudine was elusive, but progress has been made. Initially, zidovudine-resistant isolates of HIV were noted to be susceptible to stavudine, within the limits of the assays.[123,124] Lacey and Larder reported that *in vitro* passage of HIV with increasing concentrations selected a strain mutant at codon 75 (substitution of threonine for valine) of the reverse transcriptase gene which conferred sevenfold decrease in susceptibility.[125] Site directed mutagenesis into an HXB2 background confirmed the change in stavudine susceptibility and also demonstrated moderate decrease in sensitivity to didanosine and zalcitabine. Another mutation was described during *in vitro* selection, substitution of threonine for isoleucine at codon 50, which conferred 30-fold resistance to stavudine, but no apparent cross-resistance.[126]

In vivo, the situation is more complicated. Phenotypic resistance appears slowly without a consistent genotypic pattern.[127–129] The mutation at position 75 is rare in clinical isolates, and often not associated with clinical resistance.[130] The mutation at position 50 has not been reported. In an important early study that was initially cited as evidence that stavudine did not select for resistance, Lin studied 13 patients treated with stavudine for 18–22 months. Three patients had posttreatment isolates with decreased susceptibility to stavudine (fourfold to 12-fold).[128] The isolates demonstrated multiple mutations including several associated with zidovudine resistance (T215Y, K219E, K70R). Five post-treatment

Table 8-5

Summary of Major Trials Involving Stavudine With PIs or NNRIs

Study (Reference)	Design	Arms	No. of Subjects	Patients	CD4/μL at Entry	Antiviral Response[a]	Immunologic and Clinical Response[b]
de Truchis[154]	Open label	d4T/3TC bid/ indinavir 800 mg tid	144	Nucleoside experienced, protease naive. AIDS in 51%	85 (mean)	HIV RNA decrease 1.4 $\log_{10}$ at week 24. 48% <200 copies.	CD4 increase 90 cells at week 24
AG 506 [112]	Double blind RCT	d4T bid vs d4T bid + nelfinavir 500 mg tid vs d4T bid + nelfinavir 750 mg tid	308	Nucleoside experienced, d4T and protease naive (80%); naive (20%); CD4 50–500		HIV decrease 1.3–1.4 $\log_{10}$ in combination vs 0.6 in d4T at week 8. Decreasing effect at week 24.	CD4 count increase 103–106 cells in combination vs 51 on monotherapy
PACTG 338[155]	Open label RCT	ZDV/3TC vs ZDV/3TC/ritonavir vs d4T/ritonavir	298	ZDV-experienced children, d4T and PI naive.	680 (median)	8% <500 copies on ZDV/3TC vs 47% on ZDV/3TC/ritonavir vs 34% on d4T/ritonavir at week 24	No significant difference in CD4 increase at week 24
START I[118]	Open label RCT	d4T/3TC/ indinavir vs ZDV/3TC/indinavir	204	Antiretroviral naive, viral load >10000 copies	400 (median)	62% <500 copies on d4T/3TC/IND vs 54% on AZT/3TC/IND ($P = 0.21$) at 40–48 weeks. 49% <50 copies on d4t/3TC arm vs 47%.	CD4 increase 227 cells in d4T/3TC/IND vs 198 in ZDV/3TC/IND (ns). CD4 response significantly better by area under the curve on d4t/ 3TC arm ($P = 0.033$)
START II[121]	Open label RCT	d4T /ddI/indinavir vs ZDV/3TC/indinavir	205	Antiretroviral naive, viral load >10000 copies	422 (median)	61% <500 copies on d4T/ddI/IND vs 45% on AZT/3TC/IND ($P = 0.038$) at 40–48 weeks. 41% <50 copies on d4t/ddI arm vs 35%.	CD4 increase 214 cells in d4T/ddI/IND vs 142 in ZDV/3TC/IND ($P = 0.026$). CD4 response significantly better by area under the curve on d4t/ddI arm ($P = 0.001$)
Ozcombo[119]	Open label 3 arm RCT	d4T/3TC/indinavir vs d4T/ddI/indinavir vs ZDV/3TC/indinavir	109	Antiretroviral naive, viral load >30000 copies or CD4 <500 cells	285 (mean)	Proportion <50 copies at week 48 (ITT) 59% on d4T/3TC/IND vs 48% on d4T/ddI/IND vs 66% on ZDV/3TC/IND (ns).	CD4 increase 237 on d4T/3TC/IND vs 176 on d4T/ddI/IND vs 175 on ZDV/3TC/IND. No significant difference in time weighted average CD4 count increase. Higher discontinuation on d4T/ddI arm
Atlantic[156]	Open label 2 arm RCT	D4T/ddI 400 mg QD//indinavir 800 mg tid vs ddI/d4T/nevirapine 400 mg QD vs ddI/d4T/3TC	298	Antiretroviral naive viral load >500 copies and CD4 >200 cells	406 (median)	Proportion <500 copies at week 48 (ITT) 57% on d4T/ddI/IND vs 58% on d4T/ddI/NVP vs 59% on d4T/ddI/I3TC. Proportion <50 (ITT) 55% vs 54% vs 46%	Mean CD4 increase 318 cells at week 48 across all three groups. No significant difference

Table 8-5 (Continued)

Study (Reference)	Design	Arms	No. of Subjects	Patients	CD4/μL at Entry	Antiviral Response[a]	Immunologic and Clinical Response[b]
Prometheus[42,157]	Open label RCT	ritonavir 400 mg/saquinavir 400 mg/d4T vs Ritonavir/ saquinavir (d4T added if not suppressed at week 12)	208	PI and d4T naive		By ITT analysis, 69% less than 400 copies in ritonavir/saquinavir/ d4T group vs 63% ($P = 0.38$). 31% in dual PI group added nucleosides. In a CSF substudy, more patients in RTV/SQV/d4T had CSF HIV RNA <400 or less than 50 copies than in RTV/SQV group 12/13 vs 4/14 ($P = 0.001$)	No difference
DMP 043[43]	Open label single arm	d4T/3TC/efavirenz	68	Antiretroviral naive	375 (mean)	By ITT analysis, 78% less than 400 copies, 73% less than 50 copies at 72 weeks. By as treated analysis, 94% and 89% less than 400 and less than 50 copies	CD4 increase (mean) 283 cells at 72 weeks
M98-863[116]	Double blind RCT	d4T/3TC/lopinavir-ritonavir vs d4T/ 3TC/nelfinavir	653	Antiretroviral naive	260	By ITT analysis, 75% less than 400 copies in lopinavir/r group at 48 weeks group compared to 63% ($p < 0.001$) and 67% vs 52% less than 50 copies ($p < 0.001$)	
AI428-008[117]	Double blind RCT	d4T/3TC/ atazanavir vs d4T/3TC/nelfinavir	272	Antiretroviral naive	290	By ITT analysis, 67% less than 400 copies in atazanavir group at 48 weeks group compared to 59% and 59% vs 38% less than 50 copies	Lipids better in atazanavir group than in nelfinavir group
ACT 384[109]	Partially blinded RCT. Factorial design	D4T/ddI/nelfinavir AZT/3TC/ nelfinavir D4T/ ddI/efavirenz AZT/3TC/efavirenz D4T/ddI/NFV/EFV AZT/3TC/NFV/EFV	980	Antiretroviral naive	280	AZT/3TC/efavirenz associated with fewer regimen failures than other arms. No benefit to four drugs over three	
GS 903[120]	Double blind RCT	d4T/3TC/ efavirenz vs TDF/FTC/efavirenz	602	Antiretroviral naive	280	By ITT analysis, 84% less than 400 copies at 48 weeks in d4T group compared to 80%. At 144 weeks 73% less than 50 copies compared to 69% (NS)	Higher rates of neuropathy, lactic acidosis, and worse lipids in d4T group

ddI, didanosine; ZDV, zidovudine; d4T, stavudine; 3TC, lamivudine; RCT, randomized clinical trial.

[a] HIV RNA copies/μL.
[b] CD4+ T lymphocyte/μL.

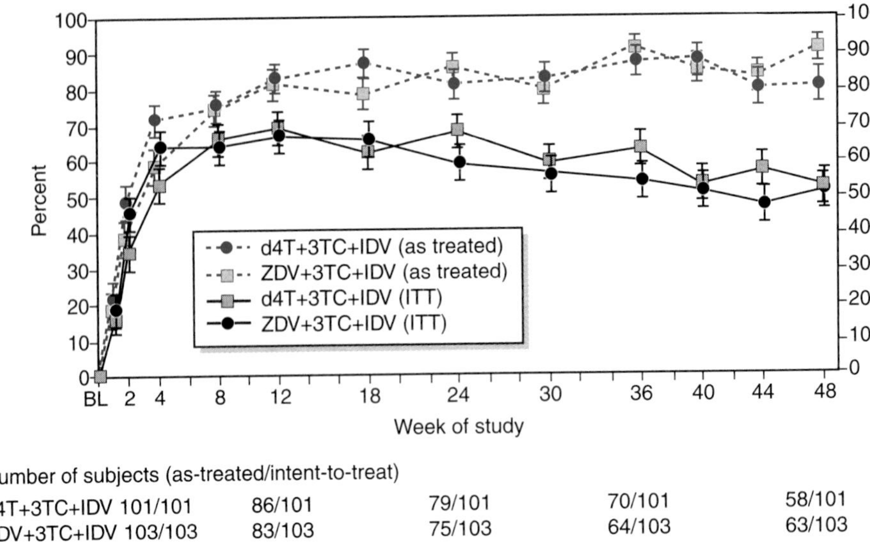

Figure 8-5 ■ Proportion (with standard error bars) of patients with HIV RNA less than 500 copies/mL by both intent-to-treat and as treated analysis among patients randomized to stavudine, lamivudine, and indinavir compared to zidovudine, lamivudine, and indinavir.

From Squires KE, Gulick R, Tebas P, et al. A comparison of stavudine plus lamivudine versus zidovudine plus lamivudine in combination with indinavir in antiretroviral-naive individuals with HIV infection: selection of thymidine analog regimen therapy (START I). AIDS 14:1591–600, 2000.

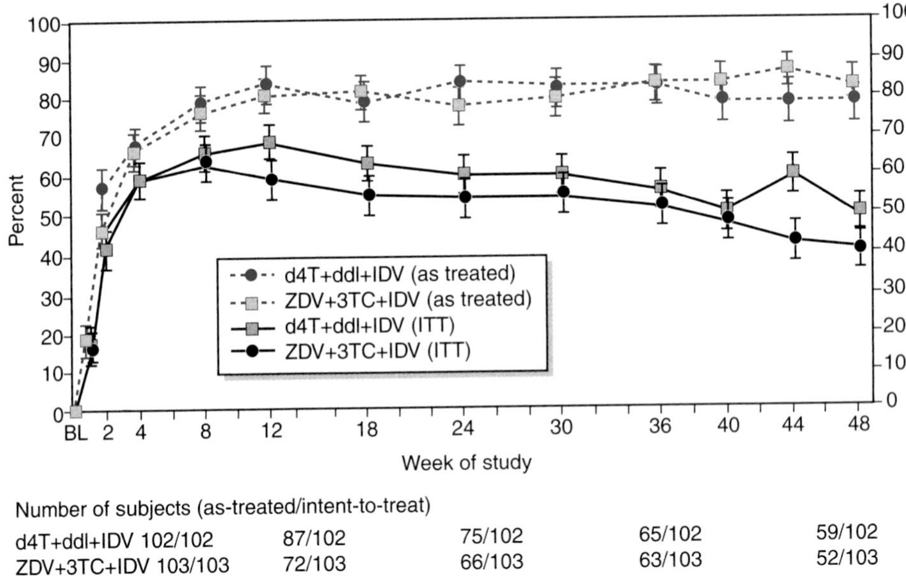

Figure 8-6 ■ Proportion (with standard error bars) of patients with HIV RNA less than 500 copies/mL by both intent-to-treat and as treated analysis among patients randomized to stavudine, lamivudine, and indinavir compared to zidovudine, lamivudine, and indinavir.

From Eron JJ Jr, Murphy RL, Peterson D, et al. A comparison of stavudine, didanosine and indinavir with zidovudine, lamivudine and indinavir for the initial treatment of HIV-1 infected individuals: selection of thymidine analog regimen therapy (START II). AIDS 14:1601–10, 2000.

isolates were resistant to zidovudine. Soriano studied 24 patients who had received 2 years of stavudine monotherapy after prolonged zidovudine use.[129] None was mutant at positions 50 or 75. However, 83% maintained zidovudine resistance mutations for more than 2 years on stavudine.

Although the clues were present in early studies, it has become clear that resistance to stavudine can develop along three pathways. The most common pathway involves the development of mutations classically associated with zidovudine resistance, including M41L, D77N, K70R, T215Y/F. Because these mutations confer resistance not only to zidovudine, but contribute to resistance to abacavir, didanosine, zalcitabine, lamivudine, and stavudine, they have been referred to as thymidine-associated mutations (TAM), or more accurately, nucleoside-associated mutations (NAM). Treatment with stavudine alone or in combination with lamivudine or didanosine may select for NAMs.[130–135] These mutations have been detected in 15–38% of stavudine failures. In contrast to zidovudine, they confer modest phenotypic resistance to stavudine, in the range of 1.9-fold change in IC_{50} in one study,[130] but this change appears to have a measurable effect of antiviral response. In another study, NAMs were detected in 38% of patients on stavudine and lamivudine compared to 50% of those on stavudine and lamivudine.[133] The presence of mutations at K70 and T215 were similar, but the zidovudine-based regimen was significantly more likely to select for M41L. This suggests that while stavudine and zidovudine select for similar mutations, the selection may be slower and less potent with stavudine.

The presence of NAMs in zidovudine-experienced patients is associated with a decreased virologic response to stavudine. In the ALTIS 2 study, magnitude of response to stavudine was associated with presence of T215Y or F mutation, number of previously used nucleosides and phenotypic sensitivity to stavudine. Modest change in IC_{50} of greater than 1.8-fold over control isolates was associated with decreased response. Purified RT from zidovudine-resistant virus shows decreased inhibition by stavudine triphosphate, providing *in vitro* correlation.[136] Interestingly, the V75T mutation may have a role in increasing pyrophosphorolysis, similar to the effect of NAMs.[137]

A second pathway is through a multidrug resistance pathway involving a signature mutation Q151M with multiple mutations. Additional mutations include A62V, V75I, F77L, F116Y, and M184V.[138–140] These strains exhibit high-level resistance to multiple nucleoside analogs including didanosine, lamivudine, stavudine, zalcitabine, and zidovudine, although tenofovir retains activity. The third pathway, described in 1998, involves insertion of two amino acids between codons 67 and 70 of RT, most often a double insertion of 6 bp coding for two threonines at codon 69.[141–144] This multidrug resistance pathway (also referred to as MDR-2) confers high-level resistance to stavudine, as well as lamivudine, zalcitabine, zidovudine, and variable resistance to abacavir and didanosine. Both the Q151M and the T69SSS pattern are selected for at lower frequency than zidovudine mutations.

The K65R mutation, selected for by tenofovir, may decrease resistance to stavudine.[145] This has been demonstrated clearly for zidovudine with reduction in the IC_{50} to the point of 'hypersusceptibility' in some instances, leading to increased use of zidovudine among patients whose virus has developed a K65R mutation. For those patients harboring a virus with K65R who are unable to tolerate zidovudine, stavudine becomes a reasonable choice for therapy in that setting.

DRUG INTERACTIONS

There are relatively few significant drug–drug interactions documented with stavudine.[146] Stavudine has no effect on the cytochrome p450 system. The most clinically relevant drug interaction is with zidovudine. Stavudine and zidovudine compete for phosphorylation by thymidine kinase.[6,28] At initial concentrations of 1 μM, this leads to decreased intracellular levels of stavudine triphosphate, although if the initial concentration of both drugs is increased to 10 μM, the concentration of stavudine triphosphate is increased relative to zidovudine triphosphate.[6,7] *In vitro*, this can result in antagonism, at least with zidovudine-resistant strains of HIV, although additive effects have been reported for some strains.[24,25] *In vivo* antagonism was demonstrated in the ACTG 290 trial.[147] This study randomized patients with greater than 12 weeks of prior zidovudine to didanosine alone, didanosine plus zidovudine, stavudine alone, or stavudine plus zidovudine. Patients in the stavudine plus zidovudine arm had decreases in their CD4 count, in contrast to modest increases in all other arms, leading to closure of the stavudine plus zidovudine arm.

In vitro, ribavirin and doxorubicin also interfere with the phosphorylation of stavudine, although the clinical relevance is unknown.[28] Co-administration with methadone results in a 27% reduction in stavudine area under the concentration curve, an amount not felt to be clinically significant.[148] Because of the potential for additive neurotoxicity, most experts would advise against the use of stavudine with zalcitibine. Other agents that cause neuropathy, including vincristine, isoniazid, ethambutol, and ethanol might be expected to have additive neurotoxicity with stavudine, although there are no clear data.

RECOMMENDATIONS FOR USE

Stavudine is a well-tolerated drug in the short term with a simple dosing regimen. It is available as capsules or a pediatric oral solution. However, its long-term toxicities limit its use in routine clinical settings. The drug may be taken fasting or with food. Stavudine should be administered at a dose of 40 mg po bid for persons weighing at least 60 kg and 30 mg po bid for adults weighing less than 30 kg. The recommended dose for children who weigh less than 30 kg is 1 mg/kg bid. Children weighing more than 30 kg should receive the adult dose. Dose adjustment is necessary for significant renal impairment. Patients with creatinine clearance of 26–50 mL/min should receive half of the usual dose (i.e., 20 mg for an adult) every 12 h. For those with creatinine clearance of 10–25 mL/min, one-half of the usual dose is given every 24 h. No formal guidelines exist for patients on dialysis, but based on the studies cited above, it is reasonable to treat patients on dialysis at the same dose as those with creatinine clearance less than 10 mL/min (i.e., 20 mg every 24 h for patients weighing >60 kg).

The major role of stavudine is in combination with lamivudine or emtricetabine as part of triple-drug combination therapy.[110,149] Clinical trial data support the combination used with protease inhibitors or non-nucleoside reverse transcriptase inhibitors. Because of the increased risk of lipoatrophy with long-term use, it is generally considered an alternative to other preferred regimens. A unique role for stavudine is its use in patients who harbor virus with the K65R mutation, and are unable to tolerate zidovudine. In many resource poor areas, fixed-dose combination of stavudine, lamivudine, and nevirapine is the most widely used regimen, and it is recommended by WHO. Clinical efficacy has been extremely good, but mitochondrial and long-term toxicities remain a concern.[80]

Peripheral neuropathy is the major short-term dose-limiting toxicity. A previous history of neuropathy, whether due to antiretrovirals or other causes, is a risk factor for neuropathy on stavudine. Careful monitoring is important if stavudine is prescribed for persons with a history of neuropathy. Care should be taken to discriminate distal symmetric painful neuropathy due to nucleosides from other causes of neuropathy.[150,151] If symptoms appear to be due to stavudine, the decision must be made whether to replace stavudine or to stop all antiretroviral drugs. While early neuropathy due to stavudine usually resolves in 1–3 weeks, neuropathy may be permanent, particularly if the drug is continued for prolonged periods in the face of worsening symptoms. Lipoatrophy is the primary long-term toxicity that limits the use of stavudine. Reversal of lipoatrophy is slow and incomplete after stopping stavudine.[88–90] If lipoatrophy or lactic acidosis are detected, stavudine should be stopped immediately.

Some experts suggest substituting stavudine for zidovudine in pregnant women who are unable to take zidovudine. The rationale is based on the fact both are thymidine analogs, the similar placental passage, similar activity in activated cells, the lack of significant animal toxicity, and lack of reported toxicity to date in pregnant women. Preliminary results from a study comparing various nucleoside analog regimens suggested that stavudine was well tolerated and at least as effective as zidovudine.[152] It is unclear whether stavudine poses increased risk of mitochondrial toxicity to infants exposed in utero, but this is a potential concern. Lactic acidosis and hepatic steatosis have been reported with the use of stavudine and didanosine during pregnancy. This combination should not be used during pregnancy.

REFERENCES

1. Mansuri MM, Starrett JE Jr, Ghazzouli I, et al. 1-(2,3-Dideoxy-beta-D-glycero-pent-2-enofuranosyl)thymine. A highly potent and selective anti-HIV agent. J Med Chem 32:461–6, 1989.
2. Bristol Myers Squibb. Package insert: Zerit (stavudine) (revised Oct 1996).
3. Moyle GJ. Stavudine: pharmacology, clinical use and future role. Exp Opin Invest Drugs 6:191–200, 1997.
4. August EM, Marongiu ME, Lin TS, Prusoff WH. Initial studies on the cellular pharmacology of 3′-deoxythymidin-2′-ene (d4T): a potent and selective inhibitor of human immunodeficiency virus. Biochem Pharmacol 37:4419–22, 1988.
5. August EM, Birks EM, Prusoft W. 3′-deoxythymidine-2′ene permeation of human lymphocyte H9 cells by nonfacilitated diffusion. Mol Pharmacol 39:246–49, 1991.
6. Ho HT, Hitchcock MJ. Cellular pharmacology of 2′,3′-dideoxy-2′,3′-didehydrothymidine, a nucleoside analog active against human immunodeficiency virus. Antimicrob Agents Chemother 33:844–9, 1989.
7. Balzarini J, Herdewijn P, De Clercq E. Differential patterns of intracellular metabolism of 2′,3′-didehydro-2′,3′-dideoxythymidine and 3′-azido-2′,3′-dideoxythymidine, two potent anti-human immunodeficiency virus compounds. J Biol Chem 264:6127–33, 1989.
8. Martin JC, Hitchcock MJ, Fridland A, et al. Comparative studies of 2′,3′-didehydro-2′,3′-dideoxythymidine (D4T) with other pyrimidine nucleoside analogues. Ann N Y Acad Sci 616:22–8, 1990.
9. Lavie A, Schlichting I, Vetter IR, et al. The bottleneck in AZT activation. Nat Med 3:922–4, 1997.
10. Hazuda D, Kuo L. Failure of AZT: a molecular perspective. Nat Med 3:836–7, 1997.
11. Hitchcock M. 2′,3′-didehydro-2′,3′-dideoxythymidine, an anti-HIV agent. Antivir Chem Chemother 2:125–32, 1991.
12. Fridland A, Connelly M, Ashmun R. Cellular pharmacology of anti-HIV agents azidothymidine (AZT) and 2′, 3′-didehydrothymidine (D4T) in human T cells. In: Int Conf AIDS, 1989.
13. Sommadossi JP. Comparison of metabolism and in vitro antiviral activity of stavudine versus other 2′,3′-dideoxynucleoside analogues. J Infect Dis 171(Suppl 2):S88–92, 1995.
14. Huang P, Farquhar D, Plunkett W. Selective action of 2′,3′-didehydro-2′,3′-dideoxythymidine triphosphate on human immunodeficiency virus reverse transcriptase and human DNA polymerases. J Biol Chem 267:2817–22, 1992.
15. Chen MS, Suttmann RT, Wu JC, Prisbe EJ. Metabolism of 4′-azidothymidine. A compound with potent and selective activity against the human immunodeficiency virus. J Biol Chem 267:257–60, 1992.
16. Lin TS, Schinazi RF, Prusoff WH. Potent and selective in vitro activity of 3′-deoxythymidin-2′-ene (3′-deoxy-2′,3′-didehydrothymidine) against human immunodeficiency virus. Biochem Pharmacol 36:2713–18, 1987.
17. Hamamoto Y, Nakashima H, Matsui T, et al. Inhibitory effect of 2′,3′-didehydro-2′,3′-dideoxynucleosides on infectivity, cytopathic effects, and replication of human immunodeficiency virus. Antimicrob Agents Chemother 31:907–10, 1987.
18. Gao WY, Shirasaka T, Johns DG, et al. Differential phosphorylation of azidothymidine, dideoxycyidine, and dideoxyinosine in resting and activated peripheral blood mononuclear cells. J Clin Invest 91:2326–33, 1993.
19. Zhu Z, Ho HT, Hitchcock MJM, Sommadossi JP. Cellular pharmacology of 2′,3′-didehydro-2′,3′-dideoxythymidine (D4T) in human peripheral blood mononuclear cells. Biochem Pharmacol 39:R15–19, 1990.
20. Milazzo L, Rusconi S, Testa L, et al. Evidence of stavudine-related phenotypic resistance among zidovudine-pretreated HIV-1-infected subjects receiving a therapeutic regimen of stavudine plus lamivudine [letter]. J Acquir Immune Defic Syndr 22:101–3, 1999.
21. Izopet J, Bicart-See A, Pasquier C, et al. Mutations conferring resistance to zidovudine diminish the antiviral effect of stavudine plus didanosine. J Med Virol 59:507–11, 1999.
22. Shulman N, Shafer R, Winters M, et al. Genotypic predictors of virologic response to stavudine after zidovudine monotherapy (ACTG 302). In: Abstracts of the 8th Conference on Retroviruses and Opportunistic Infections, Chicago, IL, 2–5 Feb 2001.
23. Calvez V, Descamps D, Valantin MA, et al. Genotypic analysis of experienced patients treated by d4T/3TC combination (ALTIS 2). In: Abstracts of the 5th Conference on Retroviruses and Opportunistic Infections, Chicago, IL, 1998.
24. Merrill DP, Moonis M, Chou TC, Hirsch MS. Lamivudine or stavudine in two- and three-drug combinations against human immunodeficiency virus type 1 replication in vitro. J Infect Dis 173:355–64, 1996.
25. Sorensen AM, Nielsen C, Mathiesen LR, et al. Evaluation of the combination effect of different antiviral compounds against HIV in vitro. Scan J Infect Dis 25:365–71, 1993.
26. Brankovan V, Tarantini K, Datema R, Chou TC. Strong synergistic anti-HIV activity of a purine and a pyrimidine nucleoside analog, ddI and d4T. In: Abstracts of the 5th International Conference on AIDS, 1989.
27. Deminie C, Bechtold C, Stock D, et al. Evaluation of d4T, ddI and BMS-186,318, in two-drug combinations against HIV replication. In: Abstracts of the 3rd Conference on Retroviruses and Opportunistic Infections, Washington, DC, 1996.
28. Back D, Haworth S, Hoggard P, et al. Drug interactions with d4T phosphorylation in vitro. In: Abstracts of the 11th International Conference on AIDS, Vancouver, BC, 1996.
29. Dudley MN, Graham KK, Kaul S, et al. Pharmacokinetics of stavudine in patients with AIDS or AIDS-related complex. J Infect Dis 166:480–5, 1992.
30. Lea AP, Faulds D. Stavudine: a review of its pharmacodynamic and pharmacokinetic properties and clinical potential in HIV infection. Drugs 51:846–64, 1996.

31. Horton CM, Dudley MN, Kaul S, et al. Population pharmacokinetics of stavudine (d4T) in patients with AIDS or advanced AIDS-related complex. Antimicrob Agents Chemother 39: 2309–15, 1995.
32. Grasela TH, Haworth SJ, Fiedler-Kelley J, Christofalo B. Population pharmacokinetic (PK) analysis of stavudine (d4T) in HIV-infected patients with CD4 counts between 50 and 500 cells/mm^3. In: Abstracts of the 11th International Conference on AIDS, Vancouver, IL, 1996.
33. Russell JW, Whiterock VJ, Marrero D, Klunk LJ. Disposition in animals of a new anti-HIV agent: 2′,3′-didehydro-3′-deoxythymidine. Drug Metab Dispos 18:153–7, 1990.
34. Kaul S, Christofalo B, Raymond RH, et al. Effect of food on the bioavailability of stavudine in subjects with human immunodeficiency virus infection. Antimicrob Agents Chemother 42:2295–8, 1998.
35. Dudley MN. Clinical pharmacokinetics of nucleoside antiretroviral agents. J Infect Dis 171(Suppl 2):S99–112, 1995.
36. Grasela DM, Stoltz RR, Barry M, et al. Pharmacokinetics of single-dose oral stavudine in subjects with renal impairment and in subjects requiring hemodialysis. Antimicrob Agents Chemother 44:2149–53, 2000.
37. Schaad HJ, Petty BG, Grasela DM, et al. Pharmacokinetics and safety of a single dose of stavudine (d4T) in patients with severe hepatic impairment. Antimicrob Agents Chemother 41: 2793–6, 1997.
38. Cretton EM, Zhou Z, Kidd LB, et al. In vitro and in vivo disposition and metabolism of 3′-deoxy-2′,3′-didehydrothymidine. Antimicrob Agents Chemother 37:1816–25, 1993.
39. Foudraine NA, Hoetelmans RM, Lange JM, et al. Cerebrospinal-fluid HIV-1 RNA and drug concentrations after treatment with lamivudine plus zidovudine or stavudine. Lancet 351:1547–51, 1998.
40. Haworth SJ, Christofalo B, Anderson RD, Dunkle LM. A single-dose study to assess the penetration of stavudine into human cerebrospinal fluid in adults. J Acquir Immune Defic Syndr 17:235–8, 1998.
41. Kline MW, Dunkle LM, Church JA, et al. A phase I/II evaluation of stavudine (d4T) in children with human immunodeficiency virus infection. Pediatrics 96(2 Pt 1):247–52, 1995.
42. Gisolf EH, Enting RH, Jurriaans S, et al. Cerebrospinal fluid HIV-1 RNA during treatment with ritonavir/saquinavir or ritonavir/saquinavir/stavudine. AIDS 14:1583–9, 2000.
43. Odinecs A, Nosbisch C, Keller RD, et al. In vivo maternal-fetal pharmacokinetics of stavudine (2′,3′-didehydro-3′-deoxythymidine) in pigtailed macaques (Macaca nemestrina). Antimicrob Agents Chemother 40:196–202, 1996.
44. Bawdon RE, Kaul S, Sobhi S. The ex vivo transfer of the anti-HIV nucleoside compound d4T in the human placenta. Gynecol Obstet Invest 38:1–4, 1994.
45. Inoue T, Tsushita K, Ito T, et al. In vitro bone marrow toxicity of nucleoside analog against human immunodeficiency virus. Antimicrob Agents Chemother 33:576–9, 1989.
46. Gogu SR, Beckman BS, Agrawal KC. Anti-HIV drugs: comparative toxicities in murine fetal liver and bone marrow erythroid progenitor cells. Life Sci 45:iii–vii, 1989.
47. Sommadosi JP. Nucleoside analogs: similarities and differences. J Infect Dis 16(Suppl 1):S7–15, 1993.
48. Cui L, Locatelli L, Xie MY, Sommadossi JP. Effect of nucleoside analogs on neurite regeneration and mitochondrial DNA synthesis in PC-12 cells. J Pharmacol Exp Ther 280:1228–34, 1997.
49. Chen CH, Vazquez Padua M, Cheng YC. Effect of anti-human immunodeficiency virus nucleoside analogs on mitochondrial DNA and its implication for delayed toxicity. Mol Pharmacol 39:625–8, 1991.
50. Browne MJ. Phase I study of 2′3′-didehydro-2′,3′-dideoxythymidine (d4T) in patients (Pts.) with AIDS or ARC. In: Abstracts of the 6th International Conference on AIDS, 1990.
51. Squires K, Sacks H, Sledz S, Murray H. Findings from a phase I study of stavudine (d4T). In: Abstracts of the 8th International Conference on AIDS, 1992.
52. Murray HW, Squires KE, Weiss W, et al. Stavudine in patients with AIDS and AIDS-related complex: AIDS clinical trials group 089. J Infect Dis 171(Suppl 2):S123–30, 1995.
53. Skowron G. Biologic effects and safety of stavudine: overview of phase I and II clinical trials. J Infect Dis 171(Suppl 2): S113–17, 1995.
54. Spruance SL, Pavia AT, Mellors JW, et al. Clinical efficacy of monotherapy with stavudine compared with zidovudine in HIV-infected, zidovudine-experienced patients. A randomized, double-blind, controlled trial. Bristol-Myers Squibb Stavudine/019 Study Group. Ann Intern Med 126:355–63, 1997.
55. Kline MW, Fletcher CV, Federici ME, et al. Combination therapy with stavudine and didanosine in children with advanced human immunodeficiency virus infection: pharmacokinetic properties, safety, and immunologic and virologic effects. Pediatrics 97(6 Pt 1):886–90, 1996.
56. Kline MW, Van Dyke RB, Lindsey JC, et al. A randomized comparative trial of stavudine (d4T) versus zidovudine (ZDV, AZT) in children with human immunodeficiency virus infection. AIDS Clinical Trials Group 240 Team. Pediatrics 101: 214–20, 1998.
57. Kline MW. Pediatric stavudine (d4T) studies. In: Abstracts of the 3rd Conference on Retroviruses and Opportunistic Infection, Washington, DC, 1996.
58. Moore RD, Wong WM, Keruly JC, McArthur JC. Incidence of neuropathy in HIV-infected patients on monotherapy versus those on combination therapy with didanosine, stavudine and hydroxyurea. AIDS 14:273–8, 2000.
59. Petersen EA, Ramirez-Ronda CH, Hardy WD, et al. Dose-related activity of stavudine in patients infected with human immunodeficiency virus. J Infect Dis 171(Suppl 2): S131–9, 1995.
60. Freiman JP, Helfert KE, Hamrell MR, Stein DS. Hepatomegaly with severe steatosis in HIV-seropositive patients. AIDS 7: 379–85, 1993.
61. Bissuel F, Bruneel F, Habersetzer F, et al. Fulminant hepatitis with severe lactate acidosis in HIV-infected patients on didanosine therapy. J Intern Med 235:367–71, 1994.
62. Brinkman K, Ter Hofstede H, Veerkamp MJ, et al. Fatal lactic acidosis following HAART containing stavudine (d4T), lamivudine (3TC) and saquinavir. In: Abstracts of the 12th International Conference on AIDS, Vancouver, BC, 1998.
63. Fortgang IS, Belitsos PC, Chaisson RE, Moore RD. Hepatomegaly and steatosis in HIV-infected patients receiving nucleoside analog antiretroviral therapy. Am J Gastroenterol 90:1433–6, 1995.
64. Sundar K, Suarez M, Banogon PE, Shapiro JM. Zidovudine-induced fatal lactic acidosis and hepatic failure in patients with acquired immunodeficiency syndrome: report of two patients and review of the literature. Crit Care Med 25:1425–30, 1997.
65. Moyle G. Toxicity of antiretroviral nucleoside and nucleotide analogues: is mitochondrial toxicity the only mechanism? Drug Saf 23:467–81, 2000.
66. Moyle G. Clinical manifestations and management of antiretroviral nucleoside analog-related mitochondrial toxicity. Clin Ther 22:911–36, 2000.
67. Pan-Zhou XR, Cui L, Zhou XJ, et al. Differential effects of antiretroviral nucleoside analogs on mitochondrial function in HepG2 cells. Antimicrob Agents Chemother 44:496–503, 2000.
68. Kakuda TN. Pharmacology of nucleoside and nucleotide reverse transcriptase inhibitor-induced mitochondrial toxicity. Clin Ther 22:685–708, 2000.
69. Chariot P, Drogou I, de Lacroix-Szmania I, et al. Zidovudine-induced mitochondrial disorder with massive liver steatosis,

myopathy, lactic acidosis, and mitochondrial DNA depletion. J Hepatol 30:156–60, 1999.
70. Brivet FG, Nion I, Megarbane B, et al. Fatal lactic acidosis and liver steatosis associated with didanosine and stavudine treatment: a respiratory chain dysfunction? [letter]. J Hepatol 32:364–5, 2000.
71. Moyle G. Mitochondrial toxicity hypothesis for lipoatrophy: a refutation. AIDS 15:413–15, 2001.
72. Brinkman K. Editorial response: hyperlactatemia and hepatic steatosis as features of mitochondrial toxicity of nucleoside analogue reverse transcriptase inhibitors. Clin Infect Dis 31:167–9, 2000.
73. Bleeker-Rovers CP, Kadir SW, van Leusen R, Richter C. Hepatic steatosis and lactic acidosis caused by stavudine in an HIV-infected patient. Neth J Med 57:190–3, 2000.
74. Gerard Y, Maulin L, Yazdanpanah Y, et al. Symptomatic hyperlactataemia: an emerging complication of antiretroviral therapy. AIDS 14:2723–30, 2000.
75. Lonergan JT, Behling C, Pfander H, et al. Hyperlactatemia and hepatic abnormalities in 10 human immunodeficiency virus-infected patients receiving nucleoside analogue combination regimens. Clin Infect Dis 31:162–6, 2000.
76. Miller KD, Cameron M, Wood LV, et al. Lactic acidosis and hepatic steatosis associated with use of stavudine: report of four cases. Ann Intern Med 133:192–6, 2000.
77. Mokrzycki MH, Harris C, May H, et al. Lactic acidosis associated with stavudine administration: a report of five cases. Clin Infect Dis 30:198–200, 2000.
78. John M, Moore CB, James IR, et al. Chronic hyperlactatemia in HIV-infected patients taking antiretroviral therapy. AIDS 15:717–23, 2001.
79. McComsey G, Maa JF. Host factors may be more important than choice of antiretrovirals in the development of lipoatrophy. AIDS Read 13:539–42, 559, 2003.
80. Hosseinipou M, Ingiliz P, Kanyama C, et al. Clinical features of lactic acidosis in Malawi. In: XVI International AIDS Conference, Toronto, Canada, 2006.
81. Saint-Marc T, Partisani M, Poizot-Martin I, et al. Fat distribution evaluated by computed tomography and metabolic abnormalities in patients undergoing antiretroviral therapy: preliminary results of the LIPOCO study. AIDS 14:37–49, 2000.
82. Carr A, Miller J, Law M, Cooper DA. A syndrome of lipoatrophy, lactic acidaemia and liver dysfunction associated with HIV nucleoside analogue therapy: contribution to protease inhibitor-related lipodystrophy syndrome. AIDS 14:F25–32, 2000.
83. Brinkman K, Smeitink JA, Romijn JA, Reiss P. Mitochondrial toxicity induced by nucleoside-analogue reverse-transcriptase inhibitors is a key factor in the pathogenesis of antiretroviral-therapy-related lipodystrophy. Lancet 354:1112–15, 1999.
84. Lichtenstein KA, Delaney KM, Ward DJ, Palella FJ. Clinical factors associated with incidence and prevalence of fat atrophy and accumulation. Antivir Ther 5(Suppl 5):61, 2000.
85. Mallal SA, John M, Moore CB, et al. Contribution of nucleoside analogue reverse transcriptase inhibitors to subcutaneous fat wasting in patients with HIV infection. AIDS 14:1309–16, 2000.
86. Saint-Marc T, Partisani M, Poizot-Martin I, et al. A syndrome of peripheral fat wasting (lipodystrophy) in patients receiving long-term nucleoside analogue therapy. AIDS 13:1659–67, 1999.
87. Heath KV, Hogg RS, Chan KJ, et al. Lipodystrophy-associated morphological, cholesterol and triglyceride abnormalities in a population-based HIV/AIDS treatment database. AIDS 15:231–9, 2001.
88. Lonergan JT, McComsey GA, Fisher RL, et al. Lack of recurrence of hyperlactatemia in HIV-infected patients switched from stavudine to abacavir or zidovudine. J Acquir Immune Defic Syndr 36:935–42, 2004.
89. McComsey GA, Ward DJ, Hessenthaler SM, et al. Improvement in lipoatrophy associated with highly active antiretroviral therapy in human immunodeficiency virus-infected patients switched from stavudine to abacavir or zidovudine: the results of the TARHEEL study. Clin Infect Dis 38:263–70, 2004.
90. McComsey GA, Paulsen DM, Lonergan JT, et al. Improvements in lipoatrophy, mitochondrial DNA levels and fat apoptosis after replacing stavudine with abacavir or zidovudine. AIDS 19:15–23, 2005.
91. Gottlieb M, Peterson D, Adler M, et al. Comparison of safety and efficacy of two doses of stavudine (Zerit, d4T) in a large simple trial in the US parallel track program. In: Abstracts of the 35th Interscience Conference on Antimicrobial Agents and Chemotherapy, San Francisco, 1995.
92. Moore RD, Keruly JC, Chaisson RE. Incidence of pancreatitis in HIV-infected patients receiving nucleoside reverse transcriptase inhibitor drugs. AIDS 15:617–20, 2001.
93. Kaul S, Dandekar KA, Schilling BE, Barbhaiya RH. Toxicokinetics of 2′,3′-didehydro-3′-deoxythymidine, stavudine (D4T). Drug Metab Dispos 27:1–12, 1999.
94. Toltzis P, Mourton T, Magnuson T. Comparative embryonic cytotoxicity of antiretroviral nucleosides. J Infect Dis 169:1100–2, 1994.
95. Schilling B, Diamond S, Proctor J, et al. Nonclinical toxicity profile of BMY 27857 (d4T, stavudine). In: Abstracts of the 8th International Conference on AIDS, 1992.
96. Minkoff H, Augenbraum M. Antiviral therapy for pregnant women. Am J Obstet Gynecol 176:478–89, 1997.
97. Griffith BP, Brett-Smith H, Kim G, et al. Effect of stavudine on human immunodeficiency virus type 1 virus load as measured by quantitative mononuclear cell culture, plasma RNA, and immune complex-dissociated antigenemia. J Infect Dis 173:1252–5, 1996.
98. Katlama C, Molina JM, Rozenbaum W, et al. Stavudine (D4T) in HIV infected patients with CD4 less than 350/mm^3: results of a double-blind randomized placebo controlled study. In: 3rd Conf Retro and Opportun Infect, Washington, DC, 1996.
99. Kuritzkes DR, Marschner I, Johnson VA, et al. Lamivudine in combination with zidovudine, stavudine, or didanosine in patients with HIV-1 infection. A randomized, double-blind, placebo-controlled trial. National Institute of Allergy and Infectious Disease AIDS Clinical Trials Group Protocol 306 Investigators. AIDS 13:685–94, 1999.
100. Katzenstein DA, Hughes M, Albrecht M, et al. Virologic and CD4+ cell responses to new nucleoside regimens: switching to stavudine or adding lamivudine after prolonged zidovudine treatment of human immunodeficiency virus infection. ACTG 302 Study Team. AIDS Clinical Trials Group. AIDS Res Hum Retroviruses 16:1031–7, 2000.
101. Pavia AT, Gathe J; BMS-019 Study Group Investigators. Clinical efficacy of stavudine (d4T, Zerit) compared to zidovudine (ZDV,Retrovir) in ZDV-pretreated HIV positive patients. In: Abstracts of the 35th Interscience Conference on Antimicrobial Agents and Chemotherapy, San Francisco, 17–20 Sep 1995.
102. Cohen CJ, Shalit P, Conant M, et al. Lamivudine (3TC) and stavudine (d4T) combination therapy: HIV viral load and CD4 changes in a retrospective study of 330 patients. In: Abstracts of the 4th Conference on Retroviruses and Opportunistic Infections, Washington, DC, 1997.
103. Katlama C, Valantin MA, Matheron S, et al. Efficacy and tolerability of stavudine plus lamivudine in treatment-naive and treatment-experienced patients with HIV-1 infection. Ann Intern Med 129:525–31, 1998.
104. Foudraine NA, de Jong JJ, Jan Weverling G, et al. An open randomized controlled trial of zidovudine plus lamivudine versus stavudine plus lamivudine. AIDS 12:1513–19, 1998.

105. Seifert RD, Stewart MB, Sramek JJ, et al. Pharmacokinetics of co-administered didanosine and stavudine in HIV-seropositive male patients. Br J Clin Pharmacol 38:405–10, 1994.
106. Pollard RB, Peterson D, Hardy D, et al. Safety and antiretroviral effects of combined didanosine and stavudine therapy in HIV-infected individuals with CD4 counts of 200 to 500 cells/mm^3. J Acquir Immune Defic Syndr 22:39–48, 1999.
107. Rutschmann OT, Opravil M, Iten A, et al. A placebo-controlled trial of didanosine plus stavudine, with and without hydroxyurea, for HIV infection. The Swiss HIV Cohort Study. AIDS 12:F71–7, 1998.
108. Molina JM, Chene G, Ferchal F, et al. The ALBI trial: a randomized controlled trial comparing stavudine plus didanosine with zidovudine plus lamivudine and a regimen alternating both combinations in previously untreated patients infected with human immunodeficiency virus. J Infect Dis 180:351–8, 1999.
109. Robbins GK, De Gruttola V, Shafer RW, et al. Comparison of sequential three-drug regimens as initial therapy for HIV-1 infection. N Engl J Med 349:2293–303, 2003.
110. DHHS Panel on Antiretroviral Guidelines for Adults and Adolescents. Guidelines for the use of antiretroviral agents in HIV-infected adults and adolescents. Available: http://aidsinfo.nih.gov 4 May 2006.
111. Gathe J Jr, Burkhardt B, Hawley P, et al. A randomized phase II study of VIRACEPT, a novel HIV protease inhibitor, used in combination with stavudine (d4T) vs. stavudine (d4T) alone. In: International AIDS Conference,Vancouver, BC, 1996.
112. Powderly W, Sension M, Conant M, et al. The efficacy of Viracept (nelfinavir mesylate, NFV) in pivotal phase II/III double-blind randomized controlled trials as monotherapy and in combination with d4T or AZT/3TC. In: 4th Conference on Retroviruses and Opportunistic Infections, Washington, DC, 1997.
113. Steigbigel RT, Cooper D, Clumeck N, et al. Indinavir with stavudine vs. IDV alone vs. stavudine alone in zidovudine experienced, HIV-infected patients. Merck Protocol 037 Study Group. In: Abstracts of the 12th International Conference on AIDS, Vancouver, BC, 1998.
114. Murphy RL. Stavudine-based multiple agent combinations: initial studies and ongoing comparative trials. Antivir Ther 3(Suppl 4):69–73, 1998.
115. Roca B, Gomez CJ, Arnedo A. A randomized, comparative study of lamivudine plus stavudine, with indinavir or nelfinavir, in treatment-experienced HIV-infected patients. AIDS 14:157–61, 2000.
116. Walmsley S, Bernstein B, King M, et al. Lopinavir–ritonavir versus nelfinavir for the initial treatment of HIV infection. N Engl J Med 346:2039–46, 2002.
117. Murphy RL, Sanne I, Cahn P, et al. Dose-ranging, randomized, clinical trial of atazanavir with lamivudine and stavudine in antiretroviral-naive subjects: 48-week results. AIDS 17:2603–14, 2003.
118. Squires KE, Gulick R, Tebas P, et al. A comparison of stavudine plus lamivudine versus zidovudine plus lamivudine in combination with indinavir in antiretroviral naive individuals with HIV infection: selection of thymidine analog regimen therapy (START I). AIDS 14:1591–600, 2000.
119. Carr A, Chuah J, Hudson J, et al. A randomised, open-label comparison of three highly active antiretroviral therapy regimens including two nucleoside analogues and indinavir for previously untreated HIV-1 infection: the OzCombo1 study. AIDS 14:1171–80, 2000.
120. Gallant JE, Staszewski S, Pozniak AL, et al. Efficacy and safety of tenofovir DF vs stavudine in combination therapy in antiretroviral-naive patients: a 3-year randomized trial. Jama 292:191–201, 2004.
121. Eron JJ Jr, Murphy RL, Peterson D, et al. A comparison of stavudine, didanosine and indinavir with zidovudine, lamivudine and indinavir for the initial treatment of HIV-1 infected individuals: selection of thymidine analog regimen therapy (START II). AIDS 14:1601–10, 2000.
122. van Leeuwen R, Katlama C, Murphy RL, et al. A randomized trial to study first-line combination therapy with or without a protease inhibitor in HIV-1-infected patients. AIDS 17:987–99, 2003.
123. Larder BA, Darby G, Richman DD. HIV with reduced sensitivity to zidovudine (AZT) isolated during prolonged therapy. Science 243:1731–4, 1989.
124. Richman DD. Susceptibilities of zidovudine-susceptible and -resistant human immunodeficency virus isolates to antiviral agents determined by using a quantitative plaque reduction assay. Am J Med 88(Suppl 5B):8S–10S, 1990.
125. Lacey SF, Larder BA. Novel mutation (V75T) in human immunodeficiency virus type 1 reverse transcriptase confers resistance to 2′,3′-didehydro-2′,3′-dideoxythymidine in cell culture. Antimicrob Agents Chemother 38:1428–32, 1994.
126. Gu Z, Gao Q, Fang H, et al. Identification of novel mutations that confer drug resistance in the human immunodeficiency virus polymerase gene. Leukemia 8(Suppl 1):S166–9, 1994.
127. Deminie C, Bechtold C, Riccardi K, et al. HIV-1 isolates from subjects on prolonged stavudine therapy remain sensitive to stavudine. In: Abstracts of the 11th International Conference on AIDS, Vancouver, BC, 1996.
128. Lin PF, Samanta H, Rose RE, et al. Genotypic and phenotypic analysis of human immunodeficiency virus type 1 isolates from patients on prolonged stavudine therapy. J Infect Dis 170:1157–64, 1994.
129. Soriano V, Dietrich U, Villalba N, et al. Lack of emergence of genotypic resistance to stavudine after 2 years of monotherapy. AIDS 11:696–7, 1997.
130. Coakley EP, Gillis JM, Hammer SM. Phenotypic and genotypic resistance patterns of HIV-1 isolates derived from individuals treated with didanosine and stavudine. AIDS 14:F9–15, 2000.
131. Pellegrin I, Izopet J, Reynes J, et al. Emergence of zidovudine and multidrug-resistance mutations in the HIV-1 reverse transcriptase gene in therapy-naive patients receiving stavudine plus didanosine combination therapy. STADI Group. AIDS 13:1705–9, 1999.
132. Schuurman R, Nijhuis M, Keulen W, et al. Selection of zidovudine resistance mutations conferring low-level resistance to stavudine occurs at low frequency in stavudine-treated patients and in vitro during prolonged selection experiments. Antivir Ther 5(Suppl 3):39–40, 2000.
133. Johnson VA, Bassett RL, Koel JL, et al. Sozrmbz-os-brartsvriAAT, 3):42–43 S. Selection of zidovudine resistance mutations by zidovudine- or stavudine-based regimens and relationship to subsequent virologic response in ACTG 370. Antivir Ther 5(Suppl 3):42–3, 2000.
134. de Mendoza C, Soriano V, Briones C, et al. Emergence of zidovudine resistance in HIV-infected patients receiving stavudine. J Acquir Immune Defic Syndr 23:279–81, 2000.
135. Moyle GJ, Gazzard BG. Differing reverse transcriptase mutation patterns in individuals experiencing viral rebound on first-line regimens with stavudine/didanosine and stavudine/lamivudine. AIDS 15:799–800, 2001.
136. Duan C, Poticha D, Stoeckli T, et al. Biochemical evidence of cross-resistance to stavudine (d4T) triphosphate in purified HIV-1 reverse transcriptase (RT) derived from a zidovudine (AZT)-resistant isolate. In: Abstracts of the 8th Conference on Retroviruses and Opportunistic Infections, Chicago, IL, 2–5 Feb 2001.
137. Selmi B, Boretto J, Navarro JM, et al. The valine-to-threonine 75 substitution in human immunodeficiency virus type 1 reverse transcriptase and its relation with stavudine resistance. J Biol Chem 276:13965–74, 2001.

138. Schmit JC, Cogniaux J, Hermans P, et al. Multiple drug resistance to nucleoside analogues and nonnucleoside reverse transcriptase inhibitors in an efficiently replicating human immunodeficiency virus type 1 patient strain. J Infect Dis 174:962–8, 1996.
139. Shafer RW, Winters MA, Iversen AK, Merigan TC. Genotypic and phenotypic changes during culture of a multinucleoside-resistant human immunodeficiency virus type 1 strain in the presence and absence of additional reverse transcriptase inhibitors. Antimicrob Agents Chemother 40:2887–90, 1996.
140. Iversen AK, Shafer RW, Wehrly K, et al. Multidrug-resistant human immunodeficiency virus type 1 strains resulting from combination antiretroviral therapy. J Virol 70:1086–90, 1996.
141. de Jong JJ, Goudsmit J, Lukashov VV, et al. Insertion of two amino acids combined with changes in reverse transcriptase containing tyrosine-215 of HIV-1 resistant to multiple nucleoside analogs. AIDS 13:75–80, 1999.
142. Larder BA, Bloor S, Kemp SD, et al. A family of insertion mutations between codons 67 and 70 of human immunodeficiency virus type 1 reverse transcriptase confer multinucleoside analog resistance. Antimicrob Agents Chemother 43:1961–7, 1999.
143. Sugiura W, Matsuda M, Matsuda Z, et al. Identification of insertion mutations in HIV-1 reverse transcriptase causing multiple drug resistance to nucleoside analogue reverse transcriptase inhibitors. J Hum Virol 2:146–53, 1999.
144. Winters MA, Coolley KL, Girard YA, et al. A 6-base pair insert in the reverse transcriptase gene of human immunodeficiency virus type 1 confers resistance to multiple nucleoside inhibitors. J Clin Invest 102:1769–75, 1998.
145. White KL, Margot NA, Ly JK, et al. A combination of decreased NRTI incorporation and decreased excision determines the resistance profile of HIV-1 K65R RT. AIDS 19:1751–60, 2005.
146. Piscitelli SC, Kelly G, Walker RE, et al. A multiple drug interaction study of stavudine with agents for opportunistic infections in human immunodeficiency virus-infected patients. Antimicrob Agents Chemother 43:647–50, 1999.
147. Havlir DV, Tierney C, Friedland GH, et al. In vivo antagonism with zidovudine plus stavudine combination therapy. J Infect Dis 182:321–5, 2000.
148. Rainey PM, McCance EF, Mitchell SM, et al. Interaction of methadone with didanosine (ddI) and stavudine (d4T). In: Abstracts of the 6th Conference on Retroviruses and Opportunistic Infection, 1999:137, abstract 371.
149. Hammer SM, Saag MS, Schechter M, et al. Treatment for adult HIV infection: 2006 recommendations of the International AIDS Society-USA panel. JAMA 296:827–43, 2006.
150. Simpson DM, Olney RK. Peripheral neuropathies associated with human immunodeficiency virus infection. Neurol Clin 10:685–711, 1992.
151. Simpson DM, Tagliati M. Nucleoside analogue-associated peripheral neuropathy in human immunodeficiency virus infection. J Acquir Immune Defic Syndr Hum Retrovirol 9:153–61, 1995.
152. Gray G, McIntyre J, Jivkov B, et al. Preliminary efficacy, safety, tolerability, and pharmacokinetics of short course regimens of nucleoside analogues for the prevention of mother-to-child transmission (MTCT) of HIV abstract TuOrB355. In: Abstracts of the XIIIth International AIDS Conference, Durban, South Africa, 2000.
153. Kline MW, Van Dyke RB, Lindsey JC, et al. Combination therapy with stavudine (d4T) plus didanosine (ddI) in children with human immunodeficiency virus infection. The Pediatric AIDS Clinical Trials Group 327 Team. Pediatrics 103:e62, 1999.
154. de Truchis P, Zucman D, Dupont C, et al. Combination therapy with D4T + 3TC + indinavir (IDV) in nucleosides-experienced HIV-infected patients: an open-label study. In: Abstracts of the 4th Conference on Retroviruses and Opportunistic Infections, Washington, DC, 1997.
155. Nachman SA, Stanley K, Yogev R, et al. Nucleoside analogs plus ritonavir in stable antiretroviral therapy-experienced HIV-infected children: a randomized controlled trial. Pediatric AIDS Clinical Trials Group 338 Study Team. JAMA 283:492–8, 2000.
156. Squires K. The Atlantic study: a randomized, open-label trial comparing two protease inhibitor (pi)-sparing anti-retroviral strategies versus a standard pi-containing regimen, final 48 week data. In: Abstracts of the XIIIth International AIDS Conference, Durban, South Africa, 2000.
157. Gisolf EH, Jurriaans S, Pelgrom J, et al. The effect of treatment intensification in HIV-infection: a study comparing treatment with ritonavir/saquinavir and ritonavir/saquinavir/stavudine. Prometheus Study Group. AIDS 14:405–13, 2000.

Chapter 9

Lamivudine

James H. Willig, MD, Joseph J. Eron Jr., MD

STRUCTURE

Lamivudine (3TC, Epivir) is the negative or *cis* enantiomer of 2′-deoxy-3′-thiacytidine that has antiviral activity against human immunodeficiency virus types 1 and 2 (HIV-1, HIV-2) and hepatitis B virus (HBV). This compound is a pyrimidine nucleoside analog that contains a sulfur atom in place of the 3′ carbon of the ribose ring (Fig. 9-1). 3TC was originally synthesized in a racemic mixture (BCH-189), and this racemic mixture was subsequently separated into positive and negative enantiomers. 3TC, the negative enantiomer, has its ribose ring in a position opposite to the ribose ring position in physiologic nucleosides and most nucleoside analogs.

MECHANISM OF ACTION AND *IN VITRO* ACTIVITY

Like all nucleoside analogs, 3TC must be metabolized to its triphosphorylated form, 3TC-triphosphate, to be an active antiviral compound. 3TC-triphosphate is a reverse transcriptase (RT) inhibitor that competes with deoxycytidinetriphosphate (dCTP), an endogenous nucleotide, for binding in the HIV RT binding site. Incorporation of 3TC-triphosphate into the elongating DNA molecule results in irreversible chain termination as 3TC lacks the 3′-hydroxyl group required for the 5′-3′ linkage required for DNA synthesis.[1] As mentioned above, 3TC was originally synthesized as a racemic mixture (BCH-189), and this mixture has potent activity *in vitro* against HIV-1 with a mean 50% inhibitory dose (IC_{50}) of 0.73 μM in an MT4 cell line assay.[2] The mixture was active against zidovudine (ZDV)-resistant isolates and had less cytotoxicity than ZDV.[2] When BCH-189 was separated into the positive and negative enantiomers, both compounds were discovered to have anti-HIV-1 activity.[3,4] The positive enantiomer, (+)-2′-deoxy-3-thiacytidine, has significantly more cytotoxicity than 3TC *in vitro*, and 3TC appeared to have more antiretroviral activity,[4,5] with a median effect in the nanomolar range in some experiments.[3] 3TC has been tested against laboratory strains of HIV-1 and HIV-2 in a variety of lymphoid cell lines, and the IC_{50} ranged from 4 to 670 nM.[6] 3TC was also highly active against HIV-1 isolates in peripheral blood mononuclear cell assays (IC_{50} 2.5–90 nM).[6] In these experiments the IC_{50} for cytotoxicity was typically 1000-fold higher. That 3TC is more active than its positive enantiomer has been ascribed to the resistance of 3TC to cleavage from the 3′ terminals of RNA/DNA complexes by 3′-5′ cellular exonucleases.[5,7] In a series of experiments, Skalski and colleagues showed that the positive enantiomer has more inhibitory activity than 3TC-TP against the HIV RT, although a novel cellular exonuclease removed the positive enantiomer at a two- to sixfold higher rate.[5] This group also showed that 3TC was more readily phosphorylated in the cell than the positive enantiomer. In addition to *in vitro* activity against

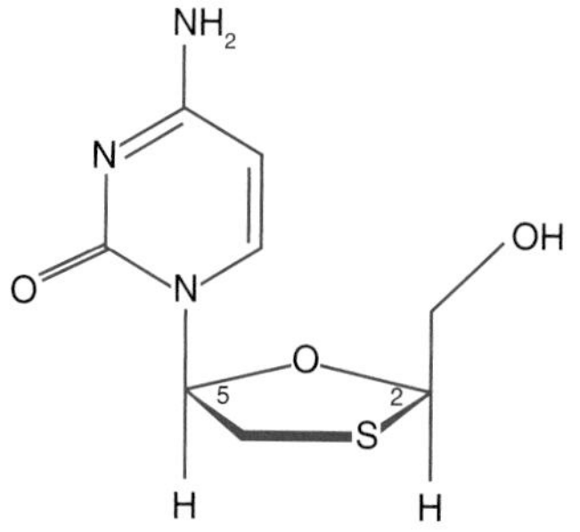

Figure 9-1 ■ Structure of *cis* enantiomer of 2′-deoxy-3′-thiacytidine (3TC).

HIV-1 and HIV-2, 3TC inhibits the HBV[8] and has antiviral activity in patients with chronic active hepatitis B.[9,10]

Lamivudine has been shown to be synergistic *in vitro* with a variety of antiretroviral agents in inhibiting HIV-1. Against ZDV-sensitive isolates and in some studies against ZDV-resistant isolates[11] 3TC has been shown to be synergistic or additive with nucleoside analogs (ZDV,[11–13] stavudine,[11,12] didanosine[12]), protease inhibitors,[11] and the non-nucleoside RT inhibitors (NNRTIs).[11,14] Three-drug combinations of 3TC/ZDV/saquinavir,[11] 3TC/ZDV/d4T,[11] 3TC/ZDV/nevirapine,[11] 3TC/ZDV/delavirdine (DLV),[14] and 3TC/ZDV/indinavir,[15–17] have also been shown to be synergistic or additive *in vitro*. 3TC/ZDV/efavirenz (EFV) has proved to be a particularly effective regimen delaying virologic failure and leading to a shorter time to viral load suppression when compared to three NRTI (nucleoside RT inhibitor) regimens (3TC/ZDV/ABC) and regimens of ddI/d4T/NFV or ddI/d4T/EFV as initial therapy.[18,19] Four-drug combination regimens (3TC/ZDV/ABC/EFV or EFV and nelfinavir combined with 3TC/ZDV and either ddI or d4T) have not proved to provide additional benefit when compared with a three-drug (3TC/ZDV/EFV) regimen as initial therapy in time to virologic failure and CD4 changes.[20,21] Two of the three NRTI combinations listed by the 2006 recommendations of the International AIDS Society-USA Panel (3TC/ZDV, 3TC/ABC and FTC/TDF) for use with either an NNRTI or ritonavir (RTV) boosted PI as initial antiretroviral regimens include 3TC[22] A trial of 3TC/ZDV/EFV versus FTC/TDF/EFV confirmed the noninferiority of the latter combination to the lamivudine containing regimen.[23]

It is of note that 3TC interferes with phosphorylation of zalcitabine (ddC),[24] most likely because these agents are both cytosine analogs. These two agents may be antagonistic against HIV-1 replication, as has been shown *in vitro* for stavudine (d4T) and ZDV, which are both thymidine analogs.[11] Neither combination is recommended as a component of highly active antiretroviral therapy (HAART).[25]

PHARMACOKINETICS

Favorable oral bioavailability was demonstrated during the initial *in vivo* studies of 3TC. When single doses of 3TC over a range of five doses (0.25–8.0 mg/kg) were given intravenously and orally to adult men who were HIV-infected, the bioavailability was 82%.[26] Food has no significant effect on the extent of 3TC absorption.[27] Other studies have shown similar oral bioavailability of tablet and oral solution formulations of 3TC,[28] although intrasubject variability in the bioavailability of the tablet was seen. The bioavailability of 3TC in infants, which was 66% in one study, is somewhat less than that seen in adults.[29]

In a phase I/II multiple-dose study, 97 subjects with acquired immunodeficiency syndrome (AIDS) or advanced HIV (median CD4+ T-lymphocyte count 128 cells/mm^3) were administered 3TC at 0.5, 1.0, 2.0, 4.0, 8.0, 12.0, and 20.0 mg/kg twice daily in sequential cohorts.[30] Pharmacokinetic parameters obtained at steady state after 2 weeks on therapy showed dose linearity with peak concentrations well above the *in vitro* IC_{90} of HIV-1, especially at the higher doses. The half-life of 3TC in serum was 3–4 h. The pharmacokinetic parameters did not change after 24 weeks of continuous dosing. Other studies, which examined single doses of 3TC, have shown that the half-life in plasma was substantially longer than in the study of Pluda et al,[30] ranging from 8 to 11 h.[28,31] 3TC clearance is dependent on weight and renal function and is not influenced by gender, disease stage, CD4+ T-lymphocyte count or race.[32] 3TC has low protein binding in plasma and freely crosses the placenta and into breast milk[33]; it appears to be concentrated in the male genital tract.[34] Similar to other drugs in its class, it appears to cross the placenta by simple diffusion and is thought to concentrate in the amniotic fluid through fetal urinary excretion.[35] 3TC clearance is prolonged in neonates compared to that in infants and older children.[33] 3TC is excreted predominantly by the kidney, with 70% excreted unchanged in the urine.[26] Dose adjustment is required with significant renal impairment (creatinine clearance <50 mL/min).[31,36] 3TC is cleared by hemodialysis, though given the large volume of distribution of 3TC no increase in dose is required once an individual with chronic renal failure begins dialysis.[36] 3TC pharmacokinetics are unchanged in individuals with moderately to severely impaired hepatic function (cirrhosis).[37]

Lamivudine enters the cell by passive diffusion[8] and appears to be phosphorylated more efficiently in resting lymphocytes than in activated cells.[38] At steady state ~15–20% of 3TC in peripheral blood mononuclear cells is in the triphosphate form (3TC-TP) and 50–55% is in the diphosphate form, (3TC-DP), making the conversion of 3TC-DP to 3TC-TP the rate-limiting step during intracellular metabolism.[39] The intracellular half-life of 3TC-TP is ~12–16 h[39,40] compared to 1.0 and 2.6 h for ZDV-TP and ddC-TP, respectively. Once-daily dosing of 300 mg of 3TC is now recommended as an acceptable dosing interval owing to these properties.

In a dose-range phase I/II study of 3TC, serum and cerebrospinal fluid (CSF) samples were obtained from some subjects and the CSF/serum drug concentration ratio was found to be low (0.06) similar to what was previously reported for ddI and ddC.[41] The concentration of 3TC in CSF relative to serum in nonhuman primates was significantly higher (41%), though levels in ventricular CSF in these animals was similar to those seen in humans.[42] In children the CSF/serum ratios were more than 0.1[41] and therefore higher than reported by van Leeuwen et al[41] in adults.[43] It is of note that because 3TC has such favorable pharmacokinetics, reaching high levels in serum, the absolute concentrations of 3TC in CSF are as high or higher than the two thymidine nucleoside analogs d4T and ZDV.[44] In addition, CSF concentrations of nucleoside analogs are relatively stable over time, unlike plasma concentrations. Therefore, CSF/serum drug ratios are highly time dependent, with higher ratios when sampling is done later in the dosing interval.[44]

The penetration of 3TC into male genital secretions has also been examined. In 70 samples from nine men on 3TC and ZDV followed over time, the median seminal fluid/blood plasma 3TC concentration ratio was 9:1, demonstrating marked accumulation of 3TC in this compartment.[34] When the steady-state relation between the seminal fluid–blood plasma 3TC concentration was examined relative to the timing of drug ingestion, the 3TC concentrations in semen were remarkably constant over time, suggesting that 3TC is either actively taken up or trapped in this compartment.[45] The semen/blood concentration ratios for 3TC are higher than for other nucleosides,[34,45,46] NNRTIs,[46,47] and single protease inhibitors[45,48,49] described to date. Whether these high concentrations of 3TC affect the likelihood of HIV-1 sexual transmission relative to other antiretroviral agents is not known.

TOXICITY

Some of the toxicity seen with nucleoside analogs results from their affinity for human DNA polymerases, although for most nucleoside analogs the affinity for this enzyme is less than that for HIV-1 RT. The relative affinity of the NRTIs for specific human DNA polymerases varies by agent and may explain in part their differing toxicities. Significant attention has been given to the potential mitochondrial toxicity of nucleoside analogs, which may relate to their affinity for DNA polymerase-γ.[50–52]

Lamivudine has limited cytotoxicity *in vitro*,[4–6] possibly owing to the low affinity of 3TC-TP for human DNA polymerases.[8,53] For each of these human enzymes the positive enantiomer has greater affinity than 3TC,[8] and these enzyme affinities offer a likely explanation for the differences in cytotoxicity between these enantiomers. There was no evidence of a neuropathic effect of 3TC in an *in vitro* model of neuron toxicity,[54] and the potential for hematologic toxicity as measured *in vitro* is low.[55]

Significant toxicity that is clearly attributable to 3TC is uncommon (the toxicities are: neutropenia, headache, and nausea). Dose-limiting toxicity was not observed in early studies of 3TC monotherapy.[26,30,41] At doses higher than currently recommended, neutropenia was observed in a small number of subjects, and a general downward trend in absolute neutrophil counts was seen.[30,41] The subjects in these studies had relatively low CD4+ T-lymphocyte counts, and individuals with low counts may be at greater risk of hematologic toxicity, as has been shown for ZDV.[56] In comparative trials, the addition of 3TC to ZDV in a double-blind placebo-controlled trial appeared to have no significant adverse effects other than those seen in subjects who were given ZDV alone.[57] In this study subjects given 3TC alone had significantly higher hemoglobin levels than the ZDV- and ZDV/3TC-treated subjects. In large clinical trials in subjects with more advanced disease and previous ZDV therapy for an average of 2 years, severe adverse effects of 3TC/ZDV were also uncommon.[58,59] In the study in which 3TC (at two doses)/ZDV was compared to ZDV alone, nausea was the most common adverse effect and was seen more commonly in the 3TC/ZDV arms (10% vs 5% of subjects), though this difference was not significant.[59] Neutropenia occurred more commonly in subjects receiving 3TC (300 mg twice daily)/ZDV, but again the differences were not significant between arms. The number of subjects with severe neutropenia was the same in the 3TC (150 twice daily)/ZDV arm and the ZDV monotherapy arm. There were no episodes of pancreatitis and only one episode of peripheral neuropathy among the 223 subjects randomized. In a larger study of subjects with relatively advanced HIV disease (median CD4+ T-lymphocyte count ~210 cells/mm) in which two doses of 3TC/ZDV were compared with ddC/ZDV, the differences in cumulative moderate and severe toxicity between the treatment arms were not significant.[58]

The contribution of 3TC to antiretroviral adverse effects that may be due to mitochondrial toxicity (e.g., lipoatrophy and lactic acidosis) is not known. Among patients with hepatitis B treated with 3TC, there was no evidence of mitochondrial toxicity on liver biopsy after 6 months of therapy, albeit the 3TC dose was lower than is commonly used to treat HIV.[60] 3TC is a preferred antiretroviral in patients with risk factors for hepatotoxiciy of antiretroviral therapy (Cirrhosis, obesity, female gender, a prior hepatotoxicity and co-infection with hepatitis B and C).[61–63] Some observational cohort studies have suggested that elevated lactate levels are more common in subjects treated with 3TC and d4T in contrast to other combinations,[64,65] but this finding has not been consistently observed.[66] An observational study found a higher rate of subcutaneous lipoatrophy and a greater increase in serum lactate at one year in those taking the nucleosides ddI/d4T versus 3TC/ABC.[67] Lamivudine has been used successfully to rechallenge patients with prior mitochondrial toxicities (symptomatic hyperlactatemia, lactic acidosis) to NRTIs regimens, including those that included 3TC.[68] In a patient with prior symptomatic lactic acidosis, reintroduction of 3TC to the antiretroviral regimen must await full recovery, preceded by careful weighing of risks and benefits, and followed by close monitoring of symptoms and lactic acid levels.[22]

Episodes of pancreatitis have been reported in pediatric patients receiving 3TC in clinical trials.[69] However, these HIV-infected children and infants had advanced HIV disease and had received or were currently receiving concomitant medications that are associated with pancreatitis. Increased frequency of pancreatitis has not been observed in subjects receiving 3TC in controlled trials in adults.

ANTIRETROVIRAL ACTIVITY AND CLINICAL EFFICACY

Multiple trials of 3TC activity and efficacy have been completed. Initially, trials of 3TC monotherapy demonstrated the antiretroviral activity of this agent. Subsequent trials have evaluated 3TC in combination with other antiretroviral agents. Some trials have evaluated the effect on the CD4+ T-lymphocyte count or virologic suppression as the primary endpoint, and others have investigated the clinical efficacy of 3TC-containing regimens. The next few sections will

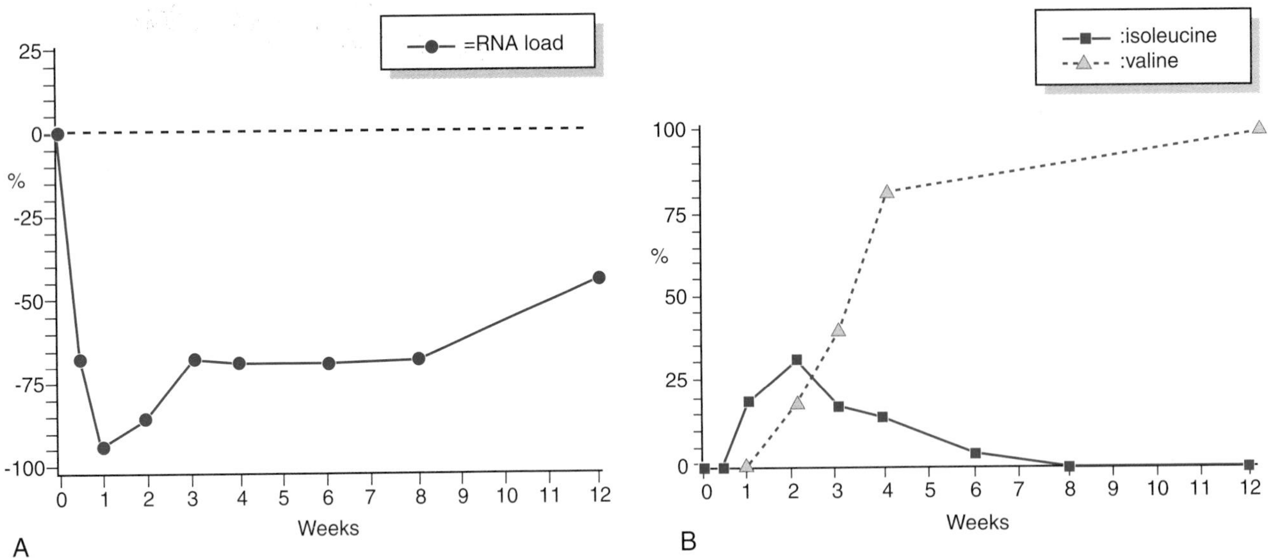

Figure 9-2 ■ (**A**) Percentage change in HIV RNA from baseline over time achieved with 3TC monotherapy in HIV-infected subjects. (**B**) Median percentage of HIV-1 variants (from 20 subjects) that contain a change in HIV-1 RT coding sequence at codon 184. Initially, mutants appear to have a substitution of isoleucine for the wild type, but these variants are rapidly replaced by variants with the methionine-to-valine change.

Adapted from Schuurman R, Nijhuis M, van Leeuwen R, et al. Rapid changes in human immunodeficiency virus type 1 RNA load and appearance of drug-resistant virus populations in persons treated with lamivudine (3TC). J Infect Dis 171:1411–19, 1995.

examine the evolution of the use of 3TC in the therapy of HIV infection.

3TC MONOTHERAPY

Trials of 3TC as a single agent were predominantly small studies that were undertaken to evaluate the pharmacokinetic parameters of the drug.[30,41,70] An initial dose-range study of patients with advanced HIV disease showed only modest evidence of virologic or immunologic activity though HIV-1 RNA was not measured at that time.[30] Short-term increases in CD4+ T-lymphocyte counts were observed at higher doses (8 and 12 mg kg^{-1} day^{-1}) but subsequently decreased to baseline after 20 weeks. A similar study performed in Europe tested doses of 3TC ranging from 0.5 to 20.0 mg/kg and showed small, short-lived increases in CD4+ T-lymphocyte counts.[41] There were also changes in other surrogate markers of HIV infections, such as p24 antigen, β_2-microglobulin, and neopterin levels. These changes persisted for a longer duration than the changes in CD4+ T-lymphocyte counts, though there was no clear dose–response effect on these parameters. Schuurman and colleagues demonstrated that 3TC administered as a single agent resulted in a rapid decrease in serum HIV-1 RNA levels with an average decrease of more than 95% in 2 weeks (Fig. 9-2A).[70] This study was also one of the first to demonstrated *in vivo* emergence of resistance to 3TC (see below). More recent trials of 3TC monotherapy have focused on comparing its antiretroviral activity to that of emtricitabine.[71,72]

Monotherapy with 3TC was also studied in 90 subjects given 300 mg twice a day in a larger clinical trial done primarily to evaluate the combination of 3TC/ZDV.[57] Lamivudine monotherapy resulted in a peak mean increase in CD4+ T-lymphocyte count of 35 cells/μL above baseline in subjects with CD4+ T-lymphocyte counts of 200–500 cells/mm^3. Mean CD4+ T-lymphocyte counts remained above baseline for ~8 months, an effect similar to that observed with ZDV monotherapy in the same study. HIV-1 RNA levels were decreased initially by a mean of 1.2 log_{10} copies/mL and remained below baseline through 52 weeks of observation (Fig. 9-3). HIV-1 RNA levels were reduced to a significantly greater extent with 3TC than with ZDV monotherapy.[57]

The limitations of 3TC monotherapy became apparent relatively early during laboratory and clinical studies of the drug. Resistance developed rapidly *in vitro*, with the initial effect of 3TC on CD4+ T-lymphocyte counts and p24 antigen levels being modest and transient.[30,73] In addition, the synergistic interactions of nucleoside analogs *in vitro* were being noted,[13,74,75] and the potential advantages of combination antiretroviral therapy were being recognized.[76,77]

Several trials have shown continued antiviral activity of 3TC despite the presence of an M184V mutation (confers high-level phenotypic drug resistance) in the HIV RT gene.[22,70,78–81] A randomized 48-week open-label pilot study of 3TC monotherapy in patients with 3TC resistant virus showed better immunological (defined as first CD4 < 350) and clinical (defined as occurrence of CDC grade B or C event) as when compared to complete therapy interruption.[82] In addition, the strategy of continuing 3TC monotherapy

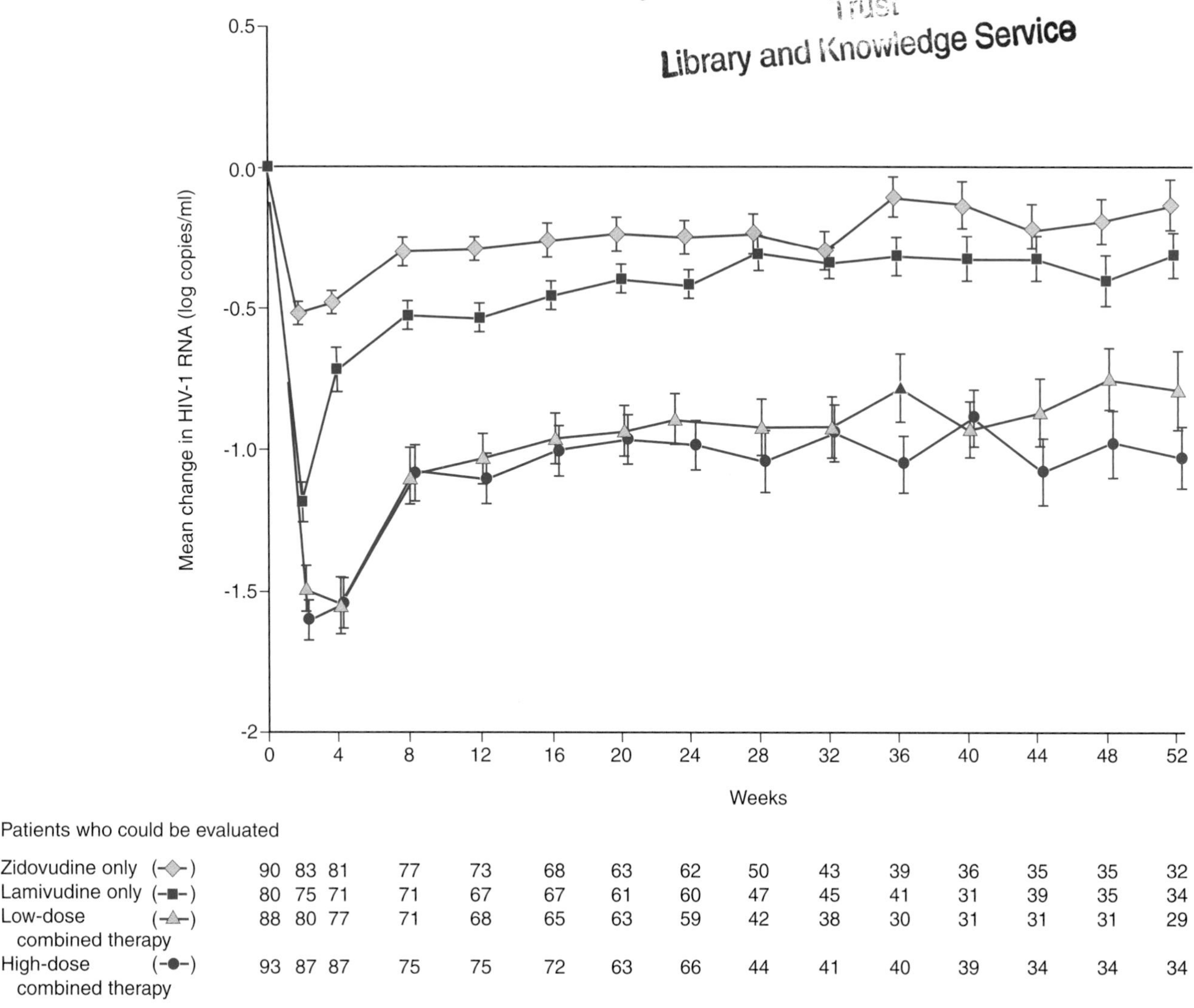

Patients who could be evaluated

Zidovudine only (-◇-)	90	83	81	77	73	68	63	62	50	43	39	36	35	35	32
Lamivudine only (-■-)	80	75	71	71	67	67	61	60	47	45	41	31	39	35	34
Low-dose combined therapy (-△-)	88	80	77	71	68	65	63	59	42	38	30	31	31	31	29
High-dose combined therapy (-●-)	93	87	87	75	75	72	63	66	44	41	40	39	34	34	34

Figure 9-3 ■ Change from baseline in HIV RNA levels over time in HIV-1-infected subjects naive to antiretroviral therapy who received ZDV alone, lamivudine (3TC) alone, or one of two doses of lamivudine in combination with ZDV. The numbers of subjects evaluated at each time point is listed below that time point.

Adapted from Eron J, Benoit S, Jemsek J, et al. Treatment with lamivudine, zidovudine or both in HIV-positive patients with 200–500 CD4+ cells/mm^3. N Engl J Med 333:1662–9, 1995.

showed benefit in the form of more favorable rates of CD4 decline, viral rebound and recovery of HIV-1 replicative capacity.[82] Based on the available data, 3TC continues to contribute antiviral activity despite existing resistance, and 3TC monotherapy is undergoing study as a 'bridging' option in HIV-1 multidrug resistant patients until the arrival of two or more active antiretrovirals.[22,78–82]

DUAL NUCLEOSIDE THERAPY

The use of 3TC in combination with ZDV resulted from a convergence of observations and treatment concepts. As outlined, the modest effect of 3TC *in vivo* and the emergence of 3TC resistance *in vitro* were apparent. The clinical toxicity of 3TC was minimal, however. Importantly, it was noted that when the mutation associated with 3TC resistance (discussed in the next section) was added to HIV-1 variants resistant to ZDV, these variants regained sensitivity to ZDV.[83] In additional experiments, it was shown that resistance to a 3TC-like compound (FTC) developed more slowly *in vitro* in the presence of FTC and ZDV.[83]

Antiretroviral Activity and Effect on CD4+ T-Lymphocyte Count

The combination of lamivudine and ZDV was evaluated in two studies of patients who had received less than 4 weeks of ZDV and no other antiretroviral therapy. Both were randomized, double-blind, placebo-controlled multicenter trials comparing 3TC/ZDV with ZDV monotherapy. 3TC monotherapy was also evaluated in one of the studies.[57] Eron and colleagues evaluated subjects with CD4+ T-lymphocyte counts of 200–500 cells/mm^3 who remained on their original blinded therapy assignment through 52 weeks.[75] Primary study endpoints included the change (from baseline) of CD4+ T-lymphocyte counts and the plasma HIV-1 RNA levels. The primary metric for analysis of immunologic and HIV-1 RNA endpoints was the time-weighted area under the curve (AUC) of all postbaseline measurements minus the baseline value.[84] Sustained CD4+ T-lymphocyte increases were seen during 52 weeks of the 3TC/ZDV combination at two doses of 3TC (150 and 300 mg twice daily); there was a peak mean increase of 79 and 78 cells/μL, respectively, with little trend toward baseline over time.[57] By week 52 the difference between the mean CD4+ T-lymphocyte count for either combination arm and ZDV monotherapy (200 mg three times a day) was more than 100 cells/mm^3. The combination arms showed a mean peak effect on HIV-1 RNA in plasma of almost 1.6 log_{10} copies/mL, whereas the peak effect of ZDV was 0.5 log_{10} copies/mL. The median time-weighted change from baseline over 24 weeks were decreases of 1.1 and 1.2 log_{10} copies/mL for the low- and high-dose 3TC/ZDV combinations, respectively, compared to a decrease of 0.3 log_{10} copies/mL for ZDV monotherapy (Fig. 9-3). It is of note that in a subset of patients who began the study with a plasma HIV-1 RNA level of 20 000 copies/mL or more and therefore had the opportunity to experience a 2 log_{10} copies/mL decrease from baseline (the lower limit of detection of the HIV-1 RNA assay was 200 copies/mL) the combination of ZDV with either dose of 3TC showed a median peak decrease of more than 2.0 log_{10} copies/mL (100-fold reduction from baseline). Over the 52 weeks of the blinded therapy phase, the 3TC/ZDV combination had a persistent ~10-fold inhibitory effect on HIV-1 RNA levels. Clinical endpoints were also examined in this study, though the size of the study limits the interpretation of this information. Significantly fewer Centers for Disease Control and Prevention (CDC) class B and C endpoints occurred during 52 weeks in patients on combination therapy compared with patients on ZDV alone (J J Eron, unpublished observations).

Katlama et al studied subjects with CD4+ T-lymphocyte counts of 100–400 randomized to one of two treatment arms: (1) ZDV 200 mg every 8 h/placebo; (2) ZDV 200 mg every 8 h/3TC 300 mg every 12 h. The initial study period was 24 weeks, after which time patients were offered open-label 3TC and ZDV and were followed for an additional 24 weeks. In this study the peak mean change in CD4+ T-lymphocyte counts from baseline was 85 cells/mm^3 at 8 weeks for ZDV/3TC and 34 cells/mm^3 at week 4 for ZDV monotherapy.[85] At 24 weeks the mean CD4+ T-lymphocyte count was 78 cells above baseline for patients on 3TC/ZDV and had decreased to nine cells below baseline in subjects on ZDV. Among the subjects who completed 24 weeks of study, 97% opted to continue on open-label 3TC and ZDV. Over the subsequent 24-week period the positive CD4+ T-lymphocyte effect of 3TC/ZDV persisted, though it declined somewhat to a mean of 48 cells above baseline at week 48. Using an immune-based capture technique,[86] HIV-1 RNA levels in plasma were evaluated in 29% of the patients. This assay measures only intact HIV-1 particles, and so a potentially smaller log reduction may be seen with this assay compared to other assays that measure HIV-1 RNA in plasma. The combination showed a 0.8 log_{10} copies/mL decrease at week 24. This antiretroviral effect persisted at 1.1 log_{10} copies/mL below baseline at week 48, though only a small number of samples were available at this time point. Despite 24 weeks of previous ZDV monotherapy the addition of 3TC to this group resulted in similar decreases in HIV-1 RNA at week 48.

These studies of 3TC and ZDV in antiretroviral treatment-naive patients yielded remarkably similar results. The 3TC/ZDV combination produced significant and prolonged effects on both CD4+ T lymphocyte counts and HIV-1 RNA levels in plasma over the 48–52 weeks of the study. These effects were clearly superior to ZDV monotherapy and were obtained with no significant increase in adverse events when compared to ZDV alone.[57,85]

The 3TC/ZDV combination was also studied in patients who had undergone previous ZDV treatment. One study compared the addition of 3TC to ZDV versus continuing ZDV alone in 223 subjects with CD4+ T-lymphocyte counts of 100–400 cells/mm^3 who had been treated with ZDV for more than 6 months. Subjects either continued ZDV 200 mg three times daily or received 3TC at 150 or 300 mg bid/ZDV. Most (54%) of the subjects were asymptomatic, with a mean CD4+ T-lymphocyte count for the group of 251 cells/mm^3. The mean duration of previous ZDV therapy was 24 months. There were significant increases in CD4+ T-lymphocytes in the patients treated with ZDV/3TC, with a mean increase in CD4+ T-lymphocytes of ~40 cells/mm^3 above baseline at 24 weeks with either dose of 3TC and remained at ~30 cells/mm^3 above baseline through 48 weeks.[59] A mean decrease in plasma HIV RNA of ~1 log_{10} copies/mL was observed in either combination-therapy arm over 24 weeks.

In a study conducted in North America in ZDV-experienced patients with CD4+ T-lymphocyte counts of 100–300 cells/mm^3, the addition of two doses of 3TC (150 and 300 mg twice daily) were compared to adding ddC.[58] Altogether, 254 subjects with a median duration of previous ZDV treatment of 20 months, a median CD4+ T-lymphocyte count of 214 cells/mm^3, and a median plasma HIV RNA level of 4.7 log_{10} copies/mL were studied. Adding 3TC to ZDV resulted in significant increases in the CD4+ T-lymphocyte counts above baseline compared to adding ddC. The median change in CD4+ T-lymphocyte count after 52 weeks on 3TC (150 mg twice daily)/ZDV was an increase of 43 cells/mm^3, whereas subjects on ddC/ZDV experienced a decrease of 30 cells/mm^3. The effects on plasma HIV-1 RNA levels were similar in all three treatment arms, with median decreases of 0.4–0.5 log_{10} copies/mL at year. There were fewer new AIDS events in the 3TC/ZDV-treated arms than in the ZDV/ddC-treated group, but this trend did not reach statistical significance. These two studies of the addition of 3TC to the treatment of ZDV-experienced patients demonstrated significant immunologic and virologic effects. They also showed that the adding 3TC to the regimen of patients already receiving

ZDV has a less potent effect than initiating the two agents simultaneously.

There has been evidence demonstrated that 3TC and ZDV can have a prolonged, though incomplete, antiretroviral effect in selected patients, even in the presence of likely 3TC resistance. In subjects treated with 3TC/ZDV for 2 years, the drugs were discontinued at the completion of the study period; the patients were then observed for 2 weeks before starting alternative antiretroviral therapy. Despite 2 years of treatment, these subjects experienced a rapid rise in HIV-1 RNA off therapy with the increases ranging from twofold to 50-fold[87] over the 2-week period; this increase suggests that a significant antiretroviral effect of 3TC/ZDV was present up to 2 years in some patients. Multiple studies have demonstrated the persistence of antiviral activity against HIV-1 and provide the rationale for recommending the continuation of 3TC or FTC in subsequent therapeutic regimens despite documented resistance to this drug, particularly in the setting of multiple regimen failures.[22,78–81]

The combination of 3TC with other nucleosides has also been evaluated. Detailed comparisons of the effects of several nucleoside regimens on HIV-1 RNA levels and CD4+ T-lymphocyte counts have been carried out by the AIDS Clinical Trials Group (ACTG). ACTG 306 enrolled subjects naive to previous treatment and who had CD4+ T-lymphocyte counts of 200–600 cells/mm^3. The patients were randomized to one of two treatment limbs: one didanosine (ddI)-based and one stavudine (d4T)-based.[88] In the ddI limb subjects were randomized to ddI monotherapy, ddI/3TC, or ZDV/3TC. In the d4T limb subjects were randomized to d4T monotherapy, d4T/3TC, or ZDV/3TC. After 24 weeks subjects on either ddI or d4T monotherapy were also given 3TC. Altogether, 299 subjects were enrolled. The median baseline plasma HIV RNA levels were ~10 000 copies/mL, and the median CD4+ T-lymphocyte counts were ~400 cells/mm^3. Using an HIV RNA assay with a lower limit of detection of 50 copies/mL, the mean $\log_{10}$ copies/mL decreases in RNA on the ddI limb at 24 weeks were 1.3, 1.2, and 1.4 for ddI, ddI/3TC, and ZDV/3TC, respectively.

None of the comparisons between treatment arms were significant. For the d4T limb the adjusted mean decreases in plasma HIV-1 RNA at 24 weeks were 0.5, 1.6, and 1.6 $\log_{10}$ copies/mL for d4T monotherapy, d4T/3TC, and ZDV/3TC, respectively. The difference between d4T and d4T/3TC was highly significant ($P = 0.001$), and the difference between d4T/3TC and 3TC/ZDV was not ($P = 0.77$). At 48 weeks the addition of 3TC to d4T and to ddI resulted in additional 0.44 and 0.79 $\log_{10}$ copies/mL adjusted decreases, respectively. After 48 weeks the decreases in HIV RNA ranged from 1.2 $\log_{10}$ copies/mL (d4T/3TC) to 1.8 $\log_{10}$ copies/mL (ddI/delayed 3TC) with both d4T/3TC and ZDV/3TC at 1.5 $\log_{10}$ copies/mL. None of the comparisons within arms were significant. During 48 weeks the CD4+ T-lymphocyte count increases were not significantly different between arms, with increases of 77–118 cells/mm^3. These results suggest that during 48 weeks in subjects with a relatively low viral load (mean HIV RNA at baseline ~10 000 copies/mL) 3TC/d4T is at least as effective at suppressing HIV RNA levels and increasing CD4+ T-lymphocyte counts as 3TC/ZDV. Data suggest that the genotypic resistance patterns for d4T and ZDV are similar, and therefore a mutational interaction between 3TC and d4T resistance similar to the 3TC–ZDV interaction may occur.[89] The antiviral activity of 3TC/ZDV compared to ddI/3TC and ddI monotherapy was more difficult to interpret, as activities over 24 and 48 weeks were quite similar. On the one hand, the similarity of the 3TC/ddI and ddI arms suggests that adding 3TC to ddI affords little benefit. On the other hand, adding 3TC to ddI after 24 weeks resulted in a 0.8 $\log_{10}$ copies/mL decrease and supports the opposite conclusion. Resistance data from this study may shed further light on the utility of the ddI/3TC combination. The overall results from this study must be interpreted with some caution. The viral load of all the subjects at baseline was low, and the results may be less applicable to individuals with high viral loads. In addition, although the censoring of change in HIV RNA levels by the lower limits of the HIV RNA assays was taken into account, these methods may be imperfect and more censoring may have occurred in the dual nucleoside arms, which perhaps narrowed the differences.

The 3TC/d4T combination has also been investigated in an open-label study.[90] In treatment-naive subjects the antiretroviral effect of 3TC/d4T over a 6-month period was similar to effects seen with ZDV/3TC in previous studies and in the ACTG 306 trial (median decrease of 1.66 $\log_{10}$ copies/mL).[88] The effect of 3TC/d4T was much less potent in nucleoside treatment-experienced subjects who had not received 3TC or d4T, with a median decrease in HIV RNA of 0.55 $\log_{10}$ copies/mL at 24 weeks.

Effect on Disease Progression and Mortality

The effect of 3TC in combination with other nucleoside analogs on HIV disease progression and mortality has now been clearly demonstrated. After completion of four of the initial studies (reviewed in previous sections) that primarily examined antiretroviral efficacy, a meta-analysis of these studies was performed in an attempt to analyze effects on disease progression.[91] This analysis, which combined data from 972 subjects, showed a beneficial effect of 3TC/ZDV on disease progression compared to the control arms in various studies. There was a 49% reduction in all clinical events with ZDV/3TC therapy and a 66% reduction in progression to new AIDS events. This difference was seen when subjects were divided into subsets by treatment history, presence of symptoms, or CD4 cell counts. Few deaths occurred in these studies, and the number of AIDS-defining endpoints was limited. These factors, coupled with the retrospective design of the analysis, limited interpretation of the results.

To examine the effect of 3TC on disease progression, a large randomized, placebo-controlled trial of the addition of 3TC to ZDV-containing nucleoside regimens was undertaken.[92] This study, referred to as the CAESAR trial to represent the locations (Canada, Australia, Europe, South Africa)

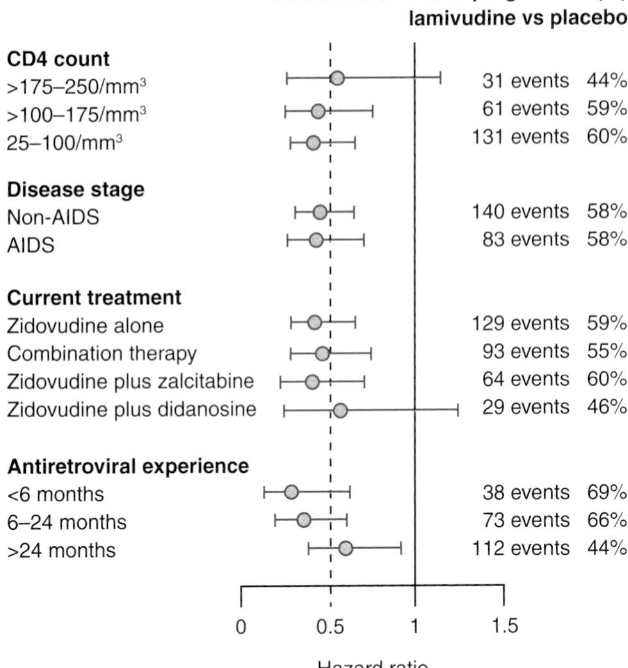

Figure 9-4 ■ Reduction in relative risk of disease progression in subjects treated with 3TC-containing combinations compared to subjects treated with placebo. Subjects entered the study on ZDV, ZDV/ddI, or ZDV/ddC and had either placebo, 3TC, or 3TC plus loviride added to this regimen. Open circle represents the percent reduction in relative risk with 95% confidence intervals represented by the horizontal lines. Observations for which the confidence interval extends across unity (1) are not statistically significant. The number of subjects in some of the categories was small, limiting the power of the observation.

Adapted from Anonymous. Randomised trial of addition of lamivudine or lamivudine plus loviride to zidovudine-containing regimens for patients with HIV-1 infection: the CAESAR trial. Lancet 349:1413–21, 1997.

where the study took place, enrolled subjects receiving ZDV alone or in combination with ddI or ddC and with a CD4+ T-lymphocyte count of 25–250 cells/mm^3. More than 1800 subjects were randomized to receive placebo, 3TC (150 mg twice daily), or 3TC/loviride (100 mg three times daily), an NNRTI. Subjects were randomized in a 1:2:1 fashion so half the subjects added 3TC alone to their ZDV-containing regimen. The median duration of antiretroviral treatment prior to study entry was 28 months, and most subjects (62%) were on ZDV alone at baseline. The study was terminated prematurely at a second interim analysis because of the statistically significant benefit of 3TC in reducing the relative risk of disease progression compared to placebo. In the final intent-to-treat analysis, the relative reduction in risk of progression to AIDS or death was 57% (relative hazard (RH) = 0.43) for 3TC-containing arms compared to placebo. There was also a 60% reduction in mortality for the 3TC-containing arms compared to placebo. The addition of loviride to the 3TC regimen appeared to offer no benefit in the overall analysis of clinical progression. When the relative risk reduction of 3TC compared to placebo was examined for various subgroups (e.g., CD4+ T-lymphocyte count, AIDS vs non-AIDS, treatment at study entry, duration of antiretroviral experience), a consistent risk reduction of ~50% was seen (Fig. 9-4). The greatest risk reduction was seen in subjects who had received less than 6 months of previous antiretroviral therapy. The CAESAR study clearly demonstrated that the antiretroviral effects of 3TC that had been seen in earlier studies are translated into clinical benefit, as suggested by smaller studies [91,93] and seen with other antiretroviral therapies.[94] Future studies of combination regimens would soon eclipse the outcomes achieved with dual NRTI regimens.

3TC IN HAART COMBINATIONS

3TC in Combination with NNRTIs

Antiretroviral Effects and Effects on CD4+ T-Lymphocyte Counts

Effect on Disease Progression and Mortality

The International AIDS Society-USA Panel and the Department of Health and Human Services Guidelines Panel 2006 recommendations for choice of initial HIV treatment regimen suggest the utilization of 2 NRTIs combined with either an nNRTI or a PI boosted with low-dose RTV.[22] The continued relevance of 3TC's and FTC's role in contemporary HIV management is validated by its inclusion in two of the three recommended choices for the dual nNRTI component of initial HAART regimens (3TC /ABC, 3TC /ZDV).[22]

3TC in Combination with Protease Inhibitors

Antiretroviral Effects and Effects on CD4+ T-Lymphocyte Counts

The demonstration of enhanced antiretroviral effect and clinical benefit of combination nucleoside therapy,[94,95] especially ZDV and 3TC,[57,92] in conjunction with the clinical development of protease inhibitors[96–99] has dramatically altered the design of clinical research trials and ultimately of recommendations for clinical practice.[100,101] HAART regimens, which most commonly consist of two nucleosides in combination with a RTV boosted protease inhibitor, or an NNRTI is the standard of care in developed countries.[22,25,102]

Multiple trials of 3TC in combination with ZDV or d4T and an unboosted protease inhibitor demonstrated the potent activity of these combinations. One of the earliest of these studies was a trial that compared 3TC/ZDV/indinavir with ZDV/3TC and with indinavir alone.[103] In this double-blind study, 97 subjects who had previously received ZDV for at least 6 months (median previous treatment for 30 months) were randomized to have 3TC added to their ZDV, to have 3TC and indinavir added, or to switch to indinavir alone. Subjects had CD4+ T-lymphocyte counts of 50–400 cells/mm^3

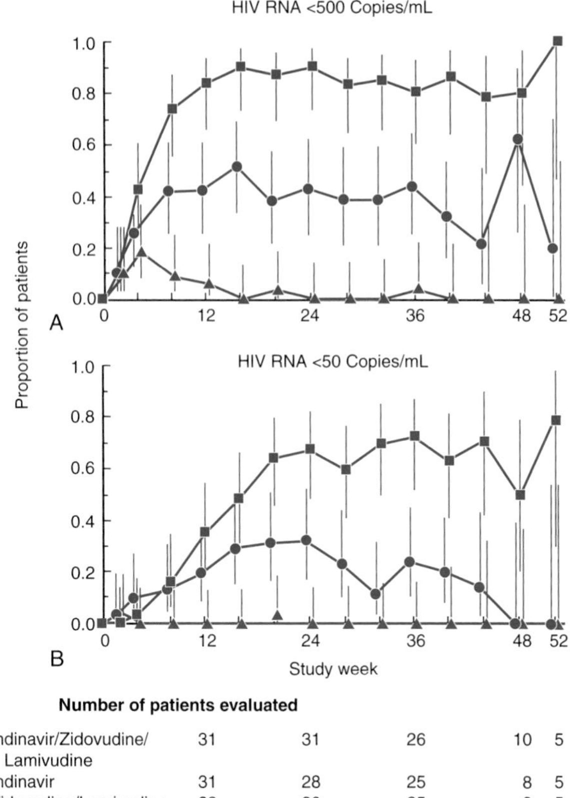

Figure 9-5 ■ Proportion of subjects who achieved HIV-1 RNA levels of less than 500 copies/mL (top graph) or 50 copies/mm (lower graph) when treated with indinavir alone, ZDV/3TC, or ZDV/3TC/indinavir. Subjects in this study had received more than 6 months of ZDV prior to randomization. The number listed below the study week is the number of patients evaluated at that study week. The diminishing number reflects the number of subjects on study long enough to have reached that time point and does not represent dropout from the study.

Adapted from Gulick RM, Mellors JW, Havlir D, et al. Treatment with a combination of indinavir, zidovudine and lamivudine in HIV-1 infected adults with prior antiretroviral use. N Engl J Med 337:734–9, 1997.

and a plasma HIV-1 level of more than 20 000 copies/mL. The median CD4+ T-lymphocyte count at entry was 144 cells/mm^3, and the median HIV-1 RNA level was 43 000 copies/mL. Subjects treated with the three-drug regimen had a more profound antiretroviral response than previously described. HIV RNA levels decreased to less than 500 copies/mL (the limit of quantification of the assay) in 90% of subjects after 24 weeks of therapy (Fig. 9-5). No subject who received only 3TC/ZDV had this level of response, whereas 43% of subjects on indinavir monotherapy were below quantification levels at 24 weeks. Approximately 70% of subjects on the three-drug therapy after 24 weeks were below detection limits when a more sensitive assay that could quantify HIV RNA in plasma to ~50 copies/mL was used (Fig. 9-5). CD4 cell changes were not significantly different between the indinavir arm and the three-drug therapy arm, although both were superior to ZDV/3TC. Follow-up of subjects on the three-drug therapy arm is ongoing, and two-thirds of subjects originally assigned to three-drug therapy have had their HIV RNA levels remain at less than 50 copies/mL through 3 years of therapy.[16,104] Similar results (although for a shorter time period) were seen with d4T/3TC and indinavir.[105]

Another trial including unboosted protease inhibitors in a population of HIV-infected individuals with more advanced disease, found the combination of 3TC/ZDV/indinavir to have pronounced antiretroviral activity.[106] In a trial design similar to the one already described,[103] subjects were enrolled with CD4+ T-lymphocyte counts of less than 50 cells/mm^3 and more than 6 months of ZDV experience. In this trial more than half of the subjects (56%) on three-drug therapy had HIV RNA levels of less than 500 copies/mL and 45% were less than 50 copies/mL after 6 months of treatment. Nelfinavir, a peptidomimetic protease inhibitor with good *in vitro* activity and a favorable toxicity profile *in vivo*, has been studied in several trials.[107–109] The largest of these trials enrolled subjects with no previous antiretroviral experience and compared 3TC/ZDV/nelfinavir to 3TC/ZDV alone with respect to the effect of treatment on HIV RNA levels and CD4+ T-lymphocyte counts.[108,109] Responses to 3TC/ ZDV/ nelfinavir were significantly better than those to 3TC/ZDV, as measured by changes in HIV RNA levels and the proportion of subjects with undetectable levels at 6 months.

The drugs 3TC and ZDV have also been studied with RTV (*see* Chapter 16), a potent protease inhibitor that has been shown to delay clinical progression in patients with advanced HIV disease.[110] Markowitz et al investigated the effects of 3TC/ZDV/RTV in acutely infected HIV-positive patients using an open-label study design.[111] This three-drug combination was highly active in the 12 patients studied for up to 240 days on therapy. The effects of 3TC/ZDV/RTV on immune response, immune function, and viral dynamics were investigated in an intensive study of ZDV-experienced subjects.[112–114] At 48 weeks the HIV RNA levels were less than 100 copies/mL in 59% (20/34 subjects), and CD4+ T-lymphocytes increased by almost 200 cells/mm^3.[113] RTV is currently most commonly used in low dose in combination with other protease inhibitors.[22]

The antiretroviral effects of 3TC/ZDV or d4T have also been demonstrated with saquinavir soft gel capsules (SQV-SGC), amprenavir, indinavir and lopinavir/RTV.[115–119] Overall, there appears to be no suggestion that the antiretroviral efficacy seen with 3TC containing PI-based regimens is better when 3TC is paired with a particular PI or with ZDV rather than d4T. Whether the antiretroviral potency of two NRTIs plus a PI is greater when one of the nucleosides is 3TC has also not been definitively demonstrated.

The utilization of RTV boosted protease inhibitors represents the current standard of care in developed countries.[22] A double-blind trial comparing HIV-infected adults not on HAART for 14 days compared 3TC/D4T/LPV-RTV versus 3TC/D4T/NFV or 3TC/D4T/nelfinavir-placebo found superior antiviral activity (persistent virologic response at 48 weeks) in the 3TC/D4T/LPV-RTV group.[120]

An open-label noninferiority study of 878 HIV-1-infected patients compared the two regimens co-formulation 3TC/ABC and LPV-RTV versus co-formulation 3TC/ABC and fosamprenavir-RTV. At 48 weeks the primary endpoints of proportion of patients reaching HIV-1 RNA levels <400 copies/mL and the proportion of discontinuations due to adverse events concluded that the fosamprenavir-RTV regimen provided similar antiviral efficacy, safety and tolerability.[121]

Lamivudine has and will continue to play an important role as part of the NRTI backbone to HAART with newer protease inhibitors and other therapeutic classes.

Effect on Disease Progression and Mortality

The positive effect of 3TC/ZDV/indinavir on the clinical outcomes of disease progression and survival was established by ACTG 320.[17] In that study the subjects had CD4+ T-lymphocyte counts of 200 cells/mm^3 or less, had been treated with at least 3 months of ZDV, were naive to 3TC and indinavir, and were randomized to receive ZDV/3TC or ZDV/3TC/indinavir. Of the 1156 subjects in the study, 38% had CD4+ T-lymphocyte counts of 50 cells/mm^3 or less and a mean HIV RNA level of 100 000 copies/mL. Stavudine could be substituted for ZDV if a subject was intolerant to ZDV. The study was halted prematurely when a predefined clinical benefit was noted at an interim analysis. In the final analysis, the proportion of subjects who progressed to a new AIDS endpoint or death was 6% (33 subjects) for 3TC/ZDV/indinavir compared to 11% (63 subjects) for 3TC ($P = 0.001$) indinavir (Table 9-1). Only eight subjects (1.4%) died on the triple-therapy arm, whereas 18 subjects (3.1%) died on 3TC/ZDV ($P = 0.04$). The results were similar when the treatment arms were compared in subjects with less than 50 CD4+ T lymphocytes/mm^3 and in subjects with counts of 50–200 cells/mm^3 at baseline (Table 9-1). Effects on CD4+ T-lymphocyte counts and HIV-1 RNA levels in plasma paralleled the clinical results. These results confirmed the clinical benefit that was anticipated from the substantial antiretroviral effects of 3TC/ZDV/indinavir seen previously.

3TC in Combination with Other RT Inhibitors

Lamivudine has been studied with two other NRTIs or with one additional NRTI and an NNRTI. A significantly larger proportion of individuals treated with 3TC in combination with ZDV and EFV had HIV RNA levels that fell below 400 copies/mL at 48 weeks than those treated with IDV/3TC/ZDV or with IDV/EFV (70% vs 48% vs 53%, respectively). The simplicity of this regimen with ZDV/3TC given twice daily without regard to meals and EFV given once daily compared with the more complex dosing of IDV-containing regimens may have contributed to the success of the 3TC/NNRTI-containing arm. 3TC has also been studied in combination with ZDV and DLV. In that study approximately two-thirds of subjects had HIV RNA levels below detectable limits at 52 weeks. This triple therapy was superior to either ZDV/3TC or DLV/ZDV.[122] Nevirapine with 3TC and ZDV has also been shown to be highly active therapy, even in individuals with HIV RNA levels of more than 100 000 copies/mL in a comparative study with NFV/3TC/ZDV.[123] A study that compared sequential three-drug regimens as initial therapy for HIV-1 infection (3TC/ZDV or ddI/d4T combined with either NFV or EFV) with a primary endpoint of length of time to failure of the second three-drug regimen, found that the combination of 3TC/ZDV/EFV resulted in a shorted time to viral suppression and significantly delayed both the first and second virologic failures.[19] This study showed no difference in CD4 increase from baseline in the different

Table 9-1 Rates of Disease Progression in the ACTG 320 Trial

Condition	ZDV/IDV/3TC (no.)	ZDV/3TC (no.)	Hazard Ratio[a]	P[b]
All subjects	577	579		
AIDS or death	33 (6%)	63 (11%)	0.50 (0.33–0.76)	0.001
Death	8 (1%)	18 (3%)	0.43 (0.19–0.99)	0.042
CD4+ count 50 cells/mm^3	219	220		
AIDS or death	23 (11%)	44 (20%)	0.49 (0.30–0.82)	0.005
Death	5 (2%)	13 (6%)	0.37 (0.13–1.04)	0.51
CD4+ count 51–200 cells/mm^3	358	359		
AIDS or death	10 (3%)	19 (5%)	0.51 (0.24–1.10)	0.08
Death	3 (1%)	5 (1%)	0.59 (0.14–2.46)	0.46

[a]Numbers in parentheses are 95% confidence intervals.
[b]Log-rank test.

Adapted from Hammer SM, Squires K, Hughes M, et al. A randomized, placebo-controlled trial of indinavir in combination with two nucleoside analogs in human immunodeficiency virus infected persons with CD4 cell counts less than or equal to 200 per cubic millimeter. N Engl J Med 337:725–33, 1997.

groups, but did show that a regimen including 3TC/ZDV delayed the occurrence of a first serious toxic effect (= grade 3, necessitating a change in regimen, $P < 0.001$ for the four-way comparison) as compared to one containing ddI/d4T.[19] More recently an open-label study successfully proved the noninferiority of FTC/TDF/EFV with 3TC/ZDV/EFV.[23] The data showed FTC/TDF/EFV achieved superior viral suppression (80% vs 70% reaching levels below 50 copies/mL), CD4 response and adverse events; but better tolerance of this regimen may explain these differences rather than intrinsic antiretroviral properties of the agents used.[22,23] Studies such as the ACTG 5202 (phase IIIB randomized, four arm study for treatment-naive patients) may help elucidate any differences that exist in these combinations when utilized as initial HIV therapy.

Lamivudine has been a key component of the HIV therapeutic approach using three nucleoside analogs. 3TC/ZDV/abacavir (ABV) has been compared to 3TC/ZDV/IDV in two randomized studies (one double-blind and one open label). In the double-blind study the two regimens were equivalent when the primary endpoint of HIV RNA levels of less than 400 copies/mL at 48 weeks was evaluated. However, in subjects with baseline HIV RNA levels higher than 100 000 copies/mL significantly fewer subjects on triple nucleoside had levels lower than 50 copies/mL at 48 weeks compared to those treated with 3TC/ZDV/IDV.[124] In contrast, when these two regimens were compared in an open-label fashion, the 3TC-containing triple-nucleoside therapy was at least as effective as 3TC/ZDV/IDV even in those with baseline HIV RNA levels of more than 100 000 copies/mL.[125] A clear suggestion from these two studies is that a convenient therapy such as 3TC/ZDV/ABV may make up with enhanced adherence what it may lose if antiretroviral potency is less. 3TC has also been tested with ddI and d4T as a triple nucleoside compared with ddI/d4T with either IDV or NVP.[126] Subjects in this study had low baseline HIV RNA levels (median 4.2 $\log_{10}$ copies/mL; interquartile range 3.8–4.8 $\log_{10}$ copies/mL). Nonetheless, there were no significant differences between treatment arms in the proportion of all subjects randomized who achieved HIV RNA levels of less than 50 copies/mm at 48 weeks. With higher viral loads (upper quartile with baseline values >4.8 $\log_{10}$ (~58 000) copies/mL) the proportions of subjects on both the 3TC- and NVP-containing arms with HIV RNA levels of less than 50 copies/mL at 48 weeks were less than with IDV (26% and 28% compared with 42%). When a less than 500 copies/mL cutoff was used, few differences were seen between arms.

The triple nucleoside regimen of 3TC/ZDV/ABC was compared to a regimen of 3TC/ZDV/EFV and 3TC/ZDV/ABC/EFV in a randomized, double-blind study (ACTG 5095) of initial HIV therapy in 1147 subjects (mean HIV-1 RNA 4.85 $\log_{10}$ or 71 434 copies/mL, mean CD4 cell count of 238 per mL). After a median follow-up of 32 weeks the data and safety monitoring board recommended to stop the triple nucleoside group and to compare its results to that of the pooled EFV groups. Virologic failure defined in this protocol as two successive HIV-1 RNA values of 200 copies/mL at 16 weeks, occurred in the 3TC/ZDV/ABC group in 21% (82 of 382) of subjects, compared to 11% (85 of 765) in the combined EFV groups. Changes in CD4 cell count and incidence of grade 3 or 4 adverse events did not differ significantly. The triple nucleoside combination of 3TC/ZDV/ABC was found to be virologically inferior (greater proportion of virologic failure, shorter time to virologic failure) than a regimen containing EFV and either 2 or 3 nucleosides.[18]

Contrary to earlier data, triple nRTI regimens are now considered inferior to both NNRTI or RTV-boosted PI regimens, and their use is limited to specific circumstances (high risk of toxicity, nonadherence to other regimens, drug interactions and others).[18,22]

Seven hundred and sixty-five of the patients from the initial ACTG 5095 were followed from Mar 2001 to Mar 2005. The group of patients on 3TC/ZDV/ABC/EFV was compared to the group on 3TC/ZDV/EFV seeking to investigate whether a four drug (three nucleosides and an nNRTI) regimen could improve antiretroviral activity. In treatment-naive patients time to virologic failure, CD4 cell increases and grade 3 or 4 adverse events were not significantly different.[127] Another randomized trial that sought to investigate the difference in outcomes in three-drug (3TC/ZDV/EFV) and four-drug (3TC/ZDV/ABC/EFV) regimens in antiretroviral-naive patients (QUAD Study) found no differences at 48 weeks in viral load suppression and CD4 increase.[128] To date there is no proven benefit of four-drug regimens over the three-drug combinations (2 NRTI and nNRTI or boosted-PI) that constitute the current standard of care.[22] At this time, a combination regimen of 3TC/ZDV/TDF is under investigation and quadruple nRTI regimens (3TC/ZDV/ABC/TDF) are considered experimental.[129,130]

3TC Co-Formulations and Dosing Strategies

The results from the open-label trial of 3TC/ZDV/ABV compared to 3TC/ZDV/IDV support the hypothesis that among treatments of similar potency a simpler regimen would be more successful. To that end, simplification of 3TC-based therapy has been an important focus of HIV clinical research. 3TC has been combined with ZDV in a fixed-dose combination (FDC) tablet. Despite reducing the pill burden by only two pills per day, this FDC tablet is widely used. Switching from separate dosing of ZDV and 3TC to the FDC ZDV/3TC combine in the setting of ongoing HAART resulted in fewer virologic failures over 16 weeks than among those who remained on separate dosing, although the number of overall failures was small.[131] The FDC 3TC/ZDV/ABV (Trizivir) has now also been developed and is approved for use in the United States, providing an acceptable HAART regimen[102] as a single pill twice a day. In a trial design similar to the one used to test the FDC ZDV/3TC, switching to the FDC ZDV/3TC/ABV from the FDC ZDV/3TC and ABV did not compromise viral suppression.[132] Changing from successful combination therapy that predominantly contained a protease inhibitor to the FDC 3TC/ZDV/ABV also appeared not to compromise activity, and it improved blood lipids and adherence to the regimen.[133] The triple nucleoside combination of ZDV/3TC/ABC was shown to be inferior to 3TC/ZDV/EFV and 3TC/ZDV/ABC/EFV and is used solely when other concomitant conditions (toxicities, noncompliance or other) inhibit the utilization of the recommended dual-class regimens.[18,22]

Data suggesting that the intracellular half-life of 3TC-TP is well above 12 h,[39] studies have been undertaken to examine 3TC given once daily. In a small study ($n = 81$) in which subjects on HAART with HIV RNA levels of less than 400 copies/mL were randomly assigned to switch to once-daily 3TC (300 mg qd) or remain on twice-daily 3TC (150 mg bid), 95% of subjects had less than 400 copies/mL on once-daily 3TC compared to 90% on the twice-daily regimen. No sustained rebounds in viral load to more than 1200 copies/mL were seen in either arm.[134]

In August 2004, the combination of lamivudine and ABV was released as a FDC once a day tablet. A trial of 265 HIV-infected subjects on twice-daily 3TC and ABC plus either a PI or NNRTI for a median time of 22 months (median viral load <50 copies/mL, median CD4 554 cells/mm) were randomized to either continuing their twice-daily 3TC/ABC regimen or receiving FDC 3TC/ABC. FDC 3TC/ABC was established as not inferior to its twice-daily counterpart in this trial.[135]

PEDIATRIC TRIALS

The antiretroviral activity and the effect of 3TC on disease progression have also been evaluated in pediatric patients. The clinical activity of 3TC plus ZDV was assessed in ACTG 300 along with two other treatments: ddI monotherapy and ddI/ZDV.[136] Didanosine and ddI/ZDV were included initially, but enrollment in the ddI/ZDV arm was stopped when the results of an earlier ACTG pediatric study (ACTG 152) suggested that treatment with ddI and ddI/ZDV I had comparable clinical efficacy. A total of 596 symptomatic children ages 6 weeks to 15 years and naive to antiretroviral treatment were enrolled. The primary endpoint was time to first progression of HIV disease or death. The 3TC/ZDV combination was significantly more effective that ddI alone in terms of both the overall combined endpoint (38 vs 15 deaths; $P < 0.001$) and survival (15 vs 3 deaths; $P = 0.004$). A mere profound effect of 3TC/ZDV on growth rates, CD4+ T-lymphocyte changes, and HIV-1 RNA levels were all consistent with the primary outcome.

As in the adult population, the combination of nucleoside analogs (including 3TC/ZDV) with a PI appears to have a more potent antiretroviral effect in HIV-infected children. In nucleoside-experienced children who had less than 4 weeks of ZDV/3TC, ZDV/3TC/ RTV had superior antiretroviral effects compared to either ZDV/3TC or d4T/RTV as measured by the proportion of subjects with HIV RNA levels less than 400 copies/mL at 48 weeks of therapy.[137] A trial evaluating the safety, tolerability and activity of three antiretroviral regimens (3TC/ZDV/nevirapine, 3TC/ZDV/ABC/nevirapine, 3TC/D4T/nevirapine/nelfinavir) in the 3-month or older age groups found that the 3TC/D4T/nevirapine/nelfinavir regimen was associated with improved long-term viral suppression.[138] Overall, the experience with 3TC in HIV-1-infected children is similar to that in adults.

LAMIVUDINE IN HEPATITIS B AND HEPATITIS B/HIV CO-INFECTION

Lamivudine was approved in 1998 by the FDA for the treatment of HBV, and has shown efficacy in several categories of HBV infected patients. In HBeAg-positive chronic hepatitis-B patient studies comparing differing doses of lamivudine to placebo, histologic, virologic, and biochemical parameters showed improvement at 1 year; and a daily dose of 100 mg a day was more effective than 25 mg a day.[139,140] Despite these improvements, lamivudine monotherapy had low rates of HBeAg seroconversion, an important goal of HBV therapy as it is associated with histological improvement, increased complication free and overall survival.[141] A combination trial of peg-interferon alfa-2a alone and in combination with lamivudine was compared with lamivudine alone in a multicenter, randomized, partially double-blind study of 814 patients.[142] The results of this trial showed no statistically significant differences in efficacy (rates of sustained HBeAg, HBsAg, virologic, and biochemical response) between peg-interferon alfa-2a alone and in combination with lamivudine, but both outperformed lamivudine alone.[142] Recent comparisons of lamivudine versus entecavir in HBeAg-positive patients have shown improved rates of HBeAg seroconversion and viral, biochemical and histologic responses favoring entecavir.[143]

Trials in HBeAg-negative patients comparing peg-interferon alfa 2a alone versus lamivudine versus both in combination have shown improved efficacy of both peg-interferon groups (regarding ability for sustained virologic, biochemical, and HBsAg response rates) and concluded that the addition of lamivudine to peg-interferon alfa 2a does not increase response rates.[144,145] Comparisons of entecavir versus lamivudine (and no prior history of therapy with nucleoside analogs) monotherapy in HBeAg-negative patients have favored entecavir therapy with improved virologic/histologic responses and higher rates of normalization of alanine aminotransferase levels.[146]

HIV–HBV co-infection are common worldwide.[147] Hepatic morbidity is significantly greater in HIV–HBV co-infected persons.[148,149] Decision to treat these patients must weigh multiple factors including both the status of HBV and the need for HAART. If 3TC is administered for HBV (approved at 100 mg per day, HIV treatment doses (150 mg bid or 300 mg per day) are recommended.[149,150] In the setting of HIV–HBV co-infection, due to the high incidence of development of 3TC resistance when this is used a monotherapy, its use is recommended as part of a combination HAART regimens including another HBV active agent (e.g., TDF).[150] Special considerations in HBV-HIV co-infected patients include HBV flares with discontinuation of 3TC or other HBV active component of HAART[149–152] and immune reconstitution mediated flares of liver disease related to a favorable response to HAART.[149,153]

A study comparing lamivudine (3 mg/kg; maximum 100 mg) to placebo in children with chronic hepatitis-B infection also found higher rates of virologic response (23% with 3TC vs 13% with placebo, $p = 0.04$) in the 3TC group.[154] 3TC therapy has also shown virologic and biochemical improvement in HBeAg-negative chronic hepatitis-B and HBsAg positive patients with clinical cirrhosis.[155,156] Further trials of 3TC in combination with other agents in pediatric HBV or HIV-HBV co-infections are needed.

In summary, the effectiveness of 3TC as monotherapy for HBV infections is inferior to that of other agents such as interferon alpha-2a or entecavir. Further trials of 3TC in combination regimens will serve to better define its goal in the therapy of HBV. In the setting of HBV-HIV co-infection, 3TC may be used as part of HAART in combination with other HIV-HBV active agents such as tenofovir. The preferred dose of lamivudine is 300 mg once daily though 150 mg twice daily can be used when clinically indicated.

RESISTANCE

High-level resistance to 3TC develops rapidly *in vitro*[83,157–159] and *in vivo*.[59,159–161] ZDV-sensitive and ZDV-resistant HIV-1 isolates passaged *in vitro* in the presence of 3TC (or a related compound 2′,3′-dideoxy-5-fluoro-3′-thiacytidine FTC or emtricitabine) (*see* Chapter 10) rapidly developed resistance to 3TC.[83,157–159] Some isolates in these experiments had more than 1000-fold decreases in sensitivity to 3TC and FTC. Sequence changes in the RT gene occurred only at codon 184, with a change from the wild-type methionine to either valine or isoleucine. Site-directed mutagenesis studies confirmed that these substitutions conveyed high-level resistance to 3TC.[83,157] The location of the 3TC resistance mutation in the RT enzyme lies within a highly conserved amino acid motif (YMDD), which is the polymerase active site of the enzyme.[162] Previous mutagenesis studies had shown that certain mutations in this location severely impaired function of the RT.[163,164] However, RNA transcriptases and RNA-dependent DNA transcriptases from many RNA viruses and retroviruses have conserved regions in their active site with a YXDD motif, where X can represent several amino acids.[165] These observations suggest that this position may 'tolerate' the most variability in this highly conserved region. Subsequent studies suggest that the HIV that is wild type at codon 184 may have a small growth advantage over virus with the M184V mutation.[166,167] M184V variants do propagate *in vitro* in the absence of 3TC selective pressure, although growth may be attenuated.[168] HIV-1 with the M184V mutation, however, appears to have a significant growth advantage over virus with the methionine to isoleucine change.[166] RT with the M184V mutation and the M184I mutation may have increased fidelity and decreased catalytic efficiency compared to wild-type RT.[167,169–171] The degree and importance of the increase in fidelity of HIV RT with the M184V mutation is uncertain, although some aspects of the treatment responses to 3TC might be explained by this phenomenon (see further ahead).

In vivo, 3TC resistance was noted to occur rapidly when this drug was administered as monotherapy,[70] and it corresponds to an increase in HIV-1 RNA levels seen after 2–4 weeks (Figs 9-2A and 9-3), although levels do not return immediately to baseline. The first mutation that appears is typically the M184I mutation. Variants with this mutation are in general rapidly replaced by resistant variants with the methionine-to-valine change (Fig. 9-2B).[70] This observation may be explained by the fact that the isoleucine change requires only one nucleotide change from the wild type, and these variants may exist in extremely low numbers even in previously untreated patients, as has been postulated for resistance mutations to nevirapine.[172] The replacement of variants with the isoleucine change by variants with valine at codon 184 may occur because viruses with the M184V mutation have a growth advantage over virus with M184I.[166]

Emergence of viral variants with 3TC resistance also occurs rapidly in subjects treated with ZDV and 3TC (Fig. 9-6).[59,161,166] By 12 weeks of therapy most subjects treated with ZDV/3TC acquire variants with 3TC resistance if they were naive to previous therapy (Fig. 9-6).[161,166] Similar emergence of resistance to 3TC has been seen in subjects who had 3TC added to chronic ZDV therapy.[59]

In contrast to dual ZDV/3TC therapy, when 3TC is used in potent three-drug combinations, emergence of 3TC resistance is delayed in most subjects.[103] The likely explanation for this observation is that with marked suppression of viral replication the rate of mutation appearance, which is a result of the error rate of the RT multiplied by the replication rate, is substantially reduced. Resistance to 3TC occurs in a small

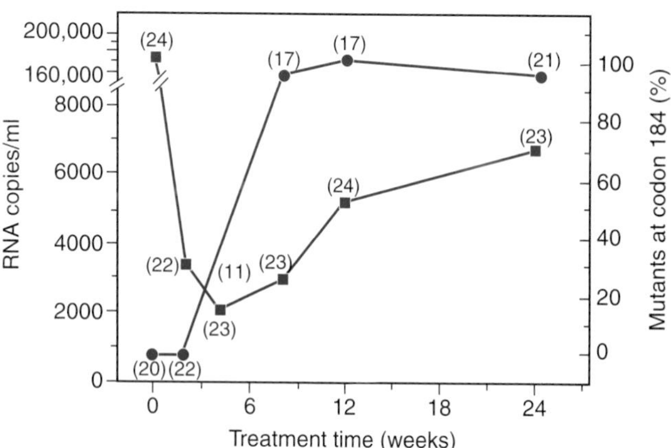

Figure 9-6 ■ The change over time in HIV-1 RNA levels in subjects treated with 3TC plus ZDV (*n*). The proportion of subjects with mutant virus at codon 184 are also shown (*l*). The numbers in parentheses represent the number of subjects contributing data at each time point.

Adapted from Larder BA, Kemp SD, Harrigan PR. Potential mechanism for sustained antiretroviral efficacy of AZT-3TC combination therapy. Science 269:696–9, 1995.

number of individuals receiving three-drug combination therapy and appears to occur in the setting of incomplete suppression of replication.[103]

Despite the rapid emergence of 3TC resistance, combination therapy with 3TC/ZDV has potent, and prolonged antiretroviral effects.[57,173] Introduction of the 3TC-resistance mutation at codon 184 into the genome of HIV-1 that contains ZDV-resistance mutations results in virions that have regained susceptibility to ZDV.[83,166] The antiretroviral and clinical effects observed when 3TC is added to ZDV therapy[58,59,92] and the fact that baseline ZDV resistance does not diminish the activity of ZDV/3TC and PI combinations[103,174] may be explained in part by this resensitization phenomenon. In addition, the prolonged effect of the ZDV/3TC combination may be due to persistent phenotypic sensitivity of HIV-1 to ZDV in treated individuals, despite the presence of ZDV resistance mutations.[173] Initiation of ZDV and 3TC simultaneously with the resultant selection of 3TC resistance would decrease the selective advantage of ZDV-resistance mutations, and indeed initial treatment with ZDV/3TC delays ZDV resistance (Fig. 9-7).[161] Subjects receiving this combination had a delay in the appearance of the codon 70 mutation, which is typically the first ZDV-resistance mutation to appear[175] and is associated with initial loss of antiretroviral activity of ZDV.[176] During a prolonged follow-up, the proportion of subjects with ZDV-resistance mutations was less when the ZDV/3TC-treated group was compared to those treated with ZDV alone.[173]

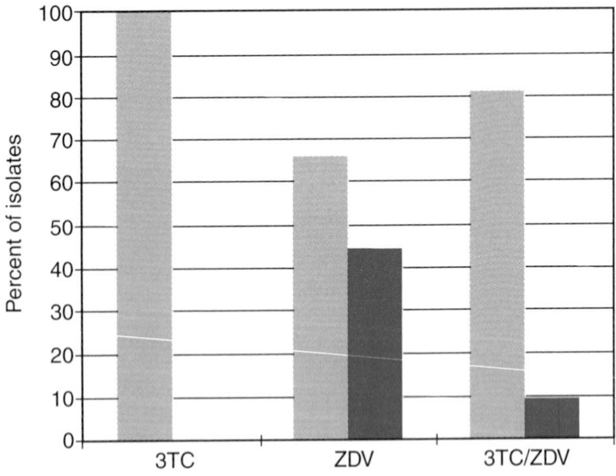

Figure 9-7 ■ Isolates were obtained from subjects treated with 3TC or ZDV alone or 3TC/ZDV as part of a larger study.[32] The percentage of HIV-1 isolates obtained at week 12 of treatment that were found to be wild type (shaded bars) or mutants (solid bars) at codon 70 of the RT gene for each treatment regimen are shown. The proportion of subjects who acquired a mutation at codon 70 when treated with 3TC/ZDV was significantly lower than the proportion seen in subjects treated with ZDV alone ($P = 0.009$).

Adapted from Kuritzkes DR, Quinn JB, Benoit SL, et al. Drug resistance and virologic response in NUCA 3001, a randomized trial of lamivudine [3TC] versus zidovudine [ZDV] versus ZDV plus 3TC in previously untreated patients. AIDS 10:975–81, 1996.

The mechanism by which 3TC resensitizes the ZDV-resistance virus is now becoming clearer. ZDV resistance has been incompletely understood. Multiple mutations in RT lead to HIV with high-level resistance to ZDV in cell culture, [177,178] although mutant RT enzymes remain sensitive to ZDV-TP, as measured by ZDV-MP incorporation.[179,180] However, the mutant RT has increased ability to remove ZDV-MP from blocked primers through a nucleotide-dependent or pyrophosphate-dependent reaction, which allows continued extension of the elongating HIV DNA and results in the phenotype of ZDV resistance.[181,182] The M184V mutation in the HIV RT impairs this rescue of chain termination[183] and therefore leads to increased susceptibility to ZDV in the presence of ZDV-resistance mutations. The resensitization of ZDV resistance by phosphonoformic acid-resistance mutations has been demonstrated to occur by this pathway.[184] The similar antiretroviral activity of 3TC/d4T when compared to 3TC/ZDV was difficult to explain if the mutational interaction of 3TC with ZDV was responsible for the enhanced activity and prolonged effect of that combination.[88] Kuritzkes and his colleagues have demonstrated that 'ZDV-resistance mutations' lead to a similar degree of resistance to d4T when inhibition of wild-type and mutant HIV RT is carefully studied.[89] Potentially, a similar mutational interaction between M184V and the thymidine-resistance mutations that lead to d4T resistance might occur, explaining the potent and prolonged activity of this dual nucleoside combination.

There may be several other mechanisms for the activity of 3TC/ZDV and 3TC/d4T combinations, which have been shown to inhibit HIV-1 replication in a synergistic manner *in vitro*.[11,13] In addition, thymidine analogs and 3TC are converted to their respective active metabolites with different avidities depending on the state of activation of the cell the drugs are entering. Thymidine analogs enter and are phosphorylated preferentially in activated lymphocytes, whereas cytosine analogs are phosphorylated more efficiently in resting lymphocytes than in activated cells.[38,185]

Despite all of the above favorable interactions between 3TC and ZDV, dual resistance to ZDV and 3TC has been clearly documented.[173,186–189] This type of resistance has usually been demonstrated in the setting of adding 3TC to prolonged ZDV therapy,[186–189] but it can also be seen with prolonged combination therapy when the two agents are initiated simultaneously.[173] The pathway to dual resistance seems variable. Mutations at RT codons 333 and 210, among others, have been implicated.[186,190]

Other pathways to 3TC resistance also exist. HIV-1 variants that are resistant to multiple nucleoside analogs, including 3TC, have been described. These variants typically have one of two mutation patterns: a family of insertions at or around codon 69[191] or a group of mutations anchored by a mutation at RT codon 151.[192] Novel mutations have been shown to be associated with low to moderate levels of 3TC resistance.[193] Mutations at codon 44 and 118 were associated with this level of 3TC resistance when a group of HIV-1 variants were examined. These mutations were typically associated with two well described thymidine-resistance mutations at codon 41 and 215. These observations were confirmed by site-directed mutagenesis,[193] and the occurrence of this pattern of mutations may be more common with a particular sequence of nucleoside administration.

The mutation that confers resistance to lamivudine at codon 184 has been shown *in vitro* to result in a low level of cross-resistance to ddI and ddC in some studies[158] but not in others.[83,159] A clinical impact of this possible low level of cross-resistance has been difficult to demonstrate. In a cross-sectional survey of HIV-1 variants from nucleoside-experienced patients in which both phenotype and genotype were determined, the presence of the M184V mutation was not associated with ddI or ddC cross-resistance.[194] However, the cutoff for phenotypic resistance was a fivefold increase in IC_{50} from the wild type, and smaller changes in IC_{50} may be clinically important for the dideoxynucleosides (ddI, d4T, ddC).

An aspect of 3TC antiretroviral activity and resistance that has yet to be fully explained is the apparent antiretroviral activity of 3TC despite emergence of the M184V mutation that results in extremely high-level resistance *in vitro*. In the initial study of 3TC monotherapy, persistent antiretroviral activity was noted after the appearance of the codon 184 mutation.[70] One treatment arm in the North American trial of 3TC/ZDV in treatment-naive individuals was 3TC monotherapy.[57] In a subset of these subjects from whom virology data were obtained, most subjects had acquired the 3TC resistance mutation at codon 184 of the RT by 12 weeks of therapy.[161] Despite this observation, the mean decrease in HIV-1 RNA in this group had not returned to baseline even after 6 months of treatment (Fig. 9-3), which suggested there was a persistent antiretroviral effect of 3TC despite the appearance of resistance. Also subjects from this study who received ZDV/3TC had more potent antiretroviral effects on average than those who received ZDV long after the appearance of 3TC resistance.[161] Explanations for these observations are speculative, though the M184V mutation may modestly decrease the replication capacity of viral variants with this mutation.[166] In addition, the M184V mutation appears to improve the fidelity of the RT enzyme in some experimental models.[167,169–171,195] Increased fidelity might be expected to decrease the appearance of mutations in progeny virus.[167] Other studies have shown persistence of antiviral activity of 3TC despite the development of a 184 mutation, and current recommendations allow for continued use of 3TC despite the presence of resistance, in salvage regimens.[22,78–82]

DRUG INTERACTIONS

Drug interactions between 3TC and other antiretroviral agents or other medications are uncommon (Table 9-2). A 43% increase in area under the concentration–time curve (AUC infinity) and a 35% decrease in renal clearance were observed when lamivudine was co-administered with trimethoprim–sulfamethoxazole compared with lamivudine alone.[196] 3TC did not significantly alter the pharmacokinetics of trimethoprim or sulfamethoxazole.

RECOMMENDATIONS FOR USE

Lamivudine is an important component of many recommended highly active antiretroviral combinations used to treat HIV infection.[18–23,25,102] The 2006 recommendations of the International AIDS Society-USA Panel note lamivudine as part of two of three recommended NRTI components of HAART in therapy-naive patients.[22] Lamivudine continues to be an important NRTI in the HIV therapeutic armamentarium, and has also been approved for treatment of HBV.

The currently recommended dose of 3TC for the treatment of HIV infection (as part of an HAART regimen) is 150 mg PO bid or 300 mg qd for adolescents and adults weighing more than 50 kg and 4 mg/kg (maximum 150 mg bid) every 12 h for adults weighing less than 50 kg. In children (3 months to 16 years old) the typical 3TC dose is 4 mg/kg every 12 hup to 300 mg daily. Dose adjustment is required for renal disease, with a 50% decrease in dose when the creatinine clearance is less than 50 mL/min (Table 9-2).[197] 3TC can be administered with or without food. Given the potency of 3TC, its ease of administration, lack of frequent toxicity, incorporation into convenient combination tablets, and infrequent drug interactions, this drug has become an important component of combination antiretroviral therapy.

Table 9-2 Important Drug Interactions and Dose Adjustment With Renal Impairment

Creatinine Clearance (mL/min)	3TC Dose
50	150 mg q12 h
30–49	150 mg q24 h
15–29	150 mg single dose, then 100 mg q24 h
5–14	150 mg single dose, then 50 mg q24 h
<5	50 mg single dose, then 25 mg q24 h

There was a 43% increase in the AUC and a 35% decrease in renal clearance when lamivudine and trimethoprim–sulfamethoxazole were co-administered, compared to lamivudine alone.

Doses for the treatment of HBV in the absence of HIV co-infection are 100 mg a day. In the presence of HIV co-infection, the HIV treatment doses should be utilized.

REFERENCES

1. Yarchoan R, Mitsuya H, Myers C, et al. Clinical pharmacology of 3′-azido-2′,3′-dideoxythymidine (zidovudine) and related dideoxynucleosides. N Engl J Med 321:726–38, 1989.
2. Soudeyns H, Yao XI, Gao Q, et al. Anti-human immunodeficiency virus type 1 activity and in vitro toxicity of 2′-deoxy-3′-thiacytidine (BCH-189), a novel heterocyclic nucleoside analog. Antimicrob Agents Chemother 35:1386–90, 1991.
3. Schinazi RF, Chu CK, Peck A, et al. Activities of the four optical isomers of 2′,3′-dideoxy-3′-thiacytidine (BCH-189) against human immunodeficiency virus type 1 in human lymphocytes. Antimicrob Agents Chemother 36:672–6, 1992.
4. Coates JA, Cammack N, Jenkinson HJ, et al. The separated enantiomers of 2′-deoxy-3′-thiacytidine (BCH 189) both inhibit human immunodeficiency virus replication in vitro. Antimicrob Agents Chemother 36:202–5, 1992.
5. Skalski V, Chang CN, Dutschman G, et al. The biochemical basis for the differential anti-human immunodeficiency virus activity of two cis enantiomers of 2′,3′-dideoxy-3′-thiacytidine. J Biol Chem 268:23234–8, 1993.
6. Coates JA, Cammack N, Jenkinson HJ, et al. (−)-2′-Deoxy-3′-thiacytidine is a potent, highly selective inhibitor of human immunodeficiency virus type 1 and type 2 replication in vitro. Antimicrob Agents Chemother 36:733–9, 1992.
7. Skalski V, Liu SH, Cheng YC. Removal of anti-human immunodeficiency virus 2′,3′-dideoxynucleoside monophosphates from DNA by a novel human cytosolic 3 + 9 :5′ exonuclease. Biochem Pharmacol 50:815–21, 1995.
8. Chang CN, Skalski V, Zhou JH, et al. Biochemical pharmacology of (+)- and (−)-2′,3′-dideoxy-3′-thiacytidine as anti-hepatitis B virus agents. J Biol Chem 267:22414–20, 1992.
9. Dienstag JL, Perrillo RP, Schiff ER, et al. A preliminary trial of lamivudine for chronic hepatitis B infection. N Engl J Med 333:1657–61, 1995.
10. Dienstag JL, Schiff ER, Wright TL, et al. Lamivudine as initial treatment for chronic hepatitis B in the United States. N Engl J Med 341:1256–63, 1999.
11. Merrill DP, Moonis M, Chou TC, et al. Lamivudine or stavudine in two- and three-drug combinations against human immunodeficiency virus type 1 replication in vitro. J Infect Dis 173:355–64, 1996.
12. Bridges EG, Dutschman GE, Gullen EA, et al. Favorable interaction of beta-L(−) nucleoside analogs with clinically approved anti-HIV nucleoside analogs for the treatment of human immunodeficiency virus. Biochem Pharmacol 51:731–6, 1996. Erratum. Biochem Pharmacol 51:1415, 1996.
13. Mathez D, Schinazi RF, Liotta DC, et al. Infectious amplification of wild-type human immunodeficiency virus from patients' lymphocytes and modulation by reverse transcriptase inhibitors in vitro. Antimicrob Agents Chemother 37:2206–11, 1993.
14. Chong KT, Pagano PJ. Synergistic inhibition of human immunodeficiency type 1 replication in vitro by two- and three-drug combination of delavirdine, lamivudine and zidovudine. Int Conf AIDS 11:1103, 1996.
15. Snyder S, D'Argenio DZ, Weislow O, et al. The triple combination indinavir-zidovudine-lamivudine is highly synergistic. Antimicrob Agents Chemother 44:1051–8, 2000.
16. Gulick RM, Mellors JW, Havlir D, et al. 3-Year suppression of HIV viremia with indinavir, zidovudine, and lamivudine. Ann Intern Med 133:35–9, 2000.
17. Hammer SM, Squires K, Hughes M, et al. A randomized, placebo-controlled trial of indinavir in combination with two nucleoside analogs in human immunodeficiency virus infected persons with CD4 cell counts less than or equal to 200 per cubic millimeter. N Engl J Med 337:725–33, 1997.
18. Gulick RM, Ribaudo HJ, Shikuma CM, et al. Triple-nucleoside regimens versus efavirenz-containing regimens for the initial treatment of HIV-1 infection. N Engl J Med 350:1850–61, 2004.
19. Robbins GK, De Grutolla V, Shafer RW, et al. Comparison of sequential three-drug regimens as initial therapy for HIV-1 infection. N Engl J Med 349:2293–303, 2003.
20. Shafer RW, Smeaton LM, Robbins GK, et al. Comparison of four-drug regimens and pairs of sequential three-drug regimens as initial therapy for HIV-1 infection. N Engl J Med 349:2304–15, 2003.
21. Gulick RM, Ribaudo HJ, Shikuma CM, et al. Three vs four-drug antiretroviral regimens for the initial treatment of HIV-1 infection: a randomized controlled trial. JAMA 296:769–81, 2006.
22. Hammer SM, Saag MS, Schechter M, et al. Treatment for adult HIV infection 2006 recommendations of the International AIDS Society-USA Panel. JAMA 296:827–43, 2006.
23. Gallant JE, DeJesus E, Arribas JR, et al. Tenofovir DF, emtricitabine, and efavirenz vs. zidovudine, lamivudine and efavirenz for HIV. N Engl J Med 354:251–60, 2006.
24. Veal GJ, Hoggard PG, Barry MG, et al. Interaction between lamivudine (3TC) and other nucleoside analogues for intracellular phosphorylation. AIDS 10:546–8, 1996.
25. Carpenter CC, Cooper DA, Fischl MA, et al. Antiretroviral therapy in adults: updated recommendations of the International AIDS Society-USA Panel. JAMA 283:381–90, 2000.
26. Van Leeuwen R, Lange JM, Hussey EK, et al. The safety and pharmacokinetics of a reverse transcriptase inhibitor, 3TC, in patients with HIV infection: a phase I study. AIDS 6:1471–5, 1992.
27. Angel J, Hussey E, Hall S, et al. Pharmacokinetics of 3TC (GR109714X) administered with and without food to HIV-infected patients. Drug Invest 6:70–4, 1993.
28. Yuen GJ, Morris DM, Mydlow PK, et al. Pharmacokinetics, absolute bioavailability, and absorption characteristics of lamivudine. J Clin Pharmacol 35:1174–80, 1995. Erratum. J Clin Pharmacol 36:373, 1996.
29. Lewis LL, Venzon D, Church J, et al. Lamivudine in children with human immunodeficiency virus infection: a phase I/II study: the National Cancer Institute Pediatric Branch-Human Immunodeficiency Virus Working Group. J Infect Dis 174:16–25, 1996.
30. Pluda JM, Cooley TP, Montaner JS, et al. A phase I/II study of 2′-deoxy-3′-thiacytidine (lamivudine) in patients with advanced human immunodeficiency virus infection. J Infect Dis 171:1438–47, 1995.
31. Heald AE, Hsyu PH, Yuen GJ, et al. Pharmacokinetics of lamivudine in human immunodeficiency virus-infected patients with renal dysfunction. Antimicrob Agents Chemother 40:1514–19, 1996.
32. Moore KH, Yuen GJ, Hussey EK, et al. Population pharmacokinetics of lamivudine in adult human immunodeficiency virus-infected patients enrolled in two phase III clinical trials. Antimicrob Agents Chemother 43:3025–9, 1999.
33. Moodley J, Moodley D, Pillay K, et al. Pharmacokinetics and antiretroviral activity of lamivudine alone or when coadministered with zidovudine in human immunodeficiency virus type 1-infected pregnant women and their offspring. J Infect Dis 178:1327–33, 1998.
34. Pereira A, Kashuba A, Fiscus S, et al. Nucleoside analogues achieve high concentrations in seminal plasma: relationship between drug concentrations and viral burden. J Infect Dis 180:2039–43, 1999.

35. Chappuy H, Trelyer JM, Jullien V, et al. Maternal-fetal transfer and amniotic fluid accumulation of nucleoside analogue reverse transcriptase inhibitors in human immunodeficiency virus-infected pregnant women. Antimicrob Agents Chemother 48:4332–6, 2004.
36. Johnson MA, Verpooten GA, Daniel MJ, et al. Single dose pharmacokinetics of lamivudine in subjects with impaired renal function and the effect of haemodialysis. Br J Clin Pharmacol 46:21–7, 1998.
37. Johnson MA, Horak J, Breuel P. The pharmacokinetics of lamivudine in patients with impaired hepatic function. Eur J Clin Pharmacol 54:363–6, 1998.
38. Gao WY, Agbaria R, Driscoll JS, et al. Divergent anti-human immunodeficiency virus activity and anabolic phosphorylation of 2′,3′-dideoxynucleoside analogs in resting and activated human cells. J Biol Chem 269:12633–8, 1994.
39. Moore KH, Barrett JE, Shaw S, et al. The pharmacokinetics of lamivudine phosphorylation in peripheral blood mononuclear cells from patients infected with HIV-1. AIDS 13:2239–50, 1999.
40. Cammack N, Rouse P, Marr CL, et al. Cellular metabolism of (−) enantiomeric 2′-deoxy-3′-thiacytidine. Biochem Pharmacol 43:2059–64, 1992.
41. Van Leeuwen R, Katlama C, Kitchen V, et al. Evaluation of safety and efficacy of 3TC (lamivudine) in patients with asymptomatic or mildly symptomatic human immunodeficiency virus infection: a phase I/II study. J Infect Dis 171:1166–71, 1995.
42. Blaney SM, Daniel MJ, Harker AJ, et al. Pharmacokinetics of lamivudine and BCH-189 in plasma and cerebrospinal fluid of nonhuman primates. Antimicrob Agents Chemother 39:2779–82, 1995.
43. Mueller BU, Lewis LL, Yuen GJ, et al. Serum and cerebrospinal fluid pharmacokinetics of intravenous and oral lamivudine in human immunodeficiency virus-infected children. Antimicrob Agents Chemother 42:3187–92, 1998.
44. Foudraine NA, Hoetelmans RM, Lange JM, et al. Cerebrospinal-fluid HIV-1 RNA and drug concentrations after treatment with lamivudine plus zidovudine or stavudine. Lancet 351:1547–51, 1998.
45. Pereira AS, Smeaton LM, Gerber JG, et al. The pharmacokinetics of amprenavir zidovudine and lamivudine in the male genital tract of HIV-1 infected men (AIDS Clinical Trial Group Study 850). J Infect Dis 35:198–204, 2002.
46. Taylor S, van Heeswijk RPG, Hoetelmans RMW, et al. Concentrations of nevirapine, lamivudine and stavudine in semen of HIV-1-infected men. AIDS 14:1979–84, 2000.
47. Reddy S, Kim J, Eron J, et al. Efavirenz (EFV) – containing antiretroviral (ARV) therapy (T) effectively reduces HIV RNA in the seminal plasma (SP) of HIV-1-infected Men (M). In: 8th Conference on Retroviruses and Opportunistic Infections, Chicago, Feb 2001, abstract 750.
48. Taylor S, Back DJ, Workman J, et al. Poor penetration of the male genital tract by HIV-1 protease inhibitors. AIDS 13:859–60, 1999.
49. Van Praag R, Weverling GJ, Portegies P, et al. Enhanced penetration of indinavir in cerebrospinal fluid and semen after the addition of low-dose ritonavir. AIDS 14:1187–94, 2000.
50. Brinkman K, Smeitink JA, Romijn JA, et al. Mitochondrial toxicity induced by nucleoside-analogue reverse-transcriptase inhibitors is a key factor in the pathogenesis of antiretroviral-therapy-related lipodystrophy. Lancet 354:1112–15, 1999.
51. Honkoop P, Scholte HR, de Man RA, et al. Mitochondrial injury: lessons from the fialuridine trial. Drug Saf 17:1–7, 1997.
52. Carr A, Miller J, Law M, et al. A syndrome of lipoatrophy, lactic acidaemia and liver dysfunction associated with HIV nucleoside analogue therapy: contribution to protease inhibitor-related lipodystrophy syndrome. AIDS 14:F25–32, 2000.
53. Hart GJ, Orr DC, Penn CR, et al. Effects of (−)-2′-deoxy-3′-thiacytidine (3TC) 5′-triphosphate on human immunodeficiency virus reverse transcriptase and mammalian DNA polymerases alpha, beta, and gamma. Antimicrob Agents Chemother 36:1688–94, 1992.
54. Cui L, Locatelli L, Xie MY, et al. Effect of nucleoside analogs on neurite regeneration and mitochondrial DNA synthesis in PC-12 cells. J Pharmacol Exp Ther 280:1228–34, 1997.
55. Dornsife RE, Averett DR. In vitro potency of inhibition by antiviral drugs of hematopoietic progenitor colony formation correlates with exposure at hemotoxic levels in human immunodeficiency virus-positive humans. Antimicrob Agents Chemother 40:514–19, 1996.
56. McLeod GX, Hammer SM. Zidovudine: five years later. Ann Intern Med 117:487–501, 1992.
57. Eron J, Benoit S, Jemsek J, et al. Treatment with lamivudine, zidovudine or both in HIV-positive patients with 200–500 CD4+ cells per cubic millimeter. N Engl J Med 333:1662–9, 1995.
58. Bartlett J, Benoit S, Johnson V, et al. Lamivudine plus zidovudine compared with zalcitabine plus zidovudine in patients with HIV infection. Ann Intern Med 125:161–72, 1996.
59. Staszewski S, Loveday C, Picazo J, et al. Safety and efficacy of lamivudine–zidovudine combination therapy in zidovudine-experienced patients: a randomized controlled comparison with zidovudine monotherapy. JAMA 276:111–17, 1996.
60. Honkoop P, de Man RA, Scholte HR, et al. Effect of lamivudine on morphology and function of mitochondria in patients with chronic hepatitis B. Hepatology 26:211–15, 1997.
61. Kontorinis N, Dieterich D. Hepatotoxicity of antiretroviral therapy. AIDS Rev 5:36–43, 2003.
62. Wit FW, Weverling GJ, Weel J, et al. Incidence of and risk factors for severe hepatotoxicity associated with antiretroviral combination therapy. J Infect Dis 186:23–31, 2002.
63. Torti C, Lapadula G, Puoti M, et al. Influence of genotype 3 hepatitis C coinfection on liver enzyme elevation in HIV-1 positive patients after commencement of a new highly active antiretroviral regimen: results from the EPOKA-MASTER Cohort. J Acquir Immune Defic Syndr 41:180–5, 2006.
64. Moore R, Keruly J, Chaisson R. Differences in anion gap with different nucleoside RTI combinations. In: 7th Conference on Retroviruses and Opportunistic Infections, San Francisco, 2000, abstract 55.
65. Chaisson RE, Keruly JC, Moore RD. Adverse effects of antiretroviral agents. In: 40th Interscience Conference on Antimicrob Agents and Chemotherapy, Toronto, Sep 2000, p 543, abstract 1882.
66. Tripuranemi NS, Smith PR, Weedon J, et al. Prognostic factors in lactic acidosis syndrome caused by nucleoside reverse transcriptase inhibitors: report of eight cases and review of the literature. AIDS Patient Care STDs 18:379–84, 2004.
67. Blanco F, Garcia-Benayas T, Jose de la Cruz J, et al. First-line therapy and mitochondrial damage: different nucleosides, different findings. HIV Clin Trials 4(1):11–9, 2003.
68. Lonergan JT, Barber RE, Mathews WC. Safety and efficacy of switching to alternative nucleoside analogues following symptomatic hyperlactatemia and lactic acidosis. AIDS 17:2495–9, 2003.
69. FDA Antiviral Drugs Advisory Committee Meeting. Lamivudine. Nov 1995.
70. Schuurman R, Nijhuis M, van Leeuwen R, et al. Rapid changes in human immunodeficiency virus type 1 RNA load and appearance of drug-resistant virus populations in persons treated with lamivudine (3TC). J Infect Dis 171:1411–19, 1995.
71. Rousseau FS, Wakeford C, Mommeja-Marin H, et al. Prospective randomized trial of emtricitabine versus lamivudine short-term monotherapy in human immunodeficiency virus-infected patients. J Infect Dis 188:1652–8, 2003.

72. Hazen R, Lanier ER. Relative anti-HIV-1 efficacy of lamivudine and emtricitabine in vitro is dependent on cell type. J Acquir Immune Defic Syndr 32:255–8, 2003.
73. Schurmann D, Bergmann F, Jautzke G, et al. Acute and long-term efficacy of antituberculous treatment in HIV-seropositive patients with tuberculosis: a study of 36 cases. J Infect 26:45–54, 1993.
74. Johnson VA, Merrill DP, Videler JA, et al. Two-drug combinations of zidovudine, didanosine, and recombinant interferon-alpha A inhibit replication of zidovudine-resistant human immunodeficiency virus type 1 synergistically in vitro. J Infect Dis 164:646–55, 1991.
75. Eron JJJ, Johnson VA, Merrill DP, et al. Synergistic inhibition of replication of human immunodeficiency virus type 1, including that of a zidovudine-resistant isolate, by zidovudine and 2′,3′-dideoxycytidine in vitro. Antimicrob Agents Chemother 36:1559–62, 1992.
76. Caliendo AM, Hirsch MS. Combination therapy for infection due to human immunodeficiency virus type 1. Clin Infect Dis 18:516–24, 1994.
77. Hirsch MS, D'Aquila RT. Therapy for human immunodeficiency virus infection. N Engl J Med 328:1686–95, 1993.
78. Quan Y, Brenner BG, Oliveira M, et al. Lamivudine can exert a modest antiviral effect against human immunodeficiency virus type 1 containing the M184V mutation. Antimicrob Agents Chemother 47:747–54, 2003.
79. Eron JJ Jr, Bartlett JA, Santana JL, et al. Persistent antiretroviral activity of nucleoside analogues after prolonged zidovudine and lamivudine therapy as demonstrated by rapid loss of activity after discontinuation. J Acquir Immune Defic Syndr 37:1581–3, 2004.
80. Campbell TB, Shulman NS, Johnson SC, et al. Antiviral activity of lamivudine in salvage therapy for multidrug-resistant HIV-1 infection. Clin Infect Dis 41:236–42, 2005.
81. Deeks SG, Hoh R, Neilands TB, et al. Interruption of treatment with individual therapeutic drug classes in adults with multidrug-resistant HIV-1 infection. J Infect Dis 192:1537–44, 2005.
82. Castagna A, Danise A, Menzo S, et al. Lamivudine monotherapy in HIV-1-infected patients harbouring a lamivudine-resistant virus: a randomized pilot study (E-184V study). AIDS 20:795–803, 2006.
83. Tisdale M, Kemp SD, Parry NR, et al. Rapid in vitro selection of human immunodeficiency virus type 1 resistant to 3′-thiacytidine inhibitors due to a mutation in the YMDD region of reverse transcriptase. Proc Natl Acad Sci USA 90:5653–6, 1993.
84. Dawson J. Comparing treatment groups on the basis of slopes, areas under-the-curve, and other summary measures. Drug Info J 28:723–32, 1994.
85. Katlama C, Ingrand D, Loveday C, et al. Safety and efficacy of lamivudine-zidovudine combination therapy in antiretroviral-naive patients: a randomized controlled comparison with zidovudine monotherapy. JAMA 276:118–25, 1996.
86. Semple M, Loveday C, Weller I, et al HIV Plasma viraemia quantification: a non-culture measurement needed for therapeutic trials. J Virol Methods 41:167–80, 1993.
87. Eron JJ Jr, Bartlett JA, Santana JL, Bellos NC, Johnson J, Keller A, Kuritzkes DR, St Clair MH, Johnson VA. Persistent antiretroviral activity of nucleoside analogues after prolonged zidovudine and lamivudine therapy as demonstrated by rapid loss of activity after discontinuation. J Acquir Immune Defic Syndr. 15;37(5):1581–3, 2004.
88. Kuritzkes D, Marschner I, Johnson V, et al. Lamivudine in combination with zidovudine, stavudine or didanosine in patients with HIV-1 infection: a randomized, double-blind, placebo-controlled trial. AIDS 13:685–94, 1999.
89. Duan C, Poticha D, Stoeckli TC, et al. Inhibition of purified recombinant reverse transcriptase from wild-type and zidovudine-resistant clinical isolates of human immunodeficiency virus type 1 by zidovudine, stavudine and lamivudine triphosphates. J Infect Dis 184:1336–40, 2001.
90. Katlama C, Valantin M, Matheron S, et al. Efficacy and tolerability of stavudine plus lamivudine in treatment-naive and treatment-experienced patients with HIV-1 infection. Ann Intern Med 129:525–31, 1998.
91. Staszewski S, Hill AM, Bartlett J, et al. Reductions in HIV-1 disease progression for zidovudine/lamivudine relative to control treatments: a meta-analysis of controlled trials. AIDS 11:477–83, 1997.
92. Anonymous. Randomised trial of addition of lamivudine or lamivudine plus loviride to zidovudine-containing regimens for patients with HIV-1 infection: the CAESAR trial. Lancet 349:1413–21, 1997.
93. Phillips AN, Eron J, Bartlett J, et al. Correspondence between the effect of zidovudine plus lamivudine on plasma HIV level/CD4 lymphocyte count and the incidence of clinical disease in infected individuals. North American lamivudine HIV working group. AIDS 11:169–75, 1997.
94. Katzenstein D, Hammer S, Hughes M, et al. The relation of virologic and immunologic markers to clinical outcomes after nucleoside therapy in HIV-infected adults with 200 to 500 CD4 cells per cubic millimeter. N Engl J Med 335:1091–8, 1996.
95. Hammer S, Katzenstein D, Hughes M, et al. A trial comparing nucleoside monotherapy with combination therapy in HIV-infected adults with CD4 cell counts from 200 to 500 per cubic millimeter. N Engl J Med 335:1081–90, 1996.
96. Erickson J, Neidhart DJ, VanDrie J, et al. Design, activity, and 2.8 Å crystal structure of a C2 symmetric inhibitor complexed to HIV-1 protease. Science 249:527–33, 1990.
97. Markowitz M, Saag M, Powderly WG, et al. A preliminary study of ritonavir, an inhibitor of HIV-1 protease, to treat HIV-1 infection. N Engl J Med 333:1534–9, 1995.
98. Danner SA, Carr A, Leonard JM, et al. A short-term study of the safety, pharmacokinetics, and efficacy of ritonavir, an inhibitor of HIV-1 protease: European–Australian Collaborative Ritonavir Study Group. N Engl J Med 333:1528–33, 1995.
99. McDonald CK, Kuritzkes DR. Human immunodeficiency virus type 1 protease inhibitors. Arch Intern Med 157:951–9, 1997.
100. Carpenter CC, Fischl MA, Hammer SM, et al. Antiretroviral therapy for HIV infection in 1997: updated recommendations of the International AIDS Society-USA panel. JAMA 277:1962–9, 1997.
101. Federal Register. HIV Infection, Principles of Therapy, NIH Panel Report; and HIV-Infected Adults, Antiretroviral Agents Use Guidelines. June 1997, p 33417.
102. Panel on Clinical Practices for the Treatment of HIV Infection: DHHS Guidelines. Guidelines for the Use of Antiretroviral Agents in HIV-Infected Adults and Adolescents, vol 2001, 2001.
103. Gulick RM, Mellors JW, Havlir D, et al. Treatment with a combination of indinavir, zidovudine and lamivudine in HIV-1 infected adults with prior antiretroviral use. N Engl J Med 337:734–9, 1997.
104. Gulick R, Mellors J, Havlir D, et al. Simultaneous vs. sequential initiation of therapy with indinair, zidovudine, and lamivudine for HIV-1 infection: 100 week follow-up. JAMA 280:35–41, 1998.
105. AVANTI Study Group. AVANTI 2: randomized, double-blind trial to evaluate the efficacy and safety of zidovudine plus lamivudine versus zidovudine plus lamivudine plus indinavir in HIV-infected antiretroviral-naive patients. AIDS 14:367–74, 2000.

106. Hirsch M, Steigbigel R, Staszewski S, et al. A randomized, controlled trial of indinavir, zidovudine, and lamivudine in adults with advanced human immunodeficiency virus type 1 infection and prior antiretroviral therapy. J Infect Dis 180:659–65, 1999.
107. Markowitz M, Conant M, Hurley A, et al. A preliminary evaluation of nelfinavir mesylate, an inhibitor of human immunodeficiency virus (HIV)-1 protease, to treat HIV infection. J Infect Dis 177(6):1533–40, 1998.
108. Powderly WG, Tebas P. Nelfinavir, a new protease inhibitor: early clinical results. AIDS 13 (Suppl 1):S41–8, 1999.
109. Saag MS, Tebas P, Sension M, et al. Randomized double-blind comparison of two nelfinavir doses plus nucleosides in HIV-infected patients (Agouron Study 511). AIDS 15:1971–8, 2001.
110. Cameron DW, Heath-Chiozzi M, Danner S, et al. Randomised placebo-controlled trial of ritonavir in advanced HIV-1 disease: the Advanced HIV Disease Ritonavir Study Group. Lancet 351:543–9, 1998.
111. Markowitz M, Vesanen M, Tenner-Racz K, et al. The effect of commencing combination antiretroviral therapy soon after human immunodeficiency virus type 1 infection on viral replication and antiviral immune responses. J Infect Dis 179:527–37, 1999.
112. Wu H, Kuritzkes DR, McClernon DR, et al. Characterization of viral dynamics in human immunodeficiency virus type 1-infected patients treated with combination antiretroviral therapy: relationships to host factors, cellular restoration, and virologic end points. J Infect Dis 179:799–807, 1999.
113. Connick E, Lederman MM, Kotzin BL, et al. Immune reconstitution in the first year of potent antiretroviral therapy and its relationship to virologic response. J Infect Dis 181:358–63, 2000.
114. Smith KY, Valdez H, Landay A, et al. Thymic size and lymphocyte restoration in patients with human immunodeficiency virus infection after 48 weeks of zidovudine, lamivudine, and ritonavir therapy. J Infect Dis 181:141–7, 2000.
115. Cohen Stuart JW, Schuurman R, Burger DM, et al. Randomized trial comparing saquinavir soft gelatin capsules versus indinavir as part of triple therapy (CHEESE study). AIDS 13:F53–8, 1999.
116. Murphy RL, Gulick RM, DeGruttola V, et al. Treatment with amprenavir alone or amprenavir with zidovudine and lamivudine in adults with human immunodeficiency virus infection: AIDS Clinical Trials Group 347 study team. J Infect Dis 179:808–16, 1999.
117. King M, Bernstein B, Kempf D, et al. Comparison of time to achieve HIV RNA <400 copies/ml and <50 copies/ml in a phase III, blinded, randomized clinical trial of ABT-378/r vs. NFV in ARV-naive patients. In: 8th Conference on Retroviruses and Opportunistic Infections, Chicago, Feb 2001, abstract 329.
118. Eron J Jr, Murphy RL, Peterson D, et al. A comparison of stavudine, didanosine and indinavir with zidovudine, lamivudine and indinavir for the initial treatment of HIV-1 infected individuals: selection of thymidine analog regimen therapy (START II). AIDS 14:1601–10, 2000.
119. Launay O, Gerard L, Morand-Joubert L, et al. Comparative antiviral activity and toxicity of nevirapine (NVP) versus lamivudine (3TC), in combination with stavudine (d4T) and indinavir (IDV), for the treatment of HIV-1-infected patients. In: 8th Conference on Retroviruses and Opportunistic Infections, Chicago, Feb 2001, abstract 326.
120. Walmsley S, Bernstein B, King M, et al. Lopinavir-ritonavir versus nelfinavir for the initial treatment of HIV infection. N Engl J Med 346:2039–46, 2002.
121. Eron J Jr, Yeni P, Gathe J Jr, et al. The KLEAN study of fosamprenavir-ritonavir versus lopinavir-ritonavir, each in combination with abacavir–lamivudine, for initial treatment of HIV infection over 48 weeks: a randomized non-inferiority trial. Lancet 368:476–82, 2006.
122. Green S, Para MF, Daly PW, et al. Interim analysis of plasma viral burden reductions and CD4 increases in HIV-1 infected patients with Rescriptor (DLV) + Retrovir (ZDV) + Epivir (3TC). In: 12th World AIDS Conference, Geneva, Jun–Jul 1998, abstract 12219.
123. Podzamczer D, Ferrer E, Consiglio E, et al. A randomized, open, multicenter trial comparing Combivir plus nelfinavir or nevirapine in HIV-infected naive patients (the combine study). In: 8th Conference on Retroviruses and Opportunistic Infections, Chicago, Feb 2001, abstract 327.
124. Staszewski S, Keiser P, Montaner J, et al. Abacavir–lamivudine–zidovudine vs indinavir–lamivudine–zidovudine in antiretroviral-naive HIV-infected adults: a randomized equivalence trial. JAMA 285:1155–63, 2001.
125. Cahn P. Potential advantages of a compact triple nucleoside regimen; efficacy and adherence with Combivir/abacavir versus Combivir/indinavir in an open-label randomised comparative study (CNAB3014). In: 40th Interscience Conference on Antimicrobial Agents and Chemotherapy, Toronto, Sep 2000, p 293, abstract 695.
126. Squires K. The Atlantic Study: a randomized, open-label trial comparing two protease inhibitor (PI) sparing anti-retroviral strategies versus a standard PI-containing regimen, final 48 week data. In: 13th International AIDS Conference, Durban, South Africa, Jun–Jul 2000, p 43, abstract LbPeB7044.
127. Gulick RM, Ribaudo HJ, Shikuma CM, et al. Three- vs four-drug antiretroviral regimens for the initial treatment of HIV-1 infection. A Randomized controlled trial. JAMA 296:769–81, 2006.
128. Orkin C, Stebbing J, Nelson M, et al. A randomized study comparing a three- and four-drug HAART regimen in first-line therapy (QUAD study). J Antimicrob Chemother 55:246–51, 2005.
129. DART virology group and trial team. Virological response to a triple nucleoside/nucleotide analogue regimen over 48 weeks in HIV-1-infected adults in Africa. AIDS 20:1391–9, 2006.
130. Moyle G, Higgs C, Teague A, et al. An open-label, randomized comparative pilot study of a single-class quadruple therapy regimen versus a 2-class regimen for individuals initiating antiretroviral therapy. Antiv Ther 11:73–8, 2006.
131. Eron JJ, Yetzer ES, Ruane PJ, et al. Efficacy, safety, and adherence with a twice-daily combination lamivudine/zidovudine tablet formulation, plus a protease inhibitor, in HIV infection. AIDS 14:671–81, 2000.
132. Fischl M, Burnside A, Farthing C, et al. Efficacy of Combivir (COM) (lamivudine 150 mg/zidovudine 300 mg) plus Ziagen (abacavir (ABC) 300 mg) bid compared to Trizivir (TZV) (3TC 150 mg/ZDV 300 mg/ABC 300 mg) bid in patients receiving prior COM plus ABC. In: 8th Conference on Retroviruses and Opportunistic Infections, Chicago, Feb 2001, abstract 315.
133. Katlama C, Clumeck N, Fenske S, et al. Use of Trizivir to simplify therapy in HAART-experienced patients with long-term suppression of HIV-RNA: TRIZAL Study (AZL30002): 24-week results. In: 8th Conference on Retroviruses and Opportunistic Infections, Chicago, Feb 2001, abstract 316.
134. Sension M, Bellos N, Johnson J, et al. Efficacy and safety of switch to 3TC 300 mg QD vs. continued 3TC 150 mg bid in subjects with virologic suppression on stable 3TC/d4T/PI therapy (COLA4005): final 24-week results. In: 8th Conference on Retroviruses and Opportunistic Infections, Chicago, Feb 2001, abstract 317.
135. Sosa N, Hill-Zabala C, Dejesus E, et al. Abacavir and lamivudine fixed-dose combination tablet once daily compared with

abacavir and lamivudine twice daily in HIV-infected patients over 48 weeks (ESS30008. SEAL). J Acquir Immune Defic Syndr 40:422–7, 2005.
136. McKinney RE Jr, Johnson GM, Stanley K, et al. A randomized study of combined zidovudine-lamivudine versus didanosine monotherapy in children with symptomatic therapy-naive HIV-1 infection: the Pediatric AIDS Clinical Trials Group Protocol 300 study team. J Pediatr 133:500–8, 1998.
137. Nachman SA, Stanley K, Yogev R, et al. Nucleoside analogs plus ritonavir in stable antiretroviral therapy-experienced HIV-infected children: a randomized controlled trial: Pediatric AIDS Clinical Trials Group 338 study team. JAMA 283:492–8, 2000.
138. Luzuriaga K, McManus M, Mofenson L, et al. A trial of three antiviral regimens in HIV-1-infected children. N Engl J Med 350:2471–80, 2004.
139. Dienstag JL, Schiff ER, Wright TL, et al. Lamivudine as initial treatment for chronic hepatitis B in the United States. N Engl J Med 341:1256–63, 1999.
140. Lai CL, Chien RN, Leung NW, et al. A one-year trial of lamivudine for chronic hepatitis B. Asia hepatitis lamivudine study group. N Engl J Med 339:61–8, 1998.
141. Niederau C, Heintges T, Lange S, et al. Long-term follow-up of HBeAg-positive patients treated with interferon alpha for chronic hepatitis B. N Engl J Med 334:1422–7, 1996.
142. Lau GK, Piratvisuth T, Luo KX, et al. Peginterferon alfa-2a, lamivudine, and the combination for HBeAg-positive chronic hepatitis B. N Engl J Med 352:2682–95, 2005.
143. Chang TT, Gish RG, de Man R, et al. A comparison of entecavir and lamivudine for HBeAg-positive chronic hepatitis B. N Engl J Med 354:1011–20, 2006.
144. Santantonio T, Niro GA, Sinisi E, et al. Lamivudine/interferon combination therapy in anti-HBe positive chronic hepatitis B patients: a controlled pilot study. J Hepatol 36:799–804, 2002.
145. Marcellin P, Lau GK, Bonino F, et al. Peginterferon alfa-2a alone, lamivudine alone and the two in combination in patients with HBeAg-negative chronic hepatitis B. N Engl J Med 351:1206–17, 2004.
146. Lai CL, Shouval D, Lok AS, et al. Entecavir versus lamivudine for patients with HBeAg-negative chronic hepatitis. N Engl J Med 354:1011–20, 2006.
147. Kellerman SE, Hanson D, McNaghten A, et al. Prevalence of chronic hepatitis B and incidence of acute hepatitis B infection in human immunodeficiency virus-infected subjects. J Infect Dis 188:571–7, 2003.
148. Thio C, Seaberg E, Skolasky R Jr, et al. HIV-1, hepatitis B virus and risk of liver related mortality in the Multicenter Cohort Study (MACS). Lancet 360:1921–6, 2002.
149. Levy V, Grant RM. Antiretroviral therapy for hepatitis B virus-HIV-coinfected patients: promises and pitfalls. CID 43:904–10, 2006.
150. Nunez M, Soriano V. Management of patients co-infected with hepatitis B virus and HIV. Lancet Infect Dis 5:374–82, 2005.
151. Bessesen M, Ives D, Condreay L, et al. Chronic active hepatitis B exacerbations in human immunodeficiency virus-infected patients following development of resistance. Clin Infect Dis 28:1032–5, 1999.
152. Soriano V, Puoti M, Bonacini M, et al. Care of patients with chronic hepatitis B and HIV co-infection: recommendations from an HIV-HBV international panel. AIDS 19:221–40, 2005.
153. Carr A, Cooper D. Restoration of immunity to chronic hepatitis B infection in HIV-infected patient on protease inhibitor. Lancet 349:995–6, 1997.
154. Jonas MM, Mizerski J, Badia IB, et al. Clinical trial of lamivudine in children with chronic hepatitis B. N Engl J Med 346:1706–13, 2002.
155. Lok AS, Hussain M, Cursano C, et al. Evolution of hepatitis B virus polymerase gene mutations in hepatitis B e antigen-negative patients receiving lamivudine therapy. Hepatology 32:1145–53, 2000.
156. Villeneuve JP, Condreay LD, Willems B, et al. Lamivudine treatment for decompensated cirrhosis resulting from chronic hepatitis B. Hepatology 31:207–10, 2000.
157. Boucher CA, Cammack N, Schipper P, et al. High-level resistance to (−) enantiomeric 2′-deoxy-3′-thiacytidine in vitro is due to one amino acid substitution in the catalytic site of human immunodeficiency virus type 1 reverse transcriptase. Antimicrob Agents Chemother 37:2231–4, 1993.
158. Gao Q, Gu Z, Parniak MA, et al. The same mutation that encodes low-level human immunodeficiency virus type 1 resistance to 2′,3′-dideoxyinosine and 2′,3′-dideoxycytidine confers high-level resistance to the (−) enantiomer of 2′,3′-dideoxy-3′-thiacytidine. Antimicrob Agents Chemother 37:1390–2, 1993.
159. Schinazi RF, Lloyd RMJ, Nguyen MH, et al. Characterization of human immunodeficiency viruses resistant to oxathiolane-cytosine nucleosides. Antimicrob Agents Chemother 37:875–81, 1993.
160. Wainberg MA, Salomon H, Gu Z, et al. Development of HIV-1 resistance to (−)2′-deoxy-3′-thiacytidine in patients with AIDS or advanced AIDS-related complex. AIDS 9:351–7, 1995.
161. Kuritzkes DR, Quinn JB, Benoit SL, et al. Drug resistance and virologic response in NUCA 3001, a randomized trial of lamivudine (3TC) versus zidovudine (ZDV) versus ZDV plus 3TC in previously untreated patients. AIDS 10:975–81, 1996.
162. Kohlstaedt LA, Wang J, Friedman JM, et al. Crystal structure at 3.5 Å resolution of HIV-1 reverse transcriptase complexed with an inhibitor. Science 256:1783–90, 1992.
163. Larder BA, Kemp SD, Purifoy DJM. Infectious potential of human immunodeficiency type 1 reverse transcriptase mutants with altered inhibitor sensitivity. Proc Natl Acad Sci USA 86:4803–7, 1989.
164. Boyer PL, Ferris AL, Hughes SH. Cassette mutagenesis of the reverse transcriptase of human immunodeficiency virus type 1. J Virol 66:1031–9, 1992.
165. Halvas EK, Svarovskaia ES, Freed EO, et al. Wild-type and YMDD mutant murine leukemia virus reverse transcriptases are resistant to 2′,3′-dideoxy-3′-thiacytidine. J Virol 74:6669–74, 2000.
166. Larder BA, Kemp SD, Harrigan PR. Potential mechanism for sustained antiretroviral efficacy of AZT-3TC combination therapy. Science 269:696–9, 1995.
167. Wainberg M, Drosopoulos W, Salomon H, et al. Enhanced fidelity of 3TC-selected mutant HIV-1 reverse transcriptase. Science 271:1282–5, 1996.
168. Miller MD, Anton KE, Mulato AS, et al. Human immunodeficiency virus type 1 expressing the lamivudine-associated M184V mutation in reverse transcriptase shows increased susceptibility to adefovir and decreased replication capability in vitro. J Infect Dis 179:92–100, 1999.
169. Feng JY, Anderson KS. Mechanistic studies examining the efficiency and fidelity of DNA synthesis by the 3TC-resistant mutant (184V) of HIV-1 reverse transcriptase. Biochemistry 38:9440–8, 1999.
170. Rezende LF, Drosopoulos WC, Prasad VR. The influence of 3TC resistance mutation M184I on the fidelity and error specificity of human immunodeficiency virus type 1 reverse transcriptase. Nucleic Acids Res 26:3066–72, 1998.
171. Hsu M, Inouye P, Rezende L, et al. Higher fidelity of RNA-dependent DNA mispair extension by M184V drug-resistant than wild-type reverse transcriptase of human immunodeficiency virus type 1. Nucleic Acids Res 25:4532–6, 1997.
172. Havlir DV, Eastman S, Gamst A, et al. Nevirapine-resistant human immunodeficiency virus: kinetics of replication and estimated prevalence in untreated patients. J Virol 70:7894–9, 1996.
173. Kuritzkes DR, Shugarts D, Bakhtiari M, et al. Emergence of dual resistance to zidovudine and lamivudine in HIV-1-infected

patients treated with zidovudine plus lamivudine as initial therapy. J Acquir Immune Defic Syndr 23:26–34, 2000.
174. Kuritzkes DR, Sevin A, Young B, et al. Effect of zidovudine resistance mutations on virologic response to treatment with zidovudine–lamivudine–ritonavir: genotypic analysis of human immunodeficiency virus type 1 isolates from AIDS clinical trials group protocol 315: ACTG Protocol 315 team. J Infect Dis 181:491–7, 2000.
175. Boucher CA, OSullivan E, Mulder JW, et al. Ordered appearance of zidovudine resistance mutations during treatment of 18 human immunodeficiency virus-positive subjects. J Infect Dis 165:105–10, 1992.
176. De Jong MD, Veenstra J, Stilianakis NI, et al. Host-parasite dynamics and outgrowth of virus containing a single K70R amino acid change in reverse transcriptase are responsible for the loss of human immunodeficiency virus type 1 RNA load suppression by zidovudine. Proc Natl Acad Sci USA 93:5501–6, 1996.
177. Larder BA, Kemp SD. Multiple mutations in the HIV-1 reverse transcriptase confer high-level resistance to zidovudine (AZT). Science 246:1155–8, 1989.
178. Kellam P, Boucher CA, Larder BA. Fifth mutation in human immunodeficiency virus type 1 reverse transcriptase contributes to the development of high-level resistance to zidovudine. Proc Natl Acad Sci USA 89:1934–8, 1992.
179. Lacey SF, Reardon JE, Furfine ES, et al. Biochemical studies of the reverse transcriptase and RNase H activities from human immunodeficiency virus strains resistant to 3′-azido-3′-deoxythymidine. J Biol Chem 267:15789–94, 1992.
180. Carroll SS, Geib J, Olsen DB, et al. Sensitivity of HIV-1 reverse transcriptase and its mutants to inhibition by azidothymidine triphosphate. Biochemistry 33:2113–20, 1994.
181. Meyer PR, Matsuura SE, Mian AM, et al. A mechanism of AZT resistance: an increase in nucleotide-dependent primer unblocking by mutant HIV-1 reverse transcriptase. Mol Cell 4:35–43, 1999.
182. Arion D, Kaushik N, McCormick S, et al. Phenotypic mechanism of HIV-1 resistance to 3′-azido-3′-deoxythymidine (AZT): increased polymerization processivity and enhanced sensitivity to pyrophosphate of the mutant viral reverse transcriptase. Biochemistry 37:15908–17, 1998.
183. Gotte M, Arion D, Parniak MA, et al. The M184V mutation in the reverse transcriptase of human immunodeficiency virus type 1 impairs rescue of chain-terminated DNA synthesis. J Viro 74:3579–85, 2000.
184. Arion D, Sluis-Cremer N, Parniak MA. Mechanism by which phosphonoformic acid resistance mutations restore 3′-azido-3′-deoxythymidine (AZT) sensitivity to AZT-resistant HIV-1 reverse transcriptase. J Biol Chem 275:9251–5, 2000.
185. Gao WY, Shirasaka T, Johns DG, et al. Differential phosphorylation of azidothymidine, dideoxycytidine, and dideoxyinosine in resting and activated peripheral blood mononuclear cells. J Clin Invest 91:2326–33, 1993.
186. Miller V, Phillips A, Rottmann C, et al. Dual resistance to zidovudine and lamivudine in patients treated with zidovudine–lamivudine combination therapy: association with therapy failure. J Infect Dis 177:1521–32, 1998.
187. Gass R, Shugarts D, Young R, et al. Emergence of dual resistance to zidovudine (ZDV) and lamivudine (3TC) in clinical HIV-1 isolates from patients receiving ZDV/3TC combination therapy. Antivir Ther 3:97–102, 1998.
188. Rusconi S, DePasquale M, Milazzo L, et al. Loss of antiviral effect owing to zidovudine and lamivudine double resistance in HIV-1 infected patients in an ongoing open-label trial. Antivir Ther 2:39–46, 1997.
189. Nijhuis M, Schuurman R, de Jong D, et al. Lamivudine-resistant human immunodeficiency virus type 1 variants (184V) require multiple amino acid changes to become co-resistant to zidovudine in vivo. J Infect Dis 176:398–405, 1997.
190. Kemp SD, Shi C, Bloor S, et al. A novel polymorphism at codon 333 of human immunodeficiency virus type 1 reverse transcriptase can facilitate dual resistance to zidovudine and L-2′,3′-dideoxy-3′-thiacytidine. J Virol 72:5093–8, 1998.
191. Larder BA, Bloor S, Kemp SD, et al. A family of insertion mutations between codons 67 and 70 of human immunodeficiency virus type 1 reverse transcriptase confer multinucleoside analog resistance. Antimicrob Agents Chemother 43:1961–7, 1999.
192. Shafer RW, Kozal MJ, Winters MA, et al. Combination therapy with zidovudine and didanosine selects for drug-resistant human immunodeficiency virus type 1 strains with unique patterns of pol gene mutations. J Infect Dis 169:722–9, 1994.
193. Hertogs K, Bloor S, De Vroey V, et al. A novel human immunodeficiency virus type 1 reverse transcriptase mutational pattern confers phenotypic lamivudine resistance in the absence of mutation 184V. Antimicrob Agents Chemother 44:568–73, 2000.
194. Miller V, Sturmer M, Staszewski S, et al. The M184V mutation in HIV-1 reverse transcriptase (RT) conferring lamivudine resistance does not result in broad cross-resistance to nucleoside analogue RT inhibitors. AIDS 12:705–12, 1998.
195. Oude Essink BB, Back NK, Berkhout B. Increased polymerase fidelity of the 3TC-resistant variants of HIV-1 reverse transcriptase. Nucleic Acids Res 25:3213–17, 1997.
196. Moore KH, Yuen GJ, Raasch RH, et al. Pharmacokinetics of lamivudine administered alone and with trimethoprim–sulfamethoxazole. Clin Pharmacol Ther 59:550–8, 1996.
197. McEvoy GK (ed). Lamivudine: American Society of Health System Pharmacists. American Hospital Formulary Service Drug Information, 1997.

Chapter 10

Emtricitabine

Michael J. Mugavero, MD, MHS, Melissa F. Wellons, MD, MHS

Emtricitabine is a pyrimidine analog with antiviral activity against human immunodeficiency virus (HIV) and hepatitis-B virus (HBV) whose activity was originally described by Schinazi et al in 1992.[1] Emtricitabine received approval from the US Food and Drug Administration (FDA) for use as a therapeutic agent for the treatment of HIV on 2 Jul 2003. Guidelines for the treatment of HIV infection by both the US Department of Health and Human Services (DHHS)[2] and the International AIDS Society-USA (IAS-USA)[3] have placed emtricitabine in the 'preferred category' of nucleoside reverse transcriptase inhibitors (NRTIs) in combination with tenofovir, zidovudine, or didanosine (IAS-USA guidelines only) for antiretroviral-naive patients initiating combination antiretroviral therapy. While emtricitabine has not received FDA approval for the treatment of HBV-infections or HIV–HBV co-infections, it is often used 'off label' in this capacity.

STRUCTURE

Emtricitabine (FTC), the negative or *cis* enatiomer of 2′,3′-dideoxy-5-fluoro-3′-thiacytidine, has antiviral activity against HIV-1, HIV-2, and HBV.[1,4] Similar to lamivudine, emtricitabine is an oxathiolane-cytosine analog and has the unusual L configuration (1-β-L) rather than the D configuration found in natural nucleosides. Unlike lamivudine, emtricitabine has a fluorine in the 5-position of its cytosine ring (Fig. 10-1).

MECHANISM OF ACTION AND *IN VITRO* ACTIVITY

Like other nucleoside analogs, emtricitabine is a prodrug that must be metabolized intracellularly to exert its activity. After entering the cell through multiple transport mechanisms, emtricitabine is phosphorylated stepwise by cellular kinases to its active 5′-triphosphate form, emtricitabine 5′-triphosphate (E-TP) (Fig. 10-2).[5–7] E-TP competitively inhibits the binding of deoxycytidine triphosphate, an endogenous deoxynucleotide triphosphate, to the reverse transcriptase (RT) binding site.[8,9] E-TP is incorporated by RT into the nascent proviral DNA chain. This incorporation causes termination of DNA synthesis because E-TP lacks a hydroxyl group in the 3′ position of its sugar moiety and therefore does not allow the 5′ to 3′ linkage required for DNA synthesis. Thus, incorporation of E-TP inhibits viral replication.[8–10]

Emtricitabine's antiviral activity has been evaluated in lymphocyte and monocyte/macrophage cell lines and peripheral blood mononuclear cell (PBMC) specimens. Emtricitabine is active against laboratory-adapted strains of HIV-1 and HIV-2 as well as clinical isolates of HIV-1, including zidovudine- and didanosine-resistant isolates. Depending on the cell type and viral isolate used, the concentration required to produce 50% inhibition (IC_{50}) of HIV ranges from 0.0014 to 1.500 μM.[1,11–15] Emtricitabine's generally low IC_{50} values are attributed to its ability to bind efficiently to the RT-DNA complex. In a kinetic analysis of RT-catalyzed

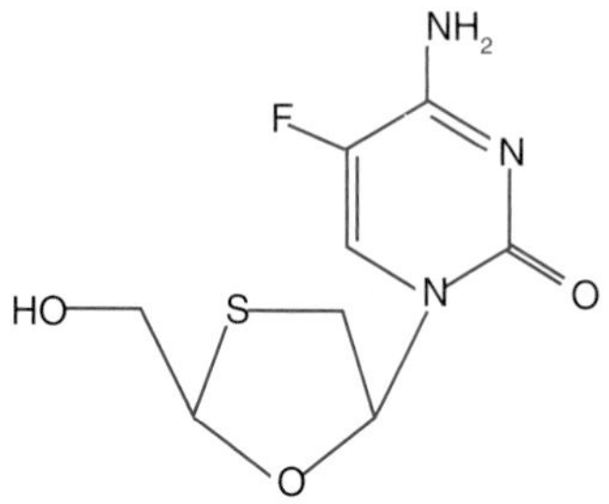

Figure 10-1 ■ Structure of emtricitabine.

DNA synthesis, E-TP bound 3.6-fold tighter to the enzyme–DNA complex (K_d, rate of dissociation) and was incorporated into nascent chain DNA (K_{pol}, rate of polymerization) 2.5-fold faster than was lamivudine 5′-triphosphate (L-TP) (Table 10-1).[16]

In addition to HIV-1 and HIV-2, emtricitabine also inhibits HBV *in vitro*. Its *in vitro* anti-HBV activity is comparable to that seen with lamivudine, inhibiting virus production with an IC_{50} of 0.01-0.04 μM. Intracellularly, emtricitabine inhibits HBV DNA synthesis with an IC_{50} of 0.16 μM.[6,17,18]

When inhibiting HIV-1, emtricitabine is synergistic *in vitro* with the nucleoside analogs zidovudine[14] and stavudine.[19] Using MT-2 cells infected with HIV-1 strain IIIB (a zidovudine-sensitive isolate), synergistic antiviral activity occurred when emtricitabine was combined with zidovudine or stavudine. Additive antiviral activity occurred when emtricitabine was combined with zalcitabine or didanosine.[19]

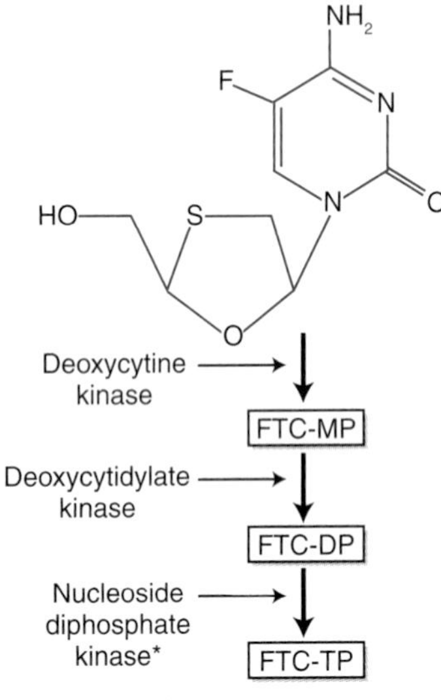

Figure 10-2 ■ Metabolism of emtricitabine.

PHARMACOKINETICS

The pharmacokinetic (PK) properties of emtricitabine have been well characterized.[20] Emtricitabine is rapidly and well absorbed following oral doses with an oral bioavailability of greater than 90%. When single doses of emtricitabine were given orally to HIV-infected volunteers over the dose range of 100–1200 mg, emtricitabine disposition followed linear kinetics, and the steady-state emitricitabine concentrations were predictable based on single-dose data. Plasma emitricitabine concentrations reached levels above the *in vitro* IC_{50} and IC_{90} values even after single-dose administration. Emtricitabine's bioavailability was not significantly affected by food intake.

Based on studies in healthy or HIV-infected adults administered emtricitabine 200 mg once daily as monotherapy or in combination with other antiretrovirals, the mean steady-state peak plasma concentration of ~2 μg/mL occurs within 2 h after the dose. The mean steady-state peak plasma area under the curve (AUC) over the 24-h dosing interval is ~7–11 h μg^{-1} mL^{-1} and mean half-life ($t_{1/2}$) is ~7.5–10 h.[20,21] Comparable PK characteristics are seen in neonates less than 3 months of age given 3 mg/kg qd,[22] and in children administered a dose of 6 mg/kg qd.[23]

Emtricitabine is excreted predominantly in the urine. Following a single oral dose, 86% of the emtricitabine dose was recovered in the urine and 13% in the feces. More than 85% of the dose was excreted in the urine as unchanged emitricitabine. The effect of renal impairment and hemodialysis on emtricitabine's PK parameters has been studied, and dose adjustments are recommended for patients with baseline creatinine clearance <50 mL/min including patients on hemodialysis.[24]

E-TP has a prolonged intracellular half-life compared to its plasma half-life and the intracellular half-life of L-TP. The estimated intracellular half-life of E-TP is 39 h,[20] compared with 16 h for L-TP (Table 10-1).[25]

Among women, emtricitabine achieves higher levels in genital tract secretions relative to plasma levels following both a single dose and at steady state (6.1-fold and 6.7-fold higher

Table 10-1 Comparison of Emtricitabine and Lamivudine

Variable	Emtricitabine	Lamivudine	Reference
In vitro activity against HIV (IC_{50} in PBMCs)[a]	0.01 μM	0.07 μM	1
Intracellular half-life ($t_{1/2}$)	39 h	16 h	20,25
Log change in HIV RNA copies/mL after 10 days of monotherapy	−1.7 $\log_{10}$	−1.5 $\log_{10}$	45
Relative substrate specificity for HIV RT (K_{pol}/K_d)[b]	1 (0.060 μM/s^{-1})	0.1 (0.0067 μM/s^{-1})	16
Relative substrate specificity for mitochondrial DNA polymerase (K_{pol}/K_d)[b]	1 (0.00014 μM/s^{-1})	100 (0.014 μM/s^{-1})	33

HIV, human immunodeficiency virus; RT, reverse transcriptase.

[a] *In vitro* activity has been variable depending on cell type and viral isolate used; most studies have shown superior *in vitro* activity with emtricitabine.

[b] K_{pol} is the rate of polymerization; K_d is the rate of dissociation.

AUC ratios, respectively).[26] This may have implications for its use in the prevention of mother-to-child transmission and in postexposure prophylaxis regimens.

During drug development, emtricitabine was hypothesized to penetrate the central nervous system because of the likely lipophilicity of its fluorine;[1] however, studies have shown that emtricitabine poorly penetrates into the cerebrospinal fluid (CSF). Animal studies have shown that emtricitabine does not effectively cross the blood–brain barrier. In monkeys, the concentration of emtricitabine in the CSF was only 4.0 ± 0.7% of the corresponding plasma emtricitabine level.[27]

TOXICITY

Emtricitabine, like other nucleoside analogs, has the potential for toxicity due to interaction with human DNA polymerases. Of particular concern is the potential for interactions with human mitochondrial DNA complexes, such as mitochondrial DNA polymerase-γ, as disruption of mitochondrial enzymes by NRTIs has been implicated as a cause of hepatic steatosis, primary lactic acidosis syndrome, myopathy, and neuropathy.[28–30] In light of this concern and because of the significant hepatotoxicity observed in subjects treated with another fluorinated nucleoside, fialuridine (FIAU),[31] emphasis has been placed on investigating emtricitabine's effects on cellular and mitochondrial DNA polymerases *in vitro* and on emtricitabine's toxicities in clinical trials.

In Vitro Studies

In investigations performed *in vitro*, E-TP does not appear to interfere significantly with cellular and mitochondrial DNA polymerase function. When the antiviral activity of E-TP against RT was compared with E-TP's activity against human (HeLa cell) DNA polymerases α, β, γ, and ε, E-TP was a weak inhibitor of each of these enzymes when compared to its inhibition of HIV RT. Apparent K_i values were 6.0 μM for polymerase-α, 17 μM for polymerase-β, 6.0 μM for polymerase-γ, and 150 μM for polymerase-ε, compared to the K_i value of 0.17 μM for HIV-1 RT.[32] When the activity of E-TP against mitochondrial DNA polymerases (pol γ) was compared with lamivudine's effect, E-TP was found to incorporate into mitochondrial DNA at a rate that was 15-fold slower than that of lamivudine (K_{pol}), while the affinity of E-TP for the enzyme–DNA complex was sevenfold weaker (K_d) (Table 10-1).[33]

Animal Studies

In short- and long-term animal toxicology studies in mice, rats, and cynomolgus monkeys, emtricitabine showed little toxicity. The only adverse outcome was mild reversible anemia.[32,34] In mice and rabbits exposed to emtricitabine in concentrations 60-fold (mice) and 120-fold (rabbits) higher than human exposures at the recommended daily dose (200 mg), emtricitabine did not adversely affect fertility or cause teratogenesis. It did not adversely affect postnatal development, neurologic development, or learning in F1 mice.[35]

Human Studies

In humans, emtricitabine does not significantly affect general behavior or neurologic, autonomic, central nervous system, cardiovascular, renal, gastrointestinal, or smooth muscle function. Selected adverse events occurring with at least a 5% frequency in controlled studies of emtricitabine include abdominal pain (8–13%), asthenia (10–16%), headache (12–22%), fever (2–8%), diarrhea (9–24%), nausea (14–20%), vomiting (8–12%), arthralgia (3–6%), depression and/or anxiety (1–7%), insomnia (0–7%), cough (4–14%), rhinitis (4–19%) and pharyngitis (4–13%).[36–40] Few serious adverse events with emtricitabine have been reported to date. Selected grade 3/4 laboratory abnormalities occurring with at least a 5% frequency in controlled studies of emtricitabine include elevated creatine kinase (11–12%), AST (3–6%), ALT (2–5%), triglycerides (9–10%), and neutropenia (5%).[36–40] In studies comparing emtricitabine and lamivudine, adverse events and grade 3/4 laboratory abnormalities, including those requiring discontinuation of study medication, are comparable and infrequent.[37] In pediatric studies, no adverse events or laboratory abnormalities occurs with a frequency greater than 5%. In children, the most common laboratory abnormalities were leucopenia (3%) and ALT elevation (3%).[41]

Skin discoloration is a unique toxicity of emtricitabine therapy that has been observed in ~3% of subjects receiving the drug in clinical trials.[42] Racial/ethnic differences in the frequency of this adverse event have been observed with skin discoloration occurring in 8% of blacks, 0.2% of whites, 2.7% of Hispanics, and 3.8% of Asians. This adverse event typically manifests as hyperpigmentation on the palms and soles, is usually of mild degree, and has not been associated with long-term toxicities to date. Discoloration of the tongue, arm, lip, and nail beds have also been observed, although this is less common (<1% frequency). The hyperpigmentation/discoloration resolves in some patients who discontinue treatment, and in some patients who continue to receive emtricitabine.[43]

Emtricitabine is a pregnancy category-B drug, and as such is acceptable to use during pregnancy.[24] Over 70 women have become pregnant during clinical trials of emtricitabine. None of the infants born to exposed mothers had congenital abnormalities.[43]

ANTIRETROVIRAL ACTIVITY AND CLINICAL EFFICACY

Emtricitabine Monotherapy

Adult volunteers, adult HIV-infected patients, and HIV-infected or HIV-exposed pediatric patients have received emtricitabine in phase I/II clinical trials. Most of these trials are PK and dose-finding trials. However, studies FTC-101[44] and FTC-102[45] also evaluated the antiviral activity of emtricitabine alone and in comparison with lamivudine. FTC-101 was a phase I/II, open-label, dose-range study of 41 treatment-naive,

HIV-infected subjects who were administered emtricitabine monotherapy at 25 mg bid, 100 mg qd, 100 mg bid, 200 mg qd, and 200 mg bid doses for 14 days.[44] Antiretroviral suppression (1.3 $\log_{10}$) occurred in all dosage cohorts, with a strong trend toward greater activity at the high doses (200 mg bid and 200 mg qd). FTC-102 was a randomized, open-label study of 81 HIV-infected patients given 10 days of monotherapy with emtricitabine or lamivudine.[45] The antiretroviral activity and safety of emtricitabine at doses of 50 mg qd, 100 mg qd, and 200 mg qd were compared with lamivudine 150 mg bid. Subjects receiving emtricitabine 200 mg qd had a significantly greater change in plasma HIV RNA, as measured by the average AUC minus baseline plasma HIV RNA level (AAUCMB) through day 11, compared with subjects treated with lamivudine ($P = 0.04$). The mean reduction in plasma HIV RNA levels was 1.7 $\log_{10}$ for subjects receiving emtricitabine, compared with 1.5 $\log_{10}$ for subjects receiving lamivudine (Table 10-1). These studies confirmed the potency of emtricitabine when used as a once-daily drug.

Emtricitabine in Three-Drug Combinations

As shown in Table 10-2, several studies have evaluated the efficacy and safety of emtricitabine in combination with other antiretrovirals.

ANRS 091/FTC-201 Study

The ANRS 091/FTC-201 study, a phase II pilot study, assessed the activity of a once-daily antiretroviral regimen that combined emtricitabine, didanosine, and efavirenz in treatment-naive subjects.[46] Among the 40 study subjects, the median baseline CD4+ T-lymphocyte count was 373 cells/mm^3, and the median baseline plasma HIV RNA was 4.8 $\log_{10}$ copies/mL. After 24 weeks of treatment, the median increase in CD4+ T-lymphocyte count was 159 cells/mm^3, and the median decrease in plasma HIV RNA was 3.4 $\log_{10}$. At 24 weeks, 98% of subjects had plasma HIV RNA levels of less than 400 copies/mL, and 93% had levels of less than 50 copies/mL. At 64 weeks the median increase in CD4+ T-lymphocyte count was 219 cells/mm^3, and 90% of subjects had plasma HIV RNA levels of less than 400 copies/mL.[47] No significant toxicities were reported during this trial.

FTC-301A Study

In the FTC-301A study, a total of 580 treatment-naive subjects were randomized to FTC or stavudine in combination with didanosine and efavirenz in a placebo-controlled study.[40] Among the 571 subjects who received study drugs and were included in analyses, mean baseline $\log_{10}$ plasma HIV RNA levels were 4.8 copies/mL and mean baseline CD4+ T-lymphocyte counts were 312 cells/mm^3 and 324 cells/mm^3 in the emtricitabine and stavudine arms respectively. Eighty-one percent of FTC treated patients and 68% of stavudine treated patients completed 48 weeks of randomized, blinded therapy. Seven percent of emtricitabine-treated patients and 13% of stavudine-treated patients discontinued study therapy due to adverse events. Four percent of patients in the emtricitabine arm and 11% of patients in the stavudine arm discontinued treatment due to virologic failure. Following a planned interim analysis by an independent data and safety monitoring board when all patients had completed 24 weeks of therapy, the double-blind comparative phase of the study was terminated and all patients in the group demonstrating lesser response were offered open-label emtricitabine. Blinding of the original treatment assignment was maintained until all patients completed their week 48 visit. Only four subjects opted to receive open-label emtricitabine, and all four patients did so on or after their week 44 study visit. After 48 weeks on study medications, the percentage of patients with plasma HIV RNA <400 copies/mL were 81% in the emtricitabine arm and 68% in the stavudine arm ($P < 0.001$), and with plasma HIV RNA <50 copies/mL were 78% and 59%, respectively ($P < 0.001$). The mean increase in CD4+ T-lymphocyte count was not significantly different between the treatment arms in on-treatment analysis (168 cells/mm^3 in the emtricitabine group and 134 cells/mm^3 in the stavudine group, $P = 0.15$). In intention-to-treat sensitivity analysis with the last CD4 count carried forward to week 48 for those subjects withdrawing from the study, a statistically significant difference in mean increase in CD4+ T-lymphocyte count between the treatment arms was observed (153 cells/mm^3 in the emtricitabine group and 120 cells/mm^3 in the stavudine group, $P = 0.02$). No difference in clinical progression, defined as development of a new clinical event included in category C of the 1993 classification of the US Centers for Disease Control and Prevention (CDC),[48] or death due to any cause, between the treatment arms was observed (1.7% in the emtricitabine group and 3.5% in the stavudine group, $P = 0.19$).

FTC-302 and FTC-303 Studies

Two randomized, equivalence (noninferiority) studies have compared the relative antiretroviral activity of emtricitabine and lamivudine. The FTC-302 trial, a double-blind, placebo-controlled study, randomized a total of 468 treatment-naive subjects to emtricitabine- or lamivudine-containing regimens.[49,50] At baseline, the mean $\log_{10}$ plasma HIV RNA levels were 4.5, and the mean CD4+ T-lymphocyte counts were 392 cells/mm^3 and 386 cells/mm^3 in the emtricitabine and lamivudine arms. During the study, 10% of subjects receiving emtricitabine and 10% receiving lamivudine experienced adverse events and withdrew from study; 12% of both groups withdrew for other reasons. After 48 weeks on study medications, the percentages of study subjects with plasma HIV RNA levels of less than 400 copies/mL and less than 50 copies/mL did not significantly differ between the two groups, (emtricitabine: 65% <400 copies/mL and 60% <50 copies/mL; lamivudine: 71% <400 copies/mL and 65% <50 copies/mL).[49] Virologic failure, defined as a lack of response (plasma HIV RNA >400 copies/mL at week 12) or loss of response (two consecutive plasma HIV RNA levels >400 copies/mL after having reached <400 copies/mL), occurred in 14% of the emtricitabine group and 10% of the lamivudine group.[51] Of note, FTC-302 was

Table 10-2 Major Phase II/III Activity and Efficacy Trials Evaluating Emtricitabine Therapy

Trial	Design	Dose	No. of Subjects	Entry Criterion	CD4+ T-Lymphocyte Count Response	Antiretroviral[a] Response	Clinical Outcomes	Comments
ANRS 091/ FTC-201[46, 47]	Open-label, single arm, qd regimen	FTC 200 mg qd, ddI 250 or 400 mg qd, EFV 600 mg qd	40	Adult, HIV-1 infected, treatment-naive, CD4 count $\geqslant$ 100 cells/mm^3, HIV RNA $\geqslant$ 5000 copies/mL	Median increase of 159 cells/mm^3 at 24 weeks, and 219 cells/mm^3 at 64 weeks	Decrease of 3.5 $\log_{10}$ at 24 weeks; 98% $\leqslant$ 400 copies/mL, 93% $\leqslant$ 50 copies/mL at 24 weeks; 90% $\leqslant$ 400 copies/mL at 64 weeks	No AIDS-defining events	Pilot study supporting the efficacy of a once-daily dosing regimen.
FTC-301A[40]	Randomized, double-blind, d4T-controlled	FTC 200 mg qd *or* d4T 30 or 40 mg bid plus ddI 250 or 400 mg qd, and EFV 600 mg qd	571	Adult, HIV-1 infected, treatment-naive, HIV RNA > 5000 copies/mL	Mean increase of 168 cells/mm^3 in the FTC arm; 134 cells/mm^3 in the d4T arm at 48 weeks in on-treatment analysis (P = 0.15)	81% $\leqslant$ 400 copies/mL, 78% $\leqslant$ 50 copies/mL at 48 weeks in the FTC arm; 68% $\leqslant$ 400 copies/mL, 59% $\leqslant$ 50 copies/mL at 48 weeks in d4T arm in ITT analysis (P < 0.001 for both)	Incident category C clinical event or death in 1.7% in FTC arm; 3.5% in d4T arm (P = 0.19)	Entirely once-daily regimen. Open-label FTC offered to subjects based on the recommendation of the independent data and safety monitoring board at a scheduled interim analysis.
FTC-302[49–52]	Randomized, double-blind, 3TC-controlled	FTC 200 mg qd *or* 3TC 150 mg bid plus d4T and nevirapine (n = 385), *or* efavirenz (n = 83)	468	Adult, HIV-infected, treatment-naive	Median increase of 191 cells/mm^3 in the FTC arm; 206 cells/mm^3 in the 3TC arm at 48 weeks	65% < 400 copies/mL, 60% < 50 copies/mL at 48 weeks in the FTC arm; 71% < 400 copies/mL, 65% < 50 copies/mL at 48 weeks in the 3TC arm (P = NS)		Supports equivalence with 3TC. Study terminated prematurely due to observed hepatoxicity attributed to nevirapine.

(Continued)

Table 10-2 (Continued)

Trial	Design	Dose	No. of Subjects	Entry Criterion	CD4+ T-Lymphocyte Count Response	Antiretroviral[a] Response	Clinical Outcomes	Comments
FTC-303/ FTC-350[38]	Randomized (2:1 switch to FTC from 3TC), open-label equivalence (noninferiority) study, responders in FTC-303 rollover to FTC-350	FTC 200 mg qd (n = 294) *or* continued 3TC 150 mg bid (n = 146) plus continued background regimen of d4T *or* ZDV and a PI *or* NNRTI	440	Adult, HIV-1 infected, on stable combination antiretroviral regimen including 3TC for at least 12 weeks, screening HIV RNA ≤ 400 copies/mL	Mean increase of 29 cells/mm^3 in the FTC arm at 48 weeks; 61 cells/mm^3 in the 3TC arm at 48 weeks (P = 0.10)	77% ≤ 400 copies/mL, 67% ≤ 50 copies/mL at 48 weeks in the FTC arm; 82% ≤ 400 copies/mL, 72% ≤ 50 copies/mL at 48 weeks in the 3TC arm (P = NS for both)		Supports equivalence with 3TC. FTC can safely and efficaciously replace 3TC in patients on stable combination antiretroviral regimens with HIV RNA ≤ 400 copies/mL.
ALIZE[39,73]	Randomized, open-label, equivalence (noninferiority) switch study	Continued PI-based combination antiretroviral regimen or switch to FTC 200 mg, ddI 250 or 400 mg qd, and EFV 600 mg qd	355	Adult, HIV-1 infected, on a combination antiretroviral regimen consisting of 1 PI and 2 NRTIs, NNRTI naive, CD4 count ≥ 100 cells/mm^3, HIV RNA ≤ 400 copies/mL for ≥ 6 months	Median increase of 16 cells/mm^3 in the switch arm at 48 weeks; 16 cells/mm^3 in the PI group at 48 weeks (P = 0.68)	91% ≤ 400 copies/mL in the switch arm at 48 weeks; 88% ≤ 400 copies/mL in the PI group at 48 weeks (P = NS)	No AIDS-defining events	NNRTI-naive patients on a PI-based regimen with HIV RNA ≤ 400 copies/mL can safely and efficaciously be switched to a regimen of FTC, ddI, and EFV.
Gilead 934[36]	Randomized, open-label, equivalence (noninferiority) study	FTC 200 mg qd and TDF 300 mg qd *or* fixed dose ZDV 300 mg and 3TC 150 mg bid; plus EFV 600 mg qd	509	Adult, HIV-1 infected, treatment-naive, HIV RNA > 10 000 copies/mL	Median increase of 190 cells/mm^3 in the FTC/TDF arm at 48 weeks; 158 cells/mm^3 in the ZDV/3TC arm at 48 weeks	81% ≤ 400 copies/mL, 77% ≤ 50 copies/mL at 48 weeks in the FTC/TDF arm; 70% ≤ 400		Difference in outcomes ascribed in part to greater number of patients discontinuing study drugs due to adverse events in

				($P = 0.002$)	copies/mL, 68% $\leqslant 50$ copies/mL at 48 weeks in the ZDV/3TC arm ($P = 0.005$ and 0.03)	the ZDV/3TC arm.
ACTG 5202	Randomized, trial of open-label RTV-enhanced ATZ *or* EFV in combination with double-blind, placebo-controlled FTC/TDF *or* ABC/3TC	Fixed dose FTC 200 mg and TDF 300 mg qd (Truvada) *or* ABC 600 mg and 3TC 300 mg qd (Epzicom) plus EFV 600 mg qd *or* ATZ 300 mg qd and RTV 100 mg qd	Adult, HIV-1 infected, treatment-naive, HIV RNA $\geqslant 1000$ copies/mL			Ongoing, comparison of safety, efficacy, and tolerability of once-daily fixed-dose NRTIs in combination with once-daily PI and NNRTI.

ddI, didanosine; EFV, efavirenz; 3TC, lamivudine; d4T, stavudine; ZDV, zidovudine; TDF, tenofovir; ABC, abacavir; ATZ, atazanavir; RTV, ritonavir; PI, protease inhibitor; NRTI, nucleoside reverse transcriptase inhibitor; NNRTI, non-nucleoside reverse transcriptase inhibitor.

terminated prematurely due to hepatotoxicity attributed to nevirapine.[52]

The FTC-303 study randomized 440 subjects on lamivudine-containing regimens with plasma HIV RNA levels of less than 400 copies/mL for at least 12 weeks to open-label emtricitabine or continued lamivudine in a 2:1 allocation.[38] At baseline, subjects had received lamivudine-containing regimens for a median of 35 months; 79% were on protease inhibitor (PI)-containing regimens, and 21% were on non-nucleoside reverse transcriptase inhibitor (NNRTI)-containing regimens. Baseline plasma HIV RNA levels were less than 50 copies/mL in 86% and 50–400 copies/mL in 14%. A significantly higher percentage of subjects receiving emtricitabine withdrew owing to adverse events compared to those receiving lamivudine (4% vs 0%). After 48 weeks on study medications, the percentages of study subjects with plasma HIV RNA levels of <400 copies/mL and <50 copies/mL were not significantly different between the two groups (emtricitabine: 77% <400 copies/mL and 67% <50 copies/mL; lamivudine: 82% <400 copies/mL and 72% <50 copies/mL). Virologic failure, defined as plasma HIV RNA levels of more than 400 copies/mL on two consecutive measurements, occurred in 7% of subjects receiving emtricitabine and 8% of subjects receiving lamivudine.

GILEAD 934 Study

In the Gilead 934 study, 517 treatment-naive subjects were randomized to tenofovir and emtricitabine (given separately) or zidovudine and lamivudine (given as fixed-dose combination combivir) in combination with efavirenz in an open-label, equivalence (noninferiority) study.[36] Of the 509 subjects that received study drugs and were included in analyses, the median baseline $\log_{10}$ plasma HIV RNA levels was 5.0 copies/mL and the median baseline CD4+ T-lymphocyte counts was 233 cells/mm^3 and 241 cells/mm^3 in the tenofovir–emtricitabine and combivir arms, respectively. After 48 weeks on study medications, the percentage of patients with plasma HIV RNA <400 copies/mL were 81% in the tenofovir–emtricitabine arm and 70% in the combivir arm ($P = 0.005$), and with plasma HIV RNA <50 copies/mL were 77% and 68% respectively ($P = 0.03$) in intention-to-treat analysis. Similar results were observed when the analyses were limited to subjects who did not have a baseline NNRTI-resistance mutations (11 patients in each arm (4%) had such mutations). The mean increase in CD4+ T-lymphocyte counts was 190 cells/mm^3 in the tenofovir–emtricitabine group and 158 cells/mm^3 in the combivir group ($P = 0.002$). There were no significant differences in viral rebound (two consecutive plasma HIV RNA levels >400 copies/mL after having reached <400 copies/mL) between the treatment arms (1% in tenofovir–emtricitabine group and 3% in combivir group, $P = 0.11$). While there was no difference in overall adverse events between treatment groups, significantly more patients in the combivir group had adverse events (mostly hematologic and gastrointestinal) that resulted in discontinuation of study medication (9% vs 4% in tenofovir–emtricitabine group, $P = 0.02$). This finding may partially explain the superior viral suppression and CD4+ T-lymphocyte count increase observed in the tenofovir–emtricitabine group. Mean adherence, as measured by pill counts, was greater among subjects in the tenofovir–emtricitabine group (90% vs 87% in the combivir group, $P = 0.04$).

PEDIATRIC TRIALS

FTC-105

In the FTC-105 study, the single dose PKs of emtricitabine at 60 and 120 mg/m^2 were evaluated in HIV-infected children from 22 months to 17 years.[23] A total of 25 children completed the study; only two children were less than 2 years of age. In this cohort, plasma emtricitabine concentrations were linear and dose-proportional over the dose range studied across all age groups. The elimination $t_{1/2}$ had a range of 9.7–11.9 h at a dose of 120 mg/m^2. Based on the AUC data at a dose of 120 mg/m^2, it was projected that a once daily emtricitabine dose of 6 mg/kg would produce plasma AUC concentrations in children comparable to that seen in adults who are given a 200 mg dose (i.e., median of ~10 h μg^{-1} mL^{-1}).

FTC-203

Based on the results of FTC-105, a therapeutic emtricitabine dose of 6 mg kg^{-7} day^{-7} was recommended for children and was evaluated in an open-label, nonrandomized phase II study, FTC-203.[41,53,54] In the FTC-203 study, a total of 71 treatment-naive and 45 treatment-experienced patients were enrolled. Treatment-naive subjects were treated with emtricitabine in combination with stavudine and lopinavir/ritonavir, while treatment-experienced subjects were treated with emtricitabine replacing lamivudine in their previous combination antiretroviral therapy regimen. Among study subjects, the mean age was 6 years, the median $\log_{10}$ plasma HIV RNA level was 4.5 copies/mL, and the median CD4+ T-lymphocyte count was 817 cells/mm^3.[41] At interim analysis, a moderate increase in emtricitabine AUC was observed with increasing age (range 8.1 h μg^{-1} mL^{-1}-14.5 h μg^{-1} mL^{-1}), but dose adjustments were not instituted based on this finding.[54] After 48 weeks on study medications, the percentage of patients with plasma HIV RNA <400 copies/mL was 93% and <50 copies/mL was 78% in the treatment-naive group. In the treatment-experienced group 87% of subjects had plasma HIV RNA <400 copies/mL and 78% had levels <50 copies/mL. Overall, study drugs were well tolerated with few adverse events and laboratory abnormalities reported. M184V was the only resistance mutation detected, occurring in four of five treatment-naive subjects (80%) and zero of three treatment-experienced subjects (0%) with virologic failure.[41]

PACTG P1021

The PACTG P1021 is an open-label phase I/II study of once-daily emtricitabine, didanosine, and efavirenz that enrolled

37 treatment-naive HIV-infected children.[55–57] Among study subjects the median age was 10.5 years, the median HIV RNA was 47 775 copies/mL, and the median CD4+ T-lymphocyte count was 310 cells/mm^3. At the initial interim analysis, FTC and ddI met protocol defined AUC targets, while EFV AUC data required an increased dose for younger patients receiving oral solution.[56] After 24 weeks on study drugs, 86% of subjects had plasma HIV RNA <400 copies/mL, 81% had levels <50 copies/mL and the median increase in the CD4+ T-lymphocyte count was 254 cells/mm^3.[55] After 96 weeks on study drugs, 85% of subjects had plasma HIV RNA <400 copies/mL, 72% had levels <50 copies/mL, and the median increase in CD4+ T-lymphocyte count was 329 cells/mm^3.[57] Overall, study medications were well tolerated. Resistance data have not yet been presented.

HBV AND HIV–HBV CO-INFECTION TRIALS

The efficacy of emtricitabine in the treatment of HBV has been evaluated *in vitro* and when given as monotherapy to HBV-infected adults in phase I, II, and III studies.[58–60] In the FTCB-301 study, 248 HBV-infected patients were randomized to emtricitabine or placebo (2:1 allocation) in a randomized, double-blind, placebo-controlled study.[60] Among emtricitabine-treated subjects, 62% had improved liver histologic findings, 54% had HBV DNA levels <400 copies/mL, and 65% had normal ALT levels after 48 weeks of treatment. These findings were all significantly superior to the placebo-treated group and are similar to published studies of adefovir and lamivudine monotherapy. Serum HBV DNA decreased by a median of 4.5 $\log_{10}$ copies/mL in the emtricitabine arm.

A high incidence of post-treatment exacerbation of HBV infection has been observed following discontinuation of emtricitabine in HBV monotherapy trials.[61] Up to 23% of subjects treated with emtricitabine experienced post-treatment exacerbations at a median of ~11 weeks following termination of therapy. Seroconversion to anti-hepatitis B e antigen (anti-HBe) does not protect against post-treatment exacerbation. Elevation in tranaminase levels was the only manifestation for most subjects (86%). Patients with bridging fibrosis and/or cirrhosis prior to initiating emtricitabine therapy appear are at higher risk for developing post-treatment exacerbation with decompensation, defined as bilirubin >2.5 mg/dL or >1 mg/dL above baseline, elevation in prothrombin time of 2 s greater than baseline, albumin <3 g/dL, or clinical decompensation. In FTCB-301, 9% of subjects with bridging fibrosis and/or cirrhosis at pre-treatment liver biopsy experienced exacerbation with decompensation (including one subject who required cadaveric liver transplantation), compared with 0% among subjects without high-grade fibrosis.[60,61]

Limited data are available regarding the efficacy and safety of emtricitabine in the management of HIV–HBV co-infected patients. Retrospective analyses have evaluated HBV virologic responses and HBV genotypic analyses among HBV surface antigen (sAg) positive patients participating in three prospective studies of emtricitabine as part of a combination antiretroviral regimen in HIV-infected treatment-naive subjects (FTC-301A, FTC-302, and MKC-401).[62,63] It is noteworthy that the antiretroviral regimens used in these studies contained no drug with activity against HBV other than emtricitabine. After 48 weeks of emtricitabine therapy, the median decrease in HBV DNA was 2.72 $\log_{10}$ copies/mL, and 59% of subjects with detectable HBV viremia at baseline had achieved an HBV DNA level <4700 copies/mL. Emtricitabine is commonly used 'off label' in the treatment of HIV–HBV co-infected patients despite limited clinical trial data and the lack of FDA approval for this indication. An HIV–HBV International Panel considered emtricitabine interchangeable with lamivudine in the treatment of HIV–HBV co-infected patients, and suggested that neither drug should be used as monotherapy given the low genetic barrier to resistance for these drugs.[64] The panel gave a strong recommendation for use of emtricitabine or lamivudine as a component of combination antiretroviral therapy in HIV–HBV co-infected patients (score A1).

Providers must use caution and monitor patients closely when changing or discontinuing emtricitabine therapy in HIV–HBV co-infected patients given the high incidence of post-treatment exacerbation of HBV seen in emtricitabine treatment trials of HBV.[61] Particularly concerning is the risk of decompensation among patients with baseline bridging fibrosis and/or cirrhosis. Liver histology results may be unavailable for many HIV–HBV co-infected patients treated with combination antiretroviral therapy. As such, providers may not be aware of patients who are at increased risk of experiencing post-treatment exacerbation of HBV with decompensation, highlighting the need for close laboratory and clinical monitoring of HIV–HBV co-infected patients after withdrawal of emtricitabine (as well as other nucleoside and nucleotide analogs with activity against HBV).

RESISTANCE

Emtricitabine-resistant HIV has been examined *in vitro* and *in vivo*. Drug resistance to emtricitabine develops rapidly and results from a single point mutation at position 184 of the highly conserved YMDD (Tyr-Met-Asp-Asp) motif of RT, the RT polymerase domain.[65] The point mutation causes methionine to be replaced by valine or isoleucine (M184V and M184I mutations). Although this mutation confers cross-resistance to lamivudine, viruses resistant to emtricitabine retain sensitivity to other nucleoside analogs and NNRTIs including zidovudine, zalcitabine, didanosine, and nevirapine.[12,13]

In Vitro Studies

In an *in vitro* comparison of lamivudine and emtricitabine by Schinazi et al, HIV-infected PBMCs were exposed to equal concentrations of lamivudine or emtricitabine and were passaged weekly. With each weekly cell passage, HIV replication increased in both cell cultures. At the third week 50% of virus replication was inhibited by emtricitabine, whereas less than 5% was inhibited by an equal concentration of lamivudine. At week 7, however, viruses passaged with either drug were more than 1000-fold resistant to both drugs. DNA sequencing of the resistant virus generated by both drugs revealed the M184V or M184I mutations in the RT YMDD motif.[13]

Tisdale et al compared the antiviral activity of emtricitabine with that of zidovudine, zalcitabine, didanosine, lamivudine, and nevirapine in drug-resistant viral mutants.[12] All viral mutants with the M184V substitution were markedly resistant to emtricitabine and lamivudine, showing a more than 1000-fold increase in IC_{50} values. The M184V substitution also led to a minor increase in the IC_{50} values for zalcitabine and didanosine but did not cause a change in susceptibility to zidovudine or nevirapine. In addition, in the presence of virus that was partially resistant to zidovudine (M41L and T215Y), the M184V substitution caused complete reversion to a zidovudine-sensitive phenotype.

In Vivo Studies

The results of resistance testing in subjects experiencing virologic relapse on emitricitabine-containing regimens suggest that wild-type virus or M184V variants occur most commonly, although data are somewhat limited given the paucity of published prospective study data. In the FTC-101 study 21% (8/38) of subjects receiving emtricitabine monotherapy in a dose range of 25 mg qd--200 mg bid for 14 days developed the M184V mutation by day 15. Five out of 10 subjects with viral rebound (50%) had the M184V mutation on genotypic analysis.[44]

Two retrospective studies have evaluated the results of genotypic resistance assays of treatment-naive subjects enrolled in clinical trials who were failing initial antiretroviral regimens containing either emtricitabine or lamivudine.[66,67] These studies have been presented as abstracts and have shown that the M184V/I mutation may occur less frequently, and that wild-type virus may occur more frequently in subjects treated with emtricitabine. These results must be interpreted with caution as the clinical trials used for these studies used different combination antiretroviral regimens, including several studies of triple NRTI regimens.

As described previously, two randomized, equivalence (noninferiority) studies have directly compared the efficacy and safety of emtricitabine and lamivudine.[38,49,50] In the FTC-302 study, 56 of 468 subjects experienced virologic failure, defined as a lack of response (plasma HIV RNA level >400 copies/mL at week 12) or loss of response (two consecutive plasma HIV RNA levels >400 copies/mL after having reached <400 copies/mL).[51] Virologic failure occurred in 14% of subjects receiving emtricitabine versus 10% of subjects receiving lamivudine. Of 56 subjects experiencing virologic failure, 25 had viruses with M184V genotype, including 10 of 33 subjects receiving emtricitabine versus 15 of 23 subjects receiving lamivudine (30% emtricitabine vs 65% lamivudine; $P = 0.01$).[51]

The FTC-303 study provides limited data regarding the emergence of M184V-resistance mutations in patients treated with emtricitabine or lamivudine given the high percentage of subjects in both treatment groups harboring this mutation in their baseline genotype.[38] Virologic failure, defined as loss of response (two consecutive plasma HIV RNA levels >400 copies/mL), occurred in 21 of 294 subjects in the emtricitabine group (7%) and 11 of 146 subjects in the lamivudine group (8%). Among patients experiencing virologic failure, performing a baseline genotype was possible for 18 of 21 subjects in the emtricitabine group and 4 of 11 patients in the lamivudine group. At baseline, the M184V-resistance mutation was seen in 16 of 18 subjects in the emtricitabine group (89%) and three of four subjects in the lamuvudine group (75%). At the time of virologic failure, genotypic resistance analysis revealed the M184V-resistance mutation in 20 of 21 subjects in the emtricitabine group (95%) and nine of 10 subjects in the lamivudine group (90%) (genotype could not be done on one subject in the lamivudine group). Only three of these mutations (two in the emtricitabine group and one in the lamivudine group) could be confirmed as new mutations.

In the FTC-301A study, 13 of 286 subjects in the emtricitabine group experienced virologic failure, defined as a lack of response (plasma HIV RNA level >400 copies/mL) or loss of response (two consecutive plasma HIV RNA levels >400 copies/mL after having reached <400 copies/mL).[40] Genotypic resistance analysis in these 13 subjects revealed an M184V/I mutation in six subjects (46%), and wild-type virus in one subject (8%). NNRTI-resistance mutations were seen in 11 subjects (85%) and K65R in one subject (8%).

In the Gilead 934 study, genotypic analysis was done on subjects with viral rebound (two consecutive plasma HIV RNA levels >400 copies/mL after having reached <400 copies/mL), with a lack of response (plasma HIV RNA level >400 copies/mL), or who discontinued the assigned study drug before 48 weeks and had a plasma HIV RNA level >400 copies/mL on their last visit.[36] Thirty-five subjects met these criteria, 12 in the tenofovir–emtricitabine group and 23 in the combivir group (genotyping of one subject in the combivir group failed due to technical reasons). Wild-type genotype was observed in three subjects in the tenofovir–emtricitabine group (25%), and five subjects in the combivir group (22%). Any M184V/I mutation was seen in two subjects in the tenofovir–emtricitabine group (17%), and seven subjects in the combivir group (30%). Any NNRTI-resistance mutation was observed in 75% (nine of 12) and 70% (16 of 23) of subjects in the respective treatment arms, and no subject in the tenofovir–emtricitabine arm had the K65R mutation.

Databases of phenotypic resistance assays from HIV-infected patient samples have been studied to evaluate differential resistance to emtricitabine and lamivudine among isolates with a variety of NRTI-resistance mutations.[68–70] Among isolates without the M184V/I mutation, resistance to emtricitabine appears to occur more commonly than resistance to lamivudine in the presence of multiple thymidine analog mutations (TAMS). Such results were not observed for other NRTI-resistance mutations in the absence of TAMS. These results are preliminary, and the clinical implications of these finding in the management of HIV-infected patients have not been studied.

When administered as monotherapy for HBV infection, emtricitabine is known to select for the M204V/I (YIDD/YMDD) mutation in the C domain of the HBV polymerase. Although this mutation confers cross-resistance to lamivudine, viruses with this mutation retain sensitivity to other antiviral drugs including adefovir and tenofovir.[71,72] In the FTCB-301 study, genotypic resistance analysis was done for all subjects with HBV DNA levels >400 copies/mL.[60] In this study, the incidence of the YMDD mutation was 13% at 48 weeks. Subjects in the FTCB-102 study had genotypic resistance testing done if their HBV DNA levels were greater than 4700 copies/mL. Among subjects who received emtricitabine at a dose of 200 mg daily, the YMDD mutation was seen in 9% of subjects at 48 weeks, and 18% of subjects at 96 weeks.[58]

DRUG INTERACTIONS

Because renal excretion of unchanged drug is the principal route of emtricitabine elimination from plasma, the potential for emtricitabine to cause metabolic drug interactions is thought to be low. In the few drug interaction studies conducted to date, emticitabine does not interact with other antiretroviral agents.[24] In the FTC-103 study, the PKs of emtricitabine in six subjects was unaffected by co-administration with either zidovudine or stavudine. In the same study, a single dose of emtricitabine caused a mild increase in the AUC and maximum concentration (C_{max}) of zidovudine (26% and 66%, respectively) but had no clinically significant effect on the PKs of stavudine.[24]

Because emtricitabine is eliminated unchanged in urine, a study was conducted that focused on potential interactions between emtricitabine and famciclovir at the site of urinary excretion. Famciclovir was chosen as a prototypical drug for this evaluation because its active form in plasma (penciclovir) is primarily eliminated in urine, and famciclovir may be commonly co-administered with emtricitabine. The results showed no clinically significant interactions between emtricitabine and famciclovir.[24]

RECOMMENDATIONS FOR USE

Emtricitabine is FDA approved for the treatment of HIV infection. In treatment guidelines, emtricitabine is in the 'preferred category' of NRTIs for the treatment of antiretroviral-naive patients initiating combination antiretroviral therapy. Emtricitabine offers once-daily dosing, and is well tolerated with infrequent treatment – limiting adverse events. The dose of emtricitabine needs to be reduced in patients with renal insufficiency, and FTC is a pregnancy category B drug. Skin discoloration is a unique toxicity to emtricitabine that has been observed in ~3% of patients with a predilection for people of color. This toxicity is usually mild in severity and does not typically lead to termination of therapy. In combination regimens, emtricitabine has displayed excellent activity when given with several other antiretroviral drugs, as documented by suppression of plasma HIV RNA levels and increases in absolute CD4+ T-lymphocyte counts. Emtricitabine resistance is caused by a single point mutation at position 184 of RT (M184V/I). Viral isolates with M184V RT mutations display high-level emtricitabine resistance and cross-resistance to lamivudine. While not FDA approved for the treatment of HBV infections and HIV–HBV co-infections, emtricitabine is often used in this capacity, typically in combination with another drug with activity against HBV in an effort to prevent the emergence of resistance (such as tenofovir in the case of HIV–HBV co-infection). HBV-infected and HIV–HBV co-infected patients must be monitored closely following discontinuation of emtricitabine therapy since post-treatment exacerbation of HBV has been observed in up to 23% of patients upon termination of therapy in HBV monotherapy trials. Patients with baseline bridging fibrosis and/or cirrhosis are at greatest risk.

REFERENCES

1. Schinazi RF, McMillan A, Cannon D, et al. Selective inhibition of human immunodeficiency viruses by racemates and enantiomers of cis-5-fluoro-1-[2-(hydroxymethyl)-1,3-oxathiolan-5-yl]cytosine. Antimicrob Agents Chemother 36:2423–31, 1992.
2. Department of Health and Human Services. Guidelines for the use of antiretroviral therapy in adults. October 5, 2005. Available: http://aidsinfo.nih.gov. 9 Feb 2006.
3. Yeni PG, Hammer SM, Hirsch MS, et al. Treatment for adult HIV infection: 2004 recommendations of the International AIDS Society-USA Panel. JAMA 292:251–65, 2004.
4. Van Roey P, Pangborn W, Schinazi RF, et al. Absolute configuration of the antiviral agent (−)-cis-5-fluoro-1-[2-(hydroxymethyl)-1,3-oxathiolan-5-yl]-cytosine. Antivir Chem Chemother 4:369–75, 1993.
5. Furman PA, Wilson LJ, Reardon JE, Painter GR. The effect of absolute configuration on the anti-HIV and anti-HBV activity of nucleoside analogues. Antivir Chem Chemother 6:345–55, 1995.
6. Furman PA, Davis M, Liotta DC, et al. The anti-hepatitis B virus activities, cytotoxicities, and anabolic profiles of the (−) and (+) enantiomers of cis-5-fluoro-1-[2-(hydroxymethyl)-1,3-oxathiolan-5-yl]cytosine. Antimicrob Agents Chemother 36:2686–92, 1992.
7. Paff MT, Averett DR, Prus KL, et al. Intracellular metabolism of (−)- and (+)-cis-5-fluoro-1-[2-(hydroxymethyl)-1,3-oxathiolan-5-yl]cytosine in HepG2 derivative 2.2.15 (subclone P5A) cells. Antimicrob Agents Chemother 38:1230–8, 1994.
8. Wilson JE, Martin JL, Borroto-Esoda K, et al. The 5′-triphosphates of the (−) and (+) enantiomers of cis-5-fluoro-1-[2-(hydroxymethyl)-1,3-oxathiolane-5-yl]cytosine equally inhibit human immunodeficiency virus type 1 reverse transcriptase. Antimicrob Agents Chemother 37:1720–2, 1993.
9. Wilson JE, Aulabaugh A, Caligan B, et al. Human immunodeficiency virus type-1 reverse transcriptase. Contribution of Met-184 to binding of nucleoside 5′-triphosphate. J Biol Chem 271:13656–62, 1996.

10. Stein DS, Moore KH. Phosphorylation of nucleoside analog antiretrovirals: a review for clinicians. Pharmacotherapy 21: 11–34, 2001.
11. Gosselin G, Schinazi RF, Sommadossi JP, et al. Anti-human immunodeficiency virus activities of the beta-L enantiomer of 2′,3′-dideoxycytidine and its 5-fluoro derivative in vitro. Antimicrob Agents Chemother 38:1292–7, 1994.
12. Tisdale M, Kemp SD, Parry NR, Larder BA. Rapid in vitro selection of human immunodeficiency virus type 1 resistant to 3′-thiacytidine inhibitors due to a mutation in the YMDD region of reverse transcriptase. Proc Natl Acad Sci USA 90:5653–6, 1993.
13. Schinazi RF, Lloyd RM, Jr, Nguyen MH, et al. Characterization of human immunodeficiency viruses resistant to oxathiolane-cytosine nucleosides. Antimicrob Agents Chemother 37:875–81, 1993.
14. Mathez D, Schinazi RF, Liotta DC, Leibowitch J. Infectious amplification of wild-type human immunodeficiency virus from patients' lymphocytes and modulation by reverse transcriptase inhibitors in vitro. Antimicrob Agents Chemother 37:2206–11, 1993.
15. Hazen R, Lanier ER. Relative anti-HIV-1 efficacy of lamivudine and emtricitabine in vitro is dependent on cell type. J Acquir Immune Defic Syndr 32:255–8, 2003.
16. Feng JY, Shi J, Schinazi RF, Anderson KS. Mechanistic studies show that (-)-FTC-TP is a better inhibitor of HIV-1 reverse transcriptase than 3TC-TP. Faseb J 13:1511–17, 1999.
17. Jansen RW, Johnson LC, Averett DR. High-capacity in vitro assessment of anti-hepatitis B virus compound selectivity by a virion-specific polymerase chain reaction assay. Antimicrob Agents Chemother 37:441–7, 1993.
18. Schinazi RF, Gosselin G, Faraj A, et al. Pure nucleoside enantiomers of beta-2′,3′-dideoxycytidine analogs are selective inhibitors of hepatitis B virus in vitro. Antimicrob Agents Chemother38:2172–4, 1994.
19. Bridges EG, Dutschman GE, Gullen EA, Cheng YC. Favorable interaction of beta-L(−) nucleoside analogues with clinically approved anti-HIV nucleoside analogues for the treatment of human immunodeficiency virus. Biochem Pharmacol51:731–6, 1996.
20. Wang LH, Begley J, St Claire RL, 3rd, et al. Pharmacokinetic and pharmacodynamic characteristics of emtricitabine support its once daily dosing for the treatment of HIV infection. AIDS Res Hum Retroviruses20:1173–82, 2004.
21. Molina JM, Peytavin G, Perusat S, et al. Pharmacokinetics of emtricitabine, didanosine and efavirenz administered once-daily for the treatment of HIV-infected adults (pharmacokinetic substudy of the ANRS 091 trial). HIV Med 5:99–104, 2004.
22. Blum MR, Ndiweni D, Chittick G, et al. Steady-state pharmacokinetic evaluation of emtricitabine in neonates exposed to HIV in utero. Presented at the 13th Conference on Retroviruses and Opportunistic Infections, Denver, 2006, abstract 568.
23. Wang LH, Wiznia AA, Rathore MH, et al. Pharmacokinetics and safety of single oral doses of emtricitabine in human immunodeficiency virus-infected children. Antimicrob Agents Chemother 48:183–91, 2004.
24. Emtricitabine (package insert). Gilead Sciences.
25. Cammack N, Rouse P, Marr CL, et al. Cellular metabolism of (−) enantiomeric 2′-deoxy-3′-thiacytidine. Biochem Pharmacol 43:2059–64, 1992.
26. Dumond J, Yeh R, Patterson K, et al. First dose and steady-state genital tract pharmacokinetics of ten antiretroviral drugs in HIV-infected women: implications for pre- and post-exposure prophylaxis. Presented at the 13th Conference on Retroviruses and Opportunistic Infections, Denver, 2006, abstract 129.
27. Frick LW, Lambe CU, St John L, et al. Pharmacokinetics, oral bioavailability, and metabolism in mice and cynomolgus monkeys of (2′R,5′S-)-cis-5-fluoro-1-[2-(hydroxymethyl)-1,3-oxathiolan-5-yl] cytosine, an agent active against human immunodeficiency virus and human hepatitis B virus. Antimicrob Agents Chemother 38:2722–9, 1994.
28. Chen CH, Cheng YC. Delayed cytotoxicity and selective loss of mitochondrial DNA in cells treated with the anti-human immunodeficiency virus compound 2′,3′-dideoxycytidine. J Biol Chem 264:11934–7, 1989.
29. Carr A, Cooper DA. Adverse effects of antiretroviral therapy. Lancet 356:1423–30, 2000.
30. Dalakas MC, Illa I, Pezeshkpour GH, et al. Mitochondrial myopathy caused by long-term zidovudine therapy. N Engl J Med 322:1098–105, 1990.
31. McKenzie R, Fried MW, Sallie R, et al. Hepatic failure and lactic acidosis due to fialuridine (FIAU), an investigational nucleoside analogue for chronic hepatitis B. N Engl J Med 333:1099–105, 1995.
32. Schinazi RF, Boudinot FD, Ibrahim SS, et al. Pharmacokinetics and metabolism of racemic 2′,3′-dideoxy-5-fluoro-3′-thiacytidine in rhesus monkeys. Antimicrob Agents Chemother 36:2432–8, 1992.
33. Feng JY, Murakami E, Zorca SM, et al. Relationship between antiviral activity and host toxicity: comparison of the incorporation efficiencies of 2′,3′-dideoxy-5-fluoro-3′-thiacytidine-triphosphate analogs by human immunodeficiency virus type 1 reverse transcriptase and human mitochondrial DNA polymerase. Antimicrob Agents Chemother 48:1300–6, 2004.
34. Frick LW, St John L, Taylor LC, et al. Pharmacokinetics, oral bioavailability, and metabolic disposition in rats of (−)-cis-5-fluoro-1-[2-(hydroxymethyl)-1,3-oxathiolan-5-yl] cytosine, a nucleoside analog active against human immunodeficiency virus and hepatitis B virus. Antimicrob Agents Chemother 37:2285–92, 1993.
35. Szczech GM, Wang LH, Walsh JP, Rousseau FS. Reproductive toxicology profile of emtricitabine in mice and rabbits. Reprod Toxicol 17:95–108, 2003.
36. Gallant JE, DeJesus E, Arribas JR, et al. Tenofovir DF, emtricitabine, and efavirenz vs. zidovudine, lamivudine, and efavirenz for HIV. N Engl J Med 354:251–60, 2006.37. Benson C, Sanne I, van der Horst C, et al. Long-term safety profile of emtricitabine (FTC) in HIV-1-infected adults. Presented at the 41st Annual Interscience Conference on Antimicrobial Agents and Chemotherapy, Chicago, 2001, abstract 1931.
38. Benson CA, van der Horst C, Lamarca A, et al. A randomized study of emtricitabine and lamivudine in stably suppressed patients with HIV. AIDS 18:2269–76, 2004.
39. Molina JM, Journot V, Morand-Joubert L, et al. Simplification therapy with once-daily emtricitabine, didanosine, and efavirenz in HIV-1-infected adults with viral suppression receiving a protease inhibitor-based regimen: a randomized trial. J Infect Dis 191:830–9, 2005.
40. Saag MS, Cahn P, Raffi F, et al. Efficacy and safety of emtricitabine vs stavudine in combination therapy in antiretroviral-naive patients: a randomized trial. JAMA292:180–9, 2004.
41. Ndiweni D, Violari A, Saez-LLorens X, et al. Once daily (qd) emtricitabine (FTC) with other antiretroviral agents (ART) in HIV-infected pediatric patients. Presented at the 7th International Congress on Drug Therapy in HIV Infection, Glasgow, UK, 2004, abstract 335.
42. Mondou E, Quinn JB, Shaw A, et al. Incidence of skin discoloration across phase 3 clinical trials of emtricitabine (FTC) in adults. Presented at the XVth International AIDS Conference, Bangkok, Thailand, 2004, abstract WePeB5916.
43. Saag MS. Emtricitabine, a new antiretroviral agent with activity against HIV and hepatitis B virus. Clin Infect Dis 42:126–31, 2006.
44. Rousseau FS, Kahn JO, Thompson M, et al. Prototype trial design for rapid dose selection of antiretroviral drugs: an example

using emtricitabine (Coviracil). J Antimicrob Chemother 48:507–13, 2001.
45. Rousseau FS, Wakeford C, Mommeja-Marin H, et al. Prospective randomized trial of emtricitabine versus lamivudine short-term monotherapy in human immunodeficiency virus-infected patients. J Infect Dis 188:1652–8, 2003.
46. Molina JM, Ferchal F, Rancinan C, et al. Once-daily combination therapy with emtricitabine, didanosine, and efavirenz in human immunodeficiency virus-infected patients. J Infect Dis 182:599–602, 2000.
47. Molina JM, Perusat S, Ferchal F, et al. Once-daily combination with emtricitabine, didanosine, and efavirenz in treatment-naive HIV-infected adults: 64 week follow-up of the ANRS091 trial. Presented at the 8th Conference on Retroviruses and Opportunistic Infections, Chicago, 2001, abstract 321.
48. Centers for Disease Control and Prevention. 1993 Revised classification system for HIV infection and expanded surveillance case definitions for AIDS among adolescents and adults. MMWR 41(RR-17):1–19, 1992.
49. van der Horst C, Sanne I, Wakeford C, et al. Two randomized, controlled, equivalence trials of emtricitabine (FTC) to lamivudine (3TC). Presented at the 8th Conference on Retroviruses and Opportunistic Infections, Chicago, 2001, abstract 18.
50. Sanne I, van der Horst C, Shaw A, et al. Two randomized, controlled, equivalence trials of emtricitabine (FTC) to lamivudine (3TC). Presented at the XIV International AIDS Conference, Barcelona, Spain, 2002, abstract TuPeB4432.
51. Sanne I, Quinn J, Harris J, et al. Genotypic analysis of HIV-1 infected ART-naive patients receiving emtricitabine (FTC) of lamivudine (3TC) in a double blind equivalence trial. Presented at the XIV International AIDS Conference, Barcelona, Spain, 2002, abstract TuPeB4433.
52. Sanne I, Mommeja-Marin H, Hinkle J, et al. Severe hepatotoxicity associated with nevirapine use in HIV-infected subjects. J Infect Dis 191:825–9, 2005.
53. Harris J, Hinkle J, Makhuli K, et al. Long-term virologic response and genotypic findings in HIV-1 infected pediatric patients receiving emtricitabine (FTC) once daily (QD). Presented at the 44th Interscience Conference on Antimicrobial Agents and Chemotherapy, Washington DC, 2004, abstract H-855.
54. Saez-LLorens X, Violari A, Ndiweni D, et al. Once-daily Emtricitabine in HIV-infected pediatric patients with other antiretroviral agents. Presented at the 10th Conference on Retroviruses and Opportunistic Infections, Boston, 2003, abstract 872.
55. McKinney R, Rodman J, Rathore M, et al. Extended follow-up and pharmacokinetics for once-daily emtricitabine, didanosine, and efavirenz for antiretroviral naive children and adolescents. Presented at the 11th Conference on Retroviruses and Opportunistic Infections, San Francisco, 2004, abstract 936.
56. McKinney R, Rathore M, Jankelovich S, et al. PACTG 1021: an ongoing phase I/II study of once-daily emtricitabine, didanosine, and efavirenz in therapy-naive or minimally treated pediatric patients. Presented at the 10th Conference on Retroviruses and Opportunistic Infections, Boston, 2003, abstract 873.
57. McKinney R, Rathore M, Hu C, et al. Phase I/II study of a once-daily regimen of emtricitabine, didanosine, and efavirenz in HIV-infected, therapy-naive children and adolescents: PACTG Protocol 1021. Presented at the 13th Conference on Retroviruses and Opportunistic Infections, Denver, 2006, abstract 17.
58. Gish RG, Trinh H, Leung N, et al. Safety and antiviral activity of emtricitabine (FTC) for the treatment of chronic hepatitis B infection: a two-year study. J Hepatol 43:60–6, 2005.
59. Gish RG, Leung NW, Wright TL, et al. Dose range study of pharmacokinetics, safety, and preliminary antiviral activity of emtricitabine in adults with hepatitis B virus infection. Antimicrob Agents Chemother 46:1734–40, 2002.
60. Lim SG, Ng TM, Kung N, et al. A double-blind placebo-controlled study of emtricitabine in chronic hepatitis B. Arch Intern Med 166:49–56, 2006.
61. Mondou E, Sorbel J, Anderson J, et al. Posttreatment exacerbation of hepatitis B virus (HBV) infection in long-term HBV trials of emtricitabine. Clin Infect Dis 41:e45–7, 2005.
62. Raffi F, Snow A, Borroto-Esoda K, et al. Anti-HBV activity of emtricitabine (FTC) in patients co-infected with HIV and hepatitis B virus. Presented at the 2nd IAS Conference on HIV Pathogenesis and Treatment, Paris, France, 2003, abstract 215.
63. Harris J, Snow A, Borroto-Esoda K, et al. Emtricitabine therapy for hepatitis infection in HIV-1 patients co-infected with hepatitis B: antiviral response and genotypic findings in antiretroviral naive patients. Presented at the 11th Conference on Retroviruses and Opportunistic Infections, San Francisco, 2004, abstract 836.
64. Soriano V, Puoti M, Bonacini M, et al. Care of patients with chronic hepatitis B and HIV co-infection: recommendations from an HIV-HBV International Panel. AIDS 19:221–40, 2005.
65. Kohlstaedt LA, Wang J, Friedman JM, Rice PA, Steitz TA. Crystal structure at 3.5 A resolution of HIV-1 reverse transcriptase complexed with an inhibitor. Science 256:1783–90, 1992.
66. Borroto-Esoda K, Harris J, Shaw A, et al. Lower incidence of the M184V mutation in patients receiving combination therapy with emtricitabine compared with lamivudine. Antivir Ther 6(Suppl 1):68, 2001.
67. Sanne I, Anderson J, Kargl D, et al. Evaluation of emtricitabine within a triple NRTI HAART regimen. Presented at the 43rd Annual Interscience Conference on Antimicrobial Agents and Chemotherapy, Chicago, 2003, abstract H-868.
68. Borroto-Esoda K, Miller M, Petropoulos C, Parkin N. A comparison of the phenotypic susceptibility profiles of emtricitabine (FTC) and lamivudine (3TC). Presented at the 44th Annual Interscience Conference on Antimicrobial Agents and Chemotherapy, Washington DC, 2004, abstract H-180.
69. Ross LL, Parkin N, Underwood MR, et al. Comparison of phenotypic effects of NRTI mutations on emtricitabine (FTC) and lamivudine (3TC). Presented at the 12th Conference on Retroviruses and Opportunistic Infections, Boston, 2005, abstract 713.
70. Ross L, Parkin N, Underwood M, et al. In a paired-sample comparison, the presence of thymidine analogue mutations, but not other common nucleoside reverse transcriptase inhibitor mutations has a differential effect on emtricitabine and lamivudine susceptibility. Presented at the 13th Conference on Retroviruses and Opportunistic Infections, Denver, 2006, abstract 602.
71. Perrillo R, Schiff E, Yoshida E, et al. Adefovir dipivoxil for the treatment of lamivudine-resistant hepatitis B mutants. Hepatology 32:129–34, 2000.
72. Ono-Nita SK, Kato N, Shiratori Y, et al. Susceptibility of lamivudine-resistant hepatitis B virus to other reverse transcriptase inhibitors. J Clin Invest 103:1635–40, 1999.
73. Molina JM, Journot V, Rozenbaum W, et al. Simplification therapy with once-daily efavirenz, emtricitabine, and didanosine in patients virologically suppressed with a protease inhibitor-based regimen: three-year follow-up of the Alize-ANRS099 trial. Presented at the Conference on Retroviruses and Opportunistic Infections, Boston, 2005, abstract K-196.

Chapter 11

Abacavir

Victoria A. Johnson, MD

STRUCTURE

Abacavir sulfate, compound 1592U89 hemisulfate ((1*S*, *cis*)-4-(2-amino-6-(cyclopropylamino)-9H-purin-9-yl)-2-cyclopentene-1-methanol sulfate (salt)(2:1)) (formerly known as 1592), also known as Ziagen or as ABC, is a carbocyclic nucleoside analog with potent and selective activity against HIV-1.[1–8] This compound contains a novel 6-cyclopropylamino-substituted purine. The structure is shown in Figure 11-1A. The compound is activated by cellular enzymes to the triphosphate derivative of the guanine analog 1144U88 ((1*R*,4*S*)-9-(4-(hydroxymethyl)-2-cyclopenten-1-yl)-guanine; (–)-carbovir), which is shown in Figure 11-1B.

IN VITRO ACTIVITY AND MECHANISMS OF ACTION

The active form of abacavir, 1144U88 triphosphate, is a potent inhibitor of HIV-1 reverse transcriptase (RT) *in vitro*, with a K_I of 0.02 μM.[1–7] In whole virus assays, abacavir has activity against HIV-1 (strain IIIB) cultured in MT-4 cells (a human leukemic cell line transformed with HTLV-1), peripheral blood mononuclear cells (PBMCs), and macrophages. The 50% inhibitory concentrations (IC_{50}s) in these cells were, respectively, 4.0, 3.7, and 0.65 μM.[5] The mean IC_{50} for abacavir against eight fresh clinical isolates of HIV-1, obtained from zidovudine-naive patients and amplified in PBMCs, was 0.26 μM (i.e., equivalent in potency to zidovudine).[1,3,5,7] Abacavir has also demonstrated synergistic activity *in vitro* against HIV-1 when used in combination with zidovudine, other nucleoside reverse transcriptase inhibitors (NRTIs) such as lamivudine and didanosine (but additive with stavudine) and non-nucleoside reverse transcriptase inhibitors (NNRTIs) such as nevirapine, and protease inhibitors (PIs) such as amprenavir.[1,5,7–9] There was no evidence for an antagonistic interaction between tenofovir and abacavir, in the presence or absence of 3TC, against wild-type and drug-resistant HIV-1 *in vitro,* to account for

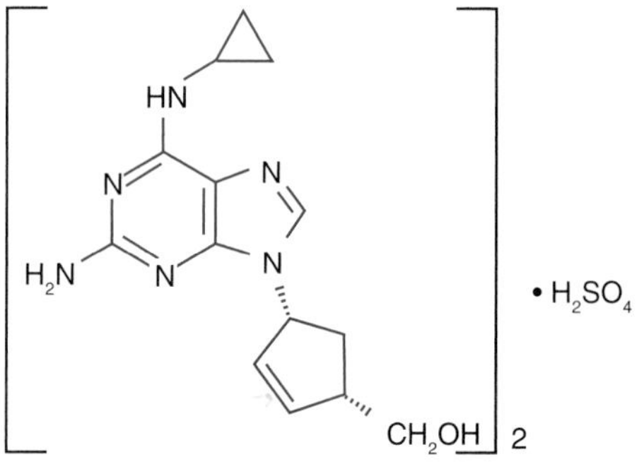

Structure of Abacavir-Sulfate

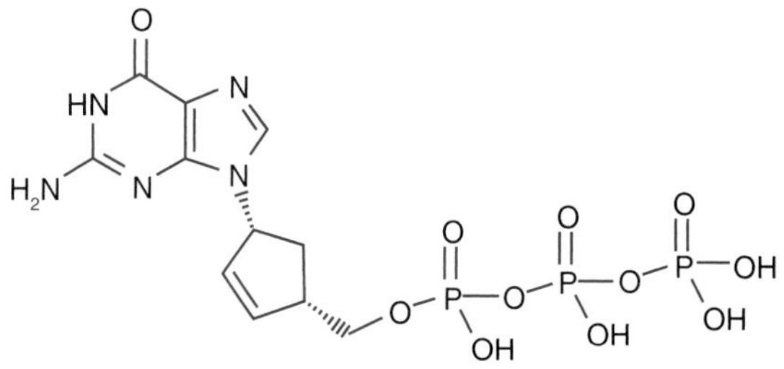

Structure of 1144U88-Triphosphate

Figure 11-1 ■ (**A**) Structure of abacavir sulfate, compound 1592U89 hemisulfate ((1*S*,*cis*)-4-(2-amino-6-(cyclo-propylamino)-9H-purin-9-yl)-2-cyclopentene-1-methanol sulfate (salt)(2:1)), also known as Ziagen, a carbocyclic nucleoside analog. The cyclopropylamino moiety of abacavir (1592U89) is important for absorption and central nervous system penetration *in vivo*. (**B**) Structure of 1144U88 triphosphate. The compound 1592U89 (abacavir sulfate) is activated by cellular enzymes to the triphosphate derivative of the guanine analog 1144U88 ((1*R*,4*S*)-9-(4-(hydroxymethyl)-2-cyclopenten-1-yl)-guanine; (–)-carbovir).

the high rate of virologic failures seen in patients initiating therapy with combined tenofovir, abacavir, and lamivudine.[10]

PHARMACOKINETICS

The cyclopropylamino moiety of abacavir is important for enhanced absorption and central nervous system penetration *in vivo* when compared to carbovir.[5,11] In contrast to the limited oral absorption of carbovir (e.g., 26% and 23% oral bioavailability in the rat and monkey, respectively), pharmacokinetic evaluation of abacavir showed good oral bioavailability (e.g., 92% and 77% in mice and monkeys, respectively).[5,12–14] In contrast to the poor brain penetration of carbovir (e.g., rat brain/plasma concentration ratios averaged 0.04), the penetration of abacavir into monkey cerebrospinal fluid (CSF) and rat brain were comparable to that of zidovudine.[5] Abacavir showed significant penetration into CSF in humans.[15] One observational cohort study (the Charter trial) in 374 highly active antiretroviral therapy (HAART)-experienced subjects with plasma and CSF viral load measurements reported a projected CSF penetration score (based on published data on CSF concentrations and/or chemical properties) that was highest for abacavir and zidovudine when compared to all other available NRTIs (including tenofovir, didanosine, zalcitabine, stavudine, lamivudine, and emtricitabine).[16]

Intracellular activation of abacavir to its active triphosphate form requires phosphorylation by cellular enzymes.[2,4,6,17] This involves a unique set of enzymes other than those involved in activation of other NRTIs that are currently approved for treatment of HIV-1 infection. Abacavir sulfate is activated intracellularly to carbovir monophosphate by a novel phosphorylation pathway[2–6] involving adenosine phosphotransferase.[18] Carbovir monophosphate is then efficiently anabolized by cellular enzymes to carbovir diphosphate, followed by anabolism to the active form carbovir triphosphate, which inhibits HIV-1 RT. The existence of this unique activation pathway enables abacavir to overcome the deficiencies of carbovir (which include low oral bioavailability and minimal brain penetration) while maintaining potent and selective anti-HIV-1 activity.[5,6] The intracellular half-life of carbovir triphosphate, produced from both abacavir and carbovir, is ~3.3 h based on previous *in vitro* studies.[2,5,19] However, more recent studies *in vivo* demonstrate that the intracellular half-life of carbovir triphosphate is much longer (20.64 h), which is possibly due to a saturation step and/or pooling of precursors (carbovir-monophosphate or carbovir-diphosphate).[20] The prolonged half-life of carbovir-triphosphate observed *in vivo* supports the administration of abacavir once daily.[20]

The main route of elimination of abacavir is metabolism, with <2% of a dose recovered as unchanged drug in urine.[15] Prolonged therapy of treatment-naive HIV-1-infected subjects over 48 weeks with combined regimens of efavirenz with either abacavir plus lamivudine, trizivir (a fixed-dose combination of Ziagen (abacavir), Retrovir (zidovudine), and Epivir (lamivudine)), or Combivir did not exhibit clinically significant changes in renal function as measured by glomerular filtration rate.[21] The catabolism of abacavir involves two pathways: glucuronidation, and carboxylation through alcohol dehydrogenase.[13,14] The metabolism of abacavir is not dependent on cytochrome P450 liver enzymes. Physiologic concentrations of human albumin or α_1-acid glycoprotein do not markedly alter the anti-HIV-1 activity of abacavir,[22] and food intake does not significantly affect abacavir bioavailability. In an initial phase I double-blind, parallel, dose-escalation trial evaluating safety and kinetics, the tablet area under the concentration time curve (AUC) at the 300 mg dose was 99% of the oral solution AUC, and administration with food lowered AUC by 5% and maximum plasma concentration by 35%.[23] The main route of metabolite excretion is renal, with 83% of a dose recovered in urine.[15]

There are no known significant drug interactions.[24,25] Abacavir demonstrated predictable pharmacokinetic characteristics when administered as single oral doses ranging from 100 to 1200 mg.[26] No significant pharmacokinetic interactions were detected after single-dose administration of abacavir in double or triple combinations with zidovudine, lamivudine, or both.[27] In multiple-dose studies, abacavir showed predictable pharmacokinetic characteristics and zidovudine co-administration had no effect on the abacavir AUC_{tau} (a parameter most closely associated with efficacy).[28] In a prospective evaluation of intracellular concentrations and pharmacokinetics of carbovir triphosphate, tenofovir diphosphate, and lamivudine triphosphate in patients receiving the triple-nucleoside regimen of tenofovir disoproxil fumarate, abacavir, and lamivudine, there was no intracellular drug interaction that could explain the suboptimal viral response seen with this regimen.[29] Changes in levels of dNTPs, carbovir-triphosphate, and tenofovir-diphosphate in purified human CD4+ and CD8+ peripheral blood T cells following treatment with tenofovir and/or abacavir and/or lamivudine *in vitro* similarly did not suggest that antagonistic drug–drug interactions occurred as the mechanism of regimen failure *in vivo*.[30]

In subjects with mild liver impairment (CNAB1006 Study), there was a 1.9-fold increase in abacavir exposure and a 1.6-fold increase in abacavir half-life in the group with liver disease. The liver disease did not modify the extent of formation of the metabolites, although the rates of formation and elimination were decreased. The CNAB1006 Study results suggested that patients with mild hepatic impairment should receive 150 mg abacavir twice daily in order to achieve an AUC equivalent to patients without liver disease receiving the recommended 300 mg twice-daily dose.[31]

The safety of abacavir and lamivudine-based HAART in 1985 treatment-naive HIV-1-infected subjects with and without hepatitis B and/or hepatitis C co-infection was examined using data from four large, randomized clinical treatment trials of abacavir plus lamivudine once daily or twice daily in combination with efavirenz or PIs. This 48-week analysis showed that these regimens were well tolerated in patients with hepatitis B and/or hepatitis C co-infection, with a similar median reduction in AST/ALT levels and a similar rate of grade 2–4 adverse events and drug-related adverse events when compared to non-co-infected subjects. Grade

2–4 increases in ALT and AST levels were more common in co-infected subjects (10.5% and 8.5%, respectively) when compared to non-co-infected subjects (1.3% and 1.3%, respectively), which was attributed to the natural history of viral hepatitis infection or to immune reconstitution leading to HBV immune-mediated response with ALT flares.[32]

Pharmacokinetics in HIV-1-Infected Infants and Children

A phase-I single-dose pharmacokinetic study evaluated two oral abacavir doses (4 and 8 mg/kg of body weight) in 22 HIV-1-infected children ages 3 months to 13 years.[33] Abacavir was rapidly absorbed, with time to peak concentration in plasma occurring within 1.5 h postdosing. Abacavir was rapidly eliminated, with a mean elimination half-life of 0.98–1.13 h. The extent of exposure to abacavir appears to be slightly lower in children than in adults, with the comparable unit doses being based on body weight.[33]

TOXICITY

In Vitro Effects

Abacavir and carbovir are less myelotoxic than either zidovudine, didanosine, or zalcitabine when tested *in vitro* using human and murine hematopoietic progenitor cells.[2,5] Carbovir triphosphate has relatively low inhibitory activity against cellular DNA polymerase γ when compared to the active triphosphates of other dideoxynucleoside analogs.[5] It is the inhibition of cellular DNA polymerase γ that has been associated with drug-induced peripheral neuropathy and mitochondrial toxicity (including lipoatrophy/lipodystrophy). Taken together, the preclinical development of abacavir sulfate was supported by both a relative lack of myelosuppressive effects and less inhibition of cellular enzymes involved in development of peripheral neuropathy and other mitochondrial toxicities.

In Vivo Effects

In clinical trials to date, the majority of adverse events were rated as mild or moderate. No specific hepatic, pancreatic, renal, or bone marrow toxicity patterns have been described. In ACTG 5095, adding abacavir to a backbone regimen of combined zidovudine plus lamivudine plus efavirenz had no consistent metabolic effects in HIV-1-infected adults as measured by fasting triglyceride and total, LDL, and HDL cholesterol, lactate, glucose, and insulin resistance measurements.[34] Mitochondrial toxicity (including lipoatrophy) occurring in association with treatment with abacavir may be lower than the risk with many other NRTIs. However, lactic acidosis and severe hepatomegaly with steatosis, including fatal cases, have been reported with the use of nucleoside analogs alone or in combination, including abacavir, zidovudine, lamivudine, and other antiretrovirals. In a Commmunity Program for Clinical Research on AIDS (CPCRA) study, 96 antiretroviral-naive subjects were enrolled and randomized to didanosine plus stavudine (n = 46) or abacavir plus lamivudine (n = 50).[35] Those subjects receiving didanosine plus stavudine experienced a decline in regional fat and total body fat when compared to increases in these parameters in subjects in the abacavir plus lamivudine arm ($P < 0.05$). Abacavir plus lamivudine therapy increased the rate of change of high-density lipoprotein cholesterol, whereas this rate decreased during didanosine plus stavudine therapy. Early and sustained increases in insulin resistance were seen only during didanosine plus stavudine therapy.[35] In lipoatrophic HIV-1-infected adults enrolled in the RAVE study, switching from a thymidine analog to abacavir or tenofovir for 48 weeks improved lipoatrophy.[36] Replacing the PI component of treatment regimens improved the lipid profile in 90 treatment-experienced subjects with controlled plasma viremia who were receiving nevirapine (n = 29), efavirenz (n = 32), or abacavir (n = 29) in the 24-month Spanish NEFA study, but did not seem to be effective for reversing body fat abnormalities.[37] After 1 year, a trend toward a lower incidence of adverse effects leading to discontinuation among those subjects receiving abacavir was seen, but also a trend toward a higher rate of virological failure was noted.

A separate 48-week, randomized, open-label study of HIV-1-infected subjects compared three abacavir-base substitution approaches in the management of dyslipidemia and peripheral lipoatrophy.[38] Subjects were receiving initial stavudine with either a PI or NNRTI and had hypercholesterolemia and/or lipoatrophy with well-controlled plasma viremia (plasma HIV-1 RNA ≤50 copies/mL). Thirty subjects were randomized to replace: (1) stavudine with abacavir; (2) PI or NNRTI with abacavir; or (3) stavudine and PI or NNRTI with abacavir plus zidovudine. Replacement of stavudine with abacavir led to modest improvements in fat mass in this study, and replacement of a PI or NNRTI with abacavir led to modest improvements in both cholesterol and triglycerides.

Gastrointestinal and Neurologic Side Effects

The most common side effects seen during abacavir therapy are gastrointestinal (GI) and neurologic. Nausea, vomiting, and diarrhea have been ascribed to abacavir therapy. Nausea is common. All of these GI complaints tend to abate over the first few weeks of abacavir therapy. Neurologic side effects are less common than GI complaints. Headache, malaise, dizziness, insomnia, and rarely paresthesias have been noted during abacavir therapy. In placebo-controlled clinical trials, only nausea, vomiting, and malaise and fatigue were statistically significant and more frequent in abacavir-containing regimens in comparison to the control regimens.

Abacavir Hypersensitivity Syndrome

Hypersensitivity reactions occurred in ~8% of 2670 patients (n = 206) receiving abacavir for the treatment of HIV-1 infection in nine clinical trials (range: 2–9%) enrolled from Nov 1999 to Feb 2002 (Abacavir FDA prescribing information). The appearance of this syndrome demands immediate discontinuation and an absolute contraindication to reinitiation of abacavir or an abacavir-containing medication (e.g., Trizivir or Epzicom). A total of 1015 cases have been described among 26 769 subjects enrolled in phase II and III clinical trials and expanded access programs.[39] The median time to onset was 11 days, with 93% of cases appearing within 6 weeks of initiation of abacavir, although reactions may occur at any time during therapy. In a risk factor meta-analysis for hypersensitivity reactions to abacavir introduction, the incidence observed was 3.7%. The odds ratios (OR) for subjects with previous HAART treatment and those of African descent were significantly lower (OR 0.41, 95% confidence intervals (CIs): 0.23, 0.72; and OR 0.51, 95% CI: 0.28, 0.92, respectively) than HAART-naive patients and other ethnic origins.[40]

The mechanism of abacavir hypersensitivity syndrome is not fully understood, but may involve an immunologic response. GlaxoSmithKline is conducting pharmacogenetic research to determine if cellular genetic DNA polymorphisms (variations) can be identified in HIV-1-infected patients who have developed hypersensitivity reactions following treatment with abacavir, in order to help predict risk of abacavir hypersensitivity in susceptible patients.[41] An association between HLA-B*5701, HLA-DR7, and HLA-DQ3 and the hypersensitivity syndrome has been reported.[42,43] A strong association between this syndrome and HLA-B*5701 carriage in Caucasians has been confirmed.[44] Conversely, a lower reported rate of suspected abacavir hypersensitivity reactions among African-American patients across five randomized controlled trials has been attributed to a lower prevalence of HLA-B*5701 among African-Americans.[45] A cutaneous patch test may help identify subjects with true abacavir hypersensitivity syndrome, since the syndrome may be difficult for clinicians to recognize.[46] HLA-B*5701 was present in all seven patch test-positive subjects with remote abacavir hypersensitivity syndrome versus one of the 11 controls tolerating abacavir ($P < 0.001$). Five of seven patch tests (71%) versus one of 11 controls (9%) ($P = 0.005$) showed significant abacavir-specific CD8+ T-cell proliferation, suggesting a direct role for HLA-B*5701-restricted CD8+ T cells in the pathophysiology of abacavir hypersensitivity syndrome.[47]

The usual presentation includes symptoms indicating involvement of multiple organ systems.[48] The most common symptoms are fever, rash, GI symptoms (nausea, vomiting, diarrhea, or abdominal pain), and malaise or fatigue. Fever is a key feature of the syndrome. Less common symptoms include respiratory symptoms (cough, sore throat, or dyspnea) and musculoskeletal complaints (myalgia, myolysis, arthralgia, edema) and headache and paresthesia. Hypotension may be present in 5% of reactions. In contrast to immunoglobulin E (IgE)-mediated anaphylactic reactions, wheezing is distinctly uncommon, and edema less common. In contrast to described reactions to NNRTIs, the rash is rarely severe, usually appearing later (e.g., 1–3 days) after the onset of the systemic symptoms, and may be absent in up to 30% of cases.[49,50] The rash is usually maculopapular or urticarial. Morbidity is related more to the systemic symptoms rather than the rash. Although the time course is variable, symptoms tend to occur in succession over the course of several days, with fever and GI symptoms appearing early and rash later. The severity of symptoms tends to increase with each dose. A delay in discontinuation of abacavir in the face of an active hypersensitivity reaction may lead to a severe reaction and even death, although the risk of a fatal reaction is far more likely in the setting of a rechallenge (see further ahead).

After discontinuation of abacavir, symptoms improve quickly and resolve over a few days, although the rash, if present, may persist longer. If abacavir is reinitiated (rechallenge), symptoms reappear within hours and may be more severe. Fever, rash, malaise, hypotension, and facial and/or throat swelling or bronchospasm have been described. Symptoms not present with the initial reaction may also appear on rechallenge and temperature elevations to 39–40°C may occur. One case report described severe anaphylactic shock after rechallenge with abacavir without preceding hypersensitivity.[51] Hypotension was present in ~25% of cases where abacavir was reinitiated after an initial reaction. Support with intravenous fluids with or without vasopressors (dopamine/dobutamine) may be necessary. Fatalities have been reported.[52] Among the reported cases where a rechallenge has been attempted, 4% of patients have died. The rechallenge reaction has occurred even at reduced doses of 100 mg abacavir. *Thus, once hypersensitivity to abacavir has been diagnosed, do not rechallenge with abacavir or an abacavir-containing medication (e.g., Trizivir or Epzicom).*

Laboratory abnormalities observed during a hypersensitivity reaction to abacavir include an increase in liver function tests and an acute, transient lymphopenia in some subjects. Occasionally, decreased platelet counts, elevated serum creatinine, and elevated creatine phosphokinase have been described. These laboratory abnormalities return to normal with prompt discontinuation of abacavir. No preexisting condition or screening laboratory abnormality has yet been identified that indicates an increased likelihood of developing this reaction.

Diagnosis of 'hypersensitivity reaction to abacavir' occurred in 2–3% of subjects assigned to the nonabacavir-treated subjects in double-blinded studies.[53] Most cases had rash alone or rash accompanied by nonspecific, mild symptoms, whereas hypersensitivity reactions to abacavir are part of a multisymptom syndrome with fever as the hallmark. Cutaneous reactions are common with other medications often prescribed to patients with HIV-1 infection, such as NNRTIs or sulfamethoxazole. The appearance or characteristics of a rash without other symptoms are not sufficiently specific to differentiate the cause in most cases. However, the morbidity associated with hypersensitivity reactions to abacavir is not related to rash, and rash is not frequently an early sign of this reaction. Thus, for patients in whom rash is the only clinical symptom, abacavir may be continued with the warning to follow the patient carefully for the development of other symptoms. The patient should be counseled to report the appearance of any additional symptoms immediately. In cases where systemic symptoms and rash are present together, differentiation may not be possible and abacavir should be discontinued. The rash of abacavir hypersensitivity is mild, but may involve mucous membranes. However, the Stevens–Johnson syndrome has *only* been reported when abacavir has been combined with NNRTIs.

In some cases, the symptoms of a hypersensitivity reaction may resemble acute infections or reactions to other medications. Keiser et al described the clinical features of diagnosed influenza infection with cases of hypersensitivity to abacavir.[54] Both rash and GI symptoms were strongly associated with the latter. Respiratory symptoms with hypersensitivity to abacavir appeared in conjunction with GI symptoms. Nevertheless, for some cases differentiation of hypersensitivity to abacavir from an acute infection can be difficult. The symptoms will increase in severity if dosing is continued. Moreover, the timing of the onset of symptoms with respect to drug exposure is critical for recognition of the syndrome. Abacavir hypersensitivity starts several days to 6 weeks after starting the drug in most cases. Furthermore, the symptoms improve after stopping abacavir. Severe reaction and fatalities have occurred when symptoms of hypersensitivity to abacavir were ascribed to another cause and the discontinuation of abacavir was delayed or rechallenge was attempted. It is important not to ascribe the symptoms of abacavir hypersensitivity to nonspecific 'flu' or 'gastroenteritis'.[49,50]

There is no evidence to indicate that interruption of abacavir administration in the absence of any symptoms (i.e., for a reason other than a side effect) increases the frequency or severity of a subsequent hypersensitivity reaction.[55,56] However, there have been cases of hypersensitivity reactions occurring within 1 day of restarting abacavir where no prior symptoms of an initial hypersensitivity reaction were recorded. This underscores the importance to advise a patient to contact the healthcare provider if abacavir is discontinued. The healthcare provider should then obtain a careful history to assure that symptoms indicating a hypersensitivity reaction were not present at the time of interruption.

Most Common Adverse Events in Adult HIV-1-Infected Subjects Enrolled in CNAA2001

A summary of clinical toxicities associated with abacavir in the CNAA2001 trial is shown in Table 11-1.[57,58] In that study, abacavir was administered as monotherapy for 4 weeks followed by randomization to therapy for 4 weeks followed in turn by randomization to zidovudine or its matching placebo for an additional 8 weeks. The most commonly reported adverse events were nausea, headache, asthenia, diarrhea, insomnia, fever, dizziness, vomiting, abdominal pain, and rash. Nausea was common, occurring in nine of 20 subjects (45%) at 300 mg PO bid. Headache occurred in eight of 20 subjects (40%) at 300 mg PO bid. A possible trend of increase in incidence of nausea and headache with increasing abacavir dose was observed. However, the small numbers of patients and the design of the study make it difficult to draw definitive conclusions about the significance of this preliminary observation. Only eight subjects (10%) withdrew from the study because of adverse events, all of which were considered possibly related to the study drug. The most common reasons for discontinuation were nausea (with or without vomiting) or hypersensitivity reaction. The latter occurred within 4 weeks of dosing. Only four subjects experienced a serious adverse event, none of which were considered related to the study drug.

Abacavir did not demonstrate any evidence of bone marrow suppression, as evidenced by the lack of abnormalities in any hematologic parameters during the study that were attributable to abacavir. Additionally, abacavir did not demonstrate any evidence of hepatic, renal, or pancreatic toxicity by biochemical analysis. Most treatment-emergent hematologic and clinical chemistry toxicities were rated as grade 1 or 2. No distinguishing pattern could be detected between the cohorts or treatment arms when clinical chemistry laboratory parameters were examined. The incidence of abnormal laboratory values was generally low, and no dose-related trends were observed. There was no evidence to indicate that abacavir used in combination with zidovudine was associated with an increase in the severity of clinical or laboratory toxicities compared with administration of the study drug alone.[57,58]

Table 11-1 Most Common Adverse Events Associated with Abacavir in the CNAA2001 Trial[a]

Toxicity	Frequency	Comment
Nausea	9/20 (45%)	A possible trend with increasing doses was noted
Headache	8/20 (40%)	A possible trend with increasing doses was noted
Asthenia	8/20 (40%)	
Diarrhea	5/20 (25%)	
Insomnia	5/20 (25%)	
Fever	4/20 (20%)	
Dizziness	2/20 (10%)	
Vomiting	3/20 (15%)	
Abdominal pain	3/20 (15%)	
Rash	1/20 (5%)	

[a]Adverse events experienced by the 300 mg bid cohort ($n = 20$ subjects) in the CNAA2001 trial, a phase I/II trial to evaluate the effects of multiple dosing of abacavir alone and in combination with zidovudine capsules. The majority of adverse events were rated as mild or moderate. The number of subjects listed experienced an event (regardless of association with abacavir) (see text).[57] This table does not specifically list the occurrence rate of the abacavir hypersensitivity reaction, which has been estimated at 3% (range 2–5%) in abacavir-treated subjects.

Safety in HIV-1-Infected Infants and Children

The side effects observed among children receiving abacavir are similar to those observed among adults. Hypersensitivity reactions to abacavir have been reported in children, and have similar frequency and clinical characteristics to those observed among adults receiving abacavir.

CLINICAL SAFETY AND EFFICACY STUDIES

Controlled clinical trials to investigate abacavir safety and antiretroviral activity have been conducted in several patient populations, including antiretroviral-naive patients as first-line treatment, NRTI- and/or PI-experienced treatment failures, and people with AIDS dementia complex. In addition to controlled clinical trials, three broad patient populations have received compassionate use/open-label treatment: adults, children, and people with severe AIDS dementia complex. More recently, studies have been conducted using once-daily abacavir formulations. Findings of several pivotal clinical trials in antiretroviral-naive and antiretroviral-experienced HIV-1-infected patients are highlighted here.

Studies Conducted in Antiretroviral-Naive HIV-1-Infected Adults

Several phase I/II controlled clinical studies were conducted to determine pharmacokinetics, safety, and antiviral activity of abacavir. A parallel, dose-ranging 12-week study (CNAA2001) was completed in 79 antiretroviral-naive HIV-1-infected adults in the United States with limited prior antiretroviral experience (<12 weeks of zidovudine therapy).[57,58] This was the first multiple-dosing study in humans. The doses of abacavir studied were 200 mg tid, 400 mg tid, 600 mg tid, or 300 mg bid. Patients received open-label abacavir monotherapy for 4 weeks, followed by 8 weeks of zidovudine (600 mg/day) or placebo in addition to abacavir. Abacavir given as monotherapy for 4 weeks resulted in median decreases in plasma HIV-1 RNA by 1.11–1.77 $\log_{10}$ copies/mL and median CD4+ T-lymphocyte count increases of 63–111 cells/μL in all groups. At week 12, median plasma HIV-1 RNA levels decreased by 1.02–2.24 $\log_{10}$ copies/mL (for abacavir monotherapy) and by 1.81–2.01 $\log_{10}$ copies/mL (for abacavir plus zidovudine). At week 12, median CD4+ T-lymphocyte counts increased by 79–195 cells/μL (for abacavir monotherapy) and by 93–142 cells/μL (for abacavir plus zidovudine). The percentage of subjects who had plasma HIV-1 RNA levels at week 12 below 400 and 40 copies/mL were 28% and 11%, respectively (abacavir monotherapy) and 69% and 22%, respectively (abacavir plus zidovudine). Eight subjects (10%) discontinued due to adverse events; nausea ($n = 4$) and hypersensitivity ($n = 3$) were the most common reasons for withdrawal; there were no fatalities. After 12 weeks of abacavir plus zidovudine or placebo, 72/79 patients were required to interrupt abacavir until essential preclinical studies were completed.

In a preliminary analysis, 43 of 72 subjects elected to restart therapy with abacavir following an interruption of up to 1 year. Six subjects received abacavir uninterrupted. During this extension phase, patients were offered open-label abacavir to use in appropriate combination antiretroviral regimens of abacavir plus either an NNRTI or a PI. The goal of this long-term open-label study was to monitor the long-term antiviral effects of abacavir therapy. Altogether, 16 of 42 subjects had plasma HIV-1 RNA levels of <400 copies/mL as extended therapy began. By the week 12 visit, 27 of 38 subjects had levels <400 copies/mL. Of 22 subjects reaching 36 weeks, 16 had viral loads <400 copies/mL. The proportions undetectable at week 24 for NRTI-only combination therapy and abacavir/PI/NNRTI were 14/18 and 9/10, respectively. Over 48 weeks of therapy, >50% of patients receiving either nucleoside-only therapy including abacavir or PI-containing therapy with abacavir were maintained below a plasma HIV-1 RNA level of 400 copies/mL. Sustained increases in CD4+ cell counts were seen in both abacavir treatment groups while on therapy, with or without PI therapy.

A second randomized, double-blind, dose-ranging clinical trial (CNAB2002) of abacavir 100, 300, and 600 mg bid was conducted in Europe.[59] A total of 60 antiretroviral-naive patients with CD4+ T-lymphocyte counts of ≥100 cells/μL and plasma HIV-1 RNA levels of ≥30 000 copies/mL received up to 24 weeks of abacavir therapy alone; 55 then went into an open-label randomized study of abacavir 300 mg bid plus other antiretrovirals for 72 weeks. At week 24, all subjects who remained on abacavir alone were switched to abacavir 300 mg bid/lamivudine 150 mg bid/zidovudine 300 mg bid or other licensed antiretrovirals as determined by their treating physician. At week 4, greater reductions in plasma HIV-1 RNA were seen in subjects receiving 300 or 600 mg abacavir twice daily (median changes −1.55 and −1.61 $\log_{10}$ copies/mL, respectively) than subjects receiving 100 mg abacavir twice daily (median change, −0.63 $\log_{10}$ copies/mL). At 24 weeks, the 300 and 600 mg twice-daily groups had a median change of plasma HIV-1 RNA of −0.70 and −1.30 $\log_{10}$ copies/mL, respectively. During the open-label phase in which zidovudine/lamivudine was added to 300 mg abacavir twice daily, a further median reduction in plasma HIV-1 RNA of 1.74 $\log_{10}$ copies/mL was seen. At week 48, a median 2.82 $\log_{10}$ drop in plasma HIV-1 RNA from randomized baseline was seen in pooled data from all abacavir-treated subjects. Sixty-five percent of patients had a plasma viral load of <400 copies/mL after 48 weeks of antiretroviral therapy (ART) containing abacavir, and 43% of patients had a plasma viral load <50 copies/mL at the same timepoint. An additional decrease in HIV-1 RNA of 2.16 $\log_{10}$ was seen during the open-label phase from the reset open-label combination baseline. Most subjects (46/55, or 87%) received abacavir combined with lamivudine 150 mg bid and zidovudine 300 mg bid since their switch to open label. Overall, this study demonstrated that abacavir 100 mg bid was inferior to 300 mg bid or 600 mg bid, with the latter two doses showing similar viral load reductions. The majority (42/47, 90%) of subjects at week 72 remained on the triple combination of abacavir/lamivudine/zidovudine, four subjects were receiving PIs in addition to the triple combination, and one subject had substituted stavudine for zidovudine. By week 72, the median change in plasma HIV-1 RNA was $-2.8 \log_{10}$ copies/mL. At week 72, 72% of subjects had a plasma HIV-1 RNA <400 copies/mL and 50% of subjects had plasma HIV-1 RNA <50 copies/mL.[60] The most frequently seen adverse experiences reported by 55 subjects during the long-term, open-label phase of the study were nausea/vomiting in 23 of the 55 (41%), malaise/fatigue in 10 (18%), headache in nine (16%), muscle pain in six (11%), GI discomfort/pain in seven (12%), sleep disorders in four (7%), and skin rashes in four (7%). These data included new adverse experiences that began once subjects switched to open-label abacavir, and not those that may have been ongoing from the randomized phase.[60]

The CNAA3003 trial investigated the effect of zidovudine and lamivudine with or without abacavir in antiretroviral-naive adults located in the USA, Spain, Belgium, and the UK.[61] This double-blind, randomized phase III study was designed to assess the safety, tolerance, and antiviral activity of abacavir/lamivudine/zidovudine over 16 weeks, as well as the safety, tolerance, and durability of the abacavir/lamivudine/zidovudine response over 48 weeks. Subjects ($n = 173$ with CD4+ T-lymphocyte counts >100 cells/μL) were randomized 1:1 to receive abacavir 300 mg bid or placebo/lamivudine 150 mg bid/zidovudine 300 mg bid. Subjects were stratified based on plasma HIV-1 RNA at screening: <10 000 copies/mL, 10 000–100 000 copies/mL, or >100 000 copies/mL. Both treatment groups had marked decreases in plasma HIV-1 RNA by week 4, which was sustained in the abacavir/lamivudine/zidovudine group. At week 16, the proportion of subjects with plasma HIV-1 RNA below the limit of detection (<400 copies/mL) was significantly superior in the abacavir/lamivudine/zidovudine group (75%) when compared to the lamivudine/zidovudine group (35%) ($P < 0.0001$ analyzed by the Cochran–Mantel–Haenzel test controlling for randomized plasma HIV-1 RNA strata). In addition, the triple combination was effective irrespective of the baseline plasma HIV-1 RNA strata. By contrast, the virologic response to lamivudine/zidovudine began to rebound toward baseline until week 16 when subjects were eligible to add abacavir plus other ART. The virologic response to lamivudine/zidovudine at week 16 was also diminished at the higher plasma HIV-1 RNA baseline strata. Mean increase in CD4+ T-lymphocyte counts was similar between the treatment groups at 16 weeks. The triple combination was generally well tolerated (3% of this group withdrew due to adverse experiences as compared to 2.5% of subjects in the lamivudine/zidovudine group).

The CNAF3007/Ecureuil open-label study evaluated the efficacy and safety of the triple nucleoside combination Combivir/abacavir versus Combivir/nelfinavir as first-line therapy in HIV-1-infected adults.[62] This randomized, open-label study in 195 HIV-1-infected adults, with plasma HIV-1 RNA 1000–500 000 copies/mL, compared Combivir/abacavir to Combivir/nelfinavir over 48 study weeks. At the intent-to-treat analysis at 48 weeks, 64% and 61% of subjects had plasma viral load <50 copies/mL in the Combivir/abacavir and Combivir/nelfinavir groups, respectively. The baseline viral load was comparable in both groups with a median of 4.2 $\log_{10}$ copies/mL (Combivir/abacavir) and 4.1 $\log_{10}$ copies/mL (Combivir/nelfinavir). The median change from baseline in plasma viral load was $-2.3 \log_{10}$ copies/mL in both groups. Median CD4+ T-lymphocyte count increases were 109 and 120 cells/μL in the Combivir/abacavir and Combivir/nelfinavir arms, respectively. Possible hypersensitivity reactions to abacavir were reported in four subjects (4%). These results suggest that Combivir/abacavir is generally well-tolerated first-line ART in HIV-1-infected adults, with comparable antiviral activity to that of a PI-containing regimen over 48 weeks.

Of 155 subjects completing 48 weeks in the CNAF3007 trial, 92 were enrolled into the CNAF3021 study to look at long-term safety and efficacy: 47 subjects initially randomized to the Combivir/abacavir group and 45 subjects to the Combivir/nelfinavir arm.[63] After a follow-up of at least 2 years post-CNAF3007 randomization (median 3 years), there was a higher proportion of patients in the Combivir/nelfinavir group (67%) than in the Combivir/abacavir group (30%) who discontinued the treatment initially attributed by randomization of the CNAF3007. In total, 11/30 patients in the Combivir/nelfinavir switched from nelfinavir to abacavir. In the intent-to-treat analyses (switch included), 76% of subjects in the Combivir/abacavir group and 71% of subjects in the Combivir/nelfinavir group had a plasma HIV-1 RNA <50 copies/mL at the single long-term entry CNAF3021 visit.

The CNA3014 study compared Combivir/abacavir to another PI-containing regimen, indinavir (800 mg tid)/abacavir in a 48-week open-label randomized study in 342 HIV-infected ART naive adults with CD4+ T-lymphocyte counts >100 cells/μL and plasma HIV-1 RNA >5000 copies/mL.[64] Subjects were stratified based on screening plasma HIV-1 RNA: >5000–100 000 copies/mL or ≥100 000 copies/mL. Results demonstrated that time to treatment failure over 48 weeks by intent-to-treat analysis was significantly longer in the abacavir/Combivir group than in the indinavir/Combivir group ($P < 0.001$). In the primary analysis (intent-to-treat, missing = failure, plasma HIV-1 RNA <400 copies/mL), the abacavir/Combivir regimen was superior. In the intent-to-treat analysis at week 48 by baseline plasma HIV-1 RNA stratum, abacavir/Combivir was more effective than indinavir/Combivir in patients with <100 000 copies/mL (70% vs 49% with plasma HIV-1 RNA <400 copies/mL). This difference was not observed in patients with plasma HIV-1 RNA >100 000 copies/mL (60% in abacavir/Combivir vs 51% in indinavir/Combivir). Sustained increases in CD4+ T lymphocytes were observed in both treatment groups over 48 weeks. Self-reported adherence to randomized treatment was significantly higher in the abacavir/Combivir group, with 72% of subjects reporting taking all of their doses or missing an average of less than one dose per week during the last month, compared with 45% of subjects in the indinavir/Combivir group ($P < 0.001$). The percentages of drug-related adverse events in the study were 65% (108/165 in abacavir/Combivir group) and 87% (142/164 in the indinavir/Combivir group). Six percent (10/165) of the subjects in the abacavir/Combivir group had a possible abacavir hypersensitivity reaction, all of which occurred during the first 6 weeks of therapy.

The KLEAN study examined two other PIs, fosamprenavir–ritonavir versus lopinavir–ritonavir, each in combination with abacavir–lamivudine.[65] This open-label, noninferiority study enrolled 878 antiretroviral-naive HIV-1-infected subjects to receive fosamprenavir–ritonavir 700 mg/100 mg twice daily or lopinavir–ritonavir 400 mg/100 mg twice daily, each with the eco-formulation of abacavir–lamivudine 600 gm/300 mg (Epzicom) once daily. Noninferiority of fosamprenavir–ritonavir to lopinavir–ritonavir was demonstrated for the primary study endpoint of proportion of subjects at week 48 achieving plasma HIV-1 RNA <400 copies/mL (95% CI around the treatment difference −4.84–7.05 was shown). At week 48, 315 of 434 (73%) subjects in the fosamprenavir–ritonavir group and 317 of 444 (71%) in the lopinavir-ritonavir group achieved plasma HIV-1 RNA <400 copies/mL. Treatment discontinuations because of an adverse event, which was another primary study endpoint, were few and occurred with similar frequency in the two treatment groups (fosamprenavir–ritonavir 53 (12%); lopinavir–ritonavir 43 (10%)). Suspected abacavir hypersensitivity was reported in 53 cases (6%); 32 (7%) in the fosamprenavir–ritonavir arm and 21 (5%) in the lopinavir–ritonavir arm.

Abacavir versus the NNRTI nevirapine combined with zidovudine/lamivudine was examined as a first-line ART for HIV-1 infection in Uganda, Africa.[66] The rationale for this safety study was that these agents might avoid drug interactions with tuberculosis therapy as described with HIV-1 PIs, plus the tolerability and toxicity of abacavir in Africa were unknown. This randomized, double-blind, 24-week trial enrolled 599 symptomatic antiretroviral-naive subjects with CD4+ T-lymphocyte counts <200 cells/μL who were either zidovudine/lamivudine (Combivir) with either 300 mg abacavir or nevirapine placebo (n = 300) or nevirapine 200 mg and abacavir placebo (n = 299) twice daily. Of 599 enrolled subjects, 569 (9%) completed 24 weeks; however, 24 (4%) died and six (1%) were lost to follow-up. Twenty subjects had serious adverse reactions (six (2%) on abacavir and 14 (4.7%) on nevirapine) (primary endpoint: hazards ratio = 4.1; 95% CI = 0.16–1.08; log rank P = 0.06). Serious adverse reactions reported in 19 of 20 patients were consistent with potential hypersensitivity reactions: similar proportions on abacavir (four of six) and nevirapine (seven of 13) had respiratory, constitutional (three with abacavir, seven with nevirapine), or GI symptoms (two with abacavir, five with nevirapine), rash (six with abacavir, 10 with nevirapine), fever (six with abacavir, nine with nevirapine), or oral/mucosal involvement (two with abacavir, five with nevirapine); but hepatic involvement was seen only in three patients on nevirapine. The remaining serious adverse reaction was asymptomatic hepatitis (nevirapine arm). In total, 14 (4.7% abacavir) and 30 (10%) nevirapine patients discontinued blinded abacavir/nevirapine (P = 0.01) due to toxicity (six (2%) abacavir vs 15 (5%) nevirapine, respectively, P = 0.05), all rash or possible hypersensitivity reactions (six with abacavir, 13 with nevirapine), or hepatotoxicity (four with nevirapine). This study concluded that abacavir had a lower discontinuation rate and a trend toward a lower rate of serious adverse reactions when compared with nevirapine in African patients initiating ART with low CD4+ T-lymphocyte counts.

The CNA30024 trial studied abacavir versus zidovudine combined with lamivudine and the NNRTI, efavirenz, in an international randomized, double-blind noninferiority clinical trial in 654 antiretroviral-naive HIV-1-infected patients in the USA, Costa Rica, Chile, Portugal, and Denmark.[67] Of 654 enrolled subjects, 649 received more than one dose of randomized study medication. A total of 503 (77%) completed ⩾48 weeks of study (78% in the abacavir group and 77% in the zidovudine group), and 145 (24%) of the subjects prematurely discontinued the study (similar for both treatment groups). The incidence of reported serious adverse events was 20% in the abacavir group and 14% in the zidovudine group. Of the 30 cases of suspected hypersensitivity reactions reported in the abacavir group, only five met the definition of a serious event. The primary study objective was the comparison of the proportion of subjects achieving plasma HIV-1 RNA ⩽50 copies/mL through 48 weeks of study: 70% of subjects in the abacavir arm versus 69% of subjects in the zidovudine group maintained confirmed plasma HIV-1 RNA levels ⩽50 copies/mL. Therefore, abacavir was found to be noninferior to zidoduvine when combined with lamivudine and efavirenz (stratified 95% CI of −6.3% to 7.9%). Furthermore, the proportion of subjects with plasma HIV-1 RNA ⩽50 copies/mL at week 48 was similar between treatment arms when stratified by screening plasma HIV-1 RNA levels of either <100 000 copies/mL (72% abacavir group vs 70% zidovudine group) or >100 000 copies/mL (67% in both treatment arms).

The ACTG 5095 study compared the triple-nucleoside regimen of abacavir plus Combivir versus NNRTI-containing (efavirenz) regimens for the initial treatment of HIV-1-infection.[68,69] This randomized, double-blind study evaluated three antiretroviral regimens for the initial treatment of subjects infected with HIV-1: zidovudine/lamivudine/abacavir, zidovudine/lamivudine plus efavirenz, and zidovudine/lamivudine/abacavir plus efavirenz. Combivir/abacavir (Trizivir) versus Combivir plus efavirenz versus Combivir/abacavir plus efavirenz. A total of 1147 subjects with a mean baseline HIV-1 RNA level of 4.85 $\log_{10}$ copies/mL and a mean CD4+ T-lymphocyte count of 238/μL were enrolled. Prespecified stopping rules led to the recommendation to stop the triple-nucleoside regimen (abacavir plus Combivir) due to virologic inferiority and allowed presentation of results in the triple-nucleoside group in comparison to pooled data from the efavirenz groups.[68] The time to virologic failure was found to be significantly shorter in the triple-nucleoside group ($P < 0.001$). After a median follow-up of 32 weeks, 82 of 382 subjects (21%) in the triple-nucleoside group and 85 of 765 (11%) in the pooled efavirenz groups had virologic failure. These differences persisted despite stratification for baseline plasma HIV-1 RNA levels in subjects either entering the study with <100 000 copies/mL (P = 0.001) or >100 000 copies/mL (P < 0.001). These differences also persisted despite stratification for baseline pretreatment CD4+ T-lymphocyte subjects of ⩾100 copies/mL (P = 0.001) or lower (P < 0.001), as well as baseline pretreatment CD4+ T-lymphocyte subjects of ⩾200 copies/mL (P = 0.004) or lower (P < 0.001). In a *post hoc* analysis, the 195 subjects in the triple-nucleoside arm who reported 100% adherence at week 12 had a higher rate of virologic failure than the 382 subjects in the pooled efavirenz arms with the same level of adherence (P < 0.001). Suspected abacavir hypersensitivity reactions were reported in 27 (7%) subjects in the triple-nucleoside group and 59 (8%) subjects in the pooled efavirenz arms. The results of the completed three versus four drug A5095 trial demonstrated no difference between the three-drug regimen of zidovudine/lamuvudine plus efavirenz versus the four-drug regimen of zidvoudine/lamivudine/abacavir plus efavirenz as initial treatment in HIV-1-infected subjects.[69] After a median 3 year follow-up, 99 (26%) of 382 and 94 (25%) of 383 patients receiving the three-drug and four-drug regimens, respectively, reached protocol-defined virologic failure; time to virologic failure was not significantly different (hazard ratio, 0.95; 97.5% CI, 0.69–1.33, P = 0.73). Overall, at least 80% of subjects had plasma HIV-1 RNA levels <50 copies/mL through 3 years of treatment. This study demonstrated that adding abacavir as a fourth initial drug to this dual-nucleoside plus NNRTI-containing regimen provided no additional benefit in a direct three versus four initial drugs comparison.

Not all abacavir-containing triple-nucleoside regimens are recommended for HIV-1-infected antiretroviral-naive subjects. Early virologic nonresponse to abacavir, tenofovir, and lamivudine was reported in the ESS30009 Study.[70] This randomized open-label, multicenter study compared tenofovir disoproxil fumarate versus the NNRTI efavirenz when both administered once daily with abacavir/lamivudine fixed combination as first-line antiHIV triple-drug therapy. A total of 340 subjects were randomized with a median baseline HIV-1 RNA level of 4.7 $\log_{10}$ copies/mL and median baseline CD4+ T-lymphocyte count of 251 cells/μL. After reports of early virologic nonresponse, an unplanned interim analysis was performed on 194 of the enrolled 340 subjects who had ⩾8 weeks of plasma HIV-1 RNA results available. Several definitions of virologic nonresponse were employed: (1) a <2.0 $\log_{10}$ copies/mL decrease in HIV-1 RNA level by study week 8; (2) a rebound of plasma HIV-1 RNA ⩾1.0 $\log_{10}$ copies/mL above the nadir; or (3) for subjects with two consecutive plasma HIV-1 RNA measurements <50 copies/mL, a subsequent increase to >400 copies/mL on two consecutive occasions. Interim results revealed that virologic nonresponse occurred in 50 (49%) of 102 subjects in the tenofovir disoproxil fumarate arm when compared to five (5%) of 92 subjects in the efavirenz arm (P < 0.001). By study week 12, genotyping of plasma HIV-1 isolates from nonresponders in the tenofovir disoproxil fumarate/abacavir/lamivudine arm detected the HIV-1 RT M184V or M184I/M/V mixtures in 40 (98%) of 41 subjects and HIV-1 RT K65R and M184V or mixtures in 22 (54%) of 41 subjects (*see section on* HIV-1 Drug Resistance). Subjects initially randomized to the tenofovir disoproxil fumarate arm were then permitted to switch to an investigator-determined second-line regimen and 131 (77%) of 171 subjects remained in follow-up. Of the 61 subjects with genotype data available at or before switching, 31 had a detectable HIV-1 RT K65R mutation. The efavirenz arm continued unaltered, and by contrast to the abacavir arm, 120 (71%) of 169 subjects achieved a plasma HIV-1 RNA level of <50 copies/mL after 48 study weeks. As mentioned previously (*see section on In Vitro* Activity and Mechanisms of Action), no drug–drug interactions to explain the virologic nonresponse of abacavir, tenofovir disoproxil fumarate, and lamivudine were found. Rather, the low genetic barrier to development of HIV-1 drug resistance is most likely to blame since this three-drug regimen exerts selective pressure with rapid development of M184V, followed by K65R in some patients. *Therefore, the combined regimen of abacavir, tenofovir disoproxil fumarate, and lamivudine for HIV-1-infection should not be used.*

The COL40263 trial evaluated the once-daily regimen of trizivir and tenofovir disoproxil fumarate in antiretroviral-naive HIV-1-infected subjects with plasma HIV-1 RNA >30 000 copies/mL.[71] The primary endpoints of this open-label, single-arm, multicenter trial were the proportion of subjects with plasma HIV-1 RNA <50 copies/mL at week 48 and the proportion of subjects with grade 3 or 4 adverse events and laboratory toxicities. Of 123 enrolled subjects, 52 (42%) discontinued study through week 48, including 14 due to adverse events, 13 lost to follow-up, and 12 with virologic nonresponse, as well as other reasons. Suspected abacavir hypersensitivity occurred in eight subjects (6.5%) within the first 3 weeks of study drug administration. Of subjects who remained on therapy over 48 weeks, 49 of 64 (77%) of subjects had plasma HIV-1 RNA levels <50 copies/mL at week 48.

The ESS40013 study tested fourdrug induction with abacavir/lamivudine/zidovudine plus the NNRTI efavirenz followed by maintenance treatment with the simplified regimen of abacavir/lamivudine/zidovudine alone in antiretroviral-naive HIV-1-infected subjects.[72] All 488 subjects received abacavir/lamivudine/zidovudine plus efavirenz during the 48-week induction phase followed by a 1:1 randomization to either the continued regimen of abacavir/lamivudine/zidovudine plus efavirenz or to simplified regimen of abacavir/lamivudine/zidovudine for the subsequent 48-week maintenance phase. No significant differences were noted in proportion of subjects with plasma HIV-1 RNA level <50 copies/mL at week 96: 79% abacavir/lamivudine/zidovudine plus efavirenz versus 77% abacavir/lamivudine/zidovudine; P = 0.75). Virologic failure occurred in 22 patients during induction and in 24 patients (16 in abacavir/lamivudine/zidovudine arm and eight in abacavir/lamivudine/zidovudine plus efavirenz group; P = 0.134) during maintenance. More subjects reported perfect adherence at week 96 in the triple therapy arm than in the four-drug arm (88.8% vs 79.6%; P = 0.057).

Studies Conducted in Antiretroviral Experienced HIV-1-Infected Adults

An abacavir open-label compassionate use program evaluated patients with advanced HIV-1 disease with CD4+ T-lymphocyte counts <100 cells/μL and plasma viral loads ⩾10000 copies/mL. From Jul. 1997 to Mar. 1998, over 2300 patients were enrolled worldwide. They were heavily pretreated with antiretrovirals at screening: 99% were on NRTI therapy, 97% were on PIs, 46% were on NNRTIs, and 75% had been on treatment for at least 1 year (unpublished data). The program did not specify the regimens selected by investigators, but included triple therapy with an NRTI and an NNRTI plus PI plus abacavir (25%). At least 38% of the patients received abacavir plus an NNRTI treatment regimen. The range of viral load responses to the therapy chosen was +1.30 to −3.68 $\log_{10}$ copies/mL in 151 patients. Overall, 25% of patients achieved a 0.5 $\log_{10}$ or greater decline in viral load. The mean change in plasma HIV-1 RNA was −0.29 $\log_{10}$ copies/mL, with a median decline of −0.18 $\log_{10}$ copies/mL. The best response among these patients was seen in those who entered the program on no prior therapy or monotherapy, in those who had higher viral loads at baseline, and in those who added at least one (and preferably two) agents at enrollment. Interestingly, what did not obviously correlate with response was the duration of prior therapy (more or less than 1 year), the CD4+ T-lymphocyte count at baseline, or the types of regimens used by category/class of agent. Abacavir is more effective in reducing viral load when the treatment history and/or disease process is less advanced. In patients with advanced disease, 25% of patients may respond to an abacavir-containing regimen, but combination with other new agents in the regimen is key. There were a total of 191 deaths during 1422 person-years of follow-up time, yielding a life expectancy of the subjects enrolled in the abacavir expanded access program of 7.4 years (95% CI: 6.6, 8.6), which is similar to that of other patients with advanced HIV-1/AIDS and other observational cohorts.[73]

Several clinical trials have looked at intensification of therapy by adding abacavir to existing therapy in order to achieve greater virologic suppression. The best results were seen in subjects without extensive prior therapy or drug resistance. The CNA3002 study was a phase II randomized, double-blind study designed to assess the potential effectiveness of abacavir in antiretroviral-experienced subjects, by adding abacavir 300 mg bid to background therapy of subjects with detectable plasma HIV-1 RNA.[74] Investigation of the usefulness of abacavir in patients previously exposed to lamivudine was another study goal. A total of 185 HIV-1-infected adults on stable background therapy for at least 12 weeks, with CD4+ T-lymphocyte counts >100 cells/μL and plasma HIV-1 RNA of 400–50000 copies/mL, were randomized to receive abacavir or placebo. At week 16, more subjects receiving abacavir plus stable background therapy had plasma HIV-1 RNA <400 copies/mL (36/92, 39%) than subjects receiving stable background therapy alone (7/93, 8%, $P < 0.001$). A similar response was seen in lamivudine-naive versus lamivudine-experienced subjects. Most subjects (73%) with the RT M184V mutation in plasma had a virologic response, as demonstrated by a >1.0 $\log_{10}$ copies/mL reduction in plasma HIV-1 RNA or ⩽400 copies/mL by week 16. However, in heavily pretreated HIV-1-infected patients examined in the Swiss HIV Cohort Study, salvage therapy with abacavir plus a NNRTI and a PI resulted in a low virologic success rate.[75] Of 23 HIV-1-infected patients with four (median) therapy changes before salvage, only 10 patients (43%) achieved a decrease of plasma HIV-1 RNA >0.5 $\log_{10}$ after 6 months of therapy. After 6 months, only two subjects had undetectable plasma HIV-1 RNA (<500 copies/mL). Only seven patients increased their CD4+ T-lymphocyte counts by >30% above baseline, whereas three patients with baseline CD4+ T-lymphocyte counts <100 cells/μL had a >30% decline. Almost all of the patients had extensive HIV-1 drug resistance-conferring mutations at study baseline.

Several studies have looked at the impact of switching treatment to abacavir-containing regimens. The TARGET study was an open-label, multicenter, single-arm clinical trial assessing the 48-week activity of a twice-daily, triple-NRTI regimen containing abacavir/lamivudine in 87 treatment-experienced, PI-naive, HIV-1-infected adults.[76] These subjects had a baseline plasma HIV-1 RNA <50000 copies/mL and CD4+ T-lymphocyte counts ⩾50 cells/μl, and had been receiving single or double NRTIs immediately before screening. The median baseline plasma HIV-1 RNA was 3.10 $\log_{10}$ copies/mL and the median CD4+ T-lymphocyte count was 506 cells/μL. In the intent-to-treat analysis at 48 weeks, plasma HIV-1 RNA was <400 copies/mL in 45 (82%) of 55 patients, and <50 copies/mL in 31 (56%) of 55 patients, respectively. Prior zidovudine or lamivudine use, as well as presence of the RT M184V mutation, did not impact virologic response. These investigators concluded that enhanced adherence by reducing the number of dosage forms to only four tablets daily translated to improved virologic response in these HIV-1-infected subjects with high CD4+ T-lymphocyte counts and relatively low plasma HIV-1 RNA levels. Similar results were obtained in 209 patients randomized to receive either trizivir versus continued HAART in the TRIZAL study (AZL30002), with subjects reporting that taking one pill twice daily was easier than in subjects in the continued HAART group ($P < 0.0001$).[77]

Other studies have looked at the impact of switching from protease-containing regimens to abacavir-based triple-nucleoside therapy in HIV-1-infected patients with either undetectable or low levels of plasma HIV-1 RNA. The CNA30017 Study concluded that replacement of a PI by abacavir in a triple-combination regimen following prolonged suppression of plasma HIV-1 RNA could afford sustained virologic suppression, significant improvements in lipid abnormalities, and enhanced ease of dosing.[78] The ESS30005 study looked at switching to the quadruple nucleoside/nucleotide regimen of trizivir plus tenofovir following early virologic failure on an initial HAART regimen containing a thymidine analog plus lamivudine in combination with a PI or NNRTI.[79] The primary endpoint was based on comparing the intent-to-treat observed proportion of patients with plasma HIV-1 <400 copies/mL at week 48. A total of 51 subjects were enrolled with a baseline median plasma HIV-1 RNA of 1972 copies/mL and a median CD4+ T-lymphocyte count of 436 cells/μL. Subjects were excluded if the screening plasma HIV-1 genotype indicated more than two NRTI-associated mutations (M41L, A62V, D67N, T69D/S, K70R, L74V/I, V75I, F77L, Y115F, F116Y, Q151M, M184V, L210W, T215Y/F, K219Q/E) or the K65R mutation. Of 51 enrolled subjects, 38 (75%) completed the study; only four of 13 who prematurely discontinued on or before week 48 had adverse events leading to premature study discontinuation, including nausea, fatigue, and cancer. The virologic response to trizivir bid and tenofovir daily was high: 87% had plasma HIV-1 RNA <400 copies/mL and 77% had plasma HIV-1 RNA <50 copies/mL at week 48 (intention-to-treat analysis (ITT) observed where those with missing data were excluded).

Studies Conducted with Once-Daily Abacavir Formulations

As described in the section on Pharmacokinetics previously, the prolonged half-life of carbovir-triphosphate observed *in vivo* supports the administration of abacavir once daily. The CNA30021 study compared the efficacy and safety of 600 mg of abacavir administered once daily as two 300 mg pills (n = 384 subjects) versus 300 mg of abacavir administered twice daily (n = 386) in combination with 300 mg of lamivudine and 600 mg of efavirenz administered once daily in antiretroviral-naive HIV-1-infected subjects of 48 weeks.[80] The baseline median CD4+ T-lymphocyte count was 262 cells/μL and the baseline median plasma HIV-1 RNA level was 4.89 $\log_{10}$ copies/mL, with 44% entering the study with viral loads >100 000 copies/mL. Abacavir administered once daily was noninferior to the twice-daily regimen, with 66% and 68% of subjects in these treatment arms, respectively, achieving a confirmed plasma HIV-1 RNA level <50 copies/mL (95% CI: −8.4%, 4.9%). Virologic failure rates were similar between the two treatment arms: 10% for once-daily abacavir and 8% for twice-daily abacavir. In 31 of 70 subjects (44%) experiencing virologic failure that had specimens with sufficient plasma viremia >400 copies/mL to yield HIV-1 genotyping results, there were more treatment-related mutations that emerged in the once-daily abacavir group (13 of 16 subjects (81%)) vs the twice-daily abacavir group (10 of 15 subjects (67%)), but this was not a statistically significant difference between the two treatment arms. The median CD4+ T-lymphocyte count increases from baseline for once-daily abacavir and twice-daily abacavir were 188 cells/μL versus 200 cells/μL, respectively. The incidence of serious adverse events was similar between the two groups. Abacavir hypersensitivity reactions were seen at similar rates in the two treatment arms: 9% for abacavir once daily versus 7% for abacavir bid. This study concluded that once-daily abacavir achieves a comparable level of viral suppression as the indicated twice-daily dosing regimen. In a separate analysis of 37 clinical trials where 9330 subjects were exposed to abacavir for at least 24 weeks, abacavir hypersensitivity frequency (501 cases or 5.1%) or severity was not influenced by once or twice-daily administration of abacavir.[81]

Abacavir in the Treatment of HIV-1-Infected Infants and Children

Abacavir is indicated for the treatment of HIV-1-infected children, age 3 months to 13 years. The dose is 8 mg/kg, up to a maximum of 300 mg bid and should be part of a multiple-drug antiretroviral treatment. Abacavir has been tested in pediatric patients in multiple studies including at least two well-controlled randomized trials. In one study of children who had previously received nucleoside therapy for HIV-1 infection, abacavir added to lamivudine and zidovudine was more efficacious in reducing plasma HIV-1 RNA than the dual combination alone.[82] In the preliminary analysis of a second study of three double nucleoside regimens, the abacavir-containing combinations, with or without nelfinavir, resulted in the greatest reduction of viral load for first-time treatment of HIV-1-infected children.[83]

HIV-1 DRUG RESISTANCE

In vitro passage of virus in abacavir does not rapidly select for resistant virus.[84–90] The first RT mutation to arise upon *in vitro* passage of HIV-1 in the presence of abacavir was M184V, and, with further passage, mutations K65R, L74V, and Y115F appeared. Although the M184V mutation alone produced only a two- to threefold shift in drug susceptibility, in combination with other mutations it produced increased abacavir resistance. Alone or in combination, these mutations conferred a maximum of about 10-fold reduction in abacavir susceptibility. In contrast, the RT M184 mutation was associated with a 100 to 1000-fold reduction in phenotypic susceptibility to lamivudine. Abacavir was not cross-resistant with zidovudine *in vitro*. Some of the abacavir-resistant recombinant viruses were cross-resistant with zalcitabine, didanosine, and stavudine.[87]

The phenotypic abacavir susceptibility of 943 clinical isolates was determined *in vitro*.[91] These isolates were from HIV-1-infected subjects many of whom had received prior combined zidovudine plus lamivudine. Abacavir susceptibility was categorized into three mutually exclusive groups: (1) susceptible (i.e., less than fourfold increase in IC_{50}); (2) intermediate resistant (i.e., four- to eightfold increase in IC_{50}); and (3) resistant (greater than eightfold increase in IC_{50}). Interestingly, 95% of the isolates were susceptible to abacavir if they were only resistant to zidovudine or lamivudine (even if the M184V was present). Most isolates (71%) that were coresistant to zidovudine and lamivudine remained susceptible to abacavir, but 25% showed intermediate susceptibility and 4% are resistant. If resistance to zidovudine, lamivudine, or zidovudine plus lamivudine was associated with other NRTI resistance, susceptibility to abacavir decreased. The decrease was more profound if resistance to one other NRTI is present. All multi-NRTI-resistant isolates (i.e., those resistant to lamivudine plus zidovudine plus all other NRTIs) showed reduced susceptibility to abacavir. For example, if there was evidence of the nucleoside multidrug-resistance mutation at RT codon 151, then less than 1% of isolates were susceptible to abacavir.

Abacavir resistance may also be conferred by the following patterns of multi-NRTI resistance-conferring HIV-1 RT mutations: (1) the multi-NRTI resistance-conferring thymidine analog-associated mutations (TAMs): M41L, D67N, K70R, L210W, T215Y/F, and K219Q/E; (2) the Q151M complex; and (3) the codon 69 insertion mutations and ZDV resistance-conferring mutations.[88,92] The M184V mutation alone does not appear to be associated with a reduced virologic response to abacavir *in vivo*.[84,93] However, the RT M184V mutation (associated with lamivudine, emtricitabine, and abacavir therapy) contributes to reduced susceptibility to abacavir when present with two or three TAMs, and is associated with impaired virologic response *in vivo*.[91,92] Moreover, the RT M184V mutation plus four or more TAMS results in no virologic response to abacavir *in vivo*.[92,93]

Several earlier clinical trials describing abacavir resistance development *in vivo* are highlighted here. The resistance profile of abacavir after monotherapy and combination therapy with zidovudine was investigated in the dose-ranging CNA2001 trial, the first trial to examine abacavir resistance *in vivo*.[57,84] The study evaluated HIV-1-infected, antiretroviral-naive subjects with CD4+ T-lymphocyte counts of 200–500 cells/μL who received four different dosing regimens of abacavir monotherapy (200 mg tid, 300 mg bid, 400 mg tid, or 600 mg tid) for 4 weeks, after which they received 8 weeks of either continued abacavir plus zidovudine placebo or combined abacavir/zidovudine. Of the subjects with detectable plasma HIV-1 RNA that could be PCR-amplified for sequence analysis at week 12, RT mutations occurred at >1 of codons K65R, L74V, or M184V in 66% of subjects receiving abacavir/placebo and in 17% of subjects receiving abacavir/zidovudine. Overall, mutations at RT codons K65R, L74V, or M184V were observed after 12 weeks in 51% of subjects assigned to the abacavir monotherapy arms (especially as double mutants), and in 11% of subjects assigned to the combined abacavir/zidovudine arm, mainly as single mutants. Small changes (two- to fourfold) in abacavir susceptibility were detected. With abacavir discontinuation, wild-type sequence occurred within 4 weeks. In a separate trial in drug-naive subjects (the CNA2002 Study), 60 subjects were randomized to 100, 300, or 600 mg abacavir twice daily.[85] Mutant viruses were not detected prior to week 12 except in one patient. While on abacavir monotherapy at weeks 6–48, a total of 21 of 43 subjects had single, double, and triple combinations of RT K65R, L74V, Y115F, and M184V mutations. The most common RT mutational pattern was L74V and M184V (11/24 cases). Twenty of 21 subjects with isolates containing abacavir-associated RT mutations reached week 48, yet achieved plasma HIV-1 RNA levels <400 copies/mL upon the addition of lamivudine/zidovudine.

The phenotypic sensitivity to abacavir in the presence of multiple genotypic mutations was correlated with viral load response in the CNAA2003 trial.[86] Abacavir was added to current NRTI therapy (defined as failing therapy with plasma HIV-1 RNA >10 000 copies/mL), CD4+ T-lymphocyte cells >100 cells/μL, and no active CDC class C problems. Patients had previously received ≥6 months stavudine, ≥6 months didanosine/zidovudine, ≥12 months zidovudine, or ≥12 months zidovudine combined with ≥6 months lamivudine. A total of 32 patients were enrolled into the study, and 23 of 32 subjects' isolates were analyzed phenotypically and genotypically. Viruses were considered susceptible (i.e., less than fourfold increase in abacavir IC_{50}), intermediate (i.e., four- to eightfold increase in abacavir IC_{50}), or resistant (i.e., greater than eightfold increase in abacavir IC_{50}). Based on mean changes in viral load response from baseline ($\log_{10}$ copies/mL) over 12 weeks, those patients with abacavir-sensitive and abacavir-intermediate viruses achieved greater peak reductions in viral load (e.g., −1.0–−2.5 $\log_{10}$ copies/mL at week 2) when compared to those patients with abacavir-resistant viruses (i.e., no reductions from baseline). The phenotypic resistance patterns also correlated with the week 4 viral load responses. However, there was a range of viral load responses within each category of abacavir phenotypic susceptibility, such that some individuals with baseline abacavir sensitivity did not achieve subsequent viral load reductions when started on abacavir *in vivo*. Phenotypic resistance to lamivudine and/or the presence of the RT M184V mutation did not necessarily preclude the virologic activity of abacavir, and patients still had virologic responses.[86,89,90,94] In general, the presence of high-level phenotypic abacavir resistance or a higher number of multiple NRTI mutations prior to initiation of therapy in a patient's virus pool predicted a poorer subsequent virologic response than in those patients harboring abacavir sensitive viruses.[86,89–91,94]

Lanier et al determined a 'clinically' relevant phenotypic resistance 'cutoff' for abacavir using the PhenoSense phenotypic assay (Monogram Biosciences) using data combined from four GlaxoSmithKline studies: CNA3001, CNA2003, CNA3002, and CNA3009.[95] In all of these studies, abacavir was added as a single agent to current therapy. The impact of baseline abacavir phenotype on virologic response to abacavir addition after 24 weeks was investigated. This study determined that plasma HIV-1 RNA response was significantly reduced when ≥4 NRTI mutations were present at baseline. Reductions in susceptibility to abacavir of >4.5-fold significantly reduced virologic response to abacavir. This result led to the 'clinical cutoff' of 4.5 as the fold change for abacavir considered to be clinically significant for patients. However, there appears to be a continuum of virologic response with increasing fold resistance to abacavir, as some subjects whose baseline isolates showing 4.5 to sevenfold reductions also responded. If the baseline susceptibility to abacavir was reduced by more than sevenfold, the virologic response was severely affected.

A more recent GlaxoSmithKline study looked at the impact of combinations of K65R, L74V, and M184V/I (i.e., mutations frequently seen during abacavir therapy) on NRTI cross-resistance in collaboration with Monogram Biosciences utilizing their large-scale clinical database of 17 633 genotyped specimens linked to phenotypic results.[96] Interestingly, all of these mutations demonstrated increased susceptibility to zidovudine, and the RT L74V and M184V mutations either alone or together were associated with increased susceptibility to tenofovir. The RT K65R mutation resulted in median fold changes about the clinical cutoff for lamivudine, didanosine, and tenofovir. The RT L74V mutation did not result in median fold changes above cutoff for any of these drugs. Having combined RT K65R and M184V mutations were associated with a greater percentage of isolates about the cutoff for abacavir, zalcitabine, didanosine, and tenofovir than the RT L74V and M184V combination.

The combination of abacavir, tenofovir, and lamivudine was associated with a high rate of early virologic nonresponse in antiretroviral-naive HIV-1-infected subjects in the ESS30009 study that led to early termination of this regimen as mentioned previously.[97] 50 of 102 (49%) abacavir/tenofovir/lamivudine-treated subjects experienced early virologic nonresponse. Paired virus samples from baseline and week 12 timepoints were analyzed from 41 subjects' isolates for genotypic and phenotypic changes by Monogram Biosciences methodology associated with early virologic nonresponse. By week 12, 98% of the 41 abacavir/tenofovir/lamivudine early virologic nonresponders studied had viruses containing M184V/I mixtures, with 54% also having K65R or K65K/R mixtures. Phenotypic resistance was not as reflective of viral response as genotypic findings. More than 54% likely developed K65R at week 12 that was missed by bulk population sequencing, since four out of four subjects had K65R detected at week 12 at minority viral variant levels by additional clonal sequencing analyses.[98] The RT mutation K70E was also identified in subjects failing abacavir/lamivudine/tenofovir.[99] This may represent an alternative resistance pathway associated with nonresponse to this regimen since the RT K65R and K70E found in viral mixtures by bulk population sequencing were not present on the same viral genome by clonal genotypic analyses.[100] It was concluded that this regimen's substandard efficacy may have resulted, in part, from a low genetic barrier to HIV drug resistance during treatment with abacavir/tenofovir/lamivudine.

The COL40263 trial investigated whether the addition of zidovudine (an agent known to not select for the RT K65R pathway) to trizivir (i.e., abacavir/zidovudine/lamivudine) would impact selection for K65R in subjects.[101] This study was initiated given the large proportion of early virologic nonresponders and high frequency of K65R and M184V mutations seen when only abacavir and lamivudine were combined with tenofovir. This open-label, multicenter trial evaluated the efficacy and safety of trizivir daily in combination with tenofovir daily over 48 weeks of study in antiretroviral-naive HIV-1-infected subjects; the study was conducted when zidovudine once daily was under clinical investigation. The study enrolled 123 subjects. Fourteen of 123 (11%) experienced protocol-defined virologic failure criteria at week 48; at baseline three of the 14 had evidence of pretherapy HIV-1 genotypic resistance by bulk population sequencing (including V118I/V, K103N, Y188F/H/L/Y, M184V, and T215A/I/S). In contrast to HIV-1 drug resistance patterns described above for tenofovir- and triple nucleoside-containing regimens where the RT K65R mutation occurred frequently, this quadruple-daily regimen of trizivir plus tenofovir selected predominantly for the NRTI TAMs mutations in these 14 isolates by both bulk viral population sequencing and by clonal genotypic analyses.[101,102] Only two of 14 (14%) last available HIV-1 genotypes examined contained the RT mutation K65R mutation in this study; one of these subjects may have been predisposed to K65R selection by the presence of K70E at study baseline.[102]

Other abacavir HIV-1 resistance studies looked at viruses derived from patients treated with abacavir/lamivudine-containing NRTI backbone regimens lacking tenofovir as a component of the HAART regimen or when used later as treatment intensification. The RT M184V and L74V mutations were most commonly selected in antiretroviral-naive subjects failing a first-line abacavir/lamivudine HAART-containing regimen.[103] In contrast, the RT K65R mutation has been reported as rarely being selected.[103] Similarly, the selection of RT L74V during therapy with abacavir/lamivudine did not signify co-selection or enhanced prevalence of RT K65R in the ZODIAC study of antiretroviral-naive HIV-1-infected subjects treated with abacavir/lamivudine/efavirenz.[104] Abacavir/lamivudine preferentially selected for M184V and L74V, even when preexisting, underlying RT K65R mutants were present at study entry. A separate study examining the role of tenofovir treatment intensification in patients with prior abacavir or didanosine therapy.[105] Although these subjects' isolates developed RT K65R or L74V/I mutations by bulk population sequencing, additional minority viral variant analyses showed that low-level RT K65R existed in 14% of the treatment-experienced patients with RT L74V/I in the absence of TAMs. Of note, these subjects did not have viruses displaying RT K65R prior to any therapy. Subsequent tenofovir treatment intensification of subjects with prior abacavir or didanosine therapy resulted in poor virological response, presumably due to expansion of a preexisting RT K65R minority variant mutant population that was selected by the first-line regimen.

DRUG INTERACTIONS

There are no known significant drug interactions in studies that have been reported to date. The pharmacology of abacavir suggests that the potential for significant drug interactions with commonly prescribed antiretroviral and opportunistic infection medications is limited.

TRIZIVIR

On 14 Nov 2000, the FDA approved Trizivir for the treatment of HIV-1 in adults and adolescents. Each dose of Trizivir is a fixed-dose tablet combination of Ziagen (abacavir), Retrovir (zidovudine), and Epivir (lamivudine), three NRTIs already approved by FDA. The recommended oral dose of Trizivir for adults and adolescents is one tablet twice daily, with no food or fluid restrictions. Trizivir is not recommended for treatment in adults or adolescents who weigh less than 40 kg because it is a fixed-dose tablet. Since Trizivir is a fixed-dose tablet and the dosage of the individual components cannot be altered, neither patients with impaired renal function and creatinine clearance <50 mL/min should receive Trizivir nor should patients with impaired hepatic function. Trizivir may be used alone or in combination with other antiretroviral agents for the treatment of HIV-1 infection, but should not be administered concomitantly with abacavir, lamivudine, zidovudine, which are already contained in Trizivir. The recommended dose is one tablet twice a day. The most common adverse events associated with the use of Trizivir in ≥5% of patients include nausea, vomiting, diarrhea, loss of appetite, weakness or tiredness, headache, dizziness, pain or tingling of the hands or feet, and muscle and joint pain. The same precautions about abacavir regarding the potential for a hypersensitivity reaction apply to Trizivir (*see section on* Recommendations for Use, Abacavir). The frequency of abacavir hypersensitivity reactions, rechallenge reactions, and hypersensitivity reaction-attributable outcomes were found to be similar with the use of abacavir or Trizivir.[106]

EPZICOM

On 2 Aug 2004, the FDA approved Epzicom for the treatment of HIV-1 in adults and adolescents. Each dose of Trizivir is a fixed-dose combination of 600 mg of Ziagen (abacavir) and 300 mg of Epivir (lamivudine), two NRTIs already approved by FDA. In Dec 2004, the European Commission approved the same fixed-dose combination under the trade name Kivexa. The fixed-dose combination was developed to reduce pill burden and dosing frequency. The recommended dose in adults is one tablet once daily with no food or fluid requirements. Bioequivalence was demonstrated of the abacavir/lamivudine fixed-dose combination tablet (Epzicom/Kivexa) in several studies.[107–109] In the ESS30008 (SEAL) study, Epzicom administered once daily was established as not being inferior to abacavir and lamivudine administered twice daily in a regimen containing an NNRTI or a PI over 48 weeks in subjects with plasma HIV-1 RNA levels <400 copies/mL and a CD4+ T-lymphocyte count >50 cells/μL.[108] In the CAL30001 study, the once-daily fixed-dose combination of abacavir/lamivudine had noninferior efficacy as measured by time-averaged change from baseline plasma HIV-1 RNA over 48 weeks when compared to abacavir twice daily and lamivudine once daily as separate entities in treatment of antiretroviral-experienced adults experiencing virologic failure.[109] It is not intended for use in pediatric patients. It should be used in combination with other antiretroviral agents for the treatment of HIV-1 infection, but should not be administered concomitantly with abacavir and lamivudine, which are already contained in Epzicom. Because it is a fixed-dose tablet, Epzicom should not be prescribed for patients requiring dosage adjustment such as those with impaired renal function and creatinine clearance <50 mL/min, those with hepatic impairment, or those experiencing dose-limiting adverse events. The most common side effects seen with Epzicom in combination with efavirenz were trouble sleeping, depression, headache, tiredness, dizziness, nausea, rash, fever, stomach pain, abnormal dreams, and anxiety. The same precautions about abacavir regarding the potential for a hypersensitivity reaction apply to Epzicom (*see section on* Recommendations for Use, Abacavir). A recently reported 12-week study (ESS101822 (ALOHA)) of abacavir/lamivudine administered once daily compared with the separate components administered twice daily did not demonstrate that the abacavir hypersensitivity reaction was higher in the once-daily abacavir/lamivudine arm than in the twice-daily arm.[110]

RECOMMENDATIONS FOR USE

Abacavir

The FDA approved nucleoside analog drug abacavir on 18 Dec 1998, for use in combination anti-HIV-1 regimens for adults and children. The drug was initially recommended to be taken twice daily, one 300 mg tablet per dose, with no food or water restrictions. Plasma HIV-1 RNA levels have been documented to fall 1.5–2.0 $\log_{10}$ with CD4+ T-lymphocyte increases of 90–145 cells/μL in antiretroviral-naive patients treated with monotherapy for 12 weeks.

Abacavir is generally well tolerated, with the most common side effects being headache, nausea, vomiting, diarrhea, and malaise. The single most important treatment-limiting condition is severe hypersensitivity (allergy) in 3–9% of patients. The hypersensitivity syndrome usually occurs during the first month of therapy: fever is the most common symptom of the syndrome. Nausea, rash, and/or malaise are also characteristic. When patients are taking multiple drugs, it is difficult to know whether fever or rash or other manifestations are due to another drug, to abacavir, or to an unrelated process. People who experience increasing nausea, abdominal pain, fever, fatigue, and/or skin rash within 6 weeks after starting abacavir should contact their doctor immediately. The major decision is whether to stop the abacavir. Symptoms increase in severity if dosing is continued. Also, interrupting and restarting after a hypersensitivity reaction may result in life-threatening return of symptoms within hours. Thus, once abacavir is stopped because of manifestations compatible with the syndrome, it should not be restarted.

For initial therapy in antiretroviral-naive patients, a regimen containing abacavir is attractive from the perspective of potency and modest pill burden (either one 300 mg pill twice daily or two 300 mg pills once daily). Whether abacavir-containing regimens are more advantageous than regimens containing other drugs in terms of long-term efficacy, safety, and tolerability still remains to be completely established. The principal limitation of choosing abacavir as a therapeutic option is the concern about abacavir hypersensitivity reactions. In some parts of the world, testing for

HLA*B5701 is performed prior to prescribing the drug. This has resulted anecdotally in a substantial reduction in the incidence of hypersensitivity reactions. Several prospective trials are underway to quantify the benefit of this approach. In the meantime, abacavir remains a reasonable choice for first-line therapy provided the patients are counseled appropriately for hypersensitivity reactions and monitored carefully for their occurrence, especially in the first 2–8 weeks of treatment.

The combined regimen of abacavir, tenofovir disoproxil fumarate, and lamivudine for HIV-1 infection should not be used due to a high rate of virologic nonresponse due to its rapid selection of drug-resistant HIV-1 virus with a low genetic barrier. Of note, the combination of abacavir plus Combivir was found to be inferior to two other efavirenz-containing regimens (Combivir/abacavir (Trizivir) plus efavirenz or Combivir plus efavirenz) as initial treatment of HIV-1 infection.

For salvage therapy, abacavir can be considered, especially for patients who may not have isolates resistant to multiple nucleoside compounds and in subjects with lower plasma HIV-1 RNA levels. The hypersensitivity syndrome associated with abacavir requires that patients and physicians be educated in the recognition and management of this event in this setting as well.

REFERENCES

1. Daluge SM, Good SS, Martin MT, et al. 1592U89 Succinate: a novel carbocyclic nucleoside with potent, selective anti-HIV activity. Presented at the 34th Interscience Conference on Antimicrobial Agents and Chemotherapy, Orlando, FL, 1994, abstract 16.
2. Faletto MB, Miller WH, Garvey EP, et al. Unique intracellular activation of a new anti-HIV agent (1S, 4R)-4-[2-amino-6-(cyclopropylamino)-9H-purin-9-yl]-2-cyclopentene-1-methanol (1592U89) in the human T-lymphoblastoid cell line CEM T4. Presented at the 34th Interscience Conference on Antimicrobial Agents and Chemotherapy, Orlando, FL, 1994, abstract 184.
3. Daluge SM, Good SS, Faletto MB, et al. 1592U89 Succinate: a potent, selective anti-HIV carbocyclic nucleoside. Antiviral Res 26:A228, 1995.
4. Faletto MB, Miller WH, Garvey EP, et al. Unique purine cross-over pathway for the potent anti-HIV agent 1592U89. Antiviral Res 26:A262, 1995.
5. Daluge SM, Good SS, Faletto MB, et al. 1592 Succinate: a novel carbocyclic nucleoside analog with potent, selective anti-HIV activity. Antimicrob Agents Chemother 41:1082, 1997.
6. Faletto MB, Miller WH, Garvey EP, et al. Unique intracellular activation of the potent antihuman immunodeficiency virus agent 1592U89. Antimicrob Agents Chemother 41:1099, 1997.
7. Tisdale M, Parry NR, Cousens D, et al. Anti-HIV activity of (1S,4R)-4-[2-amino-6-(cyclopropylamino)-9H-purin-9-yl]-2-cyclopentene-1-methanol (1592U89). Presented at the 34th Interscience Conference on Antimicrobial Agents and Chemotherapy, Orlando, FL, 1994, abstract 182.
8. Billello JA, BIlello PA, Symonds W, et al. 1592U89, a novel carbocyclic nucleoside analog with potent anti-HIV activity, is synergistic in combination with 141W94, an HIV protease inhibitor. Presented at the 4th Conference on Retroviruses and Opportunistic Infections, Toronto, ON, Canada, 1997, abstract 154.
9. St Clair MH, Millard J, Rooney J, et al. In vitro antiviral activity of 141W94 (VX-478) in combination with other antiretroviral agents. Antiviral Res 29:53, 1996.
10. Lanier ER, Hazen R, Ross L, et al. Lack of antagonism between abacavir, lamivudine, and tenofovir against wild-type and drug-resistant HIV-1. J Acquir Immune Def Syndr 39:519, 2005.
11. Ravitch JR, Jarrett JL, White HR, et al. Central nervous system penetration of the antiretroviral abacavir (1592) in human and animal models. Presented at the 5th Conference on Retroviruses and Opportunistic Infections, Chicago, 1998, abstract 636.
12. Ching SV, Ayers KM, Dornsife RE, et al. Nonclinical toxicology and in vitro toxicity studies with the novel anti-HIV agent (1592U89). Presented at the 34th Interscience Conference on Antimicrobial Agents and Chemotherapy, Orlando, FL, 1994, abstract 188.
13. Good SS, Owens BS, Faletto MB, et al. Disposition in monkeys and mice of (1S, 4R)-4-[2-amino-6-(cyclopropylamino)-9H-purin-9-yl]-2-cyclopentene-1-methanol (1592U89) succinate, a potent inhibitor of HIV. Presented at the 34th Interscience Conference on Antimicrobial Agents and Chemotherapy, Orlando, FL, 1994, abstract 186.
14. Good SS, Daluge SM, Ching SV, et al. 1592U89 Succinate: preclinical toxicological and disposition studies and preliminary clinical pharmacokinetics. Antiviral Res 26:A229, 1995.
15. McDowell JA, Chittick GE, Ravitch JR, et al. Pharmacokinetics of [^{14}C]Abacavir, a human immunodeficiency virus type 1 (HIV-1) reverse transcriptase inhibitor, administered in a single oral dose to HIV-1-infected adults: a mass balance study. Antimicrob Agents Chemother 43:2855, 1999.
16. Letendre S, Capparelli E, Best B, et al. Better antiretroviral penetration in the central nervous system is associated with lower CSF viral load. Presented at the 13th Conference on Retroviruses and Opportunistic Infections, Denver, CO, 2006, abstract 74.
17. Miller WH, Daluge SM, Garvey EP, et al. Phosphorylation of carbovir enantiomers by cellular enzymes determines the stereoselectivity of antiviral activity. J Biol Chem 267:21220, 1992.
18. Garvey E, Krenitsky TA. A novel human phosphotransferase highly specific for adenosine. Arch Biochem Biophys 296:161, 1992.
19. Parker WB, Shaddix SC, Bowdon BJ, et al. Metabolism of carbovir, a potent inhibitor of human immunodeficiency virus type 1, and its effects on cellular metabolism. Antimicrob Agents Chemother 37:1004, 1993.
20. Piliero P, Shachoy-Clark AD, Para M, et al. A study examining the pharmacokinetics of abacavir and the intracellular carbovir triphosphate (GSK Protocol CNA10905). Presented at the 43rd Interscience Conference on Antimicrobial Agents and Chemotherapy, Chicago, IL, 2003, abstract A-1797.
21. Sutherland-Phillips D, Hill-Zabala C, Brothers C, et al. Regimens containing abacavir (ABC), lamivudine (3TC), zidovudine (ZDV), and efavirenz (EFV) do not affect GRF during long-term treatment of HIV naive subjects. Presented at the 45th Interscience Conference on Antimicrobial Agents and Chemotherapy, Washington, DC, 2005, abstract H-349.
22. Bilello JA, Bilello PA, Symonds W, et al. Physiological concentrations of human albumin or α_1-acid glycoprotein do not markedly alter the anti-HIV activity of 1592U89, a novel inhibitor of the HIV-1 reverse transcriptase. Presented at the 36th Interscience Conference on Antimicrobial Agents and Chemotherapy, New Orleans, LA, 1996, abstract 18.
23. Sutherland-Phillips D, Hill-Zabala C, Brothers C, et al. Regimens containing abacavir (ABC), lamivudine (3TC), zidovudine (ZDV), and efavirenz (EFV) do not affect GFR during long-term treatment of HIV naive subjects. Presented at the 45th Interscience Conference on Antimicrobial Agents and Chemotherapy, Washington, DC, 2005, abstract H-349.

24. McDowell JA, Symonds WT, Kumar PN, et al. Initial phase I study of anti-HIV agent 1592U89: a single-dose escalation design including food effect and dosage form evaluation. Presented at the 35th Interscience Conference on Antimicrobial Agents and Chemotherapy, San Francisco, CA, 1995, abstract I-109.
25. Ravitch JR, Walsh JS, Reese MJ, et al. In vivo and in vitro studies of the potential for drug interactions involving the antiretroviral abacavir (1592) in humans. Presented at the 5th Conference on Retroviruses and Opportunistic Infections, Chicago, IL, 1998, abstract 634.
26. Kumar PN, Sweet DF, McDowell JA, et al. Safety and pharmacokinetics of abacavir (1592U89) following oral administration of escalating single doses in human immunodeficiency virus type 1-infected adults. Antimicrob Agents Chemother 43:603, 1999.
27. Symonds A, McDowell J, Chittick G, et al. The safety and pharmacokinets of GW1592U89, zidovudine, and lamivudine, alone and in combination after single dose administration in HIV infected patients. AIDS 10(Suppl 2):S23, 1996.
28. McDowell JA, Lou Y, Williams SS, et al. Multiple-dose pharmacokinetics and pharmacodynamics of abacavir alone and in combination with zidovudine in human immunodeficiency virus-infected adults. Antimicrob Agents Chemother 44:2061, 2000.
29. Hawkins T, Veikley W, St Claire RL, et al. Intracellular pharmacokinetics of tenofovir diphosphate, carbovir triphosphate, and lamivudine triphosphate in patients receiving triple-nucleoside regimens. J Acquir Immune Defic Syndr 39:406, 2005.
30. Singer S, Irlbeck D, Pruvost A, et al. Changes in levels of dNTPs, carbovir-TP, and tenofovir-DP in purified human CD4+ and CD8+ peripheral blood T cells following treatment with tenofovir +/− abacavir +/− lamivudine. Presented at the XV International Drug Resistance Workshop, Sitges, Spain, 2006, abstract 146.
31. Raffi F, Benhantou Y, Sereni D, et al. Pharmacokinetics of, and tolerability to, a single, oral 600 mg dose of abacavir in HIV-positive subjects with or without liver disease (CNAB1006 Study). Presented at the 40th Interscience Conference on Antimicrobial Agents and Chemotherapy, Toronto, ON, Canada, 2000, abstract 1630.
32. Zhao H, Hernandez J, Cutrell A, et al. Safety of abacavir (ABC) + lamivudine (3TC)-based HAART in ART-naive HIV-infected subjects with and without hepatitis B (HBV) and/or hepatitis C (HCV) co-infection. Presented at the 3rd International AIDS Society Conference on HIV Pathogenesis and Treatment, Rio de Janeiro, Brazil, 2005, abstract TuPe1.1C16.
33. Hughes W, McDowell JA, Shenep J, et al. Safety and single-dose pharmacokinetics of abacavir (1592U89) in human immunodeficiency virus type 1-infected children. Antimicrob Agents Chemother 43:609, 1999.
34. Shikuma C, Yang Y, Meyer W, et al. Metabolic analyses with A5095: effect of efavirenz against an all-nucleoside/nucleotide background. Presented at the 13th Conference on Retroviruses and Opportunistic Infections, Denver, CO, 2006, abstract 130.
35. Shlay JC, Visnegarwala F, Bartsch G, et al. Body composition and metabolic changes in antiretroviral-naive patients randomized to didanosine and stavudine vs. abacavir and lamivudine. J Acquir Immune Defic Syndr 38:147, 2005.
36. Moyle GJ, Sabin C, Cartledge J, et al. Lipid changes in a randomized, 48-weeks, open label comparative study of tenofovir DF vs. abacavir as substitutes for a thymidine analog in persons with lipoatrophy: the RAVE study. Presented at the 45th Interscience Conference on Antimicrobial Agents and Chemotherapy, Washington, DC, 2005, H-340.
37. Fisac C, Fumero E, Crespo M, et al. Metabolic benefits 24 months after replacing a protease inhibitor with abacavir, efavirenz or nevirapine. AIDS 19:917, 2005.
38. Moyle GJ, Baldwin C, Langroudi B, et al. A 48-week, randomized, open-label comparison of three abacavir-based substitution approaches in the management of dyslipidemia and peripheral lipoatrophy. J Acquir Immune Defic Syndr 33:22, 2003.
39. Hetherington S, Steel H, Naderer O. Hypersensitivity reactions during therapy with abacavir: clinical presentation and risk factors. Presented at 7th Conference on Retroviruses and Opportunistic Infections, San Francisco, 2000, abstract 60.
40. Cutrell A, Edwards A, Steel H, et al. Risk factor analysis for hypersensitivity reactions to abacavir introduction. Presented at the 1st International AIDS Society Conference on HIV Pathogenesis and Treatment, Buenos Aires, 2001, abstract 527.
41. Hetherington S, Hughes A, Mosteller M, et al. HLA-B57 and TNF-alpha variants associated with hypersensitivity reactions to abacavir among HIV-1-positive subjects. Presented at the 9th Conference on Retroviruses and Opportunistic Infections, Seattle, WA, 2002, abstract 92.
42. Mallal S, Nolan D, Witt C, et al. Association between presence of HLA-B*5701, HLA-DR7, and HLA-DQ3 and hypersensitivity to HIV-1 reverse-transcriptase inhibitor abacavir. Lancet 359:727, 2002.
43. Bowonwatanuwong C, Warren L, Mosteller M, et al. Association of HLA-B*5701 and hypersensitivity to abacavir in a sample of Thai patients. Presented at the 7th International Workshop on Adverse Drug Reactions and Lipodystrophy in HIV, Dublin, Ireland, 2005, abstract 103.
44. Mosteller M, Hughes A, Warren L, et al. Pharmacogenetic (PG) investigation of hypersensitivity to abacavir. Presented at the 16th International AIDS Conference, Toronto, ON, Canada, 2006, abstract WEPE0171.
45. Brothers C, Wannamaker P, Sutherland-Phillips D, et al. Lower reported rate of suspected hypersensitivity reactions (HSR) to abacavir (ABC) among Black patients. Presented at the 46th Interscience Conference on Antimicrobial Agents and Chemotherapy, San Francisco, CA, 2006, abstract H-1065.
46. Phillips EJ, Sullivan JR, Knowles SR, et al. Utility of patch testing in patients with hypersensitivity syndromes associated with abacavir. AIDS 15:2223, 2002.
47. Phillips EJ, Wong GA, Kaul R, et al. Clinical and immunogenetic correlates of abacavir hypersensitivity. AIDS 19:979, 2005.
48. Hetherington S. Understanding drug hypersensitivity: what to look for when prescribing abacavir. AIDS Reader 11:620, 2001.
49. Letter to clinicians regarding abacavir hypersensitivity syndrome. Research Triangle Park, NC, Glaxo Wellcome, 30 Oct 1997.
50. Hetherington S, Steel H, Lafon S, et al. Safety and tolerance of abacavir (1592, ABC) alone and in combination therapy for HIV-1 infection. Presented at the 12th World AIDS Conference, Geneva, 1998, abstract 12353.
51. Frissen P, de Vries J, Weigel H, et al. Severe anaphylactic hock after rechallenge with abacavir without preceding hypersensitivity. AIDS 15:289, 2001.
52. Escaut L, Lioter JY, Albengres E, et al. Abacavir rechallenge has to be avoided in case of hypersensitivity reaction. AIDS 13:1419, 1999.
53. Hernandez J, Cutrell A, Bonny T, et al. Diagnosis of abacavir hypersensitivity reactions among patients not receiving abacavir in two blinded studies. Presented at the 5th International Workshop on Adverse Drug Reactions and Lipodystrophy in HIV, Paris, France, 2003, abstract 134.
54. Keiser P, Andrews C, Yazdani B, et al. Comparison of symptoms of influenza A with abacavir-associated hypersensitivity reaction. Presented at the 8th Conference on Retroviruses and Opportunistic Infections, Chicago, IL, 2001, abstract 622.
55. Thompson M, Shaefer MS, Williams V, et al. Interruptions in abacavir dosing are not associated with increased risk of

hypersensitivity in the HEART (NZT4006) study. Presented at the 40th Interscience Conference on Antimicrobial Agents and Chemotherapy, Toronto, ON, Canada, 2000, abstract LB-14.
56. Loeliger AE, Steel H, McGuirk S, et al. The abacavir hypersensitivity reaction and interruptions in therapy. AIDS 15:1325, 2001.
57. Saag MS, Sonnerborg A, Torres RA, et al. Antiretroviral effect and safety of abacavir alone and in combination with zidovudine in HIV-infected adults. AIDS 12:F203, 1998.
58. McDowell JA, Symonds WT, LaFon SW; 1592U89 Clinical Trial Group. Single-dose and steady-state pharmacokinetics of escalating regimens of 1592U89 with and without zidovudine. Presented at the XIth International Conference on AIDS, Vancouver, BC, Canada, 1996, Mo.B.1140.
59. Staszewski S, Katlama C, Harrer T, et al. A dose-ranging study to evaluate the safety and efficacy of abacavir alone or in combination with zidovudine and lamivudine in antiretroviral treatment-naive subjects. AIDS 12:F197, 1998.
60. Staszewski S, Katlama C, Harrer T, et al. Abacavir (ABC, 1592) in protocol CNAB 2002 provides effective, long-term, 72 week, ART for patients on triple therapy regimens. Presented at the 12th World AIDS Conference, Geneva, Switzerland, 1998, abstract 12212.
61. Fischl M, Greenberg S, Clumeck N, et al. Safety and activity of abacavir (ABC, 1592) with 3TC/ZDV in antiretroviral naive subjects. Presented at the 12th World AIDS Conference, Geneva, Switzerland, 1998, abstract 12230.
62. Matheron S, Brun-Vezinet F, Katlama C, et al. 48-week results of the CNAF3007/Ecureuil open label study: efficacy and safety of the triple nucleoside combination abacavir/combivir versus nelfinavir/combivir as first line antiretroviral therapy in HIV-infected adults. Presented at the 5th International Congress on Drug Therapy in HIV Infection, Glasgow, Scotland, 2000, abstract 15.
63. Matheron S, Livrozet JM, Boue F, et al. Long-term safety and efficacy of two antiretroviral therapies: combivir and abacavir versus combivir and nelfinavir – ECUREUIL 2 (CNAF3021). Presented at the 2nd IAS Conference on HIV Pathogenesis and Treatment, Paris, France, 2003, abstract 556.
64. Vibhagool A; Can 3015 International Study Team. Abacavir/combivir (ABC/COM) is comparable to indinavir/combivir (IDV/COM) in HIV-1-infected antiretroviral therapy naive adults: results of a 48 week open-label study (CNA3014). Presented at the 1st International AIDS Society Conference on HIV Pathogenesis and Treatment, Buenos Aires, Argentina, 2001, abstract 063.
65. Eron J, Yeni P, Gathe J, et al. The KLEAN study of fosamprenavir-ritonavir versus lopinavir-ritonavir, each in combination with abacavir-lamivudine, for initial treatment of HIV infection over 48 weeks: a randomised non-inferiority trial. Lancet 368:476, 2006.
66. Munderi P, and The DART Trial Team. Safety of nevirapine compared to abacavir on a background of zidovudine/lamivudine as first-line antiretroviral therapy: a randomized double-blind trial. Presented at the 13th Conference on Retroviruses and Opportunistic Infections, Denver, CO, 2006, abstract 109LB.
67. DeJesus E, Herrera G, Teofilo E, et al. Abacavir versus zidovudine combined with lamivudine and efavirenz, for the treatment of antiretroviral-naive HIV-infected adults. Clinical Infect Dis 39:1038, 2004.
68. Gulick RM, Ribaudo HJ, Shikuma CM, et al. Triple-nucleoside regimens versus efavirenz-containing regimens for the initial treatment of HIV-1 infection. N Engl J Med 350:1850, 2004.
69. Gulick RM, Ribaudo HJ, Shikuma CM, et al. Three- vs four-drug antiretroviral regimens for the initial treatment of HIV-1 infection. A randomized controlled trial. JAMA 296:769, 2006.
70. Gallant JE, Rodriguez AE, Weinberg WG, et al. Early virologic nonresponse to tenofovir, abacavir, and lamivudine in HIV-infected antiretroviral-naive subjects. J Infect Dis 192:1921, 2005.
71. Cohen C, Elion R, DeJesus E, et al. Week 48 analysis of once-daily (QD) trizivir (T2V) and tenofovir DF (TDF) in antiretroviral naive subjects (COL40263). Presented at the 45th Interscience Conference on Antimicrobial Agents and Chemotherapy, Washington, DC, 2005, abstract H-521.
72. Markowitz M, Hill-Zabala, Lang J, et al. Induction with abacavir/lamivudine/zidovudine plus efavirenz for 48 weeks followed by 48-week maintenance with abacavir/lamivudine/zidovudine alone in antiretroviral-naive HIV-1-infected patients. J Acquir Immune Defic Syndr 39:257, 2005.
73. Funk ML, White AD, Cutrell A, et al. Life expectancy of patients with advanced HIV/AIDS enrolled in the abacavir expanded access program. Presented at the 40th Interscience Conference on Antimicrobial Agents and Chemotherapy (ICAAC), Toronto, ON, Canada, 2000, abstract 2042.
74. Katlama C, Clotet B, Plettenberg A, et al. The role of abacavir (ABC, 1592) in antiretroviral therapy-experienced patients: results from a randomized, double-blind trial. AIDS 14:781, 2000.
75. Khanna N, Klimkait T, Schiffer V, et al. Salvage therapy with abacavir plus a non-nucleoside reverse transcriptase inhibitor and a protease inhibitor in heavily pre-treated HIV-1 infected patients. AIDS 14:791, 2000.
76. Henry K, Wallace RJ, Bellman PC, et al. Twice-daily triple nucleoside intensification treatment with lamivudine-zidovudine plus abacavir sustains suppression of human immunodeficiency virus type 1: results of the TARGET study. J Infect Dis 183:571, 2001.
77. Katlama C, Clumeck N, Fenske S, et al. Use of Trizivir™ (abacavir, lamivudine, zidovudine) to simplify therapy in HAART-experienced subjects with long-term suppression of HIV-RNA: TRIZAL study (AZL30002) 24-week results. Presented at 8th Conference on Retroviruses and Opportunistic Infections, Chicago, IL, 2001, abstract 316.
78. Clumeck N, Goebel F, Rozenbaum W, et al. Simplification with abacavir-based triple nucleoside therapy versus continued protease inhibitor-based highly active antiretroviral therapy in HVI-1-infected patients with undetectable plasma HV-1 RNA. AIDS 15:1517, 2001.
79. Rodriguez AE, Hill-Zabala CE, Sloan LA, et al. Quadruple nucleoside/tide regimen of trizivir (TZV) + tenofovir (TDF) is effective following early virologic failure on an initial regimen containing a thymidine analog + lamivudine in combination with a protease inhibitor (PI) or non-nucleoside reverse transcriptase inhibitor (NNRTI)(ESS30005, ZIP). Presented at the 3rd IAS Conference on HIV Pathogenesis and Treatment, Rio de Janeiro, Brazil 2005, abstract WePE6.3c03.
80. Moyle GJ, DeJesus E, Cahn P, et al. Abacavir once or twice daily combined with once-daily lamivudine and efavirenz for the treatment of antiretroviral-naive HIV-infected adults. Results of the Ziagen once daily in antiretroviral combination study. J Acquir Immune Defic Syndr 38:417, 2005.
81. Brothers C, Cutrell A, Zhao H, et al. Once daily administration of abacavir is not a clinical risk factor for suspected hypersensitivity reactions in clinical trials and rash alone is not sufficient to diagnose the reaction. Presented at the 12th Conference on Retroviruses and Opportunistic Infections, Boston, MA, 2005, abstract 836.
82. Saez-Llorens X, Nelson RP, Emmanuel P, et al. A randomized, double-blind study of triple nucleoside therapy of abacavir, lamivudine, and zidovudine versus lamivudine and zidovudine in previously treated human immunodeficiency virus type 1-infected children: the CNAA3006 study team. Pediatrics 107: E4, 2001.
83. Gibb DM; PENTA 5 Executive Committee. A randomized trial evaluating three NRTI regimens with and without nelfinavir in

HIV-1 infected children: 48-week follow-up from the PENTA 5 trial. Presented at the 5th International Congress on Drug Therapy in HIV Infection, Glasgow, Scotland, 2000, abstract PL6.8.
84. Harrigan PR, Stone C, Griffin P, et al. Resistance profile of the human immunodeficiency virus type 1 reverse transcriptase inhibitor abacavir (1592U89) after monotherapy and combination therapy. J Infect Dis 181:912, 2000.
85. Miller V, Ait-Khaled M, Stone C, et al. HIV-1 reverse transcriptase (RT) genotype and susceptibility to RT inhibitors during abacavir monotherapy and combination therapy. AIDS 14:163, 2000.
86. Lanier ER, Stone C, Griffin P, et al. Phenotypic sensitivity to abacavir (1592, ABC) in the presence of multiple genotypic mutations: correlation with viral load response. Presented at the 5th Conference on Retroviruses and Opportunistic Infections, Chicago, IL, 1998, abstract 686.
87. Tisdale M, Najera I, Cousens D. Analysis of resistant variants isolated on passage with carbocyclic nucleoside analog 1592U89. J Acquir Immune Defic Hum Retrovirol 10(Suppl 3):S5, 1995.
88. Tisdale M, Alnadaf T, Cousens D. Combinations of mutations in HIV-1 reverse transcriptase required for resistance to carbocyclic nucleoside 1592U89. Antimicrob Agents Chemother 41:1094, 1997.
89. Lanier R, Danehower S, Daluge S, et al. Genotypic and phenotypic correlates of response to abacavir (ABC, 1592)(abstract 52). Antivir Ther 3(Suppl 1):36, 1998.
90. Lanier ER, Smiley ML, St Clair MH, et al. Phenotypic HIV resistance in vitro correlates with viral load response to abacavir (1592, ABC) in vivo. Presented at the 12th World AIDS Conference, Geneva, Switzerland, 1998, abstract 32289.
91. Mellors JW, Hertogs K, Peeters F, et al. Susceptibility profile (Antivirogram™) of 943 clinical HIV-1 isolates to abacavir (1592U89). Presented at the 5th Conference on Retroviruses and Opportunistic Infections, Chicago, IL, 1998, abstract 687.
92. Johnson VA, Brun-Vezinet F, Clotet B, et al. Update of the drug resistance mutations in HIV-1: Fall 2006. Top HIV Med 14:125, Aug/Sep 2006.
93. Lanier ER, Ait-Khaled M, Scott J, et al. Antiviral efficacy of abacavir in antiretroviral therapy-experienced adults harbouring HIV-1 with specific patterns of resistance to nucleoside reverse transcriptase inhibitors. Antivir Ther 9:37, 2004.
94. Rozenbaum W, Katlama C, Bentata M, et al. Intensification with abacavir (1592, ABC) reduced viral load in lamivudine/zidovudine pretreated subjects with the 184V mutation. Antivir Ther 3(Suppl 1):68, 1998.
95. Lanier ER, Hellman N, Scoot J, et al. Determination of a clinically relevant phenotypic resistance 'cutoff' for abacavir using the PhenoSense™ assay. Presented at the 8th Conference on Retroviruses and Opportunistic Infections, Chicago, IL, 2001, abstract 254.
96. Underwood M, St Clair M, Ross L, et al. Cross-resistance of clinical samples with K65R, L74V, and M184V mutations. Presented at the 12th Conference on Retroviruses and Opportunistic infections, Boston, MA, 2005, abstract 714.
97. Ross LL, Gerondelis P, Rouse EG, et al. Impact of HIV resistance mutations, drug resistance, and viral fitness on antiviral activity of tenofovir/abacavir/lamivudine in the ESS30009 study. Presented at the XIII International HIV Drug Resistance Workshop, Tenerife Sur – Costa Adeje, Canary Islands, Spain, 2004, abstract 159.
98. Rouse E, Gerondelis P, Paulsen D, et al. Clonal analysis of week 12 virologic non-responders receiving tenofovir/abacavir/lamivudine in ESS30009. Presented at 12th Conference on Retroviruses and Opportunistic Infections, Boston, MA, 2005, abstract 720.
99. Ross L, Gerondelis P, Liao Q, et al. Selection of the HIV-1 reverse transcriptase mutation K70E in antiretroviral-naive subjects treated with tenofovir/abacavir/lamivudine therapy. Presented at the XIV International HIV Drug Resistance Workshop, Quebec City, QC, Canada, 2005, abstract 92.
100. Lloyd R, Huong J, Rouse E, et al. HIV-1 RT mutations K70E and K65R are not present on the same viral genome when both mutations are detected in plasma. Presented at the 45th Interscience Conference on Antimicrobial Agents and Chemotherapy, Washington, DC, 2005, abstract H-1066.
101. Elion R, Ha B, DeJesus E, et al. Selection of HIV reverse transcriptase (RT) thymidine analogue mutations (TAMS) rather than K65R is the preferred route of resistance seen in patients with virologic failure on once-daily (QD) trizivir (TZV) and tenofovir (TDF). Presented at the 45th Interscience Conference on Antimicrobial Agents and Chemotherapy, Washington, DC, 2005, abstract H-1068.
102. Rouse E, Preble L, Elion R, et al. Comparison of clonal genotyping (CG) and population genotyping (PG) of HIV reverse transcriptase (RT) at baseline (BL) and virologic failure (VF) in patients on once-daily trizivir and tenofovir for ≤48 weeks. Presented at the 46th Interscience Conference on Antimicrobial Agents and Chemotherapy, San Francisco, CA, 2006, abstract H-1005.
103. Descamps D, Delarue S, Ait-Khaled M, et al. Rare selection of K65R mutation in naive subjects failing a first-line abacavir/lamivudine HAART containing regimen. Presented at the XIV International HIV Drug Resistance Workshop, Quebec City, QC, 2005, abstract 15.
104. Moffatt A, Gerondelis P, Stone C, et al. Population and clonal sequence analyses in HIV-1+ subjects treated with abacavir(ABC)/lamivudine(3TC)/efavirenz(EFV). Presented at the 45th Interscience Conference on Antimicrobial Agents and Chemotherapy, Washington, DC, 2005, abstract H-1067.
105. Svarovoskaia ES, Margot NA, Bae AS, et al. Allele-specific PCR shows low-level K65R in treatment-experienced patients with L74V in the absence of TAMS. Presented at XV International HIV Drug Resistance Workshop, Sitges, Spain, 2006, abstract 70.
106. Bartlett JA, Mole LA, Fusco JS, et al. Frequency of abacavir hypersensitivity reactions (HSR), rechallenge reactions, and HSR-attributable outcomes are similar with the use of ziagen or trizivir: final results from the trizivir epidemiology study. Presented at the 3rd IAS Conference on HIV Pathogenesis and Treatment, Rio de Janeiro, Brazil, 2005, abstract TuPe2.1B01.
107. Baker KL, Lou Y, Yuen G, et al. The bioequivalence and effect of food on a new once-a-day fixed-dose combination tablet of abacavir (ABC) and lamivudine (3TC). Presented at the 44th Interscience Conference on Antimicrobial Agents and Chemotherapy, Washington, DC, 2004, abstract A-458.
108. Sosa N, Hill-Zabala C, DeJesus E, et al. Abacavir and lamivudine fixed-dose combination tablet once daily compared with abacavir and lamivudine twice daily in HIV-infected patients over 48 weeks (ESS30008, SEAL). J Acquir Defic Syndr 40:422, 2005.
109. LaMarca A, Clumeck N, Plettenberg A, et al. Efficacy and safety of a once-daily fixed-dose combination of abacavir/lamivudine compared with abacavir twice daily and lamivudine once daily as separate entities in antiretroviral-experienced HIV-1-infected patients (CAL30001 study). J Acquir Immune Defic Syndr 41:598, 2006.
110. Kubota M, Cohen C, Scribner A, et al. Short-term safety and tolerability of ABC/3TC administered once-daily (QD) compared with the separate components administered twice-daily (BID): results from ESS101822 (ALOHA). Presented at the 46th Interscience Conference on Antimicrobial Agents and Chemotherapy, San Francisco, CA, 2006, abstract H-1904.

Chapter 12

Delavirdine

Lisa M. Demeter, MD, Richard C. Reichman, MD

STRUCTURE

Delavirdine (Rescriptor, previously U-90152) (Fig. 12-1) belongs to the bisheteroarylpiperazine (BHAP) class of non-nucleoside reverse transcriptase inhibitors (NNRTIs).[1–3]

MECHANISMS OF ACTION AND *IN VITRO* ACTIVITY

Delavirdine, like other NNRTIs, inhibits reverse transcriptase (RT) by binding to a hydrophobic pocket in the p66 subunit of HIV-1 RT near the catalytic site of the enzyme. The delavirdine molecule is larger than other NNRTIs, such as nevirapine and efavirenz. The average median inhibitory concentration of delavirdine against a panel of laboratory and clinical HIV-1 isolates was 0.066 μM (range <0.005 to 0.690 μM); it does not inhibit HIV-2.[2]

PHARMACOKINETICS

Delavirdine is rapidly absorbed after oral administration; its absorption is reduced by gastric hypoacidity.[4] The steady-state pharmacokinetics of delavirdine are nonlinear, leading to substantial prolongation of its apparent half-life with increasing delavirdine doses.[5,6] Delavirdine is bound extensively to plasma proteins, primarily albumin.[5,7] There is a relatively large intersubject variability in steady-state delavirdine levels.[6] The major metabolic pathway of delavirdine is *N*-dealkylation, which is mediated by cytochrome P450 3A (CYP3A). Delavirdine inhibits CYP3A activity, thereby inhibiting its own metabolism.[5] Delavirdine is excreted primarily as dealkyl delavirdine and pyridine-cleaved delavirdine in both urine and feces.[4]

DRUG INTERACTIONS

Delavirdine has important interactions with currently available protease inhibitors (PIs), which are metabolized primarily by CYP3A4 (Table 12-1). The PIs also inhibit CYP3A4 to different degrees, so these drugs have the potential to affect delavirdine metabolism. One potential advantage of delavirdine's interactions with PIs is that it may increase the levels of these drugs, allowing reduced dosing or increased regimen potency. However, such interactions can be difficult to predict, without detailed pharmacokinetic studies, and such studies have not been performed for all currently available PIs. Delavirdine significantly increased trough levels and area under the curve (AUC) of indinavir.[8–10] The recommended dose of indinavir when given in combination with delavirdine is therefore

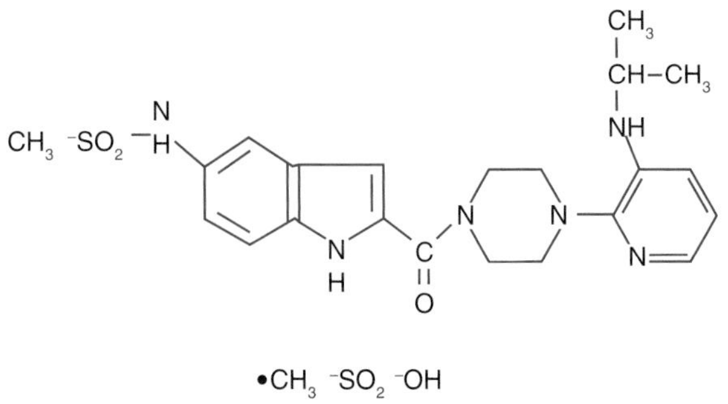

•CH_3–SO_2–OH

Figure 12-1 ■ Structure of delavirdine.

600 mg PO tid, instead of 800 mg PO tid. Delavirdine increased the trough concentration and AUC of ritonavir, nelfinavir, and amprenavir.[11–13] It is not known whether delavirdine has similar interactions with fos-amprenavir. Studies of delavirdine and saquinavir suggest that a twice-daily regimen, and a lower daily dose of saquinavir can be used.[4,14,15] The effects of delavirdine on the metabolism of the fixed dose of lopinavir/ritonavir have not been formally studied, although a small study of three HIV-1 infected patients found increases in lopinavir exposure after delavirdine addition, albeit with wide interpatient variability in the magnitude of these increases.[16]

Delavirdine also has important interactions with other drugs metabolized by cytochrome P450. Rifampin increased the oral clearance of delavirdine approximately 27-fold, leading to negligible concentrations of delavirdine in patients who received both drugs.[17] Co-administration of delavirdine and rifampin is therefore not recommended. Rifabutin increased oral clearance of delavirdine approximately fivefold, resulting in lower steady-state plasma delavirdine concentrations,[18] but delavirdine doses in excess of 600 mg tid were able to overcome this interaction.[19] Delavirdine inhibits rifabutin clearance and substantially increases rifabutin exposure.[19] Anticonvulsants such as phenobarbital, phenytoin, and carbamazepine induce CYP3A4 and therefore could potentially increase the metabolism of delavirdine. Limited unpublished data indicate that trough plasma delavirdine concentrations are reduced by concomitant administration of these agents.[4] Co-administration of delavirdine with these anticonvulsants is therefore not recommended.

A pharmacokinetic study of delavirdine and didanosine in nine HIV-infected individuals found that, under steady-state conditions, the AUCs of both drugs were reduced ~20% when the drugs were administered simultaneously rather than 1 h apart.[4,20] This effect is thought to be due to the buffering effect of the formulation of didanosine that was used, and it is not known if the same effect would be seen with nonbuffered preparations of didanosine (*see* Chapter 16).

Table 12-1 Important Drug Interactions with Delavirdine

Type of Interaction with Delavirdine
Inhibition of Delavirdine Absorption
Didanosine
Antacids
Acceleration of Delavirdine Metabolism
Carbamazepine
Phenobarbital
Phenytoin
Rifampin
Rifabutin
Inhibition of Metabolism by Delavirdine
Indinavir
Saquinavir
Nelfinavir
Lopinavir
Ritonavir
Amprenavir
Terfenadine
Astemizole
Clarithromycin
Dapsone
Rifabutin
Ergot derivatives
Alprazolam
Midazolam
Triazolam
Dihydropyridines (e.g., nifedipine)
Cisapride
Quinidine
Warfarin
Sildenafil

TOXICITY

The most frequent side effect of delavirdine is a maculopapular rash (Table 12-2). The rash characteristically occurs within 1–3 weeks after initiation of therapy and often resolves despite continuation of the drug.[21–23] The rash, which is uncommon after a month of therapy unless a prolonged interruption of treatment has intervened, is erythematous, maculopapular, and often pruritic, and involves the upper body and proximal arms, with decreasing intensity on the neck, face, trunk, and limbs.[24] It can be managed successfully in more than 90% of patients. Serious delavirdine-related skin rashes, such as erythema multiforme and Stevens–Johnson

Table 12-2 Toxicities Associated with Delavirdine

Toxicity	Frequency	Comments
Rash	18–36%	Rare after first month of therapy May be more common with higher delavirdine trough levels[21] Severe rash necessitating discontinuation of drug is uncommon (5–10%)
Hepatic enzyme elevations	Uncommon	4/30 Subjects receiving delavirdine + saquinavir had reversible increases in alanine transaminase and aspartate transaminase[8]
Neutropenia	Uncommon	Observed in 4/24 subjects receiving delavirdine + nelfinavir[12]

syndrome, are rare (~0.4%) and usually resolve after discontinuing the drug.

Occasionally, elevations of liver enzymes are seen in delavirdine recipients, most often in those who received other antiretroviral agents (Table 12-2). Significant but reversible elevations in alanine transaminase and aspartate transaminase occurred in four of 30 subjects during treatment with the combination of saquinavir and delavirdine.[8] Frank hepatitis has been rare. Neutropenia was observed in one small study of HIV-infected patients receiving nelfinavir and delavirdine, which resolved promptly after discontinuation of both drugs.[12] Another study demonstrated an increase in both cholesterol and high density lipoprotein (HDL) in patients receiving delavirdine plus two nucleosides, with more dramatic increases in cholesterol and HDL in patients receiving delavirdine in combination with a PI.[25]

EFFICACY IN CLINICAL TRIALS

The efficacy of delavirdine was evaluated initially in studies in which the drug was administered as monotherapy or in two- or three-drug combinations with zidovudine or didanosine (or both).[21,23,24,26,27] Early studies of delavirdine in combination with zidovudine or didanosine (or both) did not demonstrate consistent, clinically significant virologic benefit from inclusion of delavirdine in these regimens. Subsequent studies of the efficacy of delavirdine, when given in combination with zidovudine/lamivudine to subjects with limited nucleoside experience, or in combination with PIs as part of a salvage regimen for those with more extensive antiretroviral experience, have demonstrated that delavirdine can offer significant virologic and immunologic benefits.[28,29–33] However, none of the phase III studies has demonstrated a significant impact of delavirdine on clinical outcome (Table 12-3).

RESISTANCE OF HIV-1 TO DELAVIRDINE

In vitro passage of HIV-1 in the presence of delavirdine selects for a unique P236L mutation in RT.[34] Unlike the Y181C and K103N mutations, which confer cross-resistance to most NNRTIs, P236L sensitizes HIV-1 to nevirapine and efavirenz.[34] Mutations at codon 190, which confer resistance to nevirapine and efavirenz, cause hypersusceptibility to delavirdine.[35] In contrast to the *in vitro* studies, monotherapy with delavirdine in patients led to the rapid development of the K103N and Y181C mutants.[36] P236L occurred in fewer than 10% of patients studied. A potential explanation for the less frequent occurrence of P236L than K103N in clinical isolates is that P236L confers a substantial replication defect relative to virus with the K103N mutation.[37]

Combination therapy with various nucleoside analogs appears to influence the development of phenotypic and genotypic delavirdine resistance. The emergence of Y181C is prevented by concomitant zidovudine therapy, whereas didanosine does not appear to have this effect on Y181C.[38–40] This effect is presumably related to the fact that Y181C confers zidovudine hypersensitivity.[41] With the exception of the occasional isolate that develops the P236L mutation, it is expected that delavirdine-resistant isolates obtained from patients are also resistant to other NNRTIs such as nevirapine and efavirenz. Similarly, cross-resistance to delavirdine is frequent in isolates obtained from patients failing efavirenz or nevirapine-containing regimens. Although clinical isolates containing G190 mutations may be interpreted by resistance testing algorithms to be delavirdine sensitive, the clinical significance of this finding is uncertain.

RECOMMENDATIONS FOR USE

Indications for Use Against HIV-1 Infection

Delavirdine is approved for use in combination with other appropriate antiretroviral agents for the management of HIV-1 infection in adults when antiretroviral therapy is warranted. The drug was approved by the Food and Drug Administration (FDA) in April 1997 under the FDA's accelerated review policy that allows approval based on analysis of surrogate markers of response (e.g., changes in CD4+ T-lymphocyte counts and plasma HIV RNA concentrations) rather than clinical endpoints (e.g., disease progression or survival).

DOSING AND ADMINISTRATION

Delavirdine mesylate is available in 100 or 200 mg tablets; the recommended dose in adults is 400 mg orally tid.[22] The pharmacokinetics of delavirdine in adults older than 65 years of age have not been studied, and it is not known if dosage adjustments are necessary for this age group. Delavirdine may be taken without regard to meals. The pharmacokinetics of delavirdine in patients with hepatic or renal insufficiency have not been studied, and it is not known if dosage adjustment of this drug is necessary under these circumstances. Because it undergoes extensive hepatic metabolism, the manufacturer recommends that delavirdine be used with caution in patients with impaired hepatic function.[22] The manufacturer recommends that patients with achlorhydria take delavirdine with an acidic beverage such as cranberry or orange juice.[22] It is also recommended that delavirdine be taken at least 1 h before or after an antacid because of studies demonstrating effects of antacids on delavirdine absorption.[22]

Use of Delavirdine in Combination with Other Antiretroviral Agents

Because of the risk of developing resistance, delavirdine should be given in combination with at least two additional antiretroviral agents. Pharmacokinetic data suggest that delavirdine may increase the potency of regimens containing PIs, although more long-term data are needed on the efficacy and tolerability of such combination regimens. Patients treated with these combinations should be carefully monitored for

Table 12-3

Summary of Major Efficacy Trials Evaluating Delavirdine

Clinical Trial	Phase	Entry Criteria[a]	Prior Antiretroviral Experience	Delavirdine Dose	Treatment Arms	Outcome
Para et al[21] (ACTG 260)	I/II	CD4 200–500	<6 Months zidovudine experience; at least 50% naive	Dose chosen to achieve one of three DLV trough levels: 3–10 μM, 11–30 μM, or 31–50 μM	3–10 μM, 11–30 μM, or 31–50 μM DLV vs ZDV or ddI	Mean decline in plasma RNA at week 2 in DLV arms was 1.0 $\log_{10}$ (no significant difference among DLV arms) vs 0.67 $\log_{10}$ decline in nucleoside arm. Study stopped because RNA responses in DLV arms were not sustained beyond 8 weeks of therapy.
Friedland et al[24] (ACTG 261)	II	CD4 100–500	<6 Months nucleoside experience	400 mg tid	DLV + ZDV vs DLV + ddI vs DLV + ZDV + ddI	There was a trend in CD4 and plasma RNA responses favoring the triple therapy arm over the ZDV/ddI arm that did not achieve statistical significance. Responses in the DLV/ZDV and DLV/ddI arms were inferior to triple therapy and ZDV/ddI arms.
Freimuth et al[26] (M/0017)	II/III	CD4 <300	ZDV experience (average 1 year; <4 months of ddI)	400 mg tid	DLV/ddI vs ddI	Early RNA and CD4 response were greater in DLV/ddI arm, but these differences were not sustained. Study stopped by DSMB because of low likelihood that a significant difference in clinical outcome between the two arms would be detected.
Freimuth et al[27] (M/0021 Part I)	II/III	CD4 200–500	<6 Months	200 mg tid 300 mg tid 400 mg tid	ZDV vs ZDV/DLV (200 mg tid) vs ZDV/DLV (300 mg tid) vs ZDV/DLV (400 mg tid)	RNA and CD4 response superior in two higher DLV dose groups. Study stopped when data demonstrating inferiority of monotherapy became available.

Sargent et al[28] and Wathen et al[29] (M/0021 Part II)	II/III	CD4 200–500	<6 Months	400 mg tid	ZDV/3TC vs DLV/ZDV vs DLV/3TC/ZDV	Interim analysis showed greatest RNA and CD4 responses in the triple-therapy arm; 71% of triple-therapy arm had <400 copies/ml RNA at 24 weeks vs 29% in ZDV/3TC arm. Study closed by DSMB; final analysis pending.
Kuritzkes et al[30]	II	CD4 >200 HIV RNA > 500	3TC/ZDV, d4T, or ddI for >6 months	400 mg tid	ZDV/3TC/IDV (800 mg tid) vs ADV/DLV/IDV (600 mg tid)	73% of DLV and 58% of 3TC arms were suppressed to ≤200 copies/mL at 24 weeks (*P* = 0.29). 83% of DLV vs 48% of 3TC arms were suppressed at 48 weeks (*P* = 0.007).
Eron et al[31] (M/0074)	II	CD4 ≥ 50 HIV RNA >20 000	ZDV for <1 month; naive to 3TC, NNRTIs, PIs	400 mg tid	DLV/ZDV/IDV (600 mg tid DLV/3TC/IDV (600 mg tid) vs DLV//ZDV/3TC/ IDV (600 mg tid) vs ZDV/3TC/IDV (800 mg tid)	ITT: 43% vs 69% vs 44% vs 60%, at 48 weeks. On-treatment analyses showed 43% vs 97% vs 87.5% vs 82% were <400 copies/mL at 48 weeks.
Gulick et al[32] (ACTG 359)	II	Any CD4 HIV RNA 2000–200 000	IDV for >6 months	600 mg bid	SQV/RTV/DLV vs SQV/RTV/ADV vs SQV/RTV/ DLV/ADV vs SQV/NFV/DLV vs SQV/NFV/ADV vs SQV/NFV/ DLV/ADV	At 16 weeks, no significant differences between pooled RTV vs NFV groups (28% vs 33% with RNA <500, *P* = 0.50) or DLV vs DLV/ADV groups (40% vs 33%, *P* = 0.42). Pooled DLV groups had a greater response rate than ADV groups (40% vs 18%, *P* = 0.002).

ADV, adefovir; ddI, didanosine; DLV, delavirdine; DSMB, Data and Safety Monitoring Board; IDV, indinavir; ITT, intent-to-treat analysis; NFV, nelfinavir; NNRTIs, non-nucleoside reverse transcriptase inhibitors; PIs, protease inhibitors; SQV, saquinavir; 3TC, lamivudine; ZDV, zidovudine.

[a] CD4+ T-lymphocytes/μL, HIV RNA copies/ml.

signs of toxicity, and may benefit from monitoring plasma concentrations of delavirdine and the PI, since pharmacokinetic interactions can be unpredictable. Because of concerns about cross-resistance, patients who fail a regimen containing one NNRTI are unlikely to respond to a different NNRTI, and such a substitution is not generally recommended.

CONCLUSIONS

Delavirdine is an NNRTI with potent activity against HIV-1 *in vitro*. When studied in clinical trials alone or in combination with zidovudine or didanosine, delavirdine's efficacy has been limited. Use of delavirdine in combination with zidovudine and lamivudine may lead to greater plasma HIV RNA suppression, perhaps because of improved tolerability compared to delavirdine given in combination with zidovudine and didanosine. Because of the disappointing results from early delavirdine clinical trials and the relative paucity of data directly comparing the potency of delavirdine-containing regimens to currently used antiretroviral regimens, delavirdine is not recommended as first-line therapy. Even in treatment-experienced patients, delavirdine is rarely used because of its dosing frequency, cross-resistance to other NNRTIs, and the potential for unexpected pharmacokinetic interactions. Delavirdine has shown some promise when combined with PIs in regimens designed to take advantage of their pharmacokinetic interactions, although more data are needed before this use of the drug can be recommended.

REFERENCES

1. Romero DL, Busso M, Tan C-K, et al. Nonnucleoside reverse transcriptase inhibitors that potently and specifically block human immunodeficiency virus type 1 replication. Proc Natl Acad Sci USA 88:8806, 1991.
2. Dueweke TJ, Poppe SM, Romero DL, et al. U-90152, a potent inhibitor of human immunodeficiency virus type 1 replication. Antimicrob Agents Chemother 37:1127, 1993.
3. Dueweke TJ, Kezdy FJ, Waszak GA, et al. The binding of a novel bisheteroarylipiperazine mediates inhibition of human immunodeficiency virus type 1 reverse transcriptase. J Biol Chem 267:27, 1992.
4. Tran JQ, Gerber JG, Kerr BM. Delavirdine: clinical pharmacokinetics and drug interactions. Clin Pharmacokinet 40:207, 2001.
5. Cheng C-L, Smith DE, Carver PL, et al. Steady-state pharmacokinetics of delavirdine in HIV-positive patients: effect on erythromycin breath test. Clin Pharmacol Ther 61:531, 1997.
6. Smith PF, Dicenzo R, et al. Population pharmacokinetics of delavirdine and N-delavirdine in HIV-infected individuals. Clin Pharmacokinetics 44:99, 2005.
7. Chaput AJ, D'Ambrosio R, Morse GD. In vitro protein-binding characteristics of delavirdine and its N-dealkylated metabolite. Antiviral Res 32:81, 1996.
8. Cox SR, Ferry JJ, Batts DH, et al. Delavirdine and marketed protease inhibitors: pharmacokinetic interaction studies in healthy volunteers. In: Abstracts of the 4th Conference on Retroviruses and Opportunistic Infections, Washington, DC. Alexandria, VA: Westover Management Group; 1997, abstract 372.
9. Ferry JJ, Herman BD, Carel BJ, et al. Pharmacokinetic drug–drug interaction study of delavirdine and indinavir in healthy volunteers. J Acquir Immune Defic Syndr Hum Retrovirol 18:252, 1998.
10. Para M, Beal J, Rathburn C, et al. Potent activity with lower doses of indinavir using delavirdine in combination with zidovudine: 48 week analysis. Presented at the 39th Interscience Conference on Antimicrobial Agents and Chemotherapy, San Francisco, 1999, abstract 1985.
11. Morse GD, Shelton MJ, Hewitt RG, et al. Ritonavir pharmacokinetics during combination therapy with delavirdine. In: Abstracts of the 5th Conference on Retroviruses and Opportunistic Infections, Chicago. Alexandria, VA: Westover Management Group; 1998, abstract 343.
12. Cox SR, Schneck DW, Herman BD, et al. Delavirdine and nelfinavir: a pharmacokinetic drug–drug interaction study in healthy adult volunteers. In: Abstracts of the 5th Conference on Retroviruses and Opportunistic Infections, Chicago. Alexandria, VA: Westover Management Group; 1998, abstract 345.
13. Tran JQ, Petersen C, Garrett M, et al. Delavirdine significantly increases plasma concentrations of amprenavir in healthy volunteers. AIDS 14(Suppl 4):S92, 2000.
14. Cox SR, Batts DH, Stewart F, et al. Evaluation of the Pharmacokinetic interaction between saquinavir and delavirdine in healthy volunteers. Presented at the 4th Conference on Retroviruses and Opportunistic Infections, Washington, DC, 1997, abstract 381.
15. Cox S, Conway B, Freimuth W, et al. Pilot study of BID and TID combinations of saquinavir-SGC, delavirdine, zidvoudine, and lamivudine as initial therapy: pharmacokinetic interaction between saquinavir-SGC and delavirdine. Presented at the 7th Conference on Retroviruses and Opportunistic Infections, San Francisco, 2000, abstract 82.
16. Harris MC, Alexander C, et al. Delavirdine increases drug exposure of ritonavir-boosted protease inhibitors. AIDS 16:798, 2002.
17. Borin MT, Chambers JH, Carel BJ, et al. Pharmacokinetic study of the interaction between rifampin and delavirdine mesylate. Clin Pharmacol Ther 61:544, 1997.
18. Borin MT, Chambers JH, Carel BJ, et al. Pharmacokinetic study of the interaction between rifabutin and delavirdine mesylate in HIV-1 infected patients. Antiviral Res 35:53, 1997.
19. Cox SR, Herman BD, Batts DH, et al. Delavirdine and rifabutin: pharmacokinetic evaluation in HIV-1 patients with concentration-targeting of delavirdine. In: Abstracts of the 5th Conference on Retroviruses and Opportunistic Infections, Chicago. Alexandria, VA: Westover Management Group; 1998, abstract 344.
20. Morse GD, Fischl MA, Shelton MJ, et al. Single dose pharmacokinetics of delavirdine mesylate and didanosine in patients with human immunodeficiency virus infection. Antimicrob Agents Chemother 41:169, 1997.
21. Para MF, Meehan P, Holden-Wiltse J, et al. ACTG 260: a randomized, phase I/II, dose-ranging, trial of the anti-HIV activity of delavirdine monotherapy. Antimicrob Agents Chemother 43:1373, 1999.
22. Rescriptor package insert. La Jolla, CA: Agouron Pharmaceuticals; 2001.
23. Davey RT, Chaitt DG, Reed GF, et al. Randomized, controlled phase I/II trial of combination therapy with delavirdine (U-90152S) and conventional nucleosides in human immunodeficiency virus type 1-infected patients. Antimicrob Agents Chemother 40:1657, 1996.
24. Friedland GH, Pollard RB, Griffith B, et al. Efficacy and safety of delavirdine mesylate with zidovudine and didanosine compared with two-drug combinations of these agents in persons with CD4+ T lymphocyte counts of 100 to 500 cells/mm^3 (ACTG 261). J Acquir Immune Defic Syndr 21:281, 1999.
25. Roberts AD, Liappis AP, et al. Effect of delavirdine on plasma lipids and lipoproteins in patients receiving antiretroviral therapy. AIDS 16:1829, 2002.

26. Freimuth WW, Chuang-Stein CJ, Greenwald CA, et al. Delavirdine + didanosine combination therapy has sustained surrogate marker response in advanced HIV-1 population. In: Abstracts of the 3rd Conference on Retroviruses and Opportunistic Infections. Alexandria, VA: Westover Management Group; 1996, abstract LB8b.
27. Freimuth WW, Wathen LK, Cox SR, et al. Delavirdine in combination with zidovudine causes sustained antiviral and immunological effects in HIV-l infected individuals. In: Abstracts of the 3rd Conference on Retroviruses and Opportunistic Infections. Alexandria, VA: Westover Management Group; 1996, abstract LB8c.
28. Sargent S, Green S, Para M, et al. Sustained plasma viral burden reductions and CD4+ T lymphocyte increase in HIV-1 infected patients with Rescriptor (DLV) + Retrovir (ZDV) + Epivir (3TC). In: Abstracts of the 5th Conference on Retroviruses and Opportunistic Infections, Chicago. Alexandria, VA: Westover Management Group; 1998, abstract 699.
29. Wathen L, Freimuth W, Getchel L, et al. Use of HIV-1 RNA PCR in patients on Rescriptor (DLV) + Retrovir (ZDV) + Epivir (3TC), ZDV + 3TC, or DLV + ZDV allowed early differentiation between treatment arms. In: Abstracts of the 5th Conference on Retroviruses and Opportunistic Infections, Chicago. Alexandria, VA: Westover Management Group; 1998, abstract 694.
30. Kuritzkes DR, Bassett RL, Johnson VA, et al. Continued lamivudine versus delavirdine in combination with indinavir and zidovudine or stavudine in lamivudine-experienced patients: results of Adult AIDS Clinical Trials Group Protocol 370. AIDs 14:1553, 2000.
31. Eron J, McKinley G, LeCrerq P, et al. Potent antiviral activity using delavirdine and reduced-dose indinavir combination therapies: a 48 week analysis. Presented at the 7th Conference on Retroviruses and Opportunistic Infections, San Francisco, 2000, abstract 535.
32. Gulick RM, Hu J, Fiscus SA, et al. Randomized study of saquinavir with ritonavir or nelfinavir together with delavirdine, adefovir, or both in HIV-infected adults with virologic failure on indinavir: ACTG study 359. J Infect Dis 182:1375, 2000.
33. Gulick RM, Hu XJ, et al. Durability of response to treatment among antiretroviral-experienced subjects: 48-week results from AIDS Clinical Trials Group Protocol 359. J Infect Dis 186:626, 2002.
34. Dueweke TJ, Pushkarskaya T, Poppe SM, et al. A mutation in reverse transcriptase of bis(heteroaryl)piperazine-resistant human immunodeficiency virus type 1 that confers increased sensitivity to other nonnucleoside inhibitors. Proc Natl Acad Sci USA 90:4713, 1993.
35. Huang W, Gamarnik A, Limoli K, et al. Amino acid substitutions at position 190 of HIV-1 reverse transcriptase increase susceptibility to delavirdine and impair virus replication. J Virol 77:1512, 2003.
36. Demeter L, Shafer R, Meehan P, et al. Delavirdine susceptibilities and associated reverse transcriptase mutations in human immunodeficiency virus type 1 isolates from patients in a phase I/II trial of delavirdine monotherapy (ACTG 260). Antimicrob Agents Chemother 44:794, 2000.
37. Gerondelis P, Archer RH, Palaniappan C, et al. The P236L delavirdine-resistant HIV-l mutant is replication defective and demonstrates alterations in both RNA 5′ end- and DNA 3′ end-directed RNase H activities. J Virol 73:5803, 1999.
38. Joly V, Moroni M, Concia E, et al. Delavirdine in combination with zidovudine in treatment of HIV-1 infected patients: evaluation of efficacy and emergence of viral resistance in a randomized, comparative, phase III trial. Antimicrob Agents Chemother 44:3155, 2000.
39. Demeter LM, Meehan PM, Morse G, et al. HIV-1 drug susceptibilities and reverse transcriptase mutations in patients receiving combination therapy with didanosine and delavirdine. J Acquir Immune Defic Syndr Hum Retrovirol 14:136, 1997.
40. Demeter L, Griffith B, Bosch R, et al. HIV-1 drug susceptibilities during therapy with delavirdine (DLV) + ZDV, DLV + ddI, or DLV + ZDV + ddI. In: Abstracts of the 5th Conference on Retroviruses and Opportunistic Infections, Chicago. Alexandria, VA: Westover Management Group; 1998, abstract 706.
41. Larder BA. 3′-Azido-3′-deoxythymidine resistance suppressed by a mutation conferring human immunodeficiency virus type 1 resistance to nonnucleoside reverse transcriptase inhibitors. Antimicrob Agents Chemother 36:2664, 1992.

Chapter 13

Nevirapine

**Marianne Harris, MD, CCFP, Carlos Zala, MD,
Robert Hogg, PhD, Julio S. G. Montaner, MD**

Nevirapine (NVP) is a non-nucleoside reverse transcriptase inhibitor (NNRTI) of HIV-1. It inhibits HIV-1 replication by binding directly to reverse transcriptase (RT) in a pocket adjacent to the catalytic site of the enzyme.[1] Once NVP has bound to RT, it causes a conformational change that inactivates the enzyme, thereby preventing the polymerization of viral RNA to DNA. NVP is highly specific for HIV-1 RT and does not interfere with human DNA polymerases. NVP freely enters the cell and is active in many different cell lines, including T-lymphocytes and macrophages, well-known targets of HIV; this is in contrast to the nucleoside analogs (NRTIs), which have variable activity in different cell lines.[2,3] Unlike the NRTIs, NVP does not need to be phosphorylated intracellularly to become active; as a result, drug exposure is very consistent within and between cell lines. NVP can also bind to extracellular virion RT in the plasma. This means that the amount of cell-free viral RT is decreased, leading to a reduction in the infectivity.[4] NVP is a potent inhibitor of HIV-1, with a 90% inhibitory concentration (IC_{90}) of 60 nM.[5] The 90% inhibitory quotient for NVP (the concentration of free unbound drug in plasma relative to the IC_{90}) at trough is 113. NVP resistant HIV-1 is usually resistant to the other licensed NNRTIs (efavirenz (EFV) and delavirdine). Similarly to other NNRTIs, NVP is not active against HIV-2 isolates. NVP has no cross-resistance with any of the protease inhibitors (PIs) or NRTIs, including multinucleoside-resistant strains. NVP is available both as a tablet (200 mg) and as an oral suspension (10 mg/mL).

HUMAN PHARMACOKINETICS

Distribution

NVP is lipophilic and is nonionized at physiologic pH. Following intravenous administration to healthy adults, the apparent volume of distribution (V_{dss}) of NVP was 1.21 ± 0.09 L/kg, suggesting that NVP is readily distributed in humans. A review by Pacifici showed that neonates have a greater volume of NVP distribution in comparison with adults.[6] The $t_{1/2}$ rates were comparable for the neonate and adult, but the t_{max} of 14.8 ± 8.9 h for neonates was substantially lower than 2–4 h for adults, suggesting a lower absorption rate in neonates.[7] NVP readily crosses the placenta and is found in breast milk, and NVP has been detected in semen.[7–10] NVP is ~60% bound to plasma proteins in the plasma concentration range of 1–10 μg/mL. In contrast, intracellular NVP does not correlate with protein binding; concentrations are relatively low and remain constant over a 0–12 h interval.[11] This lower concentration of NVP in cells can be monitored by a higher P-glycoprotein expression. Moreover, penetration of NVP into the central nervous system has been extensively documented in experimental models and in animal models. NVP concentration in human cerebrospinal fluid (CSF) is 45% (±5%) of that in plasma; this ratio is approximately equal to the fraction not bound to plasma protein.[12] However, it is unknown to what extent CSF drug levels correlate to brain tissue drug levels.[13] Reduced CSF viral load has been demonstrated in patients taking NVP based regimens.[12]

Plasma Pharmacokinetics

NVP is readily absorbed (>90%) after oral administration in healthy volunteers and in HIV-1-infected adults. Absolute bioavailability in 12 healthy adults following single dose administration was >90%, whether administered as a tablet or in oral solution.[14,15] Pooled data from several studies indicate that peak plasma concentrations of 2 ± 0.4 mg/mL (7.5 mM) were reached within 4 h following a single 200 mg oral dose of NVP.[16] Following multiple doses, NVP peak concentrations appear to increase linearly in the dose range of 200–400 mg/day.[17–19] Steady-state trough NVP concentrations of 4.5 ± 1.9 mg/mL (or 17 ± 7 mM) were attained at 400 mg/day. These parameters were not altered substantially whether the drug was given with or without food or with alkaline buffers (such as antacids).[18]

It is currently recommended that NVP be administered twice a day; however, because of its long half-life at steady state (25–30 h), once-daily dosing is frequently used in clinical practice. An open-label, randomized, crossover study by van Heeswijk et al demonstrated that there was no significant difference in overall exposure to NVP (AUC) when dosed as 400 mg once daily versus 200 mg twice daily.[19] The trough level of NVP when dosed qd was ~25% lower than if dosed bid; this was still substantially above the IC_{50}. The SCAN study found that once-daily NVP was as effective and well tolerated as twice-daily NVP in patients in the early stages of HIV infection.[20] Similarly, the Atlantic study showed that a triple drug combination including two nucleosides (didanosine (ddI) and stavudine) plus NVP dosed qd, had a similar antiviral and CD4+ effect to a triple combination regimen including the same two nucleosides and a protease inhibitor (indinavir).[23]

Metabolism/Elimination

NVP is extensively metabolized via cytochrome P450 (CYP450) to several hydroxylated metabolites *in vivo* and in vitro. *In vitro* studies with human liver microsomes suggest that oxidative metabolism of NVP is mediated primarily by CYP450 isozymes from the CYP3A family, although other isozymes may also play a secondary role. CYP450 metabolism, glucuronide conjugation, and urinary excretion of glucuronidated metabolites represent the primary routes of NVP metabolism and elimination in humans.[16,17,21]

NVP has also been shown to be an inducer of CYP450 metabolic enzymes. As a result, the apparent oral clearance of NVP increases by approximately 1.5-fold to twofold from 2 to 4 weeks of dosing. Autoinduction also results in a corresponding change in the terminal-phase half-life of NVP in plasma from ~45 h (single dose) to ~25–30 h following multiple dosing.[17,21] The pharmacokinetics of NVP in patients with renal impairment is unchanged. During renal dialysis NVP is cleared from the body and repeated dosing of NVP after dialysis should be considered; patients with moderate or severe hepatic impairment (Child–Pugh score >8 ascites) are at risk of accumulating NVP, and more importantly, NVP induced liver toxicity. It is not recommended to use NVP in this setting. If NVP needs to be used in this setting, a decreased dose should be considered.[22]

A study by Hong-Brown et al has also demonstrated a decrease in protein synthesis in myocytes due to the presence of NVP in these cells. This decrease in protein synthesis is correlated with a decrease in phosphorylation levels of translation initiating proteins.[26]

Gender/Race/Age

No substantial gender or race differences have been reported in NVP pharmacokinetics across several clinical trials. In one Phase I study involving healthy volunteers (15 women, 15 men), the weight-adjusted V_{dss} of NVP was higher in women (1.54 L/kg) than in men (1.38 L/kg), suggesting that NVP was distributed more extensively in women. However, this difference was offset by a slightly shorter terminal-phase half-life in women, resulting in no significant gender difference in NVP oral clearance or plasma concentrations following either single- or multiple-dose administrations.[17] In adults, NVP pharmacokinetics do not change substantially with age (range 18–68 years). The apparent clearance rate of NVP in children reaches a maximum by the age of 1–2 years, and subsequently decreases over time. As a result, the recommended dose for children 2 months to 8 years of age is 4 mg/kg once daily for the first 14 days followed by 7 mg/kg twice daily thereafter, compared with 4 mg/kg once daily for the first 14 days followed by 4 mg/kg twice daily in children 8 years of age and older.

Human Dose-Ranging Studies

Daily doses of 12.5, 50, 200, and 400 mg were studied in adult patients with CD4+ T-lymphocyte counts <400 cells/mm^3. Dose-proportional effects were found, with the 400 mg/day dose being superior in terms of magnitude and duration of effect.[17,21] In a separate study, daily doses of 600 mg were associated with increased toxicity and no substantial gain in antiretroviral activity. The main dose-limiting toxicity observed was rash. In addition, some liver enzyme elevations and occasional somnolence were described. As a result, a dose of 400 mg daily was selected for clinical development.

TOXICITY

The most frequent drug-related adverse events reported as possibly related to NVP treatment in clinical trials include rash, fever, fatigue, headache, somnolence, nausea, liver enzyme elevations and chemical hepatitis. Rash is the most prevalent adverse event that has been attributed to NVP therapy. In four controlled, combination therapy trials with NVP, the overall incidence of rash, regardless of causal association assigned by the investigator, was 35% in the NVP group and 19% in the control group. The difference was statistically significant, for a 16% overall incidence of rash attributable to NVP.[24,25,28,29] Rashes with NVP are generally mild and self-limited, and the risk of rash is greatest within the first 6 weeks of therapy. Among NVP-treated patients in four controlled clinical trials, a total of 6.5% experienced grade 3 or 4 rash as their most severe rash event, compared to 1.3% in the controls.[27] Only 7% of patients in the NVP group discontinued because of rash, compared to 1% in the control groups, and most of them experienced a grade 3 or 4 rash. Based on 2861 NVP-treated patients in various clinical trials, nine patients were confirmed to have Stevens–Johnson syndrome (SJS), including two reported to have SJS/toxic epidermal necrolysis (TEN). This represents an overall SJS incidence of 0.3%. Although fatal cases have been reported in postmarketing surveillance, most

Guidelines for the Management of Rash

Table 13-1

Rash Description	Action with Nevirapine
Mild/moderate rash (may include pruritus)	Can continue dosing without interruption
Erythema	If rash or other suspected nevirapine toxicity occurs during lead-in, the dose should not be escalated until the rash resolves
Diffuse erythematous macular or maculopapular cutaneous eruption	If nevirapine is interrupted for >7 days, reintroduce with 200 mg/day lead-in
Urticaria	As above; however, if nevirapine is interrupted, do not reintroduce
Any rash with associated constitutional findings such as fever >39°C, myalgia/arthralgia, blistering, facial edema, oral lesions, general malaise, conjunctivitis, severely increased, liver function tests	Permanent discontinuation; no reintroduction
Severe rash	Immediate discontinuation; no reintroduction
Extensive erythematous or maculopapular rash or moist desquamation	
Angioedema	
Serum sickness-like reactions	
Stevens–Johnson syndrome	
Toxic epidermal necrolysis	

From Pollard RB, Robinson P, Dransfield K. Safety profile of nevirapine, a nonnucleoside reverse transcriptase inhibitor for the treatment of human immunodeficiency virus infection. Clin Ther 20:1071, 1998. Copyright Excerpta Medica, Inc.

cases are managed with supportive therapy, including fluid replacement and pain control. The incidence of rash in pediatric patients is no different from that in adults.[27]

To date, no factors have been identified that might predispose a patient to the development of rash. Also, the mechanism of NVP-induced rashes remains to be determined. Plasma concentrations of the drug do not correlate with the occurrence of rash, nor has a proven relationship been identified with gender, race, concomitant medications, rash history, or disease stage. The currently recommended NVP dosing regimen is 200 mg qd for 2 weeks, followed by 200 mg bid thereafter. This is based on retrospective analyses suggesting that this regimen is less frequently associated with rash. Nevertheless, patients need to be carefully warned about this potentially serious drug-related effect. In a NVP compassionate use program in the Netherlands, no rashes occurred in patients who had been pretreated with other antiretroviral agents and had plasma HIV-1 levels below the limit of detection.[30] Table 13-1 provides a set of empiric rash management guidelines developed with input from an expert panel. These guidelines provide appropriate direction for the continued use or discontinuation of NVP in the event that a patient experiences rash. A number of protocols for rash prevention, including the use of corticosteroids, antihistamines, and slower dose escalation, have been investigated. Corticosteroids do not appear to prevent NVP-related rash, and may even cause an increase in its incidence.[31,32,34] The roles of antihistamines or slower dose escalation for the prevention of NVP-related rash require further evaluation in prospective controlled trials. Whether corticosteroids or antihistamines may play a role in the treatment of NVP-related rash is also dependent on further investigations.[36]

Elevations of liver enzymes, including hepatitis, have also been reported in NVP-treated patients. Isolated gamma-glutamyl transpeptidase increases are relatively frequent; however, these are of no clinical consequence and have been attributed to liver enzyme autoinduction of NVP metabolism. Drug-induced hepatitis was reported in nine of 906 (1%) patients chronically treated with NVP in controlled clinical trials.[27] A similar result was obtained in the BI 1090 trial.[35] This was a randomized, placebo-controlled study comparing 1121 patients taking NVP plus two NRTIs with 1128 patients taking placebo plus two NRTIs over 2 years. Using an expanded hepatitis definition (including viral hepatitis), 2.8% of patients in the NVP group and 1.4% in the placebo group had hepatitis over the course of the study ($P = 0.026$). No significant difference in the incidence of serious hepatic events was observed between the two groups. The overall rate of withdrawal as a result of hepatitis in adult NVP trials has been 0.8%, but a limited number of fatal hepatitis cases associated with NVP use have been reported. Data which have aroused some concern have been reported from the blinded FTC-302 study,[37] a phase III study comparing the NRTIs emtricitabine and lamivudine, in which all patients also received stavudine and were stratified to receive either NVP or EFV, according to their baseline viral load. A total of 87% of the study subjects were black, and 59% were women. There was a high incidence of grade 3 and 4 hepatotoxicity, affecting 58 (15%) of 468 subjects, all of whom were receiving NVP, and two cases were fatal. The vast majority of cases occurred within the first 8 weeks of therapy, with a temporal association with the dose escalation of NVP from 200 to 400 mg at day 14 of treatment. A statistically significant twofold greater incidence of hepatotoxicity was noted in women. The gender-adjusted incidence of hepatotoxicity was ~11%, not dissimilar to that reported in the NVP package insert.[38] Thus current recommendations advise against initiating NVP in women with CD4+ T-lymphocyte counts >250 cells/mm^3 or men with CD4+ T-lymphocyte counts >400 cells/mm^3 to reduce the effect of adverse hepatic events.[39] Furthermore, hepatotoxicity increases with longer therapy duration and is associated with polymorphisms in the MDRI gene for the drug pump, P-glycoprotein.[40,41]

While further study is required to identify risk factors that predispose patients to develop hepatitis, it has been suggested that patients with hepatitis C co-infection may be at higher risk for developing clinical hepatitis when receiving NVP based therapy.[41,42] In turn, HBV and HCV co-infection are associated with a higher NVP trough concentration.[44] In a recent analysis of a clinical cohort (Athena study), covering ~70% of Dutch patients receiving HAART, independent risk factors associated with development of grade IV transaminase elevations were: higher baseline ALT levels (hazard ratio (HR) 1.06 per 10 units increase), chronic hepatitis B virus infection (HR 9.3), chronic hepatitis C virus infection (HR 5.2), recent start of NVP (HR 8.5) or ritonavir (HR 3.7), and female gender (HR 2.6). Furthermore, in patients chronically co-infected with hepatitis B virus, discontinuing the use of lamivudine (3TC) was associated with the development of grade 4 liver enzyme elevations (HR 4.8).[42]

To date, no previously unrecognized adverse events have been identified when using NVP in combination with different antiretrovirals, including NRTIs and PIs. Furthermore, the rate of known adverse events has not increased when NVP was used in combination with these agents. Importantly, untoward lipid abnormalities, including hyperlipidemia and lipodystrophy, have not been associated with NVP. Indeed, it has been suggested that lipid abnormalities at least partially revert following a switch from a PI to NVP.[46] In the Atlantic study, NVP-containing HAART resulted in an antiatherogenic lipid profile, with a striking increase in high-density lipoprotein (HDL) cholesterol (49%) and a significant reduction in the total over HDL cholesterol ratio (14%).[43] Recently several cases were reported where severe liver toxicity developed when NVP was given as part of a postexposure prophylaxis regimen. Although a number of potential confounders were noted in each case, it is at least likely that NVP may have contributed to the development of this serious toxicity. Until this issue is further clarified, NVP use in this setting is not recommended.[41,42,45]

CLINICAL TRIALS

Treatment-Naive Patients

The INCAS trial was among the first to illustrate that triple combination therapy was required to achieve a durable treatment response.[29] This study examined the activity, safety, and tolerance of three regimens (NVP + ZDV + ddI, NVP + ZDV, and ZDV + ddI) in 151 antiretroviral-naive HIV-1-infected patients with 200–600 CD4+ cells/mm^3. At baseline, mean plasma HIV RNA was 4.41 $\log_{10}$ copies/mL and mean CD4+ T-lymphocyte count was 374 cells/mm^3. The mean maximum viral load decrease from baseline for patients in the triple arm of the study was 2.94 $\log_{10}$ copies/mL. As shown in Figure 13-1, NVP + ZDV was associated with substantial but transient effects on virologic markers. However, NVP + ZDV + ddI was consistently superior to ZDV + ddI, providing a durable response in both virologic and immunologic markers, with 51% maintaining viral loads <20 copies/mL at 52 weeks. Raboud et al demonstrated that patients who achieve HIV-1 RNA levels <20 copies/mL were able to maintain their antiretroviral response.[47] Indeed, long-term follow-up of patients from the INCAS study demonstrated that viral suppression could be sustained with NVP-based triple-combination therapy for up to 4 years.[51] The INCAS study also

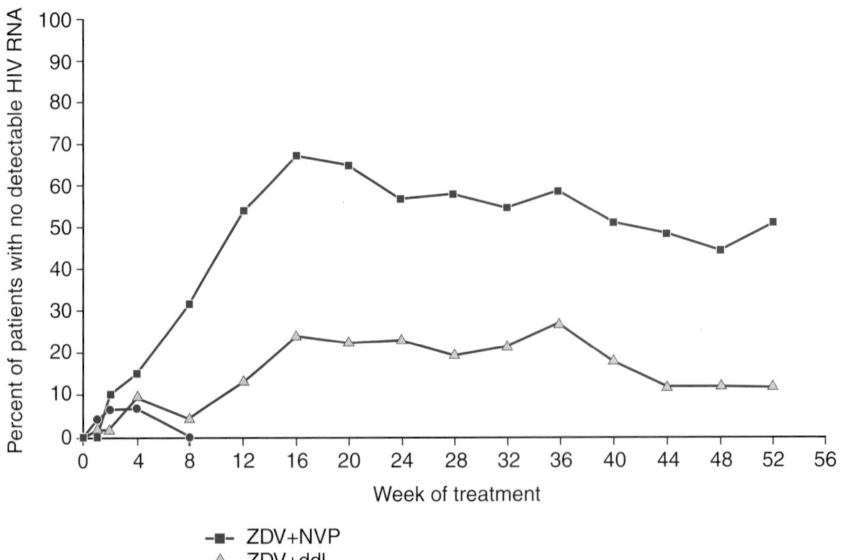

Figure 13-1 ■ INCAS: percent of patients below the limit of detection through 52 weeks of treatment (limit of detection = 20 copies/mL).

From Montaner JSG, Reiss P, Cooper D, et al (for the INCAS Study Group): A randomized, double-blind trial comparing combinations of nevirapine, didanosine, and zidovudine for HIV-infected patients. The INCAS trial. JAMA 279:930, 1998. Copyright 1998, American Medical Association.

demonstrated the need for high levels of adherence to the therapeutic regimen to achieve a sustained response. Adherence to the triple therapy regimen was associated with decreased recoverable virus and lessened the likelihood of developing resistance, whereas nonadherence was associated with virologic failure. Although the study was not designed to evaluate clinical events, fewer NVP + ZDV + ddI-treated patients (12%) had HIV progression events, compared with patients who took ZDV + ddI (25%) or NVP + ZDV (23%).[29]

The INCAS trial was the first to demonstrate the powerful potential of NVP. A cross-study evaluation, using an intent-to-treat analysis, showed that the results of the INCAS trial were consistent with those of similar triple combination regimens including PIs or the NNRTI, EFV. Two recent studies have further revealed the efficacy of NVP relative to PIs in comparative trials.[23,48] The Atlantic study, an international, multicenter, open-label, randomized trial, compared NVP + d4T + ddI with indinavir (IDV) + d4T + ddI and 3TC + d4T + ddI in antiretroviral-naive patients. This trial enrolled 298 patients with median baseline viral loads of 4.25 $\log_{10}$ copies/mL, and baseline CD4+ T-lymphocyte counts of 406 cells/mm^3. After 48 weeks, 58.4%, 57%, and 58.7% of patients in the NVP, IDV and 3TC-arms had <500 plasma HIV-1 RNA copies/mL in an intent-to-treat analysis (Not significant). After 96 weeks, these figures were 59.6%, 50.0% and 45.0%, respectively (Not significant). Looking at plasma HIV-1 RNA <50 copies/mL, figures (% undetectable) at 96 weeks in the intent-to-treat analysis were 81.8% for NVP, 79.0% for IDV and 50.9% for 3TC; the 3TC arm being inferior to the other arms (P = 0.001). The Atlantic trial showed comparable efficacy for a triple combination including NVP or a PI (IDV) (Fig. 13-2)

More recently, preliminary results from the COMBINE study have been presented. This open-label randomized study directly compared a simple twice-daily regimen of NVP + Combivir to twice-daily nelfinavir + Combivir.[48] The trial enrolled 142 HIV-infected, antiretroviral therapy-naive patients. The median baseline viral load was 59 698 copies/ml in the NVP + Combivir arm and 65 806 copies/mL in the nelfinavir + Combivir arm. The median baseline CD4+ T-lymphocyte count was also similar in the two arms, with 361 cells/mm^3 and 351 cells/mm^3 in the NVP- and nelfinavir-containing arms, respectively. After 9 months, there was no significant difference in outcome between the two arms, with 84% in the NVP + Combivir arm and 78% in the nelfinavir + Combivir arm having viral loads less than 200 copies/mL. The results remain consistent whether an on-treatment or intent-to-treat approach was used. However, using the more sensitive viral load assay with a limit of detection of 20 copies/mL, 80% of patients in the NVP arm had undetectable viral loads, significantly more than the 56% who achieved this level in the nelfinavir arm (P = 0.02). The difference between the NVP and nelfinavir arms may be explained in part, by greater adherence in the NVP arm. In summary, these two studies demonstrate that NVP-based triple-drug therapy is at least as effective as PI-based therapy in treatment-naive patients.

A substudy of the 1090 trial focused on the treatment response among treatment-naive patients with very high plasma viral load and very low baseline CD4+ T-lymphocyte count.[55] Patients were randomized to take NVP + ZDV + 3TC or placebo + ZDV + 3TC. 77 patients in the NVP + ZDV + 3TC arm had a mean baseline viral load of 138 986 copies/mL and a mean baseline CD4+ T-lymphocyte count of 101 cells/mm^3. There were 94 patients in the placebo arm, which had a mean baseline viral load of 146 332 copies/mL and a mean baseline CD4+ T-lymphocyte count of 93 cells/mm^3. Figure 13-3 demonstrates that, although response in the placebo arm of this study was very limited at 48 weeks in all viral load strata, NVP + ZDV + 3TC was as effective in patients with viral loads >500 000 copies/mL as in those with lower plasma viral load levels. Overall, 45% of patients in the NVP group had viral loads <50 copies/mL at 48 weeks using an intent-to-treat analysis, comparable to that observed

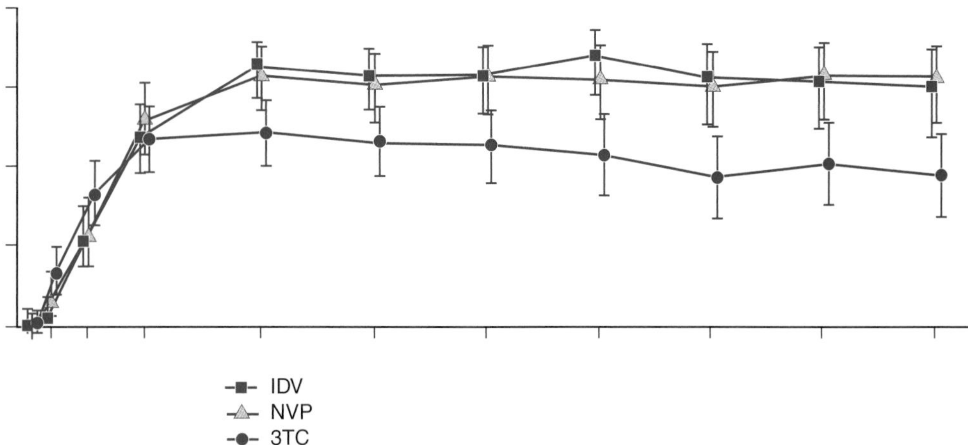

Figure 13-2 ■ Atlantic: percent of patients below limit of detection through 48 weeks of treatment (limit of detection = 50 copies/mL).

From van Leeuwen R, Katlama C, Murphy RL, et al. A randomized trial to study first-line combination therapy with or without protease inhibitor in HIV-1-infected patients. AIDS 17:987, 2003.

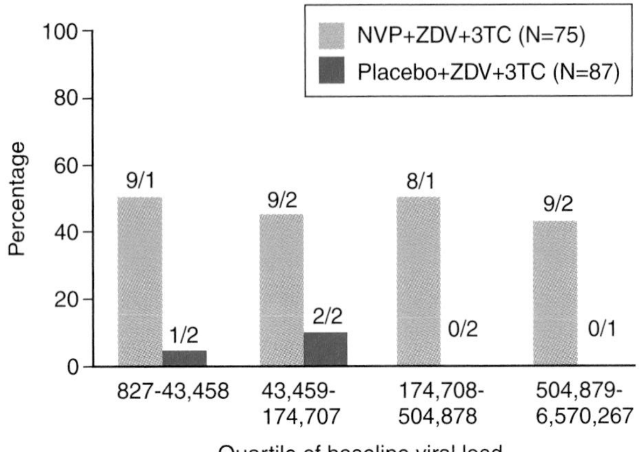

Figure 13-3 ■ BI 1090: percent of patients with sustained viral response through 48 weeks stratified by baseline viral load and CD4+ T-lymphocyte count (intent-to-treat analysis).

From Pollard R and the 1090 Team: Factors predictive of durable HIV suppression in a randomized double blind trial with nevirapine (NVP), zidovudine (ZDV) and lamivudine (3TC) in treatment-naive (ARV-n) patients with advanced AIDS. In: Abstracts of the 7th Conference on Retroviruses and Opportunistic Infections, San Francisco, 2000, abstract 517.

in the INCAS and Atlantic trials thereby confirming similar efficacy of NVP even in patients with advanced disease.[49] Of note, patients with very low CD4+ T-lymphocyte counts at baseline (<38 cells/mm^3) had a very poor response to therapy compared with those with higher CD4+ T-lymphocyte counts. Overall, these results suggest that in this particular group of patients (with very high baseline plasma viral load and very low baseline CD4+ T-lymphocyte count) the antiviral effect of the regimen was dependent on the baseline CD4+ count but independent of plasma viral load.

Additional analyses of a subset of patients within the INCAS trial indicate a statistically significant correlation between the cumulative antiviral responses achieved over 1 year and the HIV-1 RNA load in lymphoid tissue at 1 year.[56] These data, combined with similar results from a substudy of COMBINE,[50] and ATLANTIC[57] support the concept that a high level of suppression of viral replication with NVP-based therapy can lead to a sustained antiviral response in plasma and a decrease in HIV-1 RNA load in tissue reservoirs, similar to the findings reported for PI-containing regimens.

Switch Studies

There are a number of reasons why a patient successfully treated with a PI-based regimen might consider a switch to a PI-sparing regimen. Possible rationales for such a switch include an attempt to improve or arrest morphologic or metabolic changes associated with the lipodystrophy syndrome, or to improve adherence by reducing food restrictions, reducing the pill burden, or changing to a more convenient dosing schedule. Possible PI-sparing switch strategies currently tested include a switch to an NNRTI-containing regimen using EFV[53] or NVP,[54,58,59] or to a triple-NRTI regimen using abacavir.[60,61]

Negredo et al reported a randomized study of switching to NVP or EFV, or continuing with a PI-containing regimen, in 77 individuals whose HIV RNA has been suppressed below 50 copies/mL for at least 12 months (mean 29–31 months).[54] A total of 59% had clinically defined lipodystrophy as assessed by baseline DEXA scans and anthropometry. At baseline, 60% were receiving a stavudine-containing regimen (usually in combination with lamivudine), while 30% were receiving ZDV/3TC. After 24 weeks there were two cases of virologic rebound in the EFV group (n = 25) and one each in the NVP (n = 26) and PI groups (n = 26). Three patients in the EFV group stopped treatment due to neurologic toxicity. Five cases of acute hepatitis and two grade 3/4 rashes were reported in the NVP arm, one of which necessitated a change of treatment. The NVP arm experienced the greatest decline in LDL cholesterol and triglycerides, but none of the arms had experienced significant improvements in body fat distribution after 6 months.

Ruiz et al conducted a randomized study in which patients with HIV RNA less than 400 copies/mL for longer than 9 months either maintained their PI-containing regimen or switched to ddI/d4T/NVP, receiving antihistamine prophylaxis against rash during the first 15 days of therapy.[58] A statistically significant reduction in cholesterol and triglycerides occurred in the NVP group, but there was no significant improvement in body fat distribution in the NVP group. However, patient-reported quality of life was significantly better in the NVP group at week 48. In 60% of cases this was due to a simplified regimen, while 40% reported it was primarily a consequence of either reduced side effects or an improved physical status.

In summary, virologic responses in patients who switch to a NVP-based regimen are generally maintained, often associated with better adherence, and better quality of life. However, significant improvement in lipodystrophy has not been reported, with the exception of reductions in fasting triglycerides and cholesterol with NVP (but not with EFV). Switching to a PI-sparing regimen (whether NNRTI or abacavir-containing regimen) poses a significant risk of virologic rebound for patients with prior experience of mono- or dual-NRTI therapy and patients who have a history of virologic failure to any antiretroviral regimen.

PI-Experienced Patients

Introduction of a new class of agent, such as an NNRTI, is recommended when changing treatment because of virologic failure.[64] A change to lopinavir/ritonavir(r) plus an NNRTI-based therapy in NNRTI-naive patients who had failed PIs was explored in two studies, M97-765[65] and M98-957,[62] using concomitant NVP and EFV, respectively. In M97-765, 32% of participants had greater than fourfold loss of susceptibility to at least three PIs, and in M98-957, 68% had reduced susceptibility of a similar magnitude. Figure 13-4 shows the response to therapy at 96 weeks in the M97-765 study, with 49% of all patients enrolled having viral loads <50 copies/mL, using an intent-to-treat analysis and 63% having viral loads

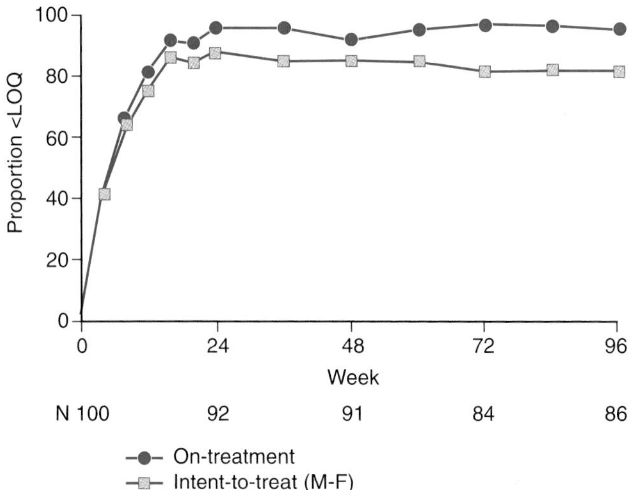

Figure 13-4 ■ M97-765: percent of patients below limit of detection through 96 weeks of treatment (limit of detection = 400 copies/mL).

From Feinberg J, Brun S, Xu Y, et al: Durable suppression of HIV + RNA after 2 years of therapy with ABT-378/ritonavir (ABT-378/r) treatment in single protease inhibitor experienced patients. In: Abstracts of the 5th International Congress on Drug Therapy in HIV Infection, Glasgow, 2000, abstract P101.

<50 copies/mL, using an on-treatment analysis. In the M98-957 study, 71% of individuals randomized to the higher lopinavir/r dose (533/133 mg bid) had HIV RNA less than 400 copies/mL at week 48, using an intent-to-treat analysis. The virologic response at week 24 was strongly associated with the number of baseline genotypic PI mutations; presence of more than seven mutations was associated with a decreased chance of suppression to below 400 copies/mL (less than 40% vs ~70% of those with six or seven baseline mutations). In these two phase II studies, 40% of patients had cholesterol greater than 300 mg/dL at week 48, and 40% had triglycerides greater than 750 mg/dL at week 48. This figure includes those individuals who had elevations to this level at baseline. Among single PI-experienced patients, the rates of cholesterol and triglyceride elevations above these levels were 29% and 26%, respectively, at 96 weeks and discontinuations because of adverse events were rare.

Of note, Rockstroh et al reported 24-week data on 40 patients receiving expanded access lopinavir/r in Germany.[63] A full 78% had received prior PIs, 78% were NNRTI-experienced, and they had taken a median of five prior NRTIs. After 24 weeks, only 36% of patients had HIV RNA less than 50 copies/mL. These results highlight the contribution of the new NRTIs or NNRTI to support lopinavir/r in PI-failing patients.

Pediatrics

NVP has also been demonstrated to be effective in pediatric populations with both advanced disease and prior PI experience.[66,67] In addition, in two separate studies of a limited number of vertically infected children, treatment with NVP plus NRTIs from an early age actually led to seroconversion in a number of individuals and to the absence of an HIV-specific cytotoxic T-lymphocyte response.[68,69] In general, NVP-based triple therapies such as NVP/ZDV/3TC and NVP/d4T/3TC are safe and well tolerated in children.[70,71] The antiviral effect of combination therapy including NVP has been evaluated in a small number of children. The PACTG 356 study assigned 52 pediatric patients to take ZDV/3TC/NVP, or ZDV/3TC/ABV/NVP, or d4T/3TC/NVP/NFV.[72] An intention-to-treat analysis revealed that significantly more children who received d4T/3TC/NVP/NFV had plasma HIV RNA levels of less than 200 copies/mL at 48 weeks (83%) and 200 weeks (72%) than children who receive the two regimens of RT inhibitors. No treatment-related adverse effects were reported among children who were receiving the four-drug combination therapy. Of note, although hepatotoxicity is most common among NVP users, this adverse effect can be readily reversed following removal of the drug.[73] Furthermore, in contrast to what has been reported in adults, hepatotoxicity seems to be less common in pediatric population.[27,74,75]

Mother-to-Child Transmission

As previously discussed, the pharmacologic profile of NVP makes it suitable for the prevention of perinatal transmission of HIV-1. NVP plasma levels remain well above the IC_{90} for NVP for up to 1 week after birth, after a single dose to the mother during labor followed by one dose to the infant 48–72 h after birth.[7] Colebunders et al demonstrated that NVP was present in breast milk within 5 days after delivery, with concentrations varying from 68% to 90%.[76] In a separate study, Musoke et al also showed that maternal plasma viral load was decreased by a median 1.3 $\log_{10}$ copies/mL 7 days after a single dose.[8] These data therefore suggested that a single dose of NVP (sdNVP) could provide a simple regimen for the prevention of mother-to-child transmission (MTCT). Two major clinical trials, HIVNET 012[77] and SAINT,[78] have investigated the use of NVP for the prevention of mother-to-child transmission in the developing world.

HIVNET 012 was conducted in a breast-feeding population in Uganda. The study randomized 645 mothers to receive either NVP (200 mg to the mother at the onset of labor and 2 mg/kg to the infant after 72 h), ZDV (600 mg at the onset of labor, and 300 mg every 3 h until delivery, with 4 mg/kg given to the infant twice daily for 7 days), or placebo. The placebo arm was discontinued after enrolling only 19 patients because a clear benefit for short-course ZDV had been demonstrated in the Thai study.[79] Figure 13-5 shows that significantly fewer infants in the NVP arm of HIVNET 012 became HIV-infected or died than in the ZDV arm. After 6–8 weeks, only 11.9% in the NVP arm were HIV-infected compared with 21.3% in the ZDV arm ($P = 0.0027$). Long-term follow-up of patients in this study found that this benefit was maintained for over 1 year although 95% were still breast-feeding at 4 months.[80] Similar results were obtained from the SAINT trial, which revealed a 13.3% rate of transmission at 6–8 weeks with NVP, compared with a 10.2% rate of transmission with ZDV + 3TC. In this trial, conducted in South Africa, the mothers received

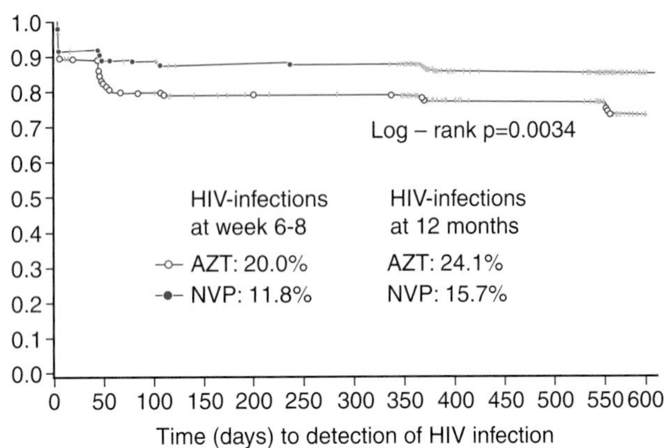

Figure 13-5 ■ HIVNET 012: Kaplan–Meier estimates of proportion of babies with HIV-free survival to 16 weeks.

From Guay LA, Musoke P, Fleming T, et al: Intrapartum and neonatal single-dose nevirapine compared with zidovudine for prevention of mother-to-child transmission of HIV-1 in Kampala, Uganda: HIVNET 012 randomised trial. Lancet 354:795, 1999.

an additional dose of NVP after delivery and infants received a fixed dose of 6 mg NVP. Mothers in the combination therapy arm underwent the same ZDV dosing schedule during labor as in the HIVNET 012 study, but also received 150 mg 3TC every 12 h during labor. Following delivery, mothers and infants received 300 mg ZDV + 150 mg 3TC twice daily, and 12 mg ZDV + 6 mg 3TC twice daily, respectively. The effect of timing of sdNVP administration to mothers and newborns was further explored in a secondary analysis of the HIVNET 024 trial. The overall rate of transmission in this study was 8.1% at 6 weeks. After adjusting for maternal and neonatal risk factors associated with HIV-1 transmission, data from 1460 women and 1480 infants showed that sdNVP remains effective in reducing HIV-1 transmission despite administration to mothers within 2 h prior to delivery. Among infants, no difference in number of HIV-1 infected were observed if they ingested NVP either less than 4 h or more than 72 h from delivery.[81a] Based on the results of these studies, among others, sdNVP to the pair mother-infant or sdNVP added to a nonsupressive regimen consisting of ZDV or ZDV + 3TC is now indicated for the prevention of MTCT in the developing world where more intensive regimens are not feasible. In those settings, sdNVP administrated within 48 h of delivery to the newborn, was still effective in reducing HIV-1 transmission among infants whose mothers did not access antiretroviral therapy during pregnancy or labor.[82a]

However, there are tradeoffs to such a feasible and simple regimen. Among them, viral resistance and drug-related toxicity have become a growing concern in HIV positive pregnant women exposed to antiretrovirals. Resistance mutations have been found in breast milk and plasma in mothers exposed to sdNVP, with prevalence rates ranging from highest to lowest order of magnitude as follows: subtype C, subtype D, and subtype A.[83–85] Recent studies have shown that a single dose of NVP to HIV-1 infected pregnant women can induce NVP resistance in 20–30% of mothers.[86] In HIV NET 012, NVP-resistant HIV-1 was detected in 70 (25%) of 279 women and 11 (46%) of 24 infants 6–8 weeks after delivery.[87] Furthermore, resistance mutations to NVP were also found 7 days after administration of sdNVP.[88] Of major concern are recent observations suggesting that exposure to sdNVP for prophylaxis of MTCT can compromise future treatment response to NNRTI-based HAART. To overcome this drawback, recent studies have explored new strategies to reduce emergence of NVP resistant mutants following sdNVP prophylaxis. Results from a prospective randomized trial in HIV infected pregnant women shows that adding a combination of 3TC and ZDV to single-dose NVP reduces the risk of emergent drug-resistant HIV-1 in both mothers and infants. In this trial, 226 mothers and 228 infants with a 6-week follow-up were evaluated. Mother–infant pairs were randomly assigned to one of three-treatment groups: (1) controls – those receiving single-dose NVP alone, during active labor, and to infants shortly after birth; (2) those receiving the NVP plus 3TC-ZDV for 4 days; and (3) those receiving this same investigational regimen for 7 days. The control group was halted early because resistance mutations were dramatically fewer in both experimental groups for both newborns and mothers. Among the mothers in the control group, 41 (60%) of 68 showed NNRTI resistance compared with eight (12%) of 67 in the 4-day group and seven (10%) of 68 in the 7-day group. Among the infants, the overall virus transmission rate was 10.5% at 6 weeks. Of note, 66% of those in the control group showed resistance mutations compared with 0% in both of the treatment groups. Whether 4 or 7 days of 3TC-ZDV is the optimum duration of therapy remains to be determined.[89,90]

The use of antepartum NVP-based HAART is an effective option to maximally suppress maternal viral load and, therefore, to minimize the risk of HIV vertical transmission. However, caution should be exercised in HIV infected pregnant women who present with CD4+ T-lymphocyte counts greater than 250 cells/mm^3 (discussed earlier). There have been at least six maternal death reports caused by liver failure related to NVP. A recent report from the Pediatric AIDS Clinical Trial Group 1022 study, identified NVP as being associated with liver toxicity in 29% (5/17) of pregnant women who had CD4+ > 250.[81]

More recently, a retrospective chart review of pregnant women who received NVP-based combination therapy suggested a relationship between NVP liver toxicity and trimester use. A significant difference was noted in the proportion of patients who developed hepatotoxicity while starting NVP in the third trimester (3/5, 60%; 95% CI: 14.66–94.73) compared with those starting NVP earlier in pregnancy (0/18, 0%; 95 CI: 0.0–18.53; $P < 0.06$).[82] Current recommendations for the use of antiretroviral drugs in pregnant HIV-1 infected women state that "nevirapine should be initiated in pregnant women with CD4 T-lymphocyte counts > 250 cells/mL only if benefit clearly outweighs risks, due to the increased risk of potentially life-threatening hepatotoxicity in women with high CD4 T-lymphocyte counts." "Women who enter pregnancy on nevirapine regimens and are tolerating them well may continue therapy, regardless of CD4 T-lymphocyte counts." (Public Health Service Task Force. Recommendations for use of antiretrovirals drugs in pregnant HIV-1 infected women for maternal health and interventions to reduce perinatal HIV-1 transmission in the United States, 24 Feb 2005) Available at http://www.aidsinfo.nih.gov.guidelines/perinatal).

Consequently, adopting combination therapy in lesser-developed countries where only monotherapy is available, as well as minimizing breast milk transmission, are present-day challenges in preventing MTCT.[92,93] Research is currently underway to devise preventive strategies as reports continue on clinical trial studies in lesser-developed countries.

DRUG INTERACTIONS

CYP450 Isoenzyme Inhibitors

Ketoconazole, a general inhibitor of CYP isoenzymes, should not be given in combination with NVP. In clinical studies, the AUC and C_{max} of ketoconazole decreased by 63% and 40%, respectively. An increase in NVP plasma levels is also possible. In a retrospective subpopulation analysis of patients in NVP clinical trials, steady-state NVP trough plasma concentrations were evaluated in patients also on cimetidine or macrolide antibiotics. Steady-state NVP trough plasma concentrations increased by 21% in patients concomitantly receiving cimetidine, and by 12% in patients concomitantly receiving macrolide antibiotics. Currently, no NVP dosage adjustments are recommended when NVP is used in combination with cimetidine or macrolide antibiotics (e.g., erythromycin, clarithromycin).[101]

CYP450 Isoenzyme Inducers

CYP450 isoenzyme inducers may be expected to bring about a decrease in plasma levels of NVP. A separate subgroup analysis detected a 16% average reduction in NVP steady-state trough plasma concentration in 19 patients receiving concomitant rifabutin. This interaction is considered not to be of clinical significance. A 37% reduction in NVP steady-state trough plasma concentration was also documented in three patients on rifampin and NVP. At this time, there are insufficient data to assess whether dosage adjustment is necessary when NVP and rifampin are co-administered. Therefore, in TB co-infected patients rifampin should not be used in combination with NVP. Concomitant use of St John's wort and NVP is to be avoided as this herbal supplement is expected to produce a substantial decrease in plasma levels of NVP.[101]

Antiretrovirals

When NVP was administered in various combinations with ZDV, ddI, and/or ddC, no substantial effect was detected on the steady-state concentrations of the NRTIs or NVP. Also, no significant drug interaction was detected between NVP and d4T. No substantial interactions between NVP and the other NRTIs, 3TC and abacavir, are anticipated because these agents use different metabolic pathways from NVP.[94,95]

Currently approved PIs are metabolized by similar CYP450 pathways. Sahai et al reported that co-administration of NVP and saquinavir hard gel capsule (SQV) led to a 27% decrease (P = 0.03) in the area under the concentration-time curve (AUC) of SQV and a 3% decrease in the NVP AUC.[96] Co-administration of NVP and ritonavir (RTV) led to an 11% decrease in the AUC for RTV but this was not statistically significant. Likewise, there was a nonsignificant decrease in NVP levels when compared to historical controls. A nonsignificant 4% increase in plasma nelfinavir levels was observed when it was dosed at 750 mg tid in combination with NVP. NVP + RTV + SQV-containing combinations have proven to be effective in PI-experienced patients. The interaction between NVP and IDV has also been extensively characterized.[97–99] In these studies, the NVP AUC was not significantly different from historical controls, whereas the mean IDV AUC decreased by approximately one-quarter to one-third. Most of the decrease in IDV AUC was attributable to those patients with the highest IDV serum levels before NVP dosing. It has been speculated, therefore, that the effect of NVP co-administration on the AUC for IDV may vary depending on the extent of prior CYP450 induction in a given patient. In general, the interaction of NVP with lopinavir, IDV, and SQV is similar in nature and extent; however, this is overcome by giving a low dose of ritonavir (as a pharmacokinetic booster of PI exposure).[100] However, as the IC_{90} of the virus increases (with increasing number of PI resistance mutations or with increasing number of PI failures) the therapeutic effect of the regimen will increase when a higher dose of the PI is used, as illustrated by the M98-957 study. In this study, a 30% dose increase of the PI was associated with a better response in patients with multiple PI failure.[62]

The interaction between NVP and EFV has recently been characterized, as a preliminary step to evaluate the efficacy and safety of this combination. A 22% decrease in the EFV AUC and a 36% decrease in the EFV C_{min} were observed when both NNRTIs were given in combination.[102] No change in NVP levels was noted relative to historical controls. The clinical significance of this interaction is not yet known, as the efficacy and safety of dual NNRTI combinations have not yet been characterized.

Other Agents

Oral contraceptives have the potential to interact with NVP. The effect of NVP on a single dose of ethinyl estradiol/norethindrone was measured, and found to significantly decrease AUC by 29% and 18%, respectively, with no effect on NVP levels.[103] It is recommended, therefore, that supplemental barrier forms of contraception be used when oral contraceptives are given in conjunction with NVP.

As a CYP450 inducer NVP has the potential, to reduce plasma levels of methadone.[91] The NNRTIs, NVP and EFV, similarly reduce plasma levels of methadone by 51% and 57%, respectively.[91,104,105] However, because methadone is dosed to achieve a certain clinical effect, it may be more informative to look at the change in methadone requirement in the presence of a CYP450 inducer. In this context, Altice et al found that methadone requirement was increased from 15 to 90 mg/day after initiation of NVP.[91]

CURRENT USE

The effectiveness of NVP has been demonstrated in treatment-naive patients, PI-experienced patients, and those with advanced disease, as well as in pediatric patients. NNRTI-based and PI-based triple combination regimens have comparable effectiveness in the treatment of antiretroviral therapy-naive patients, and this is reflected in current treatment guidelines. As discussed, NVP also plays a role in second- or third-line therapy, and as part of the PI switch strategy, as a means to simplify PI-based regimens. NVP is also singularly effective in the prevention of MTCT, but resistance mutations resulting from single-dose NVP demand necessary methods of control through combination therapy. Due to the nature of NVP as an inducer and substrate of cytochrome P450 enzymes, drug monitoring is recommended for use with PIs, methadone, oral contraceptives, and rifampicin.[106]

REFERENCES

1. Kohlstaedt LA, Wang J, Friedman JM, et al. Crystal structure at 3.5 A resolution of HIV1 reverse transcriptase complexed with an inhibitor. Science 256:1783, 1992.
2. Shirasaka T, Chokekijchai S, Yamada A, et al. Comparative analysis of anti-human immunodeficiency virus type 1 activities of dideoxynucleoside analogs in resting and activated peripheral blood mononuclear cells. Antimicrob Agents Chemother 39:2555, 1995.
3. Peterson P, Gekker F, Hu S, et al. Anti-human immunodeficiency virus type 1 activities of U-90152 and U-75875 in human brain cell cultures. Antimicrob Agents Chemother 38:2465, 1994.
4. Zhang H, Geethanjali D, Wu J, et al. Kinetic analysis of intravirion reverse transcription in the blood plasma of HIV-1 infected individuals. J Virol 70:628, 1996.
5. Shafer RW, Winters MA, Inversen AKN, et al. Genotypic and phenotypic changes during culture of a multinucleoside-resistant human immunodeficiency virus type 1 strain in the presence and absence of additional reverse transcriptase inhibitors. Antimicrob Agents Chemother 40:2887, 1996.
6. Pacifici GM. Pharmacokinetics of antivirals in neonate. Early Hum Dev 81:773, 2005.
7. Mirochnick M, Fenton T, Gagnier P, et al. Pharmacokinetics of nevirapine in human immunodeficiency virus type 1-infected pregnant women and their neonates. J Infect Dis 178:368, 1998.
8. Musoke P, Guay LA, Bagenda D, et al. A phase I/II study of the safety and pharmacokinetics of nevirapine in HIV-1-infected pregnant Ugandan women and their neonates (HIVNET 006). AIDS 13:479, 1999.
9. Taylor S, van Heeswijk RPG, Hoetelmans RMW, et al. Concentrations of nevirapine, lamivudine and stavudine in semen of HIV-1-infected men. AIDS 14:1979, 2000.
10. Glynn SL, Yazdanian M. In vitro blood–brain barrier permeability of nevirapine compared to other HIV antiretroviral agents. J Pharm Sci 87:306, 1998.
11. Almond LM, Edirisinghe D, Dalton M, et al. Intracellular and plasma pharmacokinetics of nevirapine in human immunodeficiencyvirus-infected individuals. Clin Pharmacol Ther 78:132, 2005.
12. Kearney B, Price R, Sheiner L, et al. Estimation of nevirapine exposure within the cerebrospinal fluid using CSF:plasma area under the curve ratios. In: Abstracts of the 6th Conference on Retroviruses and Opportunistic Infections, Chicago, 1999, abstract 406.
13. Price RW, Brew B, Sidtis J, et al. The brain in AIDS: central nervous system HIV-1 infection and AIDS dementia complex. Science 239:586, 1988.
14. Lamson MJ, Sabo JP, MacGregor TR, et al. Single dose pharmacokinetics and bioavailability of nevirapine in healthy volunteers. Biopharmaceutics & Drug Disposition 20:285, 1999.
15. Lamson MJ, Cort S, Sabo JP, et al. Effects of gender on the single and multiple dose pharmacokinetics of nevirapine 200 mg/d. In: Abstracts of the American Association of Pharmaceutical Sciences Meeting, Miami, 1995, abstract CS 3004.
16. Cheeseman SH, Hattox SE, McLaughlin MM, et al. Pharmacokinetics of nevirapine: initial single-rising-dose study in humans. Antimicrob Agents Chemother 37:178, 1993.
17. Cheeseman SH, Havlir D, McLaughlin M, et al. Phase I/II evaluation of nevirapine alone and in combination with zidovudine for infection with human immunodeficiency virus. J Acquir Immune Defic Syndr Hum Retrovirol 8:141, 1995.
18. Lamson MJ, Cort S, Sabo JP, et al. Effects of food or antacid on the bioavailability of nevirapine 200 mg in 24 healthy volunteers. In: Abstracts of the American Association of Pharmaceutical Sciences Meeting, Miami, 1995, abstract CS 3003.
19. van Heeswijk RPG, Veldkamp AI, Mulder JW, et al. The steady-state pharmacokinetics of nevirapine during once daily and twice daily dosing in HIV-1-infected individuals. AIDS 14:F77, 2000.
20. García F, Knobel H, Sambeat MA, et al. Comparison of twice-daily stavudine plus once- or twice-daily didanosine and nevirapine in early stages of HIV infection: the SCAN study. AIDS 14:2485, 2000.
21. Havlir D, Cheeseman SH, McLaughlin M, et al. High-dose nevirapine: safety, pharmacokinetics, and antiviral effect in patients with human immunodeficiency virus infection. J Infect Dis 171:537, 1995.
22. Lamson M, Maldonado S, Hutman H, et al. The effects of underlying renal or hepatic dysfunction on the pharmacokinetics of nevirapine (viramune). In: Abstracts of the 13th International AIDS Conference, Durban, 2000, abstract TuPeB3301.
23. van Leeuwen R, Katlama C, Murphy RL, et al. A randomized trial to study first-line combination therapy with or without protease inhibitor in HIV-1-infected patients. AIDS 17:987, 2003.
24. Carr A, Vella S, de Jong MD, et al for the Dutch–Italian–Australian Nevirapine Study Group. A controlled trial of nevirapine plus zidovudine versus zidovudine alone in p24 antigenaemic HIV-infected patients. AIDS 10:635, 1996.
25. D'Aquila RT, Hughes MD, Johnson VA, et al; National Institute of Allergy and Infectious Diseases AIDS Clinical Trials Group 241 Investigators. Nevirapine, zidovudine, and didanosine compared with zidovudine and didanosine in patients with HIV-1 infection. Ann Intern Med 124:1019, 1996.
26. Hong-Brown LQ, Brown CR, Lang CH. HIV Antiretroviral agents inhibit protein synthesis and decrease ribosomal protein S6 and 4EBP1 phosphorylation in C2C12 myocytes. AIDS Res Hum Retroviruses 21:854, 2005.
27. Pollard RB, Robinson P, Dransfield K. Safety profile of nevirapine, a nonnucleoside reverse transcriptase inhibitor for the treatment of human immunodeficiency virus infection. Clin Ther 20:1071, 1998.

28. Henry K, Erice A, Tierney C, et al. A randomized, controlled, double-blind study comparing the survival benefit of four different reverse transcriptase inhibitor therapies (three-drug, two-drug, and alternating drug) for the treatment of advanced AIDS. J Acquir Immune Defic Syndr Hum Retrovirol 19:339, 1998.
29. Montaner JSG, Reiss P, Cooper D, et al for the INCAS Study Group. A randomized, double-blind trial comparing combinations of nevirapine, didanosine, and zidovudine for HIV-infected patients. The INCAS trial. JAMA 279:930, 1998.
30. Wit FWN for the Dutch HIV-Treating Physicians. Experience with nevirapine in previously treated HIV-1 infected individuals. Antivir Ther 5:257, 2000.
31. Wit FWNM, Wood R, Horban A, et al. Prednisolone does not prevent hypersensitivity reactions in antiretroviral drug regimens containing abacavir with or without nevirapine. AIDS 15:2423, 2001.
32. Barreiro P, Soriano V, Casas E, et al. Prevention of nevirapine-associated exanthema using slow dose escalation and/or corticosteroids. AIDS 14:2153, 2000.
33. Martinez E, Blanco JL, Arnaiz JA, et al. Hepatotoxicity in HIV-1-infected patients receiving nevirapine-containing antiretroviral therapy. AIDS 15:1261, 2001.
34. Montaner JSG, Cahn P, Zala C, et al. Randomized, controlled study of the effects of a short course of prednisone on the incidence of rash associated with nevirapine in patients infected with HIV-1. JAIDS 33:41, 2003.
35. Wit FWNM, Weverling GJ, Weel J, et al. Incidence and risk factors for severe hepatotoxicity associated with antiretroviral combination therapy. J Infect Dis 186:23, 2002.
36. Robinson P. Examination of trials to prevent nevirapine (NVP)-associated rash. In: Abstracts of the 40th Interscience Conference on Antimicrobial Agents and Chemotherapy, Toronto, 2000, abstract 1554.
37. Sanne I; FTC-302 Study Investigators; FTC-302 Independent Clinical Steering Committee. Severe liver toxicity in patients receiving two nucleoside analogues and a non-nucleoside reverse transcriptase inhibitor. AIDS 14(Suppl 4):S12 (abstract PL9.3), 2000.
38. Bennett CL, Nebeker J, Lyons EA, et al. The research on adverse drug events and reports (RADAR) Project. JAMA 293:2131, 2005.
39. Leith J, Piliero P, Storfer S, et al. Appropriate use of nevirapine for long-term therapy. J Infect Dis 192:545, 2005.
40. Haas DW. Will pharmacogenomic discoveries improve HIV therapeutics? Top HIV Med 13:90, 2005.
41. Martinez E, Blanco JL, Arnaiz JA, et al. Hepatotoxicity in HIV-1 infected patients receiving nevirapine-containing antiretroviral therapy. AIDS 15:1261, 2001.
42. Wit FWNM, Weverling GJ, Weel J, et al. Incidence of and risk factors for severe hepatotoxicity associated with antiretroviral combination therapy. J Infect Dis 23–31, 2002.
43. Van der Valk M, Kastelein JJP, Murphy RL, et al. Nevirapine-containing antiretroviral therapy in HIV-1 infected patients results in an anti-atherogenic lipid profile. AIDS 15:2407, 2001.
44. Almond LM, Boffito M, Hoggard PG, et al. The relationship between nevirapine plasma concentrations and abnormal liver function test. AIDS Res Hum Retroviruses 20:716, 2004.
45. CDC. Serious adverse events attributable to nevirapine regimens for postexposure prophylaxis after HIV exposures – Worldwide, 1997-2000. MMWR 49:1153, 2001.
46. Martínez E, Conget I, Lozano L, et al. Reversion of metabolic abnormalities after switching from HIV-1 protease inhibitors to nevirapine. AIDS 13:805, 1999.
47. Raboud JM, Montaner JSG, Conway B, et al. Suppression of plasma viral load below 20 copies/ml is required to achieve a long-term response to therapy. AIDS 12:1619, 1998.
48. Podzamczer D, Ferrer E, Consiglio E, et al. A randomized, multicenter trial comparing Combivirplus nelfinavir or nevirapine in HIV-1-infected naïve patients. Antivir Ther 7:81, 2002.
49. Floridia M, Bucciardini R, Ricciardulli D, et al. A randomized, double-blind trial on the use of a triple combination including nevirapine, a nonnucleoside reverse transcriptase HIV inhibitor, in antiretroviral-naive patients with advanced disease. J Acquir Immune Defic Syndr Hum Retrovirol 20:11, 1999.
50. Podzamczer D, Ferrer E, Perez P, et al. Decrease of HIV-1 RNA levels in tonsillar lymphoid tissue of patients receiving combivir/nevirapine (CNr) or combivir/nelfinavir (CNf). In: Abstracts of the 13th International AIDS Conference, Durban, 2000, abstract TuPeB3213.
51. Robinson P, Montaner JSG; the INCAS Study Group. Long-term follow-up of patients treated with nevirapine (NVP) based combination therapy within the INCAS trial. In: Abstracts of the 12th World AIDS Conference, Geneva, 1998, abstract 12368.
52. Montaner JSG, Hogg R, Raboud J, et al. Antiretroviral treatment in 1998. Lancet 352:1919, 1998.
53. Rachlis A, Becker S, Gill J, et al. Successful substitution of protease inhibitors with Sustiva (efavirenz) in patients with undetectable plasma HIV-1 RNA levels – results of a prospective, randomized, multicenter, open-label study (DMP 266-049). Program and abstracts of the 40th Interscience Conference on Antimicrobial Agents and Chemotherapy, Toronto, ON, Canada, 17–20 Sep 2000, abstract 475.
54. Negredo E, Cruz L, Paredes R, et al. Virological, immunological, and clinical impact of switching from protease inhibitors to nevirapine or to efavirenz in patients with human immunodeficiency virus infection and long-lasting viral suppression, Clin Infect Dis 34:504, 2002.
55. Pollard R and the 1090 Team. Factors predictive of durable HIV suppression in a randomized double blind trial with nevirapine (NVP), zidovudine (ZDV) and lamivudine (3TC) in treatment-naive (ARV-n) patients with advanced AIDS. In: Abstracts of the 7th Conference on Retroviruses and Opportunistic Infections, San Francisco, 2000, abstract 517.
56. Harris M, Patenaude P, Cooperberg P, et al. Correlation of virus load in plasma and lymph node tissue in human immunodeficiency virus infection. J Infect Dis 176:1388, 1997.
57. Schacker TW, Nguyen P, Murphy R, et al. Persistent abnormalities in lymphoid tissue of persons showing good virologic response on antiretroviral therapy in all treatment arms of the Atlantic study. Presented at the HIV DART 2000, Frontiers in Drug Development for Antiretroviral Therapies, Isla Verde, PR, USA, 2000, abstract 042.
58. Ruiz L, Negredo E, Domingo P, et al. Antiretroviral treatment simplification with nevirapine in protease inhibitor-experienced patients with HIV-associated lipodystrophy: 1-year prospective follow-up of a multicenter, randomized, controlled study. JAIDS 27:229, 2001.
59. Raffi F, Esnault JL, Reliquet V, et al. The Maintavir study, substitution of a non-nucleoside reverse transcriptase inhibitor (NNRTI) for a protease inhibitor (PI) in patients with undetectable plasma HIV-1 RNA: 18 months follow-up. Program and abstracts of the 40th Interscience Conference on Antimicrobial Agents and Chemotherapy, Toronto, ON, Canada, 17–20 Sep 2000, abstract 474.
60. Opravil M, Hirschel B, Lazzarin A, et al. A randomized trial of simplified maintenance therapy with abacavir, lamivudine, and zidovudine in human immunodeficiency virus infection. J Infect Dis 185:1251, 2002.
61. Clumeck SN, Goebel F, Rozenbaum W, et al. Simplification with abacavir-based triple nucleoside therapy versus continued proteae inhibitor-based highly active antiretroviral therapy in HIV-1-infected patients with undetectable plasma HIV-1 RNA. AIDS 15:1517, 2001.

62. Danner S, Brun S, King M, et al. Lopinavir/ritonavir and efavirenz: 72-week safety and efficacy evaluation in multiple protease inhibitor-experienced patients. Program and abstracts of the 41st Interscience Conference on Antimicrobial Agents and Chemotherapy, Chicago, USA, September 22–25, 2001. Abstract 1925.
63. Rockstroh J, Brun S, Sylte J, et al. ABT-378/ritonavir (ABT-378/r) and efavirenz: one year safety/efficacy evaluation in multiple PI experienced patients. AIDS 14(Suppl 4):S29 (abstract P43), 2000.
64. Hammer SM, Saag MS, Schechter M, et al. Treatment for Adult HIV Infection: 2006 recommendations of the International AIDS Society-USA Panel. JAMA 296:827, 2006.
65. Benson CA, Deeks S, Brun S, et al. Safety and antiviral activity at 48 weeks of lopinavir/ritonavir plus nevirapine and 2 nucleoside reverse-transcriptase inhibitors in human immunodeficiency virus type 1-infected protease inhibitor-experienced patients. J Infect Dis 185:599, 2002.
66. Burchett SK, Khoury M, McIntosh K, et al. Viral load reduction (VLR) in children with advanced HIV disease treated with 4-drug antiretroviral treatment (ART) regimens including NRTIs, nevirapine (NVP), nelfinavir (NFV), and/or ritonavir (RTV) (PACTG 366). In: Abstracts of the 7th Conference on Retroviruses and Opportunistic Infections, San Francisco, 2000, abstract 698.
67. Krogstad P, Lee S, Johnson G, et al. Nucleoside-analogue reverse transcriptase inhibitors plus nevirapine, nelfinavir, or ritonavir for pretreated children infected with human immunodeficiency virus type 1. Clin Infect Dis 34:991, 2002.
68. Luzuriaga K, Bryson Y, Krogstad P, et al. Combination treatment with zidovudine, didanosine, and nevirapine in infants with human immunodeficiency virus type 1 infection. N Engl J Med 336:1343, 1997.
69. Luzuriaga K, McManus M, Catalina M, et al. Early therapy of vertical HIV-1 infection: evidence for cessation of viral replication and absence of virus-specific immunity. In: Abstracts of the 7th Conference on Retroviruses and Opportunistic Infections, San Francisco, 2000, abstract 211.
70. Lodha R, Upadhyay A, Kabra SK. Antiretroviral therapy in HIV-1 infected children. Indian Pediatr 42:789, 2005.
71. Chokephaibulkit K, Plipat N, Cressey TR, et al. Pharmacokinetics of nevirapine in HIV-infected children receiving an adult fixed-dose combination of stavudine, lamivudine, and nevirapine. AIDS 19:1495, 2005.
72. Luzuriaga K, Bryson Y, McSherry G et al. A trial of three antiretroviral regimens in HIV-1 infected children. N Engl J Med 350: 2471, 2004.
73. Shah I. Adverse effects of antiretroviral therapy in HIV-1 infected children. J Trop Pediatr 52:244–8, 2005.
74. Guidelines for the Use of Antiretroviral Agent in Pediatric HIV Infection, 3 Nov 2005. Available: http://AIDSinfo.nih.gov.
75. Ikeda T, Ch'ng TW, Oleske JM. Recommendations in pediatric antiretroviral therapy. Exp Opin Pharmacother 8:155, 2007.
76. Colebunders R, Hodossy B, Burger D, et al. The effect of highly active antiretroviral treatment on viral load and antiretroviral drug levels in breast milk. AIDS 19:1912, 2005.
77. Guay LA, Musoke P, Fleming T, et al. Intrapartum and neonatal single-dose nevirapine compared with zidovudine for prevention of mother-to-child transmission of HIV-1 in Kampala, Uganda: HIVNET 012 randomised trial. Lancet 354:795, 1999.
78. Moodley D, Moodley J, Coovadia H, et al. A multicenter randomized controlled trial of nevirapine versus a combination of zidovudine and lamivudine to reduce intrapartum and early postpartum mother-to-child transmission of human immunodeficiency virus type 1. J Infect Dis 187:725, 2003.
79. Shaffer N, Chuachoowong R, Mock PA, et al. Short-course zidovudine for perinatal HIV-1 transmission in Bangkok, Thailand: a randomised controlled trial. Lancet 353:773, 1999.
80. Jackson JB, Musoke P, Fleming T, et al. Intrapartum and neonatal single-dose nevirapine compared with zidovudine for prevention of mother-to-child transmission of HIV-1 in Kampala, Uganda: 18-month follow-up of the HIVNET 012 randomised trial. Lancet 362:859, 2003.
81. Hitti J, Frenkel LM, Stek AM, et al. Maternal toxicity with continuous nevirapine in pregnancy – results from the PACTG 1022. J Acquir Immune Defic Syndr 36:772, 2004.
81a. Chi BH, Wang L, Read JS, et al. Timing of maternal and neonatal dosing of nevirapine and the risk of mother-to-child transmission of HIV-1: HIVNET 024. AIDS 19:1857–64, 2005.
82. Joy S, Poi M, Hughes L, et al. Third-trimester maternal toxicity with nevirapine use in pregnancy. Obst Gynecol 106:1032, 2005.
82a. Antiretroviral drugs for treating pregnant women and preventing HIV infection in infants: towards universal access. Recommendations for a public health approach. 2006 version. Available at: www.who.int/hiv/pub/guidelines
83. Lee EJ, Kantor R, Zijenah L, et al. Breast-milk shedding of drug-resistant HIV-1 subtype C in women exposed to single-dose nevirapine. J Infect Dis 192:1260, 2005.
84. Eshleman SH, Hoover DR, Chen S, et al. Nevirapine (NVP) resistance in women with HIV-1 subtype C, compared with subtypes A and D, after the administration of single-dose NVP. J Infect Dis 192:30, 2005.
85. Eshleman SH, Guay LA, Wang J, et al. Distinct patterns of emergence and fading of K103N and Y191C in women with subtype A vs. D after single-dose nevirapine: HIVNET 012. J Acquir Immune Defic Syndr 40:24, 2005.
86. Eshleman SH, Jackson JB. Nevirapine resistance after single dose prophylaxis. In: Abstracts of 10th Conf Retrovir Oppor Infect, 2003, abstract 856.
87. Eshleman SH, Mracna M, Guay LA et al. Selection and fading of resistance mutations in women and infants receiving nevirapine to prevent HIV-1 vertical transmission (HIVNET 012). AIDS 15:1951, 2001.
88. Jones D, Parkin N, Hudelson SE, et al. Genetic linkage of nevirapine resistance mutations in HIV type 1 seven days after single-dose nevirapine. AIDS Res Hum Retroviruses 21:319, 2005.
89. McIntyre J. Preventing mother-to-child transmission of HIV: successes and challenges. BJOG 112:1196, 2005.
90. Ekouevi DK, Tonwe-Gold B, Dabis F. Advances in the prevention of mother-to-child transmission of HIV-1 infection in resource-limited settings. AIDS Read 15:479–80; 487–93, 2005.
91. Altice FL, Friedland GH, Cooney EL. Nevirapine induced opiate withdrawal among injection drug users with HIV infection receiving methadone. AIDS 13:957, 1999.
92. Thorne C, Newell ML. Treatment options for the prevention of mother-to-child transmission of HIV. Curr Opin Investig Drugs 6:804, 2005.
93. Chersich MF, Gray GE. Progress and emerging challenges in preventing mother-to-child transmission. Curr Infect Dis Rep 7:393, 2005.
94. MacGregor TR, Lamson MJ, Cort S, et al. Steady state pharmacokinetics of nevirapine, didanosine, zalcitabine and zidovudine combination therapy in HIV-1 positive patients. In: Abstracts of the American Association of Pharmaceutical Sciences Meeting, Miami, 1995, abstract CS 3002.
95. Skowron G, Leoung G, Hall DB, et al. Pharmacokinetic evaluation and short-term activity of stavudine, nevirapine, and nelfinavir therapy in HIV-1-infected adults. JAIDS 35:351, 2004.

96. Sahai J, Cameron W, Salgo M, et al. Drug interaction study between saquinavir (SQV) and nevirapine (NVP). In: Abstracts of the 4th Conference on Retroviruses and Opportunistic Infections, Alexandria: Westover Management Group, 1997, abstract 614.
97. Murphy RL, Sommadossi J-P, Lamson M, et al. Antiviral effect and pharmacokinetic interaction between nevirapine and indinavir in persons infected with human immunodeficiency virus type 1. J Infect Dis 179:1116, 1999.
98. Farthing C, Mess T, Ried C, et al. Ritonavir, saquinavir, and nevirapine as a salvage regimen for indinavir or ritonavir resistance. In: Abstracts of the 12th World AIDS Conference, Geneva, 1998, abstract 22356.
99. Harris M, Durakovic C, Rae S, et al. A pilot study of nevirapine, indinavir, and lamivudine among patients with advanced human immunodeficiency virus disease who had failure of combination nucleoside therapy. J Infect Dis 177:1514, 1998.
100. Ruane PJ, Tam JT, Libraty DH, et al. Salvage therapy using ritonavir/saquinavir with a non-nucleoside reverse transcriptase inhibitor after prolonged failure with indinavir or ritonavir. In: Abstracts of the 12th World AIDS Conference, Geneva, 1998, abstract 32308.
101. Viramune Product Monograph. Boehringer Ingelheim Pharmaceuticals Inc. Ridgefield, CT. April 2007.
102. Veldkamp AI, Harris M, Montaner JS, et al. The steady-state pharmacokinetics of efavirenz and nevirapine when used in combination in human immunodeficiency virus type 1-infected persons. J Infect Dis 184: 37, 2001.
103. Leitz G, Mildvan D, McDonough M, et al. Nevirapine (viramune, NVP) and ethinyl estradiol/norethindrone [Ortho-Novum 1/35 (21 pack) EE/NET] interaction study in HIV-1 infected women. In: Abstracts of the 7th Conference on Retroviruses and Opportunistic Infections, San Francisco, 2000, abstract 89.
104. Gourevitch MN, Friedland GH. Interactions between methadone and medications used to treat HIV infection: a review. Mt Sinai J Med 67:429, 2000.
105. Clarke S, Mulcahy F, Beck D, et al. Managing methadone and non-nucleoside reverse transcriptase inhibitors: guidelines for clinical practice. In: Abstracts of the 7th Conference on Retroviruses and Opportunistic Infections, San Francisco, 2000, abstract 88.
106. Milinkovic A, Martinez E. Nevirapine in the treatment of HIV. Expert Rev Anti InfectTher 2:367, 2004.

Chapter 14

Efavirenz

Schlomo Staszewski, MD

Efavirenz (EFV, Sustiva) is a human immunodeficiency virus type 1 (HIV-1) specific, non-nucleoside reverse transcriptase inhibitor (NNRTI). EFV is a noncompetitive inhibitor of HIV-1 reverse transcriptase (RT) and has no inhibitory effect on HIV-2 RT. EFV binds directly to RT and inhibits viral RNA- and DNA-dependent DNA polymerase activities by disrupting the catalytic site. Although the drug–RT–template complex may continue to bind deoxynucleoside triphosphate and to catalyze its incorporation into the newly forming viral DNA, it does so at a slower rate.[1–3]

It was approved by the US Food and Drug Administration (FDA) in 1998 for the treatment of HIV in combination with other antiretroviral medications in adults and children over 3 years of age. It is available as 200 mg capsules, 600 mg tablets, and as a liquid formulation.[4,5]

EFV plus lamivudine in combination with zidovudine, tenofovir DF, or stavudine is the preferred NNRTI-based regimen for HIV treatment-naive patients. It can also be used as part of a combination therapy for salvage regimens for treatment-experienced patients.[6]

EFV may be used with other antiretroviral agents as part of an expanded postexposure prophylaxis regimen for healthcare workers and other individuals exposed occupationally to tissues, blood, or other body fluids associated with a high risk for HIV transmission. EFV should be considered when resistance to protease inhibitors (PIs) in the source person's virus is known or suspected.[7]

EFV is an FDA pregnancy category D drug. Women should not become pregnant or breastfeed while taking EFV. Serious birth defects, mostly involving neural tube development, have been seen in children of women treated with EFV during the first trimester of pregnancy. Women must use a reliable form of barrier contraception, such as a condom, even if they also use other methods of birth control (*see section on* Pregnancy).[4,6]

STRUCTURE

EFV is chemically described as (*S*)-6-chloro-4-(cyclopropylethynyl)-1, 4-dihydro-4-(trifluoromethyl) – 2H-3, 1-benzoxazin-2-one.[3] Molecular mass of the compound is 315.68. EFV has the empirical formula $C_{14}H_9ClF_3NO_2$ and the structural formula is shown in Figure 14-1.

IN VITRO ACTIVITY AND MECHANISM OF ACTION

EFV activity is mediated predominantly by noncompetitive inhibition of HIV-1 RT. HIV-2 RT and human cellular DNA polymerases alpha, beta, gamma, and delta are not inhibited by EFV. EFV binds directly to RT and inhibits viral RNA- and DNA-dependent DNA polymerase activities by disrupting the catalytic site.[1] The 90–95% inhibitory concentration (IC_{90-95}) of EFV for wild-type laboratory strains and clinical isolates ranged from 1.7 to 25 nM.

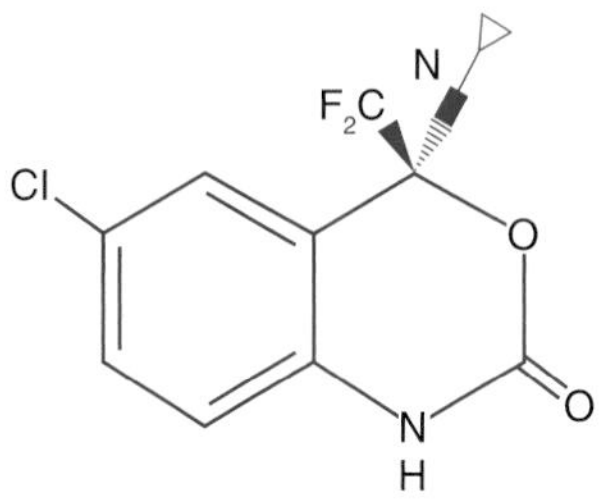

Figure 14-1 ■ Structure of EFV.

PLASMA PHARMACOLOGY

Pharmacokinetics allowing for a convenient once-daily administration makes EFV one of the first agents to be included in once-daily regimens.

Peak plasma concentrations (C_{max}) of 1.9–9.1 μM were achieved in healthy individuals within 5 h after a single oral dose of 100–1600 mg of EFV. Dose-related increases in C_{max} and area under the time–concentration curve (AUC) were seen for doses up to 1600 mg, however, as the dose increased, the absorption decreased. The increases were less than proportional suggesting diminished absorption at higher doses.[2,3]

In HIV-infected individuals, mean minimum plasma concentration levels (C_{min}), mean C_{max}, and AUC were dose proportional following 200, 400, and 600 mg daily doses. Time-to-peak plasma concentrations were ~3–5 h and steady-state plasma concentrations were attained after 6–10 days of EFV therapy.[2,4]

High-fat meals produce an increase in EFV bioavailability. In capsule form, administration of a single 600 mg dose of EFV with a high-fat/high-caloric meal resulted in a mean increase of 22% and 39% in AUC and C_{max} respectively in comparison to the plasma exposures achieved when given under fasted conditions while the tablet form was associated with a 28% increase in mean AUC and a 79% increase in mean C_{max}.[2,4]

EFV is highly protein-bound (~99.5–99.75%) to human plasma proteins, mainly albumin.[2,4] Only ~0.5% remains available as free drug. In HIV-1-infected patients who received EFV 200–600 mg once daily for at least 1 month, cerebrospinal fluid concentrations ranged from 0.26% to 1.19% (mean 0.69%) of the corresponding plasma concentration.[4,8–10] This proportion is approximately threefold higher than the free, non-protein-bound fraction of EFV in plasma.[2,4]

METABOLISM AND ELIMINATION

EFV is metabolized primarily by the hepatic cytochrome P450 isoenzymes CYP3A4 and CYP2B6 into hydroxylated, inactive metabolites. These metabolites undergo subsequent glucuronidation. EFV is an inducer of its own metabolism. Ten days of therapy with 200–400 mg of EFV daily resulted in a lower than expected accumulation of medication (22–42% lower) and a shorter terminal half-life, 40–55 h after multiple doses compared with the single-dose half-life of 52–76 h.[2]

Terminal elimination half-life is prolonged in patients with chronic liver disease. EFV is excreted principally in the feces, both as metabolites and unchanged drug. Approximately 14–34% of a radio-labeled dose of EFV was recovered in the urine (less than 1% as unchanged drug) and 16–61% of a radio-labeled dose was recovered (primarily as unchanged drug).[4,11] The effect of renal impairment on EFV elimination has not been studied to date, but it is expected to be minimal because only 1% of EFV is excreted unchanged in urine.[2,4]

Plasma concentrations of EFV may persist at therapeutic levels for 2 weeks or more after discontinuation of EFV. Although the reported half-life is 40–55 h, concentrations were found in a small group of patients tested at 0, 4, 7, and 21 days after stopping EFV therapy.[12] If drugs with a shorter half-life are stopped at the same time as EFV, this may be, in effect, EFV monotherapy for the patients. It may be advisable therefore to stop EFV at least 2 weeks before stopping other drugs to avoid the emergence of drug resistance.[12,13]

PHARMACOKINETICS, GENDER, ETHNICITY, AND RACE

It is unclear whether sex-determined pharmacokinetic differences exist. EFV clearance and volume of distribution appeared to be similar between men and women in some studies[14] while others found that females had a 25% higher mean EFV AUC.[15]

Significant associations between weight and both drug clearance and distribution have been found even after adjusting for sex and concomitant medications – those who weighed less had slower EFV clearance.[4,14]

Particular caution should be paid to patients of African origin. In clinical studies, significant associations have been found between drug clearance of EFV and race. One study showed EFV clearance to be lower in blacks and Hispanics compared to non-Hispanic white patients. The white subjects had a 32% higher drug clearance.[14] Plasma concentrations in five out of ten patients in another pharmacokinetic study had EFV elimination half-lives of longer than 100 h (114–229) although the T1/2 for EFV is 40–55 h. Four of these five were black African women. Three of these women showed therapeutic levels of greater than 1000 ng/mL 2 weeks after discontinuing EFV. The five patients with EFV half-lives within expected ranges were male Caucasians.[16]

It has been recently suggested that genetic polymorphisms are associated with differences in drug metabolism. EFV is primarily metabolized in the liver by the CYP450 2B6 enzyme and variations in this gene include the G/G, G/T, and the T/T genotypes. Haas and colleagues evaluated six allelic variants from patient DNA samples and found that the homozygous T/T genotype at position $G^{516}T$ was more prevalent in blacks (20%) than in Caucasians (3%), and was associated with greater EFV plasma exposure. The median EFV AUC drug exposure was threefold higher (130 $\mu g\ h^{-1}\ L^{-1}$) with the T/T genotype compared with 44 and 60 $\mu g\ h^{-1}\ L^{-1}$ in patients with G/G and G/T respectively. The T/T variant was also strongly associated with adverse central nervous system symptoms at week one.[17,18]

It will be necessary to investigate whether lower doses of EFV are appropriate in patients who clear the drug very slowly and/or who have very high plasma levels.

The effects of co-administration of EFV with other drugs are discussed in the section on Drug Interactions.

DRUG INTERACTIONS

Drug interaction studies have been performed with EFV and other drugs likely to be co-administered and with drugs commonly used. The effects of EFV co-administration on other drugs – plasma AUC and C_{max} – are shown in Table 14-1 and

Effect of Efavirenz on Co-administered Drug Plasma C_{max} and AUC

Table 14-1

Co-Administered Drug	Dose	Efavirenz Dose	Number of Subjects	Co-Administered Drug (% Change)	
				C_{max} (mean (90% CI))	AUC (mean (90% CI))
Atazanavir	400 mg qd with a light meal days 1–20	600 mg qd with a light meal days 7–20	27	↓(59%) (49–67%)	↓(74%) (68–78%)
	400 mg qd days 1–6, then 300 mg qd days 7–20 with ritonavir 100 mg qd and a light meal	600 mg qd 2 h after atazanavir and ritonavir days 7–20	13	↑(14%)[a] (↓17–↑58%)	↑(39%)[a] (2–88%)
Indinavir	1000 mg q8 h × 10 days	600 mg × 10 days	20		
	After morning dose			↔[b]	↓(33%)[b] (26–39%)
	After afternoon dose			↔[b]	↓(37%)[b] (26–46%)
	After evening dose			↓(29%)[b] (11–43%)	↓(46%)[b] (37–54%)
Lopinavir/ritonavir	400/100 mg q12 h × 9 days	600 mg × 9 days	11,7[c]	↔[d]	↓ (19%)[d] (↓36– ↑3%)
Nelfinavir metabolite AG-1402	750 mg q8 h × 7 days	600 mg × 7 days	10	↑(21%) (10–33%) ↓(40%) (30–48%)	↑(20%) (8–34%) ↓(37%) (25–48%)
Ritonavir	500 mg q12 h × 8 days	600 mg × 10 days	11		
	After AM dose			↑(24%) (12–38%)	↑(18%) (6–33%)
	After PM dose			↔	↔
Saquinavir SGC[e]	1200 mg q8 h × 10 days	600 mg × 10 days	12	↓(50%) (28–66%)	↓(62%) (45–74%)
Lamivudine	150 mg q12 h × 14 days	600 mg × 14 days	9	↔	↔
Zidovudine	300 mg q12 h × 14 days	600 mg × 14 days	9	↔	↔
Azithromycin	600 mg single dose	400 mg × 7 days	14	↑ (22%) (4–42%)	↔
Clarithromycin 14-OH metabolite	500 mg q12 h × 7 days	400 mg × 7 days	11	↓(26%) (15–35%) ↑(49%) (32–69%)	↓(39%) (30–46%) ↑(34%) (18–53%)
Fluconazole	200 mg × 7 days	400 mg × 7 days	10	↔	↔
Rifabutin	300 mg qd × 14 days	600 mg × 14 days	9	↓(32%) (15–46%)	↓(38%) (28–47%)
Cetirizine	10 mg single dose	600 mg × 10 days	11	↓(24%) (18–30%)	↔
Ethinyl estradiol	50 μg single dose	400 mg × 10 days	13	↔	↑(37%) (25–51%)
Lorazepam	20 mg single dose	600 mg × 10 days	12	↑(16%) (2–32%)	↑(7%) (1–14%)

(Continued)

(Continued)

Table 14-1

Co-Administered Drug	Dose	Efavirenz Dose	Number of Subjects	Co-Administered Drug (% Change)	
				C_{max} (mean (90% CI))	AUC (mean (90% CI))
Methadone	Stable maintenance 35–100 mg daily	600 mg × 14–21 days	11	↓(45%) (25–59%)	↓(52%) (33–66%)
Paroxetine	20 mg qd × 14 days	600 mg × 14 days	16	↔	↔
Sertraline	50 mg qd × 14 days	600 mg × 14 days	13	↓(29%) (15–40%)	↓(39%) (27–50%)
Voriconazole	400 mg po q12h × 1 day then 200 mg po q12h × 8 days	400 mg × 9 days	–	↓ (61%)[f]	↓(77%)[f]

↑ Indicates increase; ↓ indicates decrease; ↔ indicates no change.
[a] Compared with atazanavir 400 mg qd alone.
[b] Comparator dose of indinavir was 800 mg q8h × 10 days. Mean decreases in the C_{min} of indinavir ranged from 39% to 57%.
[c] Parallel-group design; n for efavirenz + lopinavir/ritonavir alone.
[d] C_{min} of lopinavir was significantly decreased by 39%. The pharmacokinetics of ritonavir 100 mg q12h are unaffected by concurrent efavirenz.
[e] Soft gelatin capsule.
[f] 90% CI not available.

the effects of other drugs on EFV concentrations are shown in Table 14-2.[4] As drug concentrations may be altered by co-administration with other drugs known to induce CYP3A4 activity, appropriate dose adjustments may be necessary (*see section on* Dosage).

Use of lipid lowering agents together with EFV may result in decreased plasma levels of these agents. Simvastatin (SIM), atorvastatin (ATR), and pravastatin (PRA), hydroxymethylglutaryl co-enzyme A (HMG-CoA) reductase inhibitors, are also primarily metabolized via CYP3A4.

A study of the effect of EFV investigated the effect of 600 mg/day EFV on the plasma pharmacokinetics of 40 mg/day SIM, 10 mg/day ATR and 40 mg PRA. Both healthy and HIV-infected patients were examined. Results showed that EFV reduced SIM AUC exposure by 58%, reduced ATR exposure by 43%, and decreased PRA concentrations by 40%. Neither SIM nor ATR nor PRA affected the non-steady-state EFV concentrations. Thus, the normal doses of SIM, ATR, and PRA may result in diminished antilipid efficacy when combined with EFV.[19,20]

The antituberculosis drug rifampicin decreases EFV concentrations levels and a common practice has been to increase the EFV dose to 800 mg/day.[21] Caution must be taken, however, with patients of black African origin. Recent reports noted a very severe increase in EFV concentrations in some black African patients while taking both EFV and rifampicin causing significant clinical toxicity after EFV was increased to 800 mg/day.[22,23]

Dosage

The recommended dosage for adults and adolescents is 600 mg once daily, combined with a backbone of certain NRTIs or PIs. The recommended combination for initial therapy in treatment-naive adults and adolescents according to the 10 Oct 2006 Guidelines[6] are: EFV with (lamivudine or emtricitabine) and (zidovudine or tenofovir DF) but not recommended for use in first trimester of pregnancy or in women with high pregnancy potential. The alternative regimens are: EFV with (lamivudine or emtricitabine) and (abacavir or didanosine).

It is recommended that EFV be taken on an empty stomach, at bedtime. This dosing should result in the fewest side effects. High-fat foods increase EFV levels and should be avoided before dosing.

Dose adjustments may be necessary when co-administering EFV with other PYP3A4 inducers. The manufacturer's recommended dose changes, adjustments, and comments are listed in Table 14-3.[4]

Pediatric Dosing

The recommended dose for children weighing less than 88 lbs depends on the child's weight (see Table 14-4). For children (or adults) who are not able to swallow capsules, a liquid formulation of EFV is available.[4,5,24]

Table 14-2 Effect of Co-Administered Drug on Efavirenz Plasma C_{max} and AUC

Co-Administered Drug	Dose	Efavirenz Dose	Number of Subjects	Efavirenz (% Change) C_{max} (mean (90% CI))	AUC (mean (90% CI))
Indinavir	800 mg q8 h × 14 days	200 mg × 14 days	11	↔	↔
Lopinavir/ritonavir	400/100 mg q12 h × 9 days	600 mg × 9 days	11, 12[a]	↔	↓(16%) (↓38–↑15%)
Nelfinavir	750 mg q8 h × 7 days	600 mg × 7 days	10	↔	↔
Ritonavir	500 mg q12 h × 8 days	600 mg × 10 days	9	↑ (14%) (4–26%)	↑(21%) (10–34%)
Saquinavir SGC[b]	1200 mg q8 h × 10 days	600 mg × 10 days	13	↓(13%) (5–20%)	↓(12%) (10–34%)
Azithromycin	600 mg single dose	400 mg × 7 days	14	↔	↔
Clarithromycin	500 mg q12 h × 7 days	400 mg × 7 days	12	↑(11%) (3–19%)	↔
Fluconazole	200 mg × 7 days	400 mg × 7 days	10	↔	↑(16%) (6–26%)
Rifabutin	300 mg qd × 14 days	600 mg × 14 days	11	↔	↔
Rifampin	600 mg × 7 days	600 mg × 7 days	12	↓(20%) (11–28%)	↓(26%) (15–36%)
Aluminum hydroxide 400 mg, magnesium hydroxide 400 mg, plus simethicone 40 mg	30 mL single dose	400 mg single dose	17	↔	↔
Cetirizine	10 mg single dose	600 mg × 10 days	11	↔	↓(8%) (4–11%)
Ethinyl estradiol	50 μg single dose	400 mg × 10 days	13	↔	↔
Famotidine	40 mg single dose	400 mg single dose	17	↔	↔
Paroxetine	20 mg qd × 14 days	600 mg × 14 days	12	↔	↔
Sertraline	50 mg qd × 14 days	600 mg × 14 days	13	↑(11%) (6–16%)	↔
Voriconazole	400 mg po q12 h × 1 day then 200 mg po q12 h × 8 days	400 mg × 9 days		↑ (38%)[c]	↑(44%)

↑ Indicates increase; ↓ indicates decrease; ↔ indicates no change.
[a] Parallel-group design; n for efavirenz + lopinavir/ritonavir, n for efavirenz alone.
[b] Soft gelatin capsule.
[c] 90% CI not available.

TOXICITY

The most common adverse events noted during EFV therapy are rash and central nervous system symptoms.[4,25,26] Rash generally occurs at a median 9 days after start of EFV therapy. Twenty-six percent of EFV-treated patients compared to 17% in the control arms experienced rash in controlled clinical trials. Grade 4 rash occurred only in 0.1% of patients. The rash is usually self-limiting in ~16 days. EFV should be discontinued if blistering, ulceration or desquamation occurs. Rash was reported in 46% (26/57) of pediatric patients and 2/26 experienced grade 4 rash (*see section on* Pediatric Toxicities).

Fifty-three percent of patients receiving EFV in controlled trials reported central nervous system symptoms compared to 25% of patients receiving control regimens. These symptoms included, but were not limited to, dizziness (28.1%), insomnia (16.3%), impaired concentration (8.3%), somnolence

Established Drug Interactions

Table 14-3

Drug Name	Effect	Clinical Comment
Atazanavir	↓ Atazanavir	When co-administered with Sustiva in treatment-naive patients, the recommended dose of atazanavir is 300 mg with ritonavir 100 mg and Sustiva 600 mg (all once daily). Dosing recommendations for Sustiva and atazanavir in treatment-experienced patients have not been established.
Clarithromycin	↓Clarithromycin concentration ↑14-OH metabolite concentration	Plasma concentrations decreased by Sustiva; clinical significance unknown. In uninfected volunteers, 46% developed rash while receiving Sustiva and clarithromycin. No dose adjustment of Sustiva is recommended when given with clarithromycin. Alternatives to clarithromycin, such as azithromycin, should be considered (*see* Other Drugs, following table). Other macrolide antibiotics, such as erythromycin, have not been studied in combination with Sustiva.
Indinavir	↓Indinavir concentration	The optimal dose of indinavir, when given in combination with Sustiva, is not known. Increasing the indinavir dose to 1000 mg every 8 h does not compensate for the increased indinavir metabolism due to Sustiva. When indinavir at an increased dose (1000 mg every 8 h) was given with Sustiva (600 mg once daily), the indinavir AUC and C_{min} were decreased on average by 33–46% and 39–57%, respectively, compared to when indinavir (800 mg every 8 h) was given alone.
Lopinavir/ritonavir	↓Lopinavir concentration	A dose increase of lopinavir/ritonavir to 533/133 mg (four capsules or 6.5 mL) twice daily taken with food is recommended when used in combination with Sustiva.
Methadone	↓Methadone concentration	Co-administration in HIV-infected individuals with a history of injection drug use resulted in decreased plasma levels of methadone and signs of opiate withdrawal. Methadone dose was increased by a mean of 22% to alleviate withdrawal symptoms. Patients should be monitored for signs of withdrawal and their methadone dose increased as required to alleviate withdrawal symptoms.
Ethinyl estradiol	↑Ethinyl estradiol concentration	Plasma concentrations increased by Sustiva; clinical significance unknown. Because the potential interaction of efavirenz with oral contraceptives has not been fully characterized, a reliable method of barrier contraception should be used in addition to oral contraceptives.
Rifabutin	↓Rifabutin concentration	Increase daily dose of rifabutin by 50%. Consider doubling the rifabutin dose in regimens where rifabutin is given two or three times a week.
Rifampin	↓Efavirenz concentration	Clinical significance of reduced efavirenz concentrations unknown.
Ritonavir	↑Ritonavir concentration ↓Efavirenz concentration	Combination was associated with a higher frequency of adverse clinical experiences (e.g., dizziness, nausea, paresthesia) and laboratory abnormalities (elevated liver enzymes). Monitoring of liver enzymes is recommended when Sustiva is used in combination with ritonavir.
Saquinavir	↓Saquinavir concentration	Should not be used as sole protease inhibitor in combination with Sustiva.
Sertraline	↓Sertraline concentration	Increases in sertraline dose should be guided by clinical response.

Other Potentially Clinically Significant Drug or Herbal Product Interactions with Sustiva[a]

Anticoagulants: Warfarin	Plasma concentrations and effects potentially increased or decreased by Sustiva.
Anticonvulsants: Phenytoin Phenobarbital Carbamazepine	Potential for reduction in anticonvulsant and/or efavirenz plasma levels; periodic monitoring of anticonvulsant plasma levels should be conducted.
Antifungals: Itraconazole Ketoconazole	Drug interaction studies with Sustiva and these imidazole and triazole antifungals have not been conducted. Sustiva has the potential to decrease plasma concentrations of itraconazole and ketoconazole.

(Continued)

(Continued)

Table 14-3

Drug Name	Clinical Comment
Anti-HIV protease inhibitors: Saquinavir/ritonavir combination Amprenavir.	No pharmacokinetic data are available. Sustiva has the potential to decrease serum concentrations of amprenavir
NNRTIs	No studies have been performed with other NNRTIs.
St John's wort *(Hypericum perforatum)*	Expected to substantially decrease plasma levels of efavirenz; has not been studied in combination with Sustiva.

Drugs That Should Not Be Co-administered with Sustiva

Antihistamines	Astemizole
Benzodiazepines	Midazolam, triazolam
GI motility agents	Cisapride
Antimigraine	Ergot derivatives
Antifungal	Voriconazole

[a] This table is not all-inclusive.

Pediatric Dosing

Table 14-4

Pediatric Dose to Be Administered Once Daily		
Body Weight		
kg	**lbs**	**Sustiva Dose (mg)**
10 to <15	22 to <33	200
15 to <20	33 to <44	250
20 to <25	44 to <55	300
25 to <32.5	55 to <71.5	350
32.5 to <40	71.5 to <88	400
⩾40	⩾88	600

(7.0%), abnormal dreams (6.2%), and hallucinations (1.2%). These symptoms were severe in 2.0% of patients and 2.1% of patients discontinued therapy as a result. These symptoms usually begin during the first or second day of therapy and generally resolve after the first 2–4 weeks of therapy. After 4 weeks of therapy, the prevalence of nervous system symptoms of at least moderate severity ranged from 5% to 9% in patients treated with regimens containing EFV and from 3% to 5% in patients treated with a control regimen.[4,26]

The symptoms generally improve with continued therapy and are not predictive of subsequent onset of the less frequent psychiatric symptoms. Dosing at bedtime may improve the tolerability of these nervous system symptoms. Analysis of long-term data from Study 006 for patients treated with either: EFV with zidovudine and lamivudine, or EFV with indinavir, or with indinavir and zidovudine + lamivudine, showed that beyond 24 weeks of therapy the incidences of new-onset nervous system symptoms among EFV-treated patients were generally similar to those in the indinavir-containing control arm.[4]

Patients receiving EFV should be alerted to the potential for additive central nervous system effects when EFV is used concomitantly with alcohol or psychoactive drugs.

Psychiatric Symptoms

Serious psychiatric adverse experiences have been reported in patients treated with EFV. In controlled trials of 1008 patients treated with regimens containing EFV for a mean of 2.1 years and 635 patients treated with control regimens for a mean of 1.5 years, the frequency of specific serious psychiatric events among patients who received EFV or control regimens, respectively, were: severe depression (2.4%, 0.9%), suicidal ideation (0.7%, 0.3%), nonfatal suicide attempts (0.5%, 0%), aggressive behavior (0.4%, 0.5%), paranoid reactions (0.4%, 0.3%), and manic reactions (0.2%, 0.3%). When psychiatric symptoms similar to those noted above were combined and evaluated as a group in a multivariable analysis of data from Study 006, treatment with EFV was associated with an increase in the occurrence of these selected psychiatric symptoms. Other factors associated with an increase in the occurrence of these psychiatric symptoms were history of injection drug use, psychiatric history, and receipt of psychiatric medication at study entry; similar associations were observed in both the EFV and control groups. In Study 006, onset of new serious psychiatric symptoms occurred throughout the study for both EFV-treated and control-treated patients. One percent of EFV-treated patients discontinued or interrupted treatment because of one or more of these selected psychiatric symptoms. There have also been occasional postmarketing reports of death by suicide, delusions, and psychosis-like behavior; although a causal relationship to the use of EFV cannot be determined from these reports. Patients with serious psychiatric adverse experiences should seek immediate medical evaluation to assess the possibility that the symptoms may be related to the use of EFV, and if so, to determine whether the risks of continued therapy outweigh the benefits.[4]

Lipid Changes

EFV use has been associated with hyperlipidemia either when used in combination with PIs or NRTIs. Increases from baseline in total cholesterol of 10–20% have been observed in some uninfected subjects receiving EFV. In patients treated with EFV and zidovudine with lamivudine, increases from baseline in nonfasting total cholesterol and HDL of ~20% and 25%, respectively, were observed. In patients treated with EFV and indinavir, increases from baseline in nonfasting cholesterol and HDL of ~40% and 35%, respectively, were observed. Nonfasting total cholesterol levels of 240 mg/dL and 300 mg/dL were reported in 34% and 9%, respectively, of patients treated with EFV and zidovudine with lamivudine; 54% and 20%, respectively, of patients treated with EFV and indinavir; and 28% and 4%, respectively, of patients treated with indinavir and zidovudine with lamivudine. The effects of EFV on triglycerides and LDL were not well characterized since samples were taken from nonfasting patients.[4]

Liver Enzyme Abnormalities

Liver function tests should be monitored in patients with a history of hepatitis B and/or hepatitis C. In the long-term data set from Study 006, 137 patients receiving EFV-containing regimens (median duration of therapy, 68 weeks) and 84 subjects given a control regimen (median duration, 56 weeks) were seropositive at screening for hepatitis B (surface antigen-positive) and/or C (hepatitis C antibody-positive). Among the co-infected patients, elevations in aspartate transaminase (AST) to greater than five times the upper limit of normal developed in 13% of the EFV patients and in 7% of the controls. Elevations in alanine transaminase (ALT) to greater than five times the upper limit of normal occurred in 20% of the EFV patients and in 7% of the controls. Among co-infected patients, 3% of the patients receiving EFV-containing regimens and 2% of controls withdrew from the study because of liver or biliary system disorders.[27,28]

Lipodystrophy

The exact role of EFV on body fat redistribution is still unclear. Although EFV has been associated with elevated lipid levels, there has been little data linking NNRTIs to lipodystrophy.[29–31] NNRTI combinations may even be associated with less risk of lipodystrophy, according to one study. A prospective, cross-sectional, multicenter, observational, cohort study was performed throughout Germany. The objective was to identify prevalence and risk factors associated with the HIV-associated lipodystrophy syndrome after 3 years of antiretroviral therapy (ART). A total of 221 HIV-positive patients starting ART between July and September 1996 were studied. The main outcome measure was lipodystrophy, defined as otherwise unexplained truncal fat accumulation and/or fat loss in face or extremities. The findings suggested that while stavudine use and a CD4 count below 200 cells/μL may be associated with an increased risk for the development of lipodsytrophy, NNRTIs, in contrast, may be associated with a reduced risk.[32]

In a large recent study of 925 patients, the investigators found no evidence of major differences between PI and NNRTI therapy in the risk of reported body fat changes and no evidence of an association between reported fat changes and time on NNRTI therapy relative to PI therapy in those patients who used either one therapy or the other.[33]

A substudy of clinical trial BMS-034 investigated body fat changes among those patients who started therapy with either atazanavir (ATV) or EFV each given in combination with zidovudine and lamivudine. Week 48 results showed minimal change overall in both study arms.[34] Measurements were obtained by both computed tomography (CT) scans and DEXA scans, two different technologic assessments of fat distribution. Based on the results from DEXA scanning, there were no significant differences in the overall changes observed in body fat in either arm, nor was there any significant difference between the two arms of the study. CT results aimed specifically at abdominal fat, showed only a small increase in visceral fat in both arms of the study, and an even smaller increase in subcutaneous fat. These differences in change from baseline were very similar in the two regimens.

Several other EFV-switch studies have noted either no significant changes[35,36] or improvements in fat distribution after therapy switch from a PI-based regimen to an EFV-based one.[37–39]

PEDIATRIC TOXICITIES

The principal side effect of EFV seen in children is rash, which was seen in up to 40% of children compared to 27% of adults. The rash is usually maculopapular, pruritic, and mild to moderate in severity and rarely requires drug discontinuation.

Onset is typically in the first 2 weeks of treatment. While severe rash and Stevens–Johnson syndrome have been reported, this is rare. Other reported adverse events include diarrhea, nausea, and increased aminotransferase levels.[4,26,40]

PRECAUTIONS: PREGNANCY AND IMMUNE RECONSTITUTION SYNDROME

Pregnancy

EFV is in FDA pregnancy category D; EFV may cause fetal harm when administered during the first trimester of pregnancy. No adequate and well-controlled studies have been performed in pregnant women. In prospective reports, birth defects have occurred in five of 188 live births after first-trimester maternal exposure; none were neural tube defects. Four retrospective reports identified findings consistent with neural tube defects, including meningomyelocele, in mothers exposed to EFV in their first trimester. Of note, no comment was made in these four mothers regarding use of prenatal folate administration. Although a causal relationship has not been established, similar defects have been observed in preclinical studies of EFV.[4,6]

Two methods of birth control (a barrier method in combination with a nonbarrier method such as an oral or other hormonal contraceptive) should be used to avoid pregnancy in women taking EFV. Before initiating therapy with EFV, women of childbearing potential should undergo pregnancy testing. It is recommended that EFV not be given to pregnant women except in situations in which there are no therapeutic alternatives. It is not known whether EFV is distributed into breast milk in humans; however, EFV is distributed into the milk of laboratory animals. Breastfeeding is not recommended during EFV therapy.[4]

Immune Reconstitution Syndrome

Updated information from 168 weeks of follow up from the 006 study includes data regarding immune reconstitution syndrome. This syndrome has been reported in patients treated with combination ART, including EFV. During the initial phase of combination antiretroviral treatment, patients whose immune system responds may develop an inflammatory response to indolent or residual opportunistic infections (such as *Mycobacterium avium* infection, cytomegalovirus, *Pneumocystis carinii* pneumonia, or tuberculosis), which may necessitate further evaluation and treatment.[27,28]

ADULT CLINICAL TRIALS, EFFICACY

Table 14-5 summarizes aspects of some major trials of EFV.

Study 006

Study 006 was a ground breaking trial that showed for the first time that an EFV-containing regimen with a nucleoside backbone was as effective as the gold-standard PI-containing regimen. The EFV, with NRTI combination demonstrated greater antiviral activity and better tolerance than the indinavir regimen.[26]

The study subjects were 450 patients who had not previously been treated with lamivudine or any NNRTI or PI. In this open-label study, patients were randomly assigned to one of three regimens: EFV (600 mg daily) with zidovudine (300 mg twice daily) and lamivudine (150 mg twice daily); the PI indinavir (800 mg every 8 h) with zidovudine and lamivudine; or EFV with indinavir (1000 mg every 8 h).

Suppression of plasma HIV-1 RNA to undetectable levels was achieved in more patients in the group given EFV with NRTIs than in the group given indinavir with NRTIs (70% vs 48%, $P < 0.001$). The efficacy of the regimen of EFV with indinavir was similar (53%) to that of the regimen of indinavir, zidovudine, and lamivudine. Figures 14-2 and 14-3 show the viral load reduction in all three arms. The EFV plus two NRTIs arm had a significantly greater percentage of patients with undetectable viremia (less than 400 copies and less than 50 copies/mL) than the two arms containing indinavir.

CD4 cell counts increased significantly with all combinations (range of increases, 180–201 cells/mL). More patients discontinued treatment because of adverse events in the group given indinavir and two NRTIs than in the group given EFV and two NRTIs (43% vs 27%, $P = 0.005$).

The conclusions from the 006 study were that as ART in adults, the combination of EFV with zidovudine and lamivudine has greater antiviral activity and was better tolerated than the combination of indinavir, zidovudine, and lamivudine.

BMS 034 Trial

The BMS 034 trial involved ATV versus EFV in 805 treatment-naive patients. It was a large multicenter, randomized trial of ATV versus EFV with zidovudine and lamivudine in 805 ART-naive patients.[41] Equal potency of the two regimens was a main result of this trial, with 70% of ATV recipients achieving HIV RNA less than 400 copies/mL versus 64% of EFV recipients by ITT (intent-to-treat), NC = F (noncompleters = failures) analysis (95% CI 1.2–11.7% for the difference between arms). CD4 cell count gain was comparable between the arms with the ATV arm gaining 176 cells as against 160 cells/mL in the EFV arm.

Lipid profiles were more favorable in the ATV arm, with changes of +1% versus +18% in LDL cholesterol and −9% and +23% in triglycerides in the ATV and EFV arms, respectively. Five percent of ATV patients developed jaundice or scleral icterus, a known side effect of ATV.[42]

ATV plasma concentration levels – AUC and C_{min} – are severely decreased when combined with EFV (see Table 14-1).

FOCUS Trial

In the FOCUS study,[43] saquinavir-soft gel capsules (SGC)/low-dose ritonavir was compared to EFV in a 48-week open-label study of 152 HIV-positive, ART-naive patients. Each study drug was combined with two NRTIs. The patients were randomized to receive either EFV or saquinavir (1600 mg boosted with 100 mg of ritonavir) once daily, together with two nucleoside analogs, which were not dosed once daily.

The median baseline viral load was 4.7 $\log_{10}$ and the median CD4 cell count was ~320 in each group. In the week 48 ITT analysis, 71% of those who received EFV had viral load below 50 copies (undetectable) at week 24, compared with 51% of those who received saquinavir ($P = 0.008$).

Summary of Major Trials of Efavirenz

Table 14-5

Trial	Drug Regimen	Patients	Status	Ref.
Phase I Studies				
Efavirenz-001	Efavirenz single dose 100–1600 mg	94 Healthy adult male volunteers: 70 efavirenz, 24 placebo	Completed	5
Efavirenz-002	Efavirenz multiple doses 200–400 mg qd+3–10 days	23 Healthy adult male volunteers: 17 efavirenz, 6 placebo	Completed	5
Efavirenz-019	Efavirenz 400 mg qd + NFV 750 mg tid; 14-day study	20 Healthy volunteers	Completed	38
Phase II Studies				
Efavirenz-003	Efavirenz 200, 400, 600 mg qd IDV 800, 1000, 1200 mg q8 h; 8 cohorts	+ 101 HIV-infected pts: all PI- and NNRTI-naive	Completed	13–19
Efavirenz-004	ZDV 300 mg PO bid + 3TC 150 mg PO bid + efavirenz 400 or 600 mg qd or placebo	97 HIV-infected pts; minimum 8 weeks of ZDV + 3TC	Completed	23
Efavirenz-005	ZDV 300 mg PO bid + 3TC 150 mg PO bid + efavirenz 200, 400, 600 mg qd or placebo	137 HIV-infected pts; antiretroviral drug-naive	Completed	12,22
Efavirenz-020	Blinded, 2 arms: two nucleoside agents + IDV 800 mg tid + efavirenz placebo qd **or** IDV 1000 mg tid + efavirenz 600 mg qd	184 HIV-infected pts	Completed	25
Efavirenz-024	Open-label, two strata: NFV 750 mg tid + efavirenz 600 mg qd	62 HIV-infected pts: 32 antiretroviral drug-naive, 30 nucleoside-experienced	Completed	26
Phase III Studies				
Efavirenz-006	Open-label, three arms: ZDV +3TC + efavirenz 600 mg qd, IDV 1000 mg tid + efavirenz 600 mg qd, ZDV + 3TC + IDV 800 mg tid	1236 HIV-infected pts	Ongoing (phase 3)	6, 26
ACTG 364	Blinded, three arms: two NRTI + efavirenz 600 mg qd + NFV 750 mg tid **or** two NRTIs + efavirenz 600 mg qd **or** two NRTIs + NFV 750 mg tid	196 HIV-infected pts	Completed	27
Pediatric Studies				
PACTG 382+	Open-label: one or more NRTIs +efavirenz (dose adjusted) +NFV (dose adjusted)	57 HIV-infected children	Completed	30

IDV, indinavir; NFV, nelfinavir; NRTI, nucleoside agent; PI, protease inhibitor; 3TC, lamivudine; ZDV, zidovudine.

Thirty-one percent of the saquinavir group discontinued their assigned treatment by week 24 compared to 20% of the EFV group. Eight patients stopped saquinavir due to adverse events compared to one discontinuation due to adverse events in the EFV arm.[43]

2NN Trial

The 2NN Study was a large, randomized, head-to-head comparison trial of the two NNRTIs nevirapine and EFV in 1216 ART-naive patients.[44] The subjects were assigned nevirapine 400 mg

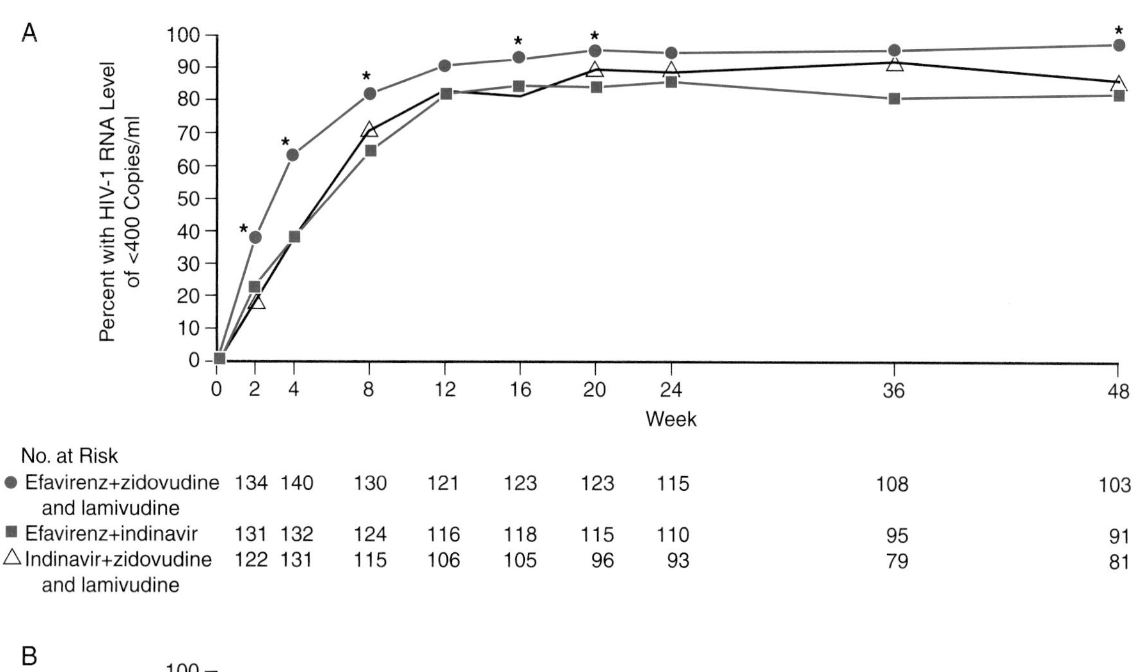

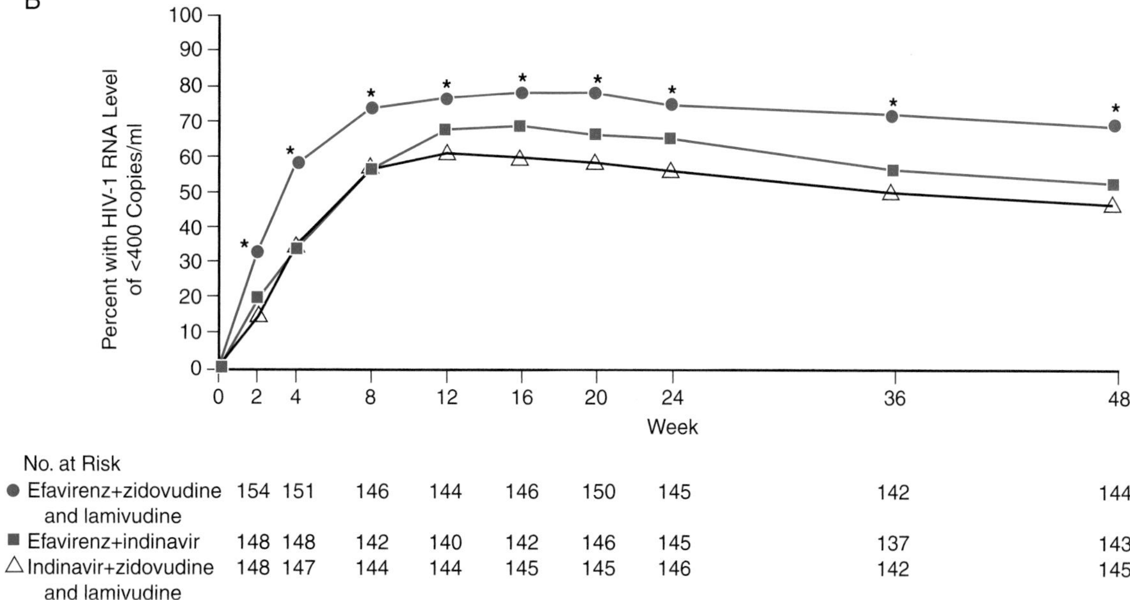

Figure 14-2 ■ Study 006 – percentage of patients with plasma HIV-1 RNA levels of less than 400 copies/mL, according to an analysis based on the treatment-received (panel A) and the ITT analysis (panel B). Asterisks denote statistically significant differences ($P < 0.05$) from indinavir plus zidovudine and lamivudine.

Redrawn from Staszewski S, Morales-Ramirez J, Tashima KT, et al. A phase III, multicenter, randomized study comparing the antiretroviral activity and tolerability of efavirenz plus indinavir, versus efavirenz plus zidovudine and lamivudine, versus indinavir plus zidovudine and lamivudine in treatment naive HIV-1 infected patients (Study 006). N Engl J Med 341:1865–73, 1999.

once daily, nevirapine 200 mg twice daily, EFV 600 mg once daily, or nevirapine (400 mg) and EFV (800 mg) once daily, with stavudine and lamivudine, for 48 weeks.

Results showed that both the NNRTIs provided similar antiviral and immunologic efficacy as first-line regimens over 48 weeks of treatment. The primary endpoint in the 2NN Study was the proportion of patients with treatment failure (less than 1 $\log_{10}$ decline in plasma HIV-1 RNA in the first 12 weeks or two consecutive measurements of more than 50 copies/mL from week 24 onward, disease progression (any new Centers for Disease Control and Prevention (CDC) grade C event or death), or change of treatment).

Treatment failure occurred in 96 (43.6%) of 220 patients given nevirapine once daily, 169 (43.7%) of 387 assigned to nevirapine twice daily, 151 (37.8%) of 400 randomized to EFV, and 111 (53.1%) of 209 patients in the nevirapine with EFV arm. The difference between nevirapine twice daily and EFV was 5.9% (95% CI −0.9–12.8). There were

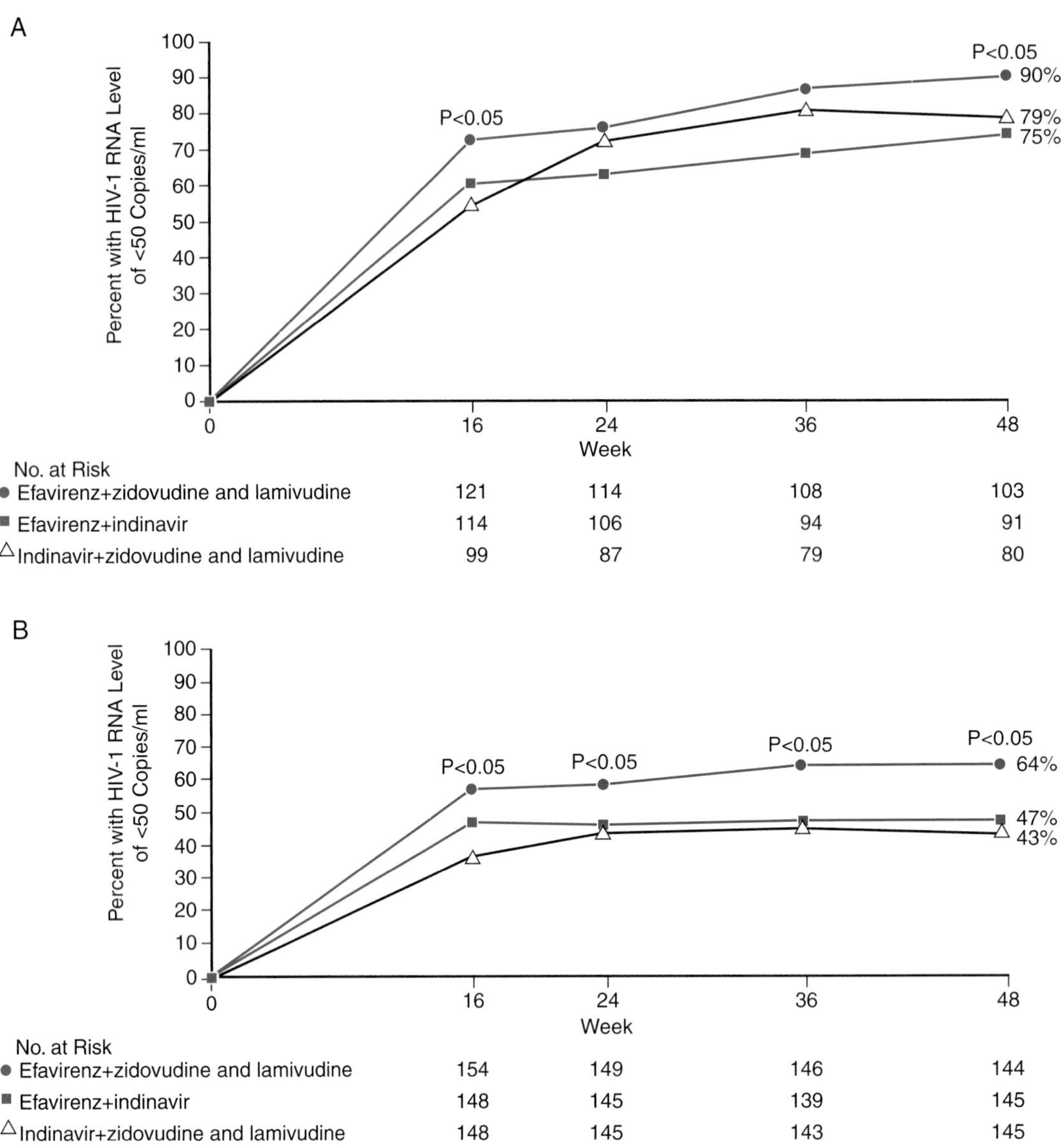

Figure 14-3 ■ Study 006 – percentage of patients with plasma HIV-1 RNA levels of less than 50 copies/mL, according to an analysis based on the treatment-received (panel A) and the ITT analysis (panel B). *P* values are for the comparison with the group given indinavir plus zidovudine and lamivudine.

Redrawn from Staszewski S, Morales-Ramirez J, Tashima KT, et al. A phase III, multicenter, randomized study comparing the antiretroviral activity and tolerability of efavirenz plus indinavir, versus efavirenz plus zidovudine and lamivudine, versus indinavir plus zidovudine and lamivudine in treatment naive HIV-1 infected patients (Study 006). N Engl J Med 341:1865–73, 1999.

no significant differences among the study groups in the proportions with plasma HIV-1 RNA concentrations below 50 copies/mL at week 48 ($P = 0.193$) or the increases in CD4 cells ($P = 0.800$).

Using both nevirapine and EFV simultaneously was associated with the highest frequency of clinical adverse events while not improving efficacy. Nevirapine used once daily resulted in significantly more hepatobiliary laboratory toxicities than EFV. Of 25 observed deaths, two were attributed to nevirapine.[45]

A pharmacokinetic substudy investigated whether any patient characteristics might have affected plasma levels. Significant findings demonstrated that nevirapine clearance (and therefore interindividual variability) was significantly affected by female gender, hepatitis B virus infection and geographic location, whereas EFV clearance was only significantly affected by concomitant nevirapine administration or geographic location and not by gender or hepatitis virus infection. Clearance of both drugs was similar throughout the study.[46]

BIKS Trial

The BIKS trial, an open-label, single-arm nonrandomized multicenter study of lopinavir/ritonavir (LPV/r) with EFV without NRTIs.[46] LPV/r was given at a dose of 533/100 mg (four capsules) bid to compensate for the drug interaction –EFV increases its clearance and results in lower drug levels.

The study enrolled 86 patients with CD4+ cell counts greater than 100 cells/mL and viral loads of greater than 5000 copies/mL who were either antiretroviral-naive or treatment-experienced but had no NNRTI experience and not more than one PI failure.

At 48 weeks, 69% of patients had viral loads less than 50 copies/mL in an ITT analysis. There was only one virologic failure and it occurred in the treatment-naive group. One-fourth of the patients discontinued the trial for reasons such as nonadherence and side effects. Grade 3 or 4 increases in cholesterol developed in 28% of subjects and equivalent increases in triglycerides developed in 13%.

The BIKS-2 study is the 2-year follow up of BIKS. Fifty-nine patients were included. At month 12 (post-week-48 follow-up), viral load of less than 400 copies/mL was achieved in 100% and 78% of the patients, and less than 50 copies/mL in 98% and 77%, in on-treatment (OT) and ITT analysis, respectively. The mean increase in CD4 cell count was +360 cells/mL (+108 cells/mL during the 12 months of follow-up) and fasting triglycerides, total cholesterol, HDL and LDL remained stable.[47]

Hippocampe – ANRS 121 Trial

The hippocampe trial was initially constructed to evaluate a first-line, nucleoside-sparing regimen consisting of an NNRTI plus a boosted-PI versus a standard-of-care nucleoside-backbone PI or NNRTI regimen in therapy-naive patients.

The primary study outcome was to be evaluation of fat loss between baseline and week 96 as measured by CT scan and anthropomorphic measurements. This main analysis was never conducted because the study was terminated early.[48]

One hundred and seventeen ARV-naive patients with a baseline viral load of greater than 5000 copies/mL and a CD4 count of greater than 350 cells/mL were randomized 2:1:1 to receive a nucleoside-sparing regimen (PI with NNRTI) (n = 60) or a standard-of-care regimen of two NRTIs with a boosted PI (n = 29) or an NNRTI (n = 28). The drugs that were chosen as percentage of the drug class were: lopinavir/ritonavir (78%) and indinavir/ritonavir (22%) for the PIs; EFV (63%) and nevirapine (37%) for the NNRTIs; and any acceptable NRTI backbone with the exception of stavudine or zalcitabine. Baseline characteristics among the groups were similar.[48]

A series of planned virologic analysis conducted at 12, 24, and 36 weeks between the nucleoside-sparing regimen group and the standard-of-care group showed that the percentage of patients with a viral load less than 400 copies/mL was not significantly different between the two groups. There were also no differences in CD4 cell count responses, adherence, or the incidence of adverse events. However, the percentage of patients with a plasma viral load less than 50 copies/mL was not only statistically different but also statistically inferior in the nucleoside-sparing regimen arm over 36 weeks of follow-up: at week 12, 37% versus 58% (P = 0.027); at week 24, 60% versus 81% (P = 0.016); and at week 36, 62% versus 79% (P = 0.046).Therefore, the study was discontinued in July 2005.[48]

Adult ACTG A5116

A5116 was a randomized, open-label study of LPV/r (533 mg/133 mg twice daily) with EFV (600 mg once daily) versus EFV with two NRTIs in subjects who received at least 18 months of a three or four drug PI- or NNRTI-based regimen as a first regimen, had plasma HIV-1 RNA levels 200 copies/mL or less, and no documented phenotypic resistance.[49] Study endpoints were virologic failure (plasma HIV-1 RNA greater than 200 copies/mL) or toxicity-related discontinuation of any component of randomized treatment.

A total of 236 patients (118 per arm) were followed a median of 110 weeks. For the EFV with two NRTI arm, 92 (78%) received zidovudine with lamivudine and 22 (19%) stavudine with 3TC.

Treatment with EFV with two NRTIs led to lower rates of regimen failure than treatment with LPV/r with EFV, due to decreased toxicity and a trend toward reduced virologic failure. Overall, 16 (7%) of the endpoints were virologic failure and 25 (11%) were toxicity-related treatment discontinuations. Low virologic failure rates were observed in both arms in this study, though there was a trend toward a higher failure rate in the LPV/r with EFV. Toxicity-related endpoints occurred more often in the LPV/r + EFV arm than the EFV with NRTI arm (17% vs 5%, respectively) due mainly to differences in triglyceride levels. Higher triglyceride and cholesterol levels were seen in the LPV/r with EFV arm with no effect seen on glucose or insulin levels. During long-term follow-up, higher CD4 cell counts occurred in the LPV/r with EFV arm but were not statistically significant.[49]

PEDIATRIC EFFICACY

According to Pediatric Guidelines, EFV is the 'strongly recommended' NNRTI for use in a combination regimen for initial treatment of children over age 3 years who can swallow capsules.[5] It is administered once daily and can be given with food (but avoid high fat meals). EFV in combination with one or two NRTIs and nelfinavir has been shown to produce sustained and durable viral suppression in a large proportion of treated children. An open-label study of EFV combined with nelfinavir and one or two NRTIs, the PACTG 382 Trial, was performed in 57 pediatric patients some as young as age 3 years.[40] In an ITT analysis, at 48 weeks of therapy, 76% of children had plasma HIV RNA levels <400 copies/mL, and 63% had HIV RNA levels <50 copies/mL. The median times to achieve those levels were 4 and 20 weeks, respectively. Therefore, children with detectable HIV-RNA greater than 50 copies/mL by the ultrasensitive RNA assay after

1 month of therapy continued to accrue some virologic benefit through 5 months of treatment with this regimen.[50]

Although there are no data in children, a PI-sparing regimen of EFV with two NRTIs has had similar efficacy in infected adults.[26] Based on these adult data, the latter PI-sparing combination offers an alternative to children when issues of adherence or use of PIs are problematic. There are currently no pharmacokinetic data available on appropriate dosage of EFV in children under age 3 years. A liquid formulation of EFV is under study to determine appropriate dosage in children under the age of 3 years or who weigh less than 13 kg, but data are not yet available.[5] In a study of children aged 3–9 years, the safety, pharmacokinetics, antiviral activity and immunologic effects of EFV liquid formulation, nelfinavir and NRTIs were studied. The combination was well tolerated.[24]

Pharmacokinetic values were similar to those observed in a previous study of older children who received EFV capsules in combination with nelfinavir and NRTIs.[40] After 48 weeks of therapy 63% of subjects had plasma HIV RNA levels of less than 400 copies/mL, and 58% had less than 50 copies/mL in an ITT analysis. CD4 cell count and percentage rose significantly over this time. Combination therapy with EFV liquid formulation, nelfinavir and NRTIs is a treatment option for HIV-infected children older than 3 years of age who are unable to take EFV capsules.[24]

DRUG RESISTANCE

The major disadvantage of currently available NNRTIs is their low genetic barrier for development of resistance. These agents only require a single mutation to confer resistance, and cross resistance often develops across the entire class. In the case of EFV, high-level resistance can occur with a single mutation (lysine to asparagine), typically in the 103 position. As a result, patients who fail this initial regimen may lose the utility of other NNRTIs and/or may transmit NNRTI-resistant virus to others.[6]

In vitro studies demonstrated that HIV-1 isolates with reduced susceptibility to EFV (>380-fold increase in IC_{90} value) emerged rapidly under *in vitro* selection. Genotypic characterization of these viruses identified mutations resulting in single amino acid substitutions L100I or V179D, double substitutions L100I/V108I, and triple substitutions L100I/V179D/Y181C in RT.[51,52] A highly EFV-resistant virus which had two mutations, the L100I and K103N,[51] produced the highest resistance to EFV of all the single amino acid substitutions.[4,51,52]

In vivo, the most frequently observed mutation develops at position K103N which confers resistance to EFV and is associated with virologic failure. It occurs in at least 90% of cases at time of treatment failure when an NNRTI mutation is present. Other mutations which decrease susceptibility to EFV occur at positions 98, 100, 101, 106, 108, 179, 181, and 188, 190, 225, and 227.[4,53,54]

Cross-resistance to EFV is likely with delavirdine (DLV)-resistant virus and also with nevirapine-resistant virus; the extent of resistance may vary depending on which mutations are present. Clinical isolates previously characterized as EFV-resistant were also phenotypically resistant *in vitro* to DLV and nevirapine compared to baseline. DLV- and/or NVP-resistant clinical viral isolates with NNRTI resistance-associated substitutions (A98G, L100I, K101E/P, K103N/S, V106A, Y181X, Y188X, G190X, P225H, F227L, or M230L) showed reduced susceptibility to EFV *in vitro*.[4] Viruses exhibiting the K103N or Y188L mutations have shown cross-resistance to all of the presently available NNRTIs (EFV, nevirapine, and DLV).[4,54,55]

CONCLUSIONS

EFV is an NNRTI with potent activity against HIV-1. It also offers the convenience of once-daily dosing. The US Department of Health and Human Services guidelines for the use of antiretroviral agents in HIV-1-infected adults and adolescents and the IAS-USA guidelines recommend that EFV, together with RT inhibitors, be the preferred NNRTI-based regimen for HIV-treatment-naive patients. It may also be used as part of a combination therapy for salvage regimens in treatment-experienced patients. Clinicians should note that resistance to EFV or nevirapine results in NNRTI-class-wide resistance. Patients who experience virologic failure with either one of these drugs are unlikely to benefit from therapy with the other. Although DLV is rarely used, DLV-experienced patients may have developed and archived resistance mutations in the past which could cause resistance to EFV.

REFERENCES

1. Young SD, Britcher SF, Tran LO, et al. L-743, 726 (DMP-266): a novel, highly potent non-nucleoside inhibitor of the human immunodeficiency virus type 1 reverse transcriptase. Antimicrob Agents Chemother 39:2602–5, 1995.
2. FDA new drug application NDA 20-972/S-019.
3. Efavirenz® (efavirenz) product information. Princeton, NJ: Bristol-Myers Squibb. Available: www.sustive.com revised Feb 2005.
4. AIDSinfo Technical version, Efavirenz. US Dept. of Health and Human Services. Available: http://aidsinfo.nih.gov.
5. Package Insert: SUSTIVA® (efavirenz) capsules and tablets. Princeton, NJ: Bristol-Myers Squibb. Based on package insert dated February 2005, 51-022486-06, 1187089; revised Apr 2005.
6. Guidelines for the Use of Antiretroviral Agents in Pediatric HIV Infection, 3 Nov 2005. Available: http://AIDSinfo.nih.gov. Working Group on Antiretroviral Therapy and Medical Management of HIV-Infected Children convened by the National Resource Center at the François-Xavier Bagnoud Center, UMDNJ, the Health Resources and Services Administration (HRSA); and the National Institutes of Health (NIH).
7. DHHS Guidelines for the Use of Antiretroviral Agents in HIV-1-Infected Adults and Adolescents, 13 Nov 2006. Available: http://AIDSinfo.nih.gov.
8. U.S. Public Health Service Guidelines for the Management of Occupational Exposures to HBV, HCV, and HIV and Recommendations for Postexposure Prophylaxis. MMWR

50(No. RR-11): 12, 2001. Available: http://www.aidsinfo.nih.gov/guidelines/health-care/HC_062901.pdf.
9. Fiske WD, Nibbelink DW, Brennan JM, et al. DMP 266 cerebrospinal fluid concentrations (CSF) after oral administration. In: 37th Interscience Conference on Antomicrobial Agents and Chemotherapy (ICAAC), Toronto, ON, Canada, 1997, abstract A-12.
10. Fiske WD, Brennan JM, Haines PJ, et al. Efavirenz (DMP 266) cerebrospinal fluid concentrations (CSF) after chronic oral administration to cynomolgus monkeys. In: 5th Conference on Retroviruses and Opportunistic Infections (CROI), Chicago, IL, USA, 1998, abstract 640.
11. Tashima KT, Caliendo AM, Ahmad M, et al. Cerebrospinal fluid human immunodeficiency virus type 1 (HIV-1) suppression and efavirenz drug concentrations in HIV-1-infected patients receiving combination therapy. J Infect Dis 180:862–4, 1999.
12. Taylor S, Allen S, Fidler S, et al. Stop study: after discontinuation of efavirenz, plasma concentrations may persist for 2 weeks or longer. In: 11th Conference on Retroviruses and Opportunistic Infections (CROI), San Francisco, CA, USA, 2004, abstract 131.
13. Ribaudo HJ, Haas DW, Tierney C, et al; Adult AIDS Clinical Trials Group Study. Pharmacogenetics of plasma efavirenz exposure after treatment discontinuation: an Adult AIDS Clinical Trials Group Study. Clin Infect Dis 42:401–7, 2006.
14. Ribaudo H, Clifford D, Gulick R, et al. Relationships between efavirenz pharmacokinetics, side effects, drug discontinuation, virologic response, and race: results from ACTG A5095/A5097s. In: 11th Conference on Retroviruses and Opportunistic Infections (CROI), San Francisco, CA, USA, 2004, abstract 132.
15. Hitti JE, Caten E, Cohn SE, et al. Sex, race and weight as covariates in the pharmacokinetics of efavirenz, indinavir and nelfinavir. In: 11th Conference on Retroviruses and Opportunistic Infections (CROI), San Francisco, CA, USA, 2004, abstract 604.
16. Taylor S, Allen S, Smit E, et al. Stop study: after discontinuation of efavirenz, plasma concentrations may persist for >2 weeks. In: 10th Conference of the British HIV Association (BHIVA), Cardiff, UK, 2004, abstract 10:O6.
17. Haas D, Ribaudo H, Kim R, et al. A common CYP2B6 variant is associated with efavirenz pharmacokinetics and central nervous system side effects: AACTG study NWCS214. In: 11th Conference on Retroviruses and Opportunistic Infections (CROI), San Francisco, CA, USA, 2004, abstract 133.
18. Haas DW, Ribaudo HJ, Kim RB, et al. Pharmacogenetics of efavirenz and central nervous system side effects: an Adult AIDS Clinical Trials Group study. AIDS18:2391–400, 2004.
19. Gerber JG, Fichtenbaum J, Rosenkranz S, et al; The ACTG A5108 team. Efavirenz is a significant inducer of simvastatin and atorvastatin metabolism: results of ACTG A5108 study. In: 11th CROI, San Francisco, CA, USA, 8–11 Feb 2004, abstract 603.
20. Gerber JG, Rosenkranz SL, Fichtenbaum CJ, et al for the AIDS Clinical Trials Group A5108 Team. Effect of efavirenz on the pharmacokinetics of simvastatin, atorvastatin, and pravastatin. JAIDS 39:307–12, 2005.
21. Pozniak AL, Miller RF, Lipman MC, et al; BHIVA Guidelines Writing Committee. BHIVA Treatment Guidelines for Tuberculosis/HIV Infection 2005. HIV Med 6(Suppl 2):62–83, 2005.
22. Brennan-Benson P, Lyus R, Harrison T, et al. Pharmacokinetic interactions between efavirenz and rifampicin in the treatment of HIV and tuberculosis: one size does not fit all. AIDS 19:1541–3, 2005.
23. Crowe G, Khoo SH. Toxic levels of efavirenz two weeks after stopping therapy. In: BHIVA Conference, Dublin, Ireland, 20–23 Apr 2005, abstract P61.
24. Starr SE, Fletcher CV, Spector SA, et al; PACTG 382 Study Team. Pediatric AIDS Clinical Trials Group. Efavirenz liquid formulation inhuman immunodeficiency virus-infected children. Pediatr Infect Dis J 21:659–63, 2002.
25. Hicks C, Hass D, Seekins D, et al; Dupont Merck Pharmaceutical Company Clinical Development Team. A phase 11, double-blind, placebo-controlled, dose ranging study to assess the antiretroviral activity and safety of DMP 266 (efavirenz, SUSTIVA™) in combination with open-label zidovudine (ZDV) with lamivudine (3TC) [DMP 266-005]. In: 5th Conference on Retroviruses and Opportunistic Infections (CROI) Chicago, Illinois, 1998, abstract 698.
26. Staszewski S, Morales-Ramirez J, Tashima KT, et al. A phase III, multicenter, randomized study comparing the antiretroviral activity and tolerability of efavirenz plus indinavir, versus efavirenz plus zidovudine and lamivudine, versus indinavir plus zidovudine and lamivudine in treatment naive HIV-1 infected patients (Study 006). N Engl J Med 341:1865–73, 1999.
27. Klein R, Struble K. US Food and Drug Administration. Sustiva labeling changes. FDA News 17 Aug 2004.
28. Tashima K, Staszewski S, Nelson M, et al. Efavirenz (Sustiva)-based HAART: 168 weeks of follow-up (3–4 yrs) of original 006 EFV pivotal study. In: XV International AIDS Conference, Bangkok, 11–16 Jul 2004, abstract TuPeB4547.
29. Tashima K, Stryker R, Skiest D, et al. Lack of clinical lipodystrophy in patients receiving efavirenz + NRTIs in study 006. In: 39th Interscience Conference on Antimicrobial Agents and Chemotherapy, San Francisco, CA, USA, 1999, abstract 1301.
30. Rickerts V, Bickel M, Tews J, et al. A case of lipodystrophy after the initiation of zidovudine, lamivudine and efavirenz in an asymptomatic HIV-1-infected patient. HIV Med 1:164–5, 2000.
31. Caso JA, Prieto Jde M, Casas E, Sanz J. Gynecomastia without lipodystrophy syndrome in HIV-infected men treated with efavirenz. AIDS 15:1447–8, 2001.
32. Mauss S, Corzillius M, Wolf E, et al; DAGNA Lipantiretroviral therapy study group. Risk factors for the HIV-associated lipodystrophy syndrome in a closed cohort of patients after 3 years of antiretroviral treatment. HIV Med 3:49–55, 2002.
33. Young J, Rickenbach M, Weber R, et al. Body fat changes among antiretroviral-naive patients on PI- and NNRTI-based HAART in the Swiss HIV cohort study. Antivir Ther 10:73–81, 2005.
34. Jemsek JG, Arathoon E, Arlotti M, et al. Body fat effects of atazanavir (ATV) and efavirenz (EFV) each combined with fixed-dose zidovudine (ZDV) and lamivudine (3TC): 48-week results from the metabolic substudy of BMS-034. In: 2nd IAS Conference on HIV Pathogenesis and Treatment; Paris, France, 13–16 Jul 2003, abstract LB-13.
35. Gharakhanian S, Salhi Y, Adda N, et al. Identification of fat redistribution/metabolic anomalies in a cohort treated by 2 NRTIs + 1 PI, and absence of significant modification following PI-substitution. In: Seventh Conference on Retroviruses and Opportunistic Infections (CROI), San Francisco, CA, USA, 30 Jan to 4 Feb 2000, abstract 46.
36. Bonnet E, Lepec R, Bluteau M, et al. Evolution of lipodystrophy syndrome and lipidic profile in HIV patients after switching from protease inhibitors to efavirenz. In: Seventh Conference on Retroviruses and Opportunistic Infections (CROI), San Francisco, CA, USA, 30 Jan to 4 Feb 2000, abstract 49.
37. Bickel M, Rickerts V, Stephan C, et al. PROTRA 1 (Protease Inhibitor Transfer Study): abacavir and efavirenz in combination as a substitute for a protease inhibitor in heavily pre-treated HIV-1 infected patients with undetectable plasma HIV-1 RNA. HIV Med 6:179–84, 2005.
38. Viciana P, Alarcon A, Martin D, et al. Partial improvement of lipodystrophy after switching from HIV-1 protease inhibitors (PI) to efavirenz (EFV). In: Seventh Conference on Retroviruses and Opportunistic Infections (CROI), San Francisco, CA, USA, 30 Jan to 4 Feb 2000, abstract 48.

39. Martinez E, Blanco JL, Garcia MA, et al. Impact of switching from HIV-1 protease inhibitors (PI) to efavirenz (EFV) in patients with lipodystrophy. In: Seventh Conference on Retroviruses and Opportunistic Infections (CROI), San Francisco, CA, USA, 30 Jan to 4 Feb 2000, abstract 50.
40. Starr SE, Fletcher CV, Spector SA, et al. Combination therapy with efavirenz, nelfinavir, and nucleoside reverse-transcriptase inhibitors in children infected with human immunodeficiency virus type 1. Pediatric AIDS Clinical Trials Group 382 Team. N Engl J Med 341:1874–81, 1999.
41. Squires K, Lazzarin A, Gatell JM, et al. Comparison of once-daily atazanavir with efavirenz, each in combination with fixed-dose zidovudine and lamivudine, as initial therapy for patients infected with HIV. J Acquir Immune Defic Syndr 36:1011–19, 2004.
42. Squires K, Thiry A, Giordano M for the AI424-034 International Study Team. Atazanavir (ATV) QD and efavirenz (EFV) QD with fixed-dose ZDV + 3TC: comparison of antiviral efficacy and safety through wk 24 (AI424-034). In: 42nd Interscience Conference on Antimicrobial Agents and Chemotherapy (ICAAC), San Diego, CA, USA, 27–30 Sep 2002, abstract H-1076.
43. Montaner JSG, Schutz M, Schwartz R, et al. Efficacy, safety and pharmacokinetics of once-daily saquinavir soft-gelatin capsule/ritonavir in antiretroviral-naive, HIV-infected patients. Med Gen Med 8:36, 2006
44. van Leth F, Phanuphak P, Ruxrungtham K, et al for the 2NN Study team. Comparison of first-line antiretroviral therapy with regimens including nevirapine, efavirenz, or both drugs, plus stavudine and lamivudine: a randomised open-label trial, the 2NN Study. Lancet 363:1253–63, 2004.
45. Kappelhoff BS, Huitema ADR, van Leth FCM, et al (for the 2NN Study Group). Nevirapine and efavirenz pharmacokinetics and covariate analysis in the 2NN Study. Antivir Ther 10:145–55, 2005.
46. Raffi F, Allavena C, Delfraissy J, et al. 48-week final results of lopinavir/r (LPV/r)-efavirenz (EFV) combination (BIKS Study). In: Program and Abstracts of the 44th Interscience Conference of Antimicrobial Agents and Chemotherapy (ICAAC), Washington, DC, 30 Oct to 2 Nov 2004, abstract H-569.
47. Allavena C, Bonnet B, Michelet C, et al. 2-year follow-up lopinavir/ritonavir (LPV/r-efavirenz (EFV)) combination. In: Program and Abstracts of the 3rd IAS Conference on HIV Pathogenesis and Treatment, Rio de Janeiro, Brazil, 24–27 Jul 2005, abstract WePe6.3C06 (poster).
48. Duvivier C, Ghosn J, Assoumou L, et al. Lower rate of virological suppression in naive patients initiating HAART with NRTI-sparing regimen compared to standard NRTI-containing regimen: results from hippocampe – ANRS 121 Trial. In: 10th European AIDS Conference (EACS), Dublin, Ireland, 17–20 Nov 2005, abstract PS1/3.
49. Fischl M, Bassett R, Collier A, et al; Adult AIDS Clinical Trials Group. Randomized, controlled trial of lopinavir/ritonavir + efavirenz vs efavirenz + 2 nucleoside reverse transcriptase inhibitors following a first suppressive 3- or 4-drug regimen in advanced HIV disease. In: 12th Conference on Retroviruses and Opportunistic Infections (CROI), Boston, MA, USA, 22–25 Feb 2005, abstract 162.
50. Spector SA, Yong FH, Cabral S, et al. Patterns of plasma human immunodeficiency virus type 1 RNA response to highly active antiretroviral therapy in infected children. J Infect Dis 182:1769–73, 2000.
51. Young SD, Britcher SF, Tran LO, et al. L-743, 726 (DMP-266): a novel, highly potent nonnucleoside inhibitor of the human immunodeficiency virus type 1 reverse transcriptase. Antimicrob Agents Chemother 39:2602–5, 1995.
52. Winslow DL, Garber S, Reid C, et al. Selection conditions affect the evolution of specific mutations in the reverse transcriptase gene associated with resistance to DMP 266. AIDS 10:1205–9, 1996.
53. Bacheler LT, Anton ED, Kudish P, et al. Human immunodeficiency virus type 1 mutations selected in patients failing efavirenz combination therapy. Antimicrob Agents Chemother 44:2475–84, 2000.
54. Bacheler L, Jeffrey S, Hanna G, et al. Genotypic correlates of phenotypic resistance to efavirenz in virus isolates from patients failing nonnucleoside reverse transcriptase inhibitor therapy. J Virol 75:4999–5008, 2001.
55. Bacheler LT. Resistance to non-nucleoside inhibitors of HIV-1 reverse transcriptase. Drug Resist Updat 2:56–67, 1999.

Chapter 15

Saquinavir

Anton Posniak, MD, FRCP, Kasha P. Singh, MBBS, FRACP

INTRODUCTION

On the 4 December 1997, the Society for Medicines Research Award for Drug Discovery was presented to Redshaw, Duncan, and Roberts for their contributions to the discovery of the HIV protease inhibitor (PI) saquinavir. Mapping of the HIV genome had revealed the existence of the virus-specified protease and this had become a target for several of the leading pharmaceutical companies.[1] A series of compounds which inhibited the protease were prepared, resulting in the synthesis of Ro 31-8959 (saquinavir) also known as compound XVI.[2] Antiviral activity was in the low nanomolar range and this, combined with a relatively clean preclinical safety profile resulted in the development of saquinavir by Hoffman–La Roche (patent #5196438). In 1995, saquinavir became the first HIV PI approved by the US Food and Drug Administration (FDA).[3] It was produced as a hard gel formulation (saquinavir-HGC), known as Invirase.

Saquinavir-HGC had poor oral bioavailability and so two further formulations were developed. In 1997, in the era when PIs were administered without ritonavir boosting, a soft gel capsule (saquinavir-SGC) marketed as Fortovase was approved for use. At the recommended dosage of 1200 mg three times daily (tid) it provided much higher plasma saquinavir concentrations and drug exposure than those attained with the conventional saquinavir-HGC formulation, administered at the recommended dosage of 600 mg tid.[4,5] Unfortunately, saquinavir-SGC was associated with an increase in gastrointestinal side effects.[6] It contained the excipient capmul which is absent in the saquinavir-HGC formulation which was probably responsible for the gastrointestinal problems seen with the saquinavir-SGC formulation. The large size of the saquinavir-SGC capsules and their need for refrigeration was also a problem. A few years later, however, low-dose ritonavir was demonstrated to significantly improve the pharmacokinetic profile of saquinavir-HGC. Saquinavir-SGC was no longer needed and production was discontinued in February 2006. In addition, the reformulation of saquinavir-HGC into a 500 mg tablet as saquinavir-500 has reduced the daily pill burden from ten tablets to four which has obvious adherence advantages. Saquinavir-500 is the only formulation of saquinavir being marketed, although saquinavir-HGC is still available for the few patients who prefer to remain on it.

CHEMICAL FORMULATION

Saquinavir is a peptide-like, hydroxyethylamine transition state analogue of the human immunodeficiency virus type 1 (HIV-l) protease. The chemical name for saquinavir mesylate is *N*-tert-butyl-decahydro-2-[2(*R*)-hydroxy-4-phenyl-3(*S*)-[[*N*-(2quinolylcarbonyl)-L-asparaginyl]amino] butyl]-(4a*S*,8a*S*)-isoquinoline-3(*S*)-carboxamide methanesulfonate with a molecular formula $C_{38}H_{50}N_6O_5$. CH_4O_3S and a molecular weight of 766.96Da.[7] The molecular weight of the free base is 670.86. The structural formula of saquinavir mesylate can be seen in Figure 15-1.

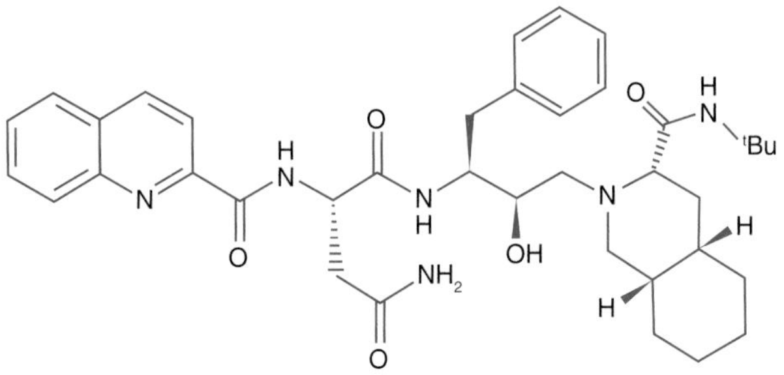

Figure 15-1 ■ The structural formula of saquinavir mesylate.

Table 15-1

Synergistic Anti-HIV Activity of Saquinavir with FDA Approved HIV-1 Agents Determined in Drug Combination Studies[15]

Saquinavir +	Mean Synergy/Antagonism Volume ($\mu M^2\%$; $n = 3$)	Interpretation <−50 $\mu M^2\%$ = antagonistic −50 to 50 $\mu M^2\%$ = Additive 550–100 $\mu M^2\%$ = Synergistic >100 $\mu M^2\%$ = Highly synergistic
Amprenavir	473/−4.5	Highly synergistic
Atazanavir	205/−0.5	Highly synergistic
Indinavir	151/−8.1	Highly synergistic
Lopinavir	224/−31	Highly synergistic
Nelfinavir	275/−8.3	Highly synergistic
Ritonavir	237/−6.9	Highly synergistic

Saquinavir mesylate is a white to off-white, very fine powder with an aqueous solubility of 2.22 mg/mL at 25°C. Saquinavir-500 as the mesylate is available as a light orange to grayish- or brownish-orange, oval cylindrical, biconvex film-coated tablet for oral administration in a 500 mg strength (as saquinavir free base). Each tablet also contains the inactive ingredients lactose, microcrystalline cellulose, povidone K30, croscarmellose sodium, and magnesium stearate. Each film coat contains hypromellose, titanium dioxide, talc, iron oxide yellow, iron oxide red, and triacetin.

IN VITRO ANTIVIRAL ACTIVITY

Saquinavir is a potent *in vitro* inhibitor of the proteases of both HIV-1 and HIV-2, with a K_i of 0.1 nM.[2,8] It has virtually no activity against various mammalian proteases, such as pepsin and cathepsin, with K_i values higher than 10 000 nM.[1] *In vitro* using the outcome measures of inhibition of HIV-1 p24 antigen production, inhibition of syncytium formation, or cell viability assays.[1–3,9,10]

Saquinavir has potent (nanomolar) anti-HIV activity against a wide variety of laboratory and clinical isolates, including: zidovudine-sensitive and zidovudine-resistant isolates; in acute and chronic infection systems; in infected T-lymphocyte lines, monocytic cell lines, and peripheral blood mononuclear cells (PBMCs). For example, in T-lymphocyte lines the range of 50% inhibitory concentration (IC_{50}) values was 0.5–7.0 nM, and the range of 90% inhibitory concentration (IC_{90}) values was 6–34 ηM. In PBMCs the IC_{50} values range from 3.5 to 10.0 nM. However, specific IC_{50} and IC_{90} values from *in vitro* experiments may not directly reflect the *in vivo* activity of saquinavir because of factors such as plasma protein binding and intracellular accumulation of drug.[5]

SAQUINAVIR IN COMBINATION WITH OTHER AGENTS

In a range of cell lines, saquinavir in combination with various other antiretroviral drugs, (compared with the activity of saquinavir alone) showed additive or synergistic activity against various strains of HIV-1 without increased cytotoxicity.[11–13] Although saquinavir and indinavir showed antagonistic activity *in vitro* against a range of clinical isolates of HIV-1 at all drug concentrations investigated,[14] recent data suggest that saquinavir is highly synergistic with other PIs (Table 15-1).

CYTOTOXICITY

Saquinavir has a high therapeutic index *in vitro* and only shows cytotoxicity at concentrations more than 1000 times higher than those producing inhibition of HIV-1.[16] In CD4 T lymphocyte cell lines, concentrations of saquinavir producing 50% toxicity (assessed by cell viability markers) ranged from 5 to 100 nmol/L. The *in vitro* effects of various concentrations of saquinavir on the development of mature virions has been assessed and has demonstrated decreasing amounts of mature particles with increasing concentrations of saquinavir from 10 nM up to 1000 nM concentrations of saquinavir. At the highest concentrations none of the virions produced had a mature appearance.[17]

In a model of chronic infection in MT-4 cells with an HIV-1 laboratory strain, 100 nM of saquinavir completely suppressed evidence of infection for 87 days. HIV-1 reemerged in this culture system when saquinavir was removed from the culture medium after a minimum of 11 days postinfection.[18]

PHARMACOKINETIC PROPERTIES

Absorption and Distribution

After administration of single 1200 mg intravenous doses of saquinavir to eight adult volunteers, the mean steady-state volume of distribution (V_d) was 700 L, suggesting that saquinavir is widely distributed in body tissues. However, concentrations of saquinavir in the cerebrospinal fluid (CSF) appear to be negligible. In 11 HIV-infected patients treated with saquinavir-HGC plus ritonavir as part of a combination therapy, a CSF:plasma saquinavir concentration ratio of ≤0.005 (0.5%) was observed in all study subjects.[19]

Protein Binding

Saquinavir is 97% bound to serum proteins, and is similar to the degree of protein binding reported with lopinavir (98–99%), nelfinavir (98%), amprenavir (90%), and indinavir (90%). Binding is predominantly to alpha-1-acid glycoprotein. Saquinavir is also a high-affinity substrate for the drug transporting protein P-glycoprotein (Pgp). Pgp binding is thought to contribute to the limited oral bioavailability of the drug.[20]

Elimination

Elimination of saquinavir is predominantly nonrenal, with ~1% of the drug excreted unchanged in the urine and 88% of the nonboosted dose eliminated in the feces as unchanged drug and metabolites. Several mono- and dihydroxylated metabolites are produced, which have no significant antiviral activity.[21]

As biliary excretion appears to be the major route of elimination, the pharmacokinetics of the drug are not expected to be markedly affected in patients with renal impairment[5] but no definitive data are available.

Metabolism

There is first-pass metabolism, predominantly by the cytochrome P450 3A4 (CYP3A4) isoenzyme in the liver and small intestine.[22,23] Drugs that induce the CYP3A4 isoenzyme such as rifampicin (rifampin), rifabutin, phenytoin and carbamazepine have the potential to decrease concentrations of saquinavir. Conversely, administration of saquinavir with drugs that inhibit CYP3A4, such as the PI ritonavir, results in an increase in the concentrations of saquinavir formulations.[24]

Bioavailability

In healthy volunteers the mean absolute bioavailability of saquinavir after a single oral 600 mg dose of the HGC formulation taken with food is only 4%. This is because of both limited absorption and extensive first-pass metabolism. The steady-state saquinavir exposure appears to be greater in HIV-infected people than in healthy volunteers.[25]

For historical interest only it was shown that the oral bioavailability of saquinavir-SGC was three to four times higher than that of the saquinavir-HGC formulation and the area under the plasma concentration–time curve (AUC) was more than eight times higher in recipients of saquinavir-SGC 1200 mg tid than after saquinavir-HGC 600 mg tid. Again, the absorption profile of saquinavir-SGC was different between healthy volunteers and patients with HIV-1 infection, with mean AUC and C_{max} values in HIV-infected patients being approximately twice those in healthy volunteers.[5,26]

Food Interactions

As was observed in pharmacokinetic investigations of the saquinavir-HGC formulation, absorption of saquinavir-500 is markedly enhanced by the presence of food especially if its fat content is high. Twenty-two HIV-infected adults were given a high fat meal (46-66 g of fat, 1070–1090 kcal) versus fasted state with three consecutive doses of 1000 mg saquinavir-500 with ritonavir 100 mg. Saquinavir PK parameters were ~70% reduced during administration under fasting conditions compared with administration following the high-fat, high-calorie meal. There was no significant change in ritonavir pharmacokinetics. The food effect seen with saquinavir-500/ritonavir in this study was less than that previously seen with saquinavir-HGC without ritonavir. Interestingly, the majority of subjects (21/22) maintained plasma saquinavir levels above the therapeutic threshold (100 ng/mL) even in the fasted state. However, saquinavir-500 and ritonavir should still be administered with food to ensure maximum therapeutic value.[27]

PHARMACOKINETICS OF SAQUINAVIR BOOSTING BY LOW-DOSE RITONAVIR

Saquinavir was one of the first antiretroviral agents for which an increase in plasma drug levels was demonstrated when given in combination with ritonavir. This was later found to be related to profound inhibition of CYP450 pathway responsible for metabolism of saquinavir and other antiretroviral medications by ritonavir. The dose regimen initially used was 400/400 mg bid saquinavir-SGC or saquinavir-HGC/ritonavir. The significant increase of saquinavir levels in the presence of ritonavir was demonstrated in an open-label, randomized, parallel, multiple-dose study involving 64 healthy HIV-1-negative volunteers who were given saquinavir-HGC (800 mg bid) alone, ritonavir (400 mg bid) alone, or a combination of saquinavir (400–800 mg bid) with ritonavir (200–400 mg bid) for 14 days.[28] Among those given saquinavir at a dose of 800 mg bid, there were overall 17-, 22-, and 23-fold increases in saquinavir (AUC-24 h) when ritonavir was administered at doses of 200, 300, and 400 mg bid, respectively.

It was later found that lower doses of ritonavir are sufficient to 'boost' saquinavir levels[29–31] and saquinavir/ritonavir is now frequently prescribed using 1000 mg of saquinavir with 100 mg of ritonavir twice daily (bid) or 2000 mg of saquinavir with 100 mg of ritonavir once daily (qd). The ritonavir should be given simultaneously in order to maximally increase saquinavir exposure.[32] Pharmacokinetics of the currently recommended dose was investigated in 24 healthy volunteers in a study that compared saquinavir-SGC/ritonavir (1000/100 mg bid) with saquinavir-HGC/ritonavir (1000/100 mg) in which each subject was given each combination separately for 10 days. Saquinavir-HGC/ritonavir led to significantly higher plasma saquinavir levels than saquinavir-SGC/ritonavir for all the pharmacokinetic variables evaluated.[33] Addition of ritonavir leads to significant increases in saquinavir exposure irrespective of whether the saquinavir-HGC or saquinavir-500 formulation is used.[31,34–37]

Increasing the dose of ritonavir above 100 mg does not improve the pharmacokinetic profile of saquinavir. A combined pharmacokinetic analysis of two dose-ranging studies

Table 15-2 Effect of Different Saquinavir/Ritonavir Regimens and Different Study Populations on Saquinavir AUC (with thanks to M Schutz Roche Valley, NJ, USA)

SQV/r Dosage, # of Subjects	Study Population	12 h AUC ($ng\ h^{-1}/mL^{-1}$)	24 h AUC ($ng\ h^{-1}/mL^{-1}$)
1000/100 bid (n = 18) 1	Healthy volunteers	20 559[a]	41 118
1000/100 bid (n = 24) 2	Western HIV+ patients	14 607[a]	29 214
1000/100 bid (n = 10) 3	Thai HIV+ patients	27 665[a]	55 330
1600/100 qd (n = 13) 4	Thai HIV+ patients		50 000[b]
1600/100 qd (n = 7) 5	Thai HIV+ patients		71 490[b]
1600/100 qd (n = 10) 6	Thai HIV+ patients		53 950[a]
1600/100 qd (n = 10) 6	Thai HIV+ patients		36 620[a]

For bid regimens, AUC_{0-24h} is estimated by doubling AUC_{0-12h}.

[a]Mean.

[b]Median.

indicates that the boosting effect on saquinavir is similar over the dose range 100–400 mg bid of ritonavir.[30] Furthermore, the combination of saquinavir/ritonavir 1000 mg/100 mg bid resulted in higher exposures to saquinavir in HIV-1 infected patients compared with the exposure to saquinavir seen historically using a saquinavir/ritonavir 400 mg/400 mg bid combination.[38] Since the toxicity of ritonavir is directly proportional to its plasma levels[39–41] use of low ritonavir doses 100–200 mg/day diminishes the potential for ritonavir-associated adverse effects such as nausea, vomiting, oral paraesthesia, taste perversion and elevated lipid levels.[40] Saquinavir does not alter the pharmacokinetic parameters of ritonavir.[29]

ONCE-DAILY PHARMACOKINETICS

Although bid dosing is currently used in clinical practice for combination saquinavir/ritonavir regimens, once-daily (qd) dosing might be a viable alternative[42] A comparison of the saquinavir exposures using the AUC for different doses and dosing regimens can be seen in Table 15-2.

CURRENT FORMULATION AND DOSING

Saquinavir is currently available as tablets containing saquinavir 500 mg and hard gelatin capsules containing saquinavir 200 mg. The recommended dose of saquinavir-HCG is 1000 mg (taken as either two 500 mg tablets or five 200 mg capsules) co-administered with 100 mg of ritonavir bid. The dose should be taken within 2 h of a full meal. Saquinavir-HGC capsules and saquinavir-500 should be stored at 15–30ºC (59–86ºF) in a tightly closed bottle. The saquinavir tablet and capsule formulations do not require refrigeration.

PHARMACOKINETICS OF SAQUINAVIR IN CHILDREN

The clinical pharmacologic characteristics of saquinavir-SGC have been investigated in HIV-1-infected children and adolescents. It was shown that the pharmacokinetics of saquinavir in children is different from that of adults. However, the study only looked at unboosted saquinavir so the relevance to today's practice is limited. PK was assessed after single-dose administration and after short- and long-term administration of 50 mg/kg saquinavir-SGC tid. The single-dose pharmacokinetics of fixed (1200 mg) versus unrestricted weight-adjusted dosing (50 mg/kg) was also investigated. Saquinavir-SGC in children resulted in lower saquinavir exposure (steady-state geometric mean AUC from time 0–24 h, 5790 ng h^{-1} mL^{-1}; steady-state concentration 8 h after drug administration (C (8 h,SS)), 65 ng/mL) and adolescents (steady-state geometric mean AUC (0–24 h), 5914 ng h^{-1} mL^{-1}) than that reported in adults treated with 1200 mg tid (steady-state geometric mean AUC (0–24 h), 21 700 ng h^{-1} mL^{-1}; C (8 h,SS), 223 ng/mL).[43]

This finding appeared to be attributable to markedly higher apparent oral clearance, potentially as a result of increased systemic clearance and reduced oral bioavailability. A significant correlation between average trough concentration and sustained viral load suppression was observed in these children. The apparent threshold for maintaining viral load suppression was a mean trough saquinavir concentration above 200 ng/mL.

SAQUINAVIR IN PREGNANCY

Saquinavir is in FDA pregnancy category B with respect to teratogenicity based on the available preclinical data. Saquinavir was not mutagenic *in vitro* in the Ames test in bacteria or in mammalian cells, and it did not induce chromosomal damage *in vitro* in PBMCs or *in vivo* in the mouse. An Antiretroviral Pregnancy Registry has been established to monitor the outcomes of pregnant women exposed to antiretroviral agents, including saquinavir (http://www.apregistry.com). It is not known whether saquinavir crosses the placenta in humans or whether it is secreted in human breast milk. It is secreted in the milk of laboratory rats.[44] There are few studies in pregnant women but there are observational data on the use of boosted saquinavir in pregnancy.

In a study of the new 500 mg saquinavir formulation at a dose of 1000 mg saquinavir with 100 mg ritonavir bd, there was no significant difference in saquinavir PK between the second and third trimester of pregnancy. This is in contrast to observations with other PIs such as nelfinavir, lopinavir and ritonavir.[44a]

LOW-DOSE BOOSTED SAQUINAVIR TWICE-DAILY (BID) IN PREGNANCY

From December 2002 to July 2005, 13 women with a total of 15 pregnancies received saquinavir-HGC with ritonavir (1000/100 mg bid) plus Combivir from a median of 21 weeks (range 13–25 weeks) until delivery. The median age of the women was 32 years (range 19–39 years); the median CD4 T-lymphocyte count at initiation of therapy was 437 cells/μL (range 237–637 cells/μL) and viral load 7901 copies/mL (range 117–55 460 copies/mL). Seven women had received HAART previously in pregnancy. One woman was switched from nevirapine/Combivir due to nevirapine-associated hepatic toxicity. All women had a HIV RNA level of <50 copies/mL at delivery. The median period of gestation was 37 weeks and 73% of women had a caesarean delivery. Sixteen HIV-negative infants including one set of twins were born during the study period. No additional resistance mutations from baseline were detected on stopping therapy post delivery.[45]

LOW-DOSE BOOSTED SAQUINAVIR ONCE-DAILY (QD) IN PREGNANCY

A cohort of 38 women pregnant women received an initial saquinavir/ritonavir dose of 1200/100 mg qd. Therapeutic drug monitoring (TDM) was used to guide the dosage of the boosted saquinavir containing therapy to maintain a saquinavir C_{min} of 100 ng/mL (24 ± 5 h post dose). Their median age was 31 years (range 21–38 years). At inclusion 15 (44.1%) women were drug naive, 33 (86.8%) had no prior PI failure, and 11 (32.3%) were already on treatment. Their median CD4 T-lymphocyte count was 508 cells/μL (range 42–1158 cells/μL) and viral load 3905 copies/mL (range <50–181 000 copies/mL). Therapy was initiated at a median of 20 weeks (range 0–35 weeks) of pregnancy and 30 (78.9%) women received zidovudine and lamivudine as their nucleosides. The saquinavir dose was increased to 1600 mg qd in two women. After a median of 17 weeks (range 3–39 weeks), 29 women had an undetectable viral load at delivery. Three women had viral loads of 110 copies/mL, 400 copies/mL and no data, respectively, but all three had started saquinavir 3–4 weeks before delivery. Mode of delivery was vaginal in 16 pregnancies and 16 by caesarean section (11 of these were for gynecological reasons). The authors reported no mother to child transmissions.[46,47]

SAQUINAVIR USE AND LIVER DISEASE

Saquinavir is metabolized by the liver, and it should be used with caution in patients with hepatic insufficiency. There are few data investigating its use in patients with chronic liver disease as patients with baseline liver function test results higher than five times the upper limit of normal were excluded from clinical studies. In the MaxCmin1 study 24/306 or 8% of patients had chronic hepatitis. No significant changes were seen in alanine transaminase (ALT) or aspartate transaminase (AST) in the boosted saquinavir or indinavir group after 48 weeks even in those who had abnormal values at baseline.[48]

DRUG INTERACTIONS

The potential for drug interactions between saquinavir and other drugs is significant because the CYP3A4 isoenzyme is a common metabolic pathway for many agents.[22] Drugs that are metabolized by or induce or inhibit the cytochrome P450 system, especially isoenzyme 3A4, may affect the metabolism, plasma levels, and systemic exposure of saquinavir. In addition, saquinavir is a mild inhibitor of cytochrome P450 enzymes and may affect the metabolism of some other drugs. Furthermore, as saquinavir is a substrate for Pglycoprotein (Pgp), drugs that modify Pgp activity may modify the pharmacokinetics of saquinavir. Similarly, saquinavir has the potential to modify the pharmacokinetics of other drugs that are substrates for Pgp.[23,49]

Antiviral Agents

Concomitant use of certain other antiretroviral agents with saquinavir may significantly increase or decrease saquinavir plasma concentrations. These antiretrovirals include delavirdine (Rescriptor), indinavir (Crixivan), nelfinavir (Viracept), and ritonavir (Norvir).[14,23] There is little clinical relevance apart from the ritonavir interaction as these drugs are rarely prescribed together. Saquinavir-HGC has no clinically significant interaction with nevirapine, lopinavir/ritonavir or with fosamprenavir/ritonavir. There is no clinical significant interaction of saquinavir with tenofovir or abacavir.

Statins

Caution should be used when any HIV PIs, especially when given with ritonavir, are used concurrently with HMG-CoA reductase inhibitors that are metabolized by the CYP3A4 pathway. The use of saquinavir with lovastatin or simvastatin is not recommended. Care should be taken when co-administration of atorvastatin, rosuvastatin, or cerivastatin is contemplated and patients should start with a low dose as the drug interaction may lead to raised concentration of statins which can cause myopathy or rhabdomyolysis.[50]

Rifampicin (Rifampin)

Recent data from a 28-day phase I clinical trial of saquinavir/ritonavir 1000 mg/100 mg bid and rifampin 600 mg qd in normal healthy volunteers showed significant hepatocellular toxicity in ~40% of patients with transaminase elevations of up to 20 times the upper limit of normal. Following drug discontinuation, clinical symptoms resolved and liver function tests returned to normal.[51] Although such an interaction has not been seen in HIV-1 patients who have had co-administration of these drugs it is recommended that rifampin should not be given to patients taking ritonavir-boosted saquinavir as part of combination antiretroviral therapy.

Efavirenz

Saquinavir levels can be significantly reduced when prescribed with efavirenz. In a previous pharmacokinetic study of the saquinavir and efavirenz interaction, it was found that efavirenz reduced the AUC of saquinavir by 62%, while the AUC of efavirenz remained almost unchanged. However, with the addition of low-dose ritonavir the decrease in saquinavir AUC was only 19%.[52] This interaction requires further investigation.

Atazanavir

A study of 18 HIV-1 patients receiving saquinavir/ritonavir switched to 1600/100 mg qd a minimum of 3 days before atazanavir (300 mg qd) was added to the regimen. Atazanavir was discontinued on day 32. Saquinavir and ritonavir pharmacokinetic parameters, with and without atazanavir were analyzed and a safety analysis was performed at screening, days 1, 11, 32, and follow-up. The addition of atazanavir to saquinavir/ritonavir increased saquinavir C_{trough}, C_{max} and $AUC_{0–24}$ by 112%, 42%, and 60%. Ritonavir C_{max} and $AUC_{0–24}$ increased by 34% and 41%. The regimen was well tolerated, with no significant change in laboratory parameters, except for the occurrence of hyperbilirubinemia. Four patients developed scleral icterus and two jaundice. Total and unconjugated bilirubin increased approximately fivefold during atazanavir therapy.[53]

In a further study, reduced doses of atazanavir administered at 150 and 200 mg qd, in the presence of low-dose ritonavir were still capable of increasing saquinavir exposure with the lowest doses limiting the occurrence of hyperbilirubinemia without unduly boosting ritonavir concentrations.[54]

Omeprazole

Proton pump inhibitors such as omeprazole can be bought as an over-the-counter medicine in many countries. The potential for them to cause significant interactions with PIs was seen with both boosted and unboosted atazanavir where significant reductions in all pharmacokinetic parameters. A study of omeprazole 40 mg qd given to 18 healthy volunteers taking saquinavir-500 with ritonavir 1000/100 mg at steady state showed a twofold increase in saquinavir C_{min} trough and AUC-12 h plasma exposure. There was no significant increase in ritonavir PK parameters. Despite the increased plasma saquinavir exposure, no clinically significant or grade 3/4 laboratory adverse events were recorded. The exact mechanism of interaction is not known but appears to be due to increased absorption as $t_{1/2}$ and time to C_{max} were not affected.[55]

A similar study in 18 HIV positive patients also showed similar increases in saquinavir levels with omeprazole without significant toxicity.[55a]

Methadone

With ritonavir-boosted saquinavir there was a small reduction in the free fraction of R-methadone.[56] However, it is not clinically significant so no methadone dose changes are required.

Oral Contraceptives

There are no data available regarding effects of saquinavir on ethyl estrogen or norethisterone levels. Saquinavir kinetics are not affected by the oral contraceptive pill.[57]

Herbal Agents

Use of saquinavir with St John's wort (*Hypericum perforatum*) or products containing St John's wort can potentially decrease saquinavir concentrations and lead to loss of virologic response and consequent resistance.[58]

Piscitelli reported that garlic supplements reduced blood levels of saquinavir by half during a 40-day study in which saquinavir was dosed at 1200 mg on days 1–4, 22–25, and 36–39 and garlic capsules were given from days 5 to 25. After a 10-day washout period from garlic treatment (saquinavir measured at day 36), trough levels of saquinavir had reached 70% of their baseline value.[59]

Others

Co-administration of certain other drugs with saquinavir may cause an increase or decrease in plasma concentrations of saquinavir or of the co-administered drug. Caution should be used when the following drugs are used concomitantly with saquinavir: calcium channel blockers, carbamazepine, clarithromycin, clindamycin, dapsone, dexamethasone, ketoconazole, phenobarbital, phenytoin, quinidine, rifabutin, and ergot derivatives.[5] Saquinavir should not be co-administered with astemizole or cisapride owing to the increased risk of cardiac arrhythmias. Other drugs, including midazolam and triazolam, can lead to prolonged sedation.

TOXICITY

In controlled studies more than 5000 patients have received saquinavir-HGC, and more than 850 patients have received saquinavir-SGC. Overall, saquinavir appears to be well tolerated. Some data are available from early studies in which saquinavir-HGC was administered as monotherapy, but most available data are from the use of saquinavir-HGC or saquinavir-SGC in combination with other antiretroviral agents. The most frequent side effects with both formulations are gastrointestinal and include diarrhea, nausea, and abdominal discomfort or pain.[60] Most treatment-related side effects have been mild. Overall, moderate or severe gastrointestinal side effects at least possibly related to treatment have occurred in 5–10% of patients receiving saquinavir-HGC and 10–20% of patients on saquinavir-SGC therapy; additional patients may have milder symptoms. Some of the GI intolerance to saquinavir-SGC was probably related to excipients in the formulation. Other toxicities that occurred in more than a few percent of patients treated included headaches, fatigue, and elevations in serum transaminases. Elevations in creatine phosphokinase have also been observed but are believed to be related to HIV-1 or other therapies, rather than to saquinavir.

Metabolic complications have been increasingly described in patients receiving PI therapy. On the basis of postmarketing surveillance reports, the FDA issued an alert in 1997 about a possible relation between PI use and the development or worsening of diabetes mellitus, hyperglycemia, and diabetic ketoacidosis; some of the reported cases occurred in persons receiving saquinavir.[61] There have also been other metabolic complications in persons receiving PIs, including body habitus changes, intraabdominal fat deposition, hypertriglyceridemia, and hypercholesterolemia.[62–67] The frequency and relation of these events to treatment with either saquinavir formulation is unknown.

Lipodystrophy

Lipoatrophy is associated with nucleoside analogue treatment especially thymidine analogs. Fat accumulation especially abdominal with an increase in waist size and abnormal waist hip ratio, buffalo hump, and breast enlargement are associated with PI use. In early studies of saquinavir larger doses of ritonavir were used from 400 to 600 mg and the prevalence of fat accumulation as assessed by physical examination was 4–14% at 5 years.[68]

An assessment of the prevalence and severity of lipodystrophy (LD) after 48 weeks was performed in the MaxCmin1 trial of indinavir/r (IDV/r) 800/100 mg bid or saquinavir/r (SQV/r) 1000/100 mg bid combined nucleosides and non-nucleosides. LD Case definition study questionnaires for patients and physicians were used at week 48. Fat accumulation severity scores were significantly higher in females ($p < 0.001$ for both), with no difference in lipoatrophy severity score ($p = 0.79$).[69]

The contribution of ritonavir to these metabolic and morphological changes was examined in a randomized pilot study evaluating the safety, tolerability, and efficacy of qd atazanavir plus saquinavir, as compared with bid ritonavir plus saquinavir, both in combination with two NRTIs.[70] Small lipid changes from baseline with atazanavir/saquinavir were not clinically significant in comparison with the prompt, marked and sustained changes of a magnitude that suggests clinical relevance that occurred in the ritonavir/saquinavir group.

Overall, it appears that saquinavir has fewer effects on fat accumulation and lipids than some of the other PIs; but as it has to be given with ritonavir, any combination it is part of may be associated with lipid and morphological changes.

Overdose

Two cases of overdose with saquinavir-HGC have been reported, but neither resulted in serious sequelae.[60] No case of overdose with saquinavir-500 has been reported.

THERAPEUTIC EFFICACY OF UNBOOSTED SAQUINAVIR

Studies using saquinavir-SGC supported the initial use of saquinavir in clinical practice and are thus important to note, even though this formulation has now been discontinued. Saquinavir-SGC was approved by the FDA in November 1997 on the basis of data from two studies: NV15355, which compared saquinavir-SGC with saquinavir-HGC in HIV-1 infected, treatment-naive patients[71], and NV15182, an open-label safety study of saquinavir-SGC in combination with other antiretroviral agents.[6] In a dose-ranging trial (NV 15107), the reduction in plasma HIV RNA levels was greater in HIV-infected patients who received saquinavir-SGC 1200 mg monotherapy tid for 8 weeks than in recipients of saquinavir-SGC 400 or 800 mg tid or saquinavir HGC 600 mg tid. The maximum median reduction in plasma HIV RNA in the saquinavir SGC 1200 mg treatment group was 1.43 $\log_{10}$ copies/mL.[72]

Several more studies of saquinavir-SGC were subsequently conducted, including the NR15503/M61005 SUN, M61003 CHEESE, NV15436 SPICE, and NR15520/M61018 TIDBID studies and the first pediatric study of saquinavir.[73–77]

In trials of saquinavir-SGC in combination with two NRTIs conducted in antiretroviral therapy-experienced adults with moderate to advanced HIV infection, plasma HIV RNA levels decreased by ~2.8 $\log_{10}$ copies/mL after 16 or 36 weeks of treatment. HIV RNA levels became undetectable (limit of detection <400 copies/mL) in 43–80% of patients. Increases in CD4 T lymphocyte cell counts also occurred (Table 15-3).

THERAPEUTIC EFFICACY OF UNBOOSTED SAQUINAVIR IN CHILDREN

The first published study to look at the use of saquinavir-SGC in children was an open-label study of HIV-infected, PI-naive children aged 3–16 years conducted in two parts, part 1 lasting 72 weeks and part 2 lasting 48 weeks. In part 1 there were 14 children who were given saquinavir-SGC (initially 33 mg/kg tid, subsequently adjusted to 50 mg/kg tid based on initial pharmacokinetics) and two nucleoside antiretroviral agents (plus nelfinavir for the five children who did not achieve a predetermined steady-state target plasma saquinavir exposure). In part 2 another 13 children received saquinavir-SGC (33 mg/kg tid) in combination with nelfinavir (30 mg/kg tid) and one or two nucleoside analogs. In part

Table 15-3

Therapeutic Efficacy of Unboosted Saquinavir-SGC(73–76)

Reference	Study Design	Treatment Regimen	Patients	Baseline HIV RNA (log_{10} copies/mL) & CD4+ count (cells/μL)	Main Efficacy Results
Sension et al(73) SUN study (NR15503/ M61005 SUN)	Open-label, single-arm study	SQV-SGC at 1200 mg tid plus ZDV (300 mg bid) and LMV (150 mg bid)	42 antiretroviral-naive HIV-1 infected	Mean baseline CD4+ 419 Mean baseline HIV-1 RNA 4.8	48w ITT, HIV-1 RNA <400: 50% HIV-1 RNA <20: 43%
Cohen Stuart et al (74) M61003 CHEESE trial	Randomized, open-label, parallel-arm study	1200 mg SQV-SGC q8h plus 300 mg ZDV bid and 150 mg LMV bid 800 mg IDV q8h, plus 300 mg ZDV bid and 150 mg LMV bid	67 HIV-1-infected with <12 months of prior ZDV experience and without prior PI or LMV therapy	Mean baseline 79 000 copies for both groups, mean baseline CD4+ counts were 310 for both groups	At 24 weeks: no significant difference between groups in terms of virologic response, but the SQV-SGC group had a better immunologic response with a rise in CD4 count of 162 versus 89 cells/mm^3 in the IDV arm.
Moyle et al75 NV15436 SPICE trial	Randomized, open-label, 4 parallel-arm study	The four treatment arms in this: (1) SQV-SGC 1200 mg tid + two NRTIs;	157 PI-naive were randomized to one of the four arms	Overall mean baseline HIV RNA of 4.8 log(10) copies/mL mean baseline CD4+ of 301 cells/μL	48w OTT (those remaining in their original arm) HIV-1 RNA <50: 61 Differences between groups not statistically significant.
		(2) NLF 750 mg tid + two NRTIs;			48w OTT HIV-1 RNA <50: 63%
		(3) SQV-SGC 800 mg tid + NLF 750 mg tid + two NRTIs; or			48w OTT HIV-1 RNA <50: 65%
		(4) SQV-SGC 800 mg tid + NLF 750 mg tid without NRTIs.			48w OTT HIV-1 RNA <50: 47%
Wheat et al76 NR15520/M61018 TIDBID	Randomized open-label study	1. SQV-SGC 1200 mg tid plus two new NRTIs	840 ARV naive or nucleoside analogue-experienced	Mean baseline HIV RNA: 4.8 mean baseline CD4+: 307	48w ITT HIV-1 RNA <50: 37%, 36%, and 35% of patients. Virologic responses in the SQV-SGC-containing BID regimens were equivalent to the SQV-SGC-containing tid regimen.
		2. SQV-SGC 1600 mg bid plus two NRTIs 3. SQV-SGC 1200 mg bid plus NLF 1250 mg bid plus one new NRTI		Mean baseline HIV RNA: 4.7 Mean baseline CD4+: 328 Mean baseline HIV RNA: 4.8 Mean baseline CD4+: 311	48w ITT HIV-1 RNA <50: 36%, 48w ITT HIV-1 RNA <50: 35%,

w, weeks; ART, antiretroviral therapy; CD4, CD4+ T-lymphocyte count (cells/mm^3); d4T, stavudine; ddi, didanoslne; EFV, efavirenz; HAART, highly active retroviral therapy; HIV RNA; Viral load (log_{10} copies/mL); LPV, lopinavil; LoQ, limit of quantitation; NRTIs, nucleoside reverse transcriptase inhibitors; PI, protease inhibitor; RTV, ritonavir; SQV-HGC saquinavir-hard gel capsules; SQV-SGC, saquinavir-soft gel capsules; ZDV, zidovudine; LMV, lamivudine; IDV, indinavir; NLF, nelfinavir; ITT, intention to treat analysis; OTT, on treatment analysis.

1, 36% of patients achieved HIV-1 RNA titers of less than 50 copies/mL at 72 weeks, in part 2 a total of 62% of patients achieved an HIV-1 RNA titer of less than 50 copies/mL.[77]

THERAPEUTIC EFFICACY OF BOOSTED SAQUINAVIR

Since the impact of ritonavir on saquinavir concentrations was first recognized using saquinavir-HGC[78] several studies have been designed to evaluate the antiviral activity of ritonavir-boosted saquinavir-SGC therapy including a number of trials at 1000 mg/100 mg bid, the dose currently licensed in Europe and North America (Table 15-4). With its better GI tolerability the hard gel formulation has also undergone further clinical trials in ritonavir-boosted regimens including those of qd regimens (Tables 15-4 and 15-5).

THERAPEUTIC EFFICACY OF TWICE-DAILY (BID) BOOSTED SAQUINAVIR

MaxCmin1 and MaxCmin2 were the first head-to-head clinical comparisons of ritonavir-boosted PI therapies to be undertaken.[79,80] Both studies were in mixed but predominantly treatment-experienced patients. MaxCmin1 showed improved efficacy of saquinavir-SGC/ritonavir 1000/100 mg compared with indinavir/ritonavir 800/100 mg by intention-to-treat analysis. Both combinations showed similar potency. Improved efficacy was related to a better tolerability profile of saquinavir/ritonavir with significantly greater number of patients with grade 3 or 4 adverse events in the indinavir/ritonavir group compared to patients in the saquinavir/ritonavir group ($p = 0.0004$).[79]

MaxCmin2 compared saquinavir/ritonavir 1000/100 mg with lopinavir/ritonavir 400/100 mg both bid with two NRTIs. Despite a longer time to virologic failure in those taking lopinavir (the primary efficacy endpoint), comparable virologic suppression and comparable grade 3 or 4 adverse event rates were observed at 48 weeks for both arms. In this study discontinuation of the assigned treatment occurred in 30% of those in the saquinavir/ritonavir arm compared with 14% in the LPV/r treated group ($p = 0.001$).[80]

Both the MaxCmin1 and MaxCmin2 trials recruited patients from all stages of treatment experience and about one-third were drug-naive making interpretation challenging because of the difficulty in matching patients for factors such as degree of resistance or adherence.

Use of the soft gel formulation of saquinavir may have also contributed to the number of patients discontinuing therapy due to gastrointestinal toxicity in MaxCmin2. MaxCmin2 was even more difficult to interpret as patients received one of two formulations of saquinavir or switched from one to the other.

THE GEMINI STUDY

This is a study of boosted saquinavir 1000 mg with ritonavir 100 bid ($n = 166$ patients) or lopinavir/ritonavir 400/100 mg bd ($n = 171$) plus FTC/Tenofovir twice daily with a follow up of 48 weeks. All study participants had to have an HIV RNA greater than 10 000 copies/ml and a CD4 count of 350 cells/mm^3 or less. The results at 24 weeks showed that similar proportion of patients in both arms (69%) had undetectable HIV/RNA to less than 50 copies per ml. The media CD4 count rise was 127 and 134 cells in the saquinavir/ritonavir and lopinavir/ritonavir arms respectively.

Six per cent of patients in the saquinavir group had virologic failure versus 1.8% of the lopinavir/ritonavir group but most virologic failures in this arm were related to poor adherence. More people stopped the lopinavir/ritonavir because of adverse events than the saquinavir. The study is for 48 weeks and the full analysis will then be performed.[80a]

THERAPEUTIC EFFICACY OF ONCE-DAILY BOOSTED SAQUINAVIR

Once-daily therapy is an attractive treatment option for many patients especially if there is potential for directly observed or supervised therapy. A range of clinical data supports the use of qd boosted saquinavir (Table 15-5). The Staccato study was the first large study of daily boosted hard gel saquinavir and the 200 patients in this study make it the largest clinical study of daily saquinavir.[88] A very low incidence (3.9%) of virologic failure was reported among patients receiving boosted saquinavir therapy who were antiretroviral therapy-naive. An absence of protease resistance mutations was also observed in this group of patients. The protease polymorphisms detected at viral load failure were similar to those seen with other boosted PIs in treatment-naive patients and are natural polymorphisms/secondary mutations that may contribute to reduced viral susceptibility in the presence of primary mutations.

There is evidence that saquinavir/ritonavir 1600 mg/100 mg qd is also of benefit in antiretroviral-experienced patients. An open-label study was conducted to evaluate the efficacy and safety of this regimen in 69 antiretroviral-experienced patients with a plasma viral load <50 copies/mL after long-term treatment with saquinavir 1400 mg bid plus two NRTIs (Table 15-5).[84] These patients were switched to a saquinavir/ritonavir 1600 mg/100 mg qd regimen while continuing their NRTIs. At 48 weeks, 63/69 patients (91%) still had a plasma viral load <50 copies/mL. In five of the remaining six patients, plasma viral load was <400 copies/mL at week 48, while one patient had an unexplained rise in viral load (to 39 500 copies/mL) that fell to <50 copies/mL 12 weeks later.[89] An increase in CD4 T lymphocyte cell count was also seen, which was significantly greater than that seen during the previous year on saquinavir bid ($p < 0.001$).[90] Saquinavir/ritonavir was well tolerated and no patients changed treatment. No significant change in the median plasma triglyceride concentration was seen following the switch. A qd boosted saquinavir/ritonavir treatment regimen that included efavirenz was evaluated in antiretroviral-experienced (two NRTIs plus PIs or non-nucleoside reverse transcriptase inhibitors (NNRTIs)) patients with extensive resistance to NRTIs.

Table 15-4

Therapeutic Efficacy – Twice Daily (BID) Boosted Saquinavir[78–82]

Reference	Study Design	Treatment Regimen	Patients	Median Baseline HIV RNA (log_{10} copies/mL & CD4+ count (cells/μL))	Main Efficacy Results
Gisolf et al[a78] Prometheus[a]	Open-label, randomized, controlled trial	SQV-HCG/RTV (400/400 mg bid)	208 PI- and d4T-naive	RNA = 4.5 CD4+ = 255	48 weeks ITT HIV <400 copies/mL: 63%
		SQV-HCG/RTV (400/400 mg) plus d4T (40 mg bid)		RNA = 4.5 CD4+ = 253	48 weeks ITT HIV <400 copies/mL: 69% (no significant difference)
Dragsted et al[79] MaxCmin1	Prospective, open-label, parallel group, randomized multicentre	SQV-SGC/RTV 1000/100 mg bid plus two NRTIs bid	ARV-naive or ARV-experience (n = 306)	RNA = 4.0 CD4+ = 272	48 weeks ITT HIV-RNA <400 copies/mL: 68%
(SQV-SGC)		IDV/RTV 800 mg/100 mg bid plus two NRTIs bids		RNA = 4.0 CD4+ = 280	48 weeks ITT HIV-RNA <400 copies/mL: 53%
Dragsted et al[80] MaxCMin2	Prospective, open-label, randomized, multicentre	SQV/RTV 1000/100 mg bid plus two or more NRTIs/non NRTIs	(n =339)	RNA = 4.4 (3.1–5.1) CD4+ = 241 (86–400)	48 weeks ITT HIV-RNA <400 copies/mL: 61%
(Mixed SQV-SGC/ SQV-HGC)		LPV/RTV 400/100 mg bid plus two or more NRTIs/non NRTIs		RNA = 4.6 (3.5–5.3) CD4+ = 239 (95–420)	48 weeks ITT HIV-RNA <400 copies/mL: 75%
Valer et al[81] Fortogene Study (SQV-SGC)	Prospective, multicentre	SQV-SGC/RTV 1000/100 mg plus two NRTIs bid	PI-experienced (n = 139)	Mean RNA = 4.9 Mean CD4+ = 368	24 weeks HIV-RNA <50 copies/mL: 60%
Piketty et al[82] (SQV-HGC)	Prospective, open-label, single-arm	SQV-HGC/RTV 1000/100 mg bid plus EFV 600 mg daily plus two NRTIs bid	SQV and EFV-naive PI experienced (n = 32)	RNA = 4.31 CD4+ = 258	24 weeks ITT HIV- <500 copies/mL: 71% HIV-RNA <50 copies/mL: 45% 48 weeks ITT HIV-RNA <500 copies/mL: 61% HIV-RNA <50 copies/mL: 58%

ART, antiretroviral therapy; CD4, CD4+ T-lymphocyte count (cells/mm^3); d4T, stavudine; ddi, didanosine; EFV, efavirenz; HAART, highly active retroviral therapy; HIV RNA; Viral load (log_{10} copies/mL); LPV, lopinavir, LoQ, limit of quantitation; NRTIs, nucleoside reverse transcriptase inhibitors; PI, protease inhibitor; RTV, ritonavir; SQV-HGC saquinavir-hard gel capsules; SQV-SGC, saquinavir-soft gel capsules; ZDV, zidovudine; IDV, indinavir; ITT, intention to treat analysis; OTT, on treatment analysis.

[a] Prometheus: intensification of study meds with reverse transcriptase inhibitors was permitted if serum HIV-RNA >400 copies/mL after 12 weeks treatment. 31 patients intensified study meds according to the protocol. 28 in the RTV/SQV group, three in the RTV/SQV/d4T group.

Table 15-5

Therapeutic Efficacy of Once Daily (QD) Boosted Saquinavir[83–88]

Reference	Study Design	Treatment Regimen	Patient Numbers and Characteristics	Median Baseline HIV RNA (log_{10} copies/mL & CD4+ count (cells/μL))	Main Efficacy Results
Montaner et al[83]	Prospective, open-label, randomized, multicentre	SQV/RTV 1600 mg/100 mg once daily plus two NRTIs bid	ARV naive (n = 159)	RNA = 4.78 CD4+ = 372	24 weeks HIV-RNA <400 copies/mL: 70% (ITT); 94% (OT)
		EFV 600 mg once- daily plus two NRTIs bid		RNA = 4.72 CD4+ = 341	24 weeks HIV-RNA <400 copies/mL: 82% (ITT); 97% (OT)
Cardiello et al[84]	Prospective, open-label, single-arm switch study from bd	SQV/RTV 1600 mg/100 mg once daily plus two NRTIs bid	ARV-experienced (n = 69)	RNA = 4.7 CD4+ = 356	48 weeks HIV-RNA <50 copies/mL: 91%
López-Cortés et al[85]	Prospective, open-label, single-arm, single centre	SQV/RTV 1200 mg/100 mg plus EFV 600 mg once daily	ARV-experienced (n = 42)	Mean RNA <50-696 000 CD4+ = 565	52 weeks HIV-RNA <50 copies/mL: 71.4%
Peytavin et al[86]	Prospective, open-label, single-arm, multicentre	SQV/RTV 1600 mg/100 mg once daily plus two NRTIs	PI-naive (n = 18)	PI-naive: RNA = 4.97 CD4+ = 219	PI naive, 12 weeks HIV-RNA dropped to 2.70 log_{10} copies/mL
			PI-experienced (n = 17)	PI-experienced: RNA = 2.3 CD4+ = 601	PI experienced, 12 weeks HIV-RNA <200 copies/mL: 64%
Mallolas et al[87]	Prospective, open-label, single-arm	SQV/RTV 1600 mg/200 mg once daily plus two NRTIs	ARV Experienced (n = 18)	RNA = 3.5 CD4+ = 479	12 weeks HIV-RNA <200 copies/mL: 85%
Ananworanich et al[88]	Prospective, open-label single-arm	SQV-HGC/RTV 1600 mg/100 once daily plus two NRTIs	ARV-naive (n = 200)	RNA = 4.7 CD4+ = 267	24 weeks ITT HIV-RNA <400 copies/mL: 96% HIV-RNA <50 copies/mL: 89%

ART, antiretroviral therapy; CD4, CD4+ T-lymphocyte count (cells/mm'); d4T, stavudine; ddi, didanoslne; EFV, efavirenz; HAART, highly active retroviral therapy; HIV RNA; Viral load (log_{10} copies/mL); LPV, lopinavil, LoQ, limit of quantitation; NRTIs, nucleoside reverse transcriptase inhibitors; PI, protease inhibitor; RTV, ritonavir; SQV-HGC, saquinavir-hard gel capsules; SQV-SGC, saquinavir-soft gel capsules; ZDV, zldovudine; IDV, indinavir; ITT, intention to treat analysis; OTT, on treatment analysis.

Table 15-6 Therapeutic Efficacy of Double Boosted Saquinavir[91–98]

Reference	Study Design	Treatment Regimen	Patient Numbers and Characteristics	Median Baseline HIV RNA ($\log_{10}$ copies/mL & CD4+ count (cells/μL))	Main Efficacy Results (Copies/mL = cps/mL)
Smith et al[91]	Prospective, open-label, single-arm	SQV 1000 mg bid plus LPV/ RTV 400 mg/100 mg bid NRTIs (EFV 600 mg plus od added at week 4 if not responding)	ARV experienced (n = 36)	RNA = 5.1 CD4+ = 91	4 weeks HIV-RNA drop of = ≥0.8 $\log_{10}$ copies/mL= 61% CD4+ increase of 16 cells/mm³
Hellinger et al[92]	Prospective, open-label, single arm, dose escalation	Initiated SQV 1000 mg bid plus LPV/RTV 400 mg/100 mg bid plus two or more NRTIs (dose individualised guided by virtual phenotype results)	LPV-naive, PI experienced (n = 28)	RNA >1000 copies/mL	24 weeks HIV-RNA <400 copies/mL: 68% (ITT), 87% (OT) HIV-RNA <50 copies/mL: 42% (ITT), 53% (OT)
Ruiz et al[93]	Prospective, open-label	SQV 1000 mg bid 400 mg/ 100 mg bid plus three NRTIs	ARV experienced (n = 24)[a]	RNA = 4.3[a] CD4+ = 322[a]	24 weeks HIV-RNA <80 copies/mL: 36%
Staszewski et al[94]	Prospective, open-label	SQV 1000 mg bid LPV/RTV 400 mg/100mg bid	All ARV-experienced: NRTI resistant, (n = 14); toxicity (n = 11); NRTI resistance and toxicity (n = 2)	RNA 113 000 copies/mL CD4+ = 192	Median 17 weeks (range 5–62) Median CD4+ increase of 73 400 mg/100 mg bid cells/mm³ Median HIV-RNA decrease of 2.7 $\log_{10}$ cps/mL
Studies of Double-Boosted Saquinavir/Lopinavir/ritonavir 1000/400/100 mg bid without NRTI					
Hellinger et al[95]	Prospective, single arm, open-label pilot study	SQV-SGC 1000 mg bid plus LPV/RTV 400 mg/100 mg bid (treatment intensification with TDF or NRTI allowed after 12 weeks)	PI naive, n = 20	Mean RNA = 4.4; CD4 = 274	48 weeks, ITT HIV RNA <50 cps/mL: 65%
Delassus et al[96]	Prospective, open-label, single-arm	SQV 1000 mg bid LPV/RTV 400 mg/100 mg bid	18	RNA = 4.57 (7900-243 000). CD4 = 223 (67-542)	24 weeks HIV RNA <50 cps/mL: 56%
Staszewski et al[97]	Prospective, open-label, single-arm	lopinavir (LPV/r) plus saquinavir (SQV) without any additional antiretroviral therapy in heavily pretreated	163	RNA = 5.2 CD4 = 164	48 weeks median HIV RNA decrease of 2.7 $\log_{10}$ cps/mL 50 had <50
Duvivier et al[98]	Prospective, open-label, single-arm	SQV/LPV/r 800/400/100 mg bid 40% of all patients in study Gp1 resistant or Gp2 intolerant to RTI s, Total 41 patients per group	25	Gp1 RNA = 4.10 CD4 = 240 Gp2 RNA <2.60 copies/mL in 71% CD4 = 294	24 weeks HIV RNA <400 cps/mL: 76%

ART, antiretroviral therapy; CD4, CD4+ T-lymphocyte count (cells/mm'); d4T, stavudine; ddi, didanoslne; EFV, efavirenz; HAART, highly active retroviral therapy; HIV RNA; Viral load ($\log_{10}$ copies/mL); LPV, lopinavil, LoQ, limit of quantitation; NRTIs, nucleoside reverse transcriptase inhibitors; PI, protease inhibitor; RTV, ritonavir; SQV-HGC, saquinavir-hard gel capsules; SQV-SGC, saquinavir-soft gel capsules; ZDV, zldovudine; IDV, indinavir; ITT, intention to treat analysis; OTT, on treatment analysis.

[a]Patients without a treatment interruption prior to therapy.

In this study, involving 42 patients, saquinavir/ritonavir 1200 mg/100 mg plus efavirenz 600 mg were administered qd (Table 15-5). After 1 year, 71.4% (30/42) of these patients had viral suppression (<50 copies/mL).[85] The authors concluded that this may be a valuable treatment option for patients unable to take NRTIs because of toxicity, as well as for those with extensive NRTI resistance.

In a prospective, open-label, noncomparative multicenter study 18 PI-naive (treatment-naive) and 17 PI-experienced subjects (NRTI pretreated) were evaluated using qd saquinavir/ritonavir 1600 mg/100 mg to dual NRTI therapy.[86] In the PI-naive patients following 3 months of therapy, plasma HIV-RNA had fallen by 2.70 $\log_{10}$ copies/mL from 4.97 $\log_{10}$ copies/mL at baseline. In the PI-experienced patients, HIV RNA levels following 3 months of therapy remained below the baseline level of 400 copies/mL. The regimen was well tolerated in all patients. Encouraging results with qd saquinavir/ritonavir (1600 mg/200 mg) were also seen in patients who previously failed a HAART regimen including saquinavir 600 mg tid (Table 15-6).[87] Of a total of 18 patients, 12 were followed up for at least 12 weeks, and their viral load fell to <200 copies/mL. More importantly, this drop in viral load was seen in 4/10 patients with the L90M mutation at baseline.

Overall, these studies show that the administration of saquinavir/ritonavir qd as part of antiretroviral therapy provides potent and durable HIV RNA suppression.

"DOUBLE BOOSTING" OF SAQUINAVIR

The application of "double boosting" has been investigated as a salvage treatment option for PI-experienced patients with multiclass drug resistance (Table 15-6). The idea is that two proteases are synergistic and may have improved efficacy in patients with a high degree of protease resistance.

The combination of lopinavir/ritonavir 400 mg/100 mg bid plus saquinavir 1000 mg bid (plus two NRTIs) resulted in increased saquinavir exposures. This was found to have positive benefits at up to 24 weeks in the salvage setting.[91] More importantly, clinical data from the PI-experienced (PIE) study has demonstrated effective viral load suppression with this combination in a population of HIV patients with limited remaining treatment options.[92] In 28 PIE (with a mean of almost three PIs), lopinavir-naive patients, 24-week results showed that 88% (19/21) of patients had effective viral load suppression (<400 copies/mL) compared with baseline median HIV RNA values of 31 100 copies/mL. The regimen was well tolerated; with grade 3 and 4 increases in cholesterol and triglycerides occurring in only three patients. The authors concluded that the high levels of exposure achieved with the double-boosted PIs may be beneficial for those patients with extensive drug resistance. An ongoing salvage study is evaluating lopinavir/ritonavir 400 mg/100 mg bid plus saquinavir 1000 mg bid with three NRTIs.[93] In an interim analysis of this combination in 24 HIV-infected patients, 36% of patients had a plasma viral load <80 copies/mL at 24 weeks. The regimen was well tolerated.

Finally, a double-boosted PI regimen of lopinavir/ritonavir plus saquinavir that does not include NRTIs has also been recently reported.[94] This regimen may be appropriate for patients with nucleoside toxicity as well as for patients with NRTI resistance. In this study, involving 27 patients (14 with multiple NRTI resistance, 11 with nucleoside toxicity and two with both resistance and toxicity), bid doses of lopinavir/ritonavir 400 mg/100 mg plus saquinavir 1000 mg were administered. After a median follow-up of 17 weeks (range 5–62 weeks), 24/27 patients were still on therapy. Median CD4 T lymphocyte cell counts had increased by 73 cells/μL from baseline and viral load decreased by a median 2.7 log. Pharmacokinetic profile monitoring of all patients after a minimum of 14 days on this regimen indicated that lopinavir/ritonavir co-administration effectively boosted saquinavir levels, with no adverse drug interactions between the two PIs. The authors concluded that a NRTI-sparing double-boosted PI regimen of saquinavir plus lopinavir/ritonavir may provide a valuable treatment option.

A number of factors make the combination of amprenavir/saquinavir/ritonavir a logical prospect for PI double boosting. Isolates with multiple PI mutations often retain susceptibility to amprenavir and saquinavir, and different key resistance mutations have been identified for these two agents.[99] In addition, a potential for antiviral synergy has been demonstrated between these agents.[23,100] PK data suggest that for saquinavir/fosamprenavir/ritonavir the optimal-dose combination is 1000/700/200 mg bid.[101] However, there are as yet no clinical data to support this regimen.

There is evidence that saquinavir boosting can be achieved with the qd PI atazanavir. The PK interactions are complex with boosting of saquinavir by both ritonavir and atazanavir which increases saquinavir elimination half-life. Importantly, this combination appears to have a favorable impact on lipid profiles.[54]

In a study of 85 patients who failed prior PI antiretroviral therapy and were then randomized to a qd saquinavir/atazanavir (1200 mg/400 mg or 1200 mg/600 mg) or bid saquinavir/ritonavir (400 mg/400 mg) regimen, durable suppression of HIV RNA and increases in CD4 T lymphocyte cell counts were observed with all three treatment regimens after 48 weeks. Total cholesterol, fasting triglycerides and fasting low-density lipoprotein cholesterol levels all fell in both saquinavir/atazanavir arms, a decrease that was not seen in the saquinavir/ritonavir arm.[102,103]

Other cohort studies have been examining the use of boosted saquinavir with atazanavir as a combination for treatment experienced patients to enhance the PI efficacy or naive patients as nucleoside sparing lipid-friendly combination. The ATSAQ study[104] enrolled 40 atazanavir-naive patients but highly treatment experienced patients with a median of three prior PIs and a median HIV viral load (range) of 3.57 $\log_{10}$ copies/mL (1.3–6.0). They had limited reverse transcriptase inhibitor options based on resistance assays and/or systemic toxicity. They were switched to atazanavir/ritonavir 300/100 mg qd with saquinavir 1000 mg bid and were given no reverse transcriptase inhibitors or other agents. The median

Saquinavir Mutations Leading to Reduced *in vitro* Susceptibility From International AIDS Society-USA 2004 Guidelines[110,111]

Table 15-7a

Resistance	Mutations
Primary saquinavir resistance or multi-PI resistance	M46I/L, G48V, V82A/F/S/T, I84V, L90M
Secondary saquinavir or multi-PI resistance	L10I/R/V, V32I, I54L/V, A71T/V, G73S, V77I, N88S

PI, protease inhibitor.

Combination of 3–4 of the Following Results in a Significant Reduction in Response

Table 15-7b

L10F/I/M/R/V, L24I
V82A/F/S/7, IISA/V
I62V, I84, K20I/M/R/T, G73S/T, L90M

MARCELIN AG 4th European HIV drug resistance workshop MAR 2006 Abst. 54.

follow-up (range) was 32 weeks (12–60) and 24/40 (60%) achieved HIV viral loads of <50 copies/mL.

Other studies which are ongoing include ASK-500 and StARS which are both looking at switches to this double-boosted regimen in virologically stable patients. In StARS 11/11 patients switching from lopinavir/ritonavir/saquinavir to atazanavir/ritonavir/saquinavir have remained virologically undetectable and have significantly improved lipid profile.[105]

However, little data exist that these combinations are of any advantage over single-boosted PIs or newer drugs such as darunavir or tipranavir, which have been shown to be useful in highly treatment experienced patients The ongoing French Centaur trial is examining this very question (M Schutz, personal communication).

RESISTANCE

Most patients with PI resistance mutations have acquired them from the use of unboosted proteases or rarely from transmitted drug resistance. In PI-naive patients who develop virologic failure on boosted saquinavir it is difficult to find mutations arising in the protease enzyme. This high genetic barrier to resistance is seen with most boosted PIs and may be due to the high concentrations of drug achieved or simply that mutations occur outside of the protease gene.

Multiple amino acid changes which can occur either at or around the active site of the HIV protease enzyme will prevent binding of saquinavir and lead to drug resistance. Studies show that when saquinavir resistance emerges *in vitro* there is an initial G48V mutation, leading to an approximately eightfold loss in sensitivity followed by an L90M mutation, causing even further loss of drug sensitivity.[106] However, when the L90M mutation, historically thought to be the key resistance mutation for saquinavir, arises alone, a less than twofold loss in sensitivity is seen.[106] In fact multiple mutations in recombinant HIV clones are needed to increase the IC_{50} by more than 10-fold compared to wild-type virus.[24]

Isolates from clinical studies that have correlated genotypic with phenotypic resistance have demonstrated a number of important mutations associated with saquinavir resistance. In one study of 78 isolates with the L90M mutation, 40% were still phenotypically sensitive defined as having an IC_{50} fold change of less than 2.5-fold to saquinavir.[107] Interestingly, 73% of isolates with the V82A/F/S/T mutation retained phenotypic sensitivity to saquinavir.

Over time, patients who remain on the same therapy with virologic failure accumulate more primary and secondary mutations[107] leading to a gradual rise in phenotypic resistance to saquinavir. In large clinical studies such as the T20 Randomization with Optimization (TORO) trials which recruited patients with a history of multiple treatment failure, the main genotypic determinants of resistance to ritonavir-boosted saquinavir were having a G48V, I84V and I54V and G73S at baseline. The L90M acted as a secondary mutation in terms of its effect on phenotype.[108]

The interpretation of these data is that no individual mutation is specific for resistance to saquinavir.[109] The main primary and secondary mutations associated with reduced susceptibility to saquinavir are in Table 15-7a. A new genotype algorithm from the Agence Nationale de Recherches sur le sida provides guidance on clinical interpretation of resistance (see Table 15.7b).

Methods of Interpreting Genotypic Resistance

For the Fortogene Spain prospective cohort, samples from 139 PI-pretreated patients were genotyped at baseline[81] The virologic response after 24 weeks of treatment with saquinavir/ritonavir 1000/100 mg bid was then correlated with a "mutation score" – the total number of mutations from eight positions (10, 48, 54, 71, 77, 82, 84, and 90), selected from International AIDS Society – USA guidelines.[110,111] Virologic response was defined as either a 1 $\log_{10}$ reduction in HIV

Genotypic cut-off levels. Adapted from Hill A, Walmsley S, Clotet B, Molts J. Analysis of genotypic and phenotypic clinical cut-off levels for tinoavir-boosted saquinavir. HIV Med 7:67, 2006.[118]

Table 15-8

Reference	Study (n)	Candidate Mutations	Rule
Valer et al[81,114]	FortoGENE Spain (n = 139)	L10I/R/V, G48V, I54V/L, A71V/T, V77I, V82A, I84V, L90M	<4 mutations: 83% response[a] ≥4 mutations: 29% response
Marcelin et al[112]	French Hospital Database (n = 72)	L24I, I62V, V82A/F/T/S, I84V, L90M	0 mutations: $-2.2 \log_{10}$ reduction[b] 1 mutation: $-1.23 \log_{10}$ reduction ≥2 mutations: $-0.27 \log_{10}$ reduction
Barreiro et al[115]	Madrid cohort (n = 53)	L10I/R/V, G48V, I54V/L, A71V/T, V77I, V82A, I84V, L90M	<5 mutations: 95% response[a] ≥5 mutations: 21% response
Morand et al[116]	ESQUIV cohort (n = 60)	L10I, K20M/R, L24I, D30N, V32I, L33F, E35D, M33I/L, M38I/L, R41K, M46I/L, I47V, G48V, I50V, F53L, I54V/T, I62V, L63P, A71I/T/V, G73S, V77I, V82A, I84V, N88S/D, L90M	≤5 mutations: 51% response[c] >5 mutations: 22% response

[a] Virological response defined as 1 $\log_{10}$ reduction in HIV RNA after 24 weeks of treatment, or HIV RNA level <400 copies/mL.
[b] Virological response measured at week 12.
[c] Virological response defined as 1 $\log_{10}$ reduction in HIV RNA after 24 weeks of treatment, or HIV RNA <50 copies/mL.

RNA or levels below 400 HIV-1 RNA copies/mL, after 24 weeks of treatment. In a multivariate analysis, patients with fewer than four of these mutations were 13 times more likely to show a virologic response to treatment.

In 72 PI-pretreated patients given saquianvir/ritonavir 800/100 mg bid (the approved dosage is 1000/100 mg bid), mutations at five key sites (L24I, I62 V, V82A/F/T/S, I84 V, and L90 M) were associated with virologic response in univariate analysis. In multivariate analysis, those with none of the above mutations showed a 2.2 $\log_{10}$ reduction in HIV RNA after 12 weeks of treatment, versus a median 1.23 $\log_{10}$ reduction for those with one mutation and a 0.27 $\log_{10}$ reduction for those with two or more of these mutations (Table 15-8).[112]

A retrospective comparison of virologic responses to three boosted PIs given to PI-pretreated patients in a large cohort from Madrid, Spain[115] also used a mutation score based on which primary and secondary mutations were present and examined virologic response. Of 52 patients treated with saquinavir/ritonavir 1000/100 mg bid, the rates of response at week 24 were 90% for those with five or fewer saquinavir mutations, versus 21% for those with more than five saquinavir mutations at baseline (Table 15-8).

In the ESQUIV study, baseline resistance was correlated with the 24-week HIV RNA response to treatment for a retrospective analysis of 60 PI-pretreated patients given saquinavir with low-dose ritonavir.[116] The French trials group the ANRS performed a retrospective, multicenter analysis of 138 PI-experienced (>6 months) patients switching to saquinavir/r 1000/100 mg bid. Genotypic resistance analysis was measured at baseline and 3 months after switch associations between baseline mutations and virologic response at 3–4 months were then analysed.[117] The median virologic response (at month 3 or 4) was $-1.48 \log_{10}$ (range, -4 to $+1.2 \log_{10}$). There were nine mutations identified that were most strongly associated with a reduced response. These were at codons 10F/I/M/R/V 15AV, 20I/M/R/T, 24 I, 62V, 73S/T, 82A/F/S/T, 84V, or 90M. It was concluded that at least four of the nine mutations are required for a significant impact on virologic response to boosted saquinavir.

Virologic response (either a 1 $\log_{10}$ reduction in HIV RNA or RNA levels under 50 copies/mL at week 24) correlated with the presence of more than five PI mutations from a list of 25 potential mutations in the univariate analysis (Table 15-8). In multivariate analysis, the strongest prediction of virologic response was the presence of three key mutations – L10I/F, L90M, and A71I/T/V, although it was not possible to calculate the response rates for patients with one, two, or all of these mutations.

There are also rules-based systems which categorize genotypes based on expert opinion and literature review.[24] This particular rules-based interpretation algorithm shows that for saquinavir, significant resistance is predicted when the following combinations of mutations are found:

1. (G48 V or I84A/V or L90 M) and one of the following group: L10F/I/R/V, K20M/R, M36I/V, I54L/T/V, L63P, A71T/V, or V82A/F/T/S; or
2. three or more of the following mutations – L10F/I/R/V, K20M/R, M36I/V, I54L/T/V, L63P, A71T/V, or V82A/F/T/S.

There are several mutations which are commonly found associated with decreased sensitivity to most currently licensed PIs such as the V82A and I84V.[111] Mostly PI cross-resistance involves mutations at positions 10 and 90, 54, 71, 77, 82, and 84.[118,120,121] In one study of 6000 clinical isolates, phenotypic cross-resistance was detected in 59–80% of samples resistant to one PI.[118,119]

Hypersusceptibility

There are four mutations, selected during treatment with other PIs, that can increase the susceptibility of HIV-1 to saquinavir *in vitro*. The D30N mutation which is seen less and less, as the use of nelfinavir with which it is associated decreases, increases the susceptibility to saquinavir, both in the presence and in the absence of L90M.[122] The I50L mutation, seen after virologic failure of unboosted atazanavir, is associated with phenotypic hypersusceptibility to saquinavir and to other PIs.[123] The I50V mutation, selected during failure of amprenavir treatment, shows increased susceptibility to saquinavir.[124] A site-directed mutagenesis analysis combined with *in vitro* competition data suggests that the V82T mutation, selected by indinavir treatment, leads to hypersusceptibility to saquinavir and has impaired replicative fitness.[125] The relevance of these data to clinical practice is not yet clear.

Phenotypic Resistance

Much of the early resistance data were derived when saquinavir was used without ritonavir. It has been difficult to define phenotype thresholds for resistance when PIs are boosted in terms of their pharmacokinetics by ritonavir.

Phenotypic assays are more expensive and have longer turnaround time compared to genotypes. However, saquinavir phenotypic cutoff levels have been extensively evaluated using Virtual Phenotype rather than an actual phenotypic assay.[113] The Virtual Phenotype is derived from a genotype by correlation with a reference database of paired genotypes and phenotypes. This methodology has been shown to have similar clinical utility to real phenotype in a randomized trial.[126] From a database of 4500 patients in cohorts and clinical trials patients treated with either unboosted or ritonavir-boosted saquinavir with a variety of other antiretrovirals had their HIV RNA response to treatment measured at 8 weeks. This was correlated with baseline adjusted saquinavir Virtual Phenotype in a multivariate analysis.[127]

The phenotypic cutoffs are given at those that will give an 80% response and a 20% response compared with wild type. These are currently set at 1.1- and 12-fold change in the IC_{50}. This is helpful to the clinician who can gauge how likely a therapy may succeed rather than have a single cutoff above which the drug is resistant and below which it is sensitive. Other phenotypic resistance cutoff levels have been calculated[82,113,114,128] (Table 15-3) but are based on smaller trials usually deriving a single clinical cutoff of around 10-fold the IC_{50}. Table 15-8 shows summary results from the main cohorts where genotypic resistance and virologic response have been correlated for treatment with saquinavir plus low-dose ritonavir.

NEW AND ONGOING STUDIES

The Gemini trial is evaluating ritonavir-boosted saquinavir 1000/100 mg compared with lopinavir/ritonavir capsules 400/100 mg in 350 treatment-naive patients.[129]

This has been fully recruited. The advantages of the Gemini trial compared with the MaxCmin2 trial include a more homogeneous patient population, an equivalent pill burden for each regimen, and a fixed-dose NRTI backbone for all participants. This study has a noninferiority design with a delta of 12% at 90% power.

BASIC is a study comparing ritonavir-boosted saquinavir 2000 mg/100 mg with boosted atazanavir 300 mg/100 mg in treatment-naive and will look at efficacy as well as effects on body fat distribution measured by CT and DEXA. It will recruit 120 patients with a 48 week follow-up.

The RAINBOW cohort has been designed to look at outcome in those prescribed the saquinavir-500 formulation. The primary endpoints of this international observational cohort study include percentage of patients with grade 3 or 4 adverse events, percentage of patients with HIV-RNA <50 and <400 copies/mL at week 24 and comparisons regarding prior therapies, country, gender, lipids, and other data. It has already recruited over 900 patients from over 80 countries.

SUMMARY

Boosted saquinavir regimens can provide potent and sustained viral suppression in HIV infected patients. While not considered a preferred first-line PI for naive patients in current IAS-USA antiretroviral guidelines, they are appropriate choices as second-line through advanced salvage therapy following failure of the preferred initial antiretroviral regimens. Saquinavir in particular, appears to be one of the better tolerated boosted PIs, with minimal effects on serum lipids. The recommended dose is saquinavir/ritonavir bid (1000 mg/ 100 mg), but data support qd (1500–2000 mg/100 mg) dosing especially in PI-naive patients. The major common clinically relevant drug interactions are relatively few but importantly include rifampicin. It has been used in pregnancy and in children with a good safety and tolerability profile. Its new formulation has lowered pill burden and improved convenience and made it more attractive to both prescribers and patients.

REFERENCES

1. Roberts NA, Martin JA, Kinchington D, et al. Rational design of peptide based proteinase inhibitors. Science 248:358, 1990.
2. Craig JC, Duncan IB, Hockley D, et al. Antiviral properties of Ro 31-8959, an inhibitor of human immunodeficiency virus (HIV) proteinase. Antiviral Res 16:259, 1991.
3. Galpin S, Roberts NA, O'Connor T, et al. Antiviral properties of the HIV-l protease inhibitor Ro-31-8959. Antivir Chem Chemother 5:43, 1994.
4. Hoffmann-La Roche. Fortivase™ (saquinavir) soft gelatin capsules. Prescribing information, 1997 (data on file).
5. Roche UK. Summary of product characteristics: invirase [online]. 2005 [cited 29 Jun 2006]. Available: http://www.rocheuk.com/ProductDB/Documents/rx/spc/Invirase_SPC.pdf
6. Gill MJ. Safety profile of soft gelatin formulation of saquinavir in combination with nucleosides in a broad patient population. NV15182 Study Team. AIDS 12:1400, 1998.
7. Ren S, Lien EJ. Development of HIV protease inhibitors: a survey. Prog Drug Res Spec:1–34, 2001.
8. Bragman K. Saquinavir: an HIV proteinase inhibitor. Adv Exp Med Biol 394:305, 1996.
9. Lazdins JK, Mestan J, Goutte G, et al. In vitro effect of alpha1-acid glycoprotein on the antihuman immunodeficiency virus (HIV) activity of the protease inhibitor CGP 61755: a comparative study with other relevant HIV protease inhibitors. J Infect Dis 175:1063, 1997.
10. Eberle J, Bechowsky B, Rose D, et al. Resistance of HIV type 1 to proteinase inhibitor Ro 31-8959. AIDS Res Hum Retroviruses 11:67, 1995.
11. Johnson VA, Merrill DP, Chou TC, Hirsch MS. Human immunodeficiency virus type 1 (HIV-1) inhibitory interactions between protease inhibitor Ro 31-8959 and zidovudine, 2′,3′-dideoxycytidine, or recombinant interferon-alpha A against zidovudine-sensitive or resistant HIV-1 in vitro. J Infect Dis 166:1143, 1992.
12. Deminie CA, Bechtold CM, Stock D, et al. Evaluation of reverse transcriptase and protease inhibitors in two-drug combinations against human immunodeficiency virus replication. Antimicrob Agents Chemother 40:1346, 1996.
13. Merrill DP, Moonis M, Chou TC, Hirsch MS. Lamivudine or stavudine in two- and three-drug combinations against human immunodeficiency virus type 1 replication in vitro. J Infect Dis 173:355, 1996.
14. Merrill DP, Manion DJ, Chou TC, Hirsch MS. Antagonism between human immunodeficiency virus type I protease inhibitors indinavir and saquinavir in vitro. J Infect Dis 176:265, 1997.
15. Heilek-Snyder G, Hill D, Palansch LA, et al. Synergistic anti-HIV activity of Saquinavir with FDA approved HIV-1 agents determined in drug combination studies. In: Proceedings of 3rd Eur Resist Workshop, Athens, Greece, 30 Mar 30 to Apr 1 2005, Abst 49.
16. Viora M, Di Genova G, Quaranta MG, et al. Lack of immunotoxicity of saquinavir (Ro 31-8959) used alone or in double or triple combination with AZT and ddC. J Clin Immunol 18:346, 1998.
17. Craig JC, Grief C, Mills JS, et al. Effects of a specific inhibitor of HIV proteinase Ro 31-8959 on virus maturation in a chronically infected promonocytic cell line. Antivir Chem Chemother 2:181, 1995.
18. Jacobsen H, Ahlborn-Laake L, Gugel R, Mous J. Progression of early steps of human immunodeficiency virus type 1 replication in the presence of an inhibitor of viral protease. J Virol 66:5087, 1992.
19. Kravcik S, Gallicano K, Roth V, et al. Cerebrospinal fluid HIV RNA and drug levels with combination ritonavir and saquinavir. J Acquir Immune Defic Syndr 21:371, 1999.
20. Mouly SJ, Paine MF, Watkins PB. Contributions of CYP3A4, P-glycoprotein, and serum protein binding to the intestinal first-pass extraction of saquinavir. J Pharmacol Exp Ther 308:941, 2004.
21. Perry C, Noble S. Saquinavir soft-gel capsule formulation a review of its use in patients with HIV infection. Drugs 55:461, 1998.
22. Van Cleef GF, Fisher EJ, Polk RE. Drug interaction potential with inhibitors of HIV protease. Pharmacotherapy 17:774, 1997.
23. Van Heeswijk RPG, Velkamp A, Mulder W, et al. Combination of protease inhibitors for the treatment of HIV-l infected patients: a review of pharmacokinetics and clinical experience. Antivir Ther 6:201, 2002.
24. Clotet B, Menedez-Arias L, Schapiro J, et al. Guide to Management of HIV Drug Resistance, Antiretroviral Pharmacokinetics and Viral Hepatitis in HIV Infected Subjects. 4th edn. Barcelona: Fundació de Lluita contra la SIDA, 2004.
25. Noble S, Faulds D. Saquinavir: a review of its pharmacology and clinical potential in the management of HIV infection. Drugs 52:93, 1996.
26. Hoffmann-La Roche. Fortivase™ (saquinavir) soft gelatin capsules. Prescribing information, 1997 (data on file).
27. Boffito M, Winston A, Fletcher C, et al. Effect of a fat-containing meal on the pharmacokinetic profile of saquinavir 500 tablet/ritonavir (SQV/r) 1000/100 mg bd in HIV infected individuals. In: 7th Int Work Clin Pharm HIV Ther, Lisbon, 20–22 Apr 2006, poster 66.
28. Hsu A, Granneman GR, Cao G, et al. Pharmacokinetic interactions between two human immunodeficiency virus protease inhibitors, ritonavir and saquinavir. Clin Pharmacol Ther 63:453, 1998.
29. Buss N, Snell P, Bock J, et al. Saquinavir pharmacokinetics following combined ritonavir and saquinavir (soft gelatin capsules) administration. Br J Clin Pharmacol 52:255, 2001.
30. Kilby J, Hill A, Buss N. The effect of ritonavir on increases in saquinavir plasma concentration is independent of ritonavir dosage: combined analysis of pharmacokinetic data from 97 subjects. HIV Med 3:1, 2002.
31. Kilby J, Sfakianos G, Gizzi N, et al. Safety and pharmacokinetics of once-daily regimens of soft-gel capsule saquinavir plus mini-dose ritonavir in human immunodeficiency virus-negative adults. Antimicrob Agents Chemother 44:2672, 2000.
32. Washington CB, Flexner C, Sheiner LB, et al; AIDS Clinical Trials Group Protocol (ACTG 378) Study Team. Effect of simultaneous versus staggered dosing on pharmacokinetic interactions of protease inhibitors. Clin Pharmacol Ther 73:406, 2003.
33. Kurowski M, Sternfeld T, Sawyer A, et al. Pharmacokinetic and tolerability profile of twice-daily saquinavir hard gelatin capsules and saquinavir soft gelatin capsules boosted with ritonavir in healthy volunteers. HIV Med 4:94, 2003.
34. Cameron D, Japour A, Xu Y, et al. Ritonavir and saquinavir combination therapy for the treatment of HIV infection. AIDS 13:213, 1999.
35. Piketty C, Race E, Castiel P, et al. Efficacy of a five-drug combination including ritonavir, saquinavir and efavirenz in patients who failed on conventional triple-drug regimen: phenotypic resistance to protease inhibitors predicts outcome of therapy. AIDS 13:F71, 1999.
36. Kurowski M, Aratesh K, Moecklinghoff C, et al. Comparative pharmacokinetics of twice-daily (BID) fortovase/ritoanvir and invirase/ritonavir. In: Proceedings of 8th Deutscher AIDS Kongress, Berlin, 4-7 Jul 2001, poster FOR 062.
37. Kurowski M, Arasteh K, Sternfeld T, et al. Comparative pharmacokinetics and short-term safety of Fortovase®/ritonavir and Invirase®/ritonavir 1000 mg/10 mg BID. In: Proceedings of 9th CROI, Washington, DC, USA, 24–28 Feb 2002, abstract 432.
38. Veldkamp A, Van Heeswijk R, Mulder J, et al. Steady-state pharmacokinetics of twice-daily dosing of saquinavir plus

ritonavir in HIV1-infected individuals. J Acquir Immune Defic Syndr 27:344, 2001.
39. Buss N, Snell P, Bock J, et al. Saquinavir pharmacokinetics following combined ritonavir and saquinavir (soft gelatine capsules) administration. Br J Clin Pharmacol 52:255, 2001.
40. Gatti G, Di Biaggio A, Casazza R. The relationship between ritonavir plasma levels and side-effects: implications for therapeutic drug monitoring AIDS 13:2083, 1999.
41. Sulkowski M, Thomas D, Chaisson R, Moore R. Hepatotoxicity associated with antiretroviral therapy in adults infected with human immunodeficiency virus and the role of hepatitis C or B virus infection. JAMA 283:74, 2000.
42. Autar RS, Boffito M, Hassink E, et al. Interindividual variability of once-daily ritonavir boosted saquinavir pharmacokinetics in Thai and UK patients. J Antimicrob Chemother 56:908, 2005.
43. Grub S, Delora P, Ludin E, et al. Pharmacokinetics and pharmacodynamics of saquinavir in pediatric patients with human immunodeficiency virus infection. Clin Pharmacol Ther 71:122, 2002.
44. Noble S, Faulds D. Saquinavir. A review of its pharmacology and clinical potential in the management of HIV infection. Drugs 52:93, 1996.
44a. Burger D, Eggink A, Ndvan dr Ende I, et al. Pharmacokinetic of Saquinavir new tablets formulation plus Ritonavir 1000/100 mg twice daily in HIV 1 infected pregnant women. Conf on Retroviruses and Opportunistic Infections, Los Angeles, 2007, Abst 741.
45. Tung MY, Khan W, Hawkins DA. The clinical outcome of using saquinavir hard-gel capsules/ritonavir (SQV/r) with two nucleosides (NRTIs) in HIV-infected pregnant women. In: Proceedings of 10th European AIDS Conference, Dublin, Ireland, 17–20 Nov 2005, abstract PE14.2/2.
46. Lopez-Cortes LF, Ruiz-Valderas R, Rivero A, et al. Therapeutic drug monitorization and efficacy of low-dose saquinavir/ritonavir QD in HIV-infected pregnant women. In: 10th European AIDS Conference, Dublin, Ireland, 17–20 Nov 2005, abstract PE14.4.1.
47. Lopez-Cortes LF, Ruiz-Valderas R, Pascual R, et al. Once-daily saquinavir-HGC plus low-dose ritonavir (1200/100 mg) in HIV-infected pregnant women: pharmacokinetics and efficacy. HIV Clin Trials 4:227, 2003.
48. Lundgren DJ, Hill A, Fox Z, et al. Hepatotoxicity of ritonavir-boosted indinavir (idv/r 800/100 mg twice daily) and saquinavir (saq/r 1000/100 mg twice daily) in a phase IV, randomized, open-label, and multicentre trial in adult HIV-1 infection: the MaxCmin1 trial. In: Proceedings of the 5th International Workshop on Adverse Drug Reactions and Lipodystrophy in HIV, Paris, 8–11 Jul 2003.:Antivir Ther 8:L83 (abstract 126), 2003.
49. Wacher VJ, Silverman JA, Zhang Y, Benet LZ. Role of P-glycoprotein and cytochrome P450 3A in limiting oral absorption of peptides and peptidomimetics. J Pharm Sci 87:1322, 1998.
50. Fichtenbaum CJ, Gerber JG, Rosenkranz SL, et al. Pharmacokinetic interactions between protease inhibitors and statins in HIV seronegative volunteers: ACTG Study A5047. AIDS 16: 569, 2002.
51. Dear Dr Letter. www.inverse.com Roche Laboratories Inc, New Jersey, 7 Feb, 2005.
52. Kurowski M, Sternfeld T, Sawyer A, et al. Minor Interaction between efavirenz and saquinavir when combined with small doses of ritonavir in a QD regimen. In: Proceedings of 8th European Conference on Clinical Aspects and Treatment of HIV-Infection, Athens, Greece, 28–31 Oct 2001, Late Breaker Poster 9.
53. Boffito M, Kurowski M, Kruse G, et al. Atazanavir enhances saquinavir hard-gel concentrations in a ritonavir-boosted once-daily regimen. AIDS 18:1291, 2004.
54. Boffito M, Maitland D, Dickinson L, et al. Pharmacokinetics (pk) of saquinavir hard gel (sqv)/ritonavir (r) in combination with different doses of atazanavir (atv) once daily (od) in HIV+ patients Int Cong Drug Therapy HIV. In: Proceedings of 7th Int Congress on Drug Therapy in HIV Infection, Glasgow, UK, 14–18 Nov 2004, abstract P272.
55. Winston A, Back D, Fletcher C, et al. Effect of omeprazole on the pharmacokinetics of saquinavir-500 mg formulation with ritonavir in healthy male and female volunteers. AIDS 20:1401, 2006.
55a. Singh K, Winston A, Dickinson L, et al. Saquinavir/ritonavir PK with omeprazole in HIV-1 infected subjects. Clin Pharm Therap (in press).
56. Gerber JG, Rosenkranz S, Segal Y, et al; ACTG 401 Study Team. Effect of ritonavir/saquinavir on stereoselective pharmacokinetics of methadone: results of AIDS Clinical Trials Group (ACTG) 401. J Acquir Immune Defic Syndr 27:153, 2001.
57. US Department of Health and Human Services. Guidelines for the use of antiretroviral agents in HIV-1-infected adults and adolescents [online]. 4 May 2006 [cited 28 Jun 2006]. Available: http://aidsinfo.nih.gov/ContentFiles/AdultandAdolescentGL.pdf
58. Tirona RG, Bailey DG. Herbal product–drug interactions mediated by induction. Br J Clin Pharmacol 61:677, 2006.
59. Piscitelli SC, Burstein AH, Welden N, et al. The effects of garlic supplements on the pharmacokinetics of saquinavir. Clin Infect Dis 34:234, 2002.
60. Saquinavir (saquinavir mesylate) capsules prescribing information. Nutley, NJ: Roche Laboratories, 1995.
61. Nightingale SL. From the Food and Drug Administration. JAMA 278:379, 1997.
62. Lo JC, Mulligan K, Tai VW, et al. "Buffalo hump" in men with HIV-l infection. Lancet 351:867, 1998.
63. Miller KD, Jones E, Yanovski JA, et al. Visceral abdominal-fat accumulation associated with use of indinavir. Lancet 351:871, 1998.
64. Henry K, Melroe H, Huebsch J, et al. Severe premature coronary artery disease with protease inhibitors. Lancet 351:1328, 1998.
65. Hengel RL, Watts NB, Lennox JL. Benign symmetric lipomatosis associated with protease inhibitors. Lancet 350:1596, 1997.
66. Carr A, Samaras K, Burton S, et al. A syndrome of peripheral lipodystrophy (LD) hyperlipidemia and insulin resistance in patients receiving HIV protease inhibitors. AIDS 12:F51, 1998.
67. Carr A, Sarnaras K, Chisholm DJ, Cooper DA. Pathogenesis of HIV-l protease inhibitor-associated peripheral lipodystrophy, hyperlipidaemia, and insulin resistance. Lancet 351:1881, 1998.
68. Cohen C, Shen Y, Rode R, et al. Effect of nucleoside (NRTI) intensification on prevalence of morphologic abnormalities (MoAs) at year 5 of ritonavir (RTV) plus saquinavir (SQV) therapy in an HIV-infected cohort. In: Proceedings from 9th CROI, Seattle, WA, USA, 24–28 Feb 2002, poster 683-T.
69. De Wit S, Wand H, Law M, et al (on behalf of the MaxCmin1 Trial Group). Prevalence of lipodystrophy and retinoid syndrome in a 48-week randomized trial to evaluate safety and efficacy of indinavir/ritonavir 800/100 mg versus saquinavir/ritonavir 1000/100 mg: the MaxCmin trial. In: 1st EACS Resistance & Pharmacology Workshop, Warsaw, Poland, 25–29 Oct 2003, poster F8/2.
70. Haas DW, Zala C, Schrader S, et al (for the Protocol AI424-009 Study Group). Therapy with atazanavir plus saquinavir in patients failing highly active antiretroviral therapy: a randomized comparative pilot trial. AIDS 17:1339, 2003.
71. Mitsuyasu RT, Skolnik PR, Cohen SR, et al. Activity of the soft gelatin formulation of saquinavir in combination therapy in antiretroviral naive patients. NV15355 Study Team. AIDS 12:FI03, 1998.

72. Lalezari J. Selecting the optimum dose for a new soft gelatine capsule formulation of saquinavir. NV15107 Study Group. J Acquir Immune Defic Syndr Hum Retrovirol 19:195, 1998.
73. Sension MG, Farthing C, Shaffer AG, et al. Challenges of antiretroviral treatment in transient and drug-using populations: the SUN study. AIDS Patient Care STDS 15:129, 2001.
74. Cohen Stuart JW, Schuurman R, Burger DM, et al. Randomized trial comparing saquinavir soft gelatin capsules versus indinavir as part of triple therapy (CHEESE study). AIDS 13:F53, 1999.
75. Moyle G, Pozniak A, Opravil M, et al. The SPICE study: 48-week activity of combinations of saquinavir soft gelatin and nelfinavir with and without nucleoside analogues: study of protease inhibitor combinations in Europe. J Acquir Immune Defic Syndr 23:128, 2000.
76. Wheat LJ, Farthing C, Cohen C, et al. Efficacy and safety of twice-daily versus three-times daily saquinavir soft gelatin capsules as part of triple combination therapy for HIV-1 infection. Antivir Ther 7:199, 2002.
77. Kline MW, Brundage IK, Fletcher CV, et al. Combination therapy with saquinavir soft gelatin capsules in children with human immunodeficiency virus infection. Pediatr Infect Dis J 20:666, 2001.
78. Gisolf EH, Jurriaans S, Pelgrom J, et al. The effect of treatment intensification in HIV-infection: a study comparing treatment with ritonavir/saquinavir and ritonavir/saquinavir/stavudine; Promet Study Group. AIDS 14:405, 2000.
79. Dragsted U, Gerstoft J, Pedersen C, et al. Randomized trial to evaluate indinavir/ritonavir versus saquinavir/ritonavir in human immunodeficiency type-1 infected patients: the MaxCmin1 trial. J Infect Dis 188:634, 2003.
80. Dragsted UB, Gerstoft J, Youle M, et al; MaxCmin2 Trial Group. A randomized trial to evaluate lopinavir/ritonavir versus saquinavir/ritonavir in HIV-1-infected patients: the MaxCmin2 trial. Antivir Ther 10:735, 2005.
80a. Raffi S, Ward D, Ruxrungtham K, et al. Saquinavir/ritonavir bid versus lopinavir/ritonavir bid plus emtricitabine/tenofovir qd as initial therapy in HIV-1 infected patients: the Gemini study 24 weeks into analysis. 4th IAS Sydney 2007, Abstract We PeB027.
81. Valer L, de Mendoza C, de Requena DG, et al (on behalf of the Fortogene Spanish Study Group). Impact of HIV genotyping and drug levels on the response to salvage therapy with saquinavir/ritonavir. AIDS 16:1964, 2002.
82. Piketty C, Race E, Castiel P, et al. Phenotypic resistance to protease inhibitors in patients who fail on highly active antiretroviral therapy predicts the outcome at 18 weeks of a five-drug combination including ritonavir, saquinavir and efavirenz. AIDS 14:626, 2000.
83. Montaner J, Saag M, Barylski C, et al. FOCUS Study: saquinavir QD regimen versus efavirenz QD regimen 24 week analysis in HIV infected patients. In: Proceedings of 41st ICAAC, Chicago, IL, USA, 16–19 Dec 2001, abstract I-670.
84. Cardiello P, Srasuebkul P, Hassink E, et al. The 48-week efficacy of once-daily saquinavir/ritonavir in patients with undetectable viral load after 3 years of antiretroviral therapy. HIV Med 6:122, 2005.
85. López-Cortés L, Ruiz-Valderas R, Viciana P, et al. Pharmacokinetics, efficacy and safety of once-daily saquinavir-sgc plus ritonavir (1,200/100 mg) and efavirenz in HIV-pretreated patients ("FrE" study). In: Proceedings of 9th CROI, Seattle, WA, USA, 24–28 Feb 2001, 2002, abstract 441-W.
86. Peytavin G, Landman R, Lamotte C, et al. Saquinavir (SQV) plasma and intracellular concentrations in a once daily dosing combination Fortovase® (SQV-SGC)-low dose ritonavir (RTV) in a prospective study (IMEA 015) in HIV-infected patients. In: Proceedings of 2nd International Workshop on Clinical Pharmacology of HIV Therapy, Noordwijk, The Netherlands, 2–4 Apr 2001, abstract 3.16.
87. Mallolas J, Blanco JL, Sarasa M, et al. Intensification therapy with saquinavir soft gel/ritonavir QD in patients failing on a saquinavir hard gel containing HAART. In: 1st IAS Conference on HIV Pathogenesis and Treatment, Buenos Aires, Argentina, 7–11 Jul 2001, abstract 675.
88. Ananworanich J, Hill A, Siangphoe U, et al; Staccato Study Group. A prospective study of efficacy and safety of once-daily saquinavir/ritonavir plus two nucleoside reverse transcriptase inhibitors in treatment-naive Thai patients. Antivir Ther 10:761, 2005.
89. Cardiello P, Srasuebkul P, Hassink E, et al. HIVNAT 001.3: the efficacy, safety and immunological changes of once-daily saquinavir soft gel capsules 1,600 mg/ritonavir 100 mg plus dual nucleosides in patients who had an undetectable viral load after 3 years of treatment. In: 9th CROI, Seattle, WA, USA, 24–28 Feb 2001, 2002, abstract 549-T.
90. Cardiello P, Van Heeswijk R, Hassink E, et al. Simplifying protease inhibitor therapy with once-daily dosing of saquinavir soft-gelatin capsules/ritonavir (1,600/100 mg): HIVNAT 001.3 study. J Acquir Immune Defic Syndr 29:464, 2002.
91. Smith G, Klein M, Gilmore N, et al. Salvage therapy for HIV infection with lopinavir/ritonavir and boosted saquinavir-SGC. In: Proceedings of Canadian Association for HIV Research (CAHR) Meeting, Toronto, ON, Canada, 31 May to 3 Jun 2001, abstract 212.
92. Hellinger J, Morris AB, Piscitelli S, et al. Pilot study of saquinavir-SGC (Fortovase, SQV) 1,000 mg twice daily and lopinavir/ritonavir(Kaletra, LPV/r) in protease inhibitor-experienced HIV+ individuals: dose escalation and combined normalised inhibitory quotient (cNIQ). In: 9th CROI, Seattle, WA, USA, 24–28 Feb 2001, 2002, abstract 451.
93. Ruiz L, Ribera E, Bonjoch A, et al. Virologic and immunological benefit of a salvage therapy that includes Kaletra plus Fortovase preceded or not by antiretroviral therapy interruption in advanced HIV-infected patients (6-month follow-up). In: 9th CROI, Seattle, WA, USA, 24–28 Feb 2001, 2002, abstract 421.
94. Staszewski S, Dauer B, Stephan C, et al. Pharmacokinetic profile monitoring as an augmentation to therapy evaluation in patients taking a simple boosted double protease inhibitor regimen of lopinavir/ritonavir plus saquinavir without reverse transcriptase inhibitors. In: Proceedings of 3rd International Workshop on Clinical Pharmacology of HIV Therapy, Washington, USA, 13 Apr 2002, abstract 2.4.
95. Hellinger J, Cohen CJ, Morris AB, et al. A pilot study of saquinavir-SGC and lopinavir/ritonavir twice daily in protease inhibitor naive HIV-positive individuals: protease inhibitor concentrations and week 48 results. In: Proceedings of 2nd IAS conference on HIV Pathogenesis and Treatment, Paris, France, 23–27 Jul 2003, poster 571.
96. Delassus JL, Mansouri R, Malbec D, et al. Lopinavir/saquinavir regimen in pre-treated protease inhibitors and reverse transcriptase inhibitors patients, with resistance or toxicity, EACS resistance & pharmacology workshop. In: 9th ECAS, Warsaw, Poland, 25–29 Oct 2003, abstract 7.4/12.
97. Staszewski S, Dauer B, Carlebach A, et al. The LOPSAQ salvage study: 48 week analysis of the full cohort treated with lopinavir (LPV/r) plus saquinavir (SQV) without any additional antiretroviral (ART) therapy. In: Program and Abstracts of the 15th International AIDS Conference, Bangkok, Thailand, 11–16 Jul 2004, abstract B10840.
98. Duvivier C, Ghosn J, Wirden M, et al. Efficacy and safety of dual boosted PI regimen without RT inhibitors in HIV-1-infected patients. In: Proceedings of 12th CROI, Boston, MA, USA, 22–25 Feb 2005, abstract 578.
99. Furfine E, Berrey M, Naderer O, et al. Virologic and pharmacokinetic rationale for a new salvage regimen: APV/saquinavir/RTV BID. In: 3rd International Workshop on Salvage

Therapy for HIV Infection, Chicago, IL, 12–14 Apr 2000, 2002, poster 16.
100. Tremblay C, Merrill DP, Chou TC, Hirsch MS. Interactions among combinations of two and three protease inhibitors against drug-susceptible and drug-resistant HIV-1 isolates. J Acquir Immune Defic Syndr 22:430, 1999.
101. Boffito M, Dickinson L, Hill A, et al. Steady-state pharmacokinetics of saquinavir hard-gel/ritonavir/fosamprenavir in HIV-1-infected patients. J Acquir Immune Defic Syndr 37:1376, 2004.
102. Haas D, Zala C, Schrader S, et al. Atazanavir plus saquinavir once daily favorably affects total cholesterol, fasting triglyceride and fasting LDL cholesterol profiles in patients failing prior therapy (trial AI424-009, week 48). In: Proceedings of 9th CROI, Seattle, WA, USA, 24–28 Feb 2001, 2002, abstract 42.
103. Haas DW, Zala C, Schrader S, et al. Therapy with atazanavir plus saquinavir in patients failing highly active antiretroviral therapy: a randomized comparative pilot trial. AIDS 17:1339, 2003.
104. Rottmann, Dauer B, Hentig N, et al. Atazanavir/ritonavir/saquinavir without an other antiretroviral drugs in PI experienced patients with no reverse transcriptase inhibitor options; a 24 wk cohort analysis. In: Proceedings of 7th Intl Cong Drug Ther HIV Infect, Glasgow, Scotland, UK, 14–18 Nov 2004, poster P21.
105. Colson A, Hellinger J, Cohen C, et al. The stars study: once daily atazanavir, low dose ritonavir and saquinavir in subjects with HIV-1 infection: 24 week efficacy and safety results. In: Proceedings of 3rd IAS, Rio De Janerio, Brazil, 24–27 Jul 2005, poster WePe12.3C20.
106. Roberts N, Craig C, Sheldon J. Resistance and cross-resistance with saquinavir and other HIV protease inhibitors: theory and practice. AIDS 12:453, 1998.
107. Parkin N, Lie Y, Hellmann N, et al. Letter. J Infect Dis 181:1864, 2000.
108. Tsai K, Heilik-Snyder G, Ravindran P et al. Changes in genotypic resistance patterns for saquinavir, lopinavir and amprenavir with rising phenotypic cut-off levels: analysis of TORO database. In: 13th International HIV Resistance Workshop, Tenerife Sur-Costa Adeje, Canary Islands, Spain, 8–12 Jun 2004, abstract 133.
109. Sune C, Brennan L, Stover DR, Klimkait T. Effect of polymorphisms on the replicative capacity of protease inhibitor-resistant HIV-1 variants under drug pressure. Clin Microbiol Infect 10:119, 2004.
110. International AIDS Society-USA [homepage on the Internet]. HIV Drug Resistance Mutations [cited Jul 2006]. Available: http://www.iasusa.org/resistance_mutations/index.html
111. Johnson V, Brun-Vezinet F, Clotet B, et al. Drug resistance mutations in HIV-1. Top HIV Med 13:4, 2005.
112. Marcelin AG, Dalban C, Peytavin G, et al. Clinically relevant interpretation of genotype and relationship to plasma drug concentrations for resistance to saquinavir–ritonavir in human immunodeficiency virus type 1 protease inhibitor-experienced patients. Antimicrob Agents Chemother 48:4687, 2004.
113. Hill A, Walmsley S, Clotet B, Molto J. Analysis of genotypic and phenotypic clinical cut-off levels for ritonavir-boosted saquinavir. HIV Med 7:67, 2006.
114. Valer L, Hill A, Gonzalez de Requena D, et al. Predictive power of single mutations, mutation score and Cmin levels for response to salvage regimens including saquinavir/r 1000/100 mg BID. In: 10th International HIV Resistance Workshop, Seville, Spain, Jun 2002, abstract 98.
115. Barreiro P, Camino N, de Mendoza C, et al. Comparison of the efficacy, safety and predictive value of HIV genotyping using distinct ritonavir-boosted protease inhibitors. Int J Antimicrob Agents 20:438, 2002.
116. Morand-Joubert L, Lacombe K, Duguit C, et al. Impact of genotypic resistance in protease inhibitor experienced patients treated by a combination including saquinavir and ritonavir. In: Proceedings of 15th IAS Conference, Bangkok, Thailand, 11–16 Jul 2004, abstract 5722.
117. Marcelin AG, Flandre P, de Mendoza C, et al. Interpretation of genotype for resistance to boosted saquinavir in HIV-1 infected protease inhibitor experienced patients. In: 4th Eur HIV Drug Resist Wkshop, Monaco, 2006, abstract 54.
118. Hertogs K, Bloor S, Kemp S, et al. Phenotypic and genotypic analysis of clinical HIV-1 isolates reveals extensive protease inhibitor cross-resistance: a survey of over 6000 samples. AIDS 14:1203, 2000.
119. Casado JL, Moreno A, Sabido R. Individualizing salvage regimens: the inhibitory quotient (Ctrough/IC50) as predictor of virologic response. AIDS 17:262, 2003.
120. Rose R, Gong Y, Greytock D, et al. Human immunodeficiency virus type 1 viral background plays a major role in development of resistance to protease inhibitors. Proc Natl Acad Sci USA 93:1648, 1996.
121. de la Carriere LC, Paulous S, Clavel F, Mammano F. Effects of human immunodeficiency virus type 1 resistance to protease inhibitors on reverse transcriptase processing, activity, and drug sensitivity. J Virol 73:3455, 1999.
122. Parkin N, Chappey C. Virologic Clinical Reference Laboratory. Discordance between genotype-based predictions of protease inhibitor susceptibility and actual phenotype in HIV-1 isolates containing mutations at positions 82 and 90: modulatory effects at secondary positions. In: 8th International HIV Resistance Workshop, Sitges, Spain, Jun 2000, abstract 152.
123. Colonno R, Friborg J, Rose R, et al. Identification of amino acid substitutions correlated with reduced atazanavir susceptibility in patients treated with atazanavir containing regimens. In: 10th International HIV Resistance Workshop, Seville, Spain, Jun 2002, abstract 004.
124. Maguire M, Shortino D, Klein A, et al. Emergence of resistance to protease inhibitor amprenavir in human immunodeficiency virus type 1 infected patients: selection of four alternative viral protease genotypes and influence of viral susceptibility to coadministered reverse transcriptase nucleoside inhibitors. Antimicrob Agents Chemother 46:731, 2002.
125. Martinez-Picado J, Savara A, Shi L, et al. Fitness of human immunodeficiency virus type 1 protease inhibitor-selected single mutants. Virology 275:318, 2000.
126. Perez-Elias M, Garcia-Arota I, Muñoz V, et al. Phenotype or Virtual Phenotype for choosing antiretroviral therapy after failure: a prospective, randomised study. Antivir Ther 8:577, 2003.
127. Bachelor LT, Winters B, Nauwelaers D, et al. Estimation of phenotypic clinical cutoffs for Virtual Phenotype™ through meta-analysis of clinical trial and cohort data. In: Proceedings of 12th International HIV Resistance Workshop, Santa Cruz, Tenerife, Spain, 8–12 Jun 2004. Antivir Ther 9:S154 (abstract 138), 2004.
128. Meynard J, Vray M, Morand-Joubert M, et al. Phenotypic or genotypic resistance testing for choosing antiretroviral therapy after treatment failure: a randomized trial. AIDS 16:727, 2002.
129. Hoffmann-La Roche. GEMINI Study – a study of saquinavir/ritonavir in treatment-naive patients with HIV-1 infection [online]. Jun 2006 [cited 3 Jul 2006]. Available: http://www.clinicaltrials.gov/ct/gui/show/NCT00105079?order=43

Chapter 16

Ritonavir

Sven A. Danner, MD, PhD

Ritonavir (RTV) is an inhibitor of the protease enzyme encoded by the human immunodeficiency virus (HIV) (Fig. 16-1). The chemical structure of the synthetic peptidomimetic antiviral agent RTV was designed based on the C^2 symmetry of this enzyme.[1,2] HIV protease cleaves the gag and gag-pol precursor molecules into smaller proteins. Without proper cleavage, the structural proteins of the virion core (p17, p24, p9, p7) and viral enzymes (reverse transcriptase (RT), integrase, protease) cannot be formed adequately, which results in the formation of immature, noninfectious virions.[3,4] Early *in vitro* studies showed equal potency of RTV and zidovudine (ZDV) on a molar basis for several laboratory HIV-1 strains in MT-4 cells and eightfold less activity against an HIV-2 strain, with a median inhibitory concentration (IC_{50}) of 0.045 μmol/L against seven clinical HIV-1 isolates in peripheral blood lymphocytes.[1] The affinity of RTV for human aspartic proteases such as renin, pepsin, cathepsin D and E, and gastricin is low; and cytotoxic effects are seen only when RTV is administered in concentrations of more than 500–1000 times those required for antiretroviral activity.[1,2]

The spectrum of antiviral activity is limited. RTV is active against human retroviruses including HIV-1 and, to a lesser degree, HIV-2.[2,3,5]

PHARMACOKINETICS

The pharmacokinetics of RTV have been studied in healthy volunteers and HIV-infected adults 18–63 years of age. The pharmacokinetics in adults above the age of 63 and in persons with kidney or liver function disturbances have not been assessed.[6] So far the results do not reveal differences in pharmacokinetics between healthy individuals and HIV-infected persons or between individuals of different gender or race.

Following oral administration, RTV is well absorbed, with peak plasma concentrations appearing within 2–4 h.[7] The maximal concentration (C_{max}) and area under the concentration–time curve (AUC) increased nonlinearly after single doses ranging from 100 to 1000 mg: The mean dose-normalized (per 100 mg) C_{max} and AUC increased from 0.416 μg/mL and 3.480 $\mu g\,h^{-1}\,mL^{-1}$ (100 mg) to 1.27 μg/mL and 12.31 $\mu g\,h^{-1}\,mL^{-1}$ (1000 mg), respectively. This points to a saturable metabolism.[7] In a phase II clinical trial, after 3 weeks of treatment with RTV monotherapy, the C_{max} and AUC varied from 5.7 μg/mL and 29.7 $\mu g\,h^{-1}\,mL^{-1}$, respectively, with a 300 mg bid dose to 11.2 μg/mL and 60.8 $\mu g\,h^{-1}\,mL^{-1}$, respectively, with a 600 mg

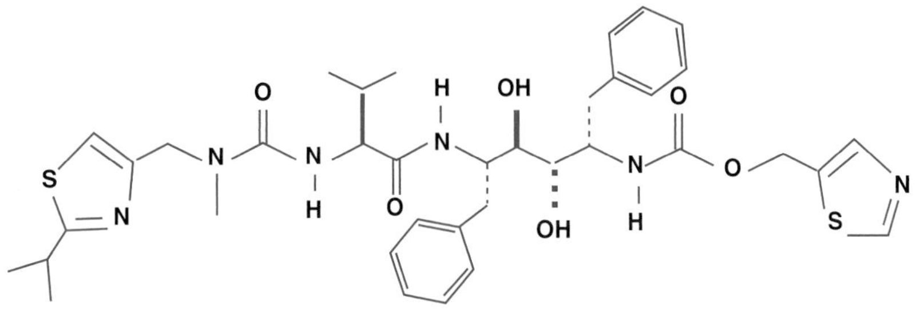

Figure 16-1 ■ Chemical structure and chemical name of ritonavir. 10-Hydroxy-2-methyl-5-(1-methylethyl)-1-[2-(1-methylethyl)-4-thiazolyl]-3,6-dioxo-8,11-bis(phenylmethyl)-2,4,7,12-tetraazatridecan-13-oic-acid,5-thiazolylmethyl ester, [5S-(5R*,8R*,10R*11R*)].
From Norvir (ritonavir) capsules and oral solution prescribing information. North Chicago, IL: Abbott Laboratories; 1996.

bid dose.[8] After oral dosing of 600 mg of ^{14}C-labeled RTV, 34% of the dose was recovered from the feces as unchanged drug, and virtually all of the RTV in the systemic circulation was unchanged, indicating an oral bioavailability of at least 60% and a small first-pass effect.[6]

Although the presence of food in the gastrointestinal tract affects the rate and extent of absorption of RTV, it does so only to a moderate degree and is dependent on the dosage form of the drug.[6] Administration of 600 mg of RTV as oral solution with food results in a delayed and decreased (~23%) peak plasma concentration and 7% decreased overall absorption when compared to administration of the same dose in the fasting state. However, the overall absorption of RTV administered as capsules seems to be increased (by ~15%) when taken simultaneously with a meal.[6]

Between 98–99% of RTV is bound to plasma proteins; most of it is bound to albumin and α_1-acid glycoprotein over a large concentration range (0.01–30 μg/mL). Currently it is not known if RTV crosses the placenta or is excreted in breast milk.[6]

The exact relation between plasma RTV concentrations and antiretroviral effects has not been determined. In patients receiving RTV 600 mg bid as an oral solution or as capsules, the plasma trough concentrations exceed the concentration of RTV (after adjustment for binding to human plasma proteins) required to inhibit 90% of detectable HIV-1 replication *in vitro*, the so-called IC_{90}.[8]

Elimination of RTV is mainly by hepatic metabolism.[6,9] In patients receiving 600 mg bid, the systemic clearance was 8.8 L/h, and the renal clearance has been reported to be less than 0.1 L/h. Plasma half-life averages 3–5 h.[6,8] In the human liver microsomes, RTV metabolism is mediated by the cytochrome P450 (CYP) subsystems 3A4 and, to a lesser degree, 2D6. As stated above, after administration of 600 mg radio-labeled RTV as an oral solution, 34% of the drug was excreted in the unchanged form, and 86% of the dose was excreted in the feces. In total, 11% of the dose was excreted in the urine, of which only 3.5% was excreted as unchanged drug.[6] There are no data available on elimination by hemodialysis or peritoneal dialysis; but given the hepatic metabolism and the high degree of binding to proteins in the plasma, it seems unlikely that substantial amounts of the drug can be eliminated via these means.

DRUG INTERACTIONS

Because RTV has a high affinity for several P450 isoenzymes, the compound exhibits clinically important drug interactions with a wide variety of other drugs. Isoenzymes CYP3A4, CYP2D6, CYP2C9, CYP2D19, and to a lesser degree CYP2A6, CYP1A2, and CYP2E1 are affected by RTV. Co-administration of RTV and drugs that are metabolized by these isoenzymes may result in competition for these enzymes, causing a decrease in metabolism and high plasma levels of the other agents. Conversely, RTV is metabolized by CYP3A4 and CYP2D6,[9] and therefore concomitant administration of RTV and drugs that induce these isoenzymes may result in decreased RTV plasma levels. Finally, RTV may increase the activity of glucuronyltransferase, and concomitant administration of RTV and drugs that are directly glucuronidated may result in loss of activity of these drugs.[6]

The manufacturer of RTV issues a regularly updated list of compounds that should not be used or be used with caution in conjunction with RTV. Pharmacokinetic interaction studies with RTV are available for some drugs (e.g., the antifungal fluconazole[10]), but for many others the recommendations are based on theoretical considerations. Table 16-1 lists recommendations for concomitant use of several drugs with RTV; this list is based on information from the manufacturer[6] and is by no means exhaustive.

The strong affinity of RTV for some P450 isoenzymes may also influence the pharmacokinetics of several other antiretroviral agents when given in combination with RTV. Concomitant administration of RTV (600 mg bid) and nucleoside analog reverse transcriptase inhibitors (NRTIs) such as didanosine (200 mg bid) or zidovudine (ZDV) (200 mg tid) over 4 days decreased the C_{max} by 16% and 27%, and decreased the AUC by 13% and 25%, respectively.[11] The manufacturer does not advocate dose adjustments of either of these antiretroviral agents.

Co-administration of RTV and the non-nucleoside reverse transcriptase inhibitor (NNRTI) nevirapine resulted in a mean nonsignificant 11% decrease in RTV AUC in 12 HIV-infected individuals[12]; the change in nevirapine pharmacokinetics also was not significant. Co-administration with another NNRTI, delavirdine, likewise had no clinically relevant effects on the steady-state pharmacokinetics of either RTV or delavirdine in a study using RTV at a reduced dose.[13]

In contrast to the co-administration of RTV and RT inhibitors, the simultaneous use of RTV and other protease inhibitors (PIs) leads to important pharmacokinetic interactions. RTV causes a highly significant increase in both the C_{max} and the AUC of saquinavir (SQV) when the two drugs are administered simultaneously. This information is useful because the oral bioavailability of SQV is poor as a result of, among other causes, an extensive first-pass effect.[14] Whereas the standard dose of SQV in combination with NRTIs is 600 mg tid, when SQV is co-administered with RTV the AUC of SQV is so greatly increased that even 400 mg bid dosing results in a 20–40-fold increase without much effect on RTV pharmacokinetics.[15,16] The soft gel capsule formulation of SQV is administered at a dosage of 1200 mg tid. However, when used with RTV, the dose administered is the same as that recommended for the older formulation of SQV: 400–600 mg bid.

The pharmacokinetics of the PI indinavir (IND) are heavily influenced by co-administration of RTV as well. In healthy volunteers, RTV increased the AUC and C_{max} of IND by 480% and 110%, respectively; even with a reduced, twice-daily dosing regimen of IND without the usual administration of the drug in the fasting state, the combination of RTV and IND yielded a comparable AUC, with higher trough and slightly lower peak levels of IND compared to the standard three-times-a-day regimen. No effects on RTV pharmacokinetics

Drug Interactions with RTV

Table 16-1

Drug Administered with RTV	Recommendation	Comments
Antifungals		
Fluconazole	No adjustment	Only small increase in C_{max} and AUC[10]
Itraconazole	Caution	
Ketoconazole	Caution	
Antimalarial and Antiprotozoals Agents		
Quinine	Caution	Threefold increase in AUC may be expected
Proguanil	No adjustment	
Chloroquine	Caution	
Primaquine	Caution	
Pyrimethamine	Caution	
Atovaquone	Caution	Possible decreased AUC as a result of enhanced glucuronidation
Antimycobacterials		
Rifabutin	Contraindicated	Large increase in AUC of rifabutin, and especially of its 25-*O*-desacetyl metabolite[6]
Rifampin	Caution	Threefold increase in AUC of rifampin, but large reduction in AUC of RTV[6]
Ethambutol	No adjustment	Anecdotal data only; no proper evaluation done
Macrolide Antibiotics		
Clarithromycin	Depends on renal function	No adjustment in patients with normal renal function; 50% dose reduction when creatinine clearance is 30–60 mL/min, 75% dose reduction when <30 mL/min
Erythromycin	Caution	Threefold increase in AUC of erythromycin to be expected
Other Antiinfectives		
Cotrimoxazole	No adjustment	20% decrease in AUC of sulfamethoxazole and 20% increase in AUC of trimethoprim expected
Metronidazole	Discouraged	Disulfiram-like reaction possible (RTV oral solution and capsules contain alcohol)
Anticoagulants		
Warfarin	Caution	Large increase in AUC of *R*-enantiomer and moderate decrease in AUC of *S*-enantiomer: monitor prothrombin time carefully
Antihistaminics		
Astemizole, terfenadine	Contraindicated	Very large increase in AUC expected
Antineoplastics		
Group I: etoposide, paclitaxel, tamoxifen, vincristine, vinblastine	Caution	These agents are metabolized by CYP3A4, so threefold or larger increase in AUC can be expected: monitor therapeutic and toxic effects carefully
Group II: cyclophosphamide, daunorubicin, doxorubicin	Caution	All these agents are metabolized by unidentified CYP isoenzymes, so changes in AUC are unpredictable: monitor therapeutic and toxic effects carefully
Cardiovascular Agents		
Group I: amiodarone, bepridil, encainide, flecainide, propafenone, quinidine	Contraindicated	
Group II: diltiazem, disopyramide, felodipine, isradipine, lidocaine, nicardipine, nifedipine, verapamil	Caution	All are metabolized by CYP3A4, so threefold or larger increase in AUC is expected
Group III: mexiletine, metoprolol, pindolol, propranolol, timolol	Caution	All are metabolized by CYP2C9/19 isoenzymes; moderate increase or decrease in AUC is to be expected

(Continued)

(Continued)

Table 16-1

Drug Administered with RTV	Recommendation	Comments
Group IV: acebutolol, digoxin, prazocin, tocainide	Caution	Metabolized by unidentified P450 isoenzymes; no data available
Antilipemic Agents		
Lovastatin, pravastatin fluvastatin, gemfibrozil	Caution	Metabolized by CYP3A4
Simvastatin	Contraindicated	Extensively metabolized by P450 isoenzymes
Clofibrate	Monitor effect	Metabolized by glucuronidation; might result in decrease of AUC
Central Nervous System Agents		
Pyroxicam	Contraindicated	
NSAIDs		
Diclofenac, ibuprofen, indomethacin	No adjustment	Only moderate increase in AUC expected
Ketoprofen, naproxen	Monitor effect	Metabolized by glucuronidation; might result in decrease of AUC
Opiate agonists		
Meperidine, propoxyphene	Contraindicated	
Alfentanyl, fentanyl	Caution	Threefold or larger increase in AUC expected
Methadone	Caution	Metabolized by unidentified P450 isoenzymes, so increase in AUC possible; also metabolized by glucuronidation, which might result in lowered AUC; net effect unknown
Codeine, morphine	Monitor effect	Metabolized by glucuronidation; might result in decrease of AUC
Anticonvulsants		
Carbamazepine	Caution	Threefold or larger increase in AUC; decrease of RTV AUC
Phenobarbital	Caution	Metabolized by unidentified P450 isoenzymes, so increase in AUC possible; decrease in RTV AUC possible
Phenytoin	Caution	Moderate increase or decrease in AUC expected; decrease in RTV AUC possible
Sedatives and hypnotics		
Alprazolam, clorazepate, diazepam, estazolam, flurazepam, midazolam, triazolam, zolpidem	Contraindicated	
Lorazepam, oxazepam, propofol, temazepam	Caution	Metabolized by glucuronidation; might result in decrease of AUC
Gastrointestinal Agents		
Dronabinol, ondansetron	Caution	Metabolized by CYP3A4: threefold or larger increase in AUC
Lansoprazole, omeprazole	No adjustment	Moderate increase or decrease in AUC to be expected
Promethazine	Caution	Metabolized by unidentified P450 isoenzymes; increase in AUC possible
Corticosteroids		
Prednisone	Caution	Metabolized by CYP3A4: threefold or larger increase in AUC
Dexamethasone	Caution	Metabolized by CYP3A4: threefold or larger increase in AUC; also, induction of CYP3A4 possible, with resulting increase in RTV clearance and lowering of plasma RTV levels
Estrogens		
Ethinyl estradiol	Increase of dose or alternative contraceptive method	RTV 500 mg bid decreased C_{max} and AUC 32% and 40%, respectively[6]

AUC, area under the time – concentration curve; NSAIDs, nonsteroidal antiinflammatory drugs.

were observed.[17] RTV also increased the AUC of the PI nelfinavir by 150%, without affecting the AUC of RTV.[18,19]

The inhibitory effect on the metabolism of other PIs has gradually become the most important and almost only use of RTV in HIV infection. However, early trials were done with RTV as the sole PI.

CLINICAL TRIALS

RTV Used As a Sole PI

Ritonavir monotherapy has been investigated in two phase I/II trials.[8,20] Danner et al in a double-blind, randomized, placebo-controlled trial, studied 84 HIV-positive patients who had no prior exposure to a PI and at least 50 CD4+ T lymphocytes per cubic microliter. They were assigned to one of four RTV dosing regimens (300, 400, 500, or 600 mg bid) or placebo for 4 weeks, then the placebo recipients were again randomized to one of the RTV regimens.[8] During the first 4 weeks, increases in CD4+ T lymphocytes and decreases in plasma HIV RNA were similar among the four RTV groups and significantly different from those in the placebo groups. Thereafter, however, a return to baseline values was noted after 16 weeks among the three lower dosage groups. In the highest dosage group, the HIV RNA load also partially increased after the nadir was reached at 4–8 weeks of treatment (1.2 $\log_{10}$ copies/mL decrease). After 32 weeks; among the patients in the 600 mg bid dosage group, the median increase from baseline in the CD4+ T-lymphocyte count was 230 cells/mL, and the mean decrease in HIV RNA was 0.81 $\log_{10}$ copies/mL. However, this last parameter was assessed with the first-generation Chiron branched-chain DNA (bDNA) assay, which had a lower limit of detection of 10 000 RNA copies/mL.[21] When a more sensitive assay was utilized, decreases in the HIV RNA load turned out to be larger; applying the Roche polymerase chain reaction (PCR) assay[22] in the two highest dose groups, a mean maximal decrease of 1.91 $\log_{10}$ copies/mL was found, in contrast to 1.1 $\log_{10}$ copies/mL when measured with the bDNA assay. Adverse events included nausea, circumoral paresthesias, and elevated transaminase and triglyceride levels. Ten withdrawals from the study were judged to be RTV related.

In another phase I/II trial, Markowitz et al studied three- and four-times-a-day dosing regimens of RTV in 62 HIV-infected patients.[20] As in the prior study, a clear increase in CD4+ T-lymphocyte count and a decreased plasma HIV RNA load were found over 12 weeks, although the responses in these dosage groups were slightly inferior to those in the 600 mg bid regimen mentioned in the previous study. In this study pharmacokinetics were studied early (days 4–11) and later (days 22–29) during RTV administration. In all dosing groups the C_{max}, minimal concentration, and AUC decreased considerably during the period between the two time points, which is in agreement with preclinical studies suggesting that RTV induces its own metabolism.[1] The spectrum of adverse events was not different from that seen in the first phase I/II study. Of the 62 patients, three withdrew because of adverse events thought to be related to RTV administration.[20]

On the basis of these two phase I/II studies, the 600 mg bid dosage was chosen for use in subsequent studies.

Use in Antiretroviral-Naive HIV-Infected Patients

Notermans et al[23] treated 33 antiretroviral-naive HIV-infected patients (31 men, two women) with a CD4+ T-lymphocyte count of more than 50 cells/mL and a plasma HIV RNA load of more than 30 000 copies/mL (Roche Amplicor) with RTV, ZDV, and lamivudine (3TC) (Table 16-2). The patients were randomized into two groups. Group I started with all three antiretroviral agents simultaneously, and group II started with RTV monotherapy for 3 weeks; ZDV and 3TC were then added (this design was chosen to investigate whether quick development of resistance against the nucleoside analogs, especially against 3TC, could be prevented by prior lowering of the HIV replication rate by a PI). A tonsillar biopsy was performed at baseline and after 2 days, 22 days, and 6 months of therapy to study changes in the HIV RNA load and lymphocyte subsets in lymphoid tissues.[24] Group I had a somewhat higher CD4+ T-lymphocyte count than group II (177 vs 134 cells/mL), but there were no differences in the baseline HIV RNA load (mean 5.3 $\log_{10}$ copies/mL) or in the Centers for Disease Control and Prevention (CDC) class of clinical HIV infection. Protease and RT gene sequencing at baseline showed only one case with a 41 and 215 RT codon change (known to confer resistance to ZDV) pretherapy, and in six cases two protease gene mutations (36, 71, or both) not known to be associated with resistance against RTV were observed. During treatment there was a quick initial rise in CD4+ T lymphocytes, with a more gradual increase with a nonsignificant, slightly better result after 24 weeks in group I (an increase in CD4+ T lymphocytes of 180 versus 99 cells/mL in group II). A protease gene codon 82 mutation (known to confer resistance to RTV) developed in only one patient on therapy who did not comply with the regimen. No new RT gene mutations developed in any of the patients. The plasma HIV RNA load showed an initial rapid decline during the first 3 weeks, followed by a slower further decline, reaching its nadir of almost 3.0 $\log_{10}$ copies/mL at week 16 (Fig. 16-2).[23] The decreased plasma viral load was mirrored in the lymphoid tissue HIV RNA load. Both the amount of HIV trapped on the surface of follicular dendritic cells and the number of actively HIV-producing mononuclear cells decreased sharply, even after 2 days of therapy, and reached a decrease of more than 3.4 and more than 2.3 log units per gram of lymphoid tissue, respectively.[24] There were many adverse events, mainly gastrointestinal in nature, prompting eight of 33 patients to withdraw from the study.

In contrast to the phase I/II studies in which RTV was administered as monotherapy, in this study the excellent HIV RNA response was maintained for at least 6 months. For example, in the RTV/ZDV/3TC study, 95% of the patients who were still on treatment after 52 weeks had no detectable

Table 16-2

Summary of Major Clinical Trials with RTV

Trial	Design	Dosage (mg)	No. of Subjects	Entry Criteria	CD4+T-Lymphocyte Count: Cells/mm^3 on Entry	CD4+T-Lymphocyte Count: Response	Antiviral Response	Comments
Danner[8]	Open-label, nonrandomized	RTV: 300, 400, 500, 600 bid	84	PI-naive	>50	Initial inc with return toward BL in lower three dose groups	A 1.2 $\log_{10}$ dec with return toward BL in lower 3 dose groups	A 1.91 $\log_{10}$ dec when PCR (vs bDNA) was used; 10 pts withdrew because of toxicity.
Markowitz[20]	Open-label, nonrandomized	RTV: 200 tid, 200 qid, 300 tid, 300 qid	62	PI-naive, VL >25 000/mL	>50 and <500	Inc of 74 cells and 83 cells at 4 and 12 week, respectively	A 0.86–1.18 $\log_{10}$ dec in VL at week 2–4; 0.5 $\log_{10}$ dec at week 12	10 Pts stopped therapy because of side effects, mostly N/V. Inc in tri-glycerides noted in some pts.
Mathez[23]	Open-label, nonrandomized	RTV 600 bid + ZDV and ddC	32	Antiretroviral-naive	50–250	150-Cell inc at week 60	A 2 $\log_{10}$ dec, sustained to 60 week	15/32 Pts discontinued treatment by week 36.
Notermans[23]	Open-label, nonrandomized	RTV 600 bid + ZDV and 3TC	33	Antiretroviral-naive, VL+ >30 000/mL	>50	180-Cell inc at week 24 in those receiving all drugs at once vs 99-cell inc in those with RTV first	A 3.0 $\log_{10}$ dec by week 16	8/33 Pts withdrew because of toxicity.
Cameron[25] (NA–Europe – Australia study)	Randomized, double blind	RTV 600 bid vs placebo; add to existing Rx	1090	ART-experienced, failing existing regimen	<101	Initial inc in CD4+ T-lymphocyte cells in Rx group; no change in placebo group	A 1.5 $\log_{10}$ dec in RTV group (not sustained), no change in placebo group	Clinical events noted in 33% of placebo group vs 16% of RTV group. Drug discontinued in 17% of RTV group vs 6% of placebo group.
Cameron[26] (RTV/SQV study)	Open-label, nonrandomized	RTV/SQV: 400/400, 600/400, 600/600 bid; 400/400 tid	141	ART-experienced, PI-naive	273[a]	+100-Cell inc by 44 week	A 80% achieved <200 copies by 44 week	The tid regimen was poorly tolerated; lower dose bid regimen best tolerated.

ART, antiretroviral therapy; bDNA, branched-chain DNA assay; BL, baseline; ddC, zalcitabine; dec, decrease; inc, increase; NA, North America; N/V, nausea/vomiting; PCR, polymerase chain reaction; PI, protease inhibitor; pts, patients; Rx, therapy; SQV, saquinavir; 3TC, lamivudine; VL, viral load; ZDV, zidovudine.

[a] Median count at baseline.

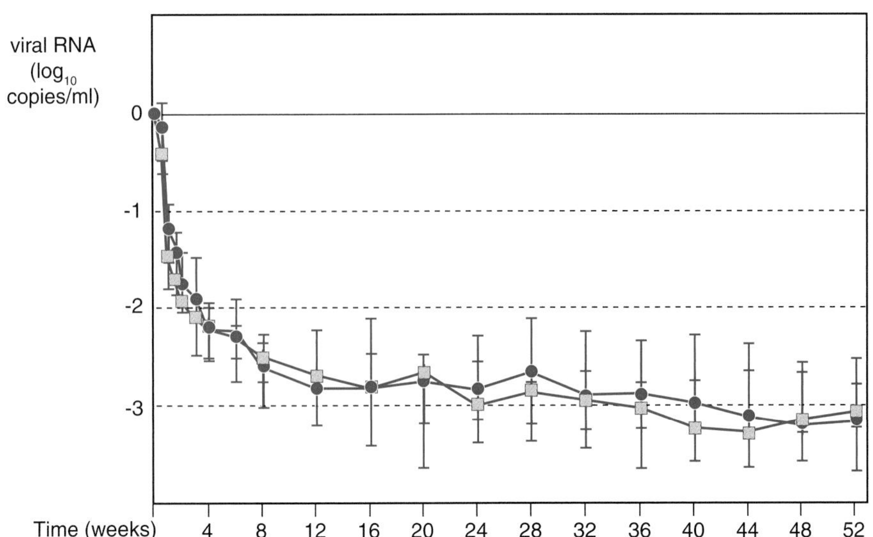

Figure 16-2 ■ Plasma log HIV RNA response (mean 6 SD) in 33 antiretroviral-naive HIV-infected patients who were treated for 52 weeks with ritonavir (RTV), zidovudine (ZDV), and lamivudine (3TC) administered simultaneously from the start of treatment (squares) or starting with RTV and adding ZDV and 3TC 3 weeks later (circles).

From Notermans D, Jurriaans S, de Wolf F, et al. Decreasing HIV-1 RNA levels in lymphoid tissue and peripheral blood during treatment with ritonavir, lamivudine and zidovudine. AIDS 12:167, 1998.

plasma HIV RNA load in the Roche Amplicor assay (S.A. Danner, unpublished results).

Saimot et al[27] evaluated the efficacy and safety of RTV in combination with stavudine (d4T) and didanosine as first-line antiretroviral treatment in an open-label study in 33 patients with 50–350 CD4+ T lymphocytes per mL. After 2 weeks of RTV induction the nucleoside analogs were added. At 12 weeks of treatment, both infectious blood cells (cells per 10^7 peripheral blood mononuclear cells (PBMCs)) and plasma HIV RNA ($\log_{10}$ copies/mL) had decreased significantly, with reductions of 2.06 and 2.14, respectively. Six patients (18%) discontinued therapy during the first 5 weeks because of adverse events.[27]

Markowitz et al treated patients presenting with primary HIV infection with ZDV/3TC/RTV or IND.[28] The time from the onset of symptoms to the start of treatment was 55 days. In the RTV-treated group, seven of 12 patients maintained their regimen for 10–16 months; in the IND group, 11 of 12 patients remained on therapy for 4–9 months. All subjects achieved undetectable levels of plasma HIV RNA (modified Chiron 2.0 assay, with a lower limit of detection of 100 copies/mL), and quantitative cultures went below the threshold of detection (0.1 $TCID_{50}/10^6$ PBMC) within months in all compliant subjects. Moreover, PBMCs isolated from semen collected from selected subjects did not express spliced or unspliced HIV-1 mRNA. No signs of viral replication could be found in lymphoid biopsy material from the sigmoid colon. The CD4+ T-lymphocyte count and the CD4/CD8 ratio increased, and reductions in env- and gag-specific antibody titers were noted.

Use in Antiretroviral-Experienced HIV-Infected Patients

In 1994, the efficacy and safety of RTV were evaluated in a 68-center North American–European–Australian study in patients with clinically advanced disease for whom there were no other treatment options. The study enrolled 1090 HIV-infected persons with a CD4+ T-lymphocyte count of less than 101 cells/mL and at least 9 months of prior antiretroviral treatment. Either RTV or placebo was added in a double-blind fashion to their existing antiretroviral medication.[25] Crossover to open RTV for any acquired immunodeficiency syndrome (AIDS) outcome was permitted after 4 months. The patients had far-advanced HIV infection, with baseline median CD4+ T-lymphocyte counts of 18 and 22 cells/mL for the RTV and placebo groups, respectively. The patients had been treated with antiretroviral drugs for a mean of 2.5 years, with an average of more than 2.5 drugs. Drug discontinuation because of adverse events occurred in 17% of the RTV group and 6% of the placebo group, mostly because of gastrointestinal symptoms during the first few weeks of the study. In the placebo group, no plasma HIV RNA-lowering effect was observed. In the RTV group, there was an initial decrease of ± 1.5 $\log_{10}$ copies/mL that was not sustained after 6 months. The study was designed with clinical endpoints (death or occurrence of a new AIDS-defining event). Death or an AIDS-defining event occurred in 85 (15.7%) versus 181 (33.1%) patients in the RTV and placebo groups, respectively ($P < 0.001$, hazard ratio 0.44%, 95% confidence interval (CI) 0.34–0.56). Although the study was not powered to detect the presumed difference in deaths, it turned out that the number of deaths differed significantly between the two groups. After a median 6.1 months of follow-up, 26 (4.8%) patients died in the RTV group versus 46 (8.4%) patients in the placebo group, a highly significant difference ($P = 0.02$, hazard ratio 0.57, 95% CI 0.35–0.91).[25]

Given the long period of prior antiretroviral treatment, it can be assumed that many patients in this study must have been nucleoside analog resistant. As a result, these patients were treated with RTV monotherapy. This is in agreement with the transient nature of the plasma HIV RNA decrease, pointing to rapid development of viral resistance against the drug. Currently, with more antiretroviral agents available, monotherapy with RTV is no longer considered acceptable even in patients with advanced disease. Because of expected rapid loss of viral susceptibility to the drug, a favorable clinical result of such a treatment must be judged remarkable. This study was instrumental in securing approval of the US Food and Drug Administration's (FDA's) New Drug Application for RTV.

Use of RTV in Pharmacologic "Boosting" of Other HIV PIs

RTV is not only an effective HIV PI, it is also one of the most powerful inhibitors of the P450 cytochrome system, especially of the isoenzyme CYP 3A4.[15,16] Because all other licensed HIV-PIs are largely metabolized by CYP3A4, RTV can be used to "boost" the efficacy of these compounds by enhancing their biologic availability.

Because RTV at its full, HIV replication suppressing dose (600mg bid) has so many side effects, and the improvement of pharmacokinetics of other co-administered PIs is so impressive, the drug is currently almost exclusively used as a "booster" for other PI's. Substantial data are available on the use of the compound in this way. RTV has been combined with SQV, IND, nelfinavir, lopinavir (LPV) (co-formulated with RTV in one capsule/tablet/liquid), amprenavir, fosamprenavir, and atazanavir. Most of the efficacy results of such trials are discussed in the respective chapters devoted to these compounds. Here a short summary is provided, mainly focusing on pharmacokinetics. Extensive reviews are written by Cooper et al[29] and by Zeldin and Petruschk.[30]

When combining RTV and another PI, two strategies can be chosen. In one the RTV dose is kept as low as possible (e.g., 100 or 200mg bid) to avoid RTV-specific side effects, accepting the fact that the plasma RTV levels will be too low to exert antiretroviral activity, and so the antiretroviral activity depends solely on the other PI. Another strategy is to administer RTV in higher doses (e.g., 400mg bid) so the drug itself inhibits HIV replication in addition to the inhibition by the other PI. The latter strategy has been used first, mainly with SQV and IND as boosted PIs. However, in order to avoid still better the RTV associated side effects, the minimal dose that is still effective in boosting (100 or 200mg daily) has become standard practice.

SQV/RTV

The combination RTV/SQV has been studied in a dose-finding clinical trial.[26,31] A total of 141 patients with a median baseline CD4+ T-lymphocyte count of 273 cells/mL and a median plasma HIV RNA load of 4.63 $\log_{10}$ copies/mL who discontinued their RT inhibitor therapy, took part in a multicenter, randomized, open-label study. The patients were randomized into four groups with various two- and three-times-a-day regimens: 400mg RTV/400mg SQV bid; 600mg RTV/400mg SQV bid; 400mg RTV/400mg SQV tid,

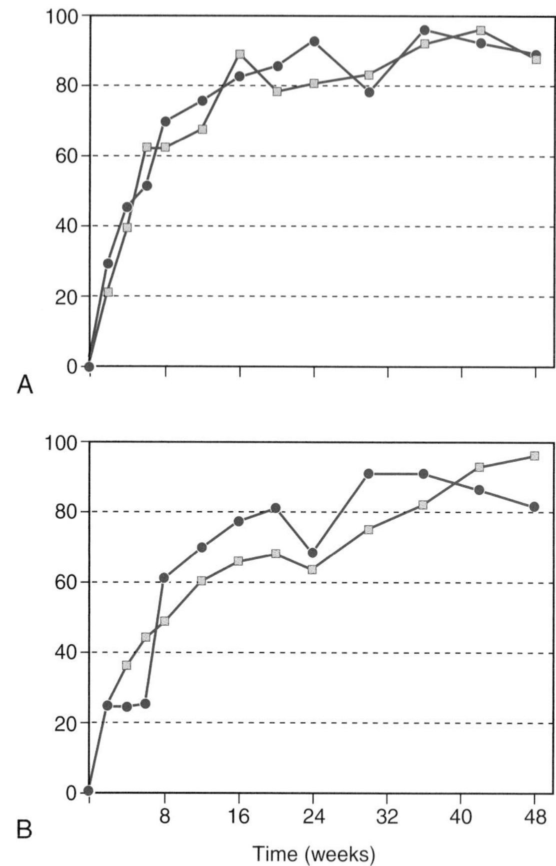

Figure 16-3 ■ Percentage of patients reaching a plasma HIV RNA load below the limit of detection (200 copies/mL) during treatment with different ritonavir–saquinavir (RTV/SQV) combinations. **(A)** Results during treatment with RTV 400mg bid/SQV 400mg bid (circles) and RTV 600mg bid/SQV 400mg bid (squares). **(B)** Results during treatment with RTV 400mg tid/SQV 400mg tid (circles) and RTV 600mg bid/SQV 600mg (squares).

From Cameron W Combining protease inhibitors for optimal HIV therapy. In: Proceedings of the Abbott Satellite Symposium During the 6th European Conference on Clinical Aspects and Treatment of HIV Infection, Hamburg, Germany, 1997, p 16.

and 600mg RTV/600mg SQV bid. All four dosage groups showed an excellent virologic and immunologic response: After 44 weeks, a median increase in CD4+ T lymphocytes to more than 100 cells/mL and a plasma RNA load decrease to less than 200 copies/mL were noted in more than 80% of the patients (intention-to-treat analysis). After 12 months, 90% of the patients on treatment still had low plasma RNA load values (Fig. 16-3). The most important difference between the four groups was tolerability: In the lowest-dose group (35 patients), few adverse events were noted, with only one discontinuation resulting from an adverse event. In seven patients who responded incompletely, d4T/3TC therapy was added at week 12, after which they also reached less than 200 copies/mL HIV RNA load.[26] Interestingly, the most important predictor of the duration of the viral response was the nadir in plasma viral load that was achieved. An HIV RNA load below 200 copies/mL at 6 months was predicted at 3 months by a level of less than 1000 copies/mL (92% positive predictive value (PPV), 75% negative predictive value (NPV); $P = 0.005$) and a level of 200 copies/mL (93% PPV, 33% NPV; $P < 0.05$).[32] This observation has been confirmed in studies with other antiretroviral drugs. For example, in the INCAS study with ZDV, didanosine (ddI), and nevirapine, the multivariate model revealed that neither the baseline plasma viral load, the viral response, the baseline CD4+ T-lymphocyte count, nor the CD4+ T lymphocyte response was independently associated with the duration of the response; rather, the nadir of the plasma viral load was highly predictive and accounted for 78% of the treatment difference in duration of suppression.[33] The favorable antiviral effect in the RTV/SQV study was even seen after 3 and 4 years of treatment, with a high virologic response in an intention-to-treat analysis.[34] At the beginning of the fourth year, 48 of 84 patients were still being treated successfully with only RTV/SQV.[35]

Another study investigating the efficacy of the RTV/SQV combination is the Dutch–Belgian Prometheus study. Combination therapy with RTV/SQV, each administered at 400 mg bid, is being compared with the same regimen plus d4T 40 mg bid.[36] Almost 200 patients who were PI and d4T-naive were enrolled. Treatment intensification with NRTIs was allowed at week 18 only when the virologic response was still unsatisfactory. In the RTV/SQV arm, more treatment intensification was seen. After 48 weeks, in patients who started treatment with a baseline serum HIV RNA concentration of more than 100 000 copies/mL treatment with RTV/SQV/d4T showed superior activity when compared with RTV/SQV alone. However, 52% of all patients on RTV/SQV never intensified their regimen and had an HIV RNA level of <400 copies/mL at week 48.

Danish investigators compared three regimens in antiretroviral-naive patients: two NRTIs plus IND, RTV, or RTV/SQV (400/400 mg bid). The RTV/SQV arm was virologically superior to the other two; toxicity in that arm compared favorably with the arm containing RTV in the standard dose.[37]

Mallolas et al found a satisfactory response after using SQV (soft gel) 1600 mg/RTV 200 mg qd as salvage treatment after failure on an SQV (hard gel) 600 mg tid-containing highly active antiretroviral therapy (HAART) regimen. After 12 weeks the viral load had dropped to less than 200 copies/mL in 12 of 14 patients.[38]

Boffito et al studied pharmacokinetics of SQV (hard gel capsules) 1000 mg bid plus RTV 100 mg bid or RTV 100 mg qd. They found that the lower dose RTV significantly reduced SQV exposure but had no influence on SQV plasma half life. This underscores the need to administer the two drugs simultaneously.[39]

Lamotte et al studied SQV/RTV once daily in a shortlasting trial, with a pharmacological endpoint at 3 months. They studied the percentage of patients with trough plasma SQV levels exceeding the inhibition of 95% of the replication *in vitro* in treatment-naive and PI-experienced patients. The percentage of success was 87 at 3 months.[40] Autar et al investigated different SQV/low RTV dose schedules and found

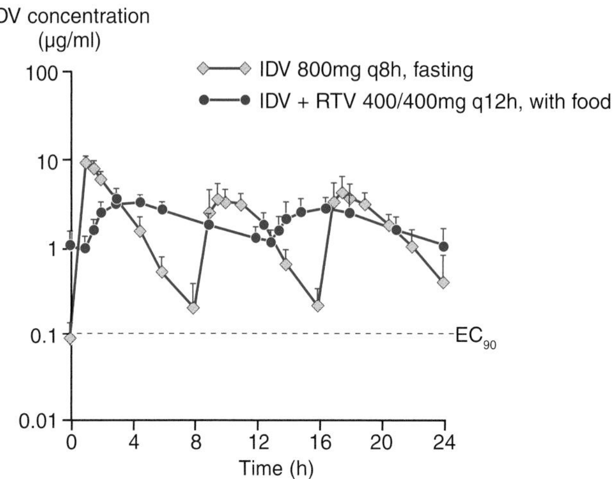

Figure 16-4 ■ Effects on indinavir pharmacokinetics of addition of ritonavir. Indinavir 800 mg tid is compared with indinavir 400 mg bid/ritonavir 400 mg bid.

From Hsu et al., Geneva, 1998.

that 2000 mg SQV combined with 100 mg RTV once daily, or 1000 mg SQV combined with 100 mg RTV twice daily were equal in important pharmacokinetic parameters. The convenience of once-daily dosing points to the 2000 SQV/100 RTV mg qd as the preferable dosing schedule.[41]

Cardiello et al switched patients who were successfully treated with SQV soft gel capsules 1400 mg bid (plus nucleoside analog RT inhibitors) to SQV/RTV (1600/100 mg qd) in order to simplify treatment. Both pharmacokinetic and virological parameters were favorable. All patients maintained SQV trough concentrations above the IC_{50}, and 93% of the patients had a plasma HIV RNA load <50 copies/mL.[42]

IND/RTV

There are ample data on the combination RTV/IND. IND, when given as the only PI, must be administered three times daily with food restriction, and the resulting plasma levels are far from ideal. Trough levels are not far above the IC_{50} for wild-type HIV, whereas peak levels are extremely high, probably contributing to the nephrolithiasis frequently seen in IND-treated patients. Combining IND with RTV makes twice-daily dosing possible, lowers the peak levels, and considerably increases the trough levels (Fig. 16-4).

In a study applying population pharmacokinetics by Burger et al IND/RTV 800/100 mg bid produced higher trough levels and more or less the same peak levels of IND as those in patients receiving a 800 mg tid IND dose. All levels measured were above the IC_{50} for wild-type HIV-1.[43]

Rockstroh et al studied 92 treatment-naive patients with a high HIV RNA load (median 220 400 copies/mL) who received two NRTIs plus RTV/IND 400/400 mg bid.[44] After 1 year, 70% had an HIV RNA load of less than 80 copies/mL in an intention-to-treat analysis; there were 29 discontinuations, eight of which were due to adverse events. No urolithiasis or flank pain had been noted. Boyd et al studied

IND/RTV 800/100 mg bid versus IND 800 mg tid in 104 patients in a randomized, open-label trial in Thailand. All patients received ZDV/3TC in addition. Efficacy was equal in both study arms, but nausea and dry mouth were more often seen in the twice-daily regimen.[45]

In a "switch study", Shulman et al showed that the viral load decreased in patients treated with IND 800 mg tid who had a detectable plasma HIV RNA load (50–50 000 copies/mL) after switching over to IND/RTV 400/400 mg bid (without a change in their NRTIs). After 3 weeks the percentage of patients with HIV RNA level of <50 copies/mL rose from 0% to 28%. After 3 weeks the NRTIs could be changed, which resulted in a 53% undetectable HIV RNA level (<50 copies/mL) after 16 weeks.[46] Whether such an intensification of IND treatment is successful depends largely on the degree of resistance against IND at the moment of intensification. Because IND and RTV have greatly overlapping resistance profiles, one can expect that this is true for both the low-dose RTV schedules (e.g., IND/RTV 800/100 mg bid) and the higher-dose RTV regimens (e.g., IND/RTV 400/400 mg bid).

Zolopa et al looked at susceptibility for IND at the start of combination therapy. They studied RTV/IDV treatment when administered to patients who failed antiretroviral therapy in routine daily practice in a multicenter cohort. In a subgroup, phenotypic analysis was done at the start. In patients with less than fourfold, four- to 25-fold, and more than 25-fold loss of susceptibility to IND, the viral responses after 24 weeks were 80%, 75%, and 20%, respectively. Apparently, boosting the IND raises the inhibitory quotient to such high levels that even moderate loss of susceptibility is compensated.[47]

Kempf et al correlated the response to such an intensification with the virtual inhibitory quotient (VIQ), which was defined as the ratio between the plasma trough level and the virtual phenotype times the serum-adjusted IC_{50} for wild-type HIV. The virtual phenotype was calculated from the genotype, and the interpretation was done by the HIV Resistance Collaborative Working Group. They found that a VIQ of more than two was the strongest predictor of successful intensification with RTV.[48]

In the ACTG 5055 protocol King et al studied the IND protein-free fraction when combined with RTV at doses of 800/200 mg qd and 400/400 mg bid.[49] Across all time points measured they found protein bound fractions of 53.4% and 51.8%, respectively. However, the percentage of IND protein binding at C_{max} was significantly lower compared with 12 h in each arm, possibly suggesting that IND protein binding is concentration dependent.

Finally, in a randomized trial SQV/RTV (1000/100 mg bid) was compared with IND/RTV (800/100 mg bid). Dragsted et al found no differences in virological outcome (25% vs 27% virological failure) after 48 weeks of treatment; however, in the IND/RTV arm more discontinuations were seen due to adverse events.[50]

LPV/RTV

LPV is coformulated with RTV in capsules (133 mg of LPV and 33 mg of RTV) and recently also in tablets (200 mg of LPV and 50 mg of RTV). RTV greatly enhances LPV pharmacokinetics, yielding LPV plasma trough levels 40- to 100-fold the IC_{50} of wild type HIV (many investigators use the so-called inhibitory quotient: Ctrough/IC_{50}). The more resistance conferring mutations an HIV strain has, the higher the $IC_{50,}$ and lower will be the inhibitory quotient (IQ). Castagna et al studied the normalized inhibitory quotient (NIQ) in a group of heavily pretreated patients whose HIV strains were expected to have been mutated extensively.[51] The NIQ was calculated by dividing each subject's IQ (LPV Ctrough/fold change in LPV susceptibility, as assessed by Virtual Phenotype) by a reference IQ (mean population LPV Ctrough/fold change in LPV $IC_{50,}$ as assessed by Virtual Phenotype). Median baseline HIV RNA load was 4.85 log copies/mL. After 48 weeks, 41% of the patients reached an undetectable viral load (>80 copies/mL). The median NIQ indeed was low (2.2) and turned out to be highly predictive of success.

Eron et al compared standard LPV/RTV (400/100 mg bid) with once-daily dosing (800/200 mg) with d4T and 3TC.[52] The IQ's for the once-daily and twice-daily dosing groups were 40- and 84-fold, respectively. After 48 weeks, there was no difference in virological outcome: in an intent-to-treat analysis (missing = failure), 74% of patients in the once-daily group and 79% of patients in the twice-daily group had HIV RNA levels of <50 copies/mL ($P = 0.70$). The very strong antiretroviral potency of the LPV/RTV combination has been demonstrated in several trials (*see also* Chapter 19).

Dragsted et al compared standard LPV/RTV (400/100 mg bid) with SQV/RTV (1000/100 mg bid) plus two or more NRTIs/NNRTIs. At 48 weeks, treatment failure occurred in 29/163 (18%) and 53/161 (33%) of patients in the LPV/r and SQV/r arms, respectively (ITT/e, $P = 0.002$, log rank test).[53]

Hicks et al reported the long-term follow-up (4 years) of 100 treatment-naive patients who were enrolled in a phase II study with different doses of LPV/RTV and who switched to a fix dose (400/100 mg bid) plus d4T and 3TC after 48 weeks. After 204 weeks, 72 patients remained on study, 70 of whom had HIV-1 RNA <50 copies/mL (70% by intent-to-treat analysis).[54] Kempf et al studied the occurrence of resistance in the phase III trial comparing LPV/RTV with nelfinavir in 653 treatment-naive patients after 108 weeks. The LPV/RTV arm was superior in virological success and no primary resistance mutations were detected in virus isolates from 51 LPV/RTV-treated subjects with available genotypes. Primary mutations related to nelfinavir resistance (D30N and/or L90M) were observed in 43 (45%) of 96 nelfinavir-treated subjects. Resistance to 3TC and d4T was also significantly higher in nelfinavir-treated versus LPV/RTV-treated subjects. These differences suggest substantially different genetic and pharmacological barriers to resistance for LPV/RTV as compared to nelfinavir.[55]

(Fos)amprenavir/RTV

Amprenavir (APV) has been combined with RTV as well to increase the trough concentration and lower the peak concentration (Fig. 16-5).

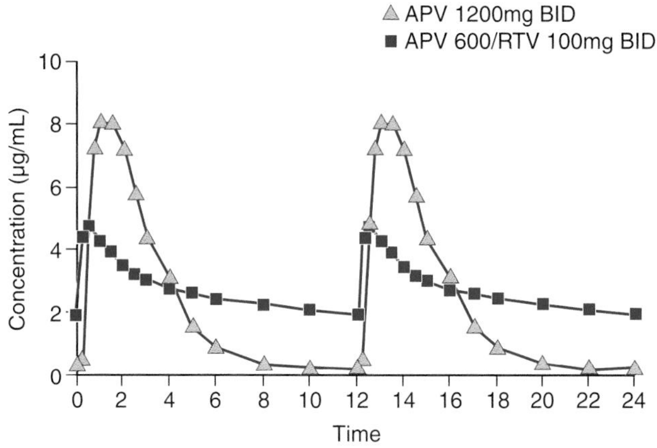

Figure 16-5 ■ Effects of ritonavir on APV pharmacokinetics. APV 1200 mg bid is compared with APV 600 mg bid/ritonavir 100 mg bid.

From Sadler, 7th Retroviral Conference, 2000, abstract 7.

Markowitz et al studied 39 individuals with primary HIV infection (mean HIV RNA load of 5.3 $\log_{10}$ copies/mL, mean CD4+ T-lymphocyte count of 503 cells/mL).[56] All patients started with an APV-based HAART regimen; 33 of them switched after a median of 48 weeks to an APV/RTV 600/100 mg bid based regimen. The adverse event profile improved, the number of "viral blips" (rises in viral loads) decreased slightly, and the plasma trough level of APV rose fivefold compared to the preswitch APV 1200 mg bid dose.[56]

Wood et al compared pharmacokinetics and tolerability of the standard APV dose (1200 mg bid) with two different APV/RTV schedules (600/100 mg bid, and 1200/200 mg qd).[57] The geometric least-square mean ratio (90% CI) of steady-state trough concentrations, compared with that of the APV 1200 mg bid regimen, was 6.08 (4.94–7.49) for the twice-daily APV/RTV regimen, and it was 4.19 (2.90–6.08) for the daily APV/RTV regimen. The regimens were well tolerated.

Katlama et al administered APV/RTV 600/100 mg bid or 600/200 mg bid to 68 patients who had been heavily pretreated. Their mean period of treatment was 7.7 years, and 68% had used more than three PIs. At 48 weeks, an intention-to-treat analysis showed a viral load of less than 200 copies/mL in 36%.[58]

Atazanavir/RTV

Cohen et al compared unboosted atazanavir (400 mg daily) with LPV/RTV (400/100 mg bid) in an open trial in 290 patients who had failed on a previous PI-containing regimen.[59] LPV/RTV resulted in a significantly greater reduction in HIV RNA than unboosted atazanavir (−2.02 vs −1.59 $\log_{10}$ copies/mL, $p < 0.001$) at week 48. However, both regimens were equally effective in subjects who had no baseline NRTI mutations. From baseline to week 48, atazanavir resulted in either no change or decreases in fasting LDL cholesterol, total cholesterol, and fasting triglycerides (−6%, −2%, and +1%), whereas LPV/RTV resulted in increases (+3%, +12%, and +53%) ($p < 0.05$, all between-treatment comparisons). Fewer patients were administered lipid-lowering therapy in the atazanavir arm (6% vs 20% for LPV/RTV).

Johnson et al also studied atazanavir in pretreated patients, but in a boosted form: they compared atazanavir/RTV (300/100 mg qd) with LPV/RTV (400/100 mg bid) and atazanavir/SQV (300/1200 mg qd), with tenofovir and another NRTI.[60] After 48 weeks, the primary efficacy endpoint (plasma HIV RNA reduction assessed by time-averaged difference) was similar for atazanavir/RTV and LPV/RTV (0.13; 97.5% CI, −0.12 to −0.39). Mean reductions from baseline were also comparable at 1.93 and 1.87 $\log_{10}$ copies/mL, respectively. The efficacy of atazanavir/SQV was lower than LPV/RTV by both these parameters. Again, the influence of the treatment on blood lipids was more favorable in the atazanavir/RTV or atazanavir/SQV group than in the LPV/RTV group.

Triple PIs Regimens

Since RTV inhibits the metabolism of all other PIs, several investigators have studied the combination of low-dose RTV and more than one other PI. Such regimens might be useful if one wants to reserve the other two classes (NRTIs and NNRTIs) for later use if necessary, or if the patient is intolerant to NRTIs and/or NNRTIs, or if the patient's viral strain has so many resistance conferring mutations that more than one PI is deemed necessary as salvage treatment, especially if the PIs used have complementary resistance profiles.

Ribera et al investigated the pharmacokinetics of SQV soft gel capsules (1000 mg bid), LPV (400 mg bid) and RTV (100 mg bid) in 40 patients in a multidrug rescue therapy study, in order to find out whether steady-state pharmacokinetics of LPV-RTV are affected by co-administration of SQV. Twenty-five patients received all three drugs, and 15 patients received only LPV/RTV. LPV concentrations were similar with or without SQV addition. SQV pharmacokinetics were comparable to those seen in other trials where SQV is the only PI boosted by RTV. There was a strong linear correlation between SQV plasma levels and RTV plasma levels, and between LPV plasma levels and RTV plasma levels. The correlation was weaker between SQV and LPV levels.[61]

Raguin et al studied the combination of APV, LPV and two different doses of RTV (200 mg daily and 400 mg daily) in heavily pretreated patients. They had a baseline HIV RNA load of 4.7 log copies/mL and, a median number of previous antiretrovirals of 7.7. After 26 weeks of treatment, 32% in the 200 mg RTV arm, and 61% in the 400 mg RTV arm had a HIV RNA load <50 copies/mL.[62] APV, but not LPV plasma concentrations were lower than expected.

De Luca et al studied the same three PIs in patients with triple drug class failure. As pharmacokinetic control patients, they used the same category of patients who had been treated with either APV/RTV or LPV/RTV at the same doses.[63] They also found a decrease in APV concentrations. The mean plasma trough concentration (C_{min}) and peak concentration

(C_{max}) of APV were 104% and 228% lower and the C_{min} of LPV was 46% lower in patients in whom the drugs were co-administered than in controls. The virologic treatment efficacy was only moderate. Mean changes from baseline HIV RNA levels and CD4+ T-lymphocyte counts after 24 weeks were −1.13 $\log_{10}$ copies/mL and +88 × 10 cells/L, respectively. When these drugs are co-administered, therapeutic drug monitoring should be employed.

Kashuba et al reported in an interim analysis the results of the ACTG 5143 protocol which likewise studied the pharmacokinetics in a fosamprenavir, LPV, and RTV combination after 2–4 weeks. They found a significant reduction in both APV and LPV exposure. As a result the study was closed to enrolment.[64]

Boffito et al added fosamprenavir (700 mg bid) to patients who were on a stable SQV/RTV (1000/100 mg bid) containing regimen. Pharmacokinetic curves were obtained at baseline, and 11 days after fosamprenavir addition. Thereafter, the dose of RTV was increased to 200 mg bid. The co-administration of fosamprenavir 700 mg bid with SQV/RTV 1000/100 mg bid resulted in a statistically nonsignificant decrease in SQV concentrations. This was compensated for by an increased RTV dose of 200 mg bid, which resulted in a statistically nonsignificant increase in SQV exposure compared with baseline. APV levels did not appear to be significantly influenced by co-administration of SQV with fosamprenavir. Fosamprenavir significantly reduced RTV exposure, but the increased RTV dose compensated for this interaction.[65]

Boosted PIs and NNRTIs

Both RTV and the currently available NNRTIs influence drug metabolism by their action on the subsystems of the hepatic P450 system. Theoretically it is not easy to predict whether the resulting change will be a decrease or an increase in the metabolism of the different substrates.

Shelton et al administered the NNRTI delarvidine to patients who were treated with the original "full" dose of RTV (600 mg bid). The C_{max}, AUC and C_{min} of RTV were increased from 50% upto 80%.[66]

Boyd et al studied the pharmacokinetic effects of efavirenz (600 mg qd) in combination with IND/RTV (800/100 mg bid). The C_{min} of IND varied greatly (>10-fold) but the values (0.32 mg/L (95% CI, 0.24–0.44)) were comparable if not slightly higher than those reported in patients with the original unboosted IND (800 mg tid).[67]

Solas et al investigated LPV pharmacokinetics in 182 HIV-1-infected patients divided in three groups: (a) patients on LPV/RTV 400/100 mg bid, without a NNRTI; (b) patients on LPV/RTV 400/100 mg bid, with either efavirenz or nevirapine; and (c) patients on LPV/RTV 533/133 mg bid, with either efavirenz or nevirapine. Both efavirenz and nevirapine lowered plasma median, C_{trough} and C_{max} levels of LPV. Increasing the LPV/RTV dose resulted in higher mean LPV values, but with a much larger interindividual variability. Thus in both NNRTI containing study arms the risk of achieving a suboptimal C_{min} of LPV was increased when compared to patients taking the standard dose of LPV/RTV without an NNRTI.[68]

Boosted PI Monotherapy

The newer PIs such as LPV and atazanavir, when pharmacologically boosted by RTV, have a relatively large therapeutic window. The daily plasma trough concentration exceeds the IC_{50} of wild type HIV 30- to 80-fold. Consequently, these compounds are very strong inhibitors of HIV replication. For that reason attempts have been made again to use them in the form of monotherapy, for example, in patients who are virologically suppressed since a long time. If this would be feasible, the advantages are clear. All other classes of antiretrovirals can be reserved for later use, the side effects of NRTIs can be avoided, and the treatment schedule will be more convenient than in most triple regimens.

Arribas et al reported the first results of treatment with only LPV/RTV 400/100 mg once daily.[69] It was a proof-of-principle small open-label randomized trial in which 42 patients who had never experienced a virologic failure and had an undetectable HIV RNA load for at least 6 months while being treated with LPV/RTV plus two NRTIs, were randomized into two groups. One group continued their triple treatment, the other group stopped the two NRTIs and continued with LPV/RTV monotherapy. After 48 weeks of follow-up, the percentage of patients remaining at <50 HIV RNA copies/mL (intention-to-treat) was 81% (64–98%) for the monotherapy group (95% CI) versus 95% (86–100%) for the triple-therapy group (95% CI, $P = 0.34$). Patients in whom monotherapy failed had significantly worse adherence than patients who remained virally suppressed on monotherapy. Monotherapy failures did not show primary resistance mutations in the protease gene and were successfully reinduced with prerandomization nucleosides. These results are encouraging but more, and longer lasting, studies are needed before such an approach can be considered reasonable.

PEDIATRIC DATA

Data on the efficacy and safety of RTV in children are scarce. Mueller et al treated 46 children who were intolerant or refractory to other antiretroviral regimens with RTV monotherapy in different dosages (liquid formula) in a phase I/II study.[70] among them, 37 completed 12 weeks of observation (median time on study 28 weeks). Six came off the study because of adverse events (three had liver enzyme elevations, and three had nausea and vomiting). Plasma HIV RNA decreased rapidly (0.5–2.0 $\log_{10}$ copies/mL) and remained below baseline up to 24 weeks. Tolerability thus seems reasonable, and these highly preliminary data point to a comparable virologic efficacy to that seen in adults.

Pediatric ACTG trial 338 compared ZDV/3TC, d4T/RTV, and ZDV/3TC/RTV in stable, antiretroviral-experienced children 2–17 years of age. The results of an interim analysis, after which the ZDV/3TC group became unblinded, are

Results of Clinical Trial Pediatric ACTG-338

Table 16-3

	Plasma HIV RNA (log_{10} copies/mL)			% Patients with Viral Load, 400 copies/mL		
Week	ZDV/3TC	Treatment B: d4T/RTV or ZDV/3TC/RTV	Treatment C: ZDV/3TC/RTV or d4T/RTV	ZDV/3TC	Treatment B: d4T/RTV or ZDV/3TC/RTV	Treatment C: ZDV/3TC/RTV or d4T/RTV
0	4.28	4.41	4.25	0	0	0
4	3.76	2.60	2.60	28	59	51
12	3.95	2.60	2.60	14	61	57

presented in Table 16-3 for 162 of the 298 children who entered the study.[71] Of the 197 children on an RTV-containing treatment arm, at 12 weeks 57% were on full dose and 10% had discontinued permanently. No clinical progression or unexpected toxicities were noted.

Chadwick et al studied early therapy with ZDV/3TC/RTV (either 350 mg/m^2 (group 1) or 450 mg/m^2 (group 2) bid) in 39 children 1–24 months of age. After 48 weeks, there were no grade 3 or 4 toxicities related to the study medication. Median RTV concentrations in group 1 were 16–57%, which were lower than predicted from adult data. Three children stopped therapy because of intolerance. Among those who could tolerate RTV, 10 of 11 in group 1 (or 91%) and seven of 17 in group 2 (or 41%) had viral loads of less than 400 copies/mL at week 48. Most virologic failures were due to poor adherence.[72]

Chadwick et al studied a regimen of RTV, ZDV and 3TC in 50 very young children, between the ages of 4 weeks and 24 months. Two sequential dosing cohorts were treated with RTV 350 or 450 mg/m^2 bid. After 16 weeks, 72% achieved an undetectable HIV RNA load (<400 copies/mL), after 104 weeks the number had decreased to 36%, mainly due to poor adherence. Apparent oral clearance of RTV was higher and the C_{min} lower than found in adults.[73]

Resino et al investigated the effects of LPV/RTV in 67 previously PI-experienced children in a multicenter prospective cohort observational study. In that study 83.5% of children had a 1 log_{10} viral load (VL) decrease including 65.6% who reached undetectable HIV RNA load (<400 copies/mL). Children with CD4+ T lymphocyte <15% ($P = 0.122$), VL <30000 ($P < 0.001$) copies/mL, and age <12 years ($P = 0.096$) achieved an earlier control of VL during the follow-up. The children with virologic failure or rebound of VL had higher baseline VL and lower CD4+ T lymphocytes/mL and had taken a greater number of drugs previous to LPV/RTV.[74]

Bergshoeff et al studied an NRTI-sparing regimen in children by administering LPV/RTV plus efavirenz in 15 children with mean age of 118 years. Efavirenz was given in the standard dose (14 mg/kg once daily) and the LPV/RTV dose was increased to 300/75 mg/m^2 twice daily because of the expected enzyme inducing effect of efavirenz. Steady-state pharmacokinetics of LPV and efavirenz were determined and compared with historical data. $AUC_{0\text{-}12}$, peak levels (C_{max}), and trough levels (C_{min}) of LPV were similar to historical data in adults and children. Efavirenz pharmacokinetics approximated previous data in adults and children. So clearly the increased LPV/RTV dose compensates enough for the enzyme-inducing effect of efvirenz.[75]

ADVERSE EVENTS

Use of RTV is accompanied by adverse events in many patients. These effects, especially gastrointestinal symptoms, occur mainly during the first few weeks of RTV treatment and are associated with high plasma trough levels of the drug. RTV induces its own metabolism, and pharmacokinetic studies show that trough levels are initially high, not reaching a steady-state level before the end of the second week of administration.[6] Addition of some NRTIs sometimes increases toxicity, especially during the first weeks of treatment. This is reflected in a relatively high dropout rate after starting on RTV during routine patient care and in controlled clinical trials.[76,77] Several measures can help improve tolerability if RTV is to be used as monotherapy. One of the most important would be gradual escalation to the full dose. Over the first 10–14 days, RTV metabolism is so slow that even a substantial dose reduction does not lead to drug levels below the IC_{90}; gradual escalation helps avoid high drug levels and resultant toxicity. In the rare situation where RTV was used as the sole PI one could start with 300 mg bid for a few days, increasing to 400 mg during the next 3 or 4 days, then 500 mg bid for 3 or 4 days, after which the full dose of 600 mg bid (not before day 12 to 14) could be administered. Careful dose escalation tailored to the symptoms in the individual, pharmacologic and nonpharmacologic interventions for side effects, and especially full disclosure to the patient of potential side effects and their transient nature would be helpful. Using these tools in a prospective study, 57 consecutive patients tolerated RTV during the first year in one study.[78]

The principal adverse effects are gastrointestinal, including nausea, diarrhea, vomiting, anorexia, abdominal pain, and taste perversion.[6] In addition, peripheral and perioral paresthesias occur frequently but are transient in nature. Asthenia and headache are noted more frequently in the RTV group in placebo-controlled monotherapy studies and even more so in studies with RTV/NRTI combinations.[6]

Substantial increases in the liver enzymes alanine transaminase and aspartate transaminase are seen in 5–6% of patients, mainly those who receive RTV plus nucleoside analogs. In one of the RTV/SQV studies, the incidence varied between 3% and 15%, depending on the dosage. In that study, a clear relation between liver toxicity and preexisting liver disease was found. Elevations of creatine phosphokinase concentrations have been reported in 1–4% of patients on RTV monotherapy or combination therapies.

As reported to date, RTV has no negative effect on hemoglobin, leukocyte count, or platelet count. On the contrary, in the phase III study in which either RTV or placebo was added to existing antiretroviral therapy, the RTV group showed improved hematologic parameters.[25,79]

Since PIs were introduced, physicians have become aware of more spontaneous bleeding episodes in patients with hemophilia than expected. Both hematomas and hemarthroses have been reported. Most cases have been described in European patients with advanced HIV infection who are receiving other multiple drugs. It is not clear if this extra bleeding tendency in hemophiliacs is associated with one or more specific PIs or with the whole class of compounds. The FDA issued a warning to care providers to monitor closely any patients with hemophilia who are taking PIs.[80]

In a substantial number of patients on RTV, hypertriglyceridemia is seen, usually to a moderate degree. Fasting triglyceride concentrations exceeding 1500 mg/dL occurred in 2–8% of patients receiving RTV as monotherapy or in combination with dideoxynucleoside agents.[6] Although occasionally extreme hypertriglyceridemia is noted that resolves quickly after cessation of RTV, the incidence of pancreatitis is not higher than expected in these patients and does not seem to be associated with elevated plasma triglyceride levels. Hypercholesterolemia has been reported in fewer than 2% of the patients receiving RTV in clinical trials.[6] Extreme hypertriglyceridemia and hypercholesterolemia seem to be dose independent, as occasionally these elevations are also seen in the very low dose RTV schedules, where RTV is used only as a pharmacologic booster for other HIV PIs.

During the last few years, the poorly understood syndrome of redistribution of fat tissue (called lipodystrophy, consisting of both lipoatrophy and lipohypertrophy) has attracted a lot of attention (*see* Chapter 72). The exact prevalence is difficult to measure, mainly because there is no standardized definition. Treatment with both NRTIs and PIs seems to be involved in the pathogenesis. In the MACS study, Kingsley et al found among HIV-positive men on no therapy or monotherapy/dual therapy a prevalence of less than 3% and 2%, respectively, but in patients on HAART it was 20%. The prevalence of lipodystrophy rose sharply during the first 2 years on HAART but remained stable thereafter.[81] The specific role of PIs in the development of this syndrome is far from clear at the moment. There are many studies on the prevalence of the syndrome, but there are few prospective data. Within the class of PIs, no differences in association with lipodystrophy between the individual PIs have been noted.

RESISTANCE

Resistance to all PIs has been produced *in vitro* by serial passage of HIV-1 in the presence of increasing drug concentrations. When this class of compounds was first introduced, physicians and patients wondered if the problems with loss of efficacy as a result of resistance, as seen during treatment with NRTIs and NNRTIs, would be observed during treatment with these highly potent replication inhibitors. In monotherapy studies with all currently available PIs, efficacy was indeed lost after a few months, and mutations in the protease gene with decreased susceptibility of the patient's HIV isolate were found. Molla et al studied clinical isolates from patients in phase I/II studies with RTV who showed virologic escape.[82] Mutations at several positions in HIV protease were found, always with a codon 82 change as the initial variation, regardless of time on therapy. Thereafter strains with more mutations were selected, with an ordered accumulation of mutations at positions 54, 71, and 36, after which other mutations were added at positions 10, 13, 20, 33, 63, 84, or 90, among others. Strains with the initial codon 82 mutation alone demonstrated only a small loss of susceptibility to RTV; but apparently the suppression of replication of these strains is incomplete enough to allow further selection of additional mutations. The occurrence of these strains with multiple mutations is unlikely to be the result of selection of preexisting strains. It is estimated that each amino acid substitution due to a single nucleotide change occurs in 1 of 10 000 bp.[83] Thus, mutants with four or more codon changes occur by chance in fewer than 1 per 10^{16} bp, which is less than the estimated life time production.[84,85] Therefore, it must be assumed that after selection of the first mutation (in the case of RTV, apparently at the protease gene codon 82) continuous selection of additional mutations takes place more easily than would be expected by chance. There is a clear relation between plasma trough levels of RTV and the selection rate, expressed as the number of mutations per week.[82]

The loss of RTV's efficacy as a result of the appearance of resistance-conferring mutations has been confirmed in other trials using combination therapy. Clavel et al found multiple mutations in the protease gene and phenotypic resistance in patients treated with ZDV/ddC/RTV. Interestingly, they found that after more than 1 year of drug exposure in all patients with a resistant plasma HIV population there were no mutations in the HIV genomes from the patient's unstimulated PBMCs.[86] Pym et al treated patients who failed virologically after prolonged SQV monotherapy by switching them to the RTV/SQV combination. Three patterns of response were seen: (1) patients who started the combination while lacking both the protease gene codon 48 and the codon 90 mutations (the two important mutations conferring resistance to SQV) showed a good, durable response; (2) patients starting with only the codon 90 mutation had a temporary response, which was lost after 16 weeks; and (3) patients starting with both SQV-induced mutations showed no response at all.[87]

Under selective drug pressure, the patient's HIV population may change not only in terms of susceptibility to the drug but also in terms of "fitness", and the two effects can work antagonistically or synergistically. Nijhuis et al isolated protease genes from patients on prolonged RTV monotherapy during phase I/II studies and introduced them into protease-deleted laboratory HIV-1 vectors via recombination. The first mutants were found to express increased drug resistance but reduced replication efficiency relative to the wild type. With prolonged treatment, variants dominated with other mutations that showed no further increase in resistance but increased replication efficiency relative to the wild type.[88]

One of the most important questions for physicians facing the initial selection of drugs for antiretroviral combination therapy in their patients is this: Suppose the initial combination fails as a result of resistance, which options remain? Because most initial treatment regimens currently contain PIs, part of this question can be rephrased as: How extensive is the phenomenon of cross-resistance in this class of compounds? Unfortunately, the initial reports about cross-resistance, mainly published after completion of short-term phase I/II studies, were more optimistic than recent results from long-term treatment periods and in routine patient care settings. Winters et al studied patients who failed long-term (1–2 years) SQV antiretroviral therapy and found that more than one-third of the patients had acquired, in addition to the codon 48 and 90 mutations, several other mutations, conferring resistance to other PIs, such as IND and RTV.[89] In contrast, in another study of 27 patients treated with either SQV monotherapy or SQV plus nucleosides, the phenomenon of cross-resistance was also demonstrated, but it was confined to a much smaller percentage (5–15%).[90] Calvez et al found, in a heavily pretreated patient population (nucleoside analogs in monotherapy and dual therapy, as well as triple regimens), that switching to the RTV/SQV combination had only a short-term effect on CD4+ T lymphocytes and the plasma HIV RNA load.[91] Also, Miller et al[92] found extensive cross-resistance to RTV and SQV after triple therapy (with IND as the PI). Unanimous agreement exists that cross-resistance between IND and RTV approaches 100%.[93]

APV seems to harbor somewhat less cross-resistance. Lo Caputo et al studied phenotypic resistance in 101 patients who were heavily PI-pretreated and who failed virologically when they were tested. The correlation coefficients between APV fold-resistance and that of individual PIs were as follows: IDV 0.23, RTV 0.42, nelfinavir 0.43, and SQV 0.31.[94]

Resistance to PIs can be caused by changes in the protease gene product, which affect binding of the inhibitor to the protease enzyme, or by changes in the substrate for the protease (i.e., the cleavage sites of the precursor polyproteins). It is conceivable that the latter changes can either facilitate or compromise the cleavage process, increasing or decreasing the degree of resistance, respectively. Considerable variation in cleavage sites has indeed been noted and has occurred in a setting of vertical transmission and during therapy with RTV or IND.[95,96]

Of particular concern are reports about simultaneous viral resistance to almost all available antiretroviral agents in patients who never had reached undetectable levels of plasma HIV RNA after nucleoside analog therapy followed by PI-containing triple regimens. Shafer et al found a specific set of 14 mutations in such patients: six in the protease gene (at condons 10, 48, 54, 63, 71, 82) and 8 in the RT gene (at codons 41, 43, 44, 67, 118, 184, 210, 215), regardless of which nucleosides and PIs had been used. The authors noted that "the striking concordance of mutations in these patients suggests that this set of RT and protease mutations provides a selective advantage in a variety of genetic contexts and in the presence of multiple different drug combinations".[97] In addition, *in vitro* studies have demonstrated that HIV-1 can readily develop resistance to several classes of antiretroviral drugs through genetic recombination of large viral genome segments, at least in the laboratory setting.[98]

Since RTV is only used as a booster at low doses (100 or 200 mg/day), resistance against the compound is no longer a relevant clinical issue. The plasma concentrations are too low to exert selective pressure on the HIV strain and the antiviral efficacy must come from other PIs.

SUMMARY AND PLACE OF RTV IN ANTIRETROVIRAL TREATMENT

RTV is highly potent. However, the specter of side effects when RTV is administered in its full dose (600 mg bid) precludes its widespread use. Instead, the compound is now being used almost exclusively as a pharmacologic booster for other PIs. A dose of 100 mg bid usually suffices to achieve the boosting effect. At those doses, side effects are minimal.

REFERENCES

1. Kempf DJ, Norbeck DW, Codacovi LM, et al. Structure-based, C^2 symmetric inhibitors of HIV protease. J Med Chem 33:2687, 1990.
2. Erickson J, Neidhart DJ, VanDrie J, et al. Design, activity, and 2.8 A crystal structure of a C^2 symmetric inhibitor complexed to HIV-1 protease. Science 249:527, 1990.
3. Kempf DJ, Marsh KC, Denissen JF, et al. ABT-538 is a potent inhibitor of human immunodeficiency virus protease and has high oral bioavailability in humans. Proc Natl Acad Sci USA 92:2484, 1995.

4. Vella S. Rationale and experience with reverse transcriptase and protease inhibitors. J Acquir Immune Defic Syndr Hum Retrovirol 10(Suppl 1):S58, 1995.
5. Markowitz M, Saag M, Powderly WG, et al. Selection and analysis of human immunodeficiency virus type 1 variants with increased resistance to ABT-538, a novel protease inhibitor. J Virol 69:701, 1995.
6. Norvir (ritonavir) capsules and oral solution prescribing information. North Chicago, IL: Abbott Laboratories; 1996.
7. Hsu A, Granneman R, Rienkiwicz K, et al. Kinetics of ABT-538, a protease inhibitor, after single oral rising doses [abstract]. Pharmacol Res 11(Suppl):400, 1994.
8. Danner SA, Carr A, Leonard JM, et al. A short-term study of the safety, pharmacokinetics, and efficacy of ritonavir, an inhibitor of HIV-1 protease. N Engl J Med 333:1528, 1995.
9. Kumar GN, Rodrigues AD, Buko AM, et al. Cytochrome P450-mediated metabolism of the HIV-1 protease inhibitor ritonavir (ABT-538) in human liver microsomes. J Pharmacol Exp Ther 277:423, 1996.
10. Cato A, Hsu A, Granneman R, et al. Assessment of pharmacokinetic interaction of the HIV-1 protease inhibitor ABT-538 and fluconazole. In: Proceedings of the 35th Interscience Conference on Antimicrobial Agents and Chemotherapy, San Francisco. Washington, DC: American Society for Microbiology; 1995, abstract 133.
11. Cato A, Hsu A, Granneman R, et al. Assessment of the pharmacokinetic interaction of the HIV-1 protease inhibitor ABT-538 and zidovudine. In: Proceedings of the 35th Interscience Conference on Antimicrobial Agents and Chemotherapy, San Francisco. Washington, DC: American Society for Microbiology; 1995, abstract 134.
12. Murphy R, Gagnier P, Lamson M, et al. Effect of nevirapine on pharmacokinetics of indinavir and ritonavir in HIV-1 infected patients. In: Proceedings of the 4th Conference on Retroviruses and Opportunistic Infections, Washington, DC. Alexandria, VA: Westover Management Group; 1997, abstract 374.
13. Cox SR, Ferry JJ, Batts DH, et al. Delavirdine and marketed protease inhibitors: pharmacokinetic interaction studies in healthy volunteers. In: Proceedings of the 4th Conference on Retroviruses and Opportunistic Infections, Washington, DC. Alexandria, VA: Westover Management Group; 1997, abstract 372.
14. Invirase (saquinavir mesylate) capsules prescribing information. Nutley, NJ: Roche Laboratories; 1995.
15. Hsu A, Granneman R, Sun E, et al. Assessment of single- and multiple-dose interactions between ritonavir and saquinavir. In: Proceedings of the XIth International Conference on AIDS, Vancouver, 1996, abstract LB.B 6041.
16. Merry C, Barry M, Mulcahy F, et al. Saquinavir pharmacokinetics alone and in combination with ritonavir in HIV-infected patients. AIDS 11:F29, 1997.
17. Hsu A, Granneman GR, Japour A, et al. Evaluation of potential ritonavir and indinavir combination bid regimens. In: Proceedings of the 37th Interscience Conference on Antimicrobial Agents and Chemotherapy, Toronto. Washington, DC: American Society for Microbiology; 1997, abstract A-57.
18. Kerr B, Lee C, Yuen G, et al. Overview of in-vitro and in-vivo drug interactions of nelfinavir mesylate, a new HIV-1 protease inhibitor. In: Proceedings of the 4th Conference on Retroviruses and Opportunistic Infections, Washington, DC. Alexandria, VA: Westover Management Group; 1997, abstract 373.
19. Burger DM, Hoetelmans RMW, Koopmans PP, et al. Clinically relevant drug interactions with antiretroviral agents. Antivir Ther 2:149, 1997.
20. Markowitz M, Saag M, Powderly WG, et al. A preliminary study of ritonavir, an inhibitor of HIV-1 protease, to treat HIV-1 infection. N Engl J Med 333:1534, 1995.
21. Pachl C, Todd JA, Kern DG, et al. Rapid and precise quantification of HIV-1 RNA in plasma using a branched DNA signal amplification assay. J Acquir Immune Defic Syndr Hum Retrovirol 8:446, 1995.
22. Mulder J, McKinney N, Christopherson C, et al. Rapid and simple PCR assay for quantification of human immunodeficiency virus type 1 RNA in plasma: application to acute retroviral infection. J Clin Microbiol 32:292, 1994.
23. Notermans D, Jurriaans S, de Wolf F, et al. Decreasing of HIV-1 RNA levels in lymphoid tissue and peripheral blood during treatment with ritonavir, lamivudine and zidovudine. AIDS 12:167, 1998.
24. Cavert W, Notermans D, Staskus C, et al. Kinetics of response in lymphoid tissue to antiretroviral therapy of HIV-1 infection. Science 276:960, 1997.
25. Cameron DW, Heath-Chiozzi M, Danner SA, et al. Prolongation of life and prevention of AIDS complications in a randomized controlled clinical trial of ritonavir in patients with advanced HIV disease. Lancet 352:543, 1998.
26. Cameron W. Combining protease inhibitors for optimal HIV therapy. In: Proceedings of the Abbott Satellite Symposium during the 6th European Conference on Clinical Aspects and Treatment of HIV Infection, Hamburg, Germany, 1997, p 16.
27. Saimot AG, Landman R, Damond F, et al. Ritonavir, stavudine (d4T), didanosine (ddI) as a triple combination treatment in antiretroviral-naive patients. In: Proceedings of the 4th Conference on Retroviruses and Opportunistic Infections, Washington, DC. Alexandria, VA: Westover Management Group; 1997, abstract 246.
28. Markowitz M, Cao Y, Vesamen M, et al. Recent HIV infection treated with AZT, 3TC and a potent protease inhibitor. In: Proceedings of the 4th Conference on Retroviruses and Opportunistic Infections, Washington, DC. Alexandria, VA: Westover Management Group; 1997, abstract LB8.
29. Cooper CL, van Heeswijk RPG, Gallicano K, Cameron DW. A review of low-dose ritonavir in protease inhibitor combination therapy. Clin Infect Dis 6:1585, 2003.
30. Zeldin RK, Petruschke RA. Pharmacological and therapeutic properties of ritonavir-boosted protease inhibitor therapy in HIV-infected patients. J Antimicrob Chemother 53:4, 2004.
31. Cameron DW, Japour AJ, Xu Y, et al. Ritonavir and saquinavir combination therapy for the treatment of HIV infection. AIDS 13:213, 1998.
32. Kempf D, Molla A, Sun E, et al. The duration of viral suppression is predicted by viral load during protease inhibitor therapy. In: Proceedings of the 4th Conference on Retroviruses and Opportunistic Infections, Washington, DC. Alexandria, VA: Westover Management Group; 1997, abstract 603.
33. Raboud JM, Montaner JSG, Rae S, et al. Predictors of duration of plasma viral load suppression. In: Proceedings of the 37th Interscience Conference on Antimicrobial Agents and Chemotherapy, Toronto. Washington, DC: American Society for Microbiology; 1997, abstract A-57.
34. Cameron DW, Xu Y, Rode R, et al. Three years follow-up and conditional outcomes survival analysis of ritonavir plus saquinavir therapy in HIV infection. In: Proceedings of the 7th Conference of Retroviruses and Opportunistic Infections, San Francisco, 2000, abstract 533.
35. Farthing C, Ryan J, Rode R, et al. Durability of ritonavir (RTV) plus saquinavir (SQV) dual protease inhibitor therapy in HIV infection: four year follow-up. In: Proceedings of the 1st IAS Conference on HIV Pathogenesis and Treatment, Buenos Aires, 2001, abstract 223.
36. Gisolf EH, Colebunders R, van Wanzeele F, et al. Treatment with ritonavir/saquinavir versus ritonavir/saquinavir/stavudine. In: Proceedings of the 5th Conference on Retroviruses and

Opportunistic Infections, Chicago. Alexandria, VA: Westover Management Group; 1998, abstract 576.
37. Kirk O, Katzenstein TL, Gerstoft J, et al. Combination therapy containing ritonavir plus saquinavir has superior short-term antiretroviral efficacy: a randomized trial. AIDS 13:F9, 1999.
38. Mallolas J, Blanco J, Sarasa M, et al. Intensification therapy with saquinavir soft gel (SSG)/ritonavir (RIT) qd in patients failing on a saquinavir hard gel (SHG) containing HAART. In: Proceedings of the 1st IAS Conference on HIV Pathogenesis and Treatment, Buenos Aires, 2001, abstract 675.
39. Boffito M, Maitland D, Dickinson L, et al. Boosted saquinavir hard gel formulation exposure in HV-infected subjects: ritonavir 100 mg once daily versus twice daily. J Antimicrob Chemother 55: 542, 2005.
40. Lamotte C, Landman R, Peytavin G, et al. Once-daily dosing of saquinavir soft-gel capsules and ritonavir combination in HIV-1 infected patients. Antivir Ther 9:247, 2004.
41. Autar RS, Ananworanich J, Apateerapong W, et al. Pharmacokinetic study of saquinavir hard gel caps/ritonavir in HIV-1 infected patients: 1600/100 mg once-daily compared with 2000/100 mg once-daily and 1000/100 mg twice-daily. J Antimicrob Chemother 54:785, 2004.
42. Cardiello PG, van Heeswijk RP, Hassink EA, et al. Simplifying protease inhibitor therapy with once-daily dosing of saquinavir soft-gelatin capsules/ritonavir (1600/100 mg): HIVNAT 001.3 study. J Acquir Immune Defic Syndr 29:464-, 2002.
43. Burger DM, Hugen PWH, Prins JM, et al. Pharmacokinetics of an indinavir/ritonavir 800/100 mg bid regimen. In: Proceedings of the 39th Interscience Conference on Antimicrobial Agents and Chemotherapy, San Francisco, 1999, abstract 363.
44. Rockstroh JK, Bergmann F, Wiesel W, et al. Efficacy and safety of twice daily first-line ritonavir/indinavir plus double nucleoside combination therapy in HIV-infected individuals. AIDS 14:1181, 2000.
45. Boyd M, Duncombe C, Newell M, et al. Indinavir/ritonavir vs indinavir in combination with AZT/3TC for treatment of HIV in nucleoside-experienced patients: a randomised, open-label trial. In: Proceedings of the 8th Conference on Retroviruses and Opportunistic Infections, Chicago, 2001, abstract 335.
46. Shulman N, Zolopa A, Havlir D, et al. Ritonavir intensification in indinavir recipients with detectable HIV RNA levels. In: Proceedings of the 7th Conference on Retroviruses and Opportunistic Infections, San Francisco, 2000, abstract 534.
47. Zolopa A, Rice H, Young B, et al. Ritonavir (RTV) boosting of indinavir (IDV) antiretroviral regimens in clinical practice: effectiveness, safety and exploration of phenotypic breakpoints. In: Proceedings of the 1st IAS Conference on HIV Pathogenesis and Treatment, Buenos Aires, 2001, abstract 678.
48. Kempf D, Hsu A, Jiang P, et al. Response to ritonavir (RTV) intensification in indinavir (IDV) recipients is highly correlated with virtual inhibitory quotient. In: Proceedings of the 8th Conference on Retroviruses and Opportunistic Infections, Chicago, 2001, abstract 523.
49. King JR, Gerber JG, Fletcher CV, et al. Indinavir protein-free concentrations when used in indinavir/ritonavir combination therapy. AIDS 19:1059, 2005.
50. Dragsted UB, Gerstoft J, Pedersen C, et al. Randomized trial to evaluate indinavir/ritonavir versus saquinavir/ritonavir in human immunodeficiency virus type 1-infected patients: the MaxCmin1 Trial. J Infect Dis 188:635, 2003.
51. Castagna A, Gianotti N, Galli L, et al. The NIQ of lopinavir is predictive of a 48-week virological response in highly treatment-experienced HIV-1-infected subjects treated with a lopinavir/ritonavir-containing regimen. Antivir Ther 9:537, 2004.
52. Eron JJ, Feinberg J, Kessler HA, et al. Once-daily versus twice-daily lopinavir/ritonavir in antiretroviral-naive HIV-positive patients: a 48-week randomized clinical trial. J Infect Dis 189:265, 2004.
53. Dragsted UB, Gerstoft J, Youle M, et al. A randomized trial to evaluate lopinavir/ritonavir versus saquinavir/ritonavir in HIV-1-infected patients: the MaxCmin2 trial. Antivir Ther 10:735, 2005.
54. Hicks C, King MS, Gulick RM, et al. Long-term safety and durable antiretroviral activity of lopinavir/ritonavir in treatment-naive patients: 4 year follow-up study. AIDS 18:775, 2004.
55. Kempf DJ, King MS, Bernstein B, et al. Incidence of resistance in a double-blind study comparing lopinavir/ritonavir plus stavudine and lamivudine to nelfinavir plus stavudine and lamivudine. J Infect Dis 189:51, 2004.
56. Markowitz M, Hurley A, Ramratnam B, et al. The safety and efficacy of a ritonavir-boosted amprenavir-based regimen after switch from amprenavir-based HAART. In: Proceedings of the 8th Conference on Retroviruses and Opportunistic Infections, Chicago, 2001, abstract 405.
57. Wood R, Eron J, Arasteh K, et al. A 42-week open-label study to assess the pharmacokinetics, antiretroviral activity, and safety of amprenavir or amprenavir plus ritonavir in combination with abacavir and lamivudine for treatment of HIV-infected patients. Clin Infect Dis 39:591, 2004.
58. Katlama C, Schneider L, Agher R, et al. Ritonavir (RTV)/amprenavir (APV) combination therapy in HIV infected patients who failed several protease inhibitor containing regimens. In: Proceedings of the 1st IAS Conference on HIV Pathogenesis and Treatment, Buenos Aires, 2001, abstract 673.
59. Cohen C, Nieto-Cisneros L, Zala C, et al. Comparison of atazanavir with lopinavir/ritonavir in patients with prior protease inhibitor failure: a randomized multinational trial. Curr Med Res Opin 21:1683, 2005.
60. Johnson M, Grinsztejn B, Rodriguez C, et al. Atazanavir plus ritonavir or saquinavir, and lopinavir/ritonavir in patients experiencing multiple virological failures. AIDS 19:685, 2005.
61. Ribera E, Lopez RM, Diaz M, et al. Steady-state pharmacokinetics of a double-boosting regimen of saquinavir soft gel plus lopinavir plus minidose ritonavir in human immunodeficiency virus-infected adults. Antimicrob Agents Chemother 48:4256, 2004.
62. Raguin G, Chene G, Morand-Joubert L, et al. Salvage therapy with amprenavir, lopinavir and ritonavir 200 mg/d or 400 mg/d in HIV-infected patients in virological failure. Antivir Ther 9:615, 2004.
63. De Luca A, Baldini F, Cingolani A, et al. Deep salvage with amprenavir and lopinavir/ritonavir: correlation of pharmacokinetics and drug resistance with pharmacodynamics. J Acquir Immune Defic Syndr 35:359, 2004.
64. Kashuba AD, Tierney C, Downey GF, et al. Combining fosamprenavir with lopinavir/ritonavir substantially reduces amprenavir and lopinavir exposure: ACTG protocol A5143 results. AIDS 19:145, 2005.
65. Boffito M, Dickinson L, Hill A, et al. Steady-state pharmacokinetics of saquinavir hard-gel/ritonavir/fosamprenavir in HIV-1-infected patients. J Acquir Immune Defic Syndr 37:1376, 2004.
66. Shelton MJ, Hewitt RG, Adams J, et al. Pharmacokinetics of ritonavir and delavirdine in human immunodeficiency virus-infected patients. Antimicrob Agents Chemother 47:1694, 2003.
67. Boyd MA, Aarnoutse RE, Ruxrungtham K, et al. Pharmacokinetics of indinavir/ritonavir (800/100 mg) in combination with efavirenz (600 mg) in HIV-1-infected subjects. J Acquir Immune Defic Syndr 34:134, 2003.
68. Solas C, Poizot-Martin I, Drogoul MP, et al. Therapeutic drug monitoring of lopinavir/ritonavir given alone or with a non-nucleoside reverse transcriptase inhibitor. Br J Clin Pharmacol 57:436, 2004.

69. Arribas JR, Pulido F, Delgado R, et al. Lopinavir/ritonavir as single-drug therapy for maintenance of HIV-1 viral suppression: 48-week results of a randomized, controlled, open-label, proof-of-concept pilot clinical trial (OK Study). J Acquir Immune Defic Syndr 40:280, 2005.
70. Mueller BU, Zuckerman J, Nelson RT Jr, et al. Update on the pediatric phase I/II study of the protease inhibitor ritonavir (ABT-538). In: Proceedings of the 4th Conference on Retroviruses and Opportunistic Infections, Washington, DC. Alexandria, VA: Westover Management Group; 1997, abstract 722.
71. Yogev R, Stanley K, Nachman RA, et al. Virologic efficacy of ZDV + 3TC vs. D4T + ritonavir (RTV) vs. ZDV + 3TC + RTV in stable, antiretroviral experienced HIV-infected children (Pediatric ACTG Trial 338). In: Proceedings of the 37th Interscience Conference on Antimicrobial Agents and Chemotherapy, Toronto. Washington, DC: American Society for Microbiology; 1997, abstract LB-6.
72. Chadwick EG, Palumbo P, Rodman J, et al. Early therapy with ritonavir (RTV), ZDV and 3TC in HIV-1-infected children 1–24 months of age. In: Proceedings of the 8th Conference on Retroviruses and Opportunistic Infections, Chicago, 2001, abstract 677.
73. Chadwick EG, Rodman JH, Britto P, et al. Ritonavir-based highly active antiretroviral therapy in human immunodeficiency virus type 1-infected infants younger than 24 months of age. Pediatr Infect Dis J 24:793, 2005.
74. Resino S, Bellon JM, Ramos JT, et al. Positive virological outcome after lopinavir/ritonavir salvage therapy in protease inhibitor-experienced HIV-1-infected children: a prospective cohort study. J Antimicrob Chemother 54:921, 2004.
75. Bergshoeff AS, Fraaij PL, Ndagijimana J, et al. Increased dose of lopinavir/ritonavir compensates for efavirenz-induced drug–drug interaction in HIV-1-infected children. J Acquir Immune Defic Syndr 39:63, 2005.
76. Clumeck N, Colebunders B, Vandercam K, et al. A comparative outcome trial of ritonavir and indinavir in HIV patients with CD4 cell count below 50. In: Proceedings of the 4th Conference on Retroviruses and Opportunistic Infections, Washington, DC. Alexandria, VA: Westover Management Group; 1997, abstract 196.
77. Gerard Y, Valette M, Ajana F, et al. Efficacy of proteinase inhibitors in combination with reverse transcriptase inhibitors: study in 177 HIV-1 infected patients in the North France AIDS Reference Center. In: Proceedings of the 4th Conference on Retroviruses and Opportunistic Infections, Washington, DC. Alexandria, VA: Westover Management Group; 1997, abstract 243.
78. Davis SM, Canniff JM, Andradas V, et al. Successful ritonavir induction: intensive patient management. In: Proceedings of the 4th Conference on Retroviruses and Opportunistic Infections, Washington, DC. Alexandria, VA: Westover Management Group; 1997, abstract 193.
79. De Wit S, Hermans P, Kabeya K, et al. Thrombocytopenia and leucopenia in HIV patients with CD4+ T lymphocyte counts below 50 treated with protease inhibitors. In: Proceedings of the 4th Conference on Retroviruses and Opportunistic Infections, Washington, DC. Alexandria, VA: Westover Management Group; 1997, abstract 200.
80. Feigal DW Jr. Dear Healthcare Provider Letter: HIV Protease Inhibitors and Patients with Hemophilia. Rockville, MD: U.S. Food and Drug Administration; 1996.
81. Kingsley L, Smit E, Riddler S, et al. Prevalence of lipodystrophy and metabolic abnormalities in the Multicenter AIDS Cohort Study (MACS). In: Proceedings of the 8th Conference on Retroviruses and Opportunistic Infections, Chicago, 2001, abstract 536.
82. Molla A, Korneyeva M, Gao Q, et al. Ordered accumulation of mutations in HIV protease confers resistance to ritonavir. Nat Med 2:760, 1996.
83. Coffin JM. HIV population dynamics in vivo: implications for genetic variation, pathogenesis, and therapy. Science 267:483, 1995.
84. Ho DD, Neumann AU, Perelson AS, et al. Rapid turnover of plasma virions and CD4 lymphocytes in HIV-1 infection. Nature 373:123, 1995.
85. Perelson AS, Neumann AU, Markowitz M, et al. HIV-1 dynamics in vivo: virion clearance rate, infected cell lifespan, and viral generation time. Science 271:1582, 1996.
86. Clavel F, Paulos S, Mathez D, et al. HIV protease sequences selected during ZDV-DDC-ritonavir triple combination. In: Proceedings of the 4th Conference on Retroviruses and Opportunistic Infections, Washington, DC. Alexandria, VA: Westover Management Group; 1997, abstract 236.
87. Pym AS, Churchill DR, Galpin S, et al. Presence of mutation at codon 90 may predict response to ritonavir/saquinavir combination in HIV seropositive patients pretreated with saquinavir monotherapy. In: Proceedings of the International Workshop on HIV Drug Resistance, Treatment Strategies and Eradication, St Petersburg, FL, 1997, abstract 84.
88. Nijhuis M, Schuurman R, De Jong D, et al. Selection of HIV-1 variants with increased fitness during ritonavir therapy. In: Proceedings of the International Workshop on HIV Drug Resistance, Treatment Strategies and Eradication, St Petersburg, FL, 1997, abstract 92.
89. Winters MA, Shapiro JM, Lawrence J, et al. Genotypic and phenotypic analysis of the protease gene in HIV-1-infected patients that failed long-term saquinavir therapy and switched to other protease inhibitors. In: Proceedings of the International Workshop on HIV Drug Resistance, Treatment Strategies and Eradication, St Petersburg, FL, 1997, abstract 17.
90. Craig C, Race E, Sheldon J, et al. A study of reduced sensitivity to inhibitors of HIV protease in virus isolates from selected patients after therapy with saquinavir. In: Proceedings of the International Workshop on HIV Drug Resistance, Treatment Strategies and Eradication, St Petersburg, FL, 1997, abstract 27.
91. Calvez V, Coutellier A, Bossi P, et al. Failure of the association of ritonavir and saquinavir in multi-experienced HIV-1-infected patients. In: Proceedings of the International Workshop on HIV Drug Resistance, Treatment Strategies and Eradication, St Petersburg, FL, 1997, abstract 76.
92. Miller V, Hertogs K, De Bethune MP, et al. Incidence of HIV-1 resistance and cross-resistance to protease inhibitors after indinavir failure: impact on subsequent ritonavir/saquinavir combination therapy. In: Proceedings of the International Workshop on HIV Drug Resistance, Treatment Strategies and Eradication, St Petersburg, FL, 1997, abstract 81.
93. Moyle GJ, Bartin SE. HIV-protease inhibitors in the management of HIV-infection. J Antimicrob Chemother 38:921, 1996.
94. Lo Caputo S, Gianotti N, Tomasoni L, et al. Phenotypic cross-resistance to amprenavir in HIV isolated from heavily pretreated patients (the Genpherex study). In: Proceedings of the 1st IAS Conference on HIV Pathogenesis and Treatment, Buenos Aires, 2001, abstract 575.
95. Bloom G, Perez E, Parikh S, et al. Comparison of gag-pol precursor cleavage in naturally arising HIV-1 variants. In: Proceedings of the International Workshop on HIV Drug Resistance, Treatment Strategies and Eradication, St Petersburg, FL, 1997, abstract 29.
96. Perez E, Lamers S, Heath-Chiozzi M, et al. Emergence of resistant protease alleles and variant gag sequences in HIV-1-infected children enrolled in protease inhibitor phase I/II clinical trials. In: Proceedings of the International Workshop on

HIV Drug Resistance, Treatment Strategies and Eradication, St Petersburg, FL, 1997, abstract 75.
97. Shafer RW, Winters MA, Merigan TC. Multiple concurrent RT and protease mutations and multidrug resistance in heavily treated HIV-1-infected patients. In: Proceedings of the International Workshop on HIV Drug Resistance, Treatment Strategies and Eradication, St Petersburg, FL, 1997, abstract 39.
98. Yusa K, Kavlick MF, Mitsuya H. HIV-1 acquires resistance to multiple classes of antiviral drugs through recombination. In: Proceedings of the 4th Conference on Retroviruses and Opportunistic Infections, Washington, DC. Alexandria, VA: Westover Management Group; 1997, abstract 585.

Chapter 17

Indinavir

Roy M. Gulick, MD, MPH

Indinavir sulfate (IDV, L-735,524; MK-639; Crixivan) is a human immunodeficiency virus type 1 (HIV-1) protease inhibitor (PI). The drug was approved by the US Food and Drug Administration (FDA) in March 1996 and is labeled for the treatment of HIV infection in combination with other antiretroviral agents.[1] Current antiretroviral guidelines no longer recommend IDV (with or without ritonavir (RTV) boosting) as initial therapy for HIV disease.[2,3] IDV/RTV may be used in some treatment-experienced patients.[4,5]

STRUCTURE

The chemical name for IDV sulfate is [1(1*S*, 2*R*),5(*S*)]-2,3,4-trideoxy-*N*-(2,3-dihydro-2-hydroxy-1H-inden-1-yl)-5-[2-[{(1,1-dimethylethyl) amino}carbonyl]4-(3-pyridinylmethyl)-1-piperazinyl]-2-(phenylmethyl) D-erythro-pentonamide sulfate (1:1) salt (Fig. 17-1).[1,6] IDV is derived from the class of hydroxyethylene peptidomimetic PIs that demonstrate potent antiretroviral activity but have poor aqueous solubility *in vitro* and inadequate oral bioavailability in animal models.[6] By incorporating a basic amine group into the structural backbone of the hydroxyethylene PIs, a new class of PIs, the hydroxyethylamine compounds, were developed. This class of compounds retains its peptide character but has improved aqueous solubility and enhanced oral bioavailability. Further improvements were achieved using a rational structure-based drug design to model and develop a series of structural analogs of these compounds in an attempt to retain potent antiretroviral activity while further improving oral bioavailability.[6–8] The modified hydroxyethylamine peptidomimetic compounds are exemplified by the HIV PI IDV.

IN VITRO ACTIVITY

IDV potently and competitively inhibits both the HIV-1 and HIV-2 aspartyl protease enzymes with KI (dissociation constant of the enzyme-inhibitor complex) values of 0.34 and 3.3 nM, respectively.[9] In concentrations higher than 10 μM, IDV did not inhibit other clinically relevant proteolytic enzymes such as the aspartyl proteases human plasma renin or human cathepsin D or the serine proteases factor Xa or elastase. IDV is a potent inhibitor of HIV-1 replication *in vitro*.[9] In cell culture systems, IDV showed potent activity against T lymphoid cell-adapted HIV variants (IIIb, MN, RFII) and a monocytotropic variant (SF162) with a 95% inhibitory concentration (IC_{95}) in the range of 12–100 nM. IDV also demonstrated potent activity against primary patient HIV isolates from peripheral blood mononuclear cells, including isolates with zidovudine

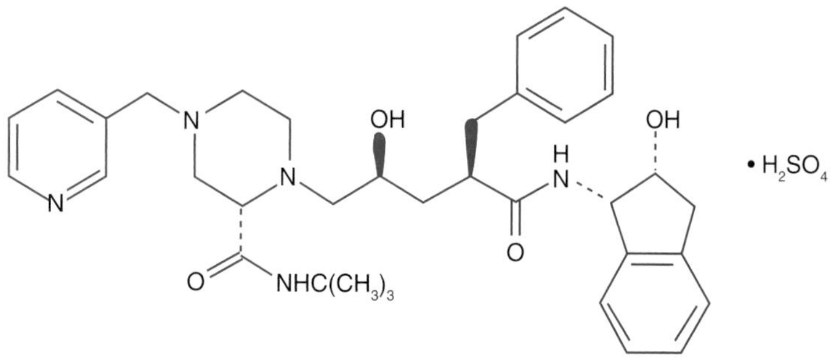

N N N OH OH H N O O NHC(CH$_3$)$_3$ • H_2SO_4

Figure 17-1 ■ Structural formula of IDV.

or non-nucleoside reverse transcriptase inhibitors (NNRTI) resistance. IDV showed synergistic *in vitro* antiviral activity in combination with zidovudine, didanosine, or an NNRTI. The combination of IDV and other PIs showed synergism to mild antagonism *in vitro*.[10] IDV demonstrated activity *in vitro* against HIV-2[11,12] and the simian immunodeficiency virus.[11]

MECHANISM OF ACTION

The HIV protease enzyme cleaves viral precursor polyproteins into structural proteins and enzymes, a step essential for the production of mature, infectious virions.[13] Retroviral proteases are unusual among proteolytic enzymes in terms of their ability to cleave protein substrates at the *N*-terminal side of proline residues. Phenylalanine–proline (Phe-Pro) residues constitute one of the important cleavage sites for the HIV-1 protease enzyme. The hydroxyethylamine peptidomimetic PIs, including IDV, were designed to mimic the Phe-Pro dipeptide transition state of the substrate protein.[6–8] These inhibitors enter the cell without intracellular processing, bind at the active site of the protease enzyme, inhibit cleavage of the viral precursor proteins, and thereby prevent maturation of the virus. Immature, noninfectious viral particles are formed in the presence of the peptidomimetic PIs. The crystal structure of IDV complexed to the HIV protease shows that binding causes closure of the flap domains of the enzyme. There are specific interactions between chemical groups of the inhibitor and the enzyme, with the lipophilic groups of IDV (except the pyridine ring) confined inside the active site of the enzyme.[14]

Adding IDV at concentrations of 500–12 000 nM to chronically HIV-infected cell culture systems decreased the amount of mature HIV proteins (p17 and p24) and increased the amount of the viral core protein precursor (p55) compared to untreated virions.[9] IDV also prevented incorporation of the HIV reverse transcriptase and integrase enzymes into viral particles. In parallel experiments, removing IDV from the cell culture medium resulted in an increase in the amount of mature viral proteins and the production of infectious virions. Thus, IDV is a reversible inhibitor of the HIV protease enzyme.

In animal studies, IDV showed antiangiogenic effects and promoted regression of Kaposi sarcoma-like lesions.[15]

PHARMACOKINETICS

Preclinical Profile

In animal models the plasma concentrations 6 h after administration of oral IDV solutions were twice the *in vitro* IC_{95}.[6,9] Oral bioavailability ranged from 14% in monkeys to 72% in dogs. IDV required an acidic pH environment for dissolution prior to absorption from the gastrointestinal tract and was less soluble at higher pH.[16] Other *in vitro* studies showed that IDV was not highly bound to plasma proteins, with the unbound drug fraction ranging from 15% in dog plasma to 56% in human plasma at drug concentrations of 81–16 300 nM.[6,9] In contrast to other PIs, the antiretroviral activity of IDV *in vitro* was similar against wild-type and PI-resistant isolates despite a fourfold increase in α_1-acid glycoprotein levels.[17] By inhibiting hepatic metabolism and clearance, RTV enhances the levels of other PIs, including IDV.[18] With concomitant RTV administration, IDV area under the curve concentration (AUC) was increased eightfold in rats.

CLINICAL PROFILE OF IDV

The first clinical study of IDV was an assessment of the safety, tolerability, and pharmacokinetics of single doses in 28 healthy volunteers.[19] Subjects were administered doses ranging from 20 to 1000 mg of the free base formulation of IDV. Plasma concentrations and urinary excretion were nonlinear, increasing more than proportionally to dose. The plasma half-life of the drug averaged 1.8–1.9 h and was not dose-dependent. Calculated free drug concentrations exceeded the *in vitro* IC_{95} through 6 h after the 700-mg dose and through 8 h following the 1000-mg dose.

To investigate the nonlinear pharmacokinetics further, 12 healthy volunteers were administered single intravenous and oral doses of IDV.[20] Although at low plasma concentrations IDV clearance was high, hepatic first-pass metabolism appeared to be saturable at higher doses of the drug (400- and 800-mg oral doses), resulting in reduced drug clearance and higher drug concentrations. In this study, oral bioavailability was estimated to be 60–65%. An intensive pharmacokinetic study in eight HIV-infected adults showed overall IDV protein binding of 61 ± 6% (range 54–70%), with considerable variability among patients.[21] The fraction of bound drug was concentration-dependent in that IDV binding was higher at the 8-h postdose concentration than at the 1-h time point.

In dose-escalation studies, IDV was given at doses of 800 mg q8h, 1000 mg q8h, and 800 mg q6h in a study of 70 HIV-positive adults.[22] The geometric mean plasma AUCs over 24 h for the three regimens were not statistically different and the 800-mg q8h dose was selected as the optimal dose. In 16 patients at the 800-mg q8h dose, the steady-state AUC was 30 691 ± 11 407 nM/h, the C_{max} was 12 617 ± 4037 nM, and the C_{min} 8-h postdose was 251 ± 178 nM.[1] There was no significant accumulation with multiple doses at 800 mg q8h. Alternative dosing of IDV at 1200 mg q12h was compared to 800 mg q8h in a combination regimen and found to have inferior virologic activity (64% vs 91% of subjects respectively had an HIV RNA level of less than 400 copies/mL at week 24) likely due to suboptimal pharmacokinetics, and this dose schedule is not recommended.[23]

In 17 patients taking IDV- or IDV/RTV-based regimens, median IDV protein binding was 64% without differences with or without RTV.[24] Another group studied 35 patients taking IDV/ritonavir at doses of 800/200 or 400/400 mg bid and found IDV was ~52% protein-bound without differences between the groups, but with significantly higher binding at peak concentrations, suggesting concentration-dependence of protein binding.[25]

FOOD EFFECTS

Administration with food high in calories, fat, and protein reduced the absorption of IDV.[19] In eight HIV-infected subjects, a 600-mg dose of IDV given with food significantly decreased absorption 30–68% compared with fasted controls with reductions in C_{max} and a delayed time to C_{max}.[26] In clinical studies of HIV-uninfected volunteers, various dose combinations of IDV/RTV were studied and adding RTV allowed twice-daily IDV dosing with food.[27,28] To explore the effects of food on IDV/RTV, nine HIV-infected patients taking IDV 800 mg/RTV 100 mg bid for at least 4 weeks were randomized to take the combination with a light meal or fasting and underwent pharmacokinetic evaluation.[29] Taking IDV/RTV in a fasted stated resulted in a 1.3-fold higher IDV C_{max} compared to administration with food ($p = 0.001$), without changes in AUC or C_{min}. The investigators hypothesized that food induced a delay in IDV absorption and suggested this as a strategy to avoid the high C_{max} concentrations that have been linked to IDV-related nephrotoxicity.

CLINICAL PROFILE OF IDV/RTV

Based on pharmacokinetics and tolerability, the optimal IDV/RTV dose appears to be 800/100 mg twice daily; this strategy increased the IDV AUC 2.3-fold and the C_{min} 10–25-fold.[28] In two clinical studies in HIV-infected subjects, the combination of IDV 800 mg/RTV 100 mg twice daily also was found to have favorable pharmacokinetic properties.[30,31] Other doses also have been explored. Solas et al reported 17 HIV-infected patients taking IDV 400 mg/RTV 200 mg bid increased the IDV C_{min} and lowered C_{max}, but was associated with toxicity.[32] Boyd and colleagues reported 19 Thai patients taking IDV 400 mg/RTV 100 mg bid but found significantly reduced AUC by 63%, C_{max} by 61% and C_{min} by 76%.[33] Wasmuth studied 16 HIV-negative volunteers who took IDV 600 mg or 400 mg/RTV 100 mg bid and reported worse tolerability in the 600-mg group, but significantly lower IDV exposure in the 400-mg group.[34] Cressey et al studied 13 HIV-infected, treatment-naive patients who started an IDV 600 mg/RTV 100 mg bid-based regimen and then reduced to IDV 400 mg after 1 month.[35] The 600 mg dose was associated with toxicity, while the 400 mg dose was associated with reductions in AUC of 54%, C_{max} by 39%, and C_{min} by 59%. Rhame compared 27 HIV-infected patients randomized to receive IDV 800 mg q8h (standard dose) versus IDV 667 mg/RTV 100 mg bid and found the RTV-boosted dosing was associated with an increased IDV AUC by 1.5-fold, C_{min} by sixfold with no change in C_{max}.[36] Once-daily dosing of IDV/RTV also has been explored but is limited by tolerability.[37–40] Zala et al described 10 patients taking an IDV 800 mg/RTV 100 mg bid-based regimen who substituted a generic formulation of IDV made in Argentina (Inhibisam, Laboratrio Richmond, Buenos Aires) and found no significant differences in IDV exposure.[41]

ELIMINATION

In one of the initial clinical studies, 1000-mg oral doses of IDV were administered to 10 healthy volunteers, and urine samples were collected and analyzed.[19,42] Seven major metabolites were identified, and glucuronidation, oxidation, and *N*-alkylation were the major metabolic pathways. The major component of drug in urine was unchanged IDV, accounting for 11% of the total dose. In follow-up experiments, single 400-mg oral doses of radiolabeled IDV were given to six healthy volunteers.[43] The major route of excretion of IDV was via feces (19% unchanged drug, 64% metabolites); the minor excretory route was via urine (9% unchanged drug, 10% metabolites); and the combined recovery was quantitative. Seven drug metabolites were identified in both plasma and urine; six oxidative metabolites and one glucuronide conjugate. The high level of metabolites in feces is consistent with biliary excretion. The cytochrome P450 (CYP) 3A4 hepatic isoform is the major enzyme responsible for formation of the oxidative metabolites[44]; intestinal CYP3A4 likely contributes relatively little to its metabolism.[45] IDV (like other PIs) serves as a substrate for the P-glycoprotein (PGP) efflux membrane transporter, which is distributed in the gastrointestinal tract, liver, kidney, blood–brain barrier, genital tract, and some CD4+ T lymphocytes.[46] The cellular pump may promote drug secretion into the intestinal lumen, enhance metabolism, or block entry into brain, testes, and some CD4+ T lymphocytes.

TISSUE PENETRATION AND RESERVOIRS

After oral administration in rats, IDV was distributed rapidly throughout the plasma and lymphatic system, with comparable concentrations.[47] Intracellular lymphocyte concentrations in HIV-infected patients are not significantly different from plasma concentrations although the intracellular elimination half-life and mean residence time of IDV were prolonged.[48] Solas et al studied 41 patients on stable IDV-based regimens and found a twofold higher IDV concentration in lymphoid tissue compared to plasma.[49]

In vitro and animal experiments showed that IDV was transported by a PGP efflux membrane transporter that is thought to limit brain (and other tissue) penetration.[46] Following intravenous administration to rats, the brain-plasma IDV-level ratio was 0.18 at steady state, suggesting limited penetration.[47] In an intensive clinical study, eight HIV-infected adults who took an IDV-containing regimen underwent sampling of cerebrospinal fluid (CSF) and plasma.[50] The mean values of free IDV in the CSF were AUC (0–8 h) 1616 nm/hr, C_{max} 294 nM, and C_{min} 122 nM, all exceeding the *in vitro* IC_{95} for IDV. Free IDV accounted for 94% of the drug in CSF and 42% in plasma. The mean ± SD CSF/plasma ratio for free IDV was 15 ± 3%. Seven of eight subjects had CSF HIV RNA levels of less than 200 copies/mL. Other population-based pharmacokinetic studies have shown similar results.[49,51–53]

CSF levels of IDV were higher when administered with RTV.[54,55] For example, in a pilot study of 13 HIV-infected patients, the addition of RTV to IDV increased IDV concentrations in the serum (C_{min} from 65 to 336 ng/mL), CSF (from 39 to 104 ng/mL), and seminal plasma (median 141–1634 ng/mL).[54] In six patients with before and after samples, RTV increased IDV levels significantly in CSF 2.4-fold and in seminal plasma by 8.0-fold. Another group found similar findings in CSF in seven patients taking IDV/RTV.[55]

Solas and colleagues found IDV concentrations were 1.9-fold higher in semen than plasma.[49] Also, Taylor et al found median seminal to plasma IDV concentration ratios ranged from 0.6 (0–2-h postdosing) to 1.4 (6–8-h postdosing), although the concentrations exceeded the IC_{95} at all time points.[56] Van Praag et al characterized IDV concentrations in two fractions of seminal plasma (testicular-prostate, seminal vesicle) and concluded IDV achieved therapeutic concentrations in both throughout the dosing interval.[57] Several groups have documented HIV RNA reduction in semen in patients taking IDV-containing regimens.[58,59]

Launay et al studied nine women taking IDV-based regimens and found IDV detectable in 93% of cervicovaginal secretions.[60] In an *ex vivo* assessment of placental transport, maternal-to-fetal clearance of IDV was significantly lower than fetal-to-maternal clearance.[61] In a study of a nursing mother taking an IDV-based regimen, breast milk drug concentrations were 90–540% of her plasma concentrations.[62]

PHARMACOKINETICS AND ANTIRETROVIRAL EFFECT

Several groups have related the plasma concentrations of IDV to its virologic effect.[63–68] Burger and colleagues prospectively followed 65 subjects on an IDV-containing regimen and observed a virologic failure rate of 37%.[63] In a multivariate analysis, a low plasma concentration of IDV was an independent predictor of failure. Similarly, Acosta and colleagues studied 43 subjects receiving IDV combination therapy and found significantly higher IDV AUC (0–8 h) in treatment-naive subjects with HIV RNA below the limit of detection, compared to those with detectable viral load levels.[64] In another study, using modeling in a treatment-naive patient population, higher IDV C_{min} values were significantly associated with virologic suppression to less than 200 copies/mL at week 24.[65] The 90% virologic response rate in this study correlated with an IDV C_{min} of 110 ng/mL. Anderson and colleagues correlated higher IDV C_{max} concentrations (>7 μg/mL) with greater CD4+ T lymphocyte increases in a group of patients with suppressed HIV RNA levels.[66] Duval et al studied 216 patients taking IDV-based regimens and found that virologic response was independently associated with full adherence, but not IDV concentration in a multivariate model (OR 8.8, $p < 0.05$).[67] A Spanish group studied 46 patients experiencing early virologic failure on an initial IDV-based regimen and found 69% had subtherapeutic IDV levels (75% of whom had no detectable levels) and found more IDV-related resistance mutations in the group with sub-optimal, but detectable IDV concentrations.[68]

Csajka and colleagues conducted a population pharmacokinetic analysis of 239 patients taking IDV with or without RTV and demonstrated significant interpatient and intra-patient variability in IDV concentrations and suggested this supported therapeutic drug monitoring (TDM).[69] Kakuda et al showed the safety and feasibility of concentration-controlled therapy in a pilot study of 11 subjects receiving an IDV-based combination regimen with dosing targeted to achieve a target trough IDV level of 0.15 mg/L.[70]

Shulman and colleagues reported 37 patients taking an IDV-based regimen with ongoing viremia who were changed to a regimen of IDV 400 mg/RTV 400 mg bid and underwent pharmacokinetic assessment.[71] The IDV/RTV regimen did not change IDV AUC, but decreased C_{max} by 57% and increased the C_{min} 3.4-fold and resulted in 21 (58%) of patients reducing HIV RNA levels to <50 copies/mL. Upon further analysis, they found a virtual inhibitory quotient (a ratio of the IDV predose concentration to the degree of virtual phenotypic resistance) was a better predictor of response than either drug resistance or drug concentration alone. The Athena study randomized 55 treatment-naive patients to an IDV-containing regimen (with or without RTV) to receive TDM results with dose adjustments based on achieved IDV concentrations versus the standard-of-care (i.e., no TDM or dose adjustment).[72] After 1 year, fewer patients in the TDM group discontinued IDV (25% vs 48%, $p = 0.07$) and there was a better virologic response.

HEPATIC OR RENAL INSUFFICIENCY

Twelve patients with clinical evidence of cirrhosis and mild to moderate hepatic insufficiency who were administered single doses of 400 mg IDV had a 60% higher mean AUC and an increased half-life of 2.8 ± 0.5 h compared to historical controls, indicating decreased metabolism of IDV.[1] Based on these results, the recommended dose in patients with mild to moderate hepatic insufficiency resulting from cirrhosis is 600 mg q8h. Bossi and colleagues studied six patients with either chronic hepatitis B or C infection who enrolled in the GENOPHAR study of TDM and were treated with IDV 400 mg/RTV 100 mg bid and reported high plasma IDV concentrations.[73] After a dose adjustment at 4 weeks to IDV 200 mg/RTV 100 mg bid, adequate IDV concentrations were maintained through 24 weeks and they suggested this was the optimal dose for co-infected patients. The pharmacokinetics have not been determined in patients with severe hepatic insufficiency or renal insufficiency, but it is assumed that because of the hepatic metabolism of the drug, substantial dose reductions for renal insufficiency are not required.[74] It is not known if IDV is dialyzable by peritoneal dialysis or hemodialysis, though case reports suggest that dosage modification may not be necessary.[75–77]

GENDER AND RACE

Gender differences in IDV metabolism were investigated in the rat, dog, and monkey and in *in vitro* studies with human microsomes.[78] Although some metabolic differences between sexes occurred in the rat and dog, no differences occurred in monkeys or in human liver microsome experiments. Using a population-based analysis of 314 patients, Dutch investigators found no difference in IDV pharmacokinetics by gender although they found dose reductions for IDV-related side effects were more common in women than men (10% vs 1%, $p < 0.01$) and suggested a subset of 10–20% of women might have higher IDV levels.[79] In other clinical studies, comparable pharmacokinetics of IDV were seen in whites and blacks, both in HIV-infected and -uninfected volunteers.[1]

PEDIATRICS

The optimal dosing of IDV in pediatric patients has not been determined. In a clinical study of 34 pediatric HIV-infected patients (age 4–15 years), IDV dosed at 500 mg/m^2 q8h had an AUC (0–8 h) of 38 742 nM/h, C_{max} 17 181 nM, and C_{min} 134 nM.[1] Compared to pharmacokinetic results in adults taking IDV 800 mg q8h, the AUC and C_{max} were higher and the C_{min} lower. Fifty percent of pediatric patients had levels of less than 100 nM compared to 10% of adults. Uncontrolled studies of IDV 500 mg/m^2 q8h in 70 children confirmed different pharmacokinetic profiles from adults.[1] Another study of 11 HIV-infected children taking 500 mg/m^2 q8h also showed a lower C_{min} and suggested that every-6-h dosing is appropriate.[80] In addition, these investigators showed that children with a small body surface area had greater AUC values than adults and suggested that dose reduction is appropriate. A Dutch study of 19 children concluded that the optimal dose to obtain IDV exposures similar to adults was 50 mg/kg of metabolic weight q8h (~600 mg/m^2), although they noted some children required higher doses.[81] Another Dutch study studied IDV 400 mg/m^2/RTV 125 mg/m^2 bid in 14 children and reported that the AUC was similar while the C_{max} was 20% lower compared to adult dosing of IDV 800 mg/RTV 100 mg bid.[82]

PREGNANCY

Kosel and colleagues reported the pharmacokinetic evaluation of 4 pregnant women in their second or third trimesters who took IDV 800 mg q8h ($n = 2$) or IDV 800 mg/RTV 200 mg bid ($n = 2$).[83] In women taking the IDV-based regimens, they found the IDV AUC decreased 52–86% in the third trimester, likely secondary to metabolic induction. However, using IDV/RTV prevented the reduction. Following childbirth, IDV levels returned to baseline.

TOXICITY

In Phase I trials the only clearly drug-related side effect of IDV was a reversible increase in indirect bilirubin.[84] Subsequent studies first documented the occurrence of nephrolithiasis.[22,85] In addition, studies of combination therapy with IDV and zidovudine first described gastrointestinal side effects.[86] In the Swiss HIV Cohort Study of 1160 patients of whom 235 (20%) received IDV, hyperbilirubinemia (odds ratio, OR 18), nephrolithiasis (OR 11) and rash (OR 2), were all significantly associated with IDV use.[87] In a French cohort of 1155 patients taking PI-based therapy, 44% of whom took IDV, IDV use was independently predictive of a serious adverse drug reaction (HR 1.7, 95% CI 1.2–2.4) and overall renal colic was the second most commonly reported event (Table 17-1).[88]

Table 17-1 Common Side Effects of Indinavir

Side Effect	Incidence (%)
Gastrointestinal disturbance	
Abdominal pain	9
Diarrhea	5
Nausea	12
Vomiting	4
Headache	6
Hyperbilirubinemia (indirect)	
Total bilirubin >2.5 mg/dL	10
Total bilirubin >5.0 mg/dL	1
Nephrolithiasis (flank pain ± hematuria)	9–43

OVERDOSE

A 5-year review of the Merck safety data base identified 79 reports of IDV overdose[89]: 15 single episodes of taking >2400 mg, 13 single extra doses <2400 mg, 43 episodes of taking extra drug doses, and eight with unknown doses. Of these, 52 (66%) had adverse events, most commonly nausea, vomiting, abdominal pain, and nephrolithiasis although most patients recovered.

CRYSTALLURIA AND NEPHROLITHIASIS

In a British cohort study of 781 patients taking IDV-based regimens over a median of 1 year, 7% developed IDV-related renal complications: groin pain, renal colic, and/or dysuria.[90] Most patients continued IDV and there was no increase in creatinine. In a Dutch cohort of 1219 patients first starting a PI-based regimen, 644 started IDV and the incidence of urologic symptoms was 8.3/100 treatment-years for IDV versus 0.8/100 treatment-years for other PIs.[91] In an Italian study of 555 patients taking IDV-based regimens, 24% had at least one episode of renal colic over 2 years and 50 (9%) stopped IDV.[92]

Crystals in the urine, most commonly composed of IDV base, occur in 32–67% of patients,[93–96] particularly in the setting of increased urine pH.[94,97] *In vitro* experiments found that IDV crystallizes in the loop of Henle[98] and this may be promoted by the presence of RTV crystals.[97] In one study, crystalluria occurred most commonly during the first 2 weeks after starting treatment and thereafter could be demonstrated in ~25% of urine sediment samples.[95] In another study of 54 patients starting IDV, 25% also had crystals seen on urinalysis.[96] A urine pH < 6 was associated with few episodes of crystals, regardless of urine specific gravity, while nearly half of patients with a urine pH >6 and a urine specific gravity >1.015 had crystalluria.

Other urinalysis abnormalities that occur commonly in the setting of crystalluria are proteinuria, hemoglobinuria, and pyuria. Also described is a more chronic lesion associated with pyuria and characterized by diffuse interstitial nephritis with eosinophilia and scarring and tubule necrosis and dilatation with crystals[99] and multinucleated histiocytes on urine cytology.[100] Case reports have linked IDV crystalluria to a foreign body giant cell reaction with acute tubulointerstitial nephritis demonstrated on renal biopsy.[101] Pyuria is common. In a Dutch cohort study of 184 patients taking IDV over a year, 35% developed pyuria at least once and of 134 evaluated, 24% had persistent pyuria.[102] Patients may experience one of several other clinical syndromes. Back or flank pain with crystalluria without nephrolithiasis or dysuria and urgency with crystalluria.[93] It is not clear if crystalluria always leads to nephrolithiasis.

Nephrolithiasis, diagnosed in the setting of flank pain with or without macroscopic or microscopic hematuria, was reported initially in 193 (9%) of 2071 patients from pooled clinical studies of IDV.[1] A total of seven of 193 patients (4%) went on to discontinue the drug, whereas others resumed therapy. However, in one series of 155 patients, 43% developed nephrolithiasis over 78 weeks.[103] In the ACTG 320 trial, the largest single clinical study of IDV, with 1156 patients randomized to zidovudine and lamivudine with or without IDV, seven patients (1%) experienced renal colic or nephrolithiasis (or both) of severe or greater intensity in the IDV group compared with no patients in the nucleoside analog group after a median follow-up of 38 weeks.[104] In a smaller clinical study with 3 years of follow-up, 12 of 33 (36%) patients ultimately experienced clinical signs of nephrolithiasis[105] and additional episodes occurred with continued therapy.[106]

Specific risks of stone formation that have been suggested include advanced age,[102] female gender,[107] concomitant hepatitis,[108,109] and living in a warm climate or exercising (because of the risk of dehydration).[110,111] Neither a prior or family history of kidney stones nor the concurrent use of acyclovir, sulfa drugs, or vitamin C has been definitively associated with developing nephrolithiasis while taking IDV.[1] One group compared 15 evaluable patients taking IDV with urologic complaints and found that 14 of 15 (90%) had a higher IDV plasma concentration than the mean in a control group of 14 asymptomatic patients taking IDV.[112] In six of these patients, the IDV dose was reduced to 600 mg q8h; plasma concentrations fell within the 95% confidence interval of the control group, and the patients remained asymptomatic. A high frequency of nephrolithiasis also has been reported in pediatric patients (29%).[1]

IDV nephrolithiasis may be difficult to demonstrate radiologically without the use of intravenous contrast dye because the stones are radiolucent.[113] In general, crystalluria and kidney stones are not associated with changes in renal function, and they can be managed with analgesics, hydration, or interruption of the drug for 1–3 days. In one series, 11 (70%) of 18 episodes of IDV-induced nephrolithiasis were successfully managed with hydration and analgesia over the first 48 h.[114] Others have recommended diuresis and acidification of the urine.[115] Of 193 patients on IDV who developed nephrolithiasis, six (3%) had hydronephrosis and six (3%) underwent stent placement.[1] However, hypertension, renal atrophy, renal failure, papillary necrosis, frank obstruction, and anuria also have been reported.[93,116–120]

Daudon and colleagues analyzed kidney stones passed from 29 referred patients taking IDV-containing regimens for periods of 1–20 weeks; they showed the stones to consist of crystals of IDV base monohydrate.[121] Seven patients had stones also containing small amounts of calcium oxalate or calcium phosphate. It is of interest that the cores of all stones analyzed were made of IDV, strongly suggesting that IDV was the promoter of stone formation. Nephrolithiasis occurs more frequently at dose of IDV higher than 2.4 g/day[122] or with IDV/RTV.[1]

In one retrospective analysis of 106 patients taking IDV, 19% experienced a sustained creatinine elevation of at least 20%, associated with low urinary specific gravity and pyuria, consistent with a crystal nephropathy.[123] All abnormalities were reversible upon discontinuing the drug. In another retrospective analysis of 72 patients, the mean serum creatinine levels increased to more than 1.3 mg/dL in 13 (18%); this increase occurred more commonly in women and was associated with pyuria and microhematuria.[107] Among 30 children taking IDV, 53% developed persistent sterile pyuria after 96 weeks and 33% had serum creatinine levels >50% above normal.[124]

BILIRUBIN AND HEPATIC TRANSAMINASE ELEVATIONS

Hyperbilirubinemia resulting from elevated indirect bilirubin (higher than 2.5 mg/dL) occurs in ~10% of patients taking IDV in pooled studies and is dose-related.[1] Unconjugated bilirubin is conjugated with glucuronic acid for biliary excretion. In an *in vitro* system, IDV inhibited uridine 5′-diphospho-glucuronosyltransferase 1A1 (UGT1A1) activity, thereby decreasing bilirubin glucuronidation and likely explaining reversible hyperbilirubinemia.[125] In a rat model, IDV competitively inhibited bilirubin UDP-glucuronosyltransferase (UGT) activity and increased plasma bilirubin levels.[126] Others demonstrated IDV potently inhibited OATP1B1, a liver-specific organic anion uptake transporter, and postulated this as the mechanism for IDV-induced hyperbilirubinemia.[127] Most commonly hyperbilirubinemia is subclinical, although occasionally mild scleral icterus occurs. Hyperbilirubinemia may resolve spontaneously and is reversible with discontinuation of the IDV. Fewer than 1% of patients have associated hepatic enzyme elevations.[1]

Patients with preexisting Gilbert's syndrome may experience the highest bilirubin values. Swiss investigators studied 96 patients and characterized the contribution of the polymorphism conferring Gilbert's syndrome (UGT1A1*28) and IDV on bilirubin levels.[128] Overall, IDV increased bilirubin levels 0.46 mg/dL and 67% of individuals homozygous for the UGT1A1*28 polymorphism had at least two episodes of bilirubin >2.5 mg/dL vs 7% without the polymorphism. It is uncommon for a patient taking IDV to have a total bilirubin level higher than 5.0 mg/dL. In Merck studies 028 and 033, ~7–8% of 302 patients receiving IDV had total serum bilirubin levels higher than 2.5 mg/dL.[86] In the ACTG 320 trial, 27 of 577 subjects (5%) taking IDV had total bilirubin more than 2.5 times the upper limit of normal, and six others (1%) had total bilirubin more than five times normal.[104]

Laboratory abnormalities other than hyperbilirubinemia are less common. One group described eight (7%) of 117 patients who developed severe hepatitis (more than 5.0 times normal or 3.5 times baseline transaminase levels) after starting IDV, although this was similar to that for a group of patients taking nucleoside analogs only; there was a threefold higher risk in patients with chronic viral hepatitis.[129] The same group followed 1161 patients taking PI-based regimen including 194 taking IDV (with or without RTV) and found 13% taking IDV had hepatic transaminases increased more than five times normal.[130] Overall, patients with viral hepatitis accounted for 63% of these cases of hepatotoxicity, however more than 85% of patients with viral hepatitis had no hepatotoxicity.

METABOLIC DISORDERS

IDV was significantly associated with hyperglycemia (hazard ratio 4.0) compared to other antiretroviral drugs.[131] The mechanism is thought to be that IDV is a relatively selective, noncompetitive inhibitor that binds one of the glucose transporters (GLUT4) involved in insulin-stimulated glucose uptake by adipocytes.[132–134] Others have suggested that IDV may interfere with insulin signaling in some cell types, but does not impair insulin secretion.[135–137] IDV acutely increases glucose and insulin levels in rats, and reduces glucose transport and insulin-induced GLUT4 activity.[138,139] A single dose of IDV given to HIV negative volunteers decreased insulin-stimulated glucose transport.[140] Two groups reported that 4-week courses of IDV in HIV-negative volunteers resulted in increased glucose production and decreased insulin sensitivity.[141,142] Dube and colleagues reported 12 HIV-infected subjects who received 2 weeks of IDV monotherapy (and then added nucleoside reverse transcriptase inhibitors (NRTI) for 6 weeks) and found fasting glucose levels increased and insulin sensitivity decreased without a compensatory increase in insulin release.[143]

IDV, like most other HIV PIs, also has been associated with increased serum lipid levels. In the Data Collection on Adverse Events of Anti-HIV Drugs (D:A:D) Study, a collaborative group of 11 cohorts following 11 205 patients, 7729 (43%) received a PI (including 2354 on IDV) and total cholesterol and triglyceride levels were highest in patients receiving RTV (with or without a second PI).[144] The Swiss Cohort Study found lopinavir/RTV was associated with fewer lipid abnormalities compared to IDV/RTV.[145] A meta analysis of three studies found no difference in triglyceride levels between groups taking dual NRTI with or without IDV.[146] The mechanism of hyperlipidemia remains unknown, although it may be due to changes in serum lipoprotein lipase activity, hepatic lipid metabolism,[147] or altered retinoid signaling[148] (*see* Chapter 71).

A fat redistribution syndrome characterized by accumulation of abdominal fat and/or loss of peripheral fat with buffalo hump, lipomas, and in women, breast enlargement, has been associated with HIV PIs[149–151] (*see* Chapter 72). The syndrome has been associated with increased serum lipid levels and insulin resistance[150,151] and is thought to be due to inhibition of sterol-regulatory element-binding protein (SREBP)-1c, a regulator of cholesterol, triglyceride, insulin and adipocyte function and differentiation.[152–154] The abdominal enlargement is characterized by an increase in visceral adipose tissue, typically without an increase in total body weight.[149] During postmarketing surveillance of 282 reports of fat redistribution in patients taking IDV reported to Merck, 159 (56%) had fat accumulation, 60 (21%) had peripheral wasting, and 63 (22%) had both.[155] Fat accumulation was more common in men and peripheral wasting more common in women. Weight gain was reported in 100% of those with fat accumulation, and weight loss was reported in 83% of those with peripheral wasting. In an Italian study, IDV exposure was significantly associated with developing both lipoaccumulation and lipoatrophy (RH 4.78 per year of exposure, $p = 0.03$).[156] Morphologic changes typically do not resolve over the short term upon discontinuing IDV.[150]

Long-term sequelae of hyperlipidemia and fat redistribution are not known, although one group found no association between IDV therapy and myocardial infarction.[157] Henry and colleagues studied 100 randomly selected patients taking an IDV-based combination regimen and found increased median levels of cholesterol (185 mg/dL, with 39% more than 200 mg/dL), triglycerides (184 mg/dL, with 12% more than 400 mg/dL), decreased median HDL levels (33 mg/dL), and a 56% rate of insulin resistance.[158] They noted that these risk factors have been associated with an increased risk of coronary heart disease and warrant risk factor modification efforts. In addition, Shankar and colleagues studied eight HIV-negative men given IDV for 4 weeks and found impaired endothelial function[159] and another group suggested IDV is associated with hypertension.[116,160] However, Henry and colleagues also reported 79 patients taking IDV with suppressed HIV RNA levels with available pretreatment C-reactive protein (CRP) levels and in 56 followed for an average of 31 months found stable or decreased CRP levels.[158] Young et al followed 11 HIV-infected patients starting IDV and found significant decreases in tissue plasminogen activator antigens, and the soluble inflammatory marker soluble TNF receptor (STNFr) and postulated that this was due to improvements in HIV-related inflammation.[161]

OTHER TOXICITIES

Gastrointestinal symptoms occur with IDV-containing regimens. In Merck studies 028 and 033 (IDV vs zidovudine vs the combination) of antiretroviral-naive patients, 4–12% of patients randomized to IDV alone reported abdominal pain, nausea, diarrhea, or vomiting of moderate or greater intensity.[86] In the same studies, 4–14% of patients randomized to zidovudine reported these symptoms, as did 4–32% of patients randomized to the combination regimen. In studies of zidovudine-experienced patients, there were no differences in gastrointestinal side effects among patients taking a combination of zidovudine and lamivudine with or without IDV.[104,162]

The FDA issued a warning letter in July 1996 noting 15 case reports of spontaneous bleeding episodes in HIV positive hemophiliacs taking HIV PIs. In a follow-up report using the FDA's postmarketing spontaneous reporting system, 39 of 67 (58%) reports of spontaneous bleeding in patients taking IDV occurred in hemophiliacs, compared to only two of 63 (3%) in hemophiliac patients taking zidovudine.[163] Bleeding episodes tended to resolve upon discontinuation of therapy but recurred in two hemophiliac patients upon rechallenge. The mechanism is not known, though it may involve a direct effect on blood vessels.[164]

IDV also has been associated with skin, hair, and nail changes, possibly due to inducing gene expression of retinal dehydrogenase (RALDH), a key enzyme involved in retinoic acid synthesis.[165] In one series of 101 patients who started an IDV-based combination regimen, 48 (57%) developed cheilitis, 34 (40%) dry skin with pruritus, five (6%) pyogenic granuloma of the toenails, and one (1%) severe alopecia.[166] A localized skin rash was described in 110 patients who started IDV where 67% of the cohort reported onset of the rash within the first 2 weeks of starting therapy, 49 (44%) reported spread that involved the whole body, 86% had associated pruritus, and 81% required symptomatic treatment with antihistamines or corticosteroids.[167] In this case series, 59% continued IDV therapy despite the presence of the rash. Stevens–Johnson syndrome is a rare complication of IDV.[168] Paronychia have also been associated with IDV in case series[169,170] with a fivefold increased risk associated with IDV treatment in one cohort study.[171] In-grown toenails also have been described with IDV/RTV.[172]

TOXICITY OF IDV/RTV

In a study of 90 treatment-naive patients who received open-label therapy with two nucleoside analogs and IDV/RTV 400/400 mg twice daily, seven (8%) patients discontinued treatment over 24 weeks because of an adverse event: increased hepatic transaminases ($n = 1$), nausea ($n = 4$), and diarrhea ($n = 2$).[173] Over the same time, 20% experienced nausea, 10% had circumoral paresthesias, 47% had a cholesterol level higher than 240 mg/dL, and 67% had a triglyceride level higher than 200 mg/dL. In a 48-week, open-label randomized study in which 106 patients received a combination regimen containing either the standard dose of IDV three times daily or IDV/RTV 800/100 mg twice daily, adverse events were evenly distributed except for nausea (48% IDV, 68% IDV/RTV; $P = 0.04$) and dry mouth (24% IDV, 46% IDV/RTV; $P = 0.02$).[174] Solas and colleagues studied 63 patients taking IDV 800 mg/RTV 100 mg bid and linked an IDV trough level of >500 ng/mL to increased toxicity ($p < 0.05$).[175] The incidence of nephrolithiasis is higher in patients receiving IDV/RTV compared to IDV.[1]

EFFICACY

Monotherapy and Dual Therapy

A 24-week randomized, blinded study (Merck 006) of IDV at either 200 or 400 mg q6h or zidovudine 200 mg q8h was conducted in 73 p24-antigenemic, mostly zidovudine-experienced HIV-positive patients.[85,176] Of the 23 patients in the 400 mg dose cohort, 21 had greater than 1 $\log_{10}$ copies/mL decreases in HIV RNA at some point over 24 weeks compared with 12 of 21 in the 200-mg group and one of 29 in the zidovudine group. A dose-escalation study (Merck 021) evaluated IDV at doses of 800 mg q8h, 1000 mg q8h, and 800 mg q6h in 70 HIV-positive patients.[22] Over 24 weeks the HIV RNA levels decreased ~2 $\log_{10}$ copies/mL, without differences among the three treatment groups.

A large Phase II study (Merck 028) compared IDV 800 mg q8h, zidovudine 200 mg q8h, or a combination of the two in 996 antiretroviral therapy-naive patients with baseline CD4-lymphocyte counts of 50–250/mm^3.[86] During the study the protocol was amended to add lamivudine to the zidovudine-containing arms. A protocol-defined interim analysis of the study found highly significant reductions in clinical progression in the IDV arms compared to the zidovudine arm; and the study was terminated early. Over a median follow-up of 1 year, reductions in the hazards of clinical progression of 70% (combination group) and 61% (IDV group) were seen over that in the zidovudine group ($P < 0.0001$). In addition, significant changes in HIV RNA and CD4-lymphocyte counts were seen in the IDV groups compared to the zidovudine group.

THREE-DRUG COMBINATION: IDV AND TWO NRTIs

A three-drug combination study (Merck 035) enrolled 97 patients with zidovudine experience without prior lamivudine or PI experience who had an HIV RNA level of 20 000 copies/mL or more. They were randomized to IDV 800 mg q8h, zidovudine 200 mg q8h/lamivudine 150 mg bid, or a combination of all three drugs.[162] At baseline, patients had taken zidovudine for a median of 31 months and had a median HIV RNA level of 43 200 copies/mL and a median CD4-lymphocyte count of 144/mm^3. At 24 weeks of follow-up, the median HIV RNA changes were −1.2 $\log_{10}$ copies/mL in the IDV group, −0.8 $\log_{10}$ copies/mL in the zidovudine/lamivudine group, and −1.8 $\log_{10}$ copies/mL in the triple combination group. At the

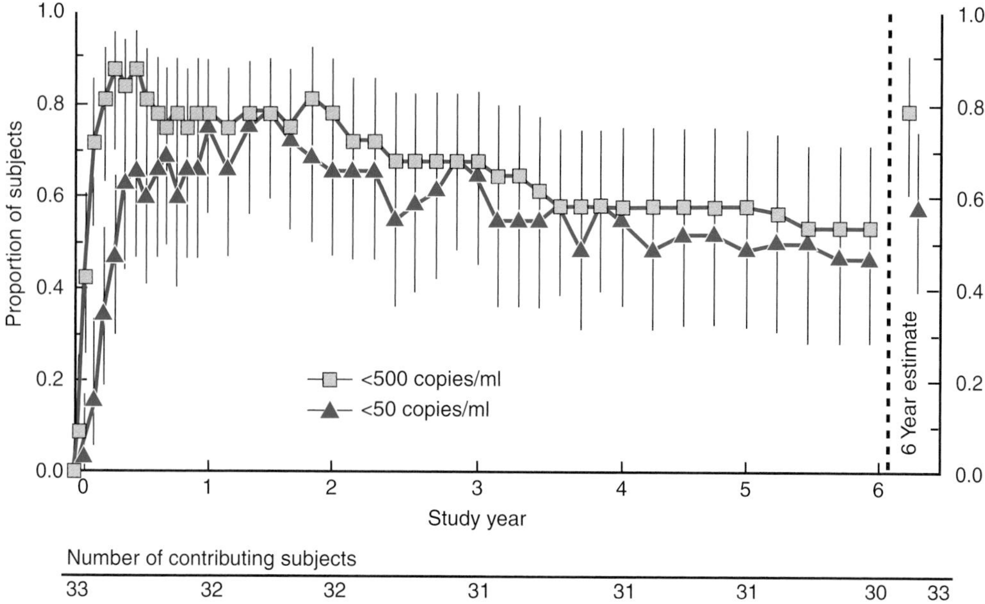

Figure 17-2 ■ Proportions (95% confidence intervals) of subjects randomized to indinavir, zidovudine, and lamivudine, with serum HIV RNA levels <500 copies/mL (squares) and <50 copies/mL (triangles) by study week over 6 years in the Merck 035 study.

Reprinted from Gulick RM, Meibohm A, Havlir D, et al. Six-year follow-up of HIV-1-infected adults in a clinical trial of antiretroviral therapy with indinavir, zidovudine, and lamivudine. AIDS 17:2345, 2003.[106]

same time, 43% of the IDV group decreased HIV RNA to less than 500 copies/mL compared with 0% of the zidovudine/lamivudine group and 90% of the triple-combination group. Most patients on triple therapy who had viral loads of less than 500 copies/mL also had levels of less than 50 copies/mL using an ultrasensitive viral load assay.

After at least 24 weeks of original therapy, all patients received triple-combination therapy and continued to be followed. The simultaneous introduction of three-drug antiretroviral therapy achieved a virologic effect superior to sequential introduction of the same three drugs.[177] Results with the triple combination were durable in most patients through 6 years of follow-up, with 53% and 47% of patients suppressing HIV RNA levels to less than 500 and less than 50 copies/mL, respectively, using an intent-to-treat analysis.[106] At the same time, the CD4-lymphocyte count increased +268 cells/mm^3 over baseline (Fig. 17-2).

A parallel study (Merck 039) enrolled 320 patients with zidovudine experience without prior lamivudine or PI experience who had 50 CD4+ T-lymphocyte cells/mm^3 or less and randomized them to IDV monotherapy, zidovudine/lamivudine, or the triple combination.[178] At baseline the mean HIV RNA was 74 353 copies/mL and the CD4+ T-lymphocyte count was 18/mm^3. The mean HIV RNA changes from baseline at 24 weeks were -0.36 $\log_{10}$ copies/mL in the IDV group, -0.25 $\log_{10}$ copies/mL in the zidovudine/lamivudine group, and -1.93 $\log_{10}$ copies/mL in the three-drug combination group. The proportion of patients with HIV RNA levels of less than 500 and less than 50 copies/mL were 3% and 2% in the IDV group, 0% and 0% in the zidovudine/lamivudine group, and 56% and 45% in the triple-drug combination group, respectively. In the 3-drug group, these results were updated through 4.5 years of follow-up with 24% (intent-to-treat) and 92% (observed) with HIV RNA levels <500 copies/mL and 22% (intent-to-treat) and 85% (observed) with HIV RNA levels <50 copies/mL.[179]

A large study of similar combination antiretroviral regimens (ACTG 320) assessed clinical endpoints.[104] In this study, 1156 patients with CD4+ T-lymphocyte counts of 200/mm^3 or less (median 86/mm^3) with zidovudine experience but without previous lamivudine or PI use were randomized to zidovudine 200 mg q8h/lamivudine 150 mg bid with or without IDV 800 mg q8h and were followed for the occurrence of a new AIDS-defining illness or death. After a median follow-up of 38 weeks, the Data and Safety Monitoring Board (DSMB) recommended stopping the study because of a significant difference between the two treatment arms: 63 patients (11%) taking the two-drug combination had a new AIDS event or death versus 33 patients (6%) on the triple-combination arm ($P = 0.001$) (Fig. 17-3). The three-drug combination of IDV/zidovudine/lamivudine demonstrated a 50% decrease in the rate of AIDS or death over the zidovudine/lamivudine regimen. A subanalysis also found a significant improvement in health-related quality of life after 24 weeks, particularly in patients with low baseline CD4+ T-lymphocyte counts.[180]

Merck 060 was a single-arm study of 199 antiretroviral-naïve patients with a CD4+ T-lymphocyte count of more than 500/mm^3 and an HIV RNA level of more than 1000 copies/mL treated with open-label zidovudine/lamivudine/IDV.[181] After 3 years, 85 (43%) subjects discontinued the study, including 15% for adverse events. Overall, 15% had nephrolithiasis, 53% (noncompleter (NC) = failure (F)) and 98% (observed) had a serum HIV RNA level of less than 400 copies/mL, and 51% (NC = F) and 93% (observed) had less than 50 copies/mL at week 96.

IDV/RTV-BASED REGIMENS

Enhancement of IDV levels by RTV allows co-administration on a twice-daily basis, with food.[27,28] and various twice-daily doses have been explored such as IDV/RTV at 800/100,

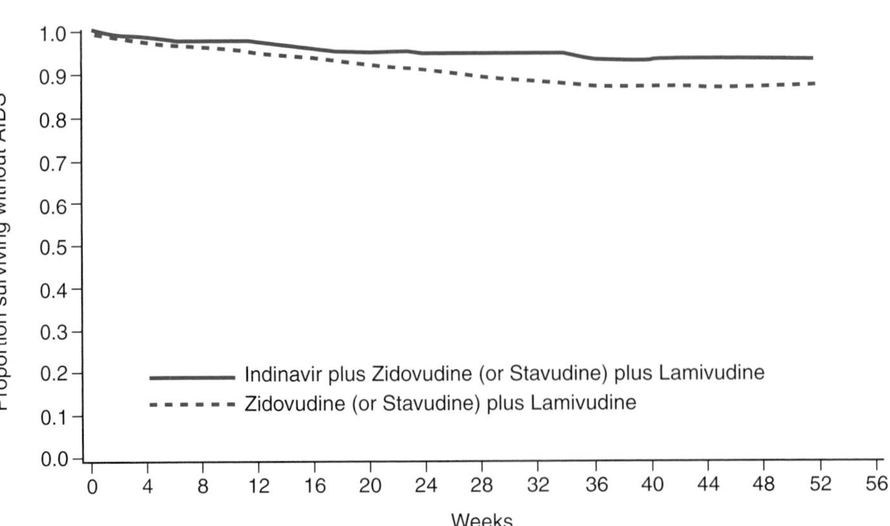

Figure 17-3 ■ Kaplan–Meier estimate of the proportion of subjects not reaching the primary study endpoint of AIDS or death in the ACTG 320 study.

From Hammer SM, Squires KE, Hughes MD, et al. A randomized placebo-controlled trial of indinavir in combination with two nucleoside analogs in human immunodeficiency virus infected persons with CD4 cell counts less than or equal to 200 per cubic millimeter. N Engl J Med 337:725, 1997; Copyright 1997, Massachusetts Medical Society.[104] All rights reserved.

800/200, 400/400, and 400/100 mg bid. An open-label single-armed study of IDV and RTV (both given at 400 mg q12h) with nucleosides explored the virologic activity of this combination in 93 treatment-naive subjects.[173] At 72 weeks, 63% and 60% had reduced HIV RNA levels to less than 500 and less than 80 copies/mL, respectively, in an intent-to-treat analysis. ACTG 5055 randomized 44 patients failing their first PI-based regimen to IDV/RTV-based regimens (either 800/200 or 400/400 mg bid) and found 55% versus 45% had HIV RNA <200 copies/mL at week 24 ($P = 0.76$) with more toxicity in the 400/400-mg group.[182] In a cohort study, Burger and colleagues found IDV/RTV dosed 800/100 or 400/400 mg bid had comparable virologic suppression rates in treatment-naive patients but found more toxicity and discontinuations in the 400/400 group.[183] Other cohort studies demonstrated IDV 800 mg/RTV 100 mg bid provided potent virologic and immunologic responses, but toxicity and drug discontinuation occurred commonly.[184,185] In a study of 323 evaluable subjects taking IDV 800 mg q8h, patients were randomized to continue or change to IDV 800 mg/RTV 100 mg bid.[186] The results at 48 weeks showed HIV RNA levels less than 500 copies/mL in 58% versus 74%, respectively (switch = failure, $P = 0.003$), with more discontinuations due to adverse events with IDV/RTV ($P < 0.001$).

In a nonrandomized study comparing IDV/RTV 800/100 or 400/100 mg bid, at 48 weeks, HIV RNA was <50 copies/mL in 77% and 64% ($p > 0.05$) but side effects leading to drug discontinuation occurred in 61% and 20% ($P < 0.0001$) and changing from 800/100 to 400/100 improved side effects in 16 of 20 patients.[187] Other pilot studies of IDV 400 mg/RTV 100 mg bid demonstrated virologic activity.[188,189] One study found IDV/RTV 400/100 dosing led to higher C_{min} and lower C_{max} than standard IDV dosing,[190] and a Thai study of this regimen reported 80 treatment-naive patients taking this dose with 67% with HIV RNA <50 copies/mL at 2 years,[191] but concerns remain about low IDV trough concentrations with this regimen. Pilot studies of once-daily regimens containing IDV 1200 mg/RTV 400 mg also have been reported,[39,40] but also raised concerns about low IDV trough concentrations. A pilot study evaluated 12 patients taking IDV/RTV-based regimens with HIV RNA <50 copies/mL who discontinued their NRTIs.[192] Over a median 78 weeks of follow-up, most patients maintained virologic suppression.

OTHER IDV STUDY RESULTS

Pediatrics

The first reported study of a PI-containing regimen in a pediatric population was a pilot study of open-label IDV 500 mg/m^2 q8h, stavudine 1 mg/kg q12h, and didanosine 90 mg/m^2 q12h in 12 nucleoside-experienced children, five of whom had received prior stavudine and didanosine.[193] During the study, the dose of IDV was increased to 500 mg/m^2 q6h when low trough levels were documented. At 48 weeks, HIV RNA decreased an average of 2.0 $\log_{10}$ copies/mL.

A Phase I/II study enrolled 54 mostly treatment-experienced children who received IDV in one of two formulations (free-base liquid suspension or sulfate salt dry-filled capsules) at one of three oral doses (250, 350, or 500 mg/m^2 q8h) for a median of 16 weeks and then added zidovudine/lamivudine.[194] During the study the suspension was found to be less bioavailable, and all children were changed to capsules. Overall, of 48 evaluable patients at 16 weeks, HIV RNA median decreases were −0.01 $\log_{10}$ copies/mL (250- and 350-mg/m^2 groups) and −0.76 $\log_{10}$ copies/mL (500-mg/m^2 group). By week 58, all children received IDV 350 mg/m^2 and at week 96, a median −0.74 HIV RNA $\log_{10}$ copies/mL was seen in 33 children completing treatment.[195]

Another study enrolled 28 children, about half of whom were treatment-experienced, who took IDV 400 mg/m^2 q8h with zidovudine/lamivudine.[196] In 70% of patients the IDV dose was increased to achieve target AUC levels. At 6 months of follow-up, 70% and 48% of subjects had HIV RNA levels less than 500 and less than 40 copies/mL, respectively. Another study randomized 25 children to receive open-label

IDV 500 mg/m² q8h with stavudine and lamivudine.[197] HIV RNA decreased to less than 400 copies/mL within 1 month in 79% of the children and was sustained through 18 months of follow-up. In ACTG 338, 24 children taking RTV-based regimens were changed to an IDV (500 mg/m² q8h)-based regimen without significant changes in virologic or immunologic responses.[198]

IDV and NNRTIs

The concomitant use of IDV and the NNRTI nevirapine has been described in several small studies,[199,200] however, giving standard doses of each resulted in 11–50% decreases in IDV levels. The combination of IDV and efavirenz also has been investigated.[201,202] The Dupont 006 study was a three-arm study of initial antiretroviral therapy, including one arm with IDV 1000 mg q8h/efavirenz 600 mg qd.[201] Of 148 initially randomized to this combination, 53% and 47% reduced HIV RNA levels to less than 500 and less than 50 copies/mL, respectively, at 48 weeks in an intent-to-treat analysis. In a nucleoside-experienced group of 184 patients randomized to IDV 1000 mg q8h/efavirenz or IDV 800 mg q8h/nucleosides, 68% and 52% had reduced HIV RNA levels (to <400 copies/mL) at 24 weeks.[202]

Comparisons to Other PIs

Older studies showed IDV-based regimens were comparable to saquinavir, RTV-, saquinavir/RTV-, or nelfinavir-based regimens.[203–205] The MaxCmin1 study randomized a mixed patient population (including treatment-naive and treatment-experienced with virologic failure or intolerance to PIs) of 306 patients to receive IDV 800 mg/RTV 100 mg bid versus saquinavir 1000 mg/RTV 100 mg bid and found at 48 weeks that virologic failure rates were comparable at ~25% (P = 0.76), but more patients had severe or greater adverse events in the IDV/RTV arm (41% vs 24%, P = 0.001).[206] A retrospective study of 107 treatment-naive patients starting IDV/RTV or lopinavir/RTV found 73% versus 88% had HIV RNA <50 copies/mL at 12 months (P = 0.001) and 29% versus 5% discontinued drugs for toxicity (P = 0.0001).[207]

Comparisons to Other Antiretroviral Regimens

The Dupont 006 study compared open-label IDV/zidovudine/lamivudine to efavirenz/zidovudine/lamivudine and IDV/efavirenz in 450 treatment-naive subjects.[201] At 48 weeks of follow-up, 48% and 43% (IDV group), 70% and 64% (efavirenz group), and 53% and 47% (IDV/efavirenz group) decreased HIV RNA levels to less than 400 and less than 50 copies/mL, respectively, in an intent-to-treat, missing equals failure analysis, favoring the efavirenz arm (P < 0.001). Results were similar at 3 years of follow-up in an extended cohort of 1266 patients, with 7–8% in each group experiencing virologic rebound of more than 50 copies mL/year.[208] Using an economic model based on this data, the efavirenz-based regimen was associated with savings of up to $11 000 over 5–15 years compared to using an IDV-based regimen.[209] In the UK Collaborative HIV Cohort Study Group, compared to 1172 patients taking efavirenz-based regimens with HIV RNA suppressed to <50 copies/mL, the rate of virologic rebound (confirmed HIV RNA >500 copies/mL) was 1.5-fold higher in 260 patients taking IDV-based regimens and twofold higher in 94 patients taking IDV/RTV.[210]

The Glaxo 3005 study enrolled 562 treatment-naive subjects to receive IDV/zidovudine/lamivudine or abacavir/zidovudine/lamivudine in a double-blind, placebo-controlled manner.[211] At week 48, ~51% had decreased HIV RNA levels to 400 copies/mL or less in each group in an intent-to-treat, missing equals failure analysis. A difference was seen in the subset of subjects who entered the study with HIV RNA of more than 100 000 copies/mL, where 45% of the IDV group versus 31% of the abacavir group reduced plasma HIV RNA levels to less than 50 copies/mL. The CNAA 3014 study had an identical design but administered the drugs in an open-label manner.[212] In this study, 342 antiretroviral-naive subjects received zidovudine/lamivudine in combination with IDV or abacavir. At 48 weeks, 50% and 50% (IDV group) and 66% and 60% (abacavir group) had reduced HIV RNA levels to less than 400 and less than 50 copies/mL, respectively. In the subjects with viral load levels of more than 100 000 copies/mL at baseline, 51% (IDV) and 60% (abacavir) had HIV RNA of less than 400 copies/mL. Self-reported adherence was better in the abacavir group, with 76% of subjects indicating that they took >95% of treatment versus 58% in the IDV group (P < 0.001).[213]

The major IDV efficacy trials are summarized in Table 17-2.

RESISTANCE

Original attempts to derive HIV resistant to IDV in vitro by serial passages of wild-type virus in cell culture in the presence of increasing concentrations of the drug were unsuccessful.[9] This led to further studies of resistance involving construction of mutant recombinant protease enzymes and assessment of their susceptibility to IDV. Using the crystal structure of the HIV protease enzyme complexed with specific PIs, single amino acid positions in the enzyme were identified as potentially important for drug binding at positions 23, 32, 47, 50, 76, 82, and 84. In the case of each recombinant enzyme with a constructed single amino acid substitution, some loss of sensitivity to the drug occurred, along with an apparent decrease in the efficiency of the enzyme. HIV variants constructed with multiple mutations had broad cross-resistance to some other PIs.[214] Similarly, viruses selected *in vitro* for high-level resistance to indinavir, RTV, or saquinavir, either separately or combined, had significant overlap in mutations and high-level cross-resistance.[215] A molecular clone carrying the eight most common substitutions demonstrated attenuation of protein processing and viral fitness.

Major Efficacy Trials of Indinavir

Table 17-2

Study	Regimen	No.	Entry Criteria	Results
Two-Drug VS Three-Drug Combinations				
Gulick et al[105,106,162,177] (Merck 035)	IDV VS ZDV+3TC VS IDV+ZDV+3TC (double blind)	97	ZDV-experienced HIV RNA >20 000 CD4 50–500	Three-drug combination superior: HIV RNA <50 in 47% at 6 years (ITT analysis)
Hirsch et al[178,179] (Merck 039)	IDV VS ZDV+3TC VS IDV+ZDV+3TC (double blind)	320	ZDV-experienced CD4 ≤50	Three-drug combination superior: HIV RNA <50 in 22% at 4.5 years (ITT analysis)
Hammer et al[104] (ACTG 320)	ZDV +3TC VS IDV+ZDV +3TC (double blind)	1156	ZDV-experienced CD4 <200	Three-drug combination superior: 50% decrease in AIDS/death over 38 weeks of follow-up (ITT analysis)
Indinavir and Ritonavir				
Lichterfeld et al[173]	Two nucleosides + IDV/RTV (400/400 mg bid) (open-label)	93	Treatment-naive HIV RNA >35 000	HIV RNA <80 in 60% at 72 weeks (ITT analysis)
Acosta et al[182] (ACTG 5055)	Nucleosides + either IDV/RTV (400/400 mg bid) or IDV/RTV (800/200 mg bid) (open label)	44	Following first PI failure	HIV RNA <200 in 45% (400/400) and 55% (800/200) at 24 weeks (ITT analysis)
Arnaiz et al[186] (best study)	Two nucleosides + either continue IDV 800 mg q8h or change to IDV/RTV 800/100 mg q12h (open-label)	323	HIV RNA <500 and CD4 >100 on IDV-based regimen	HIV RNA <500 in 74% (IDV) and 58% (IDV/RTV) at 48 weeks (ITT, switch = failure analysis); increased discontinuations due to adverse events in IDV/RTV group
Comparative Studies: Protease Inhibitors, NNRTI, Three Nucleosides				
Stazsewski et al[201,208] (Dupont 006)	ZDV+3TC+EFV VS IDV +EFV VS ZDV+3TC+IDV (open label)	450	Treatment-naive HIV RNA >10 000 CD4 >50	EFV regimen superior: HIV RNA <50 in 64% (EFV), 47% (IDV/EFV), 43% (IDV) at 48 weeks; increased dropouts in IDV group (ITT analysis); durable responses through 3.3 years
Stazsewski et al[211] (Glaxo 3005)	ZDV+3TC+ABC VS ZDV+3TC+IDV (double blind)	562	Treatment-naive HIV RNA >10 000 CD4 >100	HIV RNA <400 in 51% in both groups at week 48; with baseline HIV RNA >100 000, IDV regimen superior: HIV RNA <50 in 45% (IDV) VS 31% (ABC) (ITT analysis)
Vibhagool[212] (Glaxo 3014)	ZDV+3TC+ABC VS ZDV+3TC+IDV (open label)	342	Treatment-naive HIV RNA >5000	ABC regimen superior: HIV RNA <400 in 67% (ABC) VS 58% (IDV) at 24 weeks (ITT analysis)

ABC, abacavir; CD4 units, cells/mm^3; EFV, efavirenz; IDV, indinavir; ITT, intent-to-treat; NVP, nevirapine; RTV, ritonavir; 3TC, lamivudine; ZDV, zidovudine.

CD4 cells/mm^3; HIV RNA copies/mL.

CLINICAL STUDIES

The first study of clinical resistance to PIs was reported by Condra et al.[216] Early clinical studies of IDV using suboptimal doses (200 or 400 mg q6h) were associated with transient decreases in viral load levels, followed by subsequent rebounds.[85] Viral constructs with substitutions at positions 10, 46, 63, 82, and 84, showed that none of the single or double amino acid substitutions was associated with a loss of sensitivity to IDV or cross-resistance to other PIs, but three or more mutations resulted in a loss of IDV sensitivity and high-level cross-resistance to five other PIs.

Additional isolates from other patients on prolonged IDV treatment revealed broad phenotypic resistance to IDV and high degrees of cross-resistance to other PIs. Interestingly, the genotypic analyses revealed distinct patterns of multiple

Table 17-3 Amino Acid Substitutions in the HIV Protease

Amino Acid Position	Substitution Type
32, 82, 84, 90	Enzyme active site
10, 20, 24, 36, 46, 54, 63, 64,71	Compensatory

mutations in each case. The identified amino acid residues were of two kinds: those close to the active site of the HIV protease enzyme (positions 32, 82, 84, 90) and other "compensatory" changes (at positions 10, 20, 24, 36, 46, 54, 63, 71) (Table 17-3). These compensatory substitutions are thought to represent structural conformational changes or to promote increases in enzymatic activity to compensate for the changes in inhibitor binding.[217]

Condra and colleagues extended their observations using viral isolates from 29 additional patients from early Phase I or II studies of IDV using suboptimal doses (200 or 400 mg q6h or 600 mg q8h).[218] Development of resistance in 17 of these patients was associated with multiple variable patterns of substitutions of three to 11 amino acids in the HIV protease. No repeated pattern of changes was seen among the isolates, although substitutions at positions 46 or 82 (or both) occurred in all resistant isolates. A minimum of three mutations was required for measurable drug resistance. Changes at positions 10, 20, 24, 46, 54, 63, 64, 71, 82, 84, and 90 correlated with phenotypic IDV resistance selected *in vivo*.

Continued IDV therapy was associated with the stepwise accumulation of additional mutations and an associated increase in phenotypic resistance to IDV. In isolates from 15 patients there was some degree of cross-resistance to some other PIs, including saquinavir (63% cross-resistant), RTV (100% cross-resistant), and amprenavir (81% cross-resistant). In a subset of these subjects, the mean proportion of amino acid changes from baseline increased from 4.0% (week 0 to 24) to 7.3% (week 0 to 60), indicating continued evolution of the sequence under continued drug pressure.[219]

A second described mechanism of HIV drug resistance involves mutations in the precursor protein cleavage sites. One group described six patients on IDV-containing regimens who developed not only amino acid substitutions in the protease enzyme but also a change in the gag p7/p1 cleavage site.[220] In three of these patients the p7/p1 change occurred as early as 6–10 weeks after starting therapy. One of the patients developed a second mutation at the gag p1/p6 cleavage site. *In vitro*, recombinant viruses with protease enzyme mutations at positions 46 and 82 had a 68% reduction in replication rate. The replication rate of viruses with protease mutations was enhanced with the introduction of the gag cleavage site mutations. This compensatory mutation may confer a growth advantage to the virus and serves as an important mechanism of viral resistance. Another group described 28 patients with resistance to IDV, RTV, or saquinavir of whom 26 (93%) had one or more gag cleavage site mutations (p2/NC, NC/p1, NC/TFP).[221]

In a study of patients randomized to IDV, zidovudine/lamivudine, or the triple combination,[162,177] 26 of 31 (84%) patients on zidovudine/lamivudine developed lamivudine resistance, and 10 of 31 (32%) patients on IDV monotherapy developed IDV resistance. On the triple combination, 26 of 31 (84%) patients had HIV RNA levels that could not be amplified, implying functional drug sensitivity. However, in a substudy of six patients who experienced virologic failure while taking an IDV-based regimen on ACTG 320 and did not show primary IDV-associated mutations on bulk sequencing, one patient had evidence of the V82A substitution in nine of 30 clones at week 24[222] thus genotypic resistance can be missed with routine testing.

Not all patients experiencing virologic failure on IDV-containing regimens demonstrate resistance to IDV.[223,224] In the Trilege study, 29 patients who achieved virologic suppression on IDV-based therapy and then virologic failure after randomization to continue three drugs or change to zidovudine/IDV were characterized at the time of virologic failure, and no PI mutations were found.[223] In the ACTG 343 study, subjects who achieved virologic suppression on an IDV-based combination regimen were subsequently randomized to continue three drugs or to change to IDV monotherapy.[224] Of the 26 subjects who experienced virologic rebound (17 on three drugs, nine on IDV monotherapy), none showed evidence of IDV resistance, whereas phenotypic resistance to lamivudine was seen in 14 of 17 (82%). These findings suggest that the development of resistance to IDV may be delayed after virologic failure. In a pooled study of five IDV trials,[225] several factors were found to predict the development of resistance to IDV: a lower baseline CD4+ T-lymphocyte count, using less than a three-drug combination of antiretroviral agents, and HIV RNA levels not suppressed to below the limit of detection.

It may be possible to overcome drug resistance by enhancing drug exposure. Combining RTV with IDV leads to an increase in IDV C_{min} over the protein binding-corrected IC_{95} by 28- to 79-fold.[18,27,28] Using a panel of viruses from subjects who had experienced virologic failure on IDV-containing regimens, Condra and colleagues showed that IDV/RTV combinations of 400/400 mg or 800/100 mg had C_{min} (12 h) that exceeded the corrected IC_{95} values for half of the isolates tested and the 800/200 mg combination dose for 18 of 20 (90%) of the isolates tested.[226] Even at the 400-mg dose of RTV, the C_{min} for RTV was less than the IC_{95} value for 19 of 20 isolates, suggesting a minimal contribution by RTV to antiretroviral activity. Shulman and colleagues[71] studied 37 patients on an IDV 800 mg tid regimen with HIV RNA of 50 to 50 000 copies/mL who were changed to open-label IDV/RTV 400/400 mg bid. When given with RTV, the IDV trough concentration was 647% higher, the AUC was unchanged, and the IDV peak concentration was 57% lower than when IDV was given alone. At week 3 after the change, 21 (58%) of patients had an HIV RNA level of less than 50 copies/mL or >0.5 log copies/mL decrease, and the response correlated with a higher trough IDV concentration and less virtual phenotypic resistance at baseline. Thus, the IDV/RTV combination clearly offered benefits.

CROSS-RESISTANCE WITH OTHER PIs

Hertogs and colleagues characterized 6570 viral isolates from patients referred for resistance testing who had an HIV RNA level of at least 1000 copies/mL.[227] Among them, more than 10-fold phenotypic resistance was demonstrated in 17% to IDV, in 22% to RTV, in 25% to nelfinavir, and in 17% to saquinavir. Cross-resistance among those PIs occurred in 59–80% of the samples and a total of 11% were resistant to all four PIs. Among the 1117 isolates resistant to IDV, only five (0.4%) were fully sensitive to RTV, nelfinavir, and saquinavir. In a subset of viral isolates phenotypically resistant to at least one PI, the most frequent amino acid substitutions (>20% frequency) were at protease positions 10, 36, 46, 54, 71, 77, 82, and 90. Among isolates with phenotypic resistance to all four PIs, these substitutions and changes at positions 48 and 84 were seen. These data imply that despite unique initial mutations, a final common pathway exists for these four PIs.

Serial passage of HIV in the presence of amprenavir yielded virus with reduced sensitivity to the drug, and sequence analysis revealed the sequential accumulation of point mutations with the appearance of substitutions at positions 10, 46, 47, and 50.[228] In other experiments, a single mutation at position 50 conferred a two- to threefold reduced sensitivity to amprenavir; and a triple mutant at positions 46, 47, and 50 conferred a 14- to 20-fold reduction. The presence of mutations at 10, 46, 47, and 50 conferred a three- to fourfold loss of sensitivity to IDV. In a study of 271 viral isolates, prior exposure to IDV was associated with decreased susceptibility to amprenavir (P = 0.021) and lopinavir/RTV (P = 0.028).[229] In another study of 551 clinical isolates, IDV and atazanavir resistance were significantly correlated (R= 0.68).[230]

Results from clinical studies with the sequential use of PIs demonstrate the clinical significance of cross resistance: ACTG 333 studied patients who failed saquinavir and then started IDV and showed only modest virologic responses.[231] ACTG 359 randomized 277 patients who had failed IDV to receive saquinavir/RTV or saquinavir/nelfinavir and found only 30% of subjects had HIV RNA levels of 500 copies/mL or less at week 16, without differences between the dual PI regimens.[232] ACTG 398 randomized 481 PI-experienced patients to PI-based regimens including IDV/amprenavir and found only 31% had HIV RNA <200 copies/mL.[233] Current guidelines recommend conducting drug resistance testing in the setting of virologic failure to select the optimal next antiretroviral regimen.[2,234] Newer PIs, tipranavir[234a] and darunavir[234b], demonstrate activity against PI-resistant viruses.

DRUG INTERACTIONS

All of the HIV PIs have the potential to cause important drug interactions (Table 17-4) because of their ability to inhibit the CYP hepatic enzyme system.[2,3,235] IDV is a reversible inhibitor of the CYP3A4 enzyme isoform, a common pathway for hepatic drug metabolism; but it does not inhibit other isoforms, such as CYP1A2, 2C9, or 2E1.[236]

CONTRAINDICATED MEDICATIONS

Like other inhibitors of CYP3A4, co-administration of IDV with astemizole (Hismanal), cisapride (Propulsid), pimozide (Orap), or terfenadine (Seldane) is contraindicated because of the potential for cardiac arrhythmias; with midazolam (Versed) or triazolam (Halcion) because of the potential for prolonged sedation; or with ergot derivatives because of the potential for inducing ergotism.[1,2,237] Additionally, IDV should not be co-administered with rifampin because of an 89% reduction in IDV AUC.[1,238] Co-administration of indinavir 800 mg/RTV 100 mg bid and rifampin led to an 87% decrease in IDV levels and a 94% decrease in RTV levels.[239] Because of the marked interaction, IDV (with or without RTV) should not be given with rifampin. IDV should not be administered with St John's wort because of reductions in IDV AUC by 57% and C_{min} by 81%.[240] A constituent of St John's wort, hyperforin, induces CYP3A4, causing increased drug metabolism.[241] Co-administration of IDV with simvastatin (Zocor) or lovastatin (Mevacor) should also be avoided because their levels would be increased, with the possibility of inducing myopathy.[1,2] IDV should not be given with atazanavir due to hyperbilirubinemia caused by both drugs.[2]

INTERACTIONS WITH COMMON HIV MEDICATIONS

The IDV Pharmacokinetic Study Group performed a series of crossover studies with three dosing periods: (1) IDV alone, (2) IDV in combination with a second drug at standard dose, and (3) the second drug alone.[242] Plasma sampling after 7–10 days of drug dosing was performed with 10–14 subjects per study, and plasma drug exposures were determined. No clinically significant interactions were seen with IDV and isoniazid, fluconazole, or trimethoprim–sulfamethoxazole.[242,243] Another group studied the interaction of IDV and fluconazole in 13 patients and found a trend toward a decrease in IDV AUC, without effects on C_{max} or C_{min}, but they questioned the clinical significance of their findings.[244]

In a multidose study, co-administration of ketoconazole once daily with IDV 600 mg q8h resulted in an 18% increase in IDV AUC over that seen with IDV alone at 800 mg q8h; therefore a dose reduction in IDV is recommended.[1,245] For the same reason, itraconazole use should prompt a dose reduction in IDV to 600 mg q8h.[1] There was no significant interaction between IDV and voriconazole.[246] Co-administration with IDV increased the AUC of clarithromycin by ~47%, and the IDV C_{min} by 58% without affecting the IDV AUC or C_{max}.[247] IDV levels were not altered by co-administration with azithromycin[248] or atovaquone.[249]

Co-administration of IDV and rifabutin increased the plasma concentrations of rifabutin about twofold and reduced IDV levels ~30%.[250] A follow-up study, ACTG 365, co-administered IDV at an increased dose of 1000 mg q8h and rifabutin at a reduced dose of 150 mg qd in 18 healthy volunteers and found the IDV concentrations similar to that of

Important Drug Interactions with Indinavir OR IDV/RTV

Table 17-4

Drug	Interaction/Side Effects (Dose Change)
Contraindicated	
Astemizole (Hismanal)	Cardiac arrhythmias
Cisapride (Propulsid)	Cardiac arrhythmias
Ergot derivatives	Ergotism
Midazolam (Versed)	Extreme sedation
Pimozide (Orap)	Cardiac arrhythmias
Terfenadine (Seldane)	Cardiac arrhythmias
Triazolam (Halcion)	Extreme sedation
Not Recommended	
Atazanavir (Reyataz)	Both cause hyperbilirubinemia
Lovastatin (Mevacor)	Statin levels increased, risk of myopathy
Rifampin	Lowers IDV levels 87%; also lowers RTV levels 94%
Simvastatin (Zocor)	Statin levels increased, risk of myopathy
St John's Wort	Lowers IDV levels 57–81%
Use With Caution	
Calcium channel blockers	Increases calcium channel blocker levels
Carbamazepine (Tegretol)	Lowers IDV levels
Dexamethasone	Lowers IDV levels
Omeprazole (Prilosec)	Decreases IDV absorption –pH effect
Phenobarbital	Lowers IDV levels
Phenytoin (Dilantin)	Lowers IDV levels
Sildenafil (Viagra) and other erectile dysfunction (ED) drugs	Increases ED drug levels
Dose Change Required	
Inducers of cytochrome P450	Lowers IDV levels
Efavirenz (Sustiva)	Increase IDV dose to 1 g q8h or use IDV/RTV
Nevirapine (Viramune)	Increase IDV dose to 1 g q8h or use IDV/RTV
Rifabutin (Mycobutin)	Increase IDV dose to 1 g q8h and decrease rifabutin dose to 150 mg qd
Inhibitors of cytochrome P450	Increases IDV levels
Delavirdine (Rescriptor)	Decrease IDV dose to 600 mg q8h
Itraconazole (Sporanox)	
Ketoconazole (Nizoral)	
Protease Inhibitor Combinations	
IDV/ritonavir	IDV increased eight-fold; ritonavir no change
IDV/lopinavir/ritonavir	IDV increased (dose reduce to 400–600 mg bid)

standard dosing while rifabutin concentrations were 70–120% higher, although the clinical significance of this increase is not known.[251]

INTERACTIONS WITH NRTIS

The interaction of IDV with several NRTIs has been investigated. The IDV PK Study Group tested IDV in combination with zidovudine or stavudine and found no clinically significant interactions.[242] Another study investigated the combination of zidovudine and lamivudine and found no significant interaction with IDV.[162] The enteric-coated formulation of didanosine (ddI EC) does not interact significantly with IDV.[252] Concomitant dosing of ddI EC and IDV 1200 mg/RTV 400 mg qd with food did not decrease absorption of either ddI or IDV, although ddI exposure was slightly decreased.[253] Co-administration of abacavir did not change IDV pharmacokinetics.[254]

INTERACTIONS WITH NNRTIS

The NNRTIs are metabolized by the CYP system and have interactions with IDV. Nevirapine is an inducer of P450 metabolism and reduces the C_{max} of IDV 11% and the AUC 28%.[200] Because of this reduction it has been suggested that the IDV dose be increased to 1000 mg q8h if co-administered with nevirapine.[2] Burger and colleagues found patients taking IDV 800 mg/RTV 100 mg bid with nevirapine had 57% decreased IDV trough concentrations compared to administration without nevirapine, possibly due to effects on both PIs.[255] In contrast, delavirdine inhibits the CPY system and results in an increase in IDV levels, such that a 600-mg dose of IDV when co-adminstered with delavirdine achieves an AUC 44% greater than with IDV 800 mg alone.[256] Therefore it has been suggested that the IDV dose be reduced to 600 mg tid when the drugs are co-administered.[2] Efavirenz also induces P450 metabolism and reduces IDV levels by ~35%.[257] Increasing the dose of IDV to 1 g q8h is recommended when co-administering efavirenz[2]; this adjusted dose was superior to using IDV 1200 mg bid.[258] The addition of efavirenz to IDV 800 mg/RTV 100 mg bid in both HIV-infected and -uninfected volunteers was associated with a decrease in IDV concentrations, but trough levels remained above those seen with standard IDV dosing.[259–261]

INTERACTIONS WITH OTHER PIs

Because all the PIs are metabolized through the CPY system, they may interact with each other. In healthy volunteers, IDV increased the mean AUC and C_{max} of saquinavir approximately five- to eightfold.[262] The interaction of IDV and RTV was explored *in vitro* using human liver microsomes and *in vivo* in a rat model.[18] Co-administration of the two drugs led to an eightfold increase in the AUC (0–8 h) for IDV without a change in RTV levels. This prompted clinical combination studies of the two agents using 400 mg bid of each drug,[27] and IDV 800 mg with RTV 100 or 200 mg bid.[28] A clinical study with the combination of IDV/nelfinavir in non-HIV-infected volunteers showed that IDV raised the AUC of nelfinavir by 83%, and nelfinavir raised the AUC of IDV by 51%.[263] However, In ACTG 388, the combination of IDV 1000 mg q12h and nelfinavir led to a median IDV trough level <10 ng/mL and this dosing should not be used.[264] A "dual-boosted" combination of lopinavir/RTV and IDV 400 mg bid was co-administered to 10 HIV-infected men and did not change median lopinavir pharmacokinetic parameters although IDV levels in plasma, CSF and semen were increased.[265]

INTERACTIONS WITH OTHER MEDICATIONS

Because IDV is metabolized extensively by the liver CPY3A4 system and this isoform is involved in the metabolism of ~50% of other drugs, certain significant drug interactions may occur. A case report of a patient on a stable IDV dose who was given carbamazepine for postherpetic neuralgia developed decreased IDV levels (with therapeutic carbamazepine levels) and experienced virologic failure.[266] Similar concerns have been raised regarding phenytoin, phenobarbital, and dexamethasone.[1] Co-administration of sildenafil and IDV did not alter the IDV levels but resulted in a markedly increased sildenafil AUC compared to those of historical controls; thus a dose reduction of sildenafil is appropriate[267] and this applies to other erectile dysfunction drugs.[2] Methadone[268] and theophylline[269] metabolism were found not to be affected by IDV co-administration. Similarly, cimetidine, quinidine, and Ortho-Novum 1/35 do not require dose changes when co-administered with IDV.[1] A small case series found that four of nine subjects taking the proton pump inhibitor omeprazole had markedly decreased IDV levels, raising concern that the resultant higher pH may have led to decreased absorption of IDV.[270] ACTG 5159 explored co-administration of IDV 800 mg/RTV 100 mg bid and calcium channel blockers and found the median AUC increased for both amlodipine (+90%) and diltiazem (+22%) without effects on the PI levels, suggesting initial dose reduction of calcium channel blockers is appropriate.[271]

INTERACTIONS WITH OTHER COMPOUNDS

High-dose vitamin C (1 g qd) reduced median IDV concentrations in seven HIV-negative volunteers.[272] Double-strength grapefruit juice increased gastric pH and delayed gastric absorption of IDV, but did not effect IDV exposure,[273] while single-dose grapefruit juice did not effect IDV pharmacokinetics.[274] Herbal supplements goldenseal root[275] and milk thistle[276,277] had no effect on IDV levels. Marijuana is associated with a statistically significant decrease in IDV maximum concentrations (−14%) that is not likely to be clinically significant.[278]

RECOMMENDATIONS FOR USE

Indication

IDV is labeled for the treatment of HIV infection in combination with other antiretroviral agents.[1] Current guidelines for initial antiretroviral treatment no longer recommend IDV with or without RTV among preferred or alternative choices.

DOSAGE

IDV is formulated as a sulfate salt and is available in 100-, 200-, 333-, and 400-mg capsules; the FDA-approved dose is 800 mg (usually two 400-mg capsules) every 8 h.[1] IDV capsules are sensitive to moisture and should be stored with the desiccant that came in the original container at room temperature. For optimal absorption, IDV should be administered with water 1 h before or 2 h after a meal. Alternatively, IDV may be taken with juice, coffee, tea, or skim milk or a low-calorie, low-fat small meal. Patients taking IDV should also ensure adequate hydration by drinking at least 1.5 L (approximately six 8-ounce glasses) of liquids daily to minimize the risk of IDV-induced kidney stones.

Though not FDA-approved, the combination of IDV and RTV allows once- or twice-daily dosing of both drugs with food. Among the doses of IDV/RTV that have been investigated, 800/100 mg bid appears to be the optimal choice based on safety, tolerability, and efficacy. As noted, ensuring adequate hydration is important.

DOSE MODIFICATION

The dose of IDV should be modified depending on the administration of concurrent medications. When given in conjunction with rifabutin,[250] nevirapine,[200] or efavirenz[257] (all P450 inducers), IDV should be increased to 1000 mg q8h. Dose adjustments are not necessary when nevirapine or efavirenz is given with IDV/RTV. When given in conjunction with ketoconazole,[245] itraconazole,[1] or delavirdine[256] (P450 inhibitors), IDV should be reduced to 600 mg q8h. Similarly, for patients with mild to moderate hepatic insufficiency as a result of cirrhosis, the recommended dose of IDV is 600 mg q8h.[1]

SPECIAL POPULATIONS

Pediatric Patients

The optimal dosing regimen has not been established for pediatric patients. Ongoing studies suggest that a dose of 500 mg/m^2 q6–8h is well tolerated and has immunologic and virologic activity.[193,194,197,198] An investigational oral liquid formulation was compared to standard capsules in 12 healthy volunteers and was shown to be bioequivalent and have an acceptable taste.[279]

Pregnant Women

Current guidelines for the use of antiretroviral therapy in pregnant women emphasize that decisions regarding therapy should be the same as those for women who are not pregnant.[280,281] IDV is rated class C for use in pregnant women: "Risk cannot be ruled out. . . . However, potential benefit may justify potential risk."[1] In studies on rats, IDV was associated with an increase in the incidence of supernumerary ribs and variations of the vertebral ossification centers; and at postnatal evaluation there was delayed fur development, eye opening, undescended testis, and unilateral ophthalmia.[282] In studies of monkeys, IDV caused an exacerbation of transient physiologic hyperbilirubinemia.[1] PACTG 358 studied 16 HIV-infected pregnant women taking zidovudine, lamivudine, and IDV and found substantially decreased IDV exposure, thus IDV is not recommended in pregnancy,[1] although concomitant RTV abrogates the decrease.[83]

Postexposure Prophylaxis

IDV/RTV is recommended as an alternative choice as part of a three-drug regimen for occupational postexposure prophylaxis.[283] Certain nonoccupational exposures also may warrant postexposure prophylaxis.[284] Postexposure prophylaxis regimens should be taken for 4 weeks. However, side effects of prophylaxis regimens are common. One group described 19 health care workers taking IDV-containing prophylaxis regimens of whom seven (37%) discontinued the drugs because of intolerable side effects.[285] The risks and benefits in terms of antiretroviral effects and toxicities are unknown.

REFERENCES

1. Crixivan (indinavir sulfate): prescribing information. West Point, PA: Merck & Co; 2006.
2. Panel On Clinical Practices for the Treatment of HIV Infection, US Department of Health and Human Services. Guidelines for the use of antiretroviral agents in HIV-infected adults and adolescents. Available: http://www.aidsinfo.nih.gov 10 Oct 2006.
3. Hammer SM, Saag MS, Schechter M, et al. Treatment for adult HIV infection: 2006 recommendations of the International AIDS Society-USA panel. JAMA 296(7):827–43, 2006.
4. Palella FJ, Delaney KM, Moorman AC, et al. Declining morbidity and mortality among patients with advanced human immunodeficiency virus infection. N Engl J Med 338:853, 1998.
5. Mocroft A, Vella S, Benfield TL, et al. Changing patterns of mortality across Europe in patients infected with HIV-1: EuroSIDA study group. Lancet 352:1725, 1998.
6. Dorsey BD, Levin RB, McDaniel SL, et al. L-735,524: the design of a potent and orally bioavailable HIV protease inhibitor. J Med Chem 37:3443, 1994.
7. Roberts NA, Martin JA, Kinchington D, et al. Rational design of peptide-based HIV proteinase inhibitors. Science 248:358, 1990.
8. Huff JR. HIV protease: a novel chemotherapeutic target for AIDS. J Med Chem 34:2305, 1991.
9. Vacca JP, Dorsey BD, Schleif WA, et al. L-735,524: an orally bioavailable human immunodeficiency virus type 1 protease inhibitor. Proc Natl Acad Sci USA 91:4096, 1994.
10. Tremblay C, Merrill DP, Chou T-C, Hirsch MS. Interactions among combinations of two and three protease inhibitors against drug-susceptible and drug-resistant HIV-1 isolates. J AIDS 22:430, 1999.
11. Witvrouw M, Pannecouque C, Switzer WM, et al. Susceptibility of HIV-2, SIV, and SHIV to various anti-HIV-1 compounds: implications for treatment and postexposure prophylaxis. Antivir Ther 9:57, 2004.
12. Rodes B, Sheldon J, Toro C, et al. Susceptibility to protease inhibitors in HIV-2 primary isolates from patients failing antiretroviral therapy. J Antimicrob Chemother 57:709, 2006.
13. Kohl NE, Emini E, Schleif WA, et al. Active human immunodeficiency virus protease is required for viral infectivity. Proc Natl Acad Sci USA 85:4686, 1988.
14. Chen Z, Li Y, Chen E, et al. Crystal structure at 1.9-Å of human immunodeficiency virus (HIV) II protease complexed with L-735,524, an orally bioavailable inhibitor of the HIV proteases. J Biol Chem 21:26344, 1994.
15. Sgadari C, Barillari G, Toschi E, et al. HIV protease inhibitors are potent anti-angiogenic molecules and promote regression of Kaposi sarcoma. Nat Med 8:225, 2002.
16. Lin JH, Chen I-W, Vastag KJ, Ostovic D. pH-dependent oral absorption of L-735,524, a potent HIV protease inhibitor, in rats and dogs. Drug Metab Dispos 23:730, 1995.
17. Zhang XQ, Schooley RT, Gerber JG. The effect of increasing alpha1-acid glycoprotein concentration on the antiviral efficacy of human immunodeficiency virus protease inhibitors. J Infect Dis 180:1833, 1999.
18. Kempf DJ, Marsh KC, Kumar G, et al. Pharmacokinetic enhancement of inhibitors of the human immunodeficiency virus protease by coadministration with ritonavir. Antimicrob Agents Chemother 41:654, 1997.
19. Yeh KC, Deutsch PJ, Haddix H, et al. Single dose pharmacokinetics of indinavir and the effect of food. Antimicrob Agents Chemother 42:332, 1998.
20. Yeh KC, Stone JA, Carides AD, et al. Simultaneous investigation of indinavir nonlinear pharmacokinetics and bioavailability in healthy volunteers using stable isotope labeling technique: study design and model-independent data analysis. J Pharm Sci 88:568, 1999.

21. Anderson PL, Brundage RC, Bushman L, et al. Indinavir plasma protein binding in HIV-1-infected adults. AIDS 14:2293, 2000.
22. Steigbigel RT, Berry P, Mellors J, et al. Efficacy and safety of the HIV protease inhibitor indinavir sulfate (MK 639) at escalating dose. In: Abstracts of the 3rd Conference on Retroviruses and Opportunistic Infections, Washington, DC. Alexandria, VA: Foundation for Retrovirology and Human Health; 1996, abstract 146.
23. Haas DW, Arathoon E, Thompson MA, et al. Comparative studies of two-times-daily versus three-times-daily indinavir in combination with zidovudine and lamivudine. Protocol 054/069 study teams. AIDS 14:1973, 2000.
24. Boffito M, Hoggard PG, Reynolds HE, et al. The unbound percentage of saquinavir and indinavir remains constant throughout the dosing interval in HIV positive subjects. Br J Clin Pharmacol 54:262, 2002.
25. King JR, Gerber JG, Fletcher CV, et al. Indinavir protein-free concentrations when used in indinavir/ritonavir combination therapy. AIDS 19:1059, 2005.
26. Carver PL, Fleisher D, Zhou SY, et al. Meal composition effects on the oral bioavailability of indinavir in HIV-infected patients. Pharm Res 16:718, 1999.
27. Hsu A, Granneman GR, Cao G, et al. Pharmacokinetic interaction between ritonavir and indinavir in healthy volunteers. Antimicrob Agents Chemother 42:2784, 1998.
28. Saah AJ, Winchell GA, Nessly ML, et al. Pharmacokinetic profile and tolerability of indinavir-ritonavir combinations in healthy volunteers. Antimicrob Agents Chemother 45:2710, 2001.
29. Aarnoutse RE, Wasmuth JC, Fatkenheuer G, et al. Administration of indinavir and low-dose ritonavir (800/100mg twice daily) with food reduces nephrotoxic peak plasma levels of indinavir. Antivir Ther 8:309, 2003.
30. Van Heeswijk RP, Veldkamp AI, Hoetelmans RM, et al. The steady-state plasma pharmacokinetics of indinavir alone and in combination with a low dose of ritonavir in twice daily dosing regimens in HIV-infected individuals. AIDS 12:F95, 1999.
31. Burger D, Boyd M, Duncombe C. Pharmacokinetics and pharmacodynamics of indinavir with or without low-dose ritonavir in HIV-infected Thai patients. J Antimicrob Chemother 51:1231, 2003.
32. Solas C, Petit N, Orticoni M, et al. Experience of a combination including indinavir 400mg plus ritonavir 200mg twice daily in HIV-infected patients: pharmacokinetic data. Pathol Biol 50:565, 2002.
33. Boyd M, Mootsikapun P, Burger D, et al. Pharmacokinetics of reduced-dose indinavir/ritonavir 400/100mg twice daily in HIV-1-infected Thai patients. Antivir Ther 10:301, 2005.
34. Wasmuth JC, La Porte CJ, Schneider K, et al. Comparison of two reduced-dose regimens of indinavir (600mg vs. 400mg twice daily) and ritonavir (100mg twice daily) in healthy volunteers (COREDIR). Antivir Ther 9:213, 2004.
35. Cressey TR, Leenasirimakul P, Jourdain G, et al. Low-doses of indinavir boosted with ritonavir in HIV-infected Thai patients: pharmacokinetics, efficacy and tolerability. J Antimicrob Chemother 55:1041, 2005.
36. Rhame FS, Rawlins SL, Petruschke RA, et al. Pharmacokinetics of indinavir and ritonavir administered at 667 and 100 milligrams, respectively, every 12 hours compared with indinavir administered 800 milligrams every 8 hours in human immunodeficiency virus-infected patients. Antimicrob Agents Chemother 48:4200, 2004.
37. Mallolas J, Blanco JL, Sarasa M, et al. Dose-finding study of once-daily indinavir/ritonavir plus zidovudine and lamivudine in HIV-infected patients. J AIDS 25:229, 2000.
38. Hugen PW, Burger DM, ter Hofstede HJ, et al. Dose-finding study of a once-daily indinavir/ritonavir regimen. J AIDS 25:236, 2000.
39. Mole L, Schmidgall D, Holodniy M. A pilot trial of indinavir, ritonavir, didanosine, and lamivudine in a once-daily four-drug regimen for HIV infection. J Acquir Immune Defic Snydr 27:260, 2001.
40. Burger DM, Aarnoutse RE, Dieleman JP, et al. A once-daily HAART regimen containing indinavir + ritonavir plus one or two nucleoside reverse transcriptase inhibitors (PIPO study). Antivir Ther 8:455, 2003.
41. Zala C, Alexander CS, Ochoa C, et al. Comparable pharmacokinetics of generic indinavir (Inhibisam) versus brand indinavir (Crixivan) when boosted with ritonavir [letter]. J Acquir Immune Defic Syndr 38:363, 2005.
42. Balani SK, Arison BH, Mathai L, et al. Metabolites of L-735,524, a potent HIV-1 protease inhibitor, in human urine. Drug Metab Dispos 23:266, 1995.
43. Balani SK, Woolf EJ, Hoagland VL, et al. Disposition of indinavir, a potent HIV-1 protease inhibitor, after an oral dose in humans. Drug Metab Dispos 24:1389, 1996.
44. Chiba M, Hensleigh M, Nishime JA, et al. Role of cytochrome P450 3A4 in human metabolism of MK-639, a potent human immunodeficiency virus protease inhibitor. Drug Metab Dispos 24:307, 1996.
45. Fitzsimmons ME, Collins JM. Selective biotransformation of the human immunodeficiency virus protease inhibitor saquinavir by human small-intestinal cytochrome P4503A4. Drug Metab Dispos 25:256, 1997.
46. Kim RB, Fromm MF, Wandel C, et al. The drug transporter P-glycoprotein limits oral absorption and brain entry of HIV-1 protease inhibitors. J Clin Invest 101:289, 1998.
47. Lin JH, Chiba M, Balani SK, et al. Species differences in the pharmacokinetics and metabolism of indinavir, a potent human immunodeficiency virus protease inhibitor. Drug Metab Dispos 24:1111, 1996.
48. Hennessy M, Clarke S, Speirs JP, et al. Intracellular indinavir pharmacokinetics in HIV-infected patients: comparison with plasma pharmacokinetics. Antivir Ther 8:191, 2003.
49. Solas C, Lafeuillade A, Halfon P, et al. Discrepancies between protease inhibitor concentrations and viral load in reservoirs and sanctuary sites in human immunodeficiency virus-infected patients. Antimicrob Agents Chemother 47:238, 2003.
50. Haas DW, Stone J, Clough LA, et al. Steady-state pharmacokinetics of indinavir in cerebrospinal fluid and plasma among adults with human immunodeficiency virus type 1 infection. Clin Pharmacol Ther 68:367, 2000.
51. Martin C, Sonnerborg A, Svensson JO, Stahle L. Indinavir-based treatment of HIV-1 infected patients: efficacy in the central nervous system. AIDS 13:1227, 1999.
52. Letendre SL, Capparelli EV, Ellis RJ, McCutchan JA. Indinavir population pharmacokinetics in plasma and cerebrospinal fluid. Antimicrob Agents Chemother 44:2173, 2000.
53. Antinori A, Perno CF, Giancola ML, et al. Efficacy of cerebrospinal fluid (CSF)-penetrating antiretroviral drugs against HIV in the neurological compartment: different patterns of phenotypic resistance in CSF and plasma. Clin Infect Dis 41:1787, 2005.
54. Van Praag RM, Weverling GJ, Portegies P, et al. Enhanced penetration of indinavir in cerebrospinal fluid and semen after the addition of low-dose ritonavir. AIDS 14:1187, 2000.
55. Haas DW, Johnson B, Nicotera J, et al. Effects of ritonavir on indinavir pharmacokinetics in cerebrospinal fluid and plasma. Antimicrob Agents Chemother 47:2131, 2003.
56. Taylor S, Back DJ, Drake SM, et al. Antiretroviral drug concentrations in semen of HIV-infected men: differential penetration of indinavir, ritonavir, and saquinavir. J Antimicrob Chemother 48:351, 2001.
57. van Praag RM, Repping S, de Vries JW, et al. Pharmacokinetic profiles of nevirapine and indinavir in various fractions of seminal plamsa. Antimicrob Agents Chemother 45:2902, 2001.

58. Gupta P, Mellors J, Kingsley L, et al. High viral load in semen of human immunodeficiency virus type 1-infected men at all stages of disease and its reduction by therapy with protease and nonnucleoside reverse transcriptase inhibitors. J Virol 71: 6271, 1997.
59. Gunthard HF, Havlir DV, Fiscus S, et al. Residual human immunodeficiency virus (HIV) type 1 RNA and DNA in lymph nodes and HIV RNA in genital secretions and in cerebrospinal fluid after suppression of viremia for 2 years. J Infect Dis 183:1318, 2001.
60. Launay O, Tod M, Louchahi K, et al. Differential diffusion of indinavir and lopinavir in gential secretions of human immnodeficiency virus-infected women. Antimicrob Agents Chemother 48:632, 2004.
61. Sudharkaran S, Ghabrial H, Nation RL, et al. Differential bidirectional transfer of indinavir in the isolated perfused human placenta. Antimicrob Agents Chemother 49:1023, 2005.
62. Colebunders R, Hodossy B, Burger D, et al. The effect of highly active antiretroviral treatment on viral load and antiretroviral drug levels in breast milk [letter]. AIDS 19:1912, 2005.
63. Burger DM, Hoetelmans RM, Hugen PW, et al. Low plasma concentrations of indinavir are related to virological treatment failure in HIV-1-infected patients on indinavir-containing therapy. Antivir Ther 3:215, 1998.
64. Acosta EP, Henry K, Baken L, et al. Indinavir concentrations and antiviral effect. Pharmacotherapy 19:708, 1999.
65. Zhou XJ, Havlir DV, Richman DD, et al. Plasma population pharmacokinetics and penetration into cerebrospinal fluid of indinavir in combination with zidovudine and lamivudine in HIV-1-infected patients. AIDS 14:2869, 2000.
66. Anderson PL, Brundage RC, Kakuda TN, Fletcher CV. CD4 response is correlated with peak plasma concentrations of indinavir in adults with undetectable human immunodeficiency virus ribonucleic acid. Clin Pharmacol Ther 71:280, 2002.
67. Duval X, Mentre F, Lamotte C, et al. Indinavir plasma concentration and adherence score are codeterminant of early virologic response in HIV-infected patients of the APROCO cohort. Ther Drug Monit 27:63, 2005.
68. Gonzalez de Requena D, Gallego O, de Mendoza C. Indinavir plasma concentrations and resistance mutations in patients experiencing early virologic failure. AIDS Res Hum Retroviruses 19:457, 2003.
69. Csajka C, Marzolini C, Fattinger K, et al. Population pharmacokinetics of indinavir in patients infected with human immunodeficiency virus. Antimicrob Agents Chemother 48:3226, 2004.
70. Kakuda TN, Page LM, Anderson PL, et al. Pharmacological basis for concentration-controlled therapy with zidovudine, lamivudine, and indinavir. Antimicrob Agents Chemother 45:236, 2001.
71. Shulman N, Zolopa A, Havlir D, et al. Virtual inhibitory quotient predicts response to ritonavir boosting of indinavir-based therapy in human immunodeficiency virus-infected patients with ongoing viremia. Antimicrob Agents Chemother 46:3907, 2002.
72. Burger D, Hugen P, Reiss P, et al. Therapeutic drug monitoring of nelfinavir and indinavir in treatment-naïve HIV-1-infected individuals. AIDS 17:1157, 2003.
73. Bossi P, Peytavin G, Lamotte C, et al. High indinavir plasma concentrations in HIV-positive patients co-infected with hepatitis B or C virus treated with low doses of indinavir and ritonavir (400/100 mg twice a day) plus two nucleoside reverse transcriptase inhibitors [letter]. AIDS 17:1108, 2003.
74. Jayasekara D, Aweeka FT, Rodriguez R, et al. Antiviral therapy for HIV patients with renal insufficiency. J AIDS 21:384, 1999.
75. Fiedler R, Peinhardt R, Deuber HJ, Osten B. Antiviral therapy with lamivudine, stavudine and indinavir in a HIV positive haemodialysis patient. J Am Soc Nephrol 1059A:207, 1998.
76. Guardiola JM, Magues MA, Domingo P, et al. Indinavir pharmacokinetics in haemodialysis-dependent end-stage renal failure. AIDS 12:1395, 1998.
77. Izzedine H, Aymard G, Hamani A, et al. Indinavir pharmacokinetics in haemodialysis. Nephrol Dial Transplant 15:1102, 2000.
78. Lin JH, Chiba M, Chen I-W, et al. Sex-dependent pharmacokinetics of indinavir: in vivo and in vitro evidence. Drug Metab Dispos 24:1298, 1996.
79. Burger DM, Siebers MC, Hugen PWH, et al. Pharmacokinetic variability caused by gender: do women have higher indinavir exposure than men? [letter]. J Acquir Immune Defic Syndr 29:101, 2002.
80. Gatti G, Vigano A, Sala N, et al. Indinavir pharmacokinetics and pharmacodynamics in children with human immunodeficiency virus infection. Antimicrob Agents Chemother 44:752, 2000.
81. Burger DM, van Rossum AM, Hugen PW, et al. Pharmacokinetics of the protease inhibitor indinavir in human immunodeficiency virus type-1-infected children. Antimicrob Agents Chemother 45:701, 2001.
82. Bergshoeff AS, Fraaij PL, van Rossum AM, et al. Pharmacokinetics of indinavir combined with low-dose ritonavir in human immunodeficiency virus type 1-infected children. Antimicrob Agents Chemother 48:1904, 2004.
83. Kosel BW, Beckerman KP, Hayashi S, et al. Pharmacokinetics of nelfinavir and indinavir in HIV-1-infected pregnant women. AIDS 17:1195, 2003.
84. Deutsch P, Teppler H, Squires K, et al. Antiviral activity of L-735,524, an HIV protease inhibitor, in infected patients. In: Abstracts of the 34th International Conference on Antimicrobial Agents and Chemotherapy, Orlando. Washington, DC: American Society for Microbiology; 1994, abstract I-59.
85. Mellors J, Steigbigel R, Gulick R, et al. Antiretroviral activity of the oral protease inhibitor, MK-639, in p24 antigenemic, HIV-1 infected patients with <500 CD4/mm^3. In: Abstracts of the 35th International Conference on Antimicrobial Agents and Chemotherapy, San Francisco. Washington, DC: American Society for Microbiology; 1995, abstract I-172.
86. Lewi DS, Suleiman JM, Uip DE, et al. Randomized, double-blind trial comparing indinavir alone, zidovudine alone and indinavir plus zidovudine in antiretroviral therapy-naive HIV-infected individuals with CD4+ T-lymphocyte counts between 50 and 250/mm^3. Rev Inst Med Trop Sao Paulo 42:27, 2000.
87. Fellay J, Boubaker K, Ledergerber B, et al. Prevalence of adverse events associated with potent antiretroviral treatment: Swiss HIV Cohort Study. Lancet 358:1322, 2001.
88. Duval X, Journot V, Leport C, et al. Incidence of and risk factors for adverse drug reactions in a prospective cohort of HIV-infected adults initiating protease inhibitor-containing therapy. Clin Infect Dis 39:248, 2004.
89. Lehman HP, Benson JO, Beninger PR, et al. A five-year evaluation of reports of overdose with indinavir sulfate. Pharmacoepidemiol Drug Saf 12:449, 2003.
90. Herman JS, Ives NJ, Nelson M, et al. Incidence and risk factors for the development of indinavir-associated renal complications. J Antimicrob Chemother 48:355, 2001.
91. Dieleman JP, Sturkenboom MC, Jambroes M, et al. Risk factors for urological symptoms in a cohort of users of the HIV protease inhibitor indinavir sulfate: the ATHENA cohort. Arch Intern Med 162:1493, 2002.
92. Meraviglia P, Angeli E, Del Sorbo F, et al. Risk factors for indinavir-related renal colic in HIV patients: predictive value of indinavir dose/body mass index. AIDS 16:2089, 2002.
93. Kopp JB, Miller KD, Mican JA, et al. Crystalluria and urinary tract abnormalities associated with indinavir. Ann Intern Med 127:119, 1997.
94. Hortin GL, King C, Miller KD, Kopp JB. Detection of indinavir crystals in urine: dependence on method of analysis. Arch Pathol Lab Med 124:246, 2000.

95. Gagnon RF, Tecimer SN, Watters AK, Tsoukas CM. Prospective study of urinalysis abnormalities in HIV-positive individuals treated with indinavir. Am J Kidney Dis 36:507, 2000.
96. Gagnon RF, Alli AI, Edwardes MD, et al. Low urine pH is associated with reduced indinavir crystalluria in indinavir-treated HIV-infected individuals. Clin Nephrol 65:13, 2006.
97. Li LY, Rodriguez-Hornedo N, Heimbach T, Fleisher D. In-vitro crystallization of indinavir in the presence of ritonavir and as a function of pH. J Pharm Pharmacol 55:707, 2003.
98. Dieleman JP, Salahuddin S, Hsu YS, et al. Indinavir crystallization around the loop of Henle: experimental evidence. J Acquir Immune Defic Syndr 28:9, 2001.
99. Reilly RF, Tray K, Perazella MA. Indinavir nephropathy revisited: a pattern of insidious renal failure with identifiable risk factors. Am J Kidney Dis 38:E23, 2001.
100. Kopp JB, Falloon J, Filie A, et al. Indinavir-associated interstitial neprhitis and urothelial inflammation: clinical and cytologic findings. Clin Infect Dis 34:1122, 2002.
101. Jaradat M, Phillips C, Yum MN, et al. Acute tubulointerstitial nephritis attributable to indinavir therapy. Am J Kidney Dis 35:E16, 2000.
102. Dieleman JP, van Rossum AM, Stricker BC, et al. Persistent leukocyturia and loss of renal function in a prospectively monitored cohort of HIV-infected patients treated with indinavir. J Acquir Immune Defic Syndr 32:135, 2003.
103. Saltel E, Angel JB, Futter NG, et al. Increased prevalence and analysis of risk factors for indinavir nephrolithiasis. J Urol 164:1895, 2000.
104. Hammer SM, Squires KE, Hughes MD, et al. A randomized, placebo-controlled trial of indinavir in combination with two nucleoside analogs in human immunodeficiency virus infected persons with CD4+ T-lymphocyte counts less than or equal to 200 per cubic millimeter. N Engl J Med 337:725, 1997.
105. Gulick RM, Mellors JW, Havlir D, et al. 3-year suppression of HIV viremia with indinavir, zidovudine, and lamivudine. Ann Intern Med 133:35, 2000.
106. Gulick RM, Meibohm A, Havlir D, et al. Six-year follow-up of HIV-1-infected adults in a clinical trial of antiretroviral therapy with indinavir, zidovudine, and lamivudine. AIDS 17:2345, 2003.
107. Sarcletti M, Petter A, Romani N, et al. Pyuria in patients treated with indinavir is associated with renal dysfunction. Clin Nephrol 54:261, 2000.
108. Malavaud B, Dinh B, Bonnet E, et al. Increased incidence of indinavir nephrolithiasis in patients with hepatitis B or C infection. Antivir Ther 5:3, 2000.
109. Brodie SB, Keller MJ, Ewenstein BM, Sax PE. Variation in incidence of indinavir-associated nephrolithiasis among HIV-positive patients. AIDS 12:2433, 1998.
110. Bach MC, Godofsky EW. Indinavir nephrolithiasis in warm climates [letter]. J Acquir Immune Defic Syndr 14:296, 1997.
111. Martinez E, Leguizamon M, Mallolas J, et al. Influence of environmental temperature on incidence of indinavir-related nephrolithiasis. Clin Infect Dis 29:422, 1999.
112. Dieleman JP, Gyssens IC, van der Ende ME, et al. Urological complaints in relation to indinavir plasma concentrations. AIDS 13:473, 1999.
113. Blake SP, McNicholas MM, Raptopoulous V. Nonopaque crystal deposition causing ureteric obstruction in patients with HIV undergoing indinavir therapy. AJR Am J Roentgenol 171:717, 1998.
114. Kohan AD, Armenakas NA, Fracchia JA. Indinavir nephrolithiasis: an emerging cause of renal colic in patients with human immunodeficiency virus. J Urol 161:1765, 1999.
115. Kalaitzis C, Dimitriadis G, Tsatidis T, et al. Treatment of indinavir sulfate induced urolithiasis in HIV-positive patients. Int Urol Nephrol 34:13, 2002.
116. Cattelan AM, Trevenzoli M, Naso A, et al. Severe hypertension and renal atrophy associated with indinavir. Clin Infect Dis 30:619, 2000.
117. Tashima KT, Horowitz JD, Rosen S. Indinavir nephropathy. N Engl J Med 336:138, 1997.
118. Anglicheau D, Duvic C, Nedelec G. Sudden anuria due to indinavir crystalluria. Nephron 86:364, 2000.
119. Hanabusa H, Tagani H, Hataya H. Renal atrophy associated with long-term treatment with indinavir. N Engl J Med 340:392, 1999.
120. Dieleman JP, van der Feltz M, Bangma CH, et al. Papillary necrosis associated with the HIV protease inhibitor indinavir. Infection 29:232, 2001.
121. Daudon M, Estepa L, Viard JP, et al. Urinary stones in HIV-1-positive patients treated with indinavir. Lancet 349:1294, 1997.
122. Stein D, Drusano G, Steigbigel R, et al. Two year follow-up of patients treated with indinavir 800 mg q8h. In: Abstracts of the 4th Conference on Retroviruses and Opportunistic Infections, Washington, DC. Alexandria, VA: Foundation for Retrovirology and Human Health; 1997, abstract 195.
123. Boubaker K, Sudre P, Bally F, et al. Changes in renal function associated with indinavir. AIDS 12:F249, 1998.
124. Van Rossum AM, Dieleman JP, Fraaij PL, et al. Persistent sterile leukocyturia is associated with impaired renal function in human immunodeficiency virus type 1-infected children treated with indinavir. Pediatrics 110:e19, 2002.
125. Zhang D, Chando TJ, Everett DW, et al. In vitro inhibition of UDP glucuronosyltransferases by atazanavir and other HIV protease inhibitors and the relationship of this property to in vivo bilirubin glucuronidation. Drug Metab Dispos 33:1729, 2005.
126. Zucker SD, Qin X, Rouster SD, et al. Mechanism of indinavir-induced hyperbilirubinemia. Proc Natl Acad Sci USA 98:12671, 2001.
127. Campbell SD, de Morais SM, Xu JJ. Inhibition of human organic anion transporting polypeptide OATP 1B1 as a mechanism of drug-induced hyperbilrubinmeia. Chem Biol Interact 150:179, 2004.
128. Rotger M, Taffe P, Bleiber G, et al. Gilbert syndrome and the development of antiretroviral therapy-associated hyperbilirubinemia. J Infect Dis 192:1381, 2005.
129. Sulkowski MS, Thomas DL, Chaisson RE, Moore RD. Hepatotoxicity associated with antiretroviral therapy in adults infected with human immunodeficiency virus and the role of hepatitis C or B virus infection. JAMA 283:74, 2000.
130. Sulkowski MS, Mehta SH, Chaisson RE, et al. Hepatotoxicity associated with protease inhibitor-based antiretroviral regimens with or without concurrent ritonavir. AIDS 18:2277, 2004.
131. Brambilla AM, Novati R, Calori G, et al. Stavudine or indinavir-containing regimens are associated with an increased risk of diabetes mellitus in HIV-infected individuals. AIDS 17:1993, 2003.
132. Murata H, Hruz PW, Mueckler M. The mechanism of insulin resistance caused by HIV protease inhibitor therapy. J Biol Chem 275:20251, 2000.
133. Murata H, Hruz PW, Mueckler M. Indinavir inhibits the glucose transporter isoform Glut4 at physiologic concentrations. AIDS 16:859, 2002.
134. Hertel J, Struthers H, Horj CB, Hruz PW. A structural basis for the acute effects of HIV protease inhibitors on GLUT4 intrinsic activity. J Biol Chem 279:55147, 2004.
135. Schutt M, Meier M, Meyer M, et al. The HIV-1 protease inhibitor indinavir impairs insulin signaling in HepG2 hepatoma cells. Diabetologia 43:1145, 2000.
136. Schutt M, Meier M, Jost MM, Klein HH. The HIV protease inhibitor indinavir impairs glycogen synthesis in HepG2 hepatoma cells. Exp Clin Endocrinol Diabetes 111:16, 2003.
137. Schutt M, Zhou J, Meier M, Klein HH. Long-term effects of HIV-1 protease inhibitors on insulin secretion and insulin signaling in INS-1 beta cells. J Endocrinol 183:445, 2004.

138. Hruz PW, Murata H, Qiu H, Mueckler M. Indinavir induces acute and reversible peripheral insulin resistance in rats. Diabetes 51:937, 2002.
139. Nolte LA, Yarasheski KE, Kawanaka K, et al. The HIV protease inhibitor indinavir decreases insulin- and contraction-stimulated glucose transport in skeletal muscle. Diabetes 50:1397, 2001.
140. Noor MA, Seneviratne T, Aweeka FT, et al. Indinavir acutely inhibits insulin-stimulated glucose disposal in humans: a randomized, placebo-controlled study. AIDS 16:F1, 2002.
141. Noor MA, Lo JC, Mulligan K, et al. Metabolic effects of indinavir in healthy HIV-seronegative men. AIDS 15:F11, 2001.
142. Schwarz JM, Lee GA, Park S, et al. Indinavir increases glucose production in healthy HIV-negative men. AIDS 18:1852, 2004.
143. Dube MP, Edmondson-Melancon H, Qian D, et al. Prospective evaluation of the effect of initiating indinavir-based therapy on insulin sensitivity and B-cell function in HIV-infected patients. J Acquir Immune Defic Syndr 27:130, 2001.
144. Fontas E, van Leth F, Sabin CA, et al. Lipid profiles in HIV-infected patients receiving combination antiretroviral therapy: are different antiretroviral drugs associated with different lipid profiles? J Infect Dis 189:1056, 2004.
145. Young J, Weber R, Rickenbach M, et al. Lipid profiles for antiretroviral-naive patients starting PI- and NNRTI-based therapy in the Swiss HIV cohort study. Antivir Ther 10:585, 2005.
146. Rojas C, Coplan PM, Rhodes T, et al. Indinavir did not further increase mean triglyceride levels in HIV-infected patients treated with nucleoside reverse transcriptase inhibitors: an analysis of three randomized clinical trials. Pharmacoepidemiol Drug Saf 12:361, 2003.
147. Berthold HK, Parhofer KG, Ritter MM, et al. Influence of protease inhibitor therapy on lipoprotein metabolism. J Intern Med 246:567, 1999.
148. Lenhard JM, Weiel JE, Paulik MA, Furfine ES. Stimulation of vitamin A(1) acid signaling by the HIV protease inhibitor indinavir. Biochem Pharmacol 59:1063, 2000.
149. Miller KD, Jones E, Yanovski JA, et al. Visceral abdominal-fat accumulation associated with use of indinavir. Lancet 351:871, 1998.
150. Viraben R, Aquilina C. Indinavir-associated lipodystrophy. AIDS 12:F37, 1998.
151. Carr A, Samaras K, Burton S, et al. A syndrome of peripheral lipodystrophy, hyperlipidaemia and insulin resistance in patients receiving HIV protease inhibitors. AIDS 12:F51, 1998.
152. Caron M, Auclair M, Vigouroux C, et al. The HIV protease inhibitor indinavir impairs sterol regulatory element-binding protein-1 intranuclear locatlization, inhibits preadipocyte differentiation, and induces insulin resistance. Diabetes 50:1378, 2001.
153. Miserez AR, Muller PY, Spaniol V. Indinavir inhibits sterol-regulatory element-binding protein-1c-dependent lipoprotein lipase and fatty acid synthase gene activations. AIDS 16:1587, 2002.
154. Caron M, Auclair M, Sterlingot H, et al. Some HIV protease inhibitors alter lamin A/C maturation and stabilitiy, SREBP-1 nuclear localization and adipocyte differentiation. AIDS 17:2437, 2003.
155. Benson JO, McGhee K, Coplan P, et al. Fat redistribution in indinavir-treated patients with HIV infection: a review of post-marketing cases. J AIDS 25:130, 2000.
156. Galli M, Cozzi-Lepri A, Ridolfo AL, et al. Incidence of adipose tissue alterations in first-line antiretroviral therapy: the LipoICoNa Study. Arch Intern Med 162:2621, 2002.
157. Coplan PM, Nikas AA, Leavitt RY, et al. Indinavir did not increase the short-term risk of adverse cardiovascular events relative to nucleoside reverse transcriptase inhibitor therapy in four phase III clinical trials. AIDS 15:1584, 2001.
158. Henry K, Kitch D, Dube M, et al. C-reactive protein levels over time and cardiovascular risk in HIV-infected individuals suppressed on an indianvir-based regimen: AIDS Clinical Trials Group 5056s. AIDS 18:2434, 2004.
159. Shankar SS, Dube MP, Gorski JC, et al. Indinavir impairs endothelial function in healthy HIV-negative men. Am Heart J 150:933, 2005.
160. Cattelan AM, Trevenzoli M, Sasset L, et al. Indianvir and systemic hypertension. AIDS 15:805, 2001.
161. Young EM, Considine RV, Sattler FR, et al. Changes in thrombolytic and inflammatory markers after initiation of indinavir- or amprenavir-based antiretroviral therapy. Cardiovasc Toxicol 4:179, 2004.
162. Gulick RM, Mellors JW, Havlir D, et al. Treatment with a combination of indinavir, zidovudine, and lamivudine in HIV-infected adults with prior antiretroviral use. N Engl J Med 337:734, 1997.
163. Racoosin JA, Kessler CM. Bleeding episodes in HIV-positive patients taking protease inhibitors: a case series. Haemophilia 5:266, 1999.
164. Wilde JT. Protease inhibitor therapy and bleeding. Haemophilia 6:487, 2000.
165. Toma E, Devost D, Chow Lan N, Bhat PV. HIV-protease inhibitors alter retinoic acid synthesis. AIDS 15:1979, 2001.
166. Calista D, Boschini A. Cutaneous side effects induced by indinavir. Eur J Dermatol 10:292, 2000.
167. Gajewski LK, Grimone AJ, Melbourne KM, Vanscoy GJ. Characterization of rash with indinavir in a national patient cohort. Ann Pharmacother 33:17, 1999.
168. Teira R, Zubero Z, Munoz J, et al. Stevens–Johnson syndrome caused by indinavir. Scand J Infect Dis 30:634, 1998.
169. Bouscarat F, Bouchard C, Bouhour D. Paronychia and pyogenic granuloma of the great toes in patients treated with indinavir. N Engl J Med 338:1776, 1998.
170. Tosti A, Piraccini BM, D'Antuono A, et al. Paronychia associated with antiretroviral therapy. Br J Dermatol 140:1165, 1999.
171. Colson AE, Sax PE, Keller MJ, et al. Paronychia in association with indinavir treatment. Clin Infect Dis 32:140, 2001.
172. James CW, McNelis KC, Cohen DM, et al. Recurrent ingrown toenails secondary to indinavir/ritonavir combination therapy. Ann Pharmacother 35:881, 2001.
173. Lichterfeld M, Nischalke HD, Bergmann F, et al. Long-term efficacy and safety of ritonavir/indinavir at 400/400 mg twice a day in combination with two nucleoside reverse transcriptase inhibitors as first line antiretroviral therapy. HIV Med 3:37, 2002.
174. Boyd M, Duncombe C, Newell M, et al. Indinavir/ritonavir vs. indinavir in combination with AZT/3TC for treatment of HIV in nucleoside-experienced patients: a randomized, open-label trial. In: Abstracts of the 8th Conference on Retroviruses and Opportunistic Infections, Chicago. Alexandria, VA: Foundation for Retrovirology and Human Health; 2001, abstract 335.
175. Solas C, Basso S, Poizot-Martin I, et al. High indinavir C_{min} is associated with higher toxicity in patients on indinavir-ritonavir 800/100 mg twice-daily regimens. J Acquir Immune Defic Syndr 29:374, 2002.
176. Mellors J, Steigbigel R, Gulick R, et al. A randomized, double blind study of the oral HIV protease inhibitor, L-735,524 vs. zidovudine (ZDV) in p24 antigenemic, HIV-1 infected patients with <500 CD4 cells/mm^3. In: Abstracts of the 2nd National Conference on Human Retroviruses and Related Infections. Washington, DC: American Society for Microbiology; 1995, abstract 183.
177. Gulick R, Mellors J, Havlir D, et al. Simultaneous vs. sequential initiation of therapy with indinavir, zidovudine, and lamivudine for HIV-1 infection: 100-week follow-up. JAMA 280:35, 1998.
178. Hirsch M, Steigbigel R, Staszewski S, et al. A randomized, controlled trial of indinavir, zidovudine, and lamivudine in adults with advanced human immunodeficiency virus type 1 infection and prior antiretroviral therapy. J Infect Dis 180:659, 1999.

179. Hirsch MS, Steigbigel RT, Staszewski S, et al. Long-term efficacy, safety, and tolerability of indinavir-based therapy in protease inhibitor-naive adults with advanced HIV infection. Clin Infect Dis 37:1119, 2003.
180. Coplan PM, Cook JR, Carides GW, et al. Impact of indinavir on the quality of life in patients with advanced HIV infection treated with zidovudine and lamivudine. Clin Infect Dis 39:426, 2004.
181. McMahon D, Dinubile M, Meibohm A, et al. Long-term efficacy and tolerability of indinavir-based combination therapy in asymptomatic treatment-naïve adults with early HIV infection. In: Abstracts of the 43rd Annual Meeting of the Infectious Diseases Society of America, San Francisco, CA, 6–9 Oct 2005, abstract #798.
182. Acosta EP, Wu H, Hammer SM, et al. Comparison of two indinavir/ritonavir regimens in the treatment of HIV-infected individuals. J Acquir Immune Defic Syndr 37:1358, 2004.
183. Burger DM, Hugen PW, Aarnoutse RE, et al. A retrospective, cohort-based survey of patients using twice-daily indinavir + ritonavir combinations: pharmacokinetics, safety, and efficacy. J Acquir Immune Defic Syndr 26:218, 2001
184. Voigt E, Wickesberg A, Wasmuth JC, et al. First-line ritonavir/indinavir 100/800 mg twice daily plus nucleoside reverse transcriptase inhibitors in a German multicentre study: 48-week results. HIV Med 3:277, 2002
185. Young B, Fischl MA, Wilson HM, et al. Open-label study of a twice-daily indinavir 800-mg/ritonavir 100-mg regimen in protease inhibitor-naive HIV-infected adults. J Acquir Immune Defic Syndr 31:478, 2002.
186. Arnaiz JA, Mallolas J, Podzamczer D, et al. Continued indinavir versus switching to indinavir/ritonavir in HIV-infected patients with suppressed viral load. AIDS 17:831, 2003.
187. Konopnicki D, De Wit S, Poll B, et al. Indinavir/ritonavir-based therapy in HIV-1-infected antiretroviral therapy-naïve patients: comparison of 800/100 mg and 400/100 mg twice daily. HIV Med 6:1, 2005.
188. Justesen US, Levring AM, Thomsen A, et al. Low-dose indinavir in combination with low-dose ritonavir: steady-state pharmacokinetics and long-term clinical outcome follow-up. HIV Med 4:250, 2003.
189. Duvivier C, Myrto A, Marcelin AG, et al. Efficacy and safety of ritonavir/indinavir 100/400 mg twice daily in combination with two nucleoside analogues in antiretroviral treatment-naïve HIV-infected individuals. Antivir Ther 8:603, 2003.
190. Ghosn J, Lamotte C, Ait-Mohand H, et al. Efficacy of a twice-daily antiretroviral regimen containing 100 mg ritonavir/400 mg indinavir in HIV-infected patients. AIDS 17:209, 2003.
191. Mootsikapun P, Chetchotisakd P, Anunnatsiri S, Boonyaprawit P. Effiacy and safety of indinavir/ritonavir 400/100 mg twice daily plus two nucleoside analogues in treatment-naïve HIV-1-infected patients with CD4+ T-cell counts <200 cells/mm^3: 96-week outcomes. Antivir Ther 10:911, 2005.
192. Kahlert C, Hupfer M, Wagels T, et al. Ritonavir boosted indinavir treatment as a simplified maintenance mono-therapy for HIV infection [letter]. AIDS 18:955, 2004.
193. Kline MW, Fletcher CV, Harris AT, et al. A pilot study of combination therapy with indinavir, stavudine (d4T), and didanosine (ddI) in children infected with the human immunodeficiency virus. J Pediatr 132:543, 1998.
194. Mueller BU, Sleasman J, Nelson RP Jr, et al. A phase I/II study of the protease inhibitor indinavir in children with HIV infection. Pediatrics 102:101, 1998.
195. Jankelevich S, Mueller BU, Mackall CL, et al. Long-term virologic and immunologic responses in human immunodeficiency virus type 1-infected children treated with indinavir, zidovudine, and lamivudine. J Infect Dis 183:1116, 2001.
196. Van Rossum AM, Niesters HG, Geelen SP, et al. Clinical and virologic response to combination treatment with indinavir, zidovudine, and lamivudine in children with human immunodeficiency virus-1 infection: a multicenter study in The Netherlands. J Pediatr 136:780, 2000.
197. Vigano A, Dally L, Bricalli D, et al. Clinical and immunovirologic characterization of the efficacy of stavudine, lamivudine, and indinavir in human immunodeficiency virus infection. J Pediatr 135:675, 1999.
198. Pelton SI, Stanley K, Yogev R, et al. Switch from ritonavir to indinavir in combination therapy for HIV-1-infected children. Clin Infect Dis 40:1181, 2005.
199. Harris M, Durakovic C, Rae S, et al. A pilot study of nevirapine, indinavir, and lamivudine among patients with advanced human immunodeficiency virus disease who have had failure of combination nucleoside therapy. J Infect Dis 177:1514, 1998.
200. Murphy RL, Sommadossi JP, Lamson M, et al. Antiviral effect and pharmacokinetic interaction between nevirapine and indinavir in persons infected with human immunodeficiency virus type 1. J Infect Dis 179:1116, 1999.
201. Staszewski S, Morales-Ramirez J, Tashima K, et al. Efavirenz plus zidovudine and lamivudine, efavirenz plus indinavir, and indinavir plus zidovudine and lamivudine in the treatment of HIV infection in adults. N Engl J Med 341:1865, 1999.
202. Haas DW, Fessel WJ, Delapenha RA, et al. Therapy with efavirenz plus indinavir in patients with extensive prior nucleoside reverse-transcriptase inhibitor experience: a randomized, double-blind, placebo-controlled trial. J Infect Dis 183:392, 2001.
203. Cohen-Stuart JW, Schuurman R, Burger DM, et al. Randomized trial comparing saquinavir soft gelatin capsules versus indinavir as part of triple therapy (CHEESE study). AIDS 13:F53, 1999.
204. Katzenstein TL, Kirk O, Pederson C, et al. The Danish Protease Inhibitor Study: a randomized study comparing the virological efficacy of 3 protease inhibitor-containing regimens for the treatment of human immundeficiency virus type 1 infection. J Infect Dis 182:744, 2000.
205. Roca B, Gomez CJ, Arnedo A. A randomized, comparative study of lamivudine plus stavudine, with indinavir or nelfinavir in treatment experienced HIV infected patients. AIDS 14:157, 2000.
206. Dragsted UB, Gerstoft J, Pedersen C, et al. Randomized trial to evaluate indinavir/ritonavir versus saquinavir/ritonavir in human immunodeficiency virus type 1-infected patients: the MaxCmin1 Trial. J Infect Dis 188:635, 2003.
207. Bongiovanni M, Bini T, Chiesa E, et al. Lopinavir/ritonavir vs. indinavir/ritonavir in antiretroviral naïve HIV-infected patients: immunovirological outcome and side effects. Antiviral Res 62:53, 2004.
208. Tashima K, Staszewski S, Nelson M, et al. Durable viral suppression on EFV-based HAART: 168 weeks of follow-up. In: Abstracts of the 2004 International AIDS Society Meeting, abstract #TuPeB4547.
209. Caro JJ, O'Brien JA, Migliaccio-Walle K, Raggio G. Economic analysis of initial HIV treatment: efavirenz- versus indinavir-containing triple therapy. Pharmacoeconomics 19:95, 2001.
210. Smith CJ, Phillips AN, Hill T, et al. The rate of viral rebound after attainment of an HIV load <50 copies/ml according to specific antiretroviral drugs in use: results from a multicenter cohort study. J Infect Dis 192:1387, 2005.
211. Staszewski S, Keiser P, Montaner J, et al. Abacavir–lamivudine–zidovudine vs. indinavir–lamivudine–zidovudine in antiretroviral-naive HIV-infected adults. JAMA 285:1155, 2001.
212. Vibhagool A, Cahn P, Schechter M, et al. Triple nucleoside treatment with abacavir plus the lamivudine/zidovudine combination tablet (COM) compared to indinavir/COM in antiretroviral therapy-naive adults: results of a 48-week open-label, equivalence trial (CNA3014). Curr Med Res Opin 20:1103, 2004.
213. Cahn P, Vibhagool A, Schechter M, et al. Predictors of adherence and virologic outcome in HIV-infected patients treated

with abacavir- or indinavir-based triple combination HAART also containing lamivudine/zidovudine. Curr Med Res Opin 20:1115, 2004.
214. Tisdale M, Myers RE, Maschera B, et al. Cross-resistance analysis to human immunodeficiency virus type 1 variants individually selected for resistance to five different protease inhibitors. Antimicrob Agents Chemother 39:1704, 1995.
215. Watkins T, Resch W, Irlbeck D, Swanstrom R. Selection of high-level resistance to human immunodeficiency virus type 1 protease inhibitors. Antimicrob Agents Chemother 47:759, 2003.
216. Condra JH, Schleif WA, Blahy OM, et al. In vivo emergence of HIV-1 variants resistant to multiple protease inhibitors. Nature 374:569, 1995.
217. Schock HB, Garsky VM, Kuo LC. Mutational anatomy of an HIV-1 protease variant conferring cross-resistance to protease inhibitors in clinical trials. J Biol Chem 271:31957, 1996.
218. Condra JH, Holder DJ, Schleif WA, et al. Genetic correlates of in vivo resistance to indinavir, a human immunodeficiency virus type 1 protease inhibitor. J Virol 70:8270, 1996.
219. Brown AJL, Korber BT, Condra JH. Associations between amino acids in the evolution of HIV type 1 protease sequences under indinavir therapy. AIDS Res Hum Retroviruses 15:247, 1999.
220. Zhang YM, Imamichi H, Imamichi T, et al. Drug resistance during indinavir therapy is caused by mutations in the protease gene and in its GAG substrate cleavage sites. J Virol 71:6662, 1997.
221. Cote HC, Brumme ZL, Harrigan PR. Human immunodeficiency virus type 1 protease cleavage mutations associated with protease inhibitor cross-resistance selected by indinavir, ritonavir, and/or saquinavir. J Virol 75:589, 2001.
222. Dykes C, Najjar J, Bosch RJ, et al. Detection of drug-resistant minority variants of HIV-1 during virologic failure of indinavir, lamivudine, and zidovudine. J Infect Dis 189:1091, 2004.
223. Descamps D, Flandre P, Calvez V, et al. Mechanisms of virologic failure in previously untreated HIV-infected patients from a trial of induction maintenance therapy. JAMA 283:205, 2000.
224. Havlir DV, Hellmann NS, Petropoulos CJ, et al. Drug susceptibility in HIV infection after viral rebound in patients receiving indinavir-containing regimens. JAMA 283:229, 2000.
225. Drusano GL, Bilello JA, Stein DS, et al. Factors influencing the emergence of resistance to indinavir: role of virologic, immunologic and pharmacologic variables. J Infect Dis 178:360, 1998.
226. Condra JH, Petropoulos CJ, Ziermann R, et al. Drug resistance and predicted virologic responses to human immunodeficiency virus type 1 protease inhibitor therapy. J Infect Dis 182:758, 2000.
227. Hertogs K, Bloor S, Kemp SD, et al. Phenotypic and genotypic analysis of clinical HIV-1 isolates reveals extensive protease inhibitor cross resistance: a survey of over 6000 samples. AIDS 14:1203, 2000.
228. Partaledis JA, Yamaguchi K, Tisdale M, et al. In vitro selection and characterization of human immunodeficiency virus type 1 (HIV-1) isolates with reduced sensitivity to hydroxyethylamino sulfonamide inhibitors of HIV-1 aspartyl protease. J Virol 69:5228, 1995.
229. Paulsen D, Liao Q, Fusco G, et al. Genotypic and phenotypic cross-resistance to lopinavir and amprenavir in protease inhibitor-experienced patients with HIV viremia. AIDS Res Hum Retroviruses 18:1011, 2002.
230. Colonno RJ, Thiry A, Limoli K, Parkin N. Activities of atazanavir (BMS-232632) against a large panel of human immunodeficiency virus type 1 clinical isolates resistant to one or more approved protease inhibitors. Antimicrob Agents Chemother 47:1324, 2003.
231. Para MF, Glidden DV, Coombs RW, et al. Baseline human immunodeficiency virus type 1 phenotype, genotype, and RNA response after switching from long-term hard-capsule saquinavir to indinavir or soft-gel-capsule saquinavir in AIDS Clinical Trials Group Protocol 333. J Infect Dis 182:733, 2000.
232. Gulick RM, Hu XJ, Fiscus SA, et al. Randomized study of saquinavir with ritonavir or nelfinavir together with delavirdine, adefovir, or both in human immunodeficiency virus-infected adults with virologic failure on indinavir: AIDS Clinical Trials Group Study 359. J Infect Dis 182:1375, 2000.
233. Hammer SM, Vaida F, Bennett KK, et al. Dual vs single protease inhibitor therapy following antiretroviral treatment failure: a randomized trial. JAMA 288:169, 2002.
234. Hirsch MS, Brun-Vezinet F, Clotet B, et al. Antiretroviral drug resistance testing in adults infected with human immunodeficiency virus type 1: 2003 recommendations of an International AIDS Society-USA Panel. Clin Infect Dis 37:113, 2003.
234a. Larder BA, Hertogs K, Bloor S, van den Eynde CH, DeCian W, Wang Y, Freimuth WW, Tarpley G. Tipranavir inhibits broadly protease inhibitor-resistant HIV-1 clinical samples. AIDS 14:1943–8, 2000.
234b. Koh Y, Nakata H, Maeda K, et al. Novel bis-tetrahydrofuranylurethane-containing nonpeptidic protease inhibitor (PI) UIC-94017 (TMC114) with potent activity against multi-PI-resistant human immunodeficiency virus in vitro. Antimicrob Agents Chemother 47:3123–9, 2003.
235. Piscitelli SC, Flexner C, Minor JR, et al. Drug interactions in patients infected with human immunodeficiency virus. Clin Infect Dis 23:685, 1996.
236. Eagling VA, Back DJ, Barry MG. Differential inhibition of cytochrome P450 isoforms by the protease inhibitors, ritonavir, saquinavir, and indinavir. Br J Clin Pharmacol 44:190, 1997.
237. Rosenthal E, Sala F, Chichmanian R-M, et al. Ergotism related to concurrent administration of ergotamine tartrate and indinavir. JAMA 281:987, 1999.
238. McCrea J, Wyss D, Stone J, et al. Pharmacokinetic interaction between indinavir and rifampin. Clin Pharmacol Ther 61:152, 1997.
239. Juestesen US, Andersen AB, Klitgaard NA, et al. Pharmacokinetic interaction between rifampin and the combination of indinavir and low-dose ritonavir in HIV-infected patients. Clin Infect Dis 38:426, 2004.
240. Piscitelli SC, Burstein AH, Chaitt D, et al. Indinavir concentrations and St. John's wort. Lancet 355:547, 2000.
241. Moore LB, Goodwin B, Jones SA, et al. St. John's wort induces hepatic drug metabolism through activation of the pregnane X receptor. Proc Natl Acad Sci USA 97:7500, 2000.
242. Indinavir (MK 639) Pharmacokinetic Study Group: Indinavir (MK 639) drug interaction studies. In: Abstracts of the XIth International Conference on AIDS, Vancouver, 1996, abstract MoB174.
243. Sturgill MG, Seibold JR, Boruchoff SE, et al. Trimethoprim/sulfamethoxazole does not affect the steady-state disposition of indinavir. J Clin Pharmacol 39:1077, 1999.
244. De Wit S, Debier M, De Smet M, et al. Effect of fluconazole on indinavir pharmacokinetics in human immunodeficiency virus-infected patients. Antimicrob Agents Chemother 42:223, 1998.
245. McCrea J, Woolf E, Sterrett A, et al. Effects of ketoconazole and other P-450 inhibitors on the pharmacokinetics of indinavir. Pharm Res 13:S485, 1996.
246. Purkins L, Wood N, Kleinermans D, Love ER. No clinically significant pharmacokinetic interactions between voriconazole and indinavir in healthy volunteers. Br J Clin Pharmacol 56(Suppl 1):62, 2003.
247. Boruchoff SE, Stugill MG, Grasing KW, et al. The steady-state disposition of indinavir is not altered by the concomitant administration of clarithromycin. Clin Pharmacol Ther 67:351, 2000.
248. Foulds G, Laboy-Goral L, Wei GC, Apseloff G. The effect of azithromycin on the pharmacokinetics of indinavir. J Clin Pharmacol 39:842, 1999.

249. Emmanuel A, Gillotin C, Farinotti R, Sadler BM. Atovaquone suspension and indinavir have minimal pharmacokinetic interactions. In: Abstracts of the 12th World AIDS Conference, Geneva, 1998, abstract 12384.
250. Winchell GA, McCrea JB, Carides A, et al. Pharmacokinetic interaction between indinavir and rifabutin. Clin Pharmacol Ther 61:153, 1997.
251. Hamzeh FM, Benson C, Gerber J, et al. Steady-state pharmacokinetic interaction of modified-dose indinavir and rifabutin. Clin Pharmacol 73:159, 2003.
252. Damle BD, Mummaneni V, Kaul S, Knupp C. Lack of effect of simultaneously administered didanosine encapsulated enteric bead formulation (Videx EC) on oral absorption of indinavir, ketoconazole, or ciprofloxacin. Antimicrob Agents Chemother 46:385, 2002.
253. La Porte C, Verweij-van Wissen C, van Ewiijk N, et al. Pharmacokinetic interaction study of indinavir/ritonavir and the enteric-coated capsule formulation of didanosine in healthy volunteers. J Clin Pharmacol 45:211, 2005.
254. DiCenzo R, Forrest A, Squires KE, et al. Indinavir, efavirenz, and abacavir pharmacokinetics in human immunodeficiency virus-infected patients. Antimicrob Agents Chemother 47:1929, 2003.
255. Burger DM, Prins JM, van der Ende ME, Aarnoutse RE. The effect of nevirapine on the pharmacokinetics of indinavir/ritonavir 800/100mg bid [letter]. J Acquir Immune Defic Syndr 35:97, 2004.
256. Ferry JJ, Herman BD, Carel BJ, et al. Pharmacokinetic drug–drug interaction study of delavirdine and indinavir in healthy volunteers. J AIDS 18:252, 1998.
257. Fiske WD, Mayers D, Wagner K, et al. Pharmacokinetics of DMP 266 and indinavir multiple oral doses in HIV-1 infected individuals. In: Abstracts of the 4th Conference on Retroviruses and Opportunistic Infections, Washington, DC. Alexandria, VA: Foundation for Retrovirology and Human Health; 1997, abstract 568.
258. Squires K, Hammer S, DeGruttola V, et al. Randomized trial of abacavir (ABC) in combination with indinavir (IDV) and efavirenz (EFV) in HIV-infected patients (pts) with nucleoside analog experience (NRTI exp). In: Abstracts of the 6th Conference on Retroviruses and Opportunistic Infections, Chicago. Alexandria, VA: Foundation for Retrovirology and Human Health; 1999, abstract LB15.
259. Aarnoutse RE, Grintjes KJ, Telgt DS, et al. The influence of efavirenz on the pharmacokinetics of a twice-daily combination of indinavir and low-dose ritonavir in healthy volunteers. Clin Pharmacol 71:57, 2002.
260. Boyd MA, Aarnoutse RE, Ruxrungtham K, et al. Pharmacokinetics of indinavir/ritonavir (800/100mg) in combination with efavirenz (600mg) in HIV-1-infected subjects. J Acquir Immune Defic Syndr 34:134, 2003.
261. Aarnoutse RE, Brinkman K, Benetucci J, et al. Pharmacokinetics of indinavir/ritonavir (800/100mg twice a day) combined with efavirenz in HIV-infected patients. AIDS 18:565, 2004.
262. McCrea J, Buss N, Stone J. Indinavir-saquinavir single dose pharmacokinetic study. In: Abstracts of the 4th Conference on Retroviruses and Opportunistic Infections, Washington, DC. Alexandria, VA: Foundation for Retrovirology and Human Health; 1997, abstract 608.
263. Kerr B, Lee C, Yuen G, et al. Overview of in-vitro and in-vivo drug interaction studies of nelfinavir mesylate (NFV), a new HIV-1 protease inhibitor. In: Abstracts of the 4th Conference on Retroviruses and Opportunistic Infections, Washington, DC. Alexandria, VA: Foundation for Retrovirology and Human Health; 1997, abstract 373.
264. DiCenzo R, Forrest A, Fischl MA, et al. Pharmacokinetics of indinavir and nelfinavir in treatment-naïve, human immunodeficiency virus-infected patients. Antimicrob Agents Chemother 48:918, 2004.
265. Isaac A, Taylor S, Cane P, et al. Lopinavir/ritonavir combined with twice-daily 400mg indinavir: pharmacokinetics and pharmacodynamics in blood, CSF and semen. J Antimicrob Chemother 54:498, 2004.
266. Hugen PW, Burger DM, Brinkman K, et al. Carbamazepine-indinavir interaction causes antiretroviral therapy failure. Ann Pharmacother 34:465, 2000.
267. Merry C, Barry MG, Ryan M, et al. Interaction of sildenafil and indinavir when co-administered to HIV-positive patients. AIDS 13:F101, 1999.
268. Iribarne C, Berthou F, Carlhant D, et al. Inhibition of methadone and buprenorphine N-alkylations by three HIV-1 protease inhibitors. Drug Metab Dispos 26:257, 1998.
269. Mistry GC, Laurent A, Sterrett AT, Deutsch PJ. Effect of indinavir on the single-dose pharmacokinetics of theophylline in healthy subjects. J Clin Pharmacol 39:636, 1999.
270. Burger DM, Hugen PWH, Kroon FP, et al. Pharmokinetic interaction between the proton pump inhibitor omeprazole and the HIV protease inhibitor indinavir. AIDS 12:2080, 1998.
271. Glesby MJ, Aberg JA, Kendall MA, et al. Pharmacokinetic interactions between indinavir plus ritonavir and calcium channel blockers. Clin Pharmacol 78:143, 2005.
272. Slain D, Amsden JR, Khakoo RA, et al. Effect of high-dose vitamin C on the steady-state pharmacokinetics of the protease inhibitor indinavir in healthy volunteers. Pharmacotherapy 25:165, 2005.
273. Shelton MJ, Wynn HE, Hewitt RG, DiFrancesco R. Effects of grapefruit juice on pharmacokinetic exposure to indinavir in HIV-positive subjects. J Clin Pharmacol 41:435, 2001.
274. Penzak SR, Acosta EP, Turner M, et al. Effects of Seville orange juice and grapefruit juice on indinavir pharmacokinetics. J Clin Pharmacol 42:1165, 2002.
275. Sandhu RS, Prescilla RP, Simonelli TM, Edwards DJ. Influence of goldenseal root on the pharmacokinetics of indinavir. J Clin Pharmacol 43:1283, 2003.
276. Piscitelli SC, Formentini E, Burstein AH, et al. Effect of milk thistle on the pharmacokinetics of indinavir in healthy volunteers. Pharmacotherapy 22:551, 2002.
277. DiCenzo R, Shelton M, Jordan K, et al. Coadministration of milk thistle and indinavir in heatlhy subjects. Pharmacotherapy 23:866, 2003.
278. Kosel BW, Aweeka FT, Benowitz NL, et al. The effects of cannabiniods on the pharmacokinetics of indinavir and nelfinavir. AIDS 16:543, 2002.
279. Hugen PW, Burger DM, ter Horstede HJ, et al. Development of an indinavir oral liquid for children. Am J Health Syst Pharm 57:1332, 2000.
280. Perinatal HIV Guidelines Working Group. Public Health Service Task Force Recommendations for Use of Antiretroviral Drugs in Pregnant HIV-1 Infected Women for Maternal Health and Interventions to Reduce Perinatal HIV-1 Transmission in the United States. October 12, 2006 1-65. Available at http://aidsinfo.nih.gov/ContentFiles/PerinatalGL.pdf.
281. Safety and Toxicity of Individual Antiretroviral Agents in Pregnancy. Available: http://www.aidsinfo.nih.gov 12 Oct 2006.
282. Riecke K, Schulz TG, Shakibaei M, et al. Developmental toxicity of the HIV-protease inhibitor indinavir in rats. Teratology 62:291, 2000.
283. Updated U.S. Public Health Service Guidelines for the Management of Occupational Exposures to HIV and Recommendations for Postexposure Prophylaxis. Available: http://www.aidsinfo.nih.gov 30 Sep 2005.
284. Management of Possible Sexual, Infection-Drug-Use, or Other Nonoccupational Exposure to HIV, Including Considerations Related to Antiretroviral Therapy. Available: http://www.aidsinfo.nih.gov 21 Jan 2005.
285. Parkin JM, Murphy M, Anderson J, et al. Tolerability and side-effects of post-exposure prophylaxis for HIV infection. Lancet 355:722, 2000.

Chapter 18

Nelfinavir

Miguel A. Goicoechea, MD, Richard H. Haubrich, MD

Nelfinavir (Viracept) was the fourth protease inhibitor (PI) approved by the US Food and Drug Administration (FDA) for the treatment of human immunodeficiency virus (HIV)-infected individuals and the first PI to receive concomitant approval in both children and adults. Similar to the other drugs in its class, nelfinavir diminishes HIV replication by inhibiting the HIV-1 protease enzyme required for viral particle maturation. Nelfinavir monotherapy given for 28 days lowers levels of HIV RNA in the plasma by 1–2 $\log_{10}$ copies/mL in protease-naive patients. Like the other available PIs, nelfinavir is extensively metabolized by cytochrome P450 (CYP) including CYP3A4 and CYP2C19. Primarily CYP3A4 is inhibited at concentrations within the therapeutic range, necessitating careful attention to concomitant medication administration. Gastrointestinal side-effects can accompany nelfinavir administration, but overall the drug is well tolerated.

STRUCTURE

The development of nelfinavir is an example of 'rational' drug design, wherein computer technology is applied to design compounds based on the crystallographic structure of a target enzyme, circumventing traditional drug development, which relies on mass screening of thousands of potential compounds.[1,2] Nelfinavir is the mesylate salt of a basic amine that was designed to maximize binding and stability of the ligand to the active site of HIV protease. Its molecular weight is 663.90 (567.79 as the free base); and it is slightly soluble in water at pH 2 or lower and freely soluble in methanol, ethanol, isopropanol, and propylene glycol. It is a nonpeptidic PI (K_I 2 nM) that is active against HIV-1 and HIV-2. Computer models using evolutionary programming to predict docking of flexible ligands reproduced the structure of nelfinavir in 34 of 100 simulations.[3,4]

MECHANISM OF ACTION AND *IN VITRO* ACTIVITY

Nelfinavir blocks HIV replication by competitively inhibiting the cleavage of HIV p55 Gag and pl60 GagPol precursor polyproteins to structural proteins and enzymes by the protease enzyme. The target of nelfinavir and other PIs is the final enzymatic step required to produce mature viral progeny. HIV precursor polyproteins, transcribed and translated from cells with integrated proviral DNA, must be cleaved at eight distinct sites to produce functional, mature virions. Virions produced in the presence of nelfinavir and other PIs are defective particles, which (as seen by electron microscopy) lack the electron-dense core characteristic of mature, infectious HIV. They are unable to infect new cells and are cleared from the circulation by an unknown mechanism.[5]

The antiviral activity of nelfinavir has also been evaluated against wild-type and drug-resistant HIV-1 strains in lymphocyte cell lines and in monocyte cell culture. *In vitro*, the mean inhibitory concentration is 21 nM (range 9–60 nM) in models of acute infection that include HIV-1 strains IIIB, RF, and the clinical isolate HIV-1 RoJo.[6] During infection of a macrophage cell line with HIV-1 strain Ba-L, the inhibitory concentration is low at 23 nM. Similarly, nelfinavir has also been evaluated and found to be effective against HIV-1 strains resistant to zidovudine and non-nucleoside reverse transcriptase inhibitors (NNRTIs), including pyridinones, nevirapine, and TIBO compounds.[7,8] The 50% cytotoxic concentration ranged from 23 to 28 μM for HIV-1 RF in CEM-SS cells and HIV-IIIB in MT-2 cells, respectively, yielding a therapeutic index of 526–916.[6] This high therapeutic index of nelfinavir reflects the potent antiviral activity and relatively low cytotoxicity present in cell culture systems.

PHARMACOKINETICS

The absorption of nelfinavir has been compared across several formulations, including: 250 mg tablet, 625 mg tablet, oral powder and liquid suspension.[9] Nelfinavir (250 mg tablet) is well absorbed with an estimated oral bioavailability of 78%. Concomitant administration of food enhances both the maximum plasma concentration (C_{max}) and area under the curve (AUC) plasma concentrations two- to threefold. Fat content of meals does not influence absorption. However, in a study of healthy volunteers given a single oral dose of 1250 mg, the two formulations (250 mg and 625 mg tablet) were not bioequivalent in the fasted state.[10] The 650 mg formulation had greater absorption with an AUC and C_{max} that were 34% and 24% higher than the 250 mg formulation. Administration with a meal improved the bioavailability of the 250 mg formulation to levels comparable with the 650 mg tablets. In addition, nelfinavir pharmacokinetics after a single dose with food in healthy volunteers were similar for the oral powder and liquid suspensions compared to the 250 mg tablet formulation.[9,11]

Plasma levels and antiviral activities were determined in HIV-infected patients for nelfinavir and its metabolites during 28 days of therapy with 750 mg three times daily.[12] Nelfinavir was the major chemical species reaching a peak plasma concentration of 5.04 + 2.56 μM 2 to 5 h after dosing, followed in decreasing quantities by its metabolites hydroxyl-*t*-butylamide (M8) and 3′-methoxy-4′-hydroxynelfinavir (M1). Antiviral activity was determined in CEM-SS cells with HIV-1 RF strain and the 50% effective concentration of nelfinavir, M8, and M1 were 30, 34, and 151 nM, respectively. At steady state, the mean C_{max} and minimum plasma concentration (C_{min}) for nelfinavir were 4.96 and 1.73 μM, and corresponding values for M8 were 1.96 and 0.55 μM. Equilibrium dialysis experiments demonstrate that nelfinavir is highly bound (98%) as is the M8 metabolite (97%), indicating similar antiviral activities for nelfinavir and its M8 metabolite. Although peak levels exceed the *in vitro* inhibitory concentration by more than 100-fold, because of the large degree of protein binding, the free drug concentration exceeds the inhibitory concentrations by only several-fold. The large volume of distribution (2–7 L/kg) of nelfinavir would suggest that nelfinavir penetrates most tissues. However, like most PIs, nelfinavir does not penetrate cerebrospinal fluid (CSF). CSF concentrations were not detectable in 25 samples from six patients despite appropriate plasma concentrations.[13] Further, a study of 13 patients treated with nelfinavir-based combination therapy for at least 6 months showed decreased penetration into both genital tract (semen to plasma concentration ratio of 0.08) and lymphoid tissues (lymph node tissue to plasma concentration ratio of 0.58).[14]

The predominant metabolic pathways for nelfinavir are through the hepatic microsome P450 enzymes (CYP). Metabolism of nelfinavir by the CYP2C19 isoform leads to the formation of M8, the most common and active metabolite.[12] Subsequently, nelfinavir and M8 are both eliminated via the CYP3A4 pathway. Because CYP enzymes, in particular CYP3A4, metabolize many other drugs, inhibition of these enzymes by PIs can alter the pharmacologic activity of concomitant medications (*see section on* Drug Interactions). Nelfinavir is an inhibitor of CYP3A4, similar to saquinavir, but is a less potent inhibitor than either indinavir or ritonavir. *In vitro* assays for inhibition of other P450 isoforms by nelfinavir (CYP2C9, CYP2C8, CYP2E1, CYP2C19, CYP2D6, CYP1A2) suggests that *in vivo* effects are minimal.[15] Co-administration of low-dose ritonavir to inhibit CYP3A4 pathways is increasingly used to enhance plasma concentrations of other PIs. In a study with healthy volunteers, nelfinavir 1250 mg twice daily was given with either 100 or 200 mg ritonavir.[16] Fourteen days of ritonavir combination therapy resulted in a minor increase of the AUC of nelfinavir by 20% and 39%, respectively.

The terminal half-life of nelfinavir in the plasma is 3.5–5.0 h. Nelfinavir is excreted unchanged (22%) and as oxidative metabolites (65%) in the stool. Only 1–2% of nelfinavir is excreted in the urine. The pharmacokinetics of nelfinavir have not been studied in patients with altered renal function, but clearance of only a small fraction of the drug through the urinary system suggests that effects should be minimal. Further, no significant pharmacokinetic differences have been detected between men and women, or between African-American and Caucasian patients.[9,17] However, hepatic insufficiency has been associated with reduced CYP drug elimination and increased PI plasma concentrations.[18] Nelfinavir pharmacokinetics were studied in 119 HIV-infected individuals at steady state (74% were taking 1250 mg twice daily) of which 67 were without liver disease and hepatitis C infection (HCV), 32 were HIV-HCV co-infected without cirrhosis, and 20 were HIV-HCV co-infected with cirrhosis.[19] HIV-HCV co-infected patients with and without cirrhosis had significantly lower nelfinavir clearance than purely HIV-infected patients (28% and 58% lower, respectively; $P < 0.05$). These differences in metabolism resulted in a 2.5- and 1.3-fold increase in plasma concentrations in HIV-HCV co-infected patients with and without cirrhosis compared with patients with purely HIV infection without liver disease. In contrast, M8 concentrations were reduced in cirrhotic individuals, suggesting that CYP2C19 impairment is particularly sensitive to liver disease.

The pharmacokinetics of nelfinavir differs greatly during pregnancy, in infancy and through childhood. Studies in children (ages 2–13) have demonstrated the clearance to be two to three times greater than adults. A dose of 20–30 mg kg^{-1} day^{-1} in three divided doses in children produces plasma levels similar to those present in adults receiving a 750 mg thrice-daily regimen (~10 mg kg^{-1} day^{-1}).[20] Infants (less than 2 years) also demonstrate increased metabolism resulting in highly variable nelfinavir and M8 concentrations that are lower than what is observed in older children and adults.[21,22] In addition, nelfinavir and M8 exposure is also reduced during pregnancy either from induction of CYP3A4, or inhibition of CYP2C19, or both.[23]

TOXICITY

The most common nelfinavir-associated adverse event described in clinical trials was diarrhea or loose stools. This toxicity rarely resulted in treatment discontinuation and often resolved with or without over-the-counter antimotility agents. Data from 583 patients in two randomized, phase 3 studies support the finding that diarrhea was the most significant toxicity associated with nelfinavir.[24,25] In these studies, patients received nucleosides alone or in combination with 500 or 750 mg three times daily (Study 511) or 1250 mg twice daily of nelfinavir (Study 542). Twenty percent of patients treated with 750 mg thrice daily of nelfinavir had moderate to severe diarrhea in Study 511, compared to 3% of zidovudine (ZDV)/lamivudine (3TC)-treated patients. The two nelfinavir doses did not differ in terms of the rate of diarrhea (14% vs 20%; $P = 0.2$) and only two patients discontinued study medication while receiving the higher dosing regimen (Table 18-1). Similarly, a dose increase to 1250 mg twice a day in Study 542 also did not result in higher rates of diarrhea than with 750 mg three times daily (12% and 11%, respectively).

The overall rate of toxicity with nelfinavir compared favorably to that seen with other PI regimens (*see section on* Efficacy Trials). Although diarrhea was more common with nelfinavir use than fosamprenavir–ritonavir (16% vs 9%; $P = 0.008$)[26] or atazanavir (56% vs 15–20%; $P < 0.01$),[27] the rates of treatment discontinuation were not different. In a randomized, placebo-controlled trial comparing nelfinavir (750 mg thrice daily) with lopinavir–ritonavir (400 + 100 mg twice daily) diarrhea was the most common adverse event in both groups occurring in ~16% of patients (Table 18-1).[28]

Dyslipidemia and lipodystrophy have been associated with PI use,[29] though the clinical significance of these lipid changes remains unclear.[30] After 48 weeks of therapy, median changes in total cholesterol, low-density lipoprotein (LDL) cholesterol and triglycerides were similar between patients receiving nelfinavir and fosamprenavir[31] or fosamprenavir–ritonavir.[26] Treatment with lopinavir–ritonavir did result in greater increases in triglycerides (125 mg/dL vs 47 mg/dL; $P < 0.01$) and total cholesterol (53 mg/dL vs 48 mg/dL; $P = 0.17$) than those receiving nelfinavir, but no difference in the presence of lipodystrophy or lipoatrophy (6% vs 5%).[28] By contrast, patients who received atazanavir (400 mg daily) had significantly lower increases in baseline total cholesterol (8.6 mg/dL vs 40.5 mg/dL; at 48 weeks), fasting LDL cholesterol (5.2 mg/dL vs 22.5 mg/dL; at 56 weeks), and fasting triglycerides (9.2 mg/dL vs 53.4 mg/dL; at 48 weeks) than treatment with nelfinavir.[27]

Table 18-1

Patients with Adverse Events of Moderate or Severe Intensity[a] or Severe Laboratory Toxicity Reported in ≥2% of Patients

		Study 511[b,25]		Walmsley[b,28]	
Adverse Event	**Placebo + ZDV/3TC (*n* = 101)**	**Nelfinavir 500 mg tid + ZDV/3TC (*n* = 96)**	**Nelfinavir 750 mg tid + ZDV/3TC (*n* = 99)**	**Nelfinavir 750 mg tid + d4T/3TC (*n* = 327)**	**Lopinavir–Ritonavir 400 mg + 100 mg bid + d4T/3TC (*n* = 326)**
Clinical (%)					
Asthenia	2	1	1	3.4	4.0
Headache	2	1	1	1.8	2.5
Diarrhea	3	14	20	17.1	15.6
Vomiting	2	1	1	2.4	2.5
Nausea	4	3	7	4.6	6.7
Lipodystrophy	N/A	N/A	N/A	6	5
Laboratory (%)					
Cholesterol[c]	N/A	N/A	N/A	4.9	9.0
Triglycerides[d]	N/A	N/A	N/A	1.3	9.3
ALT or AST[e]	10	2	1	5.2	4.5

ALT, alanine transaminase; AST, aspartate transaminase; N/A, not available.

[a] Includes adverse events at least possibly related to the study drug or of unknown relation and excludes concurrent HIV conditions.
[b] Adverse events within 6 months (Study 511) and 12 months (Walmsely) of therapy initiation.
[c] Greater than 300 mg/dL.
[d] Greater than 750 mg/dL.
[e] Greater than five times upper limit of normal.

EFFICACY TRIALS

Monotherapy Studies

Two small open-label studies of escalating doses of nelfinavir monotherapy were the first to demonstrate the antiviral activity of the drug. At low doses (900 and 1200 mg/day) used in study 504,[32] five of 20 therapy-naive patients had a reduction in HIV RNA levels of 1 $\log_{10}$ copies/mL that persisted past 28 days. In Study 503, 30 patients with CD4+ T-lymphocyte counts of more than 200 cells/mm^3 received higher nelfinavir doses (1500, 2250, and 3000 total mg/day in divided thrice-daily doses).[33] These patients had median HIV RNA $\log_{10}$ decreases of 1.4, 1.0, and 1.7 copies/mL, respectively, after 28 days at the three increasing dose levels. Follow-up of 15 patients for 4 months showed the greatest HIV RNA reduction (1.5 $\log_{10}$ copies/mL) in the highest dose group.

Study 505 randomized patients to placebo or nelfinavir (500 mg vs 750 mg three times daily). Placebo patients crossed over to one of the two doses of nelfinavir after 4 weeks.[34] The 91 patients had a mean HIV RNA level of 4.9 $\log_{10}$ copies/mL and a mean CD4+ lymphocyte count of 275 cells/mm^3 at baseline. At 4 weeks the mean viral load was reduced by 0.1, 0.9, and 1.3 $\log_{10}$ copies/mm, and the CD4+ lymphocytes increased 10, 84, and 100 cells/mm^3 in the placebo, low-dose nelfinavir, and high-dose nelfinavir groups, respectively (placebo versus nelfinavir; $P < 0.01$). After 16 weeks the mean $\log_{10}$ reduction in HIV RNA was 0.6 copies/mL for the 750 mg dose group, which was significantly greater than the reduction for the 500 mg group.

Treatment-Naive Studies

Triple-therapy combinations with nelfinavir and dual nucleoside reverse transcriptase inhibitors (NRTIs) has been studied in antiretroviral naive patients and compared with regimens containing a NNRTIs, other PIs, and PIs boosted with low-dose ritonavir. The trials selected for review were well designed and most were powered to demonstrate noninferiority with nelfinavir. Although cross study comparisons are not ideal, the efficacy of nelfinavir (proportion of patients with HIV RNA < 500 copies/mL at 48 weeks) ranged from 51% to 68% of participants (Table 18-2).

Two randomized studies clarified the optimal dosing regimen for nelfinavir in combination with nucleoside analogs. In Study 511 a series of 297 therapy-naive patients with a mean baseline HIV RNA level of 5.2–5.3 $\log_{10}$ copies/mL and CD4+ lymphocyte count of 276 to 307 cells/mm^3 were randomized to nelfinavir (500 or 750 mg thrice daily)/ZDV/3TC versus ZDV/3TC alone.[25] Baseline characteristics were balanced across treatment arms. The proportions of patients at 24 weeks with HIV RNA of less than 400 copies/mL were 77% and 50% for the high-dose and low-dose nelfinavir groups, compared to 7% in the ZDV/3TC group ($P < 0.001$). Follow-up for an additional 6 months confirmed that the proportion of patients in whom HIV RNA remained undetectable at 48 weeks was significantly higher in the 750 mg group (75%) than in the 500 mg group (54%). Study 542 was a phase 3 study powered to determine equivalency between the twice-daily dosing (1250 mg twice daily) of nelfinavir to three times daily (750 mg three times daily) dosing.[9,24] A total of 323 patients received the 1250 mg twice-daily dosing and 192 patients the 750 mg thrice-daily dosing of nelfinavir in combination with stavudine (d4T) and 3TC. Mean baseline CD4+ lymphocyte count was 296 cells/mm^3 with an HIV RNA level of 5.0 $\log_{10}$ copies/mL. At 48 weeks, 61% in the 1250 mg group and 58% in the 750 mg group had achieved plasma HIV RNA levels of less than 400 copies/mL, confirming similar efficacy between dosing regimens.

Nelfinavir and the NNRTIs have been studied in two recent clinical trials. In the COMBINE study,[35] a total of 142 patients were randomized to receive either nevirapine 200 mg twice daily ($n = 72$) or nelfinavir 1250 mg twice daily ($n = 70$) plus ZDV/3TC. At 12 months, 75% of patients in the nevirapine group and 60% in the nelfinavir group had plasma HIV RNA below 200 copies/mL ($P = 0.06$). Notably, both drugs had a high incidence of study drug discontinuation due to adverse effects. Nelfinavir was discontinued in 20%, primarily due to diarrhea, and 17% discontinued nevirapine with rash and liver enzyme elevations.

ACTG 384 used a four arm factorial design to compare pairs of sequential triple therapy combinations with either nelfinavir or efavirenz combined with d4T/didanosine (ddI) or ZDV/3TC.[36] A total of 620 patients were enrolled (155 subjects each arm) of which 243 had treatment failure of their first regimen (190 were viral failures and 53 were toxicity related). For the secondary endpoint analysis, failure of the first regimen, there was a significant interaction between the treatment factors, i.e., between the selection of nucleoside backbone and the initial use of efavirenz versus nelfinavir ($P = 0.002$). Subjects who received the nucleoside combination of ZDV/3TC had a lower risk of treatment failure when combined with efavirenz versus nelfinavir (hazard ratio for failure of the first regimen, 0.39; 95% confidence interval (CI), 0.24 to 0.64). However, no significant difference in failure rates were observed when d4T/ddI was the nucleoside combination used (hazard ratio for failure of the first regimen, 0.88; 95% CI, 0.61–1.29). Although interpretation of this data is complicated by an interaction from the factorial study design, in post hoc analysis after adjustment for all six possible pair wise comparisons, the combination of efavirenz and ZDV/3TC was superior to all other triple-therapy combinations used in this study.

The NEAT study was a noninferiority study that compared 166 patients on fosamprenavir 1400 mg twice-daily with 83 on nelfinavir 1250 mg twice-daily dosed with a background combination of abacavir (ABC) and 3TC for 48 weeks.[31] The study population was generally well-balanced between arms, but patients had advanced HIV disease with 48% having a baseline CD4+ cell count less than 200 cells/mL. In intention-to-treat (ITT) analysis (missing = failure), the proportion of patients achieving a plasma HIV RNA less than 400 copies/mL was greater in the fosamprenavir group (66%) than the neflinavir group (48%) after 48 weeks of treatment. Further, over twice the numbers of patients in the nelfinavir

Table 18-2

Study	Nelfinavir Dose (mg)	Second PI or NNRTI Dose (mg)	Other Agents	Study Period (Weeks)	No.	% ARV-Naive (PI-Naive)	HIV RNA (log_{10} copies/mL) Baseline	HIV RNA (log_{10} copies/mL) At Last Follow-up	Percemt with HIV RNA< 500 (50) copies/mL at Last Visit	CD4+ Lymphocyte Count (cells/mm^3) Baseline	CD4+ Lymphocyte Count (cells/mm^3) At Last Follow-up
511[25]	Placebo		ZDV/3TC	48		100 (100)	5.2	3.8[a]	7 (4)[a]	276	371[a]
	500 tid		ZDV/3TC			100 (100)	5.3	2.9	54 (37)	307	~502
	750 tid		ZDV/3TC			100 (100)	5.2	2.3	75 (61)	283	~478
542[9,24]	750 tid		d4T/3TC	48	192	100 (100)	~5.0[b]	N/A	58 (N/A)	~296[b]	~496[b]
	1250 bid		d4T/3TC		326	100 (100)	~5.0[b]	N/A	61 (N/A)	~296[b]	~496[b]
COMBINE[35]	1250 bid		ZDV/3TC	48	70	100 (100)	5.2	3.4	60 (50) I	347	520
		NVP 200 bid	ZDV/3TC		72	100 (100)	5.1	3.2	75 (65) I	375	537
ACTG384[c, 36]	placebo	EFV 600 qd	d4T/ddI	112	155	100 (100)	5.0	N/A	69 (53)[d]	N/A	N/A
	1250 bid	placebo	d4T/ddI		155	100 (100)	5.0	N/A	77 (61)[d]	N/A	N/A
	placebo	EFV 600 qd	ZDV/3TC		155	100 (100)	4.9	N/A	31 (25)[d]	N/A	N/A
	1250 bid	placebo	ZDV/3TC		155	100 (100)	4.9	N/A	66 (51)[d]	N/A	N/A
NEAT[31]	1250 bid		ABC/3TC	48	83	100 (100)	4.9	2.6	51 (41) I	212	428
		FAPV 1400 bid	ABC/3TC		166	100 (100)	4.8	2.4	66 (55) I	214	415
Murphy[27]	1250 bid		d4T/3TC	48	91	100 (100)	4.7	2.4	53 (34) I	283	494
		ATV 400 qd	d4T/3TC		181	100 (100)	4.7	2.2	64 (35) I	294	528
		ATV 600 qd	d4T/3TC		195	100 (100)	4.7	2.1	67 (36) I	302	545
SOLO[26]	1250 bid		ABC/3TC	48	322	100 (100)	4.8	N/A	68 (53) I	177	384
		FAPV/RTV 1400/200 qd	ABC/3TC		327	100 (100)	4.8	N/A	69 (55) I	166	369
Walmsley[28]	750 tid	placebo	d4T/3TC	48	327	100 (100)	4.9	N/A	63 (52) I	258	453
	placebo	LPV/RTV 400/100 bid	d4T/3TC		326	100 (100)	4.9	N/A	75 (67) I	260	467
ACTG 364[39]	750 tid		2 NRTIs	40–48	66	0 (100)	~3.9	N/A	35 (22) I	336	~94[e]
		EFV 600 qd	2 NRTIs	40–48	65	0 (100)	~3.9	N/A	60 (44) I	343	~94[e]
	750 tid	EFV 600 qd	2 NRTIs	40–48	64	0 (100)	~3.8	N/A	74 (67) I	379	~94[e]
Roca[40]	750 tid		d4T/3TC	36	56	0 (52)	4.3	N/A	47 (N/A) A	328	35%[f]
		IDV 800 tid	d4T/3TC	36	56	0 (65)	4.6	N/A	46 (N/A) A	312	42%[f]

A, as treated; ABC, abacavir; ARV, antiretroviral; d4T, stavudine; EFV, efavirenz; FAPV, fosamprenavir; I, intent to treat; IDV, indinavir; LPV, lopinavir; NRTI, nucleoside reverse transcriptase inhibitor; NVP, nevirapine; RTV, ritonavir; SQV, saquinavir; ZDV, zidovudine; 3TC, lamivudine.

[a] After 24 weeks of therapy.
[b] Average of both arms.
[c] Only data from first regimen is presented.
[d] Number (%) of patients with failure of first regimen: virologic and toxicity-related.
[e] Increase for all groups combined.
[f] Percent with greater than 100 cell/mm^3 increase.

arm were prematurely discontinued from their randomized study drug than the fosamprenavir group due to insufficient viral load response (19% vs 7%, respectively). While the study lacked sufficient power to assess superiority of fosamprenavir, the 95% CI of 2–28% suggests a true difference between treatment groups.

In contrast, nelfinavir demonstrated equivalent efficacy with atazanavir at the currently recommended dose of 400 mg once daily.[27] A total of 467 patients were randomized in a phase 2 dose-ranging study of atazanavir (400 or 600 mg once daily) compared to nelfinavir (1250 mg twice daily), each given with d4T and 3TC. In ITT analysis (noncompletion = failure), a comparable proportion of patients on atazanavir 400 mg daily (116/156; 64%) and nelfinavir (48/80; 60%) achieved a plasma HIV RNA less than 400 copies/mL after 48 weeks of therapy. Although patients receiving 600 mg daily of atazanavir did achieve higher rates of viral control, the increased incidence of jaundice with the higher dose resulted in the decision to favor the 400 mg dose for clinical use.

Unlike the NEAT study, [31] the viral response of nelfinavir (1250 mg twice daily) in the SOLO trial[26] was similar to boosted fosamprenavir–ritonavir (1400 + 200 mg ritonavir once daily). This was a larger trial that randomized 322 patients to fosamprenavir–ritonavir and 327 to nelfinavir and again included participants largely with advanced HIV disease, having a median CD4+ T-cell count below 200 cells/mm^3. At week 48, 69% of the patients in the fosamprenavir–ritonavir group and 68% in the nelfinavir group achieved a plasma HIV RNA less than 400 copies/mL (95% CI: −6 to 8%). This equivalence was observed despite a higher adherence rate in the fosamprenavir–ritonavir once-daily group compared with the nelfinavir twice-daily group (78% vs 67%, respectively). However, in subgroup analysis of patients with pretherapy viral load above 500 000 copies/mL, more patients in the fosamprenavir–ritonavir group (73%) achieved viral control than the nelfinavir group (53%).

A large double-blind, placebo-controlled study of lopinavir–ritonavir (400 mg lopinavir + 100 mg ritonavir twice daily) compared with nelfinavir (750 mg three times daily) demonstrated superior antiviral activity of this boosted-PI combination over nelfinavir.[28] A total of 326 patients received lopinavir–ritonavir and 327 patients received nelfinavir plus d4T and 3TC for 48 weeks. Tolerability of the regimens compared favorably, except for lipid abnormalities, which were more common with lopinavir–ritonavir. In the primary analysis, patients treated with lopinavir–ritonavir had higher proportions of undetectable viral loads (less than 400 copies/mL) at week 24 than those treated with nelfinavir (79% vs 71%, respectively; $P < 0.05$). Additional follow-up showed an increasing difference in response rates with 75% of patients on lopinavir–ritonavir achieving viral suppression compared with 63% of nelfinavir-treated patients ($P < 0.001$) (Fig. 18-1). Although CD4+ T-cell increases were comparable at 48 weeks, the time to loss of viral response was greater for patients on lopinavir–ritonavir with 84% maintaining viral control compared with 66% of those taking nelfinavir, yielding a hazard ratio of 2.0 (95% CI: 1.5–2.7).

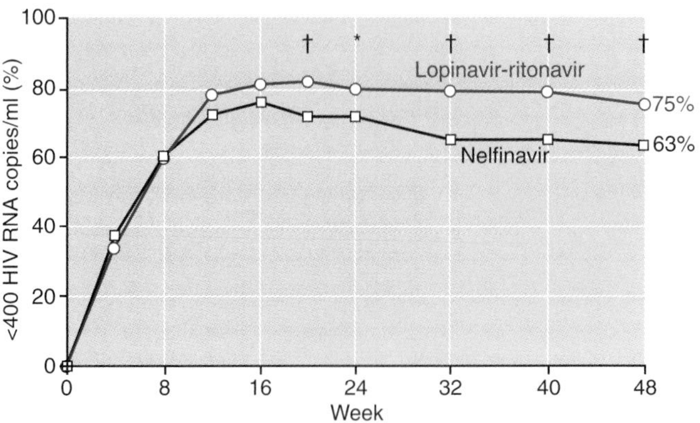

Figure 18-1 ■ Percentage of patients with plasma HIV RNA levels of fewer than 400 copies/mL. All the patients who received a study drug are included (326 in the lopinavir–ritonavir group and 327 in the nelfinavir group). The asterisk denotes $P < 0.05$ and the daggers $P < 0.001$ for the comparison between the treatment groups.

N Engl J Med, Vol. 346, 2002.[28] With kind permission from Massachusetts Medical Society©.

Treatment-Experienced Studies

Studies have evaluated nelfinavir in combination with NNRTIs and other PIs in treatment experienced patients.[37,38] However, the individual efficacy of nelfinavir in these patients is obscured by co-administration of a second PI or NNRTI. Further, some studies used companion drugs which are no longer recommended for use, i.e., adefovir and delavirdine.[37] Notwithstanding, two studies provide comparative data for nelfinavir with either an NNRTI in patients with NRTI-experience (ACTG 364),[39] or with another PI in PI-experienced patients.[40]

ACTG 364 enrolled 195 patients experiencing treatment failure (HIV RNA above 500 copies/mL) who had been treated with NRTIs only.[39] Patients were randomized to receive either efavirenz 600 mg once daily ($n = 65$) or nelfinavir 750 mg three times daily ($n = 66$) or combined efavirenz and nelfinavir ($n = 64$) plus two NRTIs. Quadruple therapy resulted in a higher rate of viral suppression than either the nelfinavir group ($P = 0.001$) or efavirenz group ($P = 0.008$) at weeks 40 and 48. Between the triple-therapy regimens, the efavirenz group had significantly higher proportions of patients who achieved a plasma HIV RNA less that 500 copies/mL than the nelfinavir group (60% vs 35%, respectively; $P = 0.004$). Baseline genotypic analyses were retrospectively examined in 140 participants. High level NRTI resistance was defined as five or more reverse transcriptase mutations. Of the patients who achieved viral control at week 40 and 48, the efavirenz group tended to have more patients with higher baseline NRTI resistance than the nelfinavir group (30% vs 19%, respectively; $P = 0.08$). Considering that the presence of NRTI-associated mutations has been associated with hypersusceptibility of HIV to NNRTIs,[41] this may have contributed to the better efficacy of efavirenz versus nelfinavir in this study.

In another randomized study nelfinavir had similar antiviral efficacy as unboosted indinavir in therapy-experienced patients.[40] Of the 112 patients that were randomized, 35% in the indinavir group and 48% in the nelfinavir group had prior PI experience. Despite a higher treatment discontinuation rate in the indinavir versus nelfinavir group (60% vs 30%; P = 0.02), both groups had similar rates of viral suppression after 9 months of therapy (46% vs 47%; P = 0.93).

SPECIAL POPULATIONS

Currently nelfinavir-based combinations are recommended as initial therapy in infants, children and pregnant women with HIV infection.[42,43] Unlike adult treatment guidelines, relatively few comparative studies exist in these populations and recommendations are largely based on efficacy studies in adults, nonrandomized phase 2 trials, pharmacokinetic data, and potential for adverse drug interactions. Nelfinavir is well tolerated during pregnancy,[44,45] its placental passage is minimal[46,47] and there is no evidence of human teratogenicity [48]. Although the recommended dose of nelfinavir is 1200 mg twice daily,[42] plasma levels are reduced during pregnancy[23,49] and therapeutic drug monitoring and dose adjustment should be considered.[50,51]

Pediatric Studies

Nelfinavir has been shown to be efficacious in infants (less than 3 months) and children (3 months to 17 years) as initial HIV therapy (Table 18-3).[52–55] PACTG 377 was a randomized, open-labeled study that evaluated the relative potency and tolerability of four treatment regimens in 181 NRTI-experienced children aged 4 months to 16 years.[53] Overall, the proportion of children with HIV RNA less than 400 copies/mL at week 48 was 41% (73 of 177). Comparisons between triple-therapy arms did not show significant differences in viral suppression between PIs (41% receiving d4T-NVP-RTV vs 30% receiving d4T–NVP–NFV) or regimens not containing an NNRTI (42% receiving d4T–3TC–NFV). However, there was significantly greater viral suppression with quadruple therapy (52% receiving d4T–3TC–NVP–NFV) compared with those receiving d4T–NVP–NFV (P = 0.048), but significant differences were not observed when compared with the other triple-therapy arms. Further, patients receiving different dosing schedules of nelfinavir (twice daily vs thrice daily) also had comparable rates of viral suppression.

A pharmacokinetic substudy of PACTG 377 evaluated drug disposition of nelfinavir thrice daily (30 mg/kg) in 45 children of varying developmental stages (ages from 8 months to 16 years) and weight, and compared these pharmacokinetic profiles with six children receiving twice-daily (55 mg/kg) nelfinavir.[56] Nelfinavir exposure was highly variable with significantly lower levels in smaller, younger patients. The AUC_{0-24h} for children who weighed greater than 25 kg and on thrice-daily dosing (8921 $\mu g\,h^{-1}\,L^{-1}$) was comparable to the AUC_{0-24h} in children weighing less than 30 kg on the twice-daily dosing (92006 $\mu g\,h^{-1}\,L^{-1}$). In contrast, children weighing less than 25 kg receiving thrice-daily dosing had significantly lower exposures (34277 $\mu g\,h^{-1}L^{-1}$) than heavier children on thrice- (P = 0.0005) or twice-daily (P = 0.012) dosing. This high degree of pharmacokinetic variability underscores the effect of maturation stage on nelfinavir metabolism which may be a rationale for routine drug monitoring in this patient population.

THERAPEUTIC DRUG MONITORING

Therapeutic drug monitoring (TDM) of PIs provides the opportunity to optimize individual drug exposure and enhance treatment responses. Several studies have demonstrated a significant relationship between nelfinavir plasma concentrations and viral response,[57–60] suggesting that nelfinavir may be a good candidate for TDM. Moreover, large interpatient variability of nelfinavir plasma levels among HIV-infected adults has been observed.[61] Trough plasma concentrations in patients taking either the 1250 mg twice-daily or 750 mg thrice-daily regimen ranged from 0.36 to 10.57 mg/L and from 0.14 to 11.74 mg/L, respectively. This yielded a high interpatient variability (coefficient of variation: 153%) and demonstrates the potential clinical utility of TDM in regimens containing nelfinavir.

Adequate plasma concentrations of nelfinavir have been shown to be predictive of short- and long-term viral suppression in antiretroviral (ARV)-naive individuals. The ATHENA study evaluated whether TDM could improve therapeutic response to PI-based therapy in ARV-naive patients.[62] A total of 147 patients were randomly selected to nelfinavir (n = 92) or indinavir (n = 55) and then were randomly assigned to either a TDM group, in which plasma PI concentrations plus dosing advice were reported to primary care providers, or to a control arm that did not receive TDM results. Among those patients receiving nelfinavir, 12.2% of the 41 patients in the TDM group had discontinued nelfinavir versus 35.3% of the 78 patients in the control group after 1 year (P = 0.01). The most common reason for treatment discontinuation was viral failure which occurred in 2.4% of TDM patients and 17.6% of control patients (P = 0.02). In a subgroup analysis of 48 patients, the minimum effective concentration of nelfinavir and its active metabolite M8 were determined.[59] A concentration ratio was calculated by dividing the concentration of an individual by the time-adjusted population value (a concentration ratio of 1.0 would be considered average). Those with viral failure (29% at 8 months) had significantly lower concentration ratios of nelfinavir than patients who achieved viral suppression (0.77 vs 0.99; P = 0.039). Similar findings were reported by Powderly et al.[63] In this study the 2-h postdose nelfinavir concentration was an independent predictor of attaining HIV RNA of less than 400 copies/mL after 48 weeks (odds ratio of response 8.1 for those with higher concentrations; P = 0.005).

One explanation for this high degree of variability in nelfinavir concentrations is that genetic differences exist among individuals which affect the pharmacokinetics of the drug. Genetic variants, or polymorphisms, of the CYP2C19 gene

Pediatric Studies

Table 18-3

Study	Age	Nelfinavir Dose (mg kg^{-1}/day^{-1} in Three Divided Doses)	Second PI or NNRTI	Other Agents	Study Period (Weeks)	Number	Number (%) with HIV RNA <500 copies/mL at Last Visit	Nelfinavir Plasma Concentrations C_{max} (ng/mL) AUC_{0-24h} (µg h^{-1}/L^{-1})
PENTA 5[a,52]	3 months to 16 years	75–90		2 NRTIs	48	30	15 (56)	N/A
		Placebo		2 NRTIs	48	25	12 (52)	N/A
Funk et al[54]	14–152 months	60		2 NRTIs	48	16	11 (69)	C_{max}(range): 1798–7900
PACTG 377[53]	4 months to 17 years		NVP/RTV	d4T	48	41	(41)	Patients <25 kg (median)[e]: AUC: 34 227 and C_{max}: 3323
		30[b]	NVP	d4T	48	44	(30)[d]	Patients >25 kg (median)[e]: AUC 89 421: and C_{max}: 4845
		30[b]	NVP	d4T/3TC	48	44	(52)[d]	Patients >30 kg (median): AUC: 92 006 and C_{max}: 6777
		30[b]		d4T/3TC	48	52	(42)	
		55[c]		d4T/3TC	48	11	(55)	
PACTG 356[55]	0.5–3.0 months	N/A	NVP	d4T/3TC	48	18	15 (83)	N/A
			NVP	ZDV/3TC	48	17	4 (24)[f]	N/A
			NVP	ZDV/3TC/ABC	48	17	7 (41)[f]	N/A

ABC, abacavir; ARV, antiretroviral; AUC, area under the plasma concentration–time curve; C_{max}, maximum plasma concentration; d4T, stavudine; N/A, not available; NRTI, nucleoside reverse transcriptase inhibitor; NVP, nevirapine; RTV, ritonavir; ZDV, zidovudine; 3TC, lamivudine.

[a]Data presented only for asymptomatic patients (arm A).
[b]Children who weighed ⩾30 kg received 27–33 mg/kg thrice-daily.
[c]Given as 55 mg/kg twice-daily.
[d]Fischer's exact P value for pairwise comparison was $P = 0.048$, for arms NFV/NVP/d4T and NFV/NVP/d4T/3TC.
[e]Nelfinavir dosed in the absence of nevirapine.
[f]$P < 0.01$ for the comparison with NFV/NVP/d4T/3TC.

can result in a poor drug metabolism phenotype resulting in an increase in drug concentrations. In ACTG 384 nelfinavir plasma exposure was associated with CYP2C19 681G→A polymorphism.[57] Individuals homozygous for AA had median 12-h AUC values that were ~36% higher than in GG homozygote individuals. There was also a trend toward more favorable viral control among slow metabolizers (GA genotype).

Although routine use of TDM in all patients is not recommended,[64] certain populations on nelfinavir-based regimens may benefit from TDM. HIV-infected children, particularly infants, have variable rates of drug metabolism related to age and developmental stage and often require higher dosing of nelfinavir compared with adults.[20,22] During pregnancy there is an increase in volume of distribution and hepatic metabolism which may result in subtherapeutic levels.[23,50] In addition, patients with liver impairment have decreased clearance of nelfinavir which may result in high plasma concentrations and increased toxicity.[19] Nelfinavir and its active metabolite M8 have a well-defined concentration-effect relationship making it an ideal candidate for TDM. However, the utility of TDM and nelfinavir may be most beneficial in certain populations with altered pharmacokinetics or when drug–drug interactions are suspected.

RESISTANCE

Nelfinavir-resistant isolates emerge after multiple passages of HIV in the presence of nelfinavir *in vitro* and, in the absence of complete viral suppression, can be isolated from patients exposed to nelfinavir for periods of weeks or more. Primary mutations are critical mutations at the substrate-binding sites that can reduce drug activity. With continued drug exposure secondary, or compensatory, mutations may be selected which may enhance viral fitness. Accumulation of these secondary mutations can lead to high-level nelfinavir resistance and cross-resistance to other PIs.

Nelfinavir resistance develops along two pathways characterized either by a D30N (without PI cross-resistance) or L90M (broad PI cross-resistance) amino acid substitution in protease. These mutations rarely occur simultaneously[65,66] and may represent mutually exclusive resistance pathways. *In vivo*, the D30N substitution is the most common mutation that emerges in the setting of nelfinavir failure.[65–68] It is associated with reduced phenotypic susceptibility (five- to 93-fold) and secondary substitutions at other codons, including: 35, 36, 46, 71, 77, and 88.[67] In ARV-naive patients, the L90M mutation is less frequent and occurs in 5–29% of clinical isolates.[65–68]

Significantly less PI cross-resistance has been observed from patients failing an initial nelfinavir-containing regimen than those receiving other PI-based regimens.[69,70] In phenotypic assays viral isolates containing D30N continued to be susceptible to amprenavir, ritonavir, indinavir, and saquinavir.[67] Despite high-level clinical resistance to nelfinavir, salvage treatment with either lopinavir, atazanavir, saquinavir, or ritonavir appeared to be preserved.[69,71,72] In contrast, patients initially treated with other PIs can develop cross-resistance to nelfinavir even in the absence of the D30N mutation. The genotypic pattern that predicts lack of clinical response or phenotypic resistance to nelfinavir is varied. In general, the greater the number of substitutions in protease, the less likely a viral response to nelfinavir salvage therapy.[73] No single amino acid mutation pattern predicted response, but patients with the L90M had poor responses.[74] Although high-level resistance PIs generally requires an accumulation of several mutations, resistance pathways associated with broad cross-resistance often contain the L90M substitution.[75] Therefore, emergence of L90M during initial nelfinavir-based therapy is likely to diminish treatment responses with subsequent PI-based regimens.

The incidence of resistance after viral failure of a non-boosted PI regimen, such as nelfinavir, was significantly higher than that of ritonavir-boosted lopinavir- and fosamprenavir-based therapies. Samples for viral phenotype and genotype were collected from study M98–863, which randomized patients to lopinavir–ritonavir versus nelfinavir plus D4T/3TC.[66] A total of 147 isolates (51 lopinavir–ritonavir, 96 nelfinavir) had resistance testing from subjects who had at least one viral load above 400 copies/mL between weeks 24 and 108. No primary PI mutations were observed in any of the lopinavir–ritonavir rebound samples compared to 43 of 96 nelfinavir samples that did contain resistance mutations. The primary PI mutations observed were D30N (65%), L90M (33%) or both (2%). The incidence of nucleoside resistance was also higher in nelfinavir treated patients. 3TC resistance occurred in 79/96 (82%) of nelfinavir isolates and 19/51 (37%) in rebound samples from patients treated with lopinavir–ritonavir ($P < 0.001$). Similarly, therapy-naive patients treated with fosamprenavir–ritonavir-based regimens had lower resistance rates than nelfinavir-treated patients for both PI (0% vs 50%; $P < 0.001$) and NRTI mutations (13% vs 69%; $P < 0.001$).[65]

These data suggest that significant differences in genetic and pharmacologic barriers to resistance exist between ritonavir-boosted PIs and nelfinavir. Indeed, the mean C_{trough} of nelfinavir (1.73 μM)[12] is only one to fivefold above its protein adjusted 50% inhibitory concentration (0.32–1.34 μM).[76] Considering that patient-derived isolates containing the D30N mutation demonstrate more than 10-fold resistance,[9] a single substitution in protease can substantially increase the likelihood of treatment failure.

DRUG INTERACTIONS

Nelfinavir is primarily metabolized by two CYP isoforms, CYP2C19 and CYP3A4,[15] and drugs that are substrates, inhibitors, or inducers of these enzymes could potentially interact with nelfinavir. Conversely, inhibition of these metabolic enzymes by nelfinavir can augment blood levels of concomitant medications metabolized by these pathways (Table 18-4). However, *in vitro* assays for inhibition of other P450 isoforms by nelfinavir (CYP2C9, CYP2C8, CYP2E1, CYP2C19, CYP2D6, CYP1A2) suggests that *in vivo* effects

Pharmacologic Interactions with Nelfinavir

Table 18-4

Co-Administered Drug	Effect on Co-Administered Drug AUC	Effect on Nelfinavir AUC	Comments
Antiretrovirals			
Nevirapine	No change	Increase by 8%	
Efavirenz	No change	Increase by 20%	
Saquinavir	Increase by 392%	Increase by 18%	Use with caution, consider TDM
Indinavir[a]	Increase by 11%	Increase by 21%	
Ritonavir[b]	No change	Increase by 20% (39%)	
Lopinavir	No data	No data	Levels of NFV likely to increase (presumed)
Amprenavir	Increase by 107%	No change	Use with caution, consider TDM
Atazanavir[c]	No data	No data	No change in NFV levels (presumed)
Tipranavir	No data	No data	—
Antifungals			
Fluconazole	No change	No change	—
Caspofungin	No change	No change	
Voriconazole	Increase (presumed)	Increase (presumed)	Use with caution and monitor for toxicities
Antimycobacterials			
Rifabutin	Increase by 207%	Decrease by 32%[d]	Use 150 mg qd or 300 mg thrice-weekly
Rifampin	No data	Decrease by 82%	Avoid concomitant use
Clarithromycin	No data	No data	
Lipid-Lowering Agents			
Simvastatin and Lovastatin	Increase by 506%	No change	Avoid concomitant use
Atorvastatin	Increase by 74%	No change	Start at lowest dose
Psychotropic Agents			
Buproprion	Increase	No change	Potential seizure risk at higher doses
Fluoxetine	No change (presumed)	Slight increase (presumed)	
Midazolam and Triazolam			Avoid concomitant use
Phenytoin	Decrease by 20–40%	Decrease (presumed)	Monitor anticonvulsant levels; consider TDM for NFV
Carbamazepine	No data	Decrease (presumed)	Monitor anticonvulsant levels; consider TDM for NFV
Miscellaneous			
Sildenafil	Increase by two- to 11-fold	No change	Start with reduced dose
Ethinyl estradiol	Decrease by 47%	No data	Use additional method
Methadone	Decrease by 43–51%	No change	Opiate withdrawal rare
St. John's wort			Avoid concomitant use
Ergotamine (various forms)			Avoid concomitant use

NFV, nelfinavir; TDM, therapeutic drug monitoring.

[a]Compared with historical data for indinavir 800 mg thrice daily and nelfinavir 750 mg twice daily.
[b]Ritonavir given as 100 mg (200 mg)/day.
[c]Atazanavir given as 400 mg/day without low-dose ritonavir.
[d]With nelfinavir given 750 mg thrice daily; no change if 1250 mg twice daily used.

are minimal and drugs metabolized by these enzymes are unlikely to be altered.[15]

Nelfinavir has been administered in combination with NRTIs, NNRTIs, and other PIs and in general has relatively few significant drug interactions with other antiretrovirals. Nucleoside analogs are not metabolized by CYP3A4, and co-administration of nelfinavir with 3TC, ZDV, d4T, tenofovir, or buffered ddI have no significant (≤35%) change in AUC or C_{max} of either the nucleoside analogs or nelfinavir.[77–79] Nevirapine and efavirenz likewise do not have clinically significant affects on nelfinavir concentrations.[80–83] In contrast, the effect of PI co-administration on nelfinavir metabolism depends on the relative potency of CYP3A4 inhibition. Combinations in which nelfinavir is the stronger inhibitor (i.e., combined with saquinavir, amprenavir, atazanavir, or indinavir) the companion PI levels are likely to increase with little change in nelfinavir concentrations. Alternatively, when nelfinavir is the weaker inhibitor (i.e., combined with ritonavir or lopinavir–ritonavir), its levels may be increased. For example, nelfinavir augments levels of soft gel saquinavir by 392% and amprenavir trough levels by 107%.[84,85] Concomitant indinavir 1200 mg twice daily and nelfinavir 1250 mg twice daily results in levels comparable to those achieved with indinavir at standard dosing (800 mg thrice daily) with no significant effect in nelfinavir levels.[86] Conversely, co-administration with low dose ritonavir at 100 and 200 mg does raise nelfinavir trough levels by 20% and 39%, respectively.[16]

Nelfinavir is a modest inhibitor of CYP3A4 and CYB2B6.[15,87] Terfenadine metabolite levels increase by almost 50% when co-administered with nelfinavir. This drug and other compounds metabolized by the CYP3A4 pathway (e.g., astemizole, cisapride, midazolam, and triazolam) should not be given with nelfinavir because of the potential for fatal cardiac arrhythmias or other adverse effects. Nelfinavir also increases rifabutin levels (207% increase in AUC). These increased levels of rifabutin are associated with a higher frequency of toxicities, such as uveitis. A 50% dose reduction of rifabutin is recommended when the drugs are given together. Dramatic elevations in simvastatin levels (506% increased AUC) and modest elevations in atorvastatin (74%) occur after nelfinavir dosing.[88] Atorvastatin should be used cautiously with nelfinavir, and simvastatin should not be used at all. *In vitro*, buproprion hydroxylation has been inhibited by nelfinavir via CYP2B6 inhibition.[87] Although the risk of seizures from buproprion increases with higher concentrations, these concerns have not yet been observed in clinical practice.[89] Fortunately, many antidepressants (including selective serotonin reuptake inhibitors and some tricyclic antidepressants) are primarily metabolized by CYP2D6 and are unlikely to have clinically significant interactions with nelfinavir.[90]

Nelfinavir can also increase the metabolism of several drugs. Co-administration can lower phenytoin levels resulting in recurrent seizures.[91] Similarly, levels of methadone may decrease necessitating an increase in methadone dose, but opiate withdrawal rarely occurs.[92] Due to induction of glucuronyl transferases, chronic dosing with nelfinavir leads to reduced (47% lower AUC) levels of ethinyl estradiol with no effect on norethindrone. Thus the dose of ethinyl estradiol may have to be increased with concurrent nelfinavir use, or a different form of contraception should be employed.

Drugs that induce the CYP3A4 enzyme can reduce plasma nelfinavir concentrations, resulting in subtherapeutic drug levels and increased risk of nelfinavir treatment failure. Rifampin is a potent inducer of CYP3A4, and multiple doses of rifampin lead to an 82% reduction (range 77–86%) in plasma nelfinavir concentrations. Rifampin should not be given with nelfinavir. Although not formally studied, it might be expected that carbamazepine, phenobarbital, and phenytoin would also lower plasma nelfinavir levels.

Some antifungals (e.g., ketoconazole and voriconazole) are inhibitors of CYP3A4 and can augment nelfinavir levels. Ketoconazole dosing increases nelfinavir levels by 35% (range 21–49%). Fluconazole is a weaker inhibitor of both CYP3A4 and CYP2C19 and results in a decrease in formation of the active metabolite M8, although the effect is unlikely to be clinically significant.[93] Co-administration of caspofungin and nelfinavir does not significantly alter the pharmacokinetics of caspofungin.[94] Finally, other drugs with less potent CYP3A4 inhibition, including macrolide antibiotics (erythromycin, clarithromycin), dapsone, and trimethoprim-sulfamethoxazole, should not affect nelfinavir concentrations.

RECOMMENDATIONS FOR USE

The recommendation for nelfinavir use as initial HIV therapy depends on the population to be treated. In nonpregnant adults, clinical trial data suggest that nelfinavir is a potent ARV agent, with 51–68% of ARV-naive patients achieving an undetectable level of HIV RNA (less than 500 copies/mL) that persists for 12 months when given in combination with two NRTIs. In these studies nelfinavir was comparable with fosamprenavir–ritonavir, unboosted-atazanavir, and nevirapine, but demonstrated less efficacy than lopinavir–ritonavir and efavirenz-based regimens. However, the modest minimum plasma concentration to 50% inhibitory concentration ratio and relative low genetic barrier to resistance raises concerns about the long-term efficacy of nelfinavir-based regimens. Indeed, nelfinavir was associated with twice the viral rebound rate in both therapy-naive and NRTI-experienced patients compared to those taking efavirenz-based regimens.[95] Further, the efficacy of nelfinavir is diminished in patients who have detectable plasma HIV RNA levels despite treatment with other PIs. Patients who failed treatment with one or more previous PIs often have reduced phenotypic susceptibility to nelfinavir (>70%), which limits the usefulness of this agent in salvage settings. Taken together, nelfinavir should not be used as first-line therapy or as salvage therapy in HIV-infected adults and should be reserved for those individuals unable to take NNRTIs or boosted-PI-based therapies.

In contrast, greater safety and pharmacokinetic data during pregnancy and in pediatric patients provides a rationale for nelfinavir use over newer (and potentially more potent) agents in these settings. The dose-response relationship of nelfinavir and the altered pharmacokinetics of these populations suggest that TDM may enhance nelfinavir response rates in these settings.

Nelfinavir has an excellent toxicity profile with mild to moderate diarrhea as the most common toxicity. Similar to other PIs, care must be taken to avoid potential drug interactions with compounds metabolized by CYP34A and CYP2C19. Although originally recommended for the treatment of HIV-infected adults at a dose of 750 mg (three 250 mg tablets) three times daily, it should now be dosed at 1250 mg (two 625 mg tablets) twice daily with a meal or a light snack to maximize bioavailability.

REFERENCES

1. Navia MA, Fitzgerald PM, McKeever BM, et al. Three-dimensional structure of aspartyl protease from human immunodeficiency virus HIV-1. Nature 337:615–20, 1989.
2. Roberts NA, Martin JA, Kinchington D, et al. Rational design of peptide-based HIV proteinase inhibitors. Science 248:358–61, 1990.
3. Appelt K, Bacquet RJ, Bartlett CA, et al. Design of enzyme inhibitors using iterative protein crystallographic analysis. J Med Chem 34:1925–34, 1991.
4. Gehlhaar DK, Verkhivker GM, Rejto PA, et al. Molecular recognition of the inhibitor AG-1343 by HIV-1 protease: conformationally flexible docking by evolutionary programming. Chem Biol 2:317–24, 1995.
5. Kohl NE, Emini EA, Schleif WA, et al. Active human immunodeficiency virus protease is required for viral infectivity. Proc Natl Acad Sci USA 85:4686–90, 1988.
6. Patick AK, Mo H, Markowitz M, et al. Antiviral and resistance studies of AG1343, an orally bioavailable inhibitor of human immunodeficiency virus protease. Antimicrob Agents Chemother 40:292–7, 1996.
7. Nunberg JH, Schleif WA, Boots EJ, et al. Viral resistance to human immunodeficiency virus type 1-specific pyridinone reverse transcriptase inhibitors. J Virol 65:4887–92, 1991.
8. Larder BA, Darby G, Richman DD. HIV with reduced sensitivity to zidovudine (AZT) isolated during prolonged therapy. Science 243:1731–34, 1989.
9. Agouron Pharmaceuticals Inc. Viracept (nelfinavir mesylate) tablets and oral powder: US prescribing information. Online. Available: http://www.pfizer.com 21 Nov 2005.
10. Kaeser B, Charoin JE, Gerber M, et al. Assessment of the bioequivalence of two nelfinavir tablet formulations under fed and fasted conditions in healthy subjects. Int J Clin Pharmacol Ther 43:154–62, 2005.
11. Regazzi MB, Seminari E, Villani P, et al. Nelfinavir suspension obtained from nelfinavir tablets has equivalent pharmacokinetic profile. J Chemother 13:569–74, 2001.
12. Zhang KE, Wu E, Patick AK, et al. Circulating metabolites of the human immunodeficiency virus protease inhibitor nelfinavir in humans: structural identification, levels in plasma, and antiviral activities. Antimicrob Agents Chemother 45:1086–93, 2001.
13. Aweeka F, Jayewardene A, Staprans S, et al. Failure to detect nelfinavir in the cerebrospinal fluid of HIV-1-infected patients with and without AIDS dementia complex. J Acquir Immune Defic Syndr Hum Retrovirol 20:39–43, 1999.
14. Solas C, Lafeuillade A, Halfon P, et al. Discrepancies between protease inhibitor concentrations and viral load in reservoirs and sanctuary sites in human immunodeficiency virus-infected patients. Antimicrob Agents Chemother 47:238–243, 2003.
15. Lillibridge JH, Liang BH, Kerr BM, et al. Characterization of the selectivity and mechanism of human cytochrome P450 inhibition by the human immunodeficiency virus-protease inhibitor nelfinavir mesylate. Drug Metab Dispos 26:609–16, 1998.
16. Kurowski M, Kaeser B, Sawyer A, et al. Low-dose ritonavir moderately enhances nelfinavir exposure. Clin Pharmacol Ther 72:123–32, 2002.
17. Scott RC, Greenberg DM, Frye J. Pharmacokinetics (PK) of nelfinavir (NFV) in African American and Caucasian HIV patients. In: Programs and Abstracts of the 40th Interscience Conference on Antimicrobial Agents and Chemotherapy, Toronto, Canada, 17–20 Sep 2000, abstract 1655.
18. Wyles DL, Gerber JG. Antiretroviral drug pharmacokinetics in hepatitis with hepatic dysfunction. Clin Infect Dis 40:174–81, 2005.
19. Regazzi M, Maserati R, Villani P, et al. Clinical pharmacokinetics of nelfinavir and its metabolite M8 in human immunodeficiency virus (HIV)-positive and HIV-hepatitis C virus-coinfected subjects. Antimicrob Agents Chemother 49:643–9, 2005.
20. Krogstad P, Wiznia A, Luzuriaga K, et al. Treatment of human immunodeficiency virus 1-infected infants and children with the protease inhibitor nelfinavir mesylate. Clin Infect Dis 28:1109–18, 1999.
21. Mirochnick M, Stek A, Acevedo M, et al. Safety and pharmacokinetics of nelfinavir coadministered with zidovudine and lamivudine in infants during the first 6 weeks of life. J Acquir Immune Defic Syndr 39:189–94, 2005.
22. Capparelli EV, Sullivan JL, Mofenson L, et al. Pharmacokinetics of nelfinavir in human immunodeficiency virus-infected infants. Pediatr Infect Dis J 20:746–51, 2001.
23. van Heeswijk RP, Khaliq Y, Gallicano KD, et al. The pharmacokinetics of nelfinavir and M8 during pregnancy and post partum. Clin Pharmacol Ther 76:588–97, 2004.
24. Johnson M, Nelson M, Peters B, et al. A comparison of BID and TID dosing of nelfinavir mesylate when given in combination with stavudine (d4T) and lamivudine (3TC) for up to 48 weeks. In: Programs and Abstracts of the 38th Interscience Conference on Antimicrobial Agents and Chemotherapy, San Diego, CA, 24–27 Sep 1998, abstract I-216.
25. Saag MS, Tebas P, Sension M, et al. Randomized, double-blind comparison of two nelfinavir doses plus nucleosides in HIV-infected patients (Agouron study 511). AIDS 15:1971–8, 2001.
26. Gathe JC Jr, Ive P, Wood R, et al. SOLO: 48-week efficacy and safety comparison of once-daily fosamprenavir/ritonavir versus twice-daily nelfinavir in naive HIV-1-infected patients. AIDS 18:1529–37, 2004.
27. Murphy RL, Sanne I, Cahn P, et al. Dose-ranging, randomized, clinical trial of atazanavir with lamivudine and stavudine in antiretroviral-naive subjects: 48-week results. AIDS 17:2603–14, 2003.
28. Walmsley S, Bernstein B, King M, et al. Lopinavir–ritonavir versus nelfinavir for the initial treatment of HIV infection. N Engl J Med 346:2039–46, 2002.
29. Sax PE, Kumar P. Tolerability and safety of HIV protease inhibitors in adults. J Acquir Immune Defic Syndr 37:1111–24, 2004.
30. Bozzette SA, Ake CF, Tam HK, et al. Cardiovascular and cerebrovascular events in patients treated for human immunodeficiency virus infection. N Engl J Med 348:702–10, 2003.
31. Rodriguez-French A, Boghossian J, Gray GE, et al. The NEAT study: a 48-week open-label study to compare the antiviral efficacy and safety of GW433908 versus nelfinavir in antiretroviral therapy-naive HIV-1-infected patients. J Acquir Immune Defic Syndr 35:22–32, 2004.
32. Moyle GJ, Youle M, Higgs C, et al. Safety, pharmacokinetics, and antiretroviral activity of the potent, specific human immunodeficiency virus protease inhibitor nelfinavir: results of a phase I/II trial and extended follow-up in patients infected with human immunodeficiency virus. J Clin Pharmacol 38:736–43, 1998.
33. Markowitz M, Conant M, Hurley A, et al. A preliminary evaluation of nelfinavir mesylate, an inhibitor of human immunodeficiency virus (HIV)-1 protease, to treat HIV infection. J Infect Dis 177:1533–40, 1998.
34. Powderly WG, Sension MG, Conant M, et al. The efficacy of viracept (nelfinavir mesylate, NFV) in pivotal phase II/III double-blind randomized controlled trials as monotherapy and in combination with d4T or AZT/3TC. In: Programs and Abstracts of the 4th Conference on Retroviruses and Opportunistic Infections, Washington, DC, 22–26 Jan 1997, abstract 370.
35. Podzamczer D, Ferrer E, Consiglio E, et al. A randomized clinical trial comparing nelfinavir or nevirapine associated to zidovudine/lamivudine in HIV-infected naive patients (the Combine Study). Antivir Ther 7:81–90, 2002.

36. Robbins GK, De Gruttola V, Shafer RW, et al. Comparison of sequential three-drug regimens as initial therapy for HIV-1 infection. N Engl J Med 349:2293–303, 2003.
37. Gulick RM, Hu XJ, Fiscus SA, et al. Randomized study of saquinavir with ritonavir or nelfinavir together with delavirdine, adefovir, or both in human immunodeficiency virus-infected adults with virologic failure on indinavir: AIDS Clinical Trials Group Study 359. J Infect Dis 182:1375–84, 2000.
38. Casado JL, Dronda F, Hertogs K, et al. Efficacy, tolerance, and pharmacokinetics of the combination of stavudine, nevirapine, nelfinavir, and saquinavir as salvage regimen after ritonavir or indinavir failure. AIDS Res Hum Retroviruses 17:93–8, 2001.
39. Albrecht MA, Bosch RJ, Hammer SM, et al. Nelfinavir, efavirenz, or both after the failure of nucleoside treatment of HIV infection. N Engl J Med 345:398–407, 2001.
40. Roca B, Gomez CJ, Arnedo A. A randomized, comparative study of lamivudine plus stavudine, with indinavir or nelfinavir, in treatment-experienced HIV-infected patients. AIDS 14:157–61, 2000.
41. Haubrich RH, Kemper CA, Hellmann NS, et al. The clinical relevance of non-nucleoside reverse transcriptase inhibitor hypersusceptibility: a prospective cohort analysis. AIDS 16: F33–40, 2002.
42. Department of Health and Human Services (US). Recommendations for use of antiretroviral drugs in pregnant HIV-1-infected women for maternal health and interventions to reduce perinatal HIV-1 transmission in the United States. Online. Available: http://aidsinfo.nih.gov/ContentFiles/PerinatalGL.pdf 9 Jan 2006.
43. Department of Health and Human Services (US). Guidelines for the use of antiretroviral agents in pediatric HIV infection. Online. Available: http://aidsinfo.nih.gov/ContentFiles/PediatricGuidelines.pdf 9 Jan 2006.
44. Reiss G, O'Brien M, Kopicko J, et al. Lack of association between pregnancy and selected gastrointestinal adverse events among women prescribed nelfinavir. J Acquir Immune Defic Syndr 26:513–4, 2001.
45. Timmermans S, Tempelman C, Godfried MH, et al. Nelfinavir and nevirapine side effects during pregnancy. AIDS 19:795–9, 2005.
46. Marzolini C, Rudin C, Decosterd LA, et al. Transplacental passage of protease inhibitors at delivery. AIDS 16:889–93, 2002.
47. Mirochnick M, Dorenbaum A, Holland D, et al. Concentrations of protease inhibitors in cord blood after in utero exposure. Pediatr Infect Dis J 21:835–8, 2002.
48. Watts DH, Covington DL, Beckerman K, et al. Assessing the risk of birth defects associated with antiretroviral exposure during pregnancy. Am J Obstet Gynecol 191:985–92, 2004.
49. Nellen JF, Schillevoort I, Wit FW, et al. Nelfinavir plasma concentrations are low during pregnancy. Clin Infect Dis 39:736–40, 2004.
50. Burger DM, Grintjes KJ, Lotgering FK, et al. Therapeutic drug monitoring of nelfinavir in pregnancy: a case report. Ther Drug Monit 26:576–8, 2004.
51. Angel JB, Khaliq Y, Monpetit ML, et al. An argument for routine therapeutic drug monitoring of HIV-1 protease inhibitors during pregnancy. AIDS 15:417–9, 2001.
52. Comparison of dual nucleoside-analogue reverse-transcriptase inhibitor regimens with and without nelfinavir in children with HIV-1 who have not previously been treated: the PENTA 5 randomised trial. Lancet 359:733–40, 2002.
53. Krogstad P, Lee S, Johnson G, et al. Nucleoside-analogue reverse-transcriptase inhibitors plus nevirapine, nelfinavir, or ritonavir for pretreated children infected with human immunodeficiency virus type 1. Clin Infect Dis 34:991–1001, 2002.
54. Funk MB, Linde R, Wintergerst U, et al. Preliminary experiences with triple therapy including nelfinavir and two reverse transcriptase inhibitors in previously untreated HIV-infected children. AIDS 13:1653–8, 1999.
55. Luzuriaga K, McManus M, Mofenson L, et al. A trial of three antiretroviral regimens in HIV-1-infected children. N Engl J Med 350:2471–80, 2004.
56. Floren LC, Wiznia A, Hayashi S, et al. Nelfinavir pharmacokinetics in stable human immunodeficiency virus-positive children: Pediatric AIDS Clinical Trials Group Protocol 377. Pediatrics 112:e220–7, 2003.
57. Haas DW, Smeaton LM, Shafer RW, et al. Pharmacogenetics of long-term responses to antiretroviral regimens containing efavirenz and/or nelfinavir: an Adult Aids Clinical Trials Group Study. J Infect Dis 192:1931–42, 2005.
58. Le Moing V, Peytavin G, Journot V, et al. Plasma levels of indinavir and nelfinavir at time of virologic response may have a different impact on the risk of further virologic failure in HIV-infected patients. J Acquir Immune Defic Syndr 34:497–9, 2003.
59. Burger DM, Hugen PW, Aarnoutse RE, et al. Treatment failure of nelfinavir-containing triple therapy can largely be explained by low nelfinavir plasma concentrations. Ther Drug Monit 25:73–80, 2003.
60. Burger DM, Bergshoeff AS, De Groot R, et al. Maintaining the nelfinavir trough concentration above 0.8 mg/L improves virologic response in HIV-1-infected children. J Pediatr 145:403–405, 2004.
61. Marzolini C, Buclin T, Decosterd LA, et al. Nelfinavir plasma levels under twice-daily and three-times-daily regimens: high interpatient and low intrapatient variability. Ther Drug Monit 23:394–8, 2001.
62. Burger D, Hugen P, Reiss P, et al. Therapeutic drug monitoring of nelfinavir and indinavir in treatment-naive HIV-1-infected individuals. AIDS 17:1157–65, 2003.
63. Powderly WG, Saag MS, Chapman S, et al. Predictors of optimal virological response to potent antiretroviral therapy. AIDS 13:1873–80, 1999.
64. Editorial Board of HIVpharmacology.com. Optimising TDM in HIV clinical care. A practical guide to performing therapeutic drug monitoring (TDM) for antiretroviral agents. Online. Available: www.HIVpharmacology.com 21 Dec 2005.
65. MacManus S, Yates PJ, Elston RC, et al. GW433908/ritonavir once daily in antiretroviral therapy-naive HIV-infected patients: absence of protease resistance at 48 weeks. AIDS 18:651–5, 2004.
66. Kempf DJ, King MS, Bernstein B, et al. Incidence of resistance in a double-blind study comparing lopinavir/ritonavir plus stavudine and lamivudine to nelfinavir plus stavudine and lamivudine. J Infect Dis 189:51–60, 2004.
67. Patick AK, Duran M, Cao Y, et al. Genotypic and phenotypic characterization of human immunodeficiency virus type 1 variants isolated from patients treated with the protease inhibitor nelfinavir. Antimicrob Agents Chemother 42:2637–44, 1998.
68. Pellegrin I, Breilh D, Montestruc F, et al. Virologic response to nelfinavir-based regimens: pharmacokinetics and drug resistance mutations (VIRAPHAR study). AIDS 16:1331–40, 2002.
69. Tebas P, Patick AK, Kane EM, et al. Virologic responses to a ritonavir–saquinavir-containing regimen in patients who had previously failed nelfinavir. AIDS 13:F23–8, 1999.
70. Kemper CA, Witt MD, Keiser PH, et al. Sequencing of protease inhibitor therapy: insights from an analysis of HIV phenotypic resistance in patients failing protease inhibitors. AIDS 15:609–615, 2001.
71. Haas DW, Zala C, Schrader S, et al. Therapy with atazanavir plus saquinavir in patients failing highly active antiretroviral therapy: a randomized comparative pilot trial. AIDS 17:1339–49, 2003.
72. Cohen C, Nieto-Cisneros L, Zala C, et al. Comparison of atazanavir with lopinavir/ritonavir in patients with prior protease

inhibitor failure: a randomized multinational trial. Curr Med Res Opin 21:1683–92, 2005.
73. Walmsley SL, Becker MI, Zhang M, et al. Predictors of virological response in HIV-infected patients to salvage antiretroviral therapy that includes nelfinavir. Antivir Ther 6:47–54, 2001.
74. Dronda F, Casado JL, Moreno S, et al. Phenotypic cross-resistance to nelfinavir: the role of prior antiretroviral therapy and the number of mutations in the protease gene. AIDS Res Hum Retroviruses 17:211–5, 2001.
75. Turner D, Schapiro JM, Brenner BG, et al. The influence of protease inhibitor resistance profiles on selection of HIV therapy in treatment-naive patients. Antivir Ther 9:301–14, 2004.
76. Molla A, Vasavanonda S, Kumar G, et al. Human serum attenuates the activity of protease inhibitors toward wild-type and mutant human immunodeficiency virus. Virology 250:255–62, 1998.
77. Boffito M, Pozniak A, Kearney BP, et al. Lack of pharmacokinetic drug interaction between tenofovir disoproxil fumarate and nelfinavir mesylate. Antimicrob Agents Chemother 49:4386–9, 2005.
78. Skowron G, Leoung G, Hall DB, et al. Pharmacokinetic evaluation and short-term activity of stavudine, nevirapine, and nelfinavir therapy in HIV-1-infected adults. J Acquir Immune Defic Syndr 35:351–8, 2004.
79. Elion R, Kaul S, Knupp C, et al. The safety profile and antiviral activity of the combination of stavudine, didanosine, and nelfinavir in patients with HIV infection. Clin Ther 21:1853–63, 1999.
80. Regazzi MB, Villani P, Maserati R, et al. Clinical pharmacokinetics of nelfinavir combined with efavirenz and stavudine during rescue treatment of heavily pretreated HIV-infected patients. J Antimicrob Chemother 45:343–7, 2000.
81. Skowron G, Leoung G, Kerr B, et al. Lack of pharmacokinetic interaction between nelfinavir and nevirapine. AIDS 12:1243–4, 1998.
82. Pfister M, Labbe L, Hammer SM, et al. Population pharmacokinetics and pharmacodynamics of efavirenz, nelfinavir, and indinavir: Adult AIDS Clinical Trial Group Study 398. Antimicrob Agents Chemother 47:130–7, 2003.
83. Villani P, Regazzi MB, Castelli F, et al. Pharmacokinetics of efavirenz (EFV) alone and in combination therapy with nelfinavir (NFV) in HIV-1 infected patients. Br J Clin Pharmacol 48:712–5, 1999.
84. Kravcik S, Sahai J, Kerr B, et al. Nelfinavir mesylate (NFV) increases saquinavir-soft gel capsule (SQV-SGC) exposure in HIV+ patients. In: Programs and Abstracts of the 4th Conference on Retroviruses and Opportunistic Infections, Washington, DC, 22–26 Jan 1997, abstract 371.
85. Morse GD, Rosenkranz S, Para MF, et al. Amprenavir and efavirenz pharmacokinetics before and after the addition of nelfinavir, indinavir, ritonavir, or saquinavir in seronegative individuals. Antimicrob Agents Chemother 49:3373–81, 2005.
86. Riddler SA, Havlir D, Squires KE, et al. Coadministration of indinavir and nelfinavir in human immunodeficiency virus type 1-infected adults: safety, pharmacokinetics, and antiretroviral activity. Antimicrob Agents Chemother 46:3877–82, 2002.
87. Hesse LM, von Moltke LL, Shader RI, et al. Ritonavir, efavirenz, and nelfinavir inhibit CYP2B6 activity in vitro: potential drug interactions with bupropion. Drug Metab Dispos 29:100–2, 2001.
88. Hsyu PH, Schultz-Smith MD, Lillibridge JH, et al. Pharmacokinetic interactions between nelfinavir and 3-hydroxy-3-methylglutaryl coenzyme A reductase inhibitors atorvastatin and simvastatin. Antimicrob Agents Chemother 45:3445–50, 2001.
89. Park-Wyllie LY, Antoniou T. Concurrent use of bupropion with CYP2B6 inhibitors, nelfinavir, ritonavir and efavirenz: a case series. AIDS 17:638–40, 2003.
90. Tseng AL, Foisy MM. Significant interactions with new antiretrovirals and psychotropic drugs. Ann Pharmacother 33:461–73, 1999.
91. Honda M, Yasuoka A, Aoki M, et al. A generalized seizure following initiation of nelfinavir in a patient with human immunodeficiency virus type 1 infection, suspected due to interaction between nelfinavir and phenytoin. Intern Med 38:302–303, 1999.
92. Hsyu PH, Lillibridge J, Daniels E, et al. Pharmacokinetic interaction of nelfinavir and methadone in intravenous drug users. Biopharm Drug Dispos 27:61–8, 2005.
93. Jackson KA, Rosenbaum SE, Kerr BM, et al. A population pharmacokinetic analysis of nelfinavir mesylate in human immunodeficiency virus-infected patients enrolled in a phase III clinical trial. Antimicrob Agents Chemother 44:1832–7, 2000.
94. Stone JA, Migoya EM, Hickey L, et al. Potential for interactions between caspofungin and nelfinavir or rifampin. Antimicrob Agents Chemother 48:4306–14, 2004.
95. Smith CJ, Phillips AN, Hill T, et al. The rate of viral rebound after attainment of an HIV load <50 copies/mL according to specific antiretroviral drugs in use: results from a multicenter cohort study. J Infect Dis 192:1387–97, 2005.

Chapter 19

Fosamprenavir and Amprenavir

Roger Paredes, MD, Lidia Ruiz, PhD, Bonaventura Clotet, MD, PhD

INTRODUCTION

Protease inhibitors (PIs) are one of the mainstays of HIV/AIDS therapy,[1] being largely responsible for the extraordinary health status improvements witnessed during the last decade in HIV-infected persons who had access to therapy.[2,3] The introduction of PIs transformed the natural history of HIV infection. Fifteen years after the description of the first AIDS cases,[4–6] PI-based therapy was the first strategy able to slow down and even reverse HIV infection progression toward severe co-morbidity, functional impairment and death. The advent of PIs in combination with two nucleoside-analog reverse transcriptase inhibitors (NRTI) led to the coining of the term "highly active antiretroviral therapy" (HAART)[7,8]; the concept that would later incorporate triple drug therapies based on non-nucleoside reverse transcriptase inhibitors (NNRTIs),[9,10] as well. The first generation of PIs exerted an unprecedented antiviral efficacy in combination with other drugs, being unambiguously clear that early PIs saved thousands of lives.[11,12] It is estimated that the increase in the use of lamivudine, indinavir, saquinavir, and ritonavir, drugs approved by the FDA in late 1995 and early 1996, was responsible for more than 90% of the drop in mortality rates from 1995 to 1998.[11] In addition, initial PI-based therapy was clearly a cost-effective strategy.[12] However, first generation PIs had four important limitations; a very high pill burden, frequent and sometimes severe or life-threatening toxicities, significant pharmacokinetic nuisances with multiple drugs, food and fluid interactions, and broad cross-family resistance, which constrained the administration of other PIs in second-line regimens.

Subsequent PI development has intended to overcome these limitations without compromising antiretroviral potency.[13] Modern PIs are even more potent than first generation PIs, but have a much more favorable adherence, tolerability, pharmacokinetic and resistance profiles. The strategy of boosting PI plasma levels with small doses of ritonavir has enabled further pharmacokinetic improvements such as once- or twice-daily administration, avoidance of food interactions and reduced pill dosing. Ritonavir boosting confers a significant enhancement to the PI resistance barrier as well. This is of clear clinical utility in first-line and salvage regimens alike, because it helps prevent the emergence of resistance and surpass acquired decreases in susceptibility. In addition, some modern PIs have particular resistance pathways, different from those of other drugs in the family. For instance, D30N mutation is characteristically selected during early nelfinavir failure in subjects infected with subtype B viruses.[14] In those with non-B viruses the first mutation is L90M.[15,16] Early atazanavir failure is due to the I50L mutation,[17] which decreases the susceptibility to atazanavir but is associated with hypersusceptibility to all other PIs. Similarly, the signature resistance mutation associated with amprenavir and fosamprenavir is I50V.[18,19] Early detection of virological failure with these PIs may permit the sequential use of other PIs in subsequent treatment lines, and this effectively widens the therapeutic arsenal against HIV infection.

Amprenavir (APV, Agenerase GlaxoSmithKline) is a PI with demonstrated antiviral efficacy and generally good tolerability when given in combination with other antiretroviral agents. It is a PI with a demonstrated antiviral efficacy and generally good tolerability when given in combination with other antiretroviral agents.[20] It also has a particular resistance profile,[20] which is different from other PIs and facilitates salvage therapy with other PIs if virological failure is detected before multiple resistance mutations accumulate. However, amprenavir has low water solubility and high lipophilicity, which results in highly variable oral bioavailability[21] and requirement of a large proportion of organic excipients to aid in gastric dissolution.[21] This, in turn, mandates a high pill burden (10 pills/day in ritonavir-boosted regimens, 16 in unboosted regimens),[22] which complicates adequate adherence and limits convenience.

Fosamprenavir (FPV, 908, Lexiva in the United States, Telzir in Canada and the European Union, GlaxoSmithKline and Vertex Pharmaceuticals)[18] is the calcium phosphate ester prodrug

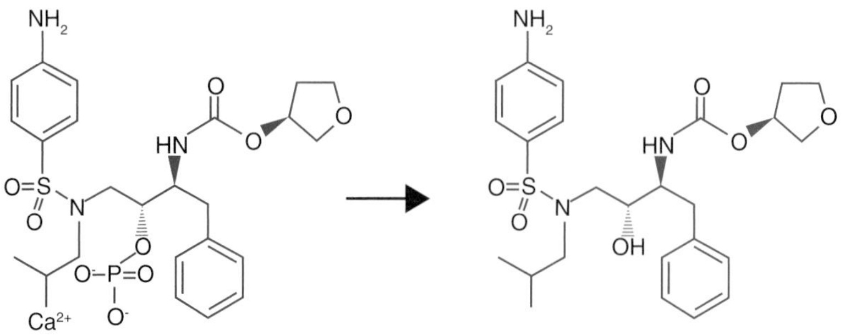

Fosamprenavir Amprenavir

Figure 19-1 ■ Structural formula of fosamprenavir (Lexiva, Telzir) and amprenavir (Agenerase).

of amprenavir (Agenerase, GlaxoSmithKline) (Fig. 19-1). Fosamprenavir was synthesized to increase the oral bioavailability of amprenavir, thus allowing a reduction in the pill burden and offering the potential for improved patient compliance. Fosamprenavir has several advantages over amprenavir, including a flexible qd dosing with ritonavir or bid dosing with or without ritonavir, a favorable tolerability profile, a low pill burden, absence of food or fluid restrictions, a particular resistance profile similar to amprenavir's and distinct from the other PIs, with I50V as the signature mutation, and demonstrated clinical efficacy in antiretroviral-naive subjects. Consequently, fosamprenavir has displaced amprenavir for the treatment of HIV-infected adults whereas amprenavir is still the treatment of choice in children. In 2005, the manufacturer of amprenavir ceased production of 150 mg capsules for adult use while the 50 mg pediatric capsule and the oral solution are still being manufactured. Studies of fosamprenavir in children are ongoing. It seems legitimate to predict that fosamprenavir will also displace amprenavir in the near future in the pediatric setting. Therefore, for the sake of clinical usefulness and durability of concepts discussed below, this chapter will focus mainly on fosamprenavir, highlighting the different aspects particular to amprenavir with respect to its prodrug, when necessary.

PHARMACOLOGY

Molecular Structure

Fosamprenavir calcium (Lexiva, Telzir) is a prodrug of the PI amprenavir (Agenerase). The chemical name of fosamprenavir calcium is (3*S*)-tetrahydrofuran-3-yl (1*S*,2*R*)-3-[[(4-aminophenyl) sulfonyl](isobutyl)amino]-1-benzyl-2-(phosphonooxy) propylcarbamate monocalcium salt. Fosamprenavir calcium is a single stereoisomer with the (3*S*)(1*S*,2*R*) configuration. The molecular formula is C25H34CaN3O9PS and has a molecular weight of 623.7. The chemical name of amprenavir is (3*S*)-tetrahydro-3-furyl*N*-[(1*S*,2*R*)-3-(4-amino-*N*isobuty lbenzenesulfonamido)-1-benzyl-2-hydroxypropyl] carbamate. Amprenavir is a single stereoisomer with the (3*S*)(1*S*,2*R*) configuration. Its molecular formula is C25H35N3O6S and has a molecular weight of 505.64. The structural formula of fosamprenavir and amprenavir is presented in Figure 19.1. Fosamprenavir and amprenavir are white to cream-colored solids with a solubility of ~0.31 and 0.04 mg/mL in water at 25°C, respectively.

Drug Forms

Fosamprenavir is commercialized in film-coated tablets for oral administration in strength of 700 mg of fosamprenavir calcium, which is equivalent to amprenavir 600 mg. Amprenavir is commercialized in two oral formulations for pediatric use: 50 mg capsules and oral solution. In 2005, amprenavir's manufacturer ceased the production of the 150 mg capsules for adult use. Amprenavir oral solution presents amprenavir solubilized with propylene glycol (Table 19-1),[18] which is a key dose-limiting factor of this presentation. The recommended daily dose of amprenavir oral solution is 22.5 mg/kg twice daily. This dose corresponds to a propylene glycol intake of 1650 mg kg^{-1} day^{-1}. Propylene glycol is a viscous, colorless liquid solvent used with many drugs with poor aqueous solubility.[23] Acceptable intake of propylene glycol for pharmaceuticals has not been established but it is known that high doses are toxic and may be especially harmful in children of age four or younger. Formerly considered safe, propylene glycol has been associated with hyperosmolality, anion gap metabolic acidosis, hemolysis, osmol gap, central nervous system depression, arrhythmias,[1,24–33] and, although less common, renal dysfunction.[34–37]

Mechanisms of Action

Amprenavir is a sulfonamide that inhibits the postranscriptional processing of Gag and Gag-Pol protein precursors, thereby arresting maturation of nascent virions and blocking their infectivity.[38–40] Amprenavir was specifically designed for anti-HIV activity and to enhance binding to the aspartate residues of the HIV-1 protease enzyme,[41] based on homology with cellular aspartyl protease[22,42] and with the aim of enhancing efficacy on viruses resistant to other PIs.[22,42] Amprenavir binds very specifically to HIV-1 and HIV-2 proteases. The inhibition constant, K_I, is 0.0003 μg/mL

Inactive Ingredients included in Fosamprenavir and Amprenavir Presentations

Table 19-1

Presentation	Inactive Ingredients
Fosamprenavir (per each 700 mg tablet)	Colloidal silicon dioxide, croscarmellose sodium, magnesium stearate, microcrystalline cellulose, and povidone K30. The tablet film coating contains hypromellose, iron oxide red, titanium dioxide, and triacetin.
Amprenavir 50 mg capsules (per each 50 mg capsule)	d-alpha tocopheryl polyethylene glycol 1000 succinate (TPGS), polyethylene glycol 400 246.7 mg, and propylene glycol 19 mg. The capsule shell contains the inactive ingredients d-sorbitol and sorbitans solution, gelatin, glycerin, and titanium dioxide. The soft gelatin capsules are printed with edible red ink. Each 50-mg amprenavir capsules contains 36.3 IU vitamin E in the form of TPGS. The total amount of vitamin E in the recommended daily adult dose of 50 mg amprenavir capsules is 1744 IU.
Amprenavir oral solution (per 1 mL)	Acesulfame potassium, artificial grape bubblegum flavor, citric acid (anhydrous) d-alpha tocopheryl polyethylene glycol 1000 succinate (TPGS), menthol, natural peppermint flavor, polyethylene glycol 400 (170 mg), propylene glycol (550 mg), saccharin sodium, sodium chloride, and sodium citrate (dihydrate). Each mL of amprenavir oral solution contains 46 IU vitamin E in the form of TPGS.

Adapted from GlaxoSmithKline. Lexiva (fosamprenavir calcium) tablets: prescribing information (US). Online. Available: http://us.gsk.com/products/assets/us_lexiva.pdf. 10 Feb 2006.

(0.6 nM) for HIV-1 and 0.0096 μg/μL (19 nM) for HIV-2 in acutely and chronically infected cells,[20,43] whereas it is higher than 0.885 μg/mL (1750 nmol/L) for human proteases.[20,43] Like other PIs, amprenavir is inactive or only weakly active against human aspartyl proteases such as renin, pepsin, and cathepsin.[38–40]

In Vitro Activity

Fosamprenavir has virtually no antiviral activity *in vitro*. The *in vitro* antiviral activity observed with fosamprenavir is due to the presence of trace amounts of amprenavir.[18] Amprenavir has a relatively high protease-binding affinity compared to other members of its class because it is more compact and has a molecular backbone that may minimize the intermolecular strain upon binding with the HIV protease. This favors tighter, more specific interaction with the catalytic aspartic acid residues and enzyme flaps. Amprenavir is highly lipophilic and rapidly accumulates within CD4+ T lymphocytes in a concentration-dependent manner. Intracellular concentrations are four times higher than extracellular concentrations, which is attributable to cytosolic protein binding. Amprenavir inhibits the HIV-1 and HIV-2 proteases competitively, with K_I values of 0.60 and 19 nM, respectively. The compound is highly selective (>5000-fold) for HIV protease versus human aspartic proteases such as renin, pepsin, and cathepsin, which have K_I values of 1750 nM, 3200 nM, and more than 10 000 nM, respectively; and it has low median cytotoxicity ($TC_{50} > 50\,\mu M$) across a wide panel of human cell lines.

Amprenavir has a potent *in vitro* antiviral activity, as evaluated against HIV-1 IIIB in both acutely and chronically infected lymphoblastic cell lines (MT-4, CEM-CCRF, H9) and in peripheral blood lymphocytes. The 50% inhibitory concentration (IC_{50}) of amprenavir ranged from 0.012 to 0.08 μM in acutely infected cells and was 0.41 μM in chronically infected cells (1 μM = 0.50 mcg/mL). Several experiments indicate that protein binding should not significantly alter the antiviral activity of amprenavir.[44] The projected minimum drug concentration, corrected for plasma protein binding, exceeded the IC_{90} of wild type HIV-1 by at least 15-fold.[45] *In vitro*, amprenavir exhibits synergistic anti-HIV-1 activity with abacavir, didanosine, zidovudine saquinavir, and additive anti-HIV-1 activity in combination with indinavir, nelfinavir, and ritonavir.[18]

Amprenavir inhibits *Giardia lamblia* at 5 μg/mL. No activity has been demonstrated against other protozoans, fungi, or bacteria, herpes simplex viruses 1 and 2, varicella-zoster virus, human cytomegalovirus, coronavirus, yellow fever virus, respiratory syncytial virus, rotavirus, influenza A virus, or rhinovirus at concentrations up to and including 100 μM. In addition, amprenavir showed no activity against human coronavirus protease or in a human papillomavirus DNA replication assay.[18,44]

Pharmacokinetics

Fosamprenavir is quickly hydrolyzed by hydrolases in intestinal epithelial cells (presumably by alkaline phosphatase[46]) into its active metabolite, amprenavir, plus an inorganic phosphate.[41] Amprenavir is rapidly absorbed into the blood with virtually no fosamprenavir available systemically thereafter.[41] Preclinical studies suggest that fosamprenavir is completely converted to amprenavir and is not absorbed.[47] Understandably, the pharmacokinetic properties of fosamprenavir and amprenavir are identical beyond this point. Both fosamprenavir and amprenavir are usually given with small doses of ritonavir. This factor modifies the pharmacokinetics

Table 19-2

Mean Pharmacokinetic Parameters of Amprenavir after Single-dose Administration of Fosamprenavir (FPV) or Amprenavir (APV) to Healthy Adult Volunteers or Adults with HIV Infection

Participants (no.)	Treatment regimen	AUC_∞ ($\mu g \times h^{-1}/mL^{-1}$)	C_{max} ($\mu g/mL$)	t_{max} (h)[a]	$t_{1/2}$ (h)
Healthy adult volunteers[63] (31)	FPV 1400 mg (2 × 700 mg tablets) fasted	19.05	4.26	1.5	
	FPV 1400 mg (2 × 700 mg tablets) fed[b]	19.37	4.51	2.0	
Adults with HIV infection[21,c] (53)	FPV 1395 mg (3 × 465 mg tablets)	22.8	4.64	2.5	7.7
	FPV 1860 mg (4 × 465 mg tablets)	42.3	7.94	2.0	7.9
	APV 1200 mg (8 × 150 mg capsules)	24.6	7.19	1.3	9.6

AUC_∞, area under the plasma amprenavir concentration–time curve from zero to infinity;
C_{max}, maximum plasma amprenavir concentration; $t_{1/2}$, elimination half-life; T_{max}, time to C_{max}.

[a] Median values.

[b] Patients received FPV with a standard high-fat meal.

[c] All patients also received abacavir 300 mg and lamivudine 150 mg twice daily.

Adapted from Chapman TM, Plosker GL, Perry CM. Fosamprenavir: a review of its use in the management of antiretroviral therapy-naive patients with HIV infection. Drugs 64:2101–2124, 2004.

of the active moiety amprenavir (Table 19-2), permits higher trough levels (which are associated with increased suppression of viral replication), lower peak levels (which reduces toxicity), and much lower pill burden and less frequent dosing intervals (which improves adherence).

Absorption

The median T_{max} of amprenavir, given as fosamprenavir, is 2.5 h (ranging between 1.5 and 4 h) whereas, when given as amprenavir, the T_{max} is between 1 and 2 h. The absorption of fosamprenavir is not affected by food. Conversely, amprenavir may be taken with or without food, but not with high-fat meals because high fat intake decreases the absorption of this drug moderately. The absolute bioavailability of amprenavir after administration of fosamprenavir has not been established.[18] The bioavailability and $t_{1/2}$ of amprenavir appears to be highly variable between patients (30–90% and 2–10 h, respectively).[41] When amprenavir is combined with ritonavir, the interindividual variations are decreased.[19] However, the relative bioavailability of amprenavir oral solution is 14% lower than that of the capsule presentation. Therefore, the recommended dose of the oral solution per body mass index is 11% higher than that for capsules.

Distribution

The first pass of amprenavir is less important than with other PIs.[19] After administration of amprenavir, the apparent volume of distribution of the drug is ~430 L in healthy adults. About 90% of amprenavir is bound to plasma proteins, primarily to α_1-acid glycoprotein. Although albumin concentrations are relatively stable among individuals, variations in α_1-acid glycoprotein concentrations may fluctuate widely and are a significant predictor of amprenavir apparent total clearance.[48] It has been suggested that differences seen in amprenavir pharmacokinetics could be due to variable α_1-acid glycoprotein concentrations *in vivo*. However, α_1-acid increases in glycoprotein concentration could also affect the intracellular concentration of PIs and, consequently, their antiviral efficacy.[49] The unbound fraction of amprenavir remains unchanged when ritonavir is added. Concentration-dependent binding was seen *in vitro* over the concentration range of 1–10 mcg/mL, with decreased binding at higher concentrations. As commented above, several experiments indicate that protein binding does not significantly alter the antiviral activity of amprenavir.[44]

Metabolism

Fosamprenavir is rapidly and almost completely hydrolyzed to amprenavir and inorganic phosphate in the gut epithelium, during absorption and before reaching the systemic circulation. Amprenavir is metabolized in the liver by the cytochrome P450 3A4 (CYP3A4) enzyme system and, to a lesser extent, by CYP2D6, CYP2C9, and CYP2C19,[44] resulting in two major metabolites from oxidation of the tetrahydrofuran and aniline moieties. Glucuronide conjugates of oxidized metabolites can be seen as minor metabolites in urine and feces. Approximately 75% and 14% of a single ^{14}C-labeled amprenavir dose was detected as metabolites in feces and urine, respectively.[43]

Elimination

The plasma elimination half-life of amprenavir is ~7.7 h.[18] Amprenavir is mostly eliminated in the feces after being metabolized into two major metabolites. Virtually no unchanged amprenavir is seen in feces. Less than 1% of the administered dose is seen in urine as unchanged amprenavir.

Pharmacokinetics in Special Populations

The pharmacokinetics of amprenavir after the administration of fosamprenavir or amprenavir have only been studied in asymptomatic adult HIV-infected patients and in healthy volunteers. Contrary to amprenavir, fosamprenavir has not been studied in patients with hepatic insufficiency. After the administration of 600 mg of amprenavir, the drugs AUC was greater in patients with moderate and severe cirrhosis compared to healthy volunteers. No pharmacokinetic differences have been observed according to gender or race in either fosamprenavir or amprenavir presentations. It is important to note that amprenavir pharmacokinetics have not been studied in patients with renal insufficiency or in people older than 65 years of age. Due to its practically nil renal elimination, this should not be a major limitation for administering fosamprenavir or amprenavir in patients with renal failure. Conversely, caution is recommended if these drugs need to be administered in elder patients.

Pharmacokinetics of fosamprenavir have not been studied in children. However, amprenavir pharmacokinetics are being investigated in the pediatric population. A phase I, open label, dose-escalating trial in 20 HIV-infected children 4 to 12 years of age,[50] evaluated four amprenavir doses of 5, 10, 15, and 20 mg/kg of body weight, administered as soft gelatin capsules. Amprenavir was rapidly absorbed, with a mean time to maximum concentration (T_{max}) occurring 0.95 to 1.58 h after dosing. The area under the concentration-time curve ($AUC_{0\rightarrow\infty}$) was dose proportional, and the mean maximum plasma concentration (C_{max}) increased linearly in a less than dose-proportional manner. Amprenavir was eliminated relatively slowly, with a mean terminal-phase half-life ($t_{1/2}$) of 6.17–8.28 h. The $t_{1/2}$, apparent total clearance and apparent volume of distribution during the elimination phase were dose independent. Considerable interpatient variability was seen for all pharmacokinetic parameters of amprenavir. The results of this study suggested that 20 mg/kg of amprenavir administered twice a day should be used in future pediatric studies. Of note, amprenavir capsules and oral solution are not interchangeable on a milligram-per-milligram basis. Also, oral solution is contraindicated in children below the age of 4 years because of the potential toxic effects of the excipient propylene glycol.[18]

Food Interactions

No significant food interactions occur with fosamprenavir or amprenavir and both drugs may be taken with or without food. However, amprenavir should preferably not be taken together with high-fat meals because they may moderately reduce the overall absorption of this drug.

Drug Interactions

Amprenavir is metabolized by, inhibits, and may induce the CYP3A4 pathway. Both fosamprenavir and amprenavir have the potential to interact with other drugs that are inducers, substrates or inhibitors of this enzyme system.[43,18] In clinical practice, fosamprenavir is usually co-administered with small doses of ritonavir with the purpose of boosting amprenavir plasma concentrations. Even at these small doses, ritonavir is a potent inhibitor of the cytochrome P450 enzyme complex, thus playing an additional role in drug–drug interactions seen with fosamprenavir. In patients receiving ritonavir-boosted fosamprenavir, it is advisable to consider ritonavir's particular interaction profile in addition to that of amprenavir.

Interactions with other PIs

Given that other PIs also inhibit the cytochrome P450, co-administration of amprenavir or fosamprenavir with other PIs will have an effect on both compounds depending on the relative effect of the co-administered drugs on CYP450 and on the particular dosing intervals of each PI. Some interactions may be of clinical benefit, whereas others are clearly detrimental. Whereas co-administration of fosamprenavir with ritonavir has the clinical purpose of boosting fosamprenavir levels and is useful at all stages of therapy, combinations of fosamprenavir/ritonavir plus another PI (the so-called double-boosted PIs) deserve special interest in salvage therapy.

1. *Ritonavir*. Co-administration of ritonavir with fosamprenavir increases plasma amprenavir AUC by approximately twofold and plasma C_{min} by four- to sixfold, compared to values obtained when fosamprenavir is administered alone. Administration of fosamprenavir 700 mg twice daily with ritonavir 100 mg twice daily results in higher plasma amprenavir concentrations,[18] with protein adjusted median ratios of C_{min}/IC_{50} and C_{min}/IC_{95} of 21.7 (range 1.19–240) and 3.21 (range 0.26–30.0), respectively. This permits smaller pill burden and wider dosing intervals.
2. *Lopinavir/ritonavir*. The co-administration of fosamprenavir/ritonavir (700/100 mg bid) with lopinavir/ritonavir (400/100 mg bid) decreases the C_{min} of both drugs by 64% and 53%, respectively, and is associated with an increase in adverse effects. However, this was not translated into worse virological response than with each individual PI in a 24-week small randomized study.[51] Current recommendation is that lopinavir/ritonavir and fosamprenavir/ritonavir should not be co-administered.
3. *Atazanavir*. In the prospective, randomized open-label COL100683 Study,[52] fosamprenavir 1400 mg qd was co-administered with atazanavir 400 mg qd with adequate tolerance. Atazanavir significantly enhanced exposure of fosamprenavir (increase in AUC, C_{max} and C_{24} by 78%, 36%, and 283%, respectively), whereas atazanavir levels were reduced (decrease in AUC, C_{max}, and C_{24} by 33%, 30%, and 57%, respectively). Another study[53] suggested that a combination of atazanavir 150 or 200 mg twice daily and fosamprenavir 700 mg twice daily with low-dose ritonavir may offer adequate C_{min} values for both drugs and may be a viable option for some treatment-experienced patients. The clinical significance of these results remains uncertain until comparative clinical studies are available but this combination deserves further study, especially in the salvage therapy setting.
4. *Saquinavir*. In a study[54] that evaluated the steady-state pharmacokinetics of saquinavir 1000 mg twice daily

(bid) and fosamprenavir 700 mg bid administered with two different doses of ritonavir (100 and 200 mg bid) in HIV-1-infected subjects, the co-administration of fosamprenavir 700 mg bid with saquinavir/ritonavir 1000/100 mg bid resulted in a statistically nonsignificant decrease in saquinavir concentrations (by 14%, 9%, and 24%, for saquinavir $(AUC)_{0-12}$, C_{max}, and C_{trough}, respectively). This was compensated for by an increased ritonavir dose of 200 mg bid, which resulted in a statistically nonsignificant increase in saquinavir exposure compared with baseline. Amprenavir levels did not appear to be significantly influenced by co-administration of saquinavir with fosamprenavir. Fosamprenavir significantly reduced ritonavir exposure, but the increased ritonavir dose compensated for this interaction.

5. *Tipranavir*. The co-administration of tipranavir/ritonavir with amprenavir/ritonavir (600/100 mg bid) decreases amprenavir's AUC and C_{min} by 44% and 55% respectively. Scarce data are available regarding interactions between tipranavir and fosamprenavir. Therefore, it is not recommended to administer the two drugs together at present. However, the C_{min} of unboosted fosamprenavir (700 mg bid) can be increased 48% when co-administered with tipranavir/ritonavir (500 mg/200 mg bid) if fosamprenavir is given together with ritonavir twice daily as fosamprenavir 1400 mg/ritonavir 200 mg bid.[55] The feasibility of this strategy awaits direct clinical comparisons, and may be suitable in certain highly antiretroviral-experienced patients as a salvage approach.

Interactions with NNRTIs

NNRTIs are potent inducers of the CYP450 system, so co-administration of PIs with NNRTIs often leads to potent interactions with high interindividual variability and outcomes that are difficult to predict. Some authors advise for therapeutic drug monitoring (TDM) if PIs and NNRTIs are to be administered together, but the clinical benefit of that approach remains unclear.

1. *Nevirapine*. There are no pharmacokinetic data available with regard to the co-administration of fosamprenavir with nevirapine. Therefore, the current recommendation is to avoid using these two compounds together.
2. *Efavirenz*. Efavirenz (600 mg qd) decreases amprenavir's C_{min} by 36% when fosamprenavir/ritonavir is given at a dose of 1400/200 mg qd. In this situation, the dose of fosamprenavir/ritonavir should be adjusted to 1400/300 mg qd. Efavirenz had no significant effect on amprenavir plasma levels when the dose of fosamprenavir/ritonavir was 700/100 mg bid.[21]

Interactions with CCR5 Inhibitors

Fosamprenavir/ritonavir has no significant effect on the pharmacokinetics of vicriviroc/ritonavir. Plasma AUC and C_{max} of the CCR5 inhibitor vicriviroc, are comparable if this drug is given with ritonavir (100 mg bid) or with fosamprenavir/ritonavir (700 mg/100 mg bid).[56] Apparently, neither modification to vicriviroc dosing, nor TDM is needed when vicriviroc is added to a ritonavir-boosted fosamprenavir regimen. No information is yet available for other CCR5 inhibitors, nor for CXCR4 inhibitors.

Interactions with Non-Antiretrovirals

Most interactions with non-antiretroviral drugs have been described with amprenavir. Since fosamprenavir is quickly metabolized to amprenavir by intestinal hydrolases and then absorbed as amprenavir, it is assumed that virtually all interactions are common to both formulations. Drugs that reduce the intestinal absorption of amprenavir by altering the intestinal pH, like the antacids, or metabolic inducers like carbamazepine or phenytoin, reduce amprenavir plasma levels, leading to a decreased antiviral efficacy of this drug. Inhibitors of amprenavir's metabolism, like the CYP450 inhibitors, increase amprenavir plasma levels, therefore increasing its toxicity. On the other hand, amprenavir's inhibition of CYP450 increases plasma drug levels of benzodiazepines, psychoactive drugs, antiarrythmics, antihypertensives, prokinetics, antihistamines, HMG CoA reductase inhibitors, certain antibacterials, antimycobacterials, oral contraceptives and oral anticoagulants. This leads to an increase in frequency and intensity of their usual adverse events. In practice, fosamprenavir is usually co-administered with ritonavir. Therefore, additional interactions of ritonavir with other non-antiretroviral compounds must be expected, as well. Clinically significant drug interactions with amprenavir are summarized in Table 19-3.

DOSING

The production of amprenavir 150 mg capsules for adult use was discontinued in 2005 and, by the time of finishing this review, the Food and Drug Administration (FDA) was studying the indication of fosamprenavir in children below 16 years of age.[18] Fosamprenavir is currently indicated in adults and children of age 16 years or older, and is not approved by the FDA for treating younger children. It is legitimate to predict that the use of amprenavir would significantly recede in children below 16 years of age, was fosamprenavir approved for treating patients in this age range.

In HIV-infected adults and in children aged 16 years or older, as well as in children aged 13 years or older who weigh 50 kg or more, fosamprenavir is approved by the FDA given in combination with small doses of ritonavir once a day (fosamprenavir 1400 mg qd with ritonavir 200 mg qd) or twice a day (fosamprenavir 700 mg bid with ritonavir 100 mg bid). Twice-a-day dosing of fosamprenavir/ritonavir is the only dosing approved for PI-experienced patients. If fosamprenavir is to be given concomitantly with efavirenz, the dose of ritonavir should be increased to 300 mg (fosamprenavir 1400 mg qd + ritonavir 300 mg qd). The FDA

Clinically relevant Interactions of Fosamprenavir with Non-antiretroviral Drugs

Table 19-3

Family	Drugs	Reason
Drugs that are contraindicated with Fosamprenavir[a]		
Antiarrhythmics	Flecainide or Propafenone[b]	Risk of serious and life-threatening reactions (e.g., cardiac arrhythmias).
Ergot derivatives	Dihydroergotamine, Ergonovine, Ergotamine, Methylergonovine	Risk of serious and life-threatening reactions (e.g., ergot toxicity with peripheral vasospasm and acral ischemia).
Neuroleptics	Pimozide	Risk of serious and life-threatening reactions (e.g., cardiac arrhythmias).
Prokinetics	Cisapride	Risk of serious and life-threatening reactions (e.g., cardiac arrhythmias).
Benzodiazepines	Midazolam or Triazolam	Risk of serious and life-threatening reactions (e.g., prolonged or increased sedation or respiratory depression).
Drugs that should not be co-administered with Fosamprenavir		
Antimycobacterials	Rifampin	Reduces amprenavir plasma concentrations by 90% when administered with nonboosted fosamprenavir. Unknown pharmacokinetics when administered with ritonavir-boosted fosamprenavir.
HMG-CoA reductase inhibitors	Lovastatin and Simvastatin	Highly dependent on CYP3A4-mediated elimination. Amprenavir-mediated CYP3A4 inhibition increases risk of rhabdomyolysis and toxic myopathy.
Herbal products	St John's Wort (*Hypericum perforatum*)	Significant reduction of amprenavir plasma concentrations, leading to suboptimal drug levels, virological failure and drug resistance.
Drugs that require dose reduction when co-administered with Fosamprenavir		
HMG-CoA reductase inhibitors	Atorvastatin	Also dependent on CYP3A4-mediated elimination, but less than lovastatin and simvastatin. Use ≤20 mg/day of atorvastatin with careful monitoring or consider other HMG-CoA reductase inhibitors such as fluvastatin, pravastatin or rosuvastatin.
Benzodiazepines	Alprazolam, Clorazepate, Diazepam, Flurazepam	Increase in benzodiazepine levels with unknown clinical significance. However, benzodiazepine dose reduction may be needed according to clinical tolerance.
Antimycobacterials	Rifabutin	Frequent blood count monitoring is warranted to detect neutropenia. Reduce dose of rifabutin by 50% if given with nonboosted fosamprenavir and by 75% (with a maximum dose of 150 mg every other day or three times weekly) if given with fosamprenavir/ritonavir.
PDE5 inhibitors	Sildenafil, Vardenafil	Increases sildenafil and vardenafil plasma levels increasing the risk of side effects, such as hypotension, blurry vision, priapism 4 h after intake. Sildenafil should be used at 25 mg every 48 h with adverse event monitoring. Vardenafil should be used with caution at doses no more than 2.5 mg every 24 or 72 h if fosamprenavir is given without or with ritonavir, respectively.
Azole antifungals	Itraconazole or Ketoconazole	Increase monitoring for adverse events due to ketoconazole or itraconazole. In patients treated with nonboosted fosamprenavir, dose reduction of ketoconazole or itraconazole below 400 mg/day may be needed. In patients treated with fosamprenavir/ritonavir, avoid doses of ketoconazole or itraconazole >200 mg/day.
Drugs that require dose increase when co-administered with Fosamprenavir		
Opioids	Methadone	Co-administration of amprenavir and methadone, decreases methadone plasma levels as well as decreases by $\frac{1}{3}$ amprenavir plasma, levels as compared with a historical cohort.
Drugs that require plasma concentration monitoring if administered with fosamprenavir		
Antiarrhythmics	Amiodarone, Lidocaine (systemic), Quinidine	Risk of cardiac arrhythmias.
Oral anticoagulants	Warfarin	Risk of bleeding. Requires close INR monitoring.

(*Continued*)

(Continued)

Table 19-3

Family	Drugs	Reason
Tricyclic antidepressants	Amitriptyline, Amoxapine, Clomipramine, Desipramine, Doxepin, Imipramine, Nortriptyline, Protriptyline, Trimipramine	Risk of serious side-effects.
Immunosuppressants	Cyclosporine, Sirolimus, Tacrolimus	Significant interactions with narrow therapeutic index. Plasma level monitoring is warranted to avoid toxicity or suboptimal immune suppression.
Other drugs with significant interactions with Fosamprenavir		
Antacids		May decrease amprenavir absorption. Antacids should be taken at least one hour before or after amprenavir. This interaction has not been evaluated with ritonavir-boosted fosamprenavir.
Calcium channel blockers	Diltiazem, Felodipine, Nifedipine, Nicardipine, Nimodipine, Verapamil, Amlodipine, Nisoldipine, Isradipine.	Risk of hypotension. Caution is warranted and clinical monitoring of patients is recommended.
Antiarrhythmic	Bepridil	Use with caution. Increased bepridil exposure may be associated with lfe-threatening reactions such as cardiac arrhythmias.
Psycoactive compounds	Trazodone	Use with caution. Dose reduction may be required.
Anticonvulsants	Carbamazepine, Phenobarbital, Phenytoin	Induce CYP3A4 and reduce amprenavir plasma concentrations, leading to suboptimal drug levels, virological failure and drug resistance.
Corticosteroids	Dexamethasone	Induces CYP3A4 and reduces amprenavir plasma concentrations.
	Fluticasone	Risk of accumulation and adverse effects. Use alternative drugs if prolonged fosamprenavir use is expected.
Oral contraceptives	Ethinyl estradiol/norethindrone	Co-administration with fosamprenavir alters hormonal levels. Alternative methods of birth control are recommended.

[a] These drugs are highly dependent on CYP3A4 for clearance, have a narrow therapeutic index, or high plasma concentrations are associated with serious and life-threatening effects.

[b] Flecainide and propafenone are contraindicated if fosamprenavir is co-administered with ritonavir. If fosamprenavir is administered without ritonavir, plasma concentration monitoring is warranted.

Based on prescribing information for LEXIVA fosamprenavir calcium.[18]

accepts the administration of fosamprenavir as a single PI without ritonavir boost at a dose of 1400 mg (two 700 mg tablets) twice a day, only for PI-naive patients. However, the European Medicines Agency (EMEA) states "Fosamprenavir must only be given with low dose ritonavir as a pharmacokinetic enhancer of amprenavir and in combination with other antiretroviral medicinal products."[57]

Fosamprenavir can be taken with or without food and, due to its virtually nil urinary elimination, dose adjustments are not required in patients with renal insufficiency. Fosamprenavir dose should be adjusted in subjects with hepatic insufficiency. Importantly, no data is available regarding the administration of ritonavir-boosted fosamprenavir in patients with hepatic insufficiency, thus ritonavir-boosted fosamprenavir should be avoided in these patients. Fosamprenavir dose should be reduced to 700 mg bid without ritonavir in patients with moderate hepatic insufficiency which is defined as a Child–Pugh score ranging from 5 to 8. Fosamprenavir should not be used in patients with severe hepatic insufficiency with Child–Pugh score from 9 to 12 due to the impossibility in reducing the dose below 700 mg and the derived risk of inducing serious hepatic toxicity or cirrhotic decompensations.

Amprenavir is generally reserved for children younger than 13 years old or in children between 13 and 16 years of age who weigh less than 50 kg. It is approved for twice-daily dosing. It is important to note that amprenavir is not FDA approved in children 4 years old or younger. Moreover, the oral solution is expressly contraindicated in this age range because of the potential toxicity derived from the high concentrations of propylene glycol, its main diluent.

In children between 4 and 12 years old and in those between 13 and 16 years of age who weigh less than 50 kg, the recommended dose of oral solution is 22.5 mg/kg bid or

17 mg/kg tid with a maximum dose of 2800 mg/day. In these age ranges, the recommended dose in capsules is 20 mg/kg bid or 15 mg/kg tid, with a maximum dose of 2400 mg/day. Children older than 16 years and those who are aged 13 years or older and weigh more than 50 kg should receive the adult dosing of fosamprenavir. Exceptionally, amprenavir oral solution may be given to adults at a dose of 1400 mg (93 mL) bid if no other options are available. However, this is no longer considered standard of care.

Importantly, amprenavir should not be given with a high-fat meal and its dose should be adjusted in patients with hepatic insufficiency. No dose adjustments are needed in patients with renal insufficiency.

CLINICAL EFFICACY

By the time of finishing this review, the main body of evidence regarding the clinical efficacy of fosamprenavir stands on four published open-label randomized studies, three performed in antiretroviral-naive patients, the NEAT study (APV30001),[58] the SOLO study (APV30002)[59,60] and the KLEAN study and one in treatment-experienced subjects, the CONTEXT study (APV30003). The NEAT and SOLO studies demonstrated the noninferiority of nonboosted and ritonavir-boosted fosamprenavir with respect to nelfinavir. The KLEAN study established the noninferiority of ritonavir-boosted fosamprenavir bid relative to ritonavir-boosted lopinavir bid. In treatment-experienced patients, ritonavir-boosted fosamprenavir failed to demonstrate clinical equivalence with lopinavir/ritonavir, in part due to limitations in the sample size of the APV30003 study.

Several trials are ongoing comparing "head-to-head" ritonavir-boosted fosamprenavir regimens to other ritonavir-boosted PIs. The ALERT study is a 48-week "head-to-head" comparison of fosamprenavir and atazanavir, each boosted with ritonavir and combined with a dual-nucleoside combination of tenofovir and emtricitabine (FTC). Results of a planned interim analysis at 24 weeks have been presented[61] suggesting virological equivalence of both regimens and an improved adverse event and metabolic profile. Several other studies have been registered to date and are currently recruiting adult (ClinicalTrials.gov identifiers NCT00144833, NCT00094523, NCT00363142, NCT00242216, NCT00122603, NCT00307502) and child participants (ClinicalTrials.gov identifiers NCT00089583, NCT00207948, NCT00071760).

Fosamprenavir versus Amprenavir in PI-Naive Patients

A small 6-week study[46] compared the plasma amprenavir pharmacokinetics of amprenavir (1200 mg bid) and fosamprenavir (at doses of 1395 mg and 1860 mg bid), in combination with abacavir 300 mg bid and lamivudine 150 mg bid in 78 PI-naive HIV-infected patients with ≤4 weeks of prior NRTI/NNRTI experience. Compared to amprenavir, both fosamprenavir dosings delivered 30% lower peak plasma concentrations, higher plasma trough concentrations (28% and 46% higher for 1395 mg and 1860 mg bid dosings, respectively) and comparable AUCs. All three regimens achieved significant and comparable plasma HIV-1 RNA reductions and CD4+ cell count increases. The adverse event profile of fosamprenavir and amprenavir was comparable. Interestingly, gastrointestinal symptoms and overall grade 2-4 drug-related adverse events appeared to be less frequent in patients receiving fosamprenavir than in those treated with amprenavir, but values were too small to reach significance.

Fosamprenavir versus Nelfinavir in Antiretroviral-Naive Patients

The NEAT Study (APV30001 Study)

The NEAT study[58] was a randomized, open-label study that compared nonboosted fosamprenavir (1400 mg bid) with nelfinavir (1250 mg bid) in 249 HIV-1-infected antiretroviral-naive subjects. Both study arms received an NRTI backbone with abacavir (300 mg bid) and lamivudine (150 mg bid). The study subjects were ethnically diverse, 31% were women and 20% had an AIDS diagnosis. Baseline median CD4+ counts were 212 cells/mm^3, being less than 50 cells/mm^3 in 18% of participants and in the range between 50 and 200 cells/mm^3 in 30% of subjects. Median baseline HIV-1 RNA was 4.83 $\log_{10}$ copies/mL, being higher than 5 log10 copies/mL in 45% of patients. Overall, 66% of patients on fosamprenavir and 52% on nelfinavir achieved virological suppression below 400 copies/mL (57% and 42% below 50 copies/mL, respectively). Whereas a similar proportion of patients experienced virological rebound (16% with fosamprenavir and 19% with nelfinavir). More patients in the nelfinavir arm (13%) did not achieve virological response through week 48 than those treated with fosamprenavir (3%). The rate of virological response was comparable in both groups for those participants with baseline HIV-1 RNA below 100000 copies/mL. However, those with higher baseline viral loads were more likely to achieve suppression below 400 copies/mL if they received fosamprenavir (67%) than if they were treated with nelfinavir (36%). Therapy discontinuation due to adverse events was similar in both groups (4% in the fosamprenavir arm and 2% in the nelfinavir arm). Grade 2-4 diarrhea was more frequent in the nelfinavir group (18% vs 5%, $p = 0.002$). In this study, unboosted fosamprenavir bid demonstrated its activity in treatment-naive patients, with overall good tolerance and a low pill burden.

The SOLO Study (APV30002 Study)

The SOLO study[59,60] was a prospective randomized open-label multicentric noninferiority trial, that compared 322 patients receiving fosamprenavir/ritonavir (1400 mg/200 mg qd) with 327 patients treated with nelfinavir 1250 mg bid, both with an NRTI backbone which included abacavir (300 mg bid) and lamivudine (150 mg bid). Subjects belonged to a total of 101 centers in the United States of America, Europe, South Africa and Australia. They were antiretroviral-naive and had a plasma HIV-1 RNA of 1000 copies/mL or higher at the study entry. The study groups were comparable at baseline, were ethnically diverse and included 27% of females. Median baseline HIV-1 RNA was 4.8 log copies/mL and median CD4+ T-cell counts were 170 cells/mm^3, with 20% of patients having CD4+ T-cell counts below 50 cells/mm^3 and 23% of patients with a prior AIDS diagnosis.

The proportion of patients achieving the primary endpoint (HIV-1 RNA suppression below 400 copies/mL at week 48, intention-to-treat (ITT) missing = failure) was 68% and 65% in the fosamprenavir/ritonavir and the nelfinavir groups, respectively. Completion of secondary endpoints was also comparable between groups, with 55% of patients receiving fosamprenavir/ritonavir and 53% of those treated with nelfinavir achieving HIV-1 RNA below 50 copies/mL at week 48. The improvement in CD4+ T-cell counts was comparable in both groups, with a median increase of 203 and 207 in the fosamprenavir/ritonavir and nelfinavir groups, respectively.

Interestingly, the rate of virological failure was higher in the nelfinavir group (17% vs 7% in the fosamprenavir/ritonavir arm) whereas the rate of nonvirologic failure was higher in patients receiving fosamprenavir/ritonavir (24%) than in those treated with nelfinavir (15%), essentially due to a higher frequency of adverse events (8% vs 5%), lost to follow-up (5% vs 2%), consent withdrawal (4% vs 3%) or other reasons (5% vs 3%). Despite this there were no significant differences across different HIV-1 RNA and CD4+ strata. Patients with HIV-1 RNA > 500 000 copies/mL and those with CD4+ T-cell counts < 50 cells/mm^3 were more likely to accomplish the primary outcome measure if they received fosamprenavir/ritonavir than if they were to be treated with nelfinavir. No patients failing fosamprenavir/ritonavir as against 50% of those failing nelfinavir developed PI-associated resistance. Furthermore, patients failing fosamprenavir/ritonavir were less likely to develop NRTI-associated resistance (13%) than those failing nelfinavir (69%). A more detailed analysis of resistance data from this study is offered below.

Roughly 40% of patients in both groups experienced grade 2–4 drug-related adverse events. Diarrhea was the only adverse event that was significantly more common in the fosamprenavir/ritonavir group. Patients treated with fosamprenavir/ritonavir were more likely to experience mostly asymptomatic grade 3 elevations in serum lipase and triglycerides. All other biochemical parameters were comparable in both groups.

SOLO and NEAT Rollover Study (APV30005)

Both SOLO and NEAT studies have been rolled over into the APV30005 study, whose main goal was to assess the long-term efficacy, adverse events and resistance profile of fosamprenavir on 120 weeks of follow-up. By the time of finishing this review, the APV30005 rollover results had only been partially published in scientific conferences[62] and were on file as a final study report by the manufacturers.[63] Essentially, this study confirms, in the long term, the results from the original studies in terms of persistent suppression of viral replication in the wide majority of patients (75% of patients with HIV-1 RNA levels <400 copies/mL at week 120, ITT analysis), good tolerability, low incidence of adverse events and laboratory abnormalities, as well as a favorable drug resistance profile with virtually no patient who failed ritonavir-boosted fosamprenavir showing amprenavir resistance mutations (*see* below for details and two exceptions).

Fosamprenavir/Ritonavir versus Lopinavir/Ritonavir in Antiretroviral-Naive Patients

The KLEAN Study (Fosamprenavir/Ritonavir versus Lopinavir/Ritonavir in Antiretroviral-Naive Patients)

The KLEAN "Kaletra vs Lexiva with Epivir and Abacavir in ART-naive patients" study[64] was an international, multicenter, open label, randomised, noninferiority trial comparing fosamprenavir/ritonavir (700 mg/100 mg bid) with lopinavir/ritonavir (400 mg/100 mg bid), each with abacavir–lamivudine (600 mg/300 mg) fixed-dose combination tablet once daily. At week 48, 73%, and 71% of subjects in the fosamprenavir/ritonavir and lopinavir/ritonavir arms, respectively, achieved the primary endpoint of the study (HIV-1 RNA suppression <400 copies/mL). These results demonstrated the noninferiority of fosamprenavir/ritonavir relative to lopinavir/ritonavir (95% CI around the treatment difference −4.84 to 7.05). The proportion of participants with HIV-1 RNA levels <50 copies/mL at week 48 was also similar between groups (66% in the fosamprenavir arm and 65% in the lopinavir/ritonavir arm). Both arms exhibited similar increases in CD4+ T-cell counts. These efficacy results remained consistent after stratifying for baseline HIV-1 RNA levels (higher or lower than 100 000 copies/mL) or CD4 counts (higher or lower than 50 copies/mm^3). The proportion of subjects with disease progression (2% and 3% in the fosamprenavir/ritonavir and lopinavir/ritonavir arms, respectively) was similar in both groups. Five deaths were reported during the study period (four in the fosamprenavir/ritonavir arm and one in the lopinavir/ritonavir arm, respectively), none of which were related to the study medication.

Only 40 patients (5%) had protocol-defined virological failure. A minority of them (31% of those with baseline and on-treatment viral genotypes and phenotypes) exhibited drug-associated resistance. Four (11%) developed PI-resistance mutations, all encoding mixtures of wild type and mutant aminoacids, including one I54I/L, two K20K/R and one I62I/V. None developed major PI-resistance mutations or viruses with reduced susceptibility to the study PIs. Only 20% of subjects with available genotypes at baseline and at failure had evidence of NRTI resistance.

The adverse event profile was comparable between groups. There were few treatment discontinuations due to adverse events (10% and 12% in fosamprenavir and lopinavir arms, respectively). Both groups had comparable changes in the lipid profile relative to baseline values. Elevation of liver enzymes was more frequent in subjects with hepatitis C virus (HCV) co-infection (12% vs 1% in the non-HCV co-infected) irrespective of the treatment arm assigned.

This study established the noninferiority of fosamprenavir/ritonavir bid (700 mg/100 mg bid) relative to lopinavir/ritonavir to treat antiretroviral-naive HIV-1 infected patients. Based on these data, current guidelines for treatment of HIV-infected adults and adolescents consider ritonavir-boosted fosamprenavir regimens as a "preferred" first-line treatment for antiretroviral-naive patients.[1]

Fosamprenavir/Ritonavir versus Atazanavir/Ritonavir in Antiretroviral-Naive Patients

The ALERT Study

The ALERT study[61] is a 48-week open-label randomized study ongoing at the time of finishing this review. The ALERT study compares fosamprenavir 1400 mg, combined with 100 mg of ritonavir (the current US product license requires 200 mg of ritonavir) versus atazanavir 300 mg once daily, with 100 mg of ritonavir, both administered with a dual-nucleoside combination of tenofovir and FTC. Data from a planned 24-week interim analysis were presented. The study included 106 antiretroviral-naive subjects, with a median baseline viral load of 4.88 log copies/mL, and a median CD4 cell count of 172 cells/mm^3. At the end of 24 weeks, both groups achieved similar virologic results. Using a missing data equals failure, ITT analysis, 89% in each arm had viral load below 400 copies/mL at week 24, and 79% in the fosamprenavir group and 83% in the atazanavir group had viral load below 50 copies/mL. Increases in CD4 counts in both groups were also similar; 126 cells/mm^3 in the fosamprenavir/ritonavir group and 156 cells/mm^3 in the atazanavir/ritonavir group. Increases in fasting plasma total cholesterol, LDL and HDL cholesterol were very modest and comparable, but triglycerides increased more substantially in the fosamprenavir arm (from 116 to 160 mg/dL, compared to an increase of 6 mg/dL in the atazanavir group). Forty-one percent of the atazanavir group experienced grade 2–4 bilirubin elevations, although no patients discontinued treatment as a result of this toxicity. No bilirubin elevations were seen in the fosamprenavir group. No other significant differences in adverse events were noted. Diarrhea occurred in 6% of fosamprenavir-treated patients and 2% of the atazanavir group. Virological failure was observed in three subjects. One of them had fourfold decrease in amprenavir susceptibility at baseline associated with mutations K20I, M46I, L63P, A71V, V77I in the protease gene. In this subject, virological failure occurred at week 20 and was associated with FTC resistance, several PI resistance mutations (K20I, M46I, I54I/L/M, L63P, A71V, V77I) and a 13-fold decrease in amprenavir susceptibility. The second subject exhibited virological failure at week 12 but only the K65R mutation in the RT gene was detected at week 24. Finally, the third subject had virological failure at week 12 but no genotypic or phenotypic resistance could be documented up to week 24. These interim results suggest comparable virological and immunological efficacy of fosamprenavir/ritonavir and atazanavir/ritonavir regimens. The improved adverse event and lipid profile in the fosamprenavir arm could be partially attributed to the use of a lower dose of ritonavir. Final results of this study at 48 weeks are awaited.

Fosamprenavir/Ritonavir versus Lopinavir/Ritonavir in Antiretroviral-Experienced Patients

The CONTEXT Study (APV30003)

This was a multicentric, randomized, three-arm, noninferiority open-label study, in which 320 participants (315 actually receiving treatment) were randomized in a 1:1:1 manner to receive fosamprenavir 1400 mg qd plus ritonavir 200 mg qd, fosamprenavir 700 mg bid along with ritonavir 100 mg bid, or lopinavir 400 mg bid with ritonavir 100 mg bid, and stratified by screening plasma HIV-1 RNA. Each regimen was administered with two active NRTIs, based on genotype analysis at study entry. This study was conducted at 103 sites in Australia, Belgium, Canada, Chile, France, Germany, Italy, Portugal, Puerto Rico, Spain, Switzerland, United Kingdom, and the United States. Eligibility criteria included HIV-1-infected males or females aged 13 years or older with: (1) a screening plasma HIV-1 RNA equal to 1000 copies/mL; (2) previous experience with one or two PIs, either used as a single PI or as part of a pharmacokinetically enhanced regimen; received at least 12 consecutive weeks of prior PI therapy (up to two prior PIs); (3) documented virologic failure on a prior PI regimen, defined as having plasma HIV-1 RNA that never went below 1000 copies/mL after at least 12 consecutive weeks of PI therapy, or initial suppression of HIV-1 RNA which subsequently rebounded to 1000 copies/mL; and (4) receiving antiretroviral therapy at study entry. The primary endpoint was the mean time-averaged change from baseline (AAUCMB) in the viral load. Secondary efficacy endpoints were: measured values and change from baseline in $\log_{10}$ plasma HIV-1 RNA over 24 and 48 weeks; proportions of subjects with plasma HIV-1 RNA levels <400 and <50 copies/mL over 24 and 48 weeks; time to treatment failure; proportion of subjects with 1 $\log_{10}$ decrease in HIV-1 RNA at 24 and 48 weeks, and measured values and change from baseline and AAUCMB in CD4+ cell count over 24 weeks and 48 weeks. Each fosamprenavir/ritonavir arm was compared to lopinavir/ritonavir and tested for noninferiority. In order to demonstrate noninferiority, the upper limit of the 97.5% CI on the difference in mean AAUCMB had to be below 0.5 $\log_{10}$ copies/mL.

All patients in this study had failed treatment with a previous PI regimen but only 65% were receiving a PI at study entry. The population enrolled mainly consisted of moderately antiretroviral-experienced patients. The median durations of prior exposure to NRTIs/PIs were 257/149 weeks for patients receiving fosamprenavir with ritonavir bid and 210/130 weeks for patients receiving lopinavir/ritonavir.

Whereas comparisons at week 24 suggested equivalence of the three regimens, at week 48, neither qd nor bid fosamprenavir/ritonavir could be considered virologically equivalent

Table 19-4 Summary of Efficacy Data from the CONTEXT (APV 30003) Study

Primary Outcome Results (ITT[E]) Mean strata-adjusted treatment difference (97.5% CI) in plasma HIV-1 RNA AAUCMBs (log_{10} copies/mL) (observed analysis)	**FAPV/RTV QD vs LPV/RTV**	**FAPV/RTV BID vs LPV/RTV**
Week 24	0.184 (−0.065, 0.433)	0.171 (−0.082, 0.424)
Week 48	0.267 (−0.017, 0.551)	0.244 (−0.047, 0.536)

Secondary Outcome Results (ITT[E]) Mean strata-adjusted treatment difference (97.5% CI) in Plasma HIV-1 RNA Changes from Baseline (log_{10}/mL)	**FAPV/RTV QD vs LPV/RTV**	**FAPV/RTV BID vs LPV/RTV**
Week 24	0.359 (−0.008, 0.725)	0.250 (−0.107, 0.608)
Week 48	0.276 (−0.088, 0.640)	0.196 (−0.182, 0.573)

	FAPV/RTV qd *N* = 105	**FAPV/RTV bid *N* = 107**	**LPV/RTV *N* = 103**
Mean Plasma HIV-1 RNA Changes (SD) from Baseline (log_{10}copies/mL)			
Week 24	−1.61 (1.21)	−1.74 (1.10)	−1.97 (1.07)
Week 48	−1.62 (1.06)	−1.72 (1.11)	−1.93 (1.07)
Proportion of subjects with plasma HIV-1 RNA <400 copies/mL (ITT RD = F)			
Baseline, *n* (%)	1 (1)	1 (1)	2 (2)
Week 24, *n* (%)	62 (59)	67 (63)	74 (72)
Week 48, *n* (%)	52 (50)	62 (58)	63 (61)
Proportion of subjects with plasma HIV-1 RNA <50 copies/mL (ITT RD = F)			
Baseline, *n* (%)	0	0	1 (1)
Week 24, *n* (%)	49 (47)	53 (50)	59 (57)
Week 48, *n* (%)	39 (37)	49 (46)	52 (50)
Proportion of subjects with plasma HIV-1 RNA at Least 1 log_{10} copies/mL below Baseline (ITT RD=F)			
Week 24, *n*	105	107	103
Proportion, *n* (%)	66 (63)	71 (66)	76 (74)
Week 48, *n*	105	107	103
Proportion, *n* (%)	58 (55)	62 (58)	71 (69)
Change from baseline in CD4+ cell counts (cells/mm^3) (observed analysis)			
Week 48, *n*	81	79	85
Week 48 median change from baseline (range)	61 (−787, 495)	81 (−255, 507)	91 (−213, 643)
CD4+ cell counts AAUCMB (cells/mm^3) (observed analysis)			
Week 48, *n*	103	105	103
Week 48 mean (sd)	55.57 (80.02)	50.96 (67.14)	65.57 (100.21)

ITT RD = F, Intention-to-treat rebound or discontinuation = failure.

to lopinavir/ritonavir bid. The mean difference in AAUCMB of fosamprenavir/ritonavir qd versus lopinavir/ritonavir was 0.267 (97.5%CI: −0.017 to 0.551). The same value for fosamprenavir/ritonavir bid versus lopinavir/ritonavir was 0.244 (97.5%CI: −0.047, 0.536). Hence, fosamprenavir/ritonavir did not demonstrate noninferiority with respect to lopinavir/ritonavir in antiretroviral-experienced patients as regards the principal study endpoint. Only fosamprenavir/ritonavir bid achieved the criteria for noninferiority for patients in the plasma HIV-1 RNA stratum between 1000 and 10000 copies/mL (Table 19-4). Regarding secondary efficacy outcomes, patients receiving lopinavir/ritonavir tended to have a better virological performance, especially in the higher baseline HIV-1 RNA strata, whereas CD4+ count outcomes did not differ between groups.

The above presented results did not demonstrate that fosamprenavir/ritonavir was virologically noninferior to lopinavir/ritonavir in PI-experienced patients. Based on these results, drug agencies consider that there are insufficient data to recommend the use of fosamprenavir with ritonavir qd in heavily pretreated patients. However, the fosamprenavir/ritonavir bid regimen provided better long-term outcomes than the qd regimen in this subject setting, and its overall pharmacokinetic profile is better. Therefore, twice-daily administration of fosamprenavir/ritonavir (700/100 mg bid) is currently recommended for treatment-experienced patients.

TOXICITY AND ADVERSE EVENTS

Fosamprenavir and amprenavir have a comparable adverse event profile. Overall, both drugs are well tolerated and safe, although adverse events may be less frequent with fosamprenavir than with amprenavir.[46] Rates of treatment discontinuation have been low (<10%) in the NEAT, SOLO, and KLEAN trials, and similar to those of the comparator regimen. Table 19-5 presents the proportion of patients who experienced select adverse events and laboratory abnormalities in the 120-week rollovers of NEAT and SOLO studies, as well as in the KLEAN study – all three in antiretroviral-naive patients – and data from the CONTEXT study in PI-experienced patients.

The most frequent adverse events seen with fosamprenavir are gastrointestinal symptoms, including abdominal pain, diarrhea, flatulence, and vomiting, with 30–50% of patients experiencing at least one gastrointestinal adverse event during fosamprenavir treatment, mainly nausea, and diarrhea.

Skin rash is less frequent, occurring in ~20% of patients in pivotal studies regardless of causality, and in less than 10% of patients in bigger and more prolonged clinical studies. Some authors have attributed most skin rashes seen in clinical trials to abacavir[41] but that is difficult to discern. Fosamprenavir-associated rash is usually maculopapular, and of mild or moderate intensity. In one study, the median onset of rash was 11 days after starting fosamprenavir and had a median duration of 2 weeks. Between 3% and 8% of patients treated with abacavir/lamivudine/fosamprenavir may experience moderate to severe rash, but severe or life-threatening skin reactions are extraordinary (less than 1%). Among 700 patients treated with fosamprenavir in clinical studies, only one case of Stevens–Johnson syndrome has been reported.[18] Fosamprenavir should be discontinued in case of severe rash, but no rash recurrences have been described in patients in whom fosamprenavir had been reintroduced.

Much more unusual adverse events include depression, mood changes, and perioral paresthesias. In phase III controlled clinical studies, the rate of treatment discontinuation was 6%, similar to comparator regimens.

Clinical data are scarce regarding the impact of fosamprenavir on fat redistribution syndromes, being mostly inferred from data collected on amprenavir. Limited preclinical data suggest that amprenavir has little effect on these parameters *in vitro*, in murine models or in healthy volunteers.[43] In addition, amprenavir did not alter adipose cell differentiation in murine cell lines.[65] Nevertheless, small studies reported significant increases in trunk fat in HIV-infected subjects after 48 weeks of therapy.[66] Insulin sensitivity, as measured by intravenous glucose tolerance test, decreased almost 40% from baseline to week 48; despite this difference, it did not achieve statistical significance.[66] Although new lipodystrophy cases have not been reported from clinical trials, US prescribing information for fosamprenavir indicates that both lipoatrophy and fat accumulation have occurred in patients receiving fosamprenavir as a component of their antiretroviral therapy.[18,41] These events include central obesity, dorsocervical fat enlargement, breast enlargement, facial wasting, and "Cushingoid appearance". There are no clinical data that suggest fosamprenavir behaves differently than other PIs in this regard.

The incidence of grade 3 and 4 laboratory abnormalities has been low in clinical trials, with similar frequency to comparator regimens (Table 19-5). In both NEAT and SOLO studies, LDL and HDL cholesterol increases were comparable in patients receiving fosamprenavir or nelfinavir. In the NEAT study, the median serum levels of triglycerides, total cholesterol, LDL cholesterol, HDL cholesterol, alanine transaminase, aspartate transaminase and lipase were within normal limits after 48 weeks of treatment. In the SOLO study there were increases in total, LDL, and HDL cholesterol levels in both study groups, but the ratio total/HDL cholesterol remained unchanged. Among the rollovers of NEAT and SOLO studies (Table 19-5), between 5% and 10% of patients had increases in transaminases of at least five times the upper limit of normality (ULN), ~10% of patients had amylase increases of at least two times the ULN. Although no direct comparisons are available, from the SOLO study, triglyceride levels above 750 mg/dL were more frequent in patients receiving ritonavir-boosted fosamprenavir than in those in the NEAT study patients treated with unboosted fosamprenavir (10% vs 4%, respectively). The incidence of hypercholesterolemia and hyperglycemia were <2% and neutropenia was seen in 3% of patients.

A more favorable adverse event and metabolic profile was recently reported from the 24-week interim analysis of the ALERT study[61]. In this study, fosamprenavir 1400 mg qd was given with 100 mg ritonavir qd, a dose smaller than the one accepted by the FDA, and was compared to atazanavir 300 mg/ritonavir 100 mg qd. Increases in fasting plasma total cholesterol, LDL and HDL cholesterol levels were very modest and comparable, but triglycerides increased more substantially in the fosamprenavir arm (from 116 to 160 mg/dL, compared to an increase of 6 mg/dL in the atazanavir group). Forty-one percent of the atazanavir group experienced grade 2–4 bilirubin elevations, although no patients discontinued treatment as a result of this toxicity. No bilirubin elevations were seen in the fosamprenavir group. No other significant differences in adverse events were noted. Diarrhea occurred in 6% of fosamprenavir-treated patients and 2% of the atazanavir group. The overall rate of grade 2–4 adverse events was smaller in the fosamprenavir/ritonavir arm (11%) than in the atazanavir/ritonavir arm (53%). The smaller ritonavir dose possibly helped decrease adverse events in subjects treated with fosamprenavir. Final results at 48 weeks are awaited to confirm these findings.

RESISTANCE TO AMPRENAVIR AND FOSAMPRENAVIR

One of the main advantages of amprenavir is its particular resistance profile, distinct from that of other PIs. Patients with

Table 19-5

Selected Adverse Events and Laboratory Abnormalities

	SOLO Study Roll-over, 120 weeks (APV30005) FPV bid $N = 211$	NEAT Study Roll-over, 120 weeks (APV30005) FPV bid $N = 112$	KLEAN Study, 48 weeks[a] FPV/RTV bid $N = 436$	KLEAN Study, 48 weeks[a] LPV/RTV $N = 443$	CONTEXT Study, 48 weeks (APV 30003) FPV/RTV qd $N = 106$	CONTEXT Study, 48 weeks (APV 30003) FPV/RTV bid $N = 106$
Drug-Related Adverse Events						
Diarrhea	11%	8%	13%	11%	31%	31%
Nausea	8%	8%	6%	5%	25%	20%
Vomiting	4%	4%	2%	2%	21%	10%
Headache	4%	2%	3%	1%	12%	25%
Fatigue	3%	2%	2%	1%	17%	9%
Rash	4%	5%	3%	<1%	8%	8%
Depression	1%	3%			11%	11%
Laboratory Abnormalities						
ALT (>5 × ULN)	9%	6%	3%	3%		4%
AST (>5 × ULN)	5%	7%	3%	2%		4%
Serum lipase (>2 × ULN)	12%	11%				5%
Triglycerides (>750 mg/dL)	10%	4%	8%	8%		
Total cholesterol (>1.6 × ULN)	1%	<1%	11%	9%		
Glucose (>250 mg/dL)	2%	2%	1%	2%		2%
Neutropenia (<750 cells/mm^3)	3%	5%	4%	5%		

[a] Abacavir hypersensitivity reaction. 6% FPV/RTV arm, 5% LPV/RTV arm. Grade 3–4 increases in creatine kinase 4% FPV/RTV arm, 6% LPV/RTV arm. Grade 3–4 increases in amylase <1% FPV/RTV arm, 2% LPV/RTV arm.

virologic failure to amprenavir, especially if virologic rebound is detected early, often do not show genotypic or phenotypic evidence of cross-resistance to other PIs like indinavir, nelfinavir or saquinavir *in vitro*, although low-level cross-resistance to ritonavir and lopinavir is sometimes noted.[41,67] On the other hand, many patients with virologic failure to other PIs may remain susceptible to amprenavir.[67] Despite fosamprenavir and amprenavir having an overlapping resistance profile, the actual incidence of PI and NRTI resistance mutations varies between them. Therefore, it is clinically meaningful to present both drugs separately.

Amprenavir

The signature resistance mutation for amprenavir is I50V.[20] This mutation is infrequently seen among other PI resistance reports. It is a minor mutation occasionally contributing to lopinavir/ritonavir failure,[68] and differs from atazanavir's signature mutation at the same position, I50L. In enzymatic assays with recombinant protease, this mutation produced an increase of 21 and 10 times, respectively, in the inhibition constants for saquinavir and indinavir. *In vivo*, as a single mutation, I50V only confers a two to threefold decrease in susceptibility to amprenavir.[69,70] I50V appears early after amprenavir failure and frequently before other minor mutations have accumulated. Since I50V confers low fitness, acquisition of high-level resistance to amprenavir sometimes requires additional substitutions in Gag p6. Insertions (P459Ins) within p6 protein, leading to partial or complete duplication of the PTAPP motif, appear to be associated with resistance to unboosted amprenavir in highly pretreated patients, particularly in the presence of mutations at codon 82 of the protease.[71] Nevertheless, such insertions are rare, especially in drug-naive individuals, being usually seen in patients treated with multiple NRTIs.[72] Mutations in HIV-1 *gag* at positions L449 and P453 are linked to I50V protease mutants *in vivo* and cause reduction of sensitivity to amprenavir and improved viral fitness *in vitro*.[73,74]

The second major mutation associated with amprenavir resistance is I84V, although this mutation is less common than I50V, I54L/M, or the V32I + I47V combination.[75] I84V is associated with reduced susceptibility to lopinavir, indinavir, nelfinavir, ritonavir, saquinavir, and tipranavir in viral isolates from PI-experienced patients.[76,77] I84V increases the inhibitory concentration of saquinavir 5.8- to 10.7-fold[78,79] although experiments in recombinant clones suggest a lesser effect on IC_{50}. The addition of V82F to I84V significantly increases resistance to ritonavir, indinavir, nelfinavir, and amprenavir.[79] *In vivo*, I84V appears as the strongest amprenavir resistance marker in PI-experienced patients,[80] particularly in the absence of resistance mutations at codon 50.[32] This mutation is also associated with reduced *in vivo* virologic responses to ritonavir-boosted amprenavir in PI-experienced patients.[78]

Mutations I54L/M and/or the combination V32I + I47V are often seen in patients failing ritonavir/amprenavir, but they usually appear in patients with further experience to PIs.[78,81] I54L/M and V32I + I47V reduce the virologic response to ritonavir-amprenavir[82] and confer cross-resistance to other PIs. As we shall see below, it is likely that these two patterns are the most common ones in patients failing ritonavir-boosted fosamprenavir.

In addition to the four main pathways of amprenavir resistance, namely I50V, I54L/M, V32I + I47V, and I84V, multiple accessory mutations are also associated with resistance to amprenavir *in vivo*, including substitutions at residues 10, 32, 46, 47, 54, 73, and 90.[75] The double mutant M46I/L plus I50V is associated *in vitro* with a fourfold increase in susceptibility to saquinavir and a two- to threefold increase in susceptibility to indinavir.[70] Significant resistance to amprenavir can be predicted when one of the following combinations of mutations is encountered[78]:

1. I84V alone;
2. I50V plus one or two mutations of the following group: L10F/I/R/V, V32I, M46I/L, I54L/V, V82I/F, or L90M; and
3. three or more mutations of the above listed group (L10F/I/R/V, V32I, M46I/L, I54L/V, V82I/F, or L90M).

A comparative analysis of rules-based algorithms found a clear association between I84V plus three or more protease-associated mutations (codons 10, 46, 54, 63, 71, 77, 82, 84, and 90), but also suggested that other mutations at codons 20, 24, 32, 33, 36, 48, 53, and 73 may also contribute to decreases in susceptibility to amprenavir.[83] Furthermore, alterations in transepithelial permeability of amprenavir and other PIs due to the G1199A or some other polymorphisms in the MDR1 gene may impact their oral bioavailability and penetration into cells and tissues of the lymphoid and central nervous systems,[84] being a cause of cell-mediated resistance to PIs. Another resistance factor, related to the geographical location of the host is that some non-subtype B strains may be naturally less sensitive to PIs, including amprenavir.[83,85] HIV-2 and SIVsm are also naturally resistant to the NNRTIs as well as the PI amprenavir.[16]

Finally, mutations K20T and N88S[86,87] and atazanavir-related I50L,[88] have been associated with hypersusceptibility to amprenavir and other PIs, particularly when other resistant mutations are present, such as L10F/I/R/V, V32I, M46I/L, I50V, I54L/V, V82I/F, or L90M.

Fosamprenavir

Fosamprenavir is the prodrug of amprenavir, which is the active metabolite interacting with the viral protease. Therefore, the resistance profile of both the drugs is superimposable. However, fosamprenavir is commonly co-administered and boosted with ritonavir. Whereas, generally speaking, the same mutations emerge whether or not the PIs are boosted with low-dose ritonavir, there may be some difference in the relative frequency of various mutations.[68] With regimens that include boosted PIs, multiple mutations may be required to result in less antiretroviral efficacy. Clinical resistance data in drug-naive patients comes mainly from the NEAT[58,88,89] and SOLO[59] studies and their respective rollovers[62] as well as from the KLEAN study.[64] Resistance analysis of the NEAT study showed that the specific mutational pathways observed at first failure on nonboosted fosamprenavir bid were either the I54L/M mutation or the V32I plus I47V mutations. These patterns were detected in virus from five (17%) of the 29 subjects studied and had been previously described in patients with resistance to amprenavir.[68] The I50V mutation was not initially detected, but the continuation of fosamprenavir despite ongoing viral replication resulted in the emergence of this mutation in one patient.[58] Amprenavir-associated mutations did not confer significant cross-resistance to indinavir, lopinavir, nelfinavir, ritonavir, or saquinavir. There was no significant difference between arms with regards to the incidence of NRTI-resistant mutations. Most patients included in the rollover of NEAT study remain virologically suppressed and, so far, resistance mutations have been detected in three additional samples with minimal cross-resistance to other PIs.[88]

In the 48 week fosamprenavir/ritonavir registration study (SOLO, APV30002) no PI resistance development was observed, and NRTI resistance to the concomitant abacavir/lamivudine therapy (13% of isolates), was substantially less common compared with the nelfinavir comparator arm (69% of isolates with NRTI resistance and 50% with PI resistance mutations).[60] This study rolled over subsequently into APV30005 to continue monitoring the long-term response to boosted fosamprenavir. Results reported out to week 120 confirmed that the cumulative incidence of abacavir resistance was 1% and that no PI resistance developed during treatment with boosted fosamprenavir,[62] with two exceptions so far.[90,91]

The first subject[90] entered the SOLO study with a baseline viral load of 392 183 copies/mL and a CD4 count of 164 cell/μL, and received a regimen of fosamprenavir/ritonavir (1400/200 mg once daily) with abacavir 300 mg and lamivudine 150 mg bid. At baseline, there was no genotypic or phenotypic resistance and only the M36I natural polymorphism was found in protease (Table 19-6). Overall, the patient went through an initial period of viral load suppression <50 copies/mL, experiencing the first confirmed virologic rebound >50 copies/mL at week 84. Low-level replication continued until week 144. At week 160, the viral load had increased to 998 copies/mL. Thereafter, the patient underwent several treatment modifications alternating between virologic suppression and low-level replication and up to the last report, remains clinically well and asymptomatic.

The second individual[91] entered the SOLO study with a baseline viral load of 606 762 copies/mL after finishing treatment for *Pneumocystis carinii* pneumonia. He was also treated with fosamprenavir/ritonavir (1400/200 mg once daily), abacavir 300 mg and lamivudine 150 mg bid, with an excellent virologic response (viral load <50 copies/mL) until week 40, before experiencing persistent low-level replication (<1000 copies/mL) until week 106. Around this time, the viral load increased to 14 195 copies/mL. A genotype

Table 19-6

Summary of Resistance Data from Individual Cases Treated with Ritonavir-Boosted Fosamprenavir and with Evidence of Evolving Amprenavir Resistance

	Case 1[89]			Case 2[90]	
RT and Protease Resistance	**Day 1**	**Week 144**	**Week 160**	**Week 0**	**Week 106**
RT					
Genotype	None	L74V, M184V	L74V, M184V	None	None
Phenotype	None	N/A	↓ susceptibility to ABC (4.5-fold), 3TC (>108-fold), ddI (1.7-fold). Retained susceptibility to LPV (4.0-fold) and ATV (0.5-fold) Marginal ↑ in susceptibility (compared to day 1) to TDF (0.9–0.3-fold), d4T (1.5–0.6-fold), ZDV (0.8–0.2-fold)	N/A	N/A
Protease					
Genotype	M36I	M36I, M46I, I50V	M36I, M46I, I50V (plus L449F in the p1/p6 cleavage site)	I47I/V, A71V, V82[a]	V32I, M46I I47V, A71V
Phenotype	None	N/A	↓ susceptibility to APV (11-fold) and RTV (6.4-fold) Marginal ↑ in susceptibility (compared to day 1) to IDV (1.1–0.4-fold), and SQV (1.4–0.8-fold)		
Replicative capacity	198% (125–314)		26% (16–41)	N/A	N/A

Genotypic data reported in this table have been obtained by either Trugene genotypic Kit or by the Monogram Biosciences Genotype Kit. Phenotypic data and replication capacity assays were preformed by Monogram Biosciences (formerly ViroLogic).

[a] V82A in patient 2 was seen in 1/62 clones at week 0 and in 1/22 at week 1.

was performed at week 106 and, retrospectively, at baseline (Table 19-6) with additional clonal analysis at baseline to detect minor variants harboring mutations.

In summary, these cases indicate that, despite being a rare event, resistance to amprenavir can also evolve in patients receiving ritonavir-boosted fosamprenavir regimens, especially in face of persistent low-level replication. Resistance mutations selected under ritonavir-boosted fosamprenavir are similar to those seen during virological failure of amprenavir or non-boosted fosamprenavir. Whereas the first case had no evidence of resistance at baseline, the preexistence of amprenavir-associated resistance mutations in the second subject suggests that baseline resistance may be an important factor driving the evolution of resistance during first-line treatment with fosamprenavir/ritonavir. Interestingly, the presence of L449F in the p1/p6 cleavage site at week 160 in the first subject and the coexistence of the amprenavir-associated I47I/V and A71V mutations with V82A at baseline in the second individual indicates, first, that mutations in *gag* cleavage sites may be acquired during active viral replication, also with boosted fosamprenavir, and, second, that either these mutations or others may importantly contribute to amprenavir resistance and virologic failure in patients receiving ritonavir-boosted fosamprenavir.

Data from the recently published KLEAN study[64] confirm the paucity of PI resistance mutations in subjects failing fosamprenavir/ritonavir or lopinavir/ritonavir. In this study, only four subjects failing either therapy (11% of failures) and only two subjects failing fosamprenavir/ritonavir exhibited PI resistance mutations. In all cases findings encoded mixtures of wild-type and mutant amino acids including one I54I/L, two K20K/R, and one I62I/V. No major resistance mutations were observed during the study. Again, only 20% of subjects developed virologic failure.

CONTRAINDICATIONS

Fosamprenavir and amprenavir are contraindicated in patients with previous significant hypersensitivity to any of their components. It is important to note that amprenavir is a sulfonamide compound. Therefore, fosamprenavir and amprenavir should be used with caution in patients with hypersensitivity to sulphonamides or derivate compounds. However, the potential for cross-sensitivity between drugs in the sulfonamide class and fosamprenavir is unknown, and there is no clinical evidence that subjects with prior sulfonamide hypersensitivity may experience more rash than those with no history of sulfonamide allergy. Fosamprenavir is also contraindicated in patients receiving one of the following drugs: antiarrhythmics (flecainide or propafenone, if fosamprenavir is administered with ritonavir), ergot derivatives (dihydroergotamine, ergonovine, ergotamine, and methylergonovine), neuroleptics (pimozide), prokinetics (cisapride), and benzodiazepines (midazolam or triazolam). See Table 19-3 for other interactions and precautions regarding the concomitant administration of fosamprenavir with other drugs. Importantly, amprenavir oral solution is contraindicated in children younger than 4 years and in adults taking disulfiram, due to its high content in propylene glycol.

CARCINOGENESIS, MUTAGENESIS, FERTILITY, AND USE OF FOSAMPRENAVIRS DURING PREGNANCY

So far, clinical studies have excluded pregnant women and no specific clinical data are available regarding fosamprenavir use during pregnancy or breast-feeding. Whereas it is unknown whether amprenavir is excreted in human milk, amprenavir is excreted into the milk of lactating rats.[18] The CDC recommends mothers should not breast-feed while taking amprenavir or fosamprenavir. Fosamprenavir and amprenavir are class-C drugs, and should not be used during pregnancy unless benefits outweigh the potential risk to the fetus. According to the manufacturer,[18] fosamprenavir embryo/fetal development studies were conducted in rats (dosed from day 6 to day 17 of gestation) and rabbits (dosed from day 7 to day 20 of gestation), with no major effects on embryo-fetal development, but with an increase in the incidence of abortion in rabbits exposed to fosamprenavir either with or without ritonavir at a dose equivalent to 0.8-0.3 times the exposure in humans. In contrast, administration of amprenavir was associated with abortions and an increased incidence of minor skeletal variations resulting from deficient ossification of the femur, humerus, and trochlea in pregnant rabbits at the tested dose; approximately one twentieth the exposure seen at the recommended human dose.

Carcinogenesis and mutagenesis studies are ongoing for fosamprenavir. Amprenavir carcinogenesis studies in male mice and rats exposed at systemic doses equivalent to two times (mice) and four times (rats) the human exposure, demonstrated an increased incidence of both benign hepatoadenoma and hepatocarcinoma, which was not observed in females. No other tumors were significantly associated with amprenavir administration in either gender or species. Similarly, no mutagenic or genotoxic effect was observed in several *in vitro* and *in vivo* assays.[18]

Fosamprenavir and amprenavir did not have any effect in the mating or fertility of male or female rats and did not affect the development and maturation of sperm from treated rats.[18] The mating and fertility of the F1 generation born to female rats given fosamprenavir was not different from control animals. However, fosamprenavir did cause a reduction in both pup survival and body weights. Surviving F1 female rats showed an increased time to successful mating, an increased length of gestation, a reduced number of uterine implantation sites per litter, and reduced gestational body weights compared to control animals.

SUMMARY: INDICATIONS FOR FOSAMPRENAVIR

Fosamprenavir has displaced amprenavir in all clinical settings except in children, where fosamprenavir studies are ongoing. Fosamprenavir has demonstrated potent and durable antiviral efficacy in antiretroviral-naive HIV-infected patients with an adequate tolerability profile, low pill burden and the possibility of once- or twice-daily administration. Its relative low pill burden may facilitate adherence and better virologic outcomes. Its active moiety, amprenavir, has a particular resistance profile, with little cross-resistance to other PIs if virologic failure is detected early. In addition, failure to ritonavir-boosted fosamprenavir is associated with extremely low incidence of PI resistance and much less NRTI resistance than with other PIs. Therefore, ritonavir-boosted fosamprenavir regimens are indicated in PI-naive patients. Current guidelines for treatment of HIV-infected adults and adolescents[1] consider ritonavir-boosted fosamprenavir regimens as a "preferred" first-line treatment for antiretroviral-naive patients.

The role of fosamprenavir is less clear for PI-experienced patients, since ritonavir-boosted regimens failed to demonstrate noninferiority with respect to lopinavir/ritonavir. The complementary resistance profile of fosamprenavir with respect to other PIs may enable, after careful examination of genotypic and/or phenotypic resistance data, successful fosamprenavir/ritonavir-based second-line or salvage regimens. In treatment-experienced patients fosamprenavir/ritonavir should only be given twice daily. Direct comparisons with other PIs, as well as clinical data on dually boosted PI combinations including fosamprenavir are awaited in order to extend the indications of this drug to other clinical settings.

REFERENCES

1. Guidelines for the Use of Antiretroviral Agents in HIV-1 Infected Adults and Adolescents. 10 Oct 2006. Available: http://aidsinfo.nih.gov/ContentFiles/AdultandAdolescentGL.pdf 12 Oct 2006.
2. Palella FJ Jr, Delaney KM, Moorman AC, et al. Declining morbidity and mortality among patients with advanced human immunodeficiency virus infection. HIV Outpatient Study Investigators. N Engl J Med 338:853–60, 1998.
3. Mocroft A, Vella S, Benfield TL, et al. Changing patterns of mortality across Europe in patients infected with HIV-1. EuroSIDA Study Group. Lancet 352:1725–30, 1998.
4. Centers for Disease Control. Diffuse, undifferentiated non-Hodgkin lymphoma among homosexual males – United States. MMWR 31:277–9, 1982.

5. Centers for Disease Control. Persistent, generalized lymphadenopathy among homosexual males. MMWR 31:249–51, 1982.
6. Centers for Disease Control. Pneumocystis pneumonia – Los Angeles. MMWR 30:250–2, 1981.
7. Hammer SM, Squires KE, Hughes MD, et al. The AIDS Clinical Trials Group 320 Study Team. A controlled trial of two nucleoside analogues plus indinavir in persons with human immunodeficiency virus infection and CD4 cell counts of 200 per cubic millimeter or less. N Engl J Med 337:725–33, 1997.
8. Gulick RM, Mellors JW, Havlir D, et al. Treatment with indinavir, zidovudine, and lamivudine in adults with human immunodeficiency virus infection and prior antiretroviral therapy. N Engl J Med 337:734–739, 1997.
9. Montaner JS, Reiss P, Cooper D, et al. A randomized, double-blind trial comparing combinations of nevirapine, didanosine, and zidovudine for HIV-infected patients: the INCAS Trial. Italy, The Netherlands, Canada and Australia Study. JAMA279:930–7, 1998.
10. Staszewski S, Morales-Ramirez J, Tashima KT, et al. The Study 006 Team. Efavirenz plus zidovudine and lamivudine, efavirenz plus indinavir, and indinavir plus zidovudine and lamivudine in the treatment of HIV-1 infection in adults. N Engl J Med 341:1865–73, 1999.
11. Duggan MG, Evans WN. Estimating the impact of medical innovation: the case of HIV antiretroviral treatments. National Bureau of Economic Research Working Paper No. 11109 February 2005. JEL No. H51, I12, I18. Available: http://www.nber.org/papers/w11109 10 Feb 2006.
12. Freedberg KA, Losina E, Weinstein MC, et al. The cost effectiveness of combination antiretroviral therapy for HIV disease. N Engl J Med 344:824–31, 2001.
13. Spaltenstein A, Kazmierski WM, Miller JF, Samano V. Discovery of next generation inhibitors of HIV protease. Curr Top Med Chem 5:1589–607, 2005.
14. Perry CM, Frampton JE, McCormack PL, et al. Nelfinavir: a review of its use in the management of HIV infection. Drugs 65:2209–44, 2005.
15. Grossman Z, Paxinos EE, Averbuch D, et al. Mutation D30N is not preferentially selected by human immunodeficiency virus type 1 subtype C in the development of resistance to nelfinavir. Antimicrob Agents Chemother 48:2159–65, 2004.
16. Parkin NT, Schapiro JM. Antiretroviral drug resistance in non-subtype B HIV-1, HIV-2 and SIV. Antivir Ther 9:3–12, 2004.
17. Weinheimer S, Discotto L, Friborg J, et al. Atazanavir signature I50L resistance substitution accounts for unique phenotype of increased susceptibility to other protease inhibitors in a variety of human immunodeficiency virus type 1 genetic backbones. Antimicrob Agents Chemother 49:3816–24, 2005.
18. GlaxoSmithKline. Lexiva (fosamprenavir calcium) tablets: prescribing information (US). Online. Available: http://us.gsk.com/products/assets/us_lexiva.pdf 10 Feb 2006.
19. Arvieux C and Tribut O. Amprenavir or fosamprenavir plus ritonavir in HIV infection. Pharmacology, efficacy and tolerability profile. Drugs 65:633–59, 2005.
20. Fung HB, Kirschenbaum HL, Hameed R. Amprenavir: a new human immunodeficiency virus type 1 protease inhibitor. Clin Ther 22: 549–72, 2000.
21. Wire MB, Ballow C, Preston SL, et al. Pharmacokinetics and safety of GW433908 and ritonavir, with and without efavirenz, in healthy volunteers. AIDS 18: 897-907, 2004.
22. Baker C, Chaturvedi PR, Hale MR, et al. Discovery of VX-175/GW433908, a novel, water-soluble prodrug of amprenavir. In: 39th Interscience Conference on Anti-microbial Agents and Chemotherapy, San Francisco, 26–29 Sep 1999, abstract 313.
23. Ezidinma NP, Fish JT, Wandschneider HL, et al. Propylene glycol associated renal toxicity from lorazepam infusions [abstract]. Crit Care Med 27:A123, 1999.
24. Arbour R, Esparis B. Osmolar gap metabolic acidosis in a 60-year-old man treated for hypoxemic respiratory failure. Chest 118:545–6, 2000.
25. Arbour RB. Propylene glycol toxicity related to high-dose lorazepam infusion: case report and discussion. Am J Crit Care 8:499–506, 1999.
26. Reynolds HN, Teiken P, Regan ME, et al. Hyperlactatemia, increased osmolar gap, and renal dysfunction during continuous lorazepam infusion. Crit Care Med 28:1631–4, 2000.
27. D'Ambrosio JA, Borchardt-Phelps P, Nolen JG, et al. Propylene glycol-induced lactic acidosis secondary to a continuous infusion of lorazepam. Pharmacotherapy 13:274, 1993.
28. Seay RE. Comment: possible toxicity from propylene glycol in lorazepam infusion. Ann Pharmacother 31:647–8, 1997.
29. Parker MG, Fraser GL, Watson DM, et al. Removal of propylene glycol and correction of increased osmolar gap by hemodialysis in a patient on high dose lorazepam infusion therapy. Intensive Care Med 28:81–4, 2002.
30. Demey H, Daelemans R, De Broe ME. Propylene glycol intoxication due to intravenous nitroglycerin [letter]. Lancet 1:1360, 1984.
31. Demey H, Daelemans R, Verpooten GA. Propylene glycol-induced side effects during intravenous nitroglycerin therapy. Intensive Care Med 1988; 14:221–6.
32. Race E, Dam E, Obry V, Paulous S, et al. Analysis of HIV cross-resistance to protease inhibitors using a rapid single-cycle recombinant virus assay for patients failing on combination therapies. AIDS 13:2061–8, 1999.
33. Doenicke A, Nebauer AE, Hoernecke R. Osmolalities of propylene glycol-containing drug formulations for parenteral use: should propylene glycol be used as a solvent? Anesth Analg 75:431–5, 1992.
34. Cawley MJ. Short-term lorazepam infusion and concern for propylene glycol toxicity: case report and review. Pharmacotherapy 21:1140–4, 2001.
35. Levy ML, Aranda M, Zelman V, et al. Propylene glycol toxicity following continuous etomidate infusion for the control of refractory cerebral edema. Neurosurgery 37:363–71, 1995.
36. Yorgin PD, Theodorou A, Al-Uzri A. Propylene glycol-induced proximal renal tubular cell injury. Am J Kidney Dis 30:134–9, 1997.
37. Morshed KM, Jain S, McMartin KE. Acute toxicity of propylene glycol: an assessment using cultured proximal tubule cells of human origin. Fundam Appl Toxicol 23:38–43, 1994.
38. Karacostas V, Nagashima K, Gonda MA, Moss B. Human immunodeficiency virus-like particles produced by a vaccinia virus expression vector. Proc Natl Acad Sci USA 86:8964–7, 1989.
39. Roberts NA, Martin JA, Kinchington D, et al. Rational design of peptide-based HIV-proteinase inhibitors. Science 248:358–61, 1990.
40. Flexner C. HIV-protease inhibitors. N Engl J Med 338:1281–92, 1998.
41. Chapman TM, Plosker GL, Perry CM. Fosamprenavir: a review of its use in the management of antiretroviral therapy-naive patients with HIV infection. Drugs 64(18):2101–24, 2004.
42. Kim EE, Baker CT, Dwyer M. Crystal structure of HIV-1 protease in complex with VX-478, a potent an orally bioavailable inhibitor of the enzyme. J Am Chem Soc 117:1181–2, 1995.
43. Noble S, Goa KL. Amprenavir: a review of its clinical potential in patients with HIV infection. Drugs 60: 1383–410, 2000.
44. Painter GR, St Clair MH, Demiranda P, et al. An overview of the preclinical development of the HIV protease inhibitor VX-478 (141W94). In: Abstracts of the 2nd National Conference on Human Retroviruses and Related Infections, Washington, DC, 1995, abstract LB5.
45. Livingstone DJ, Pazhanisamy S, Porter DJT, et al. Weak binding of VX-478 to human plasma proteins and implications

for anti-human immunodeficiency virus therapy. J Infect Dis 172:1238, 1995.

46. Wood R, Arasteh K, Stellbrink HJ, et al. Six-week randomized controlled trial to compare the tolerabilities, pharmacokinetics, and antiviral activities of GW433908 and amprenavir in human immunodeficiency virus type 1-infected patients. Antimicrob Agents Chemother 48:116–23, 2004.
47. Falcoz C, Jenkins JM, Bye C, et al. Pharmacokinetics of GW433908, a prodrug of amprenavir, in healthy male volunteers. J Clin Pharmacol 42:887–98, 2002.
48. Sadler BM, Gillotin C, Lou Y, et al. In vivo effect of alpha (1)-acid glycoprotein on pharmacokinetics of amprenavir, a human immunodeficiency virus protease inhibitor. Antimicrob Agents Chemother 45: 852–6, 2001.
49. Zhang XQ, Schooley RT, Gerber JG. The effect of increasing alpha1-acid glycoprotein concentration on the antiviral efficacy of human immunodeficiency virus protease inhibitors. J Infect Dis 180:1833–7, 1999.
50. Yogev R, Kovacs A, Chadwick EG, et al. Single-dose safety and pharmacokinetics of amprenavir (141W94), a human immunodeficiency virus type 1 (HIV-1) protease inhibitor, in HIV-infected children. Antimicrob Agents Chemother 49:336–41, 2005.
51. Collier A, Tierney C, Downey G, et al (for the Adult AIDS Clinical Trials Group Protocol 5143 Team). Randomized study of twice-daily lopinavir/ritonavir or fosamprenavir + ritonavir vs. lopinavir/ritonavir + fosamprenavir (with tenofovir DF and nucleosides) as rescue therapy. In: 12th Conference on Retroviruses and Opportunistic Infections, Boston, MA, 22–25 Feb 2005, abstract 577.
52. Clay P, Anderson P, Smith P, et al. Pharmacokinetics of once-daily fosamprenavir 1400 mg plus atazanavir 400 mg without Ritonavir in HIV-negative subjects. In: 13th Conference on Retroviruses and Opportunistic Infections, Denver, CO, 2006, abstract 587.
53. Khanlou H, Bhatti L, Farthing C. Interaction between atazanavir and fosamprenavir in the treatment of HIV-infected patients. J Acquir Immune Defic Syndr 2006; 41:124–5.
54. Boffito M, Dickinson L, Hill A, et al. Steady-state pharmacokinetics of saquinavir hard-gel/ritonavir/fosamprenavir in HIV-1-infected patients. J Acquir Immune Defic Syndr 37:1376–84, 2004.
55. Peytavin G, Marcelin A, Rouault A, et al. Therapeutic drug monitoring of boosted tipranavir with and without combination to lopinavir or fosamprenavir. In: 13th Conference on Retroviruses and Opportunistic Infections, Denver, CO, 2006, abstract 591.
56. Sansone A, Keung A, Tetteh E, et al. Pharmacokinetics of vicriviroc are not affected in combination with five different protease inhibitors boosted by ritonavir. In: 13th Conference on Retroviruses and Opportunistic Infections, Denver, CO, 2006, abstract 582.
57. European Medicines Association. Available: http://www.emea.eu.int/humandocs/PDFs/EPAR/telzir/H-534-PI-en.pdf 10 Feb 2006.
58. Rodriguez-French A, Boghossian J, Gray GE, et al. The NEAT Study: a 48-week open-label study to compare the antiviral efficacy and safety of GW433908 versus nelfinavir in antiretroviral therapy-naive HIV-1-infected patients. J Acquir Immune Defic Syndr 35:22–32, 2004.
59. Gathe JC, Ive P, Wood R, et al. SOLO: 48-week efficacy and safety comparison of once-daily fosamprenavir/ritonavir versus twice-daily nelfinavir in naive HIV-1-infected patients. AIDS 18:1529–37, 2004.
60. MacManus S, Yates PJ, Elston RC, et al. W433908/ritonavir once daily in antirretroviral therapy-naive HIV-infected patients: absence of protease resistance at 48 weeks. AIDS 18:651–5, 2004.
61. Smith K, Weinberg W, DeJesus E, et al. Efficacy and safety of once-daily boosted fosamprenavir (FPV/r) or atazanavir (ATV/r) with tenofovir (TDF)/emtricitabine (FTC) in antiretroviral-naive HIV-1 infected patients: 24-week results from COL103952 (ALERT). In: Forty-Sixth Interscience Conference on Antimicrobial Agents and Chemotherapy, San Francisco, 2006, abstract H-1670a.
62. Gathe J, Wood R, Bellos N, et al. HIV DART 2004: Frontiers in Drug Development for Antiretroviral Therapies, Montego Bay, Jamaica; 12–16 Dec 2004, abstract 61.
63. GlaxoSmithKline. Safety and Tolerability of LEXIVA® (fosamprenavir calcium) in antiretroviral-naive patients over 120 weeks. (APV30005(APV30001) Final Study Report) Data on file. Available: http://www.treathiv.com/slidekits/ppt/LEXIVA-120-WeekTolerability.ppt 10 Feb 2006.
64. Eron J Jr, Yeni P, Gathe J Jr, et al. KLEAN study team. The KLEAN study of fosamprenavir–ritonavir versus lopinavir–ritonavir, each in combination with abacavir–lamivudine, for initial treatment of HIV infection over 48 weeks: a randomised non-inferiority trial. Lancet 368:476–82, 2006.
65. Caron M, Auclair M, Sterlingot H, et al. Some HIV protease inhibitors alter lamin A/C maturation and stability, SREBP-1 nuclear localization and adipocyte differentiation. AIDS 17: 2437–44, 2003.
66. Dubé MP, Qian D, Edmondson-Melançon H, et al. Prospective, intensive study of metabolic changes associated with 48 weeks of amprenavir-based antiretroviral therapy. Clin Infect Dis 35:475–81, 2002.
67. Maguire M, Shortino D, Klein A, et al. Emergence of resistance to protease inhibitor amprenavir in human immunodeficiency virus type 1-infected patients: selection of four alternative viral protease genotypes and influence of viral susceptibility to coadministered reverse transcriptase nucleoside inhibitors. Antimicrob Agents Chemother 46:731–8, 2002.
68. Johnson VA, Brun-Vézinet F, Clotet B, et al. Update of the drug resistance mutations in HIV-1. Fall 2005 Top. HIV Med 13:125–31, 2005.
69. Partadelis JA, Yamaguchi K, Tisdale M. In vitro selection and characterization of human immunodeficiency virus type 1 isolates with reduced sensitivity to hydroxyethanylamino sulphonamide inhibitors of HIV-1 aspartyl protease. J Virol 69:5228–35, 1995.
70. Tisdale M, Mayers RE, Maschera B, et al. Cross-resistance analysis of human immunodeficiency virus type 1 variants individually selected for resistance to five different protease inhibitors. Antimicrob Agents Chemother 39:1704–10, 1995.
71. Lastere S, Dalban C, Collin G, et al. NARVAL Trial Group (ANRS 088). Impact of insertions in the HIV-1 p6 PTAPP region on the virological response to amprenavir. Antivir Ther 9:221–7, 2004.
72. Peters S, Munoz M, Yerly S, et al. Resistance to nucleoside analog reverse transcriptase inhibitors mediated by human immunodeficiency virus type 1 p6 protein. J Virol 75:9644–53, 2001.
73. Maguire MF, Guinea R, Griffin P, et al. Changes in human immunodeficiency virus type 1 Gag at positions L449 and P453 are linked to I50V protease mutants in vivo and cause reduction of sensitivity to amprenavir and improved viral fitness in vitro. J Virol 76:7398–406, 2002.
74. Bally F, Martinez R, Peters S, Sudre P, Telenti A. Polymorphism of HIV type 1 gag p7/p1 and p1/p6 cleavage sites: clinical significance and implications for resistance to protease inhibitors. AIDS Res Hum Retroviruses 16:1209–13, 2000.
75. Marcelin AG, Affolabi D, Lamotte C, et al. Resistance profiles observed in virological failures after 24 weeks of amprenavir/ritonavir containing regimen in protease inhibitor experienced patients. J Med Virol 74:16–20, 2004.

76. Kempf DJ, Isaacson JD, King MS, et al. Identification of genotypic changes in human immunodeficiency virus protease that correlate with reduced susceptibility to the protease inhibitor lopinavir among viral isolates from protease inhibitor-experienced patients. J Virol 75:7462–9, 2001.
77. Monno L, Saracino A, Scudeller L, et al. HIV-1 phenotypic susceptibility to lopinavir (LPV) and genotypic analysis in LPV/r-naive subjects with prior protease inhibitor experience. J Acquir Immune Defic Syndr 33:439–47, 1 Aug 2003.
78. Gulnik SV, Suvorov LI, Liu B, et al. Kinetic characterization and cross-resistance patterns of HIV-1 protease mutants selected under drug pressure. Biochemistry 34:9282–7, 1995.
79. Klabe RM, Bacheler LT, Ala PJ, et al. Resistance to HIV protease inhibitors: a comparison of enzyme inhibition and antiviral potency. Biochemistry 37:8735–42, 1998.
80. Paulsen D, Liao Q, Fusco G, et al. Genotypic and phenotypic cross-resistance patterns to lopinavir and amprenavir in protease inhibitor-experienced patients with HIV viremia. AIDS Res Hum Retroviruses 18:1011-9, 2002.
81. Clotet B, Menéndez-Arias L, Schapiro J, et al. Guide to management of HIV drug resistance, antiretrovirals pharmacokinetics and viral hepatitis in HIV-infected subjects. 4th edn. Badalona, Catalonia, Spain: Fundació Lluita contra la SIDA, Hospital Universitari "Germans Trias i Pujol" 2006.
82. Marcelin AG, Lamotte C, Delaugerre C, et al. Genophar Study Group. Genotypic inhibitory quotient as predictor of virological response to ritonavir–amprenavir in human immunodeficiency virus type 1-protease inhibitor-experienced patients. Antimicrob Agents Chemother 47:594–600, 2003.
83. Scudeller L, Torti C, Quiros-Roldan E, et al. GenPheRex Group of the MASTER Cohort. HIV susceptibility to amprenavir: phenotype-based versus rules-based interpretations. J Antimicrob Chemother 52:776–81, 2003.
84. Woodahl EL, Yang Z, Bui T, et al. MDR1 G1199A polymorphism alters permeability of HIV protease inhibitors across P-glycoprotein-expressing epithelial cells. AIDS 19:1617–25, 2005.
85. Kinomoto M, Appiah-Opong R, Brandful JA, et al. HIV-1 proteases from drug-naive West African patients are differentially less susceptible to protease inhibitors. Clin Infect Dis 41:243–51, 2005.
86. Martinez-Picado J, Wrin T, Frost SD, et al. Phenotypic hypersusceptibility to multiple protease inhibitors and low replicative capacity in patients who are chronically infected with human immunodeficiency virus type 1. J Virol 79:5907–13, 2005.
87. Lam E, Parkin NT. Amprenavir resistance imparted by the I50V mutation in HIV-1 protease can be suppressed by the N88S mutation. Clin Infect Dis 37:1273–4, 2003.
88. Yanchunas J Jr, Langley DR, Tao L, et al. Molecular basis for increased susceptibility of isolates with atazanavir resistance-conferring substitution I50L to other protease inhibitors. Antimicrob Agents Chemother 49:3825–32, 2005.
89. Nadler J, Rodriguez-French A, Millard J, Wannamaker P. The NEAT Study: GW433908 efficacy and safety in ART-naive subjects, final 48-week analysis. In: Program and Abstracts of the 10th Conference on Retroviruses and Opportunistic Infections, Boston, MA, 10–14 Feb 2003, abstract 177.
90. Sax PE, Xu F, Tisdale M, Elston R. First report of resistance to boosted fosamprenavir in an ART-naive subject: virologic and clinical outcome. In: 45th Interscience Conference on Antimicrobial Agents and Chemotherapy, Washington, DC, USA, 16–19 Dec 2005.
91. Schurmann D, Elston R, Xu F, et al. Evolution of resistance during first-line treatment with boosted fosamprenavir is associated with baseline mutations. AIDS 20:138–40, 2006.

Chapter 20

Lopinavir

Steven C. Johnson, MD, Daniel R. Kuritzkes, MD

Lopinavir (formerly known as ABT-378) was the first of the 'second-generation' protease inhibitors (PIs) to be approved for clinical use. Principles of rational drug design and structure-based design were used to select a compound that is active against ritonavir-resistant isolates of human immunodeficiency virus type 1 (HIV-1). In addition, lopinavir is the only approved antiretroviral agent specifically co-formulated with ritonavir, a PI that inhibits lopinavir metabolism by the cytochrome P450 3A4 enzyme. The combination of lopinavir and ritonavir is marketed under the trade name Kaletra. The initial capsule formulation contained 133.3 mg of lopinavir and 33.3 mg of ritonavir. This was replaced in 2005 with a tablet formulation (often referred to as the Meltrex formulation) containing 200 mg of lopinavir and 50 mg of ritonavir. An oral solution, containing 80 mg of lopinavir and 20 mg of ritonavir per milliliter, is also available. In the absence of other medications that produce pharmacokinetic interactions, the standard dose of lopinavir/ritonavir in adults is 400/100 mg twice daily or 800/200 mg once daily. The use of lopinavir/ritonavir in combination with other antiretroviral agents has produced excellent clinical results in both antiretroviral-naive and antiretroviral-experienced patients.

CHEMICAL STRUCTURE

Lopinavir is a *C2* symmetrical peptidomimetic inhibitor of HIV-1 protease. Chemically, the drug is designated {1*S*-[1*R**, (*R**), 3*R**, 4*R**]}-*N*-(4-{[(2,6 dimethylphenoxy)acetyl]amino}-3-hydroxy-5-phenyl-1-(phenylmethyl)pentyl)tetrahydro-*a*-(1-methylethyl)-2-oxo-1(2H)-pyrimidineacetamide (Fig. 20-1). It has a molecular weight of 628.80 Da. Development of lopinavir was based on X-ray crystallographic studies of the interaction between the first-generation inhibitor ritonavir and HIV-1 protease.[1] Binding of ritonavir to protease is strongly enhanced by interactions between the isopropylthiazolyl side chain of the P3 peripheral heterocyclic group of the molecule and the substrate-binding pocket of protease. Mutations in HIV-1 protease that lead to substitution of alanine, phenylalanine, or tyrosine for the wild-type valine at amino acid 82 disrupt these interactions, leading to a lower affinity for drug binding. To minimize the effect of resistance mutations on PI binding, modifications were introduced to the ritonavir molecule that reduced the importance of hydrophobic interactions with the side chain of Val_{82}. Replacement of the isopropylthiazolyl P3 group with a cyclic urea, and replacement of the P2′ (thiazolyl) methoxycarbonyl moiety with a dimethylphenoxyactyl group produced lopinavir.

IN VITRO ACTIVITY

Lopinavir is a potent inhibitor of HIV-1. The drug inhibits 93% of wild-type protease activity at a concentration of 0.5 nM and binds with a K_I of 1.3 pM.[1] Inhibition of HIV-1 protease by lopinavir is highly specific compared to inhibition of mammalian aspartyl proteases such as renin,

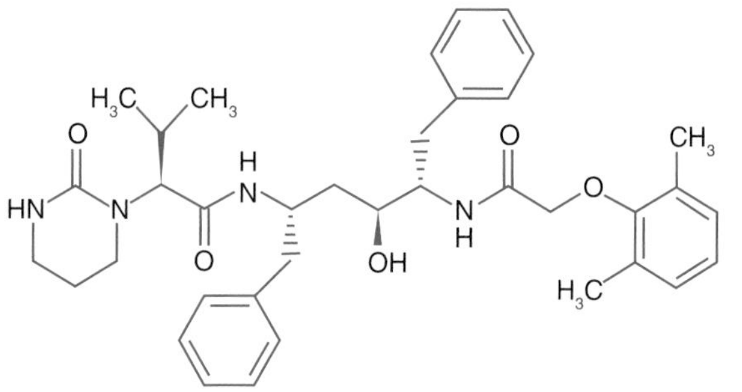

Figure 20-1 ■ Structural formula of lopinavir.

cathepsin D, and cathepsin E. Lopinavir is ~10 times more potent than ritonavir against wild-type virus. In the absence of human serum, the mean 50% effective concentration (EC_{50}) of lopinavir ranges from 10 to 27 nM (0.006–0.017 μg/mL) against HIV-1 laboratory strains and from 4 to 11 nM (0.003–0.007 μg/mL) against several clinical strains. The presence of 50% human serum increases the mean EC_{50} of lopinavir against HIV-1 laboratory strains by seven to 11-fold, resulting in values that range from 65 to 289 nM (0.04–0.18 μg/mL).[2]

PHARMACOKINETICS

When administered by itself, lopinavir achieves relatively modest plasma concentrations due to rapid metabolism by the cytochrome P450 3A4 enzyme (CYP3A4). The area under the curve (AUC) for lopinavir is greatly increased by concomitant administration of ritonavir, which inhibits the metabolism of lopinavir by CYP3A4 with a K_I of 0.013 μM.[3] In healthy volunteers, simultaneous administration of a 400-mg dose of lopinavir together with 50 mg of ritonavir increases the lopinavir AUC 77-fold over that achieved with lopinavir alone.[1] The AUC of lopinavir varies with the dose of the drug and the dose of concomitant ritonavir. In HIV-infected subjects, a 34% increase in AUC is achieved when lopinavir 400 mg bid is administered with ritonavir 100 mg bid as compared to lopinavir/ritonavir doses of 200/100 mg bid.[4]

A multiple-dose pharmacokinetic study in HIV-seropositive subjects using the 400/100 mg dose of lopinavir/ritonavir determined that at steady state the peak plasma concentration (C_{max}) of lopinavir is 9.8 ± 3.7 μg/mL, and the time to peak concentration (T_{max}) is ~4 h. The minimum steady-state concentration (C_{min}) of lopinavir in patients receiving the 400/100 mg dose twice daily is 5.5 ± 2.7 μg/mL, which exceeds the protein-binding-adjusted IC_{50} for wild-type isolates of HIV-1 by more than 30-fold.[2,4] Plasma concentrations of lopinavir and ritonavir after administration of two 200/50 mg lopinavir tablets are similar to three 133.3/33 mg lopinavir/ritonavir capsules taken after food, with less pharmacokinetic variability.[2] Once-daily dosing of 800/200 mg of lopinavir/ritonavir produces a mean lopinavir C_{max} of 11.8 + 3.7 μg/mL with a T_{max} of ~6 h. The C_{min} of lopinavir in patients receiving the 800/200 mg dose once daily is 1.7 ± 1.6 μg/mL. The 100 mg twice-daily or 200 mg once-daily dose of ritonavir achieves drug levels that are less than 7% of those achieved with the standard dose of ritonavir (600 mg bid). Therefore the observed *in vivo* activity of the lopinavir/ritonavir co-formulation is attributable almost exclusively to the lopinavir component.

Lopinavir is 98-99% bound to plasma proteins, primarily to α_1-acid glycoprotein and albumin. The extent of protein binding, which is constant throughout the therapeutic range, is similar in seronegative volunteers and HIV-infected subjects. The drug is extensively metabolized by CYP3A4. Although ritonavir is a potent inhibitor of CYP3A4, it also induces other P450 isozymes, including those responsible for its own metabolism. As a result, lopinavir trough concentrations decline somewhat over time, reaching a steady state within 10–16 days. Following a 400/100 mg dose of lopinavir/ritonavir, ~10% of administered lopinavir can be recovered from urine and 83% from feces; ~22% of the drug is excreted unchanged.[2] After multiple doses less than 3% of lopinavir is excreted unchanged in the urine. The drug exposure following a standard dose of lopinavir/ritonavir in patients on hemodialysis is similar to patients with normal renal function indicating that dosage adjustments are not necessary in the setting of diminished renal function.[5] In patients with HIV, hepatitis-C virus infection, and mild to moderate hepatic impairment, a 30% increase in lopinavir AUC and a 20% increase in C_{max} were noted when compared to HIV-infected patients with normal hepatic function.[2]

The pharmacokinetics of lopinavir/ritonavir have been studied in children aged 6 months to 12 years. A lopinavir dose of 230 mg/m^2 combined with a ritonavir dose of 57.5 mg/m^2 (using the oral solution) provides lopinavir plasma concentrations similar to those observed in adults receiving the 400/100 mg bid dose of lopinavir/ritonavir, resulting in a mean steady-state AUC of 72.6 ± 31.1 μg h^{-1} mL^{-1}, a mean C_{max} of 8.2 ± 2.9 μg/mL, a mean C_{trough} of 4.7 ± 2.9 μg/mL, and a mean C_{min} of 3.4 ± 2.1 μg/mL.[2,6]

For both adults and children, lopinavir/ritonavir drug levels can be altered by co-administration of other drugs that affect hepatic metabolism. For example, if co-administered with nevirapine or efavirenz, inducers of CYP3A4, lopinavir concentrations are reduced. In adults, increasing the dose of lopinavir/ritonavir to 600/150 mg (three tablets) twice daily or 533/133 mg (using the solution) twice daily compensates for this effect. In children when co-administered with either nevirapine or efavirenz, a lopinavir/ritonavir dose of 300/75 mg/m^2 provides lopinavir plasma concentrations similar to those observed in adults receiving the 400/100 mg dose without nevirapine or efavirenz.[6,7]

In 2005, a new tablet formulation of lopinavir/ritonavir containing 200 mg of lopinavir and 50 mg of ritonavir was approved by the FDA. This was accomplished with a novel melt extrusion technology which allows a poorly soluble compound like lopinavir/ritonavir to be dissolved in a polymer in a solvent-free environment. Studies of the new tablet formulation have documented less variability in absorption among study volunteers and also between the fed and fasted state.[8] Consequently, the new tablet can be administered with or without food. Other advantages of the new formulation include fewer pills (the standard daily dosing with four tablets is equivalent to six capsules) and the absence of a requirement for refrigeration, the latter an important limitation with the capsules.

EFFICACY

The efficacy of lopinavir/ritonavir has been examined in clinical trials in both antiretroviral-naive and antiretroviral-experienced patients. The results of the most important major clinical trials are reviewed below and summarized in Table 20-1.

Summary of Major Clinical Trials with Lopinavir/Ritonavir

Table 20-1

Study	Design	Entry Criteria	No. of Subjects	Antiviral Response	Comments
M97-720 (Murphy et al[9], Murphy et al[10])	Randomized, comparison of doses of lopinavir and ritonavir with d4T and 3TC added at week 3 (group I) or at day 0 (group II); tenofovir allowed to replace 'd4T' after year 6	Antiretroviral-naive; plasma HIV RNA level >5000 copies/mL; no CD4 cell restriction	100	59% with HIV RNA <50 copies/mL at 360 weeks (ITT, M= F)	Illustrates potency and long-term durability in antiretroviral naive subjects
M98-863 (Walmsley et al[11])	Randomized, double-blind comparison of lopinavir/ritonavir versus nelfinavir, both with d4T and 3TC	Antiretroviral-naive (no more than 14 days of any drug and no prior use of d4T or 3TC), plasma HIV RNA level >400 copies/mL; no CD4 cell restriction	653	83% of lopinavir/ritonavir-treated versus 68% of nelfinavir-treated patients reached HIV RNA<50 copies/mL at 48 weeks (on treatment analysis)	Lopinavir/ritonavir arm outperformed one of the commonly used regimens in clinical practice
KLEAN (Eron et al[12])	Randomized, open-label comparison of lopinavir/ritonavir versus fosamprenavir with ritonavir, both with abacavir and 3TC	Antiretroviral-naive, plasma HIV-1 RNA level ⩾1000 copies/mL, no CD4 cell restriction	878	ITT analysis revealed a plasma HIV-1 RNA level < 50 copies/mL in 65% of the subjects in the lopinavir/ritonavir arm and 66% in fosamprenavir the with ritonavir arm at 48 weeks	Both boosted protease inhibitor arms performed similarly with regard to virologic outcomes
ACG 5142 (Riddler et al[13])	Randomized, open-label comparison of three class-sparing regimens: lopinavir/ritonavir + EFV, lopinavir/ritonavir + 2 NRTIs, and EFV+ 2 NRTIs	Antiretroviral-naive, HIV-1 RNA level ⩾ 2000 copies/mL, no CD4 restriction	753	ITT analysis revealed a plasma HIV-1 RNA level < 50 copies/mL in 77% of subjects in the lopinavir/ritonavir + 2 NRTIs arm compared to 89% of subjects in the EFV+ 2 NRTIs arm and 83% of subjects in the lopinavir/ritonavir + EFV arm at 96 weeks	Shorter time to virologic failure for the LPV/r + 2 NRTIs arm when compared to the EFV + 2 NRTIs arm; higher rate of EFV resistance mutations in the LPV/r + EFV arm
M97-765 (Benson et al,[14] Feinberg et al[15])	Randomized study of lopinavir with one of two doses of ritonavir, with nevirapine and at least one new NRTI added at day 15	Single PI experience; HIV RNA 1000–100 000 copies/mL	70	Approximately 60% of patients achieved an HIV RNA < 400 copies/mL at 96 weeks (ITT, M = F)	Illustrates efficacy of lopinavir/ritonavir with an NNRTI in single PI failures
M98-957 (Clumeck et al[16])	Randomized trial of lopinavir/ritonavir at one of two doses with EFV and NRTIs	Failing PI-based regimen and treated with at least two PIs; NNRTI-naive; HIV RNA level >1000 copies/mL	57	56% of patients achieved an HIV RNA level <50 copies/mL at 48 weeks (ITT, M = F)	Illustrates efficacy of lopinavir/ritonavir with an NNRTI in multiple PI failures

(Continued)

(Continued)

Table 20-1

Study	Design	Entry Criteria	No. of Subjects	Antiviral Response	Comments
Study 045 (Johnson et al[17])	Randomized trial of lopinavir/ritonavir, atazanavir with ritonavir, and atazanavir with saquinavir, each with tenofovir plus an NRTI	Failed ≥ 2 prior antiretroviral regimens, CD4 > 50 cells/mm^3, HIV RNA level > 1000 copies/mL	358	Mean reductions from baseline in HIV-1 RNA levels at 48 weeks were 1.93 $\log_{10}$ copies/mL in the atazanavir with ritonavir arm, 1.55 $\log_{10}$ copies/mL in the atazanavir with saquinavir arm, and 1.87 $\log_{10}$ copies/mL in the lopinavir/ritonavir arm.	Illustrates potency of both ritonavir-boosted regimens in ARV-experienced patients
Context Study (Elston et al[18])	Randomized open label trial comparing fosamprenavir/ritonavir, dosed once daily or twice daily, versus lopinavir/ritonavir, all regimens with 2 NRTIs, in PI-experienced patients	Prior experience with ≤2 protease inhibitors with plasma HIV-1 RNA level ≥ 1000 copies/mL	320	Percent of subjects with a plasma HIV-1 RNA level <50 copies/mL at 48 weeks was 50% in the lopinavir/ritonavir arm, 46% in the twice daily fosamprenavir with ritonavir arm, and 37% in the once daily fosamprenavir with ritonavir arm	Twice daily fosamprenavir with ritonavir arm failed to show equivalence to the lopinavir/ritonavir arm; once daily fosamprenavir with ritonavir arm inferior to lopinavir/ritonavir arm
MaxCmin2 trial (Ulrik et al[19])	Randomized, open-label trial of saquinavir with ritonavir versus lopinavir/ritonavir in both ARV-naive and experienced patients	27% of subjects were ARV-naive at baseline; the remainder were ARV-experienced	339	Discontinuation of the assigned treatment occurred in 14% of those in the lopinavir/ritonavir arm versus 30% in the saquinavir with ritonavir arm	Results favor the lopinavir/ritonavir arm although the primary reason for discontinuation was adverse events.
Study 418 (Molina et al[21])	Randomized trial of lopinavir/ritonavir 800/200 mg once daily versus lopinavir/ritonavir 400/100 mg twice daily, each with tenofovir and emtricitabine	Antiretroviral naive, HIV RNA level > 1000 copies/mL, any CD4 count	190	At week 96, 57% of subjects in the once daily arm achieved an HIV-1 RNA level <50 copies/mL compared to 53% in the twice daily arm (ITT analysis with noncompleters considered failures)	Demonstrates equivalent results between once and twice daily lopinavir/ritonavir in ARV-naive patients
M98-940 (Saez-Llorens X et al [22])	Randomized trial of two doses of lopinavir/ritonavir; ARV-naive received d4T and 3TC: ARV-experienced received nevirapine plus NRTIs	Age 3 months to 12 years, HIV RNA>400 copies/mL; NNRTI-naive	100	At 48 weeks, 71% of naive and 63% of experienced subjects achieved HIV RNA <50 copies/mL (ITT analysis)	Illustrates potency and tolerability in children; also indicated effect of nevirapine to lower lopinavir/ritonavir levels

d4T, stavudine; ITT, intention-to-treat; M = F, missing=failure; NRTI, nucleoside reverse transcriptase inhibitor; PI, protease inhibitor; 3TC, lamivudine.

The antiviral activity of several dosage levels of lopinavir/ritonavir in combination with stavudine (d4T) and lamivudine (3TC) was tested in a study of 100 antiretroviral-naive adults (study M97-720).[9] Subjects initially received (1) one of two dosages of lopinavir/ritonavir (400/100 mg or 200/100 mg twice daily) alone followed by the addition of d4T and 3TC at week 3 (group I) or (2) one of two dosages of lopinavir/ritonavir (400/100 mg or 400/200 mg twice daily) together with d4T and 3TC beginning at day 0 (group II). Baseline characteristics of the enrolled patients included a median baseline CD4+ T-lymphocyte count of 398 and 310 cells/mm^3 in groups I and II, respectively, and a mean plasma HIV-1 RNA level of 4.9 $\log_{10}$ copies/mL in both groups. According to an intention-to-treat (ITT) analysis, which counted missing patients as treatment failures, a plasma HIV-1 RNA level of less than 50 copies/mL was achieved in 75% and 79% of patients in groups I and II, respectively, at 48 weeks. The CD4+ T-lymphocyte count increased by ~200–250 cells/mm^3 over this same time period. After 48 weeks, all patients in this study received lopinavir 400 mg twice daily plus ritonavir 100 mg twice daily, along with d4T and 3TC at standard doses and the study was continued to examine the long-term efficacy of this regimen. A modification at year six allowed 37 patients to replace stavudine with tenofovir. At 360 weeks (7 years), 59% of patients have maintained an HIV-1 plasma RNA level <50 copies/mL using an ITT analysis where noncompleters are counted as failures. Using an on-treatment analysis, 95% of patients have an HIV-1 plasma RNA level <50 copies/mL. Over the 7-year study, the mean CD4+ T-lymphocyte count increased by 501 cells/mm^3.[10]

A randomized, double-blind phase III study compared the efficacy of lopinavir/ritonavir with that of nelfinavir in treatment-naive patients (study M98-863).[11] Both PIs were used in combination with d4T and 3TC. Lopinavir/ritonavir was dosed at 400/100 mg twice daily; nelfinavir was dosed at 750 mg three times a day, but subjects were allowed to change to 1250 mg twice daily at approximately week 24, when data on twice-daily dosing of nelfinavir became available. At baseline the mean plasma HIV-1 RNA level and CD4+ T-lymphocyte count among the 653 participants were 4.9 $\log_{10}$ copies/mL and 259 cells/mm^3, respectively. At 48 weeks, the ITT analysis showed that a plasma HIV-1 RNA level of less than 50 copies/mL was achieved in 67% of subjects on the lopinavir/ritonavir arm versus 52% in the nelfinavir arm. An on-treatment analysis at 48 weeks confirmed the virologic superiority of the lopinavir/ritonavir arm in this study, with 83% of subjects on the lopinavir/ritonavir arm achieving a plasma HIV-1 RNA level of less than 50 copies/mL versus 68% in the nelfinavir arm. This study illustrates the potency of a lopinavir/ritonavir-containing regimen in antiretroviral-naive patients when compared to one of the unboosted PI treatment regimens commonly used in clinical practice at that time (Fig. 20-2).

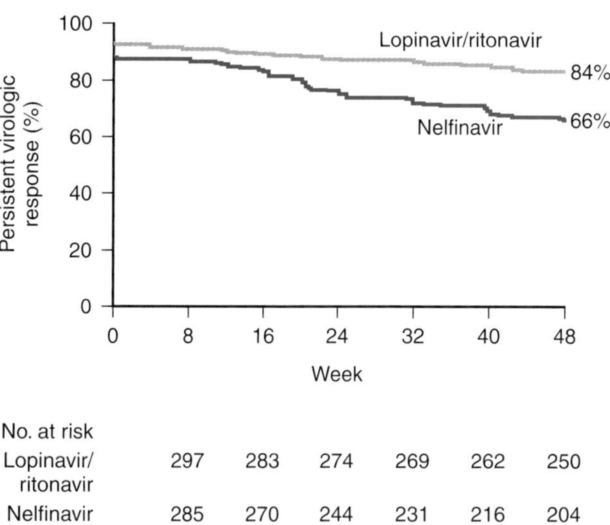

No. at risk						
Lopinavir/ ritonavir	297	283	274	269	262	250
Nelfinavir	285	270	244	231	216	204

Figure 20-2 ■ Study 863: Kaplan–Meier analysis of the time to the loss of virologic response through week 48 ($P < 0.001$ for the comparison between the two treatment groups).

Reprinted from Walmsley S, Bernstein B, King M, et al. Lopinavir/ritonavir versus nelfinavir for the initial treatment of HIV infection. N Eng J Med 346:2039, 2002.

More recently, lopinavir/ritonavir was compared to another boosted PI regimen, fosamprenavir with ritonavir, each with abacavir/lamivudine, in a prospective, randomized, open-label trial in antiretroviral-naive patients. Lopinavir/ritonavir was dosed 400/100 mg twice daily while fosamprenavir and ritonavir were dosed 700 mg twice daily and 100 mg twice daily, respectively. Baseline data for the ITT population of 878 patients included a median plasma HIV-1 RNA level of 5.07 $\log_{10}$ copies/mL and a CD4+ T-lymphocyte count of 192 cells/mm^3. At 48 weeks, an ITT analysis revealed a plasma HIV-1 RNA level <50 copies/mL in 65% of the subjects in the lopinavir/ritonavir arm and 66% in the fosamprenavir with ritonavir arm. A prospective, randomized three-arm trial (AIDS Clinical Trials Group 5142) compared lopinavir/ritonavir with two nucleoside reverse transcriptase inhibitors (NRTIs) versus efavirenz with two NRTIs versus lopinavir/ritonavir and efavirenz without NRTIs. Baseline data for the 753 subjects included a median plasma HIV-1 RNA level of 5 $\log_{10}$ copies/mL and a CD4+ T-lymphocyte count of 182 cells/mm^3. At 96 weeks, an ITT analysis revealed a plasma HIV-1 RNA level <50 copies/mL in 77% of subjects in the lopinavir/ritonavir with two NRTIs arm compared to 89% of subjects in the efavirenz with two NRTIs arm and 83% of subjects in the lopinavir/ritonavir with efavirenz arm ($P = 0.003$ for the comparison of the efavirenz with two NRTIs arm versus the lopinavir/ritonavir with two NRTIs arm). The time to virologic failure was significantly shorter for the lopinavir/ritonavir with two NRTIs arm when compared to the efavirenz with two NRTIs arm ($P = 0.006$). In addition, there was a trend for more efavirenz resistance mutations in the lopinavir/ritonavir with efavirenz arm when compared to the efavirenz with two NRTIs arm.[13]

The activity of lopinavir/ritonavir in patients failing antiretroviral therapy that included a PI with two NRTIs was evaluated in study M97-765.[14,15] Patients failing their first PI-based regimen with plasma HIV-1 RNA levels between 1000 and 100 000 copies/mL were eligible for study if they were naive to NNRTIs and to at least one NRTI. Patients received lopinavir 400 mg twice daily plus ritonavir at a dose of either 100 or 200 mg twice daily for 15 days, after which nevirapine along with at least one new NRTI were added. Seventy patients enrolled in this study. The median baseline CD4+ T-lymphocyte count and plasma HIV-1 RNA level were 349 cells/mm^3 and 4.0 $\log_{10}$ copies/mL, respectively. Prior PI use included indinavir (44%), nelfinavir (36%), saquinavir (13%), ritonavir (6%), and amprenavir (1%). Phenotypic resistance testing at study entry revealed that viruses from 32% of patients had a fourfold or more loss in susceptibility to three or more PIs. No significant difference in treatment response was observed between the two groups. At week 2, prior to the addition of nevirapine, 80% of patients had either a more than 1 $\log_{10}$ copies/mL decrease in plasma HIV-1 RNA level or achieved a plasma HIV-1 RNA level of less than 400 copies/mL. The ITT analysis at 96 weeks for the two groups combined showed that ~60% of patients achieved a plasma HIV-1 RNA of less than 400 copies/mL.[15] These results demonstrate the efficacy of lopinavir/ritonavir in antiretroviral-experienced patients. However, patients in this study had not received more than one other PI, and other approved PIs have also been effective in this setting. Moreover, activity of the treatment regimen was bolstered by adding two other effective drugs (nevirapine and a previously unused NRTI).

The use of lopinavir/ritonavir in patients with a greater degree of PI experience was assessed in another study (M98-957).[16] Patients with plasma HIV-1 RNA levels of more than 1000 copies/mL on a failing PI regimen who had been treated with at least two PIs were eligible for study if they were naive to NNRTIs. At baseline, the median plasma HIV-1 RNA level was 4.5 $\log_{10}$ copies/mL. Altogether, 68% of baseline viral isolates demonstrated a fourfold or more loss in susceptibility to three or more other PIs. Patients were randomized to receive lopinavir/ritonavir at a dose of 400/100 mg twice daily ($n = 29$) or 400/100 mg twice daily for 14 days, after which the dose was increased to 533/133 mg twice daily ($n = 28$). All patients also received efavirenz (600 mg daily) beginning at day 0. Twenty-five percent of patients also received at least one new NRTI during the first 8 weeks of the study. After week 24 the dose of lopinavir/ritonavir was changed to 533/133 mg twice daily in all patients. This change in dosing was prompted by the observation that lopinavir trough levels and the lopinavir AUC were reduced in patients who received lopinavir/ritonavir together with efavirenz, which induces lopinavir/ritonavir metabolism. The ITT analysis (missing = failure) at 48 weeks demonstrated that 56% of patients achieved a plasma HIV-1 RNA level of less than 50 copies/mL. Successful suppression of plasma HIV-1 RNA was achieved in most patients even though the mean susceptibility of lopinavir among baseline viral isolates was 16-fold higher than that of the wild-type virus. Results of this study support the concept that resistance to PIs can be overcome in part by increasing drug exposure through ritonavir-mediated inhibition of CYP3A4. Lopinavir/ritonavir was compared to atazanavir with ritonavir and atazanavir with saquinavir in a randomized, open-label 48 week trial in patients who had failed at least two prior antiretroviral regimens.[17] In this study, 358 patients with a baseline HIV RNA level >1000 copies/mL and a CD4+ T-lymphocyte count >50 cells/mm^3 were randomized 1:1:1 to atazanavir 300 mg once daily with ritonavir 100 mg once daily, atazanavir 400 mg once daily with saquinavir 1200 mg once daily, or lopinavir/ritonavir 400/100 mg twice daily, each with tenofovir and one NRTI. At week 48, the primary efficacy endpoint (plasma HIV-1 RNA reduction assessed by time-averaged difference) was similar in the lopinavir/ritonavir and atazanavir with ritonavir arms; the atazanavir with saquinavir arm was inferior. Mean reductions from baseline in HIV-1 RNA levels at 48 weeks were 1.93 $\log_{10}$ copies/mL in the atazanavir with ritonavir arm, 1.55 $\log_{10}$ copies/mL in the atazanavir with saquinavir arm, and 1.87 $\log_{10}$ copies/mL in the lopinavir/ritonavir arm.

A three-arm study compared lopinavir/ritonavir 400/100 mg twice-daily to two different dosing regimens of fosamprenavir and ritonavir, each with two NRTIs, in PI-experienced patients. Fosamprenavir was dosed at 700 mg twice daily with ritonavir 100 mg twice daily in one arm and 1400 mg once daily with ritonavir 200 mg once daily in the other arm. At 48 weeks, an HIV-1 RNA level <50 copies/mL was achieved in 50% of subjects in the lopinavir/ritonavir arm compared to 46% of subjects in the twice-daily fosamprenavir with ritonavir arm and only 37% of subjects in the once-daily fosamprenavir with ritonavir arm.[2,18]

A randomized, open-label study compared lopinavir/ritonavir to another ritonavir-boosted PI, saquinavir with ritonavir, each administered with two or more NRTIs, in both antiretroviral-naive and antiretroviral-experienced subjects (the MaxCmin2 trial). Lopinavir/ritonavir was dosed at the standard dose of 400/100 mg twice daily whereas saquinavir was dosed at 1000 mg twice daily with 100 mg of ritonavir twice daily. The 48-week analysis, by ITT, revealed treatment failure in 29/163 (18%) subjects in the lopinavir/ritonavir arm versus 53/161 (33%) in the saquinavir with ritonavir arm. The primary reason for treatment discontinuation in both arms was adverse events, which occurred more commonly in the saquinavir with ritonavir arm.[19]

When lopinavir/ritonavir was initially approved by the FDA, it was administered twice daily. A small randomized, open-label trial involving 38 antiretroviral-naive patients found comparable virologic results between 800/200 mg once-daily dosing and 400/100 mg twice-daily dosing.[20] These data led to a larger randomized, open-label trial comparing lopinavir/ritonavir 800/200 mg once daily compared with 400/100 mg twice daily, each with tenofovir and emtricitabine, in antiretroviral-naive subjects with a baseline HIV-1 RNA level subjects with a baseline HIV-1 RNA level >1000 copies/mL and any CD4+ T-lymphocyte count.[21] At baseline the median HIV-1 RNA levels were 4.8 and 4.6 $\log_{10}$ copies/mL in the once-daily and twice-daily arms, respectively. The median baseline CD4+ T-lymphocyte counts were 214 and 232 cells/mm^3 in the once-daily and twice-daily arms, respectively. Patients were randomized 3:2 with 115 patients receiving once-daily therapy and 75 patients receiving twice-daily therapy. At week 96, 57% of subjects achieved an HIV-1 RNA level

<50 copies/mL in the once-daily arm compared to 53% in the twice-daily arm (ITT analysis with noncompleters considered failures). Diarrhea was more common in the once-daily arm. This study led to the approval of lopinavir/ritonavir for once-daily dosing in antiretroviral-naive patients. Two dosage levels of lopinavir/ritonavir have been studied in treatment-naive and treatment-experienced HIV-1-infected children (study M98-940).[22] Lopinavir/ritonavir was administered every 12h at a dose of 230/57.5 mg/m^2 or 300/75 mg/m^2 in combination with d4T and 3TC (for antiretroviral-naive children) or together with nevirapine and one or two NRTIs (for antiretroviral-experienced patients). After 12 weeks, all patients received the 300/75 mg/m^2 dose. A total of 100 patients were enrolled in this study. At entry, the median plasma HIV-1 RNA level was 4.9 $\log_{10}$ copies/mL in the antiretroviral-naive group (n = 44) and 4.5 $\log_{10}$ copies/mL in the antiretroviral-experienced group (n = 56). An ITT analysis at 48 weeks showed that 84% of antiretroviral-naive subjects and 75% of antiretroviral-experienced subjects achieved a plasma HIV-1 RNA levels of less than 400 copies/mL; 71% and 63%, respectively, had plasma HIV-1 RNA levels of less than 50 copies/mL.

Novel Treatment Strategies

The use of lopinavir/ritonavir has been studied in several novel treatment strategies including monotherapy (either as initial therapy or following simplification from a combination regimen) and as part of nucleoside analog-sparing regimens. In one small study, 30 patients with a mean baseline HIV-1 RNA of 262 000 copies/mL and a CD4+ T-lymphocyte count of 169 cells/mm^3 began monotherapy with lopinavir/ritonavir dosed at either 400/100 mg or 533/133 mg twice daily. Of the 19 who completed the 48-week study, all 19 achieved an HIV-1 RNA level <400 copies/mL; 16/19 achieved an HIV-1 RNA level of <50 copies/mL (54% by an ITT analysis where noncompleters are considered failures).[23] The MONARK study randomized antiretroviral-naive subjects to either lopinavir/ritonavir monotherapy (n = 83) or lopinavir/ritonavir with zidovudine and lamivudine (n = 53). This study favored combination therapy; an on-treatment analysis at 48 weeks revealed a plasma HIV-1 RNA level of less than 50 copies/mL in 84% of subjects in the lopinavir/ritonavir monotherapy arm compared to 98% of subjects in the combination therapy arm.[24] In a study evaluating treatment simplification to boosted PI monotherapy, 42 patients without prior PI treatment failure, on lopinavir/ritonavir with two NRTIs, and with a plasma HIV-1 RNA level less than 50 copies/mL for at least 6 months, were randomized to either simplification to monotherapy with lopinavir/ritonavir 400/100 mg twice daily or continuation of the three-drug regimen. At 48 weeks after the switch, 17/21 (81%) of patients in the monotherapy arm maintained an HIV-1 RNA level <50 copies/mL.[25] A number of other studies have evaluated this approach.[26-28] However, PI monotherapy as initial therapy or as a simplification strategy should still be viewed as investigational.

Combination of PIs with NNRTIs (a nucleoside-sparing approach) is a possible treatment strategy that has been investigated in several recent trials.[13,29] In the recent ACTG trial 5142, reviewed above, an ITT analysis at 96 weeks revealed a plasma HIV-1 RNA level <50 copies/mL in 83% of subjects in the lopinavir/ritonavir and efavirenz arm compared to 77% of subjects in the lopinavir and two NRTIs arm and to 89% of subjects in the efavirenz and two NRTIs arm. There was a trend towards higher rates of efavirenz resistance in the nucleoside-sparing (lopinavir/ritonavir with efavirenz) arm when compared to the efavirenz with two NRTIs arm.[13] In another trial involving 31 antiretroviral-experienced patients with prolonged viral suppression, the combination of lopinavir/ritonavir with nevirapine was compared to lopinavir/ritonavir with two NRTIs. At 48 weeks, all patients had maintained their virologic suppression.[29]

Pediatric Efficacy Studies

Two dosage levels of lopinavir/ritonavir have been studied in treatment-naive and treatment-experienced HIV-1-infected children (study M98-940).[20] Lopinavir/ritonavir was administered every 12 h at a dose of 230/57.5 mg/m^2 or 300/75 mg/m^2 in combination with d4T and 3TC (for antiretroviral-naive children) or together with nevirapine and one or two NRTIs (for antiretroviral-experienced patients). After 12 weeks, all patients received the 300/75 mg/m^2 dose. A total of 100 patients were enrolled in this study. At entry, the median plasma HIV-1 RNA level was 4.9 $\log_{10}$ copies/mL in the antiretroviral-naive group (n = 44) and 4.5 $\log_{10}$ copies/mL in the antiretroviral-experienced group (n = 56). An ITT analysis at 48 weeks showed that 84% of antiretroviral-naive subjects and 75% of antiretroviral-experienced subjects achieved plasma HIV-1 RNA levels of less than 400 copies/mL; 71% and 63%, respectively, had plasma HIV-1 RNA levels of less than 50 copies/ml.

TOXICITY

Lopinavir/ritonavir has been generally well tolerated in clinical trials. The most commonly observed side effect is diarrhea, which is typically mild to moderate in intensity. The most significant laboratory abnormalities have been elevations in total cholesterol and triglycerides. Table 20-2 lists the most common adverse events and serious or severe (grade 3 or 4) laboratory abnormalities observed in the phase III efficacy trial that compared lopinavir/ritonavir with nelfinavir.[2,11] Pancreatitis has occurred in some patients receiving lopinavir/ritonavir, including patients who have marked hypertriglyceridemia.

The safety of lopinavir/ritonavir in the subset of patients co-infected with hepatitis B or hepatitis C virus (or both) has also been examined. Not surprisingly, liver enzyme elevations have been observed more commonly in patients with underlying hepatitis.[30,31,32] In study M97-720, patients with a positive hepatitis-B surface antigen or hepatitis C antibody had an eight-fold increased relative risk of grade 3 or 4 elevations in aspartate (AST) or alanine (ALT) transaminase on lopinavir/ritonavir.[9] A number of metabolic complications have been observed in patients receiving PIs and other antiretroviral agents. These

Table 20-2

Treatment Associated Adverse Events of Moderate or Severe Intensity and Grade 3–4 Laboratory Abnormalities Reported in Adult Patients on Study M98–863[11]

Adverse Event or Grade 3–4 Laboratory Abnormality	Lopinavir/Ritonavir 400/100 mg bid + d4T + 3TC (n = 326) (%)	Nelfinavir 750 mg tid + d4T + 3TC (n = 327) (%)
Abdominal pain	13 (4%)	10 (3.1%)
Asthenia	13 (4%)	11 (3.4%)
Headache	8 (2.5%)	6 (1.8%)
Diarrhea	51 (15.6%)	56 (17.1%)
Nausea	22 (6.7%)	15 (4.6%)
Vomiting	8 (2.5%)	8 (2.4%)
AST or ALT > 5 times upper limit of normal	14 (4.5%)	17 (5.2%)
Total cholesterol > 300 mg/dL	28 (9.0%)	16 (4.9%)
Triglycerides > 750 mg/dL	29 (9.3%)	4 (1.3%)

ALT, alanine transaminase; AST, aspartate transaminase.

Table 20-3

Drugs that should not be Co-Administered with Lopinavir/Ritonavir

Drug Class: Drug Name(s)	Clinical comment
Antihistamines: astemizole, terfenadine	Contraindicated due to risk of a life-threatening reaction such as a cardiac arrhythmia
Antimycobacterial: Rifampin, rifapentine	Induction of hepatic metabolism of lopinavir/ritonavir may lead to loss of virologic response and possible resistance
Corticosteroid (inhaled): fluticasone	Ritonavir greatly increases plasma levels of corticosteroid with reported cases of Cushing's syndrome
Ergot derivatives: ergonovine, dihydroergotamine, ergotamine, methylergonovine	Contraindicated due to risk of a life-threatening reaction such as acute ergot toxicity characterized by peripheral vasospasm with ischemia of tissues
GI motility agent: cisapride	Contraindicated due to risk of a life-threatening reaction such as a cardiac arrhythmia
Herbal products: St John's wort (*Hypericum perforatum*)	Induction of hepatic metabolism of lopinavir/ritonavir may lead to loss of virologic response or resistance
Certain HMG-CoA reductase inhibitors: lovastatin, simvastatin	Potential for serious reactions such as myopathy and rhabdomyolysis
Neuroleptic: pimozide	Contraindicated due to risk of a life-threatening reaction such as a cardiac arrhythmia
Sedative/hypnotics: midazolam, triazolam	Contraindicated due to risk of a life-threatening reaction such as prolonged or increased sedation or respiratory depression

GI, gastrointestinal; HMG-CoA, 3-hydroxy-3-methyl-glutaryl coenzyme A.

Adapted from Kaletra package insert, October 2005; Bertz R, Hsu A, Lam W, et al. Pharmacokinetic interactions between lopinavir/ritonavir (ABT-378r) and other non-HIV drugs [P291]. AIDS 14(Suppl 4):S100, 2000; Panel on Clinical Practices for Treatment of HIV infection. Department of Health and Human Services. Guidelines for the use of antiretroviral agents in HIV-1-infected adults and adolescents. Available: http://AIDSinfo.nih.gov 10 Oct 2006.

complications include diabetes mellitus, hyperlipidemia, gynecomastia, fat redistribution syndromes (including peripheral and facial wasting, dorsocervical fat pads, truncal obesity), and metabolic bone disease (osteoporosis and osteopenia). The mechanism of each of these complications and their potential association with individual antiretroviral agents, including lopinavir/ritonavir, remains unclear at this time.[33] However, lopinavir/ritonavir has clearly been shown to produce elevations in cholesterol and triglycerides and to produce modest insulin resistance in healthy volunteers.[34]

DRUG INTERACTIONS

Lopinavir and ritonavir are inhibitors of CYP3A4, although the combined formulation does not inhibit CYP3A4 as potently as does full-dose ritonavir. Lopinavir/ritonavir also inhibits CYP2D6 *in vitro* but to a lesser extent than CYP3A4. Consequently, a number of drugs are either contraindicated or require dose adjustment when used with lopinavir/ritonavir. Table 20-3 provides a list of medications that should not be co-administered with lopinavir/ritonavir.[2,35,36] Many other

Table 20-4 Established or Potential Drug Interactions Between Lopinavir/Ritonavir and Non-HIV Drugs With Suggested Adjustments in Drug Dose

Drug Class: Drug Names	Interaction with Lopinavir/Ritonavir	Adjustment of Lopinavir/Ritonavir or Concomitant Drug
Antiarrhythmics: amiodarone, bipridil, lidocaine, quinidine	Increased levels of antiarrhythmics	Therapeutic drug monitoring of the antiarrhythmics is recommended
Anticoagulant: warfarin	Warfarin levels may be affected	International normalized ratio (INR) is monitored
Anticonvulsants: carbamazepine, phenobarbital, phenytoin	Reduced levels of lopinavir	Dose adjustment unclear. Alternative anticonvulsants are used if possible
Antidepressant: trazadone	Increased levels of trazadone	Use with caution and a lower dose of trazadone should be used
Antifungals: ketoconazole, itraconazole, voriconazole	Increased levels of ketoconazole and itraconazole; reduced levels of voriconazole	High doses of ketoconazole or itraconazole not recommended; co-administration with voriconazole not recommended
Antiinfective: clarithromycin	Increased levels of clarithromycin	Clarithromycin dose is reduced in patients with renal impairment
Antimycobacterial: rifabutin	Increased levels of rifabutin	Rifabutin dose is decreased at least 75% from 300 mg/day dose
Antiparasitic: atovaquone	Potential for reduced level of atovaquone	Clinical significance unknown
Calcium channel blockers: felodipine, nifedipine, nicardipine	Potential for increased levels of these calcium channel blockers	Caution warranted when using these agents
Corticosteroid: dexamethasone	Potential for reduced level of lopinavir	Limit concomitant use
Disulfiram/metronidazole	Lopinavir/ritonavir oral solution contains alcohol	Concomitant use of lopinavir/ritonavir oral solution with these two agents may lead to a disulfiram-like reaction
PDE5 inhibitors: sildenafil, adalafil, vardenzafil	Increased levels of sildenafil, tadalafil, and vardenafil	Reduce doses and interval of all three agents (see package insert)
HMG-CoA reductase inhibitors: atorvastatin, cerivastatin	Increased levels of atorvastatin and cerivastatin likely	Use lowest possible dose or consider pravastain or fluvastatin
Immunosuppressants: cyclosporin, tacrolimus,	Increased levels of immunosuppressants likely	Therapeutic drug monitoring with rapamycin dose adjustment of immunosuppressants
Narcotic analgesics: methadone	Reduced level of methadone	Methadone dose may have to be increased
Oral contraceptive: ethinyl estradiol	Reduced level of ethinyl estradiol	Alternative or additional contraceptive measures should be used

Adapted from Kaletra package insert, October 2005; Bertz R, Hsu A, Lam W, et al. Pharmacokinetic interactions between lopinavir/ritonavir (ABT-378r) and other non-HIV drugs [P291]. AIDS 14(Suppl 4):S100, 2000; Panel on Clinical Practices for Treatment of HIV infection. Department of Health and Human Services. Guidelines for the use of antiretroviral agents in HIV-1-infected adults and adolescents. Available at http://AIDSinfo.nih.gov 10 Oct 2006.

drugs are not contraindicated but may require dose adjustment of lopinavir/ritonavir or the concomitant agent. Table 20-4 lists some of these important established or potential drug interactions.[2,35,36]

Other antiretroviral agents can also have important drug interactions with lopinavir/ritonavir, notably the NNRTIs. As mentioned above, efavirenz induces the hepatic metabolism of lopinavir/ritonavir, resulting in lower concentrations of the PI. Co-administration of efavirenz with lopinavir/ritonavir at the 400/100 mg bid dose reduces C_{min} by 40–45%, and the AUC by ~20–25%.[37] With the older capsule formulation, increasing the dose to 533 mg of lopinavir and 133 mg of the ritonavir component overcame this effect and this dose can be achieved using the liquid formulation. With the new lopinavir/ritonavir 200/50 mg tablet, increasing the dose to three tablets (600/150 mg) bid is recommended when efavirenz or nevirapine is used, especially in antiretroviral-experienced patients.[2]

Lopinavir/ritonavir has been used in combination with other PIs in the setting of extensive drug resistance or when serious nucleoside analogue toxicity (e.g., lactic acidosis) precludes the use of NRTIs. Lopinavir/ritonavir levels are reduced when co-administered with darunavir, tipranavir or fosamprenavir.[38,39] Consequently, these double-boosted PI combinations are not recommended. Additional information regarding the interaction of lopinavir/ritonavir with other antiretroviral medications is contained in Table 20-5.

Drug Interactions Between Lopinavir/Ritonavir and Other Antiretroviral Drugs with Suggested Adjustments in Durg Dose

Table 20-5

Antiretroviral Drug	Interaction with Lopinavir/Ritonavir	Suggested Adjustment of Lopinavir/Ritonavir or Concomitant Drug[a]
Tenofovir	Lopinavir/ritonavir AUC decreased 15%	No dose adjustment necessary
Nevirapine	Lopinavir/ritonavir C_{min} decreased 55%	Lopinavir/ritonavir dose increased to 3 tablets (600/150 mg) bid or oral solution (533/133 mg) bid in ARV-experienced patients
Efavirenz	Lopinavir/ritonavir AUC decreased 40%	Lopinavir/ritonavir dose increased to 3 tablets (600/150 mg) bid or oral solution (533/133 mg) bid, especially in ARV-experienced patients
Delavirdine	Lopinavir/ritonavir may be increased	Appropriate adjustment not established
Indinavir	Indinavir increased by lopinavir/ritonavir	Indinavir dosed at 600 mg bid
Nelfinavir	Nelfinavir increased and lopinavir/ ritonavir decreased	Nelfinavir dosed at 1000 mg bid; lopinavir/ ritonavir dosed at 533/133 bid
Saquinavir	Saquinavir increased by lopinavir/ritonavir	Saquinavir dosed at 1000 mg bid
Fosamprenavir	Amprenavir are decreased by lopinavir/ritonavir	Should not be co-administered
Atazanavir	Ritonavir 100 mg increases atazanavir AUC 238%	Atazanavir dosed at 300 mg daily
Tipranavir	LPV AUC and C_{min} decreased by 55 and 70%	Should not be co-administered
Darunavir	Decreased AUC of darunavir by 53%	Should not be co-administered

[a]Suggested dosages for protease inhibitors co-administered with lopinavir/ritonavir are based on preliminary pharmacokinetic observations.[2] The safety and efficacy of all such combinations have not been established.

Adapted from Kaletra package insert, October 2005; Bertz R, Hsu A, Lam W, et al. Pharmacokinetic interactions between lopinavir/ritonavir (ABT-378r) and other non-HIV drugs [P291]. AIDS 14(Suppl 4):S100, 2000; Panel on Clinical Practices for Treatment of HIV infection. Department of Health and Human Services. Guidelines for the use of antiretroviral agents in HIV-1-infected adults and adolescents. Available at http://AIDSinfo.nih.gov 10 Oct 2006.

DRUG RESISTANCE

Lopinavir was designed to be effective against HIV-1 strains resistant to other PIs, particularly ritonavir. It retains activity against many drug-resistant isolates. However, resistance to lopinavir has been observed both *in vitro* and *in vivo*. *In vitro*, serial passage of HIV-1 in the presence of lopinavir leads to the sequential appearance of the mutations I84V, L10F, M46I, T91S, V32I, and I47V in protease. Further passage of this mutant at higher lopinavir concentrations led to emergence of a V47A mutation and reversion of V32I back to wild type. The EC_{50} for lopinavir of the resulting virus was 338-fold higher than wild-type.[40] Compensatory mutations at *gag* proteolytic cleavage sites (specifically, p7/p1 and p1/p6) were necessary for *in vitro* replication of these mutants.

The relationship of specific mutations in protease to lopinavir susceptibility was explored in a detailed analysis of 112 isolates from patients failing single or multiple PI regimens.[41] Susceptibility to lopinavir was significantly correlated with the number of mutations at 11 sites (protease codons 10, 20, 24, 46, 53, 54, 63, 71, 82, 84, 90). Further work identified M46I/L, I54V/T, V82A/F mutations as having a greater contribution to lopinavir resistance than changes at other resistance-associated positions. Inclusion of additional PI resistance-associated mutations such as G16E, V32I, L33F, I47V, G48M/V, I50V, and G73T, along with previously unrecognized mutations (E34Q, K43T, Q58E, T74S, and L89I/M) in a lopinavir 'mutation score' substantially improved the correlation between genotype and phenotype (Fig. 20-3).[42] Although relatively uncommon, presence of the V47A mutation, usually in the context of other PI resistance mutations, is associated with more than 80-fold resistance to lopinavir, but hypersusceptibility to saquinavir.[43]

Lopinavir resistance is distinctly uncommon in HIV-1 from patients failing lopinavir/ritonavir when it is part of the initial treatment regimen. The lack of data reflects the generally high level of virus suppression in patients who received this drug in clinical trials. No PI resistance mutations were noted in HIV-1 sequences from 51 PI-naive patients who experienced virologic breakthrough (plasma HIV-1 RNA levels of more than 400 copies/mL) while receiving lopinavir/ritonavir together with d4T and 3TC as part of the phase III efficacy trial described above.[11,44] By comparison, isolates from 43 (45%) of 96 patients experiencing viral breakthrough while taking nelfinavir, d4T, and 3TC carried resistance mutations for nelfinavir (D30N and/or L90M). Nevertheless, individual cases of lopinavir resistance have been reported from patients failing lopinavir/ritonavir as part of an initial PI regimen.[45,46]

Accumulation of lopinavir resistance mutations occurs much more readily in the setting of preexisting partial resistance. Mutations at codons 82, 54, and 46 emerged frequently in virus from PI-experienced patients who experienced virologic failure on lopinavir/ritonavir.[47] Less common mutations including L33F, I50V, and V32I together with I47V/A also occurred. These results show that partial resistance

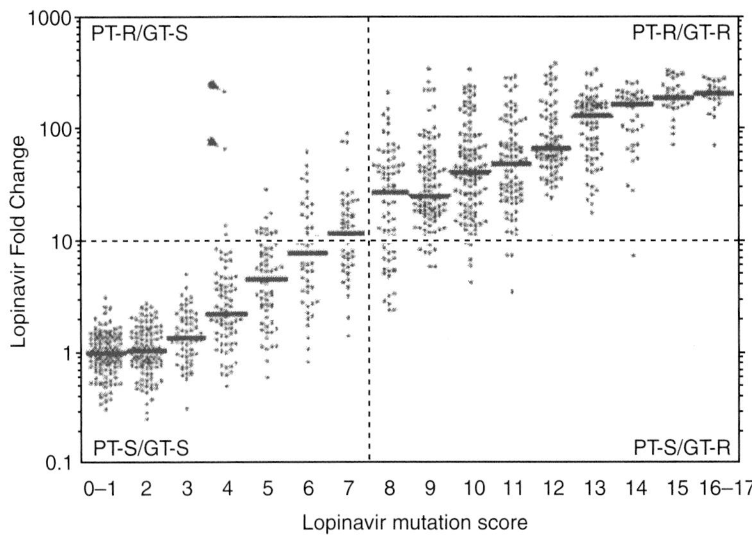

Figure 20-3 ■ Scatter plot of lopinavir susceptibility versus mutation score. Solid lines indicate median fold change in lopinavir susceptibility; dashed lines indicate boundary between susceptible/less susceptible viruses. PT, phenotype; GT, genotype; S, susceptible, R, resistant.

Reproduced from Parkin NT, Chappey C, Petropoulos CJ. Improving lopinavir genotype algorithm through phenotype correlations: novel mutation patterns and amprenavir cross-resistance. AIDS 17:955, 2003 with permission.

Table 20-6 Algorithms for Predicting Clinical Response to Lopinavir/Ritonavir

Algorithm	Possible Resistance	Resistance
IAS-USA[a]		6 or more of the following mutations: L10F/I/R/V, K20M/R, L42I, V32I, L33F, M46I/L, I47V/A, I50V, F53L, I54V/L/A/M/T/S, L63P, A71V/T, G73S, V82A/F/T/S, I84V, L90M
ANRS[b]	6 or 7 mutations from among the following: L10F/I/R/V, K20M/R, L24I, L33F, M46I/L, I50V, F53L, I54M/L/T/V, L63P, A71I/L/V/T, V82A/F/S/T, I84V, L90M	At least 8 mutations from among the following: L10F/I/R/V, K20M/R, L24I, L33F, M46I/L, I50V, F53L, I54M/L/T/V, L63P, A71I/L/V/T, V82A/F/S/T, I84V, L90M or V32I plus I47A

[a]International AIDS Society-USA. Adapted from Johnson V, Brun-Vezinet F, Clotet B, et al. Update of the drug resistance mutations in HIV-1: Fall 2005. Top HIV Med 13:125, 2005.

[b]Agence National de Recherches sur le SIDA. Adapted from Agence National de Recherches sur le SIDA. French ANRS AC11 rules (Sept 2005 update). Available: http://pugliese.club.fr/index.htm 3 March 2006.

accumulated during prior PI therapy can compromise the genetic barrier to lopinavir/ritonavir resistance.[47]

The likelihood of a clinically significant response to lopinavir/ritonavir in PI-experienced patients can be predicted by a variety of algorithms based on the number of lopinavir resistance mutations detected (Table 20-6).[48–51] The addition of plasma lopinavir levels to results of genotypic resistance test data improves the ability to predict clinical response, suggesting a possible role for therapeutic drug monitoring.[52,53]

If phenotypic resistance testing is employed, the clinical cut-off associated with full susceptibility is a less than 10-fold increase in IC_{50} relative to wild type virus; in many cases partial activity of lopinavir/ritonavir remains even in the setting of 10 to 40-fold.[48] A 10-fold increase in predicted IC_{50} also appears to be the appropriate cut-off for defining lopinavir resistance by virtual phenotype.[54]

USE DURING PREGNANCY

The lopinavir/ritonavir combination is classified as a category C drug. No treatment-related malformations were noted in studies in pregnant rats or rabbits. The drug is now one of the recommended PIs to consider as part of combination antiretroviral regimens in HIV-positive women during pregnancy.[55] Patients receiving lopinavir/ritonavir should be included in the Antiretroviral Pregnancy Registry (1-800-258-4263).

INDICATIONS FOR USE

Lopinavir/ritonavir clearly provides a potent option for initial therapy of treatment-naive patients, but a number of other regimens are also highly effective in this patient population. Factors to consider when choosing antiretroviral regimens in this setting include the inherent potency of the regimen, the results of efficacy trials to date, the ease of administration, the potential for drug toxicity and drug interactions, and the potential for drug resistance with its implications for drug sequencing. Advantages of a lopinavir/ritonavir-containing regimen include its potency and relatively low rate of significant treatment-related side effects. Moreover, the ease of administration (two tablets twice daily or four tablets once daily) may lead to high degrees of adherence. Potential disadvantages of a lopinavir/ritonavir-containing regimen as initial therapy include the significant incidence of hyperlipidemia (particularly hypertriglyceridemia) and the potential for drug interactions due to the ritonavir component. Given its high potency, lopinavir/ritonavir might be particularly useful in the subset of antiretroviral-naive patients with extremely high plasma HIV-1 RNA levels, extremely low CD4+ T-lymphocyte counts, or both. The latest treatment guidelines from the Panel on Clinical Practices for Treatment of HIV infection, convened by the Department of Health and Human Services list a lopinavir/ritonavir containing regimen as one of the preferred options in antiretroviral-naive patients.[36]

Lopinavir/ritonavir clearly has a major role in the treatment of antiretroviral-experienced patients. It is useful in patients failing an initial NNRTI-containing regimen, an initial PI-containing regimen and in those with more extensive PI experience. As with other antiretroviral agents, the use of this drug in the setting of treatment failure should be guided by the results of resistance testing. Lopinavir/ritonavir is also part of the recommended regimens for postexposure prophylaxis in both occupational and nonoccupational settings.[56,57]

REFERENCES

1. Sham H, Kempf D, Molla A, et al. ABT-378, a highly potent inhibitor of the human immunodeficiency virus protease. Antimicrob Agents Chemother 42:3218, 1998.
2. Kaletra package insert, Oct 2005.
3. Kumar G, Dykstra J, Roberts E, et al. Potent inhibition of the cytochrome P-450 3A-mediated human liver microsomal metabolism of a novel HIV protease inhibitor by ritonavir: a positive drug–drug interaction. Drug Metab Dispos 27:902, 1999.
4. Bertz R, Lam W, Brun S, et al. Multiple-dose pharmacokinetics (PK) of ABT-378/ritonavir (ABT-378/r) in HIV + subjects. Presented at the 39th Interscience Conference on Antimicrobial Agents and Chemotherapy, San Francisco, 1999, abstract 327.
5. Gupta S, Rosenkranz S, Segal Y, et al. The steady-state pharmacokinetics of efavirenz and lopinavir/ritonavir in HIV-infected persons requiring hemodialysis: AIDS Clinical Trials Group Study A5177. Presented the 13th Conference on Retroviruses and Opportunistic Infections, Denver, 2006, abstract 573.
6. Hsu A, Bertz R, Renz C, et al. Assessment of the pharmacokinetic interaction between lopinavir/ritonavir (ABT-378/r) and nevirapine (NVP) in HIV-infected pediatric subjects [P292]. AIDS 14(Suppl 4): S100, 2000.
7. Bergshoeff A, Fraaij P, Ndagijimana J, et al. Increased dose of lopinavir/ritonavir compensates for efavirenz-induced drug–drug interaction in HIV-1-infected children. JAIDS 39:63, 2005.
8. Awni W, Chiu Y, Zhu T, et al. Significantly reduced food effect and pharmacokinetic variability with a novel lopinavir/ritonavir tablet formulation. Presented at the 3rd International AIDS Society Conference on HIV Pathogenesis and Treatment, Rio de Janeiro, 2005, abstract WeOa0206.
9. Murphy R, Brun S, Hicks C, et al. ABT-378/ritonavir plus stavudine and lamivudine for the treatment of antiretroviral-naive adults with HIV-1 infection: 48-week results. AIDS 15:F1, 2001.
10. Murphy R, daSilva B, McMillan F, et al. Seven year follow-up of a lopinavir/ritonavir (LPV/r)-based regimen in antiretroviral (ARV)-naive subjects. Presented at the 10th European AIDS Clinical Society Conference/EACS, Dublin, 2005, abstract PE7.9/3.
11. Walmsley S, Bernstein B, King M, et al. Lopinavir/ritonavir versus nelfinavir for the initial treatment of HIV infection. N Eng J Med 346:2039, 2002.
12. Eron J, Yeni P, Gathe J, et al. The KLEAN Study: fosamprenavir + ritonavir (FPV/r) versus lopinavir/ritonavir (LPV/r) in antiretroviral-naive (ART-naive) HIV-1 infected adults over 48 weeks. Presented at the 16th International AIDS Conference, Toronto, 2006, abstract THLB0205.
13. Riddler S, Haubrich R, DiRienzo G, et al. A prospective, randomized, phase III trial of NRTI-, PI-, and NNRTI-sparing regimens for initial treatment of HIV-1 infection – ACTG 5142. Presented at the 16th International AIDS Conference, Toronto, 2006, abstract THLB0204.
14. Benson C, Deeks S, Brun S, et al. Safety and antiviral activity at 48 weeks of lopinavir/ritonavir plus nevirapine and 2 nucleoside reverse-transcriptase inhibitors in human immunodeficiency virus type 1-infected protease inhibitor-experienced patients. J Infect Dis 185:599, 2002.
15. Feinberg J, Brun S, Xu Y, et al. Durable suppression of HIV+ RNA after 2 years of therapy with ABT-378/ritonavir (ABT-378/r) treatment in single protease inhibitor experienced patients [P101]. AIDS 14(Suppl 4):S46, 2000.
16. Clumeck N, Brun S, Sylte J, et al. Kaletra (ABT-378/r) and efavirenz: one-year safety/efficacy evaluation and phenotypic breakpoints in multiple-PI-experienced patients. Presented at the 8th Conference on Retroviruses and Opportunistic Infections, Chicago, 2001, abstract 525.
17. Johnson M, Grinsztejn B, Rodriguez C, et al. Atazanavir plus ritonavir or saquinavir, and lopinavir/ritonavir in patients experiencing multiple virological failures. AIDS 19:685, 2005.
18. Elston R, Yates P, Tisdale M, et al. GW433908 (908)/ritonavir (r): 48 week results/in PI-experienced subjects: A retrospective analysis of virological response based on baseline genotype and phenotype. Presented at the International AIDS Confernence, Bangkok, 2004, abstract MoOrB1055.
19. Ulrik B, Gerstoft J, Youle M, et al. A randomized trial to evaluate lopinavir/ritonavir versus saquinavir/ritonavir in HIV-1-infected patients: the MaxCmin2 trial. Antivir Ther 10:735, 2005.
20. Eron J, Feinberg J, Kessler H, et al. Once-daily versus twice-daily lopinavir/ritonavir in antiretroviral-naive HIV-positive patients: a 48-week randomized clinical trial. J Infect Dis 189:265, 2004.
21. Molina J, Wilkin A, Domingo P, et al. Once-daily versus twice-daily lopinavir/ritonavir in antiretroviral-naive patients: 96 week results. Presented at the Third International AIDS Society Conference on HIV Pathogenesis and Treatment, Rio de Janeiro, 2005, abstract WePe12.3C12.
22. Saez-Llorens X, Violari A, Deetz C, et al. Forty-eight-week evaluation of lopinavir/ritonavir, a new protease inhibitor, in human immunodeficiency virus-infected children. Pediatr Infect Dis J 22:216, 2003.
23. Gathe J, Washington M, Mayberry C, et al. IMANI-1 TC3WP Single drug HAART-proof of concept study. Pilot study of the safety and efficacy of Kaletra (LPV/r) as single drug HAART in HIV+ ARV-naïve patients-interim analysis of subjects completing final 48 week data. Presented at the XV International AIDS Conference, Bangkok, 2004, abstract MoOrB1057.
24. Delfraissy J, Flandre P, Delaugerre C, et al. MONARK Trial (Monotherapy AntiRetroviral Kaletra): 48 week analysis of lopinavir/ritonavir (LPV/r) monotherapy compared to LPV/r + zidovudine/lamivudine (AZT/3TC) in antiretroviral-naive patients. Presented at the 16th International AIDS Conference, Toronto, 2006, abstract THLB0202.
25. Arribas J, Pulido F, Delgado R, et al. Lopinavir/ritonavir as single-drug therapy for maintenance of HIV-1 viral suppression. JAIDS 40:280, 2005.
26. Arribas J, Pulido F, Delgado R, et al. Lopinavir/ritonavir as single-drug maintenance therapy in patients with HIV-1

viral suppression: 48 week results of a randomized, controlled, open-label, clinical trial (OK04 Study). Presented at the 16th International AIDS Conference, Toronto, 2006, abstract THLB0203.

27. Cameron W, da Silva B, Arribas J, et al. A two-year randomized controlled clinical trial in antiretroviral-naïve subjects using lopinavir/ritonavir (LPV/r) monotherapy after initial induction treatment compared to an efavirenz (EFV) 3-drug regimen. Presented at the 16th International AIDS Conference, Toronto, 2006, abstract THLB0201.
28. Nunes E, Oliveirra M, Almeida M, et al. 48-week efficacy and safety results of simplification to single agent lopinavir/ritonavir (LPV/r) regimen in patients suppressed below 80 copies/mL on HAART-the KalMo study. Presented at the 16th International AIDS Conference, Toronto, 2006, abstract TUAB0103.
29. Negredo E, Molto J, Burger D, et al. Lopinavir/ritonavir plus nevirapine as a nucleoside-sparing approach in antiretroviral-experienced patients (NEKA study). JAIDS 38:47, 2005.
30. Arribas J, Barros C, Gonzalez-Lahoz J, et al. Treatment of HIV+ subjects co-infected with hepatitis B or C: safety and efficacy comparison of ABT-378/ritonavir (ABT-378/r) versus nelfinavir from a phase III blinded randomized clinical trial [P369]. AIDS 14(Suppl 4):S124, 2000.
32. Merviglia P, Schiavini M, Castagna A, et al. Lopinavir/ritonavir treatment in HIV antiretroviral-experienced patients: evaluation of risk factors for liver enzyme evaluation. HIV Med 5:334, 2004.
33. Schambelan M, Benson C, Carr A, et al. Management of complications associated with antiretroviral therapy for HIV-1 infection: recommendations of an International AIDS Society-USA panel. JAIDS 31:257, 2002
34. Noor MA, Parker RA, O'Mara E, et al. The effects of HIV protease inhibitors atazanavir and lopinavir/ritonavir on insulin sensitivity in HIV-seronegative healthy adults. AIDS 18:2137, 2004.
35. Bertz R, Hsu A, Lam W, et al. Pharmacokinetic interactions between lopinavir/ritonavir (ABT-378r) and other non-HIV drugs [P291]. AIDS 14(Suppl 4):S100, 2000.
36. Panel on Clinical Practices for Treatment of HIV infection. Department of Health and Human Services. Guidelines for the use of antiretroviral agents in HIV-1-infected adults and adolescents. Available: http://AIDSinfo.nih.gov 10 Oct 2006.
37. Hsu A, Isaacson J, Brun S, et al. Pharmacokinetic–pharmacodynamics analysis of lopinavir/ritonavir in combination with efavirenz and two nucleoside reverse transcriptase inhibitors in extensively pretreated human immunodeficiency virus-infected patients. Antimicrob Agents Chemother 47:350, 2003.
38. Walmsley S, Leith J, Katlama C, et al. Pharmacokinetics and safety of tipranavir/ritonavir (TPV/r) alone or in combination with saquinavir (SQV), amprenavir (APV, and lopinavir (LPV): Interim analysis of BI1182.51. Presented at the 15th International AIDS Conference, Bangkok, 2004, abstract WeOrB1236.
39. Kashuba A, Tierney C, Downey G, et al. Combining fosamprenavir with lopinavir/ritonavir substantially reduces amprenavir and lopinavir exposure: ACTG protocol A5143 results. AIDS 19:145, 2005.
40. Carrillo A, Stewart K, Sham H, et al. In vitro selection and characterization of human immunodeficiency virus type 1 variants with increased resistance to ABT-378, a novel protease inhibitor. J Virol 72:7532, 1998.
41. Kempf D, Isaacson J, King M, et al. Identification of genotypic changes in human immunodeficiency virus protease that correlate with reduced susceptibility to the protease inhibitor lopinavir among viral isolates from protease inhibitor-experienced patients. J Virol 75:7462, 2001.
42. Parkin NT, Chappey C, Petropoulos CJ. Improving lopinavir genotype algorithm through phenotype correlations: novel mutation patterns and amprenavir cross-resistance. AIDS 17:955, 2003.
43. Kagan R, Shenerovich M, Heseltine P, et al. Structural analysis of an HIV-1 protease I47A mutant resistant to the protease inhibitor lopinavir. Protein Sci 14:1870, 2005.
44. Kempf D, King M, Bernstein B, et al. Incidence of resistance in a double-blind study comparing lopinavir/ritonavir plus stavudine and lamivudine to nelfinavir plus stavudine and lamivudine. J Infect Dis 189:51, 2004.
45. Conradie F, Sanne I, Venter W, et al. Failure of lopinavir/ritonavir (Kaletra)-containing regimen in an antiretroviral-naive patient. AIDS 18:1084, 2004.
46. Friend J, Parkin N, Leigler T, et al. Isolated lopinavir resistance after virological rebound of a ritonavir/lopinavir-based regimen. AIDS 18:1965, 2004.
47. Mo H, King M, Molla A, et al. Selection of resistance in protease inhibitor-experienced, human immunodeficiency virus type 1-infected subjects failing lopinavir- and ritonavir-based therapy: mutation patterns and baseline correlates. J Virol 79:3329, 2005.
48. Kempf D, Isaacson J, King M, et al. Analysis of the virological response with respect to baseline phenotype and genotype in protease inhibitor-experienced HIV-1-infected patients receiving lopinavir/ritonavir therapy. Antivir Ther 7:165, 2002.
49. Masquelier B, Breilh D, Neau D, et al. Human immunodeficiency virus type 1 genotypic and pharmacokinetic determinants of the virological response to lopinavir/ritonavir-containing therapy in protease inhibitor-experienced patients. Antimicrob Agents Chemother 46:2926, 2002.
50. Johnson V, Brun-Vezinet F, Clotet B, et al. Update of the drug resistance mutations in HIV-1: Fall 2006. Topics in HIV Medicine 14:125, 2006.
51. Agence National de Recherches sur le SIDA. French ANRS AC11 rules (September 2005 update). Available: http://pugliese.club.fr/index.htm 3 Mar 2006.
52. Gonzalez de Requena D, Gallego O, et al. Prediction of virological response to lopinavir/ritonavir using the genotypic inhibitory quotient. AIDS Res Hum Retroviruses 20:275, 2004.
53. Marcelin AG, Cohen-Codar I, King MS, et al. Virological and pharmacological parameters predicting the response to lopinavir/ritonavir in heavily protease inhibitor-experienced patients. Antimicrob Agents Chemother 49:1720, 2005.
54. Loutfy MR, Raboud JM, Walmsley SL, et al. Predictive value of HIV-1 protease genotype and virtual phenotype on the virological response to lopinavir/ritonavir-containing salvage regimens. Antivir Ther 9:595, 2004.
55. Public Health Service Task Force. Recommendations for use of antiretroviral drugs in pregnant HIV-1-infected women for maternal health and interventions to reduce perinatal HIV-1 transmission in the United States. Available: http://AIDSinfo.nih.gov 12 Oct 2005.
56. Centers for Disease Control and Prevention. Updated US. Public Health Service guidelines for the management of occupational exposures to HIV and recommendations for postexposure prophylaxis. MMWR 54(RR-9):1. Available: http://AIDSinfo.nih.gov 30 Sept, 2005.
57. Centers for Disease Control and Prevention. Antiretroviral postexposure prophylaxis after sexual, injection-drug use, or other nonoccupational exposure to HIV in the United States. Recommendations from the US. Department of Health and Human Services. MMWR 54(RR-2):1, 2005. Available: http://AIDSinfo.nih.gov 21 Jan, 2005.

Chapter 21

Atazanavir

Graeme Moyle, MD

Atazanavir is a relatively new protease inhibitor (PI) that is dosed once daily with or without ritonavir boosting. Since its approval atazanavir has been used in patients naive to antiretroviral therapy and in those patients who are antiretroviral-experienced. Its use in deep salvage therapy is limited. The drug has a favorable lipid profile, even when boosted with low dose ritonavir. This chapter will review the preclinical and clinical experience of atazanavir with emphasis on its efficacy, safety, and resistance profile.

STRUCTURE

Atazanavir sulfate (Reyataz; BMS-232632) is an inhibitor of HIV-1 protease. It is an aza-dipeptide analog and bis(L-tert-leucine) derivative.[1] The chemical name of atazanavir is (3*S*,8*S*,9*S*,12*S*)-3,12-bis(1,1-dimethylethyl)-8-hydroxy-4,11-dioxo-9-(phenylmethyl)-6-[[4-(2-pyridinyl)phenyl]methyl]-2,5,6,10,13-pentaazatetradecanedioic acid dimethyl ester, sulfate (1:1) (Fig. 21-1).

IN VITRO ACTIVITY AND MECHANISM OF ACTION

Like other PIs, atazanavir selectively inhibits the virus-specific processing of viral gag and gag-pol polyproteins in HIV-1 infected cells, thus preventing formation of mature virions.[2] Atazanavir exhibits potent anti-HIV activity against a variety of laboratory and clinical HIV-1 isolates grown in cell culture, with a 50% effective concentration (EC_{50}; inhibition of 50% of viral replication) in the absence of human sera of 2.6–5.3 nmol/L and an EC_{90} of 9–15 nmol/L.[2] *In vitro* data suggest that atazanavir exerts more potent anti-HIV-1 protease inhibition than indinavir (EC_{50} of 5.0–28.7 nmol/L), nelfinavir (6.1–25.9 nmol/L), ritonavir (43.1–129 nmol/L), saquinavir (5.3–24.8 nmol/L), and amprenavir (16.6–54.3 nmol/L).[2] In addition, atazanavir is highly selective and has a strong affinity for HIV-1 protease with an inhibition constant (K_i) of 2.7 nmol/L.

Studies on two-drug combinations in peripheral blood mononuclear cells showed that atazanavir had additive antiviral activity with the PIs indinavir, nelfinavir, ritonavir, saquinavir, and amprenavir, as well as the nucleoside reverse transcriptase inhibitors (NRTIs) stavudine, didanosine and lamivudine.[2] Atazanavir displayed weak synergistic antiviral activity with the NRTI zidovudine. No enhanced cytotoxic effects were observed at the highest concentrations used for antiviral evaluation.

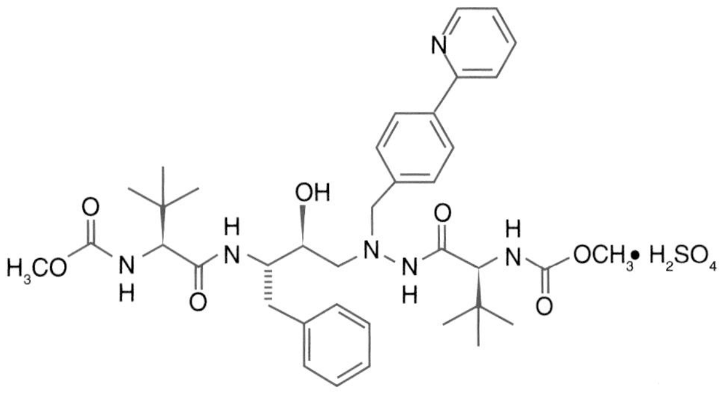

Figure 21-1 ■ The structural formula of atazanavir sulfate.

PHARMACOKINETICS

Atazanavir is rapidly absorbed in the stomach after oral administration of 400 mg qd, with a T_{max} of ~2.5 h in healthy people and 2.0 h in those infected with HIV.[3] Steady state is achieved between 4 and 8 days in both healthy volunteers and patients with HIV infection.[4] Multiple-dose administration of atazanavir results in ~2.3-fold accumulation of the drug.

The pharmacokinetics of atazanavir are nonlinear.[3–6] Indeed, in a substudy of a phase II trial of patients with HIV receiving HAART, the mean C_{max} and area under the curve (AUC) values of atazanavir 200–500 mg increased in a less than dose-proportional manner.[5] In contrast, a single-dose study in healthy volunteers demonstrated that there was a greater than dose-proportional increase in atazanavir C_{max} and AUC.[6]

Food has a significant effect on the absorption of atazanavir by enhancing its bioavailability and reducing its pharmacokinetic variability. A single 400 mg dose of atazanavir taken with a light meal (357 kcal; 8.2 g fat, 10.6 g protein) resulted in a 70% increase in AUC and a 57% increase in C_{max} relative to the fasting state.[1,7] In addition, the inter-individual variability in drug levels was reduced by 40%. Administration of a single 400 mg dose of atazanavir with a high-fat meal (721 kcal; 37.3 g fat, 29.4 g protein) resulted in a mean increase in AUC of 35% with no change in C_{max} relative to the fasting state. Thus, atazanavir should be administered with food to reduce pharmacokinetic variability and enhance bioavailability.[3]

Atazanavir is 86% bound to human serum proteins (alpha-1-acid glycoprotein and albumin).[4] Protein-binding is independent of plasma drug concentration. In a multiple dose study in HIV-infected patients dosed with atazanavir 400 mg qd with a light meal for 12 weeks, atazanavir was detected in the cerebrospinal fluid (CSF) and semen.[8] As both the semen and CSF atazanavir concentrations were greater than the EC_{50} values observed for wild-type virus after 12 weeks' treatment with atazanavir 400 mg, atazanavir should have antiviral activity in these compartments.

Atazanavir is metabolized to two oxygenated, minor metabolites by the hepatic cytochrome P450 liver complex, mainly by the 3A4 isoenzyme (CYP3A4),[3,5] which are then excreted in the bile in either free or glucuronidated forms. Additional minor metabolic pathways consist of *N*-dealkylation and hydrolysis. At clinically relevant concentrations, atazanavir is a moderate competitive inhibitor of CYP3A4 and uridine diphosphate glucuronosyl-transferase 1A1 (UGT 1A1), the enzyme involved in the liver clearance of bilirubin.

Following a single 400 mg dose of ^{14}C-atazanavir, 79% of the total radioactivity was excreted in the feces and 13% in the urine, suggesting that biliary elimination, rather than the kidneys, is a major pathway for the elimination of atazanavir and/or a fraction of the dose is unabsorbed.[9] Approximately 20% of atazanavir is excreted unchanged in the feces and 7% in the urine. The mean elimination half-life of atazanavir following a dose of 400 mg qd with a light meal in healthy volunteers and HIV-infected adult patients was ~7 h at steady state.[3] The elimination half-life of atazanavir more than doubled in healthy subjects when administered with once-daily ritonavir 100 mg and a light meal (18.1 vs 7.9 h). The increase was more modest in HIV-infected adult patients (8.6 vs 6.5 h).

A study of the pharmacokinetics of atazanavir in young (18–40 years) and elderly (~65 years of age) healthy subjects found that there were no clinically important pharmacokinetic differences due to age or gender.[3] The pharmacokinetics of atazanavir in children is being investigated. Currently, there is insufficient information to recommend a dose in pediatric patients.

As the kidneys play a minor role in the elimination of atazanavir, the dose of atazanavir does not need to be modified. In adult subjects with moderate to severe hepatic impairment, however, a 45% increase in AUC was observed in hepatically impaired subjects compared with healthy subjects after a single 400 mg dose of atanazavir.[3] The mean half-life of atazanavir in hepatically impaired subjects was 12.1 h compared to 6.4 h in healthy volunteers. As increased concentrations of atazanavir are expected in patients with moderate to severe hepatic impairment, a reduction in dose is warranted in subjects with mild to moderate hepatic impairment. Atazanavir is not recommended in patients with severe hepatic impairment. The pharmacokinetics of atazanavir in combination with ritonavir have not been studied in subjects with hepatic impairment.

DRUG INTERACTIONS

Many drug interactions with atazanavir occur via inhibition or induction of the hepatic enzymes responsible for its metabolism, i.e., CYP3A. In addition, atazanavir is an inhibitor of UGT1A1. Co-administration of atazanavir and drugs primarily metabolized by CYP3A (e.g., calcium channel blockers, HMG-CoA reductase inhibitors, immunosuppressants, and PDE5 inhibitors) or UGT1A1 (e.g., irinotecan) may therefore result in increased plasma concentrations of the co-administered drug that could increase or prolong both its therapeutic and adverse effects. Co-administration of atazanavir and drugs that induce CYP3A, such as rifampin, may decrease atazanavir plasma concentrations and reduce its therapeutic effect. Conversely, co-administration of atazanavir and drugs that inhibit CYP3A may increase atazanavir plasma concentrations. A list of drugs that should not be co-administered with atazanavir is shown in Table 21-1.

As the absorption of atazanavir requires an acidic medium, drugs that increase the gastric pH will reduce the solubility of atazanavir and may therefore decrease its plasma concentration.[3] Reduced plasma concentrations of atazanavir are thus expected if antacids, buffered medications, H_2-receptor antagonists, and proton pump inhibitors are co-administered. Indeed, it is recommended that atazanavir not be administered with any proton pump inhibitor. H_2-receptor antagonists, such as ranitidine or famotidine, can be used but only if administered 12 h away from the time of atazanavir administration. In addition, atazanavir should be given 1 h after or 2 h before antacids and buffered medications.

Drugs That Should not be Co-Administered With Atazanavir

Table 21-1

Drug Class	Specific Drugs	Reasons
Contraindicated Drug Combinations		
Benzodiazepines	Midazolam, triazolam	Potential for prolonged/increased sedation, respiratory depression
Ergot derivatives	Dihydroergotamine ergotamine, ergonovine, methylergonovine	Acute ergot toxicity (e.g., peripheral vasospasm, ischemia of extremities and other tissues)
GI motility agents	Cisapride	Potential for cardiac arrhythmias
Neuroleptics	Pimozide	Potential for cardiac arrhythmias
Unadvisable Drug Combinations		
Antimycobacterials	Rifampin	Decreases plasma concentrations and AUC of atazanavir
Antineoplastics	Irinotecan	Atazanavir may affect the metabolism of irinotecan, increasing its toxicity
Herbal products	St Johns wort (*Hypericum perforatum*)	May reduce plasma concentrations of atazanavir
HMG-CoA reductase inhibitors	Lovastatin, simvastatin	Potential for serious reactions such as myopathy
Protease inhibitors	Indinavir	Atazanavir and indinavir each associated with indirect (unconjugated) hyperbilirubinemia. No studies conducted on co-administered drugs
Proton pump inhibitors	All members	Expected to substantially decrease plasma concentrations of atazanavir

Data from Bristol-Myers Squibb Company. Reyataz® (atazanavir sulfate) capsules prescribing information. Online. Available: http://www.bms.com 2006.

EFFICACY

The therapeutic efficacy of atazanavir in combination with other antiretroviral agents for HIV infection has been investigated in controlled trials in antiretroviral (ART)-naive[10–14] or ART-experienced[15–18] patients with HIV infection.

First-Line Therapy

There are three pivotal 48-week studies (007, 008, and 034) that have studied the efficacy and safety of atazanavir regimens in drug-naive patients.[10–12] Studies 007 and 008 compared different doses of atazanavir versus nelfinavir along with a dual-NRTI backbone of didanosine (ddI) with stavudine (d4T) or lamivudine (3TC) with stavudine (d4T), respectively.[11,12] Study 034 compared atazanavir with efavirenz in combination with zidovudine + 3TC as the nucleoside backbone.[10] The phase III study (034) had a 24-week, open-label extension trial for patients who completed at least 48 weeks' treatment.[12,13] Patients continued to receive the same NRTI backbone and once-daily atazanavir 400 or 600 mg, with those previously receiving nelfinavir switched to atazanavir 400.

Study 089 is a 96-week, randomized, open-label prospective study to compare the efficacy and safety of once-daily atazanavir (400 mg) and atazanavir with ritonavir (300 mg/100 mg) both in combination with lamivudine and extended-release stavudine in ART-naive HIV patients. Patients were eligible for inclusion if their plasma HIV RNA levels were 2000 copies/mL; there were no CD4+ T-lymphocyte count restrictions.[14]

In the pivotal trials, patients were considered ART-naive if they had previously received treatment with an NRTI for 30 days and/or a non-NRTI (NNRTI) or PI for 7 days,[10,12] and no ART had been administered within 30 days of screening. Patients were eligible for inclusion in the studies if their plasma HIV RNA levels were 2000 copies/mL and CD4+ T-lymphocyte counts were 100 cells/μL or 75 cells/μL in the absence of a prior diagnosis of AIDS.[10,12] Additional inclusion criteria for the extension study included HIV RNA levels <10 000 copies/mL.[13]

Reductions in HIV viral load of ~2.5 $\log_{10}$ copies/mL were achieved by week 12 in study 034, week 16 in study 007 and week 24 in study 008.[10–12] In all three pivotal studies, the mean reductions from baseline in plasma HIV RNA levels were not significantly different between once-daily atazanavir 400 mg and two or three times-daily nelfinavir or once-daily efavirenz, although responses in both the atazanavir and efavirenz arms in study 034 were artificially low owing to defects in the blood sample tubes (Table 21-2). Viral suppression was maintained during prolonged follow-up.[13]

The proportion of patients who achieved a reduction in viral load below the limit of quantification (LOQ) at 48 weeks with atazanavir 400 mg was similar to that observed in the nelfinavir and efavirenz groups. Indeed, 64–70% of patients who received atazanavir 400 mg had HIV RNA levels <400 copies/mL compared with 53–64% with the other regimens (Table 21-2). Furthermore, in the 034 study, 32–36% of atazanavir-treated patients had an HIV RNA level <50 copies/mL compared with 34–39% in the other treatment groups. Apparent low levels of response at the <50 copies/mL level

Table 21-2

Comparison of Virologic Suppression for Atazanavir in Treatment-Naive Patients

			Mean Plasma HIV RNA Levels at Baseline (log_{10} copies/mL)		Response at 48 Weeks			Change in Plasma HIV RNA Levels from Baseline (log_{10} copies/mL)	
Study #	Description	Regimens	# Patients	Level	# Patients (ITT)	% Patients with Plasma HIV RNA < 400 copies/mL	% Patients with Plasma HIV RNA < 50 copies/mL	# Patients (OT)	Mean Decrease
007[11]	Randomized, multicenter, blinded dose-ranging study comparing safety and efficacy of atazanavir in combination with didanosine and stavudine	ATV 200 qd + ddI + d4T	104	4.72	83	61	28	67	2.57
		ATV 400 qd + ddI + d4T	103	4.60	78	64	36	64	2.42
		ATV 500 qd + ddI + d4T	110	4.77	79	59	42	60	2.53
		NFV 750 tid + ddI + d4T	103	4.81	82	56	39	65	2.33
008[12]	Randomized, multicenter, blinded[a] phase II study comparing safety and efficacy of atazanavir and nelfinavir	ATV 400 qd + 3TC + d4T	181	4.74	181	64	35	153	2.51
		ATV 600 qd + 3TC + d4T	195	4.73	195	67	36	167	2.58
		NFV 1250 bid + 3TC + d4T	91	4.73	91	53	34	80	2.31
034[10]	Randomized, double blind, double dummy, active-controlled phase III study comparing safety and efficacy of atazanavir and efavirenz	ATV 400 qd + ZDV/3TC 300/150 bid	404	4.87	404	70	32	Not recorded	2.70
		EFV 600 qd + ZDV/3TC 300/150 bid	401	4.91	401	64	37	Not recorded	2.70
044[13]	Multicenter open-label rollover/switch study (extension of study 008)	ATV 400 qd + 3TC + d4T	139	1.76	133	83	60	N/A	N/A
		ATV 600 qd + 3TC + d4T	144	1.69	139	85	56	N/A	N/A
		NFV → ATV 400 qd + 3TC + d4T	63	1.78	62	87	60	N/A	N/A
089[xx]	96-Week randomized, open-label, prospective study to compare safety and efficacy of boosted and unboosted atazanavir	ATV 400 qd + 3TC + d4T	105	5.02	105	85	70	104	
		ATV/RTV 300/100 qd + 3TC + d4T	85	4.83	95	86	75	95	

NA, not available.
[a] Blinded to atazanavir dose.

Adapted from Swainston HT, Scott LJ. Atazanavir: a review of its use in the management of HIV infection. Drugs 65:2309–36, 2005.

Table 21-3 Comparison of Immunologic Response for Atazanavir in Treatment-Naive Patients

			Mean CD4+ Lymphocyte Count at Baseline (cells/μL)		Mean Change in CD4+ Lymphocyte Count from Baseline (cells/μL)	
Study #	Description	Regimens	# Patients	CD4+	# Patients (OT)	Mean Increase
007[11]	Randomized, multicenter, blinded dose-ranging study comparing safety and efficacy of atazanavir in combination with didanosine and stavudine	ATV 200 qd +ddI + d4T	104	331	65	220
		ATV 400 qd + ddI + d4T	103	357	63	221
		ATV 500 qd + ddI + d4T	110	361	60	208
		NFV 750 tid + ddI + d4T	103	341	65	185
008[11]	Randomized, multicenter, blinded phase II study comparing safety and efficacy of atazanavir and nelfinavir	ATV 400 qd + 3TC + d4T	181	294	153	234
		ATV 600 qd + 3TC + d4T	195	302	166	243
		NFV 1250 bid + 3TC + d4T	91	283	78	211
034[10]	Randomized, double blind, double dummy, active-controlled phase III study comparing safety and efficacy of atazanavir and efavirenz	ATV 400 qd + ZDV/3TC 300/150 bid	404	286	329	176
		EFV 600 qd + ZDV/3TC 300/150 bid	401	280	314	160
044[13]	Multicenter open-label rollover/switch study (extension of study 008)	ATV 400 qd + 3TC + d4T	139	472	Not recorded	44
		ATV 600 qd + 3TC + d4T	144	524	Not recorded	43
		NFV → ATV 400 qd + 3TC + d4T	63	543	Not recorded	29

Reprinted from Swainston HT, Scott LJ. Atazanavir: a review of its use in the management of HIV infection. Drugs 65:2309–36, 2005.

are thought to be related to the use of unsuitable sampling tubes at some study sites.

In study 034, the mean increase from baseline in CD4+ T-lymphocyte count in atazanavir-treated patients were numerically greater than that with efavirenz (Table 21-3).[10] The effects of ART on CD4+ T-lymphocyte count were similar in patients receiving atazanavir and nelfinavir in studies 007 and 008.[11,12]

In study 089, the primary endpoint at week 48 was the proportion of patients with HIV RNA $<400 \log_{10}$ copies/mL. This was very similar in both arms of the study (intent-to-treat (ITT) analysis); 85% for atazanavir 400 mg vs 85% for atazanavir/ritonavir 300/100 mg (Table 21-2). Attaining HIV RNA $<50 \log_{10}$ copies/mL at 48 weeks was a secondary endpoint in the study and was achieved by 70% of patients in the atazanavir-only arm and 75% of patients in the boosted atazanavir arm. When evaluating the ITT analysis of this study, it is important to note that elevations in bilirubin were deemed a failure, and more patients went off-study owing to bilirubin elevation in the ritonavir-boosted group versus the unboosted group (8% vs 1 % respectively) thereby having significant impact on the outcomes. The mean increase in CD4+ T-lymphocyte count indicated a strong immunologic response in both arms of the study (+224 cells/mL in the atazanavir only arm versus +189 cells/mL in the boosted atazanavir arm).[14]

Salvage Therapy

Three randomized, open-label, multicenter, phase III clinical trials (043, 045, and 097) have investigated the beneficial effects and safety of atazanavir for HIV infection in patients with prior virologic failure to PI-containing regimens.[15,16,18] In study 043, patients were given once-daily atazanavir 400 mg versus twice-daily lopinavir/ritonavir 400 mg/100 mg for 24 weeks, along with a dual nucleoside backbone selected with the assistance of resistance testing.[16] Study 045 was a 48-week trial of adult patients who had failed two or more prior HAART regimens.[15] Patients were randomized to one of three groups; once-daily atazanavir 300 mg boosted with once-daily ritonavir 100 mg, once-daily atazanavir 400 mg plus once-daily saquinavir capsules 1200 mg, or twice-daily lopinavir/ritonavir 400/100 mg.[15] All treatment groups received once-daily tenofovir 300 mg plus an NRTI. Patients in study 097 received atazanavir, unboosted or boosted with ritonavir, or to their prior PI-based therapy; all groups received a backbone of two NRTIs.[18]

Patients in studies 043 and 045 had a baseline plasma HIV RNA level of 1000 copies/mL and a CD4+ T-lymphocyte count of 50 cells/μL and were highly ART experienced.[15,16] Additional inclusion criteria for study 043 were that patients were currently failing a HAART regimen containing at least one PI, and study 045 required patients to have failed at least two prior HAART regimens that included at least one drug from each ART class (PI, NRTI, and NNRTI) and have serum creatinine, lipase, ALT and AST, and total bilirubin levels of 1.5, 1.4, 3 or 1.5 times less than the upper limit of normal, respectively. In study 043, the median time of prior exposure to any NNRTI was 2.6 years in the atazanavir group and 1.6 years in the lopinavir/ritonavir group, and to any PI or NRTI in was ~2.6 years and 3.1 years, respectively, for all patients.[16]

Patients enrolled into study 097 were achieving virologic suppression with a PI-based regimen.[18] Indeed, they had had HIV RNA levels <50 copies/mL for at least 3 months and a CD4+ T-lymphocyte count >50 cells/μL.[18] Previously, patients had received a PI-containing regimen for a mean duration of 3.4 years, NRTI-based therapy for 3.9 years and an NNRTI-containing regimen for 1.3 years. Additional inclusion criteria for study 097 were that patients had received their first or second HAART regimen, and had no previous virologic failure on a PI-based regimen, and their current regimen included a PI with or without ritonavir, taken at least twice daily or with a pill burden of at least three tablets/day.

After 48 weeks of treatment in study 045, atazanavir boosted with ritonavir was as effective as lopinavir/ritonavir (Tables 21-4 and 21-5).[15] Indeed, mean reductions in plasma HIV RNA from baseline for atazanavir/ritonavir and lopinavir/ritonavir were comparable at 1.93 and 1.87 $\log_{10}$ copies/mL, respectively. Virologic suppression and comparable efficacy was maintained through to week 96, when 72% of patients in the boosted atazanavir and lopinavir/ritonavir groups achieved HIV RNA levels <50 copies/mL.[17] In addition, the mean change from baseline in HIV RNA levels at week 96 was −2.29 and −2.08 $\log_{10}$ copies/mL in the atazanavir/ritonavir and lopinavir/ritonavir groups, respectively. Efficacy of atazanavir/saquinavir was lower than that of lopinavir/ritonavir in terms of viral load reduction and increases in CD4+ T-lymphocyte count, resulting in premature discontinuation of this arm.

In study 043, 24 weeks' treatment with unboosted atazanavir demonstrated less antiviral efficacy than the boosted lopinavir/ritonavir regimen (Table 21-4).[16] Nevertheless, both regimens demonstrated significant virologic responses and ~40% of atazanavir recipients achieved HIV RNA levels of <50 copies/mL.

The results of study 097 demonstrated that patients on boosted/unboosted PIs who switched to an atazanavir-containing regimen had significantly fewer episodes of viral rebound than those who continued their prior PI treatment.[18] Significantly fewer patients in the atazanavir group experienced viral rebound at week 24 compared with the prior PI-based regimen (3% vs 8%).

VIRAL RESISTANCE

In Vitro Resistance

HIV-1 isolates with a decreased susceptibility to atazanavir have been selected *in vitro*.[3,20] After 5 months of passaging, HIV-1 isolates that were 93- to 183-fold resistant to atazanavir from three different viral strains were identified. The mutations in these HIV-1 viruses that contributed to atazanavir resistance included I50L, N88S, I84V, A71V, and M46I. Recombinant viruses containing the isoleucine to leucine substitution at amino acid residue 50 (I50L mutation) were growth impaired and displayed increased *in vitro* susceptibility to other PIs (amprenavir, indinavir, lopinavir, nelfinavir, ritonavir, and saquinavir).

The evolution to resistance seemed distinct for each of the three strains used, suggesting multiple pathways to resistance and the importance of the viral genetic background. The N88S substitution in the viral protease appeared first during the selection process in two of the three strains.[20] The I50L mutation of the HIV-1 protease gene was a key mutation in one of the strains and this substitution appears to be the signature mutation for atazanavir resistance in clinical isolates obtained from PI-naive patients.[21]

In Vivo Resistance

Differing patterns of atazanavir resistance in viral isolates from patients have been observed, depending on whether atazanavir is administered to a drug-naive or PI-experienced patient. Clinical isolates obtained from PI-naive patients who were experiencing virologic failure while receiving regimens containing once-daily atazanavir 200–600 mg had the I50L mutation.[21] The I50L substitution was observed in all isolates exhibiting phenotypic resistance to atazanavir, which were obtained from patients with virologic failure following treatment for an average of 50 weeks. The median decrease from baseline in susceptibility to atazanavir was 9.6-fold. Importantly, the mutated viruses retained *in vitro* susceptibility to all other approved PIs.

In contrast to the pattern of resistance in drug-naive patients, the mechanism of resistance to atazanavir in patients with prior PI experience relies on the loss of susceptibility caused by the accumulation of multiple "classical" PI mutations.[3,22] Thus, atazanavir-resistant isolates from treatment-experienced patients who receive atazanavir or atazanavir/ritonavir display after prior PI failure decreased susceptibility to multiple PIs. In the 045 study, the most common primary protease mutations to develop in the viral isolates of patients who failed treatment with once-daily atazanavir 300 mg and once-daily ritonavir 100 mg (together with tenofovir and an NRTI) included V32I, L33F/V/I, E35D/G, M46I/L, I50L, F53L/V, I54V, A71V/T/I, G73S/T/C, V82A/T/L, I85V,

Table 21-4

Comparison of Virologic Suppression for Atazanavir in Treatment-Experienced Patients

			Mean Plasma HIV RNA Levels at Baseline (log_{10} copies/mL)		Response at 48 Weeks			Change in Plasma HIV RNA Levels from Baseline (log_{10} copies/mL)	
Study #	Description	Regimens	# Patients	Level	# Patients (ITT)	% Patients with Plasma HIV RNA < 400 copies/mL	% Patients with Plasma HIV RNA < 50 copies/mL	# Patients (OT)	Mean Decrease
043[15]	Randomized, open-label multicenter trial to compare safety and efficacy of atazanavir and boosted lopinavir in patients with one PI failure	ATV 400 qd + 2 NRTIs[a]	150	4.18	150	59	38	150	1.67
		LPV/RTV 400/100 bid + 2 NRTIs[a]	150	4.14	150	77	54	150	2.11
045[b16]	Randomized, open-label, multicenter trial to compare safety and efficacy of atazanavir with lopinavir in patients with multiple therapy failures	ATV 300 qd + RTV 100 qd + TFV 300 qd + NRTI	120	4.44	120	56	38	120	1.87
		ATV 400 qd + SQV 1200 qd + TFV 300 qd + NRTI	115	4.42	115	38	26	115	1.67
		LPV/RTV 400/100 bid + TFV 300 qd + NRTI	123	4.47	123	58	46	123	2.11

[a] Combinations were: zidovudine + lamivudine, stavudine + lamivudine, zidovudine + didanosine, stavudine + didanosine, abacavir + didanosine, stavudine, or lamivudine.

[b] The original 2-NRTI backbone was replaced with tenovir + NRTI 2 weeks into the study. NRTI was didanosine 400 mg qd, stavudine 40 mg bid, abacavir 300 mg bid, zidovudine 300 mg bid, or lamivudine 150 mg bid.

Adapted from Swainston HT, Scott LJ. Atazanavir: a review of its use in the management of HIV infection. Drugs 65:2309–36, 2005.

Table 21-5 Comparison of Immunologic Response for Atazanavir in Treatment-Experienced Patients

			Mean CD4+ Lymphocyte Count at Baseline (cells/μL)		Mean Change in CD4+ Lymphocyte Count from Baseline (cells/μL)	
Study #	Description	Regimens	# Patients	CD4+	# Patients (OT)	Mean Increase
043[15]	Randomized, open-label multicenter trial to compare safety and efficacy of atazanavir and boosted lopinavir in patients with one PI failure	ATV 400 qd + 2 NRTIs[a]	150	288	150	94
		LPV/RTV 400/100 bid + 2 NRTIs[a]	150	261	150	121
045[b16]	Randomized, open-label, multicenter trial to compare safety and efficacy of atazanavir with lopinavir in patients with multiple therapy failures	ATV 300 qd + RTV 100 qd + TFV 300 qd + NRTI	120	317	120	110
		ATV 400 qd + SQV 1200 qd + TFV 300 qd + NRTI	115	286	115	72
		LPV/RTV 400/100 bid + TFV 300 qd + NRTI	123	283	123	121

[a] Combinations were: zidovudine + lamivudine, stavudine + lamivudine, zidovudine + didanosine, stavudine + didanosine, abacavir + didanosine, stavudine, or lamivudine.

[b] The original 2-NRTI backbone was replaced with tenovir + NRTI 2 weeks into the study. NRTI was didanosine 400 mg qd, stavudine 40 mg bid , abacavir 300 mg bid, zidovudine 300 mg bid, or lamivudine 150 mg bid.

Adapted from Swainston HT, Scott LJ. Atazanavir: a review of its use in the management of HIV infection. Drugs 65:2309–36, 2005.

and L89V/Q/M/T.[3] Other mutations that developed on boosted atazanavir treatment included E34K/A/Q, G48V, I84V, N88S/D/T, and L90M. In studies 009, 043, and 045, the I50L mutation was found in about one-third of atazanavir-resistant isolates from ART-experienced patients with virologic failure, with the most common co-emerging mutations being A71V, K45R, G73S, E34X, and L33F.[22] Generally, if multiple PI resistance mutations were present at baseline, atazanavir resistance developed through mutations associated with resistance to other PIs.[23]

Cross-Resistance

Cross-resistance has been observed among PIs. An analysis of the genotypic profiles of 943 PI-susceptible and -resistant clinical isolates found that while no single substitution or combination of substitutions was predictive of atazanavir resistance, isolates cross-resistant to multiple PIs were cross-resistant to atazanavir.[3,23] Indeed, there was high cross-resistance to atazanavir in isolates with prior PI exposure that were phenotypically and/or genotypically resistant to at least three[23,24] or four[25,26] other PIs. The median reduction in susceptibility to atazanavir compared with a reference strain was 1.6-, 2.1-, 4.0-, 6.2-, and 22-fold for isolates resistant to one, two, three, four, or five PIs, respectively.

An *in vitro* evaluation of a panel of 245 clinical samples with resistance to PIs found that cross-resistance to atazanavir was higher than that to amprenavir or lopinavir, with a 3.5-fold reduced susceptibility to indinavir, saquinavir, ritonavir, or nelfinavir compared with wild-type virus.[27]

The results of studies on the cross-resistance of atazanavir-resistant isolates have not been consistent.[3,22] Isolates resistant to atazanavir from ART-experienced patients with virologic failure were also cross-resistant to other PIs, with >90% of the isolates resistant to indinavir, lopinavir, nelfinavir, ritonavir, and saquinavir, and 80% resistant to amprenavir.[3] Isolates that contained the I50L substitution, however, displayed unchanged or increased susceptibility from baseline to lopinavir, nelfinavir, ritonavir, and saquinavir.[22]

Study 089 assessed treatment-emergent resistance in ART-naive patients. One subject in the atazanavir 400 mg arm was found to have the I50L substitution but none were found in the atazanavir/ritonavir arm.[14]

Virologic Response

Genotypic and/or phenotypic analysis of HIV-1 before initiation of boosted atazanavir therapy may help to determine atazanavir susceptibility. An analysis of the 045 study in ART-experienced patients who received boosted atazanavir or lopinavir/ritonavir investigated the association between the virologic response and the number and type of PI-resistance mutation detected at baseline.[15] The study demonstrated that both the number and type of baseline PI mutation affected response rates in treatment-experienced patients. Boosted atazanavir-treated patients with less than four mutations had a reduction in plasma HIV RNA level of 2.13 $\log_{10}$ copies/mL compared with 1.38 in those with four mutations. Similarly in the lopinavir/ritonavir-treated subjects, patients with less than four PI mutations at baseline experienced a reduction of 2.1 $\log_{10}$ copies/mL compared with 1.47 in those with four mutations. Furthermore, patients who were susceptible to atazanavir at baseline reduced their HIV RNA levels by 2.12 versus 1.17 $\log_{10}$ copies/mL in patients with virus resistant to atazanavir.

When atazanavir is used in PI-experienced patients, the genotypic inhibitory quotient (GIQ; the ratio between the C_{min} at steady state and the number of protease resistance mutations at baseline) may be the best predictor of long-term virologic response.[28–31] The GIQ determines the relationship between baseline resistance mutations, drug exposure and virologic response, and is therefore useful for therapeutic drug monitoring[32] and resistance testing[33]. In one study of PI-experienced patients who began therapy with atazanavir/ritonavir, the median GIQ was twofold higher in patients achieving undetectable viremia at 24 weeks compared with those who experienced virologic failure.[31] Other studies have also shown that the atazanavir GIQ is predictive of virologic response in ART-experienced patients following 12[28,29] or 24-week[30] treatment with unboosted atazanavir or ritonavir-boosted atazanavir[28–30]

EFFECTS ON METABOLIC PROFILE

Insulin Resistance

Insulin resistance is a component of the metabolic syndrome, which is associated with PI-containing ART.[34] Direct inhibition of the insulin-responsive glucose transporter, GLUT-4, is thought to contribute to insulin resistance. *In vitro* studies demonstrated that, unlike indinavir and ritonavir, atazanavir had little or no inhibitory activity against GLUT-4.[34,35] Moreover, data from randomized, placebo-controlled, single-[36] or multiple-dose[37] studies in healthy volunteers demonstrated that atazanavir was not associated with insulin resistance. In the same studies, ritonavir/indinavir and ritonavir/lopinavir induced insulin resistance. Using the hyperinsulinemic euglycemic clamp method to determine the insulin-stimulated glucose disposal per unit of insulin (M/I), the studies showed that there was no significant difference between the placebo, atazanavir 400 mg or atazanavir/ritonavir 300 mg/100 mg groups. In the single-dose study, the M/I was significantly lower following treatment with indinavir/ritonavir compared with atazanavir/ritonavir.[36] In the multiple-dose study, the M/I was 23% lower with lopinavir/ritonavir than with atazanavir therapy.[37]

Data from these studies *in vitro* and in healthy volunteers have been supported by study 034, which showed that there were no significant variations in the glucose metabolism in patients treated with either atazanavir- or efavirenz-containing regimens.[10] Mean fasting glucose levels were 90 mg/dL at baseline and ~94 mg/dL at week 48 in both treatment groups. Patients receiving efavirenz, however, tended to have slight increases in insulin concentrations at week 48, although these were not clinically relevant.

Lipid Profile

Generally, clinical trials in drug-naive patients have demonstrated that treatment with atazanavir results in smaller increases in total cholesterol, fasting low-density lipoprotein (LDL) cholesterol and fasting triglyceride levels than nelfinavir[11,12] or efavirenz.[10] Moreover, observed lipid changes were higher in patients treated with boosted atazanavir regimes than in regimes containing atazanavir alone (Table 21-6, Fig. 21-2).[14]

In studies 007 and 008, using stavudine-based NRTI backbones, increases in total cholesterol from baseline to 48 weeks treatment with atazanavir 400 mg qd were 5% and 7%, respectively.[11,12] The total cholesterol increases from baseline in nelfinavir-treated patients were 25% in study 007 and 28% in study 008.[11,12] Similar patterns were observed for triglycerides in studies 007 and 008 after 48-week therapy with atazanavir (+1.5% and +7%, respectively) and nelfinavir (+42% and +50%, respectively).[11,12]

In the phase III 034 trial, increases from baseline in fasting LDL (+1%) or total cholesterol (+2%), and the decrease in triglyceride levels (−9%) were not significant in the atazanavir group.[10] The mean increases in total and LDL cholesterol in the efavirenz group (+121% and +18%, respectively), however, were significantly greater than for atazanavir. Nevertheless, in both treatment arms at week 48, mean total cholesterol and LDL cholesterol levels remained within the desirable, optimal or near optimal range according to the National Cholesterol Education Program Adult Treatment Panel III guidelines.[39] The high-density lipoprotein (HDL) cholesterol levels increased in both the atazanavir and efavirenz treatment groups, but were greater with efavirenz, +24% versus +13%, respectively.

In the 089 study, increases in cholesterol and fasting triglyceride levels were observed in both arms at 48 weeks, with the exception of fasting triglyceride levels in the atazanavir arm, which decreased by 2%. In general, cholesterol increases were greater in the atazanavir/ritonavir arm than in the atazanavir only arm (15% vs 6% for total cholesterol; 23% vs 16% for fasting LDL cholesterol; and 30% vs 29% for HDL cholesterol).[14]

In ART-experienced patients, atazanavir-containing regimens tended to decrease lipid levels, while lopinavir/ritonavir therapy increased values.[15,16,40] This effect was observed in both unboosted (study 043) and boosted (study 045) use. An analysis of study 045 at 96 weeks demonstrated that this favorable effect on lipids was maintained (Table 21-7).[17]

Table 21-6

Comparison of the Effects of Different Therapy Regimens, With and Without Atazanavir, on Lipid Profiles in Treatment-Naive HIV Patients

		Total Cholesterol		Fasting LDL Cholesterol		HDL Cholesterol		Fasting Triglycerides	
Study #	Regimen	Baseline (mg/dL) [n]	Mean Change (%) [n]	Baseline (mg/dL)	Mean Change (%)	Baseline (mg/dL)	Mean Change (%)	Baseline (mg/dL)	Mean Change (%)
007[11]	ATV 400 qd + ddI + d4T	158 [101]	+7[a] [81]	101 [46]	−7[a] [35]	NA	NA	115 [57]	+2[b] [44]
	NFV 750 tid + ddI + d4T	164 [164]	+28 [82]	103 [48]	+31 [39]	NA	NA	95 [60]	+42 [46]
008[12]	ATV 400 mg qd + 3TC + d4T	168 [178]	+5[a,c] [153]	99 [136]	+5[c,d] [87]	NA	NA	128 [139]	+7[c,b] [85]
	NFV 1250 bid + 3TC + d4T	165 [91]	+25[c] [76]	97 [75]	+23[c,d] [41]	NA	NA	108 [77]	+50[c] [50]
034[e10]	ATV 400 qd + ZDV/3TC	~165 [NR]	+2[a] [NR]	~98 [NR]	+1[a] [NR]	~40 [NR]	+13[a] [NR]	~135 [NR]	−9[a] [NR]
	EFV 600 qd + ZDV/3TC	~165 [NR]	+21 [NR]	~98 [NR]	+18 [NR]	~40 [NR]	+24 [NR]	~128 [NR]	+23 [NR]
089[e14]	ATV 400 qd + 3TC + d4T	~160 [105]	+6[f] [104]	~90 [105]	+18[g] [104]	~40 [105]	+29[h] [104]	~150 [105]	−3[i] [104]
	ATV/RTV 300/100 qd + 3TC + d4T	~160 [95]	+15 [95]	~90 [95]	+23 [95]	~40 [95]	+30 [95]	~140 [95]	+26 [95]

NR, not recorded; NA, not available.
[a]$P < 0.0001$ vs active comparator.
[b]$P \leqslant 0.005$.
[c]$P < 0.01$ vs baseline.
[d]Values at 56 weeks.
[e]Baseline values estimated from a graph.
[f]$P = 0.0034$ vs active comparator.
[g]$P = 0.21$ vs active comparator.
[h]$P = 0.89$ vs active comparator.
[i]$P = 0.0004$ vs active comparator.

Adapted from Swainston HT, Scott LJ. Atazanavir: a review of its use in the management of HIV infection. Drugs 65:2309–36, 2005.

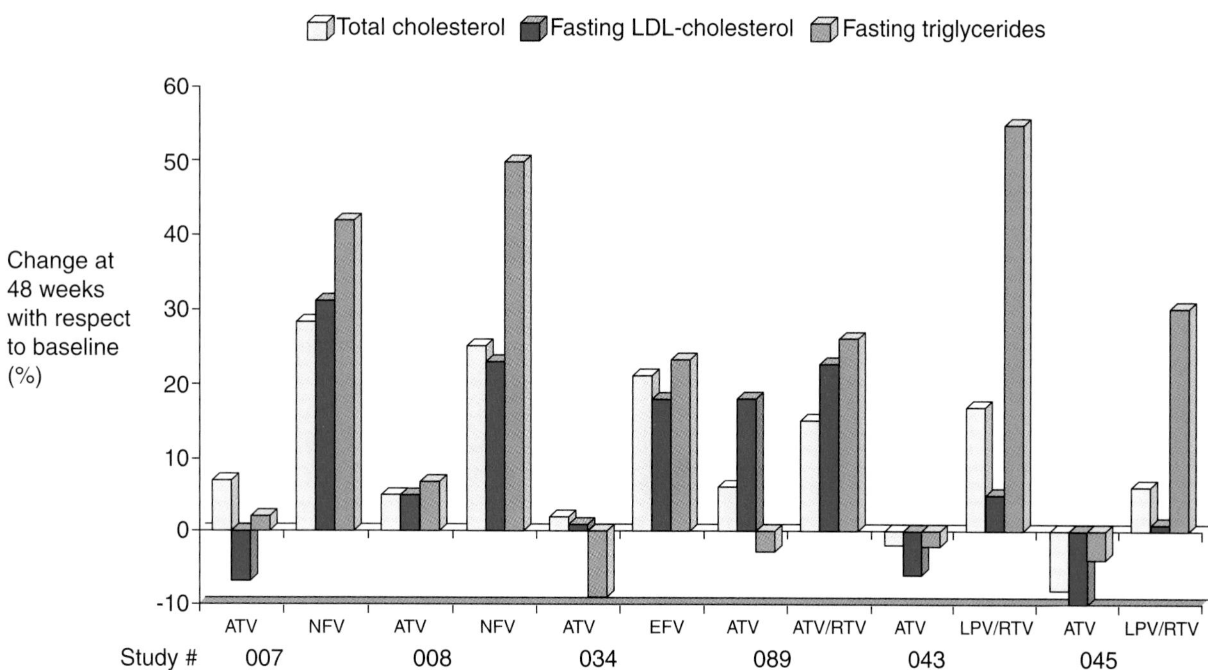

Figure 21-2 ■ Comparison of the effects of different therapy regimens, with and without atazanavir, on lipid profiles in HIV patients.

Adapted from Barreiro P, Rendon A, Rodriguez-Novoa S, Soriano V. Atazanavir: the advent of a new generation of more convenient protease inhibitors. HIV Clin Trials 6:50–61, 2005.

Table 21-7 48- and 96-Week data for Lipid Changes in Art-Experienced HIV Patients

		Total Cholesterol			Fasting Triglycerides		
Study #	**Regimen**	**Baseline (mg/dL)**	**Mean Change at 48 Weeks (%)**	**Mean Change at 96 Weeks (%)**	**Baseline (mg/dL)**	**Mean Change at 48 Weeks (%)**	**Mean Change at 96 Weeks (%)**
0043[a15]	ATV 400 qd + 2 NRTIs	NR	-2^b	NA	NR	-2^b	NA
	LPV/RTV 400/100 bid + 2 NRTIs	NR	+17	NA	NR	+55	NA
0045[c16]	ATV 300 qd + RTV 100 qd + TFV + NRTI	183	-8^b	−7	164	-4^b	−2
	LPV/RTV 400/100 bid + TFV + NRTI	178	+6	+9	163	+30	+30

NR, not recorded; NA, not available.

[a] Baseline values included in lipid profile analysis not reported.

[b] $P \leq 0.05$.

[c] Baseline values are median values.

In ART-experienced patients with HIV therapy-induced hyperlipidemia (defined as a fasting triglyceride level >500 mg/dL, total cholesterol >200 mg/dL or LDL cholesterol >130 mg/dL), switching to an atazanavir-containing regimen produced a favorable effect on the lipid profile.[41,42] Indeed, 6-month treatment with a ritonavir-boosted atazanavir-containing regimen produced significant reductions from baseline in total cholesterol (−13%), triglyceride (−21%), and non-HDL cholesterol (−14%) levels (Fig. 21-3).[42] The changes in LDL cholesterol and HDL cholesterol levels (both −5%) were not significant, although the total cholesterol to HDL cholesterol ratio decreased significantly after 12 months of therapy. Another study of 31 patients with severe hyperlipidemia who were not using lipid-lowering agents demonstrated that a switch to an unboosted atazanavir or ritonavir-boosted atazanavir regimen produced a significant improvement in HIV therapy-induced hyperlipidemia.[41] Similarly, two 48-week, randomized, open-label studies demonstrated that

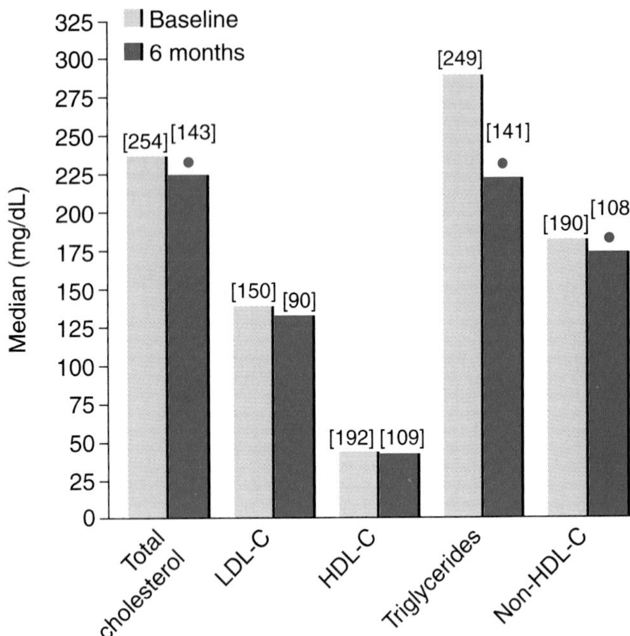

Figure 21-3 ■ Effect of switching to ritonavir-boosted atazanavir-containing therapy on the lipid profile of art-experienced patients with hyperlipidemia: summary of 6-month data.

Reproduced from Martinez E, Azuaje C, Antela A, et al. Effects of switching to ritonavir-boosted atazanavir on HIV-infected patients receiving antiretroviral therapy with hyperlipidemia (abstract no. 850 plus poster no. K-184).

patients who switched to atazanavir (boosted[18] or unboosted[43]) achieved greater reductions in their LDL cholesterol, total cholesterol, and triglyceride levels than those who continued with their prior PI-based regimen.

EFFECT ON ELECTROCARDIOGRAM

Currently, data on the potential for a pharmacodynamic interaction in humans between atazanavir and other drugs that prolong the PR interval of the electrocardiogram (ECG) are limited. However, concentration- and dose-dependent prolongation of the PR interval in the ECG has been observed in a placebo-controlled trial of healthy volunteers receiving atazanavir 400 mg.[3] In another placebo-controlled study in healthy subjects, however, atazanavir 400 mg or 800 mg had no concentration-dependent effect on the corrected QT (QTc) interval. In 1793 HIV-infected patients receiving ART regimens, QTc prolongation was comparable in the atazanavir and comparator regimens.[3] Moreover, no atazanavir-treated healthy subject or HIV-infected patient had a QTc interval >500 ms.

TOLERABILITY

Generally, atazanavir was well-tolerated in the main clinical trials in both ART-naive[10–13] and ART-experienced[15–18] patients, with 5–10% discontinuing due to adverse events. A similar proportion of ART-naive patients discontinued due to adverse events in the atazanavir 400 mg (4–6%)[10–12], efavirenz 600 mg (8%)[10], three times daily nelfinavir 750 mg (7%)[11], and twice-daily nelfinavir 1250 mg (3%)[12] groups. In trials of ART-experienced patients, discontinuation rates were similar between atazanavir and lopinavir/ritonavir groups (<1–4% vs 2–4%)[16,17] and between atazanavir and comparator PI groups (6% vs 5%).[18]

In trials of atazanavir-containing therapy in ART-naive patients, the most frequent grade 2–4 treatment-related adverse effects were jaundice/scleral icterus, nausea or rash (Table 21-8).[3] With the exception of jaundice and scleral icterus, which occurred only in patients receiving atazanavir, the type of treatment-related adverse event was similar in the atazanavir, efavirenz and nelfinavir treatment groups.[3] Moreover, atazanavir was generally well-tolerated over the longer term (median cumulative treatment time of 108 weeks).[13]

Treatments in both arms of study 089 were generally safe and well-tolerated, with few discontinuations (10% for atazanavir and 12% for atazanavir with ritonavir).[14] Adverse event-related discontinuations similarly were more common in the atazanavir with ritonavir arm (8% vs 1%) and were mainly protocol-mandated discontinuations for persistent hyperbilirubinemia, although jaundice and scleral icterus were also more common in these patients (22% and 23%, respectively, vs 7% and 13% for atazanavir, respectively).[14]

In ART-experienced patients, the tolerability profile of atazanavir[16] or ritonavir-boosted atazanavir[15,17] was similar to that of lopinavir/ritonavir (Table 21-9). In study 045, treatment-related grade 2–4 adverse events that occurred in 3% of patients in the boosted atazanavir and lopinavir/ritonavir treatment groups were lipodystrophy, nausea, fatigue, peripheral neurologic symptoms, vomiting and rash.[15] Preliminary 96-week data from study 045 indicated that boosted atazanavir was generally well-tolerated over the long term in ART-experienced patients, with the nature and incidence of adverse events similar to that observed at 48 weeks.[17]

Total bilirubin elevation is the most frequent laboratory abnormality associated with atazanavir therapy.[4] The underlying cause appears to be inhibition of the UGT 1A1 liver enzyme by atazanavir, which causes a reduction in free bilirubin concentration.[44] Moderate total bilirubin elevations were observed frequently in the first months of atazanavir therapy, although this only achieved clinical relevance (grade 3–4) in one-third of patients across studies and hyperbilirubinemia was generally reversible[10–12] and infrequently lead to treatment discontinuation (<1%). In the phase II dose-ranging trials, the incidence of bilirubin was dose-related.[11,12]

Grade 3–4 elevations in transaminase levels occurred infrequently in ART-experienced patients. These were observed in 2–6% of patients receiving an atazanavir-containing regimen,[15,16,18] 1–3% of recipients of a lopinavir/ritonavir-containing regimen,[15,16] and 2% or 5% of patients receiving a comparator PI-based regimen.[18] Nevertheless, the elevations in transaminase levels were transient and no correlation was found between bilirubin and transaminase elevations.

Table 21-8

Selected Grade 2–4 Treatment-Emergent Adverse Events[a] Reported in ≥2% of Adult Treatment-Naive Patients[b]

	Study 089		Study 034		Studies 007 and 008	
Duration	**48 Weeks[c]**		**64 Weeks[d]**		**120 Weeks[d,e]**	**73 Weeks[d,e]**
Regimen	ATV 400 qd + 3TC + d4T	ATV/RTV 300/100 qd + 3TC + d4T	ATV 400 qd + 3TC + AZT	EFV 600 qd + LMV + AZT[f]	ATV 400 qd + d4T + 3TC or ddI	NFV 750 tid or 1250 bid + d4T + 3TC or ddI
# Patients	105	95	404	401	279	191
General						
Headache	4	2	6	6	1	2
Digestive System						
Nausea	<3	<3	14	12	6	4
Jaundice/scleral icterus	1	3	7	[g]	7	[g]
Vomiting	<3	<3	4	7	3	3
Diarrhea	<3	<3	1	2	3	16
Abdominal pain	<3	<3	4	4	4	2
Nervous System						
Dizziness	<3	<3	2	7	<1	[g]
Insomnia	<3	<3	3	3	<1	[g]
Peripheral neurologic symptoms	<3	<3	<1	1	4	3
Skin and Appendages						
Rash	4	2	7	10	5	1

[a] Includes events of possible, probable, certain, or unknown relationship to treatment regimen.
[b] Based on the regimen including atazanavir.
[c] Total duration of study 96 weeks.
[d] Median time on therapy.
[e] Includes long-term follow-up.
[f] As a fixed dose combination: LMV/AZT 150/300 bid.
[g] None reported in this treatment arm.

Adapted from Bristol-Myers Squibb Company. Reyataz® (atazanavir sulfate) capsules prescribing information. Online. Available: http://www.bms.com 2006.

Table 21-9

Selected Grade 2–4 Treatment-Emergent Adverse Events[a] Reported in ≥2% of Adult Treatment-Experienced Patients[b]

	Study 045	
Duration	48 Weeks[c]	
Regimen	ATV/RTV 300/100 qd + TDF + NRTI	LPV/RTV 400/100 bid[d] + TDF + NRTI
# Patients	119	118
General		
Fever	2	[e]
Digestive System		
Jaundice/scleral icterus	9	[e]
Diarrhea	3	11
Nausea	3	2
Nervous System		
Depression	2	<1
Musculoskeletal System		
Myalgia	4	[e]

[a] Includes events of possible, probable, certain, or unknown relationship to treatment regimen.
[b] Based on the regimen including atazanavir.
[c] Median time on therapy.
[d] As a fixed dose combination.
[e] None reported in this treatment arm.

Reprinted from Bristol-Myers Squibb Company. Reyataz® (atazanavir sulfate) capsules prescribing information. Online. Available: http://www.bms.com 2006.

RECOMMENDATIONS FOR USE

Approved indications for atazanavir use vary across countries. In the United States, indications include both boosted (300 mg with 100 mg ritonavir qd) and unboosted (400 mg qd) use and both naive- and treatment-experienced use, though boosted atazanavir is preferred owing to superior antiviral efficacy. In the European Union, atazanavir in combination with low-dose ritonavir in ART-experienced patients is the only approved use.[3,45]

Atazanavir should be taken with food at least 2 h apart from antacids. Specific dosages are required in special patient populations. Atazanavir may have an advantage over other PIs because of its relatively favorable effect on lipid profiles, once-daily dosing, low capsule burden, in patients with low prior PI exposure, resistance profile at initial failure.

REFERENCES

1. Witherell G. BMS-232632 (Novartis/Bristol-Myers Squibb). Curr Opin Investig Drugs 2:340–7, 2001.
2. Robinson BS, Riccardi KA, Gong YF, et al. BMS-232632, a highly potent human immunodeficiency virus protease inhibitor that can be used in combination with other available antiretroviral agents. Antimicrob Agents Chemother 44:2093–9, 2000.
3. Bristol-Myers Squibb Company. Reyataz® (atazanavir sulfate) capsules prescribing information. Online. Available: http://www.bms.com 2006.
4. Bristol-Myers Squibb Company. BMS-232632: atazanavir briefing document May. Online. 2003.
5. O' Mara E, Piliero P, Drusano G, et al. A preliminary pharmacokinetic and pharmacodynamic evaluation of the HIV protease inhibitor BMS-232632 in a protease inhibitor-naive HIV+ population (abstract P9), 2000.
6. O' Mara E, Smith J, Olsen SJ, et al. BMS-232632: single-oral dose-safety and pharmacokinetic study in healthy volunteers (abstract I-242).
7. O' Mara E, Mummaneni V, Randall D, et al. BMS-232632: a summary of multiple dose pharmacokinetic, food effect and drug interaction studies in healthy subjects (abstract 504).
8. Randall D, Agarwala S, Mummaneni V, et al. Tissue compartment concentrations of atazanavir in cerebrospinal fluid, seminal fluid and plasma in HIV+ subjects (abstract no. 273).
9. Bristol-Myers Squibb Pharmaceuticals Ltd. Reyataz hard capsules summary of product characteristics. Online.
10. Squires K, Lazzarin A, Gatell JM, et al. Comparison of once-daily atazanavir with efavirenz, each in combination with fixed-dose zidovudine and lamivudine, as initial therapy for patients infected with HIV. J Acquir Immune Defic Syndr 36:1011–19, 2004.
11. Sanne I, Piliero P, Squires K, et al. Results of a phase 2 clinical trial at 48 weeks (AI424-007): a dose-ranging, safety, and efficacy comparative trial of atazanavir at three doses in combination with didanosine and stavudine in antiretroviral-naive subjects. J Acquir Immune Defic Syndr 32:18–29, 2003.
12. Murphy RL, Sanne I, Cahn P, et al. Dose-ranging, randomized, clinical trial of atazanavir with lamivudine and stavudine in antiretroviral-naive subjects: 48-week results. AIDS 17:2603–14, 2003.
13. Wood R, Phanuphak P, Cahn P, et al. Long-term efficacy and safety of atazanavir with stavudine and lamivudine in patients

previously treated with nelfinavir or atazanavir. J Acquir Immune Defic Syndr 36:684–92, 2004.
14. Malan N, Krantz E, David N, et al; -089 Study Group. Efficacy and safety of atazanavir with and without ritonavir in antiretroviral-naive subjects. BMS089: 48-week study results. Presentation at 13th Conference on Retroviruses and Opportunistic Infections, Denver, CO, 5–8 Feb 2006.
15. Johnson M, Grinsztejn B, Rodriguez C, et al. Atazanavir plus ritonavir or saquinavir, and lopinavir/ritonavir in patients experiencing multiple virological failures. AIDS 19:685–94, 2005.
16. Nieto-Cisneros L, Zala C, Fessel WJ, et al. Antiviral efficacy, metabolic changes and safety of atazanavir (ATV) versus lopinavir/ritonavir (LPV/RTV) in combination with two NRTIs in patients who have experienced virological failure with prior PI-containing regimen(s): 24-week results from BMSAI424-043, pp S212 (abstract 117), 2003.
17. Johnson M, De Jesus E, Grinsztejn B, et al. Long-term efficacy and durability of atazanavir (ATV) with ritonavir (RTV) or saquinavir (SQV) versus lopinavir/ritonavir (LPV/RTV) in HIV-infected patients with multiple virologic failures: 96-week results from a randomized, open-label trial, BMS AI424045 (poster PL14.4).
18. Gatell J, Salmon-Ceron D, Lazzarin A, et al; Efficacy of atazanavir (ATV) based HAART in patients switched from a stable PI or boosted PI (PI/r) treatment. Planned week 24 analysis of a phase IIIb 48-week multicenter, open-label, randomized, prospective study: the SWAN study (poster WePe6.3C15).
19. Swainston HT, Scott LJ. Atazanavir: a review of its use in the management of HIV infection. Drugs 65:2309–36, 2005.
20. Gong YF, Robinson BS, Rose RE, et al. In vitro resistance profile of the human immunodeficiency virus type 1 protease inhibitor BMS-232632. Antimicrob Agents Chemother 44:2319–26, 2000.
21. Colonno R, Rose R, McLaren C, et al. Identification of I50L as the signature atazanavir (ATV)-resistance mutation in treatment-naive HIV-1-infected patients receiving ATV-containing regimens. J Infect Dis 189:1802–10, 2004.
22. Colonno R, Parkin N, McLaren C, et al. Pathways to atazanavir resistance in treatment-experienced patients and impact of residue 50 substitutions (abstract 656).
23. Colonno RJ, Thiry A, Limoli K, Parkin N. Activities of atazanavir (BMS-232632) against a large panel of human immunodeficiency virus type 1 clinical isolates resistant to one or more approved protease inhibitors. Antimicrob Agents Chemother 47:1324–33, 2003.
24. Schnell T, Schmidt B, Moschik G, et al. Distinct cross-resistance profiles of the new protease inhibitors amprenavir, lopinavir, and atazanavir in a panel of clinical samples. AIDS 17:1258–61, 2003.
25. Colonno R, Hertogs K, Larder BA, et al; Efficacy of BMS-232632 against a panel of HIV-1 clinical isolates resistant to currently used protease inhibitors (abstract 2114).
26. Colonno R, Parkin N, McLaren C, et al. BMS-232632 sensitivity of a panel of HIV-1 clinical isolates resistant to one or more approved protease inhibitors (poster 8).
27. Schnell T, Schmidt B, Moschik G, et al. Distinct cross-resistance profiles of the new protease inhibitors amprenavir, lopinavir, and atazanavir in a panel of clinical samples. AIDS 17:1258–61, 2003.
28. Solas C, Colson P, Ravaux I, et al. Predictive factors of atazanavir response including genotypic inhibitory quotient in treatment-experienced patients (abstract 1).
29. Gonzalez de Requena D, Bonora S, Canta F, et al; Atazanavir Ctrough is associated with efficacy and safety: definition of therapeutic range (abstract 645 plus poster).
30. Gonzalez de Requena D, Bonora S, Cavechia I, et al; Atazanavir Ctrough is associated with efficacy and safety at 24 weeks: definition of therapeutic range (abstract 60 plus oral presentation).
31. Barrios A, Rendon AL, Gallego O, et al. Predictors of virological response to atazanavir in protease inhibitor-experienced patients. HIV Clin Trials 5:201–5, 2004.
32. Anderson PL, Kiser JJ. Special pharmacology topics in HIV: Therapeutic drug monitoring. Online.
33. Hirsch MS, Brun-Vezinet F, Clotet B, et al. Antiretroviral drug resistance testing in adults infected with human immunodeficiency virus type 1: 2003 recommendations of an International AIDS Society-USA Panel. Clin Infect Dis 37:113–28, 2003.
34. Wang S, Mulvey R, Elosua C, et al; Association of HIV-protease inhibitors with insulin resistance is related to potency of inhibition of GLUT4 and GLUT1 activity in adipocytes and myocytes [abstract plus poster].
35. Noor MA, Mulvey R, Wang S, et al; Maintenance of favorable in vitro metabolic profile of atazanavir when combined with low dose ritonavir (abstract no. ThOrB1356).
36. Doran DA, Jones SP, Lagathu C, et al; Mechanisms of insulin resistance in HIV-seronegative individuals acutely treated with ritonavir boosted indinavir and atazanavir regimens (abstract no. 6), pp L6, 2004.
37. Noor MA, Parker RA, O'Mara E, Grasela DM, Currie A, Hodder SL, Fiedorek FT, Haas DW. The effects of HIV protease inhibitors atazanavir and lopinavir/ritonavir on insulin sensitivity in HIV-seronegative healthy adults. AIDS 18:2137–2144, 2004.
38. Barreiro P, Rendon A, Rodriguez-Novoa S, Soriano V. Atazanavir: the advent of a new generation of more convenient protease inhibitors. HIV Clin Trials 6:50–61, 2005.
39. National Cholesterol Education Program. Third report of the expert panel on detection, evaluation, and treatment of high blood cholesterol in adults (Adult Treatment Panel III). National Institutes of Health.Available: http://www.nhlbi.nih.gov/guidelines/cholesterol 10 Mar 2006.
40. Abbott Laboratories. Norvir® (ritonavir) capsules prescribing information. Online. Available: http://www.norvir.com. 2006.
41. Mobius U, Lubach-Ruitman M, Castro-Frenzel B, et al. Switching to atazanavir improves metabolic disorders in antiretroviral-experienced patients with severe hyperlipidemia. J Acquir Immune Defic Syndr 39:174–80, 2005.
42. Martinez E, Azuaje C, Antela A, et al. Effects of switching to ritonavir-boosted atazanavir on HIV-infected patients receiving antiretroviral therapy with hyperlipidemia (abstract 850 plus poster no. K-184).
43. Sension M, Grinsztejn B, Molina J, et al. AI424067: improvement in lipid profiles after 12 weeks of switching to atazanavir from boosted or unboosted protease inhibitors in patients with no previous PI virologic failure and hyperlipidemia at baseline (abstract 858).
44. O' Mara E, Mummaneni V, Randall D, et al. Assessment of the effect of uridine diphosphate glucuronosyltransferase 1A1 genotype on indirect bilirubin elevations in healthy subjects dosed with BMS-232632 (abstract 1645).
45. Bristol-Myers Squibb Pharmaceuticals Ltd. Reyataz® hard capsules summary of product characteristics. Online. Available: http://emc.medicines.org.uk. 2006.

Chapter 22

Tenofovir

Craig J. Hoesley, MD

Tenofovir disoproxil fumarate (tenofovir DF) is the oral prodrug of tenofovir (9-[(*R*)-(2-phosphonomethoxy)propyl]adenine) (PMPA), a nucleotide (nucleoside monophosphate) analog with activity against retroviruses and hepadnaviruses. Tenofovir is an acyclic nucleoside phosphonate compound (Fig. 22-1) designed to circumvent the first phosphorylation step necessary for activation of nucleoside analogs, such as zidovudine, didanosine, stavudine, lamivudine, and abacavir.[1] The antiviral activity of unphosphorylated nucleoside analogs may be impeded by their low affinity for cellular nucleoside kinases. Tenofovir differs from the 'classic' nucleoside analogs in that it is less dependent on intracellular enzymes for activation.[2] Tenofovir DF (Viread) received FDA approval in the United States in 2001, and was approved by the European Medicines Evaluation Agency in 2002. Truvada is a fixed-dose combination of tenofovir DF and emtricitabine (FDA approved in 2004). Atripla is a fixed-dose combination of tenofovir DF, emtricitabine, and efavirenz (FDA approved July 2006).

MECHANISM OF ACTION AND *IN VITRO* ACTIVITY

Tenofovir DF is a lipophilic ester derivative of tenofovir designed to improve oral bioavailability. After oral administration and absorption tenofovir DF is rapidly cleaved by nonspecific extracellular carboxyesterases into tenofovir. Once inside cells tenofovir is metabolized by adenylate cyclase and nucleoside diphosphate kinase to tenofovir diphosphate (PMPApp), the active moiety. The antiviral effect of tenofovir is the result of selective interaction of PMPApp with the viral DNA polymerase or reverse transcriptase (RT). Based on the structural resemblance to natural deoxyadenine triphosphates (dATP), PMPApp acts as both a competitive inhibitor and an alternative substrate during the DNA polymerase chain reaction, resulting in DNA chain termination.[1]

Tenofovir has *in vitro* activity against hepadnaviruses (hepatitis B virus) and retroviruses.[3–5] The spectrum of antiretroviral activity includes HIV-1 and HIV-2, simian immunodeficiency virus (SIV), feline immunodeficiency virus, visna-maedi virus of sheep, and murine leukemia and sarcoma viruses.[6–9] *In vitro* activity against non-B HIV-1 subtypes has also been described. The mean 50% inhibitory concentration (IC_{50}) values for tenofovir against HIV-1 subtypes A, C, D, E, F, G, and O in primary peripheral blood mononuclear cell (PBMC) cultures were all within twofold of the HIV subtype B IC_{50} value (range 0.55-0.22 μM).[10]

Tenofovir has demonstrated an anti-HIV effect in both lymphocytes and macrophages.[11] The K_I value of PMPApp against HIV-1 RT is 0.022 μM, which is ~200-, 3700-, and 2700-fold lower than the K_I value against human DNA polymerases α, β, and γ, respectively.[12] Moreover, tenofovir and tenofovir DF were evaluated *in vitro* for antiviral activity (IC_{50}) and cytotoxicity (CC_{50}) using both laboratory and clinical HIV-1 strains; they were noted to have favorable selectivity indices

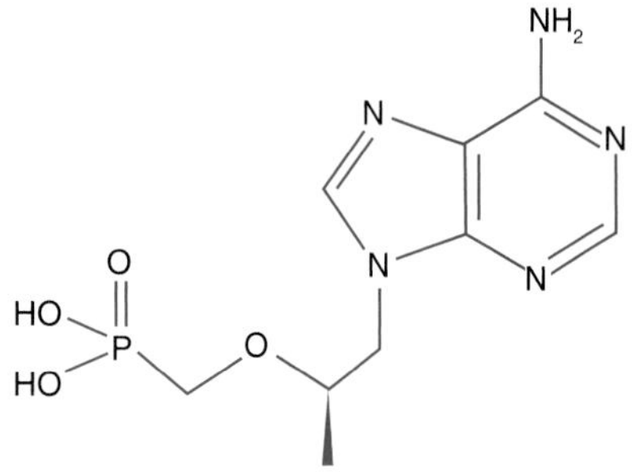

Figure 22-1 ■ Structure of tenofovir disoproxil fumarate, or 9-[(*R*)-(2-phosphonylmethoxy)propyl]adenine.

(CC_{50}/IC_{50} ratio higher than 2000).[13] The antiviral activity of tenofovir against wild-type laboratory strains of HIV-1 ranges from 0.2 to 6.0 μM.[13] *In vitro*, PMPApp (K_I 0.022 μM) is slightly less potent than the active phosphorylated metabolite of zidovudine (K_I 0.008 μM).[12] The potency of tenofovir DF monotherapy (300 mg tablet daily) was assessed in 10 antiretroviral-naive HIV-infected individuals who underwent frequent monitoring of plasma HIV-1 RNA levels over 21 days. The individual first phase decay slopes of plasma HIV-1 RNA levels from −0.24 to −0.59 $\log_{10}$ copies/mL (median − 0.40 $\log_{10}$ copies/mL) which is similar to the values previously described with ritonavir monotherapy indicating comparable potency between the two drugs. The mean reduction in viral load was 1.5 $\log_{10}$ copies/mL by day 21.[14]

In vitro analysis of MT2 cells infected with the HIV-IIIb strain were utilized to assess the activity of tenofovir in combination with a variety of other antiretroviral agents. The combination of tenofovir with zidovudine, amprenavir, and all non-nucleoside reverse transcriptase inhibitors (NNRTIs) tested demonstrated strong synergistic anti-HIV activity, whereas combinations with didanosine, adefovir, and nelfinavir resulted in minor synergistic inhibition of *in vitro* HIV replication.[15] Additive HIV inhibition was noted with tenofovir in combination with abacavir, stavudine, lamivudine, zalcitabine, ritonavir, saquinavir, and indinavir.[15,16] No tenofovir-containing combination demonstrated antagonism.

PHARMACOKINETICS

The formulation of tenofovir DF as an oral prodrug for tenofovir has allowed improved oral bioavailability. *In vitro* metabolic studies using radio-labeled tenofovir and tenofovir disoproxil fumarate in resting and activated peripheral blood lymphocytes demonstrated a more than 1000-fold higher intracellular concentration of the active PMPApp after incubation with the prodrug compared to tenofovir alone.[13] Owing to its increased cellular permeability, the anti-HIV activity of tenofovir DF is increased by 17- to 90-fold over tenofovir. The diphosphorylation of tenofovir in cells to PMPApp is independent of viral infection, and there is evidence that these active intracellular metabolites persist in cells after the drug is removed, suggesting that an antiviral effect may continue in the absence of repeated tenofovir exposure. Moreover, the long intracellular half-life of PMPApp (10 to 50 h) allows once-daily dosing. Animal models have demonstrated that ~98% of an intravenous tenofovir dose is eliminated unchanged in the urine after 24 h.[13] Tenofovir is not a substrate, or inhibitor of the CYP450 enzyme system and does not have significant binding to plasma proteins.[17]

The pharmacokinetics of tenofovir and tenofovir DF has been studied in HIV-1-infected subjects. An aqueous solution of tenofovir was administered intravenously in single doses of 1 mg/kg and 3 mg/kg, resulting in mean peak serum concentrations of 2.7 and 9.1 μg/mL, respectively.[18] Serum tenofovir concentrations declined in a biexponential manner with a terminal half-life of 7.1 h. All subjects in the higher dose (3 mg/kg) group had quantifiable serum levels up to 24 h after the initial dose. In a randomized, double-blind, placebo-controlled phase I/II study (GS-97-901) in HIV-infected individuals, the pharmacokinetics of tenofovir DF were studied at doses of 75, 150, 300, and 600 mg given in tablet form. For each dose cohort, fasting patients received a single oral dose; and after a 1-week observation period the same patients received single oral doses after ingesting a high-fat meal for 28 consecutive days. After fasting, the median peak plasma concentrations (C_{max}) of tenofovir DF were 68.6, 111, 240, and 618 ng/mL in the 75, 150, 300, and 600 mg groups, respectively. Tenofovir has a long terminal half-life in serum of ~17 h. At steady state (day 15), median C_{max} values were -80.8, 163, 303, and 633 ng/mL and area under the serum concentration time curve (AUC^{ss}) values of 717, 1613, 2937, and 6073 ng $h^{-1}mL^{-1}$ in the same dosing groups when the drug was administered in a fed state.[19] The oral bioavailability of tenofovir DF when administered with food was enhanced (~40%) and was not affected by repeated dosing. In general, tenofovir DF displayed linear pharmacokinetics over the 75 to 300 mg/day dose range and was rapidly converted to the active form (tenofovir) following oral absorption with this process facilitated by administration in the fed state.[19]

In a recent study, single-dose and steady-state pharmacokinetics of tenofovir DF (300 mg daily) were evaluated in HIV-infected children and the AUC and C_{max} were comparable to those values seen in HIV-infected adults.[20]

TOXICITY

The preclinical toxicology studies in animals (rats, dogs, monkeys) administered tenofovir over a minimum of 11 months identified the kidney and bone as potential target organs. Specifically, urinary excretion of calcium and phosphorus was increased in rats and dogs when tenofovir exposure was 11- and ninefold larger than standard human exposure, respectively; these findings were reversible and not seen when exposure was increased three- to fivefold over standard human exposure. Moreover, glucosuria and proteinuria were described in dogs and monkeys at nine- and 12-fold increased exposure but again were reversible and not present when dosing was three- to fourfold larger than standard human exposure. Decreased bone marrow density and increased parathyroid hormone secretion were noted in animals when dosing was increased nine- to 50-fold over standard human exposure. These bone toxicities were thought to be secondary to renal toxicity and were reversible with discontinuation of the drug or not seen at all when exposure was only two- to fourfold larger than standard human exposure. Other adverse effects noted in animal studies were gastritis, duodenitis, and slight elevations in liver transaminases; these findings were limited to rats in the higher dosing groups.[21]

Over 1600 HIV-infected individuals have received tenofovir DF alone or in combination with other antiretroviral agents in clinical trials, including a number of study participants who had been treated for 3 years or more. In general, tenofovir DF was well-tolerated. In a randomized, double-blind, placebo-controlled phase II study (GS-98-902), HIV-infected patients received tenofovir DF 75, 150, 300 mg or placebo once daily for 24 weeks in addition to the patient's existing stable antiretroviral regimen at the time of enrollment. At week 24, placebo patients received tenofovir DF 300 mg once daily and all treatment groups were followed for a total of 48 weeks (*see section on* Efficacy). At week 24, the number of grade 3 or 4 adverse events seen in subjects receiving tenofovir DF was similar to those receiving placebo (14-19%), and the percentage of grade 3 or 4 laboratory abnormalities was also similar amongst the treatment and placebo groups.[22] There was no evidence of dose-related increase in adverse events. In a separate randomized, double-blind, placebo-controlled phase III study (GS-99-907), HIV-infected patients received tenofovir DF 300 mg or placebo once daily for 24 weeks in addition to their existing antiretroviral regimen. At week 24, placebo recipients received tenofovir DF 300 mg once daily and were followed for a total 48 weeks (*see section on* Efficacy). As noted in the phase II study, the number of grade 3 or 4 adverse events and laboratory abnormalities were not substantially different between the placebo and treatment groups.[23] A combined list of reported grade 3 or 4 laboratory abnormalities in these studies is presented in Table 22-1.

Interestingly, there have been no grades 3 or 4 serum creatinine elevations associated with tenofovir DF administration during phase II or phase III clinical trials.[24] These findings are particularly significant given the high rate of proximal renal tubular dysfunction described with the structurally similar compound adefovir dipivoxil. The frequency of grade 3 or 4 serum hypophosphatemia in clinical trials was low (~1%) and reversible with discontinuation of treatment.[24] However, since completion of these clinical trials and with expanded use of tenofovir DF in clinical practice, there have been several small case series or case reports describing proximal renal tubular dysfunction and/or hypophosphatemia in HIV-infected patients suggesting longer follow-up may be necessary to fully assess renal toxicity.[24–26] In these studies, proximal renal tubular dysfunction was diagnosed on average 7 months after initiation of tenofovir DF therapy and resolved on average 5 weeks after discontinuation of the drug.[24] In a 3-year, randomized, multicenter, double-blind study (GS-99-903) involving 600 HIV-infected antiretroviral-naive individuals, the prevalence of grades 1, 2, and 3 serum creatinine elevations at week 144 were 4%, <1%, and 0%, respectively, in the tenofovir DF group and 2%, 0%, and <1% in the comparator (stavudine) group. Similarly, there were no differences in the prevalence of grade 1, 2, or 3 serum hypophosphatemia between the groups (4%, 3%, and <1% in the tenofovir group vs 4%, 2%, and <1% in the comparator group).[27,28] Prior adefovir dipivoxil therapy does not appear to be associated with an increased risk of nephrotoxicity.

Bone mineral density testing was performed in a small proportion of subjects participating in the phase II study mentioned above (GS-98-902) and no clinically significant decrease in bone mineral density from baseline was demonstrated in patients receiving tenofovir DF through 48 weeks.[22] Conversely, in a larger study with extended follow-up (GS-99-03, 144 weeks), a greater mean percentage decrease from baseline in bone mineral density at the lumbar spine was observed in participants receiving tenofovir DF when compared to those receiving stavudine (−2.2% vs −1.0%, respectively ($P = 0.001$)).[28] In the same trial, bone mineral density changes in the hip were similar for both groups and the number of patients who experienced bone fractures during the trial was less in the tenofovir DF group.[28]

To date, adverse events associated with mitochondrial dysfunction have not been common. Lactic acidosis has occurred

Table 22-1 Combined Grade 3 or 4 Laboratory Abnormalities Reported in GS-99-907, GS-98-902

Placebo vs Tenofovir DF 300 mg/day (0–24 Weeks)			All Tenofovir DF Recipients[a] (mean 58 Weeks)	
	Placebo	300 mg		
No. of patients	210	443	No. of patients	687
Total no. (%) with abnormal[b]	99 (47)	146 (33)	Total no. (%) with abnormality[b]	377 (55)
Creatinine kinase elevation	30 (14)	36 (8)	Creatinine kinase elevation	103 (15)
Triglyceride elevation	28 (13)	37 (8)	Triglyceride elevation	89 (13)
Amylase elevation	14 (7)	21 (5)	Amylase elevation	47 (7)
AST elevation	6 (3)	16 (4)	AST elevation	40 (3)
Glycosuria	6 (3)	12 (3)	Glycosuria	27 (4)
Serum glucose elevation	8 (4)	8 (2)	Serum glucose elevation	24 (3)
ALT elevation	4 (2)	10 (2)	ALT elevation	30 (4)
Neutropenia	3 (1)	6 (1)	Neutropenia	17 (2)

Data from Schooley R, Ruane P, Myers R, et al. Tenofovir DF in antiretroviral-experienced patients: results from a 48-week, randomized, double-blind study. AIDS 16:1257, 2002; and Squires K, Pozniak A, Pierone G, et al. Tenofovir disoproxil fumarate in nucleoside-resistant HIV-1 infection: a randomized trial. Ann Intern Med 139:313, 2003.

[a] 'All Tenofovir DF' group includes all patients in the tenofovir DF 300 mg group, those placebo recipients who later received tenofovir DF 300 mg in studies 902 and 907, and those subjects who initially received 75 or 150 mg for 24 weeks in study 902 who later received tenofovir DF 300 mg daily.
[b] Abnormalities occurring in ≥2% of patients in any group.

rarely in patients receiving tenofovir DF 300 mg daily in clinical trials and the majority of these subjects were receiving stavudine or didanosine concomitantly.[29,30] These data correlate with the *in vitro* studies suggesting tenofovir DF is less toxic to mitochondria and has less effect on mitochondrial DNA polymerase than stavudine, zalcitabine, and didanosine.[12,31]

EFFICACY

The clinical efficacy of tenofovir DF as measured by absolute CD4+ T-lymphocyte count or plasma HIV-1 RNA levels is shown in Table 22-2.

Tenofovir Disoproxil Fumarate Monotherapy

In a phase I/II randomized, double-blind, placebo-controlled, dose escalation study (GS-97-901), antiretroviral-naive and experienced adults with absolute CD4+ T-lymphocyte counts of 200 cells/mm^3 or more and plasma HIV-1 RNA levels of 10 000 copies/mL or higher were administered tenofovir DF at once-daily doses of 75, 150, 300, or 600 mg or placebo for 4 weeks.[19] Antiretroviral-naive patients receiving tenofovir DF had mean HIV-1 RNA level decreases of 0.45, 0.60, 1.57, and 1.40 $\log_{10}$ copies/mL in the 75, 150, 300, and 600 mg groups, respectively. Antiretroviral-experienced patients receiving tenofovir DF had mean HIV-1 RNA level decreases of 0.27, 0.49, 1.06, and 0.66 $\log_{10}$ copies/mL in the 75, 150, 300, and 600 mg groups, respectively. Overall, a dose-related treatment effect was observed, and individuals receiving 300 or 600 mg once daily had an overall mean HIV-1 RNA level reduction of 1.20 and 0.84 $\log_{10}$ copies/mL, respectively, compared to baseline, whereas placebo recipients experienced a 0.03 $\log_{10}$ copies/mL increase over the same period.

Combination Therapy with Tenofovir Disoproxil Fumarate

In a randomized, double-blind, placebo-controlled phase II study (GS-98-902), 189 HIV-infected patients received tenofovir DF (75, 150, 300 mg) or placebo once daily for 24 weeks in addition to the patient's existing stable antiretroviral regimen (four or fewer drugs) at the time of enrollment. At week 24, placebo patients rolled over in a blinded fashion to tenofovir DF 300 mg once daily, and all treatment groups were followed for a total of 48 weeks.[22,32] Mean baseline plasma HIV RNA levels were 3.8, 3.6, 3.6, and 3.7 $\log_{10}$ copies/mL in the placebo and the 75, 150, and 300 mg treatment groups, respectively. Study participants were highly treatment-experienced with a mean of 4.6 years on antiretroviral therapy and a baseline mean absolute CD4+ T-lymphocyte count of 374 cells/mm^3. In addition, baseline genotyping demonstrated that 94% of patients had nucleoside RT-associated mutations, 57% had protease inhibitor (PI)-associated resistant mutations, and 32% had non-nucleoside RT-associated mutations.

Through week 24, the mean change in plasma HIV RNA levels from baseline were −0.1, −0.4, −0.4, and −0.7 $\log_{10}$ copies/mL in the placebo and 75, 150, and 300 mg groups, respectively. Through week 48, the mean changes in HIV RNA levels from baseline were −0.4, −0.6, and −0.6 $\log_{10}$ copies/mL in the 75, 150, and 300 mg groups, respectively. Placebo recipients were administered tenofovir DF (300 mg) at week 24 resulting in a mean plasma HIV RNA level reduction from baseline of 0.6 $\log_{10}$ copies/mL through week 48.[22,32]

In a randomized, double-blinded, placebo-controlled phase III study (GS-99-903), 600 antiretroviral subjects were randomized to efavirenz (an NNRTI) and lamivudine with either stavudine (40 mg twice daily)/tenofovir DF placebo or tenofovir DF (300 mg once daily)/stavudine placebo.[28] The participants' baseline plasma HIV RNA levels and absolute CD4+ T-lymphocyte counts were 81 300 copies/mL and 279 cells/μL, respectively. At week 48, the intent-to-treat (ITT) analysis demonstrated equivalence with 87% of subjects in each group achieving plasma HIV RNA levels <400 copies/mL. Similarly, 82% and 81% of subjects achieved plasma HIV RNA levels <50 copies/mL in the tenofovir DF and stavudine groups, respectively. The absolute CD4+ T-lymphocyte count increased by 169 cells/μL in the tenofovir DF group compared to a 167 cells/μL increase in the stavudine group.[28]

In a separate randomized, double-blind, placebo-controlled phase III study (GS-00-907), 550 antiretroviral-experienced HIV-infected patients received tenofovir DF 300 mg once daily or placebo for 24 weeks in addition to their existing antiretroviral regimen. After week 24, placebo recipients were allowed to receive tenofovir DF for the remainder of the 48-week study period. At baseline, patients had a mean plasma HIV RNA level of 3.36 log, a mean absolute CD4+ T-lymphocyte count of 427 cells/mm^3, and had received antiretroviral therapy for a mean 5.4 years. Baseline genotypic analyses in a subset of patients ($n = 253$) demonstrated that 94% of participants had nucleoside RT-associated mutations, 58% had PI-associated resistant mutations, and 48% had non-nucleoside-associated RT mutations.[23]

Through week 24, the mean change in plasma HIV RNA levels from baseline were −0.61 and −0.03 log in the tenofovir DF and placebo groups, respectively ($P < 0.001$). In addition, 45% of tenofovir DF recipients achieved plasma HIV RNA levels <400 copies/mL compared to 13% in the placebo group ($P < 0.001$). Reduction in plasma HIV RNA levels to <50 copies/mL was seen in 22% of those receiving tenofovir DF compared to 1% of placebo recipients ($P < 0.001$). The mean change in absolute CD4+ T-lymphocyte counts from baseline were +12.6 and −10.6 cells/mm^3 in the tenofovir DF and placebo groups, respectively ($P = 0.008$). Through week 48, the prevalence of tenofovir DF recipients with plasma HIV RNA levels <400 and <50 copies/mL was 41% and 18%, respectively, suggesting a sustained response.[23]

The role of triple nucleoside analog RT inhibitor regimens for the treatment of HIV-1infection has been investigated. The once-daily triple nucleoside/nucleotide analog combination of abacavir (600 mg), lamivudine (300 mg), and tenofovir DF (300 mg) appeared advantageous relative to potency and

Table 22-2

Clinical Trials Evaluating Activity and Efficacy of Tenofovir Disoproxil Fumarate

Trial[a]	Design	Dose (mg)	No. of Subjects	Entry Criteria	Duration (Weeks)	CD4+ T-Lymphocyte Count[b]	HIV RNA[c]	
							Condition 1	Condition 2
GS-97-901	Randomized, double-blind, placebo-controlled		59	CD4 +> 200 cells/mm^3; HIV RNA > 10 000 copies/mL; ART-naive and experienced	4	Baseline: 356; NA[d]	Naive	Experienced,
		75					75 mg: −0.45 log	75 mg: −0.27 log
		150					150 mg: −0.6 log	150 mg: −0.49 log
		300					300 mg: −1.57 log	300 mg: −1.06 log
		600					600 mg: −1.40 log	600 mg: −0.66 log
GS-98-902	Randomized, double-blind, placebo-controlled	189		HIV RNA 400–100 000 copies/mL; TDF added to stable existing regimen	48	Baseline: 374; NS[d]	Week 24 Placebo: −0.1 log	Week 48 Placebo/300 mg: −0.6 log
		75					75 mg: −0.4 log	75 mg: −0.4 log
		150					150 mg: −0.4 log	150 mg: −0.6 log
		300					300 mg: −0.7 log	300 mg: −0.6 log
GS-99-903	Randomized double-blind, placebo-controlled 3TC/EFV+either d4T or TDF	300	600	HIV RNA>5000 copies/mL ART-naive	48	Baseline: 279 Week 48 TDF + 169 d4T + 167	Week 48 <400 copies/mL (ITT) d4T 87% TDF 87%	
GS-00-907	Randomized, double-blind placebo-controlled	300	552	HIV RNA 400–100 000 copies/mL; TDF added to stable existing regimen	48	Baseline: 427 Week 24 Placebo: −10.6		Baseline: 3.36 log Week 24 Placebo: −0.01 log
						300 mg: +12.6		300 mg: −0.61 log Week 48 Placebo to TDF Crossover: −0.70 log TDF: −0.56 log

ART, antiretroviral therapy; NA, not available; NS, no significant difference between placebo and treatment group; TDF, tenofovir disoproxil fumarate; 3TC, lamivudine; EFV, efavirenz, d4T, stavudine; ITT, intent to treat.

[a]Data from Barditch-Crovo P, Deeks S, Collier A, et al. Phase I/II trial of the pharmacokinetics, safety, and antiretroviral activity of tenofovir disoproxil fumarate in human immunodeficiency virus-infected adults. Antimicrob Agents Chemother 45:2773, 2001; Schooley R, Ruane P, Myers R, et al. Tenofovir DF in antiretroviral-experienced patients: results from a 48-week, randomized, double-blind study. AIDS 16:1257, 2002; Squires K, Pozniak A, Pierone G, et al. Tenofovir disoproxil fumarate in nucleoside-resistant HIV-1 infection: a randomized trial. Ann Intern Med 139:313, 2003; and Gallant J, Staszewski S, Pozniak A, et al. Efficacy and safety of tenofovir DF vs stavudine in combination therapy in antiretroviral-naïve patients. A 3-year randomized trial. JAMA 292:191, 2004.
[b]Mean change in absolute CD4+ T-lymphocyte count (cells/mm^3) from baseline.
[c]Mean change in plasma HIV RNA level from baseline ($\log_{10}$ copies/mL).
[d]Clinical trial was not powered to assess changes in CD4+ T-lymphocyte counts.

tolerability, but was associated with an unacceptably high rate of virologic failure based on preliminary data from two clinical trials which were subsequently discontinued.[33,34] Similarly, a 24-week pilot study evaluating the efficacy of once-daily didanosine EC (250 mg), lamivudine (300 mg), and tenofovir DF (300 mg) in antiretroviral-naive HIV-infected individuals demonstrated suboptimal virologic responses. At week 12, only one participant demonstrated an optimal response (defined as = 2 log reduction in plasma HIV-1 RNA level); the median change from baseline plasma HIV-1 RNA level was −0.61 log.[35] The reason for the poor performance of these regimens appears to be due to the early development of resistance, particularly the presence of the K65R and M184V mutations.[33]

In an effort to assess the efficacy of a once-daily regimen, an open-label, prospective, randomized, noninferiority study was performed in 517 HIV-1-infected, antiretroviral-naive patients comparing once-daily tenofovir DF (300 mg), emtricitabine (200 mg), and efavirenz (600 mg) to a fixed dose of zidovudine (300 mg) and lamivudine (150 mg) twice daily (Combivir) and efavirenz (600 mg) daily. Through week 48, significantly more patients in the tenofovir–emtricitabine group reached and maintained the primary end point (plasma HIV RNA of <400 copies/mL) than did those in the zidovudine–lamivudine group (84% vs 73%).[36] Significant differences were also seen in the proportion of patients with plasma HIV RNA levels <50 copies/mL (80% in the tenofovir–emtricitabine group vs 70% in the zidovudine–lamivudine group) and in increases in absolute CD4+ T-lymphocyte counts (190 vs 158 cells/mm^3, respectively).[36]

Chronic Hepatitis B Therapy in the Setting of HIV Infection

As stated previously, tenofovir DF has demonstrated *in vitro* activity against hepatitis B virus (HBV) as well as HIV. The anti-HBV efficacy of tenofovir DF in HIV co-infected individuals has been reported in several small studies with short durations of therapy, including patients with known lamivudine-associated HBV mutations.[37–39] In a retrospective analysis, 65 HIV/HBV co-infected patients who had received tenofovir DF 300 mg daily for at least 6 months as a component of antiretroviral therapy were evaluated for HBV efficacy. At baseline, 83% of the patients were hepatitis e antigen positive and 69% had documented lamivudine resistance. At 12 months, the median reduction of serum HBV DNA from baseline was 4.56 log and 2.53 log in hepatitis e antigen-positive and -negative patients, respectively, and the percentage of patients with undetectable serum HBV DNA was 30% and 82%, respectively. Four patients' serum hepatitis e antigen became negative and two of these individuals acquired serum hepatitis e antibodies.[40]

Vaginal Microbicide

Tenofovir has been formulated as a topical vaginal gel and is currently being evaluated in clinical trials as a self-adminstered mechanism to prevent HIV infection in women. A phase I study in HIV-infected and -uninfected women has demonstrated that 1% tenofovir gel is safe and well-tolerated when applied twice daily.[41] Expanded safety and effectiveness analyses, including the possibility of systemic absorption, of this product are currently being evaluated in a phase IIb clinical trial in HIV-uninfected, sexually active women.

RESISTANCE

The presence and frequency of genotypic mutations related to tenofovir DF exposure has been examined *in vitro*, and information regarding drug-resistant clinical isolates is accumulating. In the presence of tenofovir or adefovir, a K65R mutation in HIV RT has been detected during *in vitro* HIV passage experiments.[42,43] This single amino acid substitution, shown previously to be selected *in vitro* in the presence of zalcitabine, results in a three- to fourfold increase and a 12- to 15-fold increase in the IC_{50} values for tenofovir and adefovir, respectively, compared to wild-type virus.[44,45] Tenofovir exposure resulted in additional HIV RT mutations in these *in vitro* HIV passage experiments including L228R, W25R, and P272S mutations. The K70E RT mutation has been linked to adefovir exposure.

Recombinant viruses carrying the T69D RT mutation demonstrated a threefold increased IC_{50} for tenofovir compared to wild-type virus; in contrast, recombinant viruses expressing alternative RT mutations associated with multi-nucleoside drug resistance (Q151M, A62V, V75I, F77L, F116Y) showed wild-type susceptibility to tenofovir, but reduced susceptibility to zidovudine (38-fold).[44] In addition, recombinant viruses expressing both the M184V (associated with lamivudine resistance) and T215Y (associated with zidovudine resistance) mutations displayed increased susceptibility to tenofovir compared to wild-type virus.[44] In summary, *in vitro* studies suggest tenofovir may be active against HIV strains expressing one or more of the common nucleoside RT mutations. A possible explanation for these findings is tenofovir may be less efficiently removed through pyrophosphorolysis and dinucleotide synthesis in HIV strains possessing these RT mutations.[46]

In a randomized, double-blind, placebo-controlled phase II study (GS-98-902), tenofovir DF was added to background therapy in antiretroviral-experienced HIV-infected individuals (*see section on* Efficacy). In 159 participants, baseline and postbaseline (week 24, week 48, or early termination) genotypic evaluations were performed and the development of one or more new RT mutations was noted in ~40% of the study population receiving tenofovir DF at 48 weeks, but these mutations were consistent with the patient's background antiretroviral therapy and were not associated with loss of plasma HIV RNA suppression.[32] The K65R RT mutation, associated with tenofovir *in vitro*, developed in only four (2%) patients and was not linked to increasing plasma HIV RNA levels.[32] Baseline and postbaseline phenotypic analyses were performed in those subjects randomized to receive tenofovir DF 300 mg once daily (n = 54). At baseline, phenotypes revealed a mean reduced susceptibility of 1.9- and 13.8-fold over wild-type for tenofovir disoproxil fumarate and zidovidine, respectively. In regression analyses, plasma HIV RNA suppression was significantly correlated with baseline susceptibility to tenofovir disproxil fumarate ($P = 0.007$) and zidovudine ($P = 0.035$), but not to other nucleoside agents.[32] At week 48, ~50% of evaluable patients demonstrated increased susceptibility to tenofovir DF and the remaining half displayed reduced susceptibility (2.7- to 4.3-fold) to the drug. Individuals developing the K65R RT mutation ($n = 4$) showed three- to fourfold reduction in susceptibility to tenofovir DF consistent with prior *in vitro* studies.[32] As was noted in the genotypic analysis, low-level reduced susceptibility to tenofovir DF was not associated with loss of HIV RNA suppression at 48 weeks.

In a separate randomized, double-blind phase III intensification study (GS-00-907), a more detailed genotypic and phenotypic analysis was performed on a larger subset of patients. In addition to stable background antiretroviral therapy, HIV-infected patients received tenofovir DF 300 mg once daily or placebo for 24 weeks, followed by 24 weeks of open-label tenofovir DF 300 mg once daily for all patients (*see section on* Efficacy). Fifty percent ($n = 274$) and 25% ($n = 137$) of the study population were randomly assigned to the genotyping and phenotyping substudies, respectively. In participants with baseline and week 48 genotypic data, the development of mutations associated with tenofovir DF therapy occurred infrequently (3%); specifically, eight patients developed the K65R mutation, but loss of plasma HIV RNA suppression was only noted in three of these patients during the 48 week study period.[47] Moreover, only low-level reduced (less than twofold) tenofovir DF phenotypic susceptibility was associated with the presence of the K65R mutation in the majority of these patients with only one participant demonstrating greater than threefold reduced susceptibility to the drug.[47] Through week 48, the development of M41L or L210W mutations as part of at least three thymidine analog-associated mutations (TAMs) was equally common in participants receiving tenofovir DF and placebo suggesting the background antiretroviral therapy may have been responsible for the presence of these mutations.[47] In summary, the development of phenotypic or genotypic resistance to tenofovir DF was uncommon in this study of antiretroviral-experienced patients and loss of plasma HIV RNA suppression was not linked to reduced susceptibility or mutations associated with tenofovir DF therapy.

The development of resistance mutations was also investigated in a randomized, double-blinded, placebo-controlled phase III study (GS-99-903) of 600 antiretroviral subjects randomized to efavirenz and lamivudine with either stavudine (40 mg twice daily)/tenofovir DF placebo or tenofovir DF (300 mg once daily)/stavudine placebo (*see section on* Efficacy). At week 48, the K65R mutation developed in seven patients receiving tenofovir DF compared to two stavudine recipients. At week 96, only 2.7% of tenofovir DF recipients and 0.6% of stavudine recipients developed the K65R mutation and this trend was not statistically significant.[48] Of note, efavirenz resistance mutations (K103, others) preceded or accompanied the development of a K65R mutation in all cases, either with or without the M184V mutation. Among HIV-1 isolates from tenofovir DF-treated patients with a K65R mutation ($n = 8$), there were only low-level changes in tenofovir susceptibility *in vitro* (mean 1.2-fold), increased susceptibility to zidovudine (mean 0.5-fold), and no change in susceptibility to stavudine.[48]

To date, prior adefovir dipivoxil exposure has not resulted in documented reduced susceptibility to tenofovir DF.[49] In an open-label pilot study of chronic HBV infection treatment in HIV-infected patients, adefovir dipivoxil 10 mg once daily was added to existing lamividune therapy to assess for safety, efficacy, and the development of RT mutations. Despite uncontrolled HIV-1 replication in many of the subjects ($n = 35$, mean plasma HIV level 2.88 $\log_{10}$ copies/mL), no adefovir dipivoxil associated RT mutations (specifically, K65R or K70E) were observed at baseline or throughout the 48-week study period.[50] This study is limited by a relatively small study population, but the results are noteworthy given the adefovir dipivoxil dosing for chronic HBV infection is significantly lower than the dosing previously utilized in HIV clinical trials (120-250 mg daily).

DRUG INTERACTIONS

In studies designed to assess pharmacologic interactions following co-administration of tenofovir DF with lamivudine, indinavir, lopinavir/ritonavir, nelfinavir mesylate, ritonavir-boosted saquinavir mesylate, nevirapine, or efavirenz, no clinically relevant drug-drug interactions were noted. Tenofovir steady-state exposure i.e., AUC was found to be equivalent when co-administered with these agents.[51–54] Similarly, tenofovir DF co-administration with rifampin, ribavirin, and methadone does not result in significant alteration in pharmacokinetic parameters.[55–57]

Conversely, tenofovir DF co-administration with didanosine (enteric-coated capsule formulation) resulted in didanosine AUC increases of 48 and 60% in the unfed and fed state, respectively.[58] The provision of a reduced didanosine dose of 250 mg with simulataneous tenofovir DF 300 mg administration in the fasted and fed state resulted in didanosine AUCs similar to that of the reference treatment of 400 mg alone in the fasted state.[58] These data indicate that a dose reduction of didanosine is warranted when it is utilized with tenofovir DF.

A drug interaction study has also been conducted evaluating the combination of tenofovir DF (300 mg daily) with ritonavir-boosted atazanavir (ritonavir 100 mg daily, atazanavir 300 mg daily) in 10 HIV-infected volunteers. The AUC for atazanavir (300 mg daily) decreased 25% when administered with ritonavir and tenofovir DF, but the trend did not reach statistical significance.[59] Based on these data, atazanavir should not be co-administered with tenofovir DF in the absence of ritonavir boosting.

Tenofovir DF when combined with lamivudine and abacavir was an antiretroviral regimen which demonstrated poor efficacy in clinical trials.[33,34] Studies evaluating this combination of RT inhibitors for possible drug-drug interactions have been unrevealing.[60] Specifically, co-administration of abacavir and tenofovir DF in the presence or absence of lamivudine was not limited by unfavorable pharmacokinetic parameters or antagonist anti-HIV activity in *in vitro* analyses.[60] It has been proposed that the tenofovir–abacavir combination leads to the rapid emergence of K65R mutation leading to loss of antiviral response. Despite the lack of understanding of the specific mechanism leading to the previously noted poor response in clinical trials, the co-administration of tenofovir DF and abacavir should be avoided.

Tenofovir DF is primarily eliminated through renal excretion, and dosing adjustments are recommended for individuals with a baseline creatinine clearance <50 mL/min. Specifically, individuals with a creatinine clearance of 30-49 mL/min should receive tenofovir DF 300 mg every 48 h while those patients with a creatinine clearance of 10-29 mL/min should receive 300 mg twice weekly. In patients receiving hemodialysis, tenofovir DF is dosed once weekly after completion of dialysis.[61] Clinicians should monitor the prescription of concomitant drugs with overlapping toxicities and agents that may reduce renal function. The pharmacologic profile of tenofovir DF is not significantly altered in patients with moderate or severe hepatic impairment and no dose adjustments are currently recommended in the setting of hepatic insufficiency.[61]

RECOMMENDATIONS FOR USE

The efficacy of tenofovir DF in combination with other antiretroviral agents demonstrates the drug's utility in both naive and antiretroviral-experienced patients. The favorable pharmacologic profile, safety profile, and the recent availability of fixed-dose combinations (Truvada (tenofivr DF and emtricitabine) and Atripla (tenofovir DF, emtricitabine, and efavirenz)) has made tenofovir DF a popular option for HIV clinicians when prescribing initial antiretroviral therapy in patients, particularly in the setting of co-infection with HBV. In addition, the drug's favorable resistance profile and sustainable anti-HIV activity in patients with documented genotypic resistance to existing NRTI agents makes tenofovir DF an attractive option for treatment-experienced patients as well. Ritonavir boosting is required when tenofovir DF is used with atazanavir and tenofovir DF should generally not be used in combination with abacavir or didanosine, but if used with didanosine a reduced dose of didanosine (250 mg) is required.

CONCLUSIONS

Tebnofovir DF is a nucleotide analog RT inhibitor with proven *in vitro* and *in vivo* efficacy against hepadnaviruses and retroviruses. Of the three nucleotide analogs (cidofovir, adefovir dipivoxil, tenofovir disoproxil fumarate) approved for use in the United States and Europe, only tenofovir DF is approved for the treatment of HIV disease.

Tenofovir has favorable pharmacologic properties allowing for single daily dosing. The oral prodrug, tenofovir disoproxil fumarate provides improved oral bioavailability and further improvement is noted when the agent is administered in the fed state. The compound is eliminated via renal excretion and dosing adjustments are necessary in patients with renal insufficiency (specifically, creatinine clearance <50 mL/min). Co-administration of tenofovir DF and didanosine requires a reduction in the didanosine dose to 250 mg.

At dosing of 300 mg daily, tenofovir DF has anti-HIV activity as documented by suppression of plasma HIV RNA levels in antiretroviral-naive (range, 0.45-1.4 $\log_{10}$) and antiretroviral-experienced patients (range, 0.3-1.1 $\log_{10}$). Sustained antiretroviral activity has been observed up to 144 weeks. In addition, current evidence suggests tenofovir DF is efficacious and safe in the treatment of chronic HBV infection in adults, including both lamivudine-sensitive and lamivudine-resistant HBV strains.

The safety of tenofovir DF has been studied in over 1600 HIV-infected patients in clinical trials and many more patients in routine clinical care, and the drug is generally well tolerated. The preclinical toxicology studies of tenofovir in animals identified the kidney and bone as potential target organs. Interestingly, nephrotoxicity and severe serum hypophosphatemia have not been commonly noted in patients receiving tenofovir DF in clinical trials as was described in individuals receiving the structurally similar compound adefovir dipivoxil, but, with increased utility of tenofovir DF in HIV-infected patients, several small case series of proximal renal tubular dysfunction have now been published. Elevations in serum triglyceride levels, liver transaminases, and creatine kinase were observed in clinical trials, but the percentage of study participants with abnormal values was not significantly different than the frequency of these findings observed in patients receiving placebo. To date, adverse events associated with mitochondrial dysfunction (e.g., lactic acidosis) have been rare and only documented when tenofovir DF was co-administered with stavudine or didanosine. In patients with chronic HBV infection (including HIV and HBV co-infected persons), proximal renal tubular dysfunction has not been observed with lower dose adefovir dipivoxil administration.

In vitro genotypic analysis has demonstrated tenofovir DF maintains activity against most nucleoside-resistant HIV strains, but may select for a K65 HIV RT mutation resulting in three- to fourfold reduction in tenofovir susceptibility. To date, prior adefovir dipivoxil exposure has not resulted in documented reduced susceptibility to tenofovir DF.

REFERENCES

1. Naesens I, Snocek R, Andrei G, et al. HPMC (cidofovir), PMEA (adefovir), and related acyclic nucleoside phosphonate analogues: a review of their pharmacology and clinical potential in the treatment of viral infections. Antivir Chem Chemother 8:1, 1997.
2. Balzarini J, DeClerq E. 5-Phosphoribosyl 1-pyrophosphate synthetase converts the acyclic nucleoside phosphonates

9-(3-hydroxy-2-phosphonylmethoxypropyl)adenine and 9-(2-phosphonylmethoxyethyl)adenine directly to their antivirally active diphosphate derivatives. J Biol Chem 266:8686, 1991.
3. De Clerq E, Sakium T, Baba M, et al. Antiviral activity of phosphonomethoxyalkyl derivatives of purines and pyrimidines. Antiviral Res 8:261, 1987.
4. Yokota T, Konno K, Shigeta S, et al. Inhibitory effects of acyclic nucleoside phosphonate analogues on hepatitis B virus DNA synthesis in HB1611 cells. Antivir Chem Chemother 5:52, 1994.
5. Srinivas R, Robbins B, Connelly M, et al. Metabolism and in vitro antiretroviral activities of bis(pivaloyloxymethyl) prodrugs of acyclic nucleoside phosphonates. Antimicrob Agents Chemother 37:2247, 1993.
6. De Clerq E. Acyclic nucleoside phosphonates in the chemotherapy of DNA virus and retrovirus infections. Intervirology 40:295, 1997.
7. Hartmann K, Balzarini J, Higgins J, et al. In vitro activity of acyclic nucleoside phosphonate derivatives against feline immunodeficiency virus in Crandall feline kidney cells and feline peripheral blood lymphocytes. Antivir Chem Chemother 5:13, 1994.
8. Thormar H, Balzarini J, HolyA, et al. Inhibition of visna virus replication by 2', 3' -dideoxynucleosides and acyclic nucleoside phosphonate analogs. Antimicrob Agents Chemother 37:2540, 1993.
9. Haesens L, Balzarini J, Rosenberg I, et al. 9-(2-Phosphonylmethoxyethyl)-2,6-diaminopurine (PMEDAP): a novel agent with anti-human immunodeficiency virus activity in vitro and potent anti-Moloney murine sarcoma virus activity in vivo. Eur J Clin Microbiol 8:1043, 1989.
10. Palmer S, Margot N, Gilbert H, et al. Tenofovir, adefovir, and zidovudine susceptibilities of primary human immunodeficiency virus type 1 isolates with non-B subtypes or nucleoside resistance. AIDS Res Hum Retroviruses 17:1167, 2001.
11. Balzarini J, Perno C, Schols D, et al. Activity of acyclic nucleoside phosphonate analogues against human immunodeficiency virus in monocytes/macrophages and peripheral blood lymphocytes. Biochem Biophys Res Commun 178:329, 1991.
12. Cherrington J, Allen S, Bischofberger N, et al. Kinetic interaction of the diphosphates of 9-(2-phosphonylmethoxyethyl)aden ine and other anti-HIV active pure congeners with HIV reverse transcriptase and human DNA polymerase α, β, and γ. Antivir Chem Chemother 6:217, 1995.
13. Robbins B, Srinivas R, Kim C, et al. Anti-human immunodeficiency virus activity and cellular metabolism of a potential prodrug of the acyclic nucleoside phosphonate 9-R-(2-phosphonomethoxypropyl)adenine (PMPA), bis(isopropyloxymethylcarbonyl)PMPA. Antimicrob Agent Chemother 42:612, 1998.
14. Louie M, Hogan C, Hurley A, et al. Determining the relative efficacy of tenofovir diosproxil fumarate in treatment-naive chronically infected HIV-1-infected individuals. AIDS 17:1151, 2003.
15. Mulato M, Cherrington J. Anti-HIV activity of adefovir (PMEA) and PMPA in combination with other antiretroviral compounds: in vitro analyses. Antiviral Res 36:91, 1997.
16. Cherrington J, Mulato A. Adefovir (PMEA) and PMPA show synergistic or additive inhibition of HIV replication in vitro in combination with other anti-HIV agents. In: Abstracts of the 12th World AIDS Conference, Geneva, 1998, abstract 4115.
17. Kearney B, Flaherty J, Shah J. Tenofovir disoproxil fumarate: clinical pharmacology and pharmacokinetics. Clin Pharmacokinet 43:595, 2004.
18. Deeks S, Barditch-Crovo P, Lietman P, et al. Safety, pharmacokinetics, and antiretroviral activity of intravenous 9-[2-(R)-(phosphonomethoxy)propyl]adenine, a novel anti-human immunodeficiency virus (HIV) therapy, in HIV-infected adults. Antimicrob Agent Chemother 42: 2380, 1998.
19. Barditch-Crovo P, Deeks S, Collier A, et al. Phase I/II trial of the pharmacokinetics, safety, and antiretroviral activity of tenofovir disoproxil fumarate in human immunodeficiency virus-infected adults. Antimicrob Agents Chemother 45:2773, 2001.
20. Hazra R, Balis F, Tullio A, et al. Single-dose and steady-state pharmacokinetics of tenofovir disoproxil fumarate in human immunodeficiency virus-infected children. Antimicrob Agent Chemother 48:124, 2004.
21. Viread (tenofovir disoproxil fumarate) prescribing information. Gilead Sciences Inc, Forest City, California, Oct 2006.
22. Schooley R, Ruane P, Myers R, et al. Tenofovir DF in antiretroviral-experienced patients: results from a 48-week, randomized, double-blind study. AIDS 16:1257, 2002.
23. Squires K, Pozniak A, Pierone G, et al. Tenofovir disoproxil fumarate in nucleoside-resistant HIV-1 infection: a randomized trial. Ann Intern Med 139:313, 2003.
24. Izzedine H, Isnard-Bagnis C, Hulot J, et al. Renal safety of tenofovir in HIV treatment-experienced patients. AIDS 18:1074, 2004.
25. Karras A, Lafaurie M, Furco A, et al. Tenofovir-related nephrotoxicity in human immunodeficiency virus-infected patients: three cases of renal failure, Fanconi syndrome, and nephrogenic diabetes insipidus. Clin Infect Dis 36:1070, 2003.
26. Peyriere H, Reynes J, Rouanet I, et al. Renal tubular dysfunction associated with tenofovir therapy: report of 7 cases. J Acquir Immune Defic Syndr 35:269, 2004.
27. Izzedine H, Hulot J, Vittecoq D, et al. Long-term safety of tenofovir disoproxil fumarate in antitretroviral-naive HIV-1-infected patients. Data from a double-blind randomized active-controlled multicentre study. Nephrol Dial Transplant 20:743, 2005.
28. Gallant J, Staszewski S, Pozniak A, et al. Efficacy and safety of tenofovir DF vs stavudine in combination therapy in antiretroviral-naive patients. A 3-year randomized trial. JAMA 292:191, 2004.
29. Murphy M, O'Hearn M, Chou S. Fatal lactic acidosis and acute renal failure after addition of tenofovir to an antiretroviral regimen containing didanosine. Clin Infect Dis 36:1082, 2003.
30. Guo Y, Fung HB. Fatal lactic acidosis with coadminstration of didanosine and tenofovir disoproxil fumarate. Pharmacotherapy 24:1089, 2004.
31. Birkus G, Hitchcock M, Cihlar T. Assessment of mitochondrial toxicity in human cells treated with tenofovir: comparison with other nucleoside analog transcriptase inhibitors. Antimicrob Agent Chemother 46:716, 2002.
32. Margot N, Isaacson E, McGowan I, et al. Genotypic and phenotypic analyses of HIV-1 in antiretroviral-experienced patients treated with tenofovir DF. AIDS 16:1227, 2002.
33. Gallant J, Rodriguez A, Weinberg W, et al. Early virologic nonresponse to tenofovir, abacavir, and lamivudine in HIV-infected antiretroviral naive subjects. J Infect Dis 192:1921, 2005.
34. Khanlou H, Yeh V, Guyer B, Farthing C. Early virologic failure in a pilot study evaluating the efficacy of therapy containing once-daily abacavir, lamivudine, and tenofovir DF in treatment-naive HIV-infected patients. AIDS Patient Care STDS 19:135, 2005.
35. Jemsek J, Hutcherson P, Harper E. Poor virologic responses and early emergence of resistance in treatment of naive, HIV-infected patients receiving a once daily triple nucleoside regimen of didanosine, lamivudine, and tenofovir DF. In: Program and Abstracts of the 11th Conference on Retroviruses and Opportunistic Infections, Boston, 2004, abstract 51.
36. Gallant J, DeJesus E, Arribas J, et al. Tenofovir DF, emtricitabine, and efavirenz vs zidovudine, lamivudine, and efavirenz for HIV. N Engl J Med 354:251, 2006.
37. Ristig M, Crippin J, Aberg J, et al. Tenofovir disoproxil fumarate therapy for chronic hepatitis B in human immunodeficiency/hepatitis B virus-coinfected individuals for whom

interferon-alpha and lamivudine therapy have failed. J Infect Dis 186:1844, 2002.
38. Benhamou Y, Tubiana R, and Thibault V. Tenofovir disoproxil fumarate in patients with HIV and lamivudine-resistant hepatitis B. N Engl J Med 348:177, 2003.
39. Bani-Sadr F, Palmer P, Scieux C, Molina J. Ninety-six week efficacy of combination therapy with lamivudine and tenofovir in patients coinfected with HIV-1 and wild-type hepatitis B virus. Clin Infect Dis 39:1062, 2004.
40. Benhamou Y, Fleury H, Trimoulet P, et al. Anti-hepatitis B virus efficacy of tenofovir disoproxil fumarate in HIV-infected patients. Hepatology 43:548, 2006.
41. Mayer K, Mazlankowski L, Gai F, et al. Safety and tolerability of tenofovir vaginal gel in abstinent and sexually active women HIV-infected and uninfected women. AIDS 20:543, 2006.
42. Gu Z, Gao I, Fang H, et al. Identification of a mutation at codon 65 in the JKKK motif of reverse transcriptase that encodes resistance to 2′,3′-dideoxycitidine and 2′ ,3′-dideoxythiacytidine. Antimicrob Agent Chemother 38:275, 1994.
43. Gu Z, Salomon H, Cherrington J, et al. K65R mutation of human immunodeficiency virus type 1 reverse transcriptase encodes cross-resistance to 9-(2-phosphonylmethoxyethyl)adenine. Antimicrob Agent Chemother 39:1888, 1995.
44. Wainberg M, Miller M, Quan Y, et al. In vitro selection and characterization of HIV-1 with reduced susceptibility to PMPA. Antivir Ther 4:87, 1999.
45. Foli A, Sogocio K, Anderson B, et al. In vitro selection and molecular characterization of human immunodeficiency virus type 1 with reduced sensitivity to 9-[2-(phosphonomethoxy)ethyl]adenine (PMEA). Antiviral Res 32:91, 1996.
46. Naeger L, Margot N, Miller M. ATP-dependent removal of nucleoside reverse transcriptase inhibitors by human immunodefieciency virus type 1 reverse transcriptase. Antimicrob Agent Chemother 46:2179, 2002.
47. Miller M, Margot N, Lu B, et al. Genotypic and phenotypic predictors of the magnitude of response to tenofovir disoproxil fumaratetreatment in antiretroviral-experienced patients. J Infect Dis 189:837, 2004.
48. Margot N, Lu B, Cheng A, et al. Resistance development over 144 weeks in treatment-naive patients receiving tenofovir disoproxil fumarate or stavudine with lamivudine and efavirenz in study 903. HIV Med 7:442, 2006.
49. Miller M, Margot N, Lamy P, et al. Adefovir and tenofovir susceptibilities of HIV-1 after 24-48 weeks of adefovir dipivoxil therapy: genotypic and phenotypic analyses of study GS-96-408. J Acquir Immune Defic Syndr 27:450, 2001.
50. Delaugerre C, Marcelin A, Thibault V, et al. Human immunodeficiency (HIV) type 1 reverse transcriptase resistance mutations in hepatitis B virus (HBV)-HIV-coinfected patients treated for chronic HBV infection once daily with 10 milligrams of adefovir dipivoxil combined with lamivudine. Antimicrob Agent Chemother 46:1586, 2002.
51. Kearney B, Flaherty J, Wolf J, et al. Lack of clinically relevant drug-drug interactions between tenofovir DF and efavirenz, indinavir, lamivudine and lopinavir/ritonavir in healthy subjects. In: Abstracts of the 8th European Conference on Clinical Aspects and Treatment of HIV Infection, Athens, Greece, 2001, abstract 171.
52. Droste J, Kearney B, Hekster Y, Burger D. Assessment of drug–drug interactions between tenofovir disoproxil fumarate and the nonnucleoside reverse transcriptase inhibitors nevirapine and efavirenz in HIV-infected patients. J Acquir Immune Defic Syndr 41:37, 2006.
53. Chittick G, Zong J, Blum M, et al. Pharmacokinetics of tenofovir disoproxil fumarate and ritonavir-boosted saquinavir mesylate administered alone or in combination at steady state. Antimicrob Agents Chemother 50:1034, 2006.
54. Boffito M, Pozniak A, Kearney B, et al. Lack of pharmacokinetic drug interaction between tenofovir disoproxil fumarate and nelfinavir mesylate. Antimicrob Agents Chemother 49:4386, 2005.
55. Droste J, Verwejj-van Wissen C, Kearney B, et al. Pharmacokinetic study of tenofovir disoproxil fumarate combined with rifampin in healthy volunteers. Antimicrob Agents Chemother 49:680, 2005.
56. Smith P, Kearney B, Liaw S, et al. Effect of tenofovir disoproxil fumarate on the pharmacokinetics and pharmacodynamics of total, R-, and S-methadone. Pharmacotherapy 24:970, 2004.
57. Ramanathan S, Cheng A, Mittan A, et al. Absence of clinically relevant pharmacokinetic interaction between ribavirin and tenofovir in healthy subjects. J Clin Pharmacol 46:559, 2006.
58. Kearney B, Sayre J, Flaherty J, et al. Drug–drug and drug–food interactions between tenofovir disoproxil fumarate and didanosine. J Clin Pharmacol 45:1360, 2005.
59. Taburet A, Piketty C, Chazallon C, et al. Interactions between atazanavir-ritonavir and tenofovir in heavily pretreated human immunodeficiency virus-infected patients. Antimicrob Agents Chemother 28:2091, 2004.
60. Ray A, Myrick F, Vela J, et al. Lack of metabolic and antiviral drug interaction between tenofovir, abacavir, and lamivudine. Antivir Ther 10:451, 2005.
61. Kearney B, Yale K, Shah J, et al. Pharmacokinetics and dosing recommendations of tenofovir disoproxil fumarate in hepatic or renal impairment. Clin Pharmacokinet 45:1115, 2006.

Chapter 23

Enfuvirtide

J. Michael Kilby, MD

Prior to the accelerated FDA approval in 2003 of the membrane fusion inhibitor, enfuvirtide (ENF), all available antiretroviral agents were directed against one of two HIV-specific enzymes, reverse transcriptase (RT) or protease. Thus, ENF represented the first clinical agent from a novel therapeutic class in nearly eight years. The advent of an entirely distinct therapeutic class, the viral entry inhibitors, suggested the possibility of avoiding cross-resistance and shared toxicities with previous drugs, and therefore improved prospects for individuals with extensive prior treatment histories. ENF also represented the most complex synthetic peptide ever developed for large scale chemical manufacturing and the first antiretroviral agent licensed solely for administration by the parenteral route, and therefore introduced new challenges in regard to mass production, convenience and adherence, adverse event profiles and the costs of HIV care.

MECHANISM OF ACTION AND STRUCTURE

The process of HIV entry into target cells is complex, involving multiple steps; other viral entry inhibitor candidates in development are discussed in detail elsewhere in this book (Chapters 24 and 27). Briefly summarized, HIV entry into target cells begins with binding of the viral surface glycoprotein (gp120) to the CD4 molecule expressed on host target cells, particularly T helper lymphocytes. The initial interaction between the HIV-1 gp120 and CD4 triggers a conformational change in gp120 to expose a "co-receptor" binding site, with an affinity for chemokines that bind either the CKR5 or CXCR4 class of host receptors.[1–3] Following attachment of gp120 sites at both the CD4 and chemokine receptor sites, the viral transmembrane glycoprotein (gp41) undergoes a conformational change that triggers fusion of the viral and cellular membranes. The fusion step allows viral contents to be taken up by the target cell, which ultimately leads to integration into the host nucleus and production of new viral progeny (see Fig. 23-1).

Early studies of the gp41 molecular sequence revealed "heptad repeat" sequences in two regions that give the protein periodic hydrophobicity. These consensus motifs ("leucine zippers") were predictive of an alpha-helical structure within the gp41.[4,5] Synthetic peptides, originally called DP107 and DP178, corresponding to these heptad repeat sequences were found to inhibit HIV infection *in vitro*.[6,7] A series of experiments over the next several years suggested these regions of gp41 form a helical bundle or "coiled coil" structure that is critical for membrane fusion to occur. Mutations in these leucine zipper regions of gp41 were found to disrupt the "coiled coil" structure and thereby interfere with membrane fusion and infectivity. It was proposed that synthetic peptides corresponding to these alpha-helical regions had antiretroviral activity, mediated by disruption of the tertiary protein structure of the protein.[8–12]

A model of gp41 mediated membrane fusion analogous to the "spring-loaded" mechanism described for influenza virus was proposed.[13] When influenza virus first binds to a target cell, hemagglutinin goes through a conformational change, extending from a loop structure to an extended "coiled coil". This allows a "fusion peptide" to shift into a favorable position so that membrane fusion can occur. The corresponding model proposed for HIV gp41 (Fig. 23-1) is that the fusion peptide is in an unexposed position when gp41 is in its native, "nonfusogenic" state. After gp120 binds to a target cell, gp41 changes conformation, unfolding by a molecular hinge mechanism. The fusion peptide is then extended away from the virus surface and therefore better able to insert into the cell membrane. If the gp41 then returns to its native, folded ("hairpin") conformation, the result would be to pull the viral and cell membranes into close proximity in order for fusion and viral entry to occur. Based on this model, the suggested mechanism of action for these synthetic peptides is that they competitively bind to one of the heptad repeat regions when gp41 is in its extended conformation and prevent the structure from folding back onto itself. A 36-amino acid peptide (Fig. 23-2), corresponding to DP178

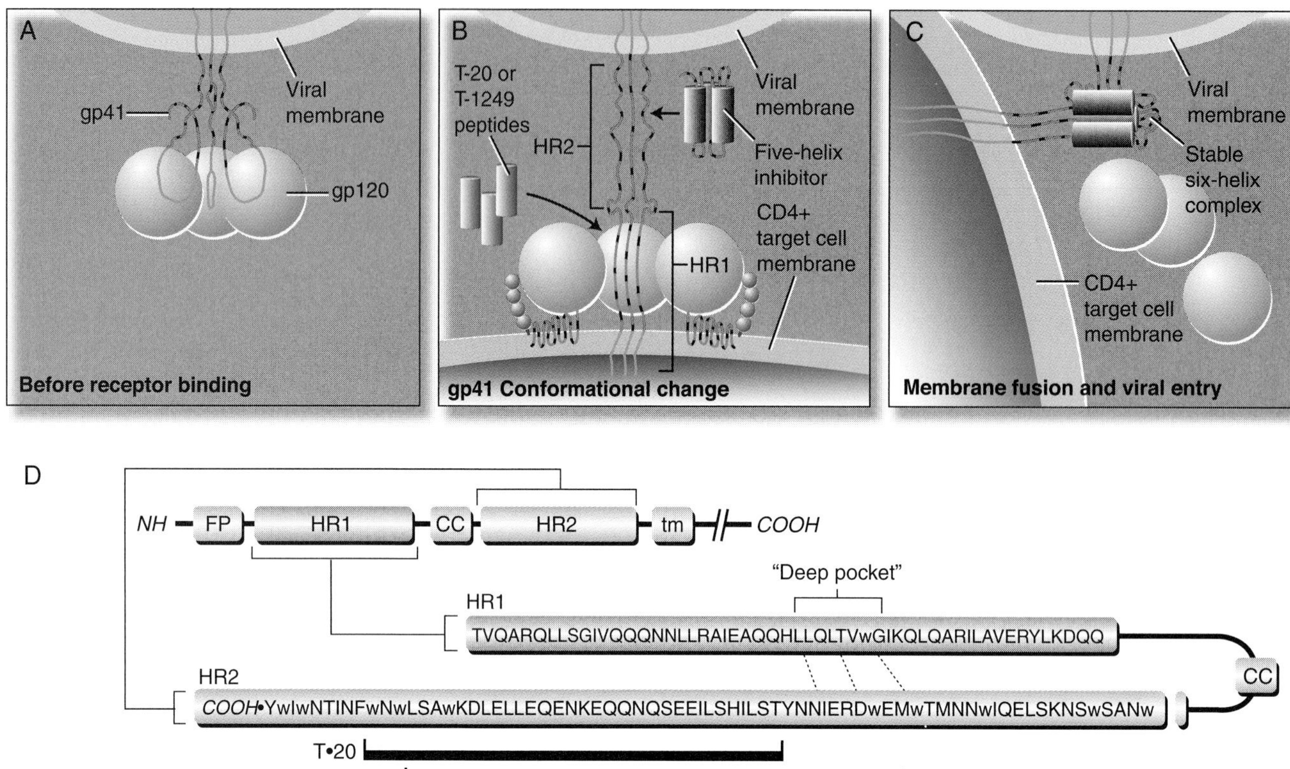

Figure 23-1 ■ Proposed model of the gp41-mediated membrane fusion step, showing sites of action for ENF, T-1249 and other fusion inhibitors in development.

From Kilby JM, Eron JJ. Novel therapies based on mechanisms of HIV-1 cell entry. N Engl J Med 348:2228–38, 2003.

and later renamed T-20, pentafuside and finally marketed as ENF (Fuzeon), was found to be a potent inhibitor of HIV-1 *in vitro*, demonstrating a 50% inhibitory concentration (IC_{50}) of 1.7 ng/mL in T cell lines.[6]

Preclinical Data

Because it is a peptide, ENF would be expected to undergo catabolism into individual amino acids already present in the body. However, detailed studies to determine the exact elimination of the drug are not available. *In vitro* experiments involving human hepatic tissues suggest that ENF initially undergoes hydrolysis to form a deamidated metabolite (abbreviated M3), and indeed this metabolite is detectable in human plasma soon after administration. *In vitro* studies suggest that ENF is not an inhibitor of CYP450 enzymes and does not appear to alter the metabolism of common substrates of CYP3A4, CYP2D6, and related hepatic enzymes. Conversely, drugs such as ritonavir and rifampin do not appear in preliminary studies to alter the pharmokinetic parameters of ENF in a clinically significant manner.[14]

ENF was not mutagenic or disruptive to chromosomes in a series of *in vitro* and animal studies. Long-term carcinogenicity studies have not been conducted. ENF had no effects on male or female fertility in rats at doses higher than the recommended human dose, relative to body surface area.[14]

PHASE I TRIAL

In the first clinical trial of a membrane fusion inhibitor,[15] the ENF peptide was administered intravenously for 14 days to 16 HIV-infected adults. Patients received ENF monotherapy in a dose-escalation protocol, in which four patients each received 3, 10, 30, and finally 100 mg, all IV twice daily. No serious adverse effects were noted during short-term administration. The median half-life of the drug was 1.83 h. The nadir drug concentrations in the highest dose group were substantially higher than the IC_{50} of the drug and the overall pharmacokinetic profile suggested that intermittent or continuous subcutaneous T-20 administration might be feasible.

The viral load results demonstrated significant, dose-related declines in plasma HIV RNA levels during intravenous T-20 treatment. There was a significant decline in plasma HIV RNA when all 16 subjects were considered together (-0.39 $\log_{10}$; $P < 0.05$). The median viral load change in plasma viral load in the 100 mg dose group was -1.96 $\log_{10}$ by day 15 (Fig. 23-3). An analysis of viral dynamics showed that

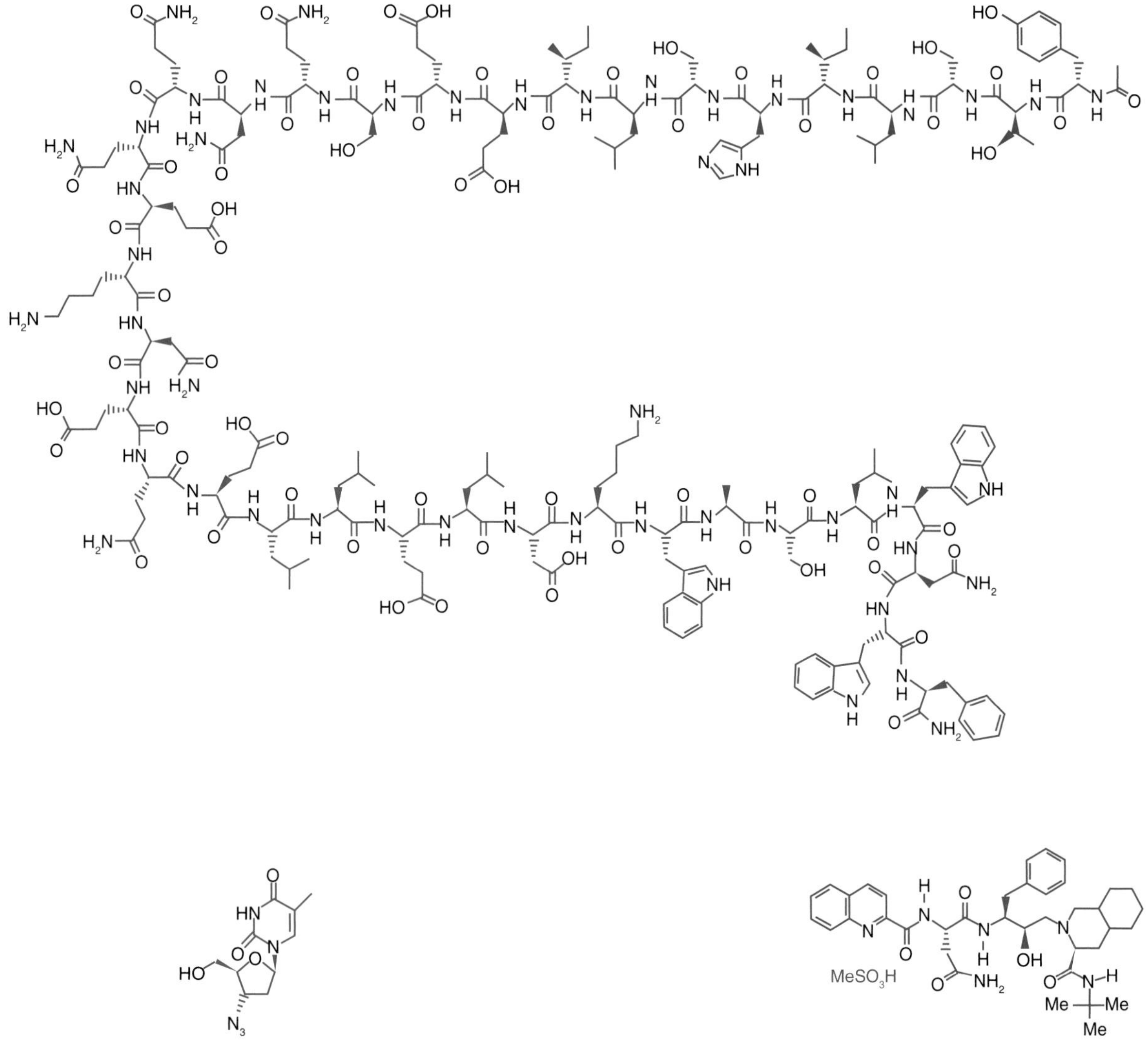

Figure 23-2 ■ Structure of enfuvirtide, a 39 amino acid membrane fusion inhibitor (top), with representative structures of orally bioavailable HIV-1 enzyme inhibitors azidothymidine (bottom left) and saquinavir (bottom right).

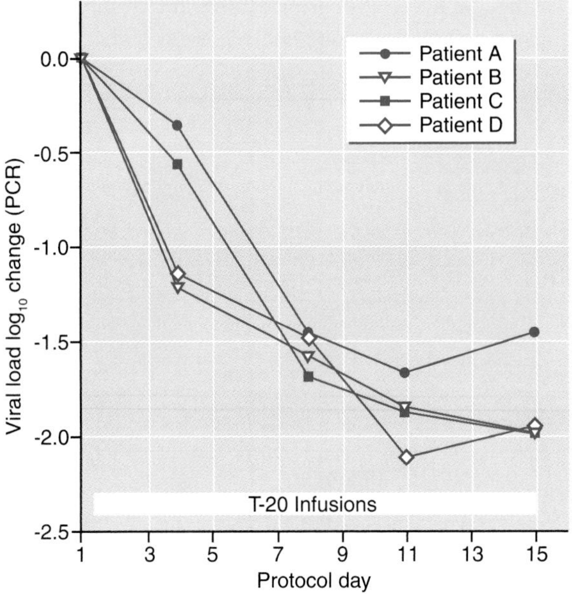

Figure 23-3 ■ Effect of ENF on viral load from phase I clinical trial.

From Kilby JM, Hopkins S, Venetta TM, et al. Potent suppression of HIV-1 replication in humans by T-20, a peptide inhibitor of gp41-medicated virus entry. Nat Med 4:1302, 1998.

the initial slope of virus decline, a measure of antiretroviral potency, was comparable to that achieved with other approved HIV therapies including three and four drug combinations of RT and protease inhibitors (PIs). Thus, these findings provided "proof-of-concept" that therapeutics targeting a viral entry event could result in safe and clinically meaningful inhibition of viral replication.

PHASE II TRIALS

The second clinical trial of ENF (TRI-003) involved 78 subjects enrolled at multiple sites around the United States.[16] This 28 day trial allowed patients to add ENF therapy to preexisting oral antiretroviral regimens. This was a dose-ranging study designed to compare continuous subcutaneous infusion (CSI) with intermittent subcutaneous injections of ENF, using escalating dose groups for each approach, in order to explore routes of administration more practical for the outpatient setting. Patients were eligible for the study if they had viral loads of >5000 copies/mL and were either on no other therapy or had not changed their antiretroviral regimen over the previous 6 weeks. Most subjects had advanced disease and extensive prior treatment histories with clinical resistance to many or all available RT and PIs, and thus the study was essentially measuring virologic responses to T-20 "functional monotherapy" in many cases.

The CSI administration route proved problematic. The continuous infusion "insulin pump" devices frequently alarmed, suggesting that efficient flow was not achieved, and inferior trough drug concentrations in all CSI groups confirmed this. More subjects also experienced local injection site reactions (see adverse effects, below) in this group than the intermittent injection group. The concerns about the CSI administration route were partially alleviated by the pharmacokinetic results in the study, which suggested that continuous subcutaneous or intravenous administration were unnecessary since twice daily subcutaneous injections provided relatively stable drug levels for over 12 h after administration. Over a 28 day administration period, dose-related reductions in plasma HIV RNA levels were demonstrated that confirmed the findings in the phase I trial. The 100 mg CSI group experienced nearly a full order of magnitude (90%) decline, while the 50 mg twice daily and the 100 mg twice daily intermittent therapy groups had greater than 90% declines. The overall trend in the higher dose groups, however, was an initial decline followed by a more gradual return toward baseline viral loads (Fig. 23-4).

Sixty-one of the initial phase II subjects plus ten other subjects who had received prior ENF therapy were later enrolled into a 48-week rollover protocol. This protocol (T20-205) evaluated the long-term effects of administering open-label ENF, at 50 mg every 12 h subcutaneously, in addition to conventional, oral, highly active antiretroviral therapy (HAART) regimens.[17] Investigators were provided with a genotypic analysis of each subject's HIV isolate at baseline to help determine an "optimized background" (OB) HAART regimen for each individual. Overall, a mean viral load decline of 1.33 $\log_{10}$ copies/mL was achieved within 14 days of ENF plus HAART, and this degree of response was maintained through the remainder of the 48-week period ($P < 0.001$ for change from baseline at 48 weeks). The mean gain in absolute CD4 T-lymphocyte count at 48 weeks was 84.9 cells/μL ($P < 0.001$ for change from baseline). Potent responses were seen with comparable frequency regardless of the presence of multidrug resistant isolates, suggesting the possibility of a substantial fusion inhibitor contribution to the durability of response to the multiagent "salvage regimens". Another phase II randomized pilot trial involved 71 patients who were protease-experienced but NNRTI-naive at entry.[18] These subjects were randomized to a salvage antiretroviral regimen (abacavir, amprenavir, low dose ritonavir, and efavirenz) alone versus the same regimen plus one of three doses of subcutaneous ENF (50, 75, or 100 mg twice daily). Although the results were considered preliminary, there was a consistent dose-related trend toward additional virologic and immunologic benefit on ENF plus HAART. The pooled ENF arms achieved a median change of $-2.27 \log_{10}$ compared with $-1.65 \log_{10}$ in the control group. Interestingly, the differential response was greater among subjects with higher viral loads

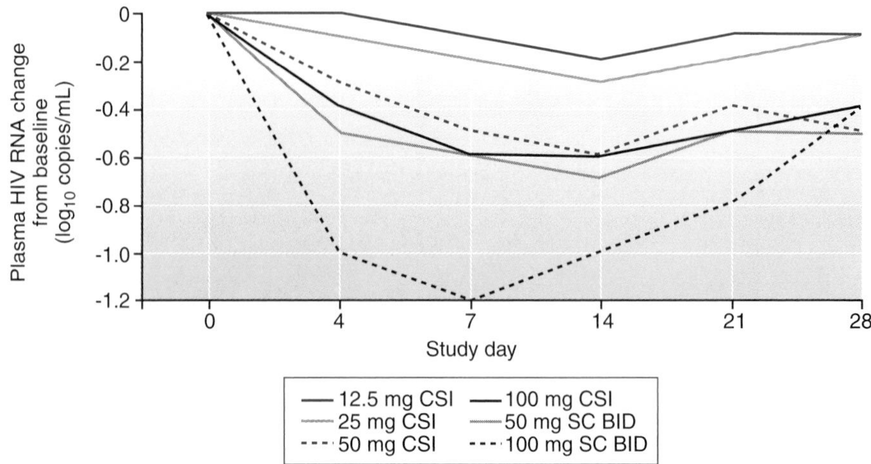

Figure 23-4 ■ Viral load changes observed when subcutaneous ENF was added to preexisting failing regimens in an open-label phase II trial.

From Kilby JM, Lalezan JP, Eron JJ, et al. The safety, plasma pharmacokinetics, and antiviral activity of subcutaneous enfuvirtide (T-20), a peptide inhibitor of gp41-medicated virus fusion, in HIV-infected adults. AIDS Res Hum Retrovirus 18:685, 2002.

(>20 000 copies/mL) at baseline (median viral load change $-2.64 \log_{10}$ vs $-1.55 \log_{10}$). The gain in CD4+ T-lymphocyte counts over 16 weeks was +10 in the control group versus +64 and +74 in the 75 and 100 mg ENF arms, respectively.

PHASE III TRIALS

ENF received accelerated FDA approval based on the results of two large phase III randomized "T-20 Versus Optimized Regimen Only" trials (TORO 1[19] and TORO 2[20]). Both trials evaluated the fusion inhibitor and OB; individualized regimens consisting of 3–5 drugs based on treatment histories, genotypic and phenotypic resistance testing) versus OB alone among patients with prior "triple class" (nucleoside RT inhibitors (NRTIs), nonnucleoside RT inhibitors (NNRTIs), and PIs) treatment experience. The two protocols combined enrolled ~1000 subjects, TORO 1 (or T20-301) at sites in the Americas (US, Canada, Brazil) and TORO 2 (or T20-302) at sites in Europe and Australia. The two trials had nearly identical designs, randomizing treatment-experienced subjects 2:1 to ENF+OB versus OB alone, and the studies had very comparable results. Therefore, their results can reasonably be presented in parallel. The primary objective of these large trials was to determine whether there is an additional decline in viral load at 24 weeks and 48 weeks on ENF therapy beyond that seen with the optimized conventional therapeutic regimens alone.

Subjects were predominantly male (~90% in both trials) and White (83% in TORO 1, 95% in TORO 2), with a median age of 42 years. Median baseline plasma viral loads and absolute CD4+ T-lymphocyte counts were >100 000 (5.1–5.2 $\log_{10}$) copies/mL and 75–100 cells/mm^3, respectively. Most subjects (75–90%) had a prior history of an AIDS-defining event. Only a minority of subjects (~20–25%) had viral isolates susceptible (by genotypic or phenotypic analyses) to three or more drugs in their chosen OB regimens, whereas a comparable proportion demonstrated *in vitro* evidence of resistance to all the OB agents they received. As expected in this context of extensive prior treatment, suboptimal clinical responses were quite common compared with typical protocols of newer agents involving treatment-naive subjects. There were significantly fewer protocol-defined cases of virologic failure between 8 and 24 weeks on the ENF-containing arms (41–48%) than the OB alone arms (63–76%) in both studies; failing subjects were provided access to open label ENF therapy. Thus, the intention-to-treat (ITT) analyses at 24 weeks and beyond likely underestimate advantages of the ENF-containing arms because of this crossover design. Nevertheless, the mean change from baseline viral load at 24 weeks was greater by nearly an order of magnitude in the ENF plus OB arm versus the OB alone arm in both protocols (−1.696 vs −0.764 in TORO 1 and −1.429 vs −0.648 in TORO 2, respectively; both differences $P < 0.001$). Whereas only a minority sustained viral load suppression below 400 copies/mL at 24 weeks overall. This favorable outcome was approximately twice as common in the arms receiving ENF plus OB versus OB alone (31.7% vs 16.4%, respectively, in TORO 1odds ratio = 3.17, $P < 0.001$); 28.4% vs 13.6%, respectively, in TORO 2 (odds ratio = 2.74; $P < 0.001$)). The time to protocol-defined failure also significantly favored the ENF arms in both studies (Fig. 23-5). Changes in absolute CD4+ T-lymphocyte counts were significantly greater for subjects receiving ENF plus OB versus OB alone in both studies (+76 vs +32 cells/mm^3, respectively, in TORO 1; +65 vs +38 cells/mm^3, respectively, in TORO 2; $P < 0.02$ for both differences). In longer term follow-up of TORO-1 and TORO-2

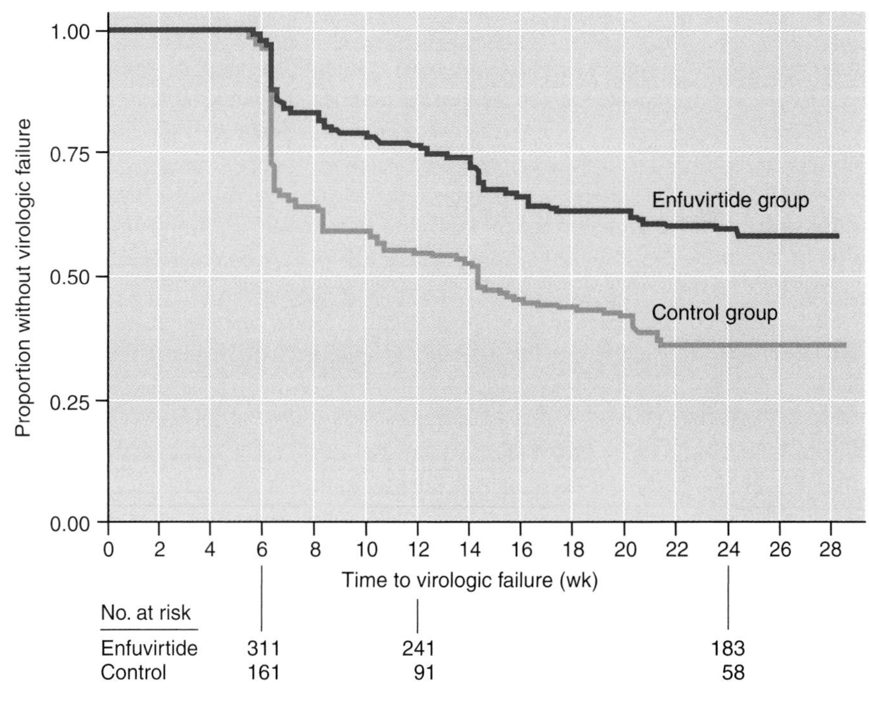

Figure 23-5 ■ Time to protocol-defined virologic failure at week 24 in the phase III TORO trial.

From Lalezari JP, Henry K, O'Hearn M, et al. Enfuvirtide, an HIV-1 fusion inhibitor, for drug-resistant HIV infection in North and South America. N Engl J Med 348:2175–85, 2003.

combined, at 48 weeks the proportion of subjects maintaining a viral load of <400 copies was 30% for ENF with OB versus 12% for OB alone.[21] At 96 weeks, 26% of those remaining on ENF with OB continued to maintain a viral load <400; subjects who had delayed addition of ENF, after experiencing virologic failure on the protocol, were at a significant long-term disadvantage compared with those initially randomized to receive ENF with OB.[22] Importantly, the achievement of >1 log decline in plasma viral load at 12 weeks on the TORO trials was a very strong predictor of beneficial responses at 24, 48, and 96 weeks of follow-up; subjects who did not experience this early response were quite unlikely to have sustained benefits (~1–3%) at later time points.[23]

PEDIATRIC EXPERIENCE

There are limited published data regarding the efficacy of ENF in HIV-infected pediatric patients. Children's Hospital Los Angeles investigators have reported on the long-term experience of 14 children (aged 4–12 years) who added on ENF 30–60 mg/m^2 bid in the setting of incomplete HIV suppression on standard antiretroviral therapy (ART) regimens. Eleven of 14 had an initial substantial virologic response, and 10 subjects (70%) maintained >1 log improvement in viral load (allowing for changes in background regimens) at 24 weeks.[24] Four subjects later experienced virologic failure (between weeks 40 and 63) in the open-label study. Of the original 14, six subjects still maintained virologic suppression >1 log below prestudy baseline at 96 weeks.[25] Preliminary pharmacokinetic results from a study involving 25 children (aged 5–16) suggests that ENF can be dosed on a per weight basis (2 mg/kg) regardless of age (>5 years), body surface area or weight.[26] The adverse experiences in these small protocols, predominantly local injection reactions, were generally comparable to the adult experience (summarized below).

PREGNANCY

There are no controlled studies of ENF in pregnant women. Animal studies have not demonstrated a risk of fetal toxicity and the agent has been classified as a category B drug. In general, recommendations for initiation of ENF in pregnant women should be similar to the considerations for women who are not pregnant, since the pvotential benefits for the mother may outweigh possible risks to the fetus. As with other ARTs, women in the first trimester may consider delaying therapy initiation or discontinuing current therapy until after week 10–12 of pregnancy. If a decision is made to prescribe ENF during pregnancy, it is recommended that the patient be enrolled into the antiretroviral pregnancy registry (1-800-258-4263).

It is not known whether ENF is excreted in human milk. When radiolabeled ENF was administered to lactating rats, radioactivity was detectable in the milk; it is unclear whether this radioactivity represents intact peptide or amino acid by-products of ENF metabolism. Regardless, due to the risks of HIV transmission and the unknown risks of ENF toxicity to the infant, mothers should be instructed not to breast-feed while receiving ENF.[14]

TOXICITY

Throughout phase I, II, and III ENF clinical trial experience, potential systemic reactions or internal organ damage associated with ENF were uncommonly reported; instead, most toxicity concerns have been related to local injection site reactions (ISRs; see Fig. 23-6). In the combined TORO 1/TORO 2 experience, the occurrence of some degree of ISR was nearly universal (~98%), typically beginning during the first week of administration and not changing in severity over the period of continued administration.[19] The majority of TORO subjects reported local induration (~90%), erythema (~90%), and nodular or cystic reactions (~75%). The majority of these local reactions were reported as mild (~40–50%) or moderate pain (~40–50%) at the injection site without limitation of usual activities. Less than 10% had limitations of usual activities or required nontopical analgesics for local discomfort, and none were hospitalized for ISRs. Less than 3% overall discontinued ENF due to ISRs during the first 24 weeks, and this figure remained <5% over more prolonged follow-up.[27]

Biopsies of typical reaction sites reveal inflammation consistent with a local hypersensitivity reaction, in a pattern resembling granuloma annulare or an interstitial granulomatous drug reaction.[28] Cutaneous biopsies of ISR lesions in the setting of more prolonged ENF administration (~80 weeks) demonstrate increases in local T lymphocytes and some evidence of angiogenesis.[29] Dermatologic findings may have variable clinical courses with different macroscopic patterns: transient infiltrative lesions, nodular lesions which resolve within 7–15 days, and sclerotic lesions persisting more than 30 days. Histologically, some lesions have an acute urticarial or vasculitic pattern with surrounding fat inflammation, whereas longer-lasting nodules may resemble scleroderma (but do not involve adnexal structures) and may slowly regress over time with rotation of injection sites. Anecdotal evidence suggests that some individuals benefit from adjuvant techniques aiming to avoid or diminish ISRs such as vigorously massaging the area immediately after injection, using smaller needles, or applying heat or ice to the site. However, data are limited to make any formal assessments regarding the risks and benefits of such manipulations.

Excluding ISRs, the overall rate of adverse events at 24 weeks in the TORO trials was roughly equivalent in the ENF with OB versus OB alone arms.[19,20] The occurrence of severe adverse events was slightly higher in the ENF with OB arms, but there were no detectable trends in terms of specific categories or organ systems (essentially individual cases of various events typically attributable to ART regimens). Peripheral neuropathy and anorexia appeared slightly more common among ENF recipients, whereas diarrhea, nausea and vomiting were more commonly reported in those receiving OB alone.

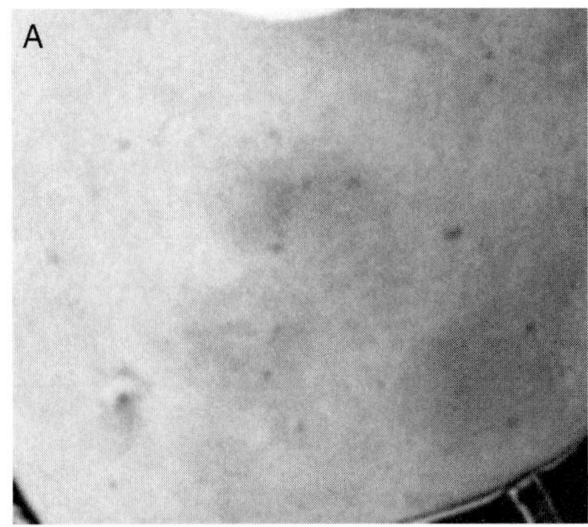

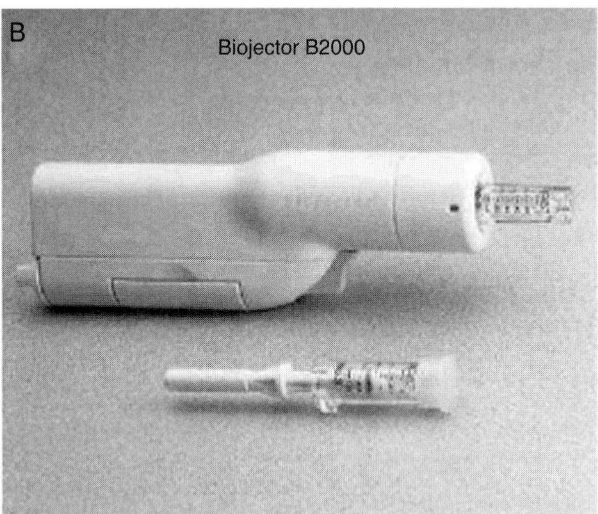

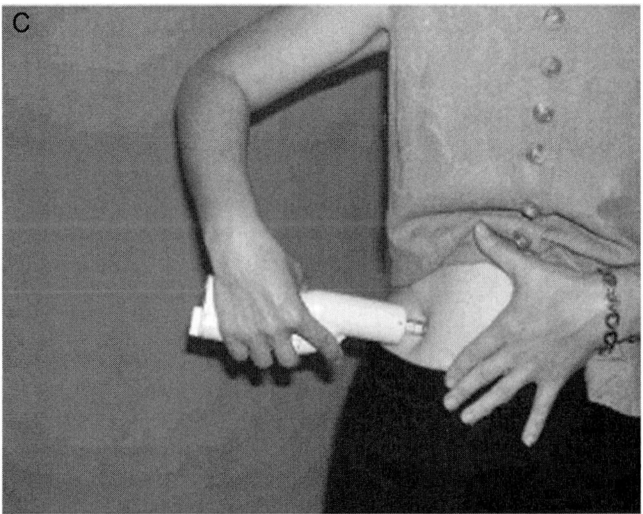

Figure 23-6 ■ (**A**) Photos of typical infection site reactions, (**B**) vial of enfuvirtide, and (**C**) the Biojector 2000 gas-powered infusion device under development.

(**A**) From Ball RA, Kinchelow T for the ISR Substudy Group. Injection site reactions with the HIV-1 fusion inhibitor enfuvirtide. J Am Acad Dermatol 49:826–31. 2003. (**B**) From Harris M, Joy R, Larsen G, et al. Enfuvirtide plasma levels and injection site reactions using a needle-free gas-powered injection system (Biojector). AIDS 20:719–23. 2006.

Systemic "hypersensitivity reactions" to ENF are apparently uncommon (two cases or <1% of TORO subjects), but have been well-substantiated and may recur with rechallenge. One TORO subject had hypersensitivity manifesting as rash, fever, nausea and vomiting whereas the other had glomerulonephritis. One case report describes successful desensitization to ENF,[30] although caution is probably warranted since one of the TORO subjects experienced severe respiratory distress during rechallenge. Whereas hypersensitivity reactions on the TORO protocols did not consistently correlate with increased circulating eosinophils, overall more subjects acquired eosinophilia in the ENF arms than in the OB only arms (~11% vs ~5%, respectively, developed >700 cells/mm^3). There was no evidence that eosinophilia was associated with clinical signs or symptoms of hypersensitivity. In terms of other safety laboratory assessments in TORO 1 and 2, there were no meaningful trends distinguishing the Grade III or IV abnormalities observed in the ENV with OB versus the OB alone arms.

One unexpected finding from the combined TORO experience that has generated discussion was the higher incidence of bacterial pneumonia among ENF recipients (50 cases (5.6% or 4.9/100 patient years) on ENF with OB vs only one in the OB alone arms (90.3% or 0.6/100 patient-years); $P = 0.02$). There was also a higher incidence of overall bacterial infections and sepsis in the ENF with OB arms compared with OB alone arms. However, after adjustments for duration of exposure (since many subjects crossed over to open-label ENF, there were more monitored patient-years on ENF with OB than in the comparator arms), these more general infectious disease differences were not statistically significant. These trends have raised speculation about whether there are unanticipated effects of the membrane fusion peptide on immunologic responses or inflammatory pathways, or whether these pulmonary infections may relate somehow to chronic subcutaneous injections. On the other hand, the prevalence of pneumonia in either the ENF with OB or the OB only arms was lower than might be anticipated based on the historical experience of patients with similar stages of HIV infection, suggesting that ENF did not result in a dramatic increase over the background rate of respiratory infections. 48-week follow-up data on the TORO populations has confirmed the same trends of adverse events discussed above but with significantly fewer treatment-related adverse events overall in those originally randomized to receive ENF.[27] Diarrhea, nausea and vomiting were slightly more common among those originally randomized to OB alone, whereas pneumonia and lymphadenopathy were conditions more common among ENF recipients. Quality of life assessments from the TORO trials demonstrated comparable outcomes regardless of treatment assignment,[31] perhaps suggesting that the challenges of self-injections and ISRs were effectively offset by other subjective benefits. "General health" quality of life subcomponent scores improved more among ENF recipients than comparators, and mental health self-assessment scores were higher among ENF recipients than comparators at 24 weeks.

PHARMACOKINETICS AND ROUTE OF ADMINISTRATION

A feature obviously unique to the peptide fusion inhibitor is its relative size (36 amino acids, see Fig. 23-2), much larger than any other antiretroviral drug and indeed one of the most complex pharmaceutical compounds ever manufactured in mass quantities. Like insulin, it is not feasible to administer this drug orally, as it would be quickly rendered inactive by oral and gastric enzymes. ENF is unique among antiretroviral agents in that evidence suggests the drug cannot enter host cells; the mechanism of viral entry inhibition likely takes place entirely in the extracellular environment. Thus, there are fewer concerns in regard to cell membrane transport or metabolism. When given parenterally, ENF has a small volume of distribution (5.48 L), low systemic clearance (1.4 L/h), and is highly bound to plasma proteins (92%).[32] The effects of hepatic or renal failure on ENF pharmacokinetics are poorly understood, but clearance does not appear to be altered substantially in the setting of mild to moderate renal insufficiency (creatinine clearance >35 mL/min). ENF and its chief metabolite do not affect levels of drugs metabolized by the cytochrome P450 system and there appear to be no significant interactions with commonly co-administered drugs such as ritonavir, boosted PIs, and rifampin.[32,33]

Other pertinent information about the pharmacokinetics of ENF was mentioned in the section on the phase I and II protocols above. After the proof of concept protocol utilizing intravenous ENF dosing (half-life 1.83 h), later studies evaluated different methods of subcutaneous administration. As described previously, CSI devices (often used as "insulin pumps" in diabetic patients) were generally ineffective, associated with weaker potency, significant local discomfort and ISRs.[16] A substantial portion of the CSI group (37%) on that phase II study switched over to intermittent subcutaneous administration, and one patient in the highest dose group (100 mg/day CSI) withdrew from the study because of infusion site pain. Two CSI subjects developed infusion site abscess or other signs of infection. The group receiving 50 mg subcutaneously twice daily had trough levels of ~1 μg/mL while the 100 mg twice daily group had trough levels in the ~1–3 μg/mL range (all higher than the *in vitro* IC_{50} for the drug). Earlier studies involving subcutaneous ENF required two injections twice daily, but a more concentrated formulation (100 mg/mL carbonate buffer) was found to be bioequivalent and more conveniently administered as one injection twice daily.[34] Notably, previous investigational formulations of T-20 sometimes reported the dose as "100 mg/90 mg deliverable" (or "50 mg/45 mg deliverable") based on the inherent imperfect delivery of medication in the syringe assembly, while the approved ENF formulation is now labeled for dosing simply as "90 mg twice daily".

Following subcutaneous injection, ENF is almost completely absorbed (apparently with only modest impact of body injection sites), with drug exposure increasing linearly and predictably over the dose range between 45 and 180 mg. Absorption is slow and protracted, which results in relatively flat steady state plasma concentrations over time. The bioavailability is high (>80%) and the elimination half-life (3.8 h) is longer than observed with IV administration.[32] When administered at the recommended dose, ENF appears to be in the plateau portion of the dose-response curve. Gender and body size do have modest affects on clearance in adults, but dose adjustments are generally not felt to be warranted based on safety and efficacy data.[32,33] As described above, data from the limited pediatric experience suggests that dosing at 2 mg/kg twice daily generally results in similar pharmacokinetics as with standard adult doses.[24]

ENF pharmacokinetic data support twice daily dosing and have invited speculation about the prospects of once daily dosing. One crossover study involving over 30 adult subjects suggested that 180 mg once daily (as two injections) is bioequivalent to 90 mg twice daily in terms of the area under the concentration curve (AUC).[35] The two approaches were associated with comparable short-term adverse events. The C_{trough} was predictably lower during the once daily phase (1.61 μg/mL) than the twice daily phase (3.77 μg/mL); importantly, 13 of the once daily subjects had C_{trough} levels less than 1 μg/mL. There was a trend toward a weaker antiretroviral effect during the once daily administration period (~1.0 log vs ~1.4 log viral load reduction from baseline to day 7, on 180 mg qd vs 90 mg bid, respectively; $P = 0.07$). Adding to concerns about further explorations of once daily dosing, assessments of ENF drug concentrations achieved with standard twice daily dosing in routine clinical settings suggest the potential for enormous interpatient variability and lower drug levels than anticipated based on experiences in closely monitored clinical trial situations.[36] Suboptimal and variable levels seen in clinical practice raise questions about the potential for diminished efficacy, as well as improved conditions for the selection of drug-resistance, with once daily administration.

The frequent occurrence of local site reactions, the general aversion of many individuals to self-injection, and the potential safety hazards of contaminated sharps in the home has prompted studies to evaluate needle-free delivery systems. One such system, the Biojector B2000 (Bioject Inc, Portland, OR) has undergone preliminary feasibility testing for ENF administration. This portable gas-powered system (Fig. 23-6) forces medication rapidly through the skin to disperse it into subcutaneous tissues, potentially with less tissue trauma and therefore lesser propensity for bleeding and pain than a needle. One pilot study demonstrated bioequivalence in ENF plasma levels over 24 h following a single dose.[37] Another observational study, involving 32 HIV-infected volunteers who had already experienced injection site reactions to ENF, assessed subjects before and after switching from standard needle injections to the Biojector gas-powered injection system.[38] ENF levels were not statistically different during the two phases (gas-powered or needle-injected) of the study, either at the predose trough or the 1 h postdose time points. Participants rated the Biojector approach significantly better than standard administration based on a predetermined scale related to ease of use ($P < 0.001$). A separate injection site rating instrument (which was also used in the TORO trials), combining a subjective self-reported score and a graded scale for objective findings (erythema, induration, pruritus, etc), also demonstrated a significant advantage in injection site reaction scores for the Biojector versus standard needle administration ($P < 0.001$). While a few subjects chose not to continue the Biojector approach because of local site reactions similar to what they had experienced with needles, the majority of subjects (>70%) opted to continue administering ENF with the needle-free system after the initial comparison phase was completed. A larger, multicenter trial to further evaluate gas-powered subcutaneous administration of ENF is underway in 2006.

RESISTANCE

Early studies involving *in vitro* passage of HIV-1 isolates in the presence of increasing ENF concentrations demonstrated selection for mutations in the first heptad repeat (HR-1) region of gp41 where the peptide was proposed to bind.[39] These observations provided important confirmation of the putative membrane fusion mechanism of action. These and later *in vitro* experiments consistently noted mutations occurring in the gp41 sequence of amino acids between 36 and 45, and in particular the relatively conserved 36–38 ("GIV") sequence.[40–42] Various mutations in the GIV region (36S, 36D, 37T, 38M) contribute to ENF resistance (often in the range of 10-fold), and the combined presence of two mutations (at positions 36 and 38 for example) may increase phenotypic resistance >100-fold.

Studies performed on viral isolates obtained from individuals with virologic failure during early clinical protocols, wherein ENF was typically given alone or as "functional monotherapy" (in the sense that it was added to completely ineffective background regimens in heavily pretreated subjects), showed clinical evidence of rather rapid selection for drug resistance, often within 2 weeks. Viral sequencing demonstrated the rapid selection for isolates containing the expected GIV region mutations as well as less well-characterized changes in other gp41 and pg120 regions.[39, 43–45] Several sources of evidence support the influence of envelope regions outside of HR-1 of gp41 on ENF sensitivity, particularly within the HR-2 region of gp41, although the mechanistic explanations for these findings are incompletely understood and a matter of some debate. There is a tremendous amount of variation in phenotypic resistance from one individual isolate to the next despite wild type codons in the primary HR-1 sequence, suggesting that other envelope areas are likely important.[42] Data from one experimental model involving site-directed mutagenesis of isolates not previously exposed to ENF suggested that chemokine co-receptor tropism (CCR5 vs CXCR4, mediated by gp120 V3 loop determinants) has substantial effects on ENF sensitivity (R5 isolates associated with a higher IC_{50} than X4 isolates) independent from the effects of GIV mutations.[40] However, studies involving R5, X4, and dual-tropic isolates obtained from clinical trial subjects receiving ENF, as well as serial isolates from individuals whose isolates evolved from R5 to X4 over time, have not supported the *in vitro* observation that baseline co-receptor tropism is an important determinant of ENF sensitivity.[42,46] Nonetheless, greater affinity for either of the gp120 co-receptors correlates with ENF resistance *in vitro*, possibly because more rapid fusion kinetics results in less opportunity for ENF to interact with its binding region.[47] Conversely, decreased gp120 co-receptor expression increases ENF sensitivity, perhaps due to slowing of the kinetics of the fusion process. Thus, there are complex interactions within the multistep viral entry process which may have potential to enhance or diminish ENF sensitivity depending on the circumstances. Notably, there is a high degree of *in vitro* synergy between ENF and experimental agents (such as CXCR4 and CCR5 blockers) with different mechanisms of inhibiting viral entry.[48,49]

In a related fashion, some HR-1 mutations conferring ENF resistance appear to slow up fusion kinetics and thereby enhance viral susceptibility to neutralizing antibodies (perhaps to antibodies targeting epitopes otherwise present only as transient intermediate structures during the viral entry process).[50] This may provide a mechanistic explanation, at least in part, for the observation that ENF resistance inversely correlates with replication capacity in growth competition assays.[51] Another potential explanation is that the highly conserved position 36 of the HR-1 gp41 region is particularly critical for normal fusion activity, and viral escape from ENF at this position may result in diminished viral infectivity and syncytium-forming activity.[52] As expected based on these observations, following ENF discontinuation viral isolates tend to revert back to wild type gp41 sequences.[53,54]

Evidence suggests there is a low genetic barrier to the rapid selection for ENF resistance, particularly when it is administered at suboptimal doses or without adequate additional potent agents.[43,54] Typically individuals with clinical drug failure have viral isolates with identifiable mutations in the HR-1 sequence. In the TORO protocols, 93% of subjects who met protocol criteria for virologic failure had demonstrable changes from pretherapy baseline within the 36–45 gp41 sequence, and this occurred in virtually all subjects who had a fourfold change in phenotypic ENF resistance.[46] Although there was a wide variation in pretreatment phenotypic ENF susceptibilities (despite wild type GIV sequences in all cases at baseline), as reported previously, having a lower pretherapy susceptibility did not predict a poor response to ENF therapy. Other studies have shown that if ENF is continued long-term in this setting of rising viral load during therapy there is evidence of ongoing selection for other resistance-conferring mutations in the HR-2 region (especially S138A coexisting with changes at position 43, amino acids that are in close proximity in the folded gp41 structure) and elsewhere, possibly compensatory changes that no longer compromise fitness to the same degree.[53,55]

In addition to the obvious importance of drug resistance emerging during therapy, the relative impact of natural polymorphisms in the gp41 sequences of viruses derived from individuals not previously treated with fusion inhibitors has been the subject of a few studies. In general it appears that the major "GIV" mutations conferring ENF resistance are uncommon (<1–3%) as naturally-occurring polymorphisms in the global community, whereas a diversity of polymorphisms in the surrounding gp41 region that may have a modest effect on ENF sensitivity may be seen in a higher percentage (~10–20%).[56–58] These potential contributors to at least mild degrees of "primary resistance" may be more common in nonclade B strains than in clade B strains.[57] One of the most common (~16% of wild type isolates) natural polymorphisms in this region, N42S, appears to confer increased sensitivity to ENF for some viral strains.[42,46]

OTHER MEMBRANE PEPTIDE CANDIDATES

Another peptide fusion inhibitor compound, corresponding to a slightly different portion of gp41 and with the same proposed mechanism of action as ENF, designated T-1249, has also been evaluated in early phase clinical protocols. T-1249 has demonstrated potency against a diversity of HIV-1 and HIV-2 isolates *in vitro*, including those with ENF resistance-conferring mutations, and has pharmacokinetics to support the possibility of once daily dosing. Phase I results of a 14-day dose-escalation trial of T-1249 monotherapy among 72 HIV-infected, treatment-experienced patients were reported.[59] Two episodes of possible drug-related serious adverse events were encountered: hypersensitivity reaction (oral ulcers, rash, and fever) and severe neutropenia. Local ISRs occurred in 40% and tended to be mild. The plasma half-life and bioavailability of T-1249 supported the possibility of once daily subcutaneous dosing, but more than one injection was required to achieve an adequate dosage. The viral load response was dose-related, with the patients receiving the highest dose experiencing a -1.40 $\log_{10}$ decline at 14 days. Another study evaluated the initial response to T-1249 in 53 subjects who had previously experienced a rising viral load while receiving ENF.[60] Despite a mean >100-fold decrease in ENF susceptibility at enrolment, there was 1.26 $\log_{10}$ viral load decline over 10 days of T-1249 therapy. Thus, there are preliminary data supporting the potential for successful sequencing of different membrane fusion inhibitors. However, at the time of this writing there are no active plans to further pursue clinical development of T-1249.

Other candidates for the next generation of peptide fusion inhibitors are in preclinical development. Recently, two peptides derived from a gp41 HR-2 sequence partially overlapping the ENF sequence have shown promising *in vitro* potency (including activity against ENF- and T-1249-resistant strains) and favorable pharmacokinetics in nonhuman primate models (*see* Chapter 27).[61] The goal is to develop sustained release formulations that might allow once weekly subcutaneous dosing.

RECOMMENDATIONS FOR USE

There are a few case reports suggesting that ENF can be attempted as part of a first-line antiretroviral regimen in exceptional circumstances, such as when patients have an aversion or intolerance to many orally administered agents.[62] Outside of these unusual anecdotal experiences, however, the typical clinical scenario for consideration of ENF injections involves patients with rather extensive prior treatment experience, comparable to the subjects evaluated in the TORO trials. This general consensus is based on a variety of factors such as, the ability to successfully suppress viral load in treatment-naive patients with increasingly convenient oral regimens, the challenges of self-injection, the nearly universal occurrence of mild ISRs (and the eventual "burnout" that can occur after enduring these side effects over years), and the costs associated with ENF therapy.

While ENF has demonstrable activity in the context of very advanced AIDS, optimal outcomes have been observed when the drug could be combined with other active agents and at a stage when the absolute CD4+ T-lymphocyte count is >100 cells and viral loads are <100 000 copies/mL.[63] Therefore, there is a clinical dilemma about the ideal placement of an ENF-containing regimen into the sequencing of HAART regimens, essentially whether to incorporate ENF after the failure of a second HAART regimen while the immune system remains reasonably intact or keep this option in reserve until there is a more urgent need for deeper salvage strategies. As discussed previously in this chapter, there is a low genetic barrier to ENF resistance when the agent is added on to failing agents or combined with "recycled" agents to which the infecting virus is already resistant, so this represents a very important clinical decision.

The large numbers of heavily treatment-experienced subjects enrolled into the TORO protocols provides important information regarding "deep salvage" treatment strategies. During the time period these protocols were screening potential subjects, the boosted PI combination lopinavir/ritonavir was either investigational or just becoming commercially available. Post hoc analyses have demonstrated that the optimal virologic outcomes in these trials occurred among subjects who received both ENF and lopinavir/ritonavir and who were previously naive (or maintained *in vitro* susceptibility) to lopinavir/ritonavir. Among these subjects, the viral load response rate (to <400 copies) was at least twofold higher among those receiving ENF with lopinavir/ritonavir versus those receiving lopinavir/ritonavir without ENF as a component of their regimens(60% vs 30% at 24 weeks[64] and 55% vs 24% at 48 weeks,[65] respectively).

Other more recent clinical trials have extended and confirmed these observations regarding the utility of combining a fusion inhibitor with a "ritonavir-boosted" PI in the setting of multiresistant virus. The RESIST trials used a design similar to TORO to evaluate boosted tipranavir (a newer PI) in addition to OB versus OB alone.[66,67] As with the TORO trials, participants in the two RESIST studies had very extensive prior treatment histories (and ~10% had previously received a fusion inhibitor). The results were analogous to the TORO trials, in that subjects who received tipranavir/ritonavir were about twice as likely to have substantial virologic responses at 24 weeks compared with those who received comparator boosted PI agents. About one quarter of all RESIST subjects received ENF in their OB regimen. When outcomes for subjects who were ENF-naive at baseline are analyzed, those who received ENF with tipranavir/ritonavir were twice as likely to have a >1 log viral load reduction at 24 weeks (~70%) than those who received tipranavir/ritonavir without ENF (~37%). This difference was seen despite evidence that ENF recipients on the RESIST trials had more advanced disease parameters at baseline compared with subjects whose caregivers chose not to include ENF in their OB salvage regimens. Similar information can be gleaned from the recent POWER trials designed to evaluate the impact of the PI, darunavir (previously referred to as TMC114, *see* Chapter 26), as part of a salvage regimen for heavily treatment-experienced patients.[68,69] These trials showed encouraging results of TMC114 relative to comparator boosted PIs, but the most consistent advantages were again seen in ENF-naive subjects who received both T-20 and TMC114. This was particularly true in POWER 2, where the proportion achieving a viral load <50 copies/mL was 64% among subjects receiving ENF plus TMC114 versus 30% who received TMC114 without ENF. In POWER 1, in contrast, the proportion of responders receiving TMC114 was essentially the same (~60%) regardless of ENF inclusion in their regimens. This discrepancy may be explained by differences in baseline viral loads and prior ENF experience. Although POWER 1 results are an exception, the overall trend from these trials with an "OB design" is that there is a substantial (twofold) advantage in the setting of extensive treatment experience for patients to receive a regimen containing a newer boosted PI agent plus a fusion inhibitor, rather than the PI agent plus other conventional agents alone.

As mentioned previously, *in vitro* experiments suggest unprecedented degrees of synergy between membrane fusion inhibitors and several of the investigational agents targeting other steps in the viral entry process. There is hope that carefully selected entry inhibitor combinations may ultimately be successful at decreasing the emergence of resistance and increasing the breadth of antiviral responses. More information on viral entry blocker combinations should be available soon, as several ongoing clinical trials of investigational viral entry inhibitors allow ENF co-administration.

Based on evolving experience, it appears prudent to consider ENF at a point when patients have developed multidrug resistant viral isolates yet while resistance testing reveals that at least one other potent drug can be paired with ENF. This can be either an active boosted PI or other potent new agent that is available for co-administration. This may mean temporarily delaying a change in HAART regimens while awaiting clinical access to new potent compounds in some situations, weighing the risks of rapid clinical deterioration against the knowledge that the response to ENF as "functional monotherapy" will have limited durability. Furthermore, as already discussed, continuing ENF in the context of ongoing viral replication appears to result in step-wise accumulation of additional resistance-conferring mutations which may further compromise future ENF use while potentially reversing theoretical benefits of the diminished replication capacity associated with the primary ENF resistance-conferring mutations.

Beyond these complex issues relating to drug sequencing strategies, there are also several practical considerations unique to ENF, primarily because it is a parenteral therapy requiring either self-administration or frequent care by skilled caregivers. In general, outside of institutionalized or sophisticated home-based care, successful long-term ENF administration using needles may be more dependent upon thoughtful selection of appropriate patients than typical all-oral ART regimens, for example with regard to adequate mental and physical functioning, emotional stability, and dedicated social support systems. Obviously, access to indoor plumbing and sanitary conditions is a basic necessity.

Finally, the cost of ENF relative to other antiretroviral agents is a major challenge. The annual cost of ENF drug and supplies alone is ~18 000–20 000 Dollars or Euros; which is currently greater than the total cost of standard three drug antiretroviral therapy. This means that the total cost of therapy (ENF with OB) may be more than doubled in most salvage therapy scenarios. This means that the drug will not be equally accessible for all individuals in need; indeed, charitable organizations and drug assistance programs with fixed budget constraints have been faced with dilemmas about trading off multiple traditional drug "slots" for one ENF "slot". However, it is also important to consider the long-term potential benefits in terms of outcomes and quality of life in the context of these economic realities. Several studies in the US and Europe have estimated an annual cost per quality-adjusted life year (QALY) for including ENF in salvage regimens. From 20 000 to 70 000 Euros/Dollars per incremental QALY gained depending upon mathematical modeling assumptions is higher than first-line ART yet less than many other acceptable life-saving medical interventions.[70–72] The current retail price for the Biojector device is $995 and another $66 per month for consumable supplies (syringes, carbon dioxide canisters).[37] While future development of a needle-free system might improve upon patient acceptability and tolerability of ENF administration, it would likely also further increase the associated costs.

REFERENCES

1. Kwong PD, Wyatt R, Robinson J. Structure of an HIV gp120 envelope glycoprotein in complex with the CD4 receptor and a neutralizing antibody. Nature 393:648–59, 1998.
2. Wyatt R, Sodroski J. The HIV-1 envelope glycoproteins: fusogens, antigens, and immunogens. Science 280:1884–8, 1998.
3. Kilby JM, Eron J. Novel therapies based on mechanisms of HIV-1 cell entry. N Engl J Med 348:2228–38, 2003.

4. Gallaher W, Ball J, Garry R, et al. A general model of the transmembrane proteins of HIV and other retroviruses. AIDS Res Hum Retroviruses 5: 431–40, 1989.
5. Delwart E, Mosialos G, Gilmore T. Retroviral envelope glycoproteins contain a "leucine zipper"-like repeat. AIDS Res Hum Retroviruses 6:703–6, 1989.
6. Wild C, Greenwell T, Matthews T. A synthetic peptide from HIV-1 gp41 is a potent inhibitor of virus-mediated cell–cell fusion. AIDS Res. Hum Retroviruses 9:1051–3, 1993.
7. Wild CT, Shugars DC, Greenwell TK, et al. Peptides corresponding to a predictive alpha-helical domain of HIV-1 gp41 are potent inhibitors of virus infection. Proc Natl Acad Sci USA 91:9770–4, 1994.
8. Chen CH, Matthews T, McDanal C, et al. A molecular clasp in HIV-1 TM protein determines the anti-HIV activity of gp41 derivatives: implication for viral fusion. J Virol 69:3771–7, 1995.
9. Wild C, Greenwell T, Shugars D, et al. The inhibitory activity of an HIV-1 peptide correlates with its ability to interact with a leucine zipper structure. AIDS Res Hum Retroviruses 11: 323–5, 1995.
10. Wild C, Oas T, McDanal C, et al. A synthetic peptide inhibitor of HIV replication: correlation between solution structure and viral inhibition. Proc Natl Acad Sci USA 89:10537–41, 1992.
11. Dubay J, Roberts S, Brody B, et al. Mutations in the leucine zipper of HIV-1 transmembrane glycoprotein affect fusion and infectivity. J Virol 65: 4748–56, 1992.
12. Wild C, Dubay JW, Greenwell T. et al. Propensity for a leucine zipper-like domain of HIV-1 gp41 to form oligomers correlates with a role in virus-induced fusion rather than assembly of the glycoprotein complex. Prco Natl Acad Sci USA 91:12676–80, 1994.
13. Carr C, Kim PS. A spring-loaded mechanism for the conformational change of influenza hemaglutinin. Cell 73: 823–32, 1993.
14. Fuzeon package insert. Roche Laboratories, Inc (Nutley, NJ) and Trimeris, Inc (Morrisville, NC); 2003–2005.
15. Kilby JM, Hopkins S, Venetta TM, et al. Potent suppression of HIV-1 replication in humans by T-20, a peptide inhibitor of gp41-mediated virus entry. Nat Med 4:1302–7, 1998.
16. Kilby JM, Lalezari JP, Eron JJ, et al. The safety, plasma pharmacokinetics, and antiviral activity of subcutaneous enfuvirtide (T-20), a peptide inhibitor of gp41-mediated virus fusion, in HIV-infected adults. AIDS Res Hum Retroviruses 18:586–93, 2002.
17. Lalezari JP, Eron JJ, Carlson M, et al. A phase II clinical study of the long-term safety and antiviral activity of enfuvirtide-based antiretroviral therapy. AIDS 17:691–8, 2003.
18. Lalezari JP, DeJesus E, Northfelt DW, et al. A controlled phase II trial assessing three doses of enfuvirtide (T-20) in combination with abacavir, amprenavir, ritonavir, and efavirenz in non-nucleside reverse transcriptase inhibitor-naive HIV-infected adults. Antivir Ther 8:279–87, 2003.
19. Lalezari JP, Henry K, O'Hearn M, et al. Enfuvirtide, an HIV-1 fusion inhibitor, for drug-resistant HIV infection in North and South America. N Engl J Med 348:2175–85, 2003.
20. Lazzarin A, Clotet B, Cooper D, et al. Efficacy of enfuvirtide in patients infected with drug-resistant HIV-1 in Europe and Australia. N Engl J Med 348:2186–95, 2003.
21. Nelson M, Arasteh K, Clotet B, et al. Durable efficacy of enfuvirtide over 48 weeks in heavily treatment-experienced HIV-1-infected patients in the T-20 versus optimized background regimen only 1 and 2 clinical trials. J Acquir Immune Defic Syndr 40:404–12, 2005.
22. Arasteh K, Lazzarin A, Clotet B. XV International AIDS Conference, Bangkok, Thailand 2004.
23. Raffi F, Katlama C, Saag MS, et al. Week 12 response to therapy as a predictor of week 24, 48, and 96 outcome in patients receiving the HIV fusion inhibitor enfuvirtide in the T-20 versus optimized regimen only (TORO) trials. Clin Infect Dis 42:870–7, 2006.
24. Church JA, Cunningham C, Hughes M, et al. Safety and antiretroviral activity of chronic subcutaneous administration of T-20 in HIV-1-infected children. Pedatr Infect Dis 21:653–9, 2002.
25. Church JA, Hughes M, Chen J, et al. Long term tolerability and safety of enfuvirtide for HIV-1-infected children. Pediatr Infect Dis 23:713–18, 2004.
26. Bellibas SE, Siddique Z, Dorr A, et al. Pharmacokinetics enfuvirtide in pediatric HIV-1-infected patients receiving combination therapy. Pediatr Infect Dis 23:1137–41, 2004.
27. Torttier B, Walmsley S, Reynes, J, et al. Safety of enfuvirtide in combination with an optimized background of antiretrovirals in treatment-experienced HIV-1-infected adults over 48 weeks. J Acquir Immune Defic Syndr 40:413–21, 2005.
28. Ball RA, Kinchelow T, ISR Substudy Group. Injection site reactions with the HIV-1 fusion inhibitor enfuvirtide. J Am Acad Dermatol 49:826–31, 2003.
29. Maggi P, Ladisa N, Cinori E, et al. Cutaneous injection site reactions to long-term therapy with enfuvirtide. J Antimicrob Chemother 53:678–81, 2004.
30. DeSimone JA, Ojha A, Pathak R, Cohn J. Successful desensitization to enfuvirtide after a hypersensitivity reaction in an HIV-1-infected man. Clin Infect Dis 15:e110–2, 2004.
31. Cohen CJ, Clumeck N, Molina JM, et al. Health-related quality of life with enfuvirtide in combination with an optimized background regimen. J Acquir Immune Defic Syndr 37:1140–6, 2004.
32. Patel IH, Zhang X, Nieforth K, Salgo M, Buss N. Pharmacokinetics, pharmacodynamics and drug interaction potential of enfuvirtide. Clin Pharmacokinet 44:175–86, 2005.
33. Mould DR, Zhang X, Nieforth K, et al. Population pharmacokinetics and exposure-response relationship of enfuvirtide in treatment-experienced HIV-1-infected patients. Clin Pharmacol Ther 77:515–28, 2005.
34. Wheeler DA, Lalezari JP, Kilby JM, et al. Safety, tolerability, and plasma pharmacokinetics of high-strength formulations of enfuvirtide (T-20) in treatment-experienced HIV-1-infected patients. J Clin Virol 30:183–90, 2004.
35. Thompson M, DeJesus E, Richmond G, et al. Pharmacokinetics, pharmacodynamics and safety of once-daily versus twice-daily dosing with enfuvirtide in HIV-infected subjects. AIDS 20:397–404, 2006.
36. Stocker H, Kloft C, Plock N, et al. Pharmacokinetics of Enfuvirtide in patients treated in typical routine clinical settings. Antimicrob Ag Chemother 50:667–73, 2006.
37. True AL, Zhang Y, Chiu YY, et al. Needle-free administration of enfuvirtide with Biojector 2000 (B2000) demonstrates pharmacokinetic bioequivalence to standard needle administration. Frontiers in Drug Development for Antiretroviral Therapies. Montego Bay, Jamaica, Dec 2004, abstract 57.
38. Harris M, Joy R, Larsen G, et al. Enfuvirtide plasma levels and injection site reactions using a needle-free gas-powered injection system (Biojector). AIDS 20:719–23, 2006.
39. Rimsky LT, Shugar DC, Matthews T. Determinants of HIV-1 resistance to gp41-derived inhibitory peptides. J Virol 72: 986–92, 1998.
40. Derdeyn CA, Decker JM, Sfakianos JN, et al. Sensitivity of HIV-1 to the fusion inhibitor T-20 is modulated by coreceptor specificity defined by the V3 loop of gp120. J Virol 74:8358–67, 2000.
41. Derdeyn CA, Decker JM, Sfakianos JN, et al. Sensitivity of HIV-1 fusion inhibitors targeted to the gp41 first heptad repeat involves distinct regions of gp41 and is consistently modulated by gp120 interactions with the coreceptor. J Virol 75:8605–14, 2001.
42. Mink M, Mosier SM, Janumpalli S, et al. Impact of HIV-1 gp41 amino acid substitutions selected during enfuvirtide treatment on gp41 binding and antiviral potency of enfuvirtide in vitro. J Virol 79:12447–54, 2005.

43. Wei X, Decker JM, Liu H, et al. Emergence of resistant HIV-1 in patients receiving fusion inhibitor (T-20) monotherapy. Antimicrob Ag Chemother 46:1896–905, 2002.
44. Heil ML, Decker JM, Sfakianos JN, et al. Determinants of HIV-1 baseline susceptibility to the fusion inhibitors enfuvirtide and T-649 reside outside the peptide interaction site. J Virol 78:7582–9, 2004.
45. Sista P, Melby T, Davison D, et al. Characterization of determinants of genotypic and phenotypic resistance to enfuvirtide in baseline and on-treatment HIV-1 isolates. AIDS 18:1787–91, 2004.
46. Melby T, Sista P, Demasi R, et al. Characterization of envelope glyocoprotein gp41 genotype and phenotypic susceptibility to enfuvirtide at baseline and on treatment in the phase III clinical trials TORO-1 and TORO-2. AIDS Res Hum Retroviruses 22:375–85, 2006.
47. Reeves JD, Gallo SA, Ahmad N, et al. Sensitivity of HIV-1 to entry inhibitors correlates with envelope/coreceptor affinity, receptor density, and fusion kinetics. Proc Natl Acad Sci USA 99:16249–54, 2002.
48. Tremblay CL, Kollmann C, Giguel F, et al. Strong in vitro synergy between the fusion inhibitor T-20 and the CXCR4 blocker AMD-3100. J Acquir Immune Defic Syndr 25:99–102, 2000.
49. Tremblay CL, Giguel F, Kollman C, et al. Anti-HIV interactions of SCH-C (SCH 351125), a CCR5 antagonist, with other antiretroviral agents in vitro. Antimicrob Agents Chemother 46:1336–9, 2002.
50. Reeves JD, Less FH, Miamidian JL, et al. Enfuvirtide resistance mutations: impact on HIV envelope function, entry inhibitor sensitivity, and virus neutralization. J Virol 79:4991–9, 2005.
51. Lu J, Sista P, Giguel F, et al. Relative replicative fitness of HIV-1 mutants resistant to enfuvirtide (T-20). J Virol 78:4628–37, 2004.
52. Kinomoto M, Yokyama M, Sato H, et al. Amino acid 36 in the HIV-1 gp41 ectodomain controls fusogenic activity: implications for the molecular mechanism of viral escape from a fusion inhibitor. J Virol 79:5996–6004, 2005.
53. Menzo S, Castagna A, Monachetti A, et al. Genotype and phenotype patterns of HIV-1 resistance to enfuvirtide during long-term treatment. Antimicrob Agents Chemother 48:3253–9, 2004.
54. Poveda E, Rodes B, Lebel-Binay S, et al. Dynamics of enfuvirtide resistance in HIV-infected patients during and after long-term enfuvirtide salvage therapy. J Clin Virol 34:295–301, 2005.
55. Xu L, Pozniak A, Wildfire A, et al. Emergence and evolution of enfuvirtide resistance following long-term therapy involves heptad repeat 2 mutations within gp41. Antimicrob Agents Chemother 49:1113–9, 2005.
56. Roman F, Gonzalez D, Lambert C, et al. Uncommon mutations at residue positions critical for enfuvirtide (T-20) resistance in enfuvirtide-naive patients infected with subtype B and non-B HIV-1 strains. J Acquir Immune Defic Syndr 33: 134–9, 2003.
57. Carmona R, Perez-Alvarez , Munoz M, et al. Natural resistance-associated mutations to enfuvirtide (T20) and polymorphisms in the gp41 region of different HIV-1 genetic forms from T20 naive patients. J Clin Virol 32:248–53, 2005.
58. Chinnadurai R, Munch J, Kirchhoff F. Effect of naturally-occurring gp41 HR1 variations on susceptibility of HIV-1 to fusion inhibitors. AIDS 19:1401–5, 2005.
59. Eron JJ, Gulick R, Merigan T, et al. Short-term safety and antiretroviral activity of T-1249, a second generation fusion inhibitor of HIV-1. J Infect Dis 189:1075–83, 2004.
60. Lalezari JP, Bellos NC, Sathasivam K, et al. T-1249 retains potent antiretroviral activity in patients who had experienced virological failure while on an enfuvirtide-containing treatment regimen. J Infect Dis 191:1155–63, 2005.
61. Delmedico M, Bray B, Cammack N, et al. Next generation HIV peptide fusion inhibitor candidates achieve potent, durable suppression of virus replication in vitro and improved pharmacokinetic properties. In: 13th Conference on Retroviruses and Opportunistic Infections, Denver, CO, 6 Feb 2006, abstract 48.
62. Bourgarit A, Lascoux C, Palmer P, et al. First-line use of enfuvirtide-containing HAART regimen with dramatic clinical and immunological improvement in three cases. AIDS 20:471–3, 2006.
63. Clotet B, Raffi F, Cooper D, et al. Clinical management of treatment-experienced, HIV-infected patients with the fusion inhibitor enfuvirtide: consensus recommendations. AIDS 18:1137–46, 2004.
64. Haubrich R, DeMasi R, Thommes JA. Improved virologic response in three-class experienced patients when an active boosted protease inhibitor is combined with enfuvirtide (ENF) [abstract]. In: 43rd Annual Meeting of the Infectious Disease Society of America, 2005.
65. Miralles GD, DeMasi R. Virologic suppression of an active boosted PI regimen is significantly enhanced by the addition of a fusion inhibitor in treatment-experienced patients [abstract]. In: 42nd Annual Meeting of the Infectious Disease Society of America, 2004.
66. Hicks C. RESIST-1: A phase 3, randomized, controlled, open-label, multicenter trial comparing tipranavir/ritonavir to an optimized comparator protease inhibitor/ritonavir regimen in antiretroviral experienced patients: 24 week data [abstract]. In: 44th Interscience Conference on Antimicrobial Agents and Chemotherapy, 2004.
67. Cahn P. 24 week data from RESIST-2: Phase 3 study of the efficacy and safety of either tripranavir/ritonavir or an optimized ritonavir-boosted standard-of-care comparator PI in a large randomized multicenter trial in treatment-experienced HIV+ patients [abstract]. In: 7th International Congress on Drug Therapy in HIV Infection, 2004.
68. Katlama C, Carvalho M, Cooper D, et al. POWER: TMC114-C213 study-week 24 analysis [abstract]. In: 3rd International AIDS Society Conference, 2005.
69. Wilkin T, Haubrich R, Steinhart C, et al. POWER 2 (TMC114-C202) week 24 efficacy analysis [abstract]. In: 45th Interscience Conference on Antimicrobial Agents and Chemotherapy, 2005.
70. Hornberger J, Green J, Wintfeld N, et al. Cost-effectiveness of enfuvirtide for treatment-experienced patients with HIV in Italy. HIV Clin Trials 6:92–102, 2005.
71. Sax PE, Losina E, Weinstein MC, et al. Cost-effectiveness of enfuvirtide in treatment-experienced patients with advanced HIV disease. J Acquir Immune Defic Syndr 39:69–77, 2005.
72. Hornberger J, Kilby JM, Wintfeld N, Green J. Cost-effectiveness of enfuvirtide in HIV therapy for treatment-experienced patients in the United States. AIDS Res Human Retro 22: 240–7, 2006.

Chapter 24

Inhibiting the Entry of R5 and X4 HIV-1 Phenotypic Variants

Shawn E. Kuhmann, PhD, Roy M. Gulick, MD, MPH, John P. Moore, PhD

Compounds that prevent HIV-1 from entering its target cells are now available as a new therapeutic drug class, the entry inhibitors. They could play an important role in treating HIV-1 infection in future years, and they may also be valuable for preventing transmission, as pre-exposure or postexposure prophylaxis and/or as a topical microbicides. This chapter will review how the entry inhibitors might be used in clinical practice.

What are these compounds, how do they act, and what aspects of HIV-1 virology and pathogenesis may influence their use clinically? In addressing these issues, emphasis should be placed on the HIV-1 phenotypic variants known as R5 (CCR5-using) and X4 (CXCR4-using) viruses, because of their implications for the design of new therapeutic strategies in general, and those based on inhibition of viral entry via CCR5 and/or CXCR4 in particular. Most transmitted strains of HIV-1 use the CCR5 co-receptor for entry into CD4+ cells. Left untreated, infection with these R5 viruses is usually fatal. The X4 or R5X4 (CCR5- and CXCR4-using) strains can instead use the CXCR4 co-receptor and are rarely transmitted, (more accurately, they rarely dominate plasma viremia in the early years of infection), but when they do become relatively prevalent they are associated with an increased rate of disease progression. This is manifested by an acceleration in the rate of CD4+ T-cell loss, particularly of naive T cells, and a reduction in the regenerative capacity of the immune system. Hence the CXCR4-using strains represent a more lethal form of HIV-1.[1–3]

As described below, there are multiple stages to the process by which HIV-1 attaches to and fuses with target cells, the different stages being susceptible to intervention by different compounds that have different mechanisms of action. Some compounds inhibit virus-cell attachment, others interfere with the subsequent co-receptor interactions that drive fusion, yet more impede the later stages of the fusion process itself.[1,4–7] Hence there has been a tendency to designate individual compounds as "attachment inhibitors", "co-receptor inhibitors", or "fusion inhibitors". To some extent, the distinction is artificial, because all the compounds inhibit the entry process, albeit in different ways (Fig. 24-1). In this chapter, the generic term "entry inhibitors" will be used to describe all compounds that prevent HIV-1 from gaining access to the interior of the target cell. However, this chapter will focus only on compounds that bind specifically to the CCR5 or CXCR4 co-receptors. Inhibitors such as the BMS-378806 family of compounds that block gp120–CD4 attachment (*see* Chapter 27),[8] and enfuvirtide (*see* Chapter 23), which prevents conformational changes in gp41 at a late stage of fusion,[7] will be reviewed in detail elsewhere in this book. Note that the BMS-378806 family and enfuvirtide are active against both R5 and X4 viruses.

There is a semantic issue relating to co-receptor usage by the phenotypic variants. In the original nomenclature devised after the identification of CXCR4 and CCR5 as the principal co-receptors for HIV-1, isolates that use CCR5 were termed R5, while those using CXCR4 were called X4. Viruses that can use either co-receptor were designated R5X4 and they are often referred to as "dual-tropic".[9] Over the past decade, however, it has been appreciated that many uncloned "dual-tropic" isolates contain a mixture of R5 and X4 viruses, rather than individual viruses that are capable of entering cells via either co-receptor.[3] A more accurate term for phenotypically mixed isolates is R5+X4, with the term R5X4 being reserved for clonal viruses that can use both CCR5 and CXCR4 at the molecular level. Because the most commonly used commercial phenotyping assay (Trofile, from Monogram Biosciences, Inc) cannot discriminate between dual-tropic clonal viruses and phenotypic mixtures, an alternative terminology has arisen to describe samples that register as positive for entry into both CCR5-expressing and

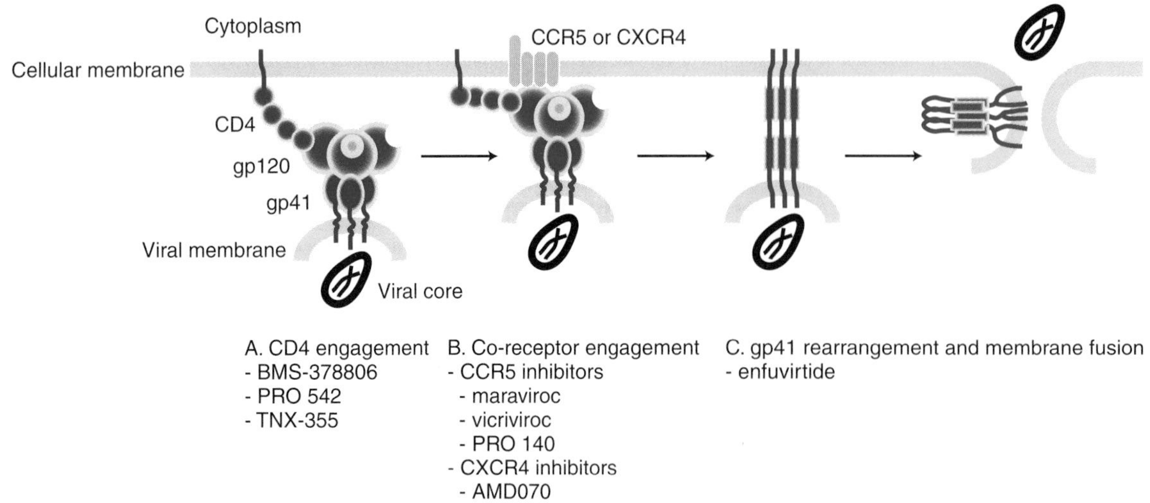

Figure 24-1 ■ A schematic depiction of the HIV-1 entry process and where in this process various inhibitors act. (A) The first stage of entry involves binding of the HIV-1 gp120 surface glycoprotein to CD4. In its native form, the HIV-1 envelope proteins consist of a trimer of gp120-gp41 hetero-dimers, the gp41 transmembrane proteins being anchored in the viral membrane. Drugs in clinical development that inhibit CD4 binding are: BMS-378806, a small molecule, PRO-542, an engineered, soluble CD4-based protein, and TNX-355, a humanized MAb to CD4. (B) The next step involves engagement of the CCR5 or CXCR4 co-receptor. The various CCR5 and CXCR4 inhibitors currently FDA-approved or in clinical development are discussed in detail in this chapter and include the small molecules maraviroc and vicriviroc directed against CCR5 and AMD070 against CXCR4, and the humanized anti-CCR5 MAb PRO 140. (C) Co-receptor binding leads to the insertion of the amino terminus of gp41 into the target cell membrane, forming a trimeric coiled-coil. Enfuvirtide acts by binding to this coiled-coil and preventing it from folding back on itself to form a six-helix bundle, an action that drives membrane fusion.

Adapted from Kuhmann SE, Moore JP. HIV-1 entry inhibitor entrances. Trends Pharmacol Sci 25:117, 2004.

CXCR4-expressing cells: "Dual/Mixed" or D/M.[10] We will not be using this terminology; instead, we will use the term R5+X4 except when making specific reference to a single virus that is known to be able to use both co-receptors (R5X4).

THE HIV-1 ENTRY PROCESS IS MEDIATED BY THE VIRAL ENVELOPE GLYCOPROTEINS

HIV-1 fuses with target cells after a series of events that are triggered by binding of the viral envelope glycoproteins to specific receptors on the cell surface.[11] The process of virus-cell attachment is usually the rate-limiting step for HIV-1 infection, just as it is for other viruses, because the negatively charged surfaces of both virions and cells create repulsive forces.[12] *In vitro*, such effects can often be overcome by experimental devices such as the use of polycations to negate the charge imbalance, or by centrifugation of virions onto the cells.[13] In the real world, however, HIV-1 uses ancillary receptors to facilitate its binding to the cell surface.[12,14,15] Several such interactions have been described, their relative importance usually being cell type-dependent.[12,14,15] Some ancillary interactions are mediated by the viral envelope glycoproteins, others by host cell-derived proteins or lipids that become incorporated into the viral membrane during egress of the virion from the cell.[12,14,15] Examples of the former type of interaction include the charge-based binding of cationic patches on the envelope glycoproteins to anionic moieties on cell surface heparan sulfate proteoglycans, and the binding of envelope glycoprotein (Env) glycans to cell surface mannose C-type lectin receptors including, but not limited to, DC-SIGN.[12,14] Alternatively, intracellular adhesion molecules (ICAM) incorporated into the virion membrane can associate with cell surface leukocyte function associated antigen-1 (LFA-1) to facilitate virus-cell attachment, particularly for the memory cells that are the preferred targets for R5 viruses.[12,15]

The ancillary interactions are neither necessary nor sufficient for triggering the events that lead to virus-cell fusion; they serve to concentrate virions on the cell surface in proximity to the fusion receptors proper, which increases the efficiency and rate of fusion, overall.[12] Irrespective of how HIV-1 attaches to cells, the fusion-related events are initiated by the sequential interaction of the viral Env complex with CD4 and a co-receptor.[11] The functional Env complex is a hetero-trimer of three gp120 surface glycoproteins, each noncovalently attached to three gp41 transmembrane glycoprotein subunits.[16–20] There may be as few as 10 Env complexes on a typical HIV-1 virion,[21] with perhaps only a single one being sufficient to mediate infection.[22] The crystal structures of the CD4-bound and free forms of gp120, together with sophisticated models of the gp120 monomer and trimer, have greatly helped an understanding of how the Env complex interacts with its receptors.[20,23–25] The structure of gp120 has been reviewed extensively elsewhere,[26,27] but in summary, gp120 contains a gp41-binding surface comprising residues in the C1 and C5 regions; a CD4-binding site (CD4bs) formed from multiple, well-conserved residues folded into proximity; a co-receptor binding site formed from elements of the V3 region and/or other, more conserved structures comprised of elements of the bridging sheet; the sequence-variable V1V2 loop structure that overlies the more conserved receptor binding sites; and 20–35 N-linked (and perhaps also several O-linked) glycan residues that are located both in the five variable regions (V1–V5) and on more conserved sites and which serve to shield the protein surface from immune recognition.[20,23–25] A key element of the CD4bs is a deep cavity that forms a contact site for an amino acid, Phe-43, protruding from a loop on CD4.[25] Due to the conformational flexibility of gp120, this cavity is probably only transiently formed in the absence of CD4 and is stabilized by CD4 engagement.[23] The binding of CD4 results in large conformational changes in other regions of gp120, including the formation of the co-receptor binding site.[23,28] BMS-378806 and related compounds inhibit the gp120–CD4 interaction, and also subsequent conformational changes involved in the formation of the co-receptor binding site.[8,29] These compounds are thought to intercalate within a cavity present in the CD4-free conformation of gp120, thereby stabilizing this conformation and inhibiting CD4 binding.[23]

The successful engagement of CD4 induces structural changes within gp120 that create, or expose, a binding site for the co-receptor.[23] The nature of the binding site on gp120 is similar for each co-receptor, but critical, and as yet ill-defined, structural differences underlie which of the two co-receptors is actually used by any given virus.[24,30,31] These changes in structure are usually created by sequence alterations in V3 that directly or indirectly affect the co-receptor-binding site.[32] The complexities of the co-receptor-binding interactions and the role of the V3 region in influencing HIV-1 phenotype have been reviewed extensively elsewhere.[32] In general, the V3 region of X4 viruses has a higher positive charge than the corresponding region of R5 viruses.[32] Changes at only a few, specific residues in V3 can sometimes be sufficient to convert an R5 virus into an X4 variant,[32] but additional changes elsewhere in gp120 are usually required to make a fully replication competent X4 virus.[33]

The engagement of the co-receptor causes structural changes in the gp41 subunits that drive membrane fusion.[1,4,5,11,34] The gp41 protein contains two segments known as the heptad-repeat (HR) regions, HR1 and HR2, which have a locally α-helical structure; the three HR1 regions of the three individual gp41 subunits form a coiled-coil structure.[6] During fusion, the interaction of HR1 with HR2 is considered to be the critical event that drags the viral and cell membranes toward one another.[6] Thus, following insertion of the gp41 fusion peptide into the host-cell membrane, the HR2 region folds back into grooves on the coiled surface of the HR1 coil to form a structure that is commonly called, and depicted as, a hairpin.[6] It is the formation of this highly stable structure, also often called the six-helix bundle, that releases enough stored energy to bring the viral and cell membranes close enough together for membrane fusion to occur.[6] Enfuvirtide, a soluble mimetic of the HR2 structure, inhibits the intermolecular association between the HR1 and HR2 domains of gp41, to sterically prevent the conformational changes needed to form the six-helix bundle.[6] Hence, fusion is arrested after the co-receptor-binding stage of the process (Fig. 24-1).

HIV-1 TROPISM: THE R5 AND X4 PHENOTYPIC VARIANTS

CCR5 and CXCR4 are the co-receptors most relevant to HIV-1 replication *in vivo*. Although at least 10 other G-protein coupled receptors (GPCRs) can mediate entry of some HIV-1 strains when they are expressed in transfected cells *in vitro*,[35,36] the use of these receptors for entry into primary CD4+ cells is rare.[37–48] Thus, the replication of HIV-1 in primary cells *in vitro* is almost always fully sensitive to inhibitors specific for CCR5 or CXCR4.[46–48] *In vivo*, individuals who lack CCR5 expression are strongly protected against HIV-1 infection.[49–51] On the rare occasions when CCR5-negative individuals become HIV-1 infected, their isolates use CXCR4 (and sometimes CCR5) but not other GPCRs to infect primary cells *in vitro*.[52–55] In general, usage of GPCRs other than CCR5 or CXCR4 does not correlate with disease progression.[40] Drug development programs aimed at blocking co-receptor binding have therefore focused only on CCR5 and CXCR4.[5,56]

Because patients can harbor HIV-1 tropism variants using either or both of the principal co-receptors, it is important to take these variants into account when making treatment decisions involving co-receptor inhibitors.[3,57] The differential replication of R5 and X4 viruses in cell types that express CCR5 and CXCR4 differently is central to an understanding of HIV-1 pathogenesis.[3,57] Indeed, as suggested, "HIV-1 infection of humans might almost be viewed as two separate diseases caused by two different lentiviruses that have different cellular tropisms: R5 HIV-1 strains, and their close cousins, the X4 viruses."[3]

It was recognized almost 20 years ago that two different HIV-1 tropism variants existed.[58–62] Isolates that formed syncytia in human peripheral blood mononuclear cells (PBMCs) were designated as syncytium inducing (SI), those that did not as NSI.[62] Viruses able to replicate in primary human monocyte-derived macrophages (MDM) were called M-tropic, those in CD4+ T-cell lines, T-tropic.[63,64] The formation of syncytia in MT-2 cells correlates well with the SI and T-tropic phenotypes, failure to do so with the NSI and M-tropic phenotypes.[65,66] The MT-2 syncytium formation assay soon became the accepted standard for routine determinations of tropism.[67–76] When CCR5 and CXCR4 were discovered, their cellular expression patterns explained tropism variants at the molecular level: CCR5 is the co-receptor for NSI/M-tropic viruses, CXCR4 for the SI/T-tropic strains.[39,77] For

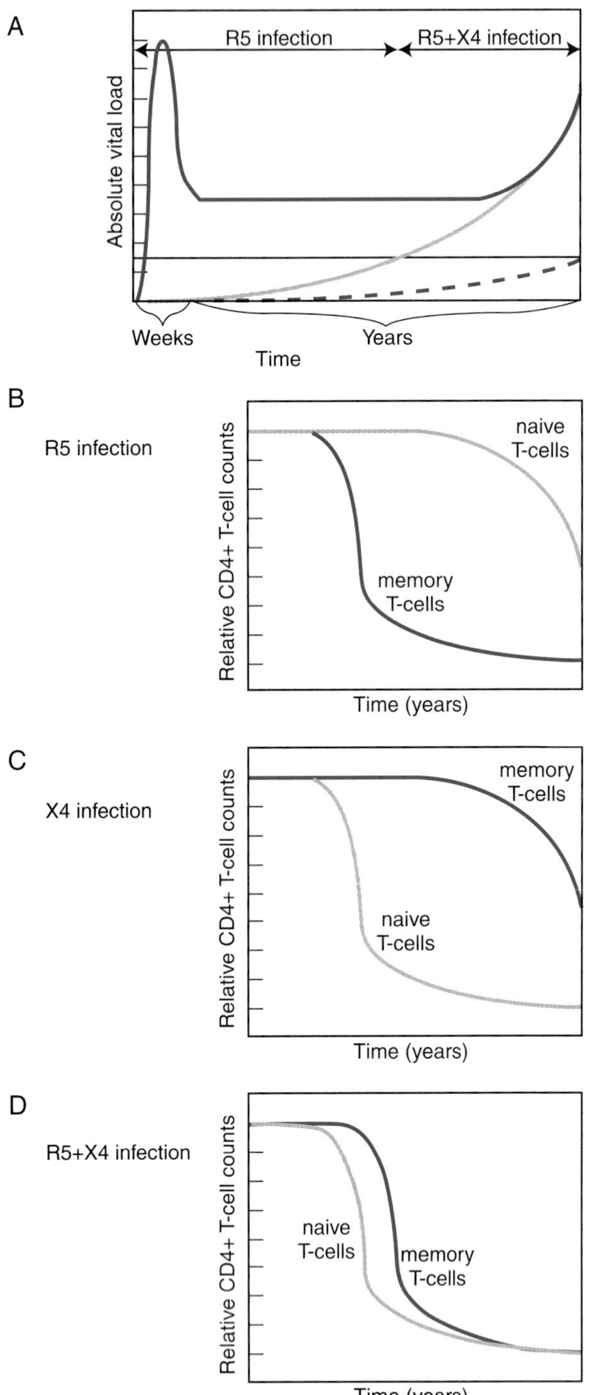

Figure 24-2 ■ Changes in R5 and X4 viral load and CD4+ T cell subsets over time, during untreated HIV-1 infection. (A) Absolute viral loads (in arbitrary units) of R5 and X4 viruses in the blood are depicted schematically over the course of HIV-1 infection. R5 viruses (dark blue lines) are shown as dominating the virus pool early, including during the primary infection phase. After acute viremia is resolved, R5 viruses reach a plateau, or set point, in the blood. X4 viruses (light blue and dashed lines) are shown to be undetectable early in infection (the horizontal line represents an arbitrary detection threshold, assuming such a threshold to be based on absolute viral load), but in rare individuals X4 viruses can be present at significant levels early in the disease course (not shown). As infection progresses, R5 viral loads increase on a time scale that correlates with disease markers (e.g., declining CD4+ T-cell counts). In another scenario (not shown), R5 viral loads may actually decrease late in infection due to depletion of the memory CD4+ T-cell pool. Two scenarios for X4 viral loads are shown. In some individuals (solid line) X4 viral loads increase to readily detectable levels on a time scale that correlates with disease progression. These individuals have a phenotypically R5+X4 infection. In other individuals (dashed line) X4 viral loads never become detectable at any stage of the disease process (pure R5 infection). (B–D) Effects of R5 and X4 infection on CD4+ T cell subsets. In this highly stylized depiction, CD4+ T cells are considered to be naive (CXCR4+CCR5−) or memory (CCR5+CXCR4+ or CCR5+CXCR4−). In panel B ("pure R5 infection"), R5 viruses deplete the memory cell pool (especially from GALT). The activation of naive CD4+ T cells to the memory phenotype renders them vulnerable to infection by R5 viruses, so over time, the naive cell pool is depleted. In panel C ("pure X4 infection"), X4 viruses rapidly deplete the naive CD4+ T cell pool without affecting memory cells. However, the expression of CXCR4 on memory CD4+ T cells is likely to render them vulnerable to X4 viruses over time, so these cells may also be eventually depleted. The "pure X4" virus infection scenario is extremely rare, and may only apply in practice to infected CCR5-d32 homozygotes. In panel D ("R5+X4 infection"), both naive and memory CD4+ T cells are depleted, leading to rapid disease progression. The schematic does not take into account changes in the proportions of R5 and X4 viruses over time. Other cell types vulnerable to HIV-1 infection, for example macrophages, are not depicted.

Reproduced from Kuhmann SE, Moore JP. The HIV-1 phenotypic variants: deadly and deadlier. J Viral Entry 1:4, 2005.

these reasons, the nomenclature system based on the R5 and X4 terminology was designed (as discussed earlier).[9]

It is essential to recognize that R5 and X4 viruses do not infect all CD4+ T cells with equal efficiency. CXCR4 is expressed on naive T cells from which CCR5 is largely absent, but, conversely, CCR5 expression is high on memory CD4+ T cells, and CXCR4 low.[78,79] This pattern of co-receptor expression is important for understanding how R5 and X4 viruses destroy the immune system at different rates. In a simplified model, R5 strains eliminate the memory CD4+ T-cell pool, and of course they also destroy the naive cells after they become activated and then express CCR5.[2,3,80,81] These events gradually erode and eventually completely destroy the T-cell mediated immune system. The targeting of naive T cells by X4 viruses has the same effect, but more rapidly; the loss of the naive T-cell pool prevents the body from responding to new pathogens (Fig. 24-2).[2,3]

The R5 and X4 viruses tend to dominate plasma viremia at different times after initial infection. Most isolates or clones from primary infection cases have the R5 phenotype with few X4.[3,39,77] Nonetheless, X4 viruses certainly can be transmitted; the rare infections that do occur in individuals homozygous for the defective CCR5-Δ32 allele involve X4 viruses.[52–55] However, the overall protection provided by CCR5-Δ32 homozygosity shows the difficulties faced by X4 viruses in establishing new infections.[49–51] The early prevalence of R5 viruses may reflect preferential transmission, but the same initial R5 dominance occurs irrespective of whether infection occurs sexually, vertically or via intravenous drug use.[3,82] Hence a compelling alternative hypothesis is that R5 viruses are more efficiently amplified soon after transmission.[3] If so, the initial target cells for viral amplification must be the same for all infection routes or, if different cells are involved, they must all favor R5 virus replication.[3]

Additional selection processes in favor of R5 viruses may operate at the level of the genital or rectal mucosa during sexual transmission. One hypothesis is that virions are transported by dendritic cells to lymph nodes where they are passed to activated memory CD4+ T cells, which express more CCR5 than CXCR4 and preferentially amplify R5 viruses.[3,83] Activated, CD4+ CCR5+ memory T cells are particularly prevalent in the gut-associated lymphoid tissue (GALT) where they normally combat food-borne pathogens.[81,84] The GALT therefore efficiently replicates R5 viruses during primary infection both in the macaque[85] and humans.[86,87] In both species, CD4+ CCR5+ T cells are substantially depleted from the GALT before this occurs in the peripheral blood, because cells of the GALT do not rapidly transit into the blood, and *vice versa*.[85,88] The preponderance of R5 viruses in GALT could, however, reflect earlier selection pressures; the GALT could be seeded with R5 viruses that had been preferentially transmitted and amplified in draining lymph nodes.[89] The rapid and selective elimination of activated memory CD4+ CCR5+ T cells from GALT by R5 viruses may suggest that tropism variants selectively deplete the subsets of CD4+ cells that express the appropriate co-receptor.[2,3,80,81] However, considerable complexities and controversies surround this issue, and direct cell killing is unlikely to be sufficient to explain viral pathogenesis, particularly for R5 viruses.[2]

Although they are rare early in infection, X4 viruses eventually become detectable in the blood of ~50% of individuals infected with subtype B viruses.[72,77,90–93] The appearance of X4 viruses at levels detectable by phenotypic assays typically takes ~5 years, but it can take much less time.[72,77,90–93] Death from AIDS does not require the appearance of X4 viruses at detectable levels in the blood, but the emergence of X4 viruses in both acute and chronic infection is associated with accelerated CD4+ T-cell count decline, and the relatively rapid onset of AIDS and death.[67–71,73–76,94] Even in chronic infection, however, it is unusual for X4 viruses to dominate plasma viremia; in most cases, the infection is phenotypically mixed (R5+X4), with the R5 component being the major contributor to the total viral load.[92,94]

It is still uncertain whether the emergence of X4 viruses is the cause or consequence of immune destruction; the interrelations between the viral phenotype and the immune system can be complex.[3] The preferential tropism of X4 and R5 viruses for naive and memory cells, respectively, has been used to model the tropism switch under *in vivo* conditions.[95] Memory T-cells divide ~10 times as often as naive cells in uninfected people. Because HIV-1 replication is more efficient in CD4+ T cells that are activated, the tropism of R5 viruses for memory cells could provide them with a quantitative advantage in early infection.[96,97] In lymphoid tissue blocks, *in vitro*, ~10-fold more R5 viruses than X4 viruses are produced on a per cell basis; their "burst-size" is higher.[98] However, during disease progression, and at low CD4 counts in particular, the division frequency of naive T cells approaches that of memory cells.[99,100] Since naive T cells are more abundant *in vivo*, particularly after R5 viruses have depleted the memory T-cell pool, this scenario provides a quantitative basis for the X4 switch late in disease.[95] Low CD4 counts may therefore both drive and arise from the late dominance of X4 viruses.[95] Such arguments underline the old cause-or-consequence controversy and imply that the R5 to X4 switch process might involve a lethal spiral.[95] Overall, R5 viruses are deadly, their X4 cousins deadlier.[57]

The tropism variants destroy the immune system in different ways, something clearly demonstrated in the macaque model. A pathogenic R5 SIV gradually, but eventually completely, depletes the memory CD4+ T-cell pool, whereas an X4 simian human immunodeficiency virus (SHIV) very rapidly destroys the entire repertoire of naive T cells in the periphery and lymphoid tissues.[80,101,102] Indeed, X4 SHIVs cause ultra-rapid progression to AIDS; the extremely rapid loss of CD4+ T-cell help for B cells even prevents the animals from developing antibody responses to viral antigens.[103] Rapid progression can also occur in a small minority of macaques infected with an R5 SIV, emphasizing the importance of host variation as an influence on the rate of disease.[104–106]

Although most R5 viruses replicate in macrophages, the R5 phenotype and macrophage tropism correlate imperfectly.[107] For example, some X4 viruses can replicate in macrophages, for reasons that probably lie in considerations of CD4+, CCR5 and CXCR4 density which are much lower on macrophages than on activated CD4+ T cells.[54,108–112] We noted earlier that R5 viruses are pathogenic even when X4 strains cannot be detected. An increased ability to replicate in macrophages is one correlate of disease progression mediated by R5 viruses.[113,114] However, it is unclear whether this is a direct consequence of HIV-1 replication in macrophages or a surrogate marker for a viral adaptation to use low CD4 and CCR5 levels more efficiently.[115] Thus, any remaining CD4+ T-cells expressing only low levels of CCR5 would also become vulnerable to more virulent R5 variants with an increased CCR5 affinity. Any increase in the ability of HIV-1 to use low CCR5 levels via an affinity increase might result in decreased susceptibility to CCR5 inhibitors and other entry inhibitors.[115,116] This point will be revisited below, because it is relevant to a consideration of when is the best time to start therapy with CCR5 inhibitors; their early use may be favored on virological grounds, as well as immunological ones, although safety issues must also be considered.[57]

Although most plasma virus is derived from CD4+ T cells, infected macrophages can sustain very high levels of virus replication.[106,117,118] Thus, in macaques infected with X4 SHIVs all the naive CD4+ T cells are rapidly eliminated to the extent that no CD4+ T cells can be detected in the peripheral blood or lymphoid tissues.[80,101,102] Yet plasma viremia levels remain extremely high because X4 viruses are produced by infected macrophages.[117,118] These cells may also be responsible for producing the even higher levels of R5 SIV that are sustained in dual-infected macaques after depletion of the CD4+ T-cell pool by an X4 SHIV.[106,119] Hence it will be useful to determine what effects CCR5 and CXCR4 inhibitors have on macrophage infection *in vivo*.

Some central questions about HIV-1 co-receptor use *in vivo* remain unanswered. For example, it is still not clear why X4 viruses emerge (or re-emerge) at high levels after several years only in some individuals and not in others. What host factors are the most relevant here? For more detailed considerations of the relationships between HIV-1 tropism and the immune system, additional reviews should be consulted.[2,3,81,84,107,120,121]

ASSAYS TO DETERMINE HIV-1 TROPISM

Given the importance of tropism as an influence on HIV-1 pathogenesis, and conceivably on treatment options, it follows that there should be accurate methods for the routine identification and quantification of tropism variants. The MT-2 syncytium formation assay indirectly measures co-receptor use because MT-2 cells express CXCR4 and CD4, but not CCR5.[3] Thus, if an isolate forms syncytia in MT-2 cells, it contains X4 or R5X4 viruses. More recently, assays using recombinant viruses have now developed to assess the co-receptor usage of clinical isolates. The Phenoscript (VIRalliance, Paris, France) and Trofile (Monogram Biosciences, Inc, South San Francisco, CA, USA) assays are available commercially.[10,122] HIV-1 *env* sequences are amplified in bulk from plasma and used to produce replication-competent viruses (Phenoscript) or replication-defective pseudoviruses (Trofile).[10,122] These viruses are used to infect target cell lines engineered to express CD4 and either CCR5 or CXCR4, the outcome being determined by activation of a reporter gene present in the cells (Phenoscript) or in the incoming viruses (Trofile).[10,122] As noted above, when a plasma sample registers as positive on both CCR5- and CXCR4-expressing cells, it usually means it contains a mixture of R5 and X4 viruses. A truly R5X4 virus cannot be distinguished from a phenotypic mixture in assays such as Phenoscript or Trofile.[3,123]

There are limitations to the present generation of tropism assays and since they could affect treatment decisions, they need to be understood. The most troublesome problem is, perhaps, the detection threshold for viruses of one phenotype in the presence of a larger amount of the other one.[57] For example, the Trofile assay can only reliably detect X4 viruses in mixtures when they constitute at least 10% of the total.[10] As an example of why this limit could cause relevant virological changes to go undetected, in a macaque that was deliberately dual-infected with an R5 SIV and an X4 SHIV the X4 component constituted ~4% of the total viral load at baseline, as measured using a highly specific, PCR-based discriminatory viral load assay.[119] It is questionable whether this animal would have registered as dual-infected using the Trofile assay, and whether that assay could have properly quantified the transient increase then decrease in the X4 component that occurred during CCR5 inhibitor therapy.[119]

The absolute sensitivity limit of the Trofile assay, i.e., the lowest viral load at which it can reliably detect the presence of viruses of either phenotype, is also an issue.[10,122] Such considerations are important, because very low plasma levels of X4 viruses may still have clinical significance, even if they cannot be readily detected and quantified.[92] An example is the accidental recruitment of a patient into a phase I trial of a CCR5 inhibitor who harbored low levels of X4 viruses; as per protocol such individuals were excluded from this study, but the screening assay (Trofile) was initially unable to detect the X4 component of the viral load.[124] In clinical practice, it would also be very important to discriminate between an absolute increase in the amount of X4 viruses during CCR5 inhibitor therapy (see further ahead), and a relative increase caused because the R5 component of a mixed R5+X4 infection is lowered by the therapy (Fig. 24-3).[57] The latter outcome would not necessarily be a bad one, but any sustained switching of co-receptor usage would certainly be unwanted. A truly useful phenotypic assay must, therefore, be able to discriminate satisfactorily between the above scenarios.

The present generation of phenotypic assays use cell lines engineered to express CCR5 or CXCR4 in combination with CD4.[10,122] Co-receptor usage on transfected cell lines and primary cells does not always correlate.[47,125–127] For example, some viruses that score as R5X4 (or R5+X4) on cell lines only use CXCR4 to enter primary CD4+ T cells.[47,126,127] A similar discordance might affect the diagnosis of resistance to CCR5 inhibitors.[128] Thus, CCR5 and CXCR4 adopt an array of conformational states on cell surfaces.[129] If the relative amounts of different configurations vary from cell to cell, there could be a cell type-specific discordance in how resistant viruses enter different cell types. The expression levels of CCR5 and CXCR4 on primary and engineered cells also differ, another potential influence on the output of phenotypic assays.[57]

Significant efforts have also been applied to defining genetic algorithms that predict tropism, the basis of a genotypic assay for CCR5 and CXCR4 use.[130–134] These methods are mostly based on analyzing the sequence of the V3 region of gp120, because a few 'signature residues' in V3 are correlated with the R5 and X4 phenotypes.[132,134,135] The predictive powers of the genotyping assays are increasing, but gp120 sequence variation is sufficient to create imperfections in phenotype-genotype correlations.[32,134] As an example of the plasticity of gp120, viruses completely resistant to small

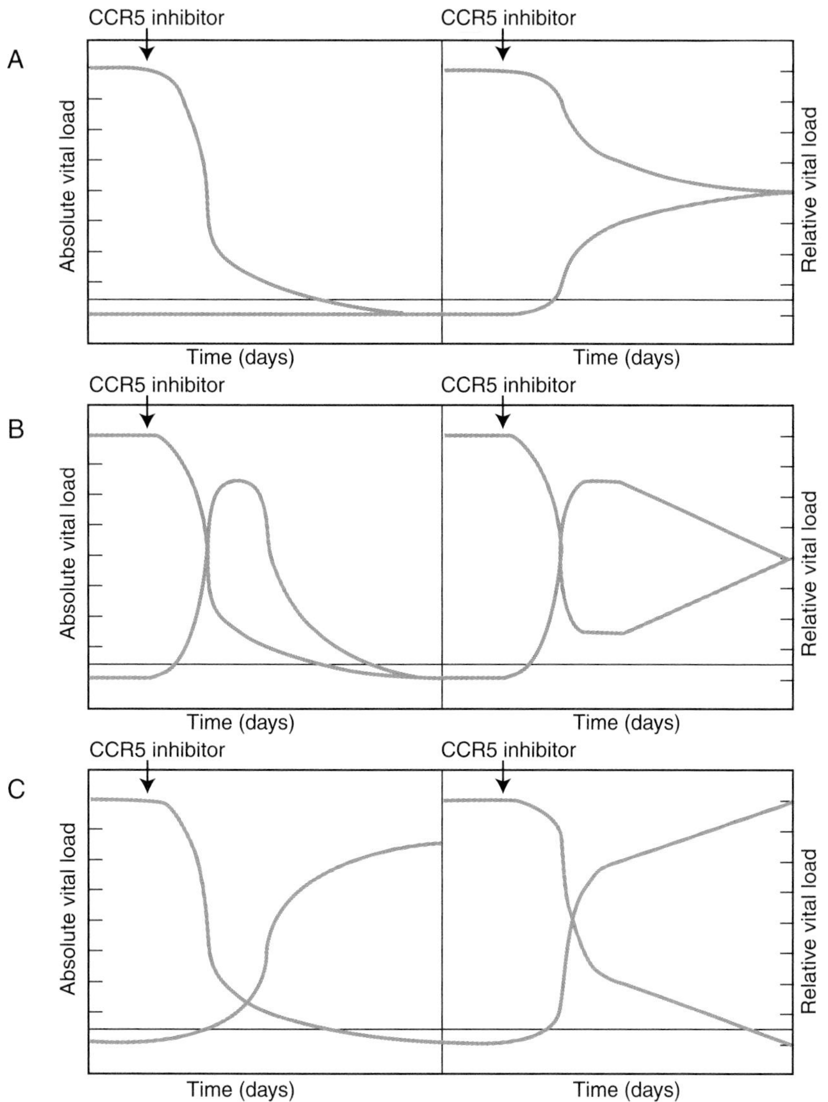

Figure 24-3 ■ Theoretical scenarios for the effects of CCR5 inhibitor therapy on R5 and X4 virus loads. In each scenario, the left panel depicts absolute viral loads (in arbitrary units), with R5 viruses high and X4 viruses undetectable. The right panel shows relative viral loads (i.e., the relative contributions of R5 and X4 viruses to the total viral load). The threshold for detection of X4 viruses in a phenotypic assay is indicated by the horizontal line. (A) The CCR5 inhibitor selectively blocks R5 virus replication and has no effect on X4 viruses. The absolute level of X4 viruses is unaffected, but because R5 viral load drops, the relative contribution of X4 viruses to the total viral load increases. In theory, this might make X4 viruses become detectable in phenotypic assays. Whether this could happen in practice is an important issue to resolve. (B) Transient increases in both absolute and relative X4 viral loads occur when the R5 viral load declines as a result of CCR5 inhibitor therapy. This scenario is similar to what was seen in two of three R5+X4 virus infected macaques treated with the R5 inhibitor CMPD 167.[119] Whether it would happen in HIV-1 infected people remains to be determined. (C) In this scenario, the therapy-induced decline in R5 viral load causes a sustained, possibly reciprocal, increase in X4 viral load. This is not a consequence of viral escape (i.e., R5 to X4 interconversion) but is due to expansion of X4 viruses into a niche vacated by R5 viruses.[3] Again, whether this will occur in clinical practice is unknown. In all three scenarios the initial X4 viral load is depicted as being below the threshold of detection in a phenotypic assay because CCR5 inhibitors are most likely to be tested clinically under these conditions. If the phenotypic assays are sensitive to changes in absolute viral load, as depicted on the left of each panel, then it should be possible to resolve between the different scenarios. However, if relative viral load has a significant influence on the clinical performance of these assays, as depicted on the right of each panel, it may not be easy to determine which scenario most applies to the clinical data. This would complicate the taking of clinical decisions. In practice, CCR5 inhibitors will not be tested as monotherapy, but we have not attempted to model the influence of other drugs that are active against both R5 and X4 viruses.

Reproduced from Kuhmann SE, Moore JP. The HIV-1 phenotypic variants: deadly and deadlier. J Viral Entry 1:4, 2005.

Co-receptor Tropism in HIV-Infected Patient Cohorts as Determined by the Trofile Assay

Table 24-1

Study	Patient Population	N	R5 only(%)	R5+X4(%)	X4 only
Brumme et al[139]	Treatment-naive	979	82	18	0.1%
Moyle et al[94]	Treatment-naive	402	81	19	Not available
Demarest et al[140]	Treatment-naive	299	88	12	0%
Moyle et al[94]	Treatment-experienced – virologic failure on first ART regimen	161	78	22	Not available
Demarest et al[140]	Treatment-experienced – not all PI-experienced	113	67	28	5%
Melby et al[141]	Heavily treatment-experienced	724	50	48	2%
Wilkin et al[142]	Heavily treatment-experienced	368	49	47	4%

molecule CCR5 inhibitors can sometimes have sequence changes in V3, and sometimes not.[128,136–138] Thus it may be very difficult to develop genetic assays of resistance to CCR5 inhibitors; signature residues for resistance may simply not exist, or their presence may be blurred by other changes within or outside V3. Additional improvements will be needed if genotypic assays are to be used routinely for co-receptor phenotype assessment in the clinic.[132]

No perfect assay for HIV-1 tropism is yet available. Whether the perceived imperfections of the present assays truly matter in routine clinical practice remains to be determined. The ongoing clinical trials of the co-receptor inhibitors may provide the answer. It will be particularly important to determine whether the low-level detection of minority viral populations that are apparently indicative of co-receptor switching have any real clinical significance.

Several population-based investigations of co-receptor tropism have been reported using the Trofile assay (Table 24-1). In general, treatment-naive populations with higher CD4 cell counts have the greatest proportion of R5 viruses; as the CD4 cell count falls, and also after the use of antiretroviral therapy, the prevalence of R5+X4 viruses increases. In a cross-sectional assessment, co-receptor tropism could be successfully determined in 979 (82%) of 1191 HIV-1-infected, treatment-naive patients from the HOMER cohort in British Columbia: of these, 82% had R5 virus, 18% had R5+X4 virus and only a single patient (<0.1%) had X4 virus.[139] Patients for whom viral phenotypes could be determined had higher HIV-1 RNA levels (130000 vs 61 000 copies/mL, $P < 0.001$), lower CD4 cell counts (260 vs 330/mm^3, $P = 0.007$), and were less often CCR5-Δ32 heterozygotes (13% vs 20%, $P = 0.007$), compared to those that yielded no phenotypic information. Individuals harboring R5+X4 viruses had higher HIV-1 RNA levels (175000 vs 120000 copies/mL, $P = 0.006$), lower CD4 cell counts (110 vs 290/mm^3, $P < 0.001$), and more often had a prior AIDS diagnosis (22% vs 11%, $P < 0.001$) than patients with only R5 viruses. In a multivariate analysis, both a higher HIV-1 RNA level and a lower CD4 cell count were associated with the presence of an R5+X4 virus. The association between R5+X4 virus and a lower CD4 cell count was particularly strong; 54% of patients with CD4 cell counts <25/mm^3 harbored an R5+X4 virus but only 7% of patients with CD4 >500/mm^3 did so.[139]

Another cross-sectional analysis was conducted on 861 patients followed at the Chelsea and Westminster Hospital in London.[94] Viral phenotypes were successfully determined for 563 (65%) of the 861 patients tested (including 19% with nonsubtype B viruses, 65% who were treatment-naive patients and 35% who had failed their first antiretroviral regimen). Tropism results were more frequently obtained from patients with higher HIV RNA levels (39325 vs 12793 copies/mL, $P < 0.001$), but less often from those whose viruses were from outside subtype B (16% vs 20%). In the 402 treatment-naive patients with tropism results, 81% had R5 virus and 19% had R5+X4 or X4 virus; in the 161 treatment-experienced patients failing their first antiretroviral regimen, 78% had R5 virus and 22% had R5+X4 or X4 virus ($P = 0.35$). Overall, only four patients (0.7%) had exclusively X4 virus. Patients with R5+X4 or X4 viruses had higher HIV-1 RNA levels (4.82 vs 4.55 $\log_{10}$ copies/mL) and lower CD4 cell counts (231 vs 307/mm^3) than those with R5 viruses; no significant associations with antiretroviral treatment experience or viral genetic subtype were seen. In a multivariate analysis, the presence of an R5 virus was significantly associated with a lower HIV-1 RNA level, a higher CD4 cell count, and a lower natural killer (NK) cell count.[94]

A cross-sectional analysis of tropism was also conducted in 412 patients enrolled in three clinical trials of a CCR5 inhibitor.[140] The group consisted of 299 treatment-naive patients and 113 patients taking a failing antiretroviral regimen. Among the treatment-naive patients, 88% had R5 viruses, the remaining 12% R5+X4 viruses, while in the experienced patients, 67% were R5, 28% R5+X4 and 5% X4. The presence of R5+X4 viruses was associated with a decreasing CD4/CD8 ratio in treatment-naive subjects ($P < 0.0001$) and with increased age ($P = 0.039$), nonwhite ethnicity ($P = 0.002$) and prior protease inhibitor (PI) treatment ($P = 0.009$) in treatment-experienced patients.[140]

Other assessments of tropism have been conducted in heavily treatment-experienced patients. From the TORO studies of enfuvirtide, 724 three-class treatment-experienced patients underwent tropism testing at baseline, of whom 50% had R5 viruses, 48% R5+X4 and 2% X4.[141] Regression analysis identified an association between R5+X4 virus and lower CD4 cell counts ($P < 0.001$), although R5+X4 viruses were also identified in 40% of patients with CD4 cell counts >200/mm^3. No association was seen between R5+X4 virus and the number of antiretroviral drugs previously taken, the baseline phenotypic sensitivity score, or the prior use of the PI, lopinavir/ritonavir (all $P > 0.5$).[141]

In the AIDS Clinical Trials Group 5211 study, heavily treatment-experienced patients were screened for tropism at baseline with results obtained from 368 participants.[142] Of these patients, 48% harbored R5 viruses, 48% R5+X4 viruses, 4% X4 viruses. There was no influence of gender on tropism; 52% of women and 51% of men harbored R5 viruses. However, R5 viruses were more common in white (52%) and Hispanic (67%) patients than in blacks (42%) ($P = 0.06$). In multivariate analysis, the presence of an R5+X4 or X4 virus was associated with a lower CD4 cell count ($P = 0.03$), but not with the HIV-1 RNA level or with drug resistance mutations, compared to when R5 viruses were present.[142]

Tropism was also determined for viruses isolated from both plasma and cerebrospinal fluid (CSF) in a cross-section of 46 patients from San Francisco, 80% of whom were treatment-naive, the remaining 20% treatment-experienced.[123] Of the plasma viruses, 83% were R5, 17% R5+X4, virtually identical to what was observed for the CSF viruses: 85% R5, 15% R5+X4. Pure X4 viruses were present in none of the plasma or CSF samples. The tropism determinations were concordant for most patients. 78% had R5 viruses and 11% had R5+X4 virus in both the plasma and CSF samples. However, tropism was discordant in five (11%) of the patients: two had R5 viruses in the plasma but R5+X4 viruses in the CSF, whereas three had R5+X4 viruses in the plasma and R5 viruses in the CSF. In principle, the discordant tropism observed in the CSF could have implications for CCR5 inhibitor therapy.[123]

THE BINDING OF GP120 TO CCR5 OR CXCR4 AS A DRUG TARGET

As noted earlier, the CD4-triggered binding of gp120 to a co-receptor is a critical stage in the fusion pathway, and it is the step that is interfered with by the class of HIV-1 drugs now referred to as co-receptor inhibitors (Table 24-2, Fig. 24-4).[56,143–145]

The binding of gp120 to CCR5 or CXCR4 involves multiple, discontinuous regions of the various proteins that form complex binding sites for one another. The co-receptor-binding site on gp120 is fully formed only after gp120 interacts with CD4.[23] The V3 region and the conserved β19 strand are the most important gp120 regions involved in CCR5 and CXCR4 binding,[24,30,31] the V3 residues contributing specificity for one co-receptor versus the other.[32]

Two distinct regions of CCR5 and CXCR4 interact with gp120, the N-terminus (Nt) and the second extracellular loop (ECL2).[146,147] There are four tyrosine residues in the CCR5 Nt, each of which can be sulfated.[148] Tyrosine sulfation, particularly at Tyr-10 and Tyr-14, is important for the efficient binding of gp120 to CCR5 or CXCR4, and viral entry, as well as for chemokine binding.[149–153]

The nature of the gp120–co-receptor interaction is probably broadly similar for CCR5 and CXCR4. Our current understanding is that the negatively charged co-receptor Nt probably associates with cationic gp120 residues in the β19 strand and near the V3 base, while ECL2 residues interact with the V3 crown.[24,32,154] However, subtle differences also need to be taken into account. Thus, V3 residues may be more important for gp120 binding to CXCR4 than to CCR5,[32] and the ECL2 region seems to play more of a role than the Nt in the gp120–CXCR4 interaction, whereas the converse may be true for gp120–CCR5 binding.[147]

The small molecule CCR5 inhibitors discussed below do not, however, directly block the gp120–CCR5 interaction. Instead, they act by inducing allosteric changes in CCR5 that render it unrecognizable by gp120.[129,155–158] The same mechanism almost certainly operates for the CXCR4 small molecule inhibitors as well, although this has not been studied in any detail. Based on mutagenesis studies and molecular modeling, the putative binding site for several small molecule CCR5 inhibitors is a small cavity formed between the transmembrane helices on the extracellular face of CCR5 and distant from the gp120 binding site.[156,159–161] Although it is likely that the details of how these inhibitors bind to this pocket differ from one compound to the next, their similar mechanisms of action imply that their binding sites are also broadly alike.[157] The comparative studies that have been performed with the investigational CCR5 inhibitors AD101, SCH-C, and TAK-779 suggest that each compound has a very similar dependence on residues that line the inhibitor-binding pocket within transmembrane helices 1, 2, 3, and 7, albeit with some compound-specific variation.[156,160,162] Mutational analyses of the binding sites for the investigational CCR5 inhibitors TAK-220 (Takeda) and CMPD 167 (Merck) indicate that they substantially overlap with those for AD101, SCH-C, and TAK-779, with additional contributions from residues in the other transmembrane helices, particularly helix 6.[159,161] Similar studies with the FDA-approved CCR5 inhibitor maraviroc have also emphasized the subtle compound-specific differences in the way these antagonists interact with CCR5.[163] In addition, some CCR5 amino acid residues may be important for the activity, but not the binding, of the small molecule inhibitors, lending support to the view that these compounds act allosterically and not competitively.[155]

Monoclonal antibodies (MAbs) such as PRO 140 are likely to act differently from the small molecules by directly impeding access of gp120 to its binding site on CCR5

Table 24-2

Co-receptor Inhibitors that have Entered Clinical Trials

Compound Name (Abbreviation)	Other Names	Manufacturer	Type of Inhibitor	Stage of Development	CYP 3A4 Interaction; RTV Effect on Compound Concentrations	Candidate Dose(s)	Maximal Virologic Activity (HIV RNA log_{10} copies/mL)[a]
AMD-070	AMD 11070	Anormed	CXCR4 – small molecule	Phase I	Under investigation	Under investigation	Unknown
AMD-3100	JM3100, SID 791	Anormed	CXCR4 – small molecule	Development terminated due to suboptimal antiretroviral activity and cardiac toxicity	Unknown		−0.9 (160 μg/kg/h) (day 11)
aplaviroc (APL)	GW 873140, AK 602, ONO 4128	GlaxoSmithKline	CCR5 – small molecule	Development terminated due to hepatoxicity	Substrate; RTV ↑ two- to sevenfold		−1.7 (600 mg bid) (day 12)
MAb004		Human Genome Sciences	CCR5 – monoclonal antibody	Phase I	None	Under investigation	Unknown
maraviroc (MVC)	UK-427 857	Pfizer	CCR5 – small molecule	FDA-approved	Substrate; RTV ↑ twofold	300 mg bid (with NVP, TPV/RTV); 150 mg bid (with other PIs/RTV); 600 mg bid (with EFV)	−1.4 (150 mg bid) −1.6 (300 mg bid) (without RTV) (day 11)
PRO 140		Progenics	CCR5 – monoclonal antibody	Phase I	None	0.5, 2.0, 5.0 mg/kg every 2 weeks	−1.9 (5 mg/kg)
SCH-C	Schering C. SCH 351125	Schering–Plough	CCRS – small molecule	Development terminated due to cardiac toxicity	Unknown		−0.7 (25 mg bid) (day 8)
vicriviroc (VCV)	SCH-D, Schering D, SCH 417690	Schering–Plough	CCR5 – Small molecule	Phase II in treatment-experienced patients	Substrate; RTV ↑ 3.5–5-fold	10 mg qd or 15 mg qd (with RTV; treatment-experienced)	−1.5 (25 mg bid) −1.6 (50 mg bid) (without RTV) −1.2 (day 14)

[a]Average viral load change from baseline when used as monotherapy; RTV, ritonavir.

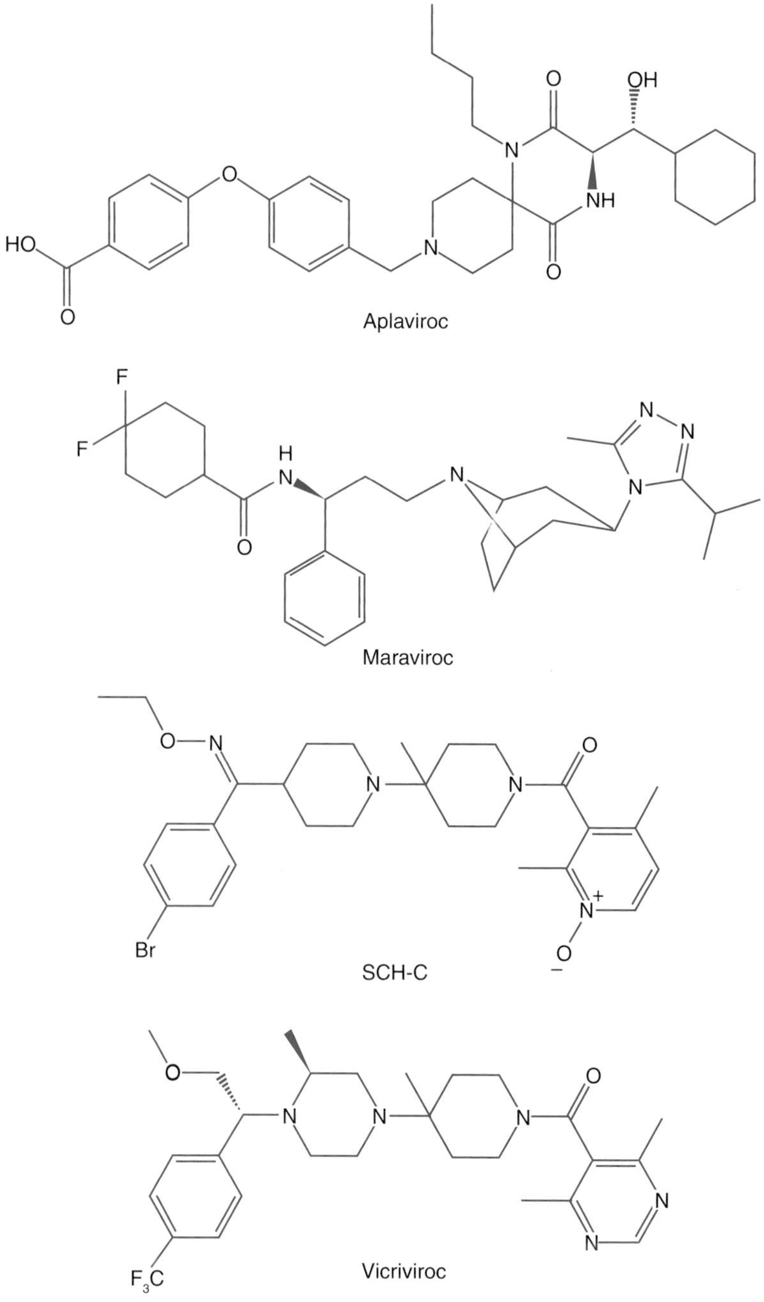

Figure 24-4 ■ The structures of four CCR5 inhibitors that have shown antiviral activity in HIV-1-infected patients.

inhibitor, although there are some uncertainties about the mechanism.[164,165] The binding site for PRO 140 is probably identical to that of the murine MAb PA14 from which it was derived by humanization; it involves residues in the CCR5 Nt and ECL-2 and so essentially overlaps the binding site on CCR5 for gp120.[147,165]

Studies of how the investigational CXCR4 inhibitor AMD3100 binds to CXCR4 suggest that the binding pocket for this inhibitor also lies within the TM helices, facing the outside of the cell.[166,167] The pocket is probably lined with several acidic residues that interact with positively charged atoms in AMD3100.[166] How AMD11070 binds to CXCR4 has not been reported, but a reasonable supposition is that it interacts with the same pocket.

A notable feature of the small molecule CCR5 inhibitors is their long half-life on the receptor, which can exceed 1 week in a cell-free system.[157] The longevity of the inhibitor-receptor complex may underlie delayed rebounds in plasma viremia seen after the cessation of therapy in both HIV-1-infected humans and in some SIV-infected macaques.[168,169] There may also be a prolonged interaction between AMD3100 and CXCR4.[170] It can reasonably be expected that PRO 140 and similar MAbs would also have a long receptor half-life as well. However, these various inhibitors do not

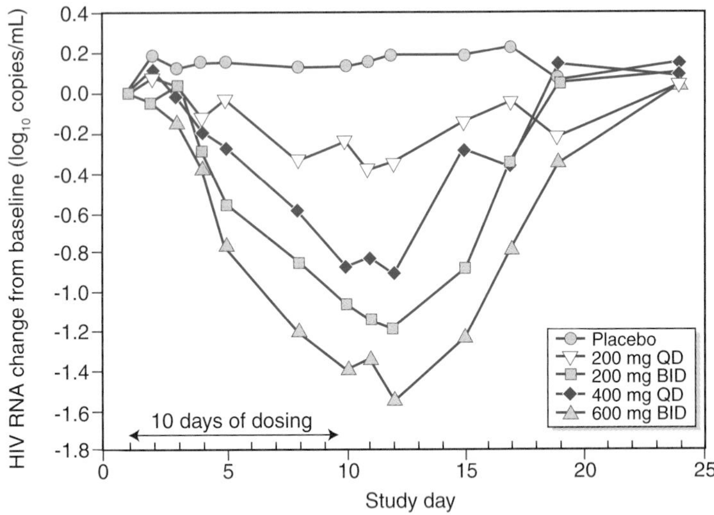

Figure 24-5 ■ Mean change in $\log_{10}$ plasma viral load over time during treatment with aplaviroc by dose group.

Reproduced from Lalezari J, Thompson M, Kumar P, et al. Antiviral activity and safety of 873140, a novel CCR5 antagonist, during short-term monotherapy in HIV-infected adults. AIDS 19:1443, 2005.

downregulate CCR5 from the cell surface, they occupy it in a way that renders it unusable by HIV-1. Because the small molecules also prevent chemokines from binding and signaling, the disruption of a feedback loop can increase the local concentration of chemokines.[171] The mechanism may be similar to that which elevates chemokine levels in cultures of CD4+ T cell from individuals with the CCR5-Δ32 allele.[172] In principle, these chemokines could either reinforce the antiviral activity of the inhibitors or, alternatively, cause immunological complications.

THE CLINICAL DEVELOPMENT OF CCR5 INHIBITORS

Several orally available small molecule CCR5 inhibitors have been evaluated in HIV-1-infected people: aplaviroc (formerly GSK-873140) from GlaxoSmithKline, maraviroc (formerly UK-427 857) from Pfizer, and SCH-C and vicriviroc (formerly SCH-D), both from Schering Plough (Fig. 24-4).[173–176] Antiviral efficacy was demonstrated for all four compounds, the mean viral load reduction at optimal dosing in 10–14 day monotherapy trials was in the range 1.5–1.7 $\log_{10}$.[173–176] This reduction is comparable to what was observed with another small molecule CCR5 inhibitor, CMPD 167, in SIV-infected macaques.[119,169] The SCH-C and aplaviroc clinical development programs have now been terminated, while maraviroc is FDA-approved and vicriviroc is in advanced clinical trials. Two humanized or human anti-CCR5 MAbs, PRO-140, from Progenics and CCR5mAb004 from Human Genome Sciences are now in phase I trials as injectable drugs.[5,56,144,177] The clinical development of all these compounds is discussed in more detail below.

Aplaviroc

Aplaviroc (APL, formerly GW 873140, AK 602, and ONO 4128) is a small-molecule spirodiketopiperazine compound that entered clinical trials. It has potent antiretroviral activity *in vitro* with an IC_{50} <4 nM, including against viruses from multiple genetic subtypes.[178] APL acts additively/synergistically *in vitro* with RTIs; PIs; enfuvirtide; other investigational CCR5 inhibitors; and investigational CXCR4 inhibitors[179] (see further ahead for a discussion of "synergy"). Like all the CCR5 small molecules, APL is an allosteric, noncompetitive inhibitor that prevents gp120 binding.[157] As noted above, the half-life of the inhibitor-CCR5 complex in a cell-free system is very long for all the small molecule drug candidates (>136 h for APL itself, slightly less for other tested compounds).[157] This may have beneficial clinical consequences; the median CCR5 receptor occupancy in eight HIV-1-negative subjects following 7 days of APL administration was 98%, and in a clinical study of 31 HIV-1-infected subjects, the half-life of APL binding to CCR5 was 122 h.[180] APL is readily absorbed orally and is a substrate for the hepatic cytochrome P450 (CYP450) 3A system.[174] The area under the curve (AUC) concentration was dose-dependent, with some accumulation observed during a 10-day clinical dosing study.[174,181]

A phase I double-blind, randomized, placebo-controlled clinical study involved 40 HIV-1-infected individuals (19 treatment-naive and 21 treatment-experienced) with only R5 virus detectable (Trofile assay), a CD4 cell count nadir >200/mm^3 and a plasma viral load >5000 RNA copies/mL who had not received antiretroviral therapy in the preceding 12 weeks. Study subjects were randomized to one of four dosing cohorts for 10 days: APL at 200 mg once or twice daily, 400 mg daily, 600 mg twice daily, or matching placebo. The baseline viral load was ~4.36 $\log_{10}$ (23 000) RNA copies/mL, the CD4 cell count was ~350/mm^3.[174]

During the 10 days of APL dosing, there was a dose-dependent decrease in viral load, ranging from a mean change of –0.46 log copies/mL (at 200 mg daily) to –1.66 log copies/mL (at 600 mg twice daily) (Fig. 24-5). The nadir HIV-1 RNA level occurred at day 12 (i.e., 2 days after discontinuation of APL dosing). Viral load reductions were comparable in treatment-naive and -experienced subjects, and no changes in CD4 cell counts were observed. The most commonly reported drug related adverse events were gastrointestinal. They were diarrhea (25–37% APL, 0% placebo), loose stools (13–38% APL, 33% placebo), and nausea and abdominal pain (13–38% APL, 11% placebo). Gastrointestinal events occurred most commonly on study day 1 and were resolved within 1–3 days while therapy was continued. In one subject in the 200 mg daily dosing group, an R5+X4 virus was detected by the Trofile assay on day 10 but only R5 viruses were present on day 24. The study investigators concluded that APL had potent antiretroviral activity and was generally well tolerated.[174]

The effects of APL on plasma chemokine and cytokine levels have also been assessed clinically.[182] A total of 30 HIV-1-negative individuals received APL (200, 600, or 800 mg) or a placebo twice daily for 7 days, while 40 HIV-1-infected subjects were given the drug at 200 mg daily or twice daily, 400 mg daily or 600 mg twice daily, or received a placebo, for 10 days. In all participants, 10 of the 11 chemokines (RANTES, MIP-1α, IL-8 and MCP-1) or Th1/Th2 cytokines (TNF-α, IFN-γ, IL-2, IL-4, IL-5, IL-10) monitored were unaffected by APL administration. MIP-1β levels did increase transiently by 1.5–2.5-fold in the APL recipients, but remained within the normal range. The study investigators concluded that APL does not induce overt, global changes in the extent of immune activation.[182]

Drug–drug interactions can be anticipated with APL because it is a CYP450 3A substrate and such interactions have now been observed clinically. Thus, APL concentrations were increased by two- to threefold and by six- to sevenfold upon co-administration of ritonavir and lopinavir/ritonavir respectively, with no change in lopinavir levels and about a 30% increase in the ritonavir concentration.[181] Similarly, co-administration of atazanavir/ritonavir and APL increased APL concentrations seven- to 17-fold without effect on atazanavir levels.[183] Conversely, efavirenz co-administration decreased APL levels by 57% with no change in efavirenz concentrations.[184] However, no such APL concentration decrease was seen with co-administration of efavirenz and fosamprenavir/ritonavir.[185] Hence pharmacokinetic boosting with ritonavir could be useful to overcome the negative impact of efavirenz. No drug–drug interactions were observed when APL and tenofovir were co-administered.[186]

In September 2005, GlaxoSmithKline announced it was stopping its phase IIb dose-ranging studies of APL in treatment-naive patients, due to the occurrence of severe hepatotoxicity in a study participant.[187] The patient was a 39-year-old man with no history of viral hepatitis and normal baseline hepatic transaminase and bilirubin levels who was randomized to receive APL 800 mg twice daily together with zidovudine/lamivudine.[188] On study day 59, he developed severe hepatotoxicity; a liver biopsy revealed a chronic inflammatory infiltrate of moderate intensity, consistent with drug-induced hepatotoxicity. Upon discontinuation of the study medications, hepatic transaminase levels returned to baseline by study day 100. Further investigation revealed that among 282 subjects receiving APL in phase IIb studies, there were three additional cases of severe hepatotoxicity. In addition, one of 26 randomly assigned, treatment-experienced individuals in a phase III trial of APL had a severe elevation in hepatic transaminases at study week 4.[188] This event led to the termination of the phase III trial, and further clinical development of APL was stopped in October 2005.[189] In total, four (1%) APL recipients had ALT levels greater than three times the upper limit of normal (ULN) and bilirubin levels greater than 1.5 times the ULN, although none developed liver failure or died.[188]

Maraviroc

Maraviroc (MVC, formerly UK-427,857) is a small-molecule cyclohexanecarboxamide compound selected from ~1000 imidazopyridine analogs that were screened for binding to CCR5.[190] MVC has potent antiretroviral activity (mean IC_{90}, 2 nM) against R5 viruses of diverse geographic origin and from multiple genetic subtypes. It is also active against isolates from both treatment-naive patients and those who had taken currently available antiretroviral drugs. As expected, MVC is inactive against X4 viruses. *In vitro*, MVC acts additively/synergistically with reverse transcriptase inhibitors (RTIs), PIs, and enfuvirtide. MVC binding to CCR5 inhibits the binding of MIP-1α, MIP-1β and RANTES, but does not itself trigger release of intracellular calcium; thus in common with the other small molecule CCR5 inhibitors, MVC is a chemokine antagonist but not a CCR5 agonist. MVC inhibits both HIV-1 gp120 binding to CCR5 (IC_{50}, 11 nM) and HIV-1 entry into host cells (IC_{50}, 0.22 nM).[190] The dissociation half-life of MVC from the CCR5 receptor is ~16 h.[191]

In animal studies, MVC was absorbed rapidly and was 40% orally bioavailable; in humans, it was 23% bioavailable and had a half-life of 13 h, allowing once or twice daily dosing.[190,192,193] MVC is moderately lipophilic, but has relatively poor membrane permeability; its transcellular transport is mediated by the P-glycoprotein pathway. In oral dose escalation studies, MVC pharmacokinetics were nonlinear, leading to greater than expected concentrations at higher doses; thus, for a 10-fold increase in dose, C_{max} increased 40-fold and AUC increased 20-fold. MVC is a substrate (but not an inducer or inhibitor) of the hepatic cytochrome P450 3A4 enzyme system, is metabolized by oxidation, and is excreted predominantly unchanged (72–94% in feces and 5–20% in urine). There was no evidence of MVC accumulation over 10 days of dosing.[173]

No cytotoxicity or adverse effects of MVC were identified in experiments using *in vitro* models of human immune system function.[190] MVC was well tolerated in small animals, with no reported significant adverse events; it inhibited the cardiac potassium hERG channel only weakly and had no effect on the QTc interval.[190,194] In cynomolgus monkeys, MVC did not affect various immune system parameters such as lymphocyte subsets, natural killer cell activity, phagocyte counts or oxidative activity; the IgM or IgG responses

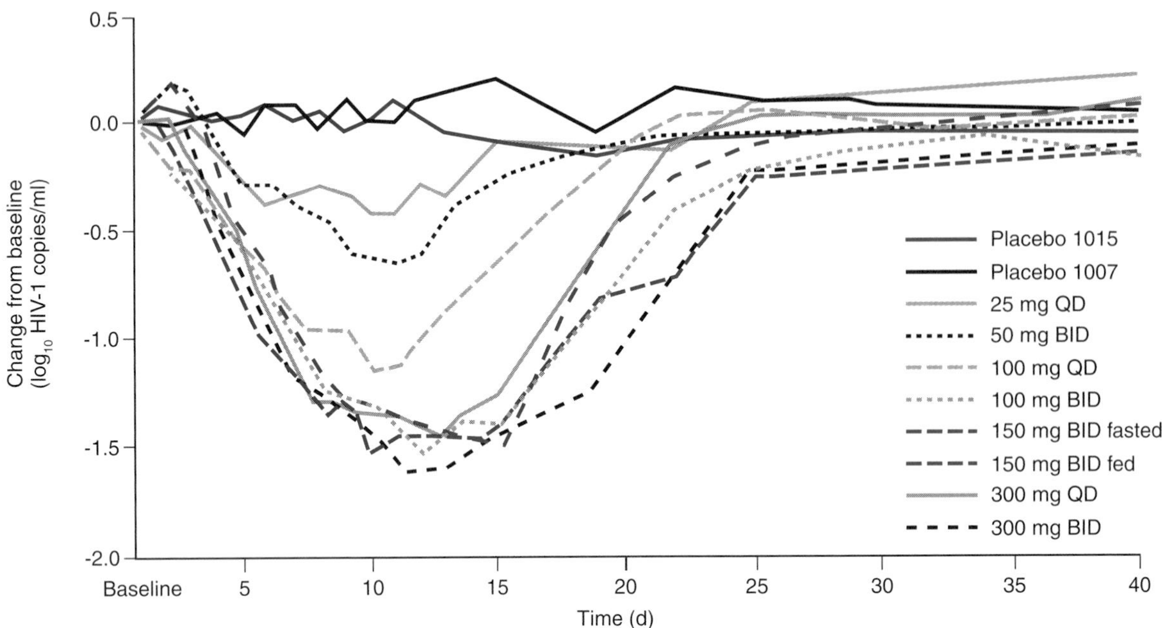

Figure 24-6 ■ Mean change in $\log_{10}$ plasma viral load over time during treatment with maraviroc by dose group.

Reproduced from Fatkenheuer G, Pozniak AL, Johnson MA, et al. Efficacy of short-term monotherapy with maraviroc, a new CCR5 antagonist, in patients infected with HIV-1. Nat Med 11:1170, 2005.

to keyhole limpet haemocyanin (KLH) were also unaltered, and MVC had no effect on the general histopathology of the immune system.[195] In a review of six clinical studies involving 195 HIV-1-infected MVC recipients, the most commonly noted treatment-related adverse events were headache, dizziness, nausea, asthenia, flatulence, and rhinitis, mostly of mild or moderate severity, with incidence rates similar to those in placebo recipients.[196] Four MVC recipients discontinued the study drug, three due to postural hypotension, the other because of elevated hepatic transaminases. There were no clinically significant changes in QTc interval in these six studies of HIV-1-infected recipients,[196] or in a formal evaluation of single-dose MVC in 61 HIV-1-negative volunteers.[197] A pharmacogenetic analysis revealed no association between 16 different CCR5 polymorphisms and blood pressure in 165 HIV-1-negative and 80 HIV-1-infected patients, suggesting that postural hypotension is not associated with CCR5 genotype.[198] An intensive study in HIV-1-negative volunteers showed that MVC at a dose of 900 mg (three times the proposed 300 mg dose) had a mild vasodilatory effect by reducing systemic vascular resistance.[199]

A single case of severe hepatotoxicity leading to liver failure occurred in a study of MVC in treatment-naive patients.[200] One subject randomized to receive MVC at 300 mg daily, together with zidovudine/lamivudine, developed a rash and severe hepatotoxicity after only four doses of the study drug. Although MVC was discontinued, isoniazid and other medications were continued and the patient was also started on lopinavir/ritonavir and parenteral paracetamol (acetaminophen). Hepatic transaminase levels worsened and the subject underwent liver transplantation on study day 16. An independent data safety monitoring board (DSMB) concluded that although MVC could not be excluded as the cause of hepatotoxicity, other medications are more likely to have been responsible. As a result, the MVC development program in both treatment-naive and treatment-experienced patients continues.[200]

Two randomized, placebo-controlled phase IIa studies were conducted to assess the short-term efficacy and safety of MVC in asymptomatic, HIV-1-infected patients with R5 viruses.[173] In total, 82 individuals were randomized to receive MVC at 25, 100, or 300 mg once daily, 50, 100, 150 mg fed and fasted, or 300 mg twice daily, or placebo for 10 days. Their mean baseline plasma viral load was 4.62 $\log_{10}$ (42 000) copies/mL, with a mean CD4 cell count of 544/mm^3. MVC resulted in a dose-dependent decrease in HIV-1 RNA levels at day 11, ranging from −0.43 log copies/mL (25 mg daily dose) to −1.60 log copies/mL (300 mg twice-daily dose) (Fig. 24-6). The mean CCR5 occupancy across the study group was >80% at day 5. The maximum viral load reduction occurred 1–4 days after MVC discontinuation. A single patient was retroactively identified as having entered the study despite the presence at baseline of R5+X4 viruses (according to the Trofile assay); there was little change in HIV-1 RNA level during therapy. Viral tropism changes were observed in two other subjects, both receiving 100 mg of MVC daily. In both cases, R5+X4 viruses were detected at day 11; in one case, only R5 viruses could be found at day 40; in the other, R5+X4 viruses persisted through day 433. As noted above, the clinical and methodological significance of such observations remain to be determined. Although food reduced the MVC C_{max} and AUC by 50–60%, C_{min} was unchanged, and the viral load reductions were similar when 150 mg of MVC was given twice daily to fed or fasting volunteers. The investigators concluded that MVC was potent, generally well tolerated, and did not require food restrictions.[173]

Drug–drug interactions between MVC and other medications can be anticipated because it is a substrate of the hepatic cytochrome P450 system.[201] A formal evaluation in HIV-1-infected patients taking various antiretroviral regimens and a single dose of 300 mg of MVC revealed that efavirenz-containing regimens reduced MVC concentrations by ~50% (n = 16), lopinavir/ritonavir-containing regimens increased MVC concentrations by about twofold (n = 5) and nevirapine increased the MVC C_{max}, but did not affect its AUC. In other studies, MVC concentrations were increased by CYP 3A4 inhibitors such as saquinavir, atazanavir, atazanavir/ritonavir, and ketoconazole, but MVC had no effect on the concentrations of zidovudine, lamivudine, tenofovir, trimethoprim, or oral contraceptive components.[192] Decreasing MVC doses by half corrected the interactions with ritonavir or ritonavir-boosted PIs (except tipranavir). MVC concentrations were decreased by CYP 3A4 inducers such as efavirenz (40–50%) and rifampin (30%), but these reductions could be overcome by doubling the MVC dose. Using lopinavir (or saquinavir)/ritonavir and efavirenz with MVC approximately halves the pharmacokinetic effect of the inhibitors. A more recent study in 12 HIV-1-negative subjects showed there was no significant interaction between MVC and tipranavir/ritonavir, and that no dose adjustment was necessary.[202]

In two phase III studies of treatment-experienced subjects with R5 viruses, MVC, when added to an optimized background antiretroviral regimen, demonstrated significantly better virologic activity than placebo with 41–48% of subjects reducing HIV RNA to <50 copies/ml at 24 weeks in the MVC groups[203,203a] These results led to FDA approval of maraviroc for treatment-experienced patients in August 2007. In a phase II clinical study however, maraviroc showed no virologic activity in subjects with X4, R5X4 or indeterminate viral phenotype.[203b] A phase III study in treatment-naive subjects compared zidovudine/lamivudine combined with either MVC given twice daily or efavirenz and found that 65% (MVC) vs. 69% (EFV) had HIV RNA levels suppressed to <50 copies/ml at 48 weeks, a difference that could not exclude a pre-specified 10% difference required to show non-inferiority of MVC.[203c]

SCH-C

Schering C (SCH-C, SCH 351125) is a small-molecule oxime-piperidine compound and investigational CCR5 inhibitor that potently inhibited R5 viruses *in vitro*, was orally bioavailable,[204] and reached clinical development.[175] However, the development of SCH-C was abandoned in favor of the structurally unrelated compound, SCH-D (vicriviroc), on the grounds that the latter was more potent and had a better selectivity among known GPCRs.

Vicriviroc

Vicriviroc (VCV, formerly SCH 417690, Schering D, SCH-D) is a small-molecule piperidine compound and investigational CCR5 inhibitor.[205,206] VCV has potent antiretroviral activity *in vitro* with mean EC_{50} and EC_{90} values of <3 and <19 nM respectively, against a panel of HIV-1 primary isolates from within and outside subtype B, and of diverse geographic origin. VCV was also active *in vitro* against strains resistant to RTIs, PIs and enfuvirtide, and also against MDR viruses. As would be anticipated, VCV did not inhibit the replication of X4 or R5+X4 viruses. Additivity/synergy was seen *in vitro* between VCV and representative HIV RTIs, PIs, and enfuvirtide.[205,207] *In vitro*, VCV inhibited signaling via MIP-1α, MIP-1β and RANTES indicating that it is a chemokine antagonist, but VCV does not itself activate signal transduction and is not a CCR5 agonist. VCV did not inhibit CYP450 hepatic enzymes *in vitro*, and no cytotoxicity was observed at VCV concentrations up to 10 μM.[205]

In dosing studies in rats and cynomolgus monkeys, VCV was 95–100% absorbed with 89–100% bioavailability.[205,206] The plasma half-life in monkeys was 3.4 h. In human plasma, 84% of VCV was protein-bound. In clinical studies with HIV-1-negative and HIV-1-infected subjects, VCV was rapidly absorbed and had high bioavailability with modest variability; its half-life of >24 h supported once or twice daily dosing.[208] When VCV was given at doses of 10, 25, and 50 mg twice daily, exposure increased in a dose-linear manner, steady state was attained by day 14 and there were no differences in pharmacokinetics between HIV-1-negative and HIV-1-infected subjects. In a clinical study of 20 HIV-negative adults given a single VCV dose (50 mg) either fasted or together with a high-fat meal, food decreased C_{max} concentrations by 58% but had no effect on the AUC. Hence co-administration of VCV with a high-fat meal decreased the rate of drug absorption, but not the overall extent of absorption, implying that VCV can be administered with or without food.[209]

VCV has a low affinity for the hERG ion channel *in vitro* and had no effect on the QTc interval in animal models.[205] In clinical studies with HIV-1-negative and HIV-1-infected individuals, neither single nor multiple doses of VCV caused a change in the QTc interval compared to placebo.[210] Phase I studies over 14 days in 47 HIV-1-infected subjects indicated that the most commonly reported adverse events were headache (28%), abdominal pain (14%), and nausea (14%).[208]

A total of 48 HIV-infected subjects who were either treatment-naive or had not received antiretroviral drugs over the prior 8 weeks, who had CCR5-tropic virus and CD4 cell counts at least 200/mm^3 were enrolled into a randomized, placebo-controlled phase IIa study to evaluate the safety and efficacy of VCV.[211] The study subjects were randomized to receive VCV at 10, 25, or 50 mg twice daily, or a matching placebo, for 14 days. The pharmacokinetic profiles showed dose proportionality with C_{min} steady state concentrations above the IC_{90}. Dose-dependent decreases in viral load at day 14 were –0.93 (10 mg), –1.49 (25 mg), and –1.62 (50 mg) log_{10} HIV RNA copies/mL, with the nadirs occurring several days after VCV dosing was discontinued. VCV therefore has a potent antiviral effect.[211]

VCV is a substrate of CYP 3A4, so drug–drug interactions can be anticipated. In a study of 46 healthy volunteers given VCV 10 mg twice daily alone or in combination with ritonavir (100, 200, or 400 mg twice daily) over 14 days, ritonavir was found to increase VCV concentrations by 3.5- to fivefold, regardless of the ritonavir dose.[212] In a similar study with 24 healthy volunteers, ritonavir and lopinavir/ritonavir increased VCV concentrations by 2.5–5.4-fold and by 2.3–4.2-fold, respectively.[213] Another study of 36 healthy volunteers given VCV 10 mg alone or together with either ritonavir 100 mg, efavirenz 600 mg or both ritonavir and efavirenz daily over 14 days revealed that ritonavir increased VCV concentrations by 2.8–5.8-fold, efavirenz decreased VCV levels by 67–81% and the combination of both ritonavir and efavirenz increased VCV concentrations by 2.0–3.8-fold.[214] In a pharmacokinetic study, eight HIV-1-negative volunteers received VCV and ritonavir for 14 days and then added a second PI, either fosamprenavir, indinavir, nelfinavir, or saquinavir for 14 days or atazanavir for 7 days.[215] There were no significant changes in VCV plasma concentrations with co-administration of any of the ritonavir-boosted PIs. In other studies, there were no interactions between VCV and either zidovudine/lamivudine[216] or tenofovir.[217]

In October 2005, Schering-Plough announced that it was discontinuing its phase II study of VCV in treatment-naive, HIV-1-infected subjects.[218] The study started in the spring of 2004 in Europe and Canada and enrolled 92 treatment-naive subjects who were randomized to receive VCV at one of three doses (25, 50, or 75 mg qd) or placebo for 14 days, and then to add zidovudine/lamivudine (or, in the placebo group, to start the standard three-drug regimen of zidovudine/lamivudine and efavirenz).[219] A review of the interim data by the independent DSMB revealed an increased rate of viral load rebound in the VCV group, leading to a recommendation that the study be stopped early. At day 14, HIV-1 RNA decreased by 0.9 $\log_{10}$ copies/mL (25 mg group), 1.2 $\log_{10}$ copies/mL (50 mg group), 1.3 $\log_{10}$ copies/mL (75 mg group), vs 0.1 $\log_{10}$ copies/mL (placebo group) ($P < 0.001$ for each VCV group vs placebo). However, at the time of study closure, the proportions of subjects with virologic rebound to >50 copies/mL were 57% (13 of 23 on 25 mg), 45% (10 of 22 on 50 mg), 22% (5 of 23 on 75 mg), vs 8% (two of 24 on zidovudine/lamivudine and efavirenz) ($P < 0.001$ for the pooled VCV groups vs the efavirenz group). All subjects with available genotypes at virologic failure demonstrated a treatment-emergent M184V substitution in reverse transcriptase (RT), associated with lamivudine resistance. The reasons for virologic failure are presently under active investigation but tolerability, pharmacokinetic parameters, or co-receptor switching to CXCR4 use did not appear to be responsible. The investigators concluded that the VCV-based regimen lacked durable virologic activity compared to the efavirenz-based regimen, in treatment-naive individuals who were starting their first antiretroviral regimen.[219]

AIDS Clinical Trials Group (ACTG) study 5211 enrolled treatment-experienced patients with R5 virus and compared VCV at one of 3 doses once-daily or placebo, each combined with an optimized background antiretroviral regimen that included ritonavir, and showed HIV RNA changes at week 24 of −1.9 (10 mg VCV), −1.7 (15 mg VCV) and −0.3 $\log_{10}$ copies/ml (placebo); the 5 mg VCV dosing arm was stopped early because of suboptimal virologic effect and more co-receptor changes.[219] A follow-up report showed durable virologic suppression at week 48 with the 10 and 15 mg VCV regimens.[220] On this study, 6 diverse malignancies occurred in subjects taking VCV; however causality could not be determined definitively. A second phase II study testing VCV at doses of 20 and 30 mg once-daily is in progress.

PRO 140

PRO 140 is a monoclonal IgG4 antibody that binds to CCR5 and inhibits HIV-1 entry.[165] Its epitope is on the external surface of CCR5 and includes elements of the second extracellular loop and the N-terminus, so its binding site on CCR5 is different from the pocket in the transmembrane helices for the small molecule inhibitors.[165] PRO 140 does not antagonize chemokine signaling via CCR5 and does not induce down-regulation of the receptor; it is neither an agonist nor a chemokine antagonist.[165] PRO 140 has potent activity (median IC_{90}, 17 nM) against the replication of R5 primary isolates from multiple genetic subtypes (A, B, C, E, F) of diverse geographic origin in both CD4+ T cells and macrophages.[221] It also inhibits primary isolates from patients with both acute and chronic HIV-1 infection.[222] As expected, PRO 140 lacks activity against X4 or most R5X4 viruses.[221] PRO 140 was first made as a murine monoclonal antibody (PA14) that was later humanized by grafting the complementarity determining region of the murine antibody onto the human IgG4 scaffold.[223] The inhibitory potencies of PA14 and PRO 140 are similar *in vitro*, and all subsequent clinical development work has been with humanized antibody. PRO 140 acts synergistically *in vitro* when combined with enfuvirtide, as well as with the small molecule CCR5 inhibitors, VCV, SCH-C, and TAK-779.[224] As discussed further below, this may be genuine, mechanism-based synergy. In a SCID-hu mouse model, PRO 140 inhibited the replication of an R5 virus, causing a viral load reduction of 1.7 $\log_{10}$ RNA copies/mL reduction over 8 days, without the emergence of resistance.[225]

The first human study of PRO 140 was a phase I, randomized, double-blind, placebo-controlled study of 20 HIV-1-negative men.[226,227] The volunteers were randomized 4:1 to receive a single intravenous dose of PRO 140 or a placebo in sequential dosing cohorts at 0.1, 0.5, 2.0, or 5.0 mg/kg. PRO 140 was generally well tolerated, with no reported clinically meaningful drug-related side effects; no significant electrocardiogram changes were observed. The serum concentrations of PRO 140 increased proportionally to the dose with a serum half-life of ~2 weeks. Dose-dependent binding of PRO 140 to CCR5 was seen with significant receptor occupancy being maintained for more than 60 days at the 5 mg/kg dose, and with no change in lymphocyte counts, plasma RANTES levels, or development of anti-PRO 140 antibodies.[226,227]

Because PRO 140 is a monoclonal antibody, significant drug–drug interactions would not be anticipated. Good agreement between viral tropism and PRO 140 susceptibility was shown using a standard virus replication assay and the commercially available Trofile assay.[228] Since their binding sites on CCR5 are different, cross-resistance between PRO 140 and the small molecule CCR5 inhibitors is likely to be minimal.[222] Escape mutants to the small molecules remain sensitive to PA14 and similar anti-CCR5 antibodies *in vitro*, which supports this prediction.[128,137,138,229]

A study in HIV-infected individuals administered single-doses of PRO 140 (0.5, 2, 5 mg/kg) or placebo and found maximal HIV RNA changes of -0.6 (0.5 mg/kg), −1.2 (2 mg/kg) and −1.8 (5 mg/kg) in the PRO 140 groups compared to −0.4 in the placebo group.[230] Further studies are planned.

Other CCR5 Inhibitors

TAK-779 (Takeda Pharmaceuticals) was the first reported small-molecule CCR5 inhibitor; it has significant activity against R5 HIV-1 strains *in vitro*, but its clinical development was compromised by its poor bioavailability.[231] TAK-652 was derived from TAK-779 and has potent activity against R5 strains *in vitro* with mean EC_{50} and EC_{90} values of 0.061 and 0.25 nM respectively, including cross-subtype activity.[232] TAK-652 acts additively/synergistically *in vitro* with RTIs, PIs, and enfuvirtide.[233] It is a chemokine receptor antagonist but does not induce CCR5 internalization or cause signal transduction.[232] A single-dose oral administration of TAK-652 (25, 50, or 100 mg) to 24 HIV-1-negative men showed that the compound was generally safe and well tolerated and that it was well absorbed. In a pharmokinetic analysis, TAK-652 had a long plasma half-life; thus the plasma concentration was 9.1 nM 24 h following administration of the 25 mg dose, suggesting that once-daily administration may be possible.[232] Further clinical development of TAK-652 can be anticipated.

The anti-CCR5mAb004 (Human Genome Sciences) is a human monoclonal antibody specific to CCR5. It binds CCR5 with an affinity of 1–2 nM, inhibiting chemokine binding without inducing intracellular signaling.[177] CCR5mAb004 inhibited HIV-1 infection *in vitro* when tested against a panel of 30 R5 viruses from subtypes A-G, including enfuvirtide-resistant strains; the median IC_{50} value was in the low nanomolar range. There was no evidence of complement-mediated lysis or antibody-dependent cell-mediated cytotoxicity when the antibody was tested *in vitro*, and it was found to have a prolonged serum half-life with ~95% bioavailability after subcutaneous administration.[177] A phase I study in HIV-1-infected subjects was initiated recently.

THE CLINICAL DEVELOPMENT OF CXCR4 INHIBITORS

Fewer CXCR4 inhibitors have been identified. One small molecule, AMD-3100 (AnorMED), completed phase I clinical trials; although it is no longer in clinical development as an HIV-1 therapeutic,[234] it is still being evaluated as a method to mobilize stem cells.[235] The orally bioavailable compound AMD11070 (AnorMED) is now in phase I trials in HIV-1-infected individuals (see further ahead) and additional orally bioavailable compounds (KRH-2731, -3140, -3955 (Kureha)) are in preclinical development.[236,237] Before it was identified as a CXCR4 antagonist, the 9-mer peptide ALX40–4C (Allelix) was tested in phase I/II clinical trials in HIV-1-infected people, although its development was discontinued several years ago, principally because of limited efficacy and the need to deliver the peptide by injection.[238]

AMD-3100

AMD-3100 (formerly JM3100 and SID 791) is a bicyclam compound that binds specifically to CXCR4.[170,239–241] *In vitro*, AMD-3100 has potent activity against X4 viruses (IC_{50}, 1–10 ng/mL) with no activity against R5 strains. It inhibits CXCR4-mediated signaling and chemotaxis, but does not change calcium flux, induce chemotaxis or trigger receptor internalization, indicating that it is a chemokine (SDF-1α) antagonist but not a CXCR4 agonist.[170,240,241] In a SCID-hu mouse model, AMD3100 administration by injection or continuous infusion significantly reduced the replication of an X4 HIV-1 strain.[242]

AMD-3100 had poor oral bioavailability of 3.9% (range 0.5–9.6%) in rats.[243] Its half-life following repeated intravenous dosing was 0.7–0.8 h. In rats and dogs, AMD-3100 was excreted primarily by the renal route following intravenous dosing, with 63–72% of the compound being recovered unchanged in the urine. Subcutaneous dosing in rats and dogs showed that maximum dose-proportional drug concentrations were achieved within 1–2 h. Dose-limiting toxicities in animals were sedation, spasms and dyspnea (rats); diarrhea and tachycardia (dogs).[243]

In the first clinical study, 13 HIV-1-negative subjects received AMD-3100 by intravenous infusion, subcutaneous injection or orally.[243] The study drug was generally well tolerated, the most commonly reported events being mild (grade 1) bloating, increased stool frequency/loose stools, and abdominal gas in the subjects who were dosed intravenously or subcutaneously. No serious adverse events or dose-limiting toxicities were identified, but a 1.5–3.1-fold increase in white blood cell counts from baseline was observed; the increase was dose-related at the lower doses of AMD-3100 and the white blood cell counts reverted to baseline within 24 h. Intravenous dosing caused a dose-proportional increase in plasma AMD-3100 concentrations, whereas subcutaneous dosing resulted in a 48% lower initial concentration peak and a median absorption of 87% compared to intravenous delivery, with identical elimination rates. No plasma AMD-3100 was detected following oral dosing.[243]

AMD-3100 was then tested in 40 HIV-1-infected subjects who were taking stable antiretroviral regimens or who were not receiving any therapy, and who had a HIV-1 RNA level >5000 copies/mL and a CD4 cell count $>50/mm^3$.[234] The

HIV-1 phenotype at baseline, assessed using the MT-2 cell assay, was SI in 30% of the patients, non-SI in 45% and not tested in the rest. Escalating doses of AMD-3100 (2.5, 5, 10, 20, 40, 80, and 160 μg/kg/h) were administered to successive cohorts by continuous infusion for 10 days. Whether to escalate the drug dose was based on meeting prespecified safety and virologic criteria. The 12 patients with SI viruses were defined as the efficacy-evaluable cohort and were enrolled at the higher dose levels. The study drug was discontinued in four patients for adverse events; premature ventricular contractions and hypocalcemia, panic attack and paresthesias, thrombocytopenia, and PICC-line infection. Adverse events leading to the temporary cessation of therapy were also observed in an additional four patients. These were bigeminy and premature ventricular contractions, orthostatic hypotension, postural tachycardia, and elevated liver enzymes. A dose-related prolonged increase (mean 2.7-fold) in white blood cell counts was also observed. Pharmacokinetic analyses showed there were dose-proportional increases in plasma AMD-3100 concentrations, with a mean half-life of 8.6 h. The median change in HIV RNA was +0.03 $\log_{10}$ copies/mL overall, and a 1 log or greater viral load decrease from baseline was not seen in any patient by study day 11. One patient receiving the highest dose (160 μg kg^{-1} h^{-1}) of AMD-3100 without other antiretroviral drugs had a viral load reduction of 0.9 $\log_{10}$ RNA copies/mL by day 11, and this suppression continued for 1 week after AMD-3100 infusion was discontinued. The investigators concluded that AMD-3100 demonstrated proof-of-concept as a CXCR4 inhibitor in this single patient, but overall had insufficient antiviral activity to be useful.[234] Further development of AMD-3100 as an antiretroviral agent was stopped, but it is still being studied clinically as a potential agent for stem cell mobilization.[244,245]

AMD-11070

AMD-070 is an investigational selective CXCR4 inhibitor currently in development. It has potent antiretroviral activity *in vitro* with an EC_{50} of 1–10 nM.[246] AMD-070 is active against X4 viruses, including strains resistant to other antiretroviral drugs, but had no activity against R5 or R5X4 viruses. Additivity/synergy was observed in combinations with RTIs, PIs, enfuvirtide and an investigational CCR5 inhibitor, AMD-887.[246,247] AMD-070 inhibits SDF-1α binding, signaling and chemotaxis without itself activating signal transduction. Unlike AMD-3100, AMD-070 is orally bioavailable.[246]

The first clinical study of AMD-070 involved 12 HIV-1-negative individuals who received single oral doses of AMD-070 ranging from 50 to 400 mg.[248] The compound was generally well tolerated, with three of 12 subjects reporting transient mild or moderate headaches; it was also well absorbed with dose-dependent pharmacokinetics. The plasma AMD-070 concentration 12 h after a single oral 400 mg dose was 79–155 nM, which is in the range of the *in vitro* EC_{90} value (125 nM). As was observed in the AMD-3100 trials, AMD-070 administration was associated with a dose-dependent leukocytosis, manifested as 1.5–2.9-fold increases in white blood cell counts[248]; the phenomenon is probably mechanism-dependent and attributable to interference with the SDF-1α/CXCR4 signaling system.[244,245] The conclusion drawn from the trial was that AMD-070 warranted further clinical testing. AMD-070 is now being evaluated in HIV-1-infected subjects in both ACTG Study A5210 and in a second trial.

KRH-2731, -3140, -3955

KRH-2731 (Kureha Inc) is an investigational CXCR4 inhibitor that inhibits X4 viruses *in vitro* with EC_{50} values in the range 1.0–4.2 nM but has no activity against R5 strains.[236] The compound inhibits SDF-1α binding and signaling via CXCR4. The binding site for KRH-2731 was probed using monoclonal antibodies to different domains of CXCR4 and involves the second and third extracellular loops. In a SCID-hu mouse model, KRH-2731 suppressed the replication of an X4 virus during 9 days of oral administration. The bioavailability in rats was 37%. However, due to *in vitro* cytotoxicity, clinical testing of this compound was not pursued.[236] Two follow-up compounds, KRH-3140 and KRH-3955 are both orally bioavailable and inhibit SDF-1 binding to the CXCR4 receptor.[237] KRH-3140 binds to the first and/or second loops of CXCR4; KRH-3955 binds to the first, second and/or third. Both compounds have potent *in vitro* antiretroviral activity with EC_{50}s of 2.2 nM (KRH-3140) and 0.2 nM (KRH-3955) and *in vivo* antiretroviral activity in a SCID-hu mouse model.[237] Clinical studies are anticipated.

THE DEVELOPMENT OF RESISTANCE TO CCR5 AND CXCR4 INHIBITORS IN VITRO, AND ITS IMPLICATIONS FOR THE CLINICAL USE OF THESE COMPOUNDS

In principle, HIV-1 could escape from a small molecule CCR5 inhibitor by using CXCR4 instead; intuitively, this seems the obvious pathway – if one door into the cell is blocked, use the other.[5] However, *in vitro* studies suggest that CXCR4 use is not the major escape pathway; the favored route is the continued use of CCR5 in an inhibitor-insensitive manner.[128,136–138,229,249] Moreover, it is now becoming clear that although R5 viruses certainly can evolve to use CXCR4 *in vitro*, the genetic pathway involved is much more complex than was first appreciated, and that intermediates in the R5 to X4 pathway suffer a significant fitness loss.[33,250] Sequence changes in V3 are usually necessary for co-receptor switching to occur, but they are often not sufficient to create fully replication-competent viruses; changes in V1/V2 are also needed to increase viral fitness.[33,250] *In vivo*, additional selection pressures, such as neutralizing antibodies and chemokines, may further suppress the replication of viruses in the pathway from CCR5 to CXCR4 use. Factors such as these might help explain why it usually takes so long for X4 viruses to emerge in most infected individuals.

The first study of small molecule CCR5 inhibitor resistance was with AD101, a precursor in the development of VCV, using the subtype B R5 primary isolate, CC1/85, as the parental, wild type virus (WTV) in activated primary lymphocyte cultures.[229] The escape mutant virus that emerged after 19 weeks was completely (>25 000-fold) resistant to AD101, but still required CCR5 for entry.[229] Mutagenesis studies proved that four amino acid changes (H308P, K305R, A316V and G321E) within the gp120 V3 region of the AD101 were necessary and sufficient to confer AD101 resistance.[136]

In a second study of similar design, viruses fully (>20 000-fold) resistant to VCV were made in activated primary lymphocytes.[128] Two related input viruses were used in a 12 to 16 week selection process: CC1/85 and CC101.6, a virus isolated from the passage 6 culture of CC1/85 with AD101.[136,229] CC101.6 was partially (about fourfold) resistant to AD101 (and also to VCV).[128,229] Clonal escape mutant viruses generated from either starting isolate remained R5 and had no sequence changes in V3; the genetic correlates of resistance remain to be identified.[128]

In a third experiment, performed at Schering Plough, SCH-C-resistant variants of JV1083, a subtype G R5 primary isolate, emerged after 14 weeks of culture in the PM1 cell line.[137] Again, the escape mutants remained CCR5-dependent. SCH-C resistance was associated with two point substitutions (I297N, K305R) and two deletions (Δ306, Δ307) in the V3 region.[137]

Viruses resistant to MVC have also been made, again using CC1/85 as input virus with PBMC as the target cells.[138] These escape mutants also still use CCR5 for entry, and two different genetic pathways to resistance have been taken by the same WTV. In one study, the resistant virus has only two sequence changes in V3, one of which is also found in the corresponding passage control virus (which has developed partial, less than fivefold, resistance to MVC) (SEK and JPM, unpublished results). A completely independent culture of the same CC1/85 virus with MVC carried out at Pfizer generated a resistant R5 variant with additional V3 changes.[138,249] The phenotypic significance of these genetic changes has not yet been fully explored.

APL-resistant viruses were generated *in vitro*, using a co-receptor-expressing cell line instead of primary lymphocytes and various R5 primary isolates as the input viruses. Under these conditions, viruses with moderate resistance to APL gradually emerged in the cultures. According to the Trofile assay, there was a 2.5- to eightfold reduction in IC_{50}, but the resistant viruses remained sensitive to higher APL concentrations; they also retained the R5 phenotype.[251] Because of methodology differences in how the resistant viruses were selected and their resistance assessed, comparisons with the above studies of resistance to similar CCR5 inhibitors are difficult, and the genetic determinants of resistance remain to be identified.

In vitro escape mutant studies involving PRO 140 have not been reported, although viral strains with a substitution at amino acid position 319 in the V3 region of gp120 had below average susceptibility to PRO 140 *in vitro*.[221] Escape from the PA14 MAb (from which PRO 140 was derived) did occur rapidly when this antibody was used to dose hu-PBL SCID mice infected with an R5 primary virus.[252] Escape from a different anti-CCR5 MAb, 2D7, *in vitro* has also been described, although the genetic pathway was not completely characterized.[253]

An escape mutant to AMD3100 was made using HIV-1 NL4–3 in the MT-4 cell line, which express CXCR4 but not CCR5.[254] After over 50 passages, the virus that emerged was fully resistant to AMD3100, but still used CXCR4 for entry, suggesting parallels to the observations made with the CCR5 inhibitors. The genetic determinants of escape from AMD3100 were not identified, but multiple changes were observed in several regions of gp120, including the V3 region.[254] No escape study involving AMD070 has yet been reported.

None of the small molecule CCR5 inhibitor-resistant viruses described above can use CXCR4 to enter primary cells.[128,136–138,229,249,251] Thus they are unable to replicate in PBMC from CCR5-Δ32 homoygotes, they are inhibited by CCR5-specific MAbs, and/or they are insensitive to AMD3100. And with one exception, they are unable to replicate in CXCR4-expressing cell lines. The outlier is one of the two VCV-resistant isolates, D1/85.16, which could replicate efficiently in U87-CD4/CXCR4 cells in an AMD3100-sensitive manner.[128] Hence some or all of the viruses present in this uncloned isolate are capable of using CXCR4 in the form present on U87-CD4/CXCR4 cells, but not in the form found on primary CD4+ T cells. D1/85.16 could not replicate in either GHOST-CXCR4 or MT4 cells. Its use of CXCR4 is, therefore, conditional and, by the classic definition, it would not be classified as an SI virus. D1/85.16 was then propagated for a short period in U87-CD4/CXCR4 cells to make the D1/85.X4 isolate which was then evaluated using primary CD4+ T cells. Compared with D1/85.16, D1/85.X4 had increased, although still only partial, sensitivity to AMD3100. Overall, the cell line-adapted D1/85.X4 virus behaves like a mixture of R5 and X4 variants, or possibly a genuinely dual-tropic R5X4 strain. In other words, this isolate retains the ability to use CCR5 for entry into primary CD4+ T cells, but some viruses are present that can now instead, or additionally, use CXCR4 to enter these cells. Without deliberate propagation of the D1/85.16 isolate on U87-CD4/CXCR4 cells, the CXCR4-using variants were either present at too low a frequency to permit a detectable level of replication in primary CD4+ T cells, or they were unable to use CXCR4 in the variant form or quantity present on these cells.[128]

The escape mutants generated under the selection pressures of AD101, SCH-C, and VCV are cross-resistant to other small molecule CCR5 inhibitors (AD101, SCH-C, VCV, CMPD 167, and MVC).[128,137,229] However, Pfizer has reported that a MVC-resistant virus retained its susceptibility (less than fivefold change in IC_{50}) to APL, VCV, and SCH-C, implying that cross-resistance among the small molecule CCR5 inhibitors is not absolutely inevitable.[249,255] Presumably, subtle differences in how different inhibitors interact with the binding pocket on CCR5 play a role here.

Invariably, all the viruses resistant to the CCR5 inhibitors remain sensitive to inhibitors of other stages of virus entry (e.g., enfuvirtide, PRO 542, BMS-378806), and to RTI and PI that act postentry (see T Ketas and JP Moore, unpublished results).[128,136–138,229,249,251] Many issues remain to be resolved experimentally, including the determination of whether, and how, the escape mutants use the inhibitor-bound form of CCR5, or alternative CCR5 conformations, for entry.

At least part of the resistance mechanism for CCR5 inhibitors seems likely to be that the escape mutant virus acquires a higher affinity for the co-receptor.[229] This property would allow the resistant virus to more effectively compete with the inhibitor for access to CCR5. An affinity increase has been documented for the AD101-resistant viruses as a rapid response to the selection pressure.[229] Thus a naturally occurring variant with a single amino acid change in V3 (H308P) was immediately selected for the input isolate.[136] The effect of this selection event was quantitatively minor compared to the development of full resistance: about fivefold compared to over 20000-fold. Nonetheless, resistance on this scale could be clinically significant. Moreover, it is possible that viruses with a higher affinity for CCR5 could have an expanded tropism and/or greater virulence if they arose *in vivo*[107]; there is some evidence from *in vitro* studies that the AD101-resistant viruses do have an increased potential for some potentially pathogenic effects.[256]

No studies of the development of resistance to the CCR5 and CXCR4 inhibitors in humans have yet been reported from short-term dosing studies, but of course resistance is to be expected in the longer term. However, resistance to the CCR5 inhibitors may not always be rapid. In one study, SIV-infected macaques were dosed twice then once daily with the small molecule CCR5 inhibitor CMPD 167.[169] Despite high residual viral loads (10^5 to 10^6 RNA copies/mL), in only one animal was there any indication of the rapid development of resistance during the period of optimal dosing.[169] In another, plasma viremia remained suppressed by the therapy for the entire 28 days of dosing, and for 21 days after it was ended.[169]

It was noted above that intermediates in the development of the X4 phenotype can suffer a fitness loss by having a reduced replication capacity in PBMC cultures.[33,250] Such viruses may also have an increased sensitivity to CCR5 inhibitors (P Pugach, SEK and JPM, unpublished results). In either case, the development of variants that continue to use CCR5 in an inhibitor-insensitive manner would be favored if the intermediates on this resistance pathway suffered less of a fitness loss. Fitness-related issues could have clinical consequences: mutations conferring resistance to RTIs or PIs often reduce replicative fitness in the absence of the inhibitor *in vitro*, and this can correlate with reduced pathogenicity *in vivo*.[257–262] When PI-resistant variants emerge and therapy with the same drug is continued, the rate of disease progression can be less than was caused by the wild type virus prior to therapy.[257–262] The *in vivo* fitness cost of resistance is further exemplified by the re-emergence of drug-sensitive variants when therapy is stopped in patients who have become resistant to RTIs and PIs.[261,263] Moreover, multidrug-resistant (MDR) viruses are transmitted inefficiently, the probability of transmission being inversely proportional to the number of resistance mutations present.[264] The evolution of resistance to the CCR5 and CXCR4 inhibitors *in vitro* appears to be a slower, more complex process than to RTIs and PIs.[128,136–138,229,263,265] Hence, if CCR5 inhibitors are combined with RTIs and PIs *in vivo*, resistance to the latter drug classes might be the first to develop. The ongoing clinical trials will provide valuable information on how resistance pathways will affect the design of CCR5 inhibitor therapy strategies.

WILL CCR5 INHIBITORS DRIVE CO-RECEPTOR SWITCHING *IN VIVO*?

A significant uncertainty about the long-term safety of the CCR5 inhibitors does not apply to conventional antiretroviral therapy (ART). Will blocking the access of R5 viruses to CCR5 cause a sustained increase in the absolute abundance of X4 viruses, and hence an increase in the rate of disease progression? The question has long been asked, but not yet answered.[5,266]

An increase in X4 virus levels in response to therapy with a CCR5 inhibitor could occur via a classic resistance pathway, but as noted above, this pathway seems disfavored, at least *in vitro*. However, a second way in which blocking CCR5 could elevate X4 virus production is the reduction of any suppressive effect that R5 viruses may have on the replication of X4 strains under *in vivo* conditions.[119] There has been speculation about such a suppression but there is no hard evidence for its existence and no real understanding of the underlying mechanism(s).[119,267] Of note is that, in two of three macaques experimentally dual-infected with R5 and X4 viruses, the administration of a small molecule CCR5 inhibitor, CMPD 167, caused a rapid, ~10-fold increase in the absolute amount of plasma X4 viruses.[119] But the effect was transient, and after 10–20 days, X4 virus levels in all three test animals were no greater than before therapy.[119] This artificial model system has limitations for understanding what might happen in dual-infected humans, yet human studies of this type will be difficult to perform.

One obvious solution to any emergence of X4 viruses during CCR5 inhibitor therapy would be the additional use of CXCR4 inhibitors, if such compounds are developed successfully.[56] Alternatively, entry inhibitors that suppress both R5 and X4 viruses might be useful (e.g., enfuvirtide or a gp120-binding compound in the BMS-378806 family). The antiviral activities of the RTIs and PIs used in conventional ART are, of course, independent of co-receptor usage, and trials of the CCR5 inhibitors in combination with RTIs and PIs are now in progress. A mathematical model was used recently to predict that the successful application of ART during advanced infection should preferentially suppress X4 virus replication and result in a reversion to the dominance of R5 viruses.[95] The basis for this prediction is that a therapy-induced reduction in the turnover of naive T cells would affect the production of X4 viruses particularly strongly.[95] The same model also suggests that CCR5 inhibitors will not promote the appearance of X4 viruses and, when given early in disease, may even delay their emergence. Again, this is because of a reduction in turnover of the naive T cells that produce X4 viruses.[95]

Whether such predictions will be accurate must await the outcome of clinical trials. However, there is already experimental support for the argument that ART preferentially suppresses X4 viruses, derived from analyses of the phenotypes and/or genotypes of viruses present in ART recipients.[268–273] At least one contradictory report also exists,[274] however, and X4 viruses can certainly persist in the latent reservoir during ART.[275,276] All of these clinical reports are, of course, subject to the aforementioned quantitative and qualitative limitations of the presently available phenotypic and genotypic assays of HIV-1 tropism.

The use of a genotypic assay suggests that X4 viruses continue to evolve slowly over time in a significant proportion of patients whose viral load is suppressed by conventional ART.[275] If this is the case, it helps place into context reports that X4 variants can be detected during CCR5 inhibitor therapy.

Some phenotypic data is now emerging from phase I and II studies of the CCR5 inhibitors, using the Trofile assay for tropism determination. In the phase I APL study of 40 subjects harboring R5 viruses, one subject randomized to the lowest dose tested (200 mg once daily) for 10 days had an R5 virus at study days 1, 5, and 24, yet R5+X4 viruses were detected transiently at study day 10.[174] He experienced a 0.5 $\log_{10}$ copies/mL HIV RNA decrease that was similar to others in the same APL dosing group. Retrospectively, he was found to have harbored R5+X4 viruses prior to entering the dosing phase of the study, but the level of X4 virus was below the limit of detection for the Trofile assay.[174] In the phase I study of MVC in 63 subjects with R5 viruses, tropism changes were observed in two subjects receiving MVC 100 mg qd for 10 days.[173] In one patient, R5+X4 viruses were detected transiently at study day 11, but only an R5 virus at study day 40. In the second patient, R5+X4 viruses were present on study day 11 and persisted through 433 days of follow-up. The 10-day virologic responses in both these patients were similar to those in other patients in the same MVC dosing groups.[124,173] In the phase II study of zidovudine/lamivudine combined with VCV vs efavirenz in treatment-naive subjects with R5 viruses, tropism shifts (i.e., R5 to R5+X4) were seen in both the VCV and efavirenz control arms.[219]

In a phase III study of enfuvirtide, 724 heavily treatment-experienced patients selected an optimal background antiretroviral regimen consisting of RT inhibitors and PIs based on resistance testing, and were then randomized 2:1 to add enfuvirtide or not (with no CCR5 inhibitor). Co-receptor tropism changes in the period until virologic failure occurred were observed in 20% of patients receiving enfuvirtide and in 13% of the control group.[141] Of these, changes from R5+X4 to R5 virus occurred in 14% of the enfuvirtide group, compared with 6% of the control group ($P = 0.04$).[141]

More time and additional studies are needed to provide an answer to whether CCR5 inhibitors do cause a switch to CXCR4 usage to any meaningful extent, and on a sustained basis. To date, the evidence that this occurs is limited, and is essentially anecdotal in nature. Nonetheless, because of the importance of this issue to the safety and success of the CCR5 inhibitors, these studies are of high priority.

THE IMMUNOLOGICAL CONSEQUENCES OF IMPAIRING CCR5 FUNCTION

CCR5 is a functional component of the immune system, so there could be immunological consequences to targeting it with antiviral drugs. Some humans and red-capped Mangabeys harbor genetic mutations in CCR5 (respectively, 32- and 24-bp deletions, notated as Δ32 and Δ24) that prevent expression of a functional protein.[51,277] This complete lack of CCR5 (CCR5-Δ32 homozygosity) has no significant adverse consequences for humans or, so far as can be discerned, their simian counterparts.[278] Several nonpathological conditions have been reported to differ subtly from the norm in humans who lack CCR5 expression, but the cohort sizes tend to be small and the effects are rarely statistically definitive.[278] An exception is the substantial increase in the rate of survival of renal allograft recipients who are CCR5-Δ32 homozygotes, compared to wild type controls.[279] Conversely, CCR5-Δ32 homozygotes appear to be at greater risk of morbidity/mortality from West Nile virus infection.[280] With that perhaps rather important exception, what has been observed in studies of CCR5-Δ32 heterozygous and homozygous individuals is generally encouraging for the development of CCR5 inhibitors, not just to treat HIV-1 infection but also for use in conditions such as rheumatoid arthritis and transplant rejection.

The genetic absence of CCR5 is, however, not the same as inhibiting the receptor's function in an organism that normally expresses it as a component of the immune system. The small molecule CCR5 inhibitors, although not the PRO 140 MAb, are chemokine antagonists, in that they inhibit signaling via CCR5 caused by the natural chemokine ligands.[56,165] Only carefully monitored human clinical trials can determine whether this matters. However, studies in CCR5 knock-out mice do clearly show that CCR5 can play a role in the normal functioning of the mammalian immune system. For example, these mice have greatly reduced survival after experimental infection of the brain with *Cryptococcus neoformans*[281]; partial defects in the clearance of *Listeria monocytogenes* from the blood[282]; reduced IFN-γ production after infection with *Leishmania donovani*[283]; an increased susceptibility to *Toxoplasma gondii*, due to decreased production of IL-12 and IFN-γ[284]; and an increased risk of developing fulminant hepatitis after lectin administration.[285] Other studies in mice raise the possibility that inhibiting CCR5 function could impair some immunological responses to viruses[280,286,287] or other antigens.[288–290] Conversely, studies in CCR5 knock-out mice have also suggested that CCR5 antagonists may be useful to treat various inflammatory conditions, such as cigarette smoke-induced emphysema, that are associated with dysregulation of Th1 cell function.[291] And CCR5 antagonists have been reported to show anticancer activity in a murine model of breast cancer.[292]

It will, therefore, be important to determine whether CCR5 inhibitors have any long-term effects on immune system function during clinical use, for example in the development of immune responses to rare pathogens. For example, if CCR5 function is important for immune responses to parasitic organisms, the incidence and severity of parasitic infections should be carefully monitored, as should the possible long-term development of other uncommon or unusual infections and malignancies. The long-term influences of CCR5 inhibitors on vaccination-induced immune responses should also be evaluated.[293] Indeed, studies of this question have been initiated.

SYNERGY BETWEEN CCR5 INHIBITORS AND OTHER INHIBITORS OF HIV-1 ENTRY *IN VITRO* MAY GUIDE THE DESIGN OF EFFECTIVE COMBINATIONS IN THE CLINIC

It is now well established from clinical studies that HIV-1 infection is best treated by the use of combinations of inhibitors with different, but complementary mechanisms of action, for reasons that are well understood. The advantages apply to RTIs and PIs, but it may be particularly relevant to the design of combinations of entry inhibitors, because of the multiple stages of the entry process and the possibility of synergy. A simple definition of synergy is that a combination of drugs gives a certain effect at lower drug concentrations than would be predicted from the sum of their individual effects. Thus synergy is any combined effect that goes beyond additivity, with which it is often confused. Assays that employ multiple cycles of viral replication can show spurious synergy.[294] A further complication is that the nonclonal nature of HIV-1 isolates sometimes means that quasispecies resistant to one inhibitor can be sensitive to a second one. Combinations of inhibitors may thus enhance the extent of inhibition, yielding spurious results in synergy analyses. For example, supraadditive inhibitions observed when entry and postentry inhibitors are combined *in vitro* may not reflect true synergy at the mechanistic level, but might instead reflect the presence in multicycle assays of viral quasispecies with different sensitivities to the different compounds (PJ Klasse and JPM, unpublished results). Supraadditive effects would, of course, still be useful in a clinical setting, no matter how they arise.

There are examples of true synergy between entry inhibitors that have rational explanations at the molecular level, and that could guide the design of particularly effective clinical combinations. A truly synergistic combination may allow dose-reductions, an efficacy increase and/or a decrease in the rate of resistance development.

The first entry inhibitor combination to be described as synergistic was enfuvirtide with a small molecule co-receptor inhibitor such as SCH-C or AMD3100.[295,296] The same results have since been observed using other small molecule CCR5 inhibitors and either enfuvirtide or another gp41-based peptide with the same mechanism of action, so the finding is clearly generalizable.[205,297,298] The accepted explanation is that the action of the CCR5 inhibitor in reducing the rate at which the viral gp120–CD4 complex can bind to CCR5 increases the duration of the period available for enfuvirtide to bind to the gp41 component of the Env complex.[299] The longer the virus remains in an enfuvirtide-sensitive state, the more likely it is to be inhibited by that drug. Hence the combination of enfuvirtide with, for example, vicriviroc could well be particularly effective in causing viral load reductions, a hypothesis that is now being evaluated clinically. The same mechanism is also likely to apply to the combination of a CXCR4 inhibitor with enfuvirtide. It has also recently been reported that an enfuvirtide-related peptide, C52L, synergizes with the BMS-378806 attachment inhibitor.[298] The underlying mechanism has not been described, but it may be similar to that for CCR5 inhibitors with enfuvirtide. The action of BMS-378806 prolongs the period for which the Env complex remains sensitive to C52L (or enfuvirtide).

The third example of synergy that most probably has an explanation at the molecular level is the combination of PRO 140 with small molecule CCR5 inhibitors.[224] These studies are still ongoing, but it seems reasonable to imagine that the binding of one or the other CCR5 ligand alters the co-receptor conformation in such a way as to facilitate the binding of the second ligand. Hence it may be possible to combine PRO 140 with a small molecule inhibitor in the clinical setting. This type of combination has an additional advantage in that the escape pathways for the MAb and the small molecule are likely to differ; the escape mutants raised to small molecule inhibitors remain sensitive to PRO 140 and other CCR5 MAbs.[128,136–138,229]

SHOULD CCR5 INHIBITORS BE USED EARLY OR LATER IN HIV-1 INFECTION?

CCR5 inhibitors do not inhibit the entry of X4 viruses, although it has been predicted they might have an indirect beneficial effect against these strains *in vivo*.[95] However, the use of CCR5 inhibitors may be contraindicated when X4 viruses are present at detectable levels, as discussed above. One logical approach is therefore to use CCR5 inhibitors early in infection, when R5 viruses dominate plasma viremia and when X4 viruses are relatively rare.[57] Starting therapy against HIV-1 infection as early as possible has always seemed sensible, but the cumulative toxicities and the risk of drug resistance associated with ART have caused a switch in thinking toward delaying the initiation of therapy.[300,301] In addition, significant safety information is already available for many current antiretroviral drugs used in the initial treatment of HIV-1 infection; this raises the bar for the testing of any new compound in treatment-naive patients. However, if the CCR5 inhibitors do transpire to be particularly safe in long-term use, it might be reasonable to revisit this issue.

An additional argument for the very early use of CCR5 inhibitors is the desirability to prevent the rapid loss of CCR5+ CD4+ T cells from the GALT during primary infection (as discussed earlier). The absence of CCR5+ CD4+ T cells from the GALT persists after their loss during primary infection, despite successful ART that restores CD4+ cell counts in the blood.[87] The availability of CCR5 inhibitors may perhaps permit improved control of HIV-1 replication in the activated, CCR5-expressing cells of the GALT. One study in the SIV-infected macaque model, albeit with tenofovir and not a CCR5 inhibitor, has suggested that the GALT can be partially preserved or restored by early therapy.[302] Overall, the early use of CCR5 inhibitors could be immunologically advantageous if drug safety issues permit this.

A third argument in favor of the early use of CCR5 inhibitors is that R5 isolates derived from late in infection tend to be less sensitive to CCR5 inhibitors than those made early.[222,303–305] The difference probably arises because of the acquisition by the virus of a higher affinity for CCR5 as disease progresses and target cells expressing the highest levels of the co-receptor become relatively scarce. However, the magnitude of the effect may not be sufficient to have much of an impact on the clinical efficacy of the compounds.

Clearly, the CCR5 inhibitors will be used for treatment-experienced patients with MDR virus given the novel mechanism of action and demonstrated activity *in vitro* against viruses resistant to the traditional antiretroviral classes (i.e., RTI, PI). An issue here is that the prevalence of X4 viruses increases over time and in treatment-experienced cohorts (see Table 24-1), rendering it increasingly likely that some patients may not benefit optimally from these inhibitors. However, provided that CCR5 inhibitors do not actually drive the sustained emergence of X4 viruses (as discussed earlier), it could still be highly beneficial to suppress the R5 component of a mixed, R5+X4, infection. The residual X4 element would presumably be no more dangerous than it would have been in the absence of the CCR5 inhibitor and it would also be suppressed by the other components of the therapeutic regimen. The use of CCR5 inhibitors in later-stage therapy does, however, raise the problem of the presence of viruses resistant to conventional therapy. This could reduce the treatment options if X4 variants did emerge as a consequence of CCR5 inhibitor therapy. Overall, patients in need of later-stage therapy are likely to have been infected for many years, increasing the chances that they will harbor X4 variants at significant levels while being less able to cope immunologically with any increase in the abundance of these viruses if this occurred during CCR5 inhibitor therapy. The ongoing clinical trials will provide information that is of critical importance for determining how best to use CCR5 inhibitors. However, as noted above, it will also be essential to develop better, more precise phenotypic or genotypic assays for detection and quantification of the R5 and X4 components of total viral load. Such assays may have to be used not only to monitor the outcome of CCR5 inhibitor therapies, but also perhaps to determine which patients should receive them. The same factors apply to CXCR4 inhibitors; again, they could benefit only patients who harbor significant levels of X4, and perhaps R5X4, viruses.

CCR5 AND CXCR4 INHIBITORS AS TOOLS TO PREVENT HIV-1 TRANSMISSION

The development of a safe, effective vaccine to prevent the transmission of HIV-1 is the single most important challenge in AIDS research, as well as one of the most important issues in international public health.[306–309] Unfortunately, progress has been slow, and an effective vaccine will not be available for widespread use in the near future. A significant contribution to the global control of AIDS may therefore be the development of vaginal or rectal microbicides that can prevent HIV-1 sexual transmission.[310–312] An alternative, or complementary, biology-based prevention measure is the use of conventional antiretroviral drugs delivered orally to uninfected, at risk individuals; i.e., preexposure prophylaxis or PrEP.[310,313] The compelling need for prevention measures such as these is highlighted by the continued, dramatic spread of HIV-1 in the countries of the developing world, in which antiretroviral therapy is still poorly available and where the AIDS pandemic takes its greatest toll.[314,315] Nearly half of the world's ~50 million HIV-1-infected people are women, and the proportion will continue to rise.[314,316–318] Women account for greater than 50% of infections in sub-Saharan Africa, where over 30% of the female populations of Zimbabwe and Botswana, aged 13–19, are known to be HIV-1-infected.[314,316–318] Among teenagers, the ratio of infected girls to boys is as high as 6:1 in Kenya, Tanzania and South Africa.[314,316–318] Sex-work is common among teenaged girls, and condom usage is low – unavailability, cost, ignorance of the benefits and customer resistance are all contributory factors here.[314,316–318] The all too frequent result is that these girls may simultaneously become HIV-infected and pregnant, giving birth to an HIV-1-infected infant.[317] In fact, 1600 infected babies are now born each day, many to teenaged mothers.[317] Epidemiologists predict that severe population decline will occur in many countries in sub-Saharan Africa and Asia as women of child-bearing age are lost to AIDS.[314–318]

Barrier contraceptive measures such as the use of the latex condom can play an important role in preventing the spread of HIV-1 and other sexually transmitted diseases; indeed, the use of condoms may be considered the best alternative to abstinence for preventing the exchange of infectious body fluids during sexual activity. Unfortunately, however, condom usage has a number of practical limitations, including the religious and cultural taboos that mitigate against their use in many parts of the world. All too often, men strongly resist the proposed use of a condom by a commercial or social sex partner who insists on condom usage, while women in stable relationships fear the stigma of being labeled barren more than they fear AIDS.[317] For many women, marriage is the single most important risk factor for HIV-1 infection;

faithfulness offers no protection unless also adopted by men.[317] Hence protection methods that are controlled by women are badly needed; topical microbicides and PrEP are potentially suitable for this role. We cannot review here all that is being done to develop these prevention methods, topics that have been reviewed elsewhere recently.[310–313] We will, however, highlight the role that CCR5- and CXCR4-specific compounds might play.

The virus-cell attachment and fusion stages of the HIV-1 replication cycle are attractive targets for the development of a mechanism-based microbicide. As noted above, CCR5 is very important for the initial establishment of infection after sexual transmission, in that CCR5-Δ32 homozygous individuals are strongly protected against all modes of HIV-1 acquisition.[3,49–51,82] It was therefore logical to determine whether the topical application of CCR5 inhibitors could protect against vaginal transmission of an R5 SHIV using the macaque model. In a pioneering study, the CCR5-reactive, chemically modified chemokine, PSC-RANTES, applied vaginally in the 0.1–1 mM range, was found to provide complete protection against vaginal challenge with a high dose of SHIV-162P3.[319] A small molecule CCR5 inhibitor, CMPD 167 from Merck, could also confer protection against the same virus, again when applied vaginally at mM concentrations.[298] The protective effect is not specific to CCR5 inhibitors, as the BMS-378806 attachment inhibitor and C52L, a gp41 peptide similar to enfuvirtide, were also active, as were inhibitor combinations.[298] Together, these results suggest that entry inhibitors in general, and a CCR5 inhibitor in particular, should be evaluated clinically as a vaginal microbicide. To date, the above compounds have not been tested against rectal transmission in the macaque model, but because other entry inhibitors are active against both routes of infection it is reasonable to assume that a CCR5 inhibitor also will be.[320,321] Although most new infections of humans involve R5 viruses, CXCR4-using strains certainly can be transmitted both sexually and by vaginal or rectal inoculation of macaques.[320,321] Hence it is prudent to also evaluate CXCR4-specific inhibitors for their protective potential in the macaque models. Studies with a small molecule CXCR4 inhibitor are now in progress, and less specific entry inhibitors have already been shown to be protective against the X4 challenge virus, SHIV-89.6P.[320,321]

The RT inhibitor tenofovir is presently being evaluated clinically for its potential for PrEP.[322] The principal concerns over PrEP in general involve safety and the development of resistance.[310,313,322] The former is a very significant issue for any drug that is going to be given to uninfected individuals over a prolonged period; the latter is also important, because resistant strains will evolve if infected individuals unknowingly receive monotherapy, compromising treatment strategies for the wider community of infected people. The small molecule CCR5 inhibitors may, perhaps, be particularly useful for PrEP for several reasons. So far, with the exception of the liver toxicity associated with APL, the safety profile of these inhibitors looks reasonable in short-term clinical studies (as discussed earlier), although longer-term studies will be required. Secondly, as discussed earlier, the development of resistance, at least *in vitro*, appears to be slow and complex, compared to that seen for RTIs and PIs. A third potential advantage is the long half-life of these compounds on CCR5,[157] which might potentially allow sustained protective effects to be achieved even if PrEP is taken intermittently, as might be the case in the real world. A small scale study in the macaque model involving oral dosing with CMPD 167 followed by vaginal challenge with SHIV-162P3 provides some support for the use of CCR5 inhibitors as PrEP; a 10-day dosing regimen postchallenge was sufficient to protect ~50% of the test macaques, with a delay in the onset of plasma viremia in the remaining animals.[323] A more prolonged dosing period would probably be more effective. Four days of dosing prior to challenge was not effective.[322]

Overall, for the reasons outlined above, there are compelling reasons for the further evaluation of entry inhibitors, and particular CCR5 inhibitors, for a role in preventing HIV-1 transmission.

Disclosure

This work was supported by grants to JPM (R01 AI41420, U19 AI65413) and RMG (AI 051966) from the NIH. JPM receives research support from Pfizer UK and Schering Plough Research Institute to study how HIV-1 escapes from small molecule CCR5 inhibitors *in vitro*. RMG receives research support from Pfizer and Schering Plough to conduct CCR5 inhibitor studies and from the AIDS Clinical Trials Group (ACTG)/NIAID/NIH to conduct studies of vicriviroc (ACTG 5211) and AMD 11070 (ACTG 5210).

REFERENCES

1. Clapham PR, McKnight A. Cell surface receptors, virus entry and tropism of primate lentiviruses. J Gen Virol 83:1809, 2002.
2. Douek DC, Picker LJ, Koup RA. T cell dynamics in HIV-1 infection. Annu Rev Immunol 21:265, 2003.
3. Moore JP, Kitchen SG, Pugach P, et al. The CCR5 and CXCR4 coreceptors – central to understanding the transmission and pathogenesis of human immunodeficiency virus type 1 infection. AIDS Res Hum Retroviruses 20:111, 2004.
4. Pierson TC, Doms RW. HIV-1 entry and its inhibition. Curr Top Microbiol Immunol 281:1, 2003.
5. Moore JP, Doms RW. The entry of entry inhibitors: a fusion of science and medicine. Proc Natl Acad Sci USA 100:10598, 2003.
6. Doms RW. Unwelcome guests with master keys: how HIV enters cells and how it can be stopped. Top HIV Med 12:100, 2004.
7. Kilby JM, Eron JJ. Novel therapies based on mechanisms of HIV-1 cell entry. N Engl J Med 348:2228, 2003.
8. Kuhmann SE, Moore JP. HIV-1 entry inhibitor entrances. Trends Pharmacol Sci 25:117, 2004.
9. Berger EA, Doms RW, Fenyö EM, et al. A new classification for HIV-1. Nature 391:240, 1998.
10. Coakley E, Petropoulos CJ, Whitcomb JM. Assessing chemokine co-receptor usage in HIV. Curr Opin Infect Dis 18:9, 2005.
11. Gallo SA, Finnegan CM, Viard M, et al. The HIV Env-mediated fusion reaction. Biochim Biophys Acta 1614:36, 2003.

12. Ugolini S, Mondor I, Sattentau QJ. HIV-1 attachment: another look. Trends Microbiol 7:144, 1999.
13. O'Doherty U, Swiggard WJ, Malim MH. Human immunodeficiency virus type 1 spinoculation enhances infection through virus binding. J Virol 74:10074, 2000.
14. Baribaud F, Pohlmann S, Doms RW. The role of DC-SIGN and DC-SIGNR in HIV and SIV attachment, infection, and transmission. Virology 286:1, 2001.
15. Tardif MR, Tremblay MJ. LFA-1 is a key determinant for preferential infection of memory CD4+ T cells by human immunodeficiency virus type 1. J Virol 79:13714, 2005.
16. Weiss CD, Levy JA, White JM. Oligomeric organization of gp120 on infectious human immunodeficiency virus type 1 particles. J Virol 64:5674, 1990.
17. Weissenhorn W, Dessen A, Harrison SC, et al. Atomic structure of the ectodomain from HIV-1 gp41. Nature 387:426, 1997.
18. Chan DC, Fass D, Berger JM, et al. Core structure of gp41 from the HIV envelope glycoprotein. Cell 89:263, 1997.
19. Lu M, Blacklow SC, Kim PS. A trimeric structural domain of the HIV-1 transmembrane glycoprotein. Nat Struct Biol 2:1075, 1995.
20. Kwong PD, Wyatt R, Sattentau QJ, et al. Oligomeric modeling and electrostatic analysis of the gp120 envelope glycoprotein of human immunodeficiency virus. J Virol 74:1961, 2000.
21. Zhu P, Chertova E, Bess J Jr, et al. Electron tomography analysis of envelope glycoprotein trimers on HIV and simian immunodeficiency virus virions. Proc Natl Acad Sci USA 100:15812, 2003.
22. Yang X, Kurteva S, Ren X, et al. Stoichiometry of envelope glycoprotein trimers in the entry of human immunodeficiency virus type 1. J Virol 79:12132, 2005.
23. Chen B, Vogan EM, Gong H, et al. Structure of an unliganded simian immunodeficiency virus gp120 core. Nature 433:834, 2005.
24. Huang CC, Tang M, Zhang MY, et al. Structure of a V3-containing HIV-1 gp120 core. Science 310:1025, 2005.
25. Kwong PD, Wyatt R, Robinson J, et al. Structure of an HIV gp120 envelope glycoprotein in complex with the CD4 receptor and a neutralizing human antibody. Nature 393:648, 1998.
26. Wyatt R, Sodroski J. The HIV-1 envelope glycoproteins: fusogens, antigens, and immunogens. Science 280:1884, 1998.
27. Poignard P, Saphire EO, Parren PW, et al. gp120: biologic aspects of structural features. Annu Rev Immunol 19:253, 2001.
28. Myszka DG, Sweet RW, Hensley P, et al. Energetics of the HIV gp120–CD4 binding reaction. Proc Natl Acad Sci USA 97:9026, 2000.
29. Guo Q, Ho HT, Dicker I, et al. Biochemical and genetic characterizations of a novel human immunodeficiency virus type 1 inhibitor that blocks gp120–CD4 interactions. J Virol 77:10528, 2003.
30. Rizzuto C, Sodroski J. Fine definition of a conserved CCR5-binding region on the human immunodeficiency virus type 1 glycoprotein 120. AIDS Res Hum Retroviruses 16:741, 2000.
31. Rizzuto CD, Wyatt R, Hernandez-Ramos N, et al. A conserved HIV gp120 glycoprotein structure involved in chemokine receptor binding. Science 280:1949, 1998.
32. Hartley O, Klasse PJ, Sattentau QJ, et al. V3: HIV's switch-hitter. AIDS Res Hum Retroviruses 21:171, 2005.
33. Pastore C, Nedellec R, Ramos A, et al. Human immunodeficiency virus type 1 coreceptor switching: V1/V2 gain-of-fitness mutations compensate for V3 loss-of-fitness mutations. J Virol 80:750, 2006.
34. Weiss CD. HIV-1 gp41: mediator of fusion and target for inhibition. AIDS Rev 5:214, 2003.
35. Berger EA, Murphy PM, Farber JM. Chemokine receptors as HIV-1 coreceptors: roles in viral entry, tropism, and disease. Annu Rev Immunol 17:657, 1999.
36. Doms RW. Chemokine receptors and HIV entry. AIDS 15: S34, 2001.
37. Willey SJ, Reeves JD, Hudson R, et al. Identification of a subset of human immunodeficiency virus type 1 (HIV-1), HIV-2, and simian immunodeficiency virus strains able to exploit an alternative coreceptor on untransformed human brain and lymphoid cells. J Virol 77:6138, 2003.
38. Lee S, Tiffany HL, King L, et al. CCR8 on human thymocytes functions as a human immunodeficiency virus type 1 coreceptor. J Virol 74:6946, 2000.
39. Connor RI, Sheridan KE, Ceradini D, et al. Change in coreceptor use coreceptor use correlates with disease progression in HIV-1-infected individuals. J Exp Med 185:621, 1997.
40. de Roda Husman AM, van Rij RP, Blaak H, et al. Adaptation to promiscuous usage of chemokine receptors is not a prerequisite for human immunodeficiency virus type 1 disease progression. J Infect Dis 180:1106, 1999.
41. Edinger AL, Hoffman TL, Sharron M, et al. Use of GPR1, GPR15, and STRL33 as coreceptors by diverse human immunodeficiency virus type 1 and simian immunodeficiency virus envelope proteins. Virology 249:367, 1998.
42. Kreisberg JF, Kwa D, Schramm B, et al. Cytopathicity of human immunodeficiency virus type 1 primary isolates depends on coreceptor usage and not patient disease status. J Virol 75:8842, 2001.
43. Pohlmann S, Lee B, Meister S, et al. Simian immunodeficiency virus utilizes human and sooty mangabey but not rhesus macaque STRL33 for efficient entry. J Virol 74:5075, 2000.
44. Sharron M, Pohlmann S, Price K, et al. Expression and coreceptor activity of STRL33/Bonzo on primary peripheral blood lymphocytes. Blood 96:41, 2000.
45. Simmons G, Wilkinson D, Reeves JD, et al. Primary, syncytium-inducing human immunodeficiency virus type 1 isolates are dual-tropic and most can use either Lestr or CCR5 as coreceptors for virus entry. J Virol 70:8355, 1996.
46. Zhang YJ, Dragic T, Cao Y, et al. Use of coreceptors other than CCR5 by non-syncytium-inducing adult and pediatric isolates of human immunodeficiency virus type 1 is rare in vitro. J Virol 72:9337, 1998.
47. Zhang YJ, Moore JP. Will multiple coreceptors need to be targeted by inhibitors of human immunodeficiency virus type 1 entry? J Virol 73:3443, 1999.
48. Zhang YJ, Zhang L, Ketas T, et al. HIV type 1 molecular clones able to use the Bonzo/STRL-33 coreceptor for virus entry. AIDS Res Hum Retroviruses 17:217, 2001.
49. Dean M, Carrington M, Winkler C, et al. Genetic restriction of HIV-1 infection and progression to AIDS by a deletion allele of the CKR5 structural gene. Hemophilia Growth and Development Study, Multicenter AIDS Cohort Study, Multicenter Hemophilia Cohort Study, San Francisco City Cohort, ALIVE Study. Science 273:1856, 1996.
50. Liu R, Paxton WA, Choe S, et al. Homozygous defect in HIV-1 coreceptor accounts for resistance of some multiply-exposed individuals to HIV-1 infection. Cell 86:367, 1996.
51. Samson M, Libert F, Doranz BJ, et al. Resistance to HIV-1 infection in Caucasian individuals bearing mutant alleles of the CCR-5 chemokine receptor gene. Nature 382:722, 1996.
52. Gorry PR, Zhang C, Wu S, et al. Persistence of dual-tropic HIV-1 in an individual homozygous for the CCR5 Delta 32 allele. Lancet 359:1832, 2002.
53. Michael NL, Nelson JA, Kewal Ramani VN, et al. Exclusive and persistent use of the entry coreceptor CXCR4 by human immunodeficiency virus type 1 from a subject homozygous for CCR5 delta32. J Virol 72:6040, 1998.
54. Naif HM, Cunningham AL, Alali M, et al. A human immunodeficiency virus type 1 isolate from an infected person homozygous for CCR5Delta32 exhibits dual tropism by infecting macrophages and MT2 cells via CXCR4. J Virol 76:3114, 2002.

55. Sheppard HW, Celum C, Michael NL, et al. HIV-1 infection in individuals with the CCR5-Delta32/Delta32 genotype: acquisition of syncytium-inducing virus at seroconversion. J Acquir Immune Defic Syndr 29:307, 2002.
56. Seibert C, Sakmar TP. Small-molecule antagonists of CCR5 and CXCR4: a promising new class of anti-HIV-1 drugs. Curr Pharm Des 10:2041, 2004.
57. Kuhmann SE, Moore JP. The HIV-1 phenotypic variants: deadly and deadlier. J Viral Entry 1:4, 2005.
58. Åsjö B, Morfeldt-Månson L, Albert J, et al. Replicative capacity of human immunodeficiency virus from patients with varying severity of HIV infection. Lancet 2:660, 1986.
59. Cheng-Mayer C, Seto D, Tateno M, et al. Biologic features of HIV-1 that correlate with virulence in the host. Science 240:80, 1988.
60. Evans LA, McHugh TM, Stites DP, et al. Differential ability of human immunodeficiency virus isolates to productively infect human cells. J Immunol 138:3415, 1987.
61. Fenyö EM, Morfeldt-Månson L, Chiodi F, et al. Distinct replicative and cytopathic characteristics of human immunodeficiency virus isolates. J Virol 62:4414, 1988.
62. Tersmette M, de Goede RE, Al BJ, et al. Differential syncytium-inducing capacity of human immunodeficiency virus isolates: frequent detection of syncytium-inducing isolates in patients with acquired immunodeficiency syndrome (AIDS) and AIDS-related complex. J Virol 62:2026, 1988.
63. Schuitemaker H, Koot M, Kootstra NA, et al. Biological phenotype of human immunodeficiency virus type 1 clones at different stages of infection: progression of disease is associated with a shift from monocytotropic to T-cell-tropic virus population. J Virol 66:1354, 1992.
64. Schuitemaker H, Kootstra NA, de Goede RE, et al. Monocytotropic human immunodeficiency virus type 1 (HIV-1) variants detectable in all stages of HIV-1 infection lack T-cell line tropism and syncytium-inducing ability in primary T-cell culture. J Virol 65:356, 1991.
65. Japour AJ, Fiscus SA, Arduino JM, et al. Standardized microtiter assay for determination of syncytium-inducing phenotypes of clinical human immunodeficiency virus type 1 isolates. J Clin Microbiol 32:2291, 1994.
66. Koot M, Vos AH, Keet RP, et al. HIV-1 biological phenotype in long-term infected individuals evaluated with an MT-2 cocultivation assay. AIDS 6:49, 1992.
67. Boucher CA, Lange JM, Miedema FF, et al. HIV-1 biological phenotype and the development of zidovudine resistance in relation to disease progression in asymptomatic individuals during treatment. AIDS 6:1259, 1992.
68. Bozzette SA, McCutchan JA, Spector SA, et al. A cross-sectional comparison of persons with syncytium- and non-syncytium-inducing human immunodeficiency virus. J Infect Dis 168:1374, 1993.
69. D'Aquila RT, Johnson VA, Welles SL, et al. Zidovudine resistance and HIV-1 disease progression during antiretroviral therapy. AIDS Clinical Trials Group Protocol 116B/117 Team and the Virology Committee Resistance Working Group. Ann Intern Med 122:401, 1995.
70. Hughes MD, Johnson VA, Hirsch MS, et al. Monitoring plasma HIV-1 RNA levels in addition to CD4+ lymphocyte count improves assessment of antiretroviral therapeutic response. ACTG 241 Protocol Virology Substudy Team. Ann Intern Med 126:929, 1997.
71. Karlsson A, Parsmyr K, Sandstrom E, et al. MT-2 cell tropism as prognostic marker for disease progression in human immunodeficiency virus type 1 infection. J Clin Microbiol 32:364, 1994.
72. Koot M, Keet IP, Vos AH, et al. Prognostic value of HIV-1 syncytium-inducing phenotype for rate of CD4+ cell depletion and progression to AIDS. Ann Intern Med 118:681, 1993.
73. Lathey JL, Hughes MD, Fiscus SA, et al. Variability and prognostic values of virologic and CD4 cell measures in human immunodeficiency virus type 1-infected patients with 200–500 CD4 cells/mm^3 (ACTG 175). AIDS Clinical Trials Group Protocol 175 Team. J Infect Dis 177:617, 1998.
74. Maas JJ, Gange SJ, Schuitemaker H, et al. Strong association between failure of T cell homeostasis and the syncytium-inducing phenotype among HIV-1-infected men in the Amsterdam Cohort Study. AIDS 14:1155, 2000.
75. Sheppard HW, Lang W, Ascher MS, et al. The characterization of non-progressors: long-term HIV-1 infection with stable CD4+ T-cell levels. AIDS 7:1159, 1993.
76. Spijkerman I, de Wolf F, Langendam M, et al. Emergence of syncytium-inducing human immunodeficiency virus type 1 variants coincides with a transient increase in viral RNA level and is an independent predictor for progression to AIDS. J Infect Dis 178:397, 1998.
77. Björndal Å, Deng H, Jansson M, et al. Coreceptor usage of primary human immunodeficiency virus type 1 isolates varies according to biological phenotype. J Virol 71:7478, 1997.
78. Bleul CC, Wu L, Hoxie JA, et al. The HIV coreceptors CXCR4 and CCR5 are differentially expressed and regulated on human T lymphocytes. Proc Natl Acad Sci USA 94:1925, 1997.
79. Ostrowski MA, Justement SJ, Catanzaro A, et al. Expression of chemokine receptors CXCR4 and CCR5 in HIV-1-infected and uninfected individuals. J Immunol 161:3195, 1998.
80. Mattapallil JJ, Douek DC, Hill B, et al. Massive infection and loss of memory CD4+ T cells in multiple tissues during acute SIV infection. Nature 434:1093, 2005.
81. Veazey RS, Lackner AA. Getting to the guts of HIV pathogenesis. J Exp Med 200:697, 2004.
82. van't Wout AB, Kootstra NA, Mulder-Kampinga GA, et al. Macrophage-tropic variants initiate human immunodeficiency virus type 1 infection after sexual, parenteral, and vertical transmission. J Clin Invest 94:2060, 1994.
83. Pope M, Haase AT. Transmission, acute HIV-1 infection and the quest for strategies to prevent infection. Nat Med 9:847, 2003.
84. Veazey R, Lackner A. The mucosal immune system and HIV-1 infection. AIDS Rev 5:245, 2003.
85. Harouse JM, Gettie A, Tan RC, et al. Distinct pathogenic sequela in rhesus macaques infected with CCR5 or CXCR4 utilizing SHIVs. Science 284:816, 1999.
86. Brenchley JM, Schacker TW, Ruff LE, et al. CD4+ T cell depletion during all stages of HIV disease occurs predominantly in the gastrointestinal tract. J Exp Med 200:749, 2004.
87. Mehandru S, Poles MA, Tenner-Racz K, et al. Primary HIV-1 infection is associated with preferential depletion of CD4+ T lymphocytes from effector sites in the gastrointestinal tract. J Exp Med 200:761, 2004.
88. Veazey RS, DeMaria M, Chalifoux LV, et al. Gastrointestinal tract as a major site of CD4+ T cell depletion and viral replication in SIV infection. Science 280:427, 1998.
89. Miller CJ, Li Q, Abel K, et al. Propagation and dissemination of infection after vaginal transmission of simian immunodeficiency virus. J Virol 79:9217, 2005.
90. de Roda Husman AM, Koot M, Cornelissen M, et al. Association between CCR5 genotype and the clinical course of HIV-1 infection. Ann Intern Med 127:882, 1997.
91. Richman DD, Bozzette SA. The impact of the syncytium-inducing phenotype of human immunodeficiency virus on disease progression. J Infect Dis 169:968, 1994.
92. Shankarappa R, Margolick JB, Gange SJ, et al. Consistent viral evolutionary changes associated with the progression of human immunodeficiency virus type 1 infection. J Virol 73:10489, 1999.
93. Tersmette M, Gruters RA, de Wolf F, et al. Evidence for a role of virulent human immunodeficiency virus (HIV) variants in

the pathogenesis of acquired immunodeficiency syndrome: studies on sequential HIV isolates. J Virol 63:2118, 1989.

94. Moyle GJ, Wildfire A, Mandalia S, et al. Epidemiology and predictive factors for chemokine receptor use in HIV-1 infection. J Infect Dis 191:866, 2005.
95. Ribeiro RM, Hazenberg MD, Perelson AS, et al. Naive and memory cell turnover as drivers of CCR5-to-CXCR4 tropism switch in human immunodeficiency virus type 1: implications for therapy. J Virol 80:802, 2006.
96. Stevenson M, Stanwick TL, Dempsey MP, et al. HIV-1 replication is controlled at the level of T cell activation and proviral integration. EMBO J 9:1551, 1990.
97. Zack JA, Arrigo SJ, Weitsman SR, et al. HIV-1 entry into quiescent primary lymphocytes: molecular analysis reveals a labile, latent viral structure. Cell 61:213, 1990.
98. Roy AM, Schweighardt B, Eckstein LA, et al. Enhanced replication of R5 HIV-1 over X4 HIV-1 in CD4(+)CCR5(+) CXCR4(+) T cells. J Acquir Immune Defic Syndr 40:267, 2005.
99. Hazenberg MD, Stuart JW, Otto SA, et al. T-cell division in human immunodeficiency virus (HIV)-1 infection is mainly due to immune activation: a longitudinal analysis in patients before and during highly active antiretroviral therapy (HAART). Blood 95:249, 2000.
100. Sachsenberg N, Perelson AS, Yerly S, et al. Turnover of CD4+ and CD8+ T lymphocytes in HIV-1 infection as measured by Ki-67 antigen. J Exp Med 187:1295, 1998.
101. Nishimura Y, Brown CR, Mattapallil JJ, et al. Resting naive CD4+ T cells are massively infected and eliminated by X4-tropic simian-human immunodeficiency viruses in macaques. Proc Natl Acad Sci USA 102:8000, 2005.
102. Nishimura Y, Igarashi T, Donau OK, et al. Highly pathogenic SHIVs and SIVs target different CD4+ T cell subsets in rhesus monkeys, explaining their divergent clinical courses. Proc Natl Acad Sci USA 101:12324, 2004.
103. Feinberg MB, Moore JP. AIDS vaccine models: challenging challenge viruses. Nat Med 8:207, 2002.
104. Edmonson P, Murphey-Corb M, Martin LN, et al. Evolution of a simian immunodeficiency virus pathogen. J Virol 72:405, 1998.
105. Kimata JT, Kuller L, Anderson DB, et al. Emerging cytopathic and antigenic simian immunodeficiency virus variants influence AIDS progression. Nat Med 5:535, 1999.
106. Kuwata T, Dehghani H, Brown CR, et al. Infectious Molecular Clones from a Simian Immunodeficiency Virus-Infected Rapid-Progressor (RP) Macaque: Evidence of differential selection of RP-specific envelope mutations in vitro and in vivo. J Virol 80:1463, 2006.
107. Gorry PR, Churchill M, Crowe SM, et al. Pathogenesis of macrophage tropic HIV-1. Curr HIV Res 3:53, 2005.
108. Cunningham AL, Li S, Juarez J, et al. The level of HIV infection of macrophages is determined by interaction of viral and host cell genotypes. J Leukoc Biol 68:311, 2000.
109. Jayakumar P, Berger I, Autschbach F, et al. Tissue-resident macrophages are productively infected ex vivo by primary x4 isolates of human immunodeficiency virus type 1. J Virol 79:5220, 2005.
110. Simmons G, Reeves JD, McKnight A, et al. CXCR4 as a functional coreceptor for human immunodeficiency virus type 1 infection of primary macrophages. J Virol 72:8453, 1998.
111. Verani A, Pesenti E, Polo S, et al. CXCR4 is a functional coreceptor for infection of human macrophages by CXCR4-dependent primary HIV-1 isolates. J Immunol 161:2084, 1998.
112. Yi Y, Isaacs SN, Williams DA, et al. Role of CXCR4 in cell-cell fusion and infection of monocyte-derived macrophages by primary human immunodeficiency virus type 1 (HIV-1) strains: two distinct mechanisms of HIV-1 dual tropism. J Virol 73:7117, 1999.
113. Li S, Juarez J, Alali M, et al. Persistent CCR5 utilization and enhanced macrophage tropism by primary blood human immunodeficiency virus type 1 isolates from advanced stages of disease and comparison to tissue-derived isolates. J Virol 73:9741, 1999.
114. Tuttle DL, Anders CB, Aquino-De Jesus MJ, et al. Increased replication of non-syncytium-inducing HIV type 1 isolates in monocyte-derived macrophages is linked to advanced disease in infected children. AIDS Res Hum Retroviruses 18:353, 2002.
115. Gorry PR, Taylor J, Holm GH, et al. Increased CCR5 affinity and reduced CCR5/CD4 dependence of a neurovirulent primary human immunodeficiency virus type 1 isolate. J Virol 76:6277, 2002.
116. Reeves JD, Gallo SA, Ahmad N, et al. Sensitivity of HIV-1 to entry inhibitors correlates with envelope/coreceptor affinity, receptor density, and fusion kinetics. Proc Natl Acad Sci USA 99:16249, 2002.
117. Igarashi T, Brown CR, Byrum RA, et al. Rapid and irreversible CD4+ T-cell depletion induced by the highly pathogenic simian/human immunodeficiency virus SHIV(DH12R) is systemic and synchronous. J Virol 76:379, 2002.
118. Igarashi T, Brown CR, Endo Y, et al. Macrophage are the principal reservoir and sustain high virus loads in rhesus macaques after the depletion of CD4+ T cells by a highly pathogenic simian immunodeficiency virus/HIV type 1 chimera (SHIV): Implications for HIV-1 infections of humans. Proc Natl Acad Sci USA 98:658, 2001.
119. Wolinsky SM, Veazey RS, Kunstman KJ, et al. Effect of a CCR5 inhibitor on viral loads in macaques dual-infected with R5 and X4 primate immunodeficiency viruses. Virology 328:19, 2004.
120. Williams KC, Hickey WF. Central nervous system damage, monocytes and macrophages, and neurological disorders in AIDS. Annu Rev Neurosci 25:537, 2002.
121. Regoes RR, Bonhoeffer S. The HIV coreceptor switch: a population dynamical perspective. Trends Microbiol 13:269, 2005.
122. Trouplin V, Salvatori F, Cappello F, et al. Determination of coreceptor usage of human immunodeficiency virus type 1 from patient plasma samples by using a recombinant phenotypic assay. J Virol 75:251, 2001.
123. Spudich SS, Huang W, Nilsson AC, et al. HIV-1 chemokine coreceptor utilization in paired cerebrospinal fluid and plasma samples: a survey of subjects with viremia. J Infect Dis 191:890, 2005.
124. Westby M, Lewis M, Whitcomb J, et al. Emergence of CXCR4-using human immunodeficiency virus type 1 (HIV-1) variants in a minority of HIV-1-infected patients following treatment with the CCR5 antagonist maraviroc is from a pretreatment CXCR4-using virus reservoir. J Virol 80:4909–20, 2006.
125. Hill CM, Kwon D, Jones M, et al. The amino terminus of human CCR5 is required for its function as a receptor for diverse human and simian immunodeficiency virus envelope glycoproteins. Virology 248:357, 1998.
126. Yi Y, Shaheen F, Collman RG. Preferential use of CXCR4 by R5X4 human immunodeficiency virus type 1 isolates for infection of primary lymphocytes. J Virol 79:1480, 2005.
127. Zhang Y, Lou B, Lal RB, et al. Use of inhibitors to evaluate coreceptor usage by simian and simian/human immunodeficiency viruses and human immunodeficiency virus type 2 in primary cells. J Virol 74:6893, 2000.
128. Marozsan AJ, Kuhmann SE, Morgan T, et al. Generation and properties of a human immunodeficiency virus type 1 isolate resistant to the small molecule CCR5 inhibitor, SCH-417690 (SCH-D). Virology 338:182, 2005.

129. Kenakin T. G-protein coupled receptors as allosteric machines. Receptors Channels 10:51, 2004.
130. Resch W, Hoffman N, Swanstrom R. Improved success of phenotype prediction of the human immunodeficiency virus type 1 from envelope variable loop 3 sequence using neural networks. Virology 288:51, 2001.
131. Jensen MA, Li FS, van't Wout AB, et al. Improved coreceptor usage prediction and genotypic monitoring of R5-to-X4 transition by motif analysis of human immunodeficiency virus type 1 env V3 loop sequences. J Virol 77:13376, 2003.
132. Jensen MA, van't Wout AB. Predicting HIV-1 coreceptor usage with sequence analysis. AIDS Rev 5:104, 2003.
133. Pillai S, Good B, Richman D, et al. A new perspective on V3 phenotype prediction. AIDS Res Hum Retroviruses 19:145, 2003.
134. Clevestig P, Pramanik L, Leitner T, et al. CCR5 use by human immunodeficiency virus type 1 is associated closely with the gp120 V3 loop N-linked glycosylation site. J Gen Virol 87:607, 2006.
135. Fouchier RA, Groenink M, Kootstra NA, et al. Phenotype-associated sequence variation in the third variable domain of the human immunodeficiency virus type 1 gp120 molecule. J Virol 66:3183, 1992.
136. Kuhmann SE, Pugach P, Kunstman KJ, et al. Genetic and phenotypic analyses of human immunodeficiency virus type 1 escape from a small-molecule CCR5 inhibitor. J Virol 78:2790, 2004.
137. Riley JP, Strizki JM. Unpublished data.
138. Westby M, Smith-Burchnell C, Mori J, et al. In vitro escape of R5 primary isolates from the CCR5 antagonist, UK-427,857 is difficult and involves continued use of the CCR5 receptor. Antivir Ther 9:S10, 2004.
139. Brumme ZL, Goodrich J, Mayer HB, et al. Molecular and clinical epidemiology of CXCR4-using HIV-1 in a large population of antiretroviral-naive individuals. J Infect Dis 192:466, 2005.
140. Demarest J, Bonny T, Vavro C, et al. HIV-1 co-receptor tropism in treatment naive and experienced subjects. In: Abstracts of the 44th Interscience Conference on Antimicrobial Agents and Chemotherapy, Washington, DC, 30 Oct to 2 Nov 2004, abstract H-1136.
141. Melby TJ, Despirito M, Demasi R, et al. HIV-1 coreceptor use in triple-class treatment-experienced patients: baseline prevalence, correlates, and relationship to enfuvirtide response. J Infect Dis 194:238–46, 2006.
142. Wilkin TJ, Su Z, Kuritzkes DR, et al. HIV type 1 chemokine coreceptor use among antiretroviral-experienced patients screened for a clinical trial of a CCR5 inhibitor: AIDS Clinical Trial Group A5211. Clin Infect Dis 44:591–5, 2007.
143. Barber CG. CCR5 antagonists for the treatment of HIV. Curr Opin Investig Drugs 5:851, 2004.
144. Kazmierski W, Bifulco N, Yang H, et al. Recent progress in discovery of small-molecule CCR5 chemokine receptor ligands as HIV-1 inhibitors. Bioorg Med Chem 11:2663, 2003.
145. Maeda K, Nakata H, Ogata H, et al. The current status of, and challenges in, the development of CCR5 inhibitors as therapeutics for HIV-1 infection. Curr Opin Pharmacol 4:447, 2004.
146. Doranz BJ, Lu ZH, Rucker J, et al. Two distinct CCR5 domains can mediate coreceptor usage by human immunodeficiency virus type 1. J Virol 71:6305, 1997.
147. Dragic T. An overview of the determinants of CCR5 and CXCR4 co-receptor function. J Gen Virol 82:1807, 2001.
148. Seibert C, Cadene M, Sanfiz A, et al. Tyrosine sulfation of CCR5 N-terminal peptide by tyrosylprotein sulfotransferases 1 and 2 follows a discrete pattern and temporal sequence. Proc Natl Acad Sci USA 99:11031, 2002.
149. Cormier EG, Persuh M, Thompson DA, et al. Specific interaction of CCR5 amino-terminal domain peptides containing sulfotyrosines with HIV-1 envelope glycoprotein gp120. Proc Natl Acad Sci USA 97:5762, 2000.
150. Cormier EG, Tran DN, Yukhayeva L, et al. Mapping the determinants of the CCR5 amino-terminal sulfopeptide interaction with soluble human immunodeficiency virus type 1 gp120–CD4 complexes. J Virol 75:5541, 2001.
151. Farzan M, Babcock GJ, Vasilieva N, et al. The role of post-translational modifications of the CXCR4 amino terminus in stromal-derived factor 1 alpha association and HIV-1 entry. J Biol Chem 277:29484, 2002.
152. Farzan M, Chung S, Li W, et al. Tyrosine-sulfated peptides functionally reconstitute a CCR5 variant lacking a critical amino-terminal region. J Biol Chem 277:40397, 2002.
153. Farzan M, Mirzabekov T, Kolchinsky P, et al. Tyrosine sulfation of the amino terminus of CCR5 facilitates HIV-1 entry. Cell 96:667, 1999.
154. Cormier EG, Dragic T. The crown and stem of the V3 loop play distinct roles in human immunodeficiency virus type 1 envelope glycoprotein interactions with the CCR5 coreceptor. J Virol 76:8953, 2002.
155. Billick E, Seibert C, Pugach P, et al. The differential sensitivity of human and rhesus macaque CCR5 to small-molecule inhibitors of human immunodeficiency virus type 1 entry is explained by a single amino acid difference and suggests a mechanism of action for these inhibitors. J Virol 78:4134, 2004.
156. Tsamis F, Gavrilov S, Kajumo F, et al. Analysis of the mechanism by which the small-molecule CCR5 antagonists SCH-351125 and SCH-350581 inhibit human immunodeficiency virus type 1 entry. J Virol 77:5201, 2003.
157. Watson C, Jenkinson S, Kazmierski W, et al. The CCR5 receptor-based mechanism of action of 873140, a potent allosteric noncompetitive HIV entry inhibitor. Mol Pharmacol 67:1268, 2005.
158. Lagane B, Ballet S, Planchenault T, et al. Mutation of the DRY motif reveals different structural requirements for the CC chemokine receptor 5-mediated signaling and receptor endocytosis. Mol Pharmacol 67:1966, 2005.
159. Castonguay LA, Weng Y, Adolfsen W, et al. Binding of 2-aryl-4-(piperidin-1-yl)butanamines and 1,3,4-trisubstituted pyrrolidines to human CCR5: a molecular modeling-guided mutagenesis study of the binding pocket. Biochemistry 42:1544, 2003.
160. Dragic T, Trkola A, Thompson DA, et al. A binding pocket for a small molecule inhibitor of HIV-1 entry within the transmembrane helices of CCR5. Proc Natl Acad Sci USA 97:5639, 2000.
161. Nishikawa M, Takashima K, Nishi T, et al. Analysis of binding sites for the new small-molecule CCR5 antagonist TAK-220 on human CCR5. Antimicrob Agents Chemother 49:4708, 2005.
162. Seibert C, Ying W, Gavrilov S, et al. Interaction of small molecule inhibitors of HIV-1 entry with CCR5. Virology 349:41–54, 2007.
163. Dorr P, Todd K, Irvine R, et al. Site directed mutagenesis studies of CCR5 reveal differences in the interactions between the receptor and various CCR5 antagonists. In: Abstracts of the 45th Annual Interscience Conference on Antimicrobial Agents and Chemotherapy, Washington, DC. 16–19 Dec 2005, abstract H-411.
164. Lee B, Sharron M, Blanpain C, et al. Epitope mapping of CCR5 reveals multiple conformational states and distinct but overlapping structures involved in chemokine and coreceptor function. J Biol Chem 274:9617, 1999.
165. Olson WC, Rabut GE, Nagashima KA, et al. Differential inhibition of human immunodeficiency virus type 1 fusion, gp120 binding, and CC-chemokine activity by monoclonal antibodies to CCR5. J Virol 73:4145, 1999.

166. Rosenkilde MM, Gerlach LO, Jakobsen JS, et al. Molecular mechanism of AMD3100 antagonism in the CXCR4 receptor: transfer of binding site to the CXCR3 receptor. J Biol Chem 279:3033, 2004.
167. De Clercq E. The bicyclam AMD3100 story. Nat Rev Drug Discov 2:581, 2003.
168. Sobieszczyk ME, Talley AK, Wilkin T, et al. Advances in antiretroviral therapy. Top HIV Med 13:24, 2005.
169. Veazey RS, Klasse PJ, Ketas TJ, et al. Use of a small molecule CCR5 inhibitor in macaques to treat simian immunodeficiency virus infection or prevent simian-human immunodeficiency virus infection. J Exp Med 198:1551, 2003.
170. Hatse S, Princen K, Bridger G, et al. Chemokine receptor inhibition by AMD3100 is strictly confined to CXCR4. FEBS Lett 527:255, 2002.
171. Xu S, Wojcik L, Strizki J. Antagonism of the CCR5 receptor by SCH-C leads to elevated beta-chemokine levels and receptor expression in chronically treated PBMC cultures. In: Abstracts of the 9th Conference on Retroviruses and Opportunistic Infections, Seattle, WA, 24–28 Feb 2002, abstract 398-T.
172. Paxton WA, Martin SR, Tse D, et al. Relative resistance to HIV-1 infection of CD4 lymphocytes from persons who remain uninfected despite multiple high-risk sexual exposure. Nat Med 2:412, 1996.
173. Fatkenheuer G, Pozniak AL, Johnson MA, et al. Efficacy of short-term monotherapy with maraviroc, a new CCR5 antagonist, in patients infected with HIV-1. Nat Med 11:1170, 2005.
174. Lalezari J, Thompson M, Kumar P, et al. Antiviral activity and safety of 873140, a novel CCR5 antagonist, during short-term monotherapy in HIV-infected adults. AIDS 19:1443, 2005.
175. Reynes J, Rouzier R, Kanouni T, et al. SCH C: safety and antiviral effects of a CCR5 receptor antagonist in HIV-1-infeted subjects. In: Abstracts of the 9th Conference on Retroviruses and Opportunistic Infections, Seattle, WA, 24–28 Feb 2002, abstract 1.
176. Schurmann D, Fatkenheuer G, Reynes J, et al. Antiviral activity, pharmacokinetics and safety of vicriviroc, an oral CCR5 antagonist, during 14-day monotherapy in HIV-infected adults. AIDS 21:1293–9, 2007.
177. Roschke V, Clark S, Branco L, et al. Characterization of a panel of novel human monoclonal antibodies that specifically antagonize CCR5 and block HIV entry. In: Abstracts of the 44th Annual Interscience Conference on Antimicrobial Agents and Chemotherapy, Washington, DC, 30 Oct to 2 Nov 2004, abstract H-213.
178. Demarest J, Shibayama S, Ferris R, et al. A novel CCR5 antagonist, 873140, exhibits potent in vitro anti-HIV activity. In: Abstracts of the XV International Conference on AIDS, Bangkok, Thailand, 11–18 Jul 2004, abstract WeOrA1231.
179. Nakata H, Koh Y, Maeda K, et al. Greater synergistic anti-HIV effects upon combinations of a CCR5 inhibitor AK602/ONO4128/GW873140 with CXCR4 inhibitors than with other anti-HIV drugs. In: Abstracts of the 12th Conference on Retroviruses and Opportunistic Infections, Boston, MA, 22–25 Feb 2005, abstract 543.
180. Sparks S, Adkison K, Shachoy-Clark A, et al. Prolonged duration of CCR5 occupancy by 873140 in HIV-negative and HIV-positive subjects. In: Abstracts of the 12th Conference on Retroviruses and Opportunistic Infections, Boston, MA, 22–25 Feb 2005, abstract 77.
181. Adkison KK, Shachoy-Clark A, Fang L, et al. The effects of ritonavir and lopinavir/ritonavir on the pharmacokinetics of a novel CCR5 antagonist, aplaviroc, in healthy subjects. Br J Clin Pharmacol 62:336–44, 2006.
182. Kitrinos K, Sparks S, Fang L, et al. Minimal to no changes in plasma chemokine/cytokine levels in HIV-negative and HIV-positive subjects following short term administration of 873140. In: Abstracts of the 45th Annual Interscience Conference on Antimicrobial Agents and Chemotherapy, Washington, DC, 16–19 Dec 2005, abstract H-1097.
183. Song I, Adkison K, Shachoy-Clark A, et al. Pharmacokinetic interaction between 873140 and atazanavir/ritonavir. In: Abstracts of the 45th Annual Interscience Conference on Antimicrobial Agents and Chemotherapy, Washington, DC, 16–19 Dec 2005, abstract A-1196.
184. Adkison K, Fang L, Shachoy-Clark A, et al. The pharmacokinetic interaction between the entry inhibitor 873140 and efavirenz in healthy adults. In: Abstracts of the 45th Annual Interscience Conference on Antimicrobial Agents and Chemotherapy, Washington, DC, 16–19 Dec 2005, abstract A-1197.
185. Adkison K, Fang L, Shachoy-Clark A, et al. Coadministration of fosamprenavir/ritonavir overcomes the effect of efavirenz induction on 873140 pharmacokinetics. In: Abstracts of the 45th Annual Interscience Conference on Antimicrobial Agents and Chemotherapy, Washington, DC, 16–19 Dec 2005, abstract A-1194.
186. Song I, Adkison K, Shachoy-Clark A, et al. Absence of pharmacokinetic drug interaction between 873140 and tenofovir disoproxil fumarate. In: Abstracts of the 45th Annual Interscience Conference on Antimicrobial Agents and Chemotherapy, Washington, DC, 16–19 Dec 2005, abstract A-1195.
187. GlaxoSmithKline, Statement to Patient Community, 15 Sep 2005.
188. Nichols W, Steel H, Bonny T. Hepatotoxicity observed in clinical trials of aplaviroc (APL, 873140). In: Abstracts of the 10th European AIDS Conference, Dublin, Ireland, 17–20 Nov 2005, abstract special presentation.
189. GlaxoSmithKline, GlaxoSmithKline terminates patient enrollment for phase 3 studies of investigational HIV entry inhibitor aplaviroc (GW873140), Press Release, 25 Oct 2005.
190. Dorr P, Westby M, Dobbs S, et al. Maraviroc (UK-427,857), a potent, orally bioavailable, and selective small-molecule inhibitor of chemokine receptor CCR5 with broad-spectrum anti-human immunodeficiency virus type 1 activity. Antimicrob Agents Chemother 49:4721, 2005.
191. Pullen S, Sale H, Napier C, et al. Maraviroc is a slowly reversible antagonist at the human CCR5 in a CRE luciferase reporter gene assay. In: Abstracts of the 13th Conference on Retroviruses and Opportunistic Infections, Denver, CO, 5–8 Feb 2006, abstract 504.
192. Abel S, Russell D, Ridgway C, et al. Overview of the drug–drug interaction data for maraviroc (MVC, UK-427,857). In: Abstracts of the 6th International Workshop on Clinical Pharmacology of HIV Therapy, Quebec, Canada, 28–30 Apr 2005, abstract 76.
193. Walker DK, Abel S, Comby P, et al. Species differences in the disposition of the CCR5 antagonist, UK-427,857, a new potential treatment for HIV. Drug Metab Dispos 33:587, 2005.
194. Mansfield R, Brunton N, Sutton M, et al. Pre-clinical assessment of the potential of UK-427,857, a CCR5 antagonist, to effect cardiac QT intervals. In: Abstracts of the XV International Conference on AIDS, Bangkok, Thailand, 11–18 Jul 2004, abstract WePeA5647.
195. Peters C, Kawabata T, Sytnin P. Assesment of immunotoxic potential of maraviroc (UK-427,857) in cynomologus monkeys. In: Abstracts of the 45th Annual Interscience Conference on Antimicrobial Agents and Chemotherapy, Washington, DC, 16–19 Dec 2005, abstract H-1100.
196. McHale M, Abel S, Russell D, et al. Overview of phase 1 and 2a safety and efficacy data of maraviroc (UK-427,857). In: Abstracts of the 3rd International AIDS Society Conference on HIV Pathogenesis and Treatment, Rio De Janeiro, Brazil, 24–27 Jul 2005, abstract TuOa0204.

197. Davis J, Hilsden F, Sudworth D, et al. A single dose study to investigate the effect of the CCR5 antagonist UK-427,857 on the QTc interval in healthy subjects. In: Abstracts of the XV International Conference on AIDS, Bangkok, Thailand, 11–18 Jul 2004, abstract TuPeB4605.
198. Penny M, Boucher M, Man M, et al. Pharmacogenetic analysis of polymorphisms in chemokine receptors CCR5 and CCR2 with respect to safety and toleration of maraviroc (UK-427,857). In: Abstracts of the 45th Annual Interscience Conference on Antimicrobial Agents and Chemotherapy, Washington, DC, 16–19 Dec 2005, abstract H-1099.
199. Russell D, Weissberger G, Wooldridge C. Investigation into the haemodynamic effects of oral maraviroc (UK-427,857) in healthy volunteers. In: Abstracts of the 10th European AIDS Conference, Dublin, Ireland, 17–20 Nov 2005, abstract LBPe4.1/10.
200. Mayer H. A case of severe hepatotoxicity. In: Targeting HIV Entry: 1st International Workshop, Bethesda, MD, 2–3 Dec 2005.
201. Muirhead G, Pozniak A, Gazzard B, et al. A novel probe drug interaction study to investigate the effect of selected ARV combinations on the pharmacokinetics of a single oral dose of UK-427,857 in HIV +ve Subjects. In: Abstracts of the 12th Conference on Retroviruses and Opportunistic Infections, Boston, MA, 22–25 Feb 2005, abstract 663.
202. Abel S, Taylor-Worth R, Ridgway C, et al. Effect of boosted tipranavir on the pharmacokinetics of maraviroc (UK-427,857) in healthy volunteers. In: Abstracts of the 10th European AIDS Conference, Dublin, Ireland, 17–20 Nov 2005, abstract LBPe4.3/15.
203. Nelson M, Fatkenheuer G, Konourina I, et al. Efficacy and safety of maraviroc plus optimized background therapy in viremic, ART-experienced patients infected with CCR5-tropic HIV-1 in Europe, Australia, and North America, 24-week results. Abstracts of the 14th Conference on Retroviruses and Opportunistic Infections, February 25–28, 2007, Los Angeles, California, abstract #104bLB.
203a. Lalezari J, Goodrich J, DeJesus E, et al. Efficacy and safety of maraviroc plus optimized background therapy in viremic ART-experienced patients infected with CCR5-tropic HIV-1 24-week results of a phase 2b/3 study in the US and Canada. Abstracts of the 14th Conference on Retroviruses and Opportunistic Infections, February 25–28, 2007, Los Angeles, California, abstract #104aLB.
203b. Mayer H, van der Ryst E, Saag M, et al. Safety and efficacy of maraviroc (MVC), a novel CCR5 antagonist, when used in combination with optimized background therapy (OBT) for the treatment of antiretroviral-experienced subjects infected with dual/mixed-tropic HIV-1: 24-week results of a phase 2b exploratory trial. Abstracts of the XVI International AIDS Conference, August 13–16, 2006, Toronto, Canada, abstract #THLB0215.
203c. Saag M, Ive P, Heera J, et al. A multicenter, randomized, double-blind, comparative trial of a novel CCR5 antagonist, maraviroc versus efavirenz, both in combination with Combivir (zidovudine[ZDV]/lamivudine [3TC]), for the treatment of antiretroviral naive patients infected with R5 HIV1: week 48 results of the MERIT study. Abstracts of the 4th International AIDS Society Conference on HIV Pathogenesis, Treatment, and Prevention, July 22-25-2007, Sydney, Australia, abstract #WESS104.
204. Strizki JM, Xu S, Wagner NE, et al. SCH-C (SCH 351125), an orally bioavailable, small molecule antagonist of the chemokine receptor CCR5, is a potent inhibitor of HIV-1 infection in vitro and in vivo. Proc Natl Acad Sci USA 98: 12718, 2001.
205. Strizki JM, Tremblay C, Xu S, et al. Discovery and characterization of vicriviroc (SCH 417690), a CCR5 antagonist with potent activity against human immunodeficiency virus type 1. Antimicrob Agents Chemother 49:4911, 2005.
206. Tagat JR, McCombie SW, Nazareno D, et al. Piperazine-based CCR5 antagonists as HIV-1 inhibitors. IV. Discovery of 1-[(4,6-dimethyl-5-pyrimidinyl)carbonyl]-4-[4-[2-methoxy-1(R)-4-(trifluoromethyl)phenyl]ethyl-3(S)-methyl-1-piperazinyl]-4-methylpiperidine (Sch-417690/Sch-D), a potent, highly selective, and orally bioavailable CCR5 antagonist. J Med Chem 47:2405, 2004.
207. Wojcik L, Gheyas F, Ogert R, et al. In vitro anti-HIV-1 activity of SCH 417690 in combination with other antiretroviral therapies and against resitant HIV-1 strains. In: Abstracts of the 45th Annual Interscience Conference on Antimicrobial Agents and Chemotherapy, Washington, DC, 16–19 Dec 2005, abstract H-1096.
208. Sansone A, Keung A, Caceres M, et al. Rising multiple-dose assessment of SCH 417690 – similar safety, tolerability, and pharmacokinetics in uninfected and HIV-infected adults. In: Abstracts of the 45th Annual Interscience Conference on Antimicrobial Agents and Chemotherapy, Washington, DC, 16–19 Dec 2005, abstract A-33.
209. Keung A, Sansone A, Caceres M, et al. Effect of food on bioavailability of SCH 417690 in healthy volunteers. In: Abstracts of the 45th Annual Interscience Conference on Antimicrobial Agents and Chemotherapy, Washington, DC, 16–19 Dec 2005, abstract A-1200.
210. Sansone A, Kraan M, Long J. QTc interval analysis of SCH 417690, a novel CCR5 inhibitor. In: Abstracts of the 45th Annual Interscience Conference on Antimicrobial Agents and Chemotherapy, Washington, DC, 16–19 Dec 2005, abstract H-1095.
211. Schuermann D, Pechardscheck C, Rouzier R, et al. SCH 417690: antiviral activity of a potent new CCR5 receptor antagonist. In: Abstracts of the 3rd International AIDS Society Conference on HIV Pathogenesis and Treatment, Rio De Janeiro, Brazil, 24–27 Jul 2005, abstract TuOa0205.
212. Seiberling M, Kraan M, Keung A, et al. Similar increase in SCH 417690 plasma exposure with coadministration of varying doses of ritonavir in healthy volunteers. In: Abstracts of the 3rd International AIDS Society Conference on HIV Pathogenesis and Treatment, Rio De Janeiro, Brazil, 24–27 Jul 2005, abstract TuPe3.1B06.
213. Saltzman M, Rosenberg M, Kraan M, et al. Pharmacokinetics of SCH 417690 administered alone or in combination with ritonavir or lopinavir/ritonavir. In: Abstracts of the 3rd International AIDS Society Conference on HIV Pathogenesis and Treatment, Rio De Janeiro, Brazil, 24–27 Jul 2005, abstract TuPe3.1B05.
214. Saltzman M, Rosenberg M, Kraan M, et al. Pharmacokinetics of SCH 417690 administered alone or in combination with ritonavir and efavirenz in healthy volunteers. In: Abstracts of the 3rd International AIDS Society Conference on HIV Pathogenesis and Treatment, Rio De Janeiro, Brazil, 24–27 Jul 2005, abstract TuPe3.1B08.
215. Sansone A, Keung A, Tetter E, et al. Pharmacokinetics of vicriviroc are not affected in combination with five different protease inhibitors boosted by ritonavir. In: Abstracts of the 13th Conference on Retroviruses and Opportunistic Infections, Denver, CO, 5–8 Feb 2006, abstract 582.
216. Guillaume M, Kraan M, Keung A, et al. The pharmacokinetics of SCH 417690 when administered alone and in combination with lamivudine/zidovudine. In: Abstracts of the 3rd International AIDS Society Conference on HIV Pathogenesis and Treatment, Rio De Janeiro, Brazil, 24–27 Jul 2005, abstract TuPe3.1B03.
217. Guillaume M, Kraan M, Soni P, et al. Pharmacokinetics of SCH 417690 administered alone or in combination with tenofovir. In: Abstracts of the 3rd International AIDS Society

Conference on HIV Pathogenesis and Treatment, Rio De Janeiro, Brazil, 24–27 Jul 2005, abstract TuPe3.1B09.
218. Greaves W, Landovitz R, Fatkenheuer G, et al. Late virologic breakthrough in treatment-naive patients on a regimen of Combivir + vicriviroc. In: Abstracts of the 13th Conference on Retroviruses and Opportunistic Infections, Denver, CO, 5–8 Feb 2006, abstract 161LB.
219. Gulick RM, Su Z, Flexner C, et al. Phase 2 study of the safety and efficacy of vicriviroc, a CCR5 inhibitor, in HIV-1-Infected, treatment-experienced patients: AIDS clinical trials group 5211. J Infect Dis 196:304–12, 2007.
220. Gulick R, Su Z, Flexner C, et al. ACTG 5211: phase II study of the safety and efficacy of vicriviroc (VCV) in HIV-infected treatment-experienced subjects: 48 week results. Abstracts of the 4th International AIDS Society Conference on HIV Pathogenesis, Treatment, and Prevention, July 22-25-2007, Sydney, Australia, abstract #TUAB102.
221. Trkola A, Ketas TJ, Nagashima KA, et al. Potent, broad-spectrum inhibition of human immunodeficiency virus type 1 by the CCR5 monoclonal antibody PRO 140. J Virol 75:579, 2001.
222. Rusert P, Kuster H, Joos B, et al. Virus isolates during acute and chronic human immunodeficiency virus type 1 infection show distinct patterns of sensitivity to entry inhibitors. J Virol 79:8454, 2005.
223. Olson WC, Tsurushita N, Hinton PR, et al. Potent, broad-spectrum inhibition of HIV-1 entry with the humanized monoclonal antibody PRO 140. In: Abstracts of the XIV International AIDS Conference, Barcelona, Spain, 7–12 Jul 2002, abstract TuP3A4363.
224. Murga JD, Franti M, Pevear DC, Maddon PJ, Olson WC. Potent antiviral synergy between monoclonal antibody and small-molecule CCR5 inhibitors of human immunodeficiency virus type 1. Antimicrob Agents Chemother 50:3289–96, 2006.
225. Franti M, Ramos L, Maloveste S, et al. In vivo control of HIV-1 replication with PRO 140, a humanized monoclonal antibody to CCR5. In: Abstracts of the XV International Conference on AIDS, Bangkok, Thailand, 11–18 Jul 2004, abstract WeOrA1230.
226. Olson W, Doshan H, Zhan C, et al. First-in-humans trial of PRO 140, a humanized CCR5 monoclonal antibody for HIv-1 therapy. In: Abstracts of the 3rd International AIDS Society Conference on HIV Pathogenesis and Treatment, Rio De Janeiro, Brazil, 24–27 Jul 2005, abstract WePe6.2C04.
227. Olson WC, Doshan H, Zhan C, et al. Prolonged coating of CCR5 lymphocytes by PRO 140, a humanized CCR5 monoclonal antibody for HIV-1 therapy. In: Abstracts of the 13th Conference on Retroviruses and Opportunistic Infections, Denver, CO, 5–8 Feb 2006, abstract 515.
228. Cormier EG, Ketas TJ, Sullivan BM, et al. Baseline viral susceptiblity to the CCR5 coreceptor inhibitor PRO 140. In: Abstracts of the 2nd International AIDS Society Conference on HIV Pathogenesis and Treatment, Paris, France, 13–16 Jul 2003, abstract 530.
229. Trkola A, Kuhmann SE, Strizki JM, et al. HIV-1 escape from a small molecule, CCR5-specific entry inhibitor does not involve CXCR4 use. Proc Natl Acad Sci USA 99:395, 2002.
230. Saag MS, Jacobson JM, Thompson M, et al. Antiviral effects and tolerability of the CCR5 monoclonal antibody PRO 140: a proof of concept study in HIV-infected individuals. Abstracts of the 4th International AIDS Society Conference on HIV Pathogenesis, Treatment, and Prevention, July 22-25-2007, Sydney, Australia, abstract #WESS201.
231. Baba M, Nishimura O, Kanzaki N, et al. A small-molecule, nonpeptide CCR5 antagonist with highly potent and selective anti-HIV-1 activity. Proc Natl Acad Sci USA 96:5698, 1999.
232. Baba M, Takashima K, Miyake H, et al. TAK-652 inhibits CCR5-mediated human immunodeficiency virus type 1 infection in vitro and has favorable pharmacokinetics in humans. Antimicrob Agents Chemother 49:4584, 2005.
233. Tremblay CL, Giguel F, Chou TC, Dong H, Takashima K, Hirsch MS. TAK-652, a novel CCR5 inhibitor, has favourable drug interactions with other antiretrovirals in vitro. Antivir Ther 10:967–8, 2005.
234. Hendrix CW, Collier AC, Lederman MM, et al. Safety, pharmacokinetics, and antiviral activity of AMD3100, a selective CXCR4 receptor inhibitor, in HIV-1 infection. J Acquir Immune Defic Syndr 37:1253, 2004.
235. Lack NA, Green B, Dale DC, et al. A pharmacokinetic-pharmacodynamic model for the mobilization of CD34+ hematopoietic progenitor cells by AMD3100. Clin Pharmacol Ther 77:427, 2005.
236. Murakami T, Yoshida A, Kumakura S, et al. A new potent and orally bioavailable X4 HIV-1 binding CXCR4 antagonist in vivo. In: Abstracts of the XV International Conference on AIDS, Bangkok, Thailand, 11–18 Jul 2004, abstract LbOrA01.
237. Tanaka Y, Okuma K, Tanaka R, et al. Development of novel orally bioavailable CXCR4 antagonists, KRH-3955 and KRH-3140: binding specificity, pharmacokinetics, and anti-HIV-1 activity in vivo and in vitro. In: Abstracts of the 13th Conference on Retroviruses and Opportunistic Infections, Denver, CO, 5–8 Feb 2006, abstract 49LB.
238. Doranz BJ, Filion LG, Diaz-Mitoma F, et al. Safe use of the CXCR4 inhibitor ALX40–4C in humans. AIDS Res Hum Retroviruses 17:475, 2001.
239. De Clercq E, Yamamoto N, Pauwels R, et al. Highly potent and selective inhibition of human immunodeficiency virus by the bicyclam derivative JM3100. Antimicrob Agents Chemother 38:668, 1994.
240. Donzella GA, Schols D, Lin SW, et al. AMD3100, a small molecule inhibitor of HIV-1 entry via the CXCR4 co-receptor. Nat Med 4:72, 1998.
241. Schols D, Struyf S, Van Damme J, et al. Inhibition of T-tropic HIV strains by selective antagonization of the chemokine receptor CXCR4. J Exp Med 186:1383, 1997.
242. Datema R, Rabin L, Hincenbergs M, et al. Antiviral efficacy in vivo of the anti-human immunodeficiency virus bicyclam SDZ SID 791 (JM 3100), an inhibitor of infectious cell entry. Antimicrob Agents Chemother 40:750, 1996.
243. Hendrix CW, Flexner C, MacFarland RT, et al. Pharmacokinetics and safety of AMD-3100, a novel antagonist of the CXCR-4 chemokine receptor, in human volunteers. Antimicrob Agents Chemother 44:1667, 2000.
244. Burroughs L, Mielcarek M, Little MT, et al. Durable engraftment of AMD3100-mobilized autologous and allogeneic peripheral-blood mononuclear cells in a canine transplantation model. Blood 106:4002, 2005.
245. Liles WC, Broxmeyer HE, Rodger E, et al. Mobilization of hematopoietic progenitor cells in healthy volunteers by AMD3100, a CXCR4 antagonist. Blood 102:2728, 2003.
246. Schols D, Claes S, Hatse S, et al. Anti-HIV profile of AMD070, an orally bioavailable CXCR4 antagonist. In: Abstracts of the 10th Conference on Retroviruses and Opportunistic Infections, Boston, MA, 10–14 Feb 2003, abstract 563.
247. Schols D, Vermeire K, Jatse S, et al. In vitro anti-HIV activity profile of AMD887, a novel CCR5 antagonist, in combination with the CXCR4 inhibitor AMD070. In: Abstracts of the 11th Conference on Retroviruses and Opportunistic Infections, San Francisco, CA, 8–11 Feb 2004, abstract 539.
248. Stone ND, Dunaway SB, Flexner C, et al. Multiple-Dose Escalation Study of the Safety, Pharmacokinetics, and Biologic Activity of Oral AMD070, a Selective CXCR4 Receptor Inhibitor, in Human Subjects. Antimicrob Agents Chemother 51:2351–8, 2007.
249. Westby M, Smith-Burchnell C, Mori J, et al. Reduced maximal inhibition in phenotypic susceptibility assays indicates

that viral strains resistant to the CCR5 antagonist maraviroc utilize inhibitor-bound receptor for entry. J Virol 81:2359–71, 2007.
250. Pastore C, Ramos A, Mosier DE. Intrinsic obstacles to human immunodeficiency virus type 1 coreceptor switching. J Virol 78:7565, 2004.
251. Labranche C, McDanal C, Harris S, et al. Analysis of in vitro derived viruses exhibiting reduced susceptibility to 873140. In: Abstracts of the 45th Annual Interscience Conference on Antimicrobial Agents and Chemotherapy, Washington, DC, 16–19 Dec 2005, abstract H-1098.
252. Olson WC, Maddon PJ. Resistance to HIV-1 entry inhibitors. Curr Drug Targets Infect Disord 3:283, 2003.
253. Aarons EJ, Beddows S, Willingham T, et al. Adaptation to blockade of human immunodeficiency virus type 1 entry imposed by the anti-CCR5 monoclonal antibody 2D7. Virology 287:382, 2001.
254. de Vreese K, Kofler-Mongold V, Leutgeb C, et al. The molecular target of bicyclams, potent inhibitors of human immunodeficiency virus replication. J Virol 70:689, 1996.
255. Westby M, Smith-Burchnell C, Hamilton D, et al. Structurally-related HIV coreceptor antagonists bind to similar regions of CCR5 but have differential activities against UK-427,857-resistant primary isolates. In: Abstracts of the 12th Conference on Retroviruses and Opportunistic Infections, Boston, MA, 22–25 Feb 2005, abstract 96.
256. Holm GH, Zhang C, Gorry PR, et al. Apoptosis of bystander T cells induced by human immunodeficiency virus type 1 with increased envelope/receptor affinity and coreceptor binding site exposure. J Virol 78:4541, 2004.
257. Barbour JD, Wrin T, Grant RM, et al. Evolution of phenotypic drug susceptibility and viral replication capacity during long-term virologic failure of protease inhibitor therapy in human immunodeficiency virus-infected adults. J Virol 76:11104, 2002.
258. Deeks SG, Barbour JD, Martin JN, et al. Sustained CD4+ T cell response after virologic failure of protease inhibitor-based regimens in patients with human immunodeficiency virus infection. J Infect Dis 181:946, 2000.
259. Deeks SG, Hoh R, Grant RM, et al. CD4+ T cell kinetics and activation in human immunodeficiency virus-infected patients who remain viremic despite long-term treatment with protease inhibitor-based therapy. J Infect Dis 185:315, 2002.
260. Deeks SG, Wrin T, Liegler T, et al. Virologic and immunologic consequences of discontinuing combination antiretroviral-drug therapy in HIV-infected patients with detectable viremia. N Engl J Med 344:472, 2001.
261. Nijhuis M, Deeks S, Boucher C. Implications of antiretroviral resistance on viral fitness. Curr Opin Infect Dis 14: 23, 2001.
262. Stoddart CA, Liegler TJ, Mammano F, et al. Impaired replication of protease inhibitor-resistant HIV-1 in human thymus. Nat Med 7:712, 2001.
263. Hammer SM. HIV drug resistance: implications for management. Top HIV Med 10:10, 2002.
264. Yerly S, Jost S, Telenti A, et al. Infrequent transmission of HIV-1 drug-resistant variants. Antivir Ther 9:375, 2004.
265. Menendez-Arias L, Este JA. HIV-resistance to viral entry inhibitors. Curr Pharm Des 10:1845, 2004.
266. Michael NL, Moore JP. HIV-1 entry inhibitors: evading the issue. Nat Med 5:740, 1999.
267. Harouse JM, Buckner C, Gettie A, et al. CD8+ T cell-mediated CXC chemokine receptor 4-simian/human immunodeficiency virus suppression in dually infected rhesus macaques. Proc Natl Acad Sci USA 100:10977, 2003.
268. Delforge ML, Liesnard C, Debaisieux L, et al. In vivo inhibition of syncytium-inducing variants of HIV in patients treated with didanosine. AIDS 9:89, 1995.
269. Ercoli L, Sarmati L, Nicastri E, et al. HIV phenotype switching during antiretroviral therapy: emergence of saquinavir-resistant strains with less cytopathogenicity. AIDS 11:1211, 1997.
270. Equils O, Garratty E, Wei LS, et al. Recovery of replication-competent virus from CD4 T cell reservoirs and change in coreceptor use in human immunodeficiency virus type 1-infected children responding to highly active antiretroviral therapy. J Infect Dis 182:751, 2000.
271. Philpott S, Weiser B, Anastos K, et al. Preferential suppression of CXCR4-specific strains of HIV-1 by antiviral therapy. J Clin Invest 107:431, 2001.
272. Pierson T, Hoffman TL, Blankson J, et al. Characterization of chemokine receptor utilization of viruses in the latent reservoir for human immunodeficiency virus type 1. J Virol 74:7824, 2000.
273. Skrabal K, Trouplin V, Labrosse B, et al. Impact of antiretroviral treatment on the tropism of HIV-1 plasma virus populations. AIDS 17:809, 2003.
274. Johnston ER, Zijenah LS, Mutetwa S, et al. High frequency of syncytium-inducing and CXCR4-tropic viruses among human immunodeficiency virus type 1 subtype C-infected patients receiving antiretroviral treatment. J Virol 77:7682, 2003.
275. Delobel P, Sandres-Saune K, Cazabat M, et al. R5 to X4 Switch of the predominant HIV-1 population in cellular reservoirs during effective highly active antiretroviral therapy. J Acquir Immune Defic Syndr 38:382, 2005.
276. van Rij RP, Visser JA, van Praag RM, et al. Both R5 and X4 human immunodeficiency virus type 1 variants persist during prolonged therapy with five antiretroviral drugs. J Virol 76:3054, 2002.
277. Chen Z, Gettie A, Ho DD, et al. Primary SIVsm isolates use the CCR5 coreceptor from sooty mangabeys naturally infected in west Africa: a comparison of coreceptor usage of primary SIVsm, HIV-2, and SIVmac. Virology 246:113, 1998.
278. de Silva E, Stumpf MP. HIV and the CCR5-Delta32 resistance allele. FEMS Microbiol Lett 241:1, 2004.
279. Fischereder M, Luckow B, Hocher B, et al. CC chemokine receptor 5 and renal-transplant survival. Lancet 357:1758, 2001.
280. Glass WG, McDermott DH, Lim JK, et al. CCR5 deficiency increases risk of symptomatic West Nile virus infection. J Exp Med 203:35, 2006.
281. Huffnagle GB, McNeil LK, McDonald RA, et al. Cutting edge: Role of C-C chemokine receptor 5 in organ-specific and innate immunity to Cryptococcus neoformans. J Immunol 163:4642, 1999.
282. Zhou Y, Kurihara T, Ryseck RP, et al. Impaired macrophage function and enhanced T cell-dependent immune response in mice lacking CCR5, the mouse homologue of the major HIV-1 coreceptor. J Immunol 160:4018, 1998.
283. Sato N, Kuziel WA, Melby PC, et al. Defects in the generation of IFN-gamma are overcome to control infection with Leishmania donovani in CC chemokine receptor (CCR) 5-, macrophage inflammatory protein-1 alpha-, or CCR2-deficient mice. J Immunol 163:5519, 1999.
284. Aliberti J, Reis e Sousa C, Schito M, et al. CCR5 provides a signal for microbial induced production of IL-12 by CD8 alpha+ dendritic cells. Nat Immunol 1:83, 2000.
285. Ajuebor MN, Aspinall AI, Zhou F, et al. Lack of chemokine receptor CCR5 promotes murine fulminant liver failure by preventing the apoptosis of activated CD1d-restricted NKT cells. J Immunol 174:8027, 2005.
286. Glass WG, Lim JK, Cholera R, et al. Chemokine receptor CCR5 promotes leukocyte trafficking to the brain and survival in West Nile virus infection. J Exp Med 202:1087, 2005.
287. Tyner JW, Uchida O, Kajiwara N, et al. CCL5–CCR5 interaction provides antiapoptotic signals for macrophage survival during viral infection. Nat Med 11:1180, 2005.

288. Amano H, Bickerstaff A, Orosz CG, et al. Absence of recipient CCR5 promotes early and increased allospecific antibody responses to cardiac allografts. J Immunol 174:6499, 2005.
289. Carvalho-Pinto C, Garcia MI, Gomez L, et al. Leukocyte attraction through the CCR5 receptor controls progress from insulitis to diabetes in non-obese diabetic mice. Eur J Immunol 34:548, 2004.
290. Wysocki CA, Jiang Q, Panoskaltsis-Mortari A, et al. Critical role for CCR5 in the function of donor CD4+CD25+ regulatory T cells during acute graft-versus-host disease. Blood 106:3300, 2005.
291. Ma B, Kang MJ, Lee CG, et al. Role of CCR5 in IFN-gamma-induced and cigarette smoke-induced emphysema. J Clin Invest 115:3460, 2005.
292. Robinson SC, Scott KA, Wilson JL, et al. A chemokine receptor antagonist inhibits experimental breast tumor growth. Cancer Res 63:8360, 2003.
293. Ng-Cashin J, Kuhns JJ, Burkett SE, et al. Host absence of CCR5 potentiates dendritic cell vaccination. J Immunol 170:4201, 2003.
294. Ferguson NM, Fraser C, Anderson RM. Viral dynamics and anti-viral pharmacodynamics: rethinking in vitro measures of drug potency. Trends Pharmacol Sci 22:97, 2001.
295. Tremblay CL, Giguel F, Kollmann C, et al. Anti-human immunodeficiency virus interactions of SCH-C (SCH 351125), a CCR5 antagonist, with other antiretroviral agents in vitro. Antimicrob Agents Chemother 46:1336, 2002.
296. Tremblay CL, Kollmann C, Giguel F, et al. Strong in vitro synergy between the fusion inhibitor T-20 and the CXCR4 blocker AMD-3100. J Acquir Immune Defic Syndr 25:99, 2000.
297. Tremblay CL, Giguel F, Guan Y, et al. TAK-220, a novel small-molecule CCR5 antagonist, has favorable anti-human immunodeficiency virus interactions with other antiretrovirals in vitro. Antimicrob Agents Chemother 49:3483, 2005.
298. Veazey RS, Klasse PJ, Schader SM, et al. Protection of macaques from vaginal SHIV challenge by vaginally delivered inhibitors of virus-cell fusion. Nature 438:99, 2005.
299. Tremblay C. Effects of HIV-1 entry inhibitors in combination. Curr Pharm Des 10:1861, 2004.
300. Carpenter CC, Cooper DA, Fischl MA, et al. Antiretroviral therapy in adults: updated recommendations of the International AIDS Society-USA Panel. JAMA 283:381, 2000.
301. Harrington M, Carpenter CC. Hit HIV-1 hard, but only when necessary. Lancet 355:2147, 2000.
302. Mattapallil JJ, Smit-McBride Z, Dailey P, et al. Activated memory CD4(+) T helper cells repopulate the intestine early following antiretroviral therapy of simian immunodeficiency virus-infected rhesus macaques but exhibit a decreased potential to produce interleukin-2. J Virol 73:6661, 1999.
303. Koning FA, Kwa D, Boeser-Nunnink B, et al. Decreasing sensitivity to RANTES (regulated on activation, normally T cell-expressed and -secreted) neutralization of CC chemokine receptor 5-using, non-syncytium-inducing virus variants in the course of human immunodeficiency virus type 1 infection. J Infect Dis 188:864, 2003.
304. Repits J, Oberg M, Esbjornsson J, et al. Selection of human immunodeficiency virus type 1 R5 variants with augmented replicative capacity and reduced sensitivity to entry inhibitors during severe immunodeficiency. J Gen Virol 86:2859, 2005.
305. Koning FA, Koevoets C, van der Vorst TJ, et al. Sensitivity of primary R5 HTV-1 to inhibition by RANTES correlates with sensitivity to small-molecule R5 inhibitors. Antivir Ther 10:231, 2005.
306. Burton DR, Moore JP. Why do we not have an HIV vaccine and how can we make one? Nat Med 4:495, 1998.
307. Garber DA, Silvestri G, Feinberg MB. Prospects for an AIDS vaccine: three big questions, no easy answers. Lancet Infect Dis 4:397, 2004.
308. Klausner RD, Fauci AS, Corey L, et al. Medicine. The need for a global HIV vaccine enterprise. Science 300:2036, 2003.
309. McMichael AJ, Hanke T. HIV vaccines 1983–2003. Nat Med 9:874, 2003.
310. Shattock RJ, Moore JP. Inhibiting sexual transmission of HIV-1 infection. Nat Rev Microbiol 1:25, 2003.
311. Stone A. Microbicides: a new approach to preventing HIV and other sexually transmitted infections. Nat Rev Drug Discov 1:977, 2002.
312. Turpin JA. Considerations and development of topical microbicides to inhibit the sexual transmission of HIV. Expert Opin Investig Drugs 11:1077, 2002.
313. Youle M, Wainberg MA. Could chemoprophylaxis be used as an HIV prevention strategy while we wait for an effective vaccine? AIDS 17:937, 2003.
314. Bertozzi S, Gutierrez JP, Opuni M, et al. Estimating resource needs for HIV/AIDS health care services in low-income and middle-income countries. Health Policy 69:189, 2004.
315. Piot P, Feachem RG, Lee JW, et al. Public health. A global response to AIDS: lessons learned, next steps. Science 304:1909, 2004.
316. Cock KM, Weiss HA. The global epidemiology of HIV/AIDS. Trop Med Int Health 5:A3, 2000.
317. Garcia-Moreno C, Watts C. Violence against women: its importance for HIV/AIDS. AIDS 14 (Suppl 3):S253, 2000.
318. Whyte B. UNAIDS estimates that half the teenagers in some African countries will die of AIDS. Bull World Health Organ 78:946, 2000.
319. Lederman MM, Veazey RS, Offord R, et al. Prevention of vaginal SHIV transmission in rhesus macaques through inhibition of CCR5. Science 306:485, 2004.
320. Tsai CC, Emau P, Jiang Y, et al. Cyanovirin-N inhibits AIDS virus infections in vaginal transmission models. AIDS Res Hum Retroviruses 20:11, 2004.
321. Tsai CC, Emau P, Jiang Y, et al. Cyanovirin-N gel as a topical microbicide prevents rectal transmission of SHIV89.6P in macaques. AIDS Res Hum Retroviruses 19:535, 2003.
322. Grant RM, Hecht FM, Warmerdam M, et al. Time trends in primary HIV-1 drug resistance among recently infected persons. JAMA 288:181, 2002.
323. Veazey RS, Springer MS, Marx PA, et al. Protection of macaques from vaginal SHIV challenge by an orally delivered CCR5 inhibitor. Nat Med 11:1293, 2005.

Chapter 25

Tipranavir

Véronique Joly, MD, Patrick Yeni, MD

INTRODUCTION

The availability of potent antiretroviral drugs, including protease inhibitors (PI), and their use in combination regimens – highly active antiretroviral therapy (HAART) – has led to a dramatic decline in the morbidity and mortality associated with human immunodeficiency (HIV) infection.[1,2] However, despite the success of HAART, there is a growing concern over the development of resistance to antiretroviral drugs. Treatment experienced patients with HIV-1 variants resistant to one or more antiretroviral agents comprise an ever larger proportion of the HIV-infected population. These patients typically have multiple PI resistance mutations conferring some level of resistance to most available PIs, including lopinavir. Furthermore, transmission of single or multidrug resistant viruses has been well documented.[3] Thus, there is an urgent need to develop new PIs with a substantial activity against resistant variants.

Tipranavir (TPV), a nonpeptidic PI with unique resistance characteristics, demonstrated potent inhibitory activity *in vitro* against variants resistant to currently available PIs, suggesting that it may offer potential therapeutic advantages in PI-experienced patients with uncontrolled viral replication.

CHEMICAL STRUCTURE

TPV is a nonpeptidic PI belonging to the class of 4-hydroxy-5, 6-dihydro-2-pyrone sulfonamides (Fig. 25-1). The chemical name of TPV is 2-pyridinesulfonamide, *N*-3-(1*R*-1-(6*R*)-5,6-dihydro-4-hydroxy-2-oxo-6-(2-phenylethyl)-6-propyl-2H-pyran-3-ylpropyl)phenyl-5-trifluoromethyl). It has a molecular weight of 602.7. It has been suggested that TPV binds to the active site of the protease enzyme with fewer hydrogen bonds than peptidic PI, resulting in increased flexibility that allows the drug to adjust to amino acid changes in the active site.[4] Other studies propose that the strong hydrogen bonding interaction with the amide backbone of the protease site Asp30 is responsible for the favorable antiviral activity of TPV against isolates with multiple PI-associated mutations.[5]

It is a white to slightly yellow solid that is freely soluble in dehydrated alcohol and propylene glycol and insoluble at pH 7.5 in aqueous buffer.

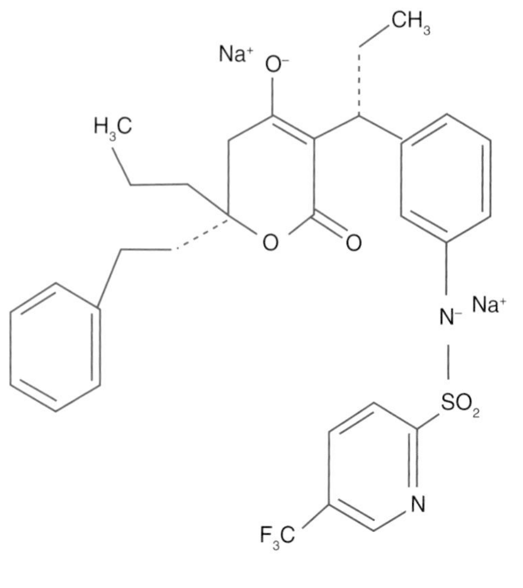

Figure 25-1 ■ Chemical structure of tipranavir.

The marketed formulation of TPV (Aptivus) is a soft gelatin capsule for oral administration. Each capsule contains TPV 250 mg.

IN VITRO ACTIVITY

TPV is a potent and selective inhibitor of HIV protease. In general, it has exhibited potent antiviral activity with 90% inhibitory concentration (IC_{90}) ranging from 0.03 to 0.18 μM.[6] When tested in human serum, protein binding decreases the activity of TPV by 3.75-fold. TPV retains *in vitro* antiviral activity against both laboratory and patient-derived isolates resistant to multiple other PIs with an IC_{90} of 0.18–0.45 μM.[7,8] TPV is also active against HIV-2.

PHARMACOKINETICS AND METABOLISM

TPV has a low solubility, resulting in limited absorption in humans. The capsules were formulated with a self-emulsifying drug delivery system (SEDDS) to achieve maximum absorption. TPV pharmacokinetics were characterized alone and in combination with ritonavir (RTV) in 95 healthy volunteers, which demonstrated that the minimum concentrations for TPV did not exceed the target threshold expected to be necessary to treat PI-resistant virus without RTV boosting.[9] TPV 500 mg bid given with RTV 200 mg bid results in close to a 50-fold increase in the morning trough of TPV concentrations compared with TPV administered without RTV, allowing to obtain levels exceeding the IC_{50} for resistant virus by 27- to 50-fold. TPV should be taken with a standard or high-fat meal, which increases the area under the curve (AUC) by ~30% and improves the gastrointestinal tolerability.[10] TPV is extensively bound to plasma proteins (>99.9%). Based on molecular weight and high protein binding, TPV is not expected to penetrate the central nervous system to an appreciable extent.

Cytochrome P450 (CYP)-3A is the major isoform that is involved in TPV metabolism *in vivo*. CYP-3A is induced by TPV and inhibited by RTV. The RTV inhibition predominates when the two drugs are co-administered. TPV metabolism is then minimal, with only trace metabolites detected and >98% of TPV remaining in the unchanged form through the dosing interval. TPV is a substrate for a weak inhibitor and a potent inducer as well of P-glycoprotein (P-gp). This is an important issue in antiretroviral therapy because P-gp can pump PIs out of cells and thus decrease antiviral efficacy. On the other hand, RTV is an inhibitor of P-gp. The clinical significance of TPV/RTV co-administration and of their interaction with P-gp is difficult to predict. Data suggest that the net effect of TPV/RTV at the proposed dose regimen (500/200 mg) is P-gp induction at steady state.[11]

About 80% of TPV is excreted in the feces. Renal clearance is negligible. TPV exhibits linear pharmacokinetics with a mean elimination half-live of 6 h at steady state.

For patients with renal impairment, no clinically significant difference in TPV clearance is expected. Close clinical and laboratory monitoring of patients with mild or moderate hepatic impairment is important. TPV is contraindicated in severe hepatic impairment.

The recommended dose of TPV is 500 mg (two 250 mg capsules or 5 mL of oral solution) co-administered twice daily with 200 mg RTV, based on BI 1182.52 study results (see further ahead).

EFFICACY

The *in vivo* antiviral efficacy of TPV in antiretroviral-naive patients was evaluated in study BI 1182.3.[12] The median change from baseline in HIV-1 RNA value over 14 days was $-0.77 \log_{10}$ when TPV was given alone at a dose of 1200 mg twice daily, and was significantly better when TPV was co-administered with RTV: $-1.43 \log_{10}$ and $-1.64 \log_{10}$ with TPV/RTV 300/200 mg and TPV/RTV 1200/200 mg twice daily, respectively.

In study BI 1182.52, three doses of TPV/RTV (500/100, 300/200, and 750/200 bid) were evaluated in patients who had previously failed at least two PI-based regimens and had one or more primary mutations. In the first 2 weeks, the current PI was replaced by TPV/RTV but the background regimen was held constant. During this 2-week functional monotherapy phase, the median HIV reductions from baseline in 216 patients were 0.9, 1.0, and 1.2 $\log_{10}$ copies/mL for TPV/RTV 500/100, 500/200 and 750/200 mg, respectively.[13] HIV-1 RNA reductions at week 24 across the doses were dependent on the number of baseline viral PI mutations. Patients in the two higher dose groups required more than one baseline viral mutation before TPV activity started to decrease. A dose–response relationship was noted for adverse events with the highest incidence of grade 3–4 gastrointestinal symptoms in the group receiving the highest dose; the grade 3–4 aspartate aminotransferase (AST) and alanine aminotransferase (ALT) were also more common in the 750/200 mg group, with almost 13% of patients experiencing this degree of elevation in ALT. Although the 750/200 mg twice-daily dose had slightly more activity, the 500/200 mg twice-daily dose was selected for further evaluation in phase III trials.

BI 1182.51 study enrolled patients who had three or four mutations at codons 33, 82, 84, and 90. The initial phase of the study was a randomized comparison of optimized background therapy and one of the four following PI regimens: TPV/RTV 500/200 mg bid, lopinavir/RTV 400/100 mg bid, amprenavir/RTV 600/100 mg bid or saquinavir/RTV 1000/100 mg bid. After day 14, TPV/RTV was added to treatment of subjects initially randomized to receive one of the three currently available PIs, with the objective of evaluating pharmacokinetic interactions between TPV/RTV 500/200 mg and a second RTV boosted PI. The first part of the study allowed a randomized 14-day comparison of TPV/RTV versus three other boosted PI regimens given as functional monotherapy. Over 14 days, plasma HIV RNA levels decreased by

Table 25-1 Selected 24-Week Treatment Outcome Data From the Combined RESIST Trials

Outcome	TPV/r + OBR (n = 582)	CPI/r + OBR (n = 577)	P
Proportion of patients with HIV RNA reduction of $\geq$1 $\log_{10}$ copies/mL	41.2%	18.9%	<0.0001
HIV RNA <400 copies/mL	34.2%	14.9%	<0.0001
HIV RNA <50 copies/mL	23.9%	9.4%	<0.0001
Median change in HIV RNA from baseline ($\log_{10}$ copies/mL)	−0.80	−0.25	<0.0001
Median absolute change in CD4+ T-lymphocyte count (cells/mm^3)	+34	+4	<0.0001

TPV/r, tipranavir/ritonavir; CPI/r, comparator-boosted protease inhibitor; OBR, optimized background regimen.

Data From: Hicks C. RESIST-1: A phase 3, randomized, controlled, open-label, multicenter trial comparing tipranavir/ritonavir (TPV/r) to an optimized comparator protease inhibitor/r (CPI/r) regimen in antiretroviral (ARV) experienced patients: 24-week data. In: 44th Interscience Conference on Antimicrobial Agents and Chemotherapy, Washington, DC, 2004, abstract H-1137a and Cahn P and the RESIST 2 Study Team. 24-week data from RESIST-2: phase 3 study of the efficacy and safety of either tipranavir/ritonavir (TPV/r) or an optimized ritonavir (RTV)-boosted standard-of-care (SOC) comparator PI (CPI) in a large randomized multicenter trial in treatment-experienced HIV+ patients. In: 7th International Congress on Drug Therapy in HIV Infection, Glasgow, 2004, abstract PL-14.3.

1.2 $\log_{10}$ copies/mL in patients taking TPV/RTV, compared with reductions <0.4 $\log_{10}$ copies/mL in each of the other boosted PI arms.[14]

The 24-week results from the two pivotal randomized, controlled, open-label studies, 'Randomized Evaluation of Strategic Intervention in multidrug resistant Subjects with Tipranavir' (RESIST) I and II led to FDA approval of TPV. RESIST I was conducted in North America and Australia while RESIST II recruited patients from Europe and Latin America. These two multicenter studies compared TPV/RTV 500/200 mg bid with a comparator PI plus RTV as booster twice daily, administered in combination with an optimized background regimen chosen on the basis of genotypic resistance testing. Patients were triple class-experienced and had failed at least two PI-based regimens. They were receiving PI treatment at the time of screening. The presence of at least one primary protease mutation at 30N, 46I/L, 48V, 50V, 82A/F/L/T, 84V, and 90 and no more than two protease mutations at codons 33, 82, 84, and 90 was required for entry into the study. The primary endpoint of the RESIST trials was the proportion of patients with two consecutive viral load measurements >1 $\log_{10}$ below baseline after 24 weeks of treatment.

There were 1483 subjects enrolled in the two RESIST trials. Characteristics of RESIST patients at baseline were as follows. Patients had received a median of four PIs, six nucleosides, and one non-nucleoside reverse transcriptase inhibitor (NNRTI). Mean baseline HIV RNA levels was 4.73 $\log_{10}$ copies/mL and mean CD4+ T-lymphocyte counts ~195/mm^3. Patients had a median of 16 baseline, nonconsensus viral protease gene mutations, including resistance associated and polymorphism mutations. Almost 40% of patients began the trial with a viral load above 100 000 copies/mL.

The comparator PI was selected by study investigators based on screening viral resistance tests and included lopinavir/ RTV (~50% of patients), amprenavir/RTV (~25% of patients), saquinavir/RTV, and indinavir/RTV. Overall, 25% of the patients in each arm used enfuvirtide. The comparator PI background regimen and enfuvirtide use were decided prior to randomization, which was stratified by comparator PI and enfuvirtide use.

Some issues need to be discussed. Although the optimal background antiretroviral therapy was predetermined before randomization, the number of subjects who had enfuvirtide predetermined as part of their optimized background treatment differed from the number of subjects who actually took enfuvirtide, due to a net loss of 25 subjects in the control arm. Some investigators, who wanted to save enfuvirtide for use with a known active PI, changed optimized background treatment once subjects were randomized in the control arm. Since there was difficulty in enrolling for the RESIST trials, the protocol was amended to allow subjects with no available active PI, as per their genotype, to enroll. Therefore, the control PI arm was not optimal for PI component in all patients.

The interim 24 week efficacy analysis contained 1159 patients of which 582 randomized to the TPV 500 mg/RTV 200 mg arm and 577 to the RTV-boosted comparator PI (CPI) arm. Week 24 results demonstrated that the proportion of treatment responders was significantly greater in the TPV group versus control group for both the RESIST studies. Treatment outcome details are shown in Table 25-1.[15,16] The proportion of treatment responders in the TPV/RTV group was similar across both RESIST I and RESIST II studies. There was no difference in the proportion of patients who developed AIDS in TPV/RTV and in CPI/RTV group.

Table 25-2 24-Week Treatment Outcome Data in Patients From the Combined RESIST Trial Assigned to LPV/r as CPI Before Randomization

Outcome	TPV/r + OBR (n = 293)	LPV/r + OBR (n = 290)	P
Proportion of patients with HIV RNA reduction of ≥1 $\log_{10}$ copies/mL			
Overall	39.6%	21.4%	<0.0001
LPV-experienced (n = 333)	35.2%	10.7%	<0.05
LPV-naive (n = 250)	45.3%	36.1%	NS
Genotypically susceptible to LPV (n = 386)	45.7%	39.6%	NS
Genotypically resistant to LPV (n = 196)	35.8%	13.1%	<0.05

NS, not significant.

Data from Cooper D, Hicks C, Cahn P et al. 24-Week RESIST Study analyses: the efficacy of tipranavir/ritonavir is superior to lopinavir/ritonavir, and the TPV/r treatment response is enhanced by inclusion of genotypically active antiretrovirals in the optimized background regimen. In: 12th Conference on Retroviruses and Opportunistic Infections. Boston, 2005, abstract 560.

Table 25-3 Selected 48-Week Treatment Outcome Data From the Combined RESIST Trials

Outcome	TPV/r + OBR (n = 746)	CPI/r + OBR (n = 737)	P
Proportion of patients with HIV RNA reduction of ≥ 1 $\log_{10}$ copies/mL	33.6%	15.3%	<0.001
HIV RNA <400 copies/mL	30.4%	13.8%	<0.0001
HIV RNA <50 copies/mL	22.8%	10.2%	<0.0001
Median change in HIV RNA from baseline ($\log_{10}$ copies/mL)	−1.14	−0.54	<0.0001
Median absolute change in CD4+ T-lymphocyte count (cells/mm^3)	+45	+21	<0.001

TPV/r, tipranavir/ritonavir; CPI/r, comparator-boosted protease inhibitor; OBR, optimized background regimen.

Data from Cahn P, Hicks C. RESIST-1 and RESIST-2 48-week meta-analyses demonstrate superiority of protease inhibitor tipranavir + ritonavir over an optimised comparator PI regimen in antiretroviral experienced patients. In: 10th European AIDS Conference; Dublin, 2005, abstract LBPS3/8.

A subgroup analysis compared patients in the TPV/r arm (n = 293, corresponding to patients for whom LPV/RTV had been chosen as optimized PI before randomization) with patients taking LPV/RTV (n = 290). Of the patients taking LPV/RTV, 42% had not taken LPV previously. At 24 weeks, 39.6% and 21.4% of the TPV/RTV and LPV/RTV treated patients achieved ≥1 $\log_{10}$ decrease in viral load from baseline, respectively. Viral loads <400 copies/mL were achieved by 34% versus 18% of the patients in the TPV/RTV and LPV/RTV groups, respectively. The results of this subgroup of subjects with resistance to comparator PI was consistent with the overall results on the primary efficacy endpoint. These differences were not statistically significant if comparisons only included patients in the LPV/r group who were LPV-naive or who had a virus that was susceptible to LPV.[17] See results in Table 25-2.

Combined analysis of the two RESIST trials at week 48 confirmed the 24 week results. The 48 week efficacy analysis evaluated the 1483 patients of which 746 randomized to the TPV 500 mg/RTV 200 mg arm and 737 to the RTV-boosted comparator arm.[18] Treatment outcome details are shown in Table 25-3.

The use of enfuvirtide led to a higher virologic and immunologic treatment response in both arms when compared to treatment response in patients who did not use it.[19,20] Details are given in Table 25-4. The difference was most striking among patients who were naive for enfuvirtide at baseline. In such patients, a virologic response (≥1 $\log_{10}$ decrease in viral load) was observed in 69.6% of patients in TPV/RTV arm versus 28.7% of patients in CPI/RTV arm, whereas respective proportions of patients with a virologic response were 27.9% and 17.6% in enfuvirtide pretreated subjects.

Table 25-4 Impact of Enfuvirtide[a] on 24-Week Treatment Outcome in the Combined RESIST Trials

	TPV/r		CPI/r	
Outcome	+ENF	−ENF	+ENF	−ENF
Achieved primary endpoint	58.9%	38.0%	27.3%	18.5%
HIV RNA <400 copies/mL	44.9%	30.2%	20.3%	13.4%
HIV RNA <50 copies/mL	30.4%	21.5%	12.5%	8.5%
Median change in HIV RNA from baseline ($\log_{10}$ copies/mL)	−2.06	−0.57	−0.40	−0.20
Median absolute change in CD4+ T-lymphocyte count (cells/mm^3)	+55	+27	+6	+3

[a]73% of patients were enfuvirtide-naive at baseline.

Data from: Tipranavir capsules, NDA 21-814. Applicant: Boehringer Ingelheim Pharmaceuticals, Inc. Anti-viral Drugs Advisory Committee (AVDAC) Briefing Document, 19 April, 2005, 1–193. Available: http://www.fda.gov/ohrms/dockets/ac/05/briefing/2005-4139b1-02-boehringer.pdf and Valdez H, McCallister S, Kohlbrenner V, et al. Tipranavir/ritonavir 500 mg/200 mg bid drives week 24 viral load below 400 copies/mL when combined with a second active drug (T-20) in protease inhibitor experienced HIV+ patients. In: 3rd IAS Conference on HIV Pathogenesis and Treatment, Rio de Janeiro, 2005, abstract WeOa0205.

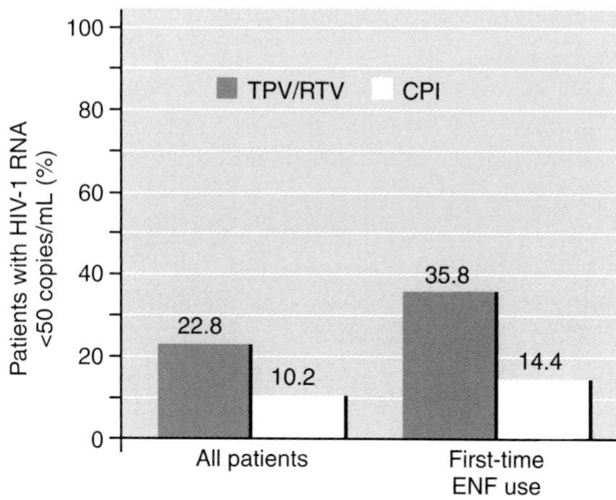

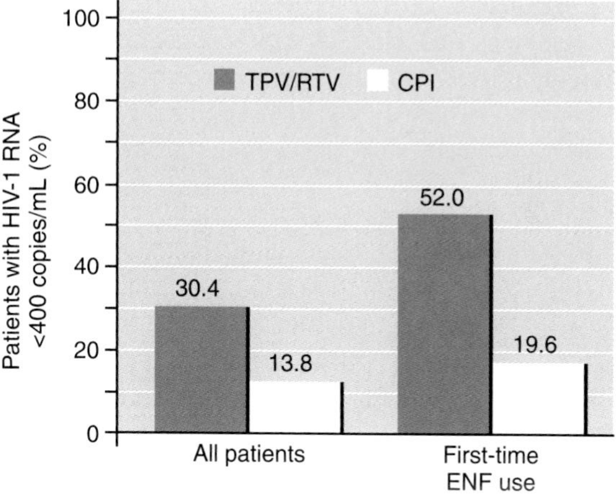

Figure 25-2 ■ RESIST-1 and -2 48 week results. Percentage of patients with plasma HIV-1 RNA below the limit of detection (<400 and <50 copies/mL) by treatment group, in all patients and in patients naive for enfuvirtide at entry into the trial. TPV, tipranavir; RTV, ritonavir; CPI, comparator protease inhibitor; ENF, enfuvirtide.

From Cahn P, Hicks C. RESIST-1 and RESIST-2 48-week meta-analyses demonstrate superiority of protease inhibitor tipranavir + ritonavir over an optimised comparator PI regimen in antiretroviral experienced patients. In: 10th European AIDS Conference, Dublin, 2005, abstract LBPS3/8.

This difference persisted at week 48. Among patients who were enfuvirtide-naive at entry and whose study regimen included enfuvirtide, 52.0% of patients taking TPV/RTV versus 19.6% taking a comparator boosted PI had an HIV-RNA <400 copies/mL at week 48. Respective proportions with viral suppression to <50 copies/mL were 35.8% and 14.4% ($P < 0.0001$ for both comparisons) (see Fig. 25-2).[18] These results show that in patients failing therapy with multiresistant virus, a goal of undetectable plasma HIV RNA may still be reasonable for a salvage regimen combining TPV/RTV to at least one drug from a new class.

TOXICITY

The most common adverse events of TPV/RTV are gastrointestinal in nature and include diarrhea, nausea, abdominal pain and vomiting. Common laboratory abnormalities

Table 25-5 Treatment-Associated Adverse Events in Patients on RESIST-1 and RESIST-2 Study (Combined from Analyses of 48-week Data)

Adverse Event or Grade 3–4 Laboratory Abnormality	TPV/r + OBR (n = 746)	CPI/r + OBR (n = 737)
Serious adverse events, per 100 patient-years	23.9	27.8
Treatment discontinuation for adverse events, per 100 patient-years	12.4	10.6
Grade 3 or 4 laboratory abnormalities (% patients)		
Elevated liver enzymes (ALT/AST)	9.7/6.1	4.2/1.8
Elevated bilirubin	0.7	0.5
Elevated total cholesterol	2.1	0.4
Elevated triglycerides	24.9	13.0

ALT alanine transaminase, AST aspartate transaminase

Data from Cahn P, Hicks C. RESIST-1 and RESIST-2 48-week meta-analyses demonstrate superiority of protease inhibitor tipranavir + ritonavir over an optimised comparator PI regimen in antiretroviral experienced patients. In: 10th European AIDS Conference; Dublin, 2005, abstract LBPS3/8.

include elevations of total cholesterol, triglycerides and liver enzymes. In the RESIST studies, the overall percentage of patients reporting study drug related adverse events of any severity and the rate of discontinuation for adverse events were higher in the TPV/RTV arm than in the CPI/RTV arm. However, the differences were reduced when results were adjusted to the length of time patients were exposed to the treatment regimens and rates of exposure-adjusted serious adverse events proved similar in the two study arms (Table 25-5). The most frequently reported severe adverse event was diarrhea. Although TPV contains a sulfonamide moiety, the potential for cross-sensitivity between sulfonamides and TPV is unknown. The incidence of rash in the TPV/RTV group was 2.1% compared to 0.9% in the comparator group. Patients with lower CD4 counts and women using estrogens appear to be at greater risk of developing rashes. Higher proportions of patients taking TPV/RTV had a grade 3 or 4 ALT elevation, a grade 3 or 4 total cholesterol increase or a grade 3 or 4 increase in triglycerides (Table 25-5). In a regression analysis, elevated baseline liver function tests, CD4+ T-lymphocyte count ⩾200 cells/mm^3 and co-infection with hepatitis B or C were risk factors for developing elevations in hepatic transaminases greater than five times the upper limit of normal.[21] The impact of changes in the plasma lipid profile on cardiovascular disease risk could not be determined over the short time frame of data presented to date.

DRUG INTERACTIONS

The drug interactions with TPV are complex due to its effects on CYP-3A and P-gp. This is further complicated by the fact that TPV needs to be administered with RTV, which has the opposite effect on CYP-3A and P-gp.

Non-Antiretroviral Drugs

Drugs that are contraindicated with TPV/RTV are essentially the same drugs that are contraindicated with other PIs and include specific drugs within the classes of antiarrhythmics, antihistamines, ergot derivatives, gastrointestinal motility agents, HMG CoA reductase inhibitors, neuroleptics and sedatives (Table 25-6). TPV/RTV may inhibit metabolism of these drugs, causing increased exposure to these agents that could result in life-threatening complications. TPV did not affect exposure to fluconazole, but increased the AUC for atorvastatin by ninefold. TPV exposure was significantly increased by fluconazole. If either atorvastatin or fluconazole are co-administered with TPV, very careful monitoring is warranted.[22,23] Administration of TPV should be separated from the dosing of antacids. The dose of rifabutine needs to be reduced by 75%.[24] Ethinyl estradiol concentrations are decreased by 50% in combination with TPV/r. Women using oral contraceptives will need to use alternative methods of nonhormonal contraception.

Antiretrovirals

The AUC for zidovudine and abacavir are both decreased by 40% when co-administered with TPV/r; a dose-dependent reduction in tenofovir C_{max} of 23–38% was shown.[25,26] The mechanism for nucleoside agent interactions with TPV and the clinical relevance of these interactions are not known. No dose adjustments are recommended at this time. Enteric-coated didanosine should not be taken within 2h of TPV/r. There was no significant pharmacokinetic interaction between TPV/r and nevirapine or efavirenz.[26,27] In healthy subjects, co-administration of TMC 125, a new NNRTI, and TPV/r is associated with a 75% decrease in TMC125 exposure, without significant alterations in TPV levels. Thus, the combination of TMC125 and TPV/r is not recommended.[28]

A significant two-way pharmacokinetic interaction occurs when TPV and RTV are co-administered. TPV concentrations are significantly elevated whereas RTV concentrations are reduced. Thus, TPV boosting is achieved with a daily RTV dose of 200mg bid.[29] The BI 1182.51 mentioned above brought information on the pharmacokinetic interactions

Table 25-6 Non-Antiretroviral Drugs With Significant Pharmacokinetic Interactions With Tipranavir

Drug Class	Drug Names	Recommendation
Antiarrhythmics	Amiodarone, bepridil, flecainide, propafenone, and quinidine	Contraindicated
Antihistamines	Astemizole, terfenadine	Contraindicated
Antimycobacterials	Rifampin	Avoid
Ergot derivatives	Dihydroergotamine, ergonovine, ergotamine, and methylergonovine	Contraindicated
Gastrointestinal motility agents	Cisapride	Contraindicated
Herbal supplements	St John's wort	Avoid
HMG CoA reductase inhibitors	Lovastatin and simvastatin	Avoid
Neuroleptics	Pimozide	Contraindicated
Sedatives/hypnotics	Midazolam and triazolam	Contraindicated

Table 25-7 Interactions between Boosted PIs and TPV/RTV

Drug	Serum AUC	C_{max}	C_{min}
Saquinavir (SQV)	Decreased by 70%	Decreased by 66%	Decreased by 81%
Amprenavir (APV)	Decreased by 45%	Decreased by 40%	Decreased by 56%
Lopinavir (LPV)	Decreased by 49%	Decreased by 43%	Decreased by 55%

AUC, area under concentration–time curve

Data from Walmsley S, Leith J, Katlama C, et al. Pharmacokinetics and safety of tipranavir/ritonavir alone or in combination with saquinavir, amprenavir or lopinavir: interim analysis of BI1182.51. In: The XV International AIDS Conference, Bangkok, 2004, abstract WeOrB1236.

between TPV and other boosted PIs. After day 14, TPV/RTV 500/100 mg was added to the treatment of subjects initially randomized to receive one of the three currently available PIs. Thus, from week 3, patients received TPV 500/100 mg and either lopinavir/RTV 400/100 mg, amprenavir/RTV 600/100 mg or saquinavir/RTV 1000/100 mg, each given twice daily. TPV's P450 induction effects resulted in dramatic reductions in the AUC, C_{max} and C_{min} concentrations of lopinavir, amprenavir and saquinavir (Table 25-7).[14] Therefore, combining these drugs with TPV/RTV is not recommended.

DRUG RESISTANCE

Resistance to TPV is complex and our knowledge regarding it is still evolving. It was anticipated from the nonpeptidic nature of TPV and the crystallographic analysis of TPV-binding interactions with the protease that this inhibitor might have activity against HIV-1 strains that have become resistant to the current peptidomimetic PIs. The antiviral activity of TPV has been assessed in *in vitro* culture for 134 clinical isolates with a wide range of resistance to currently available peptidomimetic PIs, using a phenotypic susceptibility assay. Of 105 viruses with more than 10-fold resistance to three or four PIs and an average of 6.1 PI mutations per sample, 95 (90%) had less than fourfold, eight (8%) had four- to 10-fold and only two (2%) had more than 10-fold decrease in susceptibility to TPV.[4]

In vitro studies [30] have shown that resistance to TPV develop over months. Characterization of the selected variants revealed that the first mutations to be selected were L33F and I84V in the viral protease, mutations which, when present together, conferred less than twofold resistance to TPV. At the end of the selection experiments, viruses harboring 10 mutations in the protease (L10F, I13V, V32I, L33F, M36I, K45I, I54V, A71V, V82L, I84V) as well as one mutation in the CA/SP1 gag cleavage site were selected and showed 87-fold decreased susceptibility to TPV. *In vitro*, TPV-resistant viruses had a reduced replicative capacity. Resistant isolates had a reduced sensitivity to amprenavir, atazanavir, indinavir, lopinavir, nelfinavir, and ritonavir but not saquinavir.

In vivo, determined from genotypes collected in multiple clinical studies where patients were treated with non-TPV containing PI regimens, reduced TPV virus susceptibility has been associated with 21 mutations at 16 viral protease codon

Table 25-8

Correlation Between TPV Genotypic Score and Change in Viral Load (VL) at Week 2 and Week 24.

TPV Score (N Mutations)	Change in VL at week 2		Change in VL at week 24	
	Median	N	Median	N
0 to 1	−1.25	135	−2.10	114
2 to 3	−1.37	289	−0.89	242
4 to 5	−1.40	302	−0.45	260
6 to 7	−1.27	76	−0.49	68
8 or more	−0.33	4	−0.08	4

Data from Parkin N, Chappey C. Protease mutations associated with higher or lower than expected tipranavir susceptibility based on the TPV mutation score. In: 13th Conference on Retroviruses and Opportunistic Infections, Denver, 2006, abstract 637.

positions: 10V, 13V, 20M/R/V, 33F, 35G, 36I, 43T, 46L, 47V, 54A/M/V, 58E, 69K, 74P, 82L/T, 83D, and 84V.[31,32]

The relationship between virologic response, fold change in susceptibility and genotypic profile at the 16 codons mentioned above was studied in several clinical trials of TPV, including the phase III RESIST studies, the companion trial (1182.51) for patients with more than two mutations at codons 33, 82, 84, and 90 (who were therefore not eligible for RESIST) and the phase II dose-finding trial (1182.52).[33] There was a correlation between phenotypic and genotypic susceptibility, with a substantial jump for a TPV mutation score more than seven. The TPV fold change in susceptibility was less than 2.0 for four or fewer mutations, 3.1–3.9 for five to seven mutations, and over 14 for eight or more mutations. This correlated with week 2 virologic response in that patients with seven or fewer mutations had a decrease >1.2 $\log_{10}$ copies/mL in viral load, whereas with eight or more mutations, viral load reduction was 0.33 $\log_{10}$ copies/mL (Table 25-8).

The mutation at codon 90, initially thought to be important, was not correlated with virologic response. It has to be stressed that the mutations at position 82 that are associated with resistance to other PIs (82A/F) do not appear to be involved in TPV resistance, whereas the mutations 82L/T are associated with TPV resistance.

More recently, Parkin et al confirmed the correlation between phenotype and genotypic resistance and attempted to refine the TPV mutation score. TPV fold change (FC) in phenotypic susceptibility to TPV was significantly correlated with TPV mutation score: the median FC was 3.0, 12, and 24 with a mutation score of 4, 7, and 8–9, respectively.[34] However, the variability was high within a given group of mutation score, especially for ranges thought to be clinically relevant. Analysis suggested to revise the TPV genotypic score by adding several mutations associated with lower than expected TPV FC, such as D30N, I50V, L24I or L76V, and applying weightage to certain mutations, such as I47V, I54A, V82T, or I84V.

Further studies are necessary to improve the algorithm of interpretation of TPV resistance mutations.[35,36]

CURRENT STATUS AND ONGOING STUDIES

TPV received expedited approval from the FDA on 22 Jun 2005 and EU approval on 26 Oct 2005 in HIV-1-infected adult patients who are highly treatment-experienced or have HIV-1 strains resistant to multiple PIs.

TPV is being evaluated in adult and pediatric-naive patients. It is important to study the toxicity profile in naive populations and to investigate whether the resistance profile that emerges in PI-naive patients receiving TPV differs from that in patients receiving other first PI-based regimens. Recently, Boehringer Ingelheim and the external independent Data Safety Monitoring Board (DSMB) met to review data from study 1182.33, which was designed to evaluate the efficacy and safety of TPV/RTV in treatment-naive HIV-infected patients. Following a thorough review of the 48-week data from the treatment-naive patients in this study, and considering the recommendation of the DSMB, Boehringer Ingelheim has decided to close the TPV/RTV 500/200 mg study arm in February 2006. Specifically, the rate of asymptomatic liver enzyme elevations reported in the TPV/RTV 500/200 mg study arm was higher than in the other study arms and presented a less favorable benefit-risk profile for these treatment-naive patients. The DSMB supported the continuation of the TPV/RTV 500/100 mg study arm and lopinavir/RTV comparator arm in this trial of treatment-naive patients.

RECOMMENDATIONS FOR USE

TPV is a nonpeptidic PI active against strains of HIV-1 that have reduced susceptibility to amprenavir, atazanavir, indinavir, lopinavir nelfinavir, and saquinavir. RTV co-administration is necessary to achieve plasma concentrations that are high enough to inhibit HIV-1 replication for resistant viruses. When administered with RTV 200 mg, TPV is indicated for combination antiretroviral treatment of HIV-1 infected adult patients with evidence of viral replication, who are highly treatment-experienced or have HIV-1 strains resistant to multiple PIs. The ability of TPV to suppress multidrug resistant HIV-1 replication is an important progress for the management of highly treatment-experienced patients. As the best results have been demonstrated in combination with enfuvirtide, the co-administration of these agents is encouraged and provides an opportunity of reaching undetectable plasma HIV RNA. Despite the promising efficacy results, potential safety risks associated with TPV/RTV must be kept in mind. TPV/RTV affects many drug-metabolizing enzymes, leading to clinically significant drug interactions, including deleterious interactions especially with other PIs. Other key concerns are the increased frequency of hepatotoxicity, triglycerides and total cholesterol elevations and gastrointestinal side-effects. Given these side-effects and the relatively high daily pill burden, TPV/RTV is not recommended as a first-line agent for treatment-naive patients who are infected with wild-type virus.

REFERENCES

1. Palella FJ Jr, Delaney KM, Moorman AC, et al. Declining morbidity and mortality among patients with advanced human immunodeficiency virus infection. HIV Outpatient Study Investigators. N Eng J Med 338:853, 1998.
2. Hoggs RS, Heath KV, Yip B, et al. Improved survival among HIV infected individuals following initiation of antiretroviral therapy. J Am Med Assoc 279:450, 1998.
3. Yerly S, Voras S, Rizzardi P, et al. Acute HIV infection impact on the spread of HIV and transmission of drug resistance. AIDS 15:2287, 2001.
4. Larder BA, Hertogs K, Bloor S, et al. Tipranavir inhibits broadly protease inhibitor-resistant HIV-1 clinical samples. AIDS 14:1943, 2000.
5. Schake D. How flexible is tipranavir in complex with the HIV-1 protease active site? AIDS 14:1943, 2004.
6. Washington CB, Duran GE, Man MC, et al. Interaction of anti-HIV protease inhibitors with the multidrug transporter P-glycoprotein (P-gP) in human cultured cells. J Acquir Immune Defic Syndr Hum Retrovirol 19:203, 1998.
7. Poppe SM, Stade DE, Chong KT, et al. Antiviral activity of the dihydropyrone PNU-140690, a new nonpeptidic human immunodeficiency virus protease inhibitor. Antimicrob Agents Chemother 41:1058, 1997
8. Rusconi S, La Seta Catamancio S, Citterio P, et al. Susceptibility to PNU-140690 (Tipranavir) of human immunodeficiency virus type 1 isolates derived from patients with multidrug resistance to other protease inhibitors. Antimicrob Agents Chemother 44:1328, 2000.
9. MacGregor TR, Sabo JP, Norris SH, et al. Pharmacokinetic characterization of different dose combinations of coadministered tipranavir and ritonavir in healthy volunteers. HIV Clin Trials 5:371, 2004.
10. Baldwin JR, Boron MT, Wang Y, et al. Effects of food and antacid on bioavailability of the protease inhibitor PNU-140690 in healthy volunteers. In: 5th Conference on Retroviruses and Opportunistic Infections, Chicago, 1998, abstract 649.
11. Aptivus package insert. Ridgefield, CT: Boehringer Ingelheim Pharmaceuticals, Inc; 2005.
12. McCallister S, Valdez H, Curry K, et al. A 14-day dose–response study of the efficacy, safety and pharmacokinetics of the non-peptidic protease inhibitor tipranavir in treatment-naive HIV-1 infected patients. J Acquir Immune Defic Syndr 35: 376, 2004.
13. Gathe J, Kohlbrenner VM, Pierone G, et al. Tipranavir/ritonavir demonstrates potent efficacy in multiple protease inhibitor experienced patients. BI 1182.52. In: 10th Conference on Retroviruses and Opportunistic Infections, Boston, 2003, abstract 179.
14. Walmsley S, Leith J, Katlama C, et al. Pharmacokinetics and safety of tipranavir/ritonavir alone or in combination with saquinavir, amprenavir or lopinavir: interim analysis of BI1182.51. In: The XV International AIDS Conference, Bangkok, 2004, abstract WeOrB1236.
15. Hicks C. RESIST-1: a phase 3, randomized, controlled, open-label, multicenter trial comparing tipranavir/ritonavir (TPV/r) to an optimized comparator protease inhibitor/r (CPI/r) regimen in antiretroviral (ARV) experienced patients: 24-week data. In: 44th Interscience Conference on Antimicrobial Agents and Chemotherapy, Washington, DC, 2004, abstract H-1137a.
16. Cahn P; RESIST 2 Study Team. 24-week data from RESIST-2: phase 3 study of the efficacy and safety of either tipranavir/ritonavir (TPV/r) or an optimized ritonavir (RTV)-boosted standard-of-care (SOC) comparator PI (CPI) in a large randomized multicenter trial in treatment-experienced HIV+ patients. In: 7th International Congress on Drug Therapy in HIV Infection, Glasgow, 2004, abstract PL-14.3.
17. Cooper D, Hicks C, Cahn P, et al. 24-Week RESIST Study analyses: the efficacy of tipranavir/ritonavir is superior to lopinavir/ritonavir, and the TPV/r treatment response is enhanced by inclusion of genotypically active antiretrovirals in the optimized background regimen. In: 12th Conference on Retroviruses and Opportunistic Infections, Boston, 2005, abstract 560.
18. Cahn P, Hicks C. RESIST-1 and RESIST-2 48-week meta-analyses demonstrate superiority of protease inhibitor tipranavir + ritonavir over an optimised comparator PI regimen in antiretroviral experienced patients. In: 10th European AIDS Conference; Dublin, 2005, abstract LBPS3/8.
19. Tipranavir capsules, NDA 21-814. Applicant: Boehringer Ingelheim Pharmaceuticals, Inc. Anti-viral Drugs Advisory Committee (AVDAC) Briefing Document, 19 Apri 2005, 1–193. Available: http://www.fda.gov/ohrms/dockets/ac/05/briefing/2005-4139b1-02-boehringer.pdf.
20. Valdez H, McCallister S, Kohlbrenner V, et al. tipranavir/ritonavir 500 mg/200 mg BID drives week 24 viral load below 400 copies/ml when combined with a second active drug (T-20) in protease inhibitor experienced HIV+ patients. In: 3rd IAS Conference on HIV Pathogenesis and Treatment, Rio de Janeiro, 2005, abstract WeOa0205.
21. Boehringer Ingelheim Pharmaceuticals. Tipranavir Antiviral Drugs Advisory Committee Briefing Document. Available: http://www.fda.gov/ohrms/dockets/ac/cder05.html 2005.
22. Van Heeswijk R, Sabo JP, MacGregor T, et al. The effects of tipranavir/ritonavir 500 mg/200 mg bid on the pharmacokinetics of fluconazole in healthy volunteers. In: 5th International Workshop on Clinical Pharmacology in HIV Therapy, Rome, 2004, abstract 4.8.
23. Van Heeswijk R, Sabo JP, Cooper C, et al. The pharmacokinetic interactions between tipranavir/ritonavir 500 mg/200 mg bid and atorvastatin, antacid and CYP3A4 in healthy volunteers. In: 5th International Workshop on Clinical Pharmacology in HIV Therapy, Rome, 2004, abstract 5.2.
24. Van Heeswijk R, Sabo JP, MacGregor T, et al. The pharmacokinetic interaction between single dose rifabutin and steady state tipranavir/ritonavir 500 mg/200 mg in healthy volunteers. In: 44th Interscience Conference on Antimicrobial Agents and Chemotherapy, Washington, DC, 2004, abstract A-456.

25. Philips L, Borin MT, Hopkins NK, et al. The pharmacokinetics of nucleoside reverse transcriptase inhibitors when coadministered with the HIV protease inhibitor tipranavir in HIV-1 infected patients. In: 7th Conference on Retroviruses and Opportunistic Infections. San Francisco, CA, 2000, abstract 81.
26. Roszko PJ, Curry K, Brazina B, et al. Standard doses of efavirenz, zidovudine, tenofovir and didanosine may be given with tipranavir/ritonavir. In: 3rd Conference on HIV Pathogenesis and Treatment, Paris, France, 2003, abstract 812.
27. Sabo JP, MacGregor TR, Lamson M, et al. Pharmacokinetics of tipranavir and nevirapine. A pharmacokinetic study in healthy volunteers. HIV DART 2000. In: Frontiers in drug development for antiretroviral therapies, San Juan, 2000, abstract 103.
28. Schöller M, Kraft M, Hoetelmans, et al. Significant decrease in TMC125 exposures when coadministered with tipranavir boosted with ritonavir in healthy subjects. In: 13th Conference on Retroviruses and Opportunistic Infections, Denver, 2006, abstract 583.
29. Baldwin JR, Borin MT, Ferry JJ, et al. Pharmacokinetic interaction between HIV protease inhibitor tipranavir and ritonavir. In: 39th Interscience Conference on Antimicrobial Agents and Chemotherapy, San Francisco, CA, 1999, abstract 657.
30. Doyon L, Tremblay S, Bourgon L, et al. Selection and characterization of HIV-1 showing reduced susceptibility to the non-peptidic protease inhibitor tipranavir. Antiviral Res 68:27, 2005.
31. Cooper D, Hall D, Jayaweera D, et al. Baseline phenotypic susceptibility to tipranavir/ritonavir is retained in isolates from patients with multiple protease inhibitor experience (BI 1182 52). In: 10th Conference on Retroviruses and Opportunistic Infections, Boston, 2003, abstract 596.
32. Miranda AC, Duque LM, Carvalho AP, et al. Expected tipranavir resistance in a group of 589 patients with previous exposure to protease inhibitors. In: 2nd European HIV Drug Resistance Workshop, Rome, 2004.
33. Valdez H, Hall DB, Kohlbrenner VM, et al. Non response to tipranavir is associated with pre-treatment resistance characterized by tipranavir phenotype or genotypic tipranavir score. Antiviral Therapy 10:S29, 2005.
34. Parkin N, Chappey C. Protease mutations associated with higher or lower than expected tipranavir susceptibility based on the TPV mutation score. In: 13th Conference on Retroviruses and Opportunistic Infections. Denver, 2006, abstract 637.
35. HIV-1 Genotypic Drug Resistance Interpretation's Algorithms. Available: http://www.hivfrenchresistance.org
36. www.iasusa.org

Chapter 26

Darunavir

Jose M. Gatell, MD, PhD

INTRODUCTION

Protease inhibitors (PIs) have played a crucial role in the history of antiretroviral therapy. Their use as components of highly active antiretroviral therapy (HAART) has been shown to result in durable virologic suppression and dramatic improvement in the morbidity and mortality of patients infected with the human immunodeficiency virus type 1 (HIV-1).[1–3] Thus, PIs have become cornerstones of drug treatment for HIV, whether as first-line agents for treatment-naive patients or as alternative agents for patients with a long history of antiretroviral therapy, with previous virologic failures and resistance mutations.

The emergence of drug-resistant strains of HIV-1 represents a significant threat to the efficacy of antiretroviral therapy, with increasing levels of resistance[4] and the extensive cross-resistance that exists between currently available PIs limiting the sequential use of these agents. The rational development of novel therapies, which effectively suppress viremia and address the complex problems of resistance, offers a way forward for HIV therapy.[5–7] The novel PI, darunavir (DRV; also known as TMC114 (Prezista)), was designed to be active against both wild-type HIV and strains that are resistant to currently available PIs. A lead optimization program produced a series of compounds, from which DRV was selected for development because of its favorable pharmacokinetic (PK) and antiviral profile.[6,7] As for many other PIs, the PK profile and clinical effectiveness of DRV were found to be improved by PK enhancement with low-dose ritonavir (RTV).[8]

Another important barrier to effective treatment of HIV is drug toxicity. Recently developed PIs (with the exception of tipranavir (TPV)) have been associated with fewer side effects than earlier drugs. It is anticipated that DRV will also have a favorable tolerability profile. This chapter presents an overview of the chemical and pharmacological properties and clinical development of DRV.

CHEMICAL STRUCTURE

DRV is a novel, potent, HIV-1 PI that contains a 3(*R*),3a(*S*),6a(*R*)-*bis*-tetrahydrofuranylurethane (*bis*-THF) isostere.[9] The method of synthesis of DRV was first published by Ghosh and colleagues in 2004.[10] Figure 26-1 shows the chemical structure of DRV.

Although DRV shares some structural similarities with amprenavir (APV), it binds ~100 times more tightly than APV to the HIV-1 protease (Fig. 26-2). This is due in part to the additional hydrogen bonds formed between the *bis*-THF moiety in the P2-pocket of DRV and the protease molecule.[5,7] Furthermore, DRV binds particularly tightly due to its high affinity with main-chain atoms at the bottom of the active site.[5] It has been shown that, unlike currently available PIs, DRV shows a fast association but very slow dissociation from wild-type HIV-1

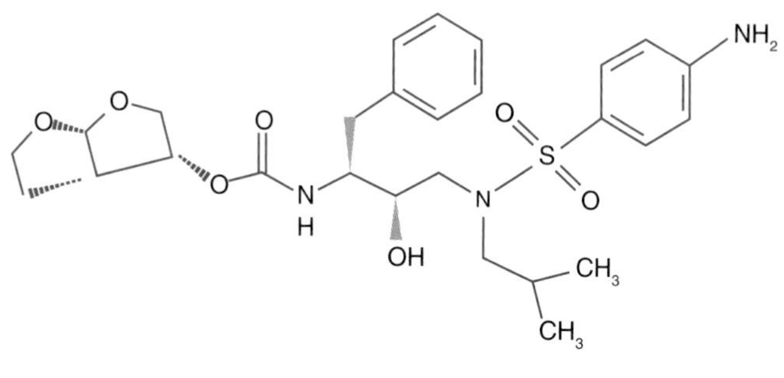

Figure 26-1 ■ Chemical structure of DRV.

Adapted from King NM, Prabu-Jeyabalan M, Nalivaika EA, et al. Structural and thermodynamic basis for the binding of TMC114, a next-generation human immunodeficiency virus type 1 protease inhibitor. J Virol 78:12012–12021, 2004.

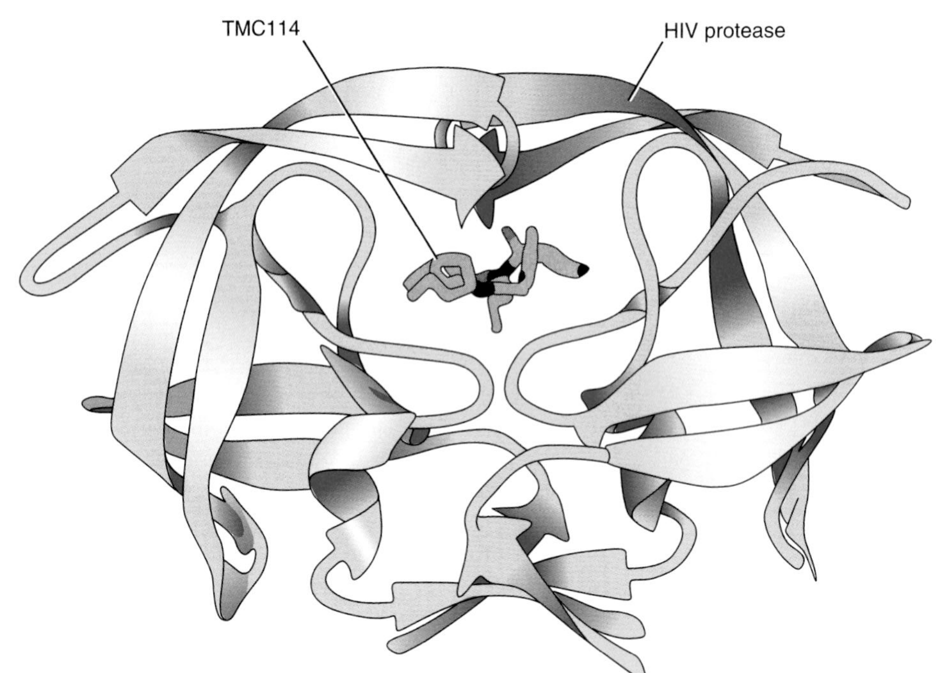

Figure 26-2 ■ DRV in the binding pocket of the HIV-1 protease dimmer, shown as ribbon diagrams.

Adapted from King NM, Prabu-Jeyabalan M, Nalivaika EA, et al. Structural and thermodynamic basis for the binding of TMC114, a next-generation human immunodeficiency virus type 1 protease inhibitor. J Virol 78:12012–12021, 2004.

protease.[11] Another characteristic of DRV is that it binds predominantly within the substrate consensus volume (the region of the enzyme's active site occupied by substrates) of HIV-1 protease. The structural shape of this volume is critical to HIV protease activity and any mutation that affects the fit of DRV would likely render the enzyme inactive, thereby preventing further viral replication. Thus, the close conformation of DRV within the substrate consensus volume may be an important factor in its low susceptibility to viral resistance.[5]

High-resolution crystallographic analysis has been performed on DRV in complexes with wild-type HIV-1 protease and the mutant proteases PR_{V82A} and PR_{I84V} that are common in drug-resistant HIV.[12] DRV forms hydrogen bonds with the conserved main-chain atoms of Asp29 and Asp30 of the protease. The close contact of DRV with the main chains of these active-site amino acids is not seen with other currently available PIs and it is believed to be critical for the potency of DRV against multiple PI-resistant HIV isolates.[9]

Furthermore, the structural flexibility of DRV indicates that small changes in the substrate consensus volume may not impair the overall ability of the drug to bind tightly to the enzyme, thus, conferring additional resilience to the effect of PI resistance-associated mutations.[5]

IN VITRO ACTIVITY

A lead optimization program resulted in DRV being identified and selected for development based on favorable PK characteristics in animals and potent *in vitro* activity against a comprehensive panel of clinical isolates of HIV representative of those found in clinical practice. De Meyer and colleagues characterized the antiviral activity of DRV against both wild-type and PI-resistant HIV.[13] Against wild-type HIV, DRV had a 50% effective concentration (EC_{50}) of 1–5 nM and an EC_{90} of 2.7–13 nM. DRV exhibited no cytotoxicity at concentrations up to 100 μM, resulting in a selectivity index of >20 000 for wild-type HIV. DRV were also active against all viruses in a panel of 19 recombinant clinical isolates that were assembled to evaluate newly synthesized compounds (the viruses carried multiple protease mutations and were resistant to an average of five other PIs with resistance defined as a fold change in EC_{50} (FC) ⩾4). Figure 26-3 shows the activity of DRV and six currently approved PIs against PI-resistant and wild-type HIV-1.[13] DRV and six approved PIs were also tested against a broad selection of several thousand HIV clinical isolates exhibiting various degrees of resistance to all commercially available PIs. DRV had significantly greater potency against the 1501 samples with PI resistance than any other tested PI (Fig. 26-4). Antiviral analyses performed on DRV by Koh and colleagues yielded similar findings to those described above.[9]

HIV-1 group M subtype B is currently predominant in the USA and Europe. However, studies have suggested that the prevalence of non-B subtypes and circulating recombinant forms may soon reach significant levels.[14,15] DRV showed similar potent activity against a range of clinically derived recombinant viruses representing HIV-1 group M subtypes A through H, and including a number of recombinant forms of HIV-1 group O.[13]

The results of *in vitro* selection experiments showed that the emergence of resistant HIV was much slower with DRV than with comparator PIs APV, nelfinavir, or lopinavir (LPV)

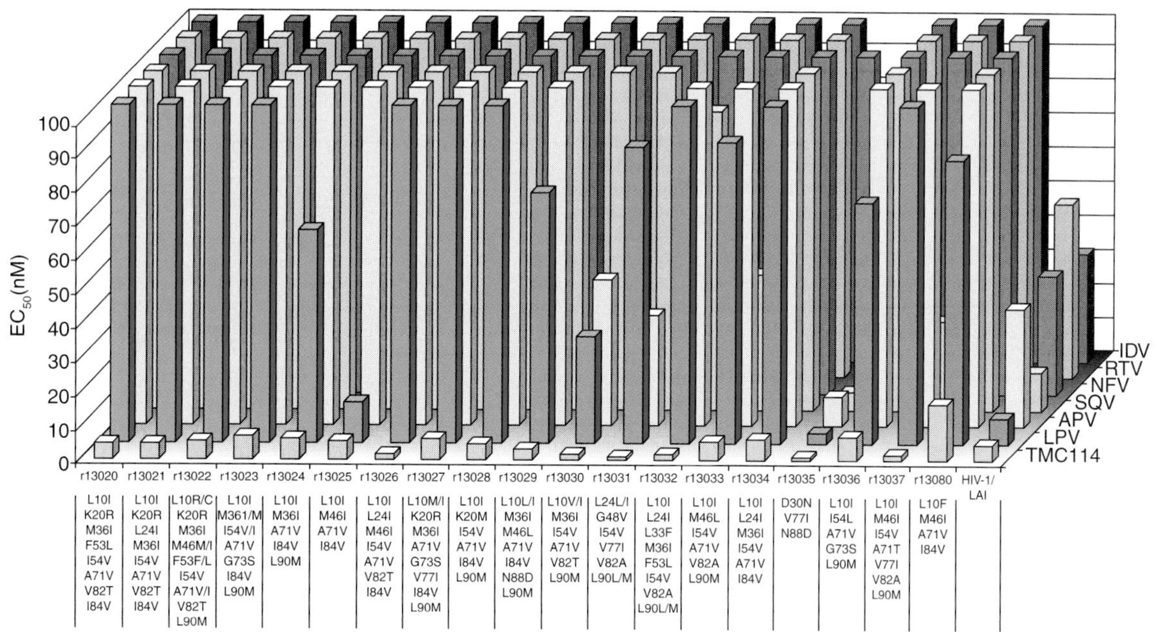

Figure 26-3 ■ Activity of DRV and currently used PIs against PI-resistant and wild-type HIV-1. Figure shows differences from the subtype B consensus at amino acid positions implicated in PI resistance according to the international AIDS Society-USA drug resistance mutation figures.

Adapted from De Meyer S, Azijn H, Surleraux D, et al. TMC114, a novel human immunodeficiency virus type 1 protease inhibitor active against protease inhibitor-resistant viruses, including a broad range of clinical isolates. Antimicrob Agents Chemother 49:2314–2321, 2005.

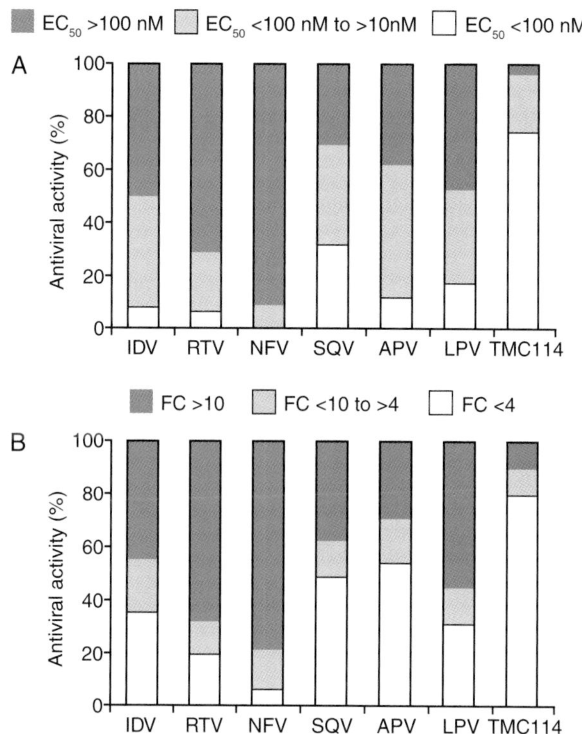

Figure 26-4 ■ Antiviral activity of different protease inhibitors tested against an panel of 1501 recent recombinant clinical isolates resistant to at least one protease inhibitor **(A)** EC_{50} range, **(B)** fold change in EC_{50} compared with wild-type.

Adapted from De Meyer S, Azijn H, Surleraux D, et al. TMC114, a novel human immunodeficiency virus type 1 protease inhibitor active against protease inhibitor-resistant viruses, including a broad range of clinical isolates. Antimicrob Agents Chemother 49:2314–2321, 2005.

(Fig. 26-5).[13] This indicates an increased genetic barrier to the development of resistance to DRV and a pathway to resistance that is different from that of other currently available PIs.

The results of these *in vitro* analyses demonstrate that DRV possesses potent activity against both wild-type and multidrug-resistant HIV-1 and illustrate its potential for the treatment of both naïve and PI-experienced patients with HIV. The rigorous resistance profiling undertaken in the design and development of DRV represents a novel and significant advancement in the identification of novel antiretrovirals.

PHARMACOKINETICS

Effect of Co-Administration with Low-Dose Ritonavir

A comparison of two randomized, multiple dose-escalating phase I trials in a total of 76 healthy volunteers concluded that co-administration of DRV and low-dose RTV (DRV/r) resulted in improved PK characteristics compared with DRV alone despite the use of lower doses of DRV.[8] Co-administration of RTV also resulted in improved safety and tolerability profiles. Both trials used an early experimental formulation of DRV as a polyethylene glycol (PEG) 400-containing oral solution. In the first trial, unboosted DRV was administered (in a placebo-controlled, double-blind manner) at doses of 400 mg twice daily, 800 mg twice daily, 800 mg three times daily and 1200 mg three times daily, while in the second (open-label) study, DRV/r was administered at doses of 200/100 mg once daily, 400/100 mg once daily, 300/100 mg twice daily, 600/200 mg once daily and

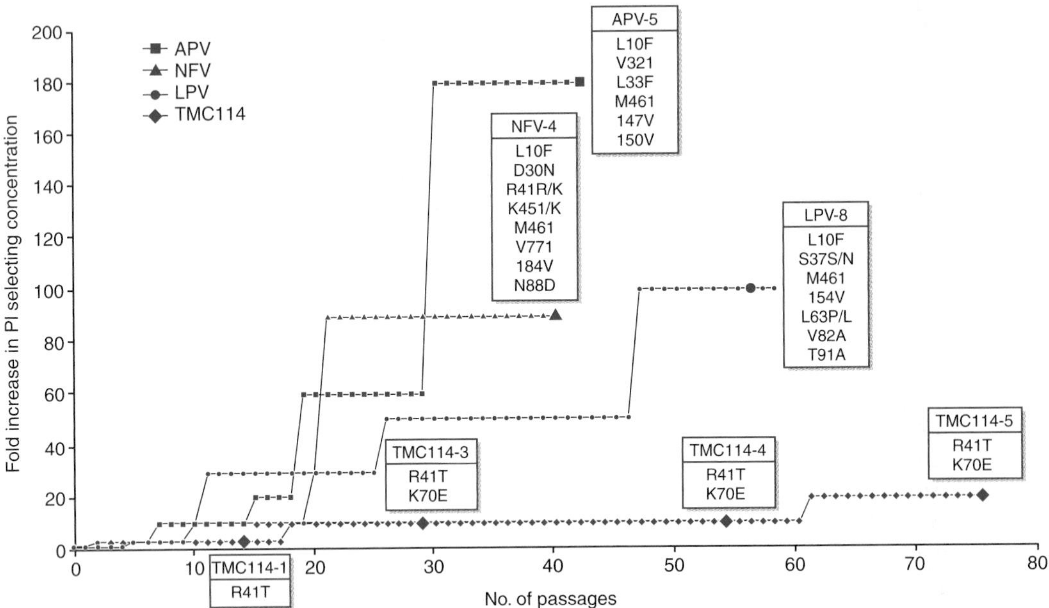

Figure 26-5 ■ *In vitro* selection of resistant HIV in the presence of nelfinavir, APV, LPV, or DRV. Selection curves have been normalized, and starting selection concentrations were 10, 20, 100, and 100 nM for DRV, LPV, APV, and nelfinavir, respectively. Each passage corresponds to 3–4 days. Passage 75 corresponds to 260 days. Genotypes of virus strains selected at defined time points (indicated by enlarged symbols) list all changes from the starting strain, HIV-1 LAI.

Adapted from De Meyer S, Azijn H, Surleraux D, et al. TMC114, a novel human immunodeficiency virus type 1 protease inhibitor active against protease inhibitor-resistant viruses, including a broad range of clinical isolates. Antimicrob Agents Chemother 49:2314–2321, 2005.

1200/200 mg once daily. DRV was rapidly absorbed with a time to maximum plasma concentration (t_{max}) achieved in less than 3 h and steady-state concentrations were reached within 3 days. Overall, mean maximum plasma concentration (C_{max}), minimum plasma concentration (C_{min}) and average steady-state plasma concentration ($C_{ss,av}$) achieved at day 14 were higher with DRV/r than with DRV alone. With DRV alone, mean C_{min} at day 14 ranged from 14 ng/mL for the lowest dose to 142 ng/mL for the highest dose. The corresponding ranges for C_{max} and $C_{ss,av}$ at day 14 were 2168–8040 ng/mL and 270–1395 ng/mL, respectively. In the RTV-boosted trial, values for C_{min} ranged from 480 to 1486 ng/mL, C_{max} from 1569 to 5453 ng/mL and $C_{ss,av}$ from 725 to 2460 ng/mL. The PK results demonstrated that the values for C_{min} and the area under the plasma concentration-time curve (AUC) at 24 h for DRV are substantially increased with the co-administration of low doses of RTV. Higher C_{min} concentrations of DRV were obtained at lower total daily doses of DRV with addition of RTV.

Most adverse events (AEs) were gastrointestinal (GI), skin, and central nervous system (CNS) disorders. There was an apparent reduction in the frequency of AEs reported in volunteers who received DRV/r compared with DRV alone (e.g., 78% of volunteers experienced diarrhea with DRV alone, compared with 30% when DRV/r was used; the GI effects were largely attributed to the PEG-containing solution).

After the determination that the co-administration of DRV with a low dose of RTV resulted in more favorable PK characteristics and tolerability profile, all further clinical development of DRV was performed with co-administration of low-dose RTV.

Effect of Food

In early studies, DRV was administered as an oral solution. However, a solid tablet formulation was developed for use in phase II dose-finding trials of DRV/r. A PK study confirmed that under fed conditions and with low-dose RTV, the tablet and oral solution of DRV meet the criteria for bioequivalence.[16] The study also showed that in the presence of low-dose RTV, the bioavailability of DRV oral tablets is greater after feeding than after fasting. It is therefore recommended that DRV tablets should be taken with food. Another study confirmed that in the presence of low-dose RTV, systemic exposure to DRV is increased by ~30% when tablets are taken after a meal than after fasting.[17] PK parameters in the study were determined after administration of a single oral dose of 400 mg of DRV in tablet formulation together with low-dose RTV under fasted conditions and with different types of food (standard breakfast, high-fat breakfast, protein-rich nutritional drink and croissant with coffee). The results demonstrated that the type of meal consumed does not affect the exposure to DRV.

Effect of Increased Intragastric pH

The effects of concomitant administration of DRV/r with drugs that inhibit gastric acid secretion and thereby elevate intragastric pH have been investigated. The combination of the proton-pump inhibitor omeprazole (20 mg daily) or the H_2-receptor antagonist ranitidine (150 mg twice daily) with DRV/r did not affect the PK characteristics of DRV after multiple dosing.[18]

EFFICACY

The efficacy of DRV/r has been studied in clinical trials in treatment-experienced, HIV-infected patients. An overview of the design and key features of trials providing clinical efficacy data is shown in Table 26-1.

In the proof-of-principle, phase IIa, controlled trials in treatment-experienced, multiple PI-resistant patients, treatment with DRV without RTV (TMC114-C201 study, unpublished) or with low-dose (100 mg) RTV (TMC114-C207) resulted in a statistically significant reduction in plasma viral load (VL) at endpoint compared with the control group.

The TMC114-C207 trial ($n = 50$) evaluated the antiviral activity of DRV/r in patients who had previously received two to four vPIs and who were on a failing NRTI- and PI-containing regimen.[19] Phenotypic and genotypic analyses were conducted on plasma samples obtained at screening and at end of therapy. At baseline, 51% of patients harbored virus that was phenotypically resistant to all PIs that were commercially available at the time of the study and only 27% had virus sensitivity to two or more PIs. Over the 14 days of treatment, DRV/r demonstrated potent antiviral activity and was active against multiple PI-resistant strains of HIV. Virologic response to DRV/r treatment was not influenced by any PI mutation or mutational pattern. Existing PIs in a non-suppressive antiretroviral regimen were replaced with DRV/r (300/100 mg twice daily, 900/100 mg daily, or 600/100 mg twice daily) or left unchanged for 14 days. The primary study endpoint of median time-averaged change in HIV-1 ribonucleic acid (RNA) from baseline was significantly greater ($P < 0.001$) for all DRV/r groups ($-0.70 \log_{10}$ copies/mL; range -0.56 to $-0.81 \log_{10}$ copies/mL) than for the control group ($-0.03 \log_{10}$ copies/mL). There were no statistically significant differences in antiretroviral activity between the three DRV/r treatment arms. The median change at day 14 was $-1.38 \log_{10}$ copies/mL for all DRV/r groups, compared with $+0.02 \log_{10}$ copies/mL for the control group. Furthermore, 40% of patients in the DRV/r groups achieved HIV RNA <400 copies/mL at some time during the 14-day treatment period, compared with only 8% in the control group.

Power 1 (TMC114-C213) and Power 2 (TMC114-C202): Patient Baseline Characteristics and Study Methods

POWER 1 and POWER 2 (Performance of TMC114/r When evaluated in treatment-experienced patients with PI Resistance) are two long-term, international, randomized, dose-finding phase IIb studies in treatment-experienced patients.[20,21] From the two trials, 97% of patients had used two or more PIs, 96% had used one or more NNRTIs and 95% had used four or more NRTIs for at least 2 months. The patient population in POWER 2 was more advanced in disease than those in POWER 1; POWER 2 patients had a longer duration of infection (13.2 vs 11.6 years), lower baseline median CD4+ T-lymphocyte count (106 vs 179 cells/μL), higher baseline VL (69% vs 59% with ⩾20 000 copies/mL) and a higher proportion of patients had ⩾3 primary PI mutations (66% vs 56%, based on IAS-USA October 2004[22]). In addition, a greater proportion of patients were infected with virus phenotypically resistant to all commercially available PIs at the time of the study in POWER 2 compared with POWER 1 (71% vs 63%), and 39% of patients in the POWER 1600/100 mg bid dose group were susceptible to one or more PI compared with 33% of POWER 2 patients in the same dose group. In each study, patients received an optimized background regimen (OBR, composed of at least two nucleoside/nucleotide reverse transcriptase inhibitors (NRTIs) with or without enfuvirtide (ENF)) plus one of four doses of DRV/r (400/100 mg once daily, 800/100 mg once daily, 400/100 mg twice daily, and 600/100 mg twice daily) or investigator-selected control PIs. The primary efficacy endpoint was confirmed virologic response (using a time-to-loss of virologic response imputation algorithm), defined as a reduction in VL of $\geqslant 1.0 \log_{10}$ compared with baseline at week 24. The primary 24-week efficacy analysis for each of the trials showed that in these patients with limited treatment options, all doses of DRV/r provided significantly higher virologic response rates and CD4+ T-lymphocyte increases compared with control PI(s), with the highest dose providing the greatest efficacy. After 24 weeks, the dose giving the greatest benefits was selected and all patients were switched to this for the remainder of each of the studies.

Primary Analysis of Pooled Data in Power 1 and Power 2

The efficacy results across the two studies were consistent and demonstrated that the dose of DRV/r that provided the best overall antiretroviral effect was 600/100 mg twice daily. This dose was selected for further study in phase III efficacy trials in treatment-experienced patients (the 800/100 mg once daily dose is currently in phase III clinical trials in treatment-naive patients). An analysis of pooled data from POWER 1 and POWER 2 ($n = 596$) showed that, in patients who received DRV/r 600/100 mg twice daily, the proportion of patients achieving $\geqslant 1 \log_{10}$ reduction in VL at week 24 was 71% compared with 21% of control PI patients (Fig. 26-6). Similarly, more patients had HIV RNA below 50 copies/mL after treatment with DRV/r 600/100 mg twice daily (48%) than with control PIs (14%; Fig. 26-7). The mean HIV RNA change from baseline at week 24 with DRV/r 600/100 mg twice daily was $-1.90 \log_{10}$ copies/mL compared with $-0.49 \log_{10}$ copies/mL for the control PIs (noncompleter considered as treatment failure; Fig. 26-8), and the mean increase in CD4+ T-lymphocyte count was 98 cells/μL for

Table 26-1 Overview of Trials Providing Clinical Efficacy and Safety Data for Darunavir

Trial Location	Design	Indication Studied/ Population	Treatment Arms	Treatment Duration	Number of Patients	Status	Efficacy Data	Safety Data
Phase IIa Proof-of-Principle Trials								
TMC114-C201 (Europe)	Phase IIa, randomized, open-label, controlled trial	HIV-1-infected, PI-experienced patients with HIV RNA >2000 copies/mL and treated with a nonsuppressive, PI-containing regimen	Control (continue screening PI-containing regimen) DRV[a] (oral solution) 400 mg bid 800 mg bid 800 mg tid 1200 mg tid	Short term (14 days)	34	Not published and not planned for publication	Median HIV RNA change ($\log_{10}$ copies/mL): −0.28 for DRV 400 mg bid, −0.59 for 800 mg bid, −0.85 for 800 mg tid, −0.79 for 1200 mg tid and +0.20 for control Median CD4+ T-lymphocyte change (cells/μL): on Day 8: −15.0 for DRV 400 mg bid; +37.5 for 800 mg bid; +25.5 for 800 mg tid; +67.0 for 1200 mg tid; +21.0 for all DRV patients; +63.5 for control	DRV was well-tolerated. Most AEs[b] were grade 1 or 2 in severity. The two most common AEs during the treatment period were diarrhea and headache. No serious AEs were reported during the treatment phase.
TMC114-C207 (Europe)	Phase IIa, randomized, open-label, controlled trial	HIV-1-infected, PI-experienced patients with HIV RNA >2000 copies/mL, CD4+ T-lymphocyte count ⩾50 cells/μL and treated with a nonsuppressive, PI-containing regimen	Control (continue screening PI-containing regimen) DRV/r[a] (oral solution) 300/100 mg bid 600/100 mg bid 900/100 mg qd	Short term (14 days)	50	Results published[19]	Median HIV RNA change ($\log_{10}$ copies/mL): −1.38 for all DRV/r groups and +0.20 for control ($P < 0.001$) Change in CD4+ T-lymphocyte count: variable; no firm conclusions could be drawn	DRV/r was well-tolerated. Most AEs were grade 1 or 2 in severity. The most commonly reported AEs with DRV/r treatment were gastrointestinal and central nervous system disorders. One serious AE of hepatotoxicity was reported in the DRV/r 600/100 mg bid group.

Phase IIb, Randomized, Controlled Trials								
TMC114-C213 (POWER 1) Europe, Brazil, Canada, Australia	Phase IIb, randomized, controlled, partially blinded, followed by open-label	HIV-1-infected, PI-, NRTI-, and NNRTI-experienced patients on a stable PI-containing regimen; HIV RNA >1000 copies/mL; ≥1 primary PI mutation; no CD4+ T-lymphocyte cell count restrictions; co-infection with hepatitis B or C allowed.	OBR[c] + CPI(s)[d] OBR + DRV/r (tablet) 400/100 mg qd 800/100 mg qd 400/100 mg bid 600/100 mg bid	Long term (at least 144 weeks[e])	318[f]	Ongoing; primary 24-week data published[20,26]	Patients with ≥1.0 $\log_{10}$ HIV RNA reduction (ITT-TLOVR)[g]: 77% for DRV/r 600/100 mg bid and 25% for CPI ($P < 0.001$) Patients with HIV RNA <50 copies/mL (ITT-TLOVR): 53% for DRV/r 600/100 mg bid and 18% for CPI ($P < 0.001$) Mean HIV RNA change ($\log_{10}$ copies/mL): −2.03 for DRV/r 600/100 mg bid and −0.63 for CPI ($P < 0.001$) Mean CD4+ T-lymphocyte increase (cells/μL): +124 for DRV/r 600/100 mg bid and +20 for CPI ($P < 0.001$)	Most common treatment-emergent AEs (≥10% of patients in all darunavir/r groups: headache (17%), diarrhea (16%), nausea (11%) and insomnia (11%); similar AE incidence with CPI except for diarrhea (29%). No relationship between DRV/r dose and AE incidence was observed.
POWER 2 (TMC114-C202) USA, Argentina	Phase IIb, randomized, controlled, partially blinded, followed by open-label	HIV-1-infected, PI-, NRTI-, and NNRTI-experienced patients on a stable PI-containing regimen; HIV RNA >1000 copies/mL; ≥1 primary PI mutation; no CD4+ T-lymphocyte cell count restrictions;	OBR + CPI(s) OBR + DRV/r (tablet) 400/100 mg qd 800/100 mg qd 400/100 mg bid 600/100 mg bid	Long term (at least 144 weeks[e])	319[h]	Ongoing; primary 24-week data published[21,27]	Patients with ≥1.0 $\log_{10}$ HIV RNA reduction (ITT-TLOVR): 62% for DRV/r 600/100 mg bid and 14% for CPI ($P < 0.001$) Patients with HIV RNA <50	Most common treatment-emergent AEs in all DRV/r groups (≥10% of patients): headache (17%), nausea (17%), diarrhea (16%), fatigue (16%) and insomnia (10%); similar AE

(Continued)

Table 26-1

(Continued)

Trial Location	Design	Indication Studied/ Population	Treatment Arms	Treatment Duration	Number of Patients	Status	Efficacy Data	Safety Data
		co-infection with hepatitis B or C excluded					copies/mL (ITT-TLOVR): 39% for DRV/r 600/100 mg bid and 7% for CPI ($P < 0.001$) Mean HIV RNA change ($\log_{10}$ copies/mL): −1.70 for DRV/r 600/100 mg bid and −0.30 for CPI ($P < 0.001$) Mean CD4+ T-lymphocyte increase (cells/μL): +59 for DRV/r 600/100 mg bid and +12 for CPI ($P < 0.01$)	incidence in control group except for diarrhea (23%), nausea (9%) and insomnia (2%). No relationship between DRV/r dose and AE incidence was observed.
Phase IIb, Open-Label Trials								
TMC114-C215 Australia, Europe, USA, Canada, Argentina, Brazil	Open-label (roll-over of TMC114-C202 and TMC114-C213+ newly recruited patients)	HIV-1-infected, PI-, NRTI-, and NNRTI-experienced patients	DRV/r 600/100 mg bid[i] + OBR (tablet)	Long term (at least 144 weeks[e])	431[j]	Ongoing; pooled C215 and C208 primary 24-week data published as POWER 3 analysis[33]	Patients with ≥1.0 $\log_{10}$ HIV RNA reduction (ITT-TLOVR): 65% Patients with HIV RNA <50 copies/mL (ITT-TLOVR): 40%	DRV/r was generally well-tolerated, with a safety profile similar to that observed in POWER 1 and 2 studies.

							Mean HIV RNA change ($\log_{10}$ copies/mL): −1.65
TMC114-C208	Open-label (roll-over of TMC114-C207and selected phase I/II trials)	HIV-1-infected, PI-experienced patients	DRV/r 600/100 mg bid[i] + OBR (tablet)	Long term (at least 144 weeks[e])	29		Mean CD4+ T-lymphocyte count increase: 80 cells/μL
Phase III Trials							
ARTEMIS (TMC114-C211) Europe, North America, Latin America, Australia, Asia-Pacific, Russia and Africa (South Africa and Uganda)	Phase III randomized, controlled, followed by open-label	HIV-1-infected, treatment-naive patients	Control (LPV/r[k] 800/200 mg daily dose (qd or bid) + fixed background regimen (tenofovir/ emtricitabine) DRV/r 800/100 mg qd + fixed background regimen (tenofovir/ emtricitabine)	Long term (at least 96 weeks)	Approximately 660	Ongoing	
TITAN (TMC114-C214) Europe, North America, Latin America, Australia, Southeast Asia, Russia and Africa	Phase III randomized, controlled, followed by open-label	HIV-1-infected, treatment-experienced, LPV/r naive patients	Control (LPV/r 400/100 mg bid + OBR [ENF not allowed]) DRV/r 600/ 100 mg bid + OBR (ENF not allowed)	Long term (at least 96 weeks)	Approximately 595	Non-inferior to lopinavir/r at week 48	Similar between groups at week 48

(*Continued*)

Table 26-1

(Continued)

Trial Location	Design	Indication Studied/ Population	Treatment Arms	Treatment Duration	Number of Patients	Status	Efficacy Data	Safety Data
Expanded Access Program (TMC114-C226) USA; other countries opening shortly	Phase III open-label	HIV-1-infected patients with limited or no treatment options due to virologic failure or intolerance to multiple antiretroviral regimens	DRV/r 600/100 mg bid + other antiretroviral drugs	Until DRV becomes commercially available		Recruiting		

[a] DRV, darunavir; DRV/r – darunavir/ritonavir.
[b] AE, adverse event.
[c] OBR, optimized background regimen.
[d] CPI, control PI.
[e] Trials are still ongoing.
[f] For POWER 1, the primary efficacy analysis used 1 Feb 2005 as the cut-off date. At that time, 318 patients were included, of which 301 had reached week 24 or discontinued earlier.
[g] ITT-TLOVR, intent to treat-time to loss of virologic response.
[h] For POWER 2, the primary efficacy analysis used 1 Feb 2005 as the cut-off date. At that time, 278 subjects were included, of which 201 had reached week 24 or discontinued earlier.
[i] After 1 Feb 2005 (release of primary efficacy analysis results of POWER 1 and 2), patients using DRV/r 400/100 mg bid in the study were switched to the recommended dose (600/100 mg bid).
[j] Of the 431 patients in TMC114-C215, 303 were newly recruited (i.e., these were patients who had not previously participated in a DRV trial and were recruited to use the recommended dose of 600/100 mg bid).
[k] LPV/r, lopinavir/ritonavir.

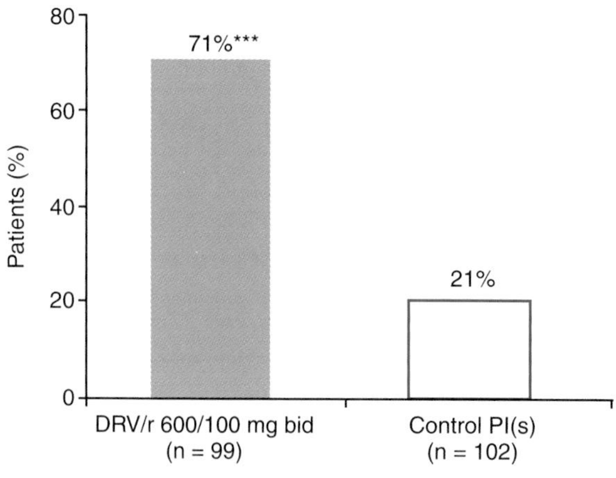

Figure 26-6 ■ POWER 1 and 2 patients with ≥1 $\log_{10}$ plasma VL reduction at week 24 (intent to treat-time to loss of virologic response).

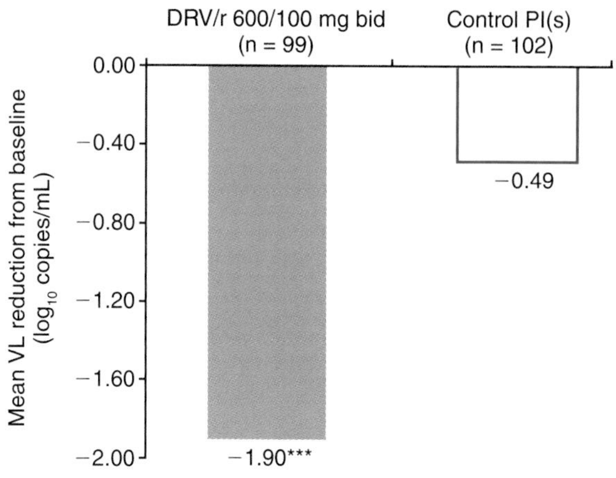

Figure 26-8 ■ Mean plasma VL reduction at week 24 in POWER 1 and 2 (noncompleter considered as failure).

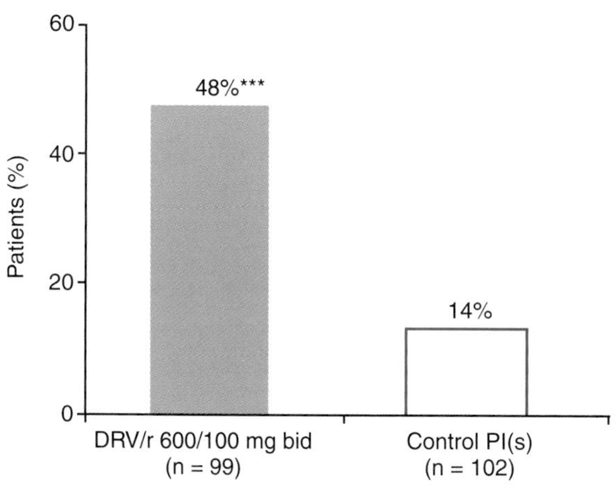

Figure 26-7 ■ POWER 1 and 2 patients with HIV RNA <50 copies/mL at week 24 (intent to treat-time to loss of virologic response).

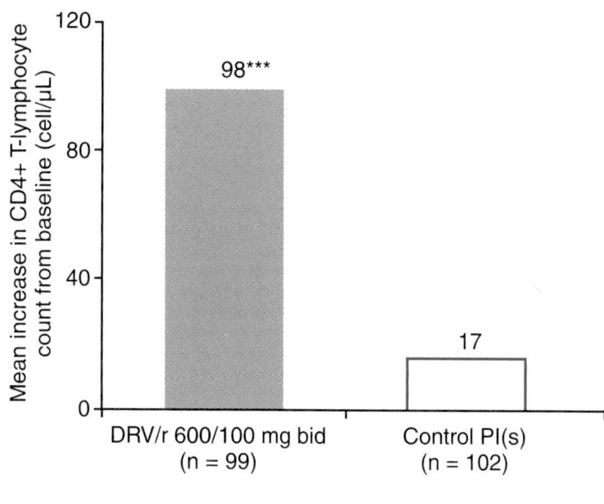

Figure 26-9 ■ Mean increase in CD4+ T-lymphocyte count at week 24 in POWER 1 and 2 (last observation carried forward).

DRV/r 600/100 mg twice daily and 17 cells/μL for the control PIs (Fig. 26-9). In both trials, discontinuations occurred earlier and more frequently in the control group than in the DRV/r groups. Discontinuations in the control group were due mainly to virologic failure (~50% of cases in each trial). Results were similar at week 48.

Influence of DRV Inhibitory Quotient on Efficacy

The high inhibitory quotients (IQs) achieved with DRV (mean values >200) provide an additional predictor of efficacy.[23] IQ is the ratio between the steady-state plasma DRV trough concentration and baseline DRV EC_{50}. When PK and pharmacodynamic analyses were performed in treatment-experienced patients who had available PK data (n = 468) from the POWER 1 and 2 studies, the IQ was found to be the strongest predictor of virologic response. The response was good when the IQ was above 435 (above 21 when adjusted for protein binding) and poorer when the IQ was below 133 (below 7 when adjusted for protein binding). The relationship between IQ and virologic response was primarily driven by the baseline DRV FC and less by DRV exposure. Based on the IQ values, all DRV/r dosing regimens would be expected to be virologically active, with the most pronounced effects for the highest dose (600/100 mg bid). This further supports the recommendation of the 600/100 mg twice daily regimen as the dose for treatment-experienced patients.

Clinical Virology

The most predictive factor of virologic outcome in the POWER studies was the FC for DRV at baseline.[24] The determinants of increased FC for DRV were explored by analyzing the influence of both the number and type of protease mutations on the virologic response at week 24, and the mutations that emerged upon virologic failure while on DRV treatment. The mutations developing in at least 10% of virologic failures (V32I, L33F, I47V, I54L, and I89V) were also associated with a diminished virologic response when present at baseline. Additional mutations associated with diminished response are V11I, G735, L76U, I84U and I50V. However, isolates harboring those mutations at baseline tended to have a higher number of PI resistance-associated mutations compared with those that did not harbor those mutations. Moreover, when introduced in a wild-type genetic background by site-directed mutagenesis, mutations V32I, L33F, I47V, or I54L, alone or in combination with one or two other PI resistance-associated mutations did not cause decreased susceptibility to DRV. Mutation I89V is currently being studied. Overall, mutations that develop after treatment failure with a DRV-containing regimen confer DRV resistance to HIV only in the background of a high number of PI resistance-associated mutations.

The isolates from virologic failures by rebound showed an 8.14-fold median FC increase for DRV.[24] Isolates from virologic failures by rebound that were sensitive to TPV at baseline remained sensitive to TPV. Since most of the baseline isolates were already resistant to the other currently approved PIs, this analysis could not be performed for these PIs. Use of eufuvintide, baseline viral load and number of active drugs in the optimised background were also predictors of response.

Predicted Effects of Treatment with DRV on Long-term Outcomes

Twenty-four-week CD4+ T-lymphocyte counts and HIV RNA data from POWER 1 and 2 have been used to predict clinical benefits of treatment with DRV/r over those of investigator-selected control PIs in terms of lower progression to AIDS or death.[25] The two methods used to predict clinical benefits were the categorization method and the regression method. The categorization method used EuroSIDA cohort data to determine the 12-month incidence of AIDS or death during HAART treatment within the CD4+ T-lymphocyte count ranges 0–50, 51–100, 101–200, 201–350, and >350 cells/μL; a weighted average of the published rates for DRV/r and control PI regimens was used to produce an overall expected rate of progression to AIDS or death for patients receiving HAART, with CD4+ T-lymphocyte counts in the different categories. This method predicted 1-year rates of progression to AIDS and death of 10.9% for control PIs and 5.9% for DRV/r, representing a reduction of 46% with DRV/r. In the regression method, data from more than 9000 patients in 14 randomized, clinical endpoint trials were used to correlate previous HIV RNA and CD4+ T-lymphocyte treatment effects with the relative risk of clinical progression. The reductions in progression predicted by the regression method were similar to the categorization method, whether HIV RNA data (55% reduction) or CD4+ T-lymphocyte data (47% reduction) were used. Thus, the effects of DRV/r in raising CD4+ T-lymphocyte counts and suppressing HIV RNA levels were predicted to lower progression rates to AIDS or death by ~47–55% compared with control PIs.

In summary, currently available clinical data suggest that DRV, administered with low-dose RTV as a PK enhancer, has potent antiviral activity and efficacy in treatment-experienced patients.

TOXICITY

Repeated doses of DRV alone or in combination with low-dose RTV have been administered to 378 healthy volunteers, resulting in a total of 12.5 patient-years of exposure. The outcome of one PK study showed that DRV/r had a more favorable safety and tolerability profile overall than DRV alone.[8] Long-term effects of co-administration on tolerability remain to be seen.

Safety data from TMC114-C207 demonstrated that DRV/r was generally well-tolerated in multiple PI-experienced patients.[19] The most commonly reported AEs were GI and CNS events of mild-to-moderate severity. Grade 3/4 treatment-emergent laboratory abnormalities were reported in 13% (5/38) of DRV/r patients and 33% (4/12) of control patients. These were mostly transient and did not require intervention; no case resulted in discontinuation of treatment. No dose–response relationship was observed for the incidence of AEs and no significant changes were observed in hematologic, biochemical or electrocardiographic parameters.

In the 24-week primary safety analyses of the POWER 1 and 2 studies, DRV/r was generally well-tolerated and there was no apparent relationship between the dose of DRV/r and frequency of AEs.[26,27] The incidence of treatment-emergent AEs and laboratory abnormalities regardless of causality from the two dose-finding phase IIb trials is summarized in Table 26-2. Due to the lack of a dose-relationship for safety and tolerability of DRV/r, primary safety data from all patients in the two trials ($n = 596$) were evaluated together in order to provide a more robust characterization of safety.

For all DRV/r dose groups, the most common treatment-emergent AEs occurring in >10% of patients were (in decreasing order of incidence); injection site reaction (25%), headache (17%), diarrhea (16%), nausea (14%), fatigue (12%), insomnia (11%), and nasopharyngitis (10%); for the control group, these were diarrhea (26%), headache (21%), injection site reaction (20%), fatigue (16%), pyrexia (12%), nausea (11%), and asthenia (10%). Injection site reaction was associated with ENF administration. A higher rate of discontinuation in the control group (63%, of which 51% were due to virologic failure and 5% due to AEs) compared with all DRV/r groups (16%, of which 7% were due to virologic failure and 6% due to AEs) meant that patients in the control group had considerably less exposure to treatment than those

Table 26-2

Incidence of Treatment-Emergent AEs and Laboratory Abnormalities (Regardless of Causality) from POWER 1 and 2 Primary Safety Analysis

	DRV/r[a] (mg)					
Incidence	400/100 qd (n = 121) (%)	800/100 qd (n = 119) (%)	400/100 bid (n = 118) (%)	600/100 bid (n = 122) (%)	All DRV/r (n = 480) (%)	Control PI(s) (n = 116) (%)
Any AE[b]	93	89	92	93	92	91
Any grade 3 or 4 AE	22	27	26	27	26	24
Grade 3–4 laboratory abnormalities						
Triglycerides	5.8	5.9	7.6	13.2	8.2	6
Total cholesterol	0.8	3.4	1.6	5	2.7	0.9
ALT[c]	0.8	0	1.7	2.5	1.3	2.6
AST[d]	1.6	0.8	1.7	2.5	1.7	4.3

[a] DRV/r, darunavir/ritonavir.
[b] AE, adverse event.
[c] ALT, alanine aminotransferase.
[d] AST, aspartate aminotransferase.

in the DRV/r groups. An analysis of the incidence of AEs per 100 patient-years of exposure was therefore performed to adjust for the shorter treatment exposure time in the control group. Adjusting for treatment exposure, the two most common AEs of headache and diarrhea (excluding injection site reaction) occurred less frequently in the DRV/r groups (23 and 25 events/100 patient-years, respectively) than in the control group (57 and 46 events/100 patient-years, respectively). The incidences of all other AEs were also lower for DRV/r than for control patients, with the exception of herpes simplex, which was more frequent in DRV/r patients, and upper respiratory tract infection, cough and nausea, which occurred at similar frequencies in both treatment arms. In POWER 1, the safety profile of patients who were co-infected with hepatitis C or hepatitis B (31/255 of all DRV/r patients and 13/63 of control patients) was comparable to the overall study population.[26] Patients with hepatitis C or hepatitis B co-infection were excluded in POWER 2.[27]

DRUG INTERACTIONS

The oxidative metabolism of DRV in humans is almost exclusively catalyzed by CYP3A4. When co-administered with low-dose RTV, DRV is a net inhibitor of CYP3A4 and therefore has the potential to increase plasma concentrations of drugs that are primarily metabolized by CYP3A4, which could increase or prolong their therapeutic and adverse effects. DRV and RTV should therefore not be co-administered with drugs that are highly dependent on CYP3A4 for clearance and for which increased plasma concentrations are associated with serious or life-threatening events (i.e., agents with a narrow therapeutic index).

Phase I clinical trials are being conducted with healthy volunteers to investigate the potential interactions between DRV/r and several other antiretrovirals (e.g., saquinavir (SQV), efavirenz (EFV), LPV/r, and indinavir), lipid-lowering agents (e.g., pravastatin), and a range of commonly prescribed drugs (e.g., paroxetine, sertraline, rifabutin, sildenafil, ketoconazole, and clarithromycin). The key findings of drug interaction studies that have been published and some preliminary results are summarized below. This is a rapidly evolving field and new findings and updates can be consulted in several websites (e.g., http://www.hiv-druginteractions.org).

Interaction with other Antiretroviral Therapies

In an open-label crossover study, a possible PK interaction between DRV/r and tenofovir was investigated in 13 healthy volunteers.[28] While systemic exposure of tenofovir increased by 22% when co-administered with DRV/r, tenofovir did not significantly influence DRV exposure.

In another study involving 23 healthy volunteers, systemic exposure to DRV was not significantly affected by co-administration of atazanavir.[29] The authors concluded that doses of up to 300 mg of atazanavir per day may be co-administered with DRV/r in HIV-1-infected patients, if the clinical need arises. Interaction with DRV seems to be irrelevant from the PK point of view. At present, co-administration of DRV with SQV or LPV seems to be not recommended. DRV can be co-administered with ENF and likely be co-administered with TMC125, EFV or nevirapine although these data are not yet definitive and studies are still ongoing.

Interaction with Atorvastatin

An open-label, randomized, one-way crossover study was conducted in 16 healthy volunteers to investigate the effect of DRV (oral solution) plus low-dose RTV on the PK of atorvastatin.[30] Low-dose atorvastatin (10 mg daily) with DRV/r (300/100 mg twice daily) resulted in exposure to atorvastatin that was 15% lower than that achieved with atorvastatin 40 mg daily alone. Thus, if atorvastatin and DRV/r must be co-administered, then atorvastatin must be given at a starting dose of 10 mg, then gradually titrated upwards as required to achieve the desired clinical response. Conversely, co-administration with pravastatin is likely to be not recommended.

Interaction with Omeprazole and Ranitidine

The effects of co-administration of omeprazole and ranitidine with DRV/r have been discussed in the PK section of this chapter.[18] Dose adjustments are not necessary when DRV/r is co-administered with omeprazole or ranitidine.

Other Potential Interactions

Most likely when co-administered with DRV/r, the dose of sildenafil should not exceed 25 mg within a period of 48 h. Co-administration of clarithromycin TMC114/r is generally well-tolerated and no dose adjustments are required.[31] However, the dose of clarithromycin must be adjusted in renally impaired patients; dose reduction by 50% for patients with creatinine clearance (CL_{CR}) of 30–60 mL/min and by 75% for patients with CL_{CR} <30 mL/min.[32] Finally, the dose of rifabutin may have to be reduced to 150 mg every other day, when given concomitantly with DRV/r although definitive data are not yet available.

USE DURING PREGNANCY AND LACTATION

At this stage, there is no sufficient data regarding the use of DRV/r in pregnant women. Until more clinical experience is available, women of childbearing potential should not receive DRV/r unless they are using adequate contraception. Plasma concentrations of ethinyl estradiol may be decreased due to induction of its metabolism by RTV, and alternative or additional contraceptive measures must be used when estrogen-based oral contraceptives are co-administered with DRV/r. A trial to investigate the effect of DRV/r on oral contraceptives is currently ongoing.

It is not known whether DRV/r is excreted in human milk; however, because of both the potential for HIV transmission and the potential for serious AEs in nursing infants, HIV-1-infected mothers should be instructed not to breast-feed if they are receiving DRV/r.

INDICATIONS FOR USE

DRV, approved by the US Food and Drug Administration (FDA) in 2006, is a potent PI with a high genetic barrier to the development of resistance. Current evidence indicates its antiretroviral efficacy among treatment-experienced, HIV-1-infected patients, particularly in patients failing one or more PI-containing regimens. In this setting, DRV/r has proven to be significantly more effective than any comparator PI (except for TPV, which was not available for evaluation in the POWER studies), even in patients with several primary PI-associated mutations (response observed in the presence of up to 10 mutations, and to a lesser degree even above 10 mutations). Moreover, in the POWER studies, DRV/r was more active than any comparator PI, even when the virus was apparently fully sensitive to the agent used. Head-to-head comparative studies with TPV are yet to be performed; it is worth noting that viral isolates emerging after DRV/r failure remain sensitive to TPV. Additionally, baseline predictors of response to DRV/r-containing regimens will need to be refined to ensure optimal use in clinical practice.

In summary, the goal of treatment for patients with advanced disease and who have had treatment failure should be virologic suppression. DRV/r can contribute substantially to this goal. Salvage therapy may further improve in the near future with the incorporation of integrase inhibitors, etravirine CCR5 co-receptor inhibitors, HIV-1 maturation inhibitors or newer reverse transcriptase inhibitors. The potential role of DRV/r in the management of a broader range of HIV-infected patients is currently being evaluated in phase III clinical trials involving treatment-naive and treatment-experienced patients who have various remaining options, or as monotherapy in virologically suppressed patients.

REFERENCES

1. Gulick RM. Assessing the benefits of antiretroviral therapy. Ann Intern Med 133:471–3, 2000.
2. Palella FJ Jr, Delaney KM, Moorman AC, et al. Declining morbidity and mortality among patients with advanced human immunodeficiency virus infection. HIV Outpatient Study Investigators. N Engl J Med 338:853–60, 1998.
3. Swanstrom R, Erona J. Human immunodeficiency virus type-1 protease inhibitors: therapeutic successes and failures, suppression and resistance. Pharmacol Ther 86:145–70, 2000.
4. Cane P, Chrystie I, Dunn D, et al. Time trends in primary resistance to HIV drugs in the United Kingdom: multicentre observational study. BMJ 331:1368–1372, 2005.
5. King NM, Prabu-Jeyabalan M, Nalivaika EA, et al. Structural and thermodynamic basis for the binding of TMC114, a next-generation human immunodeficiency virus type 1 protease inhibitor. J Virol 78:12012–21, 2004.
6. Surleraux DL, Tahri A, Verschueren WG, et al. Discovery and selection of TMC114, a next generation HIV-1 protease inhibitor. J Med Chem 48:1813–1822, 2005.
7. Surleraux DL, de Kock HA, Verschueren WG, et al. Design of HIV-1 protease inhibitors active on multidrug-resistant virus. J Med Chem 48:1965–73, 2005.

8. Hoetelmans R, van der Sandt I, De Pauw M, et al. TMC114, a next generation HIV protease inhibitor: pharmacokinetics and safety following oral administration of multiple doses with and without low doses of ritonavir in healthy volunteers. In: 12th Conference on Retroviruses and Opportunistic Infections, Boston, MA, USA, 10–14 Feb 2003, abstract 549.
9. Koh Y, Nakata H, Maeda K, et al. Novel bis-tetrahydrofuranylurethane-containing nonpeptidic protease inhibitor (PI) UIC-94017 (TMC114) with potent activity against multi-PI-resistant human immunodeficiency virus in vitro. Antimicrob Agents Chemother 47:3123–9, 2003.
10. Ghosh AK, Leshchenko S, Noetzel M. Stereoselective photochemical 1,3-dioxolane addition to 5-alkoxymethyl-2(5H)-furanone: synthesis of bis-tetrahydrofuranyl ligand for HIV protease inhibitor UIC-94017 (TMC-114). J Org Chem 69:7822–9, 2004.
11. Dierynck I, Keuleers IM, De Wit M, et al. Kinetic characterization of the potent activity of TMC114 on wild-type HIV-1 protease. In: 14th International HIV Drug Resistance Workshop, Quebec City, Canada, 7–11 Jun 2005, abstract 64.
12. Tie Y, Boross PI, Wang YF, et al. High resolution crystal structures of HIV-1 protease with a potent non-peptide inhibitor (UIC-94017) active against multi-drug-resistant clinical strains. J Mol Biol 338:341–52, 2004.
13. De Meyer S, Azijn H, Surleraux D, et al. TMC114, a novel human immunodeficiency virus type 1 protease inhibitor active against protease inhibitor-resistant viruses, including a broad range of clinical isolates. Antimicrob Agents Chemother 49:2314–21, 2005.
14. Balotta C, Facchi G, Violin M, et al. Increasing prevalence of non-clade B HIV-1 strains in heterosexual men and women, as monitored by analysis of reverse transcriptase and protease sequences. J Acquir Immune Defic Syndr 27:499–505, 2001.
15. Perrin L, Kaiser L, Yerly S. Travel and the spread of HIV-1 genetic variants. Lancet Infect Dis 3:22–7, 2003.
16. Hoetelmans R, Lefebvre E, van der Sandt I, et al. Pharmacokinetics and effect of food on TMC114, a potent next generation protease inhibitor, boosted with low-dose ritonavir. In: 5th International Workshop on Clinical Pharmacology of HIV Therapy, Rome, Italy, 1–3 Apr 2004, abstract 5.6.
17. Sekar V, Kestens D, Spinosa-Guzman S, et al. The effects of different meal types on the pharmacokinetics of TMC114 tablet formulation dosed with ritonavir in healthy volunteers. In: 10th European AIDS Conference, Dublin, Ireland, 17–20 Nov 2005, abstract PE4.1/1.
18. Sekar V, Hoetelmans R, De Marez T, et al. Pharmacokinetics of TMC114: effect of omeprazole and ranitidine. In: 6th International Workshop on Clinical Pharmacology of HIV Therapy, Quebec, Canada, 28–30 Apr 2005, abstract 2.10.
19. Arasteh K, Clumeck N, Pozniak A, et al. TMC114/ritonavir substitution for protease inhibitor(s) in a non-suppressive antiretroviral regimen: a 14-day proof-of-principle trial. AIDS 19:943–7, 2005.
20. Katlama C, Carvalho MTM, Cooper D, et al. TMC114/r outperforms investigator-selected PI(s) in 3-class-experienced patients: week 24 primary analysis of POWER 1 (TMC114-C213). In: 3rd IAS Conference on HIV Pathogenesis and Treatment, Rio de Janeiro, Brazil, 24–27 Jul 2005, abstract WeOaLB0102.
21. Wilkin T, Haubrich R, Steinhart CR, et al. POWER 2 (TMC114-C202 study) week 24 efficacy analysis. In: 45th Interscience Conference on Antimicrobial Agents and Chemotherapy, Washington, DC, USA, 16–19 Dec 2005, abstract 2860.
22. Johnson VA, Brun-Vezinet F, Clotet B, et al. Update of the drug resistance mutations in HIV-1: 2004. Top HIV Med 12:119–24, 2004.
23. Sekar V, De Meyer S, Vangeneugden T, et al. Pharmacokinetic/pharmacodynamic (PK/PD) analyses of TMC114 in the POWER 1 and POWER 2 trials in treatment-experienced HIV-infected patients. In: 13th Conference on Retroviruses and Opportunistic Infections, Denver, CO, USA, 5–8 Feb 2006, abstract J-21.
24. De Meyer S, Hill A, De Baere I, et al. Effect of baseline susceptibility and on-treatment mutations on TMC114 and control PI efficacy: preliminary analysis of data from PI-experienced patients from POWER 1 and POWER 2. In: 13th Conference on Retroviruses and Opportunistic Infections, Denver, CO, USA, 5–8 Feb 2006, abstract M-167.
25. Montaner J, Hill A, Smith C, et al. Prediction of clinical benefits of TMC114/ritonavir from treatment effects on CD4 counts and HIV RNA. In: 10th European AIDS Conference, Dublin, Ireland, 17–20 Nov 2005. abstract PE18.4/4.
26. Grinsztejn B, Arasteh K, Clotet B, et al. TMC114/r well tolerated in 3-class-experienced patients: week 24 primary analysis of POWER 1 (TMC114-C213). In: 3rd IAS Conference on HIV Pathogenesis and Treatment, Rio de Janeiro, Brazil, 24–27 Jul 2005, abstract WePeLB6.201.
27. Berger DS, Bellos N, Farthing C, et al. TMC114/r in 3-class-experienced patients: 24-week primary safety analysis of the POWER 2 Study (TMC114-C202). In: 45th Interscience Conference on Antimicrobial Agents and Chemotherapy, Washington DC, USA, 16–19 Dec 2005, abstract H-1094.
28. Hoetelmans R, Marien K, De Pauw M, et al. Pharmacokinetic interaction between TMC114/ritonavir (RTV) and tenofovir in healthy volunteers. In: 15th International AIDS Conference, Bangkok, Thailand, 11–16 Jul 2004, abstract TuPeB4634.
29. Sekar V, De Marez T, Spinosa-Guzman S, et al. Pharmacokinetic interaction between TMC114/ritonavir and atazanavir in healthy volunteers. In: 10th European AIDS Conference, Dublin, Ireland, 17–20 Nov 2005, abstract PE4.3/4.
30. Hoetelmans R, Lasure A, Koester A, et al. The effect of TMC114, a potent next-generation HIV protease inhibitor, with low-dose ritonavir on atorvastatin pharmacokinetics. In: 44th Interscience Conference on Antimicrobial Agents and Chemotherapy, Washington, DC, USA, 30 Oct-2 Nov 2004, abstract H-865.
31. Sekar V, Spinosa-Guzman S, De Pauw M, et al. The pharmacokinetic interaction between clarithromycin and TMC114/ritonavir in healthy subjects. In: Annual Meeting of the American Society for Clinical Pharmacology and Therapeutics, Baltimore, MD, USA, 8–11 Mar 2006, abstract PI-61.
32. Abbott Laboratories. Biaxin® XL (clarithromycin): summary of product characteristics. 2005. Available: http://biaxinxl.com/ 1 Jun 2006.
33. Vetter N, Van Wanzeele F, Mauss S, et al. POWER 3: 24-week analysis confirms TMC114/r efficacy and safety profile in treatment-experienced HIV patients. In: 1st Eastern European and Central Asian AIDS Conference, Moscow, Russia, 15–17 May 2006, abstract A0312.

Chapter 27

Integrase Inhibitors and Other New Drugs in Development

John J. W. Fangman, MD, Martin S. Hirsch, MD

INTRODUCTION

Since the second edition of AIDS Therapy in 2003, substantial advances have been made in the treatment of human immunodeficiency virus type 1 (HIV-1) infection. These include approval of novel classes of antiretrovirals (ARVs) such as the fusion inhibitor enfuvirtide, the CCR5 co-receptor inhibitor maraviroc, the nucleotide reverse transcriptase inhibitor tenofovir, and the integrase inhibitor raltegravir, as well as the novel protease inhibitors (PIs) atazanavir, tipranavir and darunavir. Some existing agents have been reformulated to enhance tolerability and several approved drugs have been co-formulated as well. These advances have expanded treatment options for patients with drug resistance and lowered the pill burden of many regimens, thereby facilitating improved adherence.

Despite these developments, there continues to be a pressing need for new drugs to treat HIV-1 infection. In areas where antiretroviral therapy (ART) has been widely available, the rates of drug resistance are considerable and drive demand for new agents to which viruses are susceptible. In addition, metabolic complications of ART highlight the need for drugs with improved adverse event profiles. There is also a necessity for ARV agents that can be easily and safely administered in resource-limited settings where special handling of drugs or close laboratory monitoring may not be possible.

Currently approved ARV agents target one of four steps in the HIV-1 replicative cycle: viral entry, reverse transcriptase, protease or integrase activity. New agents are being developed that target these sites as well as other sites in the HIV-1 replicative cycle. These agents can be classified as inhibitors of viral entry, intracellular replication or assembly of infectious virions (Fig. 27-1). Inhibitors of viral entry include the CCR5 chemokine co-receptor antagonist, vicriviroc, which is in advanced stages of development as well as other attachment inhibitors and novel fusion inhibitors. While next-generation nucleoside and non-nucleoside reverse transcriptase inhibitors (NNRTIs) are being tested, HIV integrase inhibitors are the most promising class of compounds being developed to inhibit intracellular replication. Agents that inhibit viral assembly that are under development include novel PIs and maturation inhibitors. Our discussion will begin with a review of integrase inhibitors and will then move to other compounds that inhibit intracellular replication, viral entry and viral assembly.

The information reported here summarizes available data on drugs that are in clinical trials, as well as some novel drugs that are in preclinical development (Table 27-1), and is not intended to be encyclopedic. Several new compounds in advanced stages of development are covered in more detail elsewhere in this text, including co-receptor inhibitors (*see* Chapter 24) and the PI darunavir (*see* Chapter 26). In addition, immune-based approaches and therapeutic vaccines are covered elsewhere (*see* Chapters 30 and 31 respectively).

INHIBITORS OF INTRACELLULAR REPLICATION

Integrase Inhibitors

Integration of HIV-1 genetic material into host DNA is essential for productive infection with HIV-1.[1] Inhibition of this process has been an attractive target for drug development since the identification of HIV-1 integrase in the 1980s. The mechanism by which integration occurs has been elucidated, and several inhibitors are in advanced stages of development. After HIV-1

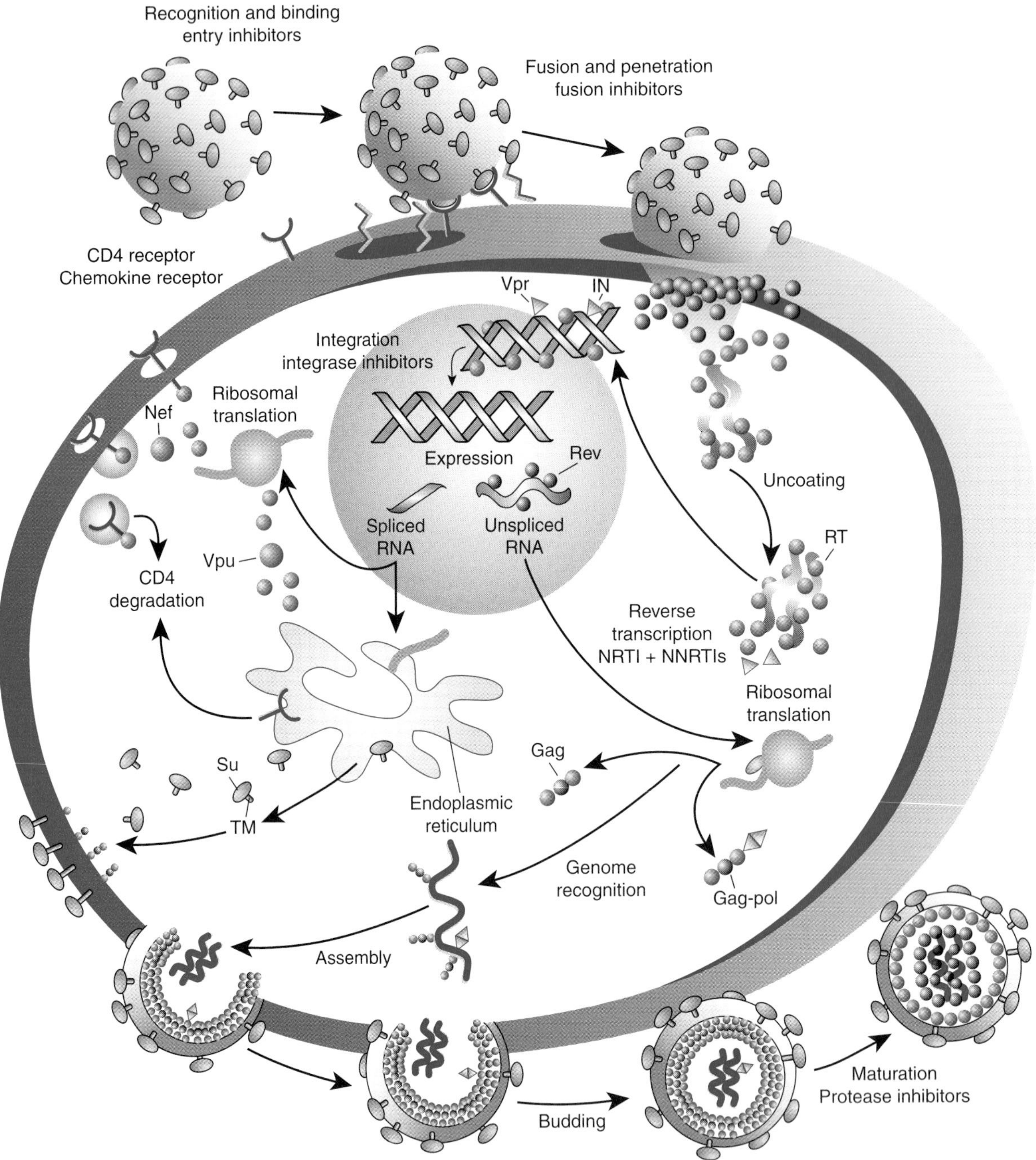

Figure 27-1 ■ HIV-1 replication cycle. Stylized representation of the HIV-1 replication cycle beginning with binding to the CD4 receptor, attachment to chemokine co-receptor (CCR5 or CXCR4), viral entry, uncoating, reverse transcription (RT), entry into nucleus, integration into host DNA, transcription of new viral RNA, translation of mRNA into virally encoded peptides, migration to cell surface, assembly, budding, and maturation mediated by a virally encoded aspartyl protease. Each of these steps is a potential target for antiretroviral drug therapy.

With permission from Pomerantz RJ, Horn DL. Twenty years of therapy for HIV-1 infection. Nat Med 2003; 9(7):867.

enters target cells, viral reverse transcriptase (RT) synthesizes a linear, double-stranded DNA copy (cDNA). Insertion of viral cDNA into the chromosomal DNA of target cells is the hallmark of retroviral infection and is a prerequisite for transcription of the HIV-1 genome and translation of viral proteins.[2,3] This process is catalyzed by the viral enzyme, integrase, which is a 288 amino acid protein derived from the 3′ end of the HIV polymerase gene. Integration of viral cDNA into host chromosomes is a multistep process that has both cytoplasmic and nuclear stages (Fig. 27-2).[4] Following reverse transcription, HIV-1 cDNA binds to integrase in the cytoplasm via interactions with specific sequences in the HIV-1 LTR region. The binding of HIV-1 cDNA to integrase catalyzes the removal of two nucleotides proximal to each 3′-end of proviral cDNA in the cytoplasm of target cells (3′-processing). After 3′-processing, integrase remains bound to HIV-1 cDNA, forming multimeric pre-integration complexes (PICs). PICs interact with a variety of viral and cellular proteins to

Table 27-1

Selected Antiretroviral Agents in Development

Agent	Manufacturer
Integrase Inhibitors	
Raltegravir (MK-0518)	Merck
Elvitegravir (GS 9137, JTK-303)	Gilead
Nucleoside Reverse Transcriptase Inhibitors	
D-d4FC (Reverset, DPC 817, dexelvucitabine)	Incyte
Elvucitabine (ACH-126,433, β-L-d4FC)	Achillion
Apricitabine (AVX-754, SPD-754, BCH-10618, (-)dOTC)	Avexa
Racivir (RCV; (+/ −)-FTC; [(+/ −)-β-2′,3′-dideoxy-5fluoro-3′-thiacytidine]	Pharmasset
Nonnucleoside Reverse Transcriptase Inhibitors	
Etravirine (TMC 125, R165335)	Tibotec/J&J
Rilpivirine (TMC 278, R278474)	Tibotec/J&J
GW678248/GW695634	GlaxoSmithKline
Attachment Inhibitors	
PRO-542	Progenics Pharmaceuticals
TNX-355	Tanox/Biogen
BMS-488043	Bristol-Myers Squibb
Fusion Inhibitors	
TR-290999 and TR291144	Trimeris
Co-receptor Inhibitors	
See Chapter 24	
Protease Inhibitors	
Brecanavir (GW640385)	GlaxoSmithKline
Maturation Inhibitors	
Bevirimat (PA-457)	Panacos

gain entry into the host nucleus. Once inside the nucleus, HIV-1 integrase catalyses insertion of viral cDNA into the host chromosome (strand transfer). Upon completion of the strand transfer process, the defects in the host cell's genome that occur during cDNA insertion are repaired. Because there is no host equivalent, HIV-1 integrase has long been recognized as a potentially attractive target for ART.[5] The development of *in vitro* assays that specifically evaluate the various steps in cDNA integration has been critical to integrase inhibitor development.[6–8] Although many compounds have been reported to inhibit its activity, development of integrase inhibitors has been plagued by difficulties identifying compounds that specifically attack this target.[9] At least four criteria need to be met in order to definitively establish that a compound targets integrase.[4] First, it should be active during the replication cycle in which integration occurs (4–16 h after infection). Second, infected cells treated with the agent should show accumulation of circular cDNA. Third, mutations in integrase should be found in resistant viruses and finally, recombinant viruses into which mutant sequences of integrase are inserted should also be resistant to the putative inhibitor. A phenotypic assay of integrase activity has been developed to identify susceptibility of integrase inhibitors using recombinant viruses that express integrase alone or in combination with protease and reverse transcriptase.[10] While lead compounds targeting each step in the process of integration into host DNA have been identified, the most promising agents currently being studied all inhibit the strand-transfer process and two different classes of strand-transfer integrase inhibitors will be reviewed here.

DKA Derivatives

Diketobutanoic acid derivatives (DKAs) were identified when molecules were screened for antiviral activity from a library of over 250 000 candidate compounds using an *in vitro* model of HIV-1 integration.[8] Structural analysis of these substances indicated a common diketo acid moiety, thus leading to their classification as DKAs. DKAs inhibit HIV-1 cDNA integrase strand-transfer function at nanomolar to micromolar concentrations.[8] The DKA L-870812 was the first integrase inhibitor to demonstrate *in vivo* antiviral activity in a simian human immunodeficiency virus (SHIV)-rhesus macaque model.[11] Because of their structural similarities, agents within this class have induced both novel integrase mutations and the potential for cross-resistance.[12,13] Biochemical modifications have improved the potency of the first generation of DKAs and second generation compounds of this class are at the leading edge of integrase inhibitor development. First generation compounds such as S-1360[14–18] and L-870,810[19–24] demonstrated potent *in vitro* activity against HIV-1 but were not pursued because of either poor bioavailability (S–1360) or hepatotoxicity in animal models (L-870,810). These DKA derivatives, however, provided proof that integrase function could be inhibited and paved the way for development of other drugs in this promising new class of compounds.

Raltegravir (MK-0518)

Raltegravir is an evolutionary descendant of the diketobutanoic acids which its developers further classify as a pyrimidinone derivative. Raltegravir has demonstrated potent *in vitro* activity against wild-type HIV-1 (IC_{90} of 33 nM ± 23 nM in 50% human serum).[25] Raltegravir maintains activity against HIV-1 regardless of virus co-receptor tropism, and is active against multidrug resistant isolates.[26] The activity of raltegravir against nonclade B HIV-1 and against HIV-2 has not been reported. Isolates that developed *in vitro* resistance to raltegravir during serial passage studies retained susceptibility to all other existing classes of ARVs. A variety of naturally occurring polymorphisms within the HIV-1 integrase gene have been identified, but mutations that confer high-level resistance to integrase inhibitors *in vitro* include T66I/O, L74M, F121Y, T125K, G140S, S230R, V249I, and C280Y. These polymorphisms have not been shown to arise

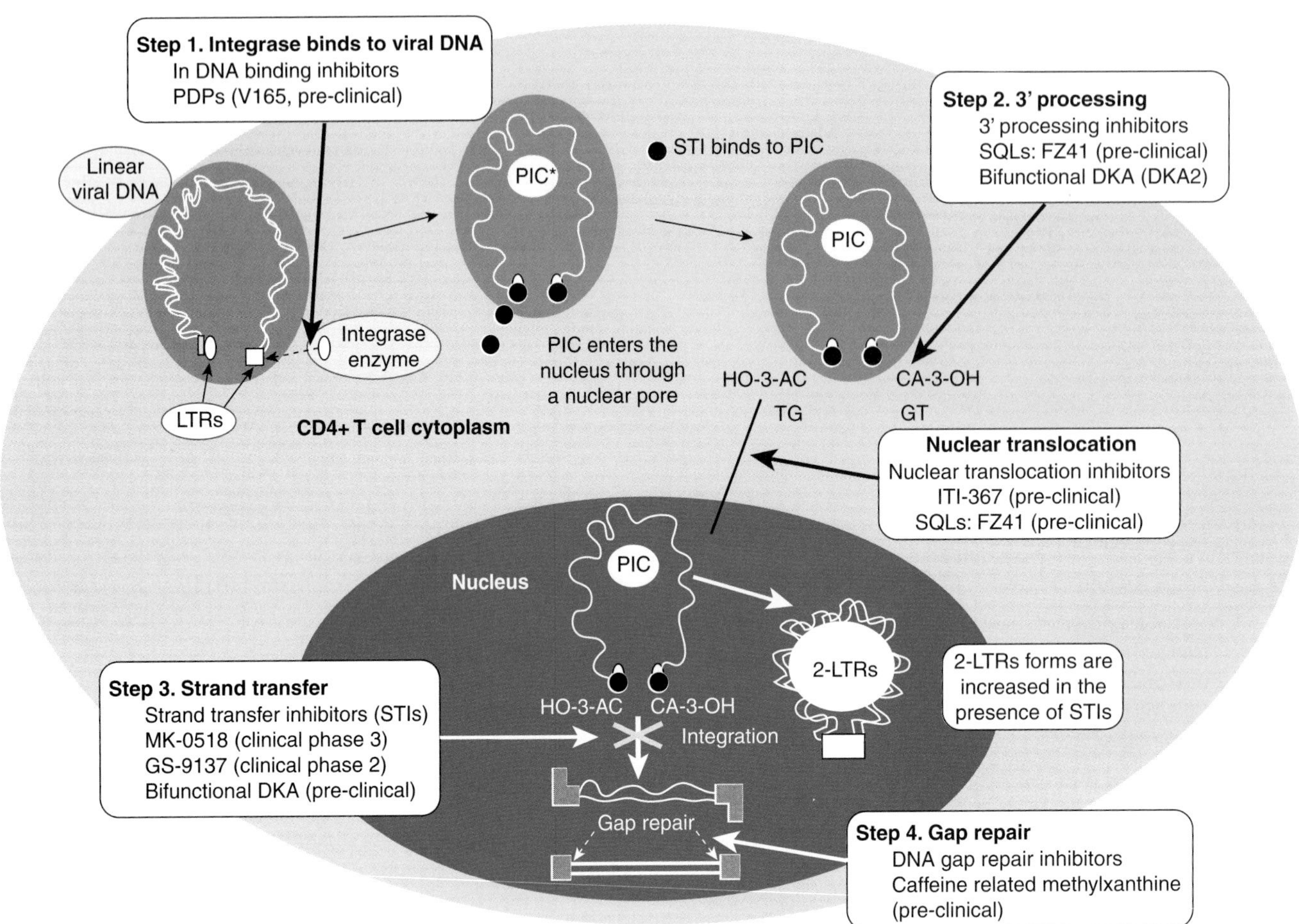

Figure 27-2 ■ HIV integration. While the linear viral DNA is still in the cytoplasm, the virally encoded integrase binds to viral DNA (step 1). The enzyme then begins to process the 3′ end of the viral DNA (step 2) prior to its translocation from the cytoplasm into the nucleus. Once inside the nucleus, the processed ends of the viral DNA integrate into host genomic DNA through the process of 'strand transfer' (step 3). Residual gaps in the DNA are repaired presumably by host-encoded gap repair enzymes (step 4). Current integrase inhibitors under study, e.g., raltegravir and elvitegravir, act at the strand transfer step (step 3). Other experimental inhibitors designed to block steps 1–4 are listed in the figure for reference.

With permission from Lataillade M Le, Kozal MJ. The Hunt for HIV-1 integrase inhibitors. AIDS Pat Care STDs 2006; 20(7): 1087.

spontaneously without prior exposure to integrase inhibitors.[27] Studies of virologic failure in subjects receiving raltegravir have demonstrated two common genetic pathways: N155H and Q148K/R/H. Additional mutations were observed in both pathways including E92Q, V151I, T97A, G163R, L74M within the N155H pathway and G140S/A, E138K within the Q148K/R/H pathway. Mutations are proximal to the catalytic center and are similar to those selected by passage of virus in the presence of drug *in vitro*. Raltegravir is metabolized by glucuronidation via UGT1A1 and does not induce or inhibit CYP3A4. Raltegravir has *in vitro* synergy with all currently available classes of ARV agents.[25]

Phase 1 studies suggested antiviral activity at a dose range between 100 and 800 mg twice daily, without regard to food intake. A phase II trial of raltegravir monotherapy assessed the antiviral activity, pharmacokinetics and tolerability in 35 treatment-naive, HIV-1-infected subjects.[25] Subjects with an HIV-1 load >5000 copies/mL and a CD4 count of >100 cells/mm^3 were randomized 4:1 to receive either 100, 200, 400, or 600 mg of raltegravir twice daily for 10 days versus placebo. HIV-1 load declined between 1.7 and 2.2 $\log_{10}$ copies/mL at the end of the study period and between 50% and 57% of treated subjects were able to achieve levels <400 copies/mL and 13–29% <50 copies/mL.[28] Pharmacokinetic analysis at the end of the study demonstrated minimum concentration (C_{min}) values for all doses studied that were greater than raltegravir's IC_{90} *in vitro*. No serious adverse events (SAEs) or grade 3 or 4 laboratory abnormalities were observed.

Interim 16-week results from a study of the antiviral activity of raltegravir in treatment-experienced subjects have been reported.[26] One hundred and sixty seven subjects with documented triple-class resistance, CD4 counts >100 cells/mm^3 and plasma HIV-1 RNA levels of >5000 copies/mL were enrolled in a trial of optimized background therapy (OBT) with raltegravir versus placebo. Study subjects were highly treatment-experienced with ~90% resistant to all available PIs and ~50% resistant to all available ARV agents, as measured by phenotyic sensitivity score (PSS). Subjects received 200, 400, or 600 mg of raltegravir versus placebo twice daily. At week 16, 65–85% of subjects receiving raltegravir had achieved an HIV-1 load <400 copies/mL and between 56% and 72% had <50 copies/mL. This compared to rates less than 20% in the OBT with placebo groups. Viral load decline was over 2 $\log_{10}$ copies/mL for all three of the arms receiving raltegravir, compared to almost 1 $\log_{10}$ copies/mL for those receiving OBT with placebo. CD4 counts increased more in the 400 mg and 600 mg raltegravir arms (100–110 cells/mm^3), compared to either the 200 mg or placebo arms (~30 cells/mm^3). Adverse event rates were comparable between the groups receiving raltegravir and placebo, and were generally mild to moderate. Twenty-four week data have confirmed sustained responses and have highlighted the importance of using raltegravir with other active agents.[29] Efficacy of raltegravir in achieving HIV-1 RNA level <400 copies/mL rose from 54–69% in participants with a PSS score of 0, to 75–84% in those with a PSS of 1-2. Similarly, addition of raltegravir to OBT with enfuvirtide in subjects who were fusion inhibitor-naive resulted in HIV-1 levels <400 copies/mL in over 90% of individuals at 24 weeks. Drug-related SAEs were reported in four subjects (pancreatitis, lacunar infarct, lipoatrophy, hepatomegaly, and metabolic acidosis, renal insufficiency and death). The first two SAEs were not attributable to raltegravir (pancreatitis was attributed to an agent in OBT and the lacunar infarct occurred in the placebo arm), but the relationship of the other SAEs to the study drug is uncertain as subjects and investigators remain blinded to the arm of the study in which they occurred. Diarrhea, nausea, fatigue, headache, and pruritus were seen at low rates in most arms but were comparable to those seen in the placebo arm. Because atazanavir is known to be an inhibitor of UGT1A1, a subgroup analysis is pending to study the potential interaction between these two compounds.

Preliminary data from two large multinational phase III trials of raltegravir have been presented.[30,31] The studies known as BENCHMRK-1 and BENCHMRK-2 (blocking integrase in treatment-experienced patients with a novel compound against HIV: Merck) were designed to evaluate virologic and immunologic responses, as well as safety and tolerability of raltegravir versus placebo, in subjects with triple-class resistant HIV-1 infection who were receiving OBT. Subjects were required to have genotypic or phenotypic evidence of resistance to one drug in the NNRTI, PI and nucleoside reverse transcriptase inhibitor (NRTI) classes along with an HIV-1 RNA level of >1000 copies/mL. OBT was investigator selected and could include investigational compounds. Individuals qualifying for inclusion were randomized 2:1 to receive 400 mg bid of raltegravir versus placebo. Persons failing virologically (defined as <1 $\log_{10}$ copies/mL or >400 copies/mL or rebound viremia after achieving an undetectable plasma HIV RNA) at week 16 were allowed to enter an open-label raltegravir arm. BENCHMRK-1 enrolled 350 patients in Europe, Asia and the Pacific, while BENCHMRK-2 recruited 349 participants in North America, Central America and South America. Subjects in both trials were predominantly male (84–91%) and averaged 44–46 years of age. Subjects in BENCHMRK-1 were predominantly Caucasian (75–81%) compared to BENCHMRK-2 (55–65%). Over 90% of subjects had AIDS, and mean CD4 counts at entry ranged from 146 to 163 cells/mm^3. Subjects were highly treatment-experienced with genotypic sensitivity score (GSS) of 0/1 in 30–33% of subjects receiving raltegravir in BENCHMRK-1 and 20–44% in BENCHMRK-2, compared to 29–41% and 26–40% for the placebo-arms of these two groups. About 20% of subjects were enfuvirtide-naive in both studies. About 27% of individuals in BENCHMRK-1 and 45% in BENCHMRK-2 were darunavir-naive compared to 25% and 50% in the placebo arms of both these trials, respectively. The 16-week data demonstrated that 77% of raltegravir-treated subjects achieved an HIV-1 level <400 copies/mL, compared to 41% and 43% in the placebo arms of BENCHMRK-1 and BENCHMRK-2, respectively. Patients receiving raltegravir demonstrated higher rates of suppression below 50 copies/mL (61% in BENCHMRK-1 and 62% in BENCHMRK-2, compared to 33% and 36% in the respective placebo arms. CD4 count rise averaged 83 cells/mm^3 in the raltegravir arm of BENCHMRK-1 and 86 cells/mm^3 in BENCHMRK-2, compared to rises of 31 and 40 cells/mm^3 in the respective placebo arms. Not surprisingly, the efficacy of raltegravir was enhanced when the OBT contained one or more additional drug with anti-HIV activity. Although subjects receiving raltegravir achieved higher rates of virologic control than those receiving placebo, the effect was magnified in those with low GSS scores or in those who were naive to either enfuvirtide or darunavir. For example, 90% of subjects receiving raltegravir who were naive to darunavir but enfuvirtide-experienced achieved an HIV-1 RNA level of <400 copies/mL compared to 55% in those with identical darunavir and enfuvirtide experience who received placebo. Like most salvage trials, adverse events (AEs) were common in all arms of the trial (81% in the BENCHMRK-1/2 arms versus 83–86% in the placebo arms). Drug-related AEs (defined as possibly, probably or definitely-related to raltegravir, placebo or OBT drug) were also common (44% in BENCHMRK-1 and 53% in BENCHMRK-2 compared to 51% and 52% in the placebo arms, respectively). Serious drug-related AEs were rare (<2.5% in all arms) as were AEs leading to discontinuation of study drugs (<3.4%). Adverse clinical experiences included gastrointestinal upset, injection site reaction, headache and fatigue, and were less frequent in the raltegravir arms of the study. Although not seen in the BENCHMRK-1 study, the raltegravir arms in BENCHMRK-2 appeared to have slightly higher rates of specific gastrointestinal disturbances such as diarrhea, abdominal distension/pain and flatulence, compared to those in the placebo arm. Grade 3–4 laboratory abnormalities were uncommon and were not more common than placebo in either trial.

The success of raltegravir in treatment-experienced patients has led the drug's developers to initiate a phase III trial comparing raltegravir to efavirenz in treatment-naive patients.[32] 24-week results from this trial have been reported.[32] The study enrolled subjects from the previous 10-day monotherapy study by adding fixed-dosed tenofovir/lamivudine to the existing bid

600, 400, 200, and 100 mg arms of raltegravir, while replacing the placebo arm with efavirenz 600 mg once daily with tenofovir and emtricitabine. Approximately 40 patients were randomized to each of the five arms in this study. Subjects were enrolled in this trial if they had no prior ART and had a CD4 count of >100 cells/mm^3 and an HIV-1 load >5000 copies/mL, with documented susceptibility to efavirenz, lamivudine and tenofovir on genotypic analysis. The study was designed to rule out non-equivalence of raltegravir-based ART compared to an efavirenz-based regimen, and assessed HIV-1 load responses, changes in CD4 cell count and safety/tolerability. Participants were primarily male (73-90%) and nonwhite (65–82%) and had comparable HIV-1 RNA levels and CD4 cell counts at entry. Rates of AIDS diagnosis varied slightly from 29% in the 400 mg arm to 43% in the 600 mg raltegravir arm. Thirty-seven percent of subjects in the efavirenz arm had AIDS at enrollment. At planned 24-week interim analysis, all four raltegravir arms demonstrated excellent virologic responses with the three highest dose arms all having plasma HIV-1 RNA levels <50 copies/mL in over 90% of subjects. The 100 mg-arm produced HIV-1 RNA levels <50 copies/mL in 87% of subjects. All arms were comparable to the 90% rates of HIV-RNA <50 copies/mL seen in the efavirenz arm. Although the clinical significance is uncertain, all four raltegravir arms had more rapid reductions of HIV-1 RNA levels compared to efavirenz, although by 24 weeks both raltegravir and efavirenz produced similar rates of virologic control. CD4 increases were comparable across arms and ranged from ~100 cells/mm^3 in the efavirenz arm to ~175 cells/mm^3 in the 100 mg raltegravir arm. Discontinuation rates were low in all arms. Side-effects were generally mild and comparable across all arms with the exceptions of headache, dizziness, and abnormal dreams, which were all more common in the efavirenz-treated subjects. SAEs were infrequent (4% in combined raltegravir group vs 3% in efavirenz arm) and none was felt to be drug related. Grade 3 or 4 laboratory abnormalities were uncommon. An analysis of the impact of raltegravir on total cholesterol and triglyceride levels in this population has been reported.[33] No change was observed in either total cholesterol or triglyceride levels in any of the raltegravir arms compared to 19 mg/dL and 47 mg/dL rises, respectively, in the efavirenz arm. This trial continues to accrue patients and additional data on efficacy, safety, toxicity and pharmacology will be forthcoming.

Next-Generation DKAs

Utilizing detailed information on structure–activity relationships in a series of viral isolates with *in vitro* resistance to various strand-transfer integrase inhibitors (including raltegravir), a series of next-generation integrase inhibitors have been identified. These compounds were derived by rational modification of a diketo acid pharmacophore to create compounds that bind tightly to the catalytic core of HIV-1 integrase, despite the fact that it contains these integrase mutations. The most promising candidate next-generation integrase inhibitor, MK-2048, retained activity against three of the four types of drug-resistant integrase mutants. The remaining viral mutant, containing integrase mutations at E138, G140, and Q148, was somewhat resistant to MK-2048, but much more resistant to current lead compounds such as raltegravir or elvitegravir. MK-2048 has demonstrated excellent *in vitro* antiviral activity with an IC_{95} of 41 nM and has demonstrated favorable pharmacokinetics in dogs and rats. Further studies of MK-2048 are planned.[34]

Quinoline Derivatives

The recognition that divalent cations were essential to the catalytic activity of HIV-1 integrase led to the identification of quinoline-derived compounds as a potential class of integrase inhibitors.[35,36] The exact mechanism by which quinoline derivatives inhibit HIV-1 integrase activity is uncertain. Studies of styrylquinoline derivatives (SQLs) suggest that they interfere with both the cytoplasmic binding of integrase to viral cDNA and the intranuclear binding to target DNA prior to strand transfer.[37] SQLs may also inhibit nuclear import of PICs.[38] SQLs inhibit replication of HIV-1 at micromolar concentrations *in vitro*.[35]

Elvitegravir (GS 9137, JTK-303)

Elvitegravir is a dihydroquinoline carboxylic acid that was derived from a quinolone antibiotic.[39] Although quinolones have no activity against HIV-1, they do share common structural motifs with DKAs, a fact that led developers to study the activity of these compounds against HIV-1 integrase. Elvitegravir inhibits the strand transfer activity of HIV-1 integrase with an IC_{50} of 8.8 nM.[40] Elvitegravir demonstrated *in vitro* activity against a variety of HIV-1 subtypes, as well as against a panel of drug-resistant clinical isolates (EC_{50} from 0.02 to 1.26 nM); elvitegravir is also active against HIV-2.[41] *In vitro* combination studies suggest that elvitegravir is synergistic or additive with available ARVs.[40] Serial passage studies of HIV-1 in the presence of elvitegravir have revealed two common pathways for the emergence of resistance *in vitro*, T66I and E92Q.[42] Important differences exist between these two pathways in that the E92Q polymorphism confers cross-resistance *in vitro* to raltegravir while the T66I results in reduced susceptibility to elvitegravir alone. A variety of secondary mutations in integrase emerge with serial passages that further reduce sensitivity to elvitegravir, including H51Y, F121Y, S147G, S153Y, E157Q, and R263K. Isolates with multiple integrase-associated mutations created through site-directed mutagenesis retained *in vitro* susceptibility to tenofovir, lopinavir/ritonavir and efavirenz.

The safety and pharmacokinetics of elvitegravir have been studied in uninfected male volunteers.[43] Thirty two subjects were randomized 3:1 to receive a single 100, 200, 400, or 800 mg dose of elvitegravir or placebo. The 400 mg group received a second dose with breakfast after an appropriate wash-out period to assess the effect of food on bioavailabilty. Maximum concentrations (C_{max}) and area under the concentration curve (AUC) increased as dose increased and plasma concentrations exceeded the EC_{90} at 12–24 h. Elvitegravir's half-life ($T_{1/2}$) was 3h. Administration of elvitegravir with food increased absorption threefold. Elvitegravir is metabolized via the cytochrome P450 system; administration of elvitegravir with 100mg of ritonavir increases AUC ~30-fold and to increase $T_{1/2}$ to ~9h.[44] No SAEs or grade 3 or 4 laboratory abnormalities were seen in this trial.

A phase 2 study of the antiviral activity, safety and tolerability of elvitegravir in HIV-1-infected persons has been reported.[44] This prospective, randomized, double-blind, placebo-controlled, monotherapy trial enrolled 40 HIV-1-infected individuals and randomized them to receive either 200, 400, or 800mg of elvitegravir twice daily, 800mg of elvitegravir once daily, or 50mg of elvitegravir once daily with 100mg of ritonavir, versus placebo for 10 days. Subjects were required to be off all ART and to have a CD4 count of ≥200 cells/mm^3 and an HIV-1 load between 10000 and 300000 copies/mL. Declines in HIV-1 load ranged from 0.89 $\log_{10}$ copies/mL for the 800mg daily group to 2.03 $\log_{10}$ copies/mL for the ritonavir-boosted 50mg group, compared to a decline of 0.13 $\log_{10}$ copies/mL seen in the placebo arm of the study. Adverse events were comparable between elvitegravir and placebo recipients, and were generally mild. The only adverse event that occurred with greater frequency in the elvitegravir groups was fatigue. Only two grade 3 laboratory abnormalities were reported in subjects receiving elvitegravir (hypertriglyceridemia and hyperamylasemia).

Preliminary data from a phase II, partially blinded (to the dose of the active agent), noninferiority trial of elvitegravir versus a comparator PI (CPI) have been presented.[45] This dose-finding study randomized 278 treatment-experienced patients to receive 20, 50, or 125mg of elvitegravir with 100mg of ritonavir versus a comparator-boosted PI with OBT. Subjects were stratified by enfuvirtide use as well and were required to have a viral load of ≥1000 copies/mL and ≥1 protease resistance mutations on resistance testing. There were no CD4 cell count exclusions. The OBT was not allowed to contain NNRTIs in any of the trial's arms and new PIs such as darunavir and tipranavir were initially not allowed to be included in the OBT of those receiving elvitegravir due to concerns about drug–drug interactions. An independent Data Safety Monitoring Board (DSMB), however, liberalized the original protocol after week 8 of the study to allow addition of darunavir or tipranavir to the OBT in the elvitegravir arms when data on potential drug–drug interactions suggested this was safe. Subjects enrolled were mostly male (86–99%) and Caucasian (66–86%) and had fairly advanced disease (mean CD4 count from 157 to 243 cells/mm^3; mean HIV-1 RNA levels were 4.47-4.71 $\log_{10}$ copies/mL. Subjects were highly treatment-experienced with about half having GSS of zero for all NRTIs in the OBT. The median number of PI mutations in the group was ~10 and most subjects were enfuvirtide-experienced (76–83%). Median numbers of ARVs in the OBT were three (including enfuvirtide). The OBT of subjects in the CPI commonly included new PIs (49% darunavir and 27% tipranavir). At week 16, only four patients had added a PI to their OBT but at week 24, this had risen substantially to 15% of those receiving elvitegravir. Analysis of preliminary data at week 8 demonstrated high rates of virologic failure in the elvitegravir 20mg-arm and the DSMB advised investigators to stop enrollment into this arm of the trial. Subjects originally randomized to receive 20mg of elvitegravir were offered open-label elvitegravir 125mg with ritonavir 100mg daily. Because the study had enrolled patients rapidly, only four subjects in the elvitegravir arms added darunavir or tipranavir before week 16. By week 24, 15% of subjects in the elvitegravir arms had added a PI to their OBT. The analysis of noninferiority was, therefore, conducted on the week-16 data (with the four patients receiving a PI prior to this point excluded from data analysis). The study's primary endpoint was the time-weighted average change in plasma HIV-1 RNA from baseline at week 24 ($DAVG_{24}$). Although subjects in the 50mg elvitegravir arm of the trial did not achieve statistically significant difference in $DAVG_{24}$, those in the 125mg group demonstrated a significant difference in virologic response compared to those in the CPI arm (−1.7 $\log_{10}$ copies/mL for elvitegravir 125mg with ritonavir 100mg versus 1.2 $\log_{10}$ copies/mL in the CPI group). There was a trend toward superior virologic outcomes with elvitegravir, with 76% of subjects in the elvitegravir 125mg-arm achieving 2 $\log_{10}$ copies/mL, compared to 51% in the CPI arm. Virologic response was maximal at 2 weeks and tended to level off by week 16 (viral load decline of 2 $\log_{10}$ copies/mL in the 125mg-arm at week 2, compared to 1.7 $\log_{10}$ copies/mL at week 16). Addition of elvitegravir to OBT with one active agent resulted in a more sustained virologic response at week 24 (−0.7 $\log_{10}$ copies/mL when 125mg elvitegravir added to OBT with no active drugs compared to −2.1 $\log_{10}$ copies/mL arm in subjects with active NRTI or first use of enfuvirtide). Although not statistically significant, mean CD4 count increase was higher in the 125mg elvitegravir arm than the CPI arm (61 cells/mm^3 versus 28 cells/mm^3). Adverse events were common in all arms of the study, as were grade 3 and 4 laboratory abnormalities (14–18% and 21–32% respectively), but there were no differences between any of the arms and rates of treatment discontinuation were rare (1–3%).

Elvitegravir is known to be metabolized both through CYP3A oxidative and glucuronidation pathways and to be a moderate inducer of CYP3A,[44] so the potential for drug–drug interactions is a concern. Pharmacokinetic studies in small groups of healthy adults did not demonstrate clinically relevant interactions between elvitegravir and either emtricitabine/tenofovir (Truvada),[46] zidovidine,[47] abacavir, didanosine, darunavir or tipranavir.[48]

Nucleoside Reverse Transcriptase Inhibitors

Although still important in the management of HIV-infected persons, current NRTIs (and the related nucleotide reverse transcriptase inhibitor, tenofovir), have toxicities that often limit their effectiveness and have also proven vulnerable to the development of resistance, fueling demand for new agents in this class. NRTI development has focused on elucidating the mechanisms of drug toxicity and identifying agents that are less toxic and retain activity in the presence of known resistance mutations.

D-d4FC (Reverset, DPC 817, Dexelvucitabine)

D-d4FC is the D-enantiomer of the cytodine analog, dideoxyfluorocytidine. Although D-d4FC was withdrawn from development, experience with the drug is instructive for development of similar compounds. Animal studies of D-d4FC suggested that it possessed good bioavailability and favorable pharmacokinetics.[49] Similarly, early human studies indicated that the agent had oral bioavailability, reasonable pharmacokinetics and antiviral activity against many viruses resistant to other nucleosides.[51–52] Clinical trials subsequently demonstrated substantial antiviral activity of D-d4FC in treatment-experienced subjects.[53–55] However, in one of these trials, interesting interactions were observed between D-d4FC and other NRTIs.[55] Viral load declines were much greater for subjects who were not receiving lamivudine or emtricitabine, suggesting a potential negative interaction between D-d4FC and other cytidine analogs. *In vitro* synergy studies had suggested that D-d4FC has additive or synergistic activity with NRTIs (zidovudine and stavudine), NNRTIs (nevirapine and efavirenz) and PIs (nelfinavir, lopinavir, and saquinavir).[56] In addition to demonstrating reduced virologic efficacy, administration of D-d4FC with didanosine was associated with a dose-dependant increased risk of pancreatitis. Among subjects in the 200 mg D-d4FC daily group who were also receiving didanosine, seven of 14 developed grade IV hyperamylasemia and several were symptomatic. Pancreatitis tended to emerge several weeks into the study and all subjects recovered completely once the D-d4FC was stopped. Although the risk was amplified when it was co-administered with didanosine, the rates of Grade IV hyperamylasemia in subjects receiving D-d4FC were judged to be unacceptably high, and, thus, further development of this compound was discontinued.

Elvucitabine (ACH-126,433, β-L-d4FC)

Elvucitabine is another cytidine analog with activity against both HIV-1 and hepatitis B virus (HBV). Elvucitabine is the L-enantiomer of D-d4FC and has demonstrated similar anti-HIV-1 activity.[57] *In vitro* studies suggest that elvucitabine is at least 10-fold more active than lamivudine and fivefold more active than emtricitabine.[58] Initial reports also suggested a low risk for mitochondrial toxicity with elvucitabine monotherapy[59] and in combination with other NRTIs.[60] Studies of elvucitabine against both wild-type HIV-1 and clinical isolates with NRTI and NNRTI resistance demonstrated IC_{50} between 0.1 and 0.3 μM; these studies included viruses with M41L, T215Y, Q151M and the NNRTI resistance mutations K103N, Y181C, and G190A.[61] Although isolates with the M184V mutation demonstrated reduced susceptibility to elvucitabine, IC_{50} only rose to 1–4 μM, an IC_{50} comparable to that of lamivudine against wild-type virus. Serial passage studies suggest that elvucitabine selects for mutations at position 184, though in an unusual way.[62] Although the development of an M184V mutation was seen, investigators more typically observed the simultaneous emergence of M184I and D237E substitutions. An *in vitro* combination study suggested synergy between elvucitabine and either zidovudine or stavudine and an additive activity when combined with didanosine.[63]

A proof of concept, open-label study of the safety and efficacy of elvucitabine has been performed.[64] Investigators recruited subjects on a failing ARV regimen with documented M184V mutations to assess the impact of substituting elvucitabine for lamivudine in their current three-drug regimen. Study subjects were randomized 25:25:10 to substitute 50 or 100 mg daily of elvucitabine for lamivudine for 28 days or to continue their baseline regimen (the control group). Investigators treated 56 subjects whose mean CD4 count was 471 cells/mm^3 and whose mean plasma HIV-1 RNA level was 10 300 copies/mL. Elvucitabine-treated subjects showed a mean decline in HIV-1 load of 0.67 and 0.78 $\log_{10}$ copies/mL for the 50 and 100 mg groups, respectively, compared to a rise of 0.01 $\log_{10}$ copies/mL for the control group. No change was seen in CD4 cell count during the study period. Unfortunately, the study was discontinued prematurely when four individuals showed signs of bone marrow suppression (as evidenced by a decline in both total white blood cell count and absolute neutrophil count). Bone marrow toxicity emerged during weeks 3 or 4 of the study and was more common in subjects receiving 100 mg/day of elvucitabine. Extrapolating from data from HBV treatment trials that used lower doses of elvucitabine, pharmacokinetic and pharmacodynamic modeling suggested that reducing both dose and frequency of administration could reduce the risk of bone marrow toxicity while maintaining antiviral activity.[65] This hypothesis has been tested in HIV-infected subjects.[66] Investigators treated 24 HIV-infected individuals with either 5 or 10 mg daily or 20 mg every other day for 21 days with lopinavir/ritonavir 400/100 mg twice daily. Plasma HIV RNA declined by 1.8 $\log_{10}$ copies/mL, 1.9 $\log_{10}$ copies/mL, and 2.0 $\log_{10}$ copies/mL at day 21 in the 5 mg daily, 10 mg daily and 20 mg every other day groups, respectively. Concentrations of elvucitabine were still three times the IC_{50} for wild-type virus at day 28. No resistance to elvucitabine was demonstrated in this study, and no hematologic or other toxicity was reported. A follow-up 7-day monotherapy study randomized 24 subjects 1:1 to receive 10 mg of elvucitabine daily or placebo.[67] Recognizing the long $T_{1/2}$ of elvucitabine, this trial called for administration of lopinavir/ritonavir twice daily for 21 days after discontinuation of the study drug to avoid development of resistance. At day 7, mean HIV-1 RNA decline was 0.85 $\log_{10}$ copies/mL and this decline continued in a concentration-dependant manner after the study drug was stopped. Elvucitabine levels remained above the IC_{50} until day 21. Mean CD4 counts rose 62 cell/mm^3 at day 7 in those receiving elvucitabine. There were no adverse events or significant laboratory abnormalities reported in this short trial and emergence of resistance was not observed. Phase II studies of elvucitabine versus lamivudine in combination with tenofovir and efavirenz are currently underway to assess the virologic and immunologic activity and safety of this compound in larger numbers of subjects.

Apricitabine (AVX-754, SPD-754, BCH-10618, (−)dOTC)

Apricitabine is the negative enantiomer of the cytidine analog racemate, dOTC and is structurally similar to lamivudine. *In vitro* studies of apricitabine against wild-type viruses demonstrated an IC_{50} between 0.02 and 4.2 μM.[68] Apricitabine retained activity against a panel of HIV-1 isolates with up to 5 thymidine-associated mutations (TAMs).[69] When tested against recombinant viruses with the M184V mutation, apricitabine's activity declined by a median of 1.8-fold and was further reduced (approximately threefold) when viruses were engineered with both the M184V mutation and 3 TAMs. Serial passage studies demonstrated the emergence of K65R, V75I, and M184V mutations.[68] K65R and V75I resulted in a 1.6- to 4.3-fold reduction in apricitabine activity. Although initial *in vitro* synergy studies of apricitabine suggested favorable interactions with lamivudine (as well as with stavudine, didanosine, zidovudine, and abacavir), subsequent studies of intracellular metabolism demonstrated a sixfold reduction in intracellular apricitabine triphosphate when administered with lamivudine.[70] This finding was particularly surprising because co-administration of apricitabine with lamivudine resulted in nearly identical plasma pharmacokinetics. Studies of co-administration with emtricitabine demonstrated similar isolated declines in intracellular apricitabine triphosphate levels,[71] and ruled out the possibility that this effect was produced by inhibition of apricitabine entry into cells.[72]

Safety and pharmacokinetics of a single dose of apricitabine were evaluated in a phase I trial in HIV-uninfected volunteers.[73] Twenty-six subjects were divided into three cohorts and received 400, 800, or 1600 mg of apricitabine. Absorption was rapid with T_{max} ranging from 1.5 to 1.7 h. Bioavailability was good and drug exposure increased with dose. Over 80% of apricitabine was eliminated unchanged in the urine, reducing concerns about interactions with ARV agents that are hepatically metabolized. Studies of intracellular pharmacokinetics of apricitabine triphosphate showed a $T_{1/2}$ of 6–7 h in target cells, supporting twice-daily dosing.[74] Absorption of apricitabine is not significantly affected by administration with food.[75]

A placebo controlled trial in treatment-naive; HIV-1 infected volunteers evaluated the pharmacokinetics, efficacy and safety of 10 days of apricitabine monotherapy.[76] Investigators treated 63 subjects, all of whom had a CD4 count >250 cells/mm^3 and plasma HIV-1 RNA level between 5000 and 100 000 copies/mL, and assigned them to receive daily doses of apricitabine ranging from 400 to 1200 mg. The groups receiving apricitabine experienced declines in HIV-1 RNA levels which ranged from 1.18 to1.65 $\log_{10}$ copies/mL, compared to ~0.18 $\log_{10}$ copies/mL for those receiving placebo. All subjects were screened for NRTI mutations at study entry and again at the completion of the trial. Four subjects demonstrated NRTI resistance at baseline (though none had an M184V mutation). When compared to subjects with wild-type virus, subjects with NRTI resistance at baseline experienced similar declines in HIV-1 RNA.[77] None of the treated subjects developed new NRTI mutations during the study. The pharmacokinetics of apricitabine were similar to those seen in uninfected volunteers.[78] Using both plasma and intracellular pharmacokinetic data from the 10-day monotherapy trial, investigators developed a mathematical model to characterize the viral dynamics of apricitabine therapy.[79] This model has been used to help investigators select 800 mg twice daily as the appropriate dose for phase II studies.

Despite encouraging data on its activity, enthusiasm for apricitabine has been tempered by the fact that development of its parent compound, dOTC, was halted because long-term administration produced a degenerative dermopathy in animals. A 52-week study of apricitabine in cynomolgus monkeys suggested that these changes were due to the (+)dOTC enantiomer.[80] The exact mechanism of this toxicity is uncertain but is probably not related to mitochondrial toxicity, as dOTC has not been shown to interfere with mitochondrial DNA expression.[81]

Racivir (RCV; (±)-FTC; ((±)-β-2′,3′-dideoxy-5fluoro-3′-thiacytidine))

Racivir is a 50:50 racemic mixture of two β-nucleoside enantiomers.[82] Both enantiomers of racivir are potent inhibitors of HIV reverse transcriptase with *in vitro* studies demonstrating EC_{90} of 0.04 μM and 0.6 μM for (−)-FTC and (+)-FTC respectively.[83] Mechanistic studies have shown that the negative enantiomer of FTC is taken up more efficiently into target cells, triphosphorylated more rapidly and degraded less readily than the positive enantiomer,[84] perhaps explaining the former's greater potency. Despite the successful licensing of (−)-FTC (emtricitabine), several distinct properties have led its developers to believe racivir will have an important role in the management of HIV infection. *In vitro* selection studies have shown that the two enantiomers of racivir select for different RT mutations. (M184V for the negative enantiomer and Y215Y for the positive). Its developers suggest that these dual pathways of resistance will reduce the likelihood of the emergence of resistance and point to the fact that racivir has a higher *in vitro* barrier to resistance with racivir compared to either lamivudine or emtricitabine[85] as grounds for moving forward with development of this compound.

Single- and multiple-dose studies of the pharmacokinetics and safety of racivir in healthy volunteers have been performed.[86] In this study, 32 subjects were randomized 4:1 to receive single 50, 100, 200, or 400 mg doses of racivir or placebo. C_{max} and AUC were dose proportional for all doses and exceeded EC_{90} for wild-type HIV. The median $T_{1/2}$ for racivir ranged from 1.8 h at 50 mg to 3.4 h at 400 mg. No SAEs were observed and side effects were generally mild (headache most commonly). At 400 mg, the C_{max} for racivir was greater than the EC_{50} for lamivudine-resistant HIV.

No studies of racivir monotherapy have been reported though the results of a 14-day, dose-escalation study of combination ART with racivir has been published.[87] In this randomized, placebo-controlled study, 25 HIV-1-infected, ART-naive subjects were randomized to receive 200, 400, or 600 mg of racivir along with standard doses of efavirenz and stavudine. The placebo group received lamvudine 300 mg daily. Racivir was administered once daily at doses of 200, 400, or 600 mg. At the end of the study, mean decreases in plasma RNA were 1.92 $\log_{10}$ copies/mL, 2.03 $\log_{10}$ copies/mL, and 2.17 $\log_{10}$ copies/mL for the 200, 400, and 600 mg racivir groups compared to 2.25 $\log_{10}$ copies/mL for the lamivudine group. All four groups displayed persistent suppression of peripheral HIV-1 RNA until day 28 (mean viral load 2.02–2.43 $\log_{10}$ copies/mL below baseline) at which time they began to return toward baseline. The most common adverse event was dizziness, which was probably attributable to efavirenz.[82]

The virologic efficacy of racivir in treating persons with documented M184V mutation has been studied.[83] Investigators randomized subjects receiving lamivudine-containing ART to substitute racivir or to continue with lamivudine for 28 days. Subjects were required to be on a stable ARV regimen for at least 60 days and to have a CD4 count of 50 cells/mm^3 with an HIV-1 RNA level of 2000 copies $\log_{10}$ copies/mL and a documented M184V mutation. Subjects were enrolled 2:1 to receive an unspecified dose of racivir versus placebo. Mean plasma HIV-1 RNA level was 4.1 $\log_{10}$ copies/mL. Viral load measurements at 28 days demonstrated a decline of 0.4 $\log_{10}$ copies/mL in those receiving racivir versus a rise of 0.14 $\log_{10}$ copies/mL in those who stayed on lamivudine. Subset analysis showed that most of the beneficial effect of racivir was observed in subjects with an M184V mutation and <3 TAMs. Mean viral load decline in these subjects was 0.7 $\log_{10}$ copies/mL, and 28% achieved a viral load of <400 copies/mL at the end of the study. Further studies of racivir as second-line therapy for patients with the M184V mutation are planned.

Non-Nucleoside Reverse Transcriptase Inhibitors

Soon after their introduction in the mid-1990s, NNRTIs assumed an important role in ART and several landmark studies established efavirenz as a preferred agent for the initial treatment of HIV-1 infection. Unfortunately, NNRTIs have demonstrated a low genetic barrier to resistance, with the most common point mutations (K103N and Y181C) rendering all three currently approved agents inactive.[88] As rates of resistance to NNRTIs in both chronically and recently infected persons increase,[85] there is a need for compounds that retain activity against viruses resistant to current NNRTIs. Development of second generation NNRTIs has been slowed by difficulties finding agents that are potent, nontoxic and maintain activity in the presence of NNRTI mutations.

TMC 125 (Etravirine, R165335)

TMC 125 was derived from the tetrahydro-imidazo[4,5, 1-jk][1,4]-benzodiazepin-2 (1H)-one and -thione (TIBO) group of compounds.[9,89] TIBO derivatives were among the first NNRTIs identified. Crystalographic analyses led to the recognition that TIBO derivatives were a new class of ARV compounds, and have allowed investigators to rationally design a series of compounds that maintain antiviral potency while expanding the spectrum of activity against viruses with resistance to first-line agents.[90] Etravirine, a derivative of diarylpyrimidine (DAPY), inhibits wild-type HIV-1 *in vitro* with an EC_{50} of 1.4 nM.[91] In contrast to other NNRTIs, etravirine has shown *in vitro* activity against HIV-2 as well, although at micromolar, rather than nanomolar, concentrations. Etravirine is equipotent against both wild-type and many NNRTI-resistant variants and retained activity against 97% of 1081 clinical isolates with NNRTI-associated mutations. It is active against a variety of HIV-1 subtypes (group M subtypes A, B, C, D, F, and H) and retains partial activity against HIV-1 group O isolates with the NNRTI mutations A98G, V179D, and Y181C. The enhanced spectrum of activity of etravirine results from multifaceted binding that produces conformational and positional stability despite changes in HIV-1 RT.[92]

Etravirine has a higher genetic barrier to resistance *in vitro* than currently available NNRTIs and requires the accumulation of multiple mutations before its activity is substantially impaired.[93] Selection experiments using increasing concentrations of etravirine resulted in the accumulation of known NNRTI-associated mutations such as L100I, Y181C, G190E M230L, and Y318F, as well as the novel mutations V179I and V179F. Etravirine is lipophilic and has limited oral absorption, but has been reformulated to improve oral bioavailability and reduce pill burden.[94] As a result, future phase III studies of etravirine are being performed with 200 mg of the tablet form of etravirine, which is bioequivalent to the previous 800 mg formulation. The absorption of etravirine is enhanced threefold when taken with food.[95] Pharmacokinetic studies of etravirine in ARV-naive, HIV-1-infected subjects demonstrated a T_{max} of 3 h and C_{max} of 93 ng/mL when dosed at 900 mg twice daily.[96] Steady-state concentrations were achieved within 5 days, at which time C_{max} averaged 418 ng/mL and C_{min} 245 ng/mL.

In a randomized, double-blind, placebo-controlled, phase II trial, seventeen treatment-naive subjects were randomized 2:1 to 900 mg of etravirine twice daily or placebo for 7 days.[96] At the end of the study, etravirine-treated subjects experienced a decrease of 1.99 $\log_{10}$ copies/mL in plasma viral load versus 0.06 $\log_{10}$ copies/mL in the placebo arm. A retrospective analysis demonstrated rates of decline in HIV-1 RNA with etravirine monotherapy that were similar to those seen with a five-drug, triple-class regimen.[97] An open-label, proof-of-concept study of subjects with documented NNRTI resistance demonstrated antiviral activity of etravirine in treatment-experienced subjects.[98] Investigators studied sixteen subjects who had a plasma HIV-1 RNA level of >2000 copies/mL while on an NNRTI-containing ARV regimen, and substituted 900 mg of etravirine twice daily for their current NNRTI (efavirenz or nevirapine). At the end of the 7 day study period, the mean decline in HIV-1 RNA was 0.89

log_{10} copies/mL. Pretreatment genotypic analysis showed an average of two different NNRTI mutations in study subjects (range 1-4). Phenotypic studies demonstrated high-level resistance to all approved NNRTIs, but preserved susceptibility to etravirine.

Recently the 24-week results of two identically designed ongoing Phase III trials of etravirine (DUET-1 and DUET-2) were reported.[99,100] Both trials enrolled adults with virologic failure on stable antiretroviral therapy, NNRTI resistance, VL > 5000 copies/ml and 3 or more PI-associated mutations. Subjects were randomly assigned to receive 200 mg of etravirine or placebo twice daily; all subjects also received darunavir/ritonavir together with investigator-selected NRTI. Enfuvirtide use was optional. Plasma viral load < 50 copies/ml was the primary endpoint.

In DUET-1, 304 subjects were randomized to etravirine and 308 to placebo.[99] At week 24, 170 (56%) in the etravirine group and 119 (39%) in the placebo group had reached the study endpoint ($p = 0.005$). Adverse events were similar in both groups, except that there were more rashes on etravirine (20% vs 10%) and more diarrhea on placebo (20% vs 12%). In DUET-2, 295 subjects were randomized to etravirine and 296 to placebo.[100] At week 24, 183 (62%) in the etravirine group and 129 (44%) in the placebo had reached the study endpoint ($p = 0.0003$). Adverse events were comparable in the two groups. In an accompanying editorial, it was suggested that by a pooled analysis of both studies, it appeared that etravirine also reduced clinical progression,[101] though this was an unplanned post-hoc analysis, utilizing data from both studies. Preliminary analyses of resistance data from DUET-1 and DUET-2 have identified 13 mutations associated with decreased virologic responses to etravirine; the concurrent presence of 3 or more mutations were necessary to substantially reduce drug efficacy.

The successes of these initial studies led the drug's developers to design a series of larger phase II/III trials of etravirine. Interim safety and tolerability data have been reported on one such study.[102] Investigators from the Etravirine-C203 trial studied individuals with a plasma HIV-1 RNA level of 1000 copies/mL, three-class experience and resistance testing that documented susceptibility to two approved ARV agents. At enrollment, subjects were randomized to receive 400, 800, or 1200 mg of etravirine twice daily versus placebo and OBT. The OBT averaged 3-4 additional drugs and was required to include compounds with anti-HIV activity identified on resistance testing. Use of enfuvirtide was allowed in the OBT. Adverse events were common in both groups (92% in pooled treatment groups versus 91% in the placebo arm). Diarrhea, headache and rash were seen most commonly, though the differences between the etravirine and placebo groups were not significant. The only SAEs reported in the treatment arms were three cases of pancreatitis (versus one in the control group), and one case of pancytopenia. Grade 3/4 laboratory abnormalities were common, but the rates were similar in subjects receiving etravirine versus placebo (35% vs 32%).

Data from a 48 week phase II placebo-controlled dose-finding trial on the efficacy and tolerability of etravirine in subjects with multidrug resistant HIV-1 infection have been reported.[103,104] At enrollment, subjects were required to have a plasma HIV RNA level of ⩾1000 copies/mL with documented NNRTI resistance and three primary PI mutations. Median baseline HIV-1 RNA was 4.7 log_{10} copies/mL and CD4 count was 100 cells/mm^3.[105] Baseline phenotypic testing showed a median fold change of 41.4 for efavirenz compared to 1.7 for etravirine. One hundred and ninety nine subjects were randomized 2:2:1 to receive either 400 or 800 mg of etravirine twice daily versus placebo, along with an optimized background regimen that could include enfuvirtide. Intention to treat analysis demonstrated HIV-1 RNA declines of 0.88 log_{10} copies/mL, 1.01 log_{10} copies/mL, and 0.14 log_{10} copies/mL in the 400 mg, 800 mg and placebo groups, respectively. Not surprisingly, response rates were better when etravirine was added to a regimen containing one or more additional agents to which the virus was sensitive. Viral load declines averaged 1.67 log_{10} copies/mL for subjects with no NNRTI mutations in the 800 mg etravirine arm compared to 0.54 log_{10} copies/mL for those with three NNRTI mutations.[104,105] Subjects receiving 400 mg and 800 mg etravirine achieved an HIV-1 RNA level of <50 copies/mL in 23% and 22% of cases, respectively, compared to 0% in the placebo arm. Virologic failure was observed in 9% of subjects in the combined etravirine arms, compared to 78% of those in placebo arm. At week 48, mean CD4 count rose by 58 and 61 cells/mm^3 respectively, in the 400 and 800 mg etravirine arms, compared to a rise of 13 cells/mm^3 in the placebo arm. Analyses of safety and tolerability of etravirine are complicated by the high rates of treatment discontinuations in the placebo arm which resulted in much shorter duration of exposure to OBT in the placebo arm (48 weeks in the etravirine arms compared to 18 weeks in those receiving placebo). Adverse events were nearly universal, with 99% of subjects in the combined etravirine groups reporting some AE. Grade 3 AEs were seen in 39% of subjects receiving etravirine versus 23% in the control arm, but Grade 4 AEs were equally common between the groups. Grade 3 or 4 AEs observed in more than three subjects receiving etravirine included four cases of pneumonia, and three cases each of abdominal pain, rash, hypertriglyceridemia, and pancreatitis. Four subjects died during the study, three in the 400 mg etravirine arm and one in the placebo arm. Only one of these (cardiopulmonary failure and myocardial infarction) was felt to be potentially attributable to etravirine. Grade 3 or 4 laboratory abnormalities were seen in 39% of the combined etravirine subjects compared to 35% in the placebo arm. Models derived from 24-week data predicted reductions in rates of progression to AIDS/death of between 31% and 39% over 1 year in persons receiving 800 mg of etravirine twice daily.[106]

Not all studies of etravirine have produced overwhelmingly positive results, however. The drug developers sought to assess the efficacy of etravirine versus investigator-selected PIs in subjects with at least one NNRTI-associated mutation but no prior PI exposure.[107] Fifty nine subjects were randomized to receive 800 mg of etravirine twice daily versus 57 who received a PI-based regimen (62% lopinavir/

ritonavir and 32% atazanavir/ritonavir). NRTI backbone was selected based on the results of resistance testing. Both NRTI and NNRTI resistance was common in both arms (~80% of participants with at least one NRTI mutation and ~70% with two or more NNRTI mutations). Despite the high number of NNRTI mutations, however, median fold change in susceptibility to etravirine at entry was only 2.0 compared to 129.8 for efavirenz. Although viral load decline in both arms of the study were comparable at 4 weeks (1.3 $\log_{10}$ copies/mL for etravirine and 1.5 $\log_{10}$ copies/mL for those receiving a PI), those receiving etravirine experienced an early virologic rebound, and the study was shut down by the study's independent DSMB. Analysis of 12 week data from the etravirine arm showed a sharp decline in efficacy of etravirine in subjects with >2 baseline TAMs and/or the M184V mutation. Viral load responses to etravirine ranged from a decline of 2 $\log_{10}$ copies/mL in those with no NRTI mutations to <0.5 $\log_{10}$ copies/mL in those with three or more. Grade 3 and 4 AEs were uncommon in this study and were comparable across both arms. Central nervous system effects were comparable, and gastrointestinal and lipid abnormalities were more common in those receiving a PI. Although the presence of multiple NNRTI mutations reduced the antiviral activity of etravirine, multivariate analysis did not suggest that presence of K103N or Y181C mutations predicted response.

Etravirine is an inducer of CYP3A4 and its AUC and C_{max} decline significantly when administered with efavirenz, nevirapine, and full-dose ritonavir.[108] Etravirine is metabolized *in vitro* by UDPGT and CYP2C.[109] Interactions with PIs include increased etravirine levels when given with indinavir and atazanavir, and reduced etravirine levels when it is administered with full-dose ritonavir. This pharmacokinetic relationship is bi-directional and levels of both indinavir and saquinavir drop substantially when co-administered with etravirine, whereas fosamprenavir levels rise, making appropriate dose adjustment advisable. Studies in healthy volunteers demonstrated no interaction between etravirine and didanosine.[110] Addition of 800 mg of etravirine twice daily to the regimens of HIV-1-infected subjects with undetectable viral loads on a stable combination ARV regimen containing saquinavir or lopinavir/ritonavir demonstrated only slightly lower C_{max} and AUC levels.[111] C_{min} for lopinavir was unaffected, arguing that the clinical impact of etravirine on lopinavir/ritonavir will be minimal. While no pharmacokinetic interaction was observed in a small study of HIV-infected subjects receiving both etravirine and TMC 124/ritonavir,[112] administration of etravirine with tipranavir/ritonavir in healthy subjects resulted in 24% decrease in AUC compared to when etravirine was administered alone.[113] Pharmacokinetic studies did not show clinically significant changes in either etravirine levels or a variety of other medications including ranitidine, omeprazole, or rifabutin. Levels of sildenafil drop substantially when given with etravirine, as do levels of clarithromycin, so the drug's developers suggest dose adjustment or alternative medications when these drugs are used.

TMC 278 (Rilpivirine, R278474)

TMC 278, another DAPY derivative, has demonstrated inhibitory activity in nanomolar concentrations against wild-type virus and laboratory-derived NNRTI resistant mutants (including double mutants such as K103N + Y181C).[90,114] Selection studies showed an increased genetic barrier to resistance for rilpivirine compared to other NNRTIs with no resistance observed after 30 days when concentrations were maintained above 40 nM/mL.[112] Resistance mutations selected included L100L/I, V106V/I, Y181Y/C, and M230M/L. Combination assays *in vitro* demonstrated no antagonism between rilpivirine and lamivudine, emtricitabine, tenofovir, efavirenz, indinavir or lopinavir. Pharmacokinetic studies in healthy, HIV-1-negative volunteers indicated dose-dependent increases in exposure to rilpivirine up to 200 mg with a median T_{max} of 4 h. For a 50 mg dose of rilpivirine, C_{max} was 247 ng/mL with a mean AUC of 7720 ng.h/mL. $T_{1/2}$ was between 34 and 55 h, suggesting that rilpivirine may be dosed once daily. Rates of adverse events in healthy volunteers were low and comparable to those observed on placebo.

The activity of rilpivirine monotherapy in ARV-naive, HIV-1-positive subjects was evaluated in a double-blind, placebo-controlled phase II trial.[115] Investigators randomized 47 subjects (mean CD4 255 cells/mm^3 and median HIV-1 RNA of 4.5 $\log_{10}$ copies/mL) to receive 25, 50, 100, or 150 mg of rilpivirine or placebo daily for 7 days. Declines in viral load of 1.3 $\log_{10}$ copies/mL, 1.2 $\log_{10}$ copies/mL, 1.1 $\log_{10}$ copies/mL, and 1.2 $\log_{10}$ copies/mL were seen for the 25, 50, 100, and 150 mg groups, respectively, versus an increase of 0.002 $\log_{10}$ in the placebo group. Overall mean increase in CD4 count in the rilpivirine-treated subjects was 55 cells/mm^3. Adverse events were uncommon (headache in 14% of rilpivirine-treated subjects vs 18% of placebo recipients), and no SAEs were reported.

Week 48 results of a large, 96-week phase II dose-finding study of rilpivirine in treatment-naive patients have been reported.[116] Investigators recruited 368 ART-naive subjects with HIV-1 RNA levels of 5000 copies/mL and no evidence of NRTI or NNRTI resistance at entry. Subjects were randomized to receive either open-label efavirenz or one of three blinded doses of rilpivirine (25, 75, or 150 mg), all given once daily. Investigators selected the NRTI backbone (75.3% received zidovudine/lamivudine and 24.7% tenofovir/emtricitabine). About one-third of the subjects were female and between 44% and 47% were Caucasian. Women of reproductive age were required to be on some type of hormonal contraception. Baseline HIV RNA levels were 4.8 $\log_{10}$ copies/mL and baseline CD4 count was 200–207 cells/mm^3. Mean age of participants was 35 years and duration of HIV infection was ~1 year. The primary endpoint for the study was the proportion of subjects with HIV-1 RNA level <50 copies/mL. Data on immunologic response, safety, and tolerability were collected as well. Virologic responses at the interim 48-week analysis were similar between all four arms of the study (77–81% in those receiving rilpivirine achieved HIV-1 RNA levels of <50 copies/mL vs 81% in efavirenz arm). Virologic responses were comparable across all arms of the study and averaged 2.6 $\log_{10}$ copies/mL. Changes in CD4 count were similar in all four groups (125–145 cells/mm^3 in those receiving rilpivirine vs 127 cells/mm^3 in the efavirenz arm). Adverse event profiles were similar, but CNS symptoms and rash were more common in the efavirenz group. Grade 3 or 4 AEs were seen in ~25% of subjects receiving rilpivirine compared to 16% in those who took efavirenz. Investigators speculated this was due to underreporting of efavirenz-related toxicity, and rates of Grade 3 or 4 laboratory abnormalities were rare and comparable between the two groups.

Administration of rilpivirine with food improved absorption with C_{max} increasing 71% and AUC 45%.[117] Rilpivirine is not metabolized by the kidney and does not appear to have an active metabolite.[114] Rilpivirine is metabolized via CYP3A4/5 and is highly protein-bound.[118] Co-administration of rilpivirine with tenofovir resulted in a significant increase of 24% in exposure to tenofovir[119]; no changes in the pharmacokinetics of rilpivirine were observed. Co-administration with lopinavir/ritonavir resulted in a 52% increase in AUC for rilpivirine, suggesting dose adjustment of rilpivirine will be necessary when the two are administered together.

GW678248/GW695634

High-throughput screening led to the identification of a series of benzophenone derivatives as potential HIV-1 therapeutic agents.[120] Analysis of structure–activity relationships resulted in the characterization of the critical determinants of effective binding to HIV-1 RT and allowed investigators to rationally design benzophenone derivatives that had nanomolar potency against HIV-1 while retaining activity against NNRTI-resistant viruses.[121] The original lead compound, GW678248, had poor oral bioavailability which investigators overcame by synthesizing an N-proprionyl sulfonamide prodrug, GW695634.[122] Although this compound is 25- to 400-fold less potent,[123] it is efficiently converted to GW678248 and results in an increase in oral bioavailability from 7% to 50%. Like most other NNRTIs, GW678248 is only active against HIV-1. *In vitro* studies of GW678248 demonstrated an IC_{50} of 1.8 nM against wild-type virus and retained activity against a panel of NNRTI-resistant mutants including L101I, K103N, V106A/I, V108I, E138K, Y181C, Y188C, P236L and the double mutants V106A-Y181C and V108I-Y181C.[124] GW678248 was active against 47 of 55 clinical isolates with NNRTI resistance.[125] Serial passage studies with GW678248 selected for K102E, V106A/I, E138K, and P236L mutations. Interestingly, viruses containing either the V106I or P236L mutations demonstrated *in vitro* resistance to nevirapine, but not to efavirenz, suggesting a possible role for efavirenz in persons experiencing virologic failure due to GW678248 resistance. Combination studies of GW678248 demonstrated *in vitro* synergy with a variety of NRTIs (AZT, d4T, TFV, ABC, 3TC) and PIs (IDV, LPV, NFV, and RTV).[125] GW695634 was also additive with nevirapine and efavirenz and antagonistic with delavirdine.

A double-blind, placebo-controlled, phase I trial assessed the safety, tolerability, and pharmacokinetics of GW695634 in healthy subjects.[126] Seven groups of 10 subjects each were randomized to receive a single dose of 10, 25, 75, 200, 400, 600, or 800 mg of GW695634 or placebo. The 200 mg group received GW695634 with a high-fat meal to assess the impact of food on absorption. Levels of GW678248 increased with increasing dose of its prodrug. T_{max} ranged from 1.00 to 3.75 h and $T_{1/2}$ was 14 h. GW695634 was rapidly converted to GW678248 and levels were not significantly increased if drug was taken with food. A subsequent randomized, double-blind, placebo-controlled trial of GW695634 evaluated the safety, tolerability and pharmacokinetics in HIV-1-infected subjects with documented NNRTI resistance.[127] Forty-six subjects were randomized to receive 100, 200, 300, or 400 mg of GW695634 orally twice daily versus placebo for 7 days. Study subjects had a median of two NNRTI-associated mutations (range 1-4, most commonly K103N and Y181C). Median baseline HIV-1 RNA levels ranged from 4.4 to 4.6 $\log_{10}$ copies/mL and CD4 T-lymphocyte counts ranged from 230 to 345 cells/mm^3. Study subjects were required to be off all ARVs for at least 4 weeks. After 7 days, median HIV-1 viral load reductions were 1.2 $\log_{10}$ copies/mL, 1.1 $\log_{10}$ copies/mL, 1.6 $\log_{10}$ copies/mL, and 1.3 $\log_{10}$ copies/mL compared to a rise of 0.14 $\log_{10}$ copies/mL in the placebo arm. In both the phase I and phase II trials, GW695634 was well tolerated and no treatment-limiting or SAEs were reported. Rash (17%), nausea (15%) and diarrhea (11%) were the most commonly seen AEs and were generally mild.

ENTRY INHIBITORS

HIV entry can be divided into three phases: attachment, co-receptor binding and membrane fusion.[128] Attachment of HIV-1 to target cells occurs when viral gp120 binds to the D1 domain of CD4 on the surface of lymphocytes and macrophages. This interaction induces conformational changes in gp120 variable region that exposes a co-receptor binding domain in its V3 region. Based on the tropism of the infecting virus, this newly exposed binding site facilitates approximation of viral and target cell membranes through interactions with either the CCR5 or CXCR4 co-receptor on the target cell. Further conformational changes in the gp120/gp41 complex lead to the insertion of gp41 into the target cell membrane, and that in turn brings the target cell and host lipid bilayers into close enough proximity that they fuse.

Attachment Inhibitors

Compounds that interfere with HIV-1 binding to CD4 were initially studied in the early 1990s with disappointing results.[129,130] Elucidation of the specific mechanism of HIV-1 replication clarified the challenges of this approach. The *Env* gene (from which both gp120 and gp41 are derived) is the region of the HIV-1 genome most prone to errors in replication. This recognition led investigators to seek conserved regions within *Env*. Several such regions have been identified and several compounds have been developed that interfere with viral-CD4 binding.

PRO-542

PRO-542 is a tetravalent fusion protein derived from the D1/D2 domains of human CD4 and the heavy and light chain constant regions of human IgG2 immunoglobulin. Electron microscopy studies of PRO-542 interactions with gp120 suggest that the drug may exert its antiviral activity through cross-linking of gp120-gp41 trimers on the virion surface.[131] PRO-542 has antiviral activity *in vitro*[132] and inhibits HIV-1 replication regardless of clade or co-receptor utilization.[133] In addition to inhibiting attachment of free virions to target cells, PRO-542 inhibits cell-associated transmission of HIV-1, suggesting a potential role as a prophylactic agent.[134] Studies of PRO-542 in a hu-PBL-SCID mouse model demonstrated inhibition of viral replication.[135] Data on potential drug interactions are limited though one study demonstrated *in vitro* synergy between PRO-542 and enfuvirtide.[136]

The initial phase I study of PRO-542 in humans was a dose-escalation trial looking at infusion of single doses of 0.2, 1, 5, or 10 mg/kg intravenously.[137] C_{max} averaged 562 ± 110 μg/mL in the 10 mg/kg group with a mean $T_{1/2}$ of 3.3 ± 0.7 days. Antibody production against PRO-542 was limited, suggesting it was not highly immunogenic. A subsequent phase I, single-dose, study of PRO-542 in twelve adults with advanced HIV-1 infection demonstrated a sustained mean decline in HIV-1 load of 0.5 $\log_{10}$ copies/mL in those who received 25 mg/kg of PRO-542 intravenously.[138] Mean $T_{1/2}$ was 2.9 days and concentrations of PRO-542 exceeded the *in vitro* IC_{50} for an average of 2 weeks after treatment. In this study, HIV-1 RNA >100 000 copies/mL and CD4 T-lymphocyte count <200 cells/mm^3 predicted benefit, suggesting a role for PRO-542 in advanced HIV-1 disease. Although data are limited, CD4 cell depletion associated with advanced HIV disease may magnify the impact of PRO-542 by limiting endogenous targets for newly released HIV-1 virions. A similar phase I trial in children demonstrated a >0.7 $\log_{10}$ copies/mL decline in viral load in four of six who received 10 mg/kg of PRO-542 intravenously four times weekly.[139] No major toxicity was seen in these trials though long-term data are limited. Current formulations of PRO-542 require intravenous administration though intramuscular and subcutaneous preparations of the drug are being developed.[140] Pharmacokinetics of PRO-542 in children displays nonlinear kinetics with doses of 20 mg/kg producing higher clearance, an observation that has been attributed to high-affinity binding of the compound.[141] Resistance to PRO-542 has not yet been described.

TNX-355

TNX-355 is a humanized, IgG4 monoclonal antibody directed against the D2 domain of CD4. Early studies of this compound indicated a target distinct from the gp120-CD4 binding site, suggesting that TNX-355 inhibited HIV-1 entry after viral attachment had occurred.[142] *In vitro* studies demonstrated comparable anti-HIV-1 activity regardless of co-receptor tropism[143] and antiviral synergy when TNX-355 was combined with enfuvirtide.[144] TNX-355 maintains *in vitro* activity against a panel of engineered isolates with enfuvirtide-associated mutations in the HR1 region of gp41.[145] Because of concerns of antibody-mediated CD4 depletion and complement activation, developers of TNX-355 chose the IgG4 isotype, known to be less immunogenic. Studies in rhesus macaques and chimpanzees have supported this approach, demonstrating immunogenicity of the humanized antibody in the former and not that latter species.[146]

A phase Ia dose-escalation study of TNX-355 evaluated the safety, pharmacokinetics, virologic and immunologic responses of various single 0.3–25 mg/kg intravenous doses in five cohorts of individuals with established HIV-1 infection. Mean peak viral load declines ranged from 0.2 $\log_{10}$ copies/mL in the lowest dose group to 1.48 $\log_{10}$ copies/mL in those receiving 10 mg/kg.[147] Persistence of HIV-1 RNA decline correlated with duration of CD4 coating by the antibody and varied from 1–2 days in the lowest to 15–27 days in the highest dose group. A transient, dose-dependant increase in CD4 cell count was observed, suggesting redistribution of CD4 cells and not a change in CD4 cell homeostasis.[148] While the majority of subjects receiving TNX-355 reported adverse events (headaches, rash, pruritus, urticaria and nasal congestion most commonly), no SAEs or drug-related laboratory abnormalities were seen. TNX-355 did not induce antibody formation. A phase Ib study looked at the impact of TNX-355 in 22 individuals with chronic HIV-1 infection.[149] Entry criteria included HIV-1 load >5000 copies/mL and CD4 counts >100 cells/mm^3 and subjects were required to be on a stable ARV regimen or to be off ARVs altogether. Subjects were randomized to receive either 10 mg/kg of TNX-355 IV weekly or a 10 mg/kg loading dose followed by 6 mg/kg every14 days. An additional three subjects who received 25 mg/kg every 14 days were also included. All three groups were treated for 9 weeks. Two-thirds of the subjects experienced a decline in HIV-1 load of 1.0 $\log_{10}$ copies/mL and 23% experienced a decline of 1.4 $\log_{10}$ copies/mL. Response was not clearly dose related and was transient with HIV-1 load returning to baseline by 9 weeks in most subjects. Phenotypic analysis showed reduced *in vitro* susceptibility to TNX-355, suggesting the development of resistance. Three subjects in this study experienced SAEs including recurrence of known depression, new-onset seizure after a vaso-vagal reaction and transient worsening of baseline renal insufficiency.

An analysis of data from a 48-week phase II, multicenter, randomized, double-blind trial comparing two doses of TNX-355 versus placebo in triple-class experienced subjects has been reported.[150] Investigators randomized 82 HIV-1 individuals with a CD4 count of >50 cells/mm^3 and a viral load of ≥10 000 copies/mL on a failing ARV regimen to receive either 10 or15 mg/kg of TNX-355 versus placebo intravenously every 14 days. Subjects in the 10 mg/kg arm received TNX-355 weekly for the first 8 weeks. All subjects received OBT. The study's primary endpoint was mean HIV-1 viral load reduction from baseline at 24 weeks. Subjects were mostly male (87%) and mean age was 46 years. While subjects were largely Caucasian, about one-third of the subjects were Latino and ~15% were of African descent. Virologic failure was defined as inability to achieve or maintain 0.5 $\log_{10}$ copies/mL decrease in HIV-1 RNA level from baseline. The study design called for subjects with virologic failure to receive open-label TNX-355 at 15 mg/kg intravenously every 2 weeks, along with a new OBT. Subjects already enrolled in the 15 mg/kg arm of the trial did not receive an increased dose of TNX-355, but they did switch OBT when virologic failure was recognized. At the planned 24-week analysis, subjects in the 10 mg/kg arm experienced a 1.16 $\log_{10}$ copies/mL drop in HIV-1 load versus 0.95 $\log_{10}$ copies/mL and 0.20 $\log_{10}$ copies/mL decline in the 15 mg/kg and placebo groups respectively. Virologic response at 48 weeks demonstrated a return toward baseline with 0.96 $\log_{10}$ copies/mL, 0.71 $\log_{10}$ copies/mL, and 0.14 $\log_{10}$ copies/mL in the 10 mg/kg, 15 mg/kg, and placebo groups respectively. Time to virologic failure was between 230 and 253 days for subjects receiving TNX-355. No subject in the placebo arm demonstrated adequate virologic response to their new OBT (100% virologic failure). Immunologic response at week 48 was significantly better in those receiving TNX-355 with mean CD4 rising (48–51 cells/mm^3 in the TNX-355 groups compared to 1 cell/mm^3 in the placebo arm). TNX-355 was well tolerated and AEs were uncommon in all arms of the trial. Grade 3 laboratory abnormalities were slightly more common in the TNX-355 groups (32–37% vs 18.5% for placebo) but Grade 4 laboratory abnormalities were comparable across all arms (7–14% in TNX-355 arms vs 18.5% for placebo). Data on potential drug–drug interactions with TNX-355 are not currently available.

BMS-488043

BMS-488043 is an orally available, small-molecule entry inhibitor that blocks the binding of HIV-1 gp120 to cellular CD4 receptors.[152] It is active *in vitro* at nanomolar concentrations and shows activity regardless of co-receptor tropism. BMS-488043 does not have activity against HIV-2 or other studied RNA viruses.[153] *In vitro* studies of resistance to BMS-488043 have identified a number of specific mutations that confer resistance, with most centering around the CD4 contact point with gp120 (M426L and M475I).[152] A phase I trial in healthy adults used an ascending, multiple-dose protocol to evaluate the pharmacokinetics of BMS-488043. In this study, four groups of healthy subjects received 400, 800, 1200, or 1800 mg of BMS-488043 every 12 h for 14 days with either a high-fat or low-fat meal.[154] Median T_{max} was 3-4 h and mean C_{max} was 2494-7136 ng/mL. Drug levels increased with a high-fat meal. BMS-488043 was well tolerated and no SAEs were reported.

A phase 1, placebo-controlled, ascending, multiple-dose study was conducted in HIV-1-infected adults with viral loads between 5000 and 500 000 copies/mL and CD4 counts of >250 cells/mm^3.[155] Participants were either ARV-naive or had been off ART for at least 16 weeks. Two groups of 15 subjects each (12 receiving drug, three placebo) received either 800 or 1800 mg of BMS-488043 versus placebo every 12 h for 8 days. Mean maximal viral load decline was 1.00 $\log_{10}$ copies/mL versus 0.3 $\log_{10}$ copies/mL for placebo. Eight of 12 BMS-488043-treated participants had a viral load decline >0.5 $\log_{10}$ copies/mL, 7/12 had a decline >1.0 $\log_{10}$ copies/mL, and 3/12 had a decline of >1.5 $\log_{10}$ copies/mL. No SAEs were observed.

Co-Receptor Blockers

The recognition that the endogenous chemokines RANTES, MIP-1α, and MIP-1β could inhibit HIV-1 replication highlighted the role of chemokine receptors in HIV pathogenesis.[156] CXCR4 (X4) and CCR5 (R5) were identified as the principal co-receptors for HIV-1 infection.[157,158] The identification of a 32 base pair deletion in the CCR5 gene (Δ32 mutation) in persons with repeated exposure to HIV-1 but no evidence of infection[159] spurred efforts to identify compounds that inhibit co-receptor binding. This approach has yielded a number of agents that are in clinical trials (discussed in Chapter 24).

Fusion Inhibitors

Enfuvirtide has been a valuable addition to the ARV armamentarium, but also presented challenges given difficulties with production, cost, administration, side-effects and a limited genetic barrier to resistance.[160] Development of the next generation of fusion inhibitors has been slow. Production of the most promising new agent in this class, T-1249, was halted in January 2004 because of formulation difficulties. Since there is an important role for fusion inhibitors in treatment-experienced patients,[143] a review of data on T-1249 and related compounds is warranted.

Next Generation Fusion Inhibitors

T-1249 is a 39 amino acid peptide composed of sequences derived from HIV-1, HIV-2, and simian immunodeficiency virus (SIV). T-1249 demonstrated potent activity against HIV-1 *in vitro* with a mean EC_{50} of 0.008 µg/mL, and retained activity against both clinical isolates and site-directed mutants with enfuvirtide-associated mutations.[161] Like enfuvirtide, T-1249 is administered by subcutaneous injection but its improved pharmacokinetic profile allows once-daily dosing. A phase I/II open-label, dose-escalation, monotherapy study of the safety and ARV activity of T-1249 was performed in 115 HIV-1-infected adults[162] Subjects in this study were highly treatment-experienced but had been off all ART for at least 14 days. Study subjects had viral loads >5000 copies/mL and mean CD4 count was 57 cells/mm^3. Total daily doses ranged from 6.25 to 192 mg. Mean maximal decline in HIV-1 RNA was dose-dependant and ranged from 0.29 $\log_{10}$ copies/mL for the lowest group to 1.96 $\log_{10}$ copies/mL in the highest. Although SAEs in those receiving T-1249 were rare (two subjects experienced allergic reactions), 57% experienced an AE (most commonly headache, fever, rash). Not surprisingly, injection-site reactions were common as well (57%). A second phase I/II study of T-1249 was conducted in 53 subjects with detectable HIV-1 viremia despite receiving an enfuvirtide-containing ARV regimen.[163] Subjects substituted daily doses of 192 mg of T-1249 for enfuvirtide during the 10-day study period, and continued their baseline ARV regimen. Median decline in HIV-1 load at day 11 was 1.26 $\log_{10}$ copies/mL.

Although not yet in clinical trials, the next generation of fusion inhibitors is under development.[164] The compounds TR-290999 and TR-291144 were developed using independent strategies to optimize potency, durability, and pharmacokinetics of the parent compound. TR-291144 displayed antiviral activity against a panel of 12 clinical isolates, with a mean IC_{50} of 7 nM. TR-290999 demonstrated even greater potency with a sevenfold improvement in IC_{50} against the same panel of clinical isolates, compared to enfuvirtide. Both compounds retained activity against isolates resistant to enfuvirtide, T-1249, and other peptide fusion inhibitors. *In vitro* studies utilizing escalating doses of enfuvirtide, T-1249, TR-290999, and TR291144, to select for resistance, demonstrated a significantly higher genetic barrier to resistance with the next generation fusion inhibitors (resistance mutations accumulated on average at 36 days for enfuvirtide and 63 days for T-1249 compared to retained activity of both TR-290999 (after 71–76 days) and TR-291144 (72–93 days).[151] As with previous studies, both TR-290999 and TR-291144 retained activity against isolates with both enfuvirtide and T-1249 resistance. Animal studies suggested that both compounds are metabolized more slowly than enfuvirtide, making weekly dosing possible, and selection experiments demonstrate a greater genetic barrier to resistance than demonstrated by earlier fusion inhibitors.

INHIBITORS OF VIRAL ASSEMBLY

Following intracellular transcription of viral RNA, HIV-1 protease cleaves HIV-1 polyproteins into functional products. Viral assembly occurs when Gag multimers complex with Gag-Pol polyproteins, viral RNA, Vif, Vpr and several host proteins. These preassembled complexes are transported to specific lipid-rich regions of the host cell where budding occurs. Following budding, virions undergo further protease-mediated structural modification, a process termed maturation. This complicated cascade of events affords several potential targets for drug development. While efforts to produce better PIs are ongoing, novel inhibitors of viral assembly, called maturation inhibitors, are entering clinical trials as well.

Protease Inhibitors

Development of the next generation of PIs has focused on expanding the spectrum of activity against resistant viruses while improving convenience and tolerability. While two new PIs have recently been FDA approved (including the nonpeptidic PI, darunavir, which is reviewed in Chapter 26), prospects for additional agents in the next several years were diminished when development of brecanavir was halted due to problems with bioavialibility.

Brecanavir (GW640385)

Brecanavir is the lead compound of a new type of PI, arylsulfonamide PI, and was identified though insights regarding structure–activity relationships of amprenavir and HIV protease. Brecanvir has demonstrated an IC_{50} of 1.1 nM against wild-type HIV-1 and retained nanomolar potency against a panel of single- and multiple-PI resistant recombinant viruses.[165,166] Although structurally similar, *in vitro* studies have demonstrated retained activity against isolates with extensive PI resistance from individuals who had failed an amprenavir-containing ARV regimen.[167] *In vitro* serial passage studies indicated two different pathways for resistance to brecanavir.[168] In a low-pressure system, Q58E and A71V mutations arose and were associated with low-level resistance to the compound. In a high-pressure assay, however, these mutations were not seen, and an A28S mutation predominated. A28S mutants were highly resistant to brecanavir but as a result had markedly impaired replication capacity. *In vitro* combination studies demonstrated additive activity with other PIs and either additive or synergistic activity with NRTIs and NNRTIs.[165] Studies in healthy volunteers demonstrated asymptomatic Grade 2-3 liver function abnormalities when ritonavir-boosted brecanavir was administered with tipranavir and this study was discontinued before detailed pharmacologic data were obtained.[169] Similar studies involving co-administration of ritonavir-boosted brecanvir and either atazanavir or lopinavir/ritonavir revealed no clinically significant pharmacokinetic interactions.

Preliminary pharmacokinetic studies in healthy volunteers demonstrated limited bioavailability ($<5\%$ when given orally).[170] Boosting with ritonavir improved bioavailability 16- to 30-fold, however. A subsequent, 2-week dose-escalation trial in healthy men and women further clarified the pharmacokinetics of brecanavir.[171] Subjects were randomized into one of six groups: unboosted brecanavir 800 mg twice daily; or brecanavir 100 or 250 mg once daily with 100 mg of ritonavir; or brecanavir 50, 150, or 300 mg twice daily with ritonavir 100 mg twice daily. Brecanavir was rapidly absorbed (T_{max} from 4.8 to 4.5 h) in all groups though steady-state levels were not achieved until day 15. Administration of brecanavir with ritonavir increased exposure 33- to 85-fold. Although once-daily dosing with ritonavir resulted in adequate trough levels for wild-type viruses, pharmacokinetic studies suggest that it should be dosed twice daily. In the multiple-dose study, 34% of subjects experienced some AEs (most commonly gastrointestinal upset, headache and dizziness though transient TSH elevations were seen in four subjects who received brecanavir).

Preliminary data from an open-label, 48-week study of ritonavir-boosted brecanavir in HIV-1-infected subjects have been reported.[172,173] Investigators enrolled 31 HIV-1-infected subjects with CD4 counts >200 cells/mm^3 and HIV-1 RNA >1000 $\log_{10}$ copies/mL and administered 300 mg of brecanavir with 100 mg ritonavir twice daily along with a standard dual NRTI backbone (27/31 received zidovudine/lamivudine). Subjects were divided into those with and without baseline PI mutations (6/31 and 25/31 respectively). On average, the subjects with baseline PI resistance had a median of two primary PI mutations and five NRTI mutations. Baseline viral load in each group was 4.2 and 5.0 $\log_{10}$ copies/mL (PI mutations vs no mutations, respectively) and median CD4 count was 389 and 264 cells/mm^3 respectively. The IC_{50} for brecanavir was assessed in each subject at baseline and ranged from 0.1 to 0.2 nM. Twenty-seven of thirty-one subjects remained in the trial at the planned 24-week analysis. At week 24, 24/31 subjects had an HIV-1 RNA level <50 copies/mL, including 5/6 with baseline PI resistant islolates. Median CD4 count rise was 84 cells/mm^3 respectively. No SAEs or clinically significant laboratory abnormalities were observed. Despite these promising results, the drug developer discontinued development when insurmountable issues with the formulation of brecanavir arose.

Maturation Inhibitors

Problems with the development of new PIs highlight the importance of developing additional classes of ARV agents. Although inhibition of protease activity has been the most productive means of inhibiting assembly of infectious virions, completion of several additional steps beyond post-translational modification of HIV polyproteins are required before infectious virions are produced. Inhibition of the maturation of virions after budding from infected CD4 lymphocytes appears to be the most promising approach to the identification of a new class of ARV compounds.

Bevirimat (PA-457)

Mechanism-blind screening assays indicated that betulinic acid derived from the plant *Syzigium claviflorum* has weak anti-HIV-1 activity.[174] Biochemical modification of the parent compound led to the identification of bevirimat (3-*O*- (3′,3′-dimethylsuccinyl) betulinic acid), a compound with nanomolar activity against HIV-1.[175] Bevirimat is active against HIV-1 isolates with resistance to NRTIs, NNRTIs and PIs though it does not inhibit HIV-2 replication.[176] Although initial observations suggested it prevented virion release,[177] bevirimat was subsequently shown to inhibit conversion of precursor capsid protein p25 to its mature form p24.[178] HIV-1 virions produced after exposure to bevirimat are structurally abnormal and noninfectious. Unlike PIs, bevirimat inhibits HIV-1 replication by binding to a specific region at the N-terminal end of the Gag-Pol precursor. Site-directed mutagenesis revealed the critical binding site for bevirimat to be in the Gag-SP1 domain.[179] This distinct mechanism of activity led to the classification of bevirimat as the first-in-class maturation inhibitor. Serial passage studies produced mutants around the Gag CA-SP1 binding site that conferred resistance to bevirimat.[180] Gag sequencing showed three substitutions at the extreme C-terminal of the capsid protein (H226Y, L231M, and L231F) and two in the SP1 region (A1V and A3V).[181] Only the A3V mutation decreased viral fitness *in vitro* and this effect was reversed when a second mutation in capsid occurred (G225S). Mutant viruses retained activity against existing classes of AR vs Combination studies have demonstrated synergy or additivity when bevirimat is combined with all tested ARVs.[182] A 10-day placebo-controlled, dose-escalation study in healthy volunteers evaluated bevirimat's safety and tolerability.[183] Subjects received 25, 50, or 100 mg of bevirimat daily. At the end of the study, mean C_{max} rose proportionally from 7.98 to 31.58 μg/mL and median AUC increased from 156.5 to 599.5 μg.h/mL. C_{min} on day 10 ranged from 5.75 to 21.57 μg/mL. Bevirimat demonstrated a prolonged half-life with $T_{1/2}$ ranging from 56.3 to 63 h. No significant AEs were observed.

A single-dose, double-blind, placebo-controlled study in 16 HIV-1-positive individuals looked at the safety and efficacy of bevirimat.[184] Enrolled subjects all had CD4 counts ⩾200 cells/mm^3 and viral loads between 5000 and 250 000 $\log_{10}$ copies/mL and were either treatment-naive or had been off ARVs for at least 4 weeks. Bevirimat produced proportional viral load reductions from 0.27 $\log_{10}$ copies/mL for the 75 mg dose to 0.51 $\log_{10}$ copies/mL for the 250 mg doses. In the 250 mg group, inhibition of HIV-1 replication from a single dose of bevirimat was seen up to 10 days after administration. A subsequent randomized, double-blind phase 2a study evaluated bevirimat in 33 HIV-1-infected subjects who were off ART.[177] Subjects were required to have a CD4 count >200 cells/mm^3 and HIV-1 RNA levels between 5000 and 250 000 $\log_{10}$ copies/mL and were randomized to receive 25, 50, 100 or 200 mg of bevirimat daily versus placebo for 10 days. Median decline in HIV-1 load ranged from a rise of 0.05 $\log_{10}$ copies/mL in the 25 mg group to a decline of 1.03 $\log_{10}$ copies/mL in the 200 mg group. Response to bevirimat correlated with both C_{max} and AUC.[185] Subgroup analysis of subjects in the 200 mg arm demonstrated a decline of 1.52 $\log_{10}$ copies/mL in subjects whose entry viral loads were <100 000 copies/mL.[177] No grade 3 or 4 AEs were observed, though one treated patient with a history of poorly-controlled diabetes and hypertension suffered a cerebrovascular accident. Isolates obtained after the completion of both of these trials demonstrated no changes in the Gag CA-SP1 cleavage site.[186] The protocol for a subsequent phase IIb trial of bevirimat in treatment-experienced patients had to be altered to allow for increased dosing when a tablet formulation proved inferior to the previous liquid formulation. Animal and human studies demonstrated little inhibition of cytochrome P450.[187] No pharmacokinetic or pharmacodynamic interaction was observed between bevirimat and atazanavir in healthy volunteers[188] and bevirimat was not teratogenic in rats and rabbits.[189]

FUTURE TARGETS

HIV drug discovery has been aided by new insights into pharmacogenomics[190] and by the development of *in vitro* models to predict potential metabolic complications[191] and drug–drug interactions[192] during the preclinical development stage. Important work is being done to identify new compounds that inhibit existing targets and additional candidate NRTIs, NNRTIs, and PIs are in development. Beyond this traditional approach to ARV drug development, new ways of attacking old targets are being elucidated. Agents such as nucleoside competing reverse transcriptase inhibitors (NcRTI)[193] and metallocarbonase PIs[194] are expanding the traditional definition of inhibitors of these viral enzymes. The search for viable RNase H inhibitors continues as well.

Identification of compounds that interfere with other HIV regulatory and accessory proteins is ongoing. Although enthusiasm for Tat inhibitors has waned, a recent study suggested that Tat inhibition may allow the host's innate RNA interference mechanisms to inhibit HIV replication.[195] In theory, inhibition of Nef, an HIV regulatory protein that causes down-regulation of CD4 and MHC-1 molecules on the surface of infected cells, may result in both reduced viral budding and more effective natural killer (NK) cell clearance of infected CD4 cells.[196] Mifepristone has been shown to interfere with the activity of Vpr,[197] a regulatory protein that is essential for the infection of macrophages and monocytes during primary HIV infection. Similarly, inhibition of Rev, a viral protein involved in movement of genetic material into and out of the nucleus of target cells, has been shown to effectively limit HIV replication *in vitro*.[198]

Other novel approaches to inhibition of HIV replication include interference with the zinc finger element found in the HIV-1 nucleocapsid. The p7 nucleocapsid protein contains two zinc fingers that are highly conserved and are important to proper packaging the genomic RNA into progeny virions. Electrophilic agents that attack the sulfur atoms in cysteine can lead to ejection of zinc and disruption of viral assembly. One particularly intriguing agent, azodicarbonamide, has been tested in HIV-infected subjects and was shown to produce up to 1.2 $\log_{10}$ copies/mL decline in viral load.[199] Development of this compound has been deferred because of a variety of potential metabolic complications seen in treated subjects.

The recognition that APOBEC3G plays a role in limiting the spread of HIV from infected cells has generated considerable excitement in its potential as a therapeutic target.[200] APOBEC3G is incorporated into budding viruses where it induces a G to A mutation that prevents transmission of affected viruses. The HIV accessory protein, Vif has been shown to interact with APOBEC3G and to initiate a cascade of events that results in the degradation of this innate host defense mechanism.[201] Investigators, therefore, hope to identify compounds that will inhibit Vif-APOBEC3G interactions.

Failure of attempts to eradicate latent virus from reservoir sites has limited antiviral approaches to date. Considerable interest has centered on ways to activate HIV-1 from latently infected CD4+ cells in order to make such cells susceptible to ART. The enzyme, histone deacetylase 1 (HDAC1) is responsible for chromatin remodeling and repression of viral gene expression.[202] Blockade of HDAC1 activity has been shown to result in activation of latently-infected CD4 cells and a recent proof-of-concept study suggested that the use of valproic acid (a known inhibitor of HDAC1 activity) can significantly reduce the reservoir of latently infected CD4 cells.[203] Clinical exploitation of such HIV activation/eradication strategies is still in its infancy and a follow-up study suggested that valproic acid treatment had no effect on decay of the latent HIV-1 reservoir.[204]

REFERENCES

1. LaFem ina RL, Schneider CL, Robbins HL, et al. Requirement of active human immunodeficiency virus type 1 integrase enzyme for productive infection of human T-lymphoid cells. J Virol 66:7414–19, 1992.
2. Taddeo B, Haseltine WA, Farnet CM. Integrase mutants of human immunodeficiency virus type 1 with a specific defect in integration. J Virol 68:8401–5, 1994.
3. Wiskerchen M, Muesing MA. Human immunodeficiency virus type 1 integrase: effects of mutations on viral ability to integrate, direct viral gene expression from unintegrated viral DNA templates, and sustain viral propagation in primary cells. J Virol 69:376–86, 1995.
4. Pommier Y, Johnson AA, Marchand C. Integrase inhibitors to treat HIV/AIDS [review] [99 refs]. Nat Rev Drug Discov 4:236–48, 2005.
5. LaFemina RL, Schneider CL, Robbins HL, et al. Requirement of active human immunodeficiency virus type 1 integrase enzyme for productive infection of human T-lymphoid cells. J Virol 66:7414-19, 1992.
6. Vink C, Banks M, Bethell R, Plasterk RH. A high-throughput, non-radioactive microtiter plate assay for activity of the human immunodeficiency virus integrase protein. Nucleic Acids Res 22:2176–7, 1994.
7. Hazuda DJ, Hastings JC, Wolfe AL, Emini EA. A novel assay for the DNA strand-transfer reaction of HIV-1 integrase. Nucleic Acids Res 22:1121–2, 1994.
8. Hazuda DJ, Felock P, Witmer M, et al. Inhibitors of strand transfer that prevent integration and inhibit HIV-1 replication in cells. Science 287:646–50, 2000.
9. Debyser Z, Pauwels R, Andries K, et al. An antiviral target on reverse transcriptase of human immunodeficiency virus type 1 revealed by tetrahydroimidazo-[4,5,1-jk] [1,4]benzodiazepin-2 (1H)-one and -thione derivatives. Proc Natl Acad Sci USA 88:1451–5, 1991.
10. Fransen S, Gupta S, Paxinos EE, et al. Integrase (IN) inhibitor susceptibility can be measured using recombinant viruses that express patient virus IN alone, or in combination with protease (PR) and reverse transcriptase (RT). In: Program and Abstracts of the 12th Conference on Retroviruses and Opportunistic Infections, Boston, 2005, abstract 725.
11. Hazuda DJ, Young SD, Guare JP, et al. Integrase inhibitors and cellular immunity suppress retroviral replication in rhesus macaques. Science 305:528–32, 2004.
12. Witvrouw M, Fikkert V, Van Remoortel B, et al. Multiple mutations in HIV-1 integrase confer resistance to the Phase 1/2 clinical trial drug S-1360. In: Program and Abstracts of the 11th Conference on Retroviruses and Opportunistic Infections, San Francisco, 2004, abstract 632.
13. Hazuda D. The potential for cross resistance between S-1360, L-870810 and other structurally diverse inhibitors of HIV-1 integrase strand transfer. In: Program and Abstracts of the 10th Conference on Retroviruses and Opportunistic Infections, Boston, 2003, abstract 140.
14. Goldgur Y, Dyda F, Hickman AB, et al. Three new structures of the core domain of HIV-1 integrase: an active site that binds magnesium. Proc Natl Acad Sci USA 95:9150–4, 1998.
15. Yoshinaga T, Sato A, Fujishita T, Fujiwara T. S-1360: in vitro activity of a new HIV-1 integrase inhibitor in clinical

development. In: Program and Abstracts of the 9th Conference on Retroviruses and Opportunistic Infections, Seattle, 2002, abstract 8.
16. Fujiwara T, Leese, Lippert, Russel. S-1360, a new HIV integrase inhibitor, repeat-dose pharmacokinetics (PK) and safety in healthy volunteers following oral administration. In: Program and Abstracts of the XIV International Conference of HIV/AIDS, Barcelona, 2002, abstract TuPeB4436.
17. Fikkert V, Hombrouck A, Van Remoortel B, et al. Multiple mutations in human immunodeficiency virus-1 integrase confer resistance to the clinical trial drug S-1360. AIDS 18:2019–28, 2004.
18. Dayam R, Sanchez T, Neamati N. Diketo acid pharmacophore. 2. Discovery of structurally diverse inhibitors of HIV-1 integrase. J Med Chem 48:8009–15, 2005.
19. Little S, Drusano G, Schooley R, et al. Antiretroviral effect of L-000870810, a novel HIV-1 integrase inhibitor, in HIV-1 infected patients. In: Program and Abstracts of the 12th Conference on Retroviruses and Opportunistic Infections, Boston, 2005, abstract 161.
20. Zhuang L, Wai JS, Embrey MW, et al. Design and synthesis of 8-hydroxy-[1,6]naphthyridines as novel inhibitors of HIV-1 integrase in vitro and in infected cells. J Med Chem 46:453–6, 2003.
21. Hazuda DJ, Anthony NJ, Gomez RP, et al. A naphthyridine carboxamide provides evidence for discordant resistance between mechanistically identical inhibitors of HIV-1 integrase. Proc Natl Acad Sci USA 101:11233–8, 2004.
22. Young S; The HIV integrase discovery team. L-870,810: a potent antiviral HIV integrase inhibitor with potential clinical utility. In: Conference Record of the 14th International AIDS Conference, Barcelona, 2002.
23. Hazuda DJ, the MRL HIV-1 drug discovery team. The identification of the active site mutations that confer resistance to structurally diverse inhibitors of HIV-1 integrase strand transfer support a general mechanism of phosphotransferase inhibition. In: Program and Abstracts of the 12th International HIV Drug Resistance Workshop, Los Cabos, Mexico, 2003, abstract 10.
24. Hazuda DJ, Young SD, Guare JP, et al. Integrase inhibitors and cellular immunity suppress retroviral replication in rhesus macaques. Science 305:528–32, 2004.
25. Morales-Ramirez JO, Teppler H, Kovacs C, et al. Antiretroviral effect of MK-0518, a novel HIV-1 integrase inhibitor, in ART-naive HIV-1 infected patients. In: Program and Abstracts of the 10th European AIDS Conference, Dublin, 2005, abstract LBPS1/6.
26. Grinsztejn B, Nguyen BY, Katlama C, et al. Potent antiretroviral effect of MK-0518, a novel HIV-1 integrase inhibitor, in patients with triple-class resistant virus. In: Program and Abstracts of the 13th Conference on Retroviruses and Opportunistic Infections, Denver, 2006, abstract 159LB.
27. Lataillade M, Chiarella J, Kozal MJ. Natural polymorphisms of the HIV-1 integrase gene and mutations associated with integrase inhibitor resistance. In: Program and Abstracts of XV International HIV Drug Resistance Workshop: Basic Principles and Clinical Implications, Sitges, Spain, 2006, abstract 23.
28. Markowitz M, Morales-Ramirez JO, et al. Antiretroviral actvity, pharmacokinetics, and tolerability of MK-0518, a novel inhibitor of HIV-1 integrase, dosed a monotherapy for 10 days in treatment-naive HIV-1-infected individuals. J Acquir Immune Defic Syndr 43:509–15, 2006.
29. Grinsztejn B, Nguyen B-Y, et al. Potent antiretroviral effect of MK-0518, a novel HIV-1 integrase inhibitor, in patients qith triple-class resistant virus.In: Program and Abstracts of the 46th Interscience Conference on Antimicrobial Agents and Chemotherapy, San Francisco, 2006, abstract H-1670b.
30. Cooper DA, Gatell J, Rockstroh J, et al (for the BENCHMRK-1 Study Goup). Results of BENCHMRK-1, a Phase III Study evaluating the efficacy and safety of Raltegravir (MK-0518), a Novel HIV-1 integrase inhibitor, in patients with triple class resistant virus. In: Program and Abstracts of the 14th Conference on Retr oviruses and Opportunistic Infections, Los Angles, abstract 105aLB, 2007.
31. Steigbigel R, Kumar P, Gotuzzo E, et al (for the BENCHMRK-2 Study Group). Results of BENCHMRK-2, a Phase III Study evaluating the efficacy and safety of Raltegravir (MK-0518), a Novel HIV-1 integrase inhibitor, in patients with triple class resistant virus. In: Program and Abstracts of the 14th Conference on Retrov iruses and Opportunistic Infections, Los Angles, abstract 105aLB, 2007.
32. Markowitz1 M, Nguyen2 B-Y, Eron J, et al. Potent antiretroviral effect of MK-0518, a Novel HIV-1 integrase inhibitor, as part of combination ART in treatment -Naive HIV-1 infected patients. In: Program and Abstracts of the XVI International AIDS Conference, Toronto, Canada, 2006, abstract THLB0214.
33. Teppler H, Azrolan N, Chen J, et al. Differential effects of MK-0518 and efavirenz on serum lipids and lipoproteins in antiretroviral therapy (ART)-naive patients (24 weeks results). In: Program and Abstracts of the 46th Interscience Conference on Antimicrobial Agents and Chemotherapy, San Francisco, 2006, abstract H-0256a.
34. Wai J, Fischer T, Embrey M, et al. Next generation inhibitors of HIV-1 integrase strand transfer inhibitor: structural diversity and resistance profiles. In: Program and Abstracts of the 14th Conference on Retroviruses and Opportunistic Infections, Los Angeles, 2007, abstract 87.
35. Mekouar K, Mouscadet JF, Desmaele D, et al. Styrylquinoline derivatives: a new class of potent HIV-1 integrase inhibitors that block HIV-1 replication in CEM cells. J Med Chem 41:2846–57, 1998.
36. Zouhiri F, Mouscadet JF, Mekouar K, et al. Structure–activity relationships and binding mode of styrylquinolines as potent inhibitors of HIV-1 integrase and replication of HIV-1 in cell culture. J Med Chem 43:1533–40, 2000.
37. Deprez E, Barbe S, Kolaski M, et al. Mechanism of HIV-1 integrase inhibition by styrylquinoline derivatives in vitro. Mol Pharmacol 65:85–98, 2004.
38. Mousnier A, Leh H, Mouscadet JF, Dargemont C. Nuclear import of HIV-1 integrase is inhibited in vitro by styrylquinoline derivatives. Mol Pharmacol 66:783–8, 2004.
39. Sato M, Motomura T, Aramaki H, et al. Novel HIV-1 integrase inhibitors derived from quinolone antibiotics. J Med Chem 49:1506–8, 2006.
40. Matsuzaki Y, Watanabe W, Yamataka K, et al. JTK-303/GS 9137, a novel small-molecule inhibitor of HIV-1 integrase: anti-HIV activity profile and pharmacokinetics in animals. In: Program and Abstracts of the 13th Conference on Retroviruses and Opportunistic Infections, Denver, 2006, abstract 508.
41. Kodama E, Shimura K, Sakagami Y, et al. In vitro antiviral activity and resistance profile of a novel HIV integrase inhibitor, JTK-303/GS-9137. In: Program and Abstracts of the 46th Interscience Conference on Antimicrobial Agents and Chemotherapy, San Francisco, 2006, abstract H-254.
42. Jones G, Ledford RM, Yu F, et al. In vitro resistance profile of HIV-1 mutants selected by the HIV-1 integrase inhibitor, GS-9137 (JTK-303). In: Program and Abstracts of the 14th Conference on Retroviruses and Opportunistic Infections, Los Angles, 2007, abstract 627.
43. Kawaguchi I, Ishikawa T, Ishibashi M and et al. Safety and pharmacokinetics of single oral dose of JTK-303/GS 9137, a novel HIV integrase inhibitor, in healthy volunteers. In: Program and Abstracts of the 13th Conference on Retroviruses and Opportunistic Infections, Denver, 2006, abstract 580.

44. DeJesus E, Berger D, Markowitz M, et al. The HIV integrase inhibitor GS-9137 (JTK-303) exhibits potent antiviral activity in treatment-naive and experienced patients. In: Program and Abstracts of the 13th Conference on Retroviruses and Opportunistic Infections, Denver, 2006, abstract 160LB.
45. Zopola AR, Mullen M, Berger D, et al. The integrase inhibitor GS-9137 demonstrates potent antiretroviral activity in treatment-experienced patients. In: Program and Abstracts of the 14th Conference on Retroviruses and Opportunistic Infections, Los Angles, 2007, abstract 143LB.
46. Ramanathan S, Skillington J, Plummer A, et al. Lack of clinically relevant drug–drug interaction between ritonavir-boosted GS-9137(GS-9137/r) and emtricitabine (FTC)/tenofovir desoproxil fumarate (TDF). In: Program and Abstracts of the XVI International AIDS Conference, Toronto, Canada, 2006, abstract TUPE0080.
47. Ramanathan S, Lagan K, Plummer A, et al. Lack of clinically relevant drug–drug interaction between ritonavir-boosted GS-9137 (GS-9137/r) and zidovudine (ZDV). In: Program and Abstracts of the XVI International AIDS Conference, Toronto, Canada, 2006, abstract TUPE0088.
48. Enejosa J; The GS-9137 Clinical Development Team. Clinical development of an HIV-1 integrase inhibitor GS-9137. In: Program and Abstracts of HIV DART 2006: Global Antiviral Journal, vol 2, Suppl 2, abstract 40.
49. Ma L, Hurwitz SJ, Shi J, et al. Pharmacokinetics of the antiviral agent beta-D-2′,3′ -didehydro-2′,3′ -dideoxy-5-fluorocytidine in rhesus monkeys. Antimicrob Agents Chemother 43:381–4, 1999.
50. Schinazi RF, Mellors J, Bazmi H, et al. DPC 817: a cytidine nucleoside analog with activity against zidovudine- and lamivudine-resistant viral variants. Antimicrob Agents Chemother 46:1394–401, 2002.
51. Geleziunas R, Gallagher K, Zhang H, et al. HIV-1 resistance profile of the novel nucleoside reverse transcriptase inhibitor beta-D-2′,3′ -dideoxy-2′,3′ -didehydro-5-fluorocytidine (Reverset). Antivir Chem Chemother 14:49–59, 2003.
52. Stuyver LJ, McBrayer TR, Schurmann D, et al. Potent antiviral effect of Reverset in HIV-1-infected adults following a single oral dose. Antivir Ther (Lond) 9:529–36, 2004.
53. Murphy RL, Schurmann D, Beard A, et al. Potent anti-HIV-1 activity of Reverset following 10 days of monotherapy in treatment-naive individuals. In: Conference Record of the 15th International AIDS Conference, Bangkok, Thailand, 2004, abstract MoOrB1056.
54. Murphy RL, Schurmann D, Levy R, et al. Tolerance and anti-HIV-1 activity of Reverset following 10 days as add-on therapy to current regimens in treatment experienced HIV-infected individuals. In: Program and Abstracts of the 44th Interscience Conference on Antimicrobial Agents and Chemotherapy, Washington DC, 2004, abstract H-1130.
55. Cohen C, Katlama C, Murphy R, et al. Antiretroviral activity and tolerability of Reverset (D-d4FC), a new fluorocytidine nucleoside analog, when used in combination therapy in treatment-experienced patients: results of phase IIb study RVT-203. In: Program and Abstracts of the Third International AIDS Society Conference on HIV Pathogenesis and Treatment, Rio de Janeiro, 2005, abstract WeOaLB103.
56. Erickson-Viitanen S, Wu JT, Shi G, et al. Cellular pharmacology of D-d4FC, a nucleoside analogue active against drug-resistant HIV. Antivir Chem Chemother 14:39–47, 2003.
57. Shi J, McAtee JJ, Schlueter Wirtz S, et al. Synthesis and biological evaluation of 2′,3′ -didehydro-2′,3′ -dideoxy-5-fluorocytidine (D4FC) analogues: discovery of carbocyclic nucleoside triphosphates with potent inhibitory activity against HIV-1 reverse transcriptase. J Med Chem 42:859–67, 1999.
58. Chen SH. Comparative evaluation of L-Fd4C and related nucleoside analogs as promising antiviral agents. Curr Med Chem 9: 899–912, 2002.
59. Lin TS, Luo MZ, Liu MC, et al. Design and synthesis of 2′,3′-dideoxy-2′,3′-didehydro-beta-L-cytidine (beta-L-d4C) and 2′,3′-dideoxy 2′,3′ -didehydro-beta-L-5-fluorocytidine (beta-L-Fd4C), two exceptionally potent inhibitors of human hepatitis B virus (HBV) and potent inhibitors of human immunodeficiency virus (HIV) in vitro. J Med Chem 39:1757–9, 1996.
60. Bridges EG, Dutschman GE, Gullen EA, Cheng YC. Favorable interaction of beta-L (−) nucleoside analogues with clinically approved anti-HIV nucleoside analogues for the treatment of human immunodeficiency virus. Biochem Pharmacol 51:731–6, 1996. Erratum. Biochem Pharmacol 51:1415, 1996.
61. Dunkle LM, Oshana SC, Cheng Y-C, et al. ACH-126,443: a new nucleoside analog with potent activity against wild-type and resistant HIV-1 and a promising pharmacokinetic and mitochondrial safety profile. In: Program and Abstracts of the 8th Conference on Retroviruses and Opportunistic Infections, Chicago, 2001, abstract 303.
62. Fabrycki J, Zhao Y, Wearne J, et al. In vitro induction of HIV variants with reduced susceptibility to elvucitabine (ACH-126,443) & Beta-L-FD4C. Antiviral Therapy 8:S1 (abstract 5), 2003.
63. Dutschman GE, Bridges EG, Liu SH, et al. Metabolism of 2′,3′-dideoxy-2′,3′-didehydro-beta-L (-)-5-fluorocytidine and its activity in combination with clinically approved anti-human immunodeficiency virus beta-D (+) nucleoside analogs in vitro. Antimicrob Agents Chemother 42:1799–804, 1998.
64. Dunkle LM, Gathe JC, Pedevillano DE, et al. Elvucitabine: potent antiviral activity demonstrated in multidrug-resistant HIV infection. Antiviral Therapy 8:S1 (abstract 2), 2003.
65. Stypinski D, Pottage JC, Gustavson LM, et al. Optimization of the therapuetic index of elvucitabine through PK/PD modeling. In: Program and Abstracts of the 5th International Workshop on Clinical Pharmacology of HIV Therapy, Rome, 2004.
66. Colucci P, Pottage J, Robison H, et al. The different clinical pharmacology of elvucitabine (beta-L-Fd4C) enables the drug to be given in a safe and effective manner with innovative dosing regimens. In: Program and Abstracts of the 45th Interscience Conference on Antimicrobial Agents and Chemotherapy, Washington DC, 2005, abstract LB-27.
67. Colucci P, Pottage J, Robison H, et al. Efficacy and novel pharmacology of elvucitabine in a 7 day placebo controlled monotherapy study. In: Program and Abstracts of the 46th Interscience Conference on Antimicrobial Agents and Chemotherapy, San Francisco, 2006, abstract LB-27.
68. Gu Z, Nguyen-Ba N, Ren C, et al. BCH-10618, a new heterosubstituted nucleoside analogue against HIV-1 infection. Antiviral Therapy 6(Suppl 1):1, 2001.
69. Bethell R, Collins P, Holdich T, Sawyer J. In vitro and in vivo antiviral activity of SPD754 against wild-type and NRTI-resistant viruses. In: Conference Record of the 15th Internation AIDS Conference, Bangkok, Thailand, 2004, abstract WePeA5642.
70. Holdich T, Shiveley LA, Sawyer J. A phase I study investigating the plasma and intracellular pharmacokinetics of SPD754 and 3TC when administered alone and in combination. In: Conference Record of the 15th International AIDS Conference, Bangkok, Thailand, 2004, abstract TuPeB4625.
71. Bethell R, Collins P, de Muys J, et al. An in vitro evaluation of the intracellular anabolism of SPD754 and FTC alone and in combination. In: Conference Record of the 15th International AIDS Conference, Bangkok, Thailand, 2004, abstract TuPeB4622.
72. Bethell R, Adams J, De Muys J, et al. Pharmacological evaluation of a dual deoxycytidine analogue combination: 3TC and SPD754. In: Program and Abstracts of the 11th Conference on Retroviruses and Opportunistic Infections, San Francisco, 2004, abstract 138.

73. Francis RJ, Lancois L, Shiveley L, Sawyer J. Pharmacokinetics (PK) of SPD754, a new cytadine analogue in healthy volunteers. In: Conference Record of the 2nd International AIDS Society Conference on HIV Pathogenesis & Treatment, Paris, 2003, abstract 528.
74. Adams J, Sawyer J, Shiveley L. Intracellular SPD754 triphosphate pharmacokinetics following administration of SPD754 capsules. In: Program and Abstracts of the 11th Conference on Retroviruses and Opportunistic Infections, San Francisco, 2004, abstract 599.
75. Smith PF, Forrest A, Adams JM, Ballow CH. Effect of food on the pharmacokinetics of (−) and (+) dOTC when administered as an oral racemate. J Clin Pharmacol 42:658–61, 2002.
76. Cahn P, Lange J, Cassetti I, et al. Anti HIV-1 activity of SPD754 a new NRTI: results of a 10 day monotherapy study in treatment naive HIV patients. In: Conference Record of the 2nd International AIDS Society Conference on HIV Pathogenesis and Treatment, Paris, 2003, abstract LB15.
77. Collins P, Shiveley L, Anderson C, Bethell R. Analysis of the genotypes of viruses isolated from patients after 10 days monotherapy with SPD754. In: Program and Abstracts of the 11th Conference on Retroviruses and Opportunistic Infections, San Francisco, 2004, abstract 526.
78. Cassetti I, Cahn P, Adams J, Brun Y, et al. Slope of viral load decline and steady state pharmacokinetics of SPD754 monotherapy administered once or twice daily in treatment-naive HIV+ individuals. In: Program and Abstracts of the 9th European AIDS Conference, Warsaw, 2003, abstract F11/4.
79. Smith P, Forrest A, et al. Disease-based model prediction of treatment response to apricitabine for viruses with reduced susceptibility. In: Program and Abstracts of the 14th Conference on Retroviruses and Opportunistic Infections, Los Angles, 2007, abstract 558.
80. Locas C, Ching S, Damment S. Safety profile of SPD754 in cynomolgus monkeys treated for 52 weeks. In: Program and Abstracts of the 11th Conference on Retroviruses and Opportunistic Infections, San Francisco, 2004, abstract 527.
81. de Muys JM, Gourdeau H, Nguyen-Ba N, et al. Anti-human immunodeficiency virus type 1 activity, intracellular metabolism, and pharmacokinetic evaluation of 2′-deoxy-3′-oxa-4′-thiocytidine. Antimicrob Agents Chemother 43:1835–44, 1999.
82. Herzmann C, Arasteh K, Murphy RL, et al. Safety, pharmacokinetics, and efficacy of (+/−)-beta-2′,3′-dideoxy-5-fluoro-3′-thiacytidine with efavirenz and stavudine in antiretroviral-naive human immunodeficiency virus-infected patients. Antimicrob Agents Chemother 49:2828–33, 2005.
83. Schinazi RF, McMillan A, Cannon D, et al. Selective inhibition of human immunodeficiency viruses by racemates and enantiomers of cis-5-fluoro-1-[2-(hydroxymethyl)-1, 3-oxathiolan-5-yl]cytosine. Antimicrob Agents Chemother 36:2423–31, 1992.
84. Feng JY, Shi J, Schinazi RF, Anderson KS. Mechanistic studies show that (-)-FTC-TP is a better inhibitor of HIV-1 reverse transcriptase than 3TC-TP. FASEB Journal 13:1511–7, 1999.
85. Richman DD, Morton SC, Wrin T, et al. The prevalence of antiretroviral drug resistance in the United States. AIDS 18:1393–401, 2004.
86. Otto MJ, Arasteh K, Schulbin H, et al. Single and multiple dose pharmacokinetics and safety of the nucleoside racivir in male volunteers. In: Program and Abstracts of Frontiers in Drug Development for Antiretroviral Therapies, HIV DART, Naples, FL, 2002.
87. Otto MJ, Arasteh K, Kreckel P, et al. Sustained anti-HIV-1 effect of racivir combined with D4T and Sustiva following a 14-day treatment of infected volunteers. In: Program and Abstracts of the 10th Conference on Retroviruses and Opportunistic Infections, Boston 2003.
88. Antinori A, Zaccarelli M, Cingolani A, et al. Cross-resistance among nonnucleoside reverse transcriptase inhibitors limits recycling efavirenz after nevirapine failure. AIDS Res Human Retroviruses 18:835–8, 2002;.
89. Pauwels R, Andries K, Desmyter J, et al. Potent and selective inhibition of HIV-1 replication in vitro by a novel series of TIBO derivatives. Nature 343:470–4, 1990.
90. Janssen PA, Lewi PJ, Arnold E, et al. In search of a novel anti-HIV drug: multidisciplinary coordination in the discovery of 4-[[4-[[4-[(1E)-2-cyanoethenyl]-2,6-dimethylphenyl]amino]-2-pyrimidinyl]amino]benzonitrile (R278474, rilpivirine).J Med Chem 48:1901–9, 2005.
91. Andries K, Azijn H, Thielemans T, et al. TMC125, a novel next-generation nonnucleoside reverse transcriptase inhibitor active against nonnucleoside reverse transcriptase inhibitor-resistant human immunodeficiency virus type 1. Antimicrob Agents Chemother 48:4680–6, 2004.
92. Das K, Clark AD Jr, Lewi PJ, et al. Roles of conformational and positional adaptability in structure-based design of TMC125-R165335 (etravirine) and related non-nucleoside reverse transcriptase inhibitors that are highly potent and effective against wild-type and drug-resistant HIV-1 variants. J Med Chem 47:2550–60, 2004.
93. Vingerhoets J, Azijn H, Fransen E, et al. TMC125 displays a high genetic barrier to the development of resistance: evidence from in vitro selection experiments. J Virol 79:12773–82, 2005.
94. Scholler M, HoetelmansR, Beets G, et al. Substantial improvements of oral bioavailability of TMC125 using new tablet formulations in healthy volunteers. In: Conference Record of the 3rd International AIDS Society Conference on HIV Pathogenesis and Treatment, Rio de Janeiro, 2005, abstract TuPe3.1B11.
95. Piscitelli SC, Baede P, Van't Klooster G, Graham N. TMC125 does not alter the lopinavir/ritonavir (LPV/RTV) pharmacokinetics in healthy volunteers. In: Program and Abstracts of the 42nd Interscience Conference on Antimicrobial Agents and Chemotherapy, San Diego, 2002, abstract A-1824.
96. Gruzdev B, Rakhmanova A, Doubovskaya E, et al. A randomized, double-blind, placebo-controlled trial of TMC125 as 7-day monotherapy in antiretroviral naive, HIV-1 infected subjects. AIDS 17:2487–94, 2003.
97. Sankatsing SU, Weverling GJ, Peeters M, et al. TMC125 exerts similar initial antiviral potency as a five-drug, triple class antiretroviral regimen. AIDS 17:2623–7, 2003.
98. Gazzard BG, Pozniak AL, Rosenbaum W, et al. An open-label assessment of ETRAVIRINE – a new, next-generation NNRTI, for 7 days in HIV-1 infected individuals with NNRTI resistance. AIDS 17:F49-54, 2003.
99. Madruga JV, Cahn P, Grinsztejn B, et al. Efficacy and safety of TMC125 (etravirene) in treatment-experienced HIV-1 infected patients in DUET-1: 24 week results from a randomized, double-blind, placebo-controlled trial. Lancet 370:29–38, 2007.
100. Lazzarin A, Campbell T, Clotet B, et al. Efficacy and safety of TMC125 (etravirine) in treatment-experienced HIV-1-infected patients in DUET-2: 24-week results from a randomized, double-blind, placebo-controlled trail. Lancet 370:39–48, 2007.
101. Hirschel B, Pernegar T. TITAN & DUET Studies Commentary. Lancet 370:3–5, 2007.
102. Woodfall B, Montaner J, Domingo p, et al. Safety and tolerability of TMC125 in 3-class-experienced HIV-infected patients: a 24-week preliminary analysis of trial TMC125-C203. In: Program and Abstracts of the 10th European AIDS Conference, Dublin, 2005, abstract LBPS3/7B.
103. Woodfall B, Nadler J, Grossman HA, et al. Efficacy and tolerability of TMC125 in HIV patients with NNRTI and PI resistance at 24 weeks: TMC125-C223. In: Program and Abstracts of the 10th European AIDS Conference, Dublin, 2005, abstract LBPS3/7A.

104. Cohen C, Steinheart CR, et al. Efficacy and safety results at 48 weeks with the novel NNRTI, ETRAVIRINE, and impact of baseline resistance on the virologic response in study TMC125-C223. In: Program and Abstracts of the XVI International AIDS Conference, Toronto, Canada, 2006, abstract TUPE 0061.
105. Vingerhoets J, Peters M, Corbett C, et al. Effect of baseline resistance on the virologic response to a novel NNRTI, ETRAVIRINE, in patients with extensive NNRTI and PI resistance: an analysis of study TMC125-c223. In: Program and Abstracts of the 13th Conference on Retroviruses and Opportunistic Infections, Denver, 2005, abstract 154.
106. Grossman H, Cohen C, Nadler J, et al. Prediction of clinical benefits of TMMC 125 from treatment effects on CD4 counts and HIV RNA. In: Program and Abstracts of the XVI International AIDS Conference, Toronto, Canada, 2006, abstract MOPE 0073.
107. Woodfall B, Vingerhoets J, Peters M, et al. Impact of NNRTI and NRTI resistance on the response to the regimen of ETRAVIRINE plus two NRTIs in study TMC125-C227. In Program and Abstracts of the 8th International Congress on Drug Therapy in HIV Infection, Glasgow, Scotland, 2006, abstract PL5.6.
108. Piscitelli S, Baede P, Graham N, Van't Klooster G. Drug interactions with TMC125, a potent next generation NNRTI. In: Program and Abstracts of the 42nd Interscience Conference on Antimicrobial Agents and Chemotherapy, San Diego, 2002, abstract A-1827.
109. Kakuda TN, Scholler-Gyure M, Woodfall BJ, et al. TMC125 in combination with other medications: summary of drug–drug interactions. In Program and Abstracts of the 8th International Congress on Drug Therapy in HIV Infection, Glasgow, Scotland, 2006, abstract PL5.2.
110. Scholler M, Hoetelmans R, Bollen S, et al. No significant interaction between TMC125 and didanosine (ddI) in healthy volunteers. In: Conference Record of the 3rd International AIDS Society Conference on HIV Pathogenesis and Treatment, Rio de Janeiro, 2005, abstract WePe3.3C16.
111. Harris M, Zala C, Ramirez S, et al. Pharmacokinetics and safety of adding TMC125 to stable regimens of saquinavir, lopinavir, ritonavir, and NRTI in HIV+ adults. In: Program and Abstracts of the 13th Conference on Retroviruses and Opportunistic Infections, Denver, 2006, abstract 575b.
112. Boffito M, Winston A, Fletcher C, et al. Pharmacokinetics and antiretroviral response to TMC114/r and TMC125 combination in patients with high level viral resistance. In: Program and Abstracts of the 13th Conference on Retroviruses and Opportunistic Infections, Denver, 2006, abstract 575c.
113. Scholler M, Kraft M, Hoetelmans R, et al. Significant decrease in TMC125 exposures when co-administered with tipranavir boosted with ritonavir in healthy subjects. In: Program and Abstracts of the 13th Conference on Retroviruses and Opportunistic Infections, Denver, 2006, abstract 583.
114. De Bethune MP, Andries K, Azijn H, et al. TMC278, a new potent NNRTI, with an increased barrier to resistance and good pharmacokinetic profile. In: Program and Abstracts of the 12th Conference on Retroviruses and Opportunistic Infections, Boston, 2005, abstract 556.
115. Goebel F, Yakovlev A, Pozniak A, et al. TMC278: potent anti-HIV activity in antiretroviral therapy-naive patients. In: Program and Abstracts of the 12th Conference on Retroviruses and Opportunistic Infections, Boston, 2005, abstract 160.
116. Pozniak A, Morales-Ramirez J, Mohapi L, et al. 48-week primary analysis of trial TMC278-C204: TMC278 demonstrates potent and sustained efficacy in ARV-naive patients. In: Program and Abstracts of the 14th Conference on Retroviruses and Opportunistic Infections, Los Angles, 2007, abstract 144LB.
117. Hoetelmans R, Van Heeswijk R, Kestens D, et al. Effect of food and multiple-dose pharmacokinetics of TMC278 as an oral tablet formulation. In: Conference Record of the 3rd International AIDS Conference on HIV Pathogenesis and Treatment, Rio de Janeiro, 2005, abstract TuPe3.1B10.
118. Van Heeswijk R, Hoetelmans R, et al. The pharmacokinetic interaction between ketoconazole and TMC278, an investigational NNRTI, in healthy volunteers. In: Program and Abstracts of the XVI International AIDS Conference, Toronto, Canada, 2006, abstract TUPE0087.
119. Hoetelmans R, Kestens D, Stevens M, et al. Pharmacokinetic interactions between the novel non-nucleoside reverse transcriptase inhibitor (NNRTI) TMC278 and tenofovir disoproxil fumarate (TDF) in healthy volunteers. In: Conference Record of the 3rd International AIDS Society Conference on HIV Pathogenesis and Treatment, Rio de Janeiro, 2005, abstract WePe3.3C15.
120. Wyatt PG, Bethell RC, Cammack N, et al. Benzophenone derivatives: a novel series of potent and selective inhibitors of human immunodeficiency virus type 1 reverse transcriptase. J Med Chem 38:1657–65, 1995.
121. Chan JH, Freeman GA, Tidwell JH, et al. Novel benzophenones as non-nucleoside reverse transcriptase inhibitors of HIV-1. J Med Chem 47:1175–82, 2004.
122. Schaller LT, Burnette T, Cowan J, et al. Prodrug strategies to deliver novel HIV-1 non-nucleoside reverse transcriptase inhibitors (NNRTIs) GW8248 and GW8635. In: Programs and Abstracts of the 43rd Interscience Conference on Antimicrobial Agents and Chemotherapy, Chicago, 2003, abstract H-872.
123. Roberts G, Porter D, Boone L, et al. Kinetic and Thermodynamic parameters for binding of the non-nucleoside inhibitors 678248 and 695634 to wild type and 12 mutants of HIV-1 reverse transcriptase. In: Program and Abstracts of the 11th Conference on Retroviruses and Opportunistic Infections, San Francisco, 2004, abstract 529.
124. Ferris RG, Hazen RJ, Roberts GB, et al. Antiviral activity of GW678248, a novel benzophenone nonnucleoside reverse transcriptase inhibitor. Antimicrob Agents Chemother 49:4046–51, 2005.
125. Hazen RJ, Harvey RJ, St Clair MH, et al. Anti-human immunodeficiency virus type 1 activity of the nonnucleoside reverse transcriptase inhibitor GW678248 in combination with other antiretrovirals against clinical isolate viruses and in vitro selection for resistance. Antimicrob Agents Chemother 49:4465–73, 2005.
126. Denning J, Kim J, Sanderson B, et al. A double-blind, parallel, randomized, placebo-controlled, single ascending dose study to investigate 695634X and 678248X safety, tolerability and pharmacokinetics following oral administration of 695634G to healthy male subjects (NN210001). In: Conference Record of the 15th International AIDS Conference, Bangkok, 2004, abstract TuPeB4480.
127. Becker S, Lalezari J, Walworth C, et al. Antiviral activity and safety of GW695634, a novel next generation NNRTI, in NNRTI-resistant HIV-1 infected patients. In: Conference Record of the 3rd International AIDS Society Conference on HIV Pathogenesis and Treatment, Rio de Janeiro, 2005, abstract WePe6.2C03.
128. Castagna A, Biswas P, Beretta A, Lazzarin A. The appealing story of HIV entry inhibitors: from discovery of biological mechanisms to drug development. Drugs 65:879–904, 2005.
129. Schooley RT, Merigan TC, Gaut P, et al. Recombinant soluble CD4 therapy in patients with the acquired immunodeficiency syndrome (AIDS) and AIDS-related complex. A phase I-II escalating dosage trial [see comment]. Ann Intern Med 112:247–53, 1990.
130. Daar ES, Li XL, Moudgil T, Ho DD. High concentrations of recombinant soluble CD4 are required to neutralize primary human immunodeficiency virus type 1 isolates. Proc Natl Acad Sci USA 87:6574–8, 1990.

131. Zhu P, Olson WC, Roux KH. Structural flexibility and functional valence of the CD4-IgG2 (Pro 542): potential for cross-linking human immunodeficiency virus type 1 envelope spikes. J Virol 75:6682–86, 2001.
132. Trkola A, Pomales AB, Yuan H, et al. Cross-clade neutralization of primary isolates of human immunodeficiency virus type 1 by human monoclonal antibodies and tetrameric CD4-IgG. J Virol 69:6609–17, 1995.
133. Trkola A, Ketas T, Kewalramani VN, et al. Neutralization sensitivity of human immunodeficiency virus type 1 primary isolates to antibodies and CD4-based reagents is independent of coreceptor usage. J Virol 72:1876–85, 1998.
134. Hu Q, Frank I, Williams V, et al. Blockade of attachment and fusion receptors inhibits HIV-1 infection of human cervical tissue. J Exp Med199:1065–75, 2004.
135. Franti M, O'Neil TO, Maddon P, et al. PRO 542 (CD4-IgG2) has a profound Impact on HIV-1 Replication in the Hu-PBL-SCID mouse model. In: Program and Abstracts of the 9th Conference on Retroviruses and Opportunistic Infections, Seattle, 2002, abstract 401.
136. Nagashima KA, Thompson DA, Rosenfield SI, et al: Human immunodeficiency virus type 1 entry inhibitors PRO 542 and T-20 are potently synergistic in blocking virus-cell and cell-cell fusion. J Infect Dis 183:1121–5, 2001.
137. Jacobson JM, Lowy I, Fletcher CV, et al. Single-dose safety, pharmacology, and antiviral activity of the human immunodeficiency virus (HIV) type 1 entry inhibitor PRO 542 in HIV-infected adults. J Infect Dis 182:326–9, 2000.
138. Jacobson JM, Israel RJ, Lowy I, et al. Treatment of advanced human immunodeficiency virus type 1 disease with the viral entry inhibitor PRO 542. Antimicrob Agents Chemother 48:423-9, 2004.
139. Shearer WT, Israel RJ, Starr S, et al. Recombinant CD4-IgG2 in human immunodeficiency virus type 1-infected children: phase 1/2 study. The Pediatric AIDS Clinical Trials Group Protocol 351 Study Team. J Infect Dis 182:1774–9, 2000.
140. Prakash K, Zhao L, Fisch D, et al. Subcutaneous and intramuscular doseage forms of the HIV-1 entry inhibitor PRO 542. In: Program and Abstracts of the 41st Annual Meeting of IDSA, San Diego, 2003, abstract 648.
141. Shearer W, DeVille J, Sampson P, et al. Non-linear pharmacokinetics of high-dose recombinant fusion protein CD4-IgG2 observed in HIV-1 infected children. In: Program and Abstracts of the 14th Conference on Retroviruses and Opportunistic Infections, Los Angles, 2007, abstract 721
142. Moore JP, Kitchen SG, Pugach P, Zack JA. The CCR5 and CXCR4 coreceptors – central to understanding the transmission and pathogenesis of human immunodeficiency virus type 1 infection.. AIDS Res Hum Retroviruses 20:111–26, 2004.
143. Haubrich R, DeMasi R, Thommes J. Improved virologic response in three-class experienced patients when an active boosted protease inhibitor is combined with enfuvirtide (ENF). In: Program and Abstracts of the 43rd Meeting of the Infectious Disease Society of America, San Francisco, 2005, abstract 785.
144. Godofsky E, Zhang X, Sorensen M, et al. In vitro antiretroviral activity of the humanized anti-CD4 monoclonal antibody, TNX-355, against CCR5, CXCR4, and dual-tropic isolates and synergy with enfuviritide. In: Program and Abstracts of the 45th Interscience Conference on Antimicrobial Agents and Chemotherapy, Washington DC, 2005, abstract LB-26/Y.
145. Weinheimer S, D'arigo K, Fung M, et al. TNX-355 is active against enfuvirtide resistant HIV. In: Program and Abstracts of the XVI International AIDS Conference, Toronto, Canada, 2006, abstract THPE 0024.
146. Boon L, Holland B, Gordon W, et al. Development of anti-CD4 MAb hu5A8 for treatment of HIV-1 infection: preclinical assessment in non-human primates. Toxicology 172:191–203, 2002.
147. Kuritzkes DR, Jacobson JM, Powderly W, et al. Safety and preclinical anti-HIV activity of an anti-CD4 mAB (TNX-355; formerly Hu5A8) in HIV-infected patients. In: 10th Conference on Retroviruses and Opportunistic Infections, Boston, 2003, abstract 13.
148. Kuritzkes DR, Jacobson J, Powderly WG, et al. Antiretroviral activity of the anti-CD4 monoclonal antibody TNX-355 in patients infected with HIV type 1. J Infect Dis 189:286–91, 2004.
149. Jacobson JM, Kuritzkes DR, Godofsky E, et al. Phase 1b study of the anti-CD4 monoclonal antibody TNX-355 in HIV-1-infected subjects:safety and antiretroviral activity of multiple doses. In: Program and Abstracts of the 11th Conference on Retroviruses and Opportunistic Infections, San Francisco, 2004, abstract 536.
150. Norris D, Morales J, Gathe J, et al. TNX-355 in combination with optimized background regimen (OBR) exhibits greater antiviral activity then OBR alone in HIV-treatent experieinced patients. In: Program and Abstracts of the 45th Interscience Conference on Antimicrobial Agents and Chemotherapy, Washington DC, 2005, abstract LB2-26/BC.
151. Davison DK, Medinas RJ, Mosier SM, et al. New fusion inhibitor peptides, TRI-999 and TRI-1144, are potent inhibitors of enfuvirtide and T-1249 resistant isolates. In: Program and Abstracts of the XVI International AIDS Conference, Toronto, Canada, 2006, abstract THPE 0021.
152. Lin PF, Ho H, Fan L, Mosier SM, et al. Inhibition mechanism of small-molecule HIV-1 attachment inhibitors. In: Program and Abstracts of the 12th Conference on Retroviruses and opportunistic infections, Boston, 2005, abstract 544.
153. Lin PF, Ho HT, Gong YF, et al. Characterization of a small molecule HIV-1 attachment inhibitor BMS-488043: virology, resistance and mechanism of action. In: Program and Abstracts of the 11th Conference on Retroviruses and opportunistic infections, San Francisco, 2004, abstract 534.
154. Hanna G, YanJ-H, Fiske W, et al. Safety, tolerability, and pharmacokinetics of a novel, small-molecule HIV-1 attachment inhibitor, BMS-488043, after single and multiple oral doses in healthy subjects. In Program and Abstracts of the 11th Conference on Retroviruses and opportunistic infections, San Francisco, 2004.
155. Hanna G, Lalezari J, Hellinger J, et al. Antiviral activity, safety, and tolerability of a novel, oral small-molecule HIV-1 attachement inhibitor, BMS-488043, in HIV-1-infected subjects. In: Program and Abstracts of the 11th Conference on Retroviruses and Opportunistic Infections, San Francisco, 2004.
156. Cocchi F, DeVico AL, Garzino-Demo A, et al. Identification of RANTES, MIP-1 alpha, and MIP-1 beta as the major HIV-suppressive factors produced by CD8+ T cells.. Science 270:1811–5, 1995.
157. Feng Y, Broder CC, Kennedy PE, Berger EA. HIV-1 entry cofactor: functional cDNA cloning of a seven-transmembrane, G protein-coupled receptor. Science 272:872–7, 1996.
158. Dragic T, Litwin V, Allaway GP, et al. HIV-1 entry into CD4+ cells is mediated by the chemokine receptor CC-CKR-5. Nature 381:667–73, 1996.
159. Liu R, Paxton WA, Choe S, et al. Homozygous defect in HIV-1 coreceptor accounts for resistance of some multiply-exposed individuals to HIV-1 infection. Cell 86:367–77, 1996.
160. Matthews T, Salgo M, Greenberg M, et al. Enfuvirtide: the first therapy to inhibit the entry of HIV-1 into host CD4 lymphocytes.. Nat Rev.Drug Discov 3:215–25, 2004.
161. Greenberg ML, Davison D, Jin L, et al. In vitro antiviral activity of T-1249, a second generation fusion inhibitor. Antiviral Therapy 7(Suppl 1):S10, 2002.
162. Eron JJ, Gulick RM, Bartlett JA, et al. Short-term safety and antiretroviral activity of T-1249, a second-generation fusion inhibitor of HIV. J Infect Dis 189:1075–83, 2004.

163. Lalezari J, Thompson M, Kumar P, et al. Antiviral activity and safety of 873140, a novel CCR5 antagonist, during short-term monotherapy in HIV-infected adults. AIDS 19:1443–8, 2005.
164. Delmedico M, Bray B, Cammack N, et al. Next generation HIV peptide fusion inhibitor candidates achieve potent, durable suppression of virus replication in vitro and improved pharmacokinetic properties. In: Program and Abstracts of the 13th Conference on Retroviruses and Opportunistic Infections, Denver, 2006, abstract 48.
165. Hazen R, St Clair M, Hanlon M, et al. GW0385. a broad spectrum, ultrapotent inhibitor of wild-type and protease-inhibitor-resistant HIV-1. In: Conference Record of the 2nd International AIDS Society Conference on HIV Pathogenesis and Treatment, Paris, 2003, abstract 541.
166. Yates P, Elston R, Tisdale M, Craig C. Genotypic and phenotypic analysis of GW640385: an assessment of the effects of specified resistance mutations alone or in combination with others in a survey of 50 viruses from protease inhibitor (PI)-experienced patients. In: Program and Abstracts of the 10th European AIDS Conference, Dublin, 2005, abstract PE3.3/3.
167. Florance A, Elston R, Johnson M, et al. Phenotypic and genotypic resistance to a new protease inhibitor, GW640385, in HIV-1 virus samples from subjects failing amprenavir. In: Program and Abstracts of the XIII International HIV Drug Resistance Workshop, Canary Islands, Spain, 2004, abstract 11.
168. Yates P, Hazen R, St Clair M, et al. In vitro selection and characterization of resistance to the new HIV protease inhibitor GW640385. In: Program and Abstracts of the XIII International Drug Resistance Workshop, Canary Islands, Spain, 2004, abstract 12.
169. Shelton MJ, Ford S, Anderson MT, et al. Overview of drug interactions between brecanavir (BCV) and other HIV protease inhibitors (PIs). In: Program and Abstracts of the XVI International AIDS Conference, Toronto, Canada, 2006, abstract TUAB105.
170. Reddy S, Ford SL, Stein DS, et al. Single-dose safety and pharmacokinetics (PK) of GW640385X [385]: an HIV-1 protease inhibitor (PI). In: Program and Abstracts of the 43rd Interscience Conference on Antimicrobial Agents and Chemotherapy, Chicago, 2003, abstract A-1800.
171. Ford S, Reddy S, Anderson M, et al. 640385, a novel HIV-1 protease inhibitor (PI): safety and pharmacokinetics (PK) of 640385 following repeat administration with and without ritonavir (RTV) in healthy subjects. In: Program and Abstracts of the 12th Conference on Retroviruses and Opportunistic Infections, Boston, 2005, abstract 563.
172. Ward D, Lalezari J, Thompson M, et al. Preliminary antiviral activity and safety of 640385/ritonavir in HIV-infected patients (study HPR10006): an 8-week analysis. In: Program and Abstracts of the 45th Interscience Conference on Antimicrobial Agents and Chemotherapy, Washington DC, 2005, abstract H-412.
173. Ward D, Lazezari J, Thomson P, et al. Preliminary antiviral activity and safety of brecanavir/ritonavir (BCV/r) in HIV-infected patients (study HPR10006); a 24 week interim analysis. In: Program and Abstracts of the XVI International AIDS Conference, Toronto, Canada, 2006, abstract CDB0376.
174. Fujioka T, Kashiwada Y, Kilkuskie RE, et al. Anti-AIDS agents, 11. Betulinic acid and platanic acid as anti-HIV principles from Syzigium claviflorum, and the anti-HIV activity of structurally related triterpenoids. J Nat Prod 57:243–7, 1994.
175. Kashiwada Y, Hashimoto F, Cosentino LM, et al. Betulinic acid and dihydrobetulinic acid derivatives as potent anti-HIV agents. J Med Chem 39:1016–7, 1996.
176. Wild CT, Kilgore NR, Reddick MS, et al. In vitro and in vivo pre-clinical analyses of PA-457, a novel betulinic acid derivative that potently inhibits HIV-1 replication. In: Conference Record of the 14th International AIDS Conference, Barcelona, 2002, abstract MoPeA3030.
177. Beatty G, Lalezari J, Eron J, et al. Safety and antiviral activity of PA-457, the first-in-class maturation inhibitor, in a 10-day monotherapy study in HIV-1 infected patients. In: Program and Abstracts of the 45th Interscience Conference on Antimicrobial Agents and Chemotherapy, Washington DC, 2005, abstract H-416d.
178. Li F, Goila-Gaur R, Salzwedel K, et al. PA-457: a potent HIV inhibitor that disrupts core condensation by targeting a late step in Gag processing. Proc Natl Acad Sci USA 100:13555–60, 2003.
179. Li F, Zoumplis D, Matallana C, et al. The determinants of activity of the HIV-1 maturation inhibitor PA-457 map to residues flanking the gag CA-SP1 cleavage site. In: Program and Abstracts of the 12th Conference on Retroviruses and Opportunistic Infections, Boston, 2005, abstract 256.
180. Salzwedel K, Goila-Gaur R, Adamson C, et al. Selection and characterization of HIV-1 isolates resistant to the maturation inhibitor PA-457. In: Conference Record of the 15th International AIDS Conference, Bangkok, 2004, abstract WeOrA1276.
181. Adamson C, Salzwedel K, Castillo A, et al. Viral resistance to PA-457, a novel inhibitor of HIV-1 maturation. In: Program and Abstracts of the 13th Conference on Retroviruses and Opportunisitic Infections, Denver, 2006, abstract 156.
182. Kilgore N, Reddick M, Zuiderhof M, et al. The first-in-class maturation inhibitor, PA-457, is a potent inhibitor of HIV-1 drug-resistant isolates and acts synergistically with approved HIV drugs in vitro. In: Program and Abstracts of the 13th Conference on Retroviruses and Opportunistic Infections, Denver, 2006, abstract 509.
183. Martin DE, Ballow C, Doto J, et al. The safety, tolerability and pharmacokinetics of multiple oral doses of PA-457, a first-in-class HIV maturation inhibitor, in healthy volunteers. In: Program and Abstracts of the 12th Conference on Retroviruses and Opportunistic Infections, Boston, 2005, abstract 551.
184. Martin D, Jacobson J, Shurmann D, et al. PA-457, the first-in-class maturation inhibitor, exhibits antiviral activity following single oral dose in HIV-1-infected patients. In: Program and Abstracts of the 12th Conference on Retroviruses and Opportunistic Infections, Boston, 2005, abstract 159.
185. Smith P, Forrest A, Beatty G, et al. Pharmacokinetics/pharmacodynamics of PA-457 in a 10-day multiple dose monotherapy trial in HIV-infected patients. In: Program and Abstracts of the 13th Conference on Retroviruses and Opportunisitic Infections, Denver, 2006, abstract 52.
186. Castillo A, Adamson C, Doto J, et al. Genotypic analysis of the gag CA-SP1 cleavage site in patients receiving the maturation inhibitor bevirimat (PA-457). In: Program and Abstracts of XV International HIV Drug Resistance Workshop: Basic Principles and Clinical Implications, Sitges, Spain, 2006, abstract 32.
187. Martin DE, Smith P, Wild T, Allaway GP. In vitro and in vivo disposition of PA-457, a novel inhibitor of HIV-1 maturation. In: Conference Record of the 15th International AIDS Conference, Bangkok, 2004, abstract WePeA5644.
188. Martin DE, Gailbrath H, Schettler J, et al. Lack of PK/PD interaction between bevirimat (PA-457) and atazanvir (ATV) in healthy volunteers. In: Program and Abstracts of the 46th Interscience Conference on Antimicrobial Agents and Chemotherapy, San Francisco 2006: Abstract A-377
189. Martin D, Alexander T, Bollinger J, et al. PA-457, a first-in-class maturation inhibitor, is non-teratogenic in rats and rabbits a 24 week interim analysis. In: Program and Abstracts of the XVI International AIDS Conference, Toronto, Canada, 2006, abstract CDA0140.
190. Haas DW. Pharmacogenomics and HIV therapeutics [comment]. J Infect Dis 191:1397–400, 2005.

191. Carr A. Toxicity of antiretroviral therapy and implications for drug development. Nat Rev Drug Discov 2:624–34, 2003.
192. Wienkers LC, Heath TG. Predicting in vivo drug interactions from in vitro drug discovery data. Nat Rev Drug Discov 4:825–33, 2005.
193. Jochmans D, Kesteleyn B, Marchland B, et al. Identification and biochemical characterization of a new class of HIV inhibitors: nucleotide-competing reverse transcriptase inhibitors. In: Program and Abstracts of the 12th Conference on Retroviruses and Opportunistic Infections, Boston, 2005, abstract 156.
194. Cigler P, Kozisek M, Rezacova P, et al. From nonpeptide toward noncarbon protease inhibitors: metallacarboranes as specific and potent inhibitors of HIV protease. Proc Natl Acad Sci USA 102:15394–9, 2005.
195. Bennasser Y, Le SY, Benkirane M, Jeang KT. Evidence that HIV-1 encodes an siRNA and a suppressor of RNA silencing. Immunity 22:607–19, 2005. Erratum. Immunity 22:773, 2005.
196. Pham HM, Arganaraz ER, Groschel B, et al. Lentiviral vectors interfering with virus-induced CD4 down-modulation potently block human immunodeficiency virus type 1 replication in primary lymphocytes. J Virol 78:13072–81, 2004.
197. Schafer E, Wagner M, Ayyavoo V. Antiviral effects of mifepristone and its analogs on HIV-1 Vpr-induced virus replication. In: Program and Abstracts of the 11th Conference on Retroviruses and Opportunistic Infections, San Francisco, 2004, abstract 544.
198. Baker TJ, Luedtke NW, Tor Y, Goodman M. Synthesis and anti-HIV activity of guanidinoglycosides. J Org Chem 65:9054–8, 2000.
199. Goebel FD, Hemmer R, Schmit JC, et al. Phase I/II dose escalation and randomized withdrawal study with add-on azodicarbonamide in patients failing on current antiretroviral therapy. AIDS 15:33–45, 2001.
200. Chiu YL, Soros VB, Kreisberg JF, et al. Cellular APOBEC3G restricts HIV-1 infection in resting CD4+ T cells. Nature 435:108–14, 2005.
201. Huthoff H, Malim MH. Cytidine deamination and resistance to retroviral infection: towards a structural understanding of the APOBEC proteins. Virology 334:147–53, 2005.
202. Ylisastigui L, Archin NM, Lehrman G, et al. Coaxing HIV-1 from resting CD4 T cells: histone deacetylase inhibition allows latent viral expression. AIDS 18:1101–8, 2004.
203. Lehrman G, Hogue IB, Palmer S, et al. Depletion of latent HIV-1 infection in vivo: a proof-of-concept study. Lancet 366:549–55, 2005.
204. Siliciano JD, Lai J, Callender M, et al. Stability of the latent reservior for HIV-1 in patients receiving valproic acid. J Infect Dis 195:833–36, 2007.

Chapter 28

HIV Resistance Testing in Clinical Practice

Charles A. B. Boucher, MD, PhD, Andrew R. Zolopa, MD, Richard T. D'Aquila, MD

INTRODUCTION

During the last decade our understanding of both the biology and the clinical relevance of human immunodeficiency virus (HIV) drug resistance has increased exponentially. There is now evidence that emergence of drug resistance to the initial highly active antiretroviral therapy (HAART) regimen is associated with an increased risk of death.[1] If drug resistance emerges to all three major drug classes (nucleoside reverse transcriptase inhibitors, non-nucleoside reverse transcriptase inhibitors (NNRTIs) and protease inhibitors (PIs)), the risk of death is substantially increased.[2]

Resistance testing is a laboratory tool that clinicians often use when making decisions about initial drug regimens, and usually use when choosing salvage regimens. In order to use resistance testing effectively in clinical practice, clinicians must understand the biology of resistance, the strengths and weaknesses of each assay, and the clinical implications of the results. Because new resistance mutations evolve, clinicians must be adept at using web-based information systems that are updated frequently.

BIOLOGY OF DRUG RESISTANCE

Evolution of Drug Resistant Viruses

In the past it was generally believed that drug resistance was an unavoidable consequence of antiretroviral (ARV) therapy.[3] This assumption was based on the knowledge that HIV replication is error prone (roughly one transcription error per every 4 Kb of transcribed cDNA), the lack of transcription proofreading enzymes, and the production of billions of viral particles every day (*see* Chapter 4). Thus, all infected individuals have potential to quickly develop an extremely heterogeneous viral population with a seemingly unlimited number of variants. As a consequence, all possible resistance patterns theoretically exist as subpopulations in untreated patients. Exposure to ARV pressure, therefore, has potential to select for the preexisting resistant subpopulation. This concept was derived from modeling based on HIV variability in initial treatment studies using suboptimal regimens such as single or double nucleoside combinations.

Mutations that confer resistance are designated in a shorthand format. The HIV gene is indicated first (for instance PR for protease), followed by a single letter abbreviation for the wild-type amino acid present at a particular location in a protein and encoded by a particular triplet of nucleotides, or codon (for instance L for leucine). The number of the amino acid/codon follows (for instance, 90). The single letter code for the new, mutant amino acid that has replaced the wild-type amino acid is given next (for instance M for methionine). The designation PR L90M, thus, indicates that the wild-type amino acid leucine at position 90 of the protease gene has been replaced with a methionine.

Mutations readily occur in HIV when patients are treated with HAART regimens that are not optimally suppressive. However, the resulting drug-resistant viruses do not necessarily have equal replicative capacity (RC) *in vitro* when compared to wild-type virus. Thus, resistant virus may not overtake wild-type virus, allowing some resistant viruses to remain as minority variants. This suggests that, in such settings, retaining drug therapy even when viral load value is above 50 copies/μL may be beneficial since the resistant virus may never achieve the viral loads that would be encountered if the wild-type repopulates as the dominant species. The less fit virus populations result in viral load values that are significantly below the pretherapy baseline level created by wild-type virus. An example of this phenomenon is the emergence of the M184V-resistant mutant selected by lamivudine monotherapy. Once this mutation appears in the viral population while patients are on lamivudine monotherapy, the HIV RNA level rebounds toward baseline but remains 0.6–0.8 log below pretherapy levels. This phenomenon of partial suppression is best explained by the classical Darwinian principle of survival of the fittest. Drug-resistant variants, preexisting as minority species owing to a reduced replicative capacity compared to wild-type virus, become dominant under conditions of drug selection pressure while the wild-type virus is suppressed by the antiviral regimen. Thus, the less fit virus predominates during therapy, but might not attain the same level of replicative success as the wild-type virus.

The risk of continuing a partially suppressive ARV regimen is the continued accumulation of additional mutations over time. As further resistance conferring mutations and compensatory mutations (i.e., those that allow the virus to compensate for the presence of the resistance conferring mutation), the replicative capacity of these variants ultimately increase leading to outgrowth of more fit viruses. Thus, poorly replicating resistant viruses can convert into viruses with higher replicative capacity that eventually can attain the original baseline.

HAART and the Genetic Barrier Principle

Clinical experience over the last decade has shown that HAART can suppress viral load to levels <50 copies/μL for many years if adherence is adequate and the original virus is susceptible to the drug regimen used. Several studies suggest that in the majority of these patients, even with very sensitive techniques, no resistant viruses can be detected and no evidence of ongoing viral evolution occurs during long periods of therapy. In these patients, there are two possible explanations for what is being observed: (1) virus is completely suppressed, or (2) resistant virus is being generated in occult reservoirs that are not being measured. The latter scenario seems less likely, however, since resistant virus should spill over from those reservoirs into the circulation and spread to other sites.

The number of mutations required to produce detectable resistance to a drug or a regimen is defined as the genetic barrier. For many drugs, such as the original NNRTI drugs or lamivudine, the genetic barrier is one to two mutations. As a consequence, the development of resistant variants occurred rapidly when these drugs were used by themselves (monotherapy) or with only one additional agent (dual therapy). Therefore, the combination of less than complete suppression of viral replication and a low genetic barrier leads to virologic failure with rapid emergence of resistant virus.

With other drugs with a higher genetic barrier, more mutations (typically three or more) are usually required to produce clinically detectable breakthrough. When these drugs are used in a typical three-drug combination, breakthrough does not occur readily, suggesting that viruses with sufficient mutations to lead to breakthrough do not ordinarily preexist in these patients. However, if viruses with one or two mutations are acquired at the time of initial transmission, or if such mutations develop due to poor adherence, further mutations can occur that will lead to regimen failure. The presence of preexisting resistance mutations, in essence, lowers the genetic barrier at the outset resulting in higher rates of regimen failure. This is also the reason why second-line, third-line, and subsequent regimens do not work as well as initial regimens and require more potent agents or those with novel mechanisms of action to more reliably achieve undetectable levels of HIV RNA.

Because regimen failure occurs more readily if the viral isolate has preexisting resistance mutations, most guidelines recommend the use of resistance testing prior to initial therapy and prior to any change in therapy. Similarly, multidrug regimens are universally recommended to create a higher genetic barrier and more completely suppress viral replication in order to prevent resistance and help assure long-term virologic success.

Resistance Mechanisms

Mutations in reverse transcriptase and protease genes produce reduced drug susceptibility through several different mechanisms. Substitutions in the amino acid sequence of binding proteins can lead to reduced binding of drug to the target protein. Such mutations can cause cross-resistance to other drugs in the class, as is observed with nucleoside and nucleotide reverse transcriptase inhibitors (NRTIs), NNRTIs, PIs, and fusion inhibitors.

Other more complex mechanisms also exist. Several common resistance-conferring mutations to NRTI agents can improve the enzymatic efficiency of the reverse transcriptase (RT)[4,5] enzyme, thereby enabling the RT to more efficiently remove the terminal nucleoside triphosphate incorporated into a growing DNA strand (excision).[6,7] In other words, the RT enzyme with the resistance-conferring mutations more efficiently “throws out” any unnatural nucleoside, i.e., the drug. This mechanism results in resistance to a broad number of nucleoside agents. An example of this type of resistance mechanism is the development of the K65R mutation.

Novel mechanisms leading to resistance to PI drugs have been identified. Changes in the PI substrate, e.g., the cleavage site, can lead to resistance to the PIs in the absence of changes in the protease itself.[8] The clinical importance of this mutation is under investigation.

Mutational Patterns and Hypersusceptibility

For most drugs, the development of resistance occurs through accumulation of mutations that lead to progressively reduced drug susceptibility. The mutations have an additive or synergistic resistance effect.[9] Generally the chance of cross-resistance to other drugs in the same class increases as the number of mutations grows.

"Thymidine-associated mutations", or TAMs pathways, are the best described pattern of mutation accumulation relevant to the thymidine analog nucleoside drugs. The most common TAMs are M41L, D67N, K70R, T215Y/F, L210W, and K219Q/E. These TAMs confer resistance not only to the drugs that select for them (zidovudine and stavudine) but also confer cross resistance to most other NRTIs, such as didanosine, tenofovir, and abacavir. Cross resistance to TAMs is critically dependent on the number of mutations. The more TAMs, the more resistance there is to more nucleoside drugs.

While more mutations usually result in more resistance, there are some exceptions to this rule. When M184V is selected by lamivudine or emtricitabine, or when Y181C is selected by the NNRTIs, or L74V selected by didanosine, the virus becomes more susceptible *in vitro* to zidovudine and stavudine. This "hypersensitization" effect is seen both when these mutations are introduced in wild-type virus and when they occur in the presence of one or more TAMs. Similarly, the M184V mutation often results in hypersusceptibility of the virus to NNRTI agents.

RESISTANCE TESTING

Two types of resistance tests are currently available. The genotypic approach looks directly for mutations. The phenotypic approach determines changes in drug sensitivity of viral constructs *in vitro*. Each technology has strengths and limitations.

For genotype testing, the most frequently used approach in assessing for resistance is population sequencing. Two tests have been approved by the FDA and the European CE Notification Body: Trugene HIV-1 genotyping assay (Bayer Healthcare, Tarrytown, NY, USA) and Viroseq genotyping assay (Abbott Laboratories, Chicago, IL, USA). The availability of FDA-approved genotype kits makes testing feasible in local and regional laboratories. Some laboratories are still using their own unique ("home-brew") assays that are not FDA approved. Less is known about the accuracy or reproducibility of such assays.

The most frequently used phenotypic assays are the Virco Vircotype (Brussels, Belgium) and the Monogram Biosciences Phenosense assay (South San Francisco, California). Several other phenotypic assays are being performed on a smaller scale in research laboratories. All of these assays are based on the creation of recombinant virus through polymerase chain reaction (PCR) amplification of the relevant viral genes from patient viruses and shuttling them into a reference virus lacking those particular genes. This approach is referred to as the recombinant virus approach. Phenotypic tests are not likely to be performed in local laboratories because of the requirement of using live virus and the associated biohazards. To safely use such virus the laboratory must have extensive expertise and sophisticated, expensive technology that is difficult to scale-up to high capacity with sufficient accuracy and reproducibility.

Currently both phenotypic and genotypic assays focus on four specific genes: protease, reverse transcriptase, integrase, and gp41 (for fusion inhibitors). Tropism assays employ phenotype-like technology using gp 120 genes. In order to perform either assay, the gene of interest must be PCR amplified first.

Amplifying the Gene of Interest

Amplification of the gene currently utilizes PCR and employs primers from highly conserved regions of the virus that anneal to sequences in the viral genome. As part of the PCR the viral RNA is transcribed into DNA in high copy number to allow sequencing (genotype) or shuttling into a recombinant expression vector (phenotype). Therefore, for each technology, the testing evaluates a representative sample of the population of circulating virus from the patient at the time the specimen was obtained. As a result, minor variants may not be detected. Adequate levels of virus must be present to be sampled (>500–1000 copies/mL of HIV RNA) in order to generate a result. For the test to be clinically useful, the patient must be taking their current regimen to accurately assess the resistance pattern, owing to the high rate of viral production and rapid overgrowth (within days) of wild-type virus once drug therapy is discontinued.

GENOTYPIC ASSAYS

Genotype assays detect changes in the cDNA sequence of the targeted HIV genes. The coding regions of genes are organized into nucleotide triplets, or codons. Each codon encodes a single amino acid of the gene product (protein). Genotypic tests indirectly measure resistance by detecting mutations in the HIV-1 genome that lead to one or more specific amino acid substitutions in proteins. The specific changes in the protein may or may not cause drug resistance. If the mutated virus has reduced susceptibility to the drug, then administration of the drug will suppress wild-type virus and select for the resistant strains. Some mutations result in "silent mutations", which are nucleic acid changes that do not alter the amino acid sequence because of the redundancy of the genetic code. While some amino acid changes result in reduction of susceptibility, others may lead to, in hypersusceptiblity, as noted above.

Specific mutations known to be associated with altered activity of a specific drug are sought in genotypic assays. These changes have been previously associated with drug resistance or hypersusceptibility. In most cases the mutations appear when virus escapes under selective pressure following exposure to that drug. Introduction of these mutations into a reference virus may produce a change in phenotype *in vitro*. In some cases these mutations may have been associated with a lack of clinical response *in vivo*, as measured by an increase in the plasma HIV RNA levels. If a large data base correlates the presence of the mutation with a poor virologic response, then that specific mutation(s) is considered to predict a lack of drug effect. The most convincing evidence that a mutation causes drug resistance occurs when both *in vitro* genotypic data and viral load response data from several independent studies confirm the association.

A

MUTATIONS IN THE REVERSE TRANSCRIPTASE GENE ASSOCIATED WITH RESISTANCE TO REVERSE TRANSCRIPTASE INHIBITORS

Nucleoside and Nucleotide Reverse Transcriptase Inhibitors (nRTIs)

Multi-nRTI Resistance: 69 Insertion Complex (affects all nRTIs currently approved by the US FDA)

M	A	▼	K	L	T	K
41	**62**	**69**	**70**	**210**	**215**	**219**
L	V	Insert	R	W	Y F	Q E

Multi-nRTI Resistance: 151 Complex (affects all nRTIs currently approved by the US FDA except tenofovir)

A	V	F	F	Q
62	**75**	**77**	**116**	**151**
V	I	L	Y	M

Multi-nRTI Resistance: Thymidine Analogue-associated Mutations (TAMs; affects all nRTIs currently approved by the US FDA)

M	D	K	L	T	K
41	**67**	**70**	**210**	**215**	**219**
L	N	R	W	Y F	Q E

Abacavir

K	L	Y	M
65	**74**	**115**	**184**
R	V	F	V

Didanosine

K	L
65	**74**
R	V

Emtricitabine

K	M
65	**184**
R	V I

Lamivudine

K	M
65	**184**
R	V I

Stavudine

M	D	K	L	T	K
41	**67**	**70**	**210**	**215**	**219**
L	N	R	W	Y F	Q E

Tenofovir

K	K
65	**70**
R	E

Zidovudine

M	D	K	L	T	K
41	**67**	**70**	**210**	**215**	**219**
L	N	R	W	Y F	Q E

B

Nonnucleoside Reverse Transcriptase Inhibitors (NNRTIs)

Efavirenz

L	K	V	V	Y	Y	G	P
100	**103**	**106**	**108**	**181**	**188**	**190**	**225**
I	N	M	I	C I	L	S A	H

Etravirine (expanded access)

V	A	L	K	V	V	Y	G
90	**98**	**100**	**101**	**106**	**179**	**181**	**190**
I	G	I	E P	I	D F	C I V	S A

Nevirapine

L	K	V	V	Y	Y	G
100	**103**	**106**	**108**	**181**	**188**	**190**
I	N	A M	I	C I	C L H	A

Figure 28-1 ■ Common point mutations conferred by use of NRTIs (**a**), NNRTIs (**b**), and PIs (**c**), mutations associated with decreased susceptibility to PIs. For each amino acid residue listed, the letter above the listing represents the wild-type virus, and the letter below the listing represents the mutation. Amino acids: A, alanine; C, cysteine; D, aspartate; E, glutamate; F, phenylalanine; G, glycine; H, histidine; I, isoleucine; K, lysine; L, leucine; M, methionine; N, asparagine; P, proline; Q, glutamine; R, arginine; S, serine; T, theronine; V, valine; W, tryptophan; Y, tyrosine. For full details of footnotes refer to article.

From International AIDS Society-USA Resistance Mutations Project Panel. Update on drug resistance mutations in HIV-1. Top HIV Med 15(4):119–127, 2007, with permission. Updates available at http://www.iasusa.org.

C **MUTATIONS IN THE PROTEASE GENE ASSOCIATED WITH RESISTANCE TO PROTEASE INHIBITORS**

Atazanavir +/– ritonavir

Position	Wild type	Substitutions
10	L	I, F, V, C
16	G	E
20	K	R, M, I, T, V
24	L	I
32	V	I
33	L	I, F, V
34	E	Q
36	M	I, L, V
46	M	I, L
48	G	V
50	I	L
53	F	L, Y
54	I	L, V, M, T, A
60	D	E
62	I	V
64	I	L, M, V
71	A	V, I, T, L
73	G	C, S, T, A
82	V	A, T, F, I
84	I	V
85	I	V
88	N	S
90	L	M
93	I	L, M

Fosamprenavir/ritonavir

Position	Wild type	Substitutions
10	L	F, I, R, V
32	V	I
46	M	I, L
47	I	V
50	I	V
54	I	L, V, M
73	G	S
76	L	V
82	V	A, F, S, T
84	I	V
90	L	M

Darunavir/ritonavir

Position	Wild type	Substitutions
11	V	I
32	V	I
33	L	F
47	I	V
50	I	V
54	I	M, L
73	G	S
76	L	V
84	I	V
89	L	V

Indinavir/ritonavir

Position	Wild type	Substitutions
10	L	I, R, V
20	K	M, R
24	L	I
32	V	I
36	M	I
46	M	I, L
54	I	V
71	A	V, T
73	G	S, A
76	L	V
77	V	I
82	V	A, F, T
84	I	V
90	L	M

Lopinavir/ritonavir

Position	Wild type	Substitutions
10	L	F, I, R, V
20	K	M, R
24	L	I
32	V	I
33	L	F
46	M	I, L
47	I	V, A
50	I	V
53	F	L
54	I	V, L, A, M, T, S
63	L	P
71	A	V, T
73	G	S
76	L	V
82	V	A, F, T, S
84	I	V
90	L	M

Nelfinavir

Position	Wild type	Substitutions
10	L	F, I
30	D	N
36	M	I
46	M	I, L
71	A	V, T
77	V	I
82	V	A, F, T, S
84	I	V
88	N	D, S
90	L	M

Saquinavir/ritonavir

Position	Wild type	Substitutions
10	L	I, R, V
24	L	I
48	G	V
54	I	V, L
62	I	V
71	A	V, T
73	G	S
77	V	I
82	V	A, F, T, S
84	I	V
90	L	M

Tipranavir/ritonavir

Position	Wild type	Substitutions
10	L	V
13	I	V
20	K	M, R
33	L	F
35	E	G
36	M	I
43	K	T
46	M	L
47	I	V
54	I	A, M, V
58	Q	E
69	H	K
74	T	P
82	V	L, T
83	N	D
84	I	V
90	L	M

MUTATIONS IN THE ENVELOPE GENE ASSOCIATED WITH RESISTANCE TO ENTRY INHIBITORS

Enfuvirtide

Position	Wild type	Substitutions
36	G	D, S
37	I	V
38	V	A, M, E
39	Q	R
40	Q	H
42	N	T
43	N	D

Maraviroc

MUTATIONS IN THE INTEGRASE GENE ASSOCIATED WITH RESISTANCE TO INTEGRASE INHIBITORS

Raltegravir (expanded access)

Position	Wild type	Substitutions
148	Q	H, K, R
155	N	H

Amino acid abbreviations: A, alanine; C, cysteine; D, aspartate; E, glutamate; F, phenylalanine; G, glycine; H, histidine; I, isoleucine; K, lysine; L, leucine; M, methionine; N, asparagine; P, proline; Q, glutamine; R, arginine; S, serine; T, threonine; V, valine; W, tryptophan; Y, tyrosine.

D

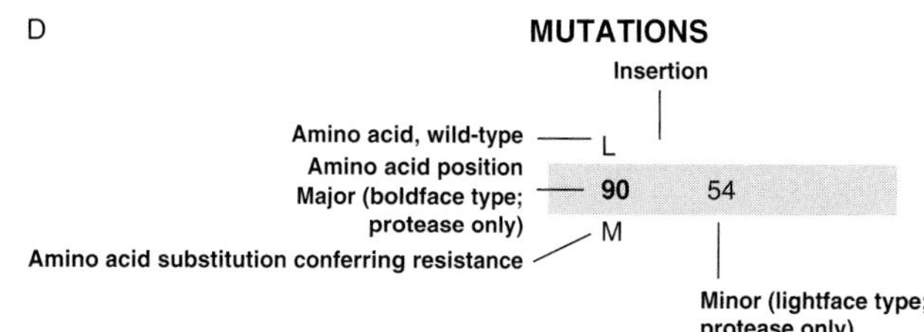

Figure 28-1 ■ (Continued)

Given the complexity of these assays, the sensitivity and specificity of assays performed by individual laboratories must be carefully and regularly assessed.[10,11] Genotypic assays are not easy to interpret when multiple mutations are present simultaneously. Summary tables and on-line resources are useful for interpreting complex patterns. Most laboratories provide interpretation in their patient result reports (Fig. 28-1).[9] Despite this complexity, many clinicians are learning how to incorporate genotypic information into their treatment strategies.

PHENOTYPIC ASSAYS

Most commercial phenotypic assays are recombinant virus assays that amplify the RT, protease, integrase and segments of the envelope genes from the predominant quasispecies of the viral RNA in the patient's plasma. These amplified fragments are inserted into a laboratory virus strain which lacks these genes. The resulting virus is then permitted to replicate in cell culture in the presence of various drug concentrations (Fig. 28-2). Viral replication is detected by emission of light induced by the activity of a luciferase gene product introduced into the laboratory viral strain as an indicator. Results are expressed as the concentration of drug required to inhibit 50% of growth (IC_{50}) and as the fold change in IC_{50} relative to a wild-type control strain.

From the example given in Figure 34-2, the patient's isolate shows a 10-fold reduction in drug susceptibility for zidovudine. In this case, the wild-type control laboratory virus requires 0.5 μM of zidovudine for an IC_{50} compared to the patient's virus which requires 5 μM concentration. In other words, to inhibit 50% of the replication of HIV in cell culture the patient sample requires 10-fold more zidovudine. Compared with a genotypic test, a phenotypic test is a more direct measure of reduced viral susceptibility to a given drug. Thus, for many clinicians, the results are easier to interpret since similar techniques are used for bacteria and fungi. Phenotypic assays are more expensive than genotypic assays, have a slower turnaround time, and are available commercially only through a small number of centralized reference laboratories worldwide. The 'biologic cut-off points' are derived by testing many clinical isolates from drug-naive subjects, then using the resulting distribution of phenotypes to define the 'normal range' of drug susceptibility (median value plus 2 SD). Much effort has been invested in developing clinical cut-off points for most available ARV agents that correlate with poor clinical response. The results from the two major commercial laboratories appear to correlate well with each other although there was more variability in RT results than protease or NNRTI results.[12,13]

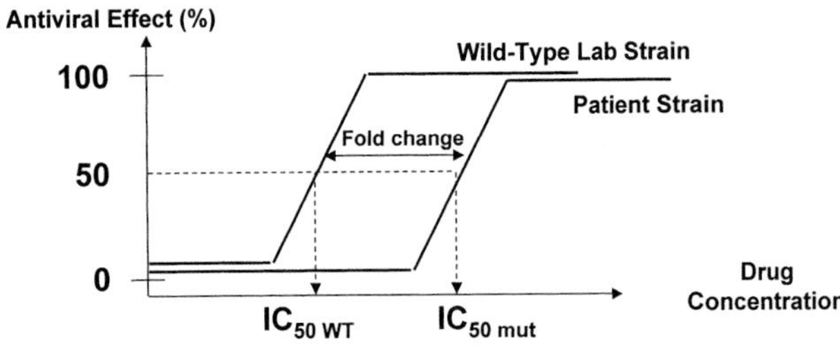

Figure 28-2 ■ Resistance (phenotype) definitions. IC_{50}, 50% inhibitory concentration; IC_{50} mut/$IC_{50\ WT}$, fold change (e.g., $IC_{50\ mu}$ 5 μM/$IC_{50\ WT}$ 0.5 μM is a 10-fold change).

Most mutations that confer resistance impair virus replicative capacity, even in the absence of drug.[3] However, compensatory mutations can accumulate and at least partially reverse the deleterious effects of other mutations on replicative capacity.[8] Evaluation of the virus's replicative capacity can be performed in research laboratories using the recombinant viruses generated during the phenotypic testing. The effects of mutations on virus replicative capacity is an active area of investigation.[14,15] However, it is difficult to translate the replication capacity values into virologic response or disease progression. Therefore, measures of replicative capacity are not yet recommended for clinical decision making.

There are no data which convincingly demonstrate a strategic advantage of genotypic testing versus phenotypic testing to enhance clinical decision making. For individual clinicians, cost and turn-around time are important considerations, as is the availability of resources (human, print, or on-line) which could assist in interpretation. Genotype tests are generally less expensive than phenotype tests and are generally preferred in earlier treatment failure (e.g., first or second regimen failure). Phenotypic tests are often preferred in settings of heavy prior ARV drug exposure where genotypes are more difficult to interpret.

CLINICAL TRIALS ASSESSING RESISTANCE ASSAYS

Multiple retrospective studies and a growing number of randomized, controlled prospective trials have demonstrated the clinical utility and cost effectiveness of resistance testing.

Retrospective analyses of monotherapy studies have demonstrated that the development of viral resistance to study drugs correlates with more rapid clinical progression.[16,17] The prognostic value of genotypic resistance testing was also illustrated in a retrospective analysis of a clinical cohort of PI-experienced patients who received saquinavir/ritonavir dual PI-based therapy.[18] Response to saquinavir/ritonavir combination therapy was best predicted by protease-resistance mutations as determined by a baseline genotype. The resistance profile explained nearly two-thirds of the variation in virologic outcomes at 12 weeks compared with an explained variance (R_2) of less than 50% based on clinical parameters alone. In multivariate models, the resistance predictors were found to be independent of clinical parameters. This study demonstrated that genotypic resistance testing provided prognostic information regarding response to dual PI therapy that could not be obtained by assessing ARV treatment history, baseline CD4+ T-lymphocyte counts, viral load, and/or clinical status.[18]

The long-term prognostic value of phenotypic resistance testing was demonstrated by a retrospective analysis of treatment-experienced patients.[19] In this clinical cohort study, the baseline phenotype provided prognostic information on virologic response at 1 year and beyond. The prognostic value of the phenotype was not limited to a particular salvage regimen and was shown to be independent of other clinical and ARV variables. Virologic response was predicted by the number of drugs to which the patient's isolate was sensitive at baseline. The phenotype was better able to discriminate clinical response than was the patient's ARV drug history.

There have been over a dozen retrospective analyses in various settings that have demonstrated the prognostic value of genotype and phenotype assays for choosing salvage therapy. The Resistance Collaborative Group used a standardized methodology and summarized many early prospective and retrospective trials.[20] The uniform finding of this review was that resistance tests, whether genotypic or phenotypic, provided prognostic information independent of other known prognostic factors, such as baseline viral load or receipt of a drug from a new ARV class. Based on multiple studies, it is now clear that resistance testing can enhance the ability to choose effective ART and that standard clinical information cannot produce comparable results.

Although retrospective studies demonstrate the value of resistance testing for achieving virologic results, these studies have not been shown to alter long-term clinical outcome. Patients whose therapy changes were guided by resistance testing had better viral load responses than patients receiving usual care without such testing.[21–23] These studies were short term (12–16 weeks). However, in one study a persistent benefit was seen through 24 weeks; in another, open-label study, benefit persisted for 3 years.[22]

In the HAVANA study, 326 heavily pretreated patients on failing ARV therapy were randomized to one of four groups: genotyping with expert advice, genotyping without expert advice, no genotypic testing but with expert advice, and no genotypic testing and no advice (standard of care).[23] In an intent-to-treat analysis, the group with both genotyping and advice had the best results: 69% achieved HIV viral loads of less than 400 copies/mL at week 24, compared with 47% of patients with expert advice, 49% of patients with genotypic testing, and 36% for those in the standard-of-care group. Interestingly, the differences in outcomes seemed to be driven by the most heavily pretreated patients. The HAVANA study demonstrates that expert advice with genotype testing provide independent, additive benefits for optimizing the selection of ARV drugs for treatment-experienced patients.

Another randomized, prospective trial assessed genotypic testing compared with standard-of-care treatment in heavily pretreated patients.[22] Adherence was assessed by patient self-reporting. In an intent-to-treat analysis at 3 months, 27% of the patients who underwent genotypic testing had viral loads of less than 500 copies/mL compared with 12% of patients who were randomized to no testing (standard of care) ($P = 0.02$). At 6 months, however, the difference was no longer statistically significant (17% vs 21%, respectively). Not surprisingly, patient adherence strongly influenced the longer-term virologic responses. This study suggested that genotype testing can be beneficial for initial selection of ART, but adherence is the strongest predictor of long-term benefit.

Not all prospective trials of resistance testing have demonstrated improvement in virologic outcomes. In the California Collaborative Treatment Group study 575 (CCTG 575), 256 PI-experienced patients who had experienced treatment failure (80% had experienced first PI failure, and 76% were NNRTI-naive) were randomized to undergo phenotypic testing or no testing (standard of care).[24] The investigators found no significant differences in virologic response between the groups in terms of change in viral load from baseline or in the proportion of patients with viral loads of less than 400 copies/mL (or 50 copies/mL) measured at 6 months and 12 months. Specifically, at 6 months, 48% of patients in both groups had less than 400 copies/mL. However, one explanation of the equivalent results in the two arms is that response to standard of care was surprisingly good. Most of the patients entering this trial were failing nelfinavir-based regimens. Almost all such patients respond well to lopinavir-ritonavir based regimens. When finding adequate salvage therapy is more complicated, results are not likely to be as good.

In a post hoc subgroup analysis of CCTG 575, patients with high degrees of baseline resistance (i.e., those with resistance to three or more PIs) were more likely to achieve viral loads of less than 400 copies/mL at 6 months if they had phenotype-testing (50% vs 17%; $P = 0.02$).

Thus, two trials of heavily pretreated patients with limited new drug options showed little benefit from resistance testing. However, testing can eliminate drugs that are unlikely to provide efficacy but provide unnecessary toxicity and expense. In the NARVAL study, patients in the standard-of-care arm received more drugs than patients who underwent resistance tests, but virologic response was no difference between the groups.[25] Resistance testing may allow the clinician the ability to be more selective and more effective at choosing drugs that have some potential for ARV efficacy.

INTERPRETATION OF RESISTANCE TEST RESULTS

The clinical interpretation of both genotypic and phenotypic tests has improved as large data bases have been developed which correlate virologic outcome with assay results. Statistical and epidemiologic techniques have also been used to develop models based on these data bases.[26] Analytic plans derived from one clinical dataset (training set) are subsequently tested on another set (testing set) are being developed. Interpretation algorithms perform more and more consistently.[27,28]

Experts are able to look at genotype results and make consistent treatment decisions when confronted with the same genotypes.[29] Most clinicians, however, rely on the interpretation which most commercial laboratories provide with their genotypic or phenotypic results.[30]

Genotypic Test Interpretation

Most commercial laboratories develop a rules-based algorithm. The "rules" that make up the algorithms are derived from expert panels and/or statistical analyses. Therefore these algorithms require regular updating. Some of these algorithms are publicly available (e.g., http://hivdb.stanford.edu/hiv/) while others are proprietary. Discrepancies have been found among the different systems. The discrepancies are seen most frequently for drugs and resistance patterns that have not been extensively studied.

Another approach to interpreting complex genotype information uses relational genotype-phenotype databases. One proprietary example of such an approach is called "virtual phenotype". In this approach the patient's genotype is matched with similar genotypes in the database that have previously been matched to phenotypes. The interpretive report includes a probabilistic estimate of a phenotype based on genotypes that match the patient's isolate at the important drug-resistant codons. It is important to note that the matches are not to a complete protease and RT sequence but only to important mutations associated with resistance as defined by experts. Currently the virtual phenotype approach is enhanced by adding information on the relationship between mutations and virologic outcomes from patient cohorts/trials rather than looking exclusively to genotype–phenotype comparison.[5,31]

Phenotypic Test Interpretation

Phenotype assay interpretation may appear to be more straightforward than genotypic assays, owing to the similarity of methodology to antimicrobial testing of bacteria that clinicians commonly use. Like antimicrobial susceptibility tests, an IC_{50} is reported. However, owing to technical issues, the primary read-out of an HIV phenotype is fold change from the wild-type IC_{50} value. The fold-change may be significantly higher than reference, thereby indicating resistance, or may be less than the wild-type reference, suggesting hypersusceptibility. Drugs with less resistance than other drugs can be identified in cases where no active alternatives seem available. From the clinician's point of view, the "cut-points" are used to distinguish active drugs from partially active drugs from inactive drugs. The fold-change cut-points are unique for each drug, depending on natural variability of the assay (assay cut-point), the achievable plasma or intracellular level of the drug, and the IC_{50} (biologic cut-point). The "clinical cut-point" is the most clinically meaningful readout, and is determined by comparing fold-change values versus virologic responses observed in clinical trials. However, not all drugs have well established clinical cut-points, leaving only the biologic and assay cut-offs available to the clinician for interpretation. More data are becoming available to demonstrate that such cut-off points correlate with likelihood of clinical response.

GUIDELINES FOR RESISTANCE TESTING: WHO SHOULD BE TESTED?

The International AIDS Society-USA (IAS-USA) (http://www.iasusa.org), the US Department of Health and Human Services (DHHS) (http://www.hivatis.org) and the EuroGuidelines Group for HIV Resistance[32] have all issued guidelines, which are summarized in Table 28-1.

Acute/Recent and Chronic Infection

In more and more areas of the world, patients are at risk for acquiring drug resistant virus when they are initially infected. Evaluations of patients experiencing acute seroconversion, the incidence has been reported to range from 5% to 15%.[33–35] Thus, resistance testing is generally recommended for patients when first diagnosed or just prior to initiation of ARV therapy, depending on the estimated prevalence of drug-resistant virus in the community.[36,37] Despite the logic of using resistance assays to assess patients when their HIV infection is first detected, there are no data which convincingly demonstrate that such testing improves virologic outcome. Thus, in 2007, most experts would recommend that resistance testing be performed at the time of initiation of therapy when deciding what therapy to initiate.

If resistance testing is not done soon after acute infection, reversion to and/or overgrowth by wild type has been documented to occur, though this is uncommon and the speed of conversion is quite variable. In situations with more rapid conversion to wild-type virus, drug-resistant mutations that emerge during drug therapy would not be detected if the initial assay was not done until many months or years after acute infection. Resistant virus typically remains archived in long-lived cells, only to reemerge when selective drug pressure is initiated. Detection of minor variants (less than 20%) can be difficult with current assays.[38]

Some data suggest that resistant mutants may persist off-drug longer than originally suspected after the initial infection. This observation could be explained by the compensatory mutations and improved fitness of viruses containing resistance-conferring mutations.[35,39]

Treatment Failures

First Regimen Failure

All three guidelines recommend resistance testing for patients who experience suboptimal viral suppression (i.e., viral loads >50 copies/μL) after 12–24 weeks of therapy (Table 28-1). The plasma specimen for resistance testing should be obtained while the patient is still receiving the failing regimen so that selection pressure is maintained when the sample is obtained. Some resistance mutations can escape detection within days to weeks of stopping therapy.

Recommendations for Using Drug-Resistance

Table 28-1

Clinical Setting/Recommendation	Rationale
Drug-Resistance Assay Recommended	
In acute HIV infection If the decision is made to initiate therapy at this time, testing is recommended prior to initiation of treatment (BIII). A genotypic assay is generally preferred (BIII).	Drug resistance testing will determine if drug-resistant virus was transmitted and will help to design initial or changed (if therapy was initiated prior to test results) regimens accordingly.
If treatment is deferred, resistance testing at this time should still be considered (CIII).	Earlier testing may be considered because of the potentially greater likelihood that transmitted resistance-associated mutations will be detected earlier in the course of HIV infection.
In chronic HIV infection: initiating therapy Drug resistance testing is recommended prior to initiation of therapy (BIII). A genotypic assay is generally preferred (BIII).	Transmitted HIV with baseline resistance to at least one drug may be seen in 6–16% of patients. Suboptimal virologic responses may be seen in patients with baseline resistant mutations.
Resistance testing earlier in the course of HIV infection may be considered (CIII).	Earlier testing may be considered because of the potentially greater likelihood that transmitted resistance-associated mutations will be detected earlier in the course of HIV infection.
In chronic HIV infection: changing therapy Drug resistance testing in the setting of virologic failure should be performed while the patient continues his/her antiretroviral drugs, or immediately (i.e., within 4 weeks) after discontinuing therapy (BII).	Determine the role of resistance in drug failure and maximize the number of active drugs in the new regimen, if indicated.
With suboptimal suppression of viral load after antiretroviral therapy initiation (BIII).	Determine the role of resistance and maximize the number of active drugs in the new regimen, if indicated.
In pregnant women Genotypic resistance testing is recommended for all pregnant women prior to initiation of therapy and for those entering pregnancy with detectable HIV RNA level while on therapy.	Optimal prevention of perinatal transmission may require initiation of antiretroviral therapy before results of resistance testing are available.
Drug Resistance Assay Not Usually Recommended After discontinuation of drugs (DIII).	Drug resistance mutations might become minor species in the absence of selective drug pressure, and available assays might not detect minor drug-resistant species. If testing is performed in this setting, the detection of drug resistance may be of value, but its absence does not rule out the presence of minor drug resistant species.
When plasma viral load $<$1 000 copies/mL (DIII).	Resistance assays cannot be consistently performed because of low HIV RNA levels; patients/providers may incur charges and not receive results.

All genotypic and phenotypic tests are difficult to perform when the viral load is less than 500–1000 copies/mL. When patients with low viral loads are subjected to resistance testing, if the virus can be amplified, sample bias may result in misleading reports because the virus sampled may not be representative.[40–42]

As more experience is gained with patients receiving common regimens, the resistance patterns resulting from drug failure are becoming more predictable. In such cases, a choice of the second regimen could logically be made based on knowledge of the initial regimen that failed. In such settings, the cost of resistance testing may not be justified.

Randomized controlled trials have demonstrated that resistance testing in the setting of the first regimen failure can improve outcome. Such testing can identify which drugs in the regimen have lost activity. Knowing which drugs in the failing regimen remain active could theoretically allow the clinician to "recycle" the still active drugs in an effort to preserve treatment options for the long term. The concept of switching only a single drug to which the virus is resistant has not been tested in clinical trials. Minor variants may exist which go undetected by the assays, and mislead the clinician to continue drugs that fail, compromising the remaining, more recently introduced agents.

Multiple Regimen Failure

Clinical trials show that resistance testing is most useful in patients who have failed multiple regimens. Resistance testing is recommended for all highly experienced patients with ARV failure prior to changing the regimen. In general, results are most reliable for agents in the patient's current regimen. Resistance that developed from prior ARV regimens may or may not be maintained. It is probably the most reasonable strategy to assume that any resistant virus detected previously will persist as archived virus and could recur under conditions of new selective pressure and contribute to treatment failure. It is therefore recommended to take the result of previous resistance testing into account.

Pregnancy and Postexposure Prophylaxis

The IAS-USA, DHHS, and EuroGuidelines explicitly recommend the use of resistance testing in pregnant women with detectable viral loads to optimize therapy for the mother and reduce the risk of perinatal transmission. Postexposure prophylaxis regimens for healthcare workers who sustain needle-stick or other high-risk exposure to HIV should also be selected with resistance testing if a sample from the source patient is available. However, initiation of prophylaxis should not be delayed while awaiting results.

Therapeutic Drug Monitoring and Inhibitory Quotient

The measurement of plasma drug levels can provide information that can logically be used with resistance testing to determine if serum levels can be obtained which can inhibit virus. The inhibitory quotient (IQ) has been proposed as a measurement to predict drug efficacy. The drug's actual concentration at the trough of the dosing interval (i.e., plasma C_{min}) is divided by IC_{50} or IC_{90}. The IQ should be a better predictor of virological response than the genotype or phenotype alone because some levels of drug resistance can be overcome by high serum levels. Several retrospective studies have shown the IQ performed as a better predictor for virologic response than either genotype or drug level alone.[43–45] Before IQ becomes more useful clinically, therapeutic drug monitoring must become more standardized (*see* Chapters 4 and 79).

CONCLUSIONS

Resistance testing is now accepted as standard procedure for patients who are initiating therapy for the first time, for patients who are failing therapy, and for all pregnant women who anticipate starting therapy.[26,46] Both genotypic and phenotypic assays can be used effectively. There is no consensus which type of assay is preferable.

REFERENCES

1. Hogg RS, Bangsberg DR, Lima VD, et al. Emergence of drug resistance is associated with an increased risk of death among patients first starting HAART. PLoS Med 3:e356, 2006.
2. Zaccarelli M, Tozzi V, Lorenzini P, et al. Multiple drug class-wide resistance associated with poorer survival after treatment failure in a cohort of HIV-infected patients. Aids 19:1081–9, 2005.
3. Coffin JM: HIV population dynamics in vivo: implications for genetic variation, pathogenesis, and therapy. Science 267:483–9, 1995.
4. Caliendo AM, Savara A, An D, et al. Effects of zidovudine-selected human immunodeficiency virus type 1 reverse transcriptase amino acid substitutions on processive DNA synthesis and viral replication. J Virol 70:2146–53, 1996.
5. Larder BA, Kemp SD. Multiple mutations in HIV-1 reverse transcriptase confer high-level resistance to zidovudine (AZT). Science 246:1155–8, 1989.
6. Arion D, Kaushik N, McCormick S, et al. Phenotypic mechanism of HIV-1 resistance to 3′-azido-3′-deoxythymidine (AZT): increased polymerization processivity and enhanced sensitivity to pyrophosphate of the mutant viral reverse transcriptase. Biochemistry 37:15908–17, 1998.
7. Meyer PR, Matsuura SE, Mian AM, et al. A mechanism of AZT resistance: an increase in nucleotide-dependent primer unblocking by mutant HIV-1 reverse transcriptase. Mol Cell 4:35–43, 1999.
8. Nijhuis M, van Maarseveen NM, Lastere S, et al. A novel substrate-based HIV-1 protease inhibitor drug resistance mechanism. PLoS Med 4:e36, 2007.
9. Johnson VA, Brun-Vezinet F, Clotet B, et al. Update of the drug resistance mutations in HIV-1: fall 2006. Top HIV Med 14:125–30, 2006.
10. Schuurman R, Brambilla D, de Groot T, et al. Underestimation of HIV type 1 drug resistance mutations: results from the ENVA-2 genotyping proficiency program. AIDS Res Hum Retroviruses 18:243–8, 2002.
11. Shafer RW, Hertogs K, Zolopa AR, et al. High degree of interlaboratory reproducibility of human immunodeficiency virus type 1 protease and reverse transcriptase sequencing of plasma samples from heavily treated patients. J Clin Microbiol 39:1522–9, 2001.
12. Qari SH, Respess R, Weinstock H, et al. Comparative analysis of two commercial phenotypic assays for drug susceptibility testing of human immunodeficiency virus type 1. J Clin Microbiol 40:31–5, 2002.
13. Zhang J, Rhee SY, Taylor J, Shafer RW. Comparison of the precision and sensitivity of the Antivirogram and PhenoSense HIV drug susceptibility assays. J Acquir Immune Defic Syndr 38:439–44, 2005.
14. Deeks SG, Wrin T, Liegler T, et al. Virologic and immunologic consequences of discontinuing combination antiretroviral-drug therapy in HIV-infected patients with detectable viremia. N Engl J Med 344:472–80, 2001.
15. Martinez-Picado J, Savara AV, Sutton L, D–Aquila RT. Replicative fitness of protease inhibitor-resistant mutants of human immunodeficiency virus type 1. J Virol 73:3744–52, 1999.
16. D'Aquila RT, Johnson VA, Welles SL, et al. Zidovudine resistance and HIV-1 disease progression during antiretroviral therapy. AIDS Clinical Trials Group Protocol 116B/117 Team and the Virology Committee Resistance Working Group. Ann Intern Med 122:401–8, 1995.
17. Japour AJ, Welles S, D'Aquila RT, et al. Prevalence and clinical significance of zidovudine resistance mutations in human

immunodeficiency virus isolated from patients after long-term zidovudine treatment. AIDS Clinical Trials Group 116B/117 Study Team and the Virology Committee Resistance Working Group. J Infect Dis 171:1172–9, 1995.

18. Zolopa AR, Shafer RW, Warford A, et al. HIV-1 genotypic resistance patterns predict response to saquinavir–ritonavir therapy in patients in whom previous protease inhibitor therapy had failed. Ann Intern Med 131:813–21, 1999.
19. Call SA, Saag MS, Westfall AO, et al. Phenotypic drug susceptibility testing predicts long-term virologic suppression better than treatment history in patients with human immunodeficiency virus infection. J Infect Dis 183:401–8, 2001.
20. DeGruttola V, Dix L, D'Aquila R, et al. The relation between baseline HIV drug resistance and response to antiretroviral therapy: re-analysis of retrospective and prospective studies using a standardized data analysis plan. Antivir Ther 5:41–8, 2000.
21. Baxter JD, Mayers DL, Wentworth DN, et al. A randomized study of antiretroviral management based on plasma genotypic antiretroviral resistance testing in patients failing therapy. CPCRA 046 Study Team for the Terry Beirn Community Programs for Clinical Research on AIDS. AIDS 14:F83–93, 2000.
22. De Luca A, Di Giambenedetto S, Cingolani A, et al. Three-year clinical outcomes of resistance genotyping and expert advice: extended follow-up of the Argenta trial. Antivir Ther 11:321–7, 2006.
23. Tural C, Ruiz L, Holtzer C, et al. Clinical utility of HIV-1 genotyping and expert advice: the Havana trial. AIDS 16:209–18, 2002.
24. Haubrich RH, Kemper CA, Hellmann NS, et al. A randomized, prospective study of phenotype susceptibility testing versus standard of care to manage antiretroviral therapy: CCTG 575. AIDS 19:295–302, 2005.
25. Meynard JL, Vray M, Morand-Joubert L. Impact of treatment guided by phenotypic or genotypic resistance tests on the response to antiretroviral therapy: a randomized trial (NARVAL, ANRS 088). Antivir Ther 5(suppl 3):67–8, 2000.
26. Weinstein MC, Goldie SJ, Losina E, et al. Use of genotypic resistance testing to guide HIV therapy: clinical impact and cost-effectiveness. Ann Intern Med 134:440-50, 2001.
27. Liu TF, Shafer RW. Web resources for HIV type 1 genotypic-resistance test interpretation. Clin Infect Dis 42:1608–18, 2006.
28. Vercauteren J, Vandamme AM. Algorithms for the interpretation of HIV-1 genotypic drug resistance information. Antiviral Res 71:335–42, 2006.
29. Zolopa AR, Lazzeroni LC, Rinehart A, et al. Accuracy, precision, and consistency of expert HIV type 1 genotype interpretation: an international comparison (The GUESS Study). Clin Infect Dis 41:92–9, 2005. PubMed ID: 15937768.
30. Salama C, Policar M, Cervera C. Knowledge of genotypic resistance mutations among providers of care to patients with human immunodeficiency virus. Clin Infect Dis 36:101–4, 2003.
31. Hales G, Birch C, Crowe S, et al. A randomised trial comparing genotypic and virtual phenotypic interpretation of HIV drug resistance: the CREST Study. PLoS Clin Trials 1:e18, 2006.
32. EuroGuidelines Group for HIV Resistance. Clinical and laboratory guidelines for the use of HIV-1 drug resistance testing as part of treatment management: recommendations for the European setting. The Euro Guidelines Group for HIV resistance. AIDS 15:309–20, 2001.
33. Wensing AM, van de Vijver DA, Angarano G, et al. Prevalence of drug-resistant HIV-1 variants in untreated individuals in Europe: implications for clinical management. J Infect Dis 192:958–66, 2005.
34. Deenan P, Martin F. Primary HIV infection, phylogenetics, and antiretroviral prevention. J Infect Dis 195:924–6, 2007. PubMed ID: 17330780.
35. Little SJ, Holte S, Routy JP, et al. Antiretroviral-drug resistance among patients recently infected with HIV. N Engl J Med 347:385–94, 2002.
36. Oette M, Kaiser R, Daumer M, et al. Primary HIV drug resistance and efficacy of first-line antiretroviral therapy guided by resistance testing. J Acquir Immune Defic Syndr 41:573–81, 2006.
37. Sax PE, Islam R, Walensky RP, et al. Should resistance testing be performed for treatment-naive HIV-infected patients? A cost-effectiveness analysis. Clin Infect Dis 41:1316–23, 2005.
38. Metzner KJ, Rauch P, Walter H, et al. Detection of minor populations of drug-resistant HIV-1 in acute seroconverters. AIDS 19:1819–25, 2005.
39. Maarseveen NM van, Wensing AMJ, de Jong D, et al. Persistence of HIV-1 variants with multiple protease inhibitior (PI) – resistance mutations in the absense of PI therapy can be explained by compensatory fixation. JID 195:399–409, 2007.
40. Gale HB, Kan VL, Shinol RC. Performance of the TruGene human immunodeficiency virus type 1 genotyping kit and OpenGene DNA sequencing system on clinical samples diluted to approximately 100 copies per milliliter. Clin Vaccine Immunol 13:235–8, 2006.
41. Hirsch MS, Conway B, D'Aquila RT, et al. Antiretroviral drug resistance testing in adults with HIV infection: implications for clinical management. International AIDS Society – USA Panel. JAMA 279:1984–91. 1998.
42. Mitsuya Y, Winters MA, Fessel WJ, et al. HIV-1 drug resistance genotype results in patients with plasma samples with HIV-1 RNA levels less than 75 copies/mL. J Acquir Immune Defic Syndr 43:56–9, 2006.
43. Duval X, Lamotte C, Race E, et al. Amprenavir inhibitory quotient and virological response in human immunodeficiency virus-infected patients on an amprenavir-containing salvage regimen without or with ritonavir. Antimicrob Agents Chemother 46:570–4, 2002.
44. Marcelin AG, Lamotte C, Delaugerre C, et al. Genotypic inhibitory quotient as predictor of virological response to ritonavir–amprenavir in human immunodeficiency virus type 1 protease inhibitor-experienced patients. Antimicrob Agents Chemother 47:594–600, 2003.
45. Winston A, Hales G, Amin J, et al. The normalized inhibitory quotient of boosted protease inhibitors is predictive of viral load response in treatment-experienced HIV-1-infected individuals. AIDS 19:1393–9, 2005.
46. Durant J, Clevenbergh P, Halfon P, et al. Drug-resistance genotyping in HIV-1 therapy: the VIRADAPT randomised controlled trial. Lancet 353:2195–9, 1999.

Chapter 29

Pharmacogenetics of Antiretroviral Agents

Catia Marzolini, PharmD, PhD, Richard Kim, MD, Amalio Telenti, MD, PhD

INTRODUCTION

Pharmacogenomics is an emerging clinical discipline that explores the interaction of drugs with genetically determined metabolic and effector pathways and has influence on disease progression, drug efficacy, and drug safety. For some associations, such as the relationship of abacavir hypersensitivity to HLA-B*5701, clinicians may be at the point where knowledge of HLA type could or should influence the choice of therapy. For other associations, the relationships are interesting and intriguing, but probably are not well enough established to warrant routine use in clinical practice. This chapter will review the current state of knowledge related to pharmacogenomics in patients with HIV infection.

There is marked interindividual variation in plasma levels, efficacy, and in susceptibility to adverse effects of antiretroviral drugs (ART). Variable drug response likely reflects the combined influence of gender, environment, disease, concurrent drugs, and genetics. In this regard, genetic variation in the genes that encode for proteins involved in the metabolism or disposition of antiretroviral drugs is a key determinant of efficacy and toxicity to HIV drugs. Drugs such as protease inhibitors (PIs) and non-nucleoside reverse transcriptase inhibitors (NNRTIs), are extensively metabolized by cytochrome P450 enzymes such as CYP3A4, CYP2C19, CYP2D6, and CYP2B6.[1,2] In addition, most PIs have been shown to be substrates of the efflux transporter P-glycoprotein, and of other cellular transporters.[3] In the section under the heading of pharmacogenetics, the influence of genetic variation in genes involved in antiretroviral drug disposition on the pharmacokinetic and pharmacodynamic of antiretroviral agents will be discussed.

Genetic susceptibility to adverse reactions (toxicogenetics) is a second area of research in the field of ART. In this section, current knowledge on genetic determinants of hypersensitivity reactions, dyslipidemia, lipodystrophy, and mitochondrial disorders, Gilbert syndrome, neuropsychological adverse events, and pancreatitis, that constitute some of the most prevalent complications of current HIV treatment will be reviewed. A third section will deal with the growing interest on genetic predictors of disease progression, and its implication for the initiation of treatment. Finally, the last section of this chapter will summarize guidelines for conducting genetic association studies, the general principles governing genetic testing in medicine, and practical aspects relevant to bringing genetic prediction to clinical use.

PHARMACOGENETICS OF ANTIRETROVIRAL AGENTS

CYP450 Metabolism

Drug metabolizing reactions are grouped into two phases; phase I reactions involve changes such as oxidation, reduction, and hydrolysis and are primarily mediated by the cytochrome P450 (CYP) family of enzymes highly expressed in organs such as the liver and intestine. Phase II reactions typically use an endogenous compound, such as glucuronic acid, glutathione or sulfate for conjugation to the drug or its phase I derived metabolite to produce a more polar product that can be excreted. Although genetic polymorphisms of phase II enzymes are well described and have been associated with disease states such as cancer,[4] they are less likely to be a major pathway for the disposition HIV drugs.[5] Accordingly, this section will focus mainly on variations in CYP enzyme-mediated metabolism and their impact on the disposition of antiretroviral drugs.

Inherited Differences in the Metabolism of Antiretroviral drugs

Table 29-1

Gene or Protein†	Allele or Variant Evaluated	Reported Consequence for Antiretroviral Drugs
CYP3A4/A5	CYP3A4*1B (-392A>G, promoter), and CYP3A4*18 (878T>C, L293P, altered activity). CYP3A5*3 (6986A>G, splice defect, severely reduced enzyme activity), and CYP3A5*6 (14690G>A, splice defect)	Possible effect on efavirenz for CYP3A4*1B and CYP3A5*3 (trend to higher AUC). No effect reported for nelfinavir. Saquinavir: metabolite ratio is lower for CYP3A5*3.
CYP2C19	CYP2C19*2 (681G>A , aberrant splice site, truncated protein, poor metabolizer)	Nelfinavir: possible trend towards higher AUC and less virologic failure. No effect reported for efavirenz.
CYP2D6	CYP2D6*3 (2549A>del, frameshift), CYP2D6*4 (1846G>A, splice defect), CYP2D6*6 (1707T>del, frameshift)	Nelfinavir: possible trend to higher plasma drug levels. Efavirenz: possible trend to higher plasma drug levels.
CYP2B6	CYP2B6*5 (1459C>T, R487C), CYP2B6*6 516TG>T, Q172H, diminished function). Additional decreased-function alleles explain extreme elevation of efavirenz plasma levels	Geometric mean of efavirenz plasma AUC is 2.3-fold higher in individuals homozygous for the CYP2B6*6 allele. Associated with increased neuropsychological toxicity. 2B6*6 allele also influences nevirapine plasma levels.

Summarized from references 15–20, 28–31, and 127

†See http:// www.imm.ki.se/CYP alleles/ for detail description of CYP alleles,[135] http:// www.hiv-pharmacogenomics.org for updated information for genetic influences on antiretroviral drugs.[133]

CYP3A

Enzymes of the *CYP3A* subfamily are the most abundantly expressed isoforms in the liver, comprising 25–40% of total hepatic P450 content[6] and thought to account for most of the monooxygenase activity present in the gastrointestinal tract.[7] Expression of CYP3A in the enterocyte of the small intestine and the liver accounts for the marked first-pass effect often observed following oral administration of its substrates. Because of its broad substrate specificity, CYP3A is involved in the metabolism of over 50% of currently used therapeutic agents, including most PIs and NNRTIs.[8] In addition to being substrates for CYP3A, most PIs are inhibitors of CYP3A4 whereas NNRTIs induce CYP3A4.

CYP3A5-mediated metabolism has wide interindividual variability reflective of both environmental factors such as drug interactions involving inhibition and induction[9,10] and genetic components.[11] Not surprisingly, a number of laboratories have looked for single nucleotide polymorphisms (SNPs) in the coding and noncoding regions of both *CYP3A4* and *CYP3A5*. Most of these appear to be uncommon (frequency <1–2%) and/or distributed to specific populations.[12] A −392A>G transition in the 5′-regulatory region of *CYP3A4* (i.e., CYP3A4*1B) occurs more frequently, particularly among those of African descent.[13] With *CYP3A5*, an A>G substitution within intron 3 (i.e., CYP3A5*3) a variant forming a truncated inactive protein is noted to be present in most subjects.[14] A rarer G>A transition in exon 7 (i.e., CYP3A5*6) also results in a splicing defect. It has been suggested that these variants may contribute to the observed interindividual variability in CYP3A activity. Several studies have been performed in order to evaluate the effect of genetic variations in *CYP3A4* on the pharmacokinetics of nelfinavir,[15–17] efavirenz,[15–18] and saquinavir[19,20] (Table 29-1). These studies indicate that CYP3A4*1B, CYP3A5*3, and CYP3A5*6 have no influence on nelfinavir and efavirenz pharmacokinetics. CYP3A5*3 polymorphism has been associated with the urinary metabolic ratio of saquinavir to its hydroxy metabolites in healthy individuals. The mean metabolic ratio was significantly lower and the clearance was higher in subjects with active CYP3A5 compared to individuals with a functionally inactive enzyme.[19,20]

CYP2C19

CYP2C19 is important in the metabolism of the PI nelfinavir. Several loss of function genetic variants exist, two variants (CYP2C19*2 and CYP2C19*3) accounting for more than 95% of poor metabolizer phenotypes. Genotypic differences are observed among populations since 2–3% of Caucasians and 4% of Africans have the poor metabolizer phenotype versus 10–25% of Asians.[21] A recent study demonstrated that nelfinavir exposure was significantly higher in treatment-naive HIV patients with GA or AA genotypes at position 681 in *CYP2C19* (i.e., CYP2C19*2) compared to the wild type.[17] This same study showed a trend toward decreased virologic failure in subjects with the GA genotype (Table 29-1).

CYP2D6

The *CYP2D6* genetic polymorphism was originally discovered as a result of differences in the pharmacokinetics and therapeutic effects of drugs metabolized by this enzyme such as codeine, dextromethorphan, metoprolol, nortriptyline, and debrisoquin.[22] Approximately 5–10% of Caucasian subjects were found to have a deficiency in their ability to oxidize the antihypertensive drug debrisoquin.[23] Subjects with poor metabolism tend to be homozygous for mutations in *CYP2D6* associated with marked loss or complete absence of enzymatic activity. However, it should also be noted that some subjects have multiple copies of *CYP2D6* resulting in an extensive metabolizer phenotype.[24] A study published by Fellay et al[15] analyzed the association between CYP2D6*3, *4, and *6, representing the most frequent inactivating mutations in Caucasians leading to a poor metabolizer phenotype, and plasma levels of nelfinavir and efavirenz in treatment-naive HIV-infected patients. Patients homozygous or heterozygous for a loss of function *CYP2D6* allele had a higher median plasma concentration of both nelfinavir and efavirenz when compared to patients with a *CYP2D6* extensive metabolizer genotype (Table 29-1).

CYP2B6

CYP2B6 was thought to be expressed at low levels and only in a fraction of human liver samples. However, CYP2B6 has gained more attention since it was shown to be significantly involved in the metabolic activation and inactivation of a number of clinically important drugs such as efavirenz.[25] A large interindividual variability in the hepatic content of CYP2B6 has been reported[26] as well as functional differences between genetic variants.[27] A number of studies have investigated for a possible role of genetic differences in *CYP2B6* as the basis for toxicity to the NNRTI efavirenz. The relationship between efavirenz pharmacokinetics, central nervous system (CNS) side effects, weight, race, and virologic response was investigated in 154 HIV-infected individuals randomized to receive efavirenz-containing regimen.[18] The authors found that a 516G>T polymorphism in exon 4 of *CYP2B6* (i.e., CYP2B6*6) was more common in African-Americans compared with Caucasians. Furthermore, efavirenz AUC was three times higher in patients with the 516 TT genotype compared to GG homozygotes or GT heterozygotes. CYP2B6 516 TT genotype was also significantly associated with increased CNS side effects during the first week of efavirenz therapy. No association was observed between the allelic variants and virologic response. A number of studies have confirmed a role for the 516G>T polymorphism for efavirenz[28–31] and nevirapine (Table 29-1).[28]

Induction of Drug Metabolizing Enzymes

In addition to genetic variations, expressed levels of CYP enzymes and drug transporters can be modulated by activation of certain nuclear receptors such as the Pregnane X Receptor (PXR).[32] In organs such as the liver, these adopted orphan receptors mediate transcriptional activation of target genes by their ability to translocate into the nucleus once activated by ligands, which include a number of HIV drugs. In the nucleus, activated receptors then heterodimerize with the 9-cis retinoic acid receptor (RXR) and bind to response elements of target genes which then initiate target gene transcription.[33] PXR has been shown to be a key factor responsible for CYP3A4, 2B6, and 2C9 transcriptional activation[34–37] as well as for the efflux transporter MDR1.[38] Of importance, it is now known that most PIs and certain NNRTIs act as PXR ligands leading to the induction of a number of phase I and II metabolic pathways. Therefore, it is not surprising that the combination of several PIs with or without NNRTIs often result in complex drug interactions. Unlike CYP enzymes, genetic variations in nuclear receptors such as PXR are rare.

Transporter Genes

Drug transporters expressed in tissues such as the intestine, liver, kidney, and brain play an important role in the absorption, distribution, and excretion of many drugs in clinical use. There are two major types of drug transporters: uptake and efflux transporters. Uptake transporters act by facilitating the translocation of drugs into cells, whereas efflux transporters function to export drugs from the intracellular to the extracellular milieu. Most efflux transporters tend to be members of the adenosine triphosphate (ATP)-binding cassette (ABC) superfamily of proteins that use energy derived from ATP hydrolysis to mediate substrate translocation across biologic membranes. Included in this class of transporters are multidrug resistance protein 1(MDR1), the multidrug resistance-associated protein (MRP) family, and the breast cancer resistance protein (BCRP). There is now increasing evidence to suggest genetic heterogeneity in drug transporters not only contribute to the observed interindividual variation in drug disposition, but also to the drug response. Numerous polymorphisms have been identified in transporters important to drug disposition.[39]

MDR1 (ABCB1)

Due to its broad substrate specificity, P-glycoprotein (P-gp), the gene product of *MDR1*, has received the greatest attention in terms of identification and characterization of SNPs. P-gp functions as a transmembrane efflux pump thereby moving drugs from the intracellular to extracellular domain; it can also act on drug molecules entrapped within the cell membrane lipid bilayer. ATP hydrolysis provides the energy for active drug transport, enabling the transporter to function against steep concentration gradients.

P-gp was first isolated from colchicine-resistant Chinese hamster ovary cells.[40] Subsequently, the gene coding for P-gp (*MDR1*) was identified because of its over-expression in tumor cells associated with an acquired cross-resistance to multiple cytotoxic anticancer agents.[41] This drug transporter was also recognized to be expressed in many normal tissues.[42] P-gp is found on the canalicular domain of hepatocytes, the apical surface of proximal tubular cells in the kidney, the brush border surface of enterocytes, the epithelium of the brain choroid plexus as well as the luminal surface of blood capillaries in the brain, the placenta, the ovaries, the testes and, of relevance to HIV therapy, in CD56+, CD8+, and CD4+ lymphocytes.[42–44] The function and tissue expression pattern for P-gp suggest that this transporter acts as a protective barrier to keep toxins out through excretion of substrate compounds into bile, urine, and the intestinal lumen and thereby limit the accumulation of such toxins or xenobiotics in organs such as the brain, gonads, and bone marrow, or in the fetus. P-gp is colocalized with the drug metabolizing enzyme CYP3A4 in the small intestine and liver suggesting that the extent of interplay between P-gp and CYP3A4 likely account for the net absorption and elimination of shared substrate drugs. Expression of P-gp at the level of the blood–brain barrier has shown to be critical to limiting the CNS entry of many drugs. Supportive evidence was obtained from animal models. A mouse strain naturally deficient in *mdr1a*, demonstrated marked sensitivity to the neurotoxic effects of ivermectin, an antiparasiticide substrate of P-gp.[45,46] The absence of P-gp in the blood–brain barrier of such mice resulted in a more than 80-fold higher brain accumulation of ivermectin.[45] Additionally, P-gp can alter oral drug absorption[47] or enhance their biliary and renal excretion.[48] P-gp has been shown to be particularly relevant to HIV therapy as PIs have been shown to be substrates of this transporter.[49]

Screening of the entire *MDR1* coding region identified a synonymous SNP in exon 26 (i.e., 3435C>T) associated with altered protein expression although the SNP does not change the encoded amino acid (Ile).[50] In the same study P-gp expression in duodenal biopsy samples among healthy Caucasians with the homozygous T allele (variant) was noted to be decreased when compared to those with the C allele (common). Subjects with the variant allele were also shown to have increased digoxin plasma concentrations after oral administration, suggesting greater drug absorption in individuals with low intestinal P-gp levels. The first study exploring associations between SNPs in *MDR1* and antiretroviral pharmacokinetic parameters was performed by Fellay et al.[15] The authors examined the influence 3435C>T on the median concentrations of nelfinavir and efavirenz in treatment-naive HIV-infected patients. Patients with the variant allele were shown to have lower nelfinavir and efavirenz levels compared to the wild type. Subsequent studies attempting to define associations between this same polymorphism in exon 26 and another in exon 21 (i.e., 2677G>T/A) and the pharmacokinetics of several PIs and efavirenz have resulted in conflicting and controversial findings (Table 29-2).[16–18,29,51–53]

In addition to drug levels, SNPs in *MDR1* may also alter the physiological protective role of P-gp and therefore influence disease.[49] Fellay et al found a relationship between expression of P-gp in peripheral blood mononuclear cells (PBMCs) of HIV-infected patients and CD4 lymphocyte response to treatment.[15] Patients with the 3435T allele in exon 26 had a significantly greater rise in CD4 cells count, 6 months after starting ART. It was hypothesized that this benefit associated with the T allele could result from an enhanced HIV PI penetration into CD4 cells. Three additional studies have reported a better virologic outcome associated with the 3435T allele.[16,17,54] However, other studies reported no virologic or immunologic effects associated with the study allele (Table 29-2).[55–57] While the exact mechanism by which SNPs in *MDR1* affect the disposition or efficacy of HIV drugs needs to be clarified, there is a growing acceptance of the fact that in many cases SNPs in MDR1 do predict response to certain HIV drugs. It should be remembered however, while P-gp is the best characterized ABC transporter, other transporters also have the potential to affect the disposition of HIV drugs (Table 29-2).

TOXICOGENETICS OF ANTIRETROVIRAL AGENTS

Drug Hypersensitivity Syndromes

The pathogenesis of a number of multisystem drug hypersensitivity reactions involves major histocompatibility complex (MHC)-restricted presentation of drug or drug metabolites to MHC molecules and/or haptenation to endogenous proteins prior to T-cell presentation.[58–60] Recent studies implicate genetic loci within the MHC in hypersensitivity reactions to abacavir and to nevirapine. Only a subset of individuals exposed to abacavir develop hypersensitivity, typically within 6 weeks of initiating therapy, and those individuals who do not develop the syndrome within this time frame remain at low risk despite ongoing therapy.[61] Non-Caucasian racial origin also decreases risk of abacavir hypersensitivity, and familial predisposition has also been reported.[62] Specific MHC alleles are strongly associated with risk of abacavir hypersensitivity.[63,64] The *HLA-B*5701* allele has an independent positive predictive value of greater than 70% and a negative predictive value greater than 90% in Caucasians, suggesting that prospective testing for susceptibility to this syndrome may represent a useful clinical test in some populations.[65] Performance of *HLA-B*5701* testing decreases for populations other than Caucasians, and according to the stringency of the case definition.[66]

Nevirapine hypersensitivity manifesting as potentially life-threatening hepatotoxicity with or without rash is also conferred by genetic factors. This syndrome is similar to abacavir hypersensitivity in that susceptible individuals develop symptoms within 6 weeks whereas continuing therapy beyond this period is not associated with increased risk.[67] The protective effect of low CD4 T-cell count in the case of nevirapine hypersensitivity [67,68] is consistent with a CD4 T-cell-dependent immune response to nevirapine-specific antigens and a participation of HLA class II alleles.[69] Human cases involving combinations of hepatitis, fever or rash have been associated with an interaction between HLA-DRB1*0101 and the percentage of CD4, whereas no associations were detected for isolated rash (Table 29-3).[69]

Table 29-2 Inherited Differences in the Transport of Antiretroviral Drugs

Gene or Protein†	Allele or Variant Evaluated	Reported Consequence for Antiretroviral Drugs
P-glycoprotein (*MDR1, ABCB1*)	3435C>T (synonymous I1145I, in linkage disequilibrium with ABCB1 1236, 2677, and IVS26+80T>C). Limited data on 61A>G (N21D), 1199G>A (S400N), other variants, or of haplotypes	Controversial issue. For nelfinavir: reported increased in cellular and plasma levels in some studies. Associated with immune recovery or less virologic failure in some studies using nelfinavir or efavirenz. No influence on indinavir, lopinavir/r, and ritonavir.
MRP2 (ABCC2)	Multiple variants analysed	No influence on cellular levels of nelfinavir.
MRP2 (ABCC2)	Multiple variants analysed	No influence on cellular levels of nelfinavir.
MRP4 (ABCC4)	No studies available (multiple variants described)	Relevant to the transport of PMEA, Azidothymidine, lamivudine, ddC, stavudine.
MRP5 (ABCC5)	No studies available (multiple variants described)	Relevant to the transport of PMEA, Azidothymidine, lamivudine, ddC, stavudine.
BCRP (ABCG2)	Multiple variants analysed	No influence on cellular levels of nelfinavir.
OAT1 (SLC22A6)	No studies available	Adefovir, Cidofovir.
OAT2 (SLC22A7)	No studies available	Azidothymidine.
OCT1 (SLC22A1)	No studies available (multiple variants described)	Azidothymidine, PIs: indinavir, saquinavir, ritonavir, nefinavir. Reduced *in vitro* uptake reduced hepatic clearance /intestinal absorption, increased susceptibility to drug–drug interaction?

Summarized from references 15–17, 51–54, 56, 57, 128, 129.
†See http://www.hiv-pharmacogenomics.org for updated information for genetic influences on antiretroviral drugs.[133]

Dyslipidemia

In considering the pharmacogenetics of ART-related dyslipidemia, it may be useful to evaluate factors that may influence lipid metabolism in the general population and may therefore potentiate the toxic effects of ART. Initial work identified the role of *APOE* and *APOC3* variants as risk factor for hyperlipoproteinemia (predominantly hypertriglyceridemia).[70–72] In addition, there is a deleterious gene–drug interaction resulting in a high risk for extreme hypertriglyceridemia when ritonavir is prescribed to individuals with unfavorable genetic profile. A recent analysis of selected allelic variants of 12 genes proposed in the literature as influencing plasma lipid levels in the general population validated five genes as contributing to ART-associated dyslipidemia.[73]

The most favorable and unfavorable *APOE/APOC3/APOA5/CETP/ABCA1* genotype resulted in median triglyceride levels of 2.6 and 4.1 mmol/L, respectively, when exposed to ritonavir. In contrast the triglyceride levels for individuals with the most favorable and unfavorable genotype were 1.37 and 2.3 mmol/L, respectively in the absence of ritonavir exposure. The most favorable and unfavorable *CETP/APOA5* genotype resulted in median HDL cholesterol levels of 1.25 and 1.11 mmol/L, respectively, with no or with a NRTI-containing regimen; and 1.5 and 1.17 mmol/L with a NNRTI-containing regimen. No genotype was significantly associated with changes in non-HDL cholesterol levels. Thus, the contribution of any single SNP on lipid levels was modest, underscoring the current understanding of genetic predisposition to dyslipidemia being a complex genetic trait. However, the magnitude of the genetic effects on dyslipidemia became apparent in the multigene analysis. A theoretical strategy of selecting the initial ART according to the results of genotyping would have the potential to reduce by 30%, the number of patients with sustained hypertriglyceridemia; and even more for individuals with unfavorable genotypes (Table 29-3).

Lipodystrophy and Mitochondrial Disorders

Lipodystrophy has been described in 25–50% of ART-treated patients. The cumulative exposure to ART has been identified as the major risk factor in multiple studies. However, lipodystrophy affects some but not all patients despite similar ART exposure, which suggests that genetic factors may be involved. A functional promoter polymorphism in *TNF-α* (-238A) has been associated with more rapid onset of lipoatrophy in some[74,75] but not all studies.[72] The functional correlates of this effect have not been characterised, although higher TNF-α levels are described among individuals carrying the -238A *TNF-α* promoter variant.[74,75] At the pathophysiological level, it is likely that cellular levels of TNF-α may modulate the threshold at which apoptosis occurs in response to toxic stimuli;[76] mechanisms are likely to be relevant in the adipose tissue.[77]

Toxicogenetics of Antiretroviral Drugs

Table 29-3

Gene or Protein†	Allele or Variant Evaluated	Reported Consequence for Antiretroviral Drugs
HLA-B, major histocompatibility complex, class I, B	HLA-B*57.1 haplotype (defined by the presence of HLAB*5701, HLA-DR7 and HLA-DQ3)	Hypersensitivity reaction to abacavir.
HLA-DR, major histocompatibility complex, class II, DR beta 1α	HLA-DRB1*0101	High negative predictive value of hypersensitivity reactions to nevirapine (fever, rash, hepatitis).
TNF-α	-238G/A TNF-α promoter polymorphism	Earlier onset lipoatrophy.
UGT1A11, UDP glycosyltransferase 1 family, polypeptide A	UGT1A1*28, Promoter region (insertion at TATA box associated with reduction in bilirubin-conjugating activity)	Gilbert's syndrome. Hyperbilirubinemia, increased levels of bilirubin in presence of atazanavir or indinavir.
APOC3, APOE	APOC3 -482 C>T, -455 T>C, 3238 C>G. APOE ε2 and ε3 haplotypes	Increased risk of hypertriglyceridemia associated with use of ritonavir. Including analysis of variants of APOA5, CETP, and ABCA1 may improve improved prediction and help in identifying also individuals at risk for low HDL cholesterol.
SPINK-1, CFTR	Multiple variants associated with cystic fibrosis and pancreatitis	Susceptibility to pancreatitis.
mtDNA	Tissue-specific mtDNA depletion may represent toxic effect of NRTI therapy on mtDNA synthesis. Possibility for accumulation of mutations in mtDNA due to gamma polymerase damage	Certain human mtDNA haplotypes (haplotype T) may increase susceptibility to peripheral neuropathy. Depletion and mutation of mtDNA likely associated with lipodystrophy.

Summarized from references 63, 64, 66, 69, 71, 72, 74, 75, 83, 102, 110, 130, 134.
† see http://www.hiv-pharmacogenomics.org for updated information for genetic influences on antiretroviral drugs toxicities, http://www.mitomap.org for detail description of polymorphisms and mutations of the human mtDNA.[134]

Defects in either the quantity or quality of mitochondrial DNA (mtDNA) has been associated with lipodystrophy, neuropathy, lactic acidosis, and with the associated complex metabolic disorders. In contrast to the nuclear genome, mtDNA may undergo quantitative and qualitative changes over an individual's lifetime, and may be influenced directly by environmental factors.[78] The effects are likely to be tissue-specific rather than general, reflecting the differing requirements of tissues for cellular energy and the differing availability of energy substrates. The putative mechanism that is invoked to explain mitochondrial toxicity of ART (and, most prominently NRTI), includes the inhibition of the gamma polymerase, the only enzyme that replicates mtDNA. Inhibition of gamma polymerase leads to depletion of mtDNA and inhibition of the transcription of proteins encoded by mtDNA, all of which represent enzymes of the electron transport system, which is involved in oxidative phosphorylation. Initiation of ART has triggered bilateral optic atrophy and blindness in HIV-infected individuals with unrecognized mitochondrial disorders such as Leber's hereditary optic neuropathy.[78–82] Underlying human variation of mtDNA, represented by common haplotypes, has been associated with differences in susceptibility to ART-related neuropathy (Table 29-3).[83]

Age has also been recognized as a risk factor for lipodystrophy and mitochondrial disorders in the setting of ART.[84] The mitochondrial hypothesis of aging postulates that accumulation of mtDNA mutations during aging leads to mitochondrial dysfunction. This in turn, is followed by increased generation of lactic acid and free oxygen radicals and additional damage to the mtDNA. A recent publication has substantially strengthened the case for the mitochondrial theory of aging. Trifunovic et al constructed knock-in mice that expressed an exonuclease-deficient gamma polymerase.[85] These 'mtDNA mutator mice' developed a three- to fivefold increase in mtDNA mutations and increased amounts of mtDNA deletions in all tissues examined; DNA polymerase activity and the amount of mtDNA expressed remained normal, but respiratory chain enzyme activity was reduced. The mtDNA mutator mice had a reduced lifespan and premature development of aging-related symptoms, including subcutaneous fat loss, weight loss, osteoporosis, anemia, and cardiomegaly. Overall, accumulation of mutations and reduction of mtDNA quantity associated with ART and against a background of aging would be a plausible mechanism explaining the complex features of lipodystrophy and associated metabolic syndrome. Detailed analysis of the mtDNA genome may help identify individuals at risk of toxicity.

Other Toxicity Issues

Unconjugated Hyperbilirubinemia

Unconjugated hyperbilirubinemia is an adverse event of therapy containing indinavir (IDV) or atazanavir (ATV).[86,87] Unconjugated bilirubin enters the hepatocyte by passive diffusion and may be facilitated through the human organic transporting polypeptide 1B1 (OATP1B1) encoded by *SLCO1B1*.[88–90] Once in the hepatocyte, bilirubin is conjugated with glucuronic acid by the microsomal enzyme UDP-glucuronosyltransferase 1A1 (UGT1A1) and excreted in the bile by MRP2 (ABCC2).[91] A polymorphism in the promoter TATA element of the gene encoding UGT1A1 (allele *UGT1A1*28*) decreases transcriptional activity and it is responsible for the unconjugated hyperbilirubinemia observed in the context of Gilbert syndrome (Table 29-3).[92,93] Nonsynonymous polymorphisms in *SLCO1B1* have been associated with differences in the function of the transporter *in vitro* [94–96] and *in vivo*.[97–101]

The additive effect of the genes described above will influence the rates of hyperbilirubinemia upon introduction of drugs such as atazanavir.[102,103] There are ethnic and racial differences in the frequency of both *UGT1A1* and *OATP1B1* variants, such that hyperbilirubinemia may occur more frequently in African and less among individuals of Japanese origin. The theoretical advantage of genotyping for *SLCO1B1* and *UGT1A1*28* before initiation of ART would contribute to the reduction of bilirubin determinations in jaundice and range from 22% to 5.0%.[103]

Neurotoxicity

As described in the section on CYP450, efavirenz and nevirapine are metabolized by CYP2B6. The best studied allele, 2B6*6 (516G>T, Gln172His), is a pharmacogenetic marker of efavirenz neuropsychological toxicity. This allele predicts adverse neuropsychological scores during the first 12 weeks after initiation of efavirenz therapy.[18] The frequency of toxicity is expected to decrease thereafter.[104] However, genotyping can also identify individuals at risk for late or persistent neuropsychological toxicity while on long-term efavirenz-containing therapy.[105] In the latter setting, the presence of the variant allele was two to three times more frequent among individuals describing sleep or mood disorders or fatigue.

Pancreatitis

Drug-induced pancreatitis has been attributed with the use of pentamidine, trimethoprim–sulfamethoxazole or didanosine.[106] Drugs may be contributing to pancreatitis by potentiating other toxic agents, a genetic predisposition, or by its action on a pancreas which was already diseased. *CFTR* (cystic fibrosis transmembrane conductance regulator) mutations have been shown to be involved in a variety of clinical conditions other than cystic fibrosis, including pancreatitis.[107,108] *SPINK-1* (serine protease inhibitor kazal-1) which encodes a trypsin inhibitor in the cytoplasm of pancreatic acinar cells is also a genetic risk factor for pancreatitis.[109] Frossard et al evaluated the frequency of *CFTR* and *SPINK-1* mutations in HIV-positive patients with clinical pancreatitis or asymptomatic elevation of serum pancreatic enzymes.[110] Among 51 patients presenting with hyperamylasemia, there were 13 carriers of *CFTR* or *SPINK-1* polymorphisms (12.7%). Those with *CFTR* or *SPINK-1* polymorphisms had a mean 648 U/L amylase levels compared to 232 U/L for those without ($P = 0.025$). Four of ten (40%) patients with clinical acute pancreatitis had *CFTR* or *SPINK-1* mutations. It was concluded that *CFTR* and *SPINK-1* mutations are frequent among HIV-positive patients suffering from acute pancreatitis. The indication to offer diagnostic genetic testing in patient with pancreatic disease has been recently considered to be any of the following: (1) recurrent attacks of acute pancreatitis for which there is no explanation, (2) unexplained chronic pancreatitis, (3) a family history of pancreatitis in a first-degree or second-degree relative, (4) an unexplained episode of acute pancreatitis in a child, and finally (5) patients with pancreatitis eligible for a research protocol.[111] A subgroup of patients that could potentially benefit are those presenting with asymptomatic elevation of amylase, in particular those with multiple risk factors (Table 29-3).

GENETICS AND OPTIMAL TIMING OF INITIATION OF TREATMENT

The rate of HIV disease progression reflects the influence of the genetic diversity of the virus as well as variation in host factors.[112] Dominant host factors identified to date include diversity in the major histocompatibility complex class I, and alleles of chemokine, chemokine receptor, and cytokine genes. MHC homozygosity, as well as specific HLA class I alleles are well-documented modifiers of infection. The most relevant alleles associated with protection are HLA-B*27 and B*57. In contrast, HLA-B*35Px, B*37, B*53, B*56, B*58, and A1-B8-DR3 have been associated with rapid progression.[113] Epistatic interactions between certain KIR (3DS1) and HLA-B alleles delay disease progression.[114] Following the discovery of the CCR5 Δ32 deletion, conferring a high level resistance to HIV infection,[115–117] extensive research has addressed the contribution of additional variants in the CCR5-CCR2 locus. Variants of the *CCR5* promoter region include a human haplotype HHE, that is associated with rapid disease progression.[118,119] In contrast, haplotypes carrying the CCR2 64I allele are associated with a favorable prognosis,[120] and possibly with some degree of protection from infection. Duplication at the locus encoding the chemokine CCL3L1 leads to gene-dose effect, that alone or in association with genetic variants determining CCR5 expression or function, defines different rates of disease progression.[121] Various cytokine variants have been reported to influence the course of HIV-1 disease through more general effects on HIV-1 pathogenesis and inflammatory homeostasis.[112] Recent work proposes new variants in cellular host factors, and in antiviral innate defense, modifying HIV-1 susceptibility with effects in the range of those of well-documented variants such as those in the CCR5/CCR2 region.[122,123] However, the contribution of any genetic variant is limited and genetic prediction needs accounting for the influence of multiple alleles.[122,124]

BRINGING GENETIC TESTING TO CLINICAL USE

The number of genetic association studies is growing rapidly, and is likely to accelerate in the future. This requires attention to the need to establish the conditions for genetic testing, including its legal and ethical aspects. In addition, there is increasing awareness that the literature of genetic association studies is fraught with false associations, thus the need to apply stricter standards, in terms of study design, statistics and quality control of genetic analysis, to prevent the promulgation of false positive results. A number of recommendations for optimal design of genetic association studies, and for conducting of clinical trials and for cohort studies are presented in Table 29-4.

An important step in the area of pharmacogenomics and genetics, has been the development of the Adult AIDS Clinical Trials Group (AACTG) Protocol A5128, approved in many

Table 29-4 Guidelines for Conducting Genetic Association Studies and for Implementation of Genetic Testing in the Clinical Setting

Conducting Genetic Association Studies	Genetic Prediction in Clinical Trials, Cohorts, and Clinical Care
1. Establish a clear distinction between candidate genes for which there is previous statistical evidence of association with the specific disease under study and genes that are proposed on the basis of a new biological hypothesis.	1. The treatment of HIV is highly standardized, and would thus allow acquisition of genetic information at a rapid pace. In clinical trials, genotype could be used as an exclusion criteria or, a posteriori, as a stratification factor.
2. Genes for which there is prior statistical evidence of association to the trait in question, (a) report the *P*-values obtained in previous studies; (b) specify any differences between the phenotypes employed in prior studies and those employed in the proposed work; and (c) specify the populations and sample size and the allelic frequencies of variants in those studies.	2. HIV-infected individuals are expected to be on life-long treatment. Treatment is frequently changed because of toxicity or failure. Thus the proposal to provide a "genetic passport" for volunteers who participate regularly in clinical trials.
3. Provide a quantitative estimate (using the cited evidence) of the prior probability that the list of genes considered contains a relevant one.	3. Cohort studies are appropriate settings for genetics projects for validation of new markers and modeling of complex traits. Thus the need to create the administrative and logistic conditions for collaborative studies by: • Assessing the unique legal and ethical conditions needed for performing this research in various cohorts and countries • Defining harmonized databases for the entry and sharing of genetic and phenotype information • Establishing adequate genotyping facilities and procedures for anonymization of patient identifiers.
4. Checklist for study design • Sampling method – is it clear how participants were selected, and are they representative of whatever population they are intended to represent? • Have issues of selection bias and population structure been considered? • Does the phenotyping method and genotyping error mean that misclassification could be extensive? • Was genotyping undertaken with the researchers masked to outcome data. • If the results depend heavily on findings in a particular subgroup, was a hypothesis about this fact specified in advance? • Is a gene dose-response effect present? • Is the study large enough to detect or exclude an association somewhat less than the size of association reported previously? • What data if any exist on whether the polymorphism is functional? • Correct the *P*-values in their results for multiple comparisons due to the multiple genes studied.	4. Clinical use of genetic data requires that genetic tests are: • Validated and standardized. • Readily interpretable • Improving outcomes, and cost-effective.

Adapted from references 112, 131, and 132

states in the USA,[125] and the NIAID-sponsored GENOMICS protocol ("Collection and use of blood for genetic and other related analyses"). The A5128 protocol facilitates that participants in past or present AACTG clinical trials contribute stored DNA for studies that were not planned when informed consent was provided. Extraction from whole blood is performed at a central laboratory, where participants' unique identifiers are replaced by randomly assigned identifiers prior to DNA storage. The GENOMICS protocol aim at providing genetic data to the Community Programs for Clinical Research on AIDS (CPCRA), with a particular interest in people of color, women, and injection drug users. Despite the negative perception of genetic research among the general public, recent studies indicate that this type of investigation is widely accepted by concerned parties such as patients, relatives of patients, and healthy study volunteers.[126]

Finally, there is much work needed before genetic testing can be brought to routine clinical care. It is unlikely that identification of multigene effects will change management of HIV-1 disease in the near future, notwithstanding this, some

Table 29-5

Genetic Prediction of Toxicity to Commonly Prescribed ART

Drug	Gene/Allele	% Population at Risk	Estimated Effects of a Universal Genotyping Policy Prior to Initiation of ART	Ref
Efavirenz	*CYP2B6*6* (and other less common loss-of-function alleles)	3% of Caucasians and 20% of blacks	• Near complete avoidance of extremely elevated plasma levels (95 Percentile) • Guided choice of initial dosing • Reduction in neuropsychological toxicity.	28, 127, 128
Ritonavir boosted PIs[†]	Selected variants of *APOE, APOC3, APOA5, CETP,* and *ABCA1*	51% of patients present unfavorable genetic background associated withsustained hypertriglyceridemia. Up to 43% of patients may carry an unfavorable genotype associated with low HDL cholesterol	• Universal genotyping and guided choice of therapy would lead to a reduction from 57% to 39% in the proportion of patients with sustained hypertriglyceridemia (>2.25 mmol/L, National Cholesterol Education Program). • Selected patients with unfavorable genotype concerning HDL would benefit from use of NNRTIs as first choice.	72, 73
Atazanavir	*UGT1A1, SLCO1B1*	The most significant allele, UGT1A1*28 is common in African-Americans ($f = 0.43$), Caucasians ($f = 0.36$–0.39), and Indians ($f = 0.35$), and less common in Japanese ($f = 0.11$), Chinese ($f = 0.16$), and Malaysians ($f = 0.19$)	• Universal genotyping and guided choice of therapy would lead to a reduction from 21.6% to 5.0% in the proportion of bilirubin determinations in jaundice range.	102, 103
Abacavir	*HLA-B*5701*	1–5% in Caucasian, less common in other populations	• Avoidance of most hypersensitivity reactions among Caucasians. • Negative predictive value remains elevated across populations, but there is a drastic decrease in sensitivity and positive predictive value for non-Caucasian populations.	63, 66
Nevirapine	*HLA-DRB1*0101*	15–22% (Caucasian) 1–18% (Asian) 3–6% (Hispanic and African-American)	• Negative predictive value of 96%. • The risk of hepatic/systemic nevirapine reaction is most significantly associated with an interaction between *HLA-DRB1*0101* and ≥25% of CD4 T cells.	69

[†]Boosted atazanavir excluded.

pharmacogenetic and toxicogenetic applications may soon contribute to patient care. In Table 29-5 we present the estimated contribution of some of these markers in limiting clinical toxicity of commonly used antiretroviral agents.

REFERENCES

1. Eagling VA, Back DJ, Barry MG. Differential inhibition of cytochrome P450 isoforms by the protease inhibitors, ritonavir, saquinavir and indinavir. Br J Clin Pharmacol 44:190, 1997.
2. Barry M, Mulcahy F, Merry C, et al. Pharmacokinetics and potential interactions amongst antiretroviral agents used to treat patients with HIV infection. Clin Pharmacokinet 36:289, 1999.
3. Kim RB. Drug transporters in HIV therapy. Top HIV Med 11:136, 2003.
4. Maruo Y, Iwai M, Mori A, et al. Polymorphism of UDP-glucuronosyltransferase and drug metabolism. Curr Drug Metab 6:91, 2005.
5. Nebert DW, Russell DW. Clinical importance of the cytochromes P450. Lancet 360:1155, 2002.
6. Shimada T, Yamazaki H, Mimura M, et al. Inter-individual variations in human liver cytochrome P-450 enzymes involved in the oxidation of drugs, carcinogens and toxic chemicals: studies with liver microsomes of 30 Japanese and 30 Caucasians. J Pharmacol Exp Ther 270:414, 1994.
7. Kolars JC, Schmiedlin-Ren P, Schuetz JD, et al. Identification of rifampin-inducible P450IIIA4 (CYP3A4) in human small bowel enterocytes. J Clin Invest 90:1871, 1992.
8. Cholerton S, Daly AK, Idle JR. The role of individual human cytochromes P450 in drug metabolism and clinical response. Trends Pharmacol Sci 13:434, 1992.
9. Thummel KE, Wilkinson GR. In vitro and in vivo drug interactions involving human CYP3A. Annu Rev Pharmacol Toxicol 38:389, 1998.
10. Fellay J, Marzolini C, Decosterd L, et al. Variations of CYP3A activity induced by antiretroviral treatment in HIV-1 infected patients. Eur J Clin Pharmacol 60:865, 2005.
11. Ozdemir V, Kalowa W, Tang BK, et al. Evaluation of the genetic component of variability in CYP3A4 activity: a repeated drug administration method. Pharmacogenetics 10:373, 2000.
12. Lamba JK, Lin YS, Schuetz EG, Thummel KE. Genetic contribution to variable human CYP3A-mediated metabolism. Adv Drug Deliv Rev 54:1271, 2002.
13. Ball SE, Scatina J, Kao J, et al. Population distribution and effects on drug metabolism of a genetic variant in the 5′ promoter region of CYP3A4. Clin Pharmacol Ther 66:288, 1999.
14. Kuehl P, Zhang J, Lin Y, et al. Sequence diversity in CYP3A promoters and characterization of the genetic basis of polymorphic CYP3A5 expression. Nat Genet 27:383, 2001.
15. Fellay J, Marzolini C, Meaden ER, et al. Response to antiretroviral treatment in HIV-1-infected individuals with allelic variants of the multidrug resistance transporter. 1. A pharmacogenetics study. Lancet 359:30, 2002.
16. Saitoh A, Singh KK, Powell CA, et al. An MDR1-3435 variant is associated with higher plasma nelfinavir levels and more rapid virologic response in HIV-1 infected children. AIDS 19:371, 2005.
17. Haas DW, Smeaton LM, Shafer RW, et al. Pharmacogenetics of long-term responses to antiretroviral regimens containing efavirenz and/or nelfinavir: an Adult Aids Clinical Trials Group Study. J Infect Dis 192:1931, 2005.
18. Haas DW, Ribaudo HJ, Kim RB, et al. Pharmacogenetics of efavirenz and central nervous system side effects: an Adult AIDS Clinical Trials Group study. AIDS 18:2391, 2004.
19. Frohlich M, Hoffmann MM, Burhenne J, et al. Association of the CYP3A5 A6986G (CYP3A5*3) polymorphism with saquinavir pharmacokinetics. Br J Clin Pharmacol 58:443, 2004.
20. Mouly SJ, Matheny C, Paine MF, et al. Variation in oral clearance of saquinavir is predicted by CYP3A5*1 genotype but not by enterocyte content of cytochrome P450 3A5. Clin Pharmacol Ther 78:605, 2005.
21. Wedlund PJ. The CYP2C19 enzyme polymorphism. Pharmacology 61:174, 2000.
22. Kroemer HK, Eichelbaum M. 'It's the genes, stupid'. Molecular bases and clinical consequences of genetic cytochrome P450 2D6 polymorphism. Life Sci 56:2285, 1995.
23. Mahgoub A, Idle JR, Dring LG, et al. Polymorphic hydroxylation of Debrisoquine in man. Lancet 2:584, 1977.
24. Johansson I, Lundqvist E, Bertilsson L, et al. Inherited amplification of an active gene in the cytochrome P450 CYP2D locus as a cause of ultrarapid metabolism of debrisoquine. Proc Natl Acad Sci USA 90:11825, 1993.
25. Ward BA, Gorski JC, Jones DR, et al. The cytochrome P450 2B6 (CYP2B6) is the main catalyst of efavirenz primary and secondary metabolism: implication for HIV/AIDS therapy and utility of efavirenz as a substrate marker of CYP2B6 catalytic activity. J Pharmacol Exp Ther 306:287, 2003.
26. Code EL, Crespi CL, Penman BW, et al. Human cytochrome P4502B6: inter-individual hepatic expression, substrate specificity, and role in procarcinogen activation. Drug Metab Dispos 25:985, 1997.
27. Lang T, Klein K, Fischer J, et al. Extensive genetic polymorphism in the human CYP2B6 gene with impact on expression and function in human liver. Pharmacogenetics 11:399, 2001.
28. Rotger M, Colombo S, Furrer H, et al. Influence of CYP2B6 polymorphism on plasma and intracellular concentrations and toxicity of efavirenz and nevirapine in HIV-infected patients. Pharmacogenetics Genomics 15:1, 2005.
29. Tsuchiya K, Gatanaga H, Tachikawa N, et al. Homozygous CYP2B6*6 (Q172H and K262R) correlates with high plasma efavirenz concentrations in HIV-1 patients treated with standard efavirenz-containing regimens. Biochem Biophys Res Commun 319:1322, 2004.
30. Hasse B, Gunthard HF, Bleiber G, Krause M. Efavirenz intoxication due to slow hepatic metabolism. Clin Infect Dis 40:e22–e23, 2005.
31. Rodriguez-Novoa S, Barreiro P, Rendon A, et al. Influence of 516G>T polymorphisms at the gene encoding the CYP450-2B6 isoenzyme on efavirenz plasma concentrations in HIV-infected subjects. Clin Infect Dis 40:1358, 2005.
32. Handschin C, Meyer UA. Induction of drug metabolism: the role of nuclear receptors. Pharmacol Rev 55:649, 2003.
33. Mangelsdorf DJ, Evans RM. The RXR heterodimers and orphan receptors. Cell 83:841, 1995.
34. Goodwin B, Moore LB, Stoltz CM, et al. Regulation of the human CYP2B6 gene by the nuclear pregnane X receptor. Mol Pharmacol 60:427, 2001.
35. Goodwin B, Hodgson E, Liddle C. The orphan human pregnane X receptor mediates the transcriptional activation of CYP3A4 by rifampicin through a distal enhancer module. Mol Pharmacol 56:1329, 1999.
36. Wang H, Faucette S, Sueyoshi T, et al. A novel distal enhancer module regulated by pregnane X receptor/constitutive androstane receptor is essential for the maximal induction of CYP2B6 gene expression. J Biol Chem 278:14146, 2003.
37. Chen Y, Ferguson SS, Negishi M, Goldstein JA. Induction of human CYP2C9 by rifampicin, hyperforin, and phenobarbital is mediated by the pregnane X receptor. J Pharmacol Exp Ther 308:495, 2004.
38. Geick A, Eichelbaum M, Burk O. Nuclear receptor response elements mediate induction of intestinal MDR1 by rifampin. J Biol Chem 276:14581, 2001.

39. Marzolini C, Tirona RG, Kim RB. Pharmacogenomics of drug transporters. In: Kalow W, Meyer UA, Tyndale RF (eds). Pharmacogenomics. Taylor & Francis, Boca Raton FL, 2005.
40. Juliano RL, Ling V. A surface glycoprotein modulating drug permeability in Chinese hamster ovary cell mutants. Biochim Biophys Acta 455:152, 1976.
41. Ueda K, Cardarelli C, Gottesman MM, Pastan I. Expression of a full-length cDNA for the human 'MDR1' gene confers resistance to colchicine, doxorubicin, and vinblastine. Proc Natl Acad Sci USA 84:3004, 1987.
42. Thiebaut F, Tsuruo T, Hamada H, et al. Cellular localization of the multidrug-resistance gene product P-glycoprotein in normal human tissues. Proc Natl Acad Sci USA 84:7735, 1987.
43. Cordon-Cardo C, O'Brien JP, Casals D, et al. Multidrug-resistance gene (P-glycoprotein) is expressed by endothelial cells at blood–brain barrier sites. Proc Natl Acad Sci USA 86:695, 1989.
44. Klimecki WT, Futscher BW, Grogan TM, Dalton WS. P-glycoprotein expression and function in circulating blood cells from normal volunteers. Blood 83:2451, 1994.
45. Schinkel AH, Smit JJ, van Tellingen O, et al. Disruption of the mouse mdr1a P-glycoprotein gene leads to a deficiency in the blood–brain barrier and to increased sensitivity to drugs. Cell 77:491, 1994.
46. Kwei GY, Alvaro RF, Chen Q, et al. Disposition of ivermectin and cyclosporin A in CF-1 mice deficient in mdr1a P-glycoprotein. Drug Metab Dispos 27:581, 1999.
47. Meerum Terwogt JM, Malingre MM, Beijnen JH, et al. Coadministration of oral cyclosporin A enables oral therapy with paclitaxel. Clin Cancer Res 5:3379, 1999.
48. Kawahara M, Sakata A, Miyashita T, et al. Physiologically based pharmacokinetics of digoxin in mdr1a knockout mice. J Pharm Sci 88:1281, 1999.
49. Marzolini C, Paus E, Buclin T, Kim RB. Polymorphisms in human MDR1 (P-glycoprotein): recent advances and clinical relevance. Clin Pharmacol Ther 75:13, 2004.
50. Hoffmeyer S, Burk O, von Richter O, et al. Functional polymorphisms of the human multidrug-resistance gene: multiple sequence variations and correlation of one allele with P-glycoprotein expression and activity in vivo. Proc Natl Acad Sci USA 97:3473, 2000.
51. Zhu D, Taguchi-Nakamura H, Goto M, et al. Influence of single-nucleotide polymorphisms in the multidrug resistance-1 gene on the cellular export of nelfinavir and its clinical implication for highly active antiretroviral therapy. Antivir Ther 9:929, 2004.
52. Colombo S, Soranzo N, Rotger M, et al. Influence of ABCB1, ABCC1, ABCC2, and ABCG2 haplotypes on the cellular exposure of nelfinavir in vivo. Pharmacogenetics Genomics 15:599, 2005.
53. Winzer R, Langmann P, Zilly M, et al. No influence of the P-glycoprotein genotype (MDR1 C3435T) on plasma levels of lopinavir and efavirenz during antiretroviral treatment. Eur J Med Res 8:531, 2003.
54. Brumme ZL, Dong WW, Chan KJ, et al. Influence of polymorphisms within the CX3CR1 and MDR-1 genes on initial antiretroviral therapy response. AIDS 17:201, 2003.
55. Haas DW, Wu H, Li H, et al. MDR1 gene polymorphisms and phase 1 viral decay during HIV-1 infection: an adult AIDS Clinical Trials Group study. J Acquir Immune Defic Syndr 34:295, 2003.
56. Nasi M, Borghi V, Pinti M, et al. MDR1 C3435T genetic polymorphism does not influence the response to antiretroviral therapy in drug-naive HIV-positive patients. AIDS 17:1696, 2003.
57. Verstuyft C, Marcellin F, Morand-Joubert L, et al. Absence of association between MDR1 genetic polymorphisms, indinavir pharmacokinetics and response to highly active antiretroviral therapy. AIDS 19:2127, 2005.
58. Zanni MP, von Greyerz S, Schnyder B, et al. HLA-restricted, processing- and metabolism-independent pathway of drug recognition by human alpha beta T lymphocytes. J Clin Invest 102:1591, 1998.
59. Schnyder B, Burkhart C, Schnyder-Frutig K, et al. Recognition of sulfamethoxazole and its reactive metabolites by drug-specific CD4+ T cells from allergic individuals. J Immunol 164:6647, 2000.
60. Park BK, Naisbitt DJ, Gordon SF, et al. Metabolic activation in drug allergies. Toxicology 158:11, 2001.
61. Hewitt RG. Abacavir hypersensitivity reaction. Clin Infect Dis 34:1137, 2002.
62. Peyrieere H, Nicolas J, Siffert M, et al. Hypersensitivity related to abacavir in two members of a family. Ann Pharmacother 35:1291, 2001.
63. Mallal S, Nolan D, Witt C, et al. Association between presence of HLA-B*5701, HLA-DR7, and HLA-DQ3 and hypersensitivity to HIV-1 reverse-transcriptase inhibitor abacavir. Lancet 359:727, 2002.
64. Hetherington S, Hughes AR, Mosteller M, et al. Genetic variations in HLA-B region and hypersensitivity reactions to abacavir. Lancet 359:1121, 2002.
65. Nolan D, Gaudieri S, Mallal S. Pharmacogenetics: a practical role in predicting antiretroviral drug toxicity? J HIV Ther 8:36, 2003.
66. Hughes AR, Mosteller M, Bansal AT, et al. Association of genetic variations in HLA-B region with hypersensitivity to abacavir in some, but not all, populations. Pharmacogenomics 5:203, 2004.
67. Stern JO, Robinson PA, Love J, et al. A comprehensive hepatic safety analysis of nevirapine in different populations of HIV infected patients. J Acquir Immune Defic Syndr 34(Suppl 1): S21–S33, 2003.
68. Patel SM, Johnson S, Belknap SM, et al. Serious adverse cutaneous and hepatic toxicities associated with nevirapine use by non-HIV-infected individuals. J Acquir Immune Defic Syndr 35:120, 2004.
69. Martin AM, Nolan D, James I, et al. Predisposition to nevirapine hypersensitivity associated with HLA-DRB1*0101 and abrogated by low CD4 T-cell counts. AIDS 19:97, 2005.
70. Behrens G, Schmidt HH, Stoll M, Schmidt RE. ApoE genotype and protease-inhibitor-associated hyperlipidaemia. Lancet 354:76, 1999.
71. Fauvel J, Bonnet E, Ruidavets JB, et al. An interaction between apo C-III variants and protease inhibitors contributes to high triglyceride/low HDL levels in treated HIV patients. AIDS 15:2397, 2001.
72. Tarr PE, Taffe P, Bleiber G, et al. Modeling the influence of APOC3, APOE, and TNF polymorphisms on the risk of antiretroviral therapy-associated lipid disorders. J Infect Dis 191:1419, 2005.
73. Arnedo M, Taffé P, Furrer H, et al. Modeling the influence of polymorphisms of several genes involved in lipid metabolism on the risk of antiretroviral therapy-associated dyslipidemia. In: 13th Conference on Retroviruses and Opportunistic Infections, Denver, Feb 2006.
74. Nolan D, Moore C, Castley A, et al. Tumour necrosis factor-alpha gene -238G/A promoter polymorphism associated with a more rapid onset of lipodystrophy. AIDS 17:121, 2003.
75. Maher B, Alfirevic A, Vilar FJ, et al. TNF-alpha promoter region gene polymorphisms in HIV-positive patients with lipodystrophy. AIDS 16:2013, 2002.
76. Thorburn A. Death receptor-induced cell killing. Cell Signal 16:139, 2004.
77. Prins JB, Niesler CU, Winterford CM, et al. Tumor necrosis factor-alpha induces apoptosis of human adipose cells. Diabetes 46:1939, 1997.
78. Wallace KB, Starkov AA. Mitochondrial targets of drug toxicity. Annu Rev Pharmacol Toxicol 40:353, 2000.

79. Luzhansky JZ, Pierce AB, Hoy JF, Hall AJ. Leber's hereditary optic neuropathy in the setting of nucleoside analogue toxicity. AIDS 15:1588, 2001.
80. Shaikh S, Ta C, Basham AA, Mansour S. Leber hereditary optic neuropathy associated with antiretroviral therapy for human immunodeficiency virus infection. Am J Ophthalmol 131:143, 2001.
81. Warner JE, Ries KM. Optic neuropathy in a patient with AIDS. J Neuroophthalmol 21:92, 2001.
82. Mackey DA, Fingert JH, Luzhansky JZ, et al. Leber's hereditary optic neuropathy triggered by antiretroviral therapy for human immunodeficiency virus. Eye 17:312, 2003.
83. Hulgan T, Haas DW, Haines JL, et al. Mitochondrial haplogroups and peripheral neuropathy during antiretroviral therapy: an adult AIDS clinical trials group study. AIDS 19:1341, 2005.
84. Nolan D, Mallal S. Effects of sex and race on lipodystrophy pathogenesis. J HIV Ther 6:32, 2001.
85. Trifunovic A, Wredenberg A, Falkenberg M, et al. Premature ageing in mice expressing defective mitochondrial DNA polymerase. Nature 429:417, 2004.
86. Boffito M, Kurowski M, Kruse G, et al. Atazanavir enhances saquinavir hard-gel concentrations in a ritonavir-boosted once-daily regimen. AIDS 18:1291, 2004.
87. Hammer SM, Squires KE, Hughes MD, et al. A controlled trial of two nucleoside analogues plus indinavir in persons with human immunodeficiency virus infection and CD4 cell counts of 200 per cubic millimeter or less. AIDS Clinical Trials Group 320 Study Team. N Engl J Med 337:725, 1997.
88. Briz O, Serrano MA, MacIas RI, et al. Role of organic anion-transporting polypeptides, OATP-A, OATP-C and OATP-8, in the human placenta-maternal liver tandem excretory pathway for foetal bilirubin. Biochem J 371:897, 2003.
89. Cui Y, Konig J, Leier I, Buchholz U, Keppler D. Hepatic uptake of bilirubin and its conjugates by the human organic anion transporter SLC21A6. J Biol Chem 276:9626, 2001.
90. Konig J, Cui Y, Nies AT, Keppler D. A novel human organic anion transporting polypeptide localized to the basolateral hepatocyte membrane. Am J Physiol Gastrointest Liver Physiol 278:G156–G164, 2000.
91. Tukey RH, Strassburg CP. Human UDP-glucuronosyltransferases: metabolism, expression, and disease. Annu Rev Pharmacol Toxicol 40:581, 2000.
92. Bosma PJ, Chowdhury JR, Bakker C, et al. The genetic basis of the reduced expression of bilirubin UDP-glucuronosyltransferase 1 in Gilbert's syndrome. N Engl J Med 333:1171, 1995.
93. Monaghan G, Ryan M, Seddon R, et al. Genetic variation in bilirubin UPD-glucuronosyltransferase gene promoter and Gilbert's syndrome. Lancet 347:578, 1996.
94. Kameyama Y, Yamashita K, Kobayashi K, et al. Functional characterization of SLCO1B1 (OATP-C) variants, SLCO1B1*5, SLCO1B1*15 and SLCO1B1*15+C1007G, by using transient expression systems of HeLa and HEK293 cells. Pharmacogenet Genomics 15:513, 2005.
95. Nozawa T, Minami H, Sugiura S, et al. Role of organic anion transporter OATP1B1 (OATP-C) in hepatic uptake of irinotecan and its active metabolite, 7-ethyl-10-hydroxycamptothecin: in vitro evidence and effect of single nucleotide polymorphisms. Drug Metab Dispos 33:434, 2005.
96. Tirona RG, Leake BF, Merino G, Kim RB. Polymorphisms in OATP-C: identification of multiple allelic variants associated with altered transport activity among European- and African-Americans. J Biol Chem 276:35669, 2001.
97. Mwinyi J, Johne A, Bauer S, et al. Evidence for inverse effects of OATP-C (SLC21A6) 5 and 1b haplotypes on pravastatin kinetics. Clin Pharmacol Ther 75:415, 2004.
98. Niemi M, Schaeffeler E, Lang T, et al. High plasma pravastatin concentrations are associated with single nucleotide polymorphisms and haplotypes of organic anion transporting polypeptide-C (OATP-C, SLCO1B1). Pharmacogenetics 14:429, 2004.
99. Niemi M, Backman JT, Kajosaari LI, et al. Polymorphic organic anion transporting polypeptide 1B1 is a major determinant of repaglinide pharmacokinetics. Clin Pharmacol Ther 77:468, 2005.
100. Niemi M, Kivisto KT, Hofmann U, et al. Fexofenadine pharmacokinetics are associated with a polymorphism of the SLCO1B1 gene (encoding OATP1B1). Br J Clin Pharmacol 59:602, 2005.
101. Nishizato Y, Ieiri I, Suzuki H, et al. Polymorphisms of OATP-C (SLC21A6) and OAT3 (SLC22A8) genes: consequences for pravastatin pharmacokinetics. Clin Pharmacol Ther 73:554, 2003.
102. Rotger M, Taffe P, Bleiber G, et al. Gilbert syndrome and the development of antiretroviral therapy-associated hyperbilirubinemia. J Infect Dis 192:1381, 2005.
103. Rotger M, Taffe P, Bleiber G, et al. Contribution of genetic polymorphisms in UGT1A1 and SCLO1B1 to the development of antiretroviral therapy assocîated hyperbilirubinemia. In: 45th International Conference on Antimicrobial Agents and Chemotherapy, Washington, 2005.
104. Adkins JC, Noble S. Efavirenz. Drugs 56:1055, 1998.
105. Lochet P, Peyriere H, Lotthe A, et al. Long-term assessment of neuropsychiatric adverse reactions associated with efavirenz. HIV Med 4:62, 2003.
106. Dassopoulos T, Ehrenpreis ED. Acute pancreatitis in human immunodeficiency virus-infected patients: a review. Am J Med 107:78, 1999.
107. Sharer N, Schwarz M, Malone G, et al. Mutations of the cystic fibrosis gene in patients with chronic pancreatitis. N Engl J Med 339:645, 1998.
108. Cohn JA, Friedman KJ, Noone PG, et al. Relation between mutations of the cystic fibrosis gene and idiopathic pancreatitis. N Engl J Med 339:653, 1998.
109. Pfutzer RH, Barmada MM, Brunskill AP, et al. SPINK1/PSTI polymorphisms act as disease modifiers in familial and idiopathic chronic pancreatitis. Gastroenterology 119:615, 2000.
110. Frossard JL, Morris MA, Wonkam A, et al. The role of CFTR and SPINK-1 mutations in pancreatic disorders in HIV-positive patients: a case control study. AIDS 18:1521, 2004.
111. Ellis I, Lerch MM, Whitcomb DC. Genetic testing for hereditary pancreatitis: guidelines for indications, counselling, consent and privacy issues. Pancreatology 1:405, 2001.
112. Telenti A, Bleiber G. Host genetics of HIV-1 susceptibility. Future Virol 1:55, 2006.
113. Carrington M, Nelson G, O'Brien SJ. Considering genetic profiles in functional studies of immune responsiveness to HIV-1. Immunol Lett 79:131, 2001.
114. Martin MP, Gao X, Lee JH, et al. Epistatic interaction between KIR3DS1 and HLA-B delays the progression to AIDS. Nat Genet 31:429, 2002.
115. Dean M, Carrington M, Winkler C, et al. Genetic restriction of HIV-1 infection and progression to AIDS by a deletion allele of the CKR5 structural gene. Hemophilia Growth and Development Study, Multicenter AIDS Cohort Study, Multicenter Hemophilia Cohort Study, San Francisco City Cohort, ALIVE Study. Science 273:1856, 1996.
116. Samson M, Libert F, Doranz BJ, et al. Resistance to HIV-1 infection in Caucasian individuals bearing mutant alleles of the CCR-5 chemokine receptor gene. Nature 382:722, 1996.
117. Huang Y, Paxton WA, Wolinsky SM, et al. The role of a mutant CCR5 allele in HIV-1 transmission and disease progression. Nat Med 2:1240, 1996.
118. Gonzalez E, Bamshad M, Sato N, et al. Race-specific HIV-1 disease-modifying effects associated with CCR5 haplotypes. Proc Natl Acad Sci USA 96:12004, 1999.
119. Mummidi S, Ahuja SS, Gonzalez E, et al. Genealogy of the CCR5 locus and chemokine system gene variants associated with altered rates of HIV-1 disease progression. Nat Med 4:786, 1998.

120. Smith MW, Dean M, Carrington M, et al. Contrasting genetic influence of CCR2 and CCR5 variants on HIV-1 infection and disease progression. Hemophilia Growth and Development Study (HGDS), Multicenter AIDS Cohort Study (MACS), Multicenter Hemophilia Cohort Study (MHCS), San Francisco City Cohort (SFCC), ALIVE Study. Science 277:959, 1997.
121. Gonzalez E, Kulkarni H, Bolivar H, et al. The Influence of CCL3L1 Gene-Containing Segmental Duplications on HIV-1/AIDS Susceptibility. Science 307:1434, 2005.
122. Bleiber G, May M, Martinez R, et al. Use of a combined ex vivo/in vivo population approach for screening of human genes involved in the Human immunodeficiency virus type 1 life cycle for variants influencing disease progression. J Virol 79:12674, 2005.
123. Telenti A. Host polymorphism in post-entry steps of the HIV-1 life cycle and other genetic variants influencing HIV-1 pathogenesis. Curr Opin HIV/AIDS 1:232, 2006.
124. O'Brien SJ, Nelson GW. Human genes that limit AIDS. Nat Genet 36:565, 2004.
125. Haas DW, Wilkinson GR, Kuritzkes DR, et al. A multi-investigator/institutional DNA bank for AIDS-related human genetic studies: AACTG Protocol A5128. HIV Clin Trials 4:287, 2003.
126. Chen DT, Rosenstein DL, Muthappan P, et al. Research with stored biological samples: what do research participants want? Arch Intern Med 165:652, 2005.
127. Rotger M, Colombo S, Cavassini M, et al. Genetic variability of CYP2B6 in individuals with extremely high efavirenz plasma concentrations. 13th Conference on Retroviruses and Opportunistic Infections,Denver, Feb 2006, L-144.
128. Haas DW, Ribaudo H, Kim RB, et al. A common CYP2B6 variant is associated with efavirenz pharmacokinetics and central nervous system side effects: AACTG Study NWCS214. In: 11th Conference on Retroviruses and Opportunistic Infections, 2004.
129. Lee-Täuber B, Décosterd L, Kerb R, Telenti A. Pharmacogenetics in infectious diseases. In: Hall IP, Pirmohamed M, (ed). Pharmacogenetics. Taylor & Francis, London, 2006, p 155.
130. Zucker SD, Qin X, Rouster SD, et al. Mechanism of indinavir-induced hyperbilirubinemia. Proc Natl Acad Sci USA 98:12671, 2001.
131. Colhoun HM, McKeigue PM, Davey SG. Problems of reporting genetic associations with complex outcomes. Lancet 361:865, 2003.
132. Freimer NB, Sabatti C. Guidelines for association studies in human molecular genetics. Hum Mol Genet 14:2481, 2005.
133. A public resource that presents host genetic information concerning HIV-1 susceptibility and treatment response. Available: http://www.hiv-pharmacogenomics.org Apr 2007.
134. A compendium of polymorphisms and mutations of the human mtDNA. Available: http://www.mitomap.org Apr 2007.
135. Precise nomenclature and functional consequences of CYP450 alleles. Available: http://www.imm.ki.se/CYPalleles Apr 2007.

Chapter 30

General Immune-Based Therapies in the Management of HIV-Infected Patients

Irini Sereti, MD, Joseph A. Kovacs, MD

The development of highly active antiretroviral drugs, especially protease inhibitors (PIs) or non-nucleoside reverse transcriptase inhibitors (NNRTIs), has resulted in the identification of potent combination regimens that have markedly improved survival and clearly serve as the mainstay of current therapy for HIV-infected patients. However, despite the profound suppression of viral replication that can be seen, the level of immune restoration and the duration of viral suppression associated with such therapies can be limited in some patients.[1,2] Further, in many additional patients adverse effects or difficulties in adhering to the rigorous medication regimens decrease the feasibility of long-term therapy with these drugs. Thus identification of effective alternative therapeutic approaches for the treatment of HIV-infected patients is essential.

Given that the vast majority of HIV-related complications, including opportunistic infections and malignancies, are a result of the immunosuppression induced by HIV, rather than being directly mediated by HIV itself, an alternative approach that can complement antiretroviral therapy is to target the immune system directly, in an effort to expand immune function, prevent further immunological deterioration, or improve the host immune response to HIV.[3–5]

A variety of immune-based approaches to the management of HIV infection have been evaluated, but to date no immunotherapy has been documented in controlled trials to have a consistent clinical benefit. Many approaches have been evaluated in a preliminary fashion in uncontrolled trials, and have limited applicability at present to the management of HIV-infected patients. This chapter will summarize approaches currently being investigated, and then focus on studies with interleukin-2 (IL-2), interferon alpha, and granulocyte-macrophage colony stimulating factor (GM-CSF), three cytokines which have been more extensively studied, have demonstrable effects on surrogate markers, and are FDA approved for other indications. IL-12 and IL-7 will also be briefly discussed.

Approaches to immune restoration have included therapy with a variety of cytokines, including IL-2,[6] IL-12,[7] IL-7, interferon alpha,[8,9] interferon gamma,[10] and GM-CSF[11] (Table 30-1); adoptive immunotherapy using peripheral blood lymphocytes or bone marrow transplants;[12–16] passive immunization with hyperimmune globulin;[17–19] and T-cell vaccination to reduce anti-CD4+ T-lymphocyte autoimmunity.[20] Studies with IL-12 in HIV-infected patients have been limited, and the potential for immunological enhancement has not been well delineated.[7] IL-7 is just entering clinical trials. In limited trials conducted in the 1980s, interferon gamma was not associated with benefit, although re-evaluation of its role in the management of certain opportunistic infections may be warranted.[10,21] IL-15, which has multiple biological effects, especially related to proliferation and homeostasis of CD8+ T-lymphocyte memory cells, has been proposed as an attractive candidate for immunotherapy but has not yet reached the clinical trial stage. Adoptive immunotherapy studies with small numbers of patients have to date shown no consistent benefit.[12–14,16] Passive immunization also failed to demonstrate consistent benefit.[17–19] Gene therapy approaches utilizing both CD4+ T-lymphocyte and CD8+ T-lymphocyte cells transduced with a variety of constructs that attempt to either improve targeting of HIV-infected cells or to protect cells from HIV infection are also underway but are at a very preliminary stage.[15,22,23]

IL-2

IL-2 is a cytokine secreted primarily by activated CD4+ T-lymphocyte helper cells.[24] It plays a crucial role in the proliferation and differentiation of a variety of cells important to host immune responses, including CD4+ T-lymphocyte helper cells, CD8+ T-lymphocyte cytotoxic cells, antibody producing B cells, natural killer cells, and monocytes/macrophages. Early *in vitro* studies demonstrated that IL-2 could restore deficient natural killer (NK) cell activity as well as cytomegalovirus (CMV) specific cytotoxicity to cells from patients with AIDS, providing a rationale for clinical trials of IL-2 in this setting.[25,26]

Early clinical trials of IL-2, which used a variety of doses and durations of treatment, as well as routes of administration, but did not provide long-term therapy, did not demonstrate any long-term immunological or clinical benefit.[27–29] Given that IL-2 can activate lymphocytes, which may facilitate replication of HIV, investigators began studies combining IL-2 with antiretroviral therapies.[30–32] These studies, which initially focused on patients with relatively intact immune systems, demonstrated that IL-2, when administered intermittently for 5 day cycles approximately every 2 months at a dose of 12–18 million international units (IU)/day by continuous intravenous infusion (CIV), resulted in substantial and sustained increases in CD4+ T-lymphocyte counts, without a concomitant effect on CD8+ T-lymphocyte cells. Based on V-beta analysis, this CD4+ T-lymphocyte cell increase was polyclonal, and was associated with an increase in the number of CD4+ T-lymphocyte cells expressing the high affinity IL-2 receptor (CD25).[30] Plasma HIV viral load measured by the branched DNA (bDNA) assay demonstrated a transient increase in some patients that peaked at the end of IL-2 therapy, and returned to baseline within a week of discontinuing IL-2.[30–33] Other similar studies noted an increase in NK cell activity, or lymphokine activated killer (LAK) cell activity, during IL-2 therapy.[34] Patients with lower CD4+ T-lymphocyte counts (who were being treated exclusively with nucleoside analogues), especially those with CD4+ T-lymphocyte counts less than 100 cells/mm^3, did not demonstrate similar CD4+ T-lymphocyte cell responses, but did exhibit more frequent increases in plasma HIV levels that were occasionally sustained.[30]

A randomized trial undertaken to evaluate these preliminary observations clearly demonstrated that intermittent IL-2 therapy can lead to a substantial and sustained increase in CD4+ T-lymphocyte counts without inducing increases in plasma viral load.[6] Sixty patients with CD4+ T-lymphocyte counts greater than 200 cells/mm^3 were randomized to receive either licensed antiretroviral drugs combined with intermittent CIV IL-2 or antiretroviral therapy alone. The control group showed a gradual decline in CD4+ T-lymphocyte cell number during the 14 months of the study (−5 cells/month), while the IL-2 group showed a mean increase of 37 cells/month ($p < 0.001$) (Fig. 30-1), with a concomitant increase in the CD4+ T-lymphocyte percent. There was no difference in the CD8+ T-lymphocyte cell number over time. Additionally, there was a substantial increase in CD4+ T-lymphocyte cells that were CD25 (high-affinity IL-2 receptor) positive, and a preferential expansion of naive CD4+ T-lymphocyte cells (Fig. 30-2). Importantly, no differences in plasma HIV levels were seen between the two groups over time (Fig. 30-1). In an extension phase in which dosing of IL-2 was individualized, the mean CD4+ T-lymphocyte count for the IL-2 group was maintained at approximately double the baseline value through the follow-up period.[6] For the control group the mean CD4+ T-lymphocyte count approached that of the IL-2 group during this extension phase.

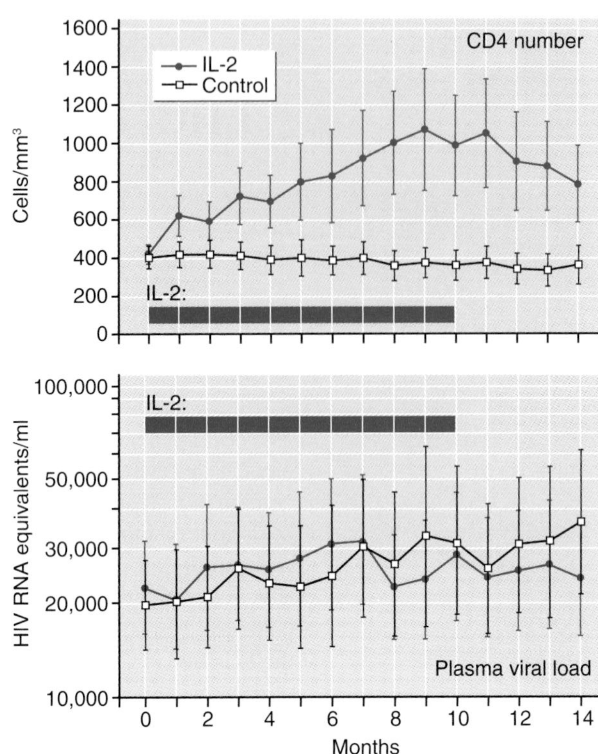

Figure 30-1 ■ Changes in mean CD4+ T-lymphocyte count (top) and viral load, as measured by the branched DNA assay (bottom), during a randomized, controlled trial of intermittent IL-2 therapy in HIV-infected patients with baseline CD4+ T-lymphocyte counts of >200 cells/mm^3. While the CD4+ T-lymphocyte count more than doubled in the IL-2 group (closed circles) compared to the control group (open squares), the viral load changes did not differ significantly between the groups. Error bars are 2 SE, which approximate the 95% confidence intervals. The shaded bars indicate the period during which IL-2 was administered (approximately every 2 months, from months 0 to 10).

Modified from Kovacs JA, Vogel S, Albert JM, et al. Controlled trial of Interleukin-2 infusions in patients infected with the human immunodeficiency virus. N Engl J Med 335:1350, 1996. Copyright 1996, Massachusetts Medical Society.

Two additional randomized trials utilizing intermittent intravenous IL-2 regimens found similar results.[35,36] In the first, IL-2 recipients also showed increased delayed type hypersensitivity responses compared to decreases in the control group.[35] The second study, which examined the relative efficacy of 3, 4, or 5 day infusions in 81 patients with more severe CD4+ T-lymphocyte depletion (baseline CD4+ T-lymphocyte counts of 100–300 cells/mm^3), found a trend toward better responses with longer therapy.[36]

While CIV IL-2 therapy is associated with substantial immunological effects, the need for continuous infusions, with the associated high cost, inconvenience, and drug toxicities as

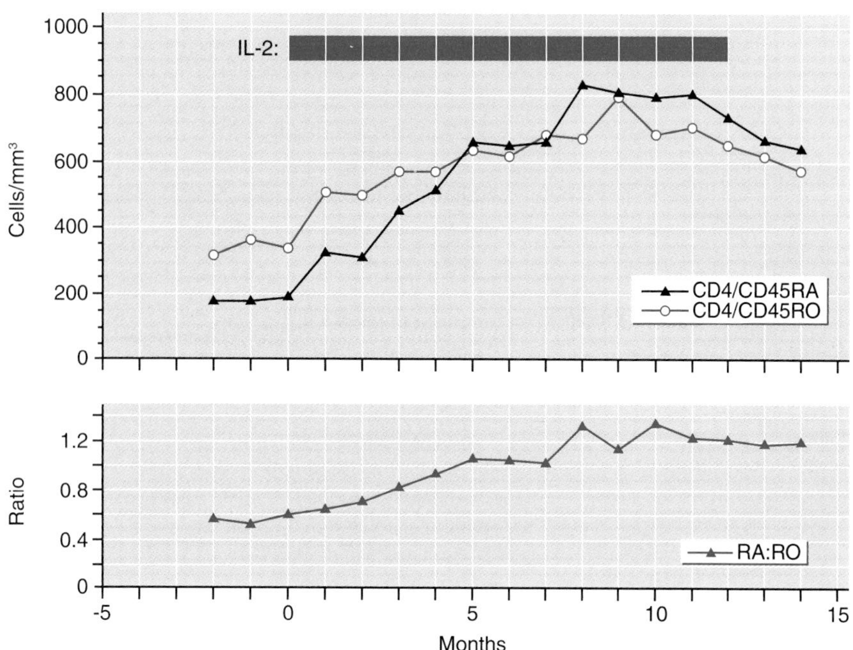

Figure 30-2 ■ Changes in naive and memory CD4+ T-lymphocyte cells in 11 patients whose CD4+ T-lymphocyte counts increased to greater than 1000 cells/mm^3 during a year of IL 2 therapy. Top panel shows the mean naive (closed triangles) and memory (open circles) CD4+ T-lymphocyte cell count during the year of IL-2 therapy, and bottom panel shows the ratio of naive to memory cells during that period. During IL-2 therapy there is an increase in both naive and memory cells, but naive cells expand preferentially, leading to an increase in the naive:memory ratio over time. Memory cells were defined as all cells that were CD45RO+; naive cells were the CD45RO– cells, which are also CD45RA+.

well as catheter related complications, has led to a focus on alternative routes of administration. Studies using subcutaneous (SC) PEG IL-2 (which is no longer being manufactured) found inadequate immunological enhancement.[35–39] However, standard IL-2 administered SC twice daily (usual starting dose, 4.5–7.5 million IU bid) is similar in activity to CIV IL-2, but is more convenient and better tolerated.[37,40,41]

A number of randomized trials have focused on optimizing the administration of SC IL-2. One study in which patients were randomized to either monthly or every other month cycles, and to two doses (1.5 or 7.5 million IU SC twice a day) of IL-2 found the higher dose induced significantly greater CD4+ T-lymphocyte responses, and that monthly therapy led to more rapid responses.[42] The inconvenience of monthly therapy probably does not warrant the more frequent dosing schedule, however. Three studies comparing three doses (1.5, 4.5, and 7.5 million IU twice a day) to antiretrovirals alone found a dose-dependent increase in CD4+ T-lymphocyte cell number, though the two higher doses both induced substantial CD4+ T-lymphocyte count increases.[43–45] In all of these randomized trials, no harmful long-term effect of IL-2 on viral load was seen; transient increases in plasma HIV RNA levels can be seen at day 5 in <5% of SC cycles.[37]

Most studies have found no evidence of enhanced viral suppression in patients receiving IL-2. However, a meta-analysis of long-term follow-up of three CIV studies suggested that IL-2 therapy led to improvements in viral load, and a controlled trial of 82 patients, over 50% of whom were receiving PI therapy, similarly suggested improved viral control in IL-2 recipients.[46,47] However, in the largest controlled trial published to date (511 patients), IL-2 therapy did not have a significant impact on viral load after 12 months.[48]

The development of highly active antiretroviral therapy (HAART) has provided the opportunity to examine the potential role of IL-2 in patients in whom a high level of viral suppression is achieved. ACTG 328 examined the effect of IL-2 in a randomized trial of PI-naive patients with baseline CD4+ T-lymphocyte counts between 50 and 350 cells/mm^3, who received 12 weeks of HAART and had suppressed plasma HIV RNA levels to less than 5000 copies/mL.[41] Median CD4+ T-lymphocyte counts were significantly higher in the IL-2 recipients (614 cells/mm^3 for SC IL-2 and 800 cells/mm^3 for initial CIV IL-2 vs 396 cells/mm^3 for controls), in the setting of good viral control (~80% of patients had <50 HIV RNA copies/mL). Similar results were observed in ANRS 079, in which patients randomized to IL-2 plus HAART had a CD4+ T-lymphocyte count increase of 865 cells/mm^3, compared to 262 cells/mm^3 in patients receiving HAART alone.[49]

Since a proportion of patients receiving HAART will be immunologic nonresponders (minimal or no increase in CD4+ T-lymphocyte count), the ability of IL-2 to increase CD4+ T-lymphocyte cell number in this setting has also been studied. In three randomized studies of patients with CD4+ T-lymphocyte counts <200–250 cells/mm^3 and viral loads <50–1000 copies/mL following 6–9 months of HAART therapy, intermittent SC IL-2 therapy induced a significant increase in CD4+ T-lymphocyte counts within 12–24 weeks.[50–52]

Table 30-1 Cytokines that are Potential Immunomodulators for the Treatment of HIV Infection

Cytokine	Trade Name	FDA-Approved Indication	Potential Additional Role in HIV Infection
Interleukin-2 Aldesleukin	Proleukin (Chiron)	Treatment of metastatic renal cell cancer or metastatic malignant melanoma:	Intermittent therapy: increase in CD4+ T-lymphocyte cell number Continuous therapy: increase in NK cell number
Interferon alpha Interferon-alpha-2a	Roferon-A (Roche)	Treatment of hairy cell leukemia, AIDS-related Kaposi sarcoma, chronic myelogenous leukemia, and chronic hepatitis C	Antiretroviral agent in patients with limited alternatives
Peginterferon alpha-2a	Pegasys (Roche)	Treatment of chronic hepatitis C	
Inteferon alpha-2b	Intron A (Schering)	Treatment of hair cell leukemia, malignant melanoma, follicular lymphoma, condylomata acuminata, AIDS-related Kaposi sarcoma, chronic hepatitis B, chronic hepatitis C	
Peginterferon alpha-2b	PEG-Intron (Schering)	Treatment of chronic hepatitis C	
GM-CSF Sargramostim	Leukine (Berlex)	Adjunctive therapy following chemotherapy or bone marrow transplantation in a variety of conditions; mobilization of hematopoietic progenitor cells	Increase in CD4+ T-lymphocyte cell number Decrease in infections
G-CSF Filgrastim	Neupogen (Amgen)	Adjunctive therapy following chemotherapy or bone marrow transplantation in a variety of conditions; mobilization of hematopoietic progenitor cells; severe chronic neutropenia	Increase in CD4+ T-lymphocyte and CD8+ T-lymphocyte cell numbers

An alternative approach to intermittent IL-2 therapy has been the continuous administration of lower doses of SC IL-2, either daily using IL-2 or twice weekly using PEG IL-2. Preliminary studies with such continuous therapy demonstrated increases in eosinophils, NK cell number, and NK and LAK cell activity, but most studies have not demonstrated an increase in CD4+ T-lymphocyte or CD8+ T-lymphocyte cell number.[38,39,53] A small study (11 patients) observed transient increases in CD4+ T-lymphocyte cell number with continuous three times per week therapy, with tachyphylaxis developing as therapy was continued.[54] A randomized study compared the effects of daily SC IL-2 (1.2 million IU m^{-2} day^{-1}) administered for 6 months to antiretroviral therapy alone in 115 patients (CD4+ T-lymphocyte counts <300 cells/mm^3).[55] Significant increases in NK and eosinophil cell number were seen in the IL-2 group. Although an early (weeks 4 and 8) increase in CD4+ T-lymphocyte cell number was seen, significant differences between the two groups were not sustained. A significant increase in the CD4+ T-lymphocyte percent and the CD4+ T-lymphocyte:CD8+ T-lymphocyte ratio was driven in part by a significant decline in the CD8+ T-lymphocyte cell number in the IL-2 group.

IL-2 administration is associated with a large number of side effects that are usually dose related, and that tend to be less frequent and less severe with SC therapy.[6,35,37,40] The most common dose-limiting toxicities are related to the constitutional symptoms that invariably occur at doses greater than 3 million IU/day; fevers, chills, rigors, sweats, muscle and joint pains, nausea and vomiting are all common.[6,40] Additional toxicities include fluid retention due to a capillary leak syndrome; elevations in hepatic enzymes and bilirubin; acalculous cholecystitis; diarrhea; renal dysfunction that is due in part to the intravascular volume depletion resulting from the capillary leak, as well as to the use of nonsteroidal antiinflammatory drugs; metabolic abnormalities, including hyponatremia, hypocalcemia, hypomagnesemia, hypoalbuminemia, and phosphate abnormalities; hypothyroidism; cardiomyopathy and congestive heart failure; neurological abnormalities; mucositis; rash, that is occasionally desquamative; and hypotension. While some of these toxicities are potentially life-threatening, such severe toxicities are rarely seen at the doses used in HIV-infected patients. Many side effects that occur can be diminished by administration of adjunctive medications (Table 30-2). Prednisone can blunt some of the toxicities (and TNF-alpha

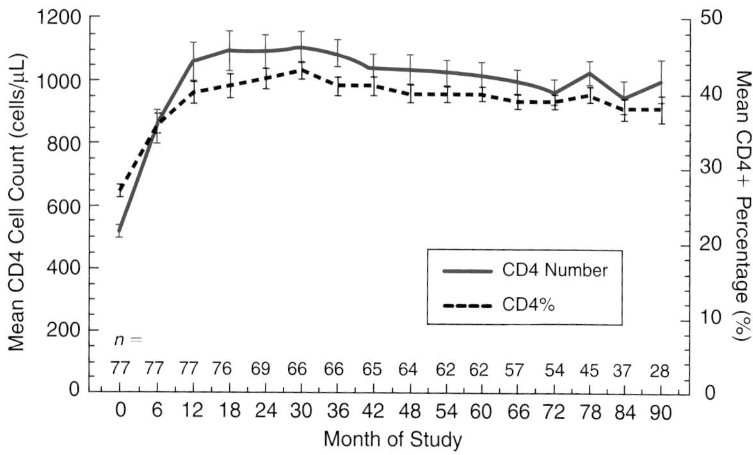

Figure 30-3 ■ Long-term changes in CD4+ T-lymphocyte number (solid line) and CD4+ T-lymphocyte percent (dashed line) for a cohort of HIV-infected patients with a mean baseline CD4+ T-lymphocyte counts of 521 cells/mm^3, who were actively participating in long-term studies of IL-2. The recent mean interval between IL-2 cycles needed to maintain these increases was 39 months.

Modified from Farel CE, Chaitt DG, Hahn BK, et al. Induction and maintenance therapy with intermittent interleukin-2 in HIV-1 infection. This research was originally published in Blood 103:3282–6, 2004. © The American Society of Hematology.

production), but also simultaneously blunts the CD4+ T-lymphocyte cell increase.[56] Most of the side effects that develop during IL-2 therapy will improve very quickly (within a few days) of discontinuing IL-2.

In patients who have demonstrated an immunological benefit from IL-2 therapy, patient inconvenience and discomfort can be decreased by individualizing the dosing regimen.[57] A strategy designed to maintain the CD4+ T-lymphocyte count above a threshold level (e.g., double the baseline value, or a count of 800 or 1000 cells/mm^3) can often result in decreasing the frequency of an IL-2 cycle to yearly or less often. A recent study of patients who had been treated intermittently with IL-2 in an individualized fashion for a mean of nearly 6 years, during which time a mean of 10 cycles were administered, found that the average recent cycling interval was 39 months.[57] This infrequent cycling was sufficient to maintain the median CD4+ T-lymphocyte count at ~1000 cells/μL (Fig. 30-3).

While substantial CD4+ T-lymphocyte count increases can be induced by intermittent IL-2, the clinical benefit of these immunological changes has not yet been demonstrated. Studies examining the function of CD4+ T-lymphocyte cells in patients receiving IL-2 suggest that the functionality of CD4+ T-lymphocyte cells pre-IL-2 and post-IL-2 appear overall to be similar.[58,59] In a substudy of ACTG 328, IL-2 treated patients did not have improved immunization responses compared to controls, despite significantly higher CD4+ T-lymphocyte cell counts. The number of substudy participants was small, however, and the two groups were not well balanced in their baseline pre-HAART characteristics.[60] In a larger randomized study of patients with higher baseline CD4+ T-lymphocyte cell counts, an improvement in antibody responses to tetatus vaccination and in proliferative responses to p24 was noted in the IL-2 group compared to controls.[49] Two studies, one a meta-analysis of three trials, found a trend toward fewer opportunistic infections in patients receiving IL-2, suggesting clinical benefit.[41,47] The true clinical efficacy of IL-2 therapy, i.e., the ability of IL-2 to prevent opportunistic infections and death, will need to be addressed in phase III studies with clinical endpoints; two such studies are currently underway, one in patients with >300 CD4+ T-lymphocyte cells/mm^3, and the other in patients with <300 CD4+ T-lymphocyte cells/mm^3 at baseline.[61,62] Evidence of clinical benefit is needed before IL-2 can be broadly recommended for the management of HIV-infected patients.

In addition to its ability to increase CD4+ T-lymphocyte counts, the potential for IL-2 to accelerate clearance of latent reservoirs of HIV has also been studied. While initial studies suggested that it was very difficult to culture HIV in a proportion of patients who had received IL-2 together with HAART therapy,[63] studies examining viral rebound following discontinuation of antiretroviral therapy found that in all patients plasma HIV levels increased, with no difference in the kinetics of rebound in IL-2 and non-IL-2 recipients.[64] Moreover, in a randomized trial of 56 patients initiating HAART, IL-2 had no effect on frequency of residual viral replication or the amount of proviral DNA.[65]

Recent studies have demonstrated that despite significant T cell proliferation during IL-2 administration, the main mechanism of CD4+ T-lymphocyte cell expansion is due to decreased T cell turnover and improved survival of CD4+ T-lymphocyte cells (Fig. 30-4).[66,67] The decreased turnover and improved survival affects predominantly CD4+ T-lymphocyte cells of naive and central memory phenotype, which are also the two subsets that are expanded preferentially by IL-2.[66–68] Among the expanded cells is a unique, polyclonal naive CD4+ T-lymphocyte cell

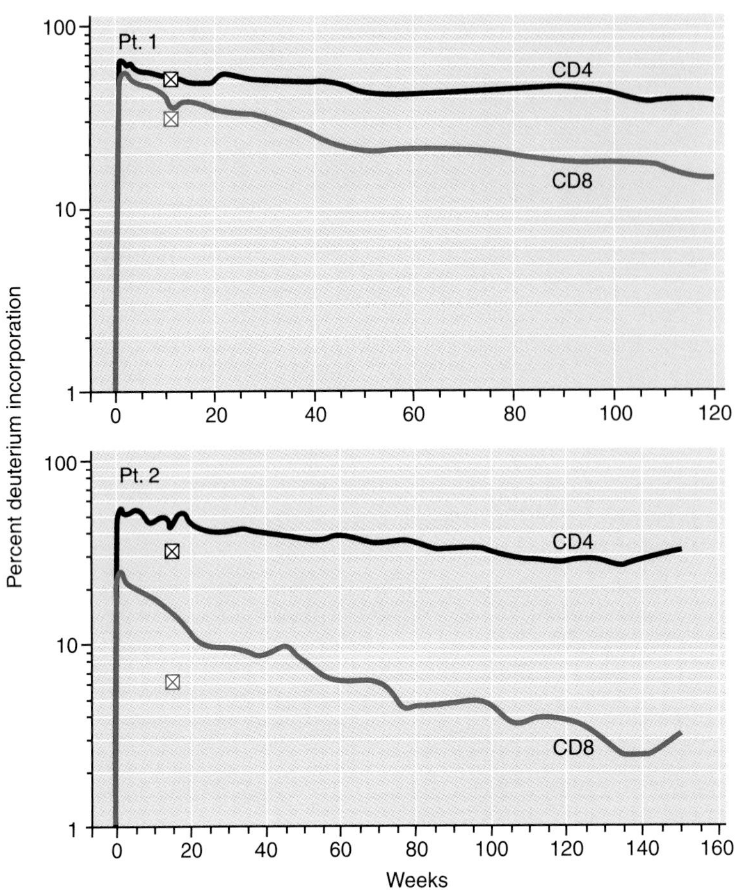

Figure 30-4 ■ Decay of label in CD4+ T-lymphocyte and CD8+ T-lymphocyte cells from two long-term IL-2 responders, illustrating the slower decay in CD4+ T-lymphocyte relative to CD8+ T-lymphocyte cells. Both patients received a 5-day infusion of deuterium-labeled glucose during an IL-2 cycle. The decay of the deuterium, which was incorporated into the DNA of cells that divided during the infusion, represents the loss of cells that divided during the IL-2 infusion. Because the y axis is on a log scale, similar decay rates will be represented by parallel lines. Both patients showed a slower loss of CD4+ T-lymphocyte cells relative to CD8+ T-lymphocyte cells, with estimated half-lives of ~3 years for CD4+ T-lymphocyte cells vs ~1 year for CD8+ T-lymphocyte cells. The open crossed symbols represent deuterium incorporation in lymph node cells, demonstrating that the peripheral blood labeling was representative of lymph node cell labeling at the same time point.

population characterized by CD25 expression (CD4+ CD45RO– CD25+) that shares some features with regulatory T cells.[68,69]

At present, IL-2 should primarily be administered during clinical trials designed to better understand the role of IL-2 in managing HIV-infected patients. If clinical benefit is documented by ongoing trials, IL-2 can potentially play a role in patients who are immunologic nonresponders to HAART therapy, as well as in patients with ongoing viral replication and declining CD4+ T-lymphocyte cell numbers. IL-2 therapy may allow periods without antiretroviral therapy or decrease the exposure to antiretroviral therapy. A pilot study (ACTG 5102) suggested that IL-2 could potentially prolong periods of antiretroviral therapy interruption by sustaining higher CD4+ T-lymphocyte counts, but this effect was not long lasting.[70] A recent structured treatment interruption trial in which patients receiving HAART were randomized to therapeutic immunization with ALVAC vCP 1433 plus HIV-LIPO-6T followed by three cycles of IL-2 or no additional therapy, found that viremia was lower and duration off-therapy was higher in the immunized/IL-2 arm.[71] The design of the study did not permit elucidation of what role, if any, IL-2 played in these responses. A more recent study of patients receiving IL-2 cycles either while remaining on continuous HAART or prior to HAART interruption showed that HIV viremia can clearly blunt the degree of CD4+ T-lymphocyte expansion that can be achieved with IL-2 but CD4+ T-lymphocyte cell expansions can still be achieved.[72] Early utilization of IL-2 (with antiretroviral therapy only during IL-2 cycles) might permit deferral of initiation of continuous antiretroviral therapy.[73] A 24-week trial of 36 patients with CD4+ T-lymphocyte counts >350 cells/mm^3 who were not receiving antiretroviral therapy found no difference in plasma HIV RNA levels, and a significant (though perhaps blunted) increase in CD4+ T-lymphocyte cell number in IL-2 recipients compared to controls.[74]

Management of IL-2 Related Toxicities

Table 30-2

Adverse Effect	Management
Constitutional symptoms (fever, chills, muscle and joint aches, fatigue)	Ibuprofen (200–600 mg q6 h) alternating with acetaminophen (650 mg q6 h); may be started prior to IL-2
Nausea/vomiting	Prochlorperazine (10 mg PO or 25 mg PR q4–6 h) or ondansetron (0.15 mg/kg IV (10 mg for 70 kg) or 8–16 mg PO q6–8 h)
Diarrhea	Loperamide (2 mg q4–6 h PO) or Lomotil (1–2 Tab. qid)
Hypotension	Increase oral fluid intake, or administer fluid bolus (e.g., 500 cc normal saline)
Mucositis	2% solution of kaolin pectate, xylocaine, and benadryl (swish prn)
Anxiety/insomnia	Lorazepam (1 mg PO q6–8 h prn); flurazepam, diphenhydramine are alternatives; avoid in patients with any mental status changes
Rash or itching	Diphenhydramine (25–50 mg PO q6 h prn) or hydroxyzine (25 mg PO tid prn)
Injection site reaction	Apply heat prn; rotate sites
Creatinine elevation	Fluids as above; discontinue meds that may be contributing, especially nonsteroidals
Hyponatremia	Follow closely for values below 130. Normal saline supplementation (50–100 cc/h) for values below 128. Discontinue IL-2 for values below 125
Hypomagnesemia	Oral magnesium supplementation
Hypocalcemia	Oral calcium supplementation (may be due to low albumin)
Dyspepsia	Ranitidine (150 mg PO q12 h) or cimetidine 300 mg PO q6 h)
Other significant toxicities or if above toxicities do not respond to therapy	Discontinue IL-2

For physicians who administer IL-2 outside a clinical trial setting, an awareness of the toxicities and management of these toxicities is essential (Table 30-2). Because of the transient viral activation that can occur, antiviral therapy should be co-administered with IL-2. Since IL-2 will result in trafficking effects on lymphocytes, with a potentially dramatic and rapid decline in lymphocytes (including CD4+ T-lymphocyte cells) in the blood during IL-2 therapy, and a marked, rapid rebound increase in lymphocytes immediately after discontinuing IL-2,[75] it is not helpful to check CD4+ T-lymphocyte counts during or immediately after IL-2 therapy. For moderate toxicities the IL-2 dose should be reduced by 3 to 6 million IU/day. Discontinuation of IL-2 will usually result in a rapid improvement in most adverse effects. While initially cycles should probably be administered approximately every other month, once a CD4+ T-lymphocyte count increase has been achieved, decreasing the frequency based on CD4+ T-lymphocyte counts can improve patient tolerability without loss of immunological benefit.[57]

IL-7

IL-7 is a cytokine that is produced by keratinocytes, epithelial cells, dendritic cells and endothelial cells in the thymus, bone marrow and lymph nodes.[76,77] IL-7 is essential for thymopoiesis and lymphocyte survival (via BCL-2 upregulation) and more recent studies suggest a critical role for IL-7 in the maturation of memory lymphocytes.[77]

Plasma levels of IL-7 were found to be elevated in lymphopenic hosts due to either HIV infection or chemotherapy and inversely correlated with CD4+ T-lymphocyte cell counts, particularly in patients with more advanced CD4+ T-lymphocyte lymphopenia, suggesting the possibility of a compensatory response.[78,79] Longitudinal analyses have demonstrated that plasma IL-7 levels decrease as CD4+ T-lymphocyte cell counts increase both after initiation of antiretroviral therapy and after recovery of lymphocytes following chemotherapy or bone marrow transplantation.[80,81] Additionally, the expression of the alpha chain of the IL-7 receptor (CD127) is decreased on both CD4+ T-lymphocyte and CD8+ T-lymphocyte cells of HIV infected patients and this decreased expression is more pronounced on CD8+ T-lymphocyte cells, particularly of the effector-activated phenotype that tend to expand in HIV infection.[82]

These observations suggest that IL-7 could be used therapeutically to improve T cell renewal and survival, and to enhance immune reconstitution in states of lymphopenia, increased T cell susceptibility to apoptosis, and memory T cell dysfunction such as HIV infection. Initial studies in nonhuman primates, including SIV-infected macaques, showed a favorable therapeutic index with biologic responses consisting of T cell proliferation as well as expansions of both CD4+ T-lymphocyte and CD8+ T-lymphocyte cells.[83–85] *In vitro* studies have suggested that IL-7 may activate latent HIV and permit infection of naive T cells by HIV,[86,87] but *in vivo* IL-7 administration to SIV-infected macaques in small studies had no effect on SIV viral load in plasma or lymph nodes.[83,85] Phase I studies of IL-7 are currently under way in both cancer and HIV infected patients.

IL-12

IL-12 is a cytokine produced primarily by antigen presenting cells that plays a critical role in generating a type 1 T helper immune response, which is characterized by preferential production of IL-2 and interferon gamma, and which plays an important role in clearing intracellular pathogens such as viruses. Single doses and multiple dose (4 week) studies of IL-12 in HIV-infected patients with a broad range of CD4+ T-lymphocyte counts showed no effect on CD4+ T-lymphocyte counts, viral load, or antigen specific lymphocyte proliferation assays.[7,88] A dose dependent increase in interferon gamma that was seen in the single dose study was not observed in the multidose study.

INTERFERON ALPHA

Interferon alpha is a cytokine produced by a variety of cells that has antiviral as well as antiproliferative and immunomodulating effects.[89] Interferon alpha is currently approved for the treatment of AIDS-related Kaposi sarcoma (KS) (discussed elsewhere), as well as hepatitis B and hepatitis C, but it also has antiretroviral effects *in vitro* as well as *in vivo*.[90] Pegylated interferon alpha has a longer half-life but similar biologic properties to unmodified interferon alpha, and is approved for treatment of chronic hepatitis C infection. Studies of unmodified interferon alpha in patients with KS demonstrated higher tumor regression rates in patients with higher baseline CD4+ T-lymphocyte counts, suggesting that this activity was related at least in part to immunomodulating rather than direct antiproliferative effects.[8,9] These studies similarly suggested that antiretroviral activity was also related to the level of immunocompetence. A randomized, placebo-controlled trial of interferon alpha (starting dose, 35 million U/day SC) in 34 asymptomatic patients with greater than 400 CD4+ T-lymphocyte cells/mm^3 and positive HIV cultures of peripheral blood mononuclear cells demonstrated antiretroviral activity, with 41% of the interferon alpha group compared to 13% of the control group developing persistently negative HIV cultures ($P = 0.05$).[91] Toxicities in the interferon alpha group were common, and included flu-like symptoms, granulocytopenia and elevated liver function tests; 35% of the interferon alpha group withdrew because of toxicities.

Subsequent uncontrolled and controlled studies of interferon alpha in combination with the nucleoside analogues zidovudine, zalcitabine, or didanosine have suggested modest enhancement of anti-HIV activities (<0.5 log decline in plasma HIV RNA levels) with regimens that included interferon alpha, but with more frequent toxicities.[92–96] Moreover, the CD4+ T-lymphocyte cell response to antiretroviral therapy appears to be blunted in patients receiving interferon alpha, presumably as a consequence of the antilymphoproliferative effect of this agent.[97] None of these studies has demonstrated an effect of interferon alpha therapy on clinical progression.[95,97,98]

Currently the role of interferon alpha in HIV-infected patients is to treat patients with KS, or with chronic hepatitis B or hepatitis C infection. Interferon alpha is not used as an antiretroviral agent although it could conceivably be considered as part of a salvage regimen. It will be important to assess the anti-HIV activity of polyethylene glycol-conjugated interferon alpha, which has greater anti-hepatitis C activity than the unmodified drug, and thus has become the treatment of choice for this infection.[99,100] Preliminary data suggests an anti-HIV effect similar to unmodified interferon alpha.[101] An intriguing retrospective study of patients diagnosed with PML in the mid 1980s suggests that interferon alpha may have activity in this disease.[102]

Immunization in an attempt to induce anti-interferon alpha antibodies (to counteract overproduction of interferon alpha) is also being studied in HIV-infected patients, though a controlled trial showed no benefit to this approach.[103]

GM-CSF

GM-CSF is a cytokine that induces proliferation and differentiation of progenitor cells of the granulocyte-macrophage pathways, as well as activation of mature cells.[104] Initial *in vitro* studies suggested that GM-CSF enhanced HIV infection, although under differing conditions viral suppression was seen. Initial clinical trials with GM-CSF were undertaken to help increase neutrophil counts, but were subsequently expanded to examine potential beneficial immunologic and antiretroviral effects. While a small uncontrolled trial (12 patients, 4 weeks of therapy)[105] found no effect on viral load or CD4+ T-lymphocyte or CD8+ T-lymphocyte cell number, a randomized open label trial (244 patients, 12 weeks of therapy) found no change in p24 antigen levels, but a 53% increase in CD4+ T-lymphocyte cell number, with a similar increase in CD8+ T-lymphocyte cell number, and consequently no change in the CD4+ T-lymphocyte : CD8+ T-lymphocyte ratio, at week 12.[106] Following discontinuation of therapy, these values were not sustained but rapidly returned to baseline. No significant difference in infections was seen between the two groups.

A subsequent randomized, placebo-controlled study (105 patients, 24 weeks of therapy) in relatively antiretroviral-naive patients (<6 months of zidovudine) with CD4+

T-lymphocyte counts under 300 cells/mm^3 or a history of an opportunistic infection found no significant difference in the incidence of opportunistic infections or survival between groups receiving GM-CSF (125 μg/m^2) or placebo.[107] A statistically significant decrease in plasma HIV levels (–0.6 log vs –0.07 log) was seen at 6 months in the GM-CSF group; in subgroup analysis, statistical significance was seen only in patients receiving nucleoside analogue monotherapy. An additional small (20 patient) placebo controlled study found a suggestion of decreasing viral load and increasing CD4+ T-lymphocyte counts in patients receiving GM-CSF.[108]

A phase III placebo-controlled trial in 309 patients with advanced disease (CD4+ T-lymphocyte counts <50 cells/mm^3 or <100 cells/mm^3 with a history of prior opportunistic infection) examined the effects of GM-CSF (250 μg three times/week for 24 weeks) on clinical endpoints (AIDS-defining opportunistic infections, bacterial pneumonia, or death).[11] No significant difference was seen in these protocol-defined endpoints, though the incidence of any infection (including skin, oropharyngeal, and urinary tract) or death was significantly less in the GM-CSF group (120 vs 104 events, $P = 0.03$). A significant increase in CD4+ T-lymphocyte cell number but not percent was also seen.

A recent randomized placebo-controlled trial of 116 patients who received GM-CSF for 16 weeks found a modest increase in viral load (+0.048 vs 0.103 log copies/mL) as well as CD4+ T-lymphocyte counts (+14 vs –6 cells/mm^3) in GM-CSF recipients compared to controls.[109]

GM-CSF was also evaluated as an adjunctive therapy during a small (33 patient) randomized structured treatment interruption trial. While there was a suggestion of a transient beneficial effect on CD4+ T-lymphocyte counts at week 4, this was not sustained at week 12.[110]

Thus, the benefit of GM-CSF as an immunomodulator in HIV-infected patients remains to be demonstrated. Studies examining the effects on AIDS-related endpoints have not shown benefit to GM-CSF therapy. While CD4+ T-lymphocyte count increases have been seen, whether this represents expansion of CD4+ T-lymphocyte cells or effects related to changes in trafficking, remains unclear. Further, while some studies suggest modest antiretroviral activity, others have not found this or seen decreases in viral load only in subsets.

A randomized, placebo-controlled trial of granulocyte colony stimulating factor (G-CSF) in 30 HIV-infected patients with CD4+ T-lymphocyte counts <350 cells/mm^3 demonstrated a transient increase in CD4+ T-lymphocyte cells, CD8+ T-lymphocyte cells, and NK cells, but no change in NK activity or plasma HIV RNA levels, and a decrease in PHA and *Candida* antigen-stimulated proliferation.[111] The CD4+ T-lymphocyte and CD8+ T-lymphocyte increases resulted from an increase in memory and activated cells.

Additional studies demonstrating clear clinical benefit are needed before either GM-CSF or G-CSF is utilized clinically in HIV-infected patients as an immunomodulator for targeting nonmyeloid cells.

IMMUNOSUPPRESSIVE THERAPY

Because immune activation may lead to an increase in HIV replication or more efficient replication, an alternative approach to immune enhancement has been to suppress the immune system in an attempt to slow HIV replication. Agents that have been used in this manner include cyclosporin A, corticosteroids, and IL-10.

While cyclosporin A did not seem to provide benefit in trials conducted in the 1980s, a recent nonrandomized trial combining 8 weeks of cyclosporin A with continuous HAART in nine acutely infected patients found that the CD4+ T-lymphocyte count increase was significantly greater than in a comparator group receiving HAART alone.[112–114] The long-term benefits of such increases are unclear; it is also unclear if such therapy will lead to higher CD4+ T-lymphocyte counts if antiretroviral therapy is discontinued. However, a 12-week randomized, placebo-controlled trial of cyclosporin A in 28 patients with chronic HIV infection and a CD4+ T-lymphocyte count of >500 cells/mm^3, about half of whom were on no antiretroviral therapy, and the other half on dual nucleoside therapy, found no changes in CD4+ T-lymphocyte counts or activation markers.[115] Small (~0.27 log) but significant increases in viral load were seen in the cyclosporin A group.

An open 1-year trial of prednisolone (0.3–0.5 mg kg^{-1} day^{-1} orally) in 44 patients with CD4+ T-lymphocyte counts of 200–800 cells/mm^3 found evidence of decreased CD4+ T-lymphocyte cell activation as well as CD4+ T-lymphocyte count increases (mean pretherapy, 421 cells/mm^3; mean first-year posttherapy, 523 cells/mm^3), without concomitant CD8+ T-lymphocyte count increases.[116] This increase occurred primarily during the first 3 months, following which the CD4+ T-lymphocyte counts decreases somewhat and remained stable during the rest of the year. Viral load remained unchanged during the year. A randomized placebo-controlled trial that was terminated prematurely (related to concerns about development of osteonecrosis) found a similar trend in CD4+ T-lymphocyte count increases, although no effect on activation or apoptosis was seen.[117] Adverse effects of corticosteroids, including potential immunosuppressive effects as well as an association with the development of avascular necrosis, must be considered in assessing the risk:benefit ratio of such therapy.[118]

IL-10 is an anti-inflammatory cytokine that in single dose studies in HIV-infected patients was shown to lead to a transient decline in plasma viral load.[119] However, a randomized, placebo controlled 39 patient trial of 3 doses of subcutaneously administered IL-10 found no significant change in plasma HIV RNA levels or CD4+ T-lymphocyte cell number during 4 weeks of therapy.[120]

ACKNOWLEDGMENT

The United States Government has been issued a patent for immunologic enhancement with intermittent IL-2 therapy, listing Dr Kovacs as one of the inventors.

REFERENCES

1. Connors M, Kovacs JA, Krevat S, et al. HIV infection induces changes in CD4+ T-cell phenotype and depletions within the CD4+ T-cell repertoire that are not immediately restored by antiviral or immune-based therapies. Nat Med 3:533–40, 1997.
2. Grabar S, Le Moing V, Goujard C, et al. Clinical outcome of patients with HIV-1 infection according to immunologic and virologic response after 6 months of highly active antiretroviral therapy. Ann Intern Med 133:401–10, 2000.
3. Lederman MM. Host-directed and immune-based therapies for human immunodeficiency virus infection. Ann Intern Med 122:218–22, 1995.
4. Sereti I, Lane HC. Immunopathogenesis of human immunodeficiency virus: implications for immune-based therapies. Clin Infect Dis 32:1738–55, 2001.
5. Letvin NL, Walker BD. Immunopathogenesis and immunotherapy in AIDS virus infections. Nat Med 9:861–6, 2003.
6. Kovacs JA, Vogel S, Albert JM, et al. Controlled trial of interleukin-2 infusions in patients infected with the human immunodeficiency virus. N Engl J Med 335:1350–6, 1996.
7. Jacobson MA, Spritzler J, Landay A, et al. A Phase I, placebo-controlled trial of multi-dose recombinant human interleukin-12 in patients with HIV infection. AIDS 16:1147–54, 2002.
8. Lane HC, Kovacs JA, Feinberg J, et al. Anti-retroviral effects of interferon-alpha in AIDS-associated Kaposi's sarcoma. Lancet 2:1218–22, 1998.
9. de Wit R, Schattenkerk JK, Boucher CA, et al. Clinical and virological effects of high-dose recombinant interferon-alpha in disseminated AIDS-related Kaposi's sarcoma. Lancet 2:1214–7, 1988.
10. Lane HC, Davey RT Jr, Sherwin SA, et al. A phase I trial of recombinant human interferon-gamma in patients with Kaposi's sarcoma and the acquired immunodeficiency syndrome (AIDS). J Clin Immunol 9:351–61, 1989.
11. Angel JB, High K, Rhame F, et al. Phase III study of granulocyte-macrophage colony-stimulating factor in advanced HIV disease: effect on infections, CD4 cell counts and HIV suppression. Leukine/HIV Study Group. AIDS 14:387–95, 2000.
12. Lane HC, Masur H, Longo DL, et al. Partial immune reconstitution in a patient with the acquired immunodeficiency syndrome. N Engl J Med 311:1099–103, 1984.
13. Lane HC, Zunich KM, Wilson W, et al. Syngenic bone marrow transplantations and adoptive transfer of peripheral blood lymphocytes combined with zidovudine in human immunodeficiency virus (HIV) infection. Ann Intern Med 113:512–9, 1990.
14. Klimas N, Patarca R, Walling J, et al. Clinical and immunological changes in AIDS patients following adoptive therapy with activated autologous CD8 T cells and interleukin-2 infusion. AIDS 8:1073–81, 1994.
15. Walker RE, Bechtel CM, Natarajan V, et al. Long-term in vivo survival of receptor-modified syngeneic T cells in patients with human immunodeficiency virus infection. Blood 96:467–74, 2000.
16. Zunich KM, Lane HC, Davey RT, et al. Phase I/II studies of the toxicity and immunogenicity of recombinant gp160 and p24 vaccines in HIV-infected individuals. AIDS Res Hum Retroviruses 8:1335, 1992.
17. Jacobson JM, Colman N, Ostrow NA, et al. Passive immunotherapy in the treatment of advanced human immunodeficiency virus infection. J Infect Dis 168:298–305, 1993.
18. Vittecoq D, Chevret S, Morand JL, et al. Passive immunotherapy in AIDS: a double-blind randomized study based on transfusions of plasma rich in anti-human immunodeficiency virus 1 antibodies vs transfusions of seronegative plasma. Proc Natl Acad Sci USA 92:1195–9, 1995.
19. Levy J, Youvan T, Lee ML. Passive hyperimmune plasma therapy in the treatment of acquired immunodeficiency syndrome: results of a 12-month multicenter double-blind controlled trial. The Passive Hyperimmune Therapy Study Group. Blood 84:2130–35, 1994.
20. Abulafia-Lapid R, Mayan S, Bentwich Z, et al. T-cell vaccination against anti-CD4+ T-Lymphocyte autoimmunity in HIV-1 subtypes B and C-infected patients – an extended open trial. Vaccine 23:2149–53, 2005.
21. Agosti JM, Coombs RW, Collier AC, et al. A randomized, double-blind, phase I/II trial of tumor necrosis factor and interferon-gamma for treatment of AIDS-related complex (Protocol 025 from the AIDS Clinical Trials Group). AIDS Res Hum Retroviruses 8:581–7, 1992.
22. Morgan RA. Genetic strategies to inhibit HIV. Mol Med Today 5:454–8, 1999.
23. Dornburg R, Pomerantz RJ. HIV-1 gene therapy: promise for the future. Adv Pharmacol 49:229–61, 2000.
24. Smith KA. Interleukin-2: inception, impact, and implications. Science 240:1169–76, 1988.
25. Siegel JP, Rook AH, Djeu JY, Quinnan GV Jr. Interleukin 2 therapy in infectious diseases: rationale and prospects. Infection 12:298–302, 1984.
26. Rook AH, Masur H, Lane HC, et al. Interleukin-2 enhances the depressed natural killer and cytomegalovirus-specific cytotoxic activities of lymphocytes from patients with the acquired immune deficiency syndrome. J Clin Invest 72:398–403, 1983.
27. Ernst M, Kern P, Flad HD, Ulmer AJ. Effects of systemic in vivo interleukin-2 (IL-2) reconstitution in patients with acquired immune deficiency syndrome (AIDS) and AIDS-related complex (ARC) on phenotypes and functions of peripheral blood mononuclear cells (PBMC). J Clin Immunol 6:170–81, 1986.
28. Lane HC, Siegel JP, Rook AH, et al. Use of interleukin-2 in patients with acquired immunodeficiency syndrome. J Biol Response Mod 3:512–6, 1984.
29. Volberding P, Moody DJ, Beardslee D, et al. Therapy of acquired immune deficiency syndrome with recombinant interleukin-2. AIDS Res Hum Retroviruses 3:115–24, 1987.
30. Kovacs JA, Baseler M, Dewar R, et al. Increases in CD4 T lymphocytes with intermittent courses of interleukin-2 in patients with human immunodeficiency virus infection: A preliminary study. N Engl J Med 332:567–75, 1995.
31. Ramachandran RV, Katzenstein D, Merigan TC. Long-term effects of interleukin-2 on CD4 cell counts in human immunodeficiency virus-infected patients [letter]. J Infect Dis 170:1044–6, 1994.
32. Schwartz DH, Skowron G, Merigan TC. Safety and effects of interleukin-2 plus zidovudine in asymptomatic individuals infected with human immunodeficiency virus. J Acquir Immune Defic Syndr 4:11–23, 1991.
33. Kovacs JA, Imamichi H, Vogel S, et al. Effects of intermittent interleukin-2 therapy on plasma and tissue human immunodeficiency virus levels and quasispecies expression. J Infect Dis 182:1063–9, 2000.
34. Mazza P, Bocchia M, Tumietto F, et al. Recombinant interleukin-2 (rIL-2) in acquired immune deficiency syndrome (AIDS): preliminary report in patients with lymphoma associated with HIV infection. Eur J Haematol 49:1–6, 1992.
35. Carr A, Emery S, Lloyd A, et al. Outpatient continuous intravenous interleukin-2 or subcutaneous, polyethylene glycol-modified interleukin-2 in human immunodeficiency virus-infected patients: a randomized, controlled, multicenter study. J Infect Dis 178:992–9, 1998.
36. de Boer AW, Markowitz N, Lane HC, et al. A randomized controlled trial evaluating the efficacy and safety of intermittent 3-, 4-, and 5-day cycles of intravenous recombinant human interleukin-2 combined with antiretroviral therapy (ART)

versus ART alone in HIV-seropositive patients with 100–300 CD4+ T cells. Clin Immunol 106:188–96, 2003.
37. Levy Y, Capitant C, Houhou S, et al. Comparison of subcutaneous and intravenous interleukin-2 in asymptomatic HIV-1 infection: a randomised controlled trial. ANRS 048 study group. Lancet 353:1923–9, 1999.
38. Teppler H, Kaplan G, Smith K, et al. Efficacy of low doses of the polyethylene glycol derivative of interleukin-2 in modulating the immune response of patients with human immunodeficiency virus type 1 infection. J Infect Dis 167:291–8, 1993.
39. Teppler H, Kaplan G, Smith KA, et al. Prolonged immunostimulatory effect of low-dose polyethylene glycol interleukin 2 in patients with human immunodeficiency virus type 1 infection. J Exp Med 177:483–92, 1993.
40. Davey RT Jr, Chaitt DG, Piscitelli SC, et al. Subcutaneous administration of interleukin-2 in human immunodeficiency virus type 1-infected persons. J Infect Dis 175:781–9, 1997.
41. Mitsuyasu R, Pollard R, Gelman R, Weng D. Prospective, randomized, controlled phase II study of highly active antiretroviral therapy (HAART) with continuous iv (CIV) or subcutaneous (SC) interleukin-2 (IL-2) in HIV-infected patients with CD4+ counts of 50–350 cells/mm^3: ACTG 328-Final results at 84 weeks. In: Abstracts of the 8th Conference on Retroviruses and Opportunistic Infections, Chicago, IL, 4–8 Feb 2001, abstract 17.
42. Davey RT Jr, Chaitt DG, Albert JM, et al. A randomized trial of high- versus low-dose subcutaneous interleukin-2 outpatient therapy for early human immunodeficiency virus type 1 infection. J Infect Dis 179:849–58, 1999.
43. Arduino RC, Nannini EC, Rodriguez-Barradas M, et al. CD4+ cell response to 3 doses of subcutaneous interleukin 2: meta-analysis of 3 Vanguard studies. Clin Infect Dis 39:115–22, 2004.
44. Losso MH, Belloso WH, Emery S, et al. A randomized, controlled, phase II trial comparing escalating doses of subcutaneous interleukin-2 plus antiretrovirals versus antiretrovirals alone in human immunodeficiency virus-infected patients with CD4+ cell counts >350/mm^3. J Infect Dis 181:1614–21, 2000.
45. Ruxrungtham K, Suwanagool S, Tavel JA, et al. A randomized, controlled 24-week study of intermittent subcutaneous interleukin-2 in HIV-1 infected patients in Thailand. Vanguard Study Group. AIDS 14:2509–13, 2000.
46. Davey RT Jr, Murphy RL, Graziano FM, et al. Immunologic and virologic effects of subcutaneous interleukin 2 in combination with antiretroviral therapy: a randomized controlled trial. JAMA 284:183–9, 2000.
47. Emery S, Capra WB, Cooper DA, et al. Pooled analysis of 3 randomized, controlled trials of interleukin-2 therapy in adult human immunodeficiency virus type 1 disease. J Infect Dis 182:428–34, 2000.
48. Abrams DI, Bebchuk JD, Denning ET, et al. Randomized, open-label study of the impact of two doses of subcutaneous recombinant interleukin-2 on viral burden in patients with HIV-1 infection and CD4+ cell counts of > or = 300/mm^3: CPCRA 059. J Acquir Immune Defic Syndr 29:221–31, 2002.
49. Levy Y, Durier C, Krzysiek R, et al. Effects of interleukin-2 therapy combined with highly active antiretroviral therapy on immune restoration in HIV-1 infection: a randomized controlled trial. AIDS 17:343–51, 2003.
50. Arno A, Ruiz L, Juan M, et al. Efficacy of low-dose subcutaneous interleukin-2 to treat advanced human immunodeficiency virus type 1 in persons with <250/μL CD4 T cells and undetectable plasma virus load. J Infect Dis 180:56–60, 1999.
51. David D, Nait-Ighil L, Dupont B, et al. Rapid effect of interleukin-2 therapy in human immunodeficiency virus infected patients whose CD4 cell counts increase only slightly in response to combined antiretroviral treatment. J Infect Dis 183:730–5, 2001.
52. Katlama C, Carcelain G, Duvivier C, et al. Interleukin-2 accelerates CD4 E cell reconstitution in HIV-infected patients with severe immunosuppression despite highly active antiretroviral therapy: the ILSTIM study – ANRS 082. AIDS 16:2027–34, 2002.
53. Jacobson EL, Pilaro F, Smith KA. Rational interleukin 2 therapy for HIV positive individuals: daily low doses enhance immune function without toxicity. Proc Natl Acad Sci USA 93:10405–10, 1996.
54. Larsen CS, Ostergard L, Moller BK, Buhl MR. Subcutaneous interleukin-2 in combination with anti-retroviral therapy for treatment of HIV-1-infected subjects. Scand J Infect Dis 32:153–60, 2000.
55. Lalezari JP, Beal JA, Ruane PJ, et al. Low-dose daily subcutaneous interleukin-2 in combination with highly active antiretroviral therapy in HIV+ patients: a randomized controlled trial. HIV Clin Trials 1:1–15, 2000.
56. Tavel JA, Sereti I, Walker RE, et al. A randomized, double-blinded, placebo-controlled trial of intermittent administration of interleukin-2 and prednisone in subjects infected with human immunodeficiency virus. J Infect Dis 188:531–6, 2003.
57. Farel CE, Chaitt DG, Hahn BK, et al. Induction and maintenance therapy with intermittent interleukin-2 in HIV-1 infection. Blood 103:3282–6, 2004.
58. Giedlin M, McGrath M, Gascon R, et al. Immunological characterization of HIV seropositive patients treated with subcutaneous Proleukin (aldesleukin) recombinant Interleukin-2. Int Conf AIDS 11:282, 1996.
59. Kelleher AD, Roggensack M, Emery S, et al. Effects of IL-2 therapy in asymptomatic HIV-infected individuals on proliferative responses to mitogens, recall antigens and HIV-related antigens. Clin Exp Immunol 113:85–91, 1998.
60. Valdez H, Mitsuyasu R, Landay A, et al. Interleukin-2 increases CD4+ lymphocyte numbers but does not enhance responses to immunization: results of A5046s. J Infect Dis 187:320–5, 2003.
61. Levy Y, Mitsuyasu R, Tambusi G, et al. CD4 count increases in patients with CD4 counts of 50–300 treated with intermittent Il-2: immunologic results from the study of IL-2 in combination with active antiretroviral therapy (SILCAAT) Trial; abstract F14/3. In: 9th European AIDS Conference (EACS), 2003, Warsaw, Poland, 2003.
62. Emery S, Abrams DI, Cooper DA, et al. and ESPRIT Study Group. The evaluation of subcutaneous proleukin (interleukin-2) in a randomized international trial: rationale, design, and methods of ESPRIT. Control Clin Trials 23:198–220, 2002.
63. Chun TW, Engel D, Mizell SB, et al. Effect of interleukin-2 on the pool of latently infected, resting CD4+ T cells in HIV-1-infected patients receiving highly active anti-retroviral therapy. Nat Med 5:651–5, 1999.
64. Davey RT Jr, Bhat N, Yoder C, et al. HIV-1 and T cell dynamics after interruption of highly active antiretroviral therapy (HAART) in patients with a history of sustained viral suppression. Proc Natl Acad Sci USA 96:15109–4, 1999.
65. Stellbrink HJ, van Lunzen J, Westby M, et al. Effects of interleukin-2 plus highly active antiretroviral therapy on HIV-1 replication and proviral DNA (COSMIC trial). AIDS 16:1479–87, 2002.
66. Kovacs JA, Lempicki RA, Sidorov IA, et al. Induction of prolonged survival of CD4+ T-lymphocytes by intermittent IL-2 therapy in HIV-infected patients. J Clin Invest 115:2139–48, 2005.
67. Sereti I, Anthony KB, Martinez-Wilson H, et al. IL-2-induced CD4+ T-cell expansion in HIV-infected patients is associated with long-term decreases in T-cell proliferation. Blood 104:775–80, 2004.
68. Sereti I, Imamichi H, Natarajan V, et al. In vivo expansion of CD4CD45RO-CD25 T cells expressing foxP3 in IL-2-treated HIV-infected patients. J Clin Invest 115:1839–47, 2005.

69. Sereti I, Martinez-Wilson H, Metcalf JA, et al. Long-term effects of intermittent interleukin 2 therapy in patients with HIV infection: characterization of a novel subset of CD4+(+)/CD25(+) T cells. Blood 100:2159–67, 2002.
70. Henry K, Katzenstein D, Cherng DW, et al. and A5102 Study Team of the AIDS Clinical Trials Group. A pilot study evaluating time to CD4 T-cell count <350 cells/mm(3) after treatment interruption following antiretroviral therapy +/− interleukin 2: results of ACTG A5102. J Acquir Immune Defic Syndr 42:140–8, 2006.
71. Levy Y, Durier C, Lascaux AS, et al. Sustained control of viremia following therapeutic immunization in chronically HIV-1-infected individuals. AIDS 20:405–13, 2006.
72. Keh CE, Shen JM, Hahn B, et al. Interruption of antiretroviral therapy blunts but does not abrogate CD4 T-Cell Responses to IL-2 administration in HIV infected patients. AIDS 20:361–9, 2006.
73. Levy Y. Cytokine-based modulation of immune function in HIV infection. Curr Opin HIV AIDS 1:69–73, 2006.
74. Youle M, Emery S, Fisher M, et al. A Randomised Trial of Subcutaneous Intermittent Interleukin-2 without Antiretroviral Therapy in HIV-Infected Patients: The UK-Vanguard Study. PLoS Clin Trials 1:e3. Epub, 2006.
75. Kovacs JA, Vogel S, Metcalf JA, et al. Interleukin-2 induced immune effects in human immunodeficiency virus-infected patients receiving intermittent interleukin-2 immunotherapy. Eur J Immunol 31:1351–60, 2001.
76. Fry TJ, Mackall CL. Interleukin-7: from bench to clinic. Blood 99:3892–904, 2002.
77. Hofmeister R, Khaled AR, Benbernou N, et al. Interleukin-7: physiological roles and mechanisms of action. Cytokine Growth Factor Rev 10:41–60, 1999.
78. Fry TJ, Connick E, Falloon J, et al. A potential role for interleukin-7 in T-cell homeostasis. Blood 97:2983–90, 2001.
79. Napolitano LA, Grant RM, Deeks SG, et al. Increased production of IL-7 accompanies HIV-1-mediated T-cell depletion: implications for T-cell homeostasis. Nat Med 7:73–9, 2001.
80. Bolotin E, Annett G, Parkman R, Weinberg K. Serum levels of IL-7 in bone marrow transplant recipients: relationship to clinical characteristics and lymphocyte count. Bone Marrow Transplant 23:783–8, 1999.
81. Fry TJ, Mackall CL. Interleukin-7: master regulator of peripheral T-cell homeostasis? Trends Immunol 22:564–71, 2001.
82. Paiardini M, Cervasi B, Albrecht H, et al. Loss of CD127 expression defines an expansion of effector CD8+ T cells in HIV-infected individuals. J Immunol 174:2900–9, 2005.
83. Beq S, Nugeyre MT, Fang RH, et al. IL-7 Induces immunological improvement in SIV-infected Rhesus Macaques under antiviral therapy. J Immunol 176:914–22, 2006.
84. Fry TJ, Moniuszko M, Creekmore S, et al. IL-7 therapy dramatically alters peripheral T-cell homeostasis in normal and SIV-infected nonhuman primates. Blood 101:2294–9, 2003.
85. Nugeyre MT, Monceaux V, Beq S, et al. IL-7 stimulates T cell renewal without increasing viral replication in simian immunodeficiency virus-infected macaques. J Immunol 171:4447–53, 2003.
86. Brooks DG, Hamer DH, Arlen PA, et al. Molecular characterization, reactivation, and depletion of latent HIV. Immunity 19:413–23, 2003.
87. Steffens CM, Managlia EZ, Landay A, Al-Harthi L. Interleukin-7-treated naive T cells can be productively infected by T-cell-adapted and primary isolates of human immunodeficiency virus 1. Blood 99:3310–8, 2002.
88. Jacobson MA, Hardy D, Connick E, et al. Phase 1 trial of a single dose of recombinant human interleukin-12 in human immunodeficiency virus-infected patients with 100–500 CD4 cells/μL. J Infect Dis 182:1070–6, 2000.
89. Baron S, Tyring SK, Fleischmann WJ, et al. The interferons. Mechanisms of action and clinical applications. JAMA 266:1375–83, 1991.
90. Ho DD, Hartshorn KL, Rota TR, et al. Recombinant human interferon alfa-A suppresses HTLV-III replication in vitro. Lancet 1:602–4, 1985.
91. Lane HC, Davey V, Kovacs JA, et al. Interferon-alpha in patients with asymptomatic human immunodeficiency virus (HIV) infection. A randomized, placebo-controlled trial. Ann Intern Med 112:805–11, 1990.
92. Fischl MA, Uttamchandani RB, Resnick L, et al. A phase I study of recombinant human interferon-alpha 2a or human lymphoblastoid interferon-alpha n1 and concomitant zidovudine in patients with AIDS-related Kaposi's sarcoma. J Acquir Immune Defic Syndr 4:1–10, 1991.
93. Krown SE, Gold JW, Niedzwiecki D, et al. Interferon-alpha with zidovudine: safety, tolerance, and clinical and virologic effects in patients with Kaposi sarcoma associated with the acquired immunodeficiency syndrome (AIDS). Ann Intern Med 112:812–21, 1990.
94. Kovacs JA, Bechtel C, Davey RT Jr, et al. Combination therapy with didanosine and interferon-alpha in human immunodeficiency virus-infected patients: results of a phase I/II trial. J Infect Dis 173:840–8, 1996.
95. Lane HC, Herpin B, Banks S, et al. Zidovudine vs alpha interferon vs the combination in patients with early HIV infection. Int Conf AIDS 8:Mo15, 1992.
96. Fischl MA, Richman DD, Saag M, et al. Safety and antiviral activity of combination therapy with zidovudine, zalcitabine, and two doses of interferon-alpha2a in patients with HIV. AIDS Clinical Trials Group Study 197. J Acquir Immune Defic Syndr Hum Retrovirol 16:247–53, 1997.
97. Haas DW, Lavelle J, Nadler JP, et al. A randomized trial of interferon alpha therapy for HIV type 1 infection. AIDS Res Hum Retroviruses 16:183–90, 2000.
98. Krown SE, Aeppli D, Balfour HH Jr. Phase II, randomized, open-label, community-based trial to compare the safety and activity of combination therapy with recombinant interferon-alpha2b and zidovudine versus zidovudine alone in patients with asymptomatic to mildly symptomatic HIV infection. HIV Protocol C91–253 Study Team. J Acquir Immune Defic Syndr Hum Retrovirol 20:245–54, 1999.
99. Zeuzem S, Feinman SV, Rasenack J, et al. Peginterferon alfa-2a in patients with chronic hepatitis C. N Engl J Med 343:1666–72, 2000.
100. Torriani FJ, Rodriguez-Torres M, Rockstroh JK, et al. Peginterferon Alfa-2a plus ribavirin for chronic hepatitis C virus infection in HIV-infected patients. N Engl J Med 351:438–50, 2004.
101. Neumann A, Wu L, McLaughlin M, et al. Differential Anti-Viral Effect of Peg-IFN on HIV and HCV in Treatment of HIV/HCV Co-Infected Patients. In: 3rd IAS Conference on HIV Pathogenesis and Treatment; 2005, Rio de Janeiro, Brazil, 2005, p WePe3.C17.
102. Huang SS, Skolasky RL, Dal Pan GJ, et al. Survival prolongation in HIV-associated progressive multifocal leukoencephalopathy treated with alpha-interferon: an observational study. J Neurovirol 4:324–32, 1998.
103. Gringeri A, Musicco M, Hermans P, et al. Active anti-interferon-alpha immunization: a European-Israeli, randomized, double-blind, placebo-controlled clinical trial in 242 HIV-1-infected patients (the EURIS study). J Acquir Immune Defic Syndr Hum Retrovirol 20:358–70, 1999.
104. Deresinski SC. Granulocyte-macrophage colony-stimulating factor: potential therapeutic, immunological and antiretroviral effects in HIV infection. AIDS 13:633–43, 1999.
105. Scadden DT, Pickus O, Hammer SM, et al. Lack of in vivo effect of granulocyte-macrophage colony-stimulating factor

on human immunodeficiency virus type 1. AIDS Res Hum Retroviruses 12:1151–9, 1996.

106. Barbaro G, Di Lorenzo G, Grisorio B, et al. Effect of recombinant human granulocyte-macrophage colony-stimulating factor on HIV-related leukopenia: a randomized, controlled clinical study. AIDS 11:1453–61, 1997.
107. Brites C, Gilbert MJ, Pedral-Sampaio D, et al. A randomized, placebo-controlled trial of granulocyte-macrophage colony-stimulating factor and nucleoside analogue therapy in AIDS. J Infect Dis 182:1531–5, 2000.
108. Skowron G, Stein D, Drusano G, et al. The safety and efficacy of granulocyte-macrophage colony-stimulating factor (Sargramostim) added to indinavir- or ritonavir-based antiretroviral therapy: a randomized double-blind, placebo-controlled trial. J Infect Dis 180:1064–71, 1999.
109. Jacobson JM, Lederman MM, Spritzler J, et al. Granulocyte-macrophage colony-stimulating factor induces modest increases in plasma human immunodeficiency virus (HIV) type 1 RNA levels and CD4+ lymphocyte counts in patients with uncontrolled HIV infection. J Infect Dis 188:1804–14, 2003.
110. Fagard C, Le Braz M, Gunthard H, et al. A controlled trial of granulocyte macrophage-colony stimulating factor during interruption of HAART. AIDS 17:1487–92, 2003.
111. Aladdin H, Ullum H, Dam Nielsen S, et al. Granulocyte colony-stimulating factor increases CD4+ T cell counts of human immunodeficiency virus-infected patients receiving stable, highly active antiretroviral therapy: results from a randomized, placebo-controlled trial. J Infect Dis 181:1148–52, 2000.
112. Andrieu J, Even P, Venet A. Effects of cyclosporin on T-cell subsets in human immunodeficiency virus disease. Clin Immunol Immunopathol 46:181–98, 1988.
113. Phillips A, Wainberg MA, Coates R, et al. Cyclosporine-induced deterioration in patients with AIDS. Can Med Assoc J 140: 1456–60, 1989.
114. Rizzardi GP, Harari A, Capiluppi B, et al. Treatment of primary HIV-1 infection with cyclosporin A coupled with highly active antiretroviral therapy. J Clin Invest 109:681–8, 2002.
115. Calabrese LH, Lederman MM, Spritzler J, et al. Placebo-controlled trial of cyclosporin-A in HIV-1 disease: implications for solid organ transplantation. J Acquir Immune Defic Syndr 29:356–62, 2002.
116. Andrieu JM, Lu W, Levy R. Sustained increases in CD4 cell counts in asymptomatic human immunodeficiency virus type 1-seropositive patients treated with prednisolone for 1 year. J Infect Dis 171:523–30, 1995.
117. Wallis RS, Kalayjian R, Jacobson JM, et al. A study of the immunology, virology, and safety of prednisone in HIV-1-infected subjects with CD4 cell counts of 200 to 700 mm(−3). J Acquir Immune Defic Syndr 32:281–6, 2003.
118. Miller KD, Masur H, Jones EC, et al. High prevalence of osteonecrosis of the femoral head in HIV-infected adults. Ann Intern Med 137:17–25, 2002.
119. Weissman D, Ostrowski M, Daucher JA, et al. Interleukin-10 decreases HIV plasma viral load: results of a phase 1 clinical trial. In: Abstracts of the 4th Conference on Retroviruses and Opportunistic Infections, 1997, abstract 37.
120. Angel JB, Jacobson MA, Skolnik PR, et al. A multicenter, randomized, double-blind, placebo-controlled trial of recombinant human interleukin-10 in HIV-infected subjects. AIDS 14:2503–8, 2000.

Chapter 31

Therapeutic Vaccines

Anna R. Thorner, MD, Dan H. Barouch, MD, PhD

INTRODUCTION

Antiretroviral therapy (ART) has proven remarkably effective at reducing acquired immunodeficiency syndrome (AIDS)-related morbidity and mortality. However, ART is unable to eradicate the virus and is associated with substantial drug-related toxicities and increasing drug resistance. It would therefore be desirable to develop immune-based therapies that enhance immune control of viral replication and reduce the requirement for ART. The goal of an HIV-1 therapeutic vaccine would be to enhance virus-specific cellular and humoral immune responses, which could in turn lead to reduced HIV-1 RNA levels, increased CD4+ T-lymphocyte counts, and delayed progression to AIDS. Several candidate therapeutic vaccines have already been evaluated for safety and immunogenicity, but no substantial clinical benefits have been demonstrated. This chapter reviews the immunologic rationale for HIV-1 therapeutic vaccines and highlights key preclinical and clinical studies to date.

IMMUNOLOGIC RATIONALE

Increasing evidence has demonstrated that adaptive immune responses are critical for control of viral replication. A therapeutic vaccine aims to enhance HIV-1-specific immunity and to improve this immune control. CD8+ T-lymphocytes exert antiviral cytolytic activity as well as other effector functions, and CD4+ T-lymphocytes provide immunologic 'help' to B cells and CD8+ T-lymphocytes.[1–3] The importance of CD8+ T-lymphocytes has been directly demonstrated by experimental depletion of CD8+ T-lymphocytes in SIV-infected rhesus macaques by monoclonal antibody administration.[4,5] Moreover, in humans with acute HIV-1 infection, potent CD8+ T-lymphocyte responses were temporally correlated with initial control of HIV-1 viremia.[6,7] Long-term nonprogressors (LTNPs) have also been shown to have vigorous HIV-1-specific CD8+ and CD4+ T-lymphocyte responses that were associated with preservation of CD4+ T-lymphocyte counts and durable control of viral replication without the use of ART.[1,8,9] T-lymphocytes from LTNPs retain a high proliferative capacity and exhibit high levels of perforin expression, suggesting the potential importance of these immune functions.[10]

Patients who initiate ART during acute HIV-1 infection typically have preserved HIV-1-specific CD4+ T-lymphocyte responses as well as detectable CD8+ T-lymphocyte responses.[2,11–13] In an observational study, supervised treatment interruptions (STIs) of HIV-1-infected individuals treated with ART during acute infection resulted in viral rebound, which in turn stimulated expansion of HIV-1-specific CD4+ and CD8+ T-lymphocyte responses and led to transiently improved virologic control during subsequent STIs.[13] Although the durability of this immune control was limited,[14] this study showed that immune-based interventions can exert detectable effects on viral replication. STI studies in chronically HIV-1-infected individuals, however, have failed to demonstrate improved control of viral replication.[15] In addition, a recent study has highlighted potential safety concerns associated with performing STIs in chronically HIV-1-infected individuals.[16] These data suggest that it may be substantially more challenging to design therapeutic vaccines for the majority of patients who are treated during chronic HIV-1 infection as compared with individuals who begin ART during acute HIV-1 infection.

The immunologic rationale of therapeutic vaccination is illustrated in Figure 31-1. As shown in Figure 31-1A, HIV-1-infected subjects treated with effective ART typically exhibit low levels of HIV-1-specific humoral and cellular immune responses and undetectable viral RNA levels. Following discontinuation of ART, HIV-1 RNA levels predictably rebound within several weeks to pretreatment 'setpoint' levels. As shown in Figure 31-1B, therapeutic vaccination in the context of suppressive ART may enhance virus-specific immune responses, which could improve

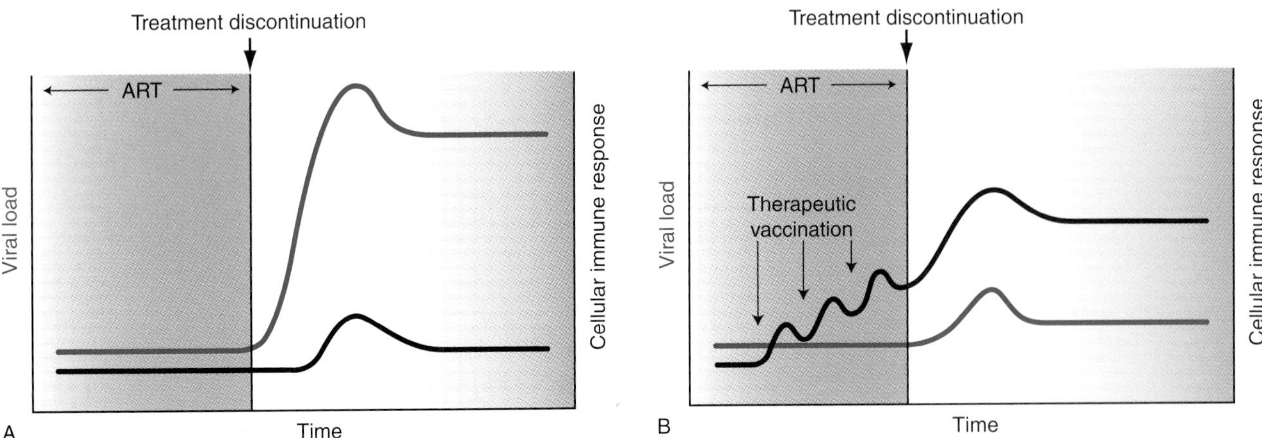

Figure 31-1 ■ Schematic depiction of rationale for therapeutic vaccination. HIV-1-specific cellular immune responses (black) and viral RNA levels (blue) in HIV-1-infected subjects on ART. (**A**) Discontinuation of ART results in predictable viral rebound with increased virus-specific cellular immune responses that fail to control the resurgent virus. (**B**) Therapeutic vaccination while on suppressive ART results in enhancement of HIV-1-specific cellular immune responses that may partially control viral rebound following withdrawal of ART.

immune control of viral replication following discontinuation of ART.

Although there is currently no evidence that HIV-1 therapeutic vaccines will afford any clinical benefit, a recent study has demonstrated the clinical utility of a therapeutic vaccine for a different virus. A live, attenuated varicella-zoster virus (VZV) vaccine has been shown to reduce the incidence and severity of illness from clinical herpes zoster as well as the incidence of postherpetic neuralgia, demonstrating that therapeutic vaccination for this persistent viral infection can result in clinical benefits.[17] Although the mechanism of action of the VZV vaccine remains to be established, it presumably involves enhancement of VZV-specific immunity. However, VZV causes latent infection without active viral replication, whereas HIV-1 causes chronic infection with persistent viral replication, and thus it will likely prove substantially more challenging to produce an HIV-1 therapeutic vaccine than a VZV therapeutic vaccine.

NONHUMAN PRIMATE STUDIES

Nonhuman primates have proven instrumental in the development of both prophylactic and therapeutic HIV-1 vaccine candidates. Although rhesus macaques cannot be infected with HIV-1, they can be infected with simian immunodeficiency virus (SIV), which leads to loss of CD4+ T-lymphocytes and clinical AIDS-like syndromes. Although significant biologic differences exist between SIV-infected rhesus macaques and HIV-1-infected humans, this animal model has proven useful for evaluating the immunogenicity and protective efficacy of candidate AIDS vaccines.

There have been several studies to date evaluating the immunogenicity and potential efficacy of therapeutic vaccines using this animal model. Early studies focused on recombinant protein subunit vaccines and whole inactivated virus vaccines. These vaccine modalities, however, have yielded disappointing results, presumably because they failed to elicit broadly reactive neutralizing antibodies and did not induce CD8+ T-lymphocyte responses. Current vaccine strategies are therefore largely focused on gene delivery technologies to augment virus-specific cellular immune responses, including recombinant virus vector-based vaccines, plasmid DNA vaccines, and dendritic cell (DC)-based vaccines.

A proof-of-concept study in the macaque model utilized a recombinant poxvirus vaccine expressing SIV structural genes (NYVAC-SIV). In rhesus macaques treated with ART following primary SIV infection, vaccination with NYVAC-SIV augmented SIV-specific CD4+ and CD8+ T-lymphocyte responses. Following discontinuation of ART, all animals exhibited viral rebound, but SIV replication was spontaneously controlled in six of eight vaccinated animals and in four of seven unvaccinated controls.[18] Although the observed virologic control following treatment discontinuation likely reflected the fact that ART was initiated during acute infection, this study nevertheless demonstrated that virus-specific immune responses could be enhanced by therapeutic vaccination. In a second study from this same group, NYVAC-SIV vaccines expressing *gag-pol-env* and *rev-tat-nef* were administered with interleukin-2 (IL-2) as an adjuvant to chronically SIV-infected macaques on ART.[19] Following treatment discontinuation, viral setpoint was significantly lower in vaccinated macaques than in control animals, and this difference persisted for at least 4 months. Viral containment in this study was also inversely correlated with vaccine-induced virus-specific CD4+ and CD8+ T-cell responses.

Therapeutic vaccine strategies utilizing plasmid DNA vaccines have focused on novel delivery approaches, given the relatively low immunogenicity of DNA vaccines in nonhuman primates and humans as compared with small animal models. One strategy involves transfecting DCs with plasmid DNA vaccines and then administering these DCs to macaques.[20] A topical DNA vaccine has also been developed and was shown to enhance SIV-specific cellular immune responses in chronically SIV-infected macaques on ART.[21] Following withdrawal of ART, vaccinated animals exhibited improved control of viral rebound as compared with unvaccinated controls. Another study demonstrated that autologous DCs pulsed with inactivated SIV enhanced virus-specific cellular immune responses and resulted in a substantial reduction in viral RNA levels in vaccinated animals as compared with unvaccinated controls.[22]

Studies in nonhuman primates have shown that several vaccine candidates can enhance virus-specific immune responses and can partially control viral rebound following discontinuation of ART. Although encouraging, translating these preclinical findings into clinical trials remains a major challenge. Studies in nonhuman primates are often designed to utilize vaccines that are based on sequences identical to those of the infecting virus. Moreover, many experimental vaccines have proven less immunogenic in humans as compared with nonhuman primates. Clinical trials are therefore critical for evaluating the potential utility of therapeutic HIV-1 vaccines.

CLINICAL STUDIES

As shown in Table 31-1, studies of therapeutic HIV-1 vaccines in humans have explored a variety of different vaccine modalities, including recombinant protein subunits, inactivated virus particles, virus-like particles, plasmid DNA vaccines, recombinant poxvirus vector-based vaccines and DC-based vaccines.[23–41] These studies have demonstrated the safety and immunogenicity of several vaccine approaches, but none of these studies have convincingly demonstrated clinically meaningful endpoints. In HIV-1-infected individuals receiving ART, vaccination with the attenuated poxvirus vectors ALVAC vCP1452 and modified vaccinia Ankara (MVA) proved safe and immunogenic.[34–36,38] The magnitude of vaccine-enhanced immune responses elicited by both of these vectors, however, was modest. Similarly, an inactivated, envelope-depleted HIV-1 preparation (Remune) was shown to be safe and immunogenic[28], but a large phase III trial failed to show any significant effect on HIV-1 viral RNA levels or progression-free survival.[27] The lack of a beneficial effect in this study may have reflected incomplete suppression of viral replication with ART prior to vaccination as well as the inability of this vaccine to elicit potent virus-specific CD8+ T-lymphocyte responses.

A randomized, double-blinded, placebo-controlled study has also recently evaluated the impact of therapeutic vaccination with ALVAC vCP1452 and/or Remune in 79 HIV-1-infected subjects treated with ART during acute infection.[39] These vaccines led to detectable increases of HIV-1-specific CD4+ and CD8+ T-cell responses, but they failed to afford any improvement in virologic control 24 weeks after discontinuation of ART. This was a disappointing result, since subjects treated during acute HIV-1 infection theoretically should be the most amenable to immune-based interventional strategies as a result of their relatively preserved immune systems. There was also no significant correlation between *gag*-specific CD4+ and CD8+ T-lymphocyte responses and viral RNA levels following discontinuation of ART in this study, suggesting that the correlates of immunity are more complex than simply the magnitude of these immune responses.

Another study has recently investigated therapeutic vaccination with ALVAC vCP1433 and HIV-1 lipopeptides (Lipo6T) together with IL-2 as an adjuvant in chronically HIV-1-infected subjects on ART. In this study, a higher percentage of vaccinees developed significant HIV-1 p24 proliferative responses and CD4+ T-lymphocyte responses as compared with controls. The breadth and magnitude of HIV-1-specific IFN-γ-producing CD8+ T-lymphocyte responses also improved in the vaccine group as compared with the control group. After treatment discontinuation, 24% of vaccinees exhibited a statistically significant reduced viral setpoint as compared with only 5% of controls, and virologic control correlated with vaccine-elicited cellular immune responses.[40]

Table 31-1 Results of Recent HIV-1 Therapeutic Vaccine Clinical Studies

Vaccine	Patient Characteristics	Results
Protein Subunits		
rgp160 (Kundu et al[23])	Chronic HIV-1 infection, CD4>400 cells/μL, not on ART; *n* = 21 vaccinees, five controls	Increased CD4+ and CD8+ T-cell responses
rgp160 (Goebel et al[24])	Chronic HIV-1 infection; CD4>200 cells/μL; some patients on ART; *n* = 103 vaccinees, 105 controls	Increased lymphoproliferative responses; no differences in CD4 counts, HIV-1 RNA levels or clinical outcomes
rgp160 (Birx et al[25])	Chronic HIV-1 infection; CD4 >400 cells/μL; not on ART; *n* = 302 vaccinees, 306 controls	Increased humoral and lymphoproliferative responses; no differences in CD4 counts, HIV-1 RNA levels or clinical outcomes
rgp120 (Schooley et al[26])	Chronic HIV-1 infection; CD4>50 cells/μL; some patients on ART; *n* = 200 vaccinees, 98 controls	Increased lymphoproliferative responses

(Continued)

(Continued)

Table 31-1

Vaccine	Patient Characteristics	Results
Inactivated Virus		
Remune (Kahn et al[27])	Chronic HIV-1 infection; CD4>300 cells/μL; some patients on ART; n = 1262 vaccinees, 1265 controls	Increased lymphoproliferative responses; no differences in CD4 percents, HIV-1 RNA levels or clinical outcomes
Remune (Robbins et al[28])	Chronic HIV-1 infection; CD4>250 cells/μL; HIV-1 RNA levels<500 copies/mL; on ART; n = 5 vaccinees, five controls	Increased lymphoproliferative responses
Virus-Like Particle		
p24 virus-like particle (Kelleher et al[29])	Chronic HIV-1 infection; CD4> 400 cells/μL; not on ART at enrollment; n = 41 vaccinees, 20 controls	No changes in humoral or lymphoproliferative responses; no differences in HIV-1 RNA levels
DNA		
DNA-nef/rev/tat (Calarota et al[30])	Chronic HIV-1 infection; some subjects on ART; n = 9 vaccinees	Increased CD8+ T-cell responses
DNA-env/rev (MacGregor et al[31])	Chronic HIV-1 infection; CD4>500 cells/μL, not on ART; n = 15 vaccinees	Increased humoral, lymphoproliferative responses; no differences in CD4 counts or HIV-1 RNA levels
DNA-HIV A (Dorrell et al[32])	Chronic HIV-1 infection; CD4>300 cells/μL; HIV-1 RNA levels<400 copies/mL; on ART; n = 10 vaccinees	Increased CD4+ and CD8+ T-cell responses in minority of subjects
DNA-nef/MultiHIV B (Blazevic et al[33])	Chronic HIV-1 infection; on ART; n = 27 vaccinees	No humoral responses; increased CD4+ and CD8+ T-cell responses
Poxvirus		
MVA-nef (Cosma et al[34])	Chronic HIV-1 infection; CD4>400 cells/μL; on ART; n = 10 vaccinees	Increased CD4+ T-cell responses
MVA-nef (Harrer et al[35])	Chronic HIV-1 infection; CD4>400 cells/μL; on ART; n = 14 vaccinees	Increased CD4+ and CD8+ T-cell responses
MVA-HIV A (Dorrell et al[36])	Chronic HIV-1 infection; CD4>300 cells/μL; HIV-1 RNA levels<50 copies/mL; on ART; n = 16 vaccinees two controls	Increased CD4+ and CD8+ T-cell responses
Poxvirus + Protein		
ALVAC vCP1452 + rgp160 (Markowitz et al[37]; Jin et al[38])	ART initiated during acute or early HIV-1 infection; HIV-1 RNA levels<50 copies/mL; n = 11 vaccinees, five controls	Increased humoral, lymphoproliferative and CD8+ T-cell responses; no differences in HIV-1 RNA levels after discontinuation of ART
Poxvirus + Inactivated Virus		
ALVAC vCP1452 ± Remune (Kinloch-de Loes et al[39])	ART initiated during acute HIV-1 infection; HIV-1 RNA levels <50 copies/mL; n = 52 vaccinees, 27 controls	Increased CD4+ and CD8+ T-cell responses; no differences in CD4 counts or HIV-1 RNA levels after discontinuation of ART
Poxvirus + Lipopeptides + IL-2		
ALVAC vCP1433 + Lipo-6T + IL-2 (Levy et al[40])	Chronic HIV-1-infection; CD4>350 cells/μL; on ART; n = 34 vaccinees, 37 controls	Increased lymphoproliferative, CD4+ and CD8+ T-cell responses; 24% vaccinees vs 5% controls had lower HIV-1 RNA levels after discontinuation of ART
Dendritic Cells + Inactivated HIV-1		
Autologous dendritic cells loaded with inactivated virus (Garcia et al[41])	Chronic HIV-1 infection; CD4>500 cells/μL; on ART; RNA levels <20 copies/mL; n = 12 vaccinees, six controls	No change in humoral or T-cell responses; decreased HIV-1 RNA levels in four subjects
Autologous dendritic cells loaded with inactivated virus (Lu et al[42])	Chronic HIV-1 infection; CD4>300 cells/μL; not on ART; n = 18 vaccinees	Increased CD4+ and CD8+ T-cell responses; reduction in HIV-1 RNA levels from baseline values in eight subjects

Another novel therapeutic vaccine approach involves the use of antigen-loaded autologous DCs. In one study, autologous DCs were pulsed with virus obtained during an initial interruption of ART and were then utilized as a therapeutic vaccine after ART was re-initiated. Following a second interruption of ART, there was a significant lengthening in mean doubling time during the viral rebound.[41] In a second study, 18 chronically HIV-1-infected individuals who were not receiving ART were treated with monocyte-derived DCs loaded with autologous inactivated HIV-1. HIV-1 RNA levels in vaccinated individuals decreased by 80% over the first 112 days, and eight subjects had virologic suppression of over 90% for at least 1 year.[42] Moreover, virologic suppression appeared to correlate with HIV-1-specific CD4+ and CD8+ T-lymphocyte responses. These results suggest that certain therapeutic vaccines can indeed exert a degree of virologic control, but these studies involved only a limited number of subjects and the clinical relevance of these observations remains unclear.

CONCLUSIONS

Clinical studies have to date shown that therapeutic vaccines are generally safe and well-tolerated in HIV-1-infected individuals. Moreover, certain vaccine regimens have also been able to enhance HIV-1-specific immune responses. It has not, however, been possible to demonstrate any convincing clinical benefits following therapeutic vaccination. It is hoped that the next generation of candidate vaccines will prove substantially more immunogenic than the ones that have been previously evaluated. For example, recombinant adenovirus vector-based vaccines and heterologous DNA prime-live vector boost regimens have been shown to be highly immunogenic in nonhuman primates as well as in clinical trials in HIV-1-uninfected individuals.[43–46] Studies are currently underway to evaluate the potential of these more immunogenic vaccine modalities as therapeutic vaccines in HIV-1-infected patients.

The goal of an HIV-1 therapeutic vaccine is to boost virus-specific immunity in HIV-1-infected individuals with the objective of allowing increased time without the need for ART. It is likely that ongoing therapeutic vaccine studies with novel vaccine strategies will be able to enhance HIV-1-specific immune responses in infected individuals, but it is possible that clinical benefits may not be realized with currently available technologies. Nevertheless, ongoing therapeutic vaccine studies will provide valuable information regarding the immunogenicity of these vaccine candidates and should increase our understanding of immune control of HIV-1.

ACKNOWLEDGMENTS

We acknowledge support from the National Institutes of Health (AI066305, AI066924, AI058727, AI060368), the Bill & Melinda Gates Foundation, and the Doris Duke Charitable Foundation.

REFERENCES

1. Rosenberg ES, Billingsley JM, Caliendo AM, et al. Vigorous HIV-1-specific CD4+ T cell responses associated with control of viremia. Science 278:1447–50, 1997.
2. Oxenius A, Price DA, Easterbrook PJ, et al. Early highly active antiretroviral therapy for acute HIV-1 infection preserves immune function of CD8+ and CD4+ T lymphocytes. Proc Natl Acad Sci USA 97:3382–7, 2000.
3. Kalams SA, Buchbinder SP, Rosenberg ES, et al. Association between virus-specific cytotoxic T-lymphocyte and helper responses in human immunodeficiency virus type 1 infection. J Virol 73:6715–20, 1999.
4. Schmitz JE, Kuroda MJ, Santra S, et al. Control of viremia in simian immunodeficiency virus infection by CD8+ lymphocytes. Science 283:857–60, 1999.
5. Jin X, Bauer DE, Tuttleton SE, et al. Dramatic rise in plasma viremia after CD8(+) T cell depletion in simian immunodeficiency virus-infected macaques. J Exp Med 189:991–8, 1999.
6. Borrow P, Lewicki H, Hahn BH, et al. Virus-specific CD8+ cytotoxic T-lymphocyte activity associated with control of viremia in primary human immunodeficiency virus type 1 infection. J Virol 68:6103–10, 1994.
7. Koup RA, Safrit JT, Cao Y, et al. Temporal association of cellular immune responses with the initial control of viremia in primary human immunodeficiency virus type 1 syndrome. J Virol 68:4650–5, 1994.
8. Cao Y, Qin L, Zhang L, Safrit J, Ho DD. Virologic and immunologic characterization of long-term survivors of human immunodeficiency virus type 1 infection. N Engl J Med 332:201–8, 1995.
9. Rinaldo C, Huang XL, Fan ZF, et al. High levels of anti-human immunodeficiency virus type 1 (HIV-1) memory cytotoxic T-lymphocyte activity and low viral load are associated with lack of disease in HIV-1-infected long-term nonprogressors. J Virol 69:5838–42, 1995.
10. Migueles SA, Laborico AC, Shupert WL, et al. HIV-specific CD8+ T cell proliferation is coupled to perforin expression and is maintained in nonprogressors. Nat Immunol 3:1061–8, 2002.
11. Lisziewicz J, Rosenberg E, Lieberman J, et al. Control of HIV despite the discontinuation of antiretroviral therapy. N Engl J Med 340:1683–4, 1993.
12. Ortiz GM, Nixon DF, Trkola A, et al. HIV-1-specific immune responses in subjects who temporarily contain virus replication after discontinuation of highly active antiretroviral therapy. J Clin Invest 104:R13–8, 1999.
13. Rosenberg ES, Altfeld M, Poon SH, et al. Immune control of HIV-1 after early treatment of acute infection. Nature 407:523–6, 2000.
14. Kaufmann DE, Lichterfeld M, Altfeld M, et al. Limited durability of viral control following treated acute HIV infection. PLOS Med 1:e36, 2004.
15. Oxenius A, Price DA, Gunthard HF, et al. Stimulation of HIV-specific cellular immunity by structured treatment interruption fails to enhance viral control in chronic HIV infection. Proc Natl Acad Sci USA 99:13747–52, 2002.
16. El-Sadr W, Neaton J, Investigators TSS. Episodic CD4-guided use of antiretroviral therapy is inferior to continuous therapy: results of the SMART study. In: 13th Conference on Retroviruses and Opportunistic Infections, Denver, CO, USA, 5–8 Feb 2006.
17. Oxman MN, Levin MJ, Johnson GR, et al. A vaccine to prevent herpes zoster and postherpetic neuralgia in older adults. N Engl J Med 352:2271–84, 2005.
18. Hel Z, Venzon D, Poudyal M, et al. Viremia control following antiretroviral treatment and therapeutic immunization during

primary SIV251 infection of macaques. Nat Med 6:1140–6, 2000.
19. Tryniszewska E, Nacsa J, Lewis MG, et al. Vaccination of macaques with long-standing SIVmac251 infection lowers the viral set point after cessation of antiretroviral therapy. J Immunol 169:5347–57, 2002.
20. Lisziewicz J, Gabrilovich DI, Varga G, et al. Induction of potent human immunodeficiency virus type 1-specific T-cell-restricted immunity by genetically modified dendritic cells. J Virol 75:7621–8, 2001.
21. Lisziewicz J, Trocio J, Xu J, et al. Control of viral rebound through therapeutic immunization with DermaVir. AIDS 19:35–43, 2005.
22. Lu W, Wu X, Lu Y, et al. Therapeutic dendritic-cell vaccine for simian AIDS. Nat Med 9:27–32, 2003.
23. Kundu SK, Katzenstein D, Moses LE, Merigan TC. Enhancement of human immunodeficiency virus (HIV)-specific CD4+ and CD8+ cytotoxic T-lymphocyte activities in HIV-infected asymptomatic patients given recombinant gp160 vaccine. Proc Natl Acad Sci USA 89:11204–8, 1992.
24. Goebel FD, Mannhalter JW, Belshe RB, et al. Recombinant gp160 as a therapeutic vaccine for HIV-infection: results of a large randomized, controlled trial. European Multinational IMMUNO AIDS Vaccine Study Group. AIDS 13:1461–8, 1999.
25. Birx DL, Loomis-Price LD, Aronson N, et al. Efficacy testing of recombinant human immunodeficiency virus (HIV) gp160 as a therapeutic vaccine in early-stage HIV-1-infected volunteers. rgp160 Phase II Vaccine Investigators. J Infect Dis 181:881–9, 2000.
26. Schooley RT, Spino C, Kuritzkes D, et al. Two double-blinded, randomized, comparative trials of 4 human immunodeficiency virus type 1 (HIV-1) envelope vaccines in HIV-1-infected individuals across a spectrum of disease severity: AIDS Clinical Trials Groups 209 and 214. J Infect Dis 182:1357–64, 2000.
27. Kahn JO, Cherng DW, Mayer K, et al. Evaluation of HIV-1 immunogen, an immunologic modifier, administered to patients infected with HIV having 300 to 549 × 10(6)/L CD4 cell counts: A randomized controlled trial. JAMA 284:2193–202, 2000.
28. Robbins GK, Addo MM, Troung H, et al. Augmentation of HIV-1-specific T helper cell responses in chronic HIV-1 infection by therapeutic immunization. AIDS 17:1121–6, 2003.
29. Kelleher AD, Roggensack M, Jaramillo AB, et al. Safety and immunogenicity of a candidate therapeutic vaccine, p24 virus-like particle, combined with zidovudine, in asymptomatic subjects. Community HIV Research Network Investigators. AIDS 12:175–82, 1998.
30. Calarota S, Bratt G, Nordlund S, et al. Cellular cytotoxic response induced by DNA vaccination in HIV-1-infected patients. Lancet 351:1320–5, 1998.
31. MacGregor RR, Boyer JD, Ugen KE, et al. First human trial of a DNA-based vaccine for treatment of human immunodeficiency virus type 1 infection: safety and host response. J Infect Dis 178:92–100, 1998.
32. Dorrell L, Yang H, Iversen AK, et al. Therapeutic immunization of highly active antiretroviral therapy-treated HIV-1-infected patients: safety and immunogenicity of an HIV-1 gag/poly-epitope DNA vaccine. AIDS 19:1321–3, 2005.
33. Blazevic V, Krohn K, Stanescu I, et al. Cell mediated immune response in HIV-1 infected subjects on HAART induced by two different DNA vaccines expressing either single gene, GTU-Nef or multigenes, GTU-MultiHIV of a subtype B-HIV-1. In: AIDS Vaccine, 29 Aug to 1 Sep 2006, Amsterdam, Netherlands, The International Society for Antiviral Research; 2006.
34. Cosma A, Nagaraj R, Buhler S, et al. Therapeutic vaccination with MVA-HIV-1 nef elicits nef-specific T-helper cell responses in chronically HIV-1 infected individuals. Vaccine 22:21–9, 2003.
35. Harrer E, Bauerle M, Ferstl B, et al. Therapeutic vaccination of HIV-1-infected patients on HAART with a recombinant HIV-1 nef-expressing MVA: safety, immunogenicity and influence on viral load during treatment interruption. Antivir Ther 10:285–300, 2005.
36. Dorrell L, Yang H, Ondondo B, et al. Expansion and diversification of virus-specific T cells following immunization of human immunodeficiency virus type 1 (HIV-1)-infected individuals with a recombinant modified vaccinia virus Ankara/HIV-1 Gag vaccine. J Virol 80:4705–16, 2006.
37. Markowitz M, Jin X, Hurley A, et al. Discontinuation of antiretroviral therapy commenced early during the course of human immunodeficiency virus type 1 infection, with or without adjunctive vaccination. J Infect Dis 186:634–43, 2002.
38. Jin X, Ramanathan M Jr, Barsoum S, et al. Safety and immunogenicity of ALVAC vCP1452 and recombinant gp160 in newly human immunodeficiency virus type 1-infected patients treated with prolonged highly active antiretroviral therapy. J Virol 76:2206–16, 2002.
39. Kinloch-de Loes S, Hoen B, Smith DE, et al. Impact of therapeutic immunization on HIV-1 viremia after discontinuation of antiretroviral therapy initiated during acute infection. J Infect Dis 192:607–17, 2005.
40. Levy Y, Gahery-Segard H, Durier C, et al. Immunological and virological efficacy of a therapeutic immunization combined with interleukin-2 in chronically HIV-1 infected patients. AIDS 19:279–86, 2005.
41. Garcia F, Lejeune M, Climent N, et al. Therapeutic immunization with dendritic cells loaded with heat-inactivated autologous HIV-1 in patients with chronic HIV-1 infection. J Infect Dis 191:1680–5, 2005.
42. Lu W, Arraes LC, Ferreira WT, Andrieu JM. Therapeutic dendritic-cell vaccine for chronic HIV-1 infection. Nat Med 10:1359–65, 2004.
43. Shiver JW, Fu TM, Chen L, et al. Replication-incompetent adenoviral vaccine vector elicits effective anti-immunodeficiency-virus immunity. Nature 415:331–5, 2002.
44. Amara RR, Villinger F, Altman JD, et al. Control of a mucosal challenge and prevention of AIDS by a multiprotein DNA/MVA vaccine. Science 292:69–74, 2001.
45. Radaelli A, Nacsa J, Tsai WP, et al. Prior DNA immunization enhances immune response to dominant and subdominant viral epitopes induced by a fowlpox-based SIVmac vaccine in long-term slow-progressor macaques infected with SIVmac251. Virology 312:181–95, 2003.
46. McConkey SJ, Reece WH, Moorthy VS, et al. Enhanced T-cell immunogenicity of plasmid DNA vaccines boosted by recombinant modified vaccinia virus Ankara in humans. Nat Med 9:729–35, 2003.

Chapter 32

Complementary and Alternative Therapies

Jason Tokumoto, MD, Donald I. Abrams, MD

BACKGROUND

Complementary and alternative medicine (CAM) can be defined as "those healthcare and medical practices that are not currently an integral part of conventional medicine".[1] Surveys on the use of CAM by HIV-infected individuals indicate that utilization of these modalities has been common from the start of the epidemic to the current era of potent antiretroviral therapy (ART).[2–7] Prior to the availability of potent ART, CAM use was focused on treating HIV and improving the immune system. Currently, the most common reasons for using CAM are (1) to relieve symptoms due to HIV infection or medications, (2) increase one's self of well-being, (3) enhance the immune system, (4) slow the progression of the disease, and (5) supplement allopathic medicine.[8–10] The latter reason is important because most HIV patients who use CAM do so in conjunction with, rather than to replace, allopathic medicine. HIV patients who take CAM are most likely to (1) be more involved in the medical decision process, (2) have a negative attitude toward ART, (3) have had HIV for a longer period of time, (4) have progression in their disease, (5) have a higher income, (6) have a higher level of education, and (7) be a female.[3,4,8,11]

One of the largest surveys on CAM use by HIV patients is the Alternative Medicine Care Outcomes in AIDS (AMCOA) study which enrolled 1675 HIV patients between 1995 and 1997. Approximately 63% of the enrollees reported taking ART and 63% reported using 1600 different types of CAM. The most common modalities were prayer (58%), garlic (53%), massage therapy (49%), meditation (46%), and acupuncture (46%).[2] More recent, smaller surveys in which at least 50% of HIV patients were on ART showed that 36-88% were on CAM.[4–6] The most common modalities were vitamins, herbs, and prayer.

One of the major concerns about CAM use by HIV patients is that many clinicians are often not aware that their patients are using CAM. In one study, 33% of clinicians were not aware that their HIV-positive patients were using complementary modalities.[3] More importantly, 25% of the patients were using CAM that had the potential for adverse effects. The two main reasons for this disconnect is the provider simply not asking and/or the patient not wanting to disclose this information for fear of losing the respect of the primary provider.

HIV care providers should be familiar with some of the common complementary and alternative agents in current use. Clinicians who care for HIV-infected individuals need to be familiar with these approaches for several reasons. First, approximately half of any HIV patient group uses them. Second, some treatments may interact with standard therapies in significant ways. Third, some CAM therapies have been shown to do harm, whereas others could conceivably show benefit. The line between standard and alternative therapy itself has blurred. When an alternative's therapeutic value is documented it rapidly becomes standard therapy.[12] Fourth, a symptom may be due to a CAM therapy and not the illness per se or from side effects of prescribed medications. Fifth, some "complementary" approaches such as nutrition, exercise, and stress reduction are logical adjuncts to therapy. Sixth, the clinician can be an important source of accurate and unbiased information on complementary therapies. Finally, since the care of the HIV patient is a long-term proposal, the physician–patient relationship is paramount. When patients see that their provider is interested in the healing approaches they are pursuing, trust and rapport deepens. There is still truth to an observation made several years earlier that "when healthcare providers take the time to get involved and learn about the panoply of alternative options, including the rationales for prescribing alternative treatments, their most frequent toxicities, and the reasons why patients are optimistic about their use; the resulting compassionate understanding, confidence, and trust could conceivably provide a significant therapeutic benefit itself for the individual with HIV infection".[13]

THE NATIONAL CENTER FOR COMPLEMENTARY AND ALTERNATIVE MEDICINE

In 1993, the National Institutes of Health (NIH) established the Office of Alternative Medicine (OAM).[14] In 1995, the office granted its first funds to investigate alternative and complementary therapies for HIV infection. Bastyr University in Seattle, a naturopathic institution, received funding to become the center for HIV CAM studies. The university established a national database cohort of HIV-infected individuals using CAM therapies.[2] They collected prevalence and follow-up information on outcome measures of patients employing a wide variety of alternative and complementary interventions. In addition, they provided seed funding to investigators conducting small pilot interventional trials in patients with HIV.

In 1998, the OAM was upgraded to the National Center for Complementary and Alternative Medicine (NCCAM). The establishment of NCCAM allowed more funds to become available for the study of CAM therapies in HIV-positive patients. The Center has awarded a number of grants to investigate promising or widely used interventions. To access current NCCAM-funded HIV/CAM clinical trials, visit their website at http://nccam.nih.gov. The existence of this program reflects the acceptance that use of complementary therapies will continue in patients with HIV despite excellent viral suppression and immune restoration with antiretroviral agents.

The NCCAM provides a concrete framework for the discussion of CAM therapies. The Center has divided the interventions into five major domains (1) alternative medical systems; (2) mind-body interventions; (3) biologic-based therapies, e.g., herbs; (4) manipulative and body-based systems, e.g., massage; and (5) energy therapies, e.g., magnets.[15] The NCCAM categorization provides a useful framework for review of available information that currently exists on the use of these various CAM interventions in the HIV population. Where data from controlled clinical trials is unavailable, a description of some widely used modalities in each category will be offered.

ALTERNATIVE MEDICAL SYSTEMS

Traditional Chinese medicine (TCM) is a system of healing that has been developed over thousands of years. TCM in various forms is a medical system which HIV-infected individuals often incorporate into their treatment regimen primarily to treat symptoms (e.g., nausea, wasting, sleep disturbances, and pain) related to HIV infection or medications. Chinese medicine involves balancing the "energy" of the body by combining primarily acupuncture, herbs, diet, exercise with an emphasis on treating the whole person rather than the disease.[16] Two individuals, each suffering from the same "disease" in Western terms, might receive very different Chinese diagnoses and medical treatments. Each individual has unique strengths, weaknesses, imbalances, and life-long patterns that affect how their body deals with HIV. The idea is to understand all of this and then effect changes in the underlying constitution of the individual by altering the flow of energy or *Qi*. TCM has been rather mysterious and ill-comprehended by Western healthcare practitioners until recently, when more have shown interest and received training in these approaches.

In spite of the highly individualized approach of Chinese medicine, standard clinical trials have been designed to test herbal formulations and acupuncture treatments in HIV. In one clinical trial, a 31-herb combination based on two preparations, Enhance and Clear Heat, was administered to patients with two or more HIV-related symptoms. Participants were randomized to receive either 28 pills of the Chinese herbal preparation or placebo daily for 12 weeks.[17] No significant changes were seen in any of the major outcome variables studied. There was a greater change in median life satisfaction in the herbal group. Another subsequent randomized, double-blind, placebo-controlled study of standard Chinese herbs showed no difference in symptoms, quality-of-life, viral load or CD4 cell counts between the herb group and placebo group.[18] The Chinese herb group had twice the frequency of gastrointestinal disturbances.

In several uncontrolled studies and anecdotal reports, formulas containing TCM ingredients such as astragalus, lingustrum, ginseng, licorice, and other Chinese herbs have shown some effectiveness against various symptoms such as fatigue, night sweats, weight loss, diarrhea, and skin rashes. In general, they did not appear to improve immune parameters or HIV viral load. In a pilot evaluation of a herbal formula called Source Qi, HIV patients with chronic pathogen-negative diarrhea experienced a modest, nonstatistically significant decrease in the average number of stools per day in each week of the 8-week open-label study.[19] Surprisingly, patients who were receiving nelfinavir-based regimens fared slightly worse than patients on other protease inhibitors (PIs). It was postulated that the known nelfinavir side effect of diarrhea could have resulted from an increased nelfinavir effect overall, perhaps due to increased nelfinavir blood levels due to a herb–drug interaction. This underscores the need to obtain data on interactions of the most commonly used Chinese herbs with antiretroviral agents.

Acupuncture is commonly used by HIV patients for pain relief, especially pain due to peripheral neuropathy. Aware of the high use of acupuncture for painful neuropathy in patients refractory to analgesics, the Community Programs for Clinical Research on AIDS designed a factorial trial of a standard acupuncture regimen and amitriptyline.[20] A total of 250 persons with HIV-related neuropathy were enrolled in the nationwide trial. There was no statistically significant difference between either of the two interventions and their placebo with regard to the effect on neuropathic pain. Because both the acupuncture intervention and the sham acupuncture produced similar relief from neuropathic pain, the investigators concluded that the acupuncture was ineffective. In truth, the sham acupuncture utilized involved insertion of needles into "alternate points" which one could argue had equal effectiveness with the experimental "true" points, making conclusions about the efficacy or lack of efficacy of acupuncture problematic. The fact that the study was conducted in the setting of a federally-funded HIV clinical trial groups, however, speaks for the viability of evaluating alternative therapies in the mainstream clinical research infrastructure.

MIND-BODY INTERVENTIONS

Mind-body interventions include meditation, prayer, hypnosis, and certain forms of art, dance or music therapy. Evidence for clinical benefits has moved some of these practices from the CAM realm into mainstream medicine. Among these are cognitive-behavioral therapies and various means of stress reduction.

Among the large survey of 1016 participants in the AMCOA study, 56% reported utilizing prayer and 33% reported being involved in spiritual activity.[2] Data from other surveys suggest that most patients have a spiritual life and regard their spiritual health as important as their physical health.[21] A number of studies in HIV-uninfected patients have shown direct relationships between religious involvement, spirituality, and positive health outcomes such as mortality, physical and mental illness, quality of life, and coping.[22] Prayer itself was shown to have a positive effect on outcome of patients in the coronary care unit (CCU).[23] In this blinded controlled trial involving 393 subjects, hospitalized patients who were prayed for by prayer groups had superior outcomes compared to those who were not. However, another study of 799 coronary care patients failed to demonstrate a clinical benefit for intercessory prayer, although it differed from the earlier trial in that patients were randomized at the time of hospital discharge rather than during their CCU stay.[24] An editorial accompanying the latter study states "the weakness of the study is that the effect explored has no basis within the current scientific paradigm. If found to be true, such an effect would indeed challenge our understanding of the universe and perhaps even overturn much accumulated scientific knowledge to date."[25]

Despite some skepticism, a systematic review of available data from randomized trials of "distant healing" found that ~57% of the 23 trials involving ~3000 patients did show a positive treatment effect.[26] Distant healing (DH) can be defined as "a conscious, dedicated act of mentation attempting to benefit another person's physical or emotional well-being at a distance".[27] A randomized, double-blind trial of DH was conducted in 40 patients with advanced AIDS at the very beginning of the HAART era.[27] Pair-matched subjects were assigned to either 10 weeks of DH or a control group. Healers included practitioners from Christian, Jewish, Buddhist, Native American and shamanic traditions as well as those practicing secular methods. Each subject in the DH group was treated by a total of ten different practitioners and each of the 40 practitioners treated a total of five patients. Baseline CD4 cell counts were less than 100/mm^3 in both arms of the study. All patients were receiving *Pneumocystis carinii* pneumonia (PCP) prophylaxis and nearly all were on PI containing antiretroviral regimens. At 6 months, a blinded chart review found that the treatment subjects had significantly fewer AIDS-defining illnesses and required less medical attention in the form of doctor visits and hospitalizations. Participants who had been in the treatment group also had significantly improved mood compared with controls. There was no effect on CD4 cell count. HIV viral load was not assessed.

A recently completed NCCAM funded study attempted to replicate these earlier findings. In this trial, 150 participants were randomized to being healed by a healer, a nurse who had been trained in DH or no healing. DH did not appear to improve various clinical outcomes in these HIV-infected patients who were taking antiretroviral combinations.[28]

Mindfulness meditation is the practice of "focusing attention and objectively acknowledging thoughts, emotions, and perceptions as they arise".[29] It appears to be effective in lowering stress. In a study of 46 HIV-infected patients of whom only 24 completed a structured, 8-week Mindfulness-Based Stress Reduction program (MBSR), the MBSR group had a significant increase in the activity and number of natural killer cells. However, there was no difference in selected psychological, endocrine, or health parameters.[29] Researchers in psychoneuroimmunology are continuing to try to demonstrate benefit from meditation. An ongoing NCCAM funded trial is evaluating the effect of MBSR versus an education control intervention on delaying the need to commence ART in naive patients with CD4 cell counts greater than 250 cells/mm^3.

BIOLOGICALLY-BASED THERAPIES

In the NCCAM classification, biologically-based therapies include herbs, special diets, and food products used therapeutically (e.g., nutraceuticals). Many of the drugs in common use, as well as a number of potent cytotoxic chemotherapy agents, are derived from the world's flora. In a comprehensive review, 63 ingredients listed in the Chinese *Materia Medica* were found to have *in vitro* activity against HIV.[30] These compounds included terpenes, flavinoids, polysaccharides, coumarins, tannins, lectins, quinolones, peptides, and other alkaloids. The natural substances were reported to have activity inhibiting reverse transcriptase, protease and integrase enzymes as well as interfering with infection at the viral cell entry level.

Surveys have shown that herbal usage by patients with HIV ranges from 21% to 68%.[2,10,11,31] In the HAART era, the main reason for using herbs is to treat co-morbidities or to alleviate symptoms due to HIV or medications rather than to treat HIV. One concern about the use of herbs is that patients may not be aware of potential herb–antiretroviral drug interactions. In a focus group study of HIV-infected individuals using CAM, all participants knew that St John's wort decreased the effectiveness of HIV medications. However,

CAM Therapies for Common Co-Morbidities and Symptoms

Table 32-1

Co-Morbidity/Symptom	CAM	Active Ingredient	Caution
Depression	St John's wort – 300–900 mg/day of 5:1 extract of flowering tops and leaves containing 0.3% hypericin[112]	Hypericin	Should not be used with protease inhibitors or non-nucleoside analogs
Hyperlipidemia	Red yeast rice (Cholestin-TM) – 1200 mg twice a day[112]	Mevinolin and other HMG-CoA reductase	One case of myositis reported
	Garlic – 1 clove or 2 g of fresh garlic or 650 mg/day of garlic powder containing 6 mg of allicin[112]	Allicin	Should not be used with saquinavir; high doses can irritate the gastrointestinal mucosa
Hypertriglyceridemia	Fish oil – 2–4 g/day of eicosapentaenoic acid and docosahexaenoic acid	Omega-3 fatty acid	
Hepatitis	Milk thistle – 175–600 mg/day of a 30:1 seed extract containing 80% silymarin[112]	Silymarin	Can decrease indinavir blood levels
Nausea	Ginger – 1 g of dried, powder root or equivalent extract containing >/= 5% gingerols and shogaols[112]	Gingerols/shogaols	Studies done primarily on morning sickness and postoperative nausea
Diarrhea	Soluble fibers – (Metamucil, Citruel, or oat bran tablets) or applesauce, pears, rice, boiled potatoes		Avoid raw fruits and vegetables, caffeinated drinks, greasy, fried foods
	Calcium supplements – 500 mg twice a day[113]		Study done on protease inhibitor-induced diarrhea
Weight loss/wasting	Dehydroepiandrosterone (DHEA) – 50 mg/day		No positive effect on CD4 cell count or HIV viral load
	Resistance exercise e.g., weight lifting		No negative effect on HIV viral load
	Protein intake of up to 1.5 g/kg of body weight per day[114]		No evidence that $>1.5\ g\ kg^{-1}\ day^{-1}$ is beneficial
Neuropathy	Acupuncture		Efficacy data inconsistent
	Cannibinoids		Smoking or orally

the participants did not know of other herbs that could interact with HIV medications. In addition, many of the participants were less concerned about safety issues when it came to CAM therapy compared to Western medicine.[32]

Herbal Preparations

Herbs Used to Treat Co-Morbidities/Symptoms

Depression is common in HIV-infected patients (see Table 32-1). St John's wort (active ingredient: hypericin) is a popular herb used for depression. The data on the efficacy of St John's wort for depression is inconsistent but available evidence suggests that specific extracts of St John's wort may be effective for mild depression.[33] St John's wort is believed to exert its effect by inhibition of the reuptake of serotonin, norepinephrine, and dopamine by neurons.[34,35] More importantly, however, studies have shown that St John's wort induces cytochrome 450 3A4 isoform and can dramatically lower indinavir levels in healthy volunteers.[36] The indinavir area under the curve was reduced by a mean of 57% and the extrapolated 8-h indinavir trough was reduced by 81%. Another study demonstrated that St John's wort lowered nevirapine levels by 20%.[37] This has led to the recommendations in 2005 by the Department of Health and Human Services (DHHS) that St John's wort not be used with protease PIs or non-nucleoside analogs.[38]

Hyperlipidemia is a major problem associated with HAART. Garlic (active ingredient: allicin) purportedly has anticholesterol activity and patients may therefore use garlic to reduce their cholesterol levels. The data on the efficacy of garlic to lower lipid levels is limited by the short duration of these studies and the different garlic preparations used in these trials.[39] NIH researchers have reported that garlic supplements sharply reduced the blood concentrations of saquinavir by 50%.[40] In a classic pharmacokinetic study, nine HIV-negative volunteers received 3 days of saquinavir. They then took garlic capsules twice daily for 3 weeks. At the ensuing analysis, it was found that the saquinavir levels had decreased by 51% and the average maximum concentrations had fallen 54%. Even after a 10 day washout without any further garlic supplementation, the blood levels of saquinavir still averaged 35% lower than baseline values. The 2005 DHHS adult antiretroviral guidelines recommend that garlic not be used with saquinavir.[38] There has also been a report of two HIV-positive patients developing significant gastrointestinal side effects from ritonavir after taking garlic.[41]

Another product that HIV-infected patients may use for hyperlipidemia is cholestin. Cholestin, produced by red yeast fermented on rice has been shown to contain nine monacolins (statins) which inhibit HMG-CoA. Two placebo-controlled trials involving 390 HIV-negative individuals showed a decrease in LDL cholesterol and triglycerides by 20-30%.[42] One case of cholestin-induced myopathy has been reported.[43] The oyster mushroom (*Pleurotus ostreatus*) is another natural source of monacolin and there is an ongoing NCCAM funded study assessing the lipid lowering effect of oyster mushrooms in HIV-positive patients with ART related hypercholesterolemia.[44]

Milk thistle (active ingredient: silymarin) is used for its hepatoprotective or hepatorestorative properties. This property is especially attractive to HIV patients co-infected with hepatitis B and/or C who may be at an increased risk to develop transaminase elevations in response to HAART. However, the current available data on the positive effect of milk thistle on the liver is inconclusive.[45] As with other herbs, milk thistle can have an effect on PI blood levels. In ten healthy individuals, milk thistle decreased mean indinavir levels by 25%.[46] Milk thistle in the dosages generally used probably should not interfere with the efficacy of PIs.

Herbs Used for Its Anti-HIV Activity

Some plant products have been investigated for their antiretroviral activity. St John's wort (hypericin) has reputed broad-spectrum antiviral effects against HIV, herpes, cytomegalovirus, and Epstein–Barr virus.[47] *In vitro*, hypericin inhibits HIV replication. However, hypericin blood levels after oral dosing were less than one-hundredth of the test-tube levels that showed anti-HIV effect. A study of high intravenous doses of hypericin was terminated because participants developed hepatotoxicity and photodermatitis.[48]

Calanolide A derived from the Malaysian rain forest tree, *Calophyllum lanigerum* has significant *in vitro* activity against HIV. Calanolide A functions like a non-nucleoside reverse transcriptase inhibitor (NNRTI). In a randomized, double-blind, placebo-controlled study, 43 HIV-infected patients who received 14 days of Calanolide A 600 mg twice a day had a mean HIV viral load reduction of $0.81\log_{10}$ from baseline when compared to the placebo group.[49]

In a recent Cochrane review that looked at nine randomized, placebo-controlled trials evaluating eight herbal products to treat HIV involving 499 HIV-positive individuals, the authors concluded that the evidence did not support the use of these products to suppress HIV infection. The authors do point out that potential benefits need to be confirmed in larger rigorous clinical trials.[50]

Herbs Used for Stimulating the Immune System

There are several herbal products used by HIV-positive individuals that are thought to stimulate the immune system such as Echinacea, mistletoe, goldenseal, shiitake and reishi mushrooms, aloe, and garlic. While each has a theoretical basis, with evidence of active ingredients and groups of vocal users and supporters, each still needs to be researched further in people with HIV infection.[51] The interactions between HIV and the immune system are so intricate that the idea of "stimulating the immune system" is an obvious oversimplification. A stimulus to CD4 cells might help the body fight infections or instead might lead to increased viral replication. Boosting certain cytokines like interleukin-2 or interleukin-12 may help the host, while boosting other cytokines such as tumor necrosis factor alpha may lead to disease progression. For example, echinacea, a member of the daisy family, is widely used in short-term pulses as prophylaxis and treatment for upper respiratory infections despite negative results from recent trials in HIV-uninfected populations.[34,35,52] Whereas, immunostimulatory effects have been demonstrated with short-term use, there is concern that long-term use of greater than 8 weeks duration may be associated with the potential for immunosuppression.[53] This theoretical concern has led some to recommend that chronic use of echinacea is contraindicated in patients with HIV infection, although no data from controlled trials is available.[35] The German E monograph also recommends that echinacea not be used in HIV-infected individuals.[54]

Vitamins

A significant segment of the HIV-infected population consumes vitamins on a daily basis.[13,55] The history of vitamins and HIV dates back to vitamin C which was one of the first interventions proposed as a potential alternative therapy. In the early days of the epidemic, prior to the availability of conventional ARTs, high dose vitamin C (up to 50 g/day) was administered by oral routes or intravenous infusion. The rationale was based on anecdotal observation of broad antiviral activity as well as *in vitro* activity demonstrated against a human retrovirus.[56,57] Patients escalated their vitamin C intake to "bowel tolerance", that is, to ingest as much vitamin C as possible, titrating the dose to the intolerability of the resultant diarrhea. Enthusiasm for this intervention in the community waned when many of the early proponents of high-dose vitamin C therapy died from the progression of their AIDS-related illness. Further interest in high dose vitamin C as an antiviral agent waned with the availability of many conventional antiretroviral agents.

Several studies have demonstrated that HIV-positive individuals had lower serum levels of vitamins A, B6, B12, and E, beta-carotene, zinc, and selenium compared to HIV-negative individuals.[58–61] Furthermore, observational studies showed that in these patients, there was a more rapid disease progression and death.[62–66] Other studies showed an association between higher intake of vitamins B, C, and multivitamins and less decrease progression and death.[67,68]

Despite the low serum levels of some vitamins and minerals in HIV patients and the high use of vitamins by these patients, there is a dearth of randomized, double-blind, placebo-controlled trials assessing the benefit of vitamin supplementation in HIV individuals. In a randomized, double-blind, placebo-controlled study done in Africa, 1078 pregnant HIV-positive patients were randomized to vitamin A only, multivitamins excluding vitamin A, multivitamins and vitamin A, or placebo.[69] After ~6 years of follow-up, the women who received multivitamins were less likely to progress to AIDS or death, had fewer upper respiratory infections, oral and gastrointestinal symptoms, rashes, and fatigue, better improvement in their CD4 cell count and lower HIV viral loads compared to the vitamin A only and placebo groups.

Symptomatic lactic acidemia due to mitochondrial toxicity from nucleoside analogs occurs in 1.5–2.5% of HIV-infected patients on regimens including nucleoside combinations.[70] Several agents such as thiamine, riboflavin, coenzyme Q, vitamins C, E, K, and L-carnitine have been used with limited success for congenital mitochondrial disease.[71] However, there is no data that supports the use of these agents in nucleoside-associated symptomatic lactic acidemia.[70]

As yet, there is no consensus and no expert guidelines on the use of vitamins in the HIV-positive population. In the absence of data from well-controlled clinical trials, HIV-infected patients are likely to benefit from a daily multivitamin as has been recommended for the general adult population.[72]

Anabolic Agents and Antiwasting Therapies

Decreased testosterone levels may play an important role in critical loss of lean body mass. Furthermore, in the HAART era, it is estimated that up to 20% of male HIV-infected patients are hypogonadal.[73] HIV-positive women who have advanced disease also have decreased testosterone levels which have been associated with loss of lean body mass.[74] Both hypogonadal and eugonadal men and hypogonadal women may turn to supplemental testosterone to counteract wasting. Testosterone can be supplemented transdermally or intramuscularly, however all require a prescription.

Some individuals who seek a testosterone-like benefit turned to dehydroepiandrosterone (DHEA) a precursor of androgenic and estrogenic steroids. The precise role of DHEA in health is unclear but serum levels decline after age 40.[75] One study demonstrated that DHEA serum levels were lower in HIV-infected patients.[76] In the lay press, DHEA has been touted to improve fatigue, mood, and libido which many HIV-infected patients desire. Data on the benefit and safety of DHEA in HIV-infected patients are limited. In a prospective, randomized, double-blind, placebo-controlled study, 32 HIV-infected patients with low DHEA serum levels were randomized to sublingual DHEA 50 mg/day for 4 months or placebo.[77] At the end of the study, the group that received DHEA had a significant improvement in their quality of life when compared to the placebo group. The DHEA was well tolerated. In another study, 29 HIV-positive women on ART were randomly assigned to receive 50 mg/day of DHEA or placebo for 6 months.[78] The women who took DHEA gained a mean 1.4 kg of weight compared to the placebo group who lost 1.2 kg, and also had improvement on multiple quality of life parameters. Of note, the DHEA group experienced a CD4 increase of 107 cells/mm^3 compared to a drop of 11 cells/mm^3 in the placebo group. A recent NCCAM-funded randomized, placebo-controlled trial investigating the antiviral, immunomodulatory and body composition effects of DHEA in individuals with undetectable HIV RNA levels was completed. Results of this study are pending.[79]

In a recent randomized, double-blind study, DHEA was shown to be helpful in treating dysthymia in HIV-infected patients. 145 HIV-infected patients with dysthymia were randomized to either DHEA or placebo for 8 weeks. Using accepted standardized depression rating scales, the DHEA group had a 56% response rate compared to 31% in the placebo group.[80]

Creatine and glutamine are two amino acid supplements utilized by HIV-infected patients for HIV-related manifestations. Creatine, utilized in doses up to 25 g/day by weight lifters, is thought to build muscle by increasing muscle phosphocreatine, an energy source.[81] In a 14-week randomized, placebo-controlled study, 40 HIV-positive patients underwent supervised resistance exercise and received either creatine or placebo.[82] Patients in the creatine group gained 2.3 kg in lean body mass compared to the exercise group, a difference which was statistically significant. There was no difference in strength. Unfortunately, the increase in muscle mass was due to fluid retention in the muscle. Glutamine also used in large doses may help heal gut mucosa in chronic diarrheal states which can cause significant weight loss. In one randomized, placebo-controlled trial, 40 g/day of glutamine plus antioxidants caused a significant increase in weight and body cell mass in AIDS patients with clinical wasting.[83]

Delta-9-tetrahydrocannibol (dronabinol), the active component of marijuana, is one of the licensed therapies available for the anorexia associated with HIV-related wasting.[84,85] The mechanism of action of cannabinoids on appetite stimulation remains unclear. The effect may be related to increasing the sensory appeal of food or decreasing satiety.[86] More recently it has also been suggested that the body's intrinsic endocannabinoids may be involved in increasing the reward effects of eating.[87] Clinical trials have demonstrated that, in a controlled residential setting, individuals inhaling marijuana increased their caloric intake and weight over time.[88]

Even with the availability of dronabinol by prescription, HIV-infected patients continue to use marijuana (smoking or ingesting) for either medical or recreational reasons.[88] In addition to improving appetite and increasing weight, other reasons cited for marijuana use is to help decrease pain, nausea, vomiting, and side effects from ART.[89] In a randomized, placebo-controlled, safety study, 67 nonwasting HIV-positive patients were randomized to receive a 3.95%-tetrahydrocannibol marijuana cigarette, a 2.5 mg dronabinol capsule or a placebo capsule three times a day for 21 days.[90] At the end of the inpatient study, there was no effect on HIV viral load, CD4 cell count, and PI blood levels. Although the study was not powered for efficacy, there was significant weight gain in both cannabinoid arms compared to placebo. The weight gain, however, was predominantly adipose tissue and not lean body mass.

Animal models and anecdotal data suggest that cannabinoids may provide relief from neuropathic pain where opioids have been generally ineffective. In a study involving 16 HIV-infected patients with neuropathic pain, smoking one 3.56%-tetrahydrocannibol marijuana cigarette three times a day for 7 days resulted in a drop in pain scores when compared to baseline scores and ten patients experienced a greater than 30% decrease in pain.[91]

In a recent randomized, double-blind, placebo-controlled, study, involving 21 HIV-negative patients, CT-3, a synthetic analog of tetrahydrocannabinol was effective in decreasing neuropathic pain when compared to placebo.[92]

MANIPULATIVE AND BODY-BASED METHODS

Chiropractic manipulation and massage are two common examples of manipulative and body-based methods. In the AMCOA study, massage was cited as the third most frequently used intervention by 54% of the 1016 first eligible participants.[2] Although many HIV-infected patients visit practitioners of these therapies for maintenance of general well-being or treatment of particular underlying musculoskeletal problems, few controlled studies have been done. In one trial, 42 HIV-infected individuals with no active medical symptoms were evaluated in a study to assess the effects of massage therapy alone or massage therapy combined with either exercise training or stress management counseling on immune function and quality of life.[93] The investigators hypothesized that immune function may become further suppressed by chronic anxiety and depression.

Patients were randomized into four groups including massage only, massage and exercise, massage and stress management, and a control group. Only the control group demonstrated an increase in CD4 cell count following the 12-week intervention, with the massage/exercise and massage/stress management cohorts sustaining a drop in CD4 counts. No significant differences were found among the groups on any of the quality-of-life measures comparing pre- and post-study values. The authors concluded that short-term massage therapy alone or combined with either exercise training or stress management counseling did not have any significant impact on immune function or quality-of-life measures and that "these alternative therapies, while not harmful, should not be used as substitutes for more conventional therapies for HIV-infected persons".[93]

ENERGY THERAPIES

Energy therapies are described as those based on activation or generation of energy fields either originating in the body or acting externally on the body. *Qi gong*, a component of TCM, is an example of an energy therapy. HIV-infected patients practice *Qi gong* which combines movement, meditation, and breathing control which enhances the flow of vital energy called *Qi*, with the intent to improve circulation and enhance immune function. An NCCAM sponsored study assessing the effect of Reiki (energy therapy) on anxiety, depression, pain, quality of life, and spiritual well-being in patients with advanced AIDS was recently completed. Results of this study are pending.

EVALUATING CAM THERAPIES

Ideally, it would be desirable to be able to investigate each widely used CAM therapy for its safety and effectiveness. The establishment of the NCCAM allows for increased guidance as well as funding in this domain, however, it remains a challenge to determine which CAM therapies should be investigated and how to go about studying them. Agents that are in widespread use that have a biological plausibility should be studied to determine if they are safe and have clinical benefit. Substances with a potential for a CAM–drug interaction with patients' prescribed antiretroviral regimens should also be investigated to rule out detrimental pharmacokinetic interactions. Although it would seem that agents should be assayed to demonstrate that they have no benefit or may, in fact, be harmful, the history of the alternative therapies movement suggests that there will always be the strong proponents of the intervention who will not accept the results of the trial. They will suggest that the preparation used in the study was the wrong one to choose, the patient population was incorrect, or there were flaws in the trial design that interfere with the interpretation of the results. The lack of standardized preparations of many CAM products does present a challenge in attempting to study the agent or reproduce the results of another investigator. One commentator lamented, "How can a herb be standardized if its active ingredients are not known and there is no suitable bioassay?"[12]

NCCAM provided a "Methodological Manifesto" to assist investigators interested in conducting clinical trials to investigate CAM therapies.[94] The document asserts that different studies may require different methodological and analytical approaches. It suggests that one use the strongest possible design and most appropriate statistical procedures and concedes that clinical trials may not be the only route to take and that observational studies may provide useful information to inform the design of subsequent controlled studies. Although alternative therapies are being tested, NCCAM warns against alternative outcomes and suggests that investigators utilize standard recognized clinical trial endpoints. NCCAM believes that existing quantitative procedures should be robust enough to analyze data generated in trials of CAM interventions and that other statistical systems are not required. Although complex complementary medical systems could be studied as "gestalts", operationally this is a challenge to study reviewers who are used to more orthodox proposals. For example, when asked to evaluate a proposed TCM intervention for patients co-infected with HIV and hepatitis C, reviewers were stymied by how to untangle the effects of the herbs from the acupuncture or *qi gong*, and how to determine which moiety of the herbal preparation was, in fact, the active part. Thus, despite all good intentions, orthodox values and mind-sets of review panels may hamper rapid increased investigation of CAM therapies. It has been suggested that even if conducted under the most rigid circumstances, results of clinical trials of CAM agents may be difficult for many conventional scientists and clinicians to embrace. The authors note that physician's adherent to the traditions of conventional medicine, when evaluating results of studies of homeopathic interventions, as an example, "reject seemingly solid evidence because it is not compatible with theory".[95]

CAUTIONS

Many who use CAM therapies automatically equate the "naturalness" of the interventions with their safety. However, in addition to herb–antiretroviral drug interactions described above, there are other reports of adverse effects from ingestion of apparently benign CAM therapies. In addition to the PI interaction, excess garlic ingestion (4 cloves/day) was implicated in the inhibition of platelet aggregation in an 87-year old man with a resultant spontaneous spinal epidural hematoma.[96] A platelet aggregation defect was also felt to be responsible for bilateral spontaneous subdural hematomas in a 37-year-old woman with a 2-year history of ingestion of 120 mg of daily gingko biloba.[97] The patient's prolonged bleeding time corrected upon discontinuation of the herb. Ginseng is also known to inhibit platelet aggregation *in vitro* and prolong both prothrombin and partial thromboplastin times in rats.[35] These effects are important in preoperative patients who may experience excessive bleeding if they do not report and discontinue these herbs before surgery. Specifically, agents known to induce qualitative platelet defects should be discontinued for at least 7 days prior to surgery.

AN INTEGRATIVE CLINICAL APPROACH

Despite the lack of strong evidence-based data from controlled clinical trials, some lifestyle modifying recommendations can be suggested to all HIV-positive patients and are discussed below. The primary care provider can integrate some of these lifestyle modifications into the patient's overall therapeutic plan. The patient, in turn, may benefit from being empowered by being able to make these potentially salubrious lifestyle modifications.

Nutrition

All HIV-infected patients should have an assessment of their nutritional status at all stages of their illness. Nutritional counseling has been associated with improved health outcomes in HIV-infected patients.[98,99] Studies have clearly shown that significant loss of muscle is associated with increased morbidity and mortality.[100–102] It is therefore important that HIV-infected patients be assessed for and maintain adequate muscle mass. People with HIV infection are believed to benefit from a higher protein, lower fat, nutrient rich diet which includes multiple sources of protein such as lean meat, cheese, fish, chicken, and nuts, whole grains, less sweets and highly refined foods.

High blood lipid levels and fat loss and/or accumulation abnormalities have been a major problem for HIV-infected patients on ART. An HIV-infected patient with hyperlipidemia should be assessed for dietary habits and the "National Cholesterol Education Program Therapeutic Lifestyle Changes (TLC)" diet should be incorporated.[103] In addition, weight reduction through dietary changes and exercise is an important therapy for decreasing lipid levels. Recently, omega-3 fatty acids in the form of fish oil consisting of 1750 mg of eicosapentaenoic acid and 1150 mg of docosahexaenoic acid a day for 16 weeks with dietary and exercise counseling was shown to reduce antiretroviral-related triglyceride levels by 19% in 52 HIV-infected patients.[104]

Food and beverages must also be free of pathogens. All animal products must be thoroughly cooked or pasteurized. "Safe kitchen" behavior means avoiding contact between uncooked animal products and foods that will not be cooked. For example, cutting up a raw chicken on a cutting board later used for salad or fresh vegetables is not safe. "Health" foods such as raw calves' liver and raw goats' milk can carry pathogens that can be a source of significant morbidity or mortality to someone with advanced HIV disease. Gourmet delights such as sushi, rare or raw meats, raw oysters, raw egg in Caesar salad and unpasteurized aged cheeses may be contaminated with helminths, yersinia, salmonella, *E. coli*, listeria, and other organisms. Many municipal water treatment systems do not filter appropriately to remove *Cryptosporidium parvum*. Thus, knowledge about local water processing procedures can help patients especially those with lower CD4 cell counts, to decide on the utility of replacing tap water with filtered water.[105]

Exercise

The two main types of exercise; aerobic and resistance exercise, have been shown to be of benefit in HIV-infected patients. A Cochrane review assessing eight studies of HIV-infected patients concluded that aerobic exercise for at least 20 min three times a week for 4 weeks was safe and led to improvement in cardiopulmonary fitness and psychological well-being.[106]

Progressive resistance exercise has been shown to help build muscle and preserve lean body mass in both men and women.[107–109] As indicated previously this is important because loss of lean body mass is associated with a poorer prognosis. One study showed regular resistance exercise lowered elevated triglyceride levels.[110]

For antiretroviral-associated central or general fat accumulation, the International AIDS Society-USA Panel encourages exercise as a nonpharmacological intervention.[70]

Addressing Emotional and Spiritual Needs

The HIV-positive individual is challenged by emotional and spiritual issues. All the aspects of dealing with a life-threatening disease, as well as all the ongoing issues of life, including career, love, sexuality, relationships, and self-worth require attention. People living with HIV often compress decades of emotional and spiritual issues into a few short months or years. Getting involved in counseling for these issues is one of the most important things an HIV-positive individual can do.

There are many approaches that can help one look for meaning and encourage self-love and self-responsibility. They provide a context for looking at all of these critical issues, with emphasis on the value of positive thinking and "attitudinal" healing. Whether these approaches provide greater peace through understanding and faith, or more directly affect the immune system awaits further study by psychoneuroimmunologists.

Many HIV-uninfected patients also want their spiritual needs addressed and welcome inquiry into this dimension, but less than 20% of physicians routinely take a spiritual history.[111] Although there is no comparable data in the HIV-positive population, in surveys inquiring about the use of CAM, up to 63% of HIV-infected patients reported involvement in a spiritual activity.[3,4,11] A patient who expresses an interest in discussing their spirituality should be acknowledged and respected by the clinician. If the clinician is uncomfortable discussing spirituality, a referral should be made to an appropriate service.

CONCLUSION

Even with the availability of potent antiretroviral combinations, individuals with HIV infection are still interested in the use of treatments complementary to their orthodox therapies, especially for treating manifestations of HIV infection where effective agents are not prescribed by their physicians. Obviously, analysis of pharmacokinetic interactions cannot be undertaken on every alternative treatment a patient with HIV infection might ingest. This increases the responsibility of the care provider to have an open and honest conversation with each patient with regard to the use of CAM therapy. The possibility of hepatic damage or drug–CAM interactions that may alter the concentrations of antiretroviral agents, including PIs and non-nucleoside analogs increases the stake in the current era of HIV therapeutics.

Providers should question their patients regarding the use of alternative and complementary interventions and counsel them as completely as possible regarding possible concerns. Taking a CAM history can be part of the medication history. To do so effectively, caregivers must stay informed about agents in widespread use, consulting available references and resources to ensure the continued well-being of HIV-infected patients utilizing CAM therapies.

REFERENCES

1. CAMBASICS. National Center for Complementary and Alternative Medicine (NCCAM), National Institute of Health. Bethesda, Maryland, p 1–5, 2007.
2. Greene KB, Berger J, Reeves C, et al. Most frequently used alternative and complementary therapies and activities by participants in the AMCOA study. J Assoc Nurses AIDS Care 10:60–73, 1999.
3. Hsiao AF, Wong MD, Kanouse DE, et al. Complementary and alternative medicine use and substitution for conventional therapy by HIV-infected patients. J Acquir Immune Defic Syndr 33:157–65, 2003.
4. Chang BL, Van Servellen G, Lombardi E. Factors associated with complementary therapy use in people living with HIV/AIDS receiving antiretroviral therapy. J Altern Complement Med 9:695–710, 2003.
5. Bica I, Tang AM, Skinner S, et al. Use of complementary and alternative therapies by patients with human immunodeficiency virus disease in the era of highly active antiretroviral therapy. J Altern Complement Med 9:65–76, 2003.
6. Kirksey, KM, Goodroad BK, Kemppainen JK, et al. Complementary therapy use in persons with HIV/AIDS. J Holistic Nursing 20:264–78, 2002.
7. Southwell H, Valdez H, Lederman M, Gripshover B. Use of alternative therapies among HIV-infected patients at an urban tertiary care center. J AIDS 31:119–20, 2002.
8. Anderson W, O'Connor B, MacGregor R, et al. Patient use and assessment of conventional and alternative therapies for HIV infection and AIDS. AIDS 7:561–566, 1993.
9. Langewitz W, Ruttimann S, Laifer G, et al. The integration of alternative treatment modalities in HIV infection: the patient's perspective. J Psychosom Res 38:687–93, 1994.
10. Fairfield KM, Eisenberg DM, Davis RB, et al. Patterns of use, expenditures, and perceived efficacy of complementary and alternative therapies in HIV- infected patients. Arch Intern Med 158:2257–64, 1998.
11. de Visser R, Ezzy D, Bartos M. Alternative or complementary? Allopathic therapies for HIV/AIDS. Altern Ther Health Med 6:44–52, 2000.
12. Goldman P. Herbal medicines today and the roots of modern pharmacology. Ann Intern Med 135:594–600, 2001.
13. Abrams DI. Alternative therapies in HIV infection. AIDS 4:1179,1990.
14. Marwick C. Alternative medicine office urged to act rapidly. JAMA 270:1400, 1993.
15. Gertz MA, Bauer BA. Caring (really) for patients who use alternative therapiesfor cancer. J Clin Oncol 19:4346–9, 2001.
16. Cohen MR. Review of HIV-related traditional Chinese medicine research. In: Standish LJ, Calabrese C, and Galantino ML, (eds). AIDS and Complementary and Alternative Medicine: Current Science and Practice, St. Louis, Missouri, Churchill-Livingstone, 2001.
17. Burack JH, Cohen MR, Hahn JA, et al. A pilot randomized controlled trial of Chinese herbal treatment for HIV-associated symptoms. J Acquir Immune Defic Syndr 12:386–93, 1996.

18. Weber R, Christen L, Loy M, et al. Randomized, placebo controlled trial of Chinese herb therapy for HIV-1 infected individuals. J Acquir Immune Defic Syndr 22:56–64, 1999.
19. Cohen MR, Mitchell TF, Bacchetti P, et al. Use of a Chinese herbal medicine for treatment of HIV-associated pathogen-negative diarrhea. Integr Med 2:79–84, 1999.
20. Shlay JC, Chaloner K, Max MB, et al. Acupuncture and amitriptyline for patient due to HIV related peripheral neuropathy. JAMA 280:1590–5, 1998.
21. Mueller PS, Plevak DJ, Rummans TA. Religious involvement, spirituality and medicine: implications for clinical practice. Mayo Clin Proc 76:1225–35, 2001.
22. Gunderson L. Faith and healing. Ann Intern Med 132:169–72, 2000.23. Byrd RC. Positive therapeutic effects of intercessory prayer in a coronary care unit population. South Med J 81:826–9, 1988.
24. Aviles JM, Whelan E Sr, Hernke DA, et al. Intercessory prayer and cardiovas-cular disease progression in a coronary care population: a randomized controlled trial. Mayo Clin Proc 76:1192–8, 2001.
25. Koenig HG. Religion, spirituality, and medicine: how are they related and what does it mean? Mayo Clinic Proc 76:1189–91, 2001.
26. Astin JA, Harkness E, Ernst E. The efficacy of 'distant healing': a systemic review of randomized trials. Ann Intern Med 132: 903–10, 2000.
27. Sicher F, Targ E, Moore D, Smith HS. A randomized, double-blind study of distant healing in a population with advanced AIDS: Report of a small scale study. West J Med 169:356–63, 1998.
28. Astin JA, Stone J, Abrams DI, Targ E (in memorium) et al. The efficacy of distant healing for HIV: results of a randomized trial. Altern Ther Health Med 12:36–41, 2006.
29. Robinson FP, Mathews HL, Witek-Janusek L. Psycho-endocrine-immune response to mindfulness-based stress reduction in individuals infected with the human immunodeficiency virus: a quasiexperimental study. J Altern Complement Med 9:695–710, 2003.
30. Chang RY, Kong XB. Meta-survey of plant and herb material as treatment for HIV(Mo.B.303). In: Abstracts of the XIth International Conference on AIDS, Vancouver, 1996, p 22.
31. Kassler WJ, Blanc P, Greenblatt R. The use of medicinal herbs by human immunodeficiency virus-infected patients. Arch Intern Med 151:2281–7, 1991.
32. Leonard B, Huff H, Merryweather B, Lim A, Mills E. Knowledge of safety and herb–drug interactions amongst HIV+ individuals: a focus group study. Can J Clin Pharmacol 11:e227–31, 2004.
33. Linde K, Mulrow CD, Berner M, Egger M. St. John's wort for depression. The Cochrane Database of Systematic Reviews, 2005.
34. Ang-Lee MK, Moss J, Yuan CS. Herbal medicines and perioperative care. JAMA 286:208–16, 2001.
35. Ernst E. The risk-benefit of commonly used herbal therapies: gingko, St. John's wort, ginseng, echinacea, saw palmetto and kava. Ann Intern Med 136:42–53, 2002.
36. Piscitelli SC, Burstein AH, Chaitt D, et al. Indinavir concentrations and St. John's wort. Lancet 355:547–8, 2000.
37. De Maat MMR, Hoetelmans RMW, van Gorp ECM, et al. A potential inter- action between St. John's wort and nevirapine? In: First International Workshop on Clinical Pharmacology of HIV Therapy, Netherlands, 2000, abstract 2.8.
38. Guidelines for the Use of Antiretroviral Agents in HIV-1-Infected Adults and Adolescents, Department and Health and Human Services (DHHS), 6 Oct 2005.
39. Ackermann RT, Mulrow CD, Ramirez G, et al. Garlic shows promise for improving some cardiovascular risk factor. Arch Intern Med 161:813–24, 2001.
40. Piscitelli SC, Burstein AH, Welden N, et al. The effect of garlic supplements on the pharmacokinetics of saquinavir. Clin Infect Dis 34:234–8, 2002.
41. Laroche M, Choudhri S, Gallicano K, Foster B. Severe gastrointestinal toxicity with concomitant ingestion of ritonavir and garlic. In: Canadian Association for HIV Research Seventh Annual Canadian Conference on HIV/AIDS, Quebec City, 1998.
42. Patrick L, Uzick M. Cardiovascular: c-reactive protein and the inflammatory disease paradigm: HMG-CoA reductive inhibitors, alpha-tocopherol, red yeast rice, and olive oil polyphenols. A review of the literature. Altern Med Rev 6:248–71, 2001.
43. Smith DJ, Olive KE. Chinese red rice-induced myopathy. South Med J 96:1265–67, 2003.
44. Abrams DI, Couey P, Shade SB, et al. Antihyperlipidemic effect of *Pleurotus Ostreatus* (Jacq.: Fr.) P. Kumm in HIV: Results of a pilot proof-of-principle clinical trial. Int J Med Mushrooms 7:339–40, 2005.
45. Jacobs BP, Dennehy C, Ramirez G, et al. Milk thistle for the treatment of liver disease: a systematic review and meta-analysis. Am J Med 113:506–15, 2002.
46. Piscitelli SC, Formentini E, Burstein AH, et al. Effect of milk thistle on the pharmacokinetics of indinavir in healthy volunteers. Pharmacotherapy 22:551–6, 2002.
47. Lavie G, Valentine F, Levin B, et al. Studies of the mechanisms of action of the antiretroviral agents hypericin and pseudohypericin. Proc Natl Acad Sci USA 86:5963–7, 1989.
48. Gulick RM, McAuliffe V, Holden-Wiltse J, et al. Phase I studies of hypericin, the active compound in St. John's wort, as an antiretroviral agent in HIV-infected adults. The AIDS Clinical Trials Group Protocol 150 and 258. Ann Intern Med 130: 510–14, 1999.
49. Sherer R, Dutta B, Anderson R, et al. A phase IB study of (+)-calanolide A In: HIV-1-Infected, Antiretroviral Therapy Naive patients. In: 7th Conference on Retrovirus and Opportunistic Infections, San Francisco, 2000.
50. Liu JP, Manheimer E, Yang M. Herbal medicines for treating HIV infection and AIDS [review]. Cochrane Database Syst Rev3:CD003937, 2005.
51. Barrett B, Kiefer D, Rabago D. Assessing the risks and benefits of herbal medicine: an overview of scientific evidence. Alternative Therapies 5:40–9, 1999.
52. Turner RB, Bauer R, Woelkart K, et al. An evaluation of *Echinacea augustifolia* in experimental rhinovirus infection. N Engl J Med 353:341–8, 2005.
53. Boulatta JI, Nace AM. Safety issues with herbal medicine. Pharmacotherapy 20:257–69, 2000.
54. Blumethal M, Busse WR, Goldberg A, Hall T, Riggins CW, Rister RS (eds). The Complete German Commission E Monographs – Therapeutic Guide to Herbal Medicines (Klein S, Rister RS, trans.). Boston: Integrative Medicine Communications; Austin, Texas: American Botanical Council; 1998.
55. Block G, Henson DE, Levine M. Vitamin C: a new look. Ann Intern Med 114:909–10, 1991.
56. Harakeh S, Jariwalla RJ, Pauling L. Suppression of human immunodeficiency virus replication by ascorbate in chronically and acutely infected cells. Proc Natl Acad Sci USA 87:7245–9, 1990.
57. Jariwalla RJ, Harakeh S. HIV suppression by ascorbate and its enhancement by glutathione precursor (PO-B-3697). In: Abstracts of the Eight International Conference on AIDS. Amsterdam; 1992, p B207.
58. Beach RS, Mantero-Atienza E, Shor-Posner G, et al. Specific nutrient abnormalities in asymptomatic HIV-1 infection. AIDS 6:701–8, 1992.
59. Coodley GO, Coodley MK, Nelson HD, Loveless MO. Micronutrient concentrations in the HIV wasting syndrome. AIDS 7:1595–600, 1993.

60. Tang AM, Smit E. Selected vitamins in HIV infection: a review. AIDS Patient Care STDs 12:263–73, 1998.
61. Fawzi W. Micronutrients and human immunodeficiency virus type 1 disease progression among adults and children. Clin Infect Dis 37(Suppl 2): S112–16, 2003.
62. Baum MK, Shor-Posner G, Lai S, et al. High risk of HIV-related mortality is associated with selenium deficiency. J Acquir Immune Defic Sydr Human Retrovirol 15:370–4, 1997.
63. Graham N, Sorensen D, Odaka N, et al. Relationship of serum copper and zinc levels to HIV-1 seropositivity and progression to AIDS. J Acquir Immune Defic Sydr Human Retrovirol 4:976–80, 1991.
64. Semba RD, Graham NMH, Caiaffa WT, et al. Increased mortality associated with vitamin A deficiency during HIV-1 infection. Arch Intern Med 153:2149–54, 1993.
65. Tang AM, Graham NMH, Semba RD, Saah AJ. Association between serum vitamin A and E levels and HIV-1 disease progression. AIDS 11:613–20, 1997.
66. Tang AM, Graham NMH, Chandra RK, Saah AJ. Low serum vitamin B12 concentrations are associated with faster human immunodeficiency virus type 1 (HIV-1) disease progression. J Nutr 127:345–51, 1997.
67. Tang AM, Graham NMH, Saah AJ. Effects of micronutrient intake on survival in human immunodeficiency virus type 1 infection. Am J Epidemiol 143:1244–56, 1996.
68. Abrams B, Duncan D, Hertz-Picciotto I. A prospective study of dietary intake and and acquired immune deficiency syndrome in HIV-seropositive homosexual men. J Acquir Immune Defic Sydr 6:949–58,1993.
69. Fawzi WW, Msamanga GI, Spiegelman D, et al. A randomized trial of multi- vitamin supplements and HIV disease progression and mortality. N Engl J Med 351:23–32, 2004.
70. Schambelan M, Benson CA, Carr A, et al. Rapid communications. Management of metabolic complications associated with antiretroviral therapy for HIV-1 infection: recommendations of an International AIDS Society-USA Panel. J AIDS 31:257–75, 2002.
71. Peterson PL. The treatment of mitochondrial myopathies and encephalo- myopathies. Biochim Biophys Acta 1271:275–80, 1995.
72. Willett WC, Stampfer MJ. What vitamins should I be taking, doctor? N Engl J Med 345:1819–24, 2001.
73. Rietschel P, Corcoran C, Stanley T, et al. Prevalence of hypogonadism among men with weight loss related to human immunodeficiency virus infection who were receiving highly active antiretroviral therapy. Clin Infect Dis 31:1240–1, 2000.
74. Grinspoon S, Corcoran C, Miller K, et al. Body composition and endocrine function in women with acquired immunodeficiency syndrome wasting. J Clin Endocrinol Metab 82: 1332–7, 1997.
75. Migeon CJ, Keller AR, Lawrence B, Shepard TH. Dehydroepiandrosterone and androsterone levels in human plasma. Effect of age and sex, day-to-day and diurnal variations. J Clin Endocrinol Metab 17:1051–62, 1957.
76. Merril CR, Harrington MG. Plasma dehydroepiandrosterone levels in HIV infection. JAMA 261:1149, 1989.
77. Piketty C, Jayle D, Leplege A, et al. Double-blind placebo-controlled trial of oral dehydroepiandrosterone in patients with advanced HIV disease. Clin Endocrinol 55:325–30, 2001.
78. Ulmar S, Feleke G, Roginsky MS. Effect of dehydroepiandrosterone (DHEA on clinical and laboratory parameters in female patients with AIDS (42373). In: Abstracts of the XIIth International Conference on AIDS, Geneva, 1998, p 848.
79. Abrams DI, Shade SB, Couey P, et al. Dehydroepiandrosterone (DHEA) effects on HIV-1 replication and host immunity: a randomized, placebo-controlled study. AIDS Res Hum Retroviruses 23:77–85, 2007.
80. Rabkin JG, McElhiney MC, Rabkin R. Placebo-controlled trial of dehydroepiandrosterone (DHEA) for treatment of non-major depression in patients with HIV/AIDS. Am J Psychiatry 163:59–66, 2006.
81. Casey A, Constantin-Teodosiu D, Howell S, et al. Creatine ingestion favorably affects performance and muscle metabolism during maximal exercise in humans. Am J Physiol 271: E31–7, 1996.
82. Sakkas GK, Mulligan K, DeSilva ML, et al. Creatine supplementation fails to augment the benefits derived from resistance exercise training in patients with HIV infection. Antiviral Ther 10:L6, 2005.
83. Shabert J, Winslow C, Shabert JK. Glutamine/antioxidant supplementation promotes gain in body cell mass in HIV patients with weight loss (42336). In: Abstracts of the XIIth International Conference on AIDS, Geneva, 1998, p 841.
84. Gorter R, Seefried M, Volberding P. Dronabinol effects on weight in patients with HIV infection. AIDS 6:1270, 1992.
85. Struwe M, Kaempfer SH, Geiger CF, et al. Effect of dronabinol on nutritional status in HIV infection. Ann Pharmaco Ther 27: 827–36, 1993.
86. Hollister LE. Hunger and appetite after single doses of marijuana, alcohol, and dextroamphetamine. Clin Pharmacol Ther 12:44–9, 1971.
87. Mechoulam R. Role of endocannabinoid receptors in health. NIDA Workshop on Clinical Consequences of Marijuana, Rockville, 2001, p 17.
88. Greenberg I, Kuehnle J, Mendelson JH, Bernstein JG. Effects of marijuana use on body weight and caloric intake in humans. Psychopharmacology (Berl) 49:79–84, 1976.
89. Furler MD, Einarson TR, Millson M, et al. Medicinal and recreational marijuana use by patients infected with HIV. AIDS Patient Care STDs. 18:215–28, 2004.
90. Abrams DI, Hilton JF, Leiser RJ, et al. Short-term effects of cannabinoids in patients with HIV-1 infection. A randomized, placebo-controlled clinical trial. Ann Intern Med 139:258–66, 2003.
91. Jay C, Shade S, Vizoso H, et al. The effect of smoked marijuana on chronic neuropathic and experimentally induced pain in HIV neuropathy: results of an open-label pilot study. In: 11th Conference on Retroviruses and Opportunistic Infections, San Francisco, 2004.
92. Karst M, Salim K, Burstein S, et al. Analgesic effect of the synthetic cannabinoid CT-3 on chronic neuropathic pain. A randomized controlled trial. JAMA 290:1757–62, 2006.
93. Birk TJ, MacArthur RD, McGrady A, et al. Lack of effect of 12 weeks of massage therapy on immune function and quality of life in HIV-infected persons. In: Abstracts of the XIth International Conference on AIDS, Vancouver, 1996, p 270, abstract Th.B 4105.
94. Levin JS, Glass TA, Kushi LH, et al. Quantitative methods in research on complementary and alternative medicine. A methodological manifesto. NIH Office of Alternative Medicine. Med Care 35:1079–94, 1997.
95. Vandenbroucke JP, De Craen AJM. Alternative medicine: a 'mirror image' for scientific reasoning in conventional medicine. Ann Intern Med 135:507–13,2001.
96. Rose KD, Croissant PD, Parliament CF, Levin MB. Spontaneous spinal epidural hematoma with associated platelet dysfunction from excessive garlic ingestion: a case report. Neurosurgery 26:880–2, 1990.
97. Rowin J, Lewis SL. Spontaneous bilateral subdural hematomas associated with chronic *Gingko biloba* ingestion. Neurology 46: 1775–6, 1996.
98. Rabeneck L, Palmer A, Knowles JB, et al. A randomized controlled trial evaluating nutrition counseling with and without oral supplementations in malnourished HIV-infected patients. J Am Diet Assoc 98:434–8, 1998.

99. McKinley MJ, Goodman-Block J, Lesser ML, Salbe AD. Improved body weight status as a result of nutrition interventions in adult HIV-positive outpatients. J Am Diet Assoc 94:1014–17, 1994.
100. Kotler D, Tierney A, Wang J, Pierson R, Jr. Magnitude of body-cell-mass depletion and the timing of death from wasting in AIDS. Am J Clin Nutr 50:444–7, 1989.
101. Suttmann U, Ockenga J, Selberg O, et al. Incidence and prognostic value of malnutrition and wasting in human immunodeficiency virus-infected outpatients. J Acquir Immune Defic Syndr 8:239–46, 1998.
102. Wheeler D, Gibert C, Launer C, et al. Weight loss as a predictor of survival and disease progression in HIV infection. J Acquir Immune Defic Syndr 18:80–5, 1998.
103. Expert Panel on Detection Evaluation and Treatment of High Blood Cholesterol in Adults. Executive summary of the third report of the National Cholesterol Education Program (NCEP) (Adult Treatment Panel III). JAMA 285:2486–97, 2001.
104. Wohl DA, Tien HC, Busby M, et al. Randomized study of the safety and efficacy of fish oil (omega-3-fatty acid) supplementation with dietary and exercise counseling for the treatment of antiretroviral therapy-associated hypertriglyceridemia. Clin Infect Dis 41:1498–504, 2005.
105. Eisenberg JNS, Wade TJ, Charles S, et al. Risk factors in HIV-associated diarrheal disease: the role of drinking water, medication, and immune status. Epidemiol Infect 128:73–81, 2001.
106. Nixon S, O'Brien K, Glazier RH, Aynan AM. Aerobic exercise interventions for adults living with HIV/AIDS. The Cochrane Library 2, 2005.
107. Grinspoon S, Corcoran C, Parlman K, et al. Effects of testosterone and progressive resistance training in eugonadal men with AIDS wasting. A randomized, controlled trial. Ann Intern Med 133:348–55, 2000.
108. Bhasin S, Storer TW, Javanbakht M, et al. Testosterone replacement and resistance exercise in HIV-infected man with weight loss and low testosterone levels. JAMA 283:763–70, 2000.
109. Agin D, Gallagher D, Wang J, et al. Effects of whey protein and resistance exercise on body cell mass, muscle strength, and quality of life in women with HIV. AIDS 15:2431–40, 2001.
110. Yarasheski K, Tebas P, Stanerson B, et al. Resistance exercise training reduces hypertriglyceridemia in HIV infected men treated with antiviral treatment. In: 7th Conference on Retroviruses and Opportunistic Infections, San Francisco, 2000, abstract 54.
111. Ellis MR, Vinson DC, Ewigman B. Addressing spiritual concerns of patients, family physicians' attitudes and practices. J Fam Pract 48:105–9, 1999.
112. McKenna DJ, (ed). Natural Dietary Supplements: A Desktop Reference. Institute for Natural Products Research; Marine on St. Croix, Minnesota, 1998.
113. Turner MJ, Angel JB, Woodend K, Giguere P. The efficacy of calcium carbonate in the treatment of protease inhibitor-induced persistent diarrhea in HIV-infected patients. HIV Clin Trials 5:19–24, 2004.
114. Shevitz AH, Knox TA. Nutrition in the era of highly active antiretroviral therapy. Clin Infect Dis 32:1769–75, 2001.

Chapter 33

Acute HIV Infection

Saurabh Mehandru, MD, Martin Markowitz, MD

INTRODUCTION

Acute infection with the human immunodeficiency virus type 1 (HIV-1) is a unique stage of the virus–host interaction. Here, the virus enters the new host, gains access to susceptible cells, disseminates, creates a pool of latently infected cells harboring infectious provirus and establishes a relentless, self-propagating, chronic infection. Acute HIV-1 infection may be associated with a transient, symptomatic illness following initial exposure. As with many other acute viral illnesses, the signs and symptoms of acute HIV-1 infection are often nonspecific and require a high index of suspicion for its recognition and diagnosis. The diagnosis is often missed due to lack of awareness on the part of both patients and healthcare providers. Identification of acute HIV-1 infection is of great importance, both from individual and public health perspectives. This chapter reviews the pathogenesis of acute HIV-1 infection and discusses clinical and laboratory aspects of diagnosis. Finally, the current concepts pertaining to the clinical management and treatment of acute HIV-1 infection are discussed.

EPIDEMIOLOGY

The HIV/AIDS pandemic continues unabated. According to estimates in 2006, there are ~40 million individuals infected with HIV-1 worldwide. This includes 17.5 million women and 2.3 million children. Approximately five million individuals acquired HIV-1 infection and an additional three million HIV-1 related deaths occurred in the year 2005 alone. Since its recognition in 1981, the AIDS epidemic has resulted in more than 25 million deaths worldwide.[1]

In the United States, the estimated number of people living with HIV-1 infection exceeds one million with ~40 000 new infections every year.[1] Men having sex with men remains the dominant mode of HIV transmission in the United States, accounting for 65% of newly diagnosed infections in 2003. However, for women living with HIV-1, heterosexual sex was the main mode of transmission. A striking feature of the HIV-1 epidemic in the United States is the high incidence of infection among African-Americans. Despite constituting 12.5% of the country's population, African-Americans accounted for ~50% of new cases as well as HIV-1-related deaths in the United States in 2003.[2]

As many as a quarter of HIV-infected individuals in the United States are unaware of their diagnosis.[3] Establishing the diagnosis, particularly during acute infection has important implications. There is ample evidence to suggest that acute HIV-1 infection is associated with a high probability of transmission.[4–8] In addition, early diagnosis provides a unique opportunity to study the natural history of this disease, with direct implications on vaccine and microbicide research. Finally, early diagnosis enables the study of the potential benefits of immediate antiretroviral therapy.[9–12]

TRANSMISSION

The majority of HIV transmissions worldwide occur across a mucosal surface[13] such as the anorectal mucosa, vaginal mucosa and less frequently, the oral mucosa.[14] HIV-receptive cells have been found in the lamina propria of rectal, cervicovaginal, foreskin, urethral, and oral epithelia in primate models.[15] Intravenous drug abuse and mother-to-child transmission also remain important routes of HIV transmission worldwide. Quite early in the AIDS epidemic, HIV was isolated from seminal secretions in infected, asymptomatic men[16] and genital secretions of infected women.[17,18] In fact, despite prolonged treatment with highly active antiretroviral therapy (HAART), HIV-1 may persist in the male and female genital tracts.[19,20]

It has been shown that host infectiousness increases as a function of the concentration of virus in the genital tract.[13,21] During acute HIV-1 infection, increased viral transmission correlates with the dramatically elevated plasma viral loads in such patients.[22,23] Higher viral loads in the blood have been associated with the transmission of HIV-1 to sexual partners of individuals with transfusion-acquired infections.[24] Acquisition of HIV-1 during pregnancy and high maternal viral load are associated with increased risk of perinatal transmission.[25] Individuals with viral loads greater than 50000 copies/mL of plasma have a more than 50-fold increased risk of transmitting the virus per sexual act, and transmission is rare among persons with levels of less than 1500 copies of HIV-1 RNA per mL of plasma.[26] Further, individuals on potent antiretroviral therapy have a significant decrease in the risk of HIV transmission to their sexual partners.[27–29]

Reproductive tract infections and other sexually transmitted diseases are strongly associated with HIV-1 transmission even when adjusted for sexual behavior.[30] Ulcerative sexually transmitted diseases such as chancroid, syphilis and herpes are associated with a significant increase in the risk of HIV for men[31] and women.[32] Other sexually transmitted diseases such as gonorrhea and chlamydia,[31–34] bacterial vaginosis,[33] urethritis,[35,36] and cytomegalovirus infection[37] are associated with increased seminal levels of HIV and hence increase the risk of transmission. Consequently, treatment of sexually transmitted diseases in the population at risk has been shown to significantly decrease the incidence of HIV-1 transmission.[38] Cervical ectopy in women[13,39] and lack of circumcision in men[33] are associated with increased risk of HIV-1 transmission.

The choice of contraceptive methods impacts on HIV transmission. Condoms are protective for both sexes.[27,40–42] In animal models, the use of hormonal contraceptives containing progesterone also increases HIV-1 transmission by mucosal thinning.[43]

Epidemiologic studies suggest that host factors may influence susceptibility to HIV-1 infection.[44–46] Individuals homozygous for a 32-bp deletion in the CCR5 molecule are relatively resistant to infection by CCR5-tropic strains of HIV-1 but not by CXCR4-tropic strains.[47] Heterozygosity for the 32-bp deletion in CCR5 results in retardation of disease progression but does not protect against infection.[48] Recent data demonstrates interindividual variation in the copy number of segmental duplication within the gene encoding for CCL3L1. CCL3L1 is the most potent known natural ligand for the CCR5 receptor, and it is a dominant HIV-1-suppressive chemokine.[49] Possession of a CCL3L1 copy number lower than the population average is associated with markedly enhanced susceptibility to HIV-1 infection.[45]

The properties of HIV-1 itself may influence transmission. To date, the two major viral types characterized are: HIV-1, the predominant HIV type throughout the world; and HIV-2, first reported and primarily found among individuals from West Africa.[50,51] Although HIV-2 shares the same modes of transmission as HIV-1, the distribution of HIV-2 remains restricted primarily to West Africa where the rates have been stable over time in contrast to the rising rates of HIV-1 infection worldwide.[52] Prospective epidemiologic studies demonstrate a large difference in transmissibility between the two types with significantly lower rates of sexual and maternal-to-infant transmission for HIV-2 than for HIV-1.[53] Within HIV-1, whether one subtype has greater transmissibility than the other remains controversial and beset by multiple confounding factors that have not yet been resolved.[54–56]

Finally, HIV-1 transmission is closely linked to complex social factors.[57] Sexual practices such as ano-receptive intercourse, frequency of sexual contact, number of sexual partners, level of education and awareness, use of recreation drugs such as crystal methamphetamine,[58] use of HAART and urologic heterogeneity all impact on HIV-1 transmission in complex and interrelated manners.[59]

IMMUNOPATHOGENESIS

Studies derived from animal models[60] and humans have provided insights into the earliest events of transmission (Fig. 33-1). The probability of transmission with each encounter is quite small (~0.001) and is related in part to the dose[21] as described above. HIV-1 can cross the mucosal barrier by a breach in the intact mucosal epithelium. Mechanisms by which HIV-1 can access susceptible cells without disruption of the mucosa have also been described. For example, transcytosis by a vesicular pathway may enable HIV-1 to cross an intact mucosal barrier and infect susceptible host T cells.[61] Another mode of entry is selective capture of CCR5-tropic HIV-1 by epithelial cells, and transfer of infection to subepithelial CCR5 expressing target T cells.[62] More recently, it has been suggested that dendritic cells could capture intraluminal antigens across intact epithelium through transepithelial dendrites using CX3CR1, a chemokine receptor.[63] It is believed that once HIV-1 enters the tissue, it is captured initially by the resident dendritic cells. These dendritic cells express CD4, CCR5, an integrin termed DC-SIGN[64,65] and other C-type lectin receptors (CLRs).[66] Recent evidence suggests these dendritic cell associated CLRs such as DC-SIGN facilitate the formation of an "infectious synapse" between dendritic cells and T cells.[67] In the regions of these synapses, dendritic cells may concentrate HIV-1, resulting in efficient transfer of infection to CD4+ T cells.[67] Based on SIV-infected macaque studies[68,69] and studies of female genital organ cultures *ex vivo*,[70] the first HIV-infected cells that could be detected were intraepithelial memory CD4+ T cells. In performing their physiological function of transferring antigens to generate an immune response, virus carrying antigen-presenting cells can disseminate infection to a large number of CD4+ T cells and serve to disseminate infection.

In the gut-associated lymphoid tissue (GALT), the largest immune organ in the body,[71] the virus finds access to a substantial pool of densely packed CCR5-expressing memory CD4+ T cells and within days of infection, culminates in a profound depletion of these cells from the lamina propria.[72–75] In addition, it has been observed that during acute HIV-1 infection gastrointestinal CD4+ T cells harbor significantly

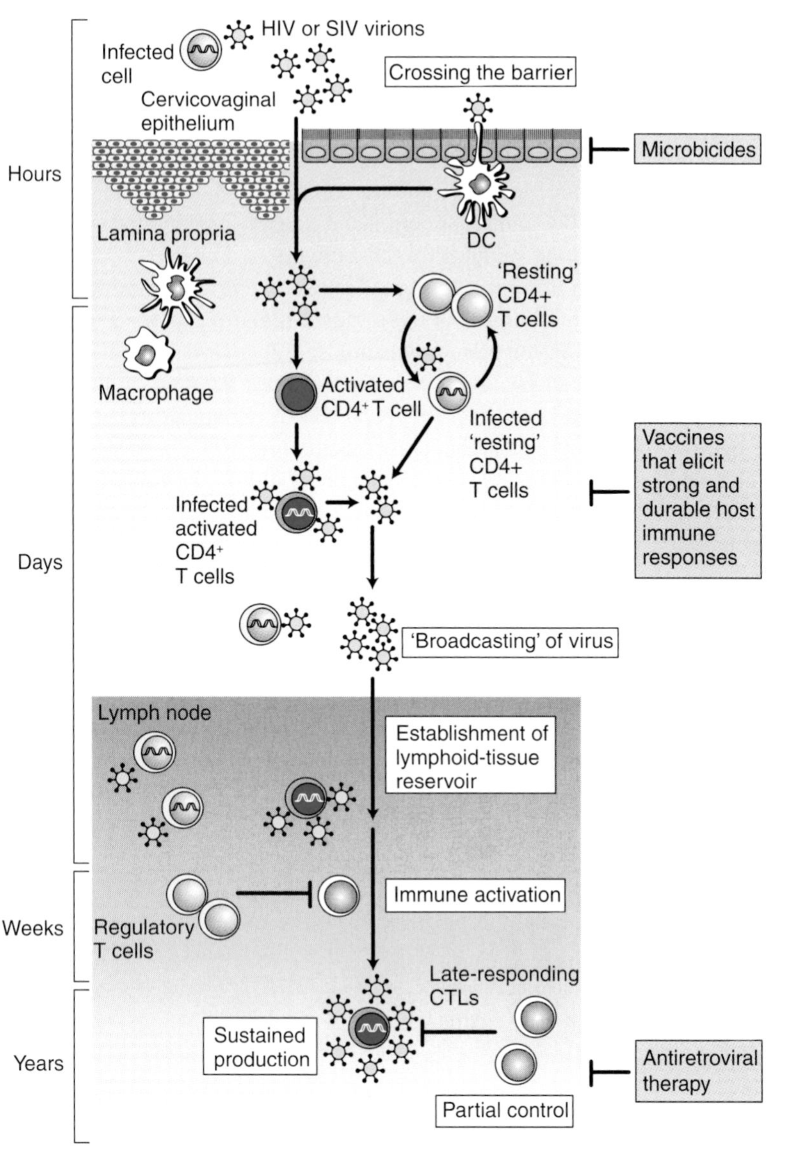

Figure 33-1 ■ Schematic representation of vaginal transmission of HIV and SIV and the subsequent stages of infection. The diagram shows the key cells and molecules and the key events in space and time for the interactions between virus and host and for maximally effective interventions. The type and activation state of CD4+ T cells is indicated by their color. In the first hours of infection, virus and/or infected cells cross the cervicovaginal mucosal barrier. Virus then becomes established at the point of entry by infecting susceptible CD4+ T cells; which, unlike cells that are truly resting, can support viral replication, because they are the most numerous target cells in the lamina propria. Expansion of infection from small founder populations of infected cells in the lamina propria then "broadcasts" the virus and infected cells, first to the draining lymph nodes and then systemically, in sufficient numbers to establish and maintain virus production in the lymphoid tissues. Immune responses are activated, but they are too late and of insufficient magnitude to eradicate infection. Immune activation supplies additional activated CD4+ T cells, which then sustain infection, and it also elicits an immunosuppressive response that blunts host defences. Nonetheless, subsequently, increasing numbers of cytotoxic T lymphocytes (CTLs) can partially control infection but cannot prevent, in the absence of therapy, the slow and continued depletion of CD4+ T cells and the eventual progression to AIDS. The interventions target vulnerabilities at the point of entry. Further reducing the size of infected founder populations in this location, using microbicides and/or a vaccine that quickly elicits large numbers of CTLs compared with the number of infected cells, could abort infection at the point of entry and/or prevent the expansion and broadcasting to distal regions that is required to establish a persistent systemic infection. SIV, simian immunodeficiency virus.

Redrawn with permission from Haase AT. Perils at mucosal front lines for HIV and SIV and their hosts. Nat Rev Immunol 2005; 5:783–92.

greater levels of proviral DNA and RNA compared to peripheral blood CD4+ T cells.[76] Therefore, it may be hypothesized that mucosal sites such as the gastrointestinal tract play a critical role in the pathogenesis of acute HIV-1 infection.[77] Substantial depletion of memory CD4+ T cells from mucosal sites within days of infection also suggests that the immunological injury due to HIV-1 is early and profound. Animal studies indicate that failure to repopulate mucosal sites with memory CD4+ T cells is associated with rapid progression.[78] However, whether this is a cause or an effect of rapid disease progression remains to be resolved.

Virology

During acute HIV-1 infection there is an initial burst of viral replication.[79] Once the basic reproductive rate or *R*0 becomes greater than or equal to 1, self propagating infection is established.[80] Virus disseminates throughout the body and quickly establishes a pool of latently infected cells[81,82] that represent a major obstacle to curing HIV-1 infection despite the availability of potent antiretroviral therapy.[83] Between 93% and 99% of virus is produced by rapid rounds of infection and destruction of activated T cells, with the rest produced by long-lived chronically infected cells such as tissue macrophages, dendritic cells, latently infected lymphocytes and release of trapped virions from lymphoid tissue.[84] During this phase of exponential viral growth, cytokines are released locally and systemically and infected individuals develop symptoms of "acute retroviral syndrome" as described below. Levels of plasma viremia at this stage are known to be in millions of copies per mL of plasma, often with an absent or evolving serologic response. The viral load then decreases substantially in temporal association with the development of HIV-1 specific immune response.[85] In a cohort of 74 individuals studied during acute and early HIV-1 infection, Schacker et al showed that inflection point in the reduction of plasma HIV-1 occurred, on average at ~117 days after infection.[86] In the majority of cases, a quasi-steady state or "setpoint" is established

3–9 months after the initial infection, predictive of long term clinical outcome[86–88] when HIV-1 production and clearance are in approximate balance.

There is conflicting information regarding HIV-1 transmission and viral variability. Early reports suggested that HIV-1 transmission was a clonal event and that an evolutionary bottleneck occurred at the level of transmission, with a single homogenous clone establishing infection in the new host.[89] Long and Overbaugh reported in a study of heterosexually acquired HIV-1 that African men ($n = 10$) and women ($n = 26$) exhibit differences in transmission events. HIV-1 infection in men was always clonal (10/10) whereas in 15 of 26 women, multiple transmitted viruses were identified.[90] Subsequent studies by this group found that women who acquired multiple viral genotypes were more likely to exhibit faster disease progression.[91] However, there is no data regarding transmissibility, that is, whether women with multiple viruses are more likely to subsequently transmit.

Studies in homosexual men have been somewhat contradictory. Again, early studies suggested that early infection was indeed clonal, based on studies of HIV-1 envelope genetic variation. Yet, Zhang et al reported that despite homogeneity in envelope, higher levels of diversity in the *gag* region were observed in primary HIV-1 infection.[92] Learn and Mullins found that eight homosexual men presenting with acute HIV-1 infection harbored more divergent envelope sequences (1.08% difference on average) than *gag* (0.81%).[93] As infection progressed envelope diversity was reduced and *gag* diversity increased. These findings support the hypothesis that in homosexual men, multiple variants can be transmitted, and perhaps, this may relate to susceptibility, subsequent transmission and perhaps clinical course. Frost and coworkers analyzed eight recently infected individuals, an estimated mean 30 days (range: 21–85) after infection and the six men who infected them. Of note, three sources were chronically infected with HIV-1 while three were newly infected. Analyses of 11–15 clones per recipient found the diversity of envelope sequences was low, a mean of 0.25% with a range of 0.18–0.34%.[94] Clinical correlations were not described. The viruses in the Frost study were much more homogenous than that published by Learn. Missing from these studies are clinical correlations. We believe that routes of transmission (oral, anal receptive versus anal insertive) and behaviors (substance use) are likely to affect these observed virologic factors.

Humoral Immunity

Humoral immunity plays a central role in clearing many viral infections. However, during acute HIV-1 infection, the neutralizing antibody response is variable,[95] weak[96–98] and frequently delayed.[85] Antibodies are often non-neutralizing,[99] being directed in part at virion debris.[100] Furthermore, the timing of neutralizing antibody detection does not correlate with peak viremia,[85,96] although this could be a function of the sensitivity of the assay used.[95] Using a sensitive recombinant viral assay, it was shown recently that host-derived neutralizing antibodies do appear early in the course of HIV-1 infection and may exert immune pressure for rapid escape. This was supported by the finding that on longitudinal assessment of viral isolates initially identified during acute and early HIV-1 infection, sequence variation developed within the viral envelope resulting in escape from neutralization.[101] Further in support of antibody induced immune pressure, Wei et al have proposed that HIV-1 may escape neutralization by modifying the carbohydrate residues associated with viral envelope.[102] Changes within this "glycan shield" impact on viral binding to neutralizing antibodies but not to host cellular receptors. Preferential transmission of neutralization sensitive virus, containing fewer N-linked glycosylation sites, has been reported by Derdeyn et al[103] in a study of subtype C HIV-1, although this may depend on subtype and mode of transmission.[94,104]

Induction of neutralizing antibodies in the context of established infection may be slow and inadequate to match viral diversity. In addition, it is clear that the virus has evolved many strategies to escape neutralization such as sequestration of critical domains, high replicative rate, and enormous sequence variation to name a few. As a result, enthusiasm for the potential of inducing neutralizing antibodies as an effective vaccine strategy waned early during the epidemic. However, many studies demonstrating that the presence of preexisting neutralizing antibodies may prevent HIV-1 or SIV infection or ameliorate the clinical course[105–109] and have reemphasized the induction of neutralizing antibodies as an effective vaccine strategy.

Cellular Immunity

There is compelling evidence to suggest that cytotoxic T Lymphocytes (CTLs) play a crucial role in the control of HIV-1 replication (*see* Fig. 33-1). During acute HIV-1 infection, a drop in plasma viremia is temporarilly associated with the appearance of virus specific CTLs.[85,110–112] In addition, there is marked expansion of oligoclonal populations of T lymphocytes in the peripheral blood of infected individuals at the time of virus containment in the early weeks after HIV-1 infection.[113] Studies done in SIV-infected macaques show a clear temporal association between the expansion of CTLs and the clearance of virus.[114–116] Perhaps the most compelling evidence demonstrating a role of virus specific CTLs arises from experiments during which antiCD8+ antibodies were used to transiently deplete CD8+ T cells from SIV-infected macaques *in vivo*.[117,118] When the duration of depletion was greater than 28 days, primary viremia was never cleared after acute infection and the SIV-infected monkeys died with a rapidly progressive AIDS-like syndrome. During chronic infection transient depletion of CD8+ T lymphocytes was associated with a substantial rise in levels of plasma viremia that returned to baseline levels coincident with the reemergence of the CD8+ T cell population. Robust CTL responses have also been shown to confer significant protection against simian immunodeficiency virus (SIV) and SHIV challenge in monkeys.[119–121]

Multiple mechanisms have been attributed to the antiviral effects of CTLs such as direct lysis of HIV-1 infected cells[122] and production of multiple soluble factors.[122,123] CTL recognition of an infected cell is based on the detection of processed viral proteins at the cell surface in the context of a major histocompatibility complex (MHC) class I molecule. Individual expression of class I molecules (grouped as A, B, and C) is genetically determined and inherited. Certain MHC class I haplotypes have predictive value for the rate of clinical disease progression. For example, heterozygosity at class I alleles, as well as the expression of the MHC class I molecules HLA-B27 and HLA-B57, in infected individuals are associated with better clinical outcomes.[124–126] On the other hand, homozygosity for class alleles and HLA-B35 is associated with a more rapid disease progression[124,127] Specific human leucocyte antigen (HLA) alleles have now also been associated with vaccine responsiveness in HIV vaccine trials[128] suggesting that certain alleles may be associated with better antigen presentation than the others. These observations underscore the importance of CTLs in containing HIV-1 replication and highlight the genetic constraints on immune control, though the mechanisms by which these interact remain obscure. CTL function is critically dependent on the presence of virus-specific T-helper cells.[129] These cells, which recognize viral protein presented in the context of an MHC class II molecule, are generated after initial antigen exposure by dendritic cells that serve to initiate this immune response.[130,131] Using sensitive assays to detect cytokine production in response to HIV-1 antigens, HIV-1 specific CD4+ T cells have been observed in infected individuals.[132,133] However, one of the hallmarks of chronic progressive infection is a dramatic reduction in the frequency of these T-helper, HIV-1 specific immune responses.[134] Long term nonprogressors on the other hand, have preserved CD4+ T-helper responses.[11] This could be explained by the finding that HIV-1 preferentially infects HIV-1 specific CD4+ T cells early in the course of infection.[135] Numerous animal and human studies demonstrate that reduction of viral load during acute infection, through antiretroviral therapy or immunization is associated with the generation of strong virus-specific T-helper responses.[11,136–139] However, some of the recent studies have shown that these responses are not durable once antiretroviral therapy is discontinued.[140]

As discussed above, virus specific CTL responses are detected in early HIV-1 infection. However, due to high replicative rate and lack of proofreading ability in the reverse transcriptase enzyme, viral escape from CTL control is well documented during acute infection.[111,112,141] Escape occurs even through single amino acid mutations in an epitope, at sites essential for MHC binding or T-cell-receptor recognition, but may also be influenced by mutations in flanking regions that affect antigen processing. Recent studies in macaques immunized with SHIV provide the most direct link between immune escape from CTLs and disease progression.[142] Immunized animals were not protected from infection but seemed to be protected from disease progression. During prolonged follow-up, one animal developed an increasing viral load which was temporally related to the emergence of a CTL escape mutation within a dominant epitope.

Innate Immunity

A growing body of evidence suggests that the function of Natural Killer (NK) cells is impaired in HIV-1 infection including reduced CC-chemokine production,[143,144] antibody-dependent cellular cytotoxicity (ADCC),[145] and changes in cytokine secretion.[146,147] A recent report where 10 subjects with acute HIV-1 infection were followed longitudinally suggests that distinct changes in the NK compartment start during acute infection.[148] There is an overall increase in NK cell number during acute HIV-1 infection with expansion of the $CD3^{neg}CD56^{dim}CD16^{pos}$ NK subset, an early depletion of $CD3^{neg}CD56^{bright}CD16^{neg}$ NK cells and a concomitant increase in the functionally anergic $CD3^{neg}CD56^{neg}CD16^{pos}$ cells. Numeric changes in NK cells are accompanied by reduced functional activity as measured by CD107a expression and cytokine secretion.

Gamma-delta T cells comprise 1–15% of peripheral blood lymphocytes.[149] In HIV-uninfected individuals, Vγ9Vd2 subset predominates in the peripheral blood while the Vd1 subset constitutes a minority of the total γd T cell population. During acute HIV-1 infection, there is a significant expansion of Vd1 and contraction of Vd2 subsets of γd T cells.[150] Inversion of the Vd2:Vd1 ratio persists during chronic HIV-1 infection. However, the clinical significance of this observation remains unclear.

NK T cells are a subset of lymphocytes that share features of both NK cells and T cells. Recent reports have indicated that during acute and early HIV-1 infection, there is a decrease in the percentage of total NK T cells as well as CD4+ NK T cells.[151] In addition, defects in NK T cell function have been observed during acute HIV-1 infection.[152]

Thus, HIV-1 infection appears to impact both adaptive and innate immunity. Understanding HIV-1 pathogenesis in the setting of both viral and host diversity is a challenge. Clearly, the virus is uniquely adapted to establish infection, avoid immune responses, be they innate or adaptive, and set up self-perpetuating, relentless infection. Such insights also indicate potential targets where the virus may be most vulnerable so that infection may be prevented or ameliorated.

CLINICAL MANIFESTATIONS

The recognition of signs and symptoms of acute infection with HIV-1 remains problematic. They are varied, inconsistent, and similar to other viral syndromes. It is estimated that 40–90% of people manifest symptoms at 2–4 weeks after infection.[153,154] The clinical features have been described in all populations at risk of HIV-1 infection, including intravenous drug users[155] and recipients of infected organs.[156] They have been described in many different countries, and in all ages. There seems to be little effect of viral clade or host ethnicity on these symptoms. It is thought that the symptoms are related to the burst of viremia that accompanies acute infection, either directly or secondarily to the immune response.[79,157,158]

Symptoms Associated with Acute HIV Infection

Table 33-1

Symptom	Incidence (%)
Fever	96
Lymphadenopathy	74
Pharyngitis	70
Rash[a]	70
Myalgias or arthralgias	54
Diarrhea	32
Headache	32
Nausea and vomiting	27
Hepatosplenomegaly	14
Weight loss	13
Thrush	12
Neurologic disorders[b]	12

[a] Including erythematous maculopapular, vesiculopapular, vasculitis, and oral/genital ulcers.
[b] Including meningoencephalitis, aseptic meningitis, peripheral neuropathy, facial palsy, Guillain–Barre syndrome, brachial neuritis, cognitive impairment, and psychosis.

Adapted from Niu MT, Stein DS, Schnittman SM. Primary human immunodeficiency virus type 1 infection: review of pathogenesis and early treatment intervention in humans and animal retrovirus infections. J Infect Dis 1993; 168:1490–501.

The first descriptions of acute HIV-1 seroconversion occurred in 1985.[159] A prospective study in Australia identified 11 men with a specific illness at the time of acute HIV-1 infection. This illness was similar to infectious mononucleosis; it was comprised of fevers, sweats, malaise, anorexia, nausea, myalgias, arthralgias, headaches, sore throat, diarrhea, generalized lymphadenopathy, a macular erythematous truncal eruption, and thrombocytopenia. In 1996, a study of 46 adults revealed that 89% of acute seroconverters developed an acute retroviral syndrome similar in nature to the above. The most common symptoms were fever, seen in 77%, sore throat, fatigue, weight loss and myalgia.[14] Seven of the patients had symptoms so severe that they required hospitalization. Fever was also a common symptom of seroconversion in studies of non-Caucasians, although the frequency was less.[160,161] A prospective study of Kenyan female sex workers reported that only 53% were symptomatic during seroconversion,[161] whereas, another study in India showed that 81% of patients with primary HIV-1 infection had fever, adenopathy, arthralgias, rash, or diarrhea.[160] The other most common symptoms are fatigue, seen in 70–90% of cases, and rash, seen in 40–80% (Table 33-1).[162] Pharyngitis, myalgias, and anorexia have also been recognized as frequent symptoms of seroconversion.[162,163] Most symptoms do not resolve until serum antibodies to HIV-1 develop.[161]

The differential diagnosis for acute HIV-1 infection is primarily comprised of infectious mononucleosis, acute hepatitis, disseminated gonorrhea, roseola, influenza, secondary syphilis, toxoplasmosis and CMV. Certain of these illnesses can be co-infections,[164] and therefore anyone presenting with a sexually transmitted disease should be evaluated for possible acute HIV infection; it should also be considered in any patient with an unexplained severe febrile illness.

One of the more suggestive and specific symptoms of the acute retroviral syndrome is the central maculopapular rash found on the trunk and face, and occasionally involving the limbs including the palms and soles (Fig. 33-2A).[162,163] The rash is painless, nonpruritic, and erythematous, with individual lesions typically 5–10 mm in diameter.[156,162–164] There are also descriptions of vesicular or pustular rashes resembling measles (Fig. 33-2B).[165,166] Histopathological evaluation of these rashes reveals a mononuclear cell infiltration mainly in the upper dermis, surrounding blood vessels and sweat ducts. Earlier studies have shown CD4+ T cells as the predominant cell type[167]; a more recent case demonstrated more CD8+ than CD4 + T cells, and CD1a+ dendritic cells were seen infiltrating the perivascular space.[166] Prior studies have demonstrated HIV-1 p24 antigens in the infiltrate, localizing to dendritic cells.[168] There is evidence of focal lymphocytic vasculitis in these biopsies, and occasional reports of palpable purpura as a presenting sign of acute infection.[169] It is thought that the interaction of CD8 + T cells with dendritic cells might be the cause of the resulting exanthem.

Mucosal involvement, in the form of ulcerations, is also fairly common and tends to be a more specific sign for acute HIV-1 infection than other signs.[170] It can involve the genitalia and oral mucosa, including the palate (Figs 33-3 and 33-4).[163] It can be associated with oral candidiasis. One study correlating symptoms with mode of transmission demonstrated that genital ulcerations are found only in those who contract the virus sexually.[171]

Acute HIV-1 infection often presents with neurological syndromes, reflecting the neurotropism of HIV-1 and the early dissemination of the virus to the central nervous system.[172–174] Facial nerve palsy,[174–176] ascending inflammatory demyelinating polyneuropathy,[177] severe myelopathy[172] and sensory ganglioneuritis[178,179] have all been reported shortly after infection. The most common neurological manifestation is aseptic meningitis, associated in some cases with a lymphocytic pleocytosis in the CSF. It has also been associated with meningoencephalitis,[180] acute psychosis,[181] and myeloradiculoneuritis.[182] The severity of neurological symptoms correlates with the amount of HIV RNA isolated from the CSF.[174] These syndromes are usually self-limiting, although there are reports of persistent impairment months later.[165,172]

Abdominal manifestations of acute HIV infection are most commonly diarrhea, nausea and vomiting, and hepatosplenomegaly.[163] There have been many reports of acute hepatitis as the presenting symptom.[183,184] Less common manifestations include an inflammatory pseudotumor of the testis,[185] pancreatitis,[186] and ulcerative esophagitis.[187]

Infants also manifest symptoms of acute seroconversion. A retrospective case-control study done in Cote d'Ivoire described the acute retroviral syndrome in infants who were infected by breastfeeding.[188] There were three dominant syndromes associated with infection; a mononucleosis-like syndrome with fevers and pharyngitis, dermatitis, and generalized lymphadenopathy. Conversely, infants who are infected

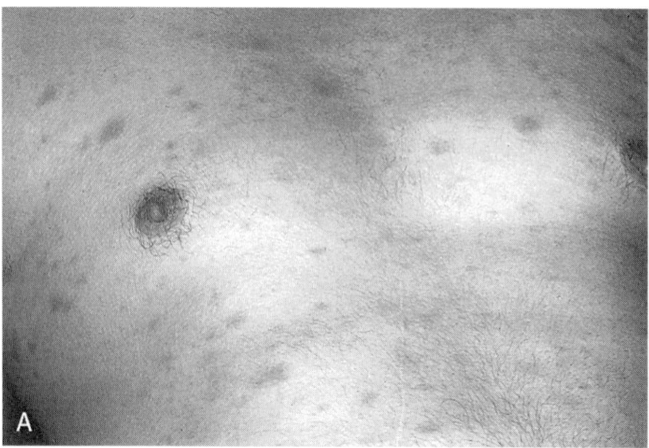

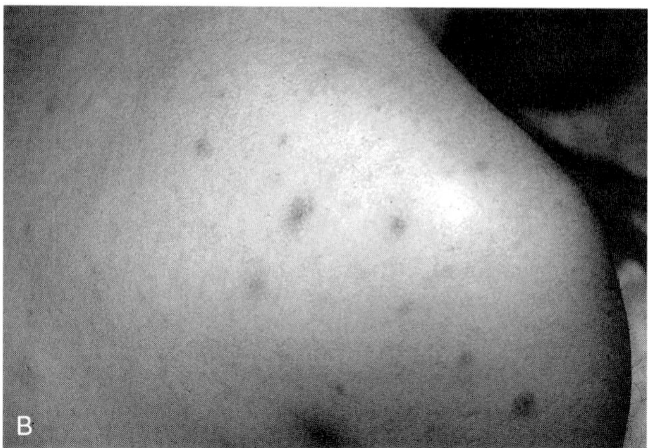

Figure 33-2 ■ (**A**) Maculopapular skin eruption in acute HIV infection. (**B**) Vesiculopapular eruption during acute HIV infection.

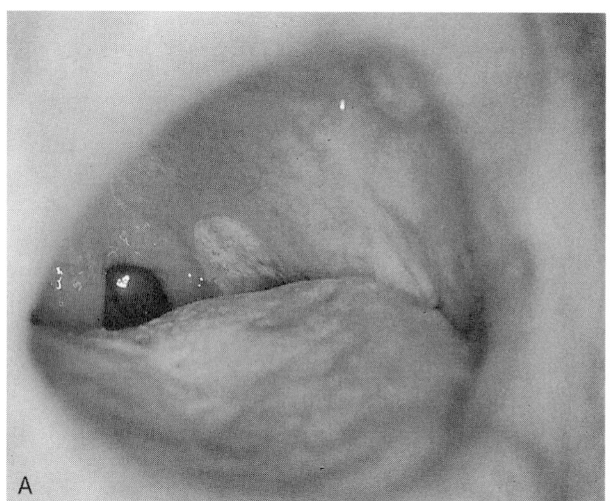

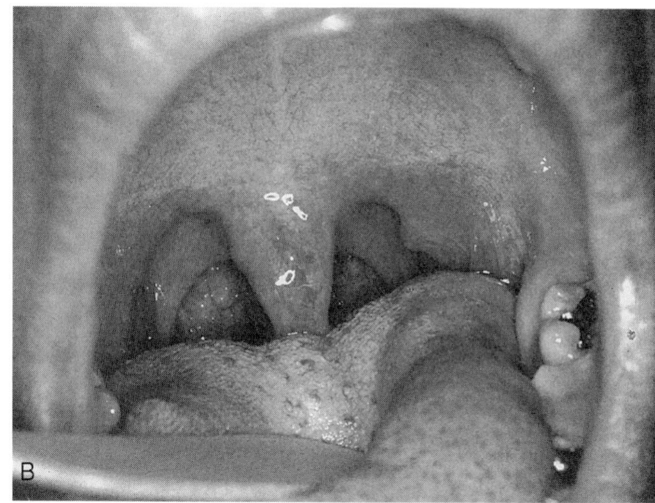

Figure 33-3 ■ (**A**) Oropharyngeal ulcer in acute HIV infection. (**B**) Thrush, diffuse oropharyngeal edema, and tonsillar erosion during acute HIV infection.

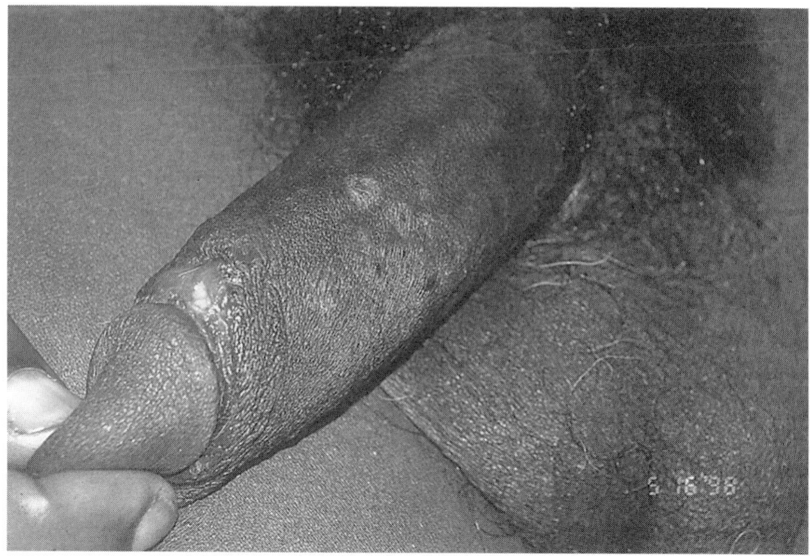

Figure 33-4 ■ Penile ulcer during HIV infection.

perinatally can be asymptomatic for prolonged periods, or may present with fever, failure to thrive, and oral candidiasis.

The most common laboratory abnormalities associated with acute HIV-1 infection are, like the signs and symptoms, quite nonspecific and may be transient. They include thrombocytopenia, lymphopenia, neutropenia, and elevated liver transaminases.[156,162,169,180] Levels of CD4+ T lymphocytes can also decrease, with inversion of the CD4+/CD8+ lymphocyte ratio as the CD8+ cytotoxic T cell population expands, sometimes dramatically.[158,180,189] Certain opportunistic infections have been associated with this immunosuppression. Herpes zoster is well described,[175] as are oral and esophageal candidiasis.[190–192]

Immune activation during acute infection, as measured by CD38 expression on T cells, has been correlated with the level of viremia.[193] In particular, the level of CD8+ T-cell activation is a strong predictor of the rate of CD4+ T-cell decline, indicating that the pathogenicity of HIV-1 in an individual host might be determined by the ability of the virus to activate the immune system.[193] Moreover, lower nadir CD4+ T-cell counts and smaller decreases in HIV-1 RNA during the first 30 days after seroconversion also predict a more rapid disease progression.[194]

Studies have demonstrated that both the duration and severity of symptoms can predict HIV-1 disease progression.[195,196] The incubation period of symptoms is also a predictor of a faster progression to AIDS. In one study, shorter incubations of fever, fatigue and myalgias were all independently associated with the rate of progression, as was a longer duration of myaglias, fever, arthralgias, fatigue, and headache.[197] It is theorized that a shorter incubation period for fever is a marker for the secretion of high levels of cytokines and thus indicates a lower degree of control of HIV replication, and a higher viral burden.[197] Further investigations into the correlation between symptoms, immunity and viral pathogenicity are warranted.

Overall, these clinical features differ greatly between individuals, and the identification of risk factors is difficult as they are often overlooked. Unfortunately, there is no combination of symptoms or physical findings that reliably distinguishes the acute HIV syndrome from other viral illnesses. As the study by Schacker et al demonstrated, only 26% of patients presenting with symptoms of seroconversion were correctly diagnosed.[14] However, the recognition of this syndrome is very important for public health, as the risk of transmission is much higher due to extremely high viral loads and continuing high-risk behavior. A recent retrospective analysis of discordant couples in Uganda demonstrated that the highest rate of HIV transmission (0.0082/coital act) was during the first 2.5 months after seroconversion.[8] Other recent studies have focused on the benefit of screening certain populations for the acute HIV syndrome. A recent study analyzed the prevalence of primary HIV infection in patients presenting with fever or other symptoms. In an urban population in the Northeastern US, 1.0% of those presenting with symptoms of a viral illness and with at least one risk factor for HIV were diagnosed with acute HIV infection.[198] Most recently, a large-scale analysis of the 2000 National Ambulatory Medical Care Survey and the 2000 National Hospital Ambulatory Medical Survey of the United States demonstrated a prevalence of acute HIV-1 infection of 0.66% in all those who presented to an ambulatory setting with fever, 0.50% in those with rash, and 0.16% in those with pharyngitis.[199] These numbers argue for increased use of nucleic acid testing (NAT) to identify the newly infected as rapidly as possible, and to improve prevention efforts in all affected populations.

DIAGNOSIS

Timely recognition of acute HIV infection is crucial both from an individual and a public health perspective (*see also* Chapter 1). The period of acute illness offers a unique opportunity to initiate early therapy and potentially alter the disease course. The high HIV-1 RNA levels seen at this stage likely correspond to high degree of infectiousness and appropriate counseling can thus potentially decrease HIV transmission.[200] The diagnosis of acute HIV infection is usually made with the help of clinical features (and exposure history, if present) in conjunction with laboratory data. An algorithm for laboratory testing is presented in Figure 33-5, and the kinetics of the appearance of various laboratory tests is depicted in Figure 33-6.

The standard enzyme-linked immunosorbent assay (ELISA) and Western blot tests that provide evidence of host immune responses to HIV cannot be used in the setting of acute HIV infection as these responses are typically not generated during the early stage of illness. Serological tests currently in use typically become positive within 22–27 days after exposure, which

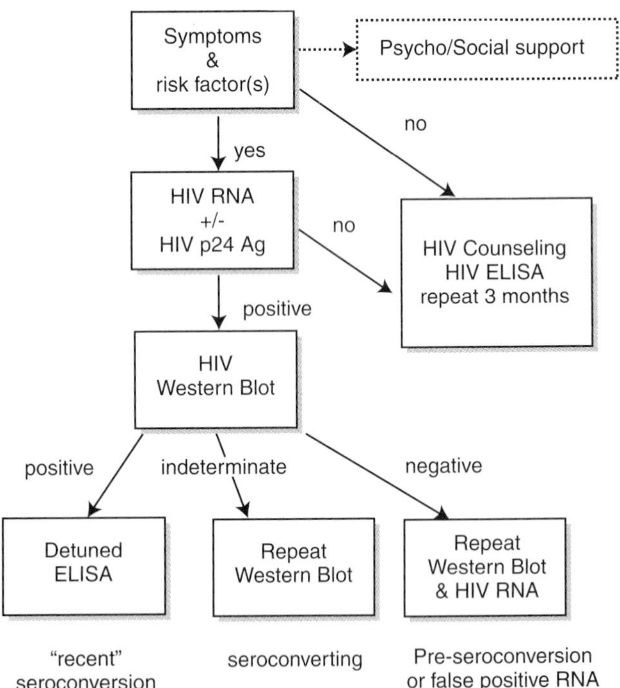

Figure 33-5 ■ Algorithm for laboratory testing for acute HIV infection.

is usually after the symptoms of acute infection have resolved and well after the time of peak viremia.[162] Thus the diagnosis of acute HIV infection must be based on detection of virus rather than on the presence of a detectable immune response to the virus. Viral culture and isolation from the infected person's plasma or peripheral blood mononuclear cells is a sensitive and specific test for the presence of HIV infection.[201,202] However, it is labor intensive, and remains a research tool and is not approved for diagnosis of acute HIV-1 infection.

The p24 antigen test, an enzyme immunoassay for a major viral core protein was the first assay available for the diagnosis of HIV infection prior to antibody seroconversion. It has high specificity in the setting of acute HIV infection[153,170,203] and is commercially available and easily performed. Prior to the approval of NATs for detection of acute HIV-1 infection in 2002, the p24 antigen test was widely available in blood banks and was routinely used for blood donor screening. Persons newly infected with HIV-1 had high p24 levels that were transiently detectable for ~40 days; beyond this period, the emergence of endogenous antibody interfered with laboratory detection and p24 sensitivity was reduced.[170] The combination of heat denaturation and signal amplification improved sensitivity of the test during early infection,[204] however sensitivity during chronic infection was still limited.

HIV NATs are highly sensitive for diagnosis of acute HIV infection and were approved by the FDA in 2002 for screening blood donors. Although not yet FDA approved for diagnosis of HIV infection in nondonor settings, judicious use of NATs has obvious advantages in specific circumstances where there is a high index of suspicion for acute HIV infection.[153] In these cases, a positive test is almost always followed by documentation of HIV antibody seroconversion. Different approaches of nucleic acid testing include nucleic acid sequence-based amplification (NASBA), signal amplification techniques – branched chain DNA (bDNA) and target amplification (Amplicor-PCR). A positive HIV RNA test in the absence of detectable antibodies establishes the presumptive diagnosis of acute HIV infection. The occurrence of false-positive results, especially

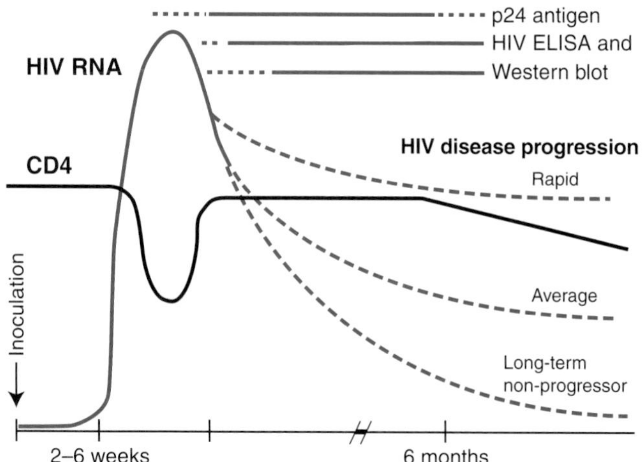

Figure 33-6 ■ Dynamics of laboratory tests during early HIV infection.

when low HIV-1 RNA levels are obtained, needs to be taken into consideration. As acute symptomatic HIV infection is associated with very high levels of HIV-1 RNA typically in the range of over 10 million copies/mL, it is generally recommended that HIV-1 RNA levels 5000 copies/mL should be regarded as false-positive tests in the setting of suspected acute HIV infection.[170] Following establishment of HIV infection, HIV-1 RNA in plasma is an excellent disease-monitoring tool, and can accurately determine the level of viral activity in an HIV-infected person, thus allowing prediction of clinical course as well as response to therapy.

The qualitative HIV-1 DNA PCR assay is an alternative to HIV-1 RNA testing for diagnosis of acute HIV infection and is commonly employed in the perinatal setting to test the exposed infant during the first 4 months to 1 year when maternally present HIV antibodies in the infant may complicate accurate serology test interpretation.[205]

Current serological methods may be modified to detect "recent" HIV infection, such as the "detuned antibody test" which can be used in a research and epidemiological setting to establish infection that has occurred in the previous 180 days.[206] This assay involves the use of the standard ELISA for HIV diagnosis that has been made less sensitive by raising the cutoff value for positivity. However this is not entirely useful in the setting of acute infection as no distinction is made between the "acute" and "recent' stage. Newer developments have led to combining the standard antibody-detecting ELISA with p24 antigen detection assay, resulting in HIV diagnosis within 16 days of infection.[207,208]

Among several proposed staging systems describing the evolution of acute HIV infection,[209,210] a recent study detailed six laboratory stages. stage I: HIV present in blood samples with only RNA assay positive; stage II: RNA and HIV-1 p24 antigen tests positive and antibody EIA nonreactive; stage III: RNA, HIV-1 antigen and HIV IgM-sensitive EIA reactive, but Western blot without HIV-1-specific bands; stage IV: as stage III, but in addition indeterminate Western blot pattern, stage V: as stage IV, but reactive Western blot pattern, except lacking p31 (*pol*) reactivity; stage VI: as stage V, but full Western blot reactivity including a p31 band.[211] Stages I–IV represent acute HIV infection, with each stage lasting ~3–5 days.

The classic clinical presentation of acute HIV infection is a mononucleosis-like illness, and hence the list of differential diagnosis is rather extensive. These include infectious mononucleosis, hepatitis, secondary syphilis, primary HSV, rubella, toxoplasmosis, disseminated gonococcal infections, and a variety of viral exanthems and enanthems. Laboratory testing may be utilized to exclude many of these infectious possibilities. Other infections may be co-transmitted along with HIV infection and also warrant appropriate investigations.

TREATMENT

An optimal management strategy for acute HIV infection has not yet been established and can only be determined by large, randomized, long-term clinical trials conducted in the current HAART era. Historically, the only randomized, placebo-controlled trials of antiretrovirals in primary HIV-1 infection were conducted before the advent of potent combination antiretroviral therapy and utilized zidovudine monotherapy in the treatment arm, which is suboptimal by current standards.[212,213] Although these trials showed that subjects in the treated arm had significant delay in development of minor opportunistic infections and less CD4+ T cell loss compared with untreated controls, these results cannot be interpreted as a true long-term benefit. In the mid-to-late 1990s, the discovery of the latent reservoir of resting CD4+ T cells with integrated HIV-1 proviral DNA[81,214] and the understanding that HAART can reduce the size of this latent reservoir[215,216] and preserve HIV-1-specific immune responses,[9,11,136,137] supported the case for early institution of therapy during primary HIV infection. Several nonrandomized studies of potent antiretroviral combination regimens used during primary HIV-1 infection have demonstrated effective suppression of viremia and improvement in immunological parameters.[9,137,217–220] One of the earliest studies conducted among individuals who started a potent PI-containing regimen within 90 days of onset of symptoms of acute HIV infection showed profound suppression of viral replication and preservation of HIV-specific CD4+ and cytotoxic T-lymphocyte responses attributable to early initiation of therapy.[9] Another study which followed a cohort of patients with primary HIV infection over 78 weeks, compared the course of those who elected immediate combination antiretroviral therapy to those who elected to delay therapy to over 26 weeks after diagnosis, and found that the immediate treatment group was associated with a decreased frequency of minor opportunistic infections and reduced progression to AIDS.[221] However with the realization that HAART is unlikely to completely eradicate the latent reservoir of infected CD4+ T cells[82] or prevent ongoing viral replication,[83,222] and the recognition of HAART-associated long-term toxicities,[223–225] the pendulum has swung away from early therapy, and the optimal timing of treatment initiation during primary HIV infection is currently an area of active investigation. One such currently enrolling multicenter randomized controlled clinical trial is AIN503/A5217, sponsored by both the Acute Infection and Early Disease Research Program and the Adult AIDS Clinical Trials Group, which is exploring the effect of early institution of therapy versus delayed therapy in altering virological setpoint and immunological surrogate markers of HIV disease progression. We believe that every effort must be made to refer newly diagnosed subjects with primary HIV infection to these and other appropriate trials.

Current Concepts

Potential Benefits of Early Therapy During Acute/Primary HIV Infection

Limiting Establishment of Latent Reservoir

The use of potent, intensified combination antiretroviral therapy has been shown to decrease the size of the latently infected pool of resting CD4+ T cells.[216] Other studies have indicated that early treatment during acute HIV, although unlikely to prevent establishment of this reservoir,[82,226] can nevertheless result in a 1–2 log reduction in the frequency of these latently infected cells.[215,227] It is hypothesized that limiting the establishment of the latent reservoir in conjunction with intensified or novel treatment strategies may allow for subsequent immune control of HIV-1 infection; however, it is unclear whether a mere reduction in latent pool size alone without complete elimination of latent infection will translate to a tangible long-term clinical benefit.

Preservation of HIV-1-Specific Immune Responses

Numerous investigators have noted that initiation of HAART during acute HIV infection led to the development of strong HIV-1-specific CD4+ T cell proliferation in response to HIV antigens.[9,11,12,136,137,228] In a prospective study of early therapy followed by treatment interruption, it was shown that five of eight patients treated early during primary HIV infection were able to achieve durable control of HIV-1 RNA levels to below 500 copies/mL for a median of 6.5 months after treatment interruption.[12] Subsequent data from the study however, indicated that the immunologic control of viremia may be transient, as only three of 14 patients were able to maintain HIV-1 RNA levels of less than 5000 copies/mL at 2 years after treatment interruption.[140] It is interesting to note that HIV-specific CD4+ and CD8+ T-cell responses remained augmented even after therapy cessation in patients who were treated early, although the magnitude of these responses did not predict duration of viremia control and clinical significance of augmented immune responses is not well defined.

Control of Viral Replication and Lowering of Viral Setpoint

Previous studies indicated that very early changes in HIV-1 RNA levels (1–2 weeks after treatment initiation) correlated well with later virologic response.[229,230] A careful analysis of first-phase decay kinetics of plasma HIV-1 RNA levels among those with acute or chronic HIV infection following treatment initiation with various regimens, indicated that the relative efficacy as measured by plasma HIV-1 RNA level decreases from day 0 to day 7 was 25% greater among those acutely infected individuals using a potent four-drug HAART regimen, while decay kinetics among chronic HIV-infected individuals were similar regardless of type of regimen.[231]

A recent study reported that patients who began HAART within 6 months of onset of acute seroconversion symptoms were only half as likely to have isolated measurable episodes of viremia (known as viral "blips") when compared to patients who started HAART during chronic infection.[232] These viral blips may represent a lower level of ongoing viral replication or less frequent release of virus from latent reservoirs among early-treated patients, although they have not been shown to be associated with treatment failure or emergence of drug resistance.[233]

Early institution of therapy in acute HIV-1 infection can also lead to a less diverse virus population.[10,89,234] The presence of a more homogenous viral population during early infection is likely to contribute to a more rapid and sustained response to antiretroviral treatment with resulting control of viral replication.[217,219,220,235] Thus, both homogeneity of the viral population as well as preserved HIV-1-specific immune responses are thought to contribute to the lowered viral setpoint seen during therapy cessation among treated patients with acute and recent HIV-1 infection. A study in which 16 individuals with acute or recent HIV-1 infection were treated with HAART for a mean of 3.2 years attempted to explore the influence of early treatment initiation on virological setpoint.[236] Although viral rebound occurred in all individuals upon treatment cessation, this was followed by a spontaneous, transient and significant reduction in log plasma HIV-1 RNA level ranging from 0.3 to 3.1 log10 copies/mL, in nearly all subjects.[236] Four of the 16 individuals maintained viral loads of less than 5000 copies/mL. Overall, the distribution of steady-state viral loads after discontinuation of drug therapy was similar to that observed in an untreated cohort of newly infected subjects followed during the pre-HAART era,[87] raising the question as to whether the virologic set point is indeed altered by early intervention. In another study of 30 individuals with acute HIV-1 infection who received continuous treatment for 24 months, 14 individuals maintained off-treatment viral loads of less than 5000 copies/mL for a median of 14 months after one to three structured therapeutic interruptions.[237] Factors that predicted a decreased viral setpoint in these individuals were low HIV-1 proviral DNA load in peripheral blood mononuclear cells and the presence of an HIV-1-specific proliferative CD4+ T-cell response before treatment interruption.[237] In summary, it appears that transient control of viremia can occur among those individuals who are treated early in the course of HIV-1 infection, and it may be possible to augment this virological response using novel immunomodulating methods.

Disadvantages of Early Therapy during Acute/Primary HIV Infection

Antiretroviral drug toxicities must be considered and weighed against the benefits of early therapy. Recent studies have shown that the risk of myocardial infarction[223] and lipodystrophy[224,238] increases over time in patients on HAART. Analysis of almost 3000 patients on HAART enrolled in clinical trials at multiple sites between 1996 and 2001 revealed that HAART-associated morbidity remained high; severe or life-threatening adverse events (11.4 per 100 patient-years) exceeded the frequency of AIDS-related events (5.6 per 100 patient-years).[225] However it must be noted that newer antiretroviral drugs such as atazanavir have been associated with lower cardiovascular, dyslipidemia-related[239] and insulin metabolism-related[240] risks. It is critical to consider the high costs involved in early initiation and maintenance on HAART as this is central to sustainability of long-term HIV infection control.[241] Early HAART initiation also commits patients to maintaining good adherence to prevent development of antiretroviral drug resistance which can severely limit future treatment options,[242,243] although comprehensive counseling and symptomatic management of adverse effects have been shown to improve adherence.

Acute HIV-1 Infection as a Window of Opportunity for Disease Modification

Despite known risk factors of antiretroviral therapy, it may be reasonable to start therapy in motivated individuals as soon as a diagnosis of HIV infection is made. The pathophysiology of acute HIV-1 infection and the impact of early combination antiretroviral therapy suggest that treatment during this period may present a unique opportunity to alter the disease course. Three immune-based interventions that have been used within the context of early therapy initiation are discussed below.

First, therapeutic immunization strategies to boost existing as well as induce *de novo* HIV-1-specific T-cell responses are currently being explored. The importance of treatment during primary infection was established in a rhesus macaque model using SIV in a study that explored the use of therapeutic immunization as an adjunct to augment immune response and sustain viral suppression following withdrawal of treatment.[138] HIV-1-specific cellular immunity appears to be generated by therapeutic vaccination among those individuals who received early treatment during acute HIV infection; however this has not translated into better virological control.[236,244,245]

A second therapeutic approach taking advantage of the early sustained viral suppression in persons with acute infection on antiretroviral therapy is the use of passively transferred human neutralizing antibodies to suppress viral rebound in these persons following cessation of antiretroviral therapy. Early antiretroviral therapy initiation among subjects with acute HIV-1 infection appeared to play a significant role in bringing about greater success in viral rebound suppression compared to a control group with untreated acute HIV-1 infection.[246,247]

Third, the specific pathophysiology of acute HIV infection resulting in extensive immune activation presents a unique opportunity for the use of immune-modulating agents during the early stage of HIV infection. Activated CD4+ T cells support massive HIV-1 replication and production with resulting rapid elimination of HIV-specific CD4+ and CD8+ T cells. Cyclosporin A (CsA) is an immune-modulating agent that selectively suppresses T cell activation by inhibiting IL-2-dependent T cell proliferation and differentiation.[248] The use of CsA in conjunction with HAART during the acute infection stage, with subsequent continuation of HAART alone in a non-randomized study showed promising results with higher percentage and absolute counts of CD4+ T cells as well as higher proportion of HIV-specific IFN-gamma-secreting CD4+ T cells seen in the CsA group.[249] A multicenter, randomized trial sponsored by AIEDRP/ACTG is currently in progress. Other immune suppressors being investigated as adjuvants to antiretroviral drugs are mycophenolate[250] and hydroxurea.[251]

Treatment Regimen

In the absence of clear evidence of long-term clinical benefit of early therapy initiation, current guidelines from the US Department of Health and Human Services (DHHS) and the International AIDS Society-USA Panel do not strongly recommend that potent antiretroviral therapy be initiated during primary infection, but state that early therapy may be considered.[252,253] Table 33-2 summarizes preferred and alternative regimens used in antiretroviral-naive HIV-1- infected persons. Triple drug regimens include efavirenz or lopinavir/ritonavir along with a backbone of lamivudine or emtricitabine with either abacavir or tenofovir. Although some four-drug regimens may achieve optimal viral suppression more rapidly than do three-drug regimens,[231] the overall superiority of a four-drug approach remains unclear and the associated increase in toxicity is an important consideration.[254]

Knowledge of viral susceptibility to currently available antiretroviral drugs is crucial for selection of an appropriate treatment regimen. Current guidelines recommend obtaining a baseline genotypic or phenotypic resistance profile of the virus in the case of acute HIV-1 infection.[252,253] The prevalence of transmitted antiretroviral drug resistance among newly diagnosed antiretroviral drug-naive individuals has ranged from 8.3% to 24.1%, with the highest rates reported among certain high-risk groups such as men who have sex with men.[255–261] Longitudinal studies of individuals with acute or primary HIV infection indicate current (2000–04) transmitted nucleos(t)ide reverse transcriptase inhibitor (NRTI) resistance rate of 12–20%, and protease inhibitor (PI) resistance rate of over 6%. A steep increase over time in transmitted non-nucleoside reverse transcriptase inhibitor (NNRTI) resistance is seen, with current estimates reported as 8–17%.[256–259,261] The relatively high prevalence of transmitted drug resistance among high-risk groups warrants judicious selection of the initial antiretroviral regimen for acute HIV infection. An important consideration when treating acute infection is whether treatment should be instituted only after the availability of viral drug susceptibility results. An acceptable approach for persons diagnosed with acute HIV-1 would be to start empiric treatment with a boosted PI-based regimen (since the antiretroviral drug resistance rate is lowest among PIs) or with an NNRTI continuing regimen and subsequent appropriate changes as necessary following availability of genotypic results.[259]

The initial regimen should provide optimal antiviral potency, which currently is regarded as reduction in plasma HIV-1 RNA levels to less than 50 copies/mL.[252,253] Although viral evolution and genotypic changes in the virus can still occur in HIV-1 reservoirs at this level of suppression, changes typically occur within genes encoding the HIV-1 envelope, rather than the reverse transcriptase and protease genes, thus preserving susceptibility to the major classes of antiretroviral agents.[82,262–264] The treatment regimen should also be sufficiently simple in order to facilitate adherence and minimize toxicity. In choosing an appropriate drug regimen, particular attention must be paid during the initial patient evaluation to the recognition of conditions that may interact with the management of HIV, particularly with respect to potential interactions of other drugs with antiretroviral agents and cardiovascular risks that may be increased by some antiretroviral drugs. Apart from

Table 33-2 Antiretroviral regimens recommended for treatment of HIV-1 infection in antiretroviral naive patients

Preferred Regimen	Alternative Regimen
NNRTI-based regimen • Efavirenz + (zidovudine or tenofovir) + (lamivudine or emtricitabine) (except during first trimester of pregnancy or in women with high pregnancy potential)	• Efavirenz + (didanosine or abacavir or stavudine) + (lamivudine or emtricitabine) (except during pregnancy, particularly the first trimester, or in women with high pregnancy potential) • Nevirapine-based regimens may be used as an alternative in adult females with CD4+ T cell counts <250 cells/mm^3 and adult males with CD4+ T cell counts <400 cells/mm^3
PI-based regimen • Lopinavir/ritonavir + zidovudine + (lamivudine or emtricitabine)	• Atazanavir, fosamprenavir, ritonavir-boosted fosamprenavir, ritonavir-boosted indinavir, nelfinavir, or ritonavir-boosted saquinavir– all used in combination with (zidovudine or stavudine or tenofovir or abacavir or didanosine) + (lamivudine or emtricitabine) • Lopinavir/ritonavir + (abacavir or stavudine or tenofovir or didanosine) + (lamivudine or emtricitabine)
Triple-NRTI-based regimen • abacavir + zidovudine + lamivudine – (only when a preferred or an alternative NNRTI- or a PI-based regimen cannot or should not be used)	

pharmacological therapy of acute HIV infection, initial emphasis should also be placed on counseling the patient with regard to the disease process, limiting the risk of secondary transmission and ensuring proper support for the patient. Following institution of therapy, close support of the patient is necessary, in order to help ensure maximum drug adherence, manage mild drug-related adverse events, monitor for toxic and life-threatening drug effects, as well as monitor for virologic and immunologic responses.

CONCLUSIONS

Identifying individuals during acute HIV-1 provides a unique opportunity to further study the pathogenesis and natural history of this disease. It allows infected individuals to enroll early into medical care programs for risk reduction counseling and access to the potential benefits of early antiretroviral treatment. Examination of individuals during acute HIV-1 infection is likely to provide novel insights into HIV-1 pathogenesis, paving the way for new approaches for effective treatment and prevention.

However, the potential clinical benefit of early initiation of antiretroviral therapy in terms of delay in death and disease progression compared to the added risk of long-term metabolic effects and emergence of drug resistance must be examined in large clinical trials.

REFERENCES

1. UNAIDS. AIDS Epidemic Update, Dec 2005.
2. Prevention CfDCa. HIV/AIDS Surveillance Report, 2004.
3. Karon JM, Fleming PL, Steketee RW, De Cock KM. HIV in the United States at the turn of the century: an epidemic in transition. Am J Public Health 91:1060–8, 2001.
4. Jacquez JA, Koopman JS, Simon CP, Longini IM Jr. Role of the primary infection in epidemics of HIV infection in gay cohorts. J Acquir Immune Defic Syndr 7:1169–84, 1994.
5. Leynaert B, Downs AM, de Vincenzi I. Heterosexual transmission of human immunodeficiency virus: variability of infectivity throughout the course of infection. European Study Group on Heterosexual Transmission of HIV. Am J Epidemiol 148:88–96, 1998.
6. Peterman TA, Stoneburner RL, Allen JR, et al. Risk of human immunodeficiency virus transmission from heterosexual adults with transfusion-associated infections. JAMA 259:55–8, 1988.
7. Pilcher CD, Tien HC, Eron JJ Jr, et al. Brief but efficient: acute HIV infection and the sexual transmission of HIV. J Infect Dis 189:1785–92, 2004.
8. Wawer MJ, Gray RH, Sewankambo NK, et al. Rates of HIV-1 transmission per coital act, by stage of HIV-1 infection, in Rakai, Uganda. J Infect Dis 191:1403–9, 2005.
9. Markowitz M, Vesanen M, Tenner-Racz K, et al. The effect of commencing combination antiretroviral therapy soon after human immunodeficiency virus type 1 infection on viral replication and antiviral immune responses. J Infect Dis 179:527–7, 1999.
10. Zhang LQ, MacKenzie P, Cleland A, et al. Selection for specific sequences in the external envelope protein of human immunodeficiency virus type 1 upon primary infection. J Virol 67:3345–3356, 1993.
11. Rosenberg ES, Billingsley JM, Caliendo AM, et al. Vigorous HIV-1-specific CD4+ T cell responses associated with control of viremia. Science 278:1447–50, 1997.
12. Rosenberg ES, Altfeld M, Poon SH, et al. Immune control of HIV-1 after early treatment of acute infection. Nature 407:523–6, 2000.
13. Royce RA, Sena A, Cates W Jr, Cohen MS. Sexual transmission of HIV. N Engl J Med 336:1072–8, 1997.
14. Schacker T, Collier AC, Hughes J, et al. Clinical and epidemiologic features of primary HIV infection. Ann Intern Med 125:257–64, 1996.
15. Hussain LA, Lehner T. Comparative investigation of Langerhans' cells and potential receptors for HIV in oral, genitourinary and rectal epithelia. Immunology 85:475–84, 1995.
16. Ho DD, Schooley RT, Rota TR, et al. HTLV-III in the semen and blood of a healthy homosexual man. Science 226:451–3, 1984.
17. Pomerantz RJ, de la Monte SM, Donegan SP, et al. Human immunodeficiency virus (HIV) infection of the uterine cervix. Ann Intern Med 108:321–7, 1988.
18. Vogt MW, Witt DJ, Craven DE, et al. Isolation of HTLV-III/LAV from cervical secretions of women at risk for AIDS. Lancet 1:525–7, 1986.
19. Dornadula G, Zhang H, VanUitert B, et al. Residual HIV-1 RNA in blood plasma of patients taking suppressive highly active antiretroviral therapy. JAMA 282:1627–32, 1999.
20. Zhang H, Dornadula G, Beumont M, et al. Human immunodeficiency virus type 1 in the semen of men receiving highly active antiretroviral therapy. N Engl J Med 339:1803–1809, 1998.
21. Gray RH, Wawer MJ, Brookmeyer R, et al. Probability of HIV-1 transmission per coital act in monogamous, heterosexual, HIV-1-discordant couples in Rakai, Uganda. Lancet 357:1149–53, 2001.
22. Pilcher CD, Eron JJ Jr, Vemazza PL, et al. Sexual transmission during the incubation period of primary HIV infection. JAMA 286:1713–14, 2001.
23. Pilcher CD, Shugars DC, Fiscus SA, et al. HIV in body fluids during primary HIV infection: implications for pathogenesis, treatment and public health. AIDS 15:837–45, 2001.
24. Lee TH, Sakahara N, Fiebig E, et al. Correlation of HIV-1 RNA levels in plasma and heterosexual transmission of HIV-1 from infected transfusion recipients. J Acquir Immune Defic Syndr Hum Retrovirol 12:427–8, 1996.
25. Keerasuntonpong A, Pitt J, Gaut PL, Daar ES. Primary human immunodeficiency virus type 1 infection in pregnancy. Obstet Gynecol 94:844, 1999.
26. Quinn TC, Wawer MJ, Sewankambo N, et al. Viral load and heterosexual transmission of human immunodeficiency virus type 1. Rakai Project Study Group. N Engl J Med 342:921–9, 2000.
27. Musicco M, Lazzarin A, Nicolosi A, et al. Antiretroviral treatment of men infected with human immunodeficiency virus type 1 reduces the incidence of heterosexual transmission. Italian Study Group on HIV Heterosexual Transmission. Arch Intern Med 154:1971–6, 1994.
28. Blower SM, Gershengorn HB, Grant RM. A tale of two futures: HIV and antiretroviral therapy in San Francisco. Science 287:650–4, 2000.
29. Katz MH, Schwarcz SK, Kellogg TA, et al. Impact of highly active antiretroviral treatment on HIV seroincidence among men who have sex with men: San Francisco. Am J Public Health 92:388–94, 2002.
30. Wasserheit JN. Epidemiological synergy. Interrelationships between human immunodeficiency virus infection and other sexually transmitted diseases. Sex Transm Dis 19:61–77, 1992.
31. Mastro TD, Satten GA, Nopkesorn T, et al. Probability of female-to-male transmission of HIV-1 in Thailand. Lancet 343:204–7, 1994.

32. Lazzarin A, Saracco A, Musicco M, Nicolosi A. Man-to-woman sexual transmission of the human immunodeficiency virus. Risk factors related to sexual behavior, man's infectiousness, and woman's susceptibility. Italian Study Group on HIV Heterosexual Transmission. Arch Intern Med 151:2411–16, 1991.
33. Kapiga SH, Shao JF, Lwihula GK, Hunter DJ. Risk factors for HIV infection among women in Dar-es-Salaam, Tanzania. J Acquir Immune Defic Syndr 7:301–9, 1994.
34. Cohen CR, Duerr A, Pruithithada N, et al. Bacterial vaginosis and HIV seroprevalence among female commercial sex workers in Chiang Mai, Thailand. AIDS 9:1093–7, 1995.
35. Moss GB, Overbaugh J, Welch M, et al. Human immunodeficiency virus DNA in urethral secretions in men: association with gonococcal urethritis and CD4 cell depletion. J Infect Dis 172:1469–74, 1995.
36. Dyer JR, Kazembe P, Vernazza PL, et al. High levels of human immunodeficiency virus type 1 in blood and semen of seropositive men in sub-Saharan Africa. J Infect Dis 177:1742–6, 1998.
37. Krieger JN, Coombs RW, Collier AC, et al. Seminal shedding of human immunodeficiency virus type 1 and human cytomegalovirus: evidence for different immunologic controls. J Infect Dis 171:1018–22, 1995.
38. Grosskurth H, Mosha F, Todd J, et al. Impact of improved treatment of sexually transmitted diseases on HIV infection in rural Tanzania: randomised controlled trial. Lancet 346:530–6, 1995.
39. Nicolosi A, Correa Leite ML, Musicco M, et al. The efficiency of male-to-female and female-to-male sexual transmission of the human immunodeficiency virus: a study of 730 stable couples. Italian Study Group on HIV Heterosexual Transmission. Epidemiology 5:570–5, 1994.
40. de Vincenzi I. A longitudinal study of human immunodeficiency virus transmission by heterosexual partners. European Study Group on Heterosexual Transmission of HIV. N Engl J Med 331:341–6, 1994.
41. Fischl MA, Dickinson GM, Scott GB, et al. Evaluation of heterosexual partners, children, and household contacts of adults with AIDS. JAMA 257:640–4, 1987.
42. Saracco A, Musicco M, Nicolosi A, et al. Man-to-woman sexual transmission of HIV: longitudinal study of 343 steady partners of infected men. J Acquir Immune Defic Syndr 6:497–502, 1993.
43. Marx PA, Spira AI, Gettie A, et al. Progesterone implants enhance SIV vaginal transmission and early virus load. Nat Med 2:1084–9, 1996.
44. Dragic T, Litwin V, Allaway GP, et al. HIV-1 entry into CD4+ cells is mediated by the chemokine receptor CC-CKR-5. Nature 381:667–73, 1996.
45. Gonzalez E, Kulkarni H, Bolivar H, et al. The influence of CCL3L1 gene-containing segmental duplications on HIV-1/AIDS susceptibility. Science 307:1434–40, 2005.
46. O'Brien SJ, Nelson GW. Human genes that limit AIDS. Nat Genet 36:565–74, 2004.
47. O'Brien TR, Winkler C, Dean M, et al. HIV-1 infection in a man homozygous for CCR5 delta 32. Lancet 349:1219, 1997.
48. Dean M, Carrington M, Winkler C, et al. Genetic restriction of HIV-1 infection and progression to AIDS by a deletion allele of the CKR5 structural gene. Hemophilia Growth and Development Study, Multicenter AIDS Cohort Study, Multicenter Hemophilia Cohort Study, San Francisco City Cohort, ALIVE Study. Science 273:1856–62, 1996.
49. Menten P, Wuyts A, Van Damme J. Macrophage inflammatory protein-1. Cytokine Growth Factor Rev 13:455–81, 2002.
50. Clavel F, Guetard D, Brun-Vezinet F, et al. Isolation of a new human retrovirus from West African patients with AIDS. Science 233:343–6, 1986.
51. Hu DJ, Dondero TJ, Rayfield MA, et al. The emerging genetic diversity of HIV. The importance of global surveillance for diagnostics, research, and prevention. JAMA 275:210–16, 1996.
52. De Cock KM, Adjorlolo G, Ekpini E, et al. Epidemiology and transmission of HIV-2. Why there is no HIV-2 pandemic. JAMA 270:2083–6, 1993.
53. Kanki PJ, Travers KU, S MB, et al. Slower heterosexual spread of HIV-2 than HIV-1. Lancet 343:943–6, 1994.
54. Hu DJ, Buve A, Baggs J, et al. What role does HIV-1 subtype play in transmission and pathogenesis? An epidemiological perspective. AIDS 13:873–81, 1999.
55. Tatt ID, Barlow KL, Nicoll A, Clewley JP. The public health significance of HIV-1 subtypes. AIDS 15(Suppl 5):S59–71, 2001.
56. Hudgens MG, Longini IM Jr, Vanichseni S, et al. Subtype-specific transmission probabilities for human immunodeficiency virus type 1 among injecting drug users in Bangkok, Thailand. Am J Epidemiol 155:159–68, 2002.
57. Aral SO, Holmes KK, Padian NS, Cates W Jr. Overview: individual and population approaches to the epidemiology and prevention of sexually transmitted diseases and human immunodeficiency virus infection. J Infect Dis 174(Suppl 2):S127–33, 1996.
58. Urbina A, Jones K. Crystal methamphetamine, its analogues, and HIV infection: medical and psychiatric aspects of a new epidemic. Clin Infect Dis 38:890–4, 2004.
59. Elford J. Changing patterns of sexual behaviour in the era of highly active antiretroviral therapy. Curr Opin Infect Dis 19:26–32, 2006.
60. Spira AI, Marx PA, Patterson BL, et al. Cellular targets of infection and route of viral dissemination after an intravaginal inoculation of simian immunodeficiency virus into rhesus macaques. J Exp Med 183:215–25, 1996.
61. Bomsel M. Transcytosis of infectious human immunodeficiency virus across a tight human epithelial cell line barrier. Nat Med 3:42–7, 1997.
62. Meng G, Wei X, Wu X, et al. Primary intestinal epithelial cells selectively transfer R5 HIV-1 to CCR5+ cells. Nat Med 8:150–6, 2002.
63. Niess JH, Brand S, Gu X, et al. CX3CR1-mediated dendritic cell access to the intestinal lumen and bacterial clearance. Science 307:254–8, 2005.
64. Geijtenbeek TB, Kwon DS, Torensma R, et al. DC-SIGN, a dendritic cell-specific HIV-1-binding protein that enhances trans-infection of T-cells. Cell 100:587–97, 2000.
65. Geijtenbeek TB, Torensma R, van Vliet SJ, et al. Identification of DC-SIGN, a novel dendritic cell-specific ICAM-3 receptor that supports primary immune responses. Cell 100:575–85, 2000.
66. Lee B, Leslie G, Soilleux E, et al. cis Expression of DC-SIGN allows for more efficient entry of human and simian immunodeficiency viruses via CD4 and a coreceptor. J Virol 75:12028–38, 2001.
67. Arrighi JF, Pion M, Garcia E, et al. DC-SIGN-mediated infectious synapse formation enhances X4 HIV-1 transmission from dendritic cells to T-cells. J Exp Med 200:1279–88, 2004.
68. Li Q, Duan L, Estes JD, et al. Peak SIV replication in resting memory CD4+ T-cells depletes gut lamina propria CD4+ T-cells. Nature 434:1148–52, 2005.
69. Mattapallil JJ, Douek DC, Hill B, et al. Massive infection and loss of memory CD4+ T-cells in multiple tissues during acute SIV infection. Nature 434:1093–7, 2005.
70. Collins KB, Patterson BK, Naus GJ, et al. Development of an in vitro organ culture model to study transmission of HIV-1 in the female genital tract. Nat Med 6:475–9, 2000.
71. Mowat AM, Viney JL. The anatomical basis of intestinal immunity. Immunol Rev 156:145–66, 1997.

72. Veazey RS, DeMaria M, Chalifoux LV, et al. Gastrointestinal tract as a major site of CD4+ T cell depletion and viral replication in SIV infection. Science 280:427–31, 1998.
73. Guadalupe M, Reay E, Sankaran S, et al. Severe CD4+ T-cell depletion in gut lymphoid tissue during primary human immunodeficiency virus type 1 infection and substantial delay in restoration following highly active antiretroviral therapy. J Virol 77:11708–17, 2003.
74. Mehandru S, Poles MA, Tenner-Racz K, et al. Primary HIV-1 infection is associated with preferential depletion of CD4+ T lymphocytes from effector sites in the gastrointestinal tract. J Exp Med 200:761–70, 2004.
75. Brenchley JM, Schacker TW, Ruff LE, et al. CD4+ T cell depletion during all stages of HIV disease occurs predominantly in the gastrointestinal tract. J Exp Med 200:749–59, 2004.
76. Mehandru S, Poles M, Horowitz A, et al. Gastrointestinal CD4+ T-cells harbor a higher viral burden than peripheral blood CD4+ T-cells in primary HIV-1 infection. Paper presented at 12th Conference on Retroviruses and Opportunistic Infections, 2005; Boston, MA, 2005.
77. Mehandru S, Tenner-Racz K, Racz P, Markowitz M. The gastrointestinal tract is critical to the pathogenesis of acute HIV-1 infection. J Allergy Clin Immunol 116:419–22, 2005.
78. Picker LJ, Hagen SI, Lum R, et al. Insufficient production and tissue delivery of CD4+ memory T-cells in rapidly progressive simian immunodeficiency virus infection. J Exp Med 200:1299–314, 2004.
79. Daar ES, Moudgil T, Meyer RD, Ho DD. Transient high levels of viremia in patients with primary human immunodeficiency virus type 1 infection. N Engl J Med 324:961–4, 1991.
80. Little SJ, McLean AR, Spina CA, et al. Viral dynamics of acute HIV-1 infection. J Exp Med 190:841–50, 1999.
81. Finzi D, Hermankova M, Pierson T, et al. Identification of a reservoir for HIV-1 in patients on highly active antiretroviral therapy. Science 278:1295–300, 1997.
82. Finzi D, Blankson J, Siliciano JD, et al. Latent infection of CD4+ T-cells provides a mechanism for lifelong persistence of HIV-1, even in patients on effective combination therapy. Nat Med 5:512–17.
83. Zhang L, Ramratnam B, Tenner-Racz K, et al. Quantifying residual HIV-1 replication in patients receiving combination antiretroviral therapy. N Engl J Med 340:1605–13, 1999.
84. Perelson AS, Neumann AU, Markowitz M, et al. HIV-1 dynamics in vivo: virion clearance rate, infected cell life-span, and viral generation time. Science 271:1582–6, 1996.
85. Koup RA, Safrit JT, Cao Y, et al. Temporal association of cellular immune responses with the initial control of viremia in primary human immunodeficiency virus type 1 syndrome. J Virol 68:4650–5, 1994.
86. Schacker TW, Hughes JP, Shea T, et al. Biological and virologic characteristics of primary HIV infection. Ann Intern Med 128:613–20, 1998.
87. Mellors JW, Munoz A, Giorgi JV, et al. Plasma viral load and CD4+ lymphocytes as prognostic markers of HIV-1 infection. Ann Intern Med 126:946–54, 1997.
88. Mellors JW, Rinaldo CR Jr, Gupta P, et al. Prognosis in HIV-1 infection predicted by the quantity of virus in plasma. Science 272:1167–70, 1996.
89. Zhu T, Mo H, Wang N, et al. Genotypic and phenotypic characterization of HIV-1 patients with primary infection. Science 261:1179–81, 1993.
90. Long EM, Rainwater SM, Lavreys L, et al. HIV type 1 variants transmitted to women in Kenya require the CCR5 coreceptor for entry, regardless of the genetic complexity of the infecting virus. AIDS Res Hum Retroviruses 18:567–76, 2002.
91. Sagar M, Lavreys L, Baeten JM, et al. Infection with multiple human immunodeficiency virus type 1 variants is associated with faster disease progression. J Virol 77:12921–6, 2003.
92. Zhang L, Rowe L, He T, et al. Compartmentalization of surface envelope glycoprotein of human immunodeficiency virus type 1 during acute and chronic infection. J Virol 76:9465–73, 2002.
93. Learn GH, Muthui D, Brodie SJ, et al. Virus population homogenization following acute human immunodeficiency virus type 1 infection. J Virol 76:11953–9, 2002.
94. Frost SD, Liu Y, Pond SL, et al. Characterization of human immunodeficiency virus type 1 (HIV-1) envelope variation and neutralizing antibody responses during transmission of HIV-1 subtype B. J Virol 79:6523–7, 2005.
95. Frost SD, Wrin T, Smith DM, et al. Neutralizing antibody responses drive the evolution of human immunodeficiency virus type 1 envelope during recent HIV infection. Proc Natl Acad Sci USA 102:18514–19, 2005.
96. Pilgrim AK, Pantaleo G, Cohen OJ, et al. Neutralizing antibody responses to human immunodeficiency virus type 1 in primary infection and long-term-nonprogressive infection. J Infect Dis 176:924–32, 1997.
97. Pellegrin I, Legrand E, Neau D, et al. Kinetics of appearance of neutralizing antibodies in 12 patients with primary or recent HIV-1 infection and relationship with plasma and cellular viral loads. J Acquir Immune Defic Syndr Hum Retrovirol 11:438–47, 1996.
98. Legrand E, Pellegrin I, Neau D, et al. Course of specific T lymphocyte cytotoxicity, plasma and cellular viral loads, and neutralizing antibody titers in 17 recently seroconverted HIV type 1-infected patients. AIDS Res Hum Retroviruses 13:1383–94, 1997.
99. Poignard P, Sabbe R, Picchio GR, et al. Neutralizing antibodies have limited effects on the control of established HIV-1 infection in vivo. Immunity 10:431–8, 1999.
100. Parren PW, Burton DR, Sattentau QJ. HIV-1 antibody – debris or virion? Nat Med 3:366–7, 1997.
101. Richman DD, Wrin T, Little SJ, Petropoulos CJ. Rapid evolution of the neutralizing antibody response to HIV type 1 infection. Proc Natl Acad Sci USA 100:4144–9, 2003.
102. Wei X, Decker JM, Wang S, et al. Antibody neutralization and escape by HIV-1. Nature 422:307–12, 2003.
103. Derdeyn CA, Decker JM, Bibollet-Ruche F, et al. Envelope-constrained neutralization-sensitive HIV-1 after heterosexual transmission. Science 303:2019–22, 2004.
104. Chohan B, Lang D, Sagar M, et al. Selection for human immunodeficiency virus type 1 envelope glycosylation variants with shorter V1-V2 loop sequences occurs during transmission of certain genetic subtypes and may impact viral RNA levels. J Virol 79:6528–531, 2005.
105. Conley AJ, Kessler JA II, Boots LJ, et al. The consequence of passive administration of an anti-human immunodeficiency virus type 1 neutralizing monoclonal antibody before challenge of chimpanzees with a primary virus isolate. J Virol 70:6751–8, 1996.
106. Ferrantelli F, Hofmann-Lehmann R, Rasmussen RA, et al. Post-exposure prophylaxis with human monoclonal antibodies prevented SHIV89.6P infection or disease in neonatal macaques. AIDS 17:301–9, 2003.
107. Hofmann-Lehmann R, Vlasak J, Rasmussen RA, et al. Postnatal passive immunization of neonatal macaques with a triple combination of human monoclonal antibodies against oral simian-human immunodeficiency virus challenge. J Virol 75:7470–80, 2001.
108. Mascola JR, Lewis MG, Stiegler G, et al. Protection of Macaques against pathogenic simian/human immunodeficiency virus 89.6PD by passive transfer of neutralizing antibodies. J Virol 73:4009–18, 1999.
109. Mascola JR, Stiegler G, VanCott TC, et al. Protection of macaques against vaginal transmission of a pathogenic HIV-1/SIV chimeric virus by passive infusion of neutralizing antibodies. Nat Med 6:207–10, 2000.

110. Borrow P, Lewicki H, Hahn BH, et al. Virus-specific CD8+ cytotoxic T-lymphocyte activity associated with control of viremia in primary human immunodeficiency virus type 1 infection. J Virol 68:6103–10, 1994.
111. Borrow P, Lewicki H, Wei X, et al. Antiviral pressure exerted by HIV-1-specific cytotoxic T lymphocytes (CTLs) during primary infection demonstrated by rapid selection of CTL escape virus. Nat Med 3:205–211, 1997.
112. Price DA, Goulder PJ, Klenerman P, et al. Positive selection of HIV-1 cytotoxic T lymphocyte escape variants during primary infection. Proc Natl Acad Sci USA 94:1890–5, 1997.
113. Pantaleo G, Demarest JF, Soudeyns H, et al. Major expansion of CD8+ T-cells with a predominant V beta usage during the primary immune response to HIV. Nature 370:463–7, 1994.
114. Yasutomi Y, Reimann KA, Lord CI, et al. Simian immunodeficiency virus-specific CD8+ lymphocyte response in acutely infected rhesus monkeys. J Virol 67:1707–11, 1993.
115. Chen ZW, Kou ZC, Lekutis C, et al. T cell receptor V beta repertoire in an acute infection of rhesus monkeys with simian immunodeficiency viruses and a chimeric simian-human immunodeficiency virus. J Exp Med 182:21–31, 1995.
116. Kuroda MJ, Schmitz JE, Charini WA, et al. Emergence of CTL coincides with clearance of virus during primary simian immunodeficiency virus infection in rhesus monkeys. J Immunol 162:5127–33, 1999.
117. Schmitz JE, Kuroda MJ, Santra S, et al. Control of viremia in simian immunodeficiency virus infection by CD8+ lymphocytes. Science 283:857–860, 1999.
118. Jin X, Bauer DE, Tuttleton SE, et al. Dramatic rise in plasma viremia after CD8(+) T cell depletion in simian immunodeficiency virus-infected macaques. J Exp Med 189:991–8, 1999.
119. Barouch DH, Santra S, Schmitz JE, et al. Control of viremia and prevention of clinical AIDS in rhesus monkeys by cytokine-augmented DNA vaccination. Science 290:486–92, 2000.
120. Amara RR, Villinger F, Altman JD, et al. Control of a mucosal challenge and prevention of AIDS by a multiprotein DNA/MVA vaccine. Science 292:69–74, 2001.
121. Shiver JW, Fu TM, Chen L, et al. Replication-incompetent adenoviral vaccine vector elicits effective anti-immunodeficiency-virus immunity. Nature 415:331–335, 2002.
122. Walker CM, Moody DJ, Stites DP, Levy JA. CD8+ lymphocytes can control HIV infection in vitro by suppressing virus replication. Science 234:1563–6, 1986.
123. Yang OO, Kalams SA, Trocha A, et al. Suppression of human immunodeficiency virus type 1 replication by CD8+ cells: evidence for HLA class I-restricted triggering of cytolytic and noncytolytic mechanisms. J Virol 71:3120–8, 1997.
124. Carrington M, Nelson GW, Martin MP, et al. HLA and HIV-1: heterozygote advantage and B*35-Cw*04 disadvantage. Science 283:1748–52, 1999.
125. Kaslow RA, Carrington M, Apple R, et al. Influence of combinations of human major histocompatibility complex genes on the course of HIV-1 infection. Nat Med 2:405–11, 1996.
126. Migueles SA, Sabbaghian MS, Shupert WL, et al. HLA B*5701 is highly associated with restriction of virus replication in a subgroup of HIV-infected long term nonprogressors. Proc Natl Acad Sci USA 97:2709–14, 2000.
127. Gao X, Nelson GW, Karacki P, et al. Effect of a single amino acid change in MHC class I molecules on the rate of progression to AIDS. N Engl J Med 344:1668–1675.
128. Kaslow RA, Rivers C, Tang J, et al. Polymorphisms in HLA class I genes associated with both favorable prognosis of human immunodeficiency virus (HIV) type 1 infection and positive cytotoxic T-lymphocyte responses to ALVAC-HIV recombinant canarypox vaccines. J Virol 75:8681–9, 2001.
129. Kalams SA, Walker BD. The critical need for CD4 help in maintaining effective cytotoxic T lymphocyte responses. J Exp Med 188:2199–204, 1998.
130. Schoenberger SP, Toes RE, van der Voort EI, et al. T-cell help for cytotoxic T lymphocytes is mediated by CD40–CD40L interactions. Nature 393:480–3, 1998.
131. Bennett SR, Carbone FR, Karamalis F, et al. Help for cytotoxic-T-cell responses is mediated by CD40 signalling. Nature 393:478–80, 1998.
132. Pitcher CJ, Quittner C, Peterson DM, et al. HIV-1-specific CD4+ T-cells are detectable in most individuals with active HIV-1 infection, but decline with prolonged viral suppression. Nat Med 5:518–25, 1999.
133. McNeil AC, Shupert WL, Iyasere CA, et al. High-level HIV-1 viremia suppresses viral antigen-specific CD4(+) T cell proliferation. Proc Natl Acad Sci USA 98:13878–83, 2001.
134. Miedema F, Meyaard L, Koot M, et al. Changing virus–host interactions in the course of HIV-1 infection. Immunol Rev 140:35–72, 1994.
135. Douek DC, Brenchley JM, Betts MR, et al. HIV preferentially infects HIV-specific CD4+ T-cells. Nature 417:95–8, 2002.
136. Oxenius A, Price DA, Easterbrook PJ, et al. Early highly active antiretroviral therapy for acute HIV-1 infection preserves immune function of CD8+ and CD4+ T lymphocytes. Proc Natl Acad Sci USA 97:3382–7, 2000.
137. Malhotra U, Berrey MM, Huang Y, et al. Effect of combination antiretroviral therapy on T-cell immunity in acute human immunodeficiency virus type 1 infection. J Infect Dis 181:121–31, 2000.
138. Hel Z, Venzon D, Poudyal M, et al. Viremia control following antiretroviral treatment and therapeutic immunization during primary SIV251 infection of macaques. Nat Med 6:1140–6, 2000.
139. Barouch DH, Craiu A, Kuroda MJ, et al. Augmentation of immune responses to HIV-1 and simian immunodeficiency virus DNA vaccines by IL-2/Ig plasmid administration in rhesus monkeys. Proc Natl Acad Sci USA 97:4192–7, 2000.
140. Kaufmann DE, Lichterfeld M, Altfeld M, et al. Limited durability of viral control following treated acute HIV infection. PLOS Med 1:e36, 2004.
141. Allen TM, O'Connor DH, Jing P, et al. Tat-specific cytotoxic T lymphocytes select for SIV escape variants during resolution of primary viraemia. Nature 407:386–90, 2000.
142. Barouch DH, Kunstman J, Kuroda MJ, et al. Eventual AIDS vaccine failure in a rhesus monkey by viral escape from cytotoxic T lymphocytes. Nature 415:335–9, 2002.
143. Fehniger TA, Herbein G, Yu H, et al. Natural killer cells from HIV-1+ patients produce C-C chemokines and inhibit HIV-1 infection. J Immunol 161:6433–8, 1998.
144. Oliva A, Kinter AL, Vaccarezza M, et al. Natural killer cells from human immunodeficiency virus (HIV)-infected individuals are an important source of CC-chemokines and suppress HIV-1 entry and replication in vitro. J Clin Invest 102:223–31, 1998.
145. Ahmad A, Morisset R, Thomas R, Menezes J. Evidence for a defect of antibody-dependent cellular cytotoxic (ADCC) effector function and anti-HIV gp120/41-specific ADCC-mediating antibody titres in HIV-infected individuals. J Acquir Immune Defic Syndr7(5):428–37, 1994.
146. Alter G, Malenfant JM, Delabre RM, et al. Increased natural killer cell activity in viremic HIV-1 infection. J Immunol 173(8):5305–11, 2004.
147. De Maria A, Fogli M, Costa P, et al. The impaired NK cell cytolytic function in viremic HIV-1 infection is associated with a reduced surface expression of natural cytotoxicity receptors (NKp46, NKp30 and NKp44). Eur J Immunol 33:2410–18, 2003.
148. Alter G, Teigen N, Davis BT, et al. Sequential deregulation of NK cell subset distribution and function starting in acute HIV-1 infection. Blood 106:3366–9, 2005.
149. Haas W, Pereira P, Tonegawa S. Gamma/delta cells. Annu Rev Immunol 11:637–85, 1993.

150. Poles MA, Barsoum S, Yu W, et al. Human immunodeficiency virus type 1 induces persistent changes in mucosal and blood gammadelta T-cells despite suppressive therapy. J Virol 77:10456–67, 2003.
151. Vasan S, Siladji E, Hogan C, et al. NKT-cells are preserved in patients beginning HAART during acute infection. In: 11th Conference on Retroviruses and Opportunistic Infections, 8–11 Feb 2004, SanFransisco, 2004.
152. Vasan S, Poles M, Horowitz A, et al. Percentage and function of NKT-cells, potential anti-HIV effector cells, are preserved by beginning HAART during acute and early HIV-1 Infection. In: 13th Conference on Retroviruses and Opportunistic Infections, 5–8 Feb 2006, Denver, Colorado.
153. Daar ES, Little S, Pitt J, et al. Diagnosis of primary HIV-1 infection. Los Angeles County Primary HIV Infection Recruitment Network. Ann Intern Med 134:25–9, 2001.
154. Lavreys L, Baeten JM, Overbaugh J, et al. Virus load during primary Human Immunodeficiency Virus (HIV) type 1 infection is related to the severity of acute HIV illness in Kenyan women. Clin Infect Dis 35:77–81, 2002.
155. Routy JP, Vanhems P, Rouleau D, et al. Comparison of clinical features of acute HIV-1 infection in patients infected sexually or through injection drug use. The Investigators of the Quebec Primary HIV Infection Study. J Acquir Immune Defic Syndr 24:425–32, 2000.
156. Huang ST, Lee HC, Liu KH, et al. Acute human immunodeficiency virus infection. J Microbiol Immunol Infect 38:65–8, 2005.
157. Clark SJ, Saag MS, Decker WD, et al. High titers of cytopathic virus in plasma of patients with symptomatic primary HIV-1 infection. N Evngl J Med 324:954–60, 1991.
158. Cossarizza A, Ortolani C, Mussini C, et al. Massive activation of immune cells with an intact T cell repertoire in acute human immunodeficiency virus syndrome. J Infect Dis 172:105–12, 1995.
159. Cooper DA, Gold J, Maclean P, et al. Acute AIDS retrovirus infection. Definition of a clinical illness associated with seroconversion. Lancet 1:537–40, 1985.
160. Bollinger RC, Brookmeyer RS, Mehendale SM, et al. Risk factors and clinical presentation of acute primary HIV infection in India. JAMA 278:2085–9, 1997.
161. Lavreys L, Thompson ML, Martin HL Jr, et al. Primary human immunodeficiency virus type 1 infection: clinical manifestations among women in Mombasa, Kenya. Clin Infect Dis 30:486–90, 2000.
162. Kahn JO, Walker BD. Acute human immunodeficiency virus type 1 infection. N Engl J Med 339:33–9, 1998.
163. Niu MT, Stein DS, Schnittman SM. Primary human immunodeficiency virus type 1 infection: review of pathogenesis and early treatment intervention in humans and animal retrovirus infections. J Infect Dis 168:1490–501, 1993.
164. Brook MG, Barnes A, Cook GC, Mabey DC. A typhus-like illness caused by acute HIV seroconversion. Postgrad Med J 67:92–3, 1991.
165. Calabrese LH, Proffitt MR, Levin KH, et al. Acute infection with the human immunodeficiency virus (HIV) associated with acute brachial neuritis and exanthematous rash. Ann Intern Med 107:849–51, 1987.
166. Kobayashi S, Segawa S, Kawashima M, et al. A case of symptomatic primary HIV infection. J Dermatol 32:137–42, 205.
167. Balslev E, Thomsen HK, Weismann K. Histopathology of acute human immunodeficiency virus exanthema. J Clin Pathol 43:201–2, 1990.
168. McMillan A, Bishop PE, Aw D, Peutherer JF. Immunohistology of the skin rash associated with acute HIV infection. AIDS 3:309–12, 1989.
169. Aggarwal M, Rein J. Acute human immunodeficiency virus syndrome in an adolescent. Pediatrics 112:e323, 2003.
170. Hecht FM, Busch MP, Rawal B, et al. Use of laboratory tests and clinical symptoms for identification of primary HIV infection. Aids 16:1119–29, 2002.
171. Vanhems P, Routy JP, Hirschel B, et al. Clinical features of acute retroviral syndrome differ by route of infection but not by gender and age. J Acquir Immune Defic Syndr 31:318–21, 2002.
172. Denning DW, Amos A, Wall RA. Oral and cutaneous features of acute human immunodeficiency virus infection. Cutis 40:171–5, 1987.
173. Ho DD, Rota TR, Schooley RT, et al. Isolation of HTLV-III from cerebrospinal fluid and neural tissues of patients with neurologic syndromes related to the acquired immunodeficiency syndrome. N Engl J Med 313:1493–7, 1985.
174. Tambussi G, Gori A, Capiluppi B, et al. Neurological symptoms during primary human immunodeficiency virus (HIV) infection correlate with high levels of HIV RNA in cerebrospinal fluid. Clin Infect Dis 30:962–5, 2000.
175. Amayo EO, Kwasa TO. HIV and acute peripheral facial nerve palsy. East Afr Med J 68:948–51, 1991.
176. Krasner CG, Cohen SH. Bilateral Bell's palsy and aseptic meningitis in a patient with acute human immunodeficiency virus seroconversion. West J Med 159:604–5, 1993.
177. Vendrell J, Heredia C, Pujol M, et al. Guillain–Barré syndrome associated with seroconversion for anti-HTLV-III. Neurology 37:544, 1987.
178. Parry GJ. Peripheral neuropathies associated with human immunodeficiency virus infection. Ann Neurol 23(Suppl): S49–53, 1988.
179. Wulff EA, Wang AK, Simpson DM. HIV-associated peripheral neuropathy: epidemiology, pathophysiology and treatment. Drugs 59:1251–60, 2000.
180. Ben-Galim P, Shaked Y, Vonsover A, Garty M. Immediate immunosuppression caused by acute HIV-1 infection: a fulminant multisystemic disease 2 days post infection. Infection 24:332–5, 1996.
181. Martel JW. Encephalitis in connection with primary HIV infection as a differential diagnosis in acute psychosis. Lakartidningen 86:1701, 1989.
182. Yasuoka C, Kikuchi Y, Yasuoka A, et al. Successful treatment of acute myeloradiculoneuritis with high-dose corticosteroids in a patient with primary HIV-1 infection. Jpn J Infect Dis 53:171–2, 2000.
183. Bramkamp GR, Holt RI, Bending JJ, et al. Hepatitis as the presenting feature of an HIV seroconversion illness. Int J STD AIDS 10:687–8, 1999.
184. Casseb JS, Caterino-de-Araujo A. Difficulties in diagnosing atypical primary HIV-1 infection: report of a case. Rev Inst Med Trop Sao Paulo 36:287–92, 1994.
185. Navai N, Yap RL, Gupta R, et al. Inflammatory pseudotumor of the testis: a novel presentation of acute retroviral syndrome. Int J Urol 12:424–6, 2005.
186. Sinicco A, Sciandra M, Di Garbo A, et al. Primary HIV infection presenting with acute pancreatitis. Scand J Infect Dis 31:423–4, 1999.
187. Fusade T, Liony C, Joly P, et al. Ulcerative esophagitis during primary HIV infection. Am J Gastroenterol 87:1523–4, 1992.
188. Rouet F, Elenga N, Msellati P, et al. Primary HIV-1 infection in African children infected through breastfeeding. AIDS 16:2303–9, 2002.
189. Gaines H, Albert J, von Sydow M, et al. HIV antigenaemia and virus isolation from plasma during primary HIV infection. Lancet 1:1317–18, 1987.
190. Dull JS, Sen P, Raffanti S, Middleton JR. Oral candidiasis as a marker of acute retroviral illness. South Med J 84:733–5, 739, 1991.
191. Kopko P, Calhoun L, Petz L. Distinguishing immunosilent AIDS from the acute retroviral syndrome in a frequent blood donor. Transfusion 39:383–6, 1999.

192. Martinez P, Munoz J, Santamaria JM, et al. Acute symptomatic HIV infection. Report of 10 cases. Enferm Infecc Microbiol Clin 10:205–10, 1992.
193. Deeks SG, Kitchen CM, Liu L, et al. Immune activation set point during early HIV infection predicts subsequent CD4+ T-cell changes independent of viral load. Blood 104:942–7, 2004.
194. Kaufmann GR, Cunningham P, Zaunders J, et al. Impact of early HIV-1 RNA and T-lymphocyte dynamics during primary HIV-1 infection on the subsequent course of HIV-1 RNA levels and CD4+ T-lymphocyte counts in the first year of HIV-1 infection. Sydney Primary HIV Infection Study Group. J Acquir Immune Defic Syndr 22:437–44, 1999.
195. Pedersen C, Lindhardt BO, Jensen BL, et al. Clinical course of primary HIV infection: consequences for subsequent course of infection. BMJ 299:154–7, 1989.
196. Vanhems P, Lambert J, Cooper DA, et al. Severity and prognosis of acute human immunodeficiency virus type 1 illness: a dose-response relationship. Clin Infect Dis 26: 323–9, 1998.
197. Vanhems P, Voirin N, Hirschel B, et al. Brief report: incubation and duration of specific symptoms at acute retroviral syndrome as independent predictors of progression to AIDS. J Acquir Immune Defic Syndr 32:542–4, 2003.
198. Pincus JM, Crosby SS, Losina E, et al. Acute human immunodeficiency virus infection in patients presenting to an urban urgent care center. Clin Infect Dis 37:1699–704, 2003.
199. Coco A, Kleinhans E. Prevalence of primary HIV infection in symptomatic ambulatory patients. Ann Fam Med 3:400–4, 2005.
200. Cates W Jr, Chesney MA, Cohen MS. Primary HIV infection – a public health opportunity. Am J Public Health 87:1928–30, 1997.
201. Ho DD, Moudgil T, Alam M. Quantitation of human immunodeficiency virus type 1 in the blood of infected persons. N Engl J Med 321:1621–5, 1989.
202. Coombs RW, Collier AC, Allain JP, et al. Plasma viremia in human immunodeficiency virus infection. N Engl J Med 321:1626–31.
203. Alter HJ, Epstein JS, Swenson SG, et al. Prevalence of human immunodeficiency virus type 1 p24 antigen in U.S. blood donors – an assessment of the efficacy of testing in donor screening. The HIV-Antigen Study Group. N Engl J Med 323:1312–17, 1990.
204. Sutthent R, Gaudart N, Chokpaibulkit K, et al. p24 Antigen detection assay modified with a booster step for diagnosis and monitoring of human immunodeficiency virus type 1 infection. J Clin Microbiol 41:1016–22, 2003.
205. Bremer JW, Lew JF, Cooper E, et al. Diagnosis of infection with human immunodeficiency virus type 1 by a DNA polymerase chain reaction assay among infants enrolled in the Women and Infants' Transmission Study. J Pediatr 129:198–207, 1996.
206. Janssen RS, Satten GA, Stramer SL, et al. New testing strategy to detect early HIV-1 infection for use in incidence estimates and for clinical and prevention purposes. JAMA 280:42–8.
207. Weber B, Fall EH, Berger A, Doerr HW. Reduction of diagnostic window by new fourth-generation human immunodeficiency virus screening assays. J Clin Microbiol 36:2235–9, 1998.
208. Ly TD, Laperche S, Courouce AM. Early detection of human immunodeficiency virus infection using third- and fourth-generation screening assays. Eur J Clin Microbiol Infect Dis 20:104–10, 2001.
209. Busch MP, Satten GA. Time course of viremia and antibody seroconversion following human immunodeficiency virus exposure. Am J Med 102:117–24, discussion 125–16, 1997.
210. McFarland W, Busch MP, Kellogg TA, et al. Detection of early HIV infection and estimation of incidence using a sensitive/less-sensitive enzyme immunoassay testing strategy at anonymous counseling and testing sites in San Francisco. J Acquir Immune Defic Syndr 22:484–9, 1999.
211. Fiebig EW, Wright DJ, Rawal BD, et al. Dynamics of HIV viremia and antibody seroconversion in plasma donors: implications for diagnosis and staging of primary HIV infection. AIDS 17:1871–9, 2003.
212. Kinloch-De Loes S, Hirschel BJ, Hoen B, et al. A controlled trial of zidovudine in primary human immunodeficiency virus infection. N Engl J Med 333:408–413, 1995.
213. Niu MT, Bethel J, Holodniy M, et al. Zidovudine treatment in patients with primary (acute) human immunodeficiency virus type 1 infection: a randomized, double-blind, placebo-controlled trial. DATRI 002 Study Group. Division of AIDS Treatment Research Initiative. J Infect Dis 178:80–91, 1998.
214. Chun TW, Carruth L, Finzi D, et al. Quantification of latent tissue reservoirs and total body viral load in HIV-1 infection. Nature 387:183–8, 1997.
215. Lori F, Jessen H, Lieberman J, et al. Treatment of human immunodeficiency virus infection with hydroxyurea, didanosine, and a protease inhibitor before seroconversion is associated with normalized immune parameters and limited viral reservoir. J Infect Dis 180:1827–32, 1999.
216. Ramratnam B, Ribeiro R, He T, et al. Intensification of antiretroviral therapy accelerates the decay of the HIV-1 latent reservoir and decreases, but does not eliminate, ongoing virus replication. J Acquir Immune Defic Syndr 35:33–7, 2004.
217. Lafeuillade A, Poggi C, Tamalet C, et al. Effects of a combination of zidovudine, didanosine, and lamivudine on primary human immunodeficiency virus type 1 infection. J Infect Dis 175:1051–5, 1997.
218. Perrin L, Yerly S, Charvier A, et al. Zidovudine plus didanosine in primary HIV-1 infection. Antivir Ther 2:5–11, 1997.
219. Lillo FB, Ciuffreda D, Veglia F, et al. Viral load and burden modification following early antiretroviral therapy of primary HIV-1 infection. AIDS 13:791–6, 1999.
220. Hoen B, Dumon B, Harzic M, et al. Highly active antiretroviral treatment initiated early in the course of symptomatic primary HIV-1 infection: results of the ANRS 053 trial. J Infect Dis 180:1342–6, 1999.
221. Berrey MM, Schacker T, Collier AC, et al. Treatment of primary human immunodeficiency virus type 1 infection with potent antiretroviral therapy reduces frequency of rapid progression to AIDS. J Infect Dis 183:1466–75, 2001.
222. Lewin SR, Vesanen M, Kostrikis L, et al. Use of real-time PCR and molecular beacons to detect virus replication in human immunodeficiency virus type 1-infected individuals on prolonged effective antiretroviral therapy. J Virol 73: 6099–103, 1999.
223. Friis-Moller N, Sabin CA, Weber R, et al. Combination antiretroviral therapy and the risk of myocardial infarction. N Engl J Med 349:1993–2003, 2003.
224. Chen D, Misra A, Garg A. Clinical review 153: Lipodystrophy in human immunodeficiency virus-infected patients. J Clin Endocrinol Metab 87:4845–56, 2002.
225. Reisler RB, Han C, Burman WJ, et al. Grade 4 events are as important as AIDS events in the era of HAART. J Acquir Immune Defic Syndr 34:379–86, 2003.
226. Chun TW, Engel D, Berrey MM, et al. Early establishment of a pool of latently infected, resting CD4(+) T-cells during primary HIV-1 infection. Proc Natl Acad Sci USA 95:8869–73, 1998.
227. Strain MC, Little SJ, Daar ES, et al. Effect of treatment, during primary infection, on establishment and clearance of cellular reservoirs of HIV-1. J Infect Dis 191:1410–18, 2005.
228. Altfeld M, Rosenberg ES, Shankarappa R, et al. Cellular immune responses and viral diversity in individuals treated during acute and early HIV-1 infection. J Exp Med 193:169–80, 2001.

229. Mittler J, Essunger P, Yuen GJ, et al. Short-term measures ofrelative efficacy predict longer-term reductions in human immunodeficiency virus type 1 RNA levels following nelfinavir monotherapy. Antimicrob Agents Chemother 45:1438–43, 2001.
230. Polis MA, Sidorov IA, Yoder C, et al. Correlation between reduction in plasma HIV-1 RNA concentration 1 week after start of antiretroviral treatment and longer-term efficacy. Lancet 358:1760–5, 2001.
231. Louie M, Hogan C, Di Mascio M, et al. Determining the relative efficacy of highly active antiretroviral therapy. J Infect Dis 187:896–900, 2003.
232. Di Mascio M, Markowitz M, Louie M, et al. Dynamics of intermittent viremia during highly active antiretroviral therapy in patients who initiate therapy during chronic versus acute and early human immunodeficiency virus type 1 infection. J Virol 78:10566–73, 2004.
233. Lee PK, Kieffer TL, Siliciano RF, Nettles RE. HIV-1 viral load blips are of limited clinical significance. J Antimicrob Chemother 57:803–5, 2006.
234. Wolinsky SM, Wike CM, Korber BT, et al. Selective transmission of human immunodeficiency virus type-1 variants from mothers to infants. Science 255:1134–7, 1992.
235. Yerly S, Kaiser L, Perneger TV, et al. Time of initiation of antiretroviral therapy: impact on HIV-1 viraemia. The Swiss HIV Cohort Study. AIDS 14:243–9, 2000.
236. Markowitz M, Jin X, Hurley A, et al. Discontinuation of antiretroviral therapy commenced early during the course of human immunodeficiency virus type 1 infection, with or without adjunctive vaccination. J Infect Dis 186:634–43, 2002.
237. Lafeuillade A, Poggi C, Hittinger G, et al. Predictors of plasma human immunodeficiency virus type 1 RNA control after discontinuation of highly active antiretroviral therapy initiated at acute infection combined with structured treatment interruptions and immune-based therapies. J Infect Dis 188: 1426–32, 2003.
238. Carr A, Samaras K, Burton S, et al. A syndrome of peripheral lipodystrophy, hyperlipidaemia and insulin resistance in patients receiving HIV protease inhibitors. AIDS 12:F51–8, 1998.
239. Cahn PE, Gatell JM, Squires K, et al. Atazanavir – a once-daily HIV protease inhibitor that does not cause dyslipidemia in newly treated patients: results from two randomized clinical trials. J Int Assoc Physicians AIDS Care (Chic Ill) 3:92–8, 2004.
240. Yan Q, Hruz PW. Direct comparison of the acute in vivo effects of HIV protease inhibitors on peripheral glucose disposal. J Acquir Immune Defic Syndr 40:398–403, 2005.
241. Levy AR, James D, Johnston KM, et al. The direct costs of HIV/AIDS care. Lancet Infect Dis 6:171–7, 2006.
242. Palella FJ Jr, Chmiel JS, Moorman AC, Holmberg SD. Durability and predictors of success of highly active antiretroviral therapy for ambulatory HIV-infected patients. AIDS 16: 1617–26, 2002.
243. Richman DD, Morton SC, Wrin T, et al. The prevalence of antiretroviral drug resistance in the United States. AIDS 18:1393–401, 2004.
244. Jin X, Ramanathan M Jr, Barsoum S, et al. Safety and immunogenicity of ALVAC vCP1452 and recombinant gp160 in newly human immunodeficiency virus type 1-infected patients treated with prolonged highly active antiretroviral therapy. J Virol 76:2206–16, 2002.
245. Kinloch-de Loes S, Hoen B, Smith DE, et al. Impact of therapeutic immunization on HIV-1 viremia after discontinuation of antiretroviral therapy initiated during acute infection. J Infect Dis 192:607–17, 2005.
246. Mehandru S., Vcelar B., O'Neil M., et al. Monoclonal antibody infusions delay HIV-1 rebound after discontinuation of antiretroviral therapy in a cohort of HIV-1 infected individuals treated during primary HIV-1 infection. Paper presented at: 13th Conference on Retroviruses and Opportunistic Infections, 2006, Denver, Colorado.
247. Trkola A, Kuster H, Rusert P, et al. Delay of HIV-1 rebound after cessation of antiretroviral therapy through passive transfer of human neutralizing antibodies. Nat Med 11: 615–22, 2005.
248. Emmel EA, Verweij CL, Durand DB, et al. Cyclosporin A specifically inhibits function of nuclear proteins involved in T cell activation. Science 246:1617–20, 1989.
249. Rizzardi GP, Harari A, Capiluppi B, et al. Treatment of primary HIV-1 infection with cyclosporin A coupled with highly active antiretroviral therapy. J Clin Invest 109:681–8, 2002.
250. Chapuis AG, Paolo Rizzardi G, D'Agostino C, et al. Effects of mycophenolic acid on human immunodeficiency virus infection in vitro and in vivo. Nat Med 6:762–8, 2000.
251. Lori F, Foli A, Groff A, et al. Optimal suppression of HIV replication by low-dose hydroxyurea through the combination of antiviral and cytostatic ("virostatic") mechanisms. AIDS 19:1173–81, 2005.
252. Guidelines for the Use of Antiretroviral Agents in HIV-1-Infected Adults and Adolescents – 6 Oct 2005. Panel on clinical practices for treatment of HIV infection, Department of Health and Human Services. Available: http://www.aidsinfo.nih.gov/Guidelines/ 4 Mar 2006.
253. Yeni PG, Hammer SM, Hirsch MS, et al. Treatment for adult HIV infection: 2004 recommendations of the International AIDS Society-USA Panel. JAMA 292:251–65, 2004.
254. Fidler S, Fraser C, Fox J, et al. Comparative potency of three antiretroviral therapy regimes in primary HIV infection. AIDS 20:247–52, 2006.
255. Boden D, Hurley A, Zhang L, et al. HIV-1 drug resistance in newly infected individuals. JAMA 282:1135–41, 1999.
256. Cane P, Chrystie I, Dunn D, et al. Time trends in primary resistance to HIV drugs in the United Kingdom: multicentre observational study. BMJ 331:1368, 2005.
257. Grant RM, Hecht FM, Warmerdam M, et al. Time trends in primary HIV-1 drug resistance among recently infected persons. JAMA 288:181–8, 2002.
258. Little SJ, Holte S, Routy JP, et al. Antiretroviral-drug resistance among patients recently infected with HIV. N Engl J Med 347:385–94, 2002.
259. Shet A, Berry L, Mohri H, et al. Tracking the prevalence of transmitted antiretroviral drug resistant HIV-1 in New York City: a decade of experience. J Acquire Immune Defic Syndr 41: 439–46, 2006.
260. Simon V, Vanderhoeven J, Hurley A, et al. Evolving patterns of HIV-1 resistance to antiretroviral agents in newly infected individuals. AIDS 16:1511–19, 2002.
261. Weinstock HS, Zaidi I, Heneine W, et al. The epidemiology of antiretroviral drug resistance among drug-naive HIV-1-infected persons in 10 US cities. J Infect Dis 189:2174–80, 2004.
262. Chun TW, Justement JS, Lempicki RA, et al. Gene expression and viral production in latently infected, resting CD4+ T-cells in viremic versus aviremic HIV-infected individuals. Proc Natl Acad Sci USA 100:1908–13, 2003.
263. Nettles RE, Kieffer TL, Kwon P, et al. Intermittent HIV-1 viremia (Blips) and drug resistance in patients receiving HAART. JAMA 293:817–829, 2005.
264. Zhang L, Chung C, Hu BS, et al. Genetic characterization of rebounding HIV-1 after cessation of highly active antiretroviral therapy. J Clin Invest 106:839–45, 2000.

Chapter 34

Occupational and Nonoccupational Exposure Management

Adelisa L. Panlilio, MD, MPH, Lisa A. Grohskopf, MD, MPH

INTRODUCTION

The primary means of preventing HIV transmission is by avoiding exposure to HIV. Nevertheless, because exposures occur, despite best intentions, additional prevention tools are needed. One element of exposure management that may offer a means of preventing infection transmission is postexposure prophylaxis (PEP) with antiretroviral agents. This chapter summarizes information relevant to the use of PEP for occupational and nonoccupational exposures, including the risk of HIV transmission associated with such exposures, the rationale for use of PEP, and a summary of United States national guidelines on the use of PEP.[1,2]

RISK OF HIV TRANSMISSION

Factors known to affect the risk of occupational HIV infection among healthcare personnel (HCP) include the following: the prevalence of HIV infection among patients; the risk of infection transmission after an exposure; and the nature and frequency of exposures. The HIV seroprevalence among patient populations has varied widely, ranging from 0% to 62%, depending on the group tested.[3] Epidemiologic and laboratory studies suggest that a variety of factors may affect the risk of HIV transmission after an occupational exposure. First, the risk of HIV infection after exposure to HIV-infected blood depends on the type of exposure. After a single percutaneous exposure, the risk of infection transmission averages 0.3% (range 0.2–0.5%), based on multiple prospective studies of HCP followed after needlestick and other percutaneous injuries involving HIV-infected sources.[3] In contrast, the risk after a mucocutaneous exposure is estimated at 0.09%, based on one seroconversion in six studies[3]; after a nonintact skin exposure, the risk is believed to be even less. The risk of infection after nonintact skin exposure has not been well quantified, as there has been no documented seroconversion documented in HCP enrolled in a prospective study after an isolated skin exposure.

The Centers for Disease Control and Prevention (CDC) assessed additional risk factors for HIV transmission through percutaneous exposures to HIV-infected blood in a case-control study.[4] This retrospective study found that the risk for HIV infection was increased with exposure to a larger quantity of blood from the source patient as indicated by a visibly bloody needle, a needle used in blood vessels, or a deep injury. These factors were suspected to be indirect measures for exposure to a larger volume of blood. The risk also was increased for exposure to blood from source patients with terminal illness, possibly due to the higher titer of HIV in blood usually seen late in the course of AIDS or other factors, such as the presence of syncytia-inducing strains of HIV. While the risk of HIV transmission from exposures that involve a larger volume of blood was not estimated, the risk may likely exceed the average risk of 0.3%, particularly when the source patient's virus load is high. Results of the case-control study must be interpreted cautiously, particularly because of the small number of case-HCP and several other limitations, including the fact that cases and controls came from different sources.

The findings and conclusions in this report are those of the authors and do not necessarily represent the views of the Centers for Disease Control and Prevention.

The use of trade names and commercial sources is for identification only and does not imply endorsement by the U.S. Department of Health and Human Services.

Table 34-1

Estimated Per-Act Risk for Acquisition of HIV, by Exposure Route[a]

Exposure Route	Risk per 10 000 Exposures to an Infected Source	Reference
Blood transfusion	9000	9
Needle-sharing injection-drug use	67	7
Receptive anal intercourse	50–300	8, 10
Percutaneous needle stick	30	3
Receptive penile–vaginal intercourse	10–20	8, 11
Mucous membrane blood splash	9	3
Insertive anal intercourse	6.5	8
Insertive penile–vaginal intercourse	5	8
Receptive oral intercourse	1	8
Insertive oral intercourse	0.5	8[b]

[a] Estimates of risk for transmission from sexual exposures assume no condom use.
[b] Source refers to oral intercourse performed on a man.

Estimates of yearly blood contacts experienced by HCP in various occupations are based on prospective observational studies or questionnaire surveys. HCP most frequently involved in performing invasive procedures, e.g., surgeons and obstetricians, tended to have the highest rates of blood contact; in general, those HCP who handle sharps/needles have the greatest potential for exposure to blood through percutaneous injuries.[3]

Nonoccupational HIV exposures, consisting primarily of sexual and injection drug use-related events, occur more frequently than occupational exposures and are responsible for a greater burden of HIV transmission worldwide.[5,6] The estimated per-act risk for HIV infection varies depending upon the type of exposure. Assuming that the source is known to be HIV-infected, receptive anal and vaginal intercourse and sharing needles during drug injection confer particularly high risk; infection rates are estimated to be 50–300, 10–20, and 67 per 10 000 contacts respectively with a known HIV-infected source (Table 34-1).[7–11] Assessment of the risk associated with a given nonoccupational exposure is often more difficult than with occupational exposures, as information about the potential source's HIV status may not be known and s/he may not be as readily available for testing.

Biologic Plausibility of HIV PEP

The mechanism by which PEP prevents HIV infection transmission is not clearly understood. Nevertheless, it is biologically plausible that infection could be prevented or ameliorated by using antiretroviral drugs. Information about primary HIV infection indicates that there is a brief "window of opportunity" during which postexposure intervention with antiretroviral agents may modify viral replication before systemic infection is established. Data from studies in animal models and *in vitro* tissue suggest that dendritic cells in the mucosa and skin may be the initial target for HIV infection or capture and have an important role in initiating HIV infection of CD4+ T-lymphocyte cells in regional lymph nodes.[12] In a primate model of simian immunodeficiency virus (SIV) infection, infection of dendritic-like cells occurred first following mucosal exposure to cell-free virus.[13] At 2 days post-inoculation, migration of these cells to regional lymph nodes occurred, and virus was detectable in the peripheral blood within 5 days. Theoretically, PEP with antiretroviral agents administered promptly after exposure may prevent or inhibit systemic infection by limiting the proliferation of virus in the initial target cells or lymph nodes.

Animal Studies

The applicability of findings from studies of PEP in animals to human exposures to HIV is limited by differences in controlled variables (e.g., choice of viral strain (based on the animal model used), inoculum size, route of inoculation, time of prophylaxis initiation, and drug regimen).[14] Most animal studies have used SIV or other nonhuman retroviruses that have different pathogenetic mechanisms from HIV-1 in humans. Furthermore, studies done to date have used higher viral inocula than are likely to be encountered in human exposures, as well as routes of exposure that may not be comparable to needlestick injuries or nonoccupational exposures. In studies of PEP in nonhuman primates, efficacy was greatest when prophylaxis was begun before or within a few hours after exposure; there was less apparent effect when drugs were begun later than 24–36 h postexposure, and when PEP was taken for shorter lengths of time. In one study performed in macaques, intravenously administered tenofovir (TDF) blocked SIV infection if administered within 24 h of intravenous viral inoculation and continued for 28 days. In comparison, only half of macaques treated for 10 days and none treated for 3 days were protected. Delaying initiation of treatment to 48 or 72 h postexposure also was less effective.[15] Another study of macaques used a combination antiretroviral regimen of zidovudine (ZDV), lamivudine (3TC), and indinavir (IDV) initiated 4 h after intravenous simian/human immunodeficiency virus (SHIV) challenge and continued for 28 days. All animals became infected but had reduced viral loads.[16]

More recently, refinements in methodology have resulted in studies that are more relevant; in particular, the mucosal exposure routes have been used and viral inocula have been reduced to levels more analogous to human exposures but sufficient to cause infection in untreated animals.[17,18] These studies provide encouraging evidence of postexposure chemoprophylactic efficacy in the experimental setting. In a study of PEP following vaginal HIV-2 exposure, all macaques administered (R)-9-(2-phosphonylmethoxypropyl) adenine (now known as TDF) for 28 days, beginning 12 h (four animals) or 36 h (four animals) after exposure were protected. Breakthrough infection was observed in one of four animals treated 72 h after exposure, providing additional support for earlier administration of PEP.[17]

Human Studies

The data used to assess the efficacy of PEP after occupational exposures in humans are largely indirect. Because seroconversion after occupational HIV exposure is uncommon, a prospective trial would have to enroll thousands of exposed HCP to achieve the statistical power necessary to demonstrate PEP efficacy. During 1987–1989, the Burroughs-Wellcome Company sponsored a prospective placebo-controlled clinical trial among HCP to evaluate PEP with 6 weeks of ZDV.[19] This trial was terminated prematurely because of low enrollment.[20] In view of current indirect evidence of PEP efficacy, it is unlikely that a placebo-controlled trial in HCP would ever be considered ethical.

The previously mentioned retrospective case-control study of HCP that assessed potential risk factors for HIV transmission after percutaneous exposure also found that use of ZDV as PEP was associated with a reduction in the risk of HIV infection by ~81% (95% CI = 43–94%).[4] ZDV was the only antiretroviral drug available for use as PEP during the period of this study.[4] Additional supportive data on the efficacy of PEP come from studies of perinatal HIV transmission. In a randomized, controlled, prospective trial (AIDS Clinical Trial Group protocol (ACTG) 076), ZDV was administered to HIV-infected pregnant women and their infants. Administration of ZDV to the mother during pregnancy, labor, and delivery and to the newborn reduced transmission by 67%.[21] This study showed that only 9–17% (depending on the assay used) of the protective effect of ZDV was explained by reduction of the HIV viral load in the maternal blood. This suggested that ZDV prophylaxis in part involves a mechanism other than the reduction of maternal viral burden.[22] Subsequent studies of various PEP regimens to prevent perinatal transmission lend further support to the role of antiretroviral agents as prophylaxis against HIV infection transmission.[23,24] The chapter on management of the pregnant patient (Chapter 35) gives additional information about prevention of perinatal transmission of HIV.

The limitations of all of these studies in animals and humans must be considered when reviewing evidence of PEP efficacy. The extent to which data from animal studies can be extrapolated to humans is largely unknown, and the exposure route for mother-to-infant HIV transmission is not similar to occupational exposures; therefore, these findings may not be directly applicable to PEP in HCP.

Human data relevant to the potential efficacy of PEP for nonoccupational exposures are limited to observational studies and registries. There is no study analogous to the case-control study in HCP cited above.[4] In general, the conclusions drawn from observational and registry data on nonoccupational exposures are limited by relatively small sample sizes and a relatively low number of seroconversions. Moreover, given the repetitive nature of the behaviors with which nonoccupational exposures are often associated, it can be difficult to determine with certainty whether a given infection resulted from the exposure for which PEP was taken. In the CDC registry of nonoccupational PEP (nPEP) use, among 785 reported exposures only one seroconversion was noted, which occurred in a person who took PEP following an insertive anal exposure. Because exposures occurred before and after the period in which nPEP was taken, it was difficult to determine whether the infection represented a true nPEP failure (CDC, unpublished data). Among 702 patients who received nPEP in a large feasibility study in San Francisco, seven seroconversions occurred. Three individuals reported no additional exposures after nPEP initiation which could have been the source of infection, though all reported other potential exposures in the 6 months prior to nPEP initiation.[25] In Australia, among 869 persons who returned 4 or more weeks postexposure for repeat HIV testing, no HIV seroconversions definitely related to treatment failure were observed.[26]

Antiretroviral Agents for PEP

Only antiretroviral agents that have been approved by the Food and Drug Administration (FDA) for treatment of HIV infection are recommended for use as PEP by the US Public Health Service. Antiretroviral agents from four classes of drugs are currently available for the treatment of HIV disease.[27] These include the nucleoside or nucleotide reverse transcriptase inhibitors (NRTIs), non-nucleoside reverse transcriptase inhibitors (NNRTIs), protease inhibitors (PIs), and a single fusion inhibitor.

TOXICITIES AND OTHER POTENTIAL RISKS OF PEP

Toxicities Associated with Antiretroviral Medications

When PEP is indicated, an important goal is completion of a 4-week PEP regimen. Toxicity and side effects among HCP have been cited as reasons why many HCP were unable to complete a full 4-week course of HIV PEP. Because all of the antiretroviral agents have been associated with side effects, the toxicity profiles of these agents, including the frequency, severity, duration, and reversibility of side effects, is an important consideration in selection of HIV PEP regimens. Table 34-2 summarizes the primary side effects and toxicities reported with use of antiretroviral agents that could be considered for use as HIV PEP. Particularly noteworthy are serious side effects reported with the use of nevirapine as PEP, including hepatotoxicity (with one instance of fulminant liver failure requiring liver transplantation); rhabdomyolysis; and a hypersensitivity syndrome.[28] Most data on adverse events have been reported primarily for persons with established HIV infection receiving prolonged antiretroviral therapy and therefore may not reflect the experience in uninfected persons who take PEP for a limited time.

At least anecdotally, antiretroviral agents appear to be tolerated more poorly by persons taking them as PEP than by HIV-infected patients taking these agents as long-term treatment. Side effects are frequently reported by persons who take antiretroviral agents as PEP.[29–37] Several investigators reported that a large proportion of HCP at their institutions did not complete a full 4 weeks of therapy because of inability to tolerate the drugs.[29–31,33,34] Data from the National

Primary Side Effects and Toxicities Associated with Antiretroviral Agents that may be Used for HIV Postexposure Prophylaxis, by Class and Agent

Table 34-2

Class and Agent	Side Effect and Toxicity
NRTIs	Class warnings: All NRTIs have the potential to cause lactic acidosis with hepatic steatosis
Zidovudine (Retrovir, ZDV, AZT)	Anemia, neutropenia, nausea, headache, insomnia, muscle pain, and weakness
Lamivudine (Epivir, 3TC)	Abdominal pain, nausea, diarrhea, rash, and pancreatitis
Stavudine (Zerit, d4T)	Peripheral neuropathy, headache, diarrhea, nausea, insomnia, anorexia, pancreatitis, elevated liver function tests (LFTs), anemia, and neutropenia
Didanosine enteric coated (Videx EC, ddI)	Pancreatitis, neuropathy, diarrhea, abdominal pain, and nausea
Abacavir (Ziagen, ABC)	Nausea, diarrhea, anorexia, abdominal pain, fatigue, headache, insomnia, and hypersensitivity reactions
Emtricitabine (Emtriva, FTC)	Headache, nausea, vomiting, diarrhea, and rash. Skin discoloration (mild hyperpigmentation on palms and soles), primarily among nonwhites
Nucleotide Analog Reverse Transcriptase Inhibitor (NtRTI)	Class warnings: NtRTIs have the potential to cause lactic acidosis with hepatic steatosis
Tenofovir (Viread, TDF)	Nausea, diarrhea, vomiting, flatulence, and headache
NNRTIs	
Nevirapine (Viramune, NVP)	Rash (including cases of Stevens–Johnson syndrome), fever, nausea, headache, symptomatic hepatitis including fatal hepatic necrosis, and elevated LFTs
Delavirdine (Rescriptor, DLV)	Rash (including cases of Stevens–Johnson syndrome), nausea, diarrhea, headache, fatigue, and elevated LFT
Efavirenz (Sustiva, EFV)	Rash (including cases of Stevens–Johnson syndrome), insomnia, somnolence, dizziness, trouble concentrating, abnormal dreaming, and teratogenicity
PIs	
Indinavir (Crixivan, IDV)	Nausea, abdominal pain, nephrolithiasis, and indirect hyperbilirubinemia
Nelfinavir (Viracept, NFV)	Diarrhea, nausea, abdominal pain, weakness, and rash
Ritonavir (Norvir, RTV)	Weakness, diarrhea, nausea, circumoral paresthesia, taste alteration, and increased cholesterol and triglycerides
Saquinavir (Fortovase, SQV)	Diarrhea, abdominal pain, nausea, hyperglycemia, and increased LFTs
Fosamprenavir (Lexiva, FOSAPV)	Nausea, diarrhea, rash, circumoral paresthesia, taste alteration, and depression
Atazanavir (Reyataz, ATV)	Nausea, headache, rash, abdominal pain, diarrhea, vomiting, and indirect hyperbilirubinemia
Lopinavir/Ritonavir (Kaletra, LPV/RTV)	Diarrhea, fatigue, headache, nausea, and increased cholesterol and triglycerides
Fusion Inhibitor	
Enfuvirtide (Fuzeon, T-20)	Local injection site reactions, bacterial pneumonia, insomnia; depression, peripheral neuropathy, and cough

Sources: Package inserts; Panel on Clinical Practices for Treatment of HIV Infection. Guidelines for the use of antiretroviral agents in HIV-infected adults and adolescents – 10, October 2006. Washington, DC: National Institutes of Health; 2005. Available at http://aidsinfo.nih.gov/contentfiles/AdultandAdolescentGL.pdf.

Surveillance for Health Care Workers system (NaSH), CDC's occupational surveillance system for occupational exposures and infections in hospitals, for June 1995 through December 2005 indicate that a large proportion (44.9%) of HCP, with at least one follow-up after starting PEP, experienced one or more drug-related symptoms. The symptoms reported most frequently were nausea (25.2%) followed by malaise/fatigue (23.1%) (CDC, unpublished data). Similar data have been reported from the Italian Registry of Antiretroviral Postexposure Prophylaxis, which includes data primarily on HCP taking PEP but also collects data on those taking PEP after nonoccupational exposures.[32] In multivariate analysis, those taking regimens that included PIs were more likely to experience PEP-associated side effects and to discontinue PEP prematurely (<28 days). In the CDC nonoccupational PEP registry, 69% of exposed persons, with at least one follow-up visit, reported at least one drug-related symptom (CDC, unpublished data). In the European Non-Occupational Post-Exposure Prophylaxis Registry, of 1418 exposed persons offered nPEP, only 164 (12%) discontinued it early and only 33% of those did so because of side effects.[38] In Australia, 72% of those taking a two-drug regimen for nPEP and 76% of those taking a three-drug regimen reported experiencing side effects; full compliance with the regimen was reported in 56% and 62% of exposures, respectively.[26]

Because side effects are frequent, and particularly because they are cited as a major reason for not completing PEP regimens as prescribed, the selection of regimens should be heavily influenced toward those that are tolerable for short-term use. In addition, all of the approved antiretroviral agents may have potentially serious drug interactions when used with certain other drugs.[39–46] For this reason, careful evaluation is required of concomitant medications, including over-the-counter medications and supplements (e.g., herbals) being used by an exposed person before prescribing PEP. Anyone receiving antiretroviral drugs should be monitored closely for toxicity (Table 34-2). PIs and NNRTIs, in general, have the most potential for significant interactions with other drugs. Current information about potential drug interactions can be found in the adult and adolescent HIV treatment guidelines[27] and in the manufacturers' package inserts.

Selection of HIV PEP Regimens

Determining which agents and how many to use as well as when to alter a PEP regimen is largely empiric.[47] In HIV-infected patients, combination regimens with three or more antiretroviral agents have proved superior to monotherapy and dual therapy regimens in reducing HIV viral load, reducing the incidence of opportunistic infections and death, and delaying onset of drug resistance in patients with established HIV infection.[27] Guidelines for the treatment of HIV infection, a condition usually involving a high total body burden of HIV, recommend the use of three or more drugs[27]; however, the applicability of these recommendations to prevention of HIV transmission using antiretroviral PEP remains unknown.

Other guidelines (e.g., New York State, European Union) recommend different HIV PEP regimens for managing occupational exposures[48,49] as do guidelines for managing nonoccupational HIV exposure.[2,38,50–54a,55,55a] The primary difference between the United States Public Health Service (USPHS) PEP recommendations for occupational HIV exposures and other PEP recommendations is the routine use of three or more drugs in PEP regimens. There are no definitive data that support the superiority of one HIV PEP regimen over another in preventing HIV transmission.

Resistance to Antiretroviral Agents

Resistance to all the currently available antiretroviral agents has been documented and cross-resistance within drug classes is frequent.[56,57] Known or suspected resistance of the source virus to antiretroviral agents, particularly to those that might be included in a PEP regimen, may influence selection of PEP regimens.[58] Despite PEP with combination drug regimens, occupational transmission of drug-resistant HIV strains, has been reported.[59–61] However, the relevance of resistance to transmission and transmissibility is still not well understood.

Determining the presence of antiretroviral drug resistance is often difficult because patients generally take more than one antiretroviral agent. Resistance testing of the source virus at the time of an exposure is impractical because the choice of the initial PEP regimen must be made before test results generally are known. Furthermore, there are no data that suggest that modification of a PEP regimen after resistance test results become available (usually 1–2 weeks) improves efficacy of PEP.[32] Resistance should be suspected in source patients when there is (1) clinical progression of disease, (2) a persistently increasing viral load, (3) a decline in CD4+ T-lymphocyte-cell count despite therapy, or (4) a lack of virologic response to therapy. A PEP regimen may need to be tailored, depending upon the drugs to which the source virus is known or suspected to be resistant.

RECOMMENDATIONS FOR USE OF PEP FOLLOWING OCCUPATIONAL AND NONOCCUPATIONAL EXPOSURES

Recommendations for Occupational PEP

The following HIV PEP recommendations (Tables 34-3 and 34-4) apply to situations in which a worker has had an exposure to a source person who has HIV infection or when information suggests that the source person is likely to be HIV-infected. These recommendations are based on the risk for HIV infection after different types of exposure and limited data regarding efficacy and toxicity of PEP. If PEP is offered and taken, and the source is later determined to be HIV-negative, PEP should be discontinued. Although concerns have been voiced about HIV-negative sources being

Table 34-3

Recommended HIV Postexposure Prophylaxis (PEP) for Percutaneous Injuries

	Infection Status of Source				
Exposure Type	**HIV-Positive, Class 1[*]**	**HIV-Positive, Class 2[*]**	**Source of Unknown HIV Status**	**Unknown Source**	**HIV-Negative**
	Asymptomatic HIV infection or known low viral load (e.g., <1500)	Symptomatic HIV infection, AIDS, acute seroconversion, or known high viral load	e.g., deceased source person with no samples available for HIV testing	e.g., a needle from a sharps disposal container	
Less severe, e.g., solid needle, superficial injury	Recommend basic 2-drug PEP	Recommend expanded ⩾3-drug PEP	Generally, no PEP warranted; however, consider basic 2-drug PEP[†] for source with HIV-risk factors[§]	Generally, no PEP warranted; however, consider basic 2-drug PEP[†] in settings in which exposure to HIV-infected persons is likely	No PEP warranted
More severe, e.g., large-bore hollow needle, deep puncture, visible blood on device, or needle used in patient's artery or vein	Recommend expanded ⩾3-drug PEP	Recommend expanded ⩾3-drug PEP	Generally, no PEP warranted; however, consider basic 2-drug PEP[†] for source with HIV-risk factors[§]	Generally, no PEP warranted; however, consider basic 2-drug PEP[†] in settings where exposure to HIV-infected persons is likely	No PEP warranted

[*] If drug resistance is a concern, obtain expert consultation. Initiation of PEP should not be delayed pending expert consultation, and, because expert consultation alone cannot substitute for face-to-face counseling, resources should be available to provide immediate evaluation and follow-up care for all exposures.

[†] The designation "consider PEP" indicates that PEP is optional; a decision to initiate PEP should be based on a discussion between the exposed person and the treating clinician of the risks versus benefits of PEP.

[§] If PEP is offered and taken and the source is later determined to be HIV-negative, PEP should be discontinued.

Table 34-4

Recommended HIV Postexposure Prophylaxis (PEP) for Mucous Membrane Exposures and Nonintact Skin* Exposures

	Infection Status of Source				
Exposure Type	**HIV-Positive, Class 1**[†]	**HIV-Positive, Class 2**[†]	**Source of Unknown HIV Status**	**Unknown Source**	**HIV-Negative**
	Asymptomatic HIV infection or known low viral load (e.g., <1500)	Symptomatic HIV infection, AIDS, acute seroconversion, or known high viral load	e.g., deceased source person with no samples available for HIV testing	e.g., splash from inappropriately disposed blood	
Small volume, e.g., few drops	Consider basic 2-drug PEP[§]	Recommend basic 2-drug PEP	Generally, no PEP warranted[¶]	Generally, no PEP warranted	No PEP warranted
Large volume, e.g., major blood splash	Recommend basic 2-drug PEP	Recommend expanded ≥3-drug PEP	Generally, no PEP warranted; however, consider basic 2-drug PEP[§] for source with HIV-risk factors[¶]	Generally, no PEP warranted; however, consider basic 2-drug PEP[§] in settings in which exposure to HIV-infected persons is likely	No PEP warranted

*For skin exposures, follow-up is indicated only if evidence exists of compromised skin integrity (e.g., dermatitis, abrasion, or open wound).

†If drug resistance is a concern, obtain expert consultation. Initiation of PEP should not be delayed pending expert consultation, and, because expert consultation alone cannot substitute for face-to-face counseling, resources should be available to provide immediate evaluation and follow-up care for all exposures.

§The designation "consider PEP" indicates that PEP is optional; a decision to initiate PEP should be based on a discussion between the exposed person and the treating clinician of the risks versus benefits of PEP.

¶If PEP is offered and taken and the source is later determined to be HIV negative, PEP should be discontinued.

in the window period for seroconversion, there have been no documented transmissions reported in the US involving such exposures.[62] Use of rapid HIV testing of source patients can facilitate making timely decisions about use of HIV PEP after occupational exposures to sources of unknown HIV status. Because most HIV exposures do not result in the transmission of HIV, potential toxicity of antiretroviral drugs must be carefully considered when prescribing PEP.

Timing and Duration of PEP

PEP should be initiated as soon as possible, preferably within hours of exposure, rather than days. If there is any question about whether to start PEP, which antiretroviral drugs to use, or whether to use a basic or expanded regimen, it may be prudent to start a basic PEP regimen immediately and not delay PEP administration. PEP regimens can be modified or stopped when additional information becomes available. Although animal studies suggest that PEP probably is substantially less effective when started more than 24–36h postexposure,[15,17] the interval after which there is no benefit from PEP for humans is undefined. Therefore, if appropriate for the exposure, PEP should be started even when the interval since exposure exceeds 36h. Initiating therapy after a longer interval (e.g., 1 week) may be considered for exposures that represent an increased risk for transmission; this may represent early treatment of HIV infection, which may be beneficial.[63] The optimal duration of PEP is unknown. Because 4 weeks of ZDV appeared protective in occupational and animal studies, PEP probably should be administered for 4 weeks, if tolerated.

Recommendations for the Selection of Drugs for HIV PEP

The process of selecting HIV PEP regimens should include a balancing of the risk for infection against the potential toxicities of the agent(s). Because all drugs recommended as HIV PEP are potentially toxic, their use is not justified for exposures that pose a negligible risk for transmission (Tables 34-3 and 34-4). In general, the regimens recommended here should be viewed as suggestions for initial HIV PEP regimens that could be changed should additional information about the source of the occupational exposure, such as possible treatment history, and antiretroviral drug resistance is obtained and/or expert consultation is provided. The doses and schedules for drugs recommended as PEP are the same as those used in the treatment of established HIV infection.[27]

Selection of the PEP regimen should consider the comparative risk represented by the exposure and information about the exposure source, including history of and response to antiretroviral therapy based on clinical response, CD4+ T-lymphocyte-cell counts, viral load measurements, and current disease stage. When the source person's virus is known or suspected to be resistant to one or more of the drugs considered for the PEP regimen, the selection of drugs to which the source person's virus is unlikely to be resistant is recommended. If this information is not immediately available, initiation of PEP, if indicated, should not be delayed; changes in the PEP regimen can be made after PEP has been started, as appropriate. Given the complexity of selecting HIV PEP regimens, persons having expertise in antiretroviral therapy and HIV transmission should be consulted whenever possible. For HCP who initiate PEP, re-evaluation of the exposed person should occur within 72h postexposure, especially as additional information about the exposure or source person becomes available.

The USPHS recommends stratifying HIV PEP regimens based on the severity of exposure and other considerations, such as concern for antiretroviral drug resistance in the exposure source (Tables 34-3 and 34-4). Most HIV exposures will warrant a two-drug regimen, using two (NRTIs) (Tables 34-3 and 34-4). Two-drug combinations that can be considered for PEP include ZDV and 3TC or emtricitabine (FTC); stavudine (d4T) and 3TC or FTC; and TDF and 3TC or FTC. In the previous USPHS guideline,[60] a combination of d4T and didanosine (ddI) was considered one of the first choice PEP regimens; but this regimen is no longer recommended because of concerns about toxicity (especially neuropathy and pancreatitis) and the availability of alternative regimens that are more tolerable.

Expanded PEP regimens consist of one of the two-drug regimens with addition of a third (or even a fourth) drug. An expanded regimen should be considered for exposures that pose an increased risk for transmission or involve a source in whom antiretroviral drug resistance is likely. The use of more than two drugs for PEP following high-risk exposures is based on demonstrated effectiveness in reducing viral burden in HIV-infected persons.[27] However, no definitive data exist that demonstrate increased efficacy of three- versus two-drug regimens as HIV PEP. Previously, indinavir (IDV), nelfinavir (NFV), efavirenz (EFV), and abacavir (ABC) were recommended as first-choice agents for inclusion in an expanded PEP regimen.[60] Now, PHS recommends that expanded PEP regimens be PI-based. The PI preferred for use in expanded PEP regimens is lopinavir/ritonavir (Kaletra™). Other PIs acceptable for use in expanded PEP regimens are atazanavir, fosamprenavir, ritonavir-boosted IDV, ritonavir-boosted saquinavir, and NFV. Although side effects may be common with the NNRTIs, EFV may be considered for expanded PEP regimens, especially when resistance to PIs in the source virus is known or suspected. EFV should be used cautiously in women of childbearing age because of the risk of teratogenicity.

Drugs that may be considered as alternatives to the above regimens, with warnings about side effects and other adverse events, are EFV and ddI with either 3TC or FTC. Although the fusion inhibitor enfuvirtide (T20) has theoretical benefits for the use in PEP since its activity occurs before viral–host cell integration, it is not recommended for routine HIV PEP because it requires twice daily subcutaneous administration. Furthermore, use of enfuvirtide has the potential for production of anti-enfuvirtide antibodies that cross react with HIV gp41. These cross-reacting antibodies, could result in a false positive enzyme-linked immunoassay (EIA) HIV antibody test. A confirmatory Western blot test would be expected to be negative in such cases. Enfuvirtide should be used only with expert consultation.

Antiretroviral drugs that are not recommended for use as PEP, due mostly to higher risk of adverse events (some serious or life threatening), include abacavir, delavirdine, and ddC, and as noted previously, the combination of ddI and d4T. Nevirapine should not be included in PEP regimens except with expert consultation because of serious side effects.

Given the complexity of choosing and administering HIV PEP, consultation with an infectious diseases specialist or other physician with experience in the use of antiretroviral agents is recommended whenever possible, if doing so will not delay the timely initiation of PEP. Some institutions have ensured appropriate consultation by requiring consultation with the hospital epidemiologist and/or infectious diseases specialist in situations where HIV PEP use is being considered or indicated. There are several situations in which this is especially important, such as management of HCP who are pregnant or breastfeeding, were exposed to treatment-experienced sources, and those experiencing drug toxicity (Boxes 34-1 and 34-2).

Follow-up of HCP Exposed to HIV

Recommendations for follow-up testing, monitoring, and counseling of exposed HCP are unchanged from earlier guidelines[60,64,65] but greater emphasis is needed on improving follow-up care. This may result in increased adherence to HIV PEP regimens, better management of associated symptoms with ancillary medications or regimen changes, improved detection of serious adverse effects, and serologic testing in a larger proportion of exposed HCP to determine if infection is transmitted after occupational exposures. Follow-up of HCP with occupational exposure to HIV should include postexposure testing, medical evaluation, and counseling regardless of whether they receive PEP. HIV-antibody testing should be performed for at least 6 months postexposure (e.g., at 6 weeks, 12 weeks, and 6 months). Extended HIV follow-up (e.g., for 12 months) is recommended for HCP who become infected with HCV following exposure to a source co-infected with HIV and HCV. It is unclear whether extended follow-up is indicated in other circumstances (e.g., exposure to a source co-infected with HIV and HCV in the absence of HCV seroconversion or for exposed persons with a medical history suggesting an impaired ability to amount an antibody response to acute infection). Although rare instances of delayed HIV seroconversion have been reported,[66,67] the infrequency of this occurrence does not warrant adding to exposed persons' anxiety by routinely extending the duration of postexposure follow-up. However, this should not preclude a decision to extend follow-up in an individual situation based on the clinical judgment of the exposed person's healthcare provider. HIV testing should be performed on any exposed person who has an illness that is compatible with an acute retroviral syndrome, regardless of the interval since exposure. When HIV infection is identified, the individual should be referred for medical management to a specialist knowledgeable in the area of HIV treatment and counseling.

HIV-antibody testing using EIA should be used to monitor for seroconversion. Direct virus assays (e.g., HIV p24 antigen EIA or tests for HIV RNA) to detect infection in exposed HCP generally are not recommended.[68] The relatively high

BOX 34-1 Situations for Which Expert* Consultation is Advised

- Delayed (i.e., later than 24–36 h) exposure report
  - the interval after which there is no benefit from PEP is undefined
- Unknown source (e.g., needle in sharps disposal container or laundry)
  - decide use of PEP on a case-by-case basis
  - consider the severity of the exposure and the epidemiologic likelihood of HIV exposure
  - do not test needles or other sharp instruments for HIV
- Known or suspected pregnancy in the exposed person
  - does not preclude the use of optimal PEP regimens
  - do not deny PEP solely on the basis of pregnancy
- Breast feeding in the exposed person
  - does not preclude the use of optimal PEP regimens
  - do not deny PEP solely on the basis of breast feeding
- Resistance of the source virus to antiretroviral agents
  - influence of drug resistance on transmission risk is unknown
  - if the source person's virus is known or suspected to be resistant to ≥1 of the drugs considered for the PEP regimen, selection of drugs to which the source person's virus is unlikely to be resistant is recommended
  - resistance testing of the source person's virus at the time of the exposure is not recommended
  - initiation of PEP should not be delayed while awaiting results of resistance testing, if obtained
- Toxicity of the initial PEP regimen
  - adverse symptoms, such as nausea and diarrhea, are common with PEP
  - symptoms often can be managed without changing the PEP regimen by prescribing antimotility and/or antiemetic agents
  - in other situations, modifying the dose interval (i.e., taking drugs after meals, administering a lower dose of drug more frequently throughout the day, as recommended by the manufacturer) may help alleviate symptoms when they occur

*Local experts and/or the National Clinicians' Post-Exposure Prophylaxis Hotline (PEPline; 1-888-448-4911)

Resources for Consultation

BOX 34-2

Occupational Exposure Management Resources

National Clinicians' Postexposure Prophylaxis Hotline (PEPline)[a]	Phone: (888) 448-4911 Internet: *http://www.ucsf.edu/hivcntr/PEPline/index.html*
CDC (reporting HIV infections in HCP and failures of PEP)	Phone: (800) 893-0485
HIV Antiretroviral Pregnancy Registry	Phone: 1-800-258-4263 (toll-free) or (910) 256-0238 FAX: (800) 800-1052 or (910) 256-0637 Write: Antiretroviral Pregnancy Registry Registries and Epidemiology, Charles River Laboratories Research Park – 1011 Ashes Drive Wilmington, NC 28405 Internet: *http://www.apregistry.com/*
Food and Drug Administration (reporting unusual or severe toxicity to antiretroviral agents)	Phone: (800) 332-1088 Write: MedWatch FDA 5600 Fishers Lane Rockville, MD 20852-9787 (910) 310-793-1935 Internet: *http://www.fda.gov/medwatch*
HIV/AIDS Treatment Information Service	Internet: *http://aidsinfo.nih.gov*

[a] Run by University of CA-San Francisco/San Francisco General Hospital staff; supported by the Health Resources and Services Administration Ryan White CARE Act and AIDS Education and Training Centers, and CDC.

rate of false-positive results of these tests in this setting could lead to unnecessary anxiety and/or treatment.[69,70] Despite the ability of direct virus assays to detect HIV infection a few days earlier than EIA, the infrequency of occupational seroconversion and increased costs of these tests do not warrant their routine use in this setting.

Monitoring and Management of PEP Toxicity

Monitoring for PEP toxicity includes testing at baseline and at 2 weeks after starting PEP. The scope of tests performed should be based on medical conditions in the exposed HCP and the toxicity of drugs included in the PEP regimen. Minimally, laboratory monitoring for toxicity should include a complete blood count and renal and hepatic function tests. Monitoring for evidence of hyperglycemia should be included for HCP whose regimens include any PI. For HCP receiving IDV, monitoring for crystalluria, hematuria, hemolytic anemia, and hepatitis also should be performed. If toxicity is noted, further diagnostic studies may be indicated and modification of the regimen should be considered after expert consultation.

Exposed HCP who choose to take PEP should be advised of the importance of completing the prescribed regimen. Information should be provided about potential drug interactions and the drugs that should not be taken with PEP, the side effects of the drugs that have been prescribed, measures to minimize these effects, and the methods of clinical monitoring for toxicity during the follow-up period. They should be advised that certain symptoms (e.g., rash, fever, back or abdominal pain, pain on urination or blood in the urine, or symptoms of hyperglycemia (increased thirst and/or frequent urination)) should be evaluated without delay.

HCP who fail to complete the recommended regimen often do so because of the side effects they experience (e.g., nausea, diarrhea). These symptoms often can be managed with antimotility and antiemetic agents or other medications that target the specific symptoms without changing the regimen. In other situations, modifying the dose interval (i.e., administering a lower dose of drug more frequently throughout the day, as recommended by the manufacturer), may facilitate adherence to the regimen. Serious adverse events should be reported to FDA's MedWatch program.

Counseling and Education

Although HIV infection following an occupational exposure occurs infrequently, the emotional impact of an exposure often is significant.[71,72] In addition, HCP are given seemingly conflicting information. Although HCP are told that there is a low risk for HIV transmission, a 4-week regimen of PEP may be recommended and they are asked to commit to behavioral measures (e.g., sexual abstinence or condom use) to prevent secondary transmission, all of which influence their lives for several weeks to months.[71] Therefore, access to persons who are knowledgeable about occupational HIV transmission and who can deal with the many concerns an HIV exposure may raise for the exposed person is an important element of postexposure management.

HIV-exposed HCP should be advised to use the following measures to prevent secondary transmission during the follow-up period, especially the first 6–12 weeks after the exposure when most HIV-infected persons are expected to seroconvert: use sexual abstinence or condoms to prevent sexual transmission and to avoid pregnancy; and refrain from donating blood, plasma, organs, tissue or semen. Exposed HCP who are breast feeding should be counseled about the risk of HIV transmission through breast milk, and discontinuation of breast feeding should be considered, especially for high-risk exposures. Additionally, some antiretroviral drugs, such as NRTIs and nevirapine are known to pass into breast milk; it is not known whether this also is true for the other approved antiretroviral drugs.

Exposed HCP should be advised to seek medical evaluation for any acute illness that occurs during the follow-up period. Such an illness, particularly if characterized by fever, rash, myalgia, fatigue, malaise, or lymphadenopathy, may be indicative of acute HIV infection but also may be due to a drug reaction or another medical condition.

Exposures for which PEP is considered appropriate, the concerned HCP should be informed that (1) knowledge about the efficacy of drugs used for PEP is limited; (2) experts recommend combination drug regimens because of increased potency and concerns about drug-resistant virus; (3) data regarding toxicity of antiretroviral drugs in persons without HIV infection or in pregnant women are limited; (4) although the short-term toxicity of antiretroviral drugs is usually limited, serious adverse events have occurred in persons taking PEP; and (5) any or all drugs for PEP may be declined or stopped by the exposed person. HCP who have HIV occupational exposures for which PEP is not recommended should be informed that the potential side effects and toxicity of taking PEP outweigh the negligible risk of transmission posed by the type of exposure.

Recommendations for Nonoccupational PEP

Formal guidelines for the use of nPEP have been published in several US States (California,[50] Massachusetts,[51] Rhode Island,[52] and New York[53]) as well as in British Columbia,[54] Australia,[54a] the United Kingdom,[55] and Europe.[55a] Among these documents, there are some variations in the specific aspects of the recommendations, such as the maximal time after an exposure that nPEP should be offered, the number of antiretroviral drugs that should be prescribed, and the specific drug regimens that should be used. This section summarizes the DHHS guidelines for the use of antiretroviral postexposure prophylaxis for nonoccupational HIV exposures, published in January 2005.[2] Guidance on the use of PEP for nonoccupational exposures occurring in children can be found in the guidelines published by the American Academy of Pediatrics.[73] The DHHS pediatric antiretroviral treatment guidelines provide dosing of antiretroviral agents in children.[74]

Considerations When Deciding Whether to Prescribe Nonoccupational PEP

The algorithm for the recommended management of nonoccupational HIV exposures is shown in Figure 34-1. The primary considerations are the characteristics of the exposure, the timing of the exposed person's presentation relative to the exposure, and the HIV status of the source. In general, PEP is only recommended for those nonoccupational exposures that are believed to confer a substantial exposure risk, in which the source is known to be HIV-infected, and in which the exposed person presents within 72 h postexposure.

When the source HIV status is unknown, but the exposed person presents within 72 h and the characteristics of the exposure are such that it would pose a substantial risk if the source were HIV-infected, the decision about use of nPEP should be made on a case-by-case basis, considering all available information about the source person and the likelihood that the exposure source is infected. If the exposure source is available for testing, use of an approved rapid HIV test kit (which will give results within minutes) is preferable. However, if the risk associated with the exposure is thought to be high, and either the source or rapid testing is not available, nPEP can be initiated and then discontinued if the source HIV status is later determined to be negative.

When the characteristics of the exposure indicate that there is not a substantial risk of infection, or when the exposed person presents more than 72 h postexposure, nPEP is not recommended. However, the absolute upper limit of time postexposure, beyond which nPEP is unlikely to be effective, is not known with certainty. Clinicians may therefore wish to consider nPEP for exposures to known HIV-infected sources which confer a serious risk of transmission, even if the exposed presents >72 h postexposure, if clinical judgment suggests that the risk of transmission far outweighs the risk of toxicity from antiretroviral medications.

Selection of an nPEP Regimen

Based upon the assumption that maximal suppression of viral replication will provide the best chance of preventing infection, the DHHS guidelines recommend three-drug regimens for nonoccupational exposures. The regimen may be selected from those currently recommended as initial therapy in infected persons.[27] These latter guidelines for treatment of HIV-infected individuals are updated several times a year, as new data on efficacy and toxicity of antiretroviral medications emerge. The current recommendations can be found at www.aidsinfo.nih.gov.

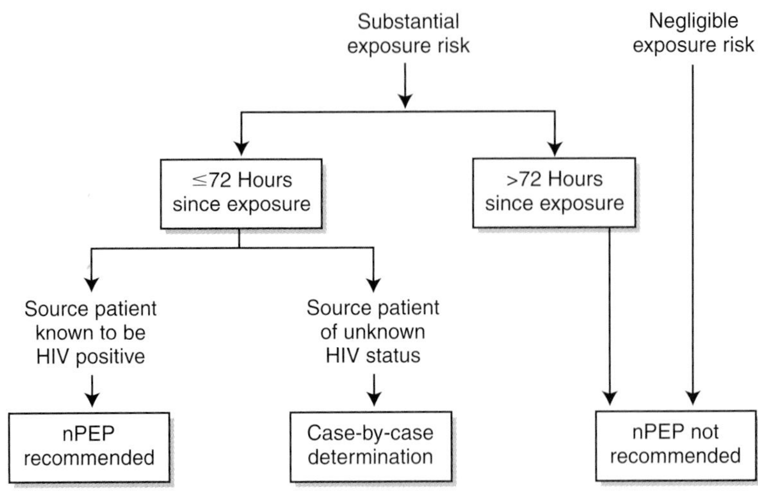

Substantial risk for HIV exposure
Exposure of
vagina, rectum, eye, mouth, or other mucous membrane, nonintact skin, or percutaneous contact
With
blood, semen, vaginal secretions, rectal secretions, breast milk, or any body fluid that is visibly contaminated with blood
When
the source is known to be HIV-infected

Negligible risk for HIV exposure
Exposure of
vagina, rectum, eye, mouth, or other mucous membrane, intact or nonintact skin, or percutaneous contact
With
urine, nasal secretions, saliva, sweat, or tears if not visibly contaminated with blood
Regardless
of the known or suspected HIV status of the source

Figure 34-1 ■ Algorithm for the evaluation and treatment of possible nonoccupational HIV exposures.

Redrawn from CDC. Antiretroviral postexposure prophylaxis after sexual, injection drug use, or other nonoccupational exposure to HIV in the United States: recommendations from the US Department of Health and Human Services. MMWR 54(RR-2):1–20, 2005.[62]

For those exposures in which the source is known to be HIV-infected, and where information regarding his or her treatment history and any resistance studies is readily available, consultation with an expert in HIV treatment is recommended in order to choose a regimen that is likely to be effective against the source virus. If this information cannot be gathered quickly, however, and if it is believed that use of nPEP is warranted, initiation of antiretrovirals should not be delayed. The nPEP regimen can be changed later if necessary.

Laboratory Testing and Follow-Up Care

Follow-up of persons with potential nonoccupational HIV exposures is similar to that of persons with occupational HIV exposure. In addition, as exposures to HIV may also involve exposure to other infections, such as gonorrhea, chlamydia, syphilis, and hepatitis B and C, additional tests for these infections also should be performed.[75] For women of childbearing potential, pregnancy testing at presentation is advisable, and may affect the choice of antiretroviral agents for PEP (EFV, for example, should not be used during pregnancy). Additional testing including, at a minimum, a complete blood count with differential, hepatic function tests, and renal function tests, should be ordered at baseline and monitored during nPEP in order to note any potential early drug toxicity. Viral load testing (HIV DNA or RNA assays) is not recommended as a component of routine postexposure follow-up. Such assays may reveal low-level viremia in persons who are uninfected, possibly leading to misdiagnosis of HIV infection.[70]

Risk Reduction Counseling

With the exception of sexual assault survivors and individuals who sustain accidental needlesticks, many nonoccupational HIV exposures occur as a result of failure to adopt risk-reduction strategies (for example, use of condoms and sterile injection equipment). In these instances, discussion of ongoing risk behaviors and counseling should be offered, regardless of whether nPEP is initiated. Patients who take nPEP should be advised that it is not 100% effective, and that they should continue to practice safe behaviors throughout the nPEP course to lower risk of transmission to others should they become infected.

Persons who engage in frequent and recurrent high-risk activities (for example, discordant sex partners who rarely use condoms or injection-drug users who often share injection equipment), would require multiple and perhaps near-continuous courses of antiretroviral medications. In these circumstances, the risk of drug toxicity becomes more serious, making use of nPEP undesirable. Under these circumstances, exposed individuals should receive intensive risk-reduction counseling in order to help them avoid future exposures.

CONCLUSION

In conclusion, PEP is an option for decreasing transmission of HIV after either occupational or nonoccupational exposure. However, the primary strategy for preventing transmission is through prevention of exposures, by adherence to safe work practices and behaviors.

REFERENCES

1. CDC. Updated Public Health Service (PHS) guidelines for the management of occupational exposures to HIV and recommendations for postexposure prophylaxis (PEP). MMWR CDC 54(RR-9), 1–17, 2005.
2. CDC. Antiretroviral postexposure prophylaxis after sexual, injection drug use, or other nonoccupational exposure to HIV in the United States: recommendations from the US Department of Health and Human Services. MMWR CDC 54(RR-2):1–20, CDC 2005.
3. Bell DM. Occupational risk of human immunodeficiency virus infection in healthcare workers: an overview. Am J Med 102(Suppl 5B):9–15, 1997.
4. Cardo D, Culver DM, Ciesielski C, et al. A case-control study of HIV seroconversion in health care workers after percutaneous exposure. New Eng J Med 337:1485–90, 1997.
5. DeCock KM, Janssen RS. An unequal epidemic in an unequal world. J Am Med Assoc 288:236–8, 2002.
6. UNAIDS/World Health Organization. AIDS epidemic update: Dec 2005. Available: http://www.searo.who.int/LinkFiles/Facts_and_Figures_PDFepiupdate2005.pdf 5 Jun 2006.
7. Kaplan EH, Heimer R. A model-based estimate of HIV infectivity via needle sharing. J Acquir Immune Defic Syndr 5:1116–18, 1992.
8. Varghese B, Maher JE, Peterman TA, et al. Reducing the risk of sexual HIV transmission: quantifying the per-act risk for HIV on the basis of choice of partner, sex act, and condom use. Sex Transm Dis 29:38–43, 2002.
9. Donegan E, Stuart M, Niland JC, et al. Infection with human immunodeficiency virus type 1 (HIV-1) among recipients of antibody-positive blood donations. Ann Intern Med 113:733–9, 1990.
10. DeGruttola V, Seage GR III, Mayer KH, et al. In factiousness of HIV between male homosexual partners. J Clinical Epidemiol 42:849–56, 1989.
11. European Study Group. Comparison of female to male and male to female transmission of HIV in 563 stable couples. BMJ 304:809–13, 1992.
12. Piguet V, Blauvelt A. Essential roles for dendritic cells in the pathogenesis and potential treatment of HIV disease. J Invest Dermatol 119:365–9, 2002.
13. Spira AI, Marx PA, Patterson BK, et al. Cellular targets of infection and route of viral dissemination after an intravaginal inoculation of simian immunodeficiency virus into rhesus macaques. J Exp Med 183:215–25, 1996.
14. Black RJ. Animal studies of prophylaxis. Am J Med 102(Suppl 5B):39–44, 1997.
15. Tsai C-C, Emau P, Follis KE, et al. Effectiveness of postinoculation (R)-9-(2-phosphonylmethoxypropyl) adenine treatment for prevention of persistent simian immunodeficiency virus SIVmne infection depends critically on timing of initiation and duration of treatment. J Virol 72:4265–73, 1998.
16. Le Grand R, Vaslin B, Larghero J, et al. Post-exposure prophylaxis with highly active antiretroviral therapy could not protect macaques from infection with SIV/HIV chimera. AIDS 14:1864–6, 2000.
17. Otten RA, Smith DK, Adams DR, et al. Efficacy of postexposure prophylaxis after intravaginal exposure of pig-tailed macaques to a human-derived retrovirus (human immunodeficiency virus type 2). J Virol 74:9771–5, 2000.
18. McClure HM, Anderson DC, Ansari AA, et al. Nonhuman primate models for evaluation of AIDS therapy. Ann NY Acad Sci 616:287–98, 1990.
19. LaFon, Lehrman SN, Barry DW. Prophylactically administered Retrovir® in health care workers potentially exposed to the human immunodeficiency virus. J Infect Dis 158:503, 1988.
20. LaFon SW, Mooney BD, McMullen JP, et al. A double-blind, placebo-controlled study of the safety and efficacy of retrovir (zidovudine, ZDV) as a chemoprophylactic agent in health care workers exposed to HIV. In: Program and Abstracts of the 30th Interscience Conference on Antimicrobial Agents and Chemotherapy. Washington, DC, American Society for Microbiology, 1990, abstract 489.
21. Connor EM, Sperling RS, Gelber R, et al. Reduction of maternal-infant transmission of human immunodeficiency virus type 1 with zidovudine treatment. N Engl J Med 331:1173–80, 1994.
22. Sperling RS, Shapiro DE, Coombs RW, et al. Maternal viral load, zidovudine treatment, and the risk of transmission of human immunodeficiency virus type 1 from mother to infant. N Engl J Med 335:1621–9, 1996.
23. Wade NA, Birkhead GS, Warren BL, et al. Abbreviated regimens of zidovudine prophylaxis and perinatal transmission of the human immunodeficiency virus. N Engl J Med 339:1409–14, 1998.
24. De Cock K, Fowler MG, Mercier E, et al. Prevention of mother-to-child HIV transmission in resource-poor countries: translating research into policy and practice. JAMA 283:1175–82, 2000.
25. Roland ME, Neilands TB, Krone MR, et al. Seroconversion following nonoccupational postexposure prophylaxis against HIV. Clin Infect Dis 41(10):1514–16, 2005.
26. Poynten M, Smith DE, Grulich AE. Final results from the Australian non-occupational post-exposure prophylaxis (NPEP) observational study. Abstract, 16th Annual Conference of the Australasian Society for HIV Medicine, Canberra, 2004.
27. Panel on Clinical Practices for Treatment of HIV Infection. Guidelines for the use of antiretroviral agents in HIV-infected adults and adolescents – 10 October 2006. Available: http://aidsinfo.nih.gov/ContentFiles/AdultandAdolescentGL.pdf5 Jul 2007.
28. CDC. Serious adverse events attributed to nevirapine regimens for postexposure prophylaxis after HIV exposures. MMWR 49:1153–6, 2001.
29. Wang SA, Panlilio AL, Doi PA, et al. HIV PEP Registry Group. Experience of healthcare workers taking post-exposure prophylaxis after occupational human immunodeficiency virus exposures: findings of the HIV Postexposure Prophylaxis Registry. Infect Control Hosp Epidemiol 21:780–5, 2000.
30. Swotinsky RB, Steger KA, Sulis C, Snyder S, et al. Occupational exposure to HIV: experience at a tertiary care center. J Occup Environ Med 40:1102–9, 1998.
31. Parkin JM, Murphy M, Anderson J, et al. Tolerability and side-effects of post-exposure prophylaxis for HIV infection. Lancet 355:722–3, 2000.
32. Puro V. Post-exposure prophylaxis for HIV infection. Italian Registry of Post-Exposure Prophylaxis. Lancet 355:1556–7, 2000.

33. Lee LM, Henderson DK. Tolerability of postexposure antiretroviral prophylaxis for occupational exposures to HIV. Drug Saf 24:587–97, 2001.
34. Russi M, Buitrago M, Goulet J, et al. Antiretroviral prophylaxis of health care workers at two urban medical centers. J Occup Environ Med 42:1092–100, 2000.
35. Garb JR. One-year study of occupational human immunodeficiency virus postexposure prophylaxis. J Occup Environ Med 44:265–70, 2002.
36. Grime PR, Risi L, Binns C, et al. Pan-Thames survey of occupational exposure to HIV and the use of post-exposure prophylaxis in 71 NHS Trusts. J Infec 42:27–32, 2001.
37. Puro V, DeCarli G, Soldani F, et al. Adverse drug reactions associated with PEP. In: Program and Abstracts of the 10th Conference on Retroviruses and Opportunistic Infections. Boston, MA, Feb 2003, Poster #711.
38. Almeda J, Marincovich B, Casabona K, et al. The European Non Occupational Post-Exposure Prophylaxis (NONOPEP) Registry: demand and use of antiretrovirals (ARV) to prevent HIV-infection. Post Exhibition: The XV International AIDS Conference: Abstract no. TuPeB4671.
39. Moyle G, Boffito M. Unexpected drug interactions and adverse events with antiretroviral drugs. Lancet 364:8–10, 2004.
40. Andrade A, Flexner C. Progress in pharmacology and drug interactions from the 10th Conference on Retroviruses and Opportunistic Infections. Hopkins HIV Rep 15:7–11, 2003.
41. de Maat MM, Ekhart GC, Huitema AD, et al. Drug interactions between antiretroviral drugs and comedicated agents. Clin Pharmacokine 42:223–82, 2003.
42. Catanzaro LM, Slish JC, DiCenzo R, Morse GD. Drug interactions with antiretrovirals. Curr HIV/AIDS Rep 1:89–96, 2004.
43. DiPerri G, Marucco DA, Mondo A, et al. Drug-drug interactions and tolerance in combining antituberculosis and antiretroviral therapy. Expert Opin Drug Saf 4:821–36, 2005.
44. Fichtenbaum CJ, Gerber JG. Interactions between antiretroviral drugs and drugs used for the therapy of the metabolic complications encountered during HIV infection. Clin Pharmacokinet 41:1195–211, 2002.
45. Piscitelli SC, Gallicano KD. Interactions among drugs for HIV and opportunistic infections. NEJM 334: 984–96, 2001.
46. University of California at San Francisco Center for HIV Information. Database of antiretroviral drug interactions. Available: http://hivinsite.ucsf.edu/InSite?page=ar-00-0213 Mar 2006.
47. Gerberding JL. Clinical practice. Occupational exposure to HIV in health care settings. N Engl J Med 348:826–33, 2003.
48. New York State Department of Health AIDS Institute. HIV prophylaxis following occupational exposure. Available: http://www.hivguidelines.org/public_html/oe/oe.pdf13 Mar 2006.
49. Puro V, Cicalini S, De Carli G, et al. Towards a standard HIV postexposure prophylaxis for healthcare workers in Europe. Euro Surveill 9:40–3, 2004.
50. California Task Force on non-occupational PEP and California Department of Health Services, Office of AIDS. Offering HIV post-exposure prophylaxis following non-occupational exposures. Recommendations for the State of California, Jun 2004. Available: http://www.dhs.ca.gov/aids/Resources/pdf/pepguidelinesfinal.pdf last accessed and checked 24 July 2007.
51. Commonwealth of Massachusetts Department of Public Health. Clinical Advisory: HIV prophylaxis for non-occupational exposures. Available: http://www.mass.gov?pageID=eohhs2terminal&L=6&L0=Home&L1=Provider&L2=Guidelines+and+Resources&L3=Guidelines+for+Clinical+Treatment&L4=Diseases+%26+Conditions&L5=HIV-AIDS&sid=Eeohhs2&b=terminalcontent&f=dph_aids_p_clinadv_non_occup_exposure&csid=Eeohhs2 Accessed 24 July 2007.
52. Merchant RC, Mayer KH, Browning CA. Nonoccupational HIV post-exposure prophylaxis: guidelines for Rhode Island from the Brown University AIDS Program and the RI Department of Health. Med Health RI 85:244–8, 2002.
53. New York State Department of Health AIDS Institute. HIV prophylaxis following non-occupational exposure including sexual assault, Dec 2005. Available: http://www.hivguidelines.org/GuideLine.aspx?pageID=78&guideLineID=2. Accessed 24 July 2007.
54. British Columbia Centre for Excellence in HIV/AIDS. Accidental Exposure Guidelines. Available:http://www.cfenet.ubc.ca/webuploads/files/06_2849_AE_Guidelines_Final.pdf. Accessed 24 July 2007.
54a. Australian Government Department of Health and Ageing. National guidelines for post exposure prophylaxis after non-occupational exposure to HIV. Available http://www.ashm.org.au/uploads/File/2007-national-NPEP-guidelines.pdf Accessed 24 July 2007.
55. Fisher M, Benn P, Evans B, et al. UK Guideline for the use of post-exposure prophylaxis for HIV following sexual exposure. Int J STD AIDS 17(2):81–92, 2006.
55a. European Non Occupational Post-Exposure Prophylaxis Group. Proposed recommendations for the management of HIV post-exposure prophylaxis after sexual, injecting drug or other exposures in Europe. Eurosurveillance Monthly 9:5–6, 2004.
56. Hirsch MS, Brun-Vézinet F D, Aquila RT, et al. Antiretroviral drug resistance testing in adult HIV-1 infection: recommendations of an international AIDS Society-USA panel. JAMA 283:2417–26, 2000.
57. Gallant JE.Antiretroviral drug resistance and resistance testing. Top HIV Med 2005 13:138–42, 2006.
58. Beltrami EM, Cheingsong R, Heneine WM, et al. Antiretroviral drug resistance in human immunodeficiency virus-infected source patients for occupational exposures to healthcare workers. Infect Control Hosp Epidemiol 24:724–30, 2003.
59. Jochimsen EM. Failures of zidovudine postexposure prophylaxis. Am J Med 102(Suppl 5B):52–5, 1997.
60. Updated U.S. Public Health Service guidelines for the management of occupational exposures to HBV, HCV, and HIV and recommendations for postexposure prophylaxis. MMWR 50(RR-11), 1–52, 2001.
61. Hawkins DA, Asboe D, Barlow K, Evans B. Seroconversion to HIV-1 following a needlestick injury despite combination post-exposure prophylaxis. J Infect 43:12–18, 2001.
62. Do AN, Ciesielski CA, Metler RP, et al. Occupationally acquired human immunodeficiency virus (HIV) infection: national case surveillance data during 20 years of the HIV epidemic in the United States. Infect Control Hosp Epidemiol 24:86–96, 2003.
63. Kinloch-de Loës S, Hirschel BJ, Hoen B, et al. A controlled trial of zidovudine in primary human immunodeficiency virus infection. N Engl J Med 333:408–13, 1995.
64. CDC. Update: provisional Public Health Service recommendations for chemoprophylaxis after occupational exposure to HIV. MMWR 45:468–72, 1996.
65. CDC. Public Health Service guidelines for the management of health-care worker exposures to HIV and recommendations for postexposure prophylaxis. MMWR 47(RR-7):1–33, 1998.
66. Ridzon R, Gallagher K, Ciesielski C, et al. Simultaneous transmission of human immunodeficiency virus and hepatitis C virus from a needle-stick injury. N Engl J Med 336:919–22, 1997.
67. Ciesielski CA, Metler RP. Duration of time between exposure and seroconversion in healthcare workers with occupationally acquired infection with human immunodeficiency virus. Am J Med 102(Suppl 5B):115–16, 1997.
68. Busch MP, Satten GA. Time course of viremia and antibody seroconversion following human immunodeficiency virus exposure. Am J Med 102(Suppl 5B):117–24, 1997.

69. Rich JD, Merriman NA, Mylonakis E, et al. Misdiagnosis of HIV infection by HIV-1 plasma viral load testing: a case series. Ann Intern Med 130:37–39, 1999.
70. Roland ME, Elbeik TA, Kahn JO, et al. HIV RNA testing in the context of nonoccupational postexposure prophylaxis. J Infect Dis 190:598–604, 2004.
71. Armstrong K, Gorden R, Santorella G. Occupational exposure of health care workers (HCWs) to human immunodeficiency virus (HIV): stress reactions and counseling interventions. Social Work in Health Care 21:61–80, 1995.
72. Meienberg F, Bucher HC, Sponagel L, et al. Anxiety in health care workers after exposure to potentially HIV-contaminated blood or body fluids. Swiss Med Wkly 132:321–4, 2002.
73. Havens PL. Committee on Pediatric AIDS. Postexposure prophylaxis in children and adolescents for nonoccupational exposure to human immunodeficiency virus. Pediatrics 111:1475–89, 2003.
74. The Working Group on Antiretroviral Therapy and Medical Management of HIV-Infected Children. Guidelines for the use of antiretroviral agents in pediatric HIV infection—26 October 2006. Available http://aidsinfo.nih.gov/contentfiles/PediatricGuidelines.pdf Accessed 24 July 2007.
75. CDC. Sexually transmitted diseases guidelines, 2002. MMWR 55(RR-11):1–94, 2006.

Chapter 35

Managing Pregnant Patients

James McIntyre, FRCOG

INTRODUCTION

The AIDS epidemic continues to affect many millions of people globally. UNAIDS estimated that there were 39.5 million people living with HIV in 2006, of which 17.7 million (almost half) were women and 2.3 million children.[1] More than 75% of these women live in sub-Saharan Africa (SSA), which is also home to most of the 700 000 new infections in children each year. Central Asia and Eastern Europe continue to see increases in new infections in women, while the epidemic appears to have stabilized more in Western Europe and the United States. In Western Europe, an increasing proportion of heterosexual infections are diagnosed in immigrants, particularly from SSA,[2–4] as may be expected with the higher prevalence rates in these countries of origin. This may impact on the care of pregnant women if they do not have full access to HIV and maternity care services.

In the United States, the absolute number of infections has decreased from a peak in 1992.[5] While most cases continue to be seen in men, the proportion of infections in women has risen from 15% in the period 1981–95 to 27% in the period 2001–04.[6] This correlates with an increase in the heterosexual mode of transmission from 10% to 30%. An additional racial skewing of the epidemic has been seen in the United States with 51% of new cases in 2001–04 occurring in blacks with a case rate in black women 21 times higher than that seen in white women (67 per 100 000 compared to 3.2 per 100 000). Although HIV infection in pregnancy is less common in some areas of the United States, these changes in the epidemiologic pattern mean that it continues to be a major concern in others.

The differences in HIV prevalence between developed and less developed countries are also seen in the rates of mother-to-child transmission (MTCT) of HIV. Although 700 000 infected children are born in the world each year, more than a decade of advances in MTCT prevention strategies has resulted in a reduction of infections in the US and Europe which make pediatric HIV infection there a relatively rare event. Transmission rates in the US have dropped to below 2%, with an estimate of only between 144 and 236 infected children born in the US in 2002.[7] Put another way, one HIV-infected child is born every minute in the less developed parts of the world, less than one a day in the most developed countries.

The counseling and care of HIV-infected pregnant women must consider the impact of the pregnancy on HIV disease, maternal health and choice of therapy, and the effect of HIV on pregnancy outcome, including the risk of MTCT of HIV. The mother's life expectancy, her longer-term parenting plans and the follow-up needs of the infant should be discussed in the counseling. The benefits and risks of specific treatments should be discussed, and recommendations for starting or continuing antiretroviral therapy during pregnancy must take into account the woman's choice, previous or current antiretroviral therapy, gestational age, maternal CD4+ T-lymphocyte count and HIV RNA level, and the potential toxicities.. Guidelines for the use of antiretrovirals in pregnancy are updated frequently, as new information becomes available, and are available on the World Wide Web, and health providers caring for HIV-infected pregnant women are advised to consult the most current applicable guidelines for up-to-date information.[8–10]

IMPACT OF PREGNANCY ON MATERNAL HEALTH

Maternal Health and HIV

Most data from the United States and Europe suggest that pregnancy does not accelerate HIV disease progression.[11–16] A similar situation has been described in Thailand.[17] Although a systematic review and meta-analysis of seven cohort studies in HIV-infected women from 1983 to 1996 suggested a weak association between death, disease progression and progression to an AIDS-defining illness and pregnancy, this association was stronger in the one study conducted in a resource-poor setting.[18] In this meta-analysis, the summary odds ratios for the risk of an adverse maternal outcome related to HIV infection and pregnancy were 1.8 (85% confidence interval (CI), 0.99–3.3) for death, 1.41 (95% CI, 0.85–2.33) for HIV disease progression and 1.63 (95% CI, 1.00–2.67) for progression to an AIDS-defining illness, although this research reflects the situation prior to widespread use of highly active antiretroviral therapy (HAART). Data from the US Women and Infants Transmission Study (WITS) over a 12-year period from 1989 to 2002 showed a 70% reduction in progression to death following AIDS associated with HAART.[19] Minkoff and colleagues studied the effect of pregnancy on progression of HIV disease in 953 women in the United States who had no additional pregnancy after the index pregnancy, compared with 329 women who had a second pregnancy subsequent to their index pregnancy. They showed no compared significant differences in the immunologic, clinical, and virologic courses of women with a subsequent pregnancy, compared to those without.[20] In a more recent cohort of 786 women with access to HAART, pregnancy was associated with a lower rate of progression to AIDS defining illnesses.[21] No benefit to maternal health has been demonstrated by pregnancy termination.

CD4+ T-lymphocyte counts drop during pregnancy in both HIV-infected and uninfected women, but will generally rebound in the postpartum period.[22–26] The drop in CD4+ counts may be more pronounced in women not receiving HAART than in those on therapy. One study in Ireland showed a decrease in CD4+ counts of 27% in those not on HAART compared to 13% on HAART.[27] The pregnancy related decrease in CD4+ count may impact on treatment decisions where CD4+ count is one of the eligibility criteria for HAART, especially where pregnant women who do not qualify for ongoing HAART will otherwise receive only shorter antiretroviral regimens for prevention of MTCT (PMTCT). This may result in "over treatment" of a significant number of women whose CD4+ counts would return to higher levels postpregnancy. It has been suggested that CD4+ percentage is less variable during pregnancy and may be a more reliable or robust measure than absolute CD4+ count in pregnant women.[28] At present, most national and international guidelines have not recommended changing to use of CD4+ percentage, and continue to use absolute CD4+ counts for treatment decisions.

HIV infection may be associated with reduced fertility, in reports from Africa and from resource-rich settings.[29–36] Birth intervals are longer in HIV-positive women in some studies, and a prolonged time to achieve conception has been associated with higher viral load.[37,38]A prospective Ugandan study showed lower rates of pregnancy and more pregnancy loss in HIV-positive compared to HIV-negative women.[39] Lowered fertility may also be associated with menstrual abnormalities in severely ill positive women with weight loss.[40]

Maternal Mortality and HIV

In developed countries the availability of specialist HIV treatment and care in pregnancy makes HIV a rare cause of maternal mortality. Pregnancy may impact more on the progression and outcome of HIV infection in less resourced settings, leading to more rapid progression to AIDS or death.[41,42] Although specific data on disease progression in pregnancy is limited, there is evidence from several studies in Africa that HIV has become a significant contributing cause of maternal mortality.[43–48] HIV/AIDS related conditions may worsen postpregnancy, manifesting in the first year after delivery and thus may be underestimated in official maternal mortality figures.[49] This postpregnancy mortality is demonstrated in several reports. In Zaire, the maternal mortality rates in HIV-infected women were ten times those of HIV-negative women[50]; with 22% of HIV-infected mothers dying during a 3-year follow-up period. In a prospective study in Malawi, the maternal mortality rate was 370 per 100000 women and the mortality rate between 6 weeks and 1 year postpartum was 341 per 100000 live births, with AIDS and anemia the major causes of postpregnancy mortality.[51]

The risk of more rapid HIV progression during and after pregnancy may be influenced by multiple factors, including nutritional and maternal genetic factors. Progression postpregnancy may be more rapid in women who have anemia during pregnancy [52] and delayed by the administration of multivitamin supplements.[53] A Kenyan study demonstrated that an increase in mortality postpregnancy was correlated with CCR5 promoter polymorphisms. This study showed a three-fold increase in death within 2 years in women (95% CI, 1.0–9.5) with the 59356 C/T genotype compared with women with the 59356 C/C genotype.[54]

In high prevalence areas, the impact of HIV on maternal mortality may be mitigated by the effect of reduced fertility in HIV-infected women. In a situation where fewer HIV-positive women become pregnant, HIV-linked mortality may be reduced or maternal mortality figures may even decline. As evidence of this, a study in the Congo has shown a 32 times higher mortality rate in HIV-infected women than uninfected, but a higher relative increase in nonpregnant than pregnant women.[55] In these settings, maternal mortality also impacts on child survival, with children more likely to die if their mothers die.[56–58] This may negate any improvements in survival of children achieved by PMTCT programs unless appropriate antiretroviral treatment for mothers is also instituted.

MTCT OF HIV

The development and implementation of strategies to prevent MTCT of HIV represents one of the most successful responses to the AIDS epidemic. Within the space of a decade, from 1994, perinatal HIV infection has been dramatically reduced in the United States, Europe and other developed world settings, and less expensive, more feasible regimens have been successfully used in less-resourced settings. Transmission rates in the US and Europe have dropped to less than 2%, with the widespread access to interventions for the PMTCT of HIV.[7] Despite this progress, more remains to be done to make interventions available to all of the 2 million HIV-infected pregnant women globally each year. Worldwide, 1800 children are infected each day and UNICEF estimates that a child dies every minute of every day from HIV infection, almost all of which is transmitted from mother to the child.[1,59] UNAIDS estimates that less than 8% of pregnant women worldwide are offered PMTCT services, dropping to under 6% in SSA, and that only 9% of HIV-infected pregnant women worldwide received antiretroviral prophylaxis for PMTCT in 2006.[1] In the 33 most affected countries, an estimated 26% of children born to HIV-infected mothers were themselves infected in 2005. Although this represents a 10% decrease from the estimated transmission rate in 2001, it illustrates the huge gap between the situation in these countries and the USA or Europe.

Factors Affecting MTCT

MTCT of HIV can occur *in utero*, during labor and delivery or through breast milk, although the bulk of transmission occurs during the intrapartum period.[60 61] These proportions of infection will change according to the availability of prevention interventions. Treating with HAART throughout pregnancy will almost eliminate antepartum and intrapartum transmission, while short-course antiretroviral interventions will have little effect on *in utero* transmission, but can dramatically reduce intrapartum transmission.[62,63] In nonbreastfeeding populations, about one-third (ranging from 20% to 60%) of transmissions appear to occur *in utero*, with the remaining two-thirds (from 40% to 80%) occurring during labor and delivery.[64–69] Evidence suggestive of intrapartum transmission includes delayed detection of HIV by culture, antigen detection, or DNA in the neonate;[66–68] later onset of clinical symptoms;[65] detection of HIV in cervicovaginal secretions of infected women that is reduced after antiretroviral therapy and has been shown to reduce transmission;[69–71] significantly higher transmission rates in the first-born twin compared to the second-born twin;[72] the association of higher transmission rates with increasing duration of ruptured membranes during labor;[73–75] and reduced transmission among women delivered by cesarean section before labor and membrane rupture.[76,77]

The risk of MTCT varies by maternal stage of disease, high viral load, low CD4+ count, use of antiretroviral therapy, mode of delivery, duration of rupture of membranes, increased genital secretion of HIV, the practice of breastfeeding and other factors such as prematurity (Table 35-1).

High viral load is the most consistently correlated factor with risk of transmission.[78–80] Other viral factors have been associated with increased risk of transmission, although less so than viral load, including viral phenotype,[81–84] and viral genotype.[85–87] It has been suggested that there may be different patterns of viral strain transmission at different times, with antepartum transmission more likely to be associated with the predominant maternal viral variant, while intrapartum transmission may be associated with minor viral variants.[88]

Table 35-1 Risk Factors for Perinatal HIV Transmission

Risk Factors
Viral Risk Factors
Viral load
Viral phenotype
Viral genotype
Maternal Risk Factors
CD4+ T-lymphocyte count
Advanced maternal disease
Lack of ARV therapy
ARV resistance
Vitamin A deficiency
STIs/other co-infections
Behavioral Risk Factors
Smoking
Substance abuse
Sexual behavior
Obstetrical Risk Factors
Vaginal delivery
Preterm delivery
Prolonged rupture of membranes
Placental disruption/abruption, chorio-amnionitis
Invasive fetal monitoring
Episiotomy/forceps
Neonatal Risk Factors
Breast milk exposure
Prematurity
Oral thrush
Gender

The role of other maternal or obstetrical factors is most obvious in the absence of antiretroviral therapy, demonstrating the importance of high viral load as a predictor of transmission. These include advanced maternal HIV infection as determined by clinical diagnosis of AIDS, low CD4+ T-lymphocyte count or percentage, longer duration of ruptured membranes before delivery, placental inflammation, and sexuallytransmitted diseases.[42,73–75,89–101]

Other maternal factors which have been implicated with an increased risk of transmission include preterm birth, maternal illicit drug use, vitamin A deficiency, female gender of the infant.[42,73,95,96,102–107] A Malawian study has suggested that microtransfusions across the placenta may play a role in increased transmission with vaginal delivery.[108]

Mode of Delivery and Transmission

Cesarean section has been shown in several studies to reduce the risk of transmission of HIV.[109] An individual patient data meta-analysis including data from 15 prospective cohorts demonstrated a significantly lower infection rate among infants delivered by scheduled cesarean section compared to other modes (emergency cesarean or vaginal delivery), with an unadjusted odds ratio (OR) of 0.45 (95% CI, 0.35–0.58) and an OR of 0.43 (95% CI, 0.33–0.56) adjusted for azidothymidine (AZT) use, maternal disease stage, and birth weight.[110] Among more than 1400 women who received AZT, most on the PACTG 076 schedule, the rate of transmission was 2% with scheduled cesarean delivery and 7% with other modes of delivery. An international randomized trial produced similar results, with a transmission rate of 1.8% among women assigned to scheduled cesarean delivery and 10.5% in those assigned to deliver vaginally (OR, 0.2, 95% CI, 0.1–0.6).[77] In an analysis stratified by AZT use, the transmission rate was 4% with scheduled cesarean delivery and 20% with vaginal delivery among those not on antiretroviral agents (adjusted OR, 0.2, 95% CI, 0–0.8), 1% with scheduled cesarean delivery, and 4% with vaginal delivery for those receiving AZT (adjusted OR 0.2, 95% CI, 0–1.7). The magnitude of the reduced transmission was similar in the two groups; but because of the small number of transmissions (six in total) in the AZT group, the difference was not statistically significant. In both studies the risk of transmission was not reduced by cesarean section performed after labor or if rupture of membranes had occurred. Neither of these studies included HIV RNA determinations or women on HAART, making it impossible to determine the potential benefit of scheduled cesarean section among women with undetectable HIV RNA or on combination therapy.

Most of the trials that demonstrate the protective effect of elective cesarean section were performed before combination antiretroviral therapy was in widespread use in developed countries. There is less evidence that cesarean section provides additional reduction in MTCT in women receiving highly active combination antiretroviral regimens who have low or undetectable maternal HIV-1 RNA levels and there does not appear to be a threshold of HIV RNA levels below which transmission does not occur. However, it has been suggested that vaginal delivery could be considered in mothers with very low or undetectable viral load. In a meta-analysis of seven prospective studies from the US and Europe there were 44 transmissions in 1020 deliveries where maternal plasma viral load was <1000 HIV RNA copies/mL at or around delivery.[111] The transmission rate for mothers on antiretroviral treatment was 1% compared to 9.8% for those on no treatment. Transmission was lower with those receiving antiretrovirals and cesarean section suggesting a protective effect of both interventions, even at very low viral loads. A cost-effectiveness analysis suggests that the MTCT rate would have to be less than 0.5% before cesarean section would be no longer cost-effective.[112] However, reported transmission rates in women on HAART with low undetectable viral loads have shown transmission rates of 0–3%[113] and elective cesarean section may not provide additional reductions in transmission. In Europe, data suggest that cesarean section may still have an additional beneficial role, even where suppressive antiretroviral therapy is available.[114,115] For those women who have access to HAART, a decision on mode of delivery should include consideration of the viral load level and clinical status. The American College of Obstetrics and Gynecology has suggested that elective cesarean section should be recommended at viral loads of >1000 copies/mL.[116] Based on current data, guidelines recommend discussing scheduled cesarean delivery with all pregnant women, emphasizing the potential benefits for women with HIV RNA levels above 1000 copies/mL and indicating the lesser probability of benefit for women with lower HIV RNA levels.[8]

Other Obstetric Factors and Transmission

Increased risks of transmission have been described with some obstetric factors, although the magnitude of risk is much less than that associated with high viral load or mode of delivery. The relative importance of these factors is likely to be much diminished where effective antiretroviral therapy is in place. The risk of MTCT is associated with the duration of rupture of membranes during labor. In a study of 505 HIV-infected women, in those with membranes that ruptured more than 4 h before delivery, the rate of transmission of HIV-1 to the infants was 25%, as compared with 14% among mothers with membranes that ruptured 4 h or less before delivery.[75] Women with low CD4+ levels were significantly more likely to transmit HIV to their offspring if the duration of rupture of membranes was 4 h or beyond.[74] In a meta-analysis of 4721 deliveries with duration of ruptured membranes before 24 h, the risk of transmission increased ~2% for every hour of rupture of membranes (ROM) up to 24 h. In women with an AIDS diagnosis the risk of transmission increased from 8% after 2 h of ROM to 31% after 24 h.[117] As artificial ROM has little obstetric benefit in normal labor, it should not be performed routinely in known HIV-positive women or areas of high HIV prevalence. Use of artificial ROM should be reserved for cases where there is fetal distress or delay in progress of labor.[118,119]

Some invasive obstetric investigations have been associated with higher risk of transmission. Penetrating or spiral scalp electrodes and the use of fetal scalp blood sampling could potentially create a portal of entry for the virus. There is little evidence that this is a significant risk factor, with few studies from high prevalence areas, where these procedures are uncommon, and little confirmation in cohorts who also have access to antiretroviral prophylaxis. In the European Collaborative Study in 19 European centers between 1984 and 1991, prior to widespread use of antiretrovirals, MTCT was higher with vaginal deliveries in which scalp electrodes, forceps, or vacuum extractors were used.[78] Viscarello et al showed no difference in transmission rates in cases where electrodes were used or not used.[120] Most current recommendations suggest the avoidance of any procedure that breaks the infant's skin, unless unavoidable for the health of the baby.

Episiotomy may increase the exposure of the infant to HIV during delivery and increase the risk of MTCT. In the European Collaborative Study between 1941 and 1991, MTCT was higher with vaginal deliveries in which episiotomy was practiced, but only in centers where these procedures were not routine.[78] In another, nonrandomized prospective cohort study among 63 HIV-positive pregnant women and their 68 infants, mothers with events involving fetal exposure to maternal blood were more likely to transmit infection.[121] Even in the presence of zidovudine therapy, episiotomy was associated with a higher rate of HIV RNA positive oropharyngeal and gastric aspirates in a French study.[122]

A Comprehensive Approach to Preventing MTCT

The World Health Organization has promoted a comprehensive approach to preventing MTCT. This includes four components: (1) primary prevention of HIV infection; (2) prevention of unintended pregnancies among HIV-infected women; (3) prevention of HIV transmission from HIV-infected mothers to their infants; and (4) care, treatment and support for HIV-infected mothers, their children and families.[123] All four of these have a role to play in preventing MTCT and optimizing care of HIV-positive women and their children. Counseling, testing and the identification of HIV-positive women is essential to provide the most appropriate care; CD4+ cell counts form a critical link between antenatal care and antiretroviral therapy (ART) services, especially for asymptomatic women. To ensure that all pregnant women who require ART are identified, efforts should be made to include CD4+ cell count measurement in the essential package of care for pregnant women.

HIV TESTING DURING PREGNANCY

Prenatal care provides an opportunity to counsel women about HIV risk and offer HIV testing. In the early years of the HIV epidemic in the United States and other countries, HIV testing was offered only to those women perceived to be "at risk" of infection. With increasing rates of infection in women and improved interventions to reduce the risk of MTCT, came recommendations that counseling about HIV infection and the benefits of testing should be "routine" in pregnancy. As early as 1995, guidelines from the CDC and leading professional associations recommended routine testing,[124,125] but uptake of testing and provision of antiretrovirals for PMTCT remained less than optimal. A review of HIV testing in pregnancy from 1994 to 1999 showed a small increase in the percentage of pregnant women tested from 41% in 1995 to 52% in 1997 and to only 60% by 1998.[126]

This relatively low uptake using an "opt-in" approach, requiring specific informed consent and request for testing, has prompted inclusion in guidelines of an "opt-out" universal approach where all pregnant women are informed that HIV testing will be performed in the routine prenatal tests, unless she declines testing.[127] A CDC review of testing strategies in 2002 showed uptake of testing in 85–98% using an opt-out approach compared to 25–83% using opt-in.[128] An opt-out approach was recommended by the US Institute of Medicine in 1999, endorsed by the American College of Obstetricians and Gynecologists (ACOG) and the American Academy of Pediatrics (AAP)[129] and included in 2003 CDC recommendations.[130] The ACOG issued guidelines in 2004 which include the use of an opt-out prenatal HIV testing approach where legally possible.[131] The ACOG also recommended a repeat offer of HIV testing in the third trimester to women in areas with high HIV prevalence, those known to be at high risk for HIV infection, and women who had declined testing earlier in pregnancy. The success of "opt-out" testing may depend on the attitude and commitment of the health workers offering the test and the community norms.[132,133] Data from a national survey in the US in 2002 show that 69% of women had been tested in pregnancy, but that testing rates were higher with higher income levels and where women reported some perceived HIV risk.[134]

Increased access to HIV testing and the changing epidemiology of the epidemic are increasing the number of women who know their HIV infection status before pregnancy. This is as high as 60–80% of HIV-positive women in the US and UK[8,3] and 38.5% in Argentina.[135] This also applies in some African countries where testing services have been in place for several years. In high HIV-prevalence, low-resource areas in Africa and Asia, the acceptance of HIV testing in pregnancy is high in many settings,[136,137] although other program challenges remain, including fear of recognition by hospital staff and difficulties in delivering results.[138,139] In other places, low uptake of testing has been a barrier to the successful implementation of some PMTCT programs.[140–142] In Botswana, uptake of HIV testing by pregnant women in the PMTCT program was initially low, estimated at only 21% of antenatal clinic attendees in 2001,[143] but the introduction of opt-out testing in 2004 increased testing to rates of over 90%.[144] Similar results have been reported in Cameroon[145] and other areas, and programs are increasingly moving to a routine, "opt-out" testing approach in both developed and developing countries.[146–148]

Women seen for the first time in late pregnancy or in labor are likely to have convergent risk factors, such as drug use or poor social circumstances, which also put them at risk of HIV infection. In some US settings women presenting in labor without a previous HIV test are two to four times more likely to be HIV-infected than women attending prenatal care.[149–151] In developing world settings, there may be less access to prenatal care and women may only attend health facilities late in pregnancy or to deliver.[119] Diagnosis during labor or early postpartum allows for interventions to reduce MTCT.[152–155]

Laboratory-based HIV tests may take too long to provide a result for women in labor and the use of rapid, on-site HIV tests allows for diagnosis in labor and implementation of antiretroviral prophylaxis.[156–159] Successful implementation of on-site rapid testing in labor has been documented in several settings,[160–162] and shown to be acceptable to most women in a large US study.[163] This study, The Mother Infant Rapid Intervention at Delivery (MIRIAD) assessed acceptability and feasibility of rapid testing in labor in six US hospitals. In these settings, 8% of women had undocumented HIV status and were eligible for rapid testing in labor, and 84%

of the almost 6000 women offered testing consented to this. The 2004 ACOG guidelines recommend rapid HIV testing for women in labor with undocumented HIV status; and if a rapid HIV test result is positive, the initiation of antiretroviral prophylaxis for PMTCT (with consent) without waiting for the results of a confirmatory test.[131] Where staffing or infrastructure makes testing difficult in labor, early postpartum diagnosis and access to antiretroviral treatment for the infant is another option.[154,164]

MANAGEMENT OF THE HIV-POSITIVE PREGNANT WOMAN

The management of a pregnant HIV-positive woman will depend on the resources available and the individual needs of the woman. Where resources permit, obstetric and medical care should be provided by a multidisciplinary team, including an HIV treatment specialist, obstetrician, pediatrician and providers of psychosocial support services. Investigations may be limited by resources, but should be as comprehensive as these allow.

Preconception Care for HIV-Infected Women

With increased access to HIV testing, increased access to ART, longer life expectancy and decreased risks of MTCT, more HIV-positive women are likely to know their HIV status before pregnancy.[3,8,165] For these women, preconception care should incorporate discussion of the stage of their HIV infection, including immune status, CD4+ count and viral load, and impact of any treatment regimen. Intensive education may be required and may best be delivered by a multidisciplinary team.[166] Pregnancy planning should take into account and discuss the risks of MTCT, interventions to reduce these risks, and the future care of the child. Contraception may be advised for a period of time to achieve the best possible maternal health status before pregnancy, and medical immunizations (e.g., hepatitis B, pneumococcal, or influenza) may be given if indicated.

ART may be started, or regimens adapted to be 'pregnancy-friendly', with the aim being maximal suppression of viral replication with agents that are also effective in reducing MTCT. Antiretrovirals with potential reproductive toxicity should be avoided where possible (e.g., efavirenz). Preconception care should also initiate appropriate prophylaxis for opportunistic infections, optimize maternal nutritional status, and screen for maternal psychological disorders or substance abuse.[8] Access for HIV-infected women to assisted reproduction technology is supported by many experts in the field, although it may be limited by local regulations or service constraints,[167–169] but successful interventions have been described in HIV-infected women in Europe and elsewhere.[170,171] In some cases, the male partner of an infected woman will not be HIV-infected, and counseling needs to focus on the risk of infection to the partner and possible ways to achieve pregnancy without increasing this risk.[166,172] Where a male partner is HIV-infected with a negative female partner, the use of sperm washing [173,168] and intracytoplasmic sperm injection (ICSI) have been reported to be successful in achieving pregnancy without exposing the HIV-negative female partner to infection.[36,174,175]

Medical Examination and Investigations

The HIV-positive pregnant woman should undergo a thorough history and physical examination to document baseline findings and to allow early identification and treatment of any complications (Table 35-2). Tuberculosis is a common opportunistic infection in HIV-positive pregnant women in many resource-poor areas and should be looked for in these settings or in recent immigrants in developed countries.[176] Depending on local policy, all HIV-positive women should be tested for tuberculosis with a skin test using intermediate strength (5-TU) purified protein derivative (PPD), unless this has been done within the previous year.

Other investigations at baseline should include fundoscopy, and neurologic examination. A pelvic examination should be undertaken, including cervical cytology, and examinations for any signs of other infections. Laboratory investigations, in addition to routine pregnancy laboratory tests, should include liver function tests, complete blood count including platelet count and lymphocyte subsets, and plasma HIV RNA viral load.

HIV-positive women are also likely to be at higher risk of other sexually transmitted infections (STIs), and, where indicated, tests for other STIs, such as *Neisseria gonorrhoeae* and *Chlamydia trachomatis* should be performed and the baseline antibody level for *T. gondii* should be determined if not previously performed. Hepatitis screening may be a routine investigation in pregnancy. Where this is not the case, hepatitis B (HBV) testing should be offered to women from high prevalence areas and hepatitis C (HCV) screening considered where intravenous drug use is common.[3,177]

Prenatal Diagnosis

Prenatal care should include a history and assessment of risk factors for familial or genetic conditions, screening for infectious diseases that may affect the fetus and folic acid supplementation. Screening for Down syndrome, neural tube defects and other chromosomal abnormalities should follow local guidelines but may present a more complex situation. A "triple test" screening combination of α-Fetoprotein, estriol, and human chorionic gonadotropin on maternal serum at 16–20 weeks gestation will detect most neural tube defects and over half the cases of Down syndrome.[178] High level ultrasound scans including assessment of nuchal translucency and anatomic ultrasound adds to the accuracy of detection. In HIV-positive women, the benefits of such testing needs to be discussed and considered carefully. One small study has demonstrated lower α-Fetoprotein in HIV-positive women on protease inhibitor (PI) treatment than in those not on

Table 35-2 Evaluation and Monitoring for the Pregnant Woman With HIV Infection

	Initial Visit	Follow-up Visits
History		
HIV history	Date of diagnosis	
	HIV signs and symptoms with special attention to history of seroconversion illness or symptoms suggesting AIDS	Every visit
	Lowest and current CD4+ T-lymphocyte cell count; highest and current HIV viral load	
	History of opportunistic infections or malignancies, or hospitalizations	Every visit
	History of genital herpes (HSV-2)	
ARV history	ARV treatment history, if any: including regimen efficacy, length of treatment, and drug switches	Every visit
	Signs and symptoms of possible toxicity and side-effects: nausea/vomiting, abdominal pain, jaundice, extreme fatigue, skin rash. Some symptoms may be similar to pregnancy symptoms and result in delay in appropriate diagnosis and management	
	Adherence to regimens	Every visit
	ARV resistance testing if performed	
Obstetric history	Number of previous pregnancies; complications and outcomes	
	Mode of delivery of previous babies	
	History of genetic disorders	
	Use of ARV prophylaxis during previous pregnancies	
	Previous liveborn children and their testing history and HIV status	
	Planned or unplanned pregnancy	
Current pregnancy	Prior contraceptive methods used, if any	
	Last menstrual period (LMP)	
	Gestational age	Every visit
	Estimated date of delivery	
	Signs or symptoms of pregnancy complications: severe nausea and vomiting, elevated blood pressure, headache, significant edema, gastrointestinal or genitourinary symptoms, persistent abdominal or back pain, vaginal discharge or bleeding, fetal movement	Every visit
	Screen for intimate partner violence	Every visit
Physical Examination		
General	Vital signs, blood pressure and weight	Every visit
	Fundoscopy, breast exam	Every visit
Gynecologic examination	Examination for perineal or vaginal lesions (condyloma, ulcerative lesions, vaginal discharge), pelvic examination, checking for cervical lesions, discharge or bleeding	
	STI screening	
Obstetric examination	Fundal height, correlating with gestational age (concordant between 18 and 30 weeks)	Every visit
	Fetal heart beat and rate, (from 16 and 19 weeks with DeLee fetal stethoscope, earlier with Doppler devices)	Every visit
	Fetal movements and position in third trimester	Every visit
Ultrasonography	Baseline scan at 18–20 weeks for confirmation of dates and detection of anomalies.	Consider follow-up ultrasonography for growth and fluid volume at 32–36 weeks

Adapted from Watts DH, Minkoff H. 2002;[435] Anderson,[38] and AIDS Education and Training Centers.[223]

PIs.[179] In the 5% of women with positive serum screening tests, some results will be explained by multiple pregnancy, or ultrasound diagnosis of a birth defect. For the others an invasive amniocentesis will be required to make a definitive diagnosis. There are concerns about the potential transmission of HIV to the fetus with amniocentesis, although the magnitude of the risk has not been clearly defined, especially with effective antiretroviral treatment in place. Reports prior to the widespread use of antiretrovirals suggested an increased risk of HIV infection, especially with late amniocentesis.[101,180] The risk is likely to be considerably reduced with the use of effective antiretroviral therapy.[181] A multicenter Italian study of HIV-infected women who underwent amniocentesis, chorionic villus sampling or cordocentesis during the second trimester of pregnancy and delivered after 1 Jan 1997 showed no significant difference in HIV-infected infants than women who had not had invasive diagnostic procedures.[182] In a Spanish program offering a combined serology screen and nuchal translucency scan assessment, 11% of 116 women screened positive, and amniocentesis undertaken in 10 women confirmed chromosomal anomalies in two.[183] No MTCT was shown in this small group.

Discussion about screening tests for fetal diagnosis for HIV-infected women should include discussion about the risks and benefits of amniocentesis and screening tests should be very carefully considered if a woman does not wish to proceed to an invasive confirmatory test if indicated, as positive screening tests in the absence of confirmatory evidence can cause significant distress. If an amniocentesis is indicated and desired by the woman, it should be performed after optimization of maternal ART, or under prophylactic cover with appropriate antiretrovirals and under direct ultrasound guidance to avoid inserting the needle through the placenta or fetal injury.[184]

Psychosocial Issues

The successful use of PMTCT interventions depends on their acceptance by pregnant women. Where the diagnosis of HIV infection is first made in pregnancy, there are challenges in helping women work through the impact of the diagnosis and then the immediate need for PMTCT prophylactic therapy.[9] An HIV diagnosis is, in itself, a traumatic event for any woman, made worse by her concerns for her unborn child, fear of transmission and guilt about putting her child at risk and sometimes a profound fear of disclosure to her sexual partner. Women with HIV may have coexistent social problems,[185,186] including gender-based violence[187–189] or be recent immigrants to the area with little family support available.[190,191] Some women, especially in high prevalence areas where awareness of HIV is widespread may be concerned that their participation in a PMTCT program may "out" them within their community, or lead to what has been called "disclosure by association".[9] In developing countries disclosure following an HIV diagnosis in pregnancy is often very low, based on women's fear of partner violence,[192] abandonment and stigmatisation in review of 17 studies in developing countries showed that between 3.5 and 14.6% of women reported a violent reaction from their male partner.[193] Alternately, an HIV diagnosis may not be the only cause of violence, but may trigger episodes of abuse in an ongoing violent relationship, and this needs to be explored with the woman.[187,194] Health providers must assess the psychosocial needs of an HIV-infected woman, including screening for depression and exposure to abuse.[195,196] Peer support, from counselors or in support groups, is an important contribution to the psychosocial support needs of these women, especially where traditional pregnancy education promoting breastfeeding and favoring vaginal delivery may appear to them to be contradictory and discriminating.

Drug use is common in HIV-infected women in some settings, both in developed countries and in parts of Asia, with 40% or more of women reporting drug use in some US cohorts.[105,197–199] The combination of pregnancy, HIV infection and drug use presents additional management challenges. Women may be less likely to seek prenatal care,[151] and be reluctant to discuss drug use because of fear of legal action, blame and stigmatization. Providers need to understand the complexity of the social situation, including the concomitant risk of violence and transactional sex, and be able to counsel in a professional and nonjudgmental manner to enable the woman to discuss her drug use and to find appropriate treatment interventions.[9] Where possible, the management of an HIV-infected drug-using woman should be undertaken in close consultation with a provider expert in drug treatment, and an experienced pediatrician. Women who are dependent on opioids should be counseled about the risks and advised to enter a methadone maintenance program. Methadone use has not been shown to have adverse effects on pregnancy, but opiate withdrawal has been associated with preterm delivery and pregnancy loss.[200] There is less experience with buprenorphine treatment for opioid dependency treatment, but adverse effects on pregnancy or on infants have not been reported to date and it may have a place in treatment in pregnancy.[201–203]

Most HIV-infected pregnant women will receive some level of ART, either for their own health or for PMTCT.[8] While there is little interaction with labor-only dosing, there may be an impact when longer ART is provided. ART may impact on recreational drug use through use of similar metabolic pathways. PIs may inhibit the metabolism of drugs such as amphetamines, ketamine, lysergic acid diethylmide (LSD), and phencyclidine (PCP).[204] Methadone is metabolized through the cytochrome P450 system and non-nucleoside reverse transcriptase inhibitors (NNRTIs) nevirapine and efavirenz may act to induce methadone metabolism and lead to withdrawal symptoms. There are some data to suggest that ritonavir and nelfinavir may have a similar effect, and PIs may induce or inhibit opiate metabolism. Toxicity, withdrawal and methadone dosages need to be monitored on an individual basis and methadone may need to be increased with the co-administration of nevirapine.[205] Both cocaine and alcohol use in pregnancy can have severe adverse fetal effects and HIV-infected women with alcohol or cocaine dependency should be advised to enter into treatment programs.

Management of Pregnancy

The management of HIV-positive women in pregnancy should be undertaken by a multidisciplinary team where possible and should include appropriate HIV care and treatment and relevant obstetric care. Where facilities allow, women who are HIV positive should have high-risk obstetric care with increased surveillance for infections and preterm labor; they should undergo targeted investigations based on any specific antiretroviral agents or opportunistic infection prophylaxis they are receiving and on their anticipated side-effects. The use of universal precautions for health workers should be mandatory to reduce the risk of occupational exposure.[119] These should include the use of gloves to handle the baby until potentially infective blood and secretions have been wiped off.

Prenatal Care

Prenatal care of HIV-positive women should include a full history and examination as detailed in Table 35-2.

The prenatal care of HIV-positive women should start with a full history of the HIV infection, including date of diagnosis and previous history of complications or opportunistic infections, and treatment in those women who were known to be positive before pregnancy. This should include details on antiretroviral drug use for treatment or in previous pregnancies for PMTCT, adherence history and any resistance testing. Pregnancy history should include details of previous pregnancies and their outcomes, any pregnancy losses, history of previous preterm delivery and mode of delivery. The HIV status of any previous children should be asked, and if not available, the mother should be encouraged to bring children for testing. Any family history of inherited diseases should be investigated.

Any current signs or symptoms of HIV-related illnesses should be noted, including thrush, weight loss, gingival disease, and peripheral neuropathy or generalized lymphadenopathy. Adverse pregnancy outcomes have been associated with weight loss during pregnancy in HIV-positive women in Tanzania.[206] Pregnancy related complications should be monitored, including elevated blood pressure, edema and any vaginal discharge or bleeding. Rates of pre-eclampsia have been reported to be lower in HIV-positive women not receiving antiretrovirals in the United Kingdom [207] but similar in HIV-positive and HIV-negative women in South Africa and Brazil. Pre-eclampsia may be increased in women on PI containing HAART.[208]

Women with HIV should be monitored for signs of preterm labor. Although there is conflicting evidence from studies on the association between antiretroviral use and preterm delivery,[209] women with HIV may also have multiple other factors which put them at risk of preterm or low birth weight babies. Studies from the United States and Europe have shown conflicting data on differences in birth weight or gestational age for untreated HIV-positive women and uninfected women and similar controls.[92,210–214] A study of 563 HIV-infected inner-city women in Atlanta did show an increase in low birth weight (adjusted OR, 1.45; 95% CI, 1.14–1.86) and preterm delivery (adjusted OR, 1.32; 95% CI, 1.04–1.70),[212] but it appears that the risk factors for adverse pregnancy outcome are similar for HIV-infected women and uninfected women[215] and this emphasizes the need for appropriate prenatal care for these women.[216]

An increase in infant mortality is associated with prematurity in European studies and with low birth weight in both infected and uninfected, exposed African children.[217,218] In developing countries, the rates of low birth weight and preterm birth appear to be increased among HIV-positive women, possibly related to nutritional differences or concurrent infections.[103] Data from Europe suggest a potential beneficial effect of AZT on birth weight and gestational age but a potential increase in preterm births among women receiving long-term PI therapy.[219–221]

Nausea and vomiting from morning sickness are common in early pregnancy, and symptoms are usually present between 6 and 16 weeks, but can persist for longer in up to one-fifth of women, and may be worsened by ART.[219,222] This may interfere with ART at this stage, increasing the risk of nonadherence with regimens or reduced drug levels. It may be possible to delay the initiation of ART until after the morning sickness has abated. Where nausea and vomiting are severe they can be treated with oral or suppository antiemetics and management of any dehydration. Drug interactions with antiretrovirals should be considered, although there are no known interactions between antiemetics and antiretrovirals.[9]

Where the symptoms cannot be controlled in early pregnancy, all antiretrovirals should be discontinued and restarted together once nausea and vomiting has resolved.[223] Hyperemesis gravidarum is defined by intractable vomiting leading to fluid and electrolyte disturbances and nutritional deficiency usually in the first trimester. These patients may require hospitalization for fluid and electrolyte replacement and ART may need to be stopped in these cases.

Laboratory Investigations

Table 35-3 shows recommended laboratory investigations for HIV-positive pregnant women, in settings of high resources, These represent the most comprehensive levels of care, Where all of these are not available, health providers will have to adjust the investigations to fit their available resources, with the most important after the HIV test being CD4+ counts and hemoglobin, and then investigations related to antiretroviral treatment monitoring.

Labor and Delivery Care

A decision on mode of delivery should be made in the prenatal period in discussion with the woman and with consideration of obstetric and HIV factors. The ACOG has suggested that elective cesarean section should be recommended at viral loads of above 1000 copies/mL.[116] Based on current data, guidelines recommend discussing scheduled cesarean delivery with all pregnant women, emphasizing the potential benefits for women with HIV RNA levels above 1000 copies/mL

Laboratory Evaluation and Monitoring for the Pregnant Woman With HIV Infection

Table 35-3

	Initial Visit	Follow-up Visits
Laboratory Investigations		
HIV	HIV test (rapid or enzyme-linked immunosorbent assay (ELISA) confirmatory test (rapid, ELISA or Western blot according to local protocol).	
	HIV viral load and CD4+ T-lymphocyte count (total and %)	Every 3 months (at least every trimester) or as indicated
	HIV resistance testing consider genotyping in acute HIV infection, virologic failure, suboptimal viral suppression on ARV therapy, or high likelihood of exposure to resistant virus based on community prevalence or source characteristics	As indicated
General	Blood group	
	Rh antibody screen	
	Complete blood count (CBC)	Every 3 months or more frequently based on ARV regimen or symptoms. Consider more frequently if on zidovudine regimen.
	Serum chemistry, electrolytes	Every 3 months or more frequently based on ARV regimen
	Liver enzymes (LFTs)	Every 3 months or more frequently based on ARV regimen. Consider LFTs more frequently with nevirapine containing therapy, recent changes in ARV therapy
	Fasting lipid measurement: consider at baseline and 3–6 months after starting PI or NNRTI regimens	As indicated, based on initial results and risks
	Pap smear Urinalysis and clean catch urine culture	As indicated
Other infections	Rubella antibody	
	Varicella IgG, if history unclear	As indicated
	Syphilis serology	As indicated
	Screening gonorrhea and chlamydia	As indicated
	Toxoplasmosis IgG: screen at initial HIV diagnosis; repeat if CD4+ T-lymphocyte <100/mm^3 and not on TMP-SMZ, or with symptoms suggestive of toxoplasmic encephalitis	As indicated
	Bacterial vaginosis screening: consider in women with previous preterm birth, or signs or symptoms of vaginitis	
	Cytomegalovirus (CMV) immunoglobulin G (IgG) if CD4+ T-lymphocyte count <100 cells/μL or if at low-risk for CMV	
	Consider HSV-2 serology, if history suggests	
Hepatitis serology	Hepatitis A (HAV) antibody (IgG)	
	Hepatitis B (HBV): HBsAg, HBcAb, HBsAb	
	Hepatitis C (HCV) antibody	
TB screening	Tuberculin skin test (PPD); (induration >5 mm is positive): obtain chest radiograph if positive	
Disease specific	G6PD level, especially if anemic	
	Consider hemoglobin electrophoresis, if anemic and/or at increased risk for hemoglobinopathies	
	Serum screening for Tay–Sachs disease, both partners if at increased risk	
	Urine toxicology screen, as indicated	As indicated
Special investigations	Diabetes screen: Glucose 1 h after 50 g glucola – 3 h oral GTT if abnormal; additional glucose monitoring may be indicated in women on PIs (consider 20 weeks screening and repeat at 24–28 weeks if on PIs)	As indicated
	Lactic acidosis investigations: If signs or symptoms suggestive of possible lactic acidosis in setting of NRTI therapy: serum lactate, electrolytes, liver enzymes; consider anion gap, CPK, amylase, lipase	
	Triple screen (HCG, unconjugated estriol, δ-fetoprotein): Voluntary; requires counseling; noninvasive test to determine risk of neural tube and abdominal wall defects, Down syndrome, and trisomy 18	

Adapted from Watts DH, Minkoff H. 2002;[435] Anderson,[38] and AIDS Education and Training Centers.[223]

and indicating the lower probability of benefit for women with lower HIV RNA levels.[8,222] Where cesarean section is performed, whether elective or emergency in HIV-infected women, they should receive prophylactic antibiotics. If it is performed after prolonged labor or prolonged ROM, longer courses of antibiotics should be considered.[224]

The potential benefit of elective cesarean section in reducing the risk of MTCT, and possible complications of the operation must be considered and discussed with pregnant women when deciding about the mode of delivery. In all women, regardless of HIV status, cesarean section carries a risk of complications five to –seven times higher than vaginal delivery,[225] mainly due to an increased risk of anesthetic complications and of postoperative infection. Factors that increase the risk of postoperative complications in the general population may be more common in HIV-positive women. They include low socioeconomic status, genital infections, malnutrition, smoking, and prolonged labor or membrane rupture. On the basis of the available evidence, cesarean section is associated with a slightly higher risk of postoperative complications in women with HIV compared to uninfected women and some studies have shown increased rates of complications in HIV-positive women compared to HIV-negative women, regardless of the mode of delivery.[226] Most have shown increases in postpartum fever, endometritis, wound infection and pneumonia.[8,227–233] Complication rates are related to the degree of immunocompromise in the mother. A South African study showed that postoperative endometritis was more common in HIV-positive than HIV-negative women, but that the severity of the condition was similar in the two groups.[234] The rates of postcesarean complications are similar to those for HIV-negative women with comparable risk factors, although women with advanced HIV disease and immunocompromise appear to be at a higher risk. The additional risk of complications does not outweigh the benefit in reduction of transmission to the infant. Elective cesarean section is more likely to result in complications than vaginal delivery but less likely than emergency cesarean section performed after labor has started or membranes ruptured. Modification of clinical practice, particularly use of prophylactic antibiotics, reduces the risk of complications.

Elective Cesarean Section in Low Resource Areas

While the use of elective cesarean section has been a major factor in reducing the rates of MTCT in well-resourced settings, it is not a feasible option in many high HIV seroprevalent, less-resourced areas. In these situations, there may be some cases that merit a lowered threshold for cesarean section. These would include any pregnancies where labor is expected to be prolonged or where other obstetric complications may be associated with increased transmission risk (e.g., abruptio placentae, preterm rupture of membranes). Depending on the available facilities, this may also apply to women with previous cesarean sections or breech presentations. The potential benefit has to be balanced against the risk to the mother, which may be higher in areas where healthcare infrastructure is less. The risks of operative and postoperative complications are often higher if the woman arrives late in labor with advanced complications requiring emergency intervention, such as intrauterine infection and sepsis. Vaginal delivery following cesarean section may carry a higher risk in these settings where skilled maternity care is scarce. An increase in HIV-related cesarean sections and a subsequent increase in repeated cesarean sections due to HIV may overload the health facilities in these settings. All of this will need to be considered when discussing local cesarean section policies.[224]

Where cesarean section is not performed, labor and delivery care should be performed in the safest possible way to reduce any additional risk of transmission. There is no evidence that shaving of the pubic areas reduces the risk of subsequent infection, on the contrary, it may increase the risk of HIV or hepatitis transmission, and should be discouraged.[224] The risk of MTCT is associated with the duration of ROM during labor. As artificial ROM has little obstetric benefit in normal labor, it should not be performed routinely in known HIV-positive women or areas of high HIV prevalence. Use of artificial ROM should be reserved for cases where there is fetal distress or delay in progress of labor.[118,119] In the case of premature ROM, with or without labor, the risk of HIV transmission must be balanced with the risk of premature delivery. There is no known contraindication to the use of short-term steroids to promote fetal lung maturity in women with HIV.

If induction of labor is indicated in a woman with HIV, it presents a management dilemma. Where cesarean section is available, induction of labor may not be desirable or necessary. In other cases, the need for induction must be balanced against the potential increased risk, and, if possible, the membranes should be left intact as long as possible. There is little information about transmission risk with induction of labor, but a prolonged period of ROM would theoretically increase the risk of transmission, especially in the absence of ongoing antiretroviral treatment.[101]

The procedure of vaginal cleansing (vaginal lavage) with chlorhexidine solution during labor was investigated as a means of reducing the risk of MTCT. In a Malawi study it was effective in reducing the risk of MTCT where membranes were ruptured for more than 4 h, but had no overall protective effect in the study group.[235] Chlorhexidine vaginal cleaning was shown to have other benefits (reduced neonatal and puerperal sepsis) without controlling for HIV status of the mother or duration of ROM.[236] A study in Kenya suggested that disinfection before the membranes were ruptured might be associated with a reduction of MTCT, especially with higher concentrations of chlorhexidine.[237]

As penetrating or spiral scalp electrodes and the use of fetal scalp blood sampling may create a portal of entry for the virus, these should be used with caution and avoided unless necessary for the health of the baby. Episiotomy may increase the exposure of the infant to HIV during delivery and increase the risk of transmission. Routine episiotomy is not recommended, and it should be reserved for those cases with a clear obstetric indication. If assisted delivery by forceps

Table 35-4 Postpartum Care for the HIV-Infected Woman and her Child

Counseling	Continuation versus discontinuation of antiretroviral therapy, depending on initial indications for therapy and maternal wishes
	Additional support for adherence to antiretroviral medications given the demands for newborn care and loss of incentive of decreasing perinatal transmission
	Counseling on infant feeding options, supporting avoidance of breastfeeding if appropriate, with education on replacement feeding.
	Psychosocial support, including mental health or substance abuse treatment services; assistance with food, housing, transportation, and legal/advocacy services if needed
	Enhanced psychosocial support during determination of infant infection status
Contraception	Contraceptive counseling, taking into consideration potential interactions of hormonal contraceptives and other maternal therapy
Clinical care	Review maternal status regarding the need for opportunistic infection prophylaxis, immunizations,
	Consider repeat CD4+ T-lymphocyte and viral load to guide treatment decisions
	Other health maintenance such as mammograms, cervical cytology
Infant	Determination of infant infection status; provision of antiretroviral prophylaxis of treatment as indicated
	Provision of infant TMP-SMZ *Pneumocystis carinii* prophylaxis beginning at 4–6 weeks of age
	Infant immunizations as recommended
Ongoing care	Referral to ongoing HIV care for mother and baby

Adapted from Watts DH, Minkoff H. 2002;[435] Anderson.[38]

or vacuum extraction is required, there is a theoretical possibility of increasing the risk of MTCT through damage to the baby's skin. Although some studies have shown an increased risk of infection with forceps deliveries or vacuum extraction, the evidence is conflicting across studies,[78,238] and may be confounded by the obstetric reason for assisted delivery, which may be an independent risk factor for transmission. There is little information on the contribution of obstetric procedures to the risk of MTCT in the presence of ART. Despite this, consideration should be given to emergency cesarean section if there is fetal distress rather than vaginal obstetric intervention.[222] This will not be possible in many instances, and where assisted delivery is required, soft vacuum cups may be preferable to metal cups or forceps.

Postpartum Care

The care provided to HIV-positive women during pregnancy should form part of a continuum of care and support for the women, their children and partners. This should ideally include; primary, obstetric, pediatric and HIV care; family planning services; mental health services; substance-abuse treatment where necessary; and ongoing psychosocial support for the woman, her children, and other family members.[113,224]

In most HIV-positive women, the postnatal course will be uncomplicated and HIV-infected women will not require special medical care. Table 35-4 lists important components of postpartum care for HIV-positive mothers. Further counseling and support may be needed and women should be warned before discharge about the signs and symptoms of infective complications. Peer counselors and supporters can be a positive influence and can help women and their families cope with postpartum stresses. Postpartum complications reported more frequently in HIV-positive women include puerperal sepsis, infected episiotomies, massive condylomata acuminata, urinary tract infections, pneumonia, fever, TB, unusual infections, and retention of urine. Infectious diseases and complications in HIV-positive women may require more aggressive antibiotic treatment.[119,239]

The decision on infant feeding choice should ideally be made in the prenatal period. HIV-positive women will need education and support for either replacement feeding or breastfeeding choices. Mothers should be counseled about the need for follow-up of the baby and availability and timing of HIV testing for children.

Appropriate family planning should be discussed in the prenatal period and discussed again postpartum. Postpartum tubal ligation should be available for those who desire this.[240] In low-resourced settings where prolonged breastfeeding is the norm, lactational amenorrhea is an important contraceptive method. Where women choose replacement feeding in these settings, additional contraception should be recommended. In some cultures, women may have a period of abstinence after the birth of the child, and may not wish to start contraceptive use before this ends, and should be informed how to access contraception when they do need it.

Continuity of antiretroviral treatment for those women on HAART is essential into the postpartum period and beyond. Adherence may be more difficult due to the physical changes of the postpartum period, and the stresses and demands of caring for a new baby, and additional support may be required at this time.[8,241] Postpartum depression may further affect adherence in some women.

Other information in health maintenance should be given to postpartum women, including nutritional advice, advice management of common HIV-related illnesses, information about gynecological infections, such as vaginal discharge and pelvic inflammatory disease and the need to seek early treatment for these, advice on cervical screening, where available, and advice on stopping smoking or alcohol and drug use.[119]

ANTIRETROVIRAL TREATMENT IN PREGNANCY

The clinical and immunologic condition of an HIV-infected pregnant woman should determine the type of therapy she requires, including the prophylaxis and management of opportunistic infections and possibly ART for her own benefit. Pregnant HIV-infected women may need to start or continue ART for their own health, or, for those women who do not yet need this, require a prophylactic regimen to reduce the risk of MTCT. In less-resourced settings, the availability of assured access to ongoing ART may influence the decision to use antiretrovirals, or the type of regimen available. While HAART may be accessible for all HIV-infected pregnant women in well-resourced settings, a range of other possible regimens, down to single-dose nevirapine monotherapy, may be the only available options in poorer countries, regardless of the clinical status or eligibility for ongoing treatment of the woman.

Where resources permit, treatment decisions and regimen choices can be made on an individual basis and tailored to the needs of the HIV-positive woman, with all available investigations. In less-resourced areas, a more public health approach may be needed and is recommended by the WHO. In these settings, the eligibility criteria for starting HAART may be based upon clinical staging and CD4+ cell count, if available, or on WHO clinical staging alone, if CD4 counts are not available.[242] Clinical staging may be more difficult in pregnant women, as assessment of weight loss may be more difficult. In this situation, health workers should take into consideration expected weight gain during pregnancy.

Antiretroviral Drug Use in Pregnancy

Although there has been increasing experience in the use of antiretrovirals in pregnant women in the last decade,[243–246] there is limited long term follow-up data available for many of the antiretroviral drugs. Any use of antiretrovirals in pregnant women, whether for maternal treatment or PMTCT, needs to consider the benefits of antiretroviral treatment compared to the possible risks to the mother, fetus or neonate.[247,248] Although pregnancy is not a barrier to the use of effective HAART regimens, it may necessitate consideration of the possible need to change antiretroviral dosing to fit with the physiological changes of pregnancy, the possible side-effects of the drugs in the mother, which may be worsened by or additive to pregnancy effects; and the potential teratogenic or short- or long-term side-effects of the drugs on the fetus or infant.[247,249,250]

On the evidence available to date, the benefits of ART during pregnancy appear to outweigh the potential side-effects or risks to mother or baby.[245,251] Antiretroviral use in pregnancy can be reported to the Antiretroviral Pregnancy Registry (http://www.APRegistry.com) and treating physicians are encouraged to report to this resource. The registry is a collaborative project of the pharmaceutical industry, pediatric and obstetric providers, the Centers for Disease Control and Prevention (CDC), and the National Institutes of Health (NIH), which collects observational data on HIV-infected pregnant women on antiretroviral treatment to determine any patterns of fetal/neonatal abnormalities. All collected information is confidential and patient names are not used. The registry had accumulated data on the use of antiretrovirals in pregnancy in 4791 women by January 2005.[252] Sufficient data existed in the database at this time to be reassuring that zidovudine, lamivudine, nevirapine, abacavir, and nelfinavir are not teratogenic.[247,253] Similar data showing no association between congenital abnormalities and antiretroviral use has been shown in a review of 3120 pregnancies in the United Kingdom.[254]

Reports of the use of HAART regimens in pregnant women in resource-constrained settings have shown a reassuring safety profile. In Brazil, HAART is now the recommended regimen for pregnant HIV-positive women, with low transmission rates described: 3.57% in one study of 297 women.[255] In Africa, antiretrovirals are increasingly available to pregnant women in some sites, through government programs, or donor programs such as MTCT-plus and the US President's Emergency Plan for AIDS Relief (PEPFAR). A report from Abidjan showed a low rate of toxicity (6/182) and no transmissions in women receiving HAART.[256] In Mozambique, the DREAM project has demonstrated successful use of HAART and replacement feeding with a transmission rate of 4% in infants reported at 4 weeks of age.[257]

Table 35-5 summarizes the available information on FDA pregnancy risk classification, passage from mother-to-infant, animal toxicity and carcinogenicity studies, human toxicity pharmacokinetics in pregnancy and any pregnancy concerns of the currently available antiretroviral drugs. As more experience is gained with the use of newer antiretrovirals in pregnant women, this safety and toxicity information may change. Providers are encouraged to obtain the most up-to-date information as needed from resources such as the US Public Health Service guidelines [258] which have a regularly updated section on antiretroviral safety in pregnancy which is available online at the AIDSinfo Web site (http://AIDSinfo.nih.gov).

Nucleoside Reverse Transcriptase Inhibitors

Zidovudine was the first antiretroviral drug shown to be efficacious in reducing the risk of MTCT and has remained one of the drugs of choice for use in pregnancy.[8,259] As more information on the safety of zidovudine and lamivudine (3TC) has been accumulated than with any of the other antiretroviral drugs, they should be included in pregnancy treatment regimens where possible. The main toxicity concern with AZT is the development of anemia and neutropenia and other NRTI drugs should be considered, rather than AZT,

Table 35-5

Antiretroviral Drugs Used During Pregnancy: Preclinical and Clinical Data

Antiretroviral Drug	FDA Pregnancy Category	Newborn/Maternal Drug Ratio	Long-Term Animal Carcinogenicity Studies	Animal Reproduction Studies	Major Toxicities	Pregnancy Dosing and Pharmacokinetics	Pregnancy Concerns
Nucleoside and nucleotide reverse transcriptase inhibitors (NRTIs)							Potential maternal and infant mitochondrial toxicity
Abacavir (ABC)	C	~1 (humans)	Positive – malignant and nonmalignant liver and thyroid tumors in female rats and preputial and clitoral gland tumors in mice and rats	Anasarca, skeletal abnormalities at 35 times human dose in rodents, not seen in rabbits	Hypersensitivity reactions in 5–8% nonpregnant with symptoms of fever, skin rash, fatigue, nausea, vomiting, diarrhea, abdominal pain. Smaller proportion potentially fatal	No significant change in PK in pregnancy. No dosing change required	Hypersensitivity rate in pregnancy not known
Didanosine (ddI)	B	0.5 (human)	Negative in lifetime rodent studies	Negative	Pancreatitis, neuropathy	Increase in clearance and decrease in area under the concentration–time curve. Clinical significance not known. No dosing change recommended	PK study (n = 14) shows no need for dose modification. Possible increased risk of lactic acidosis during pregnancy with long-term ddI/d4T together
Emtricitabine (FTC)	B	Unknown	Not complete	Negative		No pregnancy data	No studies in human pregnancy
Lamivudine (3TC)	C	1.0 (human)	Negative in lifetime rodent study	Negative	Pancreatitis increased in children	No significant change in PK in pregnancy. No dosing change required	No evidence of human teratogenicity. Well-tolerated with demonstrated short-term safety
Stavudine (d4T)	C	1.32 (humans) 0.76 (rhesus monkey)	Liver and bladder tumors in mice and rats at very high dose	Negative but decreased sternal ossification at	Peripheral neuropathy	No significant change in PK in pregnancy. No dosing	No evidence of human teratogenicity. Lactic acidosis

				high dose in rodents		change required	reported in pregnancy with long term d4T/ddI together
Tenofovir DF) (TDF)	B	Passage shown in rats and monkeys	Hepatic adenomas in female mice at high dose	Osteomalacia in juvenile animals at high dose		No pregnancy data	Monkey studies show decrease in fetal growth and reduced fetal bone porosity within 2 months of maternal therapy. Little pregnancy data available
Zalcitabine (ddC)	C	0.3–0.5 (rhesus monkey)	Thymic lymphomas in rats at 1000 times human dose	Hydrocephalus in rats at 2000 times human dose, skeletal defects and decreased weight at moderate doses	Neuropathy	No pregnancy data	Rodent studies demonstrate potential for teratogenocity. Not recommended for use in pregnancy unless no alternatives available
Zidovudine (AZT, ZDV)	C	0.85 (human)	Noninvasive vaginal tumors in rodent, possible transplacental carcinogenesis (see text)	No teratogenicity in rats, rabbits at usual dose. Increased malformations at near-lethal dose in rats	Bone marrow suppression, myopathy	Increase in clearance and decrease in area under the concentration-time curve. Clinical significance not known. No dosing change recommended	No evidence of human teratogenicity. Most well-studied ARV agent, safe for short-term
Non-nucleoside reverse transcriptase inhibitors (NNRTIs)							
Delavirdine	C	Unknown	Hepatocellular adenomas and carcinomas in male and female mice (but not rats) bladder tumors male mice	Ventricular septal defect in rodents	Rash, drug interactions	No pregnancy data	Teratogenicity in rodent studies, Not recommended in pregnancy unless no alternatives available

(*Continued*)

Table 35-5 (Continued)

Antiretroviral Drug	FDA Pregnancy Category	Newborn/Maternal Drug Ratio	Long-Term Animal Carcinogenicity Studies	Animal Reproduction Studies	Major Toxicities	Pregnancy Dosing and Pharmacokinetics	Pregnancy Concerns
Efavirenz	D	~1.0 (cynomolgous monkey, rat, rabbit)	Hepatocellular adenoma and carcinoma and pulmonary alveolar/bronchiolar adenoma in female but not male mice	Anencephaly, anophthalmia, microphthalmia, cleft palate in cynomolgous monkeys at doses similar to human doses	Rash, drug interactions	No pregnancy data	FDA Class D. Malformations in 15% of cynomolgus monkeys with first trimester dosing. 3 case reports of neural tube defects in humans after first trimester exposure. Avoid in first trimester
Nevirapine (NVP)	C	~1.0 (human)	Hepatocellular adenomas and carcinoma	Negative	Rash, drug interactions, potentially fatal hepatotoxicity. Increased risk of symptomatic, rash-associated and potentially fatal hepatotoxicity in women with CD4+ T-lymphocyte count >250/mm^3. No data as to whether pregnancy increases this risk.	No significant change in PK in pregnancy. No dosing change required	No evidence of human teratogenicity. NVP should be used in combination therapy in women with CD4+ T-lymphocyte counts >250/mm^3 only if risk outweighs benefits. Short-term safety demonstrated for single dose
Protease inhibitors (PIs)				Class effects: hyperglycemia, possible fat redistribution and lipid abnormalities, increased bleeding episodes in hemophiliacs			

Amprenavir	C	Unknown	Hepatocellular adenomas and carcinomas in male mice and rats	Negative (but deficient ossification and thymic elongation in rats and rabbits)		No pregnancy data	Insufficient data to recommend use. Oral solution contraindicated in pregnancy because of high levels of propylene glycol
Atazanavir	B	Unknown	Hepatocellular adenomas in female mice	Negative		No pregnancy data	Insufficient data to recommend use in pregnancy
Fosamprenavir	C	Unknown	Liver tumors (benign and malignant) in male rodents	Negative		No pregnancy data	Insufficient data to recommend use in pregnancy
Indinavir	C	Minimal (Humans)	Thyroid adenomas in male rats at highest dose	Negative (but extra ribs in rodents)	Kidney stones, hyperbilirubinemia, drug interactions	Lower levels shown in pregnancy with 800 mg three times a day dosing. Recommend use with ritonavir boost in pregnancy, Optimal dosing of boosted regimen not known	Theoretical concerns about kidney stones, hyperbilirubinemia in neonate from maternal exposure (but minimal transplacental passage)
Lopinavir/ritonavir (Kaletra)	C	Unknown	Hepatocellular adenomas and carcinomas in mice and rats	Negative (but delayed skeletal ossification in rats at maternally toxic doses)		Reduced plasma concentrations seen in pregnancy: increased dose may be required but no specific dosing recommendations formulated.	Limited experience in human pregnancy may need dosing adjustment
Nelfinavir	B	Minimal (humans)	Thyroid follicular adenomas and carcinomas in rats	Negative	Diarrhea, drug interactions	Adequate drug levels with 1250 mg twice daily	Extensive experience in pregnancy compared to other PIs. Recommended for pregnancy use in combination regimens

(Continued)

Table 35-5 (Continued)

Antiretroviral Drug	FDA Pregnancy Category	Newborn/Maternal Drug Ratio	Long-Term Animal Carcinogenicity Studies	Animal Reproduction Studies	Major Toxicities	Pregnancy Dosing and Pharmacokinetics	Pregnancy Concerns
Ritonavir	B	Minimal (humans)	Liver adenomas and carcinomas in male mice	Negative (but cyptorchildism in rodents)	Nausea, vomiting, diarrhea; increased triglycerides, transaminases; drug interactions	Lower levels seen in pregnancy compared to postpartum	Minimal pregnancy experience. Recommended for use as low dose 'boost' with other PIs
Saquinavir	B	Minimal (human)	Negative	Negative	Nausea, diarrhea	Adequate drug level with saquinavir 800 mg soft gel capsules boosted with 100 mg ritonavir twice daily	Well-tolerated. Use as ritonavir-boosted soft gel capsules can be considered in pregnancy
Tipranavir	C	Unknown	Not completed	Negative (but decreased ossification in rats at maternally toxic doses		No pregnancy data	No experience in human pregnancy
Fusion inhibitors							
Enfuvirtide	B	Unknown	Unknown	Negative		No pregnancy data	Minimal experience in human pregnancy. Insufficient data to recommend use in pregnancy

FDA categories:
A, adequate, well-controlled studies of pregnant women fail to demonstrate a risk to the fetus during the first trimester of pregnancy (and there is no evidence of risk during the later trimesters).
B, animal reproduction studies fail to demonstrate a risk to the fetus; adequate, well-controlled studies of pregnant women have not been conducted.
C, safety in human pregnancy has not been determined; animal studies are either positive for fetal risk or have not been conducted; and the drug should not be used unless the potential benefit outweighs the potential risk to the fetus.
D, positive evidence of human fetal risk based on adverse reaction data from investigational or marketing experiences, but the potential benefits from the use of the drug in pregnant women may be acceptable despite its potential risks.
X, studies in animals or reports of adverse reactions have indicated that the risk associated with the use of the drug for pregnant women clearly outweighs any possible benefit.
ARV, antiretroviral; ASD/VSD, atrial septal defect/ventricular septal defect; FDA, Food and Drug Administration; PK, pharmacokinetic.

Adapted from Watts and Minkoff;[435] US Public Health Service;[8] and from Best,[262] Chappuy et al.,[437,438] Mirochnick,[439] Mirochnick and Capparelli,[440] Steck,[303] Mirochnick et al.[304]

for pregnant women with severe hemoglobin levels less than 7 gm/dL. Where anemia develops in a woman on AZT therapy, it is usually associated with macrocytosis. If resources allow, treatment of the anemia, including the use of erythropoietin, can be considered, rather than stopping the drug.[38]

Other NRTI drugs which can be used in pregnancy include stavudine (d4T) and abacavir (ABC) and pharmacokinetic studies have shown that standard doses are adequate in pregnancy for these drugs.[258,260–262] There is limited data on emtricitabine (FTC) use in pregnancy, although animal toxicity data is reassuring and it is similar in structure to 3TC and is unlikely to need dosing changes. Didanosine (ddI) is not generally recommended for first line antiretroviral regimens in pregnancy, although it may be a component of second line regimens. Although animal studies have shown no risk of teratogenesis, congenital abnormalities have been described in 6.3% (13/205) of cases with first trimester exposure to ddI reported to the Antiretroviral Pregnancy Registry compared to a rate of 1.1% (2/190) among those with exposures later in pregnancy. No pattern of defects has been demonstrated and this will require further close monitoring.[252]

The antiretrovirals d4T and ddI should not be used together in pregnant women, unless the potential benefits outweigh the risks, due to an increased risk of lactic acidosis[8] with prolonged therapy, although short-term combination use appears to be safe.[263] Lactic acidosis is a relatively rare but potentially life-threatening condition, in women taking nucleoside reverse transcriptase inhibitors (NRTIs).[251,264,265] Although all NRTI drugs may cause lactic acidosis, it is more associated with ddI and d4T than AZT, 3TC, or ABC because of a greater potential for interfering with mitochondrial replication.[38] The symptoms may be nonspecific, including nausea, malaise, breathlessness, abdominal pain or discomfort, and as such, may be difficult to distinguish from pregnancy symptoms. Metabolic acidosis with elevated serum lactate and liver enzymes is common. The more widespread use of d4T as first-line antiretroviral treatment regimens in a developing countries, has been associated with higher rates of lactic acidosis than previously described in the US or Europe, and appears to be more common in women in these settings.[266] There is insufficient evidence to determine whether pregnancy increases the risk of lactic acidosis on these drugs, but symptoms of pregnancy or of other pregnancy complications maybe similar to the nonspecific symptoms of lactic acidosis. Attending practitioners need to bear this in mind and monitor carefully, including careful monitoring of electrolytes, liver function tests and possible lactate levels in the third trimester.[223] The symptoms of lactic acidosis generally improve with drug discontinuation.

There have been some reports of a possible association between NRTI-containing antiretroviral regimens and the development of mitochondrial toxicity in the newborn and mother, although the full consequences of this are not known.[267–269] There are conflicting data across studies, although the risk of severe toxicity appears to be small. Reports in a large French cohort identified 12 cases of mitochondrial dysfunction in an 18-month prospective follow-up of 4392 NRTI-exposed children.[268] In children, mitochondrial toxicity may manifest as neurologic symptoms, including febrile seizures, with or without abnormal magnetic resonance imaging or significant hyperlactatemia.[270–272] In contrast, a retrospective review of more than 16 000 HIV-exposed, uninfected infants in the United States between 1986 and 1999 showed no deaths suggestive of mitochondrial dysfunction.[273] Similarly, there was no increase in neurologic symptoms in NRTI-exposed versus placebo-exposed infants in the PETRA study in Africa,[155] or in a large cohort in the European Collaborative Study.[274] In mothers, mitochondrial toxicity may be linked to myopathy, neuropathy, cardiomyopathy, pancreatitis, hepatic steatosis and lactic acidosis.[8,275]

Nucleotide Reverse Transcriptase Inhibitors

The nucleotide reverse transcriptase inhibitor tenofovir (TDF) has become more widely used in first-line treatment regimens. There is little experience of its use in pregnancy to date, although one pharmacokinetic study has shown that maternal tenofovir concentrations are substantially lower than in adults receiving the same single dose and HIV-infected patients at steady state receiving TDF 300 mg once daily, suggesting that higher doses may be appropriate for pregnant women.[276] There are some theoretical concerns about a possible association between TDF exposure *in utero* and abnormal fetal bone development. This is based on animal data,[277] and on some reports of bone demineralization in children on chronic TDF therapy, although this is not consistent in all studies.[278,279] Further safety studies are in progress, but TDF should be used with caution in pregnancy until further information is available.

Non-Nucleoside Reverse Transcriptase Inhibitors

Nevirapine (NVP) is the NNRTI most widely used in pregnancy. The major side-effects of NVP in treatment regimens are hepatotoxicity and severe skin rash, which occur more commonly in women and in the first 2–3 months after initiation of treatment.[280,281] These complications have not been seen with the use of single dose NVP regimens for the prevention of MTCT.[63,282]

Although NVP has been extensively used in pregnancy, some reports have suggested higher rates of toxicity, including deaths,[38,283] and there have been suggestions that PI regimens may be preferable in pregnant women. NVP-related toxicity was seen in 29% of subjects (5/17) receiving NVP in the PACTG 1022 study compared to 5% (1/21) receiving nelfinavir ($P = 0.07$), including one Stevens-Johnson syndrome and one fatal fulminant hepatic failure in the NVP group.[284] All of the adverse events occurring in women with CD4 counts above 250/mm^3 in this study were NVP-associated. In the Netherlands, NVP-related toxicity was more frequent in pregnant women on HAART than in nonpregnant women, although women treated in pregnancy were more likely to have higher CD4 counts.[285] Severe toxicities were seen in 10.5% of NVP-treated pregnant women compared to 2% of PI-treated women in a Canadian observational study,[286] but in 4.7% of 189 pregnant women in a UK study, where most adverse events occurred at CD4 counts of 200–250/mm^3.[287] In contrast to these results, adverse events were less likely following initiation of NVP therapy in pregnant than nonpregnant women in another study.[288] Rates of NVP-related adverse events in Africa and Asia have been similar, reported in 10% of pregnant women in a Thai study,[289] and 8% of pregnant women receiving an NVP-containing HAART regimen for PMTCT in a study in Kisumu, Kenya.[290] In both of these reports, toxicity was similar with CD4 counts above or below 250/mm^3.

As symptoms of hepatotoxicity may be nonspecific and mimic pregnancy symptoms, clinical symptoms and hepatic transaminases (ALT and AST) should be monitored frequently, especially during the first 4 months of treatment when these toxicities are more common. If clinical symptoms occur, with raised ALT or AST, NVP should be stopped and not restarted.[8]

The use of NVP-containing HAART regimens for MTCT prophylaxis in pregnant women with higher CD4+ cell counts, who do not yet need HAART for their own health, is a cause of more concern. This is due to accumulated evidence of an increased risk of hepatic adverse events, which may be fatal and are often associated with rash, in women with pretreatment CD4 counts greater than 250 cells/mm^3 treated with NVP.[291] This increased risk has not been seen with single dose NVP regimens, and has not been linked to pregnancy. However, the use of NVP-containing antiretroviral regimens in women with higher CD4 counts is most likely to be either following guidelines to start HAART in women with CD4+ counts less than 350/mm^3, or for a PMTCT indication. A change in the NVP manufacturer's information sheet and an FDA advisory now recommends that NVP should not be used in antiretroviral treatment regimens for women with CD4 counts above 250/mm^3 unless the benefits clearly outweigh the risks.[8,292] Where there are a number of antiretrovirals available, providers may choose to start pregnant women with higher CD4+ cells on a PI regimen, but this may be a more difficult decision in resource-poor countries, where antiretroviral choices are limited and NNRTI-containing regimens are the standard first line therapy.

Where NVP regimens are used, and especially in women with CD4 counts over 250/mm^3 women should be warned about possible symptoms of toxicity, including abdominal pain, fever, and jaundice or skin rash and should have more frequent visits in the first months of treatment. Liver enzymes should be monitored at baseline, 2, 4, 8, and 12 weeks and NVP discontinued and an alternative drug substituted if ALT or AST increase to more than five times the upper limit of normal.

There are concerns over the use of efavirenz in pregnancy due to an association with neural tube defects in animal studies and a small number of reports of neural tube defects and the Dandy-Walker malformation in humans.[293,294] Although the causal relationship is not completely established, efavirenz is now classified as an FDA Pregnancy Category D drug ("Positive evidence of human fetal risk that is based on adverse reaction data from investigational or marketing experiences, but the potential benefits from the use of the drug among pregnant women might be acceptable despite its potential risks") on the basis of potential fetal harm when administered to a pregnant woman during the first trimester.[258,295] Efavirenz should not be used in the first trimester of pregnancy, or in women of child bearing potential without provision of adequate contraception, but may be an option for treatment in the second or third trimester of pregnancy. If women become pregnant while on Efavirenz therapy they should be counseled about the possible fetal risk and offered ultrasound screening.

Protease Inhibitors

PIs are a commonly used component of the combination antiretroviral regimens used in pregnancy in the USA, with over 50% of women on antiretrovirals in the WITS study after 1996 being on a PI regimen.[296] PI regimens are also more commonly being used in pregnancy HAART regimens only for PMTCT in resource-rich settings, due to the concern about NVP toxicity in women with higher CD4+ counts. In less resourced areas, PIs are generally part of second line regimens only and there is less experience in pregnancy.

Nelfinavir (NFV) and Saquinavir/ritonavir (SQV/r) have the most available safety data in pregnancy, with more experience accumulating with Lopinavir/ritonavir (LPV/r). Standard dosing is adequate for SQV/r.[297,298] Indinavir levels may be lower in pregnancy due to metabolic induction and dose changes may be indicated, although the addition of low dose ritonavir boosting may give adequate levels.[299–301] NFV levels with standard 1250 mg twice daily dosing may be very variable in pregnancy. [300,302] There are some conflicting data on LPV/r levels in pregnancy, with some studies suggesting lower levels than in postpartum women,[303] and adequate levels with increased dosing[304] but another showing adequate levels with standard dosing.[305] No data is available for pregnancy use of atazanavir or fosamprenavir in pregnancy and they should be used with caution only if no alternative regimens are available. Amprenavir oral solution is contraindicated in pregnancy, as it contains high levels of propylene glycol, which pregnant women and young children are unable to metabolize and eliminate adequately, causing severe side-effects, including lactic acidosis and respiratory depression.[38,258]

There have been concerns about the impact of PI use on pregnancy outcome.[279] Higher rates of preterm delivery have been reported in some reports of antiretroviral use in pregnancy.[285,306,307] In a US review of 233 pregnancies where a PI was used, the prematurity rate (<37 weeks' gestation) was 22.0% (95% CI, 16.9–28.0%).[297] The association with premature delivery is not consistent across studies; with an association between combination ART and preterm labor shown in Swiss and European studies but not in the WITS in the US, or in a US meta-analysis.[219,221,296,308] In a recent analysis from the WITS, there was an increase in preterm delivery in the small group of women with late use of antiretrovirals not containing zidovudine (OR, 7.9; 95% CI, 1.4–44.6), but a decrease in preterm delivery less than 37 weeks for those receiving combination therapy with zidovudine (OR, 0.5; 95% CI, 0.3–0.8). In contrast, a study at one US site of 999 women receiving ART and 3338 on no treatment, found that ART including a PI was associated with an increased risk of preterm delivery, compared with both, other combination ART (adjusted odd ratio (AOR), 1.8) and all other study patients (AOR, 2.3). In this study, exposure to a PI for more than 10 weeks increased the risk of preterm delivery less than 37 weeks.[309] In the European Collaborative Study, the prematurity rate in 4372 live births rose from 16.4% in 1985–89 to 24.9% in 2000–04, and antenatal HAART use initiated prepregnancy was strongly associated with prematurity (AOR, 2.05; 95% CI, 1.43–2.95) after controlling for other factors.[306]

In addition PIs were associated with worsening of diabetes mellitus, gestational diabetes and hyperglycemia in early studies in pregnant women.[247,251,310,311] In the US Women's Interagency HIV Study, nonpregnant women taking PI-containing regimens had a three-fold higher risk of developing diabetes mellitus than HIV-negative women or HIV-positive women taking either NRTIs or no therapy (1.35%).[312] A recent PACTG study of 161 women showed no association between PI-containing regimens and an increased risk of glucose intolerance in pregnancy, or with the sequelae of glucose intolerance.[313] Given the diabetogenic state of pregnancy and the potential complications of PIs, women receiving HAART during pregnancy should be monitored carefully for obstetric complications, and glucose levels should be monitored with the use of PIs in pregnancy.[247]

There have been suggestions that HAART use, and PI in particular, may be associated with an increased risk of preeclampsia, although there are conflicting data from studies at present and further observations are required.[207,208,250]

Adherence to Antiretroviral Regimens in Pregnancy

Adherence to HAART regimens may be taxing for pregnant women. The imperative to start antiretrovirals as soon as possible for the protection of the fetus means that some women may not have time for extensive treatment readiness education after their diagnosis of HIV infection. Their concerns about preventing transmission to a child may be counterbalanced by fears of drug toxicities and some of the side-effects of a normal pregnancy, such as nausea, vomiting and heartburn, may exacerbate drug effects. There is little information available on adherence to HAART regimens by pregnant women, although the success of antiretroviral treatment in reducing MTCT suggests that adherence is good. Some programs which have studied adherence report good levels,[314] while another study has shown a rate of 30% among HAART-treated women with HIV plasma viral loads of greater than 1000 copies/mL, and an association with reduced treatment adherence.[315] A quarter of women reported less than perfect adherence in an analysis of the PACTG 1025 study,[316] with many women having less than optimal adherence for effective use of PI regimens. Factors associated with decreased adherence included alcohol or drug use and symptoms of depression, but not age, ethnicity or type of regimen. Women with AIDS or on HAART started prior to the pregnancy were less likely to be adherent than those on HAART only for PMTCT purposes. Adherence was better in pregnancy than in the postpartum period in this analysis with 75% achieving perfect adherence during pregnancy and only 64% at 24 weeks after delivery, reinforcing the need for continued adherence counseling and support at this time. There are many demands on women in the postpartum period, and less motivation to take her treatment "for the sake of the baby", which may impact on HAART adherence.

Antiretroviral Treatment Strategies in Pregnancy

Women Who Require Antiretroviral Treatment for Their Own Health

Pregnant women who need antiretroviral treatment should start this as soon as possible.[8,9,317] While the primary purpose of this antiretroviral treatment is to benefit the mother, it will also significantly reduce the risk of MTCT, and improvements in maternal health and life expectancy can also improve child survival. Immunocompromised HIV-infected women, with low CD4 cell counts are more likely to transmit to their babies,[318] more likely to have detectable NNRTI-resistant virus following the use of NVP monotherapy[319] and their infants are more likely to die,[57,58] all of which can be improved by access to antiretroviral treatment. In the United States and Europe increasing numbers of women are aware of their HIV status prior to pregnancy and may already be on ART.[8,246] Those women already on antiretroviral treatment who become pregnant should continue with an effective antiretroviral regimen, although there may need to be some adjustment in the drugs used.[8,9,115,228,247,248,320]

Women on EFV regimens in the first trimester should change to an NVP regimen, triple NRTI regimen or a PI regimen. Change to an NVP regimen requires close monitoring for the first 3 months of treatment in women who have CD4 counts on EFV treatment above 250/mm^3. In these cases, NVP should be started at 200 mg twice daily, without a dose escalation phase. If the woman is already in the second or third trimester on EFV treatment, the drug should be continued.[321]

For women who are assessed as needing to initiate HAART during pregnancy, treatment should be started as soon as feasible. Where the woman's clinical condition allows, consideration can be given to delaying treatment until after the first trimester, to avoid early fetal exposure, but therapy should not be delayed in an ill women, as the benefits to mother and infant outweigh the possible risk to the fetus. Where the decision to treat is made late in pregnancy, treatment should also be started as soon as possible, and not delayed until postpartum, because of the high risk of MTCT.

Eligibility criteria for HAART vary across country settings. In most well-resourced settings, a CD4 count of less than 350/mm^3 is an indication to start life-long therapy, while in resource-poor settings, many guidelines recommend starting at below 200/mm.[3,8,242] This may make choice of regimen difficult for women with CD4 counts between 250 and 350, where NVP-containing regimens form the basis for first-line therapy, given the higher risk of toxicity with higher CD4 counts. However, there are also data to suggest that starting on an NVP regimen for treatment within 6 months of the use of single-dose NVP for PMTCT, which is the standard of care in many of these settings, may compromise virologic response to treatment.[322,323] These findings suggest that it may be preferable to consider starting HAART, if possible, at CD4 counts below 350/mm^3 in pregnant women with WHO stage 1 or 2 disease, who may otherwise progress to needing therapy within 6–12 months postpartum.

Women for Whom HAART is Not Yet Indicated

For women who do not yet need HAART for their own health, a choice of the most appropriate effective regimen for the prevention of MTCT should be made. This will depend upon the resources available and the woman's choice. Women who do not require HAART during pregnancy do need to be referred for continued HIV-related care. They should be assessed postpartum for eligibility for HAART and receive ongoing follow-up assessments in addition to nonantiretroviral care and treatment.

Prophylactic HAART Regimens

Where there are appropriate health service infrastructure, resources and availability of antiretrovirals; HAART regimens, started after the first trimester of pregnancy and stopped after delivery, have been recommended for all HIV-positive pregnant women for the prevention of MTCT, regardless of their need to continue with postpregnancy treatment. The use of HAART for MTCT prophylaxis aims to provide maximal viral suppression, the maximum reduction in the risk of transmission and to minimize the risk of selection of resistant virus.[247] The success of such a strategy is shown by the extremely low rates of transmission now seen in the US and Europe. In 2001–03 in Europe, 92% of HIV-infected pregnant women in the European Collaborative Study centers received ART with an overall transmission rate of 0.99% (95% CI, 0.32–2.3%).[246] In the United States, transmission rates have dropped over time from 10.4% with zidovudine monotherapy to 1–2% with HAART in the WITS.[324]

The use of these regimens in less-resourced areas, including Brazil and some African settings, has increased in the past few years. Initial reports from Cote d'Ivoire, Mozambique, Kenya and Thailand have shown a low rate of toxicity and low transmission rates in women receiving HAART.[256,257,289,290] The restricted choices of drug regimens and logistical considerations may make HAART for all HIV-positive pregnant women difficult to achieve for some time to come,[325] and treatment programs in these settings have to weigh up whether there is a significant potential benefit to providing HAART for pregnant women compared to the relatively low rates of transmission achievable through the use of short course combination regimens,[326] given the additional cost and complexity of HAART regimens.

The increased toxicity of NVP-containing HAART regimens suggests that only a conservative approach to the use of these MTCT prophylaxis is warranted, reserving it for those circumstances where the benefits clearly outweigh the risk, as suggested in the US Public Health Service guidelines.[247] Where drug choices permit such as in the United States, PI or triple NRTI regimens may be better choices for these women for PMTCT prophylaxis.

Simpler Antiretroviral Regimens

Despite major advances in increasing access to ART, HAART is still not available to many millions of HIV-infected people who need it, and will not be available for pregnant women either for treatment or prophylaxis. In these settings, simpler antiretroviral regimens may be feasible in pregnancy and can still reduce MTCT dramatically.[327] PMTCT prophylactic regimens which have been shown to be effective include the use of AZT alone or in combination with 3TC, NVP alone to mother and baby, antepartum AZT with single dose NVP to mother and baby and triple therapy regimens.[63,152,154,155,164,259,328–333]

Combination Antiretroviral PMTCT Regimens

Combination short-course regimens, where a maternal and infant NVP dose are added to an antepartum regimen of zidovudine alone or in combination with 3TC may reduce transmission to below 5% without many of the potential side-effects or logistical problems of HAART regimens for PMTCT.[332,333] This is more effective than single-dose NVP regimens, which will only reduce transmission rates to 10–15% at 6 weeks, depending on early infant feeding,[334,335] is closer to the transmission risk of less than 2% seen with HAART regimens.[7] The results of the PHPT-2 study in nonbreastfeeding mothers in Thailand, given zidovudine from 28 weeks gestation to the mother and for 1 week to the baby, and with the addition of one dose of NVP to the mother and baby, showed this combination approach to be effective in reducing transmission to 1.9% (95% CI, 0.9–3.0%) for the zidovudine with NVP to the mother and baby, and 2.8% (95% CI, 1.5–4.1%) for zidovudine with NVP to the mother only.[332] This study demonstrated no significant difference whether or not the infant NVP dose was used where mothers had received zidovudine and NVP. Results suggest, although not conclusively, that the maternal NVP dose did not add to the efficacy of the regimens where mothers had received zidovudine from 34 weeks and babies received an NVP dose.[336]

A similar approach in a breastfeeding setting in Côte d'Ivoire used a zidovudine regimen, started at 36 weeks and continued for 1 week postpartum to mother and child, with addition of one dose of NVP to mother and baby, and showed a transmission rate at 6 weeks of 6.5% (95% CI, 3.9–9.1%). When the maternal regimen was changed to zidovudine with 3TC from 32 weeks with the NVP added, the transmission rate at 6 weeks dropped to 4.7% (95% CI, 2.4–7.0%).[333]

This approach of combining an NVP dose to the mother and infant with zidovudine has become the WHO recommended regimen for those women who do not require ongoing HAART therapy in settings where HAART given only for PMTCT is not feasible or available.[317] This combination can provide a reduction in transmission to less than 5%, approximately half the rate that can be achieved by NVP alone, while avoiding some of the complexity of delivery of HAART regimens.

NVP Only Regimens

Despite the increased availability of PMTCT programs, UNAIDS estimates that only 9% of pregnant women in resource-poor countries are offered PMTCT interventions.[1] For the majority of HIV-positive women in these settings, the only available PMTCT prevention option is a single dose NVP (sdNVP) regimen.[248] First shown to be effective in the HIVNET 012 study [282] in Uganda, a single dose NVP regimen of one 200 mg at the onset of labor in mothers and one dose of 2 mg/kg given to babies within 72 h of delivery can reduce transmission rates at 4–8 weeks by close to 50%, and the introduction of this relatively simple regimen has enabled the expansion of PMTCT services in many resource-poor settings, particularly in Africa. A similar NVP regimen, with two maternal doses and one dose to infants, used in The South African Intrapartum NVP Trial (SAINT) showed a transmission rate of 12.3% (95% CI, 9.7–15.0) in the NVP group[63] and low rates of adverse effects. The safety and efficacy of NVP, alone or in short course combinations, have been further demonstrated in seven additional clinical trials reported by 2005.[63,164,332,333,337,338] In these trials, close to 5000 women and infants received NVP prophylaxis without significant side-effects, and severe toxicities, including hepatotoxicity and serious rashes were rare.[339]

The sdNVP regimen has been used in hundreds of thousands of pregnant women and their infants.[136,340] Reported transmission rates in these program settings are similar to those reported in clinical trials at between 8.7% and 22%.[319,341–346] In rural Uganda, a program providing self-administered NVP for mothers and infants demonstrated a transmission rate of 7.5% (95% CI, 0.3–16.6%),[347] showing the effectiveness of this approach even in very difficult settings. The effectiveness of the regimen is, however, dependent upon the uptake of HIV testing, which is reported as low in many programs, leading to identification and treatment of a much lesser number of HIV-positive women,[342,348,349] and even where women are identified, adherence to the NVP dose may be low[350] reducing program effectiveness.[138] Given these constraints, and the low global coverage of PMTCT programs, there have been some suggestions that NVP should be provided to all pregnant women without the need for testing.[338] This approach, promoted as an emergency response, has not been recommended by the WHO as a routine programmatic approach,[249,351] and has been rendered less attractive by the new evidence of NVP resistance following sdNVP dosing. A possible alternative approach in areas where antenatal or labor testing of mothers cannot be achieved could be the provision of sdNVP to infants of mothers of unknown HIV status. The single dose regimen in infants appears to be safe, and can be effective in reducing the risk of transmission by providing some level of postexposure prophylaxis, although it will not have any effect on the rates of *in utero* transmission.

NVP Resistance

The major concern about the use of NVP as single dose prophylaxis or in combination regimens for PMTCT is the risk of selection of NNRTI resistance mutations. The properties of NVP which confer much of its effectiveness in preventing MTCT, unfortunately, also predispose to this selection of resistance. With only one point mutation required in the viral codon, there is a low genetic barrier for NNRTI resistance, and the long half-life of the drug following even a single dose, means that there is effectively NVP monotherapy without viral suppression. NVP levels in women may remain quantifiable for up to 20 days following dosing in labor.[352]

The selection of NNRTI resistance virus following NVP use for PMTCT has been widely reported.[319,353–356] Rates of resistance detectable by standard genotyping techniques range from 15% to 75% in mothers. These rates vary with the time of sampling, being higher sooner after dosing than later, probably reflecting distinct patterns of the emergence and "fading" of resistant genotypes. The rates are also different by viral subtype. In one analysis of samples from Uganda and Malawi, rates of detectable resistance at 6–8 weeks postpartum were 69% in subtype C, 36% in subtype D, and 19% in subtype A virus, and multiple mutations were more likely to be present in subtype C.[357] Subtype may also affect the fading of different resistance mutations. Further analysis of resistance in the HIVNET 012 study showed rates of detectable resistance were similar in subtype A and D at 7 days but higher in subtype D than A at 6–8 weeks. This was attributable to two features; a faster fading of detection of Y181C mutations in women with subtype A and a faster accumulation of K103N mutations in women with subtype D.[358] Detectable resistant mutations by standard genotyping are less after 6–12 months. In a South African study resistance was detectable in 14% of women at 6 months compared to 38% at 6 weeks.[359] Other factors may affect the risk of selection of resistant virus such as; high baseline viral load, low baseline CD4 count, an increased exposure to NVP or the number of NVP doses; or the body compartment, as breast milk may have more resistant virus than plasma.[319,322,360–362]

The selection of NNRTI-resistant virus is not limited to the use of NVP alone. Resistant mutations can be detected following the use of NVP with short course zidovudine, and was found by standard genotyping techniques in mothers who had received antepartum zidovudine and intrapartum NVP in two studies; 28.4% (95% CI, 18.4–40.1%) of mothers in the DITRAME plus study,[363] and in 32% of mothers in the PHPT-2 study [322] had detectable resistant virus at 4–6 weeks postpartum. The addition of single dose NVP to other background regimens was also associated with detectable resistance in 5/39 (13%) of women on NVP-containing HAART for PMTCT in Dublin[364] and 14/95 (15%) (95% CI, 8–23%) in a substudy of the PACTG 316 study.[365]

Resistance is also commonly detectable in HIV-infected infants exposed to single dose NVP, ranging from 20% to 50%.[319,356,358,361,366–370] The patterns of mutations in children are different from those in mothers, and appear to arise most often in the child, rather than being transmitted from the mother, with Y181C mutations more commonly detected than K103N.

The emergence of NNRTI resistance may be underestimated by standard genotyping techniques, which require at least 10–20% of the viral population to have the resistant mutation for detection.[371] The use of more sensitive tests, such as real-time PCR and LigAmp has shown that resistant virus is present in up to 70% of women.[372–374]

There are concerns about the future implications of the emergence of NVP resistance following PMTCT regimens, particularly with regard to future treatment options. In many resource-constrained settings, the NNRTI drugs NVP and EFV are an important, effective and inexpensive part of first-line antiretroviral treatment regimens.[317] One study from Thailand suggested that women previously exposed to NVP for PMTCT are less likely to suppress virus to below 50 copies/mL at 6 months on NVP-containing HAART regimens, although clinical and immunologic outcomes were similar to those in unexposed women.[322] Data from women started on NVP regimens after the MASHI study in Botswana showed that sdNVP exposure was associated with significantly higher rates of virologic failure compared to unexposed women among women who started NVP-containing ART within 6 months of peripartum exposure (45.8% vs 2.9% at 12 months), but not among women starting antiretrovirals longer than 6 months after single dose NVP (12% vs 13.8% at 12 months).[323] Infants exposed to sdNVP in this study experienced a much higher rate of death or virologic failure than nonexposed infants. Although two other small descriptive studies have suggested that outcomes are similar in previously NVP exposed and unexposed women,[375,376] additional research is required on this issue. Little is known about the efficacy of repeated single dose NVP in subsequent pregnancies. Data from studies in South Africa, Cote d'Ivoire and Uganda suggest that efficacy is similar in subsequent pregnancies in women previously exposed to NVP compared to those unexposed.[377–379]

While the long-term relevance of the selection of NNRTI resistance after PMTCT regimens may not yet be clear, it would seem to be preferable to avoid this selection of resistant virus. The addition of either 4 or 7 days of zidovudine or 3TC postpartum has been shown in one study to reduce the prevalence of NNRTI resistant virus following intrapartum NVP.[380] In an analysis of 203 mothers, NNRTI resistant mutations were found in 60% (41/68) of women who received NVP alone, 12% (8/67) of those who had 4 days of zidovudine and 3TC postpartum and 10% (7/68) of those who received 7 days treatment. Additional evidence for this approach is provided in data from Abidjan, where only 1.1% NNRTI resistance was seen in women who received antepartum AZT and 3TC, and 3 days postpartum AZT and 3TC, compared to over 20% in the same population receiving AZT and NVP alone.[381] However, in this study the longer duration of antepartum and postpartum 3TC treatment resulted in 3TC resistance selection in 8.33%. The additional 4–7 day cover of the NVP "tail" of action has been included in the WHO guidelines as the preferred option to reduce the risk of resistance,[317] although other studies are in progress to determine the optimal length of treatment, given the prolonged detection of NVP up to 21 days following single dosing.[352]

A low rate of NNRTI resistance of 1.14% (CI, 0.03–6.17%) was also seen in the DITRAME PLUS study where women received zidovudine and 3TC from 32 weeks gestation, intrapartum NVP and 3 days postpartum zidovudine and 3TC. Although 3TC resistant mutations were found in 8.33% (CI, 3.66–15.7).[363] An alternative approach may be to avoid NVP dosing in mothers who have received an antepartum zidovudine course. Results from the MASHI study, although not conclusive, suggest that the maternal NVP dose may not add to the efficacy of the regimen where there is a background of antepartum zidovudine and an infant NVP dose.[336]

Infants Born to Mothers Who did not Receive Antiretroviral Drugs During Pregnancy or Labor

Where mothers have not received any antiretroviral treatment, dosing of the infant with a postexposure prophylaxis approach can still reduce the risk of MTCT. This was first shown with administration of the postpartum component of the ACTG 076 regimen, giving 6 weeks of zidovudine to infants wade. In a study in South Africa, a single infant dose of NVP given to infants of HIV-positive mothers reduced the risk of HIV infection in infants born to untreated mothers. At 12 weeks, 7.9% of those not infected at birth were infected, and NVP was slightly more effective than a 6-week course of zidovudine given to infants.[154] In a Malawi study, transmission at 6–8 weeks of age in babies who were HIV negative at birth, was 7.7% in infants who had an NVP dose and 1 week of zidovudine and 12.1% in those infants who received NVP only,[337] compared to estimates of transmission of 15–20% with no intervention. Data from Thailand suggests that a 4-week course of AZT is more effective than a 1-week course where mothers have received less than 4 weeks of antepartum treatment.[382] Based on these studies, WHO has recommended that the regimen for infant prophylaxis when the mother has not received any antiretroviral prophylaxis should be single dose NVP with 4 weeks of AZT, when possible.[317] Where this is not possible, single dose NVP or single dose NVP with 1 week of AZT should be given. The drugs should be started as soon after delivery as possible.

PROPHYLAXIS AND TREATMENT OF OPPORTUNISTIC INFECTIONS DURING PREGNANCY

As with ART, treatment and prophylaxis of opportunistic infections (OIs) during pregnancy should follow guidelines similar to those for nonpregnant women.[383,384] With more widespread use of HAART, the prevalence of severe OIs has decreased in developed countries, although this is less marked in developing countries where HAART access has been less.[176,385] This is demonstrated in the WITS, where there was a downward trend between 1989 and 2002 in the prevalence of *Mycobacterium tuberculosis*, recurrent bacterial pneumonia and herpes simplex disease, and in which HAART was associated with a 70% reduction in progression to death following AIDS.[19] The immune system restoration achieved with HAART may also enable stopping of primary or secondary OI prophylaxis.

There may be interactions between pregnancy and some OIs – affecting the symptoms, presentation and natural history of some OIs, or adversely affecting pregnancy outcome. Close monitoring of at-risk pregnant women is required, as nonspecific symptoms such as weight loss, tiredness and pain may be incorrectly attributed to pregnancy rather than to a developing infection.

Drugs frequently used for treatment or prophylaxis of OIs are summarized in Table 35-6. Immunizations for HIV-positive women in pregnancy are summarized in Table 35-7.

Several opportunistic pulmonary infections have been described in HIV-positive pregnant women. The impact of the effect of pregnancy on the course of these respiratory diseases in HIV-infected women is not well-described, and, in general, the management is similar to the nonpregnant state, although delays in diagnosing and treating may influence the course of the disease. *Pneumocystis carinii* pneumonia (PCP) may have a more aggressive course during pregnancy, increasing both the morbidity and mortality. Several case reports from the pre-HAART era illustrated the impact of PCP and the difficulties of treatment in pregnancy.[386–389] Other, more rarely described pulmonary diseases in pregnancy, include bacterial infections (*Haemophilus influenzae* and *Streptococcus pneumoniae* along with *Pseudomona aeruginosa*); fungal infections (*Cryptococcus neoformans*, *Histoplasma capsulatum*, and *Coccidioides immitis*); viral infections (CMV) and opportunistic neoplasms (Kaposi sarcoma, lymphoma).[390]

Other uncommon but potentially fatal OIs described in pregnant women include cerebral toxoplasmosis[391] and disseminated herpes zoster.[392]

Tuberculosis is a leading infectious cause of death in reproductive age women globally and is the most common OI in resource-poor settings.[393–396] A South African study conducted in Durban, investigated 101 maternal deaths occurring in 50 518 deliveries.[397] The Maternal mortality rate was 323 per 100 000 live births for HIV-infected mothers and 148 per 100 000 live births for HIV-negative mothers. The mortality rate for HIV and TB co-infection was 121/1000, three times that of TB without concurrent HIV infection. The authors concluded that 54% of maternal deaths due to TB were attributable to HIV infection.

Another common complication in SSA is malaria. Several studies have shown evidence of an association between malaria in pregnancy and HIV infection.[398–401] HIV increases the risk of malaria in women of all gravidities, although the mechanism of this association is unclear. In areas with stable malaria, HIV-positive women should have access to insecticide treated bednets, and either intermittent preventive treatment with at least three doses of sulfadoxine-pyrimethamine or daily co-trimoxazole (TMP-SMZ) prophylaxis.[402] It has been suggested that the standard recommended intermittent therapy regimens of sulphadoxine-pyrimethamine may be insufficient to clear parasitemia in these women and may need to be reassessed.[403]

OI Prophylaxis in Pregnancy

Prophylaxis against OIs is given to HIV-positive women to prevent either a primary episode of an OI (primary prophylaxis), or the recurrence of infection (secondary prophylaxis). The special situation of pregnancy may require some adaptation of recommended OI prophylactic regimens, due to the risk of fetal toxicity or teratogenesis associated with some drugs.

Primary prophylaxis for *Pneumocystis carinii* pneumonia should be offered to women with CD4+ counts below 200/mm^3, unexplained fever (higher than 100°F) for 2 weeks or more, or a history of oropharyngeal candidiasis; secondary prophylaxis should be offered to all women with previous *P. carinii* pneumonia. Primary, and probably secondary, prophylaxis may be discontinued for women on HAART with sustained elevations in their CD4+ T-lymphocyte count above 200/mm^3[404–406] Trimethoprim-sulfamethoxazole (TMP-SMZ, Septra, Bactrim, co-trimoxazole), one double-strength tablet daily, is the first choice for prophylaxis during pregnancy. Alternatives include oral dapsone 100 mg daily or aerosolized pentamidine, 300 mg monthly via Respirgard II nebulizer. Therapy may be continued up to delivery, with the infant's caregivers informed of maternal therapy so they can institute careful monitoring of bilirubin levels in the infant. There are theoretical concerns about possible teratogenicity associated with TMP-SMZ exposure in the first trimester, and aerosolized pentamidine can be considered at this time due to its lack of systemic absorption and thus lack of fetal exposure.[384] However, there is no strong evidence to suggest that TMP-SMZ causes birth defects and the benefits of prophylaxis outweigh these concerns. Primary prophylaxis may be

Drugs Used for Treatment and Prophylaxis of Opportunistic Infections During Pregnancy

Table 35-6

Drug	Pregnancy Category	Concerns Regarding Use During Pregnancy	Recommended Use During Pregnancy
Acyclovir	C	Well-tolerated	Treatment of frequent or severe symptomatic herpes outbreaks, use for prevention of recurrences at term still investigational
Amphotericin B	B	None identified	Documented invasive fungal disease
Azithromycin	B	None identified	MAC prophylaxis or treatment, *Chlamydia trachomatis* infection
Cidofovir	C	Embryotoxic and teratogenic in animals	Treatment or secondary prophylaxis of life-threatening or sight-threatening CMV
Ciprofloxacin, other quinolones	C	Arthropathy in immature animals; not teratogenic in animal studies	None
Clarithromycin	C	Teratogenic in rodents	Treatment of secondary prophylaxis of MAC only if other choices exhausted
Clindamycin	B	None identified	Secondary prophylaxis of Toxoplasma encephalitis; treatment of anaerobic bacterial infections
Dapsone	C	None identified	Alternative choice for primary or secondary PCP prophylaxis
Doxycycline, other tetracyclines	D	Incorporated into fetal bones, teeth with staining; maternal fatty liver	None
Erythromycin	B	Hepatotoxicity with erythromycin estolate, other forms acceptable	Bacterial and chlamydial infections
Ethambutol	B	Teratogenic in animals	Active tuberculosis, treatment of MAC
Fluconazole	C	Abnormal ossification, structural defects in rats, case reports of craniofacial, skeletal abnormalities in humans with prolonged *in utero* exposure	Only for documented systemic disease, not prophylaxis; not for treatment of vaginal or oral Candida
Foscarnet	C	Teratogenic in rats, rabbits	Treatment or secondary prophylaxis of life-threatening or sight-threatening CMV
Ganciclovir	C	Teratogenic in rabbits, mice	Treatment or secondary prophylaxis of life-threatening or sight-threatening CMV
Isoniazid	C	Prophylactic vitamin K recommended at birth to prevent hemorrhagic disease. Possible increase in hepatotoxicity	Active tuberculosis or prophylaxis for exposure, skin test conversion
Itraconazole	C	Teratogenic in rats, mice	Documented systemic disease
Ketoconazole	C	Teratogenic in rats, rabbits	None
Leucovorin	C/A	Not teratogenic at recommended doses	Use with pyrimethamine
Pentamidine, aerosolized	C	Embryocidal but not teratogenic in rats with systemic use; limited systemic absorption with aerosol use	Alternative primary or secondary PCP prophylaxis
Pyrimethamine	C	Teratogenic in mice, rats, hamsters; folate antagonist, use with leucovorin	Secondary prophylaxis of Toxoplasma encephalitis; alternative primary or secondary PCP prophylaxis if unable to use TMP-SMZ, dapsone, or aerosolized pentamidine
Rifabutin	B	None identified	Treatment or prophylaxis of MAC, active tuberculosis Limited experience in pregnancy
Rifampin	C	Teratogenic in mice, rats, not rabbits; no clear teratogenicity in humans; vitamin K recommended at birth to prevent hemorrhagic disease of the newborn	Active tuberculosis

(Continued)

Table 35-6

Drug	Pregnancy Category	Concerns Regarding Use During Pregnancy	Recommended Use During Pregnancy
Sulfadiazine	B	Increased jaundice, theoretical increased risk of kernicterus if used near delivery	Secondary prophylaxis of toxoplasmic encephalitis
Trimethoprim-sulfamethoxazole	C	Possible increase in congenital cardiac defects with first trimester use; increased jaundice, theoretical increased risk of kernicterus if used near delivery	Primary and secondary PCP prophylaxis

Adapted from Anderson;[38] AIDS Education and Training Centers;[223] and Watts and Minkoff,[435] US Public Health Service,[8] Mofenson.[295]

Vaccinations and immune Globulin Prophylaxis for HIV-positive Pregnant Women

Table 35-7

Product	Recommendation	Notes
Pneumococcal vaccine	Generally recommended	If not received during previous 5 years consider revaccination if initially immunized with CD4+ T-lymphocyte <200/mm³ with increase to CD4+ T-lymphocyte >200/mm³ in response to ARV treatment repeat every 5–7 years
Influenza vaccine	Generally recommended	Administer before flu season annually
Tetanus-diphtheria (Td) vaccine		Booster dose every 10 years after completion of primary series
Hepatitis B vaccine	Generally recommended for all susceptible (antiHBc-negative) patients	Three doses at 0, 1, 6 months
Hepatitis A vaccine	Generally recommended for all susceptible (antiHAV-negative) patients with chronic hepatitis C or hepatitis B	Also indicated before travel to endemic areas, in injection drug users, or in setting of a community outbreak; two doses at 0, 6 months
Enhanced potency inactivated polio vaccine	Use if not previously immunized and traveling to areas where risk for exposure is high	Note that oral polio vaccine is a live virus vaccine and is contraindicated in HIV-positive persons
Immuneglobulins	Recommended for postexposure prophylaxis in susceptible individuals	
Hyper immuneglobulins		
Varicella-zoster virus immuneglobulin (VZIG)	Recommended after significant exposure to VZV for those with undetectable antibodies to VZV or no history of either chickenpox or shingles (give within 96 h)	
Hepatitis B immuneglobulin (HBIG)	Recommended after needlestick or sexual exposure to a person with hepatitis B infection in susceptible individual (anti-HBc negative) HBIG should be given and HBV vaccine series should be started within 14 days of exposure	
Contraindicated		
Measles/Mumps/Rubella (MMR)	Contraindicated: live vaccine	
Oral polio vaccine	Contraindicated: live vaccine	
Varicella	Contraindicated: live vaccine	

Adapted from Anderson;[38] AIDS Education and Training Centers;[223] and Watts and Minkoff,[435] US Public Health Service,[8] Mofenson.[295]

safely discontinued where there is a sustained increase in CD4+ count above 200 cells/mm^3 for at least 3–6 months. Secondary prophylaxis (to prevent a recurrence) can be discontinued after a sustained CD4 cell increase above 200 cells/mm^3 for at least 6 months. Prophylaxis should be resumed if the CD4 count subsequently falls below 200 cells/mm^3.

As TMP inhibits the synthesis of metabolically active folic acid, pregnant women taking TMP-SMZ are at higher risk of folate deficiency, which increases the risk of neural tube defects in the fetus. Folate supplementation should be given to reduce the risk of neural tube defects and high doses of folate (e.g., 4 mg daily) may be recommended to overcome the folate antagonism of TMP-SMZ. Because neural tube development occurs very early in pregnancy, folate supplementation should be started at least one month before conception, if possible.

TMP-SMZ prophylaxis may have other more general benefits on pregnancy outcome in women with low CD4+ cell counts where antiretroviral treatment is not available. In a report from Zambia, women with CD4+ counts below 200/mm^3 who received TMP-SMZ had significant improvements in birth outcome compared to women who did not receive TMP-SMZ. Preterm delivery less than 34 weeks declined from 31% to 18%, clinical chorioamnionitis declined from 6.4% to 0% and perinatal mortality (within 28 days of birth) declined from 9% to 0%.[407]

United States guidelines recommend that prophylaxis for *Mycobacterium avium* complex (MAC) should be offered for CD4+ counts lower than 50 cells/mm^3 or previously documented MAC infection. Other international guidelines do not routinely recommend MAC prophylaxis. Azithromycin, 1200 mg once weekly, is the first choice for therapy during pregnancy, as in nonpregnant individuals, although some treating physicians recommend withholding the drug until after the first trimester. Clarithromycin should be avoided during pregnancy because of demonstrated teratogenicity in animals, and there is limited experience with rifabutin in pregnancy. Azithromycin with ethambutol are the preferred drugs for secondary prophylaxis (chronic maintenance therapy).

Testing for immunoglobulin G (IgG) antibodies to *Toxoplasma gondii* should be a part of antenatal testing for the pregnant woman with HIV infection. Women with negative IgG should be counseled to avoid Toxoplasma exposure, by avoiding raw or undercooked meats, unwashed or uncooked vegetables, and cat feces.[223] Toxoplasma encephalitis is usually caused by reactivation of latent *Toxoplasma gondii* infection in patients with advanced immunosuppression and with CD4 counts <100 cells/ mm^3). TMP-SMZ, as used for PCP prophylaxis, also provides prophylaxis in women who are seropositive for antibodies to *Toxoplasma gondii*. For women with previous toxoplasma encephalitis, an appropriate prophylactic regimen should be offered throughout pregnancy. TMP-SMZ may be used as primary prophylaxis during pregnancy. Prophylaxis that includes pyrimethamine generally should be deferred until after pregnancy, although pyrimethamine may be used with caution to treat active toxoplasmosis during pregnancy in sulfa-allergic patients.

Tuberculosis (TB) prophylaxis may be considered in pregnancy, in line with local guidelines, for any woman with a history of exposure to active TB or a positive purified protein derivative (PPD) skin test (≤5 mm induration). Active TB disease must be ruled out before starting prophylaxis. Isoniazid or rifampin prophylaxis can be used during pregnancy although they should be monitored closely, as pregnant women may have an increased risk of liver toxicity with isoniazid. Patients receiving isoniazid also should receive pyridoxine to reduce the risk of neurotoxicity. Because of concern about possible teratogenicity from drug exposure, clinicians may choose to delay prophylaxis until after the first trimester. Pyrazinamide should usually be avoided, especially in the first trimester, because of lack of information concerning fetal effects. For women with no evidence of active TB but exposure to multidrug-resistant TB, prophylactic therapy may best be deferred until after delivery. Treatment of active TB during pregnancy should be undertaken in consultation with obstetric and infectious disease specialists.

Prophylaxis for cytomegalovirus (CMV) disease is not recommended during pregnancy because of the potential toxicity of the drugs and limited experience with their use during pregnancy. However, for women with life-threatening or sight-threatening CMV infections during pregnancy, treatment should be provided in consultation with obstetric and infectious disease specialists. Primary prophylaxis for other conditions, including mucosal candidiasis and other fungal infections, is best avoided during pregnancy. Treatment of invasive fungal disease should be provided as it would be for a nonpregnant individual.

Where possible, immunizations should be given before pregnancy, but can be considered during pregnancy where there is high risk to the mother or fetus, and low risk of harm from the vaccine. Pneumococcal, hepatitis B, and influenza vaccines may be administered to pregnant women with the same indications as for nonpregnant individuals. Live virus vaccines such as rubella, measles, mumps, and varicella are contraindicated during pregnancy. Some vaccines may cause a transient increase in viral load and may potentially increase MTCT risk. It is advisable to defer vaccination until after ART has been commenced, which will prevent the viral load increase.[223]

INFANT FEEDING

The dramatic reduction in MTCT achieved in the United States and Europe has been partly due to the avoidance of breastfeeding in these settings.[7,408] In contrast, one-third to one-half of transmission in Africa and other low-resources settings is due to infection through breastfeeding, where replacement feeding is not easy or feasible to implement.[409,410] Transmission of HIV through breastfeeding has been well documented, both with primary infection during breastfeeding (mean ~29%, range 16–42%) and with HIV infection through pregnancy (median ~14%, range 9–32%).[89,102,411–413] Miotti et al in Malawi showed a 0.7% per month incidence of transmission from breastfeeding from 2 to 6 months of age and 0.3% incidence from 12 to 24 months, equivalent to about 3% additional risk from 12 to 24 months.[414] A randomized controlled trial comparing breastfeeding and replacement feeding in Nairobi showed a cumulative probability of HIV infection at 24 months of age of 36.7% in the breastfeeding arm and 20.5% in the formula feeding arm.[415] Forty-four percent of HIV infection in breastfed infants was attributable to breast milk. Although the 2-year mortality rates were similar in the two groups, HIV-free survival was significantly lower in the breastfeeding arm (58% vs 70%, $P = 0.02$).

HIV-positive women should be counseled about the potential risk of infection through breastfeeding. Where resources allow, and replacement feeding is acceptable, feasible, affordable, sustainable, and safe, HIV-positive women should be advised not to breastfeed. Where this is not the case, women who choose to breastfeed should be encouraged to exclusively breastfeed, without any additional solids or liquids given to the baby for 4–6 months followed by rapid weaning. Mixed feeding appears to be most likely to result in transmission.[416,417] However, achieving exclusive breastfeeding may not be easy and mothers should be supported with education on proper breastfeeding techniques, on signs, symptoms and management of breast problems such as mastitis, cracked nipples and abscesses and on the diagnosis of oral thrush or other lesions in the child.[38,418–420] If mothers choose not to breastfeed, or when they stop breastfeeding they should be given guidance and support to provide adequate infant nutrition for the first 2 years of life.[421]

Antiretrovirals and Breastfeeding

There is little information available on the use of ART in breastfeeding mothers, as breastfeeding is uncommon in women on antiretrovirals in the developed world. This situation is likely to change as treatment access improves globally, and especially in Africa, where ART may not always be linked to replacement feeding.[422]

It is possible that maternal ART may provide a benefit in this instance, in potentially reducing the risk of MTCT through breast milk. The use of HAART through the period of breastfeeding for mothers who do not yet require it for their own health, as a PMTCT strategy has also been suggested and is being investigated.[422–424] There is insufficient evidence at present to suggest that maternal ART or prophylactic antiretrovirals to mother or infant will reduce HIV transmission to infants during breastfeeding and the potential risks and benefits for antiretrovirals only to reduce transmission need to be better understood[317] before this could be recommended.

Studies of HIV-1 RNA in breast milk of mothers who received perinatal AZT monotherapy showed a reduction in breast milk RNA, with some rebound of breast milk viral load after stopping the short course zidovudine, which was associated with transmission.[425] In developed settings, triple combination therapy is used for many women only for a PMTCT indication and stopped after delivery, although it is rare for these women to breastfeed. Some less-resourced settings are using HAART PMTCT regimens, stopped after delivery, where some women will breastfeed.[256,257] There is a lack of similar data for breast milk viral load following discontinuation of combination ART regimens for PMTCT, although it is possible that a more pronounced viral rebound could occur after better viral suppression, and this may impact on breast milk transmission in this situation. This suggests that extension of HAART through the period of breastfeeding may be required. More data is needed in this regard.

Differential transfer of drugs into breast milk may select for resistant viruses. A Zimbabwean study showed that NVP resistance was more commonly found in breast milk than in plasma following sdNVP, with a different pattern of resistance mutations.[426] There may be safety concerns for infants who receive relatively high doses of antiretrovirals in breast milk over a long period of time.[427] Data from this study in Botswana showed levels of NVP in breast milk of women receiving NVP-based ART that were lower than in maternal plasma, while levels of 3TC and AZT in breast were about three-fold higher. These concerns should not be a reason at present to stop antiretroviral treatment in women who require it and are breastfeeding.

One of the advantages of NVP use for PMTCT may be the prolonged half-life of the drug and the resulting sustained suppression of breast milk viral load. In a study in Kenya, HIV transmission at 6 weeks was significantly lower in infants of women randomized to receive single dose NVP compared to those who received a short course AZT regimen. NVP was significantly more likely to decrease HIV-1 RNA in breast milk. The viral load was significantly more likely to be decreased during the first week and through the third week postpartum following single-dose NVP administration, and this was associated with a decreased transmission risk.[428] This fits with other studies which have suggested a benefit to NVP dosing in reducing postpartum transmission.[154,429]

Shapiro et al compared the levels of HIV-1 RNA and DNA in breast-milk of women in Botswana who received combination HAART (NVP, AZT and 3TC) with those in women not receiving therapy. The median time on HAART in the treated group was 98 days (range, 67–222 days). In this study, HAART suppressed cell-free HIV-1 RNA in breast milk, but did not have an effect on cell-associated HIV-1 DNA loads in breast milk.[430] The HIV-1 RNA suppression correlated with reduction in plasma viral load and HAART, although one-third of untreated mothers also had undetectable HIV-1 RNA. It is not possible to show a level of HIV RNA below which transmission does not take place.[425] It is not clear whether this reduction in cell-free virus will be sufficient to reduce breast milk transmission, which has been associated with both cell-free and cell-associated virus,[431–434] or whether longer duration of HAART would better suppress cell-associated virus. Further research is in progress to evaluate the efficacy and safety of HAART use through the period of breastfeeding.

REFERENCES

1. UNAIDS. 2006 Report on the Global AIDS Epidemic. Geneva: UNAIDS, 2006.
2. Rice BD, Payne LJ, Sinka K, et al. The changing epidemiology of prevalent diagnosed HIV infections in England, Wales, and Northern Ireland, 1997 to 2003. Sex Transm Infect 81:223–29, 2005.
3. Thorne C, Newell M-L. Managing mother-to-child transmission of HIV. Womens Health 1:1–15, 2005.
4. Hamers FF, Downs AM. The changing face of the HIV epidemic in western Europe: what are the implications for public health policies? Lancet 364:83–94, 2004.
5. Centers for Disease Control and Prevention (CDC). Twenty-five years of HIV/AIDS – United States, 1981–2006. MMWR Morb Mortal Wkly Rep 2006; 55:585–9.
6. Centers for Disease Control and Prevention (CDC). Epidemiology of HIV/AIDS – United States, 1981–2005. MMWR Morb Mortal Wkly Rep 55:589–92, 2006.
7. Centers for Disease Control and Prevention (CDC). Achievements in public health. Reduction in perinatal transmission of HIV infection – United States, 1985–2005. MMWR Morb Mortal Wkly Rep 55:592–7, 2006.
8. US Public Health Service. Public Health Service Task Force Recommendations for Use of Antiretroviral Drugs in Pregnant HIV-1-Infected Women for Maternal Health and Interventions to Reduce Perinatal HIV-1 Transmission in the United States – November 17. 2005. Available: http://www.aidsinfo.nih.gov/guidelines 17 Nov 2005.
9. The British HIV Association. Guidelines for the management of HIV infection in pregnant women and the prevention of mother-to-child transmission of HIV. London: The British HIV Association; 2005.
10. Burdge DR, Money DM, Forbes JC, et al. Canadian consensus guidelines for the care of HIV-positive pregnant women: putting recommendations into practice. CMAJ 168:1683–8, 2003.
11. Bessinger R, Clark R, Kissinger P, Rice J, Coughlin S. Pregnancy is not associated with the progression of HIV disease in women attending an HIV outpatient program. Am J Epidemiol 147:434–40, 1998.
12. Burns DN, Landesman S, Minkoff H, et al. The influence of pregnancy on human immunodeficiency virus type 1 infection: antepartum and postpartum changes in human immunodeficiency virus type 1 viral load. Am J Obstet Gynecol 178:355–9, 1998.
13. Weisser M, Rudin C, Battegay M, Pfluger D, Kully C, Egger M. Does pregnancy influence the course of HIV infection? Evidence from two large Swiss cohort studies. J Acquir Immune Defic Syndr Hum Retrovirol 17:404–10, 1998.
14. Saada M, Le Chenadec J, Berrebi A, et al. Pregnancy and progression to AIDS: results of the French prospective cohorts. SEROGEST and SEROCO Study Groups. AIDS 14:2355–60, 2000.
15. Ahdieh L. Pregnancy and infection with human immunodeficiency virus. Clin Obstet Gynecol 44:154–66, 2001.
16. Hocke C, Morlat P, Chene G, Dequae L, Dabis F. Prospective cohort study of the effect of pregnancy on the progression of human immunodeficiency virus infection. The Groupe d'Epidemiologie Clinique Du SIDA en Aquitaine. Obstet Gynecol 86:886–91, 1995.
17. Manopaiboon C, Shaffer N, Clark L, et al. Impact of HIV on families of HIV-infected women who have recently given birth, Bangkok, Thailand. J Acquir Immune Defic Syndr Hum Retrovirol 18:54–63, 1998.
18. French R, Brocklehurst P. The effect of pregnancy on survival in women infected with HIV: a systematic review of the literature and meta-analysis. Br J Obstet Gynaecol 105:827–35, 1998.
19. Charurat M, Blattner W, Hershow R, et al. Changing trends in clinical AIDS presentations and survival among HIV-1-infected women. J Womens Health (Larchmt) 3:719–30, 2004.
20. Minkoff H, Hershow R, Watts DH, et al. The relationship of pregnancy to human immunodeficiency virus disease progression. Am J Obstet Gynecol 189:552–9, 2003.
21. Tai J, Barkanic G, Udoji M, et al. The decreased risk of HIV disease progression associated with pregnancy in the HAART era is independent of durable virologic suppression and other factors that affect prognosis. In: 13th Conference on Retroviruses and Opportunistic Infections, Denver, CO, 5–8 Feb 2006, abstract 705.
22. Burns DN, Nourjah P, Minkoff H, et al. Changes in CD4+ and CD8+ cell levels during pregnancy and post partum in women seropositive and seronegative for human immunodeficiency virus-1. Am J Obstet Gynecol 174:1461–8, 1996.
23. van Benthem BH, Vernazza P, Coutinho RA, Prins M. The impact of pregnancy and menopause on CD4 lymphocyte counts in HIV-infected women. AIDS 16:919–24, 2002.
24. Tuomala RE, Kalish LA, Zorilla C, et al. Changes in total, CD4+, and CD8+ lymphocytes during pregnancy and 1 year postpartum in human immunodeficiency virus-infected women. The women and infants transmission study. Obstet Gynecol 89:967–74, 1997.
25. Temmerman M, Nagelkerke N, Bwayo J, Chomba EN, Ndinya-Achola J, Piot P. HIV-1 and immunological changes during pregnancy: a comparison between HIV-1-seropositive and HIV-1-seronegative women in Nairobi, Kenya. AIDS 9:1057–60, 1995.
26. Ekpini RA, Nkengasong JN, Sibailly T, et al. Changes in plasma HIV-1-RNA viral load and CD4 cell counts, and lack of zidovudine resistance among pregnant women receiving short-course zidovudine. AIDS 16:625–30, 2002.
27. Mulcahy F, Wallace E, Woods S, et al. CD4 counts in pregnancy do not accurately reflect the need for long-term HAART. In: 13th Conference on Retroviruses and Opportunistic Infections, Denver, CO, 5–8 Feb 2006, abstract 704b.
28. Ekouevi D, Inwoley A, Tonwe-Gold B, et al. Criteria for HAART should be revisited in HIV-infected pregnant women in resource-limited settings. In: 13th Conference on Retroviruses and Opportunistic Infections, Denver, CO, 5–8 Feb 2006, abstract 704a.
29. Fabiani M, Nattabi B, Ayella EO, Ogwang M, Declich S. Differences in fertility by HIV serostatus and adjusted HIV prevalence data from an antenatal clinic in northern Uganda. Trop Med Int Health 11:182–7, 2006.
30. Desgrees du Lou A, Msellati P, Yao A, et al. Impaired fertility in HIV-1-infected pregnant women: a clinic-based survey in Abidjan, Cote d'Ivoire, 1997. AIDS 13:517–21, 1999.
31. Gregson S, Zaba B, Garnett GP. Low fertility in women with HIV and the impact of the epidemic on orphanhood and early childhood mortality in sub-Saharan Africa. AIDS 13(Suppl A): S249–57, 1999.
32. Hunter SC, Isingo R, Boerma JT, et al. The association between HIV and fertility in a cohort study in rural Tanzania. J Biosoc Sci 35:189–99, 2003.
33. Zaba B, Gregson S. Measuring the impact of HIV on fertility in Africa. AIDS 12(Suppl 1):S41–50, 1998.
34. Zaba B, Terceira N, Mason P, Gregson S. The contribution of HIV to fertility decline in rural Zimbabwe, 1985–2000. Popul Stud (Camb) 7:149–64, 2003.
35. Lee LM, Wortley PM, Fleming PL, et al. Duration of human immunodeficiency virus infection and likelihood of giving birth in a Medicaid population in Maryland. Am J Epidemiol 151:1020–8, 2000.
36. Gilling-Smith C, Nicopoullos J, Semprini A, Frodsham L. HIV and reproductive care – a review of current practice. BJOG 116:869–78, 2006.

37. Glynn JR, Buve A, Carael M, Zaba B. Adjustment of antenatal clinic HIV surveillance data for HIV-associated differences in fertility. AIDS 13:1598–9, 1999.
38. Anderson JR. A Guide to the Clinical Care of Women with HIV. Rockville, MD: Health Services and Resources Administration; 2005.
39. Gray RH, Wawer MJ, Serwadda D, et al. Population-based study of fertility in women with HIV-1 infection in Uganda. Lancet 351:98–103, 1998.
40. Sedgh G, Larsen U, Spiegelman D, et al. HIV-1 disease progression and fertility in Dar es Salaam, Tanzania. J Acquir Immune Defic Syndr 39:439–45, 2005.
41. Deschamps MM, Pape JW, Desvarieux M, et al. A prospective study of HIV-seropositive asymptomatic women of childbearing age in a developing country. J Acquir Immune Defic Syndr 6:446–51, 1993.
42. Kumar RM, Uduman SA, Khurranna AK. Impact of maternal HIV-1 infection on perinatal outcome. Int J Gynaecol Obstet 49:137–43, 1995.
43. Department of Health SA. Second Interim Report on Confidential Enquiries into Maternal Deaths in South Africa Department of Health, Pretoria, South Africa . 1999.
44. Lema VM, Changole J, Kanyighe C, Malunga EV. Maternal mortality at the Queen Elizabeth Central Teaching Hospital, Blantyre, Malawi. East Afr Med J 82:3–9, 2005.
45. Majoko F, Chipato T, Iliff V. Trends in maternal mortality for the Greater Harare Maternity Unit: 1976 to 1997. Cent Afr J Med 47:199–203, 2001.
46. Oyieke JB, Obore S, Kigondu CS. Millennium development goal 5: a review of maternal mortality at the Kenyatta National Hospital, Nairobi. East Afr Med J 83:4–9, 2006.
47. Fawcus SR, van Coeverden de Groot HA, Isaacs S. A 50-year audit of maternal mortality in the Peninsula Maternal and Neonatal Service, Cape Town (1953–2002). BJOG 112: 1257–63, 2005.
48. McIntyre J. Mothers infected with HIV. Br Med Bull 67: 127–35, 2003.
49. McIntyre J. Maternal health and HIV. Reprod Health Matters 13:129–35, 2005.
50. Ryder RW, Nsuami M, Nsa W, et al. Mortality in HIV-1-seropositive women, their spouses and their newly born children during 36 months of follow-up in Kinshasa, Zaire. AIDS 8:667–72, 1994.
51. McDermott JM, Slutsker L, Steketee RW, et al. Prospective assessment of mortality among a cohort of pregnant women in rural Malawi. Am J Trop Med Hyg 55(1 Suppl):66–70, 1996.
52. O'Brien ME, Kupka R, Msamanga GI, et al. Anemia is an independent predictor of mortality and immunologic progression of disease among women with HIV in Tanzania. J Acquir Immune Defic Syndr 40:219–25, 2005.
53. Fawzi W, Msamanga G, Spiegelman D, Hunter DJ. Studies of vitamins and minerals and HIV transmission and disease progression. J Nutr 135:938–44, 2005.
54. John GC, Bird T, Overbaugh J, et al. CCR5 promoter polymorphisms in a Kenyan perinatal human immunodeficiency virus type 1 cohort: association with increased 2-year maternal mortality. J Infect Dis 184:89–92, 2001.
55. Le Coeur S, Khlat M, Halembokaka G, et al. HIV and the magnitude of pregnancy-related mortality in Pointe Noire, Congo. AIDS 19:69–75, 2005.
56. Zaba B, Whitworth J, Marston M, et al. HIV and mortality of mothers and children: evidence from cohort studies in Uganda, Tanzania, and Malawi. Epidemiology 16:275–80, 2005.
57. Newell ML, Coovadia H, Cortina-Borja M, et al. Mortality of infected and uninfected infants born to HIV-infected mothers in Africa: a pooled analysis. Lancet 364:1236–43, 2004.
58. Taha TE, Miotti P, Liomba G, et al. HIV, maternal death and child survival in Africa. AIDS 10:111–12, 1996.
59. The United Nations Children's Fund (UNICEF). A call to action: children, the missing face to AIDS. The Global Campaign on Children and AIDS: Unite for Children. Unite against AIDS. New York: UNICEF; 2005.
60. Mofenson LM, McIntyre JA. Advances and research directions in the prevention of mother-to-child HIV-1 transmission. Lancet 355:2237–44, 2000.
61. Newell ML. Mechanisms and timing of mother-to-child transmission of HIV-1. AIDS 12:831–7, 1998.
62. Cooper ER, Charurat M, Burns DN, et al. Trends in antiretroviral therapy and mother-infant transmission of HIV. The Women and Infants Transmission Study Group. J Acquir Immune Defic Syndr 24:45–7, 2000.
63. Moodley D, Moodley J, Coovadia H, et al. A multicenter randomized controlled trial of nevirapine versus a combination of zidovudine and lamivudine to reduce intrapartum and early postpartum mother-to-child transmission of human immunodeficiency virus type 1. J Infect Dis 187:725–35, 2003.
64. Blanche S, Tardieu M, Duliege A, et al. Longitudinal study of 94 symptomatic infants with perinatally acquired human immunodeficiency virus infection. Evidence for a bimodal expression of clinical and biological symptoms. Am J Dis Child 144:1210–15, 1990.
65. Children born to women with HIV-1 infection: natural history and risk of transmission. European collaborative study. Lancet 337:253–60, 1991.
66. Luzuriaga K, McQuilken P, Alimenti A, et al. Early viremia and immune responses in vertical human immunodeficiency virus type 1 infection. J Infect Dis 167:1008–13, 1993.
67. McIntosh K, Pitt J, Brambilla D, et al. Blood culture in the first 6 months of life for the diagnosis of vertically transmitted human immunodeficiency virus infection. The Women and Infants Transmission Study Group. J Infect Dis 170:996–1000, 1994.
68. Mock PA, Shaffer N, Bhadrakom C, et al. Maternal viral load and timing of mother-to-child HIV transmission, Bangkok, Thailand. Bangkok Collaborative Perinatal HIV Transmission Study Group. AIDS 13:407–14, 1999.
69. Clemetson DB, Moss GB, Willerford DM, et al. Detection of HIV DNA in cervical and vaginal secretions. Prevalence and correlates among women in Nairobi, Kenya. JAMA 269:2860–4, 1993.
70. Henin Y, Mandelbrot L, Henrion R, Pradinaud R, Coulaud JP, Montagnier L. Virus excretion in the cervicovaginal secretions of pregnant and nonpregnant HIV-infected women. J Acquir Immune Defic Syndr 6:72–5, 1993.
71. Chuachoowong R, Shaffer N, Siriwasin W, et al. Short-course antenatal zidovudine reduces both cervicovaginal human immunodeficiency virus type 1 RNA levels and risk of perinatal transmission. Bangkok Collaborative Perinatal HIV Transmission Study Group. J Infect Dis 181:99–106, 2000.
72. Duliege AM, Amos CI, Felton S, et al. Birth order, delivery route, and concordance in the transmission of human immunodeficiency virus type 1 from mothers to twins. International Registry of HIV-Exposed Twins. J Pediatr 126: 625–32, 1995.
73. Burns DN, Landesman S, Muenz LR, et al. Cigarette smoking, premature rupture of membranes, and vertical transmission of HIV-1 among women with low CD4+ levels. J Acquir Immune Defic Syndr 7:718–26, 1994.
74. Minkoff H, Burns DN, Landesman S, et al. The relationship of the duration of ruptured membranes to vertical transmission of human immunodeficiency virus. Am J Obstet Gynecol 173:585–9, 1995.
75. Landesman SH, Kalish LA, Burns DN, et al. Obstetrical factors and the transmission of human immunodeficiency virus type 1 from mother to child. The Women and Infants Transmission Study. N Engl J Med 334:1617–23, 1996.

76. McGowan JP, Crane M, Wiznia AA, Blum S. Combination antiretroviral therapy in human immunodeficiency virus-infected pregnant women. Obstet Gynecol 94(5 Pt 1):641–6, 1999.
77. Elective cesarean-section versus vaginal delivery in prevention of vertical HIV-1 transmission: a randomised clinical trial. The European Mode of Delivery Collaboration. Lancet 353:1035–9, 1999.
78. Risk factors for mother-to-child transmission of HIV-1. European Collaborative Study. Lancet 339:1007–12, 1992.
79. Mayaux MJ, Dussaix E, Isopet J, et al. Maternal virus load during pregnancy and mother-to-child transmission of human immunodeficiency virus type 1: the French perinatal cohort studies. SEROGEST Cohort Group. J Infect Dis 175:172–5, 1997.
80. Martinez AM, Hora VP, Santos AL, et al. Determinants of HIV-1 mother-to-child transmission in Southern Brazil. An Acad Bras Cienc 78:113–21, 2006.
81. De Rossi A, Ometto L, Masiero S, et al. Viral phenotype in mother-to-child HIV-1 transmission and disease progression of vertically acquired HIV-1 infection. Acta Paediatr Suppl 421:22–8, 1997.
82. Ometto L, Zanotto C, Maccabruni A, et al. Viral phenotype and host-cell susceptibility to HIV-1 infection as risk factors for mother-to-child HIV-1 transmission. AIDS 9:427–34, 1995.
83. Tscherning-Casper C, Vodros D, Menu E, et al. Coreceptor usage of HIV-1 isolates representing different genetic subtypes obtained from pregnant Cameroonian women. European Network for In Utero Transmission of HIV-1. J Acquir Immune Defic Syndr 24:1–9, 2000.
84. Blackard JT, Renjifo B, Fawzi W, et al. HIV-1 LTR subtype and perinatal transmission. Virology 287:261–5, 2001.
85. Renjifo B, Fawzi W, Mwakagile D, et al. Differences in perinatal transmission among human immunodeficiency virus type 1 genotypes. J Hum Virol 4:16–25, 2001.
86. Ometto L, Zanchetta M, Mainardi M, et al. Co-receptor usage of HIV-1 primary isolates, viral burden, and CCR5 genotype in mother-to-child HIV-1 transmission. AIDS 14:1721–9, 2000.
87. Philpott S, Burger H, Charbonneau T, et al. CCR5 genotype and resistance to vertical transmission of HIV-1. J Acquir Immune Defic Syndr 21:189–93, 1999.
88. Dickover RE, Garratty EM, Plaeger S, Bryson YJ. Perinatal transmission of major, minor, and multiple maternal human immunodeficiency virus type 1 variants in utero and intrapartum. J Virol 75:2194–203, 2001.
89. Ryder RW, Nsa W, Hassig SE, et al. Perinatal transmission of the human immunodeficiency virus type 1 to infants of seropositive women in Zaire. N Engl J Med 320:1637–42, 1989.
90. St Louis ME, Kamenga M, Brown C, et al. Risk for perinatal HIV-1 transmission according to maternal immunologic, virologic, and placental factors. JAMA 269:2853–9, 1993.
91. Temmerman M, Nyong'o AO, Bwayo J, et al. Risk factors for mother-to-child transmission of human immunodeficiency virus-1 infection. Am J Obstet Gynecol 172(2 Pt 1):700–5, 1995.
92. Minkoff HL, Henderson C, Mendez H, et al. Pregnancy outcomes among mothers infected with human immunodeficiency virus and uninfected control subjects. Am J Obstet Gynecol 163(5 Pt 1):1598–604, 1990.
93. Perinatal findings in children born to HIV-infected mothers. The European Collaborative Study. Br J Obstet Gynaecol 101:136–41, 1994.
94. Abrams EJ, Matheson PB, Thomas PA, et al. Neonatal predictors of infection status and early death among 332 infants at risk of HIV-1 infection monitored prospectively from birth. New York City Perinatal HIV Transmission Collaborative Study Group. Pediatrics 96(3 Pt 1):451–8, 1995.
95. Tovo PA, de Martino M, Gabiano C, et al. Mode of delivery and gestational age influence perinatal HIV-1 transmission. Italian Register for HIV Infection in Children. J Acquir Immune Defic Syndr Hum Retrovirol 11:88–94, 1996.
96. Nair P, Alger L, Hines S, et al. Maternal and neonatal characteristics associated with HIV infection in infants of seropositive women. J Acquir Immune Defic Syndr 6:298–302, 1993.
97. Van Dyke RB, Korber BT, Popek E, et al. The Ariel Project: A prospective cohort study of maternal-child transmission of human immunodeficiency virus type 1 in the era of maternal antiretroviral therapy. J Infect Dis 179:319–28, 1999.
98. Wabwire-Mangen F, Gray RH, Mmiro FA, et al. Placental membrane inflammation and risks of maternal-to-child transmission of HIV-1 in Uganda. J Acquir Immune Defic Syndr 22:379–85, 1999.
99. Sutton MY, Sternberg M, Nsuami M, et al. Trichomoniasis in pregnant human immunodeficiency virus-infected and human immunodeficiency virus-uninfected congolese women: prevalence, risk factors, and association with low birth weight. Am J Obstet Gynecol 181:656–62, 1999.
100. Fawzi W, Msamanga G, Renjifo B, et al. Predictors of intrauterine and intrapartum transmission of HIV-1 among Tanzanian women. AIDS 15:1157–65, 2001.
101. Mandelbrot L, Mayaux MJ, Bongain A, et al. Obstetric factors and mother-to-child transmission of human immunodeficiency virus type 1: the French perinatal cohorts. SEROGEST French Pediatric HIV Infection Study Group. Am J Obstet Gynecol 175(3 Pt 1):661–7, 1996.
102. Hutto C, Parks WP, Lai SH, et al. A hospital-based prospective study of perinatal infection with human immunodeficiency virus type 1. J Pediatr 118:347–53, 1991.
103. Temmerman M, Chomba EN, Ndinya-Achola J, et al. Maternal human immunodeficiency virus-1 infection and pregnancy outcome. Obstet Gynecol 83:495–501, 1994.
104. Shaffer N, Roongpisuthipong A, Siriwasin W, et al. Maternal virus load and perinatal human immunodeficiency virus type 1 subtype E transmission, Thailand. Bangkok Collaborative Perinatal HIV Transmission Study Group. J Infect Dis 179:590–9, 1999.
105. Rodriguez EM, Mofenson LM, Chang BH, et al. Association of maternal drug use during pregnancy with maternal HIV culture positivity and perinatal HIV transmission. AIDS 10:273–82, 1996.
106. Semba RD, Miotti PG, Chiphangwi JD, et al. Maternal vitamin A deficiency and mother-to-child transmission of HIV-1. Lancet 343:1593–7, 1994.
107. Burns DN, FitzGerald G, Semba R, et al. Vitamin A deficiency and other nutritional indices during pregnancy in human immunodeficiency virus infection: prevalence, clinical correlates, and outcome. Women and Infants Transmission Study Group. Clin Infect Dis 29:328–34, 1999.
108. Kwiek JJ, Mwapasa V, Milner DA, et al. Maternal–Fetal microtransfusions and HIV-1 mother-to-child transmission in Malawi. PLoS Med 3:e10, 2005.
109. Brocklehurst P. Interventions for reducing the risk of mother-to-child transmission of HIV infection. Cochrane Database Syst Rev (1):CD000102, 2002.
110. International Perinatal HIV Working Group. The mode of delivery and the risk of vertical transmission of human immunodeficiency virus type 1 – a meta-analysis of 15 prospective cohort studies. The International Perinatal HIV Group. N Engl J Med 340:977–87, 1999.
111. Ioannidis JP, Abrams EJ, Ammann A, et al. Perinatal transmission of human immunodeficiency virus type 1 by pregnant women with RNA virus loads <1000 copies/ml. J Infect Dis 183:539–45, 2001.
112. Mrus JM, Goldie SJ, Weinstein MC, Tsevat J. The cost-effectiveness of elective Cesarean delivery for HIV-infected

women with detectable HIV RNA during pregnancy. AIDS 14:2543–52, 2000.
113. US Public Health Service Task Force. Recommendations for Use of Antiretroviral Drugs in Pregnant HIV-1-Infected Women for Maternal Health and Interventions to Reduce Perinatal HIV-1 Transmission in the United States. Aug 30, 2002.
114. Kingston MA, Bowman CA. Mother to child transmission: European Collaborative Study. AIDS 15:1195–6, 2001.
115. Coll O, Fiore S, Floridia M, et al. Pregnancy and HIV infection: A european consensus on management. AIDS 16 Suppl 2:S1–18, 2002.
116. ACOG. ACOG committee opinion scheduled Cesarean delivery and the prevention of vertical transmission of HIV infection. Number 234, May 2000. Int J Gynaecol Obstet. 3:279–81, 2001.
117. The International Perinatal HIV Group. Duration of ruptured membranes and vertical transmission of HIV-1: a meta-analysis from 15 prospective cohort studies. AIDS 15:357–68, 2001.
118. World Health Organisation. Integrated Management of Pregnancy and Childbirth. Managing Complications in Pregnancy and Childbirth: A guide for midwives and doctors. WHO/RH/00.7. Geneva: World Health Organisation; 2000.
119. McIntyre JA. HIV in pregnancy: a review. Occasional paper No 2. Geneva: World Health Organisation; 1999.
120. Viscarello RR, Copperman AB, DeGennaro NJ. Is the risk of perinatal transmission of human immunodeficiency virus increased by the intrapartum use of spiral electrodes or fetal scalp pH sampling? Am J Obstet Gynecol 170:740–3, 1994.
121. Boyer PJ, Dillon M, Navaie M, et al. Factors predictive of maternal-fetal transmission of HIV-1. Preliminary analysis of zidovudine given during pregnancy and/or delivery. JAMA 271:1925–30, 1994.
122. Mandelbrot L, Burgard M, Teglas JP, et al. Frequent detection of HIV-1 in the gastric aspirates of neonates born to HIV-infected mothers. AIDS 13:2143–9, 1999.
123. World Health Organization. Strategic approaches to the prevention of HIV infection in infants. Report of a WHO meeting, Morges, Switzerland, 20–22 Mar 2002. Geneva: World Health Organization; 2002.
124. Centers for Disease Control and Prevention CDC. Public Health Service recommendations for human immunodeficiency virus counseling and voluntary testing for pregnant women. MMWR Morb Mortal Wkly Rep 1995; 44(No. RR-7).
125. AAP and ACOG statement on HIV screening. Am Fam Physician 53:1442, 1996.
126. Lansky A, Jones JL, Frey RL, Lindegren ML. Trends in HIV testing among pregnant women: United States, 1994–1999. Am J Public Health 91:1291–3, 2001.
127. Chou R, Smits AK, Huffman LH, et al. Prenatal screening for HIV: A review of the evidence for the U.S. Preventive Services Task Force. Ann Intern Med 143:38–54, 2005.
128. HIV testing among pregnant women – United States and Canada, 1998–2001. MMWR Morb Mortal Wkly Rep 51:1013–16, 2002.
129. American College of Obstetricians and Gynecologists. American Academy of Pediatrics and American College of Obstetricians and Gynecologists Joint Statement on Human Immunodeficiency Virus Screening. Washington, DC: ACOG; 1999.
130. Advancing HIV prevention: new strategies for a changing epidemic – United States, 2003. MMWR Morb Mortal Wkly Rep 52:329–32, 2003.
131. ACOG committee opinion number 304, November 2004. Prenatal and perinatal human immunodeficiency virus testing: expanded recommendations. Obstet Gynecol 104(5 Pt 1):1119–24, 2004.
132. Anderson JE, Koenig LJ, Lampe MA, et al. Achieving universal HIV screening in prenatal care in the United States: provider persistence pays off. AIDS Patient Care STDS 19:247–52, 2005.
133. Wang FL, Larke B, Gabos S, et al. Potential factors that may affect acceptance of routine prenatal HIV testing. Can J Public Health 96:60–4, 2005.
134. Anderson JE, Sansom S. HIV Testing among U.S. women during prenatal care: findings from the 2002 national survey of family growth. Matern Child Health J 2006.
135. Duran AS, Ivalo SA, Hakim A, et al. Prevention of mother to child HIV transmission. Medicina (B Aires) 6:24–30, 2006.
136. McIntyre J. Preventing mother-to-child transmission of HIV: successes and challenges. BJOG 112:1196–203, 2005.
137. Manzi M, Zachariah R, Teck R, et al. High acceptability of voluntary counselling and HIV-testing but unacceptable loss to follow up in a prevention of mother-to-child HIV transmission programme in rural Malawi: scaling-up requires a different way of acting. Trop Med Int Health 10:1242–50, 2005.
138. Stringer JS, Sinkala M, Maclean CC, et al. Effectiveness of a city-wide program to prevent mother-to-child HIV transmission in Lusaka, Zambia. AIDS 19:1309–15, 2005.
139. Giuliano M, Magoni M, Bassani L, et al. A theme issue by, for, and about Africa: results from Ugandan programme preventing maternal transmission of HIV. BMJ 331:778, 2005.
140. Shetty AK, Mhazo M, Moyo S, et al. The feasibility of voluntary counselling and HIV testing for pregnant women using community volunteers in Zimbabwe. Int J STD AIDS 16:755–9, 2005.
141. Urassa P, Gosling R, Pool R, Reyburn H. Attitudes to voluntary counselling and testing prior to the offer of Nevirapine to prevent vertical transmission of HIV in northern Tanzania. AIDS Care 17:842–52, 2005.
142. Bajunirwe F, Muzoora M. Barriers to the implementation of programs for the prevention of mother-to-child transmission of HIV: a cross-sectional survey in rural and urban Uganda. AIDS Res Ther 2:10, 2005.
143. Rakgoasi SD. HIV counselling and testing of pregnant women attending antenatal clinics in Botswana, 2001. J Health Popul Nutr 23:58–65, 2005.
144. Centers for Disease Control and Prevention (CDC). Introduction of routine HIV testing in prenatal care – Botswana, 2004. MMWR Morb Mortal Wkly Rep 53:1083–6, 2004.
145. Welty TK, Bulterys M, Welty ER, et al. Integrating prevention of mother-to-child HIV transmission into routine antenatal care: the key to program expansion in Cameroon. J Acquir Immune Defic Syndr 40:486–93, 2005.
146. Mulder-Folkerts DK, van den Hoek JA, van der Bij AK, et al. Less refusal to participate in HIV screening among pregnant women in the Amsterdam region since the introduction of standard HIV screening using the opting-out method. Ned Tijdschr Geneeskd 148:2035–7, 2004.
147. van't Hoog AH, Mbori-Ngacha DA, Marum LH, et al. Preventing mother-to-child transmission of HIV in Western Kenya: operational issues. J Acquir Immune Defic Syndr 40:344–9, 2005.
148. Perez F, Zvandaziva C, Engelsmann B, Dabis F. Acceptability of routine HIV testing ('opt-out') in antenatal services in two rural districts of Zimbabwe. J Acquir Immune Defic Syndr 41:514–20, 2006.
149. Lindsay MK, Feng TI, Peterson HB, et al. Routine human immunodeficiency virus infection screening in unregistered and registered inner-city parturients. Obstet Gynecol 77:599–603, 1991.
150. Donegan SP, Steger KA, Recla L, et al. Seroprevalence of human immunodeficiency virus in parturients at Boston City Hospital: implications for public health and obstetric practice. Am J Obstet Gynecol 167:622–9, 1992.
151. Minkoff HL, McCalla S, Delke I, et al. The relationship of cocaine use to syphilis and human immunodeficiency virus

infections among inner city parturient women. Am J Obstet Gynecol 163:521–6, 1990.
152. Guay LA, Musoke P, Fleming T, et al. Intrapartum and neonatal single-dose nevirapine compared with zidovudine for prevention of mother-to-child transmission of HIV-1 in Kampala, Uganda: HIVNET 012 randomised trial. Lancet 354:795–802, 1999.
153. Wade NA, Birkhead GS, Warren BL, et al. Abbreviated regimens of zidovudine prophylaxis and perinatal transmission of the human immunodeficiency virus. N Engl J Med 339:1409–14, 1998.
154. Gray GE, Urban M, Chersich MF, et al. A randomized trial of two postexposure prophylaxis regimens to reduce mother-to-child HIV-1 transmission in infants of untreated mothers. AIDS 19:1289–97, 2005.
155. The Petra Study Team. Efficacy of three short-course regimens of zidovudine and lamivudine in preventing early and late transmission of HIV-1 from mother to child in Tanzania, South Africa, and Uganda (Petra study): a randomised, double-blind, placebo-controlled trial. Lancet 359:1178–86, 2002.
156. Minkoff H, O'Sullivan MJ. The case for rapid HIV testing during labor. JAMA 279:1743–4, 1998.
157. Forsyth BW, Barringer SR, Walls TA, et al. Rapid HIV testing of women in labor: too long a delay. J Acquir Immune Defic Syndr 35:151–4, 2004.
158. Merhi Z, Minkoff H. Rapid HIV screening for women in labor. Expert Rev Mol Diagn 5:673–9, 2005.
159. Doyle NM, Levison JE, Gardner MO. Rapid HIV versus enzyme-linked immunosorbent assay screening in a low-risk Mexican American population presenting in labor: a cost-effectiveness analysis. Am J Obstet Gynecol 193(3 Pt 2): 1280–5, 2005.
160. Aaron E, Levine AB, Monahan K, Biondo CP. A rapid HIV testing program for labor and delivery in an inner-city teaching hospital. AIDS Read 16:22–4, 28–9, 37; discussion 30, 2006.
161. Granade TC, Parekh BS, Tih PM, et al. Evaluation of rapid prenatal human immunodeficiency virus testing in rural cameroon. Clin Diagn Lab Immunol 12:855–60, 2005.
162. Centers for Disease Control and Prevention (CDC). Rapid point-of-care testing for HIV-1 during labor and delivery-Chicago, Illinois, 2002. MMWR Morb Mortal Wkly Rep 52:866–8, 2003.
163. Bulterys M, Jamieson DJ, O'Sullivan MJ, et al. Rapid HIV-1 testing during labor: a multicenter study. JAMA 292:219–23, 2004.
164. Taha TE, Kumwenda NI, Hoover DR, et al. Nevirapine and zidovudine at birth to reduce perinatal transmission of HIV in an African setting: a randomized controlled trial. JAMA 292:202–9, 2004.
165. Agangi A, Thorne C, Newell ML. Increasing likelihood of further live births in HIV-infected women in recent years. BJOG 112:881–8, 2005.
166. Williams CD, Finnerty JJ, Newberry YG, et al. Reproduction in couples who are affected by human immunodeficiency virus: medical, ethical, and legal considerations. Am J Obstet Gynecol 189:333–41, 2003.
167. Nakhuda GS, Pena JE, Sauer MV. Deaths of HIV-positive men in the context of assisted reproduction: five case studies from a single center. AIDS Patient Care STDS 19:712–18, 2005.
168. Semprini AE, Fiore S. HIV and reproduction. Curr Opin Obstet Gynecol 16:257–62, 2004.
169. Drapkin Lyerly A, Anderson J. Human immunodeficiency virus and assisted reproduction: reconsidering evidence, reframing ethics. Fertil Steril 75:843–58, 2001.
170. Ohl J, Partisani M, Wittemer C, et al. Encouraging results despite complexity of multidisciplinary care of HIV-infected women using assisted reproduction techniques. Hum Reprod 20:6517–30, 2005.
171. Terriou P, Auquier P, Chabert-Orsini V, et al. Outcome of ICSI in HIV-1-infected women. Hum Reprod 20:2838–43, 2005.
172. Hawkins D, Blott M, Clayden P, et al. Guidelines for the management of HIV infection in pregnant women and the prevention of mother-to-child transmission of HIV. HIV Med 6 Suppl 2:107–48, 2005.
173. Sauer MV. Sperm washing techniques address the fertility needs of HIV-seropositive men: a clinical review. Reprod Biomed Online 10:135–40, 2005.
174. Garrido N, Meseguer M, Bellver J, et al. Report of the results of a 2 year programme of sperm wash and ICSI treatment for human immunodeficiency virus and hepatitis C virus serodiscordant couples. Hum Reprod 19:2581–6, 2004.
175. Mencaglia L, Falcone P, Lentini GM, et al. ICSI for treatment of human immunodeficiency virus and hepatitis C virus-serodiscordant couples with infected male partner. Hum Reprod 20:2242–6, 2005.
176. Kali PB, Gray GE, Violari A, et al. Combining PMTCT With Active Case Finding for Tuberculosis. J Acquir Immune Defic Syndr 2006.
177. Ferrero S, Bertoldi S, Lungaro P, et al. HIV-HCV co-infection during pregnancy. Minerva Ginecol 57:627–35, 2005.
178. Haddow JE, Palomaki GE, Knight GJ, et al. Prenatal screening for Down's syndrome with use of maternal serum markers. N Engl J Med 327:588–93, 1992.
179. Einstein FH, Wright RL, Trentacoste S, et al. The impact of protease inhibitors on maternal serum screening analyte levels in pregnant women who are HIV positive. Am J Obstet Gynecol 191:1004–8, 2004.
180. Tess BH, Rodrigues LC, Newell ML, et al. Breastfeeding, genetic, obstetric and other risk factors associated with mother-to-child transmission of HIV-1 in Sao Paulo State, Brazil. Sao Paulo Collaborative Study for Vertical Transmission of HIV-1. AIDS 12:513–20, 1998.
181. Maiques V, Garcia-Tejedor A, Perales A, et al. HIV detection in amniotic fluid samples. Amniocentesis can be performed in HIV pregnant women? Eur J Obstet Gynecol Reprod Biol 108:137–41, 2003.
182. Somigliana E, Bucceri AM, Tibaldi C, et al. Early invasive diagnostic techniques in pregnant women who are infected with the HIV: A multicenter case series. Am J Obstet Gynecol 193:437–42, 2005.
183. Coll O, Suy A, Hernandez S, et al. Prenatal diagnosis in human immunodeficiency virus-infected women: a new screening program for chromosomal anomalies. Am J Obstet Gynecol 194:192–8, 2006.
184. Davies G, Wilson RD, Desilets V, et al. Amniocentesis and women with hepatitis B, hepatitis C, or human immunodeficiency virus. J Obstet Gynaecol Can 25:145–48, 149–52, 2003.
185. Quinn TC, Overbaugh J. HIV/AIDS in women: an expanding epidemic. Science 308:1582–3, 2005.
186. Napravnik S, Royce R, Walter E, Lim W. HIV-1 infected women and prenatal care utilization: barriers and facilitators. AIDS Patient Care STDS 14:411–20, 2000.
187. Koenig LJ, Whitaker DJ, Royce RA, et al. Violence during pregnancy among women with or at risk for HIV infection. Am J Public Health 92:367–70, 2002.
188. Koenig LJ, Whitaker DJ, Royce RA, et al. Physical and sexual violence during pregnancy and after delivery: a prospective multistate study of women with or at risk for HIV infection. Am J Public Health 96:1052–9, 2006.
189. Dunkle KL, Jewkes RK, Brown HC, et al. Gender-based violence, relationship power, and risk of HIV infection in women attending antenatal clinics in South Africa. Lancet 363:1415–21, 2004.
190. Ades AE, Walker J, Botting B, et al. Effect of the worldwide epidemic on HIV prevalence in the United Kingdom: record

linkage in anonymous neonatal seroprevalence surveys. AIDS 13:2437–43, 1999.
191. Kropp RY, Montgomery ET, Hill DW, et al. Unique challenges to preventing perinatal HIV transmission among Hispanic women in California: results of a needs assessment. AIDS Educ Prev 17:22–40, 2005.
192. Gaillard P, Melis R, Mwanyumba F, et al. Vulnerability of women in an African setting: lessons for mother-to-child HIV transmission prevention programmes. AIDS 16:937–9, 2002.
193. Medley A, Garcia-Moreno C, McGill S, Maman S. Rates, barriers and outcomes of HIV serostatus disclosure among women in developing countries: implications for prevention of mother-to-child transmission programmes. Bull World Health Organ 82:299–307, 2004.
194. Dunkle KL, Jewkes RK, Brown HC, et al. Prevalence and patterns of gender-based violence and revictimization among women attending antenatal clinics in Soweto, South Africa. Am J Epidemiol 160:230–9, 2004.
195. Blaney NT, Fernandez MI, Ethier KA, et al. Psychosocial and behavioral correlates of depression among HIV-infected pregnant women. AIDS Patient Care STDS 18:405–15, 2004.
196. World Health Organisation. HIV-infected women and their families: psychosocial support and related issues. A literature review. Available: www.who.int/reproductive-health/publications/rhr_03_07/, 2003.
197.Thorpe LE, Frederick M, Pitt J, et al. Effect of Hard-Drug Use on CD4 Cell Percentage, HIV RNA Level, and Progression to AIDS-Defining Class C Events Among HIV-Infected Women. J Acquir Immune Defic Syndr 37:1423–30, 2004.
198. American Academy of Pediatrics Committee on Pediatric AIDS. Reducing the risk of HIV infection associated with illicit drug use. Pediatrics 117:566–71, 2006.
199. Qian ZH, Vermund SH, Wang N. Risk of HIV/AIDS in China: subpopulations of special importance. Sex Transm Infect 81:442–7, 2005.
200. New York State Department of Health AIDS Institute. HIV Guidelines. New York State Department of Health AIDS Institute. Medical Care of HIV-infected substance-using women. Available: http://www.hivguidelines.org/public_html/sub-women/sub-women.htm 23 Mar 2006. New York: New York State Department of Health AIDS Institute; 2005.
201. Lejeune C, Simmat-Durand L, Gourarier L, Aubisson S. Prospective multicenter observational study of 260 infants born to 259 opiate-dependent mothers on methadone or high-dose buprenophine substitution. Drug Alcohol Depend 2005.
202. Comer VG, Annitto WJ. Buprenorphine: a safe method for detoxifying pregnant heroin addicts and their unborn. Am J Addict 13:317–18, 2004.
203. Nocon JJ. Buprenorphine in pregnancy: the advantages. Addiction 101:608, 2006.
204. Antoniou T, Tseng AL. Interactions between recreational drugs and antiretroviral agents. Ann Pharmacother 36:1598–613, 2002.
205. Stocker H, Kruse G, Kreckel P, et al. Nevirapine significantly reduces the levels of racemic methadone and (R)-methadone in human immunodeficiency virus-infected patients. Antimicrob Agents Chemother 48:4148–53, 2004.
206. Villamor E, Dreyfuss ML, Baylin A, et al. Weight loss during pregnancy is associated with adverse pregnancy outcomes among HIV-1 infected women. J Nutr 134:1424–31, 2004.
207. Wimalasundera RC, Larbalestier N, Smith JH, et al. Preeclampsia, antiretroviral therapy, and immune reconstitution. Lancet 360:1152–4, 2002.
208. Suy A, Martinez E, Coll O, et al. Increased risk of pre-eclampsia and fetal death in HIV-infected pregnant women receiving highly active antiretroviral therapy. AIDS 20:59–66, 2006.
209. Fiore S, Newell ML, Trabattoni D, et al. Antiretroviral therapy-associated modulation of Th1 and Th2 immune responses in HIV-infected pregnant women. J Reprod Immunol 2006.
210. Johnstone FD, MacCallum L, Brettle R, et al. Does infection with HIV affect the outcome of pregnancy? Br Med J (Clin Res Ed) 96:467, 1988.
211. Selwyn PA, Schoenbaum EE, Davenny K, et al. Prospective study of human immunodeficiency virus infection and pregnancy outcomes in intravenous drug users. JAMA 261:1289–94, 1989.
212. Ellis J, Williams H, Graves W, Lindsay MK. Human immunodeficiency virus infection is a risk factor for adverse perinatal outcome. Am J Obstet Gynecol 186:903–6, 2002.
213. Rogers MF, Ou CY, Rayfield M, et al. Use of the polymerase chain reaction for early detection of the proviral sequences of human immunodeficiency virus in infants born to seropositive mothers. New York City Collaborative Study of Maternal HIV Transmission and Montefiore Medical Center HIV Perinatal Transmission Study Group. N Engl J Med 320:1649–54, 1989.
214. Goldstein PJ, Smit R, Stevens M, Sever JL. Association between HIV in pregnancy and antiretroviral therapy, including protease inhibitors and low birth weight infants. Infect Dis Obstet Gynecol 8:94–8, 2000.
215. Lambert JS, Watts DH, Mofenson L, et al. Risk factors for preterm birth, low birth weight, and intrauterine growth retardation in infants born to HIV-infected pregnant women receiving zidovudine. Pediatric AIDS Clinical Trials Group 185 Team. AIDS 14:1389–99, 2000.
216. Turner BJ, Newschaffer CJ, Cocroft J, et al. Improved birth outcomes among HIV-infected women with enhanced Medicaid prenatal care. Am J Public Health 90:85–91, 2000.
217. Wei R, Msamanga GI, Spiegelman D, et al. Association between low birth weight and infant mortality in children born to human immunodeficiency virus 1-infected mothers in Tanzania. Pediatr Infect Dis J 23:530–5, 2004.
218. Dreyfuss ML, Msamanga GI, Spiegelman D, et al. Determinants of low birth weight among HIV-infected pregnant women in Tanzania. Am J Clin Nutr 74:814–26, 2001.
219. Lorenzi P, Spicher VM, Laubereau B, et al. Antiretroviral therapies in pregnancy: maternal, fetal and neonatal effects. Swiss HIV Cohort Study, the Swiss Collaborative HIV and Pregnancy Study, and the Swiss Neonatal HIV Study. AIDS 12:F241–7, 1998.
220. Is zidovudine therapy in pregnant HIV-infected women associated with gestational age and birthweight? The European Collaborative Study. AIDS 13:119–24, 1999.
221. European Collaborative Study and the Swiss Mother and Child HIV Cohort Study. Combination antiretroviral therapy and duration of pregnancy. AIDS 14:2913–20, 2000.
222. British HIV Association. Guidelines for the management of HIV infection in pregnant women and the prevention of mother-to-child transmission. HIV Medicine 2:314–34, 2001.
223. AIDS Education and Training Centers. Clinical Manual For Management Of The HIV-Infected Adult, 2005 Edition. Section 2: Health Maintenance And Disease Prevention. Opportunistic Infection Prophylaxis. 2006. Available: http://www.aids-ed.org/aetc/aetc?page=cm-207_oipx 16 Jun 2006.
224. WHO Regional Office for Africa DoRHaR. Clinical guides for the management of pregnant women with HIV infection. Labor and delivery care for HIV-infected women. Field-testing version. Geneva: World Health Organisation, 2001.
225. Nielsen T, Hokegard KH. Postoperative cesarean section morbidity: a prospective study. Am J Obstet Gynecol 146:911–15, 1983.
226. Fiore S, Newell ML, Thorne C. Higher rates of post-partum complications in HIV-infected than in uninfected women irrespective of mode of delivery. AIDS 18:933–8, 2004.

227. Read JS, Tuomala R, Kpamegan E, et al. Mode of delivery and postpartum morbidity among HIV-infected women: the women and infants transmission study. J Acquir Immune Defic Syndr 26:236–45, 2001.
228. Lyall EG, Blott M, de Ruiter A, et al. Guidelines for the management of HIV infection in pregnant women and the prevention of mother-to-child transmission. HIV Med 2:314–34, 2001.
229. Marcollet A, Goffinet F, Firtion G, et al. Differences in postpartum morbidity in women who are infected with the human immunodeficiency virus after elective cesarean delivery, emergency cesarean delivery, or vaginal delivery. Am J Obstet Gynecol 186:784–9, 2002.
230. Bjorklund K, Mutyaba T, Nabunya E, Mirembe F. Incidence of postcesarean infections in relation to HIV status in a setting with limited resources. Acta Obstet Gynecol Scand 84:967–71, 2005.
231. Ferrero S, Bentivoglio G. Post-operative complications after cesarean section in HIV-infected women. Arch Gynecol Obstet 268:268–73, 2003.
232. Panburana P, Phaupradit W, Tantisirin O, et al. Maternal complications after Cesarean section in HIV-infected pregnant women. Aust N Z J Obstet Gynaecol 43:160–3, 2003.
233. Rowland BL, Vermillion ST, Soper DE. Scheduled cesarean delivery and the prevention of human immunodeficiency virus transmission: a survey of practicing obstetricians. Am J Obstet Gynecol 185:327–31, 2001.
234. Urbani G, de Vries MM, Cronje HS, et al. Complications associated with cesarean section in HIV-infected patients. Int J Gynaecol Obstet 74:9–15, 2001.
235. Biggar RJ, Miotti PG, Taha TE, et al. Perinatal intervention trial in Africa: effect of a birth canal cleansing intervention to prevent HIV transmission. Lancet 347:1647–50, 1996.
236. Taha TE, Biggar RJ, Broadhead RL, et al. Effect of cleansing the birth canal with antiseptic solution on maternal and newborn morbidity and mortality in Malawi: clinical trial. BMJ 315:216–19; discussion 220, 1997.
237. Gaillard P, Mwanyumba F, Verhofstede C, et al. Vaginal lavage with chlorhexidine during labour to reduce mother-to-child HIV transmission: clinical trial in Mombasa, Kenya. AIDS 15:389–96, 2001.
238. Newell ML, Gray G, Bryson YJ. Prevention of mother-to-child transmission of HIV-1 infection. AIDS 11 Suppl A:S165–72, 1997.
239. World Health Organisation. Postpartum care of the mother and newborn: a practical guide. WHO/RHT/MSM/98.3. Geneva: 1998.
240. Figueroa-Damian R, Villagrana-Zesati R. Factors associated with acceptance of postpartum tubal ligation among HIV-infected women. Salud Publica Mex 43:97–102, 2001.
241. Ickovics JR, Wilson TE, Royce RA, et al. Prenatal and postpartum zidovudine adherence among pregnant women with HIV: results of a MEMS substudy from the perinatal guidelines evaluation project. J Acquir Immune Defic Syndr 30:311–15, 2002.
242. World Health Organization . Scaling up antiretroviral therapy in resource constrained settings: treatment guidelines for a public health approach. Geneva: World Health Organization, 2003.
243. Minkoff H, Ahdieh L, Watts H, et al. The relationship of pregnancy to the use of highly active antiretroviral therapy. Am J Obstet Gynecol 184:1221–7, 2001.
244. Minkoff H. Human immunodeficiency virus infection in pregnancy. Obstet Gynecol 101:797–810, 2003.
245. Thorne C, Newell ML. The safety of antiretroviral drugs in pregnancy. Expert Opin Drug Saf 4:323–35, 2005.
246. European Collaborative Study. Mother-to-child transmission of HIV infection in the era of highly active antiretroviral therapy. Clin Infect Dis 40:458–65, 2005.
247. US Public Health Service. Public Health Service Task Force Recommendations for Use of Antiretroviral Drugs in Pregnant HIV-1-Infected Women for Maternal Health and Interventions to Reduce Perinatal HIV-1 Transmission in the United States – February 24, 2005. Available: http://www.aidsinfo.nih.gov/guidelines/ 27 Aug 2005.
248. World Health Organisation. antiretroviral drugs for treating pregnant women and preventing HIV infection in infants. Guidelines on Care, Treatment and Support for Women Living with HIV/AIDS and their Children in Resource-Constrained Settings. Geneva: World Health Organisation; 2004.
249. Newell ML. Routine provision of nevirapine to women of unknown serostatus: at best a temporary solution to prevent MTCT. Bull World Health Organ 83:228–9, 2005.
250. Watts DH. Treating HIV During pregnancy: an update on safety issues. Drug Saf 29:467–90, 2006.
251. Tuomala RE, Watts DH, Li D, et al. Improved obstetric outcomes and few maternal toxicities are associated with antiretroviral therapy, including highly active antiretroviral therapy during pregnancy. J Acquir Immune Defic Syndr 38:449–73, 2005.
252. Antiretroviral Pregnancy Registry Steering Committee. Antiretroviral Pregnancy Registry International Interim Report for 1 January 1989 through 31 January 2005. Available: www.apregistry. com. Wilmington, NC: Registry Coordinating Center; 2005.
253. Watts DH, Covington DL, Beckerman K, et al. Assessing the risk of birth defects associated with antiretroviral exposure during pregnancy. Am J Obstet Gynecol 191:985–92, 2004.
254. Townsend CL, Tookey PA, Cortina-Borja M, Peckham CS. Antiretroviral therapy and congenital abnormalities in infants born to HIV-1-infected women in the United Kingdom and Ireland, 1990 to 2003. J Acquir Immune Defic Syndr 42:91–4, 2006.
255. Joao EC, Cruz ML, Menezes JA, et al. Vertical transmission of HIV in Rio de Janeiro, Brazil. AIDS 17:1853–5, 2003.
256. Tonwe-Gold B, Ekouevi D, Rouet F, et al. Highly active antiretroviral therapy for the prevention of perinatal HIV transmission in Africa.: mother-to-child HIV transmission plus, Abidjan, Côte d'Ivoire, 2003–2004. In: 12th Conference on Retroviruses and Opportunistic Infections, Boston, MA, 22–25 Feb 2005, abstract 785.
257. Palombi L, Germano P, Liotta G, et al. HAART in pregnancy: safety, effectiveness, and protection from viral resistance: results from the DREAM cohort. In: 12th Conference on Retroviruses and Opportunistic Infections, Boston, MA, 22–25 Feb 2005, abstract 67.
258. U.S Public Health Service Task Force. Safety and Toxicity of Individual Antiretroviral Agents in Pregnancy – November 17, 2005 U.S Public Health Service Task Force, 2005.
259. Connor EM, Sperling RS, Gelber R, et al. Reduction of maternal-infant transmission of human immunodeficiency virus type 1 with zidovudine treatment. Pediatric AIDS Clinical Trials Group Protocol 076 Study Group. N Engl J Med 1994; 331:1173–80.
260. Moodley J, Moodley D, Pillay K, et al. Pharmacokinetics and antiretroviral activity of lamivudine alone or when coadministered with zidovudine in human immunodeficiency virus type 1-infected pregnant women and their offspring. J Infect Dis 178:1327–33, 1998.
261. Wade NA, Unadkat JD, Huang S, et al. Pharmacokinetics and safety of stavudine in HIV-infected pregnant women and their infants: Pediatric AIDS Clinical Trials Group protocol 332. J Infect Dis 190:2167–74, 2004.
262. Best BM, Mirochnick M, Capparelli EV, et al. Impact of pregnancy on abacavir pharmacokinetics. AIDS 20:553–60, 2006.
263. Gray G, Violari A, McIntyre J, et al. Antiviral Activity of Nucleoside Analogues During Short-Course Monotherapy or

Dual Therapy: Its Role in Preventing HIV Infection in Infants. J Acquir Immune Defic Syndr 42:169–76, 2006.
264. Mandelbrot L, Kermarrec N, Marcollet A, et al. Case report: nucleoside analogue-induced lactic acidosis in the third trimester of pregnancy. AIDS 17:272–3, 2003.
265. Sarner L, Fakoya A. Acute onset lactic acidosis and pancreatitis in the third trimester of pregnancy in HIV-1 positive women taking antiretroviral medication. Sex Transm Infect 78:58–9, 2002.
266. Boulle A, Van Cutsem G, Coetzee D, et al. Regimen durability and tolerability to 36-month duration on ART in Khayelitsha, South Africa. In: 13th Conference on Retroviruses and Opportunistic Infections, Denver, CO, 5–8 Feb 2006, abstract 66.
267. Blanche S, Tardieu M, Rustin P, et al. Persistent mitochondrial dysfunction and perinatal exposure to antiretroviral nucleoside analogues. Lancet 354:1084–9, 1999.
268. Barret B, Tardieu M, Rustin P, et al. Persistent mitochondrial dysfunction in HIV-1-exposed but uninfected infants: clinical screening in a large prospective cohort. AIDS 17:1769–85, 2003.
269. Divi RL, Leonard SL, Kuo MM, et al. Transplacentally exposed human and monkey newborn infants show similar evidence of nucleoside reverse transcriptase inhibitor-induced mitochondrial toxicity. Environ Mol Mutagen 48:201–9, 2007.
270. Landreau-Mascaro A, Barret B, Mayaux MJ, et al. Risk of early febrile seizure with perinatal exposure to nucleoside analogues. Lancet 359:583–4, 2002.
271. Tardieu M, Brunelle F, Raybaud C, et al. Cerebral MR imaging in uninfected children born to HIV-seropositive mothers and perinatally exposed to zidovudine. AJNR Am J Neuroradiol 26:695–701, 2005.
272. Giaquinto C, De Romeo A, Giacomet V, et al. Lactic acid levels in children perinatally treated with antiretroviral agents to prevent HIV transmission. AIDS 15:1074–5, 2001.
273. Dominguez K, Bertolli J, Fowler M, et al. Lack of definitive severe mitochondrial signs and symptoms among deceased HIV-uninfected and HIV-indeterminate children < or = 5 years of age, Pediatric Spectrum of HIV Disease project (PSD), USA. Ann N Y Acad Sci 918:236–46, 2000.
274. European Collaborative Study. Exposure to antiretroviral therapy in utero or early life: the health of uninfected children born to HIV-infected women. J Acquir Immune Defic Syndr 32:380–7, 2003.
275. Kamemoto LE, Shiramizu B, Gerschenson M. HIV-associated mitochondrial toxicity in pregnancy. Mitochondrion 4:153–62, 2004.
276. Rodman J, Flynn P, Shapiro D, et al. Pharmacokinetics and safety of Tenofovir Disoproxil Fumarate in HIV-1-infected pregnant women and their Infants. In: 13th Conference on Retroviruses and Opportunistic Infections, Denver, CO, Feb 5–8, 2006, abstract 708.
277. Tarantal AF, Castillo A, Ekert JE, et al. Fetal and maternal outcome after administration of tenofovir to gravid rhesus monkeys (Macaca mulatta). J Acquir Immune Defic Syndr 29:207–20, 2002.
278. Gafni R, Hazra R, Reynolds J, et al. Effect of Tenofovir Disoproxil Fumarate-containing HAART on bone mineral density in HIV-infected children. In: 13th Conference on Retrivirues and Opportunistic Infections, Denver, CO, Feb 5–8, 2006, abstract 694.
279. Giacomet V, Mora S, Martelli L, et al. A 12-month treatment with tenofovir does not impair bone mineral accrual in HIV-infected children. J Acquir Immune Defic Syndr 40:448–50, 2005.
280. Baylor MS, Johann-Liang R. Hepatotoxicity associated with nevirapine use. J Acquir Immune Defic Syndr 35:538–9, 2004.
281. Stern JO, Robinson PA, Love J, et al. A comprehensive hepatic safety analysis of nevirapine in different populations of HIV infected patients. J Acquir Immune Defic Syndr 34 Suppl 1: S21–33, 2003.
282. Guay L, Musoke P, Fleming T, et al. Intrapartum and neonatal single-dose nevirapine compared with zidovudine for prevention of mother-to-child transmission of HIV-1 in Kampala, Uganda: HIVNET 012 randomised trial. Lancet 354:795–802, 1999.
283. Lyons F, Hopkins S, Kelleher B, et al. Maternal hepatotoxicity with nevirapine as part of combination antiretroviral therapy in pregnancy. HIV Med 7:255–60, 2006.
284. Hitti J, Frenkel LM, Stek AM, et al. Maternal toxicity with continuous nevirapine in pregnancy: results from PACTG 1022. J Acquir Immune Defic Syndr 36:772–6, 2004.
285. Timmermans S, Tempelman C, Godfried MH, et al. Nelfinavir and nevirapine side effects during pregnancy. AIDS 19:795–9, 2005.
286. Money D, Khoo D, MacDonald G, et al. A Comparison of toxicity in Nevirapine- vs protease inhibitor-containing HAART regimens in pregnant women. In: 12th Conference on Retroviruses and Opportunistic Infections, Boston, MA, Feb 22–25, 2005, abstract 784.
287. Natarajan U , Pym A, Anderson J, et al. The side effect profile associated with use of Nevirapine in a cohort of pregnant women in London. In: 7th International Congress on Drug Therapy in HIV Infection, Glasgow, Scotland, Nov 14–18, 2004, abstract P190.
288. Bershoff-Matcha SJ, Mundy LM, Henry JV. Adverse events to Nevirapine therapy during pregnancy. In: 11th Conference on Retroviruses and Opportunisitc Infections, San Francisco, CA, Feb 8–11, 2004, abstract 939.
289. Phanuphak N , Apornpong T, Intarasuk S, et al. Toxicities from Nevirapine in HIV-infected males and females, including pregnant females with various CD4 cell counts. In: 12th Conference on Retroviruses and Opprtunistic Infections, Boston, MA, 22–25 Feb 2005, abstract 21.
290. Thomas T, Amornkul P, Mwidau J, et al. Preliminary findings: incidence of serious adverse events attributed to Nevirapine among women enrolled in an ongoing trial using HAART to prevent mother-to-child HIV transmission. In: 12th Conference on Retroviruses and Opportunistic Infections, Boston, MA, Feb 22–25, 2005, abstract 809.
291. Leith J, Piliero P, Storfer S, et al. Appropriate use of nevirapine for long-term therapy. J Infect Dis 192:545–6, 2005.
292. US Food and Drug Administration. FDA Public Health Advisory for Nevirapine (Viramune). 19 Jan 2005, Available: http://www.fda.gov/cder/drug/advisory/nevirapine.htm 11 Apr 2005.
293. De Santis M, Carducci B, De Santis L, et al. Periconceptional exposure to efavirenz and neural tube defects. Arch Intern Med 162:355, 2002.
294. Fundaro C, Genovese O, Rendeli C, et al. Myelomeningocele in a child with intrauterine exposure to efavirenz. AIDS 16:299–300, 2002.
295. Mofenson LM. Efavirenz reclassified as FDA pregnancy category D. AIDS Clin Care 17:17, 2005.
296. Tuomala RE, Shapiro DE, Mofenson LM, et al. Antiretroviral therapy during pregnancy and the risk of an adverse outcome. N Engl J Med 346:1863–70, 2002.
297. Morris AB, Dobles AR, Cu-Uvin S, et al. Protease inhibitor use in 233 pregnancies. J Acquir Immune Defic Syndr 40:30–3, 2005.
298. Acosta EP, Bardeguez A, Zorrilla CD, et al. Pharmacokinetics of saquinavir plus low-dose ritonavir in human immunodeficiency virus-infected pregnant women. Antimicrob Agents Chemother 48:430–6, 2004.
299. Hayashi S, Beckerman K, Homma M, et al. Pharmacokinetics of indinavir in HIV-positive pregnant women. AIDS 14:1061–2, 2000.

300. Kosel BW, Beckerman KP, Hayashi S, et al. Pharmacokinetics of nelfinavir and indinavir in HIV-1-infected pregnant women. AIDS 17:1195–9, 2003.
301. Tubiana R, Dominguez S, Perot C, et al. ARTwith Indinavir–Ritonavir (400 mg/100 mg twice daily)-containing regimen in HIV-1-infected pregnant women. In: 12th Conference on Retroviruses and Opportunistic Infections, San Francisco, CA, Feb 22–25, 2005, abstract 810.
302. van Heeswijk RP, Khaliq Y, Gallicano KD, et al. The pharmacokinetics of nelfinavir and M8 during pregnancy and post partum. Clin Pharmacol Ther 76:588–97, 2004.
303. Stek A, Mirochnick M, Capparelli E, et al. Reduced lopinavir exposure during pregnancy: preliminary results from P1026s. In: XV International AIDS Conference, Bangkok, Thailand, July 11–16, 2004. EJIAS 1:LbOrB08, 2004, abstract LbOrB08.
304. Mirochnick M, Stek A, Capparelli E, et al. Adequate Lopinavir exposure achieved with a higher dose during the third trimester of pregnancy. In: 13th Conference on Retroviruses and Opportunistic Infections, Denver, CO, Feb 5–8, 2006, abstract 710.
305. Lyons F, Lechelt M, Magaya V, et al. Adequate trough lopinavir levels with standard dosing in pregnancy. In: 13th Conference on Retroviruses and Opportunistic Infections, Denver, CO, 5–8 Feb 2006, abstract 709.
306. Thorne C, Patel D, Newell ML. Increased risk of adverse pregnancy outcomes in HIV-infected women treated with highly active antiretroviral therapy in Europe. AIDS 18:2337–9, 2004.
307. Tempelman C, Timmermans S, Godfried MH, et al. Highly active antiretroviral therapy (HAART) in HIV-positive pregnant women in the Netherlands, 1997–2003: safe, effective and with few side effects. Ned Tijdschr Geneeskd 148:2021–5, 2004.
308. Kowalska A, Niemiec T, El Midaoui A, Burkacka E. Effect of antiretroviral therapy on pregnancy outcome in HIV-1 positive women. Med Wieku Rozwoj 7(4 Pt 1):459–68, 2003.
309. Cotter AM, Garcia AG, Duthely ML, et al. Is antiretroviral therapy during pregnancy associated with an increased risk of preterm delivery, low birth weight, or stillbirth? J Infect Dis 193:1195–201, 2006.
310. Beitune PE, Duarte G, Foss MC, et al. Effect of antiretroviral agents on carbohydrate metabolism in HIV-1 infected pregnant women. Diabetes Metab Res Rev 2005.
311. Watts DH, Balasubramanian R, Maupin RT Jr, et al. Maternal toxicity and pregnancy complications in human immunodeficiency virus-infected women receiving antiretroviral therapy: PACTG 316. Am J Obstet Gynecol 190:506–16, 2004.
312. Justman JE, Benning L, Danoff A, et al. Protease inhibitor use and the incidence of diabetes mellitus in a large cohort of HIV-infected women. J Acquir Immune Defic Syndr 32:298–302, 2003.
313. Hitti J, Andersen J, McComsey G, et al. Effect of protease inhibitor-based arton glucose tolerance in pregnancy: ACTG A5084. In: 13th Conference on Retroviruses and Oppotunistic Infections, Denver CO, Feb 5–8, 2006, abstract 711.
314. Lehtovirta P, Skogberg K, Salo E, et al. Pregnancy outcome among HIV-infected women in the Helsinki metropolitan area. Acta Obstet Gynecol Scand 84:945–50, 2005.
315. Louis JM, Buhari MA, Blackwell SC, et al. Characteristics associated with suboptimal viral suppression at delivery in human immunodeficiency virus-1-infected pregnant women. Am J Obstet Gynecol 193(3 Suppl):1266–9, 2005.
316. Bardeguez A , Lindsey J, Shannon M, et al. Adherence to ART in U.S. women during and after pregnancy. In: 13th Conference on Retroviruses and Opportunistic Infections, Denver, CO,5–8 Feb 2006, abstract 706.
317. World Health Organisation. Antiretroviral drugs and the prevention of mother-to-child transmission of HIV infection in resource-limited settings. Expert consultation, Geneva, 5–6 February 2004 A summary of main points from the meeting. Available: http://www.who.int/3by5/arv_pmtct/en/ 10 Jun 2004.
318. Thorne C, Newell ML. Prevention of mother-to-child transmission of HIV infection. Curr Opin Infect Dis 17:247–52, 2004.
319. Martinson N, Morris L, Gray G, et al. HIV resistance and transmission following single-dose Nevirapine in a PMTCT cohort. In: 11th Conference on Retroviruses and Opportunistic Infections, San Francisco, CA, Feb 8–11, 2004, abstract 38.
320. Foster C, Lyall H. Current guidelines for the management of UK Infants born to HIV-1 infected mothers. Early Hum Dev 81:103–10, 2005.
321. Chersich MF, Urban MF, Venter FW, et al. Efavirenz use during pregnancy and for women of child-bearing potential. AIDS Res Ther 3:11, 2006.
322. Jourdain G, Ngo-Giang-Huong N, Le Coeur S, et al. Intrapartum exposure to nevirapine and subsequent maternal responses to nevirapine-based antiretroviral therapy. N Engl J Med 351:229–40, 2004.
323. Lockman S, Shapiro RL, Smeaton LM, et al. Response to antiretroviral therapy after a single, peripartum dose of nevirapine. N Engl J Med 356:135–47, 2007.
324. Cooper ER, Charurat M, Mofenson L, et al. Combination antiretroviral strategies for the treatment of pregnant HIV-1-infected women and prevention of perinatal HIV-1 transmission. J Acquir Immune Defic Syndr 29:484–94, 2002.
325. Chersich MF, Gray GE. Progress and emerging challenges in preventing mother-to-child transmission. Curr Infect Dis Rep 7:393–400, 2005.
326. McIntyre J. Prevention of mother-to-child transmission of HIV: treatment options. Expert Rev Anti Infect Ther 3:971–80, 2005.
327. McIntyre J. Strategies to prevent mother-to-child transmission of HIV. Curr Opin Infect Dis 19:33–8, 2006.
328. Shaffer N, Chuachoowong R, Mock PA, et al. Short-course zidovudine for perinatal HIV-1 transmission in Bangkok, Thailand: a randomised controlled trial. Bangkok Collaborative Perinatal HIV Transmission Study Group. Lancet 353:773–80, 1999.
329. Wiktor SZ, Ekpini E, Karon JM, et al. Short-course oral zidovudine for prevention of mother-to-child transmission of HIV-1 in Abidjan, Cote d'Ivoire: a randomised trial. Lancet 353:781–5, 1999.
330. Mandelbrot L, Landreau-Mascaro A, Rekacewicz C, et al. Lamivudine-zidovudine combination for prevention of maternal-infant transmission of HIV-1. JAMA 285:2083–93, 2001.
331. Lallemant M, Jourdain GKS. A trial of shortened zidovudine regimens to prevent mother-to-child transmission of human immunodeficiency virustype 1. N Engl J Med 343:982–91, 2000.
332. Lallemant M, Jourdain G, Le Coeur S, et al. Single-dose perinatal nevirapine plus standard zidovudine to prevent mother-to-child transmission of HIV-1 in Thailand. N Engl J Med 351:217–28, 2004.
333. Dabis F, Bequet L, Ekouevi DK, et al. Field efficacy of zidovudine, lamivudine and single-dose nevirapine to prevent peripartum HIV transmission. AIDS 19:309–18, 2005.
334. Leroy V, Sakarovitch C, Cortina-Borja M, et al. Is there a difference in the efficacy of peripartum antiretroviral regimens in reducing mother-to-child transmission of HIV in Africa? AIDS 19:1865–75, 2005.
335. Newell ML, Thorne C. Antiretroviral therapy and mother-to-child transmission of HIV-1. Expert Rev Anti Infect Ther 2:717–32, 2004.
336. Shapiro R, Thior I, Gilbert P, et al. Maternal single-dose nevirapine may not be needed to reduce mother-to-child HIV transmission in the setting of maternal and infant zidovudine

and infant single-dose nevirapine: results of a randomised clinical trial in Botswana. In: 12th Conference on Retroviruses and Opportunistic Infections, Boston, MA, Feb 22–25, 2005, abstract No. 74LB.
337. Taha TE, Kumwenda NI, Gibbons A, et al. Short postexposure prophylaxis in newborn babies to reduce mother-to-child transmission of HIV-1: NVAZ randomised clinical trial. Lancet 362:1171–7, 2003.
338. Stringer JS, Rouse DJ, Sinkala M, et al. Nevirapine to prevent mother-to-child transmission of HIV-1 among women of unknown serostatus. Lancet 362:1850–3, 2003.
339. McIntyre JA. Controversies in the use of nevirapine for prevention of mother-to-child transmission of HIV. Expert Opin Pharmacother 7:677–85, 2006.
340. Nuwaha FN, Karlin T, Buyse DS, Wilfert C. Prevention of mother to child transmission of HIV: from research to action. In: XIII International AIDS Conference, Barcelona, Spain, 7–12 Jul 2002, abstract TuPeF5413.
341. Sherman GG, Jones SA, Coovadia AH, et al. PMTCT from research to reality – results from a routine service. S Afr Med J 94:289–92, 2004.
342. Quaghebeur A, Mutunga L, Mwanyumba F, et al. Low efficacy of nevirapine (HIVNET012) in preventing perinatal HIV-1 transmission in a real-life situation. AIDS 18:1854–6, 2004.
343. Kiarie JN, Kreiss JK, Richardson BA, John-Stewart GC. Compliance with antiretroviral regimens to prevent perinatal HIV-1 transmission in Kenya. AIDS 17:65–71, 2003.
344. Stringer JS, Sinkala M, Chapman V, et al. Timing of the maternal drug dose and risk of perinatal HIV transmission in the setting of intrapartum and neonatal single-dose nevirapine. AIDS 17:1659–65, 2003.
345. Stringer JS, Sinkala M, Goldenberg RL, et al. Universal nevirapine upon presentation in labor to prevent mother-to-child HIV transmission in high prevalence settings. AIDS 18:939–43, 2004.
346. Ayouba A, Tene G, Cunin P, et al. Low rate of mother-to-child transmission of HIV-1 after nevirapine intervention in a pilot public health program in Yaounde, Cameroon. J Acquir Immune Defic Syndr 34:274–80, 2003.
347. Kagaayi J, Dreyfuss ML, Kigozi G, et al. Maternal self-medication and provision of nevirapine to newborns by women in Rakai, Uganda. J Acquir Immune Defic Syndr 39:121–4, 2005.
348. Teeraratkul A, Simonds RJ, Asavapiriyanont S, et al. Evaluating programs to prevent mother-to-child HIV transmission in two large Bangkok hospitals, 1999–2001. J Acquir Immune Defic Syndr 38:208–12, 2005.
349. Delva W, Temmerman M. The efficacy-effectiveness gap in PMTCT. S Afr Med J 94:796, 2004.
350. Stringer JS, Sinkala M, Stout JP, et al. Comparison of two strategies for administering nevirapine to prevent perinatal HIV transmission in high-prevalence, resource-poor settings. J Acquir Immune Defic Syndr 32:506–13, 2003.
351. Sint TT, Dabis F, Kamenga C, et al. Should nevirapine be used to prevent mother-to-child transmission of HIV among women of unknown serostatus? Bull World Health Organ 83:224–8, 2005.
352. Cressey TR, Jourdain G, Lallemant MJ, et al. Persistence of nevirapine exposure during the postpartum period after intrapartum single-dose nevirapine in addition to zidovudine prophylaxis for the prevention of mother-to-child transmission of HIV-1. J Acquir Immune Defic Syndr 38:283–8, 2005.
353. Eshleman SH, Mracna M, Guay LA, et al. Selection and fading of resistance mutations in women and infants receiving nevirapine to prevent HIV-1 vertical transmission (HIVNET 012). AIDS 15:1951–7, 2001.
354. Eshleman SH, Jones D, Guay L, et al. HIV-1 variants with diverse nevirapine resistance mutations emerge rapidly after single dose nevirapine: HIVNET 012. In: XII International HIV Drug Resistance Workshop: Basic principles and clinical implications. July 2003, Cabo San Lucas, Mexico. 2003.
355. Eshleman SH, Guay LA, Mwatha A, et al. Characterization of nevirapine resistance mutations in women with subtype A vs. D HIV-1 6–8 weeks after single-dose nevirapine (HIVNET 012). J Acquir Immune Defic Syndr 35:126–30, 2004.
356. Eshleman SH, Guay LA, Mwatha A, et al. Comparison of nevirapine (NVP) resistance in Ugandan women 7 days vs. 6–8 weeks after single-dose NVP prophylaxis: HIVNET 012. AIDS Res Hum Retroviruses 20:595–9, 2004.
357. Eshleman SH , Hoover D, Chen S, et al. Comparison of Nevirapine resistance in women with subtype C compared with subtypes A and D after single-dose NVP In: 12th Conference on Retroviruses and Oppotunistic Infections, Boston, MA, 22–25 Feb 2005, abstract 799.
358. Eshleman SH, Guay LA, Wang J, et al. Distinct patterns of emergence and fading of K103N and Y181C in women with subtype A vs. D after single-dose Nevirapine: HIVNET 012. J Acquir Immune Defic Syndr 40:24–9, 2005.
359. Morris L, Martinson N, Pillay C, et al. Persistence of nevirapine resistance mutations 6 months following single dose nevirapine. In: 15th International AIDS Conference, Bangkok, 11–16 Jul 2004, abstract ThOrB1353.
360. Eshleman SH , Guay LA, Mwatha A, et al. Extended analysis of nevirapine (NVP) resistance in women with subtype A vs. D 6–8 weeks after single dose NVP prophylaxis: HIVNET 012. In: 10th Conference on Retroviruses and Opportunistic Infections, 2/03, Boston, MA, abstract #P-40 (857).
361. Sullivan J, The SAINT Study team. South African Intrapartum Nevirapine Trial (SAINT): Selection of resistant mutations. In: XIV International AIDS Conference, Barcelona, Spain, 7–12 Jul 2002, abstract LbPeB902.
362. Lee E, Johnston E, Mateta P, et al. Breast-milk Shedding of Subtype C HIV-1 RNA Following Single-dose Nevirapine. In: 11th Conference on Retroviruses and Opportunistic Infections, San Francisco, Feb 8–11, 2004, abstract 890.
363. Chaix ML, Dabis F, Ekouevi D, et al. Addition of 3 Days of AZT+3TC Postpartum to a Short Course of AZT+3TC and Single-dose NVP Provides Low Rate of NVP resistance mutations and high efficacy in preventing peri-partum HIV-1 Transmission: ANRS DITRAME Plus, Abidjan, Côte d'Ivoire. In: 12th Conference on Retroviruses and Opportunistic Infections, Boston, MA, 22–25 Feb 2005, abstract 72LB.
364. Lyons FE, Coughlan S, Byrne CM, et al. Emergence of antiretroviral resistance in HIV-positive women receiving combination antiretroviral therapy in pregnancy. AIDS 19:63–7, 2005.
365. Cunningham CK, Chaix ML, Rekacewicz C, et al. Development of resistance mutations in women receiving standard antiretroviral therapy who received intrapartum nevirapine to prevent perinatal human immunodeficiency virus type 1 transmission: a substudy of pediatric AIDS clinical trials group protocol 316. J Infect Dis 186:181–8, 2002.
366. Eshleman SH, Lie Y, Hoover DR, et al. Association between the replication capacity and mother-to-child transmission of HIV-1, in antiretroviral drug-naive Malawian women. J Infect Dis 193:1512–15, 2006.
367. Eshleman SH, Hoover DR, Hudelson SE, et al. Development of nevirapine resistance in infants is reduced by use of infant-only single-dose nevirapine plus zidovudine postexposure prophylaxis for the prevention of mother-to-child transmission of HIV-1. J Infect Dis 193:479–81, 2006.
368. Eshleman SH, Hoover DR, Chen S, et al. Resistance after single-dose nevirapine prophylaxis emerges in a high proportion of Malawian newborns. AIDS 19:2167–9, 2005.
369. Eshleman SH, Guay LA, Mwatha A, et al. Comparison of mother-to-child transmission rates in Ugandan women with subtype A versus D HIV-1 who received single-dose nevirapine

prophylaxis: HIV Network For Prevention Trials 012. J Acquir Immune Defic Syndr 39:593–7, 2005.
370. Eshleman SH, Hoover DR, Chen S, et al. Nevirapine (NVP) resistance in women with HIV-1 subtype C, compared with subtypes A and D, after the administration of single-dose NVP. J Infect Dis 192:30–6, 2005.
371. Hammer SM. Single-dose nevirapine and drug resistance: the more you look, the more you find. J Infect Dis 192:1–3, 2005.
372. Johnson J, Li JF, Morris L, et al. Resistance Emerges in the Majority of Women Provided Intrapartum Single-dose Nevirapine. In: 12th Conference on Retroviruses and Opportunistic Infections, Boston, MA, 22–25 Feb 2005, abstract 100.
373. Palmer S, Boltz V, Martinson N, et al. Persistence of nevirapine-resistant HIV-1 in women after single-dose nevirapine therapy for prevention of maternal-to-fetal HIV-1 transmission. Proc Natl Acad Sci U S A 103:7094–9, 2006.
374. Eshleman S, Nissley D, Claasen C, et al. Sensitive Drug Resistance Assays Reveal Long-term Persistence of HIV-1 Variants with the K103N Nevirapine-resistance Mutation in Some Women and Infants after Single-dose NVP: HIVNET 012. In: 12th Conference on Retroviruses and Opportunistic Infections, Boston, MA, 22–25 Feb 2005, abstract 800.
375. Zijenah L, Kadzirange G, Rusakaniko S, et al. Community-based Generic Antiretroviral Therapy following Single-dose Nevirapine or Short-course AZT in Zimbabwe. In: 12th Conference on Retroviruses and Opportunistic Infections, Boston, MA, 22–25 Feb 2005, abstract 632.
376. Bedikou G, Viho I, Tonwe-Gold B, et al. 6-month immunological response with HAART containing Nevirapine in HIV infected women post exposure to single dose of Nevirapine for PMTCT. The MTCT-Plus Initiave in Abidjan, Côte d'Ivoire (2003–2005). In: 3rd IAS Conference on HIV Pathogenesis and Treatment, Rio de Janeiro, 24–17 Jul 2005, abstract MoOa0203.
377. Martinson N , Lupondwana P, Morris L, et al. Effectiveness of single dose nevirapine in a second pregnancy. In: 12th Conference on Retroviruses and Opportunbistic Infections, Boston, MA, 22–25 Feb 2005, abstract 103.
378. Martinson N , Ekouevi D, Gray G, et al. Effectiveness of Single-dose Nevirapine in Consecutive Pregnancies in Soweto and Abidjan. In: 13th Conference on Retroviruses and Opportunistic Infections, Denver, CO, Feb 5–8, 2006, abstract 722.
379. Eure C, Bakaki P, McConnell M, et al. Effectiveness of Repeat Single-dose Nevirapine in Subsequent Pregnancies among Ugandan Women. In: 13th Conference on Retriviruses and Opportunistic Infections, Denver, CO, Feb 5–8, 2006, abstract 125.
380. McIntyre JA , Martinson N, Gray GE, et al. Addition of short course Combivir to single dose Viramune for the prevention of mother to child transmission of HIV-1 can significantly decrease the subsequent development of maternal and paediatric NNRTI-resistant virus. In: 3rd IAS Conference on HIV Pathogenesis and Treatment, Rio de Janeiro, 24–27 Jul 2005, abstract TuFoO2O4.
381. Chaix ML, Ekouevi DK, Rouet F, et al. Low risk of nevirapine resistance mutations in the prevention of mother-to-child transmission of HIV-1: Agence Nationale de Recherches sur le SIDA Ditrame Plus, Abidjan, Cote d'Ivoire. J Infect Dis 193:482–7, 2006.
382. Lallemant M, Jourdain G, Le Coeur S, et al. A trial of shortened zidovudine regimens to prevent mother-to-child transmission of human immunodeficiency virus type 1. Perinatal HIV Prevention Trial (Thailand) Investigators. N Engl J Med 343:982–91, 2000.
383. Kaplan JE, Masur H, Holmes KK. Guidelines for preventing opportunistic infections among HIV-infected persons – 2002. Recommendations of the U.S. Public Health Service and the Infectious Diseases Society of America. MMWR Recomm Rep 51:1–52, 2002.
384. US Public Health Service. Guidelines for the Preventing Opportunistic Infections Among HIV-Infected Persons – 2002. Recommendations of the U.S. Public Health Service and the Infectious Diseases Society of America. MMWR Recomm Rep 51:1–46, 2002.
385. Wanachiwanawin D, Sutthent R, Chokephaibulkit K, et al. *Toxoplasma gondii* antibodies in HIV and non-HIV infected Thai pregnant women. Asian Pac J Allergy Immunol 19:291–3, 2001.
386. Minkoff H, deRegt RH, Landesman S, Schwarz R. *Pneumocystis carinii* pneumonia associated with acquired immunodeficiency syndrome in pregnancy: a report of three maternal deaths. Obstet Gynecol 67:284–7, 1986.
387. Gates HS Jr, Barker CD. *Pneumocystis carinii* pneumonia in pregnancy. A case report. J Reprod Med 38:483–6, 1993.
388. Albino JA, Shapiro JM. Respiratory failure in pregnancy due to *Pneumocystis carinii*: report of a successful outcome. Obstet Gynecol 83(5 Pt 2):823–4, 1994.
389. Ahmad H, Mehta NJ, Manikal VM, et al. *Pneumocystis carinii* pneumonia in pregnancy. Chest 120:666–71, 2001.
390. Saade GR. Human immunodeficiency virus (HIV)-related pulmonary complications in pregnancy. Semin Perinatol 21:336–50, 1997.
391. O'Riordan SE, Farkas AG. Maternal death due to cerebral toxoplasmosis. Br J Obstet Gynaecol 105:565–6, 1998.
392. Petrozza JC, Monga M, Oshiro BT, Graham JM, Blanco JD. Disseminated herpes zoster in a pregnant woman positive for human immunodeficiency virus. Am J Perinatol 10:463–4, 1993.
393. Diwan VK, Thorson A. Sex, gender, and tuberculosis. Lancet 353:1000–1, 1999.
394. Connolly M, Nunn P. Women and tuberculosis. World Health Stat Q 49:115–19, 1996.
395. Corbett EL, Steketee RW, ter Kuile FO, et al. HIV-1/AIDS and the control of other infectious diseases in Africa. Lancet 359:2177–87, 2002.
396. Ahmed Y, Mwaba P, Chintu C, et al. A study of maternal mortality at the University Teaching Hospital, Lusaka, Zambia: the emergence of tuberculosis as a major non-obstetric cause of maternal death. Int J Tuberc Lung Dis 3:675–80, 1999.
397. Khan M, Pillay T, Moodley JM, Connolly CA. Maternal mortality associated with tuberculosis-HIV-1 co-infection in Durban, South Africa. AIDS 15:1857–63, 2001.
398. Leroy V, Ladner J, Nyiraziraje M, et al. Effect of HIV-1 infection on pregnancy outcome in women in Kigali, Rwanda, 1992–1994. Pregnancy and HIV Study Group. AIDS 12:643–50, 1998.
399. Ladner J, Leroy V, Karita E,et al. Malaria, HIV and pregnancy. AIDS 17:275–6, 2003.
400. van Eijk AM, Ayisi JG, ter Kuile FO, et al. HIV increases the risk of malaria in women of all gravidities in Kisumu, Kenya. AIDS 17:595–603, 2003.
401. Ayisi JG, Branch OH, Rafi-Janajreh A, et al. Does infection with Human Immunodeficiency Virus affect the antibody responses to *Plasmodium falciparum* antigenic determinants in asymptomatic pregnant women? J Infect 46:164–72, 2003.
402. World Health Organisation. Malaria and HIV interactions and their implications for public health policy. Report of a Technical Consultation on Malaria and HIV Interactions and Public Health Policy Implications, 2004. Geneva, Switzerland: World Health Organisation; 2005.
403. Verhoeff FH, Brabin BJ, Hart CA, et al. Increased prevalence of malaria in HIV-infected pregnant women and its implications for malaria control. Trop Med Int Health 4:5–12, 1999.
404. Weverling GJ, Mocroft A, Ledergerber B, et al. Discontinuation of *Pneumocystis carinii* pneumonia prophylaxis after

start of highly active antiretroviral therapy in HIV-1 infection. EuroSIDA Study Group. Lancet 353:1293–8, 1999.
405. Kirk O, Lundgren JD, Pedersen C, et al. A randomized trial comparing initial HAART regimens of nelfinavir/nevirapine and ritonavir/saquinavir in combination with two nucleoside reverse transcriptase inhibitors. Antivir Ther 8:595–602, 2003.
406. Kirk O, Lundgren JD, Pedersen C, et al. Can chemoprophylaxis against opportunistic infections be discontinued after an increase in CD4 cells induced by highly active antiretroviral therapy? AIDS 13:1647–51, 1999.
407. Walter J, Mwiya M, Scott N,, et al. Cotrimoxazole prophylaxis and adverse birth outcomes among HIV-infected women in Lusaka, Zambia. In: 13th Conference on Retroviruses and Opportunistic Infections, Denver, Colorado, 5–8 Feb 2006, abstract 126.
408. European Collective Study HIV-infected pregnant women and vertical transmission in Europe since 1986. European collaborative study. AIDS 15:761–70, 2001.
409. World Health Organization. Infant feeding: a review of HIV transmission through breastfeeding. WHO/FRH/NUT/CHD/98.3. Geneva: World Health Organization; 1998.
410. Coutsoudis A, Dabis F, Fawzi W, et al. Late postnatal transmission of HIV-1 in breast-fed children: an individual patient data meta-analysis. J Infect Dis 189:2154–66, 2004.
411. Kind C, Brandle B, Wyler CA, et al. Epidemiology of vertically transmitted HIV-1 infection in Switzerland: results of a nationwide prospective study. Swiss Neonatal HIV Study Group. Eur J Pediatr 151:442–8, 1992.
412. Palasanthiran P, Ziegler JB, Stewart GJ, et al. Breast-feeding during primary maternal human immunodeficiency virus infection and risk of transmission from mother to infant. J Infect Dis 167:441–4, 1993.
413. Van de Perre P, Lepage P, Homsy J, Dabis F. Mother-to-infant transmission of human immunodeficiency virus by breast milk: presumed innocent or presumed guilty? Clin Infect Dis 15:502–7, 1992.
414. Miotti PG, Taha TE, Kumwenda NI, et al. HIV transmission through breastfeeding: a study in Malawi. JAMA 282:744–9, 1999.
415. Nduati R, John G, Mbori-Ngacha D, et al. Effect of breastfeeding and formula feeding on transmission of HIV-1: a randomized clinical trial. JAMA 283:1167–74, 2000.
416. Coutsoudis A, Pillay K, Kuhn L, et al. Method of feeding and transmission of HIV-1 from mothers to children by 15 months of age: prospective cohort study from Durban, South Africa. AIDS 15:379–87, 2001.
417. Iliff PJ, Piwoz EG, Tavengwa NV, et al. Early exclusive breastfeeding reduces the risk of postnatal HIV-1 transmission and increases HIV-free survival. AIDS 19:699–708, 2005.
418. World Health Organisation. Prevention of HIV in infants and young children: Review of evidence and WHO's activities. WHO/HIV/2002.0. Geneva: WHO, 2002.
419. Bentley ME, Corneli AL, Piwoz E, et al. Perceptions of the role of maternal nutrition in HIV-positive breast-feeding women in Malawi. J Nutr 135:945–9, 2005.
420. Magoni M, Bassani L, Okong P, et al. Mode of infant feeding and HIV infection in children in a program for prevention of mother-to-child transmission in Uganda. AIDS 19:433–7, 2005.
421. World Health Organisation. New Data on the Prevention of Mother-to-Child Transmission of HIV and their Policy Implications Conclusions and recommendations WHO Technical Consultation on Behalf of the UNFPA/UNICEF/WHO/UNAIDS Inter-Agency Task Team on Mother-to-Child Transmission of HIV. Geneva, 11–13 Oct 2000. Geneva: World Health Organisation; 2001.
422. Bulterys M, Fowler MG, Van Rompay KK, Kourtis AP. Prevention of mother-to-child transmission of HIV-1 through breast-feeding: past, present, and future. J Infect Dis 189:2149–53, 2004.
423. Gaillard P, Fowler MG, Dabis F, et al. Use of antiretroviral drugs to prevent HIV-1 transmission through breast-feeding: from animal studies to randomized clinical trials. J Acquir Immune Defic Syndr 35:178–87, 2004.
424. Maclean CC, Stringer JS. Potential cost-effectiveness of maternal and infant antiretroviral interventions to prevent mother-to-child transmission during breast-feeding. J Acquir Immune Defic Syndr 38:570–7, 2005.
425. Manigart O, Crepin M, Leroy V, et al. Effect of perinatal zidovudine prophylaxis on the evolution of cell-free HIV-1 RNA in breast milk and on postnatal transmission. J Infect Dis 190:1422–8, 2004.
426. Lee EJ, Kantor R, Zijenah L, et al. Breast-Milk shedding of drug-resistant HIV-1 Subtype C in women exposed to single-dose Nevirapine. J Infect Dis 192:1260–4, 2005.
427. Shapiro RL, Holland DT, Capparelli E, et al. Antiretroviral concentrations in breast-feeding infants of women in Botswana receiving antiretroviral treatment. J Infect Dis 192:720–7, 2005.
428. Chung MH, Kiarie JN, Richardson BA, et al. Breast milk HIV-1 suppression and decreased transmission: a randomized trial comparing HIVNET 012 nevirapine versus short-course zidovudine. AIDS 19:1415–22, 2005.
429. Jackson JB, Musoke P, Fleming T, et al. Intrapartum and neonatal single-dose nevirapine compared with zidovudine for prevention of mother-to-child transmission of HIV-1 in Kampala, Uganda: 18-month follow-up of the HIVNET 012 randomised trial. Lancet 362:859–68, 2003.
430. Shapiro RL, Ndung'u T, Lockman S, et al. Highly Active Antiretroviral Therapy Started during Pregnancy or Postpartum Suppresses HIV-1 RNA, but Not DNA, in Breast Milk. J Infect Dis 192:713–19, 2005.
431. John-Stewart G, Mbori-Ngacha D, Ekpini R, et al. Breastfeeding and Transmission of HIV-1. J Acquir Immune Defic Syndr 35:196–202, 2004.
432. Semba RD, Kumwenda N, Hoover DR, et al. Human immunodeficiency virus load in breast milk, mastitis, and mother-to-child transmission of human immunodeficiency virus type 1. J Infect Dis 180:93–8, 1999.
433. Willumsen JF, Filteau SM, Coutsoudis A, et al. Breastmilk RNA viral load in HIV-infected South African women: effects of subclinical mastitis and infant feeding. AIDS 17:407–14, 2003.
434. Richardson BA, John-Stewart GC, Hughes JP, et al. Breast-milk infectivity in human immunodeficiency virus type 1-infected mothers. J Infect Dis 187:736–40, 2003.
435. Watts DH, Minkoff H. Managing Pregnant Patients. In: Dolin R, Masur H, Saag M, Editors. AIDS Therapy. 2nd edition. New York, NY: Churchill Livingstone International, 2002.
436. Capparelli E, Rakhmanina N, Mirochnick M. Pharmacotherapy of perinatal HIV. Semin Fetal Neonatal Med 10(2):161–75, 2005.
437. Chappuy H, Treluyer JM, Jullien V, et al. Maternal-fetal transfer and amniotic fluid accumulation of nucleoside analogue reverse transcriptase inhibitors in human immunodeficiency virus-infected pregnant women. Antimicrob Agents Chemother 48(11):4332–6, 2004.
438. Chappuy H, Treluyer JM, Rey E, et al. Maternal-fetal transfer and amniotic fluid accumulation of protease inhibitors in pregnant women who are infected with human immunodeficiency virus. Am J Obstet Gynecol 191(2):558–62, 2004.
439. Mirochnick M. Antiretroviral pharmacology in pregnant women and their newborns. Ann N Y Acad Sci 918:287–97, 2000.
440. Mirochnick M, Capparelli E. Pharmacokinetics of antiretrovirals in pregnant women. Clin Pharmacokinet 43(15):1071–87, 2004.

Chapter 36

Pneumocystis Pneumonia

Laurence Huang, MD, Henry Masur, MD

During the first decade of the acquired immunodeficiency syndrome (AIDS) epidemic, Pneumocystis pneumonia (PCP) became widely recognized as the most common presenting clinical manifestation of AIDS in North America and Western Europe.[1–7] Clinicians became quite adept at monitoring CD4+ T-lymphocyte counts to determine when patients were most likely to develop PCP, and they became familiar with recognizing the initial manifestations, establishing the diagnosis, instituting therapy, and prescribing prophylaxis.[8–14]

Since the mid-1990s the AIDS epidemic has witnessed dramatic changes in the epidemiology and management of PCP. In patients with access to medical care, PCP has become a much less common disease as a result of early diagnosis of human immunodeficiency virus (HIV) disease, widespread use of anti-Pneumocystis prophylaxis, and early intervention with highly active antiretroviral therapy (HAART).[14–27] PCP continues to be common, however, in those who do not have access to medical care, do not get tested for HIV infection early in the course of their disease, elect not to treat their HIV disease consistently and aggressively, or do not respond optimally to available regimens.[22–24,26–28] Thus PCP continues to occur in North America and Western Europe, but incidence differs among patient populations depending on the availability and the quality of their long-term medical management.[22–24,26–28] PCP also occurs in patients in developing countries and its incidence appears to be greater than previously reported.[29–33]

TAXONOMY

Pneumocystis can be found in a wide variety of mammals, including rodents, horses, nonhuman primates, and humans. The organism is difficult to culture. Murine Pneumocystis can be grown with difficulty, achieving only a modest increase in number. Human Pneumocystis has never been cultivated successfully. Antigenic analysis indicates that each species of animal is infected by a distinct form of Pneumocystis.[34–36] The environmental reservoir of Pneumocystis is unknown, but humans do not appear to acquire it from other animals. Many humans appear to be infected early in life and can probably be reinfected by different human strains later in life.

Pneumocystis occurs in three distinct forms: cyst, tachyzoite, and sporozoite. Its morphology and response to the antiparasitic agent pentamidine led to its original classification as a protozoon. However, an evaluation of mRNA sequences, enzyme structure, and the cell wall suggest that it is taxonomically closer to fungi such as *Saccharomyces*, although it shares some characteristics of protozoa.

CLINICAL PRESENTATION

Pneumocystis pneumonia almost always presents as pulmonary dysfunction.[9,10,37] Although extrapulmonary or disseminated disease has been repeatedly reported in the literature, these presentations are infrequent regardless of the type of prophylaxis a patient is receiving.[38–42] When patients come to medical attention early in the course of their PCP, they typically have minimal symptoms. They often complain of a mild cough that is usually nonproductive, exertional dyspnea, or a substernal "catching". They may have a normal chest radiograph and normal arterial blood gases with no fever at this juncture, although a high-resolution computed tomography (HRCT) scan might show ground glass opacities (Fig. 36-1), and a bronchoalveolar lavage (BAL) or induced sputum specimen could contain many organisms.[9,10,37,43–46] Diagnosis and initiation of therapy at this stage clearly is associated with the best prognosis for avoiding hospitalization, complications, and death.[47–57] Patients may also present with more advanced disease, first coming to medical attention when they are on the brink of respiratory failure. Another

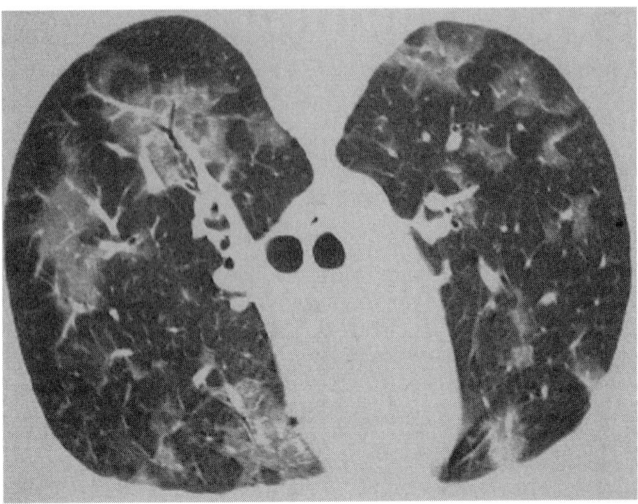

Figure 36-1 ■ Chest HRCT scan of an HIV-infected patient who had a normal chest radiograph. Chest HRCT scan reveals the characteristic ground-glass opacities of PCP.

Courtesy of L Huang.

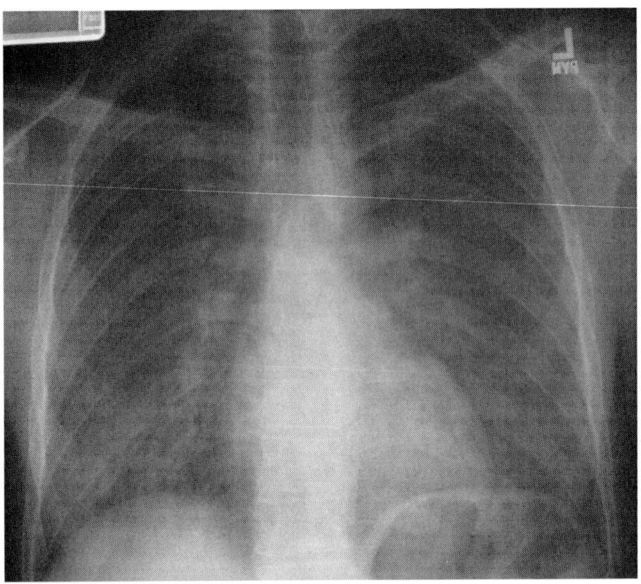

Figure 36-2 ■ Chest radiograph of an HIV-infected patient revealing the characteristic bilateral, diffuse granular opacities of PCP.

Courtesy of L Huang.

presentation of which clinicians should be aware is pneumothorax. Finding a pneumothorax in an HIV-infected patient with no other precipitating cause should raise the possibility of PCP.[58,59]

This disease most often presents with clinical and radiologic features consistent with bilateral pneumonia, manifesting with fever, nonproductive cough, shortness of breath, and the characteristic diffuse interstitial, reticular, or granular pulmonary infiltrates on chest radiography (Fig. 36-2).[43–45] Almost every conceivable radiographic pattern has been reported with PCP, including diffuse alveolar infiltrates, lobar infiltrates, nodules, cavities, upper lobe predominance, and asymmetrical patterns.[43–46,60,61] Thus clinicians must suspect PCP when pulmonary symptoms occur in any patient with HIV, regardless of radiologic appearance, especially if the patient has a low CD4+ T-lymphocyte count.

Table 36-1 Reasons Patients Develop PCP During the Era of HAART

Failure to Take Prophylaxis
Lack of awareness of HIV infection
Lack of access to healthcare
Failure of healthcare provider to prescribe prophylaxis
Failure of patient to adhere to prophylaxis
Development of PCP before recommended indicators occur

Breakthrough of Prophylaxis
Immunologic failure
Less than complete efficacy of prophylactic regimen
Drug resistance (?)

Today, patients continue to develop PCP despite the efficacy of prophylactic regimens and antiretroviral agents (Table 36-1).[22–24,26–28] One issue that has been apparent since before the era of antiretroviral therapy is that PCP occurs over a fairly wide range of CD4+ T-lymphocyte counts. Although most cases occur at CD4+ T-lymphocyte counts of less than 100 cells/μL, and 85–90% occur at CD4+ T-lymphocyte counts of less than 200 cells/μL, some occur at counts of 200–300 cells/μL and a few at CD4+ T-lymphocyte counts of more than 300 cells/μL.[3,8,24,26] A substantial fraction of these patients presenting with PCP at CD4+ T-lymphocyte counts of more than 200 cells/μL have not manifested either unexplained fever or oropharyngeal candidiasis, which are both risk factors for PCP independent of the CD4+ T-lymphocyte count.[8] Thus more sensitive laboratory or clinical indicators of disease would be useful. The HIV viral load is an independent predictor of AIDS-defining events,[62,63] and might be a logical companion measurement to the CD4+ T-lymphocyte count but how precisely to use this factor to indicate the utility of initiating PCP prophylaxis is currently unclear. A high viral load (e.g., >100 000 copies/mL) in a patient with a CD4+ T-lymphocyte count of 200–300 cells/μL would be a logical reason to consider prophylaxis. Clinical markers, including wasting, the occurrence of a previous AIDS-defining event, or the occurrence of a previous episode of pneumonia of any type, also are risk factors for PCP independent of the CD4+ T-lymphocyte count. It may be reasonable to use these indicators to initiate PCP prophylaxis before the CD4+ T-lymphocyte count falls to 200 cells/μL, especially in patients whose HIV viral load is high or whose CD4+ T-lymphocyte counts are declining rapidly. In addition, if another opportunistic infection occurred at an unusually high CD4+ T-lymphocyte count or if a prior episode of PCP occurred at a CD4+ T-lymphocyte count of more than 200 cells/μL, it is probably prudent to recommend prophylaxis despite a "high" CD4+ T-lymphocyte count.

Considerable evidence supports the concept that the CD4+ T-lymphocyte count is an accurate indicator of susceptibility to PCP even in patients receiving HAART or interleukin-2 (IL-2).[63–66] The nadir of the CD4+ T-lymphocyte fall prior to the institution of HAART or IL-2 does not influence the predictive value of counts substantially.[63]

DIAGNOSIS

A definitive diagnosis of PCP depends on recognition of organisms in pulmonary secretions or tissue. Pneumocystis from humans has never been convincingly grown in culture despite extensive efforts using various culture media, cell types, and special conditions. Detection of serum antibodies by highly specific Western blot techniques or other serologic approaches has yielded interesting epidemiologic data but has not yet been shown to be useful for diagnosing acute disease, monitoring the response to therapy, or determining the prognosis.[67–73] In one study, the measurement of plasma *S*-adenosylmethionine concentrations was found to be a sensitive test for PCP.[74] *S*-adenosylmethionine is an important biochemical intermediate in many cellular functions, and it has been shown to be depleted in laboratory animal studies of PCP. In one study, plasma *S*-adenosylmethionine concentration was undetectable in 14 of 15 HIV-infected patients with either histologically confirmed or clinically suspected PCP.[74] In addition, serial S-adenosylmethionine concentrations appeared to parallel the clinical course of PCP treatment in these patients. However, a high sensitivity and specificity of this test for PCP have been difficult for other investigators to confirm.

An approach to the diagnosis and management of PCP is outlined in Figure 36-3, and sensitivities of diagnostic procedures for PCP are summarized in Table 36-2. At most medical centers, PCP is diagnosed by detecting organisms in BAL fluid or induced sputum. Prior to the early 1980s, open lung biopsy was conventionally used to diagnose PCP.[75,76] When bronchoscopy was introduced, it became clear that bronchial washings and brushings could detect Pneumocystis in 30–70% of cases.[11,76] Bronchial washings or brushings do not sample as many alveoli as BAL, however. When BAL is properly performed (i.e., the bronchoscope is wedged in a terminal bronchiole and 10–20 mL aliquots of normal saline are instilled until 30–40 mL has been collected), this technique rarely misses cases of AIDS-associated PCP; the sensitivity of the procedure is 95–99%.[12,77] Some laboratories report that PCP may be more difficult to diagnose in aerosolized pentamidine-treated patients.[78–81] Some reports suggest that site-specific lavage (i.e., performing lavage in a radiologically affected area of the lung), preferentially lavaging the upper lobes, or performing bilateral lavage may increase the diagnostic yield.[82–84] Bilateral lavage or upper lobe lavage is not, however, performed routinely at most centers.

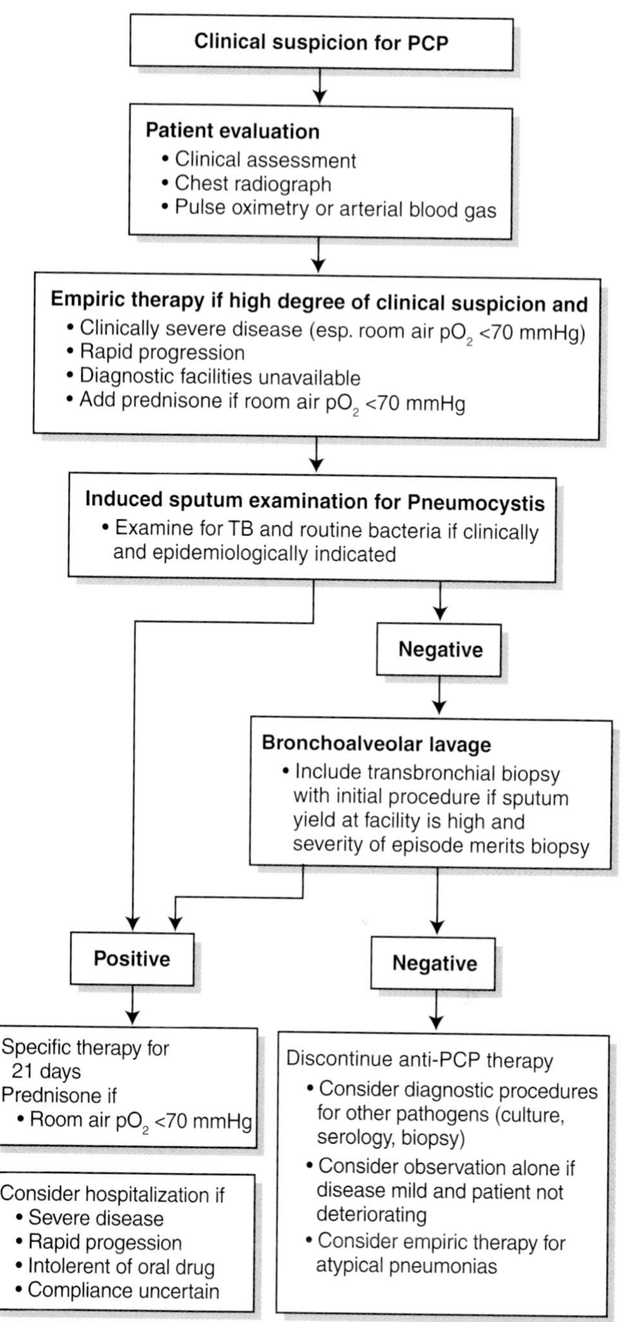

Figure 36-3 ■ Management algorithm for suspected acute Pneumocystis pneumonia (PCP). TB, tuberculosis.

BAL is a safe and well-tolerated procedure when performed by an experienced operator. Even in patients who are thrombocytopenic or neutropenic, complications are rare. Clinically significant hemorrhage is unusual, even if patients are thrombocytopenic. Many patients have a temperature elevation and perhaps a chill or rigor during the first 2–12 h following BAL. Immediately following lavage, the chest radiograph may reveal new infiltration at the site of the lavage, but such infiltrates should disappear within 24 h.

Transbronchial biopsy is rarely necessary to diagnose PCP, so it is often not performed as part of an initial diagnostic

Table 36-2 Sensitivity of Procedures to Diagnose PCP by Visualization of the Organism

Technique	Sensitivity (%)	Comment
Oral or oropharyngeal wash (gargle)	50–94	Predominantly a research tool; specificity less than 100% when combined with PCR techniques
Expectorated sputum	10–52	Rarely used
Induced sputum	55–97	Many medical centers have >80% sensitivity and 99% specificity
Nonbronchoscopic lavage	Variable	At a few centers more readily available than bronchoscopy
Bronchoscopy		
Bronchial washings	30–70	Rarely used
Bronchial brushings	30–70	Rarely used
Bronchoalveolar lavage	95–99	Procedure of choice
Transbronchial biopsy	70–90	Rarely necessary to diagnose PCP

procedure. If BAL does not reveal PCP or any other likely pathogen, bronchoscopy is often repeated, especially if the patient fails to improve on empiric therapy; and transbronchial biopsy is performed to search for processes other than PCP, such as infection with cytomegalovirus, mycobacteria, or fungi. The diagnostic yield of transbronchial biopsy for any of these processes is subject to sampling artifact because characteristically only a few small pieces of tissue are obtained. The more severe the PCP and the more tissue obtained, the higher is the diagnostic yield. At most centers it is unusual to detect PCP by transbronchial biopsy if BAL has been negative because of the high sensitivity of BAL.[77]

Open lung biopsy has a high yield of PCP detection if a large piece of tissue from an affected lobe is obtained. However, the diagnostic sensitivity of BAL and transbronchoscopic biopsy for virtually all pathogens makes open lung biopsy rarely necessary. Few medical centers perform more than a few open lung biopsies on AIDS patients per year. Patients with suspected extensive pulmonary Kaposi sarcoma comprise one of the few populations in whom open lung biopsy is likely to be useful, although even here chest CT scans and endobronchial examination usually suffice.[85,86]

Percutaneous needle aspiration is occasionally useful for obtaining tissue from focal lesions if BAL is nondiagnostic.[87,88] Although Pneumocystis occasionally is documented to cause such focal disease, in most circumstances another causative process is identified.

Bronchoscopy, an obviously invasive procedure, although safe, is uncomfortable, expensive, time-consuming, and not always readily available. Several alternative approaches to the diagnosis have been assessed.

Nonbronchoscopic alveolar lavage has been reported to have a higher diagnostic yield than induced sputum at one center.[89–91] This technique does not require an expensive bronchoscope but instead uses a disposable plastic catheter. It has been proposed that nonpulmonologists could use this technique in their offices or clinics. However, the yield of this technique is not as high as BAL in the best of circumstances; at some centers the yield has been considerably lower. Moreover, any catheter passed through the epiglottis has the potential to induce bronchospasm or vomiting and aspiration. Thus operators must be prepared to deal with airway emergencies and to be trained in conscious sedation procedures. For many nonpulmonologists, such potential complications, although rare, make this procedure imprudent for use in settings where full anesthesia or critical care support is not available.

Video-assisted thoracoscopy (VATS) with biopsy is rarely used to diagnose PCP unless an unusual manifestation such as a nodule is being evaluated. VATS can be quite helpful, however, for diagnosing other types of HIV-associated pulmonary pathology.

Detection of organisms in sputum specimens offers the advantage of a noninvasive procedure that can be easily scheduled and is less expensive to perform.[92] Expectorated sputum has a low yield and is usually not worthwhile. For patients who are intubated, tracheal aspirates also have a low yield. Saline induction of sputum produces samples that provide far superior results compared to expectorated samples. Many institutions report a diagnostic yield from induced sputum ranging from 75% to 95%.[77,93–97] Such high sensitivity requires that patients be encouraged to cough up material after nebulization with hypertonic saline and should be performed using a high-flow nebulization delivery device. High sensitivity also requires scrupulous laboratory processing of the specimen, including digestion of mucoid material, centrifugation of cellular material into a pellet, and thorough direct microscopy by an experienced observer using an appropriate stain on the microscopic slide. Many laboratories prefer a direct immunofluorescent stain that permits easy visualization of cysts or trophozoites. However, Giemsa, Diff-Quik, toluidine blue-O, and methenamine silver have been used successfully. The methenamine silver and toluidine blue-O techniques stain only cysts, whereas the Giemsa, Diff-Quik, and immunofluorescent techniques allow detection of both cysts and trophozoites.

There has been considerable interest in using the polymerase chain reaction (PCR) to detect Pneumocystis in blood,

Table 36-3 Therapy for *Pneumocystis* Pneumonia[a]

Drug	Route	Dose	Comments
First Choice			
Trimethoprim–sulfamethoxazole (TMP-SMX)	PO	Two DS tablets q8h	Six tablets qd preferred over eight tablets qd to reduce toxicity. For patients <60 kg or >100 kg, adjust dose to equivalent of trimethoprim 5 mg/kg q8h
	IV	TMP 5 mg/kg plus SMX 25 mg/kg q8h	As above; q8h regimen preferred over q6h regimen; leucovorin not indicated unless substantial cytopenia
Second Choices for Mild-Moderate PCP			
Trimethoprim plus	PO	15 mg/kg/day TMP	Less convenient than TMP-SMX
Dapsone	PO	100 mg qd	
Clindamycin plus	PO IV	300–450 mg q6-8h or 600–900 mg q6–8h	Rash, diarrhea, hepatitis, methemoglobinemia occur
Primaquine	PO	15–30 mg (base) qd	
Atovaquone	PO	750 mg bid or 1500 mg qd	For mild disease, well-tolerated
Second Choice for Severe PCP			
Pentamidine	IV	3–4 mg/kg/day	Pancreatitis, nephrotoxicity, hypoglycemia occur
Adjunctive Therapy			
Prednisone/solumedrol	PO, IV	40 mg q12 × 5 days 40 mg qd × 5 days 20 mg qd × 11 days	If room air P_{O2}, <70 mmHg or A-a O_2 gradient >35 mm Hg within 72 h of initiating therapy

A-a, alveolar arterial. DS, double strength.
[a] Total duration = 21 days.

sputum, bronchoalveolar lavage fluid, urine, or oral washings.[98–113] Several laboratories have reported that PCR can detect Pneumocystis in the serum or urine of a small fraction of patients with PCP, but the sensitivity appears to be low in these specimens.[98–100] PCR has been used more successfully to detect Pneumocystis in BAL fluid, sputum, and oral washes. Detection of Pneumocystis in an oral wash would be advantageous for diagnostic or epidemiologic studies, as such a specimen is easier to obtain than induced sputum.[105–108,110] For these specimens, PCR provides more sensitivity than staining, but false-positive results have diminished the clinical utility of currently available assays. A highly specific PCR assay might be easier to perform than tinctorial methods for some laboratories if they have already established a rigorously organized PCR laboratory for a wide variety of pathogens. However, more work is needed to develop approaches that can distinguish patients who have active pneumonitis due to Pneumocystis from patients who are colonized. Quantitative assays are currently being developed that show promise for effectively distinguishing such patients.[110] The use of PCR assays, especially with oral washes, is currently a research procedure and is not available for diagnostic purposes in most laboratories.

Nonspecific tests have been described for inclusion in the diagnostic evaluation of pulmonary dysfunction. Oxygen saturation evaluation during rest and exercise,[114] chest HRCT,[46] measurement of the diffusing capacity for carbon monoxide (DLco),[115] gallium scanning, and serum enzymes such as lactate dehydrogenase[116–118] have been studied for their ability to predict the presence of PCP. None of these tests appears to be specific and sensitive enough to warrant diagnostic use in clinical settings without subsequent microscopic confirmation.

THERAPY

To treat PCP effectively, there are three principles of cardinal importance. (1) Prompt initiation of therapy can improve prognosis. (2) Trimethoprim–sulfamethoxazole is the drug of choice for mild, moderate, or severe disease. (3) Corticosteroid therapy (prednisone or methylprednisolone) improves survival for patients with moderate or severe disease.

Initial Therapy

Because the best indicator of prognosis is the alveolar-arterial oxygen gradient at the time specific therapy is initiated,[47–52,55,56] it is logical to make prompt initiation of appropriate therapy a high priority. This obviously requires that patients be advised to come to their healthcare provider when they have any suggestive symptoms, even if such symptoms are mild, and that healthcare providers expeditiously initiate management by obtaining diagnostic tests, starting empiric therapy, or both.

Therapeutic regimens[119–127] for acute PCP are listed in Tables 36-3 and 36-4. In some situations, empirical therapy

Table 36-4

Selected Trials for Therapy of Acute PCP

Study	Eligibility	Design	No.	Drug Regimens	Failure at Day 21 (%)			Comments
					Failure of Response	Failure due to Toxicity	Death	
Safrin (ACTG 108)[125]	Confirmed PCP Symptomatic PAO_2-PaO_2 at 45 mmHg	Randomized, double-blind, 21 day course	181	TMP-SMX 2 DS PO tid (weight adjusted)	9.4	35.9	6.2	Underpowered. No statistical difference in efficacy, toxicity, mortality
				Dapsone 100 mg PO qd plus TMP 300 mg PO tid	11.9	23.7	3.4	
				Clindamycin 600 mg PO tid plus primaquine 30 mg PO qd	6.9	32.8	3.4	
Hughes[122]	Confirmed PCP Symptomatic PAO_2-PaO_2 at 45 mmHg	Randomized, double-blind, 21 day course	322	TMP-SMX 2 DS PO tid	7.0	20.0	6.0	More failures to respond with atovaquone ($P = 0.002$) but less treatment-limiting toxicity ($P = 0.001$)
				Atovaquone 750 mg (tablets) PO tid	20.0	7.0	7.0	
Dohn[123]	Confirmed PCP Symptomatic PAO_2-PaO_2 at 45 mmHg	Randomized, open-label, 21 day course	109	Pentamidine 3–4 mg IV qd	17.0	36.0	17.0	More failures to respond with atovaquone ($P = 0.18$) but less treatment-limiting toxicity ($P < 0.001$)
				Atovaquone 750 mg (tablets) PO tid	29.0	4.0	16.0	
Bozzette (CCTG)[126]	Confirmed PCP	Randomized, stratified by oxygenation, confirmed and presumed PCP	328	Standard PCP therapy				Corticosteroids reduce risk of respiratory failure at 21 days ($P = 0.004$) and death by day 84 ($P = 0.026$)
				Prednisone	0.13[a]		12.0	
				No prednisone	0.28[a]		23.0	

ACTG, AIDS Clinical Trial Group; CCTG, California Clinical Trials Group; DS, double-strength tablets; TMP-SMX, trimethoprim–sulfamethoxazole.

[a] Relative risk.

Table 36-5 DHPS Mutations Associated with Sulfonamide or Sulfone Exposure

Study Author	Year	DHPS Mutations (%)		
		Prophylaxis	No Prophylaxis	*P*-value
Ma et al[135]	1999	79	11	<0.01
Helweg-Larsen et al[134]	1999	62	11	<0.0001
Huang et al[137]	2000	80	48	<0.001
Kazanjian et al[136]	2000	76	23	<0.001
Visconti et al[140]	2001	80	27	0.031
Ma et al[141]	2002	19	4	0.017
Costa et al[251]	2003	35	25	0.39

without confirming the diagnosis may be appropriate: patients with room air P_{O2} above 80 mmHg, patients who are clinically stable, and patients who do not have prompt access to diagnostic facilities are reasonable candidates for empirical therapy.[128–130] Therapy can be administered orally if there is no evidence of gastrointestinal dysfunction and the patient adheres to the regimen. If therapy is empirical, a macrolide (e.g., azithromycin) or fluoroquinolone (e.g., levofloxacin or moxifloxacin) is often added to treat other processes that are likely to present with manifestations similar to PCP.

Trimethoprim–sulfamethoxazole is always the drug of choice unless the patient has a history of life-threatening intolerance.[119–127] In every study performed to date, including HIV-infected and HIV-uninfected patients, trimethoprim–sulfamethoxazole has been as effective as alternative drugs or more effective. Specifically, there are few patients who have a poorer clinical response to trimethoprim–sulfamethoxazole than to other drugs, except perhaps intravenous pentamidine, which has equivalent efficacy to trimethoprim–sulfamethoxazole but is more toxic.[119–121] Trimethoprim–sulfamethoxazole is well-absorbed and can be given by mouth to compliant patients who have no major gastrointestinal dysfunction and who have only mild disease. A dose of two double-strength (DS) tablets (each DS tablet contains 160 mg trimethoprim and 800 mg sulfamethoxazole) or intravenous trimethoprim 5 mg/kg with sulfamethoxazole 25 mg/kg is preferred every 8 h rather than every 6 h to reduce toxicity. There is no need to give concurrent leucovorin (there may be some reduction in efficacy, although this point is controversial and not conclusively established) unless cytopenias occur that appear to be drug-related.[131] Patients may be managed on oral therapy as outpatients if they have mild disease (room air P_{O2} above 80 mmHg), their clinical disease is not progressing rapidly, they are reliable, and they have no major gastrointestinal dysfunction.

There is evidence that Pneumocystis can develop resistance to sulfamethoxazole, the more active component of the trimethoprim–sulfamethoxazole combination.[132–147] This resistance has been suggested by sequencing the target enzyme for sulfamethoxazole, dihydropteroate synthase (DHPS), and observing nonsynonymous point mutations that have been associated with sulfa drug resistance in other microorganisms. DHPS mutations are found especially in patients who have been exposed to sulfonamides or sulfones in the past (Table 36-5). Whether the reported mutations are of a magnitude to be clinically important remains to be determined. Current reports are contradictory.[134,136,139,144,146–148] Helweg-Larsen et al reported that DHPS mutations were an independent predictor of mortality in a retrospective analysis of a Danish cohort.[134] Some subsequent studies have found that DHPS mutations were associated with an increase in morbidity but none has found an association with increased mortality.[136,139,147]

Toxicities of trimethoprim–sulfamethoxazole and other drugs are listed in Chapter 79.[13,119,120,122,124,125,149–152] A complete blood count, electrolytes, liver function tests, and creatinine should be monitored two or three times weekly to assess toxicity, as should symptoms and signs. Repeat chest radiographs and arterial blood gases are not necessary unless the patient is deteriorating or is clinically tenuous (i.e., the initial P_{O2} on room air was less than 70–80 mmHg). A chest radiograph at the end of the therapeutic course is useful for future comparison.[153] Monitoring sulfonamide levels is unnecessary except in unusual patients with unstable renal function or patients receiving renal replacement therapy.[152] A 21-day course is standard, although there is no compelling evidence that 21 days of therapy is more effective than 14 days. Trimethoprim–sulfamethoxazole pharmacokinetics are not influenced significantly by other drugs, although the dose should be adjusted if there is significant renal dysfunction.

The efficacy of trimethoprim plus dapsone for mild-to-moderate PCP is comparable to that of trimethoprim–sulfamethoxazole, and the former may be somewhat better tolerated than the latter.[125,154] This regimen is less convenient than trimethoprim–sulfamethoxazole because the dapsone must be taken once per day and the trimethoprim three times daily. Occasionally patients develop clinically important methemoglobinemia while on dapsone or hemolyze as a result of glucose-6-phosphate dehydrogenase (G6PD) deficiency. It is rarely necessary to screen for G6PD deficiency prior to initiating therapy unless there is a strong suspicion of deficiency, as might be the case for patients of Mediterranean ancestry and patients from the subtropical zones of the Eastern Hemisphere. It is not clear how many patients who are truly intolerant of trimethoprim–sulfamethoxazole can tolerate this regimen. A history of life-threatening trimethoprim–sulfamethoxazole adverse reactions should preclude the use of dapsone plus trimethoprim. For patients who do not tolerate trimethoprim–sulfamethoxazole owing to nonlife-threatening complications, dapsone–trimethoprim is a reasonable option.

Intravenous pentamidine appears to have efficacy equivalent to that of trimethoprim–sulfamethoxazole.[13,119,121,155–157] When given in a daily dose of 4 mg/kg or perhaps 3 mg/kg (the latter is less well studied),[155] the response to therapy is excellent. However, nephrotoxicity,[158] dysglycemia,[159] pancreatitis, and cardiac arrhythmias[160] (*torsade de pointes*; *see* Chapter 68) make this drug complicated to administer. A baseline electrocardiogram to assess the QT interval (*see* Chapter 68) is useful but not mandatory. If the QT interval is more than 0.48 s and cannot be corrected by normalizing electrolytes or if other drugs that substantially prolong the QT interval are used concurrently (e.g., amiodarone, sotalol, perhaps certain quinolones), a cardiologist might be consulted before administering the drug. The use of monitoring to follow QT intervals and rhythm is controversial. Patients may become hypoglycemic during therapy or even during the several weeks after therapy. This hypoglycemia may be profound and symptomatic; and it can rarely result in death.[158,159] Following acute therapy, the effects of pentamidine on the pancreas may lead to decreased insulin production and hyperglycemia, requiring chronic insulin therapy. Renal dysfunction may manifest as azotemia or tubular dysfunction. Renal dysfunction appears to be a risk factor for dysglycemia. The pancreatitis associated with pentamidine can be severe. There is some evidence that patients who have been given didanosine or zalcitabine (and perhaps stavudine) may be predisposed to pentamidine-induced pancreatitis, but this remains to be confirmed.

Aerosolized pentamidine has been used for therapy of acute PCP.[155–157] Although it is somewhat effective, especially for patients with mild disease, the relatively low response rate and high relapse rate makes it a poor option for therapy. It should almost never be used for therapy of acute disease.

Atovaquone has few life-threatening toxicities and a high degree of efficacy.[161,122,123] It is not, however, as potent as trimethoprim–sulfamethoxazole or intravenous pentamidine. In addition, steady-state levels are not reached for several days, absorption can be unpredictable, and some patients find the current liquid formulation to be unpleasant. Atovaquone absorption is improved by ingestion with a high-fat meal. Thus atovaquone has a therapeutic role for patients with mild, stable disease who have no evidence of gastrointestinal dysfunction. For this population, if neither trimethoprim–sulfamethoxazole nor trimethoprim–dapsone is tolerable, atovaquone is a good option. An intravenous preparation is not commercially available. Mutations in cytochrome *b*, the target for atovaquone, have been described.[162] Their clinical importance is unknown.

Clindamycin plus primaquine is an effective regimen that appeared comparable to trimethoprim–sulfamethoxazole and dapsone–trimethoprim in large but underpowered studies.[125,163,164] Clindamycin can be given orally or parenterally; primaquine is available only as an oral preparation. The regimen is inconvenient in that two drugs are involved. In addition, clindamycin causes a substantial amount of rash, diarrhea, and hepatic dysfunction in this population, and primaquine can be associated with G6PD deficiency-related hemolysis. This regimen is a reasonable alternative for patients with mild disease who can absorb an oral regimen and who cannot tolerate trimethoprim–sulfamethoxazole.[125,163,164]

Prednisone is part of standard therapy for patients whose initial room air P_{O2} is less than 70 mmHg or whose alveolar-arterial oxygen gradient is greater than 35 mmHg.[126,165–168] Studies show that mortality is reduced substantially in HIV-infected patients with an initial room air P_{O2} below 70 mmHg when prednisone is added to specific chemotherapy within 72 h of initial therapy. Symptomatically and in terms of oxygenation, PCP also disappears faster with prednisone than without. Whether there is an important survival benefit when prednisone is added to specific therapy for patients with initial P_{O2} values higher than 70 mmHg is unclear because the mortality in this population is low even without prednisone therapy.

There has been considerable concern about the safety of prednisone. There is, however, no convincing evidence that a 21-day course using the regimen in Table 36-3 increases the likelihood that another opportunistic infection, Kaposi sarcoma, or tuberculosis will appear or, if present, will be exacerbated. Metabolic abnormalities induced by prednisone are usually readily managed.

Acute PCP can be complicated by electrolyte abnormalities (especially syndromes of inappropriate antidiuretic hormone) or pneumothorax.[169] These complications can be managed using standard principles.

Should antiretroviral therapy be initiated or continued when patients have acute PCP? There is little information to indicate whether initiating HAART in the face of acute PCP can improve outcome.[57] It is conceivable that such therapy could improve immune function. It is also conceivable that HAART could exacerbate pulmonary dysfunction by causing a more intense inflammatory response (i.e., immune reconstitution syndrome).[170,171] In general, it is probably preferable not to initiate HAART during an episode of PCP; absorption of drugs and adherence may be erratic and could thus lead to rapid development of retroviral resistance to the HAART regimen. In addition, if multiple drugs (trimethoprim–sulfamethoxazole plus HAART) are started simultaneously it may be difficult to know to what to attribute toxicity. For patients who have been receiving HAART it may be preferable to suspend HAART therapy until the patient is stable. On the other hand, patients who are critically ill with PCP and accompanying respiratory

Approach to Patients Failing PCP Therapy

Table 36-6

Days 4–6
Repeat chest radiograph
  Assess possibility of new process
Perform or repeat bronchoscopy
  Confirm PCP
  Rule out concurrent infection or tumor
Consider Swan–Ganz catheter or lung scan
  Rule out congestive heart failure
  Consider pulmonary emboli
Consider empirical therapy for bacterial processes
  Consider quinolone for community-acquired pneumonia
Add prednisone if not already part of regimen

Days 6–8
Consider switching to
  First choice: trimethoprim–sulfamethoxazole (IV)
  Second choice: pentamidine (IV)

failure are a subset of PCP patients with a high mortality.[54,57,172] One study reported that HAART started either before or during hospitalization was an independent predictor that was associated with a lower mortality (odds ratio (OR), 0.14; 95% confidence interval (95% CI), 0.02–0.84; $P = 0.03$).[57] While the challenges of administering HAART to patients are magnified in the ICU, the subset of PCP patients who are worsening despite PCP treatment and optimal ICU care, are individuals where consideration of HAART is warranted.

Salvage Therapy

A frequent issue is how to manage patients who are not improving on their initial regimen (Table 36-6). Clinicians must understand that the median time to clinical or physiologic improvement is 4–8 days, and that the natural history of PCP is to get worse during the initial 72 h following institution of therapy unless prednisone is part of the regimen.[9,166] Thus a change in therapy before a 4- to 8-day course of therapy is premature; it is preferable to wait 6–8 days before changing agents rather than changing earlier. If a patient is deteriorating and the P_{O2} on room air approaches or falls below 70 mmHg at any point, prednisone should be added to the regimen.[173]

There have been no trials to determine the best time to switch therapy, the most effective salvage regimen, or if combination therapy (e.g., trimethoprim–sulfamethoxazole with intravenous pentamidine) is preferable to a single-drug regimen.[174] Many clinicians carefully assess the patient for concurrent pulmonary processes (i.e., bronchoscopy should be repeated after 4 days of therapy looking for pathogens other than Pneumocystis, and the patient should be carefully assessed for concurrent noninfectious processes such as heart failure, bronchospasm, or pulmonary emboli); if there is no response after 6–8 days of therapy, they switch from trimethoprim–sulfamethoxazole to intravenous pentamidine (some clinicians add subsequent drugs in preference to switching). Some clinicians prefer not to use pentamidine in patients who have been heavily exposed to didanosine or stavudine. If a patient is deteriorating or failing to improve prior to days 6–8 on a regimen other than trimethoprim–sulfamethoxazole, strong consideration should be given to using this regimen, even if desensitization is required in intensive care unit.

In terms of alternatives to trimethoprim–sulfamethoxazole or intravenous pentamidine, a clindamycin with primaquine combination has been used successfully to salvage some patients failing their initial therapy.[163] Because primaquine is available only as an oral agent, and because clindamycin alone is ineffective in animal models, many clinicians are reluctant to use clindamycin–primaquine as a salvage regimen if other options are available. Some clinicians have used aerosolized pentamidine in addition to intravenous therapy, but there are no data to indicate if this is useful or safe.

Mechanical ventilation is an appropriate option for many patients with PCP.[175–177] Patients who had a good quality of life prior to the onset of PCP and who have not received at least 6–8 days of therapy, have not received corticosteroids, or have reversible processes such as congestive heart failure or pneumothorax are reasonable candidates for mechanical ventilation if they are willing to try this mode of support and if their functional status was reasonable prior to PCP. The goals of mechanical ventilation and a realistic assessment of the prognosis must be carefully reevaluated daily. A summary of an approach to a patient who appears to be failing therapy is presented in Table 36-6.

PREVENTION

Chemoprophylaxis

Chemoprophylaxis for PCP is considered to be the standard of care for patients with CD4+ T-lymphocyte counts of less than 200 cells/μL and for patients with oropharyngeal thrush regardless of the CD4+ T-lymphocyte count.[8,13–20,178–209] Trimethoprim–sulfamethoxazole is the agent of choice; dapsone, dapsone–pyrimethamine, aerosolized pentamidine, and atovaquone can be recommended for patients who do not tolerate trimethoprim–sulfamethoxazole. Figure 36-4 summarizes an approach to prevention.

During the era prior to HAART, lifelong PCP prophylaxis was recommended; that is, once the patient's CD4+ T-lymphocyte count fell to less than 200 cells/μL or the patient had an episode of PCP, anti-PCP prophylaxis should be instituted for life.[8,13–20] Because HAART regimens have been used extensively, numerous studies have documented that neither primary nor secondary prophylaxis need be continued in patients whose CD4+ T-lymphocyte counts rise to more than 200 cells/μL as a consequence of HAART. Tables 36-7 and 36-8 summarize the reported trials that have provided extensive evidence supporting discontinuation of primary and secondary

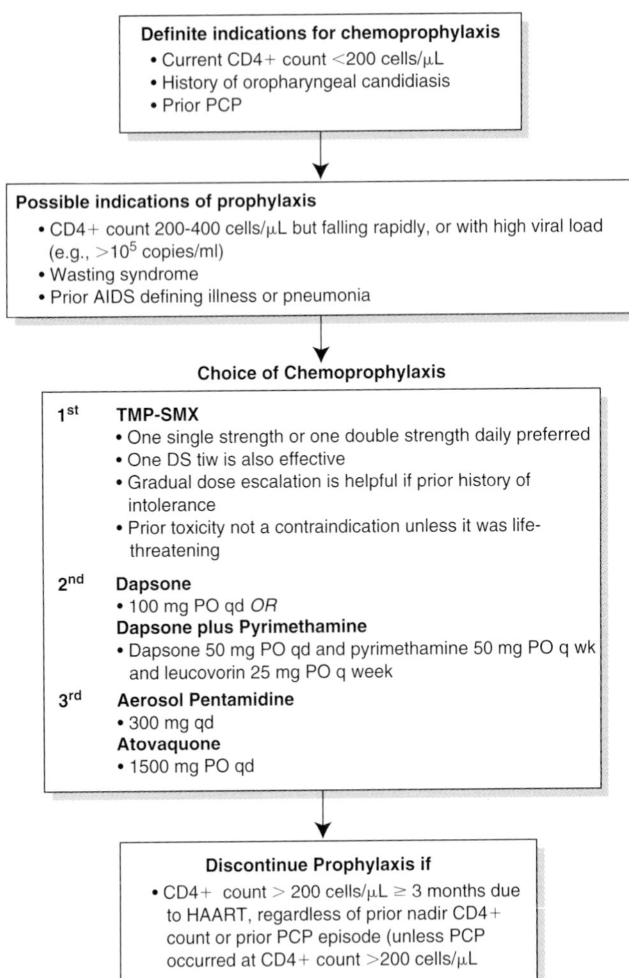

Definite indications for chemoprophylaxis
• Current CD4+ count <200 cells/μL
• History of oropharyngeal candidiasis
• Prior PCP
Possible indications of prophylaxis
• CD4+ count 200-400 cells/μL but falling rapidly, or with high viral load (e.g., >10^5 copies/ml)
• Wasting syndrome
• Prior AIDS defining illness or pneumonia
Choice of Chemoprophylaxis
1st TMP-SMX
• One single strength or one double strength daily preferred
• One DS tiw is also effective
• Gradual dose escalation is helpful if prior history of intolerance
• Prior toxicity not a contraindication unless it was life-threatening
2nd Dapsone
• 100 mg PO qd OR
Dapsone plus Pyrimethamine
• Dapsone 50 mg PO qd and pyrimethamine 50 mg PO q wk and leucovorin 25 mg PO q week
3rd Aerosol Pentamidine
• 300 mg qd
Atovaquone
• 1500 mg PO qd
Discontinue Prophylaxis if
• CD4+ count > 200 cells/μL ≥ 3 months due to HAART, regardless of prior nadir CD4+ count or prior PCP episode (unless PCP occurred at CD4+ count >200 cells/μL

Figure 36-4 ■ Algorithm for prevention of PCP. TMP-SMX, trimethoprim–sulfamethoxazole.

prophylaxis for patients whose CD4+ T-lymphocytes rise to at least 200 cells/μL.

Are all patients with CD4+ T-lymphocyte counts higher than 200 cells/μL protected from PCP without prophylaxis? As suggested above, the recommendation that prophylaxis can be safely stopped is a statistical assessment. As in the era prior to antiretroviral therapy, some patients with CD4+ T-lymphocyte counts well above 200 cells/μL develop PCP, but such cases are unusual and still support the advantage of stopping prophylaxis in terms of convenience, toxicity, ecologic pressure on microbial flora, and cost (the latter advantage is admittedly small in most cases). Furthermore, there appears to be a low incidence of community-acquired pneumonia among HIV-infected patients after discontinuation of trimethoprim–sulfamethoxazole for PCP prophylaxis.[210] There may, however, be some patients in whom prophylaxis should not be stopped.[211,212] Although there are no data to support such recommendations, clinicians might consider continuing prophylaxis in patients with high viral loads (i.e., >50 000–100 000 copies/mL), rapidly declining CD4+ T-lymphocyte counts, wasting, candidiasis, or a prior episode of PCP which developed at CD4+ T-lymphocyte counts of more than 200 cells/μL.

Trimethoprim–Sulfamethoxazole

Trimethoprim–sulfamethoxazole is clearly the drug of choice for prophylaxis because it is more effective in preventing PCP than other alternatives; moreover, it is well tolerated and inexpensive. Table 36-9 shows the results of selected trials that compared the efficacy of trimethoprim–sulfamethoxazole to aerosolized pentamidine or to dapsone, dapsone plus pyrimethamine, or atovaquone. In every large trial trimethoprim–sulfamethoxazole has demonstrated efficacy equal or superior to that of other regimens for primary or secondary prophylaxis. There are also data demonstrating that trimethoprim–sulfamethoxazole reduces the frequency of bacterial respiratory infections[185] and toxoplasmosis.[213] True breakthroughs of PCP are highly unusual for patients who are adherent to any of the recommended regimens of trimethoprim–sulfamethoxazole.[214,215] Most breakthroughs occur in patients with CD4+ T-lymphocyte counts of less than 50 cells/μL and are probably due to a poor host immune response rather than drug resistance. Logically, drug resistance is likely to occur eventually if prophylactic regimens are used widely. Until recently, as already noted (*see section on* Therapy), resistance had been impossible to detect because the human-derived organism cannot be grown *in vitro*. However, studies of DHPS genes from human isolates suggest that mutations do occur that could confer resistance.[132–147] Whether such isolates are in fact clinically resistant to trimethoprim–sulfamethoxazole prophylaxis remains to be proven.

Trimethoprim–sulfamethoxazole is associated with well-recognized toxicities (*see* Chapter 79–80), including fever, rash, pruritus, neutropenia, anemia, thrombocytopenia, hepatitis, pancreatitis, aseptic meningitis, interstitial nephritis, and crystalluria.[8,104–106,125,127] These toxicities are more likely to occur with high-dose prophylactic regimens.[8,125,127,129] A substantial number of patients must discontinue this prophylaxis because of toxicities, although minor laboratory abnormalities are not necessarily an indication to switch to less effective alternatives. Trimethoprim–sulfamethoxazole use is also associated with increased trimethoprim–sulfamethoxazole-resistant enteric bacilli and *Staphylococcus aureus*.[216]

Analyses of trials using various doses of trimethoprim–sulfamethoxazole suggest that low doses are better tolerated than high doses, although only three studies comparing various trimethoprim–sulfamethoxazole regimens have been completed in patients with HIV infection.[129,131,139] There is no evidence that a single-strength (SS) tablet once daily is less effective than a double strength (DS) tablet once daily, although there have been no studies adequately powered to prove equivalence. Thus it is reasonable to consider using an SS tablet once daily in preference to a DS tablet once daily. There has been considerable enthusiasm for intermittent regimens, such as one DS tablet three times a week. One study compared one DS tablet per day to one DS tablet three times a week for a mixed population of patients undergoing

Table 36-7

Safety of Discontinuing Primary PCP Prophylaxis in Patients with a HAART-Induced Rise in CD4+ T-lymphocyte Count to >200 cells/μL

Study	No. of Patients	Nadir CD4+ (Cells/μL)	Mean Follow-up (Months)	PCP Cases (No.)
Schneider[195]	62	85	14.0	0
Furrer[196]	262	110	11.3	0
Weverling[197]	319	123	5.0	0
Dworkin[253]	1112	146		5
Yangco[199]	131	113	18.2	0
Kirk[198]	193	117	9.6	1
Lopez Bernaldo de Quiros[204]				
Stop	233	113	20	0 (0–4.6)[a]
Continue	230	98	19	0 (0–4.3)[a]
Mussini[200]				
Stop	355		6.3	0 (0–2.5)[a]
Continue	353		6.1	0 (0–2.5)[a]

[a] 95% Confidence Interval

Table 36-8

Safety of Discontinuing Secondary PCP Prophylaxis in Patients with a HAART-Induced Rise in CD4+ T-lymphocyte Count to >200 cells/μL

Study	No. of Patients	Nadir CD4+ (Cells/μL)	%VL <50 Copies/μL	Mean Follow-up (Months)	PCP Cases (No.)
Schneider[195]	16	53	69	7.8	0
Ledergerber[205]	69	60	49		0
Koletar[206]	129	64	16	13	0
Jubault[201]	51			30	0
Furrer[252]	55	25	91	10	0
Soriano[202]	29				1
Lopez Bernaldo de Quiros[204]	99				
Stop	60	32	52	12	0
Continue	33	26	46	11	0
Mussini[207]	124				
Stop	40			9.1	0
Continue	35			7.3	0

primary and secondary prophylaxis.[139] When evaluated by intention-to-treat analysis, there was no difference in efficacy or tolerability of the two regimens. However, when evaluated by the regimen the patient was following at the time PCP developed, there were significantly more breakthroughs for patients with the intermittent regimen. This suggests that intermittent regimens may be less effective than daily regimens, but there are alternative interpretations of this trial as well.

Whether trimethoprim–sulfamethoxazole regimens that employ doses of less than one DS tablet daily provide as much efficacy for preventing toxoplasmosis or bacterial respiratory infections is uncertain. Thus it is not clear what trimethoprim–sulfamethoxazole regimen provides the best option in terms of both efficacy for all targeted pathogens and tolerability. All regimens in Figure 36–4 are reasonable. Part of the consideration of which regimen to choose involves compliance; a daily regimen may be easier for some patients

Table 36-9

Selected Trials Assessing Efficacy and Safety for PCP Prophylaxis

Study	Eligibility	Design	No.	Drug Regimen	Failure (%) PCP Breakthrough	Failure (%) Rx-Limiting Toxicity	Comments
Primary Prophylaxis							
Bozzette (ACTG 081)[180]	CD4+ <200 cells/μL No prior PCP or toxo AZT 1 month	Randomized, open-label	843	TMP-SMX 1 DS PO bid Dapsone 50 mg PO bid AP 300 mg q mo	18 17 21	27 20 4	TMP-SMX or dapsone superior to AP for CD4+ T-lymphocyte <100/cells/μL ($P = 0.4$) but not for group as whole
Schneider[181]	CD4+ <200 cells/μL No prior PCP	Randomized, open-label	260	TMP-SMX 1 SS PO qd TMP-SMX 1 DS PO qd	0 0	30 40	Both highly effective, lower dose better tolerated ($P = 0.007$)
Podzamczer[182]	CD4+ <200 cells/μL No prior PCP	Randomized	230	TMP-SMX 1 DS bid tiw, Dapsone 100 mg PO qd plus pyrimethamine 50 mg PO biw	0 6.3	9.6 9.3	TMP-SMX more effective for PCP ($P < 0.0001$) by intent-to-treat but only one episode occurred on study drug; similar toxicity ($P = 0.95$)
Bozzette[183]	CD4+ <200 cells/μL No prior PCP	Randomized, open-label	107	TMP-SMX 1 DS bid qd TMP-SMX 1 DS bid tiw	0 0	42 24	Three times weekly is better tolerated than daily with AZT
Schneider[184]	CD4+ <200 cells/μL No prior PCP	Controlled	215	TMP-SMX 1 DS qd TMP-SMX 1 SS qd AP 300 mg q mo	0 0 11	21 26 0	TMP-SMX is more effective than AP but also more toxic
Secondary Prophylaxis							
Hardy (ACTG 021)[185]	Prior PCP	Randomized, open-label	310	TMP-SMX 1 DS PO qd AP 300 mg q mo	9.1 23.1	27 4	TMP-SMX superior response rate ($P < 0.001$)
Rizzardi[186]	Prior PCP	Randomized, open-label	205	AP 300 mg q mo AP 300 mg twice/month	13.1 5.1	1 1	Efficacy difference not statistically significant

Mixed Primary and Secondary Prophylaxis							
Murphy (GW 213)[187]	TMP-SMX intolerant Prior PCP CD4+ <200/mm	Randomized, open-label	150	Atovaquone 1500 mg PO qd Atovaquone 750 mg PO qd AP 300 mg q mo	21 19 16	14 20 6	
El-Sadr (ACTG 277/CPCRA 034)[188]	TMP-SMX intolerant Prior PCP	Randomized, open-label	1057	Dapsone Atovaquone 1500 mg PO qd	18.3 15.5	27.5 26.8	Atovaquone and dapsone have similar efficacy but different toxicity profiles
Barber[189]	CD4+ <200 cells/μL ± Prior PCP	Retrospective	262	TMP-SMX – any Dapsone – any Clindamycin plus primaquine	3.4 11.0 30.7	35 13 28	Suggests clindamycin plus primaquine not highly effective at doses used
Opravil[190]	"High risk" Prior PCP CD4+ <200 cells/μL	Randomized, open-label	53	Dapsone 200 mg PO q wk plus pyrimethamine 75 mg PO q wk plus leucovorin PRN AP 300 mg q mo	4	30	Dapsone–pyrimethamine is more effective for preventing toxoplasmosis while patients receiving drug (not by intent-to-treat); but no difference for PCP
El Sadr[191]	CD4+ <200 cells/μL CD4% <15 Prior PCP	Randomized, open-label	2625	TMP-SMX DS qd TMP-SMX DS 3/wk	3.5 4.1	8.5 6.1	Trends favor daily TMP-SMX but differences not statistically significant
Dunne[192]	CD4+ <100/μL Prior PCP in 27%	Randomized, double-blind	724	Standard PCP prophylaxis plus azithromycin 1200 mg PO q wk or rifabutin 300 mg qd or both	8.2 13.1 8.5		Azithromycin associated with 50% reduction in PCP for patients who were also receiving other prophylaxis

ACTG, AIDS Clinical Trials Group; AP, aerosolized pentamidine; AZT, zidovudine; CPCRA, Community Program for Clinical Research AIDS; DS, double-strength tablets; Rx, therapy; SS, single-strength tablets; TMP-SMX, trimethoprim–sulfamethoxazole; toxo, toxoplasmosis; GW, Glaxo Wellcome.

Table 36-10 Gradual Initiation of Trimethoprim–Sulfamethoxazole Prophylaxis

Day of Regimen	Trimethoprim–Sulfamethoxazole Suspension (TMP 8 mg/ml SMX 40 mg/ml)
Procedure one[143]	Dose
1–3	1 mL PO qd
4–6	2 mL PO qd
7–9	5 mL PO qd
10–12	10 mL PO qd
13–14	20 mL PO qd
Procedure two[144]	Dose with antihistamine pretherapy days 1–6
1	1.25 mL qd
2	1.25 mL qd
3	1.25 mL qd
4	2.5 mL qd
5	2.5 mL qd
≥6	1 SS tablet qd

SS, single strength.

than a three times per week regimen. There is no evidence that daily or even intermittent leucovorin therapy is useful for preventing cytopenias.

The utility of "desensitization" regimens or gradual dose escalation of trimethoprim–sulfamethoxazole has been controversial. Two trials have been completed that compare gradual dose escalation of trimethoprim–sulfamethoxazole to immediate introduction of the full-strength dose. In both trials, gradual dose escalation resulted in a higher number of patients being able to tolerate prophylaxis at the study endpoint (12 weeks in one study and 6 months in the other).[143,144] Table 36-10 summarizes two regimens that have been studied.

An issue that frequently confronts a clinician is whether it is safe to rechallenge a patient who has previously been intolerant to trimethoprim–sulfamethoxazole. Data from the ACTG 021 study indicate that patients who have a history of nonlife-threatening toxicity are just as likely to tolerate another challenge with trimethoprim–sulfamethoxazole as are patients with no history of intolerance.[133] Thus unless a patient has a history of a life-threatening toxicity such as anaphylaxis or a desquamative skin reaction, it is reasonable to attempt to maintain that patient on trimethoprim–sulfamethoxazole again, perhaps initiating therapy with a gradual dose escalation regimen.

Dapsone

Dapsone prophylaxis is considered the best alternative for patients who cannot tolerate trimethoprim–sulfamethoxazole.[8,125–128] A daily dose of 100 mg orally may be associated with rash, fever, methemoglobinemia, or hemolysis. Patients with significant G6PD deficiency are likely to have substantial hemolysis. There is no uniform opinion as to the need to test all intended recipients of dapsone for G6PD deficiency before instituting prophylaxis or for monitoring methemoglobinemia. Many centers do not routinely do such testing unless the patient has a high probability of deficiency (i.e., subtropical zones in the Eastern Hemisphere or Mediterranean descent).

How many trimethoprim–sulfamethoxazole-intolerant patients can tolerate dapsone is unclear; 80% is a reasonable estimate.[217] Dose reduction of dapsone to improve tolerability is not recommended because doses less than 100 mg/day are considerably less effective than the full-dose regimen.

Dapsone alone has no antibacterial activity, and it is not clear if it has substantial anti-Toxoplasma activity when used without pyrimethamine. Dapsone with pyrimethamine is effective for reducing the frequency of both PCP and toxoplasmosis using either regimen listed in Figure 36-4.[125,218,130,138]

Dapsone may not be well absorbed when administered concurrently with a buffer such as is contained in some didanosine preparations. There are conflicting pharmacokinetic data about the importance of this potential interaction (*see* Chapter 79).

Pentamidine

Aerosolized pentamidine delivered by the Respirgard II nebulizer (Marquest, Englewood, CO, USA) effectively prevents PCP, especially in patients with CD4+ T-lymphocyte counts of more than 100 cells/μL,[3,8,125–128,132,133,141] but it was not as effective as trimethoprim–sulfamethoxazole or dapsone. Aerosolized pentamidine has no activity against other likely respiratory pathogens. It is well tolerated, although a few patients experience bronchospasm that may require pretreatment with albuterol. A few cases of pancreatitis have been reported to be associated with aerosolized pentamidine, but whether this association is causal or coincidental is uncertain. Uncontrolled or poorly controlled reports suggest that a monthly dose of 600 mg or biweekly doses of 300 mg may be more effective than 300 mg once per month.[134,219] Such a regimen could be tried in patients who break through the standard dose and who cannot tolerate or fail the oral regimen. Data exist for other regimens, particularly a well-studied regimen that used an ultrasonic Fisons nebulizer.[135] This nebulizer is not currently available in the United States.

When patients use a nebulizer that induces coughing, there is potential for the transmission of respiratory pathogens to staff and other patients if appropriate environmental ventilation and personal protection systems (i.e., masks) are not utilized. Outbreaks of tuberculosis associated with aerosolized pentamidine facilities have been reported. Aerosolized pentamidine has the potential to be teratogenic, so pregnant patients and healthcare workers should avoid exposure.

Atovaquone

Two trials indicate that a daily atovaquone dose of 1500 mg of the liquid suspension has efficacy comparable to that of aerosolized pentamidine[141] or oral dapsone.[136] Atovaquone has efficacy for treating Toxoplasma disease, but the effectiveness of this regimen for preventing toxoplasmosis is unknown. Atovaquone has no antibacterial activity. Atovaquone is metabolized by the cytochrome P450 system, and levels can be reduced by ritonavir-containing HAART regimens.

Atovaquone suspension has the disadvantage of a consistency that some patients find unpleasant. A regimen of 1500 mg/day is also much more expensive than other drug regimens.

Other Drugs

A variety of other drugs have some activity for preventing PCP. In a study of azithromycin prophylaxis for *Mycobacterium avium-intracellulare*, a post hoc analysis showed that patients (all of whom received standard PCP prophylaxis) receiving azithromycin had a 50% reduction in the risk of developing PCP compared to those who received no azithromycin.[140] Intravenous pentamidine has appeared to provide protection against PCP in some observational studies but not in others. Long-term intravenous administration may be associated with substantial toxicity, especially in patients heavily exposed to didanosine, zalcitabine, or stavudine. Results with clindamycin plus primaquine have been disappointing.[137]

Respiratory Isolation

Rodent studies demonstrate unequivocally that Pneumocystis is an airborne pathogen that is transmissible from healthy animals or animals with PCP to members of the same species.[220–225] Human Pneumocystis is immunologically distinct from the organisms that infect other species.[226,227] Human studies have demonstrated that immunocompromised humans with active PCP as well as healthy humans without PCP but with evidence of Pneumocystis colonization and perhaps subclinical infection may be a reservoir for human Pneumocystis.[228–242] Environmental sampling suggests that human Pneumocystis is present in random air samples, especially adjacent to humans with active PCP.[243,244] Thus it might be logical to isolate patients with active PCP from other susceptible patients.[245–249] This might be especially reasonable because there is mounting evidence that some patients with multiple episodes of PCP are infected with different strains of Pneumocystis during sequential episodes, suggesting that the disease may be due to acquisition of a new strain from the environment rather than reactivation of latent infection.[250]

Current US Public Health Service and Infectious Diseases Society of America guidelines do not recommend respiratory isolation for patients with PCP.[20] However, some institutions do attempt to isolate patients with PCP from other susceptible patients and do not place patients with PCP in hospital rooms with an immunologically susceptible roommate. This is a logical approach.

REFERENCES

1. Gottlieb MS, Schroff R, Schanker HM, et al. Pneumocystis carinii pneumonia and mucosal candidiasis in previously healthy homosexual men: evidence of a new acquired cellular immunodeficiency. N Engl J Med 305:1425–31, 1981.
2. Masur H, Michelis MA, Greene JB, et al. An outbreak of community-acquired Pneumocystis carinii pneumonia: initial manifestation of cellular immune dysfunction. N Engl J Med 305:1431–8, 1981.
3. Masur H, Ognibene FP, Yarchoan R, et al. CD4 counts as predictors of opportunistic pneumonias in human immunodeficiency virus (HIV) infection. Ann Intern Med 111:223–31, 1989.
4. Hoover DR, Graham NM, Bacellar H, et al. Epidemiologic patterns of upper respiratory illness and Pneumocystis carinii pneumonia in homosexual men. Am Rev Respir Dis 144: 756–9, 1991.
5. Munoz A, Schrager LK, Bacellar H, et al. Trends in the incidence of outcomes defining acquired immunodeficiency syndrome (AIDS) in the Multicenter AIDS Cohort Study: 1985–1991. Am J Epidemiol 137:423–38, 1993.
6. Hoover DR, Saah AJ, Bacellar H, et al. Clinical manifestations of AIDS in the era of pneumocystis prophylaxis. Multicenter AIDS Cohort Study. N Engl J Med 329:1922–6, 1993.
7. Moore RD, Chaisson RE. Natural history of opportunistic disease in an HIV-infected urban clinical cohort. Ann Intern Med 124:633–42, 1996.
8. Phair J, Munoz A, Detels R, et al. The risk of Pneumocystis carinii pneumonia among men infected with human immunodeficiency virus type 1. Multicenter AIDS Cohort Study Group. N Engl J Med 322:161–5, 1990.
9. Kovacs JA, Hiemenz JW, Macher AM, et al. Pneumocystis carinii pneumonia: a comparison between patients with the acquired immunodeficiency syndrome and patients with other immunodeficiencies. Ann Intern Med 100:663–71, 1984.
10. Stover DE, White DA, Romano PA, et al. Spectrum of pulmonary diseases associated with the acquired immune deficiency syndrome. Am J Med 78:429–37, 1985.
11. Ognibene FP, Shelhamer J, Gill V, Macher AM, et al. The diagnosis of Pneumocystis carinii pneumonia in patients with the acquired immunodeficiency syndrome using subsegmental bronchoalveolar lavage. Am Rev Respir Dis 129:929–32, 1984.
12. Golden JA, Hollander H, Stulbarg MS, Gamsu G. Bronchoalveolar lavage as the exclusive diagnostic modality for Pneumocystis carinii pneumonia. A prospective study among patients with acquired immunodeficiency syndrome. Chest 90:18–22, 1986.
13. Masur H. Prevention and treatment of pneumocystis pneumonia. N Engl J Med 327:1853–60, 1992.
14. USPHS Guidelines for prophylaxis against Pneumocystis carinii pneumonia for persons infected with human immunodeficiency virus. MMWR Morb Mortal Wkly Rep 38(Suppl 5):1–9, 1989.
15. Centers for Disease Control. Recommendations for prophylaxis against Pneumocystis carinii pneumonia for adults and adolescents infected with human immunodeficiency virus. MMWR Recomm Rep 41:1–11, 1992.
16. Centers for Disease Control. 1995 revised guidelines for prophylaxis against Pneumocystis carinii pneumonia for children infected with or perinatally exposed to human immunodeficiency virus. National Pediatric and Family HIV Resource Center and National Center for Infectious Diseases, Centers for Disease Control and Prevention. MMWR Recomm Rep 44:1–11, 1995.
17. USPHS/IDSA guidelines for the prevention of opportunistic infections in persons infected with human immunodeficiency virus: a summary. MMWR Recomm Rep 44:1–34, 1995.
18. USPHS/IDSA guidelines for the prevention of opportunistic infections in persons infected with human immunodeficiency virus. USPHS/IDSA Prevention of Opportunistic Infections Working Group. MMWR Recomm Rep 46:1–46, 1997.

19. USPHS/IDSA guidelines for the prevention of opportunistic infections in persons infected with human immunodeficiency virus. U.S. Public Health Service (USPHS) and Infectious Diseases Society of America (IDSA). MMWR Recomm Rep 48:1–59, 61–6, 1999.
20. Kaplan JE, Masur H, Holmes KK. Guidelines for preventing opportunistic infections among HIV-infected persons – 2002. Recommendations of the U.S. Public Health Service and the Infectious Diseases Society of America. MMWR Recomm Rep 51:1–52, 2002.
21. Montaner JS, Le T, Hogg R, et al. The changing spectrum of AIDS index diseases in Canada. AIDS 8:693–6, 1994.
22. Saah AJ, Hoover DR, Peng Y, et al. Predictors for failure of Pneumocystis carinii pneumonia prophylaxis. Multicenter AIDS Cohort Study. JAMA 273:1197–202, 1995.
23. Lundgren JD, Barton SE, Lazzarin A, et al. Factors associated with the development of Pneumocystis carinii pneumonia in 5,025 European patients with AIDS. AIDS in Europe Study Group. Clin Infect Dis 21:106–13, 1995.
24. Stansell JD, Osmond DH, Charlebois E, et al. Predictors of Pneumocystis carinii pneumonia in HIV-infected persons. Pulmonary Complications of HIV Infection Study Group. Am J Respir Crit Care Med 155:60–6, 1997.
25. Wallace JM, Hansen NI, Lavange L, et al. Respiratory disease trends in the Pulmonary Complications of HIV Infection Study cohort. Pulmonary Complications of HIV Infection Study Group. Am J Respir Crit Care Med 155:72–80, 1997.
26. Kaplan JE, Hanson DL, Navin TR, Jones JL. Risk factors for primary Pneumocystis carinii pneumonia in human immunodeficiency virus-infected adolescents and adults in the United States: reassessment of indications for chemoprophylaxis. J Infect Dis 178:1126–32, 1998.
27. Kaplan JE, Hanson D, Dworkin MS, et al. Epidemiology of human immunodeficiency virus-associated opportunistic infections in the United States in the era of highly active antiretroviral therapy. Clin Infect Dis 30(Suppl 1):S5–14, 2000.
28. Moorman AC, Von Bargen JC, Palella FJ, Holmberg SD. Pneumocystis carinii pneumonia incidence and chemoprophylaxis failure in ambulatory HIV-infected patients. HIV Outpatient Study (HOPS) Investigators. J Acquir Immune Defic Syndr Hum Retrovirol 19:182–8, 1998.
29. Ruffini DD, Madhi SA. The high burden of Pneumocystis carinii pneumonia in African HIV-1-infected children hospitalized for severe pneumonia. AIDS 16:105–12, 2002.
30. Madhi SA, Cutland C, Ismail K, et al. Ineffectiveness of trimethoprim–sulfamethoxazole prophylaxis and the importance of bacterial and viral coinfections in African children with Pneumocystis carinii pneumonia. Clin Infect Dis 35:1120–6, 2002.
31. Aderaye G, Bruchfeld J, Olsson M, Lindquist L. Occurrence of Pneumocystis carinii in HIV-positive patients with suspected pulmonary tuberculosis in Ethiopia. AIDS 17:435–40, 2003.
32. Worodria W, Okot-Nwang M, Yoo SD, Aisu T. Causes of lower respiratory infection in HIV-infected Ugandan adults who are sputum AFB smear-negative. Int J Tuberc Lung Dis 7:117–23, 2003.
33. Fisk DT, Meshnick S, Kazanjian PH. Pneumocystis carinii pneumonia in patients in the developing world who have acquired immunodeficiency syndrome. Clin Infect Dis 36:70–8, 2003.
34. Kovacs JA, Gill VJ, Meshnick S, Masur H. New insights into transmission, diagnosis, and drug treatment of Pneumocystis carinii pneumonia. Jama 286:2450–60, 2001.
35. Thomas CF Jr, Limper AH. Pneumocystis pneumonia. N Engl J Med 350:2487–98, 2004.
36. Redhead SA, Cushion MT, Frenkel JK, Stringer JR. Pneumocystis and Trypanosoma cruzi: nomenclature and typifications. J Eukaryot Microbiol 53:2–11, 2006.
37. Kales CP, Murren JR, Torres RA, Crocco JA. Early predictors of in-hospital mortality for Pneumocystis carinii pneumonia in the acquired immunodeficiency syndrome. Arch Intern Med 147:1413–17, 1987.
38. Telzak EE, Cote RJ, Gold JW, et al. Extrapulmonary Pneumocystis carinii infections. Rev Infect Dis 12:380–6, 1990.
39. Raviglione MC. Extrapulmonary pneumocystosis: the first 50 cases. Rev Infect Dis 12:1127–38, 1990.
40. Northfelt DW, Clement MJ, Safrin S. Extrapulmonary pneumocystosis: clinical features in human immunodeficiency virus infection. Medicine (Baltimore) 69:392–8, 1990.
41. Cohen OJ, Stoeckle MY. Extrapulmonary Pneumocystis carinii infections in the acquired immunodeficiency syndrome. Arch Intern Med 151:1205–14, 1991.
42. Ng VL, Yajko DM, Hadley WK. Extrapulmonary pneumocystosis. Clin Microbiol Rev 10:401–18, 1997.
43. Suster B, Akerman M, Orenstein M, Wax MR. Pulmonary manifestations of AIDS: review of 106 episodes. Radiology 161:87–93, 1986.
44. DeLorenzo LJ, Huang CT, Maguire GP, Stone DJ. Roentgenographic patterns of Pneumocystis carinii pneumonia in 104 patients with AIDS. Chest 91:323–7, 1987.
45. Kennedy CA, Goetz MB. Atypical roentgenographic manifestations of Pneumocystis carinii pneumonia. Arch Intern Med 152:1390–8, 1992.
46. Gruden JF, Huang L, Turner J, et al. High-resolution CT in the evaluation of clinically suspected Pneumocystis carinii pneumonia in AIDS patients with normal, equivocal, or nonspecific radiographic findings. AJR Am J Roentgenol 169:967–75, 1997.
47. Brenner M, Ognibene FP, Lack EE, et al. Prognostic factors and life expectancy of patients with acquired immunodeficiency syndrome and Pneumocystis carinii pneumonia. Am Rev Respir Dis 136:1199–206, 1987.
48. Bennett CL, Weinstein RA, Shapiro MF, et al. A rapid preadmission method for predicting inpatient course of disease for patients with HIV-related Pneumocystis carinii pneumonia. Am J Respir Crit Care Med 150(6 Pt 1):1503–7, 1994.
49. Benfield TL, Helweg-Larsen J, Bang D, et al. Prognostic markers of short-term mortality in AIDS-associated Pneumocystis carinii pneumonia. Chest 119:844–51, 2001.
50. Wachter RM, Russi MB, Bloch DA, et al. Pneumocystis carinii pneumonia and respiratory failure in AIDS. Improved outcomes and increased use of intensive care units. Am Rev Respir Dis 143:251–6, 1991.
51. Hawley PH, Ronco JJ, Guillemi SA, et al. Decreasing frequency but worsening mortality of acute respiratory failure secondary to AIDS-related Pneumocystis carinii pneumonia. Chest 106:1456–9, 1994.
52. Rosen MJ, Clayton K, Schneider RF, et al. Intensive care of patients with HIV infection: utilization, critical illnesses, and outcomes. Pulmonary Complications of HIV Infection Study Group. Am J Respir Crit Care Med 155:67–71, 1997.
53. Bedos JP, Dumoulin JL, Gachot B, et al. Pneumocystis carinii pneumonia requiring intensive care management: survival and prognostic study in 110 patients with human immunodeficiency virus. Crit Care Med 27:1109–15, 1999.
54. Nickas G, Wachter RM. Outcomes of intensive care for patients with human immunodeficiency virus infection. Arch Intern Med 160:541–7, 2000.
55. Curtis JR, Yarnold PR, Schwartz DN, et al. Improvements in outcomes of acute respiratory failure for patients with human immunodeficiency virus-related Pneumocystis carinii pneumonia. Am J Respir Crit Care Med 162(2 Pt 1):393–8, 2000.
56. Mansharamani NG, Garland R, Delaney D, Koziel H. Management and outcome patterns for adult Pneumocystis carinii pneumonia, 1985 to 1995: comparison of HIV-associated cases to other immunocompromised states. Chest 118:704–11, 2000.

57. Morris A, Wachter RM, Luce J, et al. Improved survival with highly active antiretroviral therapy in HIV-infected patients with severe Pneumocystis carinii pneumonia. AIDS 17:73–80, 2003.
58. McClellan MD, Miller SB, Parsons PE, Cohn DL. Pneumothorax with Pneumocystis carinii pneumonia in AIDS. Incidence and clinical characteristics. Chest 100:1224–8, 1991.
59. Tumbarello M, Tacconelli E, Pirronti T, et al. Pneumothorax in HIV-infected patients: role of Pneumocystis carinii pneumonia and pulmonary tuberculosis. Eur Respir J 10:1332–5, 1997.
60. Boiselle PM, Crans CA Jr, Kaplan MA. The changing face of Pneumocystis carinii pneumonia in AIDS patients. AJR Am J Roentgenol 172:1301–9, 1999.
61. Moskovic E, Miller R, Pearson M. High resolution computed tomography of Pneumocystis carinii pneumonia in AIDS. Clin Radiol 42:239–43, 1999.
62. Mellors JW, Rinaldo CR Jr, Gupta P, et al. Prognosis in HIV-1 infection predicted by the quantity of virus in plasma. Science 272:1167–70, 1996.
63. Lyles RH, Munoz A, Yamashita TE, et al. Natural history of human immunodeficiency virus type 1 viremia after seroconversion and proximal to AIDS in a large cohort of homosexual men. Multicenter AIDS Cohort Study. J Infect Dis 181:872–80, 2000.
64. Dworkin MS, Hanson DL, Kaplan JE, et al. Risk for preventable opportunistic infections in persons with AIDS after antiretroviral therapy increases CD4+ T lymphocyte counts above prophylaxis thresholds. J Infect Dis 182:611–15, 2000.
65. Dworkin MS, Williamson J, Jones JL, Kaplan JE. Prophylaxis with trimethoprim–sulfamethoxazole for human immunodeficiency virus-infected patients: impact on risk for infectious diseases. Clin Infect Dis 33:393–8, 2001.
66. Dworkin MS, Hanson DL, Navin TR. Survival of patients with AIDS, after diagnosis of Pneumocystis carinii pneumonia, in the United States. J Infect Dis 183:1409–12, 2001.
67. Peglow SL, Smulian AG, Linke MJ, et al. Serologic responses to Pneumocystis carinii antigens in health and disease. J Infect Dis 161:296–306, 1990.
68. Lundgren B, Lundgren JD, Nielsen T, et al. Antibody responses to a major Pneumocystis carinii antigen in human immunodeficiency virus-infected patients with and without P. carinii pneumonia. J Infect Dis 165:1151–5, 1992.
69. Walzer PD. Immunological features of Pneumocystis carinii infection in humans. Clin Diagn Lab Immunol 6:149–55, 1999.
70. Daly KR, Fichtenbaum CJ, Tanaka R, et al. Serologic responses to epitopes of the major surface glycoprotein of Pneumocystis jiroveci differ in human immunodeficiency virus-infected and uninfected persons. J Infect Dis 186:644–51, 2002.
71. Bishop LR, Kovacs JA. Quantitation of anti-Pneumocystis jiroveci antibodies in healthy persons and immunocompromised patients. J Infect Dis 187:1844–8, 2003.
72. Daly KR, Koch J, Levin L, Walzer PD. Enzyme-linked immunosorbent assay and serologic responses to Pneumocystis jiroveci. Emerg Infect Dis 10:848–54, 2004.
73. Daly KR, Huang L, Morris A, et al. Antibody responses to *Pneumocystis jirovecii* major surface glycoprotein. Emerg Infect Dis 2006; 12(8):1231–1237.
74. Skelly M, Hoffman J, Fabbri M, et al. S-adenosylmethionine concentrations in diagnosis of Pneumocystis carinii pneumonia. Lancet 361:1267–8, 2003.
75. Hughes WT. Current status of laboratory diagnosis of Pneumocystis carinii pneumonitis. Crit Rev Clin Lab Sci 6:145–70, 1975.
76. Stover DE, White DA, Romano PA, Gellene RA. Diagnosis of pulmonary disease in acquired immune deficiency syndrome (AIDS). Role of bronchoscopy and bronchoalveolar lavage. Am Rev Respir Dis 130:659–62, 1984.
77. Huang L, Hecht FM, Stansell JD, et al. Suspected Pneumocystis carinii pneumonia with a negative induced sputum examination. Is early bronchoscopy useful? Am J Respir Crit Care Med 151:1866–71, 1995.
78. Jules-Elysee KM, Stover DE, Zaman MB, et al. Aerosolized pentamidine: effect on diagnosis and presentation of Pneumocystis carinii pneumonia. Ann Intern Med 112:750–7, 1990.
79. Levine SJ, Masur H, Gill VJ, et al. Effect of aerosolized pentamidine prophylaxis on the diagnosis of Pneumocystis carinii pneumonia by induced sputum examination in patients infected with the human immunodeficiency virus. Am Rev Respir Dis 144:760–4, 1991.
80. Metersky ML, Catanzaro A. Diagnostic approach to Pneumocystis carinii pneumonia in the setting of prophylactic aerosolized pentamidine. Chest 100:1345–9, 1991.
81. Fahy JV, Chin DP, Schnapp LM, et al. Effect of aerosolized pentamidine prophylaxis on the clinical severity and diagnosis of Pneumocystis carinii pneumonia. Am Rev Respir Dis 146:844–8, 1992.
82. Meduri GU, Stover DE, Greeno RA, et al. Bilateral bronchoalveolar lavage in the diagnosis of opportunistic pulmonary infections. Chest 100:1272–6, 1991.
83. Chechani V, Allam AA, Haseeb MA, Kamholz SL. Pneumocystis carinii pneumonia in patients with AIDS: evaluation of lavage and staining techniques in diagnosis. J Acquir Immune Defic Syndr 4:250–3, 1991.
84. Levine SJ, Kennedy D, Shelhamer JH, et al. Diagnosis of Pneumocystis carinii pneumonia by multiple lobe, site-directed bronchoalveolar lavage with immunofluorescent monoclonal antibody staining in human immunodeficiency virus-infected patients receiving aerosolized pentamidine chemoprophylaxis. Am Rev Respir Dis 146:838–43, 1992.
85. Huang L, Schnapp LM, Gruden JF, et al. Presentation of AIDS-related pulmonary Kaposi's sarcoma diagnosed by bronchoscopy. Am J Respir Crit Care Med 153(4 Pt 1):1385–90, 1996.
86. Gruden JF, Huang L, Webb WR, et al. AIDS-related Kaposi sarcoma of the lung: radiographic findings and staging system with bronchoscopic correlation. Radiology 195:545–52, 1995.
87. Wallace JM, Batra P, Gong H Jr, Ovenfors CO. Percutaneous needle lung aspiration for diagnosing pneumonitis in the patient with acquired immunodeficiency syndrome (AIDS). Am Rev Respir Dis 131:389–92, 1985.
88. Falguera M, Nogues A, Ruiz-Gonzalez A, et al. Transthoracic needle aspiration in the study of pulmonary infections in patients with HIV. Chest 106:697–702, 1994.
89. Caughey G, Wong H, Gamsu G, Golden J. Nonbronchoscopic bronchoalveolar lavage for the diagnosis for Pneumocystis carinii pneumonia in the acquired immunodeficiency syndrome. Chest 88:659–62, 1985.
90. Mann JM, Altus CS, Webber CA, et al. Nonbronchoscopic lung lavage for diagnosis of opportunistic infection in AIDS. Chest 91:319–22, 1987.
91. Bustamante EA, Levy H. Sputum induction compared with bronchoalveolar lavage by Ballard catheter to diagnose Pneumocystis carinii pneumonia. Chest 105:816–22, 1994.
92. Huang L, Hopewell PC. Bronchoscopy versus Sputum Induction as the Initial Procedure for the Diagnosis of Pneumocystis carinii Pneumonia in Patients Infected with HIV. J Bronchol 5:163–8, 1998.
93. Pitchenik AE, Ganjei P, Torres A, et al. Sputum examination for the diagnosis of Pneumocystis carinii pneumonia in the acquired immunodeficiency syndrome. Am Rev Respir Dis 133:226–9, 1986.
94. Bigby TD, Margolskee D, Curtis JL, et al. The usefulness of induced sputum in the diagnosis of Pneumocystis carinii pneumonia in patients with the acquired immunodeficiency syndrome. Am Rev Respir Dis 133:515–18, 1986.
95. Kovacs JA, Ng VL, Masur H, et al. Diagnosis of Pneumocystis carinii pneumonia: improved detection in sputum with use of monoclonal antibodies. N Engl J Med 318:589–93, 1988.

96. Zaman MK, Wooten OJ, Suprahmanya B, et al. Rapid noninvasive diagnosis of Pneumocystis carinii from induced liquefied sputum. Ann Intern Med 109:7–10, 1988.
97. Ng VL, Gartner I, Weymouth LA, et al. The use of mucolysed induced sputum for the identification of pulmonary pathogens associated with human immunodeficiency virus infection. Arch Pathol Lab Med 113:488–93, 1989.
98. Schluger N, Godwin T, Sepkowitz K, et al. Application of DNA amplification to pneumocystosis: presence of serum Pneumocystis carinii DNA during human and experimentally induced Pneumocystis carinii pneumonia. J Exp Med 176:1327–33, 1992.
99. Lipschik GY, Gill VJ, Lundgren JD, et al. Improved diagnosis of Pneumocystis carinii infection by polymerase chain reaction on induced sputum and blood. Lancet 340:203–6, 1992.
100. Sepkowitz K, Schluger N, Godwin T, et al. DNA amplification in experimental pneumocystosis: characterization of serum Pneumocystis carinii DNA and potential P. carinii carrier states. J Infect Dis 168:421–6, 1993.
101. Chouaid C, Roux P, Lavard I, et al. Use of the polymerase chain reaction technique on induced-sputum samples for the diagnosis of Pneumocystis carinii pneumonia in HIV-infected patients. A clinical and cost-analysis study. Am J Clin Pathol 104:72–5, 1995.
102. Huang SN, Fischer SH, O'Shaughnessy E, et al. Development of a PCR assay for diagnosis of Pneumocystis carinii pneumonia based on amplification of the multicopy major surface glycoprotein gene family. Diagn Microbiol Infect Dis 35:27–32, 1999.
103. Sing A, Trebesius K, Roggenkamp A, et al. Evaluation of diagnostic value and epidemiological implications of PCR for Pneumocystis carinii in different immunosuppressed and immunocompetent patient groups. J Clin Microbiol 38:1461–7, 2000.
104. Torres J, Goldman M, Wheat LJ, et al. Diagnosis of Pneumocystis carinii pneumonia in human immunodeficiency virus-infected patients with polymerase chain reaction: a blinded comparison to standard methods. Clin Infect Dis 30:141–5, 2000.
105. Wakefield AE, Miller RF, Guiver LA, Hopkin JM. Oropharyngeal samples for detection of Pneumocystis carinii by DNA amplification. Q J Med 86:401–6, 1993.
106. Helweg-Larsen J, Jensen JS, et al. Diagnostic use of PCR for detection of Pneumocystis carinii in oral wash samples. J Clin Microbiol 36:2068–72, 1998.
107. Fischer S, Gill VJ, Kovacs J, et al. The use of oral washes to diagnose Pneumocystis carinii pneumonia: a blinded prospective study using a polymerase chain reaction-based detection system. J Infect Dis 184:1485–8, 2001.
108. Larsen HH, Masur H, Kovacs JA, et al. Development and evaluation of a quantitative, touch-down, real-time PCR assay for diagnosing Pneumocystis carinii pneumonia. J Clin Microbiol 40:490–4, 2002.
109. Huang L, Crothers K, DeOliveira A, et al. Application of an mRNA-based molecular viability assay to oropharyngeal washes for the diagnosis of Pneumocystis pneumonia in HIV-infected patients. A pilot study. J Eukaryot Microbiol 50(Suppl):618–20, 2003.
110. Larsen HH, Huang L, Kovacs JA, et al. A prospective, blinded study of quantitative touch-down polymerase chain reaction using oral-wash samples for diagnosis of Pneumocystis pneumonia in HIV-infected patients. J Infect Dis 189:1679–83, 2004.
111. Nyamande K, Lalloo UG, York D, et al. Low sensitivity of a nested polymerase chain reaction in oropharyngeal washings for the diagnosis of pneumocystis pneumonia in HIV-infected patients. Chest 128:167–71, 2005.
112. Arcenas RC, Uhl JR, Buckwalter SP, et al. A real-time polymerase chain reaction assay for detection of Pneumocystis from bronchoalveolar lavage fluid. Diagn Microbiol Infect Dis 2006.
113. Alvarez-Martinez MJ, Miro JM, et al. Sensitivity and specificity of nested and real-time PCR for the detection of Pneumocystis jiroveci in clinical specimens. Diagn Microbiol Infect Dis 2006.
114. Chouaid C, Maillard D, Housset B, et al. Cost effectiveness of noninvasive oxygen saturation measurement during exercise for the diagnosis of Pneumocystis carinii pneumonia. Am Rev Respir Dis 147(6 Pt 1):1360–3, 1993.
115. Huang L, Stansell J, Osmond D, et al. Performance of an algorithm to detect Pneumocystis carinii pneumonia in symptomatic HIV-infected persons. Pulmonary Complications of HIV Infection Study Group. Chest 115:1025–32, 1999.
116. Zaman MK, White DA. Serum lactate dehydrogenase levels and Pneumocystis carinii pneumonia. Diagnostic and prognostic significance. Am Rev Respir Dis 137:796–800, 1988.
117. Quist J, Hill AR. Serum lactate dehydrogenase (LDH) in Pneumocystis carinii pneumonia, tuberculosis, and bacterial pneumonia. Chest 108:415–18, 1995.
118. Bentsen KD, Nielsen TL, Eaftinck Schattenkerk JK, et al. Serum type III procollagen peptide in patients with Pneumocystis carinii infection. The Copenhagen-Amsterdam PCP-Prednisolone Study Group. Am Rev Respir Dis 148(6 Pt 1):1558–62, 1993.
119. Wharton JM, Coleman DL, Wofsy CB, et al. Trimethoprim–sulfamethoxazole or pentamidine for Pneumocystis carinii pneumonia in the acquired immunodeficiency syndrome. A prospective randomized trial. Ann Intern Med 105:37–44, 1986.
120. Hughes WT. Pneumocystis Carinii Pneumonitis: Boca Raton, FL: CRC Press; 1987.
121. Sattler FR, Cowan R, Nielsen DM, Ruskin J. Trimethoprim–sulfamethoxazole compared with pentamidine for treatment of Pneumocystis carinii pneumonia in the acquired immunodeficiency syndrome. A prospective, noncrossover study. Ann Intern Med 109:280–7, 1988.
122. Hughes W, Leoung G, Kramer F, et al. Comparison of atovaquone (566C80) with trimethoprim–sulfamethoxazole to treat Pneumocystis carinii pneumonia in patients with AIDS. N Engl J Med 328:1521–7, 1993.
123. Dohn MN, Weinberg WG, Torres RA, et al. Oral atovaquone compared with intravenous pentamidine for Pneumocystis carinii pneumonia in patients with AIDS. Atovaquone Study Group. Ann Intern Med 121:174–80, 1994.
124. Sattler FR, Frame P, Davis R, et al. Trimetrexate with leucovorin versus trimethoprim–sulfamethoxazole for moderate to severe episodes of Pneumocystis carinii pneumonia in patients with AIDS: a prospective, controlled multicenter investigation of the AIDS Clinical Trials Group Protocol 029/031. J Infect Dis 170:165–72, 1994.
125. Safrin S, Finkelstein DM, Feinberg J, et al. Comparison of three regimens for treatment of mild to moderate Pneumocystis carinii pneumonia in patients with AIDS. A double-blind, randomized, trial of oral trimethoprim–sulfamethoxazole, dapsone–trimethoprim, and clindamycin–primaquine. ACTG 108 Study Group. Ann Intern Med 124:792–802, 1996.
126. Bozzette SA, Sattler FR, Chiu J, et al. A controlled trial of early adjunctive treatment with corticosteroids for Pneumocystis carinii pneumonia in the acquired immunodeficiency syndrome. California Collaborative Treatment Group. N Engl J Med 323:1451–7, 1990.
127. Benson CA, Kaplan JE, Masur H, et al. Treating opportunistic infections among HIV-exposed and infected children: recommendations from CDC, the National Institutes of Health, and the Infectious Diseases Society of America. MMWR Recomm Rep 53:1–112, 2004.
128. Miller RF, Millar AB, Weller IV, Semple SJ. Empirical treatment without bronchoscopy for Pneumocystis carinii pneumonia

in the acquired immunodeficiency syndrome. Thorax 44:559–64, 1989.
129. Tu JV, Biem HJ, Detsky AS. Bronchoscopy versus empirical therapy in HIV-infected patients with presumptive Pneumocystis carinii pneumonia. A decision analysis. Am Rev Respir Dis 148:370–7, 1993.
130. Masur H, Shelhamer J. Empiric outpatient management of HIV-related pneumonia: economical or unwise? Ann Intern Med 124:451–3, 1996.
131. Safrin S, Lee BL, Sande MA. Adjunctive folinic acid with trimethoprim-sulfamethoxazole for Pneumocystis carinii pneumonia in AIDS patients is associated with an increased risk of therapeutic failure and death. J Infect Dis 170:912–17, 1994.
132. Kazanjian P, Locke AB, Hossler PA, et al. Pneumocystis carinii mutations associated with sulfa and sulfone prophylaxis failures in AIDS patients. AIDS 12:873–8, 1998.
133. Mei Q, Gurunathan S, Masur H, Kovacs JA. Failure of co-trimoxazole in Pneumocystis carinii infection and mutations in dihydropteroate synthase gene. Lancet 351:1631–2, 1998.
134. Helweg-Larsen J, Benfield TL, Eugen-Olsen J, et al. Effects of mutations in Pneumocystis carinii dihydropteroate synthase gene on outcome of AIDS-associated P. carinii pneumonia. Lancet 354:1347–51, 1999.
135. Ma L, Borio L, Masur H, Kovacs JA. Pneumocystis carinii dihydropteroate synthase but not dihydrofolate reductase gene mutations correlate with prior trimethoprim–sulfamethoxazole or dapsone use. J Infect Dis 180:1969–78, 1999.
136. Kazanjian P, Armstrong W, Hossler PA, et al. Pneumocystis carinii mutations are associated with duration of sulfa or sulfone prophylaxis exposure in AIDS patients. J Infect Dis 182:551–7, 2000.
137. Huang L, Beard CB, Creasman J, et al. Sulfa or sulfone prophylaxis and geographic region predict mutations in the Pneumocystis carinii dihydropteroate synthase gene. J Infect Dis 182:1192–8, 2000.
138. Takahashi T, Hosoya N, Endo T, et al. Relationship between mutations in dihydropteroate synthase of Pneumocystis carinii f. sp. hominis isolates in Japan and resistance to sulfonamide therapy. J Clin Microbiol 38:3161–4, 2000.
139. Navin TR, Beard CB, Huang L, et al. Effect of mutations in Pneumocystis carinii dihydropteroate synthase gene on outcome of P carinii pneumonia in patients with HIV-1: a prospective study. Lancet 358:545–9, 2001.
140. Visconti E, Ortona E, Mencarini P, et al. Mutations in dihydropteroate synthase gene of Pneumocystis carinii in HIV patients with Pneumocystis carinii pneumonia. Int J Antimicrob Agents 18:547–51, 2001.
141. Ma L, Kovacs JA, Cargnel A, et al. Mutations in the dihydropteroate synthase gene of human-derived Pneumocystis carinii isolates from Italy are infrequent but correlate with prior sulfa prophylaxis. J Infect Dis 185:1530–2, 2002.
142. Zar HJ, Alvarez-Martinez MJ, Harrison A, Meshnick SR. Prevalence of dihydropteroate synthase mutants in HIV-infected South African children with Pneumocystis jiroveci pneumonia. Clin Infect Dis 39:1047–51, 2004.
143. Morris A, Lundgren JD, Masur H, et al. Current epidemiology of Pneumocystis pneumonia. Emerg Infect Dis 10:1713–20, 2004.
144. Huang L, Crothers K, Atzori C, et al. Dihydropteroate synthase gene mutations in Pneumocystis and sulfa resistance. Emerg Infect Dis 10:1721–8, 2004.
145. Beard CB, Roux P, Nevez G, et al. Strain typing methods and molecular epidemiology of Pneumocystis pneumonia. Emerg Infect Dis 10:1729–35, 2004.
146. Stein CR, Poole C, Kazanjian P, Meshnick SR. Sulfa use, dihydropteroate synthase mutations, and Pneumocystis jirovecii pneumonia. Emerg Infect Dis 10:1760–5, 2004.
147. Crothers K, Beard CB, Turner J, et al. Severity and outcome of HIV-associated Pneumocystis pneumonia containing Pneumocystis jirovecii dihydropteroate synthase gene mutations. AIDS 19:801–5, 2005.
148. Kazanjian PH, Fisk D, Armstrong W, et al. Increase in prevalence of Pneumocystis carinii mutations in patients with AIDS and P. carinii pneumonia, in the United States and China. J Infect Dis 189:1684–7, 2004.
149. Jung AC, Paauw DS. Management of adverse reactions to trimethoprim–sulfamethoxazole in human immunodeficiency virus-infected patients. Arch Intern Med 154:2402–6, 1994.
150. Greenberg S, Reiser IW, Chou SY, Porush JG. Trimethoprim–sulfamethoxazole induces reversible hyperkalemia. Ann Intern Med 119:291–5, 1993.
151. Martin GJ, Paparello SF, Decker CF. A severe systemic reaction to trimethoprim–sulfamethoxazole in a patient infected with the human immunodeficiency virus. Clin Infect Dis 16:175–6, 1993.
152. Joos B, Blaser J, Opravil M, et al. Monitoring of co-trimoxazole concentrations in serum during treatment of pneumocystis carinii pneumonia. Antimicrob Agents Chemother 39:2661–6, 1995.
153. Datta D, Ali SA, Henken EM, et al. Pneumocystis carinii pneumonia: the time course of clinical and radiographic improvement. Chest 124:1820–3, 2003.
154. Medina I, Mills J, Leoung G, et al. Oral therapy for Pneumocystis carinii pneumonia in the acquired immunodeficiency syndrome. A controlled trial of trimethoprim–sulfamethoxazole versus trimethoprim–dapsone. N Engl J Med 323:776–82, 1990.
155. Conte JE Jr, Hollander H, Golden JA. Inhaled or reduced-dose intravenous pentamidine for Pneumocystis carinii pneumonia. A pilot study. Ann Intern Med 107:495–8, 1987.
156. Conte JE Jr., Chernoff D, Feigal DW Jr, et al. Intravenous or inhaled pentamidine for treating Pneumocystis carinii pneumonia in AIDS. A randomized trial. Ann Intern Med 113:203–9, 1990.
157. Montgomery AB, Feigal DW Jr, Sattler F, et al. Pentamidine aerosol versus trimethoprim–sulfamethoxazole for Pneumocystis carinii in acquired immune deficiency syndrome. Am J Respir Crit Care Med 151:1068–74, 1995.
158. O'Brien JG, Dong BJ, Coleman RL, et al. A 5-year retrospective review of adverse drug reactions and their risk factors in human immunodeficiency virus-infected patients who were receiving intravenous pentamidine therapy for Pneumocystis carinii pneumonia. Clin Infect Dis 24:854–9, 1997.
159. Stahl-Bayliss CM, Kalman CM, Laskin OL. Pentamidine-induced hypoglycemia in patients with the acquired immune deficiency syndrome. Clin Pharmacol Ther 39:271–5, 1986.
160. Taylor AJ, Hull RW, Coyne PE, et al. Pentamidine-induced torsades de pointes: safe completion of therapy with inhaled pentamidine. Clin Pharmacol Ther 49:698–700, 1991.
161. Falloon J, Kovacs J, Hughes W, et al. A preliminary evaluation of 566C80 for the treatment of Pneumocystis pneumonia in patients with the acquired immunodeficiency syndrome. N Engl J Med 325:1534–8, 1991.
162. Kazanjian P, Armstrong W, Hossler PA, et al. Pneumocystis carinii cytochrome b mutations are associated with atovaquone exposure in patients with AIDS. J Infect Dis 183:819–22, 2001.
163. Noskin GA, Murphy RL, Black JR, Phair JP. Salvage therapy with clindamycin/primaquine for Pneumocystis carinii pneumonia. Clin Infect Dis 14:183–8, 1992.
164. Toma E, Fournier S, Dumont M, et al. Clindamycin/primaquine versus trimethoprim–sulfamethoxazole as primary therapy for Pneumocystis carinii pneumonia in AIDS: a randomized, double-blind pilot trial. Clin Infect Dis 17:178–84, 1993.
165. Gagnon S, Boota AM, Fischl MA, et al. Corticosteroids as adjunctive therapy for severe Pneumocystis carinii pneumonia

in the acquired immunodeficiency syndrome. A double-blind, placebo-controlled trial. N Engl J Med 323:1444–50, 1990.
166. Montaner JS, Lawson LM, Levitt N, et al. Corticosteroids prevent early deterioration in patients with moderately severe Pneumocystis carinii pneumonia and the acquired immunodeficiency syndrome (AIDS). Ann Intern Med 113:14–20, 1990.
167. Nielsen TL, Eeftinck Schattenkerk JK, Jensen BN, et al. Adjunctive corticosteroid therapy for Pneumocystis carinii pneumonia in AIDS: a randomized European multicenter open label study. J Acquir Immune Defic Syndr 5:726–31, 1992.
168. The National Institutes of Health–University of California Expert Panel for Corticosteroids as Adjunctive Therapy for Pneumocystis Pneumonia. Consensus statement on the use of corticosteroids as adjunctive therapy for pneumocystis pneumonia in the acquired immunodeficiency syndrome. N Engl J Med 323:1500–4, 1990.
169. Renzi PM, Corbeil C, Chasse M, et al. Bilateral pneumothoraces hasten mortality in AIDS patients receiving secondary prophylaxis with aerosolized pentamidine. Association with a lower Dco prior to receiving aerosolized pentamidine. Chest 102:491–6, 1992.
170. Wislez M, Bergot E, Antoine M, et al. Acute respiratory failure following HAART introduction in patients treated for Pneumocystis carinii pneumonia. Am J Respir Crit Care Med 164:847–51, 2001.
171. Koval CE, Gigliotti F, Nevins D, Demeter LM. Immune reconstitution syndrome after successful treatment of Pneumocystis carinii pneumonia in a man with human immunodeficiency virus type 1 infection. Clin Infect Dis 35:491–3, 2002.
172. Morris A, Creasman J, Turner J, et al. Intensive care of human immunodeficiency virus-infected patients during the era of highly active antiretroviral therapy. Am J Respir Crit Care Med 166:262–7, 2002.
173. LaRocco A Jr, Amundson DE, Wallace MR, et al Corticosteroids for Pneumocystis carinii pneumonia with acute respiratory failure. Experience with rescue therapy. Chest 102:892–5, 1992.
174. Smego RA Jr, Nagar S, Maloba B, Popara M. A meta-analysis of salvage therapy for Pneumocystis carinii pneumonia. Arch Intern Med 161:1529–33, 2001.
175. Masur H. Management of Patients with HIV in the Intensive Care Unit. Proc Am Thorac Soc 3:96–102, 2006.
176. Morris A, Masur H, Huang L. Current issues in critical care of the human immunodeficiency virus-infected patient. Crit Care Med 34:42–9, 2006.
177. Huang L, Quartin A, Jones D, Havlir DV. Intensive Care of Patients with HIV Infection. N Engl J Med 355, 2006.
178. Ioannidis JP, Cappelleri JC, Skolnik PR, et al. A meta-analysis of the relative efficacy and toxicity of Pneumocystis carinii prophylactic regimens. Arch Intern Med 156:177–88, 1996.
179. Kovacs JA, Masur H. Prophylaxis against opportunistic infections in patients with human immunodeficiency virus infection. N Engl J Med 342:1416–29, 2000.
180. Bozzette SA, Finkelstein DM, Spector SA, et al. A randomized trial of three antipneumocystis agents in patients with advanced human immunodeficiency virus infection. NIAID AIDS Clinical Trials Group. N Engl J Med 332:693–9, 1995.
181. Schneider MM, Nielsen TL, Nelsing S, et al. Efficacy and toxicity of two doses of trimethoprim–sulfamethoxazole as primary prophylaxis against Pneumocystis carinii pneumonia in patients with human immunodeficiency virus. Dutch AIDS Treatment Group. J Infect Dis 171:1632–6, 1995.
182. Podzamczer D, Salazar A, Jimenez J, et al. Intermittent trimethoprim–sulfamethoxazole compared with dapsone–pyrimethamine for the simultaneous primary prophylaxis of Pneumocystis pneumonia and toxoplasmosis in patients infected with HIV. Ann Intern Med 122:755–61, 1995.
183. Bozzette SA, Forthal D, Sattler FR, et al. The tolerance for zidovudine plus thrice weekly or daily trimethoprim–sulfamethoxazole with and without leucovorin for primary prophylaxis in advanced HIV disease. California Collaborative Treatment Group. Am J Med 98:177–82, 1995.
184. Schneider MM, Hoepelman AI, Eeftinck Schattenkerk JK, et al. A controlled trial of aerosolized pentamidine or trimethoprim–sulfamethoxazole as primary prophylaxis against Pneumocystis carinii pneumonia in patients with human immunodeficiency virus infection. The Dutch AIDS Treatment Group. N Engl J Med 327:1836–41, 1992.
185. Hardy WD, Feinberg J, Finkelstein DM, et al. A controlled trial of trimethoprim–sulfamethoxazole or aerosolized pentamidine for secondary prophylaxis of Pneumocystis carinii pneumonia in patients with the acquired immunodeficiency syndrome. AIDS Clinical Trials Group Protocol 021. N Engl J Med 327:1842–8, 1992.
186. Rizzardi GP, Lazzarin A, Musicco M, et al. Better efficacy of twice-monthly than monthly aerosolised pentamidine for secondary prophylaxis of Pneumocystis carinii pneumonia in patients with AIDS. An Italian multicentric randomised controlled trial. The Italian PCP Study Group. J Infect 31:99–105, 1995.
187. Murphy RL, Lavelle JP, Allan JD, et al. Aerosol pentamidine prophylaxis following Pneumocystis carinii pneumonia in AIDS patients: results of a blinded dose-comparison study using an ultrasonic nebulizer. Am J Med 90:418–26, 1991.
188. El-Sadr WM, Murphy RL, Yurik TM, et al. Atovaquone compared with dapsone for the prevention of Pneumocystis carinii pneumonia in patients with HIV infection who cannot tolerate trimethoprim, sulfonamides, or both. Community Program for Clinical Research on AIDS and the AIDS Clinical Trials Group. N Engl J Med 339:1889–95, 1998.
189. Barber BA, Pegram PS, High KP. Clindamycin/primaquine as prophylaxis for Pneumocystis carinii pneumonia. Clin Infect Dis 23:718–22, 1996.
190. Opravil M, Hirschel B, Lazzarin A, et al. Once-weekly administration of dapsone/pyrimethamine vs. aerosolized pentamidine as combined prophylaxis for Pneumocystis carinii pneumonia and toxoplasmic encephalitis in human immunodeficiency virus-infected patients. Clin Infect Dis 20:531–41, 1995.
191. El-Sadr WM, Luskin-Hawk R, Yurik TM, et al. A randomized trial of daily and thrice-weekly trimethoprim–sulfamethoxazole for the prevention of Pneumocystis carinii pneumonia in human immunodeficiency virus-infected persons. Terry Beirn Community Programs for Clinical Research on AIDS (CPCRA). Clin Infect Dis 29:775–83, 1999.
192. Dunne MW, Bozzette S, McCutchan JA, et al. Efficacy of azithromycin in prevention of Pneumocystis carinii pneumonia: a randomised trial. California Collaborative Treatment Group. Lancet 354:891–5, 1999.
193. Chan C, Montaner J, Lefebvre EA, et al. Atovaquone suspension compared with aerosolized pentamidine for prevention of Pneumocystis carinii pneumonia in human immunodeficiency virus-infected subjects intolerant of trimethoprim or sulfonamides. J Infect Dis 180:369–76, 1999.
194. Chu SY, Hanson DL, Ciesielski C, Ward JW. Prophylaxis against Pneumocystis carinii pneumonia at higher CD4+ T-cell counts. JAMA 273:848, 1995.
195. Schneider MM, Borleffs JC, Stolk RP, et al. Discontinuation of prophylaxis for Pneumocystis carinii pneumonia in HIV-1-infected patients treated with highly active antiretroviral therapy. Lancet 353:201–3, 1999.
196. Furrer H, Egger M, Opravil M, et al. Discontinuation of primary prophylaxis against Pneumocystis carinii pneumonia in HIV-1-infected adults treated with combination antiretroviral therapy. Swiss HIV Cohort Study. N Engl J Med 340:1301–6, 1999.

197. Weverling GJ, Mocroft A, Ledergerber B, et al. Discontinuation of Pneumocystis carinii pneumonia prophylaxis after start of highly active antiretroviral therapy in HIV-1 infection. EuroSIDA Study Group. Lancet 353:1293–8, 1999.
198. Kirk O, Lundgren JD, Pedersen C, et al. Can chemoprophylaxis against opportunistic infections be discontinued after an increase in CD4 cells induced by highly active antiretroviral therapy? AIDS 13:1647–51, 1999.
199. Yangco BG, Von Bargen JC, Moorman AC, Holmberg SD. Discontinuation of chemoprophylaxis against Pneumocystis carinii pneumonia in patients with HIV infection. HIV Outpatient Study (HOPS) Investigators. Ann Intern Med 132:201–5, 2000.
200. Mussini C, Pezzotti P, Govoni A, et al. Discontinuation of primary prophylaxis for Pneumocystis carinii pneumonia and toxoplasmic encephalitis in human immunodeficiency virus type I-infected patients: the changes in opportunistic prophylaxis study. J Infect Dis 181:1635–42, 2000.
201. Jubault V, Pacanowski J, Rabian C, Viard JP. Interruption of prophylaxis for major opportunistic infections in HIV-infected patients receiving triple combination antiretroviral therapy. Ann Med Interne (Paris) 151:163–8, 2000.
202. Soriano V, Dona C, Rodriguez-Rosado R, et al. Discontinuation of secondary prophylaxis for opportunistic infections in HIV-infected patients receiving highly active antiretroviral therapy. AIDS 14:383–6, 2000.
203. Furrer H, Opravil M, Rossi M, et al. Discontinuation of primary prophylaxis in HIV-infected patients at high risk of Pneumocystis carinii pneumonia: prospective multicentre study. AIDS 15:501–7, 2001.
204. Lopez Bernaldo de Quiros JC, Miro JM, Pena JM, et al. A randomized trial of the discontinuation of primary and secondary prophylaxis against Pneumocystis carinii pneumonia after highly active antiretroviral therapy in patients with HIV infection. Grupo de Estudio del SIDA 04/98. N Engl J Med 344:159–67, 2001.
205. Ledergerber B, Mocroft A, Reiss P, et al. Discontinuation of secondary prophylaxis against Pneumocystis carinii pneumonia in patients with HIV infection who have a response to antiretroviral therapy. Eight European Study Groups. N Engl J Med 344:168–74, 2001.
206. Koletar SL, Heald AE, Finkelstein D, et al. A prospective study of discontinuing primary and secondary Pneumocystis carinii pneumonia prophylaxis after CD4 cell count increase to $> 200 \times 106$ /l. AIDS 15:1509–15, 2001.
207. Mussini C, Pezzotti P, Antinori A, et al. Discontinuation of secondary prophylaxis for Pneumocystis carinii pneumonia in human immunodeficiency virus-infected patients: a randomized trial by the CIOP Study Group. Clin Infect Dis 36:645–51, 2003.
208. Zellweger C, Opravil M, Bernasconi E, et al. Long-term safety of discontinuation of secondary prophylaxis against Pneumocystis pneumonia: prospective multicentre study. AIDS 18:2047–53, 2004.
209. Urschel S, Ramos J, Mellado M, et al. Withdrawal of Pneumocystis jirovecii prophylaxis in HIV-infected children under highly active antiretroviral therapy. AIDS 19:2103–8, 2005.
210. Eigenmann C, Flepp M, Bernasconi E, et al. Low incidence of community-acquired pneumonia among human immunodeficiency virus-infected patients after interruption of Pneumocystis carinii pneumonia prophylaxis. Clin Infect Dis 36:917–21, 2003.
211. Abgrall S, Matheron S, Le Moing V, et al. Pneumocystis carinii pneumonia recurrence in HIV patients on highly active antiretroviral therapy: secondary prophylaxis. J Acquir Immune Defic Syndr 26:151–8, 2001.
212. Crothers K, Huang L. Recurrence of Pneumocystis carinii pneumonia in an HIV-infected patient: apparent selective immune reconstitution after initiation of antiretroviral therapy. HIV Med 4:346–9, 2003.
213. Carr A, Tindall B, Brew BJ, et al. Low-dose trimethoprim–sulfamethoxazole prophylaxis for toxoplasmic encephalitis in patients with AIDS. Ann Intern Med 117:106–11, 1992.
214. Lundberg BE, Davidson AJ, Burman WJ. Epidemiology of Pneumocystis carinii pneumonia in an era of effective prophylaxis: the relative contribution of non-adherence and drug failure. AIDS 14:2559–66, 2000.
215. Huang L, Hecht FM. Why does Pneumocystis carinii pneumonia still occur? AIDS 14:2611–12, 2000.
216. Martin JN, Rose DA, Hadley WK, et al, Gerberding JL. Emergence of trimethoprim–sulfamethoxazole resistance in the AIDS era. J Infect Dis 180:1809–18, 1999.
217. Holtzer CD, Flaherty JF Jr, Coleman RL. Cross-reactivity in HIV-infected patients switched from trimethoprim–sulfamethoxazole to dapsone. Pharmacotherapy 18:831–5, 1998.
218. Girard PM, Landman R, Gaudebout C, et al. Dapsone–pyrimethamine compared with aerosolized pentamidine as primary prophylaxis against Pneumocystis carinii pneumonia and toxoplasmosis in HIV infection. The PRIO Study Group. N Engl J Med 328:1514–20, 1993.
219. Golden JA, Katz MH, Chernoff DN, et al. A randomized comparison of once-monthly or twice-monthly high-dose aerosolized pentamidine prophylaxis. Chest 104:743–50, 1993.
220. Hendley JO, Weller TH. Activation and transmission in rats of infection with Pneumocystis. Proc Soc Exp Biol Med 137:1401–4, 1971.
221. Walzer PD, Schnelle V, Armstrong D, Rosen PP. Nude mouse: a new experimental model for Pneumocystis carinii infection. Science 197:177–9, 1977.
222. Hughes WT. Natural mode of acquisition for de novo infection with Pneumocystis carinii. J Infect Dis 145:842–8, 1982.
223. Dumoulin A, Mazars E, Seguy N, et al. Transmission of Pneumocystis carinii disease from immunocompetent contacts of infected hosts to susceptible hosts. Eur J Clin Microbiol Infect Dis 19:671–8, 2000.
224. Gigliotti F, Harmsen AG, Wright TW. Characterization of transmission of Pneumocystis carinii f. sp. muris through immunocompetent BALB/c mice. Infect Immun 71:3852–6, 2003.
225. An CL, Gigliotti F, Harmsen AG. Exposure of immunocompetent adult mice to Pneumocystis carinii f. sp. muris by cohousing: growth of P. carinii f. sp. muris and host immune response. Infect Immun 71:2065–70, 2003.
226. Denis CM, Mazars E, Guyot K, et al. Genetic divergence at the SODA locus of six different formae speciales of Pneumocystis carinii. Med Mycol 38:289–300, 2000.
227. Demanche C, Berthelemy M, Petit T, et al. Phylogeny of Pneumocystis carinii from 18 primate species confirms host specificity and suggests coevolution. J Clin Microbiol 39:2126–33, 2001.
228. Totet A, Respaldiza N, Pautard JC, et al. Pneumocystis jiroveci genotypes and primary infection. Clin Infect Dis 36:1340–2, 2003.
229. Vargas SL, Ponce CA, Sanchez CA, et al. Pregnancy and asymptomatic carriage of Pneumocystis jiroveci. Emerg Infect Dis 9:605–6, 2003.
230. Wakefield AE, Lindley AR, Ambrose HE, et al. Limited asymptomatic carriage of Pneumocystis jiroveci in human immunodeficiency virus-infected patients. J Infect Dis 187:901–8, 2003.
231. Maskell NA, Waine DJ, Lindley A, et al. Asymptomatic carriage of Pneumocystis jiroveci in subjects undergoing bronchoscopy: a prospective study. Thorax 58:594–7, 2003.
232. Huang L, Crothers K, Morris A, et al. Pneumocystis colonization in HIV-infected patients. J Eukaryot Microbiol 50(Suppl):616–17, 2003.

233. Morris A, Kingsley LA, Groner G, et al. Prevalence and clinical predictors of Pneumocystis colonization among HIV-infected men. AIDS 18:793–8, 2004.
234. Morris A, Sciurba FC, Lebedeva IP, et al. Association of chronic obstructive pulmonary disease severity and pneumocystis colonization. Am J Respir Crit Care Med 170:408–13, 2004.
235. Totet A, Latouche S, Lacube P, et al. Pneumocystis jirovecii dihydropteroate synthase genotypes in immunocompetent infants and immunosuppressed adults, Amiens, France. Emerg Infect Dis 10:667–73, 2004.
236. de la Horra C, Varela JM, Fernandez-Alonso J, et al. Association between human-Pneumocystis infection and small-cell lung carcinoma. Eur J Clin Invest 34:229–35, 2004.
237. Vargas SL, Ponce CA, Luchsinger V, et al. Detection of Pneumocystis carinii f. sp. hominis and viruses in presumably immunocompetent infants who died in the hospital or in the community. J Infect Dis 191:122–6, 2005.
238. Respaldiza N, Montes-Cano MA, Dapena FJ, et al. Prevalence of colonisation and genotypic characterisation of Pneumocystis jirovecii among cystic fibrosis patients in Spain. Clin Microbiol Infect 11:1012–15, 2005.
239. Medrano FJ, Montes-Cano M, Conde M, et al. Pneumocystis jirovecii in general population. Emerg Infect Dis 11:245–50, 2005.
240. Beard CB, Fox MR, Lawrence GG, et al. Genetic Differences in Pneumocystis Isolates Recovered from Immunocompetent Infants and from Adults with AIDS: Epidemiological Implications. J Infect Dis 192:1815–18, 2005.
241. Miller RF, Lindley AR, Copas A, et al. Genotypic variation in Pneumocystis jirovecii isolates in Britain. Thorax 60:679–82, 2005.
242. Vidal S, de la Horra C, Martin J, et al. Pneumocystis jirovecii colonisation in patients with interstitial lung disease. Clin Microbiol Infect 12:231–5, 2006.
243. Wakefield AE. Detection of DNA sequences identical to Pneumocystis carinii in samples of ambient air. J Eukaryot Microbiol 41:116S, 1994.
244. Bartlett MS, Lee CH, Lu JJ, et al. Pneumocystis carinii detected in air. J Eukaryot Microbiol 41:75S, 1994.
245. Vargas SL, Ponce CA, Gigliotti F, et al. Transmission of Pneumocystis carinii DNA from a patient with P. carinii pneumonia to immunocompetent contact health care workers. J Clin Microbiol 38:1536–8, 2000.
246. Wohl AR, Simon P, Hu YW, Duchin JS. The role of person-to-person transmission in an epidemiologic study of Pneumocystis carinii pneumonia. AIDS 16:1821–5, 2002.
247. Miller RF, Ambrose HE, Novelli V, Wakefield AE. Probable mother-to-infant transmission of Pneumocystis carinii f. sp. hominis infection. J Clin Microbiol 40:1555–7, 2002.
248. Manoloff ES, Francioli P, Taffe P, et al. Risk for Pneumocystis carinii transmission among patients with pneumonia: a molecular epidemiology study. Emerg Infect Dis 9:132–4, 2003.
249. Rabodonirina M, Vanhems P, Couray-Targe S, et al. Molecular evidence of interhuman transmission of Pneumocystis pneumonia among renal transplant recipients hospitalized with HIV-infected patients. Emerg Infect Dis 10:1766–73, 2004.
250. Keely SP, Stringer JR, Baughman RP, et al. Genetic variation among Pneumocystis carinii hominis isolates in recurrent pneumocystosis. J Infect Dis 172:595–8, 1995.
251. Costa MC, Helweg-Larsen J, Lundgren B, et al. Mutations in the dihydropteroate synthase gene of Pneumocystis jiroveci isolates from Portuguese patients with Pneumocystis pneumonia. Int J Antimicrob Agents 22:516–20, 2003.
252. Furrer H, Opraveil M, Rossi M et al. Stop-Cox-2: is it safe to discontinue secondary PCP prophylaxis? Experience of the Swiss Cohort Study. Presented at the Conference on Retroviral Disease and Opportunistic Infection. San Francisco, 2001.
253. Dworkin MS, Hanson DL, Kaplan JE, et al. Risk for preventable opportunistic infections in persons with AIDS after antiretroviral therapy increases CD4+ T-lymphocyte counts above prophylaxis thresholds. J Infect Dis 182(2):611–5, 2000.

Chapter 37

Toxoplasmosis

José M. Miró, MD, PhD, Henry W. Murray, MD, Christine Katalama, MD

Prior to the emergence of the acquired immunodeficiency syndrome (AIDS), toxoplasmosis was largely recognized as a common, worldwide protozoal infection that produced few if any clinical manifestations in otherwise healthy, immunocompetent children and adults; at most, 20–25% of such individuals developed cervical lymphadenitis, a self-limited flu-like illness, or both. In addition, although lifelong infection was known to persist in all infected persons, it typically remained quiescent and of little consequence in the presence of intact cellular immunity.[1,2]

In three particular settings, however, toxoplasmosis did cause important clinical disease and destruction of vital tissues. In infants born to women infected with *Toxoplasma gondii* during pregnancy; in a small fraction of individuals who, when infected as children or adults, developed retinochoroiditis; and in patients with an underlying T-cell disorder (primarily AIDS) who developed a life-threatening syndrome with cerebral or disseminated disease, or both. Regarding the latter disorders, patients treated with corticosteroids or cytotoxic agents, transplant recipients, and those with immunocompromising neoplastic disorders (e.g., Hodgkin's disease) were recognized to be at risk for reactivation of previously acquired toxoplasmosis. Occasionally, such disease occurred when toxoplasma infection was acutely acquired when the child or adult was already immunosuppressed.[1–3]

Despite the relatively high prevalence of latent *T. gondii* infection in the general population[2] and its capacity to behave as an opportunistic pathogen,[1–4] toxoplasmosis was only rarely recognized in immunocompromised hosts prior to 1980. The emergence of the profound immunodeficiency of advanced human immunodeficiency virus (HIV) infection predictably and strikingly altered the clinical relevance of toxoplasmosis, especially as it relates to central nervous system (CNS) disease in patients with fully established AIDS.[5–20]

Before the highly active antiretroviral therapy (HAART) era, the incidence of *Toxoplasma* encephalitis as the initial AIDS-defining disease was 10–15% in *T. gondii* co-infected patients,[11] and without appropriate primary prophylaxis as many as one-third of patients with CD4+ T-cell counts below 100 cells/mm^3 developed CNS disease during the first year of follow-up.[21] Furthermore, in patients with previous *Toxoplasma* encephalitis, 50–80% relapsed in the following 6–12 months if chronic maintenance therapy (secondary prophylaxis) was not given.[22,23] Although the incidence of toxoplasmosis in HIV-infected patients decreased with the broad use of life-long primary and secondary prophylaxis, it was the developement of HAART in 1996 which led to a striking reduction in cases of toxoplasmosis as well as all opportunistic infections and overall reduced mortality in developed countries.[24,25] However in many resource-poor countries without access to HAART, toxoplasmosis remains a common opportunistic disease.

BIOLOGY, EPIDEMIOLOGY, TRANSMISSION

Biology

T. gondii, an obligate intracellular protozoan, exists in three forms: oocyst, tissue cyst, and tachyzoite. After inadvertent oral ingestion of oocysts or tissue cysts, techyzoites infect intestinal epithelial cells, invade mesenteric lymph nodes, and then disseminate via the blood stream to the tissues. Tachyzoites, responsible for acute toxoplasmosis, replicate intracellularly and parasitize and destroy new cells until an effective immune response develops. Surviving parasites then encyst in various tissues, including brain, retina, skeletal muscle, myocardium, and occasionally lung and thereafter usually remain quiescent for life. Years later, if T-cell-dependent immune mechanisms fail, tachyzoites may be liberated by cyst rupture, leading to reactivated infection.[1,2]

Oocysts develop in the intestinal mucosal cells of felines (domestic cats but also leopards, lions etc), the definite host. Cats become infected after ingesting cysts in raw animal tissue or

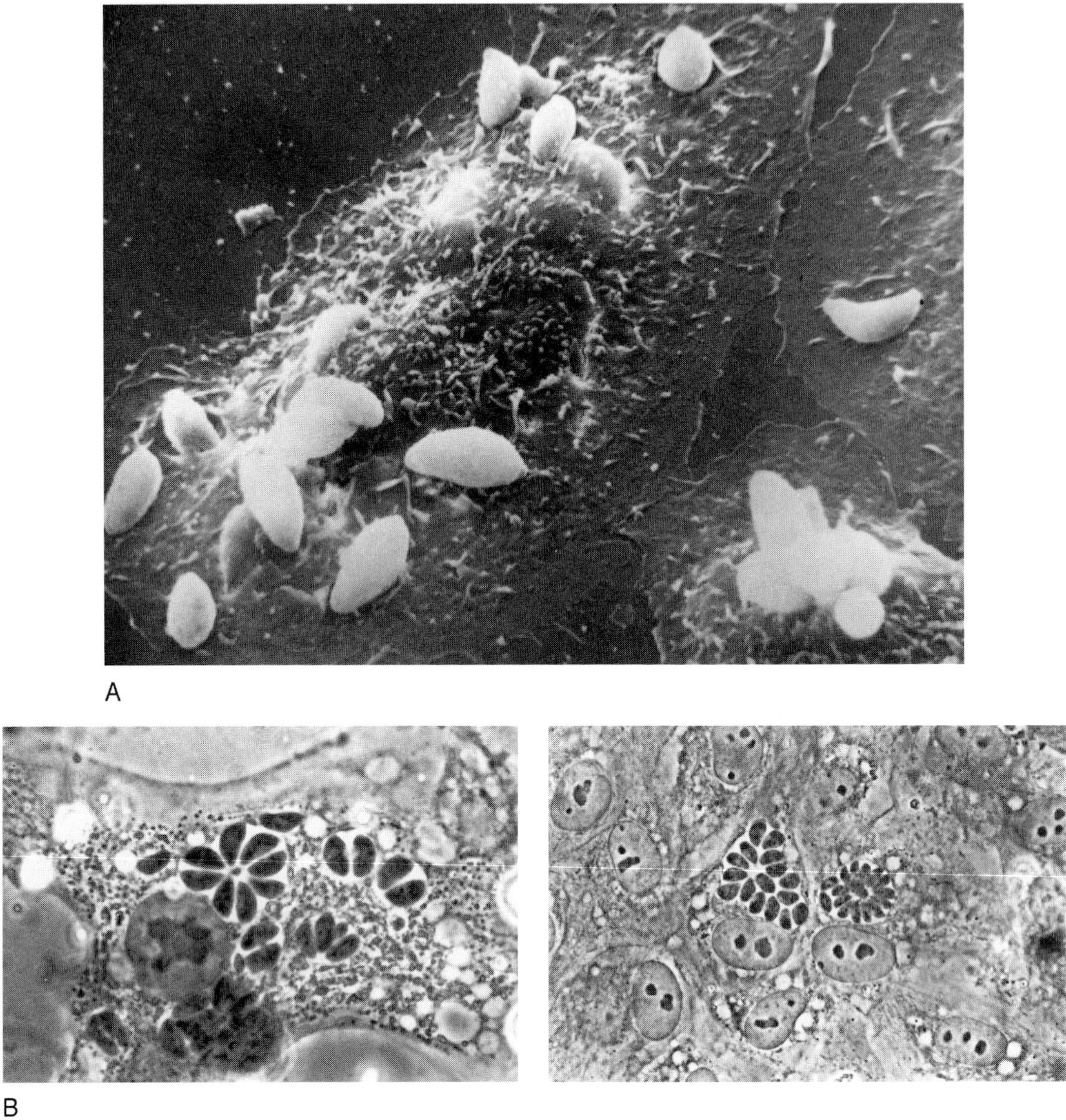

Figure 37-1 ■ (A) Scanning electron micrograph showing *Toxoplasma gondii* tachyzoites attaching to and being ingested by cultivated human monocyte-derived macrophages during *in vitro* infection. (B) Photomicrographs of unstimulated human macrophages (left) and fibroblasts (right) 20 h after in vitro infection with tachyzoites showing overt intracellular replication with up to 8–16 organisms per vacuole. At the initiation of *in vitro* infection, there had been one tachyzoite per vacuole.

(A) Photograph taken by Dr Gilla Kaplan, The Rockefeller University. From Murray HW. Immunotherapy for AIDS-associated toxoplasmosis. In: Sande MA, Root RK (eds). Contemporary Issues in Infectious Diseases, vol 9: Treatment of Serious Infections in the 1990s. New York, Churchill Livingstone, 1992, p 205. (B) Reprinted from Murray HW. Survival of intracellular pathogens within human mononuclear phagocytes. Semin Hematol 25:101, 1988.

poorly cooked meat, or they ingest oocysts shed by other felines. After 1–2 weeks, initial shedding of oocysts ceases and seldom resumes.[26] Oocysts sporulate before becoming infectious, a process favored by warm, moist conditions typical of those found in dampened soil or litter boxes. Sporulated oocysts may persist in an infectious state for a year or more.[1,2]

Tissue cysts arise in host cells in virtually any organ. Maintaining cysts in a quiescent state and controlling tachyzoites potentially liberated by periodic cyst breakdown requires mechanisms mediated by antigen-sensitized T cells and activating cytokines. Thus in previously infected individuals who subsequently become immunosuppressed or T-cell deficient, residual tissue cysts represent a ready endogenous source of tachyzoites poised to escape. Because immunologically intact and deficient individuals may develop retinochoroiditis as a manifestation of reactivated infection,[2] prevention of retinal cyst breakdown presumably requires additional mechanisms.

The tachyzoite, which can invade any nucleated cell (Fig. 37-1), is the obligate intracellular form and requires a host cell for growth and multiplication. Uncontrolled, proliferating tachyzoites rupture free from the infected host cell and probably repeatedly escape into the circulation. Replication at systemic sites then continues until immune responses develop.[1,2,4,27,28]

Epidemiology and Transmission

Virtually any animal that ingests material contaminated by oocysts or cyst-containing tissue can become infected with *T. gondii*. Undercooked pork and lamb (and less commonly venison or beef) are most frequently implicated in transmission to humans. If meat is not heated above 60ºC or frozen to below −20ºC, cysts remain viable.[2,26]

The frequency and prevalence of human *T. gondii* infection varies depending on age, dietary habits, climate, and proximity to cats. In the United States serologic prevalence is 8–40% in healthy adults and HIV-infected patients.[7,18,29,30] In other countries, seroprevalence rates in the general and HIV-infected populations are considerably higher, i.e., 70–90% (e.g., Central America, Brazil, South Pacific, France, Germany, Austria).[2,18,19] In Spain seroprevalence rates in HIV-infected patients range between 40% and 50%.[31,32] All HIV-infected individuals who are seropositive to *T. gondii* have latent infection and are at risk for developing reactivated toxoplasmosis once they become sufficiently T-cell deficient.

Seroconversion data from countries with high *T. gondii* prevalence indicate that newly acquired infection may occur in up to 1–2% of HIV-infected persons per year.[11,18,19,26] In such a setting, primary infection may be clinically severe, with diffuse, multiorgan involvement that is difficult to control despite treatment. Avoiding exposure to *T. gondii* is particularly important for all HIV-infected individuals who are *Toxoplasma*-seronegative (see further ahead).[26]

The three principal modes of human transmission of *T. gondii* are (1) ingestion of cat-derived oocysts or undercooked food containing tissue cysts; (2) transplacental spread; and (3) inadvertent infection from blood, blood products, or organ transplants.[1,2] Cats confined indoors and fed processed foods are unlikely to be a source of infection. Congenital infection,[33] occurs if the mother acquires acute infection during pregnancy. Although congenital infection has been documented in infants born to HIV-infected women who themselves had had previously controlled latent toxoplasmosis,[34,35] the risk of this complication is low.[36,37] *T. gondii* may rarely be transmitted by needlestick, transplantation of infected organs into seronegative recipients, transfusion of whole blood, or leukocytes or platelets.[1,2]

IMMUNE RESPONSE TO INFECTION AND HOST DEFENSE

In healthy individuals, tachyzoites induce humoral and cellular immune responses, reflected in IgM and then IgG antibodies followed by T cell reactivity to *T. gondii* antigen.[38–40] Both responses initially control proliferating parasites. Specific antibody opsonizes tachyzoites, enhancing killing by cytokine-stimulated cells (e.g., mononuclear phagocytes); acting with the alternative complement pathway, it also lyses the organism.[1,2,4,27]

Once CD4+ T-lymphocyte cell counts decline to below 100–150/mm^3, as many as one-third of HIV-infected patients with latent toxoplasmosis develop clinically apparent, reactivated disease within 24 months.[41] The 12-month risk of reactivation also correlates with CD4+ T-lymphocyte number. The risk is 20% with fewer than 150 cells/mm^3,[41] 25% with fewer than 100 cells/mm^3,[42] and 48% with fewer than 50 cells/mm^3.[43] Given the irreversible damage present when some patients initially present for therapy, it is clearly important to test all HIV-infected individuals for IgG antibody to *T. gondii* and to provide primary prophylaxis for all seropositive patients by the time CD4+ T-lymphocyte counts have reached 100 cells/mm^3.[18,41]

In addition to CD4+ T-lymphocyte count, in HIV-infected patients with CD4+ cell counts fewer than 200 cells/mm^3, anti-*Toxoplasma* IgG antibody titer has been reported to be an independent predictor of the occurrence of *Toxoplasma* encephalitis. In one French report, the risk appeared higher in patients with titers >150 IU/mL.[44] This association needs to be confirmed in other patient populations.

CLINICAL MANIFESTATIONS IN HIV-INFECTED PATIENTS

Acute Infection

Reactivation of latent *Toxoplasma* infection is the pathogenetic mechanism usually thought to be responsible for clinically apparent disease. There is little clinical experience with primary *T. gondii* infection in this patient population; whether an HIV-infected individual with adequate CD4 cells (e.g., >200 cells/mm^3) behaves normally and controls initial infection is not clear.[11,18,26] If infection is satisfactorily controlled and the inflammatory response is intact, one would expect that 7–21 days after initial exposure ~20% of patients would develop cervical lymphadenopathy, either asymptomatic or accompanied by a flu-like illness lasting 1–3 weeks. Additional responses (e.g., those expressed in 20–40% of otherwise healthy patients) include generalized lymphadenopathy, splenomegaly, or hepatomegaly. Transient complaints of low-grade fever, arthralgias, myalgias, headache, fatigue, sore throat, abdominal pain, or rash. Retinochoroiditis can also complicate acute infection.[1,2]

Primary toxoplasmosis acquired by patients already CD4+ T-cell deficient would likely present with more serious visceral manifestations, including pneumonitis, myositis, myocarditis, orchitis, and encephalitis (manifesting as intracerebral mass lesions).[1,2]

Reactivated Infection

Most cases of AIDS-associated toxoplasmosis appear to represent reactivation of latent infection.[18] Clinical manifestations therefore depend on where infection reactivates anatomically and the intensity of the local inflammatory response, which may vary according to the CD4+ T-lymphocyte number.[45]

The CNS (encephalitis, abscess), lung (pneumonitis), and eye (retinochoroiditis) are favored sites of symptomatic reactivated infection. CNS disease is by far the most common. Because parasites encyst in any organ and recurrent parasitemia associated with reactivation may also lead to new organ seeding, clinically apparent manifestations of extracerebral toxoplasmosis may be diverse. Indeed, autopsy studies often demonstrate multiorgan involvement not recognized antemortem; as many as 50% of patients with extracerebral disease do not have concurrent CNS lesions.[46–48]

Extracerebral Infection

Along with pneumonitis and retinochoroiditis, the following extracerebral manifestations have been reported but are not common. Endocrinopathies with pituitary or adrenal lesions (or both) and various symptoms and signs related to focal involvement of skin, peritoneum, testes, stomach, pancreas, bladder, skeletal muscle, liver, myocardium, lymph nodes, and duodenum and colon.[11,18,46–48] Occult infection can be demonstrated at autopsy in still other sites, including bone marrow, pharynx, and pericardium.[46–48] A syndrome resembling septic shock, with high fever, hypotension, respiratory symptoms or overt pneumonitis, and multiorgan failure, can also develop in response to disseminated reactivated infection.[49–51] This syndrome may be associated with thrombocytopenia and striking elevations in serum lactate dehydrogenase (LDH) levels. [49–51]

Neurologic Disease

Headache, confusion, altered mental status, and fever are presenting complaints in ~50% of patients with intracerebral infection (encephalitis with or without overt abscess). The onset of illness can be insidious or abrupt. As many as 30% have seizures as an initial manifestation, and 50–60% demonstrate focal neurologic signs.[6–11,13,18,19,52] Nuchal rigidity or other meningeal signs are unusual. High fevers and shaking chills are also unusual. Because intracerebral toxoplasmosis is typically multifocal with destructive, inflammatory mass lesions, virtually any neurologic syndrome may develop and yield motor or sensory deficits; brain stem, basal ganglia, or cerebellar dysfunction; movement disorders; an array of neuropsychiatric findings; and varying effects on the level of consciousness, including coma. Hemiparesis is the most common focal deficit among a long list of others, including cranial nerve lesions, focal seizures, aphasia, visual field losses, ataxia, dysmetria, tremor, and hemiballismus and extrapyramidal signs.[6–11,13,18,19,52] Spinal cord involvement can produce transverse myelitis or a conus medullaris syndrome.[53] Hydrocephalus, choroid plexitis, and cerebral hemorrhage may also occur.[54,55]

Eye Involvement

Ocular disease is probably the most common clinical manifestation of HIV-associated extracerebral toxoplasmosis.[56–61] In 30–60% of cases of retinochoroiditis, encephalitis is also present. [56–61] Conversely, however, relatively few patients presenting with cerebritis also have retinochoroiditis. Visual symptoms due to *Toxoplasma* retinitis include loss of visual acuity, 'floaters', and red, inflamed sclera. Ophthalmologic examination reveals yellow-white areas of full-thickness necrotizing retinitis, occasionally with hemorrhage and vascular sheathing. Lesions are predominantly unilateral. The presence of inflammation in the anterior or posterior segment, or both (hyalitis), is highly suggestive of *Toxoplasma* retinitis and occurs in 60–70% of cases. Fluorescein angiography reveals hyperfluorescence starting from the periphery and progressing toward the center of the lesions. This distinguishes *Toxoplasma* retinitis from cytomegalovirus (CMV) retinitis.[59,61] *Toxoplasma* retinitis should also be differentiated from retinitis due to varicella-zoster virus, syphilis, and fungi including *Pneumocystis jirovecii.*

Pneumonitis

Pulmonary manifestations of toxoplasmosis have accounted for up to 35% of extraneurologic *Toxoplasma* disease.[62–66] Fever and dyspnea are the most frequent symptoms, whereas cough and sputum may be absent. Chest radiographs usually show diffuse bilateral pulmonary infiltrates.[62–70] Multiple nodular densities have been reported. A rise in LDH levels has been reported to be suggestive of the diagnosis.[69] A diagnosis of pulmonary toxoplasmosis can be established by direct examination of bronchoalveolar lavage, which reveals *T. gondii* trophozoites when stained by a Giemsa or immunofluorescence technique.[70] Lung histology may also reveal tachyzoites with Giemsa staining. Disseminated *Toxoplasma* infection may manifest as acute respiratory distress syndrome associated with septic shock and thrombocytopenia.[49–51,71]

DIAGNOSIS

Routine Laboratory Test Results

Routine laboratory tests seldom yield specific information pointing to toxoplasmosis. The white blood cell (WBC) count is not characteristically abnormal, nor is the neutrophil count. CD4+ T-lymphocyte counts are rarely more than 200/mm^3. Most patients have counts less than 100/mm^3 and often less than 50 cells/mm^3.[18,26] The chest film and electrocardiogram may indicate pneumonitis or rarely myocarditis. Thrombocytopenia and elevated serum LDH values suggest the septic form of infection often associated with pneumonitis. Although not common, other routine laboratory results can reflect extracerebral involvement of the pituitary, pancreas, liver, and bladder.

Definitive Diagnosis

The definitive diagnosis of toxoplasmosis as the cause of encephalitis or extraneurologic disease requires direct demonstration of the tachyzoite form in involved tissues or in blood or other fluids. Because obtaining an appropriate sample and visualizing or isolating this organism may require invasive procedures and considerable technical expertise, few centers are prepared to cultivate *Toxoplasma* by animal inoculation or tissue culture. Standard practice has evolved to allow a presumptive diagnosis of *Toxoplasma* encephalitis acceptable in most instances (see later).[11,23,72] Establishing an empiric diagnosis of *Toxoplasma* encephalitis is considered particularly appropriate for patients with compatible neurologic disease who are not receiving prophylaxis with trimethoprim–sulfamethoxazole or pyrimethamine with dapsone and who have (1) less than 200 CD4+ T-lymphocyte cells/mm^3; (2) anti-*Toxoplasma* immunoglobulin G (IgG) antibody in the serum, and (3) a clear-cut response to empiric anti-*Toxoplasma* therapy.

Establishing a diagnosis of *Toxoplasma* retinitis is usually done by expert fundoscopic examination performed by a retinal specialist. Some syndromes are sufficiently similar to processes caused by other pathogens, so a specific diagnosis is necessary. This usually requires visualizing the organism by histology.

Serology

Cases of AIDS-related toxoplasmosis have been described in patients whose serum was reported to lack anti-*Toxoplasma* IgG.[20,72] However, in the United States and Western Europe, an undetectable IgG level is unusual if the test is performed in a reliable reference laboratory. It is not clear if there are in fact any well-documented cases in patients who were seronegative in an appropriate reference laboratory. Serum anti-*Toxoplasma* IgM antibodies are seldom detected in patients with HIV infection. Serum IgM tests are difficult to perform and poorly standardized. If toxoplasmosis is presumptively diagnosed in an AIDS patient who is IgG-seronegative, the clinician should carefully consider the possibility of an alternate diagnosis.

Although anti-*Toxoplasma* IgG is also found in cerebrospinal fluid (CSF) in 30–70% of patients with encephalitis,[6–8] its presence alone does not establish a diagnosis of intracerebral disease.[7,73] Measuring intrathecal production of IgG has been suggested to be diagnostically useful.[73] However, CSF is not routinely available because (1) many patients with intracerebral toxoplasmosis do not undergo lumbar puncture because of appropriate concern for herniation, and (2) standard CSF testing infrequently yields specific diagnostic information. Thus lumbar puncture is not part of a routine diagnostic evaluation for toxoplasmosis at most centers.

Histopathologic Findings and Culture

Free and intracellular tachyzoites can be directly visualized in Giemsa-stained cytocentrifuged preparations of CSF, bronchoalveolar lavage material, induced sputum, and peritoneal fluid as well as in bone marrow aspirates, peripheral blood or buffy coat smears, and tissue imprints (touch preparations).[1,2,11,13,19,73–77] Tachyzoites can also be detected in these materials by immunofluorescence.[76]

Peripheral blood, CSF, or any body fluid or properly obtained tissue can be used to attempt parasite isolation by intraperitoneal inoculation of mice or *in vitro* addition to cell (e.g., fibroblasts) cultures that support intracellular replication (Fig. 37-1).[1,2,18] The latter method may document the organism by microscopic examination within 2–3 days.[18,76–80] In contrast, mouse inoculation may not yield diagnostic results for up to 4–6 weeks and thus may be confirmatory but of little other clinical usefulness. Using the cell culture method (which appears to be more sensitive than microscopic examination of standard cytocentrifuge preparations),[74] parasitemia has been demonstrated in 14–38% of patients (79% in one study)[76] with intracerebral or extracerebral toxoplasmosis (or both).[18] Few centers perform cultures for *Toxoplasma*, however.

Even though biopsy of involved tissues (e.g., brain or lung) is no longer common diagnostic practice, some patients do come for organ biopsy, especially those who have failed to respond to empiric anti-*Toxoplasma* therapy. Cerebral lesions are most often approached by needle biopsy. Open excisional brain biopsy yields more satisfactory material than does needle biopsy or aspiration, but it is usually performed only if needle biopsies fail to reveal a causative process.[18]

The histologic reaction to infection may vary among organs; in the brain, it ranges from granulomatous-type changes to a modest, focal inflammatory response to evidence of severe tissue destruction with widespread necrosis.[1,2,6,8,10,18,19] Because all individuals seropositive to *T. gondii* are presumed to harbor at least some cyst forms deep in their tissues, observing a few scattered cysts in histologically quiescent sites does not necessarily establish the diagnosis of active toxoplasmosis. In contrast, finding intracellular or extracellular tachyzoites (implying cyst rupture) or numerous cysts that have provoked an inflammatory reaction is considered evidence of disease (Fig. 37-2). The sensitive peroxidase–antiperoxidase technique, which stains cysts, liberated tachyzoites, and free parasite antigen,[18] should be applied to fixed tissues that are apparently negative by routine staining.

Neuroimaging Studies

Standard Testing

In most clinical series, 10–43% of patients with *Toxoplasma* encephalitis have a solitary parenchymal lesion demonstrated by computed tomography (CT); the remaining patients have more than one lesion.[6,8,12,13,52,79,80] It is unusual in symptomatic patients to have a negative contrast enhanced CT scan (3–10%).[6,8,72,81,82] Multiple focal intracerebral lesions are typical of toxoplasmosis, especially if more sensitive magnetic resonance imaging (MRI) is used (Fig. 37-3).[18] On MRI testing, more than 80% of patients have multiple lesions.[79–89] Therefore if a single lesion is found on CT and confirmed to be solitary by MRI, lymphoma or another cause of focal

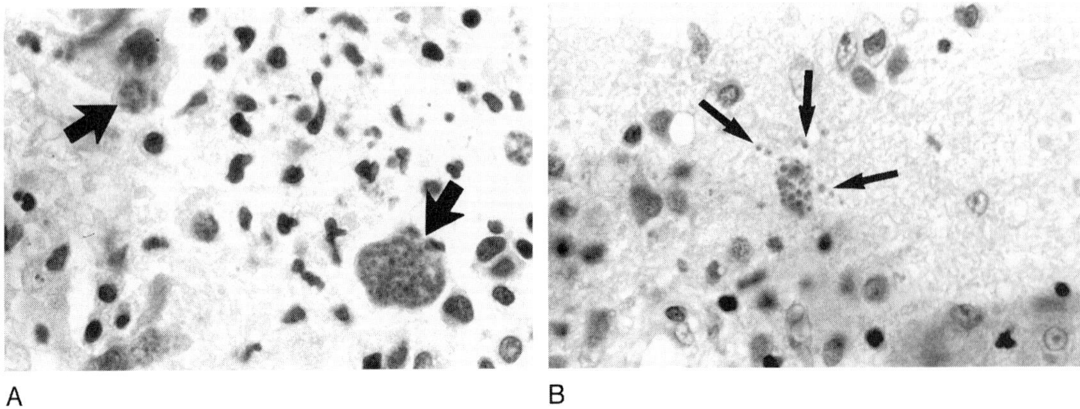

Figure 37-2 ■ Histologic appearance of reactivated intracerebral toxoplasmosis in a patient with advanced AIDS who underwent brain biopsy. (A) Section shows inflammatory response and one large and one small brain cyst (arrows). (B) Cyst breakdown with released tachyzoites (arrows) (H&E).

Reprinted from Murray HW: Immunotherapy for AIDS-associated toxoplasmosis. In: Sande MA, Root RK (eds). Contemporary Issues in Infectious Diseases, vol 9: Treatment of Serious Infections in the 1990s. New York, Churchill Livingstone; 1992, p 205.

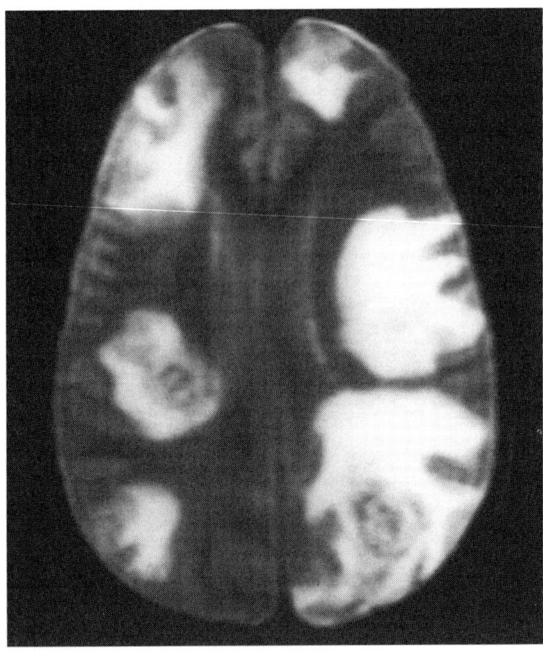

Figure 37-3 ■ Magnetic resonance image (MRI) showing multifocal brain lesions with pronounced edema in an AIDS patient with toxoplasmosis. Courtesy of Dr Henry Masur, National Institutes of Health.

brain lesions associated with AIDS should be a primary consideration, even if there is contrast enhancement.[79–89] With intracerebral toxoplasmosis, lesions are most often bilateral and contrast (ring)-enhancing (80–90%), induce a mass effect with edema, and frequently develop in the basal ganglia, thalamus, or hemispheres at the corticomedullary junction.[6,8,10,11,13,18,79–89] There is, however, no specific CT or MRI result that is accepted as absolutely diagnostic of intracerebral toxoplasmosis. For example, multifocal disease and ring-enhancing lesions can be seen in 40–50% of AIDS patients with CNS lymphoma.[83]

Functional Imaging

In an effort to sharpen the noninvasive (but still presumptive) diagnosis of toxoplasmosis, other imaging techniques have been evaluated, especially to help differentiate infection from lymphoma. There has been some experience with MR spectroscopy. Both single-photon emission computed tomography (SPECT) using thallium 201(^{201}Tl) and positron emission tomography (PET)[90–104] using labeled substrates such as 2-fluorodeoxyglucose appear useful. In patients with mass lesions on CT or MRI, the absence of increased uptake on ^{201}Tl SPECT scanning (Fig. 37-4) and decreased activity on PET scans ('cold' or hypometabolic lesions) are characteristic of infection (e.g., toxoplasmosis or other infections); lymphoma is almost invariably associated with increased uptake using these two scanning techniques.[90–104]

Small lesions (<8 mm) may be difficult to resolve with SPECT or PET scans; and although uncommon, both false-positive and false-negative results may occur.[98] Toxoplasmosis, tuberculomas, and cryptococcomas can give positive SPECT results.[96,98]

In a recent study, the combination of a high thalium index uptake and a lesion size >2 cm increased the diagnostic accuracy of SPECT for diagnosing primary CNS lymphoma.[99]

Nuclear scans are best used in the following settings: (1) those suspected of having toxoplasmosis but in whom MRI demonstrates only a solitary intracerebral lesion; (2) *Toxoplasma*-seronegative patients with multifocal enhancing lesions; and (3) the unusual individual with intracerebral disease and more than 200 CD4 cells/mm^3.[79] From a practical perspective, however, most such patients have an empiric trial of anti-*Toxoplasma* therapy for 10–14 days. If they then do not demonstrate radiologic improvement, a biopsy is performed.

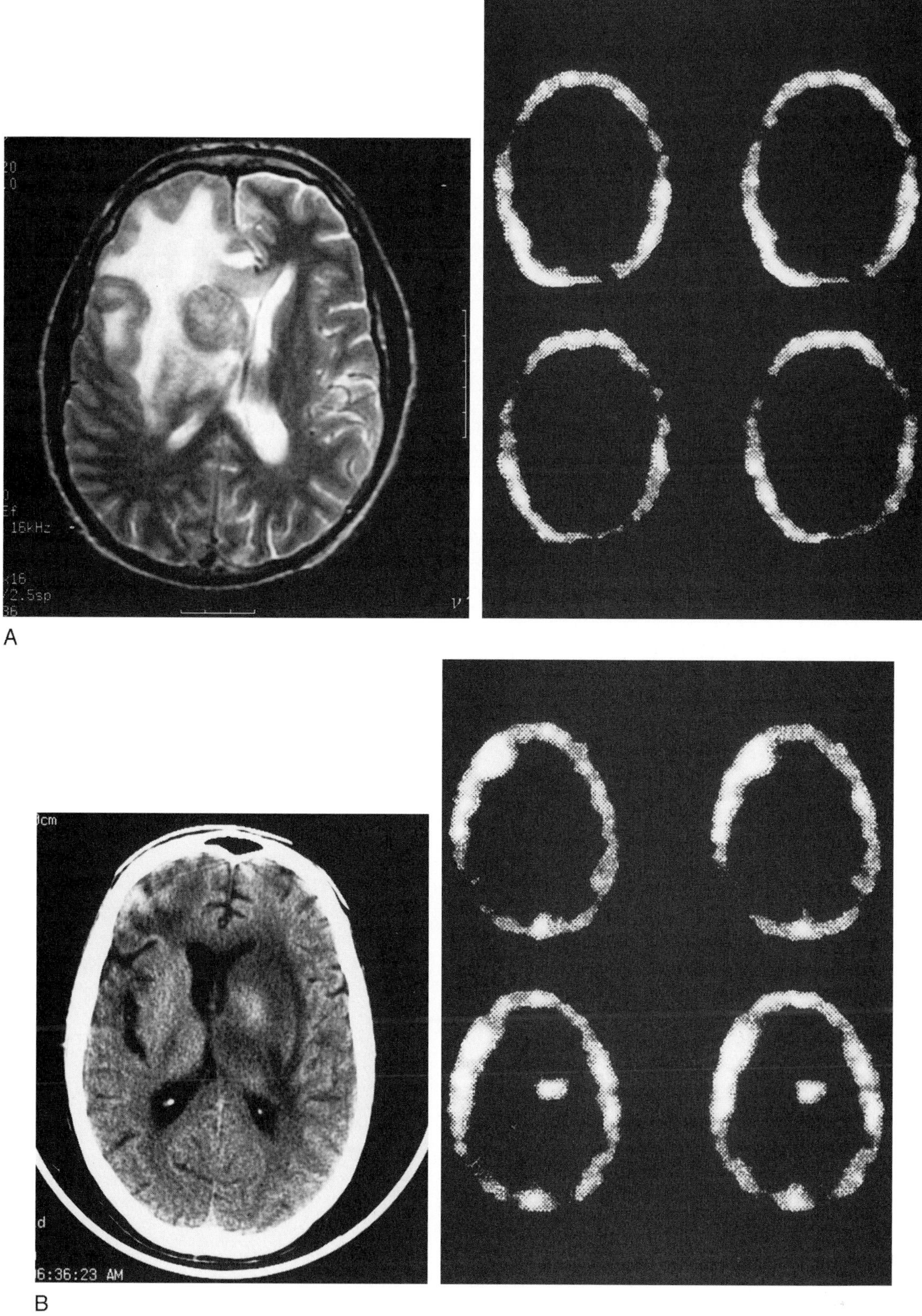

Figure 37-4 ■ Appearance of thallium-201 single-photon emission computed tomography (SPECT) scans in AIDS-related toxoplasmosis (A) versus lymphoma (B). (A) MRI showing large right-sided lesion with edema in a *Toxoplasma*-seropositive patient who responded to empiric anti-*Toxoplasma* therapy (left). SPECT scan shows no uptake at the site of the lesion (right). (B) CT scan in an AIDS patient with biopsy-documented lymphoma showing contrast-enhancing right frontal and left thalamic lesions (left), both of which demonstrate increased uptake on the SPECT scan (right).

Courtesy of Drs David Warren, James Hurley, and Josephine Rini, The New York Hospital-Cornell Medical Center.

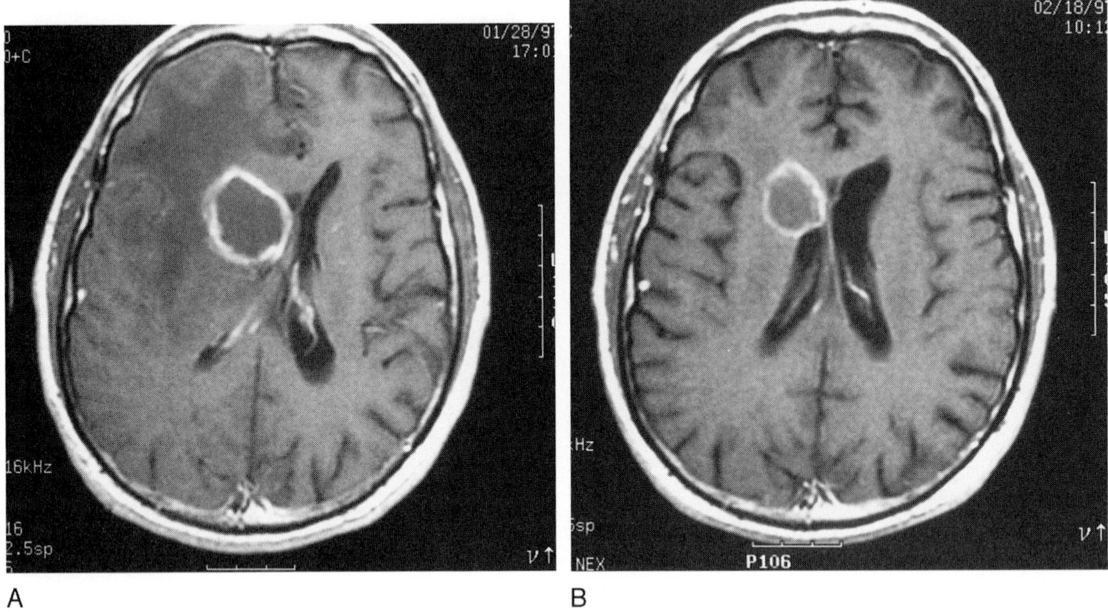

Figure 37-5 ■ Neuroradiographic response to empiric anti-*Toxoplasma* therapy in a patient with AIDS. (A) Pretreatment MRI demonstrates a solitary ring-enhancing lesion, adjacent large hypodense area of edema, and mass effect with ventricular compression and shift. *Toxoplasma* serology was positive, and lesion showed no uptake on thallium-201 SPECT scan. (B) After 3 weeks of pyrimethamine–sulfadiazine treatment, the extent of edema, mass effect, and lesion size have clearly diminished.

Courtesy of Dr David Warren, The New York Hospital-Cornell Medical Center.

Detection of *Toxoplasma* Antigen and DNA

Antigen can be detected by conventional assays in serum or urine in 25–30% patients with AIDS-related toxoplasmosis.[18,105] In contrast, depending on the material tested (CSF, blood, buffy coat, bronchoalveolar lavage fluid, aqueous humor, brain tissue), parasite DNA can be detected by the polymerase chain reaction (PCR) in an appreciably larger proportion of patients.[106–115] In those with documented or presumed encephalitis, positive PCR results using CSF have been reported in ~50% (range 40–100%) with essentially no false-negative reactions (100% specificity).[18,79,106–115] Sensitivity may be increased by simultaneously testing CSF and blood or testing CSF prior to initiating therapy. PCR results are usually negative once specific anti-*Toxoplasma* therapy has been started. PCR testing using blood or buffy coat from patients with intracerebral infection is an attractive approach to consider. In two studies, positive reactions were reported in 16–68% with occasional false-positive results.[18,112] In patients with parasitemia alone without encephalitis, PCR results using blood were positive in 84%.[72] Thus despite limitations in sensitivity and availability, the high specificity of PCR testing for *Toxoplasma* DNA makes this method of diagnosis useful if a positive result is generated.

Response to Empiric Treatment

Most patients with cerebral toxoplasmosis (65–90%) respond rapidly to two-drug treatment with pyrimethamine with either sulfadiazine or clindamycin.[2,11–13,18,20,72,79] Thus a clear-cut clinical and neuroradiographic response to empiric therapy is now considered essentially diagnostic of toxoplasmosis.[18,79] In one study, neurologic improvement was seen in 50% of patients by day 5 and in 86% by day 7; altogether, 91% showed clear evidence of a response by day 14 of treatment.[17,79] In the same study, 57% demonstrated neuroradiographic improvement at week 3.[79] Figure 37-5 illustrates such a response to empiric therapy. Therefore patients who demonstrate clinical progression or new signs during the first week of therapy and those who show no apparent improvement after 10–14 days of treatment should undergo brain biopsy.[79,98,116–118] Patients who fail to respond to 14–21 days of therapy most often have lymphoma, but as many as 25% of biopsied treatment nonresponders are still found to have toxoplasmosis as the cause of their CNS mass lesions.[98]

Corticosteroids, which have no clearly positive or negative effect on either the kinetics or extent of the overall response,[2,11] are frequently used to help manage associated increased intracranial pressure. If corticosteroids are employed, some caution should still be exercised when interpreting clinical and radiologic responses because of nonspecific antiinflammatory effects.

Role of Brain Biopsy

For diagnosis in AIDS-associated CNS toxoplasmosis, brain biopsy has evolved over the years into a secondary procedure now reserved for only a limited number of clinical situations

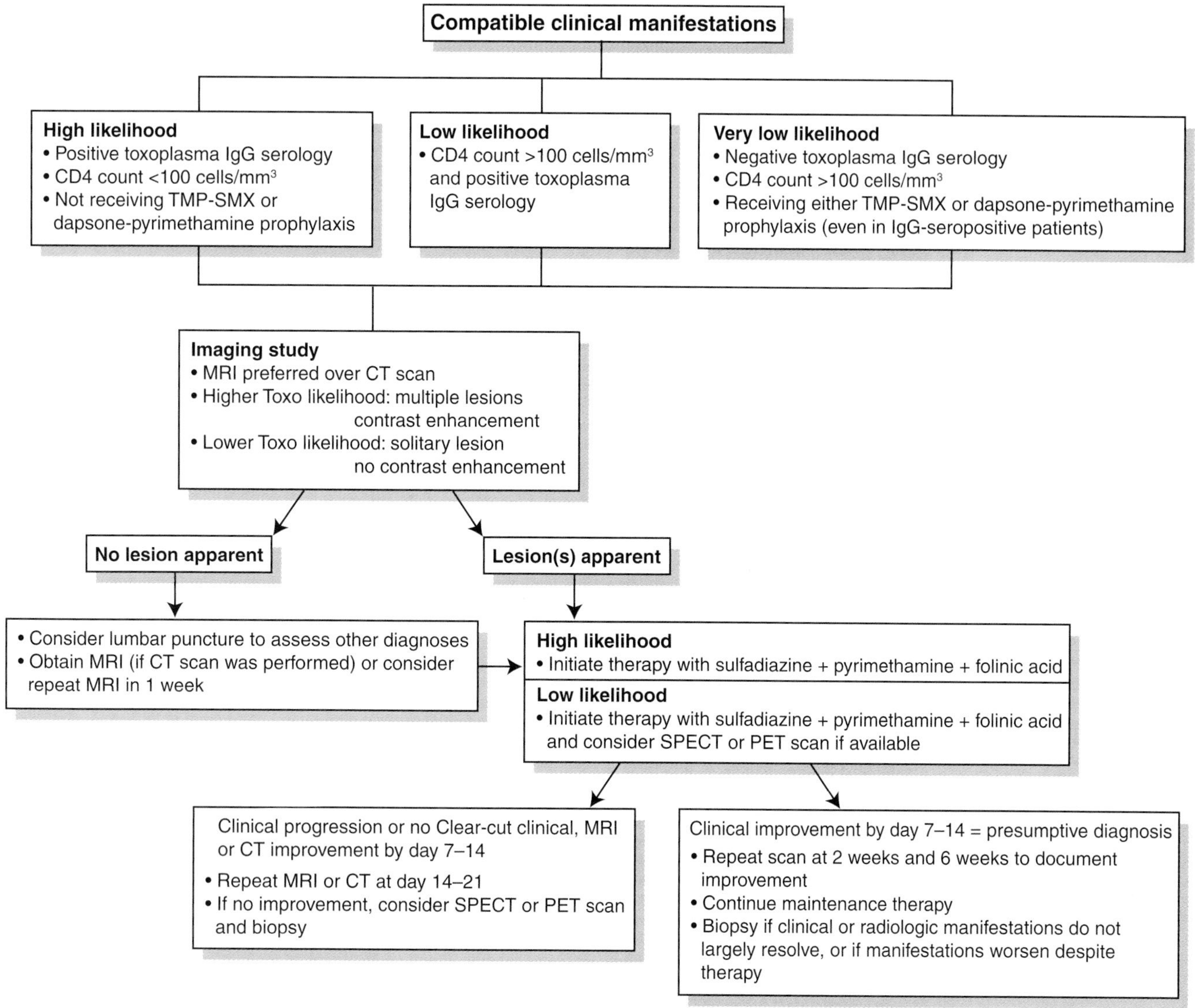

Compatible clinical manifestations
High likelihood
• Positive toxoplasma IgG serology
• CD4 count <100 cells/mm³
• Not receiving TMP-SMX or dapsone-pyrimethamine prophylaxis
Low likelihood
• CD4 count >100 cells/mm³ and positive toxoplasma IgG serology
Very low likelihood
• Negative toxoplasma IgG serology
• CD4 count >100 cells/mm³
• Receiving either TMP-SMX or dapsone-pyrimethamine prophylaxis (even in IgG-seropositive patients)
Imaging study
• MRI preferred over CT scan
• Higher Toxo likelihood: multiple lesions contrast enhancement
• Lower Toxo likelihood: solitary lesion no contrast enhancement
No lesion apparent
Lesion(s) apparent
• Consider lumbar puncture to assess other diagnoses
• Obtain MRI (if CT scan was performed) or consider repeat MRI in 1 week
High likelihood
• Initiate therapy with sulfadiazine + pyrimethamine + folinic acid
Low likelihood
• Initiate therapy with sulfadiazine + pyrimethamine + folinic acid and consider SPECT or PET scan if available
Clinical progression or no Clear-cut clinical, MRI or CT improvement by day 7–14
• Repeat MRI or CT at day 14–21
• If no improvement, consider SPECT or PET scan and biopsy
Clinical improvement by day 7–14 = presumptive diagnosis
• Repeat scan at 2 weeks and 6 weeks to document improvement
• Continue maintenance therapy
• Biopsy if clinical or radiologic manifestations do not largely resolve, or if manifestations worsen despite therapy

Figure 37-6 ■ Algorithm indicating an approach to the diagnosis and initial management of suspected toxoplasmosis.

in carefully selected patients.[98] In a decision analysis model of management strategies, similar outcomes for *Toxoplasma*-seropositive patients were assigned to early biopsy versus empiric therapy with delayed biopsy in nonresponders.[119] For *Toxoplasma*-seronegative patients with cerebral mass lesions, results from this model favored the use of early brain biopsy.[119]

Summary of Diagnosis and Initial Management

The algorithm in Figure 37-6 summarizes an overall approach to the patient with suspected cerebral toxoplasmosis.

TREATMENT

Treatment for toxoplasmosis includes primary therapy for clinically active infection followed by maintenance therapy to suppress recurrent disease for patients whose CD4+ T-lymphocyte counts do not rise above 200 cells/mm^3.[120] Recommendations for treatment,[120] which almost always involve combination agents, and summaries of selected treatment trials are shown in Table 37-1.

Primary Therapy

Conventional Treatment

Standard therapy for intracerebral toxoplasmosis consists of pyrimethamine (200 mg ×1 PO as a loading dose, then 50 (<60 kg) to 75 mg (≥60 kg) qd PO) plus sulfadiazine (1000 (<60 kg) to 1500 mg (≥60 kg) q6h PO) (Table 37-1).[12,79,119–122] For patients intolerant to sulfonamides, pyrimethamine plus clindamycin (600 mg qid, IV or PO) has been as effective in most[11–13,79,120] (but not all[121]) studies. Patients with pneumonitis, retinochoroiditis, other focal organ involvement, or disseminated infection receive the same combination

Table 37-1

Selected Treatment Trials in AIDS-Related Toxoplasmosis[a]

Trial	Design	No. of Patients	Regimen	Complete/Partial Response by Day 42 (%)	Toxicity (%)	Comments
Leport et al[122]	Open-label	35	Pyrimethamine 100–200 mg PO × 1–2, then 50–100 mg PO qd plus sulfadiazine 2–6 g PO qd plus folinic acid 5–50 mg IM qd	89[b]	71	18/24 Responders maintained relapse-free on reduced doses; 10/35 stopped at least one drug (toxicity)
Dannemann et al[12]	Randomized, open-label	59	Pyrimethamine 200 mg PO × 1, then 75 mg PO qd plus sulfadiazine 25 mg/kg q6h plus folinic acid >10 mg PO qd	70	32	Similar efficacy and toxicity in both arms
			Pyrimethamine as above plus clindamycin 1200 mg IV q6h × 21 days, then 300 mg PO q6h or 800 mg PO q8h plus folinic acid as above	65	23	
Luft et al[79]	Open-label	49	Pyrimethamine 200 mg PO × 1, then 75 mg PO qd plus clindamycin 600 mg PO q6h plus folinic acid 10 mg PO qd	75	17	86% Responders improved by day 7 of therapy
Katlama et al[121]	Randomized, open-label	299	Pyrimethamine 50 mg PO qd × 42 days, then 25 mg PO qd plus sulfadiazine 1 g PO q6h × 42 days, then 0.5 g PO q6h plus folinic acid >50 mg PO q wk	76	30	Initial efficacy similar. Relapse during maintenance phase was two times higher for clindamycin arm although less toxicity and fewer drug discontinuations
			Pyrimethamine as above plus clindamycin 600 mg PO q6h × 42 days, then 300 mg PO q6h plus folinic acid as above	68	11	

[a]Eligibility for each of these trials included clinical, neurologic, and CT or MRI results consistent with toxoplasmosis.
[b]Responses within first 8 weeks of therapy.

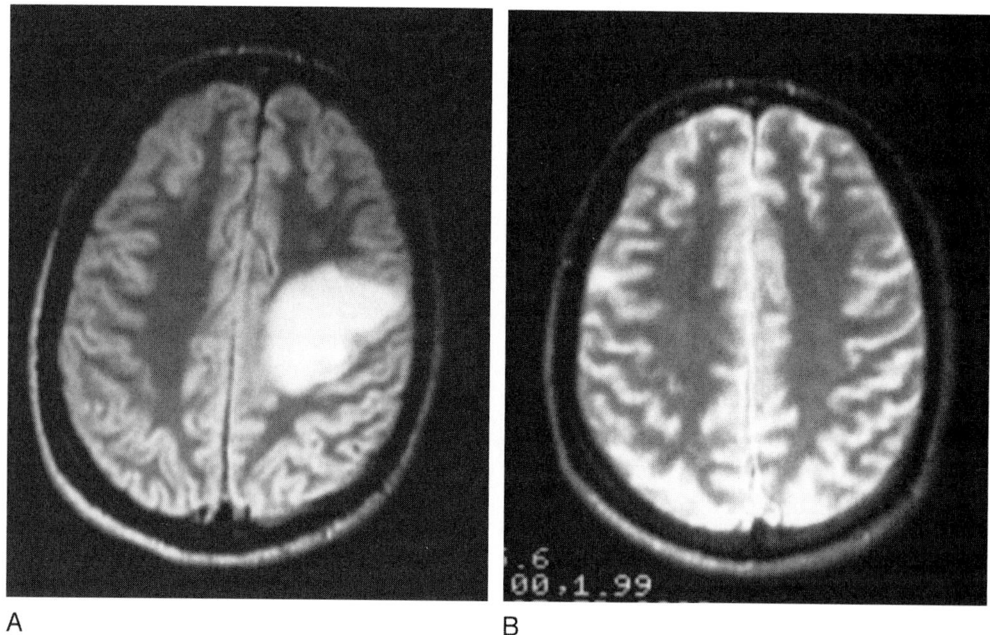

Figure 37-7 ■ Neuroradiographic (MRI) response to treatment with pyrimethamine plus clindamycin in an AIDS patient with biopsy-documented intracerebral toxoplasmosis. (A) Pretreatment scan. (B) Essentially normal MRI after 11 weeks of combination therapy.

(A) Reprinted from Murray HW. Immunotherapy for AIDS-associated toxoplasmosis. In: Sande MA, Root RK (eds). Contemporary Issues in Infectious Diseases, vol 9: Treatment of Serious Infections in the 1990s. New York, Churchill Livingstone; 1992, p 205.

regimens. Folinic acid (leucovorin calcium, 10–20 mg qd PO, although this dose can be increased 50 mg qd or higher to minimize pyrimethamine-associated toxicities) is routinely included with any pyrimethamine-containing regimen to reduce bone marrow toxicity.[18,120]

The clinical and radiologic response of patients depend on the amount of neuronal destruction at the time therapy was started, and the immune response. *Toxoplasma* have never been documented to be resistant to the drugs used for therapy.[2,11–13,79,119–122] Mortality rates in the acute phase of *Toxoplasma* encephalitis ranged between 5% and 20%. Death usually occurs due to far advanced disease at the time therapy was started, or a concurrent process.[12,121]

Most patients with retinochoroiditis also respond and show improved visual acuity within 6 weeks.[61] Patients with pneumonitis or disseminated infection have a particularly poor prognosis.[67,68] There are no evidence-based guidelines for patients with documented toxoplasmosis at any anatomic site who fail to respond promptly or develop new signs of progression during treatment and who have no evidence of an additional pathogenic process. Therapeutic choices are largely limited to using higher doses of the drugs initially selected or empirically adding one or more additional anti-*Toxoplasma* agents to the regimen.

Therapy for toxoplasmosis should continue for a minimum of 6 weeks. Most clinicians would continue therapy longer if clinical manifestations have not stabilized, or if the lesions on MRI scan have not either disappeared or remained stable for many weeks. Imaging studies should be repeated at 2 weeks to ensure that toxoplasma was the correct and the only cause of the lesions,[79,120] If the lesions are not all improving, a biopsy (or repeat biopsy) should be considered to determine if more than one process is present. If toxoplasmosis is the only proven diagnosis, and the lesions have not improved after 2–4 weeks, an alternate regimen could be used although there is no evidence such a strategy would improve prognosis. Although serial scans over subsequent months can demonstrate complete or near-complete resolution of an impressive amount of localized and multifocal disease (Fig. 37-7), repeated studies in a steadily improving patient who is receiving standard therapy are not required.

Rash and other adverse inflammatory-type reactions to sulfonamides are well recognized in HIV-infected patients.[120] In addition, sulfadiazine-treated patients may develop crystalluria, hematuria, renal colic with sludge or stones, and occasionally some degree of renal insufficiency.[123,124] A high daily fluid intake should be part of the regimen in any patient receiving sulfadiazine. The most relevant toxicity of pyrimethamine is bone marrow suppression (megaloblastic anemia, leukopenia, thrombocytopenia). Overall, as many as 40–60% of patients cannot tolerate the combination of pyrimethamine with sulfadiazine.[119] Clindamycin is well known for inducing gastrointestinal complaints and diarrhea, but it also produces rash.[12,125,126] Indeed, unacceptably high rates of diarrhea (31%) and rash (21%) developed in patients who received clindamycin alone (300 mg twice daily) in a trial of primary prophylaxis.[125] Other adverse reactions and potential drug interactions in patients receiving sulfonamides, pyrimethamine, clindamycin, dapsone, or one of the alternative agents discussed here are detailed in Chapters 78–79.

Other Regimens

Atovaquone

Hydroxynaphthoquinones are potent *in vitro* inhibitors of parasitic protozoa including *Plasmodium* and *T. gondii.* Atovaquone has been demonstrated to have good protective activity against acute murine toxoplasmosis and to reduce the viability and number of cysts in brains of chronically infected mice.[127] Atovaquone acts as an inhibitor of the mitochondrial electron transport chain of parasitic protozoa, resulting in inhibition of pyrimidine synthesis.

Several properties of atovaquone had appeared attractive particularly in patients with advanced HIV infection: a mechanism of action unrelated to folate antagonism, activity against the two most frequent opportunistic agents (*Pneumocytis jirovecii* and *T. gondii*), and a prolonged half-life (4–6 days) with a potential dosing advantage for long-term prophylaxis.

In a pilot study, atovaquone (750 mg four times per day) was given to eight patients with acute *Toxoplasma* encephalitis who were intolerant to or failed standard therapies.[128] Seven patients improved and the other remained radiographically stable. Toxicity was mild and only one patient required temporary drug discontinuation due to a rash. Atovaquone was also evaluated as salvage therapy in 93 patients with AIDS-related *Toxoplasma* encephalitis who were intolerant to or failing standard therapy with either pyrimethamine–sulfodiazine or pyrimethamine–clindamycin.[129] At the end of the 6-week acute therapy phase (750 mg four times per day), clinical improvement was noted in 52% of patients and radiologic improvement in 37%. The median survival for all patients was 189 days (Kaplan–Meier estimate).[129] Four patients had to stop therapy because of adverse events (severe rash in two cases and liver toxicity and toxic epidermal necrolysis in one case each).[129] A post hoc analysis revealed a correlation between clinical and radiologic responses and median atovaquone plasma concentrations. Plasma levels of >18.5 μg/mL were associated with an 84% response rate at 6 weeks.[129]

A published randomized phase II trial has demonstrated that the combination of atovaquone and either pyrimethamine or sulfadiazine were effective for treatment of toxoplasmic encephalitis (ACTG 237/ANRS 039).[130] Recommended doses were, atovaquone 1500 mg bid PO (with meals or oral nutritional supplements) with pyrimethamine 200 mg × 1 PO as a loading dose, then 50 (<60 kg) to 75 mg (≥60 kg) qd PO plus leucovorin 10–20 mg/day PO.[130] Atovaquone at the same dose was combined with sulfadiazine (1000–1500 mg q6h PO).[130] The role of these combination regimens needs to be better defined.

For patients intolerant to both pyrimethamine and sulfadiazine, atovaquone can be tried as a single agent.[128,129] If atovaquone is used alone, measuring plasma levels may be helpful given highly variable drug absorption among different patients. However, such levels are not readily available, and using such levels to guide practice is based on plausibility rather than extensive data.

Trimethoprim–Sulfamethoxazole

Trimethoprim–sulfamethoxazole (5 mg/kg trimethoprim plus 25 mg/kg sulfamethoxazole IV or PO bid) has been effective in two studies for treatment of *Toxoplasma* encephalitis.[131,132] A small randomized trial in 77 patients found this regimen to be as effective and better tolerated than pyrimethamine–sulfadiazine.[132]

Trimethoprim–sulfamethoxazole has the advantage over pyrimethamine–sulfadiazine that it is widely available and it is available both orally and intravenously. For patients who cannot take an oral regimen, no well-studied options exist. No parenteral formulation of pyrimethamine exists; the only available parenteral antitoxoplasma drugs are the sulfamethoxazole component of trimethoprim-sulfamethoxazole and clindamycin. Therefore, certain specialists will treat severely ill patients requiring parenteral therapy with parenteral trimethoprim-sulfamethoxazole or oral pyrimethamine plus parenteral clindamycin.

Macrolides

Clarithromycin has shown activity against *T. gondii in vitro* and in murine models. In a pilot study, clarithromycin (2 g/day) combined with pyrimethamine (75 mg/day) was given to 13 AIDS patients with *Toxoplasma* encephalitis.[133] A complete clinical response was noted in six of eight evaluable patients and a partial response in two. Five patients were withdrawn prematurely, mainly because of toxicity. Whether clarithromycin itself had a beneficial effect is unclear, as it was used in combination with higher doses of pyrimethamine than were normally used in combination with sulfadiazine or clindamycin. No further studies have evaluated prospectively the role of clarithromycin in *T. gondii* infection. Futhermore, clarithromycin doses higher than 500 mg bid have been associated with increased mortality in HIV-infected patients receiving therapy for *M. avium* infection and should not be used.[134]

Azithromycin has been reported to be active *in vitro* and in animal models. In a murine model of toxoplasmosis, prophylactic azithromycin administered alone at a high dosage was found to be only partially effective.[135] Complete protection was not seen even at a dosage of 300 mg kg^{-1} day^{-1}. In contrast, the combination of azithromycin with either sulfadiazine or pyrimethamine was synergistic; 100% and 93% survival of mice, respectively, after 30 days was observed. These findings are consistent with clinical data in humans.[136–139] Recommended doses are azithromycin 900–1200 mg/day with pyrimethamine 200 mg × 1 PO as a loading dose, then 50 (<60 kg) to 75 mg (≥60 kg) qd PO plus leucovorin 10–20 mg/day PO.[120] Adverse events have been observed (leading to discontinuation of therapy in 50% of cases) and consisted mainly of fever, rash, and increased liver enzymes.[137] In the absence of robust controlled studies comparing combination therapy with azithromycin with standard therapy, azithromycin should be used only in patients who do not respond, or are intolerant, to conventional therapy with sulfadiazine–pyrimethamine, clindamycin–pyrimethamine, atovaquone–pyrimethamine/sulfadiazine, or trimethoprim–sulfamethoxazole.[120]

Other Drugs

The following regimens have been reported to have activity in the treatment of *Toxoplasma* encephalitis in small cohorts of patients or in case reports of one or a few patients: 5-fluorouracil with clindamicyn,[140] dapsone with pyrimethamine and leucovorin,[141,142] minocycline or doxycycline combined with either pyrimethamine and leucovorin, sulfadiazine, or clarithromycin[143–148] and trimetrexate[149] have been used with success in some patients.

Corticosteroids and antiseizure drugs

Adjunctive corticosteroids (e.g., dexamethasone) should be administered when clinical evaluations indicates that there is a need to reduce intracerebral pressure, when there is considerable mass effect from focal lesions, or when seizures are intractable.[120] Patients receiving corticosteroids should be closely monitored for the development of other opportunistic infections, including CMV retinitis and tuberculosis.

Anticonvulsants should be administered to patients with demonstrated seizures, but should not be administered routinely to all patients with *Toxoplasma* encephalitis.[120] Phenobarbital or phenytoin sodium are not recommended because of potential drug interactions with antiretroviral agents. Sodium valproate is preferred. There are no clear evidence-based guidelines for how long anticonvulsants should be continued after an initial seizure. Anticonvulsants should probably be continued at least through the period of acute therapy.

Maintenance (Suppressive) Therapy

Following 6 weeks of acute therapy and a clinical and radiographic response, patients should receive life-long maintenance therapy (secondary prophylaxis or suppressive therapy) unless immune reconstitution in response to HAART therapy occurs (see further ahead). Maintenance therapy should be initiated only once CNS lesions no longer show contrast enhancement of CT/MRI.[120] Without prophylaxis, relapse rates for *Toxoplasma* encephalitis are 50–80% at 6–12 months.[7,22,23] The 1-year estimated survival probability after an episode of *Toxoplasma* encephalitis was 30%[42] in the pre-HAART (pre-1996) period but is now 77%.[52] In the current HAART era, the presence of abnormal mental status at the time of presentation is independently associated with an increased risk of death, while receiving combined antiretroviral therapy is associated with a decreased risk of death.[52]

For maintenance therapy, most clinicians maintain the acute regimen with oral dosing (Table 37-2).[13,18,120,121,150] Breakthrough can occur (10–40%). As noted above these are due to nonadherence to the drug regimen, or to severe immune deficiency. Drug resistance is thought to be rare.[13,121,150,151]

Table 37-2 Maintenance Regimens (Secondary Prophylaxis) for AIDS-Related Toxoplasmosis

Oral Drug	Suggested Regimens
Preferred Combinations[a]	
Daily treatment	
Pyrimethamine plus	25–75 mg qd
Sulfadiazine or	500–1000 mg q6h or 1 g q12h
Clindamycin	600 mg q8h
Intermittent treatment	
Pyrimethamine plus	50 mg thrice weekly
Sulfadiazine	1 g q12h thrice weekly
Other Regimens[a]	
Atovaquone alone	750 mg q6h
Pyrimethamine alone or plus	50 mg qd or 25 mg qd
Atovaquone or	750 mg q6h
Clarithromycin or	1000 mg qd
Dapsone or	100 mg twice weekly
Azithromycin	600–1800 mg qd
Pyrimethamine-sulfadoxine (Fansidar®)	25 mg/500 mg (1 tablet) twice weekly

[a]Folinic acid (10–25 mg/day) should be used with all pyrimethamine-containing regimens.

Patients with retinochoroiditis can be especially difficult to treat, either in patients with normal immunity or severe immune deficiency. In patients with treatment-responsive ocular involvement, 20% may develop recurrent retinochoroiditis (relapse) within 24 months despite continuing on pyrimethamine with either sulfadiazine or clindamycin.[61,121,120]

For maintenance regimens, treatment with pyrimethamine with sulfadiazine and leucovorin should probably be given daily. However, thrice-weekly administration (pyrimethamine, 50 mg; sulfadiazine, 1 g q12h) also appears effective.[152] Pharmacokinetic properties of sulfadiazine support its use every 12 h either in acute or maintenance therapies.[153] In patients who respond to pyrimethamine with clindamycin as primary therapy, reducing the dose of pyrimethamine to 25 mg/day but keeping clindamycin at almost full oral doses (600 mg q8h) is a reasonable approach due to the high rate of failures seen with lower doses.[18,120,121]

The ENTA study compared daily maintenance therapy comprised of pyrimethamine 25 mg with either sulfadiazine 2 g or oral clindamycin 1.2 g in 175 patients with a mean follow-up of 13 months.[121] The pyrimethamine–sulfadiazine combination appeared to be significantly more effective than the pyrimethamine–clindamycin combination, with relapse rates of 7% and 28%, respectively. The toxicity of these two combinations was lower than with acute therapy: 28% in the pyrimethamine/sulfadiazine-treated patients and 20% in the pyrimethamine/clindamycin-treated patients. Rash and fever were more frequent (12%) among pyrimethamine/sulfadiazine-treated patients, and diarrhea was more frequent (14%)

Table 37-3

Discontinuation of Maintenance Anti-*Toxoplasma* Therapy in Patients who Completed an initial Course of Therapy and had a CD4+ T Lymphocyte >200 Cells/mm^3 During More than 3 Months Due to Effective HAART

Study	No.	Relapses	Incidence/100 Patient-years (95% CI)
Denmark[159]	8	0	0 (0–47)
Madrid[161]	9	0	0 (ND)
France[162]	19	0	0 (ND)
Switzerland[162a]	22	1	4.5 (0.1–2.3)
Seven European Cohorts[163]	75	1	0.84 (0.02–4.68)
GESIDA[164]			
Stop	28	0	0 (0–4.78)
Continue	29	0	0 (0–5.19)

HAART, highly active antiretroviral therapy; ND, not done.

in those receiving pyrimethamine/clindamycin. It is of interest that hematologic toxicity with either combination was uncommon (<5%).

Table 37-2 also lists other regimens (including atovaquone with or without pyrimethamine) that decrease (but certainly do not prevent all) recurrences.[120,154–156] Among these secondary prophylactic regimens is a particularly convenient one if patients are sulfa-tolerant: a single tablet of Fansidar (pyrimethamine 25 mg plus sulfadoxine 500 mg) twice weekly. Although associated with frequent (41%) but mild to moderate allergic reactions, twice-weekly Fansidar maintained 90% of patients relapse-free at 12 months and 80% at 24 months; the probability of remaining free of *P. jirovecii* pneumonia (PCP) was also ~90% at 24 months.[156] Patients maintained on pyrimethamine–sulfadiazine, Fansidar or dapsone (but not pyrimethamine–clindamycin) also appear to be protected against PCP.[18,151,156,157] Trimethoprim–sulfamethoxazole has not been well evaluated in secondary prophylaxis. However, in a small pilot study, treatment was effective for preventing *Toxoplasma* encephalitis relapses.[158]

For patients experiencing a relapse of *Toxoplasma* encephalitis, treatment recommendations for initial therapy as outlined above should be followed.[120]

Discontinuation of Maintenance Therapy

Discontinuation of secondary prophylaxis has been evaluated in a observational studies in a small number of patients[159–162] or in studies that analyzed several small studies together as one large cohort study.[163] These data show that maintenance therapy may be safely discontinued in patients taking effective HAART who have a CD4+ T-cell count greater than 200 cells/mm^3 for at least 3–6 months. In the GESIDA clinical trial,[164] 57 patients receiving secondary prophylaxis were randomized to continue or stop maintenance therapy. The median CD4+ T-cell count before stopping prophylaxis was 407 cells/mm^3, and 86% of these HAART-treated patients had undetectable HIV-1 RNA in plasma. After a median follow-up of 30.5 months (69 person-years), there were no episodes of *Toxoplasma* encephalitis in the 28 patients who discontinued prophylaxis (95 percent confidence interval, 0–6.94 episodes per 100 person-years). The 2004 recommendations of the Centers for Disease Control, National Institutes of Health, and the HIV Medicine Association/Infectious Diseases Society of America Task Force endorse discontinuation of maintenance therapy for toxoplasmosis (Table 37-3).[120] Thus, if a patient's CD4+ T-lymphocyte count has risen to >200 cells/mm^3 for 3 months or more as a result of HAART, the patient has completed an entire course of anti-*Toxoplasma* therapy, and if the patient is asymptomatic with regard to toxoplasmosis, it appears safe to discontinue maintenance therapy so long as the CD4+ T-lymphocyte count remains over 200 cells/mm^3. Some experts suggest performing a CT or MRI scan to provide additional information supporting the safety of discontinuing secondary prophylaxis for toxoplasmosis. If CD4+ T-lymphocyte counts subsequently decline to levels below 200 cells/mm^3, prophylaxis should be reinstituted.

PRIMARY PREVENTION

Primary Prevention

It is standard practice to provide primary prophylaxis to all *Toxoplasma*-seropositive patients who are immunodeficient (Tables 37-4 and 37-5).[18,26,165] A CD4 cell count of less than 100 cells/mm^3 is widely accepted as the latest time at which prophylaxis should be initiated.[165] At this stage, 25–40% of untreated patients will develop intracerebral disease within a 1- or 2-year period.[18,21,31,41–43] In contrast, the 12-month incidence of cerebral toxoplasmosis in seropositive patients with less than 100 CD4 cells/mm^3 was reduced from 34% to 8% if one of the following agents was used: trimethoprim–sulfamethoxazole, dapsone–pyrimethamine, Fansidar, or sulfadiazine.[165]

Table 37-4

Selected Primary Prophylaxis Trials in *T. Gondii*–Seropositive Patients at Definite Risk For Reactivated Toxoplasmosis

Trial	Eligibility[a]	Design	No. of Patients[b]	Oral Regimen	Median Follow-Up	TOXO[b] (%)	Toxicity (%)	Comments and Control
Carr et al[166]	Secondary prophylaxis for PCP	Retrospective	22	TMP-SMX 2 DS biwkly	290 days	0	5	12/36 (33%) Seropositive pentamidine-treated controls developed TOXO
Girard et al[167]	CDC stage IV, <200 CD4 cells	Randomized, open-label	135	Dapsone 50 mg qd plus pyrimethamine 50 mg q plus folinic acid 25 mg q wk	539 days	4	24	28/127 (22%) Seropositive pentamidine-treated controls developed TOXO
Jacobson et al[168]	Seropositive, <200 CD4 or prior OI	Double blind, randomized, placebo controlled	264	Pyrimethamine 25 mg tiw; no folinic acid	254 days	5	27	4% Seropositive placebo-treated controls developed TOXO; 21% had toxicity. PCP prophylaxis also allowed: TMP-SMX (in 54%) and dapsone–pyrimethamine (in 12%). Increased death rate with pyrimethamine (29% vs 16%)
Opravil et al[169]	Advanced HIV or prior OI; median CD4 105–116	Randomized, open-label	120	Dapsone 200 mg q wk plus pyrimethamine 75 mg q wk; folinic acid not given routinely	543 days	3	30	Subgroup analysis vs 120 seropositive pentamidine-treated controls of whom 12% developed TOXO
Podzamczer et al[32]	<200 CD4	Randomized, open-label	131	TMP-SMX 2 DS tiw vs dapsone 100 mg biwkly plus	430 days	2	10	Groups included 65 and 66 patients. Similar efficacy and toxicity
				pyrimethamine 50 mg biwkly; no folinic acid	430 days	3	9	
Leport[21c]	Seropositive, <200 CD4	Double blind, randomized, placebo controlled	274	Pyrimethamine 50 mg tiw plus folinic acid 15 mg tiw	12 mo[d]	4	20	Placebo controls ($m = 280$): 12% developed TOXO; 7% had toxicity

CDC, Centers for Disease Control and Prevention; DS, double strength; OI, opportunistic infection; PCP, *Pneumocystis jirovecii* pneumonia; tiw, three times a week; TMP-SMX, trimethoprim–sulfamethoxazole; TOXO, toxoplasmosis.

[a]CD4 cells/mm^3

[b]Number of patients who were seropositive at study entry (and therefore at high risk for reactivated toxoplasmosis); does not necessarily indicate the total number of patients entered.

[b]Patients who developed toxoplasmosis using 'on-treatment' rather than intention-to-treat analysis. In some trials, intention-to-treat analysis did not show benefit from prophylaxis primarily because of drug adverse reactions that resulted in crossover to the other arm or discontinuation of treatment.

[c]In this trial, seropositivity to *T. gondii* was a required entry criterion.

[d]Mean follow-up period.

Table 37-5 Primary Prophylaxis to Prevent First Episode of AIDS-Related Toxoplasmosis

Oral Drug[a]	Suggested Regimens
Preferred Treatment	
TMP-SMX[b]	1 DS tablet qd Alternatives: 1 SS tablet qd, 1 DS tablet q12h tiw, or 1 DS tablet tiw
Pyrimethamine–dapsone	50 mg q wk/50 mg qd Alternatives: 25 mg + 100 mg qd biw, or 75 mg + 200 mg q wk
Other Treatments	
Pyrimethamine–sulfadoxine (Fansidar)	25 mg/500 mg (1 tablet) biw or 3 tablets once q 2 wk
Atovaquone	1500 mg qd
Atovaquone–pyrimethamine	1500 mg qd/25 mg qd

biw, twice weekly; q wk, once weekly; q 2 wk, every 2 weeks; tiw, three times per week.

[a] Folinic acid (10–25 mg/day) should be given with any pyrimethamine-containing regimen.

Numerous studies of primary prophylaxis had been carried out by 1995,[21,26,165–178] each with certain limitations and varying degrees of completeness and success, using mainly one of three regimens: trimethoprim–sulfamethoxazole, dapsone–pyrimethamine, or pyrimethamine alone.[21,32,166–169] In addition to variable drug dosages and administration schedules (ranging from daily to once-weekly), data interpretation has also been difficult because of disparate results generated by patient intolerance to the assigned drug and the use of intention-to-treat versus on-therapy analyses.[26,165–178] Additional trials have also been reported (Tables 37-4 and 37-5). Neither spiramycin, clarithromycin alone nor clindamycin with pyrimethamine is active as a primary prophylactic agent,[165,170,173,175] and current data also do not support the routine use of monotherapy with dapsone, pyrimethamine, or azithromycin.[21,31,32,165,167–169,171,172,176,178]

The doses and administration schedules of trimethoprim–sulfamethoxazole and pyrimethamine–dapsone that are recommended for PCP prophylaxis appear adequate for prevention of toxoplasmosis (Tables 37-4 and 37-5).[26,32,165] Aerosolized pentamidine does not protect against toxoplasmosis.[167,169] The optimal prophylactic regimen to prevent reactivation, using either trimethoprim–sulfamethoxazole or dapsone–pyrimethamine, has not been fully defined regarding either drug doses or daily versus intermittent administration. Although trimethoprim–sulfamethoxazole and dapsone–pyrimethamine are quite active as primary prophylaxis in *Toxoplasma*-seropositive patients with less than 100 CD4 cells/mm^3,[165] failures do occur. Fansidar can be an alternative option.[177,178] Atovaquone, with or without pyrimethamine, is thought to be a reasonable regimen in patients intolerant to the preferred treatments (Table 37-5).[165]

Discontinuing Primary Prophylaxis

In *Toxoplasma*-seropositive patients who respond to HAART with sustained increases (>3 months) in CD4 cell counts to more than 200 cells/mm^3, experience in more than 500 patients indicates that primary prophylaxis can be safely discontinued (Table 37-6).[160,164,179–183] This recommendation has been supported by several cohort studies and randomized clinical trials which except for one (GESIDA), were substudies of PCP discontinuation studies.[160,164,179–183] Susceptibility to relapse is best determined by the current CD4+ T-lymphocyte count. Following a CD4+ T-lymphocyte rise due to HAART, the absolute CD4+ T-lymphocyte count (or the percent of lymphocytes that are CD4+) is substantially more important than the prior nadir CD4+ T-lymphocyte count or the viral load. Although an occasional case of toxoplasmosis occurs at CD4+ T-lymphocyte counts of more than 100 cells/mm^3, such cases are unusual. If CD4+ T-lymphocyte counts subsequently decline to levels below 200 cells/mm^3, prophylaxis should be reinstituted.

Timing of HAART in Patients with Acute Toxoplasmosis

All patients with HIV associated toxoplasmosis need to be treated with HAART. However, no consensus has been reached regarding when to initiate HAART.[120] Patients with toxoplasmosis usually have <50 CD4+ T-lymphocyte cells/mm^3. Thus, starting HAART in the acute phase would reduce the risk of HIV disease progression or death.

Initiating HAART in patients with an acute opportunistic infection has some obvious potential disadvantages. First, antiretroviral agents and anti-*Toxoplasma* drugs often have overlapping toxicities (e.g., rash, transaminase elevations, cytopenias). Concurrent therapies also entail high pill burden which can compromise adherence. Fortunately, there are no important pharmacokinetic interactions between most antiretroviral and anti-*Toxoplasma* drugs.

Immune reconstitution inflammatory syndrome (IRIS) can potentially complicate the initial management of the opportunistic infection. However, IRIS appears to be very uncommon in patients with *Toxoplasma* encephalitis. While trials are underway to evaluate the most appropriate timing for starting HAART in this setting, the 2004 CDC/NIH

Table 37-6 Discontinuation of Primary Anti-*Toxoplasma* Prophylaxis in *T. Gondii* Co-Infected Patients who had a CD4+ T Lymphocyte >200 Cells/mm³ During More than 3 Months Due to Effective HAART

Study	No.	Mean Follow-Up (Months)	Patient-Years	Incidence/100 Patient-Years (95% CI)
HOPS[180]	146	18.2	402	0
Paris[160]	34	16.0		0
Swiss cohort-1[179]	121	11.0	109	0 (0–2.73)
Swiss cohort-2[182]	199	16.8	272	0 (0–1.10)
Eighth European Cohorts[181]	325	13.0	374	0
CIOP[183]				
Stop	115	7.2	72	0 (0–7.3)
Continue	128	6.0	72	0 (0–7.3)
GESIDA[164]				
Stop	196	24.9	400	0 (0–0.80)
Continue	185	24.9	379	0 (0–0.86)

Recommendations[120] can be usefully applied to toxoplasmosis as follows: (1) in antiretroviral-naive patients, HAART can be started after 2 weeks of therapy for toxoplasmosis; and (2) in patients with failing HAART regimens who develop toxoplasmosis, anti-*Toxoplasma* treatment should be started, HIV resistance testing should be performed and a new genotyped-based HAART regimen should be started.

Restoration of Immune Response After Initiation of HAART

Several studies have demonstrated that antigen-specific T-cell responses may require several months or longer to be regenerated in patients on HAART.[184,185] Fournier et al[186] have demonstrated in a cross-sectional study that the *in vitro T. gondii*-specific T-cell responses can be restored with HAART in severely immunosuppressed HIV-1-infected patients. This was especially true in terms of lymphoproliferative responses and production of interferon gamma, an essential cytokine for the control of *T. gondii* infection.[186] A prospective, multicenter, longitudinal study performed in Spain[187] enrolled 20 patients with acute *Toxoplasma* encephalitis who responded to anti-*Toxoplasma* treatment and started HAART and secondary prophylaxis. T-cell responses to *T. gondii* antigens were restored in most patients after at least 1 year of HAART. This study showed a correlation between the *in vitro T. gondii* lymphoproliferative responses and interferon-gamma production, and the number of CD4+ T lymphocytes. Almost all patients with more than 200 CD4+ T lymphocytes had a *T. gondii*-specific immune response. These parameters may eventually be useful for determining when anti-*Toxoplasma* therapy can safely be stopped.

These conclusions can be applied to patients living in Europe and the United States, where the majority of *T. gondii* strains can be clustered into three main clonal genotypes, type II being the most prevalent.[188] However, other geographical regions (e.g., South America) may contain different genotypes and, Ghost et al. have recently published,[188] that the HAART-induced *T. gondii* immune recovery may not be protective against re-infection with these atypical strains.

Pregnant Women and Children

Documentation of maternal *T. gondii* serologic status should be obtained at the time that pregnancy is anticipated or documented. Perinatal transmission of *T. gondii* ordinarily occurs only when the mother is parasitemic.[189] In immunologically normal women, this occurs only if acute toxoplasma infection happens during pregnancy. However, once they develop advanced HIV disease, *Toxoplasma*-seropositive pregnant women with previously quiescent chronic infection can transmit infection to the fetus.[34,35,190]

Because trimethoprim–sulfamethoxazole is thought by most experts to be safe during pregnancy, *Toxoplasma*-seropositive pregnant women with less than 100 CD4+ T-lymphocyte cells/mm³ should also receive primary prophylaxis to prevent reactivation. One recent study of 195 mother–infant pairs suggested that folate antagonists added to HAART increased the risk of congenital abnormalities.[191] However, this study needs to be confirmed. Trimethoprim–sulfamethoxazole has multiple benefits to pregnant women that should not be overlooked when assessing risk and benefit.

Pregnant women with active toxoplasmosis (e.g., encephalitis) and those who become pregnant while undergoing standard maintenance therapy (secondary prophylaxis) pose a therapeutic problem that fortunately is not frequent. Treatment of *Toxoplasma* encephalitis should be the same as in nonpregnant adults.[120,192] The dilemma is whether to use the most effective regimen for the mother, which would include pyrimethamine (posing a risk to the fetus), or to look during the first trimester for an alternative regimen without pyrimethamine. Although pyrimethamine has been associated with birth defects in animals, limited human data have not suggested an increased risk of defects, and, therefore, it can be administered to pregnant women.[193,194] Pediatric providers should be notified if sulfadiazine is continued until delivery since its use may increase the risk of neonatal hyperbilirubinemia and kernicterus.[194] In any case, appropriate consultation with specialists should be sought in these unusual situations.

Toxoplasmosis is not a common opportunistic infection in HIV-infected children. Nevertheless, children who are older than 1 year of age, who qualify for prophylaxis for PCP, and who are at risk (*Toxoplasma*-seropositive) are candidates for primary anti-*Toxoplasma* prophylaxis.[195] In practice, such children would likely already be receiving trimethoprim–sulfamethoxazole for PCP prophylaxis and, in contrast to HIV-infected adults, usually tolerate this treatment well. Alternatives to trimethoprim–sulfamethoxazole include dapsone–pyrimethamine–leucovorin or atovaquone alone.[195] Primary prophylaxis for younger children who may be immunodeficient despite high absolute CD4+ T-lymphocyte counts can also be considered if *Toxoplasma* serology is positive.

Other Preventive Measures

All HIV-infected persons should be tested for IgG antibody to *T. gondii*. Those found to be seronegative should be retested for anti-*Toxoplasma* IgG if and when the CD4+ T-lymphocyte count declines to 100/mm^3 to determine if interval infection has been acquired and primary prophylaxis is warranted.

Irrespective of the CD4 + T-lymphocyte count, seronegative individuals should also undertake measures to reduce future oral exposure to *T. gondii*.[165,196–199] All undercooked meat should be avoided, especially pork and lamb. Previously frozen meats (to −20° C for 24 h) are considered safe because tissue cysts are killed by freezing. Fruits and vegetables (potentially contaminated with oocysts from outdoor cats or other felines) should be carefully washed before being eaten uncooked. Hand washing is necessary after contact with fresh raw meat, after gardening, or after contact with soil where oocysts might have been deposited. Kitchen surfaces should also be washed after contact with raw meat. Toxoplasmosis has rarely been acquired via drinking apparently contaminated (unfiltered) water in both rural and urban settings.[165,196,197] Although there is no recommendation to boil filtered water to prevent transmission of *Toxoplasma*, it would be prudent to take such precautions if, for example, one must drink stream water to which felines have access.

Cat ownership *per se* does not appear to increase the risk of infection in HIV-positive persons,[165,198,199] so cat owners need not give up their pets. However, they should keep their current pets indoors to reduce the likelihood of the cat acquiring new infection, and cats should be fed processed or cooked foods for the same reason. Personal contact with stray cats or new cat adoption should also be avoided lest these animals (especially kittens) be recently infected and actively shed oocysts. Ideally, litter boxes should be changed daily by an HIV-negative person to prevent any excreted oocysts from having time to sporulate. Alternatively, disposable gloves followed by hand washing can be used by whoever carefully empties the litter box; some have also recommended disinfecting the litter box with boiling water after each litter change.[18,26] Because only recently infected cats excrete oocysts and usually for a limited period (less than 14 days), most long-term indoor cats do not pose a hazard to their HIV-infected owners; therefore there is no reason to test a cat's stool or serum for evidence of *T. gondii* infection. However, cats are occasionally reinfected and resume self-limited oocyst shedding-hence the importance of the preceding recommendations for all cats living in the household of an HIV-infected person.

REFERENCES

1. Kasper LH. Toxoplasma infection. Braunwald E, Fava AS, Kasper DL, Hauser SL, Longo DL, Jameson JL (eds). In: Harrison's Textbook of Medicine. New York: McGraw-Hill; 1998, p 1197.
2. Montoya JG, Remington JS. Toxoplasma gondii. In: Mandell GL, Bennett JE, Dolin R (eds). Principles and Practice of Infectious Diseases. 5th edn. Philadelphia: Churchill Livingstone; 2000, p 2858.
3. Ruskin J, Remington JS. Toxoplasmosis in the compromised host. Ann Intern Med 84:193, 1976.
4. Hunter CA, Remington JS. Immunopathogenesis of toxoplasmic encephalitis. J Infect Dis 170:1057, 1994.
5. Murray HW, Rubin BY, Masur H, et al. Impaired production of lymphokines and immune (gamma) interferon in the acquired immunodeficiency syndrome. N Engl J Med 310:883, 1984.
6. Navia BA, Petito CK, Gold JWM, et al. Cerebral toxoplasmosis complicating the acquired immune deficiency syndrome: clinical and neuropathological findings in 27 patients. Ann Neurol 19:224, 1986.
7. Luft BJ, Remington JS. Toxoplasmic encephalitis. J Infect Dis 157:1, 1988.
8. Carrazana EJ, Rossitch E, Samuels MA. Cerebral toxoplasmosis in the acquired immune deficiency syndrome. Clin Neurol Neurosurg 91:291, 1989.
9. Luft BJ, Hafner R. Toxoplasmic encephalitis. AIDS 4:593, 1990.
10. Strittmatter C, Lang W, Wiestler OD, et al. The changing pattern of human immunodeficiency virus-associated cerebral toxoplasmosis: a study of 46 postmortem cases. Acta Neuropathol (Berl) 83:475, 1992.
11. Luft BJ, Remington JS. Toxoplasmic encephalitis in AIDS. Clin Infect Dis 15:211, 1992.
12. Dannemann B, McCutchan JA, Israelski D, et al. Treatment of toxoplasmic encephalitis in patients with AIDS: a randomized trial comparing pyrimethamine plus clindamycin to pyrimethamine plus sulfadiazine. Ann Intern Med 116:33, 1992.
13. Renold C, Sugar A, Chave J-P, et al. Toxoplasma encephalitis in patients with the acquired immunodeficiency syndrome. Medicine 71:224, 1992.
14. Decker CF, Tuazon CU. Toxoplasmosis: an update on clinical and therapeutic aspects. Prog Clin Parasitol 3:21, 1993.
15. Mariuz P, Bosler EM, Luft BJ. Toxoplasmosis in individuals with AIDS. Infect Dis Clin North Am 8:365, 1994.

16. New LC, Holliman RE. Toxoplasmosis and human immunodeficiency virus (HIV) disease. J Antimicrob Chemother 33:1079, 1994.
17. Wong SY, Remington JS. Toxoplasmosis in the setting of AIDS. In: Broder S, Merigan TC, Bolognesi D (eds). Textbook of AIDS Medicine. Baltimore: Williams & Wilkins; 1994, p 223.
18. Wong SY, Israeliski DM, Remington JS. AIDS-associated toxoplasmosis. In: Sande MA, Volberding PA (eds). The Medical Management of AIDS. 4th edn. Philadelphia: WB Saunders; 1995, p 460.
19. Cohen BA. Neurologic manifestations of toxoplasmosis in AIDS. Semin Neurol 19:201, 1999.
20. Luft BJ, Chua A. Central nervous system toxoplasmosis in HIV pathogenesis, diagnosis, and therapy. Curr Infect Dis Rep 2:358, 2000.
21. Leport C, Chene G, Morlat P, et al. Pyrimethamine for primary prophylaxis of toxoplasmic encephalitis in patients with human immunodeficiency virus infection: a double-blind, randomized trial. J Infect Dis 173:91, 1996.
22. Pedrol E, Gonzalez-Clemente J, Gatell JM, et al. Central nervous system toxoplasmosis in AIDS patients: efficacy of an intermittent maintenance therapy. AIDS 4:511, 1990.
23. Cohn JA, McMeeking A, Cohen W, et al. Evaluation of the policy of empiric treatment of suspected Toxoplasma encephalitis in patients with the acquired immunodeficiency syndrome. Am J Med 86:521, 1989.
24. D'Arminio Monforte A, Cinque P, Mocroft A, et al. Changing incidence of central nervous system diseases in the EuroSIDA Cohort. Ann Neurol 55: 320, 2004.
25. Jones JL, Sehgal M, Maguire JH. Toxoplasmosis-associated deaths among human immunodeficiency virus-infected persons in the United States, 1992–1998. Clin Infect Dis. 34:1161, 2002.
26. Richards FO, Kovacs JA, Luft BJ. Preventing toxoplasmic encephalitis in persons infected with human immunodeficiency virus. Clin Infect Dis 21(Suppl 1):S49, 1995.
27. Murray HW. Immunotherapy for AIDS-associated toxoplasmosis. In: Sande MA, Root RK (eds). Contemporary Issues in Infectious Diseases, vol 9: Treatment of Serious Infections in the 1990s. New York: Churchill Livingstone; 1992, p 205.
28. Murray HW. Survival of intracellular pathogens within human mononuclear phagocytes. Semin Hematol 25:101, 1988.
29. Israelski DM, Chmiel JS, Poggensee L, et al. Prevalence of toxoplasma infection in a cohort of men at risk of AIDS and toxoplasmic encephalitis. J Acquir Immune Defic Syndr 6:414, 1993.
30. Hell KJ, Church JA, Ross L. Toxoplasma gondii seroprevalence in HIV-infected children. In: Abstracts of the 4th Conference on Retroviruses and Opportunistic Infections, Washington, DC, Jan 1996, abstract 344.
31. Mallolas J, Zamora L, Gatell JM, et al. Primary prophylaxis for Pneumocystis carinii pneumonia: a randomized trial comparing cotrimoxazole, aerosolized pentamidine and dapsone plus pyrimethamine. AIDS 7:59, 1993.
32. Podzamczer D, Salazar A, Jimenez J, et al. Intermittent trimethoprim–sulfamethoxazole compared with dapsone–pyrimethamine for the simultaneous primary prophylaxis of Pneumocystis pneumonia and toxoplasmosis in patients infected with HIV. Ann Intern Med 122:755, 1995.
33. Hohfeld P, Daffos F, Costa J-M, et al. Prenatal diagnosis of congenital toxoplasmosis with a polymerase chain reaction test on amniotic fluid. N Engl J Med 331:695, 1994.
34. Mitchell CD, Erlich SS, Mastrucci MT, et al. Congenital toxoplasmosis occurring in infants perinatally infected with human immunodeficiency virus-1. Pediatr Infect Dis J 9:512, 1990.
35. Marty P, Bongain A, Rahal A, Prenatal diagnosis of severe fetal toxoplasmosis as a result of toxoplasmic reactivation in an HIV-positive woman. Prenat Diagn 14:414, 1994.
36. Anonymous. Low incidence of congenital toxoplasmosis in children born to women infected with human immunodeficiency virus: European Collaborative Study and Research Network on Congenital Toxoplasmosis. Eur J Obstet Gynecol Reprod Biol 68:93, 1996.
37. Lefevre-Elbert V, Ciraru-Vigneron N, Garin JF, et al. Toxoplasmosis serological reactivation and parasitemia in a cohort of HIV positive pregnant women. In: Abstracts of the XIth International Conference on AIDS, Vancouver, 7–12 Jul 1996, abstract We.B.3228.
38. Yap G, Pesin M, Sher A. Cutting edge: IL-12 is required for the maintenance of IFN-gamma production in T cells mediating chronic resistance to the intracellular pathogen, Toxoplasma gondii. J Immunol 165:628, 2000.
39. Murray HW, Gellene RA, Libby DM, et al. Activation of tissue macrophages from AIDS patients: in vitro responses of AIDS alveolar macrophages to lymphokines and gamma interferon. J Immunol 135:2374, 1985.
40. Murray HW, Rubin BY, Carriero SM, et al. Human mononuclear phagocyte antiprotozoal mechanisms: oxygen-dependent vs. oxygen-independent activity against intracellular Toxoplasma gondii. J Immunol 134:1982, 1985.
41. Stellbrink HJ, Fuhrer-Burow R, Raedler A, et al. Risk factors for severe disease due to Toxoplasma gondii in HIV-positive patients. Eur J Epidemiol 9:633, 1993.
42. Oksenhendler E, Charreau I, Tournerie C, et al. Toxoplasma gondii infection in advanced HIV infection. AIDS 8:483, 1994.
43. Laing RB, Flegg PJ, Brettle RP, et al. Clinical features, outcome and survival from cerebral toxoplasmosis in Edinburgh AIDS patients. Int J STD AIDS 7:258, 1996.
44. Derouin F, Leport C, Pueyo S, et al. Predicitve value of Toxoplasma gondii antibody titres on the occurrence of toxoplasmic encephalitis in HIV infected patients. AIDS 10:1521; 1996.
45. Falangola MF, Reichler BS, Petito CK. Histopathology of cerebral toxoplasmosis in human immunodeficiency virus infection: a comparison between patients with early-onset and late-onset acquired immunodeficiency syndrome. Hum Pathol 25:1091, 1994.
46. Rabaud C, May T, Amiel C, et al. Extracerebral toxoplasmosis in patients infected with HIV: a French national survey. Medicine 73:306, 1994.
47. Hofman P, Bernard E, Michiels JF, et al. Extracerebral toxoplasmosis in the acquired immunodeficiency syndrome (AIDS). Pathol Res Pract 189:894, 1993.
48. Jautzke G, Sell M, Thalmann U, et al. Extracerebral toxoplasmosis in AIDS: histological and immunohistological findings based upon 80 autopsy cases. Pathol Res Pract 189:428, 1993.
49. Albrecht H, Skorde J, Arasteh K, et al. Disseminated toxoplasmosis in AIDS patients: report of 16 cases. Scand J Infect Dis 27:71, 1995.
50. Gandhi S, Lyubsky S, Jimenez-Lucho V. Adult respiratory distress syndrome associated with disseminated toxoplasmosis. Clin Infect Dis 19:169, 1994.
51. Lucet JC, Bailly MP, Bedos JP, et al. Septic shock due to toxoplasmosis in patients infected with the human immunodeficiency virus. Chest 104:1054, 1993.
52. Antinori A, Larussa D, Cingolani A, et al. Prevalence, associated factors, and prognostic determinants of AIDS-related toxoplasmic encephalitis in the era of advanced highly active antiretroviral therapy. Clin Infect Dis 39:1681; 2004.
53. Vyas R, Ebright JR. Toxoplasmosis of the spinal cord in a patient with AIDS: case report and review. Clin Infect Dis 23:1061, 1996.
54. Berlit P, Popescu O, Wend Y, et al. Disseminated cerebral hemorrhages as unusual manifestation of toxoplasmic encephalitis in AIDS. J Neurol Sci 143:187, 1996.
55. Falangola MF, Petito CK. Choroid plexus infection in cerebral toxoplasmosis in AIDS patients. Neurology 43:2035, 1993.

56. Weiss A, Margo CE, Ledford DK, et al. Toxoplasmic retinochoroiditis as an initial manifestation of the acquired immune deficiency syndrome. Am J Ophthalmol 101:248, 1986.
57. Friedman D. Neuro-ophthalmic manifestations of human immunodeficiency virus infection. Neurol Clin 9:55, 1991.
58. Gagliuso DJ, Teich SA, Friedman AH, et al. Ocular toxoplasmosis in AIDS patients. Trans Am Ophthalmol Soc 88:63, 1990.
59. Holland GN, Engstrom RE, Glasgow BJ, et al. Ocular toxoplasmosis in patients with the acquired immunodeficiency syndrome. Am J Ophthalmol 106:653, 1988.
60. Pivetti-Pezzi P, Accorinti M, Tamburi S, et al. Clinical features of toxoplasmic retinochoroiditis in patients with the acquired immunodeficiency syndrome. Ann Ophthalmol 26:73, 1994.
61. Cochereau-Massin I, LeHoang P, Lautier-Frau M, et al. Ocular toxoplasmosis in human immunodeficiency virus-infected patients. Am J Ophthalmol 114:130, 1992.
62. Oksenhendler E, Cadranel J, Sarfati C, et al. Toxoplasma gondii pneumonia in patients with the acquired immunodeficiency syndrome. Am J Med 88:18, 1990.
63. Schnapp L, Geaghan S, Campagna A, et al. Toxoplasma gondii pneumonitis in patients infected with the human immunodeficiency virus. Arch Intern Med 152:1073, 1992.
64. Rabaud C, May T, Lucet JC, et al. Pulmonary toxoplasmosis in patients infected with the human immunodeficiency virus: a French national survey. Clin Infect Dis 23:1249, 1996.
65. Bonilla CA, Rosa UW. Toxoplasma gondii pneumonia in patients with the acquired immunodeficiency syndrome: diagnosis by bronchoalveolar lavage. South Med J 87:659, 1994.
66. Nash G, Kerschmann RL, Nerndier B, et al. The pathological manifestations of pulmonary toxoplasmosis in the acquired immunodeficiency syndrome. Hum Pathol 25:652, 1994.
67. May T, Rabaud C, Katlama C, et al. Toxoplasmose extracerebrale au cours du SIDA: resultats d'une enquete nationale. Med Mal Infect 23:190, 1993.
68. Pomeroy C, Filice GA. Pulmonary toxoplasmosis: a review. Clin Infect Dis 14:863, 1992.
69. Pugin J, Vanhems P, Hirschel B, et al. Extreme elevations of serum lactic dehydrogenase differentiating pulmonary toxoplasmosis from Pneumocystis pneumoniae. N Engl J Med 327:1643, 1992.
70. Derouin F, Sarfati CI, Beauvais B, et al. Laboratory diagnosis of pulmonary toxoplasmosis in patients with acquired immunodeficiency syndrome. J Clin Microbiol 7:1661, 1989.
71. Buhr M, Heise W, Aarsteh K, et al. Disseminated toxoplasmosis with sepsis in AIDS. Clin Invest 70:1079, 1992.
72. Porter SS, Sande MA. Toxoplasmosis of the central nervous system in the acquired immunodeficiency syndrome. N Engl J Med 327:1643, 1992.
73. Potasman I, Resnick L, Luft BJ, et al. Intrathecal production of antibodies against Toxoplasma gondii in patients with toxoplasmic encephalitis and AIDS. Ann Intern Med 108:49, 1988.
74. Cintini C, Romani R, Magno S, et al. Diagnosis of Toxoplasma gondii infection in AIDS patients by a tissue culture technique. Eur J Clin Microbiol Infect Dis 14:434, 1995.
75. Albrecht H, Sobottka I, Stellbrink HJ, et al. Diagnosis of disseminated toxoplasmosis using a peripheral blood smear. AIDS 10:799, 1996.
76. Brouland JP, Audouin J, Hofman P, et al. Bone marrow involvement by disseminated toxoplasmosis in acquired immunodeficiency syndrome: the value of bone marrow trephine biopsy and immunohistochemistry for the diagnosis. Hum Pathol 27:302, 1996.
77. Eggers C, Gross U, Klinker H, et al. Limited value of cerebrospinal fluid for direct detection of Toxoplasma gondii in toxoplasmic encephalitis associated with AIDS. J Neurol 242:644, 1995.
78. Gadea I, Cuenca M, Benito N, et al. Bronchoalveolar lavage for the diagnosis of disseminated toxoplasmosis in AIDS patients. Diagn Microbiol Infect Dis 22:339, 1995.
79. Luft BJ, Hafner R, Korzun AH, et al. Toxoplasmic encephalitis in patients with the acquired immunodeficiency syndrome. N Engl J Med 329:995, 1993.
80. Jarvik JG, Hesselink JR, Kennedy C, et al. Acquired immunodeficiency syndrome: magnetic resonance patterns of brain involvement with pathologic correlation. Arch Neurol 45:731, 1998.
81. Levy RM, Mills CM, Posin JP, et al. The efficacy and clinical impact of brain imaging in neurologically symptomatic AIDS patients: a prospective CT/MRI study. J Acquir Immune Defic Syndr 3:461, 1990.
82. Knobel H, Guelar A, Graus F, et al. Toxoplasmic Encephalitis with Normal CT Scan and Pathologic MRI. Am J Med 99: 220, 1995.
83. Kupfer MC, Zee CS, Colletti PM, et al. MRI evaluation of AIDS-related encephalopathy: toxoplasmosis vs. lymphoma. Magn Reson Imaging 8:51, 1990.
84. Ciricillo SF, Rosenblum ML. Use of CT and MR imaging to distinguish intracranial lesions and to define the need for biopsy in AIDS patients. J Neurosurg 73:720, 1990.
85. Ciricillo SF, Rosenblum ML. Imaging of solitary lesions in AIDS. J Neurosurg 74:1029, 1991.
86. Steinmetz H, Arendt G, Hefter H, et al. Focal brain lesions in patients with AIDS: aetiologies and corresponding radiological patterns in a prospective study. J Neurol 242:69, 1995.
87. Weisberg LA, Greenbereg J, Stazio A. Computed tomographic findings in cerebral toxoplasmosis in adults. Comput Med Imaging Graph 12:379, 1988.
88. Chinn RJ, Wilkinson ID, Hall-Crasggs MA, et al. Toxoplasmosis and primary central nervous system lymphoma in HIV infection: diagnosis with MR spectroscopy. Radiology 197:649, 1995.
89. Chang L, Miller BL, McBride D, et al. Brain lesions in patients with AIDS: H-1 MR spectroscopy. Radiology 197:525, 1995.
90. Gianotti N, Marenzi R, Messa C, et al. Thallium-201 single photon emission computed tomography in the management of contrast-enhancing brain lesions in a patient with AIDS. Clin Infect Dis 23:185, 1996.
91. Ruiz A, Ganz WI, Post MJD, et al. Use of thallium-201 brain SPECT to differentiate cerebral lymphoma from Toxoplasma encephalitis in AIDS patients. Am J Neuroradiol 15:1885, 1994.
92. O'Malley JP, Ziessman HA, Kumar PN, et al. Diagnosis of intracranial lymphoma in patients with AIDS: value of ^{201}Tl single-photon emission computed tomography. Am J Roentgenol 163:417, 1994.
93. Naddaf SY, Akisik MF, Aziz M, et al. Comparison between ^{201}Tl-chloride and ^{99}Tc(m)-sestambi SPECT brain imaging for differentiating intracranial lymphoma from non-malignant lesions in AIDS patients. Nucl Med Commun 19:47, 1998.
94. D'Amico A, Messa C, Castagna A, et al. Diagnostic accuracy and predictive value of ^{201}Tl SPECT for the differential diagnosis of cerebral lesions in AIDS patients. Nucl Med Commun 18:741, 1997.
95. Lorberboym M, Estok L, Machac J, et al. Rapid differential diagnosis of cerebral toxoplasmosis and primary central nervous system lymphoma by thallium-201 SPECT. J Nucl Med 37:1150, 1996.
96. Antinori A, De Rossi G, et al. Value of combined approach with thallium-201 single-photon emission computed tomography and Epstein–Barr virus DNA polymerase chain reaction in CSF for the diagnosis of AIDS-related primary CNS lymphoma. J Clin Oncol 17:554, 1999.
97. Skiest DJ, Erdman W, Change WE, et al. SPECT thallium-201 combined with Toxoplasma serology for the presumptive

diagnosis of focal central nervous system mass lesions in patients with AIDS. J Infect 40:274, 2000.
98. Skiest DJ. Focal neurological disease in patients with acquired immunodeficiency syndrome. Clin Infect Dis 34:103, 2002.
99. Young RJ, Ghesani MV, Kagetsu NJ, DeRogatis AJ. Lesion size determines accuracy of thallium-201 brain single-photon emission tomography in differentiating between intracranial malignancy and infection in AIDS patients. Am J Neuroradiol 26:1973, 2005.
100. Pierce MA, Johnson MD, Maciunas RJ, et al. Evaluating contrast-enhancing brain lesions in patients with AIDS using positron emission tomography. Ann Intern Med 123:594, 1995.
101. Villriuger K, Jager H, Dichhgans M, et al. Differential diagnosis of CNS lesions in AIDS patients by FDG-PET. J Comput Assist Tomogr 19:532, 1995.
102. O'Doherty MJ, Barrington SF, Campbell M, et al. PET scanning and the human immunodeficiency virus-positive patient. J Nucl Med 38:1575, 1997.
103. Hoffman JM, Waskin HA, Schifter T, et al. FDG-PET in differentiating lymphoma from nonmalignant central nervous system lesions in patients with AIDS. J Nucl Med 34:567, 1993.
104. Hawkins R, Hoh C, Glaspy J, et al. Positron emission tomography scanning in cancer. Cancer Invest 12:74, 1994.
105. Letillois MF, Laigle V, Santoro F, et al. Toxoplasma gondii surface antigen-1 in sera of HIV-infected patients as an indicator of reactivated toxoplasmosis. Eur J Clin Microbiol Infect Dis 14:899, 1995.
106. Lavard I, Chouaid C, Poux P, et al. Pulmonary toxoplasmosis in HIV-infected patients: usefulness of polymerase chain reaction and cell culture. Eur Respir J 8:697, 1995.
107. Lamoril J, Molina JM, de Gouvello A, et al. Detection by PCR of Toxoplasma gondii in blood in the diagnosis of cerebral toxoplasmosis in patients with AIDS. J Clin Pathol 49:89, 1996.
108. Cingolani A, De Luca A, Ammassari A, et al. PCR detection of Toxoplasma gondii DNA in CSF for the differential diagnosis of AIDS-related focal brain lesions. J Med Microbiol 45:472, 1996.
109. Dupon M, Cazenave J, Pellegrin JL, et al. Detection of Toxoplasma gondii by PCR and tissue culture in cerebrospinal fluid and blood of human immunodeficiency virus-seropositive patients. J Clin Microbiol 33:2421, 1995.
110. Novati R, Castagna A, Morsica G, et al. Polymerase chain reaction for Toxoplasma gondii DNA in the cerebrospinal fluid of AIDS patients with focal brain lesions. AIDS 8:1691, 1994.
111. Schoondermark-van de Ven E, Galama J, Kraaijeveld C, et al. Value of the polymerase chain reaction for the detection of Toxoplasma gondii in cerebrospinal fluid from patients with AIDS. Clin Infect Dis 16:661, 1993.
112. Rodriguez JC, Martinez MM, Martinez AR, Royo G. Evaluation of different techniques in the diagnosis of Toxoplasma encephalitis. J Med Microbiol 46:597, 1997.
113. Joseph P, Calderon MM, Gilman RH, et al. Optimization and evaluation of a PCR assay for detecting toxoplasmic encephalitis in patients with AIDS. J Clin Microbiol. 40:4499, 2002.
114. Vidal JE, Colombo FA, Penalva de Oliveira AC, et al. PCR assay using cerebrospinal fluid for diagnosis of cerebral toxoplasmosis in Brazilian AIDS patients. J Clin Microbiol 42:4765, 2004.
115. Colombo FA, Vidal JE, Penalva de Oliveira AC, et al. Diagnosis of cerebral toxoplasmosis in AIDS patients in Brazil: importance of molecular and immunological methods using peripheral blood samples. J Clin Microbiol 43:5044, 2005.
116. Chappell ET, Guthrie BL, Orestein J. The role of stereotactic biopsy in the management of HIV-related focal brain lesions. Neurosurgery 30:82, 1992.
117. Mathews C, Barba D, Fullerton SC. Early biopsy versus empiric treatment with delayed biopsy of non-responders in suspected HIV-associated cerebral toxoplasmosis: a decision analysis. AIDS 9:1243, 1995.
118. Antinori A, Ammassari A, Luzzati R, et al. Role of brain biopsy in the management of focal brain lesions in HIV-infected patients. Neurology. 54:993, 2000.
119. Haverkos HW. Assessment of therapy of Toxoplasma encephalitis: the TE Study Group. Am J Med 82:907, 1987.
120. Centers for Disease Control and Prevention. Treating Opportunistic Infections Among HIV-Infected Adults and Adolescents: Recommendations from CDC, the National Institutes of Health, and the HIV Medicine Association/Infectious Diseases Society of America. MMWR; 53 (No. RR-15):1, 2004.
121. Katlama C, De Wit S, O'Doherty E, et al. Pyrmiethamine–clindamycin vs. pyrimethamine–sulfadiazine as acute and long-term therapy for toxoplasmic encephalitis in patients with AIDS. Clin Infect Dis 22:368, 1996.
122. Leport C, Raffi F, Matheron S, et al. Treatment of central nervous system toxoplasmosis with pyrimethamine/sulfadiazine combination in 35 patients with the acquired immunodeficiency syndrome. Am J Med 84:94, 1988.
123. Simon DI, Brosius FC, Rothstein DM. Sulfadiazine crystalluria revisited: the treatment of Toxoplasma encephalitis in patients with acquired immunodeficiency syndrome. Arch Intern Med 150:2379, 1990.
124. Becker K, Jablonowski H, Haussinger D. Sulfadiazine-associated nephrotoxicity in patients with the acquired immunodeficiency syndrome. Medicine (Baltimore). 75:185, 1996.
125. Jacobson MA, Besch CL, Child C, et al. Toxicity of clindamycin as prophylaxis for AIDS-associated toxoplasmic encephalitis. Lancet 339:333, 1992.
126. Katlama C. Evaluation of the efficacy and safety of clindamycin plus pyrimethamine for induction and maintenance therapy of toxoplasmic encephalitis in AIDS. Eur J Clin Microbiol Infect Dis 10:189, 1991.
127. Garaujo F, Huskingon J, Remington JS. Remarkable in vitro and in vivo activities of the hydroxynaphthoquinone, 566C80, against tachyzoites and tissue cysts of Toxoplasma gondii. Antimicrob Agents Chemother 35:293, 1991.
128. Kovacs JA, NIAID-Clinical Center Intramural AIDS Program. Efficacy of atovaquone in treatment of toxoplasmosis in patients with AIDS. Lancet 340:637, 1992.
129. Torres RA, Weinberg W, Stansell J, et al. Atovaquone for salvage treatment and suppression of toxoplasmic encephalitis in patients with AIDS. Clin Infect Dis 24:422, 1997.
130. Chirgwin K, Hafner R, Leport C, et al. Randomized phase II trial of atovaquone with pyrimethamine or sulfadiazine for treatment of toxoplasmic encephalitis in AIDS patients (ACTG 237/ANRS 039). Clin Infect Dis. 34:1243, 2002.
131. Canessa A, Del Bono V, De Leo P, et al. Cotrimoxazole therapy for Toxoplasma gondii encephalitis in AIDS patients. Eur J Clin Microbiol Infect Dis 11:125, 1992.
132. Torre D, Casari S, Speranza F, et al. Randomized trial of trimethoprim–sulfamethoxazole versus pyrimethamine–sulfadiazine for therapy of toxoplasmic encephalitis in patients with AIDS. Antimicrob Agents Chemother 42:1346, 1998.
133. Fernandes-Martin J, Leport C, Morlat P, et al. Pyrimethamine–clarithromycin combination for therapy of acute toxoplasma encephalitis in patients with AIDS. Antimicrob Agents Chemother 10:2049, 1991.
134. Cohn DL, Fisher EJ, Peng GT, et al. A prospective randomized trial of four three-drug regimens in the treatment of disseminated Mycobacterium avium complex disease in AIDS patients: excess mortality associated with high-dose

clarithromycin. Terry Beirn Community Programs for Clinical Research on AIDS. Clin Infect Dis. 29:125, 1999.
135. Remington JS. Macrolides, azalides, and streptogramins in treatment of opportunistic infections in immunocompromised patients. In: Zinner SH, Young LS, Acar JF, et al (eds). Expanding Indications for the New Macrolides, Azalides, and Streptogramins. New York: Dekker; 1997, p 189.
136. Farthing C, Rendel M, Currie B, et al. Azithromycin for cerebral toxoplasmosis. Lancet 339:437, 1992.
137. Saba J, Morlat P, Raffi F, et al. Pyrimethamine plus azithromycin for treatment of acute toxoplasmic encephalitis in patients with AIDS. Eur J Clin Microbiol Infect Dis. 12:853, 1993.
138. Wiselka MJ, Read R, Finch RG. Response to oral and intravenous azithromycin in a patient with toxoplasma encephalitis and AIDS. J Infect. 33:227, 1996.
139. Jacobson JM, Hafner R, Remington J, et al. Dose-escalation, phase I/II study of azithromycin and pyrimethamine for the treatment of toxoplasmic encephalitis in AIDS. AIDS 15:583, 2001.
140. Dhiver C, Milandre C, Poizot-Martin I, et al. 5-Fluoro-uracil-clindamycin for treatment of cerebral toxoplasmosis. AIDS 7:143, 1993.
141. Ward D. Dapsone/pyrimethamine for the treatment of toxoplasmic encephalitis. AbstrVIII IntConfAIDS 8:B133-PoB 3277, 1992.
142. Derouin F, Piketty C, Chastang C, et al. Anti-Toxoplasma effects of dapsone alone and combined with pyrimethamine. Antimicrob Agents Chemother. 35:252, 1991.
143. Lacassin F, Schaffo D, Perronne C, et al. Clarithromycin–minocycline combination as salvage therapy for toxoplasmosis in patients infected with human immunodeficiency virus. Antimicrob Agents Chemother 39:276, 1995.
144. Pope-Pegram L, Gathe J, Bohn B, et al. Treatment of presumed central nervous system toxoplasmosis with doxycycline. AbstrVII Int Conf AIDS 7:188, 1991.
145. Bockman KW, Gathe J, Stool E, et al. Utility of tetracycline derivatives in treatment of CNS toxoplasmosis. Abstr IX Int Conf AIDS 9:373, 1993.
146. Rouquet RM, Carre P, Massip P, et al. Acute respiratory distress due to *Toxoplasma gondii* in one AIDS patient. Recovery with an association pyrimethamine–doxycyclin. AbstrVIII Int Conf AIDS 8:130, 1992.
147. Hagberg L, Palmertz B, Lindberg J. Doxycycline and pyrimethamine for toxoplasmic encephalitis. Scand J Infect Dis 25:157, 1993.
148. Morris JT, Kelly JW. Effective treatment of cerebral toxoplasmosis with doxycycline. Am J Med 93:107, 1992.
149. Masur H, Polis MA, Tuazon CU, et al. Salvage trial of trimetrexate-leucovorin for the treatment of cerebral toxoplasmosis in patients with AIDS. J Infect Dis 167:1422, 1993.
150. Leport C, Tournerie C, Raguin G, et al. Long-term followup of patients with AIDS on maintenance therapy for toxoplasmosis. Eur J Clin Microbiol Infect Dis 10:191, 1991.
151. Podzamczer D, Miró JM, Bolao F, et al. Twice-weekly maintenance therapy with sulfadiazine–pyrimethamine to prevent recurrent toxoplasmic encephalitis in patients with AIDS. Ann Intern Med. 1995; 123:175.
152. Podzamczer D, Miró JM, Ferrer E, et al. Thrice-weekly sulfadiazine–pyrimethamine in HIV-infected patients. Eur J Microbiol Infect Dis 19:89, 2000.
153. Jordan MK, Burstein AH, Rock-Kress D, et al. Plasma pharmacokinetics of sulfadiazine administered twice daily versus four times daily are similar in human immunodeficiency virus-infected patients. Antimicrob Agents Chemother 48:635, 2004.
154. De Gans J, Portegies P, Reiss P, et al. Pyrimethamine alone as maintenance therapy for central nervous system toxoplasmosis in 38 patients with AIDS. J Acquir Immune Defic Syndr 5:137, 1992.
155. Katlama C, Mouthon B, Gourdon D, et al. Atovaquone as long-term suppressive therapy for toxoplasmic encephalitis in patients with AIDS and multiple drug intolerance. AIDS 10:1107, 1996.
156. Ruf B, Schurmann D, Bergmann F, et al. Efficacy of pyrimethamine–sulfadoxine in the prevention of toxoplasmic encephalitis relapses and Pneumocystis carinii pneumonia in HIV-infected patients. Eur J Clin Microbiol Infect Dis 12:325, 1991.
157. Heald A, Flepp M, Chave JP, et al. Treatment for cerebral toxoplasmosis protects against Pneumocystis carinii pneumonia in patients with AIDS. The Swiss HIV Cohort Study. Ann Intern Med 115:760, 1991.
158. Duval X, Pajot O, Le Moing V, et al. Maintenance therapy with cotrimoxazole for toxoplasmic encephalitis in the era of highly active antiretroviral therapy. AIDS 18:1342, 2004.
159. Kirk O, Lunmdgren JD, Pederson C, et al. Can chemoprophylaxis against opportunistic infections be discontinued after an increase in CD4 cells induced by highly active antiretroviral therapy? AIDS 13:1647, 1999.
160. Jubault V, Pacanowski J, Rabian C, Viard J-P. Interruption of prophylaxis for major opportunistic infections in HIV-infected patients receiving triple combination antiretroviral therapy. Ann Med Intern 151:163, 2000.
161. Soriano V, Dona C, Rodriguez-Rosado R, et al. Discontinuation of secondary prophylaxis for opportunistic infections in HIV-infected patients receiving highly active antiretroviral therapy. AIDS 4:383, 2000.
162. Zeller V, Truffot C, Agher R, et al. Discontinuation of secondary prophylaxis against disseminated Mycobacterium avium complex infection and toxoplasmic encephalitis. Clin Infect Dis 34:662, 2002.
162a. Bertschy S, Opravil M, Cavassini M et al. Discontinuation of maintenance therapy against toxoplasma encephalitis in AIDS patients with sustained response to anti-retroviral therapy. Clin Microbiol Infect 12:666, 2006.
163. Kirk O, Reiss P, Uberti-Foppa C, et al. Safe interruption of maintenance therapy against previous infection with four common HIV-associated opportunistic pathogens during potent antiretroviral therapy.Ann Intern Med 137:239, 2002.
164. Miro JM, Lopez JC, Podzamczer D, et al Discontinuation of Primary and Secondary *Toxoplasma gondii* Prophylaxis Is Safe in HIVInfected Patients after Immunological Restoration with Highly Active Antiretroviral Therapy: Results of an Open, Randomized, Multicenter Clinical Trial. Clin Infect Dis 43:79, 2006.
165. Masur H, Kaplan JE, Holmes KK; U.S. Public Health Service; Infectious Diseases Society of America. Guidelines for preventing opportunistic infections among HIV-infected persons – 2002. Recommendations of the U.S. Public Health Service and the Infectious Diseases Society of America. Ann Intern Med 137(5 Pt 2):435, 2002.
166. Carr AC, Tindall B, Brew BJ, et al. Low-dose trimethoprim–sulfamethoxazole prophylaxis for toxoplasmic encephalitis in patients with AIDS. Ann Intern Med 117:106, 1992.
167. Girard P-M, Landman R, Gaudebout C, et al. Dapsone–pyrimethamine compared with aerosolized pentamidine as primary prophylaxis against Pneumocystis carinii pneumonia and toxoplasmosis in HIV infection. N Engl J Med 328:1514, 1993.
168. Jacobson MA, Besch CL, Chikd C, et al. Primary prophylaxis with pyrimethamine for toxoplasmic encephalitis in patients with advanced human immunodeficiency virus disease: results of a randomized trial. J Infect Dis 169:384, 1994.
169. Opravil M, Hirschel B, Lazzarin A, et al. Once-weekly administration of dapsone/pyrimethamine vs. aerosolized pentamidine as combined prophylaxis for Pneumocystis carinii pneumonia and toxoplasmic encephalitis in human immunodeficiency virus-infected patients. Clin Infect Dis 20:531, 1995.

170. Leport C, Vilde JL, Katlama C, et al. Failure of spiramycin to prevent neurotoxoplasmosis in immunosuppressed patients. JAMA 255:2290, 1986.
171. Klinker H, Langmann P, Richter E. Pyrimethamine alone as prophylaxis for cerebral toxoplasmosis in patients with advanced HIV infection. Infection 24:324, 1996.
172. Torres RA, Barr M, Thorn M, et al. Randomized trial of dapsone and aerosolized pentamidine for the prophylaxis of Pneumocystis carinii pneumonia and toxoplasmic encephalitis. Am J Med 95:573, 1993.
173. Ruf B, Schurmann D, Pohle HD. Failure of clarithromycin in preventing toxoplasmic encephalitis in AIDS patients. J Acquir Immune Defic Syndr. 5:530, 1992.
174. Rizzardi GP, Lazzarin A, Musicco M, et al. Risks and benefits of aerosolized pentamidine and cotrimoxazole in primary prophylaxis of Pneumocystis carinii pneumonia in HIV-1 infected patients: a two-year Italian multicentric randomized trial. J Infect 32:123, 1991.
175. Girard PM, Lepretre A, Detruchis P, et al. Failure of pyrimethamine–clindamycin combination for prophylaxis of Pneumocystis carinii pneumonia and toxoplasmosis. Lancet 1:1459, 1989.
176. Bachmeyer C, Gorin I, Deleuze J, et al. Pyrimethamine as primary prophylaxis of toxoplasmic encephalitis in patients infected with human immunodeficiency virus: open study. Clin Infect Dis 18:479, 1994.
177. Schurmann D, Bergmann F, Albrecht H, et al. Effectiveness of twice-weekly pyrimethamine–sulfadoxine as primary prophylaxis of Pneumocystis carinii pneumonia and toxoplasmic encephalitis in patients with advanced HIV infection. Eur J Clin Microbiol Infect Dis. 21:353, 2002.
178. Payen MC, De Wit S, Sommereijns B, Clumeck N. A controlled trial of dapsone versus pyrimethamine–sulfadoxine for primary prophylaxis of Pneumocystis carinii pneumonia and toxoplasmosis in patients with AIDS. Biomed Pharmacother 51:439, 1997.
179. Furrer H, Egger M, Opravil M, et al. Discontinuation of primary prophylaxis against Pneumocystis carinii pneumonia in HIV-1-infected adults treated with combination antiretroviral therapy. Swiss HIV Cohort Study. N Engl J Med. 340:1301, 1999.
180. Yangco BG, Von Bargen JC, Moorman AC, Holmberg SD. Discontinuation of chemoprophylaxis against Pneumocystis carinii pneumonia in patients with HIV infection: HIV Outpatient Study (HOPS) Investigators. Ann Intern Med 132:201, 2000.
181. Ledergerber B, Mocroft A, Reiss P, et al. Discontinuation of secondary prophylaxis against Pneumocystis carinii pneumonia in patients with HIV infection who have a response to antiretroviral therapy: eight European study groups. N Engl J Med 18:168, 2001.
182. Furrer H, Opravil M, Bernasconi E, et al. Stopping primary prophylaxis in HIV-1-infected patients at high risk of toxoplasma encephalitis. Lancet 355:2217, 2000.
183. Mussini C, Pezzotti P, Govoni A, et al. Discontinuation of primary prophylaxis for Pneumocystis carinii pneumonia and toxoplasmic encephalitis in human immunodeficiency virus type 1-infected patients: the changes in opportunistic prophylaxis study. J Infect Dis 181:1635, 2000.
184. Ledergerber B, Egger M, Erard V, et al. AIDS-related opportunistic illnesses occurring after initiation of potent antiretroviral therapy: the Swiss HIV Cohort Study. JAMA.282:2220, 1999.
185. Li TS, Tubiana R, Katlama C, et al. Long-lasting recovery in CD4 T-cell function and viral-load reduction after highly active antiretroviral therapy in advanced HIV-1 disease. Lancet 351:1682, 1998.
186. Fournier S, Rabian C, Alberti C, et al. Immune recovery under highly active antiretroviral therapy is associated with restoration of lymphocyte proliferation and interferon-gamma production in the presence of Toxoplasma gondii antigens. J Infect Dis. 183:1586, 2001.
187. Miró JM, Lejeune M, Claramonte X, et al. Timing of reconstitution of Toxoplasma gondii-specific T-cell responses in AIDS patients with acute toxoplasmic encephalitis after starting HAART: a prospective multicenter longitudinal study. In: 10th Conference on Retroviruses and Opportunistic Infections, Boston, MA, 10–14 Feb 2003, abstract 796.
188. Ghosn J, Paris L, Ajzenberg D, et al. Atypical toxoplasmic manifestation after discontinuation of maintenance therapy in a human immunodeficiency virus type 1-infected patient with immune recovery. Clin Infect Dis. 37:e112, 2003.
189. D'Offizi G, Topino S, Anzidei G, et al. Primary *Toxoplasma gondii* infection in a pregnant human immunodeficiency virus-infected woman. Pediatr Infect Dis J 21:981, 2002.
190. Bachmeyer C, Mouchnino G, Thulliez P, Blum L. Congenital toxoplasmosis from an HIV-infected woman as a result of reactivation. J Infect 52:e55, 2006.
191. Jungmann EM, Mercey D, DeRuiter A, et al. Is first trimester exposure to the combination of antiretroviral therapy and folate antagonists a risk factor for congenital abnormalities? Sex Trans Inf 77:441, 2001.
192. Nogueira SA, Guedes AL, Machado ES, et al. Toxoplasmic encephalitis in an HIV-infected pregnant woman: successful outcome for both mother and child. Brazil J Infect Dis 6:201, 2002.
193. European Collaborative Study and Research Network on Congenital Toxoplasmosis. Low incidence of congenital toxoplasmosis in children born to women infected with human immunodeficiency virus. Eur J Obstet Gynecol Reprod Biol 68:93–96, 1996.
194. Wong S-Y, Remington JS. Toxoplasmosis in pregnancy. Clin Infect Dis 18:853, 1994.
195. Mofenson LM, Oleske J, Serchuck L, et al. Treating opportunistic infections among HIV-exposed and infected children. Recommendations from CDC, the National Institutes of Health, and the Infectious Diseases Society of America. MMWR Recomm Rep 53(RR-14):1, 2004.
196. Benenson MW, Takafuji ET, Lemon SM, et al. Oocyst-transmitted toxoplasmosis associated with ingestion of contaminated water. N Engl J Med 307:666, 1982.
197. Bowie WR, King AS, Werker DH, et al. Outbreak of toxoplasmosis associated with municipal drinking water. Lancet 350:173, 1997.
198. Wallace MR, Rossetti, Olson PE. Cats and toxoplasmosis risk in HIV-infected adults. JAMA 269:76, 1993.
199. Glaser CA, Angulo FJ, Rooney JA. Animal-associated opportunistic infections among persons infected with the human immunodeficiency virus. Clin Infect Dis 18:14, 1994.

Chapter 38

Cryptosporidia, Isospora, and Cyclospora Infections

Timothy P. Flanigan, MD, Christine A. Wanke, MD

It has only been since the recognition of the acquired immunodeficiency syndrome (AIDS) epidemic that the spore-forming protozoa that infect the gastrointestinal tract (*Cryptosporidium, Microsporidium, Isospora*, and *Cyclospora*) have been identified as significant, ubiquitous human pathogens. Initially, these pathogens were thought to cause only rare or esoteric infections; but it is now recognized that they infect both immunocompetent and immunodeficient hosts worldwide.[1–3] In many communities, infection with these parasites is the leading cause of chronic diarrheal illness. In the developing world, where more than 90% of human immunodeficiency virus (HIV)-infected patients live, diarrheal illness usually due to these protozoa is the most common opportunistic infection after tuberculosis.

The spectrum of illness caused by these enigmatic parasites is broad and is closely linked to host immunocompetence.[4] This explains why infections by these pathogens were first recognized in severely immunocompromised individuals with AIDS who presented with chronic diarrhea and wasting illness. Clearance of these intestinal pathogens is directly related to the ability to mount an effective immune response at the site of the infection, the intestinal mucosa. For example, among patients with cryptosporidiosis, the course of disease is directly related to the stage of immunodeficiency as measured by the CD4+ T-lymphocyte count.[4,5] What has become clear, with the widespread use of highly active antiretroviral therapy (HAART), is that the best therapy for some of these pathogens, such as that causing cryptosporidiosis, is augmentation of immune responses through direct suppression of HIV replication with antiretroviral agents.[6–9] The severity of illness with the two most common of these protozoal parasites, *Cryptosporidium* and *Microsporidium*, appears to be linked to improvement or deterioration of immune function related to suppression or activation of HIV. We have come full circle in that the HIV epidemic has uncovered many of the biologic, epidemiologic, and immunologic secrets of these protozoan infections among humans; and now better therapy for HIV is leading directly to curative treatment for patients with these protozoal parasites through immune restoration. This chapter deals with *Cryptosporidium, Isospora*, and *Cyclospora*. *Microsporidium* is addressed in Chapter 39. Table 38-1 highlights many of the similarities and differences among these three parasites.

CRYPTOSPORIDIUM

Clinical Presentation

Typically, acute infection with *Cryptosporidium* is characterized by watery diarrhea, crampy epigastric abdominal pain, weight loss, anorexia, malaise, and flatulence.[3,5] Diarrhea, the most noteworthy symptom, can range from a few loose bowel movements a day to more than 50 stools (more than 15 L) per day. Nausea and vomiting are common. Diarrhea and abdominal pain are usually exacerbated by eating, particularly with difficult-to-digest foods such as milk and dairy products or fatty foods. The spectrum of symptoms from infection varies widely; in fact, there are reports of asymptomatic shedding of *Cryptosporidium* for months after the primary infection.

In patients with severe immunodeficiency characterized by a CD4+ T-lymphocyte count well under 200 cells/mm^3, symptoms may begin insidiously with only mild diarrhea but then increase in severity over time. Many of these patients experience voluminous watery diarrhea, with a loss of more than 10% of total body weight. Severe malabsorption is the rule, and many patients avoid eating because it worsens the diarrhea and abdominal pain. Symptoms often remit for periods of time, but these respites are usually brief. Before the advent of HAART, most patients with AIDS never cleared the infection and so died with cryptosporidial diarrhea.

Comparison of Cryptosporidium Isospora and Cyclospora

Table 38-1

Similarities			
Biology	Protozoa Intracellular location in epithelial cells of the intestine Sporozoite infects the mucosa Spore or oocyst is shed in stool and transmits infection		
Epidemiology	Frequent cause of diarrhea in tropical regions and places with poor sanitation Acute diarrhea in children and immunocompetent hosts; chronic diarrhea in patients with AIDS		
Diagnosis	Microscopic stool examination Detection of cysts or spores requires expertise and proper stains		
	Cryptosporidium	**Isospora**	**Cyclospora**
Differences			
Morphology and fecal isolates	Oocysts: 4–6 μm, seen well with modified acid-fast stains	Oocysts: 20–30 μm, seen well on modified acid-fast stain and wet preparation	Oocysts: 8–10 μm, seen well on acid-fast stain and wet preparation
Morphology and small bowel biopsy specimens	Easily seen on light microscopy as 4 μm round blue dots on the apical membrane of the enterocyte	Easily seen on light microscopy as 20 μm oval blue enterocyte inclusions	Not seen well with light microscopy; reported with electron microscopy
Transmission	Fecal-oral, person to person, food- and water-borne	Presumably food- and water-borne	Food- and water-borne
Antibiotic treatment Acute disease	No consistently effective therapy; initiate HAART	Trimethoprim–sulfamethoxazole, one double-strength tablet twice daily for 7–10 days	Trimethoprim–sulfamethoxazole, one double-strength tablet twice daily for 7–10 days
	Consider Nitazoxanide 1000 mg PO bid for 14–21 days (Not likely effective: paromomycin 500–750 mg PO tid)	Alternative: Ciprofloxacin 500 mg PO bid 3 7–10 days	Alternative: Ciprofloxacin 500 mg PO bid 3 7–10 days
Chronic maintenance	None. Always continue and encourage HAART	Trimethoprim–sulfamethoxazole, one double-strength tablet tiw or qd	Trimethoprim–sulfamethoxazole, one double-strength tablet PO qd or tiw
		Alternative: Ciprofloxacin 500 mg PO qd	Alternative: Ciprofloxacin 500 mg PO qd

Cryptosporidial enteritis occurs in HIV-infected individuals who are immunologically competent, as determined by a normal CD4+ T-lymphocyte count. Those individuals have a clinical course similar to HIV-seronegative persons; they are able to clear the infection over a few days to a few weeks.[4,5] The median CD4+ T-lymphocyte count of individuals who develop chronic severe disease is well under 50 cells/mm^3,[5] whereas it appears that patients with CD4+ T-lymphocyte counts higher than 200 cells/mm^3 are able to clear cryptosporidial enteritis.[4]

A subset of patients with AIDS and cryptosporidiosis develop biliary tract involvement associated with right upper quadrant pain, nausea, and vomiting.[5,10] Laboratory examination is significant for elevated serum alkaline phosphatase and γ-glutamyl transferase levels. This is a difficult-to-treat complication in individuals with exceedingly low CD4+ T-lymphocyte counts and long-standing chronic cryptosporidial enteritis.[5,11] Endoscopic retrograde cholangiopancreatography (ERCP) may reveal dilatation of bile ducts with multiple luminal irregularities and distal duct strictures consistent with partial obstruction or sclerosing cholangitis.

Physical examination of individuals with cryptosporidial enteritis is usually unrevealing. Patients may have orthostatic hypotension and other signs of dehydration. Low-grade fever and mild leukocytosis are common. The abdomen is soft, with mild tenderness to palpation. Laboratory examination often reveals electrolyte disturbances consistent with diarrhea and dehydration. Fecal examination may reveal mucus, but blood and leukocytes are rarely seen. Charcot–Leyden crystals are characteristic of *Isospora belli* infection and amebiasis but not

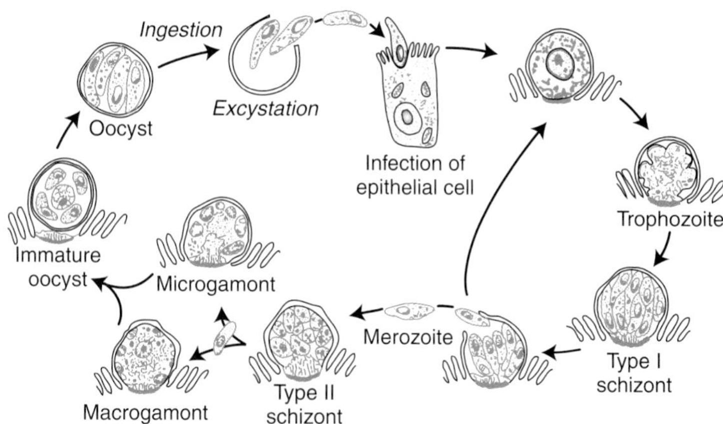

Figure 38-1 ■ Life cycle of *Cryptosporidium* species.
From Flanigan TP, Soave R. Cryptosporidiosis. Prog Clin Parasitol 3:1, 1993.

cryptosporidiosis.[2] Lactose intolerance and fat malabsorption are well documented, and the D-xylose test is abnormal. An abnormal D-xylose test correlates strongly with small intestinal infection with *Cryptosporidium* and *Microsporidium*.[12,13]

Biology

Cryptosporidium, Isospora belli, and *Cyclospora* are spore-forming sporozoa in the class of human protozoal pathogens.[1,3] Sporozoites are seen within oocysts and are the infectious form of the parasite.[14] *Cryptosporidium* infection has been identified in numerous species of animals, including mammals, fish, turkeys, and even reptiles such as rattlesnakes.[1]

Although the parasite was first described in 1907,[15] it received no clinical attention until it was recognized as a significant cause of diarrhea in domestic animals (e.g., cows, horses, pigs). The first human case was described in 1976,[16] but cryptosporidiosis was thought to be an esoteric illness until 1982, when the Centers for Disease Control (CDC) reported 21 homosexual men with severe diarrhea caused by *Cryptosporidium*.[17] It is now recognized that *Cryptosporidium* is the number one cause of protozoal diarrhea worldwide in both immunocompetent and immunodeficient persons.

Intestinal infection is initiated by ingestion of the oocysts, with subsequent excystation and release of four sporozoites from each oocyst in the gastrointestinal tract. Sporozoites implant immediately in the host epithelial cells and begin a cycle of autoinfection at the luminal surface of the epithelium. The sexual stage of the parasite results in oocysts, which are excreted in the stool and are immediately infectious to other hosts and can reinfect the same host, even without reingestion. Figure 38-1 shows the life cycle of *Cryptosporidium*. An infectious dose of *Cryptosporidium* is as low as 10 oocysts, thereby facilitating transmission.[18]

The most common site of *Cryptosporidium* infection is the small intestine, although it is frequently present in the colon and the biliary tract of persons with immunodeficiency.[2,12,13] *Cryptosporidium* infects only the epithelial surface of the mucosa; it does not invade the submucosal layer or cause ulcerations. Infection of the epithelial lining of the respiratory tract with associated cough has been reported, although it is uncommon.[1]

Cryptosporidium is a ubiquitous parasite; and transmission has been documented from animals to humans, from humans to humans (particularly in day-care centers), and from environmental sources such as water reservoirs.[1,19,20] Person-to-person transmission of *Cryptosporidium* is often underappreciated; outbreaks have been well documented in the hospital setting and in families. In Michigan, for example, 71% of families with a symptomatic child had other infected family members.[21,22] All individuals in the hospital setting with cryptosporidial diarrhea should follow enteric precautions, although isolation is not necessary to prevent roommate-to-roommate transmission.[23]

Cryptosporidium has been identified as the etiologic agent of several extensive water-borne outbreaks usually caused by surface-infected groundwater sources, often involving farm animals.[11] The oocyst is only 4 μm in diameter, making it difficult to clear through filtration, and it is resistant to routine chlorination.[19] The first documented water-borne outbreak (in San Antonio, Texas) had a 34% attack rate and was linked to sewage contamination of the well water supply, which was chlorinated but not filtered.[24] In 1987 an outbreak in Georgia resulted in an estimated 13 000 cases of cryptosporidial enteritis despite the filtered and chlorinated public supply that met the established Environmental Protection Agency guidelines.[20] Improved filtering of the water supply ultimately helped terminate the outbreak. An outbreak in Milwaukee, Wisconsin in 1993 afflicted some 375 000 residents when the spring runoff from grazing lands was not adequately filtered in the public water supply.[11,25] This massive environmental contamination led to severe illness with both small intestinal disease and biliary tract infection in HIV-infected patients with CD4+ T-lymphocyte counts under 50 cells/mm^3, and it resulted in a marked increase in morbidity and mortality in these patients.[11]

The recognition of *Cryptosporidum* as a pathogen of concern in HIV-infected patients in the resource-limited world has led to additional observations about the clinical presentation of cryptosporidial disease. Early in the HIV epidemic, cryptosporidial diarrheal illness was considered a severe and relatively untreatable disease due to an opportunisitic pathogen. The disease is more severe in those individuals in whom immune compromise was more advanced. Recently, with advances in diagnostic techniques and better surveillance, the asymptomatic carriage of cryptosporidial organisms has been recognized in a variety of settings.[26–28] In the setting of asymptomatic carriage of cryptosporidium in the noncompromised host, there are suggestive data that this carriage may compromise nutritional status in children, even in the absence of diarrheal illness.[29] Recent studies have also suggested that HIV-infected patients with severe immune compromise may carry cryptosporidial organisms asymptomatically.[30,31] The extent and impact of asymptomatic carriage of cryptosporidial organisms and the species and genotype of organisms carried asymptomatically in HIV-infected patients requires further study.

Diagnosis

The diagnosis of *Cryptosporidium* is primarily based on identifying the oocysts in stool.[32] Oocysts stain red with varying intensities with a modified acid-fast technique; this technique allows differentiation of the *Cryptosporidium* oocysts from yeasts that are similar in size and shape but not acid-fast. Oocysts can also be detected by direct immunofluorescence assays that are commercially available utilizing monoclonal antibodies raised to *Cryptosporidium* antigens.[33] In addition, an enzyme-linked immunosorbent assay may be used to detect *Cryptosporidium* in fecal specimens and tissues.[34,35] There is no consensus on the optimal oocyst detection method in fecal samples, although one comparison of a modified acid-fast stain and a fluorescein-labeled monoclonal antibody technique showed comparability for diarrheal samples but improved detection with the immunofluorescence method for formed specimens.[26,36] Cryptosporidial enteritis can also be diagnosed on small intestinal biopsy sections by identifying developmental stages, found individually or in clusters, on the brush border of the mucosal epithelial surfaces.[36] Organisms project into the lumen because of their intracellular but extracytoplasmic nature, and they appear basophilic with hematoxylin and eosin staining. Electron microscopy allows resolution of cellular detail.

While not generally available clinically at present, a number of genetic loci have been identified as targets for detection of cryptosporodial isolates as well as genotype determination. Polymerase chain reaction (PCR) methods are exquisitely sensitive for detection of organisms, either from stool samples or environmental samples. These methods may detect as few as 1–10 oocysts or as many as 80 oocysts in a gram of stool. Thus while these methods are sensitive and specific, and may ultimately be used to more readily screen large numbers of samples for presence and genotype of the cryptosporidial organisms present, there are technical issues which preclude their routine clinical use. These technical issues should be resolved and PCR based diagnostics will likely be used in clinical practice in the near future.[37]

In individuals with profuse diarrheal illness, a single tool specimen is usually adequate for the diagnosis. In individuals with less severe disease, repeat stool sampling is recommended, although there have been no controlled studies showing the utility of three consecutive stool samples as is the case for *Giardia* infection.

Treatment

Standard dogma is that there is no reliable palliative or curative treatment for severe cryptosporidiosis in immunodeficient hosts. Until the widespread use of HAART, patients with severe immunodeficiency characterized by CD4+ T-lymphocyte counts under 50 cells/mm^3 and chronic cryptosporidial diarrhea had little hope of ever eradicating the infection and living a normal life. Many of these patients were treated with intravenous hyperalimentation for life to reverse the severe wasting and chronic dehydration resulting from massive cryptosporidial infection of the small intestine.

With the availability of HAART, it is now commonplace for patients with severe diarrhea who can, to take combination antiretroviral agents and achieve viral suppression to clear *Cryptosporidium* infection.[6–9] HAART can result in complete, sustained clinical, microbiologic, and histologic resolution of HIV-associated cryptosporidiosis and microsporidiosis. Presumably, this is due to arresting HIV replication with subsequent rises in CD4+ T-lymphocyte counts and restoration of immunocompetence.

Interestingly enough, it is not clear what specific elements of the immune system are required for control of cryptosporidiosis, although clinical and experimental data implicate both humoral and cellular immunity.[38] The importance of antibody-mediated immunity is suggested by the fact that immunocompromised patients with congenital hypogammaglobulinemia may develop severe chronic disease.[39] Clinical and experimental data indicate that antibodies at the mucosal surface play an important role. For example, hyperimmune cow colostrum obtained from cows hyperimmunized with *Cryptosporidium* has been used successfully to treat individual cases of chronic disease.[40,41] In the murine model of infection, both monoclonal and polyclonal antibodies directed against sporozoite surface antigens have been successful in preventing infection.[42] In addition, experimental data in Balb-c mice infected with cryptosporidia indicate that both systemic CD4+ T-lymphocyte cells and interferon-α are important in protective immune responses.[43]

Initial treatment of individuals with *Cryptosporidium* infection should be directed toward symptomatic treatment of diarrhea. Rehydration and repletion of electrolyte losses orally or intravenously is of paramount importance. Severe diarrhea, which may be more than 10L/day in patients with AIDS, often requires intensive support. Aggressive efforts at oral rehydration should be made with Gatorade, bouillon, or oral rehydration solution that contains glucose, sodium bicarbonate, and potassium. Often intravenous repletion of fluids and electrolytes is essential to correct losses of bicarbonate, potassium, magnesium, and phosphorus. Treatment with antimotility agents often provides temporary relief and may play an important adjunctive role in therapy, but these agents are not consistently effective. Treatment with loperamide or tincture of opium often palliates symptoms of severe illness. Octreotide, a synthetic octapeptide analog of naturally occurring somatostatin that is approved for the treatment of secreting tumor-induced diarrhea, is no more effective than other oral antidiarrheal agents.[44] More than 95 interventional agents have been tried for the treatment of cryptosporidiosis with no consistent success, including drugs effective against other parasites and protozoa.

Nitazoxanide (trade name Alinia) is a synthetic antiprotozoal agent approved for oral administration for the treatment of *Giardia lamblia* and cryptosporidiosis in HIV-negative individuals. Nitazoxanide is rapidly converted to the active metabolite tizoxanide, which inhibits the enzyme dependent electron transfer reaction, which is essential to anaerobic energy metabolism. Tizoxanide directly interferes with the pyruvate: ferredoxin oxidoreductase enzyme in both Giardia and Cryptosporidium. Nitazoxanide has been approved for treatment of diarrhea due to Cryptosporidium or *Giardia lamblia* in HIV-negative children. Diarrheal symptoms resolve much more rapidly on nitazoxanide compared to placebo after 3 days of therapy (100 mg bid in pediatric patients ages 12 through 47 months, and 200 mg bid in pediatric patients ages 4 through 11 among children with cryptosporidiosis).[45] A double blind, placebo-controlled study of a 3 day course of nitazoxanide among severely malnourished pediatric patients with AIDS in Zambia resulted in similar response rates between placebo and nitazoxanide.[46] Adults with AIDS in Zambia treated with 1000 mg twice daily for 17 days had improvement in diarrhea but there was no difference in parasitologic clearance or mortality compared to placebo.[47] Adverse reactions are few (usually abdominal pain and diarrhea, which is hard to distinguish from the underlying illness). Higher doses or longer duration of therapy might prove more effective in patients with AIDS. Nonetheless, the cornerstone of therapy for cryptosporidial related disease for patients with AIDS must be HAART.

Paromomycin, a nonabsorbable aminoglycoside with *in vitro* activity against *Cryptosporidium*,[48,49] is indicated for the treatment of intestinal amebiasis. At extremely high doses paromomycin is effective in the treatment of animal models of cryptosporidiosis. The commonly used human dose (500 mg qid) is a fraction of this amount. A meta-analysis of 11 paromomycin studies reported a response rate of 67%. Relapse data are sparse, however, and the long-term success rates dropped to 33%.[50] A randomized study of paromomycin (500 mg qid × 21 days) in patients with AIDS showed it to be no more effective than placebo.[50] The high incidence of death in this trial is a clear reminder of the life-threatening nature of this infection in patients with advanced HIV disease in which immunosuppression cannot be reversed by HAART. At present there is no consistently effective pharmacologic or immunologic therapy directed specifically against *Cryptosporidium* among patients with AIDS.[2]

In HIV-positive patients who present with *Cryptosporidium*, initial efforts should be directed at restoring fluid and electrolyte balance and controlling symptoms with antidiarrheal agents. Infections with other pathogens must be ruled out because co-infection with *Clostridium difficile*, other bacterial pathogens, or some protozoa is not uncommon. Many of these co-infections respond to specific therapies. Once patients are rehydrated and electrolyte balance is restored, efforts should be directed at obtaining optimal HIV suppression with HAART.[6–9] This is certainly challenging because the symptoms of *Cryptosporidium* (including nausea, vomiting, abdominal pain, and diarrhea) may discourage all but the hardiest and most highly motivated patients from taking many pills a day. Close coaching by the physician and the patient's understanding of the importance of viral suppression, with resultant immune restoration and resolution of symptoms, is critical.

Prevention

Infection control measures are limited by resistance of the *Cryptosporidium* oocysts to common disinfectants. Ammonia, sodium hypochlorite, and formalin have been used in the laboratory setting.[1] In households, washing infected surfaces with bleach provides effective decontamination. Enteric precautions with good hygiene (e.g., hand washing) and proper disposal of contaminated materials (e.g., diapers) are important. Boiled or bottled drinking water should be considered by HIV-infected persons with CD4+ T-lymphocyte counts of less than 200 cells/mm^3 because the present drinking water purification standards do not uniformly destroy viable oocysts, and the infectious dose is small.[51] This is particularly important when surface contamination may occur in water sources such as during spring runoff or in households using well water. If personal-use water filters are utilized, they should be capable of removing particles 1 μm in diameter.[51] HIV-infected persons who travel in developing countries should meticulously avoid drinking tap water and contaminated water resources. At-risk persons should avoid contact with obvious sources of *Cryptosporidium* oocysts, such as other infected humans (especially regarding sexual practices that involve oral exposure to feces), farm animals (particularly cattle), and domestic pets that are extremely young (<6 months), have diarrhea, or have been strays.

Interestingly, in a large outpatient HIV study, patients who were receiving therapy or chemoprophylaxis for mycobacterial disease with rifabutin or clarithromycin were significantly protected against developing cryptosporidiosis. The prophylactic efficacy of either drug was 75% or more.[52] Another study, however, found rifabutin but not clarithromycin to be protective[53]; therefore the data are conflicting on this point and neither drug is currently recommended for prevention of cryptosporidiosis.

ISOSPORA

In normal hosts, symptomatic illness caused by *Isospora* is usually characterized by 3 days to 3 weeks of diarrhea, abdominal pain, and occasionally nausea, vomiting, and fever.[3] The pattern of clinical illness resulting from *Isospora* infection depends on the host's immunocompetence. It is impossible to differentiate isosporiasis from cryptosporidiosis clinically. Symptomatic illness in immunocompromised hosts, including patients with AIDS, results in protracted, severe diarrhea associated with malabsorption and dehydration.[54] Microscopic examination of the small bowel in patients infected with *Isospora* demonstrates shortened villi and infiltration of the lamina propria with inflammatory cells, particularly eosinophils.[55]

Isospora is rarely identified as a cause of AIDS-associated diarrhea in the United States and Europe (fewer than 1% of cases), whereas in Africa, Asia, Haiti, and Latin America it is a frequent cause of AIDS-related diarrhea.[3] The environmental reservoirs of *Isospora* are not well understood. There is no evidence that human *Isospora* can infect animals other than humans. All phases of the life cycle occur within the human small intestine, with the release of immature, unsporulated oocysts in the feces that are initially noninfective and then, within a few days, become infective as sporulation occurs. Transmission therefore is presumed to be via food and water contamination with human feces.

The diagnosis is made by identifying oocysts in stool by examination of a wet mount or by acid-fast staining of stool concentrates. *Isospora* is easily distinguished from *Cryptosporidium* and *Cyclospora* by its large size. Multiple stool samples may be necessary because shedding can be intermittent. Peripheral blood eosinophils and Charcot-Leyden crystals have been reported in the stool of patients with *Isospora* infection.

Treatment for *Isospora* infection (Table 38-1) is easily accomplished with a 7- to 10-day course of trimethoprim–sulfamethoxazole (one double-strength tablet twice daily), which is effective in both immunocompetent and immunodeficient hosts, including patients with AIDS.[54–56] Ciprofloxacin 500 mg PO bid is an effective alternative.[57] Most patients with AIDS relapse within 1–2 months of stopping therapy; and suppressive therapy with daily trimethoprim–sulfamethoxazole (one double-strength tablet qd or tid) or ciprofloxacin (500 mg PO qd) is recommended. It is presumed that once CD4+ T-lymphocyte counts are well over 200, suppression therapy may be discontinued.

CYCLOSPORA

The first case of human *Cyclospora* infection was reported in 1979 from Papua, New Guinea, but this protozoan did not garner much attention until 1993, when it was recognized that an acid-fast stain of stool could identify the oocysts, and therefore made the diagnosis significantly easier.[58,59] In 1996 and 1997 there was an explosive increase in cases caused by multiple outbreaks primarily from food-borne contamination.[59] Prior to 1996 there were only three reported outbreaks in the United States. From May through August of 1996, more than 1400 cases of cyclosporiasis had been reported throughout the United States and Canada, of which more than 60% were laboratory-confirmed.[60] No deaths have been reported. Outbreaks in 1996 and 1997 were due, most notably, to fresh raspberries imported from Central America, mesclun lettuce, and basil. In all probability, *Cyclospora* has been a cause of diarrheal outbreaks in the past but was unrecognized.

The parasite was not named until 1993, and many of its hosts are still unknown.[58,61] Previous underdiagnosis of *Cyclospora* has probably been due to the following factors. It is an unknown infection to many physicians; clinical laboratories do not routinely screen for *Cyclospora* unless it is requested; shedding of *Cyclospora* is intermittent; and acid-fast staining may be relatively insensitive for detecting the oocysts because of variable uptake of stains.

After ingestion of *Cyclospora*, diarrhea occurs in 1–11 days.[58,59] Diarrhea due to *Cyclospora* is similar to that induced by *Cryptosporidium* and *Isospora*, although upper gastrointestinal symptoms may initially predominate. Patients have reported watery diarrhea alternating with constipation. Nausea, abdominal cramping, anorexia, weight loss, and vomiting are frequent. The illness is self-limiting in immunocompetent individuals, although it may last for weeks. In immunocompromised hosts, particularly patients with AIDS, diarrhea is prolonged, severe, and associated with a high rate of recurrence.[61] *Cyclospora* may infect the biliary tract much like *Cryptosporidium*. The small intestine is the primary site of infection. Villous atrophy and crypt hyperplasia are found in the infected jejunum, as is common with *Cryptosporidium* and *Isospora*.

Cyclospora resembles *Isospora* in that its oocysts are excreted unsporulated and require days to weeks outside the intestinal tract for maturation and to gain infective potential.[62] The oocyst of *Cyclospora* is round, much like that of *Cryptosporidium*, and is 8–10 μm in diameter.[58,59] Early on, *Cyclospora* was called *Cryptosporidium grande*, or large *Cryptosporidium*, because of its *Cryptosporidium*-like appearance and its approximately double size. It may be necessary to use a micrometer to make the correct diagnosis. Like the oocysts of *Cryptosporidium* and *Isospora*, the oocysts of *Cyclospora* can be seen using one of many acid-fast staining techniques, including the modified Ziehl–Nielsen or the Kinyoun acid-fast stain. Stool specimens examined for ova and parasites usually are not examined for *Cyclospora* unless it is specifically requested. Alternatively, stool specimens can be fixed in 10% formalin and examined with an epifluorescence microscope, and oocytes are easily discernible by autofluorescence.[63]

Cyclospora has been implicated in water-borne outbreaks in the United States and the developing world. The methods used to prevent water-borne transmission of cryptosporidiosis should be followed to prevent *Cyclospora* infection. Transmission via contaminated raw food as well as raw beef has been reported. Raw fruits and vegetables should be washed thoroughly. In the developing world, infection may increase during the rainy season, as was documented in Nepal.[64] This would not be surprising because seasonal variation is common among other environmental protozoal infections. In Haiti, more than 10% of HIV-infected adults with chronic diarrhea have *Cyclospora* infection.[61] Much like *Isospora*, it appears to be an uncommon cause of diarrhea in adults with AIDS in the United States and Europe.

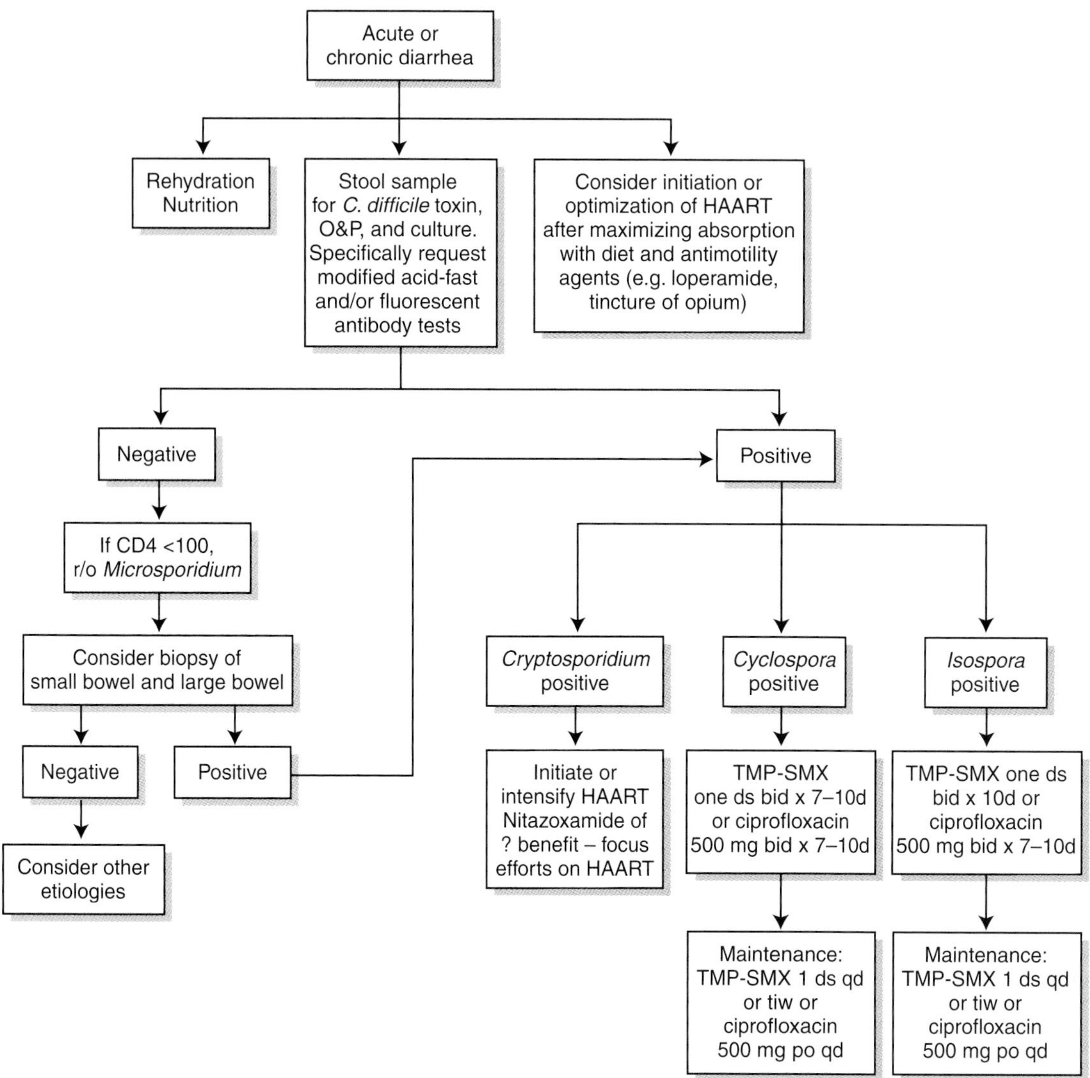

Figure 38-2 ■ Algorithm for managing cryptosporidiosis, isosporidosis, and cyclosporiasis. TMP-SMX, trimethoprim–sulfamethoxazole; DS, double strength; HAART, highly active antiretroviral therapy.

Treatment of patients with *Cyclospora* (Table 38-1) is effective using trimethoprim–sulfamethoxazole double-strength twice daily for immunocompetent and immunodeficient hosts.[61,64] Ciprofloxacin 500 mg PO bid for 10 days is an effective alternative.[57] Secondary prophylaxis with trimethoprim–sulfamethoxazole (one double-strength tablet qd or tid) or ciprofloxacin (500 mg PO qd) is effective for preventing relapse.

An algorithm for the management of infections with *Cryptosporidium, Isospora*, and *Cyclospora* is presented in Figure 38-2.

REFERENCES

1. Fayer E (ed). Cryptosporidium and Cryptosporidiosis. 2nd edn. Boca Raton, FL: CRC Press; 1997.
2. Flanigan TP, Soave R. Cryptosporidiosis. Prog Clin Parasitol 3:1, 1993.
3. Goodgame RW. Understanding intestinal spore-forming protozoa: Cryptosporidia, Microsporidia, Isospora, and Cyclospora. Ann Intern Med 124:429, 1996.
4. Flanigan TP, Whalen C, Toerner J, et al. Cryptosporidium infection and CD4 + T-lymphocyte counts. Ann Intern Med 116:840, 1992.
5. Hashmey R, Smith NH, Cron S, et al. Cryptosporidiosis in Houston, Texas: a report of 95 cases. Medicine 76:118, 1997.
6. Grube H, Ramratnam B, Ley C, et al. Resolution of AIDS associated cryptosporidiosis after treatment with indinavir. Am J Gastroenterol 92:726, 1997.
7. Milono MD, Tashima KT, Farrar D, et al. Resolution of AIDS-related opportunistic infections with HARRT. AIDS Read Winter:21, 1998.
8. Miao YM, Avad-El-Kariem FM, Franzen C, et al. Eradication of cryptosporidia and microsporidia following successful antiretroviral therapy. J AIDS 25:124, 2000.
9. Carr A, Marriott D, Field A, et al. Treatment of HIV-associated microsporidiosis and cryptosporidiosis with combination antiretroviral therapy. Lancet 351:256, 1998.
10. Ducreux M, Buffet C, Lamy P, et al. Diagnosis and prognosis of AIDS related cholangitis. AIDS 9:875, 1995.

11. Vakil NB, Schwartz SM, Buggy BP, et al. Biliary cryptosporidiosis in HIV-infected people after the waterborne outbreak of cryptosporidiosis in Milwaukee. N Engl J Med 334:19, 1996.
12. Kotler D, Francisco A, Clayton F, et al. Small intestinal injury and parasitic diseases in AIDS. Ann Intern Med 113:444, 1990.
13. Kotler D, Francisco A, Clayton F, et al. Effects of enteric parasitoses and HIV infection upon small intestinal structure and function in patients with AIDS. J Clin Gastroenterol 16:10, 1993.
14. Clark DP, Sears CL. The pathogenesis of cryptosporidiosis. Parasitol Today 12:221, 1996.
15. Tyzzer EF. A sporozoan found in the peptic glands of the common mouse. Proc Soc Exp Biol Med 5:12, 1907.
16. Nime FA, Burek JD, Page DL, et al. Acute enterocolitis in a human being infected with the protozoan Cryptosporidium. Gastroenterology 70:592, 1976.
17. Anonymous. Cryptosporidiosis: assessment of chemotherapy of males with acquired immunodeficiency syndrome (AIDS). MMWR Morb Mortal Wkly Rep 31:589, 1982.
18. DuPont HL, Chappell CL, Sterling CR, et al. The infectivity of Cryptosporidium parvum in healthy volunteers. N Engl J Med 332:855, 1995.
19. Widmer G, Carraway M, Tzipori S. Water-borne Cryptosporidium: a perspective from the U.S.A. Parasitol Today 12:109, 1996.
20. Hayes EB, Matte TD, O'Brien TR, et al. Large community outbreak of cryptosporidiosis due to contamination of a filtered public water supply. N Engl J Med 320:1372, 1989.
21. Anonymous. Cryptosporidiosis among children attending daycare centers Georgia, Pennsylvania, Michigan, California, New Mexico. MMWR Morb Mortal Wkly Rep 33:599, 1984.
22. Combee CL, Collinge ML, Britt EM. Cryptosporidiosis in a hospital-associated day care center. Pediatr Infect Dis J 5:528, 1986.
23. Bruce BB, Blass MA, Blumberg HM, et al. Risk of Cryptosporidium parvum transmission between hospital roommates. Clin Infect Dis 31:947, 2000.
24. D'Antonio RG, Winn RE, Taylor JP, et al. A waterborne outbreak of cryptosporidiosis in normal hosts. Ann Intern Med 103:886, 1985.
25. MacKenzie WR, Hoxie NJ, Proctor ME, et al. A massive outbreak in Milwaukee of Cryptosporidium infection transmitted through the public water supply. N Engl J Med 331:161, 1994.
26. Ananthasubramanian M, Ananthan S, Vennila R, Bhanu S. Cryptosporidium in AIDS patients in south India: a laboratory investigation. J Commun Dis 29:29–33, 1997.
27. Esteban JG, Aguirre C, Flores A, et al. High Cryptosporidium prevalences in healthy Aymara children from the northern Bolivian Altiplano. Am J Trop Med and Hyg 58: 50, 1998.
28. Palit A, Sur D, MitraDhar K, Saha MR. Asymptomatic Cryptosporidiosis in a periurban slum setting in Kolkata India, a pilot study. Jpn J Infect Dis 58:110, 2005.
29. Checkley W, Gilman RH, Epstein LD, et al. Asymptomatic and symptomatic cryptosporidiosis: their acute effect on weight gain in Peruvian children. Am J Epidemiol 145:156–163, 1997.
30. Pettoelle-Mantovani M, Di Martino L, Dettori G, et al. Asymptomatic carriage of intestinal cryptosporidium in immunocompetent and immunodeficient children: a prospective study. Pediatr Infect Dis J 14:1042, 1995.
31. Hooupt ER, Bushen OY, Sam NE, et al. Short report: asymptomatic cryptosporidium hominis infection among human immunodeficiency virus infected patients in Tanzania. Am J Trop Med Hyg 73:520, 2005
32. Ungar BLP. Cryptosporidium. In: Mandell GL, Bennett JE, Dolin R (eds). Principles and Practice of Infectious Diseases. 4th edn. New York: Churchill Livingstone; 1995, p 2500.
33. Sterling CR, Arrowood MD. Detection of Cryptosporidium sp. infection using a direct immunofluorescence assay. Pediatr Infect Dis J 5(Suppl):S139, 1986.
34. Ungar BLP. Enzyme-linked immunoassay for detection for Cryptosporidium antigens in fecal specimens. J Clin Microbiol 28:2491, 1990.
35. Bonnin A, Petrella T, Dubremetz JF, et al. Histopathological method for diagnosis of cryptosporidiosis using monoclonal antibodies. Eur J Clin Microbiol Infect Dis 9:664, 1990.
36. Weber R, Bryan RT, Bishop HS, et al. Threshold of detection of Cryptosporidium oocysts in human stool specimens: evidence for low sensitivity of current diagnostic methods. J Clin Microbiol 29:1323, 1991.
37. O'Conner RM, Mackay MR, Ward HD. Molecular approaches for detection, species identification and genotyping of Cryptosporidium. In: Persing DH (Editor in Chief). Molecular Microbiology Diagnostic Principles and Practice. ASM Press; Seattle, Washington 2004, pp 583–597.
38. Flanigan TP. HIV infection and cryptosporidiosis: protective immune responses. Am J Trop Med Hyg 50(Suppl):29, 1994.
39. Lasser KH, Lewin KJ, Ryning FW. Cryptosporidial diarrhea in a patient with congenital hypogammaglobulinemia. Hum Pathol 10:234, 1979.
40. Ungar BLP, Ward DJ, Fayer R, et al. Cessation of Cryptosporidium associated diarrhea in an acquired immunodeficiency syndrome patient after treatment with hyperimmune bovine colostrum. Gastroenterology 98:486, 1990.
41. Tzipori S, Robertson D, Chapman C. Remission of diarrhea due to cryptosporidiosis in an immunodeficient child treated with hyperimmune bovine colostrum. BMJ 293:2283, 1986.
42. Arrowood MJ, Mead J, Mahrt JL, et al. Effects of immune colostrum and orally administered antisporozoite monoclonal antibodies on the outcome of Cryptosporidium parvum in neonatal mice. Infect Immun 57:2283, 1989.
43. Ungar BLP, Kao TC, Burris JA, et al. Independent roles for IFN-gamma and CD4 lymphocytes in protective immunity. J Immunol 147:1014, 1991.
44. Simon DM, Cello JP, Valenzuela J, et al. Multicenter trial of octreotide in patients with refractory acquired immunodeficiency syndrome-associated diarrhea. Gastroenterology 108:1753, 1995.
45. Rossignol JF, Ayoub A, Ayers MS. Treatment of diarrhea cause by Cryptosporidium parvum: a prospective, randomized, double blind, placebo-controlled study of nitazoxanide. J Infect Dis 184:103, 2001.
46. Zulu I, Kelly P, Njobvu L, et al. Nitazoxanide for persistent diarrhoea in Zambian acquired immunodeficiency syndrome patients: a randomized-controlled trial. Aliment Pharmacol Ther 21(6):757, 2005.
47. Zulu I, Kelly P, Njobvu L, et al. A randomized-controlled trial of nitazoxanide for the syndromic treatment of AIDS related persistent diarrhoea. Gut 54(Suppl II):A104, 2005.
48. Marshall MS, Flanigan TP. Paromomycin inhibits Cryptosporidium infection of a human enterocyte cell line. J Infect Dis 165:772, 1992.
49. White AC Jr, Chappell CL, Hayat CS, et al. Paromomycin for cryptosporidiosis in AIDS: a prospective, double-blind trial. J Infect Dis 170:419, 1994.
50. Hewitt RG, Yiannoutsos CT, Higgs ES, et al. Paromomycin: no more effective than placebo for treatment of cryptosporidiosis in patients with advanced human immunodeficiency virus infection. Clin Infect Dis 31:1084, 2000.
51. Centers for Disease Control and Prevention. 1997 USPHS/IDSA guidelines for prevention of opportunistic infections in persons infected with human immunodeficiency virus. MMWR Morb Mortal Wkly Rep 46(RR-12):5, 1997.
52. Holmberg SD, Moorman AC, Von Bargen JC, et al. Possible effectiveness of clarithromycin and rifabutin for cryptosporidiosis chemoprophylaxis in HIV diseases. JAMA 279:384, 1998.
53. Fichtenbaum CJ, Zactin R, Feinberg J, et al. Rifabutin but not clarithromycin prevents cryptosporidiosis in persons with advanced HIV infection. AIDS 14:2889, 2000.

54. DeHovitz JA, Pape JW, Boncy M, et al. Clinical manifestations and therapy of Isospora belli infection in patients with the acquired immunodeficiency syndrome. N Engl J Med 315:87, 1986.
55. Keystone JS, Kozarsky P. Isospora belli, Sarcocystis species, Blastocystis hominis, and Cyclospora. In: Mandell GL, Bennett JE, Dolin R (eds) Principles and Practice of Infectious Diseases. 5th edn2. New York: Churchill Livingstone, 2000; p 2915.
56. Pape JW, Verdier RI, Johnson WD Jr. Treatment and prophylaxis of Isospora belli infection in patients with the acquired immunodeficiency syndrome. N Engl J Med 320:1044, 1989.
57. Verdier RI, Fitzgerald DW, Johnson WD Jr, Pape JW. Trimethoprim/sulfamethoxazole compared with ciprofloxacin for treatment and prophylaxis of Isospora belli and Cyclospora cayetanensis infection in HIV-infected patients: a randomized, controlled trial: brief communication. Ann Intern Med 132:885, 2000.
58. Soave R. Cyclospora: an overview. Clin Infect Dis 23:429, 1996.
59. Ortega Y, Sterling CR, Gilman RH, et al. Cyclospora species, a new protozoan pathogen of humans. N Engl J Med 328:1308, 1996.
60. Massachusetts Medical Society. Outbreak of cyclosporiasis-Northern Virginia, Washington, DC, Baltimore, Maryland, metropolitan area. MMWR Morb Mortal Wkly Rep 46:689, 1997.
61. Pape JW, Verdier RI, Boncy M, et al. Cyclospora infection in adults infected with HIV: clinical manifestations, treatment, and prophylaxis. Ann Intern Med 121:654, 1994.
62. Herwaldt BL. Cyclospora cayetanensis: a review, focusing on the outbreaks of cyclosporiasis in the 1990s: emerging infections. Clin Infect Dis 31:1040, 2000.
63. Berlin OGW, Peter JB, Gagne C, et al. Autofluorescence and the detection of Cyclospora oocysts. Emerg Infect Dis 4:127, 1998.
64. Hoge CW, Shlim DR, Ghmire M, et al. Placebo-controlled trial of clotrimoxazole for Cyclospora infections among travelers and foreign residents in Nepal. Lancet 345:691, 1990.

Chapter 39

Microsporidiosis

Louis M. Weiss, MD, MPH

Microsporidia is a nontaxonomic designation used to refer to a group of obligate, intracellular parasites belonging to the phylum Microsporidia.[1,2] The Microsporidia are ubiquitous organisms that are emerging pathogens in humans. They are most likely zoonotic or waterborne infections (or both).[3] In the immunosuppressed host (e.g., those treated with immunosuppressive drugs or infected with the human immunodeficiency virus (HIV), particularly at advanced stages of these diseases) microsporidia can produce a wide range of clinical diseases. While the most common manifestation is gastrointestinal tract infection; encephalitis, ocular infection, sinusitis, myositis, and disseminated infection are also described. These organisms have also been reported in immunocompetent individuals.

In 1857 *Nosema bombycis*, a parasite of silkworms, was the first organism identified as belonging to the order Microsporidia,[1,4] and in 1959 Microsporidia were identified as etiologic in human infection.[5] The Microsporidia are important agricultural parasites in insects, fish, laboratory rodents, rabbits, fur-bearing animals, and primates.[1,4,6] They have been described in dogs and birds kept as household pets.[6,7] In their hosts most infect the digestive tract, although reproductive, respiratory, muscle, excretory, and nervous system infections have been documented.[4,6,8,9]

The phylum Microspora contains more than 1100 species distributed into at least 150 genera, of which the following have been demonstrated to cause human disease (Table 39-1)[4,6,8,9]: *Nosema* (*N. corneum* renamed *Vittaforma corneae*[10] and *N. algerae* renamed *Bracheola algerae*)[11] *Pleistophora*, *Encephalitozoon*, *Enterocytozoon*,[12] *Septata*[13] (reclassified as *Encephalitozoon*),[14] *Trachipleistophora*[15,16] and *Brachiola*[11] (recently reclassified as *Anncaliia*).[17] In addition, the genus *Microsporidium* has been used to designate Microsporidia of uncertain taxonomic status.[6] *Vittaforma corneae*,[18] *Encephalitozoon cuniculi*,[4] *Encephalitozoon hellem*,[19] *Trachipleistophora hominis*,[15] and *Encephalitozoon intestinalis*[20,21] have been cultivated in tissue culture systems *in vitro*. *Enterocytozoon bieneusi* has not been cultivated continuously *in vitro*, although limited *in vitro* cultivation has been reported.[22] Adenovirus can mimic the

Table 39-1 Microsporidia Identified as Pathogenic to Humans

Identified in Patients with AIDS

Encephalitozoon	*Pleistophora ronneafiei*
Enc. cuniculi	*Brachiola* (now classified as Anncaliia)
Enc. hellem	*B. vesicularum*
Enc. intestinalis (previously classified as *Septata intestinalis*)	*B. (Nosema) algerae*
Enterocytozoon bieneusi	*B. (Nosema) connori*
Trachipleistophora	
T. hominis	
T. anthropopthera	

Identified in Other Patients

Encephalitzoon	*Nosema*
Enc. cuniculi	*N. ocularum*
Enc. hellem	*Vittaforma cornea* (previously classified as *Nosema corneum*)
Enc. intestinalis	*Microsporidium*
Enterocytozoon bieneusi	*M. africanus*
Pleistophora sp.	*M. ceylonesis*
Brachiola	
B. (Nosema) algerae	

cytopathologic effect of Microsporidia.[23] *N. salmonis (Nucleospora)*, an organism related to *Ent. bieneusi*, can be grown *in vitro*.[24,25] Experimental infection of simian immunodeficiency virus (SIV)-infected rhesus monkeys with *Ent. bieneusi* from human tissue has been demonstrated.[26]

Enc. hellem has been associated with superficial keratoconjunctivitis, sinusitis, respiratory disease, prostatic abscesses, and disseminated infection.[4,6,8,9] *Enc. cuniculi* has been associated with hepatitis, encephalitis, and disseminated disease.[27–30] *Encephalitozoon (Septata) intestinalis* is associated with diarrhea, disseminated infection, and superficial keratoconjunctivitis.[6,13,31] *Nosema*, *Vittaforma*, and *Microsporidium* have been associated with stromal keratitis associated with trauma in immunocompetent hosts.[9,18] *Pleistophora*, *Brachiola*, and *Trachipleistophora* have been associated with myositis.[6,11,15,32–34] *Trachipleistophora* has been associated with encephalitis and disseminated disease.[15,16,35] *Ent. bieneusi*, originally described in humans,[12] is associated with malabsorption, diarrhea, and cholangitis.[6,36]

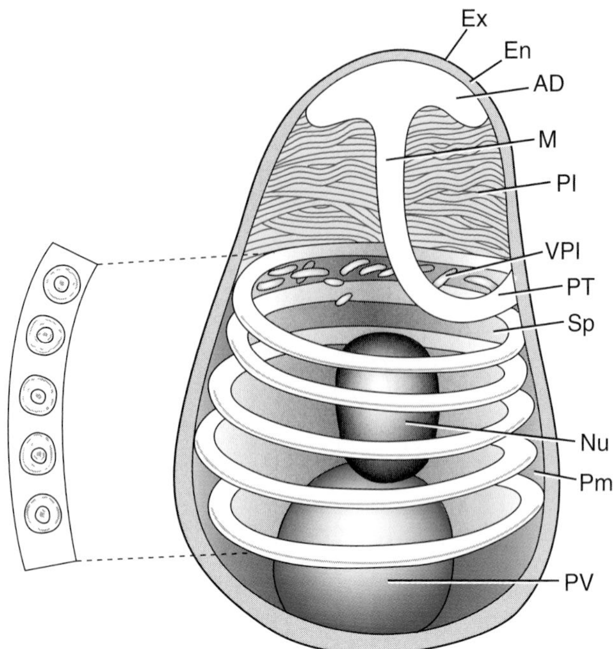

Figure 39-1 ■ Structure of a microsporidian spore. Depending on the species, the size of the spore can vary from 1 to 10 μm, and the number of polar tubule coils can vary from a few to 30 or more. Extrusion apparatus consists of the polar tube (PT), vesiculotubular polaroplast (Vpl), lamellar polaroplast (Pl), anchoring disk (AD), and manubrium (M). This organelle is characteristic of the Microsporidia. A cross section of the coiled polar tube is illustrated. The nucleus (Nu) may be single (e.g., in *Encephalitozoon* and *Enterocytozoon*) or a pair of abutted nuclei termed a diplokaryon (e.g., in *Nosema*). The plasma membrane (Pm) separates the spore coat from the sporoplasm (Sp), which contains ribosomes in a coiled helical array. En, endospore, an inner thicker electron-lucent region; Ex, exospore, an outer electron-dense region; PV, posterior vacuole, a membrane-bound structure.

Reprinted from Wittner M, Weiss LM (eds). The Microsporidia and Microsporidiosis. Washington, DC, ASM Press; 1999.

GENERAL CHARACTERISTICS

The Microsporidia are true eukaryotes, containing a nucleus with a nuclear envelope, an intracytoplasmic membrane system, chromosome separation on mitotic spindles,[37] and a Golgi apparatus.[38] Microsporidia lack mitochondria and centrioles and have prokaryote-size ribosomes[39,40] lacking a 5.8S ribosome subunit but having sequences homologous to the 5.8S region in the 23S subunit.[41] The small subunit rRNA of several Microsporidia have been sequenced and found to be significantly shorter than both eukaryotic and prokaryotic small subunit rRNA.[40,42] These rRNA genes are in a subtelomeric location on each chromosome of *Enc. cuniculi*[43,44] and lack the paromomycin binding site.[45] Sequence data of rRNA from the Microsporidia have been used to develop diagnostic polymerase chain reaction (PCR) primers and in the study of phylogenetic relations (reviewed by Weiss and Vossbrinck[42] and Weiss[46]). The karyotype of several members of the phylum Microspora has been determined by pulsed field electrophoresis. The genome size of the Microsporidia varies from 2.3 to 19.5 Mb.[6] The genomic size of the Encephalitizoonidae is less than 3.0 Mb, making them among the smallest eukaryotic nuclear genomes so far identified.[43,47,48]

Microsporidia are currently classified on the basis of ultrastructural features, including the size and morphology of the spores, number of coils of the polar tube, developmental life cycle, and the host–parasite relationship.[1,49,50] Molecular analysis of rRNA genes has begun to alter this classification system.[42,51] Antigenic differences between Microsporidia demonstrable by sodium dodecyl sulfate-polyacrylamide gel electrophoresis (SDS-PAGE) and Western blot analysis[52,53] have been used as adjunctive evidence when determining phylogenetic relationships among the Microsporidia infecting humans.[14,53] Molecular phylogenetic data indicates that the Microsporidia are related to fungi and are not "primitive eukaryotes".[54–58] Keeling has suggested that the Microsporidia are a sister group to the Zygomycota.[59]

Microsporidia form characteristic unicellular spores (Fig. 39-1) that are environmentally resistant. *Enc. cuniculi* spores remain viable for 6 days when in water and 4 weeks when dry at 22°C.[60] *Nosema bombycis* spores may remain viable for 10 years in distilled water. Spores may be killed by exposure for 30 min to 70% ethanol, 1% formaldehyde, or 2% Lysol or by autoclaving at 120°C for 10 min.[60] Whereas Microsporidia spores can be as large as 12 mm, the Microsporidia infecting humans have spores that range from 1 to 4 mm. The spore coat consists of an electron-dense, proteinaceous exospore, an electron-lucent endospore composed of chitin and protein, and an inner membrane or plasmalemma.[6,61] A defining characteristic of all Microsporidia is an extrusion apparatus that consists of a polar tube attached to the inside of the anterior end of the spore by an anchoring disc; depending on the species, it forms four to ~30 coils around the sporoplasm in the spore. During germination the polar tube rapidly everts, forming a hollow tube that brings the sporoplasm into intimate contact with the host cell. The polar tube provides a bridge to deliver the sporoplasm to the host cell. The mechanism by which the polar tube interacts with the host cell membrane is not known, but it may require the participation of host cell proteins such as actin.[62] It is possible that the sporoplasm interacts with the host cell membrane as it emerges from the polar tube. If a spore is phagocytosed by a host cell, germination occurs and the polar tube can pierce the phagocytic vacuole, delivering sporoplasm into the host cell cytoplasm. The overall process of germination and formation of the polar tube inoculates the sporoplasm directly into a host cell, functioning essentially like a hypodermic needle.[63–65]

Conditions that promote germination vary widely among species, presumably reflecting the organism's adaptation to its host and external environment.[6,66,67] Conditions that promote spore discharge include pH shifts,[68] dehydration followed by rehydration,[69] various cations[70] and anions,[71] mucin or polyanions,[72] hydrogen peroxide,[67,73] ultraviolet radiation, and the calcium ionophore A 23187.[74] Inhibitors of spore discharge include magnesium chloride, ammonium chloride, low salt concentrations, sodium fluoride, ultraviolet light, temperatures higher than 40°C, calcium channel antagonists, calmodulin inhibitors,[73] cytochalasin D, demeclocyline, and itraconozole.[73] Regardless of the stimuli required for activation, all Microsporidia appear to exhibit the same response to the stimuli (i.e., increased intrasporal osmotic pressure). This results in an influx of water into the spore accompanied by swelling of the polaroplasts and posterior vacuole prior to spore discharge. In *Brachiola (Nosema) algerae*, it has been proposed that activation brings trehalose in contact with the enzyme trehalase, causing increased osmotic pressure.[66,75–78] The polar tube then discharges from the anterior pole of the spore in an explosive reaction, occurring in less than 2 s. It has been suggested that the hollow tube is formed by a process of eversion, similar to everting the finger of a glove.[63]

EPIDEMIOLOGY

Although initially regarded as rare, Microsporidia are now believed to be common enteric pathogens that are self-limited or asymptomatic in normal hosts.[79–81] Reported prevalence rates among those with acquired immunodeficiency syndrome (AIDS) have varied between 2% and 70% depending on the symptoms of the population studied and the diagnostic technique employed.[6,8,9] Co-infection with different Microsporidia or other enteric pathogens can occur. Asymptomatic carriage can occur in immunocompromised patients. *Enc. cuniculi* isolates from various animal species have been identified and separated based on the number of tetranucleotide repeats (5′GTTT3′) in the intergenic spacer region of their rRNA genes.[82] Differences have also been found in the intergenic spacer region of rRNA genes of *Ent. bieneusi.*[83–85] Such differences have proven useful for epidemiologic identification of the environmental source of Microsporidia isolated from humans.

Serosurveys in humans have demonstrated a high prevalence of antibodies to *Enc. cuniculi* and *Enc. hellem*, suggesting that asymptomatic infection may be common.[86,87] Serologic cross-reactivity among Microsporidia has been demonstrated by immunofluorescence[88] and Western blotting.[89] Singh et al[90] found positive titers in six of 69 healthy adults in England, 38 of 89 Nigerians with tuberculosis, 13 of 70 Malaysians with filariasis, and 33 of 92 Ghanians with malaria. In another study 14 of 115 travelers returning from the tropics and none among 48 nontravelers were seropositive.[91] In a study of HIV-positive male subjects, 10 of 30 were seropositive and all had traveled to the tropics.[92] Antibodies to *Enc. intestinalis* were found among 5% of pregnant French women and 8% of Dutch blood donors[87] and antibodies to *Enc. hellem* among 5.3% of HIV-positive Czech patients.[93] These data suggest that Microsporidia are common in humans and, similar to other gastrointestinal pathogens, are associated with travel or residence in the tropics or developing nations.

It is likely that microsporidiosis is a zoonotic infectious disease.[3] *Encephalitozoon* is a widely distributed parasite of mammals and birds, and the onset of microsporidiosis has been associated with exposure to livestock, fowl, and pets.[81] *Encephalitozoon* has been described in lovebirds and budgerigars (parakeets),[7] and one case of *Enc. hellem* has been reported in a patient who had two pet lovebirds.[94] Up to 30% of dogs in animal shelters may excrete microsporidia in their stools, and *Enc. cuniculi* was etiologic in the death of Maltese puppies in a recent outbreak.[81,95] *Encephalitozoon* was found in the stools of many animals in an epidemiologic survey in Mexico. *Ent. bieneusi* has been reported in pigs,[96] dogs, birds,[97] and SIV-infected rhesus monkeys.[98] *Nosema, Brachiola* and *Vittaforma* infections are believed to be due to traumatic inoculation of environmental spores of insect pathogens into human tissue.[34]

It has been possible to transmit *Encephalitozoon* via rectal infection in rabbits, suggesting that sexual transmission may also occur.[99] *Enc. hellem* has been demonstrated in respiratory tract mucosa as well as the prostate and urogenital tract of patients, raising the possibility of respiratory and sexual transmission in humans. Although congenital transmission of *Enc. cuniculi* has been demonstrated in rabbits, mice, dogs, horses, foxes, and squirrel monkeys, no such congenital transmission has been demonstrated in humans.[100,101] It is possible that many of the microsporidia are also water-borne pathogens. Enterocytozoonidae such as *Nucleospora* (previously *Enterocytozoon*) *salmonis*[102] have been found in fish,[103] and many of the human pathogenic Microsporidia have been detected in surface water supplies.[104–108]

MICROSPORIDIAN INFECTION IN HIV-UNINFECTED PATIENTS

Levaditi et al. suggested in 1923 that microsporidians could be associated with human disease.[109] This was proven in

1973 when a 4-month-old athymic male infant died with severe diarrhea and malabsorption; at autopsy microsporidia (*N. connori*) were discovered in the lungs, stomach, small and large bowel, kidneys, adrenal glands, myocardium, liver, and diaphragm.[110] Disease due to *Encephalitozoon* was suggested by positive immunoglobulin G (IgG) and IgM indirect immunofluorescence assays (using *Enc. cuniculi*) in a 3-year-old boy with seizures and hepatomegaly.[86,91] *Encephalitozoon* sp was also reported in a 9-year-old Japanese boy with headache, vomiting, spastic convulsions, and recurrent fever.[5] *Encephalitozoon* sp have been found in the stools of patients in surveys for the etiology of diarrhea in less developed countries.[111] *Ent. bieneusi* has been identified as a cause of self-limited diarrhea in immunocompetent hosts.[79,112–116] It is seen in 1–10% of children in developing countries presenting with diarrheal syndromes,[117–121] and in patients undergoing renal, liver or bone marrow transplantation.[122–127] A *Pleistophora* sp was identified in 1985 in skeletal muscle of an HIV-negative patient with myositis and has also been described in the skeletal muscle of HIV-positive patients.[8,32,33,128] *Brachiola algerae* infection of the skin with dissemination has been seen in a patient with leukemia[129] and in a woman with rheumatoid arthritis on antibody to TNF-a.[34,130]

Two cases of corneal microsporidiosis due to *Microsporidium africanus* in Botswana and *Microsporidium ceylonesis* in Sri Lanka were described in 1973 and 1981, respectively.[131,132] Additional cases of microsporidian keratitis have been identified in immunocompetent hosts.[6] One of these organisms was classified as *N. occularum*,[132,133] and the other, which was successfully propagated *in vitro*, was named *N. corneum*[134] (now *V. cornea*).[10] Among immunologically normal patients with corneal infections, one patient required enucleation,[131] one underwent unsuccessful penetrating keratoplasty,[135] one was successfully treated with a corneal transplant,[132] and the last was maintained on a variety of topical agents without effect until keratoplasty.[134]

MICROSPORIDIAN INFECTION IN AIDS PATIENTS

Microsporidia were recognized as opportunistic pathogens causing diarrhea and wasting in AIDS patients in 1985.[12] Since then, although most reported cases have still involved diarrhea, the spectrum of diseases caused by these organisms has expanded to include keratoconjunctivitis, disseminated disease, hepatitis, myositis, sinusitis, kidney and urogenital infection, ascites, cholangitis, and asymptomatic carriage.[6,8,81]

In patients with HIV infection evaluated for diarrhea the prevalence of microsporidiosis has ranged from 7% to 50%.[136–143] Weber et al examined 1271 stool specimens from 845 HIV-infected patients in Switzerland and found Microsporidia in eight of 88 patients with chronic diarrhea, three of 57 patients with self-limited diarrhea, and none among 700 asymptomatic patients.[8] Rabeneck et al in a prospective study, found microsporidia in 29% of patients seen at an HIV primary care clinic, but there was no association with the presence of diarrhea (18/55 with diarrhea and 13/51 without diarrhea had microsporidia on duodenal biopsy).[144,145] Patients with microsporidiosis in this study had a mean CD4+ T-lymphocyte count of 113 cells/mm^3. It is thus likely, as is true for other gastrointestinal protozoa, that asymptomatic carrier states exist. During a 15-month follow-up of this study, diarrhea developed in two of the 13 asymptomatic patients and continued in the 18 symptomatic patients.[146] Kotler and Orenstein, in a study of patients presenting to a gastroenterology clinic, found that 39% of patients with HIV and diarrhea (55/141) had microsporidiosis and that the presence of microsporidia was associated with wasting, a mean CD4+ T-lymphocyte count of 28 cells/mm^3, and abnormal D-xylose tests.[147] In contrast, only 2.6% of HIV patients without diarrhea (1/38) had microsporidiosis, and this patient subsequently developed diarrhea on follow-up. Coyle et al.[148] using the polymerase chain reaction (PCR) employing primers to rRNA gene of *Ent. bieneusi*, found that 37% (25/68) of HIV patients with diarrhea and 2.3% (1/43) of HIV patients without diarrhea had microsporidiosis. The one asymptomatic patient had an abnormal D-xylose test. Based on these studies microsporidia appear to demonstrate strength of association, coherence, and reproducibility with respect to being etiologic for a diarrheal syndrome. Further evidence of the association of microsporidia with diarrhea is provided by the utility of albendazole in the treatment of microsporidian infection. Therapy with albendazole results in cure of diarrhea associated with the elimination of *Enc. intestinalis* from the stools of infected patients[149]; treatment with fumagillin has a similar effect in patients with *Ent. bieneusi* infection.[150,151]

ENTEROCYTOZOON sp

The major syndrome associated with microsporidiosis is diarrhea and wasting. This is usually due to *Ent. bieneusi* (more than 90% of cases in the United States) and occasionally *Enc. intestinalis* (in Europe this organism may be a more frequent cause of diarrhea).[21] *Ent. bieneusi* occurs most commonly when CD4+ T-lymphocyte counts are less than 50 cells/mm^3; it presents with chronic nonbloody diarrhea, anorexia, weight loss, and bloating without associated fever. Although originally thought to invade only enterocytes, it has been demonstrated that *Ent. bieneusi* can also invade cholangioepithelium.[152] When present in the cholangioepithelium this organism has been associated with sclerosing cholangitis, AIDS cholangiopathy, and cholecystitis. Interestingly, an *Ent. bieneusi*-like organism has been identified in SIV-infected rhesus monkeys as the etiologic agent of cholangitis and hepatitis.[98,153] Systemic dissemination does not appear to occur with *Ent. bieneusi*. One case report described this organism in nasal mucosa[154] and four other reports have described pulmonary involvement due to *Ent. bieneusi*,[155] however, such cases may represent contamination due to spores from gastrointestinal secretions. Reports indicate that *Ent. bieneusi* may cause self-limited infections in immunocompetent patients.[3,79] Other intestinal pathogens may occur simultaneously or sequentially with this or any other microsporidian.

This parasite has a unique intracellular developmental life cycle.[156] A characteristic feature of this organism is the presence of electron-lucent inclusions demonstrating a lamellar structure. These inclusions are closely associated with the nuclear envelope or endoplasmic reticulum (or both). The earliest intraepithelial stages of the parasite are rounded proliferative cells limited by a typical unit membrane in direct contact with the host cell cytoplasm. In these cells nuclear division is not immediately followed by cytokinesis, thus resulting in the production of multinucleate proliferative plasmodia. After the production of multiple nuclei the parasites form electron-dense disk-like structures that cluster in stacks of three to six, eventually forming the coiled portion of the polar tube. When these multinucleated sporagonial plasmodia divide by invagination of the plasmalemma, multiple spores are formed. In mature spores the polar tubule has five to seven coils that appear in two rows when seen in cross sections by transmission electron microscopy.

ENCEPHALITOZOON sp

Encephalitozoon sp are widely distributed in many animals.[81] Three members of the family Encephalitozoonidae have been associated with disease in humans: *Enc. cuniculi*, *Enc. hellem*, and *Enc. intestinalis* (previously known as *Septata intestinalis*). It appears that these microsporidia have the capacity to disseminate widely in their hosts, and involvement of most organs by these organisms has now been documented.[6,8,29,157]

Enc. intestinalis has been associated with diarrheal disease,[13] cholangitis,[158] keratoconjunctivitis, osteomyelitis of the mandible,[159] and disseminated infection[149,160] in AIDS patients. The ability of this parasite to disseminate correlates with its ability to grow in many cell types both *in vivo* and *in vitro*. Elimination of this parasite from patients with diarrhea treated with albendazole correlates with the resolution of symptoms.[149,161] The parasite develops in the cytoplasm of intestinal enterocytes, macrophages, fibroblasts, and endothelial cells of the lamina propria and in epithelial cells of the kidney and gallbladder.[13] Sporogony is tetrasporous, and tubular appendages originate from the sporont surface and terminate in an enlarged bulb-like structure. Unlike other Encephalitizoonidae, *Enc. intestinalis*-infected cells have a unique parasite-secreted fibrillar network surrounding the developing organisms, so the parasitophorous vacuole appears septate. Mature spores in cross section have a single row of four to seven coils of polar tubules.

Enc. cuniculi has been associated with hepatitis,[162] peritonitis,[163] hepatic failure,[28] disseminated disease with fever,[27,28,157] renal insufficiency, and intractable cough.[164] These infections have been reported to respond to albendazole.[27,157,164] Granulomatous encephalitis due to *Enc. cuniculi* was first described in rabbits in 1922, and cases of encephalitis and seizures due to *Enc. cuniculi* have been reported in AIDS patients.[29] *Enc. cuniculi* was identified in cerebrospinal fluid, sputum, urine, and stool specimens from a 29-year-old man with a CD4+ T-lymphocyte count of 0 cells/mm^3, and he had enhancing lesions demonstrable by both computed tomography (CT) and magnetic resonance imaging (MRI) of the brain that diminished when albendazole was administered.[29]

Enc. hellem has been reported to cause disseminated disease associated with renal failure, nephritis, pneumonia, bronchitis, and keratoconjunctivitis.[165–168] This organism is also recognized to cause infection of the nasal epithelium and is an important etiologic agent in cases of sinusitis in patients with HIV infection. Among the ocular infections due to Encephalitozoonidae reported in the literature, most have been attributed to *Enc. hellem*, including three cases originally classified as due to *Enc. cuniculi*.[9,169] The remaining cases have been due to *Encephalitozoon* sp or *Enc. intestinalis*.[170] Ocular microsporidian infection in HIV-1-infected patients has been restricted to the superficial epithelium of the cornea and conjunctiva (i.e., superficial keratoconjunctivitis) and has rarely progressed to corneal ulceration. Similar microsporidian infections are reported in contact lens wearers.[171] Patients present with bilateral punctate epithelial keratopathy and conjunctival inflammation resulting in redness, foreign body sensation, photophobia, and changes in visual acuity. Slit-lamp examination usually demonstrates punctate epithelial opacities, granular epithelial cells with irregular fluorescein uptake, conjunctival injection, superficial corneal infiltrates, and a noninflamed anterior chamber.

Enc. hellem has been cultured *in vitro* from the urine of patients with disseminated microsporidiosis[172] and those with keratoconjunctivitis.[53,173] As this organism has been found in the lung, it has been suggested that respiratory spread of this microsporidian may occur.[167] Due to the presence of this organism in the urogenital tract including the prostate, and the ability to transmit this organism by rectal inoculation in rabbits, it is possible that *Enc. hellem* may be acquired as a sexually transmitted disease.[174] *Enc. hellem* and *Enc. cuniculi* have similar developmental life cycles.[37] The genus is characterized by the presence of a phagosome-like parasitophorous vacuole. Nuclei of all stages are unpaired. Meronts divide repeatedly by binary fission. Sporonts divide into two sporoblasts that mature into spores. No tubular appendages or fibrillar networks are produced, as is seen in *Enc. intestinalis*. In cross section the mature spore has five to seven coils in single rows (Fig. 39-2).

OTHER MICROSPORIDIA

Trachipleistophora hominis is a pansporoblastic microsporidian that has been described in several patients with disseminated disease in the setting of AIDS.[15] The organism has been cultivated *in vitro*. *Trachipleistophora anthropophthera* infection has presented as encephalitis, myositis, and keratoconjunctivitis.[16,35,175] Several of these patients responded clinically to albendazole. *Brachiola vesicularum* caused myositis in an HIV-1-infected patient and responded to a regimen of albendazole and itraconozole.[11] Cases of myositis due to *Pleistophora* sp and *Brachiola algerae* have also been reported in AIDS patients.[32–34,176]

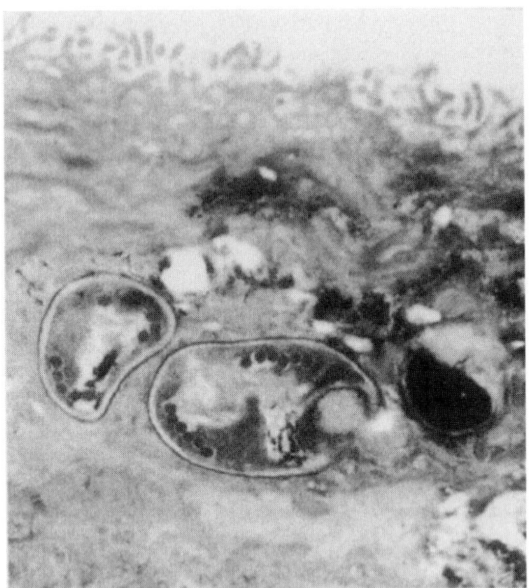

Figure 39-2 ■ Electron micrograph of conjunctival scraping demonstrating Microsporidia (*Encephalitozoon hellem*). Thick-walled spores with single nuclei and five or six coils of polar tubes are demonstrated.

Courtesy of A Cali and PM Takvorian, Rutgers University. From Weiss LM, Keohane EM. The uncommon gastrointestinal protozoa: microsporidia, Blastocystis, Isospora, Dientamoeba and Balantidium. Curr Clin Top Infect Dis 17:147, 1997.

DIAGNOSIS

Diagnostic tests for patients with suspected microsporidiosis are described in Table 39-2. In general, a urine examination should be done whenever microsporidiosis is considered, as microsporidia associated with disseminated disease such as *Encephalitozoon* and *Trachipleistophora* have invariably been present in such specimens when examined. As gastrointestinal disease with *Ent. bieneusi* is not associated with disseminated disease, this organism is not seen in the urine. For gastrointestinal disease, examination of three stools with chromotrope and chemofluorescent stains is often sufficient for diagnosis. If the stool examination is negative and the diarrhea is chronic (more than 2 months duration), endoscopy should be performed.

Effective morphologic demonstration of microsporidia by light microscopy can be accomplished by staining methods that produce differential contrast between the spores of the microsporidia and the cells and debris in clinical samples (e.g., stool) in which they are found. In addition, given the small size of the spores (1–5 mm) adequate magnification (i.e., 1000X) is required for visualization. Chromotrope 2R,[177] calcofluor white (fluorescent brightener 28),[178] and Uvitex 2B[179] have been reported to be useful as selective stains for microsporidia in stool specimens and other body fluids (Fig. 39-3). The chromotrope 2R-based method of Weber et al[177] is similar to a standard trichrome stain, but the chromotrope 2R concentration is 10-fold higher and the staining time is longer. Further modifications of this method by Ryan et al.[180] using aniline

Table 39-2 Diagnosis of Microsporidiosis

Test	Utility
Urine examination	This is often positive in cases of microsporidiosis due to microsporidia other than *Enterocytozoon* and should be done in all suspected microsporidia cases.
Stool examination	This is useful for gastrointestinal presentations. At least three stools should be examined. The combination of chromotrope and chemofluorescent stains provides the highest sensitivity and specificity.
Endoscopy	This should be considered for all patients with chronic diarrhea of more than 2 months' duration and negative stool and urine examinations. In this group endoscopy has yielded a diagnosis of microsporidia presence in up to 30% of patients. Tissue should be examined by a microsporidial stain. Touch preparations are useful for rapid diagnosis (within 24 h). If microsporidia are demonstrated to invade the lamina propria, the urine examination should be repeated, as *Encephalitozoon* are the most likely etiologic agent. In this setting albendazole has high efficacy.
PCR	This test is available as a research technique. Species identification can be performed on stool, urine, and tissue samples.
Electron microscopy	This identifies the species of microsporidia involved and is crucial for identification of new species. It is essential for the characterization of microsporidia in unusual or new locations.
Conjunctival scrapings	This has a high diagnostic yield in microsporidian keratoconjunctivitis. Urine examination should also be performed in suspected cases to screen for disseminated microsporidiosis.
Nasal scrapings	This can be useful for the diagnosis of microsporidian sinusitis. As most of the microsporidia associated with sinusitis are present in the kidneys, urine examination should be routine for suspected sinusitis cases. If these tests are negative, biopsy of nasal mucosa may be useful for diagnosis.
Serology	This is not useful for diagnosis but may be useful for epidemiologic surveys.

blue in place of fast green, and Kokoskin et al.[181] using an elevated temperature, are preferred by some laboratories. Using this stain, spores appear as 1–3 mm ovoid light pink structures with a belt-like stripe girding them diagonally and equatorially against a green or blue background. Spores can also be visualized by ultraviolet (UV) microscopy using chemofluorescent optical brightening agents such as Calcofluor white M2R (fluorescent brightener 28, Fungi-Fluor) and Uvitex 2B (Fungiqual A; Dieter Reinehr and Manfred Rembold, Spezialchemikalien fur die Medizinische Diagnostik, Kandern, Germany), which stain chitin in the spore wall (endospore layer).

Microsporidia in body fluids other than stool have been visualized with Chromotrope 2R, optical brightening agents, Giemsa, Brown–Hopps Gram stain, acid-fast staining, or Warthin–Starry silver staining. Microsporidiosis can also be diagnosed by examining biopsy material or touch preparations. In paraffin-embedded sections, microsporidial spores are discernible to experienced observers with hematoxylin and eosin and can also be seen with Chromotrope 2A or Gram (Brown–Hopps) stain. Microscopic examination of corneal tissue, obtained by gentle rubbing over the conjunctiva and cornea with a tissue swab, has revealed multiple gram-positive, oval organisms in epithelial cells. These organisms often contain a periodic acid-Schiff (PAS)-positive anterior granule. Fresh tissue may also be examined by phase-contrast microscopy, and because of their thick walls unstained spores are refractile, appearing green and possibly birefringent.

Using 50 stool specimens positive for microsporidia by transmission electron microscopy (TEM), both the chromotrope 2R and chemofluorescent brightening stains identified 100% of specimens when at least 50 high power (i.e., 1000X) fields were examined.[182] In a study employing Uvitex 2B, all of the 186 stool samples examined from 19 patients with biopsy-proven *Ent. bieneusi* infection were positive, and none of the 55 stool samples from 16 biopsy-negative patients were positive.[179] In another study Uvitex 2B staining detected microsporidia in all chromotrope 2R stain-positive samples and identified several additional samples (from three patients) as positive.[183] On re-examination, stool samples from these patients were also positive with the chromotrope 2R stain. All patients with positive duodenal biopsies were positive on stool examination by chromotrope or chemofluorescence methods. Of the six patients with negative duodenal biopsies who were identified as positive by chromotrope or chemofluorescence staining, four had confirmation of microsporidia in the stool by TEM. In infections with low numbers of spores it is likely that these noninvasive methods have a higher sensitivity than biopsy techniques. The limit of detecting microsporidia by these techniques appears to be 5×10^4 organisms/mL (500 organisms/10 mL).[182] Overall, the sensitivity of the chemofluorescent brightener-based stains is slightly higher than chromotrope-based stains (especially when low numbers of spores are present in a sample); however, the specificity of the chemofluorescent stains is lower (90% vs 100% in one study).[182] Based on an analysis of the performance characteristics of these smears, it has been suggested that chemofluorescent stains should be utilized for screening stool specimens and that all positive specimens be confirmed by a chromotrope 2R stain before being considered truly positive. Neither the chromotrope nor the chemofluorescent stains provide information on the species of microsporidia being identified. Another report notes that these stains may give false positive results due to insect microsporidia contaminating ingested food.

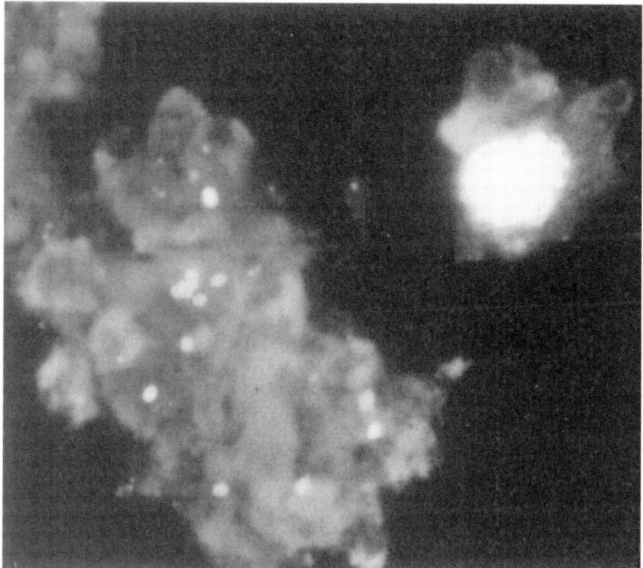

Figure 39-3 ■ Calcofluor white stain demonstrating fluorescent *Encephalitozoon hellem* spores in the urine of a patient with disseminated infection.

Courtesy of E Didier, Tulane Regional Primate Research Center. From Weiss LM, Keohane EM. The uncommon gastrointestinal protozoa: microsporidia, Blastocystis, Isospora, Dientamoeba and Balantidium. Curr Clin Top Infect Dis 17:147, 1997.

Polyclonal serum prepared to other microsporidia (*Enc. cuniculi*) has been reported to react with *Ent. bieneusi*.[89,184] Monoclonal antibodies to *Enc. hellem*,[185] *Enc. intestinalis*,[186] and *Ent. bieneusi*[187–190] have been described but are not commercially available. Diagnosis of microsporidiosis by detecting IgM antibody was reported in a case of disseminated *Enc. cuniculi* infection with encephalitis in an immunocompetent 2-year-old boy.[5] Enzyme-linked immunosorbent assay (ELISA) titers to *Enc. hellem*, *Enc. cuniculi*, and *Vit. corneae* were not useful for diagnosis in a study of 12 AIDS patients with *Ent. bieneusi*, two AIDS patients with *Enc. intestinalis*, and two immunocompetent patients with *Vit. Corneae*,[191] False-negative titers were present in seven of the patients with microsporidiosis, and half of the control patients (without clinical microsporidiosis) had positive serology to Microsporidia. This is consistent with other AIDS-associated infections in which serology has not proven useful.

Homology PCR cloning of the rRNA genes of many of the microsporidia pathogenic in humans has been accomplished and are in the GenBank database.[42,46] It has been possible to design PCR primers to these small subunit rRNA genes to identify microsporidia at the species level in clinical samples without the need for ultrastructural examination. Two main approaches have been employed in the construction of PCR primers for microsporidia: the design of universal pan-microsporidia primers and the design of species-specific primer pairs. These PCR techniques have been applied to biopsy specimens, urine, cultures, and more recently stool specimens and should greatly facilitate both diagnosis and epidemiologic studies.[192–195] See Weiss and Vossbrinck[42] for a review of the PCR tests for microsporidiosis.

TREATMENT

Immune reconstitution associated with highly active antiretroviral therapy (HAART) has been associated with the resolution of symptoms and elimination of organisms in microsporidiosis in the setting of AIDS.[196] In addition both fumagillin and albendazole have demonstrated consistent anti-microsporidial activity both *in vitro* and *in vivo*.[149,151,160,161,196–208] Despite initial reports of favorable treatment with metronidazole for intestinal infection with *Ent. bieneusi*, this drug has not been effective in other studies,[6,137,160,207,209] nor is there *in vitro* activity of metronidazole against *Enc. cuniculi*.[202] Other medications used without success in the treatment of gastrointestinal microsporidiosis are azithromycin, paromomycin (microsporidia lack the binding site for this drug), and quinacrine. Atovaquone has been anecdotally reported to have limited efficacy in microsporidiosis,[151,197,210] but there is no *in vitro* activity.[202] Sparfloxacin and chloroquine have demonstrated *in vitro* activity against microsporidia but have not been used clinically.[202] Prophylaxis with trimethoprim–sulfamethoxazole is not effective for preventing microsporidiosis, and this drug combination has no *in vitro* or *in vivo* activity against these organisms.[211] Thalidomide[212,213] and octreotide have been reported to decrease diarrhea in patients with microsporidiosis probably secondary to their effects on enterocytes. For a review of drugs used in microsporidiosis in animals see Costa and Weiss [196].

Albendazole, a benzimidazole that binds to β-tubulin, has activity against microsporidiosis (Tables 39-3 and 39-4). Albendazole is effective in inhibiting the growth of *Nosema bombycis in vitro* in *Spodoptera frugiperda* cells and *in vivo* in *Heliocoverpa zea* larvae and pupae.[201,214] *In vitro* albendazole has activity against all of the Encephalitozoonidae (*Enc. hellem, Enc. cuniculi, Enc. intestinalis*) at concentrations of less than 0.1 mg/mL, and this is true *in vivo* as well in animal models.[215–217] Data on the sequence of the Encephalitzoonidae β-tubulin genes demonstrates an amino acid sequence associated with sensitivity to benzimidazoles (e.g., albendazole) in these microsporidia.[218,219] Albendazole is poorly absorbed: Peak serum levels 2 h after an oral dose are 0.20–0.94 mg/mL, but absorption is increased if the medication is taken with food containing relatively high concentrations of fat. This drug is protein-bound (70%); is distributed in the blood, bile, and cerebrospinal fluid; and is eliminated by the kidneys. After oral administration hepatic metabolism converts albendazole to albendazole sulfoxide, which is detectable in the systemic circulation. Although side effects are rare, the following have been reported: hypersensitivity (rash, pruritus, fever),

Table 39-3

Therapy for Microsporidiosis

Organism	Drug	Dosage[a]
Enterocytozoon bieneusi	No effective commercial treatment. Oral fumagillin 60 mg/day appears effective. Albendazole[b] has resulted in clinical improvement in up to 50% of patients.	
Encephalitozoon infection (e.g., systemic, sinusitis, encephalitis, hepatitis)		
Enc. cuniculi	Albendazole	400 mg bid
Enc. hellem	Albendazole	400 mg bid
Enc. intestinalis	Albendazole	400 mg bid
Encephalitozoon keratoconjunctivitis	Fumagillin solution[c] (Fumadil B 3 mg/mL)	Two drops every 2 h for 4 days, then two drops four times a day[d]
	Patients may also need albendazole if systemic infection is present	
Trachipleistophora hominis	Albendazole	400 mg bid
Brachiola vesicularum	Albendazole	400 mg bid
	Itraconozole	400 mg qd

[a] The duration of treatment for microsporidiosis has not been established. Relapse of infection has occurred upon stopping treatment. Patients should be maintained on treatment for at least 4 weeks, and most patients should be on treatment indefinitely.
[b] Albendazole 400 mg bid.
[c] Fumidil B (fumagillin bicylohexylammonium; Mid-Continent Agrimarketing, Overland Park, KS, USA).
[d] Eyedrops should be continued indefinitely; relapse is common on stopping treatment.

neutropenia (reversible), central nervous system (CNS) effects (dizziness, headache), gastrointestinal disturbances (abdominal pain, diarrhea, nausea, vomiting), hair loss (reversible), and elevated hepatic enzymes (reversible). Albendazole is not carcinogenic or mutagenic. In animals (rats and rabbits), at dosages of 30 mg/kg it was embryotoxic and teratogenic. Thus albendazole is not recommended for use in pregnant women. There have been no well controlled studies during human pregnancy. There is a report of pseudomembranous colitis following albendazole treatment.[220]

In AIDS patients with diarrhea due to *Enc. intestinalis*, treatment with albendazole results in resolution of the diarrhea and elimination of the organism.[149,199] In cases of chronic sinusitis and disseminated infection due to *Enc. hellem*, treatment with 400 mg of albendazole twice daily resulted in resolution of symptoms and clearance of the organism.[168,221] Clinical improvement was demonstrated after albendazole treatment in a patient with disseminated *Enc. cuniculi* infection involving the CNS, conjunctiva, sinuses, kidney, and lungs.[29,164] Albendazole (400 mg bid) also resulted in clinical improvement in patients with disseminated infection with myositis due to *T. hominis* and a patient with myositis due to a *Bachiola vesicularum*.[11,15]

Albendazole treatment has not been as successful against *Ent. bieneusi* infection. Although in some patients treatment with albendazole resulted in symptomatic improvement, the organism persisted during treatment in all patients with no improvement in D-xylose absorption tests.[198,205,222] In addition,

Table 39-4 Drugs Used for Animal and Human Microsporidiosis

Drug	Organism	Disease	References
Albendazole	*Encephalitozoon cuniculi*	GI, CNS, HEP, EYE, GU	29, 149, 161, 198, 199, 207, 236, 34, 215, 223, 237
	Encephalitozoon hellem	EYE, GI, SYS, ENT	
	Encephalitozoon intestinalis	GI, EYE, SYS, GU, ENT	
	Enterocytozoon bieneusi	GI[a], BIL[a]	
	Trachipleistophora hominis	MYO	
	Brachiola algerae	MYO[a]	
	Nosema bombycis	SYS (insect host)	
Fumagillin	*Encephalitozoon hellem*	EYE	151, 197, 204, 216, 224–230
	Encephalitozoon cuniculi	EYE, SYS (murine host)	
	Encephalitozoon intestinalis	EYE	
	Enterocytozoon bieneusi	GI	
	Nosema apis	SYS (insect host)	
	Nosema kingi	SYS (insect host)	
	Octosporea muscaedomesticae	SYS (insect host)	
	Pleistophora anguillarum	Beko (fish host)	
	Loma salmonae	Gill infection (fish host)	
	Nucleospora salmonis	SYS (fish host)	
Metronidazole	*Enterocytozoon bieneusi*	GI[a]	152, 160, 209, 228, 238
	Encephalitozoon intestinalis	GI[b]	
Itraconazole	*Encephalitozoon cuniculi*	EYE[a]	11, 34, 94, 239, 240
	Brachiola vesicularum	MYO[a]	
	Brachiola algerae	MYO[a]	
Trimethoprim–sulfamethoxazole	*Enterocytozoon bieneusi*	GI[c]	211
Atovaquone	*Enterocytozoon bieneusi*	GI[c]	210, 228
	Encephalitozoon cuniculi[b]		
Furazolidone	*Enterozytozoon bieneusi*	GI[a]	228, 241, 242
Nitazoxanide	*Enterocytozoon bieneusi*	GI[a]	243
Benomyl	*Nosema* sp	SYS (insect host)	244
Toltrazuril	*Nucleospora salmonis*	SYS[c]	245
	Glugea anomala	SYS (fish host)	

Infections are in human hosts unless indicated in parentheses (i.e., insect, fish, or murine host).
BIL, cholangitis; CNS, encephalitis; ENT, sinus infections; EYE, ocular infections; GI, gastrointestinal disease (diarrhea); GU, genitourinary infections; HEP, hepatitis; MYO, myositis; SYS, systemic infection.

[a] Limited efficacy *in vivo*.
[b] No efficacy *in vitro*.
[c] No efficacy *in vivo*.
Adapted from Costa S, Weiss LM. Drug treatment of microsporidiosis. Drug Resistance Updates 3:1, 2000.

relapse occurred rapidly upon discontinuation of albendazole therapy. In a study of 29 patients with *Ent. bieneusi* infection 50% had symptomatic improvement after albendazole treatment.[198] An additional 37 patients (66 patients in total) have been treated on this protocol with similar results. Other studies have found that albendazole had no efficacy in *Ent. bieneusi* infection.[223]

Fumagillin was isolated in 1949 from *Aspergillus fumigatus*. Amebicidal effects were first noted *in vitro* against *Entamoeba histolytica*, and fumagillin was used during the 1950s to treat humans afflicted with amebiasis. Fumagillin has been used to treat honeybees infected with the microsporidian *Nosema apis*, resulting in a reduction in infected bees.[224] Fumagillin has been used to treat infections by both microsporidians and myxosporeans in various types of fish.[225–227] Toxicity has been described with the use of fumagillin in fish. Fumagillin at 0.25 and 1.0 g/kg in food for 60 days administered to rainbow trout resulted in a reduction of the hematopoietic tissue of the kidney and spleen on histologic examination and a reduction of the hematocrit in treated fish. Fumagillin and its semisynthetic analog TNP-470 have been found to have activity *in vitro* and *in vivo* against microsporidians pathogenic for humans including *Enc. cuniculi*, *Enc. hellem*, *Enc. intestinalis*, *V. corneae*, and *Ent. bieneusi*.[151,204,216,228–230] It is of concern that this agent is "static" and not "cidal." When fumagillin is discontinued *in vitro*, organisms start to grow and return to pretreatment levels. In one study, which demonstrated that fumagillin was active in cases of *Ent. bieneusi* infection, thrombocytopenia occurred in all four patients receiving fumagillin, with one patient having a grade 4 thrombocytopenia with epistaxis.[228] A dose-escalation trial of fumagillin was subsequently performed on HIV-infected patients infected with *Ent. bieneusi*.[151,197] This study employed doses of 10 mg/day for 14 days, 20 mg/day for 14 days, 40 mg/day for 14 days, and 60 mg/day for 14 days, with the patients being seen at weeks 1, 2, 4, and 6. Efficacy was assessed by the clearance of microsporidia from stool and duodenal biopsies. Of 29 patients, 21 exhibited transient clearing of parasites from their stools. These patients were in the first three dosage groups. In the 60 mg/day group, eight of 11 patients did not have spores in their stools at week 6 and remained free of them in stool specimens for a mean follow-up of 11 months. Duodenal biopsies on the same eight patients did not demonstrate microsporidia by either light or electron microscopy. A subsequent randomized trial of 12 patients treated with fumagillin (60 mg/day) also demonstrated the efficacy of this drug for the treatment of *Ent. bieneusi* enteritis.[151]

Fumagillin binds in a selective, covalent fashion to the metalloprotease methionine aminopeptidase 2 (MetAP2).[231,232] MetAP2 has been demonstrated to be the common target for other fumagillin analogs (e.g., TNP470/AGM-1470) and ovalicin. Crystallization studies have demonstrated that the specific binding site of the reactive epoxide of fumagillin and MetAP2 is a histidine residue at position 231.[232] Methionine aminopeptidase activity is essential for eukaryotic cell survival, as removal of the terminal methionine of a protein is often essential for its function and posttranslational modification (e.g., myrislyation). In microsporidia, homology PCR with sequencing of the amplicons has demonstrated the presence of MetAP2 genes in several microsporidia.[233]

Solutions of the soluble salt Fumidil B (fumagillin bicylohexylammonium, Mid-Continent Agrimarketing, Overland Park, KS, USA) applied topically have been demonstrated to be nontoxic to the cornea. Treatment of ocular microsporidiosis can be accomplished using a solution of Fumidil B (3 mg/mL) in saline (fumagillin 70 μg/mL)[200,204]; the treatment should be continued indefinitely, as recurrence is known to occur upon stopping these drops. It is of note that although clearance of microsporidia from the eye can be demonstrated, the organism is often still present systemically and can be demonstrated in the urine or in nasal smears. In such cases the use of albendazole as a systemic agent is reasonable and effective. Topical treatment with thiabendazole (0.4% suspension), a related benzimidazole, was infective in one case of keratitis due to *Enc. hellem*.[204]

Two patients with *Encephalitozoon*-like organisms have been reported to respond to imidazole (fluconazole and itraconazole) administration.[234] Yee et al. described complete improvement of a patient with *Enc. hellem* infection over a 6-week period who was given oral itraconazole (200 mg bid) after debulking the cornea.[94] Disenhouse et al. in contrast, saw no improvement in a patient with *Enc. hellem* treated with itraconazole 100 mg tid.[204] *In vitro* data have not confirmed antimicrosporidian activity for imidazole compounds. Sulfa drugs have had variable results *in vitro* and *in vivo* and are not recommended for treatment. Polymyxin B, propamidine isethionate 0.1% (Brolene), gramicidin, neomycin sulfate, and tetracycline appear to have limited efficacy for the treatment of microsporidia and should not be used except to treat secondary bacterial infections. Keratoplasty appears to provide temporary improvement in some cases, and debulking by corneal scraping may be useful in cases not responding to medical treatment. Steroids may be useful for decreasing the associated inflammatory response but have no direct action on microsporidia.

PREVENTION

Patients have developed microsporidiosis while on trimethoprim–sulfamethoxazole prophylaxis.[211] Currently, no prophylactic antiparasitic agents have been identified for these organisms. Although the epidemiology of the microsporidia that infect humans is unknown, it is likely that these are food- or waterborne pathogens; and the usual sanitary measures that prevent contamination of food and water with the urine and feces of animals should decrease the chance for infection.[235] In addition, hand washing and general good hygienic habits probably reduce the chance for contamination of the conjunctiva and cornea. The importance and prevalence of these organisms in our water supplies is an open question.

CONCLUSIONS

Since the original description of microsporidiosis in patients with AIDS in 1985, there has been a geometric increase in the number of reports describing a variety of disease entities caused by these protozoan parasites. *Enterocytozoon bieneusi* has been reported as an important cause of diarrhea and wasting syndrome as well as biliary system disease, and microsporidia of the family Encephalitozoonidae have been associated with disseminated disease, diarrhea, sinusitis, and ocular infections. There has been a dramatic increase in our ability for *in vitro* culture, to treat, and diagnose the Encephalitozoonidae. Therapy for *Ent. bieneusi* infection is still problematic and is limited by the lack of an *in vitro* culture system for this organism. It is clear that microsporidia are found in immunocompetent and immunocompromised hosts; and as our diagnostic acumen and testing improve, new disease syndromes will likely be attributed to these organisms.

REFERENCES

1. Sprague V. Systematics of the microsporidia. In: Bulla LA and Cheng TC (eds). Comparative Pathobiology Vol. 2. New York: Plenum; 1977, pp 1–510.
2. Sprague VV, Becnel JJ. Note on the name-author-date combination for the Taxon MICROSPORIDIES Balbiani, 1882, when ranked as a phylum. J Invertebr Pathol 71:91–4, 1998.
3. Mathis A, Weber R, Deplazes P. Zoonotic potential of the microsporidia. Clin Microbiol Rev 18:423–45, 2005.
4. Canning EU, Lom J. The Microsporidia of Vertebrates. London, England: Academic Press; 1986.
5. Matsubayashi H, Koide T, Mikata T, Hagiwara S. A case of Encephalitozoon-like body infection in man. Arch Pathol Lab Med 67:181–185, 1959.
6. Wittner, M Weiss LM. The Microsporidia and Microsporidiosis. Washington, DC: ASM Press; 1999, 553pp.
7. Black SS, Steinohrt LA, Bertucci DC, et al. Encephalitozoon hellem in budgerigars (Melopsittacus undulatus). Vet Pathol 34:89–98, 1997.
8. Weber R, Bryan RT, Schwartz DA, Owen RL. Human microsporidial infections. Clin Microbiol Rev 7:426–61, 1994.
9. Rastrelli, P, Didier E, Yee R. Microsporidial keratitis. Opthal Clin North Am 7:614–635, 1994.
10. Silveira H, Canning EU. Vittaforma corneae n. comb. for the human microsporidium Nosema corneum Shadduck, Meccoli, Davis & Font, 1990, based on its ultrastructure in the liver of experimentally infected athymic mice. J Eukaryot Microbiol 42:158–65, 1995.
11. Cali A, Takvorian PM, Lewin S, et al. Brachiola vesicularum, n. g., n. sp., a new microsporidium associated with AIDS and myositis. J Eukaryot Microbiol 45:240–51, 1998.
12. Desportes I, Le Charpentier Y, Galian A, et al. Occurrence of a new microsporidian: Enterocytozoon bieneusi n. g., n. sp., in the enterocytes of a human patient with AIDS. J Protozool, 32:250–245, 1985.
13. Cali A, Kotler DP, Orenstein JM. Septata intestinalis n. g., n. sp., an intestinal microsporidian associated with chronic diarrhea and dissemination in AIDS patients. J Eukaryot Microbiol 40:101–12, 1993.
14. Hartskeerl RA, Van Gool T, Schuitema AR, et al. Genetic and immunological characterization of the microsporidian Septata intestinalis Cali, Kotler and Orenstein, 1993: reclassification to Encephalitozoon intestinalis. Parasitology 110:277–85, 1995.
15. Field AS, Marriott DJ, Milliken ST, et al. Myositis associated with a newly described microsporidian, Trachipleistophora hominis, in a patient with AIDS. J Clin Microbiol 34:2803–11, 1996.
16. Yachnis AT, Berg J, Martinez-Salazar A, et al. Disseminated microsporidiosis especially infecting the brain, heart, and kidneys. Report of a newly recognized pansporoblastic species in two symptomatic AIDS patients. Am J Clin Pathol 106:535–43, 1996.
17. Franzen C, Nassonova ES, Scholmerich J, Issi IV, Transfer of the members of the genus Brachiola (microsporidia) to the genus Anncaliia based on ultrastructural and molecular data. J Eukaryot Microbiol 53:26–35, 2006.
18. Shadduck JA, Meccoli RA, Davis R, Font RL. Isolation of a microsporidian from a human patient. J Infect Dis, 162:773–6, 1990.
19. Didier PJ, Didier ES, Orenstein JM, Shadduck JA. Fine structure of a new human microsporidian, Encephalitozoon hellem, in culture. J Protozool 38:502–7, 1991.
20. Visvesvara GS, da Silva AJ, Croppo GP, et al. In vitro culture and serologic and molecular identification of Septata intestinalis isolated from urine of a patient with AIDS. J Clin Microbiol 33:930–6, 1995.
21. van Gool T, Canning EU, Gilis H, et al. Septata intestinalis frequently isolated from stool of AIDS patients with a new cultivation method. Parasitology 109:281–9, 1994.
22. Visvesvara G, Leitch GJ, Pieniazek NJ, et al. Short-term in vitro culture and molecular analysis of the microsporidian, Enterocytozoon bieneusi. J Eukaryot Microbiol 42:506–10, 1995.
23. Visvesvara GS, Leitch GJ, Wallace S, et al. Adenovirus masquerading as microsporidia. J Parasitol 82(2):316–19, 1996.
24. Wongtavatchai J, Conrad PA, Hedrick RP. In vitro characteristics of the microsporidian: Enterocytozoon salmonis. J Eukaryot Microbiol 42:401–5, 1995.
25. Docker MF, Kent ML, Hervio DML, et al. Ribosomal DNA sequence of Nucleospora salmonis Hedrick, Groff and Baxa,1991 (Microsporea: Enterocytozoonidae): implications for phylogeny and nomenclature. J Eukaryot Microbiol 44:55–60, 1997.
26. Tzipori S, Carville A, Widmer G, et al. Transmission and establishment of a persistent infection of Enterocytozoon bieneusi, derived from a human with AIDS, in simian immunodeficiency virus-infected rhesus monkeys. J Infect Dis 175(4):1016–20, 1997.
27. Orenstein JM, Gaetz HP, Yachnis AT, et al. Disseminated microsporidiosis in AIDS: are any organs spared? [letter]. AIDS 11:385–6, 1997.
28. Sheth SG, Bates C, Federman M, Chopra S. Fulminant hepatic failure caused by microsporidial infection in a patient with AIDS [letter]. AIDS 11:553–4, 1997.
29. Weber R, Deplazes P, Flepp M, et al. Cerebral microsporidiosis due to Encephalitozoon cuniculi in a patient with human immunodeficiency virus infection [see comments]. N Engl J Med 336:474–8, 1997.
30. Croppo GP, Visvesvara GS, Leitch GJ, et al. Western blot and immunofluorescence analysis of a human isolate of Encephalitozoon cuniculi established in culture from the urine of a patient with AIDS. J Parasitol 83:66–9, 1997.
31. Sheikh RA, Prindiville TP, Yenamandra S, et al. Microsporidial AIDS cholangiopathy due to Encephalitozoon intestinalis: case report and review. Am J Gastroenterol 95:2364–71, 2000.
32. Grau A, Valls ME, Williams JE, et al. Myositis caused by Pleistophora in a patient with AIDS. Med Clin (Barc) 107:779–81, 1996.

33. Chupp GL, Alroy J, Adelman LS, et al. Myositis due to Pleistophora (Microsporidia) in a patient with AIDS. Clin Infect Dis 16:15–21, 1993.
34. Coyle CM, Weiss LM, Rhodes LV 3rd, et al. Fatal myositis due to the microsporidian Brachiola algerae, a mosquito pathogen. N Engl J Med 351:42–7, 2004.
35. Vavra J, Yachnis AT, Shadduck JA, Orenstein JM. Microsporidia of the genus Trachipleistophora – causative agents of human microsporidiosis: description of Trachipleistophora anthropophthera n. sp. (Protozoa: Microsporidia). J Eukaryot Microbiol 45:273–83, 1998.
36. Pol S, Microsporidiosis and AIDS-Related Cholangitis. Med Sci 9:762–763, 1993.
37. Desportes-Livage I. Biology of microsporidia. Contrib Microbiol 6:140–65, 2000.
38. Takvorian PM Cali A. Enzyme histochemical identification of the Golgi apparatus in the microsporidian, Glugea stephani. J Eukaryot Microbiol 41:63S-64S, 1994.
39. Curgy JJ, Vavra J, Vivares C. Presence of ribosomal RNAs with prokaryotic properties in Microsporidia, eukaryotic organisms. Biol. Cell. 38:49–52, 1980.
40. Vossbrinck CR, Maddox JV, Friedman S, et al. Ribosomal RNA sequence suggests microsporidia are extremely ancient eukaryotes. Nature 326:411–14, 1987.
41. Vossbrinck CR Woese CS. Eukaryotic ribosomes that lack a 5.8S RNA. Nature 320:287–288, 1986.
42. Weiss LM Vossbrinck CR. Microsporidiosis: molecular and diagnostic aspects. Adv Parasitol 40:351–95, 1998.
43. Vivares CP Metenier G. Towards the minimal eukaryotic parasitic genome. Curr Opin Microbiol 3:463–7, 2000.
44. Brugere JF, Cornillot E, Metenier G, Vivares CP. Occurrence of subtelomeric rearrangements in the genome of the microsporidian parasite Encephalitozoon cuniculi, as revealed by a new fingerprinting procedure based on two-dimensional pulsed field gel electrophoresis [In Process Citation]. Electrophoresis 21:2576–81, 2000.
45. Katiyar SK, Visvesvara GS, Edlind TD. Comparisons of ribosomal RNA sequences from amitochondrial protozoa: implications for processing, mRNA binding and paromomycin susceptibility. Gene 152:27–33, 1995.
46. Weiss LM, Molecular phylogeny and diagnostic approaches to microsporidia. Contrib Microbiol 6:209–35, 2000.
47. Biderre C, Pages M, Metenier G, et al. On small genomes in eukaryotic organisms: molecular karyotypes of two microsporidian species (Protozoa) parasites of vertebrates. C R Acad Sci III 317:399–404, 1994.
48. Biderre C, Pages M, Metenier G, et al. Evidence for the smallest nuclear genome (2.9 Mb) in the microsporidium Encephalitozoon cuniculi. Mol Biochem Parasitol 74:229–31, 1995.
49. Sprague V, Becnel JJ, Hazard EI. Taxonomy of phylum Microspora. Crit. Rev. Microbiol 18:285–395, 1992.
50. Levine ND, Corliss JO, Cox FEG, et al. A newly revised classification of the Protozoa. J. Protozool 27:37–58, 1980.
51. Vossbrinck CR Debrunner-Vossbrinck BA. Molecular phylogeny of the Microsporidia: ecological, ultrastructural and taxonomic considerations. Folia Parasitol (Praha), 52:131–42; discussion 130, 2005.
52. Langley RC, Cali A, Somberg EW. Two-dimensional electrophoretic analysis of spore proteins of the microsporida. J Parasitol 73:910–18, 1987.
53. Didier ES, Didier PJ, Friedberg DN, et al. Isolation and characterization of a new human microsporidian, Encephalitozoon hellem (n. sp.) from three AIDS patients with keratoconjunctivitis. J. Infect. Dis 163:617–21, 1991.
54. Keeling PJ, Luker MA, Palmer JD, Evidence from beta-tubulin phylogeny that microsporidia evolved from within the fungi. Mol Biol Evol 17:23–31, 2000.
55. Keeling PJ, McFadden GI. Origins of microsporidia. Trends Microbiol 6:19–23, 1998.
56. Weiss LM, Edlind TD, Vossbrinck CR, Hashimoto T. Microsporidian molecular phylogeny: the fungal connection. J Eukaryot Microbiol 46:17S–18S, 1999.
57. Hirt RP, Logsdon JM Jr, Healy B, et al. Microsporidia are related to Fungi: evidence from the largest subunit of RNA polymerase II and other proteins. Proc Natl Acad Sci USA 96:580–5, 1999.
58. Katinka MD, Duprat S, Cornillot E, et al. Genome sequence and gene compaction of the eukaryote parasite Encephalitozoon cuniculi. Nature 414:450–3, 2001.
59. Keeling PJ. Congruent evidence from alpha-tubulin and beta-tubulin gene phylogenies for a zygomycete origin of microsporidia. Fungal Genet Biol 38:298–309, 2003.
60. Waller T. Sensitivity of Encephalitozoon cuniculi to various temperatures, disinfectants and drugs. Lab Anim 13:227–230, 1979.
61. Vavra J. Structure of the Microsporidia. In: Bulla LA Jr, Cheng TC (eds). Comparative Pathobiology. New York: Plenum; 1976, pp 1–85.
62. Foucault C, Drancourt M. Actin mediates Encephalitozoon intestinalis entry into the human enterocyte-like cell line, Caco-2. Microb Pathog 28:51–8, 2000.
63. Lom J. On the structure of the extruded microsporidian polar filament. Z Parasitenkd 38:200–213, 1972.
64. Weidner E. Cell invasion by microsporidian spores: an ultrastructural study. J Protozool 18(Suppl.):13–14, 1971.
65. Weidner E. Ultrastructural study of microsporidian invasion into cells. Z Parasitenkd 40:227–242, 1972.
66. Undeen AH. A proposed mechanism for the germination of microsporidian (Protozoa, Microspora) spores. J Theor Biol 142:223–235, 1990.
67. Lom J, Vavra J. The mode of sporoplasm extrusion in microsporidian spores. Acta Protozool 1:81–89, 1963.
68. Undeen AH, Epsky ND. In vitro and vivo germination of Nosema locustae (Microspora: Nosematidae) spores. J Invertebr Pathol 56:371–379, 1990.
69. Whitlock V, Johnson S, Stimuli for the in vitro germination of Nosema locustae (Microspora:Nosematidae) spores. J Invertebr Pathol 56:57–64, 1990.
70. Frixione E, Ruiz L, Undeen AH. Monovalent cations induce microsporidian spore germination in vitro. J Euk Microbiol 41:464–468, 1994.
71. Undeen AH, Avery SW. Effect of anions on the germination of Nosema algerae (Microspora: Nosematidae) spores. J Invertebr Pathol 52:84–89, 1988.
72. Pleshinger J. Weidner E. The microsporidian spore invasion tube. IV. Discharge activation begins with pH-triggered Ca^{2+} influx. J Cell Biol 100:1834–8, 1985.
73. Leitch GJ, He Q, Wallace S, Visvesvara GS. Inhibition of the spore polar filament extrusion of the microsporidium, Encephalitozoon hellem, isolated from an AIDS patient. J Eukaryot Microbiol 40:711–17, 1993.
74. Weidner E, Byrd W. The Microsporidian Spore Invasion Tube. II. Role of calcium in the activation of invasion tube discharge. J Cell Biol 93:970–975, 1982.
75. Undeen AH, Frixione E. The role of osmotic pressure in the germination of Nosema algerae spores. J Protozool 37: 561–567, 1990.
76. Undeen AH, Vandermeer RK. The effect of ultraviolet radiation on the germination of Nosema algerae Vávra and Undeen (Microsporida: Nosematidae) spores. J Protozool 37:194–199, 1990.
77. Undeen AH, Vandermeer RK. Conversion of intrasporal trehalose into reducing sugars during germination of Nosema algerae (Protista: Microspora) spores – a quantitative study. J Euk Microbiol 41:129–132, 1994.

78. Undeen AH, ElGazzar LM, Vandermeer RK, Narang S. Trehalose levels and trehalase activity in germinated and ungerminated spores of Nosema algerae (Microspora: Nosematidae). J Invertebr Pathol 50:230–237, 1987.
79. Weber R, Bryan RT. Microsporidial infections in immunodeficient and immunocompetent patients. Clin Infect Dis 19: 517–21, 1994.
80. Mathis A. Microsporidia: emerging advances in understanding the basic biology of these unique organisms [In Process Citation]. Int J Parasitol 30:795–804, 2000.
81. Deplazes P, Mathis A, Weber R, Epidemiology and zoonotic aspects of microsporidia of mammals and birds. Contrib Microbiol 6:236–60, 2000.
82. Didier ES, Vossbrinck CR, Baker MD, et al. Identification and characterization of three Encephalitozoon cuniculi strains. Parasitology 111:411–21, 1995.
83. Rinder H, Katzwinkel-Wladarsch S, Thomschke A, Loscher T. Strain differentiation in microsporidia. Tokai J Exp Clin Med 23:433–7, 1998.
84. Rinder H, Thomschke A, Dengjel B, et al. Close genotypic relationship between Enterocytozoon bieneusi from humans and pigs and first detection in cattle. J Parasitol 86:185–8, 2000.
85. Rinder H, Katzwinkel-Wladarsch S, Loscher T. Evidence for the existence of genetically distinct strains of Enterocytozoon bieneusi. Parasitol Res 83:670–2, 1997.
86. Bergquist NR, Stintzing G, Smedman L, et al. Diagnosis of encephalitozoonosis in man by serological tests. Br Med J (Clin Res Ed), 288:902, 1984.
87. van Gool T, Vetter JC, Weinmayr B, et al. High seroprevalence of Encephalitozoon species in immunocompetent subjects. J Infect Dis 175:1020–4, 1997.
88. Niederkorn JY, Shadduck JA, Weidner E. Antigenic cross-reactivity among different microsporidan spores as determined by immunofluorescence. J Parasitol 66:675–7, 1980.
89. Weiss LM, Cali A, Levee E, et al. Diagnosis of Encephalitozoon cuniculi infection by western blot and the use of cross-reactive antigens for the possible detection of microsporidiosis in humans. Am J Trop Med Hyg 47:456–62, 1992.
90. Singh M, Kane GJ, Mackinlay L, et al. Detection of antibodies to Nosema cuniculi (Protozoa:Microscoporidia) in human and animal sera by the indirect fluorescent antibody technique. Southeast Asian J Trop Med Public Health 13:110–13, 1982.
91. WHO parasitic diseases surveillance. Antibody to Encephalitozoon cuniculi in man. WHO Weekly Epidem Rec 58:30, 1983.
92. Bergquist R, Morfeldt-Mansson L, Pehrson PO, et al. Antibody against Encephalitozoon cuniculi in Swedish homosexual men. Scand J Infect Dis 16:389–91, 1984.
93. Pospisilova Z, Ditrich O, Stankova M, Kodym P. Parasitic opportunistic infections in Czech HIV-infected patients – a prospective study. Cent Eur J Public Health 5:208–13, 1997.
94. Yee RW, Tio FO, Martinez JA, et al. Resolution of microsporidial epithelial keratopathy in a patient with AIDS. Ophthalmology 98:196–201, 1991.
95. Snowden K, Logan K, Didier ES. Encephalitozoon cuniculi strain III is a cause of encephalitozoonosis in both humans and dogs. J Infect Dis 180:2086–8, 1999.
96. Deplazes P, Mathis A, Muller C, Weber R. Molecular epidemiology of Encephalitozoon cuniculi and first detection of Enterocytozoon bieneusi in faecal samples of pigs. J Eukaryot Microbiol 43:93S, 1996.
97. Haro M, Izquierdo F, Henriques-Gil N, et al. First detection and genotyping of human-associated microsporidia in pigeons from urban parks. Appl Environ Microbiol 71:3153–7, 2005.
98. Mansfield KG, Carville A, Shvetz D, et al. Identification of an Enterocytozoon bieneusi-like microsporidian parasite in simian-immunodeficiency-virus-inoculated macaques with hepatobiliary disease. Am J Pathol 150:1395–405, 1997.
99. Fuentealba IC, Mahoney NT, Shadduck JA, et al. Hepatic lesions in rabbits infected with Encephalitozoon cuniculi administered per rectum. Vet Pathol 29:536–40, 1992.
100. Zeman DH, Baskin GB. Encephalitozoonosis in squirrel monkeys (Saimiri sciureus). Vet Pathol 22:24–31, 1985.
101. Hunt RD, King NW, Foster HL. Encephalitozoonosis: evidence for vertical transmission. J Infect Dis 126:212–14, 1972.
102. Desportes-Livage I, Chilmonczyk S, Hedrick R, et al. Comparative development of two microsporidian species: Enterocytozoon bieneusi and Enterocytozoon salmonis, reported in AIDS patients and salmonid fish, respectively. J Eukaryot Microbiol 43:49–60, 1996.
103. Chilmonczyk S, Cox WL, Hedrick RP. Enterocytozoon salmonis n. sp. – An intranuclear microsporidium from salmonid fish. J Protozool 38:264–269, 1991.
104. Avery SW, Undeen AH. The isolation of microsporidia and other pathogens from concentrated ditch water. J Am Mosq Control Assoc 3:54–8, 1987.
105. Cotte L, Rabodonirina M, Chapuis F, et al. Waterborne outbreak of intestinal microsporidiosis in persons with and without human immunodeficiency virus infection. J Infect Dis 180:2003–8, 1999.
106. Franzen C, Muller A, Cryptosporidia and microsporidia–waterborne diseases in the immunocompromised host. Diagn Microbiol Infect Dis 34:245–62, 1999.
107. Fournier S, Liguory O, Santillana-Hayat M, et al. Detection of microsporidia in surface water: a one-year follow-up study. FEMS Immunol Med Microbiol 29:95–100, 2000.
108. Hunter PR. Waterborne outbreak of microsporidiosis [letter; comment]. J Infect Dis 182:380–1, 2000.
109. Levaditi C, Nicolau S, Schoen R. Nouvelles donnees sur L'Encephalitozoon cuniculi. C R Soc Biol 89:1157–62, 1923.
110. Margileth AM, Strano AJ, Chandra R, et al. Disseminated nosematosis in an immunologically compromised infant. Arch Pathol 95:145–50, 1973.
111. Enriquez FJ, Taren D, Cruz-Lopez A, et al. Prevalence of intestinal encephalitozoonosis in Mexico. Clin Infect Dis 26:1227–9, 1998.
112. Albrecht H, Sobottka I. Enterocytozoon bieneusi infection in patients who are not infected with human immunodeficiency virus. Clin Infect Dis 25:344, 1997.
113. Lopez-Velez R, Turrientes MC, Garron C, et al. Microsporidiosis in travelers with diarrhea from the tropics. J Travel Med 6:223–7, 1999.
114. Fournier S, Liguory O, Garrait V, et al. Microsporidiosis due to Enterocytozoon bieneusi infection as a possible cause of traveller's diarrhea. Eur J Clin Microbiol Infect Dis 17:743–4, 1998.
115. Gumbo T, Gangaidzo IT, Sarbah S, et al. Enterocytozoon bieneusi infection in patients without evidence of immunosuppression: two cases from Zimbabwe found to have positive stools by PCR. Ann Trop Med Parasitol 94:699–702, 2000.
116. Wichro E, Hoelzl D, Krause R, et al. Microsporidiosis in travel-associated chronic diarrhea in immune-competent patients. Am J Trop Med Hyg 73:285–7, 2005.
117. Bretagne S, Foulet F, Alkassoum W, et al. Prevalence of Enterocytozoon bieneusi spores in the stool of AIDS patients and African children not infected by HIV. Bull Soc Pathol Exot 86:351–7, 1993.
118. Drobniewski F, Kelly P, Carew A, et al. Human microsporidiosis in African AIDS patients with chronic diarrhea [letter]. J Infect Dis 171:515–16, 1995.
119. Gumbo T, Gangaidzo IT. Confirmation of transmission of Enterocytozoon bieneusi in South Africa. S Afr Med J 90(12):1162, 1164, 2000.

120. Endeshaw T, Kebede A, Verweij JJ, et al. Detection of intestinal microsporidiosis in diarrhoeal patients infected with the human immunideficiency virus (HIV-1) using PCR and Uvitex-2B stain. Ethiop Med J 43:97–101, 2005.
121. Leelayoova S, Subrungruang I, Rangsin R, et al. Transmission of Enterocytozoon bieneusi genotype a in a Thai orphanage. Am J Trop Med Hyg 73:104–7, 2005.
122. Sax PE, Rich JD, Pieciak WS, Trnka YM. Intestinal microsporidiosis occurring in a liver transplant recipient. Transplantation 60:617–18, 1995.
123. Guerard A, Rabodonirina M, Cotte L, et al. Intestinal microsporidiosis occurring in two renal transplant recipients treated with mycophenolate mofetil. Transplantation 68:699–707, 1999.
124. Gumbo T, Hobbs RE, Carlyn C, et al. Microsporidia infection in transplant patients. Transplantation 67:482–4, 1999.
125. Metge S, Van Nhieu JT, Dahmane D, et al. A case of Enterocytozoon bieneusi infection in an HIV-negative renal transplant recipient. Eur J Clin Microbiol Infect Dis 19:221–3, 2000.
126. Rabodonirina M, Bertocchi M, Desportes-Livage I, et al. Enterocytozoon bieneusi as a cause of chronic diarrhea in a heart-lung transplant recipient who was seronegative for human immunodeficiency virus [see comments]. Clin Infect Dis 23:114–17, 1996.
127. Kelkar R, Sastry PS, Kulkarni SS, et al. Pulmonary microsporidial infection in a patient with CML undergoing allogeneic marrow transplant. Bone Marrow Transplant 19:179–82, 1997.
128. Cali A and Takvorian PM. Ultrastructure and development of Pleistophora ronneafiei n. sp., a microsporidium (Protista) in the skeletal muscle of an immune-compromised individual. J Eukaryot Microbiol 50:77–85, 2003.
129. Visvesvara GS, Belloso M, Moura H, et al. Isolation of Nosema algerae from the cornea of an immunocompetent patient. J Eukaryot Microbiol 46:10S, 1999.
130. Cali A, Weiss LM, Takvorian PM. An analysis of the microsporidian genus Brachiola, with comparisons of human and insect isolates of Brachiola algerae. J Eukaryot Microbiol 51:678–85, 2004.
131. Pinnolis M, Egbert PR, Font RL, Winter FC, Nosematosis of the cornea: case report, including electron microscopic studies. Arch Ophthalmol 99:1044–1047, 1981.
132. Cali A, Meisler DM, Lowder CY, et al. Corneal microsporidioses: characterization and identification. J Protozool 38: 215S–217S, 1991.
133. Cali A, Meisler DM, Rutherford I, et al. Corneal microsporidiosis in a patient with AIDS. Am J Trop Med Hyg 44:463–8, 1991.
134. Davis RM, Font RL, Keisler MS, Shadduck JA. Corneal microsporidiosis. A case report including ultrastructural observations. Ophthalmology 97:953–7, 1990.
135. Ashton N, Wirasinha PA. Encephalitozoonosis (nosematosis) of the cornea. Br J Ophthalmol 57(9):669–74, 1973.
136. Deluol AM, Poirot JL, Heyer F, et al. Intestinal microsporidiosis: about clinical characteristics and laboratory diagnosis. J Eukaryot Microbiol 41:33S, 1994.
137. Eeftinck Schattenkerk JK, van Gool T, van Ketel RJ, et al. Clinical significance of small-intestinal microsporidiosis in HIV-1-infected individuals [see comments]. Lancet 337:895–8, 1991.
138. Field AS, Hing MC, Milliken ST, and Marriott DJ. Microsporidia in the small intestine of HIV-infected patients. A new diagnostic technique and a new species. Med J Aust 158:390–4, 1993.
139. Greenson JK, Belitsos PC, Yardley JH, Bartlett JG. AIDS enteropathy: occult enteric infections and duodenal mucosal alterations in chronic diarrhea [see comments]. Ann Intern Med 114:366–72, 1991.
140. Molina JM, Sarfati C, Beauvais B, et al. Intestinal microsporidiosis in human immunodeficiency virus-infected patients with chronic unexplained diarrhea: prevalence and clinical and biologic features. J Infect Dis 167:217–21, 1993.
141. Michiels JF, Hofman P, Saint Paul MC, et al. Pathological features of intestinal microsporidiosis in HIV positive patients. A report of 13 new cases. Pathol Res Pract 189:377–83, 1993.
142. van Gool T, Hollister WS, Schattenkerk WE, et al. Diagnosis of Enterocytozoon bieneusi microsporidiosis in AIDS patients by recovery of spores from faeces. Lancet 336:697–8, 1990.
143. Weber R, Bryan RT, Owen RL, et al. Improved light-microscopical detection of microsporidia spores in stool and duodenal aspirates. The Enteric Opportunistic Infections Working Group. N Engl J Med 326:161–6, 1992.
144. Rabeneck L, Gyorkey F, Genta RM, et al. The prevalence of detectable enteric organisms and microsporidia in HIV-infected patients with and without diarrhea. In: Digestive Disease Week and the 93rd Annual Meeting of the American Gastroenterlological Association. 1992: Gastroenterology.
145. Rabeneck L, Gyorkey F, Genta RM, et al. The role of Microsporidia in the pathogenesis of HIV-related chronic diarrhea [see comments]. Ann Intern Med 119:895–9, 1993.
146. Rabeneck L, Genta RM, Gyorkey F, et al. Observations on the pathological spectrum and clinical course of microsporidiosis in men infected with the human immunodeficiency virus: follow-up study. Clin Infect Dis 20:1229–1235, 1995.
147. Kotler DP, Orenstein JM. Prevalence of intestinal microsporidiosis in HIV-infected individuals referred for gastroenterological evaluation [see comments]. Am J Gastroenterol 89:1998–2002, 1994.
148. Coyle CM, Wittner M, Kotler DP, et al. Prevalence of microsporidiosis due to Enterocytozoon bieneusi and Encephalitozoon (Septata) intestinalis among patients with AIDS-related diarrhea: determination by polymerase chain reaction to the microsporidian small-subunit rRNA gene. Clin Infect Dis 23:1002–6, 1996.
149. Molina JM, Oksenhendler E, Beauvais B, et al. Disseminated microsporidiosis due to Septata intestinalis in patients with AIDS: clinical features and response to albendazole therapy. J Infect Dis 171:245–9, 1995.
150. Molina JM, Goguel J, Sarfati C, et al. Trial of oral fumagillin for the treatment of intestinal microsporidiosis in patients with HIV infection. ANRS 054 Study Group. Agence Nationale de Recherche sur le SIDA. AIDS 14:1341–8, 2000.
151. Molina JM, Tourneur M, Sarfati C, et al. Fumagillin treatment of intestinal microsporidiosis. N Engl J Med 346:1963–9, 2002.
152. Pol S, Romana CA, Richard S, et al. Microsporidia infection in patients with the human immunodeficiency virus and unexplained cholangitis. N Engl J Med 328:95–99, 1993.
153. Mansfield KG, Carville A, Hebert D, et al. Localization of persistent Enterocytozoon bieneusi infection in normal rhesus macaques (Macaca mulatta) to the hepatobiliary tree. J Clin Microbiol 36:2336–8, 1998.
154. Hartskeerl RA, Schuitema AR, van Gool T, Terpstra WJ. Genetic evidence for the occurrence of extra-intestinal Enterocytozoon bieneusi infections. Nucleic Acids Res 21:4150, 1993.
155. Sodqi M, Brazille P, Gonzalez-Canali, et al. Unusual pulmonary Enterocytozoon bieneusi microsporidiosis in an AIDS patient: case report and review. Scand J Infect Dis 36:230–1, 2004.
156. Cali A, Owen RL. Intracellular development of Enterocytozoon, a unique microsporidian found in the intestines of AIDS patients. J. Protozool 37:145–155, 1990.
157. Mertens RB, Didier ES, Fishbein MC, et al. Encephalitozoon cuniculi microsporidiosis: infection of the brain, heart, kidneys, trachea, adrenal glands, and urinary bladder in a patient with AIDS. Mod Pathol 10:68–77, 1997.

158. Willson R, Harrington R, Stewart B, Fritsche T. Human immunodeficiency virus 1-associated necrotizing cholangitis caused by infection with Septata intestinalis. Gastroenterology 108:247–51, 1995.
159. Belcher JW Jr, Guttenberg SA, Schmookler BM. Microsporidiosis of the mandible in a patient with acquired immunodeficiency syndrome. J Oral Maxillofac Surg 55: 424–6, 1997.
160. Gunnarsson G, Hurlbut D, DeGirolami PC, et al. Multiorgan microsporidiosis: report of five cases and review. Clin Infect Dis 21:37–44, 1995.
161. Weber R, Sauer B, Spycher MA, et al. Detection of Septata intestinalis in stool specimens and coprodiagnostic monitoring of successful treatment with albendazole. Clin Infect Dis 19:342–5, 1994.
162. Terada S, Rajender Reddy K, Jeffers LJ, et al. Microsporidan hepatitis in the acquired immunodeficiency syndrome. Ann Intern Med 107:61–62, 1987.
163. Gordon SC, Reddy KR, Gould EE, et al. The spectrum of liver disease in the acquired immunodeficiency syndrome. J Hepatol 2:475–84, 1986.
164. Degroote MA, Visvesvara G, Wilson ML, et al. Polymerase chain reaction and culture confirmation of disseminated Encephalitozoon cuniculi in a patient with AIDS: successful therapy with albendazole. J. Infect. Dis 171:1375–1378, 1995.
165. Schwartz DA, Bryan RT, Hewanlowe KO, et al. Disseminated microsporidiosis (Encephalitozoon hellem) and acquired immunodeficiency syndrome – autopsy evidence for respiratory acquisition. Arch. Pathol. Lab. Med 116:660–668, 1992.
166. Schwartz DA, Bryan RT, Hewanlowe KO, et al. Disseminated microsporidiosis and AIDS; pathologic evidence for respiratory transmission of Encephalitozoon infection. Int Conf AIDS. 1992.
167. Weber R, Kuster H, Visvesvara GS, et al. Disseminated microsporidiosis due to Encephalitozoon hellem: pulmonary colonization, microhematuria, and mild conjunctivitis in a patient with AIDS. Clin Infect Dis 17:415–19, 1993.
168. Visvesvara GS, Leitch GJ, da Silva AJ, et al. Polyclonal and monoclonal antibody and PCR-amplified small-subunit rRNA identification of a microsporidian, Encephalitozoon hellem, isolated from an AIDS patient with disseminated infection. J Clin Microbiol 32:2760–8, 1994.
169. Lowder CY, Meisler DM, McMahon JT, et al. Microsporidia infection of the cornea in a man seropositive for human immunodeficiency virus. Am J Ophthalmol 109:242–4, 1990.
170. Lowder CY, McMahon JT, Meisler DM, et al. Microsporidial keratoconjunctivitis caused by Septata intestinalis in a patient with acquired immunodeficiency syndrome. Am J Ophthalmol 121:715–17, 1996.
171. Theng J, Chan C, Ling ML, Tan D. Microsporidial keratoconjunctivitis in a healthy contact lens wearer without human immunodeficiency virus infection. Ophthalmology 108:976–8, 2001.
172. Visvesvara GS, Leitch GJ, Moura H, et al. Culture, electron microscopy, and immunoblot studies on a microsporidian parasite isolated from the urine of a patient with AIDS. J. Protozool 38:105s–11s, 1991.
173. Didier ES, Shadduck JA, Didier PJ, et al. Studies on ocular microsporidia. J Protozool 38:635–8, 1991.
174. Birthistle K, Moore P, Hay P. Microsporidia: a new sexually transmissable cause of urethritis [letter]. Genitourin Med 72:445, 1996.
175. Juarez SI, Putaporntip C, Jongwutiwes S, et al. In vitro cultivation and electron microscopy characterization of Trachipleistophora anthropophthera isolated from the cornea of an AIDS patient. J Eukaryot Microbiol 52:179–90, 2005.
176. Macher AR, Neafie R, Angritt P, Tuur S. Microsporidia myositis and the acquired immunodeficiency syndrome (AIDS): a four year followup. Ann Intern Med 109:343–344, 1988.
177. Weber R, Bryan RT, Owen RL, et al. Improved light-microscopal detection of microsporidia spores in stool and duodenal aspirates. New England J Med 326:161–166, 1992.
178. Vavra J, Dahbiova R, Hollister WS, Canning EU. Staining of microsporidian spores by optical brighteners with remarks on the use of brighteners for the diagnosis of AIDS associated human microsporidioses. Folia Parasitol 40: 267–72, 1993.
179. van Gool T, Snijders F, Reiss P, et al. Diagnosis of intestinal and disseminated microsporidial infections in patients with HIV by a new rapid fluorescence technique. J Clin Pathol 46(8):694–9, 1993.
180. Ryan NJ, Sutherland G, Coughlan K, et al. A new trichrome-blue stain for detection of microsporidial species in urine, stool, and nasopharyngeal specimens. J Clin Microbiol 31:3264–9, 1993.
181. Kokoskin E, Gyorkos TW, Camus A, et al. Modified technique for efficient detection of microsporidia. J Clin Microbiol 32:1074–5, 1994.
182. Didier ES, Orenstein JM, Aldras A, et al. Comparison of three staining methods for detecting microsporidia in fluids. J Clin Microbiol 33:3138–45, 1995.
183. DeGirolami PC, Ezratty CR, Desai G, et al. Diagnosis of intestinal microsporidiosis by examination of stool and duodenal aspirate with Weber's modified trichrome and Uvitex 2B strains. J Clin Microbiol 33:805–10, 1995.
184. Zierdt CH, Gill VJ, Zierdt WS. Detection of microsporidian spores in clinical samples by indirect fluorescent-antibody assay using whole-cell antisera to Encephalitozoon cuniculi and Encephalitozoon hellem. J Clin Microbiol 31:3071–4, 1993.
185. Croppo GP, Visvesvara GS, Leitch GJ, et al. Identification of the microsporidian Encephalitozoon hellem using immunoglobulin G monoclonal antibodies. Arch Pathol Lab Med 122:182–6, 1998.
186. Beckers PJA, Derks GJMM, Gool TV, et al. Encephalocytozoon (sic) intestinalis-specific monoclonal antibodies for laboratory diagnosis of microsporidiosis. J Clin Microbiol 34:282–285, 1996.
187. Achbarou A, Thellier M, Accoceberry I, et al. Production of immunological probes raised against Enterocytozoon bieneusi and Encephalitozoon intestinalis, two microsporidian species causing intestinal infections in man. J Eukaryot Microbiol 46:32S–33S, 1999.
188. Accoceberry I, Thellier M, Desportes-Livage I, et al. Production of monoclonal antibodies directed against the microsporidium Enterocytozoon bieneusi. J Clin Microbiol 37:4107–12, 1999.
189. Sheoran AS, Feng X, Kitaka S, et al. Purification of Enterocytozoon bieneusi from stools and production of specific antibodies. J Clin Microbiol 43:387–92, 2005.
190. Sheoran AS, Feng X, Singh I, et al. Monoclonal antibodies against Enterocytozoon bieneusi of human origin. Clin Diagn Lab Immunol 12:1109–13, 2005.
191. Didier E, Kotler D, Dietrich DT. Serologic studies in human microsporidosis. AIDS (7):S8, 1993.
192. Katzwinkel-Wladarsch S, Deplazes P, Weber R, et al. Comparison of polymerase chain reaction with light microscopy for detection of microsporida in clinical specimens. Eur J Clin Microbiol & Infectious Diseases 16:7–10, 1997.
193. Ombrouck C, Ciceron L, Biligui S, et al. Specific PCR assay for direct detection of intestinal microsporidia Enterocytozoon bieneusi and Encephalitozoon intestinalis in fecal specimens from human immunodeficiency virus-infected patients. J Clin Microbiol 35:652–655, 1997.

194. Fedorko DP, Nelson NA, Cartwright CP. Identification of microsporidia in stool specimens by using PCR and restriction endonucleases. J Clin Microbiol 33:1739–41, 1995.
195. Fedorko DP, Nelson NA, Didier ES, et al. Speciation of human microsporidia by polymerase chain reaction single-strand conformation polymorphism. Am J Trop Med Hyg 65:397–401, 2001.
196. Costa SF, Weiss LM. Drug treatment of microsporidiosis. Drug Resist Updat 3:384–399, 2000.
197. Molina JM, Goguel J, Sarfati C, et al. Trial of oral fumagillin for the treatment of intestinal microsporidiosis in patients with HIV infection. ANRS 054 Study Group. Agence Nationale de Recherche sur le SIDA [In Process Citation]. AIDS 14(10):1341–8, 2000.
198. Dieterich DT, Lew EA, Kotler DP, et al. Treatment with Albendazole for intestinal disease due to Enterocytozoon bieneusi in patients with AIDS. J. Infect. Dis 169:178–183, 1994.
199. Dore GJ, Marriott DJ, Hing MC, et al. Disseminated microsporidiosis due to Septata intestinalis in nine patients infected with the human immunodeficiency virus: response to therapy with albendazole. Clin Infect Dis 21:70–6, 1995.
200. Rosberger DF, Serdarevic ON, Erlandson RA, et al. Successful treatment of microsporidial keratoconjunctivitis with topical fumagillin in a patient with AIDS. Cornea 12:261–5, 1993.
201. Haque A, Hollister WS, Willcox A, Canning EU. The antimicrosporidial activity of albendazole. J Invertebr Pathol 62:171–7, 1993.
202. Beauvais B, Sarfati C, Challier S, Derouin F. In vitro model to assess effect of antimicrobial agents on Encephalitozoon cuniculi. Antimicrob Agents Chemother 38:2440–8, 1994.
203. Ditrich O, Kucerova Z, Koudela B. In vitro sensitivity of Encephalitozoon cuniculi and E. hellem to albendazole. J Eukaryot Microbiol 41:37S, 1994.
204. Diesenhouse MC, Wilson LA, Corrent GF, et al. Treatment of microsporidial keratoconjunctivitis with topical fumagillin [see comments]. Am J Ophthalmol 115:293–8, 1993.
205. Blanshard C, Peacock C, Ellis D, Gazzard B. Treatment of intestinal microsporidiosis with Albendazole. In: VII International Conference on AIDS: Science challenging AIDS, Florence, Italy: Clinical Science & Trials; 1991.
206. Franssen FF, Lumeij JT, van Knapen F, Susceptibility of Encephalitozoon cuniculi to several drugs in vitro. Antimicrob Agents Chemother 39:1265–8, 1995.
207. Molina JM, Chastang C, Goguel J, et al. Albendazole for treatment and prophylaxis of microsporidiosis due to Encephalitozoon intestinalis in patients with AIDS: a randomized double-blind controlled trial. J Infect Dis 177(5):1373–7, 1998.
208. Tremoulet AH, Avila-Aguero ML, Paris MM, et al. Albendazole therapy for Microsporidium diarrhea in immunocompetent Costa Rican children. Pediatr Infect Dis J 23: 915–18, 2004.
209. Asmuth DM, DeGirolami PC, Federman M, et al. Clinical features of microsporidiosis in patients with AIDS. Clin Infect Dis 18:819–25, 1994.
210. Anwar-Bruni DM, Hogan SE, Schwartz DA, et al. Atovaquone is effective treatment for the symptoms of gastrointestinal microsporidiosis in HIV-1-infected patients. AIDS 10:619–23, 1996.
211. Albrecht H, Sobottka I, Stellbrink HJ, Greten H. Does the choice of Pneumocystis carinii prophylaxis influence the prevalence of Enterocytozoon bieneusi microsporidiosis in AIDS patients? [letter]. AIDS 9:302–3, 1995.
212. Sharpstone D, Rowbottom A, Nelson M, Gazzard B. The treatment of microsporidial diarrhoea with thalidomide [letter]. AIDS 9:658–9, 1995.
213. Sharpstone D, Rowbottom A, Francis N, et al. Thalidomide: a novel therapy for microsporidiosis [published erratum appears in Gastroenterology 1997 Sep;113(3):1054]. Gastroenterology 112:1823–9, 1997.
214. Haque MA, Canning EU. Screening of drugs against microsporidia. Pak J Sci Ind Res 38:25–29 1995.
215. Weiss LM, Michalakakis E, Coyle CM, et al. The in vitro activity of albendazole against Encephalitozoon cuniculi. J Eukaryot Microbiol 41:65S, 1994.
216. Didier ES. Effects of albendazole, fumagillin, and TNP-470 on microsporidial replication in vitro. Antimicrob Agents Chemother 41:1541–6, 1997.
217. Didier ES, Maddry JA, Kwong CD, et al. Screening of compounds for antimicrosporidial activity in vitro. Folia Parasitol 45:129–39, 1998.
218. Edlind T, Visvesvara G, Li J, Katiyar S. Cryptosporidium and microsporidial beta-tubulin sequences: predictions of benzimidazole sensitivity and phylogeny. J Eukaryot Microbiol 41:38S, 1994.
219. Li X, Chang YH. Evidence that the human homologue of a rat initiation factor-2 associated protein (p67) is a methionine aminopeptidase. Biochem Biophys Res Commun 227:152–9, 1996.
220. Shah V, Marino C, Altice FL. Albendazole-induced pseudomembranous colitis. Am J Gastroenterol 91:1453–4, 1996.
221. Lecuit M, Oksenhendler E, Sarfati C. Use of albendazole for disseminated microsporidian infection in a patient with AIDS. J Infect Dis 19:332–333, 1994.
222. Deiterich D, Kotler D, LaFleur F, et al. Albendazole treatment of two species of microsporidial enteritis. In: VIII International Conference on AIDS and the II STD World Congress, Amsterdam: Harvard-Amsterdam Conference; 1992.
223. Leder K, Ryan N, Spelman D, Crowe SM. Microsporidial disease in HIV-infected patients: a report of 42 patients and review of the literature. Scand J Infect Dis. 30:331–8, 1998.
224. Katsnelson H, Jamieson CA. Control of Nosema disease of honeybees with fumagillin. Science 115:70–72, 1952.
225. Kano T, Fukui H. Studies on Pleistophora infection in eel, Anguilla japonica I. Experimental induction of microsporidiosis and fumagillin efficacy. Fish Pathol 16:193–200, 1982.
226. Kent M, Dawe SC. Efficacy of fumagillin DCH against experimentally induced Loma salmonae (Microsporea) infections in chinnok salmon Oncorhynchus tsawytscha. Dis Aquat Organ (20):231–5, 1994.
227. Higgins MJ, Kent ML, Moran JD, et al. Efficacy of the fumagillin analog TNP-470 for Nucleospora salmonis and Loma salmonae infections in chinook salmon Oncorhynchus tshawytscha. Dis Aquat Organ 34:45–9, 1998.
228. Molina JM, Goguel J, Sarfati C, et al. Potential efficacy of fumagillin in intestinal microsporidiosis due to Enterocytozoon bieneusi in patients with HIV infection: results of a drug screening study. The French Microsporidiosis Study Group. AIDS 11:1603–10, 1997.
229. Shadduck JA. Effect of fumagillin on in vitro multiplication of Encephalitozoon cuniculi. J Protozool 27:202–208, 1980.
230. Coyle C, Kent M, Tanowitz HB, et al. TNP-470 is an effective antimicrosporidial agent. J Infect Dis 177:515–18, 1998.
231. Griffith EC, Su Z, Niwayama S, et al. Molecular recognition of angiogenesis inhibitors fumagillin and ovalicin by methionine aminopeptidase 2. Proc Natl Acad Sci U S A 95: 15183–8, 1998.
232. Liu S, Widom J, Kemp CW, et al. Structure of human methionine aminopeptidase-2 complexed with fumagillin. Science 282:1324–7, 1998.
233. Zhang H, Huang H, Cali A, et al. Investigations into microsporidian methionine aminopeptidase type 2: a therapeutic

target for microsporidiosis. Folia Parasitol (Praha) 52:182–92, 2005.

234. Orenstein JM, Seedor J, Friedberg DN, et al. Microsporidian keratoconjunctivitis in patients with AIDS. MMWR:188–189, 1990.

235. Johnson CH, Marshall MM, DeMaria LA, et al. Chlorine inactivation of spores of Encephalitozoon spp. Appl Environ Microbiol 69:1325–6, 2003.

236. Blanshard C, Ellis DS, Tovey DG, et al. Treatment of intestinal microsporidiosis with albendazole in patients with AIDS. AIDS 6:311–13, 1992.

237. Blanshard C, Ellis DS, Dowell SP, et al. Electron microscopic changes in Enterocytozoon bieneusi following treatment with albendazole. J Clin Pathol 46:898–902, 1993.

238. Eeftinck-Schattenkerk JK, van Gool T, van Ketel RJ, et al. Clinical significance of small-intestinal microsporidiosis in HIV-1 infected individuals. Comment in: Lancet 337:1488–1489, 1991.

239. Rossi P, Urbani C, Donelli G, Pozio E. Resolution of microsporidial sinusitis and keratoconjunctivitis by itraconazole treatment. Am J Ophthalmol 127:210–12, 1999.

240. Gritz DC, Holsclaw DS, Neger RE, et al. Ocular and sinus microsporidial infection cured with systemic albendazole. Am J Ophthalmol 124:241–3, 1997.

241. Dionisio D, Manneschi LI, Di Lollo S, et al. Enterocytozoon bieneusi in AIDS: symptomatic relief and parasite changes after furazolidone. J Clin Pathol 50:472–6, 1997.

242. Dionisio D, Sterrantino G, Meli M, et al. Use of furazolidone for the treatment of microsporidiosis due to Enterocytozoon bieneusi in patients with AIDS. Recenti Prog Med 86:394–7, 1995.

243. Bicart-See A, Massip P, Linas MD, Datry A. Successful treatment with nitazoxanide of Enterocytozoon bieneusi microsporidiosis in a patient with AIDS. Antimicrob Agents Chemother 44:167–8, 2000.

244. Hsiao T. Benomyl: a novel drug for controlling a microsporidian disease of the alfalfa weevil. J Invertebr Pathol (22):303–7, 1973.

245. Schmahl G, Toukhy AE, Ghaffar FA. Transmission electron microscopicstudies on the effects of toltrazuril on Glugea anomala, Moniez, 1887 (microsporida) infecting the three-spined stickleback Gastrosteus aculeatus. Parasitol Res 76:700–706, 1990.

Chapter 40

Mycobacterium tuberculosis

Thomas E. Dobbs, MD, MPH, Michael E. Kimerling, MD, MPH

> All who mix with tuberculosis patients got infected, but remained well so long as they took care of themselves and kept the soil in a condition unfavourable for the growth of the seed.[1,2]

Speaking of physicians and nurses working in tuberculosis (TB) hospitals a century ago, when TB was a leading cause of death in the United States and Europe, the words of William Osler reflect an early recognition of the important yet undefined relationship between a TB-infected person's underlying health status (the soil) and the ability to hold in check the causative agent of TB (*Mycobacterium tuberculosis*, the seed). His words remain relevant a century later. Although most people exposed to a TB case will not become infected, the population proportion infected over time increases in high TB burden regions. While certain conditions for the growth of the seed found during Osler's time (poverty, crowding, malnutrition) remain common in these regions, other conditions have changed since 1910. The single greatest threat to treatment and control of TB today is the recent emergence of an HIV pandemic and its expanding overlay of an already well-established TB epidemic. This chapter will present the background for understanding TB co-infection in the HIV-infected patient and review the key elements to its epidemiology, diagnosis, treatment, and prevention.

TB EPIDEMIOLOGY AND CONTROL STRATEGY

Global

Mycobacterium tuberculosis infection is one of the most common infections in the world. Globally, it is estimated that one-third of the world's population is infected with TB without any evidence of disease. Infection prevalence in the Southeast Asia region is estimated at 44%; Africa, 35%; and Europe, 15%. Individual country rates vary among the highest TB incidence countries: 64% in Cambodia, 49% in Indonesia, 44% in India, 44% in Peru, 38% in South Africa, and 36% each in China, Nigeria, and Kenya.[3] Despite an available cure since the 1940s, in 1993 the World Health Organization (WHO) declared TB a global emergency, largely reflecting the neglected worldwide epidemic of undetected and untreated TB cases combined with a lack of international interest or funding for TB treatment and control.[4] This declaration followed the establishment in 1991 of a global program framework and case management strategy known as DOTS (Directly Observed Therapy, Short Course). The DOTS strategy is based on five pillars that mix technical and managerial elements, including: laboratory services to diagnose infectious cases; standardized chemotherapy using directly observed therapy; an uninterrupted supply of quality-assured drugs; and a recording/reporting system for monitoring treatment outcomes.[5] Over the last several years, the DOTS strategy has expanded to incorporate the challenges inherent to the diagnosis and care of drug-resistant cases and persons dually infected with TB and HIV.[6–9]

In 2005, WHO declared TB an emergency for Africa.[10] For 2004, an estimated 8.9 million persons developed new TB disease worldwide; 1.7 million died from TB, including 229 000 cases co-infected with HIV.[11] Among the new cases, some 8.3% were HIV-infected worldwide. However, adult co-infection rates (ages 15–49 years) are substantially higher in many countries: Cambodia, 13%; Ethiopia, 21%; Kenya, 29%; Tanzania, 36%; Mozambique, 49%; South Africa, 61%; and Zimbabwe, 69%. Surveillance data for 2003 showed an overall increase in the global TB incidence of 1% compared with 2002, impacted most strongly by the enormous increase in incidence occurring in sub-Saharan Africa, particularly in high HIV prevalence countries (adult HIV prevalence >4%). Except for the African region, TB incidence either fell or was stable elsewhere.[11–13] It is expected that TB prevalence will double in high-HIV areas of Africa to 609 per 100 000 by the year 2015 (compared with 288 in 1990).[12]

United States

As of 2000, there were an estimated 9.5–14.7 million persons with latent TB infection (LTBI) in the United States, representing 3.4–5.2% of the counted population.[14] The US TB case rate dropped an average of 5.5% per year from 1953 to 1985 (range 0–11%). From 1986 through 1992, the number of TB cases and annual US rate increased. This increase was attributed to: deterioration of the public health care infrastructure; emerging HIV epidemic; immigration from countries where TB is highly prevalent; and spread of TB within congregate settings and facilities (homeless shelters, correctional institutions, nursing homes). Since 1992, an annual decline in reported cases resumed. In 2004, there were 14 517 TB cases reported to the CDC, representing a 46% decrease since 1992. However, the number of foreign-born cases reached a new level at 54% of all cases, and for the first time, there were more Hispanic cases than non-Hispanic blacks. The TB case rate for foreign-born persons in 2004 was nearly nine times that of US-born persons (22.8 vs 2.6 per 100 000).[15] TB-HIV co-infection data is incomplete nationally due to limited testing and reporting as of 2004.

The principles and practice of TB control in the US are similar to those of the WHO. However, given the available resources and low disease burden, TB 'elimination' is the goal with an expanded emphasis on specific control components. The main components are: (1) early identification and treatment of all cases using a rifampin-based regimen, employing directly observed therapy as standard of care; (2) contact investigations around each index case, prioritized by the level of infectiousness (i.e., sputum smear positive, cavity on chest radiograph), contact risk factors (i.e., age, HIV status) and type of exposure environment (open, closed, ventilated); secondary cases are identified in this manner; (3) targeted testing of at-risk groups with treatment of LTBI to reduce the risk of subsequent disease activation; (4) infection control strategies for high-risk settings such as hospitals, health care facilities, prisons and congregate settings such as nursing homes and homeless shelters; and (5) testing of each TB isolate for the presence of drug resistance to ensure adequate therapy is used. Given the limited efficacy of the current BCG vaccination demonstrated in the US, particularly its inability to prevent infection and the limited transmission of TB in the general community, BCG vaccination is not a component of the US strategy.[14]

MYCOBACTERIUM TUBERCULOSIS AND THE *M. TUBERCULOSIS* COMPLEX

Mycobacterium tuberculosis is part of what is called the MTB complex, a six-member group of closely related pathogens distinguished by a lack of genetic diversity with a highly stable and conserved genome.[16,17] Members of the MTB complex are considered a single species as defined by DNA/DNA hybridization studies.[18,19] This complex includes *M. tuberculosis* (which is the predominate cause of human TB worldwide), *M. bovis* (which causes TB in cattle, deer, elephants, other wildlife and less frequently in humans since milk pasteurization was introduced), *M. africanuum* (which is largely limited to sub-Saharan Africa but reported in Europe and recently in the US),[20] *M. canettii* (a smooth, glossy variant of MTB and rare cause of human TB), *M. microti* (found only in voles or meadow mice) and *M. bovis* bacille Calmette-Guerin (*M. bovis* BCG, which is the live attenuated derivative of *M. bovis* used globally as the vaccine against human TB).

Clinical and Mycobacterial laboratories do not routinely distinguish between these related organisms when reporting a culture as positive growth for TB (meaning *M. tuberculosis* complex). Discrimination between them is possible, however, through various methods or combination of methods including spoligotyping, DNA fingerprinting using restriction fragment length polymorphism (RFLP) analysis, known deletion mutations, biochemical testing (niacin production, nitrate reduction), susceptibility or resistance to pyrazinamide and morphology.[18,20] The doubling time of *M. tuberculosis* and other members of the complex is ~22 to 24 h.

Evolution

Except for *M. tuberculosis* complex and *M. leprae*, most mycobacteria are commonly found in soil and water and not transmitted from person to person. Today, these so-called 'environmental' mycobacteria are collectively grouped as non-tuberculous Mycobacteria (NTM) or Mycobacteria Other Than Tuberculosis (MOTT). They include *M. avium-intracellulare* or *M. avium* complex, *M. kansasii*, *M. abscessus*, *M. chelonae* and *M. ulcerans* (Buruli ulcer disease), among several dozen validly described species.[21,22] The *M. tuberculosis* complex likely evolved to infect mammals from similar environmental sources,[18] and *M. tuberculosis* became a human pathogen some 10 000 to 15 000 years ago.[23,17] While it was believed that *M. tuberculosis* evolved from *M. bovis* (presumably after the domestication of cattle), recent analysis of the evolutionary pathway shows this is not the case. Rather, the *M. tuberculosis* lineage appears to have separated from a common ancestor before the lineage leading to *M. bovis*.[16]

Transmission

The primary means of TB transmission is person to person via the airborne route. Rarely, TB is transmitted at birth, through an open wound or across the skin through direct inoculation of infectious material. Patient-generated aerosols contain a mass of droplets expelled through talking, coughing, sneezing and singing. While most large droplets will fall to the ground quickly, smaller ones may float in the air for a long enough period to allow for droplet evaporation, yielding infectious droplet nuclei. It is these droplet nuclei of 1–5 μm in diameter that find their way to the lung alveoli where infection may be established.[24] Transmission is influenced by the concentration of organisms in the air (number of TB organisms/volume of air) and total duration of exposure, which are directly impacted by the type of exposure environment (i.e., ventilation and air exchange), characteristics of the source case (i.e., sputum smear positive for acid-fast bacilli, AFB; presence of a cavity on chest radiograph) and contact characteristics (i.e., relationship to the source case, immune status, genetic susceptibility).[25–28] In a molecular epidemiology study of clustered cases in San Francisco, 17% of secondary cases were determined to have resulted from transmission by a smear negative case. The relative transmission rate of a smear negative compared with smear positive source case was 0.22 and not impacted by HIV status.[29]

PRESENTATION OF TB IN HIV-INFECTED INDIVIDUALS

The clinical manifestations of TB are frequently altered in the setting of HIV co-infection. Typical symptoms and clinical patterns of disease are encountered in those with relatively preserved immune function.[30] As immune function deteriorates, there is a progression toward increased adenopathy, involvement of lower and middle lobes of the lung, less cavitation (Fig. 40-1), and more extrapulmonary disease.[31–35] Confirmed TB may also be found in those without any symptoms of disease.[36] The degree of immunosuppression affects the disease location as demonstrated by a progressively higher frequency of extrapulmonary involvement with advancing CD4 lymphopenia.[37] In clinical studies, pulmonary disease has been demonstrated over a wide range of CD4 counts with localized extrapulmonary disease, meningitis, and dissemination occurring with progressively lower median CD4 counts (Fig. 40-2). TB pleural effusions may occur at rates similar to those seen in patients without HIV,[38,39] although a study from South Africa demonstrated a significantly higher rate among HIV-positive patients than HIV negative (38% vs 20%).[35] Pleural effusions have been documented to occur less frequently in those with CD4 counts <200 cells/mm^3 compared to those with CD4 counts >200 (10% vs 28%).[37] Further, pulmonary disease often occurs following recent infection as documented by molecular epidemiologic studies showing HIV infection to be associated with clustering, suggesting recent transmission.[40–42]

As noted, chest radiograph findings in HIV-infected TB patients vary. Those with more advanced immunosuppression have less cavitation and a higher frequency of lymphadenopathy.[31–33] A study from Cote D'Ivoire found cavitary disease in 53% of HIV-infected TB patients with CD4 counts >200 and only 29% in those with more advanced immunosuppression. HIV-negative (control) patients had cavitary disease on 56% of chest radiographs. Additionally, there was incremental progression, with lower rates of cavitation and higher rates of lymphadenopathy, when stratified by decreasing CD4 cell counts.[32] The use of highly active antiretroviral therapy (HAART), however, has been associated with more typical CXR findings in HIV-infected patients with pulmonary TB.[43] Subclinical TB has also been described in the HIV-infected. A Tanzania study detected TB in 14 of 93 patients screened. Four of these reported no symptoms of TB and had a normal chest radiograph; the diagnosis was made by sputum culture.[36]

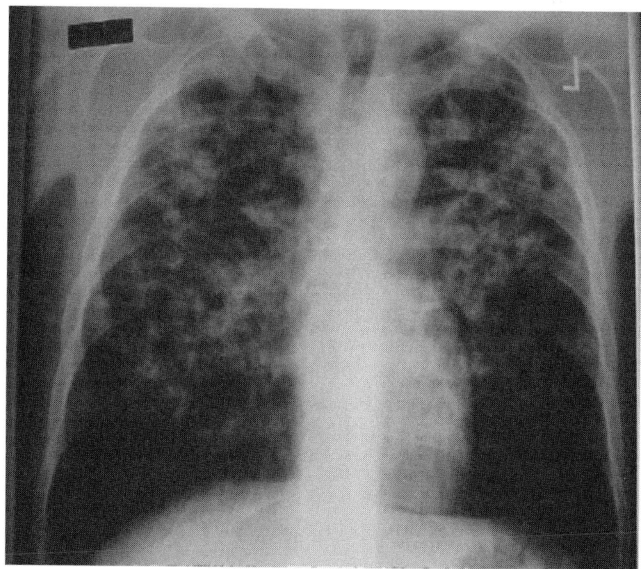

Figure 40-1 ■ Extensive bilateral pulmonary tuberculosis with upper zone predominance and lack of cavitation in a patient with advanced HIV infection (CD4 < 50).

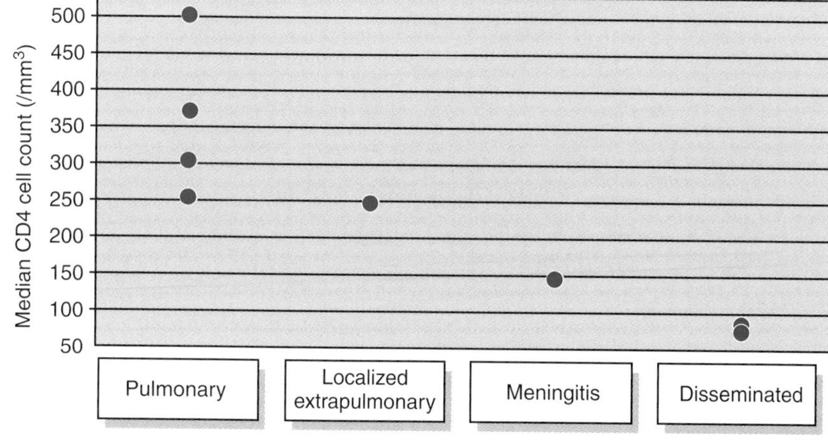

Figure 40-2 ■ Median CD4 counts (per mm^3) in different groups of human immunodeficiency virus-positive patients with tuberculosis.

Adapted from De Cock KM, Soro B, Coulibaly IM, et al. Tuberculosis and HIV infection in sub-Saharan Africa. JAMA 268:1581-7, 1992.

Several clinical studies suggest that HIV-infected patients with culture confirmed pulmonary TB are less likely to be sputum smear-positive than their HIV-negative counterparts[31,44–47]; however, this is not universally found.[48–50] The studies demonstrating no differences in smear-positivity rates utilized fluorescence microscopy. This methodology, when compared with routine Ziehl–Neelsen staining, has been shown to be more sensitive and more likely to detect bacilli in paucibacillary cases[51,52] and is not impacted by HIV status.[52] Most studies,[37,52a,52b] but not all,[48] have shown an association with lower CD4 cell counts and smear positive sputum status.

In the setting of advanced HIV infection, AFB blood cultures have been shown to be a valuable tool in the diagnosis and confirmation of disseminated TB. *M. tuberculosis* bacteremia is frequently encountered in febrile AIDS patients in areas of moderate to high endemicity, ranging from 12% to 38%.[53–55] The frequency of mycobacteremia correlates with the degree of immunosuppression. In one study of known TB patients in Los Angeles, *M. tuberculosis* was isolated from the blood of 49% (18 of 37) of patients with CD4 <100, 20% (3 of 15) with CD4 from 101 to 200, 7% (1 of 15) with CD4 from 201 to 300, and in none among eight patients with CD4 >300.[37] In two studies from Botswana and Brazil, blood culture was the sole means of diagnosis in 15% of cases.[54,56] The Botswana study involved TB suspects with cough. Overall, 22% of the study cohort was found to have a positive blood culture, including several patients also having a positive sputum culture.

EFFECT OF TB/HIV CO-INFECTION AND THE IMPACT OF HAART ON TB

TB has a deleterious effect on the natural history of HIV infection demonstrated by worse clinical outcomes and enhanced viral replication. Marked increases in viral replication are associated with active TB. Goletti et al observed five- to 160-fold increases in viral replication in patients with active disease following the diagnosis of TB.[58] TB has also been associated with increased mortality among HIV-infected individuals and may be associated with higher rates of subsequent opportunistic infections (OIs). Two European studies demonstrated significantly higher mortality rates associated with the acquisition of clinical TB, with relative risks of death of 1.34 (95% CI, 1.12-1.60)[59] and 1.5 (95% CI, 1.2-2.1).[60] A study from Uganda found higher mortality associated with pulmonary TB in HIV-infected patients (RR 1.81, 95% CI, 1.24-1.65). The mortality effect was even more pronounced for those with CD4 counts >200 (RR 3.0, 95% CI, 1.62-5.63),[61] when other OIs are less likely to occur. A study in the US comparing HIV-infected subjects with and without TB found higher mortality rates in those with TB. A trend toward a higher frequency of subsequent OIs was also found (RR 1.42, 95% CI, 0.94-2.11),[62] suggesting TB may accelerate the time course of HIV infection.

Among TB patients, mortality is consistently higher among HIV-positive than HIV-uninfected individuals.[63–65] In a study by Perriens et al of pulmonary TB,[65] 12 month survival was 69% in the HIV-infected and 98% in the HIV-negative group. TB attributable mortality was 27.8% among those with HIV. Chaisson et al, in a study from Haiti including pulmonary and extrapulmonary disease, demonstrated 33% mortality at 18 months in the HIV-positive group compared with 3% in the HIV-negative group.[64] HAART was not utilized in these studies. Diminished CD4 counts less than 100 and not using DOT have been associated with poorer survival among the HIV-TB co-infected.[66] A study of HIV-infected, smear-positive pulmonary TB cases from Uganda found anergy to tuberculin, CXR findings atypical for TB, lymphopenia, and a previous diagnosis of an HIV-associated illness all to be independent predictors of death.[67] Observational data demonstrates a large proportion of early deaths (<30 days) are attributable to TB,[68–70] while a majority of deaths beyond the first month of treatment have been attributed to causes other than TB.[69]

Impact of HAART on TB

In vitro data has demonstrated improved immunologic responses to tuberculin antigens following the initiation of HAART.[71] Such responses remain less robust in HIV-infected individuals on HAART, however, than in HIV-negative controls.[72] The improvement in immune response may be limited in those with more advanced immunosuppression prior to TB diagnosis (CD4 <50) despite an adequate response to HAART (a rise in CD4 count of 150 copies/ml from baseline at 12 months and viral load (VL) <50 at 24 weeks).[73] These data, when considered together, imply that HAART is not sufficient to restore full anti-TB cellular immune responses.[73,74] Nonetheless, HAART has been associated with improved mortality rates in those with active TB.[43]

Importantly, the use of HAART has been shown to lower the risk of developing active TB with risk reductions ranging from 80% to 92% across studies.[75–78] However, a study in South Africa demonstrated a significantly lowered incidence only in those with moderate to advanced immunosuppression, as TB manifests more frequently in those with lower CD4 counts. The incidence rate without HAART was 17.5/100 patient-years for CD4 <200 (3.4 with HAART) and 12.0/100 patient-years for CD4 between 200 and 350 (1.7 with HAART). The incidence risk ratio was not significantly reduced for CD4 values >350, although some cases were averted with HAART use.[75] This study excluded pregnant and lactating women.

Despite HAART, TB rates remain higher for those with HIV infection compared to those without HIV infection in both low and high prevalence settings.[75,79] In a large cohort analysis of HIV-infected patients across Europe and North America, among those initiated on HAART and followed for 3 years, a low baseline CD4 count, a low CD4 count at 6 months, and a viral load >400 copies/mL after 6 months of HAART were independently associated with a higher risk of developing TB [80].

While antiretroviral therapy (ART) is clearly an invaluable component of care for the individually co-infected patient and in combating the global TB epidemic, HAART alone is unlikely to reverse the high rates of TB associated with HIV infection. Extensive modeling of the potential impact of HAART on subsequent development of TB suggests that universal HAART for CD4 <200 would produce only modest reductions in the cumulative incidence of TB (22% over 20 years). Extending HAART to effectively cover 85% of those with a CD4 count up to 500 μL would result in an incidence drop of only 50% over 20 years.[81] The less than expected impact reflects the greater life expectancy of those on ART and therefore a longer opportunity to develop active TB, albeit at a lower rate than without ART.[81,74] A second model suggests that improving TB diagnosis and cure rates are the most cost-effective means of controlling TB when ART therapy is included in the control strategy.[82]

DIAGNOSIS OF DISEASE

Before TB can be diagnosed, it must be suspected. There are four steps in diagnosing TB (Fig. 40-3):

Step 1

Think TB and obtain a good medical history- The initial step is to determine if the patient has been exposed to a person with active disease, has symptoms of TB, a previous history of LTBI or active disease, and risk factors for TB. Exposure may be higher for individuals in certain professions or those living in congregate settings. Persons with TB may be symptomatic or asymptomatic, including HIV co-infected patients.[36] If the suspect patient has been treated for LTBI or previous disease, it is important to determine the drugs used and compliance with any therapy.

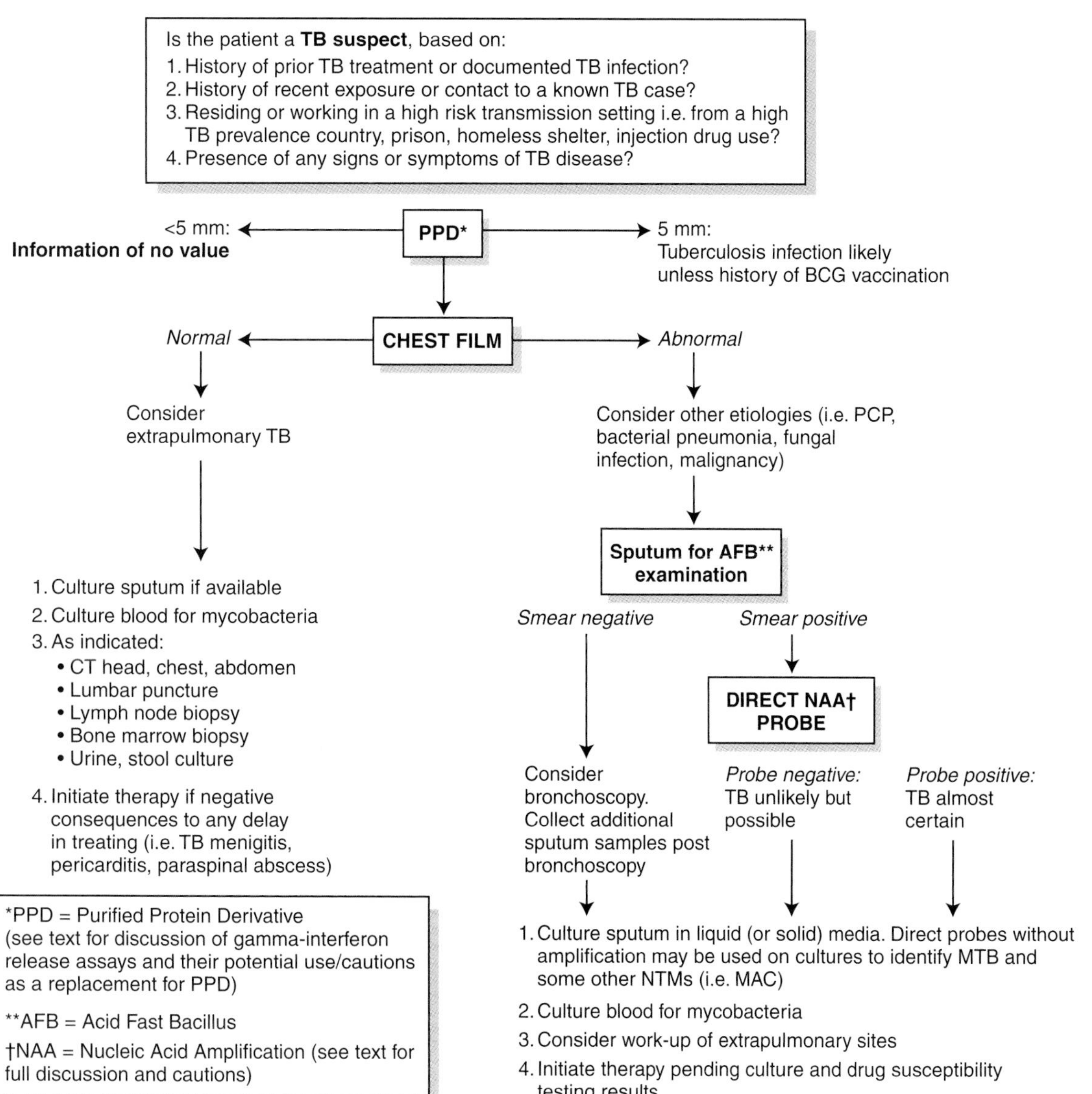

Figure 40-3 ■ Diagnostic approaches for suspected tuberculosis.

Step 2

Give the patient a tuberculin skin test (TST) using the purified protein derivative (PPD) of *M. tuberculosis*. In individuals without confirmation of disease, the TST is the primary means to determine TB infection. It relies upon the delayed-type hypersensitivity (DTH) reaction, which is promoted by interleukin-2 and interferon-gamma. Skin test conversion normally occurs within 8 weeks of infection. However, given the numerous limitations of PPD skin testing (namely cross reactivity with NTM/MOTT and BCG vaccination), recently developed serum-based gamma interferon-based release assays are increasingly available for use in some settings (see further ahead). The currently used TST consists of 0.1 mL of 5 tuberculin unit (5 TU) that is injected intradermally on the volar surface of the forearm using the Mantoux method (1 TU and 250 TU skin tests are uninterpretable with no clinical utility[83]). The induration at the injection site (not erythema) is recorded in millimeters at 48 to 72 h. Multiple puncture (Tine) PPD skin tests are not reliable,[84] and results should be confirmed with a tuberculin PPD test (except when there is blistering at the site of puncture). Up to 20% of patients with active TB who are HIV negative will have a negative PPD skin test, which may convert to positive after initiation or completion of therapy.[84–86] Patients with miliary disease are even more likely to have a negative skin test (50–70%).[85] Thus, TB should never be ruled out because of a negative PPD. Because of the window period between exposure/infection with MTB and the time to mount a DTH response, repeat PPD testing is recommended 8–10 weeks after contact with the infectious case has been broken.[87]

Because the TST result must be interpreted in the context of the estimated TB prevalence within an individual's community and the prior probability of having a true TB infection, various cut-points have been established to determine a positive result.[88–90] The cut-point for a positive PPD in an HIV-infected patient is 5 mm or greater, the same cut-point used for a recent contact to a TB case. False positives occur more often in areas with a high prevalence of NTMs and in individuals vaccinated with BCG. False negative reactions may be due to anergy and can occur in very young children or those who are very ill.[84] The booster phenomenon results when reactivity to PPD has waned over time and a PPD skin test boosts the cellular immune response. If a second TST is given, the results may be positive and misinterpreted as a new conversion. For this reason, initial two-step skin testing (a repeat TST, 2 weeks after a negative result) is recommended to establish an accurate baseline in individuals who will undergo serial TST testing due to exposure risks.[90–93]

Anergy Testing and TB

Due to its unreliability and lack of standardization, anergy testing is no longer recommended by the CDC as a routine adjunct for assessing the reaction to the PPD skin test in HIV-infected persons.[94] Nonetheless, this issue remains a point of confusion for many physicians. Anergy is the inability to mount a DTH immune response to one, several, or all skin-test antigens to which a recall response is expected due to previous exposure. Anergy therefore may be selective or general.[85] Anergy testing is done with common DTH antigens, such as Trichophyton, Candida, histoplasmin, mumps, tetanus toxoid, and tuberculin. Common causes of anergy include: infection with HIV, live viral vaccines, steroids and other immunosuppressive agents, alcoholism, stress such as major trauma, extremes of age, chronic medical conditions, and either disseminated or nondisseminated TB disease.[83,85,94,95] People with any of these conditions may have a negative PPD result even if they are clearly infected with MTB. In HIV-infected patients, the likelihood of anergy and PPD nonreactivity are greater when absolute CD4+ T-lymphocyte counts are lower. Anergy is also common in HIV-negative controls (7–23%).[96–99]

Anergy testing is not useful for interpreting a negative TST result in patients infected with HIV. HIV patients who are anergic to a standard anergy panel at initial testing may respond to these antigens on repeat testing.[95,98–100] Many people react to tuberculin but not to the test antigens, or vice versa, and the inability to mount a DTH response to one antigen does not necessarily predict anergy to other antigens.[95,96,101,102] Since both tuberculin skin testing and anergy testing are unreliable in HIV-infected persons, these tests should not be used to justify withholding treatment for TB. Further, HIV-infected individuals who are identified as contacts of an infectious pulmonary TB case, and without evidence for disease, should receive treatment for latent TB infection regardless of the TST results, particularly when the likelihood of transmission is deemed high (high proportion of contacts examined with evidence of LTBI) or when a false-negative test is suspected.[14,87,103]

Gamma Interferon-Based Release Assays to Detect TB Infection

Beyond the concern for a false-negative result in an HIV-infected person, the primary limitation of the TST is its lack of specificity, particularly its inability to discriminate between LTBI and prior BCG vaccination or infection with NTM/MOTT.[90] Consequently, serum assays have been developed based on two protein fragments, early secretory antigenic target-6 (ESAT-6) and culture filtrate protein-10 (CFP-10), not found in any BCG vaccine strain nor most MOTT, except for *M. kansasii*, *M. marinum* and *M. szulgai*.[103] The CDC issued guidelines in 2005 after FDA approval of one test, QuantiFERON-TB Gold, which uses synthesized proteins. This assay requires fresh heparinized whole blood incubated with the test antigens and measures the supernatant concentration of released interferon-gamma (IFN-γ) by ELISA. Incubation of collected blood with the antigens must occur within 12 h of collection and proper storage of the plasma for ELISA testing must be guaranteed. These requirements can limit the feasibility of the test in multiple field settings. Further, the sensitivity of the test has not been determined for immunocompromised patients (including HIV-infected) and young children. Nonetheless, the CDC has recommended its use in 'all circumstances in which the TST is currently used'.[103] Advantages of the assay are that two visits are not required for placement and reading, as for PPD, and the measurement is automated.

A second IFN-γ release assay uses isolated peripheral blood mononuclear cells rather than whole blood. The test, based on the same antigens ESAT-6 and CFP-10, employs a rapid enzyme-linked immunospot (ELISPOT) assay. Upon mixing, IFN-γ spot-forming T cells are counted. Despite improved specificity, it is not known if the assay is more sensitive than TST for LTBI detection. In a study of Zambian TB patients, the sensitivity of the assay in HIV co-infected TB patients exceeded 90%; no comparison was made with a PPD skin test. Among the study participants without evidence of TB, those who were HIV-infected had a lower median response to the ELISPOT assay than those without HIV infection.[104] This finding was attributed to a loss of CD4 T cells and again raises the issue of the accuracy of IFN-γ assays, which are T-cell-based tests, for determining LTBI status in HIV-positive individuals. Nonetheless, the technical performance of one commercial test (T-SPOT TB) has been demonstrated in HIV-infected patients with varying CD4 cell counts, but it has not been prospectively evaluated in the field for TB disease or LTBI.[105] In Senegal, while some data indicate that the ELISPOT-based assay is better than standard TST for HIV-infected persons without clinical or radiological evidence of disease (presumed LTBI), there was a significant falloff in the results as CD4 counts fell, especially below 200 cells/mm^3.[106] In a recent trial directly comparing QuantiFERON-TB Gold with T-SPOT TB, there were a significantly higher proportion of indeterminate results with QuantiFERON-TB Gold (11%) compared with T-SPOT TB (3%). Immunosuppression from cancer chemotherapy was significantly associated with an indeterminate result for both tests, while age <5 years was associated with a greater proportion of indeterminate results using QuantiFERON-TB Gold (32% vs 0%). No HIV data were presented.[107]

Step 3

Obtain a chest radiograph (CXR). The CXR is useful for determining if there is disease in the chest, and if so, its extent. A CXR, however, cannot confirm or exclude that a patient has TB disease. The problems inherent to CXR interpretation (inter and intraobserver variation) is well described in the TB literature.[96,108] CXR is also used to determine if an individual with TB disease is improving on therapy or not. Individuals with HIV co-infection may have active TB and a normal CXR. [36] Further, cavity formation is less likely as immunosuppression advances (*see section on* Presentation of TB in HIV-Infected Individuals). In children, bronchial obstruction may occur from enlarged lymph nodes and may be the only evidence of primary disease, leading to a wedge-shaped segmental or complete lung collapse.

Step 4

Obtain specimens for bacteriologic examination. Sputum specimens, material from bronchoscopy, gastric washings, or other body fluids can be stained for the presence of acid-fast bacilli (AFB) and cultured for MTB. Sputum for AFB examination should be obtained prior to bronchoscopy. Bronchoscopy is a procedure that causes significant aerosolization of the organism and is therefore a high-risk procedure with respect to transmission of TB in patients not on therapy, and individuals whose sputum smears are AFB positive are more contagious compared to those with negative smears. Since NTMs are also acid-fast, culture for MTB is the gold standard for diagnosis. For a smear to be positive, there needs to be at least 10^4 organisms per milliliter of material.

Pleural fluid from TB pleuritis is normally exudative with elevated protein concentrations, lymphocyte predominance, and <5% mesothelial cells[109] but has relatively low numbers of organisms. Pleural fluid AFB smears are therefore rarely positive, and fluid cultures are positive in only one-third of cases. Pleural biopsy is a more sensitive test and can yield a positive AFB smear, positive culture, or histology showing granulomatous inflammation with areas of caseation necrosis. Pleural biopsy histology or biopsy culture alone can each yield between 60% and 85% of cases, with histology usually a more sensitive test. The combination of histology and culture has been shown to yield ~95% of TB pleurisy cases.[110–112] Given the invasiveness of diagnosis using pleural biopsy and inherent delays awaiting culture confirmation, other means have been sought. High levels of pleural adenosine deaminase (ADA) and IFN-γ are consistently found in TB pleurisy.[109,111,113] In a recent study, both tests were demonstrated to be more sensitive for diagnosis (88% and 86%, respectively) than polymerase chain reaction testing (74%). The specificity of ADA and IFN-γ approximated or was better (86% and 97%, respectively) than their sensitivity.[113] However in low TB prevalence settings, pleural ADA levels are less specific as it may be elevated with empyemas, lymphomas, rheumatoid effusions and other infections or malignancies.[109,112] To overcome this limitation and improve utility, measurement of the isoenzyme ADA_2 has been found useful. This isoenzyme is produced only by monocytes and can be assessed by the ratio ADA_1/ADAp in pleural fluid.[112,114,115]

Because of the growth characteristics of MTB, traditional solid media culture methods take from 3 to 8 weeks to show growth or not. While commercial broth systems take only 1–3 weeks, neither culture method can readily distinguish between MTB and NTM/MOTT without further testing. Chemical testing, high performance liquid chromatography and nucleic acid probes can distinguish MTB from NTMs. Probes using nucleic acid amplification (NAA) are also available commercially for detecting MTB in clinical specimens directly, but their utility depends upon whether there are a sufficient numbers of organisms present. Consequently, not all NAA products are approved for smear-negative samples, and there is limited information on NAA performance in nonrespiratory specimens. Further, the interpretation of results can be difficult if not confirmed by culture, and interlaboratory variability is seen in test performance (in the sensitivity and specificity). CDC has published a suggested algorithm and cautions for NAA use for TB.[116] Not all laboratories have the dedicated resources, personnel and space to routinely use NAA tests, especially on clinical specimens. NAA tests can remain positive after culture conversion to negative during therapy and even after therapy is completed. Therefore, these tests should not be used to monitor treatment and cannot replace core laboratory tests of AFB staining and culture, nor clinical judgment.[116]

The utility of blood culture in diagnosing disseminated TB is well-described. Mycobacteremia is especially common in the febrile patient with advanced HIV disease (*see section on* Presentation of TB in HIV-Infected Individuals).

A decision to start (empiric) TB therapy can occur at any point during the diagnostic evaluation process, and should be made if the clinical risk of delaying therapy threatens a patient's chance of survival. However, confirmation of a TB diagnosis cannot be made without the culture or biopsy histology results. The determination of whether a patient is on adequate antituberculous therapy cannot be made until the DST results are known. Consequently, any history of exposure to another case (particularly a drug resistant case), prior TB therapy, or an assessment of nonadherence to prior therapy are key elements to determine the appropriateness of a given (empiric) regimen.

MANAGEMENT OF ACTIVE TB IN HIV-INFECTED PATIENTS

The treatment of TB in patients infected with HIV is similar to that in HIV-uninfected individuals. Recommended treatment regimens and duration of therapy are nearly identical and based on a standard four-drug regimen consisting of 2 months of isoniazid (INH), rifampin (RIF), pyrazinamide (PZA), and ethambutol (EMB), followed by 4 months of INH and RIF (Table 40-1). However, several issues complicate TB management among the HIV-infected. Potential drug–drug interactions exist between antituberculous and certain HAART regimens. Intermittent therapy can also be inappropriate for some patients with HIV co-infection, and the occurrence of paradoxical reactions (PR) and the immune reconstitution inflammatory syndrome (IRIS) can complicate treatment goals.

Each agent of the TB regimen has a unique role. INH acts on metabolically active bacilli and is the most potent bactericidal agent. RIF is bactericidal, most effective at sterilization, and helps limit the emergence of drug resistance. PZA is bactericidal against TB bacilli within macrophages in an acidic environment. In combination with INH and RIF during the first 2 months of therapy, PZA is an essential component of the recommended 6-month regimen. EMB is bacteriostatic at doses currently recommended and used primarily to prevent the emergence of resistance. EMB can usually be discontinued after the initial phase of therapy or when drug susceptibility to INH and RIF is verified.[117]

Table 40-1 **Recommended Drug Regimens for Culture-Positive Pulmonary Tuberculosis Caused by Drug-Susceptible Organisms in those Infected with HIV**

Initial Phase			Continuation Phase		
Regimen	Drugs	Interval and Doses[a] (Minimal Duration)	Regimen	Drugs	Interval and Doses (Minimal Duration)
1	INH RIF PZA EMB	Seven days/week for 56 doses (8 weeks) or 5 days/week for 40 doses	1a	INF/RIF	Seven days/week for 126 doses (18 weeks) or 5 days/week for 90 doses (18 weeks)
			1b[b]	INF/RIF	Twice weekly for 36 doses (18 weeks)
2	INH RIF PZA EMB	Seven days/week for 14 doses (2 weeks) then twice weekly for 12 doses (6 weeks) OR 5 days/week for 10 doses (2 weeks) then twice weekly for 12 doses (6 weeks)	2a[b]	INH/RIF	Twice weekly for 36 doses (18 weeks)
3	INH RIF PZA EMB	Three times weekly for 24 doses (8 weeks)	3a	INH/RIF	Three times weekly for 54 doses (18 weeks)

[a]When DOT is used, drugs may be given 5 days/week and the number of doses adjusted accordingly.
[b]Twice weekly dosing of INH/RIF not recommended for HIV-infected patients with CD4 counts <100.

Adapted from American Thoracic Society/Centers for Disease Control and Prevention/Infectious Diseases Society of America. Treatment of tuberculosis. Am J Respir Crit Care Med 167:603–62, 2003.

TB THERAPY ISSUES: DURATION, RELAPSE, REINFECTION AND INTERMITTENT THERAPY

Standard short course (6-month) TB treatment appears to be effective at rapid sterilization and cure among HIV co-infected individuals who complete therapy. Most studies have validated the 6-month regimen as appropriate, with relapse rates less than 5%.[63,64,118,119] In a study from Baltimore, Sterling et al found similarly high relapse rates among HIV-infected and uninfected individuals at 6.4% and 5.5%, respectively.[120] In a British study of HIV-TB co-infected patients, where HAART was utilized, the 2 year relapse rate was 4.1% at 2 years.[121] These findings are not universal, however. Two studies demonstrated higher relapse rates in HIV infected individuals who received 6 months of therapy in comparison with longer courses of treatment.[65,122] A study from the Democratic Republic of Congo (formerly Zaire) demonstrated a higher relapse rate at 24 months from enrollment in HIV patients treated for 6 months compared to 12 months, 9% and 1.9% respectively ($p < 0.01$), but without any survival benefit. Certain limitations, however, apply to this study. DOT was not universally implemented; twice-weekly therapy was utilized in the continuation phase, and the role of reinfection versus relapse was not assessed. Further, the duration of follow-up after completion of therapy differed between the two groups.[65] Another study from Spain demonstrated a statistically significant higher relapse rate in those receiving less than 9 months of treatment compared to those receiving more than 9 months, 24% versus 3.4% respectively ($p < 0.001$).[122] In a third study from the US comparing 6 months with 9 months of treatment (all pan-susceptible cases), relapse rates were 3.9% versus 2% respectively, a nonstatistically significant difference.[119]

Reinfection has been well described in areas of high endemicity. In a study of South African gold miners, 93% (13/14) of recurrences within the first 6 months of completing anti-TB therapy were attributable to relapse. Beyond 6 months, 52% (13/25) were attributed to reinfection. HIV-infection was found to be a risk factor for reinfection but not relapse.[123] A separate South African study from an urban population demonstrated that among those successfully completing anti-TB therapy, 77% of subsequent episodes of TB were due to reinfection rather than relapse. HIV status was not determined in this study, however.[124]

Recently published American Thoracic Society (ATS)/ Centers for Disease Control and Prevention (CDC)/Infectious Diseases Society of America (IDSA) consensus guidelines recommend standard 6-month anti-TB treatment regimens for those co-infected with HIV and TB (Table 40-1; see Table 40-2 for drug dosing).[125] However, patients with suboptimal responses, defined as sputum culture positive at the end of 2 months therapy, should be considered for a 3-month extension of the continuation phase, for a total of 9 months (Fig. 40-4). Further, all forms of TB should be treated based on the same 6-month regimen, except for TB meningitis for which 9–12 months of therapy are recommended. The American Academy of Pediatrics suggests a 9-month treatment regimen for pulmonary TB in all children co-infected with HIV[126]; 9–12 month regimens are appropriate for children with disseminated or meningeal forms of TB given the lack of specific data to support shorter treatment durations. All HIV-positive patients with TB should be treated with DOT,[125] which is especially important when any intermittent dosing regimen is applied. Short course regimens that utilize RIF throughout treatment should be utilized at all possible times as treatment outcomes are superior to those achieved by other combinations as demonstrated by higher treatment failure and relapse rates.[127] or increased mortality and delayed sterilization.[128]

Evidence suggests that intermittent dosing regimens administered less than three times a week may result in poor outcomes among certain HIV-infected groups. Acquired rifampin monoresistance has been seen in patients on twice-weekly dosing regimens.[119,129] Acquired resistance has also been observed with twice-weekly rifabutin-based regimens.[130,131] Of note, all such cases had CD4 counts less than 100. Weekly dosing of rifapentine, a long acting rifamycin with a half-life five times that of rifampin, is also contraindicated in TB-HIV co-infection. A randomized trial of HIV-related TB comparing weekly INH-rifapentine with twice-weekly INH-RIF use in the continuation phase found a higher rate of relapse in the former group, 17% (5/30) and 10% (3/31) respectively. Four of the five relapses in the INH-rifapentine group and none of the three in the INH-RIF group acquired rifampin resistance.[132] Consequently, ATS/CDC/IDSA guidelines recommend avoiding twice-weekly intermittent therapy in anyone with CD4 <100. Furthermore, rifapentine-based continuation phase regimens are contraindicated in those co-infected with TB-HIV, regardless of CD4 levels.[125]

ADMINISTRATION OF HAART DURING TB TREATMENT

Combination antiretroviral therapy has had a dramatic impact on the natural history of HIV infection, prolonging life and preventing OIs. Numerous issues, however, complicate the co-administration of HAART with anti-TB therapy. The optimal timing for initiating HAART in those co-infected with TB remains unclear. Side effect profiles overlap, making determinations of the offending agent difficult when adverse reactions do occur. Significant drug–drug interactions occur when RIF is combined with protease inhibitors (PIs) or non-nucleoside reverse transcriptase inhibitors (NNRTIs). Further, the numerous drugs and high pill burden often required to manage OIs, HIV, and TB can compromise adherence. Finally, the initiation of HAART in the setting of TB can lead to IRIS, which may be confused with the clinical worsening associated with treatment failure.

Given the complexities of co-administering HAART with anti-TB therapy, the current consensus is to delay HAART until several weeks of anti-TB therapy have been completed.[125] There are no clinical trials defining the optimal time to initiate ART, and standard guidelines are based on the underlying

Table 40-2 Dosage Recommendations for the Treatment of TB in Children[a] and Adults

	Daily Dosage		Twice-Weekly Dosage		Thrice-Weekly Dosage	
Drugs	**Children[a]**	**Adults**	**Children[a]**	**Adults**	**Children[a]**	**Adults**
Isoniazid	10–20 mg/kg Max 300 mg	5 mg/kg Max 300 mg	20–40 mg/kg Max 900 mg	15 mg/kg Max 900 mg	15 mg/kg Max 900 mg	15 mg/kg Max 900 mg
Rifampin	10–20 mg/kg Max 600 mg	10 mg/kg Max 600 mg	10–20 mg/kg Max 600 mg	10 mg/kg Max 600 mg	10 mg/kg Max 600 mg	10 mg/kg Max 600 mg
Pyrazinamide[d]	15–30 mg/kg Max 2 g	1000 mg/40–55 kg 1500 mg/56–75 kg 2000 mg/76–90 kg[e]	50 mg/kg Max 4 g	2000 mg/40–55 kg 3000 mg/56–75 kg 4000 mg/76–90 kg[e]		1500 mg/40–55 kg 2500 mg/56–75 kg 3000 mg/76–90 kg[e]
Ethambutol[b,d]	15–20 mg/kg Max 1 g	800 mg/40–55 kg 1200 mg/56–75 kg 1600 mg/76–90 kg[e]	50 mg/kg Max 4 g	2000 mg/40–55 kg 2800 mg/56–75 kg 4000 mg/76–90 kg[e]		1200 mg/40–55 kg 2000 mg/56–75 kg 2400 mg/76–90 kg[e]
Streptomycin	20–40 mg/kg Max 1 g	15 mg/kg Max 1 g	25–30 mg/kg Max 1.5 g	25–30 mg/kg Max 1.5 g	25–30 mg/kg Max 1.5 g	25–30 mg/kg Max 1.5 g
Ofloxacin[c]		600–800 mg qd		No data		No data
Levofloxacin[c]		500–1000 mg qd		No data		No data
Moxifloxacin[c]		400 mg qd		No data		No data
Ciprofloxacin[c]		750–1500 mg qd		No data		No data
Rifabutin		5 mg/kg 300 mg qd		5 mg/kg 300 mg qd	5 mg/kg 300 mg qd	5 mg/kg 300 mg qd

[a] Children are defined as being 14 years old or less.
[b] Ethambutol is not recommended for children who are too young to be monitored for changes in their vision (less than 8 years old). However, ethambutol should be considered for all children who have TB that is resistant to other drugs but susceptible to ethambutol.
[c] Quinolones are not recommended for children or during pregnancy. Also, twice weekly dosages have not been defined, although in practice are usually given the same as a daily dose.
[d] Based on estimated lean body weight.
[e] Maximum dose regardless of weight.

Adapted from American Thoracic Society/Centers for Disease Control and Prevention/Infectious Diseases Society of America. Treatment of tuberculosis. Am J Respir Crit Care Med 167:603–62, 2003.

degree of immunosuppression. Initiating HAART without delay in those with advanced immunosuppression may be beneficial as they have a high risk of subsequent OIs and OI-related death soon after the initiation of TB therapy. A retrospective study from London comparing outcomes in HIV co-infected TB patients during the pre-HAART and HAART eras demonstrated a high adverse event risk, defined as death or subsequent AIDS defining illness, within the first 2 months of TB therapy. These occurred at a rate of 139/100 person-years pre-HAART and 88/100 person-years post-HAART. Those with advanced HIV disease (CD4 <100) had a higher adverse event rate (249/100 persons-years) in the first 2 months of TB therapy. Paradoxical reactions were common in those with low CD4 counts, most often occurring 15–30 days after HAART initiation; however, the relationship to the timing of anti-TB therapy is not clear.[133]

Joint ATS/CDC/IDSA guidelines suggest initiating HAART 4–8 weeks after starting TB therapy.[125] This delay may simplify adherence issues during the initial phase of TB treatment and reduce confusion if adverse events occur. Adverse medication events, such as peripheral neuropathy, nausea and vomiting, rash, and hepatitis are commonly encountered in patients co-infected with HIV and TB. Of 183 patients studied by Dean et al, 34% had adverse reactions necessitating the discontinuation or cessation of some component of TB or HIV therapy.[121] These events are not typically specific to any drug (Table 40-3), and temporal relationships are often the only clues to which agent may be responsible. An additional advantage in delaying HAART may be to diminish the risk of IRIS (*see section on* Paradoxical Reactions and the IRIS). According to WHO guidelines, patients with CD4 counts <200 should receive HAART as soon as TB therapy is tolerated, which can be between 2 and 8 weeks. For those with CD4 counts from 200 to 350, HAART can be delayed until the initial 8 weeks of anti-TB therapy is completed. For those with CD4 counts >350, deferment of HAART is

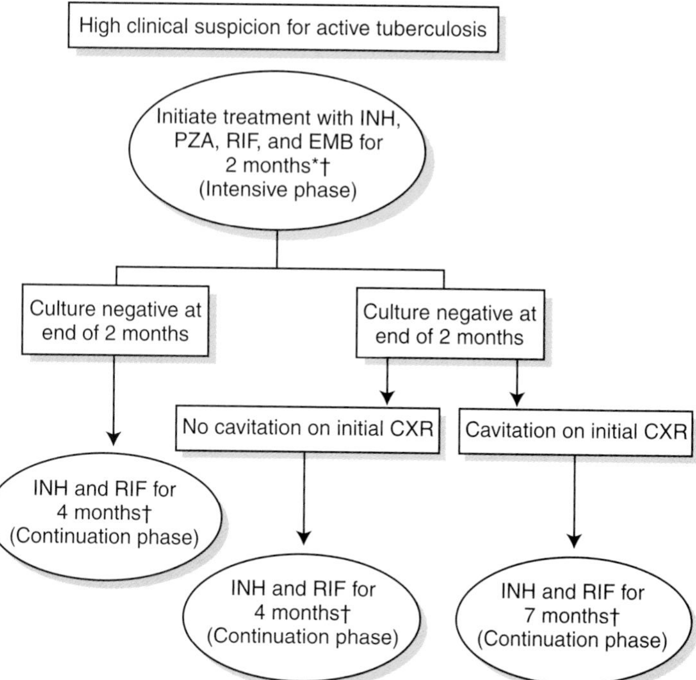

*Therapy should be administered daily for the first 2 weeks. EMB can be discontinued when results of drug susceptibility testing demonstrate no resistance to INH or RIF.
†During the intensive phase, therapy should be administered daily or thrice weekly for those with CD4 <100/μl. In the continuation phase, if CD4 <100/μl, INH and RIF should be given daily or thrice weekly too.

Figure 40-4 ■ Treatment algorithm for pulmonary tuberculosis among those with HIV infection.

Adapted from American Thoracic Society/Centers for Disease Control and Prevention/Infectious Diseases Society of America. Treatment of tuberculosis. Am J Respir Crit Care Med 167:603–62, 2003.

Drug and/or Disease-Related Adverse Events

Table 40-3

Adverse Event	Commonly Associated TB and HIV Drugs	Other Possible Etiologies Associated with HIV Disease
Hepatitis	PZA, INH, RIF, RFB, nevirapine, PIs, trimethoprim–sulfamethoxazole, PAS, ethionamide	Viral hepatitis, IRIS, CMV, EBV
Skin eruptions	PZA, INH, RIF, RFB, nevirapine, efavirenz, abacavir, trimethoprim–sulfamethoxazole, streptomycin	Eosinophilic folliculitis, scabies, psoriasis vulgaris, atopic dermatitis
Nausea and vomiting/or diarrhea	PZA, INH, RIF, RFB, AZT, ritonavir, amprenavir, indinavir, trimethoprim–sulfamethoxazole, PAS, ethionamide	Pancreatitis, HIV associated cholangiopathy, IRIS, CMV, cryptosporidiosis
Hematologic abnormalities (leukopenia, anemia, thrombocytopenia)	RIF, RFB, AZT, valgancyclovir, trimethoprim–sulfamethoxazole, INH (rare)	HIV related bone marrow suppression, ITP, autoimmune hemolytic anemia
Visual disturbances	EMB, RFB, voriconazole	CMV retinitis, IRIS, toxoplasmosis, VZV, fungal infections
Neuropathy	INH, DDC, ddI, d4T, ethionamide, dapsone	HIV-related, alcohol, CMV
Seizures	INH, cycloserine, fluoroquinolones, efavirenz	CNS lesions (lymphoma, toxoplasmosis, PML), meninigitis, HIV-associated
Flu-like syndrome	RIF (especially with intermittent therapy)	Acute HIV infection
Sleep and Psychiatric disturbances	efavirenz, cycloserine	

Table 40-4

WHO ART Recommendations for Individuals with TB Disease and HIV Co-infection

CD4 Cell Count (cells/mm^3)	ART Recommendation	Timing of ART after Initiation of TB Therapy	Comments
<200	Give ART	Between 2 and 8 weeks (as soon as TB therapy is tolerated)	ART recommended
200 to 350	Give ART	After 8 weeks	Consider ART
>350	Defer ART	Re-evaluate patient (a) after 8 weeks and (b) at end of TB therapy	Defer ART[a]
Not available/unknown	Give ART (unless patient has mild TB disease forms, then may defer)	Between 2 and 8 weeks	Consider ART[ab]

[a] Timing of ART initiation should be based on clinical judgement in relation to other signs of immunodeficiency. For extrapulmonary TB, ART should be started as soon as TB treatment is tolerated, regardless of CD4 count.
[b] If no other signs of immunodeficiency are present and patient is improving on TB treatment, ART should be started upon completion of TB treatment.

Adapted from World Health Organization. Antiretroviral Therapy for HIV Infection in Adults and Adolescents, 2006 revision.www.who.int/hiv/pub/guidelines/artadultguidelines.pdf. Accessed August, 2007.

Table 40-5

Co-administration of Rifampin with PIs[a]

	Recommended Change in Dose of Antiretroviral Drug	Recommended Change in Dose of Rifampin	Comments
Ritonavir	None	None	Ritonavir AUC[b] decreased 35%
Saquinavir/ritonavir	Saquinavir 400 mg + Ritonavir 400 mg twice-daily	None	Limited clinical experience
Lopinavir/ritonavir (Kaletra)	Kaletra 400/100 twice daily with additional ritonavir 300 mg twice daily	None	Limited clinical experience, increased risk of hepatotoxicity

[a] Due to unacceptable decreases in drug concentration of certain protease inhibitors, rifampin should not be co-administered with amprenavir (↓AUC 82%), fosamprenavir, atazanavir, indinavir (↓AUC 89 %), nelfinavir (↓AUC 82%), or unboosted saquinavir (↓AUC 84%).
[b] AUC, area under the curve.

Adapted from CDC. TB/HIV Drug interactions. Available: http://www.cdc.gov/nchstp/tb/tb_hiv_drugs/toc.htm May 2006.

recommended (Table 40-4).[134] Those on HAART prior to the diagnosis of TB should continue taking ART, although dosing adjustments or drug substitutions may be required because of drug interactions.

Major drug–drug interactions, particularly associated with RIF, complicate the management of TB-HIV co-infection when antiretroviral therapy is indicated. RIF vigorously induces the cytochrome P450 3A (CYP3A) enzyme system resulting in markedly lower concentrations of antiretroviral drugs metabolized through this pathway. Rifabutin (RFB) stimulates this pathway as well, but to a significantly lesser extent.[135] RFB, unlike RIF, is itself a substrate for the CYP3A system, and its levels are therefore altered by the administration of PIs and NNRTIs. RFB doses are generally decreased when co-administered with PIs and increased when co-administered with efavirenz. RFB can lead to significant toxicities, including uveitis, GI upset, neutropenia, and thrombocytopenia.

Special care must also be taken when rifamycins are administered with other agents. Acquired RIF monoresistance was found to be independently associated with azole use in a case-control study involving HIV-infected TB patients.[136] When used with ketoconazole, for example, RIF levels are lowered 40–50%. Concerning RFB, the use of azole antifungal agents and clarithromycin will increase the plasma levels of RFB and risk of associated toxicities.[117,137,138] Given these interactions, modifications to both anti-TB, OI and ART are required to achieve comprehensive treatment goals.

RIF administration results in significantly diminished concentrations of PIs; therefore, the use of PIs with RIF is generally contraindicated. There is some evidence, however, that suggests RIF can be used in combination with higher dose ritonavir[139], ritonavir boosted saquinavir[140], and adequately boosted lopinavir[141], as part of a HAART regimen (Table 40-5). RFB, which weakly induces CYP3A, can be dosed with all PIs except for unboosted saquinavir (Table 40-6).[142] Clinical

Table 40-6

Co-administration of Rifabutin with PIs[ab]

	Recommended Change in Dose of Antiretroviral Drug	Recommended Change in Dose of Rifabutin	Comments
Ritonavir	None	150 mg every other day or thrice weekly	Rifabutin AUC increased 430%
Amprenavir	None	150 mg daily or 300 mg thrice weekly	Rifabutin AUC increased 193%
Fosamprenavir	None	150 mg daily or 300 mg thrice weekly	Comparable to amprenavir
Atazanavir	None	150 mg every other day or thrice weekly	Rifabutin AUC increased 250%
Indinavir	1000 mg every 8 h	150 mg daily or 300 mg thrice weekly	Rifabutin AUC increased 204%; indinavir AUC decreased 32%
Nelfinavir	1000 mg every 8 h	150 mg daily or 300 mg thrice weekly	Rifabutin AUC increased 207%; nelfinavir AUC decreased 32%
Lopinavir/ritonavir (Kaletra)	None	150 mg every other day or thrice weekly	Rifabutin AUC increased 303%
Ritonavir (any dose) with saquinavir, indinavir, amprenavir, fosamprenavir, or atazanavir	None	150 mg every other day or thrice weekly	

[a] Rifabutin and saquinavir should not be used together (Saquinavir AUC↓ 43%).
[b] If CD4 count is greater than 100 cells/mm^3, may consider twice-weekly administration of rifabutin with amprenavir, fosamprenavir, indinavir, and nelfinavir.
Adapted from CDC. TB/HIV Drug interactions. Available: http://www.cdc.gov/nchstp/tb/tb_hiv_drugs/toc.htm May 2006.

Table 40-7

Co-administration of Rifabutin with Non-Nucleoside Reverse Transcriptase Inhibitors[ab]

	Recommended Change in Dose of Antiretroviral Drug	Recommended Change in Dose of Rifabutin	Comments
Efavirenz	None	450 mg daily or 600 mg thrice weekly	Rifabutin AUC decreased 38%
Nevirapine	None	300 mg daily or 300 mg thrice weekly	Rifabutin and nevirapine AUC not significantly changed

[a] Delavirdine and rifabutin should not be used together (Delavirdine AUC↓ 80%, Rifabutin AUC ↑ 100%).
[b] If CD4 count is greater than 100 cells/mm^3, may consider twice-weekly administration of rifabutin with efavirenz, and nevirapine.
Adapted from CDC. TB/HIV Drug interactions. Available: http://www.cdc.gov/nchstp/tb/tb_hiv_drugs/toc.htm May 2006.

evaluation of RFB suggests that it is as effective and well tolerated as RIF in treating TB among both HIV-negative and HIV-positive patients when incorporated into standard short course regimens.[143,144] Importantly, a 2-week washout period without RIF use is recommended to allow normalization of the CYP3A system prior to initiating PIs or NNRTIs. RFB can be immediately substituted during this interval.[125] A limiting factor to the widespread use of RFB is its cost and availability.

RFB can be used with the NNRTIs efavirenz and nevirapine, although higher doses of RFB are required when co-administered with efavirenz (Table 40-7). RIF can be administered with efavirenz, but higher doses of efavirenz may be recommended (Table 40-8). Close monitoring for efavirenz toxicity is required. Pharmacokinetic data indicate that RIF results in markedly diminished levels of nevirapine when given together.[145,146] Although limited clinical data demonstrate acceptable outcomes when the two are co-administered[146–148], this is not currently recommended unless there are no other acceptable options.

There are no significant interactions between the rifamycins and the nucleoside or nucleotide reverse transcriptase inhibitors (NRTIs) that necessitate dosing adjustments. Dosing recommendations for NNRTIs and PIs, when co-administered with RIF or RFB, are noted in Tables 40-5 to 40-8. Updated recommendations on regimen dosing and drug interactions are available on the CDC website: http://www.cdc.gov/nchstp/tb/tb_hiv_drugs/toc.htm.

Co-administration of Rifampin with Non-Nucleoside Reverse Transcriptase Inhibitors[a]

Table 40-8

	Recommended Change in Dose of Antiretroviral Drug	Recommended Change in Dose of Rifampin	Comments
Efavirenz	800 mg daily*	None	Efavirenz AUC decreased 22%.* May use 600 mg daily if higher dose not well-tolerated.
Nevirapine	200 mg twice daily	None	Nevirapine AUC decreased 37–58%. Limited, though favorable, clinical data. Use only when no other available options. May consider nevirapine 300 mg bid with close monitoring, but no safety or pharmacokinetic data.

[a]Delavirdine and rifampin should not be used together (Delavirdine AUC↓ 95%).

Adapted from CDC. TB/HIV Drug interactions. Available: http://www.cdc.gov/nchstp/tb/tb_hiv_drugs/toc.htm May 2006.

PARADOXICAL REACTIONS AND THE IRIS

Paradoxical worsening of the clinical signs and symptoms of TB associated with antituberculous therapy is a well-recognized entity, with the earliest reports dating back to 1955.[149] This phenomenon has been increasingly recognized in association with TB-HIV co-infection. Two studies have demonstrated a higher incidence of paradoxical reactions in HIV-positive patients, although neither reached statistical significance.[150,151] The introduction of HAART has further affected the incidence of new and recurrent TB symptoms through the IRIS. IRIS is a collection of inflammatory disorders associated with an improved immunologic response to occult or previously identified infections, following the administration of ART.

PRs are typically described as the worsening or development of new signs and/or symptoms after the initiation of anti-TB therapy. It is a diagnosis of exclusion; other processes such as treatment failure, drug resistance, poor compliance, drug malabsorption, drug reactions, lymphoma and other infections should be considered. PRs usually occur within the first weeks to months of treatment but may occur well into the treatment course and recur anytime during therapy.[151] The pathogenesis is not well defined, but aberrations in immune function during TB infection and an improved host immune response during TB treatment have been documented.[152,153] Improved immune function is clinically demonstrated among initially anergic patients whose skin test converts to a positive status shortly after initiating anti-TB therapy.[154]

IRIS is a well-described inflammatory process associated with preexisting OIs and the initiation of HAART. Commonly implicated pathogens include cytomegalovirus, *Cryptococcus neoformans, Toxoplasma gondii, Mycobacterium avium-complex* (MAC) *and Mycobacterium tuberculosis*. TB-associated IRIS (TB-IRIS) may be related to an improved delayed type hypersensitivity response, demonstrated by its association with restored tuberculin reactivity.[150,154–156] Improved T cell specific immune responses to TB have been demonstrated after the initiation of HAART, although the levels do not achieve that demonstrated in HIV-negative control subjects.[72] Clinical findings of IRIS often mimic worsening of the underlying condition, involving the affected organ systems (Fig. 40-5A,B). Common signs and symptoms associated with TB-IRIS include fever and new or worsening lymphadenopathy, infiltrates or pleural effusions. Of 26 IRIS cases associated with TB reported by Shelburne et al, 19 had worsening lymphadenitis, five worsening infiltrates, four worsening pleural effusions, two with protracted fevers, and one with elevated intracranial pressure associated with TB meningitis.[157] Acute renal failure has been reported in an HIV-infected individual with miliary disease and renal involvement.[158]

Paradoxical worsening of TB symptoms may be more common among HIV co-infected individuals than HIV-negative patients. In a study from London, PR occurred in 14 (28%) of 50 HIV-positive TB patients and five (10%) of 50 HIV-negative TB patients, but this difference was not statistically significant.[151] However, among HIV-positive individuals who received HAART after starting TB therapy, TB-IRIS appears to occur more frequently in those receiving HAART within 6 weeks of TB therapy initiation. Narita et al compared HIV-negative TB patients with HIV positive (not on HAART) and found a small but statistically insignificant difference between the groups (2% and 7%, respectively). Those on HAART had a high incidence of TB-IRIS at 36%.[150] A study of radiographic changes showed a higher incidence of transient worsening among HIV-positive TB patients on HAART compared with HIV-positive TB patients not on HAART and HIV-negative TB cases.[156] Again, the observed worsening of symptoms occurred early after HAART initiation at 1–5 weeks. Despite this evidence, such findings have not been universally demonstrated.[159]

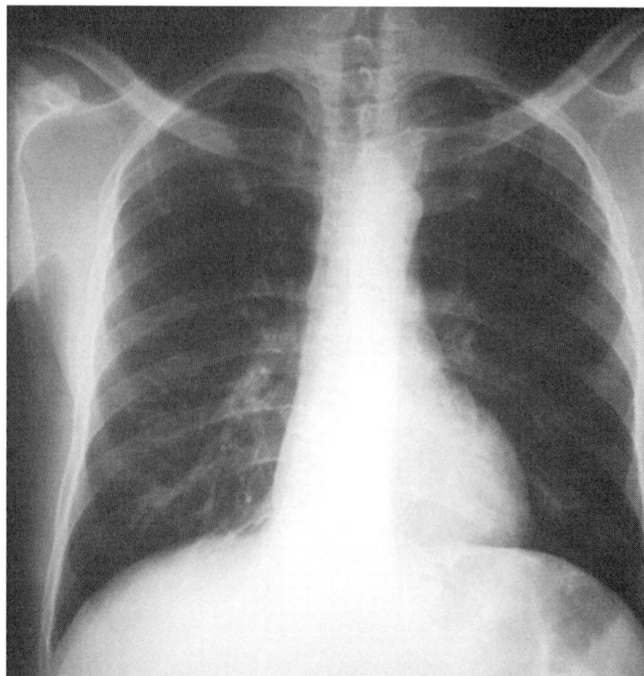

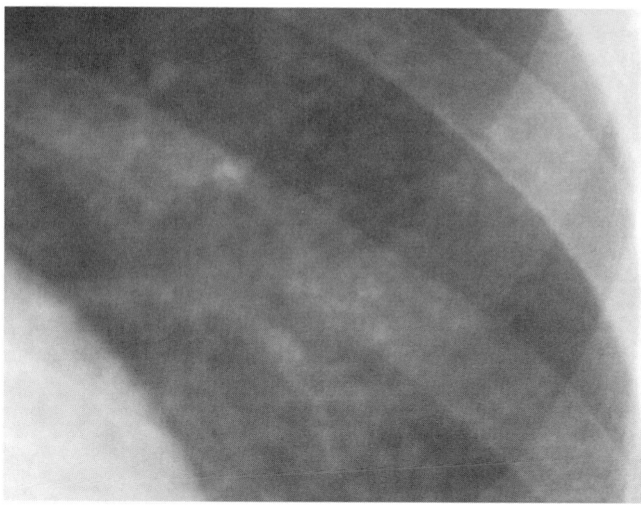

Figure 40-5 ■ (**A**) CXR of 44-year-old male with HIV infection (CD4 = 7) presenting with profound weight loss and fever. CXR is interpreted as normal. The patient's history is remarkable for a previous positive tuberculin reaction without ever receiving treatment for latent TB. Sputum specimens reveal no AFB but bronchoscopy is positive for AFB. Bronchial specimens and bone marrow aspirate yield *M. tuberculosis* on culture. (**B**) After 2 months of anti-TB treatment and HAART, the patient develops recurrent fevers and new infiltrates. CXR reveals interstitial micronodularity consistent with miliary TB. The patient is diagnosed with IRIS after treatment failure is excluded.

Risk factors for the development of TB-IRIS have been identified, including the preexisting level of immunodeficiency and the degree and rapidity of immune restoration, although these associations are not universally found. In one study, an initial CD4 count <100 was a risk factor.[160] Several studies have suggested that rapid declines in VL and prompt elevations in CD4 counts are associated with TB-IRIS.[150,157,160,161] In a study of 180 HIV-positive patients on HAART and co-infected with either TB, MAC, or *Cryptococcus neoformans*, IRIS occurred in 30% of the 86 co-infected with TB. A more robust decline in VL, initiation of HAART within 30 days of diagnosis of the OI, and being ART-naive were all independently associated with IRIS.[157] In addition, there is evidence to suggest that PR among HIV-infected and TB-IRIS may occur more commonly in those with disseminated or mixed pulmonary/extrapulmonary forms of TB.[151,159–161]

Given that IRIS is more likely to occur in patients who initiate HAART soon after the diagnosis of an OI,[151,156,157] there may be a benefit in delaying HAART during the initial phase of OI treatment. Joint CDC/ATS/IDSA guidelines for the treatment of TB suggest delaying HAART initiation until after 4–8 weeks of TB therapy. An additional consideration for delaying HAART is the overlapping side effect profiles of TB and HIV drugs.[14] Such decisions, however, must be individualized based on the needs of the particular patient. WHO guidelines for TB-HIV co-infection in resource limited settings suggest initiating HAART in those with CD4 counts <200 as soon as TB therapy is tolerated, in those with CD4 counts between 200 and 350 after 8 weeks of TB therapy, and deferring HAART in those with CD4 counts >350 (Table 40–4). These guidelines emphasize the critical necessity of administering effective TB therapy, and that this should not be compromised by the initiation of HAART.[134]

The long term consequences of PR and IRIS are unclear. In one study, the presence of IRIS was associated with improved long term viral suppression and immune function, perhaps reflecting an increased propensity for vigorous immune reconstitution.[157] Another study demonstrated a trend toward higher rates of TB relapse in those experiencing PR (33%) compared to those without PR (5%, $p = 0.06$). Of note, no relapse case had initiated HAART.[159] Current guidelines do not recommend changes in standard TB therapy in HIV-infected patients with PR or TB-IRIS.

Optimal management of HIV-positive patients with PR or TB-IRIS is not standardized. Systemic corticosteroids have been found to have a beneficial effect in those with severe symptoms. Breen et al utilized prednisolone in doses ranging from 10 to 80 mg daily with a gradual taper in patients with severe or prolonged symptoms. All responded clinically, with a median of 3 days (range 1–7 days). Three cases had recurrent PRs after discontinuing steroids, but responded again to reinitiation of steroid therapy.[151]

DRUG-RESISTANT TB

TB becomes resistant to drugs through random genetic mutations. The development of resistance to first-line antituberculous agents is a rare event, occurring once in ~10^6–10^7 organisms.[162] Among first-line agents, resistance to a particular class of agents occurs independently, is not associated with resistance to other drug classes, and develops because of the selective pressure of prior drug exposure. Patients may be infected with resistant strains of TB (primary resistance) or may develop resistance during the course of treatment (acquired resistance). Resistance to INH or RIF, the two most bactericidal anti-TB agents, precludes the most potent standard TB regimens and disallows the use of short course treatment. Multidrug-resistant TB (MDR-TB), defined by resistance to at least INH and RIF, is difficult to treat and can occur with or without resistance to other agents. Resistant organisms are most frequently encountered in the following circumstances: patients with known exposure to drug-resistant TB, those with prior treatment exposure, those who fail to convert to sputum culture negative status within 2 months of treatment, and those from geographic areas with a high prevalence of resistant TB.[117]

Historical context

Surveillance studies demonstrate that drug-resistant TB isolates occur more frequently in those with HIV.[163,164] US data from 1993 to 1996 demonstrated higher rates of drug resistance among TB patients with HIV compared to those without HIV infection. Among US born patients, HIV-infected patients had statistically significant higher rates of resistance to INH, RIF, EMB and PZA. RIF monoresistance was exceedingly rare in HIV-negative patients but was present in 2.6% of US-born HIV-positive TB patients and 2.2% of foreign-born HIV-positive TB patients. In addition, MDR-TB was significantly more common among HIV-positive patients when compared to HIV-negative patients (6.4% vs 1.4% in US-born and 4.7% vs 3.0% in foreign-born).[163] During the late 1980s and early 1990s, MDR-TB emerged as a serious public health concern in the US, with a disproportionately severe impact on HIV-positive patients in certain geographic areas. In 1991, the CDC reported large outbreaks of MDR-TB in four hospitals in Florida and New York (NYC) with a vast majority co-infected with HIV.[165] Hospital outbreaks of MDR-TB in NYC [166,167] were associated with the failure to implement standard infection control measures with the majority of cases linked by identical RFLP at one site.[167] During this same period throughout NYC, HIV infection, prior TB drug exposure and injection drug use were found to be risk factors for drug-resistant TB.[168] A prospective, multicenter study in the U.S. found prior treatment to be to the only risk factor for MDR-TB among a cohort of HIV-infected patients.[169] An international study of 11 countries also found prior TB treatment exposure to be a risk factor for developing MDR-TB, but there was no independent association between HIV-infection and MDR-TB.[170]

The preponderance of drug-resistant TB in HIV-positive patients is likely due to various factors. High risk exposure environments coupled with the increased risk of rapidly developing active disease likely accounted for a large proportion of cases in NYC. This association is demonstrated in the hospital outbreaks mentioned above[166,167] and the high rate of clustering of drug-resistant TB demonstrated by RFLP in NYC during this period.[171,172] Recent trends have also demonstrated an increasing proportion of RIF monoresistance among HIV-infected patients[136,163] and HIV infection has been found to be independently associated with acquired RIF resistance in one study.[173] RIF monoresistance had previously been considered an uncommon phenomenon and is a clear pathway for the development of MDR-TB. Ridzon and colleagues in a case-control study of 77 cases (59% HIV positive) identified antifungal therapy, diarrhea, and prior rifabutin exposure as risk factors for RIF monoresistance.[136] Furthermore, HIV infection has been associated with malabsorption of anti-TB drugs[174,175] and suboptimal serum drug concentrations, particularly RIF and EMB.[176] In a study of HIV-infected TB patients on twice-weekly therapy, lower serum levels of RFB and possibly INH were associated with acquired rifamycin resistance.[132,177] The associations between serum levels and treatment failure and drug resistance are not unique to HIV associated TB. This phenomenon has also been demonstrated in studies of drug concentrations in HIV-negative TB patients.[178,179] Rapid intestinal transit may limit the absorption of anti-TB agents, and the fecal passage of intact tablets has been reported in an HIV-infected patient being treated for TB.[117] For those unable to receive effective enteral TB therapy, some agents (INH, RIF, aminoglycosides, and fluoroquinolones) are available for parenteral administration, and this route may be appropriate in rare circumstances.

Treating MDR-TB is challenging. Among a series of 171 HIV-negative MDR-TB patients, the response rate was 56%, but this cohort represented a group of chronic patients who had been treated for a median of 6 years prior to referral for definitive therapy at an institution specializing in MDR-TB care. TB isolates in this group were resistant to a median of six drugs.[180] A more recent study of MDR-TB patients, with isolates resistant to fewer drugs, demonstrated a cure rate of 73% with medical therapy alone.[181] MDR-TB in HIV-infected individuals is associated with high and rapid mortality. In one series, a median survival time of 2.1 months was found,[182] and in another more recent study, 35% were dead at 18 months.[169] Initiating appropriate therapy without delay, therefore, is important and has been associated with improved survival.[169,183]

Extremely drug resistant TB

Extremely drug-resistant TB (XDR-TB) has emerged as a serious public health threat over the past few years. Defined as MDR-TB resistant to a fluoroquinolone and at least one of three injectable agents, capreomycin, kanamycin or amikacin,[184a] XDR-TB presents very limited treatment options by eliminating the most effective second line agents. Reminiscent of MDR-TB outbreaks in the late 1980's and early 1990's mentioned above, XDR-TB has been associated with poor outcomes and rapid death in those co-infected with HIV. A 2006 study from KwaZulu Natal, South Africa identified 53 cases of XDR-TB from a group of 221 MDR-TB cases. Fifty-two died, with a median survival of only 16 days from the establishment of XDR-TB status. Of 44 tested for HIV, all were positive. Among these, 15 were on ART[184b].

Principles of management

Recommended treatment regimens for drug resistant TB are identical for HIV-positive and HIV-negative patients, except for the required adjustment of medications and dosages as dictated by concomitant ART. For patients with resistance to INH (+/−streptomycin), CDC/ATS/IDSA consensus guidelines suggest a 6 month regimen of RIF, PZA and EMB with the consideration of adding a fluoroquinolone for those with extensive disease. For those with RIF monoresistance, INH, PZA and streptomycin (daily or thrice weekly) for 9 months has been shown to be effective. An all oral regimen of INH, EMB and a fluoroquinolone with PZA for the first 2 months could alternatively be used but requires a longer duration of therapy (minimum 12 months). An injectable agent may be added during the first 2 months for extensive disease.[14]

The treatment of MDR-TB is particularly difficult and should be managed by or in close consultation with an expert in this field. WHO guidelines[7] for selecting treatment regimens for MDR-TB follow several core principles:

1. The choice of regimen should be made based on the history of prior drug exposure.
2. The local prevalence of resistance to anti-TB agents should be taken into consideration.
3. Regimens should include at least four drugs that are almost certain to be effective for the patient's isolate, based on drug susceptibility testing.
4. Drugs should be administered at least 6 days a week.
5. Drug dosing should be based on the patient's weight.
6. An injectable agent (aminoglycoside or capreomycin) should be used for a minimum of 6 months, with at least 4 months of continued injectable therapy after culture conversion. Thrice-weekly regimens of injectable agents can be considered after the first 2–3 months.
7. Treatment should be continued for a minimum of 18 months after culture conversion.
8. DOT should be utilized throughout treatment.
9. Drug susceptibility testing, where available, should guide regimen design.
10. PZA can be used throughout the treatment course.
11. Early detection of MDR-TB and the rapid initiation of effective treatment are key elements to achieve success.

In the WHO consensus guidelines on drug-resistant TB management, drug choices are grouped into five distinct categories (Table 40-9).[7] In designing a treatment regimen, all first-line agents with preserved potency should be included. An injectable agent with preserved efficacy should also be incorporated as mentioned above. Fluoroquinolones have demonstrated a bactericidal effect against TB[184–188] and should be included if resistance testing reveals susceptibility to these agents. Susceptibility to fluoroquinolones has been shown to be an independent predictor of cure among MDR-TB patients.[181,189] The number of group 4 agents added depends on the number of agents available from the previous groups. Thiacetazone should be avoided in TB patients with HIV given its association with severe skin eruptions, including Stevens–Johnson syndrome in those with HIV. Group 5 agents should not be used routinely.

Surgical therapy, with resection of involved lung tissue, is considered as adjunctive therapy for those with MDR-TB. Surgery may be particularly useful for those with localized disease who are refractory to drug therapy. Surgical intervention for MDR-TB has been shown to be effective with low complication rates when performed at a center with expertise in this area[190] and associated with improved outcomes.[181,189] Effective anti-TB drug therapy remains a critical component, however, and in general should be given for at least 2 months prior to surgical intervention and for at least 12–24 months afterward.[7]

AntiTuberculous Drugs

Table 40-9

Group	Description	Drug
1	First-line oral antituberculosis drugs	Isoniazid Rifampicin Ethambutol Pyrazinamide
2	Injectable antituberculosis drugs	Streptomycin Kanamycin Amikacin Capreomycin Viomycin
3	Fluoroquinolones	Ciprofloxacin Ofloxacin Levofloxacin Moxifloxacin[a]
4	Oral bacteriostatic second-line antituberculosis drugs	Ethionamide Prothionamide Cycloserine Terizidone *p*-Aminosalicylic acid Thioacetazone
5	Antituberculosis drugs with unclear efficacy (not recommended by WHO for routine use in MDR-TB patients)	Clofazimine Amoxicillin/ clavulanate Clarithromycin Linezolid

[a] Moxifloxacin is the most potent anti-TB fluoroquinolone.

Adapted from World Health Organization. Guidelines for the programmatic management of drug-resistant tuberculosis. World Health Organization, WHO/HTM/TB/2006.361 Geneva, 2006.

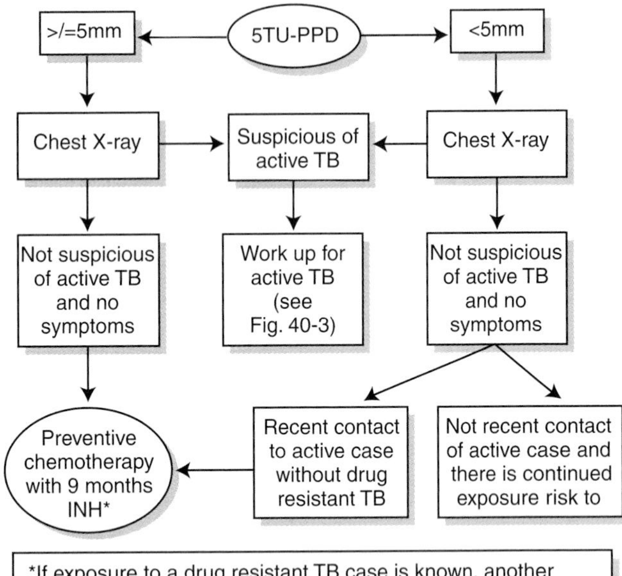

Figure 40-6 ■ Approach to the prevention of tuberculosis in HIV-infected persons.

LATENT TB INFECTION

LTBI refers to the clinical status of having been infected with TB but not having developed active disease. In immunocompetent hosts, immune responses will normally control the initial phase of primary infection but foci of quiescent mycobacteria will typically persist. HIV-positive individuals with LTBI advance to active disease much more frequently than those without HIV infection, ranging from 5% to 10% per year.[191–194] Further, they can rapidly progress to active disease upon primary infection. Active disease in HIV-infected individuals has been documented to occur as early as 1 month after exposure.[195] HIV co-infection is the single most important risk factor for the progression of LTBI to active disease.[191,193,196] It is recommended that all HIV-positive patients with either a positive PPD (>5 mm) or with recent exposure to a known case and without evidence of active TB receive a full course of treatment for latent TB infection (Fig. 40-6).[14,87,90] It is important to rapidly identify HIV-positive contacts to active cases as they are at high risk of developing active disease.[197] Joint ATS/CDC/IDSA guidelines recommend that all newly diagnosed HIV patients should receive PPD skin testing and be retested every year if indicated by exposure risk. If initial PPD skin testing was done in the setting of severe immunosuppression, repeat PPD should be performed when CD4 is greater than 200 cell/μL.[14]

Recommended Regimens for LTBI

The efficacy of INH for the treatment of tuberculin-positive HIV-positive individuals has been validated in several randomized, controlled studies, with a risk reduction for the development of active disease ranging from 36% to 78%.[193,198–200] There is conflicting evidence regarding possible mortality benefits from treating LTBI in HIV-infected patients. Pape et al demonstrated that treating LTBI in HIV-infected patients may slow the progression to death and AIDS-defining illness,[193] while others have found no such mortality benefit.[198,199] There is some evidence to support the use of INH in HIV-infected patients who are tuberculin skin test negative in high risk settings for contracting TB,[193,201] but studies have yielded inconsistent results with a relative risk of developing active disease ranging from 0.66 to 1.32.[193,198,199,202–204] A meta-analysis from 1999 suggested, however, that INH is not effective in preventing active disease in HIV-positive subjects who are tuberculin skin test negative.[205] HIV-positive patients demonstrating anergy fail to benefit from LTBI treatment[198,203] and have higher overall mortality rates than those without anergy.[198] Additionally, those with more advanced immunosuppresion (lymphopenia) have shown poorer responses to LTBI treatment.[199]

A 9-month course of daily INH is currently the preferred regimen for the treatment of LTBI in HIV-positive patients.[90] The 9-month duration of treatment is recommended based on cost-benefit considerations and extrapolation from data showing 12 months is superior to 6 months in HIV-infected patients with LTBI. In a small retrospective study from Haiti assessing LTBI therapy, longer durations of INH resulted in more durable suppression of active disease, those receiving 24–36 months achieving the greatest benefits.[206] Twice-weekly INH of 900 mg may be given by DOT for those unable to take their own medication reliably.[90] INH for the treatment of LTBI is generally well tolerated in HIV-positive patients. Toxicity necessitating the discontinuation of INH therapy in HIV disease, primarily hepatic inflammation, has ranged from 0% to 9.3% in randomized, placebo controlled studies.[193,198,199,202,203]

RIF for 4 months is an acceptable alternative for the management of LTBI in HIV-negative individuals unable to take INH or for patients exposed to an active case with INH resistant TB.[90] There are no studies demonstrating the efficacy or safety of this regimen in HIV-infected individuals, and the use of RIF is often limited by the co-administration of antiretroviral agents. RFB may be substituted for RIF, but this rationale is based solely on extrapolation from data in treating active TB.[90] Dosing adjustments may be required based on the concomitant use of other medications.

A 2-month course of RIF with PZA was recommended as an alternative treatment of LTBI in 2000, based on data from HIV-positive subjects.[199,207,208] Cases of severe hepatotoxicity were reported soon thereafter. A retrospective CDC investigation discovered a rate of significant hepatic inflammation, defined as AST above five times the upper limits of normal, of 26.4/1000 treatment initiations and a death rate of 0.9/1000 treatment initiations. Consequently this regimen is no longer recommended for routine use. [209]

WHO recommendations support the broad implementation of INH for the treatment of latent TB in those co-infected with HIV. Tuberculin skin testing may be impractical in some settings and targeted treatment may be appropriate for HIV-infected individuals in several settings: those living in areas highly endemic for TB, healthcare workers, those with household contacts with active TB, miners, prisoners, or other groups at high risk of contracting TB. The potential impact of INH therapy among HIV-infected miners was recently shown to decrease the incidence of TB by 46% among those without a prior history of TB. TST was not routinely performed in this setting.[210] An adequate evaluation to rule out active disease is an absolute prerequisite to prevent the inappropriate use of INH monotherapy for clinical TB infection.[8,211] To date, there is no evidence that LTBI treatment has led to increases in community rates of INH resistance.

The protective effects of LTBI treatment may be short-lived in areas highly endemic for TB. Mwinga et al demonstrated a durability of ~1 year following completion of LTBI treatment among HIV-infected patients in Zambia.[199] Johnson et al demonstrated a similar duration of efficacy among those receiving 6 months of INH. Those receiving INH/RIF (HR) for 3 months or INH/RIF/PZA (HRZ) for 3 months experienced a longer duration of efficacy, ranging up to 3 years.[212] In contrast, Quigley et al demonstrated a duration of protection with INH up to 2.5 years.[213]

HIV-infected patients with TB may be more likely to have recurrent TB after successful treatment of disease than HIV-negative patients, with one study demonstrating a 10-fold increase in the rate of recurrent disease.[214] Of note, all recurrent disease in this study occurred in those with advanced HIV at baseline. In a study from West Africa, a prior diagnosis of TB was found to be a significant risk factor for subsequent TB episodes in a cohort of patients on HAART (adjusted hazard ratio = 4.6).[215] The administration of INH for the prevention of recurrent disease (secondary prevention) may therefore be useful following standard treatment for active TB. Fitzgerald et al showed a reduced risk of recurrent TB in HIV-infected patients treated with 12 months of INH for secondary prevention (RR 0.18, $p = 0.03$) compared to placebo.[214] Churchyard et al demonstrated similar findings in a cohort of gold miners, with secondary preventive therapy achieving an overall 55% reduction in recurrent TB among HIV-infected individuals.[216] These findings have resulted in the consideration of lifelong preventive therapy for LTBI[199] and following the successful treatment of active TB.

PREVENTION OF PRIMARY INFECTION

HIV-infected patients appear as likely to spread TB as HIV-negative patients,[217] and both smear-negative and smear-positive patients can transmit MTB to others.[29] Spread of both susceptible and drug-resistant isolates of *M. tuberculosis* among HIV-infected persons has been reported in a variety of settings, including hospitals, prisons, shelters and group homes.[166,218–225] The common theme in these outbreaks was the rapid spread of organisms from patients with active TB to immunocompromised HIV-infected persons, who subsequently developed primary TB. These outbreaks were due to the lack of adequate infection control procedures, largely stemming from a lack of recognition of the active case.

Following the basic principles of infection control is extremely effective at preventing spread of TB among patients and from patients to health care workers.[226,227] Infection control can be divided into three components or levels: administrative controls, environmental controls and personal protection. The highest level is the administrative component, which consists of early recognition, appropriate isolation and adequate treatment of patients with or suspected of having TB.[228] Patients with abnormal chest films must be identified without delay and a decision made about the need for respiratory isolation. Some facilities with high rates of TB have developed a policy of isolation for all persons with abnormal chest films, especially those with respiratory symptoms and/or other TB risk factors, pending results of sputum smear examination and/or cultures. The implementation of an expanded three-component infection control policy at Grady Memorial Hospital in Atlanta resulted in PPD conversion rates among healthcare workers decreasing from 3.3% to 0.4% per 6-month testing intervals over 2.5 years.[229]

The decision to stop isolation, while facility-dependent, is based on the documentation of three consecutive negative smear examinations collected at 8-24 h intervals, including at least one early morning specimen.[228] For a documented smear positive TB case, the smear result should be considered in conjunction with a clinical response to antituberculous therapy, such as decreased cough and fever. For a smear-negative TB case or suspect, the clinical response is a key indicator. A repeat chest radiograph may or may not be helpful. Since smear-negative cases have been documented to spread disease, the most careful approach would be to maintain isolation for at least 2 weeks of therapy or until culture conversion is documented. For drug-resistant patients, especially those with MDR-TB, infection controllers generally prefer that such patients remain in isolation rooms until culture conversion is documented, especially given the severity and difficulty of treatment and lack of adequate secondary prevention regimens for infected contacts.[228]

Healthcare workers have been documented to have acquired TB from HIV-infected patients.[165,230] The rapid identification and isolation of TB cases and suspects is therefore critical to prevent nosocomial spread within any healthcare setting. Isolation rooms should be under negative pressure with respect to hallways, with at least six air exchanges per hour (newly constructed isolation rooms should have a minimum of 12 exchanges).[228] Upper room ultraviolet germicidal irradiation may be used as an adjunct to room ventilation and may be useful in large areas such as waiting rooms or emergency departments, where maintaining negative pressure is not feasible. Particulate respiratory air masks of the N-95 type have become the standard for use by healthcare workers. Although these protective devices should be worn by all health staff involved in TB suspect/patient care, they cannot replace adequate respiratory isolation and environmental controls.

The risk of acquiring TB from working with HIV-infected individuals was evaluated in a study of 1014 healthcare workers involved in AIDS care and research.[231] The PPD conversion rate was found to be 1.8/100 person-years, essentially the same range as reported for other health workers in general medical care. HIV-infected persons who are healthcare workers should be warned about the risk of acquiring TB in the workplace,[228] but mandatory exclusion of HIV-infected caregivers from taking care of patients with TB is not justified.[232]

ACKNOWLEDGMENTS

We would like to thank the author of the previous edition's chapter on *Mycobacterium tuberculosis*, Dr Fred Gordin, for the general outline of the current chapter. Both the section on Prevention of Primary Infection and the algorithm on diagnosing TB (Fig. 40-3) closely reflect the previous edition. We also would like to acknowledge Dr A. Edward Khan for providing the chest radiographs used. Prerna Gala and Sharon Montgomery provided much needed literature search support; Dr Ashutosh Tamhane assisted us with Figure 40-2.

REFERENCES

1. Sepkowitz KA. Tuberculosis and the health care worker: a historical perspective. Ann Intern Med 120:71–9, 1994.
2. Osler W. Hospital infection of tuberculosis as exemplified by the records of the resident staff of the Mount Vernon Hospital for Consumption and Disease of the Chest for the past fifteen years. Proc R Soc Med 3.2:137–62, 1909–10.
3. Dye C, Scheele S, Dolin P, et al. Global burden of tuberculosis: estimated incidence, prevalence, and mortality by country. JAMA 282:677–86, 1999.
4. World Health Organization. TB: a global emergency. WHO report on the TB epidemic. World Health Organization, WHO/TB/94/177, Geneva, 1994.
5. Raviglione MC, Pio A. Evolution of WHO policies for tuberculosis control, 1948–2001. Lancet 359:775–80, 2002.
6. World Health Organization and Stop TB Partnership. The Global Plan TO STOP TB 2006–2015. World Health Organization, WHO/HTM/STB/2006.35, Geneva, 2006.
7. World Health Organization. Guidelines for the programmatic management of drug-resistant tuberculosis. World Health Organization, WHO/HTM/TB/2006.361, Geneva, 2006.
8. World Health Organization. Strategic framework to decrease the burden of TB/HIV. World Health Organization. WHO/CDS/TB/2002.296, WHO/HIV_AIDS/2002.2, Geneva, 2002.
9. World Health Organization. Interim policy on collaborative TB/HIV activities. World Health Organization, WHO/HTM/TB/2004.330, WHO/HTM/HIV/2004.1, Geneva, 2004.
10. World Health Organisation (WHO). WHO declares TB an emergency in Africa: call for 'urgent and extraordinary actions' to halt a worsening epidemic, 26 Aug 2005. Available: http://www.who.int/mediacentre/news/releases/2005/ africa_emergency/en/index.html Jan 2006.
11. World Health Organization. Global tuberculosis control: surveillance, planning, and financing. WHO Report 2005, Geneva, 2006.
12. Dye C, Watt CJ, Bleed DM, et al. Evolution of tuberculosis control and prospects for reducing tuberculosis incidence, prevalence, and deaths globally. JAMA 293:2767–75, 2005.
13. Nunn P, Williams B, Floyd K, et al. Tuberculosis control in the era of HIV. Nat Rev Immunol 5:819–26, 2005.
14. American Thoracic Society/Centers for Disease Control and Prevention/Infectious Diseases Society of America. Controlling tuberculosis in the United States. Am J Respir Crit Care Med 172:1169–227, 2005.
15. CDC. Reported tuberculosis in the United States, 2004. Atlanta, GA: US Department of Health and Human Services, CDC, Sep 2005.
16. Brosch R, Banu S, Cole ST. Comparative genomics of the Mycobacterium tuberculosis complex: evolutionary insights and applications. In: Rom WN, Garay S (eds). Tuberculosis. 2nd edn. Philadelphia, PA: Williams & Wilkins; 2004, pp 65–73.
17. Sreevatsan S, Pan X, Stockbauer KE, et al. Restricted structural gene polymorphism in the Mycobacterium tuberculosis complex indicates evolutionarily recent global dissemination. Proc Natl Acad Sci 94:9869–74, 1997.
18. Cole ST. Comparative and functional genomics of the Mycobacterium tuberculosis complex. Microbiology 148:2919–28, 2002.
19. Imaeda T. Deoxyribonucleic acid relatedness among selected strains of Mycobacterium tuberculosis, Mycobacterium bovis, Mycobacterium bovis BCG, Mycobacterium microti, and Mycobacterium africanum. Int J Syst Bacteriol 35:147-–0, 1985.
20. Desmond E, Ahmed AT, Probert WS, et al. Mycobacterium africanum cases, California. Emerg Infect Dis. 10:921–3, 2004.
21. American Thoracic Society. Diagnosis and treatment of disease caused by nontuberculous mycobacteria. Am J Respir Crit Care Med 156(Suppl):S1-25, 1997.
22. Heifets L. Mycobacterial infections caused by nontuberculous mycobacteria. Semin Respir Crit Care Med 25:283–95, 2004.
23. Kapur V, Whittam TS, Musser JM. Is Mycobacterium tuberculosis 15 000 years old? J Infect Dis 170:1348–9, 1994.
24. Rieder HL. Epidemiologic Basis of Tuberculosis Control. Paris: International Union Against Tuberculosis and Lung Disease; 1999.
25. Shaw JB, Wynn-Williams N. Infectivity of pulmonary tuberculosis in relation to sputum status. Am Rev Tuberc 69:724–32, 1954.
26. Grzybowski S, Barnett GD, Styblo K. Contacts of cases of active pulmonary tuberculosis. Bull Int Union Tuberc 50:90–106, 1975.
27. Rose CE, Zerbe GO, Lantz SO, Bailey WC. Establishing priority during investigation of tuberculosis contacts. Am Rev Respir Dis 119:603–9, 1979.
28. Bailey WC, Gerald LB, Kimerling ME, et al. Predictive model to identify positive skin test results during contact investigations. JAMA 287:996–1002, 2002.
29. Behr MA, Warren SA, Salamon H, et al. Transmission of Mycobacterium tuberculosis from patients smear-negative for acid-fast bacilli. Lancet 353:444–9, 1999.
30. Theuer CP, Hopewell PC, Elias D, et al. Human immunodeficiency virus infection in tuberculosis patients. J Infect Dis 162:8–12, 1990.
31. Long R, Scalcini M, Manfreda J, et al. Impact of human immunodeficiency virus type 1 on tuberculosis in rural Haiti. Am Rev Respir Dis 143:69–73, 1991.
32. Abouya L, Coulibaly IM, Coulibaly D, et al. Radiologic manifestations of pulmonary tuberculosis in HIV-1 and HIV-2-infected patients in Abidjan, Cote d'Ivoire. Tuber Lung Dis 76:436–40, 1995.
33. Batungwanayo J, Taelman H, Dhote R, et al. Pulmonary tuberculosis in Kigali, Rwanda: impact of human immunodeficiency virus infection on clinical and radiographic presentation. Am Rev Respir Dis 146:53–6, 1992.
34. Murray JF. Cursed duet: HIV infection and tuberculosis. Respiration 57:210–20, 1990.
35. Saks AM, Posner R. Tuberculosis in HIV positive patients in South Africa: a comparative radiological study with HIV negative patients. Clin Radiol 46:387–90, 1992.

36. Mtei L, Matee M, Herfort O, et al. High rates of clinical and subclinical tuberculosis among HIV-infected ambulatory subjects in Tanzania. Clin Infect Dis 40:1500–7, 2005.
37. Jones BE, Young SM, Antoniskis D, et al. Relationship of the manifestations of tuberculosis to CD4 cell counts in patients with human immunodeficiency virus infection. Am Rev Respir Dis 148:1292–7, 1993.
38. Mlika-Cabanne N, Brauner M, Kamanfu G, et al. Radiographic abnormalities in tuberculosis and risk of coexisting human immunodeficiency virus infection: methods and preliminary results from Bujumbura, Burundi. Am J Respir Crit Care Med 152:794–9, 1995.
39. Mlika-Cabanne N, Brauner M, Mugusi F, et al. Radiographic abnormalities in tuberculosis and risk of coexisting human immunodeficiency virus infection: results from Dar-es-Salaam, Tanzania, and scoring system. Am J Respir Crit Care Med 152:786–93, 1995.
40. Small PM, Hopewell PC, Singh SP, et al. The epidemiology of tuberculosis in San Francisco: a population-based study using conventional and molecular methods. New Engl J Med 330:1703–9, 1994.
41. Alland D, Kalkut GE, Moss AR, et al. Transmission of tuberculosis in New York City: an analysis by DNA fingerprinting and conventional epidemiologic methods. New Engl J Med 330:1710–16, 1994.
42. Glynn JR, Crampin AC, Yates MD, et al. The importance of recent infection with Mycobacterium tuberculosis in an area with high HIV prevalence: a long-term molecular epidemiological study in Northern Malawi. J Infect Dis. 192:480–7, 2005.
43. Girardi E, Palmieri F, Cingolani A, et al. Changing clinical presentation and survival in HIV-associated tuberculosis after highly active antiretroviral therapy. J Acquir Immune Defic Syndr 26:326–31, 2001.
44. Klein NC, Duncanson FP, Lenox TH, et al. Use of mycobacterial smears in the diagnosis of pulmonary tuberculosis in AIDS/ARC patients. Chest 95:1190–2, 1989.
45. Elliott AM, Luo N, Tembo G, et al. Impact of HIV on tuberculosis in Zambia: a cross sectional study. BMJ 301:412–15, 1990.
46. Elliott AM, Namaambo K, Allen BW, et al. Negative sputum smear results in HIV-positive patients with pulmonary tuberculosis in Lusaka, Zambia. Tuber Lung Dis 74:191–4, 1993.
47. Nunn P, Mungai M, Nyamwaya J, et al. The effect of human immunodeficiency virus type-1 on the infectiousness of tuberculosis. Tuber Lung Dis 75:25–32, 1994.
48. Smith RL, Yew K, Berkowitz KA, et al. Factors affecting the yield of acid-fast sputum smears in patients with HIV and tuberculosis. Chest 106:684–6, 1994.
49. Finch D, Beaty CD. The utility of a single sputum specimen in the diagnosis of tuberculosis: comparison between HIV-infected and non-HIV-infected patients. Chest 111:1174–9, 1997.
50. Chheng P, Tamhane A, Natpratan C, et al. Pulmonary tuberculosis among clients visiting a voluntary confidential counseling and testing center, Cambodia. Int J Tuberc Lung Dis (Still in press).
51. Ba F, Rieder HL. A comparison of fluorescence microscopy with the Ziehl–Neelsen technique in the examination of sputum for acid-fast bacilli. Int J Tuberc Lung Dis 3:1101–5, 1999.
52. Kivihya-Ndugga LE, van Cleeff MR, Githui WA, et al. A comprehensive comparison of Ziehl–Neelsen and fluorescence microscopy for the diagnosis of tuberculosis in a resource-poor urban setting. Int J Tuberc Lung Dis 7:1163–71, 2003.
52a. Karstaedt AS, Jones N, Khoosal M, Crewe-Brown HH. The bacteriology of pulmonary tuberculosis in a population with high human immunodeficiency virus seroprevalence. Int J Tuberc Lung Dis 2:312–6, 1998.
52b. Samb B, Sow PS, Kony S, et al. Risk factors for negative sputum acid-fast bacilli smears in pulmonary tuberculosis: results from Dakar, Senegal, a city with low HIV seroprevalence. Int J Tuberc Lung Dis 3:330–6, 1999.
53. Bacha HA, Cimerman S, de Souza SA, et al. Prevalence of mycobacteremia in patients with AIDS and persistant fever. Braz J Infect Dis 8:290–5, 2004.
54. Grinsztejn B, Fandinho FC, Veloso VG, et al. Mycobacteremia in patients with the acquired immunodeficiency syndrome. Arch Intern Med 157:2359–63, 1997.
55. Archibald LK, McDonald LC, Nwanyanwu O, et al. A hospital-based prevalence survey of bloodstream infections in febrile patients in Malawi: implications for diagnosis and therapy. J Infect Dis 181:1414–20, 2000.
56. Talbot EA, Hay Burgess DC, Hone NM, et al. Tuberculosis serodiagnosis in a predominantly HIV-infected population of hospitalized patients with cough, Botswana, 2002. Clin Infect Dis 39:e1–7, 2004.
57. De Cock KM, Soro B, Coulibaly IM, et al. Tuberculosis and HIV infection in sub-Saharan Africa. JAMA 268:1581–7, 1992.
58. Goletti D, Weissman D, Jackson RW, et al. Effect of Mycobacterium tuberculosis on HIV replication: role of immune activation. J Immunol 157:1271–8, 1996.
59. Perneger TV, Sudre P, Lundgren JD, et al. Does the onset of tuberculosis in AIDS predict shorter survival?: results of a cohort study in 17 European countries over 13 years. BMJ 311:1468–71, 1995.
60. Leroy V, Salmi LR, Dupon M, et al. Progression of human immunodeficiency virus infection in patients with tuberculosis disease: a cohort study in Bordeaux, France, 1988–1994. Am J Epidemiol 145:293–300, 1997.
61. Whalen CC, Nsubuga P, Okwera A, et al. Impact of pulmonary tuberculosis on survival of HIV-infected adults: a prospective epidemiologic study in Uganda. AIDS 14:1219–28, 2000.
62. Whalen C, Horsburgh CR, Hom D, et al. Accelerated course of human immunodeficiency virus infection after tuberculosis. Am J Respir Crit Care Med 151:129–35, 1995.
63. Kassim S, Sassan-Morokro M, Ackah A, et al. Two-year follow-up of persons with HIV-1- and HIV-2-associated pulmonary tuberculosis treated with short-course chemotherapy in West Africa. AIDS 9:1185–91, 1995.
64. Chaisson RE, Clermont HC, Holt EA, et al. Six-month supervised intermittent tuberculosis therapy in Haitian patients with and without HIV infection. Am J Respir Crit Care Med 154:1034–8, 1996.
65. Perriens JH, St Louis ME, Mukadi YB, et al. Pulmonary tuberculosis in HIV-infected patients in Zaire: a controlled trial of treatment for either 6 or 12 months. New Engl J Med 332:779–84, 1995.
66. Alpert PL, Munsiff SS, Gourevitch MN, et al. A prospective study of tuberculosis and human immunodeficiency virus infection: clinical manifestations and factors associated with survival. Clin Infect Dis 24:661–8, 1997.
67. Whalen C, Okwera A, Johnson J et al. Predictors of survival in human immunodeficiency virus-infected patients with pulmonary tuberculosis. Am J Respir Crit Care Med 153:1977–81, 1996.
68. Small PM, Schecter GF, Goodman PC, et al. Treatment of tuberculosis in patients with advanced human immunodeficiency virus infection. New Engl J Med. 324:289–94, 1991.
69. Nunn P, Brindle R, Carpenter L, et al. Cohort study of human immunodeficiency virus infection in patients with tuberculosis in Nairobi, Kenya: Analysis of early (6-month) mortality. Am Rev Respir Dis 146:849–54, 1992.
70. Murray J, Sonnenberg P, Shearer SC, Godfrey-Faussett P. Human immunodeficiency virus and the outcome of treatment

for new and recurrent pulmonary tuberculosis in African patients. Am J Respir Crit Care Med 159:733–40, 1999.

71. Li TS, Tubiana R, Katlama C, et al. Long-lasting recovery in CD4 T-cell function and viral-load reduction after highly active antiretroviral therapy in advanced HIV-1 disease. Lancet 351:1682–6, 1998.
72. Schluger NW, Perez D, Liu YM. Reconstitution of immune responses to tuberculosis in patients with HIV infection who receive antiretroviral therapy. Chest 122:597–602, 2002.
73. Hsieh SM, Hung CC, Pan SC, et al. Restoration of cellular immunity against tuberculosis in patients coinfected with HIV-1 and tuberculosis with effective antiretroviral therapy: assessment by determination of CD69 expression on T cells after tuberculin stimulation. J Acquir Immune Defic Syndr 25:212–20, 2000.
74. Lawn SD, Bekker LG, Wood R. How effectively does HAART restore immune responses to Mycobacterium tuberculosis? Implications for tuberculosis control. AIDS 19:1113–24, 2005.
75. Badri M, Wilson D, Wood R. Effect of highly active antiretroviral therapy on incidence of tuberculosis in South Africa: a cohort study. Lancet. 359:2059–64, 2002.
76. Santoro-Lopes G, de Pinho AM, Harrison LH, Schechter M. Reduced risk of tuberculosis among Brazilian patients with advanced human immunodeficiency virus infection treated with highly active antiretroviral therapy. Clin Infect Dis 34:543–6, 2002.
77. Girardi E, Antonucci G, Vanacore P, et al. Impact of combination antiretroviral therapy on the risk of tuberculosis among persons with HIV infection. AIDS 14:1985–91, 2000.
78. Jones JL, Hanson DL, Dworkin MS, et al. Adult/Adolescent Spectrum of HIV Disease Group. HIV-associated tuberculosis in the era of highly active antiretroviral therapy. Int J Tuberc Lung Dis 4:1026–31, 2000.
79. Ledergerber B, Egger M, Erard V, et al. AIDS-related opportunistic illnesses occurring after initiation of potent antiretroviral therapy. JAMA 282:2220–6, 1999.
80. Girardi E, Sabin CA, d'Arminio Monforte A, et al. Incidence of Tuberculosis among HIV-infected patients receiving highly active antiretroviral therapy in Europe and North America. Clin Infect Dis 41:1772–82, 2005.
81. Williams BG, Dye C. Antiretroviral Drugs for Tuberculosis Control in the Era of HIV/AIDS. Science 301:1535–7, 2003.
82. Currie CS. Floyd K. Williams BG. Dye C. Cost, affordability and cost-effectiveness of strategies to control tuberculosis in countries with high HIV prevalence. BMC Public Health 5:130, 2005.
83. Nash DR, Douglass JE. Energy in active pulmonary tuberculosis: a comparison between positive and negative reactors and an evaluation of 5 TU and 250 TU skin test doses. Chest 77:32–7, 1980.
84. Rooney JJ Jr, Crocco JA, Kramer S, et al. Further observations on tuberculin reactions in active tuberculosis. Am J Med 60:517–22, 1976.
85. Slovis BS, Plitman JD, Haas DW. The case against anergy testing as a routine adjunct to tuberculin skin testing. JAMA 283:2003–7, 2000.
86. McMurray DN, Echeverri A. Cell-mediated immunity in anergic patients with pulmonary tuberculosis. Am Rev Respir Dis 118:827–34, 1978.
87. CDC. Guidelines for the investigation of contacts of persons with infectious tuberculosis; recommendations from the National Tuberculosis Controllers Association and CDC. MMWR 54, 2005.
88. Huebner RE, Schein MF, Bass JB Jr. The tuberculin skin test. Clin Infect Dis 17:968–75, 1993.
89. Rose DN, Schechter CB, Adler JJ. Interpretation of the tuberculin skin test. J Gen Intern Med 10:635–42, 1995.
90. CDC. Targeted tuberculin testing and treatment of latent tuberculosis infection. American Thoracic Society. MMWR 49: 1–51, 2000.
91. Thompson NJ, Glassroth JL, Snider DE, Jr, et al. The booster phenomenon in serial tuberculin testing. Am Rev Respir Dis 119:587–97, 1979.
92. Lifson AR, Grant SM, Lorvick J, et al. Two-step tuberculin skin testing of injection drug users recruited from community-based settings. Int J Tuberc Lung Dis 1:128–34, 1997.
93. Menzies D. Interpretation of repeated tuberculin tests. Boosting, conversion, and reversion. Am J Respir Crit Care Med 159:15–21, 1999.
94. CDC. Anergy skin testing and preventive therapy for HIV-infected persons: revised recommendations. MMWR 46, 1997.
95. Pesanti EL. The negative tuberculin test. Tuberculin, HIV, and anergy panels. Am J Respir Crit Care Med 149:1699–709, 1994.
96. Graham NM, Nelson KE, Solomon L, et al. Prevalence of tuberculin positivity and skin test anergy in HIV-1-seropositive and -seronegative intravenous drug users. JAMA 267:369–73, 1992.
97. Markowitz N, Hansen NI, Wilcosky TC, et al. Tuberculin and anergy testing in HIV-Seropositive and HIV-Seronegative persons. Ann Intern Med 119:185–93, 1993.
98. Caiaffa WT, Graham NM, Galai N, et al. Instability of delayed-type hypersensitivity skin test anergy in human immunodeficiency virus infection. Arch Intern Med 155:2111–17, 2005.
99. Yanai H, Uthaivoravit W, Mastro TD, et al. Utility of tuberculin and anergy skin testing in predicting tuberculosis infection in human immunodeficiency virus-infected persons in Thailand. Int J Tuberc Lung Dis 1:427–34, 1997.
100. Chin DP, Osmond D, Page-Shafer K, et al. Reliability of anergy skin testing in persons with HIV infection. The pulmonary complications of HIV infection study group. Am J Respir Crit Care Med 153:1982–4, 1996.
101. Johnson MP, Coberly JS, Clermont HC, et al. Tuberculin skin test reactivity among adults infected with human immunodeficiency virus. J Infect Dis 166:194–8, 1992.
102. Hecker MT, Johnson JL, Whalen CC, et al. Two-step tuberculin skin testing in HIV-infected persons in Uganda. Am J Respir Crit Care Med 155:81–6, 1997.
103. CDC. Guidelines for using the QuantiFERON®-TB Gold test for detecting Mycobacterium tuberculosis infection, United States. MMWR 54, 2005.
104. Chapman AL, Munkanta M, Wilkinson KA, et al. Rapid detection of active and latent tuberculosis infection in HIV-positive individuals by enumeration of Mycobacterium tuberculosis-specific T cells. AIDS 16:2285–93, 2002.
105. Dheda K, Lalvani A, Miller RF, et al. Performance of a T-cell-based diagnostic test for tuberculosis infection in HIV-infected individuals is independent of CD4 cell count. AIDS 19:2038–41, 2005.
106. Karam F, Dieye TN, Ndao CT, et al. Impact of CD4 T cell on ESAT/CFP10 interferon-g ELISPOT response amongst a cohort of HIV infected cohort without TB evidence in Dakar Senegal. In: Abstract at 10th Annual IUATLD North American Region Conference, Chicago, IL, 2006.
107. Ferrara G, Losi M, D'Amico R, et al. Use in routine clinical practice of two commercial blood tests for diagnosis of infection with Mycobacterium tuberculosis: a prospective study. Lancet 367:1328–34, 2006.
108. Toman K. Tuberculosis case-finding and chemotherapy. World Health Organization, Geneva, 1979.
109. Ferrer J. Pleural tuberculosis. Eur Respir J 10:942–7, 1997.
110. Levine H, Metzger W, Lacera D, et al. Diagnosis of tuberculous pleurisy by culture of pleural biopsy. Arch Intern Med 126:269–71, 1970.
111. Valdés L, Álvarez D, San José E, et al. Tuberculous Pleurisy. Arch Intern Med 158:2017–21, 1998.

112. Perez-Rodriguez E, Perez Walton IJ, Sanchez Hernandez JJ, et al. ADA1/ADAp ratio in pleural tuberculosis: an excellent diagnostic parameter in pleural fluid. Respir Med 93:816–21, 1999.
113. Villegas W, Labrada LA, Saravia NG. Evaluation of Polymerase Chain Reaction, Adenosine Deaminase, and Interferon- in Pleural Fluid for the Differential Diagnosis of Pleural Tuberculosis. Chest 118:1355–64, 2000.
114. Gakis C. Serum and pleural adenosine deaminase activity. Correct interpretation of the findings. Chest 99:1555–6, 1991.
115. Ungerer JP, Oosthuizen HM, Retief JH, Bissbort SH. Significance of adenosine deaminase activity and its isoenzymes in tuberculous effusions. Chest 106:33–7, 1994.
116. CDC. Update: nucleic acid amplification tests for tuberculosis. MMWR 49:593–4, 2000.
117. Khan AE, Kimerling ME. Chemotherapy of Tuberculosis. In: Schlossberg M (ed). Tuberculosis and Non-Tuberculosis Mycobacterial Infections. 5th edn. New York: McGraw-Hill; 2006, pp 77–90.
118. Kennedy N, Berger L, Curram J, et al. Randomized controlled trial of a drug regimen that includes ciprofloxacin for the treatment of pulmonary tuberculosis. Clin Infect Dis. 22:827–33, 1996.
119. El-Sadr WM, Perlman DC, Matts JP, et al. Evaluation of an intensive intermittent-induction regimen and duration of short-course treatment for human immunodeficiency virus-related pulmonary tuberculosis. Clin Infect Dis 26:1148–58, 1998.
120. Sterling TR, Alwood K, Gachuhi R, et al. Relapse rates after short-course (6-month) treatment of tuberculosis in HIV-infected and uninfected persons. AIDS 13:1899–904, 1999.
121. Dean GL, Edwards SG, Ives NJ, et al. Treatment of tuberculosis in HIV-infected persons in the era of highly active antiretroviral therapy. AIDS 16:75–83, 2002.
122. Pulido F, Pena JM, Rubio R, et al. Relapse of tuberculosis after treatment in human immunodeficiency virus-infected patients. Arch Intern Med 157:227–32, 1997.
123. Sonnenberg P, Murray J, Glynn JR, et al.P. HIV-1 and recurrence, relapse, and reinfection of tuberculosis after cure: a cohort study in South African mineworkers. Lancet 358:1687–93, 2001.
124. Verver S, Warren RM, Beyers N, et al. Rate of reinfection tuberculosis after successful treatment is higher than rate of new tuberculosis Am J Respir Crit Care Med 171:1430–5, 2005.
125. American Thoracic Society/Centers for Disease Control and Prevention/Infectious Diseases Society of America. Treatment of tuberculosis. Am J Respir Crit Care Med 167:603–62, 2003.
126. American Academy of Pediatrics. Tuberculosis. In: Pickering LJ (ed). Red book report of the Committee on Infectious Diseases, 25th edn. Elk Grove Village, IL: American Academy of Pediatrics, 2000, pp 593–613.
127. Jindani A, Nunn AJ, Enarson DA. Two 8-month regimens of chemotherapy for treatment of newly diagnosed pulmonary tuberculosis: international multicentre randomised trial. Lancet 364:1244–51, 2004.
128. Okwera A, Whalen C, Byekwaso F, et al. Randomized trial of thiacetazone and rifampin-containing regimens for pulmonary tuberculosis in HIV-infected Ugandans. Lancet 344:1323–8, 1994.
129. Nettles RE, Mazo D, Alwood K, et al. Risk factors for relapse and acquired rifamycin resistance after directly observed tuberculosis treatment: a comparison by HIV serostatus and rifamycin use. Clin Infect Dis 38:731–6, 2004.
130. CDC. Acquired rifamycin resistance in persons with advanced HIV disease being treated for active tuberculosis with intermittent rifamycin-based regimens MMWR 51:214–15, 2002.
131. Burman W, Benator D, Vernon A, et al. Acquired rifamycin resistance with twice-weekly treatment of HIV-related tuberculosis. Am J Respir Crit Care Med 173:350–6, 2006.
132. Vernon A, Burman W, Benator D, et al. Acquired rifamycin monoresistance in patients with HIV-related tuberculosis treated with once-weekly rifapentine and isoniazid. Lancet 353:1843–7, 1999.
133. Dheda K, Lampe CL, Johnson MA, et al. Outcome of HIV-associated tuberculosis in the era of highly active antiretroviral therapy.J Infect Dis 190:1670–6, 2004.
134. World Health Organization. Antiretroviral Therapy for HIV Infection in Adults and Adolescents, 2006 revision.www.who.int/hiv/pub/guidelines/artadultguidelines.pdf. Accessed August, 2007.
135. Li A, Reith M, Rasmussen A, et al. Primary human hepatocytes as a tool for the evaluation of structure–activity relationship in cytochrome P450 induction potential of xenobiotics: evaluation of rifampin, rifapentine, rifabutin. Chem Biol Interact 107:17–30, 1997.
136. Ridzon R, Whitney CG, McKenna MT, et al. Risk factors for rifampin mono-resistant tuberculosis. Am J Respir Crit Care Med 157:1881–4, 1998.
137. Trapnell CB, Narang PK, Li R, Lavelle JP. Increased plasma rifabutin levels with concomitant fluconazole therapy in HIV-infected patients. Ann Intern Med 124:573–6, 1996.
138. Narang PK, Trapnell CB, Schoenfelder JR, et al. Fluconazole and enhanced effect of rifabutin prophylaxis. New Engl J Med. 330:1316–17, 1994
139. Moreno S, Podzamczer D, Blazquez R, et al. Treatment of tuberculosis in HIV-infected patients: safety and antiretroviral efficacy of the concomitant use of ritonavir and rifampin. AIDS 15:1185–7, 2001.
140. Veldkamp AI, Hoetelmans RM, Beijnen JH. Ritonavir enables combined therapy with rifampin and saquinavir. Clin Infect Dis 29:1586, 1999.
141. la Porte C, Colbers E, Bertz R, et al. Pharmacokinetics of two adjusted dose regimens of lopinavir/ritonavir in combination with rifampin in healthy volunteers. In: 42nd Interscience Conference on Antimicrobial Agents and Chemotherapy, San Diego, CA, 2002, abstract #A-1823.
142. CDC. TB/HIV Drug interactions. Available: http://www.cdc.gov/nchstp/tb/tb_hiv_drugs/toc.htm May 2006.
143. McGregor MM, Olliaro P, Wolmarans L, et al. Efficacy and safety of rifabutin in the treatment of patients with newly diagnosed pulmonary tuberculosis. Am J Respir Crit Care Med 154:1462–1467, 1996.
144. Narita M, Stambaugh JJ, Hollender ES, et al. Use of rifabutin with protease inhibitors for human immunodeficiency virus-infected patients with tuberculosis. Clin Infect Dis 30:779–83, 2000.
145. Dean G, Back D, de Ruiter A. Effect of tuberculosis therapy on nevirapine trough plasma concentration. AIDS 13:2489–90, 1999.
146. Ribera E, Pou L, Lopez RM, et al. Pharmacokinetic interaction between nevirapine and rifampicin in HIV-infected patients with tuberculosis. J Acquir Immune Defic Synr 28:450–3, 2001.
147. Olivia J, Moreno S, Sanz J, et al. Co-administration of rifampin and nevirapine in HIV-infected patients with tuberculosis. AIDS 17:637–42, 2003.
148. Manosuthi W, Sungkanuparph S, Thakkinstian A, et al. Comparison of plasma levels of nevirapine, liver function test, virological and immunological outcomes in HIV-infected patients receiving and not receiving rifampicin: preliminary results. In: 45th Interscience Conference on Antimicrobial Agents and Chemotherapy, Washington, DC, 2005, abstract #H-414.
149. Choremis CB, Padiatellis C, Zoumboulakis D, et al. Transitory exacerbation of fever and roentgenographic findings during treatment of tuberculosis in children. Am Rev Tuberc 72:527–36, 1955.
150. Narita M, Ashkin D, Hollender ES, et al. Paradoxical worsening of tuberculosis following antiretroviral therapy in

patients with AIDS. Am J Respir Crit Care Med 158:157–161, 1998.
151. Breen RA, Smith CJ, Bettinson H, et al. Paradoxical reactions during tuberculosis treatment in patients with and without HIV co-infection. Thorax 59:704–7, 2004.
152. Ellner JJ, Wallis RS. Immunologic aspects of mycobacterial infections. Rev Infect Dis 11:S455–S459, 1989.
153. Dannenberg AM Jr Immune mechanisms in the pathogenesis of pulmonary tuberculosis. Rev Infect Dis 11:S369–S378, 1989.
154. John M, French MA. Exacerbation of the inflammatory response to Mycobacterium tuberculosis after antiretroviral therapy. Med J Australia 169:473–4, 1998.
155. French MA, Mallal SA, Dawkins RL. Zidovudine-induced restoration of cell-mediated immunity to mycobacteria in immunodeficient HIV-infected patients. AIDS 6:1293–7, 1992.
156. Fishman JE, Saraf-Lavi E, Narita M, et al. Pulmonary tuberculosis in AIDS patients: transient chest radiographic worsening after initiation of antiretroviral therapy. Am J Roentgenol 174:43–9, 2000.
157. Shelburne SA, Visnegarwala F, Darcourt J, et al. Incidence and risk factors for immune reconstitution inflammatory syndrome during highly active antiretroviral therapy. AIDS 19:399–406, 2005.
158. Jehle AW, Khanna N, Sigle JP, et al. Acute renal failure on immune reconstitution in an HIV-positive patient with miliary tuberculosis. Clin Infect Dis 38:e32–5, 2004.
159. Wendel KA, Alwood KS, Gachuhi R, et al. Paradoxical worsening of tuberculosis in HIV-infected persons. Chest 120:193–7, 2001.
160. Michailidis C, Pozniak AL, Mandalia S, et al. Clinical characteristics of IRIS syndrome in patients with HIV and tuberculosis. Antivir Ther 10:417–22, 2005.
161. Breton G, Duval X, Estellat C, et al. Determinants of immune reconstitution inflammatory syndrome in HIV type 1-infected patients with tuberculosis after initiation of antiretroviral therapy. Clin Infect Dis 39:1709–12, 2004.
162. Mitchison DA. Drug resistance in mycobacteria. Br Med Bull. 40:84–90, 1984.
163. Moore M, Onorato IM, McCray E, Castro KG. Trends in drug-resistant tuberculosis in the United States, 1993–1996. JAMA 278:833–7, 1997.
164. Gordin FM, Nelson ET, Matts JP, et al. The impact of human immunodeficiency virus infection on drug-resistant tuberculosis. Am J Respir Crit Care Med 154:1478–83, 1996.
165. CDC. Nosocomial transmission of multidrug-resistant tuberculosis among HIV-infected persons: Florida and New York, 1988–1991. MWWR 40:585–591, 1991.
166. Edlin BR, Tokars JI, Grieco MH, et al. An outbreak of multidrug-resistant tuberculosis among hospitalized patients with the acquired immunodeficiency syndrome. New Engl J Med 326:1514–21, 1992.
167. Coronado VG, Beck-Sague CM, Hutton MD, et al. Transmission of multidrug-resistant Mycobacterium tuberculosis among persons with human immunodeficiency virus infection in an urban hospital: epidemiologic and restriction fragment length polymorphism analysis. J Infect Dis 168:1052–5, 1993.
168. Frieden TR, Sterling T, Pablos-Mendez A, et al. The emergence of drug-resistant tuberculosis in New York City. New Engl J Med 328:521–6, 1993.
169. Telzak EE, Chirgwin KD, Nelson ET, et al. Predictors for multidrug-resistant tuberculosis among HIV-infected patients and response to specific drug regimens. Int J Tuberc Lung Dis 3:337–43, 1999.
170. Espinal MA, Laserson K, Camacho M, et al. Determinants of drug-resistant tuberculosis: analysis of 11 countries. Int J Tuberc Lung Dis 5:887–93, 2001.
171. Shafer RW, Small PM, Larkin C, et al. Temporal trends and transmission patterns during the emergence of multidrug-resistant tuberculosis in New York City: a molecular epidemiologic assessment. J Infect Dis 171:170–6, 1995.
172. Friedman CR, Stoeckle MY, Kreiswirth BN, et al. Transmission of multidrug-resistant tuberculosis in a large urban setting. Am J Respir Crit Care Med 152:355–9, 1995.
173. Li J, Munsiff SS, Driver CR, Sackoff J. Relapse and acquired rifampin resistance in HIV-infected patients with tuberculosis treated with rifampin- or rifabutin-based regimens in New York City, 1997–2000. Clin Infect Dis 41:83–91, 2005.
174. Berning SE, Huitt GA, Iseman MD, Peloquin CA. Malabsorption of antituberculosis medications by a patient with AIDS. New Engl J Med 327:1817–18, 1992.
175. Patel KB, Belmonte R, Crowe HM. Drug malabsorption and resistant tuberculosis in HIV-infected patients. New Engl J Med 332:336–7, 1995.
176. Peloquin CA, Nitta AT, Burman WJ, et al. Low antituberculosis drug concentrations in patients with AIDS. Ann Pharmacother. 30:919–25, 1996.
177. Weiner M, Benator D, Burman W, et al. Association between acquired rifamycin resistance and the pharmacokinetics of rifabutin and isoniazid among patients with HIV and tuberculosis. Clin Infect Dis 40:1481–91, 2005.
178. Weiner M, Burman W, Vernon A, et al. Low isoniazid concentrations and outcome of tuberculosis treatment with once-weekly isoniazid and rifapentine. Am J Respir Crit Care Med 167:1341–7, 2003.
179. Kimerling ME, Phillips P, Patterson P, et al. Low serum antimycobacterial drug levels in non-HIV-infected tuberculosis patients. Chest. 113:1178–83, 1998.
180. Goble M, Iseman MD, Madsen LA, et al. Treatment of 171 patients with pulmonary tuberculosis resistant to isoniazid and rifampin. N Engl J Med 328:527–32, 1993.
181. Tahaoglu K, Torun T, Sevim T, et al. The treatment of multidrug-resistant tuberculosis in Turkey. N Engl J Med 345:170–4, 2001.
182. Fischl MA, Daikos GL, Uttamchandani RB, et al. Clinical presentation and outcome of patients with HIV and tuberculosis caused by multiple-drug-resistant bacilli. Ann Intern Med 117:184–90, 1992.
183. Park MM, Davis AL, Schluger NW, et al. Outcome of MDR-TB patients, 1983–1993: prolonged survival with appropriate therapy. Am J Respir Crit Care Med 153:317–42, 1996.
184. Paramasivan CN, Sulochana S, Kubendiran G, et al. Bactericidal action of gatifloxacin, rifampin, and isoniazid on logarithmic- and stationary-phase cultures of Mycobacterium tuberculosis. Antimicrob Agents Chemother 49:627–31, 2005.
184a. Raviglione MC, Smith IM. XDR tuberculosis – implications for global public health. N Engl J Med 356:656–9, 2007.
184b. Gandhi NR, Moll A, Sturm AW, et al. Extensively drug-resistant tuberculosis as a cause of death in patients co-infected with tuberculosis and HIV in a rural area of South Africa. Lancet 368:1575-80, 2006.
185. Pletz MW, De Roux A, Roth A, et al. Early bactericidal activity of moxifloxacin in treatment of pulmonary tuberculosis: a prospective, randomized study. Antimicrob Agents Chemother 48:780–2, 2004.
186. Sato K, Tomioka H, Sano C, et al. Comparative antimicrobial activities of gatifloxacin, sitafloxacin and levofloxacin against Mycobacterium tuberculosis replicating within Mono Mac 6 human macrophage and A-549 type II alveolar cell lines. J Antimicrob Chemother 52:199–203, 2003.
187. Alangaden GJ, Lerner SA. The clinical use of fluoroquinolones for the treatment of mycobacterial diseases. Clin Infect Dis 25:1213–21, 1997.
188. Nuermberger EL, Yoshimatsu T, Tyagi S, et al. Moxifloxacin-containing regimens of reduced duration produce a stable

cure in murine tuberculosis. Am J Respir Crit Care Med 170:1131–4, 2004.
189. Chan ED, Laurel V, Strand MJ, et al. Treatment and outcome analysis of 205 patients with multidrug-resistant tuberculosis. Am J Respir Crit Care Med 169:1103–9, 2004.
190. Pomerantz BJ, Cleveland JC, Olson HK, Pomerantz M. Pulmonary resection for multi-drug resistant tuberculosis. J Thorac Cardiovasc Surg 121:448–53, 2001.
191. Selwyn PA, Hartel D, Lewis VA, et al. A prospective study of the risk of tuberculosis among intravenous drug users with human immunodeficiency virus infection. New Engl J Med 320:545–50, 1989.
192. Guelar A, Gatell JM, Verdejo J, et al. A prospective study of the risk of tuberculosis among HIV-infected patients. AIDS 7:1345–9, 1993.
193. Pape JW, Jean SS, Ho JL, et al. Effect of isoniazid prophylaxis on incidence of active tuberculosis and progression of HIV infection. Lancet 342:268–72, 1993.
194. Antonucci G, Girardi E, Raviglione MC, Ippolito G. Risk factors for tuberculosis in HIV-infected persons. JAMA 274:143–8, 1995.
195. Daley CL, Small PM, Schecter GF, et al. An outbreak of tuberculosis with accelerated progression among persons infected with the human immunodeficiency virus: an analysis using restriction-fragment-length polymorphisms. New Engl J Med 326:231–5, 1992.
196. Markowitz N, Hansen NI, Hopewell PC, et al. Incidence of tuberculosis in the United States among HIV-infected persons. Ann Intern Med 126:123–32, 1997.
197. Havlir DV, Barnes PF. Tuberculosis in patients with human immunodeficiency virus infection. New Engl J Med 340: 367–73, 1999.
198. Whalen CC, Johnson JL, Okwera A, et al. A trial of three regimens to prevent tuberculosis in Ugandan adults infected with the human immunodeficiency virus. N Eng J Med 337:801–8, 1997.
199. Mwinga A, Hosp M, Godfrey-Faussett P, et al. Twice weekly tuberculosis preventive therapy in HIV infection in Zambia. AIDS 12:2447–57, 1998.
200. Woldehanna S, Volmink J. Treatment of latent tuberculosis infection in HIV infected persons. The Cochrane Database of Systematic Reviews 2004, Issue 1. Art. No.: CD000171. doi: 10.1002/14651858.CD000171.pub2, 2004.
201. Gourevitch MN, Hartel D, Selwyn PA, et al. Effectiveness of isoniazid chemoprophylaxis for HIV-infected drug users at high risk for active tuberculosis. AIDS 13:2069–74, 1999.
202. Hawken MP, Meme HK, Elliott LC, et al. Isoniazid preventive therapy for tuberculosis in HIV-1 infected adults: results of a randomized controlled trial. AIDS 11:875–82, 1997.
203. Gordin FM, Matts JP, Miller C, et al. A controlled trial of isoniazid in persons with anergy and human immunodeficiency virus infection who are at high risk for tuberculosis. N Engl J Med 337:315–20, 1997.
204. Fitzgerald DW, Severe P, Joseph P, et al. No effect of isoniazid prophylaxis for purified protein derivative-negative HIV-infected adults living in a country with endemic tuberculosis: results of a randomized trial. Journal of Acquired Immune Deficiency Syndromes: J Acquir Immune Defic Syndr 28:305–7, 2001.
205. Bucher HC, Griffith LE, Guyatt GH, et al. Isoniazid prophylaxis for tuberculosis in HIV infection: a meta-analysis of randomized controlled trials. AIDS 13:501–7, 1999.
206. Fitzgerald DW, Morse MM, Pape JW, Johnson WD. Active tuberculosis in individuals infected with human immunodeficiency virus after isoniazid prophylaxis. Clin Infect Dis 31:1495–7, 2000.
207. Gordin FM, Chaisson RE, Matts JP, et al. Rifampin and pyrazinamide vs isoniazid for prevention of tuberculosis in HIV-infected persons. JAMA 283:1445–50, 2000.
208. Halsey NA, Coberly J, Desormeaux J, et al. Randomized trial of isoniazid versus rifampin and pyrazinamide for prevention of tuberculosis in HIV-1 infection. Lancet 351:786–92, 1998.
209. CDC. Adverse Event Data and Revised American Thoracic Society/CDC Recommendations Against the Use of Rifampin and Pyrazinamide for Treatment of Latent Tuberculosis Infection – United States, 2003. MMWR 52:735–9, 2003.
210. Grant AD, Charalambous S, Fielding KL, et al. Effect of routine isoniazid preventive therapy on tuberculosis incidence among HIV-infected men in South Africa. JAMA 293:2719–25, 2005.
211. World Health Organization. Preventive therapy against tuberculosis in people living with HIV. WHO Weekly Epidemiologic Record. 74:385–98, 1999.
212. Johns on JL, Okwera A, Hom DL, et al. Duration of efficacy of treatment of latent tuberculosis infection in HIV-infected adults. AIDS 15:2137–47, 2001.
213. Quigley MA, Mwinga A, Hosp M, et al. Long-term effect of preventive therapy for tuberculosis in a cohort of HIV-infected Zambian adults. AIDS. 15:215–22, 2001.
214. Fitzgerald DW, Desvarieux M, Severe P, et al. Effect of post-treatment isoniazid on prevention of recurrent tuberculosis in HIV-1-infected individuals: a randomised trial. Lancet 356:1470–4, 2000.
215. Seyler C, Slaka T, Messou E, et al. Risk factors for active tuberculosis after antiretroviral treatment initiation in Abidjan. Am J Respir Crit Care Med 172:123–7, 2005.
216. Churchyard GJ, Fielding K, Charalambous S, et al. Efficacy of secondary isoniazid preventive therapy among HIV-infected Southern Africans: time to change policy? AIDS 17:2063–70, 2003.
217. Espinal MA, Perez EN, Baez J, et al. Infectiousness of *Mycobacterium tuberculosis* in HIV-1-infected patients with tuberculosis: a prospective study. Lancet 355:275–80, 2000.
218. CDC. Drug-susceptible tuberculosis outbreak in a state correctional facility housing HIV-infected inmates: South Carolina, 1999–2000. MMWR 49:1041–4, 2000.
219. Moss AR, Hahn JA, Tulsky JP, et al. Tuberculosis in the homeless: a prospective study. Am J Respir Crit Care Med 162: 460–464, 2000.
220. Yaganehdoost A, Graviss EA, Ross MW, et al. Complex transmission dynamics of clonally related virulent Mycobacterium tuberculosis associated with barhopping by predominantly human immunodeficiency virus-positive gay men. J Infect Dis 180:1245–51, 1999.
221. CDC. HIV-related tuberculosis in a transgender network: Baltimore, Maryland and New York City Area, 1998–2000. MWWR 49:317–20, 2000.
222. Small PM, Shafer RW, Hopewell PC, et al. Exogenous reinfection with multidrug-resistant Mycobacterium tuberculosis in patients with advanced HIV infection. N Engl J Med 328:1137–44, 1993
223. Dooley SW, Villarino ME, Lawrence M, et al. Nosocomial transmission of tuberculosis in a hospital unit for HIV-infected patients. JAMA 267:2632–2364, 1992.
224. Ritacco V, DiLonardo M, Reniero A, et al. Nosocomial spread of human immunodeficiency virus-related multidrug-resistant tuberculosis in Buenos Aires. J Infect Dis 176:637–42, 1997.
225. Zolopa AR, Hahn JA, Gorter R, et al. HIV and tuberculosis infection in San Francisco's homeless adults. JAMA 272:455–61, 1994.
226. McGowan JE. Nosocomial tuberculosis: new progress in control and prevention. Clin Infect Dis 21:489–505, 1995.
227. Menzies D, Fanning A, Yuan L, et al. Hospital ventilation and risk for tuberculosis infection in Canadian health care workers. Canadian Collaborative Group in Nosocomial Transmission of TB. Ann Intern Med 133:779–89, 2000.
228. CDC. Guidelines for Preventing the Transmission of Mycobacterium tuberculosis in Health-Care Settings, 2005. MMWR 54, 2005.

229. Blumberg HM, Watkins DL, Berschling JD, et al. Preventing the nosocomial transmission of tuberculosis. Ann Intern Med 122:658–63, 1995.
230. Kenyon TA, Ridzon R, Luskin-Hawk R, et al. A nosocomial outbreak of multidrug-resistant tuberculosis. Ann Intern Med 127:32–6, 1997.
231. Zahnow K, Matts JP, Hillman, et al. Rates of tuberculosis infection in healthcare workers providing services to HIV-infected populations. Terry Beirn Community Programs for Clinical Research on AIDS. Infect Control Hosp Epidemiol 19:829–35, 1998.
232. Bayer R, Dublier NN, Landesman S, et al. The dual epidemics of tuberculosis and AIDS: ethical and policy issues in screening and treatment. Am J Public Health 83:649–54, 1993.

Chapter 41

Mycobacterium Avium Complex and Other Atypical Mycobacterial Infections

Constance A. Benson, MD, Judith S. Currier, MD

CLINICAL SYNDROMES

Mycobacterium avium complex (MAC) disease in patients with human immunodeficiency virus-1 (HIV-1) infection with acquired immunodeficiency syndrome (AIDS) and advanced immunosuppression, in the absence of potent antiretroviral therapy, is generally associated with disseminated multiorgan infection. Early symptoms may be minimal and may precede detectable mycobacteremia by several weeks.[1,2] Although mycobacteremia may be intermittent, transient, or absent, untreated disease in most patients with advanced immunosuppression progresses to clinically apparent symptoms, sustained bacteremia, and widespread infiltration of reticuloendothelial and organ tissue.[1–7] Those with established blood and widespread tissue infection report symptoms that include fever, drenching sweats, weight loss, fat and muscle-wasting, fatigue, diarrhea, and abdominal pain.[1,3–6] Localised MAC disease, while uncommon, is more often seen among patients with advanced immunosuppression who have a substantial increase in the CD4+ T-lymphocyte count (100 cells/μL or higher) and suppression of HIV-1 replication after initiation of potent combination antiretroviral therapy.[8–10] Focal lymphadenitis and fever, or other localized tissue infections caused by MAC, unaccompanied by bacteremia or disseminated tissue or organ involvement, have been described. Similarly, an inflammatory response that mimics active MAC disease may occur in those with previously established but quiescent or treated tissue infection and rapid and substantial increases in CD4+ T-lymphocyte counts after starting potent antiretroviral therapy.[8–10] Signs and symptoms of this immune recovery inflammatory syndrome may be clinically indistinguishable from those of active MAC infection but are generally unaccompanied by detectable mycobacterial replication or growth in culture or tissue samples. In patients not receiving, or who have not immunologically responded to, potent combination antiretroviral therapies, localized disease is rare. The localized syndromes described in HIV-1-infected individuals include a diarrheal malabsorption syndrome resembling Whipple's disease; cervical or mesenteric lymphadenitis; pneumonitis; pericarditis; osteomyelitis; skin, soft tissue or muscle abscesses; renal lesions; an enlarging genital ulcer; or central nervous system infection (CA Benson, personal observations).[4,11–21] Phillips and colleagues estimated the incidence of immune reconstitution inflammatory syndromes due to MAC to be 3.5% among patients with CD4+ T-lymphocyte counts less than 100 cells/μL who initiated potent combination antiretroviral therapy. The three most common presentations in their series of 45 patients included peripheral lymphadenitis, pulmonary thoracic disease and intraabdominal disease.[22] More recent reports suggest that rates of immune recovery inflammatory syndromes may be as high as 31% among patients with preexisting MAC infections who were started on and responded to potent combination antiretroviral therapy.[21]

The most frequently observed laboratory abnormalities in persons with disseminated *M. avium* disease are anemia, elevated liver alkaline phosphatase, and decreased serum albumin.[3–6,23] Neutropenia or thrombocytopenia (or both) may accompany bone marrow infiltration. Hepatomegaly, splenomegaly, or central (paratracheal, retroperitoneal, or para-aortic) lymphadenopathy may be detected on physical examination or by radiographic or other imaging studies.[3,4,24] With the exception of focal lymphadenitis, peripheral lymphadenopathy is uncommon. Other focal symptoms, signs, or laboratory abnormalities may occur in the context of the localized disease syndromes previously described.

PATHOGEN

The *M. avium* complex is comprised of two predominant species, *M. avium* and *M. intracellulare*, and several unspeciated mycobacteria.[3,25] MAC organisms are considered nonphotochromogenic, although production of yellow pigment by older colonies grown under select conditions has been reported.[26] Growth on solid media is generally slow, but growth can be detected radiometrically in liquid media within 7–10 days depending on inoculum size and laboratory conditions.[27] The colonial morphotype on solid media is determined by the glycopeptidolipid content of the cell wall, the characteristic that distinguishes serovars. Of the more than 28 identified serovars, types 1–6, 8–11, and 21 are *M. avium*, and types 7, 12–20, and 25 are *M. intracellulare*.[26,28] Types 1, 4, and 8 of *M. avium* are most frequently associated with disease in persons with AIDS in the United States and developed countries.[26,28]

Previous studies have shown that more than 95% of isolates of MAC recovered from patients with AIDS and disseminated MAC disease are *M. avium*.[29–33] In contrast, 40% of MAC isolates from HIV-uninfected individuals are *M. intracellulare*.[32] Characteristics of individual serovars and unique host genetic or immune factors may determine differences in the prevailing organisms causing disease in different hosts or geographic regions.[34]

Up to 25% of persons with AIDS and disseminated *M. avium* disease may be infected with two or more genetically distinct strains of *M. avium*.[35–37] The clinical significance of this finding is unknown, although in one study different strains recovered before and during treatment demonstrated disparate susceptibility to antimicrobial agents.[35–37] In one recent study, differences in virulence factors (as measured by invasion of gastrointestinal cells and replication in macrophages) of MAC isolates obtained from mucosal surfaces and from blood suggested that these factors may contribute to the pathogenesis of MAC infection in immunocompromised hosts.[38]

EPIDEMIOLOGY

MAC organisms can be recovered from a number of environmental reservoirs, including water, soil, domestic and farm animals, birds, foods, and some tobacco products.[33,39,40] In early studies evaluating delayed-type hypersensitivity responses to skin testing with purified protein derivative, Battey demonstrated a high prevalence of responses among persons residing in the southeastern part of the United States.[41] Studies using a more specific mycobacterial antigen derived from *M. avium*, sensitin, suggest that 7–12% of adults in the United States, Kenya, Trinidad, and Finland have been previously exposed to or infected with *M. avium*.[42] Although environmental reservoirs of *M. avium* also exist in developing countries or regions, MAC disease is uncommon among patients with AIDS in these areas.[42,43] Hypotheses suggested to explain this observation are that the high prevalence of latent or active *M. tuberculosis* infection in developing countries confers partial immunity to atypical mycobacterial infection or that biologic characteristics among local environmental serovars of MAC diminish their virulence.[4,43,44]

The environmental source of infection for individuals who develop active disease, with rare exception, is indeterminate. An epidemiologic study of MAC isolates from HIV-infected patients in Japan showed no evidence of clustering of similar isolates among patients.[45] In contrast, von Reyn et al described two small clusters of HIV-infected individuals with disseminated MAC disease from whom MAC isolates were recovered and found to be genetically identical to isolates recovered from potable water supplies in the same hospitals in which these patients had previously been hospitalized.[46] Household water supplies have also been shown to be 'contaminated' with environmental strains of *M. avium*.[47] Von Reyn and colleagues further reported an association between ingestion of raw fish, prior bronchoscopy, or treatment with granulocyte colony-stimulating factor and an increased risk of developing disseminated MAC disease.[48] Similarly, Horsburgh et al demonstrated an association between ingestion of hard cheese and an increased risk of developing MAC bacteremia.[49] In the latter two studies an association was also noted between daily showering or occupational exposure to water and a decreased risk of developing MAC bacteremia.[48,49] As these studies illustrate, however, no environmental exposure or behavior has been consistently associated with the subsequent development of MAC disease in susceptible persons; therefore behaviors aimed at avoidance of exposure cannot be expected to result in a decreased risk of developing disease for highly susceptible individuals.[50–52]

Prior to the advent of effective chemoprophylaxis and potent combination antiretroviral therapy, the incidence of disseminated MAC disease in persons with AIDS ranged from ~20% to 40%.[5,6,53,54] There has been a dramatic decline in the incidence of opportunistic infections overall and specifically in *M. avium* disease during the modern era of potent combination antiretroviral therapy. The clinical event rate in one study comparing two drugs for prophylaxis of *Pneumocystis jerovici* pneumonia in subjects intolerant of trimethoprim-sulfamethoxazole declined from 64 per 100 patient-years during the first year of follow-up to 34 per 100 patient-years during the second year; the proportion of study subjects who used protease inhibitor (PI) therapies increased from none at the beginning of the first year to 72% at the end of the second year of the study.[55] In the Centers for Disease Control and Prevention (CDC)-sponsored HIV Outpatient Study (HOPS), the overall proportion of persons followed with AIDS who had CD4+ T-lymphocyte counts of less than 100 cells/μL and who developed an opportunistic infection in 1995 was 26.9%, compared with 18.1% in 1996; the rate declined from 4.8% during the fourth quarter of 1996 to 3.0% during the second quarter of 1997 coincident with the increased use of PI therapy.[56] Although patients with low CD4 + T-cell counts remain at risk for MAC, among patients in the Johns Hopkins cohort with advanced HIV disease the proportion developing MAC has fallen from 16% before 1996 to 4% after 1996 with a rate of less than 1% in 2003.[57] Factors associated with developing MAC in the Hopkins cohort include younger age, no use of potent combination antiretroviral therapy, and enrollment before 1996. Similar rates of decrease of opportunistic infections were reported by investigators following implementation of PI therapies in Europe.[58,59] Additional studies have indicated that rates of *M. avium* disease in similar populations have declined in concert with the rates of other opportunistic infections.[60–62] Similarly, in two randomized clinical trials evaluating azithromycin or placebo for prophylaxis of MAC disease in patients on potent combination antiretroviral therapy who had an increase in their CD4+ T-lymphocyte counts from less than 50 cells/μL to more than 100 cells/μL at entry, the overall rate of MAC disease was fewer than two cases per 100 patient-years of follow-up.[61,62] These rates are considerably lower than those reported for previous years in the absence of potent antiretroviral therapy and chemoprophylaxis.

The increased susceptibility of HIV-infected persons with advanced immunosuppression to disseminated *M. avium* disease has not been fully explained. CD4+ and CD8+ T-lymphocytes, macrophages, natural killer (NK) cells, gamma delta T cells, and the host of cytokines produced by these cells in response to mycobacterial antigen stimulation represent the primary immune response to infection with MAC organisms.[63–74] Among the cytokines most central to the host immune response to MAC appear to be interleukin-12 (IL-12), interferon-γ (IFNγ), tumor necrosis factor-α (TNFα), IL-6, and IL-10.[63–74] Animal studies show that TNFα is essential for the development of protective immunity to MAC and contributes to the reduction of intracellular growth of MAC.[75,76] IL-12 stimulates IFNγ production, and both play key roles in the immune defense against MAC disease. In mice lacking these cytokines after targeted gene deletions and in humans with genetic defects of IL-12 or IFNγ production or expression, increased susceptibility to MAC infection and severe forms of disseminated MAC disease ensue.[74,77–82] IL-6 promotes *M. avium* growth, and IL-10 appears to inhibit production of TNFα and IL-12; IL-10 also down-regulates expression of co-stimulatory molecules on *M. avium*-infected monocytes, resulting in inhibition of IFNγ production.[74,83–86] Whereas *in vitro* macrophage function and response to IFNγ and the induction and expression of TNFα appear to be similar in HIV-infected individuals and HIV-uninfected controls, both HIV-infected and HIV-uninfected individuals with established MAC disease have been reported to have increased expression of IL-6, decreased production or expression of IFNγ and IL-12, and increased production of IL-10 by peripheral blood mononuclear cells.[71–74,87,88] These data suggest that, in addition to CD4+ T-lymphocyte depletion and loss of CD4+ T cells, perturbations of these cytokines are involved in the increased propensity of HIV-infected individuals to develop disseminated MAC disease. Functionally as well, untreated HIV-infected patients have significantly reduced lymphoproliferative responses to *M. avium*.[73]

MacGregor and colleagues examined immunologic factors associated with development of MAC among patients with advanced immunosuppression with and without signs and symptoms of MAC disease.[89] Subjects with disseminated MAC and asymptomatic controls with CD4+ T-lymphocyte counts of less than 50 cells/μL had similar levels of measured cytokine producing cells in bone marrow tissue including a low frequency of cells producing IL-12, TNFα, and TGF-β, however, significantly more CD8+ T cells were present among those with MAC infection compared to controls. In contrast, the group with MAC infection had significantly more CD4+ T-lymphocytes secreting IFNγ in response to MAC antigen and lower numbers of CD8+ T cells in peripheral blood than did the control group. These results suggest that ineffective MAC specific T-cell responses can persist during MAC infection. The authors speculate that the inflammatory responses to MAC that can occur shortly after initiation of potent combination antiretroviral therapy might be due to the rapid expansion of these preexisting immune responses.[89] A recent observation of a dramatic increase from baseline in PPD-specific Th1 IFNγ-producing CD4+ T cells during immune recovery inflammatory syndromes in patients with tuberculosis support this hypothesis.[90]

The most important risk factor for or predictor of the development of disseminated *M. avium* disease is advanced immunosuppression, as indicated by a CD4+ T-lymphocyte count of less than 50 cells/μL.[51–56,58–62] This remains true in patients treated with potent antiretroviral therapy.[58–62] High plasma HIV-1 RNA levels (>100 000 copies/mL) and a prior opportunistic infection, particularly cytomegalovirus disease, also contribute to the hazard of developing *M. avium* disease.[53,54,91–94]

Data regarding the relative risk of developing a specific opportunistic infection in those receiving potent combination antiretroviral therapies are limited, but as previously described, the risk has declined substantially, attributed not only to increases in CD4+ T-lymphocyte counts in response to therapy but also to more effective control of HIV-1 replication. For example, in the DACS 071 study, a retrospective analysis of the risk of developing specific opportunistic infections in patients who participated in four prospective randomized ACTG antiretroviral treatment trials, the risk of developing disseminated *M. avium* disease was reduced threefold at 24 months for those who experienced even a modest decline in the plasma HIV-1 RNA level of 0.5 $\log_{10}$ copies/mL 8 weeks following initiation of combination antiretroviral therapies that included nucleoside or non-nucleoside reverse transcriptase inhibitors (NNRTIs) (or both).[93] In an evaluation of the relationship between viral load and the occurrence of MAC disease (among other opportunistic infections), investigators from the Multicenter AIDS Cohort Study (MACS) showed that the relative hazard of developing *M. avium* disease for those with a baseline HIV-1 RNA level of 30 000–60 000 copies/mL was 1.29; it increased to 9.85 for those with a baseline HIV-1 RNA level of 60 000–90 000 copies/mL and to 14.97 for those with a baseline HIV-1 RNA of more than 90000 copies/mL.[94] HIV-1 RNA level and CD4+ T-lymphocyte count were independent predictors of risk. In the ACTG 320 trial, significant predictors of a shorter time to development of MAC disease for those treated with combination antiretroviral therapy were a 1 $\log_{10}$ copies/mL increment in baseline HIV-1 RNA with at least a 0.5 $\log_{10}$ copies/mL decrease in HIV-1 RNA at week 8 of therapy, as well as a less than 10 cell increase in CD4+ T-lymphocyte count in response to antiretroviral therapy by week 8.[60]

Aside from immunologic perturbation and the magnitude of HIV-1 replication, other physiologic factors that contribute to the risk of developing *M. avium* bacteremia and disease include colonization of the respiratory or gastrointestinal tract. Acid-fast bacilli (AFB) smears and cultures of stool or sputum may demonstrate the presence of *M. avium* prior to detection of mycobacteremia in up to 25–33% of HIV-infected individuals who subsequently develop disseminated *M. avium* disease.[95,96] Colonization of the gastrointestinal or respiratory tract, when detected, appears to have a positive predictive value approaching 60% in a profoundly immunocompromised patient population. In the ACTG 341 study of MAC pathogenesis, respiratory or gastrointestinal colonization was present in 36% of patients with disseminated infection, but in only 5% of noninfected controls with CD4 counts below 50 cells/μL.[89] However, the utility of screening cultures of these sites to detect colonization is limited because most patients are not colonized. Furthermore, when colonization can be demonstrated, it may be transient and not followed by the development of disseminated disease.[89,95,96]

Most prospective studies have not suggested differences in the incidence of *M. avium* disease according to gender, racial or ethnic group, age, or geographic distribution.[5,50,53,54,91,97] However, data collected among homosexual or bisexual men in the MACS indicated that those living in Baltimore (6.9%) or Los Angeles (5.6%) had a higher incidence of MAC disease than those in Chicago (2.6%) or Pittsburgh (0%).[91] In another study evaluating the geographic and seasonal variation in *M. avium* bacteremia among patients with AIDS receiving placebo in a randomized clinical trial of *M. avium* prophylaxis, those with the highest risk were patients in south central regions of the United States, whereas those with the lowest risk resided in northern states and Canada.[98] There also appeared to be a trend toward decreased numbers of cases in northern states during summer months compared to other seasons.

TRANSMISSION

The mode of transmission for *M. avium* infection is thought to be inhalation, aspiration, or ingestion via respiratory or gastrointestinal tract portals of entry. Support for this contention includes laboratory studies demonstrating that *M. avium* can be experimentally aerosolized from environmental sources, and that organisms recovered from environmental aerosols are genetically similar to clinical isolates.[99,100] Data that support the gastrointestinal route as the predominant portal of entry for HIV-infected patients include the not-infrequent finding of extensive infiltration of the gastrointestinal tract and intraabdominal organs in those with disseminated disease and the finding that disseminated disease rapidly follows intraoral or intrarectal challenge of the beige mouse or immunosuppressed murine or rat models with *M. avium*.[95,96,101–104] Household or close contact of those with *M. avium* disease are not at increased risk of developing disease, and isolates recovered from individuals, in general, do not appear to be genetically related, indicating that person-to-person transmission is unlikely.[35,49] However, at least one study has demonstrated multiple clusters of two or three patients infected with four genetically unique strains of *M. avium*; the investigators concluded that their data suggested a common environmental source rather than person-to-person spread.[37]

DIAGNOSIS

Disseminated *M. avium* disease is diagnosed when a compatible clinical syndrome is present coupled with the recovery of *M. avium* from cultures of blood, bone marrow, or other normally sterile tissue or body fluids. The disease may be asymptomatic or only mildly symptomatic early; in this setting low-level mycobacteremia may produce intermittently positive blood cultures, although a small proportion of patients may have extensive infiltration of bone marrow or other reticuloendothelial organs in the absence of mycobacteremia.[1,3,89,105,106]

ISOLATION OF *MYCOBACTERIUM*

Use of an Isolator (Wampole Laboratories, Cranbury, NJ, USA) or similar blood culture system and subsequent inoculation of blood into Bactec 12B liquid medium or direct inoculation of specimens into Bactec 13A bottles (Bactec; Becton-Dickinson, Sparks, MD, USA) followed by radiometric detection of growth are the most frequently employed methods for isolating *M. avium* from blood.[107] Inoculation onto solid media (e.g., Middlebrook 7H10/11 or Lowenstein–Jensen media) is most useful when quantification of mycobacteria is necessary, but adequate growth requires longer incubation. Species-specific DNA probes, high-performance liquid chromatography, or biochemical tests can be used to identify such organisms as *M. avium*, *M. intracellulare*, or other mycobacteria. Polymerase chain reaction assays for the detection of MAC species in clinical samples have not reached a level of sensitivity requisite for diagnostic clinical use.[107–109] Depending on the size of the inoculum, the average time required to cultivate and identify *M. avium* using liquid media, radiometric detection of growth, and DNA probe identification generally ranges from 7 to 14 days.[27,110,111]

Other ancillary studies that may be useful for diagnosing disseminated MAC disease for HIV-infected patients at risk include AFB smears or stool cultures, biopsies of clinically suspect tissues or organs, radiographic imaging of the abdomen or mediastinum to detect lymphadenopathy, or other studies aimed at recovery of organisms from focal infection sites. The yield of these procedures is generally dependent on the presence of symptoms, signs, or laboratory abnormalities related to the involved sites. The finding of MAC in sputum or stool in HIV-infected individuals may represent colonization rather than disease. Treatment should not be initiated based on these findings alone unless there is other evidence to indicate the presence of active disease.

SUSCEPTIBILITY TESTING

Testing *M. avium* for susceptibility to antimicrobial agents can be accomplished using conventional agar proportion, agar dilution, broth dilution, or radiometric broth macrodilution techniques. Each may produce differing results depending on the assay and laboratory conditions used. The most widely recommended method for use in clinical laboratories in the United States is radiometric broth macrodilution utilizing Bactec technology.[112] The technical performance of assays using this method has been described in detail elsewhere.[107,112,113]

The use of susceptibility test results to guide selection of initial regimens for treatment of *M. avium* disease is not uniformly adopted by all clinicians, but most would agree that such testing should be performed on clinically significant isolates recovered from tissue or blood from patients who have received or are receiving azalide or macrolide agents for therapy or chemoprophylaxis. However, the rate of background resistance may be high regardless of prior macrolide treatment. A recent study documented macrolide resistance in 17% of MAC isolates from patients with AIDS and limited or no prior macrolide exposure.[114]

In early published studies of treatment for pulmonary MAC disease in nonimmunocompromised patients, treatment with four to six drugs guided by susceptibility test results was reportedly associated with improved clinical outcome.[115] In clinical trials of patients with AIDS, a relationship between pretreatment susceptibility test results and the microbiologic and clinical responses has been demonstrated primarily for clarithromycin, azithromycin, and, less compellingly, rifabutin.[116–118] Relapses caused by clarithromycin- or azithromycin-resistant isolates have been reported when these agents are used as monotherapy during prophylaxis or treatment of *M. avium* disease, although relapse also occurs in those receiving multiple drug therapy, presumably as a result of poor adherence, poor absorption, the use of ineffective companion drugs, or drug–drug interactions. Thus far evidence indicates that *M. avium* resistance to clarithromycin is due to single-step mutations in the V domain of the 23S rRNA gene; these mutations confer cross-resistance to azithromycin and probably other macrolides.[119,120]

Clinical breakpoints for the interpretation of susceptibility test results have been proposed for clarithromycin, azithromycin, and rifabutin based on data from prospective clinical trials.[107,112] Minimum inhibitory concentrations (MICs) of 32 μg/mL or more for clarithromycin or 256 μg/mL or more for azithromycin are the suggested thresholds for determining resistance based on the Bactec method for radiometric susceptibility testing.[107,112] It has been further suggested by some that the criteria for resistance should be based on the peak concentration achieved in serum after administration of therapeutic doses of drugs; however, clarithromycin, azithromycin, and rifabutin readily penetrate cells and tissue, often to levels far exceeding the MIC of most susceptible *M. avium* organisms. *M. avium* survives and replicates within macrophages, where these levels may be highest. This point should be considered when establishing resistance breakpoints or determining the clinical significance of susceptibility test results or serum or plasma concentrations of antimycobacterial drugs.

TREATMENT OF *M. AVIUM* DISEASE

Initial Therapy

Available antimicrobial agents with demonstrated activity in human clinical trials, alone or in combination regimens, for the treatment of *M. avium* disease include clarithromycin, azithromycin, rifabutin, ethambutol, and possibly ciprofloxacin and amikacin.[1,4,116,121–132] These agents, their commonly recommended adult doses, and their most common side effects are summarized in Table 41-1.[3,4,121,133–138]

Initial treatment of *M. avium* disease consists of a combination of at least two antimycobacterial drugs to prevent or delay the emergence of resistance.[52,138] Clarithromycin or azithromycin is the preferred first agent, although data regarding the efficacy of azithromycin are more limited than for clarithromycin.[52,138] Ethambutol is the recommended second drug. A third or fourth drug selected from among rifabutin, ciprofloxacin, or parenteral amikacin may be added for those with more severe or extensive symptoms or disease.[3,4,121,127,133] Alleviation of fever and a decline in the quantity of mycobacteria in blood or tissue can be expected within 2–4 weeks after initiation of appropriate therapy; for those with widespread tissue involvement or high levels of mycobacteremia, a longer duration of treatment may be required before a clinical response is observed. Susceptibility testing is not generally recommended as a guide to initial therapy because of the lack of standardization of methods and limited correlation of results with clinical and microbiologic outcome.[112,116–118,121,138] Experts recommend testing the susceptibility of MAC isolates to clarithromycin or azithromycin for patients who fail to respond to the initial therapy, who relapse after an initial response, or who develop MAC disease while receiving a macrolide for prophylaxis, although most patients who fail clarithromycin or azithromycin prophylaxis have isolates susceptible to these drugs at the time MAC disease is detected.[139,140]

Maintenance Therapy (Secondary Prophylaxis)

Revised US Public Health Service/Infectious Disease Society of America (USPHS/IDSA) guidelines recommend that

Table 41-1 Antimycobacterial Drugs Suggested for Treatment of Disseminated Mycobacterium Avium Disease in Patients With AIDS

Drug	Adult Dose	Common Adverse Reactions	Common Drug Interactions
Initial Therapy Agents			
Clarithromycin	500 mg bid[a]	Nausea, vomiting, abdominal pain, diarrhea, dysgeusia, rash, elevated liver transaminases, hearing loss, mania(?)	Increased rifabutin levels; contraindicated with astemizole, terfenadine
Azithromycin	500–600 mg/day[a]	Diarrhea, nausea, vomiting, abdominal pain, rash, elevated liver transaminases	
Ethambutol	15 mg $kg^{-1}day^{-1}$	Nausea, vomiting, abdominal pain, diarrhea, hepatitis, optic neuritis, peripheral neuropathy (rare)	
Rifabutin	300–600 mg/day[b]	Nausea, vomiting, abdominal pain, diarrhea, rash, uveitis, brown-orange discoloration of body fluids, neutropenia, arthralgia, myositis, elevated liver transaminases	Increased clarithromycin; decreased PI levels (indinavir, saquinavir, nelfinavir, amprenavir); PIs increase rifabutin levels, dose
Secondary Agents			
Ciprofloxacin	500–750 mg bid	Nausea, vomiting, abdominal pain, diarrhea, rash, insomnia, tremors, mental status changes	Aluminum-containing antacids inhibit absorption
Amikacin	10–15 mg $kg^{-1}day^{-1}$	Ototoxicity (cochlear and vestibular), nephrotoxicity	

[a]Clarithromycin, 500 mg bid, is the dose approved by the US Food and Drug Administration (FDA) for prophylaxis and treatment of MAC disease. Azithromycin 1200 mg once per week is approved for prophylaxis of MAC disease.
[b]Rifabutin, 300 mg/day, is the dose approved by the FDA for prophylaxis of MAC disease; dose increases to 450–600 mg/day are suggested when used with efavirenz.

therapy for disseminated MAC disease in patients with AIDS be continued for life unless sustained immune recovery occurs with potent antiretroviral therapy.[52,138,141,142] The availability of potent combination antiretroviral therapy has altered the outcome of MAC disease in many individuals such that the disease can be effectively 'cured' in select patients.[143,144] Studies presented to date are summarized in Table 41-2. A nonrandomized prospective study conducted by the ACTG evaluated whether antimycobacterial therapy for disseminated MAC could be withdrawn from subjects who experienced immunologic recovery while receiving potent combination antiretroviral therapy (ART).[145] Subjects in this trial had received macrolide-based treatment for their MAC disease for at least 12 months, were asymptomatic for MAC, had received ART for at least 16 weeks, and had CD4+ T-cell counts >100 cells/μL. Forty-eight subjects were enrolled and forty-seven subjects remained MAC free, whereas 1 subject developed localized MAC osteomyelitis. The incidence of MAC infection was 1.44/100 person-years (95% confidence interval, 0.04–8.01) during the median 77 weeks of follow-up. The results of this study support the recommendation that MAC therapy can be safely withdrawn in patients who meet the entry criteria of this trial. Evaluation of small numbers of patients in several more largely observational studies also indicate that patients with established MAC disease who have completed a 12 month or longer course of MAC treatment, remain asymptomatic, and have a sustained increase in the CD4+ T-lymphocyte count to levels higher than 100 cells/μL for 6 months or longer on ART are at low risk for recurrence of MAC disease.[143,146,147] Hence the revised USPHS/IDSA guidelines now indicate that discontinuation of chronic maintenance therapy can be safely considered in patients who meet these criteria.[52,141–144,148] The guidelines also recommend reinitiation of secondary prophylaxis if the CD4+ T-lymphocyte count falls below 100 cells/μL.

REVIEW OF CLINICAL TRIALS

The early data from human clinical trials upon which the USPHS Task Force recommendations and USPHS/IDSA guidelines for treatment of disseminated *M. avium* disease are based are captured in a series of what are now largely historical studies. The majority of these were conducted prior to the availability of more potent antiretroviral drugs and combination treatment regimens. The key clinical trials that provide the evidence base for current treatment recommendations are briefly reviewed in the following text and in a summary algorithm presented as Figure 41-1.[116,122,124–128,130,149–152]

Perhaps the most important study to establish the utility of macrolide-based treatment for *M. avium* disease in individuals with AIDS is one conducted by the Canadian HIV Trials Network that compared a clarithromycin-containing regimen with a regimen containing conventional antimycobacterial drugs. In this study, 187 patients with AIDS and symptomatic *M. avium* bacteremia were randomized to receive a combination of rifampin, ethambutol, clofazimine, and ciprofloxacin or clarithromycin (1 g twice daily), ethambutol, and rifabutin (600 mg/day).[125] The clarithromycin regimen was associated with a higher proportion of patients who cleared their bacteremia (69% vs 30%; $P < 0.001$) and with improved survival (8.7 vs 5.2 months; $P < 0.001$).[125] In this study the rifabutin dose was reduced to 300 mg/day after approximately half of the patients assigned to the clarithromycin arm developed uveitis, which was attributed to a previously unrecognized drug interaction between clarithromycin and rifabutin.[153,154]

Table 41-2 Discontinuation of Secondary Prophylaxis for Disseminated MAC

Study	No.	CD4 Criteria	Viral[a] Load Criteria	Follow-Up (Months)	Relapses While CD4 >100/mm³
Aberg[143]	4	>100	<10 000	8–13	0
Shafran[148]	33	Variable	Variable	17 (median)	0[b]
Zeller[144]	26	Variable	Variable	7–58	2
Aberg[145]	48	>100	69% < 500	19	1[c]
Liao[147]	15	>100	Variable	12	0
Green [146]	15	>100	Variable	31	0

[a]Copies per milliliter.
[b]Patient relapsed after stopping HAART.
[c]MAC osteomyelitis.

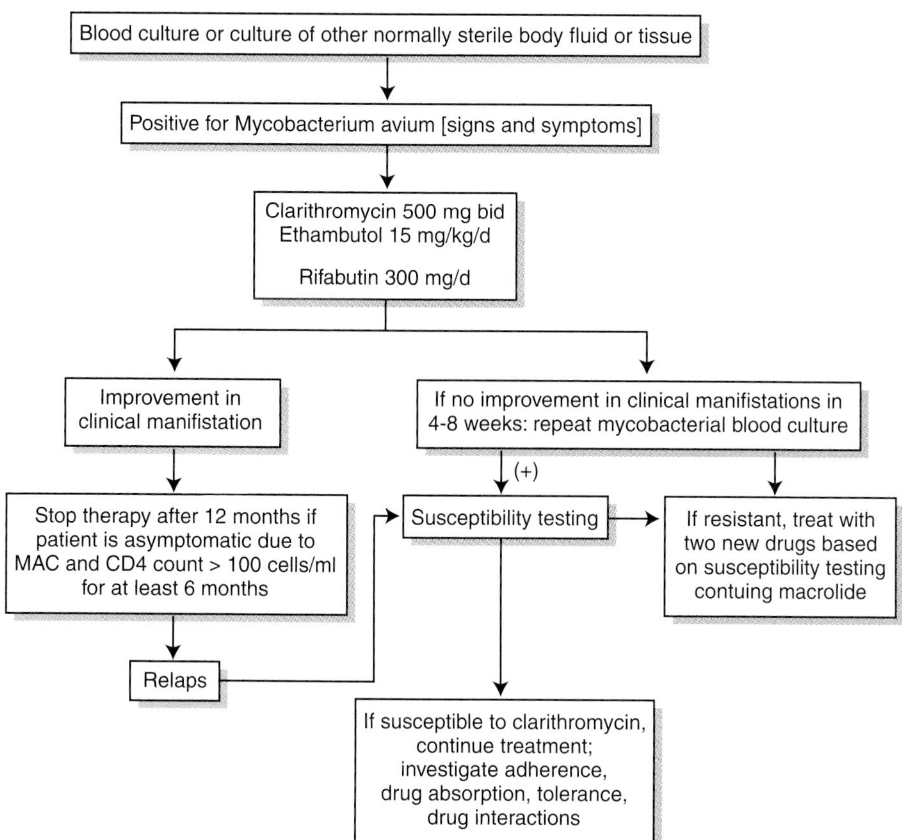

Figure 41-1 ■ Algorithm for treatment of disseminated *M. avium* complex disease in patients with AIDS.

A dose–response relationship with rifabutin was suggested by the finding that the 600 mg/day dose was associated with a higher proportion of patients who cleared their mycobacteremia but who developed uveitis than was the 300 mg/day dose.

A series of randomized clinical trials of similar design have compared combinations of two- or three-drug clarithromycin-containing regimens for treatment of MAC disease. In the first of these trials, Chaisson et al evaluated 89 patients with AIDS and *M. avium* bacteremia who were randomized to receive either clarithromycin and ethambutol or clarithromycin, ethambutol, and clofazimine.[130] Although the treatment groups were demographically and clinically comparable, there was a significant difference in baseline quantitative *M. avium* colony counts between the two arms (152 colony-forming units (CFU)/mL vs 1907 CFU/mL, respectively). The proportion of patients who cleared *M. avium* bacteremia reported improved symptoms, and relapse rates were similar.[130] However, patients randomized to the three-drug arm had a higher rate of treatment-limiting side-effects and a higher mortality rate. In a Cox proportional hazards analysis of factors associated with decreased survival, the baseline quantitative colony counts of *M. avium* in blood ($P = 0.043$) and treatment with clofazimine ($P = 0.045$) were independent predictors of decreased survival.

Dube and coinvestigators evaluated 95 patients with AIDS and MAC bacteremia who were randomized to receive either clarithromycin plus clofazimine or clarithromycin, clofazimine, and ethambutol.[128] The primary endpoint was the time to relapse. Although early clinical and microbiologic outcomes were the same for the two treatment arms, 68% of patients in the two-drug arm had relapsed by 36 weeks of therapy compared with only 12% of those on the three-drug regimen ($P = 0.004$).[128] All patients who relapsed had clarithromycin-resistant isolates recovered from blood. Ethambutol appeared to contribute to a reduced likelihood of relapse and emergence of clarithromycin-resistant *M. avium* in this study.

In a third study, 144 HIV-infected patients were randomized to receive clarithromycin, ethambutol, and rifabutin (450 mg/day) or clarithromycin plus clofazimine; 22 patients randomized to the two-drug arm relapsed compared with only 6 receiving three drugs ($P < 0.001$).[126] Of the 22 patients in the two-drug arm who relapsed, clarithromycin-resistant isolates were recovered from 21, whereas resistant isolates were found in only 2 of 6 in the three-drug arm.[126] Both groups had similar clinical responses with reduction in symptoms after 2 and 6 months of treatment, respectively.

Gordin and colleagues compared the combination of clarithromycin plus ethambutol with clarithromycin, ethambutol, and rifabutin (300 mg/day) in 198 patients with AIDS and MAC bacteremia.[127] At week 16 a total of 63% and 61% of patients in the three-drug and two-drug arms, respectively, had a bacteriologic response ($P = 0.81$), with no differences reported in clinical response or median duration of survival. Median survival duration was 439 and 398 days for the three- and two-drug arms, respectively. Moreover, no overall differences were noted with regard to the development of clarithromycin resistance; however, when only those with a bacteriologic response were included in the analysis, 2% of those receiving three drugs had a clarithromycin-resistant MAC isolate recovered during therapy compared with 14% of those receiving only clarithromycin plus ethambutol ($P = 0.055$).[127]

A fifth study evaluated 203 patients randomized to receive clarithromycin plus either ethambutol, rifabutin, or both drugs.[155] The primary endpoint was a complete microbiologic response, defined as two consecutive negative MAC blood cultures at least 1 week apart by week 12 of treatment. The proportion of patients with a complete microbiologic response at week 12 did not differ significantly among the three treatment arms. The proportion of patients with a complete microbiologic response at any time during follow-up were 55%, 46%, and 70%, respectively. The proportion who experienced a relapse on clarithromycin plus rifabutin (24%) was significantly higher than that for the three-drug regimen (6%) ($P = 0.027$) and marginally significantly higher than for clarithromycin plus ethambutol (7%) ($P = 0.057$). The rate of emergence of clarithromycin resistance was greater for clarithromycin plus rifabutin than for the other two arms. There was an overall significant difference in time to death ($P = 0.020$, log-rank test), with improved survival observed in those randomized to the three-drug arm compared to either of the two-drug arms.[155]

Finally, in a factorial study design attempting to address the potency of higher doses of clarithromycin for treatment of *M. avium* disease, Cohn et al randomized patients with AIDS and *M. avium* bacteremia to receive one of two doses of clarithromycin, 500 or 1000 mg twice daily, combined with ethambutol, and they secondarily randomized patients to receive either rifabutin or clofazimine.[129] The study was terminated early because of excess mortality observed in the higher-dose clarithromycin arm coupled with the data reported from other clinical trials indicating the lack of benefit of clofazimine and its association with increased mortality. As with the previous studies demonstrating the association of higher doses of clarithromycin with increased early mortality in patients being treated for *M. avium* disease, the cause was not apparent and the association appeared to be unrelated to adverse events, baseline clinical characteristics, or laboratory abnormalities reported in the study.[116,129]

Although comparative data are limited, in general, clarithromycin and azithromycin may be used interchangeably.[156,157] However, many experts favor the use of clarithromycin due to faster clearing of mycobacteremia and the overall greater clinical trials database demonstrating its efficacy. In the largest published comparative study to date, 246 patients with disseminated MAC disease were randomized to receive azithromycin 250 mg once daily, azithromycin 600 mg once daily, or clarithromycin 500 mg twice daily, each in combination with ethambutol.[157] The azithromycin 250 mg arm was halted after an interim analysis showed a lower rate of clearance of MAC bacteremia. At 24 weeks of therapy, the proportion of patients who experienced two consecutive negative MAC blood cultures was similar for both the azithromycin 600 mg qd (n = 68) and clarithromycin (n = 57) arms (46% and 56%, respectively; P = 0.24). The likelihood of relapse, the recovery of resistant isolates following relapse, and mortality were also similar for both treatment arms.[157]

For patients who fail to respond to initial treatment or who relapse after an initial response, many experts recommend testing *M. avium* isolates for susceptibility to clarithromycin or azithromycin, and possibly ethambutol and rifabutin, and then using these data to compose a new multidrug regimen consisting of at least two new drugs not previously used and to which the isolate is susceptible. It is unclear whether continuing clarithromycin or azithromycin in the face of resistance provides additional benefit. Preliminary results were reported from one small study in which eight patients who relapsed with a clarithromycin-resistant MAC isolate while receiving a combination of clarithromycin and clofazimine were treated with 'salvage' regimens that consisted of continuing a macrolide coupled with ethambutol and one or more additional drugs; five of eight patients had a 1 $\log_{10}$ copies/mL or more decline in mycobacterial colony counts per milliliter of blood, and two of the eight became culture-negative.[158] Because the number of drugs with activity against *M. avium* in this setting is limited, second-line regimens, if constructed in this manner, will likely require two or more of the following: ethambutol, rifabutin, ciprofloxacin, or amikacin with or without continuing a macrolide. Liposomal amikacin could also be considered.[159] Based on its lack of efficacy in randomized trials and its association with increased mortality, clofazimine should generally not be used. Other second-line agents, such as ethionamide or thiacetazone, have been anecdotally combined with these drugs, but their role in this setting is unknown.

Animal studies suggest that mefloquine and moxifloxacin have potential for the treatment of macrolide resistant MAC.[160] Mefloquine (MFQ), moxifloxacin (MXF), and ethambutol (EMB), in combination, were evaluated against both clarithromycin-resistant (CLR-R) and CLR-susceptible (CLR-S) MAC in a mouse model. After 4 weeks of treatment in mice MFQ was bactericidal, whereas MXF and EMB were bacteriostatic against both CLR-R and CLR-S MAC strains.[160] Both the combination of MFQ and EMB and the combination of MFQ and MXF significantly reduced the load of CLR-R MAC in both the liver and the spleen in the mice. Treatment with the three-drug combination resulted in an ~1 $\log_{10}$ CFU/mL reduction in CLR-R MAC in liver and spleen after 1 week, a 2.1 $\log_{10}$ reduction in CLR-R MAC after 4 weeks, and a 2.17 $\log_{10}$ CFU/mL reduction in MAC in blood. Of note, treatment of a clarithromycin-sensitive strain of MAC (MAC 101) had similar results. Telithromycin, a synthetic erythromycin derivative, has also been shown to be active against MAC in animal studies,[161,162] however drug interactions with HIV protease inhibitors may preclude the use of this drug in patients who are taking antiretroviral therapy. None of these approaches has been evaluated in controlled clinical trials in this patient population.

ADJUNCTIVE IMMUNOMODULATOR THERAPY FOR DISSEMINATED MAC DISEASE IN PATIENTS WITH AIDS

Adjunctive treatment of *M. avium* complex disease with immunomodulators remains controversial. IFNγ, TNFα, granulocyte/macrophage colony-stimulating factor (GM-CSF), and IL-12, alone or in combination with other cytokines, appear to inhibit intracellular replication or enhance *in vitro* intracellular killing of *M. avium*.[3,64–88] The use of these agents or immunomodulators that influence their production may be an attractive adjuvant treatment for those who fail more conventional antimycobacterial therapy. Some pilot human clinical trials suggest that this approach may have merit.

In a small clinical trial, HIV-infected patients with *M. avium* bacteremia were randomized to receive azithromycin alone or azithromycin plus GM-CSF for 4 weeks; preliminary results indicated that GM-CSF use was associated with enhanced monocyte activation and intracellular *M. avium* killing.[163] Holland and colleagues described their experience using IFNγ as an adjunct with antimycobacterial drugs in seven HIV-seronegative patients with disseminated *M. avium* or other nontuberculous mycobacterial infections refractory to standard therapy; the result was a reduction in clinical symptoms and quantitative mycobacteremia within 8 weeks.[82] In an anecdotal report, Wormser et al reported that five patients with AIDS and disseminated *M. avium* disease, unresponsive to conventional antimycobacterial therapy, had weight gain, reduced fever, and improvement of a number of laboratory abnormalities after the addition of dexamethasone (2 mg/day) to their antimycobacterial treatment.[164] Finally, data from a retrospective analysis comparing patients with disseminated *M. avium* disease who received standard antimycobacterial therapy plus prednisone 0.5 $mg^{-1}kg^{-1}day^{-1}$ with patients who received only antimycobacterial therapy demonstrated lower mortality, higher CD4+ T-lymphocyte counts, and greater weight gain over a 1-year observation period in those receiving adjunctive prednisone therapy.[165] The interpretation of these data may be limited, however, because other underlying disease factors and the type of and response to antiretroviral therapy were not controlled; moreover patients were not treated with standard antiretroviral or antimycobacterial therapies according to a protocol. Although these findings may be promising, the substantial improvement in immunologic function resulting from treatment with potent combination antiretroviral therapy appears to have reduced the overall incidence of 'refractory' *M. avium* disease, making this investigational approach unnecessary for most patients.

PRIMARY PROPHYLAXIS FOR DISSEMINATED MAC DISEASE IN PATIENTS WITH AIDS

The USPHS/IDSA guidelines for prevention of opportunistic infections recommend chemoprophylaxis for disseminated

MAC disease for all HIV-infected adults and adolescents who have a CD4+ T-lymphocyte count of less than 50 cells/μL (and for infants and children with similar age-adjusted CD4+ T-lymphocyte counts).[52,141] The first-line agents recommended for prophylaxis include clarithromycin 500 mg twice daily or azithromycin 1200 mg once a week. These agents also reduce the risk of respiratory bacterial infections and possibly *Pneumocystis jiroveci* pneumonia.[52,140,141,166,167] Rifabutin 300 mg/day is recommended as a second-line alternative. Although the combination of azithromycin and rifabutin was found to be more effective than either single drug in one clinical trial, the higher rate of adverse effects and cost preclude its general use.[52,140,141] Because the combination of clarithromycin/rifabutin was shown to be no more effective than clarithromycin alone, it too is not recommended for MAC chemoprophylaxis.[52,139] The clinical trials that formed the basis for these recommendations are briefly summarized in the following paragraphs. An algorithm outlining current prophylaxis guidelines is represented by Figure 41-2.

In the first of these studies, HIV-infected individuals with CD4+ T-lymphocyte counts of less than 100 cells/μL were randomized to receive clarithromycin 500 mg twice daily or placebo for prevention of *M. avium* disease; the incidence of *M. avium* bacteremia (5.6% for those randomized to clarithromycin) was reduced by 69% compared to that seen with placebo (15.5%).[166] The reduction in incidence was accompanied by an increase in the duration of survival (>700 days) for patients receiving clarithromycin versus those receiving placebo (573 days; $P < 0.01$). Of 19 isolates recovered from patients who developed *M. avium* bacteremia while on clarithromycin prophylaxis, 11 were resistant to clarithromycin; isolates from these patients had minimum inhibitory concentrations (MICs) of 512 μg/mL or more.[166] Despite the seemingly high rate of clarithromycin resistance among breakthrough isolates in this study, only 2% overall of the patients receiving clarithromycin prophylaxis developed *M. avium* disease caused by a clarithromycin-resistant organism.

In a smaller but similarly designed clinical trial, 181 HIV-infected individuals were randomized to receive either azithromycin 1200 mg once a week or placebo.[168] Of the 85 patients who received azithromycin 7 (8.2%) developed MAC disease compared to 20 (23.3%) of the 86 who received placebo ($P = 0.002$). Gastrointestinal adverse events predominated and were treatment-limiting in 8% of those randomized to azithromycin compared with 2% of those randomized to placebo ($P = 0.09$). Survival and emergence of azithromycin resistance did not differ between the two arms, although the study was not powered to detect a survival difference.

Data from these and two other studies established the superiority of clarithromycin, azithromycin, and rifabutin over placebo for prevention of MAC disease in HIV-infected patients with advanced immunosuppression.[97,166,168,169] Two additional clinical trials compared azithromycin or clarithromycin with rifabutin or combinations of azithromycin/rifabutin or clarithromycin/rifabutin.[139,140] The first evaluated azithromycin 1200 mg once a week, rifabutin 300 mg/day, or their combination in 669 HIV-infected individuals with CD4+ T-lymphocyte counts of less than 100 cells/μL at entry.[140] Of the 199 patients who received azithromycin plus rifabutin, 5 (2.5%) developed *M. avium* disease compared with 18 of 204 (8.8%) randomized to azithromycin and 25 of 207 (12.1%) randomized to rifabutin.[108] The combination

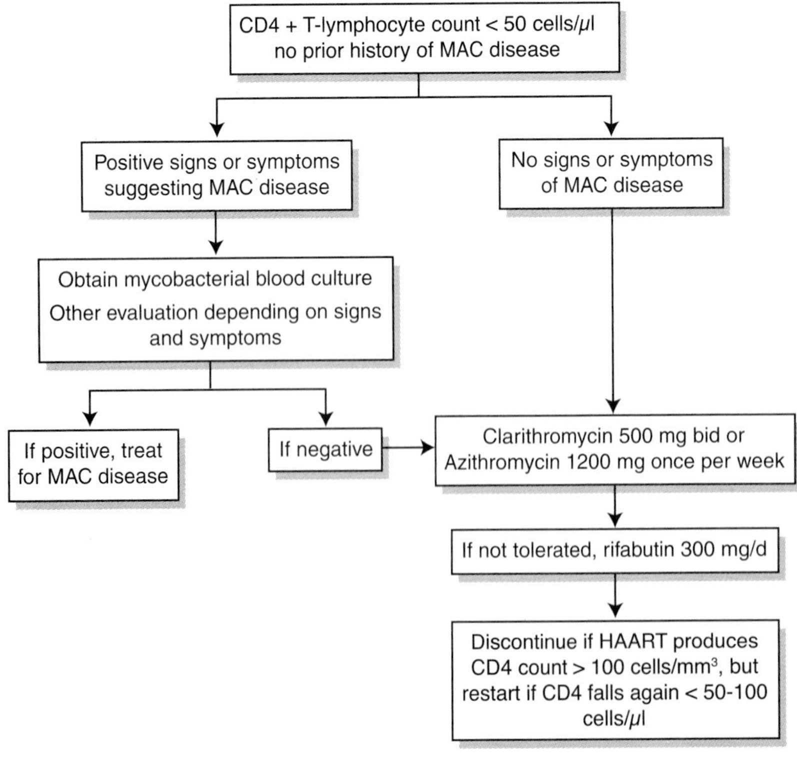

Figure 41-2 ■ Algorithm for primary chemoprophylaxis of *M. avium* complex disease in patients with AIDS.

of azithromycin and rifabutin was more effective than either single agent for reducing the occurrence of *M. avium* disease ($P < 0.001$ and 0.01, respectively, for the rifabutin and azithromycin comparisons); and azithromycin was more effective than rifabutin ($P = 0.006$). No survival differences were observed among the three treatment arms. Treatment-limiting adverse effects were more common among those receiving the two-drug combination than among those randomized to either single agent. Azithromycin- or clarithromycin-resistant *M. avium* isolates were recovered from 2 of 18 patients (11%) randomized to azithromycin and none of those randomized to the other two arms. There were no differences among the treatment arms with regard to recovery of rifabutin-resistant isolates. Rates of *P. jiroveci* pneumonia and respiratory bacterial infections were reduced for patients who received an azithromycin-containing regimen compared with those who received rifabutin alone.

In the second study, clarithromycin 500 mg twice daily was compared with rifabutin 300 mg/day and their combination in 1178 HIV-infected persons with CD4+ T-lymphocyte counts of 100 cells/μL or less at entry.[139] Of the 398 patients randomized to receive clarithromycin, 36 (9%) developed *M. avium* disease versus 59 of 391 (15%) randomized to rifabutin and 26 of 389 (7%) receiving the combination.[139] Clarithromycin and the combination were more effective than rifabutin alone ($P < 0.001$) in reducing the occurrence of *M. avium* disease, but the two clarithromycin-containing arms were equally effective. As with the previously described study, the combination of clarithromycin and rifabutin was associated with a higher rate of treatment-limiting adverse effects; gastrointestinal side-effects and uveitis predominated. No differences in survival among the three treatment arms were observed. Of the *M. avium* isolates recovered from patients who failed prophylaxis, 29% of isolates from patients randomized to clarithromycin and 25% from those randomized to the combination were resistant to clarithromycin and azithromycin; there were no differences among the treatment arms with regard to recovery of isolates resistant to rifabutin. Overall, ~2% of patients randomized to a clarithromycin-containing regimen broke through with a clarithromycin-resistant isolate.

The results of placebo-controlled trials have clearly shown that chemoprophylaxis is associated with improved survival compared to observation and serial monitoring of blood cultures. However, the availability of more potent combination antiretroviral therapies that suppress HIV replication, improve immune function, and increase CD4+ T-lymphocyte counts to levels above thresholds associated with increased risk has resulted in a marked decline in the incidence of *M. avium* disease, has altered the clinical manifestations of disease, and has improved the response to antimycobacterial therapy and mortality associated with *M. avium* disease.[55,56,58–60] Two representative randomized clinical trials have demonstrated the safety of discontinuing MAC prophylaxis for patients who have had a sustained increase in their CD4+ T-lymphocyte counts from a nadir of less than 50 cells/μL to more than 100 cells/μL while receiving potent combination antiretroviral therapies.[61,62] Currier et al studied 643 HIV-1-infected patients who met this entry criterion and who were randomized to receive azithromycin 1200 mg once weekly or placebo.[62] During a median of 16 months of follow-up, only two cases of MAC disease occurred in the placebo group and none in the azithromycin group. The calculated incidence rate in the placebo group was only 0.5 event per 100 person-years (95% confidence interval (CI), 0.06–1.83 per 100 person-years). There was no statistically significant difference in incidence for placebo versus azithromycin. In a similarly designed study conducted by El Sadr and colleagues, no cases of MAC disease occurred among 512 patients followed for a median of 12 months.[61] Based on these data, USPHS/IDSA guidelines recommend that primary prophylaxis be discontinued for patients who have responded to potent combination antiretroviral therapy with an increase in CD4+ T-lymphocyte count to levels higher than 100 cells/μL for at least 3 months.[141] For those who experience a subsequent decline in CD4+ T-lymphocyte count to less than 100 cells/μL, MAC prophylaxis should be restarted.[141] Brooks and colleagues describe the implementation of the current guidelines among a diverse cohort of patients receiving care in the United States.[170] In this study the proportion of eligible persons who discontinued primary prophylaxis against *M. avium* complex infection increased from 16.7% (in 1996) to 84.9% (in 2002). The discontinuation of primary prophylaxis was not associated with an increased risk of disseminated MAC infection.

Noting a decline in the rates of MAC just prior to the widespread availability of potent combination antiretroviral therapy in countries where MAC prophylaxis was not widely introduced, some authors question the need to immediately institute prophylaxis in newly diagnosed HIV-infected patients with CD4+ counts <50 cells/μL who are concurrently instituting potent combination antiretroviral therapy.[171] There are no currently available data to address this important question. Additionally it is unknown whether concurrent use of MAC prophylaxis has any impact on the incidence of immune reconstitution inflammatory syndromes in this setting.

DRUG INTERACTIONS AMONG AGENTS USED FOR TREATMENT OR PROPHYLAXIS OF MAC DISEASE

For those who require prophylaxis or treatment for MAC disease, the potential for significant drug interactions with agents used for prophylaxis or treatment remains problematic. The most clinically important are those occurring with drugs metabolized by the cytochrome P450 (CYP) enzyme system in the liver or intestinal tract. Clarithromycin, a potent inhibitor of the 3A4 isoenzyme of the CYP system, is associated with a bidirectional interaction with rifabutin, a moderately potent inducer of CYP 3A4. Competitive inhibition of CYP 3A4 by clarithromycin is associated with a 77% increase in rifabutin and 25-desacetyl rifabutin plasma concentrations when the two drugs are co-administered.[156,172,173] Increased rifabutin levels have been associated with the development of uveitis and other adverse effects of rifabutin.[153,174] Co-administration of rifabutin and clarithromycin also results in a 50% reduction in the clarithromycin area under the concentration curve (AUC), although there is wide individual variation.[156,172] Reduced serum or plasma concentrations may have little if any clinical impact for these drugs, which are highly concentrated in macrophages where they exert activity against replicating intracellular mycobacteria; treatment trials utilizing these agents in combination suggest that the clinical impact is small.[139,155] A similar magnitude of increase in rifabutin levels when co-administered with fluconazole appeared to enhance the efficacy of rifabutin in preventing *M. avium* disease in one study.[172,175] A comparable interaction between azithromycin and rifabutin has not been described.

Drug interactions between the protease inhibitor and NNRTI antiretroviral drugs and rifabutin or clarithromycin make management of antimycobacterial therapy and prophylaxis for MAC disease complex for those who require co-administration of these agents. Ritonavir is both a potent inhibitor and an inducer of CYP 3A4.[176] Indinavir, nelfinavir, and amprenavir (as well as the prodrug fosamprenavir) are reversible and less potent inhibitors of CYP 3A4 than ritonavir but probably produce comparable levels of inhibition.[176] Saquinavir appears to be the least potent inhibitor. Ritonavir inhibits the metabolism of clarithromycin to its 14-hydroxy metabolite; the result is an increase in the clarithromycin AUC of ~77%, a decrease in the 14-hydroxy metabolite of ~99%, and an overall increase of 35–40% in clarithromycin exposure.[177,178] Clarithromycin increases the ritonavir AUC by only ~12%. The interaction between indinavir and clarithromycin appears to be similar, producing a comparable increase in clarithromycin exposure. No dose adjustment for clarithromycin or, conversely, for ritonavir or indinavir when either is co-administered with clarithromycin, is currently recommended for patients with normal renal function. Lower doses of ritonavir used for boosting other protease inhibitor drugs are likely to have similar effect. Co-administration of atazanavir (400 mg once daily) and clarithromycin (500 mg once daily) resulted in no change in atazanavir C_{max}, a 1.28-fold increase in atazanavir AUC and a 1.91-fold increase in C_{min} ($n = 29$). C_{max}, AUC and C_{min} of clarithromycin were increased by 1.5-, 1.94-, and 2.64-fold, respectively ($n = 21$); AUC of the active metabolite (14-OH clarithromycin) decreased by 70%.[179] Increased concentrations of clarithromycin may cause QTc prolongations; therefore, the manufacturer of atazanavir recommends that a dose reduction of clarithromycin by 50% should be considered when rifabutin and clarithromycin are co-administered with atazanavir.[179] However the efficacy of this combination for the treatment of MAC has not been evaluated. Co-administration of atazanavir/ritonavir with clarithromycin has not been studied. Clarithromycin increases the C_{min} of tipranavir by more than 100%. This large increase in C_{min} is thought to be clinically relevant.[180] Patients using clarithromycin at doses higher than 500 mg twice daily with tipranavir should be carefully monitored for signs of toxicity and clarithromycin dose reduction should be instituted for patients with renal impairment.

Data fully evaluating interactions between nelfinavir, saquinavir, amprenavir, or other protease inhibitors and clarithromycin are not available. Efavirenz may induce the metabolism of clarithromycin in a manner similar to that of the protease inhibitors (i.e., resulting in a decrease in serum concentration of the parent drug but an increase in the serum concentration of the 14-hydroxy active metabolite).[141,181] Although no studies have evaluated the clinical significance of this interaction, careful monitoring is advised when these agents are used together.

The resultant interaction when ritonavir and rifabutin are co-administered is substantial. Ritonavir 500 mg every 12 h given with rifabutin 150 mg daily produces a fourfold increase in the AUC of rifabutin, a 35-fold increase in the AUC of the major metabolite, and an overall sevenfold increase in rifabutin exposure; rifabutin in this dose does not alter the AUC of ritonavir.[182,183] When used in combination with ritonavir, the dose of rifabutin should be reduced to 150 mg every other day. The interaction between rifabutin and indinavir, amprenavir, or nelfinavir is less great. Conventional doses of indinavir given concomitantly with rifabutin 300 mg/day result in an increase in the rifabutin AUC by ~204% and a decrease in the indinavir AUC by ~32%.[184] A similar magnitude of interaction has been demonstrated between nelfinavir or amprenavir and rifabutin; a dose reduction of rifabutin to 150 mg/day is recommended for patients co-administered either indinavir or nelfinavir with rifabutin.[185,186] When saquinavir (hard gel capsule formulation) in doses of 600 mg three times daily is combined with rifabutin 300 mg/day, the AUC of saquinavir is reduced by ~40%; coupled with the poor oral bioavailability of this formulation of saquinavir, the data indicate that these drugs should not be used together.[187,188] The magnitude of the interaction between rifabutin and the soft gel capsule formulation of saquinavir is unclear; these two drugs also should probably not be combined. There are sparse data characterizing the interactions of clarithromycin or rifabutin with lopinavir/ritonavir or other ritonavir-enhanced protease inhibitor combinations. Thus rifabutin in particular should be used with caution when given to patients treated with ritonavir-enhanced protease inhibitor regimens. The doses should be adjusted to at least the same levels as recommended when the protease inhibitor is used alone, and patients should be carefully monitored for rifabutin-associated toxicity.[141]

The NNRTIs are also metabolized by the CYP 3A4 isoenzyme, although as a class the drug interactions associated with them are not the same for all drugs in the class. Nevirapine and efavirenz induce CYP 3A4, whereas delavirdine inhibits this isoenzyme.[176,189,190] Pharmacokinetic interactions between all of these agents and clarithromycin have not been fully evaluated, although preliminary data for efavirenz indicate that it reduces the clarithromycin AUC by ~39% while the active metabolite was increased by 43%.[191] Rifabutin induces the metabolism of the NNRTIs. A fivefold increase in delavirdine clearance has been reported when delavirdine and rifabutin are co-administered, although interindividual variability is substantial; delavirdine inhibits rifabutin metabolism, resulting in an increased rifabutin AUC.[192] Efavirenz and rifabutin appear to induce each other's metabolism, although to what degree is unclear; data from interaction studies with rifampin suggest that rifampin reduces the efavirenz AUC by ~34%, although again there appears to be substantial interindividual variability.[189,190] A rifabutin dose adjustment to 450–600 mg/day has been suggested when it is used with efavirenz.[141,181] No dose adjustment is recommended when rifabutin and nevirapine are used in combination. When the NNRTIs are used in combination with protease inhibitors, it is unknown which level of interaction is likely to predominate among the multiple drugs. Careful monitoring of adverse effects and antiviral activity is necessary; and in many instances avoidance of rifabutin use is advisable where feasible.

MYCOBACTERIUM KANSASII INFECTION

The most common clinical manifestations of disease caused by *M. kansasii* among individuals with HIV infection include fever, pulmonary symptoms, and pulmonary infiltrates.[193–201] In a series of reported cases of *M. kansasii* disease in HIV-infected patients, the proportion of those with cavitary lung disease ranges from 0% to 53%; most of those without cavitary disease had interstitial or alveolar infiltrates on chest radiographs.[193–201] Although pulmonary disease predominates, extrapulmonary or disseminated disease occurs in a substantial proportion as well, ranging from 10% to 39%.[193–201] Although early reports suggested that the gastrointestinal tract was a common area of extrapulmonary involvement, more recent observations fail to confirm this as a frequent finding, with isolation from blood or bone marrow being the

Table 41-3

Other Atypical Mycobacterial Infections in HIV-Infected Individuals: Associated Clinical Syndromes and Suggested Treatment Regimens[210,211]

Mycobacterium Species	Clinical Syndrome	Suggested Treatment Regimen(s)
M. genovense	Disseminated multiorgan infection similar to *M. avium* (molecular techniques are required for species identification)	Clarithromycin, ethambutol, and rifamycins (amikacin and ciprofloxacin have been included in some reports with variable response)
M. scrofulaceum	Cervical lymphadenitis; disseminated disease (rare)	Surgical excision may be the treatment of choice; clarithromycin, azithromycin, rifabutin, with or without streptomycin, cycloserine, and sulfonamides appear to have activity
M. xenopi	Pulmonary nodules or diffuse reticulonodular infiltrates	Clarithromycin, ethambutol, rifabutin, streptomycin, or amikacin
M. haemophilum	Cutaneous lesions; disseminated disease (the organism grows optimally at 32°C and requires iron-containing media for optimal growth)	Isoniazid, rifampin, and ethambutol are most commonly recommended; clarithromycin, minocycline, doxycycline, ciprofloxacin, and amikacin have *in vitro* activity
M. bovis	Disseminated multiorgan disease (may be seen following bacille Calmette Gurin vaccination); cavitary pulmonary disease mimicking pulmonary tuberculosis	Isoniazid, rifampin, ethambutol, streptomycin
M. chelonei	Skin, soft tissue, bone, and joint infections with the potential for sinus tract formation	Amikacin, doxycycline, erythromycin, imipenem, tobramycin all have variable *in vitro* activity; combinations of these may be effective *in vivo*
M. fortuitum	Cutaneous lesions; soft tissue; bone; disseminated multiorgan disease; isolated central nervous system (CNS) disease	Clarithromycin, amikacin, cefoxitin, sulfonamides, doxycycline, fluoroquinolones
M. marinum	Cutaneous lesions; soft tissue; bone; usually associated with water exposure	Rifampin, ethambutol, minocycline; or clarithromycin
M. malmoense	Cavitary pulmonary disease with fever, night sweats, weight loss; CNS ring-enhancing lesions with fever, headache, neurologic symptoms	Clarithromycin or azithromycin, rifabutin, ethambutol, and ciprofloxacin have been used; resistance to isoniazid, rifampin, ethambutol demonstrated *in vitro*
M. celatum	Disseminated multiorgan disease with cavitary pulmonary lesions (in one case)	Clarithromycin, amikacin, ciprofloxacin

more common manifestation of disseminated disease. For patients who are symptomatic, fever, cough with or without sputum production, dyspnea, abdominal pain, and weight loss are reportedly the most common clinical symptoms.[193–201]

Most patients with HIV infection who develop disease caused by *M. kansasii* have CD4+ T-lymphocyte counts of less than 100 cells/μL. As with other opportunistic infections during the era of potent combination antiretroviral therapy for HIV infection, the incidence of disease caused by *M. kansasii* has declined, although there were insufficient data available at any time during the epidemic to evaluate the overall incidence of this opportunistic infection. Several reports have suggested a higher prevalence of disease caused by *M. kansasii* among individuals living in the central Midwestern portions of the United States and among injection drug users; the largest numbers of cases among patients with HIV infection in the United States have been reported from Kansas City and Chicago.[193–201]

As with other mycobacterial infections in this patient population, the diagnosis depends on the presence of a compatible clinical syndrome coupled with isolation of *M. kansasii* from respiratory secretions, blood, or other body fluids or tissue. As with *M. avium*, inoculation of specimens into Bactec 12B liquid medium or direct inoculation of specimens into Bactec 13A bottles, followed by radiometric detection of growth, is the preferred method for isolating of *M. kansasii*. Middlebrook 7H10/11 or Lowenstein-Jensen solid media can also be used. Species-specific DNA probes, high-performance liquid chromatography, or biochemical tests can also be used to identify organisms such as *M. kansasii*.

The cornerstones of combination therapy for *M. kansasii* infection are rifampin and ethambutol. Most isolates are relatively resistant to isoniazid; the latter is usually included in suggested treatment regimens, however, although its contribution is unclear. The organism is variably susceptible to other second-line antimycobacterial drugs, including clarithromycin.[200,201] *In vitro* susceptibility testing is generally recommended as a guide to therapy, although randomized clinical trials establishing a predictive relationship between *in vitro* susceptibility test results and clinical and microbiologic responses have not been reported. The recommended duration of treatment is 12–18 months for immunocompetent individuals. There are no prospective data to determine the most appropriate duration of treatment for those co-infected with HIV. As with treatment for *M. avium*, many experts would treat for 12–18 months and then discontinue it for those who have responded to potent combination antiretroviral therapy.

OTHER ATYPICAL MYCOBACTERIAL INFECTIONS IN HIV-INFECTED PATIENTS

A number of other atypical mycobacteria infrequently cause disease in HIV-infected individuals.[202] The organisms, the most commonly recognized associated clinical syndromes, and suggested treatment regimens are summarized in Table 41-3.[203–211]

REFERENCES

1. Kemper CA, Havlir D, Bartok AE, et al. Transient bacteremia due to Mycobacterium avium complex in patients with AIDS. J Infect Dis 170:488, 1994.
2. Gordin FM, Cohn DL, Sullam PM, et al. Early manifestations of disseminated Mycobacterium avium complex disease: a prospective evaluation. J Infect Dis 176:126, 1997.
3. Inderlied CB, Kemper CA, Bermudez LE. The Mycobacterium avium complex. Clin Microbiol Rev 6:266, 1993.
4. Benson CA, Ellner JJ. Mycobacterium avium complex infection and AIDS: advances in theory and practice. Clin Infect Dis 17:7, 1993.
5. Havlik Jr. JA, Horsburgh CR Jr, Metchock B, et al. Disseminated Mycobacterium avium complex infection: clinical identification and epidemiologic trends. J Infect Dis 165:577, 1992.
6. Benson CA. Disease due to the Mycobacterium avium complex in patients with AIDS: epidemiology and clinical syndrome. Clin Infect Dis 18(Suppl 3):S218, 1994.
7. Torriani FJ, McCutchan JA, Bozzette SA, et al. Autopsy findings in AIDS patients with Mycobacterium avium complex bacteremia. J Infect Dis 170:1601, 1994.
8. Cabié A, Abel S, Brebion A, et al. Mycobacterial lymphadenitis after initiation of highly active antiretroviral therapy. Eur J Clin Microbiol Infect Dis 17:812, 1998.
9. Phillips P, Kwiatkowski MB, Copland M, et al. Mycobacterial lymphadenitis associated with the initiation of combination antiretroviral therapy. J Acquir Immune Defic Syndr Hum Retrovirol 20:122, 1999.
10. Race EM, Adelson-Mitty J, Kriegel GR, et al. Focal mycobacterial lymphadenitis following initiation of protease-inhibitor therapy in patients with advanced HIV-1 disease. Lancet 351:252, 1998.
11. Packer SJ, Cesario T, Williams JH Jr. Mycobacterium avium complex infection presenting as endobronchial lesions in immunosuppressed patients. Ann Intern Med 109:389, 1988.
12. Barbaro DJ, Orcutt VL, Coldiron BM. Mycobacterium avium-Mycobacterium intracellulare infection limited to the skin and lymph nodes in patients with AIDS. Rev Infect Dis 11:625, 1989.
13. Kerns E, Benson C, Spear J, et al. Pericardial disease in patients with HIV infection. In: Abstracts of the 31st Interscience Conference on Antimicrobial Agents and Chemotherapy (ICAAC), Chicago, IL. Washington, DC: American Society for Microbiology; 1991, p 191, abstract 551.
14. Hellyer TJ, Brown IN, Taylor MB, et al. Gastro-intestinal involvement in Mycobacterium avium-intracellulare infection of patients with HIV. J Infect Dis 26:55, 1993.
15. Owen RL, Roth RI, St Hilaire RJ, et al. Pseudo Whipple's disease intestinal infection with Mycobacterium avium intracellulare (M. avium) in acquired immune deficiency syndrome (AIDS). Gastroenterology 84:1267, 1983.
16. Jacob CN, Henein SS, Heurich AE, et al. Nontuberculous mycobacterial infection of the central nervous system in patients with AIDS. South Med J 86:638, 1993.
17. Lawn SD, Bicanic TA, Macallan DC. Pyomyositis and cutaneous abscesses due to Mycobacterium avium: an immune reconstitution manifestation in a patient with AIDS. Clin Infect Dis 38:461, 2004.
18. Powles T, Thirlwell C, Nelson M, et al. Immune reconstitution inflammatory syndrome mimicking relapse of AIDS related lymphoma in patients with HIV 1 infection. Leuk Lymphoma 44:1417, 2003.

19. Salama C, Policar M, Venkataraman M. Isolated pulmonary Mycobacterium avium complex infection in patients with human immunodeficiency virus infection: case reports and literature review. Clin Infect Dis 37:e35, 2003.
20. Shelburne III SA, Hamill RJ. The immune reconstitution inflammatory syndrome. AIDS Rev 5:67, 2003.
21. Shelburne SA, Visnegarwala F, Darcourt J, et al. Incidence and risk factors for immune reconstitution inflammatory syndrome during highly active antiretroviral therapy. AIDS 19:399, 2005.
22. Phillips P, Bonner S, Gataric N, et al. Nontuberculous mycobacterial immune reconstitution syndrome in HIV-infected patients: spectrum of disease and long-term follow-up. Clin Infect Dis 41:1483, 2005.
23. Gascon P, Sathe SS, Rameshwar P. Impaired erythropoiesis in the acquired immunodeficiency syndrome with disseminated Mycobacterium avium complex. Am J Med 94:41, 1993.
24. Marinelli DL, Albelda SM, Williams TM, et al. Nontuberculous mycobacterial infection in AIDS: clinical, pathologic, and radiographic features. Radiology 160:77, 1986.
25. Wolinsky E. Nontuberculous mycobacteria and associated diseases. Am Rev Respir Dis 119:107, 1979.
26. Havlir DV, Ellner JJ. Mycobacterium avium complex. In: Mandell G, Bennett JE, Dolin R (eds). Principles and Practice of Infectious Diseases. 4th edn. New York: Churchill Livingstone; 1994, p 2250.
27. Anargyros P, Astill DS, Lim IS. Comparison of improved BACTEC and Lowenstein–Jensen media for culture of mycobacteria from clinical specimens. J Clin Microbiol 28:1288, 1990.
28. Saito H, Tomioka H, Sato K, et al. Identification of various serovar strains of Mycobacterium avium complex by using DNA probes specific for Mycobacterium avium and Mycobacterium intracellulare. J Clin Microbiol 28:1694, 1990.
29. Horsburgh Jr. CR, Cohn DL, Roberts RB, et al. Mycobacterium avium-M. intracellulare isolates from patients with or without acquired immunodeficiency syndrome. Antimicrob Agents Chemother 30:955, 1986.
30. Tsang AY, Denner JC, Brennan PJ, et al. Clinical and epidemiological importance of typing of Mycobacterium avium complex isolates. J Clin Microbiol 30:479, 1992.
31. Yakrus MA, Good RC. Geographic distribution, frequency, and specimen source of Mycobacterium avium complex serotypes isolated from patients with acquired immunodeficiency syndrome. J Clin Microbiol 28:926, 1990.
32. Guthertz LS, Damsker B, Bottone EJ, et al. Mycobacterium avium and Mycobacterium intracellulare infections in patients with and without AIDS. J Infect Dis 160:1037, 1989.
33. Horsburgh Jr. CR, Selik RM. The epidemiology of disseminated nontuberculous mycobacterial infection in the acquired immunodeficiency syndrome (AIDS). Am Rev Respir Dis 139:4, 1989.
34. Reddy VM, Parikh K, Luna-Herrera J, et al. Comparison of virulence of Mycobacterium avium complex (MAC) strains isolated from AIDS and non-AIDS patients. Microb Pathog 16:121, 1994.
35. Arbeit RD, Slutsky A, Barber TW, et al. Genetic diversity among strains of Mycobacterium avium causing monoclonal and polyclonal bacteremia in patients with AIDS. J Infect Dis 167:1384, 1993.
36. Slutsky AM, Arbeit RD, Barber TW, et al. Polyclonal infections due to Mycobacterium avium complex in patients with AIDS detected by pulsed-field gel electrophoresis of sequential clinical isolates. J Clin Microbiol 32:1773, 1994.
37. Mazurek GH, Chin DP, Hartman S, et al. Genetic similarity among Mycobacterium avium isolates from blood, stool, and sputum of persons with AIDS. J Infect Dis 176:976, 1997.
38. Ohkusu K, Bermudez LE, Nash KA, et al. Differential virulence of Mycobacterium avium strains isolated from HIV-infected patients with disseminated M. avium complex disease. J Infect Dis 190:1347, 2004.
39. Iseman MD, Corpe RF, O'Brien RJ, et al. Disease due to Mycobacterium avium-intracellulare. Chest 87(Suppl 2):139S, 1985.
40. Eaton T, Falkinham III JO, von Reyn CF. Recovery of Mycobacterium avium from cigarettes. J Clin Microbiol 33:2757, 1995.
41. Edwards LB, Palmer CE. Epidemiologic studies of tuberculin sensitivity. I. Preliminary results with purified protein derivatives prepared from atypical acid-fast organisms. Am J Hyg 68:213, 1958.
42. Gilks CF, Brindle RJ, Mwachari C, et al. Disseminated Mycobacterium avium infection among HIV-infected patients in Kenya. J Acquir Immune Defic Syndr Hum Retrovirol 8:195, 1995.
43. Morrissey AB, Aisu TO, Falkinham JO III, et al. Absence of Mycobacterium avium complex disease in patients with AIDS in Uganda. J Acquir Immune Defic Syndr 5:477, 1992.
44. von Reyn CF, Barber TW, Arbeit RD, et al. Evidence of previous infection with Mycobacterium avium–Mycobacterium intracellulare complex among healthy subjects: an international study of dominant mycobacterial skin test reactions. J Infect Dis 168:1553, 1993.
45. Otsuka Y, Fujino T, Mori N, et al. Survey of human immunodeficiency virus (HIV)-seropositive patients with mycobacterial infection in Japan. J Infect 51:364, 2005.
46. von Reyn CF, Maslow JN, Barber TW, et al. Persistent colonisation of potable water as a source of Mycobacterium avium infection in AIDS. Lancet 343:1137, 1994.
47. Montecalvo MA, Forester G, Tsang AY, et al. Colonisation of potable water with Mycobacterium avium complex in homes of HIV-infected patients. Lancet 343:1639, 1994.
48. von Reyn CF, Arbeit RD, Tosteson AN, et al. The international epidemiology of disseminated Mycobacterium avium complex infection in AIDS. AIDS 10:1025, 1996.
49. Horsburgh CR Jr, Chin DP, Yajko DM, et al. Environmental risk factors for acquisition of Mycobacterium avium complex in persons with human immunodeficiency virus infection. J Infect Dis 170:362, 1994.
50. Ostroff SM, Spiegel RA, Feinberg J, et al. Preventing disseminated Mycobacterium avium complex disease in patients infected with human immunodeficiency virus. Clin Infect Dis 21 Suppl 1:S72, 1995.
51. USPHS/IDSA Prevention of Opportunistic Infections Working Group. 1997 USPHS/IDSA guidelines for the prevention of opportunistic infections in persons infected with human immunodeficiency virus. MMWR Recomm Rep 46(RR-12):1, 1997.
52. USPHS/IDSA Prevention of Opportunistic Infections Working Group. 1999 USPHS/IDSA guidelines for the prevention of opportunistic infections in persons infected with human immunodeficiency virus. MMWR Recomm Rep 48(RR-10):1, 1999.
53. Nightingale SD, Byrd LT, Southern PM, et al. Incidence of Mycobacterium avium-intracellulare complex bacteremia in human immunodeficiency virus-positive patients. J Infect Dis 165:1082, 1992.
54. Chaisson RE, Moore RD, Richman DD, et al. Incidence and natural history of Mycobacterium avium-complex infections in patients with advanced human immunodeficiency virus disease treated with zidovudine. Am Rev Respir Dis 146:285, 1992.
55. Murphy R, El-Sadr W, Cheung T, et al. Impact of protease inhibitor containing regimens on the risk of developing opportunistic infections and mortality in the CPCRA 034/ACTG 277 Study. In: Abstracts of the 5th Conference on Retroviruses

and Opportunistic Infections, Chicago, IL. Alexandria, VA: Foundation for Retrovirology and Human Health; 1998, p 113, abstract 181.
56. Palella FJ Jr, Delaney KM, Moorman AC, et al. Declining morbidity and mortality among patients with advanced human immunodeficiency virus infection. N Engl J Med 338:853, 1998.
57. Karakousis PC, Moore RD, Chaisson RE. Mycobacterium avium complex in patients with HIV infection in the era of highly active antiretroviral therapy. Lancet Infect Dis 4:557, 2004.
58. Ledergerber B, Egger M, Erard V, et al. AIDS-related opportunistic illnesses occurring after initiation of potent antiretroviral therapy: the Swiss HIV Cohort Study. JAMA 282:2220, 1999.
59. Mocroft A, Katlama C, Johnson AM, et al. AIDS across Europe, 1994–98: the EuroSIDA study. Lancet 356:291, 2000.
60. Currier JS, Williams PL, Grimes JM, et al. Incidence rates and risk factors for opportunistic infections in a phase III trial comparing indinavir + ZDV + 3TC to ZDV + 3TC. In: Abstracts of the 5th Conference on Retroviruses and Opportunistic Infections, Chicago, IL. Alexandria, VA: Foundation for Retrovirology and Human Health; 1998, p 127, abstract 257.
61. El-Sadr WM, Burman WJ, Grant LB, et al. Discontinuation of prophylaxis for Mycobacterium avium complex disease in HIV-infected patients who have a response to antiretroviral therapy. N Engl J Med 342:1085, 2000.
62. Currier JS, Williams PL, Koletar SL, et al. Discontinuation of Mycobacterium avium complex prophylaxis in patients with antiretroviral therapy-induced increases in CD4+ cell count: A randomized, double-blind, placebo-controlled trial. Ann Intern Med 133:493, 2000.
63. Benson CA. Mycobacterium avium-intracellulare complex disease. In: Schlossberg D (ed). Tuberculosis and Nontuberculosis Mycobacterial Infections. 4th edn. Philadelphia: WB Saunders; 1999, p 351.
64. Bermudez LE. Immunobiology of Mycobacterium avium infection. Eur J Clin Microbiol Infect Dis 13:1000, 1994.
65. Bermudez LE, Young LS. Natural killer cell-dependent mycobacteriostatic and mycobactericidal activity in human macrophages. J Immunol 146:265, 1991.
66. Barnes PF, Grisso CL, Abrams JS, et al. Gamma delta T lymphocytes in human tuberculosis. J Infect Dis 165:506, 1992.
67. Katz P, Yeager H, Jr., Whalen G, et al. Natural killer cell-mediated lysis of Mycobacterium-avium complex-infected monocytes. J Clin Immunol 10:71, 1990.
68. Blanchard DK, McMillen S, Hoffman SL, et al. Mycobacterial induction of activated killer cells: possible role of tyrosine kinase activity in interleukin-2 receptor alpha expression. Infect Immun 60:2843, 1992.
69. Blanchard DK, Michelini-Norris MB, Pearson CA, et al. Mycobacterium avium-intracellulare induces interleukin-6 from human monocytes and large granular lymphocytes. Blood 77:2218, 1991.
70. Toba H, Crawford JT, Ellner JJ. Pathogenicity of Mycobacterium avium for human monocytes: absence of macrophage-activating factor activity of gamma interferon. Infect Immun 57:239, 1989.
71. MacArthur RD, Lederman MM, Benson CA, et al. Effects of Mycobacterium avium complex-infection treatment on cytokine expression in human immunodeficiency virus-infected persons: results of AIDS clinical trials group protocol 853. J Infect Dis 181:1486, 2000.
72. Tsukaguchi K, Yoneda T, Okamura H, et al. Defective T cell function for inhibition of growth of Mycobacterium avium-intracellulare complex (MAC) in patients with MAC disease: restoration by cytokines. J Infect Dis 182:1664, 2000.
73. Havlir DV, Schrier RD, Torriani FJ, et al. Effect of potent antiretroviral therapy on immune responses to Mycobacterium avium in human immunodeficiency virus-infected subjects. J Infect Dis 182:1658, 2000.
74. Vankayalapati R, Wizel B, Samten B, et al. Cytokine profiles in immunocompetent persons infected with Mycobacterium avium complex. J Infect Dis 183:478, 2001.
75. Ehlers S, Benini J, Kutsch S, et al. Fatal granuloma necrosis without exacerbated mycobacterial growth in tumor necrosis factor receptor p55 gene-deficient mice intravenously infected with Mycobacterium avium. Infect Immun 67:3571, 1999.
76. Bermudez LE, Stevens P, Kolonoski P, et al. Treatment of experimental disseminated Mycobacterium avium complex infection in mice with recombinant IL-2 and tumor necrosis factor. J Immunol 143:2996, 1989.
77. Silva RA, Pais TF, Appelberg R. Evaluation of IL-12 in immunotherapy and vaccine design in experimental Mycobacterium avium infections. J Immunol 161:5578, 1998.
78. Doherty TM, Sher A. IL-12 promotes drug-induced clearance of Mycobacterium avium infection in mice. J Immunol 160:5428, 1998.
79. Frucht DM, Holland SM. Defective monocyte costimulation for IFN-gamma production in familial disseminated Mycobacterium avium complex infection: abnormal IL-12 regulation. J Immunol 157:411, 1996.
80. Altare F, Durandy A, Lammas D, et al. Impairment of mycobacterial immunity in human interleukin-12 receptor deficiency. Science 280:1432, 1998.
81. Newport MJ, Huxley CM, Huston S, et al. A mutation in the interferon-gamma-receptor gene and susceptibility to mycobacterial infection. N Engl J Med 335:1941, 1996.
82. Holland SM, Eisenstein EM, Kuhns DB, et al. Treatment of refractory disseminated nontuberculous mycobacterial infection with interferon gamma. A preliminary report. N Engl J Med 330:1348, 1994.
83. Bermudez LE, Wu M, Petrofsky M, et al. Interleukin-6 antagonizes tumor necrosis factor-mediated mycobacteriostatic and mycobactericidal activities in macrophages. Infect Immun 60:4245, 1992.
84. Balcewicz-Sablinska MK, Gan H, Remold HG. Interleukin 10 produced by macrophages inoculated with Mycobacterium avium attenuates mycobacteria-induced apoptosis by reduction of TNF-alpha activity. J Infect Dis 180:1230, 1999.
85. Gong JH, Zhang M, Modlin RL, et al. Interleukin-10 downregulates Mycobacterium tuberculosis-induced Th1 responses and CTLA-4 expression. Infect Immun 64:913, 1996.
86. Rojas RE, Balaji KN, Subramanian A, et al. Regulation of human CD4(+) alphabeta T-cell-receptor-positive (TCR(+)) and gammadelta TCR(+) T-cell responses to Mycobacterium tuberculosis by interleukin-10 and transforming growth factor beta. Infect Immun 67:6461, 1999.
87. Johnson JL, Shiratsuchi H, Toba H, et al. Preservation of monocyte effector functions against Mycobacterium avium–M. intracellulare in patients with AIDS. Infect Immun 59:3639, 1991.
88. Johnson JL, Shiratsuchi H, Toossi Z, et al. Altered IL-1 expression and compartmentalization in monocytes from patients with AIDS stimulated with Mycobacterium avium complex. J Clin Immunol 17:387, 1997.
89. MacGregor RR, Hafner R, Wu JW, et al. Clinical, microbiological, and immunological characteristics in HIV-infected subjects at risk for disseminated Mycobacterium avium complex disease: an AACTG study. AIDS Res Hum Retroviruses 21:689, 2005.
90. Bourgarit A, Carcelain G, Martinez V, et al. Explosion of tuberculin-specific CD4 Th1 responses induces immune restoration syndrome in tuberculosis and HIV co-infected patients. In: Abstracts of the 13th Conference on Retroviruses and Opportunistic Infections, Denver, CO, 2006, abstract 797.

91. Hoover DR, Graham NM, Bacellar H, et al. An epidemiologic analysis of Mycobacterium avium complex disease in homosexual men infected with human immunodeficiency virus type 1. Clin Infect Dis 20:1250, 1995.
92. Finkelstein DM, Williams PL, Molenberghs G, et al. Patterns of opportunistic infections in patients with HIV infection. J Acquir Immune Defic Syndr Hum Retrovirol 12:38, 1996.
93. Williams PL, Currier JS, Swindells S. Joint effects of HIV-1 RNA levels and CD4 lymphocyte cells on the risk of specific opportunistic infections. AIDS 13:1035, 1999.
94. Lyles RH, Chu C, Mellors JW, et al. Prognostic value of plasma HIV RNA in the natural history of Pneumocystis carinii pneumonia, cytomegalovirus and Mycobacterium avium complex. Multicenter AIDS Cohort Study. AIDS 13:341, 1999.
95. Havlik Jr. JA, Metchock B, Thompson III SE, et al. A prospective evaluation of Mycobacterium avium complex colonization of the respiratory and gastrointestinal tracts of persons with human immunodeficiency virus infection. J Infect Dis 168:1045, 1993.
96. Chin DP, Hopewell PC, Yajko DM, et al. Mycobacterium avium complex in the respiratory or gastrointestinal tract and the risk of M. avium complex bacteremia in patients with human immunodeficiency virus infection. J Infect Dis 169:289, 1994.
97. Nightingale SD, Cameron DW, Gordin FM, et al. Two controlled trials of rifabutin prophylaxis against Mycobacterium avium complex infection in AIDS. N Engl J Med 329:828, 1993.
98. Horsburgh Jr. CR, Schoenfelder JR, Gordin FM, et al. Geographic and seasonal variation in Mycobacterium avium bacteremia among North American patients with AIDS. Am J Med Sci 313:341, 1997.
99. Fry KL, Meissner PS, Falkinham JO 3rd. Epidemiology of infection by nontuberculous mycobacteria. VI. Identification and use of epidemiologic markers for studies of Mycobacterium avium, M. intracellulare, and M. scrofulaceum. Am Rev Respir Dis 134:39, 1986.
100. Parker BC, Ford MA, Gruft H, et al. Epidemiology of infection by nontuberculous mycobacteria. IV. Preferential aerosolization of Mycobacterium intracellulare from natural waters. Am Rev Respir Dis 128:652, 1983.
101. Gray JR, Rabeneck L. Atypical mycobacterial infection of the gastrointestinal tract in AIDS patients. Am J Gastroenterol 84:1521, 1989.
102. Bermudez LE, Petrofsky M, Kolonoski P, et al. An animal model of Mycobacterium avium complex disseminated infection after colonization of the intestinal tract. J Infect Dis 165:75, 1992.
103. Brown ST, Edwards FF, Bernard EM, et al. Progressive disseminated infection with Mycobacterium avium complex after intravenous and oral challenge in cyclosporine-treated rats. J Infect Dis 164:922, 1991.
104. Orme IM, Furney SK, Roberts AD. Dissemination of enteric Mycobacterium avium infections in mice rendered immunodeficient by thymectomy and CD4 depletion or by prior infection with murine AIDS retroviruses. Infect Immun 60:4747, 1992.
105. Torriani FJ, Behling CA, McCutchan JA, et al. Disseminated Mycobacterium avium complex: correlation between blood and tissue burden. J Infect Dis 173:942, 1996.
106. Hafner R, Inderlied CB, Peterson DM, et al. Correlation of quantitative bone marrow and blood cultures in AIDS patients with disseminated Mycobacterium avium complex infection. J Infect Dis 180:438, 1999.
107. Inderlied CB. Microbiology and minimum inhibitory concentration testing for Mycobacterium avium complex prophylaxis. Am J Med 102 (5 Suppl 3):2, 1997.
108. Thierry D, Vincent V, Clement F, et al. Isolation of specific DNA fragments of Mycobacterium avium and their possible use in diagnosis. J Clin Microbiol 31:1048, 1993.
109. van der Giessen JW, Eger A, Haagsma J, et al. Rapid detection and identification of Mycobacterium avium by amplification of 16S rRNA sequences. J Clin Microbiol 31:2509, 1993.
110. Shanson DC, Dryden MS. Comparison of methods for isolating Mycobacterium avium-intracellulare from blood of patients with AIDS. J Clin Pathol 41:687, 1988.
111. Evans KD, Nakasone AS, Sutherland PA, et al. Identification of Mycobacterium tuberculosis and Mycobacterium avium–M. intracellulare directly from primary BACTEC cultures by using acridinium-ester-labeled DNA probes. J Clin Microbiol 30:2427, 1992.
112. Heifets L, Lindholm-Levy P, Libonati J, et al. Radiometric broth macrodilution method for determination of minimal inhibitory concentrations (MIC) with Mycobacterium avium complex isolates: proposed guidelines. Denver, National Jewish Center for Immunology and Respiratory Medicine, 1993.
113. Woods GL, Williams-Bouyer N, Wallace RJ Jr, et al. Multisite reproducibility of results obtained by two broth dilution methods for susceptibility testing of Mycobacterium avium complex. J Clin Microbiol 41:627, 2003.
114. Gardner EM, Burman WJ, DeGroote MA, et al. Conventional and molecular epidemiology of macrolide resistance among new Mycobacterium avium complex isolates recovered from HIV-infected patients. Clin Infect Dis 41:1041, 2005.
115. Horsburgh CR Jr, Mason III UG, Heifets LB, et al. Response to therapy of pulmonary Mycobacterium avium-intracellulare infection correlates with results of in vitro susceptibility testing. Am Rev Respir Dis 135:418, 1987.
116. Chaisson RE, Benson CA, Dube MP, et al. Clarithromycin therapy for bacteremic Mycobacterium avium complex disease. A randomized, double-blind, dose-ranging study in patients with AIDS. AIDS Clinical Trials Group Protocol 157 Study Team. Ann Intern Med 121:905, 1994.
117. Heifets L, Mor N, Vanderkolk J. Mycobacterium avium strains resistant to clarithromycin and azithromycin. Antimicrob Agents Chemother 37:2364, 1993.
118. Shafran SD, Talbot JA, Chomyc S, et al. Does in vitro susceptibility to rifabutin and ethambutol predict the response to treatment of Mycobacterium avium complex bacteremia with rifabutin, ethambutol, and clarithromycin? Clin Infect Dis 27:1401, 1998.
119. Meier A, Heifets L, Wallace RJ Jr, et al. Molecular mechanisms of clarithromycin resistance in Mycobacterium avium: observation of multiple 23S rDNA mutations in a clonal population. J Infect Dis 174:354, 1996.
120. Nash KA, Inderlied CB. Genetic basis of macrolide resistance in Mycobacterium avium isolated from patients with disseminated disease. Antimicrob Agents Chemother 39:2625, 1995.
121. Benson CA. Treatment of disseminated disease due to the Mycobacterium avium complex in patients with AIDS. Clin Infect Dis 18(Suppl 3):S237, 1994.
122. Young LS, Wiviott L, Wu M, et al. Azithromycin for treatment of Mycobacterium avium–intracellulare complex infection in patients with AIDS. Lancet 338:1107, 1991.
123. Jacobson MA, Yajko D, Northfelt D, et al. Randomized, placebo-controlled trial of rifampin, ethambutol, and ciprofloxacin for AIDS patients with disseminated Mycobacterium avium complex infection. J Infect Dis 168:112, 1993.
124. Kemper CA, Meng TC, Nussbaum J, et al. Treatment of Mycobacterium avium complex bacteremia in AIDS with a four-drug oral regimen. Rifampin, ethambutol, clofazimine, and ciprofloxacin. Ann Intern Med 116:466, 1992.
125. Shafran SD, Singer J, Zarowny DP, et al. A comparison of two regimens for the treatment of Mycobacterium avium complex bacteremia in AIDS: rifabutin, ethambutol, and clarithromycin versus rifampin, ethambutol, clofazimine, and ciprofloxacin. N Engl J Med 335:377, 1996.

126. May T, Brel F, Beuscart C, et al. Comparison of combination therapy regimens for treatment of human immunodeficiency virus-infected patients with disseminated bacteremia due to Mycobacterium avium. Clin Infect Dis 25:621, 1997.
127. Gordin FM, Sullam PM, Shafran SD, et al. A randomized, placebo-controlled study of rifabutin added to a regimen of clarithromycin and ethambutol for treatment of disseminated infection with Mycobacterium avium complex. Clin Infect Dis 28:1080, 1999.
128. Dube MP, Sattler FR, Torriani FJ, et al. A randomized evaluation of ethambutol for prevention of relapse and drug resistance during treatment of Mycobacterium avium complex bacteremia with clarithromycin-based combination therapy. J Infect Dis 176:1225, 1997.
129. Cohn DL, Fisher EJ, Peng GT, et al. A prospective randomized trial of four three-drug regimens in the treatment of disseminated Mycobacterium avium complex disease in AIDS patients: excess mortality associated with high-dose clarithromycin. Clin Infect Dis 29:125, 1999.
130. Chaisson RE, Keiser P, Pierce M, et al. Clarithromycin and ethambutol with or without clofazimine for the treatment of bacteremic Mycobacterium avium complex disease in patients with HIV infection. AIDS 11:311, 1997.
131. Wallace RJ, Jr., Brown BA, Griffith DE, et al. Clarithromycin regimens for pulmonary Mycobacterium avium complex: the first 50 patients. Am J Respir Crit Care Med 153:1766, 1996.
132. Griffith DE, Brown BA, Girard WM, et al. Azithromycin activity against Mycobacterium avium complex lung disease in patients who were not infected with human immunodeficiency virus. Clin Infect Dis 23:983, 1996.
133. Korvick JA, Benson CA. Advances in the treatment and prophylaxis of Mycobacterium avium complex in individuals infected with human immunodeficiency virus. In: Korvick JA, Benson CA (eds). Mycobacterium avium Complex Infection: Progress in Research and Treatment. New York: Dekker; 1996, p 241.
134. Clarithromycin (Biaxin) package insert/product monograph. Abbott Park: Abbott Laboratories; 1995.
135. Azithromycin (Zithromax) package insert/product monograph. New York: Pfizer; 1996.
136. Rifabutin (Mycobutin) package insert/product monograph. Kalamazoo: Pharmacia & Upjohn; 1995.
137. Benson CA, Sha BE. Management of disseminated Mycobacterium avium complex disease in HIV-infected women. In: Cotton D, Watts HD (eds). The Medical Management of AIDS in Women. New York: Wiley-Liss; 1997, p 269.
138. Masur H. Recommendations on prophylaxis and therapy for disseminated Mycobacterium avium complex disease in patients infected with the human immunodeficiency virus. Public Health Service Task Force on Prophylaxis and Therapy for Mycobacterium avium Complex. N Engl J Med 329:898, 1993.
139. Benson CA, Williams PL, Cohn DL, et al. Clarithromycin or rifabutin alone or in combination for primary prophylaxis of Mycobacterium avium complex disease in patients with AIDS: A randomized, double-blind, placebo-controlled trial. J Infect Dis 181:1289, 2000.
140. Havlir DV, Dubé MP, Sattler FR, et al. Prophylaxis against disseminated Mycobacterium avium complex with weekly azithromycin, daily rifabutin, or both. N Engl J Med 335:392, 1996.
141. USPHS/IDSA Prevention of Opportunistic Infections Working Group. 2001 USPHS/IDSA guidelines for the prevention of opportunistic infections in persons infected with human immunodeficiency virus. Available: http://www.hivatis.org 28 Nov 2001.
142. Benson CA, Kaplan JE, Masur H, et al. Treating opportunistic infections among HIV-infected adults and adolescents. Recommendations from CDC, the National Institutes of Health, and the HIV Medicine Association/Infectious Diseases Society of America. MMWR Recomm Rep 53:1, 2004.
143. Aberg JA, Yajko DM, Jacobson MA. Eradication of AIDS-related disseminated mycobacterium avium complex infection after 12 months of antimycobacterial therapy combined with highly active antiretroviral therapy. J Infect Dis 178:1446, 1998.
144. Zeller V, Jovan M, Truffaaut, et al. Discontinuing maintenance treatment for Pneumocystis pneumonia, toxoplasmic encephalitis, and disseminated Mycobacterium avium complex infection. In: Abstracts of the 1st IAS Conference on HIV Pathogenesis and Treatment, Buenos Aires, Argentina, 2001, p 302, abstract 739.
145. Aberg JA, Williams PL, Liu T, et al. A study of discontinuing maintenance therapy in human immunodeficiency virus-infected subjects with disseminated Mycobacterium avium complex: AIDS Clinical Trial Group 393 Study Team. J Infect Dis 187:1046, 2003.
146. Green H, Hay P, Dunn DT, et al. A prospective multicentre study of discontinuing prophylaxis for opportunistic infections after effective antiretroviral therapy. HIV Med 5:278, 2004.
147. Liao CH, Chen MY, Hsieh SM, et al. Discontinuation of secondary prophylaxis in AIDS patients with disseminated non-tuberculous mycobacteria infection. J Microbiol Immunol Infect 37:50, 2004.
148. Shafran SD, Gill MJ, Lalonde RG, et al. Successful discontinuation of MAC therapy following effective HAART. In: Abstracts of the 8th Conference on Retroviruses and Opportunistic Infections, Chicago, IL. Alexandria, VA: Foundation for Retrovirology and Human Health; 2001, p 208, abstract 547.
149. Chiu J, Nussbaum J, Bozzette S, et al. Treatment of disseminated Mycobacterium avium complex infection in AIDS with amikacin, ethambutol, rifampin, and ciprofloxacin. Ann Intern Med 113:358, 1990.
150. Kemper CA, Havlir D, Haghighat D, et al. The individual microbiologic effect of three antimycobacterial agents, clofazimine, ethambutol, and rifampin, on Mycobacterium avium complex bacteremia in patients with AIDS. J Infect Dis 170:157, 1994.
151. Parenti D, Ellner J, Hafner R, et al. A phase II/III trial of rifampin (RIF), ciprofloxacin (CIPRO), clofazimine (CLOF), ethambutol (ETH), amikacin (AK) in the treatment of disseminated Mycobacterium avium (MAC) infection in HIV-infected individuals. In: Abstracts of the 2nd National Conference on Human Retroviruses and Related Infections, Washington DC. Washington, DC: American Society for Microbiology; 1995, p 56, abstract 6.
152. Dautzenberg B, Truffot C, Legris S, et al. Activity of clarithromycin against Mycobacterium avium infection in patients with the acquired immune deficiency syndrome: A controlled clinical trial. Am Rev Respir Dis 144:564, 1991.
153. Shafran SD, Deschenes J, Miller M, et al. Uveitis and pseudojaundice during a regimen of clarithromycin, rifabutin, and ethambutol [letter]. N Engl J Med 330:438, 1994.
154. Hafner R, Bethel J, Power M, et al. Tolerance and pharmacokinetic interactions of rifabutin and clarithromycin in human immunodeficiency virus-infected volunteers. Antimicrob Agents Chemother 42:631, 1998.
155. Benson CA, Williams PL, Currier JS, et al. ACTG 223: an open, prospective, randomized study comparing efficacy and safety of clarithromycin (C) plus ethambutol (E), rifabutin (R) or both for treatment (Rx) of MAC disease in patients with AIDS. In: Abstracts of the 6th Conference on Retroviruses and Opportunistic Infections, Chicago, IL. Alexandria, VA: Foundation for Retrovirology and Human Health; 1999, abstract 249.

156. Ward TT, Rimland D, Kauffman C, et al. Randomized, open-label trial of azithromycin plus ethambutol vs. clarithromycin plus ethambutol as therapy for Mycobacterium avium complex bacteremia in patients with human immunodeficiency virus infection. Veterans Affairs HIV Research Consortium. Clin Infect Dis 27:1278, 1998.
157. Dunne M, Fessel J, Kumar P, et al. A randomized, double-blind trial comparing azithromycin and clarithromycin in the treatment of disseminated Mycobacterium avium infection in patients with human immunodeficiency virus. Clin Infect Dis 31:1245, 2000.
158. Dube MP, Torriani FJ, See D, et al. Successful short-term suppression of clarithromycin-resistant Mycobacterium avium complex bacteremia in AIDS. Clin Infect Dis 28:136, 1999.
159. Nelson M, Richardson S, Gazzard BS, et al. Liposomal amikacin for the treatment of non-tuberculous mycobacteria in HIV disease. In: Abstracts of the 12th World AIDS Conference, Geneva, Switzerland, 1998, p 296, abstract 22170.
160. Bermudez LE, Kolonoski P, Petrofsky M, et al. Mefloquine, moxifloxacin, and ethambutol are a triple-drug alternative to macrolide-containing regimens for treatment of Mycobacterium avium disease. J Infect Dis 187:1977, 2003.
161. Bermudez LE, Inderlied CB, Kolonoski P, et al. Telithromycin is active against Mycobacterium avium in mice despite lacking significant activity in standard in vitro and macrophage assays and is associated with low frequency of resistance during treatment. Antimicrob Agents Chemother 45:2210, 2001.
162. Bermudez LE, Yamazaki Y. Effects of macrolides and ketolides on mycobacterial infections. Curr Pharm Des 10:3221, 2004.
163. Kemper CA, Bermudez LE, Deresinski SC. Immunomodulatory treatment of Mycobacterium avium complex bacteremia in patients with AIDS by use of recombinant granulocyte-macrophage colony-stimulating factor. J Infect Dis 177:914, 1998.
164. Wormser GP, Horowitz H, Dworkin B. Low-dose dexamethasone as adjunctive therapy for disseminated Mycobacterium avium complex infections in AIDS patients. Antimicrob Agents Chemother 38:2215, 1994.
165. Graves M, Salvato P, Thompson C. MAIC and the effect of prednisone on disease progression in AIDS patients. In: Abstracts of the XI International Conference on AIDS, Vancouver, Canada, 1996, p 119, abstract Mo.B.1371.
166. Pierce M, Crampton S, Henry D, et al. A randomized trial of clarithromycin as prophylaxis against disseminated Mycobacterium avium complex infection in patients with advanced acquired immunodeficiency syndrome. N Engl J Med 335:384, 1996.
167. Currier JS, Williams P, Feinberg J, et al. Impact of prophylaxis for Mycobacterium avium complex on bacterial infections in patients with advanced human immunodeficiency virus disease. Clin Infect Dis 32:1615, 2001.
168. Oldfield EC, 3rd, Fessel WJ, Dunne MW, et al. Once weekly azithromycin therapy for prevention of Mycobacterium avium complex infection in patients with AIDS: a randomized, double-blind, placebo-controlled multicenter trial. Clin Infect Dis 26:611, 1998.
169. Moore RD, Chaisson RE. Survival analysis of two controlled trials of rifabutin prophylaxis against Mycobacterium avium complex in AIDS. AIDS 9:1337, 1995.
170. Brooks JT, Song R, Hanson DL, et al. Discontinuation of primary prophylaxis against Mycobacterium avium complex infection in HIV-infected persons receiving antiretroviral therapy: observations from a large national cohort in the United States, 1992–2002. Clin Infect Dis 41:549, 2005.
171. Lange CG, Woolley IJ, Brodt RH. Disseminated mycobacterium avium-intracellulare complex (MAC) infection in the era of effective antiretroviral therapy: is prophylaxis still indicated? Drugs 64:679, 2004.
172. Trapnell CB, Narang PK, Li R, et al. Increased plasma rifabutin levels with concomitant fluconazole therapy in HIV-infected patients. Ann Intern Med 124:573, 1996.
173. Wallace Jr. RJ, Brown BA, Griffith DE, et al. Reduced serum levels of clarithromycin in patients treated with multidrug regimens including rifampin or rifabutin for Mycobacterium avium-M. intracellulare infection. J Infect Dis 171:747, 1995.
174. Fuller JD, Stanfield LE, Craven DE. Rifabutin prophylaxis and uveitis [letter]. N Engl J Med 330:1315, 1994.
175. Narang PK, Trapnell CB, Schoenfelder JR, et al. Fluconazole and enhanced effect of rifabutin prophylaxis [letter]. N Engl J Med 330:1316, 1994.
176. Piscitelli SC, Flexner C, Minor JR, et al. Drug interactions in patients infected with human immunodeficiency virus. Clin Infect Dis 23:685, 1996.
177. Norvir (Ritonavir) package insert/product monograph. Abbott Park: Abbott Laboratories; 1996.
178. Ouellet D, Hsu A, Granneman GR, et al. Assessment of the pharmacokinetic interaction between ritonavir and clarithromycin. Clin Pharmacol Ther 59:143 (abstract PI-58), 1996.
179. Reyataz (Atazanavir) prescribing information/product monograph. Princeton: Bristol-Myers Squibb Company; 2004.
180. The Liverpool HIV Pharmacology Group. Drug interaction charts. Available: http://www.hiv-druginteractions.org 7 Nov 2005.
181. Centers for Disease Control and Prevention. Updated guidelines for the use of rifabutin or rifampin for the treatment and prevention of tuberculosis among HIV-infected patients taking protease inhibitors or nonnucleoside reverse transcriptase inhibitors. MMWR 49:185, 2000.
182. Cato A, Cavanaugh JH, Shi H, et al. Assessment of multiple doses of ritonavir on the pharmacokinetics of rifabutin. In: Abstracts of the XI International Conference on AIDS, Vancouver, Canada, 1996, p 89, abstract Mo.B.1199.
183. Sun E, Heath-Chiozzi M, Cameron DW, et al. Concurrent ritonavir and rifabutin increases the risk of rifabutin associated adverse effects. In: Abstracts of the XI International Conference on AIDS, Vancouver, Canada, 1996, p 18, abstract Mo.B.171.
184. Hamzeh F, Benson C, Gerber J, et al. Steady-state pharmacokinetic interaction of modified-dose indinavir and rifabutin. In: Abstracts of the 7th Conference on Retroviruses and Opportunistic Infections, San Francisco, CA. Alexandria, VA: Foundation for Retrovirology and Human Health; 2000, p 92, abstract 90.
185. Crixivan (Indinavir) package insert/product monograph. West Point: Merck; 1996.
186. Viracept (Nelfinavir) package insert/product monograph. La Jolla: Agouron Pharmaceuticals; 1998.
187. Invirase (Saquinavir) package insert/product monograph. Nutley: Hoffman-LaRoche; 1996.
188. Sahai J, Stewart F, Swick L, et al. Rifabutin (RBT) reduces saquinavir (SAQ) plasma levels in HIV-infected patients. In: Abstracts of the 36th Interscience Conference on Antimicrobial Agents and Chemotherapy (ICAAC), New Orleans, LA. Washington, DC: American Society for Microbiology; 1996, p 6, abstract A27.
189. Viramune (Nevirapine) package insert/product monograph. Columbus: Roxane; 1997.
190. Benson CA. Critical drug interactions with agents used for prophylaxis and treatment of Mycobacterium avium complex infections. Am J Med 102(5 Suppl 3):32, 1997.
191. Efavirenz (Sustiva) data on file. Wilmington: DuPont Merck; 1998.
192. Borin MT, Cox SR, Driver MR, et al. Effect of rifabutin on delavirdine pharmacokinetics in HIV+ patients. In: Abstracts

of the 34th Interscience Conference on Antimicrobial Agents and Chemotherapy (ICAAC), Orlando, FL. Washington, DC: American Society for Microbiology; 1994, p 81, abstract A48.
193. Bamberger DM, Driks MR, Gupta MR, et al. Mycobacterium kansasii among patients infected with human immunodeficiency virus in Kansas City. Clin Infect Dis 18:395, 1994.
194. Levine B, Chaisson RE. Mycobacterium kansasii: a cause of treatable pulmonary disease associated with advanced human immunodeficiency virus (HIV) infection. Ann Intern Med 114:861, 1991.
195. Valainis GT, Cardona LM, Greer DL. The spectrum of Mycobacterium kansasii disease associated with HIV-1 infected patients. J Acquir Immune Defic Syndr 4:516, 1991.
196. Sherer R, Sable R, Sonnenberg M, et al. Disseminated infection with Mycobacterium kansasii in the acquired immunodeficiency syndrome. Ann Intern Med 105:710, 1986.
197. Carpenter JL, Parks JM. Mycobacterium kansasii infections in patients positive for human immunodeficiency virus. Rev Infect Dis 13:789, 1991.
198. Pintado V, Fortun J, Casado JL, et al. Mycobacterium kansasii pericarditis as a presentation of AIDS. Infection 29:48, 2001.
199. Pintado V, Gomez-Mampaso E, Martin-Davila P, et al. Mycobacterium kansasii infection in patients infected with the human immunodeficiency virus. Eur J Clin Microbiol Infect Dis 18:582, 1999.
200. Graybill JR, Bocanegra R. Treatment alternatives for Mycobacterium kansasii. J Antimicrob Chemother 47:417, 2001.
201. Burman WJ, Stone BL, Brown BA, et al. AIDS-related Mycobacterium kansasii infection with initial resistance to clarithromycin. Diagn Microbiol Infect Dis 31:369, 1998.
202. Miguez-Burbano MJ, Flores M, Ashkin D, et al. Non-tuberculous mycobacteria disease as a cause of hospitalization in HIV-infected subjects. Int J Infect Dis 10:47, 2006.
203. Straus WL, Ostroff SM, Jernigan DB, et al. Clinical and epidemiologic characteristics of Mycobacterium haemophilum, an emerging pathogen in immunocompromised patients. Ann Intern Med 120:118, 1994.
204. el-Helou P, Rachlis A, Fong I, et al. Mycobacterium xenopi infection in patients with human immunodeficiency virus infection. Clin Infect Dis 25:206, 1997.
205. Hirschel B, Chang HR, Mach N, et al. Fatal infection with a novel, unidentified mycobacterium in a man with the acquired immunodeficiency syndrome. N Engl J Med 323:109, 1990.
206. Bessesen MT, Shlay J, Stone-Venohr B, et al. Disseminated Mycobacterium genavense infection: clinical and microbiological features and response to therapy. AIDS 7:1357, 1993.
207. Albrecht H, Rusch-Gerdes S, Stellbrink HJ, et al. Treatment of disseminated Mycobacterium genavense infection. AIDS 9:659, 1995.
208. Fakih M, Chapalamadugu S, Ricart A, et al. Mycobacterium malmoense bacteremia in two AIDS patients. J Clin Microbiol 34:731, 1996.
209. Tortoli E, Piersimoni C, Bacosi D, et al. Isolation of the newly described species Mycobacterium celatum from AIDS patients. J Clin Microbiol 33:137, 1995.
210. Brown BA, Wallace Jr. RJ. Infections due to nontuberculous mycobacteria. In: Mandell G, Bennett JE, Dolin R (eds). Principles and Practice of Infectious Diseases. 5th edn. Philadelphia: Churchill Livingstone; 2000, p 2630.
211. Arasteh KN, Cordes C, Ewers M, et al. HIV-related nontuberculous mycobacterial infection: incidence, survival analysis and associated risk factors. Eur J Med Res 5:424, 2000.

Chapter 42

Bartonellosis

Jane E. Koehler, MD

BARTONELLA INFECTIONS

Clinical Presentation

The spectrum of disease caused by *Bartonella* species includes cat scratch disease (*B. henselae*), bacillary angiomatosis (*B. henselae* and *B. quintana*), bacillary peliosis (*B. henselae*), endocarditis (*B. henselae*, *B. quintana*, and *B. elizabethae*), bacteremia (*B. henselae*, *B. quintana*, and *B. vinsonii* subsp *arupensis*), trench fever (*B. quintana*), meningitis/neuroretinitis (*B. henselae*, *B. grahamii*, and *B. vinsonii* subsp *arupensis*), Oroya fever (*B. bacilliformis*) and verruga peruana (*B. bacilliformis*).[1,2] *Bartonella* infections occur in both immunocompromised and immunocompetent patients, but some of the disease manifestations are related to the degree of immunocompromise (see Table 42-1). Cat scratch disease, a granulomatous lymphadenitis, usually occurs in immunocompetent individuals, or in patients early in the course of HIV infection. In contrast, bacillary angiomatosis and bacillary peliosis occur almost exclusively in severely immunocompromised individuals, especially in patients with late stage HIV infection (the median CD4 cell count in a series of patients with bacillary angiomatosis and peliosis was 22/mm^3).[3]

Bacillary angiomatosis lesions are caused by infection with *B. henselae* or *B. quintana*.[4,5] These lesions often are not recognized for several reasons: they can be impossible to distinguish clinically from Kaposi sarcoma lesions,[6] and can have very diverse presentations.[7] Bacillary angiomatosis has been described most frequently in skin (as angiomatous papules, pedunculated lesions or subcutaneous masses). These vascular proliferative lesions also occur in bone, the gastrointestinal and respiratory tracts, lymph nodes, and the central nervous system. A closely related angiomatous lesion of the liver and spleen is known as parenchymal bacillary peliosis[8] and is caused by *B. henselae*.[5]

Some manifestations of *Bartonella* infection, including endocarditis, bacteremia or meningitis, occur in patients regardless of the degree of immunocompromise. In immunocompetent individuals, cat scratch disease is usually self-limited and the need for treatment of immunocompetent patients is controversial. In contrast, *Bartonella* infections occurring in HIV-infected patients are more severe and can even be fatal,[9] and therefore all immunocompromised patients with *Bartonella* infection should be treated with appropriate antimicrobial therapy.[10]

Taxonomy

Infections with *Bartonella* were first identified in the United States because of the AIDS epidemic. In 1983, Stoler et al identified an HIV-infected patient with subcutaneous lesions.[11] They subsequently identified numerous bacilli within the lesions by electron microscopy, and treated the patient with erythromycin. The lesions resolved and little additional information became known about the causative organism until 1990, when bacterial DNA was extracted from biopsied bacillary angiomatosis tissue from HIV-infected and organ transplant patients. This molecular analysis led to identification of the organism as closely related to the agent of trench fever, *Rochalimaea quintana*.[12] The new species also was isolated from the blood of HIV-infected patients,[13] and subsequently was named *R. henselae*.[14,15] This species was thought to be the sole agent of bacillary angiomatosis until the bacilli were isolated directly from cutaneous bacillary angiomatosis lesions, and *R. quintana* also was found to cause bacillary angiomatosis in immunocompromised patients.[4]

Brenner et al found that members of the *Rochalimaea* genus were very closely related to the sole species of the genus *Bartonella*, *B. bacilliformis*, and in 1993 all *Rochalimaea* species (*R. henselae*, *R. quintana*, *R. elizabethae*, and *R. vinsonii*) were merged into the *Bartonella*

Manifestations of Bartonella Infection in HIV-Infected Patients

Table 42-1

Manifestation	Diagnostic Approach
Skin	
May resemble Kaposi sarcoma	Biopsy with W-S staining
Angiomatous nodule	
Friable vascular lesion	
Red papule	
Pedunculated lesion	
Deep subcutaneous mass	
Bone	
Extremely painful osteolysis	Biopsy with W-S staining
Lytic lesions on radiograph (technetium-positive)	
Lymph nodes	
Enlargement	Biopsy with W-S staining
Heart	
Valve vegetation	Echo, blood culture (lysis-centrifugation method or EDTA tube)
Valve insufficiency	
Blood	
Thrombosis, fever	Blood culture (echo to rule out endocarditis)
Liver/Spleen	
Hypodense lesions – CT	Biopsy with W-S staining (monitor for bleeding)
Hepatosplenomegaly – CT	
Elevated LFTs (alkaline phosphatase)	
Pancytopenia	
Thrombocytopenia	
Other	
Brain, gastrointestinal, pulmonary, others	Biopsy with W-S staining

CT, computed tomography; echo, echocardiography; LFT, liver function tests; W-S, Warthin–Starry stain.

From Koehler JE. Bartonella-associated infections in HIV-infected patients. AIDS Clin Care 7:97, 1995. Copyright 1995, Massachusetts Medical Society.

genus.[16] Another genus, *Grahamella*, was subsequently merged with *Bartonella*, adding three more species to the genus, all of which infect small mammals: *B. taylorii*, *B. grahamii*, and *B. doshiae*.[17] An additional eleven species were isolated from small mammals, including *B. clarridgeiae*, *B. tribocorum*, *B. alsatica*, *B. koehlerae*, *B. birtlesii*, *B. bovis*, *B. capreoli*, *B. chomelii*, *B. schoenbuchensis*, *B. phoceensis*, and *B. rattimassiliensis*. There are currently 19 extant species of *Bartonella*, five of which have been isolated from humans: *B. bacilliformis*, *B. elizabethae*, *B. henselae*, *B. vinsonii* subsp *arupensis*, and *B. quintana*. Only *B. henselae* and *B. quintana* have been associated with disease in HIV-infected patients.

Biology and Epidemiology

Before the bacillary angiomatosis bacillus was identified, epidemiological studies revealed that development of bacillary angiomatosis was statistically significantly associated with cat contact, cat scratches and cat bites.[18] Further investigation of household cats belonging to four patients who developed bacillary angiomatosis revealed that all seven cats of these patients were bacteremic with *B. henselae*, the same species that caused the bacillary angiomatosis in these patients.[19] Surveys of the cats in the greater San Francisco Bay area demonstrated that 41% of the 61 pet and pound cats were bacteremic with *B. henselae*, although no illness could be demonstrated in any of the infected cats.[19]

Because of this high prevalence of *B. henselae* bacteremia, and the demonstration that viable *B. henselae* could be cultured from cat fleas infesting bacteremic cats, the cat flea was suspected to be a vector of *B. henselae*. Further evidence implicating the cat flea as an arthropod vector of *B. henselae* was provided by the correlation between the increased prevalence of flea infestation and increased *B. henselae* seroprevalence in cats tested in different regions of the United States.[20] Definitive demonstration of transmission of *B. henselae* from cat to cat was provided when fleas were combed from cats bacteremic with *B. henselae* and placed on specific pathogen free cats in an arthropod-free university facility. The recipient cats developed high level *B. henselae* bacteremia within 2 weeks of experimental infestation and seroconverted several weeks later.[21]

From the initial epidemiologic study in 1993,[18] it was evident that although most of the patients had developed bacillary angiomatosis after traumatic cat contact, nearly one-third of the patients had no cat contact prior to developing bacillary angiomatosis. After the second species, *B. quintana*, was found to cause bacillary angiomatosis, it was suspected that these patients without cat contact might have developed bacillary angiomatosis infection caused by *B. quintana*. By determining the infecting species for 49 patients with bacillary angiomatosis and comparing exposures of these patients with their 96 matched controls, it was demonstrated that patients infected with *B. henselae* had a statistically significant association with cat contact including having received cat bites, cat scratches, and cat flea bites, as previously demonstrated.[5] The patients with bacillary angiomatosis caused by *B. quintana*, however, had a statistically significant exposure to the body louse and were of lower socioeconomic status than their matched controls.[5] This contemporary association between the body louse and *B. quintana* corroborates historical data demonstrating that the spread of *B. quintana* among the soldiers occurred via the body louse, causing an epidemic of trench fever affecting tens of thousands of troops in World War I.[22]

Each *Bartonella* species is believed to have one or more mammalian reservoir(s): the domestic cat for *B. henselae*, *B. koehlerae*, and *B. clarridgeiae*, the human for *B. quintana* and *B. bacilliformis*, rabbits for *B. alsatica*, cows for *B. bovis*, deer for *B. capreoli* and *B. schoenbuchensis*, and moles, voles, rats, and mice for *B. vinsonii*, *B. taylorii*, *B. doshiae*,

B. grahamii, *B. elizabethae*, and *B. tribocorum*. Arthropod vectors of *Bartonella* species have not been studied as extensively as reservoirs, but in addition to the cat flea vector (*Ctenocephalides felis*) of *B. henselae*,[21] another flea, *Xenopsylla cheopis*, transmitted *Bartonella* spp to voles.[23] The sand fly *Lutzomyia verrucarum* is the natural arthropod vector known to transmit *B. bacilliformis* among humans in the Peruvian Andes,[24] and little information is currently known about arthropod vectors of other *Bartonella* species.

Microbiology

Bartonella species are small, slowly growing, and very fastidious gram-negative rods. Five species have flagella and are motile, *B. bacilliformis*, *B. clarridgeiae*, *B. chomelii*, *B. capreoli*, and *B. schoenbuchensis*.[25] The *Bartonella* bacilli are relatively inert biochemically and are not able to oxidize glucose. *Bartonella* species are able to utilize glutamate and succinate as carbon sources, and hemin or serum supplementation of growth media permits optimal growth on artificial media.[26] The colony morphology of primary isolates differs for *B. henselae* (rough, with pitting of the agar) and *B. quintana* (smooth, without pitting of the agar).[5]

Bartonella Laboratory Diagnosis

Table 42-2

Method	Comments
Histopathology	Check for (H&E staining) Lobular, vascular proliferation Neutrophils and debris Basophilic granular material Protruberant endothelial cells Check for darkly staining bacilli (Warthin–Starry stain)
Blood culture	Lysis-centrifugation or EDTA tubes, onto fresh chocolate and rabbit blood agars Incubate in 5% CO_2 at 35°C for 21 days
Culture of tissue biopsy	Experimental Co-cultivation of endothelial cells with homogenate
Serology	Centers for Disease Control and Prevention indirect immunofluorescence antibody test

From Koehler JE: Bartonella-associated infections in HIV-infected patients. AIDS Clin Care 7:97, 1995. Copyright 1995, Massachusetts Medical Society.

DIAGNOSIS

Direct Detection

Bartonella species can be detected in biopsied bacillary angiomatosis tissue using hematoxylin and eosin (H and E) staining and optimally, the Warthin–Starry silver stain (Table 42-2). For cutaneous bacillary angiomatosis lesions, a 5 mm punch biopsy specimen usually provides adequate tissue for diagnosis (for small papules or subcutaneous nodules). The vascular proliferative changes identified by H and E staining are usually very characteristic.[27] Newly formed, capillary-sized blood vessels can be identified and are lined with protuberant endothelial cells. Adjacent to these regions of vascular proliferation are clusters of granular, amphophilic material that represent microcolonies of *Bartonella* bacteria; distinct bacilli are revealed in these granular deposits when the Warthin–Starry silver stain is used. *In situ* immunohistochemical staining also has been useful in direct visualization of *Bartonella* bacilli in biopsied tissue from bacillary angiomatosis and bacillary peliosis lesions.[28]

Culture

The extremely fastidious nature of *Bartonella* bacilli has made isolation very difficult or impossible in the clinical microbiology laboratory setting of most hospitals. Isolation is best achieved using enriched agar: optimally, heart infusion agar with 5% defibrinated rabbit blood for *B. henselae*[13] and chocolate agar (supplemented with IsovitaleX and hemoglobin) for *B. quintana*.[4] There are distinct differences in the preference of *B. quintana* and *B. henselae* for these two agar compositions.[5]

Both agar types should be inoculated with homogenized biopsied bacillary angiomatosis tissue or blood to optimize recovery of either species. Cultures should be incubated for up to 4 weeks in a CO_2-enriched (5%), moist environment; *Bartonella* colonies usually are not identifiable until 8 days after inoculation.[5] Co-cultivation of biopsied tissue with endothelial cell monolayers is usually a more sensitive technique for isolation of *Bartonella* species.[4]

Isolation from blood is optimally achieved using the lysis-centrifugation system (Wampole, Cranbury, NJ).[13] This is a primary isolation system that involves immediate centrifugation of the tube filled with 10 mL of blood, followed by plating of the pellet onto fresh agar. Many blood culture systems will not detect *Bartonella*; detection of *Bartonella* in these culture systems requires blind subbing of blood culture bottle contents onto agar or centrifuging onto endothelial cell shell vials,[29] or staining with acridine orange.[30]

Serology

A serologic test was developed by the Centers for Disease Control and Prevention (CDC), using co-cultivation of *Bartonella* species with Vero cells. This indirect immunofluorescence antibody (IFA) test has good sensitivity and specificity for detecting *Bartonella* infection in immunocompetent individuals with cat scratch disease, although it does not distinguish between *B. henselae* and *B. quintana* infection.[31] This test also appears to have utility in detecting *Bartonella* infection in immunocompromised patients with bacillary angiomatosis.[32]

In Vitro Susceptibility Testing

As for many fastidious bacteria, antibiotic susceptibility testing for *Bartonella* species is not standardized. In addition, there is little correlation between the *in vitro* susceptibilities of *Bartonella* isolates and the *in vivo* treatment experience for a number of antibiotics. This is especially true for cell wall active antibiotics such as penicillin and first generation cephalosporins. For the Fuller type strain of *B. quintana*, early studies found excellent *in vitro* susceptibility for penicillin, with an MIC_{50}/MIC_{90} of 0.024/0.035 μg/mL,[33] yet there are many reports of treatment failures and even dramatic progression of bacillary angiomatosis disease in patients receiving penicillin.[34,35] The role for routine antimicrobial susceptibility testing of *Bartonella* isolates is therefore not clear, and is currently not of practical value.

In an *in vitro* study of antimicrobial susceptibilities, 28 antibiotics were tested with 14 *Bartonella* isolates using an agar dilution method.[36] As previously demonstrated *in vitro*, the *Bartonella* strains usually were susceptible to penicillins (MIC_{90} ranging from 0.015 to 0.06 μg/mL). In addition to nine strains of *B. quintana*, the other species of *Bartonella* tested (one strain of *B. vinsonii*, one strain of *B. elizabethae* and three strains of *B. henselae*) were susceptible to erythromycin, doxycycline, and rifampin. These isolates also were susceptible to azithromycin and clarithromycin. Indeed, all *Bartonella* isolates tested to date have shown *in vitro* susceptibility to erythromycin and tetracycline, with the exception of one isolate reported by Colson et al, that had a MIC of >256 μg/mL to erythromycin and clarithromycin, but with retesting was susceptible with a MIC of 0.06 μg/mL.[37] In this patient, treatment with ciprofloxacin and rifampin was continued; a subsequent relapse isolate also was susceptible to both erythromycin and clarithromycin with a MIC of 0.06 μg/mL. The significance of this transiently elevated MIC to macrolides is unclear.

Susceptibility of ten *B. henselae* isolates to erythromycin, azithromycin, rifampin, doxycycline, ciprofloxacin, and vancomycin was evaluated using the E-test in another study.[38] Good correlation was found between the agar dilution method and E-test susceptibilities for erythromycin, azithromycin, doxycycline, and rifampin. Because the E-test is much easier to perform than the agar dilution method, susceptibility testing using the E-test may be the most practical method for determination of susceptibilities for *Bartonella* isolates.

THERAPY

Approach to Therapy – *In Vivo* Treatment Experience

Treatment of *Bartonella* infections in HIV-infected patients has not been studied systematically or in any trials, but dozens of anecdotal cases have been reported in the literature. The initially described patient with bacillary angiomatosis was treated successfully with erythromycin,[11] and the first prospectively identified case at San Francisco General Hospital, a patient with *B. quintana* osteomyelitis, was cured following treatment with 4 months of erythromycin therapy.[34] We have a cumulative experience of treating more than 50 AIDS patients with biopsy-proven bacillary angiomatosis, bacillary peliosis hepatis, and *Bartonella* bacteremia. Our experience and that of others treating bacillary angiomatosis patients, as reported in the literature, demonstrate that erythromycin and doxycycline have excellent *in vivo* activity in the treatment of bacillary angiomatosis. Additionally, tetracycline, rifampin, and newer macrolides (clarithromycin and azithromycin) seem to have *in vivo* efficacy against *Bartonella* infections in HIV-infected patients (summarized in Koehler[7] and Maurin[39]).

Anecdotal reports describe a treatment response of *Bartonella* infection to ciprofloxacin, but we have observed progression of bacillary angiomatosis during treatment with ciprofloxacin.[40] We also have isolated *Bartonella* species from patients being treated with gentamicin, trimethoprim/sulfamethoxazole, and first generation cephalosporins and therefore do not recommend treatment with these antibiotics.[5]

Several other studies provide evidence that macrolides and tetracyclines are efficacious in treatment of *Bartonella* infection. A placebo-controlled, prospective study of azithromycin treatment of immunocompetent patients with cat scratch disease was reported by Bass et al.[41] At 30 days after initiation of treatment, there was an 80% decrease in sonographically documented lymph node volume in the azithromycin-treated group compared with controls. Another placebo-controlled clinical trial for the treatment of homeless, immunocompetent patients with *B. quintana* bacteremia was conducted in France.[42] This study revealed that 7/7 patients treated with doxycycline for 28 days with gentamicin for the first 14 days had eradication of infection, but only 2/9 untreated control patients had resolution of bacteremia. Thus, although these two studies involved treatment of immunocompetent patients, they demonstrate the efficacy of antibiotics in the macrolide and tetracycline classes against *Bartonella* infections.

Recommendations For Optimal Approach to Therapy

The majority of patients with apparently focal bacillary angiomatosis actually have systemic disease: we found that half of the patients with bacillary angiomatosis were bacteremic with a *Bartonella* species.[5] Because of this, and the propensity for relapse of *Bartonella* infections treated for a short duration, we recommend that all HIV-infected patients with *Bartonella* infection receive at least three to four months of antibiotic treatment (three for uncomplicated cutaneous bacillary angiomatosis and four for osteomyelitis, bacillary peliosis or CNS involvement) (Figure 42-1). Before beginning therapy, patients with cutaneous bacillary angiomatosis should be carefully evaluated for presence of disease at another site that might require longer duration of therapy, e.g., endocarditis or osteomyelitis. Careful cardiac examination should be performed for any signs of endocarditis, and any patient with bacillary angiomatosis and a cardiac murmur should have echocardiography performed. If bony or deep soft tissue

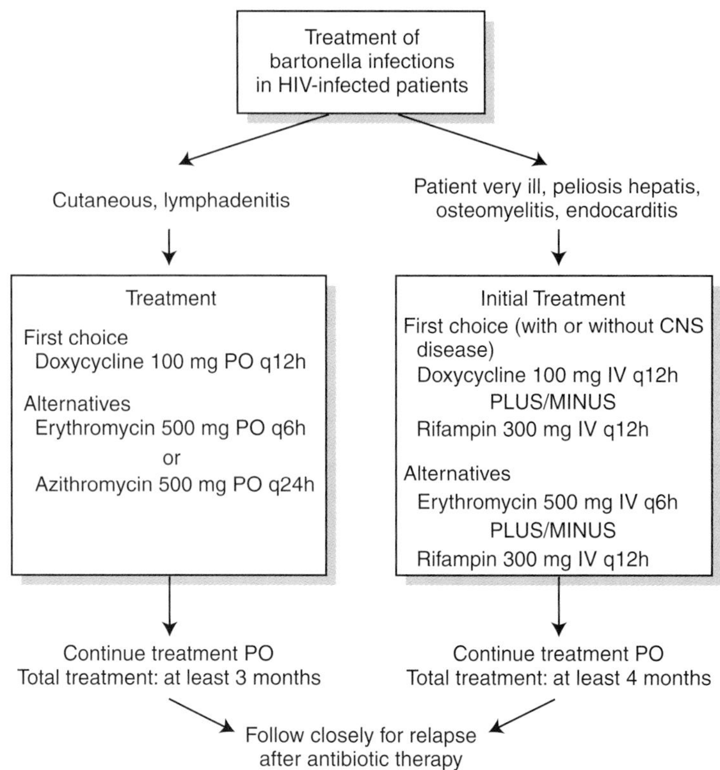

Figure 42-1 ■ Algorithm for treatment of *Bartonella* infections in HIV-infected individuals. Note that therapy or prophylaxis regimens for *Mycobacterium avium* complex that include a macrolide may treat or prevent *Bartonella* infections.

tenderness is identified on physical exam, the patient should undergo a bone scan.

Resolution of infection can be documented by abdominal CT scanning (peliosis hepatis) or ^{99m}technetium bone scans (osteomyelitis). Most patients describe improvement in symptoms of fever, anorexia and pain within one to two weeks. Cutaneous lesions usually resolve after one to two months of antibiotic treatment, although hyperpigmentation may persist at the site of bacillary angiomatosis lesions indefinitely. Hepatic lesions may require two to three months to resolve.

The drug of first choice for treatment of HIV-infected patients with bacillary angiomatosis, bacillary peliosis, or *Bartonella* bacteremia is erythromycin or doxycycline (Fig. 42-1). Erythromycin and doxycycline appear to have equivalent activity in treating bacillary angiomatosis; additionally, there does not appear to be a difference in treatment response whether bacillary angiomatosis is caused by *B. henselae* or *B. quintana*. Dosing for erythromycin should be 500 mg q6h PO or IV and for doxycycline should be 100 mg q12h PO or IV. Because of our more extensive experience with erythromycin than with other antibiotics, we usually initiate therapy for bacillary angiomatosis with erythromycin. However, doxycycline therapy is preferred over erythromycin in several settings; when *Bartonella* infection involves the CNS, or when severe gastrointestinal symptoms are present, or when the twice-daily dosing for doxycycline is likely to increase compliance.

Although the greatest numbers of HIV-infected patients have been successfully treated with erythromycin or doxycycline, other antibiotics should be considered in patients unable to tolerate either of these drugs. Experience with alternative antibiotics is very limited, but these include tetracycline, which was efficacious in an HIV-infected patient with bacillary angiomatosis,[4] or the newer macrolides. Azithromycin may be a useful alternative in patients unable to comply with two- or four-times-daily dosing with doxycycline or erythromycin. An azithromycin dose of 500 mg q24h PO was used for 28–90 days to treat five of the ten immunocompetent patients with *B. quintana* bacteremia reported by Spach et al.[46] Another report describes treatment of an immunocompromised patient with bacillary angiomatosis using azithromycin 1 gm q24h PO.[47] There are a few reports of treatment of immunocompetent patients with clarithromycin (250 mg q12h PO)[48,49], and either of these macrolides would seem to be a reasonable alternative if erythromycin cannot be used.

Intravenous therapy is recommended for patients with severe disease, especially in those patients with gastrointestinal involvement, nausea and vomiting, and in whom drug absorption may be impaired. Intravenous therapy also should be administered to patients with osteomyelitis and endocarditis. In very ill patients, treatment with combination therapy may be warranted; rifampin has demonstrated good *in vivo* activity and can be added to doxycycline or erythromycin. Treatment with rifampin alone should be avoided because of the high rate at which many bacteria develop spontaneous rifampin resistance. For patients whose infection fails to respond after 10 days of treatment, therapy should be changed to the other, first line drug, and rifampin added, or antibiotic therapy administered by the intravenous route, or both.

Toxicities, Complications and Their Management

Immunocompromised patients can develop a Jarisch–Herxheimer-like reaction after the first several doses of antibiotics for *Bartonella* infection.[4] Physicians should anticipate this possibility because it may be mistaken for an adverse drug reaction, resulting in an unnecessary change of antibiotic therapy. Patients should be informed, and those with severe respiratory or cardiovascular compromise should be monitored carefully after institution of antibiotic therapy.

Adverse reactions most frequently reported during erythromycin treatment include gastrointestinal symptoms (abdominal cramps, nausea, vomiting, and diarrhea) with either the oral or intravenous route, and thrombophlebitis with the intravenous route. Serious interactions can occur with concomitantly administered erythromycin and cisapride, cyclosporine, tacrolimus, theophylline (theophylline toxicity), warfarin (increased anticoagulation), digoxin (digoxin toxicity), and astemizole or terfenadine (torsades de pointes).[43]

Doxycycline-associated erosive esophagitis also has been well described, and most frequently occurs when a dose is taken with only a small amount of liquid, just before retiring.[44] Patients should take the evening doxycycline dose several hours before bedtime with a large amount of liquid. Doxycycline can cause gastrointestinal symptoms, dental discoloration in children, and photosensitivity reactions. Interactions of tetracyclines with oral anticoagulants may increase anticoagulation, and if given with oral contraceptive hormones may result in decreased efficacy resulting in pregnancy.[45]

PREVENTION

Environmental and Behavioral

Since the principal reservoir and vectors for *B. henselae* have been identified, some recommendations can be made to decrease the potential for human infection with this *Bartonella* species. The domestic cat is the major reservoir[19] as well as the most common vector of *B. henselae* to humans, via scratches and bites.[50,51] The arthropod vector for *B. henselae*, the cat flea, readily transmits this species between cats.[21] Although transmission of *B. henselae* to humans has never been demonstrated, control of flea infestation will decrease the potential for human exposure to *B. henselae* by reducing contamination of cat claws due to scratching and by decreasing feline infection. HIV-infected patients need not give up their pet cats, but should wash cat wounds immediately with soap and water, avoid rough play with cats and make their medical caregiver aware that they have a pet cat. If an immunocompromised individual wishes to acquire a pet cat, it preferably should be a mature cat (>1 year old); older cats are less likely to be bacteremic and less likely to scratch.[52] Testing of cats for *B. henselae* infection, or treatment of bacteremic cats, is not recommended.[52] It is not evident whether the bacterium can be eradicated from the cat, and giving the cat antibiotics incurs additional risk of scratches and bites for the owner.

B. quintana is transmitted by the body louse from human to human, and patients of low socioeconomic status are at highest risk for lice infestation.[5,46] The only current recommendation for preventing bacillary angiomatosis due to *B. quintana* is to avoid louse infestation, and caregivers should consider *Bartonella* infection in the differential diagnosis of homeless HIV-infected individuals with fever or vascular cutaneous lesions.

Approach to Prevention-Specific Drugs

Primary prophylaxis regimens for *Bartonella* infections have not been studied systematically and there is no current recommendation for primary prophylaxis. However, our case-control study of 49 patients with bacillary angiomatosis found that the macrolide class of antibiotics (e.g., erythromycin, clarithromycin) was the only class that was protective.[5] Trimethoprim/sulfamethoxazole, ciprofloxacin, dapsone, penicillin, and cephalosporin antibiotic classes were not protective against developing *Bartonella* infection. It is likely that regimens including a macrolide or rifabutin for prophylaxis or treatment of *Mycobacterium avium* complex infection will simultaneously provide prophylaxis or treatment of *Bartonella* infection.

After cessation of treatment for documented *Bartonella* infection, patients should be monitored carefully for relapse. *Bartonella* infection may recur at the same site or at a new site months later.[4] For patients who develop relapse of *Bartonella* infection, life-long secondary prophylaxis with a macrolide or doxycycline should be instituted after re-treatment.[53]

ACKNOWLEDGMENTS

Dr Koehler was supported by NIH grants R01 AI43703 and R01 AI52813, and a Burroughs Wellcome Fund Clinical Scientist Award in Translational Research.

REFERENCES

1. Koehler JE. *Bartonella*: an emerging human pathogen. In: Scheld WM, Armstrong D, Hughes JM (eds). Emerging Infections I. Washington, DC: American Society for Microbiology Press; 1998, p 147.
2. Cunningham ET Jr, Koehler JE. Ocular bartonellosis. Am J Ophthalmol 130:340–9, 2000.
3. Mohle-Boetani JC, Koehler JE, Berger TG, et al. Bacillary angiomatosis and bacillary peliosis in patients infected with human immunodeficiency virus: clinical characteristics in a case-control study. Clin Infect Dis 22:794–800, 1996.
4. Koehler JE, Quinn FD, Berger TG, et al. Isolation of *Rochalimaea* species from cutaneous and osseous lesions of bacillary angiomatosis. N Engl J Med 327:1625–31, 1992.
5. Koehler JE, Sanchez MA, Garrido CS, et al. Molecular epidemiology of *Bartonella* infections in patients with bacillary angiomatosis-peliosis. N Engl J Med 337:1876–83, 1997.

6. Berger TG, Tappero JW, Kaymen A, LeBoit PE. Bacillary (epithelioid) angiomatosis and concurrent Kaposi's sarcoma in acquired immunodeficiency syndrome. Arch Dermatol 125: 1543–7, 1989.
7. Koehler JE, Tappero JW. Bacillary angiomatosis and bacillary peliosis in patients infected with human immunodeficiency virus. Clin Infect Dis 17:612–24, 1993.
8. Perkocha LA, Geaghan SM, Yen TSB, et al. Clinical and pathological features of bacillary peliosis hepatis in association with human immunodeficiency virus infection. N Engl J Med 323:1581–6, 1990.
9. Cockerell CJ, Whitlow MA, Webster GF, Friedman-Kien AE. Epithelioid angiomatosis: a distinct vascular disorder in patients with the acquired immunodeficiency syndrome or AIDS-related complex. Lancet 2:654–6, 1987.
10. Rolain JM, Brouqui P, Koehler JE, Maguina C, et al. Recommendations for treatment of human infections caused by *Bartonella* species. Antimicrob Agents Chemother 48:1921–33, 2004.
11. Stoler MH, Bonfiglio TA, Steigbigel RT, Pereira M. An atypical subcutaneous infection associated with acquired immune deficiency syndrome. Am J Clin Pathol 80:714–8, 1983.
12. Relman DA, Loutit JS, Schmidt TM, et al. The agent of bacillary angiomatosis: an approach to the identification of uncultured pathogens. N Engl J Med 323:1573–80, 1990.
13. Slater LN, Welch DF, Hensel D, Coody DW. A newly recognized fastidious gram-negative pathogen as a cause of fever and bacteremia. N Engl J Med 323:1587–93, 1990.
14. Regnery RL, Anderson BE, Clarridge JE, et al. Characterization of a novel *Rochalimaea* species, *R. henselae sp. nov*., isolated from blood of a febrile, human immunodeficiency virus-positive patient. J Clin Microbiol 30:265–74, 1992.
15. Welch DF, Pickett DA, Slater LN, et al. *Rochalimaea henselae sp. nov.*, a cause of septicemia, bacillary angiomatosis, and parenchymal bacillary peliosis. J Clin Microbiol 30:275–80, 1992.
16. Brenner DJ, O'Connor SP, Winkler HH, Steigerwalt AG. Proposals to unify the genera *Bartonella* and *Rochalimaea*, with descriptions of *Bartonella quintana comb. nov.*, *Bartonella vinsonii comb. nov.*, *Bartonella henselae comb. nov., and Bartonella elizabethae comb. nov.,* and to remove the family *Bartonellaceae* from the order *Rickettsiales*. Int J Syst Bacteriol 43:777–86, 1993.
17. Birtles RJ, Harrison TG, Saunders NA, Molyneux DH. Proposals to unify the genera *Grahamella* and *Bartonella*, with descriptions of *Bartonella talpae comb. nov.*, *Bartonella peromysci comb. nov.*, and three new species, *Bartonella grahamii sp. nov.*, *Bartonella taylorii sp. nov.*, and *Bartonella doshiae sp. nov*. Int J Syst Bacteriol 45:1–8, 1995.
18. Tappero JW, Mohle-Boetani J, Koehler JE, et al. The epidemiology of bacillary angiomatosis and bacillary peliosis. JAMA 269:770–5, 1993.
19. Koehler JE, Glaser CA, Tappero JW. *Rochalimaea henselae* infection. A new zoonosis with the domestic cat as reservoir. JAMA 271:531–5, 1994.
20. Jameson P, Greene C, Regnery R, et al. Prevalence of *Bartonella henselae* antibodies in pet cats throughout regions of North America. J Infect Dis 172:1145–9, 1995.
21. Chomel BB, Kasten RW, Floyd-Hawkins K, et al. Experimental transmission of *Bartonella henselae* by the cat flea. J Clin Microbiol 34:1952–6, 1996.
22. Strong RP. Trench Fever: Report of Commission, Medical Research Committee, American Red Cross. Oxford: Oxford University Press; 1918.
23. von Krampitz HE. Weitere Untersuchungen an Grahamella Brumpt 1911. Zeitschr Tropenmed Parasitol 13:34–53, 1962.
24. Weinman D, Kreier JP. *Bartonella* and *Grahamella*. In: Kreier JP (ed). Parasitic Protozoa. San Diego: Academic Press; 1977, p 197.
25. Lawson PA, Collins MD. Description of *Bartonella clarridgeiae sp. nov.* isolated from the cat of a patient with *Bartonella henselae septicemia*. Med Microbiol Lett 5:64–73, 1996.
26. Myers WF, Osterman JV, Wisseman CL, Jr. Nutritional studies of *Rickettsia quintana*: nature of the hematin requirement. J Bacteriol 109:89–95, 1972.
27. LeBoit PE, Berger TG, Egbert BM, et al. Bacillary angiomatosis: the histopathology and differential diagnosis of a pseudoneoplastic infection in patients with human immunodeficiency virus disease. Am J Surg Pathol 13:909–20, 1989.
28. Reed JA, Brigati DJ, Flynn SD, et al. Immunocytochemical identification of *Rochalimaea henselae* in bacillary (epithelioid) angiomatosis, parenchymal bacillary peliosis, and persistent fever with bacteremia. Am J Surg Pathol 16:650–7, 1992.
29. La Scola B, Raoult D. Culture of *Bartonella quintana* and *Bartonella henselae* from human samples: a 5-year experience (1993 to 1998). J Clin Microbiol 37:1899–905, 1999.
30. Dougherty MJ, Spach DH, Larson AM, et al. Evaluation of an extended blood culture protocol to isolate fastidious organisms from patients with AIDS. J Clin Microbiol 34:2444–7, 1996.
31. Dalton MJ, Robinson LE, Cooper J, et al. Use of *Bartonella* antigens for serologic diagnosis of cat-scratch disease at a national referral center. Arch Intern Med 155:1670–6, 1995.
32. Tappero J, Regnery R, Koehler J. Detection of serologic response to *Rochalimaea henselae* in patients with bacillary angiomatosis (BA) by immunofluorescent antibody (IFA) testing. Presented at the 32nd Interscience Conference on Antimicrobial Agents and Chemotherapy, American Society for Microbiology, 1992.
33. Myers WF, Grossman DM, Wisseman CLJ. Antibiotic susceptibility patterns in *Rochalimaea quintana*, the agent of trench fever. Antimicrob Agents Chemother 25:690–3, 1984.
34. Koehler JE, LeBoit PE, Egbert BM, Berger TG. Cutaneous vascular lesions and disseminated cat-scratch disease in patients with the acquired immunodeficiency syndrome (AIDS) and AIDS-related complex. Ann Intern Med 109:449–55, 1988.
35. Berger TG, Koehler JE. Bacillary angiomatosis. AIDS Clin Rev 1993/1994 43–60, 1993.
36. Maurin M, Gasquet S, Ducco C, Raoult D. MICs of 28 antibiotic compounds for 14 *Bartonella* (formerly *Rochalimaea*) isolates. Antimicrob Agents Chemother 39:2387–91, 1995.
37. Colson P, Lebrun L, Drancourt M, et al. Multiple recurrent bacillary angiomatosis due to *Bartonella quintana* in an HIV-infected patient [letter]. Eur J Clin Microbiol Infect Dis 15:178–80, 1996.
38. Wolfson C, Branley J, Gottlieb T. The Etest for antimicrobial susceptibility testing of *Bartonella henselae*. J Antimicrob Chemother 38:963–8, 1996.
39. Maurin M, Raoult D. Antimicrobial susceptibility of *Rochalimaea quintana*, *Rochalimaea vinsonii*, and the newly recognized *Rochalimaea henselae*. J Antimicrob Chemother 32:587–94, 1993.
40. Tappero JW, Koehler JE. Cat scratch disease and bacillary angiomatosis [letter]. JAMA 266:1938–9, 1991.
41. Bass JW, Freitas BC, Freitas AD, et al. Prospective randomized double blind placebo-controlled evaluation of azithromycin for treatment of cat-scratch disease. Pediatr Infect Dis J 17:447–52, 1998.
42. Foucault C, Raoult D, Brouqui P. Randomized open trial of gentamicin and doxycycline for eradication of *Bartonella quintana* from blood in patients with chronic bacteremia. Antimicrob Agents Chemother 47:2204–7, 2003.
43. Sivapalasingam S, Steigbigel NH. Macrolides, clindamycin and ketolides. In: Mandell GL, Bennett JE, Dolin R (eds). Principles and Practice of Infectious Diseases. New York: Elsevier Churchill Livingstone; 2005, p 396.
44. Kikendall JW, Friedman AC, Oyewole MA, et al. Pill-induced esophageal injury. Case reports and review of the medical literature. Dig Dis and Sci 28:174–82, 1983.

45. Meyers B, Salvatore M. Tetracyclines and chloramphenicol. In: Mandell GL, Bennett JE, Dolin R (eds) Principles and Practice of Infectious Diseases. New York: Elsevier Churchill Livingstone; 2005, p 356.
46. Spach DH, Kanter AS, Dougherty MJ, et al. *Bartonella (Rochalimaea) quintana* bacteremia in inner-city patients with chronic alcoholism. N Engl J Med 332:424–8, 1995.
47. Guerra LG, Neira CJ, Boman D, et al. Rapid response of AIDS-related bacillary angiomatosis to azithromycin. Clin Infect Dis 17:264–6, 1993.
48. Bakker RC, van Heukelem H, van de Sandt MM, Bergmans AM. Visceral granulomas and pericardial effusion caused by a *Bartonella henselae* infection. Ned Tijdschr voor Geneeskd 141388–90:388–90, 1997.
49. Heizmann WR, Schalasta G, Moling O, Pegoretti S. Cat scratch disease. *Bartonella henselae* antibodies and DNA detection in regional lymphadenopathy. Dtsch Med Wochenschr 121:622–6, 1996.
50. Carithers HA. Cat-scratch disease: an overview based on a study of 1,200 patients. Am J Dis Child 139:1124–33, 1985.
51. Margileth AM. Cat scratch disease: a therapeutic dilemma. Vet Clin N Am 17:91–103, 1987.
52. Regnery RL, Childs JE, Koehler JE. Infections associated with *Bartonella* species in persons infected with human immunodeficiency virus. Clin Infect Dis 21(Suppl 1):S94–8, 1995.
53. Kaplan JE, Masur H, Holmes KK. Guidelines for preventing opportunistic infections among HIV-infected persons – 2002. Recommendations of the U.S. Public Health Service and the Infectious Diseases Society of America. MMWR Recomm Rep 51:1–52, 2002.

Chapter 43

Cryptococcosis

Judith A. Aberg, MD, William G. Powderly, MD

Disseminated cryptococcosis has been the most common life-threatening fungal infection in patients with acquired immunodeficiency syndrome (AIDS), affecting up to 8% of patients with advanced human immunodeficiency virus (HIV) infection.[1–3] In limited resource settings such as sub-Saharan Africa, the prevalence may be much higher and in one study accounted for 17% of all deaths in an AIDS cohort in Uganda.[3a] The most common manifestation is meningoencephalitis, although disseminated disease is well-described, and localized infection of many organs can occur. Carefully conducted clinical trials have helped define effective therapy for this infection, although many issues in management remain unresolved. This chapter reviews the microbiology, pathogenesis, epidemiology, clinical syndromes, and treatment of cryptococcosis in patients with AIDS.

MICROBIOLOGY

There are more than 20 known species of *Cryptococcus,*[4] but *C. neoformans* is essentially the only human pathogen, although there have been isolated case reports of infection with *Cryptococcus albidus* and *Cryptococcus laurenti. C. neoformans* is an encapsulated, round to oval yeast that reproduces by narrow-based budding. It has a surrounding polysaccharide capsule ranging from 1+ mm to more than 30+ mm when cultivated in the laboratory.[5] In its natural environment, it is smaller and poorly encapsulated. Mycelia are produced bearing basidiospores ranging from 1 to 8+ mm in its perfect state (*Filobasidiella neoformans*). *F. neoformans* has never been isolated from patients or in nature.[6] During the exponential growth phase of *Cryptococcus,* the generation or doubling time ranges from 2.5 to 6.0 h.

There are two pathogenic varieties, *C. neoformans* var *neoformans* and *C. neoformans* var *gattii,* which can be distinguished on the basis of capsular serotypes.[5,7] These two varieties differ in geographic distribution; but their growth requirements for temperature, phenol oxidase production, and capsule formation are similar. They can also be distinguished by growth characteristics on canavanine-glycine-bromthymol blue agar. The serotypes of *C. neoformans* are designated A, B, C, and D based on antigenic determinants on the polysaccharide capsule.[8] Serotypes A and D (*C. neoformans* var *neoformans*) are the most common cause of infection and are most often seen in immunocompromised hosts. Serotypes B and C (*C. neoformans* var *gattii*) are endemic in Australia and southern California, are usually isolated from normal hosts, and have a predilection for invading the central nervous system (CNS).[9,10] Although the incidence of cryptococcosis in AIDS patients appears to vary geographically, even in areas where var *gattii* is endemic, most of the isolates from patients with AIDS are var *neoformans*.[11,12] The genotypic features of *C. neoformans* were actively pursued during the 1990s, now with more than 20 genes cloned and sequenced.[13–27] Electrophoretic karyotyping has identified 12 genes in *C. neoformans* var *neoformans* compared to 13 genes in *C. neoformans* var *gattii*.[14]

PATHOGENESIS AND HOST DEFENSE MECHANISMS

It is postulated that initial infection occurs via inhalation of the basidiospores or unencapsulated forms, leading to subsequent colonization of the airways and subsequent respiratory infection.[8,28] *C. neoformans* has been isolated from the nasopharynx of ~50% of AIDS patients with cryptococcosis, whereas *C. neoformans* has not been isolated from AIDS patients without cryptococcosis.[29] The initial immune response correlates best with polymorphonuclear leukocyte activity more than macrophage activity. However, the role of pulmonary macrophages is paramount in the host's control of the yeast inoculum,[30] and complement-mediated phagocytosis appears to be the primary initial defense against cryptococcal invasion.[5] Other host–yeast interactions, such as the role of CD4+ T-lymphocyte and CD8 + T cells, as well as the role of cytokines, also appear to be important.[30–33] It is clear that the absence of an intact cell-mediated response results in ineffective ingestion and killing of the organism, leading to dissemination and increased cryptococcal burden. In murine models both CD4+ T-lymphocyte and CD8+ T cells are required to inhibit cryptococcosis. Natural killer (NK) cells also appear to have a limited role.[30,34] Specifically, interleukin-2 (IL-2)-activated T and NK cells can inhibit *C. neoformans*.[35] The role of humoral immunity in the control of cryptococcal infections is controversial. *In vitro* studies of antibodies to the soluble capsular polysaccharide of *C. neoformans* have revealed enhanced phagocytosis, increased fungicidal activity of leukocytes, and increased fungistatic activity of NK cells.[36–39] Animal models of both polyclonal and monoclonal antibody immunization have had varying results.[40–43]

Factors associated with the virulence of *C. neoformans* include its polysaccharide capsule, production of melanin, the mating type, and growth at 37°C (thermotolerance).[44–46] The polysaccharide capsule, composed mainly of glucuronoxylomannan, was the first *C. neoformans* virulence factor associated with disease.[47] There is also some evidence of an interaction between *C. neoformans* and HIV-1 *in vitro*. Soluble *C. neoformans* capsular polysaccharide is able to enhance HIV infection in cultured cells, subsequent production of HIV-1, and *in vitro* production of syncytia.[48] Additionally, a study of dual immunocytochemical staining for HIV-1 and cryptococcal antigen in brain tissue of AIDS patients showing anatomic co-localization of both pathogens suggests a possible synergistic effect of virus and yeast *in vivo*.[49]

C. neoformans is distinguished from other yeasts by its ability to assimilate urea and its possession of membrane-bound phenol oxidase enzymes, which are able to convert phenolic compounds into melanin. *C. neoformans* strains that produce melanin are more virulent in mouse models than strains that do not produce melanin.[38,39] In addition, murine cells with melanin appear more resistant to phagocytosis.[45] It is postulated that the propensity of *C. neoformans* to invade the CNS may be due to its ability to synthesize melanin from catecholamines, which are present in large concentrations there.[49]

EPIDEMIOLOGY

In the developed world prior to the use of more effective antiretroviral therapy (ART), ~5–10% of patients with AIDS developed cryptococcal meningitis. In 1991 the annual prevalence of cryptococcosis among HIV-infected patients in New York was estimated to be 6.1–8.5%.[50] There is considerable geographic variation in the prevalence of cryptococcal infection. In the United States it is more common in residents east of the Mississippi river.[51] The incidence of cryptococcosis among AIDS patients is higher in Africa and Southeast Asia than the United States, whereas it appears less often in Europe.[9] The male/female ratio among AIDS patients is essentially 1:1. Cryptococcosis in children with AIDS is less common, with a prevalence rate of ~1.4%.[52] The clinical and laboratory characteristics of cryptococcosis in children is comparable to those seen in adults.

More than three-fourths of the cases associated with AIDS develop when the CD4 T-lymphocyte count falls below 50 cells/mL.[51] Cryptococcosis is the initial AIDS-defining illness in 50–60% of patients and thus tends to be seen more commonly in patients in whom HIV infection has not yet been diagnosed. Risk factors that have been suggested for the development of cryptococcosis include black race, injection drug use, cigarette smoking, and several environmental exposures (presumed areas where pigeon droppings accumulate). No differences in demographic variables, HIV risk factors, or stage of AIDS was found in a case-controlled study. It is of note that the investigators were unable to detect an increased risk of the development of cryptococcal meningitis in patients who had received short and episodic courses of steroids.[53]

The annual incidence of invasive *C. neoformans* in the United States has declined in HIV-infected patients during the years since 1990. Between 1987 and 1992, cryptococcosis decreased from sixth to ninth place in rank order for infections associated with death in HIV-infected persons.[3] This epidemiologic trend preceded the use of highly active antiretroviral therapy (HAART) and has been temporally associated with the increased use of fluconazole since its licensure in 1990.[54] It is of note that in a large prospective, population-based surveillance study patients who had received fluconazole were significantly less likely to develop cryptococcosis, and decreases in the incidence of cryptococcosis from 1992 to 1994 were attributed to the increased use of azoles.[55] A more recent review of the Kaiser Permanente medical record database from 1981 to 2000 reported similar findings whereas the highest incidence of cryptococcosis in men occurred from 1981 to 1985 and in women from 1986 to 1990.[55a]

A 56.5% decrease in the incidence of cryptococcal meningitis was reported between 1996 and 1997 at San Francisco general hospital, correlating with a 30% increased use of potent ART that included a protease inhibitor (PI).[56] However, the decrease in incidence of crytococcosis was even more dramatic when one compared the 1995 incidence with 1996 prior to the introduction of PIs. This suggests that patients may have been receiving benefit from the use of nucleosides alone as well as the use of azoles. Furthermore, the incidence of cryptococcal meningitis had increased 30% between 1997 and 1998 and has remained constant, occurring primarily in individuals not taking potent ART.[57]

CLINICAL FEATURES AND DIAGNOSIS

CNS Disease

The most common manifestation of cryptococcosis is meningoencephalitis. The time span between the appearance of

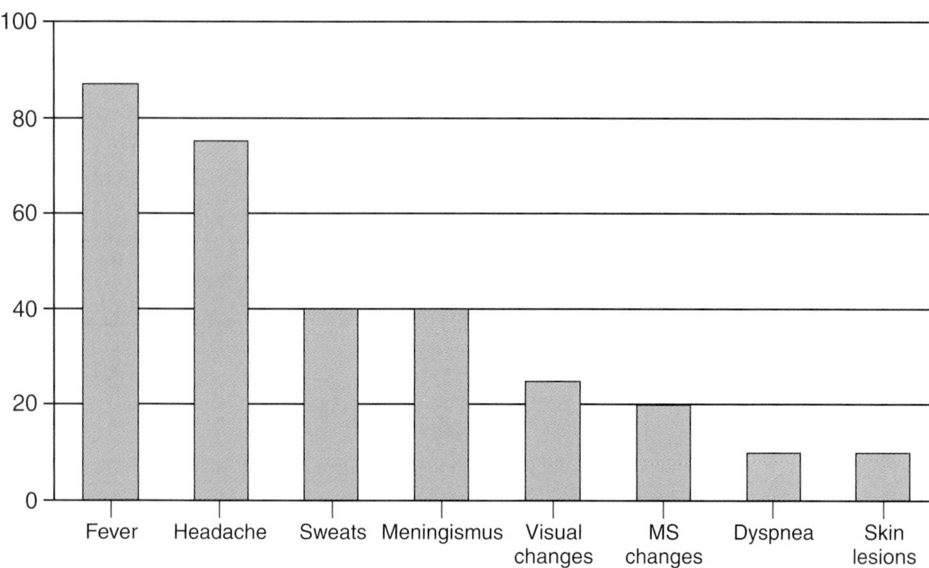

Figure 43-1 ■ Symptoms of cryptococcal meningitis. MS, mental status.

symptoms and diagnosis ranges from days to months.[58] The clinical presentation may be nonspecific (Fig. 43-1), although infection typically presents as a subacute process.[59] Symptoms may range from headache, nausea, irritability, and decline in cognitive function to frank obtundation. Physical findings may include fever and abnormal neurologic examination, with cranial nerve palsies, hyperreflexia, and papilledema. Complications of CNS infection include hydrocephalus, motor or sensory deficits, cerebellar dysfunction, seizures, and dementia. Prompt inclusion of *C. neoformans* in the differential diagnosis of acute and chronic meningitis for susceptible hosts should allow for prompt brain imaging study followed by lumbar puncture once a mass lesion has been ruled out. Although focal lesions caused by intracerebral granulomas (cryptococcomas) may be seen on computed tomography (CT) or magnetic resonance imaging (MRI), they are uncommon in patients with AIDS.[60] Acute cryptococcal meningitis in patients with AIDS is often complicated by cerebral edema. Assessment should include measuring the opening pressure by manometry in all patients. The opening pressure is usually higher than 25 cm H_2O in 60% of patients.[61] Abnormal findings in the composition of cerebrospinal fluid (CSF) include a lymphocytic pleocytosis, elevated protein, and low glucose.[59] However, as many as 20% of patients have no clear abnormality in the CSF profile despite positive cultures for *C. neoformans*. Therefore finding a normal CSF should not exclude the possibility of cryptococcal infection. Detection of CSF cryptococcal antigen by rapid diagnostic testing should prompt initiation of therapy.

Pulmonary Cryptococcosis

Although the lung is most likely the entry portal, isolated pulmonary cryptococcosis is diagnosed less frequently than meningitis in AIDS patients.[62,63] However, pulmonary involvement in the presence of disseminated disease is common. More than 10% of patients with disseminated disease may have acute respiratory failure.[64] It is unclear if disseminated disease always represents progression of pulmonary disease because many patients have no evidence of pulmonary involvement at the time of diagnosis of disseminated disease. Given the relatively nonspecific clinical signs and symptoms, variable radiographic signs, and increased frequency of other pulmonary opportunistic infections, it is likely that cryptococcal pneumonia is underdiagnosed and not recognized until dissemination. In a retrospective study aimed at determining the etiology of pulmonary symptoms in HIV-positive patients with cryptococcal meningitis, 14 of 18 patients (78%) reported respiratory symptoms within 4 months prior to the diagnosis of cryptococcal meningitis.[65] Other reviews suggest that 63% to 90% of HIV-infected patients with pulmonary cryptococcosis have concomitant extrapulmonary disease.[62,66] However, pulmonary disease may not always be cryptococcal in origin; ~15% of HIV-infected patients with proven cryptococcal disease have a second pulmonary pathogen, such as *Pneumocystis carinii, Mycobacterium tuberculosis,* or nontuberculous mycobacteria.[62,67]

In a retrospective chart review of 210 patients with cryptococcal disease,[64] independent variables predictive of acute respiratory failure included black race, lactacte dehydrogenase level of +500 IU/L, the presence of interstitial infiltrates, and the presence of cutaneous lesions. Mortality was 100% for the 19 patients in whom the respiratory failure could be attributed solely to cryptococcosis.

Patients with pulmonary cryptococcosis may present with cough, fever, malaise, shortness of breath, pleuritic pain, and an abnormal chest radiograph. Chest radiographs typically reveal focal or diffuse infiltrates similar to other opportunistic pathogens, particularly *Pneumocystis carinii* pneumonia (PCP). Other chest radiographic findings not as commonly seen include solitary subpleural nodules, mass-like infiltrates with consolidation, hilar and mediastinal adenopathy, and pleural effusions. Rarely, cavitation and empyema have been reported.[68]

Patients with apparently isolated cryptococcal pneumonia should be evaluated for cryptococcal meningitis with a lumbar puncture even in the absence of neurologic signs or symptoms. In addition, antifungal therapy should be initiated because early treatment of localized pulmonary cryptococcosis can be effective and can prevent dissemination.[69]

Other Organ Involvement

Cryptococcosis in HIV-positive patients is typically disseminated; and up to three-fourths of patients with meningitis have positive blood cultures. A small percentage of patients with cryptococcosis present initially with extrapulmonary, nonmeningeal disease, although many are subsequently found to have meningitis. Infections of the skin, joints, eye, adrenal glands, gastrointestinal tract, liver, pancreas, peritoneum, heart, prostate, and urinary tract have been described.[70–77] The prostate can serve as a reservoir of infection and is a potential source of reinfection after completion of therapy.[78] Cutaneous cryptococcosis is usually a sign of dissemination but may precede evidence of disease elsewhere by several weeks.[70,79] The lesions vary greatly and mimic many other dermatologic entities. The most typical have an appearance resembling molluscum contagiosum,[80] but cryptococcal skin disease may present as pustules, vesicles, plaques, abscesses, cellulitis, purpura, draining sinus, or subcutaneous swelling.[81]

Immune Reconstitution Inflammatory Syndrome

Unlike infections with *Mycobacterium avium* complex and cytomegalovirus, there had been few reported cases of unusual manifestations of cryptococcal disease associated with HAART. One report[82] suggested that three patients had partial immune reconstitution unmasking latent cryptococcal therapy but it is unclear if these cases truly represented immune reconstitution. Two of the patients developed cryptococcal meningitis shortly after starting HAART; both patients had nadir CD4 T-lymphocyte counts less than 50 cells/μL and CD4+ T-lymphocyte counts less than 150 cells/μL after "therapy" at the time they were diagnosed with cryptococcal meningitis. The CSF analyses were typical of those seen with cryptococcal meningitis. A third patient with a recent history of cryptococcal meningitis on itraconazole developed aseptic meningitis with leukocytosis 10 days after starting HAART. This patient's therapy was not altered, and the meningeal symptoms resolved spontaneously. There had also been two reports of cryptococcal lymphadenitis in patients receiving potent ART.[83,84]

More recently, there have been several larger case series reporting significant complications of cryptococcal-related immune reconstitution inflammatory syndrome (IRIS). Investigators from Dallas, Texas described four cases of IRIS and included a literature review of 21 additional cases.[84a] The presentations included 14 with lymphadenitis, 10 CNS complications characterized by meningitis in six and mass lesions in four as well as one pulmonary cavitary lesion. The median CD4 T-lymphocyte count at time of cryptococcal diagnosis and prior to HAART was 25 cells. The median CD4 T-lymphocyte count at time of IRIS was 197 cells and the median time to development of IRIS after cryptococcal diagnosis and initiation of HAART was 11 months (range 7 weeks to 3 years) and 7 months (range <2 weeks to 22 months), respectively. In all but one patient, the clinical manifestations resolved and four patients required anti-inflammatory medications to control their signs and symptoms.

Puthanakit and colleagues in Thailand reported an IRIS incidence of 19% among 153 symptomatic HIV-infected children of which three were attributable to cryptococcal infection.[84b] IRIS events occurred at a median of 4 weeks (range 2–31) after HAART.

Shelburne[84c] and colleagues conducted a retrospective review of 84 patients with HIV associated crypotococcal disease. Of note, the authors addressed the difficulty in diagnosing what is IRIS versus relapsed disease. For the diagnosis of the culture-negative meningitis form of IRIS, all of the following criteria had to be met: (1) the patient's condition had clinically responded to anticryptococcal therapy; (2) after the initiation of HAART, the original symptoms returned or new inflammatory symptoms developed; and (3) during the diagnostic workup for the inflammatory process, all results of cultures had to be negative, and CSF cryptococcal antigen, if still present, had to have a level that had decreased at least four-fold from the level at the initial admission to the hospital. They also included three patients who had subclinical cryptococcal disease who developed acute disease within 180 days after initiating HAART. Of the 84 patients, 59 initiated HAART and 18 (30.5%) of the 59 developed IRIS as defined above with a median time of 30 days (range 3–330 days) after HAART. Patients who developed IRIS were more likely to be antiretroviral-naive, have a higher CSF cryptocococcal antigen, higher baseline HIV viral load and to have initiated HAART within 30 days after cryptococcal diagnosis. At the time of IRIS diagnosis, these patients had higher CSF opening pressures, increased CSF WBCs and higher glucose compared with the typical presentation of acute cryptocococcal meningitis. Although there was no statistical difference in mortality at 18 months of follow-up between those who had IRIS compared with those who did not, there was a trend towards survival benefit in the IRIS group in contrast to that found by Lorthlary and colleagues.[84d] They conducted a retrospective chart review of 120 HIV-infected individuals with cryptococcal disease who initiated HAART. Ten patients developed IRIS within a median of 8 months (range 2–37 months) after HAART. Three of the 10 patients with IRIS died. They reported having unpreviously diagnosed HIV, CD4 T-lymphocyte count <7 and HAART within 2 months of cryptococcosis diagnosis were independently associated with risk of developing IRIS.

These reports have prompted some clinicians to avoid prescribing HAART within the first 2–3 months following the diagnosis of cryptococcosis; however, there is no prospective data comparing the timing of HAART and development of IRIS with outcomes to make specific recommendations. Studies are underway evaluating the timing of when to start HAART in the setting of acute opportunisitic infections which hopefully will provide valuable insight into this complication and its management.

Diagnostic Evaluation

The diagnosis is confirmed by isolating *Cryptococcus* from a sterile body site or by histopathology; the diagnosis can also be inferred by detecting cryptococcal capsular antigen in serum or CSF. The India ink stain, which outlines the polysaccharide capsule, is positive on direct examination of the CSF in ~80% of patients. Encapsulated yeasts seen after alcian blue, mucicarmine, or Gomori methenamine silver staining are diagnostic of *Cryptococcus*. Other stains, such as Fontana–Masson and periodic acid-Schiff, reveal yeast cells but are not specific for *Cryptococcus*.

Cryptococcal antigen in the CSF is produced locally in the subarachnoid space by the invading yeast and does not represent active or passive diffusion from the serum into the CNS. Soluble circulating serum cryptococcal antigen (sCRAG) has been found only in patients with substantial infection. Several commercial latex agglutination tests (LAT) kits and one enzyme-linked immunoassay (EIA) test for detection of cryptococcal antigen in serum and CSF are widely available. The detection of CRAG in serum and CSF by latex agglutination is rapid and has a sensitivity and specificity of more than 95%.[85,86] Comparative performance of four LATs and one EIA commercially available test revealed high concordance of all tests for CSF specimens, with sensitivities of 93–100% and specificities of 93–98%.[86] Pronase-containing latex tests reduce the number of false-positive sCRAGs.[86] False-positives can also occur secondary to infection with *Trichosporon beigelii*, which cross-reacts with the antigen.[87] In addition, false-positives have occurred secondary to residual disinfectant on laboratory test slides.[88] False-negatives may occur with low cryptococcal antigen concentrations. Although serum cryptococcal antigens are positive in 95–99% of cryptococcal meningitis cases, a positive result does not indicate that CNS invasion is present. Conversely, a negative sCRAG suggests that the patient is unlikely to have CNS disease; the test may be useful for screening symptomatic patients. The utility of sCRAG in asymptomatic HIV patients as a screening tool has not been adequately studied.[89] Although routine screening for cryptococcal antigen in asymptomatic patients is not recommended, if a positive titer is noted in an asymptomatic patient, therapy should be offered [89] because of the risk of its progressing to disseminated disease. The CDC is conducting a study to evaluate the utility of sCRAG in limited resource setting where the access to HAART is problematic and the incidence of cryptococcal disease is much higher than in the developed world. One could perceive that it may be a useful screen for subclinical disease at the time of initiating HAART given the potential risk of unmasking latent disease; however those studies need to be completed before recommendations for its routine use can be made.

There is little value in serial measurements of CSF and sCRAG for routine management of cryptococcal meningitis.[89a,90,91] CSF cryptococcal antigen titers should decrease after effective therapy. However, there is no evidence to support following the serum antigen serially, which shows no correlation with the outcome of antifungal therapy.[92] Management decisions should be based on an individual clinical assessment, not relying on cryptococcal antigen titers alone. There is insufficient data in interpretation of CRAG tests which become negative and subsequently become positive again, however, it is advised to caution on the side of a recurrence and begin a diagnostic work-up for recurrent disease.

TREATMENT

The reported acute mortality with treatment in patients with AIDS is 10–25%.[59,93–95] Prior to AIDS the standard therapy for cryptococcal meningitis had been to use the combination of amphotericin B and flucytosine, with a trend toward using lower doses of amphotericin B and a shorter duration of treatment.[96,97] A study of HIV-negative patients conducted by the National Institute of Allergy and Infectious Diseases (NIAID)-sponsored Mycosis Study Group (MSG)[96] compared 4 weeks of combination therapy with a 6-week course. That study was designed to randomize patients at the end of a uniform 4-week course of combination therapy. Only 91 of 181 patients initially treated were randomized. Of these 91 patients, cure or improvement was seen in 75% of those receiving 4 weeks of therapy compared with 85% of those in the 6-week cohort. There was no difference in toxicity between the two regimens. It is important to note that 31 of 80 nonrandomized patients died, giving a 17% overall acute mortality rate with this treatment for cryptococcal meningitis. The conclusions from this study were that 4 weeks of combination therapy was acceptable for patients who did not have risk factors that correlated with a high frequency of relapse.

Although there were few HIV-positive patients in the trial, one important risk factor that was predictive of relapse was immunosuppression. Thus more prolonged courses of amphotericin B and flucytosine were used initially in the AIDS epidemic. However, early reports of the experience with the amphotericin B/flucytosine regimens in patients with AIDS were not favorable. Indeed, data suggested that flucytosine was too toxic in AIDS patients and was not beneficial.[59]

The poor outcomes and increased incidence of cryptococcal meningitis in AIDS led to a search for more effective primary treatment. This became particularly relevant with the availability of the orally active antifungal triazoles fluconazole and itraconazole (Table 43-1). Initial experience with these agents was encouraging[98–101] and led to a number of controlled comparative trials (Table 43-2).

A small randomized, controlled study compared fluconazole 400 mg/day to amphotericin B with flucytosine in

Drugs used to Treat Cryptococcal Infection

Table 43-1

Agent	Usual Dose(s)	Side-Effects	Drug Interactions	Comments
Amphotericin B	Amphotericin B (deoxycholate) 0.7–1.0 mg kg^{-1} day^{-1} Liposomal amphotericin B3–6 mg kg^{-1} day^{-1} Amphotericin B lipid complex 5 mg kg^{-1} day^{-1}	Immediate hypersensitivity reactions, fever, hypotension, nausea and vomiting during administration, hypokalemia, nephropathy	Nephrotoxic drugs (e.g., aminoglycosides, pentamidine, foscarnet, cidofovir)	
Flucytosine	25 mg kg q6 h	Gastrointestinal, bone marrow suppression	Nephrotoxic drugs	Dosage must be reduced in patients with renal dysfunction
Fluconazole	400 mg day^{-1} (acute therapy); 200 mg day^{-1} (suppressive therapy)	Nausea, rash, hepatitis	Rifabutin (increased rifabutin levels); rifampin (decreased fluconazole levels) Nevriapine (NVP) (increase NVP levels)	
Itraconazole	200–400 mg bid PO	Nausea, abdominal pain, rash, headache, edema, hypokalemia	Rifamycin, ritonavir, phenobarbital, phenytoin all decrease itraconazole levels. Effect of nevirapine is unknown. The drug should not be used concomitantly with terfenadine or astemizole. Antacids, H_2-blockers decrease itraconazole absorption. Itraconazole itself acts as a moderate inhibitor of the cytochrome P450 system and can increase levels of indinavir, cyclosporin, digoxin, and phenytoin	Absorption of itraconazole is dependent on food and gastric acid and may be erratic. The newer solution is better absorbed

AIDS patients.[102] Patients were initially given amphotericin B 0.7 mg kg^{-1} day^{-1} for 7 days; the frequency was then changed to three times a week for 9 weeks. Of 14 patients randomized to fluconazole, eight failed, in contrast to no failures among those given combination therapy. Of the 16 fluconazole patients, four died; there were no deaths among six patients in the combination group. The trial was terminated early because of the higher failure and mortality rates seen in the fluconazole group. Another small study compared itraconazole 200 mg bid with amphotericin B 0.3 mg kg^{-1} day^{-1} plus flucytosine 150 mg kg^{-1} day^{-1}.[103] A 41% failure rate was reported in the itraconazole group compared to no failures in the combination group for primary treatment. More relapses were seen in the group initially treated with itraconazole.

In contrast to these apparently superior results with amphotericin B, a randomized, prospective trial conducted by the NIAID[104] comparing fluconazole to amphotericin B for treatment of acute cryptococcal meningitis in AIDS failed to show any significant differences in outcomes between the two regimens. The median dose of amphotericin B in this study was 0.4 mg/kg; flucytosine, the use of which was at the discretion of the investigators, was rarely employed. Fewer than 50% of patients in either group were successfully treated, as judged by clearance of cryptococci from their CSF cultures. However, there were hints of differences between the two regimens. Although there was no significant difference in the overall mortality between the two groups, the mortality was higher during the first 2 weeks of therapy with fluconazole. As with some other trials, the dose of amphotericin B may have been too low.

Initial therapy with azoles alone does not appear to be the most effective approach to treatment. A study comparing

Randomized Trials of Treatment of Cryptococcal Meningitis in AIDS

Table 43-2

Trial	Agents (Dose)	No. of Patients	Mycologic Response[a] (%)	Comments
Primary Infection				
Larsen et al[102]	Amphotericin B (0.7 mg kg^{-1}day^{-1}) and flucytosine (5-FC) (150 mg kg^{-1} day^{-1}) vs	7	100	Study stopped because of increased mortality in fluconazole group
	Fluconazole 200 mg qd	14	43	
De Gans et al[103]	Amphotericin B (0.3 mg kg^{-1} day^{-1}) and 5-FC (150 mg kg^{-1} day^{-1}) vs	11	100	Amphotericin B regimen superior
	Itraconazole 200 mg twice daily	14	50	
Saag et al[104]	Amphotericin (0.4 mg kg^{-1} day^{-1})[b]	63	40	No significant difference between regimens
	Fluconazole 200–400 g day^{-1}[c]	131	34	
Moskovitz et al[105]	Fluconazole 400 mg daily vs	40	41	Study confined to patients with 'good prognostic features'
	Itraconazole 200 mg twice daily	33	38	
Van der Horst et al[106]	Part A[d]			
	Amphotericin B (0.7 mg kg^{-1} day^{-1})	179	51	Difference between arms in part A were not significant (NS) ($P = 0.06$)
	vs Amphotericin B (0.7 mg kg^{-1} day^{-1}) plus 5-FC (100 mg kg^{-1} day^{-1})	202	60	
	Part B[e]			Differences in second part were NS, but the null hypothesis that fluconazole was superior could not be rejected
	Fluconazole 400 mg day^{-1} vs	151	72	
	Itraconazole 400 mg day^{-1}	155	60	
Hamill et al[107]	Amphotericin B deoxycholate (0.7 mg kg^{-1} day^{-1}) vs	87	54	All patients received 2 weeks of amphotericin followed by fluconazole for a total of 10 weeks. Differences in responses between groups were NS. More nephrotoxicity in amphotericin deoxycholate arm
	Liposomal amphotericin B (3 mg kg^{-1} day^{-1}) vs	86	63	
	Liposomal amphotericin B (6 mg kg^{-1} day^{-1})	94	54	
Suppressive Therapy				
Bozzette et al[108]	Fluconazole 200 mg day vs	34	3	Fluconazole superior
	Placebo	27	37	
Powderly et al[109]	Fluconazole 200 mg PO qd vs	119	2	Fluconazole superior ($P < 0.001$)
	Amphotericin B 1 mg kg^{-1}IV q week	88	18	
Saag et al[110]	Fluconazole 200 mg day vs	52	4	Fluconazole superior ($P = 0.003$)
	Itraconazole 200 mg day	57	23	

[a]Response is defined as mycologic clearance (CSF cultures negative) by the end of treatment (6–10 weeks depending on study; 2 weeks for part A of van der Horst study and for Hamill study) for the acute trials and as relapse rate for the suppressive trials.
[b]Median dose. Investigators were allowed to use any dose from 0.3 to 0.6 mg^{-1} kg^{-1} day. 5-FC was used in 14% of patients.
[c]Patients were treated with 200 mg initially; dose could be increased to 400 mg at the investigator's discretion.
[d]Part A was followed for the first 2 weeks of treatment.
[e]Part B was followed during weeks 3–10 of treatment.

itraconazole 200 mg bid PO and fluconazole 400 mg daily PO as primary treatment of cryptococcal meningitis in patients with AIDS showed no statistical significance in CSF sterilization between the two groups.[105] However, the study was terminated early partly because the clinical response rate was only ~40%. Thus no prospective randomized trial of triazoles given as initial therapy to unselected patients has shown a response rate higher than 50%.

In light of these data, the NIAID's MSG and AIDS Clinical Trials Group (ACTG) investigated a strategy of induction amphotericin B (for 2 weeks) followed by azole treatment. Patients with cryptococcal meningitis were randomized to receive 2 weeks of amphotericin B (0.7 mg kg day) with either flucytosine (25 mg/kg every 6 h) or matching placebo. The ACTG 159/MSG 017 study addressed two questions. Does adding flucytosine to amphotericin B as induction therapy for

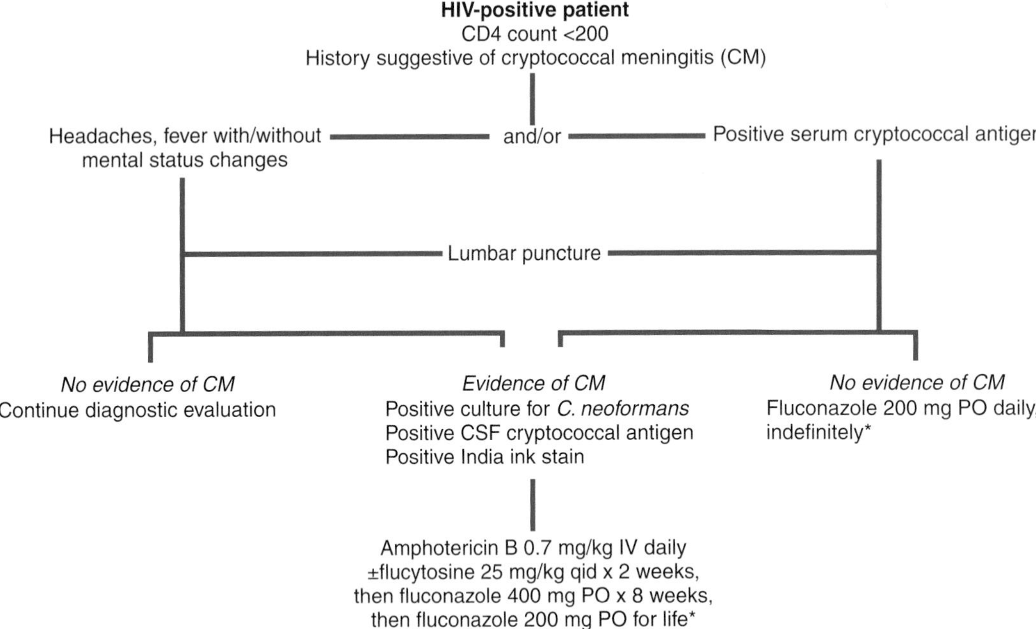

Figure 43-2 ■ Algorithm for the diagnosis and treatment of cryptococcal meningitis.

*Recent evidence suggests fluconazole secondary prophylaxis may be discontinued if the patients CD4 count rises above 100–200 cells/mL and is sustained at this level for greater than 6 months (see text).

cryptococcal meningitis improve the two- or 10-week survival compared to induction with amphotericin B alone? Is itraconazole as effective as fluconazole in suppressing relapse of cryptococcal meningitis during the maintenance phase of treatment? At the end of 2 weeks, patients who were stable or improved were again randomized to receive either fluconazole 400 mg/day or itraconazole 200 mg bid. The acute mortality with this regimen was 6%, which compares favorably with anything previously reported for cryptococcal meningitis in AIDS patients.[106] The addition of flucytosine to amphotericin B did not significantly improve the mortality rate or the clinical course. However, flucytosine was well-tolerated, and there was a trend to a better CSF sterilization rate with its use (60% of patients assigned to amphotericin B with flucytosine were culture-negative at 2 weeks, compared with 51% of patients who received amphotericin B alone). Furthermore, the use of flucytosine as initial therapy has been associated with a decreased risk of later relapse of cryptococcal meningitis. In the second (azole) phase of the MSG/ACTG trial, there was no significant difference in clinical symptoms, response rate, or mortality among patients randomized to either fluconazole or itraconazole, although trends favored fluconazole. An open-label Italian study of this strategic approach (high-dose amphotericin B followed by triazoles) was also associated with favorable outcomes.[111] Of 31 patients treated in this fashion, 29 (94%) responded to therapy, and there were no deaths resulting from cryptococcosis. Thus it is reasonable to recommend this approach as a standard one for the treatment of acute cryptococcal meningitis in AIDS (Fig. 43-2). The Infectious Diseases Society of America (IDSA) and the US Public Health Service (USPHS) in collaboration with the HIV Medicine Association released practice guidelines endorsing this strategy. In patients unable to tolerate flucytosine, amphotericin B alone is an acceptable alternative.[112,125a]

Outcome from acute cryptococcal infection is worse in patients who have abnormal mental status before treatment is initiated.[104] In addition, patients who have positive blood cultures for *C. neoformans,* high titers of cryptococcal antigen in their CSF, or a low CSF white blood cell count have generally fared worse with therapy. At this point it is not clear whether a different strategy (e.g., a more prolonged induction period with amphotericin B) is warranted for such patients.

Although the data to date suggest that azole therapy alone is not optimal initial treatment, there is still considerable interest in the possibility of a completely oral regimen. The experience with higher doses of fluconazole does not suggest that this would be sufficiently active. However, the initial experience with the combination of fluconazole (400 mg/day) with flucytosine (150 mg kg^{-1} day^{-1}) as primary treatment resulted in promising response rates in selected patients.[113] After 10 weeks of therapy, 75% of CSF cultures were negative within a median time of 23 days, which was less than previously reported times with either drug alone. Almost 30% of patients had dose-limiting adverse effects from flucytosine mandating its discontinuation. Additional studies suggest that the combination of flucytosine and high doses of fluconazole (800–2000 mg/day) are associated with initial response rates of more than 70%, comparable to those seen in trials of amphotericin B with flucytosine.[114] A small number of patients have also been treated successfully with the combination of itraconazole and flucytosine.[115] These data clearly suggest that this combination merits more extensive investigation, and that it may emerge as a useful alternative to parenteral amphotericin B-based regimens. Voriconazole may be an alternative for fluconazole refractory disease but there is insufficient data to recommend its routine use or to suggest that voriconazole may be more effective than fluconazole.

Another area of active investigation is the use of alternative formulations of amphotericin B. The use of amphotericin mixed with Intralipid has attracted some attention. In a randomized comparison of amphotericin B deoxycholate and amphotericin B/Intralipid for the treatment of AIDS-associated cryptococcal meningitis, an increased incidence of anemia and nephrotoxicity was noted in the group taking the Intralipid preparation.[116] The Intralipid preparation did reduce the incidence of infusion-related adverse reactions and was associated with a trend toward an improved mycologic cure; but given that there was no benefit in the renal toxicity or clinical outcome, its use cannot be recommended. A randomized study comparing the amphotericin B-lipid complex with amphotericin B deoxycholate in 55 HIV-positive patients with cryptococcal meningitis noted less hematologic and nephrotoxicity in the lipid complex arm.[117] There was a trend favoring 'standard' amphotericin B in terms of the mycologic outcome.

The Collaborative Exchange of Antifungal Research (CLEAR) database was queried to identify patients with cryptococcal infection who were treated with Amphotericn B Lipid Complex (ABLC).[117a] This database includes both HIV-infected and uninfected patients and ABLC may have been used first or second line. Overall, the response rate for patients with HIV infection was 58% (30/52) suggesting it is at least comparable to historical response rates of conventional amphotericin B.

Small randomized studies[118,119] of liposomal amphotericin B compared with conventional amphotericin B noted an earlier CSF sterilization rate in patients randomized to the liposomal preparation. A larger randomized comparision of amphotericin B with liposomal amphotericin B[107] found similar clinical effects but less toxicity with the liposomal product. However, given that dose-limiting toxicity is rare with 2 weeks of amphotericin B deoxycholate, the role of the much more expensive liposomal preparation is still uncertain.

One aspect of managing acute cryptococcal meningitis in AIDS patients that has become more apparent in recent years is that clinical deterioration may be due to mechanical events associated with increased intracranial pressure, and that this aspect may not respond rapidly to antifungal therapy.[120,121] Baseline pressures appear to be predictive of outcome. In the recent MSG/ACTG trial,[61] among 381 patients enrolled, pretreatment opening pressures were reported for 221. The mean opening pressure at baseline for survivors was 27.9 ± 10.0 cm H_2O; for those who died, the median pressure was 29.4 ± 17.0 cm H_2O. Among the 21 patients who died during the initial 2 weeks of therapy, 12 had had a baseline CSF pressure measured; six of these patients had a pressure of 35 cm H_2O or higher. Two of the other patients who died had opening pressures of more than 55 cm H_2O immediately prior to death. There were statistically significant differences in survival between patients whose CSF pressure was less than 19 cm H_2O and those with pressures of 25 or 35 cm H_2O or more, with survival among these with the highest pressures being significantly less than those in patients whose pressures were normal.[61]

Ten patients with HIV-associated cryptococcal meningitis complicated by elevated intracranial pressure (range 26–60 cm H_2O) were prospectively followed.[122] High-volume lumbar puncture defined as removal of 20–30 mL CSF was performed one or two times daily. All patients returned to their baseline level of consciousness following normalization of their CSF pressure, and all 10 remain alive (range 7–24 months). Eight patients eventually required placement of lumbar peritoneal shunts, only one of which has subsequently been removed.

Woodworth and colleagues[122a] reported favorable outcome in two patients who underwent ventriculoperitoneal shunts for uncontrollable intracranial hypertension without evidence of shunt infection or malfunction 12 and 16 months post-shunt placement.

These data do not prove a causal relation between the pressure and outcome, nor do they prove that lowering pressure improves the prognosis. Nevertheless, they suggest that all patients with cryptococcal meningitis should have their opening pressure measured when a lumbar puncture is performed, and strong consideration should be given to reducing such pressure (by repeated lumbar punctures, a lumbar drain, or a shunt) if the opening pressure is high (>25 cm H_2O).

Patients with AIDS and cryptococcal meningitis require lifelong maintenance therapy. This was demonstrated in a placebo-controlled, double-blind, randomized trial evaluating the effectiveness of fluconazole for maintenance therapy after successful primary treatment with amphotericin B alone or in combination with flucytosine in patients with AIDS.[108] The risk of recurrence in the placebo group was significantly higher than that in the fluconazole group. It is of note that 22% of the placebo group in that trial were found to have clinically silent, recurrent cryptococcal infection in the urinary tract after prostatic massage. Other trials have confirmed that fluconazole 200 mg/day is the most effective maintenance therapy for cryptococcal meningitis. A trial comparing fluconazole 200 mg/day and amphotericin B 1 mg kg^{-1} $week^{-1}$ for suppressive therapy of cryptococcal meningitis in AIDS patients[109] showed that the amphotericin B group had significantly more relapses, increased drug-related adverse events, and more bacterial infections, including bacteremia. A more recent comparison of fluconazole 200 mg/day versus itraconazole 200 mg/day was terminated by its Data Safety Monitoring Board after preliminary results revealed a CSF culture relapse rate of 4% in AIDS patients receiving fluconazole compared to 23% relapse in the itraconazole group.[110]

Until 2001, the USPHS and IDSA guidelines had recommended maintenance therapy with fluconazole for life.[112,123] The USPHS guidelines have revised secondary prophylaxis recommendations for most opportunistic pathogens to reflect data revealing that it is safe to discontinue secondary prophylaxis in patients who have had a sustained immunologic response on HAART.[125a] It seems reasonable to assume that it would be safe to discontinue secondary prophylaxis in patients with a history of disseminated fungal disease who have had sustained immunologic responses. There have been several case series of safely discontinuing secondary prophylaxis in patients with cryptococcal meningitis. In one study,[124] six patients with disseminated cryptococcal disease including one patient with a history of a brain abscess discontinued antifungal prophylaxis after 1 year of prophylaxis and a sustained

CD4+ T-lymphocyte count of more than 150 cells/μL (range 178–525 cells/μL) on HAART. One patient had positive CSF CRAG and sCRAG tests at the time of enrollment. In another study,[124a] six patients including three with an sCRAG titer of more than 1:8 discontinued antifungal prophylaxis after a median 11 months of HAART with a CD4+ T-lymphocyte count higher than 100 cells/μL. Four small retrospective studies found no recurrences of cryptococcosis in patients who discontinued secondary prophylaxis.[124b,c,d,e] A larger, retrospective, multicenter study reviewed charts from 100 patients who, at the time maintenance therapy was discontinued, had a median CD4 T-lymphocyte cell count of 259 cells and median plasma HIV viral load <2.30 $\log_{10}$ copies/mL.[125] The sCRAG was undetectable in 56 patients at the time of discontinuation of prophylaxis. During a median follow-up period of 28.4 months (range, 6.7–64.5; 262 person-years), four events were observed (incidence, 1.53 events per 100 person-years). Three of these patients had a CD4 T-lymphocyte cell count of >100 cells/μLand a positive sCRAG result during the recurrent episode. One patient had a CD4 T-lymphocyte count below 100 reminding us of the need to reinitiate prophylaxis at time of immunologic failure in patients who have had a history of cryptococcosis.

Thai investigators[125a] conducted a prospective, multicenter, randomized study on discontinuing secondary prophylaxis in 60 HIV-infected subjects who were successfully treated for acute cryptococcal meningitis. Subjects were randomized to continue (n = 22) or discontinue (n = 20) secondary prophylaxis when the CD4 T-lymphocyte cell count had increased to >100 cells/μL and had an undetectable HIV RNA level for 3 months on zidovudine, lamivudine, and efavirenz. At a median of 48 weeks after randomization, there were no episodes of cryptococcal meningitis in either group.

Thus, the USPHS guidelines for 2004[125b] recommend discontinuation of secondary prophylaxis if patients have successfully completed a course of initial therapy for cryptococcosis, remain asymptomatic with respect to signs and symptoms of their cryptococcosis, and have a sustained increase (i.e., >6 months) in their CD4 T lymphocyte and T-lymphoctye counts to >100–200 cells/μL following HAART. Some experts would perform a lumbar puncture to determine if the CSF were culture negative before stopping therapy even if patients were asymptomatic, but many experts do not believe this is necessary. Maintenance therapy should be restarted if the CD4 T-lymphocyte count falls to <100–200 cells/μL.

Most relapses that do occur appear to be associated with the same strain of *C. neoformans* that caused the initial infection.[126–128] In general, these strains have not been associated with changes in antifungal susceptibility (especially to fluconazole, the usual suppressive treatment). This suggests that relapse generally is due to recurrence rather than a new infection (although new infection can occur[129]) and that the major problem in such cases appears to be compliance with antifungal therapy. A small number of cases associated with the acquisition of fluconazole resistance have been reported,[130–134] as have isolated cases of cryptococcal meningitis caused by amphotericin B-resistant strains.[135] In one study, 28 isolates from 25 patients were tested for fluconazole susceptibility, and they correlated with clinical outcomes. Therapeutic failure was observed in five patients who were infected with isolates for which the fluconazole minimum inhibitory concentrations (MICs) were +16μg/mL or more.[136] Of these five patients, four died from active cryptococcal disease. Of the 20 patients with fluconazole-susceptible isolates, only two patients died, both unrelated to cryptococcal disease. These findings suggest that fluconazole susceptibility may be useful for predicting the clinical response. In addition, a previous study suggested that fluconazole susceptibility may be useful for determining if fluconazole can be used as primary therapy.[137]

Although not currently a major issue, close attention must be given to monitoring whether azole-resistant cryptococcal disease becomes a future problem. Management of these resistant cases is largely anecdotal. In one case of amphotericin B-resistant disease,[135] the patient ultimately responded well to the combination of fluconazole and flucytosine. It is possible that this combination (especially with higher azole dosages) would be effective in cases associated with azole resistance; however, the most prudent course would be to treat with amphotericin B and flucytosine and to give maintenance therapy with intermittent amphotericin B.

PREVENTION

Several studies have suggested that fluconazole can prevent many cases of cryptococcal meningitis in patients with AIDS.[51] Indeed, the declining incidence of this infection has been attributed to widespread use of fluconazole. A randomized trial comparing fluconazole 200 mg/day with clotrimazole troches for prevention of fungal infections in AIDS patients demonstrated a 2-year invasive fungal infection rate of 2.8% in the fluconazole group compared to 9.1% in the clotrimazole group, with a sevenfold reduction in the risk of cryptococcosis[138] (Table 43-3). These prospective trial data are supported by a case-controlled analysis of the effect of exposure to fluconazole on the risk of developing cryptococcal meningitis in AIDS patients.[141] A higher percentage (36%) of patients without cryptococcal meningitis had received fluconazole sometime during the preceding 6 months compared to 11% of patients with cryptococcal meningitis. Other studies have indicated that fluconazole doses lower than 200 mg/day may be effective in preventing cryptococcosis. A double-blind, randomized study comparing weekly fluconazole with daily fluconazole for the prevention of fungal infections reported equivalent effects in preventing cryptococcal disease, although the weekly regimen was less effective in suppressing oral candidiasis.[139] A study of fluconazole 200 mg three times weekly given to 231 HIV-infected individuals noted the occurrence of cryptococcal meningitis in one patient (0.4%).[142] There is also evidence that itraconazole is effective in preventing cryptococcosis. The MSG conducted a prospective, randomized trial of itraconazole 200 mg/day compared with placebo in HIV-infected patients with CD4 T- lymphocyte counts less than 150 cells/mm^3 who resided in areas endemic for histoplasmosis.[140] Cryptococcal infection occurred in one patient assigned to itraconazole

Table 43-3

Randomized Comparative Trials of Prevention of Cryptococcal Infection in HIV-Positive Patients

Trial	Agents Used	Target Populations	No. of Patients	Rates of Cryptococcal Infection (%)	Comments
Powderly et al[138]	Fluconazole, 200 mg qd vs	CD4+ T-lymphocyte count <200/mm^3	217	0.9	Fluconazole superior as prophylaxis ($P < 0.001$), but no survival benefit noted
	Clotrimazole troches 5 times daily		211	7.1	
Havlir et al[139]	Fluconazole 200 mg daily vs	CD4+ T-lymphocyte count <100/mm^3	316	0.3	Difference between two regimens not significant
	Fluconazole 400 mg once weekly		317	1.6	
McKinsey et al[140]	Itraconazole vs	CD4+ T-lymphocyte count <150/mm^3	149	0.7	Itraconazole significantly delayed cryptococcosis ($P < 0.001$); no survival benefit
	Placebo		146	5.4	
Chariyalerstak[140a]	Itraconazole vs Placebo	CD4+ T-lymphocyte <200	63 66	0 10.7	No survival benefit
Chetchotisakd[140b]	Fluconazole vs Placebo	CD4+ T-lymphocyte <100	44 46	6.8 15.2	Survival benefit in FCZ arm The number of deaths per 10000 person-days was 2.7 for the fluconazole group and 11.7 for the placebo
Smith[140c]	Itraconazole Placebo	CD4+ T-lymphocyte <300	187 187	0 0.2	High discontinuation rate: no survival benefit

compared with eight cases of cryptococcosis in patients receiving placebo. As with the fluconazole studies, no survival benefit was noted. Thus despite clear evidence of a protective effect, the overall utility of routine use of fluconazole as primary prophylaxis in advanced HIV disease is unclear. There is considerable concern that prolonged usage of fluconazole may result in acquired resistance to fluconazole, especially in *Candida* species.[143,144] The Cochrane collaboration recently conducted a review of five randomized controlled studies assessing either the use of fluconazole or itraconazole for primary prophylaxis. A meta-analysis of all 5 studies[138,140] failed to show a significant difference in mortality when compared with placebo.[144a] However, one Thai study did in fact demonstrate a survival benefit. Chetchotisakd and colleagues conducted a prospective multicenter, randomized, double-blind, placebo-controlled study of 90 HIV-infected patients with CD4 T-lymphocyte counts <100 cells. 44 received fluconazole 400 mg weekly and 46 received placebo. On an intent-to-treat basis, cryptococcal meningitis developed in 10 cases; three (6.8%) in the fluconazole group and seven (15.2%) in the placebo group. Patients in the placebo group were more likely to develop cryptococcal meningitis than those in the fluconazole group (hazard ratio = 2.23). The number of deaths per 10000 person-days was 2.7 for the fluconazole group and 11.7 for the placebo group. At this point, the recommended guidelines from the USPHS and IDSA/HIVMA for prophylaxis in patients with HIV infection do not endorse routine use of primary antifungal prophylaxis.[123] However, the survival benefit reported with the use of fluconazole 400 mg once weekly for primary prophylaxis for cryptococcal meningitis in Thailand may have implications for other resource-poor countries. Studies exploring the routine use of primary prophylaxis are warranted in resource-poor settings where the incidence of cryptococcosis is significantly higher, there is limited access to HAART and generic fluconazole or donated fluconazole is available.

FUTURE ISSUES

Several cytokines show some potential as adjunctive therapy for infection based on a number of *in vitro* and animal studies. Interferon-γ activates macrophages for fungicidal activity against *C. neoformans*.[30,33] In murine models of intraperitoneal and CNS infection with *C. neoformans*, recombinant interferon-γ improved survival, especially when combined with amphotericin B.[145,146] A randomized, double-blind, placebo-controlled, dose-range, Phase II study of the safety and antifungal activity of subcutaneous recombinant interferon-γ1b (rIFN-γ1b) in conjunction with standard therapy in patients with acute cryptococcal meningitis demonstrated no significant differences among the two doses of rIFN-γ1b compared with placebo. The CSF fungal cultures sterilization at 2 weeks was 13%, 36%, and 32% of patients in the placebo, rIFN-γ1b (100 g), and rIFN-γ1b (200 g) groups, respectively. Overall, the interferon was well-tolerated and a larger study powered to detect differences from placebo is warranted.[146a]

Tumor necrosis factor-α (TNF-α) can enhance the complement-dependent phagocytosis of *C. neoformans* by murine macrophages *in vitro*.[147] In addition, monoclonal antibodies against TNF-α enhanced mortality in response to experimental disseminated cryptococcosis.[147] IL-2 has been demonstrated to activate T cells for cytokine production of macrophages, adherence to *C. neoformans,* and inhibition of growth.[148] IL-12 alone and in combination with fluconazole significantly reduced the development of systemic cryptococcal infection in a murine infection model.[149]

Basal fungistatic anticryptococcal activity of peripheral blood monocytes for AIDS patients is significantly reduced compared to that in HIV-seronegative controls. Treatment of monocytes with granulocyte/macrophage colony-stimulating factor (GM-CSF) from AIDS patients resulted in increased fungistatic activity, and the combination of GM-CSF with fluconazole resulted in increased fungicidal activity. The effects of GM-CSF treatment in monocytes included enhanced phagocytic activity, increased superoxide anion generation, and upregulation of CD11b/CD18 expression.[150]

Monoclonal antibodies have also been investigated for their therapeutic potential. Monoclonal antibodies to *C. neoformans* glucuronoxylomannan have been demonstrated to enhance fluconazole and amphotericin B in a murine model.[151,152] In addition, a series of patients receiving serum antibody adjuvant therapy with amphotericin B for *C. neoformans* infection suggests the possibility of clinical benefit.[153] Antibody-based therapy for cryptococcal disease is currently under investigation.[154] The MSG completed a Phase I evaluation of the safety and pharmacodynamic activity of the murine-derived anticryptococcal antibody 18B7 in HIV-infected subjects who have responded to therapy for cryptococcal meningitis to determine the maximal tolerated dose. This study supports further investigation of Mab 18B7 at a dose of 1.0 mg/kg.[154a]

Although chemoprophylaxis is relatively successful in patients with AIDS, as noted above, it is not routinely recommended. An alternative strategy for prevention is to consider vaccination early during the HIV infection in the hope of eliciting a protective response. Current investigational strategies include passive antibody administration (which is likely not to be practical) and immunization with glucuronoxylomannan-tetanus toxoid conjugate.[155–157]

REFERENCES

1. Dismukes WE. Cryptococcal meningitis in patients with AIDS. J Infect Dis 157:624, 1988.
2. Powderly WG. Cryptococcal meningitis and AIDS. Clin Infect Dis 17:837, 1993.
3. Selik RM, Chu SY, Ward JW. Trends in infectious diseases and cancers among persons dying of HIV infection in the United States from 1987 to 1992. Ann Intern Med 123:933, 1995.

3a. French N, Gray K, Watrea C, et al. Cryptococcal infection in a cohort of HIV-1-infected Ugandan adults. AIDS 16:1031, 2002.

4. Kwon-Chung KJ, Bennett JE. Cryptococcosis. In: Medical Mycology. Philadelphia: Lea & Febiger, 1992, p 397.
5. Kwon-Chung KJ, Kozel TR, Edman JC, et al. Recent advances in biology and immunology of *Cryptococcus neoformans*. J Med Vet Mycol 30:133, 1992.
6. Madrenys N, De Vroey C, Raes-Wuytack C, et al. Identification of the perfect state of *Cryptococcus neoformans* from 195 clinical isolates including 84 from AIDS patients. Mycopathologia 123:65, 1993.
7. Cherniak R, Reiss E, Slodki ME, et al. Structure and antigenic activity of the capsular polysaccharide of *Cryptococcus neoformans* serotype. Ann Mol Immunol 17:10, 1980.
8. Levitz SM. The ecology of *Cryptococcus neoformans* and the epidemiology of cryptococcosis. Rev Infect Dis 13:1163, 1991.
9. Ellis DH, Pfeiffer TJ. Ecology, life-cycle, and infectious propagule of *Cryptococcus neoformans*. Lancet 336:923, 1990.
10. Speed B, Dunt D. Clinical and host differences between infections with the two varieties of *Cryptococcus neoformans*. Clin Infect Dis 21:28, 1995.
11. Rinaldi MG, Drutz DJ, Howell A, et al. Serotypes of *Cryptococcus neoformans* in patients with AIDS. J Infect Dis 153:642, 1986.
12. Shimizu RY, Howard DH, Clancy MN. The variety of *Cryptococcus neoformans* in patients with AIDS. J Infect Dis 154:1042, 1986.
13. Restrepo BI, Barbour AG. Cloning of 18S and 25S rDNAs from the pathologic fungus *Cryptococcus neoformans*. J Bacteriol 171:5596, 1989.
14. Wickes BL, Moore TDE, Kwon-Chung KJ. Comparison of the electrophoretic karyotypes and chromosomal location of ten genes in the two varieties of *Cryptococcus neoformans*. Microbiology 140:543, 1994.
15. Perfect JR, Toffaletti DL, Rude TH. The gene encoding phosphoribosylaminomidazole carboxylase (*ADE2*) is essential for growth of *Cryptococcus neoformans* in cerebrospinal fluid. Infect Immun 61:4446, 1993.
16. Parker AR, Moore TDE, Edman JC, et al. Cloning sequence analysis and expression of the gene encoding imidazole glycerol phosphate dehydratase in *Cryptococcus neoformans*. Gene 145:135, 1994.
17. Chang YC, Kwon-Chung KJ. Complementation of a capsule-deficient mutation of *Cryptococcus neoformans* restores its virulence. Mol Cell Biol 14:4912, 1994.
18. Williamson PR. Biochemical and molecular characterization of the diphenol oxidase of *Cryptococcus neoformans*: identification as a laccase. J Bacteriol 176:656, 1994.
19. Perfect JR, Rude TH, Wong B, et al. Identification of a *Cryptococcus neoformans* gene that directs expression of the cryptic Saccharomyces cerevisiae mannitol dehydrogenase gene. J Bacteriol 178:5257, 1996.
20. Lodge JK, Johnson RL, Weinberg RA, et al. Comparison of myristoyl-CoA:protein N-myristoyltransferases from three pathogenic fungi: *Cryptococcus neoformans*, Histoplasma capsulatum, and Candida albicans. J Biol Chem 269:2996, 1994.
21. Cox GM, Rude TH, Dykstra CC, et al. Actin gene from *Cryptococcus neoformans*: structure and phylogenetic analysis. J Med Vet Mycol 33:261, 1995.
22. Cruz MC, Bartlett MS, Edlind TD. In vitro susceptibility of the opportunistic fungus *Cryptococcus neoformans* to anthelmintic benzimidazoles. Antimicrob Agents Chemother 38:378, 1994.
23. Perfect JR, Rude TH, Penning LM, et al. Cloning the *Cryptococcus neoformans* TRP1 gene by complementation in Saccharomyces cerevisiae. Gene 122:213, 1992.

24. Moore TDE, Edman JC. The A mating type locus of *Cryptococcus neoformans* contains a peptide pheromone gene. Mol Cell Biol 13:1962, 1993.
25. Livi LL, Edman U, Schneider GP, et al. Cloning, expression and characterization of thymidylate synthase from *Cryptococcus neoformans*. Gene 150:221, 1994.
26. Tolkacheva T, McNamara P, Piekarz E, et al. Cloning of a *Cryptococcus neoformans* gene, GPA1, encoding a G-protein a subunit homolog. Infect Immun 62:2849, 1994.
27. Jacobson ES, Ayers DJ, Harrell AC. Genetic and phenotypic characterization of capsule mutants of *Cryptococcus neoformans*. J Bacteriol 150:1292, 1982.
28. Bulmer GS. Twenty-five years with *Cryptococcus neoformans*. Mycopathologia 109:111, 1990.
29. Sukroongreung S, Eampokalap B, Tansuphaswadikul S, et al. Recovery of *Cryptococcus neoformans* from the nasopharynx of AIDS patients. Mycopathologia 143:131, 1999.
30. Perfect JR, Granger DL, Durack DT. Effects of antifungal agents and gamma interferon on macrophage cytotoxicity for fungi and tumor cells. J Infect Dis 156:316, 1987.
31. Huffnagle GB, Yates JL, Lipscomb MF. Immunity to a pulmonary *Cryptococcus neoformans* infection requires both CD4+ and CD8+ T-cells. J Exp Med 173:793, 1991.
32. Flesch IE, Schwamberger G, Kaufman SH. Fungicidal activity of IFN-gamma activated macrophages: extracellular killing of *Cryptococcus neoformans*. J Immunol 142:3219, 1989.
33. Roseff SA, Levitz SM. Effect of endothelial cells on phagocyte-mediated anticryptococcal activity. Infect Immun 61:3818, 1993.
34. Salkowski CA, Balish E. Role of natural killer cells in resistance to systemic cryptococcosis. J Leukoc Biol 50:151, 1991.
35. Levitz SM, Dupont MP. Phenotypic and functional characterization of human leukocytes activated by interleukin-2 to directly inhibit growth of *Cryptococcus neoformans* in vitro. J Clin Invest 91:1490, 1993.
36. Miller MF, Mitchell T, Storkus WJ, et al. Human natural killer cells do not inhibit growth of *Cryptococcus neoformans* in the absence of antibody. Infect Immun 58:639, 1990.
37. Mukherjee S, Lee SC, Casadevall A. Antibodies to *Cryptococcus neoformans* glucuronoxylomannan enhance antifungal activity of murine macrophages. Infect Immun 63:573, 1995.
38. Kwon-Chung KJ, Rhodes JC. Encapsulation and melanin formation as indicators of virulence in *Cryptococcus neoformans*. Infect Immun 51:218, 1986.
39. Rhodes JC, Polacheck I, Kwon-Chung KJ. Phenoloxidase activity and virulence in isogenic strains of *Cryptococcus neoformans*. Infect Immun 36:1175, 1982.
40. Casadevall A. Antibody immunity and invasive fungal infections. Infect Immun 63:4211, 1995.
41. Gadebusch HH. Passive immunization against *Cryptococcus neoformans*. Proc Soc Exp Biol Med 98:611, 1958.
42. Mukherjee J, Lee S, Scharff MD, et al. Monoclonal antibodies to *Cryptococcus neoformans* capsular polysaccharide modify the course of intravenous infection in mice. Infect Immun 62:1079, 1994.
43. Mukherjee J, Scharff MD, Casadevall A. Protective murine monoclonal antibodies to *Cryptococcus neoformans*. Infect Immun 60:4534, 1992.
44. Murphy JW, Mosley RL, Cherniak R, et al. Serological, electrophoretic, and biological properties of *Cryptococcus neoformans* antigens. Infect Immun 56:424, 1988.
45. Wang Y, Aisen P, Casadevall A. *Cryptococcus neoformans* melanin and virulence: mechanism of action. Infect Immun 63:3131, 1995.
46. Kwon-Chung KJ, Edman JC, Wickes BL. Genetic association of mating types and virulence in *Cryptococcus neoformans*. Infect Immun 60:602, 1992.
47. Evans EE, Kessel JF. The antigenic composition of *Cryptococcus neoformans*: serologic studies with the capsular polysaccharide. J Immunol 67:109, 1951.
48. Pettoello-Mantovani M, Casadevall A, Kollmann TR, et al. Enhancement of HIV-1 infection by the capsular polysaccharide of *Cryptococcus neoformans*. Lancet 339:21, 1992.
49. Lee SC, Casadevall A. Polysaccharide antigen in brain tissue of AIDS patients with cryptococcal meningitis. Clin Infect Dis 23:194, 1996.
50. Currie BP, Casadevall A. Estimation of the prevalence of cryptococcal infection among patients infected with the human immunodeficiency virus in New York City. Clin Infect Dis 19:1029, 1994.
51. Pinner RW, Hajjeh RA, Powderly WG. Prospects for preventing cryptococcosis in persons infected with human immunodeficiency virus. Clin Infect Dis 21(Suppl 1):S103, 1995.
52. Abadi J, Nachman S, Kressle AB, Pirofski L. Cryptococcosis in children with AIDS. Clin Infect Dis 28:309, 1999.
53. Oursler KAK, Moore RD, Chaisson R. Risk factors for cryptococcal meningitis in HIV-infected patients. AIDS Res Hum Retroviruses 15:625, 1999.
54. McNeil JI, Kan VL. Decline in the incidence of cryptococcosis among HIV-infected patients. J Acquir Immune Defic Syndr Hum Retrovirol 9:206, 1995.
55. Hajjeh RA, Conn LA, Stephens DS, et al. Cryptococcosis: population-based multistate active surveillance and risk factor in human immunodeficiency virus-infected persons. J Infect Dis 179:449, 1999.
55a. Friedman GD, Fessel WJ, Udaltsova NV, Hurley LB. Cryptococcosis: the 1981–2000 epidemic. Mycoses 48:122, 2005.
56. Holtzer CD, Jacobson MA, Hadley WK, et al. Decline in the rate of specific opportunistic infections at San Francisco General Hospital, 1994–1997. AIDS 12:1931, 1998.
57. Koo JJ, Aberg JA. Increase in the rate of AIDS-related opportunistic infections at San Francisco General Hospital in the era of potent antiretroviral therapy [abstract]. Presented at the XIII International AIDS Conference, Durban, South Africa, Jul 2000.
58. Rozenbaum R, Goncalves AJR. Clinical epidemiological study of 171 cases of cryptococcosis. Clin Infect Dis 18:369, 1994.
59. Chuck SL, Sande MA. Infections with *Cryptococcus neoformans* in the acquired immunodeficiency syndrome. N Engl J Med 321:794, 1989.
60. Dismukes WE. Management of cryptococcosis. Clin Infect Dis 17(Suppl):S507, 1993.
61. Graybill JR, Sobel J, Saag M, et al. Diagnosis and management of increased intracranial pressure in patients with AIDS and cryptococcal meningitis. Clin Infect Dis 30:47, 2000.
62. Cameron ML, Bartlett JA, Gallis HA, et al. Manifestations of pulmonary cryptococcosis in patients with acquired immunodeficiency syndrome. Rev Infect Dis 13:64, 1991.
63. Clark RA, Greer DL, Valainis GT, et al. *Cryptococcus neoformans* pulmonary infection in HIV-1-infected patients. J Acquir Immune Defic Syndr Hum Retrovirol 3:480, 1990.
64. Visnegarwala F, Graviss EA, Lacke CE, et al. Acute respiratory failure associated with cryptococcosis in patients with AIDS: analysis of predictive factors. Clin Infect Dis 27:1231, 1998.
65. Driver JA, Saunders CA, Heinze-Lacey B, et al. Cryptococcal pneumonia in AIDS: is cryptococcal meningitis preceded by clinically recognizable pneumonia? J Acquir Immune Defic Syndr Hum Retrovirol 9:168, 1995.
66. Clark RA, Greer DL, Atkinson W, et al. Spectrum of *Cryptococcus neoformans* infection in 68 patients infected with human immunodeficiency virus. Rev Infect Dis 12:768, 1990.
67. Mulanovich VE, Dismukes WE, Markowitz N. Cryptococcal empyemia: case report and review. Clin Infect Dis 20:1396, 1995.
68. Darras-Joly C, Chevret S, Wolff M, et al. *Cryptococcus neoformans* infection in France: epidemiologic features of and early

prognostic parameters for 76 patients who were infected with human immunodeficiency virus. Clin Infect Dis 23:369, 1996.
69. Meyohas MC, Roux P, Bollens D, et al. Pulmonary cryptococcosis: localized and disseminated infections in 27 patients with AIDS. Clin Infect Dis 21:628, 1995.
70. Murakawa GJ, Kerschmann R, Berger T. Cutaneous cryptococcus infection and AIDS: report of 12 cases and review of the literature. Arch Dermatol 132:545, 1996.
71. Lewis W, Lipsick J, Cammarosano C. Cryptococcal myocarditis in acquired immune deficiency syndrome. Am J Cardiol 55:1240, 1985.
72. Lafont A, Wolff M, Marche C, et al. Overwhelming myocarditis due to *Cryptococcus neoformans* in an AIDS patient. Lancet 2:1145, 1987.
73. Ricciardi DD, Sepkowitz DV, Berkowitz LB, et al. Cryptococcal arthritis in a patient with acquired immune deficiency syndrome: case report and review of the literature. J Rheumatol 13:455, 1986.
74. Morinelli EN, Dugel PU, Riffenburgh R, et al. Infectious multifocal choroiditis in patients with acquired immune deficiency syndrome. Ophthalmology 100:1014, 1993.
75. Bonacini M, Nussbaum J, Ahluwalia C. Gastrointestinal, hepatic, and pancreatic involvement with *Cryptococcus neoformans* in AIDS. J Clin Gastroenterol 12:295, 1990.
76. Finazzi R, Guffanti M, Cernuschi M, et al. Unusual presentation of cryptococcosis in a patient with AIDS. Clin Infect Dis 22:709, 1996.
77. Ndimbie OK, Dekker A, Martinez AJ, et al. Prostatic sequestration of *Cryptococcus neoformans* in immunocompromised persons treated for cryptococcal meningoencephalitis. Histol Histopathol 9:643, 1994.
78. Larsen RA, Bozzette S, McCutchan JA, et al. Persistent *Cryptococcus neoformans* of the prostate after successful treatment of meningitis. Ann Intern Med 111:125, 1989.
79. Penneys NS. Skin Manifestations of AIDS. Philadelphia: JB Lippincott, 1990.
80. Concus AP, Helfand RF, Imber MJ, et al. Cutaneous cryptococcosis mimicking molluscum contagiosum in a patient with AIDS. J Infect Dis 158:897, 1988.
81. Manfredi R, Mazzoni A, Nanetti A, et al. Morphologic features and clinical significance of skin involvement in patients with AIDS-related cryptococcosis. Acta Derm Venereol 76:72, 1996.
82. Woods ML, MacGinley R, Eisen DP, Allworth AM. HIV combination therapy: partial immune reconstitution unmasking latent cryptococcal infection. AIDS 12:1491, 1998.
83. Blanche P, Gombert B, Ginsburg C, et al. HIV combination therapy: immune restitution causing cryptococcal lymphadenitis dramatically improved by anti-inflammatory therapy. Scand J Infect Dis. 30:615, 1998.
84. Lanzafame M, Trevenzoli M, Carretta G, et al. Mediastinal lymphadenitis due to cryptococcal infection in HIV-positive patients on highly active antiretroviral therapy. Chest 116:848, 1999.
84a. Skiest DJ, Hester LJ, Hardy RD. Cryptococcal immune reconstitution inflammatory syndrome: report of four cases in three patients and review of the literature. J Infect 51:e289, 2005.
84b. Puthanakit T, Oberdorfer P, Akarathum N, et al. Immune reconstitution syndrome after highly active antiretroviral therapy in human immunodeficiency virus-infected thai children. Pediatr Infect Dis J 25:53, 2006.
84c. Shelburne SA, Darcourt J, White AC, et al. The role of immune reconstitution inflammatory syndrome in AIDS-related *Cryptococcus neoformans* disease in the era of highly active antiretroviral therapy. Clin Infect Dis 40:1049, 2005.
84d. Lortholary O, Fontanet A, Memain N, et al. French Cryptococcosis Study Group. Incidence and risk factors of immune reconstitution inflammatory syndrome complicating HIV-associated cryptococcosis in France. AIDS 19:1043, 2005.
85. Currie BP, Freundlich LF, Soto MA, et al. False-negative cerebrospinal fluid cryptococcal latex agglutination tests for patients with culture-positive cryptococcal meningitis. J Clin Microbiol 31:2519, 1993.
86. Tanner DC, Weinstein MP, Fedoview B, et al. Comparison of commercial kits for detection of cryptococcal antigen. J Clin Microbiol 32:1680, 1993.
87. McManus EJ, Jones JM. Detection of a Trichosporon beigelii antigen cross reactive with *Cryptococcus neoformans* capsular polysaccharide in serum from a patient with disseminated Trichosporon infection. J Clin Microbiol 21:681, 1985.
88. Blevins LB, Fenn J, Segal H, et al. False-positive cryptococcal antigen latex agglutination caused by disinfectants and soaps. J Clin Microbiol 33:1674, 1995.
89. Feldmeser M, Harris C, Reichberg S, et al. Serum cryptococcal antigen in patients with AIDS. Clin Infect Dis 23:827, 1996.
89a. Antinori S, Radice A, Galimberti L, et al. The role of cryptococcal antigen assay in diagnosis and monitoring of cryptococcal meningitis. J Clin Microbiol 43:5828, 2005.
90. Powderly WG, Cloud GA, Dismukes WE, et al. Measurement of cryptococcal antigen in serum and cerebrospinal fluid: value in the management of AIDS-associated cryptococcal meningitis. Clin Infect Dis 18:789, 1994.
91. Powderly WG, Tuazon C, Cloud GA, et al. Serum and CSF cryptococcal antigen in management of cryptococcal meningitis in AIDS. In: Abstracts of the 4th National Conference on Human Retroviruses and Related Infections, Washington, DC. Alexandria, VA, Westover Management Group, 1997, abstract 6.
92. Aberg JA, Watson J, Segal M, Chang LW. Clinical utility of monitoring serum cryptococcal antigen (sCRAG) in patients with AIDS-related cryptococcal disease. HIV Clin Trials 1:1, 2000.
93. Zuger A, Louie E, Holzman RS, et al. Cryptococcal disease in patients with the acquired immunodeficiency syndrome: diagnostic features and outcome of treatment. Ann Intern Med 104:234, 1986.
94. Kovacs JA, Kovacs AA, Polis M, et al. Cryptococcosis in the acquired immunodeficiency syndrome. Ann Intern Med 103:533, 1985.
95. Eng RH, Bishburg E, Smith S, et al. Cryptococcal infections in the acquired immune deficiency syndrome. Am J Med 81:19, 1986.
96. Bennett JE, Dismukes WE, Duma RJ, et al. A comparison of amphotericin B alone and combined with flucytosine in the treatment of cryptococcal meningitis. N Engl J Med 301:126, 1979.
97. Dismukes WE, Cloud G, Gallis H, et al. Treatment of cryptococcal meningitis with combination of amphotericin B and flucytosine for four as compared with six weeks. N Engl J Med 317:334, 1987.
98. Dupont B, Hilmarsdottir I, Datry A, et al. Cryptococcal meningitis in AIDS patients: a pilot study of fluconazole therapy in 52 patients. In: van den Bossche H, Mackenzie DWR, Cauwenbergh G, et al (eds). Mycosis in AIDS Patients. New York: Plenum, 1990, p 287.
99. Denning DW, Tucker RM, Hanson LH, et al. Itraconazole therapy for cryptococcal meningitis and cryptococcosis. Arch Intern Med 149:2301, 1989.
100. Denning DW, Tucker RM, Hostetler JS, et al. Oral itraconazole therapy of cryptococcal meningitis and cryptococcosis in patients with AIDS. In: vanden Bossche H, Mackenzie DWR, Cauwenbergh G, et al (eds). Mycosis in AIDS Patients. New York: Plenum, 1990, p 305.
101. Robinson PA, Knirsch AK, Joseph JA. Fluconazole for life-threatening fungal infections in patients who cannot be treated with conventional antifungal therapy. Rev Infect Dis 12(Suppl 3):S349, 1990.
102. Larsen RA, Leal M, Chan L. Fluconazole compared with amphotericin B plus flucytosine for cryptococcal meningitis in AIDS. Ann Intern Med 113:183, 1990.

103. De Gans J, Portegies P, Tiessens G, et al. Itraconazole compared with amphotericin B plus flucytosine in AIDS patients with cryptococcal meningitis. AIDS 6:185, 1992.
104. Saag MS, Powderly WG, Cloud GA, et al. Comparison of amphotericin B with fluconazole in the treatment of acute AIDS-associated cryptococcal meningitis. N Engl J Med 326:83, 1992.
105. Moskovitz BL, Wiesinger B. Cryptococcal Meningitis Research Group. Randomized comparative trial of itraconazole and fluconazole for treatment of AIDS-related cryptococcal meningitis. In: Abstracts of the 1st National Conference on Human Retroviruses. Washington, DC, American Society for Microbiology, 1994, p 61.
106. Van der Horst CM, Saag MS, Cloud GA, et al: Treatment of cryptococcal meningitis associated with the acquired immunodeficiency syndrome. N Engl J Med 337:15, 1997.
107. Hamill RJ, Sobel J, el-Sadr W, et al. Randomized double-blind, trial of AmBisome (liposomal amphotericin B) and amphotericin B in acute cryptococcal meningitis in AIDS patients. In: Program and Abstracts of the 39th ICAAC, Sep 1999. San Francisco: American Society of Microbiology; 1999, abstract 1161.
108. Bozzette SA, Larsen R, Chiu J, et al. A controlled trial of maintenance therapy with fluconazole after treatment of cryptococcal meningitis in the acquired immunodeficiency syndrome. N Engl J Med 324:580, 1991.
109. Powderly WG, Saag MS, Cloud GA, et al. A controlled trial of fluconazole or amphotericin B to prevent relapse of cryptococcal meningitis in patients with the acquired immunodeficiency syndrome. N Engl J Med 326:793, 1992.
110. Saag MS, Cloud GA, Graybill R, NIAID Mycoses Study Group. A comparison of fluconazole versus itraconazole as maintenance therapy for AIDS-associated cryptococcal meningitis. Clin Infect Dis 28:291, 1999.
111. De Lalla F, Pellizzer G, Vaglia A, et al. Amphotericin B as primary therapy for cryptococcosis in AIDS patients: reliability of relatively high doses administered over a relatively short period. Clin Infect Dis 20:263, 1995.
112. Saag MS, Graybill RJ, Larsen, RA, MSG Cryptococcal Subproject. Practice guidelines for the management of cryptococcal disease. Clin Infect Dis 30:710, 2000.
113. Larsen RA, Bozzette SA, Jones BE, et al. Fluconazole combined with flucytosine for the treatment of cryptococcal meningitis in patients with AIDS. Clin Infect Dis 19:741, 1994.
114. Milefchik E, Leal M, Haubrich R, et al. A Phase II dose escalation trial of high dose fluconazole with and without flucytosine for AIDS associated cryptococcal meningitis. In: Abstracts of the 4th Conference on Retroviruses and Opportunistic Infections, Washington, DC. Alexandria, VA: Westover Management Group; 1997, abstract 5.
115. Viviani MA, Tortorano AM, Langer M, et al. Experience with itraconazole in cryptococcosis and aspergillosis. J Infect 18:151, 1989.
116. Joly V, Aubry P, Ndayiragide A, et al. Randomized comparison of amphotericin B deoxycholate dissolved in dextrose or intralipid for the treatment of AIDS-associated cryptococcal meningitis. Clin Infect Dis 23:556, 1996.
117. Sharkey PK, Graybill JR, Johnson ES, et al. Amphotericin B lipid complex compared with amphotericin B in the treatment of cryptococcal meningitis in patients with AIDS. Clin Infect Dis 22:315, 1996.
117a. Baddour LM, Perfect JR, Ostrosky-Zeichner L. Successful use of amphotericin B lipid complex in the treatment of cryptococcosis. Clin Infect Dis 40(Suppl 6):S409, 2005.
118. Coker RJ, Viviani M, Gazzarxd BG, et al. Treatment of cryptococcosis with liposomal amphotericin B (AmBisome) in 23 patients with AIDS. AIDS 7:829, 1993.
119. Leenders ACAP, Reiss P, Portegeis P, et al. Liposomal amphotericin B (AmBisome) compared with amphotericin B both followed by oral fluconazole in the treatment of AIDS-associated cryptococcal meningitis. AIDS 11:1463, 1997.
120. Denning DW, Armstrong RW, Lewis BH, et al. Elevated cerebrospinal fluid pressures in patients with cryptococcal meningitis and acquired immunodeficiency syndrome. Am J Med 91:267, 1991.
121. Malessa R, Krams M, Hengge U. Elevation of intracranial pressure in acute AIDS-related cryptococcal meningitis. Clin Investigator 72:1020, 1994.
122. Fessler RD, Sobel J, Guyot L, et al. Management of elevated intracranial pressure in patients with cryptococcal meningitis. J Acquir Immune Defic Syndr Hum Retrovirol 17:137, 1998.
122a. Woodworth GF, McGirt MJ, Williams MA, Rigamonti D. The use of ventriculoperitoneal shunts for uncontrollable intracranial hypertension without ventriculomegally secondary to HIV-associated cryptococcal meningitis. Surg Neurol 63:529, 2005.
123. USPHS/IDSA Prevention of Opportunistic Infections Working Group. Guidelines for Preventing Opportunistic Infections Among HIV Infected Persons. Recommendations of the U.S. Public Health Service and the Infectious Diseases Society of America. MMWR 51(RR8), 2002.
124. Aberg JA, Price RW, Heeren DM and Bredt B. Discontinuation of antifungal therapy for cryptococcosis following immunologic response to antiretroviral therapy. J Infect Dis 185:1179, 2002
124a. Martinez E, Garcia-Viejo MA, Marcos MA. Discontinuation of secondary prophylaxis for cryptococcal meningitis in HIV-infected patients responding to highly active antiretroviral therapy. AIDS 14:2615, 2000.
124b. Nwokolo NC, Fisher M, Gazzard BG, Nelson MR. Cessation of secondary prophylaxis in patients with cryptococcosis. AIDS 15:1438, 2001.
124c. Rollot F, Bossi P, Tubiana R, et al. Discontinuation of secondary prophylaxis against cryptococcosis in patients with AIDS receiving highly active antiretroviral therapy. AIDS 15:1448, 2001.
124d. Sheng WH, Hung CC, Chen MY, et al. Successful discontinuation of fluconazole as secondary prophylaxis for cryptococcosis in AIDS patients responding to highly active antiretroviral therapy. Int J STD AIDS 13:702, 2002.
124e. Negroni R, Helou SH, López Daneri G, et al. Successful discontinuation of antifungal secondary prophylaxis in AIDS-related cryptococcosis Rev Argent Microbiol 36:113, 2004 .
125. Mussini C, Pezzotti P, Miro J, Discontinuation of maintenance therapy for cryptococcal meningitis in patients with AIDS treated with HAART: an International, Observational Study. Clin Infect Dis 38:565, 2004.
125a. Vibhagool A, Sungkanuparph S, Mootsikapun P, et al. Discontinuation of secondary prophylaxis for cryptococcal meningitis in human immunodeficiency virus-infected patients treated with highly active antiretroviral therapy: a prospective, multicenter, randomized study. Clin Infect Dis 36:1329, 2003.
125b. Treating Opportunistic Infections Among HIV-Infected Adults and Adolescents. Recommendations from CDC, the National Institutes of Health and the HIV Medicine Association/Infectious Diseases Society of America. MMWR 53(RR15):112, 2004
126. Spitzer ED, Spitzer SG, Freundlich LF, et al. Persistence of initial infection in recurrent *Cryptococcus neoformans* meningitis. Lancet 341:595, 1993.
127. Casadevall X, Spitzer ED, Webb D, et al. Susceptibilities of serial *Cryptococcus neoformans* isolates from patients with recurrent cryptococcal meningitis to amphotericin B and fluconazole. Antimicrob Agents Chemother 37:1383, 1993.
128. Brandt ME, Pfaller MA, Hajjeh R, et al. Molecular subtypes and antifungal susceptibilities of serial *Cryptococcus neoformans* isolates in human immunodeficiency virus infected patients. J Infect Dis 174:812, 1996.

129. Haynes KA, Sullivan DJ, Coleman DC, et al. Involvement of multiple *Cryptococcus neoformans* strains in a single episode of cryptococcosis and reinfection with novel strains in recurrent infection demonstrated by random amplification of polymorphic DNA and DNA fingerprinting. J Clin Microbiol 33:99, 1995.
130. Paugam A, Dupouy-Camet J, Blanche P, et al. Increased fluconazole resistance of *Cryptococcus neoformans* isolated from a patient with AIDS and recurrent meningitis. Clin Infect Dis 19:975, 1994.
131. Birley HD, Johnson EM, McDonald P, et al. Azole drug resistance as a cause of clinical relapse in AIDS patients with cryptococcal meningitis. Int J STD AIDS 6:353, 1995.
132. Armengou A, Porcar C, Mascaro J, et al. Possible development of resistance to fluconazole during suppressive therapy for AIDS-associated cryptococcal meningitis. Clin Infect Dis 23:1337, 1996.
133. Berg J, Clancy CJ, Nguyen MH. The hidden danger of primary fluconazole prophylaxis for patients with AIDS. Clin Infect Dis 26:186, 1998.
134. Smith NH, Graviss EA, Hashmey R, et al. Multi-drug-resistant cryptococcal meningitis in an AIDS patient. In: Abstracts of the 35th Annual Meeting of the Infectious Diseases Society of America. Alexandria, VA, Infectious Diseases Society of America, 1997, abstract 529.
135. Powderly WG, Keath EJ, Sokol-Anderson M, et al. Amphotericin-B resistant *Cryptococcus neoformans* in a patient with AIDS. Infect Dis Clin Pract 1:314, 1992.
136. Aller AI, Martin-Mazuelos E, Lozano F, et al. Correlation of fluconazole MICs with clinical outcome in cryptococcal infection. Antimicrob Agents Chemother 44:1544, 2000.
137. Witt MD, Lewis RJ, Larsen RA, et al. Identification of patients with acute AIDS-associated cryptococcal meningitis who can be effectively treated with fluconazole: the role of antifungal susceptibility testing. Clin Infect Dis 22:322, 1996.
138. Powderly WG, Finkelstein D, Feinberg J, et al. A randomized trial comparing fluconazole with clotrimazole troches for the prevention of fungal infections in patients with advanced human immunodeficiency virus infection. N Engl J Med 332:700, 1995.
139. Havlir DV, Dube MP, McCutchan JA, et al. Prophylaxis with weekly versus daily fluconazole for fungal infections in patients with AIDS. Clin Infect Dis 27:1369, 1998.
140. McKinsey DS, Wheat LJ, Cloud GA, et al. Itraconazole prophylaxis for fungal infections in patients with advanced human immunodeficiency virus infection: randomized, placebo-controlled, double-blind study: National Institute of Allergy and Infectious Diseases Mycoses Study Group. Clin Infect Dis 28:1049, 1999.
140a. Chariyalertsak S, Supparatpinyo K, Sirisanthana T, Nelson KE. A controlled trial of itraconazole as primary prophylaxis for systemic fungal infections in patients with advanced human immunodeficiency virus infection in Thailand. Clin Infect Dis 34:277, 2002.
140b. Chetchotisakd P, Sungkanuparph S, Thinkhamrop B, et al. A multicentre, randomized, double-blind, placebo-controlled trial of primary cryptococcal meningitis prophylaxis in HIV-infected patients with severe immune deficiency. HIV Medicine 5:140, 2004.
140c. Smith DE, Bell J, Johnson M, et al. A randomized, double-blind, placebo-controlled study of itraconazole capsules for the prevention of deep fungal infections in immunodeficient patients with HIV infection. HIV Medicine 2:70, 2001.
141. Quagliarello VJ, Viscoli C, Visconti RI. Primary prevention of cryptococcal meningitis by fluconazole in HIV-infected patients. Lancet 345:548, 1995.
142. Singh N, Barnish MJ, Berman S, et al. Low-dose fluconazole as primary prophylaxis for cryptococcal infection in AIDS patients with CD4+ T-lymphocyte counts of < or +5100/mm^3: demonstration of efficacy in a positive, multicenter trial. Clin Infect Dis 23:1282, 1996.
143. Maenza JR, Keruly JC, Moore RD, et al. Risk factors for fluconazole-resistant candidiasis in human immunodeficiency virus-infected patients. J Infect Dis 173:219, 1996.
144. Fichtenbaum CJ, Powderly WG. Azole-resistant candidiasis. Clin Infect Dis 26:556, 1998.
144a. Chang LW, Phipps WT, Kennedy GE, Rutherford GW. Antifungal interventions for the primary prevention of cryptococcal disease in adults with HIV. Cochrane Database Syst Rev 20:CD004773, 2005.
145. Joly V, Saint-Julien L, Carbon C, et al. In vivo activity of interferon-gamma in combination with amphotericin B in the treatment of experimental cryptococcosis. J Infect Dis 170:1331, 1994.
146. Lutz JE, Clemons KV, Stevens DA. Enhancement of antifungal chemotherapy by interferon-gamma in experimental systemic cryptococcosis. J Antimicrob Chemother 46:437, 2000.
146a. Pappas PG, Bustamante B, Ticona R, et al. Recombinant interferon-gamma 1b as adjunctive therapy for AIDS-related acute cryptococcal meningitis. J Infect Dis. 2004;189:2185–91.
147. Collins HL, Bancroft GJ. Cytokine enhancement of complement-dependent phagocytosis by macrophages: synergy of tumor necrosis factor-A and granulocyte-macrophage colony-stimulating factor for phagocytosis of *Cryptococcus neoformans*. Eur J Immunol 22:1447, 1992.
148. Levitz SM. Activation of human peripheral blood mononuclear cells by interleukin-2 and granulocyte-macrophage colony-stimulating factor to inhibit *Cryptococcus neoformans*. Infect Immun 59:3393, 1991.
149. Clemons KV, Brummer E, Stevens DA. Cytokine treatment of central nervous system infection: efficacy of interleukin-12 alone and synergy with conventional antifungal therapy in experimental cryptococcosis. Antimicrob Agents Chemother 38:460, 1994.
150. Tascini C, Vecchiarelli A, Preziosi R, et al. Granulocyte-macrophage colony-stimulating factor and fluconazole enhance anti-cryptococcal activity of monocytes from AIDS patients. AIDS 13:49, 1999.
151. Mukherjee J, Feldmesser M, Scharff MD, et al. Monoclonal antibodies to *Cryptococcus neoformans* glucuronoxylomannan enhance fluconazole efficacy. Antimicrob Agents Chemother 39:1398, 1995.
152. Mukherjee J, Zuckier LS, Scharff MD, et al. Therapeutic efficacy of monoclonal antibodies to *Cryptococcus neoformans* glucuronoxylomannan alone and in combination with amphotericin B. Antimicrob Agents Chemother 38:580, 1994.
153. Gordon MA, Casadevall A. Serum therapy for cryptococcal meningitis. Clin Infect Dis 21:1477, 1995.
154. Casadevall A, Scharff MD. Return to the past: the case for antibody-based therapies in infectious diseases. Clin Infect Dis 21:150, 1995.
154a. Larsen RA, Pappas PG, Perfect J, et al and the NIAID MSG. A Phase I Evaluation of the Safety and Pharmacodynamic Activity of a Murine Derived Anti-cryptococcal Antibody 18B7 in Subjects with Treated Cryptococcal Meningitis. Antimicrobiol Agents & Chemotherapy 49:952, 2005.
155. Zebedee SL, Koduri RK, Mukherjee J, et al. Mouse-human immunoglobulin G1 chimeric antibodies with activities against *Cryptococcus neoformans*. Antimicrob Agents Chemother 38:1507, 1994.
156. Devi SJN, Schneerson R, Egan W, et al. *Cryptococcus neoformans* serotype A glucuronoxylomannan protein conjugate vaccine: synthesis, characterization and immunogenicity. Infect Immun 59:370, 1991.
157. Mukherjee J, Casadevall A, Scharff MD. Molecular characterization of the humoral responses to *Cryptococcus neoformans* infection and glucuronoxylomannan-tetanus toxoid conjugate immunization. J Exp Med 177:1105, 1993.

Chapter 44

Histoplasmosis

Lawrence J. Wheat, MD

INTRODUCTION

Histoplasmosis is a serious opportunistic infection in patients with acquired immunodeficiency syndrome (AIDS) in endemic regions of America, Africa, and Asia, although cases often are diagnosed outside the endemic regions in individuals who previously resided or traveled in endemic areas.[1] Since the introduction of potent treatment for HIV infection, the incidence of histoplasmosis has declined, and the potential for cure has improved. The clinical manifestations range from localized pulmonary disease in patients with higher CD4+ T-lymphocyte counts to widespread disseminated disease in those with more advanced HIV infection. Prompt diagnosis requires awareness of the clinical manifestations, a high index of suspicion, and familiarity with the diagnostic tests. If the diagnosis is established before the disease becomes severe, antifungal therapy with liposomal amphotericin B or itraconazole is highly effective. In patients achieving a good immunologic response to antiretroviral agents, lifelong suppressive therapy is no longer required.

CLINICAL FINDINGS

Histoplasmosis is acquired by inhalation of microconidia of the mold phase of the organism following disturbance of soil or accumulations of bird or bat droppings containing the organism. Disease manifestations following acute exposure range from asymptomatic infection in otherwise healthy individuals inhaling a small number of microconidia to life-threatening acute pulmonary disease in those inhaling a large number of spores.[2] While subclinical, nonprogressive hematogenous dissemination occurs following acute pulmonary histoplasmosis, most patients recover without treatment with development of a cell-mediated immune response during the first month following infection. Chronic pulmonary disease may occur in patients with emphysema, and progressive disseminated disease in those who are immunosuppressed. In patients with HIV infection, a similar spectrum of disease, ranging from asymptomatic or acute pulmonary infection in patients with CD4+ T-lymphocyte counts above 300 cells/mm^3 to severe progressive disseminated histoplasmosis (PDH) in those with lower CD4+ T-lymphocyte counts.

Acute Pulmonary Histoplasmosis

Manifestations of acute pulmonary histoplasmosis usually include cough and chest pain, systemic findings of headache, fever and weight loss, and infiltrates with mediastinal or hilar lymphadenopathy on chest radiogram or computed tomography (CT) scan. More diffuse infiltrates associated with respiratory insufficiency may follow heavy inoculum exposure. The majority of patients with acute pulmonary histoplasmosis recover without treatment, but the illness may be severe and recovery protracted in those with diffuse pulmonary involvement. Thus, treatment is usually indicated in patients with more severe symptoms accompanied by diffuse infiltrates, and in patients showing no improvement during the first month of infection.

Chronic Pulmonary Histoplasmosis

In contrast to the self-limited course in patients who are otherwise healthy, progressive pulmonary infection occurs in those with underlying emphysema. Radiograms and CT scans usually show cavitation, fibrosis, and pleural thickening, features suggestive of tuberculosis. The infection progresses to other areas of the lungs without treatment, and thus treatment is recommended in all cases.

Progressive Disseminated Histoplasmosis

Progressive disseminated disease occurs in 95% of cases of histoplasmosis in patients with AIDS, but localized pulmonary disease may be seen in those with CD4+ T-lymphocyte counts above 500 cells/mm^3.[3,4] About 90% of cases of PDH have occurred in patients with CD4+ T-lymphocyte counts below 200 cells/mm^3, and usually below 50 cells/mm^3. Patients present with fever, fatigue, and weight loss, and half or more exhibit respiratory symptoms. Common physical findings include hepatosplenomegaly and lymphadenopathy. The course may be rapidly fatal, but a subacute presentation over 1–3 months is more characteristic.

Radiographic abnormalities are present in half to two-thirds of cases.[3,5,6] The radiographic findings are usually diffuse and include nodular or linear opacities, or air-space disease in most cases. Calcified lymph nodes or lung lesions are noted in a third of cases, while mediastinal lymphadenopathy is uncommon (~5%).[3,6]

Patients infrequently (<10%) present with shock, respiratory insufficiency, and hepatic and renal failure.[4] The sepsis presentation represents a late manifestation, usually occurring in patients who delayed seeking care until they were severely ill. Nearly half of patients who present with a sepsis-like illness die within a week of diagnosis.

Central nervous system involvement occurs in ~15% of cases.[3,4] Patients may present with lymphocytic meningitis, focal brain lesions, or diffuse encephalitis.[7,8] Patients complain of fever and headache and often demonstrate mental status changes. Seizures or focal neurologic deficits may occur in patients with brain involvement. The cerebrospinal fluid (CSF) typically shows lymphocytic pleocytosis, protein elevation, and hypoglycorrhachia in those with meningitis. Single or multiple enhancing brain lesions may be seen by CT scans or magnetic resonance imaging (MRI) in patients with cerebral involvement. The prognosis is worse in patients with neurologic findings than in those without these complications.[3]

Gastrointestinal manifestations including diarrhea, abdominal pain, intestinal obstruction or perforation, bleeding, or peritonitis complicate ~10% of cases.[9] A spectrum of lesions, including plaques, ulcerations, pseudopolyps, small (3–8 mm) nodules, thickened intestinal folds, luminal masses, and strictures may occur anywhere along the gastrointestinal tract but are more common in the small intestine and right colon. Colonic disease may be misdiagnosed as malignancy or inflammatory bowel disease.[10] Omental and mesenteric nodules causing peritonitis and ascites have been reported. Perforation also has occurred resulting from transmural necrosis of the small intestine. Biopsies of intestinal lesions show necrotizing granulomas containing yeast forms of *Histoplasma capsulatum.*

Dermatologic findings, seen in 10% of cases, include erythematous or hyperpigmented papules, pustules, folliculitis, plaques with ulcerations, nodules, eczematous changes, erythema multiforme, and rosacea-like rashes. Skin lesions appear to be more common in patients from South America.[11] *H. capsulatum* organisms may be seen in biopsies of skin lesions, providing a rapid diagnosis. Rare manifestations include adrenal insufficiency, pericarditis, pleuritis, pancreatitis, prostatitis, and retinitis.

An immune reconstitution syndrome may be seen in patients responding to antiretroviral therapy.[12,13] Manifestations including splenic infarction, ulcerative skin lesions;[12] liver abscess, lymphadenitis, intestinal obstruction, uveitis, and arthritis.[13]

TAXONOMY

H. capsulatum var *capsulatum* is an ascomycete whose teleomorphic state is *Ajellomyces capsulatus.* It is classified in the family Arthrodermataceae, order Onygenales of the Ascomycotina. *H. capsulatum* variety *capsulatum* contains several clades, which differ in geographic distribution. Clade 2 is most common in the US, and 5 and 6 in Central and South America.[14] Other varieties include *H. capsulatum* var *duboisii* and *farciminosum*, which cause different disease syndromes than seen with *H. capsulatum* var *capsulatum* and rarely cause PDH in patients with AIDS. Although *H. capsulatum* variety *duboisii* is endemic in equatorial Africa, most infections in patients with AIDS in Africa are caused by var *capsulatum.*[1]

BIOLOGY

Histoplasma capsulatum grows as a mold in the soil and is found primarily in microfoci containing large amounts of rotted guano where birds have roosted or bats have inhabited. The mold is comprised of hyphae bearing large tuberculate macroconidia (8–14 μm in diameter), which are characteristic of *H. capsulatum,* and smaller microconidia (2–5 μm), which are the infectious form of the organism. It causes infection when conidia are inhaled. At temperatures above 35ºC *H. capsulatum* grows as a yeast measuring 2–3 $\times$ 3–4 μm in diameter. The yeast form is typically found in infected tissues. While reactivation has been proposed as the cause for PDH in AIDS, the low incidence of histoplasmosis in patients with AIDS in most endemic areas (<3%), where histoplasmin skin test positivity exceeds 50%, indicates that reactivation is rare. Pulmonary calcification, a hallmark of past histoplasmosis, was not a risk factor for clinical disease,[15] providing added evidence against reactivation. Occurrence of PDH in patients with AIDS who have calcified lesions in the lungs, rather than indicating reactivation, suggest re-infection in persons with waning immunity during progressive HIV infection.[3,4] The strongest evidence supporting reactivation was by demonstration of DNA patterns typical of Panamanian strains of *H. capsulatum* in Puerto Rican immigrants in New York City,[16] but travel information was insufficient to exclude more recent acquisition while visiting Latin America.

Cellular immunity plays a key role in defense against *H. capsulatum.*[17] With development of specific T-cell-mediated immunity, cytokines including tumor necrosis factor-alpha (TNF-α), interferon-γ, and interleukin-12 (IL-12) arm macrophages to kill the fungus and halt progression of the disease. The importance of TNF-α in defense against *H. capsulatum* is shown by the occurrence of PDH in patients with rheumatologic disorders or Crohn's disease treated with TNF-α blockers.[18] If cell-mediated immunity is impaired, an appropriate immune response to the infection cannot occur, leading to a progressive disseminated infection.

EPIDEMIOLOGY

PDH occurs in 1–5% of patients with AIDS from endemic areas. During outbreaks, however, the incidence of PDH has exceeded 25% in some US cities.[4] Rates above 5% also have been reported in some Latin American countries, as recently reviewed.[19] PDH occurs in fewer than 1% of patients from nonendemic areas. Cases reported in Europe usually were acquired in Africa, Latin America, and Asia, although there are areas in Europe where autochthonous infection may occur.[1] The incidence in the US has declined since HAART became available, and now most cases occur in patients with undiagnosed HIV infection or who are failing HAART.

MICROBIOLOGY

Growth on mycologic media at 25–30°C is slow, requiring incubation for up to 4 weeks. Mold colonies vary from white to buff brown. Definitive identification requires conversion of the mold to the yeast, demonstration of specific reactivity with anti-*H. capsulatum* antiserum (exoantigen tests), or reactivity with DNA probes specific for *Histoplasma* mRNA.

DIAGNOSIS

Diagnosis of PDH requires a high index of suspicion and an understanding of the clinical and laboratory findings.[20] The diagnosis should be suspected in patients with unexplained fever and weight loss. Radiographic findings of diffuse reticulonodular or miliary infiltrates also suggests the diagnosis.[6] Laboratory abnormalities may include anemia, thrombocytopenia, leukopenia, and hepatic enzyme elevation. A reactive hemophagocytic syndrome, consisting of fever, thrombocytopenia, and bone marrow histology exhibiting hemophagocytic phagocytosis, usually in association with markedly elevated serum lactate dehydrogenase (LDH) and ferritin, has been reported in patients with a sepsis-like presentation,[21] but is nonspecific.

LDH elevation is present in 90% of patients,[5] but may be seen in *Pneumocystis jiroveci* pneumonia and disseminated *Mycobacterium* infection. In fact, in one report *P. jiroveci* pneumonia and disseminated tuberculosis, but not PDH, were associated with LDH elevation after controlling for race and CD4+ T-lymphocyte count.[22] Ferritin elevation has been reported in PDH, but also is not specific; and while a marked elevation >10 000 ng/mL is more specific for PDH,[23] the sensitivity at that cutoff is unknown.

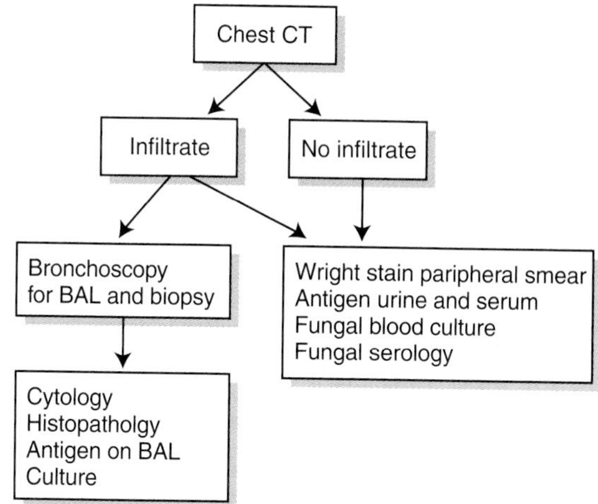

Figure 44-1 ■ Diagnostic approach.

Table 44-1 Sensitivity of Diagnostic Studies in Disseminated Histoplasmosis in Patients

Test	Percent Positive	Reference
Blood smear	12–31%	Casanova-Cardiel et al[25] Kurtin[24]
Histopathology	41%	Williams et al[26]
Antigen urine	95%	Williams et al[26]
Antigen serum	85%	Williams et al[26]
Antigen CSF	66%	Wheat et al[3]
Antigen BAL	70%	Wheat et al[27]
Serology	67%	Williams et al[26]
Culture	85%	Wheat et al[3] Williams et al[26]

In half to two-thirds of cases, pulmonary involvement is present. Bronchoscopy is recommended in such patients to assist in rapid diagnosis of PDH and exclude co-infection, which is not uncommon. An approach to evaluation in patients with pulmonary symptoms or CT abnormalities is outlined in Figure 44-1.

A battery of laboratory tests are useful for diagnosis of PDH, and their sensitivities are summarized in Table 44-1. Of note is that none of these tests are positive in all cases, and that, except for culture, positive results may be false-positive. Accordingly these tests should be used as an aid to diagnosis, in conjunction with clinical findings and corroborated by other tests, when possible.[20]

Direct Detection

Cytopathology or histopathology using a variety of techniques (Papanicolaou, Giemsa, Gram, hematoxylin and eosin, Wright, Gomori methenamine silver (GMS)) reveals yeast measuring ~3 μm in diameter, with occasional buds. Yeast may be seen by Wright stain of blood smears in up to one-third of cases with severe manifestations (Table 44-1).[21,24,25] Yeast may be identified more easily using special fungal stains such as GMS. The highest yield is from bone marrow, positive in 50–75% of patients in which the procedure is performed.[3] Overall, however, the sensitivity of histopathology is below 50%.[3,26] *Candida glabrata*, *Penicillium marneffei*, *Toxoplasma gondii*, *P. jiroveci*, and staining artifacts may be misidentified as *H. capsulatum*.

Antigen Detection

Detection of antigen in body fluids is very useful for diagnosis of PDH in patients with AIDS.[20] Antigen is detected in the urine of 95% and the serum of 85% of patients (Table 44-1).[3,26] Antigen may be detected in bronchoalveolar lavage fluid[27] and CSF[3] of patients with pulmonary or meningeal involvement. Tests for antigen may be falsely negative in patients with mild clinical manifestations or localized sites of dissemination and positive in those with systemic mycoses caused by organisms that contain cross-reactive antigens (*Blastomyces dermatitidis, Penicillium marneffei, Paracoccidioides braziliensis*). Antigen declines with effective treatment[28–30] and increases with relapse,[31] providing a useful method to monitor therapy.

Identification of false-positive results in organ transplant recipients caused by human anti-rabbit antibodies, induced in response to treatment with rabbit anti-T-lymphocyte antibody[32] led to modification of the *Histoplasma* antigen assay. Those modifications were incorporated into a second-generation *Histoplasma* assay in 2004, in which false-positivity caused by human anti-rabbit antibodies was reduced by 95%, and sensitivity in false-negative specimens improved by 73%. The second-generation assay has replaced the original assay for clinical testing at MiraVista Diagnostics. Sensitivity and specificity using the second-generation assay is assumed to be higher than previously reported,[20] and studies are in progress comparing the second-generation assay and the original assay.

The antigen test was modified in 2006 to permit quantitation, and results are expressed as ng/mL. Interassay variation is much lower in the quantitative assay than the semiquantitative assay, eliminating the need to test current versus prior specimens in the same assay to assess changes in antigen levels.

If the antigen test provides the sole basis for diagnosis, a second specimen should be tested to validate the positive result. If the initial antigen test is negative but PDH is still suspected, follow-up testing is recommended as the test may become positive with disease progression in the untreated patient.

Cultures

Histoplasma capsulatum can be isolated from blood, bone marrow, respiratory secretions, or localized lesions in up to 85% of cases,[3] with the highest yield from bronchoscopy specimens[3,26] and blood using appropriate methods.[3] Cultures of bone marrow or other involved tissues, based upon examination, laboratory findings, or CT imaging may provide a diagnosis if other tests are negative. However, isolation of *H. capsulatum* may take 4 weeks, delaying diagnosis and initiation of therapy.

Serologic Tests

High levels of IgG antibodies develop within 4–6 weeks and peak over the next few months, but may be negative in immunosuppressed individuals. Serologic tests are positive in about two-thirds of cases in patients with AIDS.[3,26] The immunodiffusion and complement fixation tests should be performed to achieve maximum sensitivity and are recommended for all patients suspected of having PDH. Complement fixation test results are expressed as titers, and positive results in serum range from 1:8 to 1:512 or more. Titers of 1:32 or more are more diagnostic of active infection; but titers of 1:8 and 1:16 should not be disregarded, as they occur in up to 20% of cases. Titers of 1:8 and 1:16 and M-precipitin bands by immunodiffusion also may represent past infection and must be interpreted cautiously to avoid misdiagnosis of PDH in patients with other infectious, inflammatory, or malignant diseases. CSF titration should begin with undiluted fluid, and any titer to be considered positive. Serologic tests may provide the sole basis for diagnosis in some cases.

Skin Tests

Histoplasmin skin testing reagents are no longer produced. Demonstration of interferon-γ production upon incubation of mononuclear cells with *Histoplasma* antigens provides a surrogate for skin test reactivity.[33]

TREATMENT

Approach to Therapy

PDH is progressive and fatal without treatment.[3] Once the diagnosis is established, a decision must be made to hospitalize the patient for intravenous therapy with amphotericin B or treat as an outpatient with itraconazole (Fig. 44-2). Key factors in this decision include severity of illness and likelihood of adherence to unsupervised treatment as an outpatient. Features correlating with poor prognosis, and favoring hospitalization, include central nervous system manifestations, hypotension, hypoxemia, dyspnea;[3] marked laboratory abnormalities including creatinine elevation and hypoalbuminemia,[34] hepatic enzyme and bilirubin elevation, LDH elevation and thrombocytopenia.[35] Additional considerations in the decision to hospitalize, which have not been shown to correlate with fatal outcome, but may still impact prognosis, include prior history of multiple opportunistic infections or poor adherence with treatment, weight loss >5% of usual weight, temperature above 40°C, hemoglobin <10 gm/dL and

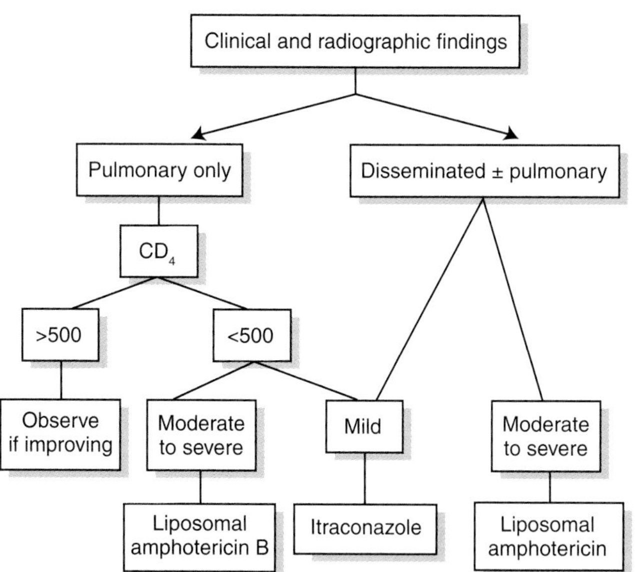

Figure 44-2 ■ Selection of therapy. (1) Criteria predicting unfavorable outcome and supporting hospitalization. (2) Medical history: prior opportunistic infection, poor adherence to therapy, relapse. (3) Clinical findings: central nervous system manifestations, hypotension, hypoxemia, dyspnea, weight loss >5% of usual weight, temperature above 40°C, concurrent opportunistic infection. (4) Laboratory findings: creatinine or bilirubin elevation >2 times normal, albumin <3 g/dL, hepatic enzyme elevation >5 times normal, LDH elevation >10 times normal, hemoglobin <10 g/dL, leukocyte count <4000/mm^3, platelet count <100 000/mm^3.

leukocyte count <4000/mm^3. Failure to improve in response to oral therapy within 2 weeks or worsening on oral therapy are additional reasons to hospitalize the patient for intravenous therapy.

Specific Drugs

Amphotericin *B*

In patients with nonlife-threatening manifestations of PDH, 98% experienced a clinical remission in response to treatment with the standard deoxycholate formulation of amphotericin B, but of those with shock or respiratory failure, nearly half died.[3] Amphotericin B also was less effective in patients with meningitis; eight of 13 patients (62%) died.[3] Often impaired renal function worsened during treatment and precluded aggressive therapy. Given the greater tolerability of the lipid preparations, the superior penetration of the liposomal formulation into the brain, and the unfavorable experience with the deoxycholate formulation, a prospective study comparing the standard formulation with liposomal amphotericin B was conducted.

Liposomal Amphotericin B

In a double-blind study enrolling patients with severe or moderately severe PDH, liposomal amphotericin B (AmBisome) was more effective than the deoxycholate formulation.[36] Clinical response by week 2 occurred in 88% of the liposomal group versus 64% of the standard treatment group. Patients receiving the liposomal preparation also defervesced more rapidly and exhibited improved survival. These findings support use of the liposomal preparation for moderately severe or severe cases. The other lipid preparations have not been studied in PDH and should not be presumed to be as effective as liposomal amphotericin B, as they exhibit different pharmacologic properties, do not penetrate brain tissue as well as the liposomal formulation, and are more nephrotoxic. Of note is that none of the amphotericin B formulations achieve detectable levels in the CSF.

Itraconazole

Oral therapy with itraconazole is effective in persons with mild illness who are not ill enough to require hospitalization.[36] Favorable response occurred in 85% of patients and fever usually resolved within a week.[37] Treatment failures occurred in those with more severe clinical manifestations and in one patient with undetectable itraconazole blood concentrations. Itraconazole does not penetrate the CSF and has not been evaluated for treatment of *Histoplasma* meningitis.

The capsule formulation was used in the studies evaluating treatment of disseminated histoplasmosis in patients with AIDS. While the solution formulation is better absorbed, and its absorption is not impaired by medications that reduce gastric acidity, its taste is objectionable to some patients, and it is less convenient because of the large number of bottles required for chronic therapy, compared to capsules. Thus, the capsule formulation is preferred. While itraconazole is generally well tolerated, except for gastrointestinal upset in some patients, more serious toxicities including hypertension, edema, and hypokalemia may occur, particularly in patients receiving high doses (600 mg/day). Itraconazole can cause heart failure and should only be used if the benefit outweighs the risk in patients with heart disease. Ventricular fibrillation caused by itraconazole-induced hypokalemia has been reported. Liver enzyme elevation is not uncommon but clinically significant hepatitis requiring discontinuation is rare. Fatal hepatitis has been reported, however.

Itraconazole blood levels vary widely, and may be subtherapeutic (trough < 0.5 μg/mL) in some patients. Itraconazole blood levels should be measured during the second week of treatment and periodically following changes in dosage, addition of interacting medications, assessment of suspected nonadherence, and evaluation of the cause for treatment failure.

Fluconazole

Fluconazole is less effective than itraconazole for treatment of PDH. Fluconazole, at a dose of 800 mg/day, induced remission in 74% of AIDS patients with mild to moderately severe manifestations of PDH (Table 44-2),[38] but one-third relapsed during suppressive treatment with 400 mg/day.[38] Furthermore, two-thirds of isolates from patients failing therapy acquired resistance to fluconazole.[39]

Outcome of Induction Therapy for Disseminated Histoplasmosis in Patients with AIDS

Table 44-2

Treatment	No.	Dose	Response (%)	Study
Amphotericin B	73	~50 mg/day	88	Wheat et al[3]
Severe disease	17		53	
Moderate	56		98	
Amphotericin B	22	$0.7\,mg\,kg^{-1}\,day^{-1} \times 14$ days	64	Johnson et al[36]
Liposomal amphotericin B	51	$3\,mg\,kg^{-1}\,day^{-1} \times 14$ days	88	Johnson et al[36]
Itraconazole	59	400 mg/day	88	Wheat et al [37]
Fluconazole	49	800 mg/day	74	Wheat et al[38]

Others

Posaconazole is active *in vitro* and highly effective in experimental infection.[40] Favorable response to posaconazole in patients without AIDS has been presented at national meetings,[41] but only one report has been published.[42]

Voriconazole appears to be less active than itraconazole, posaconazole, or ravuconazole. The MIC_{90} for isolates from patients with AIDS were 4.0 μg/mL for fluconazole, 0.25 μg/mL for voriconazole, but only 0.007 μg/mL for itraconazole, posaconazole, and ravuconazole.[42a] Furthermore, voriconazole is susceptible to development of resistance during therapy, as reported with fluconazole. Evaluating 17 pretreatment and failure isolate pairs from patients with AIDS and PDH treated with fluconazole, fourfold or greater increases in MIC were noted to voriconazole in seven (41%).[43]Although MIC for voriconazole is lower than to fluconazole, the lower voriconazole MIC is offset by its lower blood level, ~2 μg/mL versus 30 μg/mL, respectively, at the doses used in histoplasmosis. A few patients have been treated with voriconazole, with inconsistent results.[44,45] Voriconazole and posaconazole demonstrate wide variation in blood levels, which, like itraconazole, are influenced by medications that induce or inhibit cytochrome P450. Consequently, blood levels should be monitored. Although data are limited, a trough blood concentration of 0.5 μg/mL should be considered therapeutic.

Ravuconazole is highly active *in vitro*[43] but has not been studied in the experimental model or patients with histoplasmosis. The echinocandins have minimal *in vitro* or *in vivo* activity against *H. capsulatum.*[46] Nikkomycin has variable *in vitro* and *in vivo* activity in histoplasmosis but is no longer in development.[47]

Treatment of Meningitis

More aggressive therapy appears to be indicated in patients with meningitis.[8] Mortality is higher, possibly because of the limited penetration of amphotericin B and itraconazole into brain tissue and CSF. While itraconazole alone, or followed by a short course of amphotericin B is adequate in patients without meningitis, a longer course of 4–6 weeks is recommended in those with meningitis. Furthermore, the liposomal formulation may play a special role in meningitis, since it penetrates brain tissue better than other formulations. Following completion of 4–6 weeks of liposomal amphotericin B, treatment with itraconazole 200 mg twice daily or three times daily, to achieve trough concentrations of at least 1.0 μg/mL is recommended. Although fluconazole and voriconazole achieve higher concentrations in the CSF, they are less active than itraconazole against *H. capsulatum*, and in an experimental model, itraconazole was more effective for treatment of meningitis.[48] Unfortunately, data in humans are inadequate to establish the best regimen, and treatment failure remains a concern even with optimal therapy. Thus, patients with meningitis should be followed carefully for response to therapy, with demonstration of resolution of CSF abnormalities and clearance of antigen from the CSF.

Outcome of Suppressive Therapy for Disseminated Histoplasmosis in Patients with AIDS

Table 44-3

Treatment	Response		
	No.	(%)	Study
Amphotericin			
50 mg/week	21	81	McKinsey et al[49]
Itraconazole			
400 mg	42	92	Wheat et al[50]
200 mg	46	89	Hecht et al[51]
Fluconazole			
400 mg daily	36	64	Wheat et al[38]

Suppressive Treatment

A variety of regimens have been used to prevent relapse, of which itraconazole is the most effective.[49–51] The relapse rate is below 5% with itraconazole 200 mg once[51] or twice[50] daily. Fluconazole is less effective than itraconazole, relapse occurring in over one-third of cases.[38] Amphotericin B 50 mg once or twice weekly also is effective,[49] and may be appropriate in patients who fail oral suppressive therapy because of inadequate drug exposure caused by nonadherence, poor absorption, drug interactions, or antifungal resistance (Table 44-3).

Once recommended in all patients,[4] suppressive therapy is no longer required in patients with a good immunologic response to HAART.[52] Patients treated with itraconazole for at least 1 year, who received HAART for at least 6 months, who had a CD4+ T-lymphocyte count >150 cells/mm^3 and *Histoplasma* urine and serum antigen below 4 units remained relapse free with follow-up for more than 2 years after stopping suppressive therapy.[52]

Histoplasma antigen levels fall with therapy and increase with relapse.[20] An antigen increase of more than 4 ng/mL (~4 units in the semiquantitative assay) suggests recurrence and supports further laboratory evaluation and consideration of resuming induction therapy. Use of the antigen test to diagnose relapse requires measurement of antigen levels at 3- to 4-month intervals.

Recommendations for Treatment

Liposomal amphotericin B (AmBisome) 3 mg kg^{-1} day^{-1} is the treatment of choice for patients with moderately severe or severe clinical manifestations of PDH who require hospitalization (Table 44-4; Fig. 44-3). If the deoxycholate formulation of amphotericin B is used, the dose should be 0.7–1 mg/kg for 3–14 days followed by treatment with itraconazole 200 mg twice daily for 3 months, then once daily for suppressive therapy for at least 1 year. Itraconazole is recommended for patients with mild manifestations of PDH.

The capsule formulation of itraconazole should be given with food or Cola, and the solution should be given on an empty stomach for the best absorption. The oral solution formulation should be used in patients who require treatment with H^2-blockers or omeprazole, have thrush refractory to treatment with the capsules, or have low blood concentrations while receiving the capsules. The solution should be given on an empty stomach. While the solution offers advantages over the capsule, its taste is unpleasant to some patients and may contribute to treatment failure caused by poor medication adherence. Blood concentrations should be measured during the second week of therapy at the trough time following the last dose, with a target trough concentration of at least 0.5 µg/mL, including the hydroxy-itraconazole metabolite if measured.

Cytochrome P450 inducers such as rifampin,[53,54] rifabutin,[55] phenytoin,[56] and phenobarbital[57] accelerate the metabolism

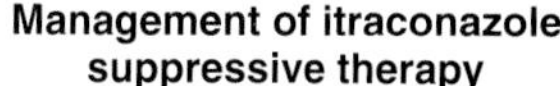

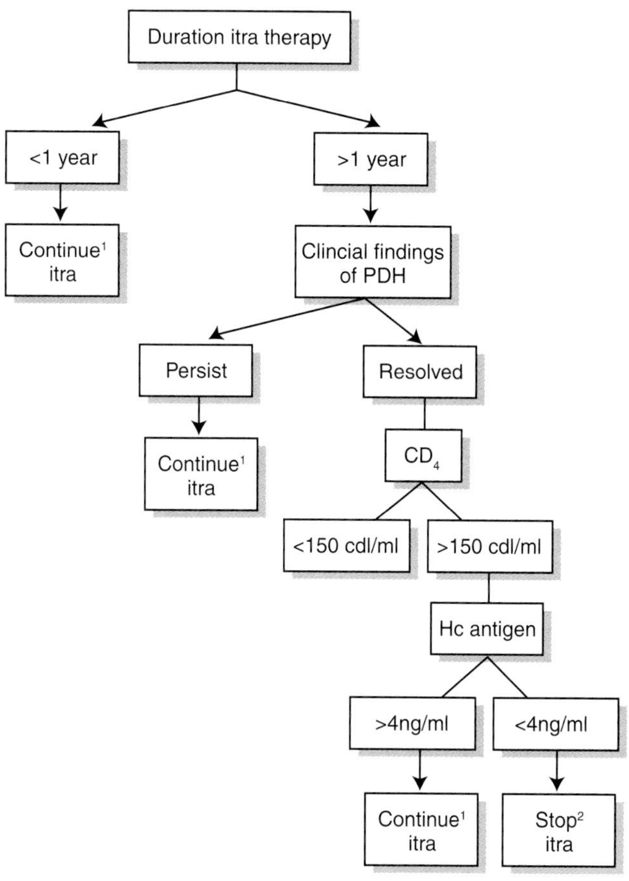

1. Continue to monitor CD_4 cell count and H. capsulalum (Hc) antigen every 3 to 4 months, and reevaluate need for suppressive therapy.
2. Continue to monitor CD_4 cell and HcAg every 3 to 4 months, and reveevaluate need to resume suppressive therapy.

Figure 44-3 ■ Determination if suppressive therapy can be stopped.[52]

Guidelines for Treatment of Disseminated Histoplasmosis in Patients with AIDS

Table 44-4

Severity	Drug	Dose	Duration
Induction			
Mild	Itraconazole	400 mg/day[a]	12 weeks
Moderate or severe	Liposomal amphotericin B	3 mg kg^{-1} day^{-1}	3–14 days
	then itraconazole	400 mg/day	12 weeks
Suppressive[b]	Itraconazole	200 mg/day	At least 1 year, CD4+ T-lymphocyte >150 cells/mm^3, and Hag <4 units, or 4 ng/mL

[a]The itraconazole capsule formulation is preferred, because of better gastrointestinal tolerability compared to the solution formulation. Itraconazole should be administered 200 mg three times daily for 3 days as a loading dose, 200 mg twice daily for 12 weeks as induction therapy, and then 200 mg once or twice daily for suppressive therapy.

[b]Suppressive therapy may be discontinued after one year in patients with CD4+ T-lymphocyte count above 150 cells/mm^3, and low antigen levels.

and reduce blood concentrations of itraconazole and should be avoided. Ritonavir increases the blood concentration of free itraconazole but reduces the concentration of its hydroxy-metabolite,[58] permitting reduction of itraconazole dosage in some patients.

Itraconazole inhibits hepatic P450 enzymes and thus slows the metabolism and increases the blood concentrations of many other drugs, including some antiretroviral agents, potentiating their toxicities. Itraconazole is contraindicated with cisapride, pimozide, quinidine, dofetilide, midazolam, triazolam, lovastatin, and simvastatin. Toxicities of other medications dependent upon P450 3A4 metabolism for clearance may be increased, necessitating careful follow-up and blood level monitoring when possible. The list of interacting medications should be reviewed with new prescriptions of itraconazole because of addition of new agents to the list.

Posaconazole 800 mg daily divided into two to four doses is the preferred alternative to itraconazole, adjusted to achieve a trough concentration of at least 0.5 μg/mL. If voriconazole is used, the recommended dosage is 200 mg twice daily and blood concentrations should be measured, striving for a trough concentration of at least 0.5 μg/mL. A higher dosage may be needed in some patients to achieve a trough concentration above 0.5 μg/mL. If patients are treated with fluconazole, a high dosage is recommended (800 mg daily in adults with normal renal function), and patients should be followed carefully for relapse. The echinocandins, alone or in combination with other antifungal agents, should not be used for the treatment of histoplasmosis.

Suppressive therapy can be safely stopped in selected patients (Fig. 44-3).[59] However, therapy should be resumed if CD4+ T-lymphocyte count falls below 100 cells/mm^3, antigen levels increase suggestive of a relapse, the patient is non-adherent to HAART, or a relapse is diagnosed.

PREVENTION

Patients with CD4+ T-lymphocyte counts below 100/mm^3 should avoid exposure to sites containing large amounts of bat or bird guano and to activities exposing them to soil. Most patients are unaware of the risk for histoplasmosis, supporting a recommendation that providers educate their patients about the risk when traveling to highly endemic areas or participating in high-risk activities exposing them to soil or guano, most notably caving. Patients with HIV infection with CD4+ T-lymphocyte counts below 500 cells/mm^3 should avoid caving; cleaning, remodeling, or demolition of buildings with accumulations of bat or bird droppings; clearing trees, digging or excavating in sites where birds have roosted. Furthermore, they should be advised to report such exposures to their physician, so that appropriate tests can be performed to diagnose PDH early, and treatment initiated promptly.

Antifungal prophylaxis is another option in patients at high risk for histoplasmosis. Itraconazole prophylaxis in persons with CD4+ T-lymphocyte counts below 150 cells/mm^3 reduced the incidence of PDH more than twofold, but had no impact on survival,[60] presumably because of the excellent outcome in patients who are followed closely in clinical trials. Nevertheless, prophylaxis may be appropriate during outbreaks of histoplasmosis, in areas where the incidence of histoplasmosis exceeded five cases per hundred patients per year, and following acute exposure. The duration of prophylaxis depends on the circumstances of exposure. For example, following a single exposure, a short course of prophylaxis, perhaps 6 to 12 weeks, should suffice. During a community-wide outbreak, prophylaxis should be continued as long as the case rate exceeds the target threshold, and CD4+ T-lymphocyte counts remain below 150 cells/mm^3.

REFERENCES

1. Antinori S, Magni C, Nebuloni M, et al. Histoplasmosis among human immunodeficiency virus-infected people in Europe: report of 4 cases and review of the literature. Medicine (Baltimore) 85:22–36, 2006.
2. Wheat LJ, Conces DJ Jr, Allen S, et al. Pulmonary Histoplasmosis Syndromes: recognition, diagnosis, and management. Semin Respir Crit Care Med 25:129–44, 2004.
3. Wheat LJ, Connolly-Stringfield PA, Baker RL, et al. Disseminated histoplasmosis in the acquired immune deficiency syndrome: clinical findings, diagnosis and treatment, and review of the literature. Medicine (Baltimore) 69:361–74, 1990.
4. Wheat J. Histoplasmosis in the acquired immunodeficiency syndrome. Curr Top Med Mycol 7:7–18, 1996.
5. McKinsey DS, Waxman MJ, Idstrom ME. Differentiation of disseminated histoplasmosis from pneumocystis pneumonia in AIDS. Infect Med 10:30–8, 1993.
6. Conces DJ Jr, Stockberger SM, Tarver RD, Wheat LJ. Disseminated histoplasmosis in AIDS: findings on chest radiographs. AJR Am J Roentgenol 160:15–9, 1993.
7. Wheat LJ, Batteiger BE, Sathapatayavongs B. *Histoplasma capsulatum* infections of the central nervous system. A clinical review. Medicine (Baltimore) 69:244–60, 1990.
8. Wheat LJ, Musial CE, Jenny-Avital E. Diagnosis and management of central nervous system histoplasmosis. Clin Infect Dis 40:844–52, 2005.
9. Kahi CJ, Wheat LJ, Allen SD, Sarosi GA. Gastrointestinal histoplasmosis. Am J Gastroenterol 100:220–31, 2005.
10. Morrison YY, Rathbun RC, Huycke MM. Disseminated histoplasmosis mimicking Crohn's disease in a patient with the acquired immunodeficiency syndrome. Am J Gastroenterol 89:1255–7, 1994.
11. Karimi K, Wheat LJ, Connolly P, et al. Differences in histoplasmosis in patients with acquired immunodeficiency syndrome in the United States and Brazil. J Infect Dis 186:1655–60, 2002.
12. Shelburne SA III, Visnegarwala F, Adams C, et al. Unusual manifestations of disseminated histoplasmosis in patients responding to antiretroviral therapy. Am J Med 118:1038–41, 2005.
13. Breton G, Adle-Biassette H, Therby A, et al. Immune reconstitution inflammatory syndrome in HIV-infected patients with disseminated histoplasmosis. AIDS 20:119–21, 2006.
14. Kasuga T, White TJ, Koenig G, et al. Phylogeography of the fungal pathogen *Histoplasma capsulatum*. Mol Ecol 12:3383–401, 2003.
15. McKinsey DS, Spiegel RA, Hutwagner L, et al. Prospective study of histoplasmosis in patients infected with human immunodeficiency virus: incidence, risk factors, and pathophysiology. Clin Infect Dis 24:1195–203, 1997.

16. Keath EJ, Kobayashi GS, Medoff G. Typing of *Histoplasma capsulatum* by restriction fragment length polymorphisms in a nuclear gene. J Clin Microbiol 30:2104–7, 1992.
17. Deepe GS Jr, Wuthrich M, Klein BS. Progress in vaccination for histoplasmosis and blastomycosis: coping with cellular immunity. Med Mycol 43:381–9, 2005.
18. Wallis RS, Broder M, Wong J, et al. Reactivation of latent granulomatous infections by infliximab. Clin Infect Dis 41(Suppl 3):S194–8, 2005.
19. Gutierrez ME, Canton A, Sosa N, et al. Disseminated histoplasmosis in patients with AIDS in Panama: a review of 104 cases. Clin Infect Dis 40:1199–202, 2005.
20. Wheat LJ. Current diagnosis of histoplasmosis. Trends Microbiol 11:488–94, 2003.
21. Koduri PR, Chundi V, Demarais P, et al. Reactive hemophagocytic syndrome: A new presentation of disseminated histoplasmosis in patients with AIDS. Clin Infect Dis 21:1463–5, 1995.
22. Butt AA, Michaels S, Kissinger P. The association of serum lactate dehydrogenase level with selected opportunistic infections and HIV progression. Int J Infect Dis 6:178–81, 2002.
23. Kirn DH, Fredericks D, McCutchan JA, et al. Marked elevation of the serum ferritin is highly specific for disseminated histoplasmosis in AIDS. AIDS 9:1204–5, 1995.
24. Kurtin PJ, McKinsey DS, Gupta MR, Driks M. Histoplasmosis in patients with acquired immunodeficiency syndrome: hematologic and bone marrow manifestations. Am J Clin Pathol 93:367–72, 1990.
25. Casanova-Cardiel LJ, Ruiz-Ordaz I. *Histoplasma capsulatum* in the peripheral blood of patients with AIDS. Report of 4 cases with an increase of lactate dehydrogenase. Rev Invest Clin 45:67–70, 1993.
26. Williams B, Fojtasek M, Connolly-Stringfield P, Wheat J. Diagnosis of histoplasmosis by antigen detection during an outbreak in Indianapolis, Ind. Arch Pathol Lab Med 118:1205–8, 1994.
27. Wheat LJ, Connolly-Stringfield P, Williams B, et al. Diagnosis of histoplasmosis in patients with the acquired immunodeficiency syndrome by detection of *Histoplasma capsulatum* polysaccharide antigen in bronchoalveolar lavage fluid. Am Rev Respir Dis 145:1421–4, 1992.
28. Wheat LJ, Connolly-Stringfield P, Blair R, et al. Effect of successful treatment with amphotericin B on *Histoplasma capsulatum* variety *capsulatum* polysaccharide antigen levels in patients with AIDS and histoplasmosis. Am J Med 92:153–60, 1992.
29. Wheat LJ, Cloud G, Johnson PC, et al. Clearance of fungal burden during treatment of disseminated histoplasmosis with liposomal amphotericin B versus itraconazole. Antimicrob Agents Chemother 45:2354–7, 2001.
30. Wheat LJ, Connolly P, Haddad N, et al. Antigen clearance during treatment of disseminated histoplasmosis with itraconazole versus fluconazole in patients with AIDS. Antimicrob Agents Chemother 46:248–50, 2002.
31. Wheat LJ, Connolly-Stringfield P, Blair R, et al. Histoplasmosis relapse in patients with AIDS: detection using *Histoplasma capsulatum* variety *capsulatum* antigen levels. Ann Intern Med 115:936–41, 1991.
32. Wheat LJ, Connolly P, Durkin M, et al. False-positive *Histoplasma* antigenemia caused by antithymocyte globulin antibodies. Transpl Infect Dis 6:23–7, 2004.
33. Vail GM, Mocherla S, Wheat LJ, et al. Cellular immune response in HIV-infected patients with histoplasmosis. J Acquir Immune Defic Syndr 29:49–53, 2002.
34. Wheat LJ, Chetchotisakd P, Williams B, et al. Factors associated with severe manifestations of histoplasmosis in AIDS. Clin Infect Dis 30:877–81, 2000.
35. Couppie P, Roussel M, Thual N, et al.Disseminated histoplasmosis: an atypical ulcerous form in an HIV-infected patient. Ann Dermatol Venereol 132:133–5, 2005.
36. Johnson PC, Wheat LJ, Cloud GA, et al. Safety and efficacy of liposomal amphotericin B compared with conventional amphotericin B for induction therapy of histoplasmosis in patients with AIDS. Ann Intern Med 137:105–9, 2002.
37. Wheat J, Hafner R, Korzun AH, et al. Itraconazole treatment of disseminated histoplasmosis in patients with the acquired immunodeficiency syndrome. AIDS Clinical Trial Group. Am J Med 98:336–42, 1995.
38. Wheat J, MaWhinney S, Hafner R, et al. Treatment of histoplasmosis with fluconazole in patients with acquired immunodeficiency syndrome. National Institute of Allergy and Infectious Diseases Acquired Immunodeficiency Syndrome Clinical Trials Group and Mycoses Study Group. Am J Med 103:223–32, 1997.
39. Wheat LJ, Connolly P, Smedema M, et al. Emergence of resistance to fluconazole as a cause of failure during treatment of histoplasmosis in patients with acquired immunodeficiency disease syndrome. Clin Infect Dis 33:1910–3, 2001.
40. Connolly P, Wheat LJ, Schnizlein-Bick C, et al. Comparison of a new triazole, posaconazole, with itraconazole and amphotericin B for treatment of histoplasmosis following pulmonary challenge in immunocompromised mice. Antimicrob Agents Chemother 44:2604–8, 2000.
41. Restrepo A, Tobon A, Clark B, et al. Salvage treatment of histoplasmosis with posaconazole. J Infect 54:319–27, 2007.
42. Clark B, Foster R, Tunbridge A, Green S. A case of disseminated histoplasmosis successfully treated with the investigational drug posaconazole. J Infect 51:e177–80, 2005.
42a. Wheat LJ, Connolly P, Smedema M, et al. Activity of newer triazoles against *Histoplasma capsulatum* from patients with AIDS who failed fluconazole. J Antimicrob Chemother 57:1235–9, 2006.
43. Wheat LJ, Connolly P, Smedema M, et al. Activity of newer triazoles against *Histoplasma capsulatum* from patients with AIDS who failed fluconazole. J Antimicrob Chemother 57:1235–9, 2006.
44. Nath DS, Kandaswamy R, Gruessner R, et al. Fungal infections in transplant recipients receiving alemtuzumab. Transplant Proc 37:934–6, 2005.
45. Hott JS, Horn E, Sonntag VK, et al. Intramedullary histoplasmosis spinal cord abscess in a nonendemic region: case report and review of the literature. J Spinal Disord Tech 16:212–5, 2003.
46. Kohler S, Wheat LJ, Connolly P, et al. Comparison of the echinocandin caspofungin with amphotericin B for treatment of histoplasmosis following pulmonary challenge in a murine model. Antimicrob Agents Chemother 44:1850–4, 2000.
47. Goldberg J, Connolly P, Schnizlein-Bick C, et al. Comparison of nikkomycin Z with amphotericin B and itraconazole for treatment of histoplasmosis in a murine model. Antimicrob Agents Chemother 44:1624–9, 2000.
48. Haynes RR, Connolly PA, Durkin MM, et al. Antifungal therapy for central nervous system histoplasmosis, using a newly developed intracranial model of infection. J Infect Dis 185:1830–2, 2002.
49. McKinsey DS, Gupta MR, Riddler SA, et al. Long-term amphotericin B therapy for disseminated histoplasmosis in patients with the acquired immune deficiency syndrome. Ann Intern Med 111:655–9, 1989.
50. Wheat J, Hafner R, Wulfsohn M, et al. Prevention of relapse of histoplasmosis with itraconazole in patients with the acquired immunodeficiency syndrome. The National Institute of Allergy and Infectious Diseases Clinical Trials and Mycoses Study Group Collaborators. Ann Intern Med 118:610–6, 1993.
51. Hecht FM, Wheat J, Korzun AH, et al. Itraconazole maintenance treatment for histoplasmosis in AIDS: a prospective, multicenter trial. J Acquir Immune Defic Syndr Hum Retrovirol 16:100–7, 1997.
52. Goldman M, Zackin R, Fichtenbaum CJ, et al. Safety of discontinuation of maintenance therapy for disseminated histoplasmosis

after immunologic response to antiretroviral therapy. Clin Infect Dis 38:1485–9, 2004.
53. Jaruratanasirikul S, Sriwiriyajan S. Effect of rifampicin on the pharmacokinetics of itraconazole in normal volunteers and AIDS patients. Eur J Clin Pharmacol 54:155–8, 1998.
54. Drayton J, Dickinson G, Rinaldi MG. Coadministration of rifampin and itraconazole leads to undetectable levels of serum itraconazole. Clin Infect Dis 18:266, 1994.
55. Benedetti MS. Inducing properties of rifabutin, and effects on the pharmacokinetics and metabolism of concomitant drugs. Pharmacol Res 32:177–87, 1995.
56. Ducharme MP, Slaughter RL, Warbasse LH, et al. Itraconazole and hydroxyitraconazole serum concentrations are reduced more than tenfold by phenytoin. Clin Pharmacol Ther 58: 617–24, 1995.
57. Albengres E, Le Louet H, and Tillement JP. Systemic antifungal agents. Drug interactions of clinical significance. Drug Saf 18:83–97, 1998.
58. Crommentuyn KM, Mulder JW, Sparidans RW, et al. Drug–drug interaction between itraconazole and the antiretroviral drug lopinavir/ritonavir in an HIV-1-infected patient with disseminated histoplasmosis. Clin Infect Dis 38:e73–5, 2004.
59. Keam SJ, Scott LJ, Curran MP. Spotlight on verteporfin in subfoveal choroidal neovascularisation. Drugs Aging 21:203–9, 2004.
60. McKinsey DS, Wheat LJ, Cloud GA, et al. Itraconazole prophylaxis for fungal infections in patients with advanced human immunodeficiency virus infection: randomized, placebo-controlled, double-blind study. National Institute of Allergy and Infectious Diseases Mycoses Study Group. Clin Infect Dis 28:1049–56, 1999.

Chapter 45

Coccidioidomycosis

Neil M. Ampel, MD

INTRODUCTION

Coccidioidomycosis is an infection caused by the dimorphic fungus *Coccidioides*. The endemic region for this mycosis is confined to the Western hemisphere from California to Argentina. Areas of endemicity tend to coincide with distinct geographic and climatic conditions, principally occurring in arid, warm regions with relatively mild winters, hot summers and with alkaline soils. In the United States, the endemic region extends from the San Joaquin Valley of California, from which the common name for coccidioidomycosis, Valley Fever, is derived, to western Texas.[1,2] The areas of highest endemicity are the southern San Joaquin Valley and the region encompassing Phoenix and Tucson in south-central Arizona.[1–3]

Recently, genetic analysis has indicated that *Coccidioides* can be divided into two species, *C. immitis* and *C. posadasii*.[4] While it is posited that *C. immitis* is geographically limited to California and *C. posadasii* is extant in other parts of the coccidioidal endemic region, this has not been established. Moreover, there are no clinical aspects of infection that distinguish these two species. Because of this, only the genus *Coccidioides* will be referred to in this chapter.

In the soil, *Coccidioides* exists as a mold in which alternating hyphal cells degenerate. The intervening live cells, called arthroconidia, may dislodge and become airborne, particularly in dry, windy conditions. If inhaled by a susceptible host, the arthroconidia can reach the alveoli and initiate infection. Once this occurs, *Coccidioides* undergoes a unique transformation among the pathogenic fungi. The outer wall rounds up and internal septations form to yield the spherule stage. These septations give rise to internal endospores. Spherules may rupture and release packets of endospores, propagating the infection within the host.

Among immunocompetent individuals, coccidioidal infection is completely asymptomatic in 60% of all cases.[5] The remainder usually present with nonspecific pulmonary symptoms. Approximately 1–5% of all patients develop chronic disease, either persistent pulmonary illness or infection disseminated beyond the thoracic cavity.[2,6] Patients who develop chronic disease may have been asymptomatic or had symptoms at the time of initial infection.

Clinical and *in vitro* studies have all indicated that cell-mediated immunity is important in host defense against coccidioidomycosis.[7–9] In particular, patients who have mild, self-limited disease usually manifest delayed-type hypersensitivity upon skin testing with coccidioidal antigens and have minimal serum antibody responses. On the other hand, patients with chronic, active disease, particularly those with disseminated infection, usually lack coccidioidal delayed-type hypersensitivity and have high serum anticoccidioidal antibody titers.[7] Because of this, it is not surprising that coccidioidomycosis is recognized as an opportunistic infection among patients with HIV infection, particularly among those living in the coccidioidal endemic areas.[10,11]

EPIDEMIOLOGY

During the early part of the HIV epidemic, coccidioidomycosis was not recognized as an opportunistic process in persons infected with HIV. One reason for this was that the initial epicenters of the HIV epidemic in North America, including the Los Angeles basin, were not in areas endemic for coccidioidomycosis and reports of cases were sporadic.[12–17] Another reason is that symptomatic coccidioidomycosis often occurs in individuals without any underlying immunodeficiency. The first series of cases of coccidioidomycosis occurring among HIV-infected persons was reported by Bronnimann and colleagues in 1987.[18] In that report, seven of 27 patients with AIDS living in southern Arizona developed symptomatic coccidioidomycosis. Six of the seven had diffuse, nodular pulmonary infiltrates, five had detectable anticoccidioidal antibodies in their sera, and all died within 14 months of the diagnosis of coccidioidomycosis. Since that report, two large case series[19,20] and one prospective study[10] have been published, expanding our understanding of the clinical expression and epidemiology of coccidioidomycosis during HIV infection.

The impact of coccidioidomycosis on patients infected with HIV infection is not geographically uniform. For example, 8.2% of all patients from Arizona reported to the Centers for Disease Control (CDC) as having AIDS had concomitant coccidioidomycosis, compared to only 0.3% nation-wide.[11] Moreover, 10% of all hospitalizations among HIV-infected persons in Arizona in 1993 included a discharge diagnosis of coccidioidomycosis and 44% of all hospitalizations for coccidioidomycosis were among HIV-infected patients.[3]

In the CDC study,[11] only 0.5% of all cases of AIDS in California were reported as having concomitant coccidioidomycosis. However, the impact of HIV infection on the development of active coccidioidomycosis appears to be significantly greater in the coccidioidal endemic areas within the state. Using data from the California State Health Department, Rutherford and colleagues found that 3.5% of patients living in Kern County, a known coccidioidal endemic area, were reported as having coccidioidomycosis as their AIDS-defining diagnosis, compared to only 0.3% for the entire state.[21]

These data indicate that coccidioidomycosis has become a major opportunistic infection in coccidioidal endemic areas. This is illustrated by the results of a prospective study from Arizona.[10] In that study, 170 HIV-infected persons who were without active coccidioidomycosis on entry were followed over time. After 41 months, 13 of these subjects developed active coccidioidomycosis, yielding an estimated cumulative incidence of ~25%. Only two risk factors, a CD4 lymphocyte count <250/μL and the clinical diagnosis of AIDS, were associated with the development of active coccidioidomycosis. Length of stay in the endemic area, a history of a prior diagnosis of coccidioidomycosis, and a positive coccidioidal skin-test were not associated with a risk of developing active coccidioidomycosis. Moreover, 11 of the 13 subjects who developed active coccidioidomycosis had either focal or diffuse pulmonary involvement. All this suggests that most clinical disease was due to primary infection.

For cases in those who have not recently resided in the endemic area, reactivation of prior infection is the mechanism of disease. In some instances, reactivation may occur years after acquisition of initial infection, as in the case of a Spanish man with HIV infection who developed cervical lymphadenitis 12 years after leaving the coccidioidal endemic zone.[22] Whether there are immunologic and epidemiologic differences between those who develop active coccidioidomycosis within the coccidioidal endemic area compared to those who develop it outside this area is not known. To date, coccidioidomycosis has not been reported as a major opportunistic infection among HIV-infected persons living in coccidioidal endemic regions outside the United States, such as in northern Mexico and focal areas of Central and South America.

The incidence of most infectious opportunistic infections has declined since the advent of potent antiretroviral therapy,[23] and it is reasonable to presume that a decline in the incidence of coccidioidomycosis among those with HIV infection has also occurred. In a retrospective analysis of cases of coccidioidomycosis in southern Arizona from 1994 through 1997,[24] a period which spans the initiation of the use of HAART, the number of cases of coccidioidomycosis among those with HIV infection declined from 77 in 1995 to 15 in 1997. While no subsequent studies have been performed, the number of cases of coccidioidomycosis among those with HIV infection seen in clinics within the endemic area appears to be lower than that observed prior to the advent of potent antiretroviral therapy. However, it is clear that coccidioidomycosis still remains a significant opportunistic infection among HIV-infected persons living within the endemic area. In one large clinic in Tucson, AZ, coccidioidomycosis was the most common cause of mortality in those with HIV infection (JK Carmichael, personal communication).

CLINICAL MANIFESTATIONS

The clinical spectrum of coccidioidomycosis among HIV-infected persons has been documented in several case series reports.[10,19,20] Diffuse pneumonia is the most common presentation. This is a devastating form of coccidioidomycosis, with a 70% mortality within 1 month.[18–20,25] It presents most often in patients with peripheral blood CD4 lymphocyte counts <50/μL, is frequently associated with fungemia, and undoubtedly represents an acute and severe form of disseminated disease. The presentation is nonspecific, with complaints of fever, night sweats, weight loss, and dyspnea. The chest radiograph reveals diffuse pulmonary nodules with increased interstitial markings, frequently described as 'reticulonodular'. In some patients, this nodularity may be striking (Fig. 45-1A), while in others, the radiographic appearance is more subtle and suggestive of *Pneumocystis* pneumonia (Fig. 45-1B). Concurrent pneumocystosis occurs in up to 30% of patients with diffuse, reticulonodular coccidioidomycosis.[19,26] Even with prompt antifungal therapy, this form of coccidioidomycosis is often rapidly fatal.[19,20]

The second most frequent presentation is focal pneumonia.[19,20] This presentation is more likely to occur in more immunocompetent patients with higher peripheral blood CD4 lymphocyte counts. Patients usually complain of cough, either nonproductive or productive of only scanty sputum, associated with pleuritic chest pain and fever. Bacterial pneumonia is usually the first diagnosis considered. However, symptoms persist despite antibiotic therapy. Clinical clues distinguishing coccidioidomycosis from bacterial pneumonia include the presence of mediastinal or hilar adenopathy and peripheral blood eosinophilia. The chest radiograph initially reveals a focal alveolar infiltrate (Fig. 45-2). Over time, usually weeks, this infiltrate may become nodular. The prognosis of focal pulmonary coccidioidomycosis in the HIV-infected patients is better than among those with diffuse pulmonary disease. In one study performed prior to the advent of potent antiretroviral therapy,[19] the median survival of those with focal pulmonary disease was 5 months, compared to 1 month in those

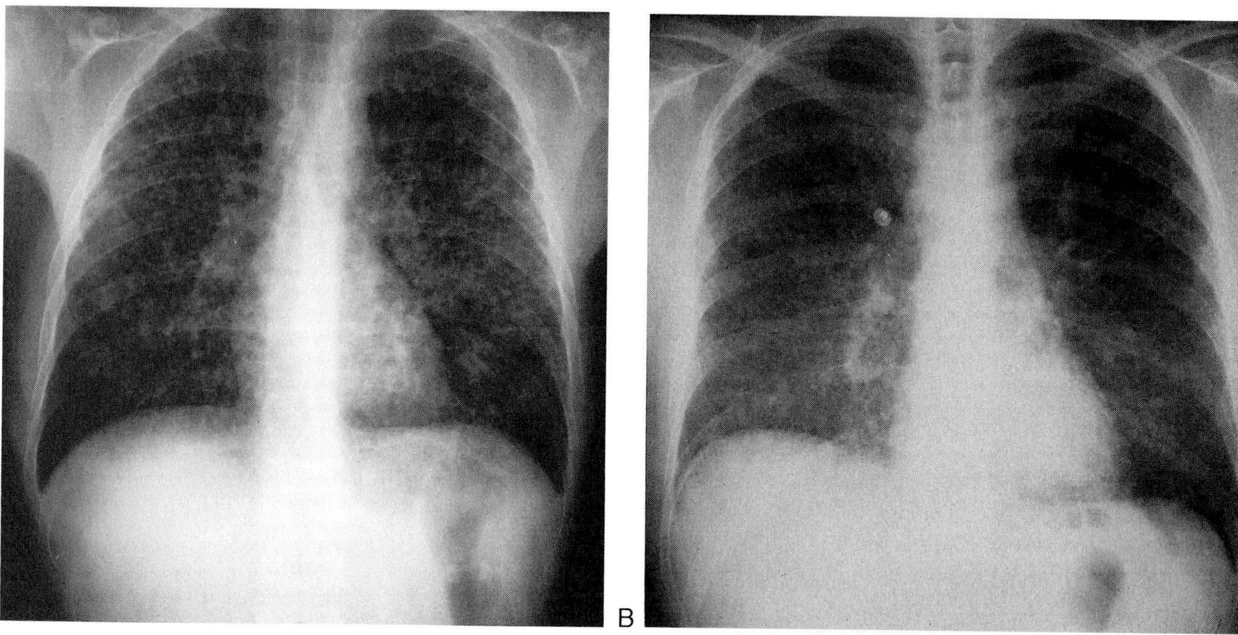

Figure 45-1 ■ Two HIV-infected patients with diffuse reticulonodular coccidioidomycosis; (**A**) chest radiograph from one patient showing diffuse nodularity; (**B**) chest radiograph from another patient revealing a finer, more reticular appearance.

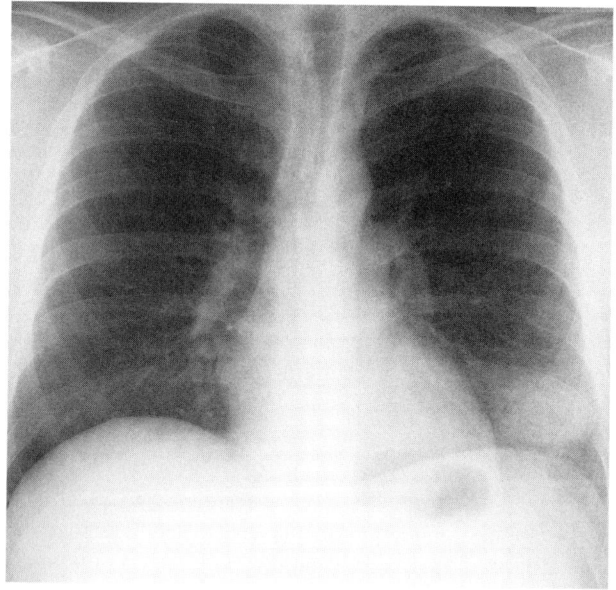

Figure 45-2 ■ Focal, primary coccidioidomycosis in a patient with HIV infection. Chest radiograph reveals a rounded infiltrate in left lower lobe.

with diffuse pulmonary disease. Currently, the survival of HIV-infected patients with focal pulmonary coccidioidomycosis who receive appropriate antifungal and antiretroviral therapy is probably not different from patients at a similar stage of HIV infection without coccidioidomycosis.

The most frequent manifestation of extrathoracic, disseminated coccidioidomycosis in the HIV-infected patient is meningitis. Coccidioidal meningitis in patients without HIV infection usually presents with headache and a decrease in mental status occurring over a period of weeks to months, usually without any other symptoms of active coccidioidomycosis.[27] The presentation is similar in the HIV-infected patient except that concurrent pulmonary involvement, particularly reticulonodular pneumonia, is more likely to be present.[20] The CSF profile of HIV-infected patients is the same as in other groups of patients. There is a lymphocytic pleocytosis with hypoglycorrhachia. The finding of eosinophils in the CSF is further suggestive. Because it is uncommon to isolate *Coccidioides* from the CSF in cases of coccidioidal meningitis, this CSF profile may be presumed to be due to tuberculous meningitis. The diagnosis of coccidioidal meningitis should always be considered in cases of lymphocytic meningitis with hypoglycorrhachia, whether within or outside the coccidioidal endemic region.

Other manifestations of disseminated coccidioidomycosis in the HIV-infected patient include cutaneous disease, lymph node involvement, and bone and joint disease. These generally present in a manner similar to that seen in patients without HIV infection, with the exception that bone and joint disease appears to be very uncommon in HIV-infected patients. Another form of disseminated coccidioidomycosis is hepatosplenic involvement, manifesting as fever, fatigue, weight loss, and an enlarged liver and spleen in association with elevated coccidioidal serologic titers. This presentation is similar to that seen with disseminated histoplasmosis in the HIV-infected patient.[28]

A unique presentation of coccidioidomycosis in the HIV-infected person is a positive serum antibody reaction without clinical manifestations of illness.[10,19] In one study, five of 13 individuals with positive coccidioidal serologic tests as their only manifestation of coccidioidomycosis subsequently developed active disease from 4 to 35 months after the positive serology was first noted. In four instances, patients developed pulmonary coccidioidomycosis, while in the fifth case, hepatosplenic coccidioidomycosis occurred. Prior use of antifungal therapy did not significantly reduce the risk of developing active coccidioidomycosis, but doses and duration of therapy varied considerably. The median peripheral blood CD4 lymphocyte count at the time of development of the positive serologic test was 89/μL, while it was 10/μL at the time of development of active disease. Most of the positive tests were of the complement-fixing type, with titers ranging from 1:2 to 1:128.[29] These data suggest that a positive coccidioidal antibody test in an HIV-infected person represents true infection with a significant risk for the development of clinically active disease.

DIAGNOSIS

The first principle in establishing the diagnosis of coccidioidomycosis in the HIV-infected patient is to consider it. Whether within or outside the endemic area, the diagnosis should be entertained in any HIV-infected patient who presents with a diffuse pneumonia, a focal pneumonia not responsive to antibacterial agents, or a lymphocytic meningitis (see Figs 45-3 and 45-4).

There are two general approaches to making the diagnosis of coccidioidomycosis in the HIV-infected patient. The first is to obtain a clinical specimen and directly examine it for the presence of *Coccidioides.* With pulmonary involvement, either an expectorated sputum or a respiratory sample obtained by bronchoscopy is useful. Direct examination of tissue from biopsy of involved tissue is often required to correctly diagnose cutaneous, lymphoid, hepatosplenic, or the rare cases of bone and joint coccidioidomycosis. For meningitis, samples of CSF infrequently reveal the presence of the fungus and the diagnosis is usually established indirectly by serology.

Once a clinical specimen is in hand, there are several tests available to detect *Coccidioides.* The KOH test is commonly used on sputum and respiratory samples. While this test is simple to perform, it has a very low yield. The Papanicolaou or Gomori-methenamine stains, particularly when used on a cell pellet obtained after centrifugation of a sample obtained by bronchoalveolar lavage (BAL), have the advantage of allowing for the identification of spherules of *Coccidioides* as well as trophozoites and cysts of *Pneumocystis.*[30] However, the yield of such cytologic stains for coccidioidomycosis may be as low as 40% in patients with HIV infection.[31] For biopsy specimens, examination of fixed samples stained by hematoxylin-eosin usually reveals the presence of spherules. The Gomori-methenamine stain, by staining spherules and endospores black, may make the organisms more easily identifiable, but is more time-consuming to perform.

Many clinicians are under the misapprehension that *Coccidioides* is fastidious and difficult to cultivate. The fungus will usually display visible colonies in culture in as few as 3–7 days on a variety of culture media.[6] Culture of respiratory samples and biopsy specimens has a high yield. In one study, culture of respiratory samples revealed the presence of *Coccidioides* in a total of 69% of cases, while lung biopsy specimens were positive in 80%.[20] Because of this, any clinical specimen suspected of containing *Coccidioides* should be cultured.

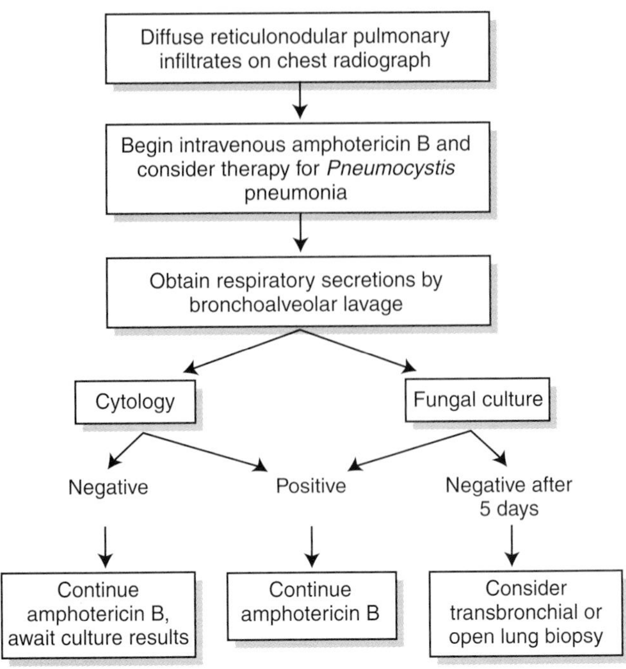

Figure 45-3 ■ Algorithm for the diagnosis and management of diffuse, reticulonodular pulmonary coccidioidomycosis in the HIV-infected patient.

Sequences unique to *Coccidioides* have been identified on the gene encoding 18S ribosomal RNA,[32] making genomic identification of the fungus within clinical specimens a possibility. While genomic identification is now used to confirm the identification of *Coccidioides* once it is visibly growing,[33] no assays are currently available for direct identification in clinical specimens. In addition, no test is clinically available to detect either antigenemia or antigenuria in coccidioidomycosis.

Without direct evidence of *Coccidioides*, detection of anticoccidioidal antibodies in the serum and CSF has been frequently used to establish the diagnosis of coccidioidomycosis. Understanding coccidioidal serology is complicated by antiquated nomenclature and changing methodology.[34,35] Two types of antibodies are recognized. Antibodies of the IgM type, first detected using the tube precipitins (TP) method, occur early in the course of disease or during acute reactivation. Serum titers of anticoccidioidal IgM antibodies do not predict outcome and they are rarely positive in the CSF in coccidioidal meningitis. On the other hand, IgG antibodies, first detected by complement fixation (CF), rise later in the course of disease, are useful in the diagnosis of meningitis, and serum and CSF titers are helpful in following the course of the disease.

Besides the TP and CF methods, latex agglutination (LA), immunodiffusion (ID), and enzyme immunoassay (EIA) are also available for detecting anticoccidioidal antibodies. The LA test is only useful for detecting IgM antibodies and has

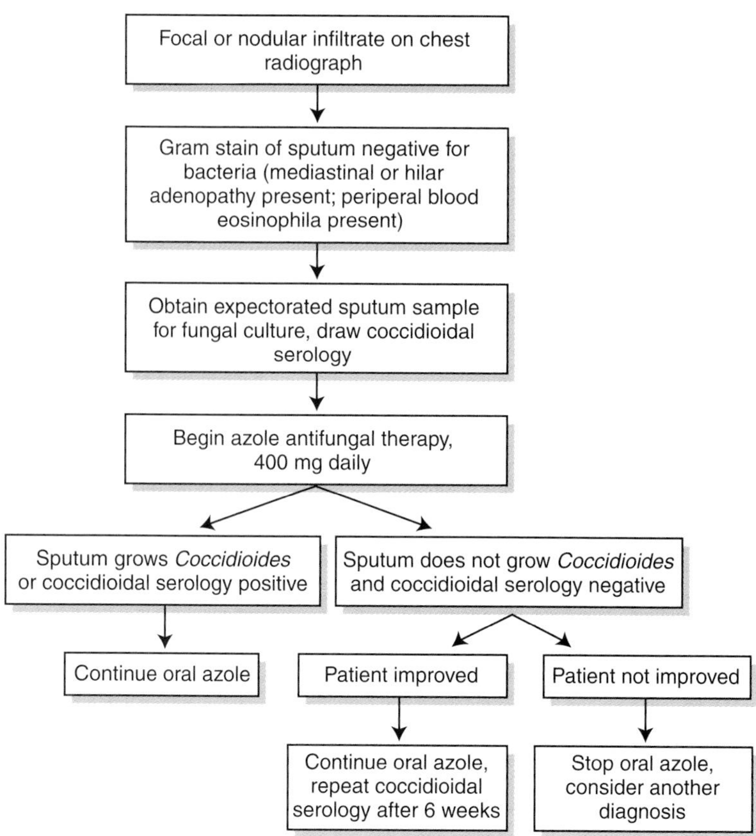

Figure 45-4 ■ Algorithm for the diagnosis and management of focal pulmonary coccidioidomycosis in the HIV-infected patient.

a high false-positive rate. Any positive result should be confirmed by another method.[34] The ID technique, which detects both TP (IDTP) and CF (IDCF) antibodies, is very sensitive and specific.[34–36] The commercially available Premier EIA (Meridian Diagnostics, Inc, Cincinnati, OH) detects both IgM and IgG antibodies and appears to be as sensitive as ID.[36–38] However false positives have been reported.[36] In addition, unlike the IDCF and CF, the IgG EIA is not expressed as a titer, making it less useful in monitoring response to therapy (Pappagianis, unpublished observations).

In individuals with HIV-infection and coccidioidomycosis, tests for anticoccidioidal antibodies in the serum are positive at the time of diagnosis in 68–100% of patients.[19,20,39] IgG type antibodies are more likely to be positive than the IgM types.[19] While some HIV-infected patients never develop positive serologic tests for coccidioidomycosis despite active infection,[39] serology remains an important diagnostic tool for most patients. It has been estimated that from 15% to 20% of patients with HIV infection and coccidioidomycosis have negative coccidioidal serologic tests, but Pappagianis has noted that only 5–7% of such samples are negative when tested in his laboratory, probably because of concentration of the serum.[35]

TREATMENT

There are currently several types of antifungal agents that are available for the treatment of coccidioidomycosis in the HIV-infected patient (see Table 45-1). The oldest is amphotericin B, a polyene macrolide initially formulated as a deoxycholate dispersion (Fungizone). Although clearly effective in the treatment of coccidioidomycosis, this formulation of amphotericin B has numerous drawbacks, including the necessity of intravenous administration and multiple adverse reactions.[40] Moreover, intravenous amphotericin B is not useful in the treatment of coccidioidal meningitis. For this form of disease, intrathecal administration is required.[41] When using intravenous amphotericin B in the deoxycholate formulation for the treatment of coccidioidomycosis, an initial daily dosage of 1.0–1.5 mg/kg should be prescribed. In recent years, several new formulations of amphotericin B have become available for clinical use, including a lipid dispersion (ABLC, ABELCET), a cholesteryl colloidal dispersion (ABCD, Amphotec), and a true liposomal preparation (Ambisome). In a recent study of murine coccidioidomycosis, deoxycholate amphotericin B was more effective in reducing fungal burden than the lipid formulations on a mg/kg basis, but higher doses of the lipid formulations could be given.[42] Clemons and colleagues observed that intravenous liposomal amphotericin B demonstrated efficacy equivalent to fluconazole in a rabbit model of coccidioidal meningitis.[43] However, this has not been confirmed in humans. Despite their reduced renal toxicity and anecdotal reports of efficacy in human coccidioidomycosis,[44] no clinical trials of lipid formulated amphotericin B have been conducted. For now, their use should continue to be reserved for those patients who are at high risk for toxicity due to the deoxycholate formulation or develop toxicity with therapy.[45]

Table 45-1

Recommendations Regarding Treatment of Coccidioidomycosis in Adult Patients Infected With HIV[a]

Type of Disease	Recommended Therapy	Alternative Therapy
Diffuse pneumonia	IV amphotericin B, 1.0–1.5 $mg\,kg^{-1}\,day^{-1}$[b]	Fluconazole or itraconazole, at least 400 mg/day[c]
Focal pneumonia	Oral fluconazole or itraconazole, at least 400 mg/day[c]	IV amphotericin B, 1.0–1.5 $mg\,kg^{-1}\,day^{-1}$ followed by oral fluconazole or itraconazole, at least 400 mg/day[c]
Meningitis	Oral fluconazole or itraconazole, beginning at 800 mg/day	Intrathecal amphotericin B[d]
Other forms of dissemination	Oral fluconazole or itraconazole, at least 400 mg/day[c]	IV amphotericin B, 1.0–1.5 $mg\,kg^{-1}\,day^{-1}$ followed by oral fluconazole or itraconazole, at least 400 mg/day[c]
Positive serology only	Oral fluconazole or itraconazole, at least 400 mg/day[c]	Observation

For all instances of coccidioidomycosis during HIV infection, life-long therapy is recommended.

[a] Assumes normal renal and hepatic function.
[b] Assumes use of the deoxycholate preparation (Fungizone).
[c] Fluconazole preferred because of better absorption, fewer drug interactions.
[d] Should be administered by someone with prior experience.

The orally absorbable azole antifungals comprise the second class of antifungal agents, of which ketoconazole, fluconazole, itraconazole, and voriconazole are currently available in the United States. Posaconazole was also recently approved for use in the United States. The use of ketoconazole for the treatment of coccidioidomycosis has largely been supplanted by the triazoles fluconazole and itraconazole. While used extensively for the treatment of coccidioidomycosis, neither fluconazole nor itraconazole is approved by the Food and Drug Administration (FDA) for this purpose.[46] In a variety of studies, both drugs have been found to be useful for the treatment of most forms of coccidioidomycosis in persons without HIV infection.[47–51] However, relapse after therapy is discontinued has been frequent for both drugs.[47,51] Fluconazole and itraconazole differ in their absorption, protein binding, and metabolism.[52] While fluconazole is well absorbed from the gastrointestinal tract and is not affected by food or gastric acid,[53] the itraconazole capsule formulation requires the presence of acid for maximum absorption, often a problem in HIV-infected persons.[54] An oral cyclodextrin solution of itraconazole has higher bioavailability,[55] but has not been studied in coccidioidomycosis.

A study directly comparing fluconazole to itraconazole, in the capsule formulation, for the management of coccidioidomycosis has been published.[56] Among the 198 subjects with various forms of chronic coccidioidomycosis, seven had concomitant HIV infection. There were no statistically significant differences between those who received fluconazole compared with those who received itraconazole after 8 months of therapy. While specific details of response among those subjects with HIV infection were not provided, HIV infection was not found to be a risk factor for failure of therapy. In this study, serum levels of itraconazole did not predict response. Given these data, either fluconazole or itraconazole appear to be appropriate choices for the treatment of coccidioidomycosis, including among those with HIV infection. Whichever azole antifungal is chosen for therapy, the initial daily dosage for the adult should be at least 400 mg[47,51] to ensure optimal response. Azole antifungals at high doses have been associated with congenital anomalies.[57] Caution is advised when treating pregnant females with these agents as therapy for coccidioidomycosis and they should be combined with effective contraception if used in any female of childbearing potential.

Voriconazole, a second-generation triazole, has been available in the United States since 2001.[58] While there are no published animal studies of its use in coccidioidomycosis and no controlled trials in humans, there are several reports indicating its apparent efficacy in cases that have failed to respond to other agents.[59–61] At this time, voriconazole may be considered in cases of coccidioidomycosis not responding to fluconazole or itraconazole. However, safety issues and drug interactions make the use of voriconazole problematic. Posaconazole is another newer triazole that was found to be very potent in a murine model of coccidioidomycosis.[62] A recently published noncomparative human trial suggests efficacy.[63]

Two reports suggest that the β-1,3-glucan-synthase inhibitor caspofungin may possess efficacy in the therapy of coccidioidomycosis.[64,65] Neither of the two reported cases were in patients with HIV infection. At this time, the use of caspofungin or any of its congeners cannot be advocated as therapy in coccidioidomycosis except in refractory cases.[45] In addition, Kuberski reported that interferon-γ administered intramuscularly at 50 μg/m^2 thrice-weekly in combination with liposomal amphotericin B resulted in eventual improvement in a critically ill patient with disseminated coccidioidomycosis who was not infected with HIV.[66]

Clinicians should be aware of interactions between antifungal agents and other medications when treating HIV-infected patients with coccidioidomycosis. Azole antifungals are both metabolized by and inhibitors of the cytochrome P450 (CYP) 3A4 enzyme system.[67] There may be bidirectional alterations of drug metabolism when azoles are combined with other drugs metabolized through this pathway. Well-recognized interactions of azoles include increases in plasma levels of warfarin, phenytoin, digoxin, statins, rifamycins, and cyclosporin. Itraconazole is a particularly potent inhibitor of CYP3A4 and a moderate inhibitor of P-glycoprotein[68] and must be used with caution when combined with drugs metabolized through these pathways.[69] For example, itraconazole increases the levels of the HIV-1 protease inhibitor ritonavir.[70] While there are no published studies on voriconazole, blood concentrations of voriconazole are markedly decreased when given with ritonavir. In addition, voriconazole levels are decreased by efavirenz and voriconazole increases the levels of efavirenz. It is recommended that voriconazole be used with caution with either ritonavir or efavirenz.

In the absence of clinical trials, the therapeutic approach to coccidioidomycosis in the patient with HIV infection must be empiric. Determinations about therapy should revolve around the extent of clinical illness, the degree of immunodeficiency, and the site of infection. Unlike the situation in patients without immunodeficiency, therapy should be considered for all forms of coccidioidomycosis in the HIV-infected patient. Currently, there are no standardized methods for antifungal susceptibility testing of *Coccidioides*.

Most HIV-infected patients who present with focal pulmonary coccidioidomycosis are clinically stable and do not require hospitalization. Given this scenario, therapy with an oral azole antifungal at an initial dosage of 400 mg each day is a reasonable approach. Response can be measured by improvement in clinical symptoms, resolution of the pulmonary process on chest radiograph and a diminution of serum anticoccidioidal CF antibody titers over time. Serum titers may be negative at the time of diagnosis, rise to a peak as the patient responds to therapy over the next weeks to months, and then fall. Hence, a rising serologic titer should not be the only factor in determining whether a patient has initially responded to therapy. Among those who respond to therapy, the initial alveolar infiltrate on chest radiograph will develop sharp, rounded borders and, in some cases, become a nodule. It is important that the initial coccidioidal pneumonia be documented, because the nodule could later be confused with a pulmonary malignancy.

Diffuse, reticulonodular pneumonia has an extremely high mortality[19,20] and requires aggressive treatment. Intravenous amphotericin B is recommended as the initial therapy. Given the significant mortality associated with this form of coccidioidomycosis in HIV-infected patients, a pertinent question is whether amphotericin B should be combined with another antifungal agent. Because azole antifungals inhibit the synthesis of fungal ergosterol while amphotericin B acts by binding to ergosterol, the combination of amphotericin B with azole antifungals is potentially antagonistic. However, *in vitro*, animal, and human data have provided no consistent evidence of such antagonism.[71] Moreover, amphotericin B and azole antifungals have been frequently combined by clinicians treating coccidioidomycosis, particularly meningitis. Hence, in patients failing to respond to amphotericin B, the addition of an azole antifungal can be considered.[45] In those patients who respond to initial amphotericin B therapy, the frequency of infusions can be slowly tapered. In all cases, once the patient is clinically stable, therapy can be changed to an oral azole antifungal alone.

The management of coccidioidal meningitis has changed dramatically since the Mycoses Study Group reported that treatment with oral fluconazole results in an ~80% response rate.[50] In that study of 50 patients, nine had concomitant HIV infection. Of these nine, three did not respond to fluconazole, with two dying and one requiring intrathecal amphotericin B. Although the two deaths were not directly related to coccidioidomycosis, both patients had evidence of continued active coccidioidal infection at the time of death. Of the six patients who responded, all required 800 mg/day of fluconazole. Four of these subjects maintained their improvement over at least 15 months, one developed hydrocephalus, and one required reinstitution of intrathecal amphotericin B.

Given these findings, treatment of coccidioidal meningitis in HIV-infected patients should begin with fluconazole at a daily dose of 800 mg. Itraconazole has also been found to have activity in coccidioidal meningitis in patients without HIV infection,[48] but no data exist on its use in the HIV-infected patient. Failure of azole antifungal therapy should lead to the use of intrathecal amphotericin B, just as it would in the patient without HIV infection. Concomitant pulmonary coccidioidomycosis, especially diffuse pulmonary involvement, is a frequent occurrence in patients with HIV infection and coccidioidal meningitis.[20] Because of this, combined intravenous amphotericin B and oral or intravenous fluconazole therapy is a reasonable choice for initial antifungal therapy in such patients. The goal of combination therapy in this situation is not to provide antifungal synergism but rather to optimally treat both manifestations of coccidioidomycosis. Once the patient has clinically responded, oral azole antifungal therapy alone can be prescribed. Therapy should be life-long[72] and daily azole antifungal doses of at least 400 mg should be maintained.

Other forms of extrathoracic disseminated coccidioidomycosis in HIV-infected patients appear to respond to antifungal therapy in a manner similar to those without HIV infection. In such cases, if the patient is severely ill and requires hospitalization, initial therapy with amphotericin B is warranted. For those who are clinically stable and are being managed as outpatients, oral azole antifungal therapy is a reasonable choice.

There are two therapeutic options for patients who present with positive coccidioidal serologic tests without evidence of active clinical disease. The first is to follow such patients over time, repeating the serologic tests every 3–4 months. If overt clinical disease develops or if the serologic titer progressively increases, antifungal therapy is warranted. The second approach is to immediately begin antifungal therapy with an oral azole antifungal at a daily dose of 400 mg. The patient should still be followed every 3–4 months for the development of clinical illness and for assessment of anticoccidioidal antibody response. With appropriate therapy, the serologic titers should diminish over time.

Any HIV-infected patient with coccidioidomycosis should be followed at intervals of approximately every 4 months to ensure control of disease. The most important test is the serum anticoccidioidal CF antibody titer. With appropriate therapy, that titer should progressively diminish over time. In most patients who clinically respond, the serum antibody titer will become undetectable. However, in some patients, it may nadir at a low but detectable level. This is acceptable if the patient is clinically well. Increasing titers, particularly up to twofold dilutions, should raise the question of treatment failure and result in a careful clinical and radiological assessment for recrudescent disease. In patients who appear to be failing azole antifungal therapy, increasing the daily dose may regain control of the infection. In other patients, amphotericin B will be required.

Currently, life-long high-dose therapy of coccidioidomycosis is recommended for the HIV-infected patient with coccidioidomycosis. However, the effect of immune reconstitution associated with potent antiretroviral therapy has not been well studied in coccidioidomycosis. Undoubtedly, there are some patients, particularly those receiving potent combination antiretroviral therapy and who have elevated CD4 lymphocyte counts, who may not require such therapy. A specific immune response to coccidioidal antigens occurs at peripheral blood CD4 lymphocyte counts above 250/μL.[73] Given this, one approach among patients with peripheral blood CD4 lymphocyte counts ⩾250/μL who are on effective antiretroviral therapy is to slowly taper the daily dose of antifungals and follow the patient's clinical course and the serum CF antibody titer closely. For example, in a patient with focal pulmonary infection, after at least 12 months of fluconazole or itraconazole therapy at 400 mg/day, the dose could be reduced to 200 mg/day. Given the high risk of relapse that occurs in coccidioidomycosis even among patients without HIV infection,[47,51] subsequent reductions in azole antifungal therapy in the HIV-infected patient should be done cautiously and many clinicians would not reduce the dosage in patients with disseminated disease at all. Relapse of disseminated disease is of particular concern in those HIV-infected patients who become nonadherent with both antiretroviral and antifungal therapy.[74] For any patient with coccidioidal meningitis, the daily azole antifungals dosage should be at least 400 mg and discontination of therapy is not advised.[72]

An immune reconstitution syndrome has been observed for several opportunistic infections after initiation of potent antiretroviral therapy in previously treatment-naive patients. This has raised a question of whether specific treatment for these infections should be instituted prior to starting antiretroviral therapy to ameliorate the impact of this phenomenon.[75] To date, no immune reconstitution syndrome has been observed with coccidioidomycosis.[76] Based on this, it is reasonable to initiate treatment for HIV infection concurrently or soon after starting therapy for coccidioidomycosis.

PREVENTION

There are few data on whether azole antifungal therapy will prevent the development of active coccidioidomycosis for HIV-infected patients living in the coccidioidal endemic area. In one retrospective study,[24] the use of azole antifungals was associated with a diminished risk of subsequent coccidioidomycosis among HIV-infected persons living in the coccidioidal endemic region who had concomitant oropharyngeal or esophageal candidiasis, but not among other groups of HIV-infected patients. Given the cost, risk of drug interactions, and the risk of the development of fungal resistance, particularly of *Candida albicans*,[77] to prevent the development of symptomatic coccidioidomycosis, azole antifungals cannot be generally recommended. For HIV-infected patients living in the coccidioidal endemic area, monitoring anticoccidioidal antibody serum tests at intervals of every 6–12 months is reasonable. The development of a new positive test would suggest possible new infection and require either close follow-up or initiation of antifungal therapy. Outside the endemic area, serial testing for anticoccidioidal antibodies is not useful. Delayed-type hypersensitivity to coccidioidal antigens does not predict the development of active coccidioidomycosis[10] and skin-testing for coccidioidomycosis, currently not available in the United States, is not recommended, either within or outside the coccidioidal endemic area.

Many persons infected with HIV are concerned about visiting areas within the coccidioidal endemic region for fear of contracting coccidioidomycosis. While it would be prudent for such persons to avoid behaviors associated with an increased risk of acquiring coccidioidomycosis, such as working closely with the desert soil or incurring extensive exposure to outdoor dust, there are no compelling data that such patients should absolutely avoid visiting this region.

REFERENCES

1. Pappagianis D. Epidemiology of coccidioidomycosis. In: McGinnis M, (ed). Current Topics in Medical Mycology. New York: Springer, 1988, p. 199–238.
2. Galgiani JN. Coccidioidomycosis. West J Med 159:153–71, 1993.
3. CDC. Coccidioidomycosis – Arizona, 1990–1995. Morbid Mortal Wkly Rep 45:1069–73, 1996.
4. Fisher MC, Koenig GL, White TJ, et al. Molecular and phenotypic description of *Coccidioides posadasii* sp. nov., previously recognized as the non-California population of *Coccidioides immitis*. Mycologia 94:73–84, 2002.
5. Smith CE, Beard RR, Whiting EG, et al. Varieties of coccidioidal infection in relation to the epidemiology and control of the diseases. Am J Public Health 36:1394–402, 1946.

6. Stevens DA. Coccidioidomycosis. N Engl J Med 332:1077–82, 1995.
7. Drutz DJ, Catanzaro A. Coccidioidomycosis. State of the art. Parts I and II. Am Rev Resp Dis 117:559–85; 727–69, 1978.
8. Ampel NM, Bejarano GC, Salas SD, et al. In vitro assessment of cellular immunity in human coccidioidomycosis: relationship between dermal hypersensitivity, lymphocyte transformation, and lymphokine production by peripheral blood mononuclear cells from healthy adults. J Infect Dis 165:710–15, 1992.
9. Corry DB, Ampel NM, Christian L, et al. Cytokine production by peripheral blood mononuclear cells in human coccidioidomycosis. J Infect Dis 174:440–3, 1996.
10. Ampel NM, Dols CL, Galgiani JN. Coccidioidomycosis during human immunodeficiency virus infection: results of a prospective study in a coccidioidal endemic area. Am J Med 94:235–40, 1993.
11. Jones JL, Fleming PL, Ciesielski CA, et al. Coccidioidomycosis among persons with AIDS in the United States. J Infect Dis 171:961–6, 1995.
12. Abrams DI, Robia M, Blumenfeld W, et al. Disseminated coccidioidomycosis in AIDS [letter]. N Engl J Med 310:986–7, 1984.
13. Kovacs A, Forthal DN, Kovacs JA, et al. Disseminated coccidioidomycosis in a patient with acquired immune deficiency syndrome. West J Med 140:447–9, 1984.
14. Roberts CJ. Coccidioidomycosis in acquired immune deficiency syndrome. Depressed humoral as well as cellular immunity. Am J Med 76:734–6, 1984.
15. Macher AM, De Vinatea ML, Koch Y, et al. Case for diagnosis. AIDS. Milit Med 151:M57–M64, 1986.
16. Wolf JE, Little JR, Pappagianis D, et al. Disseminated coccidioidomycosis in a patient with the acquired immune deficiency syndrome. Diagn Microbiol Infect Dis 5:331–6, 1986.
17. Jarvik JG, Hesselink JR, Wiley C, et al. Coccidioidomycotic brain abscess in an HIV-infected man. West J Med 149:83–6, 1988.
18. Bronnimann DA, Adam RD, Galgiani JN, et al. Coccidioidomycosis in the acquired immunodeficiency syndrome. Ann Intern Med 106:372–9, 1987.
19. Fish DG, Ampel NM, Galgiani JN, et al. Coccidioidomycosis during human immunodeficiency virus infection. A review of 77 patients. Medicine (Baltimore) 69:384–91, 1990.
20. Singh VR, Smith DK, Lawrence J, et al. Coccidioidomycosis in patients infected with human immunodefiency virus: review of 91 cases at a single institution. Clin Infect Dis 23:563–8, 1996.
21. Rutherford GW, Barrett MF. Epidemiology and control of coccidioidomycosis in California. West J Med 165:221–2, 1996.
22. Hernandez JL, Echevarria S, Garcia-Valtuille A, et al. Atypical coccidioidomycosis in an AIDS patient successfully treated with fluconazole. Eur J Clin Microbiol Infect Dis 16:592–4, 1997.
23. Palella FJ Jr, Delaney KM, Moorman AC, et al. Declining morbidity and mortality among patients with advanced human immunodeficiency virus infection. HIV Outpatient Study Investigators [see comments]. N Engl J Med 338:853–60, 1998.
24. Woods CW, McRill C, Plikaytis BD, et al. Coccidioidomycosis in human immunodeficiency virus-infected persons in Arizona, 1994–1997: incidence, risk factors, and prevention. J Infect Dis 181:1428–34, 2000.
25. Ampel NM, Ryan KJ, Carry PJ, et al. Fungemia due to *Coccidioides immitis*. An analysis of 16 episodes in 15 patients and a review of the literature. Medicine (Baltimore) 65:312–21, 1986.
26. Mahaffey KW, Hippenmeyer CL, Mandel R, et al. Unrecognized coccidioidomycosis complicating *Pneumocystis carinii* pneumonia in patients infected with the human immunodeficiency virus and treated with corticosteroids. A report of two cases. Arch Intern Med 153:1496–8, 1993.
27. Bouza E, Dreyer JS, Hewitt WL, et al. Coccidioidal meningitis. Medicine (Baltimore) 60:139–72, 1981.
28. Wheat LJ, Connolly-Stringfield PA, Baker RL, et al. Disseminated histoplasmosis in the acquired immune deficiency syndrome: clinical findings, diagnosis and treatment, and review of the literature. Medicine (Baltimore) 69:361–74, 1990.
29. Arguinchona HL, Ampel NM, Dols CL, et al. Persistent coccidioidal seropositivity without clinical evidence of active coccidioidomycosis in patients infected with human immunodeficiency virus. Clin Infect Dis 20:1281–5, 1995.
30. Thomas CF Jr, Limper AH. Pneumocystis pneumonia. N Engl J Med 350:2487–98, 2004.
31. DiTomasso JP, Ampel NM, Sobonya RE, et al. Bronchoscopic diangosis of pulmonary coccidioidomycosis: comparison of cytology, culture, and transbronchial biopsy. Diagn Microbiol Infect Dis 18:83–7, 1994.
32. Bowman BH, Taylor JW, White TJ. Molecular evolution of the fungi: human pathogens. Mol Biol Evol 9:893–904, 1992.
33. Stockman L, Clark KA, Hunt JM, et al. Evaluation of commercially available acridinium ester-labeled chemiluminscent DNA probes for culture identification of *Blastomyces dermatitidis, Coccidioides immitis, Cryptococcus neoformans, and Histoplasma capsulatum*. J Clin Microbiol 31:845–50, 1993.
34. Pappagianis D. Serology of coccidioidomycosis. Clin Microbiol Rev 3:247–68, 1990.
35. Pappagianis D. Serologic studies in coccidioidomycosis. Semin Respir Infect 16:242–50, 2001.
36. Kaufman L, Sekhon AS, Moledina N, et al. Comparative evaluation of commercial Premier EIA and microimmunodiffusion and complement fixation tests for *Coccidioides immitis* antibodies. J Clin Microbiol 33:618–9, 1995.
37. Martins TB, Jaskowski TD, Mouritsen CL, et al. Comparison of commercially available enzyme immunoassay with traditional serological tests for detection of antibodies to *Coccidioides immitis*. J Clin Microbiol 33:940–3, 1995.
38. Zartarian M, Peterson EM, de la Maza LM. Detection of antibodies to *Coccidioides immitis* by enzyme immunoassay. Am J Clin Pathol 107:148–53, 1997.
39. Antoniskis D, Larsen RA, Akil B, et al. Seronegative disseminated coccidioidomycosis in patients with HIV infection. AIDS 4:691–3, 1990.
40. Gallis HA, Drew RH, Pickard WW. Amphotericin B: 30 years of clinical experience. Rev Infect Dis 12:308–29, 1990.
41. Labadie EL, Hamilton RH. Survival improvement in coccidioidal meningitis by high-dose intrathecal amphotericin B. Arch Intern Med 146:2013–8, 1986.
42. Gonzalez GM, Tijerina R, Najvar LK, et al. Efficacies of amphotericin B (AMB) lipid complex, AMB colloidal dispersion, liposomal AMB, and conventional AMB in treatment of murine coccidioidomycosis. Antimicrob Agents Chemother 48:2140–3, 2004.
43. Clemons KV, Sobel RA, Williams PL, et al. Efficacy of intravenous liposomal amphotericin B (AmBisome) against coccidioidal meningitis in rabbits. Antimicrob Agents Chemother 46:2420–6, 2002.
44. Antony S, Dominguez DC, Sotelo E. Use of liposomal amphotericin B in the treatment of disseminated coccidioidomycosis. J Natl Med Assoc 95:982–5, 2003.
45. Galgiani JN, Ampel NM, Blair JE, et al. Coccidioidomycosis. Clin Infect Dis 41:1217–23, 2005.
46. Mirels LF, Stevens DA. Update on the treatment of coccidioidomycosis. West J Med 166:58–9, 1997.
47. Graybill JR, Stevens DA, Galgiani JN, et al. Itraconazole treatment of coccidioidomycosis. Am J Med 89:282–90, 1990.
48. Tucker RM, Denning DW, Dupont B, et al. Itraconazole therapy for chronic coccidioidal meningitis. Ann Intern Med 112:108–12, 1990.

49. Tucker RM, Galgiani JN, Denning DW, et al. Treatment of coccidioidal meningitis with fluconazole. Rev Infect Dis 12:S380–9, 1990.
50. Galgiani JN, Catanzaro A, Cloud GA, et al. Fluconazole therapy for coccidioidal meningitis. The NIAID-Mycoses Study Group. Ann Intern Med 119:28–35, 1993.
51. Catanzaro A, Galgiani JN, Levine BE, et al. Fluconazole in the treatment of chronic pulmonary and nonmeningeal disseminated coccidioidomycosis. Am J Med 98:249–56, 1995.
52. Como JA, Dismukes WE. Oral azole drugs as systemic antifungal therapy. N Engl J Med 330:263–72, 1994.
53. Blum RA, D'Andrea DT, Florentino BM, et al. Increased gastric pH and the bioavailability of fluconazole and ketoconazole. Ann Intern Med 114:755–7, 1991.
54. Lake-Bakaar G, Tom W, Lake-Bakaar D, et al. Gastropathy and ketoconazole malabsorption in the acquired immunodeficiency syndrome (AIDS). Ann Intern Med 109:471–3, 1988.
55. Buchkowsky SS, Partovi N, Ensom MH. Clinical pharmacokinetic monitoring of itraconazole is warranted in only a subset of patients. Ther Drug Monit 27:322–33, 2005.
56. Galgiani JN, Catanzaro A, Cloud GA, et al. Comparison of oral fluconazole and itraconazole for progressive, nonmeningeal coccidioidomycosis. A randomized, double-blind trial. Ann Intern Med 133:676–86, 2000.
57. Pursley TJ, Blomquist IK, Abraham J, et al. Fluconazole-induced congenital anomalies in three infants. Clin Infect Dis 22:336–40, 1996.
58. Boucher HW, Groll AH, Chiou CC, et al. Newer systemic antifungal agents: pharmacokinetics, safety and efficacy. Drugs 64:1997–2020, 2004.
59. Cortez KJ, Walsh TJ, Bennett JE. Successful treatment of coccidioidal meningitis with voriconazole. Clin Infect Dis 36:1619–22, 2003.
60. Proia LA, Tenorio AR. Successful use of voriconazole for treatment of *coccidioides* meningitis. Antimicrob Agents Chemother 48:2341, 2004.
61. Prabhu RM, Bonnell M, Currier BL, et al. Successful treatment of disseminated nonmeningeal coccidioidomycosis with voriconazole. Clin Infect Dis 39:e74–7, 2004.
62. Lutz JE, Clemons KV, Aristizabal BH, et al. Activity of the triazole SCH 56592 against disseminated murine coccidioidomycosis. Antimicrob Agents Chemother 41:1558–61, 1997.
63. Stevens DA, Rendon A, Gaona-Flores V et al. Posaconazole theraphy for chronic refractory coccidiodomycosis. Chest, June 15, 2007.
64. Antony S. Use of the echinocandins (caspofungin) in the treatment of disseminated coccidioidomycosis in a renal transplant recipient. Clin Infect Dis 39:879–80, 2004.
65. Hsue G, Napier JT, Prince RA, et al. Treatment of meningeal coccidioidomycosis with caspofungin. J Antimicrob Chemother 54:292–4, 2004.
66. Kuberski TT, Servi RJ, Rubin PJ. Successful treatment of a critically ill patient with disseminated coccidioidomycosis, using adjunctive interferon-gamma. Clin Infect Dis 38:910–2, 2004.
67. Dresser GK, Spence JD, Bailey DG. Pharmacokinetic–pharmacodynamic consequences and clinical relevance of cytochrome P450 3A4 inhibition. Clin Pharmacokinet 38:41–57, 2000.
68. Koks CH, Meenhorst PL, Bult A, et al. Itraconazole solution: summary of pharmacokinetic features and review of activity in the treatment of fluconazole-resistant oral candidosis in HIV-infected persons. Pharmacol Res 46:195–201, 2002.
69. Prentice AG, Glasmacher A. Making sense of itraconazole pharmacokinetics. J Antimicrob Chemother 56(Suppl 1):i17–22, 2005.
70. Koks CH, van Heeswijk RP, Veldkamp AI, et al. Itraconazole as an alternative for ritonavir liquid formulation when combined with saquinavir [letter]. AIDS 14:89–90, 2000.
71. Sugar AM. Use of amphotericin B with azole antifungal drugs: what are we doing? Antimicrobiol Agent Chemother 39:1907–12, 1995.
72. Dewsnupp DH, Galgiani JN, Graybill JR, et al. Is it ever safe to stop azole therapy for *Coccidioides immitis* meningitis? Ann Intern Med 124:305–10, 1996.
73. Ampel NM, Kramer LA, Kerekes KM, et al. Assessment of the human cellular immune response to T27K, a coccidioidal antigen preparation, by flow cytometry of whole blood. Med Mycol 39:315–20, 2001.
74. Mathew G, Smedema M, Wheat LJ, et al. Relapse of coccidioidomycosis despite immune reconstitution after fluconazole secondary prophylaxis in a patient with AIDS. Mycoses 46:42–4, 2003.
75. Benson CA, Kaplan JE, Masur H, et al. Treating opportunistic infections among HIV-exposed and infected children: recommendations from CDC, the National Institutes of Health, and the Infectious Diseases Society of America. MMWR Recomm Rep 53:1–112, 2004.
76. Ampel NM. Coccidioidomycosis in persons infected with HIV type 1. Clin Infect Dis 41:1174–8, 2005.
77. Maenza JR, Keruly JC, Moore RD, et al. Risk factors for fluconazole-resistant candidiasis in human immunodeficiency virus-infected patients. J Infect Dis 173:219–25, 1996.

Chapter 46

Candidiasis

Carl J. Fichtenbaum, MD, Peter G. Pappas, MD

INTRODUCTION

Oropharyngeal candidiasis (OPC) was among the initial manifestations recognized in association with human immunodeficiency virus (HIV) infection,[1,2] affecting most persons with advanced untreated HIV infection. Its importance is often obscured by the occurrence of other severe opportunistic infections seen with acquired immunodeficiency syndrome (AIDS). OPC may be a sentinel event for the detection or progression of HIV disease, presenting months or years before more severe opportunistic disease.[3–5]

Although usually associated with slight morbidity, OPC can be clinically significant. Severe OPC can interfere with the administration of medications and adequate nutritional intake and may extend to involve the esophagus.[6] Symptoms may include burning pain, altered taste sensation, and difficulty swallowing liquids and solids. Many patients are asymptomatic. Pseudomembranous candidiasis, or thrush (white plaques on the buccal mucosa, gums, or tongue), is the most common presentation for OPC. Less commonly persons have acute atrophic candidiasis (erythematous) or chronic hyperplastic candidiasis (leukoplakia) involving the tongue.

Esophageal candidiasis (EC) is usually accompanied by the presence of OPC. Typically, dysphagia and odynophagia are described. Esophageal involvement is asymptomatic in as many as 40% of patients with OPC.[6] Esophageal disease occasionally presents in the absence of clinically detectable oropharyngeal disease.

Vulvovaginal candidiasis is an important concern for women with HIV infection. Vulvar candidiasis manifests as a morbilliform rash involving the intertriginous areas with satellite lesions on the thighs. Vaginal disease generally presents as a creamy-white abnormal vaginal discharge. The vagina may appear erythematous, and white plaques are often seen. Common symptoms include pruritus, vulvar or vaginal pain, dysuria, and dyspareunia.

Invasive candidiasis typically occurs in persons with traditional risk factors (e.g., indwelling venous catheters, broad-spectrum antibacterials).[7,8] Bloodstream infections, meningitis, intra-abdominal infections, and osteomyelitis have been described, and the clinical manifestations of invasive candidiasis are similar to those of HIV-seronegative persons.

TAXONOMY AND BIOLOGY

Yeasts are fungi that grow as single cells and reproduce by budding. They are distinguished on the basis of the presence or absence of capsules, the size and shape of the yeast cells, the mechanism of daughter formation, the formation of true or pseudohyphae, and the presence of sexual spores, along with physiologic data. *Candida albicans* is the predominant causative agent of all forms of mucocutaneous candidiasis. Less frequently, *C. glabrata, C. parapsilosis, C. tropicalis, C. krusei*, and several other species cause disease. More recently, *C. dubliniesis* has been identified as a separate species distinct from *C. albicans*.[9,10]

Candida species are normal inhabitants of the human gastrointestinal tract and may be recovered from the mouths of up to one-third of normal individuals and two-thirds of those with advanced HIV disease.[11,12] Colonization with an inherently resistant organism is more common in advanced HIV infection (CD4+ T-lymphocyte counts of <50 cells/mm^3).[12] Most disease is caused by endogenous organisms of the individual, although rare cases of person-to-person transmission have been documented.[13]

MICROBIOLOGY

Candida strains affecting persons with HIV infection are typically no different from those in other immunosuppressed hosts.[14] *Candida dubliniesis* is more commonly identified in HIV-infected persons, though its clinical significance is, at this point, indistinguishable from that of *C. albicans*.[9,10] There are no detectable differences in the virulence of strains isolated from HIV-infected or HIV-uninfected persons. Recurrent disease usually results from the same species or strains of *Candida*,[14–17] and the emergence of different strains or species is more likely in persons exposed to antifungal therapy with low CD4+ T-lymphocyte counts.[18]

EPIDEMIOLOGY

Mucocutaneous candidiasis occurs in three forms among persons with HIV infection; oropharyngeal, esophageal, and vulvovaginal disease. Oropharyngeal and vulvovaginal disease are the most common forms. Historically, up to 90% of persons with advanced untreated HIV infection developed OPC, with 60% having at least one episode per year with frequent recurrences.[19–26] EC occurs less frequently (10–20%), but is the leading cause of esophageal disease.[27–29] Vaginal candidiasis has been noted in 27–60% of women, similar to the rates of oropharyngeal disease.[30–32] However, the incidence appears to be similar in HIV-infected and HIV-uninfected women.[33,34] It is notable that 75% of all women of childbearing age develop vaginal candidiasis, and 40% have a second occurrence. Few women (<5%) experience frequent recurrences (defined as four or more infections during a 12-month period).

Two factors have affected the epidemiology of mucocutaneous candidiasis. The first was the widespread use of antifungal agents, particularly the azoles. Continuous use of azoles led to a decline in the prevalence of mucosal candidiasis while leading to the emergence of refractory infections. More importantly, the introduction of highly active antiretroviral therapy (HAART) resulted in a significant decline in the incidence of a number of opportunistic illnesses (e.g., *Pneumocystis jirovecii* pneumonia and cytomegalovirus infection).[35–37] In turn, the incidence of mucocutaneous forms of candidiasis declined precipitously. For example, Cauda et al reported a significant difference in the incidence of recurrent OPC in patients treated with protease inhibitors compared with those not treated with protease inhibitors (7% vs 36%).[38] Similarly, Martins et al reported a decline in the incidence of OPC from 30% to 4% over a 1-year period in persons on HAART.[39]

A number of factors are important in the development of mucocutaneous candidiasis. The level of immunosuppression is paramount.[22] Other host factors important to the defense against *Candida* infections include blood group secretor status, salivary flow rates, epithelial barrier, antimicrobial constituents of saliva, the presence of normal bacterial flora, and local immunity.[23,40] Several studies suggest impairment of a number of anti-*Candida* host defense mechanisms in persons with HIV infection.[22,24,25] High levels of HIV-1 RNA in the plasma have been associated with increased rates of mucocutaneous candidiasis and colonization with *Candida*.[41,42] It is notable that the relationship between the level of immunosuppression and vaginal candidiasis may not be as strong. In one cross-sectional study of 833 HIV-infected and 427 HIV-uninfected women the annual incidence of vaginal candidiasis was similar in the two groups (9%).[33] There are few studies describing the incidence and prevalence of non-esophageal invasive candidiasis in HIV-infected persons. The incidence is probably less than 1%.[7,8]

DIAGNOSIS

Clinical Appearance

The diagnosis of OPC is usually made by its characteristic clinical appearance (Fig. 46-1). Recovery of an organism is not critical to the diagnosis of OPC, as oropharyngeal cultures often demonstrate *Candida* species, but frequently represent colonization.[19] The diagnosis of OPC can be confirmed by examining a 10% KOH slide preparation of a scraping of an

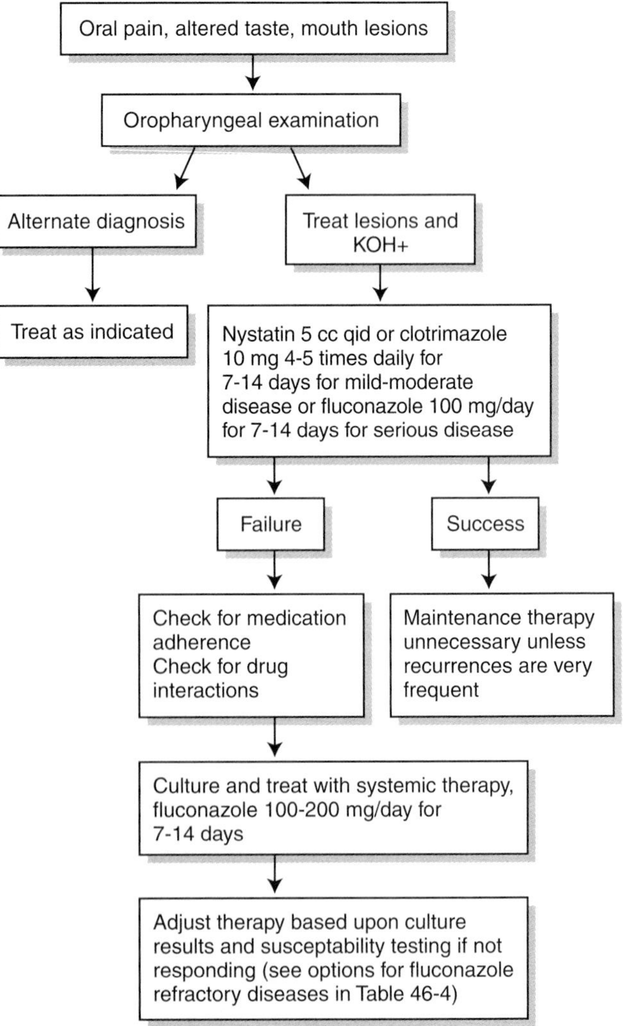

Figure 46-1 ■ Diagnosis and treatment of oral candidiasis.

active lesion, which demonstrates characteristic pseudohyphae and budding yeast. A KOH preparation is simple to perform but not mandatory for diagnosing OPC. A presumptive diagnosis of OPC can be made by visual detection of characteristic lesions, with resolution of those lesions in response to antifungal therapy. In patients with poorly responsive OPC, a culture should be obtained to look for drug resistant yeasts or those that respond poorly to certain azoles (e.g., *C. kruseii* or *C. glabrata*). Biopsies of oral lesions are rarely helpful or indicated.

A presumptive diagnosis of *Candida* esophagitis is appropriate in a patient with dysphagia or odynophagia (or both) who has OPC (Fig. 46-2). Upper endoscopy can be used to confirm esophageal involvement; a barium swallow test may be used, but it is less sensitive and specific than endoscopy. These studies are not uniformly required unless a patient fails to improve with appropriate systemic antifungal therapy.[29] If a patient with OPC does not resolve the esophageal symptoms despite resolution of the oral lesions, endoscopy is indicated to exclude other causes of esophagitis (e.g., CMV, herpes simplex virus, aphthous ulcers). The diagnosis of *Candida* esophagitis is confirmed by the presence of yeast forms on histologic examination of esophageal lesions. Specimens for culture should be obtained from patients who require endoscopy to look for drug-resistant *Candida*.

Candida vaginitis is diagnosed based on the presence of a characteristic clinical appearance and observation of yeast forms on a microscopic examination (Fig. 46-3). A KOH preparation should always be done on vaginal lesions to confirm the diagnosis of candidiasis because there are a number of other conditions that appear similar (e.g., trichomoniasis). Routine cultures are rarely helpful in the absence of KOH-positive lesions because yeasts are normal inhabitants of the vaginal mucosa. As for OPC, a culture should be prepared if a patient fails to respond to standard antifungal therapy. Vulvar disease is typically diagnosed by its characteristic appearance.

Invasive disease is diagnosed by demonstrating the presence of *Candida* from a sterile site (e.g., blood, bone biopsy, cerebrospinal fluid). Bloodstream infections are diagnosed when one or more cultures are positive for *Candida* (Fig. 46-4). In most clinical circumstances, a single positive blood culture for *Candida* should be considered significant.

Drug Resistance and Susceptibility Testing

Antifungal susceptibility testing is gradually becoming standardized. The Clinical Laboratory Standard Institute (CLSI)

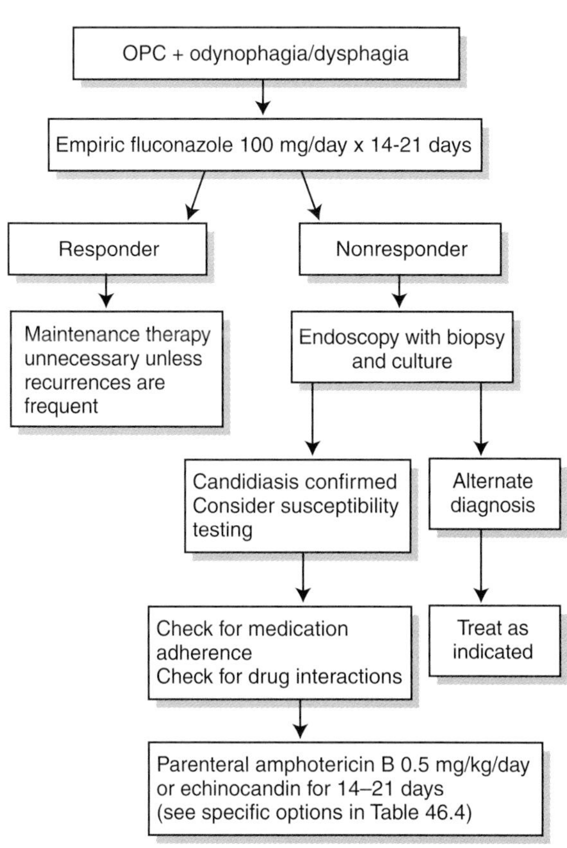

Figure 46-2 ■ Diagnosis and treatment of esophageal candidiasis.

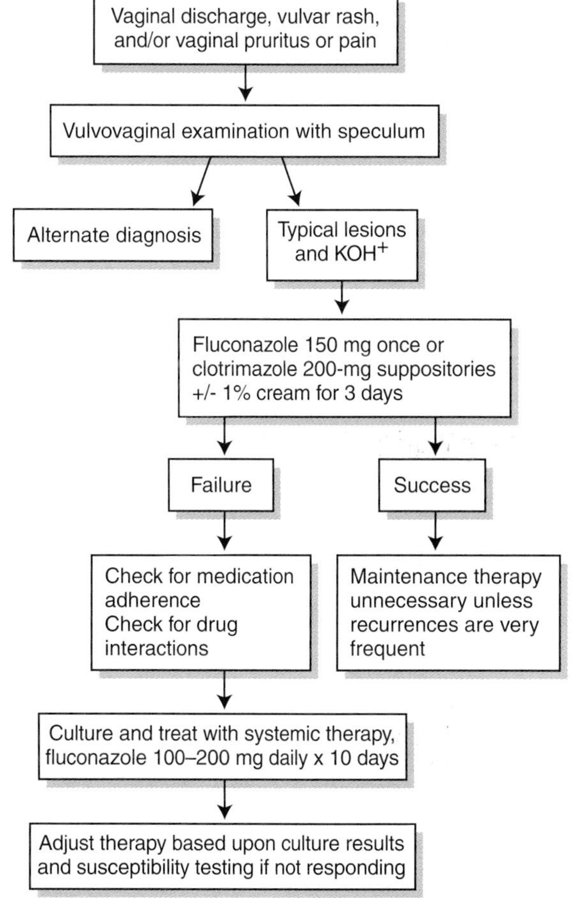

Figure 46-3 ■ Diagnosis and treatment of vaginal candidiasis.

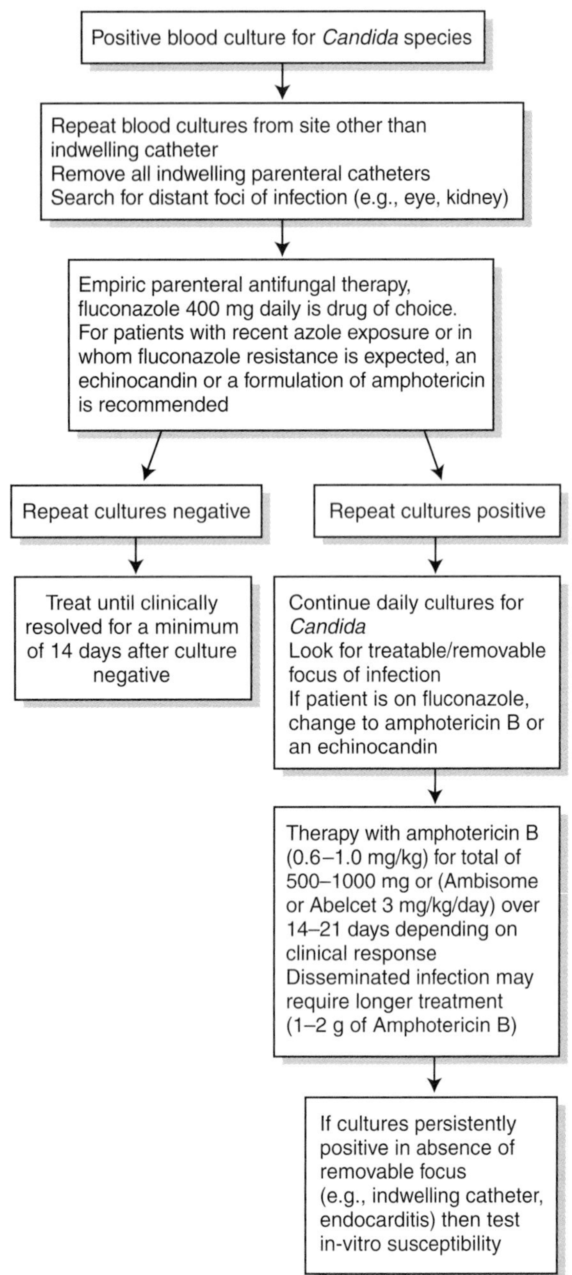

Figure 46-4 ■ Diagnosis and treatment of candidemia.

has definitions for *in vitro* susceptibilities for selected agents using standard methodologies.[43] The most common methods for *in vitro* testing are macrotube and microtiter broth dilution assays, disk diffusion tests, and the E-test. *In vitro* susceptibilities should not be used routinely to guide the choice of antifungal agents, but rather to test isolates that are clinically refractory to antifungal therapy.

There are several mechanisms that explain *in vitro* resistance to antifungal drugs, including target alteration, reduced cell permeability, and active efflux of the drug out of the cell.[44–47] Some yeasts have single drug resistance, whereas others are multidrug-resistant. Azole resistance has been demonstrated in yeasts containing alterations in the enzymes that were the target of their action or were involved in ergosterol biosynthesis. The relative incidence of the various mechanisms of resistance is unknown. Furthermore, it is not clear whether certain mechanisms of resistance may be overcome by higher dosing of the drug.

THERAPY

Numerous agents are effective against candidiasis (Table 46-1). Important factors that determine clinical response in addition to the choice of antifungal agent include the extent and severity of disease, patient adherence to the regimen, and the pharmacodynamic/pharmacokinetic properties of the drug. Treatment of OPC and vaginal candidiasis is relatively simple, with most types responding to therapy. Overall, there have been few clinical differences in randomized studies comparing topical with systemic therapy. Mild OPC or vulvovaginal disease can often be treated successfully with topical therapy. Moderate and severe episodes typically require systemic therapy. Esophagitis and other invasive disease always require systemic therapy.

ANTIFUNGAL AGENTS

There are various classes of antifungal agents: (1) the polyenes (nystatin and amphotericin B), which work by binding to ergosterol in the fungal cell membrane, inducing osmotic instability and loss of membrane integrity; (2) the azoles, including the imidazoles (clotrimazole) and triazoles (ketoconazole, itraconazole, fluconazole, voriconazole, posaconazole), which inhibit fungal cytochrome P450-dependent enzymes, resulting in impaired ergosterol biosynthesis and depletion of ergosterol from the fungal cell membrane; (3) pyrimidine synthesis inhibitors, including 5-fluorocytosine, which inhibits DNA and RNA synthesis in fungal organisms; and (4) the echinocandins (caspofungin, micafungin, and anidulafungin), which are cyclic lipopeptides that inhibit β-1,3-glucan synthase, an enzyme involved in fungal wall cell biosynthesis.

Nystatin is used in a topical preparation. The oral form is not absorbed and has minimal side effects other than dysgeusia. Clotrimazole is available as a spray, solution, and troche for oral usage. Clotrimazole has few side effects and is poorly absorbed from the gastrointestinal tract. Flucytosine is available as a tablet and has a number of associated side effects, including nausea, vomiting, diarrhea, gastrointestinal bleeding, renal insufficiency, hepatitis, thrombocytopenia, anemia, and leukopenia. Flucytosine is rarely used alone because of the rapid emergence of resistant organisms on therapy. It is sometimes used in combination with fluconazole for refractory candidiasis and has been used adjunctively for difficult-to-treat invasive candidiasis when available. When available, flucytosine levels should be obtained, with optimal levels between 50 and 100 μg/mL.

Amphotericin B is available in four parenteral forms: amphotericin B deoxycholate, liposomal amphotericin B

Therapeutic Options for Mucosal Candidiasis

Table 46-1

Medication	Dosage	Important Toxicities
Oropharyngeal Candidiasis		
Clotrimazole troches	10 mg 4–5 times/day × 7–14 days	Altered taste, GI upset
Nystatin suspension	100 000 units/cm^3 5 cc qid × 7–14 days	GI upset
Ketoconazole	200 mg/day × 7–14 days	GI upset, hepatitis, endocrine effects
Itraconazole	100 mg/day × 7–14 days	GI upset, hepatitis
Fluconazole	100 mg/day × 7–14 days	GI upset, hepatitis
Esophageal Candidiasis		
Fluconazole[a]	100 mg/day × 14–21 days	GI upset, hepatitis
Ketoconazole	400 mg/day × 14–21 days	GI upset, hepatitis, endocrine effects
Itraconazole	200 mg/day × 14–21 days	GI upset, hepatitis
Parenteral amphotericin B	0.5 mg kg^{-1} day^{-1} × 14–21 days	Renal failure, electrolyte losses, fever, chills, sweats
Lipid formulations of amphotericin B	3 mg kg^{-1} day^{-1} × 14–21 days	Fever, chills, sweats, electrolyte losses, renal insufficiency uncommon
Voriconazole	200 mg bid × 14–21 days	GI upset, hepatitis, visual impairment
Caspofungin	50–70 mg/day × 14–21 days	Fever, infusion-associated phlebitis
Micafungin	75–150 mg/day × 14–21 days	Fever, infusion-associated phlebitis
Andidulafungin	50–100 mg/day × 14–21 days	Fever, infusion-associated phlebitis
Vulvovaginal Candidiasis[b]		
Fluconazole	150 mg once	Minimal GI upset
Butoconazole		
2% Cream	5 g at bedtime × 3 days	Local irritation
2% Cream	5 g once	Local irritation
Clotrimazole		
Suppositories[c]	100 mg × 7 days	Local irritation
Suppositories[c]	200 mg × 3 days	Local irritation
1% Cream	5 g bid × 3 days	Local irritation
1% Cream	5 g/day × 7 days	Local irritation
Miconazole		
Suppositories[c]	100 mg/day × 7 days	Local irritation
2% Cream	5 g/day × 7 days	Local irritation
4% Cream	5 g at bedtime × 3 days	Local irritation
Nystatin tablets[c]	100 000 unit tablet × 14 days	Local irritation
Tioconazole 6.5% cream	4.6 g single dose	Local irritation
Terconazole		
0.4% Cream	5 g/day × 7 days	Local irritation
0.8% Cream	5 g/day × 3 days	Local irritation
Suppository 80 mg[c]	1 each day × 3 days	Local irritation

GI, gastrointestinal.

[a] Drug of choice.
[b] Nonprescription alternatives available for most topical drugs with treatment for 3–7 days.
[c] Presence of vulvar disease requires additional use of cream directly on rash for 3–7 days.

(AmBisome), amphotericin B lipid complex (Abelcet), and amphotericin B colloid dispersion (Amphotec, Amphocil). Adverse effects from the parenteral preparation include fever, chills, electrolyte disturbances, and renal insufficiency. The oral formulation is no longer commercially available.

Ketoconazole is uncommonly used as an oral formulation in the United States because of more frequent incidence of adverse effects, less predictable absorption, higher frequency of drug–drug interactions, and comparatively poor activity against *Candida* species (all relative to other available azoles), oral ketoconazole is rarely used. It is available as a tablet or cream. Oral absorption is enhanced when the gastric pH is less than 4.0. Achlorhydria has been documented in HIV-infected patients and, when present, may interfere

Important Drug Interactions with Selected Antifungal Medications

Table 46-2

Interacting Drug	Antifungal	Effect and Manifestations
Anticoagulants, oral	F, K, V	Anticoagulant levels (prolonged prothrombin time, bleeding)
Antihistamines: H_1-blockers (excluding loratadine)	I, F, K	Antihistamine levels (ventricular arrhythmias)
Carbamazepine	I	Itraconazole levels (decreased efficacy)
Contraceptives, oral	I, F, K, V	Efficacy of oral contraceptives (pregnancy)
Cyclosporin/tacrolimus	I, F, K, V	CSA/tacrolimus level (CSA/tacrolimus toxicity)
Didanosine	I, K	Complex interaction with levels of involved drugs
Digoxin	I	Digoxin levels (digitalis toxicity)
HMG-CoA inhibitors	I, F, K	HMG-CoA inhibitor levels (rhabdomyolysis)
Oral hypoglycemics	F, K	Oral hypoglycemic effect (hypoglycemia)
Isoniazid	I, F, K, V	I, F, K levels (decreased efficacy)
H_2-blockers/proton pump	I, K, V	I, K levels (decreased efficacy); V levels with omeprazole
Phenytoin	I, F, K, V	Complex (I, K, V levels; V, F, phenytoin levels)
Rifabutin	F, V	F levels (uveitis); V levels (decreased efficacy)
Rifampin	I, F, K, V	I, F, K levels (decreased efficacy)
Theophylline	I, F, K	Theophylline levels (toxicity)

F, fluconazole; I, itraconazole; K, ketoconazole; V, voriconazole; HMG-CoA, 3-hydroxy-3-methylglutaryl coenzyme A; CSA, cyclosporin A.

with ketoconazole absorption.[48] Itraconazole is a triazole compound available in a cyclodextrin suspension, capsule, or intravenous preparation. The cyclodextrin suspension has enhanced bioavailability compared to the capsule formulation. Absorption is improved when taken after a full meal. Fluconazole was the first triazole compound released in the United States. It is more completely absorbed than itraconazole or ketoconazole because its absorption is not dependent on gastric acidity or food intake. It is available in suspension, tablet, and parenteral forms. Voriconazole and posaconazole are triazoles with expanded *in vitro* activity against *Candida* species, including many fluconazole resistant strains (e.g., *C. krusei* and selected *C. glabrata*).

Results from recent clinical trials suggest that the expanded-spectrum triazoles are reasonable alternatives for mucosal candidiasis. Dupont and colleagues presented data on a blinded, randomized study of voriconazole 200 mg twice daily versus fluconazole 200 mg daily for the treatment of EC.[49] There was no difference in the number of persons with endoscopically proven cure after 2–6 weeks of therapy; 94.8% of the voriconazole group ($n = 115$) versus 90.1% of the fluconazole group ($n = 141$). In one randomized study, posaconazole 100 mg suspension/day compared favorably to fluconazole 100 mg suspension/day for treating OPC in persons with HIV infection.[50] The clinical cure rate was 92% ($n = 169$) for posaconazole versus 93% ($n = 160$) for fluconazole. Similarly, posaconazole compared favorably to fluconazole in a dose-ranging study for the treatment of oral candidiasis associated with HIV infection.[51]

In general, the side effects of ketoconazole, itraconazole, fluconazole, voriconazole, and posaconazole are similar. The more commonly reported side effects are headache, dyspepsia, diarrhea, nausea, vomiting, hepatitis, and skin rash.[52] Voriconazole can cause reversible photopsia.[49] Prolonged administration of azoles may require surveillance of liver enzymes to monitor for hepatotoxicity. There are a number of significant drug interactions with each of these medications (Table 46-2).

Caspofungin is effective for oral and EC including fluconazole-refractory disease.[53,54] In a randomized double blind study of caspofungin versus amphotericin B for the treatment of candidal esophagitis involving 128 patients, 80% of whom were HIV-infected, caspofungin was at least as effective as amphotericin B (endoscopic cure rates were 74% for caspofungin 50 mg, 89% for caspofungin 70 mg, and 63% for amphotericin B 0.5 mg/kg). Therapy was discontinued due to toxicity in 24% of patients treated with amphotericin B compared to 4% and 7%, respectively, for patients treated with caspofungin.[53] Adverse events such as fever, nausea, vomiting, flushing, and infused-vein complications are typically mild.

Micafungin is an echinocandin recently approved for the treatment of EC and prophylaxis for invasive fungal infections among stem cell transplant recipients with neutropenia. Two recently completed[54a,54b] examining micafungin in the treatment of invasive candidiasis and candidemia should result in its approval for this indication. Concerning the treatment of EC, there are three studies examining the use of micafungin in HIV-infected patients. In the first of these studies, 120 patients with EC confirmed by endoscopy were randomized to receive micafungin at incremental doses ranging from 12.5 to 100 mg daily. Endpoints included clinical and mycologic response at end of therapy and relapse of 2 weeks. The data suggested that micafungin was effective at all doses, but 75–100 mg daily were the most effective doses for healing mucosal lesions.[55] A subsequent study comparing micafungin at 50, 100, and 150 mg daily to fluconazole 200 mg daily among 245 patients with HIV-associated EC demonstrated similar observations, specifically, that micafungin at 100 and 150 mg provided efficacy comparable to fluconazole 200 mg daily (micafungin 84%, fluconazole 87%). Notably, 7% of micafungin recipients had a relapse or reinfection during the 2 week follow-up period.[56] In the last of these randomized studies, micafungin at 150 mg/day was compared to fluconazole 200 mg/day for a minimum of 14 days with 2–4 week follow-up. Over 500 patients were enrolled into this trial which resulted in a successful outcome in 87% of micafungin and 87% of fluconazole patients.[57] Relapses at 4 weeks were seen in 15% compared to 11% of micafungin and fluconazole recipients, respectively. The aggregate data from these trials suggest that micafungin is acceptable therapy for patients with primary EC.

Anidulafungin was recently approved for EC and invasive candidiasis including candidemia. The data supporting the use of anidulafungin in EC is perhaps the most robust among the echinocandins. In the largest study to date, 601 patients with esophagitis were randomized to receive either anidulafungin 50 mg daily or fluconazole 100 mg daily in a phase 3 randomized, double-blind, double-dummy trial.[58] Primary treatment duration was two to 3 weeks with either agent. As expected, *Candida albicans* was the dominant pathogen in this study, accounting for over 95% of infections in both arms of the trial. At the end of therapy, anidulafungin was as effective (97.2%) as fluconazole (98.8%) in the treatment of EC. Clinical and microbiologic response at end of therapy were similar in both arms; however, there was a higher relapse rate in the anidulafungin arm (~30% in a 6 week follow-up period compared to ~10% with fluconazole). The results of this study raise concerns about the durability of response to echinocandins among patients with EC, and this requires further investigation. Our present understanding suggests that echinocandins are very effective in the primary treatment of EC, but because of concern due to generally higher than expected relapse rates, this should lead clinicians to follow these patients carefully after a successful course of therapy.

A number of controlled trials of currently approved medications for the treatment of oral and EC are listed in Table 46-3. Response rates range from 34% to 100% in studies of treatment for oral and esophageal disease.[59–67] In clinical experience, the response rates to standard antifungal treatments are generally 75% to 95%. There are few significant differences in response to topical versus systemic therapies or among the various systemic therapies for OPC. Thus, it is reasonable to conclude that clotrimazole, ketoconazole, fluconazole, itraconazole, and voriconazole are probably equivalent as acute treatment for most cases of OPC. Mild cases of OPC can be treated with clotrimazole or nystatin initially for 7–14 days. Nonresponsive cases or patients with more severe disease should use fluconazole 100–200 mg/day or itraconazole 200 mg/day for 7–14 days.

The cure rates for vulvovaginal candidiasis range from 72% to 98% in most trials of persons without HIV infection.[68–72] Historically, treatment for vulvovaginal candidiasis consisted of topical therapy for 7 days. However, shorter courses (3 days) and single-dose therapy is often effective. Sobel et al compared a one-time dose of 150 mg of fluconazole with 7 days of topical therapy with clotrimazole (100 mg vaginal suppositories).[72] The clinical cure rate by day 35 was equivalent in the two groups (75%). Mycologic eradication rates at day 35 were 63% for the fluconazole group and 57% for the clotrimazole group. Clinical experience in women with HIV infection is generally positive with either topical or systemic therapy, but relapse rates are quite high.[32] Single-dose therapy with fluconazole is simple and effective. Among patients who fail, it is reasonable to treat with clotrimazole suppositories with or without cream for 3–7 days before using longer courses of systemic fluconazole.

The recommendation for treating nonesophageal forms of invasive candidiasis is similar to that for HIV-seronegative persons.[73] It is beyond the scope of this chapter to review all the alternative approaches to the use of systemic antifungals for invasive candidiasis. Indwelling vascular devices should be removed when possible. In uncomplicated disease, bloodstream infections may be treated with fluconazole 400 mg/day, an echinocandin, or an amphotericin B formulation for 2 weeks. The echinocandins have emerged as the agents of first choice among patients with complicated invasive candidiasis and for those with potentially resistant isolates. The lipid formulations of amphotericin B are increasingly being used to avoid the toxicity of amphotericin B deoxycholate, though there appears to be no advantage in efficacy. The typical starting dose for lipid preparations is 3 mg/kg/day. The use of these agents should be reserved for subjects intolerant of amphotericin B deoxycholate or with preexisting renal insufficiency.

REFRACTORY CANDIDIASIS

Reports of refractory OPC and esophageal disease began emerging in 1990.[12,74–91] Refractory vaginal candidiasis has remained relatively uncommon.[92] Refractory disease is defined as the failure to respond to antifungal treatment with appropriate doses for a standard duration of time (e.g., 14 days).[12,93] Fluconazole-refractory disease emerged as the focus because there was significant morbidity, treatment often required the use of parenteral agents, and fluconazole was the most commonly prescribed antifungal agent. The annual incidence of fluconazole-refractory OPC has been reported to be 4–5% in patients with advanced HIV infection during the pre-HAART era.[12,32] Like most other opportunistic infections, fluconazole-refractory OPC is less common with the widespread use of HAART. Amphotericin B-refractory disease is exceedingly uncommon.[94–97] It is of note that clinical failures may also result from inadequate drug absorption or drug interactions that decrease the levels of some antifungal medications.[48,98,99]

Refractory candidiasis tends to occur among persons with advanced HIV disease (CD4+ T-lymphocyte counts of <50 cells/mm^3) who have been exposed to lower doses of

Table 46-3

Clinical Trials for Treatment of HIV-Associated Oral and Esophageal Candidiasis

Medication	Clinical Response	Mycologic Response	Relapse Rate	Study
Oral Candidiasis				
Fluconazole				
100 mg/day × 14 days	100% (n = 16)	75%	60% at day 42	Koletar et al[60]
100 mg/day × 14 days	98% (n = 152)	65%	34% at day 42	Pons et al[26]
50 mg/day × 28 days	100% (n = 17)	87%	46% at day 30	DeWit et al[61]
200 mg/day × 14 days[a]	42% (n = 38)	NA	62%	Barchiesi et al[62]
100 mg/day × 14 days	83% (n = 94)	51%	37% at day 30	Vazquez et al[50]
100 mg/day × 14 days	83% (n = 160)	68%	38%	Nieto et al[51]
Clotrimazole				
10 mg 5×/day × 14 days	94% (n = 136)	48%	40% at day 42	Pons et al[26]
10 mg 5×/day × 14 days	65% (n = 17)	20%	14% at day 42	Koletar et al[60]
Ketoconazole				
200 mg/day × 28 days	75% (n = 16)	69%	11% at day 30	DeWit et al[61]
200 mg bid × 28 days	93% (n = 40)	73%	>80% at day 90	Smith et al[59]
200 mg/day × 14 days	60% (n = 52)	62%	80% at day 60	de Repentigny Ratelle[63]
400 mg/day × 12 days[a]	34% (n = 39)	NA	22%	Barchiesi et al[62]
Itraconazole				
200 mg/day × 14 days	71% (n = 46)	63%	80% at day 60	de Repentigny Ratelle[63]
200 mg/day × 28 days	93% (n = 46)	72%	>80% at day 90	Smith[59]
Posaconazole				
50 mg/day × 14 days	74% (n = 98)	36%	41% at day 30	Vazquez et al[50]
100 mg/day × 14 days	80% (n = 102)	37%	38% at day 30	Vazquez et al[50]
200 mg/day × 14 days	74% (n = 91)	35%	35% at day 30	Vazquez et al[50]
400 mg/day × 14 days	83% (n = 5100)	40%	36% at day 30	Vazquez et al[50]
200 mg/day × 14 days	82% (n = 169)	68%	31%	Nieto et al[51]
Esophageal Candidiasis				
Fluconazole				
100 mg/day × 21 days[b]	85% (n = 72)	NA	NA	Laine et al[64]
200 mg/day × 2–6 weeks	90% (n = 141)	NA	NA	Ally et al[49]
Itraconazole				
200 mg/day × 28 days	100% (n = 12)	NA	58% at day 60	de Repentigny Ratelle[63]
Ketoconazole				
200 mg/day × 21 days[b]	65% (n = 71)	NA	NA	Laine et al[64]
200 mg/day × 28 days	91% (n = 19)	NA	82% at day 60	de Repentigny Ratelle[63]
Voriconazole				
200 mg bid × 2–6 weeks	95% (n = 115)	NA	NA	Ally et al[49]
Caspofungin				
50 mg/day × 14 days	74%	80%	NA	Villanueva et al[53]
70 mg/day × 14 days	81%	96%	NA	
Anidulafungin				
50 mg/day × 14–21 days	99%	87%	34% at day 14	Krause et al[58]
Micafungin				
100–150 mg/day × 14–21 days	87%	88%	15% at day 28	de Wet et al[57]

NA, not available.
[a] Median duration of therapy (range 6–46 days).
[b] Treatment given for 14 days after patient was asymptomatic minimum 21 days up to 8 weeks.

antifungal agents on a continuous basis.[12] Maenza and colleagues reported a longer median duration of exposure to antifungal therapy (419 vs 118 days, $P < 0.001$) and of systemic azole therapy (272 vs 14 days, $P < 0.001$) among persons who had fluconazole-refractory OPC compared to matched controls.[78] Other factors that may predict the development of refractory candidiasis include use of prophylactic trimethoprim–sulfamethoxazole and a history of prior opportunistic

Therapeutic Options for Fluconazole – Refractory Disease

Table 46-4

Refractory Mucosal Candidiasis

Medication	Dosage
Topical Therapy	
Clotrimazole troches	100–500 mg 4–5 times daily
Gentian violet	Apply to oropharynx once (may repeat weekly as needed)
Amphotericin B oral solution[a]	100 mg/mL, 5 mL PO qid
Systemic Therapy	
Fluconazole tablets	400–800 mg PO qd or bid
5-Flucytosine	100–150 mg $kg^{-1}day^{-1}$ PO qid
Itraconazole tablets	200–400 mg PO qd or bid
Itraconazole solution[a]	40 mg/mL, 2.5–5.0 mL PO bid
Parenteral amphotericin B	0.5–1.0 mg kg^{-1} day^{-1}IV qd
Lipid formulations of amphotericin	3 mg kg^{-1} day^{-1} IV qd amphotericin B
Caspofungin	50–70 mg IV qd
Anidulafungin	100 mg IV qd
Micafungin	100–150 mg IV qd
Voriconazole	200 mg bid (IV or PO)
Adjunctive Therapy	
Potent antiretroviral therapy	RT inhibitors + protease inhibitors
GM-CSF	300 μg SC 3–5 times weekly

GM-CSF, granulocyte/macrophage colony-stimulating factor; RT, reverse transcriptase.
Duration of treatment should be a minimum of 21–28 days.
[a]Controlled study supports use of this treatment for fluconazole-refractory candidiasis.

illnesses such as *Mycobacterium avium* complex disease.[12] Similarly, chronic exposure to itraconazole results in higher rates of *in vitro* resistance, although these isolates typically remain susceptible to fluconazole.[100]

Refractory candidiasis is difficult to treat, often becoming less responsive to therapy with time. The most important step is to determine what medications and dosages have been tried and whether adherence with therapy was adequate. Removal of any interacting medications or increasing the dose of the antifungal agent is curative in some persons. Persons with OPC unresponsive to clotrimazole, nystatin, ketoconazole, or itraconazole tablets generally respond to fluconazole. Persons with OPC unresponsive to fluconazole 200 mg daily given for 2 weeks are less likely to respond to higher doses.

There are a number of options for fluconazole-refractory disease (Table 46-4). Few controlled studies of these approaches and no comparative studies have been reported. Parenteral amphotericin B or an echinocandin remain the drugs of choice for persons with severe disease or esophageal involvement. For mild to moderate fluconazole-refractory OPC, itraconazole cyclodextrin, voriconazole, or posaconazole are reasonable choices.[101–109] Treatment with protease inhibitors has been noted to result in clinical improvement in difficult-to-treat cases.[110] Protease inhibitors have also been shown to inhibit *Candida* secretory aspartic proteases demonstrating direct antifungal activity for *Candida*, though the clinical significance of this finding remains unclear.[111–113] Optimization of antiretroviral therapy (potent therapy with or without protease inhibitors) in persons with refractory disease is essential. The duration of treatment for refractory disease is based on the response, but typically a 14-day regimen is required for OPC or vaginal disease and 21–28 days for esophageal disease. Relapse rates are high in persons with refractory disease, and maintenance suppressive therapy is universally required.

PREVENTION

The most important method for preventing mucocutaneous candidiasis is reversal of the immunodeficiency associated with HIV infection. Potent antiretroviral therapy is likely the single best intervention to reduce the incidence of mucocutaneous candidiasis. Several studies have demonstrated a decline in the rate of colonization and clinical disease with the use of potent antiretroviral therapy.[38,39,41,42] This decline has been correlated with reduced HIV-1 RNA levels in plasma.[39,41,42] Other possible interventions include smoking cessation, good oral hygiene, avoidance of unnecessary antibiotics and steroids, and specific antifungal medications.

Although recurrent mucocutaneous candidiasis is frequent in persons with untreated advanced HIV infection, the indications for primary prophylactic antifungal therapy remain uncertain. A randomized study comparing clotrimazole to fluconazole demonstrated that fluconazole can prevent invasive fungal infections such as cryptococcosis and EC,[114] but there was no survival advantage in the study. Weekly fluconazole prophylaxis has also been studied for the prevention of OPC and vulvovaginal disease.[32,115,116] Schuman et al reported decreases in the incidence of both OPC (relative risk (RR) 0.50; 95% confidence interval (CI) 0.33–0.71) and vulvovaginal disease (RR 0.56; 95% CI 0.41–0.77) in a study of 323 women with moderately advanced HIV infection who took weekly doses of fluconazole 200 mg (median follow-up 29 months).[32] Thus, although one can reduce the risk of mucocutaneous candidiasis, there is no survival advantage.

The use of secondary prophylaxis should be individualized. Some experts recommend prophylaxis in persons with a prior episode of EC.[117,118] In general, persons with occasional disease or infrequent recurrences of OPC (fewer than three episodes per year) can be treated for each episode. In the largest study to address the issue of secondary prophylaxis, episodic versus continuous therapy for OPC with fluconazole among patients with advanced HIV infection and a history of oropharyngeal candidiasis, the ACTG and Mycoses Study Group recently reported the results of the study involving 829 patients (413 randomized to receive continuous fluconazole and 416 randomized to receive episodic fluconazole).[119] The primary objectives of this study were to determine the effectiveness of continuous suppressive therapy with fluconazole (200 mg po three times weekly) compared to episodic treatment for OPC, and also to determine the rates of resistant or refractory disease in both arms. After 42 months, 17 subjects (4.1%) in the continuous fluconazole arm had developed refractory OPC or EC compared to 18 subjects (4.3%) in the episodic fluconazole treatment arm. There is no difference between treatment arms with regard to the time to development of fluconazole refractory infection. Continuous fluconazole suppression was associated with fewer cases of OPC or EC (0.29 vs 1.08 episodes per patient year; $P < 0.0001$) and fewer other invasive fungal infections (15 vs 28). There were no differences in survival between the two arms. Importantly, there was no significant change in fluconazole MICs comparing baseline to end of study isolates. Also, there was no trend toward more non-*Candida albicans* isolated from patients in either arm. The conclusions of this large study suggest that continuous fluconazole suppression at doses of 200 mg three times weekly among patients with a history of OPC resulted in significantly fewer episodes of OPC and EC, numerically fewer systemic invasive fungal infections, and did not contribute to overall fungal resistance or a significant shift in causative *Candida* species compared to those who received episodic therapy. As a result of this trial, it is reasonable to conclude that continuous suppressive therapy is an effective and acceptable approach to management of this disorder.

REFERENCES

1. Gottlieb MS, Schroff R, Schanker HM. Pneumocystis carinii pneumonia and mucosal candidiasis in previously healthy homosexual men: evidence of a new acquired cellular immunodeficiency. N Engl J Med 305:1425, 1981.
2. Masur H, Michelis MA, Greene JB, et al. An outbreak of community acquired Pneumocystis carinii pneumonia: initial manifestation of cellular immune dysfunction. N Engl J Med 305:1431, 1981.
3. Klein RS, Harris CA, Small CB, et al. Oral candidiasis in high-risk patients as the initial manifestation of the acquired immunodeficiency syndrome. N Engl J Med 311:354, 1984.
4. Dodd CL, Greenspan D, Katz MH, et al. Oral candidiasis in HIV infection: pseudomembranous and erythematous candidiasis show similar rates of progression to AIDS. AIDS 5:1339, 1991.
5. Katz MH, Greenspan D, Westenhouse J, et al. Progression to AIDS in HIV-infected homosexual and bisexual men with hairy leukoplakia and oral candidiasis. AIDS 6:95, 1992.
6. Tavitian A, Raufman JP, Rosenthal LE. Oral candidiasis as a marker for esophageal candidiasis in the acquired immunodeficiency syndrome. Ann Intern Med 104:54, 1986.
7. Launay O, Lortholary O, Bouges-Michel C, et al. Candidemia: a nosocomial complication in adults with late-stage AIDS. Clin Infect Dis 26:1134, 1998.
8. Tumbarello M, Tacconelli E, de Gaetano Donati K, et al. Candidemia in HIV-infected subjects. Eur J Clin Microbiol Infect Dis 18:478, 1999.
9. Tintelnot K, Haase G, Seibold M, et al. Evaluation of phenotypic markers for selection and identification of Candida dubliniensis. J Clin Microbiol 38:1599, 2000.
10. Scholing S, Kortinga HC, Froschb M, Muhlschlegel F. The role of Candida dubliniensis in oral candidiasis in human immunodeficiency virus-infected individuals. Crit Rev Microbiol 26:59, 2000.
11. Odds FC. Candida and Candidosis. London: Ballière Tindall; 1988, p 117.
12. Fichtenbaum CJ, Koletar S, Yiannoutsos C, et al. Refractory mucosal candidiasis in advanced human immunodeficiency virus infection. Clin Infect Dis 30:749, 2000.
13. Barchiesi F, Hollis RJ, Del Poeta M, et al. Transmission of fluconazole-resistant Candida albicans between patients with AIDS and oropharyngeal candidiasis documented by pulsed-field gel electrophoresis. Clin Infect Dis 21:561, 1995.
14. Powderly WG, Robinson K, Keath EJ. Molecular typing of Candida albicans isolated from oral lesions of HIV-infected individuals. AIDS 6:81, 1992.
15. Powderly WG. Mucosal candidiasis caused by non-albicans species of Candida in HIV-positive patients. AIDS 6:604, 1992.
16. Bruatto M, Vidotto V, Marinuzzi G, et al. Candida albicans biotypes in human immunodeficiency virus type 1-infected patients with oral candidiasis before and after antifungal therapy. J Clin Microbiol 29:726, 1991.
17. Scmid J, Odds FC, Wiselka MJ, et al. Genetic similarity and maintenance of Candida albicans strains from a group of AIDS patients, demonstrated by DNA fingerprinting. J Clin Microbiol 30:935, 1992.
18. Korting HC, Ollert M, Georgii A, et al. In vitro susceptibilities and biotypes of Candida albicans isolates from the oral cavities of patients infected with human immunodeficiency virus. J Clin Microbiol 26:2626, 1988.
19. Feigal DW, Katz MH, Greenspan D, et al. The prevalence of oral lesions in HIV-infected homosexual and bisexual men: three San Francisco epidemiological cohorts. AIDS 5:519, 1991.
20. Pindborg JJ. Oral candidiasis in HIV infection. In: Robertson PB, Greenspan JS (eds). Perspectives on Oral Manifestations of AIDS. Littleton, MA, PSG Publishing, 1988, p 23.

21. Holmstrup P, Samaranayake LP. Acute and AIDS-related oral candidosis. In: Samaranayake LP, MacFarlane TW (eds). Oral Candidosis. London: Wright; 1990, p 133.
22. McCarthy GM, Mackie ID, Koval J, et al. Factors associated with increased frequency of HIV-related oral candidiasis. J Oral Pathol Med 20:332, 1991.
23. Epstein JB, Truelove EL, Izutzu KT. Oral candidiasis: pathogenesis and host defense. Rev Infect Dis 6:96, 1984.
24. McCarthy GM. Host factors associated with HIV-related oral candidiasis. Oral Surg Oral Med Oral Pathol 73:181, 1992.
25. Yeh CK, Fox PC, Ship JA, et al. Oral defense mechanisms are impaired early in HIV-1 infected patients. J Acquir Immune Defic Syndr 1:361, 1988.
26. Pons VG, Greenspan D, Koletar S, Multicenter Study Group. Comparative study of fluconazole and clotrimazole troches for the treatment of oral thrush in AIDS. J Acquir Immune Defic Syndr 6:1311, 1993.
27. Selik RM, Starcher ET, Curran JW. Opportunistic diseases reported in AIDS patients: frequencies, associations, and trends. AIDS 1:175, 1987.
28. Moore RD, Chaisson RE. Natural history of opportunistic disease in an HIV-infected urban clinical cohort. Ann Intern Med 124:633, 1996.
29. Wilcox CM, Alexander LN, Clark WS, et al. Fluconazole compared with endoscopy for human immunodeficiency virus-infected patients with esophageal symptoms. Gastroenterology 110:2803, 1996.
30. Duerr A, Sierra M, Clarke L, et al. Vaginal candidiasis among HIV-infected women. In: Proceedings of the IX International Conference on AIDS, Berlin, 1993, abstract PO-B01-0880:282.
31. Sha B, Benson C, Pottage J, et al. HIV infection in women: a six year longitudinal, observational study. In: Proceedings of the IX International Conference on AIDS, Berlin, 1993, abstract PO-B01-0891:283.
32. Schuman P, Capps L, Peng G, et al. Weekly fluconazole for the prevention of mucosal candidiasis in women with HIV infection. Ann Intern Med 126:689, 1997.
33. White MH. Is vulvovaginal candidiasis an AIDS-related illness? Clin Infect Dis 22(Suppl 2):S124, 1996.
34. Schuman P, Sobel JD, Ohmit SE, et al. Mucosal candidal colonization and candidiasis in women with or at risk for human immunodeficiency virus infection. Clin Infect Dis 27:1161, 1998.
35. Mouton Y, Alfandari S, Valette M, et al. Impact of protease inhibitors on AIDS defining events and hospitalization in 10 French AIDS reference centers. AIDS 11:F101, 1997.
36. Palella FJ, Delaney KM, Moorman AC, et al. Declining morbidity and mortality among patients with advanced human immunodeficiency virus infection: HIV Outpatient Study investigators. N Engl J Med 338:853, 1998.
37. Hammer SM, Squires KE, Hughes MO, et al. A controlled trial of two nucleosides plus indinavir in persons with human immunodeficiency infection and CD4 cell counts of 200 per cubic millimeters or less. N Engl J Med 337:725, 1997.
38. Cauda R, Tacconelli E, Tumbarello M, et al. Role of protease inhibitors in preventing recurrent oral candidosis in patients with HIV infection: a prospective case-control study. J Acquir Immune Defic Syndr 21:20, 1999.
39. Martins MD, Lozano-Chiu M, Rex JH. Declining rates of oropharyngeal candidiasis and carriage of Candida albicans associated with trends toward reduced rates of carriage of fluconazole-resistant C. albicans in human immunodeficiency virus-infected patients. Clin Infect Dis 27:1291, 1998.
40. Steele C, Leigh J, Swoboda R, Fidel PL. Growth inhibition of Candida by human oral epithelial cells. J Infect Dis 182:1479, 2000.
41. Gottfredsson M, Cox GM, Indridason OS, et al. Association of plasma levels of human immunodeficiency virus type 1 RNA and oropharyngeal Candida colonization. J Infect Dis 180:534, 1999.
42. Dios P, Ocampo A, Otero I, et al. Changes in oropharyngeal colonization and infection by Candida albicans in human immunodeficiency virus-infected patients. J Infect Dis 183:355, 2001.
43. Pfaller MA, Diekema DJ, Sheehan DJ. Interpretive breakpoints for fluconazole and Candida revisited: a blueprint for the future of antifungal susceptibility testing. Clin Microbiol Rev 19:435, 2006.
44. Hitchcock CA. Resistance of Candida albicans to antifungal agents. Biochem Soc Trans 132:1039, 1993.
45. Vanden Bossche H, Marichal P, Odds F. Molecular mechanisms of drug resistance in fungi. Trends Microbiol 2:393, 1994.
46. Ryley JF, Wilson RG, Barrett-Boe KJ. Azole resistance in Candida albicans. J Med Vet Mycol 22:53, 1984.
47. Crombie T, Falconer DJ, Hitchcock CA. Fluconazole resistance due to energy-dependent efflux in Candida glabrata. Antimicrob Agents Chemother 39:1696, 1996.
48. Lake-Bakaar G, Tom W, Lake-Bakaar D, et al. Gastropathy and ketoconazole malabsorption in the acquired immunodeficiency syndrome (AIDS). Ann Intern Med 109:471, 1988.
49. Ally R, Schurmann D, Kreisel W, et al. A randomized, double-blind, double-dummy, multicenter trial of voriconzole and fluconazole in the treatment of esophageal candidiasis in immunocompromised patients. CID 33:1447, 2001.
50. Vazquez JA, Northland R, Miller S, et al. Posaconazole compared to fluconazole for oral candidiasis in HIV-positive patients. In: Proceedings of the 40th Interscience Conference on Antimicrobial Agents and Chemotherapy, Toronto, 2000, abstract 1107.
51. Nieto L, Northland R, Pittisuttithum P, et al. Posaconazole equivalent to fluconazole in the treatment of oropharyngeal candidiasis. In: Proceedings of the 40th Interscience Conference on Antimicrobial Agents and Chemotherapy, Toronto, 2000, abstract 1108.
52. Munoz P, Moreno S, Berenguer J, et al. Fluconazole-related hepatotoxicity in patients with acquired immunodeficiency syndrome. Arch Intern Med 151:1020, 1991.
53. Villanueva A, Arathoon EG, Gotazzo E, et al. A randomized double blind study of caspofungin versus amphotericin for the treatment of candidal esophagitis. Clin Infect Dis 33:1529, 2001.
54. Keating GM, Jarvis B. Caspofungin. Drugs 61:1121, 2001.
54a. Kuse ER, Chetchotisakd P, daCunha CA et al. Micafungin versus liposomal amphotericin B for candidaemia and invasive candidosis: a phase III randomised double-blind trial. Lancet. 369(9572):1519–27, 2007.
54b. Pappas PG, Rotstein CMF, Betts R. Micafungin versus caspofungin for candidemia and other forms of candidiasis. Clin Infect Dis (in press).
55. Pettengell K, Mynhardt J, Kluyts T, et al. Successful treatment of esophageal candidiasis by micafungin: a novel systemic antifungal agent. Aliment Pharmacol Ther 20:475, 2004.
56. de Wet N, Llanos-Cuentas A, Suleiman J, et al. A randomized, double-blind, parallel-group, dose-response study of micafungin compared with fluconazole for the treatment of esophageal candidiasis in HIV-positive patients. Clin Infect Dis 39:842, 2004.
57. de Wet NT, Bester AJ, Viljoen JJ, et al. A randomized, double-blind, comparative trial of micafungin (FK463) vs. fluconazole for the treatment of esophageal candidiasis. Aliment Pharmacol Ther 21:899, 2005.
58. Krause DS, Simjee AE, van Rensburg C, et al. A randomized, double-blind trial of anidulafungin versus fluconazole for the treatment of esophageal candidiasis. Clin Infect Dis 39:770, 2004.
59. Smith DE, Midgley J, Allan M, et al. Itraconazole versus ketoconazole in the treatment of oral and esophageal candidosis in patients infected with HIV. AIDS 5:1367, 1991.

60. Koletar SL, Russell JA, Fass RJ, et al. Comparison of oral fluconazole and clotrimazole troches as treatment for oral candidiasis in patients infected with human immunodeficiency virus. Antimicrob Agents Chemother 34:2267, 1990.
61. De Wit S, Goosens H, Weerts D, et al. Comparison of fluconazole and ketoconazole for oropharyngeal candidiasis in AIDS. Lancet 1:746, 1989.
62. Barchiesi F, Giacometti A, Arzeni D, et al. Fluconazole and ketoconazole in the treatment of oral and esophageal candidiasis in AIDS patients. J Chemother 4:381, 1992.
63. De Repentigny L, Ratelle J. Comparison of itraconazole and ketoconazole in HIV-positive patients with oropharyngeal or esophageal candidiasis. Chemotherapy 42:374, 1996.
64. Laine L, Dretler RH, Conteas CN, et al. Fluconazole compared with ketoconazole for the treatment of Candida esophagitis in AIDS. Ann Intern Med 117:655, 1992.
65. Lim SG, Lee CA, Hales M, et al. Fluconazole for oropharyngeal candidiasis in anti-HIV positive hemophiliacs. Aliment Pharmacol Ther 5:199, 1991.
66. De Wit S, Urbain D, Rahir F, et al. Efficacy of oral fluconazole in the treatment of AIDS associated esophageal candidiasis. Eur J Clin Microbiol Infect Dis 10:503, 1991.
67. Chave JP, Francioli P, Hirschel B, et al. Single-dose therapy for esophageal candidiasis with fluconazole. AIDS 4:1034, 1990.
68. Kutzer E, Oittner R, Leodolter S, et al. A comparison of fluconazole and ketoconazole in the oral treatment of vaginal candidiasis: report of a double-blind multicentre trial. Eur J Obstet Gynecol Reprod Biol 29:305, 1988.
69. Van Huesden AM, Merkus HM, Corbeij RS, et al. Single-dose oral fluconazole versus single-dose topical miconazole for the treatment of acute vulvovaginal candidiosis. Acta Obstet Gynecol Scand 69:417, 1990.
70. Woolley PD, Higgins SP. Comparison of clotrimazole, fluconazole and itraconazole in vaginal candidiasis. Br J Clin Pract 49:65, 1995.
71. Anonymous. A comparison of single-dose oral fluconazole with 3-day intravaginal clotrimazole in the treatment of vaginal candidiasis: report of an international multicentre trial. Br J Obstet Gynaecol 96:226, 1989.
72. Sobel JD, Brooker D, Stein GE, et al. Single oral dose fluconazole compared with conventional clotrimazole topical therapy of Candida vaginitis. Am J Obstet Gynecol 172:1263, 1995.
73. Pappas PG, Rex JH, Sobel JD, et al. Guidelines for treatment of candidiasis. CID 38:161, 2004.
74. Baily GG, Perry FM, Denning DW, et al. Fluconazole-resistant candidosis in an HIV cohort. AIDS 8:787, 1994.
75. Boken DJ, Swindells S, Rinaldi MG. Fluconazole-resistant Candida albicans. Clin Infect Dis 17:1018, 1993.
76. Newman SL, Flanigan TP, Fisher A, et al. Clinically significant mucosal candidiasis resistant to fluconazole treatment in patients with AIDS. Clin Infect Dis 19:684, 1994.
77. White A, Goetz MB. Azole-resistant Candida albicans: report of two cases of resistance to fluconazole and review. Clin Infect Dis 19:687, 1994.
78. Maenza JR, Keruly JC, Moore RD, et al. Risk factors for fluconazole-resistant candidiasis in human immunodeficiency virus-infected patients. Clin Infect Dis 173:219, 1996.
79. Fox R, Neal KR, Leen CLS, et al. Fluconazole resistant Candida in AIDS. J Infect 22:202, 1991.
80. Kitchen VS, Savage M, Harris JRW. Candida albicans resistance in AIDS. J Infect 22:204, 1991.
81. Smith D, Boag F, Midgley J, et al. Fluconazole resistant Candida in AIDS. J Infect 23:345, 1992.
82. Willocks L, Leen CLS, Brettle RP, et al. Fluconazole resistance in AIDS patients. J Antimicrob Chemother 28:937, 1991.
83. Arilla MC, Carbonero JL, Schneider J, et al. Vulvovaginal candidiasis refractory to treatment with fluconazole. Eur J Obstet Gynaecol 44:77, 1992.
84. Sanguineti A, Carmichael JK, Campbell K. Fluconazole-resistant Candida albicans after long-term suppressive therapy. Arch Intern Med 153:1122, 1993.
85. Redding S, Smith J, Farinacci G, et al. Resistance of Candida albicans to fluconazole during treatment of oropharyngeal candidiasis in a patient with AIDS: documentation by in vitro susceptibility testing and DNA subtype analysis. Clin Infect Dis 18:240, 1994.
86. Troillet N, Durussel C, Bille J, et al. Correlation between in vitro susceptibility of Candida albicans and fluconazole-resistant oropharyngeal candidiasis in HIV-infected patients. Eur J Clin Microbiol Infect Dis 12:911, 1993.
87. Cartledge JD, Midgley J, Gazzard BG. Relative growth measurement of Candida species in a single concentration of fluconazole predicts the clinical response to fluconazole in HIV infected patients with oral candidosis. J Antimicrob Chemother 37:275, 1996.
88. Heinic GS, Stevens DA, Greenspan D, et al. Fluconazole-resistant Candida in AIDS patients. Oral Surg Oral Med Oral Pathol 76:711, 1993.
89. Quereda C, Polanco AM, Giner C, et al. Correlation between in vitro resistance to fluconazole and clinical outcome of oropharyngeal candidiasis in HIV-infected patients. Eur J Clin Microbiol Infect Dis 15:30, 1996.
90. Maenza JR, Merz WG, Romagnoli MJ, et al. Infection due to fluconazole-resistant Candida in AIDS patients: prevalence and microbiology. Clin Infect Dis 24:28, 1997.
91. Horn CA, Washburn RG, Givner LB, et al. Azole-resistant oropharyngeal and esophageal candidiasis in patients with AIDS. AIDS 9:533, 1995.
92. Arilla MC, Carbonero JL, Schneider J, et al. Vulvovaginal candidiasis refractory to treatment with fluconazole. Eur J Obstet Gynecol Reprod Biol 44:77, 1992.
93. Fichtenbaum CJ, Powderly WG. Refractory and resistant mucosal candidiasis in the acquired immunodeficiency syndrome. Clin Infect Dis 26:556, 1998.
94. Berman S, Ho M. Highly resistant esophageal candidiasis in patients with AIDS. In: Proceedings of the IX International Conference on AIDS, Berlin, 1993, abstract PO-B09-1405:369.
95. Dick JD, Merz WG, Saral R. Incidence of polyene-resistant yeasts recovered from clinical specimens. Antimicrob Agents Chemother 18:158, 1980.
96. Kwon-Chung KJ, Bennett JE. Principles of antifungal therapy. In: Medical Mycology. Philadelphia: Lea & Febiger; 1992, p 81.
97. Powderly WG, Kobayashi GS, Herzig GP, et al. Amphotericin resistant yeast infection in severely immunocompromised patients. Am J Med 84:826, 1988.
98. Blum RA, D'Andrea DT, Florentino BM, et al. Increased gastric pH and the bioavailability of fluconazole and ketoconazole. Ann Intern Med 114:755, 1991.
99. Kaltenbach G, Leveque D, Peter JD, et al. Pharmacokinetic interaction between itraconazole and rifampin in Yucatan miniature pigs. Antimicrob Agents Chemother 40:2043, 1996.
100. Goldman M, Cloud GA, Smedema M, et al. Does long-term itraconazole prophylaxis result in in vitro azole resistance in mucosal Candida albicans isolates from persons with advanced human immunodeficiency virus infection? Antimicrob Agents Chemother 44:1585, 2000.
101. Dewsnup DH, Stevens DA. Efficacy of oral amphotericin B in AIDS patients with thrush clinically resistant to fluconazole. J Med Vet Mycol 32:389, 1994.
102. Nguyen MT, Weiss PG, Labarre RC, et al. Oral amphotericin B in the treatment or oral candidiasis due to azole-resistant Candida species. In: Abstracts of the Annual Meeting of the Infectious Diseases Society of America, Orlando, 1994, abstract 287.

103. Fichtenbaum CJ, Zackin R, Rajicic N, et al. Amphotericin B oral suspension for fluconazole-resistant oral candidiasis in HIV-infected patients. AIDS 14:845, 2000.
104. Cartledge JD, Midgley J, Youle M, et al. Itraconazole cyclodextrin solution: effective treatment for HIV-related candidosis unresponsive to other azole therapy. J Antimicrob Chemother 33:1071, 1994.
105. Phillips P, Zemcov J, Mahmood W, et al. Itraconazole cyclodextrin solution for fluconazole-refractory oropharyngeal candidiasis in AIDS: correlation of clinical response with in-vitro susceptibility. AIDS 10:1369, 1996.
106. Saag MS, Fessel WJ, Kaufman CA, et al. Treatment of fluconazole refractory oropharyngeal candidiasis with itraconazole oral solution in HIV-positive patients. AIDS Res Hum Retroviruses 15:1413, 1999.
107. Moskovitz B, Wu J, Baruch A, et al. Long term safety and efficacy of itraconazole oral solution for the treatment of fluconazole refractory oropharyngeal candidiasis in HIV positive patients. In: Proceedings of the 4th Conference on Retroviruses and Opportunistic Infections, Washington, DC, Jan1997, abstract 325.
108. Ruhnke M, Schmidt-Westhausen A, Trautmann M. In vitro activities of voriconazole (UK-109,496) against fluconazole-susceptible and resistant Candida albicans isolates from oral cavities of patients with human immunodeficiency virus infection. Antimicrob Agents Chemother 41:575, 1997.
109. Hegener P, Troke PF, Fatkenheuer G, et al. Treatment of fluconazole-resistant candidiasis with voriconazole in patients with AIDS. AIDS 12:2227, 1998.
110. Zingman BS. Resolution of refractory AIDS-related mucosal candidiasis after initiation of didanosine plus saquinavir. N Engl J Med 334:1674, 1996.
111. Borg-von Zepelin M, Meyer I, Thomssen R, et al. HIV-protease inhibitors reduce cell adherence of Candida albicans strains by inhibition of yeast secreted aspartic proteases. J Invest Dermatol 113:747, 1999.
112. Naglik JR, Newport G, White TC, et al. In vivo analysis of secreted aspartyl proteinase expression in human oral candidiasis. Infect Immun 67:2482, 1999.
113. Korting HC, Schaller M, Eder G, et al. Effects of the human immunodeficiency virus (HIV) proteinase inhibitors saquinavir and indinavir on in vitro activities of secreted aspartyl proteinases of Candida albicans isolates from HIV-infected patients. Antimicrob Agents Chemother 43:2038, 1999.
114. Powderly WG, Finkelstein DM, Feinberg J, et al. A randomized trial comparing fluconazole with clotrimazole troches for the prevention of fungal infections in patients with advanced human immunodeficiency virus infection. N Engl J Med 332:700, 1995.
115. Leen CLS, Dunbar EM, Ellis ME, et al. Once-weekly fluconazole to prevent recurrence of oropharyngeal candidiasis in patients with AIDS and AIDS-related complex: a double-blind placebo-controlled study. J Infect 21:55, 1990.
116. Marriott DJE, Jones PD, Hoy JF, et al. Fluconazole once a week as secondary prophylaxis against oropharyngeal candidiasis in HIV-infected patients. Med J Aust 158:312, 1993.
117. Esposito R, Castagna A, Foppa CU. Maintenance therapy of oropharyngeal candidiasis in HIV-infected patients with fluconazole. AIDS 4:1033, 1990.
118. Agresti MB, de Bernardis F, Mondello F, et al. Clinical and mycological evaluation of fluconazole in the secondary prophylaxis of esophageal candidiasis in AIDS patients. Eur J Epidemiol 10:17, 1994.
119. Goldman M, Cloud GA, Wade KD, et al. A randomized study of the use of fluconazole in continuous versus episodic therapy in patients with advanced HIV infection and a history of oropharyngeal candidiasis: AIDS Clinical Trials Group Study 323/Mycoses Study Group Study 40. CID 41:1473, 2005.

Chapter 47

Mycoses Caused by Molds

Thomas F. Patterson, MD, John R. Graybill, MD

Infections caused by molds are uncommon but important causes of opportunistic infections in patients with advanced acquired immunodeficiency syndrome (AIDS). The most common fungal infections are due to *Candida* species and *Cryptococcus neoformans*. Less commonly seen are the endemic dimorphic mycoses, such as those due to *Histoplasma capsulatum* and *Coccidioides immitis*. The least commonly encountered mycoses in patients with HIV are the miscellaneous infections caused by organisms grouped as primary mycelial fungi, or molds.[1,2] Since the development of highly active antiretroviral therapy (HAART), infections with molds have become even less common, although mold infections due to an expanding list of organisms continue to occur.[3–13] Most often patients have advanced human immunodeficiency virus (HIV) infection with CD4+ T-lymphocyte counts usually less than 200 cells/μL (often less than 50/μL) with uncontrolled HIV viral replication. Other risk factors, such as neutropenia, injection drug use, malignancy, the use of corticosteroids or intravenous catheters, and other chronic medical illnesses, are frequently present.[14,15] The clinical presentation of these fungi ranges from sinusitis and soft pulmonary infection to localized deep tissue abscess and widely disseminated disease (Table 47-1). The possibility of a fungal infection must be considered early to allow prompt diagnosis and institution of antifungal therapy and surgical intervention as needed. Long-term suppressive therapy for these mycoses is often required because relapse is frequent. Improved antifungal therapies with excellent activity against molds, particularly the extended spectrum azoles-voriconazole and posaconazole, have been introduced which offer the potential for improved outcomes and less toxicity especially for long-term therapy. Specific guidelines for discontinuing therapy after immunologic reconstitution during HAART have not been developed due to the rarity of these infections, although approaches for the dimorphic pathogen *Penicillium marneffei* have followed the recommendations in histoplasmosis.[16]

PATHOGENS AND EPIDEMIOLOGY

The mycologic classification of molds includes dimorphic pathogens (organisms that exist in nature as molds but are seen as yeasts or yeast-like organisms in tissue), agents of hyalohyphomycosis (lightly pigmented molds) or phaeohyphomycosis (darkly pigmented molds), and Zygomycetes (fungi with wide, rarely septated hyphae). This chapter includes the dimorphic fungi *Paracoccidioides brasiliensis*, *Blastomyces dermatitidis*, *Penicillium marnefeii*, and *Sporothrix schenckii*; agents of hyalohyphomycosis (*Aspergillus*, *Fusarium*, *Pseudallescheria*, *Trichosporon*, and other less commonly encountered hyaline molds); Zygomycetes (*Rhizopus* species, and other members of the order Mucorales); and agents of phaeohyphomycosis (*Alterneria*, *Bipolaris*, *Exophiala*, and other dematiaceous molds). Agents of dermatophytosis, including *Microsporum gypseum* and *Trichophyton rubrum,* can also cause disseminated infection including invasive soft tissue disease in highly immunosuppressed patients.[7,8]

Infection by molds most commonly occurs by inhaling conidia (*B. dermatitidis*, *P. brasiliensis*, probably *P. marneffei*, *Aspergillus* species, Zygomycetes). However, intravenous injection of conidia through injection drug use (Zygomycetes, *Aspergillus* species) or direct percutaneous inoculation (*S. schenckii*, agents of phaeohyphomycosis) also occur. After infection, progression or resolution depends on the specific fungal pathogen and the immunocompetence of the patient. *Aspergillus*, Zygomycetes, and even rare fungal agents of human disease such as *Schizophyllum commune* (mushroom) have caused infection in the maxillary sinuses of patients with AIDS.[17–19]

These mycoses generally occur during late stages of AIDS, causing widely disseminated infection. Other risk factors, such as neutropenia, use of corticosteroids, cytomegalovirus infection, and chemotherapy, compound the risk of becoming infected with many molds, such as

Clinical Manifestations of Selected Mold Infections in Patients with AIDS

Table 47-1

Organism	Clinical Manifestations
Agents of Hyalohyphomycosis	
Aspergillus spp	Pulmonary, sinusitis, cutaneous, focal abscess, disseminated disease
Scedosporium apiospermum	Pneumonia, sinusitis, endocarditis, disseminated disease, meningitis
Fusarium spp	Fungemia, endocarditis, disseminated infection
Chrysosporium spp	Osteomyelitis
Trichosporon spp	Catheter-related fungemia
Geotrichum spp	Esophageal ulcer, disseminated infection
Paecilomyces spp	Disseminated infection
Penicillium decumbens and other spp	Disseminated infection
Penicillium marnefeii	Disseminated infection
Agents of Phaeohyphomycosis	
Alterneria spp	Nasal soft tissue infection, sinusitis
Exophiala spp	Esophagitis, soft tissue infection
Hormonema spp	Liver abscess
Cladophialophora bantiana	Brain abscess, pulmonary
Phialophora spp	Disseminated infection
Bipolaris spp	Endophthalmitis
Scedosporium prolificans	Disseminated infection
Scopulariopsis	Disseminated infection, brain abscess
Agents of Zygomycosis	
Rhizopus arrhizus	Orbit, soft tissue, sinus
Absidia corymbifera	Renal abscesses, pharyngeal, pulmonary
Cunninghamella bertholletiae	Soft tissue abscess
Mucor spp	Sinus

Data from Cunliffe NA, Denning DW. Uncommon invasive mycoses in AIDS. AIDS 9:411, 1995; and Minamoto GY, Rosenberg AS. Fungal infections in patients with the acquired immunodeficiency syndrome. Med Clin North Am 81:381, 1997; and case reports.[3,4,11,13,150,151]

Characteristics of Dimorphic Mycoses in Patients with AIDS

Table 47-2

Mycosis	Geographic Location	Frequency/Form
Histoplasmosis	US/Latin America	30% HIV local/disseminated infection, reticuloendothelial system
Coccidioidomycosis	Southwest US/Latin America	Locally common/primary and reactivation
Blastomycosis	US/scattered worldwide	Rare/pulmonary, disseminated
Paracoccidioidomycosis	South America	Rare/disseminated
Penicilliosis	Southeast Asia	Local 20% HIV/disseminated, pulmonary and skin
Sporotrichosis	Scattered worldwide	Uncommon/cutaneous, disseminated disease

Aspergillus. Clinical manifestations of these molds are summarized in Table 47-1.

DIAGNOSIS AND THERAPY

Diagnosis for all of these infections depends on direct demonstration of the pathogen by histopathology, culture, or serologic testing (Table 47-2). Serologic testing for antibody may be useful for some mycoses (paracoccidioidomycosis, blastomycosis, and coccidioidomycosis), but such tests may be negative in the severely immunocompromised patient and, if negative, may not be helpful. For histoplasmosis, antigen tests are a primary tool for diagnosis in clinical use. More recently, antigen tests have been developed for paracoccidioidomycosis and for blastomycosis.[20–23] Cross reactivity of these antigens with the histoplasma antigen limits the value of antigen testing to discriminate among them.[20,24] Detection of glactomannan by ELISA (Platelia EIA, BioRad, Redmond, WA) has been approved for use in invasive aspergillosis, but has not been evaluated extensively in patients with AIDS.[25,26] Another nonspecific fungal marker, β-D-glucan, which uses a limulus *Amoebocyte* lysate assay (Fungitell, Associates of Cape Cod, Falmouth, MA), is commercially available and is positive in molds (but not Zygomycetes, nor *Cryptococcus*) but has also not been validated in patients with AIDS.[27,28] Quantitative PCR testing has been used investigationally for diagnosis of histoplasmosis, blastomycosis, and coccidioidomysosis, as well as aspergillosis.[23,29–31] However, primers are not yet standardized or widely available, and PCR for molds, including aspergillosis, remains investigational.[32] A culture from any site is usually sufficient to establish a diagnosis of infection because most of these organisms do not usually cause colonization. A major exception is *Aspergillus*, which may colonize the respiratory tract and not be associated with active infection.[33,34] For aspergillosis, the underlying state of host immunity to some degree predicts a benign or invasive course. Other molds, such as *Scedosporoium prolificans*, occasionally colonize the respiratory tract or sinuses without causing invasive disease.[35] The diagnosis of invasive infection should be considered in patients with a compatible clinical syndrome.

Treatment of the invasive molds has evolved considerably in recent years. Until recently amphotericin B has been the unchallenged standard therapy for most of these organisms. Major recent developments have increased therapeutic options which have changed the drug of choice for several of the major mold pathogens. Chief among these newer agents has been voriconazole, a potent very broad spectrum triazole, which was found to be clearly superior to amphotericin B in treatment of invasive aspergillosis.[36] Voriconazole has also been found highly efficacious in treatment of phaeohyphomycosis, and may be considered the drug of choice for these infections.[37] Voriconazole is very well absorbed (>90%) and penetrates the cerebrospinal fluid at 60% of the plasma concentration.[38] Voriconazole also has some efficacy in fusariosis and against *Scedosporium apiospermum*. These uncommon infections, when localized, tend to respond to voriconazole, but are less responsive in widely disseminated infection.[37] Voriconazole has no efficacy against pathogens causing zygomycosis, but these are extremely rare in patients with AIDS. Posaconazole is another broad spectrum triazole licensed in Europe. The antifungal spectrum is similar to that for voriconazole, but whose spectrum of activity includes Zygomycetes.[39–43] There is less experience with posaconazole, although there appear to be somewhat fewer drug interactions than voriconazole and possibly less hepatic toxicity, due to its lack of hepatic metabolism.[44] Posaconazole is presently recommended as a salvage drug due to the fact it exhibits saturable absorption and is not yet available in an intravenous formulation.[45] Activity of posaconazole in salvage therapy of zygomycosis has been particularly encouraging.[39,43] There are few clinical data on either voriconazole or posaconazole for the less common dimorphic mycoses. The utility of an earlier azole, itraconazole, is limited for molds because of erratic bioavailability and toxicity.[46] The solution formulation of itraconazole improves bioavailability but there are limited data to support its use in serious mold infections, although data support the use of itraconazole in dimorphic pathogens.[47–50] Lipid formulations of amphotericin B have largely replaced amphotericin B deoxycholate for mold infections. A recent trial comparing high (10 mg kg^{-1} day^{-1}) with low (3 mg kg^{-1} day^{-1}) liposomal amphotericin B as initial therapy suggests that the high dose added nothing to the efficacy and was somewhat more toxic.[51] The echinocandins (e.g., caspofungin, micafungin, anidulafungin) have efficacy in candidiasis, for which these agents are fungicidal, but against molds they only inhibit growing *Aspergillus* mycelia.[52] Thus, these agents are used as salvage therapy for invasive aspergillosis although only caspofungin has regulatory approval for that indication.[53]

Although few randomized trials for molds have been conducted, guidelines for managing fungal infections (though mostly in non-HIV-infected patients) have been published.[48,54–58] An approach to therapy is summarized in Figure 47-1. Most important is a high index of suspicion for the diagnosis, particularly in patients with risk factors for invasive infections (e.g. steroid use, neutropenia, chemotherapy). Positive cultures from noninvasive samples (e.g., sputum, wounds, urine) may indicate infection, particularly if they are repeatedly positive. Bronchoalveolar lavage and, when appropriate, tissue biopsies should be undertaken to confirm the presence of hyphae. Culture specimens should be obtained to confirm the specific mold, as treatment options may vary.

Because aspergillosis is the most common of the filamentous pathogens, antifungal therapy with high-dose voriconazole should be initiated promptly in most patients with life-threatening disease. Voriconazole should not be used when the pathogen is an agent of zygomycosis (a rare event). Amphotericin B is an alternative, generally used at 3–5 mg/kg of liposomal amphotericin B. Exceptions are patients known to be infected with an amphotericin B-resistant pathogens such as *Aspergillus terreus* or *Scedosporium apiospermum*.[37,40,59] Adjunctive surgical resection of isolated lesions (as may occur with *Aspergillus* when lesions are juxtaposed to the pulmonary artery) or débridement of infection caused by Zygomycetes may improve outcome. Following initial therapy, long-term suppressive therapy with an oral azole is warranted for most mold infections. Long-term survival with many of these infections is uncommon unless the HIV-induced immunosuppression is corrected.

"DIMORPHIC" MYCOSES (SPOROTHRIX, PENICILLIUM, BLASTOMYCES)

Pathogen

The dimorphic mycoses are caused by fungi that are pathogenic to normal and immune hosts. These organisms tend to occur in certain limited geographic areas or have specific epidemiologic niches (Table 47-3). The mycoses caused by

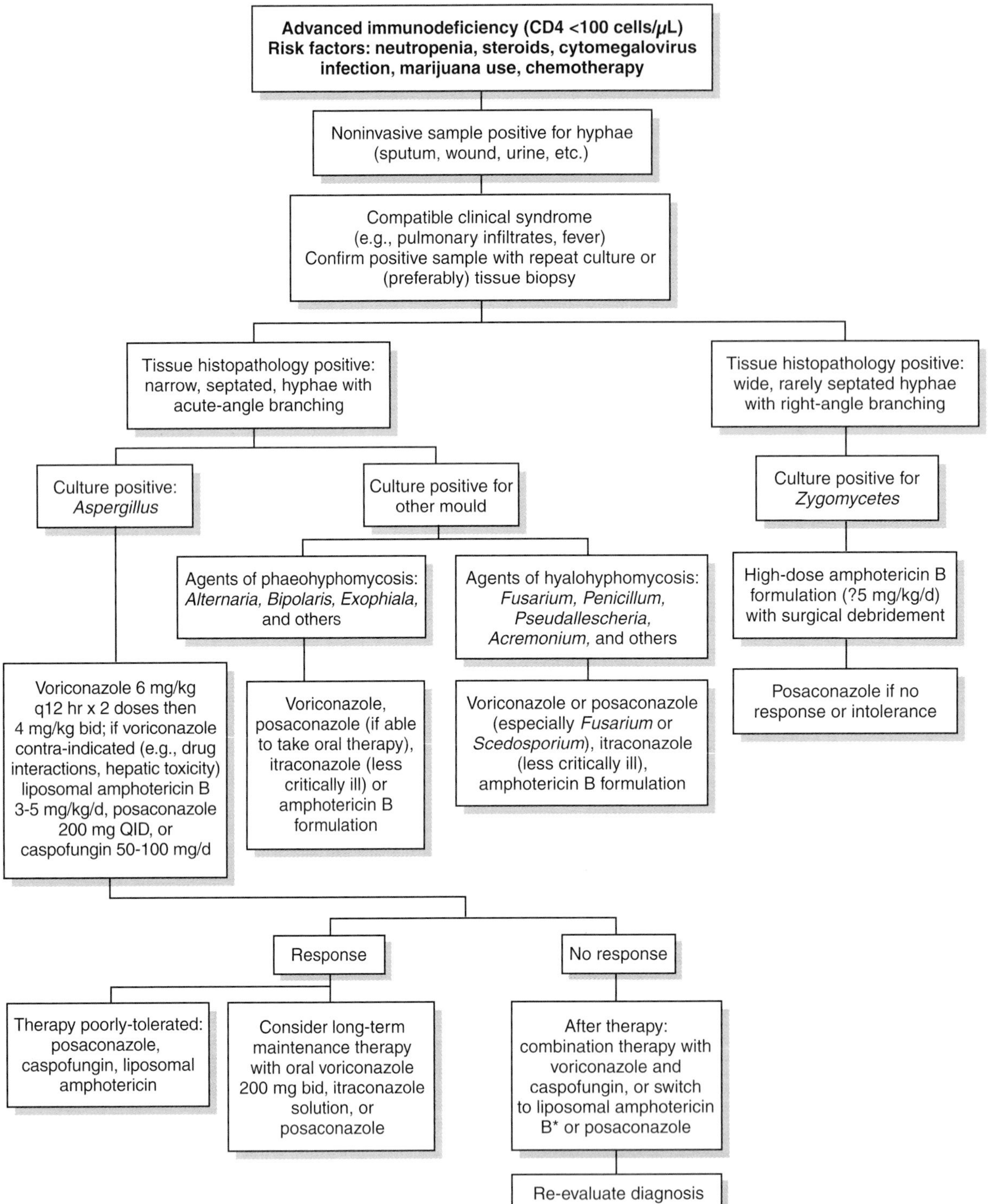

Figure 47-1 ■ Algorithm of management of invasive mold infections in patients with AIDS. *Potential for antagonism of amphotericin B and itraconazole remains controversial.

these organisms include those due to endemic fungi, histoplasmosis, coccidioidomycosis, paracoccidioidomycosis, blastomycosis, penicilliosis (caused by the fungus *Penicillium marneffei*), and sporotrichosis. Among the agents of dimorphic mycoses, *Sporothrix schenckii* does not occur in a specific geographic zone but does occur in the specific setting of exposure to contaminated vegetative material such as moss and rosebush thorns. All are dimorphic; that is, they have an infectious mycelial form in nature and a yeast or yeast-like parasitic form in humans. Histoplasmosis and coccidioidomycosis are discussed in Chapters 44 and 45, respectively.

The infectious particle is the conidium, or spore. All of the dimorphic pathogens may infect by inhalation, although *Sporothrix* infection often is due to percutaneous inoculation.[60]

Table 47-3 Diagnosis of Mold Infections in Patients with AIDS

Organism	Tissue Characteristics	Serology/Others
Agents of hyalohyphomycosis		
Aspergillus spp	Septated, acute-angle branching	Antibody not useful; galactomannan detection; PCR investigational; β-D-glucan nonspecific fungal marker; blood cultures usually negative
Other agents	Indistinguishable from *Aspergillus* spp	Serology not available for molds other than *Apsergillus* *Fusarium* may grow from blood cultures
Agents of phaeohyphomycosis	Irregular hyphae, confirm melanin with specific Masson–Fontana stain	Serology not available
Agents of zygomycosis	Wide, rarely septated hyphae	Serology not available; may not grow from homogenized tissues

Within a short time after infection occurs, the conidia are ingested by macrophages or monocytes and within hours to days the fungus converts to the parasitic form. Infection is ultimately controlled by cell-mediated immune responses. However, in patients with HIV infection, T-helper cell ($T^{H}2$) responses are depressed or ablated. The fungus may grow and spread locally or hematogenously without much restriction. In patients with AIDS the endemic mycoses are more frequently disseminated compared to their presentation in non-HIV-infected hosts. The clinical manifestations of these diseases in HIV-infected patients are summarized in Table 47-1. The geographic distributions and clinical forms are summarized in Table 47-2.

Some infections caused by dimorphic pathogens remain uncommon in patients with AIDS. For example, paracoccidioidomycosis is the major endemic mycosis in South America, but infection in patients with AIDS is rare.[11,57] When the disease does occur in AIDS patients, its presentation is distinct from that seen in normal hosts. In immunocompetent subjects paracoccidioidomycosis is associated with chronic progressive pulmonary granulomatous disease and dense fibrosis progressing over years. In patients with AIDS there is much more rapid progression, and the disease closely resembles disseminated histoplasmosis, with mucocutaneous skin lesions, miliary pulmonary infiltrates, and adrenal insufficiency being significant components. Meningitis may also occur, but fibrosis is not a major component of this form of disease. Blastomycosis is also uncommon in AIDS patients, occurring mainly as a late complication in those with advanced AIDS.[61,62] In immunocompetent hosts blastomycosis is associated with pulmonary fibrosis or skin infection; in patients with AIDS, however, there is widely disseminated infection, including meningitis.[63,64]

In contrast, penicilliosis caused by the dimorphic fungus *P. marneffei* has become the major endemic fungus of Southeast Asia, appearing particularly in southern China and northern Thailand.[12,57,65–67] Penicilliosis may occur in immunocompetent patients but more commonly is seen as an opportunistic infection of AIDS. Multisystem involvement with pulmonary, skin, and visceral lesions is similar in AIDS and nonAIDS patients. Penicilliosis is a febrile wasting disease associated with symptoms that mimic other granulomatous diseases such as tuberculosis or histoplasmosis. There are commonly seen cutaneous lesions with umbilicated centers. These lesions resemble molluscum contagiosum. Like *Histoplasma*, *P. marneffei* may be recovered in blood cultures; however, in contrast to *H. capsulatum*, the yeasts of *Penicillium* divide by fission rather than by budding, so a central zone of clearing between the yeasts may be observed.

Sporotrichosis is most commonly associated with lymphocutaneous disease in immunocompetent patients.[68] However, infection may also result from inhalation of conidia, so pulmonary infection and disseminated disease may occur. Widespread disease involving joints and the lungs and other tissues is more common in HIV-infected patients. Meningitis, which is usually rare in sporotrichosis, has been reported in a few patients with HIV infection.[9,60,69] Untreated, these pathogens may spontaneously resolve in immunocompetent patients; but in patients with immunodeficiency such as AIDS, these mycoses are commonly progressive and lethal.

Diagnosis

Table 47-3 summarizes diagnostic features of mold infections.

The fungi causing all of these dimorphic mycoses exist in nature in their mycelial forms. This is presumably related to nutritional requirements and, for *B. dermatitidis* and *P. marneffei*, may be related to animal vectors of disease (beavers and, presumably, bamboo rats, respectively). *Paracoccidioides brasiliensis* is found in certain moist tropical forest areas, but its natural habitat or vector within those zones is unclear. It has been associated with agricultural occupations (including farming) and gold mining. *Sporothrix schenckii* is also associated with outdoor activities, particularly trauma from garden exposures and sphagnum moss. Although sporotrichosis is found as far north as Canada, a number of small hyperendemic zones have been seen in tropical countries, where this infection is more common than in temperate climates.[70]

It is assumed that nutritional requirements also in large part dictate the endemic zones of these fungi. The endemic zone for blastomycosis in North America and the zone for paracoccidioidomycosis in South America largely overlap the endemic zones for histoplasmosis. However, relatively few cases of blastomycosis or paracoccidioidomycosis are associated with AIDS, whereas histoplasmosis is a major pathogen in AIDS patients. The clear rural associations of infection with *B. dermatitidis* or *P. brasiliensis* are offered as a contrast to histoplasmosis, which is seen in both urban and rural settings and is associated with construction. Late reactivation of disease appears to be less common with paracoccidioidomycosis than histoplasmosis. Another factor that may play a role in "suppressing" paracoccidioidomycosis is the frequent use of trimethoprim–sulfamethoxazole (TMP-SMX) for preventing pneumocystosis. TMP-SMX is active against *P. brasiliensis* as well, so a secondary benefit of preventing *P. brasiliensis* is theoretically possible.[71]

These dimorphic pathogens are identified by culture or presumptively by identifying distinct tissue forms on tissue samples. *B. dermatitidis*, *S. schenckii*, and *P. marneffei* grow readily as mycelia on usual fungal media such as Sabouraud dextrose agar. *P. marneffei* produces a distinctive red pigment that diffuses out into the medium and facilitates identification. Mycelial cultures may take up to a month to grow at room temperature. *P. brasiliensis* grows slowly in the mycelial phase and requires a temperature range of 18–22°C and McVeigh Morton agar to grow optimally.[71]

Although a mycologist may distinguish these dimorphic pathogens in mycelial form, the clinician encounters them more often in biopsy specimens. Infection can be diagnosed by identifying the distinctive tissue forms of the organisms. Normally the fungi are seen associated with granulomas (*P. brasiliensis*, *P. marneffei*) or mixed granuloma and pyogenic reactions (*B. dermatiditis*, *S. schenckii*). In patients with AIDS, however, there may be a much less intact granulomatous reaction.

Cultures may be prepared from sputum, cutaneous lesions, lymph nodes, or urine. Blood can be cultured by the isolator technique or using standard blood culture systems. Culture may require up to a month for growth to be detected, and it is sometimes falsely negative because of failure of the organism to convert from the parasitic form to the mycelial form *in vitro*. It is much more rapid and feasible to identify the organism in tissue using the Gomori methenamine silver stain or periodic acid-Schiff, each of which stains the cell walls. The presence of these organisms on tissue biopsy, wet mount, or culture is indicative of infection and may be associated with pulmonary or disseminated disease.[72]

Serologic testing is less useful than with histoplasmosis (which can be diagnosed with antigen testing) or coccidioidomycosis (for which positive antibody results correlate with the disease). Antibody tests, and more recently antigen tests, are available for paracoccidioidomycosis and blastomycosis.[20,22,30,57,73,74] Although the antibodies measured can be useful for diagnosis and their titers tend to rise with worsening disease, they are not protective. There is some cross reaction (especially for *B. dermatitidis*) with *H. capsulatum* and *C. immitis*.[20,73] There is a serologic test for sporotrichosis, but it is not widely used. A serologic test has been developed for *P. marneffei* disease but is still not used routinely.[75] Antibody testing may be less useful in patients with HIV infection, particularly during the late stages when antibodies are poorly produced. Fungal antibody tests are routinely available through clinical or reference laboratories. Antigen testing is clinically available only for histoplasmosis and blastomycosis (Histoplasmosis Reference Laboratory, Indianapolis, IN, USA).

Susceptibility testing of the endemic mycoses remains nonstandardized. In general, modification of the standard yeast susceptibility testing method of the Clinical Laboratory Standards Institute (formerly the National Committee for Clinical Laboratory Standards) is used, but incubation is carried out for longer periods. As a practical tool, susceptibility testing has been correlated with clinical response for *P. marneffei*, and for *H. capsulatum* for which amphotericin B, itraconazole, posaconazole, and to a lesser extent voriconazole are more potent *in vitro* than fluconazole, with corresponding clinical results.[76]

Therapy

Treatment approaches for the endemic mycoses are relatively well established, although there have been no prospective, comparative trials for any of these infections in patients with AIDS (Fig. 47-1). Experience with the dimorphic fungi in non-HIV-infected patients and results of clinical trials of HIV-infected patients with histoplasmosis and coccidioidomycosis allow some general guidelines.[48,63] First, if the patient is severely ill, amphotericin, usually a lipid formulation for improved tolerance, remains the standard therapy. Itraconazole also has activity but is used less frequently in seriously ill patients. Data to support the use of posaconazole or voriconazole for these pathogens is limited. At present, primary therapy is usually liposomal amphotericin B or amphotericin B lipid complex at 3–5 mg kg^{-1} day^{-1} or as an alternative amphotericin B at 0.7 mg kg^{-1} day^{-1}. An exception may be sporotrichosis, in which a patient may be refractory to amphotericin B but responds to itraconazole.[77]

An alternative for less seriously ill patients is itraconazole, which is administered as capsules at oral doses from 50 mg/day (*P. brasiliensis*) through 200 to 400 mg/day (for the others).[48,49,63,71,76,78] Because the drug is cleared slowly by the liver and clearance is dose-dependent, a loading dose of up to 800 mg/day may be given for the first 2–3 days. Itraconazole solution may produce serum concentrations that are double those seen with capsules, so a lower dose may be sufficient.

Because absorption of itraconazole is erratic, an intravenous form has been developed using the same vehicle. The loading dose is 200 mg twice daily for the first day, then 200 mg once daily for adults.[79,80] Before commencing itraconazole, it is important to ascertain that the patient is not receiving concurrent agents that alter the metabolism of itraconazole. For paracoccidioidomycosis and blastomycosis, the most extensive reports of treatment efficacy were accumulated from data before itraconazole had gained widespread use, and our recommendation for itraconazole is based on experience with non-HIV-infected patients. The response rate to itraconazole in non-HIV-infected patients with sporotrichosis is close to 100% for lymphocutaneous disease and more than 70% for patients with disseminated disease.[81] Alternative agents for treating the endemic mycoses include fluconazole, which has more attractive kinetics and fewer drug interactions. Fluconazole is less efficacious than itraconazole for penicilliosis, sporotrichosis, blastomycosis, histoplasmosis, and paracoccidioidomycosis.[48,76,82] There is not enough experience to make clear recommendations for either voriconazole or posaconazole for these infections.

The outcome for blastomycosis and sporotrichosis in AIDS patients is generally much worse with disseminated disease than with local pulmonary disease (blastomycosis and paracoccidioidomycosis) or cutaneous disease (sporotrichosis). Meningitis caused by *S. schenckii* is rare and does not respond well to treatment.[60] Blastomycosis in AIDS patients is strongly associated with central nervous system (CNS) involvement (46% of 24 patients), with the mortality 90% in this group.[60–62]

In these infections, patients are stabilized on "consolidation" therapy (400 mg/day itraconazole in capsular form), after which the dose may be lowered eventually to 200 mg/day for chronic suppression and prevention of relapse.[49] All of these infections are associated with relapse if treatment is interrupted. With effective antiretroviral therapy, it is possible that immune recovery will prevent relapse if treatment is discontinued. At what level of CD4 count or what duration of therapy this may be done has not been conclusively determined, but in one small study secondary prophylaxis of *P. marnefeii* infection was successfully discontinued after immune reconstitution.[16]

Prevention

There are no proven ways to eliminate the risk of infection with these dimorphic pathogens.

AGENTS OF HYALOHYPHOMYCOSIS (*ASPERGILLUS, FUSARIUM, PSEUDALLESCHERIA*)

Agents of hyalohyphomycosis are a diverse group of lightly pigmented (hyaline) molds. The most important of these organisms is *Aspergillus*, but other molds, such as *Fusarium* species, *Scedosporium apiospermum*, and *Chrysosporium* species, have also been reported occasionally in patients with advanced AIDS (Table 47-1). Since the advent of HAART, these infections have become even rarer in HIV patients. Nevertheless, they remain potential pathogens in patients with advanced AIDS and uncontrolled viral replication. They appear similar to each other and to *Aspergillus* in tissue, so cultures are needed to confirm the specific agent causing the disease. The risk factors for these infections include advanced immunodeficiency, with CD4+ T-lymphocyte counts usually less than 50/mm^3, and other alterations in host defenses, such as neutropenia, malignancy, indwelling catheters, and comorbid conditions such as diabetes mellitis.[15]

Aspergillus

Invasive aspergillosis was not defined as an opportunistic infection of AIDS because of the relative obscurity of that infection in the original cases of AIDS. Although the frequency of these infections increased for some years, they have once again become uncommon. The clinical presentation of invasive aspergillosis with AIDS includes pulmonary disease, sinusitis, cutaneous infection, localized abscesses including vertebral infection, brain abscess, and renal disease as well as widely disseminated infection.[83–88] Colonization with *Aspergillus* has been reported to occur in ~5% of AIDS patients in some series, although the rate of proven invasive disease was less than 1%.[34] The course of aspergillosis is frequently unremitting, although aggressive antifungal therapy may suppress clinical symptoms and prolong survival.[83,84] The course may not be fulminant as frequently occurs in other immunosuppressed patients, such as profoundly neutropenic patients and those undergoing bone marrow transplantation. In patients with more chronic symptoms, a high index of suspicion is needed to establish the diagnosis.[83,88]

The most common species associated with infection in most medical centers is *Aspergillus fumigatus*, though other species may be found. The usual route of infection is through inhalation of conidia, which are ubiquitous and found in air, dust, ventilation systems, plants, soil, and environmental surfaces. Cutaneous infection may also occur in association with indwelling intravenous catheters or injection drug use.[89]

The major host defenses against *Aspergillus* species are neutrophils (which inhibit conidia) and macrophages (which kill conidia).[90] Thus HIV-infected patients with impaired neutrophils, such as those undergoing cytotoxic chemotherapy, therapy for opportunistic infections that cause neutropenia, or therapy for malignancy, are at greatest risk for infection. Patients with impaired macrophage function, as occurs with the use of corticosteroids, are also at increased risk. Environmental exposures including marijuana smoke may also increase risk.[91] Some patients with HIV infection do not have other identifiable risks, so HIV infection may independently increase the risk of *Aspergillus* infection.[92]

Diagnosis

The diagnosis of invasive aspergillosis is suggested by repeated isolation of the organism from noninvasive samples

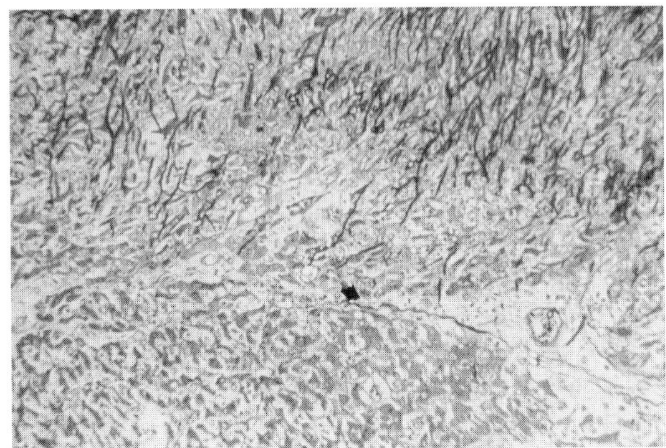

Figure 47-2 ■ Histopathologic appearance of *Aspergillus* species hyphae (silver stain).

such as sputum, particularly in a high-risk patient with compatible clinical symptoms, although cultures may be negative even with advanced infection.[34] The diagnosis is established by demonstrating hyphae in tissue samples (Fig. 47-2). The presence of hyphae consistent with *Aspergillus* on bronchoalveolar lavage samples in an HIV-infected patient with a compatible clinical syndrome is often sufficient to allow institution of empiric therapy. Evaluation of bronchoalveolar lavage and, in selected patients, a tissue biopsy are important for confirming that invasion rather than colonization is present and to determine if other opportunistic pathogens are present. A culture is necessary because other agents of hyalohyphomycosis may appear indistinguishable on a tissue biopsy. Susceptibility testing is not generally necessary, although *Aspergillus* strains resistant to amphotericin B (like *A. terreus*) or to itraconazole have been reported.[93,94]

Nonculture methods can also be used to help establish a diagnosis of invasive aspergillosis, although these methods have not been specifically validated in HIV-infected patients. Chest radiographs are usually abnormal in patients with invasive infection, but patients with ulcerative tracheobronchitis may not show pulmonary infiltrates. Radiographically invasive pulmonary aspergillosis appears most commonly as diffuse infiltrates (25%), focal infiltrates (22%), cavitary lesions (36%), bronchial aspergillosis with atelectasis (14%), and other nonspecific findings (3%).[95] Computed tomography of the chest may show an early halo or air-crescent sign, indicating the presence of infection, although these findings may be less specific in nonneutropenic patients.[96] Their presence has led some clinicians to institute therapy early in patients with neutropenia, which may improve outcomes or at least delay progression.[25]

Antigen detection of galactomannan has been introduced, particularly for patients undergoing hematopoietic stem transplantation and those with malignancies.[26,97–99] Maertens et al have summarized encouraging studies in which high-risk patients are monitored twice weekly for antigenemia and, if positive, are subjected to other confirmatory tests and treated for presumptive disease.[25] Notably in patients with fewer risk factors and with less frequent sampling the assay has been less useful. The polymerase chain reaction (PCR) has also been investigated for use in early diagnosis. Although mostly single center studies have shown good sensitivity and specificity, these assays have not been externally validated and are not standardized so that they remain investigational at the present time.[31,32] There is uncertainty over whether these methods, even if used routinely in patients at high risk for fulminating disease (leukemia, bone marrow transplant), can detect the patient who has progressive but less aggressive disease, as is more typical for the patient with AIDS. Furthermore, a large-scale screening program would be extremely costly for the few patients who might be identified.

Therapy and Prevention

Initial therapy for invasive aspergillosis should be with voriconazole, due to the significantly better responses and improved survival compared to standard amphotericin B, although limited data are available from HIV-infected patients.[36,58] Advantages of voriconazole include both oral and parenteral administration; limitations include the well known range of drug interactions for broad-spectrum triazoles along with toxicities including potentially dose-limiting hepatic toxicity, rash and an associated transient visual toxicity, which manifests as "brightness" in visual perception.[100] Alternatively, high-dose amphotericin B deoxycholate ($0.7–1.5\,mg\,kg^{-1}\,day^{-1}$) has been used in the past, but poor responses and intolerance have largely resulted in the replacement of amphotericin B with liposomal amphotericin B in invasive aspergillosis.[101]

Itraconazole has also been used, usually following an initial course of amphotericin B.[102] Response rates to itraconazole capsules at initial doses of 600 mg/day for 3 days followed by 400 mg/day produced partial responses or stabilization of symptoms in seven of the 11 AIDS patients (63%) treated.[103] However, progression of underlying disease eventually occurred in all patients. Posaconazole, an extended spectrum azole, which is an oral suspension has shown good activity and safety in *Aspergillus* infections and is currently under regulatory review.[44,104]

Other therapeutic options for *Aspergillus* include the echinocandins. This class of drug acts by inhibiting formation of the fungal cell wall and acts on the growing tips of *Aspergillus* hyphae. At present caspofungin is licensed for salvage therapy of acute invasive aspergillosis with an overall response rate of ~45%, although experience has been limited in patients with AIDS.[53] Although these drugs are administered only intravenously, their minimal toxicity and lack of meaningful drug interactions have made them attractive for use in invasive mycoses including aspergillosis. Aspergillosis is the only mycelial infection in which this class of drugs has thus far been evaluated. Clinicians often use combination therapy in desperate situations (i.e., combinations of amphotericin B with azole therapy, caspofungin, or both).[105] Whether such combination therapy is advantageous is unknown.

Although these new antifungal agents provide some basis for hope, thus far the response rates to antifungal agents in invasive aspergillosis for the highest risk patients remain dismal. If there is no response to antiretrovirals, death occurs a median of 2–4 months after diagnosis. Even if control of infection is achieved, which is seen in a limited number of patients for more than 12 months, recrudescence is common. One report demonstrated immune reconstitution syndrome resulting in bronchial obstruction due to an excessive inflammatory reponse.[106]

In patients with localized disease, surgical resection of pulmonary nodules or visceral abscesses may improve outcome. Patients with cutaneous and catheter-related infection also respond to local intervention combined with aggressive antifungal therapy. Patients with endobronchial lesions are also effectively treated with itraconazole therapy and presumably the extended spectrum azoles, voriconazole and posaconazole, as well.[107,108]

Infection with *Aspergillus* species is not readily prevented because patients are constantly exposed to conidia. Prophylaxis with antifungal agents is not indicated because of the rarity of this infection. Interestingly, one study suggested the use of sulfamethoxazole for *Pneumocystis* might have a secondary benefit of reducing aspergillosis as well.[109] However, the judicious use of steroids and the reversal of neutropenia may decrease the number of patients at risk for infection.[90]

Other Agents (*Fusarium, Scedosporium, Chrysosporium*)

An increasing number of other agents of hyalohyphomycosis have been reported to cause invasive mycoses in patients with AIDS. These organisms include a collection of hyaline molds such as *Fusarium* species, *Scedosporium apiospermum*, *Chrysosporium* species, *Geotrichum*, *Trichosporon beigelii*, and *Penicillium* species (Table 47-1).[3,4,13,110–117]

The risk factors for infection are similar to those for *Aspergillus*, and the clinical presentations of these infections may all be similar to that of invasive aspergillosis. The clinical presentations include sinusitis, pulmonary infection, localized abscesses, cutaneous infection, and (fusarium) fungemia that may be associated with disseminated infection.

In tissue, all of these organisms appear as branched, septated hyphae that are indistinguishable from those of *Aspergillus* or other hyaline molds (Fig. 47-3). Specific diagnosis requires culture of the organism from tissue. Standard treatment for most of these organisms has been amphotericin B, although some of these organisms are clinically and mycologically resistant to amphotericin B, including *Fusarium* and *Scedosporium*.[112,113,118] Posaconazole and voriconazole have both been used with success in the treatment of *Scedosporium* and *Fusarium* infections and are likely the drugs of choice for these infections.[37,42,119,120] Voriconazole appears quite effective against *Scedosporium apiospermium* (63% of 27 patients responding) but appears less effective against *Scedosporium prolificans* (two of seven patients responding).[121] Antifungal agents to prevent these mycoses are not indicated because they remain rare. Early consideration for the diagnosis and prompt initiation of therapy may improve prognosis. Lifelong suppressive antifungal therapy may be needed though improved antiretroviral therapy raises the possibility of limited duration of treatment.

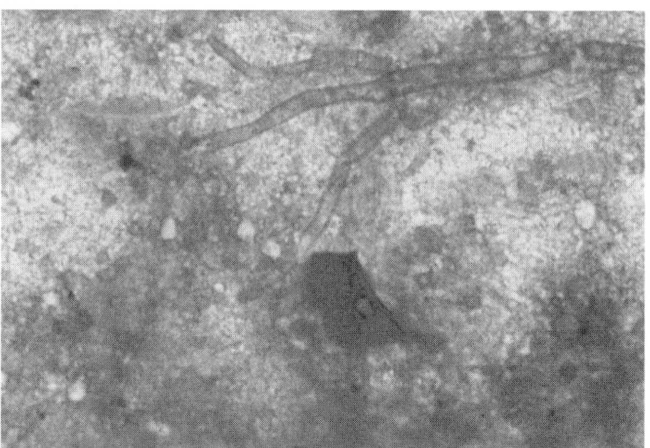

Figure 47-3 ■ Histopathologic appearance of an agent of hyalohyphomycosis in tissue (periodic acid-Schiff stain).

AGENTS OF PHAEOHYPHOMYCOSIS (*CLADOPHIALOPHORA, ALTERNERIA, EXOPHIALA*)

Pathogens

Agents of phaeohyphomycosis comprise a group of opportunistic molds that are dematiaceous, or darkly pigmented (Table 47-1).[122–132] These emerging pathogens remain rare in patients with AIDS. There are many genera of fungi in this group, but they infrequently cause infections in patients with HIV. These opportunistic fungi do not cause infections specifically in HIV-infected patients but do cause disease in certain epidemiologic settings.

As with other molds, infection usually occurs by inhalation of conidia. It usual starts in the sinuses or the lungs. Alternatively, infection may follow percutaneous inoculation.[130] Fungemia may also occur.[133]

The pathogenicity of these organisms is quite variable. In immunocompetent patients or those with minimal host defense abnormalities, phaeohyphomycosis may proceed with the development of sinusitis or pneumonia over months to years, and there may be direct invasion of the brain from the sinuses.[126] There may also be a significant component of hypersensitivity, with eosinophils and Charcot–Leyden crystals in sinus aspirates. Subcutaneous lesions may gradually enlarge over months. Colonies of the dematiaceous fungi are dark-colored. Many of these fungi, such as *Cladophialophora* species, are neurotropic and may cause brain abscesses.[129] These fungi may infect the individual at any stage of AIDS, but they are commonly associated with a more rapid course in those with late AIDS.

The organisms are found in decaying vegetation and are abundant in nature but of sufficiently low virulence that only scattered infections occur. They thrive best in an acidic, glucose-rich environment and are readily killed by polymorphonuclear leukocytes. Thus neutropenia and uncontrolled diabetes are risk factors for infection. Traumatic inoculation while gardening is a major mode of infection.

Diagnosis and Therapy

Agents of phaeohyphomycosis are characterized by production of black melanin pigment, which may be seen histopathologically and in gross lesions. The mycelia are quite variable, and identification is made by examining conidia in culture. As with endemic mycoses, the diagnosis is made by culture or biopsy. Unlike the endemic mycoses, in which the morphology of the parasitic form is distinctive, these mycoses may present with "mycelia sterilia", a mold culture that does not sporulate and thus does not allow identification. Masson–Fontana staining of tissue specimens is useful for staining the melanin in the hyphae, and it allows a specific diagnosis of an agent of phaeohyphomycosis (Fig. 47-4). Culture specimens are best obtained from normally sterile sites (e.g., biopsy of a subcutaneous lesion or sinus aspirate). These organisms may be found colonizing the respiratory tract from sputum samples, so a tissue biopsy may be needed to establish a diagnosis of invasive infection.

As with other molds, therapy has been commonly with amphotericin B. However, *in vitro* and *in vivo* activity of itraconazole and the extended spectrum azoles, posaconazole and voriconazole, has been demonstrated against many of the agents of phaeohyphomycosis, so these agents are possible alternatives, especially for patients with less serious infection and for long-term suppressive therapy.[134–136]

Itraconazole should be used at initial loading doses of 600–800 mg/day for 3 days and then continued at 400 mg/day.[137] For patients with CNS involvement, continuing a dose of 600 mg/day has controlled progression of the disease. Voriconazole and posaconazole have been clinically effective in a few patients usually as salvage therapy.[41,138,139] The new echinocandins also have activity *in vitro* against some agents of phaeohyphomycosis, but there is very limited clinical experience with them.[140,141] There are no known ways to prevent these unusual mycoses.

ZYGOMYCOSIS

Pathogens and Diagnosis (*Rhizopus species, Absidia, Mucor, Rhizomucor, Cunninghamella*)

Zygomycetes such as *Rhizopus* species, *Absidia*, *Mucor*, *Rhizomucor*, and *Cunninghamella* cause rhinocerebral disease or pneumonia in patients with diabetes, neutropenia and have recently emerged as an important pathogen in patients receiving long-term voriconazole therapy (Table 47-1).[142,143] These organisms have been reported uncommonly in patients with AIDS but may cause localized deep tissue abscesses in organs including the kidney, liver, spleen, and stomach.[144] Some of these infections progress rather slowly in patients with AIDS and respond well to surgery and to antifungal therapy with amphotericin B.[145] Disseminated infection, including infections in the CNS, may also occur; it tends to be aggressive and has a poor outcome, with mortality rates of 80% or more.[17,146,147]

Risk factors for infection include injection drug use, neutropenia, the use of corticosteroids, and diabetes. In most cases the route of infection is presumed to be through contamination of injected drugs, although inhalation of conidia is also possible.

Zygomycosis is diagnosed by demonstrating wide, rarely septated hyphae with right-angle branching in tissue (Fig. 47-5). Hematoxylin-eosin stains Zygomycete mycelia densely, usually much more than those of *Aspergillus*. However, the individual species must be identified *in vitro* in cultures, where

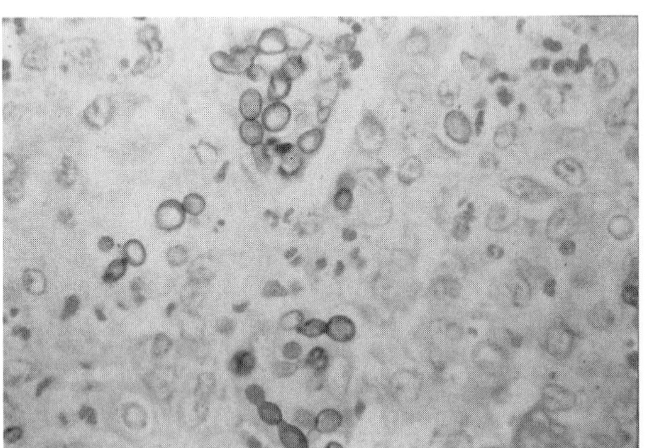

Figure 47-4 ■ Histopathologic appearance of an agent of phaeohyphomycosis in tissue (Masson–Fontana stain).

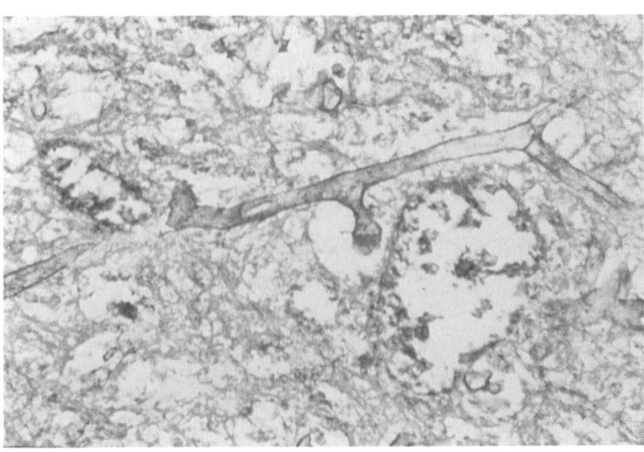

Figure 47-5 ■ Histopathologic appearance of an agent of zygomycosis in tissue (silver stain).

distinctive microscopic and macroscopic features, such as the presence or absence of rhizoids (root-like structures) or characteristics of sporangia, allow a specific diagnosis. Zygomycetes grow rapidly on culture media, usually within a day, using routine fungal media. However, when tissue is homogenized before culture, the mycelium may be broken up sufficiently that it does not grow in culture. Serologic testing is not useful for these organisms.

Therapy and Prevention

Zygomycoses have not been considered responsive to azole antifungals. Voriconazole lacks activity and its long-term use in very immunosuppressed patients has been a risk factor for infection with these organisms.[148] Posaconazole does have *in vitro* activity and has shown favorable responses usually as salvage therapy.[39,43] Specific organisms (e.g., some strains of *Absidia*) are susceptible *in vitro* to itraconazole, although clinical experience is limited. Zygomycosis is treated with surgical débridement and amphotericin B, now usually with high doses of the lipid formulations.[149] The experience in HIV-infected patients is so limited that chronic management of survivors is unclear.

This infection is rare in HIV-infected patients, and the results of treatment are mixed, with a usually poor outcome if the CNS is involved but a better outcome if the disease is localized to the skin or other organs. In some cases surgical resection is appropriate and necessary to control the infection. Specific measures to prevent these rare mycoses are not possible.

REFERENCES

1. Cunliffe NA, Denning DW. Uncommon invasive mycoses in AIDS. AIDS 9:411, 1995.
2. Perfect JR, Schell WA. The new fungal opportunists are coming. Clin Infect Dis 22(Suppl 2):S112, 1996.
3. Girija T, Kumari R, Tandon S, Bairy I, et al. Pneumonia due to Trichosporon beigelii infection in HIV positive patient–a case report. Indian J Pathol Microbiol 44:379, 2001.
4. Lovell RD, Moll M, Allen J, Cicci LG. Disseminated Paecilomyces lilacinus infection in a patient with AIDS. AIDS Read 12:212, 2002.
5. Martin CA, Roberts S, Greenberg RN. Voriconazole treatment of disseminated paecilomyces infection in a patient with acquired immunodeficiency syndrome. Clin Infect Dis 35:e78, 2002.
6. Carvalho MT, de Castro AP, Baby C, et al. Disseminated cutaneous sporotrichosis in a patient with AIDS: report of a case. Rev Soc Bras Med Trop 35:655, 2002.
7. Galhardo MC, Wanke B, Reis RS, et al. Disseminated dermatophytosis caused by Microsporum gypseum in an AIDS patient: response to terbinafine and amorolfine. Mycoses 47:238, 2004.
8. Kwon KS, Jang HS, Son HS, et al. Widespread and invasive Trichophyton rubrum infection mimicking Kaposi's sarcoma in a patient with AIDS. J Dermatol 31: 839, 2004.
9. Silva-Vergara ML, Maneira FR, De Oliveira RM, et al. Multifocal sporotrichosis with meningeal involvement in a patient with AIDS. Med Mycol 43:187, 2005.
10. Noritomi DT, Bub GL, Beer I, et al. Multiple brain abscesses due to Penicillium spp infection. Rev Inst Med Trop Sao Paulo 47:167, 2005.
11. Caseiro MM, Etzel A, Soares MC, Costa SO. Septicemia caused by Paracoccidioides brasiliensis (Lutz, 1908) as the cause of death of an AIDS patient from Santos, Sao Paulo State, Brazil–a nonendemic area. Rev Inst Med Trop Sao Paulo 47:209, 2005.
12. Carey J, Hofflich H, Amre R, et al. Penicillium marneffei infection in an immunocompromised traveler: a case report and literature review. J Travel Med 12:291, 2005.
13. Mahapatra A. Coinfection of Cryptosporidium and Geotrichum in a case of AIDS. Indian J Pathol Microbiol 48:25, 2005.
14. Ampel NM. Emerging disease issues and fungal pathogens associated with HIV infection. Emerg Infect Dis 2:109, 1996.
15. Minamoto GY, Rosenberg AS. Fungal infections in patients with acquired immunodeficiency syndrome. Med Clin North Am 81: 381, 1997.
16. Hung CC, Chen MY, Hsieh SM, et al. Discontinuation of secondary prophylaxis for penicilliosis marneffei in AIDS patients responding to highly active antiretroviral therapy. Aids 16:672, 2002.
17. Blatt SP, Lucey DR, DeHoff D, Zellmer RB. Rhinocerebral zygomycosis in a patient with AIDS. Journal of Infectious Diseases 164:215, 1991.
18. Rosenthal J, Katz R, DuBois DB, et al. Chronic maxillary sinusitis associated with the mushroom Schizophyllum commune in a patient with AIDS. Clin Infect Dis 14:46, 1992.
19. Teh W, Matti BS, Marisddaiah H, Minamoto GY. Aspergillus sinusitis in patients with AIDS: report of three cases and review. Clin Infect Dis 21:529, 1995.
20. Durkin M, Witt J, Lemonte A, et al. Antigen assay with the potential to aid in diagnosis of blastomycosis. J Clin Microbiol 42:4873, 2004.
21. Hage CA, Davis TE, Egan L, et al. Diagnosis of pulmonary histoplasmosis and blastomycosis by detection of antigen in bronchoalveolar lavage fluid using an improved second-generation enzyme-linked immunoassay. Respir Med 2006.
22. Bialek R, Ibricevic A, Aepinus C, et al. Detection of Paracoccidioides brasiliensis in tissue samples by a nested PCR assay. J Clin Microbiol 38:2940, 2000.
23. Bialek R, Feucht A, Aepinus C, et al. Evaluation of two nested PCR assays for detection of Histoplasma capsulatum DNA in human tissue. J Clin Microbiol 40:1644, 2002.
24. Wheat J, Wheat H, Connolly P, et al. Cross-reactivity in Histoplasma capsulatum variety capsulatum antigen assays of urine samples from patients with endemic mycoses. Clin Infect Dis 24:1169, 1997.
25. Maertens J, Theunissen K, Verhoef G, et al. Galactomannan and computed tomography-based preemptive antifungal therapy in neutropenic patients at high risk for invasive fungal infection: a prospective feasibility study. Clin Infect Dis 41:1242, 2005.
26. Marr KA, Balajee SA, McLaughlin L, et al. Detection of galactomannan antigenemia by enzyme immunoassay for the diagnosis of invasive aspergillosis: variables that affect performance. J Infect Dis 190:641, 2004.
27. Odabasi Z, Mattiuzzi G, Estey E, et al. Beta-D-glucan as a diagnostic adjunct for invasive fungal infections: validation, cutoff development, and performance in patients with acute myelogenous leukemia and myelodysplastic syndrome. Clin Infect Dis 39:199, 2004.
28. Ostrosky-Zeichner L, Alexander BD, Kett DH, et al. Multicenter clinical evaluation of the (1–>3) beta-D-glucan assay as an aid to diagnosis of fungal infections in humans. Clin Infect Dis 41:654, 2005.
29. Rickerts V, Bialek R, Tintelnot K, et al. Rapid PCR-based diagnosis of disseminated histoplasmosis in an AIDS patient. Eur J Clin Microbiol Infect Dis 21:821, 2002.
30. Bialek R, Cirera AC, Herrmann T, et al. Nested PCR assays for detection of Blastomyces dermatitidis DNA in paraffin-embedded canine tissue. J Clin Microbiol 41:205, 2003.

31. White PL, Linton CJ, Perry MD, et al. The evolution and evaluation of a whole blood polymerase chain reaction assay for the detection of invasive aspergillosis in hematology patients in a routine clinical setting. Clin Infect Dis 42:479, 2006.
32. Donnelly JP. Polymerase chain reaction for diagnosing invasive aspergillosis: getting closer but still a ways to go. Clin Infect Dis 42:487, 2006.
33. Perfect JR, Cox GM, Lee JY, et al. The impact of culture isolation of Aspergillus species: a hospital-based survey of aspergillosis. Clin Infect Dis 33:1824, 2001.
34. Pursell KJ, Telzak EE, Armstrong D. Aspergillus species colonization and invasive disease in patients with AIDS. Clin Infect Dis 14:141, 1992.
35. Marr KA, Carter RA, Crippa F, et al. Epidemiology and outcome of mould infections in hematopoietic stem cell transplant recipients. Clin Infect Dis 34:909, 2002.
36. Herbrecht R, Denning DW, Patterson TF, et al. Voriconazole versus amphotericin B for primary therapy of invasive aspergillosis. N Engl J Med 347:408, 2002.
37. Perfect JR, Marr KA, Walsh TJ, et al. Voriconazole treatment for less-common, emerging, or refractory fungal infections. Clin Infect Dis 36:1122, 2003.
38. Hoffman HL, Rathbun RC. Review of the safety and efficacy of voriconazole. Expert Opin Investig Drugs 11:409, 2002.
39. Greenberg RN, Mullane K, van Burik JA, et al. Posaconazole as salvage therapy for zygomycosis. Antimicrob Agents Chemother 50:126, 2006.
40. Mellinghoff IK, Winston DJ, Mukwaya G, Schiller GJ. Treatment of Scedosporium apiospermum brain abscesses with posaconazole. Clin Infect Dis 34:1648, 2002.
41. Negroni R, Tobon A, Bustamante B, et al. Posaconazole treatment of refractory eumycetoma and chromoblastomycosis. Rev Inst Med Trop Sao Paulo 47:339, 2005.
42. Raad, II, Hachem RY, Herbrecht R, et al. Posaconazole as salvage treatment for invasive fusariosis in patients with underlying hematologic malignancy and other conditions. Clin Infect Dis 42:1398, 2006.
43. van Burik JA, Hare RS, Solomon HF, et al. Posaconazole is effective as salvage therapy in zygomycosis: a retrospective summary of 91 cases. Clin Infect Dis 42:e61, 2006.
44. Raad, II, Graybill JR, Bustamante AB, et al. Safety of long-term oral posaconazole use in the treatment of refractory invasive fungal infections. Clin Infect Dis 42:1726, 2006.
45. Keating GM. Posaconazole. Drugs 65:1553, 2005.
46. Marr KA, Crippa F, Leisenring W, et al. Itraconazole versus fluconazole for prevention of fungal infections in patients receiving allogeneic stem cell transplants. Blood 103:1527, 2004.
47. Galgiani JN, Ampel NM, Catanzaro A, et al. Practice guidelines for the treatment of coccidioidomycosis. Clin Infect Dis 30:658, 2000.
48. Kauffman CA, Hajjeh R, Chapman SW, Mycoses Study Group. Practice guidelines for the management of patients with sporotrichosis. Clin Infect Dis 30: 684, 2000.
49. Supparatpinyuo K, Perriens J, Nelson KE, Sirisanthana T. A controlled trial of itraconazole to prevent relapse of Penicillium marneffei infection in patients infected with the human immunodeficiency virus. N Engl J Med 339:1739, 1998.
50. Wheat J, Sarosi G, McKinsey D, et al. Practice guidelines for the management of patients with histoplasmosis. Clin Infect Dis 30:688, 2000.
51. Cornely OA, Maertens J, Bresnik M, Herbrecht R. Liposomal amphotericin B (L-AMB) as initial therapy for invasive filamentous fungal infections (IFFI): a randomized, prospective trial of a high loading regimen vs. standard dosing (AmBiLoad Trial). Blood (ASH Annual Meeting Abstracts) 106:3222, 2005.
52. Bowman JC, Hicks PS, Kurtz MB, et al. The antifungal echinocandin caspofungin acetate kills growing cells of Aspergillus fumigatus in vitro. Antimicrob Agents Chemother 46:3001, 2002.
53. Maertens J, Raad I, Petrikkos G, et al. Efficacy and safety of caspofungin for treatment of invasive aspergillosis in patients refractory to or intolerant of conventional antifungal therapy. Clin Infect Dis 39:1563, 2004.
54. Stevens DA, Kan VL, Judson MA, et al. Practice guidelines for diseases caused by Aspergillus. Clin Infect Dis 30:696, 2000.
55. Slavin MA, Szer J, Grigg AP, et al. Guidelines for the use of antifungal agents in the treatment of invasive Candida and mould infections. Intern Med J 34:192, 2004.
56. Steinbach WJ, Stevens DA. Review of newer antifungal and immunomodulatory strategies for invasive aspergillosis. Clin Infect Dis 37(Suppl 3):S157, 2003.
57. Ruhnke M, Bohme A, Buchheidt D, et al. Diagnosis of invasive fungal infections in hematology and oncology–guidelines of the Infectious Diseases Working Party (AGIHO) of the German Society of Hematology and Oncology (DGHO). Ann Hematol 82(Suppl 2):S141, 2003.
58. Benson CA, Kaplan JE, Masur H, et al. Treating opportunistic infections among HIV-exposed and infected children: Recommendations from CDC, the National Institutes of Health, and the Infectious Diseases Society of America. MMWR Recomm Rep 53:1, 2004.
59. Steinbach WJ, Benjamin DK Jr, Kontoyiannis DP, et al. Infections due to Aspergillus terreus: a multicenter retrospective analysis of 83 cases. Clin Infect Dis 39:192, 2004.
60. Donabedian H, O'Donnell E, Olszewski C, et al. Disseminated cutaneous and meningeal sporotrichosis in an AIDS patient. Diagn Microbiol Infect Dis 18:111, 1994.
61. Pappas PG, Pottage JC, Powderly WG, et al. Blastomycosis in patients with the acquired immunodeficiency syndrome. Ann Intern Med 116:847, 1992.
62. Witzig RS, Hoadley DJ, Greer DL, et al. Blastomycosis and human immunodeficiency virus: three new cases and review. South Med J 87:715, 1994.
63. Chapman SW, Bradsher RW, Campbell GD, et al. Practice guidelines for the management of patients with blastomycosis. Clin Infect Dis 30:679, 2000.
64. Tan G, Kaufman L, Peterson EM, de la Maza LM. Disseminated atypical blastomycosis in two patients with AIDS. Clin Infect Dis 16:107, 1993.
65. Liyan X, Changming L, Xianyi Z, et al. Fifteen cases of penicilliosis in Guangdong, China. Mycopathologia 158:151, 2004.
66. Zhao DW, Zhang T, Ma DQ, et al. Disseminated Penicillium marneffei infection in acquired immunodeficiency syndrome: a case report. Chin Med J (Engl) 118:1054, 2005.
67. Vanittanakom N, Cooper CR Jr, Fisher MC, Sirisanthana T. Penicillium marneffei infection and recent advances in the epidemiology and molecular biology aspects. Clin Microbiol Rev 19:95, 2006.
68. Kauffman CA. Old and new therapies for sporotrichosis. Clin Infect Dis 21:981, 1995.
69. Penn CC, Goldstein E, Bartholomew WR. Sporothrix schenckii meningitis in a patients with AIDS. Clin Infect Dis 15:741, 1992.
70. Pappas PG, Tellez I, Deep AE, et al. Sporotrichosis in Peru: Description of an area of hyperendemicity. Clin Infect Dis 30:65, 2000.
71. Brummer E, Castaneda E, Restrepo A. Paracoccidioidomycosis: an update. Clin Microbiol Rev 6:89, 1993.
72. Lim D, Lee YS, Chang AR. Rapid diagnosis of Penicillium marneffei infection by fine needle aspiration cytology. J Clin Pathol 59:443, 2006.
73. Bialek R, Ibricevic A, Fothergill A, Begerow D. Small subunit ribosomal DNA sequence shows Paracoccidioides brasiliensis closely related to Blastomyces dermatitidis. J Clin Microbiol 38:3190, 2000.

74. Tsunemi Y, Takahashi T, Tamaki T. Penicillium marneffei infection diagnosed by polymerase chain reaction from the skin specimen. J Am Acad Dermatol 49:344, 2003.
75. Yuen KY, Wong SS, Tsang DN, Chau PY. Serodiagnosis of Penicillium marneffei infection. Lancet 344:444, 1994.
76. Supparatpinyo K, Nelson KE, Merz WG, et al. Response to antifungal therapy by human immunodeficiency virus-infected patients with disseminated Penicillium marneffei infections and in vitro susceptibilities of isolates from clinical specimens. Antimicrob Agents Chemother 37:2407, 1993.
77. Bolao F, Podzamczer D, Ventin M, Gudiol F. Efficacy of acute phase and maintenance therapy with itraconazole in an AIDS patient with sporotrichosis. Eur J Clin Microbiol Infect Dis 13:609, 1994.
78. Sharkey-Mathis PK, Kauffman CA, Graybill JR, et al. Treatment of sporotrichosis with itraconazole. Am J Med 95:279, 1993.
79. Boogaerts MA, Maertens J, Van der Geest R, et al. Pharmacokinetics and safety of a 7-day administration of intravenous itraconazole followed by a 14-day administration of itraconazole oral solution in patients with hematologic malignancy. Antimicrob Agents Chemother 45:981, 2001.
80. Caillot D. Intravenous itraconazole followed by oral itraconazole for the treatment of amphotericin-B-refractory invasive pulmonary aspergillosis. Acta Haematol 109:111, 2003.
81. Winn RE, Anderson J, Piper J, et al. Systemic sporotrichosis treated with itraconazole. Clin Infect Dis 17:210, 1993.
82. Pappas PG, Bradsher RW, Kauffman CA, et al. Treatment of blastomycosis with higher doses of fluconazole. Clin Infect Dis 25:200, 1997.
83. Lortholary O, Meyohas MC, Dupont B, et al. Invasive aspergillosis in patients with acquired immunodeficiency syndrome: report of 33 cases. French Cooperative Study Group on Aspergillosis in AIDS. Am J Med 95:177, 1993.
84. Mylonakis E, Barlam TF, Flanigan T, Rich JD. Pulmonary aspergillosis and invasive disease in AIDS – Review of 342 cases. Chest 114:251, 1998.
85. Mylonakis E, Mileno MD, Flanigan T, et al. Pulmonary invasive aspergillosis in patients infected with the human immunodeficiency virus: report of two cases. Heart Lung 27:63, 1998.
86. Mylonakis E, Paliou M, Sax PE, et al. Central nervous system aspergillosis in patients with human immunodeficiency virus infection. Report of 6 cases and review. Medicine (Baltimore) 79:269, 2000.
87. Mylonakis E, Rich J, Skolnik PR, et al. Invasive Aspergillus sinusitis in patients with human immunodeficiency virus infection. Report of 2 cases and review. Medicine (Baltimore) 76:249, 1997.
88. Mylonakis E, Rich JD, Flanigan T, et al. Muscle abscess due to Aspergillus fumigatus in a patient with AIDS. Clin Infect Dis 23:1323, 1996.
89. Smith WF, Wallace MR. Cutaneous aspergillosis. Cutis 59:138, 1997.
90. Khoo SH, Denning DW. Invasive aspergillosis in patients with AIDS. Clin Infect Dis 19(Suppl 1):S41, 1994.
91. Warris A, Verweij PE. Clinical implications of environmental sources for Aspergillus. Med Mycol 43:S59, 2005.
92. Minamoto GY, Barlam TF, Vander Els NJ. Invasive aspergillosis in patients with AIDS. Clin Infect Dis 14:66, 1992.
93. Denning DW, Venkateswarlu K, Oakley KL, et al. Itraconazole resistance in Aspergillus fumigatus. Antimicrob Agents Chemother 41:1364, 1997.
94. Steinbach WJ, Perfect JR, Schell WA, et al. In vitro analyses, animal models, and 60 clinical cases of invasive Aspergillus terreus infection. Antimicrob Agents Chemother 48:3217, 2004.
95. Miller WT Jr, Sais GJ, Frank I, et al. Pulmonary aspergillosis in patients with AIDS. Clinical and radiographic correlations. Chest 105:37, 1994.
96. Caillot D, Casasnovas O, Bernard A, et al. Improved management of invasive pulmonary aspergillosis in neutropenic patients using early thoracic computed tomographic scan and surgery. J Clin Oncol 15:139, 1997.
97. Maertens J, Theunissen K, Verbeken E, et al. Prospective clinical evaluation of lower cut-offs for galactomannan detection in adult neutropenic cancer patients and haematological stem cell transplant recipients. Br J Haematol 126:852, 2004.
98. Maertens J, Verhaegen J, Lagrou K, et al. Screening for circulating galactomannan as a noninvasive diagnostic tool for invasive aspergillosis in prolonged neutropenic patients and stem cell transplantation recipients: a prospective validation. Blood 97:1604, 2001.
99. Mennink-Kersten MA, Donnelly JP, Verweij PE. Detection of circulating galactomannan for the diagnosis and management of invasive aspergillosis. Lancet Infect Dis 4:349, 2004.
100. Patterson TF. Advances and challenges in management of invasive mycoses. Lancet 366:1013, 2005.
101. Ostrosky-Zeichner L, Marr KA, Rex JH, Cohen SH. Amphotericin B: time for a new "gold standard". Clin Infect Dis 37:415, 2003.
102. Patterson TF, Kirkpatrick WR, White M, et al. Invasive aspergillosis. Disease spectrum, treatment practices, and outcomes. I^3 Aspergillus Study Group. Medicine (Baltimore) 79:250, 2000.
103. Denning DW, Lee JY, Hostetler JS, et al. NIAID Mycoses Study Group multicenter trial of oral itraconazole therapy for invasive aspergillosis. Am J Med 97:135, 1994.
104. Raad I, Chapman S, Bradsher R, et al. Posaconazole (POS) salvage therapy for invasive fungal infections (IFI) (abstract M-699). In: Abstracts of the 44th Interscience Conference on Antimicrobial Agents and Chemotherapy, Washington, DC, 30 Oct to 2 Nov 2004.
105. Marr KA, Boeckh M, Carter RA, et al. Combination antifungal therapy for invasive aspergillosis. Clin Infect Dis 39:797, 2004.
106. Sambatakou H, Denning DW. Invasive pulmonary aspergillosis transformed into fatal mucous impaction by immune reconstitution in an AIDS patient. Eur J Clin Microbiol Infect Dis 24:628, 2005.
107. Dal Conte I, Riva G, Obert R, et al. Tracheobronchial aspergillosis in a patient with AIDS treated with aerosolized amphotericin B combined with itraconazole. Mycoses 39:371, 1996.
108. Kemper CA, Hostetler JS, Follansbee SE, et al. Ulcerative and plaque-like tracheobronchitis due to infection with Aspergillus in patients with AIDS. Clin Infect Dis 17:344, 1993.
109. Afeltra J, Meis JF, Mouton JW, Verweij PE. Prevention of invasive aspergillosis in AIDS by sulfamethoxazole. Aids 15:1067, 2001.
110. Alvarez S. Systemic infection caused by Penicillium decumbens in a patient with acquired immunodeficiency syndrome. J Infect Dis 162:283, 1990.
111. Barchiesi F, Morbiducci V, Ancarani F, et al. Trichosporon beigelii fungaemia in an AIDS patient. AIDS 7:139, 1993.
112. Eljaschewitsch J, Sandfort J, Tintelnot K, et al. Port-a-cath-related Fusarium oxysporum infection in an HIV-infected patient: treatment with liposomal amphotericin B. Mycoses 39:115, 1996.
113. Glasgow BJ, Engstrom RE Jr, Holland GN, et al. Bilateral endogenous Fusarium endophthalmitis associated with acquired immunodeficiency syndrome. Arch Ophthalmol 114:873, 1996.
114. Leaf HL, Simberkoff MS. Invasive trichosporonosis in a patient with the acquired immunodeficiency syndrome. J Infect Dis 160:356, 1989.
115. Raffanti SP, Fyfe B, Carreiro S, et al. Native valve endocarditis due to Pseudallescheria boydii in a patient with AIDS: case report and review. Rev Infect Dis 12:993, 1990.

116. Lyratzopoulos G, Ellis M, Nerringer R, Denning DW. Invasive infection due to penicillium species other than P. marneffei. J Infect 45:184, 2002.
117. Shankar EM, Kumarasamy N, Rajan R, et al. Aspergillus fumigatus, Pneumocystis jiroveci, Klebsiella pneumoniae & Mycoplasma fermentans co-infection in a HIV infected patient with respiratory conditions from Southern India. Indian J Med Res 123:181, 2006.
118. Meyer RD, Gaultier CR, Yamashita JT, et al. Fungal sinusitis in patients with AIDS: Report of 4 cases and review of the literature. Medicine 73:69, 1994.
119. Munoz P, Marin M, Tornero P, et al. Successful outcome of Scedosporium apiospermum disseminated infection treated with voriconazole in a patient receiving corticosteroid therapy. Clin Infect Dis 31:1499, 2000.
120. Nesky MA, McDougal EC, Peacock JE Jr. Pseudallescheria boydii brain abscess successfully treated with voriconazole and surgical drainage: case report and literature review of central nervous system pseudallescheriasis. Clin Infect Dis 31:673, 2000.
121. Walsh TJ, Lutsar I, Driscoll T, et al. Voriconazole in the treatment of aspergillosis, scedosporiosis and other invasive fungal infections in children. Pediat Inf Dis J 21:240, 2002.
122. Brenner SA, Morgan J, Rickert PD, Rimland D. Cladophialophora bantiana isolated from an AIDS patient with pulmonary infiltrates. J Med Vet Mycol 34:427, 1996.
123. Dhar J, Carey PB. Scopulariopsis brevicaulis skin lesions in an AIDS patient. Aids 7:1283, 1993.
124. Duggan JM, Wolf MD, Kauffman CA. Phialophora verrucosa infection in an AIDS patient. Mycoses 38:215, 1995.
125. Kanj SS, Amr SS, Roberts GD. Ramichloridium mackenziei brain abscess:report of two cases and review of the literature. Med Mycol 39:97, 2001.
126. Mukherji SK, Castillo M. Cerebral phaeohyphomycosis caused by Xylohypha bantiana: MR findings. AJR Am J Roentgenol 164:1304, 1995.
127. Nachman S, Alpan O, Malowitz R, Spitzer ED. Catheter-associated fungemia due to Wangiella (Exophiala) dermatitidis. J Clin Microbiol 34:1011, 1996.
128. Nenoff P, Gutz U, Tintelnot K, et al. Disseminated mycosis due to Scedosporium prolificans in an AIDS patient with Burkitt lymphoma. Mycoses 39:461, 1996.
129. Podnos YD, Anastasio P, De La Maza L, Kim RB. Cerebral phaeohyphomycosis caused by Ramichloridium obovoideum (Ramichloridium mackenziei): case report. Neurosurgery 45:372, 1999.
130. Revankar SG, Patterson JE, Sutton DA, et al. Disseminated phaeohyphomycosis: Review of an emerging mycosis. Clin Infect Dis 34:467, 2002.
131. Shugar MA, Montgomery WW, Hyslop NE Jr Alternaria sinusitis. Ann Otol Rhinol Laryngol 90:251, 1981.
132. Sudduth EJ, Crumbley AJ 3rd, Farrar WE. Phaeohyphomycosis due to Exophiala species: clinical spectrum of disease in humans. Clin Infect Dis 15:639, 1992.
133. Nucci M, Akiti T, Barreiros G, et al. Nosocomial outbreak of Exophiala jeanselmei fungemia associated with contamination of hospital water. Clin Infect Dis 34:1475, 2002.
134. Dixon DM, Polak A. In vitro and in vivo drug studies with three agents of central nervous system phaeohyphomycosis. Chemotherapy 33:129, 1987.
135. Al-Abdely HM, Najvar LK, Bocanegra R, Graybill JR. Antifungal therapy of experimental cerebral phaeohyphomycosis due to Cladophialophora bantiana. Antimicrob Agents Chemother 49:1701, 2005.
136. Espinel-Ingroff A. In vitro fungicidal activities of voriconazole, itraconazole, and amphotericin B against opportunistic moniliaceous and dematiaceous fungi. J Clin Microbiol 39:954, 2001.
137. Sharkey PK, Graybill JR, Rinaldi MG, et al. Itraconazole treatment of phaeohyphomycosis. J Am Acad Dermatol 23:577, 1990.
138. Al-Abdely HM, Alkhunaizi AM, Al-Tawfiq JA, et al. Successful therapy of cerebral phaeohyphomycosis due to Ramichloridium mackenziei with the new triazole posaconazole. Med Mycol 43:91, 2005.
139. Revankar SG, Sutton DA, Rinaldi MG. Primary central nervous system phaeohyphomycosis: a review of 101 cases. Clin Infect Dis 38:206, 2004.
140. Del Poeta M, Schell WA, Perfect JR. In vitro antifungal activity of pneumocandin L-743,872 against a variety of clinically important molds. Antimicrob Agents Chemother 41:1835, 1997.
141. Trinh JV, Steinbach WJ, Schell WA, et al. Cerebral phaeohyphomycosis in an immunodeficient child treated medically with combination antifungal therapy. Med Mycol 41:339, 2003.
142. Kontoyiannis DP, Lionakis MS, Lewis RE, et al. Zygomycosis in a tertiary-care cancer center in the era of Aspergillus-active antifungal therapy: a case-control observational study of 27 recent cases. J Infect Dis 191:1350, 2005.
143. Kontoyiannis DP, Wessel VC, Bodey GP, Rolston KVI. Zygomycosis in the 1990s in a tertiary-care cancer center. Clin Infect Dis 30:851, 2000.
144. Sanchez MR, Ponge-Wilson I, Moy JA, Rosenthal S. Zygomycosis and HIV infection. J. Am. Acad. Dermatol. 30:904, 1994.
145. Levy E, Bia MJ. Isolated renal mucormycosis: case report and review. J Am Soc Nephrol 5:2014, 1995.
146. Micozzi MS, Wetli CV. Intravenous amphetamine abuse, primary cerebral mucormycosis, and acquired immunodeficiency. J Forensic Sci 30:504, 1985.
147. Nagy-Agren SE, Chu P, Smith GJ, et al. Zygomycosis (mucormycosis) and HIV infection: report of three cases and review. J Acquir Immune Defic Syndr Hum Retrovirol 10:441, 1995.
148. Kauffman CA. Zygomycosis: reemergence of an old pathogen. Clin Infect Dis 39:588, 2004.
149. Perfect JR. Treatment of non-Aspergillus moulds in immunocompromised patients, with amphotericin B lipid complex. Clin Infect Dis 40 Suppl 6:S401, 2005.
150. Yao M, Messner AH. Fungal malignant otitis externa due to Scedosporium apiospermum. Ann Otol Rhinol Laryngol 110:377, 2001.
151. Sirisanthana T. Penicillium marneffei infection in patients with AIDS. Emerg Infect Dis 7:561, 2001.

Chapter 48

Herpes Simplex Virus Infections

Kimberly Y. Smith, MD, MPH, Harold A. Kessler, MD

PATHOGEN

Herpes simplex virus type 1 (HSV-1) and type 2 (HSV-2) are common pathogens in human immunodeficiency virus (HIV)-infected patients. Seroprevalence surveys of adults in the United States indicate that 50–70% of individuals are infected with HSV-1 and 15–33% with HSV-2.[1–3] HSV-2 is one of the most prevalent sexually transmitted viruses in the world. It is estimated that 50 million individuals have genital HSV infection. Genital HSV is more common in women (one in four American women) than in men (one in five American men).[4] An even higher prevalence of HSV-2, in some cases as high as 75%, has been estimated in some developing countries.[5] HSV-2 is an important public health issue worldwide due to its increasing prevalence and the fact that it has been shown to be an important cofactor in HIV transmission.[6] One study of discordant couples in Uganda showed that HSV-2-infected, HIV-negative partners had a fivefold increased risk of acquiring HIV per sexual contact, compared with HSV-2-negative partners.[7]

There are increased seroprevalence rates for both HSV-1 and HSV-2 in HIV-infected persons.[8] A European study of HIV-infected women found antibodies to HSV-1 and HSV-2 in 76% and 42%, respectively.[9] Eighty percent of HIV-infected South-African teenagers are estimated to be HSV-2 seropositive.[10] Similarly ~80% of HIV+ men who have sex with men (MSM) in the US are estimated to have genital HSV infection.[11]

In the era prior to the widespread use of highly active antiretroviral therapy (HAART) 4.4% of acquired immunodeficiency syndrome (AIDS)-defining illnesses in HIV-infected patients were due to severe HSV-1 or HSV-2 infection.[12] Several studies have shown that there is an increased incidence of HSV-related genital ulcer disease in HIV-infected women compared to HIV-infected men.[12–15] It has been noted that the overall incidence of clinically evident HSV infection in HIV-infected patients has declined, associated with the increased use of HAART.[16] Nonetheless, HSV disease continues to cause significant morbidity in HIV-infected individuals. Recent studies have demonstrated that HSV outbreaks may be associated with increased HIV replication as measured by plasma HIV RNA however these increases may be muted in patients who are on HAART. Some investigators suggest that treatment of HSV in persons co-infected with HSV and HIV could lead to delayed HIV disease progression and decreased HIV transmission particularly in settings where HAART availability is limited.[17,18] Clinical trials to evaluate this hypothesis are ongoing.

Herpes simplex virus has a double-stranded DNA enclosed in an icosahedral capsid that is surrounded by a lipid envelope. The most characteristic biologic property of these viruses is the ability to induce latency and periodically reactivate infection.[19,20] The incubation period is 2–12 days. Spread is person to person via contact with infected body secretions. Primary infection occurs following initial introduction of the virus through the skin or mucous membranes. Following local replication, the virus travels along the sensory nerves and establishes latency in the dorsal nerve root ganglia. Reactivation disease occurs when the virus travels back along the sensory nerves and replicates in the mucocutaneous region that was initially infected. Although reactivation disease is generally of shorter duration and consists of milder symptoms than primary infection, it should be noted that both primary and reactivation infections are often clinically asymptomatic.[19,20]

The most common clinical manifestation of HSV is the development of vesicular and ulcerative lesions in the orolabial and/or genital regions. HSV-1 is associated with ~70% of orolabial infections and HSV-2 with ~70% of genital infections. Symptoms are more severe and prolonged in HIV-infected patients with advanced disease than in immunocompetent patients.[19–23] Symptoms begin with painful, erythematous papules that quickly become vesicles and soon ulcerate. These ulcerations then crust and heal. In the untreated healthy host, the time course from the development of papules to healing is ~14–28 days for primary disease. The course of reactivation disease is considerably shorter. Painful, tender regional lymphadenopathy often accompanies these lesions, particularly in patients with primary infection.[10,11]

In HIV-infected patients, most morbidity is associated with HSV infections in the genital and perirectal region.[21–23] While some "initial outbreaks" represent the first symptomatic episode of recurrent disease in previously asymptomatic individuals, the first clinical presentation of HSV may be an indicator of unsafe sexual practices thus should warrant safer sex counseling. Most serious infections occur in patients with less than 200 CD4 cells/mm^3. Untreated, the time course of HSV is often prolonged. Ulcerative lesions are often present for more than 1–3 months. In patients with advanced HIV infection, recurrences become more frequent, severe, and prolonged if left untreated. Multiple ulcerations can become confluent and involve extensive areas of the perineum. Heaped-up verrucous lesions caused by HSV-2, resembling condyloma acuminata, have been reported.[24] Asymptomatic shedding of HSV-2 is more frequent and more prolonged in both HIV-infected men and women compared to HIV-uninfected patients.[25,26] Risk factors for increased HSV-2 shedding among HIV-infected men were low CD4 cell count and serum antibodies to both HSV-1 and HSV-2 compared to HSV-2 alone.[26] Notably asymptomatic shedding of HSV virus is still frequent in HIV-infected individuals who are treated with HAART despite the fact that clinical HSV outbreaks are less frequent.[27]

Proctitis caused by HSV is the most common cause of nongonococcal proctitis in MSM. It has been described primarily in HIV-infected male patients.[28–30] They usually present with fever, pruritus, rectal pain, and tenesmus. A rectal discharge or hematochezia may be present. Additionally, difficulty urinating, impotence, and the presence of sacral paresthesia may be present. External lesions and inguinal lymphadenopathy frequently accompany this syndrome. Sigmoidoscopy shows large ulcerations. Concomitant infection with *Neisseria gonorrhoeae* has also been noted.[28–30]

As with genital and perirectal disease, orolabial HSV infections are more severe and prolonged in HIV-infected patients.[23,31] Lesions can occur on any mucosal surface, most commonly the lips, palate, or gingiva. Most cases are reactivated disease and most commonly consist of one or two ulcerations. Co-infection with other pathogens such as cytomegalovirus (CMV) or *Histoplasma* has been reported.[32]

Mucocutaneous forms of HSV infection located in other parts of the body, such as herpetic whitlow or paronychia, have been reported in association with HIV infection.[33–35] As is the case for disease in the genital and orolabial regions, cutaneous disease can be more severe and prolonged than that seen in the immunocompetent host.

After mucocutaneous disease, the next most common clinical manifestation of HSV infection in HIV-infected patients is HSV esophagitis.[36–39] This AIDS-defining complication is seen usually in patients with less than 50 CD4 cells/mm^3. The symptoms are clinically indistinguishable from esophagitis caused by *Candida* species. Odynophagia or burning retrosternal pain is common. Orolabial ulcerations are present in 38–80% of patients with HSV esophagitis.[36–38] Endoscopically, most herpetic lesions are seen in the distal third of the esophagus.[36] Rare complications include esophageal strictures and perforation.[39,40]

Visceral or disseminated HSV infection in HIV-infected patients is uncommon. Case reports of hepatitis, pneumonia, or encephalitis have been noted. Most cases of HSV encephalitis are caused by HSV-1 and can be difficult to distinguish clinically from other causes of encephalitis such as CMV infection and toxoplasmosis particularly in patients with advanced HIV disease.[41] In immunocompetent patients, herpes simplex encephalitis usually occurs in the temporal lobe, whereas, in HIV-infected patients encephalitis has involved diverse areas of the brain outside the limbic system as well as the brain stem.[41] Myelitis caused by HSV has also been reported.[41]

DIAGNOSIS

Mucocutaneous vesicular ulcerative disease in patients with HIV infection can have multiple causes, including disseminated CMV, varicella-zoster virus (VZV), or disseminated cryptococcal infection; histoplasmosis; squamous cell carcinoma; or pustular dermatosis. Therefore it is important to establish a firm microbiologic diagnosis, particularly if a typical-appearing lesion does not respond to acyclovir (Fig. 48-1). The laboratory diagnosis of HSV includes culture, cytopathologic techniques, HSV antigen detection by immunologic methods, nucleic acid detection by polymerase chain reaction (PCR), and serology. Traditionally, a viral culture has been the cornerstone of the laboratory diagnosis of HSV. Specimens are most likely to yield virus if they are taken from vesicles within the first 1–2 days after formation.[19,42] Specimens for culture should be obtained from an unroofed vesicle or the base of an ulcer using a dacron tipped catheter. Contamination with stool, urine or blood should be avoided as these may lead to falsely negative results. Following inoculation into tissue culture, a cytopathic effect with ballooning degeneration and multinucleated giant cells occurs within 1–2 days. Typing for HSV-1 or HSV-2 can be done using type-specific monoclonal antibodies, although this is not important for therapy.[19,20,42] Viral isolation is especially important if acyclovir resistance is suspected because viral susceptibility testing can be performed.[43]

Cytopathologic examination of scrapings of ulcerations can be quickly performed. The Tzanck smear shows typical multinucleated giant cells characteristic of herpesvirus infection but does not differentiate HSV from VZV.[19,20,42] Additionally, it is not as sensitive as a culture, with a positivity rate of ~40–50%.

Direct identification of HSV antigens (by immunofluorescence or immunoperoxidase techniques) on the surface of cells obtained from a suspicious lesion is a newer diagnostic method suitable for the rapid diagnosis of HSV infection in

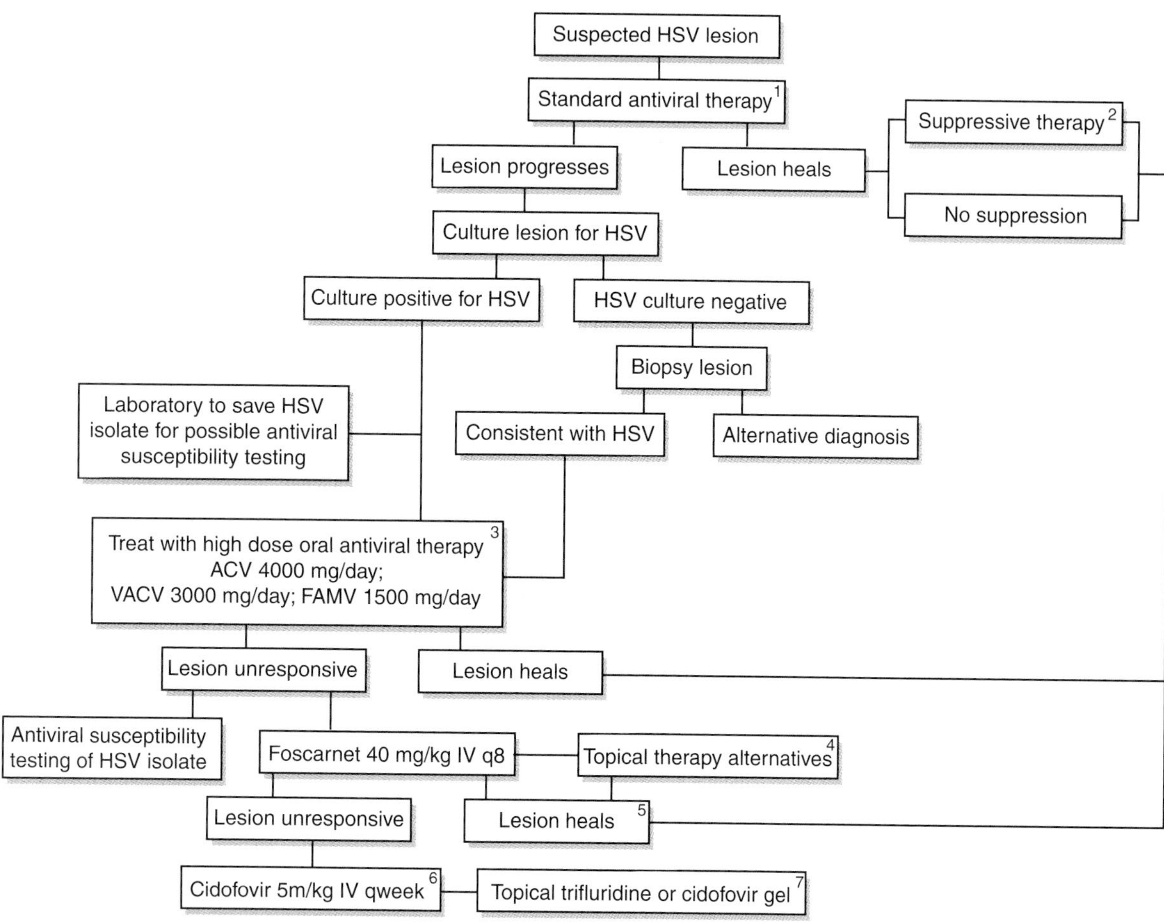

Figure 48-1 ■ Algorithm for the management of herpes simplex disease in patients with HIV infection. (1) See text for discussion of currently recommended therapies. (2) See text for discussion of management of recurrent HSV disease. (3) See text for discussion of the management of acyclovir-unresponsive HSV disease (ACV, acyclovir; FAMV, famciclovir; VACV, valacyclovir). (4) See text for discussion of trifluridine ophthalmic solution, foscarnet cream, and cidofovir gel. (5) See text for discussion of the long-term management of acyclovir-resistant HSV disease. (6) Parenteral cidofovir not currently approved for the treatment of acyclovir-resistant HSV disease; dose based on therapy for CMV infection. (7) Cidofovir gel; Food and Drug Administration approval not being pursued by the manufacturer (Gilead Sciences).

clinic settings. These tests are available via commercial labs and tend to be less expensive than viral culture or PCR. The sensitivity and specificity of these assays varies from 80% to 98% and 96% to 99% respectively.[4,44]

Sensitive type-specific serologic tests have been developed,[45] but detecting antibodies to HSV-1 or HSV-2 has no role in the diagnosis of active vesicular ulcerative disease. It does provide specific information as to whether the patient has been previously infected with the virus.

Multiple methods for *in vitro* antiviral susceptibility testing of HSV have been described including a quantitative real-time PCR (TaqMan) assay and a colorimetric yield reduction assay, ELVIRA (enzyme-linked virus inhibitor reporter assay).[43,46–48] While routine use of susceptibility testing is not indicated for the management of uncomplicated episodes of HSV disease, the availability of rapid tests may be helpful for management of episodes that appear to be unresponsive to acyclovir therapy (Fig. 48-1).

TREATMENT

Mucocutaneous Disease

Initial therapy for mucocutaneous HSV infections in HIV-infected patients is similar to that for patients who are not immunocompromised. Therapy is divided into that for primary infection and that for recurrent infection. Recurrent disease is treated either in an episodic fashion or as continuous suppressive therapy. Treatment leads to amelioration of the signs and symptoms of HSV disease and decreases the time to healing and shedding of the virus; however, individuals often remain infectious despite treatment and resolution of symptoms.

The treatment for primary infection is oral or intravenous acyclovir (Table 48-1). Therapy is given for a 7–10 day course or until the lesions have become crusted over. It has been suggested that HSV proctitis may require higher

Table 48-1 Treatment for Herpes Simplex Virus Disease in Patients with HIV Infection

Drug	Dose: Initial Disease	Dose: Recurrent Disease	Toxicity	Interactions
Acyclovir	5 mg/kg IV q8 h × 7–10 days[a] or 200–400 mg PO 5 × /day × 10–14 days	200–400 mg PO 5 ×/day × 5–10 days[b]	Phlebitis with IV formulation Reversible nephrotoxicity (rare with these doses of drug) Neurotoxicity (rare with these doses of drug in the absence of decreased renal function)	If given with nephrotoxic drugs reduce dose with decreasing CrCl Cimetidine and probenecid increase acyclovir levels
Valacyclovir	1000 mg PO bid × 7–10 days[c]	500 mg PO bid × 5–10 days	Same as for oral acyclovir Thrombotic microangiopathy (rare)[d]	Same as for acyclovir
Famciclovir	500 mg PO bid × 7–10 days[e]	500 mg PO bid × 5–10 days	No serious adverse events	If given with nephrotoxic drugs reduce dose with decreasing CrCl

CrCl, creatinine clearance.

[a] Decision on intravenous versus oral therapy based on clinical severity; switch to oral therapy as soon as a good clinical response is achieved.

[b] Intravenous therapy may initially be necessary for patients with severe oral or esophageal disease.

[c] Limited clinical data in HIV-infected patients; not approved for immunocompromised hosts.

[d] Reported in small number of patients with advanced HIV disease on prolonged high dose (8 g/day) therapy for CMV retinitis prophylaxis.

[e] Limited clinical data; not approved for treatment of initial disease.

and/or more prolonged dosing but comparative studies are not available. Alternative agents are famciclovir or valacyclovir. In patients with severe disease or who are unable to tolerate or absorb oral medications, intravenous acyclovir (5 mg/kg every 8 h) should be used. The treatment course is 7–10 days or until the lesions have crusted over. Patients can be switched to oral acyclovir to complete the course of therapy when they are clinically improved and able to tolerate oral medications.[49–52]

Recurrent disease treatment is individualized to the patient's needs. Episodic therapy is usually patient-initiated. The treatment of choice in this instance is also acyclovir. Alternate agents include famciclovir 500 mg PO twice daily or valacyclovir 500 mg PO twice daily.[50,53,54] A comparative study in HIV-infected patients with mucocutaneous HSV infection of famciclovir (500 mg PO twice daily) and acyclovir (400 mg PO five times a day) showed that there was no difference between these agents in decreasing the time to complete healing and reducing new lesion formation.[55] It should be noted that the dosage of famciclovir that was used in this trial was higher than the dosage used to treat HIV-uninfected patients, which is 125 mg PO twice daily. Studies in HIV-infected patients treated with this lower dosage have not been reported; and whether this lower dose would be equally efficacious in HIV-infected patients, particularly those with less immunosuppression, is unclear. In general, recurrent infection is treated for 5–10 days. In patients with advanced HIV infection, improvement may take up to 14 days.

Continuous suppressive therapy should be considered for patients who have frequent symptomatic recurrent infections (Table 48-2). Frequent recurrences are usually defined as three or more outbreaks during a 6-month period. Acyclovir given at a dose of 400–800 mg PO two or three times daily is the treatment of choice for suppressive therapy.[4] Alternative agents include famciclovir 250 mg PO twice daily and valacyclovir 500 mg PO twice daily or 1000 mg PO once daily.[4,56] Suppressive therapy with valacyclovir compared to placebo was associated with a 2.5-fold reduction in recurrent HSV genital HSV episodes in a study in 293 HIV-infected subjects. Valacyclovir was well tolerated with adverse event rates similar to placebo.[57] Optimization of HAART may decrease the need of continuous suppressive therapy and should form an important component of this therapeutic strategy.

Although there has not been an increase in acyclovir resistance in immunocompetent patients treated with prolonged courses of acyclovir (>6 years of therapy), there have been increasing reports of acyclovir resistance in patients with advanced HIV infection.[43,58,59] A study of patients 18 years or older with suspected genital HSV who attended 22 sexually transmitted disease (STD) and HIV clinics in the US between October 1996 and April 1998 revealed acyclovir resistant virus in 0.18% (three of 1644) HIV-negative patients

Table 48-2

Chronic Suppressive Treatment for Recurrent Herpes Simplex Virus Disease in Patients with HIV Infection

Drug	Dose	Toxicity	Interactions
Acyclovir	200 mg PO bid or 400 mg PO bid	Reversible nephrotoxicity (rare with these doses) Neurotoxicity (rare with these does in the absence of decreased renal function)	If given with nephrotoxic drugs, reduce dose with decreasing CrCl. Cimetidine and probenecid increase acyclovir levels
Valacyclovir	500 mg PO bid[a]	Same as for oral acyclovir. Thrombotic microangiopathy (rare)[b]	Same as for acyclovir
Famciclovir	250 mg PO bid[c]	No serious adverse events	If given with nephrotoxic drugs, reduce dose with decreasing CrCl

CrCl, creatine clearance.

[a] Valacyclovir 500 mg bid superior to valacyclovir 1000 mg qd.[93]

[b] Reported in small number of patients with advanced HIV disease on prolonged high dose (8 g/day) therapy for CMV retinitis prophylaxis.

[c] Limited clinical data; not approved for immunocompromised hosts.

and 5.3% (12 of 226) HIV-positive patients. Risk factors for HSV resistance included the use of oral and topical acyclovir, the duration of the current episode, a history of recurrent genital herpes, and a low CD4 cell count.[60] Treatment of HIV-infected patients with recurrent HSV disease with episodic therapy rather than continuous suppression has been advocated as a way to decrease exposure to acyclovir. Whether this reduces the likelihood of acyclovir-resistant disease has not been established.

Acyclovir-Unresponsive Disease

Although the overall incidence of acyclovir resistance remains low, there have been reports of HIV-infected patients with severe debilitating chronic mucocutaneous disease caused by acyclovir-resistant HSV.[33,43,61,62] Additionally, patients with esophagitis and visceral disease caused by acyclovir-resistant HSV have been described.[43,63,64] Typically, these patients have advanced HIV disease with less than 50 CD4 cells/mm^3. The patients with mucocutaneous disease have large, progressive, deeply ulcerated lesions that frequently develop satellite lesions. Symptoms can be present for months. Additionally, viral shedding is prolonged.[43,61,62]

Acyclovir resistance should be suspected in HIV-infected patients with mucocutaneous HSV infections that do not respond to acyclovir therapy within 14 days (Fig. 48-1). At this time, repeat cultures should be performed and the HSV isolate should be saved for antiviral susceptibility testing. Not all patients with HSV infection unresponsive to oral acyclovir have acyclovir resistance. Therefore patients should first be treated with higher doses of acyclovir (800 mg PO every 4 h five times per day). Alternatively, famciclovir or valacyclovir, which have enhanced oral bioavailability, may be tried (Fig. 48-1; Table 48-1). Continuous-infusion acyclovir (1.5–2.0 mg kg^{-1} h^{-1}) has also been reported to be beneficial for treatment of acyclovir-resistant HSV.[65,66] If these regimens fail, antiviral susceptibility testing can be performed and alternative therapy considered. Treatment of acyclovir-resistant HSV is with foscarnet[43,50,60,67–70] given intravenously at a dose of 40 mg/kg three times daily (Table 48-3). Treatment is continued until the lesions have crusted over and reepithelialized, which usually takes at least 2–3 weeks. It is interesting that following resolution of lesions caused by acyclovir-resistant HSV, recurrent infections often are caused by HSV isolates sensitive to acyclovir. This indicates that latent infection may be maintained by a virus population different from that found in the acute, cutaneous lesions.[68]

Intravenous cidofovir has been used to treat a small number of patients with acyclovir-resistant HSV disease.[71–73] Most of these patients were bone marrow transplant patients, and roughly half of the patients had foscarnet-resistant isolates in addition to acyclovir resistance. Although there was evidence of response, toxicities from cidofovir and concomitant probenecid were problematic.[71–74] A recent report of development of cidofovir-resistant HSV in three subjects receiving cidofovir for treatment of acyclovir-resistant HSV adds to the concern over use of this agent.[75] Further studies are needed to define the role of intravenous cidofovir in the treatment of HIV-infected patients with acyclovir-resistant HSV disease, and its use should be reserved for patients with disease unresponsive to acyclovir and foscarnet.

Acyclovir-resistant HSV mucocutaneous disease has also been successfully treated topically. Antiviral agents that have been used in this fashion include trifluridine, cidofovir, and foscarnet.[76–82]

Trifluridine ophthalmic solution is applied to the HSV lesions in a thin layer and covered with a nonabsorbable gauze to which polymyxin B/bacitracin ointment has been applied. Lesions are cleansed with hydrogen peroxide and gentle gauze débridement between applications. This treatment is given

Table 48-3 Treatment for Acyclovir-Resistant HSV Disease in Patients with HIV Infection

Drug	Dose	Toxicity	Interactions
Foscarnet	40 mg/kg IV q8h × 10–14 days; may require longer duration depending on rate of reepithelialization	Nephrotoxicity, electrolyte disturbances (particularly related to calcium), nausea/irritability, genital ulceration	Increased risk of nephrotoxicity if administered with other nephrotoxic drugs
Cidofovir[a]	5 mg/kg IV qweek × 2–4 weeks; may require longer duration depending on rate of reepithelialization	Nephrotoxicity (must be co-administered with probenecid); neutropenia, uveitis, alopecia, hypotony; probenecid toxic effects including rash, fever, nausea, fatigue	Increased risk of nephrotoxicity if administered with other nephrotoxic drugs; probenecid will increase levels of most drugs excreted by proximal tubules[b]
Topical Therapy			
Trifluridine	Ophthalmic solution applied to lesion tid until healed[c]	Minor local irritation including itching and stinging (uncommon)	None
Foscarnet cream 1%[d]	Apply to lesion 5 ×/day until healed	Skin ulceration, local irritation, fever	None
Cidofovir gel 1%[e]	Apply to lesion qday × 5 days; may be repeated 10 days after first application completed	Minor local irritation including pain, burning, pruritus	None

[a] Not currently approved for this indication.
[b] Zidovudine dose should be reduced by 50% of withheld on the day of infusion only. Rifampin, ketoprofen, chlorpropamide, dapsone, methotrexate, trimethoprim–sulfamethoxasole, zalcitabine and NSAIDS should be on the day of dosing only.
[c] After gentle gauze debridement of the lesion with hydrogen peroxide, a thin layer of trifluridine is applied to the lesion with overlapping of the edges, and a sterile teflon gauze covering with polymyxin-bacitracin ointment applied is used to cover the lesion. Not currently approved for this indication.
[d] Available through a compassionate-use program from the manufacturer through 1997 (Astra Pharmaceutical Products, Inc).
[e] FDA approval not being pursued by manufacturer (Gilead Sciences).

every 8 h until the lesions have reepithelialized. In a pilot study, ~30% of the patients had complete healing in a median time of 7 weeks, and 30% of the patients failed therapy. There was essentially no toxicity. However, application of the solution is unwieldy.[77]

Compared to a placebo, topical gel cidofovir at 0.3–1.0% applied once daily for 5 days was associated with decreased pain and viral shedding, and it accelerated healing of lesions. Thirty percent of the patients had complete healing within a median time of 21 days. Site reactions to the topical gel cidofovir (consisting of pain, burning, or pruritus) occurred in 23% of the patients and were not considered serious. Little systemic absorption of cidofovir occurred and then only in patients with the largest lesions.[80,81]

A pilot study using 1% foscarnet cream for treatment of acyclovir-resistant HSV in HIV-infected patients has been reported.[82] Patients were treated five times daily for ~1 month. Of these 20 patients, eight showed complete healing. There also was a decline in viral shedding and pain. Four patients developed application site reactions. Plasma foscarnet levels were not detected.[82]

In summary, treatment of acyclovir-resistant HSV disease should be individualized. Patients with extensive disease must be treated with intravenous foscarnet. The role of intravenous cidofovir is presently unknown. Patients with more limited disease may be treated with topical agents. Clearly, more experience must be gained regarding topical therapy. Additionally, improvement of the underlying immunodeficiency with potent HAART regimens may also improve the outcome of therapy in these patients.

In addition to acyclovir-resistant herpes simplex, isolates of HSV with foscarnet resistance have been described in HIV-infected patients.[80,83] Similarly to patients with acyclovir-resistant HSV, these patients also have advanced HIV disease, and they have had extensive exposure to foscarnet. The mechanism is a mutation in the DNA polymerase gene.[80] These isolates may be sensitive to acyclovir, which can be used as therapy.[80] It is of note that isolates with both foscarnet and acyclovir resistance have also been described. Treatment with cidofovir may be effective in this situation.[72,80]

Treatment of Esophagitis, Proctitis or Visceral Disease

The treatment of HSV esophagitis or proctitis is intravenous acyclovir (5 mg/kg every 8 h), oral acyclovir (400 mg every 4 h five times daily), or oral valacyclovir (500 mg every 12 h) for a 10- to 14-day course.[28,29,35,37,49,50] Concurrent use of potent HAART regimens has been associated with a reduction in recurrent symptoms and improved survival in patients with HIV-associated HSV esophagitis.[68] Visceral or central nervous system (CNS) disease is generally treated with intravenous acyclovir (10 mg/kg every 8 h) for 14–21 days.[39–41]

PHARMACOLOGY OF ANTIVIRAL AGENTS USED TO TREAT HSV

Acyclovir

Acyclovir is an acyclic nucleoside analog of guanosine with potent antiviral activity against HSV-1 and HSV-2. The drug is monophosphorylated by a herpesvirus-specific thymidine kinase (TK) to acyclovir monophosphate. Host cellular kinases then convert acyclovir monophosphate to acyclovir triphosphate, which inhibits viral DNA polymerase and incorporates into viral DNA, resulting in chain termination of the growing DNA chain.[49,50] Acyclovir resistance can occur through one of three mechanisms: (1) TK deficiency, (2) altered acyclovir affinity for TK, or (3) altered acyclovir affinity for DNA polymerase. Most (>90%) resistant isolates are characterized by TK deficiency.[43]

Acyclovir may be administered intravenously, orally, and topically. It is widely distributed in the body but only penetrates the cerebrospinal fluid at ~50% of the plasma level. Acyclovir has a half-life of ~2.5 h and is excreted through the kidneys. Dosage adjustment is needed for patients with renal failure. Acyclovir has an oral bioavailability of ~10–27% and may decrease with increasing dose. Topically applied acyclovir has no systemic absorption and has limited clinical utility.[49,51,85]

Acyclovir is an extremely well tolerated drug.[86] Phlebitis and pain occasionally follow intravenous infusion. High doses of acyclovir (30 mg kg^{-1} day^{-1}) may lead to reversible renal failure as a result of crystallization of the drug in renal tubules. Patients must be well hydrated when high doses of intravenous acyclovir are administered, and the drug should be infused over at least 1 h. Neurologic symptoms consisting of mental status changes and seizures have been reported to occur rarely and are associated with elevated acyclovir levels.[87] These symptoms resolve with discontinuation of acyclovir. Oral acyclovir has been associated with gastrointestinal disturbances, including nausea and vomiting. An erythematous maculopapular rash has uncommonly been reported to occur. A short-lived stinging or burning sensation is the only toxicity related to the topical administration of acyclovir.[49,51,85,86]

Valacyclovir

Valacyclovir is the L-valyl ester prodrug of acyclovir. Following oral administration, valacyclovir is converted to acyclovir and L-valine in the intestine and liver. The bioavailability of acyclovir following oral ingestion of a 1000 mg dose of valacyclovir is ~50%. The conversion of valacyclovir to acyclovir is more than 99%. Once converted to acyclovir, its pharmacology is that of acyclovir.[88,89]

The toxicity of valacyclovir is of special note in HIV-infected patients. A thrombotic microangiopathy syndrome similar to thrombotic thrombocytopenic purpura/hemolytic-uremic syndrome has been reported to occur in HIV-infected patients with advanced disease treated with valacyclovir at higher dosages (8 g/day) than those used for the treatment of HSV infection[90]; this information is still included as a warning in the current package insert.[90] However, there was a case report of the association of this syndrome in a patient with advanced HIV infection (CD4 count 98 cells/mm^3) who had been receiving valacyclovir at a dose of 500 mg PO twice daily for suppressive HSV therapy for 1 year.[91] Subsequent reviews have shown this syndrome to be rare in patients receiving valacyclovir for recurrent HSV. No cases of thrombotic microangiopathy were seen among the 3050 subjects in the four trials (one in HIV-infected subjects) evaluating valacyclovir for suppression of recurrent genital herpes. Patients in these studies were not severely immunocompromised.[92] Thus it seems prudent to avoid the use of valacyclovir in doses exceeding 3000 mg/day for more than a 7- to 14-day course in patients with advanced HIV disease (CD4+ T-lymphocyte counts <100 cells/mm^3). Other toxicities involving the gastrointestinal system, CNS, and kidneys are the same as those seen with acyclovir.[89,90,92]

At the present time, valacyclovir is indicated for episodic treatment of reactivated HSV infection and suppressive treatment of frequent reactivation HSV infection. The usual dose for treatment of episodic disease is 500 mg PO every 12 h in patients with normal renal function. A clinical trial comparing valacyclovir 1000 mg daily and 500 mg twice daily for suppressive therapy demonstrated that valacyclovir 500 mg twice daily was superior to valacyclovir 1000 mg daily.[93] In patients with a creatinine clearance of less than 30 mL/min, the dose should be reduced to 500 mg PO every 24 h.[90] For suppressive therapy the usual dose is 500 or 1000 mg PO once daily.[89,92]

Famciclovir

Famciclovir is the prodrug of penciclovir, an antiviral agent with excellent *in vitro* activity against HSV-1 and HSV-2. Following oral ingestion of famciclovir, the drug is metabolized by deacetylation and oxidation to penciclovir by the intestine and liver. Similarly to acyclovir, penciclovir is initially monophosphorylated by the HSV TK and then triphosphorylated by a host cellular kinase. Penciclovir triphosphate inhibits HSV DNA polymerase. Viral resistance is similar to that of acyclovir. Famciclovir is not effective in the treatment of TK-deficient mutants.[94–96]

Famciclovir is administered only orally and has penciclovir bioavailability of ~77% following a 500 mg dose (of famciclovir). Famciclovir is eliminated by the kidneys. Dose modifications must be made in patients with renal failure.[95,96] Famciclovir is well tolerated. The most common adverse events associated with it are headaches and gastrointestinal symptoms, primarily nausea and diarrhea.[96]

At the present time, famciclovir is approved for episodic treatment of reactivation HSV disease and suppressive therapy of frequent reactivation HSV disease. The usual dosage for episodic therapy is 500 mg PO twice daily for HIV-infected patients, and for suppressive therapy the usual dose is 250 mg PO twice daily. In patients with a creatinine clearance of 20–40 mL/min famciclovir should be given as 125 mg PO every 24 h, and in patients with a creatinine clearance of less than 20 mL/min the dose should be 125 mg PO every 48 h.[95,96]

Foscarnet

Foscarnet is a pyrophosphate analog that interferes with pyrophosphate binding sites on DNA polymerase. Unlike acyclovir and penciclovir, foscarnet does not require phosphorylation for its antiviral activity.[51,97] Viral isolates resistant to acyclovir and penciclovir are sensitive to and have been successfully treated with foscarnet.[98] Fortunately, resistance to acyclovir is uncommon. Recently, a surveillance network examined 3900 HSV strains isolated from 3357 patients and found the prevalence of acyclovir-resistant HSV in HIV-infected patients to be 4.2%. Notably five of 11 (38%) patients with acyclovir-resistant HSV were treated with foscarnet. Of those, two developed foscarnet resistance.[99] Foscarnet resistance caused by altered DNA polymerase has been described in HIV-infected patients. In some cases these patients can be treated successfully with acyclovir.[83] In cases of resistance to both foscarnet and acyclovir, cidofovir has been used successfully.[100]

Foscarnet is available only as an intravenous formulation; a topical cream formulation is investigational.[80] The drug penetrates the CNS. It is not metabolized and is excreted by the kidneys. Dosage adjustments are necessary for patients with decreased creatinine clearance. The normal dosage of foscarnet for treatment of HSV disease is 40 mg/kg every 8 h.[51,97,101]

The most serious toxicity associated with foscarnet is nephrotoxicity, which occurs to some degree in virtually all patients treated with foscarnet. Renal failure is generally reversible following discontinuation of foscarnet. Foscarnet chelates divalent metal ions and so may be associated with hypocalcemia, hypophosphatemia, and hypomagnesemia. CNS toxicity (consisting mainly of seizures) has been associated with elevated levels of foscarnet. Elevated liver enzymes, anemia, leukopenia, and thrombocytopenia have been associated with foscarnet usage.[97,101]

Cidofovir

Cidofovir is a monophosphate nucleotide analog of cytosine that undergoes intracellular phosphorylation to its diphosphate form by cellular kinases and blocks HSV DNA polymerase.[102] Cidofovir is active against acyclovir-resistant HSV.[103] An *in vitro* HSV-2 isolate with diminished susceptibility for cidofovir as the result of a mutation in the HSV DNA polymerase was described in 1997.[104] Recently, the first report of cidofovir resistance developing *in vivo* was published. This isolate contained multiple mutations in the DNA polymerase that had not previously been reported during *in vitro* resistance selection.[75]

Currently, cidofovir is available only as an intravenous formulation. A topical gel formulation was studied in HIV-infected patients with acyclovir-unresponsive mucocutateous HSV and was shown to accelerate healing and reduce viral shedding, however this formulation did not receive FDA approval and thus is not available commercially.[81] Other studies of cidofovir gel for treatment of genital human papilloma virus (HPV) have suggested some efficacy and are ongoing.[105] Cidofovir is given intravenously in doses of 3–5 mg/kg. Eighty percent of the drug is excreted unchanged in the urine. The plasma half-life is 2.4–3.2 h, but the intracellular half-life is 50–60 h, which is the rationale for once-weekly dosing.[102,106] Probenecid blocks the tubular secretion of cidofovir and results in increased serum levels.

The major toxicity of cidofovir is renal tubular toxicity. Proteinuria frequently occurs with high dosages of cidofovir (>3.0 mg/kg). Probenecid, which offers some protection against the renal toxicity, must be administered before and after cidofovir dosing. Saline infusions have been used to decrease nephrotoxicity. Probenecid, a sulfa-derived compound, has been associated with toxicity that includes nausea, vomiting, headaches, fevers, and flushing.[78,102]

Presently, cidofovir is approved only for treatment of CMV disease. The role of cidofovir, intravenously or topically, in the treatment of HSV disease is reserved for treatment of acyclovir- and foscarnet-resistant HSV disease.

PREVENTION

Primary prophylaxis with acyclovir to prevent acquisition of HSV is not recommended for HIV-infected patients.[4] Efforts to prevent initial exposure to HSV with latex condoms are important. Sexual contact should be avoided when lesions are present in either partner.[107]

The first step in long-term suppression of HSV disease is optimization of a potent HAART regimen. Following that step, suppression of reactivation HSV disease can be performed successfully with chronic acyclovir, valacyclovir, or famciclovir administration. The ease of treating patients episodically and the possible risk for the development of acyclovir resistance supports the recommendation that suppressive therapy be reserved for only those patients with disabling and frequent recurrences. Several investigators have suggested that chronic suppression of HSV-2 should be used more widely due to its potential public health benefit in reducing HIV transmission.[108–111] Both biological and epidemiological evidence indicate that HSV infection facilitates HIV acquisition and suppression of HSV is associated with decreases in plasma HIV-1 RNA levels.[17,108–110] It is unclear if chronic suppression of HSV disease will reduce HIV transmission or HIV disease progression in patients whose HIV is suppressed on HAART. Thus, the greatest benefit of chronic suppression for both the patient and the public may be realized in individuals who are not treated with HAART or whose virus is not suppressed despite HAART.

REFERENCES

1. Gibson JJ, Hornung CA, Alexander GR, et al. A cross-sectional study of herpes simplex virus 1 and 2 in college students: occurrence and determinants of infection. J Infect Dis 162:306, 1990.
2. Johnson RE, Nahmias AJ, Magder LS, et al. A seroepidemiologic survey of the prevalence of herpes simplex virus type 2 in the United States. N Engl J Med 321:7, 1989.
3. Siegel D, Golden E, Washington AE, et al. Prevalence and correlates of herpes simplex infections: the population based AIDS in multiethnic neighborhoods study. JAMA 268:1702, 1992.
4. CDC. Sexually transmitted diseases Treatment guidelines, 2002. MMWR 51(RR-6):1, 2002.
5. Herpes Simplex Virus Type 2 Programmatic and Research Priorities in Developing Countries, Geneva: World Health Organization; 2001. Report of a WHO/UNAIDS/LSHTM Workshop, London, 14–16 Feb 2001.
6. Wald A, Link K. Risk of human immunodeficiency virus infection in herpes simplex virus type 2-seropositive persons: a meta-analysis. J Infect Dis. 185:45, 2002.
7. Gray RH, Wawer MJ, Serwadda D, et al. Serologic HSV-2 associated with HIV acquisition/transmission in discordant couples and the general population: Rakai, Uganda. Int J STD AIDS 12:64, 2001.
8. Stewart JA, Reef SE, Pellett PE, et al. Herpes virus infection in persons infected with human immunodeficiency virus. Clin Infect Dis 21(Suppl 1):S114, 1995.
9. van Benthem BHB, Spaargaren J, van den Hoek JAR, et al. Prevalence and risk factors of HSV-1 and HSV-2 antibodies in European HIV infected women. Sex Transm Infect 77:120, 2001.
10. Auvert B, Ballard R, Campbell C, et al. HIV infection among youth in a South African mining town is associated with herpes simplex virus-2 seropositivity and sexual behaviour. AIDS 15:885, 2001.
11. Krone MR, Wald A, Tabet SR, et al. Herpes simplex virus type 2 shedding in human immunodeficiency virus-negative men who have sex with men: frequency, patterns, and risk factors. Clin Infect Dis. 30:261, 2000.
12. LaGuardia KD, White MH, Saigo PE, et al. Genital ulcer disease in women infected with human immunodeficiency virus. Am J Obstet Gynecol 172:553, 1995.
13. Anderson J, Clark RA, Watts DH, et al. Idiopathic genital ulcers in women infected with human immunodeficiency virus. J Acquir Immun Defic Syndr Hum Retrovirol 13:343, 1996.
14. Cu-Uvin S, Flanigan TP, Rich JD, et al. Human immunodeficiency virus infection and acquired immunodeficiency syndrome among North American women. Am J Med 105:316, 1996.
15. Sobel JD. Gynecologic infections in human immunodeficiency virus-infected women. Clin Infect Dis 31:1225, 2000.
16. Patton LL, McKaig R, Strauss R, et al. Changing prevalence of oral manifestations of human immuno-deficiency virus in the era of protease inhibitor therapy. Oral Surg Oral Med Oral Pathol Oral Radiol Endod 89:299, 2000.
17. Schacker T, Zeh J, Hu H et al. Changes in Plasma HIV type 1 RNA Associated with herpes simplex reactivsation and supression. J Infect. Dis 186:1718, 2002.
18. Lee V, Foley E, Barton SE, Patel R. Outbreaks of Genital Herpes: effects on plasma viral loads in individuals Recieving highly active antiretroviral therapy. J Infect. Dis 190:2057, 2004.
19. Corey L, Adams HG, Brown ZA, et al. Genital herpes simplex virus infections: clinical manifestations, course and complications. Ann Intern Med 98:958, 1983.
20. Corey L, Spear PG. Infections with herpes simplex viruses. N Engl J Med 314:686, 749, 1986.
21. Siegal FP, Lopez C, Hammer GS, et al. Severe acquired immunodeficiency in male homosexuals, manifested by chronic perianal ulcerative herpes simplex lesions. N Engl J Med 305:1439, 1981.
22. Quinnan GV Jr, Masur H, Rook AH, et al. Herpes virus infections in the acquired immunodeficiency syndrome. JAMA 252:72, 1984.
23. Safrin S, Ashley R, Houlihan C, et al. Clinical and serologic features of herpes simplex virus infection in patients with AIDS. AIDS 5:1107, 1990.
24. Tony P, Mutasim DF. Herpes simplex virus infection masquerading as condyloma acuminata in a patient with HIV disease. Br J Dermatol 134:797, 1996.
25. Augenbaum M, Feldman J, Chirgwin K, et al. Increased genital shedding of herpes simplex 2 in HIV-seropositive women. Ann Intern Med 123:845, 1995.
26. Schacker T, Zeh J, Hui-lin H, et al. Frequency of symptomatic and asymptomatic herpes simplex virus 2 reactivations among human immunodeficiency virus-infected men. J Infect Dis 170:1616, 1998.
27. Posavad CM, Wald A, Kuntz S, et al. Frequent reactivation of herpes simplex virus among HIV-1 infected patients treated with highly active antiretroiviral therapy. J Infect Dis 190:693, 2004.
28. Goodell SE, Quinn TC, Mkrtichian E, et al. Herpes simplex virus proctitis in homosexual men. N Engl J Med 308:858, 1983.
29. Quinn TC, Corey L, Chaffee RG, et al. The etiology of anorectal infections in homosexual men. Am J Med 71:395, 1981.
30. Rompalo AM. Diagnosis and treatment of sexually acquired proctitis and proctocolitis: an update. Clin Infect Dis 28(Suppl 1):S84, 1999.
31. Itin PH, Lautenschlager S, Fluckiger R. Oral manifestations in HIV infected patients: diagnosis and management. J Am Acad Dermatol 29:749, 1993.
32. Regezi JA, Eversole LR, Barker BF, et al. Herpes simplex and cytomegalovirus coinfected oral ulcers in HIV-positive patients. Oral Surg Oral Med Oral Pathol 81:55, 1996.
33. Gill MJ, Arlette J, Bucham K. Herpes simplex virus infection of the hand: a profile of 79 cases. Am J Med 84:89, 1988.
34. Norris SA, Kessler HA, Fife KH. Severe progressive herpetic whitlow caused by an acyclovir-resistant virus in a patient with AIDS. J Infect Dis 157:209, 1988.
35. Giani G, Quirino T, Sacrini F, et al. Destructive mucocutaneous phagedenic herpes simplex virus infection in an HIV-infected patient who had a partial response to interferon and ultraviolet rays. Clin Infect Dis 22:381, 1996.
36. Genereau T, Lorthollary O, Bonchaud O, et al. Herpes simplex esophagitis in patients with AIDS: report of 34 cases. Clin Infect Dis 22:926, 1996.
37. Bonacini M, Young T, Laine L. The cause of esophageal symptoms in human immunodeficiency virus infection: a prospective study of 110 patients. Arch Intern Med 151:1567, 1991.
38. Wilcox CM, Schwartz DA, Clark WS. Esophageal ulceration in human immunodeficiency virus infection: causes, response to therapy, and long term outcome. Ann Intern Med 123:143, 1995.
39. Wilcox CM. Esophageal strictures complicating ulcerative esophagitis in patients with AIDS. Am J Gastroenterol 94:339, 1999.
40. Dieckhaus KD, Hill DR. Boerhaave's syndrome due to herpes simplex virus type 1 esophagitis in a patient with AIDS. Clin Infect Dis 26:1244,1998.
41. Chretien F, Belech L, Hilton DA, et al. Herpes simplex virus type 1 encephalitis in acquired immunodeficiency syndrome. Neuropathol Appl Neurobiol 22:394, 1996.

42. Corey L, Holmes KK. Genital herpes simplex virus infections: current concepts in diagnosis, therapy, and prevention. Ann Intern Med 98:972, 1983.
43. Pottage JC Jr, Kessler HA. Herpes simplex virus resistance to acyclovir: clinical relevance. Infect Agents Dis 4:115, 1995.
44. L Verano, FJ Michalski. Herpes simplex virus antigen direct detection in standard virus transport medium by Du Pont Herpchek enzyme-linked immunosorbent assay. J Clin Microbiol 28:2555, 1990.
45. Koutsky LA, Stevens CE, Holmes KK, et al. Under diagnosis of genital herpes by current clinical and viral-isolation procedures. N Engl J Med 326:1533, 1992.
46. De la Iglesia P, Melon S, Lopez B, et al. Rapid screening tests for determining in vitro susceptibility of herpes simplex virus clinical isolates. J Clin Microbiol 36:2389, 1998.
47. Stranska R, van Loon AM, Polman M, Schuurman R. Application of real-time PCR for determination of antiviral drug susceptibility of herpes simplex virus Antimicrob. Agents Chemother 46: 2943, 2002.
48. Stranska R, Schuurman R, Scholl DR, et al. ELVIRA HSV, a yield reduction assay for rapid herpes simplex virus susceptibility testing. Antimicrob Agents Chemother 48:2331, 2004.
49. Whitley RJ, Gnann JW Jr. Acyclovir: a decade later. N Engl J Med 327:782, 1992.
50. Klepser ME, Klepser TB. Drug treatment of HIV-related opportunistic infections. Drugs 53:40, 1997.
51. Pottage JC Jr. Antifungal and antiviral therapy. In: Parrillo JE, Bone RC (eds) Critical Care Medicine: Principles of Diagnosis and Management. St Louis: Mosby Year Book; 1995, p 969.
52. Wood MJ. Antivirals in the context of HIV disease. J Antimicrob Chemother 37(Suppl B):97, 1996.
53. Sacks SL, Aoki FY, Diaz-Mitoma F, et al. Patient initiated, twice daily oral famciclovir for early recurrent genital herpes: a randomized double blind multicenter trial. JAMA 276:44, 1996.
54. Smiley ML, International Valaciclovir HSV Study Group. Valaciclovir and acyclovir for the treatment of recurrent genital herpes simplex virus infections. In: Abstracts of the 37th Interscience Conference on Antimicrobial Agents and Chemotherapy, Toronto. Washington, DC: American Society for Microbiology; 1997, abstract 1210.
55. Romanowski B, Aoki FY, Martel AY, et al. Efficacy and safety of famciclovir for treating mucocutaneous herpes simplex infection in HIV-infected individuals. AIDS 14:1211, 2000.
56. Mertz GJ, Loveless MO, Levin MJ, et al. Oral famciclovir for suppression of recurrent genital herpes simplex virus infection in women: a multicenter, double blind placebo controlled study. Arch Intern Med 157:343, 1997.
57. DeJesus E, Wald A, Warren T. et al. Valacyclovir for the suppression of recurrent genital herpes in human immunodeficiency virus-infected subjects. JID 188,1009, 2003.
58. Reyes M, Graber J, Reeves WC. Acyclovir-resistant HSV: initial results from a National Surveillance System. In: Abstracts of the 35th Annual Meeting of the Infectious Diseases Society of America, San Francisco. Alexandria, VA: Infectious Diseases Society of America; 1997, abstract 55.
59. Fife KH, Crumpacker CS, Mertz GJ, et al. Acyclovir study: recurrence and resistance of herpes simplex virus following cessation of greater than or equal to 6 years of chronic suppression with acyclovir. Infect Dis 169:1338, 1994.
60. Reyes M, et al. Acyclovir-resistant genital herpes among persons attending sexually transmitted disease and human immunodeficiency virus clinics. Arch Intern Med 163:76, 2003.
61. Erlich KS, Mills J, Chatis P, et al. Acyclovir-resistant herpes simplex virus infections in patients with the acquired immunodeficiency syndrome. N Engl J Med 320:293, 1989.
62. Chatis PA, Miller CH, Schrager LE, et al. Successful treatment with foscarnet of an acyclovir-resistant mucocutaneous infection with herpes simplex virus in a patient with acquired immunodeficiency syndrome. N Engl J Med 320:297, 1989.
63. Sacks SL, Wanklin RJ, Reece DJ, et al. Progressive esophagitis from acyclovir-resistant herpes simplex. Ann Intern Med 111:893, 1989.
64. Gateley A, Gander RM, Johnson PC, et al. Herpes simplex virus type 2 meningoencephalitis resistant to acyclovir in a patient with AIDS. J Infect Dis 161:711, 1990.
65. Engel JP, Englund JA, Fletcher CV, et al. Treatment of resistant herpes simplex virus with continuous infusion acyclovir. JAMA 263:1662, 1990.
66. Fletcher CV, Englund JA, Bean B, et al. Continuous infusion of high-dose acyclovir for serious herpes virus infections. Antimicrob Agents Chemother 33:1375, 1989.
67. Safrin S, Assauleem T, Follansbee S, et al. Foscarnet therapy for acyclovir-resistant mucocutaneous herpes simplex virus infection in 26 AIDS patients: preliminary data. J Infect Dis 161:1078, 1990.
68. Safrin S, Crumpacker C, Chatis P, et al. A controlled trial comparing foscarnet with vidarabine for acyclovir resistant mucocutaneous herpes simplex in the acquired immunodeficiency syndrome. N Engl J Med 325:551, 1991.
69. Hardy WD. Foscarnet treatment of acyclovir-resistant herpes simplex virus infection in patients with the acquired immunodeficiency syndrome: preliminary results of a controlled randomized, regimen-comparative trial. Am J Med 92(Suppl 2A):305, 1992.
70. Khurana RN, Charonis A, Samuel MA, et al. Intravenous foscarnet in the management of acyclovir-resistant herpes simplex virus type 2 in acute retinal necrosis in children. Med Sci Monit 11:CS75, 2005.
71. Lalezari JP, Drew WL, Glutzer E, et al. Treatment with intravenous (s)-1-(3-hydroxy-2-phosphonylmethoxypropyl)cytosine of acyclovir-resistant mucocutaneous infection with herpes simplex virus in a patient with AIDS. J Infect Dis 170:550, 1994.
72. Chen Y, Scieux C, Garrait V, et al. Resistant herpes simplex virus type 1 infection: an emerging concern after allogeneic stem cell transplantation. Clin Infect Dis 31:927, 2000.
73. LoPresti AE, Levine JF, Munk GB, et al. Successful treatment of an acyclovir- and foscarnet-resistant herpes simplex virus type 1 lesion with intravenous cidofovir. Clin Infect Dis 26:512, 1998.
74. Martinez CM, Luks-Golger DB. Cidofovir use in acyclovir-resistant herpes infection. Ann Pharmacother 31:1519, 1997.
75. Wyles DL, Patel A, Madinger N, et al. Development of herpes simplex disease in patients who are receiving cidofovir. Clin Infect Dis 41:676, 2005.
76. Birch CJ, Tyssen DP, Tacheddjian G, et al. Clinical effects and in vitro studies of trifluorothymidine combined with interferon for treatment of drug resistant and sensitive herpes simplex virus infections. J Infect Dis 166:108, 1992.
77. Kessler HA, Hurwitz C, Farthing C, et al. Pilot study of topical trifluridine for the treatment of acyclovir-resistant mucocutaneous herpes simplex disease in patients with AIDS (ACTG 172). J Acquir Immun Defic Syndr 12:147, 1996.
78. Amiu AR, Robinson MR, Smith DD, et al. Trifluorothymidine 0.5% ointment in the treatment of acyclovir resistant mucocutaneous herpes simplex in AIDS [letter]. AIDS 10:1051, 1996.
79. Snoeck R, Andrei G, DeClercq E, et al. A new topical treatment for resistant herpes simplex infections [letter]. N Engl J Med 327:968, 1993.
80. Snoeck R, Andei G, Gerard M, et al. Successful treatment of progressive mucocutaneous infection due to acyclovir and foscarnet resistant herpes simplex virus with (S)-1-(3-hydroxy-2-phosphonylmethoxypropyl)cytosine (HPMPC). Clin Infect Dis 18:570, 1994.
81. Lalezari J, Schacker T, Feinberg J, et al. A randomized, double blind, placebo-controlled study of cidofovir gel for the

treatment of acyclovir-unresponsive mucocutaneous herpes simplex virus infections in patients with AIDS. J Infect Dis 17:862, 1997.
82. Javaly K, Wohlfeiler M, Kalayjian R, et al. Treatment of mucocutaneous herpes simplex virus infections unresponsive to acyclovir with topical foscarnet cream in AIDS patients: a phase I/II study. J Acquir Immune Defic Syndr 21:301, 1999.
83. Safrin S, Kemmerly S, Plotkin B, et al. Foscarnet-resistant herpes simplex virus infection in patients with AIDS. J Infect Dis 169:193, 1994.
84. Bini EJ, Micale PL, Weinshel EH. Natural history of HIV-associated esophageal disease in the era of protease inhibitor therapy. Dig Dis Sci 45:1301, 2000.
85. Bras AP, Sitar DS, Aoki FY. Comparative bioavailability of acyclovir from oral valacyclovir and acyclovir in patients treated for recurrent genital herpes simplex virus infection. Can J Clin Pharmacol. Winter 8(4):207, 2001.
86. Tilson HH, Engl CR, Andrews EB. Safety of acyclovir: a summary of the first ten years experience. J Med Virol 41(Suppl 1): 67, 1993
87. Haefeli WE, Schoenberger RAZ, Weiss P, et al. Acyclovir-induced neurotoxicity: concentration-side effect relationship in acyclovir overdose. Am J Med 94:212, 1993.
88. Weller S, Blum MR, Doucette M, et al. Pharmacokinetics of acyclovir prodrug valaciclovir after escalating single and multiple-dose administration to normal volunteers. Clin Pharmacol Ther 54:595, 1993.
89. Jacobson MA, Gallant J, Wang LH, et al. Phase 1 trial of valaciclovir, the L-valyl ester of acyclovir, in patients with advanced human immunodeficiency virus disease. Antimicrob Agents Chemother 38:1534, 1994.
90. Valtrex (valcyclovir hydrochloride) package Insert. Research Triangle Park, NC: GlaxoSmithKline; 2005.
91. Rivaud E, Massiani MA, Vincent F, et al. Valacyclovir hydrochloride therapy and thrombotic thrombocytopenic purpura in an HIV-infected patient. Arch Intern Med 160:1707, 2000.
92. Tyring SK, Baker D, Snowden W. Valacyclovir for herpes simplex virus infection: long-term safety and sustained efficacy after 20 years' experience with acyclovir. JID 186:S40, 2002.
93. Conant MA, Schacker TW, Murphy RL, et al. Valaciclovir versus acyclovir for herpes simplex infection in HIV-infected individuals: two randomized trials. Int J STD AIDS 13:12, 2002.
94. Earnshaw DL, Bacon TH, Darlison SJ, et al. Mode of antiviral action of penciclovir in MRC-5 cells infected with herpes simplex virus type 1 (HSV-1), HSV-2, and varicella-zoster virus. Antimicrob Agents Chemother 36:2747, 1992.
95. Pue M, Benet LZ. Pharmacokinetics of famciclovir in man. Antiviral Chem Chemother 4(Suppl 1):47, 1993.
96. Saltzman R, Jurewicz R, Boon R. Safety of famciclovir in patients with herpes zoster and genital herpes. Antimicrob Agents Chemother 38:2454, 1994.
97. Oberg B. Antiviral effects of phosphonoformate (PFA, foscarnet sodium). Pharmacol Ther 40:213, 1989.
98. Charis P, Miller C, Schrager L, Crumpacker C. Successful treatment with foscarnet of an acyclovir resistant mucocutaneous infection of herpes simplex virus in a patient with acquired immunodeficiency syndrome. N Engl J Med 320:297.
99. Danve-Szatanek, C, Aymard M., Thouvenor D, et al. Surveillance network for herpes simplex virus resistance to antiviral drugs: 3 year follow-up. J Clin Micro 242, 2004.
100. Blot NP, Shneider P, Young P, et al. Treatment of an acyclovir and foscarnet resistant herpes simplex virus infection with cidofovir in a child after unrelated bone marrow transplant. Bone Marrow Transplant 26:903.
101. Jacobson MA. Review of the toxicities of foscarnet. J Acquir Immune Defic Syndr 5(Suppl 2):511, 1992
102. Lea AP, Bryson HM. Cidofovir. Drugs 52:225, 1996.
103. Martinez CM, Luks-Golger DB. Cidofovir use in acyclovir resistant herpes infection. Ann Phamacother 1997; 31:1519–21.
104. Mendel DB, Tai CY, Barkhimer DB, et al. Characterization of an in vitro selected herpes simplex virus type 2 (HSV-2) strain with decreased susceptibility to cidofovir. In: Abstracts of the 4th Conference on Retroviruses and Opportunistic Infections. Alexandria, VA: Westover Management Group; 1997, abstract 681.
105. Snoeck R, Bossens M, Parent D, et al. Phase II double-blind, placebo-controlled study of the safety and efficacy of cidofovir topical gel for the treatment of patients with human papillomavirus infection. Clin Infect Dis 33:597, 2001.
106. Cundy KC, Petty BG, Flaherty J, et al. Clinical pharmacokinetics of cidofovir in human immunodeficiency virus-infected patients. Antimicrob Agents Chemother 39:1247, 1995.
107. Benson CA. Kaplan JE. Masur H. et al. National Institutes of Health. Infectious Diseases Society of America. Treating opportunistic infections among HIV-infected Adults and Adolescents: Recommendations from CDC, the National Institutes of Health, and the Infectious Diseases Society of America. MorbMortal Wkly Rep. Recomm Rep 53(RR-15):1, 2004. Erratum. Morb Mortal Wkly Rep 54(12):311, 2005.
108. Celum CL, Robinson NJ, Cohen MS. Potential effect of HIV-1 antiretroviral and herpes simplex virus type 2 antiviral therapy on transmission and acquisition of HIV type 1 infection. J Infect Dis 191(Suppl 1):S107, 2005.
109. Corey L. Wald A, Celum CL, Quinn TC. The effects of herpes simplex virus-2 on HIV acquisition and transmission: a review of two overlapping epidemics. J Acquir Immune Defic Syndr 35:435.
110. Wald A and Corey L. How does herpes simplex virus 2 influence human immunodeficiency virun infection and pathogenesis? J Infect Dis 187:1509.

Chapter 49

Varicella-Zoster Virus Infections

John W. Gnann Jr, MD

Diseases caused by all human herpesviruses, including varicella-zoster virus (VZV), occur with increased frequency in patients with human immunodeficiency virus (HIV) infection.[1,2] Among HIV-seropositive children, primary VZV infection (varicella or chickenpox) is associated with a higher rate of complications than is seen among immunocompetent children. An association between recurrent VZV disease (herpes zoster or shingles) and acquired immunodeficiency syndrome (AIDS) has been noted since the onset of the pandemic. As with herpes simplex virus (HSV) infections and tuberculosis, herpes zoster can occur in HIV-infected individuals with relatively high CD4+ T-lymphocyte counts and may be the initial opportunistic infection.[3] In most HIV-seropositive patients, herpes zoster presents as a self-limited cutaneous eruption in a dermatomal distribution. A variety of complications have been described that are associated with increased morbidity and occasional mortality. A unique feature of herpes zoster in patients with HIV infection is a propensity for multiple recurrences.

VZV INFECTIONS

Pathogenesis of VZV Infections

Varicella

Humans are the only reservoir for VZV. Primary infection occurs when a susceptible individual is exposed to airborne virus via the respiratory route. Patients with chickenpox are contagious for ~2 days prior to rash onset and 4–5 days thereafter. Varicella is most often acquired following exposure to another person with active chickenpox, but infection can also result from close exposure to a patient with herpes zoster. Varicella is highly infectious, and attack rates of 60–90% have been observed among household contacts. VZV in airborne droplets enters the susceptible host via mucosal surfaces of the conjunctivae, oropharynx, or upper respiratory tract, then undergoes an initial round of replication in cervical lymph nodes. When local immune responses are overcome, primary viremia occurs with widespread dissemination of VZV to the reticuloendothelial system. Following additional cycles of replication, a second viremic phase occurs ~1 week after the initial viremia and is accompanied by the onset of clinical symptoms. VZV localizes to endothelial cells of cutaneous capillaries and then extends to epithelial cells of the epidermis where replication results in formation of the characteristic vesicles. In the normal host, viremia and new vesicle formation continue for 3–5 days until humoral and cellular immune responses appear.

There is no convincing evidence that varicella acts as a cofactor to accelerate the progression of HIV disease. Although VZV can transactivate long terminal repeat (LTR) sequences of HIV *in vitro*, clinical studies have not demonstrated an impact of varicella on CD4+ T-lymphocyte counts.[4] This is important because use of a live varicella vaccine in HIV-infected children could not be considered if VZV functioned as a cofactor.

Herpes Zoster

As VZV replicates in the skin during acute varicella, some virions are transported via sensory nerves to the corresponding dorsal root ganglia where latent infection is established. VZV periodically reactivates and undergoes limited gene expression, but replication is suppressed by immunity before any clinical symptoms result. The specific immune responses that limit reactivation of VZV in the sensory ganglia are not well defined. In general, the most important factor that predisposes to the development of herpes zoster is a decline or suppression of VZV-specific cellular immunity, which occurs naturally with aging or can be induced by immunosuppressive illness or therapy. Following reactivation and replication in the ganglion, VZV moves via axonal transport along the sensory nerve to the skin where the virus again replicates in epithelial cells, producing the characteristic dermatomal vesicular rash of herpes zoster. In contrast to the varied lesion stages seen in varicella, most zoster lesions are in similar stages of development.

Investigators initially described herpes zoster as an early sentinel marker of HIV seropositivity.[3] Although herpes zoster can occur in patients with any CD4+ lymphocyte count, the incidence is higher among individuals with advanced HIV disease.[5–7] In a survey of 175 cases reported from an American cohort, the incidence of herpes zoster was substantially higher in patients with CD4+ lymphocyte counts of less than 100 cells/mm^3 (4.1% annually) than in patients with counts of more than 500 cells/mm^3 (2.2% annually).[8] Unlike most other opportunistic infections, herpes zoster continues to occur at increased frequency despite successful initiation of highly active antiretroviral therapy (HAART).[9] Some conflicting data exist, but prednisone therapy probably does not significantly increase the risk of herpes zoster in HIV-infected patients.[10]

Herpes zoster was originally considered a marker for rapid progression of HIV disease. However, larger studies controlled for age and for CD4+ T-lymphocyte counts have clearly demonstrated that the development of herpes zoster is not significantly associated with the rate of disease progression to AIDS.[7,11,12]

As has previously been observed with infections caused by cytomegalovirus (CMV) and mycobacteria, immune reconstitution following initiation of HAART may be associated with an increased frequency of VZV reactivation in both adults and children.[13–16] Between 4 and 16 weeks after beginning combination antiretroviral therapy (containing a protease inhibitor (PI) or non-nucleoside reverse transcriptase inhibitor (NNRTI)), the risk of herpes zoster increases two- to fourfold from baseline. In one study, 24 (8%) of 316 patients beginning combination antiretroviral therapy developed herpes zoster after a mean of 5 weeks.[15] During the 6 months following the start of combination antiretroviral therapy, the incidence of herpes zoster exceeds 90 episodes per 1000 person-years.[13,15] The percentage of CD8+ lymphocytes at baseline and the magnitude of their increase at 1 month after initiation of drug therapy is strongly associated with an increased risk of herpes zoster.[13,15,16] The immunologic mechanisms that account for this observation are not fully understood.[17] The clinical presentation and natural history of herpes zoster in the setting of immune reconstitution does not differ from that seen in other HIV-infected patients.[13,15]

Epidemiology of VZV Infections

Varicella

Until the recent widespread adoption of varicella vaccination, chickenpox epidemics occurred annually in the United States (US) during the late winter and early spring, with numbers of cases peaking in March. During the prevaccine era ~3.8 million cases of varicella occurred each year in the US, which is approximately equal to the annual birth cohort. About 50–60% of varicella cases occurred in children between the ages of 5 and 9 years, and 90% of cases were in children under 15 years of age. Serologic surveys demonstrated that more than 95% of the US population had been infected by VZV by age 20. Introduction of the varicella vaccine in the US in 1995 has resulted in striking changes in the epidemiology of chickenpox and a dramatic decline in incidence. By monitoring vaccine usage and disease activity at three sentinel sites, the Centers for Disease Control and Prevention (CDC) showed that vaccine coverage among preschool-age children increased from 40% in 1997 to 70% in 1999.[18] Between 1995 and 1999 the varicella incidence declined 80% in the surveillance areas, accompanied by an attenuation of disease seasonality. The greatest decline in incidence was seen in children aged 1–4 years.[18]

Herpes Zoster

The annual incidence of herpes zoster in the US has been estimated at 1.5–3.5 cases per 1000 population.[19] An incidence of 2.0 cases per 1000 persons would project to almost 600 000 cases of herpes zoster annually in the US. Increasing age is clearly the most important risk factor for the development of herpes zoster. There is a significant increase in the age-specific incidence of herpes zoster beginning at around age 55; individuals over 75 years of age have a herpes zoster incidence of ~10 cases per 1000 person-years.[19,20] These figures predict that an immunocompetent individual living to be 70 years of age has a 10–20% risk of developing herpes zoster at some point during his or her lifetime. Shingles occurs with equal frequency in men and women, and there is no seasonal association.

The other well-defined risk factor for herpes zoster is altered cell-mediated immunity, as seen in patients with lymphoproliferative malignancies, organ transplant recipients, and AIDS patients. Results from several prospective studies have confirmed the incidence rates for herpes zoster in HIV-infected individuals to be ~30–50 cases per 1000 person-years.[6–8,21,22] In a surveillance study conducted in San Francisco, the incidence of herpes zoster among HIV-seropositive men was 29.4 cases per 1000 person-years, compared with 2.0 cases per 1000 person-years among a control group of HIV-seronegative gay men.[23] HIV infection was associated with an increased relative risk (RR) of herpes zoster in all age groups (RR 16.9; 95% confidence interval (CI) 8.7–32.6).[23] The cumulative proportion of men developing herpes zoster increased linearly; by 12 years after the diagnosis of HIV infection, 30% of the patients had developed herpes zoster. Among patients with herpes zoster, 22% experienced more than one episode of shingles.[23] In a similar prospective study conducted in The Netherlands, the incidence of herpes zoster among HIV-seropositive patients was 51.5 cases per 1000 person-years, with a 41% cumulative incidence over 10 years; in the HIV-seronegative control population, the zoster incidence was 3.31 cases per 1000 person-years, with a 10-year cumulative incidence of 3%.[7] Prospective studies in

Uganda yielded similar results.[22] These observations confirm that the incidence of herpes zoster is ~15-fold higher among HIV-infected individuals than among age-matched seronegative controls. As a corollary, the possibility of HIV infection should be considered in otherwise healthy patients less than 55 years of age who present with herpes zoster. In African populations where the prevalence of HIV infection is high, more than 90% of patients presenting with a new diagnosis of herpes zoster were found to be HIV infected.[24]

Clinical Presentation

Varicella

Varicella is usually a benign disease in healthy children, although symptoms are frequently more severe in adolescents and adults. Symptoms develop after an incubation period of ~15 days. The appearance of the rash is sometimes preceded by a brief (1–2 days) prodrome of fever, malaise, headache, and anorexia. Cutaneous lesions begin as pink macules that quickly become papular and evolve into fragile vesicles 1–4 mm in diameter surrounded by a zone of erythema. The lesions first appear on the head, progress to the trunk, and finally to the extremities. The rash of varicella is characterized by rapid evolution of lesions over 8–12 h and by successive crops of new lesions. Consequently, lesions at all stages of development are present simultaneously. New vesicle formation continues for 2–4 days, accompanied by pruritus, fever, headache, malaise, and anorexia. The rash peaks at about the fifth day with a lesion count of ~250–500 (lower in children under 5 years of age and higher in adults). With the influx of inflammatory cells, vesicles pustulate and then crust. The scabs detach after 1–3 weeks, and the lesions usually heal without scarring.

Varicella does not appear to be unusually severe in most HIV-seropositive children.[25–27] However, the natural history of varicella in this population is difficult to ascertain from the literature, as most published reports are based on retrospective studies of hospitalized patients or referral populations that likely overestimate the frequency of complications. The clinical presentation of varicella is similar to that seen in immunocompetent children, although some investigators have reported a longer duration of new lesion formation and higher median lesion counts.[28] In a prospective, case-controlled study of 30 HIV-infected children with chickenpox, 29 of the cases were scored as mild or moderate in severity, even among the children who received no treatment with acyclovir.[4] The only serious complication was one severe case of varicella pneumonia.[4] The manifestations of varicella were judged to be less severe in HIV-infected children than in children with acute leukemia.[4]

A variety of varicella complications in HIV-infected children have been reported, although reliable incidence figures are not available. An inverse correlation between CD4+ T-lymphocyte counts and complication rates has been suggested, but not substantiated in other studies. Cutaneous complications of varicella may include hemorrhagic skin lesions or bacterial superinfections. Visceral dissemination of VZV may manifest by disseminated intravascular coagulopathy, pneumonitis, hepatitis, or encephalitis.[29] Deaths attributable to chickenpox in patients with HIV infection are rare and are usually due to pneumonitis.[30]

Following an episode of varicella, HIV-infected children are at high risk for persistent or recurrent VZV infections.[4,25,31] In a few reported cases, the cutaneous lesions of primary varicella failed to heal and remained VZV culture-positive; this was usually associated with a very low CD4+ T-lymphocyte count.[29] More often, children develop recurrent cutaneous VZV infections months to years after the primary infection. In a population of 480 HIV-infected children, 117 episodes of VZV infection were identified in 73 patients.[29] Of the 73 children, 38 (53%) had recurrent VZV infections; the mean interval from the first to second episode was 17 months. Among 22 children with primary varicella who were followed for 24 months, 10 (45%) had recurrent VZV disease. CD4+ T-lymphocyte counts were no different between children who experienced recurrences and those who did not. Five of the recurrences were classic herpes zoster, and the other five were described as 'recurrent varicella' with a widespread cutaneous rash.[29] In most cases 'recurrent varicella' probably results from VZV reactivation and is actually generalized cutaneous zoster (as has been previously described in other immunocompromised populations), although true reacquisition due to failed immune responses occurs occasionally. Seroconversion following varicella was documented by enzyme-linked immunosorbent assay (ELISA) testing of acute and convalescent sera in six of eight HIV-infected children.[32]

About 95% of HIV-infected adults have antibody against VZV as a result of childhood varicella, and antibody levels are well preserved even in patients with advanced AIDS. However, when chickenpox does occur in HIV-infected adults, the disease may produce significant morbidity, including VZV pneumonia.[33] In a series of five HIV-seropositive adults with varicella, three had uncomplicated courses, one had possible central nervous system (CNS) involvement, and one had possible CNS infection plus hepatitis and thrombocytopenia.[34] All five patients improved with acyclovir therapy. Four developed VZV antibody, and one had herpes zoster 2 years after varicella.[34] Recurrent varicella-like eruptions, as described above in children, have also been reported in adults.[35]

Herpes Zoster

Herpes zoster presents as a painful cutaneous eruption in a dermatomal distribution.[36] The inflammatory changes that occur as latent VZV reactivates in the sensory ganglion, produce discomfort in the corresponding dermatome. The patient may report sensations ranging from mild itching or tingling to severe pain that precedes the development of the skin lesions by 1–5 days (or rarely weeks). The cutaneous eruption, appearing in the skin segment innervated by a single sensory ganglion, is unilateral and does not cross the midline (Fig. 49-1A). Overlap of lesions into adjacent dermatomes occurs in 20% of cases. The most common sites for herpes

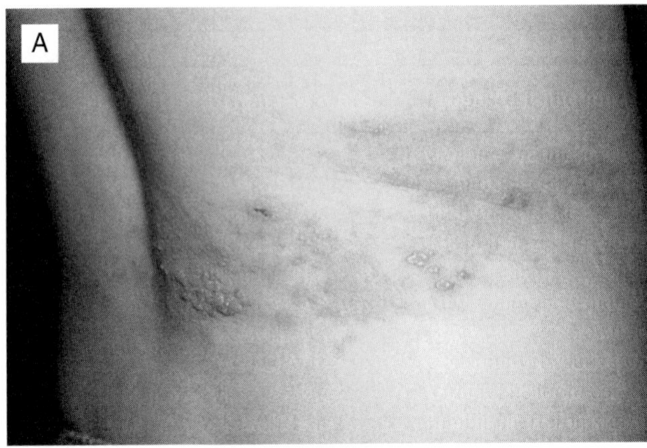

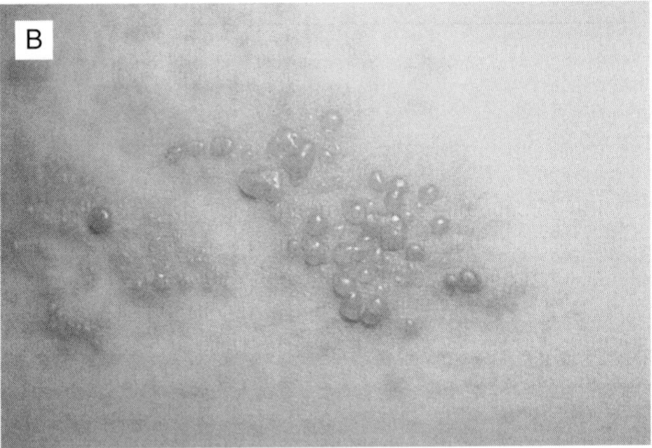

Figure 49-1 ■ Typical cutaneous eruption of herpes zoster. A, Shingles involving the right T-10 dermatome. B, Vesicles characteristic of early VZV infection.

zoster are the thoracic dermatomes (50% of cases), followed by cranial nerve (15%), cervical (15%), lumbar (15%), and sacral (5%) dermatomes. During the acute phase of herpes zoster, most patients experience dermatomal pruritus and pain, which can be quite severe. Patients may also complain of headache, photophobia, and malaise, but significant fever is rare. Skin changes begin with an erythematous maculopapular rash followed by the appearance of clear vesicles (Figs. 49-1A&B). New vesicle formation typically continues for 3–5 days followed by lesion pustulation and scabbing. Bacterial superinfection of the cutaneous lesions occurs in 10–15% of cases.[3,6] Skin lesions heal within 2–4 weeks, often leaving skin scarring and permanent pigmentation changes. In rare cases, patients develop dermatomal neuralgic pain but do not progress to the cutaneous eruption phase, a condition termed "*zoster sine herpete*". In the normal host, the most frequent complication of herpes zoster is chronic pain, called postherpetic neuralgia (PHN). The incidence and the duration of PHN are markedly increased in elderly individuals.

Patients with deficiencies of cell-mediated immunity, including AIDS, have a high incidence of herpes zoster and an increased likelihood of complications. Most cases of herpes zoster in HIV-seropositive patients are clinically similar to shingles seen in the immunocompetent host, although distinctive features such as frequent recurrences and atypical lesions are well described. Herpes zoster involving multiple nonadjacent dermatomes has occasionally been observed in HIV-infected patients.[3,37] A high frequency of herpes zoster involving the first division of the trigeminal nerve (herpes zoster ophthalmicus, or HZO) among HIV-infected patients was reported from both the US[38] and Africa.[39] However, prospective studies have shown that ~15% of herpes zoster cases in HIV-seropositive patients involve cranial dermatomes, which is similar to the frequency seen in immunocompetent patients.[6,37] Because of the prominent symptoms and cosmetic issues associated with facial herpes zoster, patients with HZO may be more likely to seek care. Studies conducted in Ethiopia and Miami showed that 81 of 85 (95%) and 29 of 112 (26%) patients, respectively, presenting with HZO were found to be HIV seropositive.[38,39] HZO warrants aggressive antiviral therapy to prevent ocular complications such as conjunctivitis, keratitis (both acute and chronic), iritis, and uveitis.[40]

Patients infected with HIV have a much higher frequency of recurrent shingles than is seen in either immunocompetent persons or other populations of immunocompromised patients. About 20–30% of HIV-infected patients develop one or more subsequent episodes of herpes zoster, which may involve the same or different dermatomes.[6] The probability of a recurrence of zoster within 1 year of the index episode is ~12%.[41]

Whereas, herpes zoster is uncommon in healthy children, shingles is frequently diagnosed in HIV-infected children.[4,42] In a prospective study, eight of 30 HIV-infected children with documented varicella subsequently developed herpes zoster.[4] The average interval between varicella and zoster was ~24 months,[4,42] although intervals as short as 2 months have been reported. A low CD4+ T-lymphocyte count at the onset of varicella has been reported to correlate strongly with an increased risk of subsequent herpes zoster.[4] Investigators at the National Cancer Institute reported a series of 11 HIV-seropositive children with frequently recurring herpes zoster, averaging five episodes per child over 25 months. Of the 58 discrete episodes documented, 29 were characterized as localized herpes zoster, nine cases involved multiple dermatomes, and 20 cases had cutaneous dissemination; there were no cases of visceral dissemination and no deaths.[42]

VZV can cause atypical skin lesions in HIV-seropositive patients that are not characteristic of either classic varicella or herpes zoster.[43] Aberrant presentations include disseminated varicella-like lesions, disseminated verrucous or hyperkeratotic lesions, disseminated ecthymatous lesions, and disseminated pinpoint papules.[44,45] The most common atypical manifestation in HIV-seropositive patients is multiple hyperkeratotic lesions, measuring 3–20 mm in diameter, that follow no dermatomal distribution and may be chronic, persisting for months or years (Fig. 49-2A). A second dermatologic variant is ecthymatous VZV lesions, presenting with multiple large (10–30 mm) punched-out ulcerations with a central black eschar and a peripheral rim of vesicles (Fig. 49-2B). The atypical appearance of these lesions may be linked

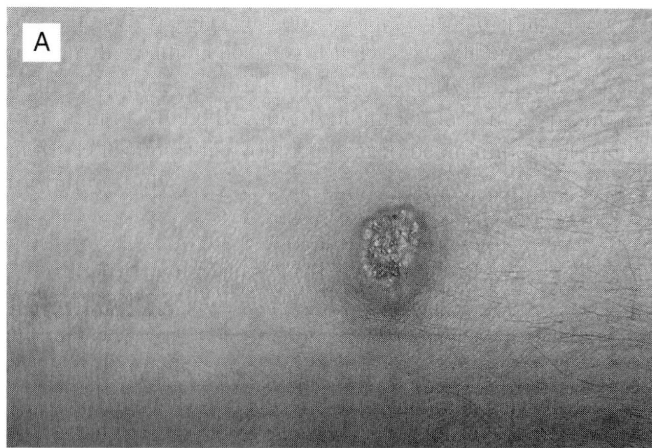

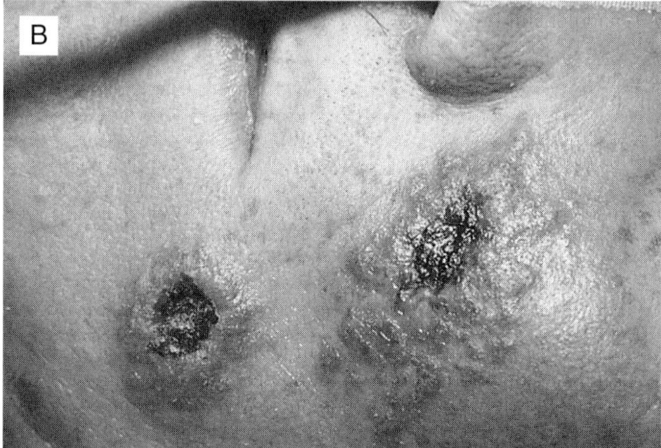

Figure 49-2 ■ Atypical cutaneous lesions caused by acyclovir-resistant VZV. (**A**) Hyperkeratotic nodule on the forearm. (**B**) Facial echthymatous ulcerations with rim of vesicles.

to abnormal expression of VZV glycoproteins.[46] Making the correct diagnosis requires a high index of suspicion, with confirmation provided by viral culture or lesion biopsy. Importantly, a significant number of these atypical verrucous or ecthymatous lesions are caused by acyclovir-resistant strains of VZV. VZV isolates obtained from these atypical lesions should routinely be submitted for antiviral susceptibility testing.

Most herpes zoster-related complications occur in patients with CD4+ lymphocyte counts of less than 200 cells/μL.[6,37] A review of 23 cases of VZV dissemination in patients with HIV infection documented that most of these patients experienced zoster involving several contiguous dermatomes, extensive local skin necrosis, and cutaneous dissemination of lesions.[47,48] Visceral dissemination of VZV to lung or liver has rarely, if ever, been documented as a complication of herpes zoster in AIDS patients.[42,47]

The frequency of PHN does not appear to differ markedly between HIV-infected and HIV-seronegative patients with herpes zoster. About 10–15% of HIV-seropositive patients report PHN as a complication following herpes zoster.[6] The primary predictors for chronic pain are older age and severity of pain at presentation.[49]

The primary target organ for herpes zoster dissemination in patients with HIV infection is the CNS.[50,51] CNS involvement may occur simultaneously with the cutaneous eruption, follow the acute episode of herpes zoster by weeks or months, or occur in patients with no documented history of cutaneous herpes zoster.[52] A variety of neurologic syndromes attributed to VZV infection have been described in HIV-infected patients, including multifocal leukoencephalitis, ventriculitis, myelitis, and myeloradiculitis, optic neuritis, cranial nerve palsies and focal brain stem lesions, and aseptic meningitis.[6,53–58] A chronic, progressive form of VZV encephalitis attributed to small vessel vasculopathy has been diagnosed in several AIDS patients.[59] Virtually all of these diagnoses of VZV neurologic diseases were made in AIDS patients with markedly depleted CD4+ lymphocytes. Approximately 30–40% of these patients had no recognized recent history of cutaneous VZV infection. In cases in which antecedent herpes zoster had been diagnosed, the skin lesions often preceded the neurologic symptoms by months.

Acute retinal necrosis (ARN) caused by VZV has previously been described in immunocompetent patients. More aggressive variants of this disease have been recognized in patients with AIDS and have been termed varicella-zoster virus retinitis (VZVR), progressive outer retinal necrosis (PORN), or rapidly progressive herpetic retinal necrosis (RPHRN).[60,61] The RPHRN syndrome is seen almost exclusively in AIDS patients with CD4+ lymphocyte counts of less than 100 cells/μL.[60,62–64] This form of VZV retinitis may occur concurrently with active herpes zoster or, more frequently, develops weeks or months after the acute episode of herpes zoster has resolved. RPHRN can occur after HZO or after herpes zoster involving a remote dermatome. The retinitis begins with multifocal necrotizing lesions involving the peripheral retina. Most patients present with unilateral involvement, but progression to bilateral disease occurs frequently.[60,61] The funduscopic examination reveals granular, yellowish, nonhemorrhagic lesions that rapidly extend and coalesce, often resulting in retinal detachment. There is a relative lack of intraocular inflammatory changes. RPHRN rapidly progresses to confluent full-thickness retinal necrosis (which differs from the slow progression seen with CMV retinitis) and results in blindness in 75–85% of involved eyes.[60,62] The etiologic role of VZV in most cases of RPHRN has been established by demonstrating the virus by culture or the polymerase chain reaction (PCR) from choroid, vitreous fluid, and retinal biopsies[65,66] HSV occasionally causes an identical syndrome.[60,67]

DIAGNOSIS OF VZV INFECTIONS

The appearance of varicella is quite distinctive, and a clinical diagnosis is usually accurate and reliable (Fig. 49-3). The presentation of an unvaccinated child with mild constitutional symptoms, a diffuse vesicular rash, and no history of chickenpox is strongly suggestive of the diagnosis, especially if there has been a documented exposure within the previous 2 weeks. Herpes zoster, with its characteristic vesicular rash, is also readily diagnosed on the basis of clinical appearance,

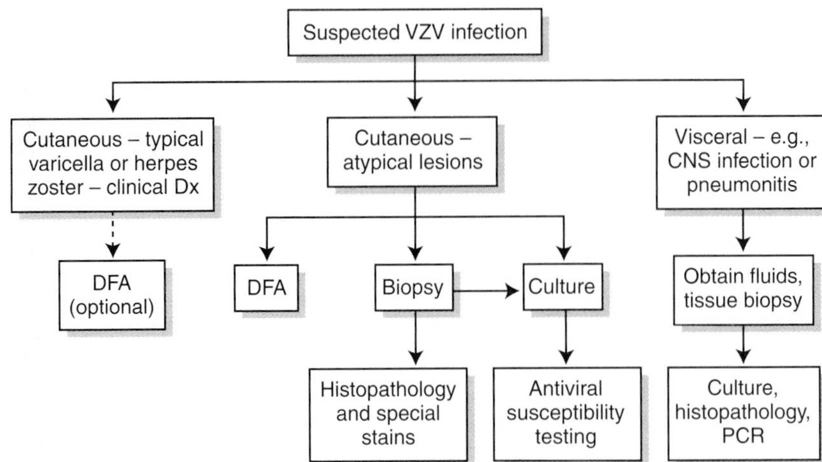

Figure 49-3 ■ Diagnostic approach to VZV infections in HIV-seropositive patients. DFA, direct fluorescent antigen (test).

although the diagnosis may be initially obscure in patients who present with dermatomal neuralgic pain prior to the development of skin lesions. The skin disease most commonly confused with herpes zoster is zosteriform HSV infection, which appears in a dermatome-like distribution (most commonly in the sacral area) and may closely mimic the appearance of shingles.

Serologic techniques can be used to determine susceptibility to VZV infection and to document rising antibody titers in patients with acute varicella. Serum immunoglobulin G (IgG) becomes detectable several days after the onset of varicella, with titers peaking at 2–3 weeks, so routine serologic tests provide only a retrospective diagnosis. Acute infection can be confirmed by VZV-specific serum IgM titers, but antigen detection techniques are usually faster and more reliable. Patients with herpes zoster are VZV seropositive at the time of disease onset, although most show a significant rise in antibody titer during the convalescence phase.[68] Elevated antibody titers in CSF can be measured to support the diagnosis of VZV CNS infection. A variety of methods have been used to detect VZV antibodies, but most laboratories have now adopted an ELISA or a latex agglutination (LA) assay for VZV serodiagnosis. The ELISA is capable of detecting IgG or IgM responses, is a reliable indicator of immune status following natural infection, and is readily automated. However, the ELISA may not be sufficiently sensitive to measure vaccine-induced immunity.[69] The LA assay is rapid, simple, inexpensive, and highly sensitive, but cannot be automated or used to detect IgM. The fluorescent antibody to membrane antigen (FAMA) test is also highly sensitive but not widely available.

Unlike HSV or CMV, VZV is not shed asymptomatically. Consequently, demonstration of VZV virions, antigens, or nucleic acids in tissues (other than sensory ganglia) or body fluids is diagnostic of active disease. VZV can be identified in infected tissues by histopathology or electron microscopy, but visualization of multinucleated giant cells with inclusion bodies or herpesvirus virions does not distinguish between VZV and HSV. Immunohistochemical staining of viral antigens can provide a more specific diagnosis. Direct fluorescent antigen (DFA) staining using fluorescein-conjugated monoclonal antibodies to detect VZV glycoproteins in infected epithelial cells is especially helpful for making a rapid diagnosis when the clinical presentation is atypical (Fig. 49-3). This simple, rapid technique is more sensitive than virus culture, especially in later stages of VZV infection when virus isolation becomes more difficult.[68] In a population of 92 HIV-infected adults with suspected herpes zoster, DFA and viral culture were positive in 85 of 92 (92%) and 60 of 92 (65%) patients, respectively.[68] To perform the DFA assay, epithelial cells are scraped from the base of a vesicle or ulcer with a scalpel blade, smeared on a glass slide, fixed with cold acetone, stained with fluorescein-conjugated monoclonal antibodies, and then examined using a fluorescence microscope. By using virus-specific monoclonal antibodies, HSV can be readily distinguished from VZV, making DFA staining a much more powerful technique than a simple Tzanck preparation.

The use of the PCR to detect VZV nucleic acids in clinical specimens has emerged as an important diagnostic tool and has replaced viral culture in many settings.[70,71] The PCR overcomes the difficulties inherent in culturing labile VZV and has been used successfully to detect viral DNA in cerebrospinal fluid (CSF) from patients with VZV encephalitis[53,72,73] and in ocular fluids and tissues from VZV retinitis cases.[66,74]

In the past, viral culture has been the benchmark method for diagnosing active VZV infection. VZV can be cultured by inoculating vesicular fluid onto monolayers of human fetal diploid kidney or lung cells. Unlike HSV, VZV is extremely labile, and every effort should be made to minimize the time spent for specimen transport and storage. Ideally, fluid should be aspirated from clear vesicles using a tuberculin syringe containing 0.2 mL of medium, inoculated directly into tissue culture at the bedside (or taken immediately to the laboratory), and then incubated at 36°C in 5% CO_2 atmosphere. If no vesicles or pustules are available for aspiration, the clinician should carefully remove overlying debris or crusts from

Antiviral Drugs for VZV Infections in AIDS Patients

Table 49-1

Drug	Indication	Dose[a]	Major Toxicities
Acyclovir	Varicella or herpes zoster	20 mg/kg (or 800 mg) PO five times daily until healed (>7 days)	None; minor nausea or headache
	Disseminated or visceral VZV infection	10 mg/kg IV q8 >7 days	Nephrotoxicity (rare), CNS disturbances (rare)
Famciclovir	Herpes zoster	500 mg PO q8h until healed (>7 days)	None; minor nausea or headache
Valacyclovir	Herpes zoster	1.0 g q8h until healed (>7 days)	? Associated with TTP/HUS; minor nausea or headache
Foscarnet	Acyclovir-resistant VZV infections	60–90 mg/kg IV q12h until healed (>10 days)	Nephrotoxicity (common), electrolyte disturbances (common), seizures, arrhythmias, anemia, genital ulcers

HUS, hemolytic-uremic syndrome; TTP, thrombotic thrombocytopenic purpura.

[a]Doses given are for adults with normal renal function.

the freshest lesions available, swab the underlying ulcers, and place the swab directly into viral transport medium for rapid delivery on ice to the laboratory. Characteristic cytopathic effects are usually seen in tissue culture in 3–7 days, although cultures should be held for 14 days before they are declared negative. The culture process can be accelerated by using centrifugation cultures in shell vials. Identification of the isolate can be confirmed by staining the monolayer with VZV-specific monoclonal antibodies. In general, viral culture for VZV is highly specific but slow, insensitive, and expensive. Culture remains essential if *in vitro* susceptibility testing of the VZV isolate is desired.

Diseases caused by strains of VZV resistant to acyclovir have been reported in a substantial number of HIV-seropositive patients. Resistance, which never occurs in immunocompetent patients, is usually seen in severely immunocompromised patients with extensive previous exposure to acyclovir or similar drugs. *In vitro* studies of acyclovir-resistant isolates have documented a variety of mutations in the thymidine kinase gene that result in production of an enzyme that is truncated and nonfunctional or has altered substrate specificity. Patients with VZV infections who fail to respond to conventional antiviral therapy or who present with chronic atypical lesions should have specimens submitted to a reference laboratory for VZV culture and drug-susceptibility testing. Isolates that are resistant to acyclovir are usually also resistant to drugs with similar mechanisms of action, including penciclovir and ganciclovir. VZV resistance to foscarnet and cidofovir, drugs that utilize different mechanisms of action, are rare.[75,76]

Diagnosing VZV infection of the CNS can be difficult, especially when there is no concomitant cutaneous disease. Examination of the CSF usually reveals a moderate lymphocytic pleocytosis, normal to moderately elevated protein, and normal glucose. The PCR for VZV DNA in CSF should be positive in more than 75% of cases.[52] In one series of 34 HIV-infected patients with VZV neurologic complications, the mean CSF white blood cell count was 126/μL, the mean protein concentration was 230 mg/dL, and the PCR was positive for VZV in all cases.[50] In patients with chronic VZV encephalitis, magnetic resonance imaging (MRI) may show a characteristic picture of multifocal lesions located in deep white matter and at the gray-white matter junction.[52,53,59]

THERAPY OF VZV INFECTIONS

Treatment of Varicella

Chickenpox is associated with low rates of morbidity and mortality among immunocompetent children, and supportive care is usually sufficient. Astringent soaks and antipyretics (e.g., acetaminophen) provide symptomatic relief. Aspirin (possibly associated with Reye syndrome) and nonsteroidal antiinflammatory drugs (possibly associated with an increased risk of necrotizing fasciitis) should be avoided. Trimming fingernails closely helps prevent bacterial superinfections caused by scratching the lesions. If bacterial cellulitis develops, antibiotics may be required. Oral acyclovir has been evaluated for treatment of uncomplicated varicella in immunocompetent children, adolescents, and adults. In these studies, initiation of acyclovir therapy within 24 h of rash onset reduced the time to cessation of new lesion formation, the number of lesions, and constitutional symptoms, including fever. The dose of oral acyclovir for chickenpox is 20 mg/kg (up to a maximum of 800 mg) five times daily (Table 49-1). Unlike acyclovir, valacyclovir, and famciclovir are not available as suspensions and have not been evaluated extensively for treatment of varicella, although the properties of these drugs suggest that they should be at least as effective as acyclovir. No controlled prospective

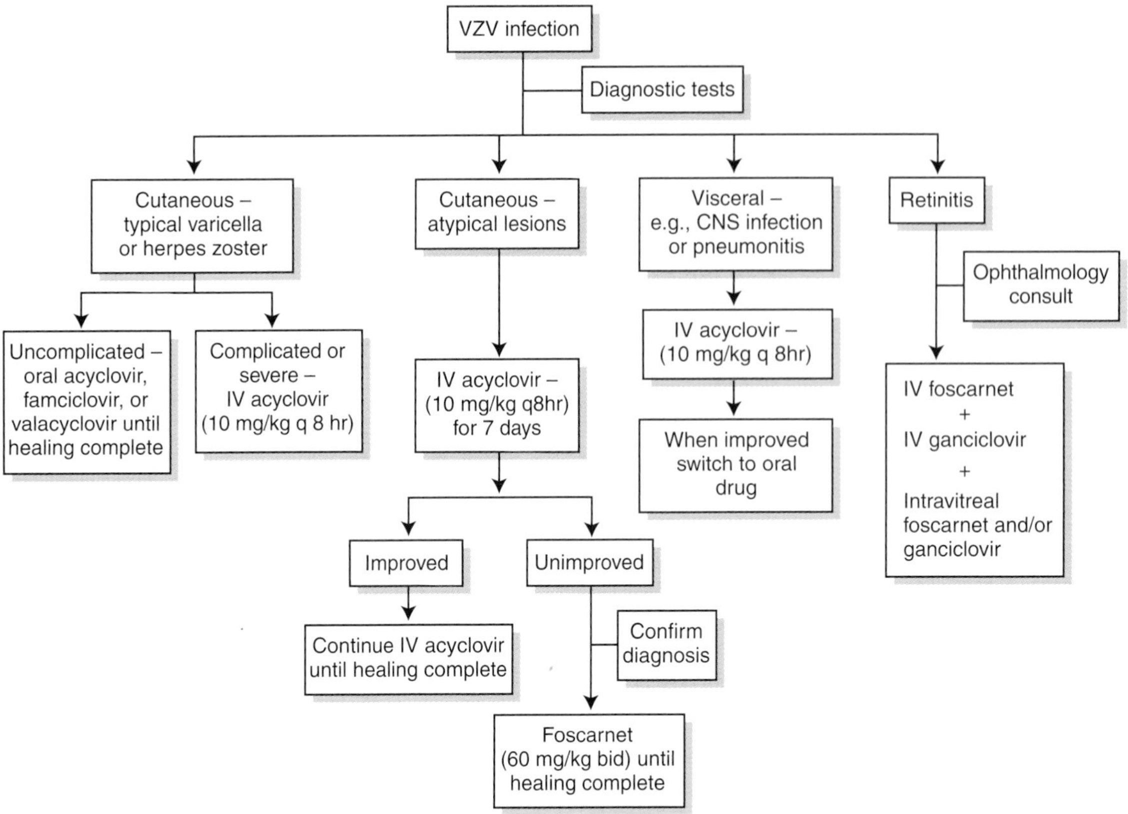

Figure 49-4 ■ Approach to therapy of VZV infections in HIV-seropositive patients.

studies of antiviral therapy for chickenpox in HIV-infected children have been reported, so recommendations must be derived from anecdotal experience or from data derived in other populations (Fig. 49-4). Most clinicians prescribe oral antiviral therapy, reserving intravenous acyclovir for patients with unusually severe or complicated infections.[4,29,77]

Treatment of Herpes Zoster

Three oral antiviral drugs are currently approved in the US for treating herpes zoster (Table 49-1). In the normal host, acyclovir, valacyclovir, and famciclovir have all been demonstrated to reduce the duration of viral shedding, decrease days of new lesion formation, accelerate the events of cutaneous healing, and limit the duration of pain when therapy is initiated within 72 h of the onset of herpes zoster.[78–80] Because of their superior pharmacokinetic properties, valacyclovir and famciclovir are currently considered the preferred drugs for herpes zoster.[81,82] Appropriate supportive care can help make patients with herpes zoster more comfortable. Skin lesions should be kept clean and dry to reduce the risk of bacterial superinfection. Astringent soaks (e.g., aluminum sulfate) may be soothing. Most patients with acute herpes zoster have significant pain and usually require treatment with opioid analgesics.

Prospectively acquired data to guide clinicians when selecting antiviral therapy for herpes zoster in HIV-seropositive patients are currently limited (Fig. 49-4). Nearly 300 HIV-infected patients with herpes zoster were enrolled in controlled studies comparing orally administered acyclovir (800 mg five times daily) with sorivudine (40 mg once daily).[41,83] Times to cessation of new vesicle formation, total crusting, and resolution of zoster-associated pain were 3–4 days, 7–8 days, and ~60 days, respectively.[41] Although sorivudine was not commercially developed, these studies clearly confirmed the efficacy and safety of oral antiviral therapy for herpes zoster in patients with HIV infection. Famciclovir was judged to be effective and safe for herpes zoster in AIDS patients when evaluated in a small, open-label clinical trial.[84] Valacyclovir has not been systematically evaluated as a treatment for herpes zoster in HIV-infected patients, although anecdotal clinical experience suggests therapeutic benefit. Long-term administration of antiherpesvirus drugs to prevent recurrences of herpes zoster is not routinely recommended.

The value of anti-VZV therapy in patients presenting with herpes zoster of more than 72 h duration has not been determined. Patients who have signs of ongoing VZV replication (evidenced by new vesicle formation) may benefit from antiviral therapy even when initiated after 72 h of illness. Patients who have HZO should also be treated to reduce the risk of serious ocular complications, even when presenting beyond 72 h. Antiviral therapy is unlikely to be useful for patients whose lesions are crusted or scabbed. Because of the documented risk of relapsing infection, VZV disease in HIV-seropositive patients should be treated until all lesions are completely resolved, which is often longer than the standard 7–10 day course. What impact anti-VZV therapy may have on the risk of subsequent complications such as CNS infection or retinitis is unknown. Adjunctive therapy of herpes zoster with corticosteroids has not been evaluated in HIV-infected patients and is not currently recommended.[85] The effect of therapy on *zoster sine herpete* is also not established, although some clinicians advocate a trial of antiviral therapy in an attempt to ameliorate symptoms.

Most clinicians select intravenous acyclovir as the drug of choice to treat severe or complicated herpes zoster in HIV-infected patients, although this approach has not been studied in a prospective fashion. The literature contains case reports documenting successful therapy of neurologic complications, including myelitis, with intravenous acyclovir.[86,87] Some investigators have recommended intravenous acyclovir for initial therapy of HZO in HIV-infected patients, although oral therapy appears adequate in most cases.

Optimal antiviral therapy for VZV-induced, RPHRN remains undefined. Responses to intravenous acyclovir or ganciclovir have been inconsistent and disappointing with 49–67% of involved eyes progressing to no light perception.[61,88] Several case reports have documented improved preservation of vision in patients treated with a combination of intravenous ganciclovir alongwith foscarnet, with or without intravitreal antiviral drugs.[89–94] Cidofovir has also been used successfully in a small number of patients.[95,96] The optimal duration of induction therapy and options for long-term antiviral maintenance therapy have not been established.

Management of Acyclovir-Resistant VZV Infections

The first acyclovir-resistant isolate of VZV was recovered from an HIV-infected child in 1988.[97] Additional case reports have provided a better picture of the characteristic features of disease caused by acyclovir-resistant VZV.[98,99] Virtually all cases have been described in AIDS patients with very low CD4+ T-lymphocyte counts, and most patients had been treated previously with acyclovir. Most isolates resistant to acyclovir are also resistant to valacyclovir, famciclovir, penciclovir, and ganciclovir, all of which depend on viral thymidine kinase for activation. A strong association exists between acyclovir-resistant VZV and the presence of atypical skin lesions.[97,98] One report described four HIV-seropositive adults undergoing chronic suppressive acyclovir therapy who developed disseminated hyperkeratotic papules that failed to respond to acyclovir.[98] *In vitro* susceptibility testing confirmed that the VZV isolates were acyclovir-resistant, with a mean IC_{50} for acyclovir of 20 µg/mL, compared with 0.75 µg/mL for reference strain VZVOka.[98] Patients with chronic or atypical VZV-positive lesions merit a thorough evaluation for the possibility of acyclovir-resistant virus. In addition, the possibility of acyclovir resistance should be strongly considered in patients who develop VZV disease while undergoing suppressive ganciclovir therapy for CMV disease.

The drug of choice for treatment of acyclovir-resistant VZV disease is foscarnet, a viral DNA polymerase inhibitor that is not dependent on thymidine kinase for activation.[100] In a series of 13 patients with AIDS and acyclovir-resistant VZV infection treated with intravenous foscarnet, 10 patients (77%) had complete lesion healing after a mean of 17.8 days of therapy.[100] Of the 10 responding patients, five subsequently had a herpes zoster recurrence after a median of 110 days. Most cases of disease caused by acyclovir-resistant VZV have been limited to cutaneous involvement, although a few instances of visceral infection caused by acyclovir-resistant VZV have been reported, including cases of retinal necrosis[101] and meningoradiculitis.[102]

Fortunately, VZV isolates resistant to both acyclovir and foscarnet have been encountered infrequently.[75] The molecular biology of these dually resistant isolates has not been fully explored, but a mutation in the viral DNA polymerase could account for both acyclovir and foscarnet resistance.[76] Cidofovir would likely retain activity against these isolates and could be tried in patients with disease caused by dually resistant VZV, although there are no data available to validate this approach.

Although the mechanisms that lead to the development of acyclovir resistance are incompletely understood, clinical data indicate that many cases are associated with inadequate dosing of acyclovir for either acute therapy or long-term suppression, possibly allowing selection of thymidine kinase-deficient mutants. Clinicians using acyclovir or related drugs for treatment of varicella or herpes zoster in AIDS patients should utilize the full therapeutic dose (which is higher than the dose required to treat HSV infections) and continue therapy until VZV lesions have completely resolved (Table 49-1).

PREVENTION OF VZV INFECTIONS

Serologic Testing

The presence of serum VZV-specific IgG indicates that an individual has previously been infected or vaccinated and is not at risk for primary varicella. The more sensitive latex agglutination assay (rather than ELISA) must be used to detect serum IgG reliably after varicella vaccination. The magnitude of the anti-VZV antibody titer does not predict risk for developing herpes zoster. Serologic surveys have shown that ~95% of HIV-infected adults have VZV antibodies. Children or adults with no clinical history of chickenpox, herpes zoster, or varicella vaccination can be tested to determine susceptibility.

Varicella Vaccine

A live, attenuated varicella vaccine containing VZVOka strain has been available for use in the US since 1995. The varicella vaccine is safe and effective for healthy children. The vaccine provides 70–90% protection against infection and 95% protection against severe disease for at least 10 years.[103,104] Investigations of the role of varicella vaccine in HIV-seropositive persons are ongoing. In a study of 41 HIV-infected children with relatively well-preserved immunity, varicella vaccine was well tolerated and did not affect the HIV viral load.[105] Two months after the second dose of vaccine, 60% of recipients had detectable serum anti-VZV antibody, and 83% had a positive response in a lymphocyte proliferation assay against VZV antigen.[105] On the basis of these data and in view of the potential morbidity caused by chickenpox, advisory groups now recommend that HIV-seropositive children who are asymptomatic and not significantly immunosuppressed (CDC immunologic category 1) should receive varicella vaccine.[69,106,107] Little information is available regarding the safety and efficacy of varicella vaccination in HIV-seropositive adults. HIV-seronegative/VZV-seronegative household contacts of HIV-seropositive/VZV-seronegative individuals should be vaccinated.[108] A vaccine containing an increased dose of VZVOka has been shown to significantly reduce the frequency and severity of herpes zoster in older immunocompetent adults, but has not been evaluated in HIV-seropositive patients.[109]

Postexposure Prophylaxis

Persons infected with HIV who are VZV seronegative should receive prophylactic treatment after close exposure to an individual with active VZV disease. The goal is to prevent or modify symptomatic chickenpox. Three options can be considered: passive immunoprophylaxis with immune globulin; chemoprophylaxis with an antiviral drug (e.g., acyclovir); or postexposure vaccination.

Passive Immunoprophylaxis

Advisory committees have recommended administration of varicella-zoster immune globulin (VZIG) to VZV-seronegative/HIV-seropositive children or adults who have a recognized close exposure to VZV (to a patient with either chickenpox or herpes zoster).[106–108] In many cases VZIG administration does not prevent infection in the susceptible host but delays the onset of varicella and reduces the severity of the resulting illness.[29] Placebo-controlled trials in other (non-AIDS) immunocompromised children have demonstrated that VZIG ameliorates the severity of chickenpox and reduces the risk of disseminated infection by ~75%. For maximal efficacy, VZIG must be given as soon as possible after exposure (within 96 h). VZIG is administered by deep intramuscular injection at a dose of 125 units/10 kg (to a maximum of 625 units). Intravenous immunoglobulin (IVIG) also contains substantial amounts of VZV-specific IgG and can be used if VZIG is not immediately available. Unfortunately, if the VZV exposure is unrecognized (which is often the case), the opportunity for VZIG administration is missed. The efficacy of VZIG prophylaxis in HIV-seropositive children or adults has not been evaluated prospectively. Licensed VZIG is currently nearly depleted. However, a new investigational varicella-zoster immune globulin (VariZIGTM) is available from FFF Enterprises (Temecula, California) through an IND submitted to FDA.[110]

Chemoprophylaxis

Prophylactic administration of acyclovir following VZV exposure has been studied to a limited extent in susceptible immunocompetent children, but not in children with HIV infection. In studies of healthy children conducted in Japan, varicella developed in 16% of the children prophylactically treated with acyclovir and in 100% of the children in the control group.[111] About 80% of children prophylactically treated with acyclovir subsequently seroconverted, indicating VZV infection without significant disease.[112] However, additional data are required before this approach can be routinely recommended in either immunocompetent or immunocompromised populations. A suggested (but unvalidated) regimen is acyclovir 200 mg orally four or five times daily for 21 days beginning 5 days after exposure.[108]

Postexposure Vaccination

Small clinical trials in immunocompetent populations have shown that postexposure immunization of susceptible children and adults can prevent varicella.[113,114] Administration of varicella vaccine to a VZV-seronegative individual within 3–4 days of VZV exposure provides a protective (or partially protective) immune response. Up to one-half of patients receiving a postexposure vaccination may still develop some signs or symptoms of chickenpox, but the disease manifestations are usually mild. This approach may be appropriate for HIV-infected patients who are asymptomatic and not significantly immunosuppressed but has not been evaluated prospectively. In appropriate populations, postexposure VZV vaccination may prove to be more effective and less expensive than preemptive antiviral therapy.

REFERENCES

1. Stewart JA, Reef SE, Pellett PE, et al. Herpesvirus infections in persons infected with human immunodeficiency virus. Clin Infect Dis 21(Suppl 1):S114, 1995.
2. Vafai A, Berger M. Zoster in patients infected with HIV: a review. Am J Med Sci 321:372, 2001.
3. Tyndall MW, Nasio J, Agoki E, et al. Herpes zoster as the initial presentation of human immunodeficiency virus type 1 infection in Kenya. Clin Infect Dis 21:1035, 1995.
4. Gershon AA, Mervish N, LaRussa P, et al. Varicella-zoster virus infection in children with underlying human immunodeficiency virus infection. J Infect Dis 176:1496, 1997.
5. Holmberg S, Buchbinder SP, Conley LJ, et al. The spectrum of medical conditions and symptoms before acquired immunodeficiency syndrome in homosexual and bisexual men. Am J Epidemiol 141:395, 1995.
6. Glesby MJ, Moore RD, Chaisson RE. Clinical spectrum of herpes zoster in adults infected with human immunodeficiency virus. Clin Infect Dis 21:370, 1995.
7. Veenstra J, Krol A, Van Praag RME, et al. Herpes zoster, immunological deterioration, and disease progression. AIDS 9:1153, 1995.
8. Engels EA, Rosenberg PS, Biggar RJ. Zoster incidence in human immunodeficiency virus-infected hemophiliacs and homosexual men, 1984–1997. District of Columbia Gay

Cohort Study; Multicenter Hemophilia Cohort Study. J Infect Dis 180:1784, 1999.
9. Vanhems P, Voisin L, Gayet-Ageron A, et al. The incidence of herpes zoster is less likely than other opportunistic infections to be reduced by highly active antiretroviral therapy. J Acquir Immune Defic Syndr 38:111, 2005.
10. Keiser P, Jodcus J, Horton H, et al. Prednisone therapy is not associated with increased risk of herpetic infections in patients infected with human immunodeficiency virus. Clin Infect Dis 23:201, 1996.
11. Alliegro MB, Dorrucci M, Pezzotti P, et al. Herpes zoster and progression to AIDS in a cohort of individuals who seroconverted to human immunodeficiency virus. Clin Infect Dis 23:990, 1996.
12. McNulty A, Li Y, Radtke U, et al. Herpes zoster and the stage and prognosis of HIV-1 infection. Genitourin Med 73:467, 1997.
13. Martinez E, Gatell J, Moran Y, et al. High incidence of herpes zoster in patients with AIDS soon after therapy with protease inhibitors. Clin Infect Dis 27:1510, 1998.
14. Aldeen T, Hay P, Davidson F, et al. Herpes zoster infection in HIV-seropositive patients associated with highly active antiretroviral therapy. AIDS 12:1719, 1998.
15. Domingo P, Torres OH, Ris J, et al. Herpes zoster as an immune reconstitution disease after initiation of combination antiretroviral therapy in patients with human immunodeficiency virus type-1 infection. Am J Med 110:605, 2001.
16. Tangsinmankong N, Kamchaisatian W, Lujan-Zilbermann J, et al. Varicella zoster as a manifestation of immune restoration disease in HIV-infected children. J Allergy Clin Immunol 113:742, 2004.
17. French MA, Price P, Stone SF. Immune restoration disease after antiretroviral therapy. AIDS 18:1615, 2004.
18. Seward J, Watson B, Peterson C, et al. Decline in varicella incidence and hospitalizations in sentinel surveillance areas in the United States, 1995–2000. Presented at the Fourth International Conference on Varicella, Herpes Zoster, and Post-Herpetic Neuralgia, LaJolla, CA, 2001, abstract 11.
19. Insinga RP, Itzler RF, Pellissier JM, et al. The incidence of herpes zoster in a United States administrative database. J Gen Intern Med 20:748, 2005.
20. Donahue JG, Choo PW, Manson JE, et al. The incidence of herpes zoster. Arch Intern Med 155:1605, 1995.
21. Moore PS, Gao SJ, Dominguez G, et al. Primary characterization of a herpesvirus agent associated with Kaposi's sarcoma. J Virol 70:549, 1996.
22. Morgan D, Mahe C, Malamba S, et al. Herpes zoster and HIV-1 infection in a rural Ugandan cohort. AIDS 15:223, 2001.
23. Buchbinder SP, Katz MH, Hessol NA, et al. Herpes zoster and human immunodeficiency virus infection. J Infect Dis 166:1153, 1992.
24. Naburi AE, Leppard B. Herpes zoster and HIV infection in Tanzania. Int J STD AIDS 11:254, 2000.
25. Derryck A, LaRussa P, Steinberg S, et al. Varicella and zoster in children with human immunodeficiency virus infection. Pediatr Infect Dis J 17:931, 1998.
26. Rongkavilit C, Mitchell CD, Nachman S. Varicella zoster infection in HIV-infected children. Paediatr Drugs 2:291, 2000.
27. Geoghagen M, Pierre R, Evans-Gilbert T, et al. Tuberculosis, chickenpox and scabies outbreaks in an orphanage for children with HIV/AIDS in Jamaica. West Indian Med J 53:346, 2004.
28. Zampogna JC, Flowers FP. Persistent verrucous varicella as the initial manifestation of HIV infection. J Am Acad Dermatol 44:391, 2001.
29. von Seidlein L, Gilette SG, Bryson Y, et al. Frequent recurrence and persistence of varicella-zoster virus infections in children infected with human immunodeficiency virus type 1. J Pediatr 128:52, 1996.
30. Popara M, Pendle S, Sacks L, et al. Varicella pneumonia in patients with HIV/AIDS. Int J Infect Dis 6:6, 2002.
31. Gershon AA. Prevention and treatment of VZV infections in patients with HIV. Herpes 8:32, 2001.
32. Kelley R, Mancao M, Sawyer M, et al. Varicella in children with perinatally acquired human immunodeficiency virus infection. J Pediatr 124:271, 1994.
33. Fraisse P, Faller M, Rey D, et al. Recurrent varicella pneumonia complicating an endogenous reactivation of chickenpox in an HIV-infected adult patient. Eur Respir J 11:776, 1998.
34. Wallace MR, Hooper DG, Pyne JM, et al. Varicella immunity and clinical disease in HIV-infected adults. South Med J 87:74, 1994.
35. Baran J, Khatib R. Recrudescence of initial cutaneous lesions after crusting of chickenpox in an adult with advanced AIDS suggests prolonged local viral persistence. Clin Infect Dis 24:741, 1997.
36. Gnann JW Jr, Whitley RJ. Clinical practice. Herpes zoster. N Engl J Med 347:340, 2002.
37. Veenstra J, van Praag RM, Krol A, et al. Complications of varicella zoster virus reactivation in HIV-infected homosexual men. AIDS 10:393, 1996.
38. Sellitti TP, Huang AJW, Schiffman J, et al. Association of herpes zoster ophthalmicus with acquired immunodeficiency syndrome and acute retinal necrosis. Am J Ophthalmol 116:297, 1993.
39. Bayu S, Alemayehu W. Clinical profile of herpes zoster ophthalmicus in Ethiopians. Clin Infect Dis 24:1256, 1997.
40. Chern KC, Conrad D, Holland GN, et al. Chronic varicella-zoster virus epithelial keratitis in patients with acquired immunodeficiency syndrome. Arch Ophthalmol 116:1011, 1998.
41. Gnann JW, Crumpacker CS, Lalezari JP, et al. Sorivudine versus acyclovir for treatment of dermatomal herpes zoster in human immunodeficiency virus-infected patients: results from a randomized, controlled clinical trial. Antimicrob Agents Chemother 42:1139, 1998.
42. Freifeld AG, Marchigiani D, Lewis L, et al. Frequently recurrent zoster in children with AIDS. Presented at 35th ICAAC, San Francisco, 1995, abstract H90.
43. Cohen JI, Brunell PA, Straus SE, et al. Recent advances in varicella-zoster virus infection. Ann Intern Med 130:922, 1999.
44. Kimya-Asadi A, Tausk FA, Nousari HC. Verrucous varicella zoster virus lesions associated with acquired immunodeficiency syndrome. Int J Dermatol 39:77, 2000.
45. Castanet J, Rodots S, Lacour JP, et al. Chronic varicella presenting as disseminated pinpoint-sized papules in a man infected with the human immunodeficiency virus. Dermatology 192:84, 1996.
46. Nikkels AF, Rentier B, Piérard GE. Chronic varicella-zoster virus skin lesions in patients with human immunodeficiency virus are related to decreased expression of gE and gB. J Infect Dis 176:261, 1997.
47. Cohen PR, Beltrani VP, Grossman ME. Disseminated herpes zoster in patients with human immunodeficiency virus infection. Am J Med 84:1076, 1988.
48. Cohen PR, Grossman ME. Clinical features of human immunodeficiency virus-associated disseminated herpes zoster virus infection-a review of the literature. Clin Exp Dermatol 14:273, 1989.
49. Harrison RA, Soong S, Weiss HL, et al. A mixed model for factors predictive of pain in AIDS patients with herpes zoster. J Pain Symptom Manage 17:410, 1999.
50. De La Blanchardiere A, Rozenberg F, Caumes E, et al. Neurological complications of varicella-zoster virus infection in adults with human immunodeficiency virus infection. Scand J Infect Dis 32:263, 2000.
51. Gnann JW Jr. Varicella-zoster virus: atypical presentations and unusual complications. J Infect Dis 186:S91, 2002.

52. Iten A, Chatelard P, Vuadens P, et al. Impact of cerebrospinal fluid PCR on the management of HIV-infected patients with varicella-zoster virus infection of the central nervous system. J Neurovirol 5:172, 1999.
53. Brown M, Scarborough M, Brink N, et al. Varicella zoster virus-associated neurological disease in HIV-infected patients. Int J STD AIDS 12:79, 2001.
54. Manian FA, Kindred M, Fulling KH. Chronic varicella-zoster virus myelitis without cutaneous eruption in a patient with AIDS: report of a fatal case. Clin Infect Dis 21:986, 1995.
55. Kenyon LC, Dulaney E, Montone KT, et al. Varicella-zoster ventriculo-encephalitis and spinal cord infarction in a patient with AIDS. Acta Neuropathol (Berl) 92:202, 1996.
56. Liu JZ, Brown P, Tselis A. Unilateral retrobulbar optic neuritis due to varicella zoster virus in a patient with AIDS: a case report and review of the literature. J Neurol Sci 237:97, 2005.
57. Franco-Paredes C, Bellehemeur T, Merchant A, et al. Aseptic meningitis and optic neuritis preceding varicella-zoster progressive outer retinal necrosis in a patient with AIDS. AIDS 16:1045, 2002.
58. Moulignier A, Pialoux G, Dega H, et al. Brain stem encephalitis due to varicella-zoster virus in a patient with AIDS. Clin Infect Dis 20:1378, 1995.
59. Gilden DH, Kleinschmidt-DeMaster BK, LaGuardia JJ, et al. Neurologic complications of the reactivation of varicella-zoster virus. New Engl J Med 342:635, 2000.
60. Ormerod LD, Larkin JA, Margo CA, et al. Rapidly progressive herpetic retinal necrosis: a blinding disease characteristic of advanced AIDS. Clin Infect Dis 26:34, 1998.
61. Moorthy RS, Weinberg DV, Teich SA, et al. Management of varicella zoster virus retinitis in AIDS. Br J Ophthalmol 81:189, 1997.
62. Batisse D, Eliaszewicz M, Zazoan L, et al. Acute retinal necrosis in the course of AIDS: study of 26 cases. AIDS 10:55, 1996.
63. Miller RF, Brink NS, Cartledge J, et al. Necrotising herpetic retinopathy in patients with advance HIV disease. Genitourin Med 73:462, 1997.
64. Purdy KW, Heckenlively JR, Church JA, et al. Progressive outer retinal necrosis caused by varicella-zoster virus in children with acquired immunodeficiency syndrome. Pediatr Infect Dis J 22:384, 2003.
65. Garweg J, Böhnke M. Varicella-zoster virus is strongly associated with atypical necrotizing herpetic retinopathies. Clin Infect Dis 24:603, 1997.
66. Short GA, Margolis TP, Kuppermann BD, et al. A polymerase chain reaction-based assay for diagnosing varicella-zoster virus retinitis in patients with acquired immunodeficiency syndrome. Am J Ophthalmol 123:157, 1997.
67. Kashiwase M, Sata T, Yamauchi Y, et al. Progressive outer retinal necrosis caused by herpes simplex virus type 1 in a patient with acquired immunodeficiency syndrome. Ophthalmology 107:790, 2000.
68. Dahl H, Marcoccia J, Linde A. Antigen detection: the method of choice in comparison with virus isolation and serology for laboratory diagnosis of herpes zoster in human immunodeficiency virus-infected patient. J Clin Microbiol 35:345, 1997.
69. American Academy of Pediatrics Committee on Infectious Diseases. Varicella vaccine update. Pediatrics 105:136, 2000.
70. Stranska R, Schuurman R, de Vos M, et al. Routine use of a highly automated and internally controlled real-time PCR assay for the diagnosis of herpes simplex and varicella-zoster virus infections. J Clin Virol 30:39, 2004.
71. O'Neill HJ, Wyatt DE, Coyle PV, et al. Real-time nested multiplex PCR for the detection of herpes simplex virus types 1 and 2 and varicella zoster virus. J Med Virol 71:557, 2003.
72. Burke DG, Kalayjian RC, Vann VR, et al. Polymerase chain reaction and clinical significance of varicella-zoster virus in cerebrospinal fluid from human immunodeficiency virus-infected patients. J Infect Dis 176:1080, 1997.
73. Cinque P, Bossolasco S, Vago L, et al. Varicella-zoster virus (VZV) DNA in cerebrospinal fluid of patients infected with human immunodeficiency virus: VZV disease of the central nervous system or subclinical reactivation of VZV infection? Clin Infect Dis 25:634, 1997.
74. Danise A, Cinque P, Vergani S, et al. Use of polymerase chain reaction assays of aqueous humor in the differential diagnosis of retinitis in patients infected with human immunodeficiency virus. Clin Infect Dis 24:1100, 1997.
75. Fillet A-M, Visse B, Caumes E, et al. Foscarnet-resistant multidermatomal zoster in a patient with AIDS. Clin Infect Dis 21:1348, 1995.
76. Visse B, Dumont B, Huraux JM, et al. Single amino acid change in DNA polymerase is associated with foscarnet resistance in a varicella-zoster virus strain recovered from a patient with AIDS. J Infect Dis 178(Suppl 1):S55, 1998.
77. Arvin AM. Antiviral therapy for varicella and herpes zoster. Semin Pediatr Infect Dis 13:12, 2002.
78. Wood MJ, Kay R, Dworkin RH, et al. Oral acyclovir therapy accelerates pain resolution in patients with herpes zoster: a meta-analysis of placebo-controlled trials. Clin Infect Dis 22:341, 1996.
79. Beutner KR, Friedman DJ, Forszpaniak C, et al. Valaciclovir compared with acyclovir for improved therapy for herpes zoster in immunocompetent adults. Antimicrob Agents Chemother 39:1546, 1995.
80. Tyring S, Barbarash RA, Nahlik JE, et al. Famciclovir for the treatment of acute herpes zoster: effects on acute disease and post-herpetic neuralgia: a randomized, double-blind, placebo-controlled trial. Ann Int Med 123:89, 1995.
81. Tyring SK, Beutner KR, Tucker BA, et al. Antiviral therapy for herpes zoster: randomized, controlled clinical trial of valacyclovir and famciclovir therapy in immunocompetent patients 50 years and older. Arch Fam Med 9:863, 2000.
82. Benson CA, Kaplan JE, Masur H, et al. Treating opportunistic infections among HIV-exposed and infected children: recommendations from CDC, the National Institutes of Health, and the Infectious Diseases Society of America. MMWR Recomm Rep 53:1, 2004.
83. Bodsworth NJ, Boag F, Burdge D, et al. Evaluation of sorivudine (BV-araU) versus acyclovir in the treatment of acute localized herpes zoster in human immunodeficiency virus-infected adults. J Infect Dis 176:103, 1997.
84. Sullivan M, Skiest D, Signs D, et al. Famciclovir in the management of acute herpes zoster (HZ) in the HIV-positive patients. Presented at the Fourth Conference on Retroviruses and Opportunistic Infections, Washington, DC, 1997, abstract 704.
85. Whitley RJ, Weiss H, Gnann JW, et al. Acyclovir with and without prednisone for the treatment of herpes zoster. A randomized, placebo-controlled trial. The National Institute of Allergy and Infectious Diseases Collaborative Antiviral Study Group. Ann Intern Med 125:376, 1996.
86. de Silva SM, Mark AS, Gilden DH, et al. Zoster myelitis: improvement with antiviral therapy in two cases. Neurology 47:929, 1996.
87. Lionnet F, Pulik M, Genet P, et al. Myelitis due to varicella-zoster virus in 2 patients with AIDS: successful treatment with acyclovir. Clin Infect Dis 22:138, 1996.
88. Johnston WH, Holland GN, Engstrom RE, et al. Recurrence of presumed varicella-zoster virus retinopathy in patients with acquired immune deficiency syndrome. Am J Ophthalmol 116:42, 1993.
89. Scott IU, Luu KM, Davis JL. Intravitreal antivirals in the management of patients with acquired immunodeficiency syndrome with progressive outer retinal necrosis. Arch Ophthalmol 120:1219, 2002.

90. Galindez OA, Sabates NR, Whitacre MW, et al. Rapidly progressive outer retinal necrosis caused by varicella zoster virus in a patient infected with human immunodeficiency virus. Clin Infect Dis 22:149, 1996.
91. Perez-Blazquez E, Traspas R, Mendez MI, et al. Intravitreal ganciclovir treatment in progressive outer retinal necrosis. Am J Ophthalmol 124:418, 1997.
92. Ciulla TA, Rutledge BK, Morley MG, et al. The progressive outer retinal necrosis syndrome: successful treatment with combination antiviral therapy. Ophthalmic Surg Lasers 29:198, 1998.
93. Spaide RF, Martin DF, Teich SA, et al. Successful treatment of progressive outer retinal necrosis syndrome. Retina 16:479, 1996.
94. Meffert SA, Kertes PJ, Lim PL, et al. Successful treatment of progressive outer retinal necrosis using high-dose intravitreal ganciclovir. Retina 17:560, 1997.
95. Schliefer K, Gumbel HO, Rockstroh JK, et al. Management of progressive outer retinal necrosis with cidofovir in a human immunodeficiency virus-infected patient. Clin Infect Dis 29:684, 1999.
96. Zambarakji HJ, Obi AA, Mitchell SM. Successful treatment of varicella zoster virus retinitis with aggressive intravitreal and systemic antiviral therapy. Ocul Immunol Inflamm 10:41, 2002.
97. Pahwa S, Biron K, Lim W, et al. Continuous varicella-zoster infection associated with acyclovir resistance in a child with AIDS. J Am Med Assoc 260:2879, 1988.
98. Jacobson MA, Berger TG, Fikrig S, et al. Acyclovir-resistant varicella zoster virus infection after chronic oral acyclovir therapy in patients with the acquired immunodeficiency syndrome (AIDS). Ann Intern Med 112:187, 1990.
99. Bernhard P, Obel N. Chronic ulcerating acyclovir-resistant varicella zoster lesions in an AIDS patient. Scand J Infect Dis 27:623, 1995.
100. Breton G, Fillet AM, Katlama C, et al. Acyclovir-resistant herpes zoster in human immunodeficiency virus-infected patients: results of foscarnet therapy. Clin Infect Dis 27:1525, 1998.
101. Wunderli W, Miner R, Wintsch J, et al. Outer retinal necrosis due to a strain of varicella-zoster virus resistant to acyclovir, ganciclovir, and sorivudine. Clin Infect Dis 22:864, 1996.
102. Snoeck R, Gérard M, Sadzot-Delvaux C, et al. Meningoradiculitis due to acyclovir-resistant varicella-zoster virus in a patient with AIDS [letter]. J Infect Dis 168:1330, 1993.
103. Vazquez M, LaRussa PS, Gershon AA, et al. The effectiveness of the varicella vaccine in clinical practice. N Engl J Med 344:955, 2001.
104. White CJ. Varicella-zoster virus vaccine. Clin Infect Dis 24:753, 1997.
105. Levin MJ, Gershon AA, Weinberg A, et al. Immunization of HIV-infected children with varicella vaccine. J Pediatr 139:305, 2001.
106. Centers for Disease Control. Prevention of varicella. Update recommendations of the Advisory Committee on Immunization Practices (ACIP). MMWR 48:1, 1999.
107. Kaplan JE, Masur H, Holmes KK. Guidelines for preventing opportunistic infections among HIV-infected persons – 2002. Recommendations of the U.S. Public Health Service and the Infectious Diseases Society of America. MMWR Recomm Rep 51:1, 2002.
108. Kaplan JE, Masur H, Holmes KK, et al. An overview of the 1999 US Public Health Service/Infectious Diseases Society of America guidelines for preventing opportunistic infections in human immunodeficiency virus-infected persons. Clin Infect Dis 30(Suppl 1):S15, 2000.
109. Oxman MN, Levin MJ, Johnson GR, et al. A vaccine to prevent herpes zoster and postherpetic neuralgia in older adults. N Engl J Med 352:2271, 2005.
110. VariZIG™, MMWR Early release, 24 Feb 2006/55;1–2.
111. Asano Y, Yoshikawa T, Suga S, et al. Postexposure prophylaxis of varicella in family contacts by oral acyclovir. Pediatrics 92:219, 1993.
112. Suga S, Yoshikawa T, Ozaki T, et al. Effect of oral acyclovir against primary and secondary viraemia in incubation period of varicella. Arch Dis Child 69:639, 1993.
113. Salzman MB, Garcia C. Postexposure varicella vaccination in siblings of children with active varicella. Pediatr Infect Dis J 17:256, 1998.
114. Watson B, Seward J, Yang A, et al. Postexposure effectiveness of varicella vaccine. Pediatrics 105:84, 2000.

Chapter 50

Cytomegalovirus Disease

Paul D. Griffiths, MD, DSc, Michael A. Polis, MD, MPH

Cytomegalovirus (CMV) is a common infection in the general community, with 60% of adults in developed countries typically seropositive, rising to 90–100% in developing countries and in poorer socioeconomic groups within developed countries. CMV is highly immunogenic and a considerable proportion of the human immune response is directed to keeping this virus suppressed into latency. It follows that end-organ disease due to CMV occurs late in the course of human immunodeficiency virus (HIV) infection, once HIV has progressively damaged immune capability. The increased use of highly active antiretroviral therapy (HAART) for the treatment of HIV infection has led to improved immunocompetence and a decrease in the incidence of opportunistic infections, including CMV, in persons with HIV infection.[1] Immune reconstitution due to HAART is the most important therapeutic intervention for prevention and for long-term management of established CMV disease in persons with HIV infection. However, CMV-associated diseases are still seen for a variety of reasons (see Table 50-1).

PATHOGEN

CMV was first isolated in 1956 using the 'new technology' of cell culture *in vitro*. The only cells to support growth were human fibroblasts and the evolution of cytopathic effect in these cells was slow. This slow growth became part of the definition of the *Betaherpesvirinae* subfamily of *Herpesviridae* of which CMV is the prototype member. This slow growth *in vitro,* coupled with the absence of overt disease in people with normal immunity and restriction of disease to those with impaired immunity such as the fetus or allograft recipient, led to the impression that CMV is a virus of low inherent pathogenicity. The application of more modern technology in the form of quantitative polymerase chain reaction (PCR) to measure changes in viral load directly in humans[2] has shown that this impression is false and is an artifact of propagating the virus in fibroblasts *in vitro*.

Studies of CMV titer measured in the urine of children with congenital CMV first reported in 1975 that CMV disease was associated with a high viral load.[3] The implication from this report, that CMV disease developed once a threshold value of viral load had been crossed, was confirmed in 1997 in renal allograft patients when multivariate statistical analyses showed that a high viral load explained the previously recognized risk factors of viremia (detected by cell culture) and seropositive donor serostatus.[4] The same was true when CMV viral load was measured in the blood of renal transplant recipients and the measurement of such viremia (viremia throughout this chapter refers to virus detected in the blood by PCR) completely replaced detection of CMV in urine because viremia has a closer correlation with disease events.[5–7] Viremia was also strongly associated with CMV disease in liver transplant patients and stem cell transplant patients where

Table 50-1 Some Reasons Patients Continue to Present with CMV End-Organ Disease in the Era of HAART

Not Taking HAART
Unaware of HIV infection
Lack of access to healthcare
Unwilling to take medication
Failure of HAART
HIV resistance
Poor compliance

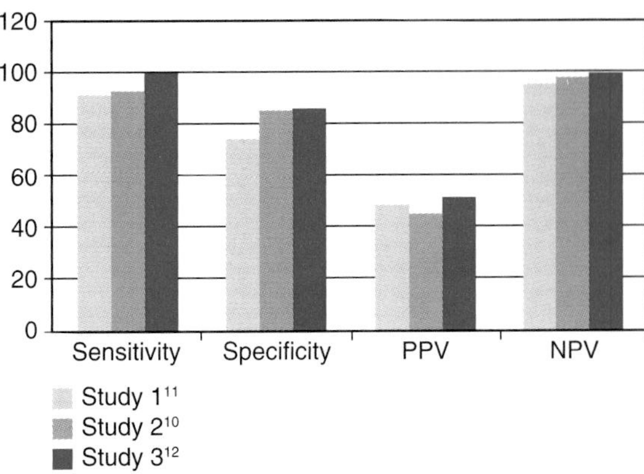

Figure 50-1 ■ Prognostic value of PCR assays defined in the pre-HAART era by three independent laboratories. PPV, positive predictive value; NPV, negative predictive value.

it again explained the previously recognized risk factors.[8,9] These principles of CMV pathogenesis in the immunocompromised host transferred directly to acquired immunodeficiency syndrome (AIDS) patients when, in 1997, three groups[10–12] simultaneously reported that viremia preceded CMV retinitis (see Fig. 50-1). However, there is one differentiating feature between these groups of immunocompromised hosts; in AIDS patients, CMV crosses the blood–organ barrier to preferentially cause clinically relevant retinal disease whereas this is uncommon in allograft recipients. Specifically, 85% of AIDS patients with CMV end-organ disease have retinitis (with ~10% having enteritis and the remaining patients having neurological disease); whereas, retinitis occurs in less than 5% of allograft recipients.[13,14] This striking difference between these groups of patients remains unexplained. Nevertheless, it is important to consider the concept of viremic dissemination of CMV in AIDS patients with retinitis because viremia is the route by which the virus reaches the contralateral eye and other organs.

Direct measurements have been made of the turnover of CMV in serial samples of viremic patients and reveal that CMV replicates with rapid dynamics.[2] Specifically, in patients with primary CMV infection, the dynamics are essentially equivalent to those of primary HIV infection.[15] One important difference from HIV replication however, is that CMV DNA polymerase has a proofreading activity so that many replicative cycles are required to select for resistance to drugs such as ganciclovir (GCV). Strains resistant to GCV frequently coexist with wild type strains in clinical samples. These strains compete in the laboratory so that, in the absence of ganciclovir, the wild type outcompetes the mutant, leading to failure to identify resistant subpopulations.[16]

IMMUNOLOGY

CMV virus-encoded proteins within cells are marked by ubiquitination and so targeted for degradation within the proteosome. The resulting short peptides are transported by TAP (the transporter associated with antigen presentation) through to the lumen of the endoplasmic reticulum (ER). There they associate with the heavy chains of HLA class I molecules and progress through the trans-Golgi region to be presented as mature complexes at the plasma membrane. Thus, the cytotoxic T-lymphocyte (CTL) sees a virus-specific peptide presented in the context of an HLA class I molecule. Molecules which become misfolded in the ER are reexported back into the cytosol where they are degraded in the proteosome. The signal peptides derived from this natural cycling of HLA class I molecules are presented by HLA class E molecules at the plasma membrane and provide a negative signal to natural killer (NK) and other cells which thereby sense that HLA turnover is normal within the cell.

Cytomegalovirus interferes with this pathway at several points (see Fig. 50-2). First, a phosphoprotein termed pp65 phosphorylates the major immediate early antigen of CMV so that this cannot be degraded in the proteosome.[17] This may explain why pp65 is the immunodominant protein of CMV seen by the cell-mediated immune system, rather than the major immediate early protein which is the first protein to be made in the cell. This might represent a mechanism of the virus to divert immune responses away from important proteins and toward others that are less able to control CMV infection. Protein US6 blocks TAP, protein US3 binds to HLA class I molecules and sequesters them in the ER, protein US2 and protein US11 mimic the natural cellular pathway that reexports class I molecules into the cytosol leading to their degradation.[18–22] These proteins act in a coordinated temporal fashion, with pp65 being a structural protein of the virus released by uncoating, so that it is active as soon as the virus enters the cell, US3 being active at immediate early times and US6, US2, and US11 being active at early times. Thus, before the onset of DNA replication, CMV has taken over the cell and effectively prevented its recognition by the CTL. However, the cell is still susceptible to attack from NK cells and macrophages which sense the reduced display of HLA class I (missing self hypothesis). CMV has evolved genes to combat these responses as well. Gene *UL18* contains an HLA class I homolog (presumably captured from the human genome millions of years ago) which is presented at the plasma membrane and provides an inhibitory signal to macrophages through the CD85j receptor.[23,24] Another HLA class I homolog is encoded by gene *UL142* which provides a negative signal to NK cells through an unknown molecule.[25] Gene *UL40* contains a 9 amino acid peptide which is identical to the signal peptide of HLA class I molecules. This is presented by HLA-E, so mimicking the natural authentic signal which NK cells sense through the CD94 receptor, and provides an inhibitory signal by upregulating HLA-E.[26,27]

In addition to these negative signals, CMV interferes with natural positive signals given to NK cells via their G2D receptor. Gene *UL16* is expressed and binds to natural gene products (dubbed UL binding proteins) as well as *MICA* and *MICB* which normally provide a positive signal to the NK cell through the G2D receptor.[28] The protein from gene

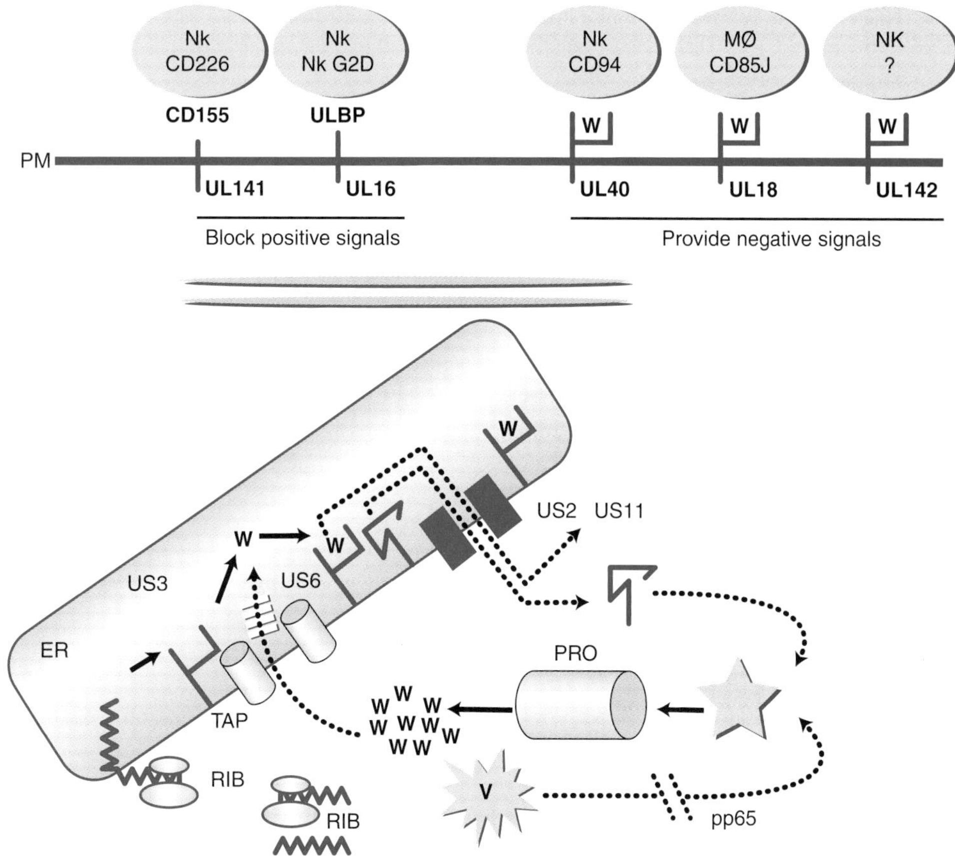

Figure 50-2 ■ Immune evasion mechanisms of CMV. RIB, ribosome; PRO, proteasome; ER, endoplasmic reticulum; TAP, transporter associated with antigen presentation; PM, plasma membrane.

UL141 binds CD155, so preventing it from giving an activating signal through CD226.[26]

The net result of all of these immune evasion genes is that CMV can replicate in cells relatively free from attack from the CTL, NK, and macrophage components of the immune system. The induction phase of the immune system is fully active and a considerable proportion of the host immune response is directed toward CMV-encoded epitopes. For example, using tetramer reagents, typically 1% of CTLs recognize a single peptide from pp65 protein.[29] In normal individuals, a stand-off occurs between this high incidence of CTLs and the sequestered nature of CMV replicating in relatively protected cells. However, when HIV progressively damages the effectiveness of CTLs, CMV gains the upper hand and can replicate to high levels causing viremia and subsequent dissemination in the bloodstream.

Several authors have described CMV-specific cell-mediated immune responses which correlate with protection against CMV viremia[30] or delayed progression of retinitis.[31] These cells include a broad range of antigenic diversity repertoire and degree of differentiation;[31] immediate-early specific, interferon gamma (IFNγ) producing CD8+ T-lymphocyte cells,[32,32] IFNγ CD4+ T-lymphocyte cells[33] or ELISpot positive results, but not IFNγ production[30] were each reported to be associated with a better prognosis. Furthermore, some others[32] reported maintenance of large populations of CMV-specific CD8+ T-lymphocyte cells in the absence of specific CD4+ T-lymphocyte cells. Thus, it is not possible to identify at this time, the immune correlates of protection against CMV infection and disease.

EPIDEMIOLOGY OF CMV END-ORGAN DISEASE

In HIV-infected persons, as with most other opportunistic infections associated with HIV infection, CMV disease appears in a previously infected host. This may be due to reactivation of the latent virus although reinfection with a different strain is an additional mechanism. Although more than 90% of persons with HIV infection have antibodies to CMV, indicating prior infection, the clinical manifestations of CMV disease do not generally present until the CD4+ T-lymphocyte count drops below 100 cells/μL.[34–36] In a multicenter observational cohort of 1002 HIV-infected persons with fewer than 250 CD4+ T lymphocytes per microliter receiving zidovudine, disease due to CMV developed in 109 persons.[14] Kaplan–Meier estimates of the proportion of persons who developed CMV disease was 21.4% at 2 years for persons entering the study with fewer than 100 CD4+ T lymphocytes per microliter and 10.3% for persons with initial counts higher than 100 cells/μL. A smaller study of 135 persons with fewer than 250

CD4+ T lymphocytes per microliter found the Kaplan–Meier estimate for the development of CMV retinitis to be 42% within 27 months for the group with fewer than 50 CD4+ T lymphocytes per microliter.[37] Of the 26 persons developing CMV retinitis, 24 had CD+ T-lymphocyte counts of less than 50 cells/μL before developing CMV retinitis; the other two persons had counts of 60 and 160 cells/μL 7 and 11 months before the diagnosis, respectively. The mean time from the first CD4+ T-lymphocyte count of less than 50 cells/μL until the diagnosis of CMV retinitis was 13.1 months. Since 1990, when cases of *Pneumocystis carinii* (now termed *Pneumocystis jiroveci)* pneumonia (PCP) reported to the CDC began to decrease owing to the widespread use of prophylaxis to prevent PCP, cases of AIDS-defining CMV retinitis increased. (Total cases of CMV retinitis, however, did not decrease.) A prospective cohort of 844 men were followed before the development of an AIDS-related opportunistic infection. Among those who received PCP prophylaxis, CMV disease was the initial AIDS-related opportunistic infection in 9.4% of men compared to 3.1% of men who did not receive PCP prophylaxis. The lifetime occurrences of CMV disease were 44.9% and 24.8% in those groups, respectively.[38]

Disease due to primary infection with CMV is rarely recognized in persons with HIV infection. More than 90% of persons with AIDS in the United States have evidence of prior infection with CMV.[39] Reactivation of the latent infection may result in systemic signs and symptoms such as fevers, myalgias, leukopenia, and weight loss in addition to symptoms attributable to end-organ disease.

GENERAL LABORATORY DIAGNOSIS

The diagnosis of CMV in organs such as the colon and lung requires the identification of characteristic histopathologic findings of the pathognomonic 'owl's eye' intranuclear and smaller intracytoplasmic inclusion bodies on tissue specimens.

Viremia with CMV is common in asymptomatic persons with low CD4+ T-lymphocyte counts (i.e., 50–100 cells/μL). In addition, in the absence of clinical disease, rare cells containing CMV inclusion bodies may be seen on histopathologic specimens even when other pathogens are causing organ dysfunction. In these cases, there are many examples where patients recovered with treatment for the other pathogen but no treatment for CMV. Thus for most syndromes CMV disease should be diagnosed only when many typical CMV inclusion-containing cells are seen with an associated inflammatory response in the appropriate clinical setting. Because of the difficulty in obtaining appropriate tissue specimens, the diagnosis of retinitis due to CMV is not determined by histopathologic findings but by the characteristic appearance of a hard or fluffy exudate often associated with hemorrhage and perivascular sheathing in the retina.

Data on the use of a qualitative CMV-specific polymerase chain reaction (PCR) on whole blood suggests that this test may be both sensitive and specific for the development of CMV disease. In a prospective cohort of 97 HIV-infected persons with fewer than 50 CD4+ T lymphocytes per microliter followed every 3 months with CMV PCR, 16 of 27 persons (59%) who were CMV-positive by PCR at baseline developed CMV disease within 12 months compared with only three of 70 persons (4%) who were initially CMV negative.[12] In a cohort of 94 HIV-infected individuals without CMV disease at baseline, a qualitative plasma CMV PCR was more sensitive and specific (89% and 75%, respectively) than either urine CMV cultures (85% and 29%, respectively) or leukocyte cultures (38% and 74%, respectively) for the identification of persons developing CMV disease within 12 months.[11] Quantitative CMV PCR was able to increase the specificity of the assay at some cost to the sensitivity.

In an analysis of 619 persons with AIDS who participated in a study of the efficacy of oral GCV for the prevention of CMV disease, CMV DNA was quantitated by PCR.[40] A positive baseline plasma CMV DNA PCR was associated with a 2.5-fold risk of death, and each log increase in CMV DNA load was associated with a 3.1-fold increased risk for CMV disease and a 2.2-fold increase in mortality ($P < 0.001$ for both).[40] Commercial PCR assays for CMV are currently available, but these study data have not translated into widespread clinical use in HIV-infected persons. The identification of persons at high risk for the development of CMV disease may allow the development of preemptive therapeutic strategies to prevent end-organ disease due to CMV; but because of the overwhelming impact of HAART in the management of persons with advanced HIV infection, such strategies are of marginal use at present. A prospective study (ACTG 5030) is assessing the utility of plasma PCR for preemptive therapy and its results are awaited with interest.

NATURAL HISTORY AND ORGAN-SPECIFIC DIAGNOSIS

Retinitis

Retinitis due to CMV results from the hematogenous dissemination of CMV after reactivation of a latent CMV infection.[34] Progression of the infection within the retina is generally to contiguous cells. Lesions near the macula or optic nerve (zone 1) commonly produce complaints of decreased visual acuity or defects in the visual field. Retinal lesions at least 1500 μm from the edge of the optic nerve and at least 3000 μm from the center of the fovea (zones 2 and 3) or anterior to the equator of the eye may be asymptomatic or present with the complaint of 'floaters' or loss of peripheral vision. CMV retinitis is not associated with pain or photophobia.

Visual loss due to CMV retinitis occurs in several ways. Direct infection of the retinal cells by CMV causes retinal necrosis, which may result in a visual field defect or scotoma, depending on where in the retina the lesion occurs. This permanent, irreversible loss of vision is not amenable to therapy and depends on the location and extent of the retinal necrosis. Normal central vision may be preserved if the macula is not involved. Second, retinal involvement of the area near the

Table 50-2

Clinical Event Rates (Per Person-Year of Follow-Up) Reported from a Prospective Cohort of 271 Patients with CMV Retinitis

HAART Era	Progression of Retinitis[199]	Contralateral Eye Involvement[200]	Retinal Detachment[200]
Pre-HAART	3.0	0.40	0.50
HAART	0.10	0.07	0.06
(CD4+ T lymphocyte <50)	(0.58)	(0.34)	(0.30)
(CD4+ T lymphocyte >200)	(0.02)[200]	(0.02)[201]	(0.02)

macula may produce edema in the macula and loss of central visual acuity. The macular edema and loss of visual acuity are potentially reversible if recognized and treated promptly before the retinal cells are infected. Third, after infection with CMV and subsequent retinal necrosis, the retina is left as a thin, atrophic tissue that is susceptible to breaks and detachment.[41] Retinal detachment occurs commonly in persons with CMV retinitis and presents with the sudden onset of floaters, flashing lights, loss of visual field, and decreased visual acuity. Retinal detachments can be repaired; but owing to the nature of the atrophic retinal tissue they frequently recur. Data from 681 patients with CMV retinitis reported substantial visual loss on follow-up. Events per 100 eye-years ranged from 51.7 to 97.7 for loss of visual acuity to worse than 20/40 and 18.9 to 49.1 for acuity worse than 20/200.[42]

Recent data show that the incidence of progression of retinitis, retinal detachments, and involvement of the contralateral eye is markedly reduced in persons receiving HAART (see Table 50-2). Nevertheless, CMV retinitis, whether acute or long-standing, continues to significantly affect quality of life when measured formally.[43]

Data from randomized controlled trials using standard treatment with GCV, foscarnet, or cidofovir showed that the median time to relapse after successful initial therapy of CMV retinitis, in the absence of HAART, ranges from 50 to 120 days.[44–46]

Because of the difficulty of obtaining retinal tissue for histopathologic examination, CMV retinitis is diagnosed based on the appearance of the characteristic perivascular fluffy yellow-white retinal infiltrate that is often associated with retinal hemorrhage. The portion of the vessels near the lesion may appear to be sheathed. Occasionally, the lesions present with a granular, rather than fluffy, appearance.[34] Progression of retinitis is in a characteristic 'brushfire' pattern, with a granular, white leading edge advancing before an atrophic, gliotic scar. Progression is irregular and occurs in fits and starts. In a study performed before the availability of HAART using serial, masked retinal photographs, the median progression rate at which disease approached the fovea in 17 untreated patients was found to be 24.0 μm/day compared with a median progression rate of 11.5 μm/day in 14 patients treated with GCV.[47] Patients with AIDS and CMV retinitis, who are not being treated with HAART and have not reconstituted their immune system, usually have minimal inflammation of the vitreous. CMV retinitis usually presents unilaterally but, untreated, becomes bilateral in most cases. Retinitis in a CMV-seronegative individual would make a diagnosis of CMV retinitis highly improbable.

Other ocular lesions that occur in HIV-infected persons are in the differential diagnosis of CMV retinitis.[48] Cotton-wool spots are microinfarctions of the retinal nerve fiber layer that occur commonly in persons with HIV infection and may present similar to an early CMV retinitis.[49] These small, white lesions do not affect vision and spontaneously regress over several weeks. In the setting of an HIV-infected person with fewer than 100 CD4+ T lymphocytes per microliter, it is critical to ensure that lesions that appear to be cotton-wool spots regress and do not progress as would be expected with CMV retinitis. Acute retinal necrosis, caused by herpes zoster, presents with either peripheral retinal vascular occlusion overlying a white, necrotic retina or, when more central vessels are involved, ischemia due to central vascular occlusion.[50] Intraocular lymphomas may present with small retinochoroidal infiltrates, optic nerve head swelling, and vascular sheathing. Toxoplasmic chorioretinitis may be unifocal or multifocal but is usually associated with a moderate to severe inflammatory reaction in the vitreous, which helps differentiate it from CMV retinitis.[51] *Pneumocystis jiroveci* chorioretinitis appears as multifocal, white-yellow raised choroidal lesions with minimal inflammation.[52] Other, rare causes of ocular disease in persons with HIV infection include syphilis, *Mycobacterium tuberculosis*, *Cryptococcus*, and *Candida* infections, and histoplasmosis.[53]

Gastrointestinal Disease

CMV Esophagitis

Esophagitis due to CMV is a common cause of odynophagia in persons with AIDS.[53] *Candida* more characteristically causes dysplasia. CMV esophagitis occurs in ~10% of persons with AIDS who develop CMV disease,[14] but is much less common than *Candida* esophagitis. The definitive diagnosis of CMV esophagitis is established by biopsy evidence of CMV with an inflammatory response in the appropriate clinical setting. The presence of extensive large, shallow ulcers of the distal esophagus is the hallmark of the disease. Pathologically, the large intranuclear inclusion bodies characteristic of CMV can be seen in the endothelial cells at the edge of the ulcer and are required to confirm the diagnosis.[54] Immunohistochemical stains may add to the sensitivity of routine hematoxylin and eosin staining for CMV. Culturing CMV from a biopsy or brushing of the esophagus is not sufficient to establish the diagnosis of CMV esophagitis because many persons with low CD4+ T-lymphocyte counts are viremic and have positive cultures for CMV in the absence of clinical disease.[55] Furthermore, adding viral culture and brush cytology to routine multiple biopsies with standard histopathology does not increase diagnostic sensitivity.[56]

The differential diagnosis of CMV esophagitis includes esophagitis due to herpes simplex, reflux or peptic ulcer disease, histoplasmosis, Kaposi sarcoma, lymphoma, HIV infection, *M. tuberculosis* infection, and rarely *Mycobacterium avium-intracellulare* complex infection, cryptosporidial infection, and *Pneumocystis jiroveci* pneumonia.[57] Because of the relative prevalence of *Candida* esophagitis in this population, many clinicians treat esophageal symptoms empirically, especially in the presence of oral thrush. Empiric therapy usually consists of fluconazole for presumptive *Candida* esophagitis, endoscoping only those persons who fail to respond.[58] Both CMV or *Candida* esophagitis most commonly present with CD4+ T-lymphocyte counts of less than 50 cells/μL; however, persons with esophageal candidiasis, but not CMV, can present with counts between 50 and 400 cells/μL.[36,45]

CMV Gastroduodenitis

Cytomegalovirus may be an under-recognized cause of peptic ulcers in AIDS patients, in whom it is found more frequently than in association with *Heliobacter pylori.*[59]

CMV Colitis

Colitis due to CMV occurs in fewer than 10% of persons with AIDS in whom disease due to CMV is diagnosed.[14] Fever, weight loss, anorexia, abdominal pain, debilitating diarrhea, and malaise are frequently present. Extensive hemorrhage and perforation can be life-threatening complications.[60] The symptoms are nonspecific and may be similar to those due to other gastrointestinal pathogens, such as *Cryptosporidium, Microsporidium, Cyclospora cayetanensis, Mycobacterium avium* complex, *Giardia lamblia, Entamoeba histolytica, Salmonella*, and *Shigella* or the gastrointestinal involvement seen with lymphoma or Kaposi sarcoma. The radiographic manifestations of CMV colitis are nonspecific and may mimic the findings of other inflammatory bowel conditions, including ulcerative colitis.[61] Colonoscopic or rectal biopsy with histopathologic identification of characteristic intranuclear inclusions is required for diagnosis. Identification of CMV by culture or even on histopathologic specimens may not be sufficient to implicate CMV; frequently multiple pathogens may coexist and must be considered in persons with advanced HIV infection.[62]

Pneumonitis

Although CMV can be cultured routinely from throat washings, pulmonary secretions, bronchoalveolar lavage specimens, and autopsy lung tissue, CMV is seldom implicated antemortem as an isolated pathogen causing pneumonitis in persons with HIV infection.[63] Foci of CMV inclusion bodies and pneumonitis are often found at autopsy. In one study from San Francisco, although CMV was cultured from bronchial alveolar lavage fluid or transbronchial biopsy specimens in 54 of 111 patients diagnosed with their first episode of PCP, the presence of CMV had no impact on the long-term survival, acute death rate, or length of hospital stay.[64] Of 17 persons with biopsy-diagnosed CMV pneumonitis, no clinical, radiographic, or histologic findings distinguished persons with CMV as the sole pathogen from those with other, concomitant pathogens.[65]

Pneumonitis due to CMV generally presents as an interstitial pneumonitis in an individual with advanced HIV infection. Shortness of breath, dyspnea on exertion, a nonproductive cough, and hypoxemia are characteristic. CMV pneumonitis should be diagnosed only in the setting of pulmonary infiltrates by identifying multiple CMV inclusion bodies in lung tissue of appropriate clinical specimens in the absence of other pathogens that are more commonly associated with pneumonitis in this population, such as *P. jiroveci, M. tuberculosis, Histoplasma capsulatum, Coccidioides immitis, Cryptococcus neoformans,* or bacterial pathogens such as *Streptococcus pneumoniae* or *Haemophilus influenzae.* Treatment should be considered for persons with histologic evidence of CMV infection who do not respond to treatment of other pathogens.

Neurologic Disease

Cytomegalovirus has been found to be associated with various neurologic infections in persons with HIV infection, particularly ventriculoencephalitis[66–72] and ascending polyradiculopathy.[73–76] Ventriculoencephalitis usually occurs in advanced HIV infection in persons with a prior CMV disease diagnosis. Patients typically present with lethargy, confusion, and fever; but the clinical presentation may overlap that of HIV encephalitis. The cerebrospinal fluid (CSF) generally shows a pleocytosis that may be polymorphonuclear, low to normal glucose levels, and normal to elevated protein levels. PCR techniques are superior to culture for detection of CMV in CSF.[67,72] Periventricular enhancement of computed tomography (CT) or magnetic resource imaging (MRI) scales are suggestive of CMV ventriculoencephalitis rather than HIV-related neurologic disease.

Polyradiculopathy caused by CMV is characterized by urinary retention and progressive bilateral leg weakness.[73–76] The clinical symptoms generally progress over several weeks to include loss of bowel and bladder control and flaccid paraplegia. A spastic myelopathy has been reported, and sacral paresthesia may occur. The CSF often shows a pleocytosis that is usually polymorphonuclear, hypoglycorrhachia, and elevated protein levels. PCR techniques are superior to culture for detection of CMV in CSF.

Although CMV is found in the central nervous system (CNS) in up to 25% of persons in autopsy studies,[66,71,77] the incidence of overt CMV neurologic disease antemortem appears to be low.

Other CMV-Associated Diseases

CMV Adrenalitis

Involvement of the adrenal glands with CMV is frequently reported in autopsy studies of persons with HIV infection, with the involvement documented in as many as 64 of 83 (77%)[78] and 42 of 71 (59%)[77] persons in two autopsy studies. Patients rarely manifest adrenal insufficiency by laboratory or clinical parameters. Adrenalitis due to CMV is uncommonly diagnosed premortem, but hypoadrenalism is occasionally documented in persons with CMV disease by the cosyntropin stimulation test.[79]

CMV Hepatitis and Biliary Disease

Although CMV involvement of the liver and biliary tract is often seen in autopsy specimens, clinical hepatitis due to CMV is rare in persons with HIV infection.[14] Biliary tract or hepatic involvement by CMV may present with right upper quadrant pain and elevated alkaline phosphatase, but infections with *Cryptosporidium* and *M. avium-intracellulare* complex are more common causes. In one series of 66 consecutive persons with AIDS and first-episode gastrointestinal CMV disease, 22 patients presented with esophagitis, 28 with colitis, nine with sclerosing cholangitis, and only two with acute hepatitis.[80]

THERAPY

Specific therapies for CMV disease are summarized in Table 50-3. Drug susceptibilities and pharmacokinetic values are summarized in Table 50-4. The chemical formulas of the drugs are shown in Figure 50-3.

Specific Treatments

The US Food and Drug Administration (FDA) has approved seven approaches to CMV therapy for patients with HIV (Table 50-5). Oral GCV is no longer available having been replaced by valganciclovir (VGCV) oral prodrug, and we will give the equivalent dose of VGCV where appropriate.

Ganciclovir

Initial Therapy with Intravenous GCV

The first major advance in the treatment for CMV disease was the development of GCV, an agent highly specific for human herpesviruses. GCV is a nucleoside analog whose activity depends on inhibition of herpesvirus DNA polymerases. It requires phosphorylation in CMV-infected cells (see Fig. 50-4), and most strains of CMV resistant to GCV are unable to phosphorylate GCV. The CMV UL97 open reading frame codes for a protein kinase capable of phosphorylating GCV in CMV-infected cells.[81,82] When treatment for disease is stopped, viral spread and progression of disease characteristically begin again.[35] Prior to the introduction of HAART, lifelong daily therapy was required, most often intravenously through an indwelling catheter. An oral formulation of GCV was used, but was poorly absorbed (less than 10% bioavailable) and not as clinically effective as the intravenous formulation.[83,84]

When given intravenously by a 1-h infusion, the standard 5 mg/kg dose of GCV reaches a maximum concentration in the plasma at the end of infusion of ~6 μg/mL (24 μM).[84] Trough levels 11 h after infusion are ~1 μg/mL (4 μM). The initial distribution half-life ($t_{1/2}$) is ~0.76 h, and the terminal elimination $t_{1/2}$ is 3.60 h.[84] Most studies report that for human CMV isolates the 50% inhibition (ID_{50}) of viral plaque formation is attained by concentrations of GCV between 0.4 and 11.0 μM.[35,85]

GCV was licensed by the FDA in 1988. The recommended dosing of GCV for the treatment of CMV retinitis in persons with AIDS is 5 mg/kg IV twice daily for a 14- to 21-day induction period followed by a 5 mg/kg daily indefinite maintenance phase. The terms 'induction' and 'maintenance' may be misnomers inasmuch as progression of CMV retinitis is regularly seen during the maintenance phase with GCV and foscarnet (Table 50-3). Patients with progression during the maintenance phase are routinely retreated with the twice-daily regimen. GCV at 1000 mg PO thrice daily was approved for maintenance therapy of CMV retinitis but was not recommended for persons whose central visual acuity would be threatened if progression of disease should occur. VGCV was licensed by the FDA in 2001 and is the oral anti-CMV agent of choice.

In a compilation of clinical data, treatment with GCV resulted in the improvement or stabilization of CMV retinitis in 80–90% of patients.[86] The median time to clinical progression in these uncontrolled studies appeared to be as long as 145 days from the diagnosis of CMV retinitis while continuing some maintenance therapy with GCV. One large, uncontrolled series reported the outcomes of 105 immunocompromised (primarily AIDS) patients who were treated with GCV for CMV retinitis. Analysis of a subset of these patients selected for their ability to tolerate a prolonged course of therapy and who had high-dose maintenance therapy (25–35 mg kg^{-1} $week^{-1}$) after induction therapy showed that the mean time to progression of retinitis was 18 weeks. This result, however, is based on subset analysis; these patients were selected for their ability to tolerate a prolonged course of relatively high-dose GCV without the development of neutropenia. The results of other trials indicate that with standard doses of both agents there is no difference in the rate of progression of CMV retinitis in AIDS patients treated with either GCV or foscarnet.[45,46,87] Clinical examination

Table 50-3

Therapies for AIDs-associated CMV Retinitis Defined in Pre-HAART ERA

Parameter	Ganciclovir IV	Foscarnet IV	Combined GCV IV/FOS IV	VGCV PO	GCV Implant	Cidofovir IV	Intravitreal Fomivirsen
Median time to first retinitis progression	47–104 days	53–93 days	129 days	160 days	216–226 days	64–120 days	71 days
Induction regimen	5 mg/kg q12h for 14–21 days	90 mg/kg q12h for 14–21 days or 60 mg/kg q8h for 14–21 days	FOS 90 mg/kg IV q12h and GCV 5 mg/kg IV qd, both for 14–21 days	900 mg PO bid for 14–21 days	Intraocular implantation via pars plana of GCV (4.5 mg) implant; requires concomitant VGCV therapy	5 mg/kg q wk for 2 weeks with probenecid and IV fluids before and after therapy	Intravitreal injection of 0.05 mL (330 μg) q 2 weeks for 2 doses
Maintenance	5 mg/kg qd	90–120 mg/kg qd	FOS 90–120 mg/kg and GCV 5 mg/kg IV each qd	900 mg PO qd	Requires replacement q 5–8 months	5 mg/kg q 2 weeks	0.05 mL q 4 weeks
Adverse effects	Neutropenia, thrombocytopenia, catheter sepsis	Nephrotoxicity, electrolyte abnormalities, catheter sepsis, genital ulceration	Same as GCV and FOS	Same as GCV	Surgical complications transient blurred vision, infection, hemorrhage	Nephrotoxicity, uveitis, hypotony	Abnormal or blurred vision, eye pain, ocular inflammation
Comments	Higher doses may be used for refractory disease Dosage should be adjusted for creatinine clearance <70 mL/min	Dosage should be adjusted based on recent creatinine clearance Requires hydration with 0.9% saline to reduce nephrotoxicity	Dosages of either may be increased based on prior drug experience	Consider as standard for both induction and maintenance unless concomitant GI disease may reduce absorption	Oral VGCV recommended to prevent systemic CMV disease	Requires dose reduction to 3 mg/kg for increase in serum creatinine by 0.3–0.4 mg/dL	Limited to persons with refractory disease
Main toxicities, side effects	Requires IV therapy Bone marrow toxicity	Requires IV therapy Renal toxicity	Requires frequent infusions; toxicities of both agents. Both drugs incompatible in the same infusion fluid	Bone marrow toxicity. Therapeutic failure due to GI disease or poor compliance	Surgical risks No coverage for systemic disease unless VGCV also given	Requires IV therapy Renal toxicity hypotony	Requires intravitreal therapy

FOS, foscarnet; GCV, ganciclovir; VGCV, valganciclovir.

Table 50-4 Reported Anti-CMV Drug Susceptibility and Pharmacokinetic Values

		Plasma Concentration (μg/mL)		Intravitreal Concentration (μg/mL)		Half-life (h)		
Drug	(μg/mL)	C_{max}	C_{min}	C_{max}	C_{min}	Plasma	Intracellular	Intravitreal
Ganciclovir	1.50						16.5[a]	13.3
5 mg/kg		8.2	0.05	0.6–1.8	0.2			
1000 mg PO tid		1.2	0.23					
200 μg, Intravitreal				17.9	NA			
4.5 mg intraocular device				0.69–7.40	0.69–7.40			
Valganciclovir[b]	1.50							
900 mg PO bid		5.6	NA			4.1		
Foscarnet	120.00							
90 mg/kg IV q12h		181	16		57	3.4		32
2400 μg intravitreal				269	NA			
Cidofovir	0.63							
5 mg/kg q2wk[c]		25	NA			3.2	65[b]	

C_{max}, maximum concentration; C_{min}, minimum concentration; ED_{50}, drug concentration that inhibits by 50% the *in vitro* replication of clinical CMV isolates obtained from patients who have not been treated with the drug; NA, not available.

[a]Ganciclovir triphosphate.

[b]Ganciclovir levels measured.

[c]Co-administered with probenecid 4 g PO over 8 h.

tends to overestimate the time to progression compared with data based on rigorous photographic endpoints.[84,86,88,89]

The results of a randomized, controlled trial comparing GCV with delayed therapy using strictly graded retinal photographs demonstrated that retinitis progressed while on GCV within a median of 50.5 days, compared with the progression on delayed therapy, which occurred within a median of 15 days.[46] Similarly, the results of the Studies of the Ocular Complications of AIDS (SOCA) trial demonstrated that the median time to progression of CMV retinitis while on GCV was 56 days.[87]

In an open study of GCV for the treatment of CMV esophagitis, among 10 evaluable patients treated with an induction regimen of 2.5 mg/kg IV q8h or 5 mg/kg IV q12h for 10 days, five persons had a good response, three had a partial response, and two had no response to therapy.[53] In general, in the absence of HAART, there is a high rate of relapse of CMV esophagitis in persons who receive intermittent therapy. The decision about whether to use daily, lifelong treatment or intermittent, high-dose therapy for esophagitis due to CMV must be individualized. Maintenance therapy should be considered, particularly after a relapse (Fig. 50-5).

GCV has been evaluated in a multicenter, double-blind, placebo-controlled trial for the treatment of CMV colitis in persons with AIDS.[90] Although the trial lasted only 14 days and was too short to demonstrate colonic healing and resolution of diarrhea, colonoscopy scores reflecting inflammation and positive cultures for CMV from the colon and urine significantly decreased in patients on the GCV arm. Most experienced clinicians recommend that treatment for CMV colitis should be given for 3–6 weeks. Unlike CMV retinitis, because the cells lining the gastrointestinal tract regenerate rapidly, therapy can often wait for the development of moderate to severe symptoms to justify the use of a systemic therapy with considerable toxicities. As with esophagitis, maintenance therapy is not necessarily required but should be strongly considered after a relapse. In a randomized, controlled trial of 48 patients with biopsy-proven gastrointestinal CMV disease comparing intravenous GCV ($n = 22$) with intravenous foscarnet ($n = 26$), 73% of subjects had a good or complete clinical response to a 2- to 4-week trial of either drug, with more than 83% of the subjects demonstrating an endoscopic response.[91]

The utility of GCV therapy in the treatment of CMV in other organ systems is not proven by randomized controlled trials. Although the combination of GCV with high-dose intravenous immunoglobulin has been suggested to be more effective than GCV alone in the treatment of CMV pneumonitis in bone marrow transplant recipients using historical controls,[92,93] the addition of intravenous immunoglobulin has not shown any benefit over GCV alone in persons with AIDS.[94] The response of pneumonitis to intravenous GCV has been reported to be better than 60%.[65] Response is probably better when patients are treated before the disease is

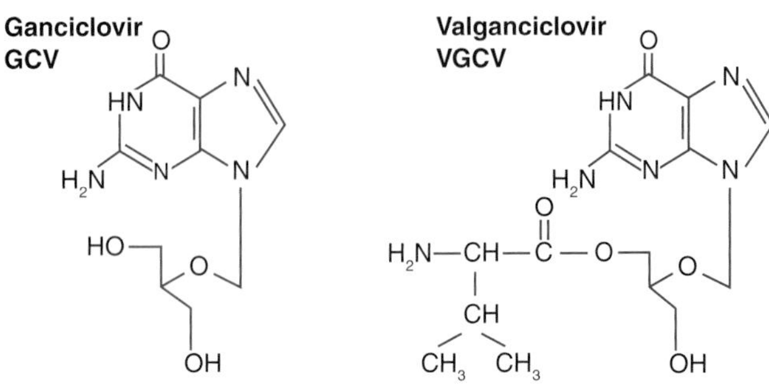

Fomivirsen

5'-d-[G*C*G*T*T*T*G*C*T*C*T*T*C*T*T*C*T*T*G*C*G]-3'
Sodium salt
* = racemic phosphorothioate

Foscarnet
PFA

Cidofovir
CDV

Figure 50-3 ■ Chemical formulas of drugs used to treat CMV disease.

Anti-CMV Agents

Table 50-5

Drug	Year of FDA Approval
Ganciclovir IV	1988
Foscarnet IV	1991
Ganciclovir capsules	1994[a]
Ganciclovir implant	1996
Cidofovir IV	1996
Fomivirsen injectable	1998
Valganciclovir	2001

[a]No longer distributed in the USA after June 2005.

severe. The role for maintenance therapy for CMV pneumonitis has not been established (Fig. 50-6). Many clinicians recommend such maintenance, however, as long as the CD4+ T-lymphocyte count remains below 100–150 cells/μL. For neurologic disease, initiating therapy promptly is critical for an optimal clinical response. Most clinicians treat CMV neurologic disease with GCV. Some data suggest that combination therapy with GCV and foscarnet is best for stabilizing or improving the response (Figs 50-7 and 50-8).[95]

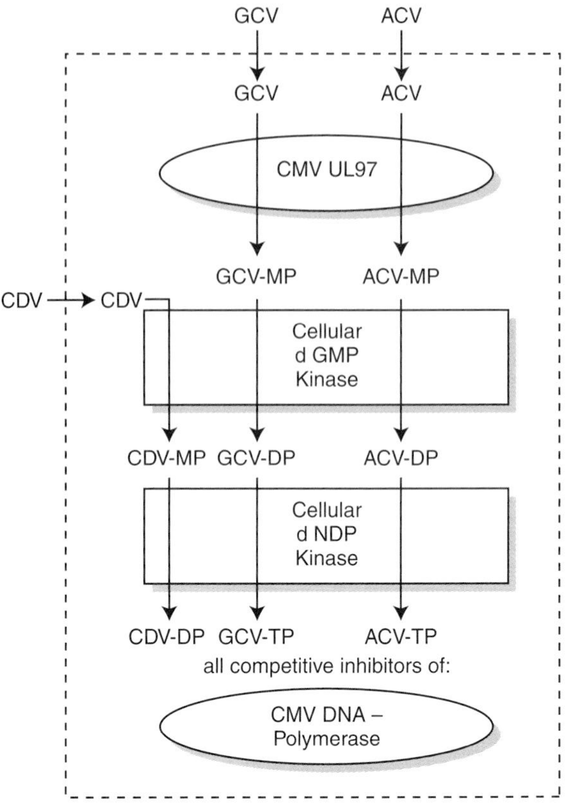

Figure 50-4 ■ Anabolism of drugs with activity against CMV in humans.

Cytomegalovirus viremia may be associated with subclinical involvement of other organ systems. Treatment of viremia in the absence of attributable clinical disease is not recommended. Treatment of CMV viremia when no other pathogen has been identified after thorough investigation is rarely warranted in patients with fever or wasting.

Neutropenia and thrombocytopenia are the major dose-limiting toxicities of GCV therapy (Table 50-3). Because GCV and zidovudine are both myelosuppressive, it is difficult to administer these agents concurrently.[96] In one study, only 18% of 29 persons with CMV disease were able to tolerate full doses of GCV with 600 mg of zidovudine daily.[97] In the randomized trial comparing initial therapy with GCV versus foscarnet for the treatment of CMV retinitis, 14 of 127 (11%) patients required switching from GCV to foscarnet: nine of 14 for progression of retinitis but only one of 14 for drug toxicity.[87] Limited *in vitro* data suggest that the antiretroviral activity of both zidovudine and didanosine may be antagonized by GCV.[97]

Intravitreal GCV

Intravitreal injections of GCV have been used for the treatment of CMV retinitis in persons unable or unwilling to tolerate systemic therapy with GCV or foscarnet.[98–100] The concentration of GCV in intravitreal fluid immediately after injection has been as high as 65 μM.[99] Concentrations higher than the ID_{50} for most strains of CMV can be maintained

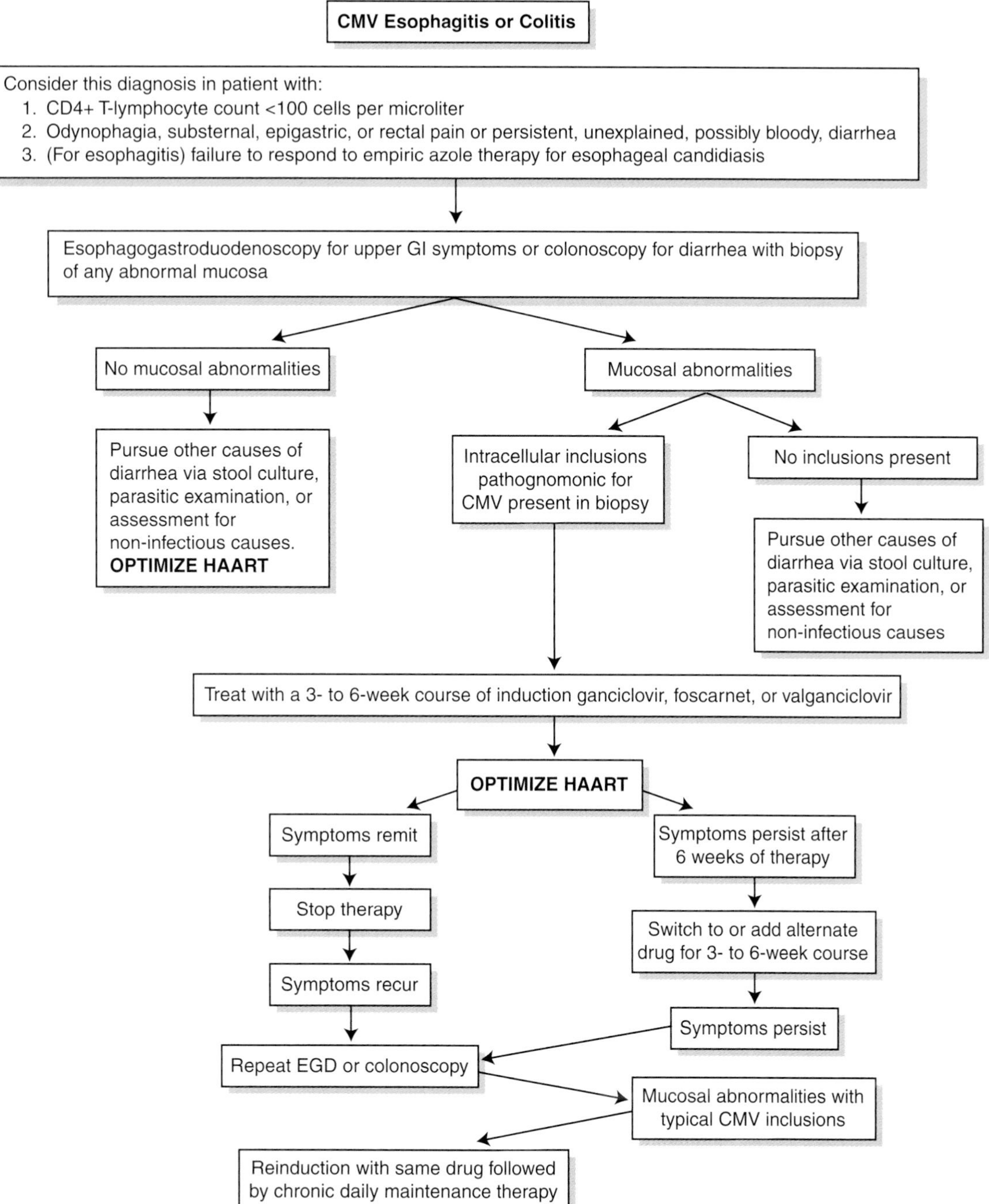

Figure 50-5 ■ Algorithm for diagnosing and treating CMV gastrointestinal (GI) disease. EGD, esophagogastroduodenoscopy.

for 60 h after a single 400 μg injection.[100] Two injections of 400 μg of GCV per week are given for 2–3 weeks during an induction period, followed by weekly maintenance injections. Alternatively, a single 2 mg injection may be given weekly. This alternative therapy effectively prevents the progression of CMV retinitis without the systemic toxicity of GCV and without significant toxicity to the retina. However, adjunctive systemic therapy is recommended to protect other organs (including the contralateral eye) from viremic spread. Rarely, retinal detachment, intraocular infection, intravitreal hemorrhage, or damage to the lens occurs. One retrospective case series from the pre-HAART era reported that retinal detachment was less common among patients who received intravitreal infections compared to systemic maintenance therapy.[101] This difference might be explained by high intraocular drug concentrations decreasing the area of retina involved with retinitis, so decreasing the risk of detachments.

GCV Intraocular Device

Local administration of GCV can be accomplished using a GCV intraocular device, licensed by the FDA for the

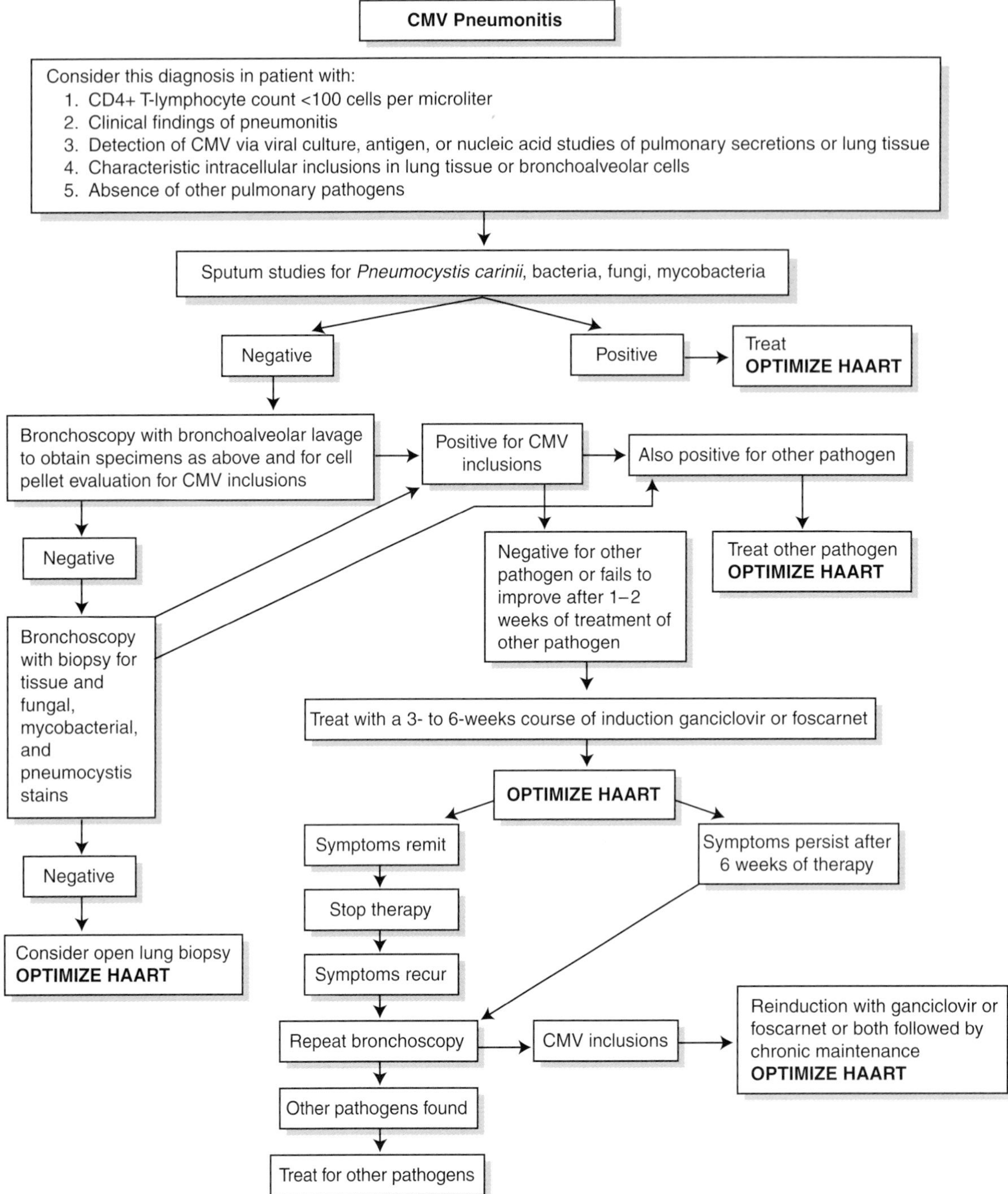

Figure 50-6 ■ Algorithm for diagnosing and treating CMV pulmonary disease.

treatment of CMV retinitis in 1996. This implant device releases GCV into the vitreous cavity at a rate of ~1.40 μg/h for a period of 6–9 months. It is surgically implanted in the affected eye during a simple outpatient surgical procedure. Recovery time is generally of the order of several days, but persons tend to have decreased visual acuity in the implanted eye for 4 weeks.[102] In a randomized, controlled clinical trial patients with peripheral CMV retinitis received either immediate implantation of the device or were closely monitored; the median time to progression of retinitis was 15 days in eyes of the delayed treatment group (n = 16) compared with 226 days in the immediate treatment group (n = 14) ($P < 0.00001$).[102] In eight persons in whom vitreous levels of GCV were obtained, the mean vitreous drug level was 4.1 μg/mL, roughly four times the concentration in the eye obtained with intravenous GCV. The major complications of the trial included the risk of CMV retinitis development in the fellow eye (estimated at 50% at 6 months) and the development of visceral CMV disease in 31% of patients. Seven late retinal detachments occurred in this study, but because

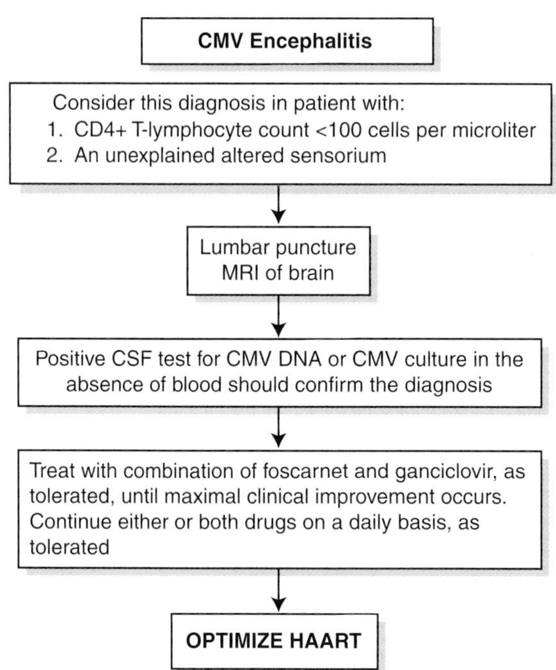

Figure 50-7 ■ Algorithm for diagnosing and treating CMV encephalitis.

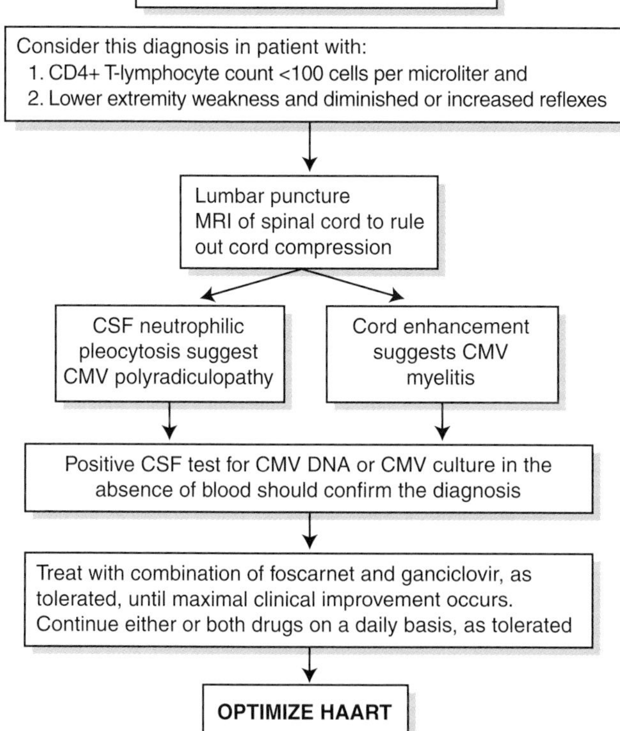

Figure 50-8 ■ Algorithm for diagnosing and treating CMV polyradiculopathy or myelitis.

retinal detachment occurs in those with treated and untreated CMV retinitis[41,103,104] it appears that an increased rate of early, surgically associated retinal detachment may be balanced by a decreased rate of late retinal detachments due to better control of the CMV retinitis.

A randomized, controlled clinical trial compared the use of intravenous GCV with that of two GCV implant devices releasing GCV at different rates.[105] The median time to progression of retinitis was 191 days (71 eyes) and 221 days (75 eyes) with the two implants, compared with 71 days (76 eyes) with intravenous GCV ($P < 0.001$). Extraocular CMV disease occurred more commonly in persons with the implant devices than in those receiving intravenous GCV (10.3% vs 0%; $P = 0.04$). Vitreous hemorrhage, which was generally transient, occurred in 7.8% of eyes. Endophthalmitis was reported in three eyes. Retinal detachments were reported in 11.9% of eyes receiving implants compared with 5.1% of the eyes of persons receiving intravenous GCV. There was no indication of a significant difference in mortality between the groups on this study.[105]

To evaluate the efficacy of oral GCV in combination with the GCV implant to control the development of extraocular and fellow-eye CMV disease, a multicenter, three-arm randomized clinical trial comparing the use of the implant alone versus the implant with co-administration of oral GCV (1500 mg PO thrice daily) versus standard intravenous GCV was conducted.[106] In 377 patients with AIDS and CMV retinitis restricted to one eye, after 6 months of treatment the development of extraocular CMV disease or CMV retinitis in the fellow-eye was 37.8%, 22.4%, and 17.9% in the three groups, respectively, a statistically significant finding comparing either the combination or the intravenous GCV groups with the implant-alone group. Progression of retinitis was also decreased by systemic therapy, consistent with the possibility that some progressions may be caused by exogenous viremic reinfections.[107] It is of note that the rate of development of Kaposi sarcoma was similarly decreased, occurring in 11.3%, 2.7%, and 1.5% of the three groups, respectively. This is the first time that use of an antiviral agent in a randomized clinical trial decreased the incidence of Kaposi sarcoma. Doses of VGCV currently used include 450 mg bid and 900 mg od.

Complications seen with use of the GCV implant are associated with the insertion procedure and include retinal detachment and, rarely, serious intraocular hemorrhage or infection. The incidence of surgical complications may decrease with increased familiarity with the procedure. Persons may have multiple devices implanted to control CMV retinitis once the GCV is spent. It is controversial whether to perform scheduled surgical replacement of these devices at 5–8 months after implantation or to replace them once the CMV disease progresses. The implant device is especially useful in individuals who are unable or incapable of administering daily intravenous therapy. It can be used in individuals who require temporary therapy for CMV retinitis while waiting for a response after initiating HAART, although oral VGCV is probably preferable. Finally, because of the increased intraocular levels of GCV achieved with the implant device compared to systemic administration of GCV, it may be useful in persons who do not respond to systemic GCV. In those circumstances it may be prudent to treat with intravitreal GCV initially to determine if higher levels of GCV would be useful or if high-level resistance to GCV is present.

Oral VGCV

VGCV was approved for both induction and maintenance therapy of CMV retinitis in 2001.[108] Induction therapy for CMV retinitis is 900 mg PO bid for 2–3 weeks followed by indefinite maintenance therapy of 900 mg PO daily. The oral administration of 900 mg of VGCV results in serum GCV levels approximating those obtained with 5 mg/kg IV (Fig. 50-9).[109] The results of a randomized, open-label controlled study of 160 patients with AIDS and newly diagnosed CMV retinitis randomized to receive either VGCV or intravenous GCV at the standard doses were reported.[110] After 4 weeks of either oral VGCV or intravenous GCV, all patients in the study received VGCV maintenance therapy at a dose of 900 mg daily. Among each group of 79 subjects, seven had progression of their CMV retinitis at 4 weeks determined by a masked review of retinal photographs. Two persons in the intravenous GCV arm and one person in the VGCV arm died. Notably, detection of CMV by PCR at week 4 was similar in the two arms. The median time to progression of retinitis in the VGCV-alone arm was 160 days, compared with 125 days in the intravenous GCV to VGCV arm, which is much longer than the median times observed in similar randomized trials conducted before the introduction of HAART (Fig. 50-10). The incidence of adverse events in the two study arms was similar (Table 50-6). VGCV, owing to its better bioavailability, has entirely supplanted the use of oral GCV as well as a major portion of the use of intravenous GCV.

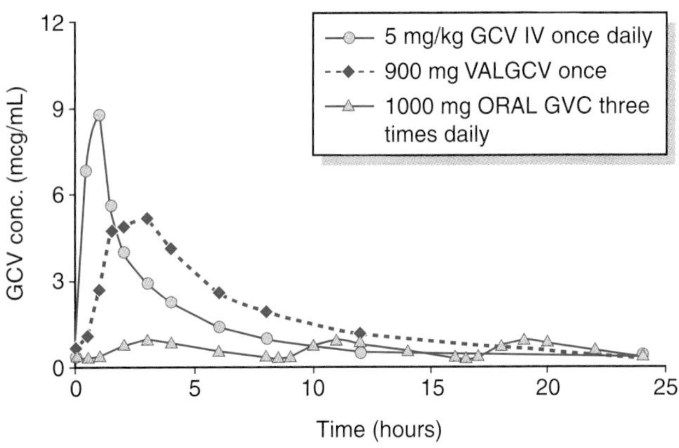

Figure 50-9 ■ Ganciclovir plasma concentration–time profiles in HIV+/CMV+ patients.

Foscarnet

Intravenous Administration

Foscarnet, or trisodium phosphonoformate hexahydrate, was approved by the FDA in 1991. The recommended regimen for CMV retinitis in persons with AIDS is 90 mg/kg IV q12h for an induction period of 2–3 weeks followed by an indefinite 90 mg/kg IV daily for maintenance (Table 50-3). As with GCV, the terms ‘induction’ and ‘maintenance’, though commonly used, may be misnomers; the half-lives of both GCV and foscarnet are both relatively short, and therapeutic drug levels against CMV of each may not be maintained during most of the day during the ‘maintenance’ phase of therapy. This probably accounts for the routine progression of CMV retinitis while on the ‘maintenance’ phase of therapy with either agent. Patients experiencing progression of CMV retinitis during the maintenance phase are routinely retreated with ‘induction’ doses of foscarnet.

Foscarnet is an antiviral agent with activity against CMV and other human herpesviruses as well as HIV. Foscarnet inhibits DNA polymerases of all herpesviruses and prevents chain elongation by occupying the binding site for pyrophosphate. Foscarnet prevents cleavage of pyrophosphate from adenine triphosphate and, unlike GCV, does not require phosphorylation in virally infected cells.[35] In addition to having inhibitory activity against the DNA polymerases of herpes simplex 1 and 2 and CMV, foscarnet has activity against the reverse transcriptase of HIV.[111–113]

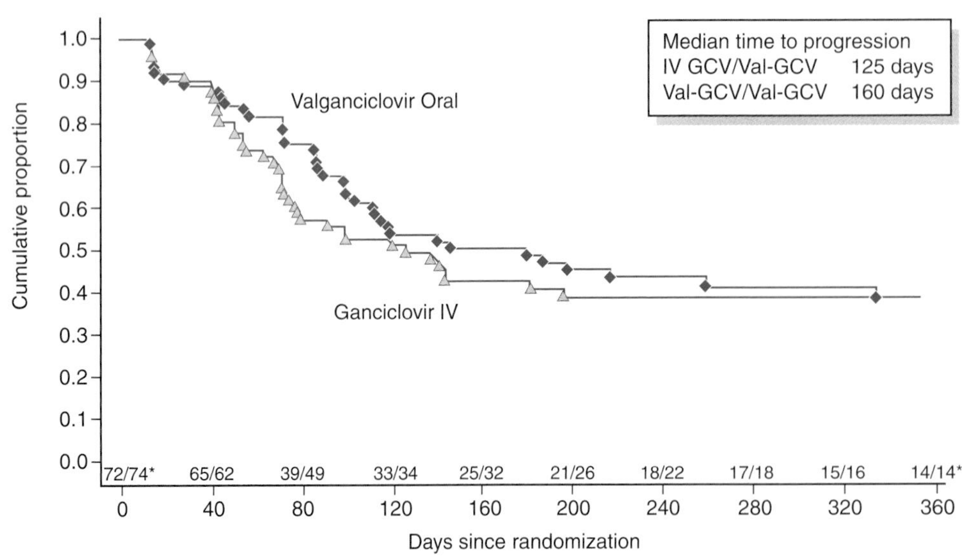

Figure 50-10 ■ CMV retinitis maintenance therapy: IV ganciclovir vs oral valganciclovir. Time to progression determined by retinal photography.

Table 50-6

IV Ganciclovir vs Oral Valganciclovir: Adverse Events

Adverse Event	IV GCV (n = 79)	Val-GCV (n = 79)
Diarrhea	8 (10%)	13 (16%)
Nausea	11 (14%)	6 (8%)
Vomiting	8 (10%)	6 (8%)
Catheter related	9 (11%)	2 (3%)
Neutropenia	5 (6%)	5 (6%)
<500 cells/dL	10 (13%)	12 (15%)
<500–750 cells/dL	0	1 (1%)
Platelets <50 000/dL	0	1 (1%)

Oral preparations of foscarnet have been absorbed poorly and have resulted in plasma concentrations that are inadequate to inhibit herpesvirus or HIV replication.[114] In humans, pharmacokinetic studies have been performed using both intermittent and continuous foscarnet infusions. Administration of foscarnet 60 mg/kg (or less depending on creatinine clearance) every 8 h to eight patients with AIDS and CMV retinitis resulted in a mean plasma $t_{1/2}$ of 4.5 h and steady-state peak plasma concentrations ranging between 272 and 876 μM, well above the drug concentrations that inhibit *in vitro* viral replication by 50% (ID_{50}) of susceptible viruses. Trough concentrations of 57–225 μM were sometimes lower than susceptible virus ID_{50} values. Plasma clearance was directly related to renal function; two patients with impaired creatinine clearance had delayed clearance and higher plasma concentrations of foscarnet.[115]

Continuous infusion of foscarnet (0.14–0.19 mg $kg^{-1} min^{-1}$ for 8–21 days) in 13 patients with HIV infection and generalized lymphadenopathy or AIDS resulted in a mean plasma $t_{1/2}$ of 6.8 h.[116] At steady state, 79–92% of the dose was excreted unchanged in the urine. After 8 days, small amounts of foscarnet could still be measured in the urine of all patients; and in one patient trace amounts were measurable 2.3 years after infusion. Persistent urinary levels are probably due to slow release from bone. CSF levels of foscarnet measured in five subjects found a mean CSF/plasma concentration ratio of 43%. Four of the subjects, however, had elevated CSF protein, suggesting a preexisting meningeal barrier defect.[116]

Prior to the availability of HAART, lifelong treatment of disease was generally required. The major toxicities of foscarnet are its effects on renal function and serum electrolytes. The need for concurrent or preadministration of a saline solution to minimize renal dysfunction requires a longer infusion period than with GCV.[117] Therefore foscarnet should be infused over at least 1 h with an infusion pump. This is especially true when other nephrotoxic agents are also being administered. Frequent monitoring of serum creatinine, creatinine clearance, and serum electrolytes is required.

Uncontrolled trials initially demonstrated the efficacy of foscarnet in the treatment of CMV retinitis in AIDS patients.[118–120] In a randomized, controlled trial of foscarnet, 24 AIDS patients with CMV retinitis who were not in immediate danger of losing central visual acuity were entered onto a trial with a 1:1 assignment to either an immediate or delayed treatment group.[45] Among those patients, 13 received immediate induction therapy with foscarnet (60 mg IV q8h for 21 days followed by 90 mg IV daily as maintenance therapy), and 11 patients were assigned to delayed therapy. The endpoint of the trial was defined as the time when any evaluable lesion progressed 750 μm (one-half the diameter of the optic disk) over a 750 μm front or when any new retinal lesion due to CMV appeared. The mean time to progression of retinitis was 13.3 weeks (median 7.5 weeks) in the foscarnet group versus 3.2 weeks (median 3.0 weeks) in the delayed therapy group from endpoints determined from retinal photographs obtained weekly and read at a masked reading center. Patients in the delayed therapy arm received foscarnet when retinitis progressed. This trial design became the model by which other trials of therapeutic agents for CMV retinitis were tested. Persons receiving immediate therapy with foscarnet frequently had conversion of CMV blood and urine cultures from positive to negative, whereas conversion of cultures in those not receiving therapy was a rare event. Although foscarnet only delayed the progression of retinitis in most patients on maintenance therapy, progression could generally be halted by another induction course of foscarnet or by increasing the maintenance dose.

In the SOCA study comparing foscarnet and GCV directly, no difference in the time to progression of CMV retinitis was found between the two arms, with a median time to progression of 59 days in the foscarnet arm and 56 days in the GCV arm.

Clinical cohort studies have reported the clinical utility of foscarnet against gastrointestinal infections due to CMV.[80,91,121] In one study in patients with AIDS, 18 episodes of esophagitis and 27 episodes of colitis were treated with foscarnet, 20 mg/kg over 10–30 min followed by a continuous infusion of 200 mg/kg over 24 h for a total of 3 weeks of therapy.[121] Symptoms and mucosal ulcerations resolved in 15 of 16 episodes of esophagitis in which therapy was completed, for a response rate of 94%. Three patients had a relapse of CMV esophagitis at 1, 4, and 7 months after therapy; two of these cases were successfully retreated with foscarnet and remained in remission 9 months later. Of the remaining 12 patients, eight died a mean 5.8 months later without recurrence of esophagitis, suggesting that maintenance therapy may not be necessary for sustained remission of CMV esophagitis.

Of 18 initial episodes of CMV colitis in which foscarnet therapy was completed, 11 had a complete response, six had a partial response, and one had no response. In the six with partial responses, other pathogens were also present. Therefore, 11 of 12 initial episodes of colitis due to CMV alone responded to foscarnet for a response rate of 92%. Two patients with relapses responded to either foscarnet or GCV. The one case that did not respond to foscarnet also failed to respond to GCV.[121] Similar rates of response were found with intermittent infusions of foscarnet.[80]

In comparison, 42 immunocompromised (primarily AIDS) patients treated with GCV for upper (esophagitis and gastritis) and lower (enteritis and colitis) CMV gastrointestinal disease had a response rate of 83%. Some of these patients received maintenance or repeat therapy as a result of disease relapses.[86] In a randomized, controlled trial of 48 patients with biopsy-proven gastrointestinal CMV disease comparing intravenous GCV and foscarnet, equivalent clinical and endoscopic responses to a 2- to 4-week trial of either was seen.[91]

The utility of foscarnet therapy in the treatment of CMV pneumonitis, CNS disease, viremia, or other infections due to CMV is largely anecdotal. Data suggest efficacy rates similar to those for GCV.[92]

Foscarnet is not commonly associated with neutropenia and can usually be administered along with zidovudine (Table 50-1).[45,87] Elevations in serum creatinine are perhaps the most common laboratory abnormality encountered and occur more frequently when other nephrotoxic agents are administered at the same time. These elevations are almost always reversible with reduction or discontinuation of therapy. In one study[117] elevations in serum creatinine of more than 25% over baseline occurred in 66% of 56 episodes of CMV infection treated with foscarnet. Acute renal failure requiring temporary hemodialysis occurred in one instance. In this same report, a series of 27 patients were prehydrated with 2.5 L of normal saline per day before and during the administration of foscarnet. Only one patient in this group developed an elevated serum creatinine level. Autopsy of one patient revealed acute tubular necrosis, suggesting it as one mechanism of foscarnet-associated renal toxicity. The major toxicities of foscarnet in the randomized immediate versus delayed treatment study included abnormalities in serum electrolytes, neutropenia (>500 cells/μL), increased red blood cell transfusion requirements, nausea that required discontinuation of therapy in two instances, and seizures.[45] The seizures occurred in the setting of preexisting toxoplasmic encephalitis in one patient and cryptococcal disease in the other. In the third instance the patient had a known idiopathic seizure disorder and suffered a seizure after initiation of foscarnet therapy. The occurrence of seizures in this study suggests that foscarnet may lower the seizure threshold in those who are already predisposed.[45,87] Seizures have also been reported in several patients with elevated serum levels of foscarnet due to administration of inappropriately large doses. In a randomized trial comparing initial therapy of foscarnet with GCV for the treatment of CMV retinitis, 39 of 107 (36%) patients required switching from foscarnet to GCV, 22 of 39 for drug-related toxicity, and nine of 39 for progression of retinitis,[87] demonstrating that foscarnet is generally less well tolerated than GCV.

Low serum ionized calcium was reported in six patients from one study immediately after foscarnet infusion, although total serum calcium remained normal.[122] The combination of foscarnet with intravenous pentamidine was associated with severe hypocalcemia in four patients with AIDS and *P. jiroveci* pneumonia. After discontinuing one of the drugs, the serum calcium level returned to normal in three patients, but the fourth patient died with severe hypocalcemia.[123] Other less commonly occurring adverse experiences associated with foscarnet therapy include genital and oral ulcerations, generalized cutaneous rash, and nephrogenic diabetes insipidus.

Intravitreal Administration

Intravitreal injections of foscarnet have also been used to treat CMV retinitis in persons unable or unwilling to tolerate systemic foscarnet.[124] Foscarnet, 2400 μg per injection given twice weekly for 2–3 weeks during an induction period followed by weekly maintenance injections, is similar to that of GCV. This alternative therapy appears to be as effective and safe as intravitreal GCV for preventing the progression of CMV infection, but there are few published long-term data available.

Cidofovir

Initial Studies

Cidofovir, a nucleotide analog with activity against all herpesviruses, was licensed for the treatment of CMV retinitis in 1996. Though the terminal $t_{1/2}$ of cidofovir is ~2.6 h, a fraction of the drug appears to be excreted in a slow elimination phase, suggesting that phosphorylated metabolites of cidofovir may have long intracellular half-lives.[125] Early data suggested that clinically tolerated effective doses of cidofovir could be administered as infrequently as every 2 weeks.[126,127] Nephrotoxicity was found to be a relatively common toxicity of cidofovir therapy, and it was necessary to administer saline hydration and large doses of probenecid around the time of infusion of cidofovir to block the uptake of cidofovir by the proximal renal tubular cells.[126,127] Cidofovir is a substrate for human organic anion transporter, which explains the high concentration of the drug, and resulting toxicity, in the kidney.[128] This transporter is expressed in brain tissue[128] and, if also expressed in the eye, could explain why cidofovir is a potent treatment for CMV retinitis but not extraocular CMV disease.

Two randomized, clinical trials have been conducted comparing intravenous cidofovir with deferred therapy in persons with advanced HIV infection and peripheral CMV retinitis (Table 50-3).[44,129] In the first trial, using a previously established trial design,[45,46] persons were randomized to receive immediate therapy ($n = 25$) with cidofovir 5 mg/kg IV (with probenecid on the day of infusion, 2 g PO 3 h prior to infusion and 1 g 2 h and 8 h after infusion) weekly for 2 weeks for induction therapy, then every 2 weeks for maintenance, or deferred treatment ($n = 23$) until progression of retinitis. Progression of retinitis was documented by masked reading of retinal photographs. The median time to progression of CMV retinitis was 120 days in the immediate treatment group compared with 22 days in the deferred treatment group ($P < 0.001$). Asymptomatic neutropenia and proteinuria occurred in 15% and 12% of patients, respectively. Cidofovir was discontinued in 10 of 41 patients (24%) because of treatment-limiting nephrotoxicity. Mild to moderate constitutional symptoms or nausea occurred in 23 of 41 patients (56%), but they were treatment-limiting in only three (7%).

Using similar eligibility criteria, the second trial randomized patients to: (1) deferred treatment (n = 26); (2) high-dose treatment using the same dose of cidofovir as in the first trial (n = 12); and (3) low-dose treatment with cidofovir 5 mg/kg weekly for 2 weeks then 3 mg/kg every 2 weeks for maintenance.[129] Probenecid was given on the day of cidofovir administration using the same regimen as the first trial. The median time to progression was 21 days in the deferred treatment group and 64 days in the low-dose treatment group; progression had not yet recurred in the high-dose treatment group at the time of data closure. Patients receiving cidofovir in this trial developed a significant incidence of proteinuria and reactions to probenecid; the data suggested that the use of probenecid, hydration, and careful monitoring of patients receiving cidofovir may have minimized but not prevented nephrotoxicity.[129] Four patients on this trial were noted to have ocular hypotony, defined as an intraocular pressure (IOP) of less than 5 mmHg and a decrease in IOP of at least 50% from baseline.

Another report has raised a concern about the development of iritis in association with the administration of cidofovir.[130] Iritis, defined as an increase in anterior chamber cells accompanied by photophobia, redness, pain, or blurred vision, occurred in 11 of 43 persons (26%) receiving cidofovir in three medical centers. Most patients with iritis were successfully managed with topical corticosteroids and cycloplegics and were able to continue to receive cidofovir. The development of iritis in association with cidofovir was potentially confounded by the use of protease inhibitors in 10 of the 11 persons with iritis, suggesting that the inflammatory response may be a therapeutic response to the institution of HAART rather than drug toxicity due to cidofovir.[130] It is of note that four of the 11 patients with iritis also developed hypotony. The hypotony was associated with clinically significant events including choroidal or retinal detachments, a macular fold, or a reduction in visual acuity in five of the six eyes (two persons had bilateral hypotony). Another case series reported that cidofovir was a significant risk factor for developing immune recovery.[131]

The data from the two randomized clinical trials suggest that cidofovir is at least as effective as GCV or foscarnet for controlling CMV retinitis, but it has not been compared directly to these agents in controlled clinical trials, and the results of analysis of the time-to-progression curves were somewhat different in the different studies.[44–46,129] The incidence of treatment-limiting toxicities of cidofovir (or probenecid) may be greater than those of GCV or foscarnet, but the convenience of an every-2-week therapy compared with daily intravenous therapy and the need to maintain a chronic indwelling catheter for foscarnet is a major advantage for the use of cidofovir (Table 50-3). Close monitoring of renal function and ocular pressure are required when administering cidofovir.

Few clinical data on the efficacy of cidofovir for extraocular CMV disease are available. Intravenous cidofovir appears to be ineffective in suppressing CMV viremia.[44,127,129] Treatment of extraocular CMV diseases with cidofovir should not be routinely attempted.

Intravitreal Administration

Similar to GCV and foscarnet, cidofovir has been administered by the intravitreal route.[132] Cidofovir, 20 μg intravitreally (with probenecid, as with intravenous administration of cidofovir) was administered to 32 eyes of 22 patients at 5- to 6-week intervals for a mean follow-up period of 15.3 weeks (range 5–44 weeks). Only two of 32 eyes developed progression of CMV retinitis during the study period. Mild iritis developed after 14 of 101 injections (14%) but responded within 2 weeks to topical steroids and cycloplegics. Two cases of hypotony (6%) requiring treatment discontinuation and associated with significant visual loss, one irreversible, occurred. The incidence of visual loss from hypotony precludes the routine intravitreal use of cidofovir.

Intravitreal Fomivirsen

Fomivirsen is an oligonucleotide antisense compound that can only be administered intravitreally. It is indicated in persons with CMV retinitis intolerant of or resistant to other therapies.[133] It consists of phosphorothioate linkages between each nucleotide, so that human enzymes cannot readily degrade it. Fomivirsen is given by intravitreal injections of 0.05 mL (330 μg) every 2 weeks for two doses, then every 4 weeks. Contraindications include hypersensitivity to fomivirsen or receipt of intravenous or intravitreal administration of cidofovir within the previous 2–4 weeks. Side effects include abnormal or blurred vision, eye pain, ocular inflammation, and increased intraocular pressure. In persons with unilateral, peripheral CMV retinitis, treatment with fomivirsen 165 μg weekly for 3 weeks and then every other week resulted in a median time-to-disease progression of 71 days compared to 14 days for persons in whom therapy was delayed until the CMV retinitis progressed. In persons with sight-threatening, refractory CMV retinitis, treatment with fomivirsen 330 μg weekly for 2–3 weeks and then every 2–4 weeks resulted in a median time-to-disease progression of 90 days, significantly delaying disease progression.[134]

DRUG RESISTANCE

With the increased use of GCV in the pre-HAART era, especially with oral GCV, GCV-resistant CMV was reported with increasing frequency.[135] In one study of 72 CMV-viremic AIDS patients treated with GCV for CMV disease and followed prospectively for the development of GCV-resistant CMV, no resistant strains of CMV were found in 31 randomly chosen patients before therapy or seven culture-positive patients treated for less than 3 months.[136] After 3 months of therapy, only 20% of persons remained culture-positive; five of 13 (38%) randomly chosen positives, or 8% overall, were found to have GCV-resistant strains with an IC_{50} higher than 12 μM. However, there appears to be a decreasing sensitivity of strains of CMV to GCV in persons receiving the drug for extended periods, suggesting that the progressive shortening of the time between relapses of CMV retinitis may be due in part to decreasing sensitivity of the virus.[137] In a cohort of persons with CMV retinitis followed at a single site, CMV developed resistance to GCV at a rate of ~11% at 6 months and 28% at 9 months of continuous therapy with GCV.[138] Low-level GCV resistance (IC_{50} 8–30 μM) is mediated by mutations in the *UL97* viral phosphotransferase gene, whereas high-level GCV resistance ($IC_{50} > 30\,\mu M$) is mediated predominantly by combined *UL97* and *UL54* viral DNA polymerase gene mutations.[139]

Treatment with foscarnet has been successful for GCV-resistant CMV retinitis.[140] The development of foscarnet-resistant strains of CMV is directly related to duration of therapy; they appeared at a rate of ~26% after 6 months and 37% after 9 months of continuous therapy in one study[141] and 13% and 24% at the same time-points in another study.[142] Unlike GCV, foscarnet does not require viral phosphotransferase to be activated, so low-level GCV-resistant isolates are usually sensitive to foscarnet.[143] Resistance to foscarnet is mediated by mutations in the CMV polymerase gene but at a site distinct from those that mediate high-level resistance to GCV and cidofovir.[143] Most isolates of CMV resistant to GCV and cidofovir are likely to be sensitive to foscarnet, but at least one mutation confers resistance to all three drugs.[144]

Resistance mutations in the CMV polymerase gene causing resistance to GCV overlap those of cidofovir, suggesting that persons with CMV with high-level resistance to GCV are probably also resistant to cidofovir. Strains of CMV with low-level resistance to GCV (due to CMV *UL97* mutations) are susceptible to cidofovir.[145] Foscarnet may be used for strains of CMV resistant to GCV and cidofovir.[146]

Most patients with resistant strains of CMV in the eye also have concomitant CMV viremia with the same strain containing the same mutations.[147] The positive predictive value of detecting viremia is too low to be useful clinically under these circumstances, but the negative predictive value of getting a negative PCR result in a patient with suspected resistance is good enough to exclude the diagnosis.[148]

The best means of preventing the emergence of CMV resistance is to maintain effective HAART regimens so that the number of replicative cycles of CMV is suppressed to a minimum.

All of these results of the incidence of CMV resistance came from the pre-HAART era where clinical samples were passaged in fibroblast cell cultures *in vitro*. Under these circumstances, as explained earlier, wild-type strains often outcompete the resistant strains in the absence of GCV so that the laboratory reports state, correctly, that the culture contains wild-type CMV whereas the patient harbors a mixed population. Several molecular methods can be used to detect resistant strains of CMV in clinical material.[144,149]

Salvage Therapy For CMV Retinitis

Despite continued therapy with prolonged maintenance doses of therapeutic agents, most persons with CMV retinitis develop progression of their disease. Simple progressions can be treated with reinduction doses of any of the agents, though successive progressions of retinitis occur at progressively shorter intervals. In a CMV retinitis retreatment trial, there appeared to be no benefit when switching from GCV to foscarnet or from foscarnet to GCV in individuals who developed early progression of their CMV retinitis.[150] Higher doses of GCV have been safely administered, though often in conjunction with colony-stimulating factors to prevent neutropenia. Doses up to 10 mg/kg IV twice daily can be given and may overcome low-level resistance due to protein kinase mutations but are not likely to overcome high-level resistance due to polymerase mutations.[146,151] Higher doses of foscarnet and cidofovir are difficult to administer owing to the potential for nephrotoxicity of these agents.

In persons intolerant of intravenous therapy, the GCV implant may be useful for treating progressive disease. It should be used with caution, however, in individuals who have received intravenous GCV for an extended period and may be resistant to GCV. In these individuals, it may be prudent to administer a test dose of intravitreal GCV and monitor the response prior to subjecting patients to the surgical procedure of inserting the implant.

Laboratory data have suggested that the co-administration of GCV and foscarnet have synergistic activity against CMV,[152] prompting initiation of a clinical trial of this combination for persons whose CMV retinitis progressed through continued monotherapy with either GCV or foscarnet.[150] In this controlled clinical trial, patients with progressive CMV retinitis were randomized to receive high-dose GCV ($n = 94$), high-dose foscarnet ($n = 89$), or a combination regimen of standard doses of GCV and foscarnet ($n = 96$). Persons receiving the combination regimen had a longer time to progression (median 4.3 months) compared with persons receiving GCV (2.0 months) or foscarnet (1.3 months) ($P < 0.001$). Though persons did not have any significant laboratory toxicities associated with the combination therapy compared with either monotherapy, there was a significant adverse effect on quality of life in persons receiving combination therapy due to the requirement for two intravenous infusions daily.[150]

The possibility that GCV and foscarnet are synergistic *in vivo* has been tested directly in a randomized clinical trial in transplant recipients.[153] Patients were followed post-transplant with twice-weekly PCR tests for viremia and were recruited when two consecutive PCRs showed viremia. A total of 48 patients were randomized and the two treatment groups were well matched at baseline, including the baseline median viral load of CMV. They were randomized to receive GCV at the full dose (5 mg/kg bid) or GCV at the same dose given once a day together with foscarnet given at half the normal dose, i.e. 90 mg/kg. The primary end point of the proportion of patients who were PCR negative by day 14 was not increased in the group receiving the combination; in fact, there was a strong trend in favor of those receiving GCV. Furthermore, significantly more adverse events were identified in the patients receiving the combination. The absence of a demonstrable effect of synergism *in vivo* suggests that this is not an explanation for the improved control of CMV retinitis seen in the SOCA trial and favors the possibility that the survival benefit may have been attributable to the anti-HIV activity of foscarnet and/or the presence of CMV resistance against GCV at baseline in these pretreated patients.

NEW ANTI-CMV AGENTS

The current therapies for CMV infection all suffer from significant toxicities and limited efficacy.[154] A number of novel, potentially effective compounds are in preclinical and clinical evaluation. Unfortunately, none of these agents is sufficiently advanced in its development to suggest that it may be available within the next 2 years.[155] An orally bioavailable benzimidazole riboside 1263W94 (maribavir) has potent, selective activity *in vitro* against CMV by inhibiting CMV DNA synthesis via a mechanism that does not require phosphorylation and does not involve DNA polymerase. Clinical CMV isolates resistant to GCV appear to be susceptible to 1263W94,[156] an agent in Phase II studies in stem cell transplant patients.

PREVENTION

Primary Disease

In the first prospective, double-blind study to be completed for prophylaxis of CMV disease, 725 HIV-infected persons with advanced disease were randomized to receive either oral GCV (1 g PO three times daily) or placebo.[157] At 18 months, CMV disease, retinitis, and colitis occurred, respectively, in 39%, 39%, and 4% of persons receiving placebo but in only 20%, 18%, and 2%, respectively, of patients treated with GCV. A second study failed to show that oral GCV was beneficial, but this study was limited by lack of routine ophthalmologic examinations and perhaps a lower rate of ascertainment of endpoints.[158] There is no role for acyclovir or its prodrug valaciclovir, in the therapy or prevention of CMV disease in persons with HIV infection.[159]

The 2001 US Public Health Service (USPHS)/Infectious Disease Society of America (IDSA) guidelines for the prevention of opportunistic infections in persons infected with HIV recommended that prophylaxis with oral GCV be considered an option for HIV-infected patients who are CMV seropositive with fewer than 50 CD4+ T lymphocytes per microliter, but that it should not be considered the standard of care.[160] Despite some indications that primary prophylaxis could prevent disease, this intervention was not recommended because: (1) long-term vision does not differ in patients who receive prophylaxis compared to those whose disease is treated when it occurs; (2) the regimen is expensive; (3) the regimen requires taking 12 large tablets per day, which is difficult for adherence; (4) chronic therapy would be likely to induce resistance; and (5) chronic therapy would be associated with toxicities such as cytopenia. The availability of VGCV offers a drug that would be easier to take (i.e., fewer pills per day). However, the impact of chronic therapy for primary prophylaxis on long-term vision as well as cost, adherence, toxicity, and resistance remain issues that are likely to deter health-care providers and patients from undertaking primary prophylaxis with this agent. Furthermore, HAART has effectively reduced the incidence of CMV end-organ disease so that many more patients would have to receive prophylaxis in order for one person to have CMV disease prevented. If patients at especially high risk could be identified among those with very low CD4+ T-lymphocyte counts (e.g., by quantitative PCR) then primary prophylaxis (or preemptive therapy) might be more attractive.

The most important intervention to prevent CMV disease is maintenance of the individual's CD4+ T-lymphocyte count above 100 cells/μL, with the use of HAART.

Secondary Disease (Maintenance Therapy)

As already noted, once CMV retinitis occurs, it is likely to recur promptly in patients with persistently low CD4+ T-lymphocyte counts unless maintenance therapy is administered. CMV disease of other organs is also likely to recur, although the limited data available suggest that recurrence is not as frequent as with retinitis. The maintenance regimens recommended are listed in Table 50-3.

Some individuals with advanced HIV infection and CMV retinitis who have had immune reconstitution in response to potent antiretroviral therapy manifested by sustained increases in their CD4+ T-lymphocyte counts to more than 100–150 cells/μL have discontinued their maintenance CMV therapy and have not had progression of disease for up to 12 months (Table 50-7).[161–169] Follow-up of these case series has suggested that the progression of CMV retinitis can be delayed or prevented for more than 5 years with judicious use of potent antiretroviral therapy.[170] Guidelines recommended that discontinuation of maintenance therapy for CMV retinitis should be considered in patients with sustained increases in CD4+ T-lymphocyte counts to these levels[160] and this recommendation has been supported by ongoing clinical experience.[171,172] Decisions to discontinue therapy should be made in consultation with an ophthalmologist and should evaluate factors such as the magnitude and duration of the CD4+ T-lymphocyte count increase, the anatomic location and extent of the retinitis, vision in the contralateral eye, and the availability of regular ophthalmologic evaluation. Relapses have generally, but not exclusively, occurred when the CD4+ T-lymphocyte counts have dropped below 50 cells/μL.[173] Relapses have occurred in persons with CD4+ T-lymphocyte counts higher than 100 cells/μL as well, but to date such relapses have been highly unusual.[172,174,175] Dissemination of CMV to the contralateral eye can occur, even in patients given HAART and systemic anti-CMV treatment. A rate of 26.1% per person per year of follow-up was reported from

Table 50-7

Follow-Up of Patients With CMV Retinitis Who Discontinued Maintenance Therapy Due to Immune Reconstitution

Study	No. of Patients	CD4+ T-Lymphocyte Count (cells/μL) Required for Inclusion in Study	CD4+ T-Lymphocyte Count (cells/μL) Median Count at Study Entry	Median Duration of HAART at Study Entry (Months)	Median Duration of Follow-Up (Months)	Relapses (No.)
Tural[166]	7	>150	233	NR	9	0
MacDonald[165]	22	>50	161	NR	16	3
Whitcup[169]	14	>150	315	NR	18	0
Jabs[162]	15	>100	297	17.0	8	0
Jouan[163]	48	>75	239	18.0	11	2
Berenguer[161]	36	>100	287	17.5	21	1

HAART, highly active antiretroviral therapy; NR, not reported.

one series of 376 patients. Benefit from HAART was seen only in the subset who developed a >50 cells/μL increase in CD4+ T-lymphocyte count to exceed 100 cells. Most contralateral eye involvement occurred in the first 6 months following the initial diagnosis of CMV retinitis.[176]

IMMUNE RECOVERY UVEITIS

The ability to discontinue specific anti-CMV therapy is not without its problems. The immune reconstitution associated with the use of HAART has also been associated with the development of an immune recovery-associated uveitis.[177,178] This entity is characterized by posterior segment inflammation, including vitreitis, papillitis, and optic disk and macular edema. Clinically important complications of immune-recovery uveitis include cataract, epiretinal membrane formation and loss of visual acuity.[171] This entity is common in persons with CMV retinitis who have substantial increases in their CD4+ T-lymphocyte counts. Immune recovery uveitis is seen in patients who do, or do not, continue with anti-CMV therapy after making an immune response to HAART.[172] One study diagnosed this problem in 19 of 30 patients (63%) responding to HAART with an annual incidence of 83 per 100 person-years.[177] A second study found evidence of intraocular inflammation in 22 of 23 eyes, with CMV retinitis in 16 patients who discontinued CMV therapy after responding to HAART.[178] A third study found immune recovery uveitis much less frequently; only six persons among 33 responding to HAART were found to have immune recovery uveitis, for an incidence of 11 per 100 person-years.[179] This lower rate may be related to a less dramatic response to HAART in this population and the retrospective nature of the study.[179]

SCREENING FOR DISEASE DUE TO CMV

There is no consensus regarding the screening of persons for CMV disease. The diseases rarely occur in persons with more than 100 CD4+ T lymphocytes per microliter,[14,36,37] so screening these persons seems not to be cost- or time-effective. Screening blood and urine cultures for CMV has poor specificity and poor sensitivity for detecting persons who will subsequently develop CMV disease[55,180] and PCR also has a low positive predictive value in the HAART era. The early diagnosis of CMV colitis or esophagitis before the onset of moderate to severe symptoms is unlikely to benefit most patients because, due to the toxicities of the agents available for treatment, most patients tolerate mild disease before beginning therapy. Additionally, because the cells that line the colon and esophagus reproduce rapidly, delayed treatment with GCV or foscarnet usually produces no permanent morbidity.

The early diagnosis of CMV retinitis is more important. Because retinal cells do not regenerate, delay in diagnosis can lead to spread of the disease and permanent loss of vision. Early diagnosis is critical to the management of CMV retinitis. Many experts recommend a baseline dilated ophthalmologic examination by the time the CD4+ T-lymphocyte count falls below 100 cells/μL. Because most persons with CMV retinitis present with some symptoms (either vision changes or 'floaters') it is most important to query patients about any subtle visual changes, discuss with susceptible persons the early signs of CMV disease, and bring them to the attention of their health-care provider. Some experienced clinicians recommend to their patients that they test their own visual fields using standard grids, and others have dilated ophthalmologic examinations performed on their patients with low CD4+ T-lymphocyte counts every 2–3 months. Whether these routines are better than close questioning about visual symptoms is unknown.

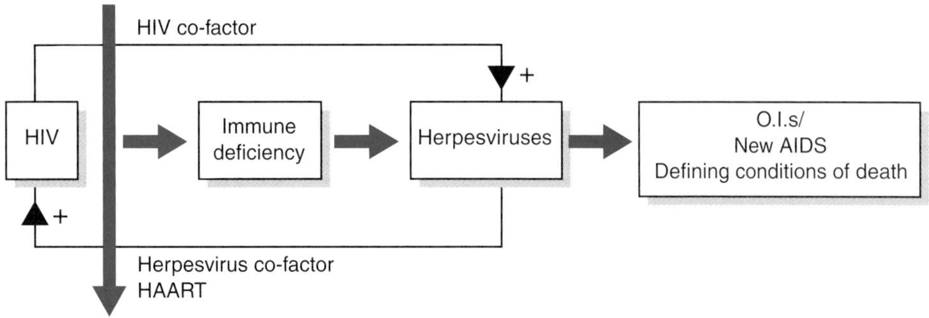

Figure 50-11 ■ Opportunistic and cofactor relationships between CMV and HIV. OIs, opportunistic infections.

CONTRIBUTION OF CMV TO MORTALITY IN PERSONS WITH AIDS

We tend to think of the relationship between HIV and CMV as following the linear pathway shown in Figure 50-11. Thus, HIV replication causes progressive immune deficiency that allows CMV to reactivate, replicate to high levels and cause opportunistic diseases such as CMV retinitis. However, there is an additional, more subtle, relationship between these two viruses as shown by the circular pathway shown in Figure 50-11. Once reactivated, CMV could interact with HIV to drive its pathogenicity while HIV could theoretically do the same for CMV, driving this virus to cause retinitis. Importantly, the ability of CMV to cause opportunistic disease may be completely dissociated from its ability to act as a co-factor, so we should look for evidence for both of these actions in natural history and therapeutic clinical trials.

There are at least six different ways that the two viruses could interact together.[181] The first three lead to activation of latent HIV. CMV could activate HIV gene expression by co-infecting the same cell and using its transactivators to stimulate HIV latent provirus. Alternatively, CMV could replicate in a bystander cell, releasing cytokines which, through signal transduction, could achieve the same end point of activating latent HIV provirus. Finally, in the special case where HIV is latent in a T-memory cell specific for CMV, release of the CMV cognate antigen for this cell from a bystander cell could lead to activation of the provirus. The other three mechanisms allow CMV to alter the tropism of HIV. If CMV and HIV infect the same cell, then HIV could bud from the plasma membrane acquiring the surface glycoproteins of CMV. This virion would then not be restricted by the CD4+ T-lymphocyte molecule but could infect any cell in the body that CMV was normally able to infect. Once this pseudotype had gained access to new cells, HIV would replicate autonomously. Alternatively, CMV could infect a bystander cell, increasing the expression of CD4+ T lymphocyte so rendering the cell susceptible to HIV infection; this has not been described for CMV but has been described for human herpesvirus 6.[182] Finally, CMV could express an alternative receptor for HIV as such has been shown for the Fc-receptor encoded by CMV which allows HIV coated in non-neutralizing antibody to gain access to fibroblasts, cells which are not normally tropic for HIV.[183] Likewise, gene *US28* of CMV is a chemokine receptor which can substitute for CCR5 allowing HIV to enter cells.[184] In addition to these six specific mechanisms, CMV could worsen the prognosis for HIV-infected individuals because of its general immunosuppressive, immune evasion, and immunomodulatory effects.

Irrespective of the precise mechanisms, there is evidence from the pre-HAART era that CMV was associated with a worse outcome for HIV-infected individuals. One study of hemophiliacs reported that an increased proportion developed AIDS if they were CMV seropositive after differences in age had been controlled using Cox proportional hazards models,[185] although this difference was not observed in a second large study.[186] Persistent secretion of CMV in the semen predicted AIDS development, after changes in baseline CD4+ T-lymphocyte count had been controlled using Cox proportional hazards models.[187] Patients who presented with first episode CMV retinitis had a significantly increased risk of mortality if they had above average CMV viral load at the time of presentation, even though all patients in the cohort were treated with GCV.[188] At that time, it was not possible to be sure that this was not just an indirect association with high viral loads of HIV, but Spector and colleagues subsequently showed that the death rate was driven much more by changes in CMV viral load than by changes in HIV viral load.[189] Finally, Kovacs and colleagues showed that infants born to HIV-positive mothers had an increased risk of developing HIV disease if they were CMV-infected.[190] Interestingly, HIV viral load was a risk factor among the CMV seronegatives only, suggesting that the presence of CMV overwhelmed the predictive value of HIV viral load.

When HAART was introduced, it was possible that its clinical benefit against CMV retinitis could be due to HAART decreasing CMV viremia or decreasing the risk associated with viremia, i.e., it might allow CMV viremia to continue but block the ability of the virus to cross the blood–retina barrier. A natural history study showed that the introduction of HAART completely abolished CMV viremia, presumably by giving patients back their preexisting CMV-specific immunity.[191]

Thus, the effect of HAART has been to both reduce the immune deficiency caused by CMV and to interfere with the ability of CMV to act as a putative cofactor to drive HIV

Table 50-8

Association Between CMV Viremia and Progression of AIDS

Factors	Progression to new AIDS-defining condition						Mortality					
	Univariable Models		Multivariable Baseline Covariates		Multivariable Covariates Measured Over Follow-Up		Univariable Models		Multivariable Baseline Covariates		Multivariable Covariates Measured Over Follow-Up	
	Relative Rate	***P*-Value**	**Relative Rate**	***P*-Value**	**Relative Rate**	***P*-Value**	**Relative Rate**	***P*-Value**	**Relative Rate**	***P*-Value**	**Relative Rate**	***P*-Value**
CMV DNA												
At baseline	2.11	0.005	1.94	0.02			2.87	0.004	2.06	0.07		
Over follow-up	4.97	0.0001			2.35	0.002	12.63	0.0001			4.69	0.0001
CD4+ T-Lymphocyte Count												
At baseline	0.95	0.03	0.98	0.49			0.94	0.10	0.99	0.82		
Over follow-up	0.86	0.0001			0.92	0.004	0.80	0.0001			0.86	0.003
HIV RNA Level												
At baseline	1.51	0.0001	1.50	0.0003			2.13	0.0004	2.03	0.002		
Over follow-up	1.77	0.0001			1.42	0.005	2.02	0.0001			1.38	0.07

pathogenicity (Figure 50-11). It is possible therefore that the dramatic clinical benefit and durable response to HAART might be partially explained by inhibition of the putative cofactor effect. To evaluate this, a prospective natural history study monitored the introduction of HAART in a cohort of patients who had ever had a CD4+ T-lymphocyte count less than 100. They were followed for an average of 36 months to determine whether the presence of CMV viremia detected by PCR was still predictive of mortality and, using multivariable statistical models, to determine the relative impact of HIV viral load and CD4+ T-lymphocyte count.

In summary, samples were collected for CMV PCR testing whenever HIV viral load and CD4+ T-lymphocyte counts were measured. Baseline and time updated multivariate models were used to examine the covariates of CMV PCR, CD4+ T-lymphocyte count, and HIV viral load. The results are summarized in Table 50-8 and show that CMV viremia is significantly associated with progression to a new AIDS defining event, and that this effect is statistically independent of CD4+ T-lymphocyte count and HIV RNA levels. The results also show that mortality was driven by the presence of CMV viremia and by the CD4+ T-lymphocyte count and that, once these two factors had been controlled, the HIV viral load had no further contribution to make to the risk analysis. The summary of the multivariable analysis of the covariates measured over follow-up are thus consistent with the hypothesis that HIV provides the context that allows CMV viremia, in the presence of a low CD4+ T-lymphocyte count, to contribute to the mortality of patients. We continue to suggest that the interpretation that CMV infection (although clinically silent) is the cause of death, should be subject to a double-blind randomized placebo-controlled trial of a drug with activity against CMV because it remains possible that the presence of CMV viremia may be an indirect marker of some underlying immune deficiency that is not captured by measurement of the CD4+ T-lymphocyte count. However, it is interesting to note that, in the pre-HAART era and in the HAART era, there is evidence from cohort studies that those who are treated for CMV have an improved survival benefit.[189,192,193] These studies confirm that CMV viremia is a risk factor for mortality, independent of HIV viral load, and CD4+ T-lymphocyte count.[189,192,193]

Before 1988 the survival of individuals diagnosed with CMV retinitis in conjunction with HIV infection ranged from 1 to 6 months.[89,152,194,195] With the increasing familiarity with the diagnosis of this CMV disease and the availability of GCV after 1988 to treat it, survival after diagnosis of CMV retinitis increased from 5 to 13 months.[87,194,196] Two of these studies have suggested a survival benefit in patients treated with GCV compared with untreated patients or patients not responding to GCV. Holland et al reported that patients treated with GCV survived a median of 7 months compared with untreated patients, who survived a median of only 2 months.[194] Jabs et al reported that patients who responded to treatment with GCV had a median survival of 10.0 months, compared with a median survival of only 2.3 months among patients who did not have a complete response.[197] A retrospective study evaluating the effect of foscarnet on survival found no difference in the median survival time from the diagnosis of CMV retinitis between patients treated with GCV (8 months, $n = 56$) and those treated with foscarnet (9 months, $n = 21$).[196] In a randomized clinical trial of initial therapy with GCV compared with foscarnet for the treatment of CMV retinitis, persons randomized to the foscarnet arm of the trial ($n = 107$) had a significantly increased survival (12.6 months) compared with those randomized to the GCV arm (8.5 months, $n = 127$).[87] This increase in survival was not confounded by the differential use of specific antiretroviral agents. A long-term follow-up of the randomized foscarnet trial independently corroborated the extended survival of foscarnet-treated persons with a median survival of that cohort of 13.5 months.[198] Much of this survival difference will change based on the use of more HAART for HIV infection. At present, the use of HAART has enabled persons with CMV retinitis and AIDS to discontinue therapy for CMV retinitis; the median survival in persons with CMV retinitis who have responded to HAART has not yet been determined, though it appears to be longer than 6 years.[170]

REFERENCES

1. Kaplan JE, Hanson D, Dworkin MS, et al. Epidemiology of human immunodeficiency virus-associated opportunistic infections in the United States in the era of highly active antiretroviral therapy. Clin Infect Dis 30:S5, 2000.
2. Emery VC, Cope AV, Bowen EF, et al. The dynamics of human cytomegalovirus replication in vivo. J Exp Med 190:177, 1999.
3. Stagno S, Reynolds DW, Tsiantos A, et al. Comparative serial virologic and serologic studies of symptomatic and subclinical congenitally and natally acquired cytomegalovirus infections. J Infect Dis 132:568, 1975.
4. Cope AV, Sweny P, Sabin C, et al. Quantity of cytomegalovirus viruria is a major risk factor for cytomegalovirus disease after renal transplantation. J Med Virol 52:200, 1997.
5. Meyers JD, Ljungman P, Fisher LD. Cytomegalovirus excretion as a predictor of cytomegalovirus disease after marrow transplantation: importance of cytomegalovirus viremia. J Infect Dis 162:373, 1990.
6. Kidd IM, Fox JC, Pillay D, et al. Provision of prognostic information in immunocompromised patients by routine application of the polymerase chain reaction for cytomegalovirus. Transplantation 56:867, 1993.
7. Hassan-Walker AF, Kidd IM, Sabin C, et al. Quantity of human cytomegalovirus (CMV) DNAemia as a risk factor for CMV disease in renal allograft recipients: relationship with donor/recipient CMV serostatus, receipt of augmented methylprednisolone and antithymocyte globulin (ATG). J Med Virol 58:182, 1999.
8. Cope AV, Sabin C, Burroughs A, et al. Interrelationships among quantity of human cytomegalovirus (HCMV) DNA in blood, donor–recipient serostatus, and administration of methylprednisolone as risk factors for HCMV disease following liver transplantation. J Infect Dis 176:1484, 1997.
9. Gor D, Sabin C, Prentice HG, et al. Longitudinal fluctuations in cytomegalovirus load in bone marrow transplant patients: relationship between peak virus load, donor/recipient serostatus, acute GVHD and CMV disease. Bone Marrow Transplant 21:597, 1998.
10. Dodt KK, Jacobsen PH, Hofmann B, et al. Development of cytomegalovirus (CMV) disease may be predicted in

HIV-infected patients by CMV polymerase chain reaction and the antigenemia test. AIDS 11:F21, 1997.
11. Shinkai M, Bozzette SA, Powderly W, et al. Utility of urine and leukocyte cultures and plasma DNA polymerase chain reaction for identification of AIDS patients at risk for developing human cytomegalovirus disease. J Infect Dis 175:302, 1997.
12. Bowen EF, Sabin CA, Wilson P, et al. Cytomegalovirus (CMV) viraemia detected by polymerase chain reaction identifies a group of HIV-positive patients at high risk of CMV disease. AIDS 11:889, 1997.
13. Whitley RJ, Jacobson MA, Friedberg DN, et al. Guidelines for the treatment of cytomegalovirus diseases in patients with AIDS in the era of potent antiretroviral therapy: recommendations of an international panel. International AIDS Society-USA. Arch Intern Med 158:957, 1998.
14. Gallant JE, Moore RD, Richman DD, et al. Incidence and natural history of cytomegalovirus disease in patients with advanced human immunodeficiency virus disease treated with zidovudine. The Zidovudine Epidemiology Study Group. J Infect Dis 166:1223, 1992.
15. Emery VC, Hassan-Walker AF, Burroughs AK, et al. Human cytomegalovirus (HCMV) replication dynamics in HCMV-naive and -experienced immunocompromised hosts. J Infect Dis 185:1723, 2002.
16. Emery VC, Griffiths PD. Prediction of cytomegalovirus load and resistance patterns after antiviral chemotherapy. Proc Natl Acad Sci USA 97:8039, 2000.
17. Gilbert MJ, Riddell SR, Plachter B, et al. Cytomegalovirus selectively blocks antigen processing and presentation of its immediate-early gene product. Nature 383:720, 1996.
18. Ahn K, Gruhler A, Galocha B, et al. The ER-luminal domain of the HCMV glycoprotein US6 inhibits peptide translocation by TAP. Immunity 6:613, 1997.
19. Lehner PJ, Karttunen JT, Wilkinson GW, et al. The human cytomegalovirus US6 glycoprotein inhibits transporter associated with antigen processing-dependent peptide translocation. Proc Natl Acad Sci USA 94:6904, 1997.
20. Tirosh B, Iwakoshi NN, Lilley BN, et al. Human cytomegalovirus protein US11 provokes an unfolded protein response that may facilitate the degradation of class I major histocompatibility complex products. J Virol 79:2768, 2005.
21. Wiertz EJ, Jones TR, Sun L, et al. The human cytomegalovirus US11 gene product dislocates MHC class I heavy chains from the endoplasmic reticulum to the cytosol. Cell 84:769, 1996.
22. Jones TR, Wiertz EJ, Sun L, et al. Human cytomegalovirus US3 impairs transport and maturation of major histocompatibility complex class I heavy chains. Proc Natl Acad Sci USA 93:11327, 1996.
23. Chapman TL, Heikeman AP, Bjorkman PJ. The inhibitory receptor LIR-1 uses a common binding interaction to recognize class I MHC molecules and the viral homolog UL18. Immunity 11:603, 1999.
24. Park B, Oh H, Lee S, et al. The MHC class I homolog of human cytomegalovirus is resistant to down-regulation mediated by the unique short region protein (US)2, US3, US6, and US11 gene products. J Immunol 168:3464, 2002.
25. Wills MR, Ashiru O, Reeves MB, et al. Human cytomegalovirus encodes an MHC class I-like molecule (UL142) that functions to inhibit NK cell lysis. J Immunol 175:7457, 2005.
26. Tomasec P, Braud VM, Rickards C, et al. Surface expression of HLA-E, an inhibitor of natural killer cells, enhanced by human cytomegalovirus gpUL40. Science 287:1031, 2000.
27. Wang EC, McSharry B, Retiere C, et al. UL40-mediated NK evasion during productive infection with human cytomegalovirus. Proc Natl Acad Sci USA 99:7570, 2002.
28. Wu J, Chalupny NJ, Manley TJ, et al. Intracellular retention of the MHC class I-related chain B ligand of NKG2D by the human cytomegalovirus UL16 glycoprotein. J Immunol 170:4196, 2003.
29. Gillespie GM, Wills MR, Appay V, et al. Functional heterogeneity and high frequencies of cytomegalovirus-specific CD8(+) T lymphocytes in healthy seropositive donors. J Virol 74:8140, 2000.
30. Weinberg A, Tierney C, Kendall MA, et al. Cytomegalovirus-specific immunity and protection against viremia and disease in HIV-infected patients in the era of highly active antiretroviral therapy. J Infect Dis 193:488, 2006.
31. Sacre K, Carcelain G, Cassoux N, et al. Repertoire, diversity, and differentiation of specific CD8 T cells are associated with immune protection against human cytomegalovirus disease. J Exp Med 201:1999, 2005.
32. Stone SF, Price P, Khan N, et al. HIV patients on antiretroviral therapy have high frequencies of CD8 T cells specific for immediate early protein-1 of cytomegalovirus. AIDS 19:555, 2005.
33. Bronke C, Palmer NM, Jansen CA, et al. Dynamics of cytomegalovirus (CMV)-specific T cells in HIV-1-infected individuals progressing to AIDS with CMV end-organ disease. J Infect Dis 191:873, 2005.
34. Bloom JN, Palestine AG. The diagnosis of cytomegalovirus retinitis. Ann Intern Med 109:963, 1988.
35. Drew WL. Cytomegalovirus infection in patients with AIDS. Clin Infect Dis 14:608, 1992.
36. Crowe SM, Carlin JB, Stewart KI, et al. Predictive value of CD4 lymphocyte numbers for the development of opportunistic infections and malignancies in HIV-infected persons. J Acquir Immune Defic Syndr 4:770, 1991.
37. Pertel P, Hirschtick R, Phair J, et al. Risk of developing cytomegalovirus retinitis in persons infected with the human immunodeficiency virus. J Acquir Immune Defic Syndr 5:1069, 1992.
38. Hoover DR, Saah AJ, Bacellar H, et al. Clinical manifestations of AIDS in the era of pneumocystis prophylaxis. Multicenter AIDS Cohort Study. N Engl J Med 329:1922, 1993.
39. Jacobson MA, Mills J. Serious cytomegalovirus disease in the acquired immunodeficiency syndrome (AIDS). Clinical findings, diagnosis, and treatment. Ann Intern Med 108:585, 1988.
40. Spector SA, Wong R, Hsia K, et al. Plasma cytomegalovirus (CMV) DNA load predicts CMV disease and survival in AIDS patients. J Clin Invest 101:497, 1998.
41. Freeman WR, Henderly DE, Wan WL, et al. Prevalence, pathophysiology, and treatment of rhegmatogenous retinal detachment in treated cytomegalovirus retinitis. Am J Ophthalmol 103:527, 1987.
42. Holbrook JT, Jabs DA, Weinberg DV, et al. Visual loss in patients with cytomegalovirus retinitis and acquired immunodeficiency syndrome before widespread availability of highly active antiretroviral therapy. Arch Ophthalmol 121:99, 2003.
43. Kempen JH, Martin BK, Wu AW, et al. The effect of cytomegalovirus retinitis on the quality of life of patients with AIDS in the era of highly active antiretroviral therapy. Ophthalmology 110:987, 2003.
44. Lalezari JP, Stagg RJ, Kuppermann BD, et al. Intravenous cidofovir for peripheral cytomegalovirus retinitis in patients with AIDS. A randomized, controlled trial. Ann Intern Med 126:257, 1997.
45. Palestine AG, Polis MA, De Smet MD, et al. A randomized, controlled trial of foscarnet in the treatment of cytomegalovirus retinitis in patients with AIDS. Ann Intern Med 115:665, 1991.
46. Spector SA, Weingeist T, Pollard RB, et al. A randomized, controlled study of intravenous ganciclovir therapy for cytomegalovirus peripheral retinitis in patients with AIDS. AIDS Clinical Trials Group and Cytomegalovirus Cooperative Study Group. J Infect Dis 168:557, 1993.

47. Holland GN, Shuler JD. Progression rates of cytomegalovirus retinopathy in ganciclovir-treated and untreated patients. Arch Ophthalmol 110:1435, 1992.
48. De Smet MD. Differential diagnosis of retinitis and choroiditis in patients with acquired immunodeficiency syndrome. Am J Med 92:17S, 1992.
49. O'Donnell JJ, Jacobson MA. Cotton-wool spots and cytomegalovirus retinitis in AIDS. Int Ophthalmol Clin 29:105, 1989.
50. Engstrom RE Jr, Holland GN, Margolis TP, et al. The progressive outer retinal necrosis syndrome. A variant of necrotizing herpetic retinopathy in patients with AIDS. Ophthalmology 101:1488, 1994.
51. Holland GN, Engstrom RE Jr, Glasgow BJ, et al. Ocular toxoplasmosis in patients with the acquired immunodeficiency syndrome. Am J Ophthalmol 106:653, 1988.
52. Dugel PU, Rao NA, Forster DJ, et al. *Pneumocystis carinii* choroiditis after long-term aerosolized pentamidine therapy. Am J Ophthalmol 110:113, 1990.
53. Wilcox CM, Diehl DL, Cello JP, et al. Cytomegalovirus esophagitis in patients with AIDS. A clinical, endoscopic, and pathologic correlation. Ann Intern Med 113:589, 1990.
54. Dieterich DT, Wilcox CM. Diagnosis and treatment of esophageal diseases associated with HIV infection. Practice Parameters Committee of the American College of Gastroenterology. Am J Gastroenterol 91:2265, 1996.
55. Zurlo JJ, O'Neill D, Polis MA, et al. Lack of clinical utility of cytomegalovirus blood and urine cultures in patients with HIV infection. Ann Intern Med 118:12, 1993.
56. Wilcox CM, Rodgers W, Lazenby A. Prospective comparison of brush cytology, viral culture, and histology for the diagnosis of ulcerative esophagitis in AIDS. Clin Gastroenterol Hepatol 2:564, 2004.
57. Wilcox CM. Esophageal disease in the acquired immunodeficiency syndrome: etiology, diagnosis, and management. Am J Med 92:412, 1992.
58. Porro GB, Parente F, Cernuschi M. The diagnosis of esophageal candidiasis in patients with acquired immune deficiency syndrome: is endoscopy always necessary? Am J Gastroenterol 84:143, 1989.
59. Chiu HM, Wu MS, Hung CC, et al. Low prevalence of *Helicobacter pylori* but high prevalence of cytomegalovirus-associated peptic ulcer disease in AIDS patients: Comparative study of symptomatic subjects evaluated by endoscopy and CD4 counts. J Gastroenterol Hepatol 19:423, 2004.
60. Dieterich DT, Rahmin M. Cytomegalovirus colitis in AIDS: presentation in 44 patients and a review of the literature. J Acquir Immune Defic Syndr 4:S29, 1991.
61. Frager DH, Frager JD, Wolf EL, et al. Cytomegalovirus colitis in acquired immune deficiency syndrome: radiologic spectrum. Gastrointest Radiol 11:241, 1986.
62. Smith PD, Lane HC, Gill VJ, et al. Intestinal infections in patients with the acquired immunodeficiency syndrome (AIDS). Etiology and response to therapy. Ann Intern Med 108:328, 1988.
63. Wallace JM, Hannah J. Cytomegalovirus pneumonitis in patients with AIDS. Findings in an autopsy series. Chest 92:198, 1987.
64. Jacobson MA, Mills J, Rush J, et al. Morbidity and mortality of patients with AIDS and first-episode *Pneumocystis carinii* pneumonia unaffected by concomitant pulmonary cytomegalovirus infection. Am Rev Respir Dis 144:6, 1991.
65. Rodriguez-Barradas MC, Stool E, Musher DM, et al. Diagnosing and treating cytomegalovirus pneumonia in patients with AIDS. Clin Infect Dis 23:76, 1996.
66. Petito CK, Cho ES, Lemann W, et al. Neuropathology of acquired immunodeficiency syndrome (AIDS): an autopsy review. J Neuropathol Exp Neurol 45:635, 1986.
67. Arribas JR, Clifford DB, Fichtenbaum CJ, et al. Level of cytomegalovirus (CMV) DNA in cerebrospinal fluid of subjects with AIDS and CMV infection of the central nervous system. J Infect Dis 172:527, 1995.
68. Arribas JR, Storch GA, Clifford DB, et al. Cytomegalovirus encephalitis. Ann Intern Med 125:577, 1996.
69. Holland NR, Power C, Mathews VP, et al. Cytomegalovirus encephalitis in acquired immunodeficiency syndrome (AIDS). Neurology 44:507, 1994.
70. Kalayjian RC, Cohen ML, Bonomo RA, et al. Cytomegalovirus ventriculoencephalitis in AIDS. A syndrome with distinct clinical and pathologic features. Medicine (Baltimore) 72:67, 1993.
71. Morgello S, Cho ES, Nielsen S, et al. Cytomegalovirus encephalitis in patients with acquired immunodeficiency syndrome: an autopsy study of 30 cases and a review of the literature. Hum Pathol 18:289, 1987.
72. Wolf DG, Spector SA. Diagnosis of human cytomegalovirus central nervous system disease in AIDS patients by DNA amplification from cerebrospinal fluid. J Infect Dis 166:1412, 1992.
73. Behar R, Wiley C, McCutchan JA. Cytomegalovirus polyradiculoneuropathy in acquired immune deficiency syndrome. Neurology 37:557, 1987.
74. McCutchan JA. Cytomegalovirus infections of the nervous system in patients with AIDS. Clin Infect Dis 20:747, 1995.
75. Miller RF, Fox JD, Thomas P, et al. Acute lumbosacral polyradiculopathy due to cytomegalovirus in advanced HIV disease: CSF findings in 17 patients. J Neurol Neurosurg Psychiatry 61:456, 1996.
76. So YT, Olney RK. Acute lumbosacral polyradiculopathy in acquired immunodeficiency syndrome: experience in 23 patients. Ann Neurol 35:53, 1994.
77. McKenzie R, Travis WD, Dolan SA, et al. The causes of death in patients with human immunodeficiency virus infection: a clinical and pathologic study with emphasis on the role of pulmonary diseases. Medicine (Baltimore) 70:326, 1991.
78. Bricaire F, Marche C, Zoubi D, et al. Adrenocortical lesions and AIDS. Lancet 1:881, 1988.
79. Greene LW, Cole W, Greene JB, et al. Adrenal insufficiency as a complication of the acquired immunodeficiency syndrome. Ann Intern Med 101:497, 1984.
80. Blanshard C. Treatment of HIV-related cytomegalovirus disease of the gastrointestinal tract with foscarnet. J Acquir Immune Defic Syndr 5:S25, 1992.
81. Littler E, Stuart AD, Chee MS. Human cytomegalovirus UL97 open reading frame encodes a protein that phosphorylates the antiviral nucleoside analogue ganciclovir. Nature 358:160, 1992.
82. Sullivan V, Talarico CL, Stanat SC, et al. A protein kinase homologue controls phosphorylation of ganciclovir in human cytomegalovirus-infected cells. Nature 358:162, 1992.
83. Drew WL, Ives D, Lalezari JP, et al. Oral ganciclovir as maintenance treatment for cytomegalovirus retinitis in patients with AIDS. Syntex Cooperative Oral Ganciclovir Study Group. N Engl J Med 333:615, 1995.
84. Sommadossi JP, Bevan R, Ling T, et al. Clinical pharmacokinetics of ganciclovir in patients with normal and impaired renal function. Rev Infect Dis 10:S507, 1988.
85. Faulds D, Heel RC. Ganciclovir. A review of its antiviral activity, pharmacokinetic properties and therapeutic efficacy in cytomegalovirus infections. Drugs 39:597, 1990.
86. Buhles WC Jr, Mastre BJ, Tinker AJ, et al. Ganciclovir treatment of life- or sight-threatening cytomegalovirus infection: experience in 314 immunocompromised patients. Rev Infect Dis 10:S495, 1988.
87. Studies of Ocular Complications of AIDS Research Group A. Mortality in patients with the acquired immunodeficiency

syndrome treated with either foscarnet or ganciclovir for cytomegalovirus retinitis. Studies of Ocular Complications of AIDS Research Group, in collaboration with the AIDS Clinical Trials Group. N Engl J Med 326:213, 1992.

88. Jacobson MA, O'Donnell JJ, Mills J. Foscarnet treatment of cytomegalovirus retinitis in patients with the acquired immunodeficiency syndrome. Antimicrob Agents Chemother 33:736, 1989.
89. Palestine AG, Rodrigues MM, Macher AM, et al. Ophthalmic involvement in acquired immunodeficiency syndrome. Ophthalmology 91:1092, 1984.
90. Dieterich DT, Kotler DP, Busch DF, et al. Ganciclovir treatment of cytomegalovirus colitis in AIDS: a randomized, double-blind, placebo-controlled multicenter study. J Infect Dis 167:278, 1993.
91. Blanshard C, Benhamou Y, Dohin E, et al. Treatment of AIDS-associated gastrointestinal cytomegalovirus infection with foscarnet and ganciclovir: a randomized comparison. J Infect Dis 172:622, 1995.
92. Emanuel D, Cunningham I, Jules-Elysee K, et al. Cytomegalovirus pneumonia after bone marrow transplantation successfully treated with the combination of ganciclovir and high-dose intravenous immune globulin. Ann Intern Med 109:777, 1988.
93. Reed EC, Bowden RA, Dandliker PS, et al. Treatment of cytomegalovirus pneumonia with ganciclovir and intravenous cytomegalovirus immunoglobulin in patients with bone marrow transplants. Ann Intern Med 109:783, 1988.
94. Jacobson MA, O'Donnell JJ, Rousell R, et al. Failure of adjunctive cytomegalovirus intravenous immune globulin to improve efficacy of ganciclovir in patients with acquired immunodeficiency syndrome and cytomegalovirus retinitis: a phase 1 study. Antimicrob Agents Chemother 34:176, 1990.
95. Anduze-Faris BM, Fillet AM, Gozlan J, et al. Induction and maintenance therapy of cytomegalovirus central nervous system infection in HIV-infected patients. AIDS 14:517, 2000.
96. Hochster H, Dieterich D, Bozzette S, et al. Toxicity of combined ganciclovir and zidovudine for cytomegalovirus disease associated with AIDS. An AIDS Clinical Trials Group Study. Ann Intern Med 113:111, 1990.
97. Medina DJ, Hsiung GD, Mellors JW. Ganciclovir antagonizes the anti-human immunodeficiency virus type 1 activity of zidovudine and didanosine in vitro. Antimicrob Agents Chemother 36:1127, 1992.
98. Cantrill HL, Henry K, Melroe NH, et al. Treatment of cytomegalovirus retinitis with intravitreal ganciclovir. Long-term results. Ophthalmology 96:367, 1989.
99. Henry K, Cantrill H, Fletcher C, et al. Use of intravitreal ganciclovir (dihydroxy propoxymethyl guanine) for cytomegalovirus retinitis in a patient with AIDS. Am J Ophthalmol 103:17, 1987.
100. Schulman J, Peyman GA, Horton MB, et al. Intraocular 9-([2-hydroxy-1-(hydroxymethyl) ethoxy] methyl) guanine levels after intravitreal and subconjunctival administration. Ophthalmic Surg 17:429, 1986.
101. Young S, McCluskey P, Minassian DC, et al. Retinal detachment in cytomegalovirus retinitis: intravenous versus intravitreal therapy. Clin Experiment Ophthalmol 31:96, 2003.
102. Martin DF, Parks DJ, Mellow SD, et al. Treatment of cytomegalovirus retinitis with an intraocular sustained-release ganciclovir implant. A randomized controlled clinical trial. Arch Ophthalmol 112:1531, 1994.
103. Jabs DA, Enger C, Haller J, et al. Retinal detachments in patients with cytomegalovirus retinitis. Arch Ophthalmol 109:794, 1991.
104. Kempen JH, Jabs DA, Dunn JP, et al. Retinal detachment risk in cytomegalovirus retinitis related to the acquired immunodeficiency syndrome. Arch Ophthalmol 119:33, 2001.
105. Musch DC, Martin DF, Gordon JF, et al. Treatment of cytomegalovirus retinitis with a sustained-release ganciclovir implant. The Ganciclovir Implant Study Group. N Engl J Med 337:83, 1997.
106. Martin DF, Kuppermann BD, Wolitz RA, et al. Oral ganciclovir for patients with cytomegalovirus retinitis treated with a ganciclovir implant. Roche Ganciclovir Study Group. N Engl J Med 340:1063, 1999.
107. Bowen EF, Emery VC, Wilson P, et al. Cytomegalovirus polymerase chain reaction viraemia in patients receiving ganciclovir maintenance therapy for retinitis. AIDS 12:605, 1998.
108. Anonymous. Valganciclovir, a more potent oral therapy for CMV retinitis in AIDS, approved by FDA. Clin Infect Dis 32, 2001.
109. Brown F, Banken L, Saywell K, et al. Pharmacokinetics of valganciclovir and ganciclovir following multiple oral dosages of valganciclovir in HIV- and CMV-seropositive volunteers. Clin Pharmacokinet 37:167, 1999.
110. Martin DF, Sierra-Madero J, Walmsley S, et al. A controlled trial of valganciclovir as induction therapy for cytomegalovirus retinitis. N Engl J Med 346:1119, 2002.
111. Eriksson B, Oberg B, Wahren B. Pyrophosphate analogues as inhibitors of DNA polymerases of cytomegalovirus, herpes simplex virus and cellular origin. Biochim Biophys Acta 696:115, 1982.
112. Ostrander M, Cheng YC. Properties of herpes simplex virus type 1 and type 2 DNA polymerase. Biochim Biophys Acta 609:232, 1980.
113. Sandstrom EG, Kaplan JC, Byington RE, et al. Inhibition of human T-cell lymphotropic virus type III in vitro by phosphonoformate. Lancet 1:1480, 1985.
114. Sjovall J, Karlsson A, Ogenstad S, et al. Pharmacokinetics and absorption of foscarnet after intravenous and oral administration to patients with human immunodeficiency virus. Clin Pharmacol Ther 44:65, 1988.
115. Aweeka F, Gambertoglio J, Mills J, et al. Pharmacokinetics of intermittently administered intravenous foscarnet in the treatment of acquired immunodeficiency syndrome patients with serious cytomegalovirus retinitis. Antimicrob Agents Chemother 33:742, 1989.
116. Sjovall J, Bergdahl S, Movin G, et al. Pharmacokinetics of foscarnet and distribution to cerebrospinal fluid after intravenous infusion in patients with human immunodeficiency virus infection. Antimicrob Agents Chemother 33:1023, 1989.
117. Deray G, Martinez F, Katlama C, et al. Foscarnet nephrotoxicity: mechanism, incidence and prevention. Am J Nephrol 9:316, 1989.
118. Fanning MM, Read SE, Benson M, et al. Foscarnet therapy of cytomegalovirus retinitis in AIDS. J Acquir Immune Defic Syndr 3:472, 1990.
119. Lehoang P, Girard B, Robinet M, et al. Foscarnet in the treatment of cytomegalovirus retinitis in acquired immune deficiency syndrome. Ophthalmology 96:865, 1989.
120. Walmsley SL, Chew E, Read SE, et al. Treatment of cytomegalovirus retinitis with trisodium phosphonoformate hexahydrate (Foscarnet). J Infect Dis 157:569, 1988.
121. Nelson MR, Connolly GM, Hawkins DA, et al. Foscarnet in the treatment of cytomegalovirus infection of the esophagus and colon in patients with the acquired immune deficiency syndrome. Am J Gastroenterol 86:876, 1991.
122. Jacobson MA, Gambertoglio JG, Aweeka FT, et al. Foscarnet-induced hypocalcemia and effects of foscarnet on calcium metabolism. J Clin Endocrinol Metab 72:1130, 1991.
123. Youle MS, Clarbour J, Gazzard B, et al. Severe hypocalcaemia in AIDS patients treated with foscarnet and pentamidine. Lancet 1:1455, 1988.

124. Diaz-Llopis M, Espana E, Munoz G, et al. High dose intravitreal foscarnet in the treatment of cytomegalovirus retinitis in AIDS. Br J Ophthalmol 78:120, 1994.
125. Cundy KC, Petty BG, Flaherty J, et al. Clinical pharmacokinetics of cidofovir in human immunodeficiency virus-infected patients. Antimicrob Agents Chemother 39:1247, 1995.
126. Lalezari JP, Drew WL, Glutzer E, et al. (S)-1-[3-hydroxy-2-(phosphonylmethoxy)propyl]cytosine (cidofovir): results of a phase I/II study of a novel antiviral nucleotide analogue. J Infect Dis 171:788, 1995.
127. Polis MA, Spooner KM, Baird BF, et al. Anticytomegaloviral activity and safety of cidofovir in patients with human immunodeficiency virus infection and cytomegalovirus viruria. Antimicrob Agents Chemother 39:882, 1995.
128. Cihlar T, Lin DC, Pritchard JB, et al. The antiviral nucleotide analogs cidofovir and adefovir are novel substrates for human and rat renal organic anion transporter 1. Mol Pharmacol 56:570, 1999.
129. Studies of the Ocular Complications of AIDS Research Group in collaboration with AIDS Clinical Trial Group. Parenteral cidofovir for cytomegalovirus retinitis in patients with AIDS: the HPMPC periperhaeral cytomegalovirus retinitis trial. Ann Intern Med 126:264, 1997.
130. Davis JL, Taskintuna I, Freeman WR, et al. Iritis and hypotony after treatment with intravenous cidofovir for cytomegalovirus retinitis. Arch Ophthalmol 115:733, 1997.
131. Song MK, Azen SP, Buley A, et al. Effect of anti-cytomegalovirus therapy on the incidence of immune recovery uveitis in AIDS patients with healed cytomegalovirus retinitis. Am J Ophthalmol 136:696, 2003.
132. Rahhal FM, Arevalo JF, Chavez dlP, et al. Treatment of cytomegalovirus retinitis with intravitreous cidofovir in patients with AIDS. A preliminary report. Ann Intern Med 125:98, 1996.
133. De Smet MD, Meenken CJ, van den Horn GJ. Fomivirsen – a phosphorothioate oligonucleotide for the treatment of CMV retinitis. Ocul Immunol Inflamm 7:189, 1999.
134. Perry CM, Balfour JA. Fomivirsen. Drugs 57:375, 1999.
135. Erice A, Chou S, Biron KK, et al. Progressive disease due to ganciclovir-resistant cytomegalovirus in immunocompromised patients. N Engl J Med 320:289, 1989.
136. Drew WL, Miner RC, Busch DF, et al. Prevalence of resistance in patients receiving ganciclovir for serious cytomegalovirus infection. J Infect Dis 163:716, 1991.
137. Studies of Ocular Complications of AIDS Research Group A. Cytomegalovirus (CMV) culture results, drug resistance and clinical outcome in patients with AIDS and CMV retinitis treated with foscarnet or ganciclovir. J Infect Dis 50, 1997.
138. Jabs DA, Enger C, Dunn JP, et al. Cytomegalovirus retinitis and viral resistance: ganciclovir resistance. CMV Retinitis and Viral Resistance Study Group. J Infect Dis 177:770, 1998.
139. Smith IL, Cherrington JM, Jiles RE, et al. High-level resistance of cytomegalovirus to ganciclovir is associated with alterations in both the UL97 and DNA polymerase genes. J Infect Dis 176:69, 1997.
140. Jacobson MA, Drew WL, Feinberg J, et al. Foscarnet therapy for ganciclovir-resistant cytomegalovirus retinitis in patients with AIDS. J Infect Dis 163:1348, 1991.
141. Jabs DA, Enger C, Forman M, et al. Incidence of foscarnet resistance and cidofovir resistance in patients treated for cytomegalovirus retinitis. The Cytomegalovirus Retinitis and Viral Resistance Study Group. Antimicrob Agents Chemother 42:2240, 1998.
142. Weinberg A, Jabs DA, Chou S, et al. Mutations conferring foscarnet resistance in a cohort of patients with acquired immunodeficiency syndrome and cytomegalovirus retinitis. J Infect Dis 187:777, 2003.
143. Erice A, Gil-Roda C, Perez JL, et al. Antiviral susceptibilities and analysis of UL97 and DNA polymerase sequences of clinical cytomegalovirus isolates from immunocompromised patients. J Infect Dis 175:1087, 1997.
144. Chou S, Lurain NS, Thompson KD, et al. Viral DNA polymerase mutations associated with drug resistance in human cytomegalovirus. J Infect Dis 188:32, 2003.
145. Smith IL, Cherrington JM, Jiles RE, et al. High-level resistance of cytomegalovirus to ganciclovir is associated with alterations in both the UL97 and DNA polymerase genes. J Infect Dis 176:69, 1997.
146. Baldanti F, Underwood MR, Stanat SC, et al. Single amino acid changes in the DNA polymerase confer foscarnet resistance and slow-growth phenotype, while mutations in the UL97-encoded phosphotransferase confer ganciclovir resistance in three double-resistant human cytomegalovirus strains recovered from patients with AIDS. J Virol 70:1390, 1996.
147. Hu H, Jabs DA, Forman MS, et al. Comparison of cytomegalovirus (CMV) UL97 gene sequences in the blood and vitreous of patients with acquired immunodeficiency syndrome and CMV retinitis. J Infect Dis 185:861, 2002.
148. Jabs DA, Martin BK, Forman MS, et al. Cytomegalovirus (CMV) blood DNA load, CMV retinitis progression, and occurrence of resistant CMV in patients with CMV retinitis. J Infect Dis 192:640, 2005.
149. Bowen EF, Johnson MA, Griffiths PD, et al. Development of a point mutation assay for the detection of human cytomegalovirus UL97 mutations associated with ganciclovir resistance. J Virol Methods 68:225, 1997.
150. Studies of Ocular Complications of AIDS Research Group ACTG. Combination foscarnet and ganciclovir therapy vs monotherapy for the treatment of relapsed cytomegalovirus retinitis in patients with AIDS: the Cytomegalovirus Retreatment Trial. Arch Ophthalmol 23, 1996.
151. Smith IL, Cherrington JM, Jiles RE, et al. High-level resistance of cytomegalovirus to ganciclovir is associated with alterations in both the UL97 and DNA polymerase genes. J Infect Dis 176:69, 1997.
152. Henderly DE, Freeman WR, Causey DM, et al. Cytomegalovirus retinitis and response to therapy with ganciclovir. Ophthalmology 94:425, 1987.
153. Mattes FM, Hainsworth EG, Geretti AM, et al. A randomized, controlled trial comparing ganciclovir to ganciclovir plus foscarnet (each at half dose) for preemptive therapy of cytomegalovirus infection in transplant recipients. J Infect Dis 189:1355, 2004.
154. Griffiths PD. Therapeutic patents for cytomegalovirus. Exp Opin Therap Pat 13:319, 2003.
155. Martinez A, Castro A, Gil C, et al. Recent strategies in the development of new human cytomegalovirus inhibitors. Med Res Rev 21:227, 2001.
156. McSharry JJ, McDonough A, Olson B, et al. Inhibition of ganciclovir-susceptible and -resistant human cytomegalovirus clinical isolates by the benzimidazole L-riboside 1263W94. Clin Diagn Lab Immunol 8:1279, 2001.
157. Spector SA, McKinley GF, Lalezari JP, et al. Oral ganciclovir for the prevention of cytomegalovirus disease in persons with AIDS. Roche Cooperative Oral Ganciclovir Study Group. N Engl J Med 1996;334:1491–7.
158. Brosgart CL, Louis TA, Hillman DW, et al. A randomized, placebo-controlled trial of the safety and efficacy of oral ganciclovir for prophylaxis of cytomegalovirus disease in HIV-infected individuals. Terry Beirn Community Programs for Clinical Research on AIDS. AIDS 12:269, 1998.
159. Feinberg JE, Hurwitz S, Cooper D, et al. A randomized, double-blind trial of valaciclovir prophylaxis for cytomegalovirus disease in patients with advanced human immunodeficiency virus infection. AIDS Clinical Trials Group Protocol

204/Glaxo Wellcome 123-014 International CMV Prophylaxis Study Group. J Infect Dis 177:48, 1998.
160. USPHS I. 2001 USPHS/IDSA guidelines for the prevention of opportunistic infections in persons infected with human immunodeficiency virus. USPHS/IDSA 2001.
161. Berenguer J, Gonzalez J, Pulido F, et al. Discontinuation of secondary prophylaxis in patients with cytomegalovirus retinitis who have responded to highly active antiretroviral therapy. Clin Infect Dis 34:394, 2002.
162. Jabs DA, Bolton SG, Dunn JP, et al. Discontinuing anticytomegalovirus therapy in patients with immune reconstitution after combination antiretroviral therapy. Am J Ophthalmol 126:817, 1998.
163. Jouan M, Saves M, Tubiana R, et al. Discontinuation of maintenance therapy for cytomegalovirus retinitis in HIV-infected patients receiving highly active antiretroviral therapy. AIDS 15:23, 2001.
164. Macdonald JC, Torriani FJ, Morse LS, et al. Lack of reactivation of cytomegalovirus (CMV) retinitis after stopping CMV maintenance therapy in AIDS patients with sustained elevations in CD4 T cells in response to highly active antiretroviral therapy. J Infect Dis 177:1182, 1998.
165. Macdonald JC, Karavellas MP, Torriani FJ, et al. Highly active antiretroviral therapy-related immune recovery in AIDS patients with cytomegalovirus retinitis. Ophthalmology 107:877, 2000.
166. Tural C, Romeu J, Sirera G, et al. Long-lasting remission of cytomegalovirus retinitis without maintenance therapy in human immunodeficiency virus-infected patients. J Infect Dis 177:1080, 1998.
167. Vrabec TR, Baldassano VF, Whitcup SM. Discontinuation of maintenance therapy in patients with quiescent cytomegalovirus retinitis and elevated CD4+ counts. Ophthalmology 105:1259, 1998.
168. Whitcup SM, Fortin E, Nussenblatt RB, et al. Therapeutic effect of combination antiretroviral therapy on cytomegalovirus retinitis. JAMA 277:1519, 1997.
169. Whitcup SM, Fortin E, Lindblad AS, et al. Discontinuation of anticytomegalovirus therapy in patients with HIV infection and cytomegalovirus retinitis. JAMA 282:1633, 1999.
170. Sklar PA, Agyemang AF, Monastra R, et al. Five-year follow up of a cohort of profoundly immunosuppressed patients discontinuing therapy for cytomegalovirus retinitis. AIDS 18: 567, 2004.
171. Goldberg DE, Smithen LM, Angelilli A, et al. HIV-associated retinopathy in the HAART era. Retina 25:633, 2005.
172. Wohl DA, Kendall MA, Owens S, et al. The safety of discontinuation of maintenance therapy for cytomegalovirus (CMV) retinitis and incidence of immune recovery uveitis following potent antiretroviral therapy. HIV Clin Trials 6:136, 2005.
173. Torriani FJ, Freeman WR, Macdonald JC, et al. CMV retinitis recurs after stopping treatment in virological and immunological failures of potent antiretroviral therapy. AIDS 14:173, 2000.
174. Crum NF, Blade KA. Cytomegalovirus retinitis after immune reconstitution. AIDS Read 15:186, 2005.
175. Johnson SC, Benson CA, Johnson DW, et al. Recurrences of cytomegalovirus retinitis in a human immunodeficiency virus-infected patient, despite potent antiretroviral therapy and apparent immune reconstitution. Clin Infect Dis 32:815, 2001.
176. Kempen JH, Jabs DA, Wilson LA, et al. Incidence of cytomegalovirus (CMV) retinitis in second eyes of patients with the acquired immune deficiency syndrome and unilateral CMV retinitis. Am J Ophthalmol 139:1028, 2005.
177. Karavellas MP, Plummer DJ, Macdonald JC, et al. Incidence of immune recovery vitritis in cytomegalovirus retinitis patients following institution of successful highly active antiretroviral therapy. J Infect Dis 179:697, 1999.
178. Robinson MR, Reed G, Csaky KG, et al. Immune-recovery uveitis in patients with cytomegalovirus retinitis taking highly active antiretroviral therapy. Am J Ophthalmol 130:49, 2000.
179. Nguyen QD, Kempen JH, Bolton SG, et al. Immune recovery uveitis in patients with AIDS and cytomegalovirus retinitis after highly active antiretroviral therapy. Am J Ophthalmol 129:634, 2000.
180. Salmon D, Lacassin F, Harzic M, et al. Predictive value of cytomegalovirus viraemia for the occurrence of CMV organ involvement in AIDS. J Med Virol 32:160, 1990.
181. Griffiths PD. Studies of viral co-factors for human immunodeficiency virus in vitro and in vivo. J Gen Virol 79(Pt 2): 213, 198.
182. Lusso P, Garzino-Demo A, Crowley RW, et al. Infection of gamma/delta T lymphocytes by human herpesvirus 6: transcriptional induction of CD4 and susceptibility to HIV infection. J Exp Med 181:1303, 1995.
183. McKeating JA, Griffiths PD, Weiss RA. HIV susceptibility conferred to human fibroblasts by cytomegalovirus-induced Fc receptor. Nature 343:659, 1990.
184. Pleskoff O, Treboute C, Brelot A, et al. Identification of a chemokine receptor encoded by human cytomegalovirus as a cofactor for HIV-1 entry. Science 276:1874, 1997.
185. Webster A, Lee CA, Cook DG, et al. Cytomegalovirus infection and progression towards AIDS in haemophiliacs with human immunodeficiency virus infection. Lancet 2:63, 1989.
186. Rabkin CS, Hatzakis A, Griffiths PD, et al. Cytomegalovirus infection and risk of AIDS in human immunodeficiency virus-infected hemophilia patients. National Cancer Institute Multicenter Hemophilia Cohort Study Group. J Infect Dis 168:1260, 1993.
187. Detels R, Leach CT, Hennessey K, et al. Persistent cytomegalovirus infection of semen increases risk of AIDS. J Infect Dis 169:766, 1994.
188. Bowen EF, Wilson P, Cope A, et al. Cytomegalovirus retinitis in AIDS patients: influence of cytomegaloviral load on response to ganciclovir, time to recurrence and survival. AIDS 10:1515, 1996.
189. Spector SA, Hsia K, Crager M, et al. Cytomegalovirus (CMV) DNA load is an independent predictor of CMV disease and survival in advanced AIDS. J Virol 73:7027, 1999.
190. Kovacs A, Schluchter M, Easley K, et al. Cytomegalovirus infection and HIV-1 disease progression in infants born to HIV-1-infected women. Pediatric Pulmonary and Cardiovascular Complications of Vertically Transmitted HIV Infection Study Group. N Engl J Med 341:77, 1999.
191. Deayton J, Mocroft A, Wilson P, et al. Loss of cytomegalovirus (CMV) viraemia following highly active antiretroviral therapy in the absence of specific anti-CMV therapy. AIDS 13:1203, 1999.
192. Jabs DA, Holbrook JT, Van Natta ML, et al. Risk factors for mortality in patients with AIDS in the era of highly active antiretroviral therapy. Ophthalmology 112:771, 2005.
193. Wohl DA, Zeng D, Stewart P, et al. Cytomegalovirus viremia, mortality, and end-organ disease among patients with AIDS receiving potent antiretroviral therapies. J Acquir Immune Defic Syndr 38:538, 2005.
194. Holland GN, Sison RF, Jatulis DE, et al. Survival of patients with the acquired immune deficiency syndrome after development of cytomegalovirus retinopathy. UCLA CMV Retinopathy Study Group. Ophthalmology 97:204, 1990.
195. Jacobson MA, O'Donnell JJ, Porteous D, et al. Retinal and gastrointestinal disease due to cytomegalovirus in patients with the acquired immune deficiency syndrome: prevalence, natural history, and response to ganciclovir therapy. Q J Med 67:473, 1988.
196. Harb GE, Bacchetti P, Jacobson MA. Survival of patients with AIDS and cytomegalovirus disease treated with ganciclovir or foscarnet. AIDS 5:959, 1991.

197. Jabs DA, Enger C, Bartlett JG. Cytomegalovirus retinitis and acquired immunodeficiency syndrome. Arch Ophthalmol 107:75, 1989.
198. Polis MA, deSmet MD, Baird BF, et al. Increased survival of a cohort of patients with acquired immunodeficiency syndrome and cytomegalovirus retinitis who received sodium phosphonoformate (foscarnet). Am J Med 94:175, 1993.
199. Jabs DA, Van Natta ML, Thorne JE, et al. Course of cytomegalovirus retinitis in the era of highly active antiretroviral therapy: 1. Retinitis progression. Ophthalmology 111:2224, 2004.
200. Jabs DA, Van Natta ML, Thorne JE, et al. Course of cytomegalovirus retinitis in the era of highly active antiretroviral therapy: 2. Second eye involvement and retinal detachment. Ophthalmology 111:2232, 2004.

Chapter 51

Epstein–Barr Virus and Kaposi Sarcoma-Associated Herpesvirus

Eric Johannsen, MD

Epstein–Barr virus (EBV), the agent of infectious mononucleosis, is associated with the HIV-related syndromes of oral hairy leukoplakia (OHL) and non-Hodkgin lymphoma (NHL), including primary CNS lymphoma and Burkitt-like anaplastic lymphomas. In other populations, it has been implicated in the pathogenesis of post-transplant lymphoproliferative disease, nasopharyngeal carcinoma, and some forms of Hodgkin's disease. An infectious etiology was long suspected for Kaposi sarcoma (KS) based on epidemiologic evidence. The identification of a herpesvirus, closely related to EBV, in KS biopsies has revolutionized our understanding of this disease. Information on this virus, called human herpesvirus 8 or KS-associated herpesvirus (KSHV), has accumulated at an astounding rate. The complete sequence of the virus was published just 2 years after its discovery. KSHV has subsequently been linked to other forms of neoplasia: primary effusion lymphoma (PEL) and the multicentric form of Castleman's disease (MCD). EBV and KSHV, like all herpesviruses, can switch to a latent form of infection in which most of the viral genes are not expressed and the genome is maintained in the nucleus by cellular machinery. It is well established that the EBV genes expressed during latent infection of B lymphocytes drive them to proliferate and are almost certainly responsible for EBV's association with malignancy. The pathophysiology of KSHV-related diseases is less completely understood, but expression of viral genes during latency appears to play a prominent role. The natural history and pathophysiology of these two viruses and implications for therapy are discussed in this chapter.

TAXONOMY

Human herpesviruses have diverged to fill unique biologic niches, but all employ the same basic replication mechanisms. Latent infection permits herpesviruses to persist quiescently in their hosts for decades and, from an evolutionary standpoint, has placed them among the most successful of human parasites. Five of the eight known human herpesviruses infect >90% of the population. Based on genomic organization and biologic characteristics, EBV and KSHV belong to the gammaherpesviridae subfamily of herpesviruses (Fig. 51-1). Their genomes are ~170 kb in size and encode ~90 proteins each. About 60 of these proteins are derived from the common ancestral gammaherpesvirus from which EBV and KSHV diverged ~100 million years ago.[1] A substantial fraction of the nonancestral proteins are expressed during latency (Fig. 51-2), underscoring the importance of latent infection for the adaptation of each virus to its biologic niche.

The two strains of EBV, type I and type II, show an overall divergence of <4%, and are indistinguishable on clinical grounds or by commercially available serologic tests.[2] Infection with type I EBV is far more prevalent in most populations, although type II is more common among HIV-infected patients as is co-infection with type I and II. Five major subtypes of KSHV have been designated A–E.[3,4] Unlike the situation with EBV, KSHV subtypes demonstrate distinct geographic distribution: A and C predominate in Europe with C extending to Asia and the Americas as well, B is predominately in Africa, and D and E are restricted to Oceania or Amerindian populations.[4,5] It is not currently known if these subtypes differ significantly in their biologic properties.

EBV

Natural History

EBV is transmitted by contact with the oral secretions of infected persons. Primary infection in children is generally asymptomatic, whereas many adults and adolescents experience the typical symptoms of infectious mononucleosis: fever, lymphadenopathy, and pharyngitis. The virus replicates within the oropharynx and spreads to B lymphocytes by binding to the C3d complement protein receptor (also known as CR2 or CD21). EBV induces a growth transformation of infected B lymphocytes, and these proliferating B cells incite a brisk cytotoxic T-cell response. It is these reactive T cells that account for the atypical lymphocytosis or 'mononucleosis' of acute infection and are ultimately responsible for containing the infection.

After resolution of primary infection EBV, like all herpesviruses, establishes a persistent latent infection in the host and is able to reactivate periodically. Latent infection occurs in B lymphocytes, and is characterized by cessation of most viral gene expression and maintenance of the viral genome as a circular episome by cellular machinery. *In vitro*, lymphocytes latently infected with EBV are growth transformed into lymphoblastoid cell lines (LCLs) and can be propagated indefinitely. *In vivo*, EBV growth transformation of B lymphocytes is controlled by specific cytotoxic T-lymphocytes, but can result in lymphoproliferative disease in the immunosuppressed. Approximately 1 in 10^6 lymphocytes is latently infected with EBV and serves as the reservoir for reactivation. Virions released from lymphocytes undergo lytic replication in the oral epithelium and are shed in the saliva of seropositive individuals.

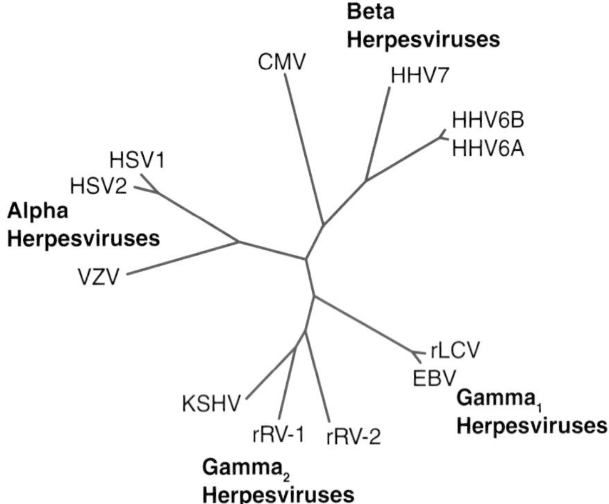

Figure 51-1 ■ Phylogenetic tree of human herpesviruses based on a comparison of amino acid sequences of the viral DNA polymerase. The alpha and beta subfamily groupings are labeled. EBV belongs to the lymphocryptovirus (or $\gamma 1$) genus of gammaherpesviruses and is most closely related to other (nonhuman) lymphocryptoviruses. KSHV belongs to the rhadinovirus (or γ_2) genus of gammaherpesviruses and is most closely related to other (nonhuman) rhadinoviruses. Primate species are infected by two distinct genogroups of rhadinoviruses termed RV1 and RV2. KSHV is a member of RV1. As yet no human RV2 rhadinovirus has been identified. Comparison of the phylogenetic tree of host organisms (not shown) to the rhadinovirus tree reveals a similar branching pattern. This suggests that a common primate ancestor was infected with an ancestral rhadinovirus which cospeciated with its host. The divergence of γ_1 and γ_2 herpesviruses is even more ancient. Abbreviations: rRV-1 rhesus rhadinovirus genogroup RV1, rRV-2 rhesus rhadinovirus genogroup RV2.

Epidemiology

Seroepidemiologic studies show >95% of the adults are infected with EBV. In developing countries, primary infection occurs in infancy or early childhood, but in affluent populations of industrial countries, as many as one third of infections occur in adolescence or early adulthood. With the exception of vertical HIV transmission, EBV infection precedes HIV infection. Studies in children who acquired HIV infection by vertical transmission reveal that EBV seroconversion, at

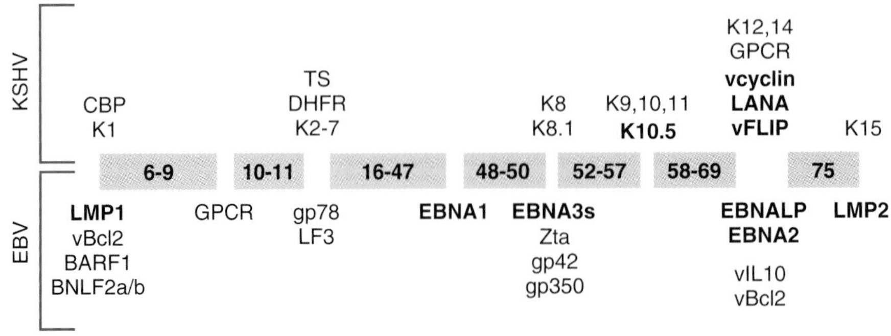

Figure 51-2 ■ EBV and KSHV genes are shown schematically in the order in which they are encoded in their respective genomes. Homologous genes found in large co-linear blocks are shown in reverse type and numbered using their KSHV ORF designations for simplicity. Between these conserved blocks of genes are inserted genes unique to each virus. Genes unique to KSHV are shown at the top and those unique to EBV are below. Genes expressed during latent infection comprise a substantial portion of these unique genes and are shown in bold faced type. The prefix 'v' refers to a viral homolog of a cell gene. CBP, complement binding protein; DHFR, dihydrofolate reductase; TS, thymidylate synthetase; GPCR, G-protein coupled cytokine receptor; LMP, latent membrane protein; EBNA, EBV nuclear antigen. n.b., the EBV and KSHV vGPCRs are not homologs of the same cytokine receptor.

least in this HIV-positive population, did not have appreciable effect on clinically important parameters such as CD4 count or viral load.[6,7] Moreover, primary infection appears to be largely asymptomatic, although one study noted an increased incidence of hepatosplenomegaly. By contrast, many studies have shown significant increases in the frequency of oral shedding of EBV by HIV-positive persons.[6,8,9] As previously stated, type II EBV infection, rare outside of Africa and New Guinea, is present in about half of the HIV-positive population and at least half of these are co-infected with type I and II. In nonendemic areas, acquisition of type II EBV infection appears to be closely linked to sexual behavior.[10,11]

Pathogenesis/Molecular Biology

Multiple factors probably account for the interaction of HIV and EBV infections. First, persons with AIDS have 10–20 times as many circulating EBV-infected B cells. T lymphocytes from these patients have been shown to suppress EBV-positive B cells less effectively than do T cells from HIV-negative controls.[12] Increased salivary shedding of EBV in the HIV population indicates that control of lytic infection is also impaired. Host factors also appear to be important as evidenced by the observation that HIV-positive persons with the 3′A allele of the stromal cell-derived growth factor 1 (SDF-1) chemokine have a twofold increased risk of NHL in the heterozygous state and a fourfold increase when the host is homozygous.[13,14] The chemokine receptor 5 variant CCR5Δ32 and the chemokine receptor 2 variant CCR2-64I, which are protective against progression to AIDS, were investigated in one study. The study found that the CCR5Δ32 allele conferred a threefold lower risk of developing NHL, but carrying the CCR2-64I had no effect on NHL risk.[13]

EBV-associated disease is distinctive because it is largely caused by latent infection not by viral replication. OHL, caused by extensive EBV lytic replication in oral epithelium, represents a notable exception. Although viral particles are not produced, latent EBV infection of B lymphocytes is not passive. In fact, EBV expresses two membrane proteins (LMP1 and LMP2), six nuclear proteins (EBV nuclear antigens or EBNAs), two untranslated RNAs (EBERs), and multiple micro-RNAs during latency.[15] It is these viral proteins that transform B lymphocytes into LCLs, and are almost certainly responsible for EBV's association with malignancy. Genetic analysis and biochemical techniques have begun to define the mechanisms by which these viral genes work.[16] LMP1 is the major viral oncogene and induces a growth promoting signal that mimics a constitutively active form of the B-cell surface molecule CD40. The nuclear protein EBNA-1 ensures that the viral episome is maintained by cell machinery. A second nuclear protein, EBNA-2 is a powerful activator of transcription which targets downstream elements of the Notch signaling pathway to induce expression of both viral and cellular genes, including *c-myc*. The function of the remaining four nuclear proteins is less completely understood, but they may modulate the effects of EBNA-2.

The expression of all 10 latent EBV genes, referred to as type III latency, induces a potent immune response and is only seen in the peripheral blood of normal hosts during infectious mononucleosis. After resolution of primary infection, more restricted latent gene expression is observed. Continued EBNA-1 expression assures maintenance of the viral genome and, because EBNA-1 can inhibit its own processing for presentation on class I MHC molecules, does not incite a significant immune response.[17] The EBERs and LMP2 also continue to be expressed and, though they appear to have no direct role in lymphocyte transformation, they may be important for the biology of EBV *in vivo*. For example, LMP2 has been shown to interact with signaling proteins downstream of the B cell receptor to prevent B cell activation. Since this signal frequently induces lytic replication, LMP2 may act to maintain EBV in a latent state of infection.[18] Reversion to type III latency likely occurs at some low frequency since normal individuals maintain lifelong strong cytotoxic T-cell responses against type III latency antigens. In fact, a recent study suggested that type III latency is frequently observed in tonsillar B cells of normal hosts.[19] In immunocompromised hosts, the balance between immune clearance and B cell proliferation is disturbed. The lymphoproliferative syndromes seen in these hosts probably represent the *in vivo* equivalent of LCL transformation.

Primary Infection

For obscure reasons, primary EBV infection is accompanied ~90% of the time by the appearance of antibodies that react with antigens found on sheep, horse, and beef erythrocytes. Detection of these so-called heterophile antibodies forms the basis for commercial assays such as the Monospot test.[20] Heterophile antibodies can be found in 5–10% of the healthy adult population, and in the setting of immune dysregulation by HIV, the rate may be even higher. In children, the only HIV-positive population likely to be EBV-naive, primary EBV infection is heterophile negative in about one-half of cases. When diagnostic uncertainty exists, specific antibodies to EBV proteins can be measured.

Immunoglobulin M (IgM) antibodies to viral capsid antigen (VCA) are present in 90% of acute infections and absent in the general population, thus their presence is essentially diagnostic of primary infection.[20,21] By contrast, a fourfold rise in VCA IgG titers can only be demonstrated in 10–20% of cases because titers are generally already high upon initial presentation. Measurement of other antibodies is probably of limited clinical utility. One possible exception is that seroconversion to anti-EBNA antibodies occurs relatively late and can be used to confirm recent EBV infection in a patient previously documented to be anti-VCA positive and anti-EBNA negative.[22] Although virus can be cultured from the saliva, this assay is of little clinical use since it is slow, unable to distinguish acute infection from the viral shedding seen in healthy adults, and not generally available. Because primary HIV infection can closely mimic primary EBV infection, measurement of an HIV viral load should always

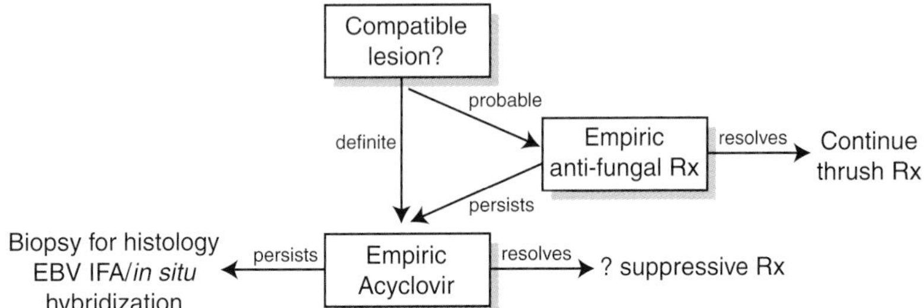

Figure 51-3 ■ Diagnostic approach to oral hairy leukoplakia. IFA, immunofluorescence assay.

be considered in any person presenting with symptoms suggestive of infectious mononucleosis.[23]

Oral Hairy Leukoplakia

OHL presents as a corrugated or 'hairy' white lesion on the lateral surface of the tongue that is not removed by gentle scraping. It is a nonmalignant lesion caused by unchecked lytic replication of EBV.[24,25] OHL is seen in ~20% of persons with asymptomatic HIV infection and becomes more common with advanced disease.[26] Development of OHL is itself associated with a more rapid progression to AIDS and death after controlling for CD4 count.[27,28] It is also seen in other immunosuppressed persons, including bone marrow and solid organ transplant recipients.[29,30] OHL can very rarely be seen in the absence of immunosuppression, nevertheless, its presence demands that HIV be excluded.[31] The diagnosis of OHL is generally based on the typical appearance of the lesions in the appropriate clinical setting (Fig. 51-3). The differential includes oral candidiasis which can be distinguished by its ease of removal from the tongue and/or an empiric trial of antifungal therapy. Biopsy for histology and *in situ* hybridization or immunofluorescence staining for EBV is rarely necessary, but will confirm the diagnosis. PCR detection of EBV in 'oral scrapes' is neither sensitive nor specific for OHL.[32]

Persons with OHL are frequently asymptomatic and lesions spontaneously resolved in 37% of a cohort followed for 1 year.[33] The incidence of OHL has decreased since the advent of HAART and antiretroviral therapy should be sufficient in most cases.[34] Further selection of therapy for OHL is based on data from small case series as large placebo-controlled trials are unlikely to ever be completed. An early study by Resnick et al treated six of 13 OHL patients with acyclovir (3.2 g/day for 20 days), and observed regression in five.[35] All five recurred with cessation of therapy, and no spontaneous regressions were seen in the seven who refused therapy. Other authors have reported similar results.[36–38] Desciclovir (750 mg/day), an analog of acyclovir, produced a similar complete response followed by relapse in eight patients treated by Greenspan et al.[39] Foscarnet and ganciclovir which also inhibit EBV replication, have been associated with resolution of OHL in the context of treatment of cytomegalovirus-related disease.[40,41] Less impressive results were seen in a study of acyclovir for CMV prophylaxis, 19 of 32 (59%) who had OHL on entry improved on acyclovir versus 13 of 30 (43%) in the placebo group.[42] Moreover, there appeared to be no prophylactic benefit: the incidence of new OHL in the placebo group was 16% compared to 14% in the acyclovir group (118 patients in each group).

Topical therapy of OHL has also met with some success. Treatment with 25% podophyllum resin in one study resulted in remissions lasting 2–28 weeks.[43] A second observer-blinded study demonstrated marked improvement (relative to the untreated side) within 2 days of a single application.[44] Side effects were minimal, and consisted of slight burning or pain and transient dysgusia.

NHL

NHL is an AIDS-defining illness and persons with AIDS have an ~100-fold increased risk of NHL (see also Chapter 60).[45,46] Because the incidence of NHL has not decreased as dramatically as opportunistic infections, it is responsible for a greater proportion of the AIDS attributable morbidity and mortality in the era of HAART.[47–51] Risk of NHL is consistently associated with low CD4 count, but increasing age, and male sex have also been implicated.[48,49,51] Selective loss of EBV reactive T cells may promote the clonal expansion of EBV-infected B lymphocytes and, in conjunction with other factors, result in lymphoma. Indeed, loss of EBNA1 reactive CD4+ and CD8+ T cells has been documented in AIDS patients with NHL.[52] Other factors such as polyclonal B-cell expansion from chronic antigenemia may explain higher rates, particularly of Burkitt lymphoma, seen in less immunocompromised HIV-infected persons.[53]

HIV infection is associated with two types of EBV-related B-cell lymphomas. The first, diffuse large cell lymphoma (DLCL), bears a striking resemblance to post-transplant lymphoproliferative disease (PTLD). As with PTLD, it occurs in the setting of profound immunosuppression; those with the lowest CD4 counts for the longest time are at greatest risk. Presentation as primary CNS lymphoma is frequent and essentially all CNS lymphomas are EBV positive, whereas about two-thirds of DLCL outside the CNS is EBV positive.[54] The frequency of type I verses type II EBV in these tumors roughly parallels the increased prevalence of type II EBV infection seen in the HIV-positive population.[55–57] The pattern of EBV latent gene expression in DLCL and PTLD resemble that seen in LCLs.[58–60] Both diseases probably represent EBV-driven B-cell proliferation that has escaped immune control.

The second EBV-related B-cell lymphoma seen in HIV infection, Burkitt-like lymphoma, generally occurs early in the course of HIV infection and is EBV positive 30–40% of the time.[54,61] Presentation at multiple extranodal sites and aggressive growth are the norm. The tumors contain the typical *c-myc* translocations of Burkitt lymphomas.[62] As with classic Burkitt lymphoma, the precise role of EBV in pathogenesis is not clear. When present, EBV episomes are monoclonal, implying that EBV infection preceded tumor expansion.[63] However, latent EBV gene expression in these tumors is restricted to EBNA-1 and the EBERs which are expressed do not have well-established oncogenic properties.

The diagnosis of EBV-related NHL generally rests on the histology and *in situ* hybridization for EBV gene products of appropriate biopsy material. Amongst solid organ and bone marrow transplant recipients, a consistent correlation between serum EBV viral load and risk of PTLD is observed.[64–68] Limited data suggest that this correlation extends to DLCL in HIV-positive patients.[69] Not surprisingly many persons without DLCL have detectable amounts of EBV DNA in their serum. Moreover, EBV serum viral load can correlate poorly with clinical response during treatment.[70] Further studies are required before a role for serum EBV PCR can be entertained in HIV-infected patients.

The approach to CNS mass lesions in AIDS is presented in Figure 51-1. Because the magnetic resonance imaging (MRI) and computed tomography (CT) appearance of primary CNS lymphoma are not sufficiently specific to exclude infectious etiologies, single photon computed tomography (SPECT) or positron emission tomography (PET) scanning may be desirable.[71,72] Unlike the results seen for serum, PCR for EBV DNA in the cerebrospinal fluid (CSF) has high sensitivity and specificity (>90%).[73–75] It has been suggested that the combination of PET scanning and EBV PCR may avoid the need for most biopsies.[71] However, as primary CNS lymphoma is seen only in the profoundly immunosuppressed, this diagnosis should be confirmed by biopsy in patients with CD4 counts >100/μL.

The prognosis of AIDS-related DLCL had been quite poor, but has improved significantly with the advent of HAART.[49,76–78] Treatment of NHL outside the CNS begins with a complete staging workup including: complete blood count (CBC), lactate dehydrogenase (LDH), CT of abdomen, pelvis, and chest, bone marrow biopsy, and lumbar puncture (to exclude concurrent leptomeningeal disease). Systemic chemotherapy is required, even in cases that appear to be localized. A complete discussion of NHL chemotherapy is presented in Chapter 60, but several points are worth noting here. In general, dose-reduced chemotherapy regimens have produced similar response rates and less myelosuppression and infectious complications than standard doses.[79,80] Similarly, the anti-CD20 monoclonal antibody rituximab which has established efficacy and safety for treatment of NHL in HIV-negative patients, failed to improve clinical outcome in a phase III trial of AIDS-associated NHL.[81–83] Although rituximab administration appeared to improve response rates, this was offset by an increase in infectious complications not seen in earlier phase II trials. It remains possible that select patients, particularly those with the most preserved immune function, may benefit from dose intensified chemotherapy or rituximab administration. Treatment of primary CNS lymphoma remains problematic with reported median survival rates <2 months.[84] Radiation therapy can increase median survival to ~4 months and dramatically improve quality of life. The role of systemic chemotherapy for primary CNS disease remains to be defined.

Perhaps the most controversial aspect of treatment of EBV-associated lymphoma is the role of antiviral therapy. Despite strong evidence that latent EBV infection is central to the pathogenesis of these malignancies, interest in antiviral therapy persists. Several justifications for this interest have been advanced. First, PTLD in pediatric patients frequently occurs in the setting of primary EBV infection. The use of acyclovir (or similar agents) in this setting may limit the extent of spread of the virus to the B-cell compartment. It has also been argued that lytic gene expression, reported in some tumors,[85] may allow antivirals to act against some fraction of EBV-positive tumor cells. Several investigators report successful treatment of EBV-associated lymphomas with regimens that include acyclovir, foscarnet, or ganciclovir, though no well-controlled trials exist to support or refute this practice.[86–89] A retrospective study by Fong et al, suggested that acyclovir may find a role in the prevention of EBV-associated lymphoma.[90] They found patients receiving high, low or intermittent doses, or no acyclovir developed NHL at a rate of 7%, 16%, and 25% respectively. The distribution of CNS lymphoma (3%, 9%, and 5%) did not correlate with acyclovir exposure, and the proportion of non-CNS lymphomas that were EBV positive was not determined. An earlier study found no decrease in NHL associated with acyclovir exposure.[91] Such a prophylactic effect, if confirmed by prospective trial, would be surprising in light of earlier data that acyclovir treatment has no effect on number of circulating EBV-positive B-cells.[92]

One antiviral drug that has shown activity against EBV during latent infection is hydroxyurea. *In vitro* this drug can eliminate EBV genomes from tissue culture cell lines. Slobod et al reported a limited response to hydroxyurea in two patients with primary CNS lymphoma.[93]

Other EBV-Associated Diseases

Lymphoid interstitial pneumonitis is characterized by diffuse interstitial pulmonary infiltrates. It occurs primarily in children infected with HIV, but can also be seen in adults. EBV proteins and DNA have been detected in biopsy specimens from affected children.[94]

EBV genomes have also been found in leiomyosarcoma biopsies from children with AIDS.[95] The authors were able to demonstrate that these tumors expressed the EBV receptor (CD21) and did not find any evidence that EBV was associated with smooth muscle tumors of HIV-negative patients.

Two other EBV-associated diseases deserve mention. Nasopharyngeal carcinoma (NPC), a disease endemic in southern China and among the Inuit, is strongly associated with EBV infection.[2] There does not appear to be an appreciably increased incidence of NPC in the HIV-positive population. Hodgkin disease, particularly the mixed cellularity and lymphocyte depleted forms, has also been linked to EBV infection. There is probably a modest increase in risk for HIV-positive persons in whom the disease tends to follow a more aggressive course.[96]

KSHV

Epidemiology

Although advances in the molecular biology of KSHV have outpaced our understanding of its natural history, epidemiologic studies were critical to establishing an infectious etiology for KS. A transmissible agent had long been suspected and intensive investigation had even uncovered ultrastructural evidence for a herpesvirus in KS tissue.[97] However, repeated efforts failed to isolate a pathogen. This changed in 1994 when Chang, Moore, and colleagues, using a novel technique called representational difference analysis, succeeded in isolating two DNA sequences from KS tumors that ultimately proved to be from KSHV.[98] They later stated that epidemiologic evidence was a critical determinant of their decision to continue to search for a 'KS agent'.[99] Particularly compelling were surveillance data from the CDC which established that men who have sex with men (MSM) were 20 times more likely to present with KS than similarly immunodeficient hemophiliac men.[100,101] Remarkably, much of what we know about the natural history of KSHV infection in HIV-positive persons, could be deduced from study of the epidemiology of KS. Infection with the KS agent is relatively uncommon in the general population, and it is transmitted by sexual or parasexual practices common amongst MSM, but inefficiently transmitted by blood or blood products.

The identification of a specific pathogen enabled investigators to prove the same virus was associated with all forms of KS: classic, endemic, AIDS, and transplant related.[98,102] The diversity of assays used to measure KSHV antibodies has made estimating KSHV seroprevalence anything but straightforward. For example, assays that measure antibodies to latent KSHV antigens yield prevalence rates consistently lower than assays that measure antibodies to lytic antigens. Nevertheless, it can be safely stated that KSHV infection is not ubiquitous and displays distinct geographic variation. The KSHV seropositivity in the general population of the US and Western Europe is in the range of 1–5%.[103–105] In certain regions of Mediterranean countries where classic KS is found this increases to 10–20%,[105–107] and may be as high as 30–80% in parts of sub-Saharan Africa.[108–114] In Western countries, KSHV seroprevalence among HIV-negative MSM is ~11–20% and rises to the 30–54% range in HIV-positive MSM, but amongst other HIV risk groups is comparable to that seen in the general population.[104,115–117] One retrospective study found that a cohort of HIV-positive MSM seroconverted to KSHV at a median of 33 months prior to the development of KS.[103]

Although a receptor for KSHV has recently been identified, the precise mode of transmission of KSHV remains unclear.[118] The marked geographic variation in seroprevalence indicates that transmission is inefficient relative to herpesviruses such as EBV. In endemic countries, acquisition in childhood appears to be common, indicating that the mode of transmission may be different than in the MSM population. The observed clustering in families suggests transmission between siblings or from mother to child may occur.[119,120] Although reported, neither vertical transmission nor transmission through breastfeeding appears to be the major mode of transmission because seroconversion occurs predominately after the age of two.[121,122] Studies of MSM cohorts have suggested HIV positivity, increasing number of sexual partners, a history of a partner with KS, orogenital sex, and even use of inhaled amyl nitrate capsules were independent risk factors for KSHV seroconversion.[116,123–127] In heterosexual populations, birth in Africa appears to be the strongest risk factor.[124] Some studies have observed elevated rates of KSHV positivity at STD clinics or amongst female sex workers, though other studies did not find evidence for heterosexual transmission.[104,105,124,128,129] KSHV DNA was found in the semen of HIV-infected persons, but was not in samples from healthy donors.[130] However, viral loads appear to be about two logs higher in saliva than in semen, breast milk, or blood, and infectious virions have been recovered from saliva specimens.[131,132] These findings are most consistent with salivary transmission of KSHV.

Pathogenesis/Molecular Biology

In addition to KS, KSHV has been linked to two lymphoproliferative disorders: MCD and PEL.[133–135] An abundance of molecular evidence supports a central role for KSHV in their pathogenesis. First, within the limits of available assays, KSHV seroconversion precedes development of these diseases.[103,129] In HIV-positive persons, KSHV viremia was associated with a ninefold increased risk of developing KS and high KSHV viral load correlates with clinical symptoms of MCD.[136,137] KSHV genomes are present in the spindle cells of KS lesions, in PEL cells, and in plasmablasts found in the mantle zone of MCD.[133,135,138–140] Terminal repeat analysis of the KSHV genome reveals that KSHV infection of PEL and most KS spindle cells occurs prior to neoplastic expansion.[141] There is good reason to believe that the presence of KSHV early in the evolution of these tumors reflects a causal relationship.

The KSHV genome contains a large number of candidate genes to explain KSHV's relationship to neoplastic transformation (Fig. 51-2). Many genes, including *K1*, *K9* (*vIRF*), *K12*/kaposin, and *vGPCR*, were shown to have transforming properties in standard assays, before there was any consensus as to which genes were expressed in KSHV-associated neoplasms. Because KSHV genomes are present as latent

Table 51-1 Patterns of latent EBV gene expression[15,16]

Latency pattern	*LMP-1*	*LMP-2*	*EBNA-1*	*EBNA-2* *EBNA-LP*	*EBNA-3s*	*EBERs*	Occurrence
Type I	—	—	+	—	—	+	Burkitts lymphoma
Type II	+	+	+	—	—	+	NPC Hodgkin disease peripheral T-cell lymphoma
Type III	+	+	+	+	+	+	Infectious mononucleosis LCL XLPD, PTLD
—	—	+	+	—	—	+	Healthy carrier

For historical reasons, nomenclature of latent EBV gene expression derives from patterns of gene expression seen in EBV-related tumors.
Abbreviations: *LMP*, latent membrane protein; *EBNA*, EBV nuclear antigen; *EBER*, EBV encoded *RNA*; NPC nasopharyngeal carcinoma; LCL, lymphoblastoid cell line; XLPD, X-linked lymphoproliferative disease; PTLD, post-transplant lymphoproliferative disease.

episomes in KS lesions and PEL cells, there is general agreement that latent gene products are the primary mediators of KSHV pathogenesis in these diseases.[142] Four latency proteins, LANA, vFLIP, v-cyclin, and K12/kaposin are expressed in KS cells and a fifth, K10.5/LANA2 is expressed in PEL cells.[142–147] The mechanisms by which these gene products may contribute to pathogenesis are summarized in Table 51-1. It should be noted that because no *in vitro* model exists for evaluating the importance of KSHV genes in oncogenesis comparable to the LCL system used for EBV, there is no accepted standard for determining which KSHV genes mediate human disease. About 1–5% of KS spindle and PEL cells express some lytic proteins and some authors feel that lytic infection also plays an important role. The evidence is most compelling for v-IL6 which has been shown to play a critical paracrine role in promoting PEL growth and for vGPCR which produces KS-like lesions in a transgenic mouse model.[148,149]

Attempting to understand the pathogenesis of latent KSHV infection by analogy to EBV can only succeed to a point. The divergence between these two viruses is vastly greater in the latent genes than the divergence between lytic, particularly structural, genes (Fig. 51-2). Only one KSHV latent gene, *LANA*, has a clearly established EBV functional homolog. LANA has been demonstrated to be a sequence-specific DNA binding protein that recognizes a GC-rich sequence found in the terminal repeat region of the genome. It appears to function in a manner analogous to EBNA-1 in maintenance of the viral genome.[150,151] LANA is also reported to have other functions not shared by EBNA-1.[152–154] Further study is required to determine the importance and specific role of the other KSHV genes expressed in latency.

Primary Infection

A clearer picture of KSHV primary infection is beginning to emerge. Andreoni et al identified six putative cases of primary KSHV infection (seronegative with KSHV DNA in blood or saliva by PCR) among 86 children evaluated for a febrile syndrome in a KSHV endemic area. All had fever and five had a maculopapular rash that began on the face and spread to the trunk and extremities. Sore throat was also seen in five children and none had cervical lymphadenopathy or oral ulcers. Seroconversion was confirmed in all three children for whom convalescent serum was obtained. KSHV seroconversion in a prospective cohort of 108 HIV-negative adults was associated with mild symptomatology, including: cervical/submental lymphadenopathy (three of five), diarrhea (two of five), localized rash on face (one of five), or ankle (one of five), and fatigue (one of five). One patient was completely asymptomatic. By contrast, Casper et al found lymphadenopathy in four of 15 (27%) KSHV seroconverters compared with 5% lymphadenopathy in controls to be the symptom in a cohort of 378 HIV-negative men.[155] Only one case of KSHV seroconversion in an HIV-positive person has been reported to date. Using banked serum samples Oksenhendler et al documented KSHV seroconversion in a 43-year-old man who had presented 5 weeks previously with fever, arthralgia, cervical mass, and splenomegaly.[156] Interestingly, although pathologic examination of the cervical nodes revealed foci of KS, the patient never developed clinically evident KS, despite 9 years of follow-up.

Kaposi Sarcoma

KS was initially described in 1872 as a rare, indolent tumor occurring in elderly men of Mediterranean descent (classic KS). Subsequently the disease was found to be endemic in portions of eastern Africa. Endemic KS was more aggressive, often presented in children with lymphadenopathy instead of skin lesions, and was frequently fatal. KS was later seen in organ transplant recipients; and its occurrence at an unexpectedly high rate amongst MSM heralded the HIV epidemic. Although the distribution of cases of classic KS is probably attributable to KSHV seroprevalence in these regions, the environmental or genetic cofactors that produce

Table 51-2 Viral gene expression in KSHV-related neoplasia[180–185]

Class	Gene Product	Proposed Function	KS	MCD	PEL
Latent	LANA	Genome maintenance	+	+	+
Latent	v-cyclin	Stimulates cell division via cyclin dependent kinases	+	+	+
Latent	vFLIP	Inhibit apoptosis	+	+	+
Latent	Kaposin A Kaposin B	A can transform rodent fibroblasts B may stabilize cytokine mRNAs	+	+	+
Latent	K10.5/LANA2	May inhibit p53-induced apoptosis	–	+	+
Lytic	K2/vIL-6	B lymphocyte growth factor	–	+/–	+/–
Lytic	vGPCR	Constitutively active G protein coupled cytokine receptor	+/–	+/–	+/–
Lytic	K8	Viral replication, cell cycle arrest	–	+/–	–
Lytic	K9/vIRF-1	Inhibit interferon signaling; can transform rodent fibroblasts	–	+/–	–
Lytic	K10/vIRF4	Inhibit interferon signaling	–	+/–	–

LANA, latency associated nuclear antigen. The prefix v refers to a viral homolog of a cell gene. + expressed in most or all cells, +/– expressed in a minority of cells, – expressed in <1% of cells.

the more aggressive endemic form of KS are unknown. Even immunodeficiency is not the straightforward risk factor that it appears to be. AIDS patients in the Gambia rarely present with KS, despite the high seroprevalence of KSHV in this region. Interestingly, HIV-2 infection is much more common in this region than HIV-1 infection, yet most reported cases of KS are in AIDS patients infected with HIV-1.[108]

Whether KS represents a true malignancy or a semimalignant angioproliferation is still a contested issue. The histology of these lesions is complex, being composed of spindle cells, endothelial cells, extravasated erythrocytes, and a variable inflammatory infiltrate. Examination of spindle cells, the neoplastic component of KS lesions, for clonality has produced conflicting results. The finding of polyclonal spindle cells by some investigators suggests KS is an angioproliferation, whereas reports of spindle cell monoclonality are more consistent with a true malignancy.[141,157–159] One potentially unifying explanation for these discrepant observations is that KS initiates as a polyclonal proliferation with a propensity to evolve into a true malignancy. In support of this theory is that late (nodular) KS has been more frequently monoclonal.

A detailed description of the treatment of KS is presented in Chapter 59. As with EBV-associated disease, the role of antiviral therapy is unclear. *In vitro* studies have established that foscarnet, ganciclovir, and cidofivir can inhibit KSHV replication, whereas acyclovir does not.[160–163] Several studies have reported a reduced rate of KS lesion appearance in patients taking ganciclovir or foscarnet, but not in those taking acyclovir.[91,164–167] Surprisingly, two small studies found foscarnet administration to be associated with KS lesion regression.[168,169] Another study demonstrated patients receiving intravenous foscarnet or ganciclovir still had detectable levels of KSHV in the peripheral blood mononuclear cells.[170] Larger studies are required to define a role for antiviral agents in the treatment of KSHV disease. A recent report suggested that it may be possible to disrupt KSHV latent infection: glycyrrhizic acid downregulated LANA and induced apoptosis in PEL cell lines.[171] Whether this can be translated into clinical practice remains to be seen.

Primary Effusion Lymphoma

PEL, once termed body cavity based lymphoma, represents a rare HIV-associated disease that presents as a malignant effusion in the pleural, pericardial, or peritoneal space. PEL cells are consistently KSHV positive and frequently co-infected with EBV.[133] Five latent genes are expressed in most PEL tumor cells and a small fraction also express the early lytic genes *v-IL6* and *vGPCR* (Table 51-2). The establishment of PEL cell lines from clinical samples has been an invaluable tool for the study of KSHV in the laboratory. Fixed PEL cells form the basis for most serologic tests for KSHV latent antibodies. Induction of KSHV replication in PEL cell lines produces infectious virus and allows the detection of antibodies to lytic gene products.

Multicentric Castleman's Disease

Angiofollicular lymphoid hyperplasia or Castleman's disease consists of two distinct clinical entities with similar histology.[172] The localized form presents as a solitary mass and excision is generally curative. By contrast, MCD presents with diffuse lymphadenopathy and constitutional symptoms and is an aggressive, usually fatal disorder. Biopsies of MCD have shown KSHV to be present in mantle zone large immunoblastic B cells of these lesions.[146] Those diagnosed with MCD are at increased risk of subsequent development of lymphoma or KS. HIV infection is associated with MCD, and 75% of HIV-positive MCD patients subsequently develop KS.[173] In contrast to other KSHV-associated neoplasia, MCD is clearly a polyclonal disorder.[174] It has been associated with high levels of IL-6 which is thought to play an important paracrine role in stimulating growth.[136,175–177] The increased rate of lytic KSHV infection in MCD may permit the lytic *vIL-6* gene and other lytic genes to play a greater role in the pathogenesis of MCD.[178,179] There are no data in the literature regarding the use of antiviral agents for the treatment of MCD. Because lytic infection is more prominent in MCD lesions, this would appear to be an important avenue for future study.

REFERENCES

1. McGeoch DJ, Cook S, Dolan A, et al. Molecular phylogeny and evolutionary timescale for the family of mammalian herpesviruses. J Mol Biol 247:443–58, 1995.
2. Rickinson A, Kieff E. Epstein–Barr virus. In: Knipe D, Howley P, Griffin D, et al, (eds). Fields Virology. Philadelphia: PA Williams & Wilkins; 2001, pp 2575–2628.
3. Zong JC, Ciufo DM, Alcendor DJ, et al. High-level variability in the ORF-K1 membrane protein gene at the left end of the Kaposi's sarcoma-associated herpesvirus genome defines four major virus subtypes and multiple variants or clades in different human populations. J Virol 73:4156–70, 1999.
4. Biggar RJ, Whitby D, Marshall V, et al. Human herpesvirus 8 in Brazilian Amerindians: a hyperendemic population with a new subtype. J Infect Dis 181:1562–8, 2000.
5. Hayward GS. KSHV strains: the origins and global spread of the virus. Semin Cancer Biol 9:187–99, 1999.
6. Jenson H, McIntosh K, Pitt J, et al. Natural history of primary Epstein–Barr virus infection in children of mothers infected with human immunodeficiency virus type 1. J Infect Dis 179:1395–404, 1999.
7. Pedneault L, Lapointe N, Alfieri C, et al. Natural history of Epstein–Barr virus infection in a prospective pediatric cohort born to human immunodeficiency virus-infected mothers. J Infect Dis 177:1087–90, 1998.
8. Luxton JC, Williams I, Weller I, Crawford DH. Epstein–Barr virus infection of HIV-seropositive individuals is transiently suppressed by high-dose acyclovir treatment. AIDS 7:1337–43, 1993.
9. Ferbas J, Rahman MA, Kingsley LA, et al. Frequent oropharyngeal shedding of Epstein–Barr virus in homosexual men during early HIV infection. AIDS 6:1273–8, 1992.
10. Yao QY, Croom-Carter DS, Tierney RJ, et al. Epidemiology of infection with Epstein–Barr virus types 1 and 2: lessons from the study of a T-cell-immunocompromised hemophilic cohort. J Virol 72:4352–63, 1998.
11. van Baarle D, Hovenkamp E, Dukers NH, et al. High prevalence of Epstein–Barr virus type 2 among homosexual men is caused by sexual transmission. J Infect Dis 181:2045–9, 2000.
12. Birx DL, Redfield RR, Tosato G. Defective regulation of Epstein–Barr virus infection in patients with acquired immunodeficiency syndrome (AIDS) or AIDS-related disorders. N Engl J Med 314:874–9, 1986.
13. Rabkin CS, Yang Q, Goedert JJ, et al. Chemokine and chemokine receptor gene variants and risk of non-Hodgkin's lymphoma in human immunodeficiency virus-1-infected individuals. Blood 93:1838–42, 1999.
14. Dean M, Jacobson LP, McFarlane G, et al. Reduced risk of AIDS lymphoma in individuals heterozygous for the CCR5-delta32 mutation. Cancer Res 59:3561–4, 1999.
15. Kieff E, Rickinson AB. Epstein–Barr virus and its replication. In: Knipe D, Howley P, Griffin D, et al, (eds). Fields Virology. Philadelphia: PA Lippincott-Raven; 2001, pp 2511–74.
16. Cohen JI. Epstein–Barr virus infection. N Engl J Med 343:481–92, 2000.
17. Levitskaya J, Sharipo A, Leonchiks A, et al. Inhibition of ubiquitin/proteasome-dependent protein degradation by the Gly-Ala repeat domain of the Epstein–Barr virus nuclear antigen 1. Proc Natl Acad Sci USA 94:12616–21, 1997.
18. Longnecker R. Epstein–Barr virus latency: LMP2, a regulator or means for Epstein–Barr virus persistence? Adv Cancer Res 79:175–200, 2000.
19. Babcock JG, Hochberg D, Thorley-Lawson AD. The expression pattern of Epstein–Barr virus latent genes in vivo is dependent upon the differentiation stage of the infected B cell. Immunity 13:497–506, 2000.
20. Evans AS, Niederman JC, Cenabre LC, et al. A prospective evaluation of heterophile and Epstein–Barr virus-specific IgM antibody tests in clinical and subclinical infectious mononucleosis: Specificity and sensitivity of the tests and persistence of antibody. J Infect Dis 132:546–54, 1975.
21. Henle W, Henle G, Niederman JC, et al. Antibodies to early antigens induced by Epstein–Barr virus in infectious mononucleosis. J Infect Dis 124:58–67, 1971.
22. Henie G, Henle W, Horwitz CA. Antibodies to Epstein–Barr virus-associated nuclear antigen in infectious mononucleosis. J Infect Dis 130:231–9, 1974.
23. Schacker T, Collier AC, Hughes J, et al. Clinical and epidemiologic features of primary HIV infection. Ann Intern Med 125:257–64, 1996.
24. Greenspan JS, Greenspan D, Lennette ET, et al. Replication of Epstein–Barr virus within the epithelial cells of oral 'hairy' leukoplakia, an AIDS-associated lesion. N Engl J Med 313:1564–71, 1985.
25. Triantos D, Porter SR, Scully C, Teo CG. Oral hairy leukoplakia: clinicopathologic features, pathogenesis, diagnosis, and clinical significance. Clin Infect Dis 25:1392–6, 1997.
26. Feigal DW, Katz MH, Greenspan D, et al. The prevalence of oral lesions in HIV-infected homosexual and bisexual men: three San Francisco epidemiological cohorts. AIDS 5:519–25, 1991.
27. Greenspan D, Greenspan JS, Hearst NG, et al. Relation of oral hairy leukoplakia to infection with the human immunodeficiency virus and the risk of developing AIDS. J Infect Dis 155:475–81, 1987.
28. Katz MH, Greenspan D, Westenhouse J, et al. Progression to AIDS in HIV-infected homosexual and bisexual men with hairy leukoplakia and oral candidiasis. AIDS 6:95–100, 1992.
29. Epstein JB, Sherlock CH, Greenspan JS. Hairy leukoplakia-like lesions following bone-marrow transplantation. AIDS 5:101–2, 1991.
30. Greenspan D, Greenspan JS, de Souza Y, et al. Oral hairy leukoplakia in an HIV-negative renal transplant recipient. J Oral Pathol Med 18:32–4, 1989.
31. Wurapa AK, Luque AE, Menegus MA. Oral hairy leukoplakia: a manifestation of primary infection with Epstein–Barr virus? Scand J Infect Dis 31:505–6, 1999.
32. Scully C, Porter SR, Di Alberti L, et al. Detection of Epstein–Barr virus in oral scrapes in HIV infection, in hairy leukoplakia, and in healthy non-HIV-infected people. J Oral Pathol Med 27:480–2, 1998.
33. Katz MH, Greenspan D, Heinic GS, et al. Resolution of hairy leukoplakia: an observational trial of zidovudine versus no treatment. J Infect Dis 164:1240–1, 1991.
34. Patton LL, McKaig R, Strauss R, et al. Changing prevalence of oral manifestations of human immuno-deficiency virus in the era of protease inhibitor therapy. Oral Surg Oral Med Oral Pathol Oral Radiol Endod 89:299–304, 2004.
35. Resnick L, Herbst JS, Ablashi DV, et al. Regression of oral hairy leukoplakia after orally administered acyclovir therapy. JAMA 259:384–8, 1988.
36. Glick M, Pliskin ME. Regression of oral hairy leukoplakia after oral administration of acyclovir. Gen Dent 38:374–5, 1990.
37. Laskaris G, Laskaris M, Theodoridou M. Oral hairy leukoplakia in a child with AIDS. Oral Surg Oral Med Oral Pathol Oral Radiol Endod 79:570–1, 1995.

38. Naher H, Helfrich S, Hartmann M, Freese UK. EBV replication and therapy of oral hairy leukoplakia using acyclovir. Hautarzt 41:680–2, 1990.
39. Greenspan D, De Souza YG, Conant MA, et al. Efficacy of desciclovir in the treatment of Epstein–Barr virus infection in oral hairy leukoplakia. J Acquir Immune Defic Syndr 3:571–8, 1990.
40. Newman C, Polk BF. Resolution of oral hairy leukoplakia during therapy with 9-(1,3-dihydroxy-2-propoxymethyl)guanine (DHPG). Ann Intern Med 107:348–50, 1987.
41. Albrecht H, Stellbrink HJ, Brewster D, Greten H. Resolution of oral hairy leukoplakia during treatment with foscarnet. AIDS 8:1014–16, 1994.
42. Youle MS, Gazzard BG, Johnson MA, et al. Effects of high-dose oral acyclovir on herpesvirus disease and survival in patients with advanced HIV disease: a double-blind, placebo-controlled study. European–Australian Acyclovir Study Group. AIDS 8:641–9, 1994.
43. Lozada-Nur F, Costa C. Retrospective findings of the clinical benefits of podophyllum resin 25% sol on hairy leukoplakia. Clinical results in nine patients. Oral Surg Oral Med Oral Pathol 73:555–8, 1992.
44. Gowdey G, Lee RK, Carpenter WM. Treatment of HIV-related hairy leukoplakia with podophyllum resin 25% solution. Oral Surg Oral Med Oral Pathol Oral Radiol Endod 79:64–7, 1995.
45. Goedert JJ, Cote TR, Virgo P, et al. Spectrum of AIDS-associated malignant disorders. Lancet 351:1833–9, 1998.
46. Cote TR, Biggar RJ, Rosenberg PS, et al. Non-Hodgkin's lymphoma among people with AIDS: incidence, presentation and public health burden. AIDS/Cancer Study Group. Int J Cancer 73:645–50, 1997.
47. Appleby P, Beral V, Newton G, Reeves G. Highly active antiretroviral therapy and incidence of cancer in human immunodeficiency virus-infected adults. J Natl Cancer Inst 92:1823–30, 2000.
48. Matthews GV, Bower M, Mandalia S, et al. Changes in acquired immunodeficiency syndrome-related lymphoma since the introduction of highly active antiretroviral therapy. Blood 96:2730–4, 2000.
49. Besson C, Goubar A, Gabarre J, et al. Changes in AIDS-related lymphoma since the era of highly active antiretroviral therapy. Blood 98:2339–44, 2001.
50. Grulich AE. AIDS-associated non-Hodgkin's lymphoma in the era of highly active antiretroviral therapy. J Acquir Immune Defic Syndr 21(Suppl 1):S27–30, 1999.
51. Kirk O, Pedersen C, Cozzi-Lepri A, et al. Non-Hodgkin lymphoma in HIV-infected patients in the era of highly active antiretroviral therapy. Blood 98:3406–12, 2001.
52. Piriou E, van Dort K, Nanlohy NM, et al. Loss of EBNA1-specific memory CD4+ and CD8+ T cells in HIV-infected patients progressing to AIDS-related non-Hodgkin lymphoma. Blood 106:3166–74, 2005.
53. Grulich AE, Wan X, Law MG, et al. B-cell stimulation and prolonged immune deficiency are risk factors for non-Hodgkin's lymphoma in people with AIDS. AIDS 14:133–40, 2000.
54. Hamilton-Dutoit SJ, Raphael M, Audouin J, et al. In situ demonstration of Epstein–Barr virus small RNAs (EBER 1) in acquired immunodeficiency syndrome-related lymphomas: correlation with tumor morphology and primary site. Blood 82:619–24, 1993.
55. Boyle MJ, Sewell WA, Sculley TB, et al. Subtypes of Epstein–Barr virus in human immunodeficiency virus-associated non-Hodgkin lymphoma. Blood 78:3004–11, 1991.
56. Gunthel CJ, Ng V, McGrath M, et al. Association of Epstein–Barr virus types 1 and 2 with acquired immunodeficiency syndrome-related primary central nervous system lymphomas. Blood 83:618–19, 1994.
57. van Baarle D, Hovenkamp E, Kersten MJ, et al. Direct Epstein–Barr virus (EBV) typing on peripheral blood mononuclear cells: no association between EBV type 2 infection or superinfection and the development of acquired immunodeficiency syndrome-related non-Hodgkin's lymphoma. Blood 93:3949–55, 1999.
58. Hamilton-Dutoit SJ, Rea D, Raphael M, et al. Epstein–Barr virus-latent gene expression and tumor cell phenotype in acquired immunodeficiency syndrome-related non-Hodgkin's lymphoma. Correlation of lymphoma phenotype with three distinct patterns of viral latency. Am J Pathol 143:1072–85, 1993.
59. Rea D, Delecluse HJ, Hamilton-Dutoit SJ, et al. Epstein–Barr virus latent and replicative gene expression in post-transplant lymphoproliferative disorders and AIDS-related non-Hodgkin's lymphomas. French Study Group of Pathology for HIV-associated Tumors. Ann Oncol 5:113–16, 1994.
60. Brink AA, Dukers DF, van den Brule AJ, et al. Presence of Epstein–Barr virus latency type III at the single cell level in post-transplantation lymphoproliferative disorders and AIDS related lymphomas. J Clin Pathol 50:911–18, 1997.
61. Subar M, Neri A, Inghirami G, et al. Frequent c-myc oncogene activation and infrequent presence of Epstein–Barr virus genome in AIDS-associated lymphoma. Blood 72:667–71, 1988.
62. Chaganti RS, Jhanwar SC, Koziner B, et al. Specific translocations characterize Burkitt's-like lymphoma of homosexual men with the acquired immunodeficiency syndrome. Blood 61:1265–8, 1983.
63. Neri A, Barriga F, Inghirami G, et al. Epstein–Barr virus infection precedes clonal expansion in Burkitt's and acquired immunodeficiency syndrome-associated lymphoma. Blood 77:1092–5, 1991.
64. Savoie A, Perpete C, Carpentier L, et al. Direct correlation between the load of Epstein–Barr virus-infected lymphocytes in the peripheral blood of pediatric transplant patients and risk of lymphoproliferative disease. Blood 83:2715–22, 1994.
65. Rooney CM, Loftin SK, Holladay MS, et al. Early identification of Epstein–Barr virus-associated post-transplantation lymphoproliferative disease. Br J Haematol 89:98–103, 1995.
66. Rowe DT, Qu L, Reyes J, et al. Use of quantitative competitive PCR to measure Epstein–Barr virus genome load in the peripheral blood of pediatric transplant patients with lymphoproliferative disorders. J Clin Microbiol 35:1612–15, 1997.
67. Lucas KG, Burton RL, Zimmerman SE, et al. Semiquantitative Epstein–Barr virus (EBV) polymerase chain reaction for the determination of patients at risk for EBV-induced lymphoproliferative disease after stem cell transplantation. Blood 91:3654–61, 1998.
68. Green M, Bueno J, Rowe D, et al. Predictive negative value of persistent low Epstein–Barr virus viral load after intestinal transplantation in children. Transplantation 70:593–6, 2000.
69. Laroche C, Drouet EB, Brousset P, et al. Measurement by the polymerase chain reaction of the Epstein–Barr virus load in infectious mononucleosis and AIDS-related non-Hodgkin's lymphomas. J Med Virol 46:66–74, 1995.
70. Yang J, Tao Q, Flinn IW, et al. Characterization of Epstein–Barr virus-infected B cells in patients with posttransplantation lymphoproliferative disease: disappearance after rituximab therapy does not predict clinical response. Blood 96:4055–63, 2000.
71. Antinori A, De Rossi G, Ammassari A, et al. Value of combined approach with thallium-201 single-photon emission computed tomography and Epstein–Barr virus DNA polymerase chain reaction in CSF for the diagnosis of AIDS-related primary CNS lymphoma. J Clin Oncol 17:554–60, 1999.
72. Hoffman JM, Waskin HA, Schifter T, et al. FDG-PET in differentiating lymphoma from nonmalignant central nervous system lesions in patients with AIDS. J Nucl Med 34:567–75, 1993.
73. Cinque P, Brytting M, Vago L, et al. Epstein–Barr virus DNA in cerebrospinal fluid from patients with AIDS-related primary lymphoma of the central nervous system. Lancet 342:398–401, 1993.

74. Cingolani A, Gastaldi R, Fassone L, et al. Epstein–Barr virus infection is predictive of CNS involvement in systemic AIDS-related non-Hodgkin's lymphomas J Clin Oncol 18:3325–30, 2000.
75. Broccolo F, Iuliano R, Careddu AM, et al. Detection of lymphotropic herpesvirus DNA by polymerase chain reaction in cerebrospinal fluid of AIDS patients with neurological disease. Acta Virol 44:137–43, 2000.
76. Ratner L, Lee J, Tang S, et al. Chemotherapy for human immunodeficiency virus-associated non-Hodgkin's lymphoma in combination with highly active antiretroviral therapy. J Clin Oncol 19:2171–8, 2001.
77. Vaccher E, Spina M, di Gennaro G, et al. Concomitant cyclophosphamide, doxorubicin, vincristine, and prednisone chemotherapy plus highly active antiretroviral therapy in patients with human immunodeficiency virus-related, non-Hodgkin lymphoma. Cancer 91:155–63, 2001.
78. Gerard L, Galicier L, Maillard A, et al. Systemic non-Hodgkin lymphoma in HIV-infected patients with effective suppression of HIV replication: persistent occurrence but improved survival. J Acquir Immune Defic Syndr 30:478–84, 2002.
79. Levine AM. Acquired immunodeficiency syndrome-related lymphoma: clinical aspects. Semin Oncol 27:442–53, 2000.
80. Clayton A, Mughal T. The changing face of HIV-associated lymphoma: what can we learn about optimal therapy in the post highly active antiretroviral therapy era? Hematol Oncol 22:111–20, 2004.
81. Kaplan LD, Lee JY, Ambinder RF, et al. Rituximab does not improve clinical outcome in a randomized phase 3 trial of CHOP with or without rituximab in patients with HIV-associated non-Hodgkin lymphoma: AIDS-Malignancies Consortium Trial 010. Blood 106:1538–43, 2005.
82. Coiffier B, Haioun C, Ketterer N, et al. Rituximab (anti-CD20 monoclonal antibody) for the treatment of patients with relapsing or refractory aggressive lymphoma: a multicenter phase II study. Blood 92:1927–32, 1998.
83. Coiffier B, Lepage E, Briere J, et al. CHOP chemotherapy plus rituximab compared with CHOP alone in elderly patients with diffuse large-B-cell lymphoma. N Engl J Med 346:235–42, 2002.
84. Bower M, Fife K, Sullivan A, et al. Treatment outcome in presumed and confirmed AIDS-related primary cerebral lymphoma. Eur J Cancer 35:601–4, 1999.
85. Pallesen G, Hamilton-Dutoit SJ, Rowe M, et al. Expression of Epstein–Barr virus replicative proteins in AIDS-related non-Hodgkin's lymphoma cells. J Pathol 165:289–99, 1991.
86. Raez L, Cabral L, Cai JP, et al. Treatment of AIDS-related primary central nervous system lymphoma with zidovudine, ganciclovir, and interleukin 2. AIDS Res Hum Retroviruses 15:713–19, 1999.
87. Brockmeyer NH, Pohl G, Mertins L. Combination of chemotherapy and antiviral therapy for Epstein–Barr virus-associated non-Hodgkin's lymphoma of high grade malignancy in cases of HIV infection. Eur J Med Res 2:133–5, 1997.
88. Oertel SH, Ruhnke MS, Anagnostopoulos I, et al. Treatment of Epstein-Barr virus-induced posttransplantation lymphoproliferative disorder with foscarnet alone in an adult after simultaneous heart and renal transplantation. Transplantation 67:765–7, 1999.
89. Schmidt W, Anagnostopoulos I, Scherubl H. Virostatic therapy for advanced lymphoproliferation associated with the Epstein–Barr virus in an HIV-infected patient. N Engl J Med 342:440–1, 2000.
90. Fong IW, Ho J, Toy C, et al. Value of long-term administration of acyclovir and similar agents for protecting against AIDS-related lymphoma: case-control and historical cohort studies. Clin Infect Dis 30:757–61, 2000.
91. Ioannidis JP, Collier AC, Cooper DA, et al. Clinical efficacy of high-dose acyclovir in patients with human immunodeficiency virus infection: a meta-analysis of randomized individual patient data. J Infect Dis 178:349–59, 1998.
92. Yao QY, Ogan P, Rowe M, Wood M, Rickinson AB. Epstein–Barr virus-infected B cells persist in the circulation of acyclovir-treated virus carriers. Int J Cancer 43:67–71, 1989.
93. Slobod KS, Taylor GH, Sandlund JT, et al. Epstein–Barr virus-targeted therapy for AIDS-related primary lymphoma of the central nervous system. Lancet 356:1493–4, 2000.
94. Andiman WA, Eastman R, Martin K, et al. Opportunistic lymphoproliferations associated with Epstein–Barr viral DNA in infants and children with AIDS. Lancet 2:1390–3, 1985.
95. McClain KL, Leach CT, Jenson HB, et al. Association of Epstein–Barr virus with leiomyosarcomas in children with AIDS. N Engl J Med 332:12–18, 1995.
96. Spina M, Vaccher E, Nasti G, Tirelli U. Human immunodeficiency virus-associated Hodgkin's disease. Semin Oncol 27:480–8, 2000.
97. Giraldo G, Beth E, Buonaguro FM. Kaposi's sarcoma: a natural model of interrelationships between viruses, immunologic responses, genetics, and oncogenesis. Antibiot Chemother 32:1–11, 1983.
98. Chang Y, Cesarman E, Pessin MS, et al. Identification of herpesvirus-like DNA sequences in AIDS-associated Kaposi's sarcoma. Science 266:1865–9, 1994.
99. Moore PS, Chang Y. Kaposi's sarcoma (KS), KS-associated herpesvirus, and the criteria for causality in the age of molecular biology. Am J Epidemiol 147:217–21, 1998.
100. Beral V, Peterman TA, Berkelman RL, Jaffe HW. Kaposi's sarcoma among persons with AIDS: a sexually transmitted infection? Lancet 335:123–8, 1990.
101. Albrecht H, Helm EB, Plettenberg A, et al. Kaposi's sarcoma in HIV infected women in Germany: more evidence for sexual transmission. A report of 10 cases and review of the literature. Genitourin Med 70:394–8, 1994.
102. Moore PS, Chang Y. Detection of herpesvirus-like DNA sequences in Kaposi's sarcoma in patients with and without HIV infection. N Engl J Med 332:1181–5, 1995.
103. Gao SJ, Kingsley L, Hoover DR, et al. Seroconversion to antibodies against Kaposi's sarcoma-associated herpesvirus-related latent nuclear antigens before the development of Kaposi's sarcoma. N Engl J Med 335:233–41, 1996.
104. Kedes DH, Operskalski E, Busch M, et al. The seroepidemiology of human herpesvirus 8 (Kaposi's sarcoma-associated herpesvirus): distribution of infection in KS risk groups and evidence for sexual transmission. Nat Med 2:918–24, 1996.
105. Simpson GR, Schulz TF, Whitby D, et al. Prevalence of Kaposi's sarcoma associated herpesvirus infection measured by antibodies to recombinant capsid protein and latent immunofluorescence antigen. Lancet 348:1133–8, 1996.
106. Whitby D, Luppi M, Barozzi P, et al. Human herpesvirus 8 seroprevalence in blood donors and lymphoma patients from different regions of Italy. J Natl Cancer Inst 90:395–7, 1998.
107. Calabro ML, Sheldon J, Favero A, et al. Seroprevalence of Kaposi's sarcoma-associated herpesvirus/human herpesvirus 8 in several regions of Italy. J Hum Virol 1:207–13, 1998.
108. Ariyoshi K, Schim van der Loeff M, Cook P, et al. Kaposi's sarcoma in the Gambia, West Africa is less frequent in human immunodeficiency virus type 2 than in human immunodeficiency virus type 1 infection despite a high prevalence of human herpesvirus 8. J Hum Virol 1:193–9, 1998.
109. Mayama S, Cuevas LE, Sheldon J, et al. Prevalence and transmission of Kaposi's sarcoma-associated herpesvirus (human herpesvirus 8) in Ugandan children and adolescents. Int J Cancer 77:817–20, 1998.
110. Bestetti G, Renon G, Mauclere P, et al. High seroprevalence of human herpesvirus-8 in pregnant women and prostitutes from Cameroon. AIDS 12:541–3, 1998.

111. Bourboulia D, Whitby D, Boshoff C, et al. Serologic evidence for mother-to-child transmission of Kaposi sarcoma-associated herpesvirus infection. JAMA 280:31–2, 1998.
112. Sitas F, Carrara H, Beral V, et al. Antibodies against human herpesvirus 8 in black South African patients with cancer. N Engl J Med 340:1863–71, 1999.
113. Gessain A, Mauclere P, van Beveren M, et al. Human herpesvirus 8 primary infection occurs during childhood in Cameroon, Central Africa. Int J Cancer 81:189–92, 1999.
114. Chatlynne LG, Ablashi DV. Seroepidemiology of Kaposi's sarcoma-associated herpesvirus (KSHV). Semin Cancer Biol 9:175–85, 1999.
115. Schulz TF. KSHV (HHV8) infection. J Infect 41:125–9, 2000.
116. Pauk J, Huang ML, Brodie SJ, et al. Mucosal shedding of human herpesvirus 8 in men. N Engl J Med 343:1369–1377, 2000.
117. Perna AM, Bonura F, Vitale F, et al. Antibodies to human herpes virus type 8 (HHV8) in general population and in individuals at risk for sexually transmitted diseases in Western Sicily. Int J Epidemiol 29:175–9, 2000.
118. Akula SM, Pramod NP, Wang FZ, Chandran B. Integrin alpha-3beta1 (CD 49c/29) is a cellular receptor for Kaposi's sarcoma-associated herpesvirus (KSHV/HHV-8) entry into the target cells. Cell 108:407–19, 2002.
119. Guttman-Yassky E, Kra-Oz Z, Dubnov J, et al. Infection with Kaposi's sarcoma-associated herpesvirus among families of patients with classic Kaposi's sarcoma. Arch Dermatol 141:1429–34, 2005.
120. Mbulaiteye SM, Pfeiffer RM, Whitby D, et al. Human herpesvirus 8 infection within families in rural Tanzania. J Infect Dis 187:1780–5, 2003.
121. Lyall EG, Patton GS, Sheldon J, et al. Evidence for horizontal and not vertical transmission of human herpesvirus 8 in children born to human immunodeficiency virus-infected mothers. Pediatr Infect Dis J 18:795–9, 1999.
122. Brayfield BP, Phiri S, Kankasa C, et al. Postnatal human herpesvirus 8 and human immunodeficiency virus type 1 infection in mothers and infants from Zambia. J Infect Dis 187:559–68, 2003.
123. Dukers NH, Renwick N, Prins M, et al. Risk factors for human herpesvirus 8 seropositivity and seroconversion in a cohort of homosexual men. Am J Epidemiol 151:213–24, 2000.
124. Smith NA, Sabin CA, Gopal R, et al. Serologic evidence of human herpesvirus 8 transmission by homosexual but not heterosexual sex. J Infect Dis 180:600–6, 1999.
125. Martin JN, Ganem DE, Osmond DH, et al. Sexual transmission and the natural history of human herpesvirus 8 infection. N Engl J Med 338:948–54, 1998.
126. Goudsmit J, Renwick N, Dukers NH, et al. Human herpesvirus 8 infections in the Amsterdam Cohort Studies (1984–1997): analysis of seroconversions to ORF65 and ORF73. Proc Natl Acad Sci USA 97:4838–43, 2000.
127. Blackbourn DJ, Osmond D, Levy JA, Lennette ET. Increased human herpesvirus 8 seroprevalence in young homosexual men who have multiple sex contacts with different partners. J Infect Dis 179:237–9, 1999.
128. Sosa C, Klaskala W, Chandran B, et al. Human herpesvirus 8 as a potential sexually transmitted agent in Honduras. J Infect Dis 178:547–51, 1998.
129. Lennette ET, Blackbourn DJ, Levy JA. Antibodies to human herpesvirus type 8 in the general population and in Kaposi's sarcoma patients. Lancet 348:858–61, 1996.
130. Howard MR, Whitby D, Bahadur G, et al. Detection of human herpesvirus 8 DNA in semen from HIV-infected individuals but not healthy semen donors AIDS 11:F15–19, 1997.
131. LaDuca JR, Love JL, Abbott LZ, et al. Detection of human herpesvirus 8 DNA sequences in tissues and bodily fluids. J Infect Dis 178:1610–15, 1998.
132. Vieira J, Huang ML, Koelle DM, Corey L. Transmissible Kaposi's sarcoma-associated herpesvirus (human herpesvirus 8) in saliva of men with a history of Kaposi's sarcoma. J Virol 71:7083–7, 1997.
133. Cesarman E, Chang Y, Moore PS, et al. Kaposi's sarcoma-associated herpesvirus-like DNA sequences in AIDS-related body-cavity-based lymphomas. N Engl J Med 332:1186–91, 1995.
134. Nador RG, Cesarman E, Chadburn A, et al. Primary effusion lymphoma: a distinct clinicopathologic entity associated with the Kaposi's sarcoma-associated herpes virus. Blood 88:645–56, 1996.
135. Soulier J, Grollet L, Oksenhendler E, et al. Kaposi's sarcoma-associated herpesvirus-like DNA sequences in multicentric Castleman's disease. Blood 86:1276–80, 1995.
136. Oksenhendler E, Carcelain G, Aoki Y, et al. High levels of human herpesvirus 8 viral load, human interleukin-6, interleukin-10, and C reactive protein correlate with exacerbation of multicentric castleman disease in HIV-infected patients. Blood 96:2069–73, 2000.
137. Engels EA, Biggar RJ, Marshall VA, et al. Detection and quantification of Kaposi's sarcoma-associated herpesvirus to predict AIDS-associated Kaposi's sarcoma. AIDS 17:1847–51, 2003.
138. Li JJ, Huang YQ, Cockerell CJ, Friedman-Kien AE. Localization of human herpes-like virus type 8 in vascular endothelial cells and perivascular spindle-shaped cells of Kaposi's sarcoma lesions by in situ hybridization. Am J Pathol 1996; 148:1741–8.
139. Kennedy MM, Cooper K, Howells DD, et al. Identification of HHV8 in early Kaposi's sarcoma: implications for Kaposi's sarcoma pathogenesis. Mol Pathol 51:14–20, 1998.
140. Boshoff C, Schulz TF, Kennedy MM, et al. Kaposi's sarcoma-associated herpesvirus infects endothelial and spindle cells. Nat Med 1:1274–8, 1995.
141. Judde JG, Lacoste V, Briere J, et al. Monoclonality or oligoclonality of human herpesvirus 8 terminal repeat sequences in Kaposi's sarcoma and other diseases. J Natl Cancer Inst 92:729–36, 2000.
142. Decker LL, Shankar P, Khan G, et al. The Kaposi sarcoma-associated herpesvirus (KSHV) is present as an intact latent genome in KS tissue but replicates in the peripheral blood mononuclear cells of KS patients. J Exp Med 184:283–8, 1996.
143. Katano H, Sato Y, Kurata T, et al. High expression of HHV-8-encoded ORF73 protein in spindle-shaped cells of Kaposi's sarcoma. Am J Pathol 155:47–52, 1999.
144. Staskus KA, Zhong W, Gebhard K, et al. Kaposi's sarcoma-associated herpesvirus gene expression in endothelial (spindle) tumor cells. J Virol 71:715–19, 1997.
145. Blasig C, Zietz C, Haar B, et al. Monocytes in Kaposi's sarcoma lesions are productively infected by human herpesvirus 8. J Virol 71:7963–8, 1997.
146. Dupin N, Fisher C, Kellam P, et al. Distribution of human herpesvirus-8 latently infected cells in Kaposi's sarcoma, multicentric Castleman's disease, and primary effusion lymphoma. Proc Natl Acad Sci USA 96:4546–51, 1999.
147. Kellam P, Bourboulia D, Dupin N, et al. Characterization of monoclonal antibodies raised against the latent nuclear antigen of human herpesvirus 8. J Virol 73:5149–55, 1999.
148. Chatterjee M, Osborne J, Bestetti G, et al. Viral IL-6-induced cell proliferation and immune evasion of interferon activity. Science 298:1432–5, 2002.
149. Jensen KK, Manfra DJ, Grisotto MG, et al. The human herpes virus 8-encoded chemokine receptor is required for angioproliferation in a murine model of Kaposi's sarcoma. J Immunol 174:3686–94, 2005.
150. Ballestas ME, Chatis PA, Kaye KM. Efficient persistence of extrachromosomal KSHV DNA mediated by latency-associated nuclear antigen. Science 284:641–4, 1999.

151. Cotter MA, Robertson ES. The latency-associated nuclear antigen tethers the Kaposi's sarcoma-associated herpesvirus genome to host chromosomes in body cavity-based lymphoma cells. Virology 264:254–64, 1999.
152. Friborg J, Kong W, Hottiger MO, Nabel GJ. p53 inhibition by the LANA protein of KSHV protects against cell death. Nature 402:889–94, 1999.
153. Lim C, Sohn H, Gwack Y, Choe J. Latency-associated nuclear antigen of Kaposi's sarcoma-associated herpesvirus (human herpesvirus-8) binds ATF4/CREB2 and inhibits its transcriptional activation activity. J Gen Virol 81:2645–52, 2000.
154. Renne R, Barry C, Dittmer D, et al. Modulation of cellular and viral gene expression by the latency-associated nuclear antigen of Kaposi's sarcoma-associated herpesvirus. J Virol 75:458–68, 2001.
155. Casper C, Wald A, Pauk J, et al. Correlates of prevalent and incident Kaposi's sarcoma-associated herpesvirus infection in men who have sex with men. J Infect Dis 185:990–3, 2002.
156. Oksenhendler E, Cazals-Hatem D, Schulz TF, et al. Transient angiolymphoid hyperplasia and Kaposi's sarcoma after primary infection with human herpesvirus 8 in a patient with human immunodeficiency virus infection. N Engl J Med 338:1585–90, 1998.
157. Delabesse E, Oksenhendler E, Lebbe C, et al. Molecular analysis of clonality in Kaposi's sarcoma. J Clin Pathol 50:664–8, 1997.
158. Rabkin CS, Janz S, Lash A, et al. Monoclonal origin of multicentric Kaposi's sarcoma lesions. N Engl J Med 336:988–93, 1997.
159. Gill PS, Tsai YC, Rao AP, et al. Evidence for multiclonality in multicentric Kaposi's sarcoma. Proc Natl Acad Sci USA 95:8257–61, 1998.
160. Kedes DH, Ganem D. Sensitivity of Kaposi's sarcoma-associated herpesvirus replication to antiviral drugs. Implications for potential therapy. J Clin Invest 99:2082–6, 1997.
161. Medveczky MM, Horvath E, Lund T, Medveczky PG. In vitro antiviral drug sensitivity of the Kaposi's sarcoma-associated herpesvirus. AIDS 11:1327–32, 1997.
162. Neyts J, De Clercq E. Antiviral drug susceptibility of human herpesvirus 8. Antimicrob Agents Chemother 41:2754–6, 1997.
163. Cannon JS, Hamzeh F, Moore S, et al. Human herpesvirus 8-encoded thymidine kinase and phosphotransferase homologues confer sensitivity to ganciclovir. J Virol 73:4786–93, 1999.
164. Jones JL, Hanson DL, Chu SY, et al. AIDS-associated Kaposi's sarcoma. Science 267:1078–9, 1995.
165. Glesby MJ, Hoover DR, Weng S, et al. Use of antiherpes drugs and the risk of Kaposi's sarcoma: data from the Multicenter AIDS Cohort Study. J Infect Dis 173:1477–80, 1996.
166. Mocroft A, Youle M, Gazzard B, et al. Anti-herpesvirus treatment and risk of Kaposi's sarcoma in HIV infection. Royal Free/Chelsea and Westminster Hospitals Collaborative Group. AIDS 10:1101–5, 1996.
167. Martin DF, Kuppermann BD, Wolitz RA, et al. Oral ganciclovir for patients with cytomegalovirus retinitis treated with a ganciclovir implant. Roche Ganciclovir Study Group. N Engl J Med 340:1063–70, 1999.
168. Morfeldt L, Torssander J. Long-term remission of Kaposi's sarcoma following foscarnet treatment in HIV-infected patients. Scand J Infect Dis 26:749–52, 1994.
169. Robles R, Lugo D, Gee L, Jacobson MA. Effect of antiviral drugs used to treat cytomegalovirus end-organ disease on subsequent course of previously diagnosed Kaposi's sarcoma in patients with AIDS. J Acquir Immune Defic Syndr Hum Retrovirol 20:34–8, 1999.
170. Humphrey RW, O'Brien TR, Newcomb FM, et al. Kaposi's sarcoma (KS)-associated herpesvirus-like DNA sequences in peripheral blood mononuclear cells: association with KS and persistence in patients receiving anti-herpesvirus drugs. Blood 88:297–301, 1996.
171. Curreli F, Friedman-Kien AE, Flore O. Glycyrrhizic acid alters Kaposi sarcoma-associated herpesvirus latency, triggering p53-mediated apoptosis in transformed B lymphocytes. J Clin Invest 115:642–52, 2005.
172. Herrada J, Cabanillas F, Rice L, et al. The clinical behavior of localized and multicentric Castleman disease. Ann Intern Med 128:657–62, 1998.
173. O'Leary JJ, Kennedy MM, McGee JO. Kaposi's sarcoma associated herpes virus (KSHV/HHV 8): epidemiology, molecular biology and tissue distribution. Mol Pathol 50:4–8, 1997.
174. Soulier J, Grollet L, Oksenhendler E, et al. Molecular analysis of clonality in Castleman's disease. Blood 86:1131–8, 1995.
175. Cannon JS, Nicholas J, Orenstein JM, et al. Heterogeneity of viral IL-6 expression in HHV-8-associated diseases. J Infect Dis 180:824–8, 1999.
176. Kim JE, Kim CJ, Park IA, et al. Clinicopathologic study of Castleman's disease in Korea. J Korean Med Sci 15:393–8, 2000.
177. Mori Y, Nishimoto N, Ohno M, et al. Human herpesvirus 8-encoded interleukin-6 homologue (viral IL-6) induces endogenous human IL-6 secretion. J Med Virol 61:332–5, 2000.
178. Parravinci C, Corbellino M, Paulli M, et al. Expression of a virus-derived cytokine, KSHV vIL-6, in HIV-seronegative Castleman's disease. Am J Pathol 151:1517–22, 1997.
179. Katano H, Sato Y, Kurata T, et al. Expression and localization of human herpesvirus 8-encoded proteins in primary effusion lymphoma, Kaposi's sarcoma, and multicentric Castleman's disease. Virology 269:335–44, 2000.
180. Moore P, Chang Y. Kaposi's sarcoma-associated herpesvirus. In: Knipe D, Howley P, Griffin D, et al (eds). Fields Virology. Philadelphia: PA Lippincott-Raven; 2001, pp 2803–33.
181. Schulz TF. The pleiotropic effects of Kaposi's sarcoma herpesvirus. J Pathol 208:187–98, 2006.
182. Jenner RG, Alba MM, Boshoff C, Kellam P. Kaposi's sarcoma-associated herpesvirus latent and lytic gene expression as revealed by DNA arrays. J Virol 75:891–902, 2001.
183. Katano H, Sata T. Human herpesvirus 8-virology, epidemiology and related diseases. Jpn J Infect Dis 53:137–55, 2000.
184. Parravicini C, Chandran B, Corbellino M, et al. Differential viral protein expression in Kaposi's sarcoma-associated herpesvirus-infected diseases: Kaposi's sarcoma, primary effusion lymphoma, and multicentric Castleman's disease. Am J Pathol 156:743–9, 2000.
185. Chiou CJ, Poole LJ, Kim PS, et al. Patterns of gene expression and a transactivation function exhibited by the vGCR (ORF74) chemokine receptor protein of Kaposi's sarcoma-associated herpesvirus. J Virol 76:3421–39, 2002.

Chapter 52

Human Herpesvirus-6 and Herpesvirus-7 Infections

David W. Kimberlin, MD, John W. Gnann Jr, MD

In 1986 a novel virus was isolated from six patients with lymphoproliferative syndromes, two of whom were also infected with the human immunodeficiency virus (HIV).[1] Molecular and structural characterization of the new virus revealed an icosahedral core structure of 162 capsomeres, indicating that it was a herpesvirus. Because of the initial belief that the new virus selectively infected freshly isolated human B cells, the virus was given the name human B-lymphotropic virus.[1] Subsequent investigation revealed a broader cell tropism, with notable T-cell lymphotropism.[2] For this reason, current nomenclature refers to this virus as human herpesvirus-6 (HHV-6).

Four years after the discovery of HHV-6, Frenkel and colleagues isolated another novel virus from the CD4+ T lymphocytes of a healthy adult.[3] Designated human herpesvirus-7 (HHV-7), this new virus is closely related to HHV-6,[4] exhibiting partial antigenic cross-reactivity with HHV-6.[5,6] In 1994 DNA from the eighth member of the human herpesvirus family was isolated from Kaposi sarcoma lesions of HIV-infected individuals. Human herpesvirus-8, or Kaposi sarcoma-associated herpesvirus, is discussed in Chapter 51.

Thus in less than a decade the number of known human herpesviruses increased from five to eight. New technologic advances (peripheral blood mononuclear cell (PBMC) culture, representational difference analysis) and the emergence of the acquired immunodeficiency syndrome (AIDS) epidemic converged to create the circumstances necessary for this remarkable pace of discovery. Two of the three new herpesviruses were initially isolated from AIDS patients, and all three may prove to cause disease in severely immunocompromised persons. This chapter reviews the current knowledge of HHV-6 and HHV-7 biology and the possible impact of these viruses in HIV-infected persons. Although much work is needed to elucidate fully the clinical implications of co-infection with HHV-6 or HHV-7 in HIV-infected persons, preliminary data suggest that an enhanced appreciation of these new herpesviruses may expand the understanding of HIV infection and disease progression. Moreover, such lines of investigation may ultimately provide information on which therapeutic strategies for disease intervention can be based.

HUMAN HERPESVIRUS-6

Since its discovery in AIDS patients, HHV-6 has been implicated as a possible pathogen in HIV-infected persons or a cofactor in HIV disease progression. As researchers investigated and characterized HHV-6 in HIV-infected adults, Yamanishi and colleagues pursued its association with disease in immunocompetent children, discovering in 1988 that HHV-6 caused the common childhood disease exanthem subitum (roseola).[7] As with all herpesviruses, HHV-6 establishes latency following primary infection during childhood, and reactivation from latency can result in active viral replication in both immunocompromised and immunocompetent persons.

Virology

Classification

HHV-6 is a member of the Herpesviridae family. Genomic analysis places HHV-6 among the β-herpesviruses, along with human cytomegalovirus (CMV) and HHV-7. Similarities with respect to amino acid sequences, gene organization, and putative protein functions suggest that HHV-6 is closely related to both CMV and HHV-7.[3,8,9] On the basis of DNA restriction analysis, *in vitro* tropism studies, and antigenic relations defined by reactivities of monoclonal antibodies, HHV-6 can be separated into two variants: variant A (HHV-6A) and variant B (HHV-6B).[10] Characteristic HHV-6A isolates include GS (the original isolate) and U 1102 (isolated from a Ugandan AIDS patient).[1,11] The prototypic HHV-6B isolate is Z 29, isolated from a Zairian AIDS patient.[12] The intravariant nucleotide sequence homology ranges from 97% to 100% and the intervariant homology from 94% to 96%.[13,14]

Although the first isolate of HHV-6 (GS) was a variant A strain, only HHV-6B strains have been definitively proven to cause disease (exanthem subitum during childhood, as described later). At the current time it is unclear if HHV-6A causes any disease. Variant A strains of HHV-6 are mainly isolated from AIDS patients or persons with lymphoproliferative disorders, whereas HHV-6B strains are primarily recovered from patients with exanthem subitum.

Viral Composition

Virion Structure

An enveloped virus, HHV-6 has an icosahedral nucleocapsid consisting of 162 capsomeres.[15] The capsid diameter measures 95–105 nm, with the diameter of the nucleoid being 60–80 nm. The nucleocapsid is surrounded by a dense, prominent tegument 25–40 nm thick.[15] Extracellular enveloped virions range from 160 to 200 nm, comparable to that of herpes simplex virus.

Genomic Structure and Genetic Content

Contained within the nucleocapsid of HHV-6 is a linear, double-stranded DNA molecule of 160–162 kb (Fig. 52-1). The genome consists of a 143–145 kb unique sequence (U) flanked by direct repeats, DRL (left) and DRR (right), of 8–9 kb and interrupted by three intermediate repeats (R1, R2, and R3) in the immediate-early A (IE-A) region.[16,17] The variation in length is due to the heterogeneous (het) region at the left end of both DR elements.[18,19] The genomic organization of the U region of HHV-6 is similar to that of the unique long (UL) region of CMV and is co-linear to that of HHV-7. The mean G + C content is 43%.[8,16,18] The complete nucleotide sequences of HHV-6A (U 1102) and of HHV-6B (Z29 and HST) have been reported.[16,17,20] The genomes contain 119 distinct open reading frames likely to encode proteins.[20] Nine open reading frames of HHV-6A do not have counterparts in HHV-6B.[16] The genes in the U region are termed U1 to U100 and open reading frames within the direct repeats are designated DR1 to DR7, whereas the nine open reading frames unique to HHV-6B are termed B1 to B9.[21] The overall nucleotide sequence identity between HHV-6A and HHV-6B is 90%.[20]

Protein Properties

More than 30 polypeptides encoded by HHV-6 have been identified in virions and infected cells.[22,23] The molecular weight of these proteins ranges from 30 000 to 200 000, and the proteins include six or seven glycoproteins.

In Vitro Biologic Properties

HHV-6 exhibits predominantly CD4+ T-lymphocyte tropism.[2,24] It can be isolated from CD4+ CD8− and CD3+ CD4+ mature T lymphocytes but not from CD4+ CD8+, CD4− CD8−, or CD3− T cells.[24] Additionally, HHV-6 can be propagated in CD4+ CD8+, CD4+ CD8−, and CD3+ CD4+ cells with mature phenotypes and rarely in CD4+ CD8+ human cord blood mononuclear cells (CBMCs).[24] CD46 serves as the receptor for HHV-6,[25] and is present on the membrane of all nucleated cells. For HHV-6A, the complex of glycoprotein H (encoded by the HHV-6 gene *U48*), glycoprotein L (encoded by the HHV-6 gene *U82*), and glycoprotein Q (encoded by the HHV-6 gene *U100*) is the viral ligand for human CD46.[26] Glycoprotein H is the component responsible for binding at the short consensus repeat domains SCR2 and SCR3 of CD46.[27] The HIV-1 receptors and co-receptors CD4, CXCR4, and CCR5 are not receptors for HHV-6.[28,29]

Consistent with the ubiquity of the CD46 receptor, HHV-6 infects a multitude of tissues in the body, including brain,[30–32] liver,[33–35] tonsils,[36] salivary glands,[37] and endothelium.[38] At the organ level, co-infection with HHV-6 and HHV-7 results in increased quantities of HHV-6 viral genome.[39] Likewise, reactivation of HHV-6 by infection with HHV-7 has been achieved *in vitro*.[40]

Efficient HHV-6 replication in primary cell culture requires both prior mitogen activation of primary T cells, as provided by phytohemagglutinin (PHA),[1,12] and full progression of the cell cycle, as demonstrated by the requirement for interleukin-2 (IL-2).[41] Mitogenic anti-CD3 monoclonal antibodies can also enhance HHV-6 replication.[42]

The HHV-6A and HHV-6B strains have both been adapted by serial passage to replicate in continuous cell lines. Established human cell lines that support HHV-6A replication include those of T cell (including the T-lymphoblastoid cell line HSB-2), B-cell, megakaryocyte, and glial cell lineages, as well as transformed cervical epithelial cells.[19] HHV-6B strains replicate well in the Molt-3 T cell line and the T-cell lymphoma line MT-4.[41,43]

The cytopathic effect (CPE) of HHV-6 is first visible in culture 3–5 days following infection. The CPE is characterized by refractile enlargement of some of the lymphocytes and occasional multinucleated cells. Lytic degeneration of the infected cells occurs following the development of CPE.

Epidemiology

Geographic Distribution

Seroprevalence studies of HHV-6 infection have demonstrated remarkable reproducibility from widely separated regions of the globe. With rare exceptions,[44] the prevalence of antibodies to HHV-6 is high among populations throughout the world.

Incidence and Prevalence of Infection

Epidemiologic studies in normal children have shown that most primary HHV-6 infections occur within the first year of

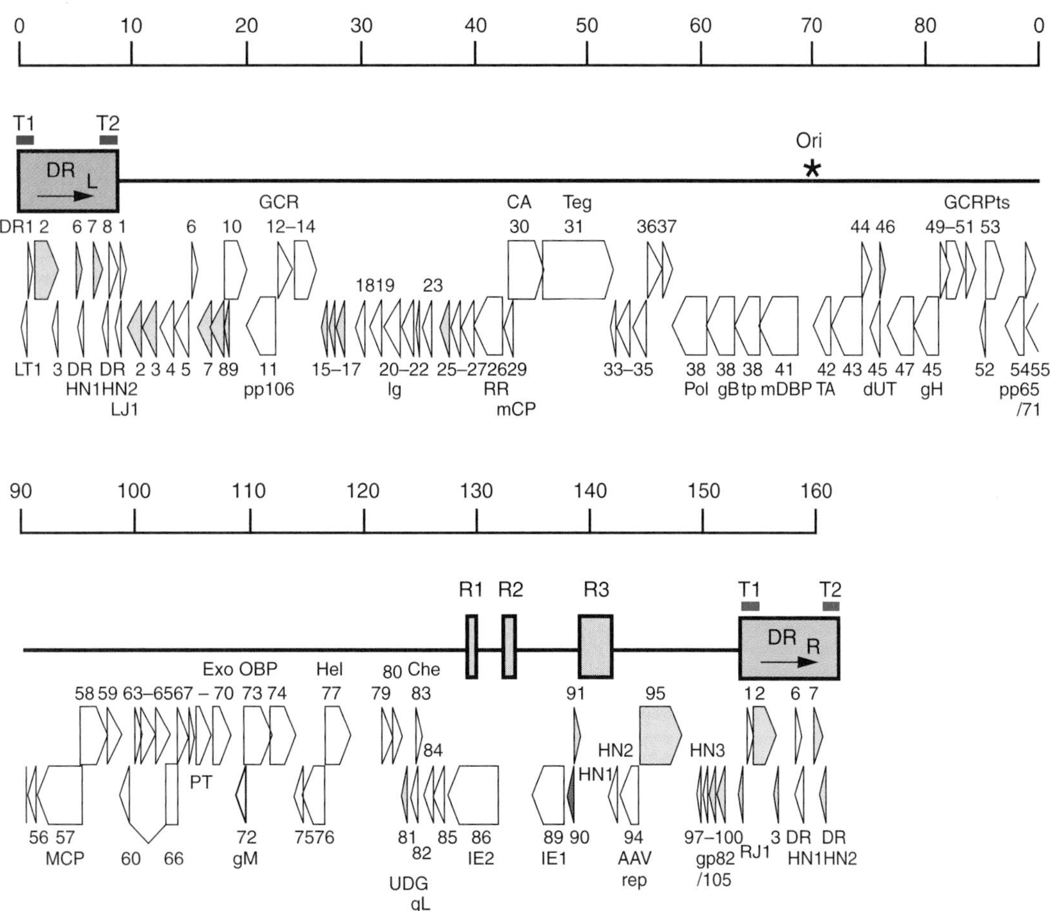

Figure 52-1 ■ Predicted ORF organization of HHV-6 strain HST. Repeat regions (DRL, DRR, R1, R2, and R3) are boxed; telomeric repeat regions (T1 and T2) are denoted by striped bars; UR is indicated by a solid line. Protein coding regions are indicated as open arrows and are numbered DR1, DR2, DR3, DR6, DR7, DR8, DRHN1, and DRHN2 within the direct repeats and HN1, HN2, HN3, and U1 to U100 (excluding U78, U88, U92, U93, and U96) within the UR. The Ori is indicated by an asterisk. The *US22* gene family is shaded. GCR, G-protein-coupled receptor; Ig, Ig immunoglobulin superfamily; RR, large subunit of ribonucleotide reductase; mCP, minor capsid protein; CA, capsid assembly protein; Teg, tegument protein; Pol, DNA polymerase; tp, transport protein; mDBP, major single-stranded DNA binding protein; TA, conserved herpesvirus transactivator; dUT, dUTPase; Pts, protease/assembly protein; pp. 65/71, phosphoprotein 65/71K; MCP, major capsid protein; PT, phosphotransferase; Exo, exonuclease; OBP, origin binding protein; Hel, helicase; UDG, uracil-DNA glycosylase; Che, chemokine; AAV rep1, adeno-associated virus replication protein homolog.

From Isegawa Y, Mukai T, Nakano K, et al. Comparison of the complete DNA sequences of human herpesvirus 6 variants A and B. J Virol 73:8053, 1999.

life.[45,46] HHV-6 immunoglobulin G (IgG) can be detected in more than 90% of neonates,[47,48] reflecting both the high seroprevalence of HHV-6 among adults[48,49] and the active transport of HHV-6 IgG across the placenta.[46] The prevalence of HHV-6 IgG drops significantly by 4–6 months of life as maternal antibodies decline, then increases through the third year of life and remains high into adulthood.[45,46,48] The highest geometric mean titers of HHV-6 antibody occur during the first 3 years of life, indicating a predominant clustering of primary infections in infants and toddlers.[46,49] More than 90% of normal children become infected with HHV-6 by 12 months of life,[48] and virtually 100% acquire infection by 3 years of age.[49]

Transmission

Although the mode(s) of transmission of HHV-6 has yet to be proven definitively, most children probably acquire infection through contact with the secretions of adult caretakers shedding the virus in saliva.[37,50–52] Reports of culture isolation of HHV-6 from the saliva of healthy adults[50,52] and adult patients infected with HIV[52] document salivary shedding in more than 85% of persons. Viral shedding in saliva is intermittent,[53] and the serum antibody titer to HHV-6 does not correlate with the ability to isolate HHV-6 from saliva samples.[52] HHV-6 DNA can be detected by polymerase chain reaction (PCR) in saliva or PBMCs of more than 90%

of healthy individuals.[54,55] Using *in situ* hybridization and immunohistochemical staining, HHV-6 DNA and HHV-6 protein expression have been demonstrated in tissue from submandibular glands,[37] parotid glands,[37] salivary glands,[51] and bronchial glands.[51] Although breast milk is unlikely to be an important source of early HHV-6 infection,[56] several reports suggest that HHV-6 may infect an infant congenitally or perinatally.[57–60] Definitive proof of such transmission, however, remains elusive.

Pathogenesis

Viral Replication and Latency

Analysis of pathologic specimens reveals that HHV-6 can infect a wide variety of cell and tissue types. During acute infection, infection of lymphocytes, macrophages, histiocytes, endothelial cells, and epithelial cells occurs, with CD4+ T lymphocytes being the predominant target cell type in the blood. The cell target of HHV-6 in the oropharynx during primary infection remains under investigation. Persistent HHV-6 infection can occur in salivary glands and brain tissue,[30,31,37,61] and HHV-6 has been shown to establish latency in mononuclear cells[62,63] and early bone marrow progenitor cells.[64] Low concentrations of HHV-6 DNA can be found in PBMCs from healthy individuals.

Immune Responses to HHV-6 Infection

Humoral Immune Response

The protective effect of antibody is suggested by the epidemiology of HHV-6 infection. As noted above, passively acquired maternal antibody wanes over the first 6 months of infancy; and during the next 6 months of life the number of children acquiring HHV-6 for the first time approaches 90%.[48] This finding suggests that maternal antibody provides protection against primary HHV-6 infection. Additionally, during primary HHV-6 infection the clearance of viremia coincides with the appearance of HHV-6B-specific neutralizing antibody,[65] again suggesting the importance of the humoral arm of the immune response to HHV-6.

Following primary HHV-6 infection, IgM-neutralizing antibodies appear within 5–7 days. Maximum IgM titers appear at 2–3 weeks, and the titers then decline and reach undetectable levels after 2 months.[66] Host IgG responses following primary HHV-6 infection develop 7–10 days following the febrile period.[67] Serologic evidence of previous infection manifested by HHV-6 IgG is maintained indefinitely.

Cellular Immune Response

The T-cell immune responses against HHV-6 infection are readily identified in healthy adult populations, and HHV-6-specific T-cell clones have been isolated.[68,69] Moreover, the importance of the cellular component of the host immune response in maintaining latency is suggested by the increased frequency of HHV-6 reactivation in solid organ transplant recipients.[70] Complete understanding of the role of cellular immunity in primary HHV-6 infection and in viral reactivation from latency awaits further investigation.

Clinical Relevance of HHV-6

The only disease for which HHV-6B has been shown definitively to be the causative agent is exanthem subitum (roseola), a common disease of childhood.[7,67] In addition, HHV-6B is a major cause of emergency room visits and hospitalizations for infants and young children.[58] HHV-6 produces a spectrum of neurologic diseases as well, including encephalitis and febrile seizures.[71–73]

Clinical Relevance in Relation to HIV Infection

In Vitro Data

Because HHV-6 was initially isolated from two HIV-positive patients and exhibits CD4+ cell tropism, it was hypothesized that HHV-6 may act as a cofactor in the acceleration of HIV infection to AIDS in patients co-infected with the two viruses. Initial evaluation of possible interactions between HHV-6 and HIV led to the discovery that the viruses can simultaneously infect the same CD4+ T lymphocytes under experimental conditions.[2,74] Studies evaluating the impact of HHV-6 co-infection on active HIV viral replication *in vitro* have yielded contradictory results, with some investigations documenting enhanced HIV replication,[74–76] whereas others reported inhibition of HIV replication.[12,77–80] HHV-6 infection in the presence of HIV *tat* results in significantly higher HIV long terminal repeat (LTR) activation than that observed by *tat* or HHV-6 alone, indicating that HHV-6 and *tat* interact synergistically.[81,82] Effects of co-infection on HHV-6 replication are less impressive: HHV-6 replication is unaffected[78,80] or slightly inhibited[77] in cells co-infected with HIV. However, expression of HIV-1 *tat* inhibits HHV-6 replication more dramatically, as shown by a 3.6- to 15.4-fold reduction in yield of infectious virus.[81]

HHV-6 induces expression of CD4 receptor molecules on the cell membranes of infected lymphocytes, hematopoietic progenitor cell lines, natural killer cells, and lymphoid tissue *ex vivo*, rendering them susceptible to co-infection with HIV.[83–89] *In vitro* studies demonstrate that such co-infection leads to accelerated cellular apoptosis.[74,85] Transactivation of the CD4 promoter by the IE1 and IE2 proteins of HHV-6 is responsible for this enhanced CD4 receptor expression.[90] HHV-6 has been shown to downregulate the HIV-1 co-receptor CXCR4 *in vitro*,[29,91] although expression of both CXCR4 and CCR5 are not affected by HHV-6 in an *ex vivo* propagation system.[92] HHV-6 replication enhances the production of the CCR5 ligand RANTES,[89,92,93] thus providing a mechanism for the selective blockade of CCR5-tropic but not CXCR4-tropic HIV-1 replication by HHV-6.[92]

Perhaps most interestingly, numerous investigators have demonstrated that HHV-6 can trans-activate the LTR promoter of HIV.[74,75,81,94–104] Such transcriptional activation occurs in an NF-κB- or Spl-binding-site-dependent manner.[75,95,97,102,104] Co-expression of HIV-1 *tat* transactivating protein produces enhanced transcriptional activation.[75,81] Transactivation of the HIV LTR is accomplished by both HHV-6A and HHV-6B, although HHV-6B induction requires T cells to be stimulated, whereas induction by HHV-6A can occur in either stimulated or resting T cells.[95]

Loci of HHV-6A that are capable of HIV-1 LTR transactivation are depicted in Figure 52-1.[19] These loci contain homologs of the CMV *UL36-38* and CMV *US22* gene families,[95–100] a portion of the putative DNA polymerase accessory protein,[103] putative IE genes,[96] and sequences of unknown function.[95,102]

In Vivo Data

The consequence of HHV-6 on HIV infection *in vivo* has been inadequately evaluated. Of the few published clinical reports that have evaluated the potential interaction between these two viruses from epidemiologic and pathologic perspectives, conflicting results have emerged. In a study of the prevalence of HHV-6 seropositivity in a cohort of HIV-1-infected patients, the frequency of HHV-6 seropositivity was significantly lower in patients who had a slower decline in CD4 cells, compared to patients with rapidly declining CD4+ T-lymphocyte counts and to the general population.[105] This finding suggests a role for HHV-6 co-infection in the progression of HIV-1 disease. HHV-6 DNA has been detected primarily in HIV-infected patients with high CD4+ T-lymphocyte counts in some studies[75,106,107] and primarily in patients with low CD4+ T-lymphocyte counts in others.[108] A small longitudinal study of HIV-infected patients has demonstrated that HHV-6 reactivation was followed by a temporary decrease in CD4+ T-lymphocyte counts and by a progressive, dramatic loss of CD4 cells during the following 18 months.[109]

HHV-6 DNA is present in the peripheral lymph nodes and spleens of recent HIV-1 seroconverters at a frequency and distribution similar to that of control tissues from individuals not infected with HIV.[110] In patients with advanced HIV disease, however, HHV-6 can disseminate widely to visceral organs, including the lungs of patients who died of pneumonitis.[111–113] AIDS patients have significantly higher HHV-6 viral loads in these visceral organs than do patients who are not infected with HIV.[113] Furthermore, HIV-infected patients whose organs are co-infected with HHV-6 have higher concentrations of HIV proviral DNA in those organs, compared with HIV-infected persons who are not co-infected with HHV-6.[39,75]

HHV-6 DNA has been detected by PCR in the colonic mucosa of HIV-seropositive patients with diarrhea undergoing intestinal biopsy.[114] A study involving serologic evaluation of Romanian children with nonprogressive HIV disease found that current or recent HHV-6 infection appeared to be associated with the development of pneumonitis,[115] although other reports have not correlated HHV-6 with respiratory disorders in HIV-infected patients.[116] HHV-6 has been correlated with pneumonitis in other immunocompetent and immunocompromised pediatric populations, however.[117] Several reports have documented the presence of HHV-6 antigens and DNA in retinal lesions from patients with AIDS-associated retinitis, with CMV or HIV-1 usually being present concomitantly.[118–122] *In vitro* studies have proven that HIV-1 and HHV-6 are capable of simultaneously infecting corneal epithelial cells.[123] Several studies have suggested that HHV-6 can be detected infrequently from cerebrospinal fluid of HIV-infected persons, although its pathogenicity in such settings has been called into question and may relate to co-pathogens such as CMV.[124–126]

Although the studies cited above suggest that HHV-6 plays a role as cofactor in HIV disease progression, other reports have found no correlation between HHV-6 infection and the course of the HIV infection.[127–132] Investigations in animal models have also failed to demonstrate a clinical consequence of simultaneous infection with HHV-6 and HIV.[133]

With limited exceptions,[59,115] each of the *in vivo* studies to date involved only adult patients. Because HHV-6 establishes latency following primary infection during childhood, an inherent difficulty with clinical evaluations of the possible interaction(s) between HHV-6 and HIV-1 is distinguishing causality. That is, it is difficult to determine if HHV-6 reactivation results in progression of HIV-1 disease, or if progression of HIV-1 disease (with its corresponding decline in immunoregulatory function) results in reactivation of HHV-6. In an effort to assess the impact of primary HHV-6 acquisition on HIV viral dynamics and disease course, Thai and Japanese investigators evaluated 227 infants born to HIV-infected women. The cumulative infection rates of HHV-6 at 6 and 12 months of age were significantly lower in HIV-infected children (11% and 33%, respectively) than in uninfected children (28% and 78%, respectively; $P < 0.001$).[59] Similar findings have been observed by one of the authors of this chapter in an analysis of specimens obtained from patients enrolled in the National Institutes of Health (NIH)-sponsored Women and Infants Transmission Study (WITS). HIV-infected infants without HHV-6 co-infection had lower rates of HIV disease progression at 12 months of life than did co-infected patients (42% vs 100%; $P < 0.05$), suggesting an association of HHV-6 infection and progression of HIV disease in children with vertically acquired HIV infection.[59]

Diagnosis

Diagnosis of HHV-6 infection is accomplished both serologically and virologically. As with other herpesvirus infections for which latency is established, documentation of primary infection is less difficult than establishing viral reactivation. In general, a fourfold or greater rise in anti-HHV-6 antibody titer between acute and convalescent serum samples suggests that active viral replication has occurred. Detection of HHV-6 IgM in infants and young children is a reliable marker of primary infection, although extrapolation to adults is problematic because IgM can be detected during HHV-6 reactivation.[134] In organ transplant recipients, reactivation of HHV-6 can produce IgM neutralizing antibody responses that persist for 2–3 months and then become undetectable 5–6 months after transplantation.[66] Furthermore, avidity of IgG antibodies to HHV-6, as determined by elution with urea, can distinguish between primary and recurrent infection: with primary infection low-avidity antibody is detected that matures to high avidity within 5 months, whereas with recurrent infection high-avidity antibody is present from the time of viral reactivation from latency.[135]

Detection of HHV-6 by viral culture provides indisputable evidence of active HHV-6 infection. Likewise, detection of HHV-6 DNA in cell-free plasma specimens suggests the presence of active HHV-6 replication *in vivo*,[136,137] as does detection by reverse transcriptase (RT)-PCR assay.[138]

Prevention and Treatment

Given the ubiquity of HHV-6 during early childhood and the lack of an effective vaccine, prevention of primary HHV-6 infection is not feasible. However, prevention of HHV-6 reactivation from latency with antiviral therapy may be possible. Data suggesting such a possibility come from investigations in stem cell and organ transplant recipients receiving acyclovir[139] or ganciclovir.[140–142] Whether similar beneficial effects of acyclovir prophylaxis of HHV-6 reactivation can be demonstrated in HIV-infected patients remains to be determined.

Antiviral susceptibility patterns of HHV-6 closely resemble those of CMV. Several investigators have analyzed the *in vitro* sensitivity of HHV-6 to antiviral agents currently used to treat herpesvirus infections.[143–150] HHV-6 multiplication is readily inhibited by foscarnet, cidofovir, and ganciclovir at levels that are easily achievable in the plasma of humans. Although acyclovir also has an inhibitory effect against HHV-6, it is much less active than the other antiviral agents listed above. Maribavir (1263W94) and other benzimidazole ribonucleosides are not active against HHV-6, even though they have significant activity against CMV.[151] The orally bioavailable lipid analogs of cidofovir, hexadecyloxypropyl-CDV, and octadecyloxyethyl-CDV, have even greater activity against HHV-6 and other herpesviruses than does the parent (unmodified) cidofovir.[152] Despite these *in vitro* findings, there have been no controlled prospective clinical evaluations of antiviral therapy for HHV-6 infections, and only anecdotal reports of ganciclovir, foscarnet, or cidofovir suggesting benefit in the transplant population exist in the literature.[153–160] Mutations conferring resistance of HHV-6 to ganciclovir, cidofovir, and foscarnet have been described.[150,161,162]

HUMAN HERPESVIRUS-7

In 1990 Frenkel and colleagues discovered another new herpesvirus, HHV-7 in cultures of CD4+ T lymphocytes.[3] As with HHV-6, growth of HHV-7 *in vitro* requires co-cultivation of activated CD4+ T cells with fresh PBMCs or cord blood mononuclear cells (CBMCs). Such activation can be achieved utilizing the polyclonal T-cell mitogen PHA in addition to IL-2. Although the potential for *in vivo* interaction between HHV-7 and HIV exists, a paucity of data precludes even preliminary speculation in this regard. Therefore, this review of HHV-7 is relatively brief, focusing on basic knowledge from which possible interactions with HIV may be postulated.

Biologic Properties

As with HHV-6, HHV-7 exhibits CD4+ T-lymphocyte tropism,[3,9] with the CD4 cell surface molecule being a critical component of the HHV-7 receptor.[163] Specifically, selective, progressive downregulation of the surface membrane expression of CD4 was observed in human CD4+ T cells during the course of HHV-7 infection. Addition of murine monoclonal antibodies directed against CD4 or the recombinant soluble form of human CD4 resulted in dose-dependent inhibition of HHV-7 infection in primary CD4+ T lymphocytes. In the same study, a marked reciprocal interference was observed between HHV-7 and HIV, with prior exposure of CD4+ T cells to HHV-7 dramatically interfering with infection by both primary and *in vitro*-passaged HIV-1 isolates. Similarly, persistent infection with HIV-1 or treatment with the soluble form of gp 120 rendered CD4+ T-cells resistant to HHV-7 infection.[163]

The HIV-1 co-receptors CXCR4 and CCR5 are not receptors for HHV-7.[29,164] Two studies found that HHV-7 downregulates CXCR4 by a mechanism independent of CD4,[29,165] whereas one study failed to confirm this observation.[164] If true, such downregulation would provide further *in vitro* evidence suggesting interference of HIV replication by HHV-7. HHV-7 inhibits HIV-1 infection in cells of the mononuclear phagocytic lineage, despite its inability to replicate actively in such cells.[166] HHV-7 can provide a transactivating function, mediating reactivation of HHV-6 from latency;[167] and co-infection with HHV-6 and HHV-7 within an organ results in increased quantities of HHV-7 viral genome.[39]

Epidemiology

Primary HHV-7 infection usually occurs during childhood, although the age of infection appears to be somewhat later than the very early age documented for HHV-6. In one study, the mean age at which HHV-7 seroconversion occurred was 17 months versus a mean age of 11 months for HHV-6.[168] Most adults have serologic evidence of prior HHV-7 infection.[169]

Transmission

Data suggest that the salivary glands may be the site of HHV-7 replication and transmission. Among blood donors in Germany, HHV-7 DNA was detected by PCR in 95.5% of saliva specimens and 66.1% of blood buffy coat specimens.[170] HHV-7 DNA was detected by PCR in 75% of the salivary glands of Italian patients with parotid tumors and in 55% of salivary samples from healthy adults.[171] In the same Italian study, HHV-7 DNA was detected with similar frequency in saliva from donors with the common cold or recurrent aphthous ulcerations, but saliva specimens from HIV-infected patients harbored HHV-7 with higher frequency (81%) and increased viral load.[171] Among healthy adults in Japan, HHV-7 DNA was detected by PCR in 89.7% of saliva samples, and the viral load detected in saliva remained constant over time.[53] In addition to persistent replication in salivary gland tissue, HHV-7 establishes latency in peripheral blood T cells.[172]

Clinical Relevance of HHV-7

As yet HHV-7 has not been definitively shown to cause a specific disease. The strongest data for the association of HHV-7 with clinical disease implicate it as a cause of first or second episodes of exanthem subitum.[168,173] HHV-7 may also be associated with febrile seizures and other neurologic manifestations as well as with minor upper respiratory tract infections.[71,73,173–176]

With limited exceptions, knowledge of specific viral interactions between HHV-7 and HIV *in vivo* is almost completely lacking. HHV-7 is detected more frequently and in greater amounts in the saliva of HIV-infected persons, as described above.[171] Lymph node tissue from HIV-infected persons also is more likely to demonstrate immunohistochemical evidence of HHV-7 infection than that of HIV-negative patients.[177] However, HHV-7 cell load and detection rate do not correlate with HIV-1 plasma load, suggesting that HHV-7 infection may not be stimulated by nor interact with HIV-1 infection.[178]

Treatment

In vitro analysis suggests that foscarnet and cidofovir are most active against HHV-7, with ganciclovir and penciclovir having less activity and acyclovir showing no activity.[145,179] A study of ganciclovir therapy in renal transplant recipients failed to demonstrate any effect of treatment on the incidence of HHV-7 viremia, suggesting that HHV-7 may be resistant to ganciclovir *in vivo*.[180]

CONCLUSIONS

Investigations of the recently discovered herpesviruses HHV-6 and HHV-7 have yielded intriguing suggestions of *in vivo* interactions with HIV. Systematic evaluation of such potential interactions has not yet been carried out in a definitive manner. It is likely that such research will enhance our understanding of the natural history of HIV infection and could provide avenues for improved therapeutic strategies. The potential for HHV-6 and HHV-7 to cause significant opportunistic infections in HIV-infected persons also requires additional investigation.

REFERENCES

1. Salahuddin SZ, Ablashi DV, Markham PD, et al. Isolation of a new virus, HBLV, in patients with lymphoproliferative disorders. Science 234:596, 1986.
2. Lusso P, Markham PD, Tschachler E, et al. In vitro cellular tropism of human B-lymphotropic virus (human herpesvirus-6). J Exp Med 167:1659, 1988.
3. Frenkel N, Schirmer EC, Wyatt LS, et al. Isolation of a new herpesvirus from human CD4+ T cells. Proc Natl Acad Sci USA 87:748, 1990.
4. Mukai T, Isegawa Y, Yamanishi K. Identification of the major capsid protein gene of human herpesvirus 7. Virus Res 37:55, 1995.
5. Wyatt LS, Rodriguez WJ, Balachandran N, Frenkel N. Human herpesvirus 7: antigenic properties and prevalence in children and adults. J Virol 65:6260, 1991.
6. Frenkel N, Wyatt LS. HHV-6 and HHV-7 as exogenous agents in human lymphocytes. Dev Biol Stand 76:259, 1992.
7. Yamanishi K, Okuno T, Shiraki K, et al. Identification of human herpesvirus-6 as a causal agent for exanthem subitum. Lancet 1:1065, 1988.
8. Lawrence GL, Chee M, Craxton MA, et al. Human herpes virus 6 is closely related to human cytomegalovirus. J Virol 64:287, 1990.
9. Berneman ZN, Ablashi DV, Li G, et al. Human herpesvirus 7 is a T-lymphotropic virus and is related to, but significantly different from, human herpesvirus 6 and human cytomegalovirus. Proc Natl Acad Sci USA 89:10552, 1992.
10. Anonymous. Human herpesvirus-6 strain groups: a nomenclature. Arch Virol 129:363, 1993.
11. Downing RG, Sewankambo N, Serwadda D, et al. Isolation of human lymphotropic herpesviruses from Uganda. Lancet 2:390, 1987.
12. Lopez C, Pellett P, Stewart J, et al. Characteristics of human herpesvirus-6. J Infect Dis 157:1271, 1988.
13. Aubin JT, Collandre H, Candotti D, et al. Several groups among human herpesvirus 6 strains can be distinguished by Southern blotting and polymerase chain reaction. J Clin Microbiol 29:367, 1991.
14. Aubin JT, Agut H, Collandre H, et al. Antigenic and genetic differentiation of the two putative types of human herpes virus 6. J Virol Methods 41:223, 1993.
15. Biberfeld P, Kramarsky B, Salahuddin SZ, Gallo RC. Ultrastructural characterization of a new human B lymphotropic DNA virus (human herpesvirus 6) isolated from patients with lymphoproliferative disease. J Natl Cancer Inst 79:933, 1987.
16. Gompels UA, Nicholas J, Lawrence G, et al. The DNA sequence of human herpesvirus-6: structure, coding content, and genome evolution. Virology 209:29, 1995.
17. Isegawa Y, Mukai T, Nakano K, et al. Comparison of the complete DNA sequences of human herpesvirus 6 variants A and B. J Virol 73:8053, 1999.
18. Lindquester GJ, Pellett PE. Properties of the human herpesvirus 6 strain Z29 genome: G + C content, length, and presence of variable-length directly repeated terminal sequence elements. Virology 182:102, 1991.
19. Pellett PE, Black JB. Human herpesvirus 6. In: Fields BN, Knipe DM, Howley PM, et al, (eds). Fields Virology. 3rd edn. Philadelphia: PA Lippincott-Raven; 1996, p. 2587.
20. Dominguez G, Dambaugh TR, Stamey FR, et al. Human herpesvirus 6B genome sequence: coding content and comparison with human herpesvirus 6A. J Virol 73:8040, 1999.
21. De Bolle L, Naesens L, De Clercq E. Update on human herpesvirus 6 biology, clinical features, and therapy. Clin Microbiol Rev 18:217, 2005.
22. Balachandran N, Amelse RE, Zhou WW, Chang CK. Identification of proteins specific for human herpesvirus 6-infected human T cells. J Virol 63:2835, 1989.
23. Shiraki K, Okuno T, Yamanishi K, Takahashi M. Virion and nonstructural polypeptides of human herpesvirus-6. Virus Res 13:173, 1989.
24. Takahashi K, Sonoda S, Higashi K, et al. Predominant CD4 T-lymphocyte tropism of human herpesvirus 6-related virus. J Virol 63:3161, 1989.

25. Santoro F, Kennedy PE, Locatelli G, et al. CD46 is a cellular receptor for human herpesvirus 6. Cell 99:817, 1999.
26. Mori Y, Yang X, Akkapaiboon P, et al. Human herpesvirus 6 variant A glycoprotein H-glycoprotein L-glycoprotein Q complex associates with human CD46. J Virol 77:4992, 2003.
27. Santoro F, Greenstone HL, Insinga A, et al. Interaction of glycoprotein H of human herpesvirus 6 with the cellular receptor CD46. J Biol Chem 278:25964, 2003.
28. Lusso P, Gallo RC, DeRocco SE, Markham PD. CD4 is not the membrane receptor for HHV-6. Lancet 1:730, 1989.
29. Yasukawa M, Hasegawa A, Sakai I, et al. Down-regulation of CXCR4 by human herpesvirus 6 (HHV-6) and HHV-7. J Immunol 162:5417, 1999.
30. Chan PK, Ng HK, Hui M, Cheng AF. Prevalence and distribution of human herpesvirus 6 variants A and B in adult human brain. J Med Virol 64:42, 2001.
31. Donati D, Akhyani N, Fogdell-Hahn A, et al. Detection of human herpesvirus-6 in mesial temporal lobe epilepsy surgical brain resections. Neurology 61:1405, 2003.
32. Luppi M, Barozzi P, Maiorana A, et al. Human herpesvirus 6 infection in normal human brain tissue. J Infect Dis 169:943, 1994.
33. Harma M, Hockerstedt K, Lautenschlager I. Human herpesvirus-6 and acute liver failure. Transplantation 76:536, 2003.
34. Ishikawa K, Hasegawa K, Naritomi T, et al. Prevalence of herpesviridae and hepatitis virus sequences in the livers of patients with fulminant hepatitis of unknown etiology in Japan. J Gastroenterol 37:523, 2002.
35. Ozaki Y, Tajiri H, Tanaka-Taya K, et al. Frequent detection of the human herpesvirus 6-specific genomes in the livers of children with various liver diseases. J Clin Microbiol 39:2173, 2001.
36. Roush KS, Domiati-Saad RK, Margraf LR, et al. Prevalence and cellular reservoir of latent human herpesvirus 6 in tonsillar lymphoid tissue. Am J Clin Pathol 116:648, 2001.
37. Fox JD, Briggs M, Ward PA, Tedder RS. Human herpesvirus 6 in salivary glands. Lancet 336:590, 1990.
38. Caruso A, Rotola A, Comar M, et al. HHV-6 infects human aortic and heart microvascular endothelial cells, increasing their ability to secrete proinflammatory chemokines. J Med Virol 67:528, 2002.
39. Emery VC, Atkins MC, Bowen EF, et al. Interactions between beta-herpesviruses and human immunodeficiency virus in vivo: evidence for increased human immunodeficiency viral load in the presence of human herpesvirus 6. J Med Virol 57:278, 1999.
40. Tanaka-Taya K, Kondo T, Nakagawa N, et al. Reactivation of human herpesvirus 6 by infection of human herpesvirus 7. J Med Virol 60:284, 2000.
41. Black JB, Sanderlin KC, Goldsmith CS, et al. Growth properties of human herpesvirus-6 strain Z29. J Virol Methods 26:133, 1989.
42. Kikuta H, Lu H, Tomizawa K, Matsumoto S. Enhancement of human herpesvirus 6 replication in adult human lymphocytes by monoclonal antibody to CD3. J Infect Dis 161:1085, 1990.
43. Ablashi DV, Balachandran N, Josephs SF, et al. Genomic polymorphism, growth properties, and immunologic variations in human herpesvirus-6 isolates. Virology 184:545, 1991.
44. Yadav M, Umamaheswari S, Ablashi DV. Low prevalence of antibody to human herpesvirus-6 (HHV-6) in Kadazans. Southeast Asian J Trop Med Public Health 21:259, 1990.
45. Farr TJ, Harnett GB, Pietroboni GR, Bucens MR. The distribution of antibodies to HHV-6 compared with other herpesviruses in young children. Epidemiol Infect 105:603, 1990.
46. Yoshikawa T, Suga S, Asano Y, et al. Distribution of antibodies to a causative agent of exanthem subitum (human herpesvirus-6) in healthy individuals. Pediatrics 84:675, 1989.
47. Knowles WA, Gardner SD. High prevalence of antibody to human herpesvirus-6 and seroconversion associated with rash in two infants. Lancet 2:912, 1988.
48. Leach CT, Sumaya CV, Brown NA. Human herpesvirus-6: clinical implications of a recently discovered, ubiquitous agent. J Pediatr 121:173, 1992.
49. Brown NA, Sumaya CV, Liu CR, et al. Fall in human herpesvirus 6 seropositivity with age. Lancet 2:396, 1988.
50. Harnett GB, Farr TJ, Pietroboni GR, Bucens MR. Frequent shedding of human herpesvirus 6 in saliva. J Med Virol 30:128, 1990.
51. Krueger GR, Wassermann K, De Clerck LS, et al. Latent herpesvirus-6 in salivary and bronchial glands. Lancet 336:1255, 1990.
52. Levy JA, Ferro F, Greenspan D, Lennette ET. Frequent isolation of HHV-6 from saliva and high seroprevalence of the virus in the population. Lancet 335:1047, 1990.
53. Fujiwara N, Namba H, Ohuchi R, et al. Monitoring of human herpesvirus-6 and -7 genomes in saliva samples of healthy adults by competitive quantitative PCR. J Med Virol 61:208, 2000.
54. Cone RW, Huang ML, Ashley R, Corey L. Human herpesvirus 6 DNA in peripheral blood cells and saliva from immunocompetent individuals. J Clin Microbiol 31:1262, 1993.
55. Aberle SW, Mandl CW, Kunz C, Popow-Kraupp T. Presence of human herpesvirus 6 variants A and B in saliva and peripheral blood mononuclear cells of healthy adults. J Clin Microbiol 34:3223, 1996.
56. Takahashi K, Sonoda S, Kawakami K, et al. Human herpesvirus 6 and exanthem subitum. Lancet 1:1463, 1988.
57. Dunne WM Jr, Demmler GJ. Serological evidence for congenital transmission of human herpesvirus 6. Lancet 340:121, 1992.
58. Hall CB, Long CE, Schnabel KC, et al. Human herpesvirus-6 infection in children. A prospective study of complications and reactivation. N Engl J Med 331:432, 1994.
59. Kositanont U, Wasi C, Wanprapar N, et al. Primary infection of human herpesvirus 6 in children with vertical infection of human immunodeficiency virus type 1. J Infect Dis 180:50, 1999.
60. Dahl H, Fjaertoft G, Norsted T, et al. Reactivation of human herpesvirus 6 during pregnancy. J Infect Dis 180:2035, 1999.
61. Jarrett RF, Clark DA, Josephs SF, Onions DE. Detection of human herpesvirus-6 DNA in peripheral blood and saliva. J Med Virol 32:73, 1990.
62. Yoshikawa T, Suzuki K, Ihira M, et al. Human herpesvirus 6 latently infects mononuclear cells but not liver tissue. J Clin Pathol 52:65, 1999.
63. Kondo K, Kondo T, Okuno T, et al. Latent human herpesvirus 6 infection of human monocytes/macrophages. J Gen Virol 72:1401, 1991.
64. Luppi M, Barozzi P, Morris C, et al. Human herpesvirus 6 latently infects early bone marrow progenitors in vivo. J Virol 73:754, 1999.
65. Asano Y, Yoshikawa T, Suga S, et al. Viremia and neutralizing antibody response in infants with exanthem subitum. J Pediatr 114:535, 1989.
66. Suga S, Yoshikawa T, Asano Y, et al. IgM neutralizing antibody responses to human herpesvirus-6 in patients with exanthem subitum or organ transplantation. Microbiol Immunol 36:495, 1992.
67. Ueda K, Kusuhara K, Hirose M, et al. Exanthem subitum and antibody to human herpesvirus-6. J Infect Dis 159:750, 1989.
68. Yakushijin Y, Yasukawa M, Kobayashi Y. T-cell immune response to human herpesvirus-6 in healthy adults. Microbiol Immunol 35:655, 1991.
69. Yasukawa M, Yakushijin Y, Furukawa M, Fujita S. Specificity analysis of human CD4+ T-cell clones directed against human herpesvirus 6 (HHV-6), HHV-7, and human cytomegalovirus. J Virol 67:6259, 1993.
70. Singh N, Carrigan DR. Human herpesvirus-6 in transplantation: an emerging pathogen. Ann Intern Med 124:1065, 1996.
71. Kimberlin DW, Whitley RJ. Human herpesvirus-6: neurologic implications of a newly-described viral pathogen. J Neurovirol 4:474, 1998.

72. Chan PK, Ng HK, Hui M, et al. Presence of human herpesviruses 6, 7, and 8 DNA sequences in normal brain tissue. J Med Virol 59:491, 1999.
73. Yoshikawa T, Ihira M, Suzuki K, et al. Invasion by human herpesvirus 6 and human herpesvirus 7 of the central nervous system in patients with neurological signs and symptoms. Arch Dis Child 83:170, 2000.
74. Lusso P, Ensoli B, Markham PD, et al. Productive dual infection of human CD4+ T lymphocytes by HIV-1 and HHV-6. Nature 337:370, 1989.
75. Knox KK, Carrigan DR. Active HHV-6 infection in the lymph nodes of HIV-infected patients: in vitro evidence that HHV-6 can break HIV latency. J Acquir Immune Defic Syndr Hum Retrovirol 11:370, 1996.
76. Ensoli B, Lusso P, Schachter F, et al. Human herpes virus-6 increases HIV-1 expression in co-infected T cells via nuclear factors binding to the HIV-1 enhancer. EMBO J 8:3019, 1989.
77. Levy JA, Landay A, Lennette ET. Human herpesvirus 6 inhibits human immunodeficiency virus type 1 replication in cell culture. J Clin Microbiol 28:2362, 1990.
78. Asada H, Klaus-Kovtun V, Golding H, et al. Human herpesvirus 6 infects dendritic cells and suppresses human immunodeficiency virus type 1 replication in coinfected cultures. J Virol 73:4019, 1999.
79. Bonura F, Perna AM, Vitale F, et al. Inhibition of human immunodeficiency virus 1 (HIV-1) by variant B of human herpesvirus 6 (HHV-6). New Microbiol 22:161, 1999.
80. Pietroboni GR, Harnett GB, Farr TJ, Bucens MR. Human herpes virus type 6 (HHV-6) and its in vitro effect on human immunodeficiency virus (HIV). J Clin Pathol 41:1310, 1988.
81. Di Luca D, Secchiero P, Bovenzi P, et al. Reciprocal in vitro interactions between human herpesvirus-6 and HIV-1 Tat. AIDS 5:1095, 1991.
82. Garzino-Demo A, Chen M, Lusso P, et al. Enhancement of TAT-induced transactivation of the HIV-1 LTR by two genomic fragments of HHV-6. J Med Virol 50:20, 1996.
83. Lusso P, Malnati MS, Garzino-Demo A, et al. Infection of natural killer cells by human herpesvirus 6. Nature 362:458, 1993.
84. Lusso P, De Maria A, Malnati M, et al. Induction of CD4 and susceptibility to HIV-1 infection in human CD8+ T lymphocytes by human herpesvirus 6. Nature 349:533, 1991.
85. Schonnebeck M, Krueger GR, Braun M, et al. Human herpesvirus-6 infection may predispose cells to superinfection by other viruses. In Vivo 5:255, 1991.
86. Mayne M, Cheadle C, Soldan SS, et al. Gene expression profile of herpesvirus-infected T cells obtained using immunomicroarrays: induction of proinflammatory mechanisms. J Virol 75:11641, 2001.
87. Vignoli M, Furlini G, Re MC, et al. Modulation of CD4, CXCR-4, and CCR-5 makes human hematopoietic progenitor cell lines infected with human herpesvirus-6 susceptible to human immunodeficiency virus type 1. J Hematother Stem Cell Res 9:39, 2000.
88. Lusso P, Garzino-Demo A, Crowley RW, Malnati MS. Infection of gamma/delta T lymphocytes by human herpesvirus 6: transcriptional induction of CD4 and susceptibility to HIV infection. J Exp Med 181:1303, 1995.
89. Grivel JC, Santoro F, Chen S, et al. Pathogenic effects of human herpesvirus 6 in human lymphoid tissue ex vivo. J Virol 77:8280, 2003.
90. Flamand L, Romerio F, Reitz MS, Gallo RC. CD4 promoter transactivation by human herpesvirus 6. J Virol 72:8797, 1998.
91. Hasegawa A, Yasukawa M, Sakai I, Fujita S. Transcriptional down-regulation of CXC chemokine receptor 4 induced by impaired association of transcription regulator YY1 with c-Myc in human herpesvirus 6-infected cells. J Immunol 166:1125, 2001.
92. Grivel JC, Ito Y, Faga G, et al. Suppression of CCR5- but not CXCR4-tropic HIV-1 in lymphoid tissue by human herpesvirus 6. Nat Med 7:1232, 2001.
93. Caruso A, Favilli F, Rotola A, et al. Human herpesvirus-6 modulates RANTES production in primary human endothelial cell cultures. J Med Virol 70:451, 2003.
94. Horvat RT, Wood C, Balachandran N. Transactivation of human immunodeficiency virus promoter by human herpesvirus 6. J Virol 63:970, 1989.
95. Horvat RT, Wood C, Josephs SF, Balachandran N. Transactivation of the human immunodeficiency virus promoter by human herpesvirus 6 (HHV-6) strains GS and Z-29 in primary human T lymphocytes and identification of transactivating HHV-6(GS) gene fragments. J Virol 65:2895, 1991.
96. Martin ME, Nicholas J, Thomson BJ, et al. Identification of a transactivating function mapping to the putative immediate-early locus of human herpesvirus 6. J Virol 65:5381, 1991.
97. Geng YQ, Chandran B, Josephs SF, Wood C. Identification and characterization of a human herpesvirus 6 gene segment that trans activates the human immunodeficiency virus type 1 promoter. J Virol 66:1564, 1992.
98. Kashanchi F, Thompson J, Sadaie MR, et al. Transcriptional activation of minimal HIV-1 promoter by ORF-1 protein expressed from the SalI-L fragment of human herpesvirus 6. Virology 201:95, 1994.
99. Nicholas J, Martin ME. Nucleotide sequence analysis of a 38.5-kilobase-pair region of the genome of human herpesvirus 6 encoding human cytomegalovirus immediate-early gene homologs and transactivating functions. J Virol 68:597, 1994.
100. Thompson J, Choudhury S, Kashanchi F, et al. A transforming fragment within the direct repeat region of human herpesvirus type 6 that transactivates HIV-1. Oncogene 9:1167, 1994.
101. Thomson BJ, Weindler FW, Gray D, et al. Human herpesvirus 6 (HHV-6) is a helper virus for adeno-associated virus type 2 (AAV-2) and the AAV-2 rep gene homologue in HHV-6 can mediate AAV-2 DNA replication and regulate gene expression. Virology 204:304, 1994.
102. Wang J, Jones C, Norcross M, et al. Identification and characterization of a human herpesvirus 6 gene segment capable of transactivating the human immunodeficiency virus type 1 long terminal repeat in an Sp1 binding site-dependent manner. J Virol 68:1706, 1994.
103. Zhou Y, Chang CK, Qian G, et al. trans-activation of the HIV promoter by a cDNA and its genomic clones of human herpesvirus-6. Virology 199:311, 1994.
104. McCarthy M, Auger D, He J, Wood C. Cytomegalovirus and human herpesvirus-6 trans-activate the HIV-1 long terminal repeat via multiple response regions in human fetal astrocytes. J Neurovirol 4:495, 1998.
105. Chen H, Pesce AM, Carbonari M, et al. Absence of antibodies to human herpesvirus-6 in patients with slowly-progressive human immunodeficiency virus type 1 infection. Eur J Epidemiol 8:217, 1992.
106. Fairfax MR, Schacker T, Cone RW, et al. Human herpesvirus 6 DNA in blood cells of human immunodeficiency virus-infected men: correlation of high levels with high CD4 cell counts. J Infect Dis 169:1342, 1994.
107. Fabio G, Knight SN, Kidd IM, et al. Prospective study of human herpesvirus 6, human herpesvirus 7, and cytomegalovirus infections in human immunodeficiency virus-positive patients. J Clin Microbiol 35:2657, 1997.
108. Blazquez MV, Madueno JA, Jurado R, et al. Human herpesvirus-6 and the course of human immunodeficiency virus infection. J Acquir Immune Defic Syndr Hum Retrovirol 9:389, 1995.

109. Iuliano R, Trovato R, Lico S, et al. Human herpesvirus-6 reactivation in a longitudinal study of two HIV-1 infected patients. J Med Virol 51:259, 1997.
110. Madea B, Roewert HJ, Krueger GR, et al. Search for early lesions following human immunodeficiency virus type 1 infection. A study of six individuals who died a violent death after seroconversion. Arch Pathol Lab Med 114:379, 1990.
111. Corbellino M, Lusso P, Gallo RC, et al. Disseminated human herpesvirus 6 infection in AIDS. Lancet 342:1242, 1993.
112. Knox KK, Carrigan DR. Disseminated active HHV-6 infections in patients with AIDS. Lancet 343:577, 1994.
113. Clark DA, Ait-Khaled M, Wheeler AC, et al. Quantification of human herpesvirus 6 in immunocompetent persons and post-mortem tissues from AIDS patients by PCR. J Gen Virol 77:2271, 1996.
114. Gautheret A, Monfort. L, Poirel L, et al. Human cytomegalovirus, human herpesvirus-6 and human herpesvirus-7 DNA in colonic mucosa from HIV-seropositive patients with diarrhea. XI International Conference on AIDS, Vancouver, Canada, 1996.
115. Nigro G, Luzi G, Krzysztofiak A, et al. Detection of IgM antibodies to human herpesvirus 6 in Romanian children with nonprogressive human immunodeficiency virus disease. Pediatr Infect Dis J 14:891, 1995.
116. Portolani M, Fabio G, Pecorari M, et al. Search for human herpesvirus 6 and human cytomegalovirus in bronchoalveolar lavage from patients with human immunodeficiency virus-1 and respiratory disorders. J Med Virol 48:179, 1996.
117. Hammerling JA, Lambrecht RS, Kehl KS, Carrigan DR. Prevalence of human herpesvirus 6 in lung tissue from children with pneumonitis. J Clin Pathol 49:802, 1996.
118. Reux I, Fillet AM, Agut H, et al. In situ detection of human herpesvirus 6 in retinitis associated with acquired immunodeficiency syndrome. Am J Ophthalmol 114:375, 1992.
119. Qavi HB, Green MT, SeGall GK, et al. Transcriptional activity of HIV-1 and HHV-6 in retinal lesions from AIDS patients. Invest Ophthalmol Vis Sci 33:2759, 1992.
120. Qavi HB, Green MT, Pearson G, Ablashi D. Possible role of HHV-6 in the development of AIDS retinitis. In Vivo 8:527, 1994.
121. Qavi HB, Green MT, Lewis DE, et al. HIV-1 and HHV-6 antigens and transcripts in retinas of patients with AIDS in the absence of human cytomegalovirus. Invest Ophthalmol Vis Sci 36:2040, 1995.
122. Fillet AM, Reux I, Joberty C, et al. Detection of human herpes virus 6 in AIDS-associated retinitis by means of in situ hybridization, polymerase chain reaction and immunohistochemistry. J Med Virol 49:289, 1996.
123. Qavi HB, Xu B, Green MT, et al. Morphological and ultrastructural changes induced in corneal epithelial cells by HIV-1 and HHV-6 in vitro. Curr Eye Res 15:597, 1996.
124. Quereda C, Corral I, Laguna F, et al. Diagnostic utility of a multiplex herpesvirus PCR assay performed with cerebrospinal fluid from human immunodeficiency virus-infected patients with neurological disorders. J Clin Microbiol 38:3061, 2000.
125. Bossolasco S, Marenzi R, Dahl H, et al. Human herpesvirus 6 in cerebrospinal fluid of patients infected with HIV: frequency and clinical significance. J Neurol Neurosurg Psychiatry 67:789, 1999.
126. Cinque P, Vago L, Dahl H, et al. Polymerase chain reaction on cerebrospinal fluid for diagnosis of virus-associated opportunistic diseases of the central nervous system in HIV-infected patients. AIDS 10:951, 1996.
127. Brown NA, Kovacs A, Lui CR, et al. Prevalence of antibody to human herpesvirus 6 among blood donors infected with HIV. Lancet 2:1146, 1988.
128. Essers S, Schwinn A, ter Meulen J, et al. Seroepidemiological correlations of antibodies to human herpesviruses and human immunodeficiency virus type 1 in African patients. Eur J Epidemiol 7:658, 1991.
129. Fox J, Briggs M, Tedder RS. Antibody to human herpesvirus 6 in HIV-1 positive and negative homosexual men. Lancet 2:396, 1988.
130. Spira TJ, Bozeman LH, Sanderlin KC, et al. Lack of correlation between human herpesvirus-6 infection and the course of human immunodeficiency virus infection. J Infect Dis 161:567, 1990.
131. Gautheret A, Aubin JT, Fauveau V, et al. Rate of detection of human herpesvirus-6 at different stages of HIV infection. Eur J Clin Microbiol Infect Dis 14:820, 1995.
132. Dorrucci M, Rezza G, Andreoni M, et al. Serum IgG antibodies to human herpesvirus-6 (HHV-6) do not predict the progression of HIV disease to AIDS. Eur J Epidemiol 15:317, 1999.
133. Gobbi A, Stoddart CA, Locatelli G, et al. Coinfection of SCID-hu Thy/Liv mice with human herpesvirus 6 and human immunodeficiency virus type 1. J Virol 74:8726, 2000.
134. Fox JD, Ward P, Briggs M, Irving W, Stammers TG, Tedder RS. Production of IgM antibody to HHV6 in reactivation and primary infection. Epidemiol Infect 104:289, 1990.
135. Ward KN, Gray JJ, Joslin ME, Sheldon MJ. Avidity of IgG antibodies to human herpesvirus-6 distinguishes primary from recurrent infection in organ transplant recipients and excludes cross-reactivity with other herpesviruses. J Med Virol 39:44, 1993.
136. Huang LM, Kuo PF, Lee CY, et al. Detection of human herpesvirus-6 DNA by polymerase chain reaction in serum or plasma. J Med Virol 38:7, 1992.
137. Secchiero P, Carrigan DR, Asano Y, et al. Detection of human herpesvirus 6 in plasma of children with primary infection and immunosuppressed patients by polymerase chain reaction. J Infect Dis 171:273, 1995.
138. Norton RA, Caserta MT, Hall CB, et al. Detection of human herpesvirus 6 by reverse transcription-PCR. J Clin Microbiol 37:3672, 1999.
139. Wang FZ, Dahl H, Linde A, et al. Lymphotropic herpesviruses in allogeneic bone marrow transplantation. Blood 88:3615, 1996.
140. Rapaport D, Engelhard D, Tagger G, et al. Antiviral prophylaxis may prevent human herpesvirus-6 reactivation in bone marrow transplant recipients. Transpl Infect Dis 4:10, 2002.
141. Tokimasa S, Hara J, Osugi Y, et al. Ganciclovir is effective for prophylaxis and treatment of human herpesvirus-6 in allogeneic stem cell transplantation. Bone Marrow Transplant 29:595, 2002.
142. Wang FZ, Linde A, Hagglund H, et al. Human herpesvirus 6 DNA in cerebrospinal fluid specimens from allogeneic bone marrow transplant patients: does it have clinical significance? Clin Infect Dis 28:562, 1999.
143. Agut H, Collandre H, Aubin JT, et al. In vitro sensitivity of human herpesvirus-6 to antiviral drugs. Res Virol 140:219, 1989.
144. Russler SK, Tapper MA, Carrigan DR. Susceptibility of human herpesvirus 6 to acyclovir and ganciclovir. Lancet 2:382, 1989.
145. Yoshida M, Yamada M, Chatterjee S, et al. A method for detection of HHV-6 antigens and its use for evaluating antiviral drugs. J Virol Methods 58:137, 1996.
146. Yoshida M, Yamada M, Tsukazaki T, et al. Comparison of antiviral compounds against human herpesvirus 6 and 7. Antiviral Res 40:73, 1998.
147. Burns WH, Sandford GR. Susceptibility of human herpesvirus 6 to antivirals in vitro. J Infect Dis 162:634, 1990.

148. Manichanh C, Grenot P, Gautheret-Dejean A, et al. Susceptibility of human herpesvirus 6 to antiviral compounds by flow cytometry analysis. Cytometry 40:135, 2000.
149. Amjad M, Gillespie MA, Carlson RM, Karim MR. Flow cytometric evaluation of antiviral agents against human herpesvirus 6. Microbiol Immunol 45:233, 2001.
150. De Bolle L, Manichanh C, Agut H, et al. Human herpesvirus 6 DNA polymerase: enzymatic parameters, sensitivity to ganciclovir and determination of the role of the A961V mutation in HHV-6 ganciclovir resistance. Antiviral Res 64:17, 2004.
151. Williams SL, Hartline CB, Kushner NL, et al. In vitro activities of benzimidazole D- and L-ribonucleosides against herpesviruses. Antimicrob Agents Chemother 47:2186, 2003.
152. Williams-Aziz SL, Hartline CB, Harden EA, et al. Comparative activities of lipid esters of cidofovir and cyclic cidofovir against replication of herpesviruses in vitro. Antimicrob Agents Chemother 49:3724, 2005.
153. Bethge W, Beck R, Jahn G, et al. Successful treatment of human herpesvirus-6 encephalitis after bone marrow transplantation. Bone Marrow Transplant 24:1245, 1999.
154. Johnston RE, Geretti AM, Prentice HG, et al. HHV-6-related secondary graft failure following allogeneic bone marrow transplantation. Br J Haematol 105:1041, 1999.
155. Mookerjee BP, Vogelsang G. Human herpes virus-6 encephalitis after bone marrow transplantation: successful treatment with ganciclovir. Bone Marrow Transplant 20:905, 1997.
156. Paterson DL, Singh N, Gayowski T, et al. Encephalopathy associated with human herpesvirus 6 in a liver transplant recipient. Liver Transplant Surg 5:454, 1999.
157. Rieux C, Gautheret-Dejean A, Challine-Lehmann D, et al. Human herpesvirus-6 meningoencephalitis in a recipient of an unrelated allogeneic bone marrow transplantation. Transplantation 65:1408, 1998.
158. Yoshida H, Matsunaga K, Ueda T, et al. Human herpesvirus 6 meningoencephalitis successfully treated with ganciclovir in a patient who underwent allogeneic bone marrow transplantation from an HLA-identical sibling. Int J Hematol 75:421, 2002.
159. Zerr DM, Gupta D, Huang ML, et al. Effect of antivirals on human herpesvirus 6 replication in hematopoietic stem cell transplant recipients. Clin Infect Dis 34:309, 2002.
160. Denes E, Magy L, Pradeau K, et al. Successful treatment of human herpesvirus 6 encephalomyelitis in immunocompetent patient. Emerg Infect Dis 10:729, 2004.
161. Manichanh C, Olivier-Aubron C, Lagarde JP, et al. Selection of the same mutation in the U69 protein kinase gene of human herpesvirus-6 after prolonged exposure to ganciclovir in vitro and in vivo. J Gen Virol 82:2767, 2001.
162. Safronetz D, Petric M, Tellier R, et al. Mapping ganciclovir resistance in the human herpesvirus-6 U69 protein kinase. J Med Virol 71:434, 2003.
163. Lusso P, Secchiero P, Crowley RW, et al. CD4 is a critical component of the receptor for human herpesvirus 7: interference with human immunodeficiency virus. Proc Natl Acad Sci USA 91:3872, 1994.
164. Zhang Y, Hatse S, De Clercq E, Schols D. CXC-chemokine receptor 4 is not a coreceptor for human herpesvirus 7 entry into CD4(+) T cells. J Virol 74:2011, 2000.
165. Secchiero P, Zella D, Barabitskaja O, et al. Progressive and persistent downregulation of surface CXCR4 in CD4(+) T cells infected with human herpesvirus 7. Blood 92:4521, 1998.
166. Crowley RW, Secchiero P, Zella D, et al. Interference between human herpesvirus 7 and HIV-1 in mononuclear phagocytes. J Immunol 156:2004, 2004.
167. Katsafanas GC, Schirmer EC, Wyatt LS, Frenkel N. In vitro activation of human herpesviruses 6 and 7 from latency. Proc Natl Acad Sci USA 93:9788, 1996.
168. Torigoe S, Kumamoto T, Koide W, et al. Clinical manifestations associated with human herpesvirus 7 infection. Arch Dis Child 72:518, 1995.
169. Secchiero P, Berneman ZN, Gallo RC, Lusso P. Biological and molecular characteristics of human herpesvirus 7: in vitro growth optimization and development of a syncytia inhibition test. Virology 202:506, 1994.
170. Wilborn F, Schmidt CA, Lorenz F, et al. Human herpesvirus type 7 in blood donors: detection by the polymerase chain reaction. J Med Virol 47:65, 1995.
171. Di Luca D, Mirandola P, Ravaioli T, et al. Human herpesviruses 6 and 7 in salivary glands and shedding in saliva of healthy and human immunodeficiency virus positive individuals. J Med Virol 45:462, 1995.
172. Black JB, Pellett PE. Human herpesvirus 7. Rev Med Virol 9:245, 1999.
173. Tanaka K, Kondo T, Torigoe S, et al. Human herpesvirus 7: another causal agent for roseola (exanthem subitum). J Pediatr 125:1, 1994.
174. Kimberlin DW. Human herpesviruses 6 and 7: identification of newly recognized viral pathogens and their association with human disease. Pediatr Infect Dis J 17:59, 1998.
175. van den Berg JS, van Zeijl JH, Rotteveel JJ, et al. Neuroinvasion by human herpesvirus type 7 in a case of exanthem subitum with severe neurologic manifestations. Neurology 52:1077, 1999.
176. Caserta M, Hall CB, Schnabel K, D'Heron N. Human herpesvirus-7 (HHV-7) infection in U.S. children. Pediatr Res 39:168A, 1996.
177. Kempf W, Muller B, Maurer R, et al. Increased expression of human herpesvirus 7 in lymphoid organs of AIDS patients. J Clin Virol 16:193, 2000.
178. Boutolleau D, Bonduelle O, Sabard A, et al. Detection of human herpesvirus 7 DNA in peripheral blood reflects mainly CD4+ cell count in patients infected with HIV. J Med Virol 76:223, 2005.
179. Zhang Y, Schols D, De Clercq E. Selective activity of various antiviral compounds against HHV-7 infection. Antiviral Res 43:23, 1999.
180. Brennan DC, Storch GA, Singer GG, et al. The prevalence of human herpesvirus-7 in renal transplant recipients is unaffected by oral or intravenous ganciclovir. J Infect Dis 181:1557, 2000.

Chapter 53

International Parasitic Infections

Matthew B. Laurens, MD, MPH, Roberto Badaró, MD, PhD, Sanjay Mehta, MD, Constance A. Benson, MD, Miriam K. Laufer, MD, MPH

INTRODUCTION

HIV and parasitic infections share a common geographic distribution in many tropical areas where the burden of disease is greatest. All the organisms discussed in this section can act as pathogens in immuncompetent as well as immunocompromised hosts. The effect of HIV-associated immunosuppression on tropical parasitic infections does not follow a uniform pattern. HIV co-infection influences the clinical presentation, accuracy of diagnosis, and response to therapy, but the extent of the interactions varies by pathogen.

The diagnosis and therapy of parasitic disease in patients with HIV infection presents specific challenges that apply to most infections. The clinical presentation may overlap with other opportunistic infections, making diagnosis difficult, especially in regions of scarce medical resources. Serologic tests decrease in sensitivity and specificity with HIV progression. In addition, there is concern about the interaction between antiparasitic agents and antiretroviral therapy. The latter issue has not yet been sufficiently explored as the widespread availability of antiretroviral therapy where tropical parasitic diseases are common represents a relatively recent phenomenon.

Some of the common parasitic diseases found in those living with HIV are covered in other chapters, including toxoplasmosis (Chapter 37), cryptosporidia, isospora, cyclospora infections (Chapter 38), and microsporidiosis (Chapter 39). This chapter will focus on those parasitic infections not usually acquired in the United States or Western Europe where differences in epidemiology, clinical manifestations, pathology, therapy, or prognosis in HIV-positive populations have been established. These diseases include Chagas' disease, leishmaniasis, malaria, and schistosomiasis.

CHAGAS' DISEASE (*TRYPANOSOMA CRUZI* INFECTION)

Trypanosoma cruzi, causative agent of Chagas' disease, is the third most common parasitic infection in humans, after malaria and schistosomiasis. It is found throughout South America and is transmitted by the reduviid bug and less frequently by blood transfusion or organ transplantation.[1,2] In the immunocompetent host, primary infection is associated with nonspecific illness. In less than 5% of infected individuals, chronic disease develops in the myocardium, colon, or esophagus, causing cardiomyopathy or a megasyndrome. More commonly, the parasite remains in the host in an indeterminate phase that is clinically undetectable.

Clinical Presentation

During immunosuppression, *T. cruzi* infection in the indeterminate phase may reactivate as the parasites replicate within the host and cause end-organ disease. In people living with HIV infection, this usually occurs when CD4+ T-lymphocyte counts fall below 200–300 cells/mm^3. The most common site of reactivation for HIV-infected patients is the central nervous system (CNS); patients present with a meningoencephalitis syndrome.[3–10] Trypanosome invasion of the brain forms chagoma masses, causing patients to present with headache, fever, cognitive changes, and seizures. Focal neurological impairments resulting from chagomas include tremors, hemiparesis, cranial nerve abnormalities, and aphasia.[11]

After the central nervous system, the second site most commonly affected during reactivation is the heart.[12] Cardiac reactivation manifests as acute myocarditis or cardiomyopathy. In patients who already have cardiac damage due to chronic infection, reactivation can lead to

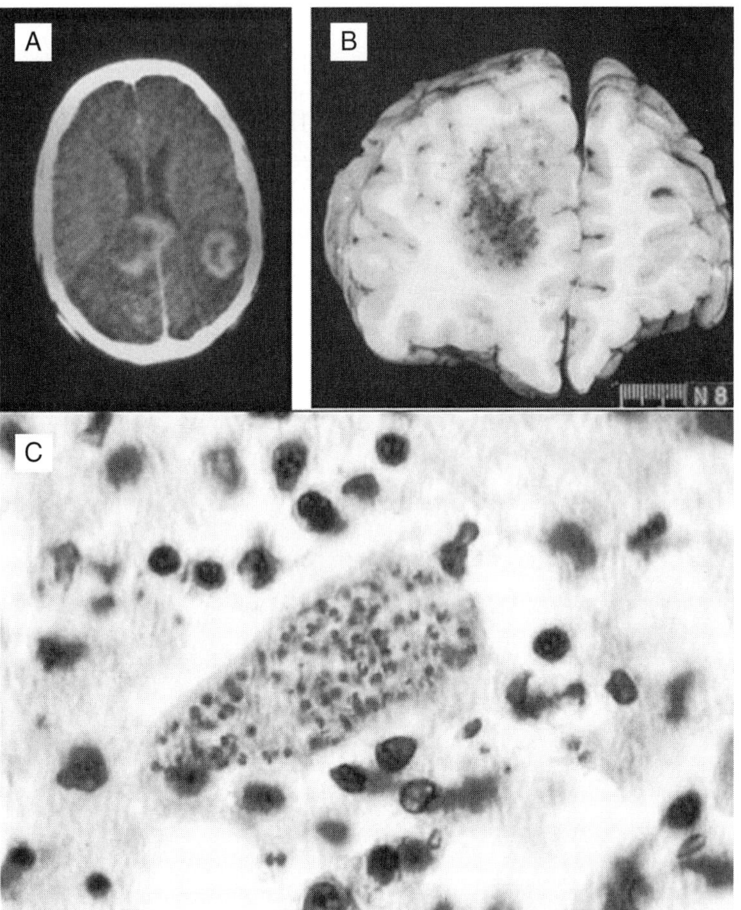

Figure 53-1 ■ Central nervous system Chagas' disease in a patient. **(A)** CT scan showing large ring enhancing mass lesion. **(B)** Coronal section of brain of same patient showing lesion with old hemorrhage within the white matter. **(C)** Hematoxylin and eosin stain of brain biopsy from the same patient showing many amastigotes residing within a glial cell.

Photograph provided by Dr Roberto Badaró, Dr Anastacio Queiroz de Souza, and Dr Marcelo Ferreira Federal University of Bahia, Salvador, Brazil.

new, acute inflammation or worsening congestive heart failure.[13,14] Signs and symptoms of systemic infection may also be present. Reactivation of cardiac disease may occur with or without neurological disease.

Histopathologically, microglial nodules and multifocal gliosis with nests of amastigotes can be seen in brain tissue (Fig. 53-1). Cardiac involvement may manifest as a mild inflammatory reaction with focal, intrafascicular or endomysial infiltrates, and amastigotes with localized or diffuse inflammation can also be demonstrated in the bridging fibrous fascicles from endocardial and epicardial tissue (Fig. 53-2).

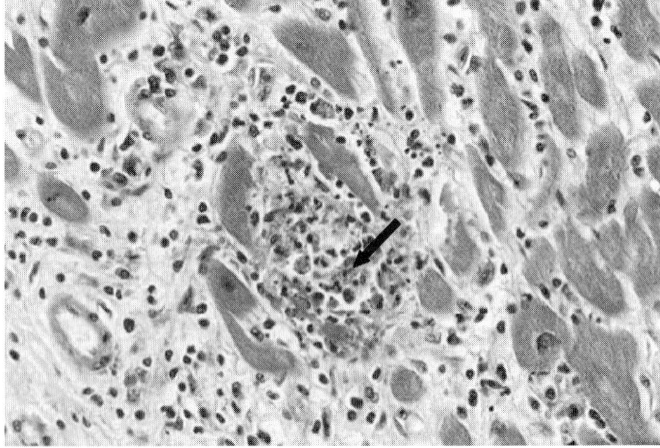

Figure 53-2 ■ Photograph of heart muscle biopsy in a patient with advanced Chagas' disease and myocarditis. Inflammatory cells can be seen infiltrating the muscle. Black arrow is directed at the intracellular amastigote form of *Trypanosoma cruzi*.

Photograph provided by Dr Roberto Badaró, Dr Anastacio Queiroz de Souza, and Dr Marcelo Ferreira Federal University of Bahia, Salvador, Brazil.

Diagnosis

Definitive diagnosis of *T. cruzi* requires demonstration of the organisms. Microscopy of blood smears is most useful during the acute stage and in symptomatic reactivation of chronic infection, when large numbers of parasites circulate in the bloodstream. In a phase contrast microscope, the motility of live trypomastigotes can easily be seen on a wet mount. In addition to Giemsa-stained blood smears, parasites may also be visualized in lymph nodes, bone marrow, pericardial fluid, intestinal mucosa, cerebrospinal fluid, and CNS mass lesions (Fig. 53-3). Certain microbiological tests, such as xenodiagnosis (recovering the parasite after inoculation of laboratory-raised insect vectors) or blood culture in liquid medium are more sensitive than direct visualization methods, but may take 2–8 weeks to become positive and are available only in highly specialized research settings.[15] When reactivation is suspected, patients may require therapy while awaiting the

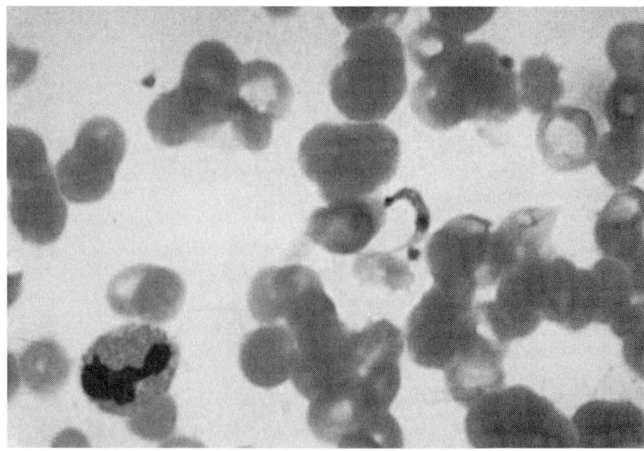
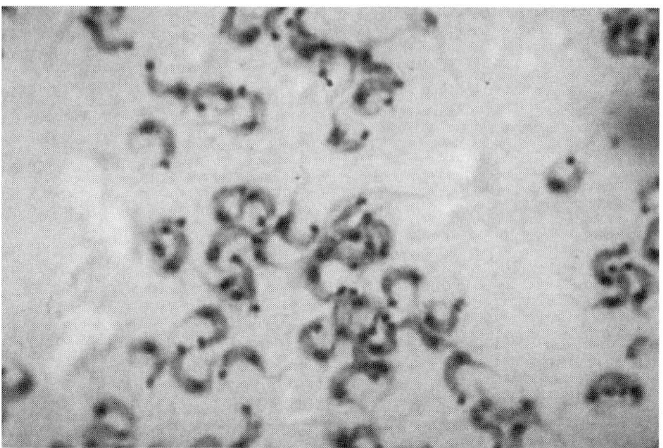

Figure 53-3 ■ Diagnosis of *Trypansoma cruzi* infection from clinical specimens. **(A)** Photograph of a blood smear revealing the trypomastigote form of *Trypansoma cruzi*. **(B)** Photograph of cerebrospinal fluid from a patient with CNS disease.

Photographs provided by Dr Roberto Badaró, Dr Anastacio Queiroz de Souza, and Dr Marcelo Ferreira Federal University of Bahia, Salvador, Brazil.

results of definitive testing. Because of their increased sensitivity, these tests are most useful in the chronic stages of *T. cruzi* infection, when the level of parasitemia is low, and in detection of indeterminate infection. Polymerase chain reaction (PCR) of blood also has been shown to be an extremely sensitive method to detect trypanosomes in the blood but it is not yet available in most clinical facilities.[16,17]

Serological tests to detect IgG antibody responses to *T. cruzi* are useful for diagnosis of chronically infected patients, to screen blood donors, and for seroepidemiological studies. IgM detection does not differentiate exposure from infection, and both IgM and IgG may be absent in HIV patients with trypanosomiasis.[18,19] Multiple tests are available in endemic areas and several ELISA-based tests can be found in the United States. In the absence of therapy, the IgG remains positive for life, although the level may fall below the threshold of detection in advanced HIV disease. For this reason, the diagnosis of Chagas' disease should not be discarded based on negative serological tests if the patient comes from an endemic region and has clinical findings compatible with Chagas' disease. In such cases, direct parasitological testing (e.g., microscopic examination of blood or CSF for trypomastigotes) is the best diagnostic strategy.

In cases of CNS reactivation, the cerebrospinal fluid (CSF) profile is consistent with encephalitis. Typically, there is a mild pleocytosis (<100 cells/mL) with lymphocyte predominance. CSF protein levels are also elevated. Microscopy may also be employed to screen the CSF in patients with suspected CNS Chagas' disease.

Chagas' disease shares a similar presentation to toxoplasmosis when it presents in the CNS, making this differentiation difficult. Chagomas have a predilection for subcortical white matter, with occasional gray matter involvement. The infection tends to cause extensive, diffuse hemorrhage.[20] In contrast, cerebral toxoplasmosis is usually found in the cerebral cortex and basal ganglia.[18,21] The differential diagnosis in endemic areas includes other entities such as lymphoma, bacterial abscesses, and tuberculosis. PCR plus microscopy of CSF or brain biopsy is often necessary to establish the etiology unequivocally.

Treatment

The two effective treatment regimens of Chagas' disease is indicated during acute infection and in the case of reactivation. Although the role of therapy during the chronic or indeterminate phase is unclear, treatment is often recommended in cases of infection of less than 10 years' duration and without overt cardiomyopathy, megacolon, or megaesophagus.[22] Treatment under these conditions is administered in the hope of limiting progression to end-organ damage. The two effective treatment regimens are nifurtimox (8–10 mg kg^{-1} day^{-1} divided three times per day) for 90–120 days or benznidazole (5–7 mg kg^{-1} day^{-1} in two divided doses) for 30–90 days. Children 1–10 years of age require 15–20 mg kg^{-1} day^{-1} and 12–16 year olds should be given 12.5–15 mg kg^{-1} day^{-1}, divided in four doses. The pediatric dose of benznidazole is 10 mg kg^{-1} day^{-1} in two doses. Common side effects of benzidazole include hypersensitivity, bone marrow depression, and peripheral neuropathy, and may require suspension of treatment with benznidazole. Weight loss, GI distress, and psychiatric disturbance may result from treatment with nifurtimox.[23] No interaction between antitrypanosomal drugs and antiretroviral drugs has been reported. Availability of these drugs varies by country. Only nifurtimox, produced by Bayer in Germany, is available in the United States. This drug can be obtained from the Centers for Disease Control and Prevention (CDC) Drug Service. Benznidazole is produced in Brazil by Roche.

Therapy of reactivation disease is considered successful if there is resolution of parasitemia or parasitic tissue infection. With successful treatment, the IgG can become negative, but seroconversion may not be a reliable indicator of cure: in the presence of HIV co-infection antibody may decrease over time despite persistence of active infection. People living with HIV may be at risk for incomplete cure and recurrent reactivation disease. Although no studies have investigated secondary prophylaxis rigorously, it is standard practice in Brazil to administer secondary prophylaxis after reactivation disease with benznidazole at 5 mg kg^{-1} day^{-1} three times per week for life. Benznidazole is highly toxic and difficult to tolerate for long-term administration. Other alternatives include allopurinol or triazole derivatives, although their efficacy has not been documented.[11,12] A proposed algorithm for the diagnosis and treatment of Chagas' disease is shown in Figure 53-4.

Primary prophylaxis for Chagas' disease is not utilized: the efficacy of such prophylaxis is unknown, and there is no convenient and well-tolerated agent that is likely to be effective.[18]

Prognosis

Even with therapy, people with HIV co-infection and CNS reactivation rarely survive beyond 3 months. In small case series, outcomes appear to be improved with treatment early in the course of the disease.[12] In Brazil, Chagas' disease was added to the list of AIDS-defining illnesses in 2004.[10] Antiretroviral therapy in addition to antitrypanosomal agents may improve the outcomes of chagasic meningoencephalitis and reactivation cardiac disease and should be utilized. There are no reports yet of related immune reconstitution syndromes.

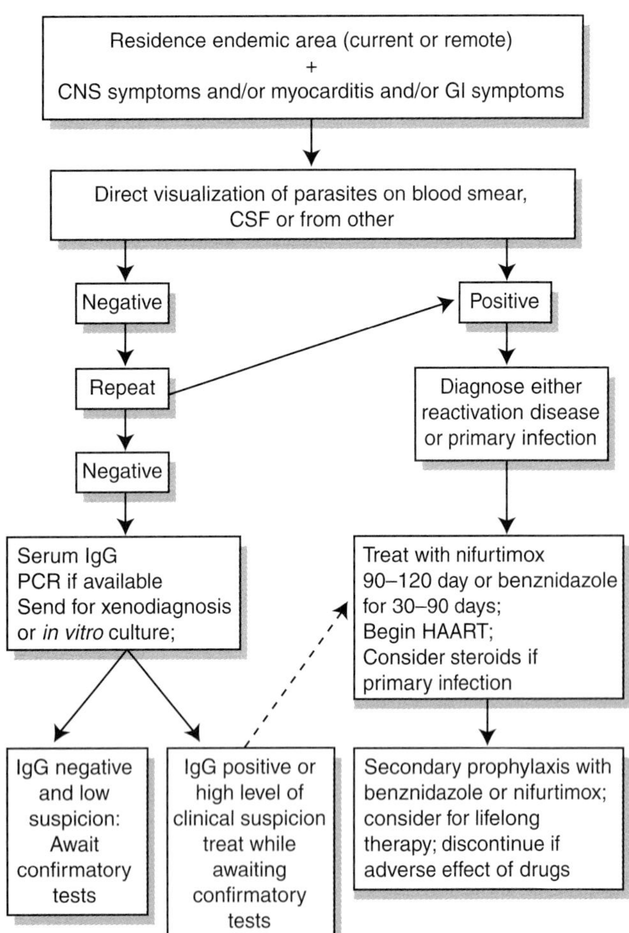

Figure 53-4 ■ Algorithm for diagnosis of management of trypanosomiasis in HIV-infected individuals.

LEISHMANIASIS

Leishmania species are obligate intracellular parasites that cause a broad spectrum of clinical disease in man that can generally be classified as visceral, mucosal, or cutaneous leishmaniasis. Visceral leishmaniasis (VL) is caused by *L. infantum* (in Europe, the Middle East, and Africa), *L. donovani* (in Asia) or *L. chagasi* (in South America) and is the clinical form that has the strongest interaction with HIV co-infection. It is spread by insect vectors and via blood, usually due to needle sharing among intravenous drug users.[24,25] Asymptomatic infection is very common and the incubation period from initial disease to infection is 2–6 months or longer. A minority of immunocompetent patients with subclinical infection progress to develop symptomatic disease. In contrast, symptomatic disease is frequent when severely immunosuppressed patients become infected. The interaction between HIV and Leishmania has been best described in Europe where diagnostic resources are available. In the other regions where HIV and Leishmania coexist, notably Brazil and east Africa, less data are available.[26]

Clinical Presentation

With HIV-associated immunosuppression, exposed individuals progress to VL more frequently than immunocompetent hosts. HIV-infected patients may present with unusual manifestations. HIV co-infection increases the risk of VL 100- to 1000-fold in endemic areas of Europe, where the disease is found predominantly in HIV-co-infected patients with CD4+ T-lymphocyte cell counts less than 200 cells/mm^3.[27,28] The triad of fever, hepatomegaly, and splenomegaly is the typical manifestation found in HIV-infected patients with CD4+ T-lymphocyte cell counts >50 cells/mm^3. Fever alone may be the presenting symptom of VL among patients with extremely low CD4+ T-lymphocyte cell counts. Anemia, thrombocytopenia, and leucopenia are common manifestations of symptomatic disease, even when the classic triad is absent.[29,30] Through uncontrolled hematogenous dissemination, the pathogens are able to infect atypical locations, leading to unusual clinical manifestations. Lesions have been documented to involve the gastrointestinal and respiratory tracts, peritoneum, pleura, eyes, skin, and tonsils.[29,31–33] Skin lesions of disseminated VL may mimic Kaposi sarcoma (Fig. 53-5).[34,35] Strains that only cause cutaneous infection in normal hosts may visceralize when HIV co-infection is present.[36]

Although VL is not an AIDS-defining illness, symptomatic disease usually occurs in patients with very low CD4+ T-lymphocyte counts. The presentation of leishmaniasis often coincides with other opportunistic infections, and thus clinicians should consider the possibility that VL is not the only process responsible for a complex clinical syndrome.[27]

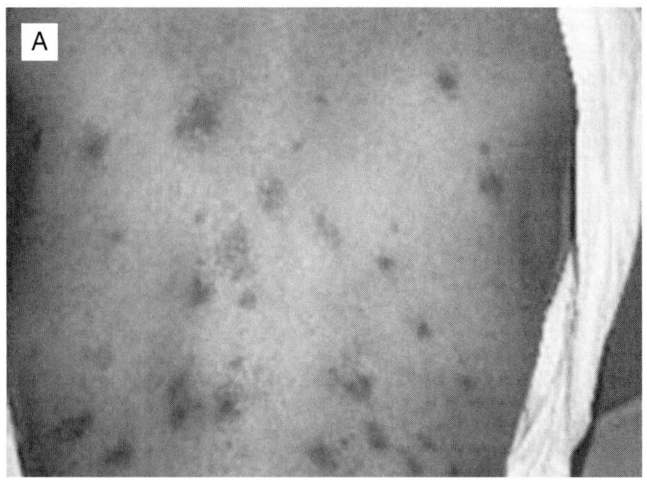

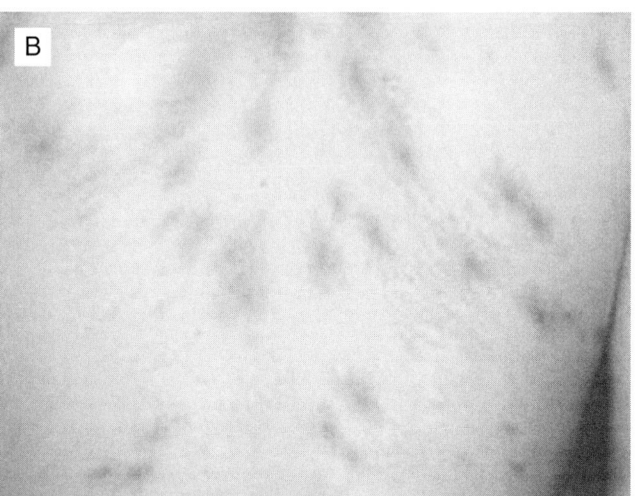

Figure 53-5 ■ Photographs of patients with HIV and Leishmania co-infection. **(A)** Photograph of a patient with HIV and visceral leishmaniasis with unusual skin manifestations mimicking Kaposi sarcoma. **(B)** Photograph of a patient with HIV who developed PKDL.

Photographs provided by Dr Roberto Badaró, Dr Anastacio Queiroz de Souza, and Dr Marcelo Ferreira Federal University of Bahia, Salvador, Brazil.

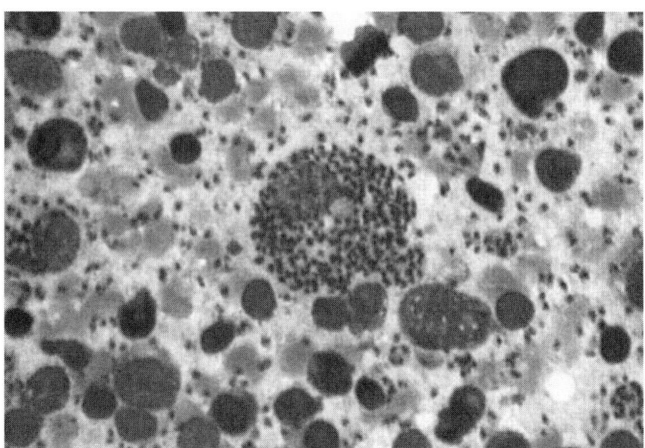

Figure 53-6 ■ Photograph of a splenic aspirate of a HIV- and Leishmania-co-infected patient stained with Giemsa showing the heavy burden of parasites within a single macrophage, and in the surrounding tissue.

Photograph provided by Dr Roberto Badaró, Dr Anastacio Queiroz de Souza, and Dr Marcelo Ferreira Federal University of Bahia, Salvador, Brazil.

In studies from Europe, when the diagnosis of VL was made, 42–68% of patients had additional concurrent opportunistic infections.[28]

Diagnosis

The gold standard for diagnosis of leishmaniasis is the demonstration of amastigotes on bone marrow, liver, or spleen biopsy (Fig. 53-6). Where possible, bone marrow aspirate is preferred over spleen aspirate for safety concerns. Specimens from individuals with low CD4+ T-lymphocyte cell counts are more frequently positive by this method compared to patients with higher CD4+ T-lymphocyte cell counts due to the higher parasite burden.[29] With advanced HIV disease, hypocellular bone marrow may make the diagnosis more difficult since these organisms are found intracellularly. PCR tests of blood can also be useful although these tests are not standardized for sensitivity or specificity.[37,38] PCR can also be used to speciate the organism.[39] In individuals with low CD4+ T-lymphocyte cell counts, staining of the buffy coat of the blood or a blood culture with Leishmania-specific media (Schneiders or NNN media) may be used for diagnosis.[40,41] In cases of disseminated disease with infection in atypical locations, the organisms may only be visible at the sites of disseminated disease.[29]

The three main serological assays utilized for diagnosing leishmaniasis include the indirect immunoflourescent antibody test (IFAT), ELISA to detect antibodies to the cloned antigen rK39, and Western blot.[28] If the tissue diagnosis cannot be obtained, at least two different serological tests should be used in HIV-positive persons. Leishmanial antigens should be freshly prepared to increase sensitivity.[27] A summary of diagnostic methods for leishmaniasis in the presence of HIV co-infection is found in Table 53-1.

Treatment

The available therapies for VL include amphotericin B, the antimony compounds (sodium stibogluconate (SSG) and meglumine) and miltefosine. These drugs can be used either alone or in combination. The antimonials ($20\,\mathrm{mg\,kg^{-1}\,day^{-1}}$ IM or IV for 28 days) have been the standard treatment for leishmaniasis but they have lost their efficacy in some regions, notably in south Asia, due to the emergence of resistance.

In the HIV-co-infected population, drug-associated toxicities are severe and can be fatal. Where Leishmania retain

Table 53-1

Diagnostic methods for cases of *Leishmania*/HIV co-infection

Method	% Positive
Microscopic examination of bone marrow smear	86[27]
Microscopic examination of blood smear	45[27]
Microscopic examination of tissue smear (skin, GI tract, liver, spleen)	87[27]
Hemoculture using Schneider's or Novy–McNeal–Nicolle (NNN) media	72–87[40,52]
IFAT (indirect immunoflourescence antibody test)	11–58[27,40,99,100]
ELISA (anti-rK39)	22–60[27,99,100]
Western blot	71[27]

susceptibility to antimonials, these drugs are as effective as amphotericin B. In HIV-co-infected patients in Europe, cure rates were ~75% in both the meglumine arm and the amphotericin B arm in a study among subjects who were able to complete the full course of therapy. However, in a series of studies from Spain, 19/63 (30%) HIV-positive patients who were assigned to the meglumine arm were unable to complete therapy due to adverse side effects.[42,43] In Africa, the adverse reactions may be even more severe. In Ethiopia, SSG was associated with a 90% cure rate, but a 6% death rate in the first month of therapy among HIV-infected participants. In the miltefosine arm of this study, poorer efficacy was observed, yet only 1% died in the first month of therapy.[44] The higher risk of death is attributed to antimonial toxicity, although the precise causes of death were not identified. SSG is produced by GlaxoSmithKline and can be obtained in the United States through the CDC Drug Service. Meglumine is made by Aventis in France but is not available in the US.

The best-tolerated treatment option for HIV-positive individuals is the liposomal formulation of amphotericin B ($3\,mg\,kg^{-1}\,day^{-1}$).[42] Several dosing schedules have been shown to be effective including administration for 10 days or for 5 days followed by doses on day 14 and 21. It has minimal toxicity and is usually as effective as or more effective than other options. In Europe, where leishmaniasis occurs almost exclusively as a complication of immunosuppression, liposomal amphotericin B or amphotericin B lipid complex is the standard therapy. Amphotericin B lipid complex is licensed in the United States as first-line therapy for VL.

In resource-limited settings where leishmaniasis is endemic, antileishmanial drugs cannot be widely used due to prohibitively high costs and the requirement for intravenous administration. A new treatment option, miltefosine ($2.5\,mg\,kg^{-1}\,day^{-1}$ for 28 days) is an oral therapy for VL that is effective against organisms resistant to the antimony compounds. Miltefosine is effective in immunocompetent hosts,[45] but efficacy in HIV-co-infected hosts has not been well-documented. A small study in Ethiopia showed miltefosine to be less effective, although better tolerated, than the antimonial compounds in HIV-positive individuals.[44] In a review of the cases of compassionate use for HIV-infected individuals who had contraindications to amphotericin B or failed previous therapy, miltefosine was associated with a 41% cure rate. It was also well tolerated, with no dose-limiting side effects.[46] Other isolated case reports have demonstrated miltefosine efficacy with HIV co-infection either alone or in combination with other agents.[47,48] Miltefosine has significant reproductive toxicity. It cannot be used in pregnant women and women are recommended to use effective contraception during and for 2 months after therapy. It is produced by Zentaris in Germany and has been distributed in Europe on a compassionate use protocol, but is not currently available in the United States.

Prognosis

Regardless of the choice of therapy, the long-term outcomes of patients with VL and HIV co-infection are poor. When an effective drug is administered, the initial cure rate assessed after 4 weeks may be as high as 75% among co-infected patients who complete therapy.[42] However, relapse is frequent following treatment. VL that is initially cured may relapse in 60–90% of HIV-co-infected patients in the first year.[24,28,30] Relapses usually occur at the initial site of infection. Cutaneous disease after treatment of VL is a well-recognized but poorly understood phenomenon called post-kala-azar dermal leishmaniasis (PKDL), usually occurring several years after therapy (see Figure 53.5). In HIV-co-infected patients, PKDL may occur within months after treatment and can present with both visceral and cutaneous disease.[49,50]

During a relapse, amastigotes are more difficult to visualize than during the initial infection. Leishmania nucleic acid material can be detected in the blood for years after therapy and thus their detection via PCR has poor specificity for clinical relapse.[37,51] The preferred examination is a blood culture because a positive result during post-treatment follow-up is associated with a 76% risk of clinical relapse.[52]

Prophylaxis, best studied with liposomal amphotericin B but also possible with antimonials, decreases the relapse rate.[30,53] At this time, there is no consensus as to exactly which population should be targeted for secondary prophylaxis and for how long it should be administered. Some recommend prolonged prophylaxis until immune reconstitution has been achieved as marked by CD4+ T-lymphocyte count remaining above 200–350 cells/mm^3.[24,54]

Although it is not currently used in any HIV staging criteria, leishmaniasis is considered an indication to begin highly active antiretroviral therapy (HAART) because it is a marker of advanced HIV disease. Successful treatment of VL is associated with a decrease in HIV viral load,[55] but there is no evidence that this is associated with disease progression. Co-infected individuals are at risk for progression to death, but the presence of VL is not an independent risk factor for death among patients with AIDS.[56,57] The diagnosis and treatment algorithm for leishmaniasis is shown in Figure 53-7.

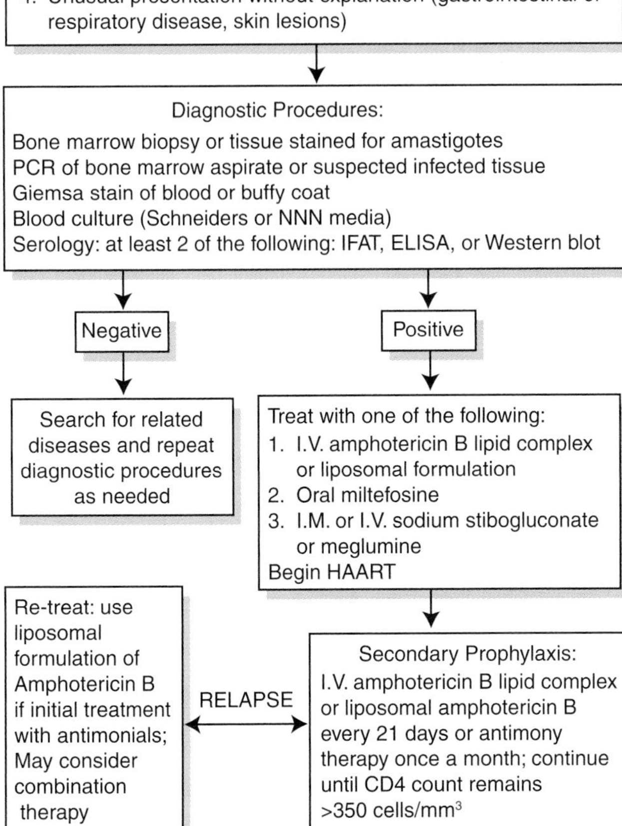

Figure 53-7 ■ Algorithm for diagnosis and management of leishmaniasis when suspected in HIV-infected individuals.

Prevention

Leishmaniasis can be prevented in the HIV-positive population through reduction of exposure and restoration of immune function among people in endemic areas infected with HIV. Needle exchange programs prevent the transmission of leishmaniasis in the intravenous drug user population and vector control decreases transmission from phlebotomine sand flies. Antiretroviral therapy prevents the transition from latent asymptomatic infection to clinical disease.[58] Increased availability of antiretroviral therapy has led to a decrease in disease burden of leishmaniasis in Europe.[59] A large cohort study in France examined the impact of combination antiretroviral therapy on the occurrence of VL and found that patients treated with HAART had a 59% reduction in the risk of developing active VL compared to patients who did not receive HAART.[60] Once clinical disease occurs, HAART does not improve the response to therapy. However, HAART did reduce the rate of relapse in Italy in one study from 64% (before HAART) to 36% (after HAART).[59] The ability of HAART to prevent relapse after appropriate therapy has not been confirmed in another European cohort.[61]

MALARIA

Four *Plasmodium* species; *falciparum, vivax, ovale*, and *malariae* cause human malaria. *P. falciparum* causes the most lethal form of the disease and is found in many regions of sub-Saharan Africa where HIV prevalence rates are high. *Falciparum* malaria is also found in southeast Asia, the Pacific, and South America. Malaria meets the definition of an opportunistic infection for patients with HIV infection; symptomatic disease occurs more commonly, and disease is more severe.

Clinical Presentation

In regions of high malaria transmission, children experience multiple malaria infections and eventually achieve a state of semi-immunity by late childhood: they may become infected with the parasite but the parasitemia is low and they are partially protected against disease. Because people usually acquire HIV infection in adulthood, the development of partial immunity typically occurs prior to any impairment of the immune system. Studies from Uganda and Malawi show that adults with HIV-associated immunosuppression in high transmission areas may be at slightly increased risk of developing clinical disease compared with HIV-negative or less immunocompromised groups.[62–64] However, these studies found no difference in severity of disease or mortality.

In the era before HAART became more widely available, very few data were available about the effect of HIV infection on the acquisition of immunity during childhood due to the poor survival of HIV-infected children. Now that antiretroviral programs in Africa include children, more information should become available in this population. Whether or not children treated with HAART will be able to develop partial immunity to malaria will be elucidated.

For pregnant women, HIV augments the severity of malaria. During pregnancy, even women who have acquired immunity become more vulnerable to malaria again. Parasites that infect the placenta express new antigens to which the primigravid woman's immune system has never been exposed. This leads to increased rates of parasitemia, symptomatic disease, and anemia. Placental malaria is also associated with adverse outcomes in the newborn, most notably intrauterine growth retardation.[65] In women with an intact immune system, this vulnerability decreases with subsequent pregnancies, due to acquisition of immunity to the placental form of the parasite.[66] Women with HIV infection who are pregnant for the first time have higher rates of parasitemia and malaria disease than those without HIV infection. With subsequent pregnancies, women with HIV have delayed acquisition of parity-specific immunity, such that their rate of decrease in susceptibility to malaria with subsequent pregnancies is slower than in pregnant women who are HIV uninfected.[67] The rate of adverse outcomes in newborns among mothers who had both HIV and malaria infection during pregnancy is higher than with either infection alone.[68]

The evidence is conflicting as to whether pregnancy increases the risk of maternal-to-child transmission of HIV.[69–72]

Among those with no preexisting immunity to malaria, HIV infection is associated with increased risk of severe disease and mortality. This has been demonstrated in South Africa, where residents became infected with malaria during rare outbreaks or travel to endemic neighboring countries. Adults with HIV infection are more likely to experience severe complications of malaria including acidosis, renal failure, anemia, and coma, than HIV-uninfected adults with malaria. The malaria case fatality rate is also significantly higher for patients with HIV infection compared with uninfected; 20% versus 4% in a rural health center[73] and 5% versus 0% in a large referral hospital.[74] HIV infection in children is associated with higher risk of hypoglycemia and coma during episodes of malaria. Although no studies have been conducted among HIV-infected travelers who become infected with malaria, it is expected that their clinical presentation would resemble the disease patterns described from this malaria-naive population.

Diagnosis

The definitive diagnosis of malaria infection is based on a thick and thin blood smear demonstrating malaria parasites. Thick smears are more sensitive than thin smears to detect low level parasitemia, but thin smears are used to identify the species. In patients with no preexisting immunity to malaria, infection almost always causes disease. In contrast, individuals with partial immunity to malaria may have infection without disease. In areas of high transmission, asymptomatic infection usually occurs with lower parasite density (e.g., $<3000/mm^3$).[62,64] However, there is no definitive test to distinguish asymptomatic parasitemia from clinical disease. A positive malaria smear should always be treated appropriately, as described below. For adults who are from endemic areas, it is important to continue to pursue other diagnoses, particularly HIV-associated opportunistic infections, even when the malaria smear is positive.

Therapy

The treatment of choice for uncomplicated malaria in Africa and Asia is artemisinin-based combination therapy such as artemether–lumefantrine, mefloquine–artesunate, or piperaquine–dihydroartemisinin. In developed countries, where these medications are often unavailable, recommended treatments are atovaquone–proguanil (four tablets of 250 mg atovaquone/100 mg proguanil per day for 3 days, taken with milk or a fatty meal) mefloquine for cases outside of Asia (750 mg PO followed by 500 mg PO 12 h later) or quinine (650 mg IV or PO every 8 h for 7 days) with doxycycline (100 mg PO twice a day) or clindamycin (20 mg/kg divided three times a day for 7 days). The World Health Organization (WHO) defines severe malaria and a malaria illness with one or more of the following clinical or laboratory criteria: impaired consciousness/coma, severe normocytic anemia, renal failure, pulmonary edema, acute respiratory distress syndrome, circulatory shock, disseminated intravascular coagulation, spontaneous bleeding, acidosis, hemoglobinuria, jaundice, repeated generalized convulsions or parasitemia >5%. For severe disease, parenteral quinine or artesunate should be administered, followed by oral medication after stabilization. In cases of severe disease, patients who are treated with quinidine gluconate should receive a loading dose of 10 mg/kg over 1–2 h. This loading dose should be decreased or omitted if the patient has already received quinine, quinidine, or mefloquine. If quinidine is not available, clinicians may contact the manufacturer (Eli Lilly 800-545-5979) or the CDC Malaria Hotline (770-488-7788). Intravenous artesunate is only available in the United States through the CDC. A proposed malaria treatment algorithm for *P. falciparum* is shown in Figure 53-8.

Cases of severe malaria require hospitalization, usually in an intensive care unit setting. Patients with uncomplicated malaria, especially with HIV infection, warrant hospitalization for directly observed therapy and monitoring of clinical response. Malaria-naive, HIV-positive patients are at high risk for severe disease and complications. The best route of drug administration has not been studied in this population. Because of the risks associated with intravenous quinidine administration, patients with uncomplicated disease can be treated with oral medication but closely monitored for signs and symptoms of severe disease. Any deterioration in the respiratory, metabolic, renal, or neurological status should prompt a change to intravenous medication and management as severe disease.

There is currently expanding interest in the interaction between antimalarial medications and antiretroviral therapy. While the potential for interactions exists, very few have been thoroughly explored.[75] Of special concern are the PIs and some NNRTIs that inhibit cytochrome P450 enzymes. PIs and nevirapine may slow the elimination of halofantrine and lumefantrine. Halofantrine has a narrow therapeutic window and an increased concentration may lead to prolonged *Q-T* intervals. Lumefantrine does not have this toxicity, however it may be prudent to avoid lumenfantrine administration in patients on PI or nevirapine-containing regimens. Ritonavir or boosted PI regimens may interfere with the elimination of quinine and quinidine, leading to increased risk of cardiac toxicity. If possible, quinine and quinidine should be avoided in patients also receiving ritonavir. If no alternative is available, patients on ritonavir therapy who are administered quinine require intensive care unit monitoring for cardiac arrhythmias associated with quinine toxicity.

Prognosis

The response to antimalarial therapy is not affected by HIV status or CD4+ T-lymphocyte count in studies conducted in areas of high malaria transmission.[76,77] HIV-infected and malaria-experienced patients with acute malaria can be treated using standard procedures that apply to the general population. Because they are at higher risk for severe disease and death, patients with HIV infection and acute malaria

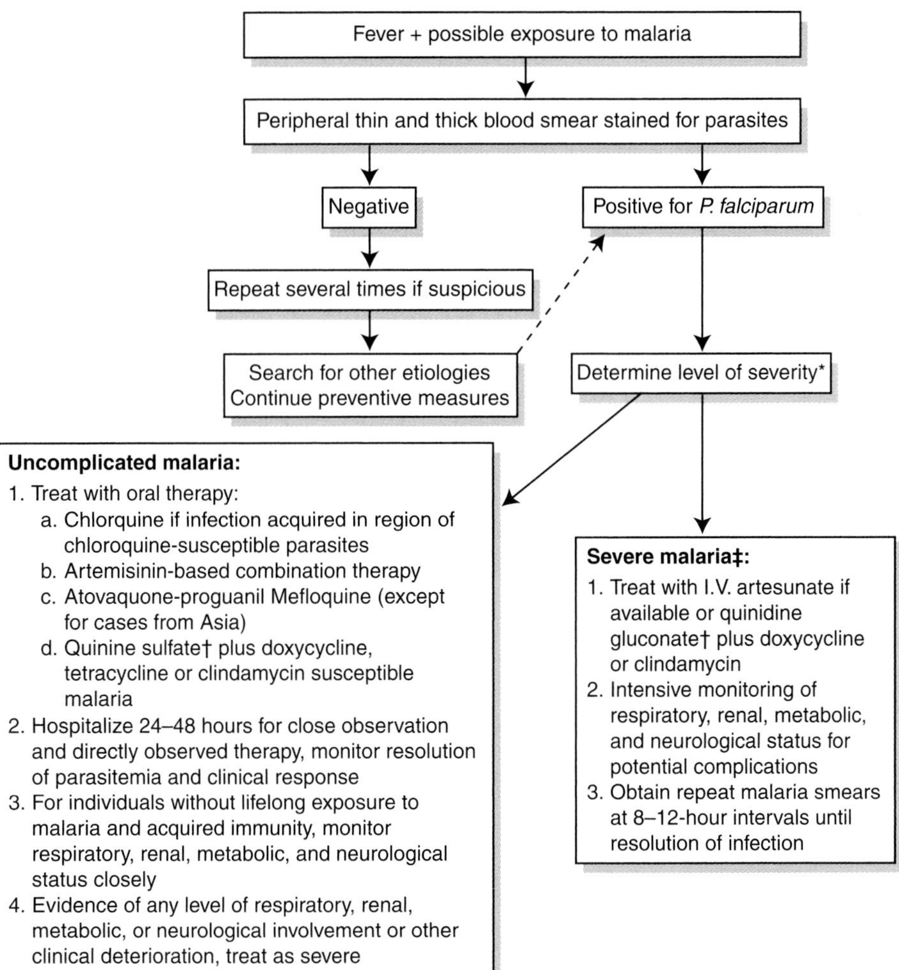

Fever + possible exposure to malaria
Peripheral thin and thick blood smear stained for parasites
Negative
Positive for *P. falciparum*
Repeat several times if suspicious
Search for other etiologies
Continue preventive measures
Determine level of severity*
Uncomplicated malaria:
1. Treat with oral therapy:
a. Chlorquine if infection acquired in region of chloroquine-susceptible parasites
b. Artemisinin-based combination therapy
c. Atovaquone-proguanil Mefloquine (except for cases from Asia)
d. Quinine sulfate† plus doxycycline, tetracycline or clindamycin susceptible malaria
2. Hospitalize 24–48 hours for close observation and directly observed therapy, monitor resolution of parasitemia and clinical response
3. For individuals without lifelong exposure to malaria and acquired immunity, monitor respiratory, renal, metabolic, and neurological status closely
4. Evidence of any level of respiratory, renal, metabolic, or neurological involvement or other clinical deterioration, treat as severe
Severe malaria‡:
1. Treat with I.V. artesunate if available or quinidine gluconate† plus doxycycline or clindamycin
2. Intensive monitoring of respiratory, renal, metabolic, and neurological status for potential complications
3. Obtain repeat malaria smears at 8–12-hour intervals until resolution of infection
*Diagnosis of severe malaria includes one or more of the following clinical criteria: impaired consciousness/coma, severe normocytic anemia, renal failure, pulmonary edema, acute respiratory distress syndrome, circulatory shock, disseminated intravascular coagulation, spontaneous bleeding, acidosis, hemoglobinuria, jaundice, repeated generalized convulsions, and/or parasitemia of >5%
‡Physicians can contact the CDC Malaria Hotline for assistance with management of any malaria case: 770-488-7788
†Quinine and quinidine should be used with caution in patients on protease inhibitors

Figure 53-8 ■ Algorithm describing diagnosis and management of malaria in HIV-infected individuals.

who do not have partial immunity warrant special care and attention. Such patients would include outbreak situations in areas without annual malaria transmission and travelers who contract malaria. Intensive monitoring for renal, neurological, or metabolic disease should be instituted to detect and treat potential complications. Therapeutic efficacy has not been systematically studied in malaria-naive patients with HIV infection, so malaria smears should be obtained at regular intervals to assure resolution of the infection in this population.

Acute malaria infection is associated with a transient rise in HIV viral load. The viral load returns to baseline several weeks after effective therapy.[77a] Viral load testing should therefore not be conducted during an acute malaria episode. Malaria infection has not been shown to increase progression of HIV disease, despite the brief increase in viral replication. However, a mathematical model suggested that where malaria and HIV are both highly prevalent, malaria-induced elevations in viral load may lead to more rapid spread of HIV infection.[78]

Prevention

The prevention of malaria for individual patients involves personal protective measures such as the use of an insecticide-treated bednet and antimalarial prophylaxis. Because pregnant women are at increased risk for malaria, the practice of intermittent presumptive therapy (IPT) has been adopted by many endemic countries. IPT involves administering treatment doses of antimalarial therapy to pregnant women two to three times during pregnancy. The administration of IPT twice during pregnancy is less effective in preventing placental malaria among HIV-infected women compared to uninfected.[79] Because better prevention was obtained when a monthly dose was administered, women who are known to be HIV infected should receive more frequent dosing of

IPT. In areas where HIV infection is high among pregnant women, more frequent administration of IPT may be adopted as standard practice. Most malaria-endemic countries promote the use of insecticide-treated bednets for children under 5 years of age and pregnant women regardless of HIV status. All travelers to malaria-endemic regions should be encouraged to use personal insecticide, sleep under insecticide treated bednets and take prophylactic medication. The role of antimalarial prophylaxis and bednets for HIV-infected older children and adults in malaria-endemic areas has not been established.

Trimethoprim–sulfamethoxazole (TMP-SMZ) prophylaxis is widely used among the HIV-infected population in Africa, both before and during antiretroviral therapy. In addition to its antibacterial effects, TMP-SMZ has the added benefit of being an effective antimalarial preventive agent. Even in the face of high rates of antifolate-resistant malaria, individuals receiving daily TMP-SMZ prophylaxis have much lower rates of malaria infection.[80] Therefore, women on daily TMP-SMZ prophylaxis do not need to receive IPT during pregnancy.

SCHISTOSOMIASIS

Schistosomiasis or bilharzia is a disease caused by *Schistosoma* worms. The main three disease-causing species in humans are *S. haematobium*, affecting the urinary system, *S. mansoni*, and *S. japonicum*, both causing gastrointestinal and hepatic disease. The acute infection of schistosomiasis (Katayama fever) is characterized by a febrile syndrome and is mostly seen in travelers after primary infection. The chronic form is due to eggs trapped in mostly perivesicular and hepatic tissues but also in ectopic tissues. These eggs stimulate granulomatous inflammation that is subsequently replaced by fibrosis.

Clinical Presentation

The clinical presentation of schistosomiasis in HIV-infected individuals may actually be milder than in the HIV-uninfected population. Hematuria, the hallmark presentation of urinary schistosomiasis, may occur less frequently among HIV-infected individuals.[81] In addition, the quantity of eggs shed in the urine or stool may be lower among patients with HIV,[81,82] although this association is not found consistently.[83] The decreased rate of symptomatic disease and egg burden has been attributed to impaired T-cell function leading to decreased granulomatous formation. These granulomas are necessary for the passage of eggs from the tissue into the urinary and gastrointestinal lumen. Hepatic fibrosis due to chronic *S. mansoni* infection has not been shown to be altered by HIV status.[84]

Because schistosomiasis causes chronic infection, it may trigger immune reconstitution disease after treatment with antiretroviral therapy. To date, only two cases have been reported: one with enteritis[85] and the other with eosinophilia and liver disease[86] in African patients with remote histories of exposure to *Schistosoma* infection. As antiretroviral therapy becomes more widely available in Africa and awareness of this syndrome increases, more cases may be appreciated.

Diagnosis

Direct detection of schistosomal eggs is the method of choice for diagnosing the disease and is reliable in the HIV-infected population. Eggs may be demonstrated in urine or stool. Schistosomal antigens can be detected with labeled monoclonal antibodies in the serum or urine. These can be detected with HIV co-infection.[87] Some antibody-based assays are available, but may be unreliable in the presence of HIV infection. False-positive results may occur due to nonspecific cross reactivity.[88] The serologic tests may fail to detect evidence of infection due to the impaired inflammatory response.[89]

Treatment

Treatment of schistosomiasis in the HIV population reflects the standard regimen for treatment of *Schistosoma* infection. For chronic schistosomiasis, 40 mg/kg^{-1} is give orally, usually divided into two doses. In populations with high egg burdens and reinfection rates or if the infection is with *S. japonicum*, a dose of 60 mg/kg may be used, with the dose divided in three and spaced by several hours to reduce side effects. Acute schistosomiasis is treated with 40 mg/kg of praziquantel together with steroids to reduce the hypersensitivity reaction. Four to 6 weeks later, the same dose of praziquantel is repeated since the immature worms present during acute infection are not susceptible to the drug. Possible side effects are mild and include dizziness/drowsiness, nausea, vomiting, rash, and fever. The only contraindication to praziquantel use is ocular cysticercosis. Praziquantel is not known to interfere with antiretroviral therapy. Surgery should be considered for large granulomas.

Prognosis

Chronic helminth infection leads to activation of a type 2 immune response, which includes B cell proliferation, antibody production and eosinophil proliferation. By weighting the immune response in this manner, the concern arose that helminth infection would promote HIV disease progression by decreasing the type 1 immune response. Clinical studies failed to show a consistent alteration in viral load associated with treatment of schistosomiasis, possibly due to differences in *Schistosoma* species, timing to treatment, and follow-up period.[90–92]

STRONGYLOIDIASIS

The intestinal nematode *Strongyloides stercoralis* is endemic in Southeast Asia, Latin America, sub-Saharan Africa, and the southeastern United States. The organism has the unique ability to replicate within a human host, leading to chronic disease that can last for years. Female worms reside in the small intestine and deposit eggs into the intestinal lumen. Offspring can develop into infective larvae that penetrate the intestinal mucosa and travel to the lungs to perpetuate infection. Hyperinfection, characterized by a heavy burden of organisms in the lungs, and disseminated disease, with organisms found at ectopic sites, can occur in individuals who are treated with corticosteroids or who have HTLV-1 infection. Despite the frequent detection of *Strongyloides* infection among people living with HIV in Africa and South America, HIV does not appear to predispose to severe disease.[93] Some investigators hypothesize that HIV-associated immunosuppression promotes the maturation of larvae into free-living adults rather than into the infectious forms that migrate throughout the host. Increased proportion of free-living adult worms compared to the infective larvae in clinical specimens was associated with lower CD4+ T-cell counts among people living with HIV in Uganda.[94]

Screening is indicated in HIV-infected individuals who reside in or have been exposed to endemic areas if they require corticosteroid therapy. It should also be considered in these patients prior to the initiation of antiretroviral therapy because disseminated strongyloidiasis has been reported as a cause of immune reconstitution syndrome.[95–97] Ivermectin (200 μg kg^{-1} day^{-1} for 2 days) is the drug of choice to treat strongyloidiasis and is effective in cases of HIV co-infection.[98]

OTHER PARASITIC INFECTIONS

The effect of HIV infection on some tropical parasitic diseases have not been sufficiently explored to allow comment on the interaction of the two infections. These organisms include onchocercosis, nonfalciparum malaria, guinea worm, and filariasis.

REFERENCES

1. Riarte A, Luna C, Sabatiello R, et al. Chagas' disease in patients with kidney transplants: 7 years of experience 1989–1996. Clin Infect Dis 29:561–7, 1999.
2. Dodd RY. Transmission of parasites and bacteria by blood components. Vox Sang 78(Suppl 2):239–42, 2000.
3. Leiguarda R, Roncoroni A, Taratuto AL, et al. Acute CNS infection by *Trypanosoma cruzi* (Chagas' disease) in immunosuppressed patients. Neurology 40:850–1, 1990.
4. Ferreira MS, Nishioka SA, Rocha A, et al. Acute fatal *Trypanosoma cruzi* meningoencephalitis in a human immunodeficiency virus–positive hemophiliac patient. Am J Trop Med Hyg 45:723–7, 1991.
5. Rosemberg S, Chaves CJ, Higuchi ML, et al. Fatal meningoencephalitis caused by reactivation of *Trypanosoma cruzi* infection in a patient with AIDS. Neurology 42:640–2, 1992.
6. Rocha A, Ferreira MS, Nishioka SA, et al. *Trypanosoma cruzi* meningoencephalitis and myocarditis in a patient with acquired immunodeficiency syndrome. Rev Inst Med Trop Sao Paulo 35:205–8, 1993.
7. Villanueva MS. Trypanosomiasis of the central nervous system. Semin Neurol 13:209–18, 1993.
8. Rocha A, de Meneses AC, da Silva AM, et al. Pathology of patients with Chagas' disease and acquired immunodeficiency syndrome. Am J Trop Med Hyg 50:261–8, 1994.
9. Silva N, O'Bryan L, Medeiros E, et al. *Trypanosoma cruzi* meningoencephalitis in HIV-infected patients. J Acquir Immune Defic Syndr Hum Retrovirol 20:342–9, 1999.
10. Madalosso G, Pellini AC, Vasconcelos MJ, et al. Chagasic meningoencephalitis: case report of a recently included AIDS-defining illness in Brazil. Rev Inst Med Trop Sao Paulo 46:199–202, 2004.
11. Walker M, Kublin JG, Zunt JR. Parasitic central nervous system infections in immunocompromised hosts: malaria, microsporidiosis, leishmaniasis, and African trypanosomiasis. Clin Infect Dis 42:115–25, 2006.
12. Ferreira MS, Nishioka SA, Silvestre MT, et al. Reactivation of Chagas' disease in patients with AIDS: report of three new cases and review of the literature. Clin Infect Dis 25:1397–400, 1997.
13. Sartori AM, Shikanai-Yasuda MA, et al. Follow-up of 18 patients with human immunodeficiency virus infection and chronic Chagas' disease, with reactivation of Chagas' disease causing cardiac disease in three patients. Clin Infect Dis 26:177–9, 1998.
14. Sartori AM, Lopes MH, Benvenuti LA, et al. Reactivation of Chagas' disease in a human immunodeficiency virus-infected patient leading to severe heart disease with a late positive direct microscopic examination of the blood. Am J Trop Med Hyg 59:784–6, 1998.
15. Braz LM, Amato N, V, Carignani FL, De Marchi CR. *Trypanosoma cruzi* parasitemia observed in immunocompromised patients: the importance of the artificial xenodiagnosis. Rev Inst Med Trop Sao Paulo 43:113–5, 2001.
16. Kirchhoff LV, Votava JR, Ochs DE, Moser DR. Comparison of PCR and microscopic methods for detecting *Trypanosoma cruzi*. J Clin Microbiol 34:1171–5, 1996.
17. Portela-Lindoso AA, Shikanai-Yasuda MA. Chronic Chagas' disease: from xenodiagnosis and hemoculture to polymerase chain reaction. Rev Saude Publica 37:107–15, 2003.
18. Prata A. Clinical and epidemiological aspects of Chagas disease. Lancet Infect Dis 1:92–100, 2001.
19. Tanowitz HB, Kirchhoff LV, Simon D, et al. Chagas' disease. Clin Microbiol Rev 5:400–19, 1992.
20. Di Lorenzo GA, Pagano MA, Taratuto AL, et al. Chagasic granulomatous encephalitis in immunosuppressed patients. Computed tomography and magnetic resonance imaging findings. J Neuroimaging 6:94–7, 1996.
21. Yoo TW, Mlikotic A, Cornford ME, Beck CK. Concurrent cerebral American trypanosomiasis and toxoplasmosis in a patient with AIDS. Clin Infect Dis 39:e30–e34, 2004.
22. Viotti R, Vigliano C, Lococo B, et al. Long-term cardiac outcomes of treating chronic Chagas disease with benznidazole versus no treatment: a nonrandomized trial. Ann Intern Med 144:724–34.
23. Rodriques CJ, de Castro SL. A critical review on Chagas disease chemotherapy. Mem Inst Oswaldo Cruz 97:3–24, 2002.
24. Cruz I, Nieto J, Moreno J, et al. Leishmania/HIV co-infections in the second decade. Indian J Med Res 123:357–88, 2006.
25. Desjeux P. The increase in risk factors for leishmaniasis worldwide. Trans R Soc Trop Med Hyg 95:239–43, 2001.
26. Wolday D, Berhe N, Akuffo H, et al. Emerging Leishmania/HIV co-infection in Africa. Med Microbiol Immunol (Berl) 190:65–7, 2001.
27. Desjeux P, Alvar J. Leishmania/HIV co-infections: epidemiology in Europe. Ann Trop Med Parasitol 97(Suppl 1):3–15, 2003.
28. Alvar J, Canavate C, Gutierrez-Solar B, et al. Leishmania and human immunodeficiency virus coinfection: the first 10 years. Clin Microbiol Rev 10:298–319, 1997.
29. Rosenthal E, Marty P, del GP, et al. HIV and Leishmania coinfection: a review of 91 cases with focus on atypical locations of Leishmania. Clin Infect Dis 31:1093–5, 2000.

30. Pasquau F, Ena J, Sanchez R, et al. Leishmaniasis as an opportunistic infection in HIV-infected patients: determinants of relapse and mortality in a collaborative study of 228 episodes in a Mediterreanean region. Eur J Clin Microbiol Infect Dis 24:411–18, 2005.
31. Meenken C, van Agtmael MA, Ten Kate RW, et al. Fulminant ocular leishmaniasis in an HIV-1-positive patient. AIDS 18:1485–6, 2004.
32. Munoz-Rodriguez FJ, Padro S, Pastor P, et al. Pleural and peritoneal leishmaniasis in an AIDS patient. Eur J Clin Microbiol Infect Dis 16:246–8, 1997.
33. Gobels K, Feldt T, Oette M, et al. Visceral leishmaniasis presenting as subcutaneous nodules in a HIV-positive patient. Eur J Clin Microbiol Infect Dis 22:329–31, 2003.
34. Gonzalez-Beato MJ, Moyano B, Sanchez C, et al. Kaposi's sarcoma-like lesions and other nodules as cutaneous involvement in AIDS-related visceral leishmaniasis. Br J Dermatol 143:1316–18, 2000.
35. Gallego MA, Aguilar A, Plaza S, et al. Kaposi's sarcoma with an intense parasitization by Leishmania. Cutis 57:103–5, 1996.
36. Gramiccia M. The identification and variability of the parasites causing leishmaniasis in HIV-positive patients in Italy. Ann Trop Med Parasitol 97(Suppl 1):65–73, 2003.
37. Maurya R, Singh RK, Kumar B, et al. Evaluation of PCR for diagnosis of Indian kala-azar and assessment of cure. J Clin Microbiol 43:3038–41, 2005.
38. Garcia-Garcia JA, Martin-Sanchez J, Gallego M, et al. Detection of Leishmania infection by using non-invasive markers in asymptomatic human immunodeficiency virus-infected patients. J Clin Microbiol 2006.
39. Salotra P, Sreenivas G, Pogue GP, et al. Development of a species-specific PCR assay for detection of *Leishmania donovani* in clinical samples from patients with kala-azar and post-kala-azar dermal leishmaniasis. J Clin Microbiol 39:849–54, 2001.
40. Lopez-Velez R, Laguna F, Alvar J, et al. Parasitic culture of buffy coat for diagnosis of visceral leishmaniasis in human immunodeficiency virus-infected patients. J Clin Microbiol 33:937–9, 1995.
41. Martinez P, de l, V, Laguna F, et al. Diagnosis of visceral leishmaniasis in HIV-infected individuals using peripheral blood smears. AIDS 7:227–30, 1993.
42. Laguna F, Videla S, Jimenez-Mejias ME, et al. Amphotericin B lipid complex versus meglumine antimoniate in the treatment of visceral leishmaniasis in patients infected with HIV: a randomized pilot study. J Antimicrob Chemother 52:464–8, 2003.
43. Laguna F, Lopez-Velez R, Pulido F, et al. Treatment of visceral leishmaniasis in HIV-infected patients: a randomized trial comparing meglumine antimoniate with amphotericin B. Spanish HIV-Leishmania Study Group. AIDS 13:1063–9, 1999.
44. Ritmeijer K, Dejenie A, Assefa Y, et al. A comparison of miltefosine and sodium stibogluconate for treatment of visceral leishmaniasis in an Ethiopian population with high prevalence of HIV infection. Clin Infect Dis 43:357–64, 2006.
45. Sundar S, Jha TK, Thakur CP, et al. Oral miltefosine for Indian visceral leishmaniasis. N Engl J Med 347:1739–46, 2002.
46. Sindermann H, Engel KR, Fischer C, Bommer W. Oral miltefosine for leishmaniasis in immunocompromised patients: compassionate use in 39 patients with HIV infection. Clin Infect Dis 39:1520–3, 2004.
47. Schraner C, Hasse B, Hasse U, et al. Successful treatment with miltefosine of disseminated cutaneous leishmaniasis in a severely immunocompromised patient infected with HIV-1. Clin Infect Dis 40:e120–4, 2005.
48. Belay AD, Asafa Y, Mesure J, Davidson RN. Successful miltefosine treatment of post-kala-azar dermal leishmaniasis occurring during antiretroviral therapy. Ann Trop Med Parasitol 100:223–7, 2006.
49. Nandy A, Addy M, Maji AK, Guha SK. Impact of a co-factor on the dynamics of *Leishmania donovani* infection: does HIV infection encourage the recurrence of visceral leishmaniasis following post-kala-azar dermal leishmaniasis? Ann Trop Med Parasitol 98:651–4, 2004.
50. Bittencourt A, Silva N, Straatmann A, et al. Post-kala-azar dermal leishmaniasis associated with AIDS. Braz J Infect Dis 6:313–16, 2002.
51. Cruz I, Canavate C, Rubio JM, et al. A nested polymerase chain reaction (Ln-PCR) for diagnosing and monitoring *Leishmania infantum* infection in patients co-infected with human immunodeficiency virus. Trans R Soc Trop Med Hyg 96(Suppl 1):S185–9, 2002.
52. Riera C, Fisa R, Ribera E, et al. Value of culture and nested polymerase chain reaction of blood in the prediction of relapses in patients co-infected with Leishmania and human immunodeficiency virus. Am J Trop Med Hyg 73:1012–15, 2005.
53. Lopez-Velez R, Videla S, Marquez M, et al. Amphotericin B lipid complex versus no treatment in the secondary prophylaxis of visceral leishmaniasis in HIV-infected patients. J Antimicrob Chemother 53:540–3, 2004.
54. Berenguer J, Cosin J, Miralles P, et al. Discontinuation of secondary anti-Leishmania prophylaxis in HIV-infected patients who have responded to highly active antiretroviral therapy. AIDS 14:2946–8, 2000.
55. Berhe N, Wolday D, Hailu A, et al. HIV viral load and response to antileishmanial chemotherapy in co-infected patients. AIDS 13:1921–5, 1999.
56. Alvar J. Leishmaniasis and AIDS co-infection: the Spanish example. Parasitol Today 10:160–3, 1994.
57. Russo R, Laguna F, Lopez-Velez R, et al. Visceral leishmaniasis in those infected with HIV: clinical aspects and other opportunistic infections. Ann Trop Med Parasitol 97(Suppl 1): 99–105, 2003.
58. De La RR, Pineda JA, Delgado J, et al. Influence of highly active antiretroviral therapy on the outcome of subclinical visceral leishmaniasis in human immunodeficiency virus-infected patients. Clin Infect Dis 32:633–5, 2001.
59. Russo R, Nigro L, Panarello G, Montineri A. Clinical survey of Leishmania/HIV co-infection in Catania, Italy: the impact of highly active antiretroviral therapy (HAART). Ann Trop Med Parasitol 97(Suppl 1):149–55, 2003.
60. del GP, Mary-Krause M, Pradier C, et al. Impact of highly active antiretroviral therapy on the incidence of visceral leishmaniasis in a French cohort of patients infected with human immunodeficiency virus. J Infect Dis 186:1366–70, 2002.
61. Villanueva JL, Alarcon A, Bernabeu-Wittel M, et al. Prospective evaluation and follow-up of European patients with visceral leishmaniasis and HIV-1 coinfection in the era of highly active antiretroviral therapy. Eur J Clin Microbiol Infect Dis 19:798–801, 2000.
62. French N, Nakiyingi J, Lugada E, et al. Increasing rates of malarial fever with deteriorating immune status in HIV-1-infected Ugandan adults. AIDS 15:899–906, 2001.
63. Whitworth J, Morgan D, Quigley M, et al. Effect of HIV-1 and increasing immunosuppression on malaria parasitaemia and clinical episodes in adults in rural Uganda: a cohort study. Lancet 356:1051–6, 2000.
64. Laufer MK, van Oosterhout JJ, Thesing PC, et al. Impact of HIV-associated immunosuppression on malaria infection and disease in Malawi. J Infect Dis 193:872–8, 2006.
65. Steketee RW, Wirima JJ, Hightower AW, et al. The effect of malaria and malaria prevention in pregnancy on offspring birthweight, prematurity, and intrauterine growth retardation in rural Malawi. Am J Trop Med Hyg 55(1 Suppl):33–41, 1996.
66. Steketee RW, Nahlen BL, Parise ME, Menendez C. The burden of malaria in pregnancy in malaria-endemic areas. Am J Trop Med Hyg 64(Suppl 1–2):28–35, 2001.

67. van Eijk AM, Ayisi JG, ter Kuile FO, et al. HIV increases the risk of malaria in women of all gravidities in Kisumu, Kenya. AIDS 17:595–603, 2003.
68. ter Kuile FO, Parise ME, Verhoeff FH, et al. The burden of co-infection with human immunodeficiency virus type 1 and malaria in pregnant women in sub-saharan Africa. Am J Trop Med Hyg 71(Suppl 2):41–54, 2004.
69. Inion I, Mwanyumba F, Gaillard P, et al. Placental malaria and perinatal transmission of human immunodeficiency virus type 1. J Infect Dis 188:1675–8, 2003.
70. Gallagher M, Malhotra I, Mungai PL, et al. The effects of maternal helminth and malaria infections on mother-to-child HIV transmission. AIDS 19:1849–55, 2005.
71. Brahmbhatt H, Kigozi G, Wabwire-Mangen F, et al. The effects of placental malaria on mother-to-child HIV transmission in Rakai, Uganda. AIDS 17:2539–41, 2003.
72. Ayisi JG, van Eijk AM, Newman RD, et al. Maternal malaria and perinatal HIV transmission, western Kenya. Emerg Infect Dis 10:643–52, 2004.
73. Grimwade K, French N, Mbatha DD, et al. HIV infection as a cofactor for severe falciparum malaria in adults living in a region of unstable malaria transmission in South Africa. AIDS 18:547–54, 2004.
74. Cohen C, Karstaedt A, Frean J, et al. Increased prevalence of severe malaria in HIV-infected adults in South Africa. Clin Infect Dis 41:1631–7, 2005.
75. Khoo S, Back D, Winstanley P. The potential for interactions between antimalarial and antiretroviral drugs. AIDS 19: 995–1005, 2005.
76. Kamya MR, Gasasira AF, Yeka A, et al. Effect of HIV-1 infection on antimalarial treatment outcomes in Uganda: a population-based study. J Infect Dis 193:9–15, 2006.
77. Van Geertruyden JP, Mulenga M, Mwananyanda L, et al. HIV-1 immune suppression and antimalarial treatment outcome in Zambian adults with uncomplicated malaria. J Infect Dis 194:917–25, 2006.
77a. Kublin JG, Patnaik P, Jere CS, et al. Effect of Plasmodium falciparum malaria on concentration of HIV-1-RNA in the blood of adults in rural Malawi: a prospective cohort study. Lancet January 15; 365(9455):233–40, 2005.
78. bu-Raddad LJ, Patnaik P, Kublin JG. Dual infection with HIV and malaria fuels the spread of both diseases in sub-Saharan Africa. Science 314:1603–6, 2006.
79. Filler SJ, Kazembe P, Thigpen M, et al. Randomized trial of 2-dose versus monthly sulfadoxine–pyrimethamine intermittent preventive treatment for malaria in HIV-positive and HIV-negative pregnant women in Malawi. J Infect Dis 194:286–93, 2006.
80. Mermin J, Lule J, Ekwaru JP, et al. Effect of co-trimoxazole prophylaxis on morbidity, mortality, CD4-cell count, and viral load in HIV infection in rural Uganda. Lancet 364:1428–34, 2004.
81. Mwanakasale V, Vounatsou P, Sukwa TY, et al. Interactions between *Schistosoma haematobium* and human immunodeficiency virus type 1: the effects of coinfection on treatment outcomes in rural Zambia. Am J Trop Med Hyg 69:420–8, 2003.
82. Karanja DM, Colley DG, Nahlen BL, et al. Studies on schistosomiasis in western Kenya. I. Evidence for immune-facilitated excretion of schistosome eggs from patients with *Schistosoma mansoni* and human immunodeficiency virus coinfections. Am J Trop Med Hyg 56:515–21, 1997.
83. Kallestrup P, Zinyama R, Gomo E, et al. Schistosomiasis and HIV-1 infection in rural Zimbabwe: implications of coinfection for excretion of eggs. J Infect Dis 191:1311–20, 2005.
84. Mwinzi PN, Karanja DM, Kareko I, et al. Short report: evaluation of hepatic fibrosis in persons co-infected with *Schistosoma mansoni* and human immunodeficiency virus 1. Am J Trop Med Hyg 71:783–6, 2004.
85. de SS, Walsh J, Brown M. Symptomatic *Schistosoma mansoni* infection as an immune restoration phenomenon in a patient receiving antiretroviral therapy. Clin Infect Dis 42:303–4, 2006.
86. Fernando R, Miller R. Immune reconstitution eosinophilia due to schistosomiasis. Sex Transm Infect 78:76, 2002.
87. Kallestrup P, Zinyama R, Gomo E, et al. Schistosomiasis and HIV in rural Zimbabwe: efficacy of treatment of schistosomiasis in individuals with HIV coinfection. Clin Infect Dis 42:1781–9, 2006.
88. Kern W, Kirsten C, Forster P, et al. Specificity of routine parasite serological tests in autoimmune disorders, neoplastic disease, EBV-induced mononucleosis, and HIV infection. Klin Wochenschr 65:898–905, 1987.
89. Joseph S, Jones FM, Laidlaw ME, et al. Impairment of the *Schistosoma mansoni*-specific immune responses elicited by treatment with praziquantel in Ugandans with HIV-1 coinfection. J Infect Dis 190:613–8, 2004.
90. Kallestrup P, Zinyama R, Gomo E, et al. Schistosomiasis and HIV-1 infection in rural Zimbabwe: effect of treatment of schistosomiasis on CD4 cell count and plasma HIV-1 RNA load. J Infect Dis 192:1956–61, 2005.
91. Lawn SD, Karanja DM, Mwinzia P, et al. The effect of treatment of schistosomiasis on blood plasma HIV-1 RNA concentration in coinfected individuals. AIDS 14:2437–43, 2000.
92. Brown M, Kizza M, Watera C, et al. Helminth infection is not associated with faster progression of HIV disease in coinfected adults in Uganda. J Infect Dis 190:1869–79, 2004.
93. Lucas SB. Missing infections in AIDS. Trans R Soc Trop Med Hyg 84(Suppl 1):34–8, 1990.
94. Viney ME, Brown M, Omoding NE, et al. Why does HIV infection not lead to disseminated strongyloidiasis? J Infect Dis 190:2175–80, 2004.
95. Kim AC, Lupatkin HC. *Strongyloides stercoralis* infection as a manifestation of immune restoration syndrome. Clin Infect Dis 39:439–40, 2004.
96. Lanzafame M, Faggian F, Lattuada E, et al. Strongyloidiasis in an HIV-1-infected patient after highly active antiretroviral therapy-induced immune restoration. J Infect Dis 191:1027, 2005.
97. Brown M, Cartledge JD, Miller RF. Dissemination of *Strongyloides stercoralis* as an immune restoration phenomenon in an HIV-1-infected man on antiretroviral therapy. Int J STD AIDS 17:560–1, 2006.
98. Torres JR, Isturiz R, Murillo J, et al. Efficacy of ivermectin in the treatment of strongyloidiasis complicating AIDS. Clin Infect Dis 17:900–2, 1993.
99. Houghton RL, Petrescu M, Benson DR, et al. A cloned antigen (recombinant K39) of *Leishmania chagasi* diagnostic for visceral leishmaniasis in human immunodeficiency virus type 1 patients and a prognostic indicator for monitoring patients undergoing drug therapy. J Infect Dis 177:1339–44, 1998.
100. Medrano FJ, Canavate C, Leal M, et al. The role of serology in the diagnosis and prognosis of visceral leishmaniasis in patients coinfected with human immunodeficiency virus type-1. Am J Trop Med Hyg 59:155–62, 1998.

Chapter 54

Hepatitis B Infection and GB Virus C

Ruth Berggren, MD, Holly Murphy, MD

HEPATITIS B VIRUS

Pathogen

Hepatitis B virus (HBV) is a hepatotropic DNA virus of the family hepadnaviridae. It is a 40–42 nm virion enclosed by a lipoprotein envelope bearing three envelope glycoproteins, or surface antigens.[1] Inside the envelope is a nucleocapsid containing the viral genome, as well as a DNA polymerase. The viral genome consists of partially double stranded, relaxed-circular DNA.[2] There are eight HBV genotypes (A through H) with distinct geographic distributions and variable response rates to therapy.[3,4] The genome possesses four open reading frames: preS-S, preC, P, and X. The presurface–surface (preS-S) encodes three surface antigens including HBsAg, which is the most abundant of the three. The second open reading frame is the precore–core region (preC), which encodes hepatitis B core antigen (HBcAg) and hepatitis B e antigen (HBeAg). HBeAg is secreted into the blood and is used as a marker for unresolved infection, though its function is not well known. PreC mutations result in HBeAg-negative infections which are clinically well-documented, seen in up to 33% of hepatitis B surface antigen (HBsAg) carriers, associated with high rates of relapse, and less favorable outcomes in response to interferon-alpha treatment.[1,5] The third open reading frame, or P coding region, encodes a polyfunctional enzyme which is a viral polymerase for DNA synthesis and a reverse transcriptase as well.[1] Finally, the X open reading frame encodes viral X protein (HBx) which regulates host and viral gene expression, and has been implicated in the development of hepatocellular carcinoma (HCC).[1,6]

The Viral Life Cycle

HBV binds to cell surface receptors and is internalized by hepatocytes. Core particles are transported to the nucleus, where their genomes are modified into covalently closed circles (cccDNA). CccDNA is transcribed into mRNA which is transported to the cytoplasm and translated into viral surface, core, polymerase, and X proteins. Subsequently assembled viral particles incorporate viral RNA which is then reverse transcribed into viral DNA.[2] Core particles either bud off the host cell membrane to infect other cells, or are transported back to the nucleus where they are converted back to cccDNA and maintain a stable intranuclear pool of templates allowing persistent infection.[7] Four antivirals, (nucleoside analogs lamivudine and emtricitabine; nucleotide analogs adefovir and tenofovir) originally developed to inhibit the reverse transcriptase inhibitor of HIV-1, potently inhibit HBV replication. The existence of these dually active drugs provides expanded opportunities for HBV therapy, as well as simplified regimens, in HIV-co-infected patients. Two additional nucleoside analogs, entecavir and telbuvidine, are active against HBV and have no therapeutic role for treatment of HIV.[8,9,9a] Unfortunately, therapy must be prolonged as cccDNA evades the action of the drugs until the replication phases of the viral life cycle.

Pathogenesis

HBV is not directly cytotoxic to hepatocytes. Rather, liver injury occurs as a result of cytotoxic CD8+ T-lymphocyte cell (CTL) responses to the viral antigens that are displayed on hepatocyte surfaces. Aminotransferases rise with hepatocyte death. Not surprisingly, immunocompromised hosts with HBV often have mild acute hepatitis B infections, but high rates of chronicity.[2,7] Over 90% of normal adults and 75% of normal infants will resolve acute infection with HBV without therapy. Those who do not resolve acute infection are defined as chronic carriers if they demonstrate serum HBsAg positivity for over 6 months.[6]

Both cellular and humoral immune responses are implicated in control of infection and development of protective immunity. Anti-HBsAg antibodies (anti-HBS) are produced in response to recombinant envelope antigen and confer protective immunity. These antibodies are found in persons who recover from acute HBV and also in those who have been immunized with recombinant HBV vaccine.[1]

In HIV-infected patients, as in chronic HBV carriers, desirable anti-HBV cell-mediated immune responses, including CTL (which are believed to play a central role in viral clearance), are blunted. Nevertheless, chronic inflammation from unresolved viral infection generates inflammatory and profibrotic cytokines (such as TNF-alpha and interferon gamma) as well as proteases, free radicals and natural killer cell activity which contribute to the development of chronic liver damage, fibrosis, cirrhosis, and end-stage liver disease (ESLD).[6,10] Individuals with chronic HBV infection have a 100 times higher risk of HCC compared to noncarriers.[11] Mechanisms for the provocation of HCC by HBV are not well understood. Though cirrhosis is a predisposing factor for HCC, 30–50% of HCC associated with HBV occurs in patients who do not have cirrhosis, and HCC can occur in long-term carriers who have cleared HBsAg. Chronically infected patients should be screened every 6 months for HCC using liver ultrasonography as well as serum alpha-fetoprotein (AFP).[6,7] Note that use of both screening modalities is warranted by the imperfect sensitivity and specificity of either test alone; the positive predictive value of AFP is no higher than 30%.[6]

Epidemiology

Globally, there are some 370 million persons persistently infected with HBV,[4,12] with 2–4 million individuals estimated to be co-infected with HIV and chronic HBV.[12] HBV is endemic in Asia, sub-Saharan Africa, and the South Pacific.[1,6,12] In the United States and Western Europe, there is evidence for chronic HBV co-infection among 6–14% of all HIV-infected persons. Co-infection rates differ according to risk group, with HBV found in 4–6% of HIV-infected heterosexuals, 9–17% of men who have sex with men (MSM), and 7–10% of injection drug users (IDU).[12] HBV shares routes of transmission with HIV and hepatitis C (HCV), and is transmitted percutaneously via needlestick injuries, injection drug use, or by blood transfusions, sexual or mucous membrane exposure, and perinatal exposure. However, HBV differs from HIV and HCV in the efficiency by which various exposures result in disease transmission. For example, HBV is 100 times more infectious than HIV from a percutaneous exposure, and HBV is transmitted perinatally and sexually with greater ease than HCV.[12]

Natural History

The clinical manifestations of acute HBV infection are often clinically undetectable, but may include nausea, vomiting, fatigue, fever, arthralgias, and right-upper quadrant abdominal pain followed by jaundice.[13] In the outpatient HIV clinical setting, chronic HBV commonly presents as asymptomatic disease with HBsAg positivity and elevated alanine aminotransferase (ALT). These patients may demonstrate poor tolerance to certain antiretroviral medications, palmar erythema, gynecomastia, cutaneous spider angiomata, and/or hepatomegaly. Later, ESLD manifests with the onset of ascites, jaundice, encephalopathy, coagulopathy, esophageal varices, and/or caput medusa. Extrahepatic manifestations of HBV include vasculitis, glomerulonephritis, and polyarteritis nodosa.[1,13] Co-infected patients may be at a higher risk of developing HCC than HBV-monoinfected patients,[14,15] but screening recommendations for HCC in this population are similar to those in monoinfected persons: AFP and hepatic ultrasound should be performed every 6 months.[7,13,15]

Most (95%) acute HBV infections are resolved by the host immune response (Fig. 54-1). Initially there are high levels of serum HBV DNA, and HBeAg is measurable. In those who resolve infection, HBeAg is eventually lost; antibody to HBeAg (anti-HBe) appears, with a concomitant reduction of HBV DNA to fewer than 10^5 copies/mL, normalization of aminotransferase levels, and reduction of necroinflammation.[6] HBeAg to anti-HBe conversion is frequently preceded by an ALT flare.[16] However, fulminant or chronic persistent hepatitis may develop due to incompletely defined host and viral factors. Persistence of HBV occurs more often with the HBV/Ae genotype than others. Fulminant hepatitis is associated with HBV/Bj accompanied by lack of HBeAg and a precore mutation.[4] In HIV-negative patients with chronic HBV, 25% will develop serious complications of HBV during their lifetime.[7]

Some 0.5–2.5% of chronic carriers clear HBsAg yearly and then develop anti-HBs.[16,17] Up to half of these people will still have low levels of HBV DNA detectable by PCR, the significance of which is not well understood. About 20% of HBV-infected patients will develop cirrhosis as a result of

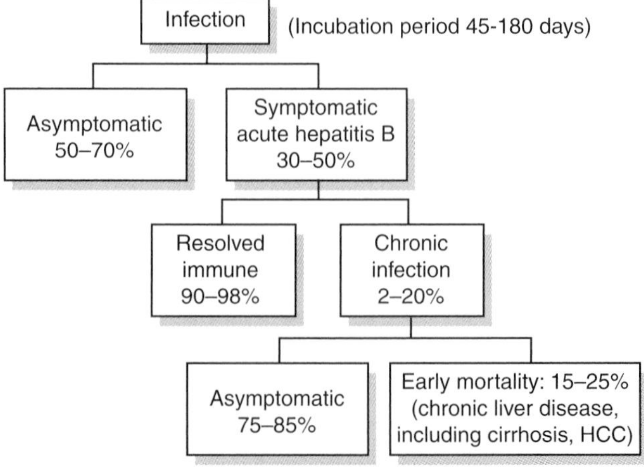

Figure 54-1 ■ Outcome of HBV infection in monoinfected adults.

the chronic carrier state.[2] The 5- and 10-year survival rates for HBV patients with compensated cirrhosis are 84% and 68%, respectively. The annual incidence of HCC in HBV carriers with cirrhosis ranges from 3% to 10%.[16]

When a patient with HBV infection worsens, or when a test for HBeAg is negative in the presence of active liver disease, hepatitis D (HDV) infection should be considered. HDV is an RNA-containing defective passenger virus which cannot replicate in the absence of HBV. The results of treatment in HBV/HDV-infected persons have been disappointing.[7] There is no specific therapy for HDV, which is unfortunate, because disease progression is more rapid with combined infections than with HBV infection alone.[1]

Impact of HIV on the Natural History of HBV

Patients with HIV/HBV infection have substantial liver-related mortality (Fig. 54-2) Co-infected persons have more severe liver disease and higher liver-related mortality rates than do HBV-monoinfected persons.[7,18,19,9,20] Analysis of the multicenter AIDS Cohort Study found a 17 times higher liver-related mortality rate in co-infected patients compared with HBV-monoinfected individuals.[18] HIV/HBV-co-infected patients also have higher levels of HBV DNA and lower rates of HBeAg seroconversion.[6,7,21,22] Moreover, the tolerability of HIV medications can be adversely affected by the presence of HBV co-infection.[7,23–25] The incidence of serious drug-related hepatotoxicity in HIV/HBV-co-infected persons can be as much as nine times higher than for HIV-monoinfected persons.[26] Antiviral drugs can cause liver injury directly, or they can lead to immunologically mediated liver injury by effecting immune reconstitution in immunocompromised individuals.[7,27]

With the advent of highly active antiretroviral therapy (HAART), and greatly improved survival of patients with HIV infection, chronic liver disease due to hepatitis B or C co-infection has now become a major cause of morbidity and mortality for patients with HIV.[28–31] It is important, therefore, to screen all HIV-infected persons for viral hepatitis co-infection, and to provide hepatitis A and B vaccines to those who are not immune.[13,7] The presence of HBV infection at initial screening of an HIV-infected person will critically affect the timing and choice of antiretroviral regimen,[32] as well as long-term clinical management (*see section on* Treatment).

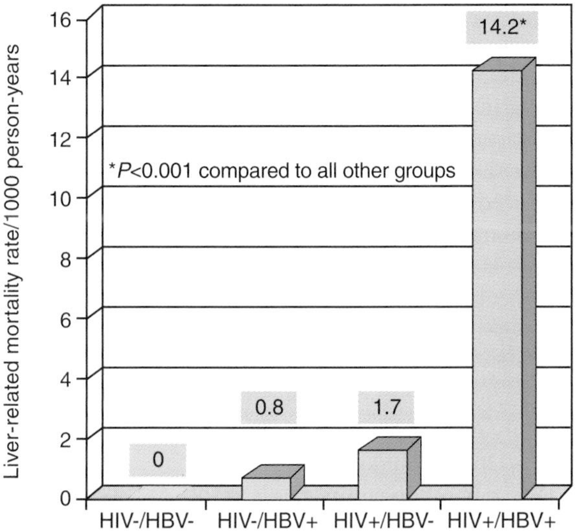

Figure 54-2 ■ Liver-related mortality rates in HIV/HBV-co-infected subjects.

Diagnosis

The optimal testing strategy for HBV in HIV-infected persons is not well-defined.[13] In screening HIV patients, it is important to understand the serological markers that distinguish between acute, chronic, and resolved HBV infection. One must also remember the distinct pattern displayed by individuals with the preCore mutation, and that immunocompromised hosts sometimes display aberrant serology. The usual markers of acute infection include hepatitis B core IgM, HBsAg, HBeAg, and HBV DNA>10^5 copies/mL (Figs 54-3 and 54-4).[1] Individuals with chronic infection are so defined if they remain HBsAg positive for greater than 6 months. The other markers of chronic infection are HBeAg, anti-HBe antibody negativity, HBV DNA>10^5 copies/mL and (usually) elevated ALT. Individuals chronically infected with the HBV preCore mutant will be HBeAg negative with

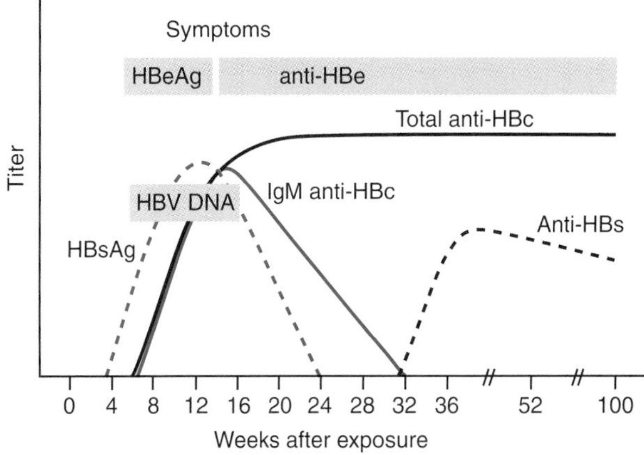

Figure 54-3 ■ Acute hepatitis B virus infection with recovery: Typical serologic course.

Reproduced from the CDC.

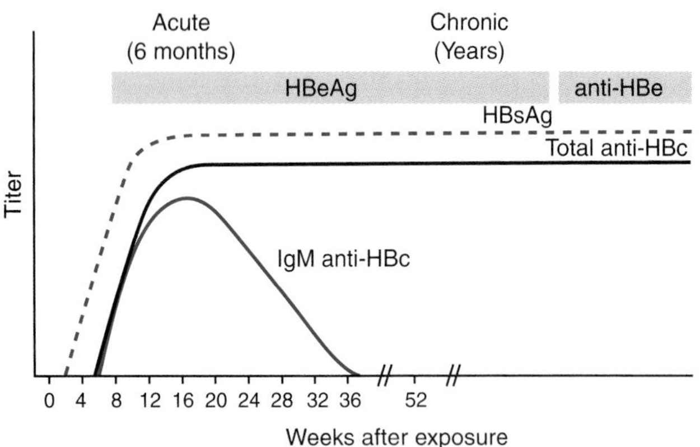

Figure 54-4 ■ Progression of chronic hepatitis B virus infection: Typical serologic course.

Reproduced from the CDC.

elevated ALT and elevated HBV DNA levels. Markers of resolved infection are anti-HBe antibody positivity, negative HBeAg, loss of HBsAg, normal ALT, and HBV DNA $< 10^5$ copies/mL. The aberrant serology sometimes noted in HIV-infected persons is characterized by the presence of HBV DNA in persons without HBsAg, in whom anti-HBc is the only serological marker of infection.[33–36]

Treatment

HBV-specific treatment is recommended for co-infected patients with a positive HBeAg or HBV DNA levels >105 copies/mL and liver disease (elevated ALT and/or fibrosis seen by liver biopsy).[7] Ideally, the goal of therapy should be the resolution of infection as defined by the disappearance of HBsAg and the appearance of anti-HBs (antibodies against HBsAg). However, this goal is rarely achieved as cccDNA evades available drugs. Failing cure, patients can still benefit from the more modest goal of halting the progression of fibrosis while preventing ESLD or HCC. Antiviral therapy can be used to maximally suppress HBV replication for as long as possible. There are five parameters that may be monitored prospectively for treatment response: HBV DNA, HBeAg, HBsAg, ALT, and liver histology.[7] A currently accepted surrogate marker for successful anti-HBV treatment is clearance of serum HBV DNA. Alternatively, if HBV DNA PCR is not available, anti-HBe antibodies are considered markers of successful treatment response in individuals who were HBeAg-positive prior to therapy.[8]

There is no uniform treatment recommendation for the management of HBV in the setting of HIV.[13] Because of limited data about the safety and efficacy of chronic HBV treatment in co-infected persons, current guidelines are based on consensus opinion.[7] The approved drugs for treatment of HBV include pegylated interferon-alpha 2a, as well as non-pegylated interferon alpha 2a or 2b[37] (nearly all practitioners choose the pegylated formulation of interferon alpha due to more favorable outcomes and dosing schedule)[38–40] the nucleoside analogs lamivudine or entecavir,[5,14,41–45] or the nucleotide analog, adefovir dipivoxil.[8,46,47] Not approved for HBV by regulatory agencies, but clearly efficacious are the nucleotide analog tenofovir (approved for HIV, and closely related to adefovir)[47–52] and the nucleoside analog emtricitabine (also developed for HIV, and related to lamivudine)[53–55]. (Telbivudine has not been studied in co-infected patients to date.) Of these active drugs, lamivudine, emtricitabine, and tenofovir have dual activity against HIV and HBV. While entecavir was initially not noted to have anti-HIV activity, there are a few cases reported in which coinfected patients treated with entecavir monotherapy had reductions in HIV viremia and subsequently developed the HIV resistance mutation M184V, conferring HIV resistance to lamivudine and emtricitabine. While the significance of these few reports is not yet well understood, experts advise the avoidance of entecavir monotherapy in coinfected persons.[56] When used in co-infected persons, entecavir should be given with a full HAART regimen.[56a] A summary of therapeutic options for HBV in HIV/HBV-co-infected patients, including regulatory agency approval status and dosing schedules, is listed in Table 54-1.

The first drug approved for chronic hepatitis B in monoinfected persons was interferon-alpha 2b.[9] For monoinfected persons, interferon alpha is more efficacious in HBeAg+ than in HBeAg− persons.[7] In HIV/HBV-co-infected patients, the response rate to therapy with interferon (14.3%) is inferior to that seen in HBV-monoinfected patients, who achieve a 36–45% remission rate after 4 months of treatment.[1,9,57] Moreover, interferon therapy requires subcutaneous injections and presents many side effects. Pegylated interferon alpha requires less frequent injections, and is more effective against HBV than nonpegylated interferon.[9,58] While rigorous trials of this drug in co-infected patients are lacking, some experts feel that certain variables favor the treatment of HBV/HIV-co-infected patients with pegylated interferon. These variables include: HBeAg positivity, elevated aminotransferases, high CD4+ T-lymphocyte counts, absence of advanced liver disease, no need for HAART, and absence of psychiatric disorders.[8] Co-infected patients are more commonly treated with oral medications because dual-purpose drugs directed against both viruses permit a tolerable, simplified regimen. Monotherapy for HBV with oral nucleoside analogs presents a significant risk of drug resistance development. For example, mutations in the active site of HBV polymerase/reverse transcriptase targeted by lamivudine (*YMDD* mutations), develop at a rate of 15% per year. In HIV/HBV-co-infected patients, these mutations are more rapidly selected, at a rate of 50% after 2 years, and 90% after 4 years.[8,59] *YMDD* mutations can also be elicited by emtricitabine, which is closely related to lamivudine. Fortunately, the nucleotide analogs tenofovir and adefovir have demonstrated *in vivo* activity against *YMDD* mutant viruses.[7]

Table 54-2 summarizes some of the larger trials for co-infected patients.

A currently accepted algorithm for treatment of HBV in co-infected patients starts with serological assessment of

Therapeutic Options for HBV in HIV Co-Infected Patients

Table 54-1

Drug	Approval for HBV[a]	Active vs HIV	Dose in HIV-Infected Patients
Interferon-α-2b	Yes	Yes	5–6 × 10^6 U sq qd or 9–10 × 10^6 U sq 3x/week
Peginterferon-α-2a	Yes	Yes	180 μg sq qwk × 48 weeks
Lamivudine	Yes	Yes	100 mq PO qd[c]
Adefovir	Yes	No	10 mg PO qd
Entecavir	Yes	No	0.5–1.0 mg PO qd
Tenofovir	No	Yes	300 mg PO qd
Emtricitabine	No	Yes	200 mg PO qd
Peginterferon-α-2b	No	Yes	1.5 μg/kg sq qwk (max 100 μg/week)
Telbivudine[d]	Yes	No	600 mg PO pd

[a]By the United States Food and Drug Administration.
[b]For HIV the does of lamivudine is 150 mg bid.
[c]Lower dose in lamivudine-naive subjects.
[d]Not studied in HIV patients. High rate of HBV resistance to lamivudine and entecavir elicited by this drug when drug when given as monotherapy.

patients who are HBsAg positive (Fig. 54-5). These individuals should be screened for HBeAg, anti-HBe, and quantitative plasma HBV DNA PCR. A liver biopsy is not required, but may be considered if there is no immediate indication for HIV treatment, in patients with normal ALT, or with low levels of HBV DNA (10^4 copies/mL). Furthermore, liver biopsy may be useful if alternate, co-existing morbidities (like steatosis or opportunistic infections) are suspected.

In treatment-naive patients whose HIV disease does not warrant initiation of HAART, HBV treatment should consist of pegylated interferon or adefovir. The guiding principle is to avoid monotherapy using the dual purpose drugs (lamivudine, emtricitabine, or tenofovir) in this setting, to prevent development of HIV resistance mutations to these drugs. For HBeAg-negative individuals who do not require HAART, adefovir monotherapy may be initiated.[8] Pegylated interferon may be used for e-antigen negative cases, however, the response rate is less favorable than for e-antigen positive cases, with a higher rate of relapse. Using adefovir in co-infected individuals theoretically could lead to cross-resistance to tenofovir, as adefovir does inhibit HIV replication at higher doses. However, such cross-resistance has yet to be demonstrated clinically.[9,60] If entecavir is used in coinfection, it should be used in the context of a full HAART regimen to avoid HIV resistance mutation M184V.

In patients who require simultaneous treatment of HIV and HBV, consensus opinion suggests that HAART should be initiated including tenofovir with either lamivudine or emtricitabine in addition to a third HIV specific drug.[8,9] This opinion prevails despite the existence of a black box warning stating that tenofovir is not indicated for the treatment of chronic hepatitis B virus infection, and that the safety and efficacy of tenofovir have not been established in patients co-infected with HBV and HIV. Severe exacerbations of HBV have been reported in patients who are co-infected with HBV and have discontinued tenofovir.[9] The rationale for the consensus opinion relates to the known high rate of development of HBV resistance to lamivudine monotherapy in co-infected individuals, as well as clinical evidence of potent anti-HBV activity by tenofovir.[9,56] There is at least one clinical trial in HIV/HBV-co-infected individuals examining the strategy of tenofovir with lamivudine compared with either drug alone among lamivudine-naive or experienced patients. This small study ($N = 59$), compared dual to monotherapy for HBV. At week 24 among naive subjects, combination therapy with tenofovir was superior to monotherapy, and there was no difference between the tenofovir versus lamivudine monotherapy arms.[61] The study also supports either adding or switching to tenofovir in lamivudine-experienced patients who have lamivudine resistance. If only HIV treatment is indicated, one should include at least one anti-HBV drug in the HAART regimen to avoid flares in aminotransferases that can be seen in co-infected persons undergoing HAART-mediated immune reconstitution.[8] Monotherapy with dual purpose drugs (emtricitabine, lamivudine, and tenofovir) should be avoided to prevent the selection of HIV resistance mutations.[56]

Patients with HBV viremia who have been taking lamivudine-containing HAART without a second HBV active drug for more than 2 years may be presumed to have lamivudine resistance mutations. These individuals have been shown to benefit from the addition of tenofovir,[61] but not emtricitabine (due to cross resistance with lamivudine). They are also likely to benefit from the addition of adefovir, which will treat HBV without altering HIV viral load. There is concern for elicitation of HIV resistance mutations from the use of entecavir, as previously noted.

In the absence of clinical data to guide treatment duration, and especially in settings where access to serologic testing is not always possible, one approach is to continue HBV therapy indefinitely in HIV-infected persons. There are documented cases of fulminant hepatitis and liver enzyme flares in co-infected patients whose lamivudine-containing regimens were changed to regimens without an HBV active drug.[62,56] Published guidelines on management of opportunistic

Table 54-2

Selected clinical trials evaluating treatment of HBV in HIV co-infected patients

Study Reference	Size "N"	Treatment Regimen	Comparator	Mean ↓ in HBV DNA	Seroconversion Anti-HBe or Loss HBeAg	Seroconversion Anti-HBS or Loss HBSAg	Comments
Schmutz, 2006	75	TDF after LAM failure	TDF + LAM in naives	3 $\log_{10}$↓	36% vs. 24% Not significant	4% vs. 6% Not significant	Small study, 2 yr follow up
Benhamou, 2006	65	TDF	eAg+ vs. eAg−	4.6 log↓ vs. 2.5log↓	HBV DNA became undetect. in 82% of eAg− and 30% of eAg+		TDF works in precore mutants and in LAM resistant HBV
Stephan, 2005	31	TDF	Hi replicative Lo replicative	5.37 log↓	N = 2 became HBeAg−	N = 1 became sAg negative	No TDF resistance noted
Benhamou, 2006	35	ADF added to LAM	None	5.9 log↓ At 108 weeks	N = 2 became HBeAg−, Compared with 43% in HBV monoinfected patients		29/35 patients followed × 144 wks. No HIV ADF resistance mutations seen
DiMartino, 2002	26	IFN-α	HIV+ vs HIV−	7(27%) HIV+ vs. 56% HIV− Undet.	N = 4 (15%) HBeAg seroconversion at 3 years vs. 52% HBeAg seroconversion in HIV−	N = 1 became sAg negative	HIV+ responders had higher CD4, higher ALT; worse fibrosis vs. nonresponders
Dore, 1999	122	LAM	Placebo	2.7 log↓ At 52 weeks, vs. no ↓	N = 7 (22%) for LAM, vs. 0/7 for placebo with eAg seroconversion		Follow up limited to 52 wks. Study confirms dual action of LAM
Pessoa, 2005	68	ETV + LAM (in LAM experienced)	Placebo + LAM	3.7 log↓ At 24 weeks, vs. no ↓			Mean follow up of 40 weeks, adverse events comparable with placebo
Gish, 2005 (HBV mono-infection study only)	98	FTC	25 mg, 100 mg, 200 mg	2.4 log↓ 3.1 log↓ 2.9 log↓ (Wk 48)	eAg loss seen in 36% 38% 50% respectively	SAg loss in 0% 0% 3% respectively	Resistance develops more slowly to FTC, compared with LAM. Potent antiviral response seen for 2 yrs. 200 mg dose was chosen for future studies

Data from (1) Schmutz G, et al. Combination of tenofovir and lamivudine versus tenofovir after lamivudine failure for therapy of hepatitis B in HIV-coinfection. AIDS 20(15):1951–54, 2006; (2) Benhamou Y, et al. Anti-hepatitis B virus efficacy of tenofovir disoproxil fumarate in HIV-infected patients. Hepatology 43(3):548–55, 2006; (3) Stephan C, et al. Impact of tenofovir-containing antiretroviral therapy on chronic hepatitis B in a cohort co-infected with human immunodeficiency virus. J Antimicrob Chemother 56(6):1087–93, 2005; (4) Benhamoub Y, et al. Safety and efficacy of adefovir dipivoxil in patients infected with lamivudine-resistant hepatitis B and HIV-1. J Hepatol 44(1):62–7, 2006; (5) Di Martino V. et al. Influence of HIV infection on the response to interferon therapy and the long-term outcome of chronic hepatitis B. Gastroenterology 123(6):1812–22, 2002; (6) Dore GJ, et al. Dual efficacy of lamivudine treatment in human immunodeficiency virus/hepatitis B virus-coinfected persons in a randomized, controlled study (CAESAR). The CAESAR Coordinating Committee. J Infect Dis 180(3):607–13, 1999; (7) Pessoa W, et al., Entecavir in HIV/HBV-co-infected patients: safety and efficacy in a phase II study (ETV-038). In: 12th Conference on Retroviruses and Opportunistic Infections, Boston, MA, USA, 2005; (8) Gish RG, et al. Safety and antiviral activity of emtricitabine (FTC) for the treatment of chronic hepatitis B infection: a two-year study. J Hepatol 43(1):60–6, 2005.

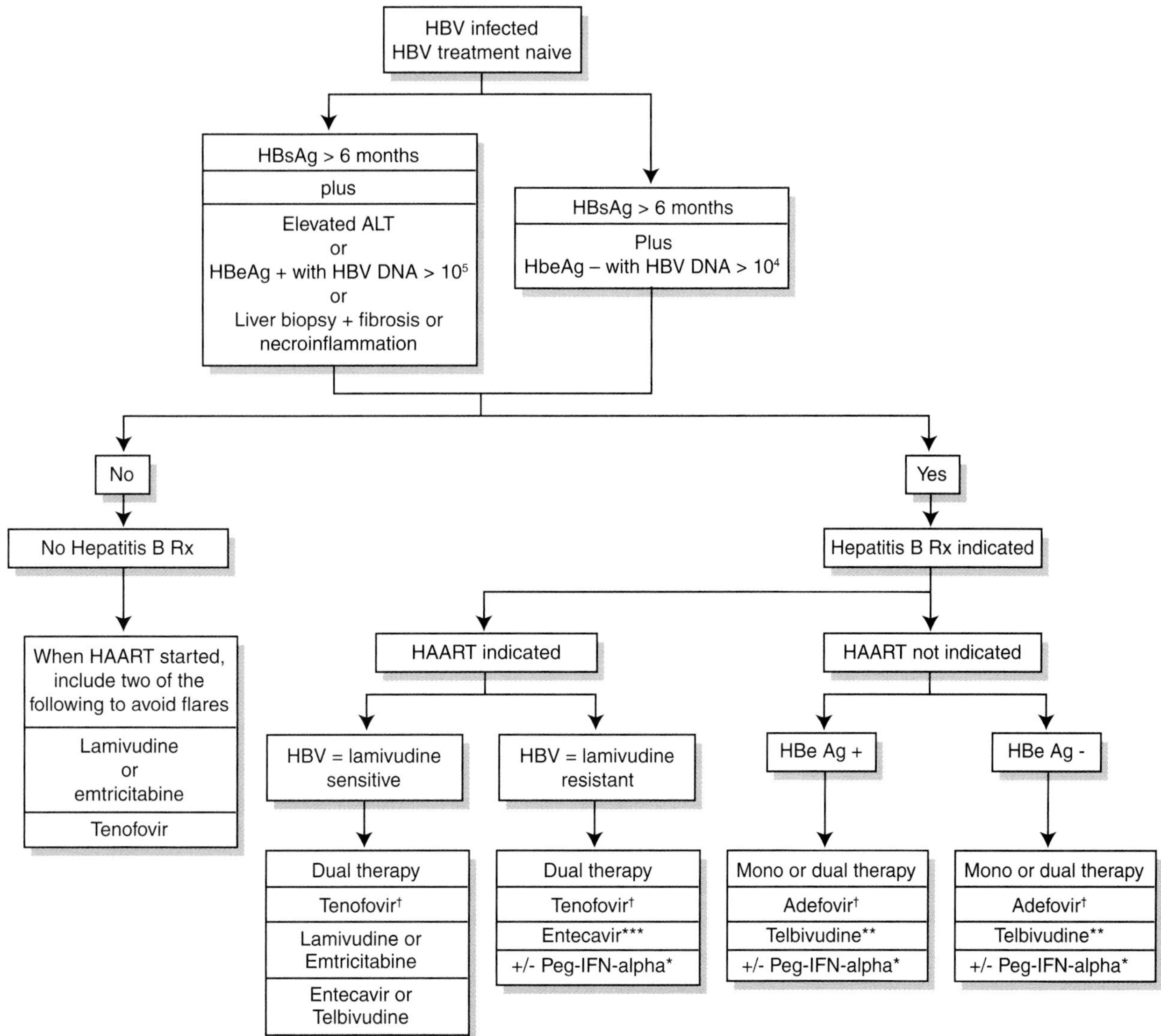

Figure 54-5 ■ Algorithm for treatment of hepatitis B in HIV-infected patients. The optimal duration for HBeAg negative persons is not known. Patients who become e antigen negative and anti-e-positive on therapy should be treated for a minimum of 12 months beyond the E antigen seroconversion. Patients who require HIV therapy should continue HBV therapy even if seroconversion to anti-HBe has taken place.

infections in HIV recommend that HBeAg positive, HIV/HBV-co-infected patients who become HBeAg negative and anti-HBeAg positive should be treated for a minimum of 1 year beyond HBeAg seroconversion.[13] For individuals who are HBeAg negative at the outset, there is no information on optimal treatment duration.[13]

Several newer drugs are being investigated for HBV treatment in clinical trials. These include nucleoside analogs telbivudine (now approved for HBV monotherapy), clevudine, elvucitabine, and valtorcitabine, none of which possess anti-HIV activity, as well as one more nucleoside analog, DAPD, which is active against both viruses.[8] Regardless of the regimen used, all chronically HBV infected persons should be counseled to avoid alcohol consumption to minimize further liver damage.

Prevention

All HIV-infected persons should be screened for HBV infection with HbsAg, HbsAb, and anti-HbcAb. Nonimmune persons should receive the HBV vaccine series. Those individuals with isolated anti-HBcAb should also be vaccinated, as the majority of these patients are not immune to hepatitis B infection.[62a] Partners of patients who are HBsAg positive should be offered vaccination as well.[63] Unfortunately, HIV-infected subjects have a lower seroconversion rate and less durable response to the HBV vaccine series compared to HIV-uninfected persons.[64,65] Not surprisingly, the individuals with CD4+ T-lymphocyte counts over 500 respond better than those with CD4+ T-lymphocyte between 200 and 500.[66] Limited data suggest that doubling the number of hepatitis B vaccinations in HIV-infected patients might improve the anti-HBS response. However, even with additional dosing of vaccine, the antibody response is short lived. A more effective strategy would be to strive to immunize patients at higher CD4+ T-lymphocyte counts. In a study by the United States military, HAART was found to improve vaccine efficacy independently of CD4+ T-lymphocyte count. Of 24 individuals with clinical vaccine failures, 23 were not on HAART at the time of vaccination. Co-infection with HCV also predicts HBV vaccine failure,[65,67] and further strategies to improve HBV vaccine immunogenicity in HIV-infected persons are needed.[67] Recent guidelines state that HIV-infected patients with a CD4 count >350 cells/mm^3 should be vaccinated with 40 micrograms (twice the usual dose) of vaccine at 0, 1, and 6 months. The vaccine response may be evaluated 4 weeks after the series completion; a second series should be considered in those who have not attained anti-HBSAb >10 IU/ml.[62a]

Despite the ready availability of HBV vaccine in industrialized nations for many years, numerous agencies continue to report low coverage rates of vulnerable populations in HIV clinics. In France, a study of 1849 patients showed that among those not infected with HBV, only 10.3% had received three doses of the vaccine.[68] Similarly low coverage rates for at risk populations have been reported in North America and Australia as well.[69,70] These data suggest that a sizable population exists in whom enhanced HBV vaccination strategies could be studied. Hepatitis A vaccine is especially important in nonimmune persons with chronic liver disease, in order to prevent potentially fulminant acute Hepatitis A infection in these individuals.

The Role of Liver Transplantation

Orthotopic liver transplants have been offered to a limited number of HIV/HBV-co-infected subjects with ESLD. Because of complicated interactions between antiretroviral drugs and immunosuppressants, careful monitoring, dose adjustments, and a multidisciplinary group of care providers are required to care for these patients. While data remain limited, the evidence suggests that HIV infection is not a valid reason to withhold organ transplantation from individuals who could potentially benefit from this life-prolonging procedure.[71–73] In one study, the 12-, 24-, and 36-month survival rates after liver transplant in HIV-infected persons were 87%, 73%, and 73% respectively, compared with 86.6%, 81.2%, and 78% in HIV-negative persons.[71] In HIV/HBV patients, HBV recurrence after transplant can be prevented with combination prophylaxis using hepatitis B immune globulin and antivirals.[74] A number of centers across the United States are performing solid organ transplants in HIV-infected individuals with carefully designed standard protocols and prospective monitoring. These studies will answer important questions that remain regarding patient selection and clinical management of solid organ transplantation in HIV-infected persons.[72–75]

HEPATITIS G VIRUS/GB VIRUS C

Virology

Although GBV-C is a nonpathogenic virus, it commonly co-infects persons with HIV, and may influence HIV disease pathogenesis. Hepatitis G virus (HGV) and GB virus subtype C (GBV-C) are two different isolates of the same virus. The 'GB-agent' was described in 1967 after inoculation of marmosets with serum from a surgeon with post-transfusion non-A, non-B hepatitis.[76] Initially, two viruses, GBV type A and type B, were identified through analysis of the marmoset serum. However, these viruses were later determined to be marmoset viruses.[77] The same group identified a related virus in human serum that they called GBV-C.[77] Another group subsequently reported on a virus isolated from a patient with cryptogenic hepatitis and patients with non-A to non-E hepatitis that they termed HGV.[78] There is 96% homology between the genomes of HGV and GBV-C, which are also closely related to HCV.[79] Later work showed not only that the surgeon 'GB' did not harbor HGV/GBV-C, but also that the virus is not associated with hepatitis, suggesting that both are misnomers. For clarity, the term GBV-C will be used to designate this virus in this chapter.

GBV-C is a flavivirus, phylogenetically most closely related to HCV with ~30% amino acid homology.[79] Like HCV, it has a single-stranded RNA genome that is ~9400 nucleotides long. The viral polyprotein is processed by cellular and viral proteases into eight or more proteins.[80] Whereas HCV replicates primarily in hepatocytes, GBV-C replicates in CD4+ T lymphocytes and CD8+ T lymphocytes as well as in B lymphocytes.[81–83] The GBV-C major envelope glycoprotein, E2, is not as extensively glycosylated[77,80] as in HCV and the HCV hypervariable region, thought to be involved in immune escape and viral persistence, is lacking. In longitudinal studies, fewer than 1% of immunocompetent individuals with GBV-C viremia display detectable GBV-C antibody titers.[80] Over 75% of GBV-C infected individuals will naturally clear this virus.

Phylogenetic analysis reveals six major GBV-C genotypes that correlate with distinct ethnicity or geographic locations.[84,85] The first genotype described is confined to sub-Saharan Africa. Populations from India, North Africa, and Europe are primarily infected with genotype 2. Genotype 3 represents most of the GBV-C sequences from East Asia. Genotype 4 is unique to

Southeast Asia, genotype 5 was discovered in South Africa, and genotype 6 was isolated in Indonesia.[85] Genomic sequencing and phylogenetic analysis suggest that the virus is ancient,[84] and that it likely originated in Africa.[86]

Diagnosis, Animal Models, and *In Vitro* Culture

Diagnostic tests for GBV-C are used in research, and are not clinically useful tools. The presence of GBV-C RNA in serum by nucleic acid amplification indicates active infection.[77,78] Quantification is achieved using branched chain DNA assays,[87] real-time (TaqMan) polymerase chain reaction[88,89] and terminal dilution methods.[90] Accurate detection of GBV-C viremia may require the use of primers from multiple genome regions.[91] Anti-E2 antibody appearance is temporally related to clearance of GBV-C viremia, appears protective against reinfection,[92] and is only rarely detectable during viremia.[93] There is evidence that E2 antibody titers in serum decline over time; ~5% of HIV-uninfected individuals and 29% of HIV-infected individuals lose antibody over a 10.7-year period.[94]

Nonhuman primate models in China have been used for studying GBV-C replication and pathogenesis[95–98] though there are several failed attempts to infect chimpanzees and macaques.[99] An *in vitro* system has been developed using peripheral blood mononuclear cells (PBMCs) to culture some isolates of GBV-C.[81]

Epidemiology, Natural History and Clinical Relevance

Epidemiology and Transmission of GBV-C

Infection with GBV-C is extremely common and widely dispersed among human populations even extending to highly isolated populations in Papua New Guinea and Central Africa. Approximately 2% of healthy blood donors in the United States have GBV-C detectable in their blood and 16% have detectable GBV-C E2 antibody.[100,101] Prevalence of active infection among immunocompetent individuals worldwide ranges from 2% to 15%, with the highest rates reported from Africa.[102,103] Thousands of different standard primer sets used for detection of GBV-C RNA by nested RT-PCR may account for the wide variability in prevalence noted in published studies.[91]

GBV-C is transmitted sexually, vertically, and by exposure to contaminated blood. Among GBV-C viremic individuals, the virus has been detected in saliva and semen.[104] Transmission of GBV-C by sexual and vertical routes appears to be more efficient than that of HIV or HCV.[105] Among hemophiliacs treated with documented amounts of nonvirus-inactivated clotting factor, the rate of GBV-C infection (40.3%) was less than that of HIV (56.3%) and HCV (98.6%) and did not increase with increasing amounts of clotting factor, suggesting there may be host factors that prevent parenteral transmission of GBV-C.[106] Among chronically HCV-infected individuals, 15–20% have active GBV-C infection and up to 70% are E2 antibody positive.[80,101] Relatively low rates of GBV-C viremia among HCV-infected individuals, despite evidence for extensive GBV-C exposure, imply greater GBV-C clearance in HCV.[99] The conservation of T cell epitopes between HCV and GBV-C may provide some immunological protection,[99] this is one hypothesis regarding these observations. It has been hypothesized (or Expert opinion hypothesizes) that conservation of T cell epitopes between HCV and GVV-C may provide some immunological protection.

Epidemiology of GBV-C in HIV Disease

Due to shared modes of transmission, GBV-C co-infection among HIV-infected individuals is not uncommon. Several large trials of HIV-infected individuals reveal rates of 17–42% with GBV-C viremia and another 19–57% with detectable antibody to E2.[93,107–110] The highest prevalence rates of GBV-C have been noted in two cohort studies of homosexual men: 85% in the Multicenter AIDS Cohort Study (39% GBV-C viremic and 46% E2 positivity) and 83% in the Amsterdam Cohort Series of Homosexual Men (42% GBV-C viremic and 41% E2 positivity).[93,108] Aside from two studies of HIV/HCV-co-infected hemophiliacs where GBV-C viremia was 17% (n = 131)[111] and 26.8% (n = 41),[112] prospective studies of GBV-C among large cohorts of HIV/HCV-co-infected individuals are lacking. Higher clearance among intravenous drug users may be explained by HCV co-infection.[80,99] Overall, HIV-infected individuals have less GBV-C clearance (~50%) than seen among other populations.[80] GBV-C RNA clearance, and E2 antibody clearance occurs with interferon treatment for HCV, though some studies report this to be a transient phenomenon.[87,88]

Evidence for GBV-C clearance with interferon therapy raises the concern that eradication of GBV-C during HCV treatment could negatively impact HIV disease progression. This theoretical concern has not been supported by early studies. A retrospective study of 130 HIV/HCV-co-infected subjects enrolled in a multicenter randomized trial (ACTG 5071) studying the efficacy of standard interferon alpha with ribavirin versus pegylated interferon with ribavirin treatment for chronic HCV infection documented 85% (111/130) GBV-C infection: 40 GBV-C RNA-positive subjects and 71 subjects with antibody to E2. After completion of 24 weeks of treatment, GBV-C RNA clearance was documented among 50% of GBV-C viremic individuals. Sustained clearance was found in 31% of subjects and was not associated with changes in HIV load or with CD4+ T-lymphocyte cell counts.[113] This study also found that co-infection with GBV-C genotype 2 was associated with significantly higher CD4+ T-lymphocyte cell counts; an observation worthy of further study. Other reports have suggested that GBV-C clearance with interferon therapy for HCV is modest and transient and therefore may not have substantial implications for HIV disease outcomes.[114,115] Jarvis et al. observed that GBV-C clearance was associated with HCV clearance among HIV/

HCV-co-infected individuals suggesting a possible link between clearances of the two viruses.[116]

Clinical Relevance of GBV-C in HIV Disease

Despite persistent GBV-C viremia among patients with acute or chronic hepatitis, this virus is not associated with liver disease or any other pathology.[117] Though transmission of GBV-C by blood transfusion has been documented, GBV-C screening is not recommended by the FDA.

Two reports suggesting that GBV-C may be beneficial in HIV disease[112,118] sparked investigations to determine the association between GBV-C status and HIV disease progression. Six of nine studies of survival among GBV-C/HIV-co-infected individuals provide epidemiologic evidence for a survival benefit with GBV-C infection. A Japanese study of HIV-infected hemophiliacs treated with either zidovudine (AZT) or AZT with didanosine ($n = 41$) showed delayed AIDS diagnosis and death among GBV-C RNA-positive subjects compared to GBV-C RNA-negative individuals.[112] A study of GBV-C infection among blood donors in Paris with early HIV disease ($n = 95$) showed that GBV-C viremic subjects had higher baseline CD4+ T-lymphocyte cell counts ($p = 0.02$), delayed progression to AIDS ($p = 0.05$) and improved survival ($p = 0.02$)[89] compared to subjects without GBV-C viremia. A study of HIV-infected subjects, most of whom received HAART, found higher mortality among the GBV-C RNA-negative group compared with the GBV-C RNA-positive group (relative risk 3.5), an effect most pronounced at lower CD4+ T-lymphocyte counts.[119] Another report provided data on a cohort[118] stratified before and after introduction of HAART. These data showed a survival benefit for GBV-C RNA-positive individuals ($p < 0.001$) that remained significant even with HAART.[110] An inverse relationship was found between GBV-C viral load and HIV viral load ($r = -0.3$, $p < 0.001$) but there was no correlation between GBV-C viral load and CD4+ T-lymphocyte count.[110]

Analysis of data from the Multicenter AIDS Cohort Study (MACS) included GBV-C status among men at early (12–18 months) and late (5–6 years) time points after HIV seroconversion, censoring at 1996 to exclude bias attributed to HAART.[93] GBV-C viremia at the late, but not the early time point was associated with survival. Individuals positive for GBV-C RNA at 5–6 years after HIV seroconversion were 2.78 times more likely to survive than those without detectable GBV-C RNA at that time point ($p = 0.006$). The effect remained significant after controlling for CD4+ T-lymphocyte cell count and HIV viral load at both time points. Loss of GBV-C RNA at 5–6 years after HIV seroconversion was associated with the highest mortality compared to persistent GBV-C viremia and persistent GBV-C RNA-negativity.

Efforts to better understand GBV-C clearance include a cohort study of over 800 HIV-infected and uninfected women in Africa.[99] Preliminary results from this cohort of mostly immunocompetent women with multiple measurements of GBV-C RNA over 5.5 years suggest that intermittent loss of viremia is rare, but the rate of GBV-C clearance is significant and does not differ by HIV status. For HIV-infected women with GBV-C clearance, the average CD4+ T-lymphocyte cell count was greater than 300 cells.[99]

A study of 320 HIV-infected homosexual men in the Netherlands observed a beneficial effect ($p < 0.0001$) of persistent GBV-C infection on survival, with (hazard ratio (HR) of death ranging from 0.52 to 0.57.[108] Weaknesses of the study include missing data for CD4+ T-lymphocyte cell counts and HIV viral loads, as well as unknown HIV seroconversion dates for 62% of the subjects. The association between the loss of GBV-C RNA over time and decreased survival, however, is in agreement with other studies.

Three studies failed to find an association between GBV-C viremia and improved survival. Birk et al. used death from AIDS rather than all-cause mortality as the outcome of interest. GBV-C RNA status was determined within 0.75 years after HIV seroconversion and subjects were followed for a median of 7.0 years (range 1–12). There was no significant difference in AIDS-related death by GBV-RNA status ($p = 0.6$).[120] Bjorkman et al studied GBV-C status within 2 years of HIV diagnosis among 230 HIV-infected subjects in association with survival for a median of 4.3 years (range 1.6–8.8). Baseline GBV-C status was not associated with survival ($p = 0.12$). Consistent with the findings of others, loss of GBV-C RNA over time without E2 seroconversion was associated with increased all-cause mortality in this HAART-naive cohort ($p = 0.018$).[109] There was no association between GBV-C status and mortality among women enrolled in a perinatal transmission study in the Gambia. However the majority of subjects in the study were infected with HIV-2.[121] Two studies found no significant association between GBV-C status and mother-to-child transmission of HIV.[122,123]

To assess evidence regarding GBV-C status and outcomes in HIV disease, a meta-analysis of 11 prospective studies testing for both GBV-C RNA and GBV-C E2 antibody with death as a primary outcome was performed.[124] Results were grouped by whether GBV-C was measured within 2 years of HIV seroconversion ('early') or not ('late'). GBV-C status within the first 2 years after HIV seroconversion was not associated with survival, however, detectable GBV-C viremia more than 5 years after HIV seroconversion was associated with a significant reduction in the hazard for mortality (HR 0.41; 95% CI 0.23, 0.69). Taken together, the data suggest that persistent infection with GBV-C may be the key to the association between GBV-C and survival. Importantly, none of the studies analyzed (all observational) could imply direct causality for prolonged survival due to GBV-C.[124]

Bjorkman and colleagues hypothesized that the loss of GBV-C viremia with HIV progression may be due to suppression of GBV-C replication by HIV viremia, rather than GBV-C clearance. They longitudinally tested GBV-C/HIV co-infected, HAART-naive subjects ($n = 28$) for HIV and GBV-C viral loads prior to and subsequent to initiating HAART. They found that median GBV-C RNA titers increased significantly when HIV replication was suppressed on HAART

($p = 0.05$), and continued to increase with prolonged HIV suppression ($p = 0.002$). Among six subjects with HAART interruptions, GBV-C viral load decreased as HIV replication resumed after a median time of 1.8 years off-therapy ($p = 0.03$).[125] These data support a direct interaction between replication of the two viruses that is yet poorly understood.

SUMMARY

Available data indicate that the effect of GBV-C infection status on mortality in HIV disease changes over time and suggest that persistently detectable GBV-C RNA may be protective in HIV disease. GBV-C clearance without E2 seroconversion occurs frequently among HIV-infected individuals and is poorly understood. These data do not provide evidence for a causal relationship between GBV-C and improved survival. Whether maintenance of GBV-C viremia is protective or GBV-C loss is simply a marker of an unknown host immune mechanism associated with HIV disease progression or representative of CD4+ T-lymphocyte cell loss can not be explained by observational studies. A number of studies with *in vitro* data supporting biological mechanisms for these findings have been published, and are ongoing.[126–131]

Epidemiologic and *in vitro* data indicate that persistent viremia with this common, nonpathogenic virus is associated with a survival benefit in HIV-infected individuals.

The literature to date does not support GBV-C RNA testing as a prognostic index. Though understanding of the possible protective mechanisms of GBV-C is lacking, a protective effect would likely be multifactorial; related to some combination of direct antiviral effects, changes in chemokines resulting in decreased HIV co-receptor density on PBMCs and, perhaps, decreased Fas-mediated lymphocyte apoptosis.[58–63] Reproducible nonhuman primate models of GBV-C and GBV-C/SIV co-infection would advance the understanding of GBV-C in HIV disease.

Due to the complex interactions between HIV, GBV-C, and HCV, a better understanding of GBV-C may lead to advances in HIV and/or HCV research and management. For clinicians managing HIV/HCV-co-infected individuals, recent data show that GBV-C clearance with pegylated interferon and ribavirin is not harmful to HIV disease progression in the short term.[113,114] The question of whether interferon treatment for HIV/HCV/GBV-C-infected individuals may result in GBV-C clearance impacting deleteriously on HIV disease progression in the long term remains unanswered. Though epidemiologic data suggests that interferon therapy leads to modest and sometimes transient clearance of GBV-C, further studies of GBV-C in the context of clinical trials with longer follow-up periods are needed.

REFERENCES

1. Lee WM. Hepatitis B virus infection. N Engl J Med 337:1733–45, 1997.
2. Ganem D, Prince AM. Hepatitis B virus infection – natural history and clinical consequences. N Engl J Med 350:1118–29, 2004.
3. Kao JH. Hepatitis B viral genotypes: clinical relevance and molecular characteristics. J Gastroenterol Hepatol 17:643–50, 2002.
4. Ozasa A, Tanaka Y, Orito E, et al. Influence of genotypes and precore mutations on fulminant or chronic outcome of acute hepatitis B virus infection. Hepatology (Baltimore, MD) 44:326–34, 2006.
5. Lai CL, Shouval D, Lok AS, et al. Entecavir versus lamivudine for patients with HBeAg-negative chronic hepatitis B. N Engl J Med 354:1011–20, 2006.
6. Lok AS, McMahon BJ. Chronic hepatitis B. Hepatology (Baltimore, MD) 34:1225–41, 2001.
7. Soriano V, Puoti M, Bonacini M, et al. Care of patients with chronic hepatitis B and HIV co-infection: recommendations from an HIV-HBV International Panel. AIDS (London, England) 19:221–40, 2005.
8. Nunez M, Soriano V. Management of patients co-infected with hepatitis B virus and HIV. Lancet Infect Dis 5:374–82, 2005.
9. Thio CL, Sulkowski MS, Thomas DL. Treatment of chronic hepatitis B in HIV-infected persons: thinking outside the black box. Clin Infect Dis 41:1035–40, 2005

9a. Kim JW, Park SH, Louie SG. Telbivudine: a novel nucleoside analog for chronic hepatitis B. Ann Pharmacother 40:472–8, 2006.

10. Baron JL, Gardiner L, Nishimura S, et al. Activation of a nonclassical NKT cell subset in a transgenic mouse model of hepatitis B virus infection. Immunity 16:583–94, 2002.
11. Beasley RP. Hepatitis B virus. The major etiology of hepatocellular carcinoma. Cancer 61:1942–56, 1988.
12. Alter MJ. Epidemiology of viral hepatitis and HIV co-infection. Journal of hepatology 44(1 Suppl):S6–9, 2006.
13. Benson CA, Kaplan JE, Masur H, et al. Treating opportunistic infections among HIV-exposed and infected children: recommendations from CDC, the National Institutes of Health, and the Infectious Diseases Society of America. MMWR Recomm Rep 53(RR-15):1–112, 2006.
14. Shire NJ, Sherman KE. Management of hepatitis B virus in HIV-positive patients. Minerva gastroenterologica e dietologica 52:67–87, 2006.
15. Puoti M, Bruno R, Soriano V, et al. Hepatocellular carcinoma in HIV-infected patients: epidemiological features, clinical presentation and outcome. AIDS (London, England) 18:2285–93, 2004.
16. Chu CM. Natural history of chronic hepatitis B virus infection in adults with emphasis on the occurrence of cirrhosis and hepatocellular carcinoma. J Gastroenterol Hepatol 15(Suppl): E25–30, 2000.
17. Kato Y, Nakao K, Hamasaki K, et al. Spontaneous loss of hepatitis B surface antigen in chronic carriers, based on a long-term follow-up study in Goto Islands, Japan. J Gastroenterol 35:201–5, 2000.
18. Thio CL, Seaberg EC, Skolasky R, Jr., et al. HIV-1, hepatitis B virus, and risk of liver-related mortality in the Multicenter Cohort Study (MACS). Lancet 360:1921–6, 2002.
19. Puoti M, Spinetti A, Ghezzi A, et al. Mortality for liver disease in patients with HIV infection: a cohort study. J Acquir Immune Defic Syndr (1999) 24:211–17, 2000.
20. Konopnicki D, Mocroft A, de Wit S, et al. Hepatitis B and HIV: prevalence, AIDS progression, response to highly active antiretroviral therapy and increased mortality in the EuroSIDA cohort. AIDS (London, England) 19:593–601, 2005.
21. Bodsworth N, Donovan B, Nightingale BN. The effect of concurrent human immunodeficiency virus infection on chronic hepatitis B: a study of 150 homosexual men. J Infect Dis 160:577–82, 1989.

22. Housset C, Pol S, Carnot F, et al. Interactions between human immunodeficiency virus-1, hepatitis delta virus and hepatitis B virus infections in 260 chronic carriers of hepatitis B virus. Hepatology (Baltimore, MD) 15:578–83, 1992.
23. den Brinker M, Wit FW, Wertheim-van Dillen PM, et al. Hepatitis B and C virus co-infection and the risk for hepatotoxicity of highly active antiretroviral therapy in HIV-1 infection. AIDS (London, England) 14:2895–902, 2000.
24. De Luca A, Bugarini R, Lepri AC, et al. Coinfection with hepatitis viruses and outcome of initial antiretroviral regimens in previously naive HIV-infected subjects. Arch Intern Med 162:2125–32, 2002.
25. Saves M, Vandentorren S, Daucourt V, et al. Severe hepatic cytolysis: incidence and risk factors in patients treated by antiretroviral combinations. Aquitaine Cohort, France, 1996–1998. Groupe dEpidemiologie Clinique de Sida en Aquitaine (GECSA). AIDS (London, England) 13:F115–21, 1999.
26. Wit FW, Weverling GJ, Weel J, Jurriaans S, Lange JM. Incidence of and risk factors for severe hepatotoxicity associated with antiretroviral combination therapy. J Infect Dis 186:23–31, 2002.
27. Pol S, Lebray P, Vallet-Pichard A. HIV infection and hepatic enzyme abnormalities: intricacies of the pathogenic mechanisms. Clin Infect Dis 38(Suppl 2):S65–72, 2004.
28. Weber R, Sabin CA, Friis-Moller N, et al. Liver-related deaths in persons infected with the human immunodeficiency virus: the D:A:D study. Arch Inter Med 166:1632–41, 2006.
29. Lewden C, Salmon D, Morlat P, et al. Causes of death among human immunodeficiency virus (HIV)-infected adults in the era of potent antiretroviral therapy: emerging role of hepatitis and cancers, persistent role of AIDS. Int J Epidem 34:121–30, 2005.
30. Salmon-Ceron D, Lewden C, Morlat P, et al. Liver disease as a major cause of death among HIV infected patients: role of hepatitis C and B viruses and alcohol. J Hepatol 42:799–805, 2005.
31. Jain MK, Skiest DJ, Cloud JW, Jain CL, Burns D, Berggren RE. Changes in mortality related to human immunodeficiency virus infection: comparative analysis of inpatient deaths in 1995 and in 1999–2000. Clin Infect Dis 36:1030–8, 2003.
32. Matthews GV, Bartholomeusz A, Locarnini S, et al. Characteristics of drug resistant HBV in an international collaborative study of HIV-HBV-infected individuals on extended lamivudine therapy. AIDS (London, England) 20:863–70, 2006.
33. Grob P, Jilg W, Bornhak H, et al. Serological pattern 'anti-HBc alone': report on a workshop. J Med Virol 62:450–5, 2000.
34. Hofer M, Joller-Jemelka HI, Grob PJ, Luthy R, Opravil M. Frequent chronic hepatitis B virus infection in HIV-infected patients positive for antibody to hepatitis B core antigen only. Swiss HIV Cohort Study. Eur J Clin Microbiol Infect Dis 17:6–13, 1998.
35. Silva AE, McMahon BJ, Parkinson AJ, et al. Hepatitis B virus DNA in persons with isolated antibody to hepatitis B core antigen who subsequently received hepatitis B vaccine. Clin Infect Dis 26:895–7, 1998.
36. Lok AS, Lai CL, Wu PC. Prevalence of isolated antibody to hepatitis B core antigen in an area endemic for hepatitis B virus infection: implications in hepatitis B vaccination programs. Hepatology (Baltimore, MD) 8:766–70, 1988.
37. Leung N. Treatment of chronic hepatitis B: case selection and duration of therapy. J Gastroenterol Hepatol 17:409–14, 2002.
38. Cooksley WG. Treatment of hepatitis B with interferon and combination therapy. Clin Liver Dis 8:353–70, 2004.
39. ter Borg MJ, van Zonneveld M, Zeuzem S, et al. Patterns of viral decline during PEG-interferon alpha-2b therapy in HBeAg-positive chronic hepatitis B: relation to treatment response. Hepatology (Baltimore, MD) 44:721–7, 2006.
40. Wursthorn K, Lutgehetmann M, Dandri M, et al. Peginterferon alpha-2b plus adefovir induce strong cccDNA decline and HBsAg reduction in patients with chronic hepatitis B. Hepatology (Baltimore, MD) 44:675–84, 2006.
41. Kanwal F, Farid M, Martin P, et al. Treatment alternatives for hepatitis B cirrhosis: a cost-effectiveness analysis. Am J Gastroenterol 101:2076–89, 2006.
42. Robinson DM, Scott LJ, Plosker GL. Entecavir: a review of its use in chronic hepatitis B. Drugs 66:1605–22, 2006.
43. Hache C, Villeneuve JP. Lamivudine treatment in patients with chronic hepatitis B and cirrhosis. Expert opin Pharmacother 7:1835–43, 2006.
44. Sherman M, Yurdaydin C, Sollano J, et al. Entecavir for treatment of lamivudine-refractory, HBeAg-positive chronic hepatitis B. Gastroenterology 130:2039–49, 2006.
45. Chang TT, Gish RG, de Man R, et al. A comparison of entecavir and lamivudine for HBeAg-positive chronic hepatitis B. N Engl J Med 354:1001–10, 2006.
46. Benhamou Y, Bochet M, Thibault V, et al. Safety and efficacy of adefovir dipivoxil in patients co-infected with HIV-1 and lamivudine-resistant hepatitis B virus: an open-label pilot study. Lancet 358:718–23, 2001.
47. Benhamou Y. Treatment algorithm for chronic hepatitis B in HIV-infected patients. J Hepatol 44(1 Suppl):S90–4, 2006.
48. Dore GJ, Cooper DA, Pozniak AL, et al. Efficacy of tenofovir disoproxil fumarate in antiretroviral therapy-naive and experienced patients coinfected with HIV-1 and hepatitis B virus. J Infect Dis 189:1185–92, 2004.
49. Lada O, Benhamou Y, Cahour A, Katlama C, Poynard T, Thibault V. In vitro susceptibility of lamivudine-resistant hepatitis B virus to adefovir and tenofovir. Antivir Ther 9:353–63, 2004.
50. Ristig MB, Crippin J, Aberg JA, et al. Tenofovir disoproxil fumarate therapy for chronic hepatitis B in human immunodeficiency virus/hepatitis B virus-coinfected individuals for whom interferon-alpha and lamivudine therapy have failed. The J Infect Dis 186:1844–7, 2002.
51. Stephan C, Berger A, Carlebach A, et al. Impact of tenofovir-containing antiretroviral therapy on chronic hepatitis B in a cohort co-infected with human immunodeficiency virus. J Antimicrob Chemother 56:1087–93, 2005.
52. Nelson M, Portsmouth S, Stebbing J, et al. An open-label study of tenofovir in HIV-1 and Hepatitis B virus co-infected individuals. AIDS (London, England) 17:F7–10, 2003.
53. Levy V, Grant RM. Antiretroviral therapy for hepatitis B virus-HIV-coinfected patients: promises and pitfalls. Clin Infect Dis 43:904–10, 2006.
54. Xu XW, Chen YG. Current therapy with nucleoside/nucleotide analogs for patients with chronic hepatitis B. Hepatobiliary Pancreat Dis Int 5:350–9, 2006.
55. Lim SG, Krastev Z, Ng TM, et al. Randomized, double-blind study of emtricitabine (FTC) plus clevudine versus FTC alone in treatment of chronic hepatitis B. Antimicrob Agents Chemother 50:1642–8, 2006.
56. Hirsch M. Entecavir surprise. N Engl J Med 356, 2007.
56a. The HBV Drug Entecavir – Effects on HIV-1 replication and resistance. N Engl J M 356:2614–21, 2007.
57. Puoti M, Airoldi M, Bruno R, et al. Hepatitis B virus co-infection in human immunodeficiency virus-infected subjects. AIDS reviews 4:27–35, 2002.
58. Cooksley WG, Piratvisuth T, Lee SD, et al. Peginterferon alpha-2a (40 kDa): an advance in the treatment of hepatitis B e antigen-positive chronic hepatitis B. J Viral Hepat 10:298–305, 2003.
59. Thibault V, Benhamou Y, Seguret C, et al. Hepatitis B virus (HBV) mutations associated with resistance to lamivudine in patients coinfected with HBV and human immunodeficiency virus. J Clin Microbiol 37:3013–6, 1999.

60. Benhamou Y. Antiretroviral therapy and HIV/hepatitis B virus coinfection. Clin Infect Dis 38(Suppl 2):S98–103, 2004.
61. Nelson M, Bhagani S, Fisher M, et al. A 48-week study of tenofovir or lamivudine or a combination of tenofovir and lamivudine for the treatment of chronic hepatitis B in HIV/HBV-co-infected individuals. In: 13th Conference on Retroviruses and Opportunistic Infections. Denver, CO, USA; 2006.
62. Bessesen M, Ives D, Condreay L, Lawrence S, Sherman KE. Chronic active hepatitis B exacerbations in human immunodeficiency virus-infected patients following development of resistance to or withdrawal of lamivudine. Clin Infect Dis 28:1032–5, 1999.
62a. DHHS-IDSA Guidelines for the Prevention and Treatment of Opportunistic Infections in HIV-Infected Adults.
63. Aberg JA, Gallant JE, Anderson J, et al. Primary care guidelines for the management of persons infected with human immunodeficiency virus: recommendations of the HIV Medicine Association of the Infectious Diseases Society of America. Clin Infect Dis 39:609–29, 2004.
64. Pasricha N, Datta U, Chawla Y, et al. Poor responses to recombinant HBV vaccination in patients with HIV infection. Trop Gastroenterol 26:178–82, 2005.
65. Zhang W, Chaloner K, Tillmann HL, et al. Effect of early and late GBV-C viremia on survival of HIV-infected individuals: a meta-analysis. HIV Med 7 173–180, 2006.
65a. Landrum M, Rasnake M, Bradley W, Murray C, Dolan M, Agan B. The clinical efficacy of hepatitis B vaccine in HIV-1-infected individuals. In: 13th Conference on Retroviruses and Opportunistic Infections, Denver, CO, USA, 2006.
66. Rey D, Krantz V, Partisani M, et al. Increasing the number of hepatitis B vaccine injections augments anti-HBs response rate in HIV-infected patients. Effects on HIV-1 viral load. Vaccine 18:1161–5, 2000.
67. Gandhi RT, Wurcel A, Lee H, et al. Response to hepatitis B vaccine in HIV-1-positive subjects who test positive for isolated antibody to hepatitis B core antigen: implications for hepatitis B vaccine strategies. J Infect Dis 191:1435–41, 2005.
68. Salmon D, Larsen C, Pialoux G, et al. HBV/HIV Co-infection and HBV vaccination in a national hospital survey. In: 13th Conference on Retroviruses and Opportunistic Infections, Denver, CO, 2006, abstract #839.
69. Remis RS, Dufour A, Alary M, et al. Association of hepatitis B virus infection with other sexually transmitted infections in homosexual men. Omega Study Group. Am J Pub Health 90:1570–4, 2000.
70. Winstock AR, Anderson CM, Sheridan J. National survey of HIV and hepatitis testing and vaccination services provided by drug and alcohol agencies in Australia. Med J Aust 184:560–2, 2006.
71. Ragni MV, Belle SH, Im K, et al. Survival of human immunodeficiency virus-infected liver transplant recipients. J Infect Dis 188:1412–20, 2003.
72. Roland ME, Stock PG. Solid organ transplantation is a reality for patients with HIV infection. Curr HIV/AIDS Rep 3:132–8, 2006.
73. Roland ME, Stock PG. Liver transplantation in HIV-infected recipients. Seminars Liver Dis 26:273–84, 2006.
74. Terrault NA, Carter JT, Carlson L, Roland ME, Stock PG. Outcome of patients with hepatitis B virus and human immunodeficiency virus infections referred for liver transplantation. Liver Transpl 12:801–7, 2006.
75. Norris S, Taylor C, Muiesan P, et al. Outcomes of liver transplantation in HIV-infected individuals: the impact of HCV and HBV infection. Liver Transpl 10:1271–8, 2004.
76. Deinhardt F, Holmes AW, Capps RB, Popper H. Studies on the transmission of human viral hepatitis to marmoset monkeys. I. Transmission of disease, serial passages, and description of liver lesions. J Exp Med 125:673–88, 1967.
77. Simons JN, Leary TP, Dawson GJ, et al. Isolation of novel virus-like sequences associated with human hepatitis. Nat Med 1:564–9, 1995.
78. Linnen J, Wages J Jr, Zhang-Keck ZY, et al. Molecular cloning and disease association of hepatitis G virus: a transfusion-transmissible agent. Science 271:505–8, 1996.
79. Leary TP, Muerhoff AS, Simons JN, et al. Sequence and genomic organization of GBV-C: a novel member of the flaviviridae associated with human non-A–E hepatitis. J Med Virol 48:60–7, 1996.
80. Stapleton JT. GB virus type C/Hepatitis G virus. Semin Liver Dis 23:137–48, 2003.
81. Fogeda M, Navas S, Martin J, et al. In vitro infection of human peripheral blood mononuclear cells by GB virus C/Hepatitis G virus. J Virol 73:4052–61, 1999.
82. Handa A, Brown KE. GB virus C/hepatitis G virus replicates in human haematopoietic cells and vascular endothelial cells. J Gen Virol 81(Pt 10):2461–9, 2000.
83. George SL, Varmaz D, Stapleton JT. GB Virus C Replicates in Primary T and B Lymphocytes. J Infect Dis 193:451–4, 2006.
84. Smith DB, Basaras M, Frost S, et al. Phylogenetic analysis of GBV-C/hepatitis G virus. J Gen Virol 81:769–80, 2000.
85. Muerhoff AS, Dawson GJ, Desai SM. A previously unrecognized sixth genotype of GB virus C revealed by analysis of5'-untranslated region sequences. J Med Virol 78:105–11, 2006.
86. Muerhoff AS, Leary TP, Sathar MA, et al. African origin of GB virus C determined by phylogenetic analysis of a complete genotype 5 genome from South Africa. J Gen Virol 86:1729–35, 2005.
87. Tillmann HL, Manns MP. GB virus-C infection in patients infected with the human immunodeficiency virus. Antiviral Res 52:83–90, 2001.
88. George SL, Xiang J, Stapleton JT. Clinical isolates of GB virus type C vary in their ability to persist and replicate in peripheral blood mononuclear cell cultures. Virology 316:191–201, 2003.
89. Lefrere JJ, Roudot-Thoraval F, Morand-Joubert L, et al. Carriage of GB virus C/hepatitis G virus RNA is associated with a slower immunologic, virologic, and clinical progression of human immunodeficiency virus disease in coinfected persons. J Infect Dis 179:783–9, 1999.
90. Xiang J, Wunschmann S, Schmidt W, et al. Full-length GB virus C (hepatitis G virus) RNA transcripts are infectious in primary CD4-positive T cells. J Virol 74:9125–33, 2000.
91. Souza IE, Allen JB, Zhang W, et al. Primer selection influences GBV-C viremia detection rates and epidemiological outcomes in HIV-positive populations In: The 3rd International AIDS Society Conference on HIV Pathogenesis and Treatment, Rio de Janeiro, 2005.
92. Thomas DL, Vlahov D, Alter HJ, et al. Association of antibody to GB virus C (hepatitis G virus) with viral clearance and protection from reinfection. J Infect Dis 177:539–42, 2000.
93. Williams CF, Klinzman D, Yamashita TE, et al. Persistent GB virus C infection and survival in HIV-infected men. N Engl J Med 350:981–90, 2004.
94. Stapleton JT, Williams CF, Xiang J. GB virus type C: a beneficial infection? J Clin Microbiol 42:3915–9, 2004.
95. Bukh J, Kim JP, Govindarajan S, et al. Experimental infection of chimpanzees with hepatitis G virus and genetic analysis of the virus. J Infect Dis 177:855–62, 1998.
96. Wang XT, Zhuang H, Li HM, et al. Macaca mulatta as an animal model for HGV infection. Zhonghua Weishengwuxue He Mianyixue Zazhi 17:363–5, 1997.
97. Mao PY, He HX, Hong SW, et al. Study on the experimental infection of hepatitis G virus in rhesus monkey. Zhonghua Shiyan He Linchuang Bingduxue Zazhi 12:258–60, 1998.

98. Ren H, Zhu FL, Cao MM, et al. Hepatitis G virus genomic RNA is pathogenic to Macaca mulatta. World J Gastroenterol 11:970–5, 2005.
99. Stapleton JT (personal Communication February 7, 2006).
100. Dawson GJ, Schlauder GG, Pilot-Matias TJ, et al. Prevalence studies of GB virus-C infection using reverse transcriptase-polymerase chain reaction. J Med Virol 50:97–103, 1996.
101. Tacke M, Schmolke S, Schlueter V, et al. Humoral immune response to the E2 protein of hepatitis G virus is associated with long-term recovery from infection and reveals a high frequency of hepatitis G virus exposure among healthy blood donors. Hepatology 26:1626–33, 1997.
102. Tuveri R, Perret JL, Delaporte E, et al. Prevalence and genetic variants of hepatitis GB-C/HG and TT viruses in Gabon, equatorial Africa. Am J Trop Med Hyg 63:192–8, 2000.
103. Casteling A, Song E, Sim J, et al. GB virus C prevalence in blood donors and high risk groups for parenterally transmitted agents from Gauteng, South Africa. J Med Virol 55:103–8, 1998.
104. Bourlet T, Berthelot P, Grattard F, et al. Detection of GB virus C/hepatitis G virus in semen and saliva of HIV type-1 infected men. Clin Microbiol Infect 8:352–7, 2002.
105. Ramia S, Mokhbat J, Sibai A, Klayme S, Naman R. Exposure rates to hepatitis C and G virus infections among HIV-infected patients: evidence of efficient transmission of HGV by the sexual route. Int J STD AIDS 15:463–6, 2004.
106. Kupfer B, Ruf T, Matz B, et al. Comparison of GB virus C, HIV, and HCV infection markers in hemophiliacs exposed to non-inactivated or inactivated factor concentrates. J Clin Virol 34:42–7, 2005.
107. Rey D, Vidinic-Moularde J, Meyer P, et al. High prevalence of GB virus C/hepatitis G virus RNA and antibodies in patients infected with human immunodeficiency virus type 1. Eur J Clin Microbiol Infect Dis 19:721–4, 2000.
108. Van der Bij AK, Kloosterboer N, Prins M, et al. GB virus C coinfection and HIV-1 disease progression: The Amsterdam Cohort Study. J Infect Dis 191:678–85, 2005.
109. Bjorkman P, Flamholc L, Naucler A, et al. GB virus C during the natural course of HIV-1 infection: viremia at diagnosis does not predict mortality. AIDS 18:877–86, 2004.
110. Tillmann HL, Heiken H, Knapik-Botor A, et al. Infection with GB virus C and reduced mortality among HIV-infected patients. N Engl J Med 345:715–24, 2001.
111. Yeo AE, Matsumoto A, Hisada M, et al. Effect of hepatitis G virus infection on progression of HIV infection in patients with hemophilia. Multicenter Hemophilia Cohort Study. Ann Intern Med 132:959–63, 2000.
112. Toyoda H, Fukuda Y, Hayakawa T, et al. Effect of GB virus C/hepatitis G virus coinfection on the course of HIV infection in hemophilia patients in Japan. J Acquir Immune Defic Syndr Hum Retrovirol 17:209–13, 1998.
113. Schwarze-Zander C. GB virus-C clearance in HIV-HCV co-infected patients receiving interferon and ribavirin treatment. In: 1st International Workshop on HIV and Hepatitis Coinfection, Amsterdam, The Netherlands, 2004.
114. Lau DT, Miller KD, Detmer J, et al. Hepatitis G virus and human immunodeficiency virus coinfection: response to interferon-alpha therapy. J Infect Dis 180:1334–7, 1999.
115. Cheng PN, Jen CM, Young KC, et al. High-dose interferon-alpha 2b plus ribavirin combination therapy for GB virus-C/hepatitis G virus infection – a study in patients with chronic hepatitis C. Hepatogastroenterology 50:449–52, 2003.
116. Jarvis LM, Bell H, Simmonds P, et al. The effect of treatment with alpha-interferon on hepatitis G/GBV-C viraemia. The CONSTRUCT Group. Scand J Gastroenterol 33:195–200, 1998.
117. Alter HJ, Nakatsuji Y, Melpolder J, et al. The incidence of transfusion-associated hepatitis G virus infection and its relation to liver disease. N Engl J Med 336:747–54, 1997.
118. Heringlake S, Ockenga J, Tillmann HL, et al. GB virus C/hepatitis G virus infection: a favorable prognostic factor in human immunodeficiency virus-infected patients? J Infect Dis 177:1723–6, 1998.
119. Xiang J, Wunschmann S, Diekema DJ, et al. Effect of coinfection with GB virus C on survival among patients with HIV infection. N Engl J Med 345:707–14, 2001.
120. Birk M, Lindback S, Lidman C. No influence of GB virus C replication on the prognosis in a cohort of HIV-1-infected patients. AIDS 16:2482–5, 2002.
121. Kaye S, Howard M, Alabi A, et al. No observed effect of GB virus C coinfection on disease progression in a cohort of African woman infected with HIV-1 or HIV-2. Clin Infect Dis 40:876–8, 2005.
122. Weintrob AC, Hamilton JD, Hahn C, et al. Active or prior GB virus C infection does not protect against vertical transmission of HIV in coinfected women from Tanzania. Clin Infect Dis 38:e46–8, 2004.
123. Barqasho B, Naver L, Bohlin AB, Lindgren S, Hultgren C, Birk M. GB virus C coinfection and vertical transmission in HIV-infected mothers before the introduction of antiretroviral prophylaxis. HIV Med 5:427–30, 2004.
124. Zhang W, Chaloner K, Tillmann HL, Williams CF, Stapleton JT, Effect of early and late GBV-C viremia on survival of HIV-infected individuals: a meta-analysis. HIV Med 7:173–80, 2006.
125. Bjorkman P, Letelier Molnegren V, Marshall A, Flamholc L, Guner N, Widell A. Enhanced Replication of GB Virus C in HIV-infected Patients Receiving HAART. In: 13th Conference on Retroviruses and Opportunistic Infections, Denver, 2006.
126. Xiang J, et al. Inhibition of HIV-1 replication by GB virus C infection through increases in RANTES, MIP-1alpha, MIP-1beta, and SDF-1. Lancet 363:2040–6, 2004.
127. Nattermann J, et al. Regulation of CC chemokine receptor 5 in hepatitis G virus infection. Aids 17:1457–62, 2003.
128. Jung S, et al. HIV entry inhibition by the envelope 2 glycoprotein of GB virus C. Aids 21:645–47, 2007.
129. Kaufman TM, McLinden JH, Xiang J, Engel AM, Stapleton JT. The GBV-C envelope glycoprotein E2 does not interact specifically with CD81. Aids 21:1045–48, 2007.
130. Nunnari G, et al. Slower progression of HIV-1 infection in persons with GB virus C co-infection correlates with an intact T-helper 1 cytokine profile. Ann Intern Med 139:26–30, 2003.
131. Moekemeyer M, Heiken H, Schmidt R. Decreased Fas Expression on Natural Killer Cells in GBV-C Co-infected HIV-1 Patients. In: 13th Conference on Retroviruses and Opportunistic Infections (Denver, 2006).

Chapter 55

Hepatitis C Infection

Mark S. Sulkowski, MD

Human immunodeficiency virus (HIV)-infected persons have an increased incidence of hepatitis C and an accelerated course of chronic liver disease, leading to a relatively high incidence of liver-related morbidity and mortality in the era of highly effective antiretroviral therapy (ART). Accordingly, the US Public Health Service (USPHS), Infectious Diseases Society of America (IDSA), American Association for the Study of Liver Diseases and the European Consensus panel have published guidelines on the management of HCV infection in persons with HIV.[1–4] In this chapter, the pathogen, epidemiology/natural history, diagnosis, treatment, and prevention are discussed. Emphasis is placed on clinical issues of greatest importance to the HIV-infected patient.

PATHOGEN

The hepatitis C virus (HCV) is a spherical, enveloped RNA virus, classified within the *Hepacivirus* genus of the Flaviviridae family. The positive-sense, single-stranded, ~9.6-kb RNA genome contains a single large (~3000-amino acid) open reading frame flanked by 3 + 9 and 5 + 9 untranslated regions.[5] The open reading frame encodes for at least 10 proteins including four structural proteins (core protein, envelope proteins E1 and E2, NS2A) and six nonstructural proteins (*cis*-active Zn^2 + 1-dependent proteinase, serine proteinase, NTPase, RNA helicase, NS3 proteinase cofactor and RNA-dependent RNA polymerase).

Replication of HCV chiefly occurs in the cytoplasm of hepatocytes, although some studies have suggested that replication may occur in some other cell types, such as B cells, T cells, and monocytes. In chronically infected humans, mathematic models of HCV kinetics suggest that up to 1.0×10^{12} virions are produced daily with a half-life of ~2.5 h.[6] This high level of virion turnover coupled with the lack of proofreading by the RNA polymerase results in the rapid accumulation of mutations, estimated at a rate of 0.90×10^{-3} 1.92×10^{-3} base substitutions per year.[7,8] Consequently, within each infected person, HCV exists as a quasispecies, a group of closely related variants that typically share 91–99% sequence identity. HCV sequences from different individuals may have less than 60% RNA identity, and six major genotypes have been identified.[9] HCV strains are further classified into subtypes that typically share 75–85% nucleotide sequence identity.[10,11] Although the natural history of HCV genotypes does not seem to vary, there are dramatic intergenotypic differences in responsiveness to interferon-based therapies.

EPIDEMIOLOGY AND NATURAL HISTORY

Epidemiology

Hepatitis C virus is transmitted chiefly by percutaneous exposure to blood. Although transfusion of contaminated blood and blood products was once a major source of HCV transmission, HCV transmission by administration of clotting factors diminished in the United States and Europe during the mid-1980s because of viral inactivation procedure and use of recombinant products.[12] In addition, during the early 1990s when blood donations were routinely screened for HCV antibody, the incidence of post-transfusion HCV infection dropped to less than 1:100 000 per unit transfused in the United States.[13] After 1999 the risk of transfusion transmission of HCV declined even further (1:1.8 million per unit transfused) because of routine screening of donations for HCV RNA.[14] Injection drug use is the leading route of HCV transmission in the United States. Indeed, worldwide, 50–90% of injection drug users are HCV infected as a consequence of sharing contaminated needles and drug-use equipment.[12,15,16]

The HCV can also be transmitted between sexual partners and from mother to the infant.[17] A higher than expected HCV prevalence is frequently found in persons reporting high-risk sexual practices (e.g., multiple sexual partners), and 15–20% of persons with acute hepatitis C have an anti-HCV-positive partner or admit having had multiple sexual partners during the 6 months before illness onset, in the absence of other risk factors for infection.[18] In addition, in one study women attending a clinic for sexually transmitted diseases (STDs) were threefold more likely to have HCV infection if their sexual partner was HCV infected.[19] On the other hand, in at least five studies the prevalence of HCV infection was less than 2% among long-term sexual partners of HCV-infected individuals.[20–24] Furthermore, a higher than expected prevalence of HCV infection has been found in only a few studies of men who have sex with men (MSM).[25,26] However, recent reports suggest that HIV-infected men engaging in unprotected, traumatic sexual acts with other men may be at increased risk for the sexual transmission of hepatitis C.[27–30] Taken together, although there is evidence that HCV may be transmitted sexually, heterosexual intercourse appears to be a relatively inefficient mode of transmission.

The HCV infection occurs in ~2–5% of infants born to HCV-positive mothers.[17] However, the incidence of mother–infant transmission increases approximately threefold if the mother is co-infected with HIV.[31–33] In addition, in one study an increased rate of HIV transmission was found among infants born to mothers who were co-infected with HIV and HCV.[34]

Because of shared routes of transmission, HCV and HIV co-infection is common. In the United States there are thought to be 150 000–300 000 persons co-infected with HCV and HIV, representing 15–30% of the estimated 1 000 000 individuals with HIV infection.[35] Similar data have been reported from Europe; 33% of more than 3000 patients with HIV infection followed in the EuroSIDA cohort study had evidence of HCV infection.[36] However, the prevalence of HCV/HIV co-infection varies depending on the route of HIV infection (Fig. 55-1). HCV is ~10-fold more likely than HIV to be transmitted by an accidental needlestick exposure and is acquired more readily than HIV by injection drug users.[37,38] Thus 50–90% of persons who acquire HIV from injecting drugs are also HCV infected. Similarly, more than 50% of hemophiliacs who were exposed to unscreened, nonheat-treated blood products had HCV/HIV co-infection.[39] HCV infection is less common (~10%) in men who acquired HIV infection from same-sex intercourse.[37,40]

Natural History

After acute infection, ~15% of individuals clear virus from the blood and presumably have fully recovered from infection.[41,42] The remaining 70–85% of acutely infected persons have viremia that persists for life. In some chronically infected persons, alanine aminotransferase (ALT) levels are persistently elevated or normal. However, in most persons they fluctuate and are poor predictors of liver disease.[43] Some persistently infected persons develop hepatic fibrosis that progresses to cirrhosis, liver failure, or hepatocellular carcinoma.[44] The probability of cirrhosis after 20 years of infection is estimated to be 5–25%, depending on the population studied.[44–46] After cirrhosis has developed, the rates of progression to liver failure and hepatocellular carcinoma are estimated to be ~2–4% and 1–7% per year, respectively.[47]

Unfortunately, disease progression for an individual patient cannot be predicted by currently available laboratory tests. The magnitude or the pattern of ALT elevation does not correlate well with disease outcome.[48] Unlike the HIV RNA level, which is highly correlated with HIV disease progression, the HCV RNA level is not closely associated with the outcome of hepatitis C.[41,49] The best tool for evaluating the stage of infection is liver biopsy, but even liver histology is an imperfect indicator of the ultimate disease course.[50,51]

HIV Infection Impact on Hepatitis C Progression

Infection with HIV has been reported to exacerbate several steps in the natural history of hepatitis C. First, HIV-infected persons were less likely to have cleared viremia than those

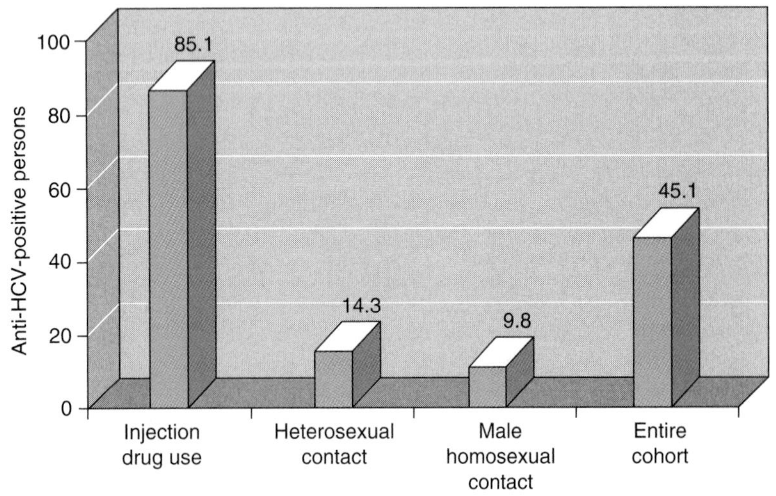

Figure 55-1 ■ Prevalence of anti-HCV in HIV-infected persons receiving medical care in the Johns Hopkins HIV clinic ($n = 1742$) according to reported risk factor for HIV infection. Sulkowski MS, et al. Ann Intern Med 138:197–207, 2003.

without HIV.[41,52] HIV infection has also been associated with a higher HCV RNA viral load and a more rapid progression of HCV-related liver disease.[53–58] As early as 1993, Eyster and colleagues reported that HCV RNA levels were higher in people with hemophilia who became HIV infected than in those who remained HIV negative, and liver failure occurred exclusively in HIV/HCV-co-infected patients.[56] More recently, among 1816 HCV-positive men with hemophilia who were prospectively monitored, Goedert and colleagues estimated the 16-year cumulative incidence of end-stage liver disease (ESLD) among men with and without HIV to be 14.0% and 2.6%, respectively.[57] Furthermore, among those men with HIV/HCV co-infection, the ESLD risk increased 8.1-fold with HBsAg positivity, 2.1-fold with CD4+ T-lymphocyte cell counts below 200 cells/mm^3, and 1.04-fold per additional year of age. Similarly, among HCV-infected persons who chiefly acquired HCV from injection drug use, Pol and co-workers found that HIV co-infection was an independent risk factor for the development of cirrhosis.[58] Finally, the effect of HIV on HCV was summarized in a meta-analysis of studies by Graham and co-workers that assessed the correlation between HIV co-infection and the progression of HCV-related liver disease. HIV co-infection was associated with a relative risk of ESLD of 6.14 and a relative risk of cirrhosis of 2.07 when compared with HCV monoinfection.[55]

Given these data, and as survival among patients with HIV increases because of the use of potent antiretroviral therapies and prevention of traditional opportunistic pathogens, HCV-related morbidity and mortality among HIV-infected individuals can be expected to increase. Gebo and co-workers evaluated rates of admission at the Johns Hopkins University Hospital, Baltimore, Maryland, from 1995 to 2000 among HIV-infected patients and found that admissions for liver-related complications among HCV-positive patients increased nearly fivefold from 5.4 to 26.7 admissions per 100 person-years during that time.[59] Similarly, among 23441 HIV-infected North American and European patients followed in the Data Collection on Adverse Events of Anti-HIV Drugs (D:A:D) study, liver disease was the second leading cause of death, with an incidence of 0.23 cases per 100 person-years follow-up behind HIV/AIDS (0.59 cases per 100 person-years) and ahead of cardiovascular disease (0.14 cases per 100 person-years).[60] Accordingly, in the era of potent ART, HCV-related liver disease is a major cause of hospital admissions and deaths among HIV-infected persons.

HCV Infection Impact on HIV Disease Progression

There are conflicting reports about the effect of HCV infection on the natural history of HIV disease. In a prospective study of 416 HIV seroconverters the 51.4% who were HCV co-infected had an HIV progression rate similar to those without HCV infection.[61] Among 1742 patients, Sulkowski and co-workers found that HCV infection was not independently associated with progression to AIDS or death after adjusting for exposure to highly active antiretroviral therapy (HAART) and HIV suppression.[37] Similarly, HCV infection was not associated with progression to AIDS or death after controlling for important confounding conditions among 10481 HIV-infected individuals followed in 100 US centers or among 5957 HIV-infected patients observed in the EuroSIDA cohort.[36,62] Conversely, Sabin and co-workers found that HIV/HCV-co-infected hemophiliacs with HCV genotype 1 infection experienced a more rapid progression to AIDS and death than did those infected with other genotypes.[63] Among 3111 patients receiving potent ART, Greub and colleagues reported that HCV-infected persons had a modestly increased risk of progression to a new AIDS-defining event or death, even among the subgroup with continuous suppression of HIV replication.[64]

Interestingly, Greub and co-workers also found that the magnitude of the CD4+ T-lymphocyte cell increase following effective anti-HIV therapy was significantly less than that observed in HCV-uninfected persons, suggesting that HCV co-infection may blunt immune recovery following HAART.[64] However, at least four other studies have failed to detect any significant impact of HCV infection on immunological or virological response to ART.[36,37,62,65]

HCV Co-Infection and HAART-Associated Hepatotoxicity

Antiretroviral drugs, such as zidovudine, nevirapine, and HIV-1 protease inhibitors, have been associated with hepatotoxicity, which may interrupt HIV therapy and cause significant morbidity and mortality.[66–70] Some but not all studies suggest that drug-induced hepatotoxicity may be more common among patients with HIV/HCV co-infection, particularly with the use of HIV-1 protease inhibitors and antituberculosis drugs.[71] The mechanism of enhanced drug-induced hepatotoxicity among co-infected patients is unknown but may be the result of underlying HCV-related liver disease or immune reconstitution with enhanced cytolytic anti-HCV immune activity.[72–74] Although co-infected patients may be at increased risk for the development of hepatotoxicity, 88% of a large cohort of HCV-co-infected patients prospectively studied did not experience significant hepatotoxicity following HAART, and no irreversible outcomes were observed among the patients experiencing toxicity.[68]

Furthermore, recent studies suggest that the suppression of HIV replication and prevention or reversal of immunosuppression due to effective ART may be associated with decreased risk of liver disease progression and liver-related mortality. Indeed, Qurishi and co-workers found that ART significantly reduced long-term liver-related mortality among 285 patients followed for ~10 years.[75] In addition, several retrospective cohort studies have observed a decreased risk of cirrhosis among HIV/HCV-co-infected persons effectively treated with ART.[76,77] Thus, the available evidence suggests that ARTs can be safely administered to HIV-infected patients with chronic hepatitis C; however, serum liver enzymes should be closely monitored in these patients. Although there are currently no established guidelines for the management of antiretroviral-associated hepatotoxicity, some studies have suggested that it is not necessary to discontinue ART unless patients are symptomatic or develop significant elevations in liver enzymes (>5–10 times the upper limit of the normal range).[78]

DIAGNOSIS

All HIV-infected persons should be screened for HCV infection because of the high prevalence of HCV infection in this group.[3] HCV screening should be done with enzyme immunoassays (EIA) licensed for the detection of antibody to HCV in blood.[79] Patients with positive anti-HCV results by EIA should have confirmatory testing performed using assays to detect HCV RNA such as reverse transcriptase-polymerase chain reaction (RT-PCR).[1] The detection of HCV RNA in a person with a positive anti-HCV result indicates current infection. However, because some persons with chronic HCV infection experience intermittent viremia, a single undetectable HCV RNA result must be interpreted cautiously. Anti-HCV titers may decline to undetectable levels in persons with advanced immunodeficiency (CD4+ T-lymphocyte count + <100/mm^3).[80] Likewise, in patients with acute HCV infection, anti-HCV EIA may remain undetectable for weeks.[81] Thus HCV RNA should be assessed in the blood when HCV infection is suspected in persons with negative anti-HCV results. The clinical significance of quantitative HCV RNA level (i.e., viral load) in HIV-infected patients is not known and should not be interpreted based on the well-described relation of HIV viral load and HIV disease progression.[82]

MANAGEMENT

All HIV-infected individuals with chronic HCV infection should be counseled to prevent liver damage and HCV transmission and should be evaluated for chronic liver disease and considered for anti-HCV treatment (Table 55-1). Because alcohol ingestion, particularly in quantities of more than 50 g (four drinks) per day, accelerates the progression of liver disease and significantly increases the risk of cirrhosis, all HIV/HCV-infected patients should be advised to abstain from alcohol use.[4,77,83] Counseling regarding household and sexual practices to prevent HIV transmission also should be effective to prevent HCV transmission.

The HIV-infected patients with chronic HCV infection who are susceptible to hepatitis A virus (HAV) or hepatitis B virus (HBV) infections should be vaccinated because most of these patients have risk factors for acquiring HAV and HBV infection.[17] In addition, HCV-infected patients with chronic liver disease who become infected with HAV are at increased risk for fulminant hepatitis.[84]

The HIV/HCV-co-infected patients should be evaluated for the presence of chronic liver disease. Assessments of disease severity should include a history and physical examination to look for signs and symptoms of chronic liver disease, measurement of blood albumin, prothrombin time, direct bilirubin assay, and platelet count to determine hepatic function; evaluation of liver histology by biopsy is appropriate in many patients. Measurements of the serum ALT level and HCV RNA level are important to establish that the infection is ongoing, but these tests provide only limited information regarding HCV disease severity. The liver biopsy provides important information about HCV-related disease activity and fibrosis stage and may exclude alternative causes of liver disease. Most studies indicate that liver biopsy can be safely performed in HIV-infected individuals.[85] However, liver biopsy is an expensive and invasive procedure and may be difficult to perform in many settings where HIV-infected persons are encountered. Accordingly, noninvasive tests for determining liver disease stage have been developed and, despite limited validation data, are increasingly used to evaluate viral hepatitis-related liver disease (Table 55-2).[29,66,86–92]

Treatment

In mid-2007, the standard treatment for hepatitis C in persons with and without HIV co-infection is peginterferon-alpha-2a or 2b plus ribavirin (Box 55-1).[1,3,4] Two distinct benefits have been attributed to HCV treatment. First, it is possible to eradicate the infection, referred to as a sustained virologic response (undetectable HCV RNA at the end of treatment and 6 months later). Marcellin and colleagues reported that 96% of patients with no detectable HCV RNA 6 months after therapy maintained their virologic response and experienced sustained histologic improvement during long-term follow-up.[93] Similarly, Lau and co-workers reported that five patients with 6-month post-treatment virologic responses also had favorable clinical and histologic outcomes 6–13 years after therapy, with no detectable HCV RNA in the serum and liver tissue.[94]

A second potential benefit of HCV treatment is a reduction in the risk of liver failure and liver cancer.[95–97] Although there are relatively few data linking HCV treatment to long-term outcomes, it is important to note that this benefit does not appear to be restricted to patients with sustained virologic response. These preliminary data form the basis for treating patients at the greatest risk for ESLD (e.g., those with advanced hepatic fibrosis) to prevent hepatic decompensation without regard to virologic response. If substantiated, this approach could be especially pertinent to HIV/HCV-co-infected patients who generally have more liver disease, lower sustained virologic response, and limited access to orthotopic liver transplantation compared to HCV-infected adults without HIV.[98]

However, current HCV treatment is associated with significant morbidity. Accordingly, published guidelines recommend the treatment of hepatitis C in patients co-infected with HIV, in whom the likelihood of serious liver disease and a treatment response are judged to outweigh the risk of morbidity from the adverse effects of therapy.[1,3,4] On the basis of the findings of three, large randomized, controlled trials, initial treatment of hepatitis C in most HIV-infected persons should be peginterferon-alpha-2a or 2b plus ribavirin for 48 weeks duration (Table 55-3).[99–102]

Table 55-1 Strength of Evidence for Recommendations for the Management of HCV in HIV-Infected Patients[1]

Recommendation	Strength of Evidence[a]
• Anti-HCV testing should be performed in all HIV-infected patients	Grade III
• HCV RNA testing should be performed to confirm HCV infection in HIV-infected patients who are seropositive for anti-HCV, as well as in those who are seronegative and have evidence of unexplained liver disease	Grade III
• HCV should be treated in the HIV/HCV-co-infected patient in whom the likelihood of serious liver disease and a treatment response are judged to outweigh the risk of morbidity from the adverse effects of therapy	Grade III
• Initial treatment of HCV in most HIV-infected patients consists of peginterferon-alpha plus ribavirin for 48 weeks	Grade III
• Given the high likelihood of adverse events, HIV/HCV-co-infected patients on HCV treatment should be monitored closely	Grade III
• Ribavirin should be used with caution in patients with limited myeloid reserves and in those taking zidovudine or stavudine. When possible, patients receiving didanosine should be switched to an equivalent antiretroviral before beginning ribavirin	Grade III
• HIV-infected patients with decompensated liver disease may be candidates for orthotopic liver transplantation	Grade III

[a]Quality of evidence on which the recommendation is based: I, randomized, controlled trials; II-1, controlled trials without randomization; II-2, cohort or case-control analytic studies; II-3, multiple time series, dramatic uncontrolled experiments; III, opinions of respected authorities, descriptive epidemiology.

Table 55-2 Noninvasive Markers of HCV-Related Liver Disease

Marker	Components	Model	Sensitivity/Specificity for Advanced Fibrosis, %
AST/ALT ratio[132]	AST/ALT	Ratio > 1	53/100
Forns test[133]	Platelets GGT Cholesterol	7.811 − 3.131 ln(platelet count (10^9 cells/L)) + 0.781 ln(GGT (UI/L)) + 3.467 ln(age (years)) − 0.014 (cholesterol (mg/dL))	94/51
AST-platelet ratio index (APRI)[86]	AST Platelets	(AST level × upper limit of normal)/(platelet count (10^9 cells/L)) × 100	41/95
FibroSURE/ FibroTest[134]	GGT Haptoglobin Bilirubin Apolipoprotein A Alpha-2-macroglobulin	Proprietary	87/59
FIBRO*Spect II*[135]	Hyaluronic acid TIMP-1 Alpha-2-macroglobulin	Proprietary	83/66
FibroScan[87]	Transient elastography pulse-echo ultrasound acquisitions to measure liver stiffness	N/A	88/74

HCV Treatment Algorithm in HIV-Infected Persons[131]

BOX 55 -1

Assessment Before Starting Therapy

- Review HIV disease status including CD4+ T-lymphocyte count, HIV RNA level, use of ART and active opportunistic diseases.
- Examine comorbid conditions such as depression, drug and alcohol use, and cardiopulmonary disease, and cytopenias.
- Consider a liver biopsy to confirm the diagnosis of hepatitis C virus (HCV), assess the grade and stage of disease, and rule out other diagnoses. In situations where a liver biopsy is contraindicated or patient declines, therapy can be given without a pretreatment liver biopsy.
- Measure serum HCV RNA to document that viremia is present.
- Test for HCV genotype to help determine the probability of virologic response.
- Measure blood counts, thyroid stimulating hormone (TSH) and aminotransferases to establish a baseline for these values.
- Counsel the patient about the relative risks and benefits of treatment. Side effects should be thoroughly discussed.

Criteria for Starting Therapy

HCV treatment should be routinely offered to persons in whom the potential benefits of therapy are judged to outweigh the potential risks including (but not limited) to persons with:

- HCV genotype 2 or 3 infection
- HCV genotype 1 infection with low HCV RNA level (<800 000 IU/mL)
- Significant hepatic fibrosis (bridging fibrosis or cirrhosis)
- Stable HIV infection not requiring antiretroviral therapy
- Acute HCV infection (<6–12 months duration)
- Cryoglobulinemic vasculitis
- Cryoglobulinemic membranoproliferative glomerulonephritis
- Strong motivation to treat their HCV infection

Recommended Regimens

- Hepatitis C genotype 1 or 4, 5, 6
  Peginterferon alfa-2a 180 mcg by subcutaneous injection weekly or peginterferon alfa-2b 1.5 mg/kg by subcutaneous injection weekly plus ribavirin by mouth twice daily (<75 kg or 165 lbs body weight, 600 mg qAM and 400 qPM; ≥75 kg or 165 lbs body weight, 600 mg qAM and 600 qPM)
  Treatment duration: 48 weeks
- Hepatitis C genotype 2 or 3
  Peginterferon alfa-2a 180 mcg by subcutaneous injection weekly or peginterferon alfa-2b 1.5 mg/kg by subcutaneous injection weekly plus ribavirin by mouth twice daily (fixed dose, 400 mg qAM and 400 qPM)
  Treatment duration: 48 weeks

Monitoring During Therapy

- Measure blood counts and aminotransferases at weeks 2 and 4, and at 4- to 8-week intervals thereafter. Consider the concurrent administration of filgrastim in the management of interferon-associated neutropenia.
- Measure HIV RNA, absolute CD4+ T-lymphocyte cell count and percentage CD4 at 12-week intervals.
- Adjust the dose of ribavirin downward (by 200 mg at a time) if significant anemia occurs (hemoglobin less than 10 g/dL or hematocrit <30%) and stop ribavirin if severe anemia occurs (hemoglobin <8.5 g/dL or hematocrit <26%). Consider the concurrent administration of epoetin-alpha (40 000 IU by subcutaneous injection weekly) in the management of treatment-related anemia.
- Evaluate for neuropsychiatric complications monthly (depression screen). Consider use of antidepressants and/or consultation with a mental health provider.
- Measure TSH levels every 12 weeks during therapy.
  - Measure HCV RNA by PCR at 12 weeks.
    If HCV RNA has not decreased by 2 $\log_{10}$ from baseline or become undetectable, consider stopping therapy.
    If HCV RNA is negative continue therapy for at least an additional 36 weeks.
    If HCV RNA is detectable but >2 $\log_{10}$ below baseline, repeat HCV RNA testing at 24 weeks of therapy.
  - Measure HCV RNA by PCR at 24 weeks.
    If HCV RNA[A10] is negative, continue therapy for at least an additional 24 weeks.
    If HCV RNA is detectable, consider stopping therapy.
- Reinforce the need to practice strict birth control during therapy and for 6 months thereafter.
- At the end of therapy, test HCV RNA by PCR to assess whether there is an end-of-treatment response.

(Continued)

Assessment After Therapy

- Measure aminotransferases every 2 months for 6 months.
- Six months after stopping therapy test for HCV RNA by PCR. If HCV RNA is still negative, the chance for a long-term virologic response is very high; relapses have rarely been reported after this point.

Contraindications to Therapy

Treatment with peginterferon plus ribavirin should not be routinely administered to persons in whom the potential risks of therapy are judged to outweigh the potential benefits including (but not limited to) persons with:

- Pregnancy or who are not willing to use birth control
- Advanced AIDS with insufficient suppression of HIV replication. HCV treatment may be considered following the successful implementation of antiretroviral therapy
- Hepatic decompensation (e.g. coagulopathy, hyperbilirubinemia, encephalopathy, ascites). Liver transplantation, where feasible, should be the primary treatment option for patients with decompensated liver disease.
- Severe, uncontrolled comorbid medical conditions (e.g. cancer or cardiopulmonary disease)
- Severe, active depression with suicidal ideation. HCV treatment may be considered following the successful implementation of psychiatric care
- Significant hematologic abnormality (e.g. hemoglobin $<10.5\,g/dL$, absolute neutrophil count $<1000/mm^3$, platelet count $<50{,}000/mm^3$). HCV treatment may be considered following the correction of hematologic abnormalities (e.g. treatment of underlying causative conditions and/or use of hematopoietic growth factors)
- Renal insufficiency (creatinine >2.5). In such persons, HCV treatment with peginterferon alone may be considered
- Sarcoidosis due to increased risk of severe disease exacerbation with interferon therapy
- Active, uncontrolled autoimmune conditions (e.g., systemic lupus erythematosus or rheumatoid arthritis) due to increased risk of severe disease exacerbation with interferon therapy.
- Patients with contraindications to the use of ribavirin (e.g., unstable cardiopulmonary disease, pre-existing anemia unresponsive to erythropoietin, renal failure, or hemoglobinopathy) can be treated with peginterferon alfa (2a or 2b) monotherapy. However, decreased SVR rates are expected among patients not receiving ribavirin.
- Persons with modifiable contraindications to HCV treatment should be reassessed at regular intervals to assess candidacy for therapy.
- Active injection drug use does not represent a contraindication to HCV treatment; treatment of active IDUs should be considered on a case-by-case basis taking into account comorbid conditions, adherence to medical care and risk of re-infection. Management of HCV-infected IDUs is enhanced by linking IDUs to drug-treatment programs.
- Alcohol use negatively impacts HCV disease progression and treatment; therefore, alcohol abstinence is strongly recommended before and during antiviral therapy. A history of alcohol abuse is not a contraindication to therapy.

Modified from 2007 Guidelines for Management of HIV Related Opportunistic Infections, www.aidsinfo.nih.gov

Adult AIDS Clinical Trials Group

In study 5071 of the Adult AIDS Clinical Trials Group (AACTG), Chung et al randomized 133 HCV-infected adults to a dose-escalating regimen of oral ribavirin plus peginterferon-alpha-2a or standard interferon-alpha-2a for 48 weeks.[99] Most patients enrolled in the trial were male Caucasians. At baseline, the median CD4+ T-lymphocyte count was relatively high (greater than 450 cells/mm^3). Most patients were receiving ART and were infected with HCV genotype 1 and had a high level of hepatitis C viremia.

The sustained virologic response (SVR) was higher in patients who received peginterferon compared to those who received standard interferon (27% vs 12%, $P < 0.03$). Among patients treated with peginterferon with ribavirin, the SVR was lower in those infected with HCV genotype 1 (14%) than in those infected with genotype 2 or 3 (73%). The relatively low SVR in patients with HCV genotype 1 was the result of both a low rate of viral suppression on treatment (29% at the end of therapy) and a high rate of virologic relapse (53%) after the discontinuation of therapy. Similar to HIV-negative patients, the pattern of early virologic response to therapy (at 12 weeks) was highly predictive of a lack of an SVR. In addition, there was a histologic response (defined as decreased necroinflammatory activity on paired liver biopsy) in 35% of patients who had an insufficient viral response after 24 weeks of therapy but had not yet discontinued treatment. The safety and tolerability of peginterferon-alpha-2a plus ribavirin was similar to that previously observed among patients with hepatitis C not co-infected with HIV. Overall, 12% of patients discontinued therapy prematurely, mainly as a result of neuropsychiatric side effects.

Agence Nationale de Recherche sur le Sida (ANRS RIBAVIC) Study

In the RIBAVIC study, Carrat et al randomized 412 co-infected patients to ribavirin plus either peginterferon-alpha-2b or standard interferon-alpha-2b.[103] At baseline, the median CD4+ T-lymphocyte cell count of enrolled patients

Table 55-3

Comparison of Four Randomized Controlled Trials of Peginterferon Plus Ribavirin in HIV/HCVCo-infected Patients[99,100,103]

Parameter	APRICOT	ACTG A5071	ANRS HCO2 RIBAVIC
Number of subjects	868	133	412
Country	Multinational	United States	France
Regimen			
• Peginterferon	Peginterferon-alpha-2a 180 μg/week	Peginterferon-alpha-2a 180 μg/week	Peginterferon-alpha-2b 1.5 $\mu g\, kg^{-1}$ $week^{-1}$
• Ribavirin	800 mg/day	Dose escalated from 600 to 800 to 1000 mg/day at 4-week intervals	800 mg/day
• Duration	48 weeks	48 weeks	48 weeks
Baseline Characteristics			
• White, %	79	33	93
• Mean CD4+ T-lymphocyte cell count, cells/mm^3	530	474	482
• Undetectable HIV-1 RNA, %	60	60	67
• On ART, %	84	86	83
• Bridging fibrosis or cirrhosis, %	16	11[a]	39
• Genotype 1, %	61	77	59
• HCV RNA > 800 000 IU/mL, %	72	83[b]	Not reported
SVR by Genotype, %			
• 1	29	14	Not reported
• 1 & 4	Not reported	Not reported	17
• 2 & 3	62	73	44

ACTG, AIDS Clinical Trials Group; ANRS, National AIDS Research Agency (France); ART, antiretroviral therapy.

[a]Patients with cirrhosis.

[b]HCV RNA > 1 million IU/mL.

was >475 cells/mm^3 and most patients were receiving potent ART and had an HIV RNA level below the limit of detection (<400 copies/mL). Most patients were male, Caucasian, and infected with HCV genotype 1.

There was a higher SVR in patients treated with peginterferon-alpha-2b with ribavirin compared with those treated with standard interferon with ribavirin (27% vs 19%). Among patients infected with HCV genotype 1 or 4, the SVR was 17% and 6% in the pegylated and standard interferon groups, respectively. In both treatment groups, the SVR in those with HCV genotype 2 or 3 infection was similar and higher than observed in genotype 1 infection (~44%). The safety profile of peginterferon with ribavirin in the RIBAVIC study was similar to that documented in patients with hepatitis C alone. However, 17% of patients prematurely discontinued therapy; because of an adverse event or laboratory abnormality (~30% experienced a grade 4 (life-threatening) adverse event). Severe adverse events included: psychiatric events, liver failure, pneumonia or sepsis, symptomatic hyperlactemia (related to didanosine use), and liver enzyme elevations. Although oral candidiasis and increased lipodystrophy were observed in ~15% of patients, no new AIDS-defining illnesses developed.

APRICOT Study

In the AIDS PEGASYS Ribavirin International Co-infection Trial (APRICOT), 868 co-infected patients were treated with standard interferon-alpha-2a with ribavirin or peginterferon-alpha-2a with ribavirin or placebo for 48 weeks.[100] Most patients were male Caucasians. At baseline, patients had mean CD4+ T-lymphocyte cell counts above 500 cells/mm^3 and only 7% had a CD4+ T-lymphocyte count 200 cells/mm^3. Most patients were receiving potent ART and over half had an HIV RNA level below detection limits (<50 copies/mL). Approximately 60% of patients were infected with HCV genotype 1, 72% had a high HCV RNA level (>800 000 IU/mL), and 16% had histologic evidence of bridging fibrosis or cirrhosis.

The SVR was higher in patients receiving peginterferon-alpha-2a with ribavirin than in the other groups. Among patients treated with peginterferon with ribavirin, there was a lower SVR rate in those infected with genotype 1 compared with genotypes 2 or 3 (29% vs 62%). Baseline HCV viral load was a strong predictor of SVR in patients infected with genotype 1 (18% with a viral load > 800 000 IU/mL vs 61% with a viral load = 800 000 IU/mL). Conversely, in those patients infected with genotype 2 or 3, the level of HCV viremia did not influence the SVR. In multivariate analysis, SVR was independently associated with genotype and HCV viral load but not with factors related to HIV disease (e.g., HIV RNA level or CD4+ T-lymphocyte cell count) or its treatment with antiretroviral drugs. Similar to other studies, early virologic response after 12 weeks of therapy was highly predictive of treatment failure; only 2% of patients treated with peginterferon-alpha-2a plus ribavirin who failed to achieve at least a 2 $\log_{10}$ decrease in HCV RNA level had a SVR.

There were serious adverse events in 17% of patients, which led to discontinuation of therapy in 12%. Peginterferon dose reduction because of neutropenia occurred in 27% of patients and 12% used filgrastim to treat neutropenia. Similarly, ribavirin dose reduction as a result of anemia occurred in 18% of patients and 10% used epoetin-alpha to treat anemia. AIDS-defining events occurred in 1% of patients, including the development of esophageal candidiasis, herpes zoster, and presumptive progressive multifocal leukoencephalopathy. The mean CD4+ T-lymphocyte cell decline during therapy was 157 cells/mm^3 while the mean CD4+ T-lymphocyte percentage increase was 3%. Interestingly, among persons with detectable HIV RNA at baseline, peginterferon-alpha-2a was associated with a modest reduction (~0.7 $\log_{10}$) in HIV viremia, suggesting potential clinical benefit. On the other hand, Mauss et al reported that 14 of 133 patients with cirrhosis who were enrolled in the APRICOT study had hepatic decompensation during treatment, of whom six died.[104] Importantly, half of these cases occurred in patients with baseline evidence of hepatic insufficiency (Child-Pugh B cirrhosis), and laboratory markers of advanced liver disease, such as increased total bilirubin and alkaline phosphatase levels and decreased platelet count, were strongly associated with liver failure during hepatitis C therapy. These data strongly indicate that HCV therapy should be withheld from co-infected patients with evidence of decompensated (Childs B or C) cirrhosis.

Adverse Effects of Peginterferon with Ribavirin Therapy

Interferon alpha therapy is associated with many adverse effects, most of which are relatively minor, treatable with adjunctive therapies, and in most cases reversible with discontinuation of therapy.[105,106] With the first several doses of interferon alpha most (60–90%) patients experience influenza-like symptoms (e.g., fever, malaise, tachycardia, chills, headache, arthalgia, myalgia). However, these symptoms usually subside after the first several injections, and their intensity may be ameliorated by acetaminophen or nonsteroidal antiinflammatory drugs (NSAIDs). Fatigue, malaise, anorexia, weight loss, skin rash, and reversible alopecia can occur months into therapy.

Additionally, neuropsychiatric side effects (irritability, insomnia, mood, and cognitive changes) are observed in 25–60% of patients but generally can be managed effectively with pharmacologic agents. Rarely, depression is severe, and suicides have been reported in persons taking interferon alpha.[107–109] Interferon-associated thyroid dysfunction occurs in ~4% of patients and may take the form of thyroiditis, hypothyroidism, or hyperthyroidism.[110] With careful monitoring of thyroid function (thyroid-stimulating hormone) during therapy, this condition is rarely symptomatic; however, the thyroid dysfunction may be irreversible, and long-term thyroid replacement therapy may be required. Interferon may also cause neutropenia, mild anemia, and thrombocytopenia, adverse events that are often minor and may respond to dose reduction or the administration of filgrastim (granulocyte colony-stimulating factor).[111]

Ribavirin also causes side effects. During the first 4 weeks of therapy ~80% of patients develop a dose-related hemolytic anemia.[112] With interferon-alpha-2b and ribavirin combination therapy, the hemoglobin level usually decreases by 2–3 g/dL, sometimes associated with fatigue, shortness of breath, and headache. In rare circumstances anemia occurs more rapidly and has caused angina and myocardial infarction. Thus, ribavirin should be used cautiously in persons with preexisting cardiac disease, and older patients or those with significant cardiac risk factors should undergo pretreatment cardiac testing. Ribavirin-associated anemia is reversible with dose reduction or discontinuation (or both). In addition, epoetin-alpha can effectively increase the hemoglobin level in HIV-infected and HIV-uninfected patients experiencing ribavirin-associated anemia.[113,114] Ribavirin-induced anemia may be a greater problem in HIV-co-infected patients owing to the high prevalence of anemia and limited myeloid reserves that may exist as a result of co-morbid diseases or concurrent drug toxicity.[115] Ribavirin may also be associated with rash, pruritus, nasal congestion, cough, and gout. Importantly, ribavirin causes birth defects and must not be administered to pregnant women or men intending to conceive. All men and women receiving ribavirin therapy must be counseled to use two forms of effective contraception during therapy and for a period of 6 months after discontinuation because of the long half-life of ribavirin.

ART and HCV Therapy

The management of co-infected patients is complicated by possible drug–drug interactions between ribavirin, a guanosine nucleoside analog, and nucleoside analogs used to treat HIV. *In vitro*, ribavirin inhibits the anti-HIV activity of pyrimidine 2′,3′-dideoxynucleosides, including zidovudine, zalcitabine, and stavudine by inhibiting their intracellular phosphorylation.[116–118] By contrast, Rodriguez-Torres et al found that ribavirin had no significant effect on the plasma pharmacokinetics or intracellular phosphorylation of lamivudine, stavudine, and zidovudine in patients taking peginterferon-alpha-2a with ribavirin or placebo.[119]

By inhibiting inosine monophosphate dehydrogenase (IMPDH), ribavirin increases the intracellular conversion of the nucleoside analog, didanosine, to its active metabolite, which enhances its activity against HIV infection *in vitro*, but might be associated with an increased risk of mitochondrial toxicity.[120–122] Furthermore, among patients with cirrhosis enrolled in the APRICOT study, patients receiving didanosine were fourfold more likely to decompensate than those not on the drug.[104] Similarly, in the RIBAVIC study, 11 cases of symptomatic mitochondrial toxicity were observed in patients receiving didanosine.[102] Accordingly, didanosine is strictly contraindicated in persons taking ribavirin.

In addition to pharmacokinetic interactions, the prescription of multiple medications in co-infected patients on ART and peginterferon with ribavirin therapy creates the potential for synergistic or additive drug-related toxicity. For example, zidovudine use might be associated with bone marrow suppression, leading to neutropenia and anemia, which could exacerbate neutropenia and hemolytic anemia associated with peginterferon therapy. Indeed, Brau and co-workers reported that the incidence of anemia requiring ribavirin dose reduction was substantially greater in patients treated with interferon/ribavirin with zidovudine compared with those not on zidovudine.[123] In one study, however, epoetin-alpha (40 000 IU weekly) effectively increased hemoglobin levels in patients taking zidovudine.[113] Thus, patients receiving zidovudine should be closely monitored for anemia after the initiation of HCV therapy and, if anemia develops, treated with epoetin alpha. Alternatively, if possible, zidovudine should be discontinued before treatment of hepatitis C.

Despite the uncertainties and limitations of currently available HCV treatment strategies, HCV treatment may be beneficial for some HCV/HIV-co-infected persons. However, many HIV-infected patients have co-morbid conditions, such as major depressive illness, cytopenias, and active illicit drug or alcohol use, which may prevent or complicate interferon alpha with ribavirin therapy. HCV treatment in co-infected patients should be coordinated by healthcare providers with experience treating both HIV and HCV disease.

Novel Therapies for the Treatment of HCV

The development of targeted antiviral therapy is based on the identification and selection of molecules with a high affinity for binding to specific functional sites within HCV particles, RNA, or proteins that result in the interruption of the virus life cycle. The development and selection of these molecules requires a detailed understanding of the three-dimensional structure of the HCV target, such as several of the enzymes critical to viral replication or parts of the internal ribosome entry site. The two most promising targets include the NS3 serine protease, which is a major catalyst in posttranslational polyprotein processing, and the NS5B RNA-dependent RNA polymerase, the enzyme that is crucial for RNA replication. The recent development of *in vitro* HCV cell culture infection systems that allow for the propagation of HCV will undoubtedly facilitate the evaluation of candidate antiviral agents.[124] The development of NS3 serine protease inhibitors has been problematic because the active site of the enzyme is long, shallow, and exposed, making interaction with small inhibitors difficult. One promising compound in this class, BILN 2061, reduced HCV replication by at least 2–3 $\log_{10}$ IU/mL in the majority of 31 patients with HCV genotype 1 after only 2 days of administration and was well tolerated.[125] However, further development of BILN 2061 has been halted due to animal studies that suggest that the agent might cause cardiac toxicity. Two additional HCV protease inhibitors have since progressed to phase II clinical trials in HIV-uninfected patients in the United States and Europe.[126,127] In addition, antiviral agents targeting the RNA-dependent RNA polymerase (RdRp), encoded by NS5B, are in human studies.[128]

Although new agents specifically targeting hepatitis C have entered human studies in 2006, significant questions regarding the safety, tolerability, efficacy, and resistance profiles of each investigational drug and drug class remain unanswered. Early clinical studies suggest that these novel agents will initially be used in combination with peginterferon with or without ribavirin. To date, studies of novel HCV therapies have not been conducted among persons co-infected with HIV. Access to novel anti-HCV agents will be a critical step in adequately addressing the burden of HCV-related liver disease in HIV-infected persons.

Management of Advanced Liver Disease

There are few guidelines to direct management of HIV/HCV-co-infected patients with cirrhosis. It is important to look for evidence of hepatic dysfunction, portal hypertension, encephalopathy, ascites, and hepatocellular carcinoma, since patients with hepatic decompensation are not candidates for interferon-based therapy. In the era of effective HIV therapy, multiple centers in the United States and Europe are investigating the feasibility of liver transplantation in HIV/HCV-co-infected persons with ESLD.[98,129,130] However, due to limited access to organs and expertise, most HCV-HIV-co-infected patients with decompensated liver disease are not likely to receive liver transplantation.

PREVENTION

Infection with HCV currently cannot be prevented by vaccination or administration of immune globulin. HCV infection can be avoided by adhering to counseling typically provided to HIV-infected persons to prevent HIV transmission.[17] In particular, HIV-infected MSM should be educated regarding the risk of sexual transmission of hepatitis C in the context of unprotected, traumatic sexual practices. Furthermore, patients should be counseled to stop using injection drugs, and those who continue to inject drugs should be counseled to use safer injection practices to reduce harm.

REFERENCES

1. Strader DB, Wright T, Thomas DL, Seeff LB. Diagnosis, management, and treatment of hepatitis C. Hepatology 39:1147–71, 2004.
2. Soriano V, Puoti M, Sulkowski M, et al. Care of patients with hepatitis C and HIV co-infection. AIDS 18:1–12, 2004.
3. Benson CA, Kaplan JE, Masur H, et al. Treating opportunistic infections among HIV-infected adults and adolescents. MMWR 53:1–112, 2004.
4. Alberti A, Clumeck N, Collins S, et al. Short statement of the first European consensus conference on the treatment of chronic hepatitis B and C in HIV-coinfected patients. J Hepatol 42: 615–24, 2005.
5. Choo QL, Richman KH, Han JH, et al. Genetic organization and diversity of the hepatitis C virus. Proc Natl Acad Sci USA 88:2451–55, 1991.
6. Neumann AU, Lam NP, Dahari H, et al. Hepatitis C viral dynamics in vivo and the antiviral efficacy of interferon-alpha therapy. Science 282:103–7, 1998.
7. Ogata N, Alter HJ, Miller RH, Purcell RH. Nucleotide sequence and mutation rate of the H strain of hepatitis C virus. Proc Natl Acad Sci USA 88:3392–96, 1991.
8. Abe K, Inchauspe G, Fujisawa K. Genomic characterization and mutation rate of hepatitis C virus isolated from a patient who contracted hepatitis during an epidemic of non-A, non-B hepatitis in Japan. J Gen Virol 73:2725–29, 1992.
9. Koizumi K, Enomoto N, Kurosaki M, et al. Diversity of quasispecies in various disease stages of chronic hepatitis C virus infection and its significance in interferon treatment. Hepatology 22:30–5, 1995.
10. Simmonds P, Holmes EC, Cha T-A, et al. Classification of hepatitis C virus into six major genotypes and a series of subtypes by phylogenetic analysis of the NS-5 region. J Gen Virol 74:2391–99, 1993.
11. Zein NN, Rakela J, Krawitt EL, et al. Hepatitis C virus genotypes in the United States: epidemiology, pathogenicity, and response to interferon therapy. Ann Intern Med 125:634–9, 1996.
12. Armstrong GL, Wasley A, Simard EP, et al. The prevalence of hepatitis C virus infection in the United States, 1999 through 2002. Ann Intern Med 144:705–14, 2006.
13. Donahue JG, Munoz A, Ness PM, et al. The declining risk of post-transfusion hepatitis C virus infection. N Engl J Med 327:369–73, 1992.
14. Busch MP, Glynn SA, Stramer SL, et al. A new strategy for estimating risks of transfusion-transmitted viral infections based on rates of detection of recently infected donors. Transfusion 45:254–64, 2005.
15. Thomas DL, Vlahov D, Solomon L, et al. Correlates of hepatitis C virus infections among injection drug users in Baltimore. Medicine 74:212–20, 1995.
16. Villano SA, Vlahov D, Nelson KE, et al. Incidence and risk factors for hepatitis C among injection drug users in Baltimore, Maryland. J Clin Microbiol 35:3274–77, 1997.
17. Centers for Disease Control and Prevention. Recommendations for prevention and control of hepatitis C virus (HCV) infection and HCV-related chronic disease. MMWR 47:1–39, 1998.
18. Alter MJ, Kruszon-Moran D, Nainan OV, et al. The prevalence of hepatitis C virus infection in the United States, 1988 through 1994. N Engl J Med 341:556–62, 1999.
19. Thomas DL, Zenilman JM, Alter HJ, et al. Sexual transmission of hepatitis C virus among patients attending sexually transmitted diseases clinics in Baltimore: an analysis of 309 sex partnerships. J Infect Dis 171:768–75, 1995.
20. Everhart JE, Di Bisceglie AM, Murray LM, et al. Risk for non-A, non-B (type C) hepatitis through sexual or household contact with chronic carriers. Ann Intern Med 112:544–5, 1990.
21. Gordon SC, Patel AH, Kulesza GW, et al. Lack of evidence for the heterosexual transmission of hepatitis C. Am J Gastroenterol 87:1849–51, 1992.
22. Osmond DH, Padian NS, Sheppard HW, et al. Risk factors for hepatitis C virus seropositivity in heterosexual couples. JAMA 269:361–5, 1993.
23. Osmond DH, Charlebois E, Sheppard HW, et al. Comparison of risk factors for hepatitis C and hepatitis B virus infection in homosexual men. J Infect Dis 167:66–71, 1993.
24. Eyster ME, Alter HJ, Aledort LM, et al. Heterosexual co-transmission of hepatitis C virus (HCV) and human immunodeficiency virus (HIV). Ann Intern Med 115:764–8, 1991.
25. Melbye M, Biggar RJ, Wantzin P, et al. Sexual transmission of hepatitis C virus: cohort study (1981–9) among European homosexual men. BMJ 301:210–2, 1990.
26. Buchbinder SP, Katz MH, Hessol NA, et al. Hepatitis C virus infection in sexually active homosexual men. J Infect 29: 263–9, 1994.
27. Rauch A, Rickenbach M, Weber R, et al. Unsafe sex and increased incidence of hepatitis C virus infection among HIV-infected men who have sex with men: the Swiss HIV Cohort Study. Clin Infect Dis 41:395–402, 2005.
28. Zylberberg H, Pol S. Reciprocal interactions between human immunodeficiency virus and hepatitis C virus infections. Clin Infect Dis 23:1117–25, 1996.
29. de Lédinghen V, Douvin C, Kettaneh A, et al. Diagnosis of hepatic fibrosis and cirrhosis by transient elastography in HIV/hepatitis C virus-coinfected patients. J Acquir Immune Defic Syndr 41:175–9, 2006.
30. Gotz HM, van Doornum G, Niesters HG, et al. A cluster of acute hepatitis C virus infection among men who have sex with men–results from contact tracing and public health implications. AIDS 19:969–74, 2005.
31. Thomas DL, Villano SA, Riester KA, et al. Perinatal transmission of hepatitis C virus from human immunodeficiency virus type 1-infected mothers. J Infect Dis 177:1480–8, 1998.
32. Mast EE, Hwang LY, Seto DS, et al. Risk factors for perinatal transmission of hepatitis C virus (HCV) and the natural history of HCV infection acquired in infancy. J Infect Dis 192: 1880–9, 2005.
33. Gibb DM, Goodall RL, Dunn DT, et al. Mother-to-child transmission of hepatitis C virus: evidence for preventable peripartum transmission. Lancet 356:904–7, 2000.
34. Hershow RC, Riester KA, Lew J, et al. Increased vertical transmission of human immunodeficiency virus from hepatitis C virus-coinfected mothers. J Infect Dis 176:414–20, 1997.
35. Sherman KE, Rouster SD, Chung R, Rajicic N. Hepatitis C Virus prevalence among patients infected with Human Immunodeficiency Virus: a cross-sectional analysis of the US adult AIDS Clinical Trials Group. Clin Infect Dis 34:831–7, 2002.
36. Rockstroh JK, Mocroft A, Soriano V, et al. Influence of hepatitis C virus infection on HIV-1 disease progression and response to highly active antiretroviral therapy. J Infect Dis 192: 992–1002, 2005.
37. Sulkowski MS, Moore RD, Mehta SH, et al. Hepatitis C and progression of HIV disease. JAMA 288:199–206, 2002.
38. Kiyosawa K, Sodeyama T, Tanaka E, et al. Hepatitis C in hospital employees with needlestick injuries. Ann Intern Med 115:367–9, 1991.
39. Makris M, Preston FE, Triger DR, et al. Hepatitis C antibody and chronic liver disease in haemophilia. Lancet 335:1117–19, 1990.
40. Donahue JG, Nelson KE, Munoz A, et al. Antibody to hepatitis C virus among cardiac surgery patients, homosexual men, and intravenous drug users in Baltimore, Maryland. Am J Epidemiol 134:1206–11, 1991.
41. Thomas DL, Astemborski J, Rai RM, et al. The natural history of hepatitis C virus infection: host, viral, and environmental factors. JAMA 284:450–6, 2000.

42. Farci P, Shimoda A, Coiana A, et al. The outcome of acute hepatitis C predicted by the evolution of the viral quasispecies. Science 2000; 288:339–44.
43. Mehta SH, Netski D, Sulkowski MS, et al. Liver enzyme values in injection drug users with chronic hepatitis C. Dig Liver Dis 37:674–80, 2005.
44. Tong MJ, El-Farra NS, Reikes AR, Co RL. Clinical outcomes after transfusion-associated hepatitis C. N Engl J Med 332:1463–6, 1995.
45. Kenny-Walsh E. Clinical outcomes after hepatitis C infection from contaminated anti-D immune globulin. Irish Hepatology Research Group. N Engl J Med 340:1228–33, 1999.
46. Seeff LB, Hollinger FB, Alter HJ, et al. Long-term mortality and morbidity of transfusion-associated non-A, non-B, and type C hepatitis: A National Heart, Lung, and Blood Institute collaborative study. Hepatology 33:455–63, 2001.
47. Fattovich G, Giustina G, Degos F, et al. Morbidity and mortality in compensated cirrhosis C: a follow-up study of 384 patients. Gastroenterology 112:463–72, 1997.
48. Rai R, Wilson LE, Astemborski J, et al. Severity and correlates of liver disease in hepatitis C virus-infected injection drug users. Hepatology 35:1247–55, 2002.
49. Fanning L, Kenny E, Sheehan M, et al. Viral load and clinicopathological features of chronic hepatitis C (1b) in a homogeneous patient population. Hepatology 29:904–7, 1999.
50. Perrillo RP. The role of liver biopsy in hepatitis C. Hepatology 26(3 Suppl 1):57S–61S, 1997.
51. Bravo AA, Sheth SG, Chopra S. Liver biopsy. N Engl J Med 344:495–500, 2001.
52. Mehta SH, Cox A, Hoover DR, et al. Protection against persistence of hepatitis C. Lancet 359:1478–83, 2002.
53. Thomas DL, Astemborski J, Vlahov D, et al. Determinants of the quantity of hepatitis C virus RNA. J Infect Dis 181: 844–51, 2000.
54. Darby SC, Ewart DW, Giangrande PL, et al. Mortality from liver cancer and liver disease in haemophilic men and boys in UK given blood products contaminated with hepatitis C. Lancet 350:1425–31, 1997.
55. Graham CS, Baden LR, Yu E, et al. Influence of human immunodeficiency virus infection on the course of hepatitis C virus infection: a meta-analysis. Clin Infect Dis 33:562–9, 2001.
56. Eyster ME, Diamondstone LS, Lien JM, et al. Natural history of hepatitis C virus infection in multitransfused hemophiliacs: effect of coinfection with human immunodeficiency virus. The Multicenter Hemophilia Cohort Study. J Acquir Immune Defic Syndr 6:602–10, 1993.
57. Goedert JJ, Eyster ME, Lederman MM, et al. End-stage liver disease in persons with hemophilia and transfusion-associated infections. Blood 100:1584–89, 2002.
58. Pol S, Lamorthe B, Thi NT, et al. Retrospective analysis of the impact of HIV infection and alcohol use on chronic hepatitis C in a large cohort of drug users. J Hepatol 28:945–50, 1998.
59. Gebo KA, Diener-West M, Moore RD. Hospitalization rates differ by hepatitis C status in an urban HIV cohort. J Acquir Immune Defic Syndr 34:165–73, 2003.
60. Weber R, Friis-Møller N, Sabin C, et al. HIV and non-HIV-related deaths and their relationship to immunodeficiency: the D:A:D Study. In: Program and Abstracts of the 12th Conference on Retroviruses and Opportunistic Infections, Boston, MA, 22–25 Feb 2005, abstract 595.
61. Dorrucci M, Pezzotti P, Phillips AN, et al. Coinfection of hepatitis C virus with human immunodeficiency virus and progression to AIDS. J Infect Dis 172:1503–8, 1995.
62. Sullivan PS, Hanson DL, Teshale EH, et al. Effect of hepatitis C infection on progression of HIV disease and early response to initial antiretroviral therapy. AIDS 20:1171–9, 2006.
63. Sabin CA, Telfer P, Phillips AN, et al. The association between hepatitis C virus genotype and human immunodeficiency virus disease progression in a cohort of hemophilic men. J Infect Dis 175:164–8, 1997.
64. Greub G, Ledergerber B, Battegay M, et al. Clinical progression, survival, and immune recovery during antiretroviral therapy in patients with HIV-1 and hepatitis C virus coinfection: the Swiss HIV Cohort Study. Lancet 356:1800–5, 2000.
65. Chung RT, Evans SR, Yang Y, et al. Immune recovery is associated with persistent rise in hepatitis C virus RNA, infrequent liver test flares, and is not impaired by hepatitis C virus in co-infected subjects. AIDS 16:1915–23, 2002.
66. Sulkowski MS, Thomas DL, Mehta SH, et al. Hepatotoxicity associated with nevirapine or efavirenz-containing antiretroviral therapy: role of hepatitis C and B infections. Hepatology 35:182–9, 2002.
67. Sulkowski MS, Mehta SH, Chaisson RE, et al. Hepatotoxicity associated with protease inhibitor-based antiretroviral regimens with or without concurrent ritonavir. AIDS 18: 2277–84, 2004.
68. Sulkowski MS, Thomas DL, Chaisson RE, Moore RD. Hepatotoxicity associated with antiretroviral therapy in adults infected with human immunodeficiency virus and the role of hepatitis C or B virus infection. JAMA 283:74–80, 2000.
69. den Brinker M, Wit FW, Wertheim-van Dillen PM, et al. Hepatitis B and C virus co-infection and the risk for hepatotoxicity of highly active antiretroviral therapy in HIV-1 infection. AIDS 14:2895–902, 2000.
70. Wit FW, Weverling GJ, Weel J, et al. Incidence of and risk factors for severe hepatotoxicity associated with antiretroviral combination therapy. J Infect Dis 186:23–31, 2002.
71. Sadaphal P, Astemborski J, Graham NM, et al. Isoniazid preventive therapy, hepatitis C virus infection, and hepatotoxicity among injection drug users infected with *Mycobacterium* tuberculosis. Clin Infect Dis 33:1687–91, 2001.
72. Stern JO, Robinson PA, Love J, et al. A comprehensive hepatic safety analysis of nevirapine in different populations of HIV infected patients. J Acquir Immune Defic Syndr 34(Suppl 1): S21–S33, 2003.
73. Aranzabal L, Casado JL, Moya J, et al. Influence of liver fibrosis on highly active antiretroviral therapy-associated hepatotoxicity in patients with HIV and hepatitis C virus coinfection. Clin Infect Dis 40:588–93, 2005.
74. Wyles DL, Gerber JG. Antiretroviral drug pharmacokinetics in hepatitis with hepatic dysfunction. Clin Infect Dis 40: 174–81, 2005.
75. Qurishi N, Kreuzberg C, Lutchters G, et al. Effect of antiretroviral therapy on liver-related mortality in patients with HIV and hepatitis C virus coinfection. Lancet 362:1708–13, 2003.
76. Brau N, Salvatore M, Rios-Bedoya CF, et al. Slower fibrosis progression in HIV/HCV-coinfected patients with successful HIV suppression using antiretroviral therapy. J Hepatol 44: 47–55, 2006.
77. Benhamou Y, Bochet M, Di MV, et al. Liver fibrosis progression in human immunodeficiency virus and hepatitis C virus coinfected patients. The Multivirc Group. Hepatology 30: 1054–8, 1999.
78. Sulkowski MS, Thomas DL. Hepatitis C in the HIV-infected person. Ann Intern Med 138:197–207, 2003.
79. Thio CL, Nolt KR, Astemborski J, et al. Screening for hepatitis C virus in human immunodeficiency virus-infected individuals. J Clin Microbiol 38:575–7, 2000.
80. George SL, Gebhardt J, Klinzman D, et al. Hepatitis C virus viremia in HIV-infected individuals with negative HCV antibody tests. J Acquir Immune Defic Syndr 31:154–62, 2002.
81. Cox AL, Netski DM, Mosbruger T, et al. Prospective evaluation of community-acquired acute-phase hepatitis C virus infection. Clin Infect Dis 40:951–8, 2005.

82. Mellors JW, Rinaldo CRJ, Gupta P, et al. Prognosis in HIV-1 infection predicted by the quantity of virus in plasma. Science 272:1167–70, 1996.
83. Wiley TE, McCarthy M, Breidi L, Layden TJ. Impact of alcohol on the histological and clinical progression of hepatitis C infection. Hepatology 28:805–9, 1998.
84. Vento S, Garofano T, Renzini C, et al. Fulminant hepatitis associated with hepatitis A virus superinfection in patients with chronic hepatitis C. N Engl J Med 338:286–90, 1998.
85. Poles MA, Dieterich DT, Schwarz ED, et al. Liver biopsy findings in 501 patients infected with human immunodeficiency virus (HIV). J Acquir Immune Defic Syndr Hum Retrovirol 11:170–7, 1996.
86. Wai CT, Greenson JK, Fontana RJ, et al. A simple noninvasive index can predict both significant fibrosis and cirrhosis in patients with chronic hepatitis C. Hepatology 38: 518–26, 2003.
87. Castera L, Vergniol J, Foucher J, et al. Prospective comparison of transient elastography, Fibrotest, APRI, and liver biopsy for the assessment of fibrosis in chronic hepatitis C. Gastroenterology 128:343–50, 2005.
88. Myers RP, Benhamou Y, Imbert-Bismut F, et al. Serum biochemical markers accurately predict liver fibrosis in HIV and hepatitis C virus co-infected patients. AIDS 17:721–5, 2003.
89. imbert-Bismut F, Ratziu V, Pieroni L, et al. Biochemical markers of liver fibrosis in patients with hepatitis C virus infection: a prospective study. Lancet 357:1069–75, 2001.
90. Macias J, Giron-Gonzalez JA, Gonzalez-Serrano M, et al. Prediction of liver fibrosis in human immunodeficiency virus/ hepatitis C virus coinfected patients by simple non-invasive indexes. Gut 55:409–14, 2006.
91. Nunes D, Fleming C, Offner G, et al. HIV infection does not affect the performance of noninvasive markers of fibrosis for the diagnosis of hepatitis C virus-related liver disease. J Acquir Immune Defic Syndr 40:538–44, 2005.
92. Kelleher TB, Mehta SH, Bhaskar K, et al. Prediction of hepatic fibrosis in HIV/HCV co-infected patients using serum fibrosis markers: the SHASTA index. J Hepatol 43:78–84, 2005.
93. Marcellin P, Boyer N, Gervais A, et al. Long-term histologic improvement and loss of detectable intrahepatic HCV RNA in patients with chronic hepatitis C and sustained response to interferon-α therapy. Ann Intern Med 127:875–81, 1997.
94. Lau DTY, Kleiner DE, Ghany MG, et al. 10-Year follow-up after interferon-alpha therapy for chronic hepatitis C. Hepatology 28:1121–7, 1998.
95. Effect of interferon-alpha on progression of cirrhosis to hepatocellular carcinoma: a retrospective cohort study. International Interferon-alpha Hepatocellular Carcinoma Study Group. Lancet 351:1535–9, 1998.
96. Nishiguchi S, Shiomi S, Nakatani S, et al. Prevention of hepatocellular carcinoma in patients with chronic active hepatitis C and cirrhosis. Lancet 357:196–7, 2001.
97. Lim R, Knight B, Patel K, et al. Antiproliferative effects of interferon alpha on hepatic progenitor cells in vitro and in vivo. Hepatology 43:1074–83, 2006.
98. Ragni MV, Belle SH, Im K, et al. Survival of human immunodeficiency virus-infected liver transplant recipients. J Infect Dis 188:1412–20, 2003.
99. Chung RT, Andersen J, Volberding P, et al. Peginterferon alfa-2a plus ribavirin versus interferon alfa-2a plus ribavirin for chronic hepatitis C in HIV-coinfected persons. N Engl J Med 351:451–9, 2004.
100. Torriani FJ, Rodriguez-Torres M, Rockstroh JK, et al. Peginterferon alfa-2a plus ribavirin for chronic hepatitis C virus infection in HIV-infected patients. N Engl J Med 351:438–50, 2004.
101. Laguno M, Murillas J, Blanco JL, et al. Peginterferon alfa-2b plus ribavirin compared with interferon alfa-2b plus ribavirin for treatment of HIV/HCV co-infected patients. AIDS 18: F27–F36, 2004.
102. Carrat F, Bani-Sadr F, Pol S, et al. Pegylated interferon alfa-2b vs standard interferon alfa-2b, plus ribavirin, for chronic hepatitis C in HIV-infected patients: a randomized controlled trial. JAMA 292:2839–48, 2004.
103. Carrat F, Bani-Sadr F, Pol S, et al. Pegylated interferon alfa-2b vs standard interferon alfa-2b, plus ribavirin, for chronic hepatitis C in HIV-infected patients: a randomized controlled trial. JAMA 292:2839–48, 2004.
104. Mauss S, Valenti W, Depamphilis J, et al. Risk factors for hepatic decompensation in patients with HIV/HCV coinfection and liver cirrhosis during interferon-based therapy. AIDS 18: F21–F25, 2004.
105. Schaefer M, Schmidt F, Folwaczny C, et al. Adherence and mental side effects during hepatitis C treatment with interferon alfa and ribavirin in psychiatric risk groups. Hepatology 37:443–51, 2003.
106. Fried MW. Side effects of therapy of hepatitis C and their management. Hepatology 2002; 36:S237–S244.
107. Grassi L, Mondardini D, Pavanati M, et al. Suicide probability and psychological morbidity secondary to HIV infection: a control study of HIV-seropositive, hepatitis C virus (HCV)-seropositive and HIV/HCV-seronegative injecting drug users. J Affect Disord 64:195–202, 2001.
108. El Serag HB, Kunik M, Richardson P, Rabeneck L. Psychiatric disorders among veterans with hepatitis C infection. Gastroenterology 123:476–82, 2002.
109. Fireman M, Indest DW, Blackwell A, et al. Addressing tri-morbidity (hepatitis C, psychiatric disorders, and substance use): the importance of routine mental health screening as a component of a comanagement model of care. Clin Infect Dis 40(Suppl 5):S286–S291, 2005.
110. Deutsch M, Dourakis S, Manesis EK, et al. Thyroid abnormalities in chronic viral hepatitis and their relationship to interferon alfa therapy. Hepatology 26:206–10, 1997.
111. Soza A, Everhart JE, Ghany MG, et al. Neutropenia during combination therapy of interferon alfa and ribavirin for chronic hepatitis C. Hepatology 36:1273–9, 2002.
112. Sulkowski MS, Wasserman R, Brooks L, et al. Changes in haemoglobin during interferon alpha-2b plus ribavirin combination therapy for chronic hepatitis C virus infection. J Viral Hepat 11:243–50, 2004.
113. Sulkowski MS, Dieterich DT, Bini EJ, et al. Epoetin alfa once weekly improves anemia in HIV/hepatitis C virus-coinfected patients treated with interferon/ribavirin: a randomized controlled trial. J Acquir Immune Defic Syndr 39:504–6, 2005.
114. Afdhal NH, Dieterich DT, Pockros PJ, et al. Epoetin alfa maintains ribavirin dose in HCV-infected patients: a prospective, double-blind, randomized controlled study. Gastroenterology 126:1302–11, 2004.
115. Moore RD. Human immunodeficiency virus infection, anemia, and survival. Clin Infect Dis 29:44–9, 1999.
116. Vogt MW, Hartshorn KL, Furman PA, et al. Ribavirin antagonizes the effect of azidothymidine on HIV replication. Science 235:1376–9, 1987.
117. Hoggard PG, Kewn S, Barry MG, et al. Effects of drugs on 2′,3′-dideoxy-2′,3′-didehydrothymidinephosphorylationinvitro. Antimicrob Agents Chemother 41:1231–6, 1997.
118. Baba M, Pauwels R, Balzarini J, et al. Ribavirin antagonizes inhibitory effects of pyrimidine 2′,3′-dideoxynucleosides but enhances inhibitory effects of purine 2′,3′-dideoxynucleosides on replication of human immunodeficiency virus in vitro. Antimicrob Agents Chemother 31:1613–17, 1987.
119. Rodriguez-Torres M, Torriani FJ, Soriano V, et al. Effect of ribavirin on intracellular and plasma pharmacokinetics of nucleoside reverse transcriptase inhibitors in patients with human immunodeficiency virus-hepatitis C virus coinfection: results

of a randomized clinical study. Antimicrob Agents Chemother 49:3997–4008, 2005.

120. Fleischer R, Boxwell D, Sherman KE. Nucleoside analogues and mitochondrial toxicity. Clin Infect Dis 38:e79–e80, 2004.
121. Balzarini J, Lee CK, Herdewijn P, De Clercq E. Mechanism of the potentiating effect of ribavirin on the activity of 2′,3′-dideoxyinosine against human immunodeficiency virus. J Biol Chem 266:21509–14, 1991.
122. Salmon-Ceron D, Chauvelot-Moachon L, Abad S, et al. Mitochondrial toxic effects and ribavirin. Lancet 357: 1803–4, 2001.
123. Brau N, Rodriguez-Torres M, Prokupek D, et al. Treatment of chronic hepatitis C in HIV/HCV-coinfection with interferon alpha-2b+ full-course vs. 16-week delayed ribavirin. Hepatology 39:989–98, 2004.
124. Lohmann V, Korner F, Koch J, et al. Replication of subgenomic hepatitis C virus RNAs in a hepatoma cell line. Science 285:110–13, 1999.
125. Lamarre D, Anderson PC, Bailey M, et al. An NS3 protease inhibitor with antiviral effects in humans infected with hepatitis C virus. Nature 426:186–9, 2003.
126. Lin K, Perni RB, Kwong AD, Lin C. VX-950, a novel hepatitis C virus (HCV) NS3-4A protease inhibitor, exhibits potent antiviral activities in HCv replicon cells. Antimicrob Agents Chemother 50:1813–22, 2006.
127. Malcolm BA, Liu R, Lahser F, et al. SCH 503034, a mechanism-based inhibitor of hepatitis C virus NS3 protease, suppresses polyprotein maturation and enhances the antiviral activity of alpha interferon in replicon cells. Antimicrob Agents Chemother 50:1013–20, 2006.
128. Tedaldi EM. New drug targets for HIV and hepatitis C virus coinfection. Clin Infect Dis 41(Suppl 1):S101–S104, 2005.
129. Neff GW, Bonham A, Tzakis AG, et al. Orthotopic liver transplantation in patients with human immunodeficiency virus and end-stage liver disease. Liver Transpl 9:239–47, 2003.
130. Duclos-Vallee JC, Vittecoq D, Teicher E, et al. Hepatitis C virus viral recurrence and liver mitochondrial damage after liver transplantation in HIV-HCV co-infected patients. J Hepatol 42:341–9, 2003.
131. Sulkowski MS. Treatment algorithm for the management of hepatitis C in HIV-coinfected persons. J Hepatol 44(1 Suppl): S49–S55, 2006.
132. Lok AS, Ghany MG, Goodman ZD, et al. Predicting cirrhosis in patients with hepatitis C based on standard laboratory tests: results of the HALT-C cohort. Hepatology 42:282–92, 2005.
133. Forns X, Ampurdanes S, Llovet JM, et al. Identification of chronic hepatitis C patients without hepatic fibrosis by a simple predictive model. Hepatology 36:986–92, 2002.
134. Imbert-Bismut F, Ratziu V, Pieroni L, et al. Biochemical markers of liver fibrosis in patients with hepatitis C virus infection: a prospective study. Lancet 357:1069–75, 2001.
135. Cales P, Oberti F, Michalak S, et al. A novel panel of blood markers to assess the degree of liver fibrosis. Hepatology 42:1373–81, 2005.

Chapter 56

Sexually Transmitted Human Papillomavirus Infection

William Bonnez, MD

Human papillomaviruses (HPVs) represent a large group of viruses that infect mostly the squamous epithelia of the body. They cause latent, asymptomatic infections as well as neoplasms that range from benign warts to malignant squamous cell carcinoma, particularly of the cervix. A subgroup of HPVs has a predilection for the anogenital tract (Table 56-1). Because these genital HPVs are mostly sexually transmitted, they are likely to be encountered in the human immunodeficiency virus (HIV)-infected population; immunosuppression and immunodeficiencies tend to be associated with HPV diseases that are more florid and difficult to eradicate or control than in the immunocompetent host. Consequently, sexually transmitted HPV diseases in the HIV-infected patient create management problems for the practitioner. This chapter describes the resources and approaches that are available.

PATHOGEN

HPVs are circular, double-stranded DNA, nonenveloped viruses that belong to the *Papillomavirus* genus of the Papillomaviridae family. The nucleic acid is enclosed in a 55 nm diameter icosahedral capsid composed of 72 pentamers. One strand of the DNA encodes all the open reading frames (ORFs). The genome can be divided in three parts. The first is a noncoding region, or upstream regulatory region (URR) that contains the origin of replication as well as a promoter sequence and binding sites for various viral and cellular regulatory proteins. Downstream of the URR is a group of 'early' ORFs (E1, E2, E4, E5, E6, and E7) that encode for nonstructural

Table 56-1 Genital HPV Types and Their Disease Association

Disease	HPV Types: Frequent Association[a]	HPV Types: Less-Frequent Association
Condylomata acuminata	6, 11	30,[b] 42, 43, 44, 45,[b] 51,[b] 54, 55, 70[b]
Intraepithelial neoplasias		
Unspecified		30,[b] 34, 39,[b] 40, 53, 57, 59,[b] 61, 62, 64, 66,[b] 67,[b] 68,[b] 69, 71, 72, 82[b]
Low grade	6, 11	16,[b] 18,[b] 31,[b] 33,[b] 35,[b] 42, 43, 44, 45,[b] 51,[b] 52,[b] 74,[c] 86, 87, 89, 90, 91
High grade	16,[b] 18[b]	6, 11, 31,[b] 33,[b] 35,[b] 39,[b] 42, 44, 45,[b] 51,[b] 52,[b] 56,[b] 58,[b] 66[b]
Cervical (and other genital) carcinomas	16,[b] 18[b]	31,[b] 33,[b] 35,[b] 39,[b] 45,[b] 51,[b] 52,[b] 56,[b] 58,[b] 59,[b] 66,[b] 68,[b] 70,[b] 73,[b] 82[b]
Recurrent respiratory papillomatosis	6, 11	

[a] The distinction between frequent and less frequent is arbitrary in many instances. Large descriptive statistics of HPV type distribution by disease are not available for the majority of HPV types. Moreover, many HPV types have been looked for or identified only once.
[b] Types with high malignant potential or only isolated in one or a few lesions that were malignant.
[c] Type first recovered from immunosuppressed or HIV-infected patients.

proteins. E1 is involved in viral replication, as is E2, which also regulates viral expression. E4 produces an abundant cytoplasmic protein that associates with the intermediate filament network but whose role is obscure. E5 is believed to contribute to malignant transformation, a role that has been well established for E6 and E7 of high-risk oncogenic HPVs. The E6 protein binds to p53, a major tumor suppressor protein, and induces its degradation. Similarly, the E7 protein binds and inactivates other tumor suppressor molecules, the retinoblastoma protein (pRB) and pRB-associated proteins. Both p53 and pRB exert essential control on cellular replication and apoptosis. E6 and E7 also interact with many other cellular proteins. The late ORFs are the third component of the genome and are made up of two ORFs, L1 and L2, encoding for structural proteins: the major and minor capsid proteins, respectively. In malignant lesions, HPV DNA is typically found integrated into the host genome. This integration always disrupts the E2 ORFs but never the E6 and E7 ORFs, which become unregulated.

The classification of HPVs is based on genotypes rather than serotypes. HPV types are distinct if they share less than 90% of the DNA sequence homology for the L1 ORF with one another. More than 200 HPV types have been identified so far, and 10 types have been characterized. Each type tends to be associated with a particular tissue specificity, pathology, and oncogenic risk (Table 56-1).

Thus three main groups of HPV diseases can be delineated. The first consists of cutaneous warts, which include the common warts found on hands and soles, deep plantar warts, and flat warts. HIV infection increases the prevalence of these lesions; they are not discussed further here.

The second group corresponds to epidermodysplasia verruciformis, a rare genodermatosis. It first manifests in late childhood as flat wart-like lesions, plaques, or pityriasis versicolor-like lesions that in the sun-exposed areas have a high risk of evolving into malignant squamous cell carcinomas in the fourth and fifth decades. The immunosuppression of HIV infection may cause a phenocopy of the disease.[1]

The third group includes the genital or mucosal HPV diseases. They involve the external genitalia and anus and, in the female, the vagina and cervix as well. Their manifestations can be subclinical or full-blown, the latter being the only state relevant to treatment. The diseases range from the typically benign warts (or condylomas) to preinvasive and invasive cancers (squamous cell carcinomas and, for the cervix, adenocarcinomas). The precursors of cancer are called intraepithelial neoplasias (also improperly named dysplasias).

Although condylomas or warts can be present on the vagina, cervix, or anal canal, anogenital (venereal) warts usually refer to exophytic lesions of the external anogenital area; they are also called condylomata acuminata (singular, condyloma acuminatum). Condylomata acuminata may on occasion be extremely large (giant condylomas). They may then adopt a locally invasive behavior and be called condylomatous carcinomas or Buschke–Löwenstein tumors.

The intraepithelial neoplasias are a group of conditions defined by the proliferation in the anogenital stratified epithelium of basaloid (basal-appearing) cells with an excess of often abnormal mitotic figures (dyskaryosis). Three grades are recognized, from the less to the more severe, based schematically on the proportion of the epithelium involved in this process. Thus the process involves up to the lower third of the epithelium in grade 1 (I), more than one-third but less than two-thirds in grade 2 (II), and more than two-thirds in grade 3 (III). In carcinoma *in situ* (CIS), a form of intraepithelial neoplasia grade 3, the full thickness of the epithelium is involved. Breakage of the basement membrane by this cellular proliferation represents invasion and the ultimate stage of evolution of an intraepithelial neoplasia: squamous cell carcinoma. Originally devised for the cervix (Fig. 56-1), this simple histologic classification scheme is also used for other locations, giving rise to various acronyms: CIN for cervical intraepithelial neoplasia, VAIN for the vagina, VIN for the vulva, PIN for the penis, and AIN for the anus. Other conditions developing on the external genitalia are simply clinical variants of intraepithelial neoplasias. They include bowenoid papulosis (pigmented papules with a condylomatous cytoarchitecture); Bowen disease (CIS presenting as a flat, red to brown plaque, with well-demarcated borders and a scaly surface); and erythroplasia of Queyrat (Bowen disease of the glans penis). Condylomas and intraepithelial neoplasias of the cervix typically arise in the transformation zone, the virtual space between the location of the squamocolumnar-epithelial junction at birth and the current location of this junction, which with age recedes toward the endocervix. Similarly, in the anus, it is in the area of squamous metaplasia, at the junction of the squamous and glandular epithelium, that one finds AIN and carcinomas.

If only based on the fact that they are in part caused by the same HPV types, these diseases are related. Another relation, histopathologic, has been particularly well documented for the cervix, where a lesion may progress from condyloma or CIN 1 to CIN grades 2 and 3, and cancer. This progression is not necessarily steady, it may not even occur, some of its stages may be missed, and up to grade 3 it may revert. Importantly, the risk of progression or regression is related to the HPV type causing the process, molecular variants within HPV types, HPV viral load and persistence, as well as possibly other factors such as smoking, use of oral contraceptives, immunogenetics, diet, and co-infections. Figure 56-1 illustrates the relation between HPV type and disease grade in greater detail in the case of the uterine cervix involvement.

Two minor groups of diseases are related to the genital HPV diseases because they are caused by the same HPV types and are mostly sexually transmitted: recurrent respiratory papillomatosis and oral condylomas. Although risk factors for the acquisition of recurrent respiratory papillomatosis include receptive oral sex in adults and vaginal delivery in children, for unclear reasons the disease seems to be rare in HIV-infected individuals. Oral HPV diseases include condylomas resulting from sexual transmission. Only histology helps distinguish them from other oral benign HPV-associated lesions such as squamous papillomas and verruca vulgaris.[2] Heck disease (focal epithelial hyperplasia), an uncommon florid oral

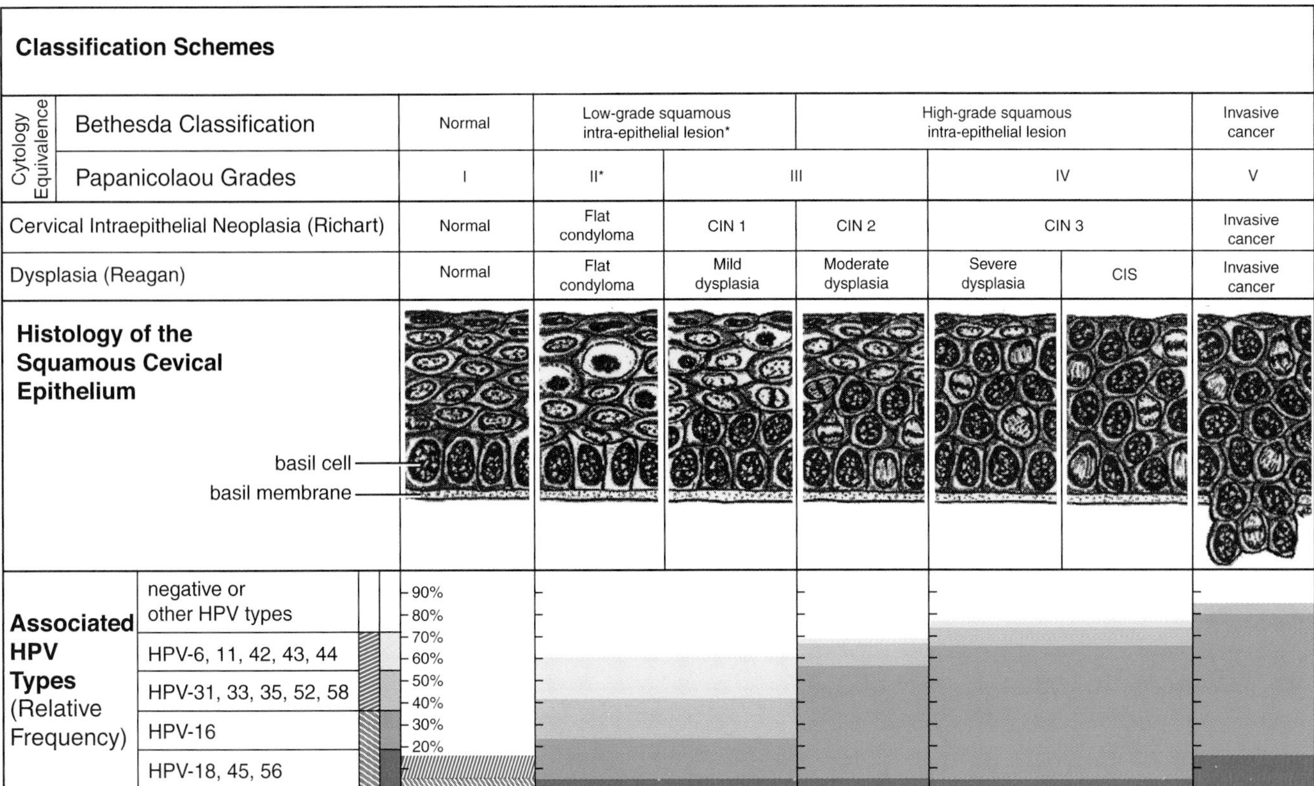

Figure 56-1 ■ Nomenclature, histologic features, and distribution of associated HPV types in HPV-related cervical lesions. The dysplasia and the cervical intraepithelial neoplasia classifications are primarily histologic classifications that are also used for cytology, whereas the Bethesda classification is designed mainly for cytology (see text for details). Not shown are benign cell changes, reactive changes, atypical squamous cells of unknown significance (ASCUS).

papillomatosis predominantly caused by HPV type 13, has been described in HIV patients associated with HPV32.[2]

Anogenital HPV infections are particularly common in the general population, but the prevalence varies with the method of diagnosis and, as would be expected for agents that are mostly sexually transmitted, the age of the population. For example, in one study, using a polymerase chain reaction (PCR) assay, 49% of women between the ages of 20 and 25 years had HPV in their cervix, in contrast to 34% of women 26–50 years of age.[3] Based on cytology, the rates fall to ~1–5% depending on age and diagnostic criteria.[4] It is estimated that ~1% of the population has condyloma acuminatum.[4] These numbers exemplify the large size of the virus reservoir in the population at large. Sexual transmission is by far the major mode of dissemination and although direct evidence is lacking, it is probably more efficient if the infection causes full-blown disease rather than latency or subclinical disease.

Three types of anogenital HPV diseases are clearly overrepresented in the HIV-seropositive population compared to the seronegative population: condyloma acuminatum, AIN (in men, and in women to a lesser extent), and CIN (Table 56-2).[5–19]

A large population survey has shown that in patients who have AIDS, the relative risks of *in situ* or invasive squamous cell carcinomas are increased in several anatomic locations: cervix, vulva/vagina, anus (both genders), penis, and (men only) tonsils and conjunctiva.[14]

These findings are consistent with the observation that HIV infection is associated with anogenital infections involving high-risk rather than low-risk HPV genotypes, and with more persistent and high HPV viral loads.[7,12,15–27] Other factors, such as smoking and young age, independently contribute to the risk of anogenital HPV infection and disease.[11,15,28] Although anal intercourse is a risk factor for anal HPV infection and disease in men and women, high prevalence of these conditions still exist in its absence.[29,30]

The nature of the link between HIV and HPV infections seems to be behavioral and immunologic, but the details are not well defined. Because both infections are sexually transmitted, it is obvious that they share some of the same behavioral risk factors. However, if oral sex seems to be a risk factor for adult-onset recurrent respiratory papillomatosis in the general population, it is not clear why this entity is not more common in HIV-infected patients.[31] HIV infection depresses the immune defenses that control HPV infections. Accordingly, the more severe the HIV infection (as measured by the progression to AIDS, CD4+ cell count, or HIV viral load) the higher is the risk of finding high-risk HPV DNA in the anogenital tract, condylomata acuminata, or preinvasive squamous cell carcinomas in the cervix and anus of men and women.[32–35] It is also not surprising that because of the

Table 56-2 **Selected Epidemiologic Data on the Relationship Between HPV Disease and HIV**

	Number of Individuals with Pathology/Total (%)		
Population and Pathology	**HIV+**	**HIV−**	**Odds Ratio[a]**
Homosexual Men[342]			
With history of anal warts	28/48 (58%)	13/44 (30%)	3.3[a]
With history of penile warts	4/49 (8%)	7/46 (15%)	0.5
Presence of anal warts	12/49 (24%)	6/45 (13%)	2.1
Presence of anal HPV DNA[b]	13/49 (26%)	3/47 (6%)	5.3[a]
Homosexual Men with Anogenital Warts[10]			
With abnormal anal cytology	159/346 (46%)	26/261 (10%)	7.7[a]
With anal HSIL	8/346 (2.3%)	0/261 (0%)	+∞[a]
STD Clinic Population, Haiti[343]			
Anogenital warts	43/374 (11.4%)	28/548 (5.1%)	2.4[a]
Women with anogenital warts[344]	**22/253 (8.7%)**	**8/660 (1.2%)**	**7.8[a]**
Women[345]			
With LSIL[d]	33/135 (94.3%)	8/101 (7.9%)	3.5[a]
With HSIL	15/135 (11.1%)	1/101 (0.9%)	12.5[a]
Women, IVDA[d,346]			
With presence of cervical HPV DNA[e]	30/53 (57%)	7/55 (13%)	8.9[a]
With presence of anal HPV DNA[e]	40/52 (77%)	28/50 (56%)	2.6[a]

[a] Indicates a p value less than 0.05.
[b] By a combination of dotblot and Southern blot.
[c] SIL, squamous intraepithelial lesion; LSIL, low-grade SIL, HSIL, high-grade SIL.
[d] IVDA, intravenous drug abuser.
[e] By PCR assay.

HIV-induced immunosuppression, HPV diseases in these patients tend to be more severe and intractable, and they recur more frequently.[36–45]

This simple biologic explanation is not sufficient, however, otherwise the risk of invasive cervical cancer should rise as patients progress to AIDS. On the basis of that expectation, in 1993 the Centers for Disease Control and Prevention (CDC) had included cervical cancer as an AIDS-defining illness.[46] The failure for the expectation to materialize clearly has been a surprise. It has since been reasoned that because cervical cancer takes about a decade to develop in the general population, the limited survival of HIV patients did not permit a sufficient number of cervical cancers to occur for the trend to be detected. This interpretation is losing much strength because larger surveys still did not detect a trend.[14,47] It has been also proposed that intensified screening programs in combination with improved antiretroviral treatments might have curbed the progression of CIN to invasive cancer. However, the introduction of highly active antiretroviral therapy (HAART) had no effect on the incidence of invasive cervical carcinoma in an Italian cohort study.[48] In Africa where cervical cancer screening programs and antiretroviral therapy (ART) are rarely available, the increase in the incidence of cervical cancers in the HIV population has been much more limited, when present, than in the developed world.[49,50] We do not know if, when noted, this increase correlates with the degree of immunosuppression or some important covariates.[51,52] Some of those covariates might be independent of the stage of HIV disease and be linked to the possible direct enhancing role of HIV proteins on HPV oncogenesis, or the seeming ability of HPV16, the most oncogenic HPV, to evade the immune system.[53,54] Some have argued for abandoning the characterization of cervical cancer as an AIDS-defining cancer, but this does not change the need for attentive screening for HPV-related anogenital cancers in the HIV population.[55]

DIAGNOSIS

All available treatment modalities are directed at eradicating HPV disease rather than HPV infection. Therefore, disease diagnosis is more relevant than proving HPV infection. To detect HPV disease, the clinician depends on clinical methods, cytology, colposcopy, and histology. It is clear that the diagnosis of HPV infection and the typing of its agents are likely to play an important role in the future. Because HPVs cannot yet be grown and propagated *in vitro*, the diagnosis of HPV infection depends on the detection of HPV DNA. Serology is useful in epidemiology but has no place in clinical practice.

Clinical Diagnosis

Diagnosis of anogenital HPV diseases in HIV-infected patients requires a history and physical examination. The history should focus on symptoms of the anogenital area (itching, discomfort, pain, bleeding, change of appearance) and inquiries about changes that affect sexual intercourse, urination, and defecation. Anorectal symptoms are particularly common in patients with AIN grade 3 and minimally invasive anal cancer, and should not be ignored.[56] If a diagnosis has already been established, one should assess its psychological impact and note the treatment received for the present condition and possible previous occurrences. To ensure future treatment compliance, it is wise to inquire about the patient's experience with prior treatment. It is also important to document how the diagnosis was made (e.g., clinically, cytologically, biopsy), because it may be open to revision. A sexual history should identify age at first intercourse, number of past and present sexual partners, sexual practices, and use of barrier methods of contraception and sexually transmitted disease (STD) prevention. The history and treatment of other STDs should be also recorded as well as the histories of warts, intraepithelial neoplasias, or cancers in the sexual partners.

The physical examination of the male patient is typically carried out with the subject leaning back against the end of the examining table and standing in front of the seated clinician. For the anal examination the patient turns back, legs apart, the torso bent and applied against the table. A tilting, proctologic examination table is helpful, if available. Alternatively, the patient can be examined in lateral decubitus and genuflected. For the female, the entire examination is conducted with the patient in the lithotomy position, legs placed in stirrups. Good lighting is essential. The examiner should wear gloves; the use of aprons, gown, mask, and eye-protective equipment should be tailored to the circumstances of the examination and to the additional procedures performed. Physical examination of the external genitalia can be augmented by the application for 1–5 min of gauzes soaked in 3–5% acetic acid (white vinegar). This is most helpful for detecting small or maculopapular HPV lesions because they tend to be acetowhite, particularly on the nonkeratinized ('mucosal') epithelia. However, acetowhitening is not a specific test when used alone and treatment should only be directed at papular lesions consistent with warts. The use of a magnifying glass or, better, a colposcope assists the diagnosis further. An anoscopic examination should be done if there are anal symptoms, a history of anal-receptive intercourse, or perianal warts (*see section on* Therapy).[57] Anoscopic diagnosis requires some familiarity, and proper evaluation should be left to experts. The diagnosis can be aided with a colposcope and prior application of 1% acetic acid, a procedure called high-resolution anoscopy.[58] Because lesions rarely extend beyond the pectinate line, a sigmoid examination is not routinely indicated.[59,60] In women, a speculum examination of the vagina and cervix should be done to at least rule out gross abnormalities and obtain a Papanicolaou (Pap) smear, if indicated (*see section on* Prevention). Application of acetic acid and use of a colposcope aid the diagnosis considerably, but such skills are usually beyond those of the primary care practitioner. The visual inspection of the anus, vagina, and cervix should be completed by a digital examination. An examination of the oral cavity should be considered to exclude associated oral warts. Whenever the proper diagnosis is in doubt, especially if intraepithelial neoplasia or cancer is in the differential diagnosis, a biopsy should be considered. This particularly applies to pigmented lesions and anal, vaginal, or cervical lesions. The use of anatomic diagrams to document the lesions is strongly recommended because they facilitate subsequent evaluations.

Cytology and Colposcopy

Cervical cytology in the form of the Pap smear is an important tool for detecting and managing HPV diseases of the cervix. Several methods and instruments have been designed to collect the cervical cells. Ideally, one uses a wooden Ayre spatula. The longer lip is placed in the cervical os, and the spatula is rotated 360º. A Dacron swab or, better, an endocervical brush is then introduced in the os and rotated 180º. The material collected on the spatula and on the brush are then respectively smeared and rolled on the same side of a glass slide bearing the patient's identification. The slide is immediately exposed to a fixative, either with a spray or by immersion in a transport jar filled with alcohol. A Cervex brush ('broom') substitutes advantageously for the Ayre spatula and brush when the cells are collected for liquid-based cytology (ThinPrep; AutoCyte). This newer technology allows better preparation of the sample, increases the sensitivity for the detection of squamous intraepithelial lesion (SIL), but is more costly and time-consuming than traditional cytology, which it has largely supplanted.[61,62] Figure 56-1 illustrates the correspondence between the various histologic and cytologic classification schemes for HPV cervical lesions. The Bethesda classification, established in 1988, and revised in 1992 and 2001, calls for establishing the adequacy of the sample, categorizing the cytology, and recommending management and follow-up (http://www.bethesda2001.cancer.gov).[63] Squamous cell abnormalities fall into four categories: (1) atypical squamous cells (a) of undetermined significance (ASC-US), or (b) but high-grade squamous intraepithelial lesion (HSIL) cannot be excluded (ASC-H) (both subcategories used to be grouped as atypical squamous cells of unknown significance (ASCUS); (2) low-grade squamous intraepithelial lesion (LSIL); (3) HSIL and (4) squamous cell carcinoma. The sensitivity and specificity of the Pap smear for the detection of CIN in HIV-seropositive and HIV-seronegative women appear to be similar.[64,65] The Pap smear is not a diagnostic test, but because it is inexpensive and can be repeated frequently it remains an excellent, so far essential, screening tool.

Colposcopy plays a role in the evaluation of an abnormal Pap smear. In that context, it has two connected purposes; the visual identification of lesions and the selection of biopsy sites for histologic confirmation. The colposcope is simply a binocular microscope with a long focal length (300–350 mm) and its own light source that permits detailed inspection of the cervix exposed with a vaginal speculum. With its complete implementation, the colposcopic examination includes application of 5% acetic acid and possibly an iodine (Lugol) solution (Schiller test). Lesion identification is based on one of several scoring systems that rely on elements such as color, shape of the margins, and vessel appearance. If abnormalities are present, colposcopy should be supplemented by biopsies for a more reliable histologic diagnosis. The performance characteristics of colposcopy in HIV-seropositive women might not be as good as in HIV-seronegative women.[65]

Cytologic screening has been extended to the anal canal. The technique requires introduction of a Dacron swab moistened with saline or water, or a cervical cytobrush, into the anal canal more than 2 cm from the anal margin.[66] The swab is rotated as it is withdrawn and then rolled over a glass slide or shaken in a liquid cytology transportation medium (ThinPrep; Auto Cyte) vial bearing the patient's identification. The slide is promptly fixed and processed as for a Pap smear. The test can be self-administered.[67] The sensitivity and specificity of anal cytology for the diagnosis of AIN (excluding ASCUS) in HIV-seropositive homosexual men are 46% and 81%, respectively.[68] Therefore, as for the cervix, anal cytology should be viewed more as a screening tool than a diagnostic tool. Anal cytology screening for SIL in HIV-positive and HIV-negative homosexual and bisexual men appears to be cost-effective when theoretical models are analyzed.[69,70] Nevertheless, as appealing and promising as it is, it cannot be widely recommended at this time for several reasons.[71,71a] The interpretation of anal cytology and histology suffers from poor to moderate inter- and intraobserver reliability.[72] There is a lack of clinically validated screening strategies adapted to the various populations at risk. We also do not know the natural evolution of high-grade anal SIL, which also are prone to recur after treatment.[73] In addition, the medical and surgical treatment options are limited yet their selection is not codified or validated by comparative studies. Furthermore, their impact on the prevention of anal cancer is largely unknown. Another difficulty is the need to train physicians on how to evaluate, biopsy, and treat a cytology-positive patient with anoscopy under magnified optics (high-resolution anoscopy).

Histology

Histologic diagnosis is used to confirm the diagnosis of HPV disease. The histologic material may be an operative sample or a biopsy specimen obtained by scalpel, scissors, punch, forceps, or electrosurgical or laser excision. Buffered formalin is the fixative of choice if subsequent *in situ* hybridization techniques are contemplated. Although diagnostic criteria are well recognized, particularly for the cervix, sampling variations, the size and condition of the sample, and intra- and interobserver variabilities can still affect the accuracy of the diagnosis. Furthermore interobserver reproducibility of cervical histology is no better than that of cervical cytology and is only moderate with both techniques.[74] Anal cytology and histology suffer from the same limitations.[72]

Nucleic Acid Detection Assays

Nucleic acid detection assays permit the diagnosis of HPV infection and typing of the virus. The material submitted for analysis can be cells collected from scraping, cervical lavage, or tissue. The Hybrid Capture II assay (Digene Diagnostics) is the only test approved by the US Food and Drug Administration (FDA) that is available to the practitioner. This proprietary assay is based on liquid phase hybridization. Cells or DNA extracted from the tissue sample are denatured in an alkaline solution. Two pools of RNA probes are added in parallel. Probes in pool A hybridize low-risk HPV types (6, 11, 42, 43, 44), whereas in pool B they hybridize high-risk HPV types (16, 18, 31, 33, 35, 39, 45, 51, 52, 56, 58, 59, 68). The hybrid DNA–RNA is immobilized by an antibody coating the wells of a microtiter plate and is recognized by an antibody conjugated to alkaline phosphatase that generates a chemoluminescent signal. The assay is rapid, resilient to cross-contamination, and quantitative. Investigators have also developed various assays based on the PCR for HPV DNA detection and typing. The Hybrid Capture II assay and PCR have comparable sensitivities, but PCR is more type-specific.[75,76] HPV DNA testing has been recommended in the management of ASCUS.[77] Since 2003, HPV DNA testing is also approved by the FDA to be used simultaneously with liquid-based cytology in women who are 30 years and older. The place of HPV typing for the anus is not established, but does not appear to be promising.[78]

THERAPY

This section focuses on condyloma acuminatum, a condition whose treatment and management are amenable to direct intervention by the primary care practitioner. Intraepithelial neoplasias and cancer, which mostly concern the cervix and anus, typically necessitate specialized care; only those aspects that are relevant for the primary care practitioner are discussed here.

Approach to Therapy

Condyloma Acuminatum

A wide variety of options are available for the treatment of condyloma acuminatum; unfortunately, none is satisfactory. Treatments are often ineffective, painful, and costly. Therefore it is important to discuss with the patient the goals and limitations of treatment.

Goals of Therapy

The psychological effect of condyloma acuminatum in the general population tends to be overlooked, yet it is an important reason for seeking treatment.[79] In fact, about half of the patients report a significant psychosexual impact either before or after treatment.[80–83] It is not known if the HIV-seropositive population is similarly affected, or if the social stigma of an additional STD is a reason for seeking treatment.

In the general population three-fourths of patients are asymptomatic, and treatment is initiated for cosmetic reasons.[84] There are no data on the frequency and nature of symptoms in HIV-seropositive patients, but symptoms such as itching and less frequently burning, pain, discomfort, discharge, bleeding, and dyspareunia may be indications for treatment. In pregnant women, warts may partially obstruct the birth canal or compromise hemostasis and repair of lacerations and incisions after delivery.

Treatment should be directed at the disease, not the infection, although the latter may be more extensive than the former.[85–87] Current treatments are considered ineffective for eliminating HPV infection. For example, laser vaporization of the entire mucosal surface of the lower genital tract of women with histologic evidence of HPV infection failed to eradicate the infection in most patients, and it was associated with severe morbidity.[88] Similar disappointing results have been obtained in men.[89]

No information is available on the prevalence of condyloma acuminatum and other anogenital HPV diseases in the sexual partners of HIV-seropositive patients with condyloma acuminatum. However, several studies in the general population have indicated that 40–70% of sexual partners of patients with anogenital HPV disease have lesions, which are macroscopic in half the cases.[90,91] Treating the male partner of women with CIN or subclinical genital HPV infection has failed to have an impact on the patient's condition.[88,92] Whether the reverse situation wherein treating the female partner helps the male patient is unknown. At present, the CDC does not advocate tracing and treating sexual partners for HPV disease.[93] The sexual partners of HIV-seropositive patients are more likely to be evaluated for HPV disease when traced for HIV infection or other STDs.

There is an association between condyloma acuminatum and the presence of cervical or anal intraepithelial neoplasias and cancer in HIV patients.[94] As yet there is no other evidence to indicate that treatment of condyloma acuminatum, even intra-anal, has an effect on these conditions. Vulvar and penile cancers are too rare for studies to be able to gauge an effect from treating condyloma acuminatum. Thus so long as one can be reassured that it is condyloma acuminatum, not intraepithelial neoplasia or cancer, cancer prevention should not be a reason for treating condyloma acuminatum.

Risks of Therapy

Frequent but usually transient adverse effects can be expected for the various treatment modalities of condyloma acuminatum. Permanent complications are rarer and include scarring and loss of tissue. Little is known of the psychosexual impact of the various therapies. Because recurrences or incomplete responses to treatment are common, some patients are exposed to several therapeutic attempts that increase the cumulative risk of durable side-effects. Costs, which can be particularly high with certain forms of treatment, are another concern.

Therapeutic abstention is definitely an option to consider, provided one is confident that the patient has only condylomata acuminata, not intraepithelial neoplasia or cancer, and that regular follow-up is possible. Although HIV-seropositive patients may have more recalcitrant and longer-standing disease than their HIV-seronegative counterparts, this is not uniformly the case.[36,41] The natural history of condyloma acuminatum is poorly known, especially among those who are HIV seropositive. In the nonimmunocompromised host, the experience with the placebo recipients in controlled clinical trials suggests that one can expect a 5–20% rate of spontaneous resolution of condyloma acuminatum within 3–4 months.[95–100]

Other Anogenital HPV Diseases

The three general principles that apply to the management of intra-anal warts and anogenital intraepithelial neoplasias are simple. First is the need to make a tissue diagnosis. Biopsies are essential, but sampling errors are a problem. For example, cervical punch biopsies of the cervix may underdiagnose HPV disease in HIV-seropositive women.[101] The second principle is to apply the proper treatment, which should be left to experts.[102] The third, extremely important principle is to follow the patient on a regular basis. In at least half of the HIV-seropositive patients treated for CIN, disease recurs, with a risk that increases with the falling CD4+ cell count, and disease involvement of the margins of the resected tissue.[37,42,44,45,103] Recurrence is also the typical outcome for anal HSIL lesions.[73] Screening is part of the management for cervical HPV diseases.[104]

Effect of HIV Antiviral Treatment on HPV Disease

The effect of antiretroviral treatment (HAART in particular) on the natural history of anogenital HPV diseases is confusing. The conflicting data have been recently reviewed by Heard and colleagues.[105] In summary, HAART might improve the resolution of genital warts and of vulvar neoplasia.[106] The effect on CIN varies for reasons that are still unclear from nonexistent to favorable. HAART generally does not correlate with a positive outcome of HPV-associated anal disease.[107–111] The incidence of oral warts appears unaffected or increased with HAART.[112]

Available Treatment Modalities

Treatment modalities for condyloma acuminatum are many, a reflection of the limitations of them all.[113] To choose among them is complicated by the relative paucity of well conducted comparative trials. Even some commonly used treatments have never been submitted to a double-blind, placebo-controlled, randomized trial. The most commonly used or best studied treatment modalities are emphasized in this section. The available information presented has been derived from studies done largely, if not exclusively, in immunocompetent patients. For the most part, one can only extrapolate this knowledge to the HIV-positive population, remembering that a successful treatment response may be less frequent, recurrences more common, disease more extensive, and side-effects different.[114,115] Table 56-3 summarizes practical information on the drugs commonly used to treat condyloma acuminatum.

Laser therapy, electrosurgery, and cryotherapy are the three most common approaches offered for the treatment of CIN or AIN. Cold-blade surgery is sometimes required. Choosing among these therapies is guided by personal experience, reported case series, availability of equipment, and some technical considerations. A limited but growing experience with some of these approaches in the HIV-seropositive population has been reported.

The CDC, the National Institutes of Health (NIH), and the Infectious Diseases Society of America (IDSA) have issued human papillomavirus diseases treatment recommendations for HIV-infected adults and adolescents.[102]

Podophyllin/Podofilox

Podophyllin is a natural product extracted from the rhizome of *Podophyllum peltatum* or *P. emodi*. The two major groups of compounds found in podophyllin resin are flavonols and lignans. The antiwart activity is limited to the lignans and principally to podophyllotoxin, which represents ~10% of the preparation.[116] Podofilox is now the generic name of podophyllotoxin. Like colchicine, it binds tubulin and inhibits microtubule polymerization.[116] This causes disruption of the mitotic spindle and mitosis, and there is disruption of the other cellular functions dependent on the integrity of microtubules. In addition, podofilox may directly damage HPV DNA.[117]

Table 56-3 describes how podophyllin and podofilox are used and prescribed for treatment of condyloma acuminatum. Being a purified, standardized product, podofilox has a more predictable effect than podophyllin. It is also more active and less toxic on a weight basis, permitting the drug to be applied by the patient.[116,118] The toxicity of podophyllin is well documented.[116,118] In addition to the local side-effects listed in Table 56-3, the medication can be readily absorbed through the skin and cause systemic side-effects including nausea, vomiting, sometimes irreversible motor and sensory neuropathies, seizures, coma, and death. The drug can also be toxic to the bone marrow, the lungs, and the kidneys. It is contraindicated during pregnancy, because of its mutagenic and abortifacient properties. Skin biopsies obtained after application of podophyllin should be interpreted with great caution. The drug causes skin necrosis, and the presence of large keratinocytes with disrupted chromatin (podophyllin cells) or mitoses can be misinterpreted for intraepithelial neoplasia.[119,120] Podophyllin has been associated with contact dermatitis caused by the benzoin vehicle or guaiacum wood contaminants. Podofilox is much less toxic than podophyllin.[116,118]

Since the 1940s there have been many reports on the use and efficacy of podophyllin and, later, podofilox for the treatment of anogenital warts.[116,118] The efficacy can be best ascertained from the many randomized comparative trials. Reported rates of a complete response to podophyllin vary widely, from 22% to 100%, but mostly range from 35% to 50%. They are inferior to those of the other standard forms of treatment (excisional surgery, electrodesiccation, cryotherapy, podofilox). Recurrences are common (typically 40–70%), so the net complete response rates are even lower, ranging from 25% to 45% (the longer the follow-up and the larger the HPV viral load, the higher the recurrences rate).[121] Overall, podofilox is more effective than podophyllin, but the complete response rates associated with its use range from 20% to 100%, typically 60–70%; and recurrences are common (30–50%), bringing the net complete response rate to a common range of 30–50%.[116,118,122] Prophylactic application of podofilox after the lesions disappear does prevent recurrences.[123] Podofilox 0.5% self-applied once a day for 3 consecutive days a week for 8 weeks after condylomata acuminata had been eradicated with either podofilox or cryotherapy resulted in only two of 21 patients (19%) having recurrences. In contrast, 12 of 24 patients (50%) treated with only the vehicle recurred. The durability of this effect is unknown. The abandoning of podophyllotoxin in favor of podofilox has been argued in view of the ease of application, and the toxicity and efficacy data.[116,118]

Information on the use of podophyllin or podofilox in HIV-seropositive patients is limited. Beck et al treated 31 patients with anal condylomas using 5% podophyllin and found a 26% recurrence rate at a mean 12 months later.[124] Orkin and Smith observed worse results in their study; 17 of their 21 patients (81%) treated with podophyllin failed.[125] Podofilox has also been associated with a poor outcome. After a single cycle of podofilox 0.5% solution applied twice a day for 3 consecutive days, eight of 18 HIV-seronegative patients (45.5%) were free of condylomata acuminata after 6 months of follow-up compared to only one of 15 HIV-seropositive patients ($P = 0.02$).[40] Podophyllin has been used successfully in the eradication of bowenoid papulosis in a 9-year-old child who had previously failed to respond to imiquimod.[126]

Bi- and Trichloroacetic Acids

Bichloroacetic and trichloroacetic (TCA) acids have long been used, predominantly by gynecologists, but also by proctologists. They induce acid hydrolysis, which is responsible for their keratolytic action. They may bind to the cellular proteins, acting as a cauterizing, fixative agent.[127] They also readily destroy HPV DNA. Only one of 14 condyloma acuminatum patients (7%) treated *in vitro* by TCA yielded HPV DNA by PCR.[117] Table 56-3 lists dosages and administration of bichloroacetic acid and TCA, and their side-effects. Discomfort, ulcerations, and scabbing are some of the adverse reactions

Table 56-3

Common Drugs Used for the Treatment of Condyloma Acuminatum

Drug	Formulations[a]	Presentations	Typical Dosing Regimen	Common Potential Toxicities	Comments
Podophyllin	Podophyllum (USP)[a] Podocon-25 Podofin	 15 mL bottle 15 mL bottle	qwk, ≤6 applications with a cotton-tipped applicator	Itching Pain Inflammation Chemical burns Ulcerations Scarring Contact dermatitis Systemic penetration and toxicities are possible if large doses are delivered	Applied by the practitioner Application on healthy skin is to be avoided; may use protective ointment (e.g., zinc oxide-based paste) Do not treat more than 10 cm^2 of skin area or overapply the drug Do not leave medication on for more than 24 h. Best to wash-off by the end of the day Not to be used in pregnant women, and discouraged for nursing women
Podofilox (podophyllo-toxin)	Condylox 0.5% solution* or gel*	3.5 mL bottle with cotton-tipped applicators or 3.5 g gel tube	Therapeutic: bid applications, × 3 consecutive days/week, ≤4 cycles Suppressive: qd applications, × 3 consecutive days/week, ≤8 cycles	Same as with podophyllin No contact dermatitis	Self-applied, after demonstration of technique and lesions to be treated Application on healthy skin is to be avoided; may use protective ointment when using the solution (e.g., zinc oxide-based paste) Do not treat more than 10 cm^2 of skin area or apply more than 0.5 mL of the drug Effectiveness and safety beyond 8 weeks has not been determined for suppressive use Not to be used in pregnant women, and discouraged for nursing women
Bi- and trichloroacetic acids	Bichloracetic acid 80% Tri-Chlor 80%	10 mL bottle 15 mL bottle	qwk, ≤6 applications with a cotton-tipped applicator or wooden stick	Itching Pain Inflammation Chemical burns Ulcerations Scarring	Applied by the practitioner Application on healthy skin is to be avoided; may use protective ointment (e.g., zinc oxide-based paste) or buffer the excess acid with talcum powder or bicarbonate soda Can be used in pregnant and nursing women
5-Fluorouracil	Efudex 5% cream Fluroplex 1% cream and solution	25 g tube 30 g tube or 30 mL bottle	Many different regimens have been recommended from bid to qowk (see the literature.[131–142] Applied externally with the fingers (finger cots may be used) or internally with a vaginal applicator	Itching Pain Inflammation Chemical burns Ulcerations Mucosal denudation Scarring Contact dermatitis	Self-applied; fingers should be washed afterward Use is discouraged in pregnant women

(Continued)

Table 56-3 (Continued)

Drug	Formulations[a]	Presentations	Typical Dosing Regimen	Common Potential Toxicities	Comments
Interferon (IFN) injection				Fever Chills Malaise Headache Myalgia Fatigue	Intralesional injection is the most effective. IFN is injected at the base of the lesion Systemic injection is done either subcutaneously or intramuscularly Systemic reactions are usually mild with the intralesional injections. They may be blunted by taking acetaminophen or a nonsteroidal antiinflammatory agent prior to the injection Monitoring of complete blood count and liver enzymes is recommended when systemic reactions are anticipated
IFN-αn3	Alferon N[a]	5 MIU/vial	250 000 IU/wart (total ≤ 2.5 MIU[b]) biw, ≤ 8weeks[271]		
IFN-α-2b	Intron A[a]	10 MIU/vial	1 MIU/wart (≤5 warts), tiw, x3wk[210,272–277]		
IFN-α-2a	Roferon-A	Various formulations	See the literature[c,248,249,278]		
IFN-β-1a	Avonex	6.6 MIU/vial	See the literature[279,280]		
IFN-γ-1b	Actimmune	3 MIU/vial	See the literature[281,282]		
IFN-β-1b	Betaseron	9.6 MIU/vial	See the literature[274]		
Imiquimod	Aldara 5% cream[a]	box of 12 single-use 250 mg packets	qod applications, ×3/week, ≤16weeks	Itching Burning Erythema Erosion Excoriation Edema	Self-applied; fingers should be washed afterwards Anogenital area should be washed 6–10 h after cream application No data available about use in nursing or pregnant women The cream weakens condoms and diaphragms; sex should be avoided the day the cream is applied

qd, once daily, bid, twice daily; qod, every other day; qwk, once weekly; biw, twice weekly; tiw, 3 times per week; qowk, every other week.

[a] These products have been approved by the FDA for the treatment of condyloma acuminatum.

[b] MIU, million international units.

[c] References are given only for studies using intralesional injections. Studies on other routes of administration are reported elsewhere.[261,283]

that occur in about two-thirds of the patients.[128,129] They are more common than with cryotherapy. Widely used, these agents have been submitted to limited evaluation, and only TCA has been compared to other standard therapies.[128–130] TCA appears to be equivalent to cryotherapy in terms of the complete response rate (~65–80%) and recurrence rate, with about half of the patients remaining free of disease.[128] Acids are safe for the treatment of pregnant women.

5-Fluorouracil and Nucleoside Derivatives

5-Fluorouracil (5-FU) is a pyrimidine antagonist. A structural analog of thymidine, it interferes with the synthesis of DNA and to a lesser extent of RNA by blocking the methylation of deoxyuridylic acid into thymidylic acid. Dividing cells are particularly sensitive to its action, and the compound has been widely used topically by dermatologists to treat diverse conditions.

Various topical regimens with 5-FU have been applied for the treatment and prophylaxis of condyloma acuminatum, vaginal warts, and intraepithelial neoplasias of the vagina and cervix.[131–142] 5-FU has been applied twice daily to weekly for durations ranging from a few days to 10 weeks. The frequency and nature of the side-effects depend on the regimens used and the sites treated. Pain, itching, burning, and hyperpigmentation are the most common local adverse reactions, affecting approximately half of the patients. More serious reactions have also been noted, such as contact and allergic dermatitis and chronic vaginal ulcerations,[143–146] which has discouraged many practitioners from using this drug. Twice-weekly applications are much better tolerated than daily applications, without an apparent difference in efficacy.[140] Reportedly, fair-skinned individuals are particularly prone to local side-effects.[147] Rarer but significant complications should be mentioned: leukopenia, thrombocytopenia, toxic granulations, and eosinophilia as well as the development of vaginal adenosis and vaginal clear cell carcinoma.[148] Administration of 5-FU has not been associated with congenital malformations, but the safety of this drug during pregnancy is not established.[149]

Intrameatal warts seem to be particularly responsive to 5-FU treatment, usually administered daily for 3–14 days.[133,134,150] Krebs observed that 16 of 20 patients (80%) with vaginal warts had a long-term (median 16 months) complete response after treatment with bedtime application of 1.5 g of 5% 5-FU cream once a week for 10 weeks.[139] Similarly, intravaginal or vulvar 5-FU prophylaxis against recurrences after treatment of vaginal and vulvar warts, respectively, appeared to be effective in HIV-uninfected patients.[138,151] In the HIV population, a placebo-controlled trial evaluated the efficacy of 1% 5-FU gel in 60 women with intravaginal warts, all of whom were receiving zidovudine 250 mg three times a day.[152] The 5-FU preparation was self-administered for 4 weeks: every other day 3 times a week at bedtime by deep intravaginal application of 4 mL. Sixteen weeks after treatment initiation the complete response rates were 83.4% in the 5-FU group and 13.3% in the placebo group. Side-effects included mild erythema, vaginal erosion, and edema. No patients dropped out of the study.

Anecdotal case series suggest that 5-FU might be useful for treatment of anogenital intraepithelial neoplasias in the general population, a claim that remains to be evaluated properly.[153] In addition, 5% 5-FU cream, applied daily, has been used successfully in combination with 5% imiquimod cream three times a week for treatment of AIN grade 3 lesions in an HIV-positive man.[154] Better evidence supports the use of 5-FU as secondary prophylaxis of CIN in HIV patients.[155] In the ACTG 200 trial, 101 HIV-positive women who had undergone ablative or excisional treatment for CIN were randomized to receive either topical vaginal 5% 5-FU cream (2 g) self-administered twice a week or nothing. Of the 50 (28%) women in the 5-FU group, 14 developed CIN recurrences compared to 24 of 51 (47%) in the observation group ($P < 0.05$). Moreover, in the 5-FU group recurrences tended to appear later and were more likely to be CIN grade 1 than CIN grade 2 or 3.

Cidofovir (Vistide), or (*S*)-1-(3-hydroxy-2-phosphonylmethoxypropyl)cytosine, is an acyclic nucleotide analog that is available for treatment of cytomegalovirus (CMV) retinitis. Intralesional injection of the compound has been found effective in a small number of patients, HIV-infected or not, with cutaneous warts, condylomata acuminata, oral warts, recurrent respiratory papillomatosis, VIN, and upper digestive HPV tumors.[156–165] A topical gel formulation of 1% cidofovir gel (Forvade) has been evaluated in a Phase II trial for treating condyloma acuminatum in immunocompetent patients.[166] It was administered daily for 5 days every other week for up to six cycles. One-third of the patients were randomized to receive placebo. At the end of the treatment period (12 weeks), 9 of 19 (47%) patients treated with cidofovir had a complete response compared to none of 11 patients in the placebo group ($P = 0.01$). In an open, nonrandomized trial including HIV-infected patients, cidofovir (1% in Beeler base) led to a complete response rate of condylomata acuminata of 32% (9 of 27), compared to 100% (20 of 20) of those treated with electrocautery.[167] Those patients failing cidofovir were given electrocautery. Relapse rate was low in this group (3.7%) compared to the group treated with electrocautery alone (55%).

Various strengths (0.3%, 1%, 3%) of cidofovir gel applied daily for 5 or 10 days every other week for up to three cycles were evaluated in an open Phase I/II study conducted in HIV-positive patients with anogenital warts.[159] Overall, seven of 46 (15%) patients had a complete response. All treatment regimens appeared equipotent. Topical 1% cidofovir cream was compared to placebo in a small randomized study of condyloma acuminatum in HIV-infected patients.[168] Partial clearance (>50% of wart area) was noted in half (three of six) of the cidofovir recipients, but in none of the six placebo recipients. Electrocautery was compared to 1% cidofovir gel (given daily 5 days a week, for up to 6 weeks) or 1% cidofovir gel (daily 5 days a week for 2 weeks) following electrocautery within 1 month for the treatment of condyloma acuminatum in HIV-infected patients.[169] Electrosurgery alone achieved a 93% (27 of 29) complete response rate, compared to 76% (20 of 26) for cidofovir alone, and 100% (19 of 19) for the combined regimen. Cidofovir 1% gel was also administered three times every other day on biopsy-proven CIN grade 3 lesions in 15 immunocompetent women.[170] One month later the cervix was excised, and seven of 15 (47%) of the specimens showed complete histologic resolution; four of them also demonstrated disappearance of HPV DNA. Topical cidofovir 1% has been associated with complete eradication of recurrent VIN grade 3 lesions in an HIV-negative woman. A 1% cream preparation was used to obtain the resolution of recalcitrant oral papillomatosis in an AIDS patient. Cidofovir gel or cream is currently not available commercially but can be made up by a pharmacist upon request.[171] Cidofovir is a potential carcinogen, and caution should be exercised with its use.[161]

Cryotherapy

Cryotherapy is one of the most common forms of treatment for anogenital HPV diseases and other dermatologic conditions. Solid carbon dioxide (carbonic ice; boiling temperature –78.5°C), nitrous oxide (–89.5°C), and especially liquid nitrogen (–196°C) are the principal cryogenic agents. Cold can be applied with cryogenic pencils or cotton swabs, but the most common modes of delivery are sprays for external lesions and cryoprobes of various sizes for internal lesions. Cryoprobes carry the potential risk of virus transmission, which is avoided with sprays.[172] Cryotherapy techniques are varied and empiric.[173–175] A common approach is to spray or cool the wart for 20 to 30 s until a 1–2 mm ice halo forms around the lesion. Some practitioners allow the lesion to thaw completely and then freeze it again.

Cold injury causes necrosis of the tissue but little HPV DNA destruction.[117,176] The patient experiences a brief stinging sensation followed by numbness. Upon thawing, about half of the patients report discomfort: itching, burning, or pain.[177,178] Uterine cramping follows cervical cryotherapy. Aggressive treatment may cause blisters and pronounced edema and should be avoided. One-fourth of the patients treated for condyloma acuminatum have skin discoloration at the treatment site 6 months later.[177]

The efficacy of cryotherapy for the treatment of condyloma acuminatum has been demonstrated in several open studies.[128,129,179–188] Unfortunately, although it is a common approach, there have been few randomized comparative trials. This makes it difficult to define confidently the role of cryotherapy. Typically, 65–85% of patients have a complete response with a 20–40% recurrence rate. When recurrences are taken into account, the complete response rate with cryotherapy is ~60%, which makes it a better choice than podophyllin and podofilox, equivalent to TCA, but slightly inferior to electrosurgery. Cryotherapy is particularly well suited for the care of meatal warts and the pregnant patient.

Along with electrosurgery and laser surgery, cryotherapy is used to treat internal HPV diseases (condylomas and intraepithelial neoplasias). These three techniques appear to have similar efficacies.[189,190] Compared to laser therapy, cryotherapy of the cervix is more painful and associated with longer symptomatic bleeding and vaginal discharge.[191] The cervix can be treated with cryotherapy during pregnancy.[192]

Cold-Blade Surgery

Surgical excision is one of the simplest radical approaches to the treatment of condyloma acuminatum. Thomson and Grace described the current technique developed for the treatment of anal warts.[193] The skin is disinfected and the base of the lesion is infiltrated with an anesthetic such as lidocaine. The resultant swelling aids in demarcating the margins of the lesion. Epinephrine (1:100000) may be added to the anesthetic to give better hemostatic control. The lesion is excised with curved (iridectomy) scissors, and bleeding is controlled by pressure with a gauze and application of 30% TCA or another hemostatic agent. The procedure is remarkably well tolerated. After the brief stinging pain of the anesthesia, little is felt by the patient, who later may experience mild local discomfort or itching. Frank pain is rare.[194] Slight bleeding of the wound is often noted but is self-limited. Hypopigmentation, the most common long-term complication, occurs in a small number of patients, and hypertrophic scarring is rare.[195] A variation of cold-blade surgery is the use of micro-resectors for internal lesions.[196]

Net complete response rates vary from 46% to 92% with cold-blade surgery.[193,194,197–202] Typically, the procedure is reserved for patients with few lesions, and this potential selection bias may contribute to the excellent efficacy of this technique. Cold-blade surgery is often used in combination with other therapies such as podophyllin, fulguration (electrosurgery), or both, with no evidence that outcomes are improved. In HIV-seropositive patients, cold-blade surgery has been combined with fulguration for the treatment of anal condylomas. Results of these open, retrospective case series have been mixed. Beck et al found a recurrence rate of only 4% in 27 patients followed for a mean of 1 year.[124] Miles et al treated 24 patients; of the 15 available for follow-up 1 month later, seven required additional treatment.[203] The addition of systemic interferon-γ does not lower the recurrence rate.[204] Wound healing after anorectal surgery for condylomata acuminata is usually not a problem in the HIV-seropositive patient, although it may be significantly delayed in the more severely immunocompromised patients (CD4+ count >50 cells/μL) or those with anal cancer.[205,206]

Cold-blade surgery applied to the treatment of cervical HPV diseases is known as conization.[207] It consists of excising a large cone of the cervix that includes the endocervix (the exocervix forms the base of the cone). Conization is now being largely replaced by less aggressive treatment options: electrosurgery, laser surgery, cryotherapy. Even for the rare indications of conization such as endocervical CIN or microinvasion, adapted laser and electrosurgical techniques (laser or loop electrosurgical excision cone biopsy) have replaced the traditional scalpel excision. As with all surgical procedures that generate biologic fluids potentially infected with HIV, the operator should wear gloves, apron or gown, mask, and eye protection.

Electrosurgery and Infrared Coagulation

Electrosurgical techniques are diverse and not necessarily interchangeable.[208] Depending on the number of electrodes used, contact (or not) with the lesion, and the type, intensity, frequency, and wave-shape of the current delivered; one recognizes, in an unfortunately often muddled nomenclature; electrofulguration (electrodesiccation), electrocoagulation, electrosection, and electrocautery. Although electrosurgery is often used in the treatment of HPV diseases by surgeons and dermatologists, it has undergone very little rigorous evaluation.

Vuori et al reported that 58 of 100 patients treated with electrocoagulation had a complete response.[209] One important randomized study compared cryotherapy, 20% podophyllin, and electrodesiccation.[187] All three treatments were administered weekly until complete response was evident or for up to 6 weeks. Electrosurgery was the best treatment, with 83 of 88 patients (94%) having a complete response; cryotherapy was the next best, with 68 complete responses in 86 patients (79%), followed by podophyllin, with 26 complete responses in 63 patients (41%) (all differences were statistically significant). A 3- to 5-month follow-up indicated that only about a fifth of the patients treated with electrosurgery or cryotherapy had any recurrence, compared to two-fifths of those treated with podophyllin. The intralesional administration of interferon-α as adjuvant to electrosurgery may reduce the rate of recurrence. In one study, patients treated with electrocautery were randomized to receive 5 million units of interferon (IFNα2b) in each lesion site (up to a total dose of 25 million units) for 2–3 days, or nothing.[210] Thirty-one percent of the 22 interferon-treated patients had recurrences, compared to 45% of the 11 non-interferon-treated patients ($P = 0.03$). In another study, patients treated for anal condylomas with surgical excision and electrosurgery were randomized to receive the addition of 500 000 units of IFNαn3 or saline in each quadrant of the anal canal.[211] After a mean follow-up of 16 weeks, three of the 25 interferon recipients (12%) had recurrences as compared to seven of 18 saline recipients (39%) ($P = 0.07$). Interestingly, half of the patients in this study were HIV seropositive. They exhibited the same favorable response to interferon as the seronegative patients. Thirty-eight HIV-seropositive patients with anogenital warts were treated with electrocautery and IFNβ (3 million units/day IM for 10 days) and then were randomized to receive IFNβ as maintenance three times a week for 1 or 3 months.[212] No significant differences in recurrence rates were observed between the two groups.

Electrosurgical procedures on the external genitalia are painful, but effective topical anesthesia could be obtained with EMLA cream (lidocaine and prilocaine) in 90% of men and 40% of women.[213] Another complication is scarring.[187]

Over the past decade electrosurgical techniques have emerged as among the most popular approaches for the management of CIN.[214] These techniques, which come in several varieties, are known as large loop excision of the transitional zone (LLETZ) or the loop electrosurgical excision procedure (LEEP).[215,216] They provide a diagnostic specimen and a therapeutic procedure in one intervention. Under the proper indications, ~95% of treatment-naive patients remain free of disease regardless of CIN grade in the absence of HIV infection. However, recurrences are much more common in the HIV-infected patients.[44,45] Local anesthesia is typically required, but these procedures are well tolerated, with minimal subsequent pain, bleeding, and vaginal discharge. Fertility does not seem to be affected.[217] Electrosurgical procedures should be avoided on a pregnant cervix. Chang et al have used high-resolution anoscopy followed by excisional biopsy and electrosurgery to treat anal HSIL.[73] All eight HIV-seronegative men had a complete resolution sustained for a mean 2.5 years. In contrast, only six of 29 HIV-seropositive men had a persistent complete response for a mean of 2 years.

Electrosurgery, like laser surgery, emits a plume of smoke that must be evacuated because, as discussed in the next section, it poses a potential infectious risk to the operator and assistants.[218,219]

Thermal ablation of condyloma acuminatum can be achieved with an infrared coagulator, an instrument that delivers pulsed far-infrared light through a guide applied to the lesion.[220] It has the advantages of outpatient use (after local anesthesia), of providing good hemostasis, and of not releasing smoke. A recent study has shown that the results seem similar to those of electrocautery for the management of anal HSIL in HIV-seropositive patients.[73,221] Of the 68 male patients studied after the first treatment, 35% were free of HSIL a median of 474 days later.[221] Of the 44 patients who failed, 36 were treated a second time, yielding a 42% complete response rate. Fifteen patients who had failed the second treatment agreed for a third treatment, and 60% had a complete response at a median of 739 days of follow-up.

Laser Surgery

Lasers are optical devices that generate a powerful beam of monochromatic and highly collimated light (the electromagnetic waves have the same wavelength, travel in parallel planes, and are in phase). Various types of medical lasers are available. The pulse dye, argon, and KTP lasers have been used for the treatment of HPV disease, but the one that is best adapted to anogenital surgery is the CO_2 laser.[222–227] Its infrared wavelength (10 600 nm) is well absorbed by water, which converts the energy to heat. That heat is responsible for vaporizing the lesion. A focused, narrow, high-energy beam is used for cutting and excision. A defocusing device allows a broader spot, convenient for tissue destruction and ablation. The lower energy density of the beam causes less tissue vaporization but more thermal conductive damage ('brushing' technique), resulting in coagulation of the cellular proteins; it can also be used for hemostasis. A pulsed output provides greater control for the operator. The laser light can be delivered through a handheld device, which is convenient for external lesions, or more commonly through the colposcope by a set of mirrors and lenses.

Laser surgery is applicable to the full range of anogenital HPV diseases.[147,223–228] Typically, laser procedures are conducted under topical anesthesia (EMLA cream or injectable anesthetics), but general anesthesia is required in some patients because of pain or the extent of the lesions. In addition to pain in the external genitalia, bleeding, discharge, tissue swelling, dysuria, meatal stenosis, and scarring occur in up to one-fourth of patients.[147,195,229–232] For vaginal and cervical procedures, symptomatic bleeding and vaginal discharge are minimal, usually lasting less than a week.[191] Pregnancy is not a contraindication to laser surgery.

Laser surgery and electrocoagulation generate smoke that contains HPV DNA; it can be found in the surgeon's upper respiratory tract and on the walls of the surgical suite.[218,219,233,234] It represents a true infectious risk because laser surgeons appear to be at increased risk of developing hand and nasopharyngeal warts.[235] In addition to the protections already customary for surgeons working with HIV-infected individuals (gloves, gown, mask, and goggles), a smoke evacuation system should be used.

Although the general principles of laser surgery are well defined, the technique is difficult to evaluate from the literature because individual techniques and skills vary appreciably. A review of laser surgery for the treatment of condyloma acuminatum in retrospective case series and randomized comparative trials in the general population indicates that the more rigorous the evaluation the poorer is the efficacy.[85,195,204,229–232,236–251] Although laser surgery provides an immediate complete response in 90–100% of patients, in the better designed studies 50–65% of the patients experience a relapse. Systemic interferon therapy has been given as an adjuvant to laser surgery to prevent wart recurrence. The results have been inconsistent, with either doubling of the net complete response rate[246,248,252] or no effect.[204,249,250]

There are few strict comparative studies of laser surgery versus electrosurgery or cryotherapy for treating CIN. The available data suggest that all these techniques yield similar results.[189–191,214,253–255] CO_2 laser surgery has been evaluated for the treatment of condylomata acuminata in 19 HIV-seropositive men.[256] Eleven patients had a complete response (58%). In this retrospective study, 32 of 45 (71%) HIV-seronegative patients also became disease-free. Laser surgery has been used for the treatment of oral HPV lesions in HIV-infected patients.[257] The main limitations of laser surgery are cost and the availability of a skilled practitioner.

Photodynamic laser therapy relies on the laser light to activate selectively the cytotoxicity of a photosensitizing compound applied topically (5-aminolevulinic acid, 5-ALA) or systemically (e.g., meso-tetra(m-hydroxyphenyl) porphyrin (m-THPP) or 5-ALA). Photodynamic laser therapy is a technique in development whose application for the treatment of condyloma acuminatum and CIN has so far been limited.[258–260]

Interferon and Cytokine Inducers

Interferons comprise a group of cytokines recognized for their immunomodulatory, antitumor, and antiviral properties. There are three main classes of these proteins: α, β, and γ. IFNα and IFNβ (type I IFN) share the same cellular receptor and some physicochemical properties.[261,262] IFNγ is distinct (type II IFN).

Interferons are produced in cell cultures (e.g., IFNβ, IFNαn1, IFNαn3) or by recombinant technology (e.g., IFNα2a, IFNα2b, IFNα2c), as full, truncated, consensus, or hybrid gene products. Because they have been used extensively to treat various diseases, their clinical adverse effects are well recognized. These effects are in part dose-related and are typically reversible upon cessation of the drug. The most common symptoms include fever, chills, malaise, headache, myalgia, and fatigue, which occur several hours after administration but rarely persist beyond 24 h. Acetaminophen or nonsteroidal antiinflammatory agents, if taken at the time of drug administration, can blunt these side-effects. Side-effects wane with repeated administration of the drug. More serious side-effects include lethargy, confusion, anxiety, depression, weight loss, anorexia, nausea, vomiting, alopecia, insomnia, and peripheral neuropathies. Biologic alterations may be noted, particularly neutropenia, thrombocytopenia, a rise in serum transaminases, and occasionally anemia and hypertriglyceridemia. Antibodies may form, possibly compromising efficacy. Interferons are contraindicated during pregnancy.

Interferons are some of the best studied treatments for HPV disease. These investigations have examined various diseases, various interferon classes, different dosages and schedules of administration, and different routes of administration.

For the treatment of condyloma acuminatum, the topical route has been generally disappointing.[263–266] The excellent results of Syed et al with a natural IFNα cream or gel are unusual in this respect.[267–269] The application of an IFNβ gel after excisional or ablative therapy for genital warts might be effective for preventing recurrence.[270] Topical IFN preparations are not available in the United States. The best and more consistent results have been obtained with intralesional interferon.[210,248,249,261,271–283] The limitations of this approach include fastidiousness, a limit on the number of lesions that can be treated at one session, and the pain associated with the injection. Other side-effects are usually minimal. The most important obstacle raised against intralesional interferon in HIV-infected patients is the report by Douglas et al.[284] They administered, in up to three warts per patient, 1 million IU of IFNα2a three times a week for 4 weeks. After a 16-week follow-up, none of the eight HIV-seropositive patients had a complete response compared to 11 of 21 HIV-seronegative patients (52%) ($P = 0.01$).

Systemic administration of interferon for the treatment of condyloma acuminatum has been largely ineffective when evaluated in randomized, rigorous studies. There is little reason to believe that it would be more effective in HIV-seropositive patients.[261] As mentioned in previous sections, interferons have been used in combination with other treatment modalities. They also have been extensively evaluated when used with cryotherapy or podophyllin, and their effect has been disappointing.[177,178,285] Interferons have also been used for the treatment of CIN. The experience remains largely unconvincing of their efficacy and role in the management of this condition.[286–289] In contrast to these poor results with standard IFN, the limited results obtained with the new long-acting, pegylated IFNs are intriguing. Brockmeyer et al administered pegylated IFNα2b (PEG-IFN) 80μg subcutaneously once a week, for 24 weeks, to a group of 12 HIV-infected subjects with condylomata acuminata, and followed them for 6 months.[290] Of 10 evaluable patients, four had a complete response, and another four had a major response. In contrast, all 10 patients in a control, untreated group had disease progression ($P < 0.001$). PEG-IFN also appeared to enhance the effect of HAART on HIV viral load reduction.

Imiquimod(1-(2-methylpropyl)-1*H*-imidazo[4,5-*c*]quinolin-4-amine) is an imidazoquinolineamine derivative with immunomodulating properties. In particular, it is an inducer of IFNα and other cytokines.[291–294] The drug has demonstrated excellent activity as a topical preparation for the treatment of condyloma acuminatum. It has been approved for that indication by the FDA as a 5% cream (Aldara). In one double-blind, randomized study 108 patients were treated with a 5% cream or vehicle, every other day three times a week for up to 8 weeks.[295] At the end of therapy no patients in the vehicle group had a complete response compared to 37% in the imiquimod group ($P < 0.001$). Only three of 16 patients (19%) had recurrences within 10 weeks of follow-up. In another study patients were randomized to self-apply 5% imiquimod, 1% imiquimod, or placebo cream with the same frequency but for up to 16 weeks.[98] The complete response rates were 50% (54 of 109), 21% (21 of 102), and 11% (11 of 100), respectively. The differences between the 5% imiquimod group and either of the two other groups were statistically significant ($P < 0.001$). The response was much better in females than in males irrespective of treatment. The recurrence rates in the three groups were 13%, 0%, and 10%, respectively. A similar randomized, double-blind trial was conducted to evaluate daily rather than thrice-weekly imiquimod self-administration.[296] At the end of the 16-week treatment period the complete response rates were 52% (49 of 94) in the 5% imiquimod group, 14% (13 of 90) in the 1% imiquimod group, and 4% (3 of 95) in the placebo cream group ($P < 0.0001$). As in the previous trial, women responded better than men; for instance, in the 5% imiquimod group there was a complete response rate of 64% (27 of 42) in women compared to 42% (22 of 52) in men. A fourth randomized trial was done in men to evaluate self-application of 5% imiquimod cream three times a week, once daily, twice daily, or three times a day.[297] Complete response rates at 16 weeks were similar in all four groups (ranging from 24% to 35%) without evidence of a dose–response effect. As in the previous trials, the magnitude of the side-effects was directly related to the dose and they were most severe with more frequent application than with daily application. A dose-range study was also done to determine the optimal dosing for the treatment of foreskin-associated warts in uncircumcised men.[298] Imiquimod cream 5%, every other day three times a week was best, yielding a 62% complete response rate. These results were consolidated in a large open-label multicenter trial conducted in patients with condyloma acuminatum.[299] The overall complete clearance rate at week 32 for the subjects who adhered to the protocol was 57% (235 of 413) for males and 66% (503 of 768) for females. When looking at all the participants, the sustained clearance rate at 6 month was 33% (311 of 943).

Imiquimod has been evaluated in HIV-infected patients for the treatment of condyloma acuminatum. A randomized, placebo-controlled study enrolled 97 men and three women with CD4+ cell counts higher than 99 cells/μL.[300] Patients were self-treated with 5% imiquimod cream every other day, three times a week for up to 16 weeks. Two-thirds ($n = 65$) were randomized to imiquimod and one-third ($n = 35$) to placebo. Tolerance was similar to that in immunocompetent hosts, but the complete response rate was poor: 11% in the imiquimod group and 6% in the placebo group ($P = 0.49$). However, 38% of patients receiving imiquimod had at least 50% or more wart clearance, compared to 14% of the placebo recipients ($P = 0.01$). In another comparative study of mostly male patients with anogenital warts, 31% (23 of 75) of HIV-seropositive patients were free of disease at the end of standard treatment, compared to 62% (31 of 50) of HIV-seronegative patients.[301] At a 3-month follow-up visit, the recurrence rates of the HIV-seropositive and HIV-seronegative patients were 17% and 6%, respectively. When used after surgical removal of condyloma acuminatum, imiquimod decreased the recurrence rate from 65% (13 of 20) in a nontreated group to 20% (4 of 20).

Intra-anal application of imiquimod 5% cream three times a week for up to 16 weeks resulted in at least a partial response in 10 HIV-seropositive patients with AIN.[302] Imiquimod has also been beneficial in preventing recurrences after electrocautery of intra-anal warts in HIV-seronegative[303] and HIV-seropositive[304] males. Imiquimod was delivered as suppositories or through anal gauze tampons. There is now a growing literature on the treatment of female external genital intraepithelial neoplasias with imiquimod.[292–294]

Side-effects of imiquimod are local and include itching and burning sensations, as well as erythema, erosion, and swelling. All are well tolerated by the patients, especially at the FDA-approved dosing of three times a week.

Other Modalities

Retinoids (e.g., tretinoin, isotretinoin, etretinate) are synthetic derivatives of retinol, a vitamin A analog.[305] They increase desquamation and inhibit the proliferation of keratinocytes, including cells infected by HPV.[306] This and the observation that vitamin A and other vitamins may play a role in the etiology of CIN led to the evaluation of these compounds for the treatment and prophylaxis of anogenital HPV diseases.[307,308] Isotretinoin given to eight subjects, 1 mg/kg PO for 6 weeks, had no effect on their condylomata acuminata.[309] Similarly, 0.05% tretinoin cream was found ineffective for the topical treatment of anogenital warts.[310] Retinoids were found to be more successful for the treatment of CIN. Meyskens et al randomized 301 women with CIN grade 2 or 3 to receive cervical caps with sponges containing 1 mL of

0.372% tretinoin cream or vehicle. The treatment was applied daily for 4 days the first month and daily for 2 days at months 3 and 6. Tretinoin was effective at reducing the grade of CIN grade 2 (43% for tretinoin compared to 27% for the vehicle; $P = 0.04$) but not of CIN grade 3.[311] Vaginal discharge was the most severe side-effect. Only anecdotal evidence supports the use of retinoids in HIV-seropositive men or women with intraepithelial neoplasia.[312,313] A Phase III study to compare oral isotretinoin to observation for the treatment of LSIL in HIV-seropositive women (ACTG 293) failed to show any difference.[314]

Cimetidine is a histamine receptor antagonist for which several claims of efficacy for the treatment of cutaneous warts have dissipated with the negative results of randomized, double-blind studies.[315] It is thus unlikely that the case report of cimetidine successfully treating condyloma acuminatum in the presence of HIV infection can be confirmed.[316]

Recommendations for Optimal Approach to Therapy

Condyloma Acuminatum

Table 56-4 summarizes the suggested treatment approaches to condyloma acuminatum in the HIV-infected patient. These recommendations are tentative and are largely derived from the experience reviewed above. They incorporate some of the guidelines published by the CDC, the NIH, and the IDSA for the treatment of human papillomavirus diseases in the general population[317] and in HIV-infected adults and adolescents.[102] Various other treatment guidelines for the general population have been issued.[283,318–320] They should give the reader a sense of the uncertainties attached to any treatment recommendations.

In addition to efficacy and tolerance, cost is a factor to consider when choosing a treatment. Several cost-effectiveness analyses have been reported, and their assumptions are sufficiently arguable and their conclusions sufficiently conflicting that their general usefulness is limited. However, they may help practitioners determine the most cost-effective options in their own practice. Often convenience and availability are the deciding factors, but the treatment methods are not necessarily interchangeable. If the patient is pregnant, cryotherapy or TCA is the treatment of choice. If few lesions are present, one should consider scissor excision. Large, numerous lesions may be best treated by laser surgery.

In HIV-infected patients with condyloma acuminatum, it is important to ensure proper follow-up, particularly if a patient has failed several treatments, so that preinvasive malignancies can be detected. Such monitoring should be integrated into the management of the HIV infection. One must also realize that treatment failure is not a strong predictor of resistance to future, even identical treatments.[177,178,221,257]

Other HPV Diseases

As a general principle, the management of intraepithelial neoplasias is best left in the hands of the expert. First, the diagnosis is established, and then the patient is advised, with referral as necessary. Figure 56-2 offers a suggested approach for the management of anal HPV diseases.[16–19,102] Note that anal cytology is not yet a validated procedure, and it is incorporated into the algorithm simply to indicate how it might be used.[70,321]

Consensus guidelines have been issued by the American Society for Colposcopy and Cervical Cytopathology for the management of women with cervical cytological and histologic abnormalities.[77,322] These guidelines also apply to the HIV-infected population.[102] CIN grade 1 lesions, which are particularly common in HIV-infected women, seem to progress only infrequently and do not appear to warrant a management different from those in immunocompetent women.[323] The largely empirical nature of these schemes leaves room for variations.[324] Cryotherapy and LEEP are less expensive and less technically demanding than laser surgery.[214,325] Other considerations apply as well. Cervical LEEP is contraindicated during pregnancy. Cryotherapy may not be optimal if the lesion extends toward the endocervix, is large, or cannot be covered by the cryoprobe. Laser surgery may have an advantage if the lesions are particularly large or extend to the vaginal fornices. LEEP, which is the preferred mode of therapy, is not only conservative to the cervix but has the unique advantage of providing a tissue sample that allows diagnostic verification.

Patient Advice and Support

The psychosexual impact of genital warts is well recognized in the general population but not in the HIV-infected subset. The patient may be referred to resources available to the HIV-infected population for advice and support as well as to resources devoted to HPV diseases. One such resource is the CDC, and for HIV/AIDS hotline is accessible at 1-800-232-4636. Another is the American Social Health Association (ASHA) hotline at 1-800-227-8922 (Monday through Friday, 9:00 a.m. to 6:00 p.m., EST).

PREVENTION

Approach to Prevention

The measures taken by health practitioners to prevent nosocomial transmission of HIV to other patients are adequate for HPVs. Disposable material should not be reused; instruments are sterilized and surfaces decontaminated with a 1:10 household bleach (5.25% sodium hypochlorite) solution. As mentioned earlier, special precautions must be taken by the operator during electrosurgery and laser surgery.

The best method of prevention is screening. At this point screening with the Pap smear can only be recommended for HPV cervical disease. Table 56-5 summarizes several of the current cervical cancer screening recommendations.[93,326–328] The CDC has issued screening and treatment recommendations for the HIV-infected population that support the guidelines currently established in the general population.[102,329]

Table 56-4

Suggested Approaches to the Treatment of Sexually Transmitted HPV Diseases

	Treatment Options	
Type of Wart or Lesion	**First line**	**Second line**
Condylomata acuminata	Podofilox[a] Imiquimod[a] Cryotherapy Trichloroacetic acid Scissor excision (if few and small lesions)	Electrosurgery Laser surgery Cidofovir, topical *Third line* Interferon
Oral warts	Cryotherapy Electrosurgery Laser surgery	Cold-blade excision
Urethral meatus warts	Cryotherapy Podofilox[a] 5-Fluorouracil	Podofilox[a] Electrosurgery
Anal warts (and AIN grade 1)	Cold-blade surgery Cryotherapy Trichloroacetic acid	Electrosurgery Infrared coagulation Laser surgery Imiquimod
Vaginal warts	Cryotherapy (liquid nitrogen spray, not a cryoprobe) Trichloroacetic acid 5-Fluorouracil (secondary prophylaxis)	Laser surgery
Cervical warts	Electrosurgery (LEEP) Cryotherapy Laser surgery	
Intraepithelial neoplasia of the external genitalia	Cold-blade surgery Electrosurgery Laser surgery Cryotherapy (penis)	Imiquimod *Third line* Cidofovir, topical
Anal intraepithelial neoplasia (grades 2 and 3)	Cold-blade surgery Electrosurgery Laser surgery Cryotherapy Trichloroacetic acid	Electrosurgery Infrared coagulator Cold-blade surgery[b]
Vaginal intraepithelial neoplasia	Laser surgery	5-Fluorouracil (secondary prophylaxis)
Cervical intraepithelial neoplasia	Electrosurgery (LEEP) Cryotherapy Laser surgery	Cidofovir, topical

[a] These treatments are applied by the patient for home-based therapy.
[b] Typically done with micro-resectors.
Additional management information can be found in the text and at http://www.cdc.gov/std/treatment/ and http://www.cdc.gov/mmwr/preview/mmwrhtml/rr5315a1.htm.[317,329]

Prophylaxis

The use of condoms and other barrier methods is recommended to prevent HIV and other sexually transmitted infections.[317] A meta-analysis of 20 studies suggested condoms may not prevent HPV infection, but may reduce genital warts, CIN grades 2 and 3, and cervical cancer.[330] Recently, a prospective study of 84 college-aged women, 100% consistent condom use was associated with a 2.4-fold reduction in the risk of acquiring genital HPV infection.[331] It was also associated with the absence of incident SIL compared to 14 cases in those women who used condoms less consistently or never. The effect of condom use on HPV clearance was also shown in a randomized study of 125 couples of women with CIN and

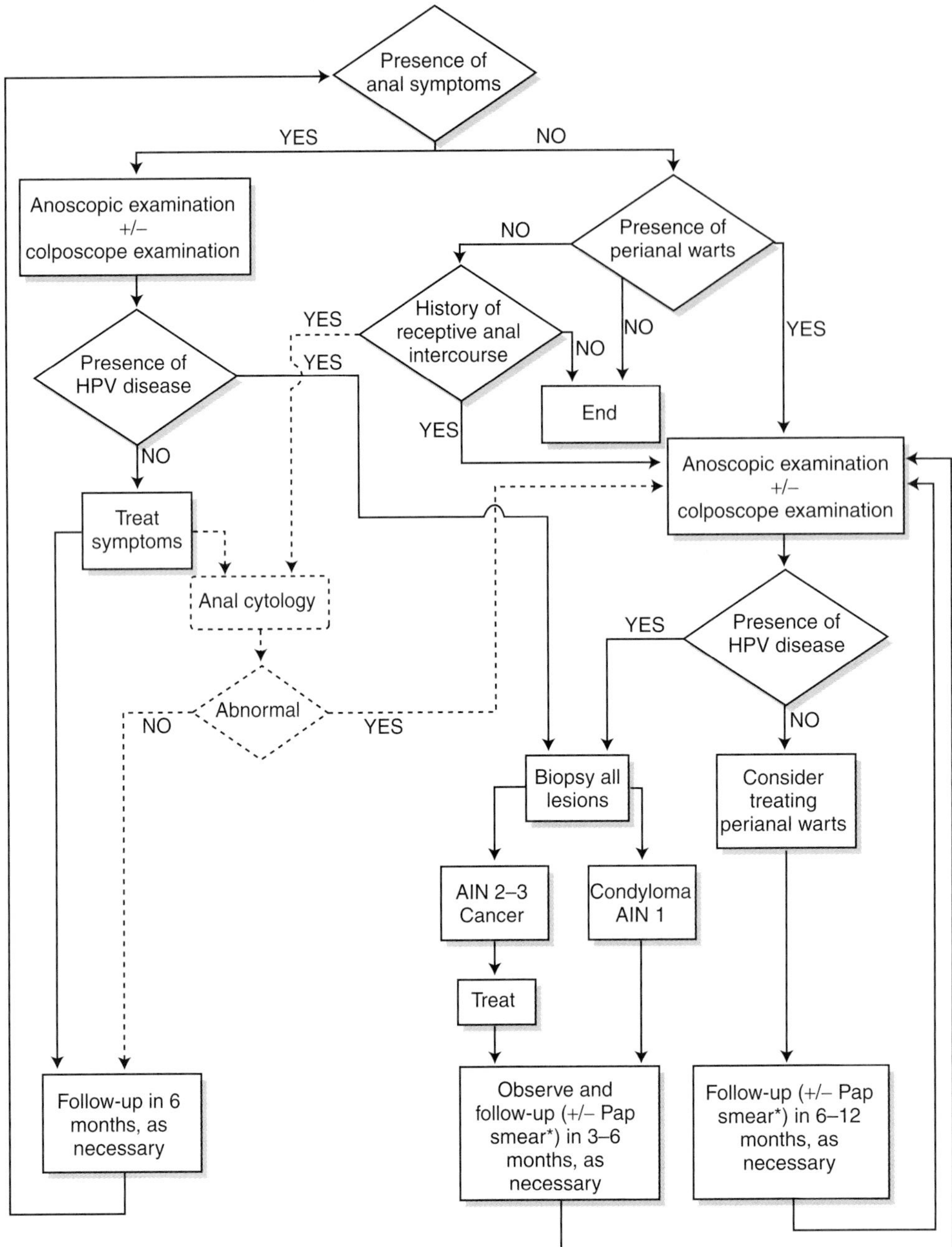

Figure 56-2 ■ Suggested management of anal HPV diseases. The dashed pathways and asterisk refer to the potential place of anal cytology, a tool that remains to be validated.

their male sexual partners. There was a greater rate of CIN (1.5-fold) and HPV DNA clearance (5.7-fold) in the women from the couples assigned to condom use.[332] Similarly, there was a faster (×1.9) rate of clearance of HPV-associated flat lesions in the males.[333] Consistent with a barrier effect to infection, the clearance effect of condoms in males was seen only in the couples with concordant HPV types (hazard ratio 2.63).[334] These data argue for encouraging the use of condoms not only for primary, but also the secondary prevention of genital HPV infections.

Spermicidal agent may have a weak protective effect.[335] There are no effective microbicide agents currently available. Smoking should be discouraged because it may lead HPV infection to progress to condyloma acuminatum.[28,336] There are no available primary chemoprophylaxis methods for HPV infections or diseases. 5-FU is effective for the secondary prophylaxis of CIN in HIV-infected women (*see section on* Therapy).[155]

Vaccines

A quadrivalent vaccine directed against HPV types 6, 11, 16, and 18 (GARDASIL; Merck) has been approved in June 2006 in several Latin American countries and in the United

Summary of Cervical Cancer Screening Guidelines

Table 56-5

When to Begin Pap Test Screening?	
USPSTF & ACS	Approximately 3 years after a woman begins having sexual intercourse, but no later than 21 years old
How Often?	
USPSTF	Every 3 years (regardless of the cervical cytology technique used)
ACS	1. Annually with conventional cytology OR 2. At or after age 30, women who have had three consecutive, technically satisfactory normal/negative cytology results may be screened every 2–3 years UNLESS a. They have a history of *in utero* diethylstilbestrol (DES) exposure b. Are HIV positive c. Are immunocompromised by organ transplantation, chemotherapy, or chronic corticosteroid treatment
When to Discontinue Screening?	
USPSTF	At age 65 in women who have had normal results previously and who are not otherwise at high risk for cervical cancer
ACS	At age 70 years or older in women with an intact cervix and who have had three or more documented, consecutive, technically satisfactory, normal/negative cervical cytology tests, and no abnormal/positive cytology tests within the 10-year period prior to age 70 EXCEPTIONS: a. Women who have not been previously screened b. Women for whom information about previous screening is unavailable c. Women for whom past screening is unlikely d. Women with a history of: (1) cervical cancer; (2) *in utero* exposure to diethylstilbestrol (DES) e. Women who are immunocompromised (e.g., due to organ transplantation, HIV infection, chemotherapy, or chronic corticosteroid treatment) f. Women who have tested positive for HPV DNA
Screening After Hysterectomy	
USPSTF & ACS	Not necessary if (total) hysterectomy was for benign disease
Screening with HPV DNA Testing (Hydrid Capture II Test for High-Risk HPV)	
USPSTF	Not recommended
ACS	It should be used, with cytology, only at age 30 or older and not more frequently than every 3 years
Additional Guidelines	
ACOG	Yearly testing using cytology alone remains an acceptable screening plan
CDC	Women who have external genital warts do not need to have Pap tests more frequently than women who do not have warts, unless otherwise indicated

Abbreviations, references, and web-based sources:
American Cancer Society (ACS)[326] – http://caonline.amcancersoc.org/cgi/content/short/52/6/342
US Preventive Services Task Force (USPSTF)[327] – http://www.ahrq.gov/clinic/3rduspstf/cervicalcan/cervcanrr.htm; http://www.ahrq.gov/clinic/uspstf/uspscerv.htm
American College of Obstetrics and Gynecology (ACOG)[328]
Centers for Disease Control and Prevention (CDC)[93] – http://www.cdc.gov/std/treatment/

States for the prevention of cervical cancer, CIN, vulvar and vaginal intraepithelial neoplasias grades 2 and 3, cervical adenocarcinoma *in situ*, and genital warts on females aged 9 through 26 years. This vaccine, which is made of HPV virus-like particles, was shown to give 100% efficacy against HPV16 cervical infection.[337] A subsequent study, done with the current quadrivalent formulation showed that the vaccine was 90% effective in preventing either infection with HPV types 6, 11, 16, and 18, or cervical or external genital disease.[338] More extensive, just published data[338a–d], support the effectiveness, tolerability, and safety of this vaccine. A similar vaccine, limited to HPV16 and HPV18 (CERVARIX; GSK), is currently in development and has shown similar results.[339,340] HPV16 and HPV18 are the cause of ~70% of cervical cancers.[341] They are also associated with anal squamous carcinomas and subsets of penile cancers. Therefore, the availability of an HPV vaccine is a major addition to the prevention of HPV disease, and full use should be made of it for the approved indications. The place of HPV immunization in populations other than those approved, especially the HIV-infected population is unclear at present.

CONCLUSION

Sexually transmitted HPV diseases are a substantial problem in the HIV-infected population because they are frequent and can progress to various anogenital cancers. Longer survival may mean a greater chance for some lesions to progress to cancer. Unfortunately, our means of detecting, treating, and preventing these diseases are presently deficient. Although these diseases are caused by a viral infection, none of the treatments so far available is truly antiviral. A drug development effort needs to be fostered. Management and screening strategies have been developed in the general population largely by an empiric approach, but their multiplicity is an invitation to conduct more scientific prospective evaluations to identify the best approaches, both in the general population and in HIV-infected patients. Finally, HPV vaccines that are very effective at preventing the major genital HPV infections and diseases are a major step forward toward eventual control of the disease.

REFERENCES

1. Orth G. Human papillomaviruses associated with epidermodysplasia verruciformis in non-melanoma skin cancers: guilty or innocent? J Invest Dermatol 125:xii-xiii, 2005.
2. Bonnez W. Editorial comment: issues with HIV and oral human papillomavirus infections. AIDS Reader 12:174–6, 2002.
3. Ley C, Bauer HM, Reingold A, et al. Determinants of genital human papillomavirus infection in young women. J Natl Cancer Inst 83:997–1003, 1991.
4. Koutsky L. Epidemiology of genital human papillomavirus infection. Am J Med 102:3–8, 1997.
5. Northfelt DW, Swift PS, Palefsky JM. Anal neoplasia. Pathogenesis, diagnosis, and management. Hematol Oncol Clin North Am 10:1177–87, 1996.
6. Robinson WR, Morris CB. Cervical neoplasia. Pathogenesis, diagnosis, and management. Hematol Oncol Clin North Am 10:1163–76, 1996.
7. Sun X-W, Kuhn L, Ellerbrock TV, et al. Human papillomavirus infection in women infected with the human immunodeficiency virus. N Engl J Med 337:1343–49, 1997.
8. Palefsky JM, Holly EA, Ralston ML, Jay N, Berry JM, Darragh TM. High incidence of anal high-grade squamous intra-epithelial lesions among HIV-positive and HIV-negative homosexual and bisexual men. AIDS 12:495–503, 1998.
9. Aynaud O, Piron D, Barrasso R, Poveda JD. Comparison of clinical, histological, and virological symptoms of HPV in HIV-1 infected men and immunocompetent subjects. Sex Transm Infect 74:32–4, 1998.
10. Palefsky JM, Holly EA, Ralston ML, et al. Anal squamous intraepithelial lesions in HIV-positive and HIV-negative homosexual and bisexual men: prevalence and risk factors. J Acquir Immune Defic Syndr Hum Retrovirol 17:320–6, 1998.
11. Palefsky JM, Minkoff H, Kalish LA, et al. Cervicovaginal human papillomavirus infection in human immunodeficiency virus-1 (HIV)-positive and high-risk HIV-negative women. J Natl Cancer Inst 91:226–36, 1999.
12. Ellerbrock TV, Chiasson MA, Bush TJ, et al. Incidence of cervical squamous intraepithelial lesions in HIV-infected women. JAMA 283:1031–7, 2000.
13. Moscicki AB, Ellenberg JH, Vermund SH, et al. Prevalence of and risks for cervical human papillomavirus infection and squamous intraepithelial lesions in adolescent girls: impact of infection with human immunodeficiency virus. Arch Pediatr Adolesc Med 154:127–34, 2000.
14. Frisch M, Biggar RJ, Goedert JJ. Human papillomavirus-associated cancers in patients with human immunodeficiency virus infection and acquired immunodeficiency syndrome. J Natl Cancer Inst 92:1500–10, 2000.
15. Palefsky JM, Holly EA, Ralston ML, et al. Prevalence and risk factors for anal human papillomavirus infection in human immunodeficiency virus (HIV)-positive and high risk HIV-negative women. J Infect Dis 183:383–91, 2001.
16. de Sanjose S, Palefsky J. Cervical and anal HPV infections in HIV positive women and men. Virus Res 89:201–11, 2002.
17. Vukasin P. Anal condyloma and HIV-associated anal disease. Surg Clin North Am 82:1199–211, vi, 2002.
18. Abbasakoor F, Boulos PB. Anal intraepithelial neoplasia. Br J Surg 92:277–90, 2005.
19. Fox PA. Human papillomavirus and anal intraepithelial neoplasia. Curr Opin Infect Dis 19:62–6, 2006.
20. Klein RS, Ho GYF, Vermund SH, et al. Risk factors for squamous intraepithelial lesions on Pap smear in women at risk for human immunodeficiency virus infection. J Infect Dis 170:1404–9, 1994.
21. Critchlow CW, Surawicz CM, Holmes KK, et al. Prospective study of high grade anal squamous intraepithelial neoplasia in a cohort of homosexual men: influence of HIV infection, immunosuppression and human papillomavirus infection. AIDS 9:1255–62, 1995.
22. Hillemanns P, Ellerbrock TV, McPhillips S, et al. Prevalence of anal human papillomavirus infection and anal cytologic abnormalities in HIV-seropositive women. AIDS 10:1641–1647, 1996.
23. Langley CL, Benga-De E, Critchlow CW, et al. HIV-1, HIV-2, human papillomavirus infection and cervical neoplasia in high-risk African women. AIDS 10:413–17, 1996.
24. St. Louis ME, Icenogle JP, Manzila T, et al. Genital types of papillomavirus in children of women with HIV-1 infection in Kinshasa, Zaire. Int J Cancer 54:181–4, 1993.
25. Ahdieh L, Munoz A, Vlahov D, et al. Cervical neoplasia and repeated positivity of human papillomavirus infection in human immunodeficiency virus-seropositive and -seronegative women. Am J Epidemiol 151:1148–57, 2000.
26. Friedman HB, Saah AJ, Sherman ME, et al. Human papillomavirus, anal squamous intraepithelial lesions, and human immunodeficiency virus in a cohort of gay men. J Infect Dis 178:45–52, 1998.
27. Heard I, Tassie JM, Schmitz V, et al. Increased risk of cervical disease among human immunodeficiency virus-infected women with severe immunosuppression and high human papillomavirus load. Obstet Gynecol 96:403–409, 2000.
28. Minkoff H, Feldman JG, Strickler HD, et al. Relationship between smoking and human papillomavirus infections in HIV-infected and -uninfected women. J Infect Dis 189:1821–8, 2004.
29. Piketty C, Darragh TM, Da Costa M, et al. High prevalence of anal human papillomavirus infection and anal cancer precursors among HIV-infected persons in the absence of anal intercourse. Ann Intern Med 138:453–9, 2003.
30. Durante AJ, Williams AB, Da Costa M, et al. Incidence of anal cytological abnormalities in a cohort of human immunodeficiency virus-infected women. Cancer Epidemiol Biomarkers Prev 12:638–42, 2003.
31. Derkay CS. Recurrent respiratory papillomatosis. Laryngoscope 111:57–69, 2001.
32. Conley LJ, Ellerbrock TV, Bush TJ, et al. HIV-1 infection and risk of vulvovaginal and perianal condylomata acuminata and intraepithelial neoplasia: a prospective cohort study. Lancet 359:108–13, 2002.
33. Palefsky JM. Cervical human papillomavirus infection and cervical intraepithelial neoplasia in women positive for human immunodeficiency virus in the era of highly active antiretroviral therapy. Curr Opin Oncol 15:382–8, 2003.

34. Harris TG, Burk RD, Palefsky JM, et al. Incidence of cervical squamous intraepithelial lesions associated with HIV serostatus, CD4+ cell counts, and human papillomavirus test results. JAMA 293:1471–6, 2005.
35. Palefsky JM, Holly EA, Efirdc JT, et al. Anal intraepithelial neoplasia in the highly active antiretroviral therapy era among HIV-positive men who have sex with men. AIDS 19:1407–14, 2005.
36. McMillan A, Bishop PE. Clinical course of anogenital warts in men infected with human immunodeficiency virus. Genitourin Med 65:225–8, 1989.
37. Wright TC Jr, Koulos J, Schnoll F, et al. Cervical intraepithelial neoplasia in women infected with the human immunodeficiency virus: outcome after loop electrosurgical excision. Gynecol Oncol 55:253–8, 1994.
38. Palefsky JM. Anal human papillomavirus infection and anal cancer in HIV-positive individuals: an emerging problem. AIDS 8:283–95, 1994.
39. Heard I, Bergeron C, Jeannel D, et al. Papanicolaou smears in human immunodeficiency virus-seropositive women during follow-up. Obstet Gynecol 86:749–53, 1995.
40. Kilewo CD, Urassa WK, Pallangyo K, et al. Response to podophyllotoxin treatment of genital warts in relation to HIV-1 infection among patients in Dar es Salaam, Tanzania. Int J STD AIDS 6:114–16, 1995.
41. von Krogh G, Wikström A, Syrjänen K, Syrjänen S. Anal and penile condylomas in HIV-negative and HIV-positive men: clinical, histological and virological characteristics correlated to therapeutic outcome. Acta Dermatol Venereol (Stockholm) 75:470–4, 1995.
42. Fruchter RG, Maiman M, Sedlis A, et al. Multiple recurrences of cervical intraepithelial neoplasia in women with the human immunodeficiency virus. Obstet Gynecol 87:338–44, 1996.
43. Cappiello G, Garbuglia AR, Salvi R, et al. HIV infection increases the risk of squamous intra-epithelial lesions in women with HPV infection – an analysis of HPV genotypes. Int J Cancer 72:982–6, 1997.
44. Heard I, Potard V, Foulot H, et al. High rate of recurrence of cervical intraepithelial neoplasia after surgery in HIV-positive women. J AIDS 39:412–18, 2005.
45. Gilles C, Manigart Y, Konopnicki D, et al. Management and outcome of cervical intraepithelial neoplasia lesions: a study of matched cases according to HIV status. Gynecol Oncol 96:112–18, 2005.
46. Anonymous. 1993 revised classification system for HIV infection and expanded surveillance case definition for AIDS among adolescents and adults. MMWR 41:1–19, 1992.
47. Frisch M, Biggar RJ, Engels EA, et al. Association of cancer with AIDS-related immunosuppression in adults. JAMA 285:1736–45, 2001.
48. Dorrucci M, Suligoi B, Serraino D, et al. Incidence of invasive cervical cancer in a cohort of HIV-seropositive women before and after the introduction of highly active antiretroviral therapy. J Acquir Immune Defic Syndr 26:377–380, 2001.
49. Beral V, Newton R. Overview of the epidemiology of immunodeficiency-associated cancers. J Natl Cancer Inst Monogr 1998:1–6.
50. La Ruche G, Ramon R, Mensah-Ado I, et al. Squamous intraepithelial lesions of the cervix, invasive cervical carcinoma, and immunosuppression induced by human immunodeficiency virus in Africa. Dyscer-CI Group. Cancer 82:2401–8, 1998.
51. Sitas F, Pacella-Norman R, Carrara H, et al. The spectrum of HIV-1 related cancers in South Africa. Int J Cancer 88:489–92, 2000.
52. Strickler HD, Burk RD, Fazzari M, et al. Natural history and possible reactivation of human papillomavirus in human immunodeficiency virus-positive women. J Natl Cancer Inst 97:577–86, 2005.
53. Clarke B, Chetty R. Postmodern cancer: the role of human immunodeficiency virus in uterine cervical cancer. Mol Pathol 55:19–24, 2002.
54. Strickler HD, Palefsky JM, Shah KV, et al. Human papillomavirus type 16 and immune status in human immunodeficiency virus-seropositive women. J Natl Cancer Inst 95:1062–71, 2003.
55. Bower M, Mazhar D, Stebbing J. Should cervical cancer be an acquired immunodeficiency syndrome-defining cancer? J Clin Oncol 24:2417–19, 2006.
56. Forti RL, Medwell SJ, Aboulafia DM, et al. Clinical presentation of minimally invasive and in situ squamous cell carcinoma of the anus in homosexual men. Clin Infect Dis 21:603–7, 1995.
57. Schlappner OLA, Schaffer EA. Anorectal condylomata acuminata: a missed part of the condyloma spectrum. Can Med Assoc J 118:172–3, 1978.
58. Jay N, Berry JM, Hogeboom CJ, et al. Colposcopic appearance of anal squamous intraepithelial lesions: relationship to histopathology. Dis Colon Rectum 40:919–28, 1997.
59. McMillan A. Sigmoidoscopy – a necessary procedure in the routine investigation of homosexual men? Genitourin Med 63:44–6, 1987.
60. Parker BJ, Cossart YE, Thompson CH, et al. The clinical management and laboratory assessment of anal warts. Med J Austral 147:59–63, 1987.
61. McGoogan E. Liquid-based cytology: the new screening test for cervical cancer control. J Fam Plann Reprod Health Care 30:123–5, 2004.
62. Davey E, Barratt A, Irwig L, et al. Effect of study design and quality on unsatisfactory rates, cytology classifications, and accuracy in liquid-based versus conventional cervical cytology: a systematic review. Lancet 367:122–32, 2006.
63. Solomon D, Davey D, Kurman R, et al. The 2001 Bethesda System: terminology for reporting results of cervical cytology. JAMA 287:2114–19, 2002.
64. Wright TC Jr, Ellerbrock TV, Chiasson MA, et al. Cervical intraepithelial neoplasia in women infected with human immunodeficiency virus: prevalence, risk factors, and validity of Papanicolaou smears. New York Cervical Disease Study. Obstet Gynecol 84:591–7, 1994.
65. Branca M, Rossi E, Alderisio M, et al. Performance of cytology and colposcopy in diagnosis of cervical intraepithelial neoplasia (CIN) in HIV-positive and HIV-negative women. Cytopathology 12:84–93, 2001.
66. Northfelt DW. Anal neoplasia in persons with HIV infection. AIDS Clin Care 8:63–6, 1996.
67. Cranston RD, Darragh TM, Holly EA, et al. Self-collected versus clinician-collected anal cytology specimens to diagnose anal intraepithelial neoplasia in HIV-positive men. J AIDS 36:915–20, 2004.
68. Palefsky JM, Holly EA, Hogeboom CJ, et al. Anal cytology as a screening tool for anal squamous intraepithelial lesions. J Acquir Immune Defic Syndr Hum Retrovirol 14:415–22, 1997.
69. Fairley CK, Chen S, Tabrizi S, et al. Influence of quartile of menstrual cycle on pellet volume of specimens from tampons and isolation of human papillomavirus. J Infect Dis 166: 1199–200, 1992.
70. Goldie SJ, Kuntz KM, Weinstein MC, et al. The clinical effectiveness and cost-effectiveness of screening for anal squamous intraepithelial lesions in homosexual and bisexual HIV-positive men. JAMA 281:1822–9, 1999.
71. Palefsky JM. Anal squamous intraepithelial lesions in human immunodeficiency virus-positive men and women. Semin Oncol 27:471–9, 2000.
71a. Kaplan JE, Masur H, Holmes KK. Guidelines for preventing opportunistic infections among HIV-infected persons. 2002.

Recommendations of the U.S. Public Health Service and the Infectious Diseases Society of America. MMWR Recomm Rep. 51:1–52, 2002.
72. Colquhoun P, Nogueras JJ, Dipasquale B, et al. Interobserver and intraobserver bias exists in the interpretation of anal dysplasia. Dis Colon Rectum 46:1332–6; discussion 1336–8, 2003.
73. Chang GJ, Berry JM, Jay N, et al. Surgical treatment of high-grade anal squamous intraepithelial lesions: a prospective study. Dis Colon Rectum 45:453–8, 2002.
74. Stoler MH, Schiffman M, Group ASCoUS-L-gSILTSA. Interobserver reproducibility of cervical cytologic and histologic interpretations. Realistic estimates from the ASCUS-LSIL Triage Study. JAMA 285:1500–5, 2001.
75. Peyton CL, Schiffman M, Lorincz AT, et al. Comparison of PCR- and hybrid capture-based human papillomavirus detection systems using multiple cervical specimen collection strategies. J Clin Microbiol 36:3248–54, 1998.
76. Anonymous. Human papillomavirus testing for triage of women with cytologic evidence of low-grade squamous intraepithelial lesions: baseline data from a randomized trial. The Atypical Squamous Cells of Undetermined Significance/ Low-Grade Squamous Intraepithelial Lesions Triage Study (ALTS) Group. J Natl Cancer Inst 92:397–402, 2000.
77. Wright TC Jr, Cox JT, Massad LS, et al. Conference AS-SC. 2001 Consensus Guidelines for the management of women with cervical cytological abnormalities[see comment]. JAMA 287:2120–9, 2002.
78. Fox PA, Seet JE, Stebbing J, et al. The value of anal cytology and human papillomavirus typing in the detection of anal intraepithelial neoplasia: a review of cases from an anoscopy clinic. Sex Transm Infect 81:142–6, 2005.
79. Maw RD, Reitano M, Roy M. An international survey of patients with genital warts: perceptions regarding treatment and impact on lifestyle. Int J STD AIDS 9:571–8, 1998.
80. Persson G, Gösta Dahlöf L, Krantz I. Physical and psychological effects of anogenital warts on female patients. Sex Transm Dis 20:10–13, 1993.
81. Voog E, Löwhagen GB. Follow-up of men with genital papilloma virus infection. Psychosexual aspects. Acta Dermatol Venereol (Stockholm) 72:185–6, 1992.
82. Filiberti A, Tamburini M, Stefanon B, et al. Psychological aspects of genital human papillomavirus infection: a preliminary report. J Psychosom Obstet Gynaecol 14:145–52, 1993.
83. Sheppard S, White M, Walzman M. Genital warts: just a nuisance? Genitourin Med 71:194–5, 1995.
84. Chuang T-Y, Perry HO, Kurland LT, Ilstrup DM. Condyloma acuminatum in Rochester, Minn, 1950–1978. I. Epidemiology and clinical features. Arch Dermatol 120:469–475, 1984.
85. Ferenczy A, Mitao M, Nagai N, et al. Latent papillomavirus and recurring genital warts. N Engl J Med 313:784–8, 1985.
86. Ward KA, Winter PC, Walsh M, et al. Detection of human papillomavirus by the polymerase chain reaction in histologically normal penile skin adjacent to penile warts. Sex Transm Dis 21:83–8, 1994.
87. Boxman ILA, Hogewoning A, Mulder LHC, et al. Detection of human papillomavirus types 6 and 11 in pubic and perianal hair from patients with genital warts. J Clin Microbiol 37:2270–3, 1999.
88. Riva JM, Sedlacek TV, Cunnane MF, Mangan CE. Extended carbon dioxide laser vaporization in the treatment of subclinical papillomavirus infection of the lower genital tract. Obstet Gynecol 73:25–30, 1999.
89. Carpiniello VL, Zderic SA, Malloy TR, Sedlacek T. Carbon dioxide laser therapy of subclinical condyloma found by magnified penile surface scanning. Urology 29:608–10, 1987.
90. Höckenström T, Jonassen F, Knutsson F, et al. High prevalence of cervical dysplasia in female consorts of men with genital warts. Acta Dermatol Venereol (Stockholm) 67:511–16, 1987.
91. Barrasso R. HPV-related genital lesions in men. In: Munoz N, Bosch FX, Shah KV, Meheus A (eds). The Epidemiology of Cervical Cancer and Human Papillomavirus. Lyon, France: International Agency for Research on Cancer; 1992, pp 85–92.
92. Krebs H-B, Helmkamp BF. Does the treatment of genital condylomata in men decrease the treatment failure rate of cervical dysplasia in the female sexual partner? Obstet Gynecol 76:660–3, 1990.
93. Sexually transmitted diseases treatment guidelines 2002. Centers for Disease Control and Prevention. MMWR Recomm Rep 51:1–78, 2002.
94. Anonymous. Human papillomaviruses. IARC Monographs on the Evaluation of Carcinogenic Risks to Humans 94:1–379, 1995.
95. Schonfeld A, Nitke S, Schattner A, et al. Intramuscular human interferon-β injections in treatment of condylomata acuminata. Lancet i:1038–42, 1984.
96. Reichman RC, Oakes D, Bonnez W, et al. Treatment of condyloma acuminatum with three different alpha interferon preparations administered parenterally: a double-blind, placebo-controlled trial. J Infect Dis 162:1270–6, 1990.
97. Group CICS. Recurrent condylomata acuminata treated with recombinant interferon alfa-2a. A multicenter double-blind placebo-controlled clinical trial. JAMA 265:2684–87, 1991.
98. Edwards L, Ferenczy A, Eron L, et al. Self-administered topical 5% imiquimod cream for external anogenital warts. Arch Dermatol 134:25–30, 1998.
99. Syed TA, Ahmadpour OA, Ahmad SA, Ahmad SH. Management of female genital warts with an analog of imiquimod 2% in cream: a randomized, double-blind, placebo-controlled study. J Dermatol 25:429–33, 1998.
100. Syed TA, Hadi SM, Qureshi ZA, et al. Treatment of external genital warts in men with imiquimod 2% in cream. A placebo-controlled, double-blind study. J Infect 41:148–51, 2000.
101. Del Priore G, Gilmore PR, Maag T, et al. Colposcopic biopsies versus loop electrosurgical excision procedure cone histology in human immunodeficiency virus-positive women. J Reprod Med 41:653–7, 1996.
102. Benson CA, Kaplan JE, Masur H, et al. Treating opportunistic infections among HIV-exposed and infected children: recommendations from CDC, the National Institutes of Health, and the Infectious Diseases Society of America. MMWR Recomm Rep 53:1–112.
103. Cuthill S, Maiman M, Fruchter RG, et al. Complications after treatment of cervical intraepithelial neoplasia in women infected with the human immunodeficiency virus. J Reprod Med 40:823–8, 1995.
104. Kaplan JE, Masur H, Holmes KK. Guidelines for preventing opportunistic infections among HIV-infected persons – 2002. Recommendations of the U.S. Public Health Service and the Infectious Diseases Society of America. MMWR Recomm Rep 51:1–52, 2002.
105. Heard I, Palefsky JM, Kazatchkine MD. The impact of HIV antiviral therapy on human papillomavirus (HPV) infections and HPV-related diseases. Antiviral Ther 9:13–22, 2004.
106. Massad LS, Silverberg MJ, Springer G, et al. Effect of antiretroviral therapy on the incidence of genital warts and vulvar neoplasia among women with the human immunodeficiency virus. Am J Obstet Gyn 190:1241–8, 2004.
107. Fox P, Stebbing J, Portsmouth S, et al. Lack of response of anal intra-epithelial neoplasia to highly active antiretroviral therapy. AIDS 17:279–80, 2003.
108. Horster S, Thoma-Greber E, Siebeck M, Bogner JR. Is anal carcinoma a HAART-related problem? Eur J Med Res 8:142–6, 2003.

109. Stadler RF, Gregorcyk SG, Euhus DM, et al. Outcome of HIV-infected patients with invasive squamous-cell carcinoma of the anal canal in the era of highly active antiretroviral therapy. Dis Colon Rectum 47:1305–9, 2004.
110. Bower M, Powles T, Newsom-Davis T, et al. HIV-associated anal cancer: has highly active antiretroviral therapy reduced the incidence or improved the outcome? J AIDS 37:1563–5, 2004.
111. Diamond C, Taylor TH, Aboumrad T, et al. Increased incidence of squamous cell anal cancer among men with AIDS in the era of highly active antiretroviral therapy. Sex Transm Dis 32:314–20, 2005.
112. Greenspan D, Gange SJ, Phelan JA, et al. Incidence of oral lesions in HIV-1-infected women: reduction with HAART. J Dent Res 83:145–50, 2004.
113. Lacey CJ. Therapy for genital human papillomavirus-related disease. J Clin Virol 32(Suppl 1):S82–90, 2005.
114. De Panfilis G, Melzani G, Mori G, et al. Relapses after treatment of external genital warts are more frequent in HIV-positive patients than in HIV-negative controls. Sex Transm Dis 29:121–5, 2002.
115. de la Fuente SG, Ludwig KA, Mantyh CR. Preoperative immune status determines anal condyloma recurrence after surgical excision. Dis Colon Rectum 46:367–73, 2003.
116. Longstaff E, von Krogh G. Condyloma eradication: self-therapy with 0.15–0.5% podophyllotoxin versus 20–25% podophyllin preparations – an integrated safety assessment. Regul Toxicol Pharmacol 33:117–37, 2001.
117. Zhu W-Y, Blauvelt A, Goldstein BA, et al. Detection with the polymerase chain reaction of human papillomavirus DNA in condylomata acuminata treated in vitro with liquid nitrogen, trichloroacetic acid, and podophyllin. J Am Acad Dermatol 26:710–14, 1992.
118. von Krogh G, Longstaff E. Podophyllin office therapy against condyloma should be abandoned. Sex Transm Infect 77:409–12, 2001.
119. Sullivan M, King LS. Effects of resin of podophyllum on normal skin, condylomata acuminata and verruca vulgares. Arch Dermatol Syphil 56:30–47, 1947.
120. Wade TR, Ackerman AB. The effects of resin of podophyllin on condyloma acuminatum. Am J Dermatopathol 6:109–22, 1984.
121. De Marco F, Di Carlo A, Poggiali F, et al. Detection of HPV in genital condylomata: correlation between viral load and clinical outcome. J Exp Clin Cancer Res 20:377–83, 2001.
122. Lacey CJ, Goodall RL, Tennvall GR, et al. Randomised controlled trial and economic evaluation of podophyllotoxin solution, podophyllotoxin cream, and podophyllin in the treatment of genital warts. Sex Transm Infect 79:270–5, 2003.
123. Bonnez W, Elswick RK Jr, Bailey-Farchione A, et al. Efficacy and safety of 0.5% podofilox solution in the treatment and suppression of anogenital warts. Am J Med 1994;96:420–5.
124. Beck DE, Jaso RG, Zajac RA. Surgical management of anal condylomata in the HIV-positive patient. Dis Colon Rectum 33:180–3, 1990.
125. Orkin BA, Smith LE. Perineal manifestations of HIV infection. Dis Colon Rectum 35:310–14, 1992.
126. Godfrey JC, Vaughan MC, Williams JV. Successful treatment of bowenoid papulosis in a 9-year-old girl with vertically acquired human immunodeficiency virus. Pediatrics 112:e73–6, 2003.
127. Weiner M, Semah D, Schewach-Millet M, Cesarini J-P. Preclinical and clinical evaluation of topical acid products for skin tumors. Clin Pharmacol Ther 33:77–83, 1983.
128. Godley MJ, Bradbeer CS, Gellan M, Thin RNT. Cryotherapy compared with trichloroacetic acid in treating genital warts. Genitourin Med 63:390–2, 1987.
129. Abdullah AN, Walzman M, Wade A. Treatment of external genital warts comparing cryotherapy (liquid nitrogen) and trichloroacetic acid. Sex Transm Dis 20:344–5, 1993.
130. Gabriel G, Thin RNT. Treatment of anogenital warts: comparison to trichloroacetic acid and podophyllin versus podophyllin alone. Br J Vener Dis 59:124–6, 1983.
131. Nel WS, Fourie ED. Immunotherapy and 5% topical 5–fluoro-uracil ointment in the treatment of condylomata acuminata. S Afr Med J 47:45–9, 1973.
132. Haye KR. Treatment of condyloma acuminata with 5 per cent 5–fluorouracil (5-FU) cream. Br J Vener Dis 50:466, 1974.
133. Dretler SP, Klein LA. The eradication of intraurethral condyloma acuminata with 5 per cent 5-fluorouracil cream. J Urol 113:195–8, 1975.
134. von Krogh G. 5-fluoro-uracil cream in the successful treatment of therapeutically refractory condylomata acuminata of the urinary meatus. Acta Dermatol Venereol (Stockholm) 56:297–301, 1976.
135. Wallin J. 5-fluorouracil in the treatment of penile and urethral condylomata acuminata. Br J Vener Dis 53:240–3, 1977.
136. von Krogh G. The beneficial effect of 1% 5-fluorouracil in 70% ethanol on therapeutically refractory condylomas in the preputial cavity. Sex Transm Dis 5:137–140, 1978.
137. Pareek S. Treatment of condyloma acuminatum with 5% 5-fluorouracil. Br J Vener Dis 55:65–6, 1979.
138. Krebs H-B. Prophylactic topical 5-fluorouracil following treatment of human papillomavirus-associated lesions of the vulva and vagina. Obstet Gynecol 68:837–41, 1986.
139. Krebs H-B. Treatment of vaginal condylomata acuminata by weekly topical application of 5-fluorouracil. Obstet Gynecol 70:68–71, 1987.
140. Krebs H-B. Treatment of extensive vulvar condylomata acuminata with topical 5-fluorouracil. South Med J 83:761–4, 1990.
141. Pride G. Treatment of large lower genital tract condylomata acuminata with topical 5-fluorouracil. J Reprod Med 35:384–7, 1990.
142. Bergman A, Nalick R. Genital human papillomavirus infection in men. Diagnosis and treatment with a laser and 5-fluorouracil. J Reprod Med 36:363–6, 1991.
143. Shelley WB, Shelley ED. Scrotal dermatitis caused by 5-fluorouracil (Efudex). J Am Acad Dermatol 19:929–31, 1988.
144. Goette DK, Odom RB. Allergic contact dermatitis to topical fluorouracil. Arch Dermatol 113:1058–61, 1977.
145. Mansell PWA, Litwin MS, Ichinose H, Krementz ET. Delayed hypersensitivity to 5-fluorouracil following topical chemotherapy of cutaneous cancers. Cancer Res 35:1288–94, 1975.
146. Krebs H-B, Helmkamp BF. Chronic ulcerations following topical therapy with 5-fluorouracil for vaginal human papillomavirus-associated lesions. Obstet Gynecol 78:205–8, 1991.
147. Reid R. The management of genital condylomas, intraepithelial neoplasia, and vulvodynia. Obstet Gynecol Clin North Am 23:917–91, 1996.
148. Goodman A, Zukerberg LR, Nikrui N, Scully RE. Vaginal adenosis and clear cell carcinoma after 5-fluorouracil treatment for condylomas. Cancer 68:1628–32, 1991.
149. Odom LD, Plouffe L Jr, Butler WJ. 5-fluorouracil exposure during the period of conception: report on two cases. Obstet Gynecol 163:76–7, 1990.
150. de Benedictis JT, Marmar JL, Praiss DE. Intraurethral condylomata acuminata: management and a review of the literature. J Urol 118:767–9.
151. Reid R, Greenberg MD, Lörincz AT, et al. Superficial laser vulvectomy. IV. Extended laser vaporization and adjunctive 5-fluorouracil therapy of human papillomavirus-associated vulvar disease. Obstet Gynecol 76:439–48, 1990.
152. Syed TA, Quresh ZA, Ahmad SA, Shahida M. Management of intravaginal warts in HIV-infected women with a dual

combination therapy: 5-fluorouracil (1%) in injectable hydrophylic gel and zidovudine 250 mg. Natl HIV Prev Conf Abstracts 105, 1999.
153. Sillman FH, Sedlis A, Boyce JG. A review of lower genital intraepithelial neoplasia and the use of topical 5-fluorouracil. Obstet Gynecol Surv 40:190–220, 1985.
154. Pehoushek J, Smith KJ. Imiquimod and 5% fluorouracil therapy for anal and perianal squamous cell carcinoma in situ in an HIV-1-positive man. Arch Dermatol 137:14–16, 2001.
155. Maiman M, Watts DH, Andersen J, et al. Vaginal 5-fluorouracil for high-grade cervical dysplasia in human immunodeficiency virus infection: a randomized trial. Obstet Gynecol 94:954–61, 1999.
156. van Cutsem E, Snoeck R, van Ranst M, et al. Successful treatment of a squamous papilloma of the hypopharynx-esophagus by local injections of (S)-1-(3-hydroxy-2-phosphonylmethoxypropyl) cytosine. J Med Virol 45:230–5, 1995.
157. Snoeck R, van Ranst M, Andrei G, et al. Treatment of anogenital papillomavirus infections with an acyclic nucleoside phosphonate analogue. N Engl J Med 333:943–4, 1995.
158. Snoeck R, Wellens W, Desloovere C, et al. Treatment of severe recurrent laryngeal papillomatosis by local injections of (S-1-(3-hydroxy-2-phosphonylmethoxypropyl)cytosine (Cidofovir). Antiviral Res 30:A25, 1996.
159. Douglas J, Corey L, Tyring S, et al. A phase I/II study of cidofovir topical gel for refractory condyloma acuminatum in patients with HIV infection. In: Abstracts 4th Conf Retrovir Opportun Infect; Foundation for Retroviral and Human Health 1997, p 677.
160. Dancey DR, Chamberlain DW, Krajden M, et al. Successful treatment of juvenile laryngeal papillomatosis-related multicystic lung disease with cidofovir: case report and review of the literature. Chest 118:1210–14, 2000.
161. Koonsaeng S, Verschraegen C, Freedman R, et al. Successful treatment of recurrent vulvar intraepithelial neoplasia resistant to interferon and isotretinoin with cidofovir. J Med Virol 64:195–8, 2001.
162. Martinelli C, Farese A, Mistro AD, et al. Resolution of recurrent perianal condylomata acuminata by topical cidofovir in patients with HIV infection. J Eur Acad Dermatol Venereol 15:568–9, 2001.
163. Stragier I, Snoeck R, De Clercq E, et al. Local treatment of HPV-induced skin lesions by cidofovir. J Med Virol 67:241–5, 2002.
164. Toro JR, Sanchez S, Turiansky G, Blauvelt A. Topical cidofovir for the treatment of dermatologic conditions: verruca, condyloma, intraepithelial neoplasia, herpes simplex and its potential use in smallpox. Dermatol Clin 21:301–9, 2003.
165. Husak R, Zouboulis CC, Sander-Bahr C, et al. Refractory human papillomavirus-associated oral warts treated topically with 1–3% cidofovir solutions in human immunodeficiency virus type 1-infected patients. Br J Dermatol 152:590–1, 2005.
166. Snoeck R, Bossens M, Parent D, et al. A double-blind, placebo-controlled study of cidofovir gel for human papillomavirus (HPV)-associated genital warts. In: Abstracts 11th International Conference on Antiviral Research, Washington, DC; International Society on Antiviral Research 1998, p 27.
167. Coremans G, Margaritis V, Snoeck R, et al. Topical cidofovir (HPMPC) is an effective adjuvant to surgical treatment of anogenital condylomata acuminata. Dis Colon Rectum 46:1103–8, 2003.
168. Matteelli A, Beltrame A, Graifemberghi S, et al. Efficacy and tolerability of topical 1% cidofovir cream for the treatment of external anogenital warts in HIV-infected persons. Sex Transm Dis 28:343–6, 2001.
169. Orlando G, Fasolo MM, Beretta R, et al. Combined surgery and cidofovir is an effective treatment for genital warts in HIV-infected patients. AIDS 16:447–50, 2002.
170. Snoeck R, Noel JC, Muller C, et al. Cidofovir, a new approach for the treatment of cervix intraepithelial neoplasia grade III (CIN III). J Med Virol 60:205–9, 2000.
171. Calista D. Resolution of recalcitrant human papillomavirus gingival infection with topical cidofovir. Oral Surg Oral Med Oral Pathol Oral Radiol Endodont 90:713–15, 2000.
172. Jones SK, Darville JM. Transmission of virus particles by cryotherapy and multi-use caustic pencils: a problem to dermatologists? Br J Dermatol 121:481–6, 1989.
173. Kuflik EG, Lubritz RR, Torre D. Cryotherapy. Dermatol Clin 2:319–32, 1984.
174. Dachow-Siwiec E. Technique of cryotherapy. Clin Dermatol 3:185–8, 1985.
175. Hatch KD. Cryotherapy. Baillière's Clin Obstet Gynaecol 9:133–43, 1995.
176. Grimmett RH. Liquid nitrogen therapy. Arch Dermatol 83:563–7, 1961.
177. Bonnez W, Oakes D, Bailey-Farchione A, et al. A randomized, double-blind, placebo-controlled trial of systemically administered alpha-, beta-, or gamma-interferon in combination with cryotherapy for the treatment of condyloma acuminatum. J Infect Dis 171:1081–9, 1995.
178. Bonnez W, Oakes D, Bailey-Farchione A, et al. A randomized, double-blind trial of parenteral low dose versus high dose interferon-alpha in combination with cryotherapy for treatment of condyloma acuminatum. Antiviral Res 35:41–52, 1997.
179. Ghosh AK. Cryosurgery of genital warts in cases in which podophyllin treatment failed or was contraindicated. Br J Vener Dis 53:49–53, 1977.
180. Balsdon MJ. Cryosurgery of genital warts. Br J Vener Dis 54:352–3, 1978.
181. Simmons PD, Langlet F, Thin RNT. Cryotherapy versus electrocautery in the treatment of genital warts. Br J Vener Dis 57:273–4, 1981.
182. Dodi G, Infantino A, Moretti R, et al. Cryotherapy of anorectal warts and condylomata. Cryosurgery 19:287–8, 1982.
183. Bergman A, Bhatia NN, Broen EM. Cryotherapy for treatment of genital condylomata during pregnancy. J Reprod Med 29:432–5, 1984.
184. Bashi SA. Cryotherapy versus podophyllin in the treatment of genital warts. Int J Dermatol 24:535–6, 1985.
185. Sand PK, Shen W, Bowen LW, Ostergard DR. Cryotherapy for the treatment of proximal urethral condyloma acuminatum. J Urol 137:874–6, 1987.
186. Matsunaga J, Bergman A, Bhatia NN. Genital condylomata acuminata in pregnancy: effectiveness, safety and pregancy outcome following cryotherapy. Br J Obstet Gynaecol 94:168–72, 1987.
187. Stone KM, Becker TM, Hadgu A, Kraus SJ. Treatment of external genital warts: a randomised clinical trial comparing podophyllin, cryotherapy, and electrodesiccation. Genitourin Med 66:16–19, 1990.
188. Damstra RJ, van Vloten WA. Cryotherapy in the treatment of condylomata acuminata: a controlled study of 64 patients. J Dermatol Surg Oncol 17:273–6, 1991.
189. Cox JT. Management of cervical intraepithelial neoplasia. Lancet 353:857–9, 1999.
190. Martin-Hirsch PL, Paraskevaidis E, Kitchener H. Surgery for cervical intraepithelial neoplasia. Cochrane Database Syst Rev CD001318, 2000.
191. Wetchler SJ. Treatment of cervical intraepithelial neoplasia with the CO_2 laser: laser versus cryotherapy. A review of effectiveness and cost. Obstet Gynecol Surv 39:469–73, 1984.
192. Bergman A, Matsunaga J, Bhatia NN. Cervical cryotherapy for condylomata acuminata during pregnancy. Obstet Gynecol 69:47–50, 1987.
193. Thomson JPS, Grace RH. The treatment of perianal and anal condylomata acuminata. J R Soc Med 71:180–5, 1978.

194. Jensen SL. Comparison of podophyllin application with simple surgical excision in clearance and recurrence of perianal condylomata acuminata. Lancet 2:1146–8, 1985.
195. Duus BR, Philipsen T, Christensen JD, et al. Refractory condylomata acuminata: a controlled clinical trial of carbon dioxide laser versus conventional surgical treatment. Genitourin Med 61:59–61, 1985.
196. Myer CM 3rd, Willging JP, McMurray S, Cotton RT. Use of a laryngeal micro resector system. Laryngoscope 109:1165–6, 1999.
197. Gollock JM, Slatford K, Hunter JM. Scissor excision of anogenital warts. Br J Vener Dis 58:400–1, 1982.
198. Khawaja HT. Treatment of condyloma acuminatum. Lancet i:208–9, 1986.
199. Khawaja HT. Podophyllin versus scissor excision in the treatment of perianal condylomata acuminata: a prospective study. Br J Surg 76:1067–8, 1989.
200. Simmons PD, Thompson JPS. Scissor excision of penile warts: case report. Genitourin Med 62:277–8, 1986.
201. McMillan A, Scott GR. Outpatient treatment of perianal warts by scissor excision. Genitourin Med 63:114–15, 1987.
202. Bonnez W, Oakes D, Choi A, et al. Therapeutic efficacy and complications of excisional biopsy of condyloma acuminatum. Sex Transm Dis 23:273–6, 1996.
203. Miles AJG, Mellor CH, Gazzard B, et al. Surgical management of anorectal disease in HIV-positive homosexuals. Br J Surg 77:869–71, 1990.
204. Zouboulis CC, Büttner P, Orfanos CE. Systemic interferon gamma as adjuvant therapy for refractory anogenital warts: a randomized clinical trial and meta-analysis of the available data. Arch Dermatol 128:1413–14, 1992.
205. Burke EC, Orloff SL, Freise CE, et al. Wound healing after anorectal surgery in human immunodeficiency virus-infected patients. Arch Surg 126:1267–71, 1991.
206. Lord RVN. Anorectal surgery in patients infected with human immunodeficiency virus – Factors associated with delayed wound healing. Ann Surg 226:92–9, 1997.
207. Jones HW III. Cone biopsy in the management of cervical intraepithelial neoplasia. Clin Obstet Gynecol 26:968–79, 1983.
208. Odell RC. Electrosurgery: principles and safety issues. Clin Obstet Gynecol 38:610–20, 1995.
209. Vuori J, Alfthan O, Pyrrhönen S, et al. Treatment of condyloma acuminata in male patients. Eur Urol 3:213–15, 1977.
210. Tiedemann K-H, Ernst T-M. Kombinationstherapie von rezidivierenden Condylomata acuminata mit Elektrokaustik und Alpha-2-Interferon. Akt Dermatol 14:200–4, 1988.
211. Fleshner PR, Freilich MI. Adjuvant interferon for anal condyloma – a prospective, randomized trial. Dis Colon Rectum 37:1255–9, 1994.
212. Orani AM, Fossati M, Bolis D, et al. Efficacy and safety evaluation on combination therapy with systemic interferon beta and electrocautery in the anogenital warts treatment of HIV-seropositive patients. Int Conf AIDS 9: abstract PO-B08-1326, 1993.
213. Hallen A, Ljunghall K, Wallin J. Topical anesthesia with local anesthetic (lidocaine and prilocaine, EMLA) cream for cautery of genital warts. Genitourin Med 63:316–19, 1987.
214. Wright TC, Richart RM, Ferenczy A. Electrosurgery for HPV-related diseases of the lower genital tract. New York, NY: Arthur Vision; 1991.
215. Wright TC Jr, Gagnon S, Richart RM, Ferenczy A. Treatment of cervical intraepithelial neoplasia using the loop electrosurgical excision procedure. Obstet Gynecol 79:173–8, 1992.
216. Prendiville W. Large loop excision of the transformation zone. Clin Obstet Gynecol 38:622–39, 1995.
217. Bigrigg A, Haffenden DK, Sheehan AL, et al. Efficacy and safety of large-loop excision of the transformation zone. Lancet 343:32–4, 1994.
218. Sawchuk WS, Weber PJ, Lowy DR, Dzubow LM. Infectious papillomavirus in the vapor of warts treated with carbon dioxide laser or electrocoagulation: detection and protection. J Am Acad Dermatol 21:41–9, 1989.
219. Bergbrant I-M, Samuelsson L, Olofsson S, et al. Polymerase chain reaction for monitoring human papillomavirus contamination of medical personnel during treatment of genital warts with CO_2 laser and electrocoagulation. Acta Dermatol Venereol (Stockholm) 74:393–5, 1994.
220. Bekassy Z, Weström L. Infrared coagulation in the treatment of condyloma accuminata in the female genital tract. Sex Transm Dis 14:209–12, 1987.
221. Goldstone SE, Kawalek AZ, Huyett JW. Infrared coagulator: a useful tool for treating anal squamous intraepithelial lesions. Dis Colon Rectum 48:1042–54, 2005.
222. Herd RM, Dover JS, Arndt KA. Basic laser principles. Dermatol Clin 15:355–72, 1997.
223. Dover JS, Arndt KA, Dinehart SM, et al. Guidelines of care for laser surgery. J Am Acad Dermatol 41:484–95, 1999.
224. Hruza GJ. Laser treatment of warts and other epidermal and dermal lesions. Dermatol Clin 15:487–506, 1997.
225. Reid R. Laser surgery of the vulva. Obstet Gynecol Clin North Am 18:491–510, 1991.
226. Ferenczy A. Laser treatment of genital human papillomavirus infections in the male patient. Obstet Gynecol Clin North Am 18:525–35, 1991.
227. Bhatta KM. Lasers in urology. Lasers Surg Med 16:312–30, 1995.
228. Dorsey JH. Laser surgery for cervical intraepithelial neoplasia. Obstet Gynecol Clin North Am 18:475–89, 1991.
229. Bellina JH. The use of the carbon dioxide laser in the management of condyloma acuminatum with eight-year follow-up. Am J Obstet Gynecol 147:375–8, 1983.
230. Calkins JW, Masterson BJ, Magrina JF, Capen CV. Management of condylomata acuminata with the carbon dioxide laser. Obstet Gynecol 59:105–8, 1982.
231. Krogh J, Beuke H-P, Miskowiak J, et al. Long-term results of carbon dioxide laser treatment of meatal condylomata acuminata. Br J Urol 65:621–3, 1990.
232. Bar-Am A, Shilon M, Peyser MR, et al. Treatment of male genital condylomatous lesions by carbon dioxide laser after failure of previous nonlaser methods. J Am Acad Dermatol 24:87–9, 1991.
233. Garden JM, O'Banion MK, Shelnitz LS, et al. Papillomavirus in the vapor of carbon dioxide laser-treated verrucae. JAMA 259:1199–1202, 1988.
234. Kashima HK, Kessis T, Mounts P, Shah K. Polymerase chain reaction identification of human papillomavirus DNA in CO_2 laser plume from recurrent respiratory papillomatosis. Otolaryngol Head Neck Surg 104:191–5, 1991.
235. Gloster HM Jr, Roenigk RK. Risk of acquiring human papillomavirus from the plume produced by the carbon dioxide laser in the treatment of warts. J Am Acad Dermatol 32:436–441, 1995.
236. Baggish MS. Carbon dioxide laser treatment for condylomata acuminata venereal infections. Obstet Gynecol 55:711–15, 1980.
237. Ferenczy A. Using the laser to treat vulvar condylomata acuminata and intraepidermal neoplasia. Can Med Assoc J 128:135–7, 1983.
238. Kryger-Baggesen N, Larsen JF, Pedersen PH. CO_2-laser treatment of condylomata acuminata. Acta Obstet Gynecol Scand 63:341–3, 1984.
239. Ferenczy A. Treating genital condyloma during pregnancy with the carbon dioxide laser. Am J Obstet Gynecol 148:9–12, 1984.
240. Reid R. Superficial laser vulvectomy. I. The efficacy of extended superficial ablation for refractory and very extensive condylomas. Am J Obstet Gynecol 151:1047–52, 1985.

241. Baggish MS. Improved laser techniques for the elimination of genital and extragenital warts. Am J Obstet Gynecol 153:545–50, 1985.
242. Krebs H-B, Wheelock JB. The CO_2 laser for recurrent and therapy-resistant condylomata acuminata. J Reprod Med 30:489–92, 1985.
243. Graversen PH, Baggi P, Rosenkilde P. Laser treatment of recurrent urethral condylomata acuminata in men. Scand J Urol Nephrol 24:163–6, 1990.
244. Larsen J, Petersen CS. The patient with refractory genital warts in the STD-clinic. Dan Med Bull 37:194–5, 1990.
245. Geraci A, Thomas G, Lavigne J, Levy M. Relative efficacy of laser versus radio-frequency ablation of anogenital condylomata. Int Conf AIDS 6:2020 (abstract), 1990.
246. Hohenleutner U, Landthaler M, Braun-Falco O. Postoperative adjuvante Therapie mit Interferon-alfa-2b nach Laserchirurgie von Condylomata acuminata. Hautarzt 41:545–8, 1990.
247. Petersen CS, Bjerring P, Larsen J, et al. Systemic interferon alpha-2b increases the cure rate in laser treated patients with multiple persistent genital warts: a placebo-controlled study. Genitourin Med 67:99–102, 1991.
248. Reid R, Greenberg MD, Pizzuti DJ, et al. Superficial laser vulvectomy. V. Surgical debulking is enhanced by adjuvant systemic interferon. Am J Obstet Gynecol 166:815–20, 1992.
249. Group CICS. Randomized placebo-controlled double-blind combined therapy with laser surgery and systemic interferon-alpha 2a in the treatment of anogenital condylomata acuminatum. J Infect Dis 167:824–9, 1993.
250. Nieminen P, Aho M, Lehtinen M, Vesterinen E, Vaheri A, Paavonen J. Treatment of genital HPV infection with carbon dioxide laser and systemic interferon alpha-2b. Sex Transm Dis 21:65–9, 1994.
251. Klutke JJ, Bergman A. Interferon as an adjuvant treatment for genital condyloma acuminatum. Int J Gynaecol Obstet 49:171–4, 1995.
252. Hoyme UB, Hagedorn M, Schindler AE, et al. Effect of adjuvant imiquimod 5% cream on sustained clearance of anogenital warts following laser treatment. Infect Dis Obstet Gynecol 10:79–88, 2002.
253. Morris M, Tortolero-Luna G, Malpica A, et al. Cervical intraepithelial neoplasia and cervical cancer. Obstet Gynecol Clin North Am 23:347–410, 1996.
254. Townsend DE, Richart RM. Cryotherapy and carbon dioxide laser management of cervical intraepithelial neoplasia: a controlled comparison. Obstet Gynecol 61:75–8, 1983.
255. Mathevet P, Dargent D, Roy M, Beau G. A randomized prospective study comparing three techniques of conization: cold-knife, laser, and LEEP. Gynecol Oncol 54:175–9, 1994.
256. Carrozza PM, Merlani GM, Burg G, Hafner J. CO_2 laser surgery for extensive, cauliflower-like anogenital condylomata acuminata: retrospective long-term study on 19 HIV-positive and 45 HIV-negative men. Dermatology 205:255–9, 2002.
257. Convissar RA. Laser palliation of oral manifestations of human immunodeficiency virus infection. J Am Dent Assoc 133:591–8, 2002.
258. Abdel-Hady ES, Martin-Hirsch P, Duggan-Keen M, et al. Immunological and viral factors associated with the response of vulval intraepithelial neoplasia to photodynamic therapy. Cancer Res 61:192–6, 2001.
259. Stefanaki IM, Georgiou S, Themelis GC, et al. In vivo fluorescence kinetics and photodynamic therapy in condylomata acuminata. Br J Dermatol 149:972–6, 2003.
260. Wang XL, Wang HW, Wang HS, et al. Topical 5-aminolaevulinic acid-photodynamic therapy for the treatment of urethral condylomata acuminata. Br J Dermatol 151:880–5, 2004.
261. Rockley PF, Tyring SK. Interferons alpha, beta and gamma therapy of anogenital human papillomavirus infections. Pharmacol Ther 65:265–87, 1995.
262. Parmar S, Platanias LC. Interferons: mechanisms of action and clinical applications. Curr Opin Oncol 15:431–9, 2003.
263. Vesterinen E, Meyer B, Cantell K, Purola E. Topical treatment of flat vaginal condyloma with human leukocyte interferon. Obstet Gynecol 64:535–8, 1984.
264. Vesterinen E, Meyer B, Purola E, Cantell K. Treatment of vaginal flat condyloma with interferon cream. Lancet i:157, 1984.
265. Keay S, Teng N, Eisenberg M, et al. Topical interferon for treating condyloma acuminata in women. J Infect Dis 158:934–9, 1988.
266. Frega A, Stentella P, Direnzi F, et al. Assessment of self application of four topical agents on genital warts in women. J Eur Acad Dermatol Venereol 8:112–15, 1997.
267. Syed TA, Cheema KM, Khayyami M, et al. Human leukocyte interferon-alpha versus podophyllotoxin in cream for the treatment of genital warts in males. A placebo-controlled, double-blind, comparative study. Dermatology 191:129–32, 1995.
268. Syed TA, Khayyami M, Kriz D, et al. Management of genital warts in women with human leukocyte interferon-alpha vs. podophyllotoxin in cream: a placebo-controlled, double-blind, comparative study. J Mol Med 73:255–8, 1995.
269. Syed TA, Ahmadpour OA. Human leukocyte derived interferon-alpha in a hydrophilic gel for the treatment of intravaginal warts in women: a placebo-controlled, double-blind study. Int J Sex Trans Dis AIDS 9:769–72, 1998.
270. Gross G, Rogozinski T, Schofer H, et al. Recombinant interferon beta gel as an adjuvant in the treatment of recurrent genital warts: results of a placebo-controlled double-blind study in 120 patients. Dermatology 196:330–4, 1998.
271. Friedman-Kien A, Eron LJ, Conant M, et al. Natural interferon alfa for treatment of condylomata acuminata. JAMA 259:533–8, 1988.
272. Vance JC, Bart BJ, Hansen RC, et al. Intralesional recombinant alpha-2 interferon for the treatment of patients with condyloma acuminatum or verruca plantaris. Arch Dermatol 122:272–7, 1986.
273. Eron LJ, Judson F, Tucker S, et al. Interferon therapy for condylomata acuminata. N Engl J Med 315:1059–64, 1986.
274. Reichman RC, Oakes D, Bonnez W, et al. Treatment of condyloma acuminatum with three different interferons administered intralesionally: A double-blind, placebo-controlled trial. Ann Intern Med 108:675–9, 1988.
275. Welander CE, Homesley HD, Smiles KA, Peets EA. Intralesional interferon alfa-2b for the treatment of genital warts. Am J Obstet Gynecol 162:348–54, 1990.
276. Douglas JM Jr, Eron LJ, Judson FN, et al. A randomized trial of combination therapy with intralesional interferon alpha-2b and podophyllin versus podophyllin alone for the therapy of anogenital warts. J Infect Dis 162:52–9, 1990.
277. Bart BJ, Vance JC, Krywonis N, et al. Treatment of condylomata acuminata: comparing intralesional alpha-2b interferon combined with liquid nitrogen to liquid nitrogen alone. J Invest Dermatol 90:545, 1988.
278. Handley JM, Horner T, Maw RD, et al. Subcutaneous interferon alpha 2a combined with cryotherapy vs cryotherapy alone in the treatment of primary anogenital warts: a randomised observer blind placebo controlled study. Genitourin Med 67:297–302, 1991.
279. Bornstein J, Pascal B, Zarfati D, et al. Recombinant human interferon-beta for condylomata acuminata: a randomized, double-blind, placebo-controlled study of intralesional therapy. Int J Sex Trans Dis AIDS 8:614–21, 1997.
280. Dinsmore W, Jordan J, O'Mahony C, et al. Recombinant human interferon-beta in the treatment of condylomata acuminata. Int J Sex Trans Dis AIDS 8:622–8, 1997.
281. Trizna Z, Evans T, Bruce S, et al. A randomized phase II study comparing four different interferon therapies in patients with

recalcitrant condylomata acuminata. Sex Transm Dis 25:361–5, 1998.
282. Gaspari AA, Zalka A. Interferon gamma immunotherapy for generalized verrucosis in the setting of chronic immunodeficiency. J Am Acad Dermatol 38:286–7, 1998.
283. Beutner KR, Wiley DJ, Douglas JM, et al. Genital warts and their treatment. Clin Infect Dis 28:S37–S56, 1998.
284. Douglas JM, Rogers M, Judson FN. The effect of asymptomatic infection with HTLV-III on the response of anogenital warts in intralesional treatment with recombinant alpha-2 interferon. J Infect Dis 154:331–4, 1986.
285. Armstrong DK, Maw RD, Dinsmore WW, et al. A randomised, double-blind, parallel group study to compare subcutaneous interferon alpha-2a plus podophyllin with placebo plus podophyllin in the treatment of primary condylomata acuminata. Genitourin Med 70:389–93, 1994.
286. Yliskoski M, Cantell K, Syrjänen K, Syrjänen S. Topical treatment with human leukocyte interferon of HPV 16 infections associated with cervical and vaginal intraepithelial neoplasia. Gynecol Oncol 36:353–7, 1990.
287. Bornstein J, Ben-David Y, Atad J, et al. Treatment of cervical intraepithelial neoplasia and invasive squamous cell carcinoma by interferon. Obstet Gynecol Surv 48:251–60, 1993.
288. Rotola A, Costa S, Di Luca D, et al. Beta-interferon treatment of cervical intraepithelial neoplasia: a multicenter clinical trial. Intervirology 38:325–31, 1995.
289. Gonzalez-Sanchez JL, Martinez-Chequer JC, Barahona-Bustillos E, Andrade-Manzano AF. Randomized placebo-controlled evaluation of intramuscular interferon beta treatment of recurrent human papillomavirus. Obstet Gynecol 97:621–4, 2001.
290. Brockmeyer NH, Poffhoff A, Bader A, et al. Treatment of condylomata acuminata with pegylated interferon alfa-2b in HIV-infected patients. Eur J Med Res 11:27–32, 2006.
291. Garland SM. Imiquimod. Curr Opin Infect Dis 16:85–9, 2003.
292. Skinner RB Jr. Imiquimod. Dermatol Clin 21:291–300, 2003.
293. Burns CA, Brown MD. Imiquimod for the treatment of skin cancer. Dermatol Clin 23:151–64, 2005.
294. Chang YC, Madkan V, Cook-Norris R, et al. Current and potential uses of imiquimod. South Med J 98:914–20, 2005.
295. Spruance S, Douglas J, Hougham A, et al. Multicenter trial of 5% imiquimod (IQ) cream for the treatment of genital and perianal warts. In: Abstracts 33rd Interscience Conf Antimicrob Chemother; American Society of Microbiology, 1993, p 1432.
296. Beutner KR, Tyring SK, Trofatter KF Jr, et al. Imiquimod, a patient-applied immune-response modifier for treatment of external genital warts. Antimicrob Agents Chemother 42:789–94, 1998.
297. Fife KH, Ferenczy A, Douglas JM Jr, et al. Treatment of external genital warts in men using 5% imiquimod cream applied three times a week, once daily, twice daily, or three times a day. Sex Transm Dis 28:226–31, 2001.
298. Gollnick H, Barasso R, Jappe U, et al. Safety and efficacy of imiquimod 5% cream in the treatment of penile genital warts in uncircumcised men when applied three times weekly or once per day. Int J Sex Trans Dis AIDS 12:22–8, 2001.
299. Garland SM, Sellors JW, Wikstrom A, et al. Imiquimod 5% cream is a safe and effective self-applied treatment for anogenital warts – results of an open-label, multicentre Phase IIIB trial. Int J STD AIDS 12:722–9, 2001.
300. Gilson RJ, Shupack JL, Friedman-Kien AE, et al. A randomized, controlled, safety study using imiquimod for the topical treatment of anogenital warts in HIV-infected patients. Imiquimod Study Group. AIDS 13:2397–404, 1999.
301. Cusini M, Salmaso F, Zerboni R, et al. 5% Imiquimod cream for external anogenital warts in HIV-infected patients under HAART therapy. Int J STD AIDS 15:17–20, 2004.
302. Kreuter A, Hochdorfer B, Stucker M, et al. Treatment of anal intraepithelial neoplasia in patients with acquired HIV with imiquimod 5% cream. J Am Acad Dermatol 50:980–1, 2004.
303. Kaspari M, Gutzmer R, Kaspari T, et al. Application of imiquimod by suppositories (anal tampons) efficiently prevents recurrences after ablation of anal canal condyloma. Br J Dermatol 147:757–9, 2002.
304. Kreuter A, Brockmeyer NH, Weissenborn SJ, et al. 5% imiquimod suppositories decrease the DNA load of intra-anal HPV types 6 and 11 in HIV-infected men after surgical ablation of condylomata acuminata. Arch Dermatol 142:243–4, 2006.
305. Orfanos CE, Ehlert R, Gollnick H. The retinoids. A review of their clinical pharmacology and therapeutic use. Drugs 34:459–503, 1987.
306. Eckert RL, Agarwal C, Hembree JR, et al. Human cervical cancer. Retinoids, interferon and human papillomavirus. Adv Exp Med Biol 375:31–44, 1995.
307. Schneider A, Shah K. The role of vitamins in the etiology of cervical neoplasia: an epidemiological review. Arch Gynecol Obstet 246:1–13, 1989.
308. Mitchell MF, Hittelman WK, Lotan R, et al. Chemoprevention trials and surrogate end point biomarkers in the cervix. Cancer 76:1956–77, 1995.
309. Olsen EA, Kelly FF, Vollner RT, et al. Comparative study of systemic interferon alfa-n1 and isotretinoin in the treatment of resistant condylomata acuminata. J Am Acad Dermatol 20:1023–30, 1989.
310. Handley J, Dinsmore W. Topical tretinoin in the treatment of anogenital warts. Sex Transm Dis 19:181, 1992.
311. Meyskens FL Jr, Surwit E, Moon TE, et al. Enhancement of regression of cervical intraepithelial neoplasia II (moderate dysplasia) with topically applied all-trans-retinoic acid: a randomized trial. J Natl Cancer Inst 86:539–43, 1994.
312. Ampel NM, Stout ML, Garewal HS. Persistent ulcer associated with human papillomavirus type 33 in a patient with AIDS: successful treatment with isotretinoin. Rev Infect Dis 12:1004–7, 1990.
313. Del Priore G, Herron MM. Retinoids for vulvar dysplasia in the HIV-infected patient. Int J Gynaecol Obstet 55:77–8, 1996.
314. Robinson WR, Andersen J, Darragh TM, et al. Isotretinoin for low-grade cervical dysplasia in human immunodeficiency virus-infected women. Obstet Gynecol 99:777–84, 2002.
315. Rogers CJ, Gibney MD, Siegfried EC, et al. Cimetidine therapy for recalcitrant warts in adults: is it any better than placebo? J Am Acad Dermatol 41:123–7, 1999.
316. Wargon O. Cimetidine for mucosal warts in an HIV positive adult. Austral J Dermatol 37:149–50, 1996.
317. Anonymous. Sexually transmitted diseases treatment guidelines 2002. MMWR 51:1–82, 2002.
318. Anonymous. 1998 guidelines for the treatment of sexually transmitted diseases. MMWR 47:1–116, 1998.
319. Beutner KR, Reitano MV, Richwald GA, Wiley DJ. External genital warts – Report of the American Medical Association Consensus Conference. Clin Infect Dis 27:796–806, 1998.
320. von Krogh G, Lacey CJ, Gross G, et al. European course on HPV associated pathology: guidelines for primary care physicians for the diagnosis and management of anogenital warts. Sex Transm Infect 76:162–8, 2000.
321. Volberding P. Looking behind: time for anal cancer screening. Am J Med 108:674–5, 2000.
322. Wright TC Jr, Cox JT, Massad LS, Cet al. 2001 consensus guidelines for the management of women with cervical intraepithelial neoplasia. Am J Obstet Gynecol 189:295–304, 2003.
323. Massad LS, Evans CT, Minkoff H, et al. Natural history of grade 1 cervical intraepithelial neoplasia in women with human immunodeficiency virus. Obstet Gynecol 104:1077–85, 2004.

324. Maiman M. Management of cervical neoplasia in human immunodeficiency virus-infected women. J Natl Cancer Inst Monogr 23:43–9, 1998.
325. Montz FJ. Management of high-grade cervical intraepithelial neoplasia and low-grade squamous intraepithelial lesion and potential complications. Clin Obstet Gynecol 43:394–409, 2000.
326. Saslow D, Runowicz CD, Solomon D, et al. American Cancer Society guideline for the early detection of cervical neoplasia and cancer. CA Cancer J Clin 52:342–62, 2002.
327. US Preventive Services Task Force. Screening for cervical cancer. In: AHRQ Publication No. 03–515A, January 2003. Rockville, MD: Agency for Healthcare Research and Quality; 2003.
328. ACOG Practice Bulletin. Cervical cytology screening. Number 45. Int J Gynaecol Obstet 83:237–47, 2003.
329. Kaplan JE, Masur H, Holmes KK, USPHS, Infectious Disease Society of America. Guidelines for preventing opportunistic infections among HIV-infected persons – 2002. Recommendations of the U.S. Public Health Service and the Infectious Diseases Society of America. MMWR 51:1–52, 2002.
330. Manhart LE, Koutsky LA. Do condoms prevent genital HPV infection, external genital warts, or cervical neoplasia? A meta-analysis. Sex Transm Dis 29:725–35, 2002.
331. Winer RL, Hughes JP, Feng Q, et al. Condom use and the risk of genital human papillomavirus infection in young women. N Engl J Med 354:2645–54, 2006.
332. Hogewoning CJ, Bleeker MC, van den Brule AJ, et al. Condom use promotes regression of cervical intraepithelial neoplasia and clearance of human papillomavirus: a randomized clinical trial. Int J Cancer 107:811–16, 2003.
333. Bleeker MC, Hogewoning CJ, Van Den Brule AJ, et al. Penile lesions and human papillomavirus in male sexual partners of women with cervical intraepithelial neoplasia. J Am Acad Dermatol 47:351–7, 2002.
334. Bleeker MC, Berkhof J, Hogewoning CJ, et al. HPV type concordance in sexual couples determines the effect of condoms on regression of flat penile lesions. Br J Cancer 92:1388–92, 2005.
335. Hildesheim A, Brinton LA, Mallin K, et al. Barrier and spermicidal contraceptive methods and risk of invasive cervical cancer. Epidemiology 1:266–72, 1990.
336. Feldman JG, Chirgwin K, Dehovitz JA, Minkoff H. The association of smoking and risk of condyloma acuminatum in women. Obstet Gynecol 89:346–50, 1997.
337. Koutsky LA, Ault KA, Wheeler CM, et al. A controlled trial of a human papillomavirus type 16 vaccine. N Engl J Med 347:1645–51, 2002.
338. Villa LL, Costa RL, Petta CA, et al. Prophylactic quadrivalent human papillomavirus (types 6, 11, 16, and 18) L1 virus-like particle vaccine in young women: a randomised double-blind placebo-controlled multicentre phase II efficacy trial. Lancet Oncol 6:271–8, 2005.
338a. Garland SM, Hernandez-Avila M, Wheeler CM, et al. Quadrivalent vaccine against human papillomavirus to prevent anogenital diseases. N Engl J Med 356:1928–43, 2007.
338b. Koutsky LA. Quadrivalent vaccine against human papillomavirus to prevent high-grade cervical lesions. N Engl J Med 356:1915–27, 2007.
338c. Ault KA. Effects of prophylactic human papillomavirus L1 virus-like particle vaccine on risk of cervical intraepithelial neoplasia grade 2, grade 3 and adenocarcinoma in situ: a combined analysis of four randomised clinical trials. Lancet 369:1861–8, 2007.
338d. Joura EA, Leodolter S, Hernandez-Avila M, et al. Efficacy of a quadrivalent prophylactic human papillomavirus (types 6, 11, 16 and 18) L1 virus-like-particle vaccine against high-grade vulval and vaginal lesions: a combined analysis of three randomised trials. Lancet 369: 1693–702, 2007.
339. Harper DM, Franco EL, Wheeler C, et al. Efficacy of a bivalent L1 virus-like particle vaccine in prevention of infection with human papillomavirus types 16 and 18 in young women: a randomised controlled trial. Lancet 364:1757–65, 2004.
340. Harper DM, Franco EL, Wheeler CM, et al. Sustained efficacy up to 4.5 years of a bivalent L1 virus-like particle vaccine against human papillomavirus types 16 and 18: follow-up from a randomised control trial. Lancet 367:1247–55, 2006.
341. Munoz N, Bosch FX, Castellsague X, et al. Against which human papillomavirus types shall we vaccinate and screen? The international perspective. Int J Cancer 111:278–85, 2004.
342. Kiviat N, Rompalo A, Bowden R, et al. Anal human papillomavirus infection among human immunodeficiency virus-seropositive and -seronegative men. J Infect Dis 162:358–61, 1990.
343. Mellon LR, Gélin-Charlot C, Grand'Pierre R, et al. Prevalence of STDs among HIV+ and HIV− patients in an STD clinic in Haiti. Int Conf AIDS 10:459C (abstract), 1994.
344. Chirgwin KD, Feldman J, Augenbraun M, et al. Incidence of venereal warts in human immunodeficiency virus-infected and uninfected women. J Infect Dis 172:235–8, 1995.
345. Rezza G, Giuliani M, Branca M, et al. Determinants of squamous intraepithelial lesions (SIL) on Pap smear: the role of HPV infection and of HIV-1-induced immunosuppression. DIANAIDS Collaborative Study Group. Eur J Epidemiol 13:937–43, 1997.
346. Williams AB, Darragh TM, Vranizan K, et al. Anal and cervical human papillomavirus infection and risk of anal and cervical epithelial abnormalities in human immunodeficiency virus-infected women. Obstet Gynecol 83:205–11, 1994.

Chapter 57

JC Virus Neurologic Infection

Sunil Chauhan, MD, MsPH, Colin D. Hall, MBChB

Progressive multifocal leukoencephalopathy (PML) was initially described by Astrom and colleagues in 1958,[1] as a complication of chronic leukemia and Hodgkin's disease. It has since been recognized in an increasing number of conditions associated with impairment in human cellular immunity. It became more prevalent with the more aggressive use of therapeutic immunosuppressive agents in the 1960s and 1970s, but was still regarded as a rare disease until the AIDS epidemic, with its resulting large pool of immune-compromised patients. PML is an AIDS-defining illness and one of the common opportunistic infections of the brain in this population, occurring in up to 8% of patients at autopsy.[2–5] Before the availability of highly active antiretroviral therapy (HAART), it was reported as the presenting manifestation of HIV infection in 10–55% of case series.[6–8] While there are no clear figures on the incidence and prevalence of PML following the introduction of HAART, the disease continues to occur, although probably at a reduced rate. The incidence and prevalence in resource-poor settings, such as sub-Saharan Africa, is unknown. PML is rare in pediatric AIDS but does occur.[9]

In 1971, Padgett and colleagues isolated the viral agent etiologically responsible for PML from the brain of an infected patient, and named it JC virus (JCV), from the initials of the patient.[10] JCV is a polyomavirus. It is similar to the other human polyomavirus, BK, and to simian immunodeficiency virus 40 (SV40). JCV is ubiquitous in humans and is usually acquired by adolescence, and over 70% of the adult population generate a humoral response.[11,12] The precise mode of transmission is not established, although it is suspected to be via the respiratory tract.[1]

There are no known symptoms associated with the initial infection with JCV, and the only known clinical manifestations of PML are the results of nervous system involvement. Its clinical presentation is quite variable, depending on the size and location of the lesions. It presents with the insidious onset and progression of neurological dysfunction, generally without fever or headache. It is primarily a disease of white matter, but may at times involve gray matter structures, and may therefore result in a wide spectrum of neurological symptoms and signs.

The most common initial clinical findings reported in AIDS patients with PML include painless progressive monoparetic or hemiparetic limb weakness and/or sensory loss, gait difficulty, and visual disturbance (Table 57-1). Subtle or overt alteration of mental status may accompany other manifestations; occasionally the initial presentation may be of encephalopathy without focal findings. Prior to HAART, the course was generally rapidly progressive over weeks, leading to coma with vegetative signs and death, but the prognosis has improved considerably with effective antiretroviral therapy (ART).

DIAGNOSIS

Diagnosis of PML is primarily based on clinical findings and a compatible magnetic resonance imaging (MRI) picture (Figs 57-1 and 57-2). The diagnosis is confirmed by establishing the presence of JCV and ruling out other opportunistic infections.

The clinical presentation is dependent on the location of active infection. Because this may involve any area of the brain, brain stem, and/or cerebellum, PML must be considered in any patient presenting with central nervous system disease. Abnormalities on computed tomography (CT) are typically hypodense white matter lesions without mass effect. Only rarely do these lesions enhance with contrast. MRI is more sensitive than CT and will typically show greater involvement.[14–16] Lesions on MRI are primarily but not exclusively of white matter, and appear as single or multiple large or small bright areas on T2-weighted images, again generally without contrast enhancement or mass effect (Fig. 57-2). T1-weighted images are invariably of low density. However, it is not always possible to exclude other lesions, including lymphoma and

Table 57-1

Neurological Manifestations of PML

Neurological Manifestations of PML
Focal deficit (monoparesis or hemiparesis)
Gait disturbances (ataxia)
Visual field deficits
Cognitive disturbances
Speech difficulties (aphasia and dysarthria)
Sensory disturbances
Seizure
Cranial nerve deficits

HIV encephalitis, on MRI. Immune restoration syndrome, which may give contrast-enhancing white matter lesions with or without the presence of PML, may also create confusion in the radiological diagnosis.[13]

Further, while MRI is of paramount importance as a diagnostic tool, there is no evidence that the number or size of the lesions found has any prognostic significance.[14] Magnetic resonance spectroscopy is an additional diagnostic tool.[15] Typically, spectroscopy shows an elevated choline to creatine ratio, but this is not a specific finding.

Routine testing for antibodies to JCV is not of value in establishing the diagnosis of PML. Immunoglobulin G antibody identification by hemagglutination inhibition is positive in most healthy adults worldwide. The titer does not rise with active disease, and there is generally a lack of immunoglobulin M antibody in either serum or cerebrospinal fluid (CSF), indicating PML results from reactivation of a latent infection.[12]

Routine CSF analysis is generally unhelpful. Although some elevation of cell count, protein, and immunoglobulin may be found,[3] it is not clear whether this occurs more often than in HIV-infected patients without PML.[16]

Before the advent of CSF JCV polymerase chain reaction (PCR) analysis the definitive diagnosis was dependent on pathologic examination of brain tissue. The typical appearance on biopsy is of multiple areas of demyelination at the corticomedullary junction, extending in severe cases into large areas of white matter (Fig. 57-3). In advanced disease, gray matter may also be involved. The oligodendrocytes have large, deeply staining nuclei, many with inclusions and with large numbers of virions (Fig. 57-4). Reactive astrocytosis is generally present, and there may be giant astrocytes similar to those found in glioblastoma multiforme.[17] Neurons are not infected. HIV-infected patients have a higher incidence of very large, confluent lesions, with prominent necrosis and a higher incidence of marked perivascular inflammatory infiltrates, compared to patients with other causes of immune compromise.[18]

Stereotactic brain biopsy offers less morbidity than open biopsy and is generally the preferred procedure,[19,20] but may not always give adequate tissue for definitive microscopic diagnosis. The use of *in situ* hybridization techniques[21] and immunocytochemistry increases the diagnostic potential of stereotactic biopsy, and these are useful adjunctive diagnostic tools.[22,23] Utilizing PCR, JCV DNA has been identified in the brains of HIV-infected patients with and without PML, and in uninfected control brains. This presumably reflects indolent infection of brain tissue, and suggests that PCR of brain biopsy tissue is too sensitive for specific diagnosis of active disease.[24–26]

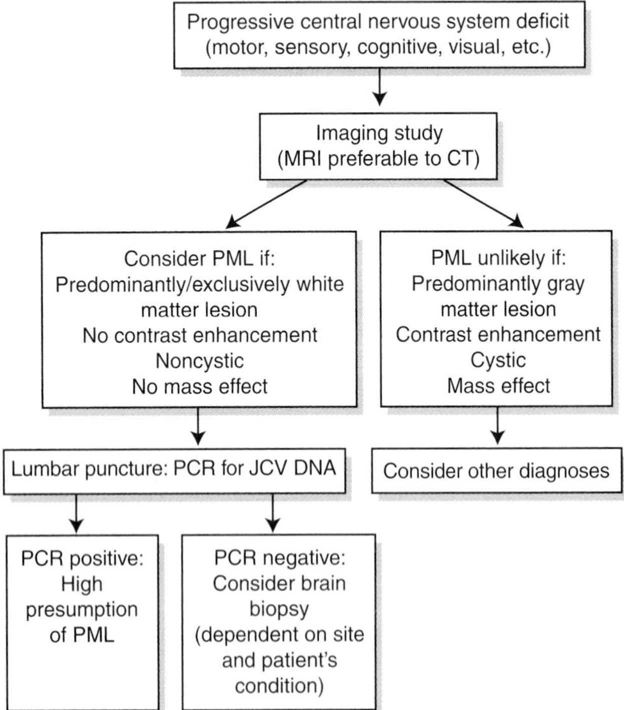

Figure 57-1 ■ Diagnostic algorithm for progressive multifocal leukoencephalopathy (PML).

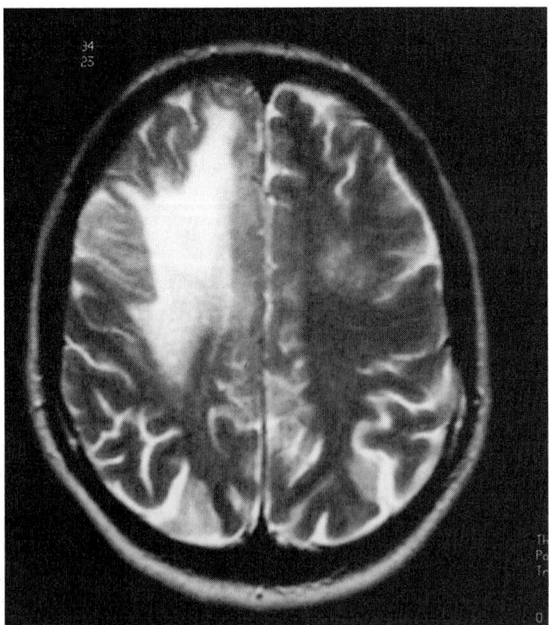

Figure 57-2 ■ T2-weighted MRI scan of the brain in a patient with PML. There is a large lesion in the right anterior hemisphere, with smaller lesions in the left frontal lobe and both occipital lobes.

In an effort to spare the patient the need for brain biopsy, much work has been done on analysis of easily accessible body fluids to provide a reliable method for diagnosis. It is clear that the kidney may act as a viral reservoir in healthy populations; in different series, 20–80% of urine samples from healthy adults have yielded isolates of JCV.[27,28] PCR in urine is thus unsuitable for diagnosis of disease. The same is true of evaluation of peripheral blood. Fifteen percent of samples from healthy subjects without immune compromise will yield positive JCV PCR.[29] In addition, Tornatore et al detected JCV DNA in lymphocytes of 89% of patients with PML and in 38% of asymptomatic HIV-positive patients.[30] Dubois et al found JCV DNA in lymphocytes of over 40% of HIV-infected patients without PML.[31]

Much greater specificity has been achieved through the evaluation of CSF. Weber et al identified JCV DNA in CSF from each of three HIV-infected patients with PML but in none of 30 HIV-infected patients without PML.[32] Later, the same group reported CSF analysis from 28 patients with PML and 82 HIV-infected patients without PML. JCV DNA was detected in 82% of the PML patients and none of the controls.[33] De Luca and colleagues evaluated CSF from 19 patients with clinical PML and 83 patients with advanced HIV disease but no evidence of PML. Nested PCR had 74% sensitivity and 100% specificity, with no positive results in the patients without PML.[34] McGuire et al, using conditions optimized to detect one viral copy in 50 μg CSF, reported both sensitivity and specificity of 92%.[35] Thus it is now accepted, even for clinical trials, that a firm diagnosis of PML can be reached based on typical clinical and radiological appearance along with a positive JCV DNA analysis in CSF. Brain biopsy confirmation would then only be required if the CSF evaluation was negative, if the clinical picture was atypical, or if there was concern about a concomitant condition, such as lymphoma. Current treatment trials are based on this algorithm. It is generally accepted that greater than 90% of patients with PML will have positive JCV PCR in the CSF, and this does not occur in normal subjects or HIV-infected patients without PML. However, a number of studies have demonstrated that all CSF samples will not be positive, so in cases with a high clinical suspicion and an initially negative PCR, repeat CSF evaluation may be helpful. A further complication in interpreting the CSF results is the observation in a number of trials that treatment with HAART may be associated with disappearance of JCV from the CSF.[36,37] The JCV viral load in the CSF also appears to be of prognostic value, the higher the number of copies, the worse the prognosis.[38,39]

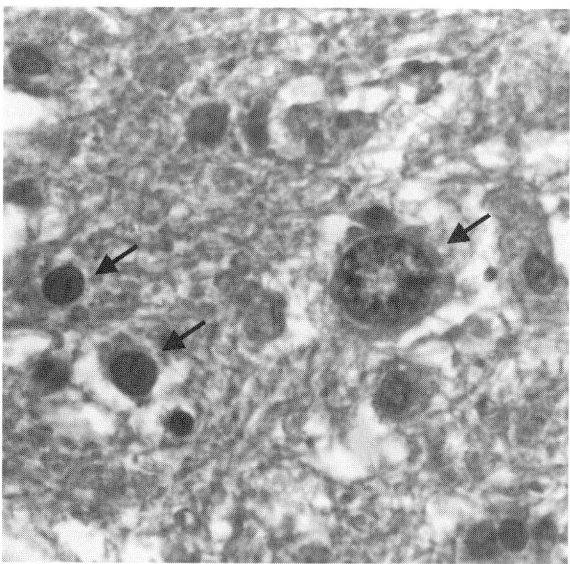

Figure 57-4 ■ Hyperchromatic, enlarged nuclei of infected oligodendrocytes (small arrows) and atypical bizarre astrocyte (large arrow) (×150).

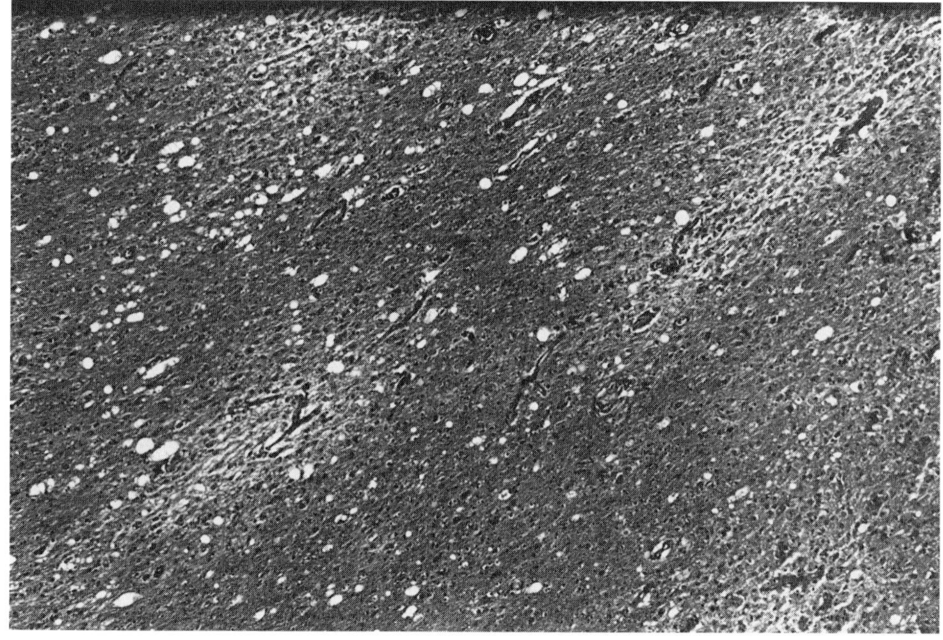

Figure 57-3 ■ Multiple foci of demyelination unaccompanied by significant inflammatory infiltrate (×45).

PCR for JCV is available commercially through the laboratories listed in Table 57-2.

It is recognized among clinicians that there are occasional cases that appear clinically and radiographically to be typical of PML, but which do not have JCV PCR positivity in the CSF or in areas of demyelinating brain tissue. It is not clear whether these may be due to JCV mutation which is not detected by current probes, or whether it is due to a different as yet unidentified virus.

THERAPY

Other than the maintenance of immune function, there are no measures for prophylaxis or prevention of PML.

Before the advent of ART, the prognosis for HIV-infected patients who develop PML was grave. Median survival from diagnosis has generally been from 2.6 to 4 months.[18,37,40] Wiley and colleagues have theorized that the prognosis may be worse in HIV infection because JCV, in addition to its direct toxicity, may increase ingress to the brain of HIV-infected macrophages.[41] However, ~10% of HIV-infected patients had a more protracted course, with stabilization over months or years and occasionally with apparent reduction or resolution of lesions.[42,43] Based on retrospective and prospective cohort studies and individual case reports, there is good evidence that treatment with HAART has resulted in improvement in the survival of patients with PML.[44–48] Maximization of ART is therefore a clear goal in treatment. Despite this, a significant number of treated patients still succumbed to PML. In addition there are a number of reports of patients who developed PML after the institution of ART, perhaps related to the immune reconstitution syndrome.[49–51] This inconsistent and incomplete response to ART, in addition to the emergence of ART resistance, mandate the continued search for more specific and effective therapy aimed at JCV. Such therapy would also be of great value in the 20% of PML patients who are not HIV-infected. A recent reminder of this possibility was the emergence of PML in a patient with Crohn's disease treated with natalizumab, a humanized monoclonal antibody which binds to the adhesion molecule alpha 4 integrins, and two patients with multiple sclerosis who were being treated with a combination of natalizumab and interferon-β1a.[52,53]

The infrequency of PML before the AIDS pandemic precluded the development of adequately controlled studies, and therapeutic measures were based on anecdotal case reports using agents with theoretical potential efficacy. A number of such agents have been tried and some suggested benefit in single cases or small series. Despite the increase in cases, controlled studies have remained a rarity, and to date there has been no convincing evidence of improvement other than that associated with ART administration. As all patients should be treated with maximized ART, any current and future studies of specific therapy must also account for the beneficial effects of HAART. The prognostic factors for PML are listed in Table 57-3.

Completed Studies

Immune compromise is a common factor in the development of PML. In the AIDS population, antiretroviral agents, by improving immune function, might be expected to have the potential to reverse or retard the progression of disease. There is strong evidence to support this, both from uncontrolled case reports and from incidence studies of populations before and after the era of HAART. In 1988, Fiala et al first reported improvement in an AIDS patient with suspected PML following the administration of zidovudine (AZT).[54] In 1990, Conway et al reported a case of biopsy-proven PML in an AIDS patient with marked improvement following AZT administration.[55] Britton and colleagues reported that 7/26 patients stabilized or showed improvement on ART alone.[56] Not all investigators reported positive results in the pre-HAART era.[57] The ACTG 243 study, primarily designed to evaluate cytosine arabinoside (Ara-C) (see further ahead),

Table 57-2 Laboratories offering JCV PCR

Molecular Microbiology
Mayo Medical Laboratories
Mayo Clinic
200 First Street SW
Rochester, MN 55905
(Tel. 1-800-533-1710)

Diagnostic Virology Laboratory
University of Colorado Health Sciences Center
4200 East 9th Avenue
Room MS 1632
Denver, CO 80220
(Tel. 303-372-8182)

Virolab, Inc
1204 10th Street
Berkeley, CA 94710
(Tel. 510-524-6201)

Table 57-3 Prognostic Factors for PML

Favorable Factors	Unfavorable Factors
High CD4 count and low HIV RNA (serum and CSF)[39, 47, 118] PML patient naive to antiretrovirals[119] Presence of cytotoxic T-cell activity against JCV T and VP1 proteins[120–122]	High CSF viral load[123] HIV-positive patient on antiretrovirals.

encouraged the use of moderately high-dose (900 mg/day) AZT in combination with another antiretroviral, generally didanosine (ddI) or zalcitabine (ddC), in each of its three arms. There was no control arm against which to compare the effects of ART, but the mean survival in the three arms, ~3 months, suggests there was no significant improvement over historical survival figures.[37]

Several studies have now indicated improved survival in AIDS-associated PML patients treated with ART.[46,58–63] Dworkin, on review of 415 cases, found improved survival with ART in general, particularly when the regimen included a protease inhibitor. Beringuer reported a median survival of over 2 years in 118 PML patients treated with HAART, with neurological improvement in many. In 101 patients, Antoniri also found marked improvement in survival with HAART treatment.[64,65] Clifford, in a descriptive study of 57 HAART treated PML patients, found a median survival of greater than 46 weeks. Cinque, Miralles, De Luca, and Albrecht each reported series with considerable neurologic improvement and a more favorable outcome. Overall, these different studies reported improvement in mean survival varying from 46 weeks to 2.2 years. Thus while there remains a dearth of prospective controlled studies, the evidence is overwhelming that HAART is beneficial.

Therapeutic agents with specific anti-JC activity are listed in Table 57-4. Adenine arabinoside[66,67] and iododeoxyuridine[68] have been unsuccessful in altering the clinical course of PML. Isolated reports and small case studies suggested encouraging results with Ara-C, which has fairly powerful antiviral effects in cell culture studies.[69] These reports suggested some patients benefited from intravenous treatment, some from intrathecal, and some from combination, and they included both HIV-infected patients and those with other reasons for immune compromise.[56,70–75]

Not all investigators have reported positive effects from Ara-C.[76–78] To address the question, the Neurologic AIDS Research Consortium, in conjunction with the AIDS Clinical Trials Group, designed a three-arm study (ACTG 243) to compare the efficacy of high-dose ART alone to ART with either intravenous or intrathecal Ara-C (Table 57-5). The study was terminated in June 1993 after interim analysis demonstrated no benefit in either the intravenous or the intrathecal arm, and Ara-C, which has major bone marrow toxicity, cannot currently be recommended as therapy when delivered by intravenous or intraventricular injection.[37] It has recently been suggested that there may be a role for Ara-C in combination with HAART (D Clifford, personal communication), but this remains purely speculative.

On the theory that PML is the result of activated JCV-infected B lymphocytes gaining access to the brain, and because heparin sulfate in animal models prevents activated lymphocytes from crossing the blood–brain barrier,[79] Major et al reported initial encouraging results in an uncontrolled trial of low-dose heparin sulfate in HIV-infected patients with PML.[12,13] Subjects treated with 5000 units of subcutaneous heparin twice a day did appear to form fewer new lesions than a control group, but numbers were too small for statistical significance (S Houff, personal communication).

Alpha-Interferon

Based on its beneficial effect on the treatment of other papillomaviruses, including human papillomavirus associated genital warts and laryngeal papillomatosis,[80,81] and on its effect on SV40 suppression *in vitro*,[82] alpha-interferon has also been postulated as therapy for PML. There are reports of efficacy of alpha-interferon in nonAIDS PML.[83,84] The two reports in AIDS patients have not been encouraging. In an uncontrolled, open-label multicenter study, Berger et al treated 15 patients with biopsy-confirmed PML with up to 18 million units of

Table 57-4 Therapeutic Agents with Anti-JC Activity

- Cidofovir
- Cytarabin
- Topotecan (derivative of camptothecin)
- Immunotherapy (IFN alpha, IFN beta, IL-2)
- Phenothiazine derivatives, e.g, Chlorpromazine
- Serotonin receptor (5-HT2A) antagonist, e.g., Mirtazepine, Cyproheptadine

Table 57-5 Trials of OF PML Therapy

Study	Study Design	Result	Comment
Hall et al[37](ACTG 243)	Open label, three arms ARVs alone (AZT + ddl/ddC) ARVs + IV Ara-C ARVs + IT Ara-C	No efficacy	Only prospective, biopsy-confirmed study of PML to date
Marra et al[96] (ACTG 363)	Open label, cidofovir + HAART	No clear benefit	24 patients; 11 died from PML
Royal et al[110]	Open label, topotecan	No clear benefit	11 patients; 7 died from PML

AraC, cytosine arabinoside; ARVs, antiretrovirals; AZT, zidovudine; ddC, dideoxycytidine; ddl, didanosine; HAART, highly active antiretroviral therapy; IT, intrathecal; PML, progressive multifocal leukoencephalopathy.

alpha-interferon per day by subcutaneous injection.[85] Although two patients appeared to stabilize during treatment, there was reason to believe both had the protracted form of the disease described in 10% of AIDS patients, rather than response to the medication. Counihan et al treated four AIDS patients with pathologically confirmed PML with 5–10 million units of subcutaneous alpha-interferon per day for 4–12 weeks and noted no clinical response.[86] Recently, McArthur presented a retrospective analysis of the Johns Hopkins University experience with alpha-interferon in HIV infection.[87] Forty patients were treated with 3 million units per day. Although there was an initial impression that survival was improved, multivariate analysis demonstrated that the difference was entirely explained by the concomitant use of HAART.[88]

Beta-Interferon

Nath reported on one patient with multidrug-resistant HIV infection and a clinical course compatible with PML, but without tissue biopsy or positive CSF JC PCR and who was treated with beta-interferon 44 micrograms subcutaneously three times a week for 4 months. There was no evidence of a therapeutic effect.[89]

Cidofovir

Cidofovir is a nucleoside analog that is highly active *in vitro* against mouse and primate polyomaviruses, including SV40.[90] It also has demonstrable *in vivo* antiviral effect against papillomavirus-induced condylomata.[91] It has therapeutic effect in an animal model of cytomegalovirus encephalitis[92] and in cytomegalovirus retinitis in humans,[93,94] suggesting it crosses the blood–brain barrier. Although it has not been shown to have efficacy against JCV *in vitro*, and indeed showed cellular toxicity,[95] it was felt there was enough reason to evaluate its effects in PML.

There have been a number of reports on the use of cidofovir in PML with AIDS. The treatment regimens have been similar across studies. For example, in ACTG 363 cidofovir was given as 5 mg/kg intravenously, over 1 h.[96] Three doses of probenecid were given orally with each administration, 1.5 g given 3 h prior to infusion, 750 mg given 2 h postinfusion and again given 8 h postinfusion. The infusion was weekly for the first two doses, then every other week for a total of 13 doses. Most communications are case reports purporting success in one or two cases.[97–101] The concomitant antiretrovirals used in these studies have not been consistent, and both the degree of disability and the time between diagnosis and treatment have been varied. The lesson of Ara-C shows that case reports of improvement must be treated with a healthy degree of skepticism. To address this an open-label study to evaluate safety of cidofovir, ACTG 363 entered 24 subjects within 90 days of the onset of symptoms of PML.[96] Seventeen were receiving ART. Survival at 12 weeks was 54%. Twelve of the subjects died, 11 from progressive PML. Only 13 patients were able to continue to week 8 of the study. Two of these showed improvement of greater than 25%. This is not convincingly better than in historical controls. Two European studies showed slightly more promise. Gasnault reviewed the French Hospital Database on HIV, in patients with both proven and presumptive PML.[102] Twenty-two patients were treated with ART alone and 24 with ART and cidofovir. For the period between 4 and 12 months after PML diagnosis, the cidofovir-treated group had a significantly better survival rate. There was no difference in the neurological deficit, or in JC virus DNA clearance from the CSF. De Luca, in a multicenter observational study, reviewed 27 patients treated with ART alone and 16 with ART and cidofovir with a median follow-up of 132 weeks. Twenty-four percent of the HAART alone group and 57% of the ART with cidofovir group had improved after 2 months, and 87% of cidofovir-treated reached undetectable JC virus DNA in the CSF as compared to 42% of those who received ART alone. The 1-year cumulative probability of survival was 0.61 with cidofovir and 0.29 without (log-rank test, $P = 0.02$).[103,104] In an attempt to resolve the discrepancies between studies, De Luca conducted a meta-analysis of data from six cohorts including the three above, comprising in total of 372 HIV-infected patients diagnosed after 1995 and treated with ART with or without cidofovir. Estimated 1 year survival was 0.56 and when follow-up was started at the time of cidofovir, cidofovir was not associated with either improvement of survival or severity of disability.[105] Thus, the conclusion is that cidofovir does not show efficacy sufficient to merit its recommendation in HIV-associated PML.

Topoisomerase Inhibitors

JCV has tissue tropism for oligodendrocytes and to a lesser extent for astrocytes, but not for neurons. The primary determinant of this neurotropism is believed to be the glial-restricted expression of the viral early protein.[106,107] One step in this early DNA replication is dependent on the recruitment of the cellular enzyme topoisomerase 1. The enzyme binds to one of the DNA strands and causing a nick in the strand allows the helix to swivel, releasing topologic strain. The topoisomerase inhibitor camptothecin and its analogs have been shown to block SV40 and JCV replication *in vitro*,[108] and camptothecin and topotecan inhibit JCV DNA replication in glioma cells.[109] Controlled clinical studies have been designed using the camptothecin analogs topotecan and 9-amino-camptothecin. Topotecan has less protein binding than camptothecin, and reaches CSF levels which are 30% of those in blood. Royal et al have reported on the results of treatment of 11 patients.[110] Three appeared to respond to therapy. Hematological adverse events were common, and one patient died of accidental topotecan overdosage. In a smaller treatment trial of topotecan, Houff found a high degree of toxicity with no clear benefit (S Houff, personal communication). Further controlled study is clearly required before this toxic therapy can be recommended.

Interleukin-2

Przepiorka et al recently reported on a patient with low grade lymphoma without HIV infection who developed PML and responded to treatment with continuous infusion of interleukin-2 at 0.5 MU $m^{-2} day^{-1}$.[95,111] The improvement had persisted for over a year after therapy was terminated. There was complete resolution of symptoms, and a general improvement in immune parameters. The investigators suggested the improvement was due to upregulation of cytokines by interleukin-2. Buckanovich also described improvement in PML following interleukin-2 therapy, in an HIV-negative patient with refractory Hodgkin's disease.[112] While this observation may merit further study only two patients have been reported, without HIV infection, and this cannot be recommended as routine therapy.

Phenothiazine Derivatives

Pho et al have demonstrated that JC virus enters the cell via clathrin-dependent endocytosis.[113] They demonstrated the dose-dependent effect of chlorpromazine (*in vitro*) in inhibition of JCV spread through the tissue via the inhibition of clathrin-dependent endocytosis.[114] The low dose of chlorpromazine increases the spread of infection and high dose may increase the Parkinsonian side-effects. Atwood and colleagues have demonstrated that chlorpromazine inhibits the endocytic pathway used by JCV to infect glial cells *in vitro*, and that nontoxic doses of chlorpromazine are effective at inhibiting JCV multiplication and spread in a tissue culture model, raising the possibility that serotonin reuptake inhibitors could have a therapeutic role *in vivo*.[115]

Serotonin (5-Hydroxytryptamine; 5-HT) Receptor Blockade

JCV needs 5-HT2a receptors to infect human glial cells and medications that have antagonistic effects on 5-HT2a have a potential role in prophylaxis or treatment of PML.[116] O'Hara and Antwood have described the role of mirtazepine and cyprohepatadine as antagonists to 5-HT2a receptor, which might be worthy of study in therapy of JCV infection.[117]

RECOMMENDATIONS

PML remains one of the most devastating opportunistic infections in AIDS. It is important to rule out treatable infections of the brain, including toxoplasmosis, lymphoma, cytomegalovirus, syphilis, cryptococcosis, and other fungal infections. This will generally be possible by evaluating the clinical presentation in combination with CSF analysis and neuroradiologic evaluation. Confirmatory diagnosis of PML by brain biopsy is now rarely required, even in the setting of clinical trials. In the face of a negative PCR, the decision to proceed to brain biopsy must be individually based on the patient's clinical condition, the likelihood of missing a treatable condition, and the site of the lesion(s), with the concomitant danger of biopsy.

The first approach to treatment should be to maximize the patient's ability to resist progression by the use of HAART. There is no information on whether there is any advantage to any particular HAART regimen. The response to HAART plus the fact that up to 10% of patients will have a more protracted course, even without therapy, allows us to offer some hope. However, PML in this setting remains an incurable and generally progressive disease, there is no clear alternative or adjunctive therapy that has proven helpful, and more effective treatments are desperately needed.

REFERENCES

1. Astrom KE, Mancall EL, Richardson EP Jr. Progressive multifocal leuko-encephalopathy; a hitherto unrecognized complication of chronic lymphatic leukemia and Hodgkin's disease. Brain 81:93–111, 1958.
2. Lang W, Miklossy J, Deruaz GP, et al. Neuropathology of the acquired immune deficiency syndrome (AIDS): a report of 135 consecutive autopsy cases from Switzerland. Acta Neuropathol (Berl) 77:379–90, 1989.
3. Berger JR, et al. Progressive multifocal leukoencephalopathy associated with human immunodeficiency virus infection. A review of the literature with a report of sixteen cases. Ann Intern Med 107:78–87, 1987.
4. Petito CK, et al. Neuropathology of acquired immunodeficiency syndrome (AIDS): an autopsy review. J Neuropathol Exp Neurol 45:635–46, 1986.
5. Krupp LB, et al. Progressive multifocal leukoencephalopathy: clinical and radiographic features. Ann Neurol 17:344–9, 1985.
6. Levy RM, Bredesen DE, Rosenblum ML. Neurological manifestations of the acquired immunodeficiency syndrome (AIDS): experience at UCSF and review of the literature. J Neurosurg 62:475–95, 1985.
7. Li A. Symptomatology and Clinical Course in AIDS patient with Progressive Multifocal Leukoencephalopathy. In: XI International Conference on AIDS, Vancouver, 1996.
8. Whiteman ML, et al. Progressive multifocal leukoencephalopathy in 47 HIV-seropositive patients: neuroimaging with clinical and pathologic correlation. Radiology 187:233–40, 1993.
9. Berger JR, et al. Progressive multifocal leukoencephalopathy in HIV-1-infected children. AIDS 6:837–41, 1992.
10. Padgett BL, et al. Cultivation of papova-like virus from human brain with progressive multifocal leucoencephalopathy. Lancet 1:1257–60, 1971.
11. Walker DL, Padgett BL, The epidemiology of human polyoma viruses. In: Sever JL, Madden DL (eds). Polyomaviruses and Human Neurological Diseases, New York: Alan R Liss; 1983, p 99.
12. Major EO, Amemiya K, Tornatore CS, et al. Pathogenesis and molecular biology of progressive multifocal leukoencephalopathy, The JC virus induced demyelinating diseases of the human brain. Clinic Microbiol Rev 5: 49–73, 1992.
13. Collazos J, et al. Contrast-enhancing progressive multifocal leukoencephalopathy as an immune reconstitution event in AIDS patients. AIDS 13:1426–8, 1999.
14. Post MJ, et al. Progressive multifocal leukoencephalopathy in AIDS: are there any MR findings useful to patient management and predictive of patient survival? AIDS Clinical Trials Group, 243 Team. Am J Neuroradiol 20:1896–906, 1999.
15. Chang L, et al. Brain lesions in patients with AIDS: H-1 MR spectroscopy. Radiology 197:525–31, 1995.
16. Hall CD, et al. Cerebrospinal fluid analysis in human immunodeficiency virus infection. Ann Clin Lab Sci 22:139–43, 1992.
17. Walker DL. Progressive multifocal leukoencephalopathy: an opportunistic viral infection of the central nervous system. Ch16 pp 307-329 In: Vinken PJ & Bruyn GW (eds.) Handbook of Clinical Neurology.Volume 34. Elsevier North-Holland Biomedical Press 1978.

18. Kuchelmeister K, et al. Progressive multifocal leukoencephalopathy (PML) in AIDS: morphological and topographical characteristics. Verh Dtsch Ges Pathol 75: 189–90, 1991.
19. MacArthy RD, Nandi P, McMillen L, et al. CT guided brain biopsy findings in HIV infected persons: a retrospective review of 44 cases at Urban medical center. In: XI International Conference on AIDS, 1996.
20. Chappell ET, Guthrie BL, Orenstein J. The role of stereotactic biopsy in the management of HIV-related focal brain lesions. Neurosurgery 30:825–9, 1992.
21. Greenlee JE, Keeney PM. Immunoenzymatic labelling of JC papovavirus T antigen in brains of patients with progressive multifocal leukoencephalopathy. Acta Neuropathol (Berl) 71:150–3, 1986.
22. Aksamit AJ. Treatment of non-AIDS progressive multifocal leukoencephalopathy with cytosine arabinoside. J Neurovirol 7:386–90, 2001.
23. Hulette CM, Downey BT, Burger PC. Progressive multifocal leukoencephalopathy. Diagnosis by in situ hybridization with a biotinylated JC virus DNA probe using an automated Histomatic Code-On slide stainer. Am J Surg Pathol 15:791–7, 1991.
24. Elsner C, Dorries K. Evidence of human polyomavirus BK and JC infection in normal brain tissue. Virology 191:72–80, 1992.
25. Quinlivan EB, et al. Subclinical central nervous system infection with JC virus in patients with AIDS. J Infect Dis 166:80–5, 1992.
26. White FA, 3rd, et al. JC virus DNA is present in many human brain samples from patients without progressive multifocal leukoencephalopathy. J Virol 66:5726–34, 1992.
27. Agostini HT, Ryschkewitsch CF, Stoner GL, Genotype profile of human polyomavirus JC excreted in urine of immunocompetent individuals. J Clin Microbiol 34:159–64, 1996.
28. Martin JD, Padgett DL, Walker DL. Characterization of tissue culture-induced heterogeneity in DNAs of independent isolates of JC virus. J Gen Virol 64 (Pt 10):2271–80, 1983.
29. Seth P, Diaz F, Major EO. Advances in the biology of JC virus and induction of progressive multifocal leukoencephalopathy. J Neurovirol 9:236–46, 2003.
30. Tornatore C, et al. Detection of JC virus DNA in peripheral lymphocytes from patients with and without progressive multifocal leukoencephalopathy. Ann Neurol 31:454–62, 1992.
31. Dubois V, et al. JC virus genotypes in France: molecular epidemiology and potential significance for progressive multifocal leukoencephalopathy. J Infect Dis 183:213–17, 2001.
32. Weber T, et al. Progressive multifocal leukoencephalopathy diagnosed by amplification of JC virus-specific DNA from cerebrospinal fluid. AIDS 8:49–57, 1994.
33. Weber T, et al. Specific diagnosis of progressive multifocal leukoencephalopathy by polymerase chain reaction. J Infect Dis 169:1138–41, 1994.
34. de Luca A, et al. Improved detection of JC virus DNA in cerebrospinal fluid for diagnosis of AIDS-related progressive multifocal leukoencephalopathy. J Clin Microbiol 34:1343–6, 1996.
35. McGuire D, et al. JC virus DNA in cerebrospinal fluid of human immunodeficiency virus-infected patients: predictive value for progressive multifocal leukoencephalopathy. Ann Neurol 37:395–9, 1995.
36. Giudici B, et al. Highly active antiretroviral therapy and progressive multifocal leukoencephalopathy: effects on cerebrospinal fluid markers of JC virus replication and immune response. Clin Infect Dis 30:95–9, 2000.
37. Hall CD, et al. Failure of cytarabine in progressive multifocal leukoencephalopathy associated with human immunodeficiency virus infection. AIDS Clinical Trials Group 243 Team. N Engl J Med 338:1345–51, 1998.
38. Gasnault J, et al. Prolonged survival without neurological improvement in patients with AIDS-related progressive multifocal leukoencephalopathy on potent combined antiretroviral therapy. J Neurovirol 5:421–9, 1999.
39. Yiannoutsos CT, et al. Relation of JC virus DNA in the cerebrospinal fluid to survival in acquired immunodeficiency syndrome patients with biopsy-proven progressive multifocal leukoencephalopathy. Ann Neurol 45:816–21, 1999.
40. Karahalios D, et al. Progressive multifocal leukoencephalopathy in patients with HIV infection: lack of impact of early diagnosis by stereotactic brain biopsy. J Acquir Immune Defic Syndr 5:1030–8, 1992.
41. Wiley CA, et al. Human immunodeficiency virus (HIV) and JC virus in acquired immune deficiency syndrome (AIDS) patients with progressive multifocal leukoencephalopathy. Acta Neuropathol (Berl) 76:338–46, 1988.
42. Berger JR, Mucke L. Prolonged survival and partial recovery in AIDS-associated progressive multifocal leukoencephalopathy. Neurology 38:1060–5, 1988.
43. Berger JR, et al. Progressive multifocal leukoencephalopathy in patients with HIV infection. J Neurovirol 4:59–68, 1998.
44. Price RW, Yiannoutses DB, Clifford DB, et al. Neurological outcomes in late HIV infection: adverse impact of neurological impairment on survival and protective effect of antiviral therapy. AIDS Clinical Trial Group and Neurological AIDS Research Consortium study team. AIDS 13:1677–85, 1999.
45. Tashima K, F.D, Elliot NC, et al. Resolution of AIDS-related opportunistic infections with addiction of protease inhibitor treatment. In: 4th Conference on Retroviruses and Opportunistic Infections. 1997, Washington, DC. Alexandria, VA: Westover Management Group.
46. Tassie JM, et al. Survival improvement of AIDS-related progressive multifocal leukoencephalopathy in the era of protease inhibitors. Clinical Epidemiology Group. French Hospital Database on HIV. AIDS 13:1881–7, 1999.
47. De Luca A, Giancola ML, Ammassari A, et al. The effect of potent antiretroviral therapy and JC virus load in cerebrospinal fluid on clinical outcome of patients with AIDS-associated progressive multifocal leukoencephalopathy. J Infect Dis 182:1077–83, 2000.
48. Bethany E, A.C, Flaningan TP, et al. Prolonged remission of AIDS-associated progressive multifocal leukoencephalopathy with combined antiretroviral therapy. In: XI International Conference on AIDS, Vancouver, 1996.
49. Safdar A, et al. Fatal immune restoration disease in human immunodeficiency virus type 1-infected patients with progressive multifocal leukoencephalopathy: impact of antiretroviral therapy-associated immune reconstitution. Clin Infect Dis 35:1250–7, 2002.
50. Miralles P, et al. Inflammatory reactions in progressive multifocal leukoencephalopathy after highly active antiretroviral therapy. AIDS 15:1900–2, 2001.
51. Hoffmann C, et al. Progressive multifocal leucoencephalopathy with unusual inflammatory response during antiretroviral treatment. J Neurol Neurosurg Psychiatry 74:1142–4, 2003.
52. Kleinschmidt-DeMasters BK, Tyler KL. Progressive multifocal leukoencephalopathy complicating treatment with natalizumab and interferon beta-1a for multiple sclerosis. N Engl J Med 353:369–74, 2005.
53. Van Assche G, et al. Progressive multifocal leukoencephalopathy after natalizumab therapy for Crohn's disease. N Engl J Med 353:362–8, 2005.
54. Fiala M, et al. Responses of neurological complications of AIDS to 3′-azido-3′-deoxythymidine and 9-(1,3-dihydroxy-2-propoxymethyl) guanine. I. Clinical features. Rev Infect Dis 10:250–6, 1988.
55. Conway B, Halliday WC, Brunham RC. Human immunodeficiency virus-associated progressive multifocal leukoencephalopathy: apparent response to 3′-azido-3′-deoxythymidine. Rev Infect Dis 12:479–82, 1988.

56. Britton CB, Miller JR, Sisti M, et al. Analysis of outcome and response to intrathecal Ara-C in 26 patients. In: Neuroscience of HIV Infection: Basic and Clinical Frontiers, Amsterdam, 1992.
57. Garrote FJ, et al. The inefficacy of zidovudine (AZT) in progressive multifocal leukoencephalopathy (PML) associated with the acquired immunodeficiency syndrome (AIDS). Rev Clin Esp 187:404–7, 1990.
58. Miralles P, et al. Treatment of AIDS-associated progressive multifocal leukoencephalopathy with highly active antiretroviral therapy. AIDS 12:2467–72, 1998.
59. Albrecht H, et al. Highly active antiretroviral therapy significantly improves the prognosis of patients with HIV-associated progressive multifocal leukoencephalopathy. AIDS 12:1149–54, 1998.
60. Berenguer J, et al. Clinical course and prognostic factors of progressive multifocal leukoencephalopathy in patients treated with highly active antiretroviral therapy. Clin Infect Dis 36:1047–52, 2003.
61. Dworkin MS, et al. Progressive multifocal leukoencephalopathy: improved survival of human immunodeficiency virus-infected patients in the protease inhibitor era. J Infect Dis 180:621–5, 1999.
62. Clifford DB, et al. HAART improves prognosis in HIV-associated progressive multifocal leukoencephalopathy. Neurology 52:623–5, 1999.
63. Cinque P, Casari S, Bertelli D. Progressive multifocal leukoencephalopathy, HIV, and highly active antiretroviral therapy. N Engl J Med 339:848–9, 1998.
64. Antinori A, et al. Clinical epidemiology and survival of progressive multifocal leukoencephalopathy in the era of highly active antiretroviral therapy: data from the Italian Registry Investigative Neuro AIDS (IRINA). J Neurovirol 9(Suppl 1):47–53, 2003.
65. Antinori A, et al. Epidemiology and prognosis of AIDS-associated progressive multifocal leukoencephalopathy in the HAART era. J Neurovirol 7:323–8, 2001.
66. Wolinsky JS, et al. Progressive multifocal leukoencephalopathy: clinical pathological correlates and failure of a drug trial in two patients. Trans Am Neurol Assoc 101:81–2, 1976.
67. Rand KH, et al. Adenine arabinoside in the treatment of progressive multifocal leukoencephalopathy: use of virus-containing cells in the urine to assess response to therapy. Ann Neurol 1:458–62, 1977.
68. Tarsy D, et al. 5-Iodo-2′-deoxyuridine (IUDR; NSC-39661) given intraventricularly in the treatment of progressive multifocal leukoencephalopathy. Cancer Chemother Rep 57:73–8, 1973.
69. Zaky DA, et al. Varicella-zoster virus and subcutaneous cytarabine: correlation of in vitro sensitivities to blood levels. Antimicrob Agents Chemother 7:229–32, 1975.
70. Bauer WR, Turel AP Jr, Johnson KP. Progressive multifocal leukoencephalopathy and cytarabine. Remission with treatment. JAMA 226:174–6, 1973.
71. Portegies P, et al. Response to cytarabine in progressive multifocal leucoencephalopathy in AIDS. Lancet 337:680–1, 1991.
72. O'Riordan T, et al. Progressive multifocal leukoencephalopathy – remission with cytarabine. J Infect 20:51–4, 1990.
73. Nicoli F, et al. Efficacy of cytarabine in progressive multifocal leucoencephalopathy in AIDS. Lancet 339:306, 1992.
74. Lidman C, et al. Progressive multifocal leukoencephalopathy in AIDS. AIDS 5:1039–41, 1991.
75. Marriott PJ, et al. Progressive multifocal leucoencephalopathy: remission with cytarabine. J Neurol Neurosurg Psychiatry 38:205–9, 1975.
76. Urtizberea JA, Flament-Saillour M, Clair B, et al. Cytarabine for progressive multifocal leukoencephathy in AIDS patients. In: International Conference AIDS. 1993.
77. Antinori A, et al. Failure of cytarabine and increased JC virus-DNA burden in the cerebrospinal fluid of patients with AIDS-related progressive multifocal leucoencephalopathy. AIDS 8:1022–4, 1994.
78. Horn GV, Bastian FO, Moake JL. Progressive multifocal leukoencephalopathy: failure of response to transfer factor and cytarabine. Neurology 28:794–7, 1978.
79. Houff SA, et al. Involvement of JC virus-infected mononuclear cells from the bone marrow and spleen in the pathogenesis of progressive multifocal leukoencephalopathy. N Engl J Med 318:301–5, 1988.
80. Howley PM, Schlegel R. The human papillomaviruses. An overview. Am J Med 85:155–8, 1988.
81. Finter NB, et al. The use of interferon-alpha in virus infections. Drugs 42:749–65, 1991.
82. Yamamoto K, Yamaguchi N, Oda K. Mechanism of interferon-induced inhibition of early simian virus 40(SV40) functions. Virology 68:58–70, 1975.
83. Colosimo C, et al. Alpha-interferon therapy in a case of probable progressive multifocal leukoencephalopathy. Acta Neurol Belg 92:24–9, 1992.
84. Steiger MJ, et al. Successful outcome of progressive multifocal leukoencephalopathy with cytarabine and interferon. Ann Neurol 33:407–11, 1993.
85. Berger JR, Pall L, McArthur J, et al. A pilot study of recombinant alpha 2a interferon in the treatement of AIDS-related PML. Neurology 42 (Supp 3):257, 1992.
86. Counihan T, Venna N, Craven D. Alpha interferon in AIDS-related progressive multifocal leukoencephalopathy. J Neuro-AIDS 1:79, 1996.
87. Huang SS, et al. Survival prolongation in HIV-associated progressive multifocal leukoencephalopathy treated with alpha-interferon: an observational study. J Neurovirol 4:324–32, 1998.
88. Geschwind MD, Skolosky RI, Royal WS, McArthur JC. The relative contributions of HAART and alpha-interferon for therapy of progressive multifocal leukoencephalopathy in AIDS. J Neurovirol 7:353–7, 2001.
89. Nath A, Venkataramana DS, Reich D, Major E. Progression of PML despite treatment with beta-interferon in a patient with HIV infection. J Neurovirol 11(Suppl 2):112, 2005.
90. Andrei G, et al. Activities of various compounds against murine and primate polyomaviruses. Antimicrob Agents Chemother 41:587–93, 1997.
91. Snoeck R, et al. Treatment of anogenital papillomavirus infections with an acyclic nucleoside phosphonate analogue. N Engl J Med 333:943–4, 1995.
92. Neyts J, et al. Efficacy of (S)-1-(3-hydroxy-2-phosphonylmethoxypropyl)-cytosine and 9-(1,3-dihydroxy-2-propoxymethyl)-guanine in the treatment of intracerebral murine cytomegalovirus infections in immunocompetent and immunodeficient mice. Eur J Clin Microbiol Infect Dis 12:269–79, 1993.
93. Lalezari J, Kemper C, Stagg R, et al. A randomized controlled study of the safety and efficacy of intravenous cidofovir (CDV, HPMPC) for the treatment of relapsing CMV retinitis in patients with AIDS. In: XI International Conference on AIDS, Vancouver, 1996.
94. Polis MA, et al. Anticytomegaloviral activity and safety of cidofovir in patients with human immunodeficiency virus infection and cytomegalovirus viruria. Antimicrob Agents Chemother 39:882–6, 1995.
95. Hou J, Major EO. The efficacy of nucleoside analogs against JC virus multiplication in a persistently infected human fetal brain cell line. J Neurovirol 4:451–6, 1998.
96. Marra CM, et al. A pilot study of cidofovir for progressive multifocal leukoencephalopathy in AIDS. AIDS 16:1791–7, 2002.
97. Dodge RT. A case study: the use of cidofovir for the management of progressive multifocal leukoencephalopathy. J Assoc Nurses AIDS Care 10:70–4, 1999.

98. Happe S, et al. Cidofovir (vistide) in therapy of progressive multifocal leukoencephalopathy in AIDS. Review of the literature and report of 2 cases. Nervenarzt 70:935–43, 1999.
99. Cardenas RL, Cheng KH, Sack K. The effects of cidofovir on progressive multifocal leukoencephalopathy: an MRI case study. Neuroradiology 43:379–82, 2001.
100. Roberts MT, Carmichael A, Lever AM. Prolonged survival in AIDS-related progressive multifocal leucoencephalopathy following anti-retroviral therapy and cidofovir. Int J Antimicrob Agents 21:347–9, 2003.
101. Zimmermann T, et al. Successful treatment of AIDS-related PML with HAART and cidofovir. Eur J Med Res 6:190–62, 2001.
102. Gasnault J, et al. Cidofovir in AIDS-associated progressive multifocal leukoencephalopathy: a monocenter observational study with clinical and JC virus load monitoring. J Neurovirol 7:375–81, 2001.
103. De Luca A, et al. Cidofovir added to HAART improves virological and clinical outcome in AIDS-associated progressive multifocal leukoencephalopathy. AIDS 14:F117–21, 2000.
104. De Luca A, et al. Potent anti-retroviral therapy with or without cidofovir for AIDS-associated progressive multifocal leukoencephalopathy: extended follow-up of an observational study. J Neurovirol 7:364–8, 2001.
105. De Luca A, Gasnaut J, Cinque P, et al. Survival and neurological outcome with or without cidofovir in AIDS-related progressive multifocal leukoencephalopathy on HAART: a multicohort analysis. J Neurovirol 11(Suppl 2):77–78, 2005.
106. Small JA, et al. The early region of human papovavirus JC induces dysmyelination in transgenic mice. Cell 46:13–8, 1986.
107. Raj GV, Khalili K. Transcriptional regulation: lessons from the human neurotropic polyomavirus, JCV. Virology 213:283–91, 1995.
108. Tsao YP, et al. Interaction between replication forks and topoisomerase I-DNA cleavable complexes: studies in a cell-free SV40 DNA replication system. Cancer Res 53:5908–14, 1993.
109. Kerr DA, et al. Inhibition of human neurotropic virus (JCV) DNA replication in glial cells by camptothecin. Virology 196:612–18, 1993.
110. Royal W 3rd, et al. Topotecan in the treatment of acquired immunodeficiency syndrome-related progressive multifocal leukoencephalopathy. J Neurovirol 9:411–19, 2003.
111. Przepiorka D, et al. Successful treatment of progressive multifocal leukoencephalopathy with low-dose interleukin-2. Bone Marrow Transplant 20:983–7, 1997.
112. Buckanovich RJ, et al. Nonmyeloablative allogeneic stem cell transplantation for refractory Hodgkin's lymphoma complicated by interleukin-2 responsive progressive multifocal leukoencephalopathy. Ann Hematol 81:410–13, 2002.
113. Pho MT, Ashok A, Atwood WJ. JC virus enters human glial cells by clathrin-dependent receptor-mediated endocytosis. J Virol 74:2288–92, 2000.
114. Baum S, et al. Early events in the life cycle of JC virus as potential therapeutic targets for the treatment of progressive multifocal leukoencephalopathy. J Neurovirol 9(Suppl 1):32–7, 2003.
115. Atwood WJ. A combination of low-dose chlorpromazine and neutralizing antibodies inhibits the spread of JC virus (JCV) in a tissue culture model: implications for prophylactic and therapeutic treatment of progressive multifocal leukencephalopathy. J Neurovirol 7:307–10, 2001.
116. Roth BL. Regulation of serotonin receptor expression: relevance for the pharmacotheray of PML. J Neurovirol 11(Suppl 2):79, 2005.
117. O'Hara BAW. Misrtazepine and cyprohepatadine block JCV infection by antagonizing 5HT2A receptors. J Neurovirol 11(Suppl 2):113, 2005.
118. Garcia De Viedma D, et al. JC virus load in progressive multifocal leukoencephalopathy: analysis of the correlation between the viral burden in cerebrospinal fluid, patient survival, and the volume of neurological lesions. Clin Infect Dis 34:1568–75, 2002.
119. Wyen C, et al. Progressive multifocal leukencephalopathy in patients on highly active antiretroviral therapy: survival and risk factors of death. J Acquir Immune Defic Syndr 37:1263–8, 2004.
120. Koralnik IJ, et al. Association of prolonged survival in HLA-A2+ progressive multifocal leukoencephalopathy patients with a CTL response specific for a commonly recognized JC virus epitope. J Immunol 168:499–504, 2002.
121. Weber T, et al. Immune response in progressive multifocal leukoencephalopathy: an overview. J Neurovirol 7:311–17, 2001.
122. Du Pasquier RA, et al. JCV-specific cellular immune response correlates with a favorable clinical outcome in HIV-infected individuals with progressive multifocal leukoencephalopathy. J Neurovirol 7:318–22, 2001.
123. Bossolasco S, et al. Prognostic significance of JC virus DNA levels in cerebrospinal fluid of patients with HIV-associated progressive multifocal leukoencephalopathy. Clin Infect Dis 40:738–44, 2005.

Chapter 58

Sexually Transmitted Infections

Lara B. Strick, MD MSc, Christina M. Marra, MD, Connie L. Celum, MD, MPH

INTRODUCTION

The importance of the bidirectional relationship between human immunodeficiency virus (HIV)-1 and other sexually transmitted infections (STIs) has become better understood over the past 15 years since the notion of 'epidemiologic synergy' between STIs and HIV-1 was first proposed.[1,2] Ulcerative and nonulcerative STIs increase the risk of HIV-1 acquisition and transmission and may impact the natural history of HIV-1 infection. Similarly, HIV-1 influences the risk of acquisition, natural history, clinical presentation, and the management of STIs in HIV-infected persons. The multiple and complex epidemiologic and clinical interrelationships between HIV-1 and STIs suggests that effective STI control may be important for HIV-1 prevention.

HIV/STI CO-INFECTION

Diagnosis of HIV in the Setting of STIs

Given the overlap in risks associated with HIV and STIs, diagnosis of an STI should prompt testing for HIV-1, and be used as an opportunity for risk reduction counseling. A particularly severe or atypical presentation of an STI can be a diagnostic clue to HIV-1 infection; neurosyphilis, persistent deep herpetic ulcerations, severe genital warts, and perhaps severe pelvic inflammatory disease (PID) or tuboovarian abscess should increase the clinical suspicion for co-infection with HIV-1. However, most clinical presentations of STIs in HIV-infected persons are no different than among immunocompetent persons and thus typical symptoms and manifestations of STIs should not deter HIV-1 testing. The prevalence and incidence of HIV-1 tends to be higher among sexually transmitted disease (STD) clinic attendees compared to the general population.[3–5] In the US, the overall prevalence of HIV-1 in some urban STD clinic settings has been 1–2%, but is even higher in persons with additional HIV risk factors such as injection drug use or men who have sex with men (MSM).[4,6–9] Consequently, STD clinics play a key role in the identification of HIV-infected persons and more than a quarter of publicly funded HIV counseling and testing occurs in STD clinics in the US.[6] Once HIV is diagnosed, many STD clinics refer patients to HIV specialty clinics, but some STD clinics have begun to provide ongoing HIV care.

STIs and Primary HIV Prevention

Numerous epidemiologic studies have shown that STIs, particularly ulcerative STIs, are associated with increased risk for HIV-1 acquisition.[1,2,10–18] Identification and treatment of STIs is considered by most to be an important strategy for the primary prevention of HIV-1. In the community-level randomized trial conducted in Mwanza, Tanzania, improved STI diagnosis and syndromic management reduced HIV-1 incidence by 42% (risk ratio (RR) 0.58; 95% confidence interval (CI), 0.42–0.79; $P = 0.007$).[19] However, two other community-based randomized trials conducted in Rakai and Masaka, Uganda, found that mass treatment for STIs and improved STI management with community education, respectively, did not result in reduced HIV-1 incidence, despite reduced STI rates in the intervention arms.[20–22] The contradictory results between these community STI trials may in part be due to differences in the interventions tested as well as the stage of the HIV-1 epidemic with Uganda having a more mature HIV-1 epidemic with higher HIV-1 prevalence (16% and 10% in Rakai and Masaka, respectively), fewer numbers of sexual partners, and lower prevalence of curable STIs compared to Mwanza.[1,23–27] Symptomatic STIs may have a more substantial impact on HIV-1 dynamics; in Rakai, symptomatic genital ulcer disease (GUD) (adjusted RR 3.14; 95% CI, 1.98–4.98) and genital discharge or dysuria in men (RR 2.44; 95% CI, 1.17–5.12) were associated with HIV-1 acquisition. However, the majority of incident HIV-1 cases occurred in persons who did not report symptoms and the majority of persons who reported symptoms did not have a curable STI.[11] Monthly antibiotic prophylaxis with azithromycin given to female sex workers (FSW) in a randomized trial conducted in Nairobi, Kenya reduced the incidence of STI, but not the incidence of HIV-1 infection.[28]

In these community-based trials, only curable bacterial STIs were treated and no targeted herpes simplex virus type-2 (HSV-2) interventions were included, even though HSV-2 prevalence was very high in the general population (e.g., 43–47% in women and 13–21% in men) in Mwanza, Rakai, and Masaka[26] and 70% in HIV-uninfected FSW in Nairobi.[28] In summary, treatment of curable STIs may have played a role in HIV prevention in earlier HIV-1 epidemics, and remains an important priority to reduce adverse reproductive sequelae and burden of STI-associated disease. Recently HSV-2 interventions have become a major focus for HIV-1 prevention.[29,30]

Diagnosis of STIs in the Setting of HIV

HIV-infected persons should be tested for STIs even in the absence of symptoms, since HIV-1 is associated with high STI prevalence rates in many populations.[31–37] Since STIs frequently are asymptomatic, the Centers for Disease Control and Prevention (CDC) recommends screening all HIV-infected persons for STIs at regular intervals and offering treatment based on syndromic diagnoses and laboratory testing.[37,38] Detection of an incident STI (e.g., early syphilis or gonorrhea) in a person with known HIV infection may be an indicator of recent high-risk sexual behavior[34,39,40] which should prompt risk reduction counseling and, if appropriate and available, additional prevention interventions.

The high incidence of new STI among known HIV-infected persons is concerning.[39–44] For example, among 316 HIV-infected women in the US with CD4+ T-lymphocyte cell counts of 300 cells/mm^3, 25% were diagnosed with an STI during a median follow-up of 2 years.[41] More concerning are data from the Hlabisa district of KwaZulu Natal, South Africa where the prevalence of HIV-1 is 22%, it is estimated that of the 24.9% of women infected with an active STI, 48% are asymptomatic, 50% are symptomatic but do not seek care, and only 1.7% are both symptomatic and seek treatment,[45] which highlights why STIs are difficult to control, even in HIV-infected persons.

STIs and Secondary HIV Prevention

The role of STIs in the transmission of HIV-1 has been a public health focus for secondary HIV-1 prevention efforts.[40,46,47] Few studies have been conducted to assess predictors of HIV-1 transmission, including STIs, due to logistics of longitudinal HIV-discordant couple studies. The best data come from analysis of monogamous HIV-discordant couples from the Rakai STI trial, which indicated that serum HIV-1 level was the strongest predictor of sexual HIV-1 transmission and that genital ulcers, primarily due to HSV-2, were associated with increased risk of HIV-1 transmission.[48] STIs are often associated with increased genital shedding of HIV-1[49–59] which may correlate with increased HIV-1 infectiousness, although this has not been directly studied. Following appropriate antimicrobial treatment of the specific STI, HIV-1 RNA levels in genital secretions are reduced.[49,58,60–64] The effect of STIs on HIV-1 transmission risk is likely greater from males to females.[1,15,65] The CDC and the World Health Organization (WHO) promote STI control in persons with known HIV infection as an important component of secondary HIV prevention programs to decrease HIV transmission,[38,66] however, successful implementation of STI control efforts have been variable.

GENITAL ULCER DISEASE

Since early in the HIV-1 epidemic, GUD due to syphilis, chancroid, or herpes simplex virus (HSV) and much less commonly due to lymphogranuloma venereum (LGV) and granuloma inguinale, was recognized as a factor for sexual acquisition and transmission of HIV-1 and is thought to have fueled the rapid spread of HIV-1 in sub-Saharan Africa.[2,12,65,67,68] Epidemiologic studies have indicated that GUD increases HIV-1 acquisition by two- to sevenfold.[11,13–17,69–71] Among the ulcerative STIs, HSV-2 appears to have the strongest and most consistent link to HIV-1 acquisition across continents and populations.[10,18] Ulcerative STIs can provide a portal of entry for HIV by disrupting the normal mucosal barrier and cause local inflammation with increased presence of HIV-1 target cells at the site of infection.[68,72]

Observational studies also have found that GUD increases the likelihood of HIV-1 transmission,[73,74] although fewer studies have been conducted to assess predictors of HIV-1 infectiousness. GUD increased the probability of HIV-1 transmission fourfold on a per-contact basis among monogamous HIV-1 discordant heterosexual couples from Rakai, Uganda, after controlling for serum HIV-1 RNA in the index partner.[73] HIV-1 has been detected by culture and PCR in genital ulcerations and sometimes in higher levels than in blood.[52,53,58,75,76] In a study of women in the Ivory Coast, successful treatment of GUD reduced the amount of genital HIV-1 detected after 1 week to levels similar to women who did not have GUD.[53] A high level of HIV-1 RNA in the genital tract is thought to increase the likelihood of HIV-1 transmission, although the threshold for transmission and correlation of genital HIV-1 levels with risk for HIV-1 transmission has not been determined, whereas serum HIV-1 levels have been shown to be a strong predictor of sexual HIV-1 transmission.[48]

Clinical diagnosis to determine the specific etiology of GUD is often inaccurate even by experienced STI clinicians,[77–80] and some patients with genital ulcers may have more than one infection.[79–81] In addition, some genital ulcers are caused by trauma or other non-STI etiologies, such as Behçet's. When possible, the evaluation of all patients with GUD should include syphilis serology, darkfield microscopy, HSV culture, PCR or serology, and culture for *Haemophilus ducreyi*. However, even after diagnostic testing, at least 25% of persons with GUD lack a laboratory-confirmed etiology[79,81] and management should be based on clinical presentation and local epidemiology. In Africa, an increasing proportion of genital ulcers are due to HSV-2 rather than bacterial causes,[82,83] resulting in frequent failure of syndromic management of GUD, which usually does not include antiviral therapy.[84] The ideal management of GUD in resource-poor countries needs to be re-evaluated, especially in settings with high HIV-1 prevalence, given that HSV-2 is the most common cause of GUD.[85]

Syphilis – *Treponema pallidum*

Epidemiology of Syphilis

The recent steep rise in the rates of early syphilis in the United States and Europe is a growing public health concern. With effective treatment available, the implementation of public health measures and the response to acquired immunodeficiency syndrome (AIDS), the rates of early syphilis reached a nadir in 2000 in the US, with most cases occurring in African-Americans living in the Southeast.[86,87] Despite efforts to eliminate the disease, syphilis rates in the US and Europe have recently increased, particularly among MSM. Outbreaks of syphilis among MSM have occurred in many major US cities, including Los Angeles, Chicago, New York, Boston, Miami, Seattle, and San Francisco,[33,88–94] cities in Europe[95–98] and Australia.[99] The increased rates of syphilis among MSM are consistent with reports of increased high-risk sexual behavior[33,87,100] perhaps due to waning fear of HIV, better health with the advent of effective antiretroviral therapy[101] and growing apathy toward safe sex messages.[102]

A substantial proportion of early syphilis is associated with HIV infection.[103–106] In 2002, it was estimated that 25% of primary and secondary syphilis cases in the US occurred in persons infected with HIV-1.[104] The overlap of the HIV-1 and syphilis epidemics is particularly marked among MSM.[97,104,105,107] In Seattle, Los Angeles, and San Francisco, over 50% of MSM diagnosed with early syphilis were co-infected with HIV-1[88,91,108] and the odds of HIV-1 infection were from 3.9- to 8.5-fold higher in men with syphilis compared to those without syphilis.[103,105,107] Therefore, all persons presenting with syphilis should be offered HIV-1 testing and persons diagnosed with HIV-1 should be screened for syphilis.

Interaction between Syphilis and HIV-1

Laboratory research supports an association between syphilis and HIV-1 acquisition and transmission.[109,110] Epidemiologic studies also lend further support for the role of syphilis in HIV-1 acquisition. Among STD clinic attendees in Miami in the early 1990s, patients with primary or secondary syphilis acquired HIV-1 at a rate almost sixfold higher (12.8 vs 2.3 cases per 100 person-years) than patients who never had syphilis and 18% of all HIV-1 seroconversions were attributable to newly acquired syphilis.[3] In the past decade, less epidemiologic data have been published that support a relationship between syphilis and HIV-1 acquisition and transmission.

Effect of Syphilis on HIV-1

Syphilis activates the cellular immune system[109,111–113] and *in vitro* has been demonstrated to increase replication of HIV-1.[110] One study of 41 co-infected persons found that the treatment of syphilis was associated with an increase in CD4+ T-lymphocyte cells (mean 66 cell/mm^3; $P = 0.02$) and a decrease in HIV-1 RNA (mean -0.261 RNA $\log_{10}$ copies/mL; $P = 0.04$) compared to pretreatment levels.[114] Another study found that plasma HIV-1 RNA levels were higher during primary or secondary syphilis compared with presyphilis levels by a mean of 0.22 RNA $\log_{10}$ copies/mL ($P = 0.02$).[115] However, a retrospective study comparing persons with early syphilis to persons presyphilis and postsyphilis treatment, and controls with nonsystemic STIs (e.g., gonorrhea and chlamydia) found that early syphilis had little effect on plasma HIV-1 RNA levels.[116] Treatment of syphilis did not reduce the plasma HIV viral load and had a modest or no effect on CD4+ T-lymphocyte cell counts.[115,116] Therefore, it is still debatable whether syphilis has a significant clinical impact on the course of HIV-1 infection.

Clinical Presentation and Natural History of Syphilis in HIV-Infected Persons

Data are conflicting about whether HIV-1 infection affects the clinical manifestation of syphilis. There have been several case reports of aggressive or atypical syphilis in HIV-infected persons,[117–122] but larger controlled trials have observed only minor or no significant differences in the clinical manifestations of early syphilis between HIV-1-infected and HIV-1-uninfected persons.[123–125] In a prospective, randomized, multicenter study of early syphilis in the US, the median number of ulcers and percentage of persons with multiple ulcers having primary syphilis was greater among the 53 HIV-infected persons. However, no other differences in clinical manifestations were noted in comparison to the 200 HIV-negative controls.[125] A study of 677 men from Malawi showed that HIV-infected persons had impaired healing of genital ulcers ($P = 0.003$), of which 29% were due to syphilis.[126]

Several studies suggested more rapid progression of syphilis in HIV-infected persons since they more often have secondary syphilis at the time of presentation and occasionally have concomitant manifestations of primary and secondary syphilis.[127–131] In a case-control study, 53% of patients with HIV-1 presented with secondary syphilis compared to 33% of patients without HIV-1 infection ($P = 0.01$).[128] In the US prospective study referenced above, 25% of HIV-infected persons with secondary syphilis presented with concomitant chancres compared with only 14% of HIV-uninfected persons.[125] It was not possible to determine whether the HIV-infected persons truly progressed more rapidly to secondary stage, had delayed healing of primary chancres, or sought healthcare earlier. In contrast to these results, Gourevitch and co-workers did not find that the stage of syphilis at the time of presentation was associated with HIV status.[123]

Diagnosis of Syphilis in HIV-Infected Persons

Most experts believe that syphilis serologies are accurate and reliable in the vast majority of HIV-infected individuals and can be used for the diagnosis of syphilis and for monitoring the response to treatment in the usual manner.[66,125,132–135] Nonetheless, occasionally HIV-infected persons can have atypical syphilis serologic results, with higher titers or more biologic false-positives.[123,136–140] The higher rate of biologic false-positive rapid plasma reagin (RPR) may be due to injection drug use, rather than HIV infection itself.[133,138] Infrequently, lower titers, delayed seroreactivity, and false-negatives have been reported in primary, and less commonly, in secondary syphilis.[141–144] When syphilis serology and clinical presentation do not correspond, other diagnostic tests for syphilis should be used, such as direct microscopy with dark-field examination or fluorescent antibody staining of exudate, or in difficult diagnostic cases, biopsy.[66,143]

Neurosyphilis

T. pallidum invades the central nervous system early in the course of disease, but only persists in a subset of persons who are at higher risk for developing neurosyphilis. Unfortunately, it is impossible to predict which patients are at greater risk for persistence. Some studies suggest that HIV-infected persons have higher likelihood of neurosyphilis, including symptomatic and asymptomatic meningitis, ocular disease, and meningovasculitis.[145–148] In the absence of neurologic symptoms, 9–58% of HIV-infected persons with serologic evidence of syphilis have neurologic involvement.[128,149–151] In a recent study of 326 persons with early and late syphilis, 72% of whom were HIV-infected, those with serum RPR titers of $\geqslant$1:32 and CD4+ T-lymphocyte cell counts of $\leqslant$350 cells/mm^3 were more likely to have laboratory-defined neurosyphilis.[152]

At any syphilis stage, if neurologic symptoms are present, persons should be treated for neurosyphilis. Examination of the CSF prior to treatment of neurosyphilis establishes a baseline for later evaluation of the CSF to determine response to treatment (Fig. 58-1). Some experts recommend CSF examination before treatment of HIV-infected persons with early syphilis regardless of neurologic signs or symptoms, because HIV-infected patients with early syphilis may be at higher risk for developing neurosyphilis after appropriate treatment.[129–131,159–164] If CSF results are abnormal then treatment for neurosyphilis should be initiated (Fig. 58-1 and Table 58-1). Most experts agree that all HIV-infected persons with late latent syphilis, tertiary syphilis, or syphilis of unknown duration should undergo a lumbar puncture and treatment decisions should be based on the CSF examination (Fig. 58-1).[66]

A reactive CSF-VDRL is considered diagnostic of neurosyphilis, but can be falsely negative in up to 70% of neurosyphilis cases.[153] Thus, the diagnosis may need to be based on CSF pleocytosis or elevated protein concentration. Because CSF abnormalities, including mild pleocytosis and elevated protein levels, are common in patients with HIV infection alone,[154,155] the clinical significance of such CSF abnormalities in HIV-infected persons with syphilis is often difficult to interpret. However, many experts recommend that HIV-infected persons with syphilis who have a CSF white blood cell count above 20 cells/μL be treated for neurosyphilis, even if the CSF-VDRL is nonreactive. The CSF fluorescent treponemal antibody (FTA) and FTA-absorbed (FTA-ABS) tests are more sensitive, although less specific for neurosyphilis, and can be used to help rule out the diagnosis of neurosyphilis when the CSF-VDRL is nonreactive.[156–158]

Treatment of Syphilis and Serologic Response to Therapy in HIV-Infected Persons

Early Syphilis (Primary, Secondary, or Early Latent)

Most HIV-1-infected persons with early syphilis respond to standard benzathine penicillin G (BPG) therapy as is recommended for HIV-1-uninfected persons.[123,124] Some experts choose to treat HIV-1-infected persons with early syphilis more aggressively, with 2.4 million units weekly for 3 weeks, due to concerns that the recommended single injection of 2.4 million units of BPG may not be adequate,[66,131] although there is no evidence that three weekly doses are any more effective than standard therapy for early syphilis.

Given the higher risk for treatment failure and neurologic involvement among HIV-1-infected persons,[129,160,165] careful follow-up is essential. HIV-1-infected patients with early syphilis should be clinically and serologically evaluated for treatment response at 3, 6, 9, 12, and 24 months after therapy.[66] As with HIV-1-uninfected patients, HIV-1-infected persons with clinical treatment failure or titers that do not decrease fourfold within 6–12 months after therapy, should undergo CSF examination and re-treatment as indicated by CSF findings (Fig. 58-1). If the CSF is normal, most experts would treat with intramuscular BPG 2.4 million units once a week for 3 weeks; whereas, abnormal CSF should prompt treatment for neurosyphilis.[66] The management of penicillin allergy is the same for HIV-1-infected and HIV-1-uninfected patients.

Alternatives to penicillin have not been well studied in HIV-1-infected persons and should be used with caution. The CDC recommends doxycycline 100 mg twice a day for 14 days as second-line treatment for early syphilis if a person

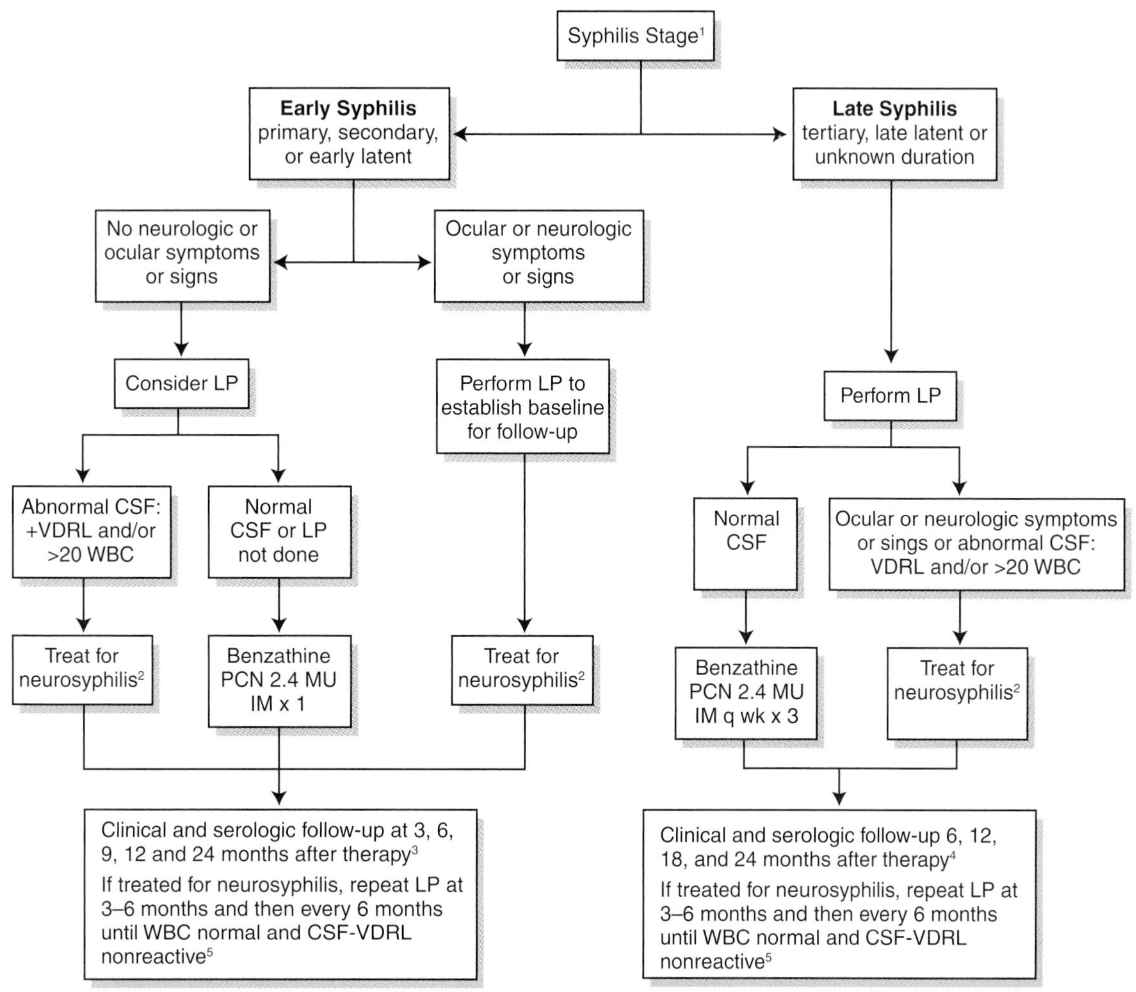

LP, lumbar puncture; CSF, cerebrospinal fluid; PCN, penicillin; MU, million units
[1]Syphilis stage is determined by clinic manifestations and RPR or VDRL titer.
[2] Treat neurosyphilis with aqueous crystalline penicillin or procaine penicillin plus probenecid [See Table 58-1]
[3]Serologic failure is defined as non-treponemal titers that increase by 4-fold at any time or that do not decrease 4-fold within 6-12 months of therapy.
[4]Serologic failure is defined as non-treponemal titers that rise 4-fold at any time or fail to decline 4-fold by 12-24 months after therapy.
[5]Neurosyphilis treatment failure is indicated by new or worsening neurologic or ocular symptoms or signs, increase in CSF WBC, 4-fold increase in CSF-VDRL titer at any time or failure of CSF WBC to normalize or CSF-VDRL to become nonreactive 2 years after therapy.

Figure 58-1 ■ Algorithm for the management of syphilis in the setting of HIV infection.

is penicillin allergic or refuses a parenteral regimen.[66] A retrospective study comparing BPG to doxycycline for the treatment of persons with early syphilis, a minority of whom were HIV-infected, found no difference in the time to serologic response.[166] In a small study of HIV-1-infected persons, the serologic response rates for persons with early syphilis treated with BPG and doxycycline were also similar.[114] Other options for treating early syphilis include 1 g of intramuscular or intravenous ceftriaxone daily for 10 days. A single oral 2 g dose of azithromycin had been a promising alternative treatment, but treatment failure and identification of azithromycin-resistant isolates indicate that azithromycin should not be used for the treatment of syphilis.[167–169]

Most studies suggest that the serological response after treatment for early syphilis is no different in HIV-1-infected and HIV-1-uninfected persons. A study in Baltimore showed a similar rate of decline in RPR titer during the 12-month period after standard treatment for early syphilis among HIV-1-infected and HIV-1-uninfected patients and baseline serum RPR titer and CD4+ T-lymphocyte cell count did not predict clinical failure.[128] Similarly, a case-control study in New York City found no difference in serological response 6 months after treatment for secondary syphilis in HIV-1-infected and HIV-1-uninfected persons, though the HIV-1-infected persons with primary syphilis were less likely to have at least a fourfold decrease in RPR titers.[170]

Table 58-1

Therapy for Selected STIs in Patients With HIV-1 Infection

Disease	Drug	Regimen	Comments
Syphilis			
Early syphilis (primary, secondary, or early latent)	Benzathine penicillin G	2.4 MU IM × 1 dose	Consider LP to rule out neurosyphilis; some experts recommend 2.4 MU IM every week × 3
	Doxycycline	100 mg PO bid × 14 days	Recommended second-line therapy if penicillin allergic; strongly consider desensitization
	Ceftriaxone	1 g IM/IV qd × 14 days	Less well studied, especially in HIV-infected persons
Late syphilis (tertiary or late latent) or unknown duration	Benzathine penicillin G	2.4 MU IM q week × 3	LP indicated
	Doxycycline	100 mg PO bid × 28 days	Recommended second-line therapy if penicillin allergic; strongly consider desensitization
Neurosyphilis	Aqueous penicillin G	18–24 MU IV qd × 10–14 days	Can be administered as 3–4 MU q4h or as continuous infusion; if penicillin allergic, desensitize if possible
	Procaine penicillin	2.4 MU IM qd × 10–14 days plus probenecid 500 mg PO qid × 10–14 days	Only use if compliance can be ensured; contraindicated if sulfa allergy
	Ceftriaxone	2 g IV qd × 10–14 days	May be an acceptable alternative, particularly in setting of early syphilis
Lymphogranuloma Venereum	Doxycycline	100 mg PO bid × 21 days	
	Erythromycin base	500 mg PO qid × 21 d	Not preferred due to problems with adherence and gastrointestinal intolerance
Chancroid	Azithromycin	1 g PO × 1 dose	
	Ceftriaxone	250 mg IM × 1 dose	
	Ciprofloxacin	500 mg PO bid × 3 days	Isolates with intermediate resistance reported
	Erythromycin base	500 mg PO tid × 7 days	Isolates with intermediate resistance reported; some recommend in the setting of HIV infection due to less data with other antibiotics
Herpes Simplex Virus			
Episodic therapy	Acyclovir	400 mg PO tid × 5–10 days	Can increase up to 800 mg PO 5/day
	Valacyclovir	500 mg PO bid × 5–10 days	Can increase up to 1.0 g PO tid
	Famciclovir	500 mg PO bid × 5–10 days	Can increase up to 750 mg PO tid
Suppression	Acyclovir	400 mg PO bid	Can increase up to 800 mg PO tid if frequent breakthroughs
	Valacyclovir	500 mg PO bid	Slightly lower efficacy with 1 g PO qd
	Famciclovir	500 mg PO bid	
Severe disease (disseminated, central nervous system)	Acyclovir	5–10 mg/kg IV q8h	For encephalitis, use 10 mg/kg IV q8h
Acyclovir resistant	Foscarnet	40 mg/kg IV q8h	Should be managed in consultation with a specialist
Gonorrhea			
Cervicitis, urethritis, proctitis, pharyngitis	Cefixime	400 mg PO × 1 dose	If chlamydia not ruled out, empirically treat for both gonorrhea and chlamydia
	Ceftriaxone	125 mg IM × 1 dose	Not recommended for pharyngitis
	Ciprofloxacin	500 mg PO × 1 dose	Use for conjunctivitis
	Ofloxacin	400 mg PO × 1 dose	Increased prevalence of quinolone resistance in Hawaii and Southeast Asia and among MSM

(*Continued*)

(Continued)

Table 58-1

Disease	Drug	Regimen	Comments
Chlamydia			
Cervicitis, urethritis, or NGU	Azithromycin	1 g PO × 1 dose	Test of cure not necessary unless symptoms persist
	Doxycycline	100 mg PO bid × 7 days	
	Ofloxacin	300 mg PO bid × 7 days	
	Erythromycin base	500 mg PO qid × 7 days	
	Erythromycin ethylsuccinate	800 mg PO qid × 7 days	
	Levofloxacin	500 mg PO qd × 7days	
Trichomonas	Metronidazole	2 g PO × 1 or 500 mg PO bid × 7 days	Better adherence with single dose therapy; tinidazole is an alternative, where available, if metronidazole resistant
Persistent Urethritis	Metronidazole and	2 gm PO × 1 dose	
	Erythromycin base	500 mg PO qid × 7 days	
	Erythromycin ethylsuccinate	800 mg PO qid × 7 days	
Pelvic Inflammatory Disease	Cefoxitin	2 g IV q6h plus doxycycline 100 mg IV/PO q12h	When clinically improved, may complete 14-day course with oral doxycycline and consider adding metronidazole if abscess present
	Cefotetan	2 g IV q12h plus doxycycline 100 mg IV/PO q12h	Same as above
	Ampicillin/Sulbactam	3 g IV q6h plus doxycycline 100 mg IV/PO q12h	Same as above
	Clindamycin	900 mg IV q8h plus gentamicin 2 mg/kg IV × 1 then 1.5 mg/kg IV q8h	Gentamicin may be dosed once daily; when clinically improved, may complete 14-day course with oral clindamycin
	Ofloxacin	400 mg IV/PO bid × 14 days	Consider adding metronidazole
	Levofloxacin	500 mg IV/PO qd × 14 days	Consider adding metronidazole
Granuloma Inguinale	Doxycycline	100 mg PO bid for ⩾3 week	Continue until lesions heal; consider adding an aminoglycoside
	TMP-SMX	1 DS tab PO bid × ⩾3 weeks	
	Erythromycin base	500 mg PO qid × ⩾3 weeks	
	Azithromycin	1 g PO q week ⩾3 weeks	
	Ciprofloxacin	750 mg PO bid × ⩾3 weeks	
Bacterial Vaginosis	Metronidazole	500 mg PO bid × 7 days	Metronidazole 2 g PO × 1 is less efficacious
	Metronidazole gel 0.75%	One applicator (5 g) intravaginally qd or bid × 5 days	
	Clindamycin cream 2%	One applicator (5 g) intravaginally qhs × 7 days	Less efficacious; May weaken some condoms
	Clindamycin ovules	100 g intravaginally qhs × 3 days	Same as above
	Clindamycin	300 mg PO bid × 7 days	Less efficacious

LP, lumbar puncture; MU, million units; TMP-SMX, trimethoprim–sulfamethoxazole; NGU, nongonococcal urethritis.

Late Syphilis (Late Latent Syphilis, Tertiary Syphilis) or Syphilis of Unknown Duration

HIV-1-infected persons with tertiary syphilis, late latent syphilis or syphilis of unknown duration without evidence of neurosyphilis should be treated with 2.4 million units BPG intramuscularly once a week for 3 weeks and then clinically and serologically evaluated at 6, 12, 18, and 24 months after therapy.[66] If at any time neurological symptoms develop, nontreponemal titers rise fourfold, or if in 12–24 months the nontreponemal titer does not decline fourfold, CSF examination should be repeated and treatment further determined based on CSF findings. Because nonpenicillin regimens have not been well investigated in HIV-infected persons, these should be used with caution. The management of penicillin allergy is the same for HIV-1-infected and HIV-1-uninfected patients; desensitize to penicillin if possible. If indicated, doxycycline 100 mg twice daily for 28 days is an alternative regimen, but compliance should be closely monitored.[66]

The serological response after treatment for late syphilis is no different in HIV-1-infected and HIV-1-uninfected persons. Among women in Zaire treated for late syphilis, the percentage of HIV-1-infected women with at least a fourfold decline in the RPR titer by 2 years was similar to HIV-uninfected women, regardless of the baseline RPR titer.[171]

Neurosyphilis

Regardless of the stage of disease, if CSF abnormalities consistent with neurosyphilis are found (reactive CSF-VDRL or elevated CSF WBC), the patient should be treated for neurosyphilis with 18–24 million units of aqueous penicillin G intravenously divided into 3–4 million units every 4 h or as a continuous infusion for 10–14 days (Fig. 58-1 and Table 58-1). If compliance can be ensured, 2.4 million units of procaine penicillin intramuscularly can be given daily along with probenecid 500 mg orally four times per day for 10–14 days as an easier outpatient alternative. Ceftriaxone may also be an acceptable alternative to penicillin in HIV-1-infected persons with neurosyphilis in early disease.[66]

After neurosyphilis treatment, CSF should be reexamined after 3–6 months and then every 6 months thereafter until the abnormalities resolve; normalization of CSF protein in HIV-1-infected patients often does not occur. Failure of protein to normalize should not prompt re-treatment.[172] Resolution of CSF abnormalities may be slower after neurosyphilis treatment in HIV-1-infected patients.[172,173] In one study, HIV-1-infected persons were 2.5 times less likely to revert to a nonreactive CSF-VDRL compared to HIV-1-uninfected persons, and 3.7 times less likely if the CD4+ T-lymphocyte cell count was ≤200 cells/mm^3.[172] Another study found that at 24 weeks after treatment, although the CSF-VDRL titer decreased or reverted to nonreactive in only four of 11 persons with neurosyphilis, *T. pallidum* was not detected by PCR or isolated by rabbit-infectivity testing in any CSF specimens after treatment.[164] Despite clinical resolution of symptoms, two participants had no improvement in any of the tested parameters, including serum RPR titer, CSF-VDRL titer, CSF white cell count and CSF protein concentration, and one person relapsed, despite high-dose penicillin therapy.

Chancroid – *Haemophilus ducreyi*

The prevalence of chancroid is decreasing worldwide and HSV-2 is now a much more common cause of GUD than chancroid.[85,174–177] In the 1980s and early 1990s, chancroid was a cofactor for HIV acquisition and transmission, when the prevalence of chancroid was high in sub-Saharan Africa.[178–180] The clinical presentation of chancroid in HIV-1-infected persons is similar to HIV-1-uninfected persons, although there have been reports of atypical presentations, longer incubation period, slower ulcer healing, and greater number of ulcers in the setting of HIV-1 infection.[181–183] The management of chancroid in HIV-1-infected patients is the same as HIV-1-uninfected persons (Table 58-1), however, occasionally HIV-1-infected patients may require a longer treatment course and treatment failure has been reported.[184] Most persons with chancroid are treated syndromically, since the bulk of disease occurs in the developing world where chancroid culture and PCR are rarely available.

LGV – *Chlamydia trachomatis* Serovars L1–L3

Epidemiology of LGV and HIV-1

LGV, a previously rare STI in the Western world, has had a recent resurgence. There have been several outbreaks of anorectal LGV among MSM in Europe and the US and 57–87% of the cases were found to be co-infected with HIV-1.[185–190] In Amsterdam, HIV seropositivity was found to be the strongest risk factor for LGV infection compared to MSM without any chlamydial infection (OR, 9.3; 95% CI, 4.4–20.0).[191] Many LGV cases had several other concomitant STIs diagnosed and reported high-risk sexual behavior.[186,189]

Clinical Presentation, Diagnosis, and Treatment of LGV in Persons with HIV-1 Infection

LGV is an STI caused by *Chlamydia trachomatis* (CT) serovars L1–L3 that classically presents with inguinal buboes associated with a genital ulcer or papule. Among MSM, LGV often presents with rectal manifestations ranging from mild constipation and rectal discharge, perianal ulcerations, to severe fistulous proctitis resulting in permanent scarring. During an outbreak in the Netherlands, ulcerative proctitis was visualized in all nine men who underwent sigmoidoscopy.[186]

To diagnose LGV, rectal swabs can be tested for CT by PCR and if positive, the sample can be submitted for genotyping to identify LGV by the CDC's chlamydia laboratory. A positive chlamydia serology is supportive of the diagnosis, and although not specific can help identify probable cases when genotyping is not available. The recommended treatment of LGV is doxycycline 100 mg for 21 days (Table 58-1).[66]

Genital Herpes – HSV-2

Epidemiology and Presentation of HSV-2 in the Setting of HIV-1

HSV-2 infection is one of the most common co-infections with HIV-1,[176,192–194] occurring in 50–90% of HIV-infected persons, with the highest prevalence among African heterosexuals and MSM from the Americas.[12,176,195–198] Anogenital herpes was one of the first opportunistic infections described in persons with AIDS.[199] Among HIV-1-infected persons, especially those with low CD4+ T-lymphocyte cell counts, genital herpes can present with more severe, chronic herpetic lesions.[85,200] Yet, as with immunocompetent individuals, most HIV-infected persons with HSV-2 are asymptomatic.[201,202] HSV-2 increases HIV-1 acquisition[10,18] and HIV-1 transmission.[29,73,203] The effect of HSV-2 on HIV-1 transmission will be ascertained through an ongoing proof-of-concept randomized trial of HSV-2 suppression in HIV-discordant couples.

Diagnosis and Treatment of HSV-2 in HIV-Infected Persons

Clinical diagnosis of genital HSV-2 in HIV-1-infected persons is unreliable.[77,80] An accurate diagnosis of HSV-2 can be made by culture or PCR of lesions or by IgG-based type-specific serology. Once a diagnosis is established, nucleoside analogs (acyclovir, valacyclovir, and famciclovir) decrease the frequency and severity of both HSV-2 recurrences and asymptomatic HSV-2 reactivation (Table 58-1). They are effective, safe, well-tolerated drugs in the setting of HIV-1 infection.[204–207] Studies are underway to determine whether HSV-2 suppression decreases HIV-1 acquisition and transmission. Studies have already demonstrated that HSV-2 suppression significantly reduces HIV-1 levels in the blood which may slow HIV-1 disease progression, and in the genital tract which could result in decreased HIV-1 infectiousness,[29,58,208–210] thus associated with both potential clinical and public health benefits (*see* Chapter 47 for more detail on HSV-2, HIV-1 co-infection).

NONULCERATIVE STIS

Nonulcerative STIs, specifically gonococcal, chlamydial, and trichomonal infections, have been reported to increase risk of HIV-1 acquisition, but to a lesser extent compared to the ulcerative STI.[2,15] However, due to the high prevalence of these infections in some populations, nonulcerative STI may be a significant factor in the HIV epidemic globally. Nonulcerative STIs increase the risk of HIV acquisition in the range of 1.5- to 5-fold,[1,2,11,14,15,211–214] perhaps due to recruitment of CD4+ T lymphocytes and increased levels of proinflammatory cytokines.

Nonulcerative STIs are also a risk factor for sexual transmission of HIV-1, after controlling for sexual exposure as demonstrated in African FSWs.[14,215] In a nested case-control study of Zairian FSWs, women with gonorrhea (GC), CT, and *Trichomonas vaginalis* (Tv) had higher risk of HIV-1 seroconversion with an adjusted OR of 4.8 (95% CI, 2.4–9.8) for GC, 3.6 (95% CI, 1.4–9.1) for CT and 1.9 (95% CI, 0.9–4.1) for Tv.[215] Nonulcerative STIs are associated with increased numbers of CD4+ T-lymphocyte inflammatory cells in the endocervix.[216] Women with cervicitis have higher HIV-1 RNA concentrations in cervical secretions,[50,54,56,217] and treatment for cervicitis results in significant decreases in cervicovaginal HIV-1 shedding.[53,62] Similarly in men, nonulcerative STIs, particularly gonococcal urethritis, increase seminal HIV-1 levels[61,71,218–222] and seminal HIV levels are reduced after effective treatment for urethritis.[61,63]

Neisseria gonorrhoeae, CT and PID

Clinical Presentation of Gonorrhea, Chlamydia, and PID in Persons with HIV-1

The presentation of GC and CT infection in HIV-1-infected individuals is the same as in HIV-1-uninfected persons; they cause urethritis and proctitis in men and urethritis, cervicitis, and PID in women. Less commonly, GC can also cause pharyngitis, conjunctivitis, or disseminated infection. PID, typically caused by GC, CT, or mixed aerobic and anaerobic organisms, can result in long-term sequelae in women, including infertility, ectopic pregnancies, and chronic abdominal pain. The microbiology and clinical presentation of PID do not seem to be altered significantly by HIV-1 infection.[223] However, early studies reported a higher proportion of tubo-ovarian abscesses in HIV-1-infected women sometimes requiring surgical intervention, associated with a lower CD4+ T-lymphocyte count in one study.[224–227] Of note, women with HIV-1 infection may not have an elevated white blood cell count at baseline as a diagnostic clue of PID.[223,226] Given the possible increased likelihood of a tubo-ovarian abscess in HIV-1-infected women, clinicians should have a low threshold to do an abdominal ultrasound of an HIV-1-infected woman with lower abdominal pain and a presumptive diagnosis of PID.

Diagnosis and Treatment of GC, CT, and PID in Persons with HIV-1

Newer diagnostic methods, utilizing nucleic acid amplification techniques (NAATs), are more sensitive than older methods for the diagnosis of urethritis and cervicitis in persons with and without HIV-1.[228] NAATs for GC and CT have not been approved by the Food and Drug Administration (FDA) for rectal specimens or oropharyngeal specimens due to limited clinical evaluation as well as potential cross-reactivity with other *Neisseria* species, which are common commensal organisms in the oropharynx. Thus, culture is still the diagnostic method of choice for oropharyngeal and rectal CT and GC, since Gram stain is insensitive.[229,230] In a small study, PCR for chlamydial infection was found to have high specificity in rectal specimens.[231]

Treatment for urethritis has been found to be equally effective in HIV-1-infected and HIV-1-uninfected person.[232] Recent studies have also found that HIV-infected persons responded equally well to standard antibiotic regimens for PID when compared to HIV-uninfected persons and were not at a higher risk for surgery.[224,233–235] Thus, in the setting of HIV, the CDC recommendations for GC and CT infections and PID are the same for HIV-infected and HIV-uninfected persons (Table 58-1).[66]

Trichomonas – *Trichomonas vaginalis*

Epidemiology of Trichomonas and HIV-1

Trichomonas vaginalis is a protozoa that, although frequently asymptomatic, can cause vaginitis in women and urethritis in men.[236,237] Tv is the most common nonviral STI worldwide and is estimated to infect 170 million people annually.[238] Since Tv is not a reportable STI in the US, prevalence estimates are based on clinic surveys and from selected populations, sometimes utilizing poor diagnostic techniques (e.g., wet mount only).[239] Wet mount has a sensitivity of 58% when compared to culture[240] and culture has a sensitivity of 70% when compared to PCR.[241] Prevalence estimates of Tv infection have varied considerably from 3% to 48%, depending on the population studied.[31,32,217,242–248] The first US population-based prevalence estimates of trichomoniasis among young adults from a cross-sectional analysis of Wave III of the prospective cohort of the National Longitudinal Study of Adolescent Health indicates an overall prevalence of 2.3% with the highest prevalence (10.5%) among black women.[249]

Trichomonas is prevalent among HIV-infected persons and other individuals with high-risk sexual behavior[31,237,243,250–252] and is particularly common among African-American women with HIV-1 infection.[217] Some studies have reported that 36% of HIV-infected women have recurrent Tv, but studies have difficulty in distinguishing re-infection versus persistent infection, and often have not characterized the degree to which male partners, who often have asymptomatic trichomonal infection, were treated.[250,251] Tv also has high seroprevalence (~10%) among women in parts of Africa.[253] A nested case-control study from Africa reported a twofold (95% CI, 1.1–3.6) increased risk for Tv among 215 HIV-infected pregnant women compared to HIV-uninfected pregnant women.[252]

Few studies have estimated the prevalence of trichomoniasis among men. Although Tv is recognized as a common cause of morbidity in women, its role in men is often ignored since most infections are asymptomatic. Among men attending US STD clinics, 3–12% were infected with trichomonas by culture.[254–256] Tv is more frequently recovered from men with symptomatic urethritis with rates ranging from 10% to 21%.[53,63,222,257–259] A minority of men with Tv have urethral inflammation and are leukocyte esterase positive by urine dipstick.[260] Tv is probably more common among men than has been generally appreciated.

Interaction between Trichomonas and HIV-1

Several cross-sectional studies have indicated an association between Tv and HIV-1 acquisition.[53,215,253] There was approximately a twofold (95% CI, 1.74–2.55, $P<0.001$) increased risk of HIV-1 acquisition among women with Tv infection in Zimbabwe.[253] In a prospective cohort study of 1579 HIV-1-seronegative FSW, the adjusted hazard ratio for Tv infection and risk of HIV-1 acquisition was 1.52 (95% CI, 1.04–2.24).[214] Since the majority of persons with Tv are asymptomatic or have subclinical infection,[45] they are likely to continue to be sexually active and prolonged carriage of Tv could lead to a protracted period of interaction between trichomonas and HIV-1. Moreover, Tv is actually cytotoxic to urogenital epithelial cells,[261–263] disrupting the integrity of the urogenital epithelium with punctate hemorrhages.[264] Tv can be associated with persistent inflammation in the genital tract even 3 weeks after successful antibiotic therapy due to persistent local inflammatory cytokines.[222] Tv also has the capacity to degrade secretory leukocyte protease inhibitor, a product known to block HIV cell attachment.[265] *In vitro,* HIV-1 can attach to trichomonads[266] and it has been theorized that in this manner HIV-1 could be carried across the urogenital epithelium facilitating exposure to target cells for HIV.[264] Tv is implicated as a cofactor for HIV-1 transmission and diagnosis and treatment of Tv is being studied as a means of HIV-1 prevention.

Clinical Presentation of Trichomonas in HIV-Infected Persons

T. vaginalis causes lower genital tract infection, including vaginitis, cervicitis, and urethritis, that has been associated with adverse pregnancy outcomes, such as premature rupture of membranes, preterm delivery, and low birth weight in HIV-1-infected women.[252,267,268] In HIV-1-infected women, trichomonal infection has also been associated with PID[269] and there are case reports of extragenital infection.[270,271] Urethritis attributable to Tv can be associated with more severe symptoms (e.g., dysuria and urethral discharge) in the setting of HIV-1 infection.[237] A cross-sectional study suggested that Tv prevalence was inversely correlated with CD4+ T-lymphocyte cell count,[53] but more recent cohort studies found no association between Tv incidence and CD4+ T-lymphocyte count.[243,250,251,272]

Treatment of Trichomonas in HIV-1-Infected Persons

Despite reports of more severe Tv symptoms in persons with HIV-1, it does not appear to affect clearance of Tv infection with standard doses of metronidazole (Table 58-1).[63] Importantly, although metronidazole is included as part of the syndromic management of vaginal discharge, it is not routinely used for syndromic management of urethritis in men. The addition of metronidazole for syndromic management of urethritis in males cleared 95% of culture-positive trichomonal infections compared to 54% of the placebo group. In areas of high Tv prevalence, the addition of metronidazole to either the first-line syndromic treatment or for initial treatment failures of male urethritis should be considered.[63,222,237,252]

Bacterial Vaginosis

Epidemiology of Bacterial Vaginosis and HIV-1

Whether bacterial vaginosis (BV) should be considered an STI or represents a change in vaginal flora primarily among sexually active women is controversial. BV is a common gynecologic infection, characterized by alterations in the vaginal microflora with loss of the normal lactobacilli that can lead to poor obstetric and gynecologic outcomes such as PID, endometritis, preterm delivery, and postabortion infection. In sub-Saharan Africa, the prevalence of both HIV-1 and BV are high.[273,274] Cross-sectional and case-control studies have demonstrated a higher prevalence of HIV-1 infection in persons with BV.[273,275–279] In Rakai, Uganda, HIV-1 prevalence was 14.2% among women with normal vaginal flora and 26.7% among those with severe BV (RR 1.51; 95% CI, 1.25–1.81; $P < 0.0001$).[273] A 5-year longitudinal study of a large cohort from four US cities of HIV-infected women with a high-risk HIV-uninfected control group, revealed that there was a higher prevalence of BV in HIV-infected women, especially at lower CD4+ T-lymphocyte counts, but that this was due to persistent rather than incident infections.[280] The Women's Interagency HIV Study (WIHS), the Heart and Estrogen/Progestin Replacement Study (HERS) cohort and a cohort in Mombasa, which included high-risk HIV-uninfected control groups, did not confirm the association between HIV-seropositivity and BV,[35,281,282] although HAART was associated with a lower prevalence of BV (adjusted OR 0.54; 95% CI, 0.38–0.77).[282] Therefore, it is unclear whether the higher prevalence of BV seen in HIV-infected persons is related to increased BV acquisition or more persistent BV.

Diagnosis of BV in HIV-Infected Persons

The diagnosis of BV is based on clinical Amsel criteria (malodorous vaginal discharge and increased vaginal pH) or by Gram stain using the Nugent score to classify severity of microflora alterations and quantity of lactobacilli. In HIV-infected women the Amsel criteria poorly predicted a diagnosis of BV in comparison to the gold standard, the Nugent score.[283]

Interaction between Bacterial Vaginosis and HIV-1

Unlike other nonulcerative vaginal infections, BV is not associated with significant inflammatory changes, yet there is some evidence that abnormal vaginal flora typical of BV facilitates the acquisition of HIV.[273,284–286] Longitudinal data from FSW and antenatal populations in Kenya and Malawi, respectively, found that BV increases HIV-1 acquisition by two- to fourfold.[285,286] Although HIV-infected women in Malawi were found to have a higher prevalence of BV by Nugent criteria than HIV-uninfected women (adjusted OR 1.29; 95% CI, 1.08–1.55), incidence of BV was similar.[280] A recent report from the Rakai cohort indicated that women with preexisting BV by Gram stain were not more likely to acquire HIV-1.[287]

Microbiologic data support a role of BV in the acquisition of HIV-1. H_2O_2-producing *Lactobacillus acidophilus* have been shown to have direct virucidal activity against HIV-1 *in vitro*.[288] The maintenance of a low vaginal pH by these bacteria may reduce CD4+ T-lymphocyte cell activation.[289] Studies are underway to determine if treatment of BV and recolonization of the vagina with Lactobacilli decreases the risk of HIV-1 acquisition.

Some studies indicate that BV may increase HIV-1 infectiousness. Specifically, BV was significantly associated with levels of HIV-1 RNA in the female genital tract of HIV-infected women when diagnosed by Amsel criteria (adjusted OR 3.7; 95% CI, 1.4–10.0)[290] or by the presence of BV-associated bacteria after adjusting for plasma HIV-1 viral load.[291] Lysates of *Gardnerella vaginalis* and certain anaerobic bacteria, frequently isolated from the vagina of women with BV, have been found to increase HIV-1 expression by activating HIV-1 transcription.[292,293] *In vitro* studies indicate that BV-associated microflora enhance HIV-1 expression via a soluble HIV-inducing factor as well as other cytokines.[294–297]

Clinical Presentation and Treatment of BV in HIV-Infected Persons

Immunocompromised women with low CD4+ T-lymphocyte cell counts tend to have more severe BV by both clinical and Gram stain criteria.[276,277,287,298] In the Rakai, Uganda STI trial, severe BV increased in parallel with HIV-1 viral load.[287] In the prospectively followed HERS cohort of women, HIV-infected women were also more likely to have persistent BV (adjusted OR 1.49; 95% CI, 1.18–1.89), especially when the CD4+ T-lymphocyte cell count was <200 cells/mm^3.[280] The utility and benefits of treating asymptomatic BV has not been demonstrated, since when treated, many women do not achieve a cure (Table 58-1). HIV-1-infected women are even less likely to be cured compared to HIV-uninfected women (28% vs 52%; $P < 0.001$).[232]

CONCLUSION

The high prevalence of STIs in persons with HIV-1 infection is of increasing importance given the association of bacterial, viral, and protozoal STIs with increased risk of HIV-1 acquisition and HIV-1 infectiousness. For some STIs, HIV-1 affects their clinical presentation, natural history, and management. The recent increases in LGV and early syphilis among MSM in multiple cities demonstrates how the ease of travel has widened sexual networks, creating a need for greater collaboration of researchers, providers, and public health officials across geographic boundaries.[299] Given the synergistic interrelation between HIV-1 and STIs, emphasis on the recognition, treatment, and prevention of STIs is warranted for primary and secondary HIV-1 prevention to reduce the role of STIs in HIV-1 acquistion and transmission.

REFERENCES

1. Fleming DT, Wasserheit JN. From epidemiological synergy to public health policy and practice: the contribution of other sexually transmitted diseases to sexual transmission of HIV infection. Sex Transm Infect 75:3–17, 1999.
2. Wasserheit JN. Epidemiological synergy. Interrelationships between human immunodeficiency virus infection and other sexually transmitted diseases. Sex Transm Dis 19:61–77, 1992.

3. Otten MW Jr, Zaidi AA, Peterman TA, et al. High rate of HIV seroconversion among patients attending urban sexually transmitted disease clinics. AIDS 8:549–53, 1994.
4. Harawa NT, Douglas J, McFarland W, et al. Trends in HIV prevalence among public sexually transmitted disease clinic attendees in the Western region of the United States (1989–1999). J Acquir Immune Defic Syndr 37:1206–15, 2004.
5. Mehta SH, Gupta A, Sahay S, et al. High HIV prevalence among a high-risk subgroup of women attending sexually transmitted infection clinics in Pune, India. J Acquir Immune Defic Syndr 41:75–80, 2006.
6. Centers for Disease Control and Prevention. HIV counseling and testing in publicly funded sites annual report 1997–1998, Atlanta, 2001.
7. Weinstock H, Dale M, Gwinn M, et al. HIV seroincidence among patients at clinics for sexually transmitted diseases in nine cities in the United States. J Acquir Immune Defic Syndr 29:478–83, 2002.
8. Weinstock H, Dale M, Linley L, et al. Unrecognized HIV infection among patients attending sexually transmitted disease clinics. Am J Public Health 92:280–3, 2002.
9. Weinstock H, Sweeney S, Satten GA, et al. HIV seroincidence and risk factors among patients repeatedly tested for HIV attending sexually transmitted disease clinics in the United States, 1991 to 1996. STD Clinic HIV Seroincidence Study Group. J Acquir Immune Defic Syndr Hum Retrovirol 19:506–12, 1998.
10. Freeman EE, Weiss HA, Glynn JR, et al. Herpes simplex virus 2 infection increases HIV acquisition in men and women: systematic review and meta-analysis of longitudinal studies. AIDS 20:73–83, 2006.
11. Gray RH, Wawer MJ, Sewankambo NK, et al. Relative risks and population attributable fraction of incident HIV associated with symptoms of sexually transmitted diseases and treatable symptomatic sexually transmitted diseases in Rakai District, Uganda. Rakai Project Team. AIDS 13:2113–23, 1999.
12. Greenblatt RM, Lukehart SA, Plummer FA, et al. Genital ulceration as a risk factor for human immunodeficiency virus infection. AIDS 2:47–50, 1988.
13. Nelson KE, Eiumtrakul S, Celentano D, et al. The association of herpes simplex virus type 2 (HSV-2), *Haemophilus ducreyi,* and syphilis with HIV infection in young men in northern Thailand. J Acquir Immune Defic Syndr Hum Retrovirol 16:293–300, 1997.
14. Plummer FA, Simonsen JN, Cameron DW, et al. Cofactors in male–female sexual transmission of human immunodeficiency virus type 1. J Infect Dis 163:233–9, 1991.
15. Rottingen JA, Cameron DW, Garnett GP. A systematic review of the epidemiologic interactions between classic sexually transmitted diseases and HIV: how much really is known? Sex Transm Dis 28:579–97, 2001.
16. Serwadda D, Gray RH, Sewankambo NK, et al. Human immunodeficiency virus acquisition associated with genital ulcer disease and herpes simplex virus type 2 infection: a nested case-control study in Rakai, Uganda. J Infect Dis 188:1492–7, 2003.
17. Telzak EE, Chiasson MA, Bevier PJ, et al. HIV-1 seroconversion in patients with and without genital ulcer disease. A prospective study. Ann Intern Med 119:1181–6, 1993.
18. Wald A, Link K. Risk of human immunodeficiency virus infection in herpes simplex virus type 2-seropositive persons: a meta-analysis. J Infect Dis 185:45–52, 2002.
19. Grosskurth H, Mosha F, Todd J, et al. Impact of improved treatment of sexually transmitted diseases on HIV infection in rural Tanzania: randomised controlled trial. Lancet 346:530–6, 1995.
20. Kamali A, Quigley M, Nakiyingi J, et al. Syndromic management of sexually-transmitted infections and behaviour change interventions on transmission of HIV-1 in rural Uganda: a community randomised trial. Lancet 361:645–52, 2003.
21. Quigley MA, Kamali A, Kinsman J, et al. The impact of attending a behavioural intervention on HIV incidence in Masaka, Uganda. AIDS 18:2055–63, 2004.
22. Wawer MJ, Sewankambo NK, Serwadda D, et al. Control of sexually transmitted diseases for AIDS prevention in Uganda: a randomised community trial. Rakai Project Study Group. Lancet 353:525–35, 1999.
23. Grosskurth H, Gray R, Hayes R, et al. Control of sexually transmitted diseases for HIV-1 prevention: understanding the implications of the Mwanza and Rakai trials. Lancet 355:1981–7, 2000.
24. Korenromp EL, White RG, Orroth KK, et al. Determinants of the impact of sexually transmitted infection treatment on prevention of HIV infection: a synthesis of evidence from the Mwanza, Rakai, and Masaka intervention trials. J Infect Dis 191(Suppl 1):S168–78, 2005.
25. Orroth KK, Korenromp EL, White RG, et al. Comparison of STD prevalences in the Mwanza, Rakai, and Masaka trial populations: the role of selection bias and diagnostic errors. Sex Transm Infect 79:98–105, 2003.
26. Orroth KK, Korenromp EL, White RG, et al. Higher risk behaviour and rates of sexually transmitted diseases in Mwanza compared to Uganda may help explain HIV prevention trial outcomes. AIDS 17:2653–60, 2003.
27. White RG, Orroth KK, Korenromp EL, et al. Can population differences explain the contrasting results of the Mwanza, Rakai, and Masaka HIV/sexually transmitted disease intervention trials? A modeling study. J Acquir Immune Defic Syndr 37:1500–13, 2004.
28. Kaul R, Kimani J, Nagelkerke NJ, et al. Monthly antibiotic chemoprophylaxis and incidence of sexually transmitted infections and HIV-1 infection in Kenyan sex workers: a randomized controlled trial. JAMA 291:2555–62, 2004.
29. Corey L, Wald A, Celum CL, et al. The effects of herpes simplex virus-2 on HIV-1 acquisition and transmission: a review of two overlapping epidemics. J Acquir Immune Defic Syndr 35:435–45, 2004.
30. Celum CL, Robinson NJ, Cohen MS. Potential effect of HIV type 1 antiretroviral and herpes simplex virus type 2 antiviral therapy on transmission and acquisition of HIV type 1 infection. J Infect Dis 191:S107–14, 2005.
31. Bersoff-Matcha SJ, Horgan MM, Fraser VJ, et al. Sexually transmitted disease acquisition among women infected with human immunodeficiency virus type 1. J Infect Dis 178:1174–7, 1998.
32. Bunnell RE, Dahlberg L, Rolfs R, et al. High prevalence and incidence of sexually transmitted diseases in urban adolescent females despite moderate risk behaviors. J Infect Dis 180:1624–31, 1999.
33. Chen SY, Gibson S, Katz MH, et al. Continuing increases in sexual risk behavior and sexually transmitted diseases among men who have sex with men: San Francisco, Calif, 1999–2001, USA. Am J Public Health 92:1387–8, 2002.
34. Kalichman SC, Rompa D, Cage M. Sexually transmitted infections among HIV seropositive men and women. Sex Transm Infect 76:350–4, 2000.
35. McClelland RS, Lavreys L, Katingima C, et al. Contribution of HIV-1 infection to acquisition of sexually transmitted disease: a 10-year prospective study. J Infect Dis 191:333–8, 2005.
36. Monteiro CA, Bachmann LH, Desmond RA, et al. Incidence and risk factors for sexually transmitted infections among women in an Alabama HIV clinic. AIDS Res Hum Retroviruses 20:577–83, 2004.
37. Phipps W, Stanley H, Kohn R, et al. Syphilis, chlamydia, and gonorrhea screening in HIV-infected patients in primary care,

San Francisco, California, 2003. AIDS Patient Care STDS 19:495–8, 2005.
38. Centers for Disease Control and Prevention. HIV prevention through early detection and treatment of other sexually transmitted diseases – United States. MMWR Morb Mortal Wkly Rep 47:1998.
39. Erbelding EJ, Chung SE, Kamb ML, et al. New sexually transmitted diseases in HIV-infected patients: markers for ongoing HIV transmission behavior. J Acquir Immune Defic Syndr 33:247–52, 2003.
40. Zenilman JM, Erickson B, Fox R, et al. Effect of HIV posttest counseling on STD incidence. JAMA 267:843–5, 1992.
41. Capps L, Peng G, Doyle M, et al. Sexually transmitted infections in women infected with the human immunodeficiency virus. Terry Beirn Community Programs for Clinical Research on AIDS (CPCRA). Sex Transm Dis 25:443–7, 1998.
42. Golden MR, Rompalo AM, Fantry L, et al. Early intervention for human immunodeficiency virus in Baltimore Sexually Transmitted Diseases Clinics. Impact on gonorrhea incidence in patients infected with HIV. Sex Transm Dis 23:370–7, 1996.
43. Munoz-Perez MA, Rodriguez-Pichardo A, Camacho Martinez F. Sexually transmitted diseases in 1161 HIV-positive patients: a 38-month prospective study in southern Spain. J Eur Acad Dermatol Venereol 11:221–6, 1998.
44. Osewe PL, Peterman TA, Ransom RL, et al. Trends in the acquisition of sexually transmitted diseases among HIV-positive patients at STD clinics, Miami 1988–1992. Sex Transm Dis 23:230–3, 1996.
45. Wilkinson D, Abdool Karim SS, Harrison A, et al. Unrecognized sexually transmitted infections in rural South African women: a hidden epidemic. Bull World Health Organ 77:22–8, 1999.
46. McClelland RS, Baeten JM. Reducing HIV-1 transmission through prevention strategies targeting HIV-1-seropositive individuals. J Antimicrob Chemother 57:163–6, 2006.
47. Otten MW Jr, Zaidi AA, Wroten JE, et al. Changes in sexually transmitted disease rates after HIV testing and posttest counseling, Miami, 1988 to 1989. Am J Public Health 83:529–33, 1993.
48. Quinn TC, Wawer MJ, Sewankambo N, et al. Viral load and heterosexual transmission of human immunodeficiency virus type 1. Rakai Project Study Group. N Engl J Med 342:921–9, 2000.
49. Ballard R, Htun Y, Dangor Y, et al. HIV and genital ulcer disease: determinants of HIV shedding from persons and consequences of therapy. In: International Society for Sexually Transmitted Disease Research, Denver, CO, 1999, abstract #055.
50. Clemetson DB, Moss GB, Willerford DM, et al. Detection of HIV DNA in cervical and vaginal secretions. Prevalence and correlates among women in Nairobi, Kenya. JAMA 269:2860–4, 1993.
51. Fiscus SA, Vernazza PL, Gilliam B, et al. Factors associated with changes in HIV shedding in semen. AIDS Res Hum Retroviruses 14(Suppl 1):S27–31, 1998.
52. Gadkari DA, Quinn TC, Gangakhedkar RR, et al. HIV-1 DNA shedding in genital ulcers and its associated risk factors in Pune, India. J Acquir Immune Defic Syndr Hum Retrovirol 18:277–81, 1998.
53. Ghys PD, Fransen K, Diallo MO, et al. The associations between cervicovaginal HIV shedding, sexually transmitted diseases and immunosuppression in female sex workers in Abidjan, Cote d'Ivoire. AIDS 11:F85–93, 1997.
54. Kreiss J, Willerford DM, Hensel M, et al. Association between cervical inflammation and cervical shedding of human immunodeficiency virus DNA. J Infect Dis 170:1597–601, 1994.
55. Lawn SD, Subbarao S, Wright TC Jr, et al. Correlation between human immunodeficiency virus type 1 RNA levels in the female genital tract and immune activation associated with ulceration of the cervix. J Infect Dis 181:1950–6, 2000.
56. Mostad SB. Prevalence and correlates of HIV type 1 shedding in the female genital tract. AIDS Res Hum Retroviruses 14(Suppl 1):S11–15, 1998.
57. Mostad SB, Kreiss JK. Shedding of HIV-1 in the genital tract. AIDS 10:1305–15, 1996.
58. Schacker T, Ryncarz AJ, Goddard J, et al. Frequent recovery of HIV-1 from genital herpes simplex virus lesions in HIV-1-infected men. JAMA 280:61–6, 1998.
59. Wright TC Jr, Subbarao S, Ellerbrock TV, et al. Human immunodeficiency virus 1 expression in the female genital tract in association with cervical inflammation and ulceration. Am J Obstet Gynecol 184:279–85, 2001.
60. Baeten JM, Overbaugh J. Measuring the infectiousness of persons with HIV-1: opportunities for preventing sexual HIV-1 transmission. Curr HIV Res 1:69–86, 2003.
61. Cohen MS, Hoffman IF, Royce RA, et al. Reduction of concentration of HIV-1 in semen after treatment of urethritis: implications for prevention of sexual transmission of HIV-1. AIDSCAP Malawi Research Group. Lancet 349:1868–73, 1997.
62. McClelland RS, Wang CC, Mandaliya K, et al. Treatment of cervicitis is associated with decreased cervical shedding of HIV-1. AIDS 15:105–10, 2001.
63. Price MA, Zimba D, Hoffman IF, et al. Addition of treatment for trichomoniasis to syndromic management of urethritis in Malawi: a randomized clinical trial. Sex Transm Dis 30: 516–22, 2003.
64. Wang CC, McClelland RS, Reilly M, et al. The effect of treatment of vaginal infections on shedding of human immunodeficiency virus type 1. J Infect Dis 183:1017–22, 2001.
65. Hayes RJ, Schulz KF, Plummer FA. The cofactor effect of genital ulcers on the per-exposure risk of HIV transmission in sub-Saharan Africa. J Trop Med Hyg 98:1–8, 1995.
66. Centers for Disease Control and Prevention. Sexually transmitted diseases treatment guidelines 2002. MMWR Recomm Rep 51:1–78, 2002.
67. Holmberg SD, Stewart JA, Gerber AR, et al. Prior herpes simplex virus type 2 infection as a risk factor for HIV infection. JAMA 259:1048–50, 1988.
68. Stamm WE, Handsfield HH, Rompalo AM, et al. The association between genital ulcer disease and acquisition of HIV infection in homosexual men. JAMA 260:1429–33, 1988.
69. Cameron DW, Simonsen JN, D'Costa LJ, et al. Female to male transmission of human immunodeficiency virus type 1: risk factors for seroconversion in men. Lancet 2:403–7, 1989.
70. Mertens TE, Hayes RJ, Smith PG. Epidemiological methods to study the interaction between HIV infection and other sexually transmitted diseases. AIDS 4:57–65, 1990.
71. Royce RA, Sena A, Cates W Jr, et al. Sexual transmission of HIV. N Engl J Med 336:1072–8, 1997.
72. Piot P, Laga M. Genital ulcers, other sexually transmitted diseases, and the sexual transmission of HIV. BMJ 298:623–4, 1989.
73. Gray RH, Wawer MJ, Brookmeyer R, et al. Probability of HIV-1 transmission per coital act in monogamous heterosexual, HIV-1-discordant couples in Rakai, Uganda. Lancet 357:1149–53, 2001.
74. Latif AS, Katzenstein DA, Bassett MT, et al. Genital ulcers and transmission of HIV among couples in Zimbabwe. AIDS 3:519–23, 1989.
75. Kreiss JK, Coombs R, Plummer F, et al. Isolation of human immunodeficiency virus from genital ulcers in Nairobi prostitutes. J Infect Dis 160:380–4, 1989.
76. Plummer FA, Wainberg MA, Plourde P, et al. Detection of human immunodeficiency virus type 1 (HIV-1) in genital ulcer

exudate of HIV-1-infected men by culture and gene amplification. J Infect Dis 161:810–1, 1990.
77. DiCarlo RP, Martin DH. The clinical diagnosis of genital ulcer disease in men. Clin Infect Dis 25:292–8, 1997.
78. Morse SA, Trees DL, Htun Y, et al. Comparison of clinical diagnosis and standard laboratory and molecular methods for the diagnosis of genital ulcer disease in Lesotho: association with human immunodeficiency virus infection. J Infect Dis 175:583–9, 1997.
79. Risbud A, Chan-Tack K, Gadkari D, et al. The etiology of genital ulcer disease by multiplex polymerase chain reaction and relationship to HIV infection among patients attending sexually transmitted disease clinics in Pune, India. Sex Transm Dis 26:55–62, 1999.
80. Dangor Y, Ballard RC, da LEF, et al. Accuracy of clinical diagnosis of genital ulcer disease. Sex Transm Dis 17:184–9, 1990.
81. LaGuardia KD, White MH, Saigo PE, et al. Genital ulcer disease in women infected with human immunodeficiency virus. Am J Obstet Gynecol 172:553–62, 1995.
82. Johnson LF, Coetzee DJ, Dorrington RE. Sentinel surveillance of sexually transmitted infections in South Africa: a review. Sex Transm Infect 81:287–93, 2005.
83. Paz-Bailey G, Rahman M, Chen C, et al. Changes in the etiology of sexually transmitted diseases in Botswana between 1993 and 2002: implications for the clinical management of genital ulcer disease. Clin Infect Dis 41:1304–12, 2005.
84. Wolday D, Z GM, Mohammed Z, et al. Risk factors associated with failure of syndromic treatment of sexually transmitted diseases among women seeking primary care in Addis Ababa. Sex Transm Infect 80:392–4, 2004.
85. Gresenguet G, Weiss HA, Frost E, et al. Aetiology of genital ulcer disease among women in Ghana and Central African Republic: randomised trial of episodic acyclovir treatment in addition to syndromic management (ANSR 1212 Study). In: 16th Meeting of the International Society for Sexually Transmitted Diseases Research, Amsterdam, The Netherlands, 2005, abstract M0-605.
86. Centers for Disease Control and Prevention. Primary and secondary syphilis – United States, 2002. MMWR Morb Mortal Wkly Rep 52:1117–20, 2003.
87. Wolitski RJ, Valdiserri RO, Denning PH, et al. Are we headed for a resurgence of the HIV epidemic among men who have sex with men? Am J Public Health 91:883–8, 2001.
88. Centers for Disease Control and Prevention (CDC). Resurgent bacterial sexually transmitted disease among men who have sex with men – King County, Washington, 1997–1999. MMWR Morb Mortal Wkly Rep 48:773–7, 1999.
89. Centers for Disease Control and Prevention. Outbreak of syphilis among men who have sex with men – southern California, 2000. JAMA 285:1285–7, 2001.
90. Bronzan R, Echavarria L, Hermida J, et al. Syphilis among men who have sex with men in Miami–Dade County, Florida. In: 2002 National STD Prevention Conference, San Diego, CA, 4–7 March, abstract 292.
91. Chen JL, Kodagoda D, Lawrence AM, et al. Rapid public health interventions in response to an outbreak of syphilis in Los Angeles. Sex Transm Dis 29:277–84, 2002.
92. Ciesielski C, Beidinger H. Emergence of primary and secondary syphilis among men who have sex with men in Chicago and relationship to HIV infection. In: The 7th Conference on Retroviruses and Opportunistic Infections; Chicago, IL, 30 Jan to 2 Feb 2000, abstract 470.
93. Cohen DE, Mayer KH, Fever JC, et al. Increasing rates of syphilis and gonorrhea among men who have sex with men at a Boston community health center, 1997–1999. In: The 38th Annual Meeting of the Infectious Diseases Society of America, Alexandria, VA, 2000, abstract 538.
94. Centers for Disease Control and Prevention. Primary and Secondary syphilis among men who have sex with men – New York City, 2001 MMWR 2002, 51: (38) 853.
95. Abraham B, Marih L, Thevenet S, et al. Outbreak of syphilis among HIV-infected patients: descriptive data from a Parisian hospital. Sex Transm Dis 32:718–9, 2005.
96. Doherty L, Fenton KA, Jones J, et al. Syphilis: old problem, new strategy. BMJ 325:153–6, 2002.
97. Marcus U, Kollan C, Bremer V, et al. Relation between the HIV and the re-emerging syphilis epidemic among MSM in Germany: an analysis based on anonymous surveillance data. Sex Transm Infect 81:456–7, 2005.
98. Righarts AA, Simms I, Wallace L, et al. Syphilis surveillance and epidemiology in the United Kingdom. Euro Surveil 9: 21–5, 2004.
99. Debattista J, Dwyer J, Anderson R, et al. Screening for syphilis among men who have sex with men in various clinical settings. Sex Transm Infect 80:505–8, 2004.
100. Dodds JP, Nardone A, Mercey DE, et al. Increase in high risk sexual behaviour among homosexual men, London 1996–8: cross sectional, questionnaire study. BMJ 320:1510–1, 2000.
101. Kravcik S, Victor G, Houston S, et al. Effect of antiretroviral therapy and viral load on the perceived risk of HIV transmission and the need for safer sexual practices. J Acquir Immune Defic Syndr Hum Retrovirol 19:124–9, 1998.
102. Stall RD, Hays RB, Waldo CR, et al. The Gay '90s: a review of research in the 1990s on sexual behavior and HIV risk among men who have sex with men. AIDS 14(Suppl 3):S101–14, 2000.
103. Blocker ME, Levine WC, St Louis ME. HIV prevalence in patients with syphilis, United States. Sex Transm Dis 27:53–9, 2000.
104. Chesson HW, Heffelfinger JD, Voigt RF, et al. Estimates of primary and secondary syphilis rates in persons with HIV in the United States, 2002. Sex Transm Dis 32:265–9, 2005.
105. Paz-Bailey G, Meyers A, Blank S, et al. A case-control study of syphilis among men who have sex with men in New York City: association with HIV infection. Sex Transm Dis 31:581–7, 2004.
106. Quinn TC, Cannon RO, Glasser D, et al. The association of syphilis with risk of human immunodeficiency virus infection in patients attending sexually transmitted disease clinics. Arch Intern Med 150:1297–302, 1990.
107. Wong W, Chaw JK, Kent CK, et al. Risk factors for early syphilis among gay and bisexual men seen in an STD clinic: San Francisco, 2002–2003. Sex Transm Dis 32:458–63, 2005.
108. Centers for Disease Control and Prevention (CDC) Trends in primary and secondary syphilis and HIV infections in men who have sex with men – San Francisco and Los Angeles, California, 1998–2002. MMWR Morb Mortal Wkly Rep 53:575–8, 2004.
109. Sellati TJ, Wilkinson DA, Sheffield JS, et al. Virulent *Treponema pallidum*, lipoprotein, and synthetic lipopeptides induce CCR5 on human monocytes and enhance their susceptibility to infection by human immunodeficiency virus type 1. J Infect Dis 181:283–93, 2000.
110. Theus SA, Harrich DA, Gaynor R, et al. *Treponema pallidum*, lipoproteins, and synthetic lipoprotein analogues induce human immunodeficiency virus type 1 gene expression in monocytes via NF-kappaB activation. J Infect Dis 177:941–50, 1998.
111. McBroom RL, Styles AR, Chiu MJ, et al. Secondary syphilis in persons infected with and not infected with HIV-1: a comparative immunohistologic study. Am J Dermatopathol 21:432–41, 1999.
112. Norgard MV, Arndt LL, Akins DR, et al. Activation of human monocytic cells by *Treponema pallidum* and *Borrelia burgdorferi* lipoproteins and synthetic lipopeptides proceeds via a

pathway distinct from that of lipopolysaccharide but involves the transcriptional activator NF-kappa B. Infect Immun 64:3845–52, 1996.
113. Van Voorhis WC, Barrett LK, Koelle DM, et al. Primary and secondary syphilis lesions contain mRNA for Th1 cytokines. J Infect Dis 173:491–5, 1996.
114. Kofoed K, Gerstoft J, Mathiesen LR, et al. Syphilis and human immunodeficiency virus (HIV)-1 coinfection: influence on CD4 T-cell count, HIV-1 viral load, and treatment response. Sex Transm Dis 33:143–8, 2006.
115. Buchacz K, Patel P, Taylor M, et al. Syphilis increases HIV viral load and decreases CD4 cell counts in HIV-infected patients with new syphilis infections. AIDS 18:2075–9, 2004.
116. Sadiq ST, McSorley J, Copas AJ, et al. The effects of early syphilis on CD4 counts and HIV-1 RNA viral loads in blood and semen. Sex Transm Infect 81:380–5, 2005.
117. Ajithkumar K. Unusual skin ulceration in an HIV-positive patient who had cutaneous syphilis and neurosyphilis [letter]. Br J Dermatol 138:366–7, 1998.
118. Guerrero AF, Straight TM, Eastone J, et al. Gastric syphilis in an HIV-infected patient. AIDS Patient Care STDS 19:281–5, 2005.
119. Oette M, Hemker J, Feldt T, et al. Acute syphilitic blindness in an HIV-positive patient. AIDS Patient Care STDS 19: 209–11, 2005.
120. Radolf JD, Kaplan RP. Unusual manifestations of secondary syphilis and abnormal humoral immune response to *Treponema pallidum* antigens in a homosexual man with asymptomatic human immunodeficiency virus infection. J Am Acad Dermatol 18:423–8, 1988.
121. Regal L, Demaerel P, Dubois B. Cerebral syphilitic gumma in a human immunodeficiency virus-positive patient. Arch Neurol 62:1310–11, 2005.
122. Sands M, Markus A. Lues maligna, or ulceroglandular syphilis, in a man infected with human immunodeficiency virus: case report and review. Clin Infect Dis 20:387–90, 1995.
123. Gourevitch MN, Selwyn PA, Davenny K, et al. Effects of HIV infection on the serologic manifestations and response to treatment of syphilis in intravenous drug users. Ann Intern Med 118:350–5, 1993.
124. Rolfs RT, Joesoef MR, Hendershot EF, et al. A randomized trial of enhanced therapy for early syphilis in patients with and without human immunodeficiency virus infection. The Syphilis and HIV Study Group. N Engl J Med 337:307–14, 1997.
125. Rompalo AM, Joesoef MR, O'Donnell JA, et al. Clinical manifestations of early syphilis by HIV status and gender: results of the syphilis and HIV study. Sex Transm Dis 28:158–65, 2001.
126. Behets FM, Liomba G, Lule G, et al. Sexually transmitted diseases and human immunodeficiency virus control in Malawi: a field study of genital ulcer disease. J Infect Dis 171:451–5, 1995.
127. Gutierrez-Galhardo MC, do Valle GF, Sa FC, et al. Clinical characteristics and evolution of syphilis in 24 HIV+ individuals in Rio de Janeiro, Brazil. Rev Inst Med Trop Sao Paulo 47:153–7, 2005.
128. Hutchinson CM, Hook EW 3rd, Shepherd M, et al. Altered clinical presentation of early syphilis in patients with human immunodeficiency virus infection. Ann Intern Med 121: 94–100, 1994.
129. Johns DR, Tierney M, Felsenstein D. Alteration in the natural history of neurosyphilis by concurrent infection with the human immunodeficiency virus. N Engl J Med 316:1569–72, 1987.
130. Katz DA, Berger JR. Neurosyphilis in acquired immunodeficiency syndrome. Arch Neurol 46:895–8, 1989.
131. Musher DM. Syphilis, neurosyphilis, penicillin, and AIDS. J Infect Dis 163:1201–6, 1991.
132. Gwanzura L, Latif A, Bassett M, et al. Syphilis serology and HIV infection in Harare, Zimbabwe. Sex Transm Infect 75:426–30, 1999.
133. Rusnak JM, Butzin C, McGlasson D, et al. False-positive rapid plasma reagin tests in human immunodeficiency virus infection and relationship to anti-cardiolipin antibody and serum immunoglobulin levels. J Infect Dis 169:1356–9, 1994.
134. Sordillo EM, Hoehl B, Belch J. False-negative fluorescent treponemal tests and confirmation of syphilis infection. J Infect Dis 178:294–5, 1998.
135. Terry PM, Page ML, Goldmeier D. Are serological tests of value in diagnosing and monitoring response to treatment of syphilis in patients infected with human immunodeficiency virus? Genitourin Med 64:219–22, 1988.
136. Augenbraun MH, DeHovitz JA, Feldman J, et al. Biological false-positive syphilis test results for women infected with human immunodeficiency virus. Clin Infect Dis 19:1040–4, 1994.
137. Glatt AE, Stoffer HR, Forlenza S, et al. High-titer positive nontreponemal tests with negative specific treponemal serology in patients with HIV infection and/or intravenous substance use. J Acquir Immune Defic Syndr 4:861–4, 1991.
138. Hernandez-Aguado I, Bolumar F, Moreno R, et al. False-positive tests for syphilis associated with human immunodeficiency virus and hepatitis B virus infection among intravenous drug abusers. Valencian Study Group on HIV Epidemiology. Eur J Clin Microbiol Infect Dis 17:784–7, 1998.
139. Joyanes P, Borobio MV, Arquez JM, et al. The association of false-positive rapid plasma reagin results and HIV infection. Sex Transm Dis 25:569–71, 1998.
140. Rompalo AM, Cannon RO, Quinn TC, et al. Association of biologic false-positive reactions for syphilis with human immunodeficiency virus infection. J Infect Dis 165:1124–6, 1992.
141. Blum L, Bachmeyer C, Caumes E. Seronegative secondary syphilis in an HIV-infected patient. Clin Exp Dermatol 30:158–9, 2005.
142. Erbelding EJ, Vlahov D, Nelson KE, et al. Syphilis serology in human immunodeficiency virus infection: evidence for false-negative fluorescent treponemal testing. J Infect Dis 176:1397–400, 1997.
143. Hicks CB, Benson PM, Lupton GP, et al. Seronegative secondary syphilis in a patient infected with the human immunodeficiency virus (HIV) with Kaposi sarcoma. A diagnostic dilemma. Ann Intern Med 107:492–5, 1987.
144. Kuznetsov AV, Burgdorf WH, Prinz JC. Latent syphilis confirmed by polymerase chain reaction in 2 HIV-positive patients with inconclusive serologic test results. Arch Dermatol 141:1169–70, 2005.
145. Berger JR. Neurosyphilis in human immunodeficiency virus type 1-seropositive individuals. A prospective study. Arch Neurol 48:700–2, 1991.
146. Katz DA, Berger JR, Duncan RC. Neurosyphilis. A comparative study of the effects of infection with human immunodeficiency virus. Arch Neurol 50:243–9, 1993.
147. McLeish WM, Pulido JS, Holland S, et al. The ocular manifestations of syphilis in the human immunodeficiency virus type 1-infected host. Ophthalmology 97:196–203, 1990.
148. Zellan J, Augenbraun M. Syphilis in the HIV-infected patient: an update on epidemiology, diagnosis, and management. Curr HIV/AIDS Rep 1:142–7, 2004.
149. Dowell ME, Ross PG, Musher DM, et al. Response of latent syphilis or neurosyphilis to ceftriaxone therapy in persons infected with human immunodeficiency virus. Am J Med 93:481–8, 1992.

150. Holtom PD, Larsen RA, Leal ME, et al. Prevalence of neurosyphilis in human immunodeficiency virus-infected patients with latent syphilis. Am J Med 93:9–12, 1992.
151. Marra CM, Maxwell CL, Smith SL, et al. Cerebrospinal fluid abnormalities in patients with syphilis: association with clinical and laboratory features. J Infect Dis 189:369–76, 2004.
152. Marra CM, Maxwell CL, Smith SL, et al. Risk factors for neurosyphilis [latebreaker abstract]. In: 2002 National STD Prevention Conference, San Diego, CA, 4–7 Mar.
153. Hart G. Syphilis tests in diagnostic and therapeutic decision making. Ann Intern Med 104:368–76, 1986.
154. Marra CM, Gary DW, Kuypers J, et al. Diagnosis of neurosyphilis in patients infected with human immunodeficiency virus type 1. J Infect Dis 174:219–21, 1996.
155. Marshall DW, Brey RL, Cahill WT, et al. Spectrum of cerebrospinal fluid findings in various stages of human immunodeficiency virus infection. Arch Neurol 45:954–8, 1988.
156. Davis LE, Schmitt JW. Clinical significance of cerebrospinal fluid tests for neurosyphilis. Ann Neurol 25:50–5, 1989.
157. Marra CM, Critchlow CW, Hook EW 3rd, et al. Cerebrospinal fluid treponemal antibodies in untreated early syphilis. Arch Neurol 52:68–72, 1995.
158. Marra CM, Tantalo LC, Maxwell CL, et al. Alternative cerebrospinal fluid tests to diagnose neurosyphilis in HIV-infected individuals. Neurology 63:85–8, 2004.
159. Bayne LL, Schmidley JW, Goodin DS. Acute syphilitic meningitis. Its occurrence after clinical and serologic cure of secondary syphilis with penicillin G. Arch Neurol 43:137–8, 1986.
160. Berry CD, Hooton TM, Collier AC, et al. Neurologic relapse after benzathine penicillin therapy for secondary syphilis in a patient with HIV infection. N Engl J Med 316:1587–9, 1987.
161. Lanska MJ, Lanska DJ, Schmidley JW. Syphilitic polyradiculopathy in an HIV-positive man. Neurology 38:1297–301, 1988.
162. Musher DM, Hamill RJ, Baughn RE. Effect of human immunodeficiency virus (HIV) infection on the course of syphilis and on the response to treatment. Ann Intern Med 113:872–81, 1990.
163. Tramont EC. Syphilis in the AIDS era. N Engl J Med 316:1600–1, 1987.
164. Gordon SM, Eaton ME, George R, et al. The response of symptomatic neurosyphilis to high-dose intravenous penicillin G in patients with human immunodeficiency virus infection. N Engl J Med 331:1469–73, 1994.
165. Lukehart SA, Hook EW 3rd, Baker-Zander SA, et al. Invasion of the central nervous system by *Treponema pallidum*: implications for diagnosis and treatment. Ann Intern Med 109:855–62, 1988.
166. Ghanem KG, Erbelding EJ, Cheng WW, et al. Doxycycline compared with benzathine penicillin for the treatment of early syphilis. Clin Infect Dis 42:e45–9, 2006.
167. Centers for Disease Control and Prevention. Azithromycin treatment failures in syphilis infections – San Francisco, California, 2002–2003. MMWR Morb Mortal Wkly Rep 53:197–8, 2004.
168. Lukehart SA, Godornes C, Molini BJ, et al. Macrolide resistance in *Treponema pallidum* in the United States and Ireland. N Engl J Med 351:154–8, 2004.
169. Holmes KK. Azithromycin versus penicillin G benzathine for early syphilis. N Engl J Med 353:1291–3, 2005.
170. Telzak EE, Greenberg MS, Harrison J, et al. Syphilis treatment response in HIV-infected individuals. AIDS 5:591–5, 1991.
171. Goeman J, Kivuvu M, Nzila N, et al. Similar serological response to conventional therapy for syphilis among HIV-positive and HIV-negative women. Genitourin Med 71:275–9, 1995.
172. Marra CM, Maxwell CL, Tantalo L, et al. Normalization of cerebrospinal fluid abnormalities after neurosyphilis therapy: does HIV status matter? Clin Infect Dis 38:1001–6, 2004.
173. Marra CM, Longstreth WT Jr, Maxwell CL, et al. Resolution of serum and cerebrospinal fluid abnormalities after treatment of neurosyphilis. Influence of concomitant human immunodeficiency virus infection. Sex Transm Dis 23:184–9, 1996.
174. Chen CY, Ballard RC, Beck-Sague CM, et al. Human immunodeficiency virus infection and genital ulcer disease in South Africa: the herpetic connection. Sex Transm Dis 27:21–9, 2000.
175. Mertz KJ, Trees D, Levine WC, et al. Etiology of genital ulcers and prevalence of human immunodeficiency virus coinfection in 10 US cities. The Genital Ulcer Disease Surveillance Group. J Infect Dis 178:1795–8, 1998.
176. Weiss H. Epidemiology of herpes simplex virus type 2 infection in the developing world. Herpes 11(Suppl 1):25A–35A, 2004.
177. Kharsany AB, Mahabeer Y, Connolly C, et al. Changing aetiology of genital ulcer disease (GUD) in STD clinic attenders with a rising HIV prevalence (Abstract ThOr (728)). In: 13th International AIDS Conference, Durban, South Africa, 9–14 Jul.
178. Hanson S, Sunkutu RM, Kamanga J, et al. STD care in Zambia: an evaluation of the guidelines for case management through a syndromic approach. Int J STD AIDS 7:324–32, 1996.
179. Htun Y, Morse SA, Dangor Y, et al. Comparison of clinically directed, disease specific, and syndromic protocols for the management of genital ulcer disease in Lesotho. Sex Transm Infect 74(Suppl 1):S23–8, 1998.
180. O'Farrell N, Hoosen AA, Coetzee KD, et al. Genital ulcer disease in men in Durban, South Africa. Genitourin Med 67: 327–30, 1991.
181. King R, Choudhri SH, Nasio J, et al. Clinical and in situ cellular responses to *Haemophilus ducreyi* in the presence or absence of HIV infection. Int J STD AIDS 9:531–6, 1998.
182. Kimani J, Bwayo JJ, Anzala AO, et al. Low dose erythromycin regimen for the treatment of chancroid. East Afr Med J 72:645–8, 1995.
183. Quale J, Teplitz E, Augenbraun M. Atypical presentation of chancroid in a patient infected with the human immunodeficiency virus. Am J Med 88:43N–4N, 1990.
184. Hartmann AA, Elsner P, Burg G. Intravenous single-dose ceftriaxone treatment of chancroid. Dermatologica 183:132–5, 1991.
185. Halioua B, Bohbot JM, Monfort L, et al. Ano-rectal lymphogranuloma venereum: 22 cases reported in a sexually transmitted infections center in Paris. Eur J Dermatol 16:177–80, 2006.
186. Nieuwenhuis RF, Ossewaarde JM, Gotz HM, et al. Resurgence of lymphogranuloma venereum in Western Europe: an outbreak of *Chlamydia trachomatis* serovar l2 proctitis in The Netherlands among men who have sex with men. Clin Infect Dis 39:996–1003, 2004.
187. van Krosigk A, Meyer T, Jordan S, et al. Dramatic increase in lymphogranuloma venereum among homosexual men in Hamburg. J Dtsch Dermatol Ges 2:676–80, 2004.
188. Williams D, Churchill D. Ulcerative proctitis in men who have sex with men: an emerging outbreak. BMJ 332:99–100, 2006.
189. Lymphogranuloma venereum among men who have sex with men – Netherlands, 2003–2004. MMWR Morb Mortal Wkly Rep 53:985–8, 2004.
190. LGV reported in Europe and the U.S. AIDS Clin Care 17:77, 2005.
191. Van der Bij AK, Spaargaren J, Morre SA, et al. Diagnostic and clinical implications of anorectal lymphogranuloma venereum in men who have sex with men: a retrospective case-control study. Clin Infect Dis 42:186–94, 2006.

192. Enzensberger R, Braun W, July C, et al. Prevalence of antibodies to human herpesviruses and hepatitis B virus in patients at different stages of human immunodeficiency virus (HIV) infection. Infection 19:140–5, 1991.
193. Gwanzura L, McFarland W, Alexander D, et al. Association between human immunodeficiency virus and herpes simplex virus type 2 seropositivity among male factory workers in Zimbabwe. J Infect Dis 177:481–4, 1998.
194. Obasi A, Mosha F, Quigley M, et al. Antibody to herpes simplex virus type 2 as a marker of sexual risk behavior in rural Tanzania. J Infect Dis 179:16–24, 1999.
195. Auvert B, Ballard RC, Campbell C, et al. HIV infection among youth in South African mining town is associated with herpes simplex virus-2 seropositivity and sexual behaviour. AIDS 15:885–98, 2001.
196. Mbizvo M, Mashu A, Chipato T, et al. Trends in HIV-1 and HIV-2 prevalence and risk factors in pregnant women in Harare, Zimbabwe. Cent Afr J Med 42:14–21, 1996.
197. Mostad SB, Kreiss JK, Ryncarz AJ, et al. Cervical shedding of herpes simplex virus in human immunodeficiency virus-infected women: effects of hormonal contraception, pregnancy, and vitamin A deficiency. J Infect Dis 181:58–63, 2000.
198. Sanchez J, Volquez C, Totten P, et al. The etiology and management of genital ulcers in the Dominican Republic and Peru. Sex Transm Dis 29:559–67, 2002.
199. Siegal FP, Lopez C, Hammer GS, et al. Severe acquired immunodeficiency in male homosexuals, manifested by chronic perianal ulcerative herpes simplex lesions. N Engl J Med 305:1439–44, 1981.
200. Bagdades EK, Pillay D, Squire SB, et al. Relationship between herpes simplex virus ulceration and CD4+ cell counts in patients with HIV infection. AIDS 6:1317–20, 1992.
201. Schacker T, Zeh J, Hu HL, et al. Frequency of symptomatic and asymptomatic herpes simplex virus type 2 reactivations among human immunodeficiency virus-infected men. J Infect Dis 178:1616–22, 1998.
202. Strick LB, Wald A, Celum C. Management of HSV-2 infection in HIV-1 infected persons. Clin Infect Dis 43(30):347–56, 2006.
203. Freeman EE, Glynn JR. Factors affecting HIV concordancy in married couples in four African cities. AIDS 18:1715–21, 2004.
204. Conant MA, Schacker TW, Murphy RL, et al. Valaciclovir versus aciclovir for herpes simplex virus infection in HIV-infected individuals: two randomized trials. Int J STD AIDS 13:12–21, 2002.
205. DeJesus E, Wald A, Warren T, et al. Valacyclovir for the suppression of recurrent genital herpes in human immunodeficiency virus-infected subjects. J Infect Dis 188:1009–16, 2003.
206. Romanowski B, Aoki FY, Martel AY, et al. Efficacy and safety of famciclovir for treating mucocutaneous herpes simplex infection in HIV-infected individuals. Collaborative Famciclovir HIV Study Group. AIDS 14:1211–17, 2000.
207. Schacker T, Hu HL, Koelle DM, et al. Famciclovir for the suppression of symptomatic and asymptomatic herpes simplex virus reactivation in HIV-infected persons. A double-blind, placebo-controlled trial. Ann Intern Med 128:21–8, 1998.
208. Mole L, Ripich S, Margolis D, et al. The impact of active herpes simplex virus infection on human immunodeficiency virus load. J Infect Dis 176:766–70, 1997.
209. Schacker T, Zeh J, Hu H, et al. Changes in plasma human immunodeficiency virus type 1 RNA associated with herpes simplex virus reactivation and suppression. J Infect Dis 186:1718–25, 2002.
210. Nagot N, Ouedraogo A, Mayaud P, et al. Impact of HSV-2 suppressive therapy on HIV-1 genital shedding and plasma viral load: a proof of concept randomised double-blind placebo controlled trial (ANRS 1285a Trial). In: The 13th Conference of Retroviruses and Opportunistic Infections, Denver, CO, 5–8 Feb, abstract 33LB.
211. Sturm PD, Moodley P, Khan N, et al. Aetiology of male urethritis in patients recruited from a population with a high HIV prevalence. Int J Antimicrob Agents 24(Suppl 1):S8–14, 2004.
212. Lazzarin A, Saracco A, Musicco M, et al. Man-to-woman sexual transmission of the human immunodeficiency virus. Risk factors related to sexual behavior, man's infectiousness, and woman's susceptibility. Italian Study Group on HIV Heterosexual Transmission. Arch Intern Med 151:2411–16, 1991.
213. Kapiga SH, Vuylsteke B, Lyamuya EF, et al. Evaluation of sexually transmitted diseases diagnostic algorithms among family planning clients in Dar es Salaam, Tanzania. Sex Transm Infect 74(Suppl 1):S132–8, 1998.
214. McClelland RS, Lavreys L, Hassan WM, et al. Infection with *T. vaginalis* increases the risk for HIV-1 acquisition. In: The 13th Conference of Retroviruses and Opportunistic Infections, Denver, CO, 5–8 Feb, abstract 131.
215. Laga M, Manoka A, Kivuvu M, et al. Non-ulcerative sexually transmitted diseases as risk factors for HIV-1 transmission in women: results from a cohort study. AIDS 7:95–102, 1993.
216. Levine WC, Pope V, Bhoomkar A, et al. Increase in endocervical CD4 lymphocytes among women with nonulcerative sexually transmitted diseases. J Infect Dis 177:167–74, 1998.
217. Sorvillo F, Kerndt P. *Trichomonas vaginalis* and amplification of HIV-1 transmission. Lancet 351:213–14, 1998.
218. Sadiq ST, Taylor S, Copas AJ, et al. The effects of urethritis on seminal plasma HIV-1 RNA loads in homosexual men not receiving antiretroviral therapy. Sex Transm Infect 81:120–3, 2005.
219. Moss GB, Overbaugh J, Welch M, et al. Human immunodeficiency virus DNA in urethral secretions in men: association with gonococcal urethritis and CD4 cell depletion. J Infect Dis 172:1469–74, 1995.
220. Eron JJ Jr, Gilliam B, Fiscus S, et al. HIV-1 shedding and chlamydial urethritis. JAMA 275:36, 1996.
221. Winter AJ, Taylor S, Workman J, et al. Asymptomatic urethritis and detection of HIV-1 RNA in seminal plasma. Sex Transm Infect 75:261–3, 1999.
222. Hobbs MM, Kazembe P, Reed AW, et al. *Trichomonas vaginalis* as a cause of urethritis in Malawian men. Sex Transm Dis 26:381–7, 1999.
223. Barbosa C, Macasaet M, Brockmann S, et al. Pelvic inflammatory disease and human immunodeficiency virus infection. Obstet Gynecol 89:65–70, 1997.
224. Kamenga MC, De Cock KM, St Louis ME, et al. The impact of human immunodeficiency virus infection on pelvic inflammatory disease: a case-control study in Abidjan, Ivory Coast. Am J Obstet Gynecol 172:919–25, 1995.
225. Bukusi E, Stevens CE, Cohen CR. Impact of HIV on acute pervic inflammatory disease in a Nairobi out-patient clinic. In: Abstracts of the XI International Conference on AIDS, Vancouver, Canada, abstract 1618.
226. Hoegsberg B, Abulafia O, Sedlis A, et al. Sexually transmitted diseases and human immunodeficiency virus infection among women with pelvic inflammatory disease. Am J Obstet Gynecol 163:1135–9, 1990.
227. Korn AP, Landers DV, Green JR, et al. Pelvic inflammatory disease in human immunodeficiency virus-infected women. Obstet Gynecol 82:765–8, 1993.
228. Peralta L, Durako SJ, Ma Y. Correlation between urine and cervical specimens for the detection of cervical *Chlamydia trachomatis* and *Neisseria gonorrhoeae* using ligase chain reaction in a cohort of HIV infected and uninfected adolescents. J Adolesc Health 29:87–92, 2001.

229. Johnson RE, Newhall WJ, Papp JR, et al. Screening tests to detect *Chlamydia trachomatis* and *Neisseria gonorrhoeae* infections – 2002. MMWR Recomm Rep 51:1–38; quiz CE1–4, 2002.
230. Sherrard J, Barlow D. Gonorrhoea in men: clinical and diagnostic aspects. Genitourin Med 72:422–6, 1996.
231. Golden MR, Astete SG, Galvan R, et al. Pilot study of COBAS PCR and ligase chain reaction for detection of rectal infections due to *Chlamydia trachomatis*. J Clin Microbiol 41:2174–5, 2003.
232. Moodley P, Wilkinson D, Connolly C, et al. Influence of HIV-1 coinfection on effective management of abnormal vaginal discharge. Sex Transm Dis 30:1–5, 2003.
233. Bukusi EA, Cohen CR, Stevens CE, et al. Effects of human immunodeficiency virus 1 infection on microbial origins of pelvic inflammatory disease and on efficacy of ambulatory oral therapy. Am J Obstet Gynecol 181:1374–81, 1999.
234. Cohen CR, Sinei S, Reilly M, et al. Effect of human immunodeficiency virus type 1 infection upon acute salpingitis: a laparoscopic study. J Infect Dis 178:1352–8, 1998.
235. Irwin KL, Moorman AC, O'Sullivan MJ, et al. Influence of human immunodeficiency virus infection on pelvic inflammatory disease. Obstet Gynecol 95:525–34, 2000.
236. Fouts AC, Kraus SJ. *Trichomonas vaginalis*: reevaluation of its clinical presentation and laboratory diagnosis. J Infect Dis 141:137–43, 1980.
237. Price MA, Miller WC, Kaydos-Daniels SC, et al. Trichomoniasis in men and HIV infection: data from 2 outpatient clinics at Lilongwe Central Hospital, Malawi. J Infect Dis 190:1448–55, 2004.
238. Gerbase AC, Rowley JT, Heymann DH, Berkley SF. Global prevalence and incidence estimates of selected curable STDs. Sex Transm Infect 74(Suppl 1):S12–16, 1998.
239. Sorvillo F, Smith L, Kerndt P, et al. *Trichomonas vaginalis*, HIV, and African-Americans. Emerg Infect Dis 7:927–32, 2001.
240. Wiese W, Patel SR, Patel SC, et al. A meta-analysis of the Papanicolaou smear and wet mount for the diagnosis of vaginal trichomoniasis. Am J Med 108:301–8, 2000.
241. Madico G, Quinn TC, Rompalo A, et al. Diagnosis of *Trichomonas vaginalis* infection by PCR using vaginal swab samples. J Clin Microbiol 36:3205–10, 1998.
242. Cu-Uvin S, Hogan JW, Warren D, et al. Prevalence of lower genital tract infections among human immunodeficiency virus (HIV)-seropositive and high-risk HIV-seronegative women. HIV Epidemiology Research Study Group. Clin Infect Dis 29:1145–50, 1999.
243. Cu-Uvin S, Ko H, Jamieson DJ, et al. Prevalence, incidence, and persistence or recurrence of trichomoniasis among human immunodeficiency virus (HIV)-positive women and among HIV-negative women at high risk for HIV infection. Clin Infect Dis 34:1406–11, 2002.
244. Wilson TE, Minkoff H, DeHovitz J, et al. The relationship of cocaine use and human immunodeficiency virus serostatus to incident sexually transmitted diseases among women. Sex Transm Dis 25:70–5, 1998.
245. Bell TA, Farrow JA, Stamm WE, et al. Sexually transmitted diseases in females in a juvenile detention center. Sex Transm Dis 12:140–4, 1985.
246. Shuter J, Bell D, Graham D, et al. Rates of and risk factors for trichomoniasis among pregnant inmates in New York City. Sex Transm Dis 25:303–7, 1998.
247. Cotch MF, Pastorek JG 2nd, Nugent RP, et al. Demographic and behavioral predictors of *Trichomonas vaginalis* infection among pregnant women. The Vaginal Infections and Prematurity Study Group. Obstet Gynecol 78:1087–92, 1991.
248. Vazquez F, Palacio V, Vazquez JA, et al. Gonorrhea in women prostitutes: clinical data and auxotypes, serovars, plasmid contents of PPNG, and susceptibility profiles. Sex Transm Dis 18:5–9, 1991.
249. Miller WC, Swygard H, Hobbs MM, et al. The prevalence of trichomoniasis in young adults in the United States. Sex Transm Dis 32:593–8, 2005.
250. Niccolai LM, Kopicko JJ, Kassie A, et al. Incidence and predictors of reinfection with *Trichomonas vaginalis* in HIV-infected women. Sex Transm Dis 27:284–8, 2000.
251. Sorvillo F, Kovacs A, Kerndt P, et al. Risk factors for trichomoniasis among women with human immunodeficiency virus (HIV) infection at a public clinic in Los Angeles County, California: implications for HIV prevention. Am J Trop Med Hyg 58:495–500, 1998.
252. Sutton MY, Sternberg M, Nsuami M, et al. Trichomoniasis in pregnant human immunodeficiency virus-infected and human immunodeficiency virus-uninfected Congolese women: prevalence, risk factors, and association with low birth weight. Am J Obstet Gynecol 181:656–62, 1999.
253. Mason PR, Fiori PL, Cappuccinelli P, et al. Seroepidemiology of *Trichomonas vaginalis* in rural women in Zimbabwe and patterns of association with HIV infection. Epidemiol Infect 133:315–23, 2005.
254. Borchardt KA, Al-Haraci S, Maida N. Prevalence of *Trichomonas vaginalis* in a male sexually transmitted disease clinic population by interview, wet mount microscopy, and the InPouch TV test. Genitourin Med 71:405–6, 1995.
255. Joyner JL, Douglas JM Jr, Ragsdale S, et al. Comparative prevalence of infection with *Trichomonas vaginalis* among men attending a sexually transmitted diseases clinic. Sex Transm Dis 27:236–40, 2000.
256. Krieger JN, Verdon M, Siegel N, et al. Risk assessment and laboratory diagnosis of trichomoniasis in men. J Infect Dis 166:1362–6, 1992.
257. Watson-Jones D, Mugeye K, Mayaud P, et al. High prevalence of trichomoniasis in rural men in Mwanza, Tanzania: results from a population based study. Sex Transm Infect 76:355–62, 2000.
258. Morency P, Dubois MJ, Gresenguet G, et al. Aetiology of urethral discharge in Bangui, Central African Republic. Sex Transm Infect 77:125–9, 2001.
259. Pepin J, Sobela F, Deslandes S, et al. Etiology of urethral discharge in West Africa: the role of *Mycoplasma genitalium* and *Trichomonas vaginalis*. Bull World Health Organ 79:118–26, 2001.
260. Jackson DJ, Rakwar JP, Bwayo JJ, et al. Urethral *Trichomonas vaginalis* infection and HIV-1 transmission. Lancet 350:1076, 1997.
261. Alderete JF, Pearlman E. Pathogenic *Trichomonas vaginalis* cytotoxicity to cell culture monolayers. Br J Vener Dis 60:99–105, 1984.
262. Gilbert RO, Elia G, Beach DH, et al. Cytopathogenic effect of *Trichomonas vaginalis* on human vaginal epithelial cells cultured in vitro. Infect Immun 68:4200–6, 2000.
263. Rasmussen SE, Nielsen MH, Lind I, et al. Morphological studies of the cytotoxicity of *Trichomonas vaginalis* to normal human vaginal epithelial cells in vitro. Genitourin Med 62:240–6, 1986.
264. Guenthner PC, Secor WE, Dezzutti CS. *Trichomonas vaginalis*-induced epithelial monolayer disruption and human immunodeficiency virus type 1 (HIV-1) replication: implications for the sexual transmission of HIV-1. Infect Immun 73:4155–60, 2005.
265. Draper D, Donohoe W, Mortimer L, et al. Cysteine proteases of *Trichomonas vaginalis* degrade secretory leukocyte protease inhibitor. J Infect Dis 178:815–9, 1998.
266. Rendon-Maldonado J, Espinosa-Cantellano M, Soler C, et al. *Trichomonas vaginalis*: in vitro attachment and internalization of HIV-1 and HIV-1-infected lymphocytes. J Eukaryot Microbiol 50:43–8, 2003.

267. Cotch MF, Pastorek JG, 2nd, Nugent RP, et al. *Trichomonas vaginalis* associated with low birth weight and preterm delivery. The Vaginal Infections and Prematurity Study Group. Sex Transm Dis 24:353–60, 1997.
268. Minkoff H, Grunebaum AN, Schwarz RH, et al. Risk factors for prematurity and premature rupture of membranes: a prospective study of the vaginal flora in pregnancy. Am J Obstet Gynecol 150:965–72, 1984.
269. Moodley P, Wilkinson D, Connolly C, et al. *Trichomonas vaginalis* is associated with pelvic inflammatory disease in women infected with human immunodeficiency virus. Clin Infect Dis 34:519–22, 2002.
270. Borczuk AC, Hagan R, Chipty F, et al. Cytologic detection of *Trichomonas esophagitis* in a patient with acquired immunodeficiency syndrome. Diagn Cytopathol 19:313–16, 1998.
271. Duboucher C, Noel C, Durand-Joly I, et al. Pulmonary coinfection by *Trichomonas vaginalis* and *Pneumocystis* sp. as a novel manifestation of AIDS. Hum Pathol 34:508–11, 2003.
272. Magnus M, Clark R, Myers L, et al. *Trichomonas vaginalis* among HIV-infected women: are immune status or protease inhibitor use associated with subsequent *T. vaginalis* positivity? Sex Transm Dis 30:839–43, 2003.
273. Sewankambo N, Gray RH, Wawer MJ, et al. HIV-1 infection associated with abnormal vaginal flora morphology and bacterial vaginosis. Lancet 350:546–50, 1997.
274. Govender L, Hoosen AA, Moodley J, et al. Bacterial vaginosis and associated infections in pregnancy. Int J Gynaecol Obstet 55:23–8, 1996.
275. Cohen CR, Duerr A, Pruithithada N, et al. Bacterial vaginosis and HIV seroprevalence among female commercial sex workers in Chiang Mai, Thailand. AIDS 9:1093–7, 1995.
276. Royce RA, Thorp J, Granados JL, et al. Bacterial vaginosis associated with HIV infection in pregnant women from North Carolina. J Acquir Immune Defic Syndr Hum Retrovirol 20:382–6, 1999.
277. Taha TE, Gray RH, Kumwenda NI, et al. HIV infection and disturbances of vaginal flora during pregnancy. J Acquir Immune Defic Syndr Hum Retrovirol 20:52–9, 1999.
278. Mbizvo ME, Musya SE, Stray-Pedersen B, et al. Bacterial vaginosis and intravaginal practices: association with HIV. Cent Afr J Med 50:41–6, 2004.
279. Myer L, Denny L, Telerant R, et al. Bacterial vaginosis and susceptibility to HIV infection in South African women: a nested case-control study. J Infect Dis 192:1372–80, 2005.
280. Jamieson DJ, Duerr A, Klein RS, et al. Longitudinal analysis of bacterial vaginosis: findings from the HIV epidemiology research study. Obstet Gynecol 98:656–63, 2001.
281. Greenblatt RM, Bacchetti P, Barkan S, et al. Lower genital tract infections among HIV-infected and high-risk uninfected women: findings of the Women's Interagency HIV Study (WIHS). Sex Transm Dis 26:143–51, 1999.
282. Warren D, Klein RS, Sobel J, et al. A multicenter study of bacterial vaginosis in women with or at risk for human immunodeficiency virus infection. Infect Dis Obstet Gynecol 9:133–41, 2001.
283. Sha BE, Chen HY, Wang QJ, et al. Utility of Amsel criteria, Nugent score, and quantitative PCR for *Gardnerella vaginalis, Mycoplasma hominis, and Lactobacillus* spp. for diagnosis of bacterial vaginosis in human immunodeficiency virus-infected women. J Clin Microbiol 43:4607–12, 2005.
284. Hillier SL. The vaginal microbial ecosystem and resistance to HIV. AIDS Res Hum Retroviruses 14(Suppl 1):S17–21, 1998.
285. Martin HL, Richardson BA, Nyange PM, et al. Vaginal lactobacilli, microbial flora, and risk of human immunodeficiency virus type 1 and sexually transmitted disease acquisition. J Infect Dis 180:1863–8, 1999.
286. Taha TE, Hoover DR, Dallabetta GA, et al. Bacterial vaginosis and disturbances of vaginal flora: association with increased acquisition of HIV. AIDS 12:1699–706, 1998.
287. Gray RH, Wawer MJ, Kiwanuka N, et al. Is bacterial vaginosis a cause or a consequence of HIV infection? Studies from Rakai, Uganda. In: 11th Conference on Retroviruses and Opportunistic Infections, San Francisco, CA, 8–11 Feb, abstract 146.
288. Klebanoff SJ, Coombs RW. Viricidal effect of *Lactobacillus acidophilus* on human immunodeficiency virus type 1: possible role in heterosexual transmission. J Exp Med 174:289–92, 1991.
289. Hill JA, Anderson DJ. Human vaginal leukocytes and the effects of vaginal fluid on lymphocyte and macrophage defense functions. Am J Obstet Gynecol 166:720–6, 1992.
290. Cu-Uvin S, Hogan JW, Caliendo AM, et al. Association between bacterial vaginosis and expression of human immunodeficiency virus type 1 RNA in the female genital tract. Clin Infect Dis 33:894–6, 2001.
291. Sha BE, Zariffard MR, Wang QJ, et al. Female genital-tract HIV load correlates inversely with *Lactobacillus* species but positively with bacterial vaginosis and *Mycoplasma hominis*. J Infect Dis 191:25–32, 2005.
292. Hashemi FB, Ghassemi M, Roebuck KA, et al. Activation of human immunodeficiency virus type 1 expression by *Gardnerella vaginalis*. J Infect Dis 179:924–30, 1999.
293. Hashemi FB, Ghassemi M, Faro S, et al. Induction of human immunodeficiency virus type 1 expression by anaerobes associated with bacterial vaginosis. J Infect Dis 181:1574–80, 2000.
294. Al-Harthi L, Roebuck KA, Olinger GG, et al. Bacterial vaginosis-associated microflora isolated from the female genital tract activates HIV-1 expression. J Acquir Immune Defic Syndr 21:194–202, 1999.
295. Olinger GG, Hashemi FB, Sha BE, et al. Association of indicators of bacterial vaginosis with a female genital tract factor that induces expression of HIV-1. AIDS 13:1905–12, 1999.
296. Sturm-Ramirez K, Gaye-Diallo A, Eisen G, et al. High levels of tumor necrosis factor-alpha and interleukin-1beta in bacterial vaginosis may increase susceptibility to human immunodeficiency virus. J Infect Dis 182:467–73, 2000.
297. Cohn JA, Hashemi FB, Camarca M, et al. HIV-inducing factor in cervicovaginal secretions is associated with bacterial vaginosis in HIV-1-infected women. J Acquir Immune Defic Syndr 39:340–6, 2005.
298. Moodley P, Connolly C, Sturm AW. Interrelationships among human immunodeficiency virus type 1 infection, bacterial vaginosis, trichomoniasis, and the presence of yeasts. J Infect Dis 185:69–73, 2002.
299. Fenton KA, Imrie J. Increasing rates of sexually transmitted diseases in homosexual men in Western Europe and the United States: why? Infect Dis Clin North Am 19:311–31, 2005.

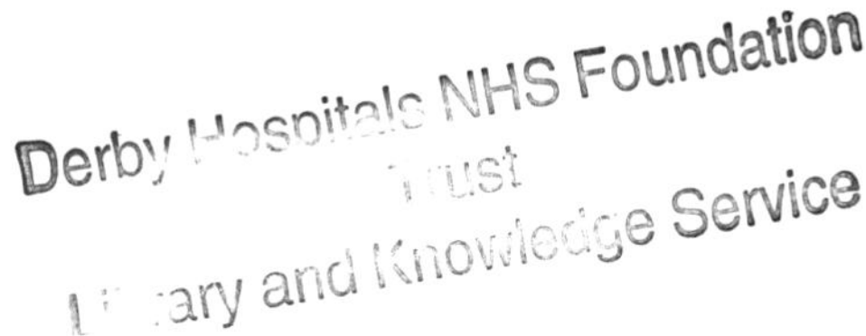

Chapter 59

Kaposi Sarcoma

Susan E. Krown, MD

Kaposi sarcoma (KS) was one of the first opportunistic diseases described in association with the acquired immune deficiency syndrome (AIDS).[1] Despite a decline in its incidence, which began before the introduction of potent antiretroviral regimens for human immunodeficiency virus-1 (HIV-1) but which has accelerated since their widespread introduction in 1996,[2] KS continues to be the most frequently diagnosed AIDS-associated neoplasm and a cause of significant morbidity and occasional mortality in HIV-infected patients. The rapid decline in KS incidence that followed the introduction of potent antiretroviral regimens for HIV and the observed regression of established KS lesions after their use may be a consequence of a decrease in the production of KS-stimulatory cytokines and viral proteins associated with poorly controlled HIV infection. Alternatively or in addition, effective antiretroviral therapy might permit the development of an effective immune response against human herpesvirus 8 (HHV-8), also known as the KS-associated herpesvirus (KSHV), the virus required for development of KS. The emergence of drug-resistant HIV strains and intolerance or lack of adherence to effective antiviral regimens make it difficult to know whether the decreased incidence of KS in developed countries will continue. In addition, the incidence of KS remains high in parts of the world where effective antiretroviral therapy is not widely available and where the incidence of HIV and HHV-8 co-infection is high.[3]

KS most commonly presents with lesions on the skin that may be widely disseminated from the outset, although other sites may be initially involved. Although the course of KS is quite variable, in some patients KS not only disseminates in the skin but also involves the oral cavity and visceral organs, especially the lungs and gastrointestinal (GI) tract, and it is often complicated by lymphedema of the lower extremities, and, less commonly the face, trunk, upper extremities, and genitalia. Depending on its location and severity, KS can cause serious functional disability. KS lesions of the feet may be painful and limit mobility. Oral KS may cause difficulty eating and speaking. Edema may be associated with ulceration, infection, pain, and reduced mobility. GI KS may be asymptomatic but sometimes causes bleeding, pain, and obstruction. Pulmonary KS can cause respiratory insufficiency; and untreated pulmonary KS was associated in one study with a median survival of only 2.1 months.[4] Even in the absence of symptomatic visceral disease or edema, KS often impairs the quality of life when it causes disfigurement, leads to social isolation, or serves as a visual reminder of an AIDS diagnosis.

Several treatment options are available for KS, and the choice is dictated by the extent of disease, the rate of disease progression, and the presence and severity of symptoms affecting function and quality of life. The choice of treatment may also be influenced by the severity of the underlying HIV infection and the presence of co-morbid opportunistic complications of HIV infection. KS usually presents multifocally, without a defined 'primary' lesion, so staging according to a standard T(umor)/N(ode)/M(etastasis) classification is not appropriate. In addition to tumor extent, immune status and the presence of systemic manifestations of HIV infection are relevant to the prognosis of HIV-infected patients with KS. The most commonly applied staging classification for KS, which takes these factors into account, is the TIS system proposed in 1989 by the AIDS Clinical Trials Group (ACTG) Oncology Committee[5] (Table 59-1). This staging system divides patients into good-risk or poor-risk groups according to extent of tumor, immune system status measured by CD4+ T-lymphocyte count, and symptoms of systemic HIV-associated illness. An analysis of 294 consecutive patients entered into eight ACTG KS therapy trials between 1989 and 1995 showed that each of the TIS variables was significantly associated with survival.[6] In a multivariate analysis, the level of CD4+ T lymphocytes and tumor extent were the only significant factors predicting survival.[6] In this analysis, a CD4 T-lymphocyte count of 150/μL provided better discrimination between good- and

Table 59-1 AIDS-Associated Kaposi Sarcoma Staging and Prognosis

ACTG Prognostic Categories[a]	Validation Studies: Pre-HAART[b]	Validation Studies: Post-HAART[c]
	Univariate Analyses	
T: Tumor extent	**Median survival:**	**3-Year survival:**
T_0: Confined to skin and/or lymph nodes minimal (non-nodular) oral cavity lesions	T_0: 27 mos $P < 0.001$ T_1: 15 mos	T_0: 85% $P = 0.007$ T_1: 69%
T_1: Extensive oral KS and/or symptomatic tumor-associated edema or ulceration and/or non-nodal visceral KS	I_0: 40 mos $p < 0.001$ I_1: 13 mos	I_0: 83% $P = 0.06$ I_1: 71%
I: Immune status I_0: CD4 count ≥200/μL I_1: CD4 count <200/μL	S_0: 22 mos $P = 0.04$ S_1: 16 mos	S_0: 83% $P = 0.003$ S_1: 63%
	Multivariate Analyses	
S: HIV-related systemic illness S_0: KPS[e] ≥70; no B symptoms;[f] no AIDS-defining illnesses or thrush S_1: KPS <70; B symptoms; any AIDS-defining illness or thrush	T_0I_0: Not reached[d] T_0I_0: 35 mos $P < 0.001$ $T_{any}I_1$: 13 mos	T_0S_0 : 88% T_1S_0: 80% $P = 0.0001$ T_0S_1: 81% T_1S_1: 53%

[a]Adapted from Krown SE, Metroka C, Wernz JC, Kaposi's sarcoma, in the acquired immune deficiency syndrome: a proposal for uniform evaluation, response and staging criteria. J Clin Oncol 7: 1201, 1989.
[b]Adapted from Krown WE, Testa MA, Huang J. AIDS-related Kaposi sarcoma: propective validation of the AIDS clinical trial group staging classification. J Clin Oncol 15: 3085, 1997.
[c]Adapted from Nasti G, Talamini R, Antinori A, et al. AIDS-related Kaposi sarcoma evaluation of potential new prognostic factors and assessment of the AIDS clinical trial group staging system in the HAART era – the Italian Cooperative Group on AIDS and Tumors and the Italian Cohort of Patients Naive From Antiretrovirals. J Clin Oncol 21: 2876, 2003.
[d]For this analysis, I_0 was defined as a CD4 lymphocyte count of ≥150 cells/μL and I_1 was defined as a CD4 lymphocyte count of <150 cells/μL, which gave better discrimination between the good- and poor-risk groups than the previous cut-off point of 200 cells/μL.
[e]KPS, Karnofsky performance status.
[f]B symptoms are unexplained night sweats or fever, >10% unexplained weight loss, or unexplained diarrhea lasting 2 weeks or more.

poor-risk groups than the originally recommended cut-off point of 200 cells/μL. A more recent multivariate analysis of prognostic factors conducted after the introduction of highly active antiretroviral therapy (HAART) identified extent of KS and systemic HIV-associated symptoms as the most important predictors of survival, and established pulmonary KS as a particularly poor prognostic feature.[7] Little information exists, however, about the factors predicting response to KS therapy or if TIS staging is a useful guide to the choice of therapy. Studies are underway to determine whether either the HIV-1 viral RNA level or the HHV-8 DNA level adds to the predictive value of TIS staging with respect to survival or response to treatment.

DIAGNOSIS

Although a presumptive diagnosis of KS may be based on visual identification of typical red or violaceous skin or oral lesions in a patient at risk (Fig. 59-1), biopsy of at least one lesion is important for establishing the diagnosis and distinguishing KS from other pigmented skin lesions such as bacillary angiomatosis.[8] A diagnosis of GI or pulmonary KS may be more difficult to establish. KS may occur throughout the GI tract and sometimes occurs in the absence of cutaneous or oral disease.[9] Although estimates of the frequency of GI KS have ranged from 40% at the time of KS diagnosis to 80% in autopsy series,[10,11] it is frequently asymptomatic, and there is no evidence that the presence of asymptomatic GI lesions adversely affects prognosis or response to treatment. Therefore, it is currently recommended that patients be evaluated for the presence of GI KS only when symptoms (e.g., pain, occult or gross bleeding, dysphagia, obstructive signs) are present. Endoscopy is generally required for diagnosis, as KS lesions are often submucosal and not easily visualized on contrast radiographs or scans, which are nondiagnostic. Upper or lower GI endoscopy (or both) permits direct visualization of the red lesions in the esophagus, stomach, duodenum, or colon; digital rectal examination often discloses lesions in the anorectal area. Although endoscopic biopsy of typical KS lesions may confirm the diagnosis pathologically, superficial biopsies sometimes yield only normal mucosa, especially when the lesions are not ulcerated. In the presence of pathologically confirmed KS elsewhere in the body, however, the visual identification of typical lesions in the GI tract can be considered presumptive evidence of GI KS.

Pulmonary KS is generally seen as a late complication of KS, but on rare occasions the lung is the initial or sole site of KS. KS may present as intrathoracic adenopathy or involve the pleural surfaces, the lung parenchyma, and the bronchial tree. Pulmonary KS usually, but not invariably, causes symptoms that may include dyspnea, cough, or hemoptysis, although gross bleeding is uncommon. The radiographic picture may include enlarged hilar and mediastinal lymph nodes, pleural effusions, diffuse interstitial or alveolar infiltrates, poorly defined nodules, or some combination of these

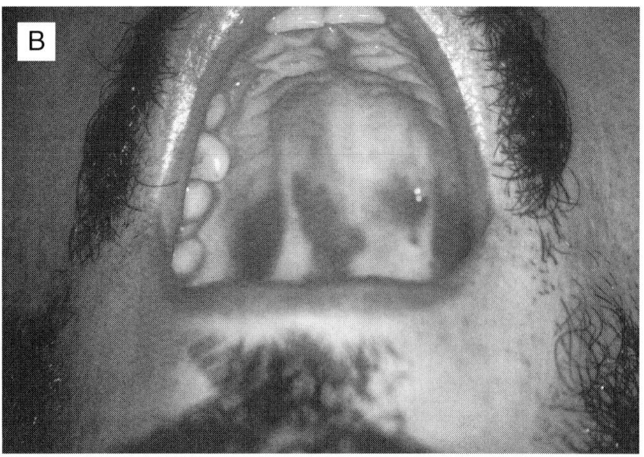

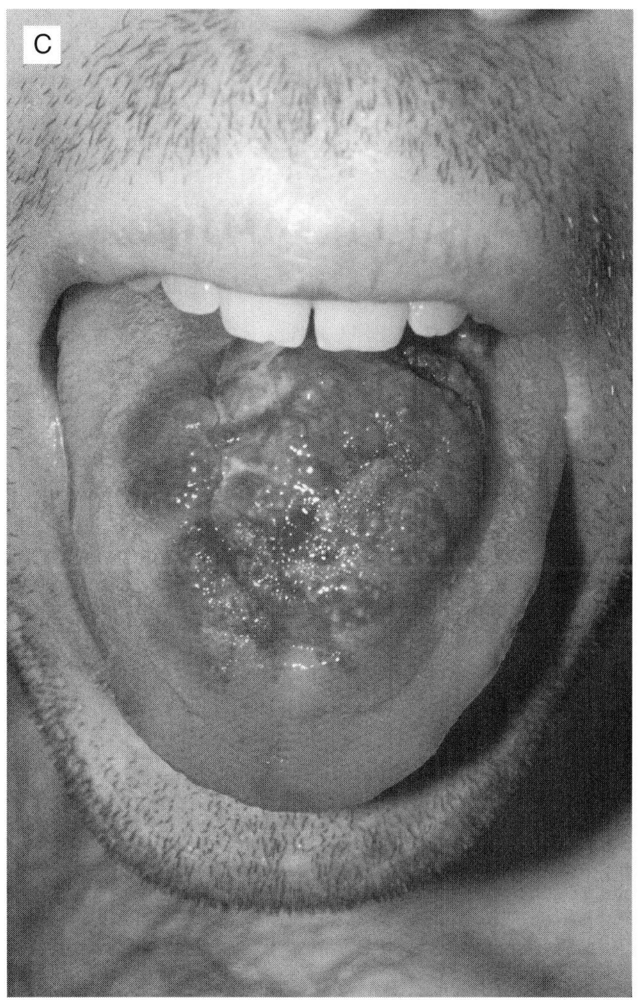

Figure 59-1 ■ (A) Cutaneous KS. Note multiple, pale macules on the back and darker red nodules on the posterior arms. (B) KS of the hard palate. Note both flat and nodular areas of involvement. (C) Nodular, exophytic KS of the tongue.

features (Fig. 59-2A), although some patients with endobronchial lesions have normal plain films despite prominent respiratory symptoms.[12] Bronchoscopy is the diagnostic procedure of choice because it allows direct visualization of red endobronchial lesions (when present), and coexisting infectious diseases can be diagnosed or excluded. When endobronchial lesions are not present, however, a definitive diagnosis of KS may not be possible, as transbronchial biopsies often do not yield diagnostic tissue.[13] Gallium (or combined gallium–thallium) scanning has been advocated as a technique to distinguish pulmonary KS from other neoplastic or infectious conditions.[14] KS has been reported to be gallium-negative and thallium-positive, whereas infections or other inflammatory diseases of the lung typically show the opposite pattern. In practice, however, thallium scanning is not widely used and false-negative gallium scans have been documented in patients with various opportunistic infections. A negative gallium scan alone is therefore not sufficient to exclude infectious causes of an abnormal radiograph, particularly in a febrile patient. In an afebrile patient with an established KS diagnosis, however, a negative gallium scan together with a negative infection workup (including bronchoscopy) and compatible radiographs may be accepted as presumptive evidence of pulmonary KS. Rarely, open lung biopsy or computed tomography (CT)-guided needle biopsy is required to establish a diagnosis of pulmonary KS, particularly when the differential diagnosis suggests other neoplasms or infections. CT scans offer better definition of pulmonary KS involvement than plain radiographs[12] and are helpful for following the response to treatment, especially in patients with poorly defined lesions on routine films. Typically, KS nodules show a peribronchovascular distribution on CT and are larger than one centimeter in diameter (Fig. 59-2B).[15]

THERAPY OF AIDS-ASSOCIATED KS

Management of HIV Infection

A successful KS management strategy includes optimal antiretroviral therapy for the stage of HIV infection and prophylaxis for, and prompt recognition and treatment of, opportunistic infections. There are several reasons to believe that HIV suppression is a critical component of KS management. The observation that KS sometimes regresses after initiation of potent antiretroviral regimens suggests that in some cases a decrease in immunosuppression, pathologic immune activation, and/or HIV replication may be sufficient to control KS. Although it is attractive to speculate that the development of anti-KSHV immune reconstitution accounts for KS regression, in one study a sustained increase in anti-KSHV-specific CD8+ T-lymphocyte cell responses required more than 12 months of antiretroviral therapy,[16] whereas KS regression often occurs much earlier, so other mechanisms may be involved. KS spindle cell proliferation *in vitro* is stimulated by inflammatory cytokines,[17,18] whose production is increased in the setting of acute opportunistic infections and active HIV replication. It has also been suggested that the HIV Tat protein may stimulate KS lesion development and growth. Tat has been shown to act synergistically with growth factors to increase KS cell proliferation *in vitro*[19,20] and to accelerate formation of KS-like tumors in

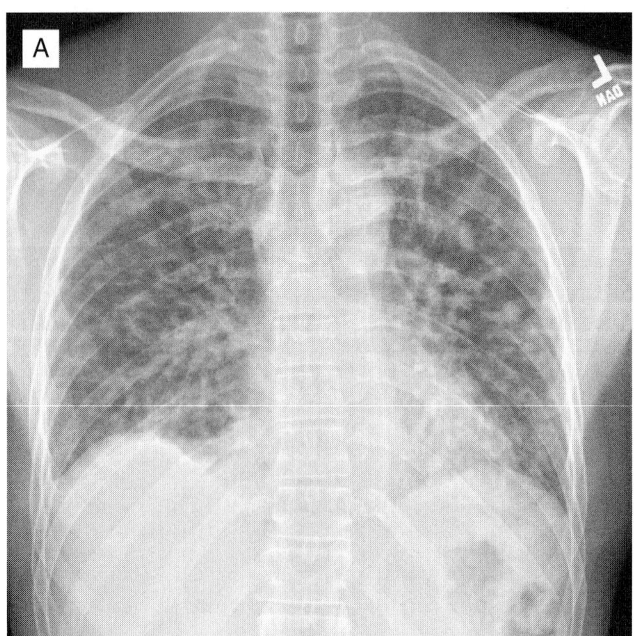

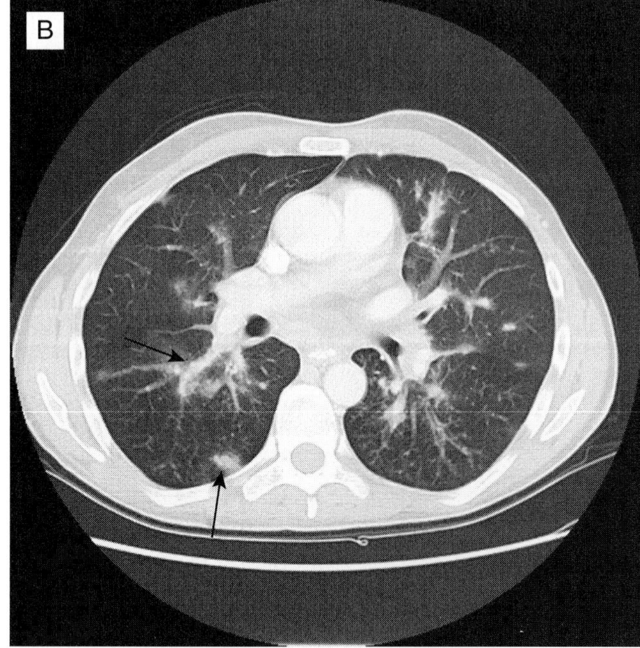

Figure 59-2 ■ (A) Chest radiograph from a patient with biopsy-proven pulmonary KS, showing bilateral reticular-nodular opacities; discrete nodules are more evident in the left lateral lung. (B) CT image of the chest from a patient with pulmonary KS showing scattered peripheral nodular opacities, extensive nodularity along the bronchovascular bundles and increased interstitial markings.

transgenic mice that express the KSHV G protein-coupled receptor (GPCR), a virally encoded chemokine receptor that is believed to play an important role in the development of KS.[21] Additionally, direct angiogenesis-inhibitory effects of certain protease inhibitors have been described in experimental models.[22] Although there is no evidence that potent antiretroviral regimens that do not include an HIV-1 protease inhibitor are less effective than protease inhibitor-containing regimens in their ability to prevent KS development,[23] there is conflicting and largely anecdotal data on the relative efficacy of protease inhibitor-based and non-nucleoside reverse transcriptase inhibitor-based antiretroviral regimens in controlling established KS.[24,25]

The foregoing observations support optimization of HIV suppression as part of the management strategy for all patients presenting with KS. In the setting of a relatively low tumor burden and the absence of highly symptomatic or life-threatening KS, a trial of antiretroviral therapy can be considered before specific anti-KS therapy is instituted. It should be emphasized, however, that successful control of HIV replication does not invariably lead to KS regression, and specific KS therapy may need to be administered. Although there is only anecdotal evidence that antiretroviral therapy alone leads to regression of advanced KS in the absence of concomitant chemotherapy,[26] there is clearer evidence that potent antiretroviral therapy prolongs the time to treatment failure for patients receiving local or systemic KS therapy.[27,28] Additionally, in a small proportion of patients, KS lesions may initially develop or progress more rapidly after starting effective potent antiretroviral therapy; this is considered a manifestation of the immune reconstitution inflammatory syndrome.[29–31]

Local Therapy

For limited, slowly progressive disease without life-threatening organ involvement, local therapy aimed at the control of individual lesions is suitable in some cases. Local approaches are most appropriate for patients who have relatively few, small lesions but may also be suitable for patients with more widespread disease who have contraindications to systemic therapy but in whom control of certain lesions for cosmetic or functional reasons is needed.

Several studies that investigated topical application of a 9-*cis*-retinoic acid (alitretinoin; Panretin) gel[32,33] provided the basis for US Food and Drug Administration (FDA) approval of this agent for KS treatment. In one vehicle-controlled trial in which cutaneous lesions were treated two to four times daily, 35% of patients who received a 12-week course of 0.1% 9-*cis*-retinoic acid gel and 18% of patients treated with the vehicle gel showed an objective response ($P = 0.002$). The responses were partial in all but one patient. With longer treatment, additional responses were observed with 9-*cis*-retinoic acid gel. Application-site reactions (erythema, pain, pruritus, flaking, desquamation, crusting, swelling) were common but were rarely severe.[33]

Before the introduction of 9-*cis*-retinoic acid gel, the most commonly used local approaches were liquid nitrogen cryotherapy[34] and intralesional injections of vinblastine.[35] There are few published studies on response rates or the characteristics of lesions best suited to these types of local therapy. In one study[35] a single intralesional injection of vinblastine was administered to 33 lesions in 11 patients. The size of the treated lesions was not specified. Of the 33 injected lesions, 20 (61%) showed complete clinical response, and nine others (27%) showed partial regression. Raised (papular or nodular) lesions became macular after treatment, but nearly all the lesions healed with postinflammatory hyperpigmentation. Of 12 regressed lesions observed 4–7 months after treatment, five (42%) had relapsed, and three of four biopsy specimens from persistently 'regressed' lesions showed histologic evidence of residual KS. Transient (≤2 min) pain was associated with injection and was followed, after 6–48 h, by more severe aching pain that was generally relieved by non-narcotic analgesics. In another study[34] liquid nitrogen therapy was given to 61 lesions in 20 evaluable subjects. Each lesion received an average of three treatments (range one to eight) at 2- to 3-week intervals to allow for healing of local blisters. The average area of the treated lesions was relatively small, 68 mm^2 (range 10–230 mm^2). Based on the area of the residual tumor, 80% of the lesions showed a complete response, and 7% showed partial regression. An independent evaluation of pre- and post-treatment color slides for 44 lesions, however, was interpreted as complete absence of residual KS in 50% and partial response in 27% of lesions. Overall cosmetic results were scored as complete (normal skin) in 20.5% and partial (>50% improvement) in 50%. At a 6-month follow-up in 13 of the 20 subjects, only one showed progressive KS in a treated area. In addition to local blistering and crusting, no significant side effects were reported other than short-lived (≤1 h) local pain relieved by acetaminophen.

Several other locally injected agents have also been tested in small clinical trials, including recombinant interferon-alpha (IFN-α),[36] recombinant granulocyte/macrophage colony-stimulating factor (GM-CSF),[37] recombinant platelet factor 4,[38] and human chorionic gonadotropin.[39] Although all of these agents have been shown to induce local KS regression, there are no convincing data to support their superiority over the more commonly used local agents. Local injections of vinblastine and the sclerosing agent Sotradecol[40] have also been reported to induce regression of oral KS lesions. Local treatments have the advantage of inducing few systemic side effects and can often be completed quickly, yielding acceptable cosmetic results in some patients. The benefits of local treatment are confined to the treated lesions, however, and there is no evidence that local lesion control inhibits the development of new lesions elsewhere, so systemic therapy is often preferable for long-term disease control. Lesions may recur at treated sites, and local side effects may include pain, eschar formation, and hyper- or hypopigmentation.

Radiation Therapy

Radiation therapy (RT) is most often used to treat KS of the skin and oral cavity and less frequently to treat visceral KS.

A review of the literature on RT for KS reveals no uniform 'standard' approach.

In a prospectively randomized trial, Stelzer and Griffin[41] compared treatment of individual KS skin lesions with 6MeV electrons given as 800cGy in one fraction (a frequently recommended regimen[42]), 2000cGy in 10 fractions over 2 weeks, or 4000cGy in 20 fractions over 4 weeks to the palpable tumor with a 2cm margin. Complete resolution of the palpable lesion was significantly better for the fractionated (2000 or 4000cGy) regimens (79% and 83%) than for the single-dose (800cGy) regimen (50%); and complete resolution of residual pigmentation was significantly better for the 4000cGy regimen (43%) than for the 2000 or 800cGy regimen (8% for each). The 4000cGy regimen also led to a significantly longer median duration of lesion control (43 weeks) than 2000cGy (26 weeks) or 800cGy (13 weeks). Acute toxicity was somewhat higher in the 4000cGy lesions, but this was limited to mild erythema, dry desquamation, local alopecia, and hyperpigmentation. These data suggest that the type of RT should be individualized based on the intent of treatment and the overall health status of the patient. If long-term cosmesis is the primary objective, a 4000cGy regimen over a protracted course is optimal. However, for lesions of lesser cosmetic importance or for treating extremely ill or symptomatic patients who have limited mobility or a short overall life expectancy, a more rapid fractionation regimen may produce acceptable local results without the need for repeated treatment visits over many weeks. In addition, the 4000cGy regimen was subsequently reported in one patient to be associated with a radiation recall reaction when bleomycin was administered, whereas there was no reaction in other lesions in the same patient that had been treated with 800 or 2000cGy.[43] Thus for patients in whom a future need for systemic chemotherapy is anticipated, the more rapid fractionation regimens may be associated with a lower risk of recall reactions.

RT of more extensive KS, such as diffusely involved extremities, with or without edema, usually requires larger photon fields. Severe local reactions (skin erythema, pain, desquamation of the skin on the soles of the feet) were observed in five of seven patients who received 2000cGy to the feet over 2 weeks.[44] Berson et al[42] observed a lower incidence of high-grade local reactions with a single 800cGy fraction to treat KS of the foot. Stelzer (personal communication) suggested, however, that lower doses per fraction and a planned rest period may allow delivery of higher total doses without severe acute reactions and may avoid later radiation-induced edema from subcutaneous fibrosis. Although KS-associated edema is often reduced with RT, its resolution is rarely complete.[42,44]

Although oral KS has also been treated successfully with RT, patients with HIV infection have sometimes been noted to have unusual radiation sensitivity of normal tissues. Oral radiation using 4MeV photons at 180cGy daily for 9 days (total 1620cGy), was reported by Chak et al[44] to be associated with severe mucositis, mouth dryness, and altered sense of taste, which was decreased but not eliminated by lowering the total dose to 1400cGy. Berson et al[42] also reported a high incidence of severe mucositis when the oropharynx was treated with high-dose fractions (180–400cGy) to total doses of 2000–2400cGy. The severity was decreased by using 150cGy fractions to a total dose of 1500cGy.[42] Stelzer (personal communication) has advocated using 150cGy fractions 5 days a week for 10 doses to the oral cavity, followed by a 1-week scheduled break in therapy to reduce the risk of mucositis. Patients may then be given as many as five additional fractions, depending on tolerance. Tumor shrinkage is rapid with oral RT and can induce rapid relief of symptoms from bulky lesions. Systemic therapy is also effective for many patients with oral KS, so the decision to choose local RT or systemic therapy may depend on whether other indications for systemic KS treatment coexist with the oral disease.

Although chemotherapy is a more common approach to symptomatic lung or GI tract involvement, RT has also been used to treat selected patients with visceral KS. Berson et al[42] reported responses in 88% of patients treated with involved field photons to GI lesions located mainly in the anorectum, and they described relief of obstructive symptoms in two patients with upper GI lesions. Rapid subjective improvement has also been reported[42,45] in patients with pulmonary KS who received whole-lung radiation, generally in 150cGy fractions to total doses of 900–1500cGy. Meyer[45] reported a significant reduction in hemoptysis and need for supplemental oxygen, but only 28% of patients with radiographic abnormalities showed a 50% or more reduction in measurable lesions.

IFN Therapy

IFNs have the potential to influence many of the complex processes involved in the growth of KS[17,46] through their antiviral effects and multiple effects on cell growth and function. Recombinant IFNs-α2a (Roferon-A) and α2b (Intron-A) were approved for the treatment of certain patients with AIDS-associated KS on the basis of studies performed before the introduction of antiretroviral drugs. The approved doses were therefore based on the results of studies of IFN as a single agent in which extremely high doses (e.g., 36 million units daily, or 30 million units/m^2 three times a week) were required to achieve KS regression. The use of such doses was often complicated by fatigue, malaise, anorexia, and hepatotoxicity. In those early studies the overall tumor response rates were ~30%. Responses were usually observed only in patients with CD4+ T-lymphocyte counts of 200/μL or more who had no history of opportunistic infection and who lacked other signs and symptoms of advanced HIV infection. In patients with these 'good risk' features, regression of extensive cutaneous, oral, or GI KS was sometimes observed.[47] Median response durations were 6–12 months for partial responders and up to 2 years among complete responders.

Subsequently, IFN was generally administered in combination with antiretroviral agents and at lower doses. Although combined IFN and chemotherapy regimens have been poorly tolerated and have not yielded superior therapeutic results,[48–50] improved results have been described when IFN-α was combined, at lower doses than those used for monotherapy, with nucleoside reverse transcriptase inhibitors. Several phase I studies that combined IFN-α with zidovudine demonstrated KS response rates exceeding 40% in patients treated with IFN-α doses ranging from 4 million to 18 million IU/day.[51–53] These high response rates were confirmed in a phase II trial of the combination, which used a daily IFN dose of 18 million IU and a zidovudine dose of 100 mg every 4 h.[54] The IFN-α–zidovudine combination induced KS regression in 25–30% of patients with CD4+ T-lymphocyte counts less than 200/μL,[51,54] whereas fewer than 10% of such patients responded to high-dose IFN-α monotherapy.[48] Although the dose-limiting neutropenia frequently seen with the combination[51–54] could be prevented or reversed by administration of GM-CSF,[55,56] later trials evaluated IFN in combination with less myelosuppressive antiretroviral drugs. In one such trial (ACTG 206) patients were randomly assigned to receive IFN-α at a dose of either 1 million or 10 million IU/day together with standard doses of didanosine. Similar rates of objective tumor regression were observed in both dosage groups, but the lower dose was significantly better tolerated.[57] More recently, a phase I study conducted by the AIDS Malignancy Consortium (AMC 004) evaluated the safety and maximum tolerated dose of IFN-α2b in combination with protease inhibitor-based combination antiretroviral therapy.[58] Dose-limiting toxicities were neutropenia and malaise. The maximum tolerated IFN dose was 5 million IU/day. The median CD4+ T-lymphocyte count increased from 260/μL at baseline to a maximum on-study value of 359/μL. In six patients with paired baseline and on-study values, the median HIV RNA level decreased from 20 179 copies/mL to a minimum on-study value of 309 copies/mL. Of 13 patients whose KS response could be evaluated, five (38%) showed objective tumor regression. Responses occurred in both HAART-experienced and HAART-naive subjects.[58]

Maximal responses to IFN-α, alone or combined with antiretroviral therapy, often require 6 months or more of treatment. Thus despite documented activity in some patients with visceral disease, IFN probably should not be considered for treating patients with rapidly progressive KS, particularly those with symptomatic visceral involvement. Because responses to IFN may persist for several years, however, it can be considered for patients with more slowly progressive KS when rapid relief of symptoms is not urgently required. It remains to be seen whether IFN combined with potent antiretroviral regimens will prove superior to other available KS therapies for certain subsets of patients. Polyethylene glycol-conjugated (PEG) IFN-α has a long half-life, requires only weekly administration, and has been tolerated in HIV+ patients with hepatitis C; it may prove more acceptable to patients who find it difficult to adhere to a frequent injection schedule, but has not yet been tested in KS.

Chemotherapy

Chemotherapy is indicated for patients with advanced or rapidly progressive KS that causes medical or functional impairment. This group includes patients with extensive or symptomatic cutaneous disease, extensive oral disease, symptomatic tumor-associated edema, pulmonary KS, or symptomatic GI KS. The goals of such therapy are to rapidly induce durable regression of widespread, disfiguring, or disabling lesions; control or reverse life-threatening visceral disease; reduce functional impairment caused by edema or mucocutaneous disease; and achieve these benefits with agents that have an acceptable side-effect profile. In addition, because such patients often have an advanced HIV infection, chemotherapy should not interfere with delivery of treatment with antiretroviral drugs or treatment and prophylaxis for other opportunistic complications of AIDS. It should be noted, however, that most trials of chemotherapeutic agents were conducted in patients with extremely low CD4+ T-lymphocyte counts, and a low CD4+ T-lymphocyte count should not preclude systemic therapy when its use is otherwise warranted.

A wide variety of single chemotherapeutic agents and drug combinations have shown activity against AIDS-related KS. Only three such agents; liposomal daunorubicin (DaunoXome), liposomal doxorubicin (Doxil), and paclitaxel (Taxol), have been reviewed and approved by the FDA specifically for KS treatment. Although these three drugs are now considered standard treatments for KS, knowledge of earlier treatment regimens may be valuable in resource-limited settings where the newer drugs may not be available.

Single agents with reported activity include etoposide,[59–64] vinblastine,[65] vincristine,[66] bleomycin,[57–69] and doxorubicin,[70–72] each of which has been studied alone or as part of combination regimens in multiple clinical trials. In addition, single clinical trials have indicated anti-KS activity for teniposide,[73] vinorelbine,[74] and epirubicin.[75] Despite their demonstrated activity, with reported objective response rates as high as 76%, and averaging over 40%, disease control by these agents has often been limited by their toxicities, the most common of which are alopecia, mucositis, and neutropenia with etoposide and doxorubicin; neutropenia with vinblastine; peripheral neuropathy from vincristine; and fever and cutaneous and cumulative pulmonary toxicities from bleomycin. High cumulative doses of doxorubicin are also associated with cardiac toxicity. The reported response rates and response durations for these agents are difficult to interpret or compare, as patient characteristics and response definitions varied from study to study, the use of antiretroviral therapy and infection prophylaxis was inconsistent, the methods of disease documentation and response definitions were often ambiguous and inconsistently applied, and with rare exception the studies were not controlled.

Before the introduction of liposomal anthracyclines and paclitaxel, combination chemotherapy was generally considered to induce higher response rates than single-agent therapy but at the expense of increased toxicity, which often limited long-term use. Nonetheless, by the early 1990s combination therapy was considered the standard of care. The ABV regimen[71] combining doxorubicin (Adriamycin), bleomycin, and vincristine, was most commonly used in the United States.

Several variations of the ABV regimen were used, with and without concomitant antiretroviral therapy and hematopoietic growth factor support,[71,72,76–80] but the most commonly used regimen was doxorubicin 20 mg/m^2, bleomycin 10 U/m^2, and vincristine 1 mg, administered every 2 weeks. Other frequently used combinations included bleomycin and vincristine,[81,82] which was more widely used than ABV as a standard regimen outside the United States, and vinblastine alternating with vincristine on a weekly schedule.[83] Several more-intensive chemotherapy regimens were tested,[84,85] but they generally induced unacceptable toxicity without a corresponding increase in therapeutic activity or response duration. The results of trials with chemotherapy combinations have been extensively reviewed elsewhere;[46,86,87] their use has largely been supplanted by the liposomal anthracyclines and paclitaxel. Although high response rates, averaging in excess of 60%, were reported for these regimens, the same caveats described for interpretation of the reported results for single-agent therapy apply to the combination regimens. Notably, much lower response rates were observed for combination chemotherapy when these regimens were tested in randomized, controlled trials in comparison with liposomal anthracyclines in which more stringent response criteria were applied (discussed later). In addition, all of these regimens were tested before the introduction of HAART; their activity in combination with current antiretroviral regimens is unknown.

The first chemotherapeutic agents approved by the FDA specifically for treatment of advanced AIDS-related KS were Doxil and DaunoXome.[87,88–99] The liposomal formulations prolong the circulating half-life of the anthracyclines (hours vs minutes for the unencapsulated drugs), increase drug concentrations in tumor tissue, and modify their toxicities.[98,100,101] Neutropenia is frequently induced by these agents,[90,91,102,103] but alopecia, nausea, and vomiting, which are common after administration of free doxorubicin, are uncommon with the liposomal agents.[102,104,105] Anthracycline-induced cardiac toxicity has been observed rarely after administration of high cumulative doses to patients with KS,[98,106,107] but maximum safe cumulative doses have not been defined. Doxil (but not DaunoXome) treatment has sometimes been associated with the hand-foot syndrome (palmar-plantar erythrodysesthesia).[108] This reaction, consisting of painful erythema and desquamation of the palms and soles, is generally associated with chemotherapeutic agents administered by continuous infusion. It is believed that the markedly increased serum half-life (~48 h) associated with the PEG-coated liposome used to formulate Doxil simulates a continuous drug infusion, whereas the uncoated liposome used to formulate DaunoXome has a $t_{1/2}$ of only ~4 h. Both Doxil and DaunoXome administration, on occasion, have been complicated by acute infusional reactions characterized by back or chest pain, a sensation of choking, and intense flushing.[109] The latter reaction usually occurs within minutes of starting treatment and generally subsides quickly after stopping the drug infusion.

Doxil was approved in 1995 for treatment of advanced KS after failure or intolerance of combination chemotherapy. Tumor response rates of 27% and 48%, respectively, were documented depending on whether a global disease assessment was used as the response criterion or the response was based on changes in selected indicator lesions. The median response durations were 2.4 and 2.3 months, respectively, from the time a partial response was recorded by these two assessment methods. Significantly, the lesions of some patients whose tumors had progressed on regimens containing conventional (unencapsulated) doxorubicin responded subsequently to Doxil. In practice, however, Doxil is most often used as first-line chemotherapy. The recommended dose and treatment schedule for Doxil is 20 mg/m^2 as a slow (30–60 min) intravenous infusion every 3 weeks. DaunoXome was approved in 1996 for first-line chemotherapy of advanced KS based on a randomized comparison with a standard ABV regimen[102] (described later). The labeled response rate is 23%, lasting a median of 3.7 months from the time a partial response was documented. The approved dose is 40 mg/m^2 every 2 weeks. Escalation to 60 mg/m^2 has sometimes induced responses in patients who did not respond or who relapsed after treatment at the lower dose. The 60 mg/m^2 dose has also proven effective for patients with pulmonary KS.[99] Objective response rates reported in the literature for these agents have varied widely. Some early reports in relatively small numbers of patients suggested that response rates might be as high as 70–90% even in previously treated patients.[88–92,95–98] Larger multicenter trials that applied strict response criteria, however, have documented response rates between 25% and 59%.[94,102,103,110] Although strictly defined response rates may be somewhat lower than originally believed, many patients experience palliation of KS-associated symptoms without achieving 50% tumor regression. At the time these studies were conducted, standard evaluation criteria for KS did not specifically address clinical benefits of treatment (e.g., pain relief, increased mobility associated with reduced edema). A joint National Cancer Institute (NCI)/FDA/AMC initiative has attempted to address this gap. Revised evaluation criteria have been developed that quantitatively evaluate changes in KS-associated signs and symptoms that affect patient function and quality of life.[111] These clinical benefit assessments are now being tested prospectively. Additionally, a double-blind, randomized trial of Doxil and DaunoXome, with the primary aim of documenting clinical benefit in symptomatic KS patients, demonstrated clinical benefit (relief of KS-associated symptoms) in 80% of Doxil-treated patients and 63% of DaunoXome-treated patients, which were higher than the objective tumor response rates of 55% and 32%, respectively.[112]

Several prospectively randomized studies performed in the early 1990s, before the introduction of potent combination antiretroviral regimens, compared liposomal anthracyclines with conventional combination chemotherapy (Table 59-2). One study compared Doxil 20 mg/m^2 with ABV every 2 weeks. A significantly higher response rate was observed with Doxil (46%) than with ABV (25%).[103] A comparison of DaunoXome 40 mg/m^2 with ABV every 2 weeks showed comparable response rates, which were 25% and 28%,

Randomized Trials of Liposomal Anthracyclines vs Combination Chemotherapy in AIDS-Related Kaposi Sarcoma

Table 59-2

Treatments Compared	Dose and Schedule	Number Entered (Number Evaluable)	Objective Response Rate (Complete + Partial)	Reference
Liposomal Daunorubicin (DaunoXome)	40 mg/m^2 q2wk	117 (116)	25%	Gill et al[102]
			P = NS	
vs				
ABV[a]	A: 10 mg/m^2 q2wk B: 15 U q2wk V: 1 mg q2wk	115 (111)	28%	
Liposomal Doxorubicin (Doxil)	20 mg/m^2 q2wk	133 (133)	46%	Northfelt et al[103]
			$P < 0.001$	
vs				
ABV	A: 20 mg/m^2 q2wk B: 10 mg/m^2 q2wk V: 1 mg q2wk	125 (125)	25%	
Liposomal Doxorubicin (Doxil)	20 mg/m^2 q3wk	121 (116)	59%	Stewart et al[110]
			$P < 0.001$	
vs				
BV	B: 15 IU/m^2 q3wk V: 2 mg q3wk	120 (102)	23%	

[a]A: doxorubicin (Adriamycin); B: bleomycin; V: vincristine; NS: no significant difference; q: every; wk: weeks.

respectively.[102] A third study compared Doxil (20 mg/m^2) with the combination of bleomycin (15 U/m^2) and vincristine (2 mg).[110] Each regimen was given every 3 weeks. A significantly higher response rate was observed among patients who received Doxil (59%) than among those who received bleomycin and vincristine (23%).[110] In each of the three studies, patients who received the liposomal anthracycline showed a significantly lower incidence of peripheral neuropathy, nausea, and vomiting than those who received combination therapy. Doxil induced more neutropenia than bleomycin and vincristine, and more mucositis than ABV, but it was less likely than ABV to cause significant alopecia and severe neutropenia. Response rates in each of these randomized trials were considerably lower than those reported previously for both the liposomal anthracyclines (in uncontrolled trials) and for the standard combination regimens (in both single-arm and randomized studies); but as noted before, objective response rates are not necessarily the equivalent of clinical benefit.

To determine if Doxil might be more effective as part of a combination chemotherapy regimen, a randomized, multicenter trial (ACTG 286) compared biweekly Doxil alone (at a dose of 20 mg/m^2) to Doxil (at the same dose and schedule) in combination with bleomycin (10 U/m^2) and vincristine (1 mg) in patients with advanced KS who had received no prior chemotherapy. The two regimens induced almost identical response rates of similar duration, but the combination regimen induced significantly more and earlier toxicity than Doxil alone and was associated with a more rapid decline in quality of life.[93]

Although the studies leading to the FDA approvals of liposomal anthracyclines were conducted before the introduction of HAART, subsequent studies have specifically examined the efficacy of Doxil combined with these potent antiretroviral regimens. In one study of 54 patients, complete or partial KS responses were observed in 81.5% of patients after a median of 8 weeks.[113] CD4+ T-lymphocyte counts increased to a similar degree both in study patients and matched pairs with HIV-1 infection but without KS. In another study, 28 patients with moderate to advanced KS who were either HAART-naive or failing on their HAART regimen were randomly assigned to receive a new HAART regimen alone, or a new HAART regimen with Doxil.[114] At 48 weeks, a significantly higher response rate was observed among the patients who received combined therapy than among those who received HAART alone (76% vs 20%, P = 0.003). Ten patients who received HAART only eventually required Doxil treatment; seven of these had developed KS progression within the first 3 months of HAART monotherapy.[114]

Several studies have also shown paclitaxel to be highly active against KS. Paclitaxel is a mitotic spindle poison that promotes microtubulin formation[115] and leads to mitotic arrest.[116] Paclitaxel also inhibits cell chemotaxis and invasion induced by angiogenic factors.[117] HHV-8, the virus implicated in the development of KS, encodes a homolog of cellular Bcl-2, an antagonist of apoptosis, and both viral and cellular Bcl-2 mRNAs have been identified in KS biopsies.[118] Pertinently, paclitaxel has been shown to promote apoptosis and to downregulate Bcl-2 protein expression in KS cells *in vitro* and KS-like lesions in mice.[119] Two studies that used different doses and schedules of paclitaxel administration, but a similar planned dose intensity, were performed in patients with advanced, symptomatic KS, many of whom had visceral disease and tumor-associated edema.[120–122] Many of the patients had previously undergone systemic treatment for KS, and most had low CD4+ T-lymphocyte counts (median = 20/μL). Doses of 135 mg/m^2 every 3 weeks or 100 mg/m^2 every 2 weeks, each of which was administered as a 3-h infusion, induced objective response rates of 69% and 59%, respectively, in a total of 85 patients. Median response durations were 7–10 months from the start of treatment. Lesion regression was accompanied by alleviation of KS-associated edema and pain and an improved performance status; but treatment was complicated by significant myalgias, neutropenia, and alopecia in a high proportion of patients. Neutropenia was ameliorated by granulocyte colony-stimulating factor (G-CSF). On the basis of these findings, the FDA approved paclitaxel as second-line chemotherapy for advanced AIDS-related KS.

In addition to the adverse events noted above, paclitaxel may also cause peripheral neuropathy, a particular concern in HIV-infected patients, and was reported to induce excessive and unexpected toxicity in two patients who had previously tolerated the drug, when combined with a new antiretroviral drug regimen that included delavirdine and saquinavir.[123] Although a pharmacologic interaction between antiretroviral agents that inhibit cytochrome P450 enzymes and paclitaxel, which is metabolized by these enzymes, was hypothesized as the basis for this apparent interaction, a limited pharmacokinetic study failed to demonstrate any effect of indinavir, ritonavir, saquinavir, or nevirapine on paclitaxel metabolism.[124] The potential may exist to improve the efficacy and safety of paclitaxel, for example through the use of large macromolecule taxanes that prolong tumor exposure to active drug and minimize systemic exposure,[125] or by the addition of agents that inhibit cytoprotective pathways that are induced by paclitaxel[126] and activated in KS lesions.[127]

KS PATHOBIOLOGY AND ITS IMPLICATIONS FOR INVESTIGATIONAL THERAPY

Although several systemic and local approaches have proved effective in controlling the growth of KS lesions, a need still exists for more effective, less toxic therapeutic agents. Existing treatments are not invariably effective. In addition, KS may recur after effective treatment, and many of the available treatments are toxic or have the potential to interact pharmacologically with other drugs used to treat HIV infection and its non-neoplastic complications. Also, as the life expectancy of HIV-infected individuals increases, there is concern about the potential long-term consequences of treatment with cytotoxic drugs.

Recent advances in understanding the pathogenesis of KS and its relation to HIV infection have provided a framework for the rational development of more effective treatment strategies and underlie most current investigational approaches to this tumor. Although KS pathogenesis is as yet incompletely understood, studies of HHV-8 gene expression have provided insights into potential mechanisms by which the virus may induce KS lesion development, and these provide potential treatment targets.

As with other herpesviruses, HHV-8 expresses some genes during latency and others during lytic replication. A remarkable and unique feature of the viral genome is the presence of a large number of human gene homologs that encode proteins involved in cell-cycle regulation and signaling. During latent infection, three major genes are expressed that encode: a latency-associated nuclear antigen (LANA-1), which inhibits p53, thereby inhibiting apoptosis;[128] a viral cyclin, which prevents cell-cycle arrest by cyclin-dependent kinases and pRB;[129] and a viral FAS-ligand interleukin-1B-converting enzyme inhibitory protein (vFLIP) that protects latently-infected cells from apoptosis by preventing activation of the Fas death receptor pathway.[130] During HHV-8 lytic replication, additional gene products are transcribed that correspond to cellular proteins involved in cell-cycle progression, apoptosis, proliferation and immune regulation. These include the K1 protein, a viral Bcl-2 homolog, a viral GPCR (vGPCR), a viral homolog of interleukin (IL)-6, viral macrophage inflammatory proteins (vMIPs), and viral interferon regulatory factors.[131–135] Notably, mice transfected with the vGPCR develop vascular tumors resembling KS,[136] suggesting a key role in KS lesion development. Additionally, cells transfected with the vGPCR secrete vascular endothelial growth factor (VEGF),[135] an angiogenic growth factor that is overexpressed in KS lesions,[137] and show activation of the VEGF-receptor 2.[138] Expression of the vGPCR and K1 also activate nuclear factor κB (NFκB), which induces transcription of a number of angiogenic and proinflammatory mediators including VEGF and matrix metalloproteinases (MMP)-9.[131,133,134,139] Many of the proteins encoded by the HHV-8 genome are capable of inhibiting the human immune response to the virus. For example, vFLIP, by inhibiting activation of Fas, has been shown to block killing of HHV-8-infected cells by cytotoxic T cells;[140] vMIP-II may restrict recruitment of Th1 lymphocytes to HHV-8-infected cells;[141] K1 may prevent class 2 major histocompatibility complex (MHC)-mediated T cell activation by HHV-8;[142] and K3 and K5 block cell surface display of class 1 MHC molecules on the cell surface by enhancing their endocytosis.[143]

KS lesions are histologically pleomorphic and characterized by the presence of spindle cells, dilated vascular spaces containing extravasated erythrocytes, and mononuclear inflammatory cells. Most of the spindle cell population is infected with HHV-8. The majority of cells are latently infected, but a small subset expresses lytic cycle genes[144] and produce viral progeny.[145] The origin of the spindle cells has been the subject of controversy. Although recent data indicate that HHV-8 can infect both lymphatic and blood vessel cells *in vitro*, gene expression microarrays suggest that the neoplastic cells within KS biopsies are most closely related to lymphatic endothelial cells.[146] Spindle cells derived from KS lesions have been shown to express a variety of angiogenic/inflammatory cytokines and growth factors, which include VEGF, basic fibroblast growth factor (bFGF), interleukin-1 (IL-1), and IL-6, among others,[147,148] although recent data indicate that not all of these are overexpressed compared to normal skin.[146] However, KS cells overexpress receptors for multiple cytokines, including those for which the ligand is not overexpressed, suggesting that various cytokines may promote KS growth through autocrine or paracrine mechanisms.[146] KS cells also proliferate in response to exogenously administered cytokines, including IL-1, IFN-γ, IL-6, and tumor necrosis factor (TNF), which are present in excess in the serum of patients with poorly controlled HIV infection.[149] KS cells also overexpress MMPs,[150] which are enzymes involved in the destruction of extracellular matrix proteins required for angiogenesis and metastasis, and express high levels of the vitronectin receptor $\alpha_v\ \beta_3$, a vascular integrin that is strongly upregulated on activated endothelium.[151]

Although HIV infection is neither necessary nor sufficient to induce the development of KS, the presence of HIV infection is associated with an increased incidence of the tumor and alteration of its natural history. Along with several of the proteins encoded by HHV-8, the immunosuppression associated with HIV infection may contribute to an ineffective immune response directed against HHV-8. In addition, acute HIV infection of CD4+ T-lymphocyte cells results in extracellular release of the HIV transactivator protein Tat, which stimulates the *in vitro* growth of spindle cells derived from KS lesions.[152] KS-derived spindle cells become responsive to Tat's growth-promoting effects only in the presence of inflammatory cytokines and growth factors, which also stimulate spindle cell proliferation and migration.[152] In addition to their autocrine production by KS cells, the activated T cells and monocytes of individuals with poorly controlled HIV infection produce many of these factors. The Tat protein may mediate angiogenesis through two distinct regions: an RGD (Arg-Gly-Asp) region, which induces migration and invasion of KS by binding to integrins that are strongly expressed on KS-derived spindle cells, and a basic region, which allows release of a soluble form of bFGF that promotes vascular cell growth.[153] Tat is also capable of augmenting the angiogenesis-promoting activity of IFN-γ on endothelial cells, transactivating the IL-6 promoter, inducing phosphorylation of the Flk-1/KDR VEGF receptor, and increasing MMP-9 expression by monocytes, which may facilitate breakdown of tissue matrix and permit migration of growing tumor and vascular endothelial cells.[152–155] To what extent these Tat-mediated activities occur in patients with KS is not known, however.

Potential targets for KS therapy

BOX 59-1

- Angiogenic cytokines and growth factors (cellular/viral)
- Growth factor receptors
- Downstream signaling intermediates of growth factors and their receptors
- Endothelial cell proliferation
- Matrix metalloproteinase inhibitors
- Vascular integrins
- HHV-8 viral genes/proteins
- HIV (Tat; immunosuppression)

Attempts are being made to translate the growing understanding of KS pathogenesis into more effective targeted therapy (Box 59-1). The role of antiretroviral therapy directed against HIV has been discussed earlier in this chapter. Given the essential role of HHV-8 in KS development, attempts to target this virus are obvious. However, as HHV-8 is present primarily in latent form in the majority of cells in KS lesions, it is not surprising that attempts to treat established KS lesions with standard antiherpesvirus agents, which inhibit late lytic genes but not latent or early lytic genes, have met with only sporadic success. Anecdotal reports of KS regression after treatment with cidofovir[156,157] and foscarnet[158] have been published. However, despite studies demonstrating that cidofovir was one of the most active drugs against HHV-8 *in vitro*,[159–161] a prospective trial of cidofovir in seven KS patients failed to demonstrate antitumor activity or a decrease in HHV-8 virus load in the blood.[162] Nonetheless, administration of ganciclovir and foscarnet has been associated with a decreased subsequent risk of developing KS,[163–166] suggesting a potential role for agents of this type in KS prophylaxis. Given the toxicities of these drugs, however, and the difficulties in predicting who will develop KS, this approach is not currently feasible; the development of more accurate methods to detect HHV-8 infection and of better tolerated, orally bioavailable antiherpesvirus drugs may make this a more feasible approach, and could someday have practical implications where HHV-8 seroprevalence is high and where KS is a leading cause of cancer morbidity.

A more indirect approach targeting HHV-8 has been suggested by the observation that valproic acid, an orally bioavailable histone deacetylase inhibitor used as an anticonvulsant and mood stabilizer, could induce HHV-8 lytic gene expression in latently infected BCBL-1 cells at clinically achievable concentrations.[167] Expression of lytic viral genes could have therapeutic benefits for several reasons. First, induction of lytic infection could directly lead to cell death. Second, the cytotoxic T cell response to herpesviruses commonly targets viral lytic antigens, so induction of HHV-8 into lytic infection might make KS subject to cytotoxic T cell killing. The potential efficacy of this approach is currently being tested in a clinical trial.

Finally, HHV-8 viral genes represent unique, tumor-specific targets, and compounds directed against viral genes should have high selectivity and potentially less toxicity than agents targeting cellular proteins. Studies performed to evaluate HHV-8 expression profiles in KS biopsy samples showed that mRNAs for LANA, v-cyclin, vFLIP, kaposin (K1), and vIRF1 were consistently present in KS biopsies from 21 patients, whereas vGPCR and viral thymidine kinase (TK) were present in only a subset.[168] These findings form the basis for potential targeted therapies, and active screening for agents that target these widely expressed viral gene products is underway.

In addition to targeting HHV-8, there is a wealth of agents under investigation that have the potential to target factors induced by the virus, and which establish the angiogenic-inflammatory milieu required for KS development. Among the agents with reported anti-KS activity in preliminary studies are thalidomide,[169] which may limit angiogenesis through inhibition of TNF and through TNF-independent mechanisms; systemically administered 9-*cis*-retinoic acid;[170] COL-3, an MMP inhibitor;[171,172] IL-12,[173] which induces production of IFN-γ, stimulates growth of T cells and natural killer (NK) cells, promotes Th1-type helper T cell responses and inhibits angiogenesis; and TNP-470,[174,175] an inhibitor of endothelial cell proliferation.

Other targeted therapeutic approaches include agents that interfere with tyrosine kinase-mediated transmembrane receptor signals for angiogenic growth factors. The example of a recent study with imatinib mesylate is considered here in detail, as it exemplifies the rationale behind this approach. Various observations suggest that both the platelet-derived growth factor receptor (PDGF-R) and c-kit play important roles in KS development. KS spindle cells express PDGF-Rs and their ligand, PDGF, is expressed by a distinct subpopulation of KS spindle cells.[176,177] KS spindle cell growth *in vitro* is arrested in PDGF-depleted medium, which can be reversed by addition of recombinant PDGF.[176,178] PDGF also induces expression of VEGF by KS spindle cells.[179] KSHV infection of dermal microvascular endothelial cells (DMVEC) results in upregulation of the c-kit receptor;[180] and KSHV-infected DMVEC proliferate in response to the c-kit ligand (stem-cell factor), which is constitutively expressed by DMVEC;[180] c-kit expression in KS lesions has been also been demonstrated by immunohistochemistry.[181]

Based on these observations, Koon and colleagues conducted a pilot study of imatinib in patients with AIDS/KS.[182] Imatinib is an orally bioavailable tyrosine kinase signal transduction inhibitor approved by the FDA for treatment of chronic myeloid leukemia (CML) and gastrointestinal stromal tumor (GIST). In preclinical studies, imatinib was found to be a potent inhibitor of BCR-ABL (involved in CML), as well as the c-kit receptor (activated in GIST) and PDGF-R. Gleevec has also shown activity against dermatofibrosarcoma protuberans and hypereosinophilic syndrome, which are dependent on the PDGF pathway.

In this study, partial responses were observed in five of 10 patients. In four patients from whom tumor biopsies were available, inhibition of PDGF-R expression and its downstream effector, extracellular receptor kinase (ERK), a member of the mitogen-activated protein kinase (MAPK; MEK) family was demonstrated. At the imatinib dose tested, which had been well tolerated in other clinical settings, six patients required dosage reduction because of diarrhea.[182] As imatinib is a substrate for the CYP3A4 and CYP2D6 cytochrome p450 isoforms, this could have been a result of pharmacologic interactions between imatinib and antiretroviral drugs, many of which induce and/or inhibit CYP3A4. These preliminary observations are being extended in a phase II clinical trial.

Additional approaches to KS treatment may include the use of antisense oligonucleotides or antibodies directed against growth factors implicated in KS pathogenesis (e.g., PDGF, VEGF, IL-6),[183] and agents directed against endothelial cell surface molecules expressed preferentially on proliferating vasculature, such as the $\alpha_v \beta_3$ integrin.[184] Although the multiple growth factors and receptors implicated in KS pathogenesis have disparate functions, they share a number of downstream signaling intermediates such as phosphatidylinositol 3-kinase (PI3K) and members of the MAPK family. The availability of specific receptor inhibitors and inhibitors of signaling intermediates, such as the mammalian target of rapamycin (mTOR), provide an opportunity to test the importance of these pathways in KS pathogenesis *in vivo*. For example, it has been reported recently that when sirolimus (rapamycin), which binds to and downregulates mTOR, was substituted for cyclosporin and mycophenolate mofetil to prevent graft rejection in kidney allograft recipients who developed KS, all 15 patients treated showed complete KS regression within 3 months.[185] Finally, a number of the growth factor pathways involved in KS activate NF-κB *in vitro*, which could be a therapeutic target. This is supported by observations that tumors associated with γ-herpesviruses (HHV-8, Epstein–Barr virus (EBV)) exhibit high constitutive NF-κB nuclear activity and that inhibition of NF-κB induces apoptosis.[186–188] The proteasome inhibitor bortezomib, an agent approved for use in the treatment of multiple myeloma, blocks NF-κB function and induces apoptosis in a wide variety of tumors,[189] and agents of this type can be considered as candidates for future trials in KS.

TREATMENT STRATEGY

Regression and symptom palliation of KS can be achieved with many drugs and techniques. Although long-term tumor regression has been achieved, in some patients the benefits of treatment may be temporary and KS treatment is not considered curative. The choice of therapy must be individualized. Factors to consider include the overall severity of the KS, the presence of specific KS-associated symptoms (e.g., edema, pain, dyspnea), the rate of KS progression, and the patient's treatment history. Individual patient goals and concerns (e.g., cosmetic issues or the desire to avoid particular treatment side effects) also require consideration. In addition, the degree to which the underlying HIV infection can be controlled, performance status, and the presence of

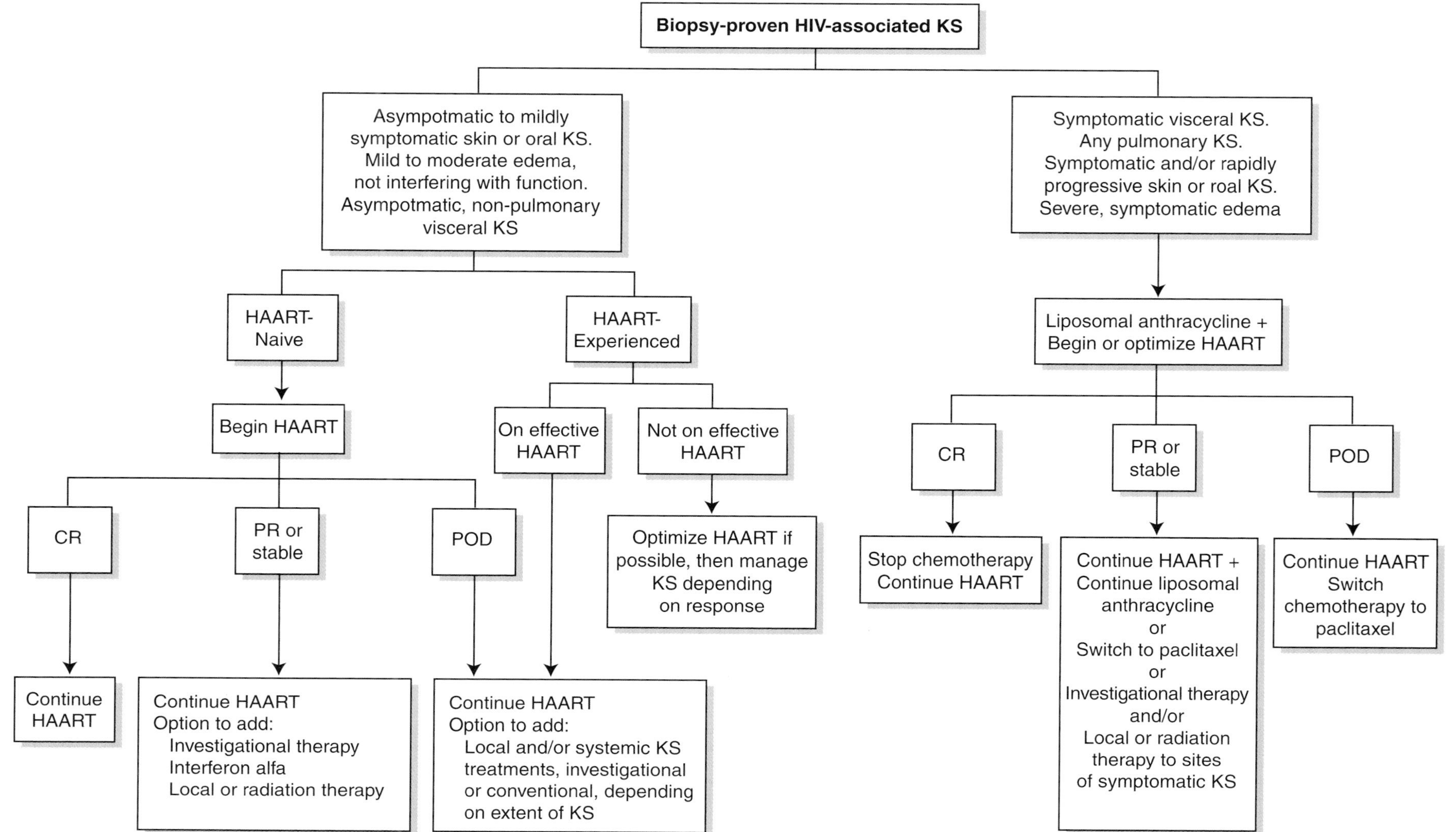

Figure 59-3 ■ Decision tree for management of KS. Antiretroviral therapy should be modified as required to manage HIV. There are no data to suggest, however, that changing antiretroviral therapy is a useful strategy to control progressive KS when HIV infection is otherwise well controlled.

concomitant conditions (e.g., neuropathy, wasting, chronic infections, abnormal hematologic, cardiac, hepatic, or pulmonary function) may also influence the therapeutic approach. A successful KS treatment strategy requires appropriate supportive care, including nutritional support, pain control, and hematopoietic colony stimulating factors to reverse treatment-associated anemia and neutropenia, in addition to standard treatments for HIV infection and treatment and prophylaxis of its non-neoplastic complications. Although adverse drug interactions have, on occasion, been described,[123] chemotherapeutic agents and standard antiretroviral regimens have, for the most part, been safely combined. As a rule, KS treatment and state-of-the-art antiretroviral regimens should be used concurrently, as effective HIV control appears to be associated with better KS response and response duration. Whenever possible, however, it may be prudent to avoid zidovudine, which may cause excessive hematologic suppression and increase the need for hematopoietic growth factors.

Figure 59-3 provides a decision tree for treatment of KS. This is intended as a general guide to the choice of therapy and, depending on the overall condition of the patient and the coexistence of multiple KS-related problems, various treatment approaches may have to be used sequentially or concurrently. In addition to standard KS treatments, the decision tree includes the option of referring patients for participation in investigational drug trials. This option should be considered especially for patients with relatively early KS whose lesions have not responded to HAART. Given the many drug trials that are based on the growing understanding of KS pathogenesis, together with the significantly poorer survival of patients with advanced KS even in the HAART era,[7] participation in such trials should be considered prior to the development of advanced, symptomatic disease when chemotherapy may be the only treatment option. In the long term, it is likely that early intervention, possibly with combinations of agents that influence the pathogenesis of this neoplasm, will provide the most effective approach to KS management.

REFERENCES

1. Centers for Disease Control. Kaposi's sarcoma and Pneumocystis pneumonia among homosexual men – New York City and California. MMWR Morb Mortal Wkly Rep 30:305, 1981.
2. Jones JL, Hanson DL, Dworkin MS, et al. Incidence and trends in Kaposi's sarcoma in the era of effective antiretroviral therapy. J Acquir Immune Defic Syndr 24:270, 2000.
3. Mbulaiteye SM, Katabira ET, Wabinga H, et al. Spectrum of cancers among HIV-infected persons in Africa: The Uganda AIDS-Cancer Registry Match Study. Int J Cancer 118:985, 2005.
4. Kaplan LD, Hopewell PC, Jaffe H, et al. Kaposi's sarcoma involving the lung in patients with the acquired immunodeficiency syndrome. J Acquir Immune Defic Syndr 1:23, 1988.
5. Krown SE, Metroka C, Wernz JC. Kaposi's sarcoma in the acquired immune deficiency syndrome: a proposal for uniform evaluation, response and staging criteria. J Clin Oncol 7:1201, 1989.
6. Krown WE, Testa MA, Huang J. AIDS-related Kaposi's sarcoma: prospective validation of the AIDS Clinical Trials Group staging classification. J Clin Oncol 15:3085, 1997.
7. Nasti G, Talamini R, Antinori A, et al. AIDS-related Kaposi's sarcoma: evaluation of potential new prognostic factors and assessment of the AIDS Clinical Trial Group staging system in the HAART era – the Italian Cooperative Group on AIDS and Tumors and the Italian Cohort of Patients Naive From Antiretrovirals. J Clin Oncol 21:2876, 2003.
8. Adal KA, Cockerell CJ, Petri WA Jr, et al. Cat scratch disease, bacillary angiomatosis, and other infections due to Rochalimaea. N Engl J Med 330:1509, 1994.
9. Barrison IG, Foster S, Harris JW, et al. Upper gastrointestinal Kaposi's sarcoma in patients positive for HIV antibody without cutaneous disease. BMJ 296:92, 1988.
10. Danzig JB, Brandt LJ, Reinus JF, et al. Gastrointestinal malignancy in patients with AIDS. Am J Gastroenterol 8:715, 1991.
11. Laine L, Amerian J, Rarick M, et al. The response of symptomatic gastrointestinal Kaposi's sarcoma to chemotherapy: a prospective evaluation using an endoscopic method of disease quantification. Am J Gastroenterol 85:959, 1990.
12. White DA. Pulmonary complications of HIV-associated malignancies. Clin Chest Med 17:755, 1996.
13. Meduri G, Stover D, Lee M, et al. Pulmonary Kaposi's sarcoma in the acquired immune deficiency syndrome: clinical, radiographic, and pathologic manifestations. Am J Med 81:11, 1986.
14. Lee V, Fuller J, O'Brien M, et al. Pulmonary Kaposi sarcoma in patients with AIDS: scintigraphic diagnosis with sequential thallium and gallium scanning. Radiology 180:409, 1991.
15. Edinburgh KJ Jasmer RM, Huang L, et al. Multiple pulmonary nodules in AIDS: usefulness of CT in distinguishing among potential causes. Radiology 214:427, 2000.
16. Bourboulia D, Aldam D, Lagos D, et al. Short- and long-term effects of highly active antiretroviral therapy on Kaposi's sarcoma-associated herpesvirus immune responses and viraemia. AIDS 18:485, 2004.
17. Karp JE, Pluda JM, Yarchoan R. AIDS-related Kaposi's sarcoma: a template for the translation of molecular pathogenesis into targeted therapeutic approaches. Hematol Oncol Clin North Am 10:1031, 1996.
18. Miles SA. Pathogenesis of AIDS-related Kaposi's sarcoma: evidence of a viral etiology. Hematol Oncol Clin North Am 10:1011, 1996.
19. Ensoli B, Barillari G, Salahuddin SZ, et al. Tat protein of HIV-1 stimulates growth of cells derived from Kaposi's sarcoma lesions of AIDS patients. Nature 345:84, 1990.
20. Ensoli B, Gendelman R, Markham P, et al. Synergy between basic fibroblast growth factor and HIV-1 Tat protein in induction of Kaposi's sarcoma. Nature 371:674, 1994.
21. Guo H-G, Pati S, Sadowska M, et al. Tumorigenesis by human herpesvirus 8 vGPCR is accelerated by human immunodeficiency virus type 1 Tat. J Virol 78:9336, 2004.
22. Monini P, Sgadari C, Barillari G, et al. HIV protease inhibitors: antiretroviral agents with anti-inflammatory, anti-angiogenic and anti-tumour activity. J Antimicrob Chemother 51:207, 2003.
23. Portsmouth S, Stebbing J, Gill J, et al. A comparison of regimens based on non-nucleoside reverse transcriptase inhibitors or protease inhibitors in preventing Kaposi's sarcoma. AIDS 17:F17, 2003.
24. Ridolfo AL, Corbellino M, Tosca N, et al. Is switching protease inhibitor-based effective antiretroviral therapy safe in patients with AIDS-associated Kaposi's sarcoma? AIDS 18:1224, 2004.
25. Bani-Sadr F, Fournier S, Molina JM. Relapse of Kaposi's sarcoma in HIV-infected patients switching from a protease inhibitor to a non-nucleside reverse transcriptase inhibitor-based highly active antiretroviral therapy regimen. AIDS 17:1580, 2003.
26. Krown SE. Highly active antiretroviral therapy in AIDS-associated Kaposi's sarcoma: implications for the design of therapeutic trials in patients with advanced, symptomatic Kaposi's sarcoma. J Clin Oncol 22:399, 2004.

27. Bower M, Fox P, Fife K, et al. Highly active anti-retroviral therapy (HAART) prolongs time to treatment failure in Kaposi's sarcoma. AIDS 13:2105, 1999.
28. Holkova B, Takeshita K, Cheng DM, et al. Effect of highly active antiretroviral therapy on survival in patients with AIDS-associated pulmonary Kaposi's sarcoma treated with chemotherapy. J Clin Oncol 19:3848, 2001.
29. Weir A, Wainsbrough-Jones M. Mucosal Kaposi's sarcoma following protease inhibitor therapy in an HIV-infected patient. AIDS 11:1895, 1997.
30. Connick E, Kane MA, White IE, et al. Immune reconstitution inflammatory syndrome associated with Kaposi sarcoma during potent antiretroviral therapy. Clin Infect Dis 39:1852, 2004.
31. Bower M, Nelson M, Young AM, et al. Immune reconstitution inflammatory syndrome associated with Kaposi's sarcoma. J Clin Oncol 23:5224, 2005.
32. Duvic M, Friedman-Kien AE, Looney DJ, et al. Topical treatment of cutaneous lesions of acquired immunodeficiency syndrome-related Kaposi sarcoma using alitretinoin gel: results of phase 1 and 2 trials. Arch Dermatol 136:1461, 2000.
33. Walmsley S, Northfelt DW, Melosky B, et al. Treatment of AIDS-related cutaneous Kaposi's sarcoma with topical alitretinoin (9-cis-retinoic acid) gel. J Acquir Immune Defic Syndr 22:235, 1999.
34. Tappero JW, Berger TG, Kaplan LD, et al. Cryotherapy for cutaneous Kaposi's sarcoma (KS) associated with acquired immune deficiency syndrome (AIDS): a phase II trial. J Acquir Immune Defic Syndr 4:839, 1991.
35. Boudreaux AA, Smith LL, Cosby CD, et al. Intralesional vinblastine for cutaneous Kaposi's sarcoma associated with acquired immunodeficiency syndrome: a clinical trial to evaluate efficacy and discomfort associated with injection. J Am Acad Dermatol 28:61, 1993.
36. Depuy J, Price M, Lynch G, et al. Intralesional interferon-alpha and zidovudine in epidemic Kaposi's sarcoma. J Am Acad Dermatol 28:966, 1993.
37. Boente P, Sampaio C, Brandáo MA, et al. Local perilesional therapy with rhGM-CSF for Kaposi's sarcoma. Lancet 341:1154, 1993.
38. Staddon A, Henry D, Bonnem E. A randomized dose finding study of recombinant platelet factor 4 (rPF4) in cutaneous AIDS-related Kaposi's sarcoma [abstract]. Proc Am Soc Clin Oncol 13:50, 1994.
39. Gill PS, Lunardi-Iskandar Y, Louie S, et al. The effects of preparations of human chorionic gonadotropin on AIDS-related Kaposi's sarcoma. N Engl J Med 335:1261, 1996.
40. Lucatoro FM, Sapp JP. Treatment of oral Kaposi's sarcoma with a sclerosing agent in AIDS patients: a preliminary study. Oral Surg Oral Med Oral Pathol 75:192, 1993.
41. Stelzer KJ, Griffin TW. A randomized prospective trial of radiation therapy for AIDS-associated Kaposi's sarcoma. Int J Radiat Oncol Biol Phys 27:1057, 1993.
42. Berson AM, Quivey JM, Harris JW, Wara WM. Radiation therapy for AIDS-related Kaposi's sarcoma. Int J Radiat Oncol Biol Phys 19:569, 1990.
43. Stelzer KJ, Griffin TW, Koh WJ. Radiation recall skin toxicity with bleomycin in a patient with Kaposi sarcoma related to acquired immune deficiency syndrome. Cancer 71:1322, 1993.
44. Chak LY, Gill PS, Levine AM, et al. Radiation therapy for acquired immunodeficiency syndrome-related Kaposi's sarcoma. J Clin Oncol 6:863, 1988.
45. Meyer JL. Whole-lung irradiation for Kaposi's sarcoma. Am J Clin Oncol 16:372, 1993.
46. Krown SE. Acquired immunodeficiency syndrome-associated Kaposi's sarcoma: biology and management. Med Clin North Am 81:471, 1997.
47. Real FX, Krown SE, Oettgen HF. Kaposi's sarcoma and the acquired immunodeficiency syndrome: treatment with high and low doses of recombinant leukocyte A interferon. J Clin Oncol 4:544, 1986.
48. Evans LM, Itri LM, Campion M, et al. Interferon-alpha 2a in the treatment of acquired immunodeficiency syndrome-related Kaposi's sarcoma. J Immunother 10:39, 1991.
49. Krigel RL, Slywotzky CM, Lonberg M, et al. Treatment of epidemic Kaposi's sarcoma with a combination of interferon-α2b and etoposide. J Biol Response Mod 7:359, 1988.
50. Shepherd FA, Evans WK, Garvey B, et al. Combination chemotherapy and α-interferon in the treatment of Kaposi's sarcoma associated with acquired immune deficiency syndrome. Can Med Assoc J 139:635, 1988.
51. Krown SE, Gold JWM, Niedzwiecki D, et al. Interferon-α with zidovudine: safety, tolerance, and clinical and virologic effects in patients with Kaposi's sarcoma associated with the acquired immunodeficiency syndrome (AIDS). Ann Intern Med 112:812, 1990.
52. Fischl MA, Uttamchandani R, Resnick L, et al. A phase I study of recombinant human interferon alfa-n1 and concomitant zidovudine in patients with AIDS-related Kaposi's sarcoma. J Acquir Immune Defic Syndr 4:1, 1991.
53. Kovacs JA, Deyton L, Davey R, et al. Combined zidovudine and interferon-α therapy in patients with Kaposi's sarcoma and the acquired immunodeficiency syndrome (AIDS). Ann Intern Med 111:280, 1989.
54. Fischl MA, Finkelstein DM, He W, et al. A phase II study of recombinant human interferon-α2a and zidovudine in patients with AIDS-related Kaposi's sarcoma. J Acquir Immune Defic Syndr Hum Retrovir 11:379, 1996.
55. Scadden DT, Bering HA, Levine JD, et al. Granulocyte-macrophage colony-stimulating factor mitigates the neutropenia of combined interferon alfa and zidovudine treatment of acquired immune deficiency syndrome-associated Kaposi's sarcoma. J Clin Oncol 9:802, 1991.
56. Krown SE, Paredes J, Bundow D, et al. Interferon-α, zidovudine and granulocyte-macrophage colony-stimulating factor: a phase I trial in patients with Kaposi's sarcoma associated with the acquired immunodeficiency syndrome (AIDS). J Clin Oncol 10:1344, 1992.
57. Krown SE, Li P, VonRoenn JH, et al. Efficacy of low-dose interferon with antiretroviral therapy in Kaposi's sarcoma: a randomized phase II AIDS clinical trials group study. J Interferon Cytokine Res 22:295, 2002.
58. Krown SE, Lee JY, Lin L, et al. A phase I trial of protease inhibitor-based antiretroviral therapy with recombinant interferon alfa-2b in patients with HIV-related Kaposi's sarcoma. J Aquired Immun Defic Syndr 41:149, 2006.
59. Laubenstein LJ, Krigel RL, Odajnyk CM, et al. Treatment of epidemic Kaposi's sarcoma with etoposide or a combination of doxorubicin, bleomycin and vinblastine. J Clin Oncol 2: 1115, 1984.
60. Bakker PJM, Danner SA, Lange JMA, Veenhof KHN. Etoposide for epidemic Kaposi's sarcoma: a phase II study. Eur J Cancer Clin Oncol 24:1047, 1988.
61. Paredes J, Kahn JO, Tong WP, et al. Weekly oral etoposide in patients with Kaposi's sarcoma associated with human immunodeficiency virus infection: a phase I multicenter trial of the AIDS Clinical Trials Group. J Acquir Immune Defic Syndr Hum Retrovirol 9:138, 1995.
62. Schwartsmann G, Sprinz E, Kromfield M, et al. Clinical and pharmacokinetic study of oral etoposide in patients with AIDS-related Kaposi's sarcoma with no prior exposure to cytotoxic therapy. J Clin Oncol 15:2118, 1997.
63. Bufill JA, Grace WR, Astrow AB. Phase II trial of prolonged, low-dose, oral VP-16 in AIDS-related Kaposi's sarcoma (KS) [abstract]. Proc Am Soc Clin Oncol 11:47, 1992.
64. Evans SR, Krown SE, Testa MA, et al. A phase II evaluation of low-dose oral etoposide for the treatment of relapsed or

progressive AIDS-related Kaposi's sarcoma: an ACTG clinical study. J Clin Oncol 20: 3236, 2002.
65. Volberding PA, Abrams DI, Conant M, et al. Vinblastine therapy for Kaposi's sarcoma in the acquired immunodeficiency syndrome. Ann Intern Med 103:335, 1985.
66. Mintzer DM, Real FX, Jovino L, et al. Treatment of Kaposi's sarcoma and thrombocytopenia with vincristine in patients with acquired immunodeficiency syndrome. Ann Intern Med 102:200, 1985.
67. Caumes E, Guermonprez G, Katlama C, et al. AIDS-associated mucocutaneous Kaposi's sarcoma treated with bleomycin. AIDS 6:1483, 1992.
68. Lassoued K, Clauvel JP, Katlama C, et al. Treatment of the acquired immune deficiency syndrome-related Kaposi's sarcoma with bleomycin as a single agent. Cancer 66:1869, 1990.
69. Remick SC, Reddy M, Herman D, et al. Continuous infusion bleomycin in AIDS-related Kaposi's sarcoma. J Clin Oncol 12:1130, 1994.
70. Fischl MA, Krown SE, O'Boyle KP, et al. Weekly doxorubicin in the treatment of patients with AIDS-related Kaposi's sarcoma. J Acquir Immune Defic Syndr 6:259, 1993.
71. Gill PS, Rarick M, McCutchan JA, et al. Systemic treatment of AIDS-related Kaposi's sarcoma: results of a randomized trial. Am J Med 90:427, 1991.
72. Gill PS, Akil B, Colletti P, et al. Pulmonary Kaposi's sarcoma: clinical findings and results of therapy. Am J Med 87:57, 1989.
73. Schwartzmann G, Sprinz E, Kronfeld M, et al. Phase II study of teniposide in patients with AIDS-related Kaposi's sarcoma. Eur J Cancer 27:1637, 1991.
74. Nasti G, Errante D, Talamini R, et al. Vinorelbine is an effective and safe drug for AIDS-related Kaposi's sarcoma: results of a phase II study. J Clin Oncol 18:1550, 2000.
75. Shepherd FA, Burkes RL, Paul KE, Goss PE. A phase II study of 4′-epirubicin in the treatment of poor-risk Kaposi's sarcoma and AIDS. AIDS 5:305, 1991.
76. Cadranel JL, Kammoun S, Chevret S, et al. Results of chemotherapy in 30 AIDS patients with symptomatic pulmonary Kaposi's sarcoma. Thorax 49:958, 1994.
77. Gill PS, Rarick MU, Espina B, et al. Advanced acquired immune deficiency syndrome-related Kaposi's sarcoma: results of pilot studies using combination chemotherapy. Cancer 65:1074, 1990.
78. Gill PS, Miles SA, Mitsuyasu RT, et al. Phase I AIDS Clinical Trials Group (075) study of adriamycin, bleomycin and vincristine in the treatment of AIDS-related Kaposi's sarcoma. AIDS 8:1695, 1994.
79. Gill PS, Bernstein-Singer M, Espina BM, et al. Adriamycin, bleomycin and vincristine chemotherapy with recombinant granulocyte-macrophage colony-stimulating factor in the treatment of AIDS-related Kaposi's sarcoma. AIDS 6:1477, 1992.
80. Mitsuyasu RT, Gill P, Paredes J, et al. Combination chemotherapy, adriamycin, bleomycin, vincristine (ABV) with dideoxyinosine (ddI) or dideoxycytidine (ddC) in advanced AIDS-related Kaposi's sarcoma (ACTG 163) [abstract 822]. Proc Am Soc Clin Oncol 14:289, 1995.
81. Gompels MM, Hill A, Jenkins P, et al. Kaposi's sarcoma in HIV infection treated with vincristine and bleomycin. AIDS 6:1175, 1992.
82. Gill PS, Rarick M, Bernstein-Singer M. Treatment of advanced Kaposi's sarcoma using a combination of bleomycin and vincristine. Am J Clin Oncol 13:315, 1990.
83. Kaplan L, Abrams D, Volberding P. Treatment of Kaposi's sarcoma in acquired immunodeficiency syndrome with an alternating vincristine–vinblastine regimen. Cancer Treat Rep 70:1121, 1986.
84. Gelmann EP, Longo D, Lane HC, et al. Combination chemotherapy of disseminated Kaposi's sarcoma in patients with the acquired immune deficiency syndrome. Am J Med 82:456, 1987.
85. Sloand E, Kumar PN, Pierce PF. Chemotherapy for patients with pulmonary Kaposi's sarcoma: benefit of filgrastim (G-CSF) in supporting dose administration. South Med J 86:1219, 1993.
86. Lee F-C, Mitsuyasu RT. Chemotherapy of AIDS-related Kaposi's sarcoma. Hematol Oncol Clin North Am 10:1051, 1996.
87. Krown SE, Northfelt DW, Osoba D, et al. Use of liposomal anthracyclines in Kaposi's sarcoma. Semin Oncol 6(Suppl 13):36, 2004.
88. Simpson JK, Miller RF, Spittle MF. Liposomal doxorubicin for treatment of AIDS-related Kaposi's sarcoma. Clin Oncol 5:372, 1993.
89. James ND, Coker RJ, Tomlinson D, et al. Liposomal doxorubicin (Doxil): an effective new treatment for Kaposi's sarcoma in AIDS. Clin Oncol 6:294, 1994.
90. Bogner JR, Kronawitter U, Rolinski B, et al. Liposomal doxorubicin in the treatment of advanced AIDS-related Kaposi's sarcoma. J Acquir Immune Defic Syndr 7:463, 1994.
91. Harrison M, Tomlinson D, Stewart S. Liposomal-entrapped doxorubicin: an active agent in AIDS-related Kaposi's sarcoma. J Clin Oncol 13:914, 1995.
92. Goebel F-D, Goldstein D, Goos M, et al. Efficacy and safety of Stealth liposomal doxorubicin in AIDS-related Kaposi's sarcoma. Br J Cancer 73:989, 1996.
93. Mitsuyasu R, VonRoenn J, Krown S, et al. Comparison study of liposomal doxorubicin (Dox) alone or with bleomycin and vincristine (DBV) for treatment of advanced AIDS-associated Kaposi's sarcoma (AIDS-KS): AIDS Clinical Trial Group (ACTG) protocol 286 [abstract 191]. Proc Am Soc Clin Oncol 16:55a, 1997.
94. Northfelt DW, Dezube BJ, Thommes JA, et al. Efficacy of pegylated-liposomal doxorubicin in the treatment of AIDS-related Kaposi's sarcoma after failure of standard chemotherapy. J Clin Oncol 15:653, 1997.
95. Money-Kyrle JF, Bates F, Ready J, et al. Liposomal daunorubicin in advanced Kaposi's sarcoma: a phase II study. Clin Oncol (R Coll Radiol) 5:367, 1993.
96. Presant CA, Scolaro M, Kennedy P, et al. Liposomal daunorubicin treatment of HIV-associated Kaposi's sarcoma. Lancet 341:1242, 1993.
97. Chew T, Jacobs M, Huckabee M, et al. A phase II clinical trial of DaunoXome (VS103, liposomal daunorubicin) in Kaposi's sarcoma of AIDS patients [abstract WS-B15-3]. Int Conf AIDS 9:58, 1993.
98. Gill PS, Espina BM, Muggia F, et al. Phase I/II clinical and pharmacokinetic evaluation of liposomal daunorubicin. J Clin Oncol 13:996, 1995.
99. Tulpule A, Yung RC, Wernz J, et al. Phase II trial of liposomal daunorubicin in the treatment of AIDS-related pulmonary Kaposi's sarcoma. J Clin Oncol 16:3369, 1998.
100. Brenner DC. Liposomal encapsulation: making old and new drugs do new tricks. J Natl Cancer Inst 81:13, 1989.
101. Northfelt DW, Martin FJ, Working P, et al. Doxorubicin encapsulated in liposomes containing surface-bound polyethylene glycol: pharmacokinetics, tumor localization, and safety in patients with AIDS-related Kaposi's sarcoma. J Clin Pharmacol 36:55, 1996.
102. Gill PS, Wernz J, Scadden DT, et al. Randomized phase II trial of liposomal daunorubicin (DaunoXome) versus doxorubicin, bleomycin, vincristine (ABV) in AIDS-related Kaposi's sarcoma. J Clin Oncol 14:2353, 1996.
103. Northfelt DW, Dezube B, Thommes JA, et al. Pegylated liposomal doxorubicin versus doxorubicin, bleomycin, and vincristine in the treatment of AIDS-related Kaposi's sarcoma: results

of a randomized phase III clinical trial. J Clin Oncol 16:2445, 1998.

104. Cowens JW, Creaven PJ, Greco WR, et al. Initial clinical (phase I) trial of TLC D-99 (doxorubicin encapsulated in liposomes). Cancer Res 53:2796, 1993.

105. Wagner D, Kern WV, Kern P. Liposomal doxorubicin in AIDS-related Kaposi's sarcoma: long term experiences. Clin Invest 72:417, 1994.

106. Berry G, Billingham M, Alderman E, et al. The use of cardiac biopsy to demonstrate reduced cardiotoxicity in AIDS Kaposi's sarcoma patients treated with pegylated liposomal doxorubicin. Ann Oncol 9:711, 1998.

107. Ross M, Gill PS, Espina BM, et al. Liposomal daunorubicin (DaunoXome) in the treatment of advanced AIDS-related Kaposi's sarcoma: results of a phase II study [abstract PoB 3123]. Int Conf AIDS 8:B107, 1992.

108. Gordon KB, Tajuddin A, Guitart J, et al. Hand-foot syndrome associated with liposome-encapsulated doxorubicin therapy. Cancer 75:2169, 1995.

109. Uziely B, Jeffers S, Isaacson R, et al. Liposomal doxorubicin: antitumor activity and unique toxicities during two complementary phase I studies. J Clin Oncol 13:1777, 1995.

110. Stewart JSW, Jablonowski H, Goebel FD, et al. Randomized comparative trial of pegylated liposomal doxorubicin versus bleomycin and vincristine in the treatment of AIDS-related Kaposi's sarcoma: International Pegylated Liposomal Doxorubicin Study Group. J Clin Oncol 16:683, 1998.

111. Feigal EG, VonRoenn J, Justice R, et al. Kaposi's sarcoma response criteria: issues identified by the National Cancer Institute, Food and Drug Administration, and the AIDS Malignancy Consortium [abstract 24]. J Acquir Immune Defic Syndr Hum Retrovirol 14:A22, 1997.

112. Henry D, Cooley T, Volberding P, et al. Final results of a phase III randomized trial of doxil vs DaunoXome in patients with AIDS-related Kaposi's sarcoma (KS) [abstract 1640]. Proc Am Soc Clin Oncol 21:411a, 2002.

113. Lichterfeld M, Qurishi N, Hoffmann C, et al. Treatment of HIV-1-associated Kaposi's sarcoma with pegylated liposomal doxorubicin and HAART simultaneously induces effective tumor remission and CD4+ T cell recovery. Infection 33:140, 2005.

114. Martin-Carbonero L, Barrios A, Saballs P, et al. Pegylated liposomal doxorubicin plus highly active antiretroviral therapy versus highly active antiretroviral therapy alone in HIV patients with Kaposi's sarcoma. AIDS 18:1737, 2004.

115. Schiff PB, Fant J, Horwitz SB. Promotion of microtubule assembly in vitro by Taxol. Nature 277:665, 1979.

116. Schiff PB, Horwitz SB. Taxol stabilizes microtubules in mouse fibroblast cells. Proc Natl Acad Sci USA 77:1561, 1980.

117. Belotti D, Vergani V, Drudis T, et al. The microtubule-affecting drug paclitaxel has antiangiogenic activity. Clin Cancer Res 2:1843, 1996.

118. Opalenik SR, Browning PJ. Human herpesvirus 8 (HHV-8) encodes a bcl-2 homologue that is expressed in Kaposi's sarcoma [abstract 42]. J Acquir Immune Defic Syndr Hum Retrovirol 14:A26, 1997.

119. Sgadari C, Toschi E, Palladino C, et al. Mechanism of paclitaxel activity in Kaposi's sarcoma. J Immunol 165:509, 2000.

120. Saville MW, Lietzau J, Pluda JM, et al. Treatment of HIV-associated Kaposi's sarcoma with paclitaxel. Lancet 346:26, 1995.

121. Welles L, Saville MW, Lietzau J, et al. Phase II trial with dose titration of paclitaxel for the therapy of human immunodeficiency virus-associated Kaposi's sarcoma. J Clin Oncol 16:1112, 1998.

122. Gill PS, Tulpule A, Espina BM, et al. Paclitaxel is safe and effective in the treatment of advanced AIDS-related Kaposi's sarcoma. J Clin Oncol 17:1876, 1999.

123. Schwartz JD, Howard W, Scadden DT. Potential interaction of antiretroviral therapy with paclitaxel in patients with AIDS-related Kaposi's sarcoma [letter]. AIDS 13:283, 1999.

124. Nannan Panday VR, Hoetelmans RM, van Heeswijk RP, et al. Paclitaxel in the treatment of human immunodeficiency virus 1-associated Kaposi's sarcoma–drug–drug interactions with protease inhibitors and a nonnucleoside reverse transcriptase inhibitor: a case report study. Cancer Chemother Pharmacol 43:516, 1999.

125. Singer JW, Shaffer S, Baker B, et al. Paclitaxel poliglumex (XYOTAX; CT-2103): an intracellularly targeted taxane. Anticancer Drugs 16:243, 2005.

126. McDaid HM, Lopez-Barcons L, Grossman A, et al. Enhancement of the therapeutic efficacy of taxol by the mitogen-activated protein kinase kinase inhibitor CI-1040 in nude mice bearing human heterotransplants. Cancer Res 65:2854, 2005.

127. Sharma-Walia N, Krishnan HH, Naranatt PP, et al. ERK1/2 and MEK1/2 induced by Kaposi's sarcoma-associated herpesvirus (human herpesvirus 8) early during infection of target cells are essential for expression of viral genes and for establishment of infection. J Virol 79:10308, 2005.

128. Friborg J Jr, Kong W, Hottiger MO, et al. p53 inhibition by the LANA protein of KSHV protects against cell death. Nature 402:889, 1999.

129. Swanton C, Mann DJ, Fleckenstein B, et al. Herpes viral cyclin/Cdk6 complexes evade inhibition by CDK inhibitor proteins. Nature 390:184, 1997.

130. Irmler M, Thome M, Hahne M, et al. Inhibition of death receptor signals by cellular FLIP. Nature 388:190, 1997.

131. Samaniego F, Pati S, Karp JE, et al. Human herpesvirus 8 K1-associated nuclear factor-kappa B-dependent promoter activity: role in Kaposi's sarcoma inflammation? J Natl Cancer Inst Monogr (28)15–23, 2001.

132. Sarid R, Sato T, Bohenzky RA, et al. Kaposi's sarcoma-associated herpesvirus encodes a functional bcl-2 homologue. Nat Med 3:293, 1997.

133. Dourmishev LA, Dourmishev AL, Palmeri D, et al. Molecular genetics of Kaposi's sarcoma-associated herpesvirus (human herpesvirus-8) epidemiology and pathogenesis. Microbiol Mol Biol Rev 67:175, 2003.

134. Jenner RG, Boshoff C. The molecular pathology of Kaposi's sarcoma-associated herpesvirus. Biochim Biophys Acta 1602:1, 2002.

135. Bais C, Santomasso B, Coso O, et al. G-protein coupled receptor of Kaposi's sarcoma-associated herpesvirus is a viral oncogene and angiogenesis activator. Nature 391:86, 1998.

136. Yang TY, Chen SC, Leach MW, et al. Transgenic expression of the chemokine receptor encoded by human herpesvirus 8 induces an angioproliferative disease resembling Kaposi's sarcoma. J Exp Med 191:445, 2000.

137. Weindel K, Marme D, Weich HA. AIDS-associated Kaposi's sarcoma cells in culture express vascular endothelial growth factor. Biochem Biophys Res Commun 183:1167, 1992.

138. Bais C, Van Geelen A, Eroles P, et al. Kaposi's sarcoma associated herpesvirus G protein-coupled receptor immortalizes human endothelial cells by activation of the VEGF receptor-2/KDR. Cancer Cell 3:131, 2003.

139. Wang L, Wakisaka N, Tomlinson CC, et al. The Kaposi's sarcoma-associated herpesvirus (KSHV/HHV-8) K1 protein induces expression of angiogenic and invasion factors. Cancer Res 64:2774, 2004.

140. Djerbi M, Screpanti V, Catrina AL, et al. The inhibitor of death-receptor signaling, FLICE-inhibitory protein defines a new class of tumor progression factors. J Exp Med 190:1025, 1999.

141. Weber KS, Grone HJ, Rocken M, et al. Selective recruitment of Th2-type cells and evasion from a cytotoxic immune

response mediated by viral macrophage inhibitory protein-II. Eur J Immunol 31:2458, 2001.

142. Lee BS, Alvarez X, Ishido S, et al. Inhibition of intracellular transport of B cell antigen receptor complexes by Kaposi's sarcoma-associated herpesvirus K1. J Exp Med 192:11, 2000.
143. Coscoy L, Ganem D. Kaposi's sarcoma-associated herpesvirus encodes two proteins that block cell surface display of MHC class I chains by enhancing their endocytosis. Proc Natl Acad Sci USA 97:8051, 2000.
144. Staskus KA, Zhong W, Gebhard K, et al. Kaposi's sarcoma-associated herpesvirus gene expression in endothelial (spindle) tumor cells. J Virol 71:715, 1997.
145. Orenstein JM, Alkan S, Blauvelt A, et al. Visualization of human herpesvirus type 8 in Kaposi's sarcoma by light and transmission electron microscopy. AIDS 11:F35, 1997.
146. Wang H-W, Trotter MWB, Lagos D, et al. Kaposi sarcoma herpesvirus-induced cellular reprogramming contributes to the lymphatic endothelial gene expression in Kaposi sarcoma. Nat Genet 36:687, 2004.
147. Ensoli B, Nakamura S, Salahuddin SZ, et al. AIDS Kaposi's sarcoma derived cells express cytokines with autocrine and paracrine growth effects. Science 243:223, 1989.
148. Miles SA, Rezai AR, Salazar-Gonzales JF, et al. AIDS Kaposi sarcoma-derived cells produce and respond to interleukin 6. Proc Natl Acad Sci USA 87:4068, 1990.
149. Samaniego F, Markham PD, Gendleman R, et al. Vascular endothelial growth factor and basic fibroblast growth factor present in Kaposi's sarcoma (KS) are induced by inflammatory cytokines and synergize to promote vascular permeability and KS lesion development. Am J Pathol 152:1433, 1998.
150. Meade-Tollin LC, Way D, Witte MH. Expression of multiple matrix metalloproteinases and urokinase type plasminogen activator in cultured Kaposi sarcoma cells. Acta Histochem 101:305, 1999.
151. Barillari G, Sgadari C, Palladino C, et al. Inflammatory cytokines synergize with the HIV-1 Tat protein to promote angiogenesis and Kaposi's sarcoma via induction of basic fibroblast growth factor and the alpha v beta 3 integrin. J Immunol 163:1929, 1999.
152. Fiorelli V, Barillari G, Toschi E, et al. IFN-gamma induces endothelial cells to proliferate and to invade the extracellular matrix in response to the HIV-1 Tat protein: implications for AIDS-Kaposi's sarcoma pathogenesis. J Immunol 162:1165, 1999.
153. Ganju RK, Munshi N, Nair BC, et al. Human immunodeficiency virus tat modulates the Flk-1/KDR receptor, mitogen-activated protein kinases, and components of focal adhesion in Kaposi's sarcoma cells. J Virol 72:6131, 1998.
154. Ambrosino C, Ruocco MR, Chen X, et al. HIV-1 Tat induces the expression of the interleukin-6 (IL6) gene by binding to the IL6 leader RNA and by interacting with CAAT enhancer-binding protein beta (NF-IL6) transcription factors. J Biol Chem 272:14883, 1997.
155. Kumar A, Dhawan S, Mukhopadhyay A, et al. Human immunodeficiency virus-1-tat induces matrix metalloproteinase-9 in monocytes through protein tyrosine phosphatase-mediated activation of nuclear transcription factor NF-kappaB. FEBS Lett 462:140, 1999.
156. Mazzi R, Parisi SG, Sarmati L, et al. Efficacy of cidofovir on human herpesvirus 8 viraemia and Kaposi's sarcoma progression in two patients with AIDS. AIDS 15:2061, 2001.
157. Fife K, Gill J, Bourboulia D, et al. Cidofovir for the treatment of Kaposi's sarcoma in an HIV-negative homosexual man. Br J Dermatol 141:1148, 1999.
158. Morfeldt L, Torssander J. Long-term remission of Kaposi's sarcoma following foscarnet treatment in HIV-infected patients. Scand J Infect Dis 26:749, 1994.
159. Medveczky MM, Horvath E, Lund T, Medveczky PG. In vitro antiviral drug sensitivity of the Kaposi's sarcoma-associated herpesvirus. AIDS 11:1327, 1997.
160. Kedes DH, Ganem D. Sensitivity of Kaposi's sarcoma-associated herpesvirus replication to antiviral drugs: implications for potential therapy. J Clin Invest 99:2082, 1997.
161. Neyts J, De Clercq E. Antiviral drug susceptibility of human herpesvirus 8. Antimicrob Agents Chemother 41:2754, 1007.
162. Little RF, Merced-Galindez F, Staskus K, et al. A pilot study of cidofovir in patients with Kaposi sarcoma. J Infect Dis 187:149, 2003.
163. Jones JL, Hanson DL, Chu SY, et al. AIDS-associated Kaposi's sarcoma [letter]. Science 267:1078, 1995.
164. Mocroft A, Youle M, Gazzard B, et al. Anti-herpesvirus treatment and risk of Kaposi's sarcoma in HIV infection: Royal Free/Chelsea and Westminster Hospitals collaborative group. AIDS 10:1101, 1996.
165. Glesby MJ, Hoover DR, Weng S, et al. Use of antiherpes drugs and the risk of Kaposi's sarcoma: data from the Multicenter AIDS Cohort Study. J Infect Dis 173:1477, 1996.
166. Martin DF, Kuppermann BD, Wolitz RA, et al. Oral ganciclovir for patients with cytomegalovirus retinitis treated with a ganciclovir implant. Roche Ganciclovir Study Group. N Engl J Med 340:1063, 1999.
167. Shaw RN, Arbiser JL, Offermann MK. Valproic acid induces human herpesvirus 8 lytic gene expression in BCBL-1 cells [letter]. AIDS 14:899, 2000.
168. Dittmer DP. Transcription profile of Kaposi's sarcoma-associated herpesvirus in primary Kaposi's sarcoma lesions as determined by real-time PCR arrays. Cancer Res 63:2010, 2003.
169. Krown SE. Management of Kaposi sarcoma: the role of interferon and thalidomide. Curr Opin Oncol 13:374, 2001.
170. Miles SA, Dezube B, Lee JY, et al. Antitumor activity of oral 9-cis-retinoic acid in HIV infected patients with Kaposi's sarcoma: a multicenter trial of the AIDS Malignancy Consortium. AIDS 16:421, 2002.
171. Cianfrocca M, Cooley TP, Lee JY, et al. Matrix metalloproteinase inhibitor COL-3 in the treatment of AIDS-related Kaposi's sarcoma: a phase I AIDS Malignancy Consortium study. J Clin Oncol 20:153, 2002.
172. Dezube BJ, Krown SE, Lee JY, et al. Matrix metalloproteinase inhibitor COL-3 in the treatment of AIDS-related Kaposi's sarcoma: a phase II AIDS Malignancy Consortium Study. J Clin Oncol 24:1389, 2006.
173. Little RF, Pluda JM, Wyvill KM, et al. Activity of subcutaneous interleukin-12 in AIDS-related Kaposi sarcoma. Blood 107:4650, 2006.
174. Dezube BJ, VonRoenn JH, Holden-Wiltse J, et al. Fumagillin analog in the treatment of Kaposi's sarcoma: a phase I AIDS Clinical Trial Group study; AIDS Clinical Trial Group No. 215 Team. J Clin Oncol 16:1444, 1998.
175. Pluda JM, Wyvill KK, Lietzau J, et al. A phase I trial administering the angiogenesis inhibitor TNP-470 (AGM-1470) to patients (pts) with HIV-associated Kaposi's sarcoma (KS) [abstract 13]. J Acquir Immune Defic Syndr Hum Retrovirol 14:A19, 1997.
176. Sturzl M, Roth WK, Brockmeyer NH, et al. Expression of platelet-derived growth factor and its receptor in AIDS-related Kaposi sarcoma in vivo suggests paracrine and autocrine mechanisms of tumor maintenance. Proc Natl Acad Sci USA 89:7046, 1992.
177. Sturzl M, Brandstetter H, Zietz C, et al. Identification of interleukin-1 and platelet-derived growth factor-B as major mitogens for the spindle cells of Kaposi's sarcoma: a combined in vitro and in vivo analysis. Oncogene 10:2007, 1995.
178. Roth WK, Werner S, Schirren CG, et al. Depletion of PDGF from serum inhibits growth of AIDS-related and sporadic Kaposi's sarcoma cells in culture. Oncogene 4:483, 1989.

179. Cornali E, Zietz C, Benelli R, et al. Vascular endothelial growth factor regulates angiogenesis and vascular permeability in Kaposi's sarcoma. Am J Pathol 149:1851, 1996.
180. Moses AV, Jarvis MA, Raggo C, et al. Kaposi's sarcoma-associated herpesvirus-induced upregulation of the c-kit proto-oncogene, as identified by gene expression profiling, is essential for the transformation of endothelial cells. J Virol 76:8383, 2002.
181. Pantanowitz L, Dezube BJ, Pinkus GS, et al. Histological characterization of regression in acquired immunodeficiency syndrome-related Kaposi's sarcoma. J Cutan Pathol 31:26, 2004.
182. Koon HB, Bubley GJ, Pantanowitz L, et al. Imatinib-induced regression of AIDS-related Kaposi's sarcoma. J Clin Oncol 23:982, 2005.
183. Ensoli B, Markham P, Kao V, et al. Block of AIDS-Kaposi's sarcoma (KS) cell growth, angiogenesis and lesion formation in nude mice by antisense oligonucleotide targeting basic fibroblast growth factor. J Clin Invest 94:1736, 1994.
184. Varner JA, Cheresh DA. Tumor angiogenesis and the role of vascular cell integrin $\alpha_v \beta_3$. Important Adv Oncol 69–87, 1996.
185. Stallone G, Schena A, Infante B, et al. Sirolimus for Kaposi's sarcoma in renal-transplant recipients. N Engl J Med 352:1317, 2005.
186. Cahir-McFarland ED, Davidson DM, Schauer SL, et al. NF-kappa B inhibition causes spontaneous apoptosis in Epstein-Barr virus-transformed lymphoblastoid cells. Proc Natl Acad Sci USA 97:6055, 2000.
187. Keller SA, Schatttner EJ, Cesarman E. Inhibition of NF-kappaB induces apoptosis of KSHV-infected primary effusion lymphoma cells. Blood 96:2537, 2000.
188. Brown HJ, Song MJ, Deng H, et al. NF-kappaB inhibits gammaherpesvirus lytic replication. J Virol 77:8532, 2003.
189. Goy A, Gilles F. Update on the proteasome inhibitor bortezomib in hematologic malignancies. Clin Lymphoma 4:230, 2004.

Chapter 60

Non-Hodgkin Lymphoma

Richard F. Little, MD, Stefania Pittaluga, MD, Robert Yarchoan, MD

INTRODUCTION

Non-Hodgkin lymphoma (NHL) is a broad term encompassing many neoplasms of lymphocytes, and along with Hodgkin lymphoma (HL) is the most commonly occurring hematologic malignancy in the United States.[1] Compared to the general population, the incidence of NHL and HL in persons with human immunodeficiency virus (HIV) infection is markedly elevated.[2] In 1985 the US Centers for Disease Control (CDC) included biopsy-confirmed NHL of high-grade pathologic type (diffuse, undifferentiated) and of B-cell or unknown immunologic phenotype, in the setting of HIV infection, as a case definition for acquired immunodeficiency syndrome (AIDS).[3] AIDS-related lymphoma (ARL) is one of the most lethal complications of HIV infection,[4] although its prognosis has improved since the introduction of highly active antiretroviral therapy (HAART).[5,6]

The prognosis for ARL is worse than that for similar lymphomas occurring in non-AIDS patients.[6–8] Recently, HAART has been associated with changes in the epidemiology and natural history of these tumors. Therapeutic approaches have become more similar to non-HIV NHL. Pre-HAART, the therapeutic goal was frequently palliation, since the prospects for long-term survival were generally poor. In the HAART era, certain subsets of patients with AIDS and lymphoma may have outcomes equivalent to those of their counterparts in the general population.[9,10] Consequently, curative intent treatment is appropriate for many, if not most, patients with ARL. Lymphoma cure depends on achieving a complete remission of the tumor without subsequent recurrence, and recurrence is a major cause of treatment failure in lymphoma. Identification of patients most likely to have a favorable outcome is informed on the basis of the underlying AIDS and appropriate tumor classification. Optimal treatment planning must take these features into account.

NHL encompasses a broad spectrum of lymphocyte neoplastic diseases. In non-AIDS patients, optimal management and prognosis are dependent on the specific lymphoma type. In ARL, the specific lymphoma type has until recently been less relevant to either treatment or to prognosis. Lymphoma classification incorporates morphologic, immunophenotypic, and clinical features. Recent advances in identifying the presumed cell of origin from which specific lymphoma types derive have helped in unraveling the underlying biology of various lymphomas and distinguishing various lymphoma subtypes. This information helps place into perspective the finding that while lymphomas occurring in AIDS share similarities with HIV-unrelated lymphomas, they also have distinguishing epidemiologic and clinical features (Table 60-1).

There is increasing evidence that in the HAART era, consolidation of ARL into a 'catch-all' quasidiagnostic label may be less useful than in the pre-HAART era. Also, it appears that lymphoma-specific disease features are of relatively greater prognostic importance than in the pre-HAART era.[5,10] In order to confirm this early observation, inclusion of appropriate diagnostic refinement and subset analysis in clinical trails of ARL will be essential. In non-AIDS, outcome is critically dependent on appropriate histology guided treatment. In the HAART era, this may prove to be the case for ARL.

The World Health Organization Classification of Tumors has broadened the original CDC spectrum of lymphomas associated with HIV infection, as listed in Table 60-2. These lymphomas can have markedly different clinical characteristics and prognosis, and understanding these differences is essential toward optimal management, clinical trial development, and disease surveillance.

EPIDEMIOLOGY

Early after AIDS was recognized as a new disease, it was apparent that NHL was one of the complicating opportunistic illnesses. In contrast to AIDS-related Kaposi sarcoma (KS) which occurred

Table 60-1 Characteristics of Peripheral Aggressive Lymphoma in AIDS and Non-AIDS

Characteristic	AIDS	Non-AIDS
% of cancers	20–30%	5%
Proportion of all NHL with aggressive histologic features	90%	50%
High grade	75%	10%
Extranodal involvement	40–80%	40%
Leptomeningeal involvement	17%	10%
% NHL primary brain	20% (pre-HAART)	2%
'B' symptoms	⩾80%	<30%
Age at onset	Second to third decade	Fifth to sixth decade

From Clifford et al,[20] National Cancer Institute,[35] Biggar,[158] and Jones et al.[59]

Table 60-2 Categories of HIV-Associated Lymphoma

Lymphomas Also Occurring in Immunocompetent Patients
Burkitt lymphoma
Diffuse large B-cell lymphoma
  Centroblastic
  Immunoblastic
Extranodal marginal zone B-cell lymphoma of mucosa-associated lymphoid tissue type (MALT lymphoma)
Peripheral T-cell lymphoma
Classical Hodgkin lymphoma

Lymphomas Occurring More Specifically in HIV+ Patients
Primary effusion lymphoma
Plasmablastic lymphoma of the oral cavity
Lymphomas Also Occurring in Other Immunodeficiency States
Polymorphic B-cell lymphomas (PTLD-like)

From Jaffe ES, Harris NL, Stein H, Vardiman JW (eds). World Health Organization Classification of Tumors: Pathology & Genetics: Tumors of Haematopoietic and Lymphoid Tissues. Lyon: IARC Press; 2001.

with greatest excess among men who had sex with other men (MSM), the risk of NHL appeared to be unrelated to the HIV risk acquisition factors.[2,11] In the pediatric population, the incident cases were ~300-fold greater than observed in general population, although since NHL is a rare pediatric disease, there were not a great number of cases.[2] However, in young adults aged 20–40 years, the incident cases were found to be over 70-fold greater than expected, leading to ~3000 cases by 1989 compared to the ~50 cases expected for the period. In addition, although not an AIDS-defining condition, it became clear that the incidence of HL was increased. There is an eight- to 10-fold increase of HL in HIV-infected compared to the noninfected population. HL is the most common non-AIDS-defining cancer among individuals with HIV infection.[12,13]

Epidemiologic features of ARL have been modified by the introduction of HAART. Most studies have shown ARL to have decreased in incidence by ~50% since HAART,[6,14] although the proportion of AIDS-defining illness (ADI) that is due to lymphoma appears to be somewhat increased, owing to the relatively greater decrease in other ADIs.[15,16] Also, lymphoma is now nearly equal to or exceeds KS as the leading malignant AIDS-defining event.[17–20] Where HAART is readily available, cancer has overall become the leading cause of death in HIV-infected persons, and NHL is the leading cause of cancer-related death in AIDS.[21,22]

The risk of developing ARL is inversely related to CD4+ cell count and in populations where HAART is widely used, the proportion of individuals with low CD4+ cells is reduced, resulting in a decrease in ARL incidence.[20] Also, the use of HAART has resulted in a change in the relative distribution of ARL subtypes. This appears to be explained in part by the observation that there is a correlation between CD4+ cell count and the risk of developing a specific ARL type.[17,23] Most studies show that only those lymphoma subtypes that are most associated with advanced immune depletion are particularly decreased in incidence in the HAART era, though there is no complete agreement in the data.[5,6,17]

The greatest decrease in incidence has been seen in the immunoblastic variant of diffuse large B-cell lymphomas (DLBCL), a subtype strongly associated with advanced CD4+ cell count depletion and Epstein–Barr virus (EBV) infection. This variant accounted for ~60% of all ARL prior to HAART,[2] and has substantially decreased in incidence so that since HAART was introduced, the immunoblastic variant

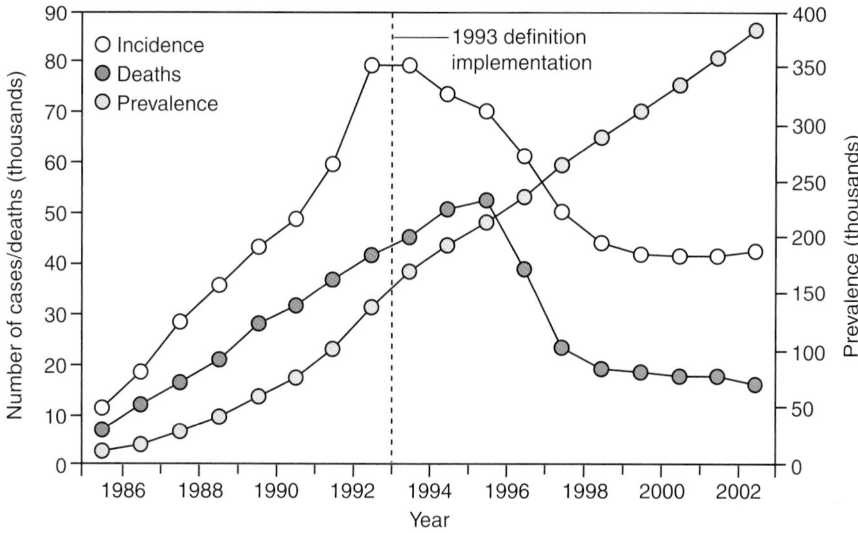

Figure 60-1 ■ Incidence, deaths, and prevalence of AIDS in the United States.

From Centers for Disease Prevention and Control. AIDS Surveillance – General Epidemiology (through 2003). Atlanta: CDC; 2003.

represents ~30% of cases.[17] However, caution should be taken in the interpretation of such data because there is no uniform agreement among pathologists as to what establishes the diagnosis of immunoblastic lymphoma. Prior to HAART, AIDS-related primary central nervous system lymphomas (AR-PCNSLs), which are virtually all of the immunoblastic variant, accounted for ~20% of all ARLs.[2] Since the introduction of HAART, tumor has decreased in incidence by ~70%.[6] Interestingly, this subtype is nearly always EBV associated.

In a large retrospective review, Besson and colleagues reported a statistically nonsignificant increase in AIDS-related B-cell lymphoma (AR-BL) in the HAART era from 17.7% to 26.8% of cases.[6] DLBCL cases were decreased from 79% to 63.4% of overall ARL cases. A notable finding from these data is that within CD4+ cell strata, no overall change in ARL incidence was seen, suggesting that the overall decrease in ARL incidence with HAART is due to a decreased population of individuals with low CD4+ cell counts. However, there is evidence that factors in addition to absolute CD4+ cell counts are likely involved in the complex changes in incidence of various lymphoma subtypes. As yet, with only less than one decade of data available for analysis, it may be too soon to fully appreciate the effects of HAART on tumor epidemiology in HIV infection.

While most data show that the incidence of the centroblastic DLBCL variant and Burkitt lymphoma (BL) has remained relatively stable since HAART was introduced,[17,24] some studies report an increase in DLBCL and a decrease in Burkitt.[5] Lim and colleagues identified a shift in the ratio of cases favoring the more likely occurrence of DLBCL over other subtypes by a factor of ~3.5 in the HAART era in Southern California. This result is somewhat unexpected as DLBCL occurs with lower CD4+ cell counts than the BLs, and this result illustrates the complexity of the epidemiology and HAART effect.[5] These interesting data underscore the uncertainly at present regarding the epidemiology in ARL, and also highlights the importance of rigorous lymphoma subset and variant classification.

Unlike EBV-associated ARL, which occur most frequently in the setting of low CD4+ cell counts, HIV HL tends to occur while the CD4+ cells are relatively intact, even though the vast majority are also EBV associated.[25] In contrast to the EBV-associated NHL, HL appears not to have decreased, and if anything to have increased in incidence in the HAART era.[17,20] Such epidemiological discrepancies underscore the differences in tumor pathophysiology, the role of EBV in HL and NHL, and the complex interaction between the immune system and viral oncogenesis.

It remains to be seen how the overall burden of cancer in HIV-infected individuals will be affected by HAART. Although the risk of ARL and other AIDS-defining malignancies per patient-year has decreased with HAART, the at-risk population of persons with AIDS in the United States has grown by more than 50% since the introduction of HAART (Fig. 60-1). Since as yet no person has been cured of HIV infection, but treatment advances have translated into substantially increased longevity, this trend may be predicted to continue. Consequently, the prevalence of persons living with HIV/AIDS is likely to increase further. Moreover, as these individuals age, there may be an increased risk of developing NHL as is the case in the general population. It is conceivable that the future will bring new challenges to the medical oncology community and their infectious disease consultants if the absolute number of HIV-infected individuals with cancer increases commensurate with the already documented increase in AIDS prevalence.[26]

PATHOGENESIS

Lymphoma pathogenesis is a complex process that has not been fully unraveled. Clues to lymphomagenesis can be found from a synthesis of the various data available from epidemiologic, histologic, genetic, and molecular studies. For example, it has long been established that patients with congenital or acquired immune dysfunction have an increased risk of developing lymphoma, and that these are frequently viral associated.[27] Additionally, pathogenic mechanisms have been informed by advances in the ability to identify the putative normal cellular counterpart from which the various lymphoma types derive. As the normal lymphocyte transits through the lymph node, the specific immune microenvironment is reflected by cell surface markers. Identification of such markers can be used to postulate the point when malignant transformation took place relative to passage through the nodal germinal center. This ontological information has helped to segregate lymphoma subsets into biologically and clinically relevant distinct entities.[28,29] The specific histogenic pathways give rise to distinct biological and clinical patterns specific to the ARL subtypes (Table 60-3).[30–32] Modification of the host immune microenvironment likely affects histogenesis, in part explaining the changing epidemiologic and clinical patterns of ARL in the HAART era.[33]

Over 80% of the NHL cases in HIV-infected patients are aggressive B-cell lymphomas,[34] in contrast to the HIV-unrelated cases where less than 15% are of this type (Table 60-1).[35] ARL are frequently associated with oncogenic gamma-herpesviruses, as is commonly the case with other immunosuppression-related lymphoproliferative disorders.[26,27] Moreover, those ARLs associated with advanced immune depletion are more likely to be viral associated, whereas those that occur with higher CD4+ counts are less likely to be viral associated.[30,33,36–38] As mentioned above, an exception to this is HL, which typically occurs prior to AIDS onset, and yet 80% or more are EBV associated.[25,39,40] Also, it is possible that as yet undiscovered viral associations may be involved for those ARLs not currently known to be associated with oncogenic viruses. For example, the putatively oncogenic Simian virus 40 (SV40) has reportedly been found in association with some ARLs,[41] although epidemiological analysis has not supported this as an etiologic agent in NHL.[42]

The association with gamma-herpesvirus infection in ARL invokes the possibility that these are lymphoproliferations that develop as immune control against the virus is lost. However, immunosuppression alone does not adequately explain why lymphoma is increased in HIV infection. Complex molecular events are involved in lymphomagenesis and in many cases, a series of events must occur for lymphomas to develop. The immunosuppression of AIDS may act in part to permit expansion of virally infected cells, especially those that express immunogenic markers, and thus increase the chance of subsequent genetic events that lead to frank lymphoma. As one example, EBV appears to rescue from apoptosis germinal center B-cells that have otherwise accumulated fatal somatic hypermutations.[43] EBV proteins such as LMP1 and LMP2A can mimic the function of the B-cell receptors CD40 and BCR that are vital to cell survival. EBV may transform cells in part by overcoming loss of these cell proteins, providing a major role of the virus in the pathogenesis of HL and posttransplantation lymphomas.[44] Such transformed cells also have an increased chance of developing other abnormalities without being destroyed by apoptosis.

Other factors that have been invoked in AIDS lymphomagenesis include chronic immune stimulation and cytokine dysregulation associated with HIV infection, and the response to these disturbances is in part dependent on innate host immune characteristics. For example, chemokines that are involved in normal B-lymphocyte maturation and proliferation are often dysregulated in patients with HIV. Also, certain gene variants of the chemokine receptor CCR5 and the CXC chemokine ligand-12 (stromal cell-derived factor-1) affect the risk of NHL in AIDS, independently of any potential protection from HIV itself.[45,46] The finding that receptor variants affect lymphoma risk is consistent with the concept that HAART modification of immune dysregulation can through this mechanism affect lymphomagenesis and ARL epidemiology. A number of additional considerations support the role of immune microenvironment on ARL.

Since the subtype of ARL is dependent on histogenic origin, factors that influence B-cell transit through the lymph node are important to tumor biology.[30,31] This provides another mechanism by which HIV can affect lymphoma histogenesis. As HIV disease advances, lymph node architecture is substantially altered.[47] The nodal architecture to some degree reflects the effect of HIV on shortened T-cell survival and consequent changes in B-cell function.[48] Also, the stage of HIV infection influences cytokine levels and these in turn are associated with the relative composition of germinal center cells and mature B-cells within the nodes and periphery.[49,50] Thus, immune status, B-cell migration through the germinal center, and histogenesis may be intrinsically related. HAART can delay progression of HIV disease, and thus preserve nodal architecture, potentially influencing these relationships as reflected in the changing patterns of ARL epidemiology.

Gene expression profiling using DNA array technology provides strong evidence supporting the role of immune environment on ARL biology and epidemiology. Approximately 50–70% of ARL are DLBCL.[5,51–53] Gene expression profiling has identified at least three major ontogenetically distinct DLBCL subtypes in non-AIDS.[54] These subtypes have distinct tumor biology and clinical behavior. AIDS DLBCLs have similar gene expression patterns, except that a higher proportion of AIDS cases express the T-cell leukemia-1 proto-oncogene.[55] Disruption of the immune microenvironment promotes expression of this oncogene.[56,57] The increased incidence and aggressiveness of DLBCL in AIDS may thus be due to impaired immunosurveillance affecting expression of specific genes rather than changes in the overall gene expression pattern associated with prognosis of the various DLBCL subtypes. The decreased risk of developing ARL and improvements in ARL prognosis with HAART may in turn be related to changes in the expression of this oncogene. Whether expression of this oncogene influences development of specific DLBCL subtypes is not known.

Further evidence that the immune microenvironment influences tumor biology is the finding that the expression pattern of oncogenic viruses such as EBV can be modified by cytokines relevant to HIV disease stage. For example, interleukin-10 can induce the expression of LMP-1, demonstrating that this major transforming gene can be induced by extracellular signals.[58] As HIV disease progresses, T-helper type II (THII) cytokines such as IL-10 become elevated,[59] potentially promoting viral oncogenesis through its effects

Table 60-3 CLINICAL AND BIOLOGIC FEATURES OF ARL

Histology	Immunophenotype and Pathobiological Markers (percentage of cases)					Oncogenic Virus (percentage of cases)					Outcome	
	CD20	CD10	BCL-2	BCL-6	c-MYC	EBV	KSHV	CD4+ Count	Age Peak	Since Infection	Interval Pre-HAART	HAART
Burkitt	~100	> 90	0	100	100	<50	0	May be well preserved	10–19 years	May be early event	Poor	Poor
Diffuse large b-cell												
Centroblastic	~100	> 60	Rare	>75	0–50	<30	0	Moderate	>40 years	May be early event	Fair	Improved
Immunoblastic	Variable/ positive	0	90	<50	0	>80	0	Usually low		Generally late event	Poor	Improved
Primary effusion	Rare (dim)	0	0	0	0	70	100	Usually low		Generally late event	Poor	Poor
Plasmablastic of the oral cavity	Rare	0	0	0	0	>70	0	Usually low		Generally late event	Poor	Poor
	CD20	**CD30**	**CD15**	**CD45**	**Reed–Sternberg Cells**							
Hodgkin lymphoma												
Classic	Usually negative	Usually positive	Usually positive	Usually negative	Always present	>75	0	Usually well preserved		May be early event	Moderate	Moderate/ improved
Lymphocyte predominant	Positive	Rare positive	Negative	Positive	L&H cells							
Multicentric Castleman disease	Polyclonal plasmacytosis with KSHV+/Lambda+ B-cells; reactive CD20+ B-cells present					0	100[a]	Can be high			Poor	Poor

[a] Less than 60% in HIV unrelated cases.

Adapted from Lim et al,[5] Little et al,[9] Gaidano et al,[23,144] and Jaffe et al.[160]

on viral latency patterns and giving rise to those tumors more likely to be associated with poor prognosis.[30,31]

Additional evidence that HAART has influenced ARL histogenesis comes from studies of the BCL-2 antiapoptotic protein. BCL-2 is one of the pathobiological markers predictive of poor prognosis in NHL, and appears to track with DLBCL arising from nongerminal center B-cells.[29,60–63] Some evidence suggests that since HAART was introduced, fewer ARL over-express BCL-2 and that this may partially explain the improved prognosis, though not all data agree on this.[8,9] Thus, while several lines of evidence support the notion that HAART has improved ARL prognosis through its effect on tumor histogenesis and subsequent tumor biology, this concept is not proven. As mentioned above, AR-PCNSL, which is universally EBV-associated and associated with profound immune depletion, rarely occurs with successful HAART. Table 60-3 summarizes the major pathobiological and viral markers that distinguish the chief ARL subtypes and immune correlates.

The discovery in 1993 of the KS-associated herpes virus (KSHV, also known as human herpes virus-8 or HHV-8),[64] has further informed the relationship between viral oncogenesis and immune function. KSHV is the etiologic agent of primary effusion lymphoma (PEL), described later in this chapter. These lymphomas appear to derive from postgerminal center preterminally differentiated B-cells with an absence of the other genetic lesions commonly found in other ARLs, a feature associated with advanced immune depletion (Table 60-3).[30,65,66] KSHV appears to be a causative oncogenic virus in these tumors, which primarily involve the body cavities as lymphomatous effusions.[67] The particular association of this tumor with HIV infection and its presentation in the body cavities may in part be explained by a number of interesting properties of KSHV (Fig. 60-2). HIV can promote KSHV infectivity of new cells.[68] KSHV encodes for hypoxia response elements, and can be activated by hypoxia. The virus may then enter lytic replication when an infected cell enters body cavities, which are relatively hypoxic.[69,70] This environmental stimulus could potentially result in activation of lytically expressed KSHV oncogenes including viral BCL-2 (vBCL-2), and proangiogenic factors such as viral interleukin-6 and others.[69–73] The KSHV-encoded G protein-coupled receptor, which is constitutively active, upregulates vascular endothelial growth factor perhaps contributing to the characteristic accumulation of body cavity effusions, thus further promoting the hypoxic environment that may be conducive to this tumor's relatively niche-specific growth. Since PEL can present occasionally as solid lymphoma, these mechanisms do not fully explain the tumor biology, and other mechanisms are also important.

Plasmablastic lymphoma of the oral cavity, initially described as a rapidly growing tumor localized to the oral cavity or the jaw, is typically seen only in HIV-infected patients.[74] Morphologically these are similar to DLBCL, but do not express CD20 and expression of the leukocyte common antigen is minimal or absent. The tumor cells react with the plasma cell characteristic antibody VS38c and also frequently with the CD79a antibody, both B-cell markers. They variably express cytoplasmic immunoglobulin and a monoclonal rearrangement of the immunoglobulin heavy chain gene, confirming the clonal B-cell origin, and the plasmacellular differentiation of these neoplasms. Most are EBV associated. B-cell histogenic markers confirm a postgerminal center origin,[31] consistent with the poor prognosis the diagnosis generally implies. In the HAART era, there is evidence of improved outcome and that diffuse involvement of the lymphoma in multiple sites and organs may occur.[75–78]

HL in HIV (HIV-HL) has several biologic and clinical characteristics distinguishing it from classical HL in the general population.[25,79] HIV-HL is EBV associated in 80% or more of cases, whereas in the general population less than 50% of cases are EBV associated. HIV-HL is most often of the mixed cellularity type without substantial mediastinal involvement, whereas in the general population HL is

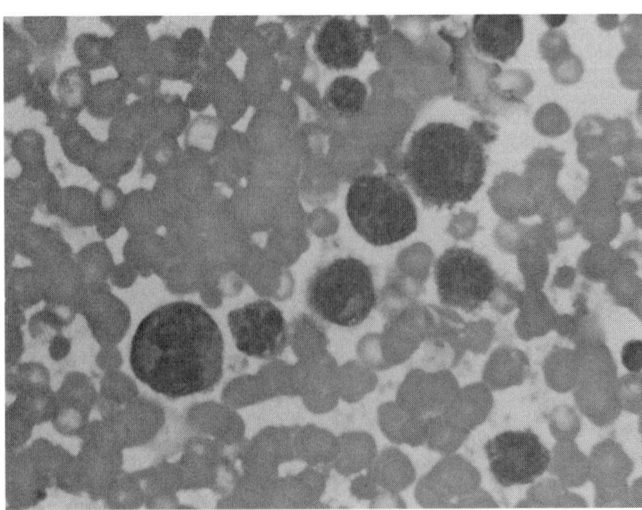

Figure 60-2 ■ CT scan findings and effusion showing primary effusion lymphoma in a patient with AIDS.

most often the nodular sclerosis histologic subtype, and often presents with bulky mediastinal enlargement. HIV-HL is more likely to present with advanced stage disease in younger patients than expected in HL occurring in the general population, and to be more likely associated with extranodal involvement and 'B' symptoms (unexplained weight loss, fevers, and drenching night sweats).[40] The Reed–Sternberg cells of HIV-HL appear to derive from postgerminal center B-cells and although they express CD40, they are not surrounded by CD40 ligand-positive (CD40L+) reactive T lymphocytes, which are thought to regulate the disease phenotype through CD40/CD40L interactions in cases occurring outside HIV.[80] The EBV-encoded LMP-1, which being functionally homologous to CD40, may contribute in part to the modulation of the HIV-HL phenotype.

PERIPHERAL ARL: CLINICAL FEATURES

General

ARL is a serious complication of AIDS and is associated with poorer survival than similar lymphomas in the general population.[6,7,81] Moreover, ARL is one of the more rapidly lethal of AIDS-defining events, though the prognosis of certain histologic types has substantially improved in the HAART era.[4,5] Since the introduction of HAART, median ARL survival has improved from 2–11 months to ~2 years, but this does not extend to all ARL subtypes.[5,6,82,83] Some small studies have shown AR-DLBCL progression-free survival to be about equivalent to non-AIDS lymphoma counterparts.[9] Emphasizing the emerging importance of histologic subtype in ARL, Lim and colleagues found that improved survival since HAART is restricted to DLBCL and that Burkitt prognosis remains poor since the advent of HAART.[5] The median survival of patients with DLBCL in the HAART era appears to be greater than 40 months compared to less than 6–18 months pre-HAART, whereas median survival for Burkitt remains at ~6 months across eras.[5,82] This finding potentially highlights that in the HAART era, lymphoma-specific disease features have become more important.

Presentation, Diagnosis, Staging

The initial presentation for ARL can in some cases be subtle, while in other cases the diagnosis is immediately suspected. The initial level of suspicion of a diagnosis of ARL is in part dependent on the lymphoma type, the extent or stage of lymphoma involvement, and the organ systems impaired. Early in the disease course, only subtle nonspecific abnormalities may be present, and a broad differential diagnosis is appropriately entertained. Early findings in patients with ARL include diffuse minimal adenopathy, low-grade fevers, and perhaps minor hematologic and/or biochemical abnormalities more suggestive of intercurrent viral or bacterial infection than malignancy.

More advanced cases can present with bulky adenopathy, either as solitary or diffusely involved anatomic sites, and often including extranodal sites. The presenting symptoms and signs are related to the anatomic location of tumor involvement, and virtually any anatomic location can be involved, a feature that distinguishes ARL from the majority of non-AIDS NHL cases. Elevations in the serum lactate dehydrogenase (LDH) are often found in aggressive lymphoma, and have prognostic implications.[84] Patients can present with severe constitutional symptoms referred to as 'B' symptoms characterized by drenching night sweats, unexplained fevers, and unexplained weight loss in excess of 10% of the body weight.[85]

Lymphoma can cause varying degrees of organ dysfunction which can at times be severe and life-threatening. Organ dysfunction can result from direct effects of tumor involvement or indirectly from tumor lysis syndrome. This latter complication should be suspected when there is evidence of lactic acidosis with concomitant hyperuricemia, hyperkalemia, hyperphosphatemia, and hypocalcemia. Patients may rapidly develop renal failure. Patients with tumor lysis syndrome require management in intensive care settings. Patients with severe organ dysfunction or symptoms may require urgent hospitalization and prompt consultation with surgeons, hematopathologists, and medical oncologists.

The diagnosis of lymphoma is made by biopsy of an affected area. Often it is readily obvious what site should be biopsied, but occasionally this can be a difficult issue, given that it is not uncommon to find enlarged lymph nodes in HIV infection unrelated to lymphoma. Due to the invasive nature of diagnostic procedures, there is often reticence in early disease to begin a tumor workup until after a trial of empiric antimicrobial therapy followed by a watch and wait approach. In such cases, progression of symptoms and clinical findings may then prompt a more aggressive evaluation. Additionally, in cases of ARL with clinically unimpressive adenopathy, the most easily accessible lymph node targeted for biopsy may reveal only HIV-related hyperplasia and not lymphoma. Such cases can be difficult to diagnose, and it is important to avoid becoming overly complacent on the basis of an unrevealing initial biopsy, especially if this has been performed by needle aspiration of a lymph node targeted primarily because of easy accessibility. Such cases are not uncommon, and a balance must be reached between overly aggressive diagnostic maneuvers and the potential that a lymphoma could worsen in its prognostic features during a period of observation.

Early in the AIDS epidemic, the prognosis for ARL was often very poor, and early diagnosis did not generally confer a clinical advantage. Consequently, aggressive diagnostic maneuvers were not always appropriate. With current treatments and improved outcomes, a more aggressive search for lymphoid malignancy may be more reasonable, especially when signs and symptoms discussed above persist after a minimal empiric course of antibiotics or watchful waiting. In cases with a high suspicion for lymphoma, early biopsy may be preferable. Whenever feasible, excision node biopsy is favored over needle procedures which may not preserve the architectural features useful in diagnostic evaluation. Often the affected lymph nodes will not be markedly enlarged, and identification of the biopsy target most likely to yield a diagnosis of lymphoma can be subjective. If the initially biopsied node shows only hyperplasia, further efforts to search for lymphoma should be considered, and this may necessitate an invasive surgical procedure. Occasionally, disease may be confined to the bone marrow and bone marrow biopsy should be considered when suspicion is high and lymph node biopsy alone is unrevealing.

Once the diagnosis of lymphoma has been made, it is important to adequately define clinically relevant immunophenotypic markers, such as CD20, and to complete a lymphoma staging workup. Because 17% or more of peripheral lymphoma cases in AIDS also involve the central nervous system, staging for all ARL should include brain magnetic resonance imaging (MRI) and lumbar puncture for cytological assessment of the cerebrospinal fluid (CSF).[86,87] If MRI is not readily available, contrast computed tomography (CT) can be used to rule out mass lesions, but has the disadvantage of potentially missing small lesions within the brain. Also, MRI can identify leptomeningeal involvement, though sensitivity may be low.[88] Flow cytometry studies on the CSF can identify occult leptomeningeal lymphoma, and where available may be useful toward ruling out this sanctuary site for lymphoma.[89] Additional studies to complete lymphoma staging include CT scans of the chest, abdomen, and pelvis and bone marrow biopsy (Table 60-4). Additional studies prior to treatment initiation include complete blood count and chemistries to assess LDH, renal and hepatic function. Routine cardiac assessment should include an ECG, and if the patient has received prior anthracycline-based chemotherapy, the cardiac ejection fraction should be measured with an echo or multiple gated acquisition (MUGA) scan. CD4+ cell enumeration should be obtained at lymphoma diagnosis, since it is of prognostic importance. Fluorodeoxyglucose-positron emission tomography (FDG-PET) scans should be obtained if possible prior to therapy to identify sites of lymphoma. This can be particularly useful in assessing response in the case of residual masses seen on restaging CT scans, and early FDG-PET normalization has prognostic as well as therapeutic implications.[90,91]

Table 60-4 Ann Arbor Staging System

Stage	Description
I IE	Single node region or lymphoid structure or single extranodal organ or site
II IIE	Two or more nodes on the same side of the diaphragm or single nodal site with extranodal extension
III	Nodal regions or lymphoid structure on both sides of the diaphragm
IIIE	Or localized involvement of an extralymphatic organ
IIIS	Or spleen
IIISE	Or both
IV	Bone marrow or liver or extranodal sites beyond those designated as ‘E’

Designate absence of constitutional symptoms with A; presence of symptoms: B (fever, sweats, unexplained weight loss greater than 10% of body weight).

From Carbone PP, Kaplan HS, Musshoff K, et al. Report of the Committee on Hodgkin’s Disease Staging Classification. Cancer Res 31:1860–1, 1971.

Therapy

Chemotherapy in ARL

Prior to the 1996 introduction of HAART, low- and standard-dose chemotherapy resulted in equivalent survival in ARL, but toxicity was not acceptable with the standard-dose regimens.[82] Because it resulted in better quality of life and prospects for longer-term survival were poor, low-dose chemotherapy was adopted as the standard of care. Also, prior to HAART, lymphoma-specific disease features appeared to be of relatively little predictive value in predicting outcome as compared to the underlying AIDS disease features.[92] Consequently, therapy was not tailored to the specific lymphoma type, in contrast to the non-AIDS setting where outcome is dependent on lymphoma classification and the regimen selected for the specific class. In the HAART era, it appears that lymphoma-specific disease features are relatively more important and that therapy appropriate to the specific lymphoma subtype may also be important.[5] The current practice of administering the same therapy for DLBCL and BLs in AIDS may explain why the prognosis of BL has not improved in the HAART era (Table 60-3). However, data are not yet available to fully confirm these impressions, and evolving standards of care will almost certainly change as further research progresses.

Standard curative intent therapy for lymphoma in the non-AIDS setting is based on anthracycline-containing regimens administered with sufficient dose-intensity to optimize the curative potential of the regimen.[93,94] This also appears to be the case for ARL in the HAART era. There is evidence that patients who have well-controlled HIV infection on HAART tolerate higher dose-intensity of chemotherapy and to have better lymphoma outcomes than those in whom HIV infection is not amenable to control.[95] Selected therapies commonly used for ARL in the HAART era are listed in Tables 60-5 and 60-6.

In non-AIDS, dose-intensive regimens for BL are associated with a high cure rate, whereas CHOP (cyclophosphamide, doxorubicin, vincristine, and prednisone) or similar regimens are associated with poor outcome. As mentioned, the current standard of care does not distinguish the lymphoma types in AIDS, but there is increasing interest in exploring dose-intensive regimens for AIDS-Burkitt as used in the non-AIDS setting.[96,97] Other regimens may also prove to be of value in AIDS-Burkitt. For example, preliminary data

Table 60-5 Commonly Used Regimens for ARL in the HAART Era

Regimen	Drugs	Comments
R-CHOP	Rituximab 375 mg/m^2 IV day 1 Cyclophosphamide 750 mg/m^2 IV day 1 Doxorubicin 50 mg/m^2 IV day 1 Vincristine 1.4 mg/m^2 IV day 1 (maximum 2 mg) Prednisone 50 mg/m^2 PO days 1–5	Treatment is repeated every 21 days. As noted in the discussion, rituximab appears to be associated with excess treatment related death, and must be used with caution. Rituximab may be omitted if there is concern for toxicity, especially in those with CD4+ cells < 50/mm^3. (Omission of rituximab does not imply that other changes should be made to the regimen) Treatment is continued for 2 cycles after complete response, for a total of 6–8 cycles of therapy. Restaging is done after the fourth and sixth cycles. It is becoming more common to restage after cycle 2, and if a CR is documented, to stop after cycle 4
Kaplan et al[8]	Filgrastim 5 µg/kg daily day 4 until neutrophil 10 000/mm^3	
R-CDE	Rituximab 375 mg/m^2 IV day 1	Treatment is repeated very 28 days for a maximum of 6 cycles. Rituximab may be omitted if there is concern for toxicity. However, the data suggests that rituximab adds substantial activity to this regimen. (Omission of rituximab does not imply that other changes should be made to the regimen)
	Cyclophosphamide 187.5–200 mg m^{-2} day^{-1} days 1–4 CIV	Infection prophylaxis with trimethoprim/sulfamethoxazole PO three times weekly and fluconazole 100 mg PO daily
	Doxorubicin 12.5 mg m^{-2} day^{-1} days 1–4 CIV	
	Etoposide 60 mg/m^{-2} day^{-1} days 1–4 days CIV	
	Filgrastim 5 µg kg^{-1} day^{-1}, subcutaneous injection day 6 until neutrophil recovery	
Spina et al[107]	Methotrexate 12 mg or Cytarabine 50 mg by intrathecal injection	Methotrexate given day 1 each cycle; Cytarabine D1 and D4 of cycles 1 and 2 for patients with Burkitt lymphoma or bone marrow involvement
Dose Adjusted EPOCH	Etoposide 50 mg m^{-2} day^{-1} CIV days 1–4	Rituximab not well studied with this regimen in AIDS. Preliminary data suggests equivalence with EPOCH alone, though fewer cycles to complete response may be required. Ongoing randomized trial of R-EPOCH versus EPOCH followed by R may provide definitive information
	Doxorubicin 10 mg m^{-2} day^{-1} CIV days 1–4	In the original phase II trial, antiretroviral therapy was suspended until completion of all chemotherapy cycles. In the ongoing randomized trail of R-EPOCH versus EPOCH followed by rituximab, HAART is generally co-administered
	Vincristine 0.4 mg m^{-2} day^{-1} CIV days 1–4 (no cap)	
	Cyclophosphamide 187.5–375 mg m^{-2} day^{-1} IV day 5 (see comment for adjustment)	Cycle 1 cyclophosphamide dose CD4+ cell dependent: if CD4+ <100, cyclophosphamide 187 mg/m^2; otherwise 350 mg/m^2. Subsequent cycles adjust up or down in increments of 187 mg/m^2 depending on ANC nadir of ≤500/mm^3 or not. Maximum dose 750 mg/m^2. Note that after a reduction, if ANC >500 mg/m^2 per dose is increased by 187 mg/m^2 (e.g. dose reductions not permanent)
	Prednisone 60 mg/m^2 PO daily days 1–5	
	Filgrastim 5 µg/kg subcutaneous injection day 6 until neutrophil recovery > 5000	Infection prophylaxis with trimethoprim/sulfamethoxazole PO three times weekly; MAC prophylaxis is CD4+ cells < 75/mm^3
Little et al[9]	Methotrexate 12 mg IT days 1 and 5 cycles 3–6	

suggest that CHOP-like regimens combined with rituximab may be active in AIDS-Burkitt.[98] As yet, such patients should most likely be treated on a research protocol in order to confirm the findings of small early reports.

There is evidence that if HIV is suppressed by HAART, patients may have a favorable outcome of lymphoma therapy regardless of the CD4+ cell count at lymphoma diagnosis, in contrast to the pre-HAART era where low CD4+ cells

Table 60-6 Selected Regimens and Outcome for AIDS-Related Lymphoma

Course of Therapy			Number of Evaluable Patients	Median CD4+ Cells/mm^3 at Baseline	HAART	Complete Response Rate (%)	Median Overall or Progression Free (PFS) Survival (Months)		Author
m-BACOD	Randomized	Low dose	94	100	Pre-HAART	41	8.75	$P = 0.56$	Kaplan et al[82]
		Standard dose	81	107	Pre-HAART	52	7.75		
CHOP	Not Randomized	Low Dose	40	138	HAART required	30	PFS ~ 15		Ratner et al[81]
		Standard Dose	23	122	HAART required	48	Not reached at 6.5 months median follow up		
EPOCH		Dose adjusted	39	198	HAART suspended	74	Not reached: 60% at median follow-up of 53 months		Little et al[9]
CDE			43	90	Pre-HAART	47	6.8		Sparano et al[108]
			55	227	During HAART era	44	13.7		
R-CDE			74	161	76% received HAART with R-CDE	70	Not reached: 65% at median follow up of 23 months		Spina et al[107]
CHOP vs R-CHOP	Randomized	Rituximab	99	130	HAART required	57.6	34.8	$P = 0.76$	Kaplan et al[8]
		No Rituximab	50	147	During (required)	47	27.5		

m-BACOD, methotrexate, bleomycin, doxorubicin, cyclophosphamide, vincristine, dexamethasone; CHOP, cyclophosphamide, doxorubicin, vincristine, prednisone; EPOCH, etoposide, prednisone, vincristine, cyclophosphamide, doxorubicin; CDE, cyclophosphamide, doxorubicin, etoposide; R, rituximab.

almost universally implied a poorer prognosis.[82,99,100] As the prognostic weight of CD4+ cells lessens, a greater role for the international prognostic index (IPI) score for lymphoma is emerging,[8,101] Prior to the HAART era, the IPI score appeared of little relevance to prognosis. The IPI is based on factors such as age, stage, biochemical abnormalities, and performance status. As such, treatment delays can result in a worsening of the IPI score and hence prognosis. This concept reinforces the need for timely diagnosis in the HAART era.

Patients with advanced AIDS and HIV that is not amenable to long-term control may not be as likely to benefit from newer treatment strategies. However, these patients can sometimes gain additional years and high-quality survival,[9] so appropriately directed treatment with curative intent should be considered for these patients as well. In the past, many physicians shied away from this approach, but the cumulative experience with such patients indicates that curative therapy is often warranted. Certain circumstances bode for palliative therapy only, and these cases may best be decided in concert with oncologists who are experienced in the treatment of AIDS-associated malignancies.

The single most important advance in non-ARL therapy since introduction of CHOP chemotherapy has been rituximab.[102–104] Rituximab is a monoclonal anti-CD20 antibody that targets B-cells expressing this protein, and also makes them more susceptible to the lympholytic effects of chemotherapy.[105] In the non-AIDS setting, the addition of rituximab leads to improved outcome when added to standard chemotherapy regimens and has become the standard of care for almost all lymphoma types expressing CD20 antigen.[106]

The issue of whether to add rituximab to cytotoxic chemotherapy is more complex in ARL. A trial in which all patients received HAART and CHOP and were randomized to receive rituximab or not, failed to reach the targeted 50% improvement in complete response rate.[8] Moreover, the treatment-related death rate was 14% in the rituximab group compared to 2% in the CHOP alone group. The excess toxicity in the rituximab arm appeared to be particularly problematic in those with advanced immune depletion. Sixty percent of these treatment-related deaths occurred in those with <50 CD4+ cells/mm^3. Other studies have also suggested that rituximab adds toxicity to chemotherapy. Spina and colleagues reported pooled results from three phase II trials of rituximab and infusional CDE (cyclophosphamide, doxorubicin and etoposide given over 96 h by continuous intravenous infusion), which also suggested that rituximab conferred a degree of added toxicity to the regimen.[107] However, this analysis provided evidence that the addition of rituximab was associated with improved outcome compared to previous experience with CDE alone.[108] Moreover, the improvement did not appear to be explained by HAART. The complete response rate with R-CDE in the pooled studies was 70% whereas previous studies had reported complete responses of 47% pre-HAART and 44% in the HAART era. Additional information about rituximab has been from studies of the EPOCH regimen. When rituximab was added to the infusional EPOCH regimen, preliminary results suggest that toxicity appears higher, but it is uncertain whether this is due to a modification of the initial chemotherapy doses from that used in the earlier trial, or rituximab, or both.[98] Outcomes with EPOCH and R-EPOCH appear similar, though as yet the data are not sufficient to state this with certainty.

As can be seen, there is currently some controversy and concern regarding the use of rituximab in ARL. At the same time, it is also important to recognize that there appears to be some advantage to giving it. Although the previously mentioned randomized R-CHOP versus CHOP trial did not show a statistically significant difference in ARL outcome, the actual numerical difference was similar to that seen in randomized trials of non-AIDS DLBCL that targeted a more modest response effect,[109] raising the question of whether the ARL trial targeted too high an improvement. This issue was discussed in a panel on controversies in the treatment of ARL at the NCI-sponsored Ninth International Conference on Malignancies in AIDS and Other Immunodeficiencies held September 2005 in Rockville, Maryland. There was a general consensus expressed by the panelists that rituximab may have a role in the treatment of ARL but that care be taken when considering it, especially in patients with fewer than 50 CD4+ cells mm^3.[110] Additionally it was noted that such patients should be considered as high risk for infectious complications and routinely administered antibiotic prophylaxis if given rituximab-based immunotherapy for ARL, based on recent randomized trials showing efficacy of antibiotic prophylaxis in reducing complications of episodic febrile neutropenia in cancer patients receiving chemotherapy.[111,112] Thus, while the use of rituximab was generally felt by the panelists to be useful in ARL, especially those with higher CD4+ cell counts,[113] it should be noted that this recommendation is not universally accepted and is not as fully based on scientific data as in the non-AIDS setting. The recommendations should not be taken to supersede the judgment of treating physicians expert in the management of ARL. Also, physicians should be alert for new data and changes in the recommended practice.

HAART in ARL

There has been some debate as to whether HAART should be administered concomitantly with chemotherapy in ARL or delayed until after completion of antilymphoma therapy. Both approaches have been investigated, but there are no direct comparisons upon which to base rigorous conclusions. There are pros and cons to both approaches, as summarized in Table 60-7. These issues can only be considered indirectly through available data from a variety of trials, most of which had other primary endpoints and were not focused primarily on this issue.

The NCI-sponsored AIDS Malignancy Consortium conducted one of the first trials assessing the feasibility of co-administering HAART and chemotherapy in ARL. Treatment included stavudine, lamivudine, and indinavir with either low-dose or standard-dose CHOP.[81] Patients were sequentially entered first onto the low-dose then onto the standard-dose CHOP arms. Pharmacokinetic data showed an apparent slowing of cyclophosphamide clearance by ~50% in these patients compared to historic controls who were not receiving antiretroviral therapy. However, there were no apparent effects on levels of doxorubicin or indinavir. The authors felt that there was no obvious increase in toxicity, but this issue was somewhat subjective as there was no control group. However, in support of this observation, a retrospective analysis of 44 patients treated with a variety of regimens, including CHOP and similar regimens, found that those patients who were responding to HAART long-term had better chemotherapy tolerance and outcome compared to patients either naive to HAART or failing HAART.[95] A multi-institutional trial of CDE that spanned the pre-HAART and HAART eras showed a similar response rate between the two eras, but less chemotherapy-associated toxicity and improved overall survival in the HAART era.[108] The previously mentioned pooled R-CDE trial included HAART in 76% of the patients, and in univariate analysis, a low or undetectable HIV viral load was associated with better overall survival.[107] Thus, these studies indicate that there are no apparent problems with HAART co-administration on lymphoma outcome. Moreover, the ability of patients to maintain low viral loads in the referenced studies provides credible evidence that chemotherapy does not necessarily impair HAART adherence during chemotherapy.

At the same time, there is evidence that good responses to lymphoma therapy can be obtained without concomitant HAART. In a phase II trail of dose-adjusted EPOCH, favorable

Table 60-7 Considerations for Using HAART Concomitantly or Suspending it During Chemotherapy for ARL

Concomitant	Sequential
Protect CD4+ cells and prevent AIDS progression	No protective effect on CD4+ cells; minimal CD4+ cell loss due to HIV during chemotherapy; major chemotherapy-induced CD4+ cell loss
Improved chemo tolerance	PK and toxicity interactions
Decrease in HIV-related pro-lymphoma factors	HAART adherence adversely affected
Protease inhibitors block PGP/MDR receptors	NRTI stabilize mitochondrial membrane blocking apoptosis
HIV proteins such as VPR can block apoptosis	HIV proteins such as Tat increase apoptosis

results were found when HAART was omitted until the completion of chemotherapy.[9] These results, along with the CDE trials, suggest that HAART is not operative in response induction, but they highlight the importance of HAART in controlling the subsequent course of AIDS and improving long-term survival. Of course, if patients have decreased toxicity with HAART and are thus able to maintain appropriate dose-schedule chemotherapy cycles, there may be an association with improved responses with HAART co-administration.

Taken in sum, it appears that a reasonable case can be made to either administer HAART concomitantly with chemotherapy or to delay it until the end of chemotherapy. Although decisions for the best approach should be made in regards to each individual patient, there was general agreement during discussions at the previously mentioned Ninth International Conference on Malignancies in AIDS and Other Immunodeficiencies regarding controversies in ARL that a reasonable recommendation for standard practice would be to concurrently administer HAART and chemotherapy if a patient is already on a stable HAART regimen. However, if a patient is not on HAART at the commencement of chemotherapy, most participants felt that waiting to start HAART later would be a reasonable strategy.[110] The viewpoint was expressed that HAART initiation and its acute induction of cytochrome enzymes is more likely to cause or provoke toxicity than in the case where a patient is already on a stable regimen of HAART. However, it was emphasized that avoidance of excessively myelotoxic agents such as zidovudine and careful monitoring for a variety of effects such as atazanavir-related hyperbilirubinemia is essential. Hyperbilirubinemia can be associated with excessive toxicity for numerous chemotherapy agents. Given the panoply of anti-HIV drugs, the potential for adverse or unexpected effects owing to drug combinations is difficult to rigorously study, and a simplified alternative approach may be to omit HAART during the period of combination lymphoma chemotherapy.[114]

AR-PCNSL: CLINICAL FEATURES

General

AR-PCNSL is a devastating complication of AIDS. Patients may initially present with subtle personality changes obvious only to those who know the patient well. Progression of the presenting clinical findings in AR-PCNSL typically takes only days to a few weeks and patients can develop headaches, seizures, focal neurological deficits, aphasia, lethargy, confusion, delirium, psychosis, or obtundation.[115] By contrast, progression of such symptoms in PCNSL in the immunocompetent population may take months.[116] Additionally, patients with AR-PCNSL may initially present with constitutional symptoms such as fevers, night sweats, weight loss, anorexia, and fatigue that may be ascribed to advanced AIDS in the absence of other findings suggestive of CNS pathology. Nearly all cases of AR-PCNSL occur in patient with advanced immune suppression when the CD4+ cells are less than 50/mm^3.

Diagnosis and Staging

MRI of the brain should be obtained in all cases suggestive of CNS pathology. Often CT scans are obtained instead at the time of initial presentation because logistically they may be easier and faster to schedule. Although CT scans can identify larger lesions and reliably inform safety of performing a lumbar puncture, small parenchymal brain lesions may not be seen on CT, and so MRI should be performed at some point in the evaluation. Although some cases show only unifocal abnormalities, 30–70% of cases show multifocal enhancing lesions with contrast CT (Fig. 60-3).[115] MRI will demonstrate lesions that appear hypointense or isointense on T1-weighted images, with variable intensity on T2-weighted images.

With CT or MRI studies alone, it is not possible to distinguish AR-PCNSL from toxoplasmosis infection in the brain, the most likely cause of intracranial mass lesions in AIDS.[117] Therefore, additional diagnostic studies that may include brain biopsy should be undertaken as soon as possible. Whenever possible, steroid administration should be delayed until after the biopsy, because the lympholytic effect of steroids can obscure the diagnosis.[118] In addition, patients can have coexisting cerebral infection and brain lymphoma. Thus, although biopsy is considered the gold standard for diagnosis in AR-PCNSL, at times the results can be difficult to interpret.

It is not uncommon for biopsy to be deferred in patients with advanced AIDS who present with an intracerebral mass lesion. Since the risk of toxoplasma abscess is high, often a

Table 60-8 Use of FBV-DNA Detection in CSF by PCR and SPECT Thallium for the Diagnosis of AIDS-Related PNCSL

	Sensitivity	Specificity	Positive Predictive Value	Negative Predictive Value
SPECT and EBV-DNA	76.9	100	100	85.7
SPECT and/or EBV-DNA	100	88.9	86.7	100

From Antinori A, De Rossi G, Ammassari A, et al. Value of combined approach with thallium-201 single-photon emission computed tomography and Epstein–Barr virus DNA polymerase chain reaction in CSF for the diagnosis of AIDS-related primary CNS lymphoma. J Clin Oncol 17:554–60, 1999.

period of observation to assess the effects of empiric antibiotic therapy will be undertaken. If there is a response, then the lesion is presumed to be infectious in etiology. In the case of no response or progression, oncologists are faced with administering definitive therapy in the absence of biopsy. This is one of the very rare situations where this is acceptable oncologic practice. It is also of concern that during the observation period, the patent's clinical status can continue to deteriorate. Recent advances in diagnostic strategies may be useful in making more rapid and reliable AR-PCNSL diagnosis.

Nearly 100% of AR-PCNSL are EBV associated, and EBV DNA detection by PCR in the CSF is highly predictive that a mass brain lesion is PCNSL in AIDS.[119–123] In addition, nuclear medicine studies such as SPECT-thallium and FDG-PET scans are highly specific and sensitive for malignant conditions, including lymphoma.[124–127] Antorini and colleagues have shown that when EBV PCR from the spinal fluid and SPECT thallium scans are combined in the evaluation, the results can be used to reliably predict whether a cerebral mass is lymphoma or not (Table 60-8).[128] When both tests are positive, the positive predictive value is ~100% that the lesion is lymphoma. Conversely, if both tests are negative the likelihood for lymphoma is slim. Some authorities have appropriately cautioned that these results be used carefully since the confidence intervals in the studies were rather wide.[115] Additionally, this study was done in the pre-HAART era, and some have called into question whether these associations remain valid in the HAART era.[129] However, when biopsy is not feasible or the biopsy results are inconclusive because of prior steroids or presence of infectious abscess concurrent with lymphoma, oncologists can consider this information in planning whether to initiate definitive therapy. In cases where waiting for empiric toxoplasmosis treatment to fail and the risk of lymphoma growth is likely to promote clinical deterioration, some argue in favor of proceeding with the specific lymphoma therapy on the basis of these results, thus avoiding the potential decline in performance status and prognosis associated with treatment delay in this disease.[130]

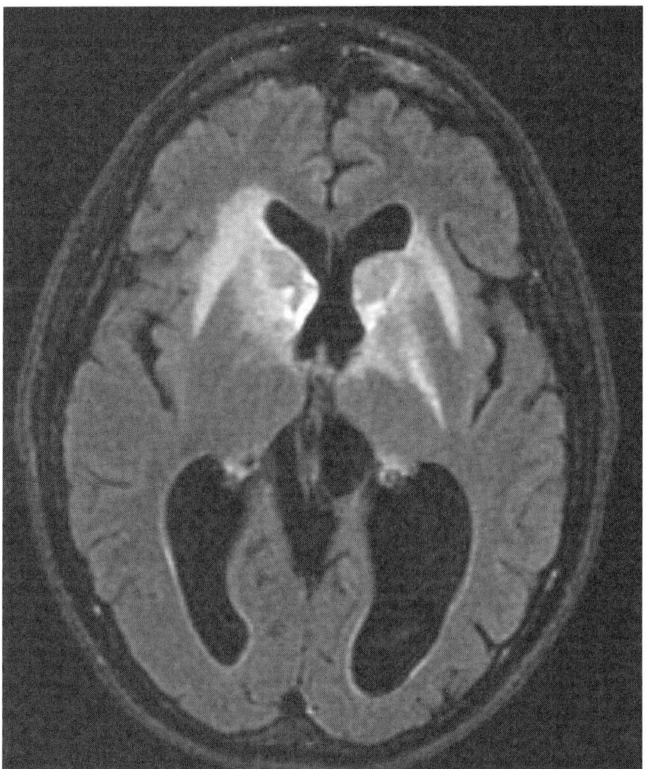

Figure 60-3 ■ MRI in a patient with AIDS-related primary central nervous system lymphoma.

Once the diagnosis of PCNSL has been established, staging workup should be performed in consultation with a medical oncologist. It is important to rule out peripheral lymphoma involvement. The finding of extracerebral lymphoma denotes by definition that the central nervous system involvement is metastatic, rather than primary, and substantially alters the treatment. Although the search for lymphoma outside the CNS is typically of low yield,[115,131] most oncologists recommend performing a complete evaluation. Additional staging involves spinal MRI with gadolinium and lumbar puncture. Often the CSF will have elevated protein and cytology will reveal only a nonspecific pleocytosis. Flow cytometric evaluation of the CSF may reveal clinically occult disease in this setting.[89] Ophthalmologic evaluation should be performed in all patients to rule out intraocular lymphoma. Given the high risk for infectious ocular co-morbidity in this population, periodic surveillance of the retinas is indicated until adequate immune recovery has occurred.

Treatment

Whole brain radiotherapy is typically utilized for treatment of AR-PNCSL. In the non-AIDS setting, there has been a shift toward chemotherapy-based treatment in PCNSL.[132,133]

Chemotherapy-based approaches have been developed for PCNSL outside the setting of AIDS in part because long-term PCNSL survivors are otherwise at risk for severe delayed neurocognitive decline following whole-brain radiotherapy (WBRT).[134,135] Prior to HAART, high-dose chemotherapy appeared to prolong survival in few patients and was excessively toxic for most.[136] Only recently have investigators begun to explore the use of chemotherapy-based treatment for AR-PNCSL in the HAART era. Because AR-PCNSL is quite responsive to WBRT, this was without question the optimal therapy pre-HAART, since patients were unlikely to survive long enough to develop late radiation-related neurotoxicity. The median survival was less than 4 months, owing to progressive AIDS complications or recurrent brain lymphoma.[137] Longer-term survival with HAART introduces the potential that survival with AR-PCNSL will be long enough for patients to develop these late-occurring radiation-related effects. Therefore, exploration of treatments that apply in non-AIDS to determine whether they will be applicable to AR-PCNSL seems reasonable. There are insufficient data to conclude that a chemotherapy approach in AR-PCNSL will benefit this population. The National Cancer Institute and National Institute of Allergy and Infectious Disease have initiated a collaborative trial in the National Institutes of Health Clinical Research Center to further evaluate the use of EBV and nuclear medicine studies in diagnosing AR-PCNSL and on the use of high-dose methotrexate with rituximab and HAART in patients with AR-PCNSL to provide preliminary data on the feasibility of this approach.

HL: CLINICAL FEATURES

HIV-HL is typically associated with more aggressive clinical features compared with the HIV-unrelated setting. HIV-HL more often presents with unfavorable histologic subtypes and advanced-stage disease.[79] Most patients, even prior to the HAART era, had relatively well preserved CD4+ cells at HL diagnosis and did not have a prior AIDS diagnosis. Although reported response rates are typically high, survival was generally short owing to recurrent HL or progressive AIDS following chemotherapy.[25,79] In the HAART era, there has been improved survival that appears to be primarily related to better HIV therapy, and its potential effect on more favorable HL features at presentation.[138]

The clinical presentation for HL and staging is essentially the same as that for ARL, except that it is not necessary to evaluate the CNS as part of routine staging. Contrary to NHL, LDH is not a sensitive biochemical marker for HL.

In part because HIV-HL is a rare and complex disease in which patients with different stages and types may respond differently to therapy, there is no clear treatment standard that dictates one Hodgkin regimen as being superior to others. In general, combination ABVD (doxorubicin, bleomycin, vincristine, dacarbazine) is recommended in non-AIDS as the standard of care in HL based on randomized trials comparing this to other regimens.[139,140] It is difficult to assess superiority of one regimen over another in HIV infection because there are no reported randomized trails available.

KSHV-RELATED LYMPHOPROLIFERATIVE DISEASE

KSHV is associated with three diseases: KS, PEL, and multicentric Castleman's disease (MCD).[141–143] PEL and MCD are both rare B-cell lymphoproliferative disorders (Table 60-3). PEL is associated with KSHV in 100% of cases, and EBV in 70% or more of cases. Nearly 100% of HIV-related MCD cases are KSHV associated, and ~50% of HIV-unrelated MCD are KSHV associated.[144] PEL, also known as body cavity lymphoma owing to its predilection to form as lymphomatous effusions in the serous body spaces (Fig. 60-2), is frequently seen in the setting of concomitant KS. It generally remains confined to the site of initial presentation, but also can involve nodal tissue and the bone marrow. MCD can involve multiple nodes, the sizes of which are often unimpressive. The syndrome can be characterized by fevers, cytopenias, hemolysis, multiple organ dysfunctions, fluid retention, coagulopathy, and other infectious complications. Many of the clinical and biochemical features of MCD appear to be mediated by interleukin-6, which can be cellular or viral (KSHV) in origin (Fig. 60-4).[145–147]

Both PEL and MCD are serious diseases for which there is no standard treatment. The median survival for PEL is less than 6 months and the median survival for MCD is generally less than 2 years.[83,148,149] Chemotherapeutic approaches for each of these diseases can result in responses, but remissions are often of short duration. Rituximab has been reported to be of some use in MCD.[150] Monoclonal antibody to interleukin-6 may also be of promise in this condition.[151,152] Other investigative approaches for these diseases involve the use of targeted therapy including antiangiogenesis approaches and drugs such as ganciclovir to exploit KSHV-encoded genes for potential oncolytic effect.[26,153,154]

SUPPORTIVE CARE

Patients undergoing combination antilymphoma chemotherapy should routinely receive prophylaxis against *Pneumocystis jeroveci* pneumonia (PCP), regardless of HIV serostatus or CD4+ cell count, and remain on it for several months post-therapy or until the CD4+ cells are stable above 200/mm^3.[155] Additionally, prophylaxis against *Mycobacterium avium* complex (MAC) is recommended by some for patients with CD4+ cells less than 100/mm^3 since further immunosuppression is associated with chemotherapy.[9] As mentioned above, prophylaxis against bacterial sepsis during periods of neutropenia is currently recommended, especially for patients receiving rituximab.[110–112] Fluconazole prophylaxis is recommended by some authorities during antilymphoma therapy.[107] Most authorities recommend preemptive use of filgrastim in patients with HIV receiving combination chemotherapy to help avoid or shorten periods of neutropenia.[8,9,107]

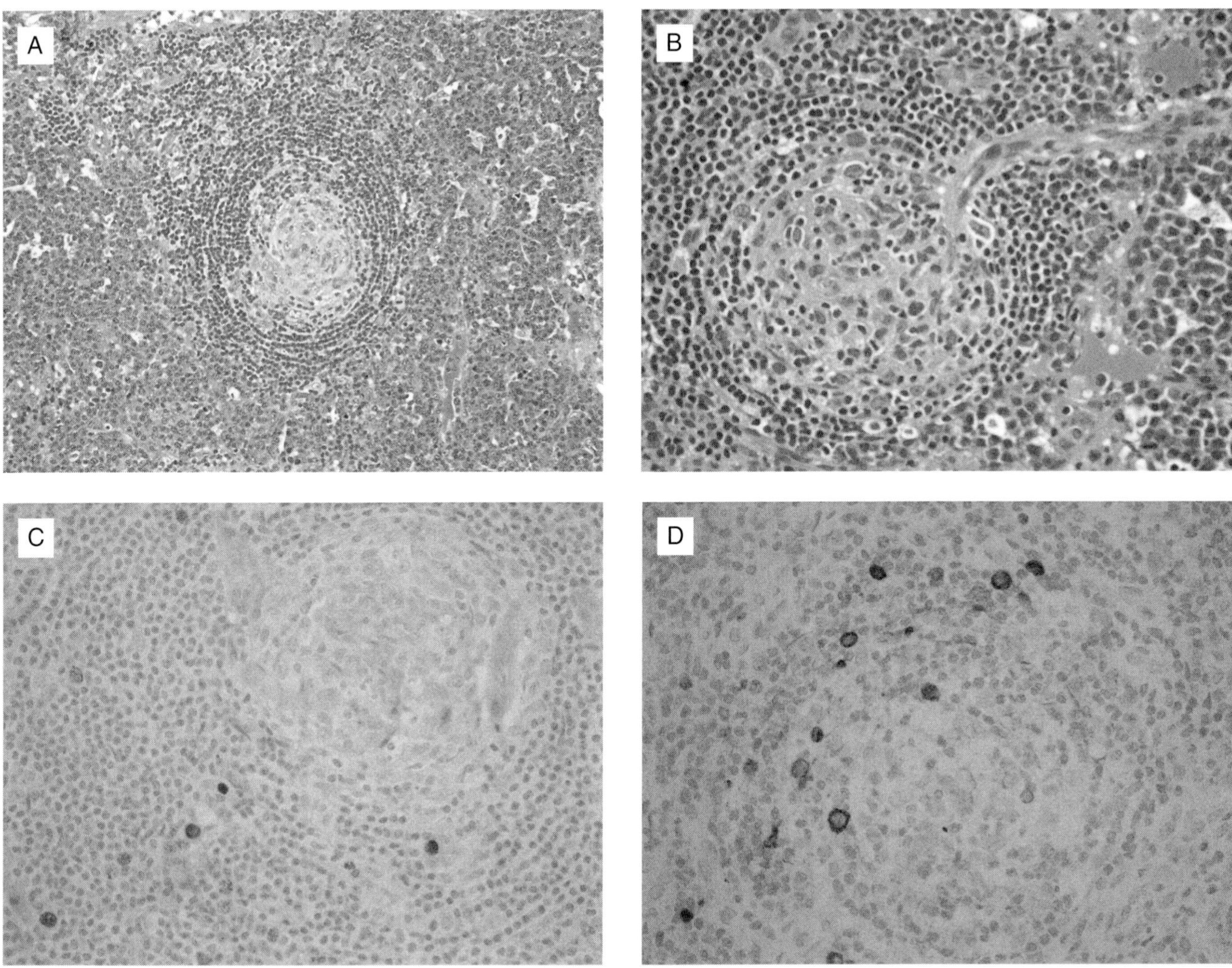

Figure 60-4 ■ Histopathologic stains of KSHV-related multicentric Castleman's disease in HIV-infected patients showing (**A**) H&E stain of involved node and at (**B**) higher magnification; and immunohistochemistry showing mononuclear cells positive for (**C**) LANA and (**D**) viral IL-6.

FUTURE PROSPECTS

The availability of HAART has created new opportunities and challenges in treating patients with ARL and HL. Additionally, some diseases such as KSHV-related MCD are being recognized more and might be seen with increasing prevalence in the HAART era. Determination of whether various lymphoma subtypes should be treated with equivalent type-specific regimens to those used in the non-AIDS setting is a current area of research. Michelle Spina and colleagues in Italy are initiating a study of dose-intensive methotrexate-based chemotherapy for AIDS-BL that is likely to substantially add to the understanding of these issues. Further evaluation of the potential for CHOP-based therapy with rituximab in AIDS-Burkitt also appears warranted. Such CHOP regimens are better tolerated than the dose-intensive methotrexate regimens, and if effective, would represent an advance for AIDS-Burkitt. The NCI-sponsored AIDS Malignancy Consortium is conducting a randomized trial of R-EPOCH versus EPOCH followed by rituximab maintenance, which will help to further define the role of rituximab in ARL, possibly including for Burkitt. Evaluation of CHOP given every 14 days (CHOP-14) in ARL is also a priority being initiated by Spina and colleges in Italy. In non-AIDS-related lymphoma, some randomized data indicates that high-risk elderly patients have superior outcome when treated with CHOP-14, compared to standard 21-day cycles.[156] Moreover, the role of rituximab in CHOP-14 is an important area to be investigated for ARL, and precedent in non-AIDS again suggests that this is likely to represent an advance, notwithstanding toxicity concerns in the AIDS population.[157]

The frequent associations with oncogenic viruses in ARL and immunosuppression-related lymphoproliferations create opportunities to consider novel pathogenesis-based approaches in ARL.[26,130] Viral genes and products offer unique targets for potential therapeutic exploitation. Interfering RNA, antiangiogenesis approaches, histone modulation, and other novel therapies are under active laboratory and clinical study in malignancies associated with HIV infection and AIDS. Basic and translational research in this field provides a unique opportunity to explore new approaches that may be advantageous in advancing oncology and related medical fields.

REFERENCES

1. Morton LM, Wang SS, Devesa SS, et al. Lymphoma incidence patterns by WHO subtype in the United States, 1992–2001. Blood 107:265–76, 2006.
2. Beral V, Peterman T, Berkelman R, Jaffe H. AIDS-associated non-Hodgkin lymphoma. Lancet 337:805–9, 1991.
3. MMWR. Current Trends Revision of the Case Definition of Acquired Immunodeficiency Syndrome for National Reporting – United States. Atlanta: Centers for Disease Control; 1985, Report No. 34.
4. Mocroft AJ, Lundgren JD, d'Armino Monforte A, et al. Survival of AIDS patients according to type of AIDS-defining event. The AIDS in Europe Study Group. Int J Epidemiol 26:400–7, 1997.
5. Lim ST, Karim R, Nathwani BN, et al. AIDS-related Burkitt's lymphoma versus diffuse large-cell lymphoma in the pre-highly active antiretroviral therapy (HAART) and HAART eras: significant differences in survival with standard chemotherapy. J Clin Oncol 23:4430–8, 2005.
6. Besson C, Goubar A, Gabarre J, et al. Changes in AIDS-related lymphoma since the era of highly active antiretroviral therapy. Blood 98:2339–44, 2001.
7. Fisher RI, Gaynor ER, Dahlberg S, et al. Comparison of a standard regimen (CHOP) with three intensive chemotherapy regimens for advanced non-Hodgkin's lymphoma. N Engl J Med 328:1002–6, 1993.
8. Kaplan LD, Lee JY, Ambinder RF, et al. Rituximab does not improve clinical outcome in a randomized phase III trial of CHOP with or without rituximab in patients with HIV-associated non-Hodgkin's lymphoma: AIDS-malignancies consortium trial 010. Blood 106:1538–43, 2005.
9. Little RF, Pittaluga S, Grant N, et al. Highly effective treatment of acquired immunodeficiency syndrome-related lymphoma with dose-adjusted EPOCH: impact of antiretroviral therapy suspension and tumor biology. Blood 101:4653–9, 2003.
10. Lim S-T, Karim R, Tulpule A, et al. Prognostic factors in HIV-related diffuse large-cell lymphoma: before versus after highly active antiretroviral therapy. J Clin Oncol 23:8477–82, 2005.
11. Beral V, Peterman TA, Berkelman RL, Jaffe HW. Kaposi's sarcoma among persons with AIDS: a sexually transmitted infection? Lancet 335:123–8, 1990.
12. Grulich AE, Li Y, McDonald A, et al. Rates of non-AIDS-defining cancers in people with HIV infection before and after AIDS diagnosis. AIDS 16:1155–61, 2002.
13. Dal Maso L, Franceschi S. Epidemiology of non-Hodgkin lymphomas and other haemolymphopoietic neoplasms in people with AIDS. Lancet Oncol 4:110–19, 2003.
14. Kirk O, Pedersen C, Cozzi-Lepri A, et al. Non-Hodgkin lymphoma in HIV-infected patients in the era of highly active antiretroviral therapy. Blood 98:3406–12, 2001.
15. Matthews GV, Bower M, Mandalia S, et al. Changes in acquired immunodeficiency syndrome-related lymphoma since the introduction of highly active antiretroviral therapy. Blood 96:2730–4, 2000.
16. Dore GJ, Li Y, McDonald A, et al. Impact of highly active antiretroviral therapy on individual AIDS-defining illness incidence and survival in Australia. J Acquir Immune Defic Syndr 29:388–95, 2002.
17. International Collaboration on HIV and Cancer. Highly active antiretroviral therapy and incidence of cancer in human immunodeficiency virus-infected adults. J Natl Cancer Inst 92:1823–30, 2000.
18. Gayet-Ageron A, Baratin D, Marceillac E, et al. The AIDS epidemic in Lyon: patient characteristics and defining illnesses between 1985 and 2000. HIV Med 5:163–70, 2004.
19. Grulich AE, Li Y, McDonald AM, et al. Decreasing rates of Kaposi's sarcoma and non-Hodgkin's lymphoma in the era of potent combination anti-retroviral therapy. AIDS 15:629–33, 2001.
20. Clifford GM, Polesel J, Rickenbach M, et al. Cancer risk in the Swiss HIV Cohort Study: associations with immunodeficiency, smoking, and highly active antiretroviral therapy. J Natl Cancer Inst 97:425–32, 2005.
21. Bonnet F, Lewden C, May T, et al. Malignancy-related causes of death in human immunodeficiency virus-infected patients in the era of highly active antiretroviral therapy. Cancer 101: 317–24, 2004.
22. Lewden C, Salmon D, Morlat P, et al. Causes of death among human immunodeficiency virus (HIV)-infected adults in the era of potent antiretroviral therapy: emerging role of hepatitis and cancers, persistent role of AIDS. Int J Epidemiol 34: 121–30, 2005.
23. Gaidano G, Pastore C, Lanza C, et al. Molecular pathology of AIDS-related lymphomas. Biologic aspects and clinicopathologic heterogeneity. Ann Hematol 69:281–90, 1994.
24. Beral V, Jaffe H, on behalf of the International Collaboration on HIV and Cancer. HIV-related malignancies in developing countries. In: 9th International Conference on Malignancies in AIDS and Other Acquired Immunodeficiencies, Bethesda, 2005, p S5.
25. Rubio R. Hodgkin's disease associated with human immunodeficiency virus infection. A clinical study of 46 cases. Cooperative Study Group of Malignancies Associated with HIV Infection of Madrid. Cancer 73:2400–7, 1994.
26. Yarchoan R, Tosato G, Little RF. Therapy insight: AIDS-related malignancies – the influence of antiviral therapy on pathogenesis and management. Nat Clin Pract Oncol 2:406–15; quiz 23, 2005.
27. Little RF, Yarchoan R. Treatment of gammaherpesvirus-related neoplastic disorders in the immunosuppressed host. Semin Hematol 40:163–71, 2003.
28. Rosenwald A, Wright G, Chan WC, et al. The use of molecular profiling to predict survival after chemotherapy for diffuse large-B-cell lymphoma. N Engl J Med 346:1937–47, 2002.
29. Lossos IS, Czerwinski DK, Alizadeh AA, et al. Prediction of survival in diffuse large-B-cell lymphoma based on the expression of six genes. N Engl J Med 350:1828–37, 2004.
30. Carbone A, Gaidano G, Gloghini A, et al. Differential expression of BCL-6, CD138/syndecan-1, and Epstein–Barr virus-encoded latent membrane protein-1 identifies distinct histogenetic subsets of acquired immunodeficiency syndrome-related non-Hodgkin's lymphomas. Blood 91:747–55, 1998.
31. Carbone A, Gloghini A, Larocca LM, et al. Expression profile of MUM1/IRF4, BCL-6, and CD138/syndecan-1 defines novel histogenetic subsets of human immunodeficiency virus-related lymphomas. Blood 97:744–51, 2001.
32. Dalla-Favera R. Mechanisms of genetic lesions in AIDS-associated lymphoma. In: The Seventh International Conference on Malignancies in AIDS and Other Immunodeficiencies, Bethesda, 2003, abstract S13.
33. Little RF. AIDS-related non-Hodgkin's lymphoma: etiology, epidemiology, and impact of highly active antiretroviral therapy. Leuk Lymphoma 44(Suppl 3):S63–8, 2003.
34. Levine AM. Lymphoma complicating immunodeficiency disorders. Ann Oncol 5(Suppl 2):29–35, 1994.
35. National Cancer Institute sponsored study of classifications of non-Hodgkin's lymphomas: summary and description of a working formulation for clinical usage. The Non-Hodgkin's Lymphoma Pathologic Classification Project. Cancer 49: 2112–35, 1982.

36. Carbone A, Gloghini A. AIDS-related lymphomas: from pathogenesis to pathology. Br J Haematol 130:662–70, 2005.
37. Knowles DM. Etiology and pathogenesis of AIDS-related non-Hodgkin's lymphoma. Hematol Oncol Clin North Am 10:1081–109, 1996.
38. Gaidano G, Dalla-Favera R. Molecular pathogenesis of AIDS-related lymphomas. Antibiot Chemother 46:117–24, 1994.
39. Bellas C, Santon A, Manzanal A, et al. Pathological, immunological, and molecular features of Hodgkin's disease associated with HIV infection. Comparison with ordinary Hodgkin's disease. Am J Surg Pathol 20:1520–4, 1996.
40. Tirelli U, Errante D, Dolcetti R, et al. Hodgkin's disease and human immunodeficiency virus infection: clinicopathologic and virologic features of 114 patients from the Italian Cooperative Group on AIDS and Tumors. J Clin Oncol 13:1758–67, 1995.
41. Vilchez RA, Lopez-Terrada D, Middleton JR, et al. Simian virus 40 tumor antigen expression and immunophenotypic profile of AIDS-related non-Hodgkin's lymphoma. Virology 342:38–46, 2005.
42. Engels EA, Viscidi RP, Galloway DA, et al. Case-control study of simian virus 40 and non-Hodgkin lymphoma in the United States. J Natl Cancer Inst 96:1368–74, 2004.
43. Mancao C, Altmann M, Jungnickel B, Hammerschmidt W. Rescue of 'crippled' germinal center B cells from apoptosis by Epstein–Barr virus. Blood 106:4339–44, 2005.
44. Bechtel D, Kurth J, Unkel C, Kuppers R. Transformation of BCR-deficient germinal-center B cells by EBV supports a major role of the virus in the pathogenesis of Hodgkin and posttransplantation lymphomas. Blood 106:4345–50, 2005.
45. Rabkin CS, Yang Q, Goedert JJ, et al. Chemokine and chemokine receptor gene variants and risk of non-Hodgkin's lymphoma in human immunodeficiency virus-1-infected individuals. Blood 93:1838–42, 1999.
46. Dean M, Jacobson LP, McFarlane G, et al. Reduced risk of AIDS lymphoma in individuals heterozygous for the CCR5-delta32 mutation. Cancer Res 59:3561–4, 1999.
47. Pantaleo G, Menzo S, Vaccarezza M, et al. Studies in subjects with long-term nonprogressive human immunodeficiency virus infection. N Engl J Med 332:209–16, 1995.
48. Lane PJ, Gaspal FM, Kim MY. Two sides of a cellular coin: CD4(+)CD3− cells regulate memory responses and lymph-node organization. Nat Rev Immunol 5:655–60, 2005.
49. Beniguel L, Begaud E, Cognasse F, et al. Identification of germinal center B cells in blood from HIV-infected drug-naive individuals in Central Africa. Clin Dev Immunol 11:23–7, 2004.
50. Gray CM, Morris L, Murray J, et al. Identification of cell subsets expressing intracytoplasmic cytokines within HIV-1-infected lymph nodes. AIDS 10:1467–75, 1996.
51. Kaplan LD, Abrams DI, Feigal E, et al. AIDS-associated non-Hodgkins lymphoma in San Francisco. JAMA 261:719–24, 1989.
52. Knowles DM, Chamulak GA, Subar M, et al. Lymphoid neoplasia associated with the acquired immunodeficiency syndrome (AIDS): The New York University Medical Center experience with 105 patients (1981–1986). Ann Intern Med 108:744–53, 1988.
53. Tirelli U, Spina M, Vaccher E, et al. Clinical evaluation of 451 patients with HIV related non-Hodgkin's lymphoma: experience on the Italian cooperative group on AIDS and tumors (GICAT). Leuk Lymphoma 20:91–6, 1995.
54. Bea S, Zettl A, Wright G, et al. Diffuse large B-cell lymphoma subgroups have distinct genetic profiles that influence tumor biology and improve gene expression-based survival prediction. Blood.
55. Patrone L, Henson SE, Teodorovic J, et al. Gene expression patterns in AIDS versus non-AIDS-related diffuse large B-cell lymphoma. Exp Mol Pathol 74:129–39, 2003.
56. Said JW, Hoyer KK, French SW, et al. TCL1 oncogene expression in B cell subsets from lymphoid hyperplasia and distinct classes of B cell lymphoma. Lab Invest 81:555–64, 2001.
57. Teitell M, Damore MA, Sulur GG, et al. TCL1 oncogene expression in AIDS-related lymphomas and lymphoid tissues. Proc Natl Acad Sci USA 96:9809–14, 1999.
58. Kis LL, Takahara M, Nagy N, et al. IL-10 can induce the expression of EBV-encoded latent membrane protein-1 (LMP-1) in the absence of EBNA-2 in B-lymphocytes, in Burkitt lymphoma-, and in NK-lymphoma derived cell lines. Blood 107:2928–35, 2005.
59. Maggi E, Mazzetti M, Ravina A, et al. Ability of HIV to promote a TH1 to TH0 shift and to replicate preferentially in TH2 and TH0 cells. Science 265:244–8, 1994.
60. Gascoyne RD, Adomat SA, Krajewski S, et al. Prognostic significance of Bcl-2 protein expression and Bcl-2 gene rearrangement in diffuse aggressive non-Hodgkin's lymphoma. Blood 90:244–51, 1997.
61. Wilson WH, Grossbard ML, Pittaluga S, et al. Dose-adjusted EPOCH chemotherapy for untreated large B-cell lymphomas: a pharmacodynamic approach with high efficacy. Blood 99:2685–93, 2002.
62. Hermine O, Haioun C, Lepage E, et al. Prognostic significance of bcl-2 protein expression in aggressive non-Hodgkin's lymphoma. Groupe d'Etude des Lymphomes de l'Adulte (GELA). Blood 87:265–72, 1996.
63. Natkunam Y, Lossos IS, Taidi B, et al. Expression of the human germinal center-associated lymphoma (HGAL) protein. A new marker of germinal center B cell derivation. Blood 105:3979–86, 2005.
64. Chang Y, Cesarman E, Pessin M, et al. Identification of herpesvirus-like DNA sequences in AIDS-associated Kaposi's sarcoma. Science 266:1865–9, 1994.
65. Fais F, Gaidano G, Capello D, et al. Immunoglobulin V region gene use and structure suggest antigen selection in AIDS-related primary effusion lymphomas. Leukemia 13:1093–9, 1999.
66. Carbone A, Gloghini A, Cozzi MR, et al. Expression of MUM1/IRF4 selectively clusters with primary effusion lymphoma among lymphomatous effusions: implications for disease histogenesis and pathogenesis. Br J Haematol 111:247–57, 2000.
67. Nador RG, Cesarman E, Chadburn A, et al. Primary effusion lymphoma: a distinct clinicopathologic entity associated with the Kaposi's sarcoma-associated herpes virus. Blood 88: 645–56, 1996.
68. Aoki Y, Tosato G. HIV-1 Tat enhances KSHV infectivity. Blood.
69. Davis DA, Rinderknecht AS, Zoeteweij JP, et al. Hypoxia induces lytic replication of Kaposi sarcoma-associated herpesvirus. Blood 97:3244–50, 2001.
70. Haque M, Davis DA, Wang V, et al. Kaposi's sarcoma-associated herpesvirus (human herpesvirus 8) contains hypoxia response elements: relevance to lytic induction by hypoxia. J Virol 77:6761–8, 2003.
71. Jarviluoma A, Koopal S, Rasanen S, et al. KSHV viral cyclin binds to p27KIP1 in primary effusion lymphomas. Blood 104:3349–54, 2004.
72. Widmer I, Davis D, Haque M, et al. KSHV viral BCL-2 (ORF16) promoter region is activated by hypoxia. In: 7th International Conference on Malignancies in AIDS and Other Immunodeficiencies, Bethesda, 2003. abstract 48.
73. Bais C, Santomasso B, Coso O, et al. G-protein-coupled receptor of Kaposi's sarcoma-associated herpesvirus is a viral oncogene and angiogenesis activator. Nature 391:86–9, 1998.
74. Delecluse HJ, Anagnostopoulos I, Dallenbach F, et al. Plasmablastic lymphomas of the oral cavity: a new entity associated with the human immunodeficiency virus infection. Blood 89:1413–20, 1997.

75. Nasta SD, Carrum GM, Shahab I, et al. Regression of a plasmablastic lymphoma in a patient with HIV on highly active antiretroviral therapy. Leuk Lymphoma 43:423–6, 2002.
76. Chetty R, Hlatswayo N, Muc R, et al. Plasmablastic lymphoma in HIV+ patients: an expanding spectrum. Histopathology 42:605–9, 2003.
77. Lester R, Li C, Galbraith P, et al. Improved outcome of human immunodeficiency virus-associated plasmablastic lymphoma of the oral cavity in the era of highly active antiretroviral therapy: a report of two cases. Leuk Lymphoma 45:1881–5, 2004.
78. Schichman E. HIV and plasmablastic lymphoma manifesting in sinus, testicles, and bones: A further expansion of the disease spectrum. Am J Hematol 77:291–5, 2004.
79. Andrieu JM, Roithmann S, Tourani JM, et al. Hodgkin's disease during HIV1 infection: the French registry experience. French Registry of HIV-associated Tumors. Ann Oncol 4: 635–41, 1993.
80. Carbone A, Gloghini A, Larocca LM, et al. Human immunodeficiency virus-associated Hodgkin's disease derives from post-germinal center B cells. Blood 93:2319–26, 1999.
81. Ratner L, Lee J, Tang S, et al. Chemotherapy for human immunodeficiency virus-associated non-Hodgkin's lymphoma in combination with highly active antiretroviral therapy. J Clin Oncol 19:2171–8, 2001.
82. Kaplan LD, Straus DJ, Testa MA, et al. Low-dose compared with standard-dose m-BACOD chemotherapy for non-Hodgkin's lymphoma associated with human immunodeficiency virus infection. National Institute of Allergy and Infectious Diseases AIDS Clinical Trials Group. N Engl J Med 336:1641–8, 1997.
83. Simonelli C, Spina M, Cinelli R, et al. Clinical features and outcome of primary effusion lymphoma in HIV-infected patients: a single-institution study. J Clin Oncol 21: 3948–54, 2003.
84. Rossi G, Donisi A, Casari S, et al. The international prognostic index can be used as a guide to treatment decisions regarding patients with human immunodeficiency virus-related systemic non-Hodgkin lymphoma (in process citation). Cancer 86:2391–7 (MEDLINE record in process), 1999.
85. Carbone PP, Kaplan HS, Musshoff K, et al. Report of the committee on Hodgkin's disease staging classification. Cancer Res 31:1860–1, 1971.
86. Enting RH, Esselink RA, Portegies P. Lymphomatous meningitis in AIDS-related systemic non-Hodgkin's lymphoma: a report of eight cases. J Neurol Neurosurg Psychiatry 57: 150–3, 1994.
87. Ziegler JL, Beckstead JA, Volberding PA, et al. Non-Hodgkin's lymphoma in 90 homosexual men. Relation to generalized lymphadenopathy and the acquired immunodeficiency syndrome. N Engl J Med 311:565–70, 1984.
88. Yousem DM, Patrone PM, Grossman RI. Leptomeningeal metastases: MR evaluation. J Comput Assist Tomogr 14: 255–61, 1990.
89. Hegde U, Filie A, Little RF, et al. High incidence of occult leptomeningeal disease detected by flow cytometry in newly diagnosed aggressive B-cell lymphomas at risk for central nervous system involvement: the role of flow cytometry versus cytology. Blood 105:496–502, 2005.
90. Little R, Dunleavy K, Grant N, et al. Phase II study of abbreviated treatment (short-course) with EPOCH and rituximab (EPOCH-R) in AIDS-related lymphoma (ARL): preliminary results on the role of rituximab in treatment. In: American Society of Hematology, San Diego, 2003, abstract 1494.
91. Zinzani PL, Magagnoli M, Chierichetti F, et al. The role of positron emission tomography (PET) in the management of lymphoma patients [see comments]. Ann Oncol 10:1181–4, 1999.
92. Straus DJ, Huang J, Testa MA, et al. Prognostic factors in the treatment of human immunodeficiency virus-associated non-Hodgkin's lymphoma: analysis of AIDS Clinical Trials Group protocol 142 – low-dose versus standard-dose m-BACOD plus granulocyte-macrophage colony-stimulating factor. National Institute of Allergy and Infectious Diseases. J Clin Oncol 16:3601–6, 1998.
93. Feugier P, Van Hoof A, Sebban C, et al. Long-term results of the R-CHOP study in the treatment of elderly patients with diffuse large B-cell lymphoma: A study by the Groupe d'Etude des Lymphomes de l'Adulte. J Clin Oncol 23:4117–26, 2005.
94. Bociek RG. Adult Burkitt's lymphoma. Clin Lymphoma 6: 11–20, 2005.
95. Antinori A, Cingolani A, Alba L, et al. Better response to chemotherapy and prolonged survival in AIDS-related lymphomas responding to highly active antiretroviral therapy. AIDS 15:1483–91, 2001.
96. Wang ES, Straus DJ, Teruya-Feldstein J, et al. Intensive chemotherapy with cyclophosphamide, doxorubicin, high-dose methotrexate/ifosfamide, etoposide, and high-dose cytarabine (CODOX-M/IVAC) for human immunodeficiency virus-associated Burkitt lymphoma. Cancer 98:1196–205, 2003.
97. Cortes J, Thomas D, Rios A, et al. Hyperfractionated cyclophosphamide, vincristine, doxorubicin, and dexamethasone and highly active antiretroviral therapy for patients with acquired immunodeficiency syndrome-related Burkitt lymphoma/leukemia. Cancer 94:1492–9, 2002.
98. Dunleavy K, Wayne A, Little R, et al. The addition of rituximab to dose-adjusted EPOCH with HAART suspension is highly effective and tolerable in AIDS-related lymphoma (ARL) and allows the delivery of abbreviated chemotherapy. In: Annual Meeting American Society of Hematolgoy, 16 Nov 2005; Miami: Blood; 2005, abstract 930.
99. Lascaux AS, Hemery F, Goujard C, et al. Beneficial effect of highly active antiretroviral therapy on the prognosis of AIDS-related systemic non-Hodgkin lymphomas. AIDS Res Hum Retroviruses 21:214–20, 2005.
100. Bower M, Gazzard B, Mandalia S, et al. A prognostic index for systemic AIDS-related non-Hodgkin lymphoma treated in the era of highly active antiretroviral therapy. Ann Intern Med 143:265–73, 2005.
101. Hoffmann C, Tiemann M, Schrader C, et al. AIDS-related B-cell lymphoma (ARL): correlation of prognosis with differentiation profiles assessed by immunophenotyping. Blood 106:1762–9, 2005.
102. McKelvey EM, Gottlieb JA, Wilson HE, et al. Hydroxyldaunomycin (Adriamycin) combination chemotherapy in malignant lymphoma. Cancer 38:1484–93, 1976.
103. Sehn LH, Donaldson J, Chhanabhai M, et al. Introduction of combined CHOP plus rituximab therapy dramatically improved outcome of diffuse large B-cell lymphoma in British Columbia. J Clin Oncol 23:5027–33, 2005.
104. Sehn LH, Connors JM. Treatment of aggressive non-Hodgkin's lymphoma: a north American perspective. Oncology (Williston Park) 19(4 Suppl 1):26–34, 2005.
105. Alas S, Bonavida B. Rituximab inactivates signal transducer and activation of transcription 3 (STAT3) activity in B-non-Hodgkin's lymphoma through inhibition of the interleukin 10 autocrine/paracrine loop and results in down-regulation of Bcl-2 and sensitization to cytotoxic drugs. Cancer Res 61:5137–44, 2001.
106. Maloney DG. Immunotherapy for non-Hodgkin's lymphoma: monoclonal antibodies and vaccines. J Clin Oncol 23:6421–8, 2005.
107. Spina M, Jaeger U, Sparano JA, et al. Rituximab plus infusional cyclophosphamide, doxorubicin, and etoposide in HIV-associated non-Hodgkin lymphoma: pooled results from 3 phase 2 trials. Blood 105:1891–7, 2005.
108. Sparano JA, Lee S, Chen MG, et al. Phase II trial of infusional cyclophosphamide, doxorubicin, and etoposide in patients

with HIV-associated non-Hodgkin's lymphoma: an Eastern Cooperative Oncology Group Trial (E1494). J Clin Oncol 22:1491–500, 2004.
109. Coiffier B, Lepage E, Briere J, et al. CHOP chemotherapy plus rituximab compared with CHOP alone in elderly patients with diffuse large-B-cell lymphoma. N Engl J Med 346: 235–42, 2002.
110. Kaplan L, Spina M, Little RF, Levine AM. Roundtable: Controversies in the Management of AIDS Lymphoma. In: 9th International Conference on Malignancies in AIDS and Other Acquired Immunodeficiencies: Basic, Epidemiologic and Clinical Research, Bethesda, 2005, pp 26–27.
111. Bucaneve G, Micozzi A, Menichetti F, et al. Levofloxacin to prevent bacterial infection in patients with cancer and neutropenia. N Engl J Med 353:977–87, 2005.
112. Cullen M, Steven N, Billingham L, et al. Antibacterial prophylaxis after chemotherapy for solid tumors and lymphomas. N Engl J Med 353:988–98, 2005.
113. Spina M, Tirelli U. Rituximab for HIV-associated lymphoma: weighing the benefits and risks. Curr Opin Oncol 17: 462–5, 2005.
114. Scadden DT. AIDS lymphomas: beginning of an EPOCH? Blood 101:4647, 2003.
115. Kasamon YL, Ambinder RF. AIDS-related primary central nervous system lymphoma. Hematol Oncol Clin North Am 19:665–87, vi–vii, 2005.
116. Ciacci JD, Tellez C, VonRoenn J, Levy RM. Lymphoma of the central nervous system in AIDS. Semin Neurol 19: 213–21, 1999.
117. Portegies P, Solod L, Cinque P, et al. Guidelines for the diagnosis and management of neurological complications of HIV infection. Eur J Neurol 11:297–304, 2004.
118. Deangelis LM, Hormigo A. Treatment of primary central nervous system lymphoma. Semin Oncol 31:684–92, 2004.
119. MacMahon EM, Glass JD, Hayward SD, et al. Epstein–Barr virus in AIDS-related primary central nervous system lymphoma. Lancet 338:969–73, 1991.
120. Antinori A, Ammassari A, De Luca A, et al. Diagnosis of AIDS-related focal brain lesions: a decision-making analysis based on clinical and neuroradiologic characteristics combined with polymerase chain reaction assays in CSF. Neurology 48:687–94, 1997.
121. Cingolani A, De Luca A, Larocca LM, et al. Minimally invasive diagnosis of acquired immunodeficiency syndrome-related primary central nervous system lymphoma. J Natl Cancer Inst 90:364–9, 1998.
122. Yarchoan R, Jaffe ES, Little R. Diagnosing central nervous system lymphoma in the setting of AIDS: a step forward [editorial; comment]. J Natl Cancer Inst 90:346–7, 1998.
123. Cingolani A, Gastaldi R, Fassone L, et al. Epstein–Barr virus infection is predictive of CNS involvement in systemic AIDS-related non-Hodgkin's lymphomas. J Clin Oncol 18: 3325–30, 2000.
124. Lorberboym M, Estok L, Machac J, et al. Rapid differential diagnosis of cerebral toxoplasmosis and primary central nervous system lymphoma by thallium-201 SPECT. J Nucl Med 37:1150–4, 1996.
125. Ruiz A, Ganz WI, Post MJ, et al. Use of thallium-201 brain SPECT to differentiate cerebral lymphoma from toxoplasma encephalitis in AIDS patients. AJNR Am J Neuroradiol 15:1885–94, 1994.
126. Villringer K, Jager H, Dichgans M, et al. Differential diagnosis of CNS lesions in AIDS patients by FDG-PET. J Comput Assist Tomogr 19:532–6, 1995.
127. Hoffman JM, Waskin HA, Schifter T, et al. FDG-PET in differentiating lymphoma from nonmalignant central nervous system lesions in patients with AIDS. J Nucl Med 34: 567–75, 1993.
128. Antinori A, De Rossi G, Ammassari A, et al. Value of combined approach with thallium-201 single-photon emission computed tomography and Epstein–Barr virus DNA polymerase chain reaction in CSF for the diagnosis of AIDS-related primary CNS lymphoma. J Clin Oncol 17:554–60, 1999.
129. Ivers LC, Kim AY, Sax PE. Predictive value of polymerase chain reaction of cerebrospinal fluid for detection of Epstein–Barr virus to establish the diagnosis of HIV-related primary central nervous system lymphoma. Clin Infect Dis 38:1629–32, 2004.
130. Yarchoan R, Little R. Immunosuppression-related malignancies. In: DeVita VT, Hellman S, Rosenberg SA (eds). Cancer Principles and Practice of Oncology. 7th edn. Philadelphia PA: Lippincott; 2005, pp 2247–63.
131. Ambinder RF, Lee S, Curran WJ, et al. Phase II intergroup trial of sequential chemotherapy and radiotherapy for AIDS-related primary central nervous system lymphoma. Cancer Ther 1:215–21, 2003.
132. Deangelis LM, Yahalom J. Primary central nervous system lymphoma. In: Vincent T, Devita J, Hellman S, Rosenberg SA, (eds). Cancer Principles and Practice of Oncology. 7th edn. Philadelphia PA: Williams & Wilkins; 2005, pp 2012–20.
133. Pels H, Schmidt-Wolf IGH, Glasmacher A, et al. Primary central nervous system lymphoma: results of a pilot and phase II study of systemic and intraventricular chemotherapy with deferred radiotherapy. J Clin Oncol 21:4489–95, 2003.
134. Correa DD, DeAngelis LM, Shi W, ed al. Cognitive functions in survivors of primary central nervous system lymphoma. Neurology 62:548–55, 2004.
135. Omuro AMP, Ben-Porat LS, Panageas KS, et al. Delayed neurotoxicity in primary central nervous system lymphoma. Arch Neurol 62:1595–600, 2005.
136. Forsyth PA, Yahalom J, DeAngelis LM. Combined-modality therapy in the treatment of primary central nervous system lymphoma in AIDS. Neurology 44:1473–9, 1994.
137. Deangelis LM, Yahalom J, Rosenblum M, Posner JB. Primary CNS lymphoma: managing patients with spontaneous and AIDS-related disease. Oncology (Huntingt) 1:52–62, 1987.
138. Spina M, Rossi G, Gabarre J, et al. HAART influences the presenting characteristics and improves the outcome of patients (pts) with Hodgkin's disease and HIV infection (HD-HIV). In: 2005 ASCO Annual Meeting, Orlando, 2005, abstract 6584.
139. Straus DJ, Portlock CS, Qin J, et al. Results of a prospective randomized clinical trial of doxorubicin, bleomycin, vinblastine, and dacarbazine (ABVD) followed by radiation therapy (RT) versus ABVD alone for stages I, II, and IIIA nonbulky Hodgkin disease. Blood 104:3483–9, 2004.
140. Meyer RM, Gospodarowicz MK, Connors JM, et al. Randomized comparison of ABVD chemotherapy with a strategy that includes radiation therapy in patients with limited-stage Hodgkin's lymphoma. National Cancer Institute of Canada Clinical Trials Group and the Eastern Cooperative Oncology Group. J Clin Oncol 23:4634–42, 2005.
141. Cesarman E, Chang Y, Moore PS, et al. Kaposi's sarcoma-associated herpesvirus-like DNA sequences in AIDS-related body-cavity-based lymphomas. N Engl J Med 332:1186–91, 1995.
142. Moore PS, Chang Y. Detection of herpesvirus-like DNA sequences in Kaposi's sarcoma in patients with and without HIV infection. N Engl J Med 332:1181–5, 1995.
143. Cesarman E, Knowles DM. The role of Kaposi's sarcoma-associated herpesvirus (KSHV/HHV-8) in lymphoproliferative diseases. Semin Cancer Biol 9:165–74, 1999.
144. Gaidano G, Pastore C, Gloghini A, et al. Human herpesvirus type-8 (HHV-8) in haematopoietic neoplasia. Leuk Lymphoma 24:257–66, 1997.
145. Brandt SJ, Bodine DM, Dunbar CE, Nienhuis AW. Dysregulated interleukin-6 expression produces a syndrome resembling Castleman's syndrome. J Clin Invest 86:592–9, 1990.

146. Nicholas J, Ruvolo VR, Burns WH, et al. Kaposi's sarcoma-associated human herpesvirus-8 encodes homologues of macrophage inflammatory protein-1 and interleukin-6. Nat Med 3:287–92, 1997.
147. Aoki Y, Jaffe ES, Chang Y, et al. Angiogenesis and hematopoiesis induced by Kaposi's sarcoma-associated herpesvirus-encoded interleukin-6. Blood 93:4034–43, 1999.
148. Frizzera G, Peterson BA, Bayrd ED, Goldman A. A systemic lymphoproliferative disorder with morphologic features of Castleman's disease: clinical findings and clinicopathologic correlations in 15 patients. J Clin Oncol 3:1202–16, 1985.
149. Hengge UR, Ruzicka T, Tyring SK, et al. Update on Kaposi's sarcoma and other HHV8 associated diseases. Part 2: pathogenesis, Castleman's disease, and pleural effusion lymphoma. Lancet Infect Dis 2:344–52, 2002.
150. Marcelin AG, Aaron L, Mateus C, et al. Rituximab therapy for HIV-associated Castleman disease. Blood 102:2786–8, 2003.
151. Nishimoto N, Sasai M, Shima Y, et al. Improvement in Castleman's disease by humanized anti-interleukin-6 receptor antibody therapy. Blood 95:56–61, 2000.
152. Nishimoto N, Kanakura Y, Aozasa K, et al. Humanized anti-interleukin-6 receptor antibody treatment of multicentric Castleman's disease. Blood 106:2627–32, 2005.
153. Aoki Y, Tosato G. Role of vascular endothelial growth factor/vascular permeability factor in the pathogenesis of Kaposi's sarcoma-associated herpesvirus-infected primary effusion lymphomas. Blood 94:4247–54, 1999.
154. Brown HJ, McBride WH, Zack JA, Sun R. Prostratin and bortezomib are novel inducers of latent Kaposi's sarcoma-associated herpesvirus. Antivir Ther 10:745–51, 2005.
155. Browne MJ, Hubbard SM, Longo DL, et al. Excess prevalence of *Pneumocystis carinii* pneumonia in patients treated for lymphoma with combination chemotherapy. Ann Intern Med 104:338–44, 1986.
156. Pfreundschuh M, Truemper L, Kloess M, et al. 2-weekly or 3-weekly CHOP chemotherapy with or without etoposide for the treatment of elderly patients with aggressive lymphomas: results of the NHL-B2 trial of the DSHNHL. Blood 2004.
157. Pfreundschuh M, Kloess M, Schmits R, et al. Six, not eight cycles of bi-weekly CHOP with rituximab (R-CHOP-14) is the preferred treatment for elderly patients with diffuse large B-cell lymphoma (DLBCL): results of the RICOVER-60 trial of the German High-Grade Non-Hodgkin Lymphoma Study Group (DSHNHL). In: American Society of Hematology, 16 Nov 2005; Miami: Blood; 2005, abstract 13.
158. Biggar RJ. Survival after cancer diagnosis in persons with AIDS. J Acquir Immune Defic Syndr 39:293, 2005.
159. Jones SE, Fuks Z, Bull M, et al. Non-Hodgkin's lymphomas. IV. Clinicopathologic correlation in 405 cases. Cancer 31:806–23, 1973.
160. Jaffe ES, Harris NL, Stein H, Vardiman JW (eds). World Health Organization Classification of Tumors: Pathology & Genetics: Tumors of Haematopoietic and Lymphoid Tissues. Lyon: IARC Press; 2001.

Chapter 61

Wasting Syndrome

Jens J. Kort, MD, PhD, Fred R. Sattler, MD

INTRODUCTION

At the onset of the AIDS epidemic, weight loss and muscle wasting were so intimately linked with HIV infection that AIDS was often referred to as "slim disease" in parts of the world.[1,2] In 1987, the United States Centers for Disease Control (CDC) defined HIV wasting syndrome as an involuntary weight loss of >10% along with either chronic diarrhea or opportunistic complications (infections or cancer).[3] Prior to the mid-1990s and before highly active antiretroviral therapy (HAART) became available, AIDS wasting syndrome (AWS) was the initial AIDS-defining diagnosis in up to one-third of patients.[4]

With the introduction of HAART, survival improved[5–7] along with a decline in the incidence of AIDS indicator conditions, including opportunistic infections and Kaposi sarcoma.[8,9] National surveillance data from the CDC,[10] the Multicenter AIDS Cohort Study (MACS),[11] and the Adult and Adolescent Spectrum of HIV Disease (ASD) Project[12] showed a decline in the incidence in AWS from 7% to 8% of adults and adolescents in 1997 and 1998, respectively (CDC), a decline in AWS cases from 22 cases per 1000 person-years in 1994–95 to 13.4 cases per 1000 person-years in 1996–99 (MACS), and a decline in AWS cases of 30.2 cases per 1000 person-years in 1992 to 11.9 cases per 1000 person-years in 1999 (ASD). However, data from the Nutrition for Healthy Living (NFHL) cohort, which enroled 713 participants between 1995 and 2003, showed that weight loss and wasting were still common in HIV-infected persons receiving HAART, with approximately one-third of the cohort meeting at least one definition of wasting. Weight loss ⩾10% from baseline was associated with a four- to sixfold increase in mortality.[13]

More recent data from the NFHL cohort demonstrate a 50% increase in the 6-month risk of ⩾5% unintentional weight loss during the later HAART years (1998–2003) compared to the early HAART years (1995–97).[14] Data from four intervention studies involving 2382 HIV-infected patients suggest that weight loss of as little as 5% over a period of 4 months predicts an increased risk of death and opportunistic infections.[15] These findings support the clinical importance of a 5% weight loss occurring over 4–6 months.

Weight loss in HIV infection appears to occur in equal frequency in women and men.[16,17] Early in the AIDS epidemic, episodes of rapid weight loss were reported during secondary infections including bacterial infections such as sinusitis and major opportunistic infections. Weight loss was primarily due to inadequate intake of caloric energy during these infections but was not fully recovered following resolution of the infections.[18,19]

However, there is considerable variability in the clinical presentation of HIV wasting. Experimental clinical models indicate that with fasting, fat tissue is predominantly lost until subjects have little body fat at which time lean body mass (LBM) is progressively lost.[20,21] With cachexia, muscle mass is primarily lost from the outset.

In HIV infection, wasting is characterized by loss of LBM, especially skeletal muscle, but loss of fat also occurs. Further, muscle wasting may occur without loss of weight[22,23] and wasting in HAART-treated patients may be subtle and not easily assessed because these patients are also predisposed to lipodystrophy (loss of fat in the extremities and central fat accumulation). Finally, unlike men, women lose body fat at all stages of wasting disproportionately to men.[24]

PATHOPHYSIOLOGY

Weight loss in HIV-infected individuals is a complex multifactorial process. Three key mechanisms contribute individually or in combination to wasting in HIV infection: (1) malnutrition due to inadequate intake of caloric energy as may occur with vomiting, diarrhea, malabsorption, or lack of appetite; (2) cachexia due to infection with HIV *per se*, secondary infections or malignancy; and (3) fat wasting (lipoatrophy). It is important to differentiate these causes of wasting since they have different prognoses and may require different treatments. Indeed, with severe muscle wasting, there is an increased risk for opportunistic complications and early fatality.[25–29] Thus, a search for the underlying cause should be sought expeditiously so that specific treatments can be implemented.

Malnutrition with Impaired Intake of Caloric Energy

Inadequate calorie intake has been a consistent contributing factor for muscle wasting, particularly during periods of rapid weight loss[18,19] that are often associated with opportunistic infections.[30,31] Of importance, nearly two decades ago, Forbes showed in fasting and overfeeding human experiments that the ratio of ΔLBM/ΔWt is low (mostly fat loss) during starvation but when the percent of body fat reaches ~15%, the ratio increases exponentially indicating a primary loss of lean tissue.[20,21] Thus, mild to moderate malnutrition results primarily in fat loss, whereas severe malnutrition is associated with substantial losses of lean tissue.

Mild increases in resting energy expenditure (REE) of 8–11% is a common finding in patients with asymptomatic HIV infection.[30–31,33] Increases greater than 25% have been reported in patients with AIDS.[30,32,34,35–37] While a decrease in caloric energy intake causes a decrease in REE in uninfected persons, elevated REE persists in HIV-infected persons despite a decrease in caloric intake, which accelerates the negative energy balance.[38] In addition, reduced levels of physical activity can result in loss of lean tissue and may perpetuate HIV wasting.

Gastrointestinal Dysfunction

In the NFHL cohort, 88% of patients experienced at least one abnormality in gastrointestinal (GI) function.[13] Diarrhea was the most frequent complaint and has been reported in up to 80% of AIDS patients from North America and Europe, and almost 100% of patients in developing countries.[39–41] In many cases, a specific pathogen may be identified.[42,43] In chronic diarrhea, lasting more than 30 days, parasitic infections due to organisms such as *Crytosporidium parvum, Isospora belli, Cyclospora, Microspora, Giardia lamblia,* and *Entamoeba histolytica* predominate.[42–44] Diarrhea due to common enteropathogenic bacteria, including *Salmonella, Shigella, Campylobacter, Clostridium difficile*, or adherent *E. coli* species are usually intermittent and resolve with therapy in patients receiving HAART and the effects on nutrition are therefore short-lived.

Malabsorption with or without diarrhea is often associated with progressive weight loss, malabsorption of carbohydrates, fat and micronutrients, and has been observed in patients at all stages of HIV infection.[39,45] Data from the Multicenter AIDS Cohort indicate that the association between diarrhea and loss of LBM is weak,[46] suggesting that malabsorption may be more important than diarrhea in wasting. In some patients with AIDS, a cause of GI symptoms and malabsorption cannot be found, which suggests a diagnosis of 'HIV enteropathy'.[47] The pathogenesis of HIV enteropathy is not well understood, since HIV does not directly infect enterocytes, but the elimination of CD4+ T-lymphocyte in the lamina propria, and ultrastructural changes in the gut mucosa suggest indirect mechanisms of HIV induced enteropathy along with direct HIV gp120-induced cytotoxic effects on intestinal epithelial cells.[48,49]

Cachexia Due to Catabolic Disorders

Infection due to HIV *per se* or secondary opportunistic infections and AIDS-related malignancies are frequently associated with systemic inflammation and dysregulation of proinflammatory cytokines. These infections are associated with increased production of TNF-α, IL-1, IL-6, and shedding of soluble TNF-α receptor I and II or release of IL-1Ra from the Golgi apparatus into the systemic circulation.[50–53] In animals, administration of TNF-α, IL-1β, IL-6, or IFN-γ produced significant weight loss.[54,55] In patients with HIV, weight loss has been correlated with serum levels of TNF-α, IL-1, IL-6, or IL-1RA.[56–59] In addition, IL-1β is elevated during opportunistic infections, and can produce clinical and biochemical abnormalities of cachexia.[60] Elevated levels of IL-6 and TNF-α measured in blood have also been correlated with concurrent opportunistic infections in patients with AIDS[61] and IL-6 levels correlated with weight loss in these patients.[62] Further, data from the NFHL cohort demonstrated that loss of LBM and increased REE in HIV-infected patients may occur without loss of weight despite HAART over longer periods of time and was correlated with the level of peripheral blood mononuclear cell-derived production of TNF-α and IL-1β[71]

Complex interactions between multiple cytokines may be involved in the metabolic abnormalities in HIV infection. However, the biology of these mediators makes it difficult to establish a causal relationship between levels of key proinflammatory cytokines such as TNF-α and IL-1 and HIV wasting. For example, secretion of TNF-α and IL-1 is episodic, tightly regulated and these cytokines have short plasma half-lives in the range of minutes. TNF-α and IL-1 act in a paracrine or juxtacrine manner at the cellular level. Thus, blood levels may not reflect tissue effects of cytokines and assessment of levels of these mediators in blood are complicated by their binding to soluble receptors or inhibitors (i.e., sTNFR-1 and -2, IL-1Ra), which often circulate in concentrations of 10-1000-fold in excess of the free cytokines.[63–65]

In addition, unsuppressed HIV replication has been associated with elevated levels of proinflammatory cytokines and correlated with the degree of wasting.[53,57] In 835 patients entering AIDS Clinical Trials Group (ACTG) studies, plasma

HIV levels prior to initiating study therapy predicted subsequent weight loss. Indeed, for subjects with HIV RNA <10000, 10000–100000, and >100000 copies/mL, the cumulative weight loss was on average 6.8%, 10.6%, and 18.4% at 1 year, respectively, and 9.4%, 20.6%, and 38.6% at 2 years, respectively. Furthermore, in 33 HIV-infected patients with a history of prior weight loss (10.5 ± 6.4 kg over 461 ± 304 days) and a median plasma HIV RNA viral load of 46 887 copies/mL (range <200–510 070), plasma HIV RNA levels correlated with the absolute amount and percentage of weight loss as well as the difference in body mass index (BMI) at the prior maximal and minimal recorded weights ($r = 0.7, 0.67, 0.69$, respectively, $P = 0.0001$ for the comparisons).[57] Together, these studies suggest that HIV viral load is closely linked to HIV wasting and measures of inflammation in patients with HIV in the absence of malnutrition or other apparent causes. Thus, assessment of HIV plasma RNA viral load is an important diagnostic tool in the workup of HIV-infected patients with loss of LBM.

The exact mechanism resulting in the loss of skeletal muscle is not well understood, but may be associated with inadequate intake of essential amino acids, systemic inflammation, inactivity, metabolic abnormalities, or hormonal dysregulation. Clinical studies utilizing stable isotopes indicate that muscle serves as a substrate reservoir of amino acids to support increased turnover of systemic protein.[66] Indeed 10^8 to 10^9 CD4+ T-lymphocytes turn over each day during uncontrolled HIV infection.[67] As a result, breakdown and release of amino acids from skeletal muscle to support the synthesis of proteins for new lymphocytes may exceed myofibrillar protein synthesis resulting in a net loss of muscle protein.[68]

Dysregulation of muscle amino acid metabolism in AIDS, including a lower rate of muscle protein synthesis,[68] and altered muscle protein catabolism is only partially corrected by treatment with HAART.[69] In fact, high levels of plasma HIV RNA were associated with impaired synthesis of myofibrillar proteins and indirect evidence of increased muscle proteolysis. HAART decreased plasma HIV RNA levels from a median of 155 828 copies/mL to 100 copies/mL, which was associated with significant increase in skeletal muscle protein synthesis and lean tissue along with a decrease in muscle proteolysis.

Muscle protein metabolism may be further deranged by specific treatments for HIV. In particular, muscle mitochondrial DNA (mtDNA) is reduced in HIV-infected, ART-naive patients, but to a greater degree in nucleoside reverse transcriptase inhibitors (NRTI)-containing HAART-treated patients, along with an increase in cytochrome oxidase-negative muscle fibers.[69] Thus, HIV and certain NRTIs may contribute to muscle pathology during wasting, but reducing the level of HIV replication with HAART is likely to improve net anabolic balance of skeletal muscle protein synthesis.[70]

Collectively, these data are consistent with the pathognomonic feature of persistent immune activation despite suppression of HIV replication with current HAART, and support the concept that persisting excess production of local proinflammatory cytokines and /or viral factors result in a long-term cumulative negative effect on energy balance and protein metabolism.

Lipoatrophy, Metabolic and Endocrine Abnormalities

Multiple metabolic abnormalities of protein[36] and lipid[72] turnover, as well as insulin resistance and diabetes mellitus have been associated with HIV infection.[73–75] Lipodystrophy (disordered fat metabolism) has been reported in 13–83% of HAART recipients,[76–79] with ~8–14% experiencing lipoatrophy,[80–82] which complicates the assessment of wasting since it may be difficult to ascertain whether thin extremities are due to loss of muscle or fat, or a combination of both.

Accumulating evidence implicates NRTIs including stavudine (d4T) and to a lesser extent zidovudine (AZT), in the pathogenesis of lipoatrophy.[79,83–85] Inhibition of the mtDNA polymerase-γ by zalcitabine (ddC), didanosine (ddI), and d4T leads to impairment of mtDNA synthesis, mitochondrial toxicity, and death of fat cells.[86] Recent data suggest that peripheral as well as central fat loss is a characteristic of long-term therapy with HAART (at least 6 years), even in the absence of d4T-containing antiretroviral regimens.[87]

Decreased serum testosterone levels were observed in as many as 30–50% of HIV-infected men in the pre-HAART era and were associated with lower CD4+ T-lymphocyte numbers and decreased survival.[88–91] The prevalence of hypogonadism in HIV-infected men in the post-HAART era appears to be in the range of 20%.[92–95] Decreased testosterone levels in HIV infection is most commonly due to inadequate testicular stimulation by luteinizing hormone (LH) from the pituitary gland (hypogonadotropic hypogonadism).[88–91,96] Hypogonadism and decreased testosterone levels in men with HIV may be due to malnutrition, severe illness,[97,98] depression, or treatment with opiates, megestrol acetate, anabolic steroids, or even testosterone *per se*,[89,99,100] though is usually not the cause of wasting. However, low testosterone levels may be associated with loss of weight, muscle mass, and decreased exercise capacity[101,102] and although usually secondary to a remedial cause, hypogonadism may complicate efforts to restore muscle mass. Further, defects in other anabolic mediators, including resistance to growth hormone (GH) and decreased hepatic production of insulin-like growth factor 1 (IGF-1) have been associated with HIV wasting but as with androgen deficiency are unlikely to be primary causes of wasting.[98,103]

Finally, regulated energy homeostasis may be adversely affected in patients with psychiatric illness and depression resulting in impaired appetite, an important contributor to weight loss. Neuroendocrine circuits, emotions, and behavior are linked with the hormones, leptin,[104] ghrelin,[105] and α-melanocyte-stimulating hormone,[106] which control body weight,[107] Understanding the neuroendocrinology of energy homeostasis and emotions will likely contribute to new therapeutic strategies for psychiatric illnesses affecting body weight.

CLINICAL PRESENTATION AND DIAGNOSTIC TOOLS

A progressive and unexplained loss of weight in patients with HIV infection should prompt an expeditious search for clinical evidence of one or more of the three key contributing mechanisms described in the prior section. Table 61-1 provides several definitions for wasting, including time-dependent weight loss, along with body cell mass (BCM) and BMI criteria.[15,74,108] The gender-specific BCM thresholds for wasting may not be evident by weight loss but are revealed by body composition analysis. For patients with suspected wasting, a comprehensive history and physical examination should be performed, along with a careful weight history, assessment of diet and caloric energy intake, and review of potential psychosocial contributing factors (Table 61-2). Since loss of lean tissue has important prognostic implications, assessment of body composition may be useful adjunct for diagnosis and evaluating the severity of wasting and is helpful in monitoring the course of therapy.

Weight History

Weight history should be carefully reviewed to assess the amount and rate of weight loss. Ideally, all weights should be obtained under standardized conditions using the same calibrated scale with patients lightly clothed in underwear, socks, and gown and without jewelry. Calculation of the BMI (weight in kilograms divided by height in square meters) is useful in comparing patients with non-HIV-infected populations such as NHANES III.[109] Declines in body weight with a new BMI $<18.5\,kg/m^2$ in adults with HIV infection may be associated with a greater risk for complications and defines a state of HIV-associated wasting (Table 61-1). Whereas, changes in body weight and BMI if based on self-reported history or weights not obtained under carefully standardized conditions may be inaccurate and may not reflect the true magnitude of HIV wasting due to malnutrition or cachexia.

Diet History

An assessment of the intake of total caloric energy as well as macronutrients (carbohydrates, proteins, and fats) and use of dietary supplements or even the lack of access to food should be assessed.

Clinical History

A careful search should be made for factors, which might impair or decrease ingestion of caloric energy, including early satiety, nausea and vomiting, painful oral or esophageal ulcerations, gastroesophageal reflux disease (GERD), gastric dysmotility, or other upper GI (UGI) abnormalities. In addition, changes in taste due to medications may impair appetite. Diarrhea and malabsorption secondary to less common causes such as small bowel tumors, folate, or vitamin B_{12} deficiencies, autoimmune disease, or pancreas insufficiency also need to be considered. Therapies to treat HIV and its complications may be associated with GI side-effects and may lead to impaired intake of caloric energy.

One of the most important aspects of the clinical history is recent evidence of incompletely controlled viral replication, which may result in an inflammatory response, an increase in REE, net loss of skeletal muscle protein and cachexia.[23,27,110] Similarly, isolated fever or symptoms of a subclinical opportunistic infection or malignancy could also cause wasting due to systemic proinflammatory state, and thus even minor symptoms such as chronic cough, abdominal discomfort, or visual problems (e.g., 'floaters') should be carefully evaluated as harbingers of occult infections or tumors.

Table 61-1 Criteria for HIV Wasting

Diagnostic Measure	Must Meet One of the Criteria for AWS
Body weight (BW)	10% nonvoluntary weight loss over 12 months[a] >10% weight loss from pre-illness maximum or >5% in the previous 6 months[b] >5% nonvoluntary weight loss over 4 months[c]
Body cell mass (BCM)	Men: BCM < 35% of total BW with BMI $<27\,kg/m^2$[a] Women: BCM < 23% of total BW with BMI $<27\,kg/m^2$[a]
Body mass index (BMI)	Men or women: BMI $<18.5\,kg/m^2$[b] or Weight < 90% of IBW[b]

[a] Adapted from Polsky B, Kotler D, Steinhart C: HIV-associated wasting in the HAART era: guidelines for assessment, diagnosis and treatment. AIDS Pat Care STDs 15:411, 2001.
[b] Adapted from Grinspoon S, Mulligan K: Weight loss and wasting in patients infected with human immunodeficiency virus. Clin Infect Dis 36(Suppl 2):S69, 2003.
[c] Adapted from Wheeler DA, Gibert CL, Launer CA, et al: Weight loss as a predictor of survival and disease progression in HIV infection. Terry Beirn Community Programs for Clinical Research on AIDS. J Acquir Immune Defic Syndr Hum Retrovirol 18:80, 1998.

Diagnostic Work-Up of Wasting Syndrome in HIV Infection

Table 61-2

Diagnostic Group	Comment
Weight history	Amount and rate of weight loss Serial standardized weight (gown, underclothing) on regularly calibrated scale Body mass index calculation (weight(kg)/height(m)^2)
Diet history	Calculation of current and recent total and macronutrient energy intake Assessment of appetite, supplements consumed, and access to food
Clinical History	Virologic and immunologic control of HIV infection Opportunistic infections and malignancies Factors that decrease oral intake due to oral or upper GI pathology Nausea, vomiting, diarrhea, dyspepsia, change in taste Oral, gingival, dental, and odontogenic pathologies Endocrine abnormalities: hypogonadism, thyroid dysfunction, adrenal insufficiency, diabetes mellitus Hyperlactatemia, or lactic acidosis Malabsorption
Medication history	Various GI side-effects
Body composition	Dual-energy X-ray absorptiometry (DEXA), bioelectrical impedance analysis (BIA), and anthropometry
Psychosocial history	Screen for depression and dementia; consideration of other psychiatric disorders

Anorexia due to IL-1β or TNF-α systemic spillover may precede other clinical symptoms of an opportunistic infection by days or weeks. In the absence of clinical evidence of malnutrition or infections and tumors associated with cachexia, metabolic complications including lipoatrophy may be important confounding factors in the assessment of wasting and may or may not coincide with lactic acidosis and weight loss.[111] However, weight loss due to lactic acidosis is often rapid, and accompanied by abdominal pain and fatigue.[81,111]

Endocrine abnormalities such as hyperthyroidism, type I diabetes, adrenal insufficiency, and hypogonadism may be associated with weight loss. Although low testosterone *per se* is usually not a cause of weight loss and is often a result of weight loss,[95,96] it is important to identify overt hypogonadism, since repletion of skeletal muscle and other components of lean tissue is difficult in the absence of adequate androgen status. Free serum testosterone is thought to be a more accurate measure of bioavailable testosterone, particularly in HIV-infected men, in whom sex hormone-binding globulin is increased.[112] Unfortunately, clinically available tracer analog assays underestimate true levels of free testosterone as measured by more accurate and expensive equilibrium dialysis[113] or mass spectroscopy. Thus, low free testosterone levels in the presence of normal total testosterone levels may result in a false diagnosis of hypogonadism and unnecessary use of replacement therapy, which may result in permanent hypogonadism.

Decreased libido, erectile dysfunction, and irregular menses are more likely due to chronic infection, adverse effects of medications, or depression and should not be used to justify androgen therapy.[24,93,94] Thus, a total testosterone level by routine laboratory platform assays is the most cost-efficient and reliable way to initially assess men for hypogonadism.

Body Composition Analysis

Morbidity and mortality due to loss of weight is directly associated with the depletion of lean tissue and not fat. Thus, estimates of the different components of the body mass provide important clues for diagnosis and help to anticipate and monitor response to interventions for wasting syndromes.[15,114,115] Arguably the most important measure of involuntary weight loss is a decline in BCM, defined as the cells, which metabolize glucose, utilize oxygen and produce carbon dioxide.[116] Although substantial progress has been made in technologies to accurately measure body composition, there has been no consensus toward an optimal practical approach to evaluate HIV wasting. Figure 61-1 provides an overview of different models of body composition, and diagnostic tools to measure body composition.

1. *Anthropometry* is an inexpensive technique to assess body composition. For example, serial measurements of mid-arm circumference by tape measure and triceps skinfolds with calipers may be used to assess changes in arm muscle mass. The technique is relatively easy to perform but its accuracy depends on serial measurements by the same operator with rigorous attention to landmarks and consistent use of the calipers and tape measures. Anthropometry also utilizes regression equations to estimate whole-body composition based on measurements in healthy individuals, which may not reflect those with HIV wasting. Measurements in patients with lipoatrophy are particularly difficult to interpret.

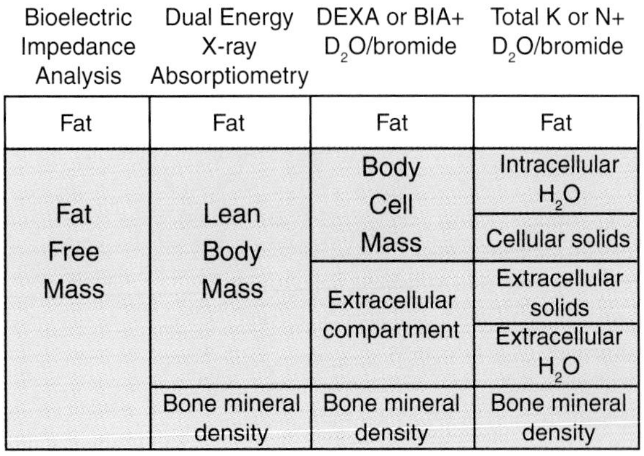

Bioelectric Impedance Analysis	Dual Energy X-ray Absorptiometry	DEXA or BIA+ D_2O/bromide	Total K or N+ D_2O/bromide
Fat	Fat	Fat	Fat
Fat Free Mass	Lean Body Mass	Body Cell Mass	Intracellular H_2O
			Cellular solids
		Extracellular compartment	Extracellular solids
			Extracellular H_2O
	Bone mineral density	Bone mineral density	Bone mineral density

Figure 61-1 ■ Methods to analyze body composition.

2. *Bioelectrical impedance analysis* (BIA) is a widely used 'low tech' means to assess body composition. BIA provides assessment of a two-compartment model, based on the differential impedance (resistance and reactance) to a low intensity electrical current through tissue compartments.[117,118] Differences in body shape and inconsistent positioning of electrodes limits the accuracy of BIA. Further, BIA only directly measures fat free mass (FFM), and not LBM or BCM although the latter can be derived by regression equations using other methods to assess body composition. Fat mass is derived by subtraction of FFM from total body weight and is not directly measured. Thus, use of BIA in patients with lipodystrophy requires validation of the test in that population based on other more accurate tests of body composition (e.g., total potassium counting). Regardless, BIA is convenient and widely used.[117,119,120] Further, low phase angle measurements derived by BIA have been reported to be predictive of adverse outcomes, when assessed longitudinally in patients with HIV infection.[121,122]
3. *Dual-energy X-ray absorptiometry* (DEXA) may be used to assess three body compartments through differential absorption of X-rays at two intensities to accurately quantify LBM, fat and bone mineral density (BMD).[123–125] However, DEXA, like BIA, is unable to accurately distinguish changes in tissue hydration from changes in FFM or LBM. Thus, DEXA is most precise when used with stable isotopes such as D_2O or NaBr to assess total body and extracellular fluid status, respectively. Since DEXA is the standard method to diagnose osteopenia and osteoporosis, the test is widely available, relatively inexpensive, and associated with low exposure to radiation (about one-tenth of a standard chest radiograph).

   Significant differences in the measurements of FFM between DEXA, BIA, and skin fold thickness have been demonstrated in patients with HIV wasting. For example, BIA overestimates FFM compared with DEXA in patients with greater body fat, suggesting that standard BIA equations may not be accurate for assessing FFM in some patients with HIV.[114]
4. *Measures of four body compartments* provide estimates of the BCM, which if decreased, is a reliable, functional measure of lean tissue wasting. Indirect estimates of the BCM may be obtained by measurement of total body potassium and total body nitrogen but those methods remain limited to a few research centers. It is noteworthy that formulas to determine BCM or intracellular water with BIA are based on measurements utilizing these analytically validated techniques in HIV-infected patients.[126,127]
5. *Imaging techniques* such as computerized tomography (CT), have proven valuable to determine regional changes in muscle and fat from limited (due to radiation exposure) cross-sectional examinations of the extremities and trunk and is particularly valuable in patients with lipodystrophy.[76,128,129] Magnetic resonance imaging (MRI) is reputed to be the most accurate body imaging technique to delineate the anatomy, structure and size of various tissues, and to assess muscle and fat cross-sectional areas or volume[130] and wasting.[131] It is arguable whether MRI is superior to CT for assessing quantitative and qualitative regional changes in muscle or fat, but MRI provides no radiation exposure and is usually more expensive than CT. In the research setting, MRI in conjunction with ^{31}P-MRS, near infrared spectroscopy (NIRS), and functional measurements of muscle strength and contraction provides detailed analysis of abnormal muscle metabolism and function.[132–134]

Psychosocial History

Because energy homeostasis may be adversely affected in patients with psychiatric illness, psychological evaluation should be undertaken to determine if depressive disorders may be linked with impaired appetite and weight loss.

THERAPEUTIC OPTIONS

In considering treatment options for HIV wasting, potential contributing factors must first be addressed. Conditions that lead to inadequate calorie intake, including impaired taste and appetite, nausea, vomiting, diarrhea, and malabsorption as well as depression and anxiety should be treated. Nutritional counseling should be offered to improve dietary intake. Most importantly, optimal suppression of HIV replication with HAART should be achieved, and balanced carefully with HAART-related toxicities. Rapid diagnosis and treatment of acute illnesses including opportunistic infections and malignancies must be facilitated. Figure 61-2 outlines a stepwise approach for the management of HIV wasting. Pharmacological interventions should be aimed at reversing loss of lean tissue and restoring muscle mass and functional

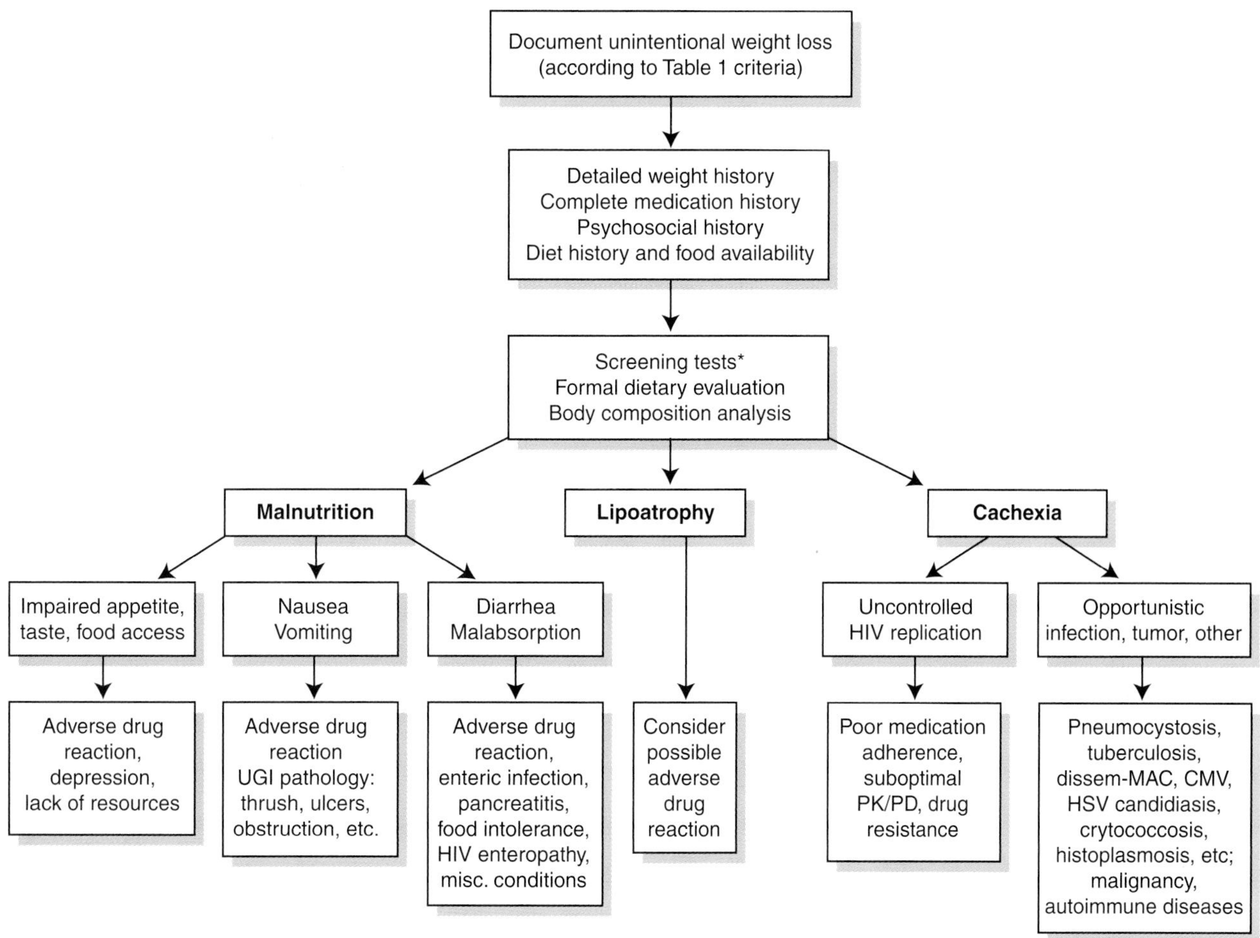

Figure 61-2 ■ Algorithm for workup of wasting syndrome.

capacity to improve quality of life and reduce mortality due to HIV wasting.

Optimizing Nutrition and Calorie Intake

Nutritional supplements,[135–137] enteral[127,138,139] or parenteral feeding[140,141] may increase protein synthesis[36] and nitrogen balance[142] and LBM in some HIV-infected patients. Despite a body of data, there are no established HIV-specific recommendations for daily intake of caloric energy and macronutrients. Individual requirements may vary depending on levels of REE or physical activity.[143,144] Protein intake of greater than 1.5 g/kg has been utilized in AWS,[142,143] based on data from other catabolic disorders, whereby protein intake in this range has been necessary to achieve a positive nitrogen balance.[145]

Specific formulas, including supplemental glutamine,[135] polymeric diet,[137] β-hydroxy-β-methylbutyrate,[136] or whey-protein[146] have been assessed, but the benefits of these supplements have not been established in blind, controlled studies. Advancement in understanding of the molecular mechanisms regulating muscle protein degradation in cachexia has fostered interest in proteasome inhibition by pharmacological or nutritional intervention,[147,148] including the use of dietary eicosapentaenoic acid (EPA) in cancer cachexia.[149,150] However, there have been no controlled clinical trials with EPA in patients with AWS to date.

Selection of specific supplements should be based on tolerability and cost. However, it is important to recognize that nutritional supplements often do not increase total caloric intake since there may be a compensatory decrease in the intake of selected foods,[151] they may be costly, and associated with early satiety or diarrhea.

PHARMACOLOGIC THERAPIES

Appetite Stimulants

Because reduction in caloric energy intake is a contributing factor to HIV-associated wasting, therapies (e.g., megestrol acetate or dronabinol) to stimulate appetite may be considered (Table 61-3).

Megestrol acetate (MA) is an oral synthetic progestational agent that is a powerful appetite stimulant approved by the FDA in 1993 for the treatment of anorexia, cachexia, or unexplained weight loss in patients with HIV. The mechanism whereby MA increases appetite may be related to its inhibitory effects on TNF-α for lipids and fat tissue[152,153] and other cytokines.[154,155] In two double-blind placebo-controlled studies,[156,157] MA convincingly increased weight. Similar effects occurred when the agent was combined with testosterone,[158] dronabinol,[159] cyproheptadine,[160] or nandrolone decanoate.[161] However, approximately two-thirds of the gains in weight were attributable to increases in fat mass.

MA at doses of 160 mg/day to 800 mg/day was generally well-tolerated. The most common adverse effect has been hypogonadism. Thus, suppression of serum testosterone levels may account for the gains in fat and may inhibit accrual of lean tissue despite increases in total calorie intake. MA also has glucocorticoid activity and may suppress the pituitary-adrenal axis, resulting in low cortisol levels and even frank adrenal insufficiency,[158,161–164] hyperglycemia,[165,166] occasional Cushing syndrome[166] and a steroid withdrawal syndrome.[162–164] The risk of these abnormalities appears to be greater with higher doses given over longer periods of time. Further, MA-treated patients may require glucocorticoid replacement during periods of illness or stress. In a recent comprehensive meta-analysis of published clinical trials with MA, data for HIV patients were insufficient to define the optimal dose of megestrol.[167]

Dronabinol (δ-9-tetrahydrocannabinol) is the principal psychoactive component of marijuana, and apart from its effect on mood, has some antinausea and appetite stimulating properties. Oral dronabinol is almost completely absorbed and undergoes extensive first pass metabolism in the liver with only 10–20% of the initial dose reaching systemic circulation. Because of its high lipid solubility and CNS penetration, the CNS side-effects may be dose-limiting. Dronabinol has been evaluated in pilot studies[168,169] and a larger randomized placebo-controlled phase III trial in patients with HIV wasting,[170,171] which were the basis for its FDA approval for the treatment of anorexia in AIDS patients.[172] In the randomized clinical trial, dronabinol improved appetite, increased caloric intake, but weight gain did not occur in most patients.[171] Whereas, 43% of dronabinol-treated patients experienced toxicities, primarily neurologic in nature including euphoria, dizziness, somnolence, and abnormal thinking versus 13% with placebo. Finally, a combination of MA and dronabinol showed no benefit over MA treatment alone.[159]

Marijuana has been shown to stimulate appetite and suppresses nausea.[173–175] Small studies of inhaled marijuana have shown short-term improvements of appetite in HIV-infected patients, but compelling evidence that it produces weight gain are lacking.[175–177] Although no significant effect on plasma HIV viral load, CD4+ T-lymphocyte cell count, or protease inhibitor levels occurred during a short course of inhaled marijuana,[178,179] there was a 50-fold increase in systemic HIV RNA viral load, in tetrahydrocannabinol treated (compared with placebo) severe combined immunodeficient mice, engrafted with human peripheral blood leukocytes and HIV infection.[180] The lack of consistent weight gain, neurologic toxicities, potential for addiction, and possible unfavorable immunologic properties suggest limited utility of dronabinol or tetrahydrocannabinol for the treatment of HIV wasting.

Cyproheptadine, an antihistamine, antiserotoninergic agent, which stimulates appetite, was compared with MA in 14 HIV-infected patients (seven in each arm) with weight loss ≥5 kg over 12 weeks.[160] Weight gain in both study arms was associated with increases in daily caloric intake. However, only three of seven subjects in the cyproheptadine arm (12 mg/day) compared with five of seven in the MA arm gained weight.

Of the appetite-stimulating agents tested for treatment of HIV wasting, MA was better tolerated than dronabinol, and produced more robust weight gain than dronabinol or cyproheptadine. However, with MA most of the weight gain has been in fat mass, and hypogonadism and suppression of the adrenal axis are frequent side-effects. The addition of testosterone replacement does not improve gains in LBM, when compared to MA treatment alone, but preserves sexual function in men with HIV wasting.[158].

Anabolic Agents

The observation that depletion of lean tissue continues in a substantial number of patients despite HAART and appetite stimulants are ineffective in restoring LBM has fostered interest in agents, which target anabolic protein metabolism for the treatment of HIV wasting. This group of anabolic agents includes testosterone (intramuscular or transdermal), anabolic steroids including nandrolone decanoate (intramuscular),

Table 61-3 Pharmacotherapy of HIV Wasting Targeting Appetite: Clinical Trials

Agent, Author	Dose	N[a]	Study Duration (Weeks)	Weight (Mean Change)	Lean Body Mass (Mean Change)	Appetite	Adverse Events
Megestrol Acetate							
Summerbell et al[160]	160 mg/day	14	12	+3.6 kg[c]	Not done	↑	↑Glucose
Von Roenn et al[157,b]	100 mg/day	61	12	+0.86 ± 1.9	−0.14 kg[d]		Impotence
	400 mg/day	53	12	+1.9 ± 0.6 kg	+0.68 kg[d]		
	800 mg/day	53	12	+3.5 ± 0.6 kg	+1.1 kg[d]	↑	Hypogonadism
Oster et al[156, b]	800 mg/day	42	12	+4.2 kg	No change	↑	
Timpone et al[159, b]	750 mg/day	39	12	+6.5 ± 1.1 kg	Not done	↑	
Batterham and Garsia[161]	400 mg/day	14	12	+10.2 ± 4.5 kg	+2.76 ± 0.55 kg[e]	↑	↓ Cortisol
Mulligan et al[158, b]	800 mg/day	38	12	+5.3 kg	+3.3 kg[d]	↑	↓ Cortisol, ↓ Testosterone
Dronabinol							
Struwe et al[169, b]	5 mg bid	5	5	+0.5 kg[f]	Not done	↑	Euphoria[g], thinking
Beal et al[170, b]	2.5 mg bid	88	6	+0.1 kg	Not done	=	Abnormalities[g]
Beal et al[171] follow-up		93	52	+1.4 ± 3.5 kg[f]	Not done	=	Somnolence[g]
Timpone et al[159]	2.5 mg bid	47	12	No change	Not done	=	Dizziness, anxiety[g]
Cyproheptadine							
Summerbell et al[160]	12 mg/day	14	12	+3.1 kg[h]	Not done	↑	None

[a] Number of subjects included in analysis.
[b] Randomized, double-blind, placebo-controlled trial.
[c] In 5 of 7 patients.
[d] Measured by bioelectrical impedance analysis (BIA).
[e] Fat free mass measured by BIA.
[f] Not significantly different from baseline ($P > 0.05$).
[g] Dose-related, reversible with 2.5 mg daily.
[h] In 3 of 7 patients.

oxandrolone (oral), and oxymetholone (oral), and growth factors, e.g., recombinant human GH, and IGF-1.

Testosterone

Ten randomized placebo-controlled trials have been conducted in patients with HIV-associated wasting to evaluate the effectiveness of testosterone therapy alone, with or without exercise or MA, and in comparison with nandrolone (Table 61-4). In a crossover study, 200 mg of parenteral testosterone therapy every 2 weeks compared with placebo produced no difference in weight, but quality of life was significantly improved during therapy with testosterone.[181] In another study, 300 mg of testosterone enanthate given every 3 weeks versus placebo for 6 months in HIV-infected men with wasting and low testosterone levels, resulted in significant increases in LBM (1.9 kg), FFM (2 kg), muscle mass (2.4 kg), and quality of life in patients receiving testosterone.[182]

Testosterone enanthate (100 mg weekly) with or without resistance exercise was compared with placebo in hypogonadal HIV-infected men with wasting.[183] There were significant increases in weight in the testosterone alone (2.6 kg) and exercise alone (2.2 kg) arms, increased strength with each intervention except placebo, and significant increases in thigh muscle mass in testosterone containing arms (2.3 kg testosterone alone; 2.6 kg testosterone with exercise). These data suggested that the combination of testosterone and resistance exercise did not produce greater gains in weight and lean muscle mass than either intervention alone. In a similar study, the effects of testosterone and resistance training were evaluated in a 2 × 2 factorial design in eugonadal HIV-infected men.[184] Increases in arm and leg muscle mass were similar in the testosterone and resistance exercise groups. HDL cholesterol levels decreased significantly in the testosterone arms compared to placebo but significantly increased with exercise.

Because low testosterone levels have been observed in as many as 60% of HIV-infected women with wasting,[24,185] three randomized placebo-controlled trials investigated safety, tolerability, and effect of transdermal testosterone replacement therapy on weight and muscle mass in HIV-infected women with low serum testosterone levels and HIV wasting.[186–188] In the first of these studies, testosterone at 150 mcg/day for 12 weeks when compared to placebo produced significant weight gain of 1.9 ± 0.7 kg and improved social functioning, which was superior to the results with supraphysiologic testosterone (300 mcg/day).[186] In five out of six previously amenorrheic patients receiving 150 mcg/day testosterone, menses resumed, and there were no adverse effects such as hirsutism, abnormal liver tests or lipid abnormalities. In a 6-month randomized placebo-controlled trial, transdermal testosterone via a 4 mg patch administered twice weekly (150 mcg/day) resulted in a significant improvement in strength of the major muscle groups of the upper and lower body and trend toward an increase in muscle mass (1.4 ± 0.6 kg, $P = 0.08$) as estimated by urinary creatinine excretion.[187] However, in a third study, 300 mcg/day of transdermal testosterone produced no improvements in FFM, fat mass, muscle strength, and quality of life after 6 months of study therapy.[188] It is not possible to explain these disparate results other than it may be that the level of androgen deficiency, degree of muscle wasting, dose of testosterone or duration of study therapies affected outcomes.

Nandrolone

Nandrolone decanoate is a long acting injectable, nonaromatizable synthetic derivative of testosterone. In one open-label study, nandrolone decanoate at 100 mg biweekly produced significant mean increases in weight of 0.14 kg/week, LBM by 3 kg and improvement of quality of life after 16 weeks in 17 HIV subjects with wasting and who had previously failed to gain weight with a nutritional intervention program.[189] In a rigorous placebo-controlled 21 day study conducted on a metabolic ward, nandrolone decanoate at 60 or 200 mg/week produced significant increases in nitrogen retention compared to placebo in HIV-infected men with wasting and low or low-normal testosterone levels.[190] In 10 subjects who completed open-label therapy for 12 weeks, significant gains in weight (4.9 ± 1.2 kg), LBM (3.1 ± 0.5 kg), and improvements in treadmill exercise performance were achieved. In the largest placebo-controlled study of nandrolone, subjects with HIV wasting were randomized to nandrolone decanoate at 150 mg/week or placebo for 12 weeks.[191] After 12 weeks, LBM by DEXA increased by 1.6 ± 0.3 kg for the recipients of nandrolone compared to 0.4 ± 0.3 kg with placebo ($P < 0.05$). Further, treatment with nandrolone was associated with greater improvements in perceptions of health and sexual function than placebo.

In the trial cited earlier comparing nandrolone decanoate with MA and diet counseling, significant weight gain occurred after 12 weeks with diet counseling (1.1 ± 0.4 kg), nandrolone decanoate (100 mg every 2 weeks, 4 ± 1.7 kg), and MA (10.2 ± 4.5 kg).[161] Weight accrual with nandrolone decanoate was mostly due to increases in FFM (3.5 ± 2 kg, 88%) compared to 2.8 ± 0.6 kg (27%) gain in FFM with MA, and no significant gains in FFM with diet counseling alone. A small open-label study ($n = 9$) with a combination of nandrolone decanoate (100 mg every 15 days) with MA (400 mg daily) in HIV-infected men with wasting produced gains in weight of 11.9 ± 9.1 kg, gains in FFM of 5.1 ± 4.1 kg, and improvements in muscle strength and Karnofsky performance without significant gains in fat mass after 16 weeks.[192] However, adrenal suppression and decreases in testosterone levels occurred in some subjects.

In the largest multicenter randomized double-blind placebo-controlled trial of androgen therapies for wasting, 303 subjects with HIV wasting were randomized to nandrolone decanoate (150 mg biweekly) and testosterone (250 mg biweekly, as a mixture of 30 mg propionate, 60 mg phenylpropionate, and 100 mg decanoate) or placebo.[193] Of the 303 enroled subjects, 152/157 in the nandrolone arm, 59/66 in the testosterone arm and 77/80 in the placebo arm completed the 12-week study period. Nandrolone was superior to testosterone and placebo

Table 61-4

Therapies Targeting Skeletal Muscle Protein Metabolism: Testosterone and Anabolic Steroids

Agent, Author, and Dose	N[a]	Study Duration (Weeks)	Weight (Mean Change)	LBM, or FFM (Mean Change)	Strength, or Exercise Capacity	Adverse Events
Testosterone (T)						
Coodley and Coodley[181] T cypionate 200 mg biweekly	35	12	No change	Not done	Trend ↑	
Grinspoon et al[182,b] Enanthate 300 mg every 3 weeks	43	26	+1.6 ± 5.8 kg	+1.9 ± 3.4 kg	No change	↓Sex hormone binding globulin
Dobs (1999)[243b] T transscrotal patch 6 mg/day	110	12	No change	No change[c]	Not done	
Bhasin et al[183,b] T enanthate 100 mg/week	49	16	+2.6 kg	+2.3 kg	↑	↑Hemoglobin
Grinspoon et al[184,b] T enanthate 200 mg/week	43	12	+2.6 ± 2.5 kg	+4.4 ± 2.2 kg	↑	↓HDLchol ↓LH, FSH
Miller et al[186] (women) 150 μg/day	18	12	1.9 ± 0.7 kg	No change	No change	
Transdermal T 300 μg/day	18	12	No change	No change	No change	
Choi et al[188,b] (women) Transdermal T 300 μg/day	44	24	No change	No change	No change	
Dolan et al[187,b] (women) Transdermal T 150 μg/day	52	26	No change	Trend increase of muscle mass	↑	
Mulligan et al[158,b] Megestrol acetate 800 mg daily and T 200 mg biweekly	59	12	+5.3 kg	+3.3 kg	Not done	↓Cortisol
Nandrolone Decanoate (ND)						
Strawford et al[190] ND 65 mg/week or 200 mg/week	10	15	+4.9 ± 1.2 kg	+3.1 ± 0.5 kg	↑	
Batterham et al[161] ND, 100 mg biweekly	14	12	+4 ± 1.7 kg	+3.5 ± 2.0 kg	Not done	
Storer et al[191,b] ND 150 mg biweekly	82	12	Not reported	+1.6 ± 0.3 kg	No change	↓Testosterone ↓LH, FSH
Cuerda et al[192] ND 100 mg every 15days plus megestrol acetate 400 mg daily	7	16	+11.9 ± 9.1 kg	+5.1 ± 4.1 kg*	↑	Adrenal suppression ↓Testosterone hyperglycemia ↑AST, GGT
Mulligan (2005)[244b] women ND 100 mg biweekly	33	12	+4.6 kg	+3.5 kg	Not done	↑HCT, hirsutism hoarseness
Gold et al[193,b] ND 150 mg biweekly	152	12	+2.1 ± 2.2 kg	+1.6 ± 3 kg	Not done	
Testosterone 250 mg biweekly	59	12	+0.9 ± 2.1 kg	+0.8 ± 1.9 kg	Not done	

(Continued)

Table 61-4 (Continued)

Agent, Author, and Dose	N[a]	Study Duration (Weeks)	Weight (Mean Change)	LBM or FFM (Mean Change)	Strength, or Exercise Capacity	Adverse Events
Oxandrolone						
Berger et al[194,b]	63	16	No change	No change	No change	
Oxandrolone 5 mg/day, oxandrolone 15 mg/day						
Strawford et al[198,b]						
Oxandrolone						
No oxandrolone	11	8	+6.7 ± 2 kg	+6.9 ± 1.7 kg	↑	↑LFTs, ↓HDLchol
Resistance exercise + replacement testosterone, ±20 mg/day oxandrolone	11	8	+4.2 ± 2.8 kg	+3.8 ± 2.9 kg	↑	↓LH, ↓FSH
Earthman et al[195]						
Oxandrolone (20 mg/day)						
Mwamburi et al[199]	25	18	+2.6 ± 3.0 kg	+3.0±2.9 kg	Not done	
Oxandrolone (10 mg bid) vs megestrol acetate 800 mg daily	33	8	+2.5 ± 2.4 kg	+1.4 ± 1.9 kg	Not done	↑LFTs
Oxymetholone						
Hengge et al[200,b]						
Oxymetholone 50 mg tid	14	12	+5.7 ± 3.7 kg	Not done	Not done	
± ketotifen 50 mg daily	16	12	+3.0 ± 0.5 kg	Not done	Not done	
Hengge et al[201,b] 50 mg bid	25	16	+3.5 ± 0.7 kg	+2.9 ± 0.5 kg	Not done	↑LFTs, ↓Testosterone
Oxymetholone 50 mg tid	27	16	+3.0 ± 0.5 kg	+1.8 ± 0.8 kg	Not done	↓LH, FSH

LBM, lean body mass; FFM, fat free mass.

[a] Number of subjects included in analysis.
[b] Randomized, double-blinded, placebo-controlled trial.
[c] Body cell mass was determined.

for increasing weight (2.1 ± 2.2, 0.9 ± 2.1, and 0.5 ± 3.1 kg) and patient perception of treatment benefit. Gains in FFM measured by BIA were significantly different from placebo, but not different between nandrolone (1.6 ± 3.0 kg) and testosterone groups (0.8 ± 1.9 kg). The 50 subjects with low free serum testosterone levels (<42 pmol/L), and $n = 15$ with low total testosterone levels (<12.1 nmol/L) at baseline responded to these agents similarly to those with higher levels.

Oxandrolone

Oxandrolone is a synthetic derivative of testosterone that is orally absorbed without HIV-specific FDA labeling indications but is approved by the agency for persons unable to maintain body weight even if the cause is unknown. In a double-blind placebo-controlled trial, oxandrolone at 5 and 15 mg/day produced no significant weight gain in 46 patients with HIV wasting after 16 weeks of treatment, but the group receiving 5 mg/day oxandrolone maintained their weight, those receiving 15 mg/day gained weight, and the placebo group lost weight.[194] Oxandrolone at 20 mg/day induced a mean gain in BCM (3.7 ± 3 kg) and LBM (3.0 ± 2.9 kg) in 25 HIV-infected patients on HAART with AWS in an open-label study after an average of 18 weeks of therapy.[195] One subject discontinued oxandrolone due to elevation of liver tests. Other studies have reported BCM gains of 2.2 kg in HIV patients with wasting given oxandrolone over 16 weeks[196] and 3 kg after 12 weeks,[197] but the gain in BCM by BIA in the latter study was not statistically significant.

In a carefully conducted placebo-controlled study, oxandrolone at 20 mg/day produced significant gains in LBM in eugonadal HIV-infected subjects with wasting (11 per arm), all of whom concomitantly received 100 mg/week intramuscular testosterone and progressive resistance exercise (PRE).[198] After 8 weeks, LBM by DEXA scanning increased by 6.9 ± 1.7 kg in the oxandrolone arm and 3.8 ± 2.9 kg in the placebo arm ($P < 0.05$), suggesting that oxandrolone enhanced the effects of PRE. Muscle strength also increased more in the oxandrolone arm when compared to placebo. Serum LH and follicle-stimulating hormone (FSH) were suppressed and serum testosterone levels were somewhat lowered but still within the normal range in study subjects. HDL cholesterol declined with oxandrolone and one participant discontinued oxandrolone due to elevated liver tests.

Treatment with MA (800 mg/day) was compared with oxandrolone (10 mg twice daily) for 2 months in 40 patients with HIV wasting.[199] Mean weight gain (2.8 kg vs 2.5 kg) and mean gain in LBM by BIA (0.8 kg vs 1.4 kg) were similar in the treatment arms. Seven of 18 study subjects in the MA arm experienced nausea, vomiting, bloating, decrease in libido, interruption of menses, or hyperglycemia and five of 15 subjects in the oxandrolone arm had elevations of liver tests more than three times the upper limit of normal.

Oxymetholone

Oxymetholone, an orally bioavailable 17-α-alkylated dihydrotestosterone derivative, was administered alone at 50 mg thrice daily and in combination with ketotifen to block TNF-α in HIV patients with wasting.[200] The average weight gain after 30 weeks was ~6 kg. Karnofsky performance and quality of life measures also improved. The effects were similar in both arms, suggesting that ketotifen provided little additional benefit. In a double-blind placebo-controlled randomized follow-up trial, oxymetholone 50 mg three times daily or 50 mg twice daily was compared to placebo in eugonadal AIDS patients with wasting and receiving HAART.[201] The 50 mg twice-daily dose resulted in the largest increase in FFM (2.9 ± 0.5 kg) and BCM (3.8 ± 0.4 kg) by BIA after 16 weeks. Twenty-seven and 35% of subjects in the twice-daily and thrice-daily dosing arms, respectively, developed ALT increases more than five times the baseline values.

Treatment with anabolic steroids significantly increased LBM, exercise capacity and muscle strength, but the magnitude of these effects varied widely, dependent on the drug and heterogeneity of the study population with wasting. Long-term effects of anabolic steroids have not been studied, and it remains unclear whether increases in LBM and strength correlate with more relevant improvements in physical functioning and survival.[202] Replacement doses of testosterone may improve sexual functions in hypogonadal men and improve amenorrhea in women with low testosterone levels. Suppression of the gonadal axis is common with all anabolic androgens including generic testosterone, whereas decreases in HDL cholesterol, increases in hemoglobin, occurrence of abnormal liver function tests (LFTs) and hyperglycemia have been mostly observed with supraphysiologic doses of testosterone and with the anabolic steroids. The C17α-alkylated anabolic steroids (oxymetholone, stanozol, methyltestosterone, metandienone, danazol, norethandrolone, fluoxymesterone) have been associated with hepatotoxicity when given long-term in non-HIV subjects.[203] Hypogonadal men receiving testosterone or synthetic analogs for greater than 3–4 months should undergo regular prostate examination and prostate-specific antigen (PSA) monitoring. Long-term therapy with these agents may produce irreversible suppression of the hypothalamic-pituitary-gonadal axis, resulting in permanent hypogonadism and need for life-long androgen replacement therapy.

Recombinant Human Growth Hormone

Recombinant human growth hormone (rhGH)has increased nitrogen and potassium balance[34] and augmented LBM in HIV-infected patients with wasting,[204–207] sustained LBM in AIDS patients during acute opportunistic infections,[208] and improved exercise capacity in patients with HIV-associated wasting receiving HAART.[209] Four randomized, placebo-controlled trials evaluated either the effect of rhGH alone[210,211] or combination of rhGH with IGF-1,[212,213] treatment of HIV-associated wasting over 3 months (Table 61-5). In the pivotal registration trial, an average dose of 6 mg rhGH/day (0.1 mg kg^{-1} day^{-1}) produced significant gains in LBM and weight (3 ± 3 kg and 1.6 ± 3.7 kg), decreases in fat mass (1.7 ± 1.7 kg), and improved aerobic exercise capacity

Table 61-5

Therapies Targeting Protein Anabolic Metabolism: Recombinant Human Growth Hormone and IGF-1

Agent, Author, and Dose	N[a]	Study Duration (Weeks)	Weight (Mean Change)	LBM, or FFM (Mean Change)	Strength, or Exercise Capacity	Adverse Events
Schambelan et al[210,b]						
placebo	71	12	No change	No change	No change	
0.1 $mgkg^{-1}$ day^{-1} rhGH[c]	69	12	+1.6 ± 3.7 kg	+3 ± 3 kg	↑	Fluid retention, hyperglycemia
Lee et al[213,b]						
0.34 mg bid rhGH plus 5 mg bid IGF-1[d]	80	12	No change	No change	No change	Edema, arthralgias
Waters et al[212,b]						
placebo	11	12	No change	No change	No change	
1.4 $mgday^{-1}$ rhGH	11	12	No change	No change	↑	Edema
5 mg bid IGF-1	4	12	No change	No change	No change	
rhGH + IGF-1	9	12	No change	3.2 ± 0.6 kg	No change	Arthralgias, myalgias
Moyle et al[211,b]						
placebo	203	12	No change	No change	No change	
0.1 $mgkg^{-1}$ daily rhGH	178	12	+3 kg	+4.0 kg	↑	Carpal tunnel, edema gynecomastia, hyperglycemia
0.1 $mgkg^{-1}$ every other day rhGH	206	12	+2.2 kg	+3.1 kg	↑	

[a] Number of subjects included in analysis.
[b] Randomized, double-blind, placebo-controlled trial.
[c] Recombinant human growth hormone administered subcutaneously.
[d] Insulin-like growth factor 1 administered subcutaneously.

in the rhGH arm ($n = 90$).[210] Body composition was analyzed by DEXA and D_2O/bromide dilution and showed that a portion of the gains in LBM were likely due to accumulation of total and extracellular water and improvements in treadmill performance appeared to be lost when corrected for the increases in body mass.

In two other trials, treatment with rhGH at 0.34 mg twice daily[213] and 1.4 mg once daily.[212] were combined with IGF-1 (5 mg twice daily). Although significant increases in FFM, calculated by skin fold thickness[213] and LBM determined by DEXA[212] occurred after 6 weeks of treatment in the groups receiving rhGH alone or the combination of rhGH with IGF-1, these gains were not sustained after 12 weeks of therapy. The authors interpreted the results that the rhGH doses were possibly too low and IGF-1 provided no additional benefits.

In the largest multinational trial with 757 study subjects, every-other-day versus daily dosing of rhGH (0.1 mg/kg body weight up to maximum of 6 mg/kg of body weight per dose) was compared with placebo in patients with HIV wasting and who mostly were receiving HAART (87.6%).[211] After 12 weeks of treatment, mean body weight increased by 2.2 and 3 kg in alternate day and daily treatment groups, respectively, which were significantly greater than changes in the placebo group. LBM by DEXA increased by 3.1 and 4.0 kg in the respective rhGH treatment groups and fat mass, predominantly truncal, decreased. Median maximum work output by cycle ergometry increased by 2.4 and 2.6 kJ in the respective rhGH treatment groups. Fluid retention, hyperglycemia, carpal tunnel syndrome, gynecomastia were more common in subjects receiving daily than every other day rhGH. Total cholesterol was significantly reduced with the daily rhGH compared to placebo. General health, social behavior, attention, reasoning, and problem-solving improved significantly with both active treatment groups. During open-label extension of the trial, further increases in LBM were observed in both rhGH treatment groups (mean increases 3.7 and 7.8 kg respectively) after 48 weeks.

In the only study that prospectively compared the effects of an anabolic androgen (nandrolone decanoate at 150 mg/week) with rhGH at 6 mg/day, 86 subjects were randomized to one of these interventions or nandrolone placebo.[191] Treatment with open-label rhGH produced increases in LBM of 2.5 ± 0.3 kg, which was similar to increases with nandrolone (1.6 ± 0.3 kg, $P > 0.05$) but rhGH produced greater decreases in body fat. Treatment with rhGH was more often discontinued because of toxicities and greater increases in extracellular water. Whereas, nandrolone was associated with greater improvements in perception of healthy sexual function than rhGH.

In a study of rhGH (4 mg every other day) for treatment of 30 patients with lipodystrophy, arm and leg fat decreased significantly by DEXA after 12 and 24 weeks of study therapy along with increases in LBM.[215] It is noteworthy that all of the changes in lean and fat tissue were lost after 12 weeks of washout (study week 36). Regardless, care must be taken when selecting rhGH for therapy of wasting in subjects predisposed to lipoatrophy since the therapy may aggravate the loss of appendicular fat. Further, in other populations, rhGH is associated with worsening insulin resistance, impaired glucose tolerance and new onset diabetes during the first several months of treatment.[214–217] Because patients receiving HAART are at risk of insulin resistance related to lipodystrophy, consideration should be given to this potential complication in patients already at risk for diabetes and cardiovascular morbidity.

In patients with HIV-associated wasting, GH resistance, namely, increased GH levels and decreased IGF-1 levels, has been observed.[103] In contrast, patients who developed visceral fat accumulation and loss of subcutaneous fat during HAART show decreased levels of GH,[218] whereas, otherwise "healthy" HIV-infected individuals usually have normal GH levels.[219] Thus, endogenous GH secretion responds to changes in nutrition and body composition, and treatment for a GH-resistant state, such as HIV-associated wasting, or a relative GH deficiency state, such as lipodystrophy, may require different dosing of rhHG.

Overall, studies utilizing pharmacologic doses of rhGH corroborate significant short-term beneficial effects on body composition, including the gain of LBM (albeit a portion of the gains may have been due to fluid accumulation) and loss of fat mass (both central and extremity fat), improvements in physical function and quality of life. There are insufficient data about the optimal dosing regimens, and the derangements of glucose metabolism and lack of durability of effects on body composition is disconcerting. Further, there is little evidence in patients with HIV or other populations that rhGH increases muscle mass despite enhancements in LBM. Initial studies of GH releasing hormone[220] or a synthetic GH releasing factor[221] in HIV-infected patients with lipodystrophy showed encouraging results with partial reversal of fat accumulation, gains in LBM and absence of adverse effects on insulin and glucose metabolism.

Cytokine Modulator

Agents that inhibit TNF-α, such as pentoxifylline,[222] fish oil,[223] and thalidomide[224] have been investigated for the treatment of HIV wasting. Pentoxifylline failed to produce weight gain in HIV or cancer patients with wasting,[225,226] and fish oil supplementation (MaxEPA, 18 g/day) did not lead to weight gain in a placebo-controlled trial of 16 evaluable HIV-infected patients with wasting.[227] Thalidomide produced weight gain in three randomized placebo-controlled trials in HIV wasting,[228–230] including a gain of ~1 kg in FFM after 12 weeks of treatment at 100 mg four times a day, or after 8 weeks at 100 and 200 mg/day. The optimal dose of thalidomide has not been defined and adverse events including teratogenicity, dose-related somnolence, and peripheral neuropathy preclude its common use.[230,231] Thus, thalidomide should be reserved for patients failing other therapies such as testosterone, anabolic steroids, or rhGH.

Exercise

Muscle wasting is associated with poor physical function in patients with HIV.[232,233] While aerobic exercise training

Table 61-6

PRT for AIDS Wasting

Author, Intervention	N[a]	Study Duration (Weeks)	Weight (Mean Change)	LBM, or FFM (Mean Change)	Strength or Exercise Capacity	Quality of Life
Roubenoff and Wilson,[239]						
wasting	6	16	+3.9 kg	+2.6 ± 1.2 kg	↑	Not done
no wasting	15	16	No change	+1.1 ± 1.9 kg	No change	
PRT, three times a week on stationary pneumatic resistance equipment for 8 weeks, followed by 8 weeks of usual activity						
Strawford et al,[190,b]						
no oxandrolone	11	8	+4.2 ± 2.8 kg	+3.8 ± 2.9 kg	↑	No change
20 mg/day oxandrolone	11	8	+6.7 ± 2.0 kg	+6.9 ± 1.7 kg	↑	No change
PRT three-times a week on weight-stack isotonic exercise equipment, plus replacement testosterone (100 mg/week) ± oxandrolone						
Sattler et al,[131]						
nandrolone weekly	15	12	+3.2 ± 2.7 kg	+3.9 ± 2.3 kg	↑	Not done
nandrolone + exercise	15	12	+4.0 ± 2.0 kg	+5.2 ± 5.7 kg	↑↑	Not done
PRT three-times a week with free weights, one repetition maximum strength of upper and lower body muscle groups						
Bhasin et al,[183,b]						
exercise alone	11	16	+2.2 kg	+2.0 ± 0.9 kg	↑	No change
testosterone alone	15	16	+2.6 kg	+2.9 ± 1.0 kg	↑	No change
testosterone + exercise	11	16	No change	+1.6 ± 0.8 kg	↑	No change
2 × 2 factorial design including placebo arm (n = 12, not shown), PRT three times a week, one-repetition maximum strength of upper and lower body muscle groups						
Grinspoon et al,[184,b]						
exercise alone	10	12	No change	+2.3 ± 2.2 kg	No change	
testosterone alone	10	12	+2.7 ± 2.6 kg	+4.2 ± 2.3 kg	↑	
testosterone + exercise	11	12	+2.5 ± 2.5 kg	+4.6 ± 2.1 kg	↑	
2 × 2 factorial design, including placebo arm (n = 12) PRT three times a week, isometric strength testing of upper and lower body muscle groups						
Agin et al[146] (women)						
exercise	10	14	No change	+1.6 ± 2.4 kg	↑	↑
whey protein + exercise	10	14	No change	+1.4 ± 2.0 kg	↑	↑

[a] Number of subjects included in analysis.
[b] Randomized, double-blind, placebo-controlled trial.

primarily alters muscle cell mitochondrial and cytosolic enzyme activities, progressive resistance exercise training (PRT) increases contractile protein,[234,235] leading to increases in muscle mass and strength. Early studies in HIV-infected patients showed gains in weight and aerobic capacity with a combination of bicycle and resistance exercises,[236] and weight gain with PRT in patients recovering from *Pneumocystis jiroveci* pneumonia.[237] Since then, open-label[238,239] and randomized controlled trials[131,146,183,184,198] have demonstrated benefits of PRT, including gains in LBM, muscle mass, strength, and exercise capacity in HIV-infected men and women (Table 61-6).[146] PRT alone increased FFM and maximal voluntary skeletal muscle strength in eugonadal men[184] and hypogonadal men.[183] Of note, in another study PRT improved LBM and strength in patients with HIV infection with or without wasting but was more effective in improving physical functioning in patients with wasting.[239]

Testosterone treatment did not augment the benefits of PRT but lowered HDL cholesterol in one study.[183] Whereas, treatment with oxandrolone produced significant additional gain in LBM by DEXA during PRT (6.9 ± 1.7 kg by DEXA) compared with PRT alone (3.8 ± 2.9 kg).[199] Conversely, PRT with nandrolone decanoate increased the gains in LBM (5.2 ± 5.7 kg) by DEXA compared to therapy with nandrolone alone (3.9 ± 2.3 kg) after 12 weeks, although these subjects did not have documented wasting.[131] In addition, the gains in strength were substantially greater in the PRT arm.

In addition to increasing muscle mass as observed with testosterone, anabolic steroids, or rhGH, PRT specifically improves muscle contractility, specific tension, and reduces hypertriglyceridemia.[240] Resistance exercise is, therefore, a valuable adjunct for the treatment of HIV wasting but requires adherence to a long-term training regimen, access to facilities or trainers, and frailty *per se* may present difficult barriers for some patients.[241,242]

SUMMARY

Detection and management of HIV wasting is an important goal in persons with HIV, as a body of epidemiologic data demonstrates that loss of weight and LBM remain common problems in HIV-infected patients despite HAART, indicating that suppression of HIV replication alone may not provide complete protection against weight loss and wasting. Further, wasting remains an independent predictor of morbidity and mortality in persons with HIV infection. Therefore, it is important to identify and expeditiously manage risk factors for wasting, including[1] inadequate nutrition,[2] suboptimal control of HIV infection or active secondary infections and malignancies, which promote muscle catabolism and anorexia, and[3] metabolic derangements of glucose, lipid, and protein homeostasis.

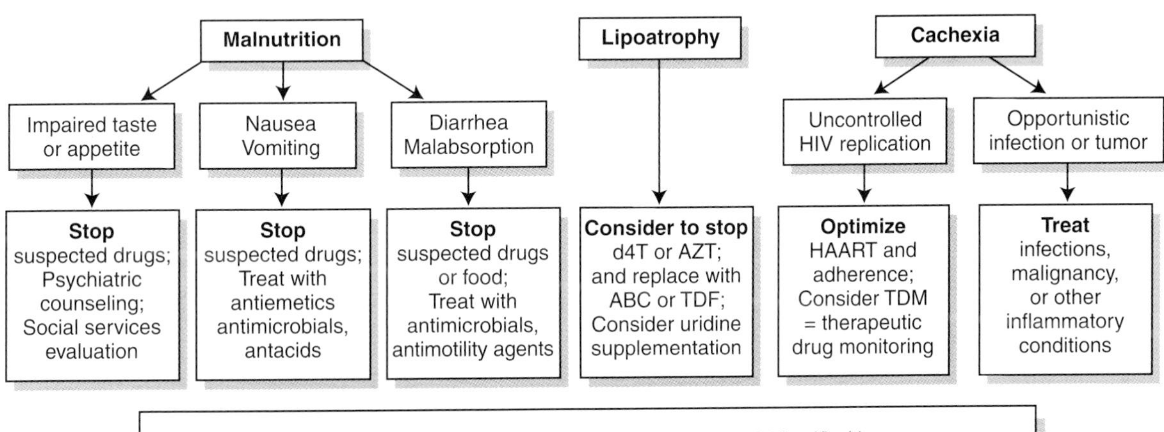

Figure 61-3 ■ Algorithm for treatment of wasting syndrome.

Fortunately, substantial advances have been made in understanding of the pathogenesis of HIV wasting along with an expanded availability of new diagnostic modalities and treatment strategies. An approach to the diagnostic workup for specific causes of HIV-associated wasting is shown in Figure 61-2. Careful standardized monitoring of weight is the first step in early detection of wasting followed by assessment of body composition to refine whether predominantly lean or fat tissue is being lost. A consideration of three major categories for wasting including cachexia, malnutrition, and lipoatrophy has proven clinically useful. Given the multifactorial nature of HIV wasting and differences in clinical presentation, treatment options should be tailored to the individual patient as suggested in the stepwise treatment algorithm of Figure 61-3. In all patients, intake of macronutrients, especially protein, and total calories should be optimized. Appetite stimulation with MA may be used in some patients but should only be prescribed for a limited time and patients should be carefully monitored for suppression of gonadal function, adrenal insufficiency, and hyperglycemia. Of the anabolic therapies, testosterone replacement is appropriate for hypogonadal men, whereas, for wasting syndrome, parenteral nandrolone or oral oxandrolone may be considered in women and men without hypogonadism. rhGH is an alternative for patients who have failed testosterone or anabolic steroids but its effects on augmenting muscle mass are less well defined and may aggravate extremity fat loss. These therapeutic interventions have been shown to be effective in reversing HIV wasting. However, the long-term beneficial effects on physical function and survival have not been demonstrated with these interventions. Further, because of potentially serious adverse effects and substantial costs, there is limited utility for long-term continuous use of MA and anabolic agents including synthetic steroids and rhGH. Exercise regimens are relatively safe, can be combined with nutritional and anabolic strategies, but require substantial patient motivation and effort as well as access to training facilities to be effective. Thus, exploring new treatment strategies for long-term management of wasting that are safe and produce durable and functionally meaningful responses are important goals to improve quality of life for persons infected with HIV.

REFERENCES

1. Serwadda D, Mugerwa RD, Swankambo NK, et al. Slim disease: a new disease in Uganda and its association with HTLV-III infection. Lancet 19:849, 1985.
2. Mhiri C, Belec L, Di Costanzo B, et al. The slim disease in African patients with AIDS. Trans R Soc Trop Med Hyg 86:303, 1992.
3. Centers for Disease Control. Revision of the CDC surveillance case definition of acquired immunodeficiency syndrome. MMWR 36(Suppl 1):3S, 1987.
4. Weiss PJ, Wallace MR, Olson PE, et al. Change in the mix of AIDS – defining conditions. N Engl J Med 329:1962, 1993.
5. Hogg RS, Heath KV, Yib B, etal. Improved survival among HIV-infected individuals following initiation of antiretroviral therapy. JAMA 279:450, 1998.
6. Detels, R, Munoz R, McFarlane G, et al. Effectiveness of potent antiretroviral therapy on time to AIDS and death in men with known HIV infection duration. Multicenter AIDS Cohort Study Investigators. JAMA 280:1497, 1998.
7. Lichtenstein K, Armon C, Buchacz K, et al. Early, uninterrupted antiretroviral therapy is associated with improved outcomes and fewer toxicities in the HIV outpatient study. In: 13th Conference on Retroviruses and Opportunistic Infections, Denver, 2006, abstract 769.
8. Mocroft A, Sabin CA, Youle M, et al: Changes in AIDS-defining illnesses in a London clinic, 1987–1998. J Acquir Immune Defic Syndr 21:401, 1999.
9. Moore RD, Chaisson RE. Natural history of HIV infection in the era of combination antiretroviral therapy. AIDS 13:1933, 1999.
10. Jones JL, Hanson DL, Dworkin MS, et al. Surveillance for AIDS-defining opportunistic illnesses, 1992–1997. MMWR CDC Surveill Summ 48:1, 1999.
11. Smit E, Skolasky RL, Dobs RS, et al. Changes in the incidence and predictors of wasting syndrome related to human immunodeficiency virus infection, 1987–1999. Am J Epidemiol 156:211, 2002.
12. Dworkin MS, Williamson, JM, Adult/Adolescent Spectrum of HIV disease Project. AIDS wasting syndrome: trends, influence on opportunistic infections, and survival. J Acquir Immune Defic Syndr 33:267, 2003.
13. Wanke C, Silva M, Knox TA, et al. Weight loss and wasting remain common complications in individuals infected with HIV in the era of highly active antiretroviral therapy. Clin Infect Dis, 31:803, 2000.
14. Tang AM, Jacobson DL, Spiegelman D, et al. Increasing risk of 5% or greater unintentional weight loss in a cohort of HIV-infected patients, 1995 to 2003. J Acquir Immune Defic Syndr 40:70, 2005.
15. Wheeler DA, Gibert CL, Launer CA, et al. Weight loss as a predictor of survival and disease progression in HIV infection. Terry Beirn Community Programs for Clinical Research on AIDS. J Acquir Immune Defic Syndr Hum Retrovirol 18:80, 1998.
16. Nahlen BL, Chu SY, Nwanyanwu OC, et al. HIV wasting syndrome in the United States. AIDS 7:183, 1993.
17. Melnick SL, Sherer R, Louis TA, et al. Survival and disease progression according to gender of patients with HIV infection. JAMA 272:1915, 1994.
18. Grunfeld C, Pang M, Shimizu L, et al. Resting energy expenditure, caloric intake and short-term weight change in human immunodeficiency virus infection and the acquired immunodeficiency syndrome. Am J Clin Nutr 55:455, 1992.
19. Macallan DC, Noble C, Baldwin C, et al. Prospective analysis of patterns of weight change in stage IV HIV infection. Am J Clin Nutr 58:417, 1993.
20. Forbes GB, Kreipe RE, Lipinski B. Body composition and energy cost of weight gain. Hum Nutr Clin Nutr 36:485, 1982.
21. Forbes GB. Survival during fasting. JAMA 250:1026, 1983.
22. Roubenoff R, Heymsfield SB, Kehayias JJ, et al. Standardization of nomenclature of body composition in weight loss. Am J Clin Nutr. 66:192, 1997.
23. Roubenoff R, Freeman LM, Smith DE. Adjuvant arthritis as a model of inflammatory cachexia. Arthritis Rheum 40: 534, 1997.
24. Grinspoon S, Corcoran C, Miller K, et al. Body composition and endocrine function in women with acquired immunodeficiency syndrome wasting. J Clin Endocrinol Metab 82:1332, 1997. Erratum. J Clin Endocrinol Metab 82: 3360, 1997.
25. Kotler DP, Tierney AR, Wang J, Pierson RN Jr. Magnitude of body-cell-mass depletion and the timing of death from wasting in AIDS. Am J Clin Nutr 50:444, 1989.

26. Palenicek JP, Graham NM, He YD, et al. Weight loss prior to clinical AIDS as a predictor of survival. J Acquir Immune Defic Syndr Hum Retrovirol 10:366, 1995.
27. Suttmann U, Ockenga J, Selberg O, et al. Incidence and prognostic value of malnutrition and wasting in human immunodeficiency virus-infected patients. J Acquir Immune Defic Syndr Hum Retrovirol 8:239, 1995.
28. Hoots WK, Mahoney E, Donfield S, et al. Are there clinical and laboratory predictors of 5-year mortality in HIV-infected children and adolescents with hemophilia? J Acquir Immune Defic Syndr Hum Retrovirol 18:349, 1998.
29. Morley JE, Thomas DR, Wilson MM. Cachexia: pathophysiology and clinical relevance. Am J Clin Nutr 83:735, 2006.
30. Melchior J-C, Raguin G, Boulier A, et al. Resting energy expenditure in human immunodeficiency virus infected patients: comparison between patients with and without secondary infections. Am J Clin Nutr 57:614, 1993.
31. Sharpstone DR, Ross HM, Gazzard BG. The metabolic response to opportunistic infections in AIDS. AIDS 10: 1529, 1996.
32. Melchior J-C, Salmon D, Rigaud D, et al. Resting energy expenditure is increased in stable, malnourished HIV-infected patients. Am J Clin Nutr 53:437, 1991.
33. Hommes MJ, Romijn JA, Endert E, Sauerwein HP. Resting energy expenditure and substrate oxidation in human immunodeficiency virus (HIV)-infected asymptomatic men: HIV affects host metabolism in the early asymptomatic stage. Am J Clin Nutr 54:311, 1991.
34. Mulligan K, Grunfeld C, Hellerstein MK, et al. Anabolic effects of recombinant human growth hormone in patients with wasting associated with human immunodeficiency virus infection. J Clin Endocrinol Metab 77:956, 1993.
35. Macallan DC, Noble C, Baldwin C, et al. Energy expenditure and wasting in human immunodeficiency virus infection. N Engl J Med 333:83, 1995.
36. Macallan DC, McNurlan MA, Milne E, et al. Whole-body protein turnover from leucine kinetics and the response to nutrition in human immunodeficiency virus infection. Am J Clin Nutr 61:818, 1995.
37. Grunfeld C, Kotler DP. Pathophysiology of the AIDS wasting syndrome. AIDS Clin Rev 191–224, 1992.
38. Grunfeld C. What causes wasting in AIDS? N Eng J Med 333:123, 1995.
39. Dworkin B, Wormser GP, Rosenthal, WS, et al. Gastrointestinal manifestations of the acquired immunodeficiency syndrome: a review of 22 cases. Am J Gastroenterol 80:774, 1985.
40. May GR, Gill MJ, Church DL, Sutherland LR. Gastrointestinal symptoms in ambulatory HIV-infected patients. Dig Dis Sci 38:1388, 1993.
41. Quinn TC, Piot P, McCormick JB, et al. Serologic and immunologic studies in patients with AIDS in North America and Africa. JAMA 257:2617, 1987.
42. Bartlett JG, Belitsos PC, Sears CL. AIDS enteropathy. Clin Infect Dis 15:726, 1992.
43. DuPont HL, Marshall GD: HIV-associated diarrhoea and wasting. Lancet 346:352, 1995.
44. Dieterich DT, Lew EA, Kotler, DP, et al. Treatment with albendazole for intestinal disease due to Enterocytozoon bieneusi in patients with AIDS. J Infect Dis 169:178, 1994.
45. Ehrenpreis ED, Ganger DR, Kochvar GT, et al. D-xylose malabsorption: characteristic finding in patients with the AIDS wasting syndrome and chronic diarrhea. J Acquir Immune Defic Syndr 5:1047, 1992.
46. Graham NM, Munoz A, Bacellar H, et al. Clinical factors associated with weight loss related to infection with the human immunodeficiency virus type 1 in the Multicenter AIDS Cohort Study. Am J Epidemiol 137:439, 1993.
47. Kotler, DP, Gaetz HP, Lange M, et al. Enteropathy associated with the acquired immunodeficiency syndrome. Ann Intern Med. 101:421, 1984.
48. Swaggerty, CL, Frolov AA, McArthur MJ, et al. The envelope glycoprotein of simian immunodeficiency virus contains an enterotoxin domain. Virology 277:250, 2000.
49. Maresca M, Mahfoud R, Garmy N, et al. The virotoxin model of HIV-1 enteropathy: involvement of GPR15/Bob and galactosylceramide in the cytopathic effects induced by HIV-1 gp120 in the HT-29-D4 intestinal cell line. J Biomed Sci 10:156, 2003.
50. Godfried MH, van der Poll T, Weverling GJ, et al. Soluble receptors for tumor necrosis factor as predictor of progression to AIDS in asymptomatic human immunodeficiency virus type I infection. J Infect Dis 169:739, 1994.
51. Rautonen J, Rautonen N, Martin NL, et al. Serum interleukin-6 concentrations are elevated and associated with elevated tumor necrosis factor-alpha and immunoglobulin G and A concentrations in children with HIV infection. AIDS 5:1319, 1991.
52. Scott-Algara D, Vuillier F, Marasescu M, et al. Serum levels of IL-2, IL-1 alpha, TNF-alpha, and soluble receptor of IL-2 in HIV-1-infected patients. AIDS Res Hum Retroviruses 7: 381, 1991.
53. Lederman MM, Kalish LA, Asmuth D, et al. 'Modeling' relationships among HIV-1 replication, immune activation and CD4+ T-cell losses using adjusted correlative analyses. AIDS 14: 951, 2000.
54. Hellerstein MK, Meydani SN, Meydani M, et al. Interleukin-1 induced anorexia in the rat: influence of prostaglandins. J Clin Invest 84:228, 1989.
55. Tracey KJ, Cerami A. The role of cachectin/tumor necrosis factor in AIDS. Cancer Cells 1:62, 1989.
56. Stein TP, Koerner B, Schluter MD, et al. Weight loss, the gut and the inflammatory response in AIDS patients. Cytokine 9:143, 1997.
57. Rivera S, Briggs W, Quian D, Sattler FR. Levels of ribonucleic acid are quantitatively related to prior weight loss in human immunodeficiency virus associated wasting. J Acquir Immune Defic Syndr Hum Retorvirol 17:411, 1998.
58. Belec L, Meillet D, Hernvann A, et al. Differential elevation of circulating interleukin-1 beta, tumor necrosis factor alpha, and interleukin-6 in AIDS-associated cachectic states. Clin Diagn Lab Immunol 1:117, 1994.
59. Rimaniol AC, Zylberberg H, Zarvala F, Viard JP. Inflammatory cytokines and inhibitors in HIV infection: correlation between interleukin-1 receptor antagonist and weight loss. AIDS 10:1349, 1996.
60. Feingold KR, Grunfeld C. Role of cytokines in inducing hyperlipidemia. Diabetes 41(Suppl 2):97, 1992.
61. Havlir DV, Torriani FJ, Schrier RD, et al. Serum interleukin-6 (IL-6), IL-10, tumor necrosis factor (TNF) alpha, soluble type II TNF receptor, and transforming growth factor beta levels in human immunodeficiency virus type 1-infected individuals with Mycobacterium avium complex disease. J Clin Microbiol 39:298, 2001.
62. van Lettow M, van der Meer JW, West CE, et al. Interleukin-6 and human immunodeficiency virus load, but not plasma leptin concentration, predict anorexia and wasting in adults with pulmonary tuberculosis in Malawi. J Clin Endocrinol Metab 90:4771, 2005.
63. Rogy MA, Coyle SM, Oldenburg HS, et al. Persistently elevated soluble tumor necrosis factor receptor and interleukin-1 receptor antagonist levels in critically ill patients. J Am Coll Surg 178:132, 1994.
64. Suttmann U, Selberg O, Gallati H, et al. Tumor necrosis factor receptor levels are linked to the acute-phase response and malnutrition in human-immunodeficiency-virus-infected patients. Clin Sci 86:461, 1994.

65. Godfried MH, Romijn JA, van der Poll T, et al. Soluble receptors for tumor necrosis factor are markers for clinical course but not for major metabolic changes in human immunodeficiency virus infection. Metabolism 44:1564, 1995.
66. Lacey JM, Wilmore DW. Is glutamine a conditionally essential amino acid? Nutr Rev 48:297, 1990.
67. Perelson AS, Neumann, AU, Markowitz M, et al. HIV-1 dynamics in vivo: virion clearance rate, infected cell life-span, and viral generation time. Science 271:1582, 1996.
68. Yarasheski KE, Zachwieja JJ, Gischler J, et al. Increased plasma gln and Leu Ra and inappropriately low muscle protein synthesis rate in AIDS wasting. Am J Physiol 275: E577, 1998.
69. Maagaard A, Holberg-Petersen M, Kollberg G, et al. Mitochondrial DNA in peripheral blood does not reflect the mitochondrial status in skeletal muscle in HIV-infected patients. In: 13th Conference on Retroviruses and Opportunistic Infections, Denver, 2006, abstract 753.
70. Ferrando SJ, Rabkin JG, Lin SH, McElhiney M. Increase in body cell mass and decrease in wasting are associated with increasing potency of antiretroviral therapy for HIV infection. AIDS Patient Care STDS 19:216, 2005.
71. Roubenoff R, Grinspoon S, Skolnik PR, et al. Role of cytokines and testosterone in regulating lean body mass and resting energy expenditure in HIV-infected men. Am J Physiol Endocrinol Metab 283:E138, 2002.
72. Hellerstein MK, Grunfeld C, Wu K, et al. Increased de novo hepatic lipogenesis in human immunodeficiency virus infection. J Clin Endocrinol Metab 76:559, 1993.
73. Valcour VG, Shikuma CM, Shiramizu BT, et al. Diabetes, insulin resistance, and dementia among HIV-1-infected patients. J Acquir Immune Defic Syndr 38:31, 2005.
74. Grinspoon S, Mulligan K. Weight loss and wasting in patients infected with human immunodeficiency virus. Clin Infect Dis 36(Suppl 2):S69, 2003.
75. El-Sadr WM, Mullin, CM, Carr A, et al. Effects of HIV disease on lipid, glucose and insulin levels: results from a large antiretroviral-naive cohort. HIV Med 6:114, 2005.
76. Miller J, Carr A, Emery S, et al. HIV lipodystrophy: prevalence, severity and correlates of risk in Australia. HIV Med 4:293–301, 2003.
77. Tsiodras S, Mantzoros C, Hammer S, Samore M. Effects of protease inhibitors on hyperglycemia, hyperlipidemia, and lipodystrophy: a 5-year cohort study. Arch Intern Med 160:2050, 2000.
78. Lichtenstein KA, Ward DJ, Moorman AC, et al. Clinical assessment of HIV-associated lipodystrophy in an ambulatory population. AIDS 15:1389, 2001.
79. Saint-Marc T, Partisani M, Poizot-Martin I, et al. A syndrome of peripheral fat wasting (lipodystrophy) in patients receiving long-term nucleoside analogue therapy. AIDS 13:1659, 1999.
80. Martinez E, Mocroft A, Garcia-Viejo MA, et al. Risk of lipodystrophy in HIV-1-infected patients treated with protease inhibitors: a prospective cohort study. Lancet 357:592, 2001.
81. Worm D, Kirk O, Andersen O. Clinical lipoatrophy in HIV-1 patients on HAART is not associated with increased abdominal girth, hyperlipidaemia or glucose intolerance. HIV Med 3:239, 2002.
82. Sattler F. Body habitus changes related to lipodystrophy. Clin Infect Dis 36(Suppl 2):S84, 2003.
83. Galli M, Ridolfo AL, Adorni F, et al. Body habitus changes and metabolic alterations in protease inhibitor-naive HIV-1-infected patients treated with two nucleoside reverse transcriptase inhibitors. J Acquir Immune Defic Syndr 29:21, 2002.
84. Amin J, Moore A, Carr A, et al. Combined analysis of two-year follow-up from two open-label randomized trials comparing efficacy of three nucleoside reverse transcriptase inhibitor backbones for previously untreated HIV-1 infection. OzCombo 1 and 2. HIV Clin Trials 4:252, 2003.
85. Chene G, Angelini E, Cotte L, et al. Role of long-term nucleoside analog therapy in lipodystrophy and metabolic disorders in human immunodeficiency virus-infected patients. Clin Infect Dis 34:649, 2002.
86. McComsey GA, Walker UA. Role of mitochondria in HIV lipoatrophy: insight into pathogenesis and potential therapies. Mitochondrion 4:111, 2004.
87. Hansen AB, Lindegaard B, Obel N, et al. Pronnounced lipoatrophy in HIV-infected men receiving HAART for more than 6 years compared with the background population. HIV Med 7:38, 2006.
88. Dobs AS, Dempsey MA, Landenson PW, Polk BF. Endocrine disorders in men infected with human immunodeficiency virus. Am J Med 84:611, 1988.
89. Grinspoon SK, Bilezikian JP. HIV disease and the endocrine system. N Engl J Med 327:1360, 1992.
90. Lefrere JJ, Laplanche JL, Vitecoq D, et al. Hypogonadism in AIDS. AIDS 2:135, 1988.
91. Croxson TS, Chapman WE, Miller KL, et al. Changes in the hypothalamic-pituitary-gonadal axis in human deficiency virus-infected homosexual men. J Clin Endocrinol Metab 68:317, 1989.
92. Rietschel P, Corcoran C, Stanley T, et al. Prevalence of hypogonadism among men with weight loss related to human immunodeficiency virus infection who were receiving highly active antiretroviral therapy. Clin Infect Dis 31:1240, 2000.
93. Crum NF, Furtek KJ, Olson PE, et al. A review of hypogonadism and erectile dysfunction among HIV-infected men during the pre- and post-HAART eras: Diagnosis, pathogenesis, and management. AIDS Pat Care STDs 19:655, 2005.
94. Crum-Cianflone N, Bavarao M, Hale B, et al. Prevalence and risk factors of hypogonadism among HIV-infected men. In: 13th Conference on Retroviruses and Opportunistic Infections, Denver, 2006, abstract 775.
95. Klein RS, Lo Y, Santoro N, Dobs RS. Androgen levels in older men who have or who are at risk of acquiring HIV infection. Clin Infect Dis 41:1794, 2005.
96. Grinspoon S. Androgen deficiency and HIV infection [eEditorial commentary]. Clin Infect Dis 41:1804, 2005.
97. Woolf PD, Hamill RW, McDonald JV, et al. Transient hypogonadotrophic hypogonadism caused by critical illness. J Clin Endocrinol Metab 60:444, 1985.
98. Dobs AS, Few WL 3rd, Blackman MR, et al. Serum hormones in men with human immunodeficiency virus-associated wasting. J Clin Endocrinol Metab 81:4108, 1996.
99. Wagner G, Rabkin JG, Rabkin R. Illness stage, concurrent medications, and other correlates of low testosterone in men with HIV illness. J Acquir Immune Defic Syndr Hum Retrovirol 8:204, 1995.
100. Smith CG, Asch RH. Drug abuse and reproduction. Fertil Steril 48:355, 1987.
101. Coodley GO, Loveless MO, Nelson HD, Coodley MK. Endocrine function in the HIV wasting syndrome. J Acquir Immune Defic Syndr 7:45, 1994.
102. Grinspoon S, Corcoran C, Lee K, et al. Loss of lean body and muscle mass correlates with andogren levels in hypogonadal men with acquired immunodeficiency syndrome and wasting. J Clin Endocrinol Metab 81:4051, 1996.
103. Frost RA, Fuhrer J, Steigbigel R, et al. Wasting in the acquired immune deficiency syndrome is associated with multiple defects in the serum insulin-like growth factor system. Clin Endocrinol (Oxf) 44:501, 1996.
104. Zhang Y, Proenca R, Maffei M, et al. Positional cloning of the mouse obese gene and its human homologue. Nature 372:425, 1994.

105. Nakazato M, Murakami N, Date Y, et al. A role for ghrelin in the central regulation of feeding. Nature 409:194, 2001.
106. Eberle AN. Propriomelanocortin and the melanocortin peptides. In: Cone RD (ed). The Melanocortin Receptors. New Jersey: Humana Press; 2000, pp 3–67.
107. Kishi T, Elmquist JK. Body weight is regulated by the brain: a link between feeding and emotion. Molec Psychiatry 10: 132, 2005.
108. Polsky B, Kotler D, Steinhart C. HIV-associated wasting in the HAART era: guidelines for assessment, diagnosis and treatment. AIDS Pat Care STDs 15:411, 2001.
109. Kuczmarski RJ. Bioelectrical impedance analysis measurements as part of a national nutrition survey. Am J Clin Nutr 64(Suppl):453S, 1996.
110. Mulligan K, Tai VW, Schambelan M. Energy expenditure in human immunodeficiency virus infection. N Engl J Med 336:70, 1997.
111. Carr A, Miller J, Law M, Cooper DA. A syndrome of lipoatrophy, lactic acidemia, and liver dysfunction associated with HIV nucleoside analogue therapy: contribution to protease inhibitor-related lipodystrophy syndrome. J Acquir Immune Defic Syndr 14:F25, 2000.
112. Martin ME, Benassayag C, Amiel C, et al. Alterations in the concentrations and binding properties of sex steroid binding protein and corticosteroid-binding globulin in HIV+patients. J Endocrinol Invest 15:597, 1992.
113. Snyder PJ. Hypogonadism in elderly men – what to do until the evidence comes. N Engl J Med 350:440, 2004.
114. Corcoran C, Anderson EJ, Burrows B, et al. Comparison of total body potassium with other techniques for measuring lean body mass in men and women with AIDS wasting. Am J Clin Nutr 72:1053, 2000.
115. Kotler D. Challenges to diagnosis of HIV-associated wasting. J Acquir Immunodefic Syndr 37(Suppl 5):S280, 2004.
116. Moore FD, Boyden CM. Body cell mass and limits of hydration of the fat-free body: their relation to estimated skeletal weight. Ann NY Acad Sci. 110:62, 1963.
117. Kushner RF, Gudivaka R, Schoeller DA. Clinical characteristics influencing bioelectrical impedance analysis measurements. Am J Clin Nutr. 64(Suppl 3):423S, 1996.
118. Kotler DP, Burastero, S, Wang J, Pierson RN Jr. Prediction of body cell mass, fat-free mass, and total body water with bioelectrical impedance analysis: effects of race, sex, and disease. Am J Clin Nutr 64(Suppl 3):489S, 1996.
119. Swanson B, Keithley JK. Bioelectrical impedance analysis (BIA) in HIV infection: principles and clinical applications. J Assoc Nurses AIDS Care 9:49, 1998.
120. Polsky B, Kotler D, Steinhart C. Treatment guidelines for HIV-associated wasting. HIV Clin Trials 5:50, 2004.
121. Ott M, Fischer H, Polat H, et al. Bioelectrical impedance analysis as a predictor of survival in patients with human immunodeficiency virus infection. J Acquir Immunodefic Syndr Hum Retrovirol 9:20, 1995.
122. Schwenk A, Beisenherz A, Romer K, et al. Phase angle from bioelectrical impedance analysis remains an independent predictive marker in HIV-infected patients in the era of highly active antiretroviral treatment. Am J Clin Nutr 72:496, 2000.
123. Ellis KJ. Human body composition: in vivo methods. Physiol Rev 80:649, 2000.
124. Svendsen OL, Haarbo J, Hassager C, Christiansen C. Accuracy of measurements of body composition by dual-energy X-ray absorptiometry in vivo. Am J Clin Nutr. 57:605, 1993.
125. Hansen RD, Raja C, Aslani A, et al. Determination of skeletal muscle and fat-free mass by nuclear and dual-energy X-ray absorptiometry methods in men and women aged 51–84 y (1–3). Am J Clin Nutr.70:228, 1999.
126. Kotler DP, Rosenbaum K, Allison D, et al. Validation of bioimpedance analysis as a measure of change in body cell mass as estimated by whole-body counting of potassium in adults. J Parenter Enteral Nutr 23:345, 1999.
127. Kotler DP, Tierney AR, Ferraro R, et al. Enteral alimentation and repletion of body cell mass in malnourished patients with acquired immunodeficiency syndrome. Am J Clin Nutr 53:149, 1991.
128. Saint-Marc T, Partisani M, Poizot-Martin I, et al. Fat distribution evaluated by computed tomography and metabolic abnormalities in patients undergoing antiretroviral therapy: preliminary results of the LIPOCO study. AIDS 14: 37, 2000.
129. Gellett LR , Haddon L, Maskell GF. CT appearances of HIV-related lipodystrophy syndrome. Br J Radiol 74:382, 2001.
130. Yang Y, Sitoh YY, OoTha N, Paton NI. Facial fat volume in HIV-infected patients with lipoatrophy. Antivir Ther 10:575, 2005. Erratum. Antivir Ther 10:778, 2005.
131. Sattler FR, Jaque SV, Schroeder ET, et al. Effects of pharmacological doses of nandrolone decanoate and progressive resistance training in immunodeficient patients infected with human immunodeficiency virus. J Clin Endocrinol Metab 84:1268, 1999.
132. Edwards RH, Gibson H, Roberts N, et al. Magnetic resonance spectroscopy and imaging of muscle – a physiological approach. Int J Sports Med 13(Suppl 1):S143, 1992.
133. Johansen KL, Schubert T, Doyle J, et al. Muscle atrophy in patients receiving hemodialysis: effects on muscle strength, muscle quality, and physical function. Kidney Int 63: 291, 2003.
134. Kemp GJ, Crowe AV, Anijeet HK, et al. Abnormal mitochondrial function and muscle wasting, but normal contractile efficiency, in haemodialysed patients studied non-invasively in vivo. Nephrol Dial Transplant19:1520, 2004.
135. Shabert JK, Winslow C, Lacey JM, Wilmore DW. Glutamine-antioxidant supplementation increases body cell mass in AIDS patients with weight loss: a randomized double-blind controlled trial. Nutrition 15:860, 1999.
136. Clark RH, Feleke G, Din M, et al. Nutritional treatment for acquired immune deficiency virus-associated wasting using beta-hydroxy beta-methylbutyrate, glutamine, and arginine: a randomized, double-blind, placebo-controlled study. J Parent Enteral Nutr 24:133, 2000.
137. Charlin V, Carrasco F, Sepulveda C, et al. Nutritional supplementation according to energy and protein requirements in malnourished HIV-infected patients. Arch Latinoam Nutr 52:267, 2002.
138. Cappell MS, Godil A. A mutlticenter case-controlled study of percutaneous endoscopic gastrostomy in HIV-seropositive patients. Am J Gastroenterol 88:2059, 1993.
139. Ockenga J, Suttmann U, Selberg O, et al. Percutaneous endoscopic gastrostomy in AIDS and control patients: risk and outcome. Am J Gastroenterol 91:1817, 1996.
140. Kotler DP, Tierney AR, Culpepper-Morgan JA, et al. Effect of home total parenteral nutrition on body composition in patients with acquired immunodeficiency syndrome. J Parenter Enteral Nutr 14:454, 1990.
141. Melchior J, Chastang C, Gelas P, et al. Efficacy of 2-month total parenteral nutrition in AIDS patients: a controlled randomized prospective trial. AIDS 10:379, 1996.
142. Selberg O, Suttmann U, Melzer A, et al. Effect of increased protein intake and nutritional status on whole-body protein metabolism of AIDS patients with weight loss. Metabolism 44:1159, 1995.
143. Coyne-Meyers K, Trombley LE. A review of nutrition in human immunodeficiency virus infection in the era of highly active antiretroviral therapy. Nutr Clin Pract 19:340, 2004.
144. McDermott AY, Shevitz A, Must A, et al. Nutrition treatment for HIV wasting: a prescription for food as Medicine. Nutr Clin Pract 18:86, 2003.

145. Macias, WL, Alaka KJ, Murphy MH, et al. Impact of the nutritional regimen on protein catabolism and nitrogen balance in patients with acute renal failure. J Parenter Enteral Nutr 20:56, 1996.
146. Agin D, Kotler DP, Papandreou D, et al. Effects of whey protein and resistance exercise on body composition and muscle strength in women with HIV infection. Ann NY Acad Sci 904:607, 2000.
147. Lee SJ, McPherron AC. Regulation of myostatin activity and muscle growth. Proc Natl Acad Sci USA 98:9306, 2001.
148. McPherron AC, Lee SJ. Double muscling in cattle due to mutation in the myostatin gene. Proc Natl Acad Sci USA 67:12457, 1997.
149. Whitehouse AS, Smith HJ, Drake JL, Tisdale MJ. Mechanism of attenuation of skeletal muscle protein catabolism in cancer cachexia by eicosapentaenoic acid. Cancer Res 61:3604, 2001.
150. Wigmore SJ, Barber MD, Ross JA. Effect of oral eicosapentaenoic acid on weight in patients with pancreatic cancer. Nutr Cancer 36:177, 2000.
151. Chelebowski RT, Beall G, Lilligton L, et al. Nutritional intervention in the course of HIV disease. Nutrition 11(Suppl 2):250, 1995.
152. Hamburger AW, Parnes H, Gordan GB, et al. Megestrol acetate-induced differentiation of 3T3-L1 adipocytes in vitro. Semin Oncol 15(Suppl 1): 76, 1988.
153. Beck SA, Tisdale MS. Effect of megestrol acetate on weight loss induced by tumor necrosis factor alpha and a cachexia-inducing tumor (MAC16) in NMRI mice. Br J Cancer 62:420, 1990.
154. Yeh SS, Wu SY, Levine DM, et al. The correlation of cytokine levels with body weight after megestrol acetate treatment in geriatric patients. J Gerontol A Biol Sci Med Sci 56:M48, 2001.
155. Lambert CP, Flynn MG, Sullivan DH, Evans WJ. Effects of megestrol acetate on circulating interleukin-15 and interleukin-18 concentrations in healthy elderly men. J Gerontol A Biol Sci Med Sci 59:855, 2004.
156. Oster MH, Enders SR, Samuels SJ, et al. Megestrol acetate in patients with AIDS-related cachexia. Ann Intern Med 121:393, 1994.
157. Von Roenn JH, Armstrong D, Kotler DP, et al. Megestrol acetate in patients with AIDS-related cachexia. Ann Int Med 121:393, 1994.
158. Mulligan K, Zackin R, Von Roenn JH, et al (ATCG313). 2006 (submitted). With J Clin Endocrinal Metab 92:563, 2007. Testosterone replacement during treatment with megestrol acetate does not enhance lean tissue accrual in men with HIV-associated weight loss: a randomized, double-blind, multicenter trial (ACTG313). 2006 (submitted).
159. Timpone JG, Wright DJ, Li N, et al. The safety and pharmacokinetics of single agent and combination therapy with megestrol acetate and dronabinol for the treatment of HIV-wasting syndrome. AIDS Res Hum Retroviruses 13:305, 1997.
160. Summerbell CD, Youle M, McDonald V, et al. Megestrol acetate versus cyproheptadine in the treatment of weight loss associated with HIV infection. Int J STD AIDS 3:278, 1992.
161. Batterham MJ, Garsia R. A comparison of megestrol acetate, nandrolone decanoate and dietary counseling for HIV associated weight loss. Int J Androl 24:232, 2001.
162. Engelson ES, Pi-Sunyer FX, Kotler DP. Effects of megestrol acetate therapy on body composition and circulating testosterone concentrations in patients with AIDS. AIDS 9:1107, 1995.
163. Loprinzi CL, Jensen MD, Jiang NS, Schaid DJ. Effect of megestrol acetate on the human pituitary-adrenal axis. Mayo Clini Proc 67:1160, 1992.
164. Leinung MC, Liporace R, Miller CH. Induction of adrenal suppression by megestrol acetate in patients with AIDS. Ann Intern Med 122:843, 1995.
165. Henry K, Rathgaber S, Sullivan C, McCab K. Diabetes mellitus induced by megestrol acetate in a patient with AIDS and cachexia. Ann Intern Med 116:53, 1992.
166. Mann M, Koller E, Murgo A, et al. Glucocorticoidlike activity of megestrol. A summary of Food and Drug Administration experience and a review of the literature. Arch Intern Med 157:1651, 1997.
167. Berenstein EG, Ortiz Z. Megestrol acetate for the treatment of anorexia-cachexia syndrome. Cochrane Database Syst Rev (2) 4:1–37, 2005.
168. Gorter R, Seefried M, Volberding P. Dronabinol effects on weight in patients with HIV infection. AIDS 6:127, 1992.
169. Struwe M, Kaempfer SH, Geiger CJ, et al. The effect of dronabinol on nutritional status in HIV infection. Ann Pharmacother 27:827, 1993.
170. Beal JE, Olson R, Laubenstein L, et al. Dronabinol as a treatment for anorexia associated with weight loss in patients with AIDS. J Pain Symptom Manage 10:89, 1995.
171. Beal JE, Olsen R, Lefkowitz L, et al. Long-term efficacy and safety of dronabinol for acquired immunodeficiency syndrome-associated anorexia. J Pain Symptom Manage. 14:7, 1997.
172. Food and Drug Administration. Unimed's Marinol (dronabinol) gains indication for anorexia in AIDS patients. FDA Rep 4:14, 1993.
173. Greenberg I, Kuehnle J, Mendelson JH, Bernstein JG. Effects of marijuana use on body weight and caloric intake in humans. J Psychopharm (Berlin) 49:79, 1976.
174. Vinciguerra V, Moore T, Brennan E. Inhalation marijuana as an antiemetic for cancer chemotherapy. NY State J Med 88:525, 1988.
175. Foltin RW, Fishman MW, Pippen PA, Kelly TH. Behavioral effects of cocaine alone and in combination with ethanol or marijuana in humans. Drug Alcohol Depend 32:93, 1993.
176. Haney M. Effect of smoked marijuana in healthy and HIV+ marijuana smokers. J Clin Pharmacol 42(Suppl 11):34S, 2002.
177. Haney M, Rabkin J, Gunderson E, Foltin RW. Dronabinol and marijuana in HIV(+) marijuana smokers: acute effects on caloric intake. Psychopharmacology (Berl) 181:170, 2005.
178. Abrams, DI, Hilton JF, Leiser RJ, et al. Short-term effects of cannabinoids in patients with HIV-1 infection: a randomized, placebo-controlled clinical trial. Ann Intern Med 139:258, 2003.
179. Kosel BW, Aweeka FT, Benowitz NL, et al. The effect of cannabinoids on the pharmacokinetics of indinavir and nelfinavir. AIDS 16:543, 2002.
180. Roth MD, Tashkin DP, Whittaker KM, et al. Tetrahydrocannabinol suppresses immune function and enhances HIV replication in the huPBL-SCID mouse. Life Sci 77:1711, 2005.
181. Coodley GO, Coodley MK. A trial of testosterone therapy for HIV-associated weight loss. AIDS 11: 1347, 1997.
182. Grinspoon S, Corcoran C, Askari H, et al. Effects of androgen administration in men with the AIDS wasting syndrome. A randomized, double-blind, placebo-controlled trial. Ann Intern Med 129:18, 1998.
183. Bhasin S, Storer TW, Javanbakht M, et al. Testosterone replacement and resistance exercise in HIV-infected men with weight loss and low testosterone levels. JAMA 283:763, 2000.
184. Grinspoon S, Corcoran C, Parlman K, et al. Effect of testosterone and progressive resistance training in eugonadal men with AIDS wasting. A randomized, controlled trial. Ann Intern Med 133:348, 2000.
185. Huang JS, Wilkie SJ, Dolan S, et al. Reduced testosterone levels in human immunodeficiency virus-infected women with weight loss and low weight. Clin Infect Dis 36:499, 2003.
186. Miller K, Corcoran C, Armstrong C, et al. Transdermal testosterone administration in women with acquired immunodeficiency syndrome wasting: a pilot study. J Clin Endocrinol Metab 83:2717, 1998.

187. Dolan S, Wilkie S, Aliabadi N, et al. Effects of testosterone administration in human immunodeficiency virus-infected women with low weight: a randomized placebo-controlled study. Arch Intern Med 164:897, 2004.
188. Choi HH, Gray, PB, Storer TW, et al. Effects of testosterone replacement in human immunodeficiency virus-infected women with weight loss. J Clin Endocrinol Metab 90: 1531, 2005.
189. Gold J, High HA, Li Y, et al. Safety and efficacy of nandrolone decanoate for treatment of wasting in patients with HIV infection. AIDS 10:745, 1996.
190. Strawford A, Barbieri T, Neese R, et al. Effects of nandrolone decanoate therapy in borderline hypogonadal men with HIV-associated weight loss. J Acquir Immune Defic Syndr Hum Retrovirol 20:137, 1999.
191. Storer TW, Woodhouse LJ, Sattler F, et al. A randomized, placebo-controlled trial of nandrolone decanoate in human immunodeficiency virus-infected men with mild to moderate weight loss with recombinant human growth hormone as active reference treatment. J Clin Endocrinol Metab 90: 4474, 2005.
192. Cuerda C, Zugasti A, Breton I, et al. Treatment with nandrolone decanoate and megestrol acetate in HIV-infected men. Nutr Clin Pract 20: 93, 2005.
193. Gold J, Batterham MJ, Rekers H, et al. Effects of nandrolone decanoate compared with placebo or testosterone on HIV-associated wasting. HIV Med 7:146, 2006.
194. Berger JR, Pall L, Hall CD, et al. Oxandrolone in AIDS-wasting myopathy. AIDS 10:1657, 1996.
195. Earthman CP, Reid PM, Harper IT, et al. Body cell mass repletion and improved quality of life in HIV-infected individuals receiving oxandrolone. J Parenter Enteral Nutr 26: 357, 2002.
196. Fisher A, Abbaticola M. The Oxandrolone Study Group. The effects of oxandrolone on the body composition in patients with HIV-associated weight loss. In: 5th Conference on Retroviruses and Opportunistic Infections, Chicago, 1998.
197. Poles M, Meller J, Lin A, et al. Oxandrolone as a treatment for HIV-associated weight loss: a one year follow up. In: 37th Interscience Conference on Antimicrobial Agents and Chemotherarapy, Toronto, 1997.
198. Strawford A, Barbieri T, Van Loan M, et al. Resistance exercise and supraphysiologic androgen therapy in eugonadal men with HIV-related weight loss. JAMA 281:1282, 1999.
199. Mwamburi DM, Gerrior J, Wilson IB, et al. Comparing megestrol acetate therapy with oxandrolone therapy for HIV-related weight loss: Similar results in 2 months. Clin Infect Dis 38:895, 2004.
200. Hengge UR, Baumann M, Maleba R, et al. Oxymetholone promotes weight gain in patients with advanced human immunodeficiency virus (HIV-1) infection. Br J Nutr 75:129, 1996.
201. Hengge UR, Stocks K, Wiehler H, et al. Double-blind, randomized, placebo-controlled phase III trial of oxymetholone for the treatment of HIV wasting. AIDS 17:699, 2003.
202. Johns K, Beddall MJ, Corrin RC. Anabolic steroids for the treatment of weight loss in HIV-infected individuals. Cochrane Database Syst Rev 4:1, 2005.
203. Orr R, Fiatarone Singh MF. The anabolic androgenic steroid oxandrolone in the treatment of wasting and catabolic disorders: review of efficacy and safety. Drugs 64:725, 2004.
204. Krentz AJ, Koster FT, Crist DM, et al. Anthropometric, metabolic, and immunological effects of recombinant human growth hormone in AIDS and AIDS-related complex. J Acquir Immune Defic Syndr 6:245, 1993.
205. Cominelli S, Raguso CA, Karsegard L, et al. Weight-losing HIV-infected patients on recombinant human growth hormone for 12 wk: a national study. Nutrition 18:583, 2002.
206. Jager H, Knechten H, Moll A, et al. Treatment of HIV-associated wasting with recombinant human growth hormone: monitoring of body composition changes by bioelectrical impedance analysis (BIA). Eur J Med Res 7:103, 2002.
207. Klauke S, Fisher H, Rieger A, et al. Use of bioelectrical impedance analysis to determine body composition changes in HIV-associated wasting. Int J STD AIDS 16:307, 2005.
208. Paton NI, Newton PJ, Sharpstone DR, et al. Short-term growth hormone administration at the time of opportunistic infections in HIV-positive patients. AIDS 13:1195, 1999.
209. Evans WJ, Kotler DP, Staszewski S, et al. Effect of recombinant human growth hormone on exercise capacity in patients with HIV-associated wasting on HAART. AIDS Read 15: 301, 2005.
210. Schambelan M, Mulligan K, Grunfeld C, et al. Recombinant human growth hormone in patients with HIV-associated wasting: a randomized, placebo-controlled trial. Ann Intern Med 125:873, 1996.
211. Moyle GJ, Daar ES, Gertner JM, et al. Growth hormone improves lean body mass, physical performance, and quality of life in subjects with HIV-associated weight loss or wasting on highly active antiretroviral therapy. J Acquir Immune Defic Syndr 35:367, 2004.
212. Waters D, Danska J, Hardy K, et al. Recombinant human growth hormone, insulin-like growth factor I, and combination therapy in AIDS-associated wasting: a randomized double-blind, placebo-controlled trial. Ann Intern Med 125: 865, 1996.
213. Lee PD, Pivarnik JM, Bukar JG. A randomized, placebo-controlled trial of combined insulin-like growth factor I and low dose growth hormone therapy for wasting associated with human immunodeficiency virus infection. J Clin Endocrinol Metab. 81:2968, 1996. Erratum. J Clin Endocrinol Metab 81:3696, 1996.
214. Engelson ES, Glesby MJ, Mendez D. Effect of recombinant human growth hormone in the treatment of visceral fat accumulation in HIV infection. J Acquir Immune Defic Syndr 30:379, 2002.
215. Marcus R, Butterfield G, Holloway L. Effect of short term administration of recombinant human growth hormone to elderly people. J Clin Endocrinol Metab 70:519, 1990.
216. Johannsson G, Marin P, Lonn L, et al. Growth hormone treatment of abdominally obese men reduces abdominal fat mass, improves glucose and lipoprotein metabolism, and reduces diastolic blood pressure. J Clin Endocrinol Metab 82: 727, 1997.
217. Blackman MR, Sorkin JD, Munzer T, et al. Growth hormone and sex steroid administration in healthy aged women and men: a randomized controlled trial. JAMA 288:2282, 2002.
218. Rietschel PR, Hadigan C, Corcoran C, et al. Assessment of growth hormone dynamics in human immunodeficiency virus-related lipodystrophy. J Clin Endocrinol Metab 86: 504, 2001.
219. Heijligenberg R, Sauerwein HP, Brabant G, et al. Circadian growth hormone secretion in asymptomatic human immune deficiency virus infection and acquired immunodeficiency syndrome. J Clin Endocrinol Metab 81:4028, 1996.
220. Koutkia P, Canavan B, Breu J, et al. Growth hormone-releasing hormone in HIV-infected men with lipodystrophy: a randomized controlled trial. JAMA 292:210, 2004.
221. Falutz J, Allas S, Kotler D, et al. A placebo-controlled, dose-ranging study of growth hormone releasing factor in HIV-infected patients with abdominal fat accumulation. AIDS 19:1279, 2005.
222. Dezube PJ, Pardee AB, Chapman B, et al. Pentoxifylline decreases tumor necrosis factor expression and serum triglycerides in people with AIDS. NIAID AIDS Clinical Trials Group. J Acquir Immune Defic Syndr 6:787, 1993.
223. Endres S, Ghorbani R, Kelley VE, et al. The effect of dietary supplementation with n-3 polyunsaturated fatty acids on the

synthesis of interleukin-1 and tumor necrosis factor by mononuclear cells. N Engl J Med 320:265, 1989.
224. Moreira AL, Sampaio EP, Zmuidzinas A, et al. Thalidomide exerts its inhibitory action on tumor necrosis factor alpha by enhancing mRNA degradation. J Exp Med. 177:1675, 1993.
225. Landman D, Sarai A, Sathe SS. Use of pentoxifylline therapy for patients with AIDS-related wasting: a pilot study. Clin Infect Dis 18:97, 1994.
226. Goldberg RM, Loprinzi CL, Mailliard JA, et al. Pentoxifylline for treatment of cancer anorexia and cachexia: a randomized, double-blind, placebo-controlled trial. J Clin Oncol 13: 2856, 1995.
227. Hellerstein MK, Wu K, McGrath M, et al. Effects of dietary n-3 fatty acid supplementation in men with weight loss associated with the acquired immunodeficiency syndrome: relation to indices of cytokine production. J Acquir Immune Defic Syndr Hum Retrovirol 11:258, 1996.
228. Klausner JD, Makonkawkeyoon S, Akarasewi P, et al. The effect of thalidomide in the pathogenesis of human immunodeficiency virus type 1 and M. tuberculosis infection. J Acquir Immune Defic Syndr Hum Retrovirol 11:247, 1996.
229. Reyes-Teran G, Sierra-Madero JG, Martinez del Cerro V, et al. Effects of thalidomide on HIV-associated wasting syndrome: a randomized, double-blind placebo-controlled clinical trial. AIDS 10:1501, 1996.
230. Kaplan G, Thomas S, Fierer DS, et al. Thalidomide for the treatment of AIDS-associated wasting. AIDS Res Hum Retroviruses 16:1345, 2000.
231. Matthews SJ, McCoy C. Thalidomide: a review of approved and investigational uses. Clin Ther 25:342, 2003.
232. Wilson IB, Cleary PD. Clinical predictors of declines in physical functioning in persons with AIDS: results of a longitudinal study. J Acquir Immune Defic Syndr Hum Retrovirol 16: 343, 1997.
233. Corcoran C, Grinspoon S. Treatments for wasting in patients with the acquired immunodeficiency syndrome. N Engl J Med 340:1740, 1999.
234. Lambert CP, Evans WJ. Adaptations to aerobic and resistance exercise in the elderly. Rev Endocr Metab Disord 6:137, 2005.
235. Goldspink G. Gene expression in muscle in response to exercise. J Muscle Res Cell Motil 24:121, 2003.
236. Elliot DL, Goldberg L, Coodley GO. Physical conditioning among HIV-positive men. Med Sci Sports Exerc 24:838, 1992.
237. Spence DW, Galantino ML, Mosberg KA, Zimmerman SO. Progressive resistance exercise: effect on muscle function and anthropometry of a select AIDS population. Arch Phys Med Rehabil 71:644, 1990.
238. Roubenoff R, McDermott A, Weiss L, et al. Short-term progressive resistance training increases strength and lean body mass in adults infected with human immunodeficiency virus. AIDS 13:231, 1999.
239. Roubenoff R, Wilson IB. Effect of resistance training on self-reported physical functioning in HIV infection. Med Sci Sports Exerc. 33:1811, 2001.
240. Yarasheski KE, Tebas P, Stanerson B, et al. Resistance exercise training reduces hypertriglyceridemia in HIV-infected men treated with antiretroviral therapy. J Appl Physiol 90: 133, 2001.
241. Macarthur RD, Levine SD, Birk TJ. Supervised exercise training improves cardiopulmonary fitness in HIV-infected persons. Med Sci Sports Exerc 25:684, 1993.
242. Smith BA, Neidig JL, Nickel JT, et al. Aerobic exercise: effects on parameters related to fatigue, dyspnea, weight and body composition in HIV-infected adults. AIDS 15:693, 2001.
243. Dobs AS, Confrancesco J, Nolten WE, et al. The use of a transscrotal testosterone delivery system in the treatment of patients with weight loss related to human immunodeficiency virus infection. Am J Med 107:126, 1999.
244. Mulligan K, Zackin R, Clark RA, et al. Effect of nandrolone decanote therapy on weight and lean body mass in HIV-infected women with weight loss: a randomized, double-bind, placebo-controlled, multicenter trial. Arch Intern Med 165:578, 2005.

Chapter 62

Neurological Disease

Serena S. Spudich, MD, Richard W. Price, MD

Human immunodeficiency virus (HIV)-1 infection, and particularly its late stage of severe immunodeficiency (acquired immunodeficiency syndrome, AIDS), renders the nervous system susceptible to an array of neurological disorders. In the aggregate, these can afflict virtually every component of the nervous system, manifest therefore in a variety of clinical syndromes, and contribute importantly to both morbidity and mortality. This chapter aims to provide a general view of the approach to diagnosis of these disorders. Because several of the specific neurological diseases are discussed in detail in other chapters of this volume, individual disorders are considered here chiefly in relation to issues of differential diagnosis, with greater detail confined to some of the disorders not considered elsewhere. Several recent and older reviews also discuss the individual neurological complications in more detail and provide useful, more extensive reference sections.[1–8] Discussion of specific therapies is also limited in this chapter to reduce redundancy.

The frequency of neurological complications of HIV-1 infection has changed considerably in the past 10 years in the developed world, where there has been a marked reduction related to the widespread use of highly active antiretroviral therapy (HAART) and other measures.[9–17] Despite this overall decrease in incidence, the spectrum of disorders afflicting those who progress to severe immunosuppression is similar to that earlier in the epidemic, with some exceptions. This chapter maintains its principal focus on these "late-stage" HIV-1-infected patients. However, as clinics follow increasing numbers of HIV-1-infected patients who do not progress to this stage of susceptibility, the frequency of encountering more "ordinary" neurological diseases similar to those affecting HIV-1-uninfected peers will rise. For these patients, the approach to neurological diagnosis will follow that of the general neurology text, rather than the algorithms presented here. Additionally, these algorithms should be followed with the usual caution that diagnosis must be carefully individualized not only with respect to variability of presenting symptoms and signs, but also recognizing that simple formulas can hardly be applicable to a patient who may present with an unusual manifestation of a common disease or a truly rare condition. Also, these diagrams necessarily present diagnostic pathways as if they are linear, when, in fact, parallel processing of several avenues is a more common and sensible approach.

GENERAL APPROACH TO DIAGNOSIS

Despite the variety of neurological diseases in those with HIV-1 infection, a diagnostic approach is based upon three principal variables; (1) the neuroanatomical localization of the lesion(s), (2) the temporal course of onset and evolution, and (3) the constellation of background risks affords a firm starting point and logical evaluation sequence that usually leads to timely and precise diagnosis. The first of these variables, i.e., neuroanatomical localization, also provides the organizing principal of this chapter with individual conditions considered within anatomical categories. The value of this approach rests on two central considerations: first, different disease processes, including opportunistic infections, have predilections for damaging particular structures within the nervous system – the principal of selective vulnerabilities – in predictable patterns and thus cause anatomically defined syndromes; second, anatomic localization guides further diagnostic evaluation, most importantly neuroimaging in the case of the central nervous system (CNS) and electrophysiological testing in diseases of the peripheral nervous system (PNS).

Figure 62-1 diagrams the first steps in this anatomic approach. The clinical history usually provides a first approximation of the neuroanatomical localization (e.g., language difficulty related to dysfunction of the dominant cerebral hemisphere or numbness of both feet suggesting polyneuropathy) and the formulation of an initial neuroanatomic hypothesis. This is then tested by the neurological examination. The combination of these two bedside components usually allows not only a tentative localization but also initial consideration of the most likely diagnoses,

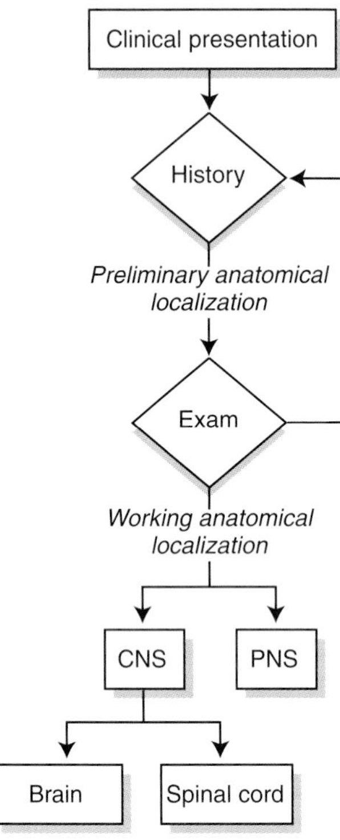

Figure 62-1 ■ Initial approach to neurological diagnosis in HIV-1 infection. PNS, peripheral nervous system.

separating CNS and PNS diseases (and those of muscle, which we have grouped with the PNS). CNS disease can be further subdivided into those affecting the brain or spinal cord.

The second diagnostic element – the time course of the evolution of symptoms and signs – is also often critical to diagnosis and management. The utility of this variable has a pathobiological basis, since individual disease processes evolve over characteristic time frames, as summarized in Table 62-1. Hence, the temporal profile narrows the different possibilities. It also importantly guides the pace of diagnostic evaluation and therapeutic intervention. For example, 5 months of gradually worsening gait in a patient who walks comfortably but stiffly (as seen in the vacuolar myelopathy variant of the AIDS dementia complex) may warrant either no or only elective spinal magnetic resonance imaging (MRI). By contrast, 3 days of back pain and 4h of leg weakness, as might accompany spinal epidural abscess, demands emergency imaging. As outlined below, the three most common causes of focal brain lesions tend to evolve at different, although overlapping, rates. This relates to the time scales of the replication of the invading organisms or of tumor cells in concert with the tempo and strength of immune responses, and can provide an initial clue to which is most likely. Exceptions to the subacute progression of most AIDS-related CNS diseases can relate to secondary developments, such as seizures, that can dramatically punctuate the course of either macroscopic or microscopic brain diseases. Hemorrhage into focal brain lesions, although far less common, can also accelerate presentation. For these reasons it is always important to define the time course of the illness and be certain that it is explained by the diagnoses being considered.

The patient's risk background is the third important variable in determining probability of differential diagnosis. The most important factor in this category is the stage of systemic HIV-1 infection and resultant immunosuppression. Severe compromise of cell-mediated immunity so importantly increases vulnerability to a particular group of disorders that they come to dominate the course of late infection and, hence, diagnostic probabilities. If patients presenting with subacute onset of focal cerebral dysfunction have less than 50 CD4+ T lymphocytes per mm^3 in blood, then more than the great majority will have one of three conditions: CNS toxoplasmosis, primary CNS lymphoma (PCNSL), or progressive multifocal leukoencephalopathy (PML). Earlier stages of HIV-1 infection may result in higher risk of certain autoimmune disorders, including demyelinating peripheral neuropathies.

Other background factors (including the risks that led to acquisition of HIV-1 infection) also confer risks of specific neurological conditions that may not directly relate to HIV. For example, an active intravenous drug abuser may develop pyogenic infections such as epidural abscess or bacterial endocarditis with septic cerebral emboli, or a sexually active individual in a high-risk group may be prone to acquiring syphilis and its potential neurological complications. For this reason, it is important to define both the stage of HIV-1 infection and other background risks in each patient presenting with neurological disease.

Another important contributor to "risk background" in terms of diagnosis of neurological disease in an HIV-infected patient is antiretroviral treatment status. The importance of "non-HIV-1-related" neurological diseases in treated patients with preserved immunity was emphasized earlier. Another potential implication of the larger number of treated patients with preserved immunity is that clinicians may encounter major opportunistic infections or the AIDS dementia complex at CD4+ T-lymphocyte counts higher than those reported for most such patients in earlier eras. In part this simply relates to development of this expanding population – despite continued low probabilities, the susceptible group is larger. Some differences may also relate to recovery of immune function after antiretroviral therapy. Restoration of CD4+ T-lymphocyte counts may not be followed by reconstitution of completely protective immunity against opportunistic diseases. On the other hand, effective restoration of immunity may impact on disease phenotype if vigorous host responses cause immunopathological injury. Apparent development or progression of infectious or autoimmune disorders after initiation of HAART may be due to aberrant immune responses in the setting of rapid changes in the quantity of and repertoire of circulating T cells. Such conditions seem to differ in natural history from their well-recognized counterparts occurring at extreme immunosuppression, and thus have been termed "immune reconstitution" or "restoration" diseases (IRD), or the "immune restoration inflammatory syndrome".[18–21] These disorders have proved difficult to systematically characterize, in part due to heterogeneity of clinical setting and presentation. Furthermore, based on clinical presentation alone, it may be difficult to define whether a condition relates truly to

Table 62-1

Typical Features of Major CNS Processes in AIDS

	Clinical Features				Neuroimaging Features	
Lesion Type	**Temporal Progression**	**Level of Alertness**	**Fever**	**Number of Lesions**	**Characteristic Imaging Appearance**	**Lesion Location**
Cerebral toxoplasmosis	Days	Reduced	Possible	Multiple	Mass effect, edema, ring-enhancing target sign	Basal ganglia, cortex eccentric
Primary CNS lymphoma	Days/weeks	Variable	Absent	One/few	Mass effect, irregular, ring- or wholly-enhancing	Periventricular, subependymal
Progressive multifocal leukoencephalopathy	Weeks	Preserved	Absent	One/multiple	No mass effect, bright on T_2 and dark on T_1, no enhancement	White matter, involving U-fibers, subcortical
AIDS dementia complex	Weeks/months	Preserved	Absent	None/diffuse	Brain atrophy, diffuse bright patches on T_2, no mass effect, no enhancement	Deep white matter, involving U-fibers, subcortical
CMV encephalitis	Days/weeks	Reduced	Common	Few/diffuse	T_2 bright signal or enhancement	Ventricular ependyma
Cryptococcal meningitis	Days/weeks	Variable	Possible	None/diffuse	Dilated perivascular spaces, enlarged ventricles	Basal ganglia

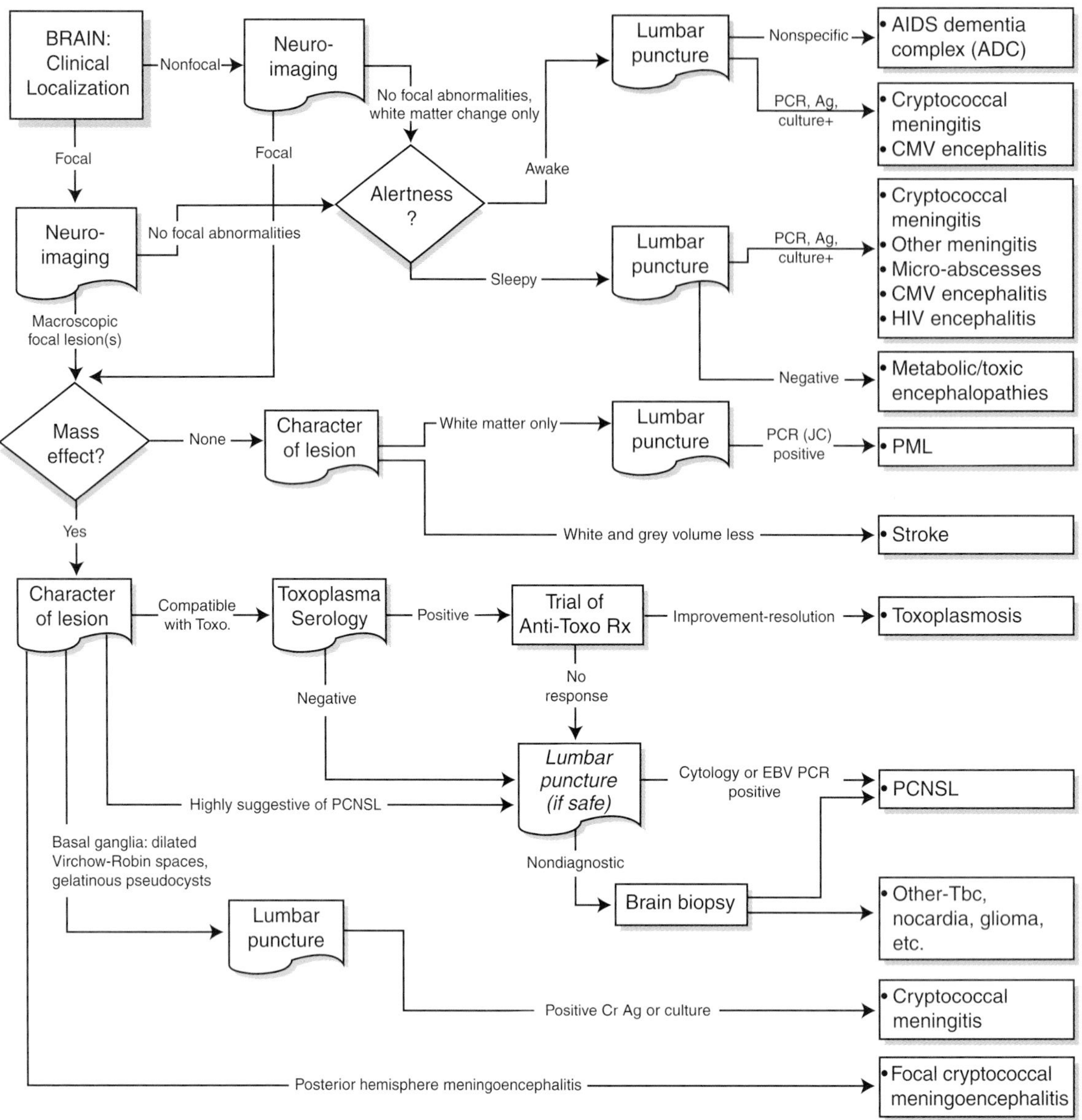

Figure 62-2 ■ Diagnostic approach to brain diseases in late HIV-1 infection. Ag, antigen; CMV, cytomegalovirus; Cr Ag, cryptococcal antigen; HSV, herpes simplex virus; PCR, polymerase chain reaction; Tbc, tuberculosis.

an unusual inflammatory response or simply to occurrence of a typical disease that happens to manifest soon after initiation of therapy. Such syndromes generally present within the first 3 months of HAART, mainly occur when HAART is initiated at CD4+ T-lymphocyte counts below 100 cells/μL, and have clinical features distinct from the usual natural history of opportunistic infections or autoimmune diseases in AIDS. In these conditions, addition of antiinflammatory agents such as corticosteroids may be of therapeutic benefit, though this has not yet been rigorously examined and there are no proven guidelines for management. Altered presentation of disorders involving the nervous system in the setting of immune reconstitution have recently been reported, including cryptococcal meningitis,[22–24] PML,[25–27] mycobacterial infections,[28–31] autoimmune demyelinating neuropathies,[32,33] polymyositis,[34] and herpes zoster,[35] among others. Although some of these disorders warrant further characterization prior to considering them entities distinct from their typical presentations, IRD in the setting of both cryptococcal meningitis and PML has been consistently observed and likely represent new manifestations of familiar disorders in the context of partially "restored" immunity, and will be discussed below. It is likely that the scope of these immune reconstitution disorders observed in the nervous system will continue to expand as more patients with advanced immunosuppression are treated with HAART.

NONFOCAL BRAIN DISEASES

Figure 62-2 depicts a general algorithm for diagnosis of brain disease in AIDS. The upper third of this figure concentrates

AIDS Dementia Complex Staging

Table 62-2

ADC Stage	Characteristics
Stage 0 (normal)	Normal mental and motor function
Stage 0.5 (equivocal/subclinical)	Either minimal or equivocal symptoms of cognitive or motor dysfunction characteristic of AIDS dementia complex, or mild signs (snout response, slowed extremity movements) but without impairment of work or capacity to perform activities of daily living (ADL). Gait and strength are normal
Stage 1 (mild)	Unequivocal evidence (symptoms, signs, neuropsychological test performance) of functional intellectual or motor impairment characteristic of ADC but able to perform all but the more demanding aspects of work or ADL. Can walk without assistance
Stage 2 (moderate)	Cannot work or maintain the more demanding aspects of daily life but able to perform basic activities of self-care. Ambulatory but may require a single prop
Stage 3 (severe)	Major intellectual incapacity (cannot follow news or personal events, cannot sustain complex conversation, considerable slowing of all output) or motor disability (cannot walk unassisted, requiring walker or personal support, usually with slowing and clumsiness of arms as well)
Stage 4 (end stage)	Nearly vegetative. Intellectual and social comprehension and responses are at a rudimentary level. Nearly or absolutely mute. Paraparetic or paraplegic with double incontinence

Adapted from Price R, Brew B: The AIDS dementia complex. J Infect Dis 158:1079, 1988; and Sidtis JJ, Price RW: Early HIV-1 infection and the AIDS dementia complex. Neurology 40:323, 1990.

upon disorders that characteristically lack focal features. These conditions present with "diffuse" alterations in cognition and symmetrical motor dysfunction that is not readily explained by one or a few macroscopic focal brain lesions. There is no aphasia, apraxia, or agnosia to provide discrete cortical localization, nor hemiparesis or dysmetria to point to a lesion in a cerebral or cerebellar hemisphere. Sensory abnormalities are usually absent or reflect coincident neuropathy. These nonfocal disorders can be further segregated clinically into those in which cognition is altered in the face of preserved alertness and those in which these two elements are altered in parallel. The most important disorder in the first category is the AIDS dementia complex (ADC).

AIDS Dementia Complex

ADC is a syndrome of cognitive and motor dysfunction that has also been designated by several other synonymous terms, including HIV-associated cognitive-motor complex and the shorter terms AIDS dementia or HIV dementia.[36,37] Its pediatric counterpart, which is not discussed in detail here, is most often called HIV encephalopathy.[38,39] We prefer the term AIDS dementia complex for the adult form because it is simple and emphasizes that cognitive impairment is the predominating difficulty, yet also implies that this is not the only clinical manifestation and is usually accompanied by abnormal motor function and, at times, characteristic behavior abnormalities as well.[40,41]

ADC is believed to be caused by HIV-1 itself, rather than by another opportunistic organism, although the detailed mechanistic links between the virus and brain injury remain speculative.[8,42–48] ADC is characteristically a late complication of HIV-1 infection and, particularly in its more severe form, occurs in the same context as the major clinical AIDS-defining opportunistic infections. Table 62-2 outlines the ADC staging scheme that is used to describe patients' disease severity based on their functional capacity in cognitive and motor spheres.[49,50]

On the basis of its central clinical features that include impairment of attention and concentration, slowing of mental speed and agility, concomitant slowing of motor speed and apathetic behavior, ADC has been classified among the subcortical dementias.[51–54] More detailed description of its clinical features is available elsewhere.[7,41,55,56] Although Figure 62-2 depicts the process of diagnosis as largely exclusionary (nonfocal neuroimaging and nonspecific lumbar puncture findings), the diagnosis should be pursued principally on the basis of its positive features, which include characteristic mental and motor findings. Additionally, although the character of the clinical abnormalities is consistent through the spectrum of its severity, it is useful to segregate the approach to diagnosis in those with milder (stage 0.5 or 1) ADC from those with more severe (stages 2–4) affliction. The major differential diagnoses often diverge in these two settings.

Mild ADC

Patients with mild ADC usually complain of difficulties with concentration and attention. They lose their train of thought in conversation or need to reread paragraphs of

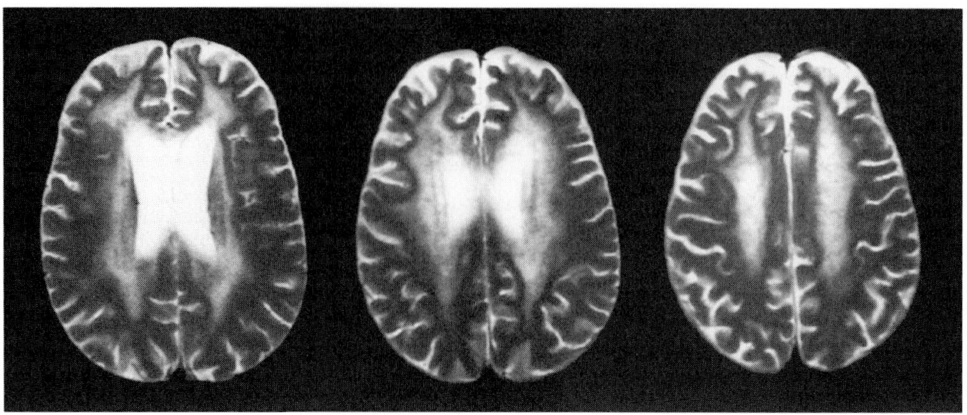

Figure 62-3 ■ MRI images of patient with stage 2 ADC. The T2-weighted images show brain atrophy and striking increase in signal (white) in the white matter that is most prominent centrally, less so peripherally and spares the U fibers posteriorly. The hyperintensity likely represents breakdown of the blood–brain barrier and increased water content.

a book. Complex tasks previously performed "reflexively" now are more labored and take longer. Patients need to keep lists of formerly routine daily chores. These difficulties become intrusive and require compensatory strategies or changes in activities. These complaints can be similar to those of depression or of hypochondriasis. Diagnosis in these milder patients can, as a result, center on the question of whether or not there is indeed "organic" brain disease, rather than pursuit of the other nonfocal diagnoses shown in Figure 62-2. The presence of motor symptoms or signs may help support the diagnosis of ADC. These patients often have slowing of rapid finger movements (such as repeated opposing of the thumb and index tips), toe tapping and walking, along with hyperactive deep tendon reflexes and development of "release" reflexes, most notably a snout response. If there is doubt regarding either the presence or pattern of cognitive changes, formal evaluation by a neuropsychologist familiar with this condition may be helpful.[57]

Severe ADC

In patients with more severe ADC (stage 2 or above), neurological abnormalities are more distinct. These patients cannot live comfortably without some help from others. They are usually clearly mentally slow and perform tasks requiring concentration (reversing a five-letter word or subtracting serial 7s) either slowly or inaccurately. Motor findings are also more evident and may include more marked slowing or unsteadiness of gait. Abnormal reflexes are more prevalent. When alertness is completely preserved, the diagnosis is usually evident unless there is concern that cognitive difficulty relates to earlier, static brain disease. However, manifestations of some other conditions may overlap, and for this reason neuroimaging is justified to screen for other disorders that may present similarly. For example, PCNSL that involves the frontal white matter bilaterally may cause cognitive slowing without notable focal or lateralizing signs. Cytomegalovirus (CMV) encephalitis can also be confused with ADC as described below.

Laboratory Diagnosis

ADC is fundamentally a clinical diagnosis that relies on recognition of the characteristic profile of cognitive and motor impairment in the absence of confounding causes. Laboratory tests are performed chiefly to rule out other conditions, though certain findings may provide evidence that suggests this diagnosis. Most important in this regard are neuroimaging and cerebrospinal fluid (CSF) examination.

While neuroimaging is usually performed to detect evidence of alternative conditions, it may sometimes be helpful in supporting an ADC diagnosis. Most ADC patients have some degree of atrophy, detected by either computed tomography (CT) or MRI.[58,59] Unfortunately, this is not diagnostically entirely specific or sensitive, since it is also found in those without clinical ADC and may be common in certain risk groups more broadly, such as substance abusers. Nonetheless, those with severe ADC usually have marked brain atrophy, with the exception of those who present with a brief, subacute course in whom atrophy may be inconspicuous or absent. Somewhat more specific are changes in white matter with increased water content noted on T_2-weighted, proton density, or FLAIR sequences.[60] Most common are regional changes in white matter signal, ranging from diffuse to more circumscribed "fluffy" patches of increased signal (see Fig. 62-3). If present, these tend to be more common in more severe disease, and thus are less useful in mild ADC. More recently, magnetic resonance spectroscopy (MRS) has shown abnormalities in ADC that may eventually prove useful in diagnosis and characterization of ADC.[61–64] This method has not yet been tested for individual case diagnosis, but rather for clinical trials to characterize patient groups so that sensitivity and specificity for clinical application awaits further study.

CSF examination has much the same purpose as neuroimaging, primarily to screen for other disorders including cryptococcal and other meningitides, neurosyphilis, or viral encephalitis using culture, tests for antigens, and polymerase chain reaction (PCR) amplifications. It would be helpful if CSF could be used to confirm an ADC diagnosis. However, while CSF is very often abnormal, the abnormalities are not diagnostically specific. Among routine assessments, CSF protein and cell counts are frequently elevated in ADC, but these abnormalities are common in early asymptomatic systemic HIV-1 infection, especially in patients not on HAART, and may also be found in subjects with alternate diagnoses such as neurosyphilis. A number of markers of macrophage activation have been observed to be elevated in ADC, but also are not diagnostically specific. Early studies showed elevations in neopterin, beta-2-microglobulin, and quinolinic acid[65–67] and more recent reports show elevations of monocyte chemoattractant protein-1 (MCP-1), other cytokines, and related inflammatory markers,[68,69] but these factors are also elevated in other conditions, and their practical application to clinical diagnosis has not been carefully evaluated. In certain situations they might be useful (e.g., in diagnosis of stage 1 ADC or in distinguishing active ADC from residual injury or other static encephalopathy), but diagnostic guidelines using these tests have not been defined.

Extensive evidence supports the notion that CSF HIV-1 is compartmentalized from that in plasma, with distinct resistance genotypes and phenotypes, chemokine receptor utilization of viral quasispecies, and envelope sequences as detected by viral sequencing and cloning or heteroduplex tracking assays in the two fluids.[70–72] The concept that CSF compartmentalization might reflect CNS-specific HIV-1 infection, combined with availability of quantitative HIV-1 nucleic acid amplification in CSF, has raised the question of whether viral load measurement in this compartment might help in diagnosis.[73] Though there may be a correlation of CSF HIV-1 concentration with ADC severity and HIV encephalitis pathologically,[74] this correlation applies only to patients with more advanced immunosuppression.[75–77] In those with higher CD4+ T-lymphocyte counts, CSF viral loads may also be elevated without neurological abnormalities; additionally, CNS opportunistic infections may be accompanied by increased CSF viral load.[73] Thus the CSF viral load cannot be used by itself for ADC diagnosis. There may be situations where CSF HIV-1 measurement may be useful, either for diagnosis (e.g., in the face of low CD4+ T-lymphocyte count or when the CSF viral load is higher than that of plasma) or for tracking responses to therapy. However, clear guidelines are not yet defined, and CSF viral load is not a routine part of clinical practice.

Treatment

It is clear from epidemiological studies that antiretroviral therapy can prevent ADC, and experience from limited coordinated trials and individual cases indicates that treatment can arrest or reverse the condition.[7,10,15,78–88] Early studies demonstrated that zidovudine monotherapy had both therapeutic and preventative effects on ADC. Because formal clinical trials of ADC are now very difficult to implement, reports describing responses to contemporary combination antiretroviral therapy are largely anecdotal. Nonetheless, if one (1) uses the early experience with monotherapy as proof of concept, (2) extends the advantage of multidrug therapy on systemic disease to treating the CNS, (3) extrapolates from the therapeutic reduction of CSF viral load to effects on brain parenchymal infection, and (4) calls upon anecdotal (including our own personal) experience, there is a reasonable basis for considering HAART to be an effective avenue of treatment for ADC. More at issue now are refinements of therapy to better target the CNS, particularly the question of whether it is necessary that each of the components of a multidrug regimen penetrate well into the brain. Whereas several of the current nucleoside (including zidovudine, abacavir, and stavudine) and non-nucleoside (nevirapine) reverse transcriptase inhibitors penetrate relatively well (though with extracellular fluid exposures that may still be only about one-third that of plasma), most of the protease inhibitors do not.[89–102] Indinavir and lopinavir are the most notable exceptions, and, in general, penetration of this class is increased by ritonavir boosting to the extent that it increases plasma concentrations. On the other hand, judging from CSF HIV responses, patients seem to respond to regimens with one or more poorly penetrating drugs, and the need for such drug penetration may vary in different types of patients. Also, drug levels in CSF do not necessarily indicate exposure and intracellular effects on the critical target cells, including particularly brain macrophages. As a result, in the absence of clearer guidelines, we recommend that drugs for symptomatic ADC patients be selected with the following general priorities: (1) assure susceptibility of virus isolates to the individual drugs just as in treatment of systemic infection, including susceptibility to CSF isolates in cases with prior drug exposure and suspected "compartmentalized" infection; (2) use an aggressive regimen, usually with four or more drugs, including nucleosides; and, finally (3) where possible, choose at least two drugs with more favorable CNS penetration including those listed above.

Additional approaches to treat ADC can be grouped under the category of adjuvant treatments. These range from various forms of symptom management (e.g., cautious neuroleptics or mood stabilizers to relieve behavioral symptoms and signs) to efforts at attenuating the disease process by interfering with various endogenous neurotoxic pathways. The latter has led to clinical trials of candidate neuroprotective agents without firm evidence of efficacy.[103–105]

Other Nonfocal Brain Disorders

Most nonfocal brain disorders complicating HIV-1 infection other than ADC are accompanied by concomitant depression of both alertness and cognition. Overall, the most common in this category are the toxic encephalopathies related to sedative, narcotic, and other CNS-acting medications. Metabolic encephalopathies are also common and relate to failure of systemic organs – hypoxia, renal or hepatic failure, and the like.

Among opportunistic infections, the most common "nonfocal" infection causing general confusion with a picture similar to metabolic encephalopathy is CMV encephalitis.[106–113] Like other organ afflictions with this herpesvirus, CMV encephalitis is becoming rare in patients taking HAART. Additionally, its clinical spectrum has not been sharply defined. Autopsy studies earlier in the AIDS epidemic showed histological evidence of CMV infection in about one quarter of brains.[114–117] However, the extent to which these lesions, some quite mild, contributed to clinical abnormalities was uncertain in many cases. On the other hand, it is also clear that some patients develop severe CMV encephalitis with distinct morbidity and mortality. Thus the key issue was not whether CMV caused symptomatic brain infection in AIDS, but rather what was the importance of the milder end of the spectrum. Also, CMV infection can coincide with ADC, and it may be difficult to discern which process is responsible for particular clinical manifestations. Clinical-pathologic studies have pointed out certain features that associate with CMV encephalitis. These include subacute onset, frank confusion or delirium, hyponatremia, and, more specifically, periventricular abnormalities on MRI (increased water signal or enhancement with contrast). Some patients have distinct focal features, including nystagmus, ataxia, and ocular motor palsies, indicating brain stem involvement; seizures are likely more common than with ADC. Unusual cases of CMV have more prominent focal features and may even have focal lesions detected on neuroimaging that exceed 1 cm in diameter.[118] CSF may vary from bland fluid to pleocytosis with polymorphonuclear or mononuclear predominance and high protein. Diagnosis has been revolutionized by nucleic acid amplification techniques, and detection of CMV DNA provides a sensitive test.[106,119–123] Most, but not all, patients have CMV disease in other organs, which often helps to support the diagnosis. Therapy is with one or more of the anti-CMV drugs discussed elsewhere in this volume.

Other diseases that cause widespread microscopic pathology may present a similar picture, including the encephalitic form of cerebral toxoplasmosis that presents without distinct focality and may be accompanied by a nearly normal CT scan.[124,125] This is usually a fulminant infection associated with multiple microabscesses, with little inflammatory or tissue reaction. In cases of rapid-onset encephalitis of this type, empiric antitoxoplasma therapy may be justified while diagnostic evaluation is underway. Diffuse CNS dysfunction may also be caused by disseminated intravascular coagulation in the septic or otherwise gravely ill patient. Herpes simplex encephalitis in the AIDS patient may also present as a diffuse encephalopathy and differ from the characteristic focal encephalitis of the immunocompetent patient.[119,126–129] Neuroimaging may be negative. PCR amplification of HSV in the CSF is likely the most sensitive diagnostic tool, but test results are often delayed; if this diagnosis is suspected, empiric therapy with intravenous acyclovir may be warranted until results are available.

Meningitis and Headache

As in other settings, meningitis in AIDS may present with confusion and altered consciousness as the predominating manifestations. In the case of pyogenic bacterial meningitis caused by *Listeria monocytogenes* or *Streptococcus pneumoniae*, which are more common complications of HIV in developing regions,[130] headache and stiff neck are usually present and push the clinician to lumbar puncture. However, these findings may be less conspicuous or even absent at onset in cryptococcal meningitis, the most common meningitis in this setting. Frequently there is only a mild inflammatory reaction in the CSF compared to the burden of microorganisms recovered (*see* Chapter 43).[131] Hence, even relatively low suspicion of the latter should trigger lumbar puncture and analysis for cryptococcal antigen, along with diagnostic studies for bacteria and other fungi, particularly when the CD4+ T-lymphocyte count is low. Recently, CNS cryptococcal disease with predominant inflammatory characteristics has been described in the setting of immune reconstitution on HAART. Within 6 weeks of starting potent HAART, some patients with previously undetected disease develop clinically apparent, rapidly progressive meningitis characterized by neck stiffness, headache, nausea, vomiting, and a prominent CSF pleocytosis.[24] Unusual manifestations of cryptococcal disease have been observed in patients with a known cryptococcal diagnosis by culture or antigen positivity, started on HAART soon after antifungal treatment.[22] IRD in these patients was characterized by various forms of sterile inflammation, including clinical syndromes of meningismus, headache, nausea, vomiting, increased intracranial pressure, and lack of organisms on CSF culture. Hypothesized mechanisms for these presentations include an atypical response to a previously clinically latent infection, or an enhanced (and immonopathological) response to the presence of low-grade cryptococcal antigenemia in the CSF. These syndromes present a departure from the more typical indolent course of cryptococcal meningitis, and have raised issues of when to initiate HAART in patients with known cryptococcal disease.[132]

CSF abnormalities such as a mild mononuclear pleocytosis (10–400 cells/μL) and elevated protein, accompanied by a variable degree of overt symptoms may be seen in patients with HIV-1 infection and neurosyphilis. Syphilis is now endemic in many metropolitan areas in the developed world[133,134] and is a major co-infection for patients with HIV.[135] The clinical presentations of neurosyphilis include meningeal involvement with prominent cranial neuropathies, meningovascular disease with stroke, uveitis from ocular disease, dementia from general paresis, and ataxia and neuropathic pain from tabes dorsalis.[136] Of these, HIV-infected patients most commonly present with meningeal or ocular syphilis. Diagnosis of neurosyphilis is accomplished mainly by obtaining CSF in subjects found to have a positive serum rapid plasma reagin (RPR) test, examining the fluid for positive VDRL and RPR titers.[137] Unfortunately, CSF VDRL is only 30–70% sensitive in cases of neurosyphilis,[138,139] so more conservative algorithms use diagnostic criteria of a positive serum RPR and elevated CSF protein or white blood cells in the setting of HIV-1 infection. As we have noted, CSF abnormalities in HIV-1-infected patients may be difficult to interpret, primarily because many (mostly not on HAART) with seemingly asymptomatic HIV have pleocytosis and elevated protein, likely due to HIV itself. As a result, new, specific methods are needed to define the patient truly afflicted with neurosyphilis, in order to prioritize appropriate therapy which involves 10–14 days of IV or IM penicillin. A recent report has suggested that detection of an elevated proportion of B lymphocytes in the CSF, in combination with measurement of CSF fluorescent treponemal antibody (FTA), may be more sensitive than CSF VDRL and more specific than the presence of pleocytosis for diagnosis of neurosyphilis.[140]

Mycobacterium tuberculosis is a major cause of meningitis, neurological morbidity, and death in regions where tuberculosis is endemic or epidemic, though less common in the Western world.[130,141,142] The typical presentation of tuberculous (TB) meningitis pursues a somewhat protracted course (days to weeks), with CSF demonstrating increased lymphocyte predominance, elevated protein levels, and low glucose. Recent studies of TB meningitis in HIV-infected patients have demonstrated that HIV-infected patients may have more extrameningeal TB, more infarcts, and fewer meningeal signs and symptoms than seen in the typical course of disease. Furthermore, CSF may demonstrate either acellularity, neutrophil predominance, or normal protein in more than 10% of AIDS patients with TB meningitis.[141,142] Treatment requires evaluation for drug-resistant strains in some areas, multidrug therapy, and in some cases ventriculoperitonal shunting for hydrocephalus, though this has not been shown to be of clear overall benefit.[143]

Although headache is a common symptom in AIDS, many patients with this complaint do not suffer bacterial or fungal infections.[144–150] As discussed above, in some individuals with HIV-1 infection lumbar puncture will detect a pleocytosis sufficient to warrant the designation of "aseptic meningitis". However, use of this term for a relatively common laboratory finding in otherwise asymptomatic individuals can be problematic, and one should probably distinguish patients who develop meningitic symptoms and exhibit these types of CSF findings from those in whom they are incidental. In an earlier report, Hollander divided patients who presented with headache and CSF pleocytosis into two groups, those with an acute presentation and those with a more chronic course.[151] Because of the high prevalence of asymptomatic pleocytosis in HIV-1 infection, the relationship between elevated CSF cells and headache is not always clear, and in some the symptom and the laboratory finding may indeed be unrelated.[152] In our own studies of treatment interruption in which we have noted a resurgence of HIV-1 in CSF accompanying that in plasma, we have been struck not only by the robust lymphocytic cell response but also by the fact that this response is clinically silent.[153] No formal study has addressed the question of whether headache in HIV-1 infection responds to HAART, though pleocytosis without other causes characteristically resolves after institution of HAART in parallel with clearing of CSF virus.[71,154] Further complicating this issue, a clinically similar headache can manifest in HIV-1-infected patients in the absence of pleocytosis; this was common enough to have been designated "HIV headache".[155,156] This headache can have a migrainous quality with periodicity, photophobia, and nausea. Treatment is empiric and may include agents active in prophylaxis of migraine, such as anticonvulsants, tricyclics, or calcium channel blockers.

FOCAL BRAIN DISEASES

The diagnosis of macroscopic brain disorders begins with clinical recognition of symptoms and signs that indicate the presence of focal brain dysfunction. These include hemispheric (hemiparesis, hemianopsia, aphasia, and apraxia) or brain stem-cerebellar (vertigo, ataxia, diplopia, bilateral pyramidal signs, and the like) dysfunction. Symptoms and signs may be prominent or subtle, and more than one focal lesion affecting "eloquent" brain structures may confuse exact localization. The first step in evaluation is usually neuroimaging both to confirm the presence of detectable focal lesions and to further define their character (see Fig. 62-2). Only rarely will focal lesions escape detection by MRI; in such patients either the imaging is done too early to discern abnormalities (e.g., the rare patient with PML at its earliest stage), or the abnormalities are microscopic and below the limit of image detection. Some metabolic disorders may present with focal features (e.g., nonketotic, hyperglycemic hyperosmolar encephalopathy). In addition, microscopic disease, encephalitis, or meningitis can cause seizures that transiently expand the zone of physiologic dysfunction beyond that caused by the lesion itself, with residual focal deficits that are slow to clear.

Among the focal brain disorders afflicting AIDS patients, PCNSL, cerebral toxoplasmosis, and PML are most common, and most diagnostic efforts relate to distinguishing these three diseases. Since neurological symptoms and signs are determined by localization, the particular deficits are not helpful in their segregation. However, each of the three tends to have a different temporal profile (see Table 62-1). In general, toxoplasmosis evolves most rapidly, presenting within a few days after the onset of symptoms. PCNSL usually evolves somewhat more slowly, with 1 to 3 weeks separating the onset of first symptoms and presentation to the physician. PML advances even more slowly and may take several weeks to a few months before the patient seeks medical evaluation. Associated constitutional symptoms also tend to differ. Patients with toxoplasmosis are more often febrile, appear generally ill, and are lethargic or sleepy; they also more commonly complain of headache. This contrasts with both the PCNSL and PML patients, who are constitutionally asymptomatic unless they suffer an additional overt infection.

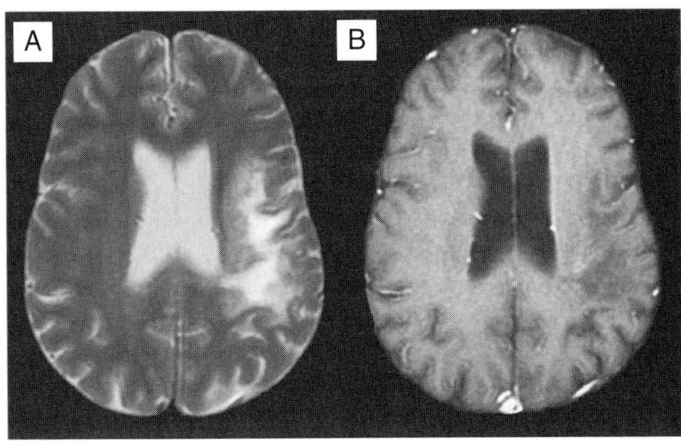

Figure 62-4 ■ MRI of patient with PML. (**A**) T_2-weighted image shows a large area of increased signal in the left hemisphere (right side of image). (**B**) T_1-weighted image shows the same lesion in its densest parts, but now with decreased attenuation (dark).

Progressive Multifocal Leukoencephalopathy

Despite these clinical differences, neuroimaging is needed to further define diagnosis of these focal disorders. MRI usually readily identifies PML.[156–160] PML is caused by JC virus brain infection and is characterized by demyelination and loss of tissue rather than an expanding mass effect.[161,162] Areas of demyelination that follow death of infected oligodendrocytes coalesce to leave behind areas of lost white matter and even cavitation. PML lesions usually begin as small foci that expand concentrically, either singly or in several sites. Inflammation and surrounding edema is usually absent or scant, and consequently the typical MRI of PML shows one or more lesions afflicting predominantly or exclusively the white matter in which there is increased signal (white) on T_2-weighted images but diminished signal (black) on T_1-weighted images (see Fig. 62-4). Lesions have a predilection to involve the white matter adjacent to the cortex but can be located anywhere. When contrast enhancement is present (likely in <10% of cases), it tends to have a delicate, lacy appearance. There are two principal differential diagnoses to consider with this type of scan result, both of which are usually easily eliminated by correlation with the clinical presentation and by observing their evolution over time. The first is ADC, which can be associated with focal white matter changes. However, ADC characteristically involves deeper white matter, lesions usually are not black on T_1-weighted images, and, most importantly, localized image abnormalities are not accompanied by corresponding focal neurological deficits. The second is cerebral infarction. However, in the latter, the gray matter is also affected, the distribution of the lesion follows a vascular territory, and the clinical evolution occurs in hours rather than weeks.

A common clinical question in these patients is, "What level of diagnostic certainty is necessary for clinical management of PML?" For the typical case in which the MRI shows the abnormalities outlined above (confirmed by an experienced neuroradiologist) and these imaging findings can be correlated with the clinical picture, a clinical diagnosis of PML is highly probable and may not require further diagnostic testing. CSF examination should probably be done routinely to eliminate diagnostic surprises such as neurosyphilis or vasculitis, depending upon the individual patient's findings. CSF also allows PCR confirmation of local JC virus infection detected in the CSF with ~75% sensitivity but very high specificity for PML,[163–168] though the sensitivity of this test may be lower in the setting of HAART.[169] If other measures fail and the case is atypical, brain biopsy should be undertaken for final confirmation.

There is no proven specific treatment for PML. However, remission has been clearly documented. Early in the epidemic, Berger and colleagues noted spontaneous remission in the absence of treatment, and following a number of case reports documenting remission in PML patients treated with HAART,[170] retrospective studies comparing the outcome of this opportunistic infection before and after HAART have demonstrated that about half of PML patients do well after starting HAART, with arrest of progression and an element of improvement in some.[171–175] Radiographic improvement has also been documented by MRI.[176] The theoretical interpretation of this response, which is in keeping with earlier reports of PML remission in non-AIDS patients, is that HAART restores the host's capacity to mount an effective immune response to JC virus. The current standard of therapy for PML therefore begins with institution or modification of HAART, which is then assessed by the standard measures of viral load reduction and CD4+ T-lymphocyte cell increase.

For those cases that fail to respond, the remaining treatment options are experimental. Unfortunately, the history of PML includes reports of several therapies that initially showed promise but failed when examined prospectively in a larger trial.[177] Most recently, interest has centered upon the use of cidofovir, an antiviral active against CMV. Studies of this drug in PML have been uncontrolled and the results are conflicting; a recent prospective multicenter trial found no benefit of cidofovir in terms of neurological examination score after 8 weeks of treatment.[178–181]

In the setting of immune reconstitution, new phenotypes of CNS disease referable to infection with JC virus have been described. Neurological deficits due to PML may occur around the time of immune reconstitution, either newly developing after HAART, or worsening in the context of immune restoration with increased CD4+ T-lymphocyte counts.[25,182,183] On MRI scans, these lesions may appear typical of PML in location and morphology, but may also show edema, mass effect, and peripheral enhancement with gadolinium, suggesting a local immune reaction and breakdown of the blood–brain barrier and inflammation. This inflammatory nature of PML immune reconstitution disease has been confirmed by biopsies demonstrating an atypical inflammatory reaction (perivascular lymphomonocytic infiltration of CD8+ T-lymphocyte suppressor cells and CD20+ B cells) in cerebral white matter in patients with PML who had dramatic clinical worsening soon after HAART was

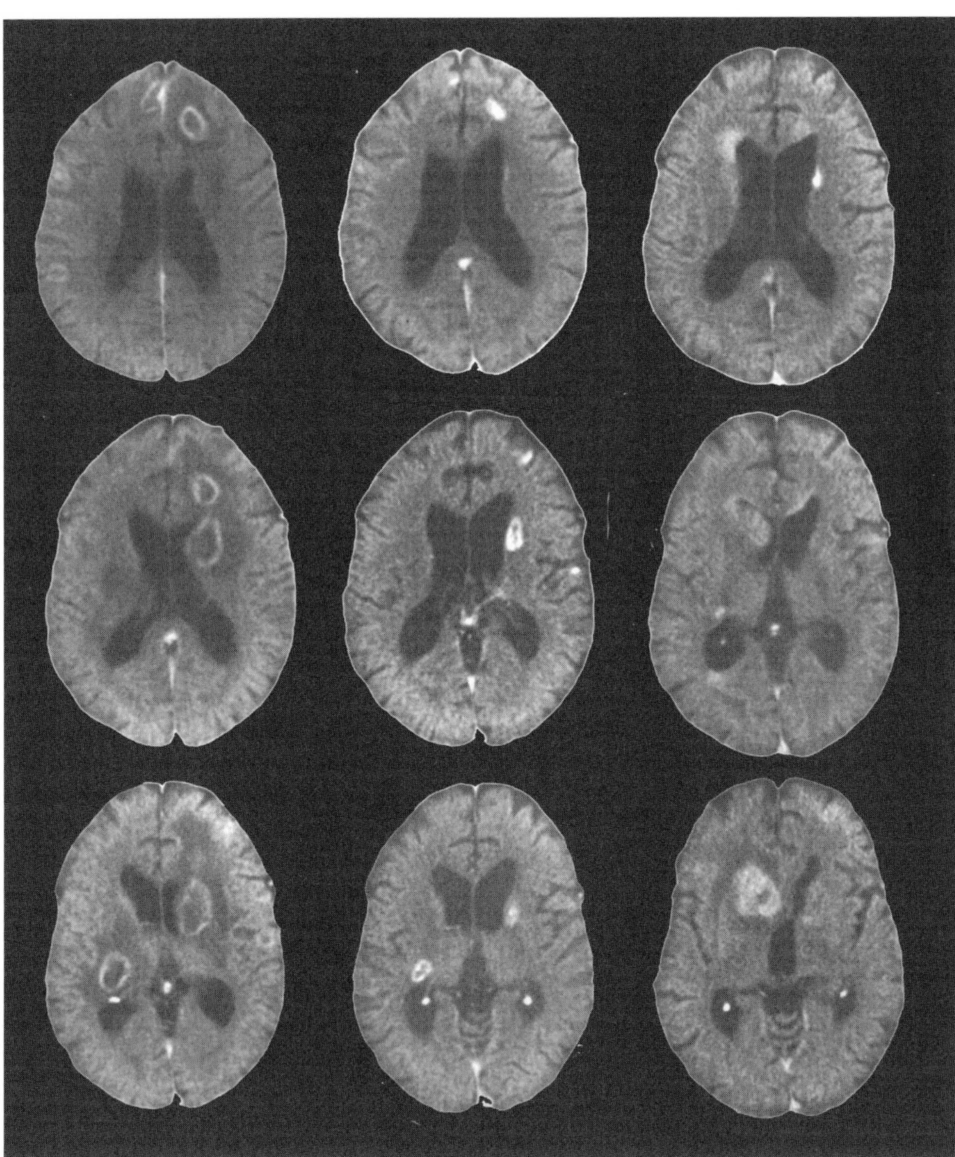

Figure 62-5 ■ CT scans with contrast of patient who initially presented with toxoplasmosis (**A–C**) with multiple ring-enhancing lesions. Ten months later (**D–F**) the response to empiric therapy was very evident with marked shrinkage of the lesions, most of which still showed contrast enhancement. Four months later he presented with different neurological symptoms (**G–I**) and with multiple brain lesions that had a different morphology (including more diffuse contrast enhancement and spread along the lateral ventricle walls). This new entity was found to be primary CNS lymphoma.

initiated.[26] Finally, a recent report describes two patients with known PML who had paradoxical fatal worsening after initiating HAART. Because of atypical presentations, fulminant progression, and negative JC virus PCR from the CSF, brain biopsies were performed, demonstrating dramatic lymphocytic infiltrates and JC virus detected in brain tissue through PCR.[27] In several of these reports, antiinflammatory therapy with corticosteroids was administered as adjunctive therapy to HAART, but did not seem to alter the course of disease. The paradox of immune reconstitution disease is especially manifest in these examples of progression of PML in the setting of HAART, since otherwise the prognosis of this disease has been overall dramatically improved in the era of combined antiretroviral therapy.

A recent report has expanded the cellular tropism of JC virus beyond the oligodendrocyte to the granule cell layer of the cerebellum, suggesting that diffuse cerebellar dysfunction and atrophy in patients with AIDS may be mediated by cytolytic neuronal infection by JC virus even in the absence of demyelinating lesions.[184,185]

Cerebral Toxoplasmosis and PCNSL

The other two common focal brain lesions, cerebral toxoplasmosis and PCNSL, in contrast to PML, usually are defined radiologically as having mass effect (an expansion of tissue) with surrounding edema. Figure 62-2 outlines an approach to diagnosis of focal mass lesions that is aimed particularly at the early diagnosis of brain lesions other than toxoplasmosis. Because cerebral toxoplasmosis is nearly always due to reactivated *Toxoplasma gondii* infection, greater than 95% of such patients have detectable serum antibody to this organism.[125,186–188] Hence, if the radiographic character of the lesion(s) is compatible with toxoplasmosis and the blood serology is positive, the patients are subjected to a trial of antitoxoplasma therapy. They improve clinically within days to (at most) 2 weeks, and this is followed with radiographic documentation (Fig. 62-5). Typically, neuroimaging shows contrast-enhancing lesions (usually multiple, but they can be single) involving the cortex or deep gray nuclei (basal ganglia and thalamus); the lesions often have a border of strong

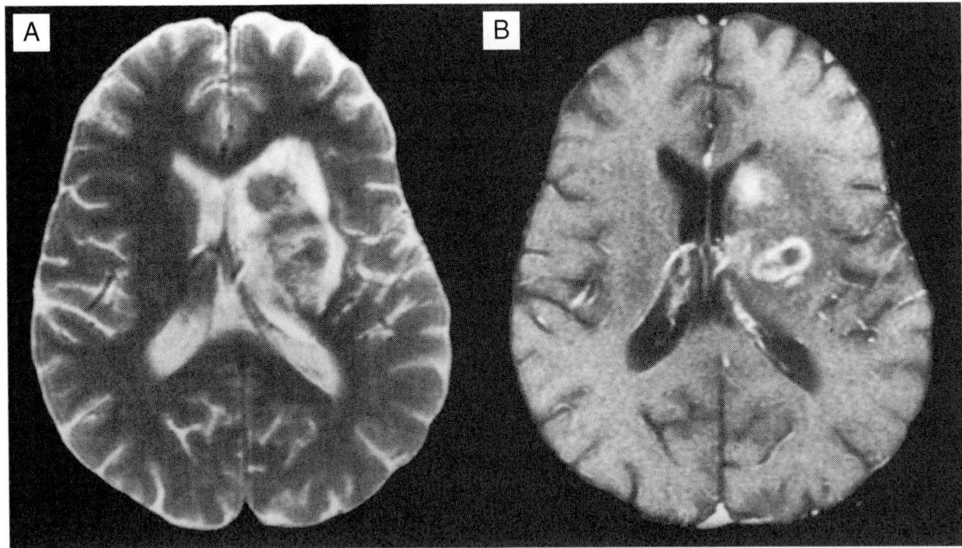

Figure 62-6 ■ MRI scan of PCNSL. (**A**) T_2-weighted image showing large, deep multilobed lesion with surrounding edema. (**B**) Contrast-enhanced MRI showing variable enhancement of the lesion, diffuse in the anterior portion with an area of ring enhancement more posteriorly.

contrast enhancement, and there may be an "eccentric target" sign.[189,190] Because prophylaxis against *Pneumocystis carinii* pneumonia with trimethoprim–sulfamethoxazole is also active in preventing cerebral toxoplasmosis, this variable is also considered in the probability of this diagnosis.[163] Indeed, its widespread use, and more recently the use of HAART, has reduced the incidence of cerebral toxoplasmosis.[13] However, it is still a prevalent disorder in many settings, chiefly in individuals who have not been receiving ongoing medical care.[191]

Because the outcome of PCNSL is likely influenced by how early diagnosis is made and treatment started, it is important to pursue this diagnosis aggressively. In this respect, it is not reasonable to simply undertake a trial of toxoplasmosis therapy in all AIDS patients with mass lesions, as had been recommended by some in the past. In patients with negative toxoplasma blood serology, neuroimaging abnormalities that suggest PCNSL or with radiographically and clinically atypical features, we advocate early brain biopsy, though usually after CSF examination if lumbar puncture is judged to be safe. Imaging abnormalities that favor PCNSL include deep lesions involving the white matter, including the corpus callosum; subependymal extension of lesions along the ventricular walls; and diffuse or weak contrast enhancement rather than the ring-like appearance of toxoplasmosis (Figs 62-5 and 62-6).[190,192] In most settings, brain biopsy is necessary for certain diagnosis of PCNSL. PCR detection of Epstein–Barr virus (EBV) DNA sequences in CSF has been reported to enhance diagnosis, perhaps to the point of substituting for biopsy.[4,163,193,194] However, the accuracy of this test through different commercial laboratories needs to be confirmed by more extended experience. Conventional cytology is much less commonly helpful.[195]

Focal CNS lesions may be better defined by metabolic imaging through either positron emission tomography (PET) with labeled deoxyglucose to measure active tissue metabolism, single-photon emission computed tomography (SPECT) to detect metabolically linked cerebral blood flow, or MRS to detect different tissue metabolite profiles.[63,89,196–202] By PET and SPECT, PCNSL lesions are characteristically "active" with increased uptake of the tracer, while toxoplasmosis lesions are characteristically "cold" by these techniques. Despite the fact that the results of these scanning techniques can be impressive in the individual case, specificity is not absolute, although combining results of radionuclide imaging with PCR detection of EBV has been shown to be highly specific in certain settings.[193]

Although in the pre-HAART era, mean survival in those with PCNSL was only a few months from diagnosis, survival has improved in subjects who have immune restoration on antiretroviral therapy.[203–205] Whole-brain irradiation, the previous mainstay of palliative therapy, leads to leukoencephalopathy in patients who survive long-term. Thus, chemotherapy regimens, including high-dose intravenous methotrexate, are now under study in combination with HAART for treatment of this condition.[206,207]

Other Focal Lesions

The etiologic range of more uncommon focal brain lesions in patients with advanced immunosuppression includes infections due to typical and atypical bacterial organisms including *Staphylococcus* and *Streptococcus* species, fungi, and parasites.[3,208] The general approach to their diagnosis usually includes search for particular susceptibilities or involvement of other organs more easily accessible to culture or biopsy. Where this fails, early brain biopsy should be considered. This remains an essential tool for diagnosis of unusual focal brain lesions as well as in most cases of PCNSL, and is often the fastest and surest approach to such disorders as *Mycobacterium tuberculosis*,[208–211] nocardia,[209,210,212,213] glioma[214,215]; macronodular CMV lesions,[216] *Aspergillus*,[217,218] or the rare abscesses due to *mucor*, *candida*, or *entamoeba*.

Many clinicians are unduly wary of resorting to brain biopsy. However, when used selectively, its morbidity is low[126,219,220] and the most frequent disappointment is failure of biopsy to establish diagnosis.

Cryptococcal meningitis can also be complicated by focal brain lesions of several types. One of these relates to the dilatation of the perivascular (Virchow–Robin) spaces at the base of the brain by organisms and capsular debris. These may be small and give rise to a mottled appearance of the diencephalon on MRI, particularly with T_2 weighting.[221] Larger lesions justify the term gelatinous pseudocysts, and may range from a solitary cystic appearance to bubbly lesions that encompass the entire basal ganglia.[222] Because they are not associated with inflammation, these lesions do not elicit contrast enhancement, and they resolve with treatment of the meningitis. Although cryptococcal granulomas (cryptococcoma) are unusual in AIDS patients, we have encountered six patients with another characteristic type of inflammatory lesion that develops as a delayed complication of cryptococcal meningitis.[223] Patients characteristically present with focal seizures and, subsequently, focal neurological deficits. MRI shows a characteristic pattern of linear deep sulcal enhancement and underlying edema that extends into the white matter. There is a predilection for the posterior hemispheres – the parietal and occipital lobes. Biopsy has shown cortical invasion by the cryptococci and local inflammation. However, the MRI findings are sufficiently distinct in this setting to allow clinical diagnosis without biopsy. This complication can occur while patients are on maintenance therapy, and the CSF cryptococcal antigen titer is usually lower than at the time of the patient's initial presentation with meningitis. Although four of the six patients responded well to changes in therapy, two progressed despite all therapeutic efforts.

Stroke is unusual in those with HIV-1 infection,[223–226] although it may become more common as the infected population survives to a more susceptible age and if the lipid abnormalities accompanying therapy predispose to cerebrovascular disease. This diagnosis is suspected when the onset of neurological deficit is acute.[227,228] In younger AIDS patients who are otherwise well, the causes of stroke include a miscellany of relatively uncommon conditions.[229] Cerebral vasculitis can complicate varicella-zoster virus (VZV), usually manifesting as delayed hemiplegia contralateral to trigeminal herpes zoster, although other distributions of both rash and cerebral infarction can occur.[230–232] The diagnosis is suspected by the setting of recent zoster and supported by the finding of cerebral infarction and vascular occlusion or narrowing on magnetic resonance, CT, or conventional angiography. CSF PCR may also be helpful.[233,234] The effect of treatment is uncertain, although usually anti-VZV therapy is given either alone or in combination with anticoagulants or corticosteroids. Septic embolism, invasive fungal vasculitis (most commonly caused by *Aspergillus*), and neurosyphilis can also occur in this setting, and patients may also develop the more common cerebrovascular diseases that afflict the general population. For those still using illicit drugs, cocaine and amfetamines may cause either infarction or cerebral hemorrhage. When patients are more systemically ill, nonbacterial thrombotic endocarditis and other coagulopathic strokes may occur. Although AIDS patients frequently exhibit laboratory abnormalities that may predispose to stroke (e.g., protein S deficiency), the role of these serologic changes to clinical stroke is uncertain.[235]

MYELOPATHIES

Diagnostic considerations of myelopathies echo those of brain diseases. The starting point is recognizing that the localization of disease is in the spinal cord, and the next step involves separation of nonsegmental from focal myelopathies (Fig. 62-7).

Vacuolar and Other Nonsegmental Myelopathies

The nonsegmental myelopathies are distinguished by their "diffuse" rather than focal character. In these patients there is no discrete level below which abnormalities are distinct and above which signs are absent. Rather, there is gradual shading toward increasing abnormality caudally, and, hence, the legs are more affected than the arms. Motor abnormalities tend to predominate, and, when sensory symptoms or signs are present, they involve distal loss of sensation, usually without any changes over the trunk. Right–left asymmetries are usually minor or absent. Bladder and bowel dysfunction tend to occur late.

The most common myelopathy of this type in AIDS is the vacuolar myelopathy, which was defined as a component of ADC.[236–238] The reason that this myelopathy is included within the larger ADC syndrome relates to the frequency with which clinical myelopathy and cognitive deficits coexist, and the observation that abnormalities may not be confined to the spinal cord even in those patients in whom cognition is spared; for example, a brisk jaw jerk is common in vacuolar myelopathy. However, despite this overlap, many patients present with a strongly predominating picture of spastic or spastic-ataxic gait that may progress to paraparesis or paraplegia with minor or no cognitive deficit. Pathologically, the spinal cord shows a characteristic vacuolated or foamy appearance of the white matter, most notably affecting the lateral and posterior columns. This pathology is indistinguishable from that of subacute combined degeneration caused by vitamin B_{12} deficiency, although these patients have normal B_{12} levels. While developing in the setting of advanced HIV infection, vacuolar changes do not correlate with productive spinal cord infection.[239–243] Thus, the etiology and pathogenesis of vacuolar myelopathy remain a matter of speculation.[238,244]

Myelopathy is common in those who progress to late AIDS, either as an overt, symptomatic disease or in milder, subclinical form as evidenced by hyperactive knee jerks and mildly slow or clumsy walking. The ankle jerks may be less brisk in some patients because concomitant neuropathy is common. The disorder is usually gradually progressive and

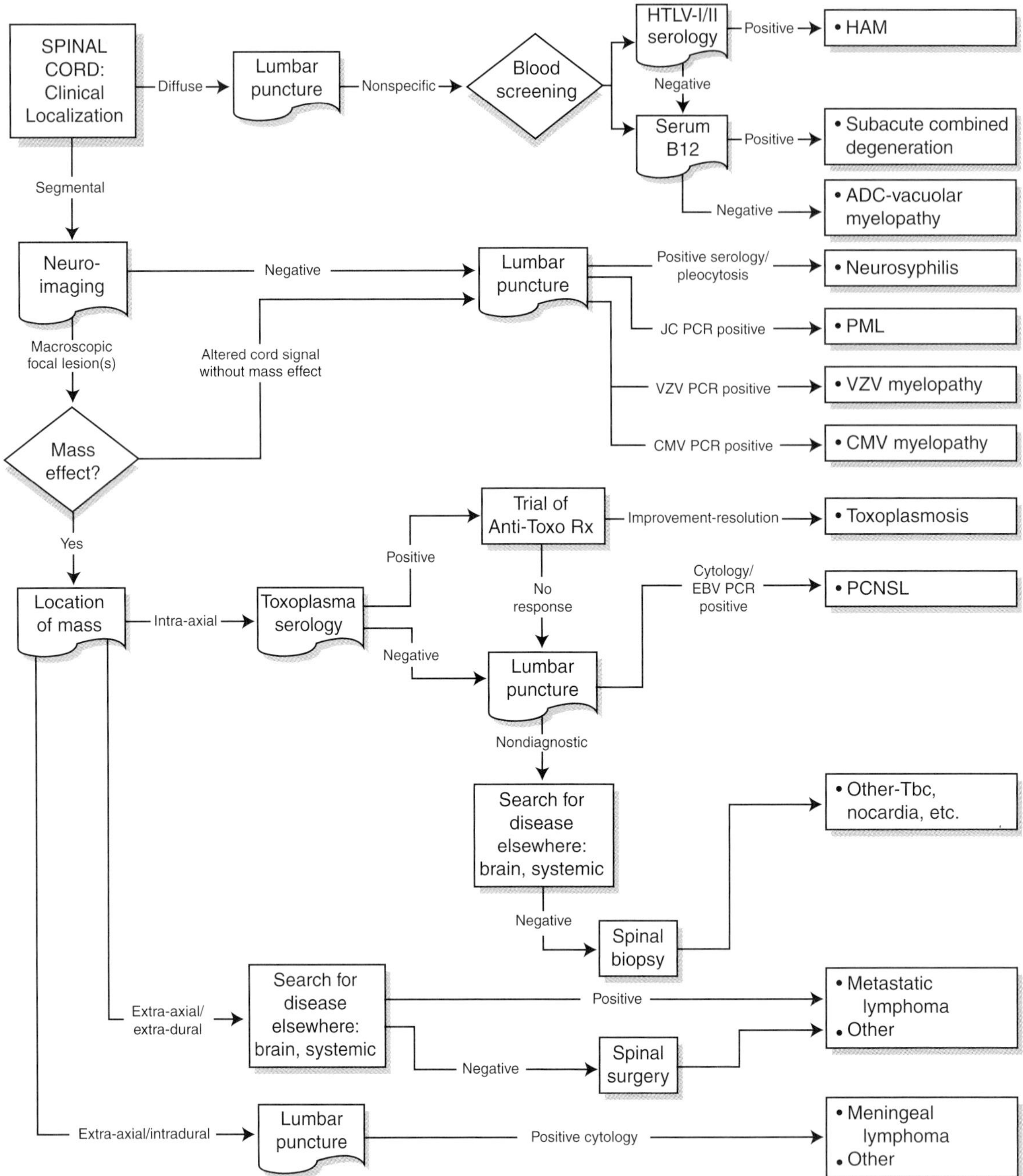

Figure 62-7 ■ Diagnostic approach to spinal cord diseases in late HIV-1 infection. HAM, HTLV-1B-associated myelopathy; Tbc, tuberculosis; VZV, varicella-zoster virus.

may exacerbate with severe coincident infections, resolving partially afterward. Because there is no distinct laboratory marker, this is a clinical diagnosis. MRI is usually normal or detects only spinal cord atrophy. In typical cases, diagnostic imaging is not imperative;[245] however, if there is reason to suspect a focal lesion then MRI should be done. Lumbar puncture is performed to rule out other conditions rather than to confirm the diagnosis. Among the principal differential diagnoses are the myelopathies associated with HTLV-1 (called HTLV-1-associated myelopathy or HAM, or tropical spastic paraparesis, TSP, or the combined HAM/TSP) and HTLV-2.[246–252] Except for cases of more rapid onset following transfusion, HAM is clinically similar to vacuolar myelopathy, although spasticity can be more severe early in the course and low back pain more frequent. Diagnosis usually relies on serologic studies showing antibodies to these other retroviruses in blood and CSF, and unlike vacuolar myelopathy, HTVLV-1/2 myleopathies are not associated with low blood CD4+ T-lymphocyte cells. Treatment with interferon has shown some effect in the non-AIDS HAM patient. However, there are no clear studies of treatment-induced improvement in coinfected patients. Vitamin B_{12} deficiency should be ruled out.

There is some controversy regarding whether vacuolar myelopathy responds to antiretroviral therapy in a fashion similar to the cognitive impairment of ADC. Because vacuolar pathology does not correlate with local productive HIV-1 infection of the spinal cord, there is also theoretical reason to suspect that this mode of treatment would not be effective.[253,254] However, the lack of seeming efficacy in past experience might relate to the low potency of antiviral therapies available at the time. This issue needs to be re-examined in the current era of HAART. We have seen examples of patients with clinical diagnosis of vacuolar myelopathy and recent onset who have improved remarkably following contemporary combination antiviral drug treatment. Although this therapeutic issue needs careful study, in the absence of conclusive data, we pursue the optimistic path of treating such patients aggressively with antiviral drug combinations as discussed above for ADC in general.

Focal (Segmental) Myelopathies

Focal myelopathies are much less common than vacuolar myelopathy. Although most of these are caused by the same diseases that cause focal lesions in brain, there are a few causes that are more specific or common to the spinal cord in HIV-1-infected patients. The most common of these is VZV, which characteristically complicates cutaneous herpes zoster after a variable delay (days to a week or two, rarely several weeks or months).[255,256] The focal myelopathy due to VZV usually is centered at or near the spinal cord segment corresponding to the dermatomal zoster rash and is caused by direct viral infection that enters at the dorsal root entry zone and then extends centrifugally. This explains localization in some to a partial or complete hemicord (Brown–Sequard) syndrome. Pathologically there may be both parenchymal infection and infectious vasculitis with infarction; the latter likely accounts for the abruptness of onset in many cases. Diagnosis is usually suspected on the basis of the combined temporal and spatial (spinal segment) relationship to the rash. Clinical severity varies from transverse myelitis to subclinical hyperactive reflexes and Babinski sign on the side of the rash. Because of the rapid evolution of the condition and its rarity, the effects of treatment are not well established. However, in the absence of adequate data, aggressive anti-VZV treatment seems appropriate. Spinal MRI may show a focal cord lesion with little or no mass effect but with focal edema that extends above and below the central location of pathology. CSF may exhibit a mononuclear pleocytosis, although this can also be present with uncomplicated herpes zoster. PCR detection of VZV DNA sequences in CSF may also be helpful,[257,258] although again interpretation may be tainted by very recent cutaneous herpes zoster, which might also cause a positive CSF PCR. Thus the clinical presentation is the principal basis of diagnosis, and the laboratory is of ancillary value.

The diagnostic approach to the other focal myelopathies is similar to that of their counterparts in the brain. It relies heavily upon neuroimaging, chiefly spinal MRI.[259,260] As outlined in Figure 62-7, the cross-sectional location of the mass lesion divides the major diagnostic categories into three anatomic groups: intraaxial, extraaxial/intradural, and extraaxial/extradural. While intraaxial (within the spinal cord) lesions are uncommon, toxoplasmosis and PCNSL are the most frequent,[261–263] and the diagnostic evaluation follows the same path as with brain lesions. Because both may be part of a multifocal process, brain imaging may also be helpful in revealing clinically silent lesions that may be more characteristic or accessible. Both of these diseases usually show contrast enhancement. In toxoplasma seropositive patients, a trial of therapy may establish diagnosis while either cytologic assessment or PCR detection of EBV sequences may confirm the presence of PCNSL. When these measures fail, direct biopsy may be required.

The most common extraaxial/extradural lesions in HIV-1-infected patients are caused by metastatic lymphoma.[264,265] This diagnosis is usually established by tissue sampling from another site. Without this, needle or open biopsy is required. An important differential in the intravenous drug user is pyogenic epidural abscess, which requires rapid evaluation and commencement of antibiotic therapy and, usually, surgical drainage. These patients usually present with an acute (hours) or subacute (days) history, back pain, and leukocytosis or elevated erythrocyte sedimentation rate, although each of these elements may be minor or absent in some. Neuroimaging also usually distinguishes these diseases.

Metastatic lymphoma can also present with primary meningeal involvement causing back pain, patchy or ascending radiculopathies, or cranial nerve palsies; in some of these cases compressive or invasive myelopathy may be part of the picture.[266] Spinal MRI reveals thickened nerve roots and nodular enhancing lesions within the dura. CSF cytology usually establishes the diagnosis. CMV polyradiculopathy may also be accompanied by spinal cord involvement and clinical myelopathy, and even with a similar MRI picture of enlarged nerve roots.[267] However, the CSF profile is usually different, as described below.

NEUROPATHIES

Figure 62-8 outlines a diagnostic approach to the more common neuropathies that complicate HIV-1 infection. The starting point again is with clinical localization based upon the history and examination. Anatomic localization can divide patients into four groups, the first two relating to polyneuropathies with either sensory or motor abnormalities predominating and the third and fourth encompassing more focal processes – sacral ascending polyradiculopathy and asymmetrical radiculopathies and neuropathies. Myopathies are included with the motor localization in Figure 62–8, but they are discussed separately below.

Sensory Polyneuropathies

The sensory polyneuropathies are the most common neuropathies complicating AIDS, and characteristically present with

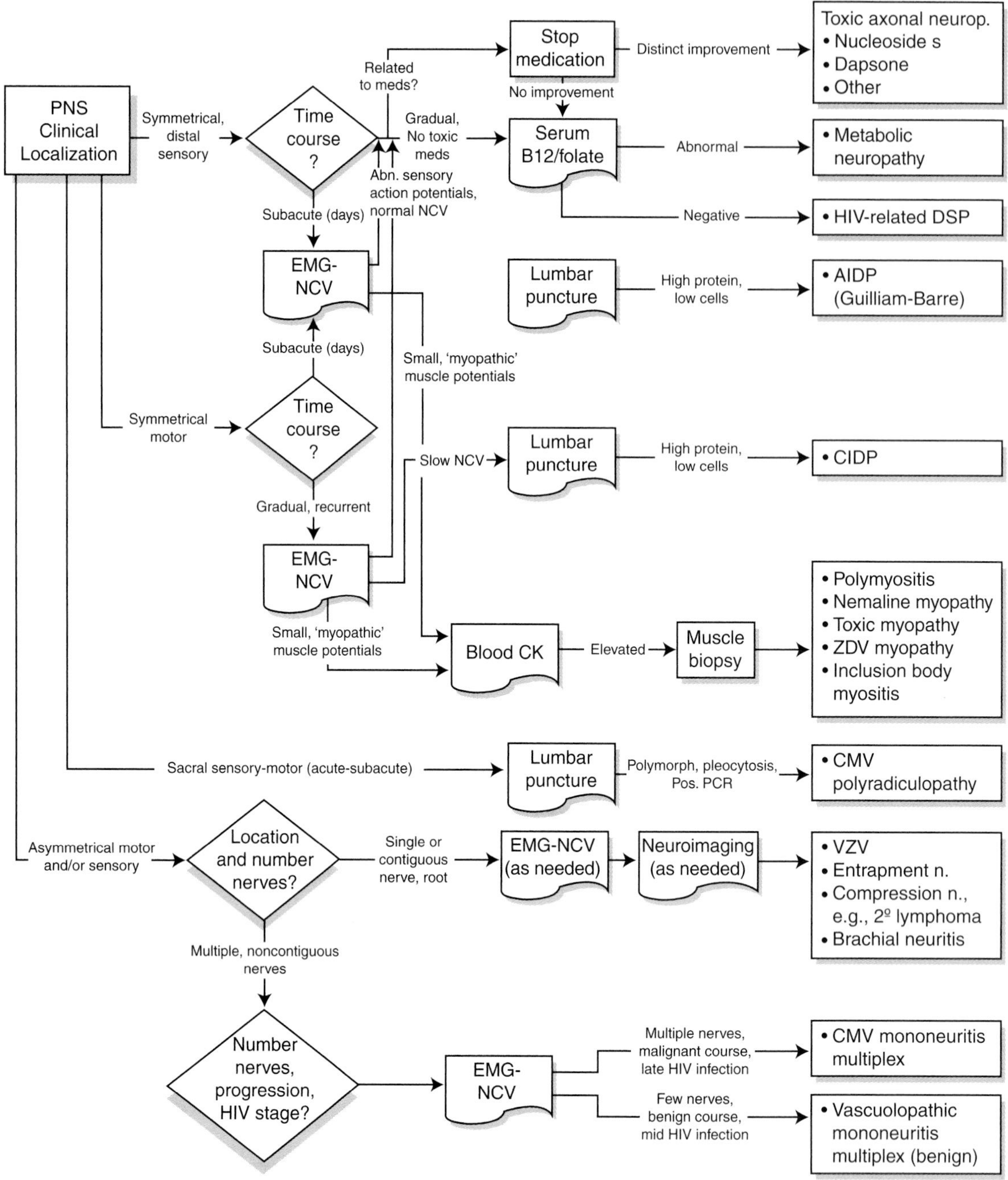

Figure 62-8 ■ Diagnostic approach to PNS and muscle diseases in HIV-1 infection. AIDP, acute idiopathic demyelinating polyneuropathy; CIDP, chronic idiopathic demyelinating polyneuropathy; CK, creatine kinase; DSP, distal sensory polyneuropathy; EMG, electromyography; NCV, nerve conduction velocity.

distal sensory symptoms – paresthesias, numbness, or pain that begins in the toes or feet and extends proximally.[268,269] With greater severity the fingertips and hands may be included. These symptoms are usually symmetrical or show only minor asymmetries and evolve in a length-dependent fashion; initial symptoms indicate preferential affliction of the most distal portions of the longest nerves.

The most important neuropathy of this type is the distal sensory polyneuropathy (DSP, specifically termed HIV-related DSP) that appears to be caused in some way by the retrovirus itself.[270,271] The pathogenesis of HIV-related DSP is still a matter of speculation because it does not clearly result from direct viral infection of the nerves themselves. A cytokine-mediated toxic pathway has been hypothesized in this disorder similar to that invoked to explain brain injury in ADC.[272] The principal targets of this pathogenetic process are the axon and sensory ganglion cell body rather than the myelin sheath. Hence it is classified among the axonal, rather than demyelinating, neuropathies.

Although severity may vary, the presentation of HIV-related DSP is fairly stereotyped, and diagnosis can be based on symptoms and signs. Symptoms of paresthesias and pain usually markedly overshadow disability caused by loss of either sensory or motor function. Thus, unless pain is severe, patients walk normally and suffer little or no evident imbalance despite demonstration on examination of mildly impaired distal sensation (cold, pin, scratch, vibration, and position) and depressed or absent ankle jerks. Recently a neuropathy screening tool applicable to diagnosis of HIV-related DSP even in resource-limited settings has been developed and validated.[273] Characteristically, the earliest sensory symptoms are perceived in the toes or the anterior plantar surface (the ball) of the foot. With progression the level rises to the foot, to the ankle, or beyond. The degree of accompanying pain is curiously variable; patients with equal degrees of sensory loss may have very different levels of pain. Most frequently the pain is described as "burning" or "tingling" in type, but sometimes "tightness" is noted. When severe, all skin contact in the affected zone is abhorrent, and patients may not be able to wear shoes, tolerate foot contact with bedclothes, or walk. Some patients also experience superimposed, intermittent "shooting" or "electric" pains.

Treatment usually focuses on symptom relief. However, as more individuals are maintained on successful antiviral therapy without viremia or progressive immunosuppression, the incidence may be declining, though this issue needs additional study.[14] Another exception to the purely symptomatic approach has been the use of recombinant human nerve growth factor (NGF), a trophic factor involved in development and maintenance of sensory nerves; results of an initial trial suggest that NGF may have afforded some symptomatic benefit but the trial failed to document nerve regeneration as assessed by cutaneous nerve density in skin biopsies.[274]

At present the first approach to symptom relief has been with gabapentin given three times a day in escalating dosage.[275–277] Next in line for longer-term management are the tricyclic antidepressants, generally started at low doses (e.g., 10–25 mg of amitriptyline or nortriptyline at bedtime) and gradually increased; this conservative dosing approach avoids early experience of side effects that may lead patients to abandon treatment before an adequate trial.[278] Other antiseizure medications, including carbamazapine, phenytoin, or lamotrigine[279] may be effective for symptom relief (though only the latter seems to have no interactions with antiretroviral medications). For others, narcotic analgesics may be necessary.

The second most frequent sensory polyneuropathy is that caused by a group of the antiretroviral nucleosides – zalcitabine, didanosine, and stavudine, in descending order of neurotoxic frequency.[280–286] Whereas some patients with this type of toxic neuropathy complain of "aching" or "deep" pain across the top of the foot rather than the tingling or burning pain of HIV-related DSP, most describe symptoms that are indistinguishable from the latter. This is not surprising because this toxic neuropathy also targets axons. Because of these similar symptoms, diagnosis may rely on a clear history either of onset that is temporally linked to initiation of one of these drugs or of clinical improvement after their discontinuation, perhaps after an initial period of "coasting". The distinction between spontaneous HIV-related DSP and nucleoside neuropathy may be of major importance in some patients for whom the toxic neuropathy precludes use of one or more of these active nucleosides as part of drug combinations when alternatives are limited. It is possible that neuropathy is attributed to these nucleosides by patients or their clinicians more often than is justified, although there is no doubt that a substantial number of patients also have major difficulty with these drugs. Other than stopping the offending drug, symptomatic management is the same as HIV-related DSP. Among other drugs commonly prescribed for AIDS patients, dapsone can also cause toxic neuropathy, but this usually occurs after longer exposure and affects motor more than sensory function.[287] A variety of other medications and chemotherapeutic agents (including isoniazid (INH), high-dose vitamin B_6, cisplatin, and thalidomide) are also complicated by toxic neuropathy. Patients therefore need to be queried regarding both their orthodox and supplementary medications. A vasculitic neuropathy responsive to corticosteroids may present in a manner similar to axonal polyneuropathy.[288] Painful polyneuropathy can also complicate the diffuse infiltrative lymphocytosis syndrome; this syndrome also includes Sjögren-like manifestations and may improve with antiretroviral therapy.[289] Hepatitis C may also cause symmetrical polyneuropathy, and the role of this common co-infection in polyneuropathy in those with HIV is difficult to define.[290]

In general, electromyography and nerve conduction studies (EMG/NCS) are not necessary for routine diagnosis of these axonal neuropathies. They do not distinguish HIV-related DSP from nucleoside toxicity. However, if there is any question of whether complaints of distal extremity pain do or do not relate to neuropathy, or if there are atypical features such as motor weakness, functionally important sensory loss, or major asymmetries in symptoms or signs, then EMG and NCS may be very helpful.

Motor Polyneuropathies

Because the common axonal neuropathies of HIV-1 infection rarely cause motor impairment, when patients present with weakness, other diagnoses need to be pursued. The most common types of polyneuropathy causing symmetrical motor weakness relate to underlying demyelination.[268] Presentation may be either acute/subacute (Guillain–Barré syndrome, GBS, or acute idiopathic demyelinating polyneuropathy) or chronic (chronic idiopathic demyelinating polyneuropathy, CIDP).[271,291] Typically these disorders manifest with weakness that begins distally, most often in the feet. Reflexes are lost, although they may be preserved at initial presentation of acute idiopathic demyelinating polyneuropathy despite weakness, and sensory abnormalities are absent or inconspicuous in relation to the degree of weakness. When severe, these neuropathies can eventuate in ventilatory compromise and may also be accompanied by autonomic instability. Electrodiagnostic studies, when performed after a few weeks, show the characteristic decline in nerve conduction velocity. It is generally thought that these neuropathies have an autoimmune basis and resemble counterparts that occur in the absence of HIV-1 infection. One atypical feature that has been emphasized is the presence of more frequent CSF pleocytosis in the HIV-1 setting, but whether this suggests a pathogenetic difference or simply reflects the high background incidence of pleocytosis accompanying HIV-1 infection generally is uncertain. Although these neuropathies characteristically occur during the earlier phase of HIV-1 infection (even in the setting of acute infection), when CD4+ T-lymphocyte cells are above 200/mm^3, they can also complicate more advanced infection. Two recent reports suggest that GBS might also manifest itself during the early stages of immune reconstitution after initiation of HAART.[32,33] Regardless of setting, treatment follows guidelines for non-HIV-associated demyelinating neuropathies and includes intravenous immunoglobulin and plasma exchange, along with supportive therapies.[268,292,293]

Sacral Ascending Polyradiculopathy

One of the most dramatic and devastating neuropathies complicating HIV-1 is the ascending polyradiculitis caused by CMV infection.[108,267,294,295] This characteristically begins abruptly, evolves relatively rapidly over days, and is often fatal if not treated. Most commonly the initial abnormalities localize to sacral and lumbar nerve roots with sensory, motor, and autonomic dysfunction. Back pain is also common. Patients develop impaired bladder and bowel function, sacral sensory loss, and ascending leg weakness and sensory loss early in the course. These abnormalities then progress rostrally to involve the trunk and the arms. Pathologically, the nerve roots and then the spinal cord are involved in CMV infection and inflammatory reaction. The CSF shows a characteristic, and indeed virtually pathognomonic, neutrophil-predominant pleocytosis – a pattern otherwise rare in AIDS. CMV can also be cultured and its nucleic acid sequences detected by amplification techniques in CSF. However, treatment should be started on clinical grounds and not delayed until these specialized results are available, because outcome depends upon how soon treatment starts. Spinal MRI is usually not necessary but when done may show inflammatory arachnoiditis with contrast enhancement and thickening of the nerve roots.[267] This disease most commonly complicates CMV infection that has manifested clinically elsewhere (e.g., the eye or gastrointestinal tract) but can occur as the first clinical presentation of CMV disease. Like other manifestations of CMV infection, the incidence of this condition has decreased markedly. While optimal treatment is uncertain, and in most cases must take into account previous or ongoing treatment of CMV infection of other organs, most now recommend some type of combined drug therapy. Those treated successfully may not only stop progressing but experience a degree of recovery.[296]

Focal Radiculopathies and Neuropathies

HIV-1 infection, through the course of its evolution, can be complicated by a variety of focal neuropathies and radiculopathies. These present with asymmetrical motor and sensory symptoms and signs. Diagnostic evaluation depends upon their localization and their pattern of deficits. This begins with clear delineation of whether abnormalities can be attributed to involvement of a single nerve or nerve root, or whether several contiguous or spatially separate nerves are afflicted. This may be evident from the history and examination or may require electrodiagnostic studies for additional clarification and precision. As in other neurological complications, the stage of HIV-1 infection is an important variable because early in infection the diagnostic probabilities, with a few relatively uncommon exceptions, parallel those of the general population, whereas in late-stage disease complications of HIV-1 assume increasing importance. Cervical and lumbar radiculopathies complicating cervical and lumbar spine degeneration and disk herniation, and entrapment neuropathies such as carpel tunnel syndrome, may occur in the HIV-1-infected patient just as in the uninfected patient.

Among the neuropathic complications occurring earlier in infection that are more specific to patients with HIV-1 infection are brachial neuritis and metastatic systemic lymphoma. The first of these is thought to be an autoimmune disorder but is otherwise pathogenetically obscure. It may complicate or follow shortly upon primary infection and seroconversion or occur later during the "asymptomatic" phase.[297] Onset and evolution are subacute, and the disorder is usually unilateral, presenting as painful weakness in a distribution beyond that of a single root or nerve. Systemic lymphoma complicating early HIV-1 infection can cause a variety of nerve dysfunctions. Just as in systemic lymphoma in the non-AIDS patient, this cancer can compress nerve roots either by epidural extension from bony disease or by infiltration into neural foramina and the epidural space.[264,298] Most frequently there is the sequential development of local or radicular pain, followed by segmental nerve deficit and finally by spinal cord compression. It is important to establish diagnosis in the early phases in order to prevent irreparable nerve or spinal cord injury and also to more specifically relieve pain. Neuroimaging is usually an essential component of diagnosis. Meningeal lymphomatosis may present with radicular or cranial nerve dysfunction.[299]

Recurrent VZV infection (herpes zoster) is perhaps the most common radiculopathy in the mid-phase of HIV-1 infection, but usually remains a diagnostic question only for the period between the onset of discomfort and the appearance of the characteristic rash. Although radicular pain may develop without rash (*zoster sine herpete*), this is unusual. Cutaneous zoster can also be complicated by myelopathy as described earlier.

Isolated unilateral or bilateral facial palsy has been recognized as a complication of AIDS from early in the epidemic.[265] This may occur in the presence or absence of CSF pleocytosis, and examples have been reported both in the early and late phases of HIV-1 infection. The course appears to be similar to that of individuals without HIV infection.[300–302]

Also important among the focal neuropathies that associate with HIV-1 are at least two types of mononeuritis multiplex (a disorder afflicting multiple independent peripheral nerves).[303] One of these occurs earlier (CD4+ T-lymphocyte count >200 cells/mm^3) in the course of HIV-1 infection, results in less severe deficits, and appears to be self-limiting.[304] It is presumed to have an immunopathologic basis and involve microvascular occlusions. Cryoglobulinemia has also been reported to associate with a vasculitic mononeuritis multiplex in an HIV-infected patient.[305] The more severe type of mononeuritis multiplex occurs when CD4+ T-lymphocyte counts are low (usually <50 cells), assumes a more malignant course, and is caused by CMV infection.[295,306] This disease has a penchant for affecting nerves supplying proximal muscles of the shoulder girdle. In the absence of treatment, it is often fatal. Diagnosis is usually made on clinical grounds, and treatment is with anti-CMV therapy either with one or more drugs depending upon previous CMV infections and treatments. Because diagnosis may be difficult or slow, patients should be treated aggressively on the basis of the clinical presentation alone. Hepatitis can also cause vasculitic neuropathy in those with or without HIV infection.[307]

MYOPATHIES

Several types of myopathies have been described complicating AIDS. They may have inflammatory (polymyositis) and noninflammatory pathology, including nemaline rod myopathy.[308–313] In both instances patients usually present with progressive proximal muscle weakness. Corticosteroid treatment has been the principal treatment of inflammatory myopathy and has been advocated by some for the noninflammatory myopathy as well. Zidovudine used to be the most common cause of myopathy in AIDS patients, but this now seems to be uncommon at current dosing and duration.[314–320] The pathogenesis likely relates to an effect of this nucleoside upon muscle mitochondria, and some biopsies show ragged red fibers with abnormal-appearing mitochondria. Inclusion body myositis has also been associated with HIV infection.[321] Diagnosis of myopathy is established by clinical features (pattern of proximal weakness, preservation of reflexes), laboratory findings (elevated creatinine kinase levels in blood), electrodiagnostic studies (small, brief "myopathic" potentials), and histologic analyses. The tests performed and their interpretation depend upon the clinical setting, severity and correlations among these different findings. Pyogenic infection, usually caused by *Staphylococcus aureus*, may cause severe myositis, and several other opportunistic infections, including *T. gondii*, *Cryptococcus neoformans*, and *Mycobacterium avium*, have been reported to involve muscle, but usually with less severe or silent clinical manifestations.[268,322]

CONCLUSIONS

On first consideration, the array of neurological diseases complicating HIV-1 infection and AIDS appears overwhelmingly complex. Although the algorithms outlined in the figures may also give this initial impression, with crossing lines and multiple tests, the range of common disorders is actually relatively narrow and diagnosis straightforward. Following a route from anatomic diagnosis through targeted laboratory testing will lead to a confirmed or high-probability presumptive diagnosis to guide therapy in perhaps 90% or more of cases. These will be made up largely of the common diseases discussed here. In the remaining 10% or so, diagnosis may be more difficult either because the clinical presentation is atypical or because the patient actually has a rarer condition. Finally, in a few patients diagnosis will turn out to be something previously unreported or will elude all efforts, because the complete map of neurological diseases complicating HIV-1 has not been drawn in detail. This should lead the clinician to a continuous sense of discovery and challenge in these patients, for whom exact diagnosis may importantly prolong the duration and the quality of life. Even when treatment is not available, informed prognosis allows patients, their families, and their caregivers to accurately plan the future. Although neurological disability often leads to therapeutic nihilism because of the patient's momentary incapacity, this is not always justified and should not take place in the face of diagnostic ignorance.

REFERENCES

1. Harrison MJG, McArthur JC. AIDS and Neurology. New York: Churchill Livingstone; 1995.
2. Berger JR, Levy RM. AIDS & the Nervous System. 2nd edn. Philadelphia, PA: Lippincott-Raven; 1997.
3. Marra CM. Bacterial and fungal brain infections in AIDS. Semin Neurol 19:177–84, 1999.
4. Ammassari A, Cingolani A, Pezzotti P, et al. AIDS-related focal brain lesions in the era of highly active antiretroviral therapy. Neurology 55:1194–200, 2000.
5. Brew BJ. HIV Neurology. New York: Oxford University Press; 2001.
6. McArthur JC, Brew BJ, Nath A. Neurological complications of HIV infection. Lancet Neurol 4:543–55, 2005.
7. Navia B, Price RW. An overview of the clinical and biological features of the AIDS dementia complex. In: Gendelman HE, Grant I, Everall I, et al (eds). The Neurology of AIDS, 2nd edn. Oxford: Oxford University Press; 2005, pp 339–56.
8. Gendelman HE, Grant I, Everall I, et al. The Neurology of AIDS, 2nd edn. Oxford: Oxford University Press; 2005.
9. Detels R, Tarwater P, Phair JP, et al. Effectiveness of potent antiretroviral therapies on the incidence of opportunistic infections before and after AIDS diagnosis. AIDS 15:347–55, 2001.
10. d'Arminio Monforte A, Cinque P, Mocroft A, et al. Changing incidence of central nervous system diseases in the EuroSIDA cohort. Ann Neurol 55:320–28, 2004.
11. Lee LM, Karon JM, Selik R, et al. Survival after AIDS diagnosis in adolescents and adults during the treatment era, United States, 1984–1997. JAMA 285:1308–15, 2001.
12. Berrey MM, Schacker T, Collier AC, et al. Treatment of primary human immunodeficiency virus type 1 infection with potent antiretroviral therapy reduces frequency of rapid progression to AIDS. J Infect Dis 183:1466–75, 2001.
13. Sacktor N, Lyles RH, Skolasky R, et al. HIV-associated neurologic disease incidence changes: Multicenter AIDS Cohort Study, 1990–1998. Neurology 56:257–60, 2001.
14. Maschke M, Kastrup O, Esser S, et al. Incidence and prevalence of neurological disorders associated with HIV since the

introduction of highly active antiretroviral therapy (HAART). J Neurol Neurosurg Psychiatry 69:376–80, 2000.
15. d'Arminio Monforte A, Duca PG, Vago L, et al. Decreasing incidence of CNS AIDS-defining events associated with antiretroviral therapy. Neurology 54:1856–9, 2000.
16. Brew BJ, Dore G. Decreasing incidence of CNS AIDS defining events associated with antiretroviral therapy. Neurology 55:1424, 2000.
17. Lanska DJ. Epidemiology of human immunodeficiency virus infection and associated neurologic illness. Semin Neurol 19:105–11, 1999.
18. Behrens GM, Meyer D, Stoll M, Schmidt RE. Immune reconstitution syndromes in human immuno-deficiency virus infection following effective antiretroviral therapy. Immunobiology 202:186–93, 2000.
19. DeSimone JA, Pomerantz RJ, Babinchak TJ. Inflammatory reactions in HIV-1-infected persons after initiation of highly active antiretroviral therapy. Ann Intern Med 133:447–54, 2000.
20. Gea-Banacloche JC, Clifford Lane H. Immune reconstitution in HIV infection. AIDS 13(Suppl A):S25–38, 1999.
21. Kaplan JE, Hanson D, Dworkin MS, et al. Epidemiology of human immunodeficiency virus-associated opportunistic infections in the United States in the era of highly active antiretroviral therapy. Clin Infect Dis 30(Suppl 1):S5–14, 2000.
22. Jenny-Avital ER, Abadi M. Immune reconstitution cryptococcosis after initiation of successful highly active antiretroviral therapy. Clin Infect Dis 35:e128–33, 2002.
23. Skiest DJ, Hester LJ, Hardy RD. Cryptococcal immune reconstitution inflammatory syndrome: report of four cases in three patients and review of the literature. J Infect 51:e289–97, 2005.
24. Woods ML 2nd, MacGinley R, Eisen DP, Allworth AM. HIV combination therapy: partial immune restitution unmasking latent cryptococcal infection. AIDS 12:1491–94, 1998.
25. Collazos J, Mayo J, Martinez E, Blanco MS. Contrast-enhancing progressive multifocal leukoencephalopathy as an immune reconstitution event in AIDS patients. AIDS 13:1426–28, 1999.
26. Miralles P, Berenguer J, Lacruz C, et al. Inflammatory reactions in progressive multifocal leukoencephalopathy after highly active antiretroviral therapy. AIDS 15:1900–2, 2001.
27. Safdar A, Rubocki RJ, Horvath JA, et al. Fatal immune restoration disease in human immunodeficiency virus type 1-infected patients with progressive multifocal leukoencephalopathy: impact of antiretroviral therapy-associated immune reconstitution. Clin Infect Dis 35:1250–7, 2002.
28. Crump JA, Tyrer MJ, Lloyd-Owen SJ, et al. Miliary tuberculosis with paradoxical expansion of intracranial tuberculomas complicating human immunodeficiency virus infection in a patient receiving highly active antiretroviral therapy. Clin Infect Dis 26:1008–9, 1998.
29. Sumner CJ, Newman M, Jay CA. Recurrent myelopathy after HAART in a patient with spinal mycobacterial infection. Neurology 61:139–40, 2003.
30. Lawn SD, Wood C, Lockwood DN. Borderline tuberculoid leprosy: an immune reconstitution phenomenon in a human immunodeficiency virus-infected person. Clin Infect Dis 36: e5–6, 2003.
31. Visco-Comandini U, Longo B, Cuzzi T, et al. Tuberculoid leprosy in a patient with AIDS: a manifestation of immune restoration syndrome. Scand J Infect Dis 36:881–3, 2004.
32. Piliero PJ, Fish DG, Preston S, et al. Guillain–Barre syndrome associated with immune reconstitution. Clin Infect Dis 36: e111–14, 2003.
33. Makela P, Howe L, Glover S, et al. Recurrent Guillain–Barre syndrome as a complication of immune reconstitution in HIV. J Infect 44:47–9, 2002.
34. Calza L, Manfredi R, Colangeli V, et al. Polymyositis associated with HIV infection during immune restoration induced by highly active anti-retroviral therapy. Clin Exp Rheumatol 22:651–2, 2004.
35. Domingo P, Torres OH, Ris J, Vazquez G. Herpes zoster as an immune reconstitution disease after initiation of combination antiretroviral therapy in patients with human immunodeficiency virus type-1 infection. Am J Med 110:605–9, 2001.
36. Organization WH. 1990 World Health Organization consultation on the neuropsychiatric aspects of HIV-1 infection. AIDS 4:935–6, 1990.
37. Janssen RS, Cornblath DR, Epstein LG, et al. Human immunodeficiency virus (HIV) infection and the nervous system: report from the American Academy of Neurology AIDS Task Force. Neurology 39:119–22, 1989.
38. Belman AL. Infants, children and adolescents. In: Berger JR, Levy RM (eds). AIDS and the Nervous System. 2nd edn. Philadelphia, PA: Lippincott-Raven; 1997, pp 223–53.
39. Mintz M. Clinical features and treatment interventions for human immunodeficiency virus-associated neurologic disease in children. Semin Neurol 19:165–76, 1999.
40. Price RW. Management of the Neurological Complications of HIV-1 and AIDS. In: Sande MA, Volberding PA (eds). The Medical Management of AIDS. 6th edn. Philadelphia, PA: WB Saunders; 1999, 217–40.
41. Navia BA, Jordan BD, Price RW. The AIDS dementia complex: I. Clinical features. Ann Neurol 19:517–24, 1986.
42. Epstein LG, Gendelman HE. Human immunodeficiency virus type 1 infection of the nervous system: pathogenetic mechanisms. Ann Neurol 33:429–36, 1993.
43. Price RW. Neurological complications of HIV infection. Lancet 348:445–52, 1996.
44. Zheng J, Gendelman HE. The HIV-1 associated dementia complex: a metabolic encephalopathy fueled by viral replication in mononuclear phagocytes. Curr Opin Neurol 10:319–25, 1997.
45. Wesselingh SL, Thompson KA. Immunopathogenesis of HIV-associated dementia. Curr Opin Neurol 14:375–9, 2001.
46. Kaul M, Garden GA, Lipton SA. Pathways to neuronal injury and apoptosis in HIV-associated dementia. Nature 410:988–94, 2001.
47. Nath A, Berger J. HIV Dementia. Curr Treat Options Neurol 6:139–51, 2004.
48. Gonzalez-Scarano F, Martin-Garcia J. The neuropathogenesis of AIDS. Nat Rev Immunol 5:69–81, 2005.
49. Price RW, Brew BJ. The AIDS dementia complex. J Infect Dis 158:1079–83, 1988.
50. Sidtis JJ, Price RW. Early HIV-1 infection and the AIDS dementia complex. Neurology 40:323–6, 1990.
51. Benson DF. The spectrum of dementia: a comparison of the clinical features of AIDS/dementia and dementia of the Alzheimer type. Alzheimer Dis Assoc Disord 1:217–20, 1987.
52. Gray F. Dementia and human inmmunodeficiency virus infection. Rev Neurol (Paris) 154(Suppl 2):S91–8, 1998.
53. Lopez OL, Smith G, Meltzer CC, Becker JT. Dopamine systems in human immunodeficiency virus-associated dementia. Neuropsychiatry Neuropsychol Behav Neurol 12:184–92, 1999.
54. Castellon SA, Hinkin CH, Myers HF. Neuropsychiatric disturbance is associated with executive dysfunction in HIV-1 infection. J Int Neuropsychol Soc 6:336–47, 2000.
55. McArthur JC, Selnes OA. Human immunodeficiency virus-associated dementia. In: Berger JR, Levy RM (eds). AIDS and the Nervous System. 2nd edn. Philadelphia, PA: Lippincott-Raven; 1997, pp 527–67.
56. Price RW. The AIDS dementia complex and human immunodeficiency virus type 1 infection of the central nervous system. In: Aminoff MJ, Goetz CG (eds). Handbook of Clinical Neurology, Systemic Diseases, Part III. Amsterdam: Elsevier Science; 1998, pp 235–60.
57. Sidtis JJ. Evaluation of the AIDS dementia complex in adults. Res Publ Assoc Res Nerv Ment Dis 72:273–87, 1994.

58. Dal Pan GJ, McArthur JH, Aylward E, et al. Patterns of cerebral atrophy in HIV-1-infected individuals: results of a quantitative MRI analysis. Neurology 42:2125–30, 1992.
59. Gelman BB, Guinto FC Jr. Morphometry, histopathology, and tomography of cerebral atrophy in the acquired immunodeficiency syndrome. Ann Neurol 32:31–40, 1992.
60. Post MJ. Fluid-attenuated inversion-recovery fast spin-echo MR: a clinically useful tool in the evaluation of neurologically symptomatic HIV-positive patients. AJNR Am J Neuroradiol 18:1611–16, 1997.
61. Tracey I, Carr CA, Guimaraes AR, et al. Brain choline-containing compounds are elevated in HIV-positive patients before the onset of AIDS dementia complex: a proton magnetic resonance spectroscopic study. Neurology 46:783–8, 1996.
62. Moller HE, Vermathen P, Lentschig MG, et al. Metabolic characterization of AIDS dementia complex by spectroscopic imaging. J Magn Reson Imaging 9:10–8, 1999.
63. Ernst T, Itti E, Itti L, Chang L. Changes in cerebral metabolism are detected prior to perfusion changes in early HIV-CMC: a coregistered (1)H MRS and SPECT study. J Magn Reson Imaging 12:859–65, 2000.
64. Chang L, Ernst T, Leonido-Yee M, et al. Cerebral metabolite abnormalities correlate with clinical severity of HIV-1 cognitive motor complex. Neurology 52:100–8, 1999.
65. Brew BJ, Bhalla RB, Paul M, et al. Cerebrospinal fluid neopterin in human immunodeficiency virus type 1 infection. Ann Neurol 28:556–60, 1990.
66. Heyes MP, Brew BJ, Saito K, et al. Inter-relationships between quinolinic acid, neuroactive kynurenines, neopterin and beta 2-microglobulin in cerebrospinal fluid and serum of HIV-1-infected patients. J Neuroimmunol 40:71–80, 1992.
67. McArthur JC, Nance-Sproson TE, Griffin DE, et al. The diagnostic utility of elevation in cerebrospinal fluid beta 2-microglobulin in HIV-1 dementia. Multicenter AIDS Cohort Study. Neurology 42:1707–12, 1992.
68. Conant K, McArthur JC, Griffin DE, et al. Cerebrospinal fluid levels of MMP-2, 7, and 9 are elevated in association with human immunodeficiency virus dementia. Ann Neurol 46:391–8, 1999.
69. Kelder W, McArthur JC, Nance-Sproson T, et al. Beta-chemokines MCP-1 and RANTES are selectively increased in cerebrospinal fluid of patients with human immunodeficiency virus-associated dementia. Ann Neurol 44:831–5, 1998.
70. Strain MC, Letendre S, Pillai SK, et al. Genetic composition of human immunodeficiency virus type 1 in cerebrospinal fluid and blood without treatment and during failing antiretroviral therapy. J Virol 79:1772–88, 2005.
71. Spudich SS, Huang W, Nilsson AC, et al. HIV-1 chemokine coreceptor utilization in paired cerebrospinal fluid and plasma samples: a survey of subjects with viremia. J Infect Dis 191:890–8, 2005.
72. Harrington PR, Haas DW, Ritola K, Swanstrom R. Compartmentalized human immunodeficiency virus type 1 present in cerebrospinal fluid is produced by short-lived cells. J Virol 79:7959–66, 2005.
73. Brew BJ, Pemberton L, Cunningham P, Law MG. Levels of human immunodeficiency virus type 1 RNA in cerebrospinal fluid correlate with AIDS dementia stage. J Infect Dis 175: 963–6, 1997.
74. Cinque P, Vago L, Ceresa D, et al. Cerebrospinal fluid HIV-1 RNA levels: correlation with HIV encephalitis. AIDS 12: 389–94, 1998.
75. Ellis RJ, Hsia K, Spector SA, et al. Cerebrospinal fluid human immunodeficiency virus type 1 RNA levels are elevated in neurocognitively impaired individuals with acquired immunodeficiency syndrome. HIV Neurobehavioral Research Center Group. Ann Neurol 42:679–88, 1997.
76. McArthur JC, McClernon DR, Cronin MF, et al. Relationship between human immunodeficiency virus-associated dementia and viral load in cerebrospinal fluid and brain. Ann Neurol 42:689–98, 1997.
77. Price RW, Staprans S. Measuring the "viral load" in cerebrospinal fluid in human immunodeficiency virus infection: window into brain infection? Ann Neurol 42:675–8, 1997.
78. Baldeweg T, Catalan J, Lovett E, et al. Long-term zidovudine reduces neurocognitive deficits in HIV-1 infection. AIDS 9:589–96, 1995.
79. Brouwers P, Moss H, Wolters P, et al. Effect of continuous-infusion zidovudine therapy on neuropsychologic functioning in children with symptomatic human immunodeficiency virus infection. J Pediatr 117:980–5, 1990.
80. Chiesi A, Vella S, Dally LG, et al. Epidemiology of AIDS dementia complex in Europe. AIDS in Europe Study Group. J Acquir Immune Defic Syndr Hum Retrovirol 11:39–44, 1996.
81. Filippi CG, Sze G, Farber SJ, et al. Regression of HIV encephalopathy and basal ganglia signal intensity abnormality at MR imaging in patients with AIDS after the initiation of protease inhibitor therapy. Radiology 206:491–8, 1998.
82. Gray F, Belec L, Keohane C, et al. Zidovudine therapy and HIV encephalitis: a 10-year neuropathological survey. AIDS 8:489–93, 1994.
83. Portegies P. Review of antiretroviral therapy in the prevention of HIV-related AIDS dementia complex (ADC). Drugs 49(Suppl 1):25–31; discussion 38–40, 1995.
84. Price RW. Management of AIDS dementia complex and HIV-1 infection of the nervous system. AIDS 9(Suppl A):S221–36, 1995.
85. Sacktor NC, Lyles RH, Skolasky RL, et al. Combination antiretroviral therapy improves psychomotor speed performance in HIV-seropositive homosexual men. Multicenter AIDS Cohort Study (MACS). Neurology 52:1640–7, 1999.
86. Schmitt FA, Bigley JW, McKinnis R, et al. Neuropsychological outcome of zidovudine (AZT) treatment of patients with AIDS and AIDS-related complex. N Engl J Med 319:1573–8, 1988.
87. Sidtis JJ, Gatsonis C, Price RW, et al. Zidovudine treatment of the AIDS dementia complex: results of a placebo-controlled trial. AIDS Clinical Trials Group. Ann Neurol 33:343–9, 1993.
88. Eggers C, Hertogs K, Sturenburg HJ, et al. Delayed central nervous system virus suppression during highly active antiretroviral therapy is associated with HIV encephalopathy, but not with viral drug resistance or poor central nervous system drug penetration. AIDS 17:1897–906, 2003.
89. Simone IL, Federico F, Tortorella C, et al. Localised 1H-MR spectroscopy for metabolic characterisation of diffuse and focal brain lesions in patients infected with HIV. J Neurol Neurosurg Psychiatry 64:516–23, 1998.
90. Albright AV, Erickson-Viitanen S, O'Connor M, et al. Efavirenz is a potent nonnucleoside reverse transcriptase inhibitor of HIV type 1 replication in microglia in vitro. AIDS Res Hum Retroviruses 16:1527–37, 2000.
91. Burger DM, Kraaijeveld CL, Meenhorst PL, et al. Penetration of zidovudine into the cerebrospinal fluid of patients infected with HIV. AIDS 7:1581–7, 1993.
92. Brew BJ. Neurological efficacy of stavudine, zidovudine, and lamivudine. Lancet 352:402, 1998.
93. Collier A, Marra C, Coombs R. Cerebrospinal fluid (CSF) HIV RNA levels in patients on chronic indinavir therapy. In: Abstracts of the Infectious Diseases Society of America, 35th Annual Meeting, San Francisco, 13–16 Sep 1997, abstract 22.
94. Foudraine NA, Hoetelmans RM, Lange JM, et al. Cerebrospinal-fluid HIV-1 RNA and drug concentrations after treatment with lamivudine plus zidovudine or stavudine. Lancet 351:1547–51, 1998.
95. Enting RH, Foudraine NA, Lange JM, et al. Cerebrospinal fluid beta2-microglobulin, monocyte chemotactic protein-1, and soluble tumour necrosis factor alpha receptors before and after

treatment with lamivudine plus zidovudine or stavudine. J Neuroimmunol 102:216–21, 2000.
96. Gisslen M, Svennerholm B, Fuchs D, Hagberg L. Neurological efficacy of stavudine, zidovudine, and lamivudine. Lancet 352:402–3, 1998.
97. Gisolf EH, Enting RH, Jurriaans S, et al. Cerebrospinal fluid HIV-1 RNA during treatment with ritonavir/saquinavir or ritonavir/saquinavir/stavudine. AIDS 14:1583–9, 2000.
98. Lanier ER, Sturge G, McClernon D, et al. HIV-1 reverse transcriptase sequence in plasma and cerebrospinal fluid of patients with AIDS dementia complex treated with Abacavir. AIDS 15:747–51, 2001.
99. Portegies P. HIV-1, the brain, and combination therapy. Lancet 346:1244–5, 1995.
100. Thomas SA, Segal MB. The transport of the anti-HIV drug, 2′,3′-didehydro-3′-deoxythymidine (D4T), across the blood–brain and blood–cerebrospinal fluid barriers. Br J Pharmacol 125:49–54, 1998.
101. Zhang L, Price R, Aweeka F, et al. Making the most of sparse clinical data by using a predictive-model-based analysis, illustrated with a stavudine pharmacokinetic study. Eur J Pharm Sci 12:377–85, 2001.
102. Letendre SL, Capparelli EV, Ellis RJ, McCutchan JA. Indinavir population pharmacokinetics in plasma and cerebrospinal fluid. The HIV Neurobehavioral Research Center Group. Antimicrob Agents Chemother 44:2173–5, 2000.
103. A randomized, double-blind, placebo-controlled trial of deprenyl and thioctic acid in human immunodeficiency virus-associated cognitive impairment. Dana Consortium on the Therapy of HIV Dementia and Related Cognitive Disorders. Neurology 50:645–51, 1998.
104. Clifford DB. Human immunodeficiency virus-associated dementia. Arch Neurol 57:321–4, 2000.
105. Navia BA, Dafni U, Simpson D, et al. A phase I/II trial of nimodipine for HIV-related neurologic complications. Neurology 51:221–8, 1998.
106. Cinque P, Cleator GM, Weber T, et al. Diagnosis and clinical management of neurological disorders caused by cytomegalovirus in AIDS patients. European Union Concerted Action on Virus Meningitis and Encephalitis. J Neurovirol 4:120–32, 1998.
107. Cohen B, Dix R. Cytomegalovirus and other herpesviruses. In: Berger J, Levy R (eds). AIDS and the Nervous System. 2nd edn. Philadelphia, PA: Lippincott-Raven; 1997, 595–639.
108. Fuller GN. Cytomegalovirus and the peripheral nervous system in AIDS. J Acquir Immune Defic Syndr 5(Suppl 1):S33–6, 1992.
109. Holland NR, Power C, Mathews VP, et al. Cytomegalovirus encephalitis in acquired immunodeficiency syndrome (AIDS). Neurology 44:507–14, 1992.
110. Kalayjian RC, Cohen ML, Bonomo RA, Flanigan TP. Cytomegalovirus ventriculoencephalitis in AIDS. A syndrome with distinct clinical and pathologic features. Medicine (Baltimore) 72:67–77, 1993.
111. McCutchan JA. Clinical impact of cytomegalovirus infections of the nervous system in patients with AIDS. Clin Infect Dis 21(Suppl 2):S196–201, 1995.
112. Salazar A, Podzamczer D, Rene R, et al. Cytomegalovirus ventriculoencephalitis in AIDS patients. Scand J Infect Dis 27:165–9, 1995.
113. Setinek U, Wondrusch E, Jellinger K, et al. Cytomegalovirus infection of the brain in AIDS: a clinicopathological study. Acta Neuropathol (Berl) 90:511–15, 1995.
114. Bell JE. The neuropathology of adult HIV infection. Rev Neurol (Paris) 154:816–29, 1998.
115. Gray F, Belec L, Geny C, Schouman-Claeys E. Diagnosis of diffuse encephalopathies in adults with HIV infection. I. Presse Med 22:1226–31, 1993.
116. Miller RF, Lucas SB, Hall-Craggs MA, et al. Comparison of magnetic resonance imaging with neuropathological findings in the diagnosis of HIV and CMV associated CNS disease in AIDS. J Neurol Neurosurg Psychiatry 62:346–51, 1997.
117. Petito CK, Cho ES, Lemann W, et al. Neuropathology of acquired immunodeficiency syndrome (AIDS): an autopsy review. J Neuropathol Exp Neurol 45:635–46, 1986.
118. Masdeu JC, Small CB, Weiss L, et al. Multifocal cytomegalovirus encephalitis in AIDS. Ann Neurol 23:97–9, 1988.
119. Cinque P, Vago L, Dahl H, et al. Polymerase chain reaction on cerebrospinal fluid for diagnosis of virus-associated opportunistic diseases of the central nervous system in HIV-infected patients. AIDS 10:951–8, 1996.
120. Arribas JR, Clifford DB, Fichtenbaum CJ, et al. Level of cytomegalovirus (CMV) DNA in cerebrospinal fluid of subjects with AIDS and CMV infection of the central nervous system. J Infect Dis 172:527–31, 1995.
121. Bestetti A, Pierotti C, Terreni M, et al. Comparison of three nucleic acid amplification assays of cerebrospinal fluid for diagnosis of cytomegalovirus encephalitis. J Clin Microbiol 39:1148–51, 2001.
122. Gozlan J, el Amrani M, Baudrimont M, et al. A prospective evaluation of clinical criteria and polymerase chain reaction assay of cerebrospinal fluid for the diagnosis of cytomegalovirus-related neurological diseases during AIDS. AIDS 9:253–60, 1995.
123. Zhang F, Tetali S, Wang XP, et al. Detection of human cytomegalovirus pp67 late gene transcripts in cerebrospinal fluid of human immunodeficiency virus type 1-infected patients by nucleic acid sequence-based amplification. J Clin Microbiol 38:1920–5, 2000.
124. Gray F, Gherardi R, Wingate E, et al. Diffuse "encephalitic" cerebral toxoplasmosis in AIDS. Report of four cases. J Neurol 236:273–7, 1989.
125. Navia B, Petito C, Gold J, et al. Cerebral toxoplasmosis complicating the acquired immune deficiency syndrome: clinical and neuropathological findings in 27 patients. Ann Neurol 19:224–38, 1986.
126. Nielsen CJ, Gjerris F, Pedersen H, et al. Brain biopsy in AIDS. Diagnostic value and consequence. Acta Neurochir (Wien) 127:99–102, 1994.
127. Cinque P, Vago L, Marenzi R, et al. Herpes simplex virus infections of the central nervous system in human immunodeficiency virus-infected patients: clinical management by polymerase chain reaction assay of cerebrospinal fluid. Clin Infect Dis 27:303–9, 1998.
128. Chretien F, Belec L, Hilton DA, et al. Herpes simplex virus type 1 encephalitis in acquired immunodeficiency syndrome. Neuropathol Appl Neurobiol 22:394–404, 1996.
129. Hamilton RL, Achim C, Grafe MR, et al. Herpes simplex virus brainstem encephalitis in an AIDS patient. Clin Neuropathol 14:45–50, 1995.
130. Hakim JG, Gangaidzo IT, Heyderman RS, et al. Impact of HIV infection on meningitis in Harare, Zimbabwe: a prospective study of 406 predominantly adult patients. AIDS 14:1401–7, 2000.
131. Saag MS, Graybill RJ, Larsen RA, et al. Practice guidelines for the management of cryptococcal disease. Infectious Diseases Society of America. Clin Infect Dis 30:710–8, 2000.
132. Torok ME, Day JN, Hien TT, Farrar JJ. Immediate or deferred antiretroviral therapy for central nervous system opportunistic infections? AIDS 19:535–6, 2005.
133. Klausner JD, Kent CK, Wong W, et al. The public health response to epidemic syphilis, San Francisco, 1999–2004. Sex Transm Dis 32:S11–8, 2005.
134. Ashton M, Sopwith W, Clark P, et al. An outbreak no longer: factors contributing to the return of syphilis in Greater Manchester. Sex Transm Infect 79:291–3, 2003.

135. Marra CM. Syphilis and human immunodeficiency virus: prevention and politics. Arch Neurol 61:1505–8, 2004.
136. Marra CM. Neurosyphilis. Curr Neurol Neurosci Rep 4:435–40, 2004.
137. Luger AF, Schmidt BL, Kaulich M. Significance of laboratory findings for the diagnosis of neurosyphilis. Int J STD AIDS 11:224–34, 2000.
138. Hart G. Syphilis tests in diagnostic and therapeutic decision making. Ann Intern Med 104:368–76, 1986.
139. Hook EW 3rd, Marra CM. Acquired syphilis in adults. N Engl J Med 326:1060–9, 1992.
140. Marra CM, Tantalo LC, Maxwell CL, et al. Alternative cerebrospinal fluid tests to diagnose neurosyphilis in HIV-infected individuals. Neurology 63:85–8, 2004.
141. Karstaedt AS, Valtchanova S, Barriere R, Crewe-Brown HH. Tuberculous meningitis in South African urban adults. QJM 91:743–7, 1998.
142. Schutte CM. Clinical, cerebrospinal fluid and pathological findings and outcomes in HIV-positive and HIV-negative patients with tuberculous meningitis. Infection 29:213–17, 2001.
143. Nadvi SS, Nathoo N, Annamalai K, et al. Role of cerebro-spinal fluid shunting for human immunodeficiency virus-positive patients with tuberculous meningitis and hydrocephalus. Neurosurgery Online 47:644–9; discussion 649–50, 2000.
144. Lipton RB, Feraru ER, Weiss G, et al. Headache in HIV-1-related disorders. Headache 31:518–22, 1991.
145. Lorenz KA, Shapiro MF, Asch SM, et al. Associations of symptoms and health-related quality of life: findings from a national study of persons with HIV infection. Ann Intern Med 134:854–60, 2001.
146. Graham CB 3rd, Wippold FJ 3rd. Headache in the HIV patient: a review with special attention to the role of imaging. Cephalalgia 21:169–74, 2001.
147. Gifford AL, Hecht FM. Evaluating HIV-infected patients with headache: who needs computed tomography? Headache 41:441–8, 2001.
148. Hewitt DJ, McDonald M, Portenoy RK, et al. Pain syndromes and etiologies in ambulatory AIDS patients. Pain 70:117–23, 1997.
149. Singer EJ, Kim J, Fahy-Chandon B, et al. Headache in ambulatory HIV-1-infected men enrolled in a longitudinal study. Neurology 47:487–94, 1996.
150. Berger JR, Stein N, Pall L. Headache and human immunodeficiency virus infection: a case control study. Eur Neurol 36:229–33, 1996.
151. Hollander H, Stringari S. Human immunodeficiency virus-associated meningitis. Clinical course and correlations. Am J Med 83:813–16, 1987.
152. Hollander H, McGuire D, Burack JH. Diagnostic lumbar puncture in HIV-infected patients: analysis of 138 cases. Am J Med 96:223–8, 1994.
153. Price RW, Paxinos EE, Grant RM et al. Cerebrospinal fluid response to structured treatment interruption after virological failure. AIDS 15:1251–9, 2001.
154. Staprans S, Marlowe N, Glidden D, et al. Time course of cerebrospinal fluid responses to antiretroviral therapy: evidence for variable compartmentalization of infection. AIDS 13:1051–61, 1999.
155. Brew BJ, Miller J. Human immunodeficiency virus-related headache. Neurology 43:1098–100, 1993.
156. Holloway RG, Kieburtz KD. Headache and the human immunodeficiency virus type 1 infection. Headache 35:245–55, 1995.
157. Post MJ, Yiannoutsos C, Simpson D et al. Progressive multifocal leukoencephalopathy in AIDS: are there any MR findings useful to patient management and predictive of patient survival? AIDS Clinical Trials Group, 243 Team. Am J Neuroradiol 20:1896–906, 1999.
158. Thurnher MM, Thurnher SA, Muhlbauer B, et al. Progressive multifocal leukoencephalopathy in AIDS: initial and follow-up CT and MRI. Neuroradiology 39:611–18, 1997.
159. Trotot PM, Vazeux R, Yamashita HK, et al. MRI pattern of progressive multifocal leukoencephalopathy (PML) in AIDS. Pathological correlations. J Neuroradiol 17:233–54, 1997.
160. von Giesen HJ, Neuen-Jacob E, Dorries K et al. Diagnostic criteria and clinical procedures in HIV-1 associated progressive multifocal leukoencephalopathy. J Neurol Sci 147:63–72, 1997.
161. Berger JR, Pall L, Lanska D, Whiteman M. Progressive multifocal leukoencephalopathy in patients with HIV infection. J Neurovirol 4:59–68, 1997.
162. Tornatore C, Berger JR, Houff SA, et al. Detection of JC virus DNA in peripheral lymphocytes from patients with and without progressive multifocal leukoencephalopathy. Ann Neurol 31:454–62, 1992.
163. Antinori A, Ammassari A, De Luca A, et al. Diagnosis of AIDS-related focal brain lesions: a decision-making analysis based on clinical and neuroradiologic characteristics combined with polymerase chain reaction assays in CSF. Neurology 48:687–94, 1992.
164. Garcia de Viedma D, Alonso R, Miralles P, et al. Dual qualitative-quantitative nested PCR for detection of JC virus in cerebrospinal fluid: high potential for evaluation and monitoring of progressive multifocal leukoencephalopathy in AIDS patients receiving highly active antiretroviral therapy. J Clin Microbiol 37:724–8, 1999.
165. Hammarin AL, Bogdanovic G, Svedhem V, et al. Analysis of PCR as a tool for detection of JC virus DNA in cerebrospinal fluid for diagnosis of progressive multifocal leukoencephalopathy. J Clin Microbiol 34:2929–32, 1996.
166. Matsiota-Bernard P, De Truchis P, Gray F, et al. JC virus detection in the cerebrospinal fluid of AIDS patients with progressive multifocal leucoencephalopathy and monitoring of the antiviral treatment by a PCR method. J Med Microbiol 46:256–9, 1996.
167. Yiannoutsos CT, Major EO, Curfman B, et al. Relation of JC virus DNA in the cerebrospinal fluid to survival in acquired immunodeficiency syndrome patients with biopsy-proven progressive multifocal leukoencephalopathy. Ann Neurol 45:816–21, 1999.
168. Bossolasco S, Calori G, Moretti F, et al. Prognostic significance of JC virus DNA levels in cerebrospinal fluid of patients with HIV-associated progressive multifocal leukoencephalopathy. Clin Infect Dis 40:738–44, 2005.
169. Marzocchetti A, Di Giambenedetto S, Cingolani A, et al. Reduced rate of diagnostic positive detection of JC virus DNA in cerebrospinal fluid in cases of suspected progressive multifocal leukoencephalopathy in the era of potent antiretroviral therapy. J Clin Microbiol 43:4175–7, 2005.
170. Berger JR, Mucke L. Prolonged survival and partial recovery in AIDS-associated progressive multifocal leukoencephalopathy. Neurology 38:1060–5, 2005.
171. Albrecht H, Hoffmann C, Degen O, et al. Highly active antiretroviral therapy significantly improves the prognosis of patients with HIV-associated progressive multifocal leukoencephalopathy. AIDS 12:1149–54, 1998.
172. Baldeweg T, Catalan J. Remission of progressive multifocal leucoencephalopathy after antiretroviral therapy. Lancet 349:1554–5, 1997.
173. Berger JR, Concha M. Progressive multifocal leukoencephalopathy: the evolution of a disease once considered rare. J Neurovirol 1:5–18, 1995.
174. Domingo P, Guardiola JM, Iranzo A, Margall N. Remission of progressive multifocal leucoencephalopathy after antiretroviral therapy. Lancet 349:1554–5, 1997.
175. Garrels K, Kucharczyk W, Wortzman G, Shandling M. Progressive multifocal leukoencephalopathy: clinical and MR

response to treatment. AJNR Am J Neuroradiol 17:597–600, 1996.
176. Miralles P, Berenguer J, Garcia de Viedma D, et al. Treatment of AIDS-associated progressive multifocal leukoencephalopathy with highly active antiretroviral therapy. AIDS 12:2467–72, 1998.
177. Hall CD, Dafni U, Simpson D, et al. Failure of cytarabine in progressive multifocal leukoencephalopathy associated with human immunodeficiency virus infection. AIDS Clinical Trials Group 243 Team. N Engl J Med 338:1345–51, 1998.
178. Houston S, Roberts N, Mashinter L. Failure of cidofovir therapy in progressive multifocal leukoencephalopathy unrelated to human immunodeficiency virus. Clin Infect Dis 32:150–2, 2001.
179. Happe S, Besselmann M, Matheja P, et al. Cidofovir (vistide) in therapy of progressive multifocal leukoencephalopathy in AIDS. Review of the literature and report of 2 cases. Nervenarzt 70:935–43, 1999.
180. De Luca A, Fantoni M, Tartaglione T, Antinori A. Response to cidofovir after failure of antiretroviral therapy alone in AIDS-associated progressive multifocal leukoencephalopathy. Neurology 52:891–2, 1999.
181. Marra CM, Rajicic N, Barker DE, et al. A pilot study of cidofovir for progressive multifocal leukoencephalopathy in AIDS. AIDS 16:1791–7, 2002.
182. Cinque P, Bossolasco S, Brambilla AM, et al. The effect of highly active antiretroviral therapy-induced immune reconstitution on development and outcome of progressive multifocal leukoencephalopathy: study of 43 cases with review of the literature. J Neurovirol 9(Suppl 1):73–80, 2003.
183. Cinque P, Koralnik IJ, Clifford DB. The evolving face of human immunodeficiency virus-related progressive multifocal leukoencephalopathy: defining a consensus terminology. J Neurovirol 9(Suppl 1):88–92, 2003.
184. Du Pasquier RA, Corey S, Margolin DH, et al. Productive infection of cerebellar granule cell neurons by JC virus in an HIV+ individual. Neurology 61:775–82, 2003.
185. Koralnik IJ, Wuthrich C, Dang X, et al. JC virus granule cell neuronopathy: a novel clinical syndrome distinct from progressive multifocal leukoencephalopathy. Ann Neurol 57:576–80, 2005.
186. Grant IH, Gold JW, Rosenblum M, et al. *Toxoplasma gondii* serology in HIV-infected patients: the development of central nervous system toxoplasmosis in AIDS. AIDS 4:519–21, 1990.
187. Belanger F, Derouin F, Grangeot-Keros L, Meyer L. Incidence and risk factors of toxoplasmosis in a cohort of human immunodeficiency virus-infected patients: 1988–95. HEMOCO and SEROCO Study Groups. Clin Infect Dis 28:575–81, 1999.
188. Israelski DM, Chmiel JS, Poggensee L, et al. Prevalence of *Toxoplasma* infection in a cohort of homosexual men at risk of AIDS and toxoplasmic encephalitis. J Acquir Immune Defic Syndr 6:414–8, 1993.
189. Brightbill TC, Post MJ, Hensley GT, Ruiz A. MR of *Toxoplasma* encephalitis: signal characteristics on T2-weighted images and pathologic correlation. J Comput Assist Tomogr 20:417–22, 1996.
190. Laissy JP, Soyer P, Tebboune J, et al. Contrast-enhanced fast MRI in differentiating brain toxoplasmosis and lymphoma in AIDS patients. J Comput Assist Tomogr 18:714–18, 1994.
191. Antinori A, Larussa D, Cingolani A, et al. Prevalence, associated factors, and prognostic determinants of AIDS-related toxoplasmic encephalitis in the era of advanced highly active antiretroviral therapy. Clin Infect Dis 39:1681–91, 2004.
192. Hawkins CP, McLaughlin JE, Kendall BE, McDonald WI. Pathological findings correlated with MRI in HIV infection. Neuroradiology 35:264–8, 1993.
193. Antinori A, De Rossi G, Ammassari A, et al. Value of combined approach with thallium-201 single-photon emission computed tomography and Epstein–Barr virus DNA polymerase chain reaction in CSF for the diagnosis of AIDS-related primary CNS lymphoma. J Clin Oncol 17:554–60, 1999.
194. d'Arminio Monforte A, Cinque P, Vago L, et al. A comparison of brain biopsy and CSF-PCR in the diagnosis of CNS lesions in AIDS patients. J Neurol 244:35–9, 1997.
195. DeAngelis LM. Primary central nervous system lymphoma: a new clinical challenge. Neurology 41:619–21, 1991.
196. Ernst TM, Chang L, Witt MD, et al. Cerebral toxoplasmosis and lymphoma in AIDS: perfusion MR imaging experience in 13 patients. Radiology 208:663–9, 1998.
197. Chang L, Ernst T. MR spectroscopy and diffusion-weighted MR imaging in focal brain lesions in AIDS. Neuroimaging Clin N Am 7:409–26, 1997.
198. Catafau AM, Sola M, Lomena FJ, et al. Hyperperfusion and early technetium-99m-HMPAO SPECT appearance of central nervous system toxoplasmosis. J Nucl Med 35:1041–3, 1994.
199. Hoffman JM, Waskin HA, Schifter T, et al. FDG-PET in differentiating lymphoma from nonmalignant central nervous system lesions in patients with AIDS. J Nucl Med 34:567–75, 1993.
200. Lorberboym M, Estok L, Machac J, et al. Rapid differential diagnosis of cerebral toxoplasmosis and primary central nervous system lymphoma by thallium-201 SPECT. J Nucl Med 37:1150–4, 1996.
201. Lorberboym M, Wallach F, Estok L, et al. Thallium-201 retention in focal intracranial lesions for differential diagnosis of primary lymphoma and nonmalignant lesions in AIDS patients. J Nucl Med 39:1366–9, 1998.
202. Skiest DJ, Erdman W, Chang WE, et al. SPECT thallium-201 combined with *Toxoplasma* serology for the presumptive diagnosis of focal central nervous system mass lesions in patients with AIDS. J Infect 40:274–81, 2000.
203. Skiest DJ, Crosby C. Survival is prolonged by highly active antiretroviral therapy in AIDS patients with primary central nervous system lymphoma. AIDS 17:1787–93, 2003.
204. McGowan JP, Shah S. Long-term remission of AIDS-related primary central nervous system lymphoma associated with highly active antiretroviral therapy. AIDS 12:952–4, 1998.
205. Hoffmann C, Tabrizian S, Wolf E, et al. Survival of AIDS patients with primary central nervous system lymphoma is dramatically improved by HAART-induced immune recovery. AIDS 15:2119–27, 2001.
206. Cheung MC, Pantanowitz L, Dezube BJ. AIDS-related malignancies: emerging challenges in the era of highly active antiretroviral therapy. Oncologist 10:412–26, 2005.
207. Lamontagne F, Lukiana T, Moulinier A, et al. Dramatic Improvement of Survival in AIDS-related Primary Central Nervous System Lymphoma with Combined High Dose Intravenous Methotrexate and HAART. In: 13th Conference on Retrovirology and Opportunisitic Infections, Denver, CO, 2006.
208. Vidal JE, Penalva de Oliveira AC, Bonasser Filho F, et al. Tuberculous brain abscess in AIDS patients: report of three cases and literature review. Int J Infect Dis 9:201–7, 2005.
209. Farrar DJ, Flanigan TP, Gordon NM, et al. Tuberculous brain abscess in a patient with HIV infection: case report and review. Am J Med 102:297–301, 1997.
210. Folgueira L, Delgado R, Palenque E, Noriega AR. Polymerase chain reaction for rapid diagnosis of tuberculous meningitis in AIDS patients. Neurology 44:1336–8, 1994.
211. Corti ME, Villafane MF, Yampolsky CG, Schtirbu RB. Brain abscess due to *Mycobacterium* tuberculosis in a patient with AIDS: report of a case and review of the literature. Int J Infect Dis 9:225–7, 1994.

212. Jones N, Khoosal M, Louw M, Karstaedt A. Nocardial infection as a complication of HIV in South Africa. J Infect 41:232–9, 2000.
213. Kim J, Minamoto GY, Grieco MH. Nocardial infection as a complication of AIDS: report of six cases and review. Rev Infect Dis 13:624–9, 1991.
214. Neal JW, Llewelyn MB, Morrison HL, et al. A malignant astrocytoma in a patient with AIDS: a possible association between astrocytomas and HIV infection. J Infect 33:159–62, 1996.
215. Vannemreddy PS, Fowler M, Polin RS, et al. Glioblastoma multiforme in a case of acquired immunodeficiency syndrome: investigation of a possible oncogenic influence of human immunodeficiency virus on glial cells. Case report and review of the literature. J Neurosurg 92:161–4, 2000.
216. Dyer JR, French MA, Mallal SA. Cerebral mass lesions due to cytomegalovirus in patients with AIDS: report of two cases. J Infect 30:147–51, 1995.
217. Mylonakis E, Paliou M, Sax PE, et al. Central nervous system aspergillosis in patients with human immunodeficiency virus infection. Report of 6 cases and review. Medicine (Baltimore) 79:269–80, 2000.
218. Stevens DA. Management of systemic manifestations of fungal disease in patients with AIDS. J Am Acad Dermatol 31: S64–7, 1994.
219. Viswanathan R, Ironside J, Bell JE, et al. Stereotaxic brain biopsy in AIDS patients: does it contribute to patient management? Br J Neurosurg 8:307–11, 1994.
220. Andrews BT, Kenefick TP. Neurosurgical management of the acquired immunodeficiency syndrome. An update. West J Med 158:249–53, 1993.
221. Miszkiel KA, Hall-Craggs MA, Miller RF, et al. The spectrum of MRI findings in CNS cryptococcosis in AIDS. Clin Radiol 51:842–50, 1996.
222. Garcia CA, Weisberg LA, Lacorte WS. Cryptococcal intracerebral mass lesions: CT-pathologic considerations. Neurology 35:731–4, 1985.
223. McGuire D, Bromley E, Aberg J, et al. Focal posterior hemisphere invasive cryptococcal encephalitis: a distinct neuroimaging entitity complicating cryptococcal meiningitis in AIDS [abstract]. Ann Neurol 41:467, 1997.
224. Berger JR, Harris JO, Gregorios J, Norenberg M. Cerebrovascular disease in AIDS: a case-control study. AIDS 4:239–44, 1990.
225. Connor MD, Lammie GA, Bell JE, et al. Cerebral infarction in adult AIDS patients: observations from the Edinburgh HIV Autopsy Cohort. Stroke 31:2117–26, 2000.
226. Davies J, Everall IP, Weich S, et al. HIV-associated brain pathology in the United Kingdom: an epidemiological study. AIDS 11:1145–50, 1997.
227. Engstrom JW, Lowenstein DH, Bredesen DE. Cerebral infarctions and transient neurologic deficits associated with acquired immunodeficiency syndrome. Am J Med 86:528–32, 1989.
228. Gillams AR, Allen E, Hrieb K, et al. Cerebral infarction in patients with AIDS. AJNR Am J Neuroradiol 18:1581–5, 1997.
229. Roquer J, Palomeras E, Knobel H, Pou A. Intracerebral haemorrhage in AIDS. Cerebrovasc Dis 8:222–7, 1998.
230. Morgello S, Block GA, Price RW, Petito CK. Varicella-zoster virus leukoencephalitis and cerebral vasculopathy. Arch Pathol Lab Med 112:173–7, 1988.
231. Hilt DC, Buchholz D, Krumholz A, et al. Herpes zoster ophthalmicus and delayed contralateral hemiparesis caused by cerebral angiitis: diagnosis and management approaches. Ann Neurol 14:543–53, 1983.
232. Picard O, Brunereau L, Pelosse B, et al. Cerebral infarction associated with vasculitis due to varicella zoster virus in patients infected with the human immunodeficiency virus. Biomed Pharmacother 51:449–54, 1997.
233. Gilden DH, Kleinschmidt-DeMasters BK, Wellish M, et al. Varicella zoster virus, a cause of waxing and waning vasculitis: the New England Journal of Medicine case 5–1995 revisited. Neurology 47:1441–6, 1996.
234. Kleinschmidt-DeMasters BK, Amlie-Lefond C, Gilden DH. The patterns of varicella zoster virus encephalitis. Hum Pathol 27:927–38, 1996.
235. Thirumalai S, Kirshner HS. Anticardiolipin antibody and stroke in an HIV-positive patient. AIDS 8:1019–20, 1994.
236. Petito C, Navia B, Cho E, et al. Vacuolar myelopathy pathologically resembling subacute combined degeneration in patients with acquired immunodeficiency syndrome (AIDS). N Engl J Med 312:874–9, 1985.
237. Navia BA, Cho ES, Petito CK, Price RW. The AIDS dementia complex. II. Neuropathology. Ann Neurol 19:525–35, 1986.
238. Di Rocco A. Diseases of the spinal cord in human immunodeficiency virus infection. Semin Neurol 19:151–5, 1999.
239. Dal Pan GJ, Glass JD, McArthur JC. Clinicopathologic correlations of HIV-1-associated vacuolar myelopathy: an autopsy-based case-control study. Neurology 44:2159–64, 1994.
240. Petito CK, Vecchio D, Chen YT. HIV antigen and DNA in AIDS spinal cords correlate with macrophage infiltration but not with vacuolar myelopathy. J Neuropathol Exp Neurol53:86–94, 1994.
241. Rosenblum M, Scheck AC, Cronin K, et al. Dissociation of AIDS-related vacuolar myelopathy and productive HIV-1 infection of the spinal cord. Neurology 39:892–6, 1989.
242. Schmidbauer M, Budka H, Okeda R et al. Multifocal vacuolar leucoencephalopathy: a distinct HIV-associated lesion of the brain. Neuropathol Appl Neurobiol 16:437–43, 1990.
243. Shepherd EJ, Brettle RP, Liberski PP, et al. Spinal cord pathology and viral burden in homosexuals and drug users with AIDS. Neuropathol Appl Neurobiol 25:2–10, 1999.
244. Di Rocco A, Bottiglieri T, Werner P, et al. Abnormal cobalamin-dependent transmethylation in AIDS-associated myelopathy. Neurology 58:730–5, 2002.
245. Chong J, Di Rocco A, Tagliati M, et al. MR findings in AIDS-associated myelopathy. AJNR Am J Neuroradiol 20:1412–16, 1999.
246. Nakagawa M, Izumo S, Ijichi S, et al. HTLV-I-associated myelopathy: analysis of 213 patients based on clinical features and laboratory findings. J Neurovirol 1:50–61, 1995.
247. Nakagawa M, Nakahara K, Maruyama Y, et al. Therapeutic trials in 200 patients with HTLV-I-associated myelopathy/tropical spastic paraparesis. J Neurovirol 2:345–55, 1996.
248. Kitze B, Puccioni-Sohler M, Schaffner J, et al. Specificity of intrathecal IgG synthesis for HTLV-1 core and envelope proteins in HAM/TSP. Acta Neurol Scand 92:213–17, 1995.
249. Kitze B, Brady JN. Human T cell lymphotropic retroviruses: association with diseases of the nervous system. Intervirology 40:132–42, 1997.
250. Izumo S, Umehara F, Kashio N, et al. Neuropathology of HTLV-1-associated myelopathy (HAM/TSP). Leukemia 11(Suppl 3):82–4, 1997.
251. Murphy EL, Fridey J, Smith JW, et al. HTLV-associated myelopathy in a cohort of HTLV-I and HTLV-II-infected blood donors. The REDS investigators. Neurology 48:315–20, 1997.
252. Lehky TJ, Flerlage N, Katz D, et al. Human T-cell lymphotropic virus type II-associated myelopathy: clinical and immunologic profiles. Ann Neurol 40:714–23, 1996.
253. Geraci A, Di Rocco A, Liu M, et al. AIDS myelopathy is not associated with elevated HIV viral load in cerebrospinal fluid. Neurology 55:440–2, 2000.
254. Di Rocco A, Tagliati M. Remission of HIV myelopathy after highly active antiretroviral therapy. Neurology 55:456, 2000.
255. Devinsky O, Cho ES, Petito CK, Price RW. Herpes zoster myelitis. Brain 114(Pt 3):1181–96, 1991.

256. Gray F, Belec L, Lescs MC, et al. Varicella-zoster virus infection of the central nervous system in the acquired immune deficiency syndrome. Brain 117(Pt 5):987–99, 1994.
257. Cinque P, Bossolasco S, Vago L, et al. Varicella-zoster virus (VZV) DNA in cerebrospinal fluid of patients infected with human immunodeficiency virus: VZV disease of the central nervous system or subclinical reactivation of VZV infection? Clin Infect Dis 25:634–9, 1997.
258. Burke DG, Kalayjian RC, Vann VR, et al. Polymerase chain reaction detection and clinical significance of varicella-zoster virus in cerebrospinal fluid from human immunodeficiency virus-infected patients. J Infect Dis 176:1080–4, 1997.
259. Thurnher MM, Post MJ, Jinkins JR. MRI of infections and neoplasms of the spine and spinal cord in 55 patients with AIDS. Neuroradiology 42:551–63, 2000.
260. Quencer RM, Post MJ. Spinal cord lesions in patients with AIDS. Neuroimaging Clin N Am 7:359–73, 1997.
261. Resnick DK, Comey CH, Welch WC, et al. Isolated toxoplasmosis of the thoracic spinal cord in a patient with acquired immunodeficiency syndrome. Case report. J Neurosurg 82:493–6, 1995.
262. Henin D, Smith TW, De Girolami U, et al. Neuropathology of the spinal cord in the acquired immunodeficiency syndrome. Hum Pathol 23:1106–14, 1992.
263. Fairley CK, Wodak J, Benson E. Spinal cord toxoplasmosis in a patient with human immunodeficiency virus infection. Int J STD AIDS 3:366–8, 1992.
264. Levy RM, Bredesen DE, Rosenblum ML. Neurological manifestations of the acquired immunodeficiency syndrome (AIDS): experience at UCSF and review of the literature. J Neurosurg 62:475–95, 1985.
265. Snider WD, Simpson DM, Nielsen S, et al. Neurological complications of acquired immune deficiency syndrome: analysis of 50 patients. Ann Neurol 14:403–18, 1983.
266. Chamberlain MC, Dirr L. Involved-field radiotherapy and intra-Ommaya methotrexate/cytarabine in patients with AIDS-related lymphomatous meningitis. J Clin Oncol 11:1978–84, 1993.
267. Eidelberg D, Sotrel A, Vogel H et al. Progressive polyradiculopathy in acquired immune deficiency syndrome. Neurology 36:912–16, 1986.
268. Simpson D, Tagliati M. Neuromuscular syndromes in human immunodeficiency virus disease. In: Berger J, Levy R (eds). AIDS and the Nervous System. 2nd edn. Philadelphia, PA: Lippincott-Raven; 1997, pp 189–221.
269. Verma A. Epidemiology and clinical features of HIV-1 associated neuropathies. J Peripher Nerv Syst 6:8–13, 2001.
270. Rizzuto N, Cavallaro T, Monaco S, et al. Role of HIV in the pathogenesis of distal symmetrical peripheral neuropathy. Acta Neuropathol (Berl) 90:244–50, 1995.
271. Cornblath DR, McArthur JC. Predominantly sensory neuropathy in patients with AIDS and AIDS-related complex. Neurology 38:794–6, 1988.
272. Wesselingh SL, Glass J, McArthur JC et al. Cytokine dysregulation in HIV-associated neurological disease. Adv Neuroimmunol 4:199–206, 1994.
273. Cherry CL, Wesselingh SL, Lal L, McArthur JC. Evaluation of a clinical screening tool for HIV-associated sensory neuropathies. Neurology 65:1778–81, 2005.
274. McArthur JC, Yiannoutsos C, Simpson DM, et al. A phase II trial of nerve growth factor for sensory neuropathy associated with HIV infection. AIDS Clinical Trials Group Team 291. Neurology 54:1080–8, 2000.
275. Newshan G. HIV neuropathy treated with gabapentin. AIDS 12:219–21, 1998.
276. Nicholson B. Gabapentin use in neuropathic pain syndromes. Acta Neurol Scand 101:359–71, 2000.
277. Tremont-Lukats IW, Megeff C, Backonja MM. Anticonvulsants for neuropathic pain syndromes: mechanisms of action and place in therapy. Drugs 60:1029–52, 2000.
278. Max MB. Treatment of post-herpetic neuralgia: antidepressants. Ann Neurol 35(Suppl):S50–3, 1994.
279. Simpson DM, McArthur JC, Olney R, et al. Lamotrigine for HIV-associated painful sensory neuropathies: a placebo-controlled trial. Neurology 60:1508–14, 2003.
280. Adkins JC, Peters DH, Faulds D. Zalcitabine. An update of its pharmacodynamic and pharmacokinetic properties and clinical efficacy in the management of HIV infection. Drugs 53:1054–80, 1997.
281. Blum AS, Dal Pan GJ, Feinberg J, et al. Low-dose zalcitabine-related toxic neuropathy: frequency, natural history, and risk factors. Neurology 46:999–1003, 1996.
282. Berger AR, Arezzo JC, Schaumburg HH, et al. 2′,3′-dideoxycytidine (ddC) toxic neuropathy: a study of 52 patients. Neurology 43:358–62, 1993.
283. Fichtenbaum CJ, Clifford DB, Powderly WG. Risk factors for dideoxynucleoside-induced toxic neuropathy in patients with the human immunodeficiency virus infection. J Acquir Immune Defic Syndr Hum Retrovirol 10:169–74, 1995.
284. Moyle GJ, Sadler M. Peripheral neuropathy with nucleoside antiretrovirals: risk factors, incidence and management. Drug Saf 19:481–94, 1998.
285. Rana KZ, Dudley MN. Clinical pharmacokinetics of stavudine. Clin Pharmacokinet 33:276–84, 1997.
286. Simpson DM, Tagliati M. Nucleoside analogue-associated peripheral neuropathy in human immunodeficiency virus infection. J Acquir Immune Defic Syndr Hum Retrovirol 9:153–61, 1995.
287. Waldinger TP, Siegle RJ, Weber W, Voorhees JJ. Dapsone-induced peripheral neuropathy. Case report and review. Arch Dermatol 120:356–59, 1984.
288. Bradley WG, Verma A. Painful vasculitic neuropathy in HIV-1 infection: relief of pain with prednisone therapy. Neurology 47:1446–51, 1996.
289. Moulignier A, Authier FJ, Baudrimont M, et al. Peripheral neuropathy in human immunodeficiency virus-infected patients with the diffuse infiltrative lymphocytosis syndrome. Ann Neurol 41:438–45, 1997.
290. Estanislao LB, Morgello S, Simpson DM. Peripheral neuropathies associated with HIV and hepatitis C co-infection: a review. AIDS 19(Suppl 3):S135–9, 2005.
291. Cornblath DR, Griffin JW, Tennekoon GI. Immunoreactive myelin basic protein in cerebrospinal fluid of patients with peripheral neuropathies. Ann Neurol 20:370–2, 1986.
292. Saperstein DS, Katz JS, Amato AA, Barohn RJ. Clinical spectrum of chronic acquired demyelinating polyneuropathies. Muscle Nerve 24:311–24, 2001.
293. Lindenbaum Y, Kissel JT, Mendell JR. Treatment approaches for Guillain-Barre syndrome and chronic inflammatory demyelinating polyradiculoneuropathy. Neurol Clin 19:187–204, 2001.
294. Kolson DL, Gonzalez-Scarano F. HIV-associated neuropathies: role of HIV-1, CMV, and other viruses. J Peripher Nerv Syst 6:2–7, 2001.
295. Said G, Lacroix C, Chemouilli P, et al. Cytomegalovirus neuropathy in acquired immunodeficiency syndrome: a clinical and pathological study. Ann Neurol 29:139–46, 1991.
296. So YT, Olney RK. Acute lumbosacral polyradiculopathy in acquired immunodeficiency syndrome: experience in 23 patients. Ann Neurol 35:53–8, 1994.
297. Calabrese LH, Proffitt MR, Levin KH, et al. Acute infection with the human immunodeficiency virus (HIV) associated with acute brachial neuritis and exanthematous rash. Ann Intern Med 107:849–51, 1987.

298. Berger JR, Flaster M, Schatz N, et al. Cranial neuropathy heralding otherwise occult AIDS-related large cell lymphoma. J Clin Neuroophthalmol 13:113–18, 1993.
299. Enting RH, Esselink RA, Portegies P. Lymphomatous meningitis in AIDS-related systemic non-Hodgkin's lymphoma: a report of eight cases. J Neurol Neurosurg Psychiatry 57:150–3, 1994.
300. Schot LJ, Devriese PP, Hadderingh RJ, et al. Facial palsy and human immunodeficiency virus infection. Eur Arch Otorhinolaryngol S498–500, 1994.
301. Murr AH, Benecke JE Jr. Association of facial paralysis with HIV positivity. Am J Otol 12:450–1, 1991.
302. Casanova-Sotolongo P, Casanova-Carrillo P. Association of peripheral facial paralysis in patients with human immunodeficiency virus infection. Rev Neurol 32:327–30, 2001.
303. So Y, Olney R. The natural history of mononeuropathy multiplex and simplex in patients with HIV infection [abstract]. Neurology 41(Suppl):374, 1991.
304. Lipkin WI, Parry G, Kiprov D, Abrams D. Inflammatory neuropathy in homosexual men with lymphadenopathy. Neurology 35:1479–83, 1985.
305. Stricker RB, Sanders KA, Owen WF, et al. Mononeuritis multiplex associated with cryoglobulinemia in HIV infection. Neurology 42:2103–5, 1992.
306. Roullet E, Assuerus V, Gozlan J, et al. Cytomegalovirus multifocal neuropathy in AIDS: analysis of 15 consecutive cases. Neurology 44:2174–82, 1994.
307. Said G, Lacroix C. Primary and secondary vasculitic neuropathy. J Neurol 252:633–41, 2005.
308. Wulff EA, Simpson DM. Neuromuscular complications of the human immunodeficiency virus type 1 infection. Semin Neurol 19:157–64, 1999.
309. Simpson DM, Bender AN. Human immunodeficiency virus-associated myopathy: analysis of 11 patients. Ann Neurol 24:79–84, 1988.
310. Nordstrom DM, Petropolis AA, Giorno R, et al. Inflammatory myopathy and acquired immunodeficiency syndrome. Arthritis Rheum 32:475–9, 1989.
311. Miro O, Grau JM, Pedrol E. Distinct light microscopic changes in HIV-associated nemaline myopathy. Neurology 53:241–2, 1999.
312. Gherardi RK. Skeletal muscle involvement in HIV-infected patients. Neuropathol Appl Neurobiol 20:232–7, 1994.
313. Bailey RO, Turok DI, Jaufmann BP, Singh JK. Myositis and acquired immunodeficiency syndrome. Hum Pathol 18:749–51, 1987.
314. Arnaudo E, Dalakas M, Shanske S, et al. Depletion of muscle mitochondrial DNA in AIDS patients with zidovudine-induced myopathy. Lancet 337:508–10, 1991.
315. Casademont J, Barrientos A, Grau JM, et al. The effect of zidovudine on skeletal muscle mtDNA in HIV-1 infected patients with mild or no muscle dysfunction. Brain 119(Pt 4):1357–64, 1996.
316. Dalakas MC, Illa I, Pezeshkpour GH, et al. Mitochondrial myopathy caused by long-term zidovudine therapy. N Engl J Med 322:1098–105, 1990.
317. Manji H, Harrison MJ, Round JM, et al. Muscle disease, HIV and zidovudine: the spectrum of muscle disease in HIV-infected individuals treated with zidovudine. J Neurol 240:479–88, 1993.
318. Masanes F, Pedrol E, Grau JM, et al. Symptomatic myopathies in HIV-1 infected patients untreated with antiretroviral agents – a clinico-pathological study of 30 consecutive patients. Clin Neuropathol 15:221–5, 1996.
319. Morgello S, Wolfe D, Godfrey E, et al. Mitochondrial abnormalities in human immunodeficiency virus-associated myopathy. Acta Neuropathol (Berl) 90:366–74, 1995.
320. Peters BS, Winer J, Landon DN, et al. Mitochondrial myopathy associated with chronic zidovudine therapy in AIDS. Q J Med 86:5–15, 1993.
321. Dalakas MC. Inflammatory, immune, and viral aspects of inclusion-body myositis. Neurology 66:S33–8, 2006.
322. Gherardi R, Baudrimont M, Lionnet F, et al. Skeletal muscle toxoplasmosis in patients with acquired immunodeficiency syndrome: a clinical and pathological study. Ann Neurol 32:535–42, 1992.

Chapter 63

AIDS Psychiatry

Alex Thompson, MD, MBA, Benjamin C. Silverman, BA, Andrew Angelino MD, Glenn J. Treisman, MD, PhD

INTRODUCTION

HIV infection is spread through intimate contact, which involves specific behaviors that place patients at risk. Since the late 1980s, prevention programs have focused on education for populations at risk for HIV, and those who are unable to change behaviors despite education often suffer from vulnerabilities, like major psychiatric illness, impulsivity, or cognitive limitations. Those same vulnerabilities often prove to be major obstacles to effective treatment. It takes organization, support, and education to participate in the antiretroviral treatment necessary to suppress this disease. Being able to guide each patient to his or her highest level of functioning goes a long way toward promoting disease suppression. For that reason, HIV care providers need familiarity with the psychiatric problems commonly present in those with HIV and AIDS. This chapter will present descriptions and practical management approaches to the psychiatric problems frequently encountered in the care of HIV patients.

THE ROLE OF PSYCHIATRIC ILLNESS IN HIV TRANSMISSION

Prior to the mid-1980s, the public was relatively unaware of the risk factors related to both contracting and transmitting HIV. As education improved, individuals learned to protect themselves by avoiding the risky behaviors well understood to transmit the virus.[1,2] Historically, risk reducing measures have included screening donors and donated blood products, abstinence from sex or safe sexual practices, and using clean needles for injection drugs. Due to these public health efforts, much of the developed world understands the transmission routes and risk factors of HIV and AIDS. Despite this, vulnerable populations of people continue to engage in activities that place them at risk for contracting and transmitting HIV.

Individuals with severe mental illness (such as recurrent major depression, bipolar affective disorder, and schizophrenia) and substance abuse problems (also a psychiatric problem) make up a large part of this vulnerable population. Between 3% and 23% of adults with severe mental illness are HIV positive, compared to 0.6% of the population in the United States.[3] Those with severe mental illness are at risk for contracting HIV through high-risk sexual and drug use behavior. A 1996 epidemiologic study of 2864 patients receiving medical care for HIV found a 1-year prevalence of ~50% for psychiatric illness, with only 27.2% using a psychotropic medication.[4] In the outpatient HIV clinic at Johns Hopkins Hospital (Moore Clinic), just over half of the patients who seek medical care have a major psychiatric disorder other than substance abuse (75% have a substance abuse disorder).[5,6]

Patients with HIV/AIDS and mental illness often lack the capacity to adhere to complicated medication regimens.[7,8] Additionally, we now know that HIV infection carries its own psychiatric sequelae, such as AIDS mania and dementia, compounding the disease manifestations and containment efforts in certain patients. In effect, AIDS has become a psychiatric epidemic, in which those individuals at greatest risk of exposure to and spread of the virus are mentally ill patients who are unable to incorporate preventive, educational, or medical measures into their lives. Treatment of co-morbid psychiatric illness can improve patient care and therapeutic outcomes, effectively fighting the spread of the AIDS epidemic.

PSYCHIATRIC FORMULATION

A thorough psychiatric formulation, like its counterpart in any medical field, allows the physician to develop a comprehensive treatment plan that addresses all the problems of the patients, therefore increasing the chances of treatment success. Psychiatric diagnosis is limited by the lack of chemical, genetic, and radiological tests assisting in the placement of presenting signs and symptoms under a diagnostic label that guides evidence-based treatment. This situation makes a comprehensive formulation guiding overall treatment vital. One method of organizing the complicated clinical details which the patients present has been described.[9] It is a formulation that involves looking at the details of a comprehensive history, mental state exam, and physical exam so as to develop a formula that encompasses four different vantages, or perspectives. Those perspectives are (1) the disease, (2) the dimension, (3) the behavior, and (4) the life story.

The Disease

The disease perspective assumes that some psychiatric disorders represent the results of specific deficits in brain function, such as a lesion. This perspective categorizes patients into distinct groups, based upon the presence of defining characteristics of an illness. Disease reasoning implies the presence of a lesion or pathophysiologic etiology to explain the presenting signs and symptoms that are common across patient populations. There are a few psychiatric diseases despite the lack of identified lesions (this is an area of controversy). The idiopathic forms of schizophrenia, recurrent major depression, and bipolar disorder are likely to be related to specific disease states of focal brain function. Some of these conditions can be modeled using lesions in the brains of animals, but the models remain incomplete. Panic-like anxiety may fall in this category also. The recognition of disease states in psychiatry, guides research and empirical treatment of conditions that have a major impact on the well-being and self-care of patients.

The Dimension

The dimensional perspective takes into account individual variations in psychological determinants, such as extraversion or intelligence. Dimensional characteristics of humans include height, weight, and skin color. It is the same for personality characteristics and intelligence. Recognizing that your patient may, in fact, be mildly mentally retarded by asking questions about schooling, special education, and prior testing may go a long way toward helping clinicians craft a productive treatment plan. It goes the same for recognizing patient personality types such as introverted and extraverted, stable and unstable, and how these features of a person affect the care plan. It is clear that these features are related to risky behaviors and the ability to adapt to the constraints of HIV infection.

The Behavior

This perspective presumes that some patients have disorders based on specific goal-directed behaviors that interfere with other types of functioning. This approach assumes that certain behaviors are conditioned, that is, that they are entrained by rewards and consequences until they become automatic. Addictions to drugs and alcohol, eating disorders and other behaviors are the result of appetite-based drives and cravings. Many patients are in the HIV clinic as a direct result of something they did while trying to accomplish an altogether different goal. The drive for these behaviors seems overwhelming to patients, who feel that they 'cannot help it' when they use drugs, eat too much, or compulsively starve themselves, or go out to look for anonymous sexual partners of a particular sort. The behaviors are 'shaped' by a complex set of internal and external rewards and consequences that ultimately result in specific behavioral actions. Changing behavior is one of the most difficult and critical aspects to improving the life of patients.

The Life Story

The events of a person's life have a profound impact on the way diseases, personalities, and behaviors are expressed. One must evaluate psychiatric disorders within the context of the life that they occur in and appreciating that story and understanding its interplay with the patient's personality, motivated behaviors, and illnesses, allows you the opportunity to help them change course. This is the part of psychiatry that understands that a person who was molested as a child may have trust issues as an adult, or that someone who grew up in an oppressive environment may have difficulty with figures of authority. The psychological makeup of a person develops in large part from their experience.

PSYCHIATRIC TREATMENT

The treatment plan for each patient must be informed by the following:

1. the diagnosis and available treatments;
2. the availability of treatment for a particular patient;
3. the patient's ability to engage in and tolerate the treatment and its side effects; and
4. the interactions the psychiatric treatment may have with other treatments (for instance, will the antidepressant interact with a protease inhibitor).

Unfocused, symptomatic treatment is less desirable than diagnostically driven treatment. For instance, providing anxiety-relieving benzodiazepines (like alprazolam) to treat a patient's anxiety is far less productive than diagnosing a panic disorder (if it is present), educating the patient about it, and treating with an antidepressant (like sertraline). Understanding the patient and diagnosis creates the opportunity to evaluate the benefit of treatment compared with the side effects of the treatment. The process of illness education and discussion of risks and benefits of treatment is critical when developing a therapeutic alliance with the patient. The therapeutic alliance serves the purpose of bringing patients back to the clinic and promoting their adherence to the medications and other treatments prescribed.[10,11]

In many psychiatric conditions, available evidence supports a number of treatment options (like cognitive behavioral therapy, medication, or a combination of the two). There is no evidence that one antidepressant is more effective than others at treating major depression in HIV-positive patients. Therefore, clinicians have the option to initiate treatment with any approved antidepressant. Similarly, data often show similar success rates for medication and behavioral therapy-based treatment options. In panic disorder, the literature suggests that cognitive behavioral treatments, including exposure/desensitization therapy, and medications have similar efficacy.[12–14] Combination treatment with cognitive behavioral therapy and medication may have even greater success.[15] The availability of treatments may have a large impact on what is chosen for your patient. For instance, is cognitive behavioral therapy available for a patient with a depression or anxiety disorder and does his insurance cover it? Can he or she engage in therapy or make use of it? Does the treating clinician have time to provide the labor-intensive therapy? These questions realistically guide the psychiatric treatment.

MEDICATION INTERACTIONS

Patients living with HIV and AIDS routinely have complicated medical regimens, involving multiple antiretroviral and antimicrobial drugs. As a result, rational treatment of psychiatric disorders in these patients requires careful consideration of potential drug interactions. Like patients with other chronic medical conditions, HIV-positive patients may have delayed absorption, metabolism, and excretion of medications, as well as diminished renal and hepatic clearance. These differences can complicate treatment decisions and worsen medication interactions.

Decisions regarding medications require some understanding of the cytochrome P450 metabolism of both antiretrovirals and psychiatric medications. All antiretrovirals beside the nucleoside reverse transcriptase inhibitors (NRTIs) and fusion inhibitor, enfuvirtide, are metabolized by the CYP system. HIV protease inhibitors (PIs), such as lopinavir and ritonavir, typically inhibit the CYP 3A4 and 2D6 isoenzymes. Non-nucleoside reverse transcriptase inhibitors (NNRTIs), including nevirapine and efavirenz, generally induce these same systems.[16–20] Fortunately, in spite of these theoretical drug interactions, there are few clinically significant adverse reactions, likely because most medications utilize multiple metabolic pathways. At the same time, real increases in plasma concentrations may have little or no clinical impact as a result of the wide therapeutic indices of many medications. Many documented interactions involve ritonavir, which appears to be one of the most powerful inhibitors of the CYP 3A and 2D6 isoenzymes. The clinical relevance of most potential interactions remains largely unknown, necessitating the need for close observation of patients with co-administration of these drug classes.[21,22] While this is an area that needs additional research, we are hopeful that the improved mental health and medication adherence that can result from the use of psychotropics outweighs the potential impact on antiretroviral blood levels.[23]

MAJOR PSYCHIATRIC SYNDROMES AND THEIR TREATMENT

Demoralization and Major Depression

Depression is the most common psychiatric complaint in the HIV clinic. Depression is a symptom, but is often treated in the literature as a diagnostic category. The complaint of depression should generate a differential diagnosis that includes many psychiatric conditions, including subcortical dementia and delirium, but we will focus on major depression (endogenous depression or melancholia) and demoralization. Major depression and demoralization commonly occur in patients infected with HIV. Both conditions present with low mood. Major depression and its associated changes in mood, self-attitude, and vital sense, represents a form of organic brain dysfunction in the domain of affect, fitting best into the disease category. On the other hand, demoralization is a low mood that can be understood as a response to stresses and life events. Unlike major depression, demoralization is a ubiquitous human experience. People get sad, have sleep and appetite disturbances, and may even contemplate suicide when loved ones die or serious stresses (such as a physically debilitating medical illness) occur.

Major Depression

Major depression is the most common psychiatric disease in the HIV clinic. It is best thought of as a disease of the brain. In clinical descriptions, major depression presents with persistent low mood, a diminished sense of vitality, poor self-attitude, and a loss of pleasure associated with activities that are usually enjoyable. Additionally, there are often neurovegetative changes such as alterations in sleep (increased or decreased), appetite (increased or decreased), and energy that accompany major depressions. The low mood may present as irritability or anger instead of obvious sadness, or even as flatness or lack of emotions. Patients also experience a low self-attitude such that they view themselves as dysfunctional, shoulder guilt inappropriately, and feel worthless. This may lead them to conclude they are unworthy of continued existence and contemplate death passively or actively. In addition, there is often affective (essentially the facial manifestation of the internal mood; the way they look) blunting, psychomotor retardation, and cognitive symptoms such as poor concentration and memory. Major depressions can have concurrent psychotic symptoms. In such cases, it is common to uncover mood-congruent persecutory delusions or auditory hallucinations with negative themes.

In the HIV clinic, major depression may be harder to evaluate. Sadness, low mood, and feelings of illness are important descriptors, yet these are common symptoms in the chronically ill patient with HIV. It is often the anhedonia, that is, the loss of pleasure associated with pleasurable activities, that is most easily assessed. Patients will say that they no longer enjoy visiting family, or that sports are no longer interesting to them. Nothing seems to bring joy. Each patient must be asked what he or she ordinarily likes or enjoys, and patients with major depression will often say that these things have lost their interest or their usual pleasure.

Demoralization

Demoralization is best understood as an adjustment reaction to a stressful event. The chronological relationship to an event is not the distinguishing factor between demoralization and major depression. Many patients trace the start of a major depression back to a catalyzing event. The distinguishing factors are related to self-attitude changes, neurovegetative changes, and thoughts of death. In other words, when demoralized, a patient has low mood and some functional impairment yet lacks the defining characteristics of a major depression. Demoralized patients may report feeling 'normal' when their attention is diverted away from the inciting event. At the same time, they may become overwhelmed with grief or sadness when reminded of the distressful situation. Similarly, patients with demoralization are able to distinguish between their event-specific feelings of sadness and their own self worth.[24] Demoralized patients retain the ability to find joy in usual activities if they are distracted from the inciting event or circumstances that led to their depressed mood. Patients with major depression have impairment in their ability to experience joy in any circumstances. Whereas major depression is a disease of the brain, demoralization is a disorder of mood based on circumstances.

Prevalence and Risk

In a study at the Hopkins Moore clinic, approximately one-half of HIV-positive patients with depressive symptoms suffered from major depression, while the other half experienced demoralization or adjustment disorder, as defined in the Diagnostic and Statistical Manual of Mental Disorders.[25,26] Overall, studies have shown the prevalence rates of major depression in HIV-positive patients to be between 15% and 40%.[27–29]

Major depression is a risk factor for acquiring HIV. Epidemiologic data show a correlation between risky behaviors in HIV-negative individuals and higher scores on screening tools for psychological distress.[30] Another study revealed a sevenfold increase in the lifetime prevalence of mood disorders among nonsubstance-abusing patients who presented for HIV testing when compared to the general population.[31] Furthermore, researchers have clearly identified major depression as a risk factor for unsafe behaviors, such as substance abuse, that may lead to HIV infection.[32–34]

The literature has shown marked decreases in antiretroviral compliance among HIV-infected patients suffering from major depression compared to infected individuals who are free from mental illness.[35,36] Treatment of co-morbid depression appears to improve adherence to antiretroviral regimens[37] and therapeutic outcomes.[38] Unfortunately, data show that over half of HIV-positive patients reporting a major depressive disorder do not receive antidepressant therapy.[39] In one clinic study, early recognition and treatment of major depression with both pharmacotherapy and psychotherapy helped 85% of patients and restored half of them to baseline.[40]

Treatment of Major Depression

Antidepressant drugs are targeted to treat the underlying chemical imbalance in the brain that is associated with major depression (see Fig. 63-1). Patients with HIV/AIDS are prescribed antidepressants more often than any other class of psychotropics.[41] Antidepressants include selective serotonin reuptake inhibitors (SSRIs), tricyclic antidepressants (TCAs), monoamine oxidase inhibitors (MAOIs), and other atypical drugs (bupropion, venlafaxine, duloxetine, mirtazipine, and trazodone). The development of SSRIs brought to market a class of antidepressants that were relatively easy to use, had limited side effects, and were safer in overdose. Though not more effective than tricyclics or MAOIs, the newer antidepressants offered primary care (and specialist) physicians the opportunity to treat the depressions seen so often in their clinics. To date, studies have shown no antidepressant more effective than others in treating depression among HIV-positive patients as a group. For that reason, much of the discussion here is generally related to the treatment of depression in all patients. In general, side effect profiles can guide the selection of an antidepressant agent because of their similar efficacies as a whole. For example, the side effects of TCAs can be capitalized on to treat an HIV-positive patient who is underweight, has diarrhea, and sleeping problems. Table 63-1[42] provides a list of antidepressants, dose ranges, and clinically important side effects and benefits (aside from antidepressant effects).

General Considerations

Successful antidepressant treatment requires consistent patient adherence and titration to an adequate therapeutic dose. We cannot overemphasize the importance of close follow-up with patients suffering from depression. It is not appropriate to diagnose a depression (with its inherent risk of suicide), start a medication (that may be initially agitating and cause other side effects prior to any benefit) and have the patient follow-up in 3 to 4 weeks. Close follow-up (initially weekly) gives the opportunity to provide support, stability, and close observation of any side effects that might warrant action. In order to minimize side effects, clinicians should start therapy at low doses and slowly increase to full doses or therapeutic serum levels (available for some of the tricyclic antidepressants). If a patient experiences any intolerable side effects, he may have already stopped the medicine (this is important to ask). If changing medications due to side effects, drugs in the same class still have the potential to offer improved response and decreased adverse reactions.[43] At the same time, patients experiencing relief of depressive symptoms and annoying but

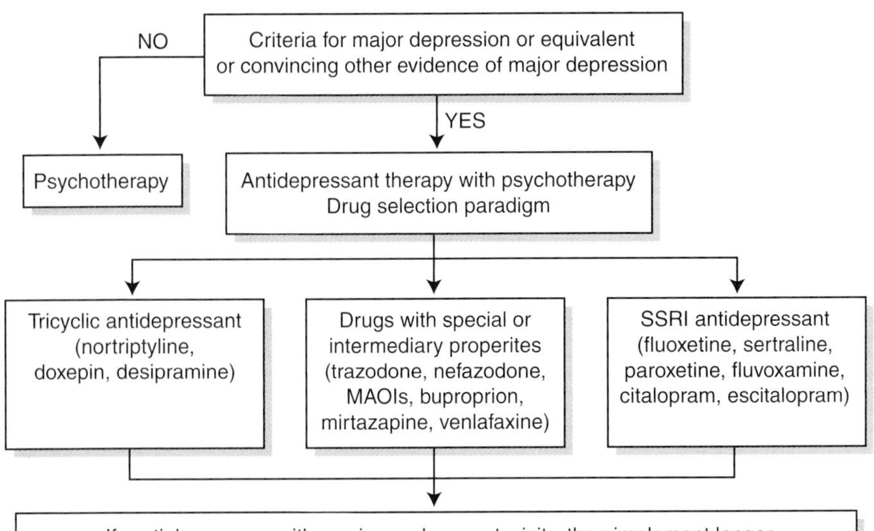

Figure 63-1 ■ Algorithm for pharmacologic treatment of depression.

Table 63-1 Clinically Useful Information About Commonly Prescribed Antidepressants

Drug	Starting Dose	Therapeutic Dose	Important Clinical Information
Nortriptyline (Pamelor)	25 mg q hs	50–150 mg q hs	Promotes sleep, weight gain, and decreases diarrhea. Less anticholinergic side effects than its parent compound, amitriptyline. May be effective for chronic pain syndromes. Well-established therapeutic drug level (50–150 ng/mL). We usually treat toward a level of 80–120 ng/mL
Desipramine (Norpramin)	25 mg q hs	100–300 mg q hs	Promotes sleep, weight gain, and decreases diarrhea. Less anticholinergic side effects than its parent compound, imipramine. Drug levels can be monitored (though not well established) with efficacy found from 75 to >200 ng/mL
Imipramine (Tofranil)	25 mg q hs	50–300 mg q hs	Promotes sleep, weight gain, and decreases diarrhea. Drug levels can be monitored (though not well established) and are given as imipramine and desipramine with efficacy >200 ng/mL
Amitriptyline (Elavil)	25–100 mg q hs	50–300 mg q hs	Promotes sleep, weight gain, and decreases diarrhea. May be effective for chronic pain conditions. Drug levels can be monitored but are not well established. Labs usually provide a combination level of amitriptyline and nortriptyline with total levels of 125–210 ng/mL as effective
Clomipramine (Anafranil)	25 mg q hs	150–250 mg q hs	Promotes sleep, weight gain, and decreases diarrhea. Drug levels can be monitored with efficacy somewhere between 160 and 200 ng/mL. The most serotonergic of the tricyclics. FDA approved for obsessive compulsive disorder but not major depression
Doxepin (Sinequan)	25 mg q hs	75–300 mg q hs	Promotes sleep, weight gain, and decreases diarrhea. Drug levels are not well established. Doxepin is the most antihistaminergic of the tricyclics and can be very

(Continued)

(Continued)

Table 63-1

Drug	Starting Dose	Therapeutic Dose	Important Clinical Information
			helpful in pruritic skin conditions. It comes in a 5% cream that is indicated for the treatment of lichen simplex chronicus
Fluoxetine (Prozac)	10–20 mg q am	20–80 mg q am	Considered the most stimulating of the SSRIs. The long half life limits possibility of a withdrawal syndrome. May be effective for noncompliant patients due to its long half-life and a once-weekly dosing option
Sertraline (Zoloft)	25–50 mg q am	50–200 mg q am	Wide therapeutic dose ranges allow for many titration options. It has limited drug interactions and is well tolerated
Citalopram (Celexa)	20 mg q am	20–60 mg q am	It is touted as having less GI and sexual side effects than other SSRIs and is easily dosed
Escitalopram (Lexapro)	10 mg q am	10–20 mg q am	The s-enantiomer of citalopram, this medicine is effective for depression and anxiety disorders. It is touted as having less GI and sexual side effects than other SSRIs
Paroxetine (Paxil)	20 mg q hs (extended release: 25 mg q hs)	20–50 mg q hs (extended release: 25–50 mg q hs)	Of the SSRIs, paroxetine appears to be the most sedating and anticholinergic. Of the SSRIs, it appears most likely to cause a withdrawal syndrome
Fluvoxamine (Luvox)	50 mg q hs	100–300 mg q hs	Though an SSRI, this is used primarily in the treatment of obsessive compulsive disorder
Venlafaxine (Effexor)	75 mg/day in divided doses (extended release: 37.5–75 mg q am)	75–300 mg q am (extended release: 150–225 mg/day)	Affects both serotonin and norepinephrine (like tricyclics) with no anticholinergic side effects. May be effective in chronic pain syndromes. Like paroxetine, be wary and warn patients of a withdrawal syndrome composed of GI distress, headaches, and anxiety. Potential to elevate blood pressure must be considered in hypertensive patients
Mirtazepine (Remeron)	15 mg q hs	15–45 mg q hs	Very useful for chronically ill patients as main side effects are sedation and weight gain. There are risks of serious hematologic problems (agranulocytosis, neutropenia) (1.1 in 1000) that must be considered in HIV-positive patients
Trazodone (Desyrel)	50–100 mg q hs	50–150 mg q hs for sleep; 200–600 mg q hs for depression	Primarily used as a nonbenzodiazepine sleeping agent. Reaching therapeutic doses to treat depression is difficult due to sedation and orthostasis. There is a risk of priapism
Bupropion (Wellbutrin)	100 mg bid (extended release: 100–150 mg q am)	300–450 mg/day in divided doses (extended release: 300–400 mg/day in divided doses)	Structurally similar to amfetamine, it has been found effective in ADHD, smoking addiction, and has very few sexual side effects. Is often used as an adjunct agent to other antidepressants (such as treating the sexual side effects of SSRIs). Can cause anxiety and psychosis. There is a dose-related risk of seizures (0.1% up to 300 mg/day and 0.4% at 400 mg daily)
Duloxetine (Cymbalta)	20 mg bid	20–30 mg bid	The most recently approved antidepressant. It is approved for the treatment of depression and diabetic neuropathy and may be beneficial in other chronic pain syndromes
BLACK BOX WARNINGS	*All antidepressants*: Suicidality in children and adolescents		

tolerable side effects such as insomnia, constipation, or sexual dysfunction should be encouraged and receive adjunctive treatments (e.g., trazodone for insomnia or increased water and fiber intake for constipation). A full trial of an antidepressant is 6 to 8 weeks at a standard therapeutic dose.[44–46] After this time, patients experiencing minimal or partial relief of symptoms should be considered for higher doses, a different medicine, or an augmenting agent. Lithium addition is the augmenting strategy best supported by evidence. Other promising augmenting agents include triiodothyronine, pindolol, and DHEA.[47]

Selective Serotonin Reuptake Inhibitors

As a group, SSRIs have broad clinical indications, including major depression (fluoxetine, sertraline, paroxetine, citalopram, escitalopram), bulimia (fluoxetine), panic disorder (fluoxetine, sertraline, paroxetine), obsessive compulsive disorder (fluoxetine, fluvoxamine, sertraline, paroxetine), generalized anxiety disorder (paroxetine, escitalopram), posttraumatic stress disorder (sertraline, paroxetine), social phobia (sertraline, paroxetine), and premenstrual dysphoric disorder (fluoxetine, sertraline, paroxetine). Common side effects include anxiety, restlessness (akathisia), nausea, diarrhea (increased gastric motility), insomnia, and sexual dysfunction (including decreased arousal or erections, delayed ejaculation, and anorgasmia). Randomized clinical trials have noted fluoxetine most effective of the SSRIs in treating major depression in HIV-positive patients. However, paroxetine, sertraline, and citalopram have also demonstrated clinical efficacy.[48]

A small number of studies have examined the combination of SSRIs and antiretrovirals for drug interactions. Fluoxetine has been shown to increase concentrations of ritonavir with co-administration.[49] At the same time, researchers examining a series of five cases of serotonin syndrome concluded that co-administered ritonavir increased levels of fluoxetine through inhibition of CYP 2D6.[50] Although no evidence exists addressing interactions between other SSRIs and antiretrovirals, adverse reactions are possible with all combinations through the potential for CYP450 inhibition, necessitating careful observation of all HIV-positive patients taking SSRIs.[51,52] However, SSRIs differ in their pharmacokinetics and potential inhibitory effect on CYP450, possibly making certain drugs, such as citalopram and escitalopram, better choices in patients taking numerous medications.[53]

Tricyclic Antidepressants

Clinicians most commonly employ TCAs for the treatment of depression (amitriptyline, imipramine, desipramine, doxepin, nortriptyline, protriptyline, trimipramine) and obsessive compulsive disorder (clomipramine). The TCAs last introduced to the market before SSRIs are probably the best tolerated and easiest to use. There is a tendency to underdose TCAs and therefore blood levels are particularly useful in these agents to avoid toxicity and to make sure patients are adequately treated. Unlike most other antidepressants, the serum levels of TCAs are useful and predict response. The TCAs we use most frequently are doxepin, nortriptyline, and desipramine, listed here from most to least sedating. TCAs likely act through reuptake inhibition of norepinephrine and serotonin, though their mechanisms are not entirely clear. Side effects are anticholinergic (decreased gastric motility, dry mouth, urinary retention, and blurry vision), antihistaminergic (sedation and weight gain), and antiadrenergic (hypotension and orthostasis). Cardiac conduction abnormalities (prolonged QT interval) may cause death in overdose and warrant an EKG prior to starting these medicines. Studies show TCAs to be as effective as other antidepressants in HIV-positive patients.[54,55] Although no published reports have demonstrated interactions between TCAs and antiretrovirals, the potential for adverse reactions requires close observation of patients receiving both medication types. In one case report, fluconazole, an antifungal agent commonly prescribed to HIV-positive patients, caused increased serum concentrations of nortriptyline.[56]

Atypical Antidepressants

Additional antidepressant options with demonstrated effectiveness for treating depressed HIV patients include mirtazipine,[57] nefazodone,[58] trazodone, bupropion,[59] and the psychostimulants methylphenidate and dextroamfetamine.[60–63] The novel antidepressant mirtazipine has demonstrated effectiveness in HIV-positive patients and a valuable tendency to promote appetite and sleep. Nefazodone improves depression in HIV-positive patients, but is used infrequently due to the black box warning related to life-threatening liver failure. Trazodone is often used as a nonaddictive sleeping aid, though co-administered antiretrovirals may complicate its use in HIV-positive patients. In a study of HIV-free individuals, co-administered ritonavir slowed the clearance of trazodone and resulted in nausea, dizziness, and hypotension, including one episode of syncope.[64] Bupropion effectively improves depression in HIV-positive patients but carries a risk of seizures. Although one study indicated decreased hydroxylation of bupropion with co-administration of ritonavir, nelfinavir, and efavirenz,[65] a case series of 10 patients found no increased occurrence of seizures (no seizures reported).[66] Psychostimulants such as methylphenidate and dextroamfetamine have been shown to improve energy, mood, and severe fatigue in HIV-positive patients. The use of these drugs must be judicious given the potential for diversion and the availability of many effective antidepressants. From our clinical experience, other antidepressant agents, including venlafaxine and duloxetine, improve mood in HIV-positive patients, but they have not been directly studied in this population.

Bipolar Disorder

In general, patients with bipolar disorder experience episodes of hypomania or mania, along with periods of major depressions. Hypomanic patients have expansive or irritable moods, excessive energy, decreased need for sleep, a subjective sense of 'racing thoughts' and pressured (rapid and hard to interrupt) speech. The self attitude of the patient is grandiose and his activities are often driven, dangerous, and lead to unfortunate consequences due to excess spending, sexual indiscretions, and over commitment.

The Diagnostic and Statistical Manual of Mental Disorders (DSM-IV) distinguishes between mania and hypomania based on the length of time symptoms have lasted (7 versus 4 days) and the degree of impairment.[67] We prefer to rely on the presence of psychotic features to define this distinction. Those psychotic symptoms would include a formal thought disorder, perceptual abnormalities, and delusions. The thought disorder is manifest as a loosening of associations so that the speech is not just pressured, but presents a train of thought that is derailed and illogical. Auditory hallucinations are common in manic patients as are fixed, false, idiosyncratic beliefs that have a theme of grandiosity (being a prophet, religious leader, secret agent, powerful doctor, etc).

According to the DSM-IV, a mixed state is defined as meeting criteria for both a major depression and mania in the same week. Clinically, it may be easier to understand a mixed state as containing the low mood, poor self attitude, and poor outlook of a major depression in the setting of racing thoughts, pressured speech, increased energy, and profound irritability. Bipolar disorder type I refers to patients who have manias either with or without major depressions. Patients diagnosed with bipolar disorder type II have episodes of hypomanias interspersed with major depressions. Patients experiencing only hypomanias sufficient to interfere in their lives would be diagnosed with a nonspecific bipolar disorder.

Like major depression, bipolar disorder increases the risk of acquiring HIV and complicates its treatment. Patients experiencing hypomanias or manias are more likely to engage in the unsafe sexual and substance abuse behaviors that place one at risk for exposure to HIV.[68] As we have discussed, being in the midst of a major depression or mania makes it very hard to adhere to a HIV treatment regimen.

AIDS Mania

Patients without any personal or family history of bipolar disorder often develop a manic syndrome in late-stage HIV infection. This would be considered a secondary mania related etiologically to the underlying HIV infection and its related neurologic sequelae. Termed AIDS mania, this syndrome is clinically distinct from bipolar mania in symptoms, course, and treatment. It is associated with more irritability, pressured speech, and is typically associated with late-stage disease, AIDS dementia, and significant cognitive impairment.[69–71] Patients with AIDS mania are particularly difficult to treat. Mood stabilizers frequently cause delirium requiring the use of low-dose antipsychotic agents. Aggressive regimens of highly active antiretroviral therapy (HAART) may result in significant improvement.[72] Acute mania obstructs patients' compliance with HAART; however, antipsychotics often remain a necessary part of treatment.

Treatment of Bipolar Disorder

The maintenance treatment of bipolar disorder refers to the use of mood stabilizers to prevent manias and depressions. Evidence-based mood stabilizers indicated for maintenance treatment of bipolar disorder include lithium, valproic acid, carbamazepine, lamotrigine, and olanzapine.[73] The treatment of acutely manic patients and those in mixed states should be considered a psychiatric emergency and usually requires hospitalization. Mania and mixed states are treated with mood stabilizers in combination with typical or atypical neuroleptics. Prior to the use of lithium and the anticonvulsants, antipsychotics were used as acute treatment and maintenance therapies in patients with bipolar disorder. Of the newer antipsychotics, olanzapine is FDA indicated for this use. The other atypical neuroleptics (quetiapine, risperidone, ziprasidone, and aripiprazole) are indicated for the acute treatment of manias and mixed states and may be used as maintenance therapies in some patients. This is important to consider in the HIV-positive patient who may have complicated health problems precluding the use of lithium or anticonvulsants. Table 63-2[42] provides a list of mood stabilizers, dose ranges, and clinically important side effects and benefits.

Lithium

Lithium should be considered the benchmark when looking at evidence-based mood stabilizers in the treatment of acute manic episodes and bipolar disorder maintenance.[74–76] Lithium has a narrow therapeutic window and carries many side effects including nausea, vomiting, diarrhea, polyuria, polydipsia, weight gain, dose-related tremor, delirium, nephrotoxicity (nephrogenic diabetes insipidus), and thyroid dysfunction (hypothyroidism). As a result, clinicians must carefully titrate lithium doses to a therapeutic serum level (0.8–1.2 meq/L) and watch thyroid and kidney function closely. Any decrease in glomerular clearance (due to NSAIDs, dehydration, HIV-related kidney disease, or nephrotoxic drugs) quickly can lead to lithium intoxication. One benefit of lithium is its lack of metabolism by the liver and lack of interactions with antiretrovirals and antibiotics.

Anticonvulsants

Well-studied anticonvulsants for the treatment of acute manias, mixed states, and maintenance of bipolar disorder include valproic acid and carbamazepine.[77–79] Valproic acid may cause sedation, weight gain, hair loss, dose-related tremor, ataxia, nystagmus, delirium, thrombocytopenia, temporary increases in serum transaminases, hepatitis, and less commonly, hemorrhagic pancreatitis. Although studies suggest that valproic acid may interfere with zidovudine glucuronidation and metabolism, no evidence has shown clinically important interactions when co-administered with antiretrovirals.[80] Carbamazepine has greatest efficacy in combination with lithium or valproate in treating acute mania and bipolar disorder. Because its metabolism is autoinduced, carbamazepine requires close monitoring as it is started. Side effects include sedation, weight gain, tremor, and the potential for bone marrow

Table 63-2 Clinically Useful Information About Commonly Prescribed Mood Stabilizers

Drug	Starting Dose	Therapeutic Dose	Important Clinical Information
Lithium	150–300 mg bid	900–1500 mg daily in divided doses (varies greatly based on renal function)	Few interactions with drugs due to lack of metabolism. May cause nephrogenic diabetes insipidus, hypothyroidism, leukocytosis, and cardiac conduction abnormalities. Levels are well established (0.6–1.2 meq/L) and should be checked frequently until stable. Lithium usually takes 5 days to equilibrate in the body. Toxicity presents with confusion, worsening of tremor, and GI distress
Valproic acid	250 mg bid	1000–2000 mg in divided doses (max dose is 60 mg kg^{-1} day^{-1} in divided doses)	May cause liver function test abnormalities and thrombocytopenia. It can cause stomach distress, ataxia, and a tremor. A common side effect that may be beneficial for chronically ill patients is weight gain. Therapeutic drug levels are well established (80–120 μ/mL) and help guide therapy and concerns about toxicity
Carbamazepine (Tegretol)	100–200 mg bid	600–1600 mg in divided doses	As noted previously, CBZ autoinduces its metabolism so levels must be monitored closely. Therapeutic drug levels are well established (8–12 μ/mL). Hemogram counts need to be monitored regularly due to the idiosyncratic risk of agranulocytosis. This medicine is a common cause of SIADH. There is a risk of dermatologic reaction in 4% with the possibility of severe rash
Lamotrigine (Lamictal)	25 mg daily for 2 weeks	200–400 mg once daily or in divided doses	Due to the risk of a Stevens–Johnson rash, there is a specific dosing regimen (25 mg daily for 2 weeks, then 50 mg daily for 2 weeks) that limits the speed of titration. If given with valproic acid, the dose of lamotrigine must be halved in this titration regimen. Overall, it is quite well tolerated and free from interactions. Unfortunately, there are not well-established therapeutic drug levels
BLACK BOX WARNINGS	*Lithium*: Lithium toxicity is closely related to levels and facilities for checking levels should be readily available prior to starting treatment *Valproic acid*: Hepatotoxicity, pancreatitis, and teratogenicity *Carbamazepine*: Aplastic anemia *Lamotrigine*: Life-threatening rash		

suppression (idiosyncratic agranulocytosis) requiring complete blood count monitoring during use. Both carbamazepine and lamotrigine have shown unusual interactions with antiretrovirals.[82] Clinical evidence has shown ritonavir to cause carbamazepine toxicity through CYP 3A4 inhibition. Another report, however, demonstrated antiretroviral failure due to the CYP induction effects of carbamazepine.[81] Although lamotrigine does not utilize the CYP system, co-administration of ritonavir decreases its blood levels without any apparent clinical implications. Lamotrigine has been shown effective in the maintenance treatment of bipolar disorder.[82,83] Its use is eased by the lack of routine blood monitoring. There is a risk of a severe rash that is related to the speed with which the dose is increased. For that reason, there is a manufacturer-specified dosing regimen that must be followed.

Other atypical anticonvulsants have been tested extensively as treatments for bipolar disorder. While some of them, such as gabapentin and topiramate, may work effectively as adjunctive therapies for bipolar disorder,[84,85] little evidence supports their use alone for acute mania or maintenance of bipolar disorder.

Antipsychotics

Antipsychotic or neuroleptic medications often provide faster relief of acute mania than mood stabilizers. Typical or first-generation antipsychotics, such as haloperidol and fluphenazine, are potently antidopaminergic and have the potential to cause extrapyramidal side effects including acute dystonias, akathisia, and parkinsonism. The risk for tardive dyskinesia increases the longer these medications are administered and are of major concern in older patients and those with cognitive impairment (often a problem with HIV-positive patients). The extrapyramidal side effects are often prevented or treated with anticholinergic medications such as diphenhydramine, benztropine, or trihexyphenidyl.

Second-generation or atypical antipsychotics are called such as they interact with other neurotransmitter systems (like serotonin) besides dopamine. For that reason, these drugs (which include risperidone, olanzapine, quetiapine, ziprasidone, and aripiprazole) are less likely to cause extrapyramidal symptoms (EPS) and tardive dyskinesia. They are considered first-line treatments for acute manias and mixed states. Unfortunately, there are a number of metabolic complications (weight gain, elevated cholesterol, and hyperglycemia) that may prove as difficult to manage over the long-term as tardive dyskinesia. Antipsychotics will be addressed in more detail below.

Schizophrenia

Schizophrenia is the disorder of mental life more clearly thought to be a disease. It presents as a syndrome with an epidemiology that is consistent through the world. Patients present with disorganized speech (a formal thought disorder), disorganized behavior (purposeless movements, catatonia), perceptual abnormalities, and delusions (the positive or criteria A symptoms from the DSM IV-TR). The most disabling symptoms (called negative or the criteria B symptoms) include social withdrawal, apathy, and general dysfunction in all social areas of interaction (like work, family, and school).

Unfortunately, patients with schizophrenia generally receive poor medical care, and are often involved in coercive sexual behaviors and substance use, rendering them vulnerable to HIV infection. Patients with schizophrenia have an increased risk for getting HIV and are poorly adherent to treatment for their medical conditions in general.

While patients with schizophrenia may also have affective symptoms (major depression is a common co-morbid condition and grandiose delusions are not uncommon), the longitudinal clinical picture is different than that of an affective illness. With the onset of these symptoms, the patient does not ever return to his or her level of premorbid functioning. It was this characteristic observed by Emil Kraepelin when he first made the distinction between schizophrenia and bipolar disorder (he termed them dementia praecox and manic depressive insanity, respectively).

The positive symptoms make up the term 'psychotic' and are effectively treated with neuroleptics. Unfortunately, the negative symptoms are relatively resistant to treatment. The atypical antipsychotics, namely clozapine, seem to be more effective than other medications at treating negative symptoms but this is not a universal phenomen in clozapine-treated patients. There are no major differences between the treatment of schizophrenia in HIV- and non-HIV-positive patients.

Treatment of Schizophrenia

As with the medication management of the other mental illnesses in patients with HIV, side effect profiles and drug–drug interactions motivate treatment decisions. There is no conclusive evidence that one antipsychotic drug is more effective than another for the acute treatment of psychosis or maintenance therapy in schizophrenia. Patients with HIV appear to be more sensitive to neuroleptic-induced extrapyramidal side effects than uninfected patients.[86–88] Due to the potential for dangerous increases in their serum levels, clozapine and pimozide are contraindicated with the potent CYP inhibitor, ritonavir. Clinical observation is important when using other neuroleptics like chlorpromazine, haloperidol, olanzapine, and risperidone in concert with CYP inhibitors.[21]

We would recommend first-line treatment with an atypical neuroleptic as they have less potential for extrapyramidal side effects and are usually well tolerated. Clozapine has been used effectively in HIV-positive patients[89] but its use is certainly complicated by the risk of agranulocytosis and the required blood count monitoring. Noncompliance is a special problem in schizophrenic patients with HIV. While there is no specific evidence regarding the use of decanoate preparations in HIV-positive patients, these long-acting forms of haloperidol, fluphenazine, and risperidone, can be very useful in the long-term stabilization of schizophrenic patients (Table 63-3).[42]

Substance Abuse and Addiction

Like other psychiatric conditions, substance abuse increases the risk of acquiring HIV and complicates its treatment. As previously noted, there is a high rate of substance abuse disorders present in patients seeking treatment for HIV. Substance abuse disorders themselves pose an independent risk for HIV transmission, apart from the danger present due to sharing needles.[90–92] When considering substance abuse and HIV-positive patients, it is important to understand addiction as a behavior motivated both by internal and external forces. Identifying substance abuse as a motivated behavior guides the treatment critical for psychological and medical improvement in HIV-positive and substance-addicted patients.

The Motivated Behavior of Substance Addiction

The motivated behavior of drug addiction arises out of a cycle of both internally motivated drives and externally reinforced rewards. The positive reinforcement of addictive behaviors from environmental and internal rewards leads to their intense craving, frequent repetition, and progressive amplification. The external circuit plays an important role in initiating substance use and leading to disordered behavior, but the internal cycle creates and maintains the physiologic setting for addiction.

The presence of an internal reward and drive distinguishes motivated behaviors (like eating, sleeping, sexual activity, and drug use) from other actions and activities. Most behaviors are

Clinically Useful Information About Commonly Prescribed Antipsychotics

Table 63-3

Drug	Starting Dose	Therapeutic Dose	Important Clinical Information
Risperidone (Risperdal)	0.5–1 mg bid	4–6 mg daily once or in divided doses	The only atypical to come in a decanoate form. Also comes in an orally dissolvable tablet that is excellent for acute agitation in that it can not be 'cheeked' and avoids an injection
Olanzapine (Zyprexa)	5–10 mg daily	15–30 mg daily once or in divided doses	May be given intramuscularly for acute agitation with less risk of extrapyramidal side effects than the typical neuroleptics. Also comes in an orally dissolvable tablet that is excellent for acute agitation in that it can not be 'cheeked' and avoids an injection. Sedation and weight gain are common side effects. Metabolic complications including hyperglycemic crises, diabetes, and high cholesterol are appearing in patients
Quetiapine (Seroquel)	25–100 mg bid	400–600 mg daily in divided doses (with max of 800 mg daily)	It is very sedating and has a low incidence of extrapyramidal side effects. Though the practice is questionable, it is being used as a nonbenzodiazepine sleep agent in patients without chronic psychotic illnesses
Ziprasidone (Geodon)	20 mg bid	40–80 mg twice daily (with a max of 80 mg twice daily)	Though all neuroleptics (typical and atypical) have an associated risk of QT prolongation, ziprasidone carries a black box warning for QT prolongation. it comes in an intramuscular form for acute agitation
Aripiprazole (Abilify)	10–15 mg qd	15–30 mg daily (max dose of 30 mg daily)	The newest of the atypical neuroleptics, it can be effective and may have less metabolic complications than other atypicals like olanzapine
Clozapine (Clozaril)	12.5 mg qd or bid	300–450 mg daily in divided doses with a max of 900 mg daily	Clozapine is generally considered to be the most effective antipsychotic in treatment refractory patients. Its use is limited by significant orthostasis, tachycardia, weight gain, and drooling. Those side effects require a slow titration often difficult to do in an outpatient setting. In addition, the risk of agranulocytosis requires blood counts weekly for the first 6 months and twice weekly for the next 6 months. Those white counts must be reported on a special form to a pharmacy weekly for the medicine to be dispensed
Haloperidol (Haldol)	0.5–5 mg qd or bid	5–20 mg daily once or in divided doses (max dose is 100 mg daily)	Haloperidol is the classic typical, high-potency neuroleptic. It comes in an elixir and can be given orally, intravenously, or intramuscularly. In medically ill delirious patients with agitation, we recommend small doses (0.5 mg) intravenously. It also comes in a decanoate form. As with other typical neuroleptics, extrapyramidal side effects may develop and should be watched for closely
Fluphenazine (Prolixin)	0.5–5 mg qd or bid	5–20 mg daily once or in divided doses (max dose is 100 mg daily)	This medication is similar in potency and efficacy to haloperidol. It comes in an elixir and can be given intramuscularly as well as orally. It comes in a decanoate form. As with all typical neuroleptics, extrapyramidal side effects may develop
BLACK BOX WARNINGS	*All atypicals*: Elderly patients with dementia-related psychosis treated with atypical antipsychotic drugs are at an increased risk of death compared to placebo *Clozapine*: In addition to the above warning, also has black box warnings related to agranulocytosis, seizures, myocarditis, and orthostatic hypotension *Ziprasidone*: Prolonged QT interval		

conditioned by external factors, such as the approval of parents and peers, status and material success, and more directly, access to food, water, shelter, and other necessities. The motivated behaviors, however, link internally to the reward circuitry of the brain, causing individuals to develop drive states for these activities. Substances of abuse strongly activate the reward circuits in the mesolimbic dopaminergic system, located primarily in the mid-brain, including the ventral tegmental area, the nucleus accumbens, and the medial forebrain bundle. Dopamine acts as the main neurotransmitter in this system, though serotonin, norepinephrine, glutamate, and gamma-aminobutyric acid (GABA) also play important roles.

Activation of the internal reward circuits by substance abuse leads to the physiologic cycle of addiction. After satiation, addicts experience intense cravings for drugs of abuse as a way of repetitively invoking the sensations of internal reward. The frequency of drug use increases in order to maintain these feelings for as long as possible. As physiologic tolerance develops, substance abusers require larger quantities of drugs to achieve the same rewards. Likewise, physiologic dependence leads to withdrawal symptoms when substance abusers abstain from use, further discouraging disruption of the addiction cycle. Over time, patients develop an overwhelming and out of control internal drive to propagate their substance use behavior, devoting increasing resources to the pursuit of drugs and consuming all of their assets, including time, money, employment, and relationships.

This syndrome of addiction independently places patients at increased risk for contracting HIV. As their addictions intensify, substance abusers engage in increasingly risky behaviors. Motivated drives quickly overcome reasonable judgment and patients knowingly share needles with HIV-positive individuals and engage in prostitution for drugs and money. Several studies have demonstrated the role of prostitution as a risk factor for transmission of HIV, as well as other sexually transmitted diseases.[93,94]

Treatment of Substance Use Disorders

Because addiction increases the risk of HIV transmission and interferes with antiretroviral compliance,[95] optimal care of HIV infection in substance abusers requires direct treatment of their addictive behaviors as well. In general, substance abuse treatment involves four steps: detoxification, rehabilitation, treatment of co-morbid psychiatric conditions, and relapse prevention.

Detoxification

Initially, clinicians must wait for patients to recover from states of acute intoxication before assessing additional treatment needs and beginning to combat their addictive behaviors. Unfortunately, there are no specific medication options for patients withdrawing from stimulants or hallucinogens. The detoxification from alcohol and sedative-hypnotics (barbiturates and benzodiazepines) can be life threatening and therefore require benzodiazepine tapers. While the detoxification from opiates is not life threatening, it is a miserable experience that can cause medical problems due to vomiting, diarrhea, and poor intake. The internal drive to relieve that distress is so strong, patients are limited in their ability to participate in recovery work if actively withdrawing. For that reason, it is advocated a detoxification strategy that includes a narcotic with the adjunctive antispasmodic, dicyclomine, and pain reliever, methocarbamol. As a narcotic, buprenorphine in either an intramuscular or sublingual form can also be used successfully.

Rehabilitation and Treatment of Co-Morbid Conditions

After detoxification, rehabilitation utilizes externally derived responses to encourage patients to stop using drugs and to enter treatment programs. The foundation of this is in group-based psychotherapy (like Alcoholics Anonymous) that creates social networks positively reinforcing abstinence and stigmatizing addictive behaviors. Typically, 12-step programs like Alcoholics Anonymous utilize peer pressure and stepwise treatment goals to provide positive external responses to an addictive-free lifestyle.

As rehabilitation begins, clinicians must evaluate and treat substance-addicted patients for co-morbid psychiatric conditions that have the potential to interfere with recovery. Primary care physicians and mental health providers should not hesitate to utilize pharmacotherapy for psychiatric co-morbidities. In general, the potential for psychiatric conditions to obstruct substance use recovery usually outweighs the risk of using psychotropic medications.

Relapse Prevention

As duration of abstinence in a patient increases, rehabilitation efforts gradually extend to long-term relapse prevention measures. In general, relapse prevention focuses on replacement of drug-seeking and substance use behaviors with activities designed to promote a higher quality of life, as well as the creation of a drug-free personal environment. Essentially, patients receive vocational and social rehabilitation to aid them in establishing new employment and relationships. Additionally, patients should continue long-term group therapy to maintain external positive feedback of their new lives and to provide this same reinforcement as an encouraging example to others.

Interactions between Substances of Abuse and Antiretrovirals

The concurrent use of benzodiazepines (which depend on either CYP 3A4 or glucuronidation for metabolism) and antiretrovirals can lead to serious side effects.[96,97] The CYP inhibitors ritonavir and delavirdine (as well as other HIV protease inhibitors) can increase plasma levels of certain benzodiazepines such as alprazolam, midazolam, and triazolam, potentially leading to oversedation and death. On the other hand, antiretrovirals that increase the activity of glucuronidation, such as ritonavir and nelfinavir, can lower the concentrations of oxazepam, lorazepam, and temazepam, causing acute withdrawal and life-threatening autonomic instability.

Clinicians have reported overdoses secondary to interactions between the rave drugs methylenedioxymethamfetamine (MDMA, also known as ecstasy) and gamma-hydroxybutyrate (GHB) and protease inhibitors. Additionally, ritonavir and other protease inhibitors may inhibit the metabolism of amfetamines, ketamine, diethylmide (LSD), and phencyclidine (PCP) through the CYP system. Antiretrovirals also have the potential to interact with methadone, a medication commonly administered to HIV-positive patients in substance abuse treatment programs. The body metabolizes methadone primarily though CYP 3A4, and induction of these enzymes by efavirenz, nevirapine, ritonavir, and lopinavir/ritonavir can cause opiate withdrawal.[98–102] Significant interactions between heroin, cocaine, tetrahydrocannabinol (THC), and ethanol and antiretroviral agents have not been described. Importantly, consumption of alcohol uniquely affects HIV-positive patients by escalating the risk of liver disease progression in patients co-infected with hepatitis C and decreasing adherence to medication in a temporal and dose-dependent fashion.[103,104]

Personality Disorder

When addressing matters of personality in patients with HIV, we broadly consider two categories of temperament based on work by Eysenck and Rachman: introversion and extraversion.[105] Introverted individuals are avoidant of negative consequences, focused on the future more than the present, and place greater importance on function and thoughts than feelings. Extraverted individuals, on the other hand, are reward sensitive, focused on the present more than the future, and place utmost importance on their feelings (to such an extent that they may feel overwhelmed by them).

As expected from these descriptions, introverted individuals tend to avoid risky or hazardous behaviors, but have increased vulnerability to obsessions, compulsions, and anxieties. Based on their nature, introverts have less risk for contracting HIV because of their avoidance of risky situations, fear of medical consequences, and anxiety over health in general. Our experience is that introverted patients make up a minority of HIV patients presenting for psychiatric care. Extraverted temperaments increase the risk of HIV contraction through higher rates of substance abuse,[106] as well as impulsive, risky behaviors.[107–110] In fact, a large number of patients seen in STD clinics have extraverted characteristics, indicating increased risk for HIV in individuals with this disposition.[111]

Emotionally unstable, extraverted patients are often difficult to engage in treatment. Initially, they appear genuinely committed to their healthcare and well-being, even demanding particular services from their providers, such as specific medications or assistance with legal and social issues. Because of their focus on feelings and the present, however, this attitude toward treatment can change quickly. Extraverts are extremely vulnerable to noncompliance and abandonment of relationships with their healthcare providers. For instance, extraverted patients commonly sign out of the hospital against medical advice, in spite of clear health risks, because their feelings so strongly cloud their judgment.

Treatment of Personality Disorders

Changing personality is not easy, and usually starts with a focus on behavior. Clinicians often dislike these patients, and the patients often use this dislike to manipulate healthcare workers. They also tend to divide staff by appealing for sympathy to one staff member while disparaging another. Clinicians often feel helpless in the face of the constantly changing demands and behaviors that the characterize personality-disorder, and may feel their treatment is futile. Once it is clear that the personality of a patient (or pervasive style of interacting with other adults and life situations) is hindering his or her treatment, the clinician has the opportunity and the power to change things for the better.

A key to the treatment of the personality disordered patient in the HIV clinic is for the healthcare provider to establish himself/herself as a stable responder to the behaviors of the patient. The focus stays on behavior and not on feelings, and on what the patient must do to get the rewards that are set up as part of the treatment. The care provider does not alter treatment plans based on the patient's tumult of the day. One works with the patient to design a treatment plan based around rewards important to the patient and consistent with what the care provider determines to be in the patient's best interest. Rewards for treatment compliance may be as simple as reading a poem or as complicated as filling out government forms or offering another trial of HAART. Chiding, anger, and other forms of punishment have limited ability to motivate any change in the extraverted, personality-disordered patient. Extraverted patients are remarkably reward sensitive, but remarkably consequence insensitive, and often continue high-risk sexual behaviors in spite of their personal experience with the consequences of previous STDs.[112] Clinicians can optimize the treatment of extraverted patients from the outset by creating treatment contracts in which patients agree to make certain changes to improve their health in exchange for desired services by the provider. This manner of interacting described sounds, and is, paternalistic. Unfortunately, that is necessary in the cases where a patient's personality prevents him from comprehending the benefits of abstaining from drug use, adhering to antiretroviral medications, and avoiding risky behaviors.

Psychological Reactions to Life Events

Events in our lives change the way we perceive events, and the meanings we attach to the actions of other people, and even our own existence. As described above, patients with early misuse at the hands of trusted figures will have a variety of difficulties with relationships in adult life. It is equally important to recognize the impact of current events on patients. Grief, demoralization, and hopelessness often accompany the diagnosis of HIV, as well as events that mark progression and treatment failure. The need to treat hepatitis C may provoke profound hopelessness in a person doing well with HIV who may feel like they cannot stand one more medical problem. The term PTSD is often a shorthand description of a person who is overwhelmed by the events of a life that seems out of control and in a downward spiral. Patients benefit from an understanding of the forces at work in their lives, and often benefit from the kinds of therapy that provide a sense of mastery of life and insight into how to do better.

While there are over 100 kinds of described psychotherapy, all of them are directed at mastering the problems of life and of learning ways to deal with emotionally distressing circumstances. The therapist is socially sanctioned as a purveyor of help. The interaction between the two that improves the life of the patient is psychotherapy. All doctor–patient interactions contain elements of psychotherapy. Supportive psychotherapy is critical to the improvement of patients with HIV. There is an almost endless possibility of demoralizing events facing patients diagnosed with HIV. With empathy and close follow-up, you provide support and develop a plan that has improvement as a goal. Cognitive-behavioral therapy will allow a patient to master ideas and behaviors that help them to cope with distressing emotions and experiences. Just listening to patients and validating the distress they feel will allow the opportunity to help patients change.

Patients often come asking for treatments that produce a quick fix for their feelings of distress. They simply cannot go on unless they receive a medication that makes them feel better. This method of coping leads to a life of chaos and dysfunction. Rather than focusing on feeling better, patients need to focus on getting better. The relationship with a well prepared and sympathetic provider allows this change to take place.

SUMMARY

Waking daily with the awareness that one has an incurable disease brings a stress to make the stoutest of us flinch. The experience of treating patients with HIV and AIDS can be just as daunting. Patients have often been marginalized and cast off by their friends, their families, and even themselves. They are offered treatments that have as a collective goal suppression of HIV, not cure. Healthcare providers work with patients whose behavioral and personality vulnerabilities may leave them ungrateful and noncompliant. They often have mental illnesses that contributed to their infection and hinder their ongoing treatment. Despite these barriers to care, care givers have a huge impact on the quality of life and function of patients. It has been shown that patients treated for psychiatric disorders have improved outcomes. The key to treatment is to fully evaluate every patient and to treat all the psychiatric barriers to effective HIV care. This includes recognition of mental illness such as depression, treatment plans that are adapted to personality problems, and collaborative treatment for addictions. Patients are often hopeless, and it is the therapeutic optimism that clinicians bring through their experiences and successes that persuades hopeless patients to cooperate with treatment. As they improve, they will begin to recognize the possibility of a better future and life, but the clinician must remain a buttress against old patterns of behavior.

REFERENCES

1. Holtgrave DR. Causes of the decline in AIDS deaths, United States, 1995–2002: prevention, treatment, or both? Int J STD AIDS 16:777–81, 2005.
2. Fishman M, Lyketsos CG, Treisman G. Mood disorders in HIV infection. Int Rev Psychiatry 8:267–76, 1996.
3. Meade CS, Sikkema KJ. HIV risk behavior among adults with severe mental illness: a systematic review. Clin Psychol Rev 25:433–57, 2005.
4. Bing EG, Burnam MA, Longshore D, et al. Psychiatric disorders and drug use among human immunodeficiency virus-infected adults in the United States. Arch Gen Psychiatry 58:721–8, 2001.
5. Treisman G, Fishman M, Lyketsos C, McHugh PR. Evaluation and treatment of psychiatric disorders associated with HIV infection. Res Publ Assoc Res Nerv Ment Dis 72:239–50, 1994.
6. Lyketsos CG, Hanson A, Fishman M, et al. Screening for psychiatric morbidity in a medical outpatient clinic for HIV infection: the need for a psychiatric presence. Int J Psychiatry Med 24:103–13, 1994.
7. Singh N, Squier C, Sivek C, et al. Determinants of compliance with antiretroviral therapy in patients with human immunodeficiency virus: prospective assessment with implications for enhancing compliance. AIDS Care 8:261–9, 1996.
8. Bartlett JA. Addressing the challenges of adherence. J Acquir Immune Defic Syndr 29(Suppl 1):S2–10, 2002.
9. McHugh PR, Slavney PR. The Perspectives of Psychiatry. 2nd edn. Baltimore, MD: Johns Hopkins University Press; 1998.
10. Tsasis P. Adherence assessment to highly active antiretroviral therapy. AIDs Patient Care STDs 15: 109–15, 2001.
11. Murphy DA, Roberts KJ, Martin DJ, et al. Barriers to antiretroviral adherence among HIV-infected adults. AIDS Patient Care STDs 14: 47–58, 2000.
12. Barlow DH, Gorman JM, Shear MK, Woods SW. Cognitive-behavioral therapy, imipramine, or their combination for panic disorder: a randomized, controlled trial. JAMA 283:2529–36, 2000.
13. Van Balkom A, Bakker A, Spinhoven P, et al. A meta-analysis of the treatment of panic disorder with or without agoraphobia: a comparison of psychopharmacological, cognitive-behavioral, and combination treatments. J Nerv Ment Dis 185: 510–16, 2000.
14. Otto MW, Deveney C. Cognitive-behavioral therapy and the treatment of panic disoder: efficacy and strategies. J Clin Psychiatry 66(Suppl 4):28–32, 2005.
15. Roy-Byrne PP, Craske MG, Stein MB, et al. A randomized effectiveness trial of cognitive-behavioral therapy and medication for primary care panic disorder. Arch Gen Psychiatry 62:290–8, 2005.
16. von Moltke LL, Greenblatt DY, Grassi JM, et al. Protease inhibitors as inhibitors of human cytochromes P450: high risk associated with ritonavir. J Clin Pharmacol 38:106–11, 1998.
17. von Moltke LL, Greenblatt DY, Granda BW et al. Inhibition of cytochrome P450 isoforms by nonnucleoside reverse transcriptase inhibitors. J Clin Pharmacol 41:85–91, 2001.
18. Deeks SG, Smith M, Holodniy M, Kahn JO. HIV-1 protease inhibitors: a review for clinicians. JAMA 277:145–53, 1997.
19. Barry M, Mulcahy F, Merry C, et al. Pharmacokinetics and potential interactions amongst antiretroviral agents used to treat patients with HIV infection. Clin Pharmacokinet 36:289–304, 1999.
20. Piscitelli SC, Flexner C, Minor JR, et al. Drug interactions in patients infected with HIV. Clin Infect Dis 23:685–93, 1996.
21. Tseng AL, Foisy M. Significant interactions with new antiretrovirals and psychotropic drugs. Ann Pharmacother 33:461–73, 1999.

22. Ferrando SJ, Wapenyi K. Psychopharmacological treatment of patients with HIV and AIDS. Psychiatr Q 73: 33–49, 2002.
23. Himelhoch S, Moore RD, Treisman G, Gebo KA. Does the presence of a current psychiatric disorder in AIDS patients affect the initiation of antiretroviral treatment and duration of therapy? J Acquir Immune Defic Syndr 37:1457–63, 2004.
24. Lindemann E. Symptomatology and management of acute grief. Am J Psychiatry 101:141–8, 1944.
25. Lyketsos CG, Hanson A, Fishman M, et al. Screening for psychiatric morbidity in a medical outpatient clinic for HIV infection: the need for a psychiatric presence. Int J Psychiatry Med 24:103–13, 1994.
26. American Psychiatric Association. Diagnostic and Statistical Manual of Mental Disorders. 3rd edn, revised. Washington, DC: American Psychiatric Association; 1987.
27. Atkinson JH Jr, Grant I, Kennedy CJ, et al. Prevalence of psychiatric disorders among men infected with human immunodeficiency virus: a controlled study. Arch Gen Psychiatry 45:859–64, 1988.
28. Perkins DO, Stern RA, Golden RN, et al. Mood disorders in HIV infection: prevalence and risk factors in a nonepicenter of the AIDS epidemic. Am J Psychiatry 151:233–6, 1994.
29. Treisman GJ, Fishman M, Schwartz J, et al. Mood disorders in HIV infection. Depress Anxiety 7:178–87, 1998.
30. Hartgers C, Van Den Hoek JAR, Coutinho RA, Van Der Pligt J. Psychopathology, stress and HIV-risk injecting behaviour among drug users. Br J Addict 87:857–65, 1992.
31. Perry S, Jacobsberg LD, Fishman B, et al. Psychiatric diagnosis before serological testing for the human immunodeficiency virus. Am J Psychiatry 147:89–93, 1990.
32. Regier DA, Farmer ME, Rae DS, et al. Comorbidity of mental disorders with alcohol and other drug abuse. JAMA 264:2511, 1990.
33. Hutton HE, Lyketsos CG, Zenilman JM, et al. Depression and HIV risk behaviors among patients in a sexually transmitted disease clinic. Am J Psychiatry 161:912–14, 2004.
34. McDermott BE, Sautter FJ, Winstead DK, Quirk T. Diagnosis, health beliefs, and risk of HIV infection in psychiatric patients. Hosp Community Psychiatry 45:580–5, 1994.
35. Singh N, Squier C, Sivek C, et al. Determinants of compliance with antiretroviral therapy in patients with human immunodeficiency virus: prospective assessment with implications for enhancing compliance. AIDS Care 8:261–9, 1996.
36. Paterson DL, Swindells S, Mohr J, et al. Adherence to protease inhibitor therapy and outcomes in patients with HIV infection. Ann Int Med 133:21–30, 2000.
37. Yun LW, Maravi M, Kobayashi JS, et al. Antidepressant treatment improves adherence to antiretroviral therapy among depressed HIV-infected patients. J Acquir Immune Defic Syndr 38:432–8, 2005.
38. Himelhoch S, Moore RD, Treisman G, Gebo KA. Does the presence of a current psychiatric disorder in AIDS patients affect the initiation of antiretroviral treatment and duration of therapy? J AIDS 37:1457–63, 2004.
39. Vitiello B, Burnam MA, Bing EG, et al. Use of psychotropic medications among HIV-infected patients in the United States. Am J Psychiatry 160:547–54, 2003.
40. Lyketsos CG, Fishman M, Hutton H, et al. The effectiveness of psychiatric treatment for HIV-infected patients. Psychosomatics 38:423–32, 1997.
41. Bing EG, Burnam MA, Longshore D, et al. Psychiatric disorders and drug use among human immunodeficiency virus-infected adults in the United States. Arch Gen Psychiatry 58:721–8, 2001.
42. Micromedex(r) Healthcare Series (electronic version). Thomson Micromedex, Greenwood Village, CO, USA. Online. Available: http://www.thomsonhc.com 1 April 2006.
43. Thase ME, Blomgren SL, Birkett MA, et al. Fluoxetine treatment of patients with major depressive disorder who failed initial treatment with sertraline. J Clin Psychiatry 58:16–21, 1997.
44. Glassman AH, Perel JM, Shostak M, et al. Clinical implications of imipramine plasma levels for depressive illness. Arch Gen Psychiatry 34:197–204, 1977.
45. Asberg M, Cronholm B, Sjoqvist F, Tuck D. Relationship between plasma level and therapeutic effect of nortriptyline. BMJ 3:331–4, 1971.
46. Ziegler VE, Clayton PJ, Taylor JR, et al. Nortriptyline plasma levels and therapeutic response. Clin Pharmacol Ther 20: 458–63, 1976.
47. Coryell W. Augmentation strategies for inadequate antidepressant response: a review of placebo controlled studies. Ann Clin Psychiatry 12:141–6, 2000.
48. Caballero J, Nahata MC. Use of selective serotonin-reuptake inhibitors in the treatment of depression in adults with HIV. Ann Pharmacother 39:141–5, 2005.
49. Ouellet D, Hsu A, Qian J, et al. Effect of fluoxetine on pharmacokinetics of ritonavir. Antimicrob Agents Chemother 42:3107–12, 1998.
50. DeSilva KE, Le Flore DB, Marston BJ, Rimland D. Serotonin syndrome in HIV-infected individuals receiving antiretroviral therapy and fluoxetine. AIDS 15:1281–5, 2001.
51. Baker GB, Fang J, Sinha S, Coutts RT. Metabolic drug interactions with selective serotonin reuptake inhibitor (SSRI) antidepressants. Neurosci Biobehav Rev 22:325–33, 1998.
52. Hemeryck A, Belpaire FM. Selective serotonin reuptake inhibitors and cytochrome P-450 mediated drug–drug interactions: an update. Curr Drug Metab 3:13–37, 2002.
53. Gutierrez MM, Rosenberg J, Abramowitz W. An evaluation of the potential for pharmacokinetic interaction between escitalopram and the cytochrome P450 3A4 inhibitor ritonavir. Clin Ther 25:1200–10, 2003.
54. Elliott AJ, Uldall KK, Bergam K, et al. Randomized, placebo-controlled trial of paroxetine versus imipramine in depressed HIV-positive outpatients. Am J Psychiatry 155:367–72, 2003.
55. Rabkin JG, Rabkin R, Harrison W, Wagner G. Effect of imipramine on mood and enumerative measures of immune status in depressed patients with HIV illness. Am J Psychiatry 151:516–23, 1994.
56. Gannon RH, Anderson ML. Fluconazole–nortriptyline drug interaction [letter]. Ann Pharmacother 26:1456–57, 1992.
57. Elliott AJ, Roy-Byrne PP. Mirtazapine for depression in patients with human immunodeficiency virus. J Clin Psychopharmacol 20:265–7, 2000.
58. Elliott AJ, Russo J, Bergam K, et al. Antidepressant efficacy in HIV-seropositive outpatients with major depressive disorder: an open trial of nefazodone. J Clin Psychiatry 60:226–31, 1999.
59. Currier MB, Molina G, Kato M. A prospective trial of sustained-release bupropion for depression in HIV-seropositive and AIDS patients. Psychosomatics 44:120–5, 2003.
60. Fernandez F, Levy JK, Samley HR, et al. Effects of methylphenidate in HIV-related depression: a comparative trial with desipramine. Int J Psychiatry Med 25:53–67, 1995.
61. Wagner GJ, Rabkin JG, Rabkin R. Dextroamfetamine as a treatment for depression and low energy in AIDS patients: a pilot study. J Psychosomatic Res 42:407–11, 1997.
62. Wagner GJ, Rabkin R. Effects of dextroamfetamine on depression and fatigue in men with HIV: a double-blind, placebo-controlled trial. J Clin Psychiatry 61:436–40, 2000.
63. Breitbart, W, Rosenfeld B, Kaim M, Funesti-Esch J. A randomized, double-blind, placebo-controlled trial of psychostimulants for the treatment of fatigue in ambulatory patients with human immunodeficiency virus. Arch Internal Med 161: 411–20, 2001.

64. Greenblatt DJ, von Moltke LL, Harmatz JS, et al. Short-term exposure to low-dose ritonavir impairs clearance and enhances adverse effects of trazodone. J Clin Pharmacol 43:414–22, 2003.
65. Hesse LM, von Moltke LL, Shader RI, Greenblatt DJ. Ritonavir, efavirenz, and nelfinavir inhibit CYP2B6 activity in vitro: potential drug interactions with bupropion. Drug Metab Dispos 29:100–2, 2001.
66. Park-Wyllie LY, Antoniou T. Concurrent use of bupropion with CYP2B6 inhibitors, nelfinavir, ritonavir and efavirenz: a case series. AIDS 17:638–40, 2003.
67. American Psychiatric Association. Diagnostic and Statistical Manual of Mental Disorders. 4th edn, text revision. Washington, DC: American Psychiatric Association; 2000.
68. McKinnon K, Cournos F, Sugden R, et al. The relative contributions of psychiatric symptoms and AIDS knowledge to HIV risk behaviors among people with severe mental illness. J Clin Psychiatry 57:506–13, 1996.
69. Lyketsos CG, Schwartz J, Fishman M, Treisman G. AIDS mania. J Neuropsychiatry Clin Neurosci 9:277–9, 1997.
70. Ellen SR, Judd FK, Mijch AM, Cockram A. Secondary mania in patients with HIV infection. Aust NZ J Psychiatry 33: 353–60, 1999.
71. Lyketsos CG, Hanson AL, Fishman M, et al. Manic episodes early and late in the course of HIV. Am J Psychiatry 150: 326–7, 1993.
72. Mijch AM, Judd FK, Lyketsos CG, et al. Secondary mania in patients with HIV infection: are antiretrovirals protective? J Neuropsychiatry Clin Neurosci 11:475–80, 1999.
73. Taylor MJ, Goodwin GM. Long-term prophylaxis in bipolar disorder. CNS Drugs 20:303–10, 2006.
74. Baastrup PC, Schou M. Lithium as a prophylactic agent: its effect against recurrent depressions and manic-depressive psychosis. Arch Gen Psychiatry 16:162–72, 1967.
75. Baastrup PC, Poulsen JC, Schou M, et al. Prophylactic lithium: double blind discontinuation in manic-depressive and recurrent-depressive disorders. Lancet 2:326–30, 1970.
76. Suppes T, Baldessarini RJ, Faedda GL, Tohen M. Risk of recurrence following discontinuation of lithium treatment in bipolar disorder. Arch Gen Psychiatry 48:1082–8, 1991.
77. Bowden CL, Brugger AM, Swann AC, et al. Efficacy of divalproex vs. lithium and placebo in the treatment of mania. JAMA 271:918–24, 1994.
78. Pope HG Jr, McElroy SL, Keck PE, Hudson JI. Valproate in the treatment of acute mania: a placebo controlled study. Arch Gen Psychiatry 48:62–8, 1991.
79. Denicoff KD, Smith-Jackson EE, Disney ER, et al. Comparative prophylactic efficacy of lithium, carbamazepine, and the combination in bipolar disorder. J Clin Psychiatry 58:470–8, 1997.
80. Liedtke M, Lockhart S, Rathbun RC. Anticonvulsant and antiretroviral interactions. Ann Pharmacother 38:482–9, 2004.
81. Hugen PW, Burger DM, Brinkman K, et al. Carbamazepine–indinavir interaction causes antiretroviral therapy failure. Ann Pharmacother 34:465–70, 2000.
82. Bowden CL, Calabrese JR, McElroy SL, et al. The efficacy of lamotrigine in rapid cycling and non-rapid cycling patients with bipolar disorder. Biol Psychiatry 45:953–8, 1999.
83. Ichim L, Berk M, Brook S. Lamotrigine compared with lithium in mania: a double-blind randomized controlled trial. Ann Clin Psychiatry 12:5–10, 2000.
84. Letterman L, Markowitz JS. Gabapentin: a review of published experience in the treatment of bipolar disorder and other psychiatric conditions. Pharmacotherapy 19:565–72, 1999.
85. Marcotte D. Use of topiramate, a new anti-epileptic, as a mood stabilizer. J Affect Disord 50:245–51, 1998.
86. Hriso E, Kuhn T, Masdeu JC, Grundman M. Extrapyramidal symptoms due to dopamine-blocking agents in patients with AIDS encephalopathy. Am J Psychiatry 148:1558–61, 1991.
87. Hollander H, Golden J, Mendelson T, Cortland D. Extrapyramidal symptoms in AIDS patients given low-dose metoclopramide or chlorpromazine. Lancet ii:1186, 1985.
88. Edelstein H, Knight RT. Severe parkinsonism in two AIDS patients taking prochlorperazine. Lancet ii:341–2, 1987.
89. Lera G, Zirulnik J. Pilot study with clozapine in patients with HIV-associated psychosis and drug-induced parkinsonism. Mov Disord 14:128–31, 1999.
90. Chaisson MA, Stoneburner RL, Hildebrandt DS, et al. Heterosexual transmission of HIV-1 associated with the use of smokable free-base cocaine (crack). AIDS 5:1121–6, 1991.
91. Edlin BR, Irwin KL, Faruque S, et al. (Multicenter Crack Cocaine and HIV Study Team) Interesting epidemics–crack cocaine use and HIV infection among inner-city young adults. N Engl J Med 331:1422–7, 1994.
92. Nuttbrock L, Rosenblum A, Magura S, et al. The association between cocaine use and HIV/STDs among soup kitchen attendees in New York City. J AIDS 25:86–91, 2000.
93. Astemborski J, Vlahov D,Waren D, et al. The trading of sex for drugs or money and HIV seropositivity among female intravenous drug users. Am J Public Health 84:382–7, 1994.
94. Windle M. The trading of sex for money or drugs, sexually transmitted diseases (STDs), and HIV-related risk behaviors among multisubstance using alcoholic inpatients. Drug Alcohol Depend 49:33–8, 1997.
95. Chesney M. Factors affecting adherence to antiretroviral therapy. Clin Infect Dis 30(Suppl 2):S171–6, 2000.
96. Wynn G, Cozza K, Zapor M, et al. Antiretrovirals, Part III: Antiretrovirals and drugs of abuse. Psychosomatics 46:79–87, 2005.
97. Antoniou T, Tseng AL. Interactions between recreational drugs and antiretroviral agents. Ann Pharmacother 36:1598–613, 2002.
98. Altice F, Friedland G, Cooney E. Nevirapine induced opiate withdrawal among injection drug users with HIV infection receiving methadone. AIDS 13:957–62, 1999.
99. Beauverie P, Taburet AM, Dessalles MC, et al. Therapeutic drug monitoring of methadone in HIV-infected patients receiving protease inhibitors [letter]. AIDS 12:2510–11, 1998.
100. Pinzani V, Faucherre V, Peyreire H, Blayac JP. Methadone withdrawal symptoms with nevirapine and efavirenz [letter]. Ann Pharmacother 34:405–7, 2000.
101. McCance-Katz EF, Farber S, Selwyn PA, O'Connor A. Decrease in methadone levels with nelfinavir mesylate [letter]. Am J Psychiatry 157:481, 2000.
102. Bart PA, Rizzardi PG, Gallant S, et al. Methadone blood concentrations are decreased by the administration of abacavir plus amprenavir. Ther Drug Monit 23:553–5, 2001.
103. Kresina TF, Flexner CW, Sinclair J, et al. Alcohol use and HIV pharmacotherapy. AIDS Res HumRetroviruses 18: 757–70, 2002.
104. Braithwaite RS, McGinnis KA, Conigliaro J, et al. A temporal and dose-response association between alcohol consumption and medication adherence among veterans in care. Alcohol Clin Exp Res 29: 1190–7, 2005.
105. Eysenck HJ, Rachman S. The Causes and Cures of Neurosis. San Diego, CA: Robert R Knapp; 1965, pp 14–28.
106. Nace EP, Davis CW, Gaspari JP. Axis II comorbidity in substance abusers. Am J Psychiatry 148:118–20, 1991.
107. Zubenko GS, George AW, Soloff PH, Schulz P. Sexual practices among patients with borderline personality disorder. Am J Psychiatry 144:748–52, 1987.
108. Sacks MH, Perry S, Graver R, et al. Self-reported HIV-related risk behaviors in acute psychiatric inpatients: a pilot study. Hosp Community Psychiatry 41:1253–5, 1990.

109. Brooner RK, Greenfield L, Schmidt CW, Bigelow GE. Antisocial personality disorder and HIV infection among intravenous drug abusers. Am J Psychiatry 150:53–8, 1993.
110. Perkins DO, Davidson EJ, Leserman J, et al. Personality disorder in patients infected with HIV: a controlled study with implications for clinical care. Am J Psychiatry 150:309–15, 1993.
111. Wells BWP. Personality study of VD patients: using the psychoticism, extroversion, neuroticism inventory. Br J Vener Dis 46:498–501, 1970.
112. O'Campo P, Deboer M, Faden RR, et al. Prior episode of sexually transmitted disease and subsequent sexual risk reduction practices. Sex Transm Dis 19:326–30, 1992.

Chapter 64

Dermatologic Disease

Arturo Saavedra-Lauzon, MD, PhD, Richard A. Johnson, MD

Cutaneous disorders occur nearly universally during the course of HIV disease as a result of acquired immunodeficiency or related to treatment. Management of dermatologic conditions in HIV disease is a very broad subject, overlapping many other medical specialties.[1] Individuals who have access to highly active antiretroviral therapy (HAART), in most cases those living in North America, Western Europe, and Australia, have a markedly altered course of HIV disease if immune restoration is achieved. In most cases, there is a marked reduction in the incidence of opportunistic infections (OIs) and neoplasms (ONs). Globally, however, more than 95% of those HIV-infected individuals have no access to any medical interventions. Despite estimates by the World Health Organization that at least 4.4 million people in sub-Saharan Africa (the region with the highest number of people living with HIV/AIDS) were in need of treatment with antiretroviral therapy in 2003, only ~100 000 people were on therapy.[2] Consequently, many of the cutaneous manifestations associated with HIV disease become chronic and progressive. Furthermore, the incidence and severity of cutaneous manifestations of HIV, including molluscum contagiosum, herpes simplex, oropharyngeal candidiasis, secondary syphilis, papular pruritic eruptions and seborrheic dermatitis among others, may serve as indicators of CD4+ T-lymphocyte counts and CD4:CD8 ratios, particularly in the developing world.[3]

DIAGNOSIS

Clinical findings are often adequate for diagnosis of the majority of cutaneous disorders occurring in HIV-infected persons. With more advanced immunodeficiency, the clinical value of the gross appearance of a cutaneous lesion may be limited. Lesional skin biopsy is often the most rapid and sensitive method for diagnosis of any dermatosis. Infectious agents can be detected both histologically and immunologically by appropriate cultures and stains. A 6- or 8-mm punch biopsy is usually sufficient. An adequate portion of the tissue is sent for histopathologic evaluation by routine methods and also by special stains for fungi, mycobacteria, and bacteria. When indicated, the remaining tissue can be cultured for aerobic and anaerobic bacteria, mycobacteria, and fungi. When histopathology and culture are negative, polymerase chain reaction (PCR) can be helpful in establishing the diagnosis, particularly in the case of mycobacterial disease.

ACUTE HIV INFECTION (PRIMARY RETROVIRAL SYNDROME)

Mucocutaneous findings in acute HIV infection include "rash" (50–60%; Fig. 64-1), oral candidiasis (17%), oral ulcers (10–20%), and genital ulcers (5–15%).[4,5] Individuals with problematic rash or ulceration(s) should be treated symptomatically, as well as with HAART. Though it is important to recognize and treat a variety of sexually transmitted disease that may be co-transmitted with acute HIV infection, studies report that between 34% and 60% of genital ulcers have no proven etiological agent and may be related to HIV-mediated aphthous ulceration. In up to 12% of cases, mixed etiologies may be responsible for genital ulceration.[6] Symptomatic candidiasis can be treated with topical or systemic anticandidal therapy (*see section on* Cutaneous Candidiasis).

CUTANEOUS DISORDERS OCCURRING WITH HIV DISEASE

Pruritus and Pruritic Eruptions in HIV Disease

Pruritus, a common complaint in patients with late symptomatic and advanced HIV disease, is a surrogate cutaneous marker for disease progression, occurring commonly in patients with

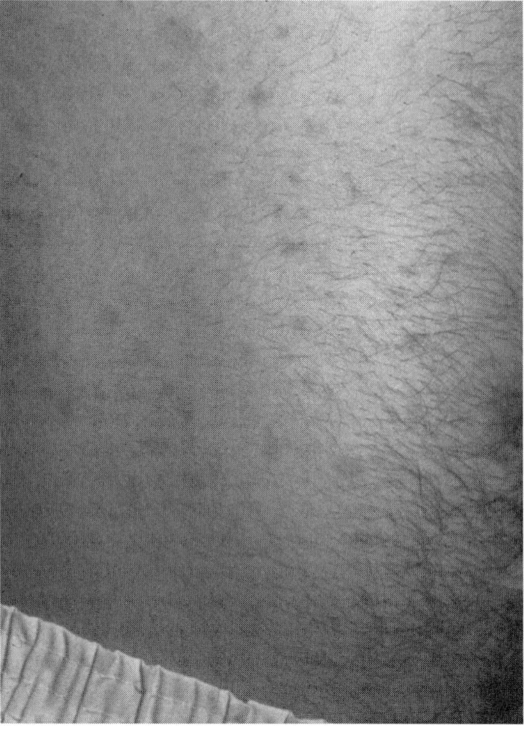

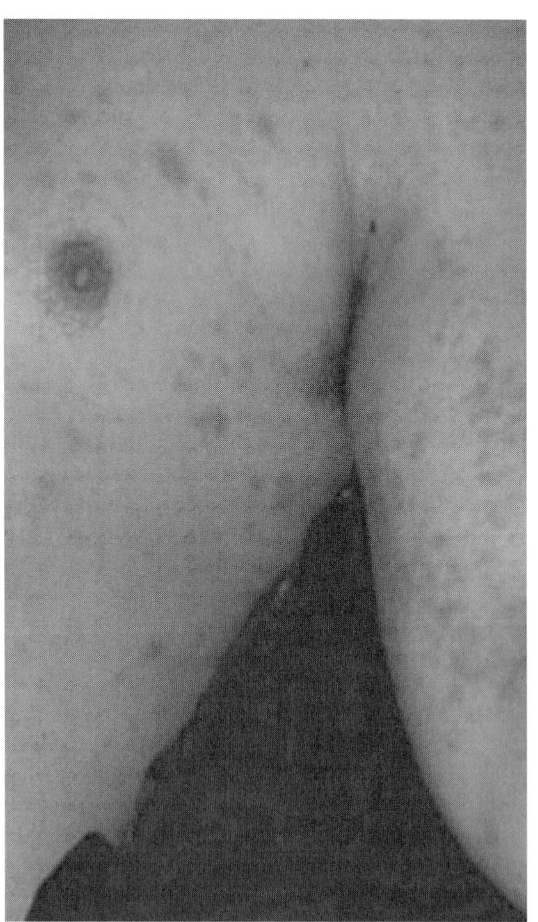

Figure 64-1 ■ Acute retroviral syndrome: exanthem.

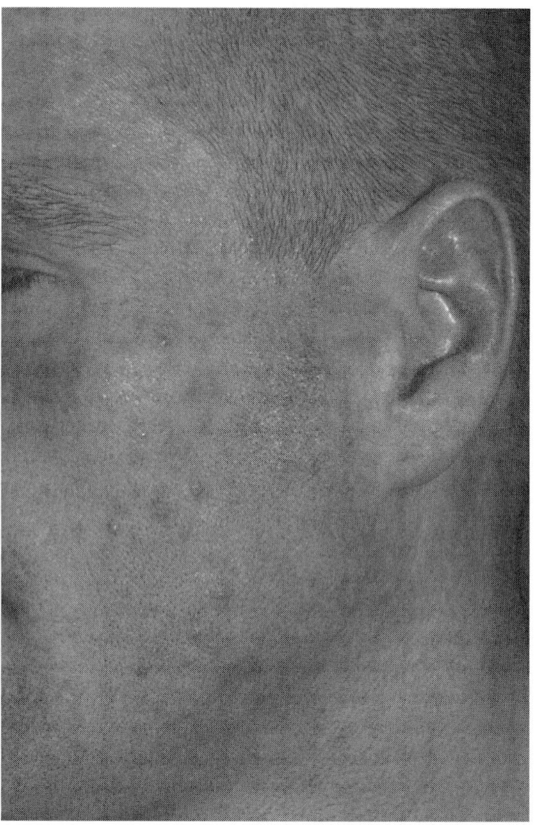

Figure 64-2 ■ Eosinophilic folliculitis: IRIS.

CD4+ T-lymphocyte counts less than 50 cells/μL compared with those with counts over 250 cells/μL.[7] In most cases, primary or secondary dermatoses rather than metabolic disorders are the cause of pruritus.[8] The differential diagnosis of primary pruritic skin disorders includes eosinophilic folliculitis (EF) (Fig. 64-2), papular pruritic eruption of HIV, adverse cutaneous drug eruptions, atopic dermatitis, xerosis, dermatographism, allergic contact dermatitis, scabies, and insect bites.[9] Much less commonly, systemic and metabolic disorders such as lymphoma, renal failure, viral hepatitis (hepatitis B or C), or obstructive liver disease are associated with pruritus in the absence of cutaneous findings, i.e., "metabolic" pruritus.[10]

An atopic diathesis (characterized by personal or family history of atopic dermatitis, asthma, and allergic rhinitis), which exists in up to 20% of the general population, may become manifest in individuals with advanced HIV disease and pruritus. Changes secondary to chronic rubbing and scratching include excoriations, atopic dermatitis, lichen simplex chronicus, and prurigo nodularis (Fig. 64-3). Up to 50% of HIV-infected individuals are *Staphylococcus aureus* nasal carriers. Secondary *S. aureus* infection (impetiginization, furunculosis, or cellulitis) is very common in any of these traumatized lesions. Ichthyosis vulgaris and xerosis are common in advanced HIV disease and may be associated with mild pruritus.

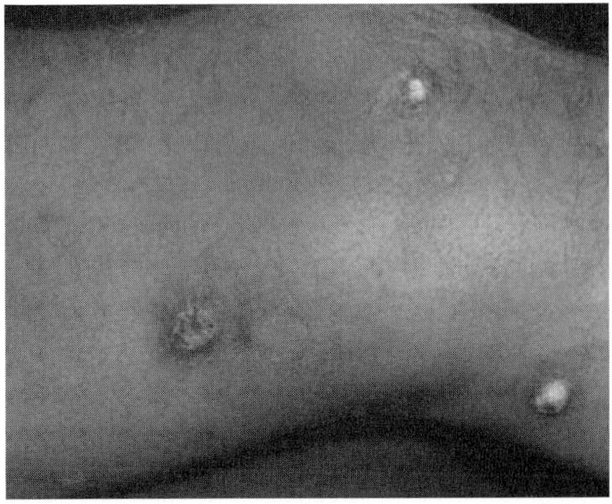

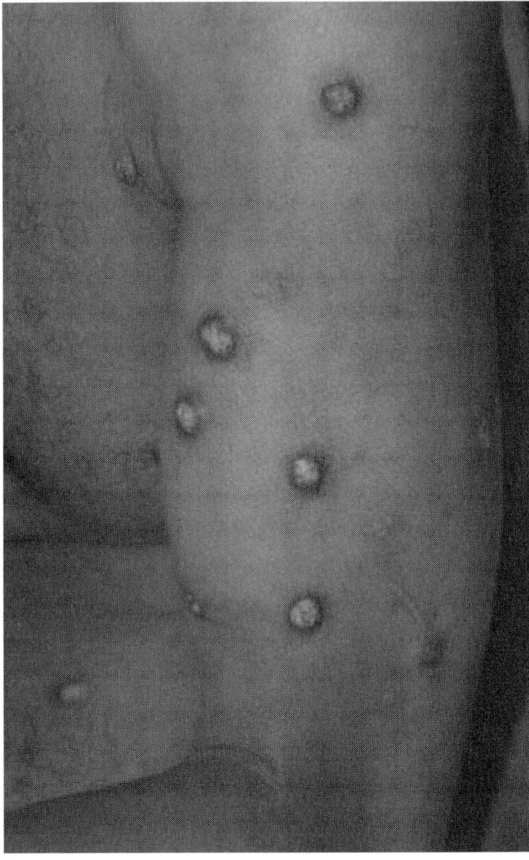

Figure 64-3 ■ Prurigo nodularis.

The protease inhibitors (especially indinavir) frequently cause xerosis with or without eczematous dermatitis, which may be associated with mild or moderate pruritus (*see section on* Adverse Cutaneous Drug Reactions). These changes occur relatively soon after initiation of therapy, presenting with xerosis (dry skin) with or without eczematous dermatitis or nummular eczema. Exanthematous drug eruptions such as those caused by trimethoprim–sulfamethoxazole (TMP-SMX) occur relatively suddenly and are easily associated with a newly prescribed drug.

Scabies can present with significant pruritus but few cutaneous findings in HIV disease in the early course of infestation (*see section on* Crusted (Norwegian) Scabies). Conversely, in individuals with advanced disease, pruritus may be minimal, resulting in delayed diagnosis. In these cases, the clinical presentation is of a generalized eczematous or psoriasiform dermatosis, i.e., hyperkeratotic or crusted (Norwegian) scabies.

Insect bites especially those of mosquitos can become very large, 1–2 cm, presenting as few or multiple pruritic papules or nodules on exposed skin sites. Severely symptomatic insect bites may require corticosteroid therapy applied topically, or given intralesionally or orally (usually a 1 week tapered course).

Therapy

Control of pruritus is of great importance, in that scratching or rubbing the skin both causes as well as compounds the eczematous dermatitis. Oral doxepin is an excellent antipruritic agent taken at bedtime, the adult dosing varying from 10 to 200 mg. Many other less sedating antihistaminic agents are also effective for daytime or bedtime dosing. Gabapentin may also be helpful in dosages between 300 and 1800 mg/day, which can be titrated over a month according to symptoms. In recalcitrant cases, as is seen in prurigo nodularis, thalidomide in doses ranging from 33 to 200 mg/day, has been shown to be beneficial. Neurological examination is essential, as up to one-third of patients may develop peripheral neuropathy.[11]

Eosinophilic Folliculitis

EF is a chronic dermatosis occurring in persons with advanced HIV disease or in those with immune restoration associated with HAART. The etiology and pathogenesis are unknown. Symptoms of EF usually occur when the CD4+ T-lymphocyte cell count is under 100 cells/μL; however, with HAART, EF occurs initially, recurs, or flares as immune restoration occurs and viral load levels fall (Fig. 64-2). As association with nadir in CD4+ T-lymphocyte counts less than 70 cells/μL has also been noted.[12]

The pruritus associated with EF is often intense, more so in individuals with an atopic diathesis. Even early in the course of EF, with few lesions present, pruritus can be the most bothersome symptom, especially by disturbing sleep. Clinically, small pink-to-red, edematous, folliculocentric papules (and much less commonly pustules) occur symmetrically above the nipple line on the chest, proximal arms, head, and neck. The lesions have the appearance of small insect bites (papular urticaria). Rubbing, scratching, and excoriation soon alter primary lesions with the appearance of excoriations, excoriated papules, lichen simplex chronicus, and prurigo nodularis. In individuals with darker skin, postinflammatory hyperpigmentation often produces significant cosmetic disfigurement. Any of these secondary changes can become infected with *S. aureus*, or less commonly, group A streptococcus. Once significant immune restoration has been achieved with HAART, EF resolves.

Although subjective and objective findings of early EF are nearly pathognomonic, subacute or chronic EF may have many secondary changes, which make a clinical diagnosis tentative. In these cases, diagnosis of EF should be confirmed by the histologic findings. Peripheral eosinophilia is common in HIV-associated EF, in some cases, up to 35%.[13]

Therapy

The most effective therapy for EF is prednisone. Beginning with an initial dose of 70 mg PO, prednisone is tapered by 10 or 5 mg over 7 or 14 days; established lesions resolve, new lesions do not occur, and pruritus resolves. In the majority of persons with successfully treated EF, lesions and pruritus recur within a few weeks after prednisone has been discontinued. In those with severe symptoms, prednisone can be given on alternate days or weekly.

Several orally administered agents have been reported to be effective in treatment of EF. Oral isotretinoin is effective and safe in treatment of EF, usually 40 mg bid until lesions and symptoms resolve, then tapered to 40 mg daily for several weeks, and then to 20 mg daily or 40 mg qod.[14] Isotretinoin can raise serum triglyceride levels, which are often high in HIV-infected persons; serum lipid should be monitored regularly. Isotretinoin (as well as protease inhibitors) commonly causes cheilitis, eczematous dermatitis, and xerosis; these adverse effects can usually be managed with "moisturizing" agents and corticosteroid ointment.

Phototherapy with ultraviolet radiation (UVR), using ultraviolet A (UVA), ultraviolet B (UVB) with or without topical or systemic psoralen is considered to be a safe topical treatment modality in HIV-infected persons.[15] UVR does not appear to have a significant deleterious effect on HIV viral load.[16] UVB phototherapy of EF, given by skilled technicians to compliant patients, is effective in suppressing both lesions and symptoms. Compliance is an issue for many individuals in that treatment is usually given three times per week for 4–8 weeks, subsequently reducing the frequency of treatment as the skin clears.

High-potency topical corticosteroid preparations may reduce the formation of new EF lesions and cause established lesions to resolve, thus providing symptomatic relief. New lesions occur once corticosteroids are discontinued. There is a significant risk of cutaneous atrophy if corticosteroids are applied chronically. Tacrolimus ointment 0.1% has been reported to be effective.[16] Sedating antihistamines such as doxepin are most effective for symptomatic control of nocturnal pruritus; nonsedating antihistamines are ineffective in controlling pruritus.

Unlike EF, acne does not appear to be exacerbated by HIV.[17] However, acne has been observed in those treated with androgel for hypogonadism in HIV disease.

Papular Pruritic Eruption of HIV

Papular pruritic eruption of HIV (PPE) represents significant morbidity to the HIV-infected individual, particularly in sub-Saharan Africa. It has been classified with other pruritic disorders in HIV disease in the spectrum of EF and nonspecific pruritus. The prevalence is estimated between 12% and 46% in Africans and Haitians, and the disease is only rarely observed in Europe and North America. The positive predictive value of PPE for HIV infection is ~85%.[18] In addition, it appears to be a marker of severe immunosuppression as over 80% of patients with this disorder have counts less than 100 cells/μL.[19]

The primary lesion is a firm urticarial papule (though sterile pustules have been described as well) and displays variable erythema distributed symmetrically on the trunk and extremities and less commonly on the face. It is occasionally but not always folliculocentric and may be associated with excoriations, postinflammatory hyperpigmentation and scarring which result from the intense pruritus caused by the disease. A recent report from studies in Uganda has suggested that PPE is a hypersensitivity reaction to arthropod bites based on histopathologic evaluation of skin biopsies. The authors proposed changing the name of this disorder to "arthropod-induced prurigo of HIV."[18]

Therapy

PPE is particularly difficult to treat and is only moderately responsive to antihistamines and topical steroids. UVB appears to be the most effective therapy, though its utility is limited by the lack of treatment centers in resource-poor settings where the prevalence is highest. Studies with more advanced or costly alternatives are lacking.

Atopic Dermatitis (Eczematous Dermatitis)

Eczematous dermatitis is managed by treating underlying causes such as xerosis, adverse cutaneous drug reactions, scabies, or metabolic pruritus. Potent corticosteroids or tacrolimus 0.1% ointment are the most effective topical agents for treatment of eczematous dermatitis. High potency, short-term dosing usually minimizes the use of topical corticosteroid preparations. In more severe cases, a 1–2 week tapered course of prednisone is indicated, beginning at an initial dose of 70 mg in adults. For patients with dermatitis recurring after prednisone, phototherapy is effective and safe (*see section on* Pruritus and Pruritic Eruptions in HIV Disease).[20]

Psoriasis Vulgaris

The prevalence of psoriasis vulgaris in HIV-infected individuals may be somewhat higher than that of the general population; that of psoriatic arthritis, however, is higher, correlating with the presence of HLA-B27. The onset of psoriatic lesions may be prior to or following HIV infection. Onset of psoriasis in an individual at risk for HIV disease may be an indication for HIV serotesting. Psoriasis and Reiter's syndrome may coexist in the same patient, suggesting the two disorders may be part of a spectrum of clinical manifestations of one disease. Psoriasis with onset following HIV infection has been observed to improve more so with HAART than psoriasis noted prior to HIV infection.

In a cohort of 50 HIV-infected individuals with psoriasis, one-third of psoriasis cases were presumed to have occurred prior to HIV infection (group I) and two-thirds after infection (group II). Group I had a lower mean age of onset (19 years vs 36 years) and more commonly had a family history of psoriasis. The clinical patterns of psoriasis (Fig. 64-4a–c) were reported to be plaque type (78%), inverse (37%), guttate (29%), palmoplantar (8%), erythrodermic (14%), and pustular (8%). Palmoplantar and inverse pattern psoriasis were more common in group II; severe psoriasis occurred in one quarter of these patients. Psoriasis tended to become more severe as the degree of immunodeficiency increased, but did not affect survival.

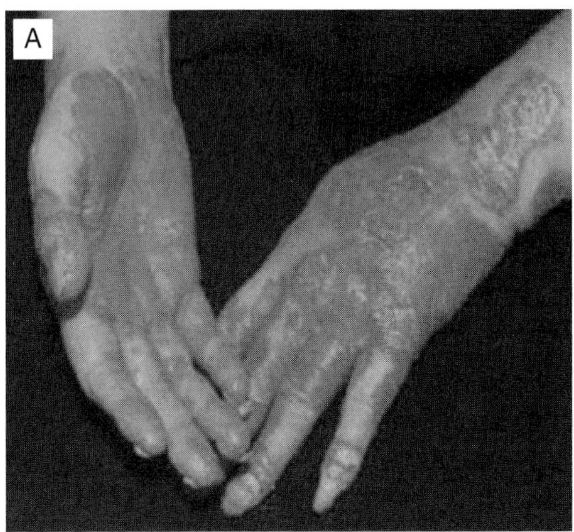

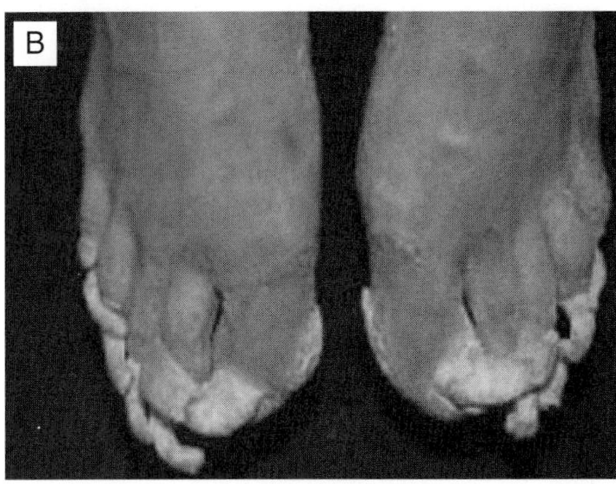

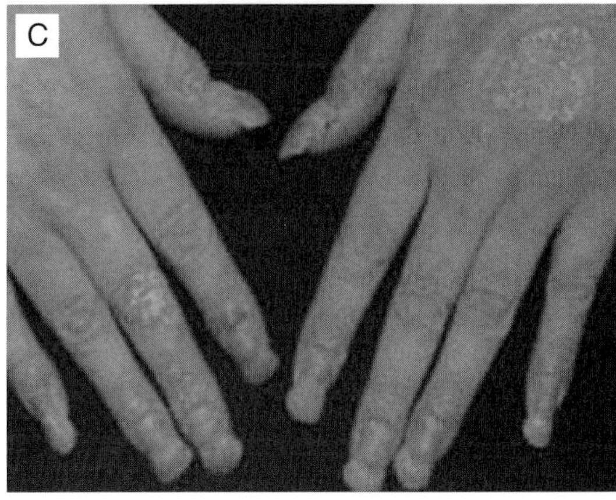

Figure 64-4 ■ Psoriasis vulgaris: hands (**a**), feet (**b**), nails (**c**).

Therapy

Topical agents may be effective in management of limited psoriasis, i.e., corticosteroids, calcipotriene, or retinoids. Tacrolimus and pimecrolimus ointment may be effective for psoriasis occurring in naturally occluded skin (inverse pattern psoriasis) such as in the axilla, submammary region, and anogenital sites. Subacute or chronic use of corticosteroids to these sites causes cutaneous atrophy, striae, and/or erosions.

For more widespread disease, phototherapy with UVB, narrow band UVB (311 nm), or psoralen UVA (PUVA) is safe and effective (*see section on* Eosinophilic Folliculitis). Photosensitizing agents such as sulfa drugs can cause phototoxic or photoallergic reactions in an individual treated with phototherapy.

Oral therapy with retinoids such as acitretin, methotrexate, and cyclosporin is indicated for persons with psoriasis that is unresponsive to topical steroids and phototherapy. Oral or intramuscular methotrexate given weekly is effective for psoriatic arthritis. Systemic therapy requires careful monitoring of lipids, complete white cell count and liver function tests. Successful treatment of psoriasis and psoriatic arthritis with biologics such as etanercept and infliximab in the HIV-host exists in the form of case reports.[21]

Erythroderma

Erythroderma in HIV disease may be related to drug hypersensitivity, atopic dermatitis, psoriasis vulgaris, photosensitivity dermatitis, the hypereosinophilic syndrome and cutaneous T-cell lymphoma. In addition, rare infections such as histoplasmosis and coexistent HTLV-I infection may present as erythroderma in the HIV host.[22]

Xerosis and Ichthyosis

Xerosis and acquired ichthyosis are very common in HIV-infected individuals, occurring in up to 30% of those with advanced disease. These disorders are more common during the winter months associated with low relative humidity. Several factors are involved in the pathogenesis including chronic illness, malnutrition, atopic diathesis with ichthyosis vulgaris, wasting syndrome, protease inhibitor therapy, or HIV infection itself.

Therapy

Xerosis is best treated with application of "emollient" creams after bathing. Products with hydroxy acids are keratolytic and hydrophilic. In persons with chronic xerosis, eczematous dermatitis can occur within fissures in areas of hyperkeratosis, i.e., eczema craquelé or asteatotic eczema (*see section on* Atopic Dermatitis (Eczematous Dermatitis)).

Photosensitivity

Idiopathic photosensitivity is an increasingly recognized phenomenon in HIV disease, and may be the presenting complaint.[23,24] African-American ethnicity and HAART appear to be independent risk factors for development of disease, which presents mostly as lichenoid or eczematous dermatitis.[25] The most common types of photosensitivity in HIV disease are related to drug therapy. Drug-induced photosensitivity reactions are of two types; phototoxic, which occurs in all individuals and is essentially an exaggerated sunburn response (erythema, edema, vesicles, e.g., TMP-SMX), and photoallergic, which involves an immunologic response in which the eruption is papular, vesicular, eczema-like, and occurs only in previously sensitized individuals. Drug-induced photosensitivity reactions are most commonly caused by UVA, and to a much lesser extent UVB. Photosensitivity in HIV disease appears to be a manifestation of advanced disease (*see section on* Porphyria Cutanea Tarda).[26]

Three patterns of phototoxic reactions occur: immediate erythema and urticaria, delayed sunburn-type pattern developing within 16–24 h or later (48–72 h), or delayed (72–96 h) melanin pigmentation. Clinically, phototoxic reactions are an "exaggerated sunburn", presenting as erythema, edema, and blister formation (e.g., pseudoporphyria). Marked brown epidermal melanin pigmentation may occur in the course of the eruption; gray dermal melanin pigmentation develops with certain drugs (chlorpromazine and amiodarone). After repeated exposure, some scaling and lichenification can develop. The reaction is confined exclusively to areas exposed to light.

In photoallergic drug hypersensitivity, the drug present in the skin absorbs protons and forms a photodrug, which then binds to a soluble or membrane-bound protein to form an antigen. Since photoallergy depends on individual immunologic reactivity, it develops in only a small percentage of persons exposed to drugs and light. Clinically, acute photoallergic reactions present as eczematous dermatitis or as lichen planus-like (lichenoid) eruptions. In chronic drug photoallergy, marked scaling, lichenification (thickening), and pruritus/scratching mimic atopic dermatitis or chronic allergic contact dermatitis. Photoallergic eruptions are confined primarily to areas exposed to light, but may spread to adjacent nonexposed skin; therefore, they are not as circumscribed as phototoxic reactions.

Therapy

In management of photosensitivity, a photosensitizing agent should be identified and discontinued if possible. If the offending drug cannot be discontinued, sunlight should be avoided; sunscreen and protective clothing should be recommended. Phototoxic drug reactions disappear after cessation of the drug. Photoallergic drug reactions can persist for months or years after the drug is discontinued (known as persistent light reaction or chronic actinic dermatitis). In severe cases of photoallergic dermatitis topical or systemic corticosteroids or other agents such as nonsteroidal antiinflammatory drugs (NSAIDs) or pentoxifylline are indicated.[27]

Pigmentary Disorders

Postinflammatory hyper- and hypopigmentation are the most common disorders affecting HIV-infected individuals. With the exception of light skinned individuals of northern European heritage, significant lightening or darkening of skin color occurs following any type of inflammatory dermatosis or infection. In addition to pigmentary alterations, significant atrophic or hypertrophic scarring can follow herpes zoster. This alteration in normal skin color results in significant cosmetic disfigurement, especially when it occurs on highly visible sites such as the face, neck, and upper extremities. If the dermatosis is chronic, the pigmentary change can become persistent and progressive. If the dermatosis resolves, the pigmentary disorder can take from months to years to gradually fade to uniform pigmentation.

Therapy

The primary goal in management of these pigmentary disorders is to treat the primary skin disorder. Topical preparations containing 4% hydroquinone may be helpful in treating postinflammatory hyperpigmentation.

APHTHOUS ULCERS

Recurrent and/or persistent aphthous ulcers (AUs) complicate advanced HIV disease, arising in the mouth, oropharynx, and esophagus (*see* Chapter 65). AU-like lesions occur on the external genitalia during the course of acute HIV infections. AU of the upper mouth and esophagus frequently cause moderate to severe pain, impairing eating and speaking, and are associated with significant weight loss. The incidence appears to be reduced with HAART.

Therapy

Individual AUs of the anterior mouth and oropharynx usually respond to intralesional triamcinolone injection; deeper lesions, however, cannot be treated with this effective, low-risk modality. Prednisone is usually quite effective in treatment of persistent AUs; most AUs resolve with an initial dose of 70 mg tapered by 10 or 5 mg/day. In persons in whom prednisone is contraindicated or ineffective, thalidomide 50–200 mg HS is an effective alternative medication.[28] The most common adverse events occurring with thalidomide are neutropenia, rash, and peripheral sensory neuropathy.

CUTANEOUS MANIFESTATIONS OF SYSTEMIC DISORDERS OCCURRING IN HIV DISEASE

Porphyria Cutanea Tarda and Pseudoporphyria

Porphyria cutanea tarda (PCT) in HIV disease is most often associated with an underlying hepatopathy (hepatitis C virus (HCV) infection, alcoholism, or hepatitis B virus (HBV) infection).[29] The HIV virus is thought to inhibit the cytochrome oxidase system, thereby affecting porphyrin metabolism.[30] In one study, 40% of patients ($n = 33$) with advanced HIV disease had increased urinary porphyrin excretion; 31 patients were herpes simplex virus (HSV)-seropositive; four patients had urine and stool porphyrin excretion patterns that were classic for PCT.[31] No study patient, however, had clinical evidence of PCT. Thus, porphyrin studies are recommended for HIV-infected individuals with photosensitivity. Clinically, PCT presents with blisters, erosions, crusts, milia on the dorsum of the hands as a manifestation of photosensitivity. Hyperpigmentation and hypertrichosis often occur on the face.

Therapy

PCT is managed by removal of hepatotoxins, especially alcohol. Biochemical remission can be achieved by depletion of iron stores with weekly or biweekly phlebotomy of 500 mL of blood until the hemoglobin is reduced to 10 g. Chloroquine can be effective in persons with anemia.

Pseudoporphyria (pseudo-PCT) occurs in the absence of abnormalities of porphyrin metabolism, is usually drug-induced, and is characterized clinically by blisters and/or erosions on the dorsum of the hands. The most common drugs associated with pseudo-PCT are NSAIDs such as naproxen, ibuprofen, oxaprozin, and nabumetone. Other drugs implicated include tetracyclines, nalidixic acid, dapsone, amiodarone, bumetanide, cyclosporine, furosemide, chlorthalidone, hydrochlorthiazide, pyridoxine. UVA in phototherapy or tanning beds can induce pseudo-PCT. Pseudo-PCT also occurs in the setting of chronic renal failure with hemodialysis.

Vasculitis

Cutaneous and systemic vasculitis of many etiologies have been reported to occur in HIV disease, including adverse cutaneous drug reaction, erythema elevatum diutinum, cytomegalovirus (CMV) infection, polyarteritis nodosa, and Kawasaki's disease, lymphomatoid granulomatosis, and possibly HIV infection itself.[32] Causative drugs should be discontinued if possible. Most other causes are not specifically treatable. Systemic immunosuppressive therapy may be indicated in some cases.

Autoimmunie Disorders

Immune reconstitution following therapy with HAART may exacerbate or induce autoimmune disorders. Generally, immunosuppression caused by HIV infection improves conditions such as systemic lupus erythematosus. Systemic, tumid and discoid lupus have been reported soon after initiation of HAART.[33,34] Though tumid and discoid lupus may respond to antimalarials such as hydroxychloroquine 200 mg orally twice a day, systemic lupus usually requires systemic immuno suppression. Immune reconstitution may also induce vitiligo and sarcoid.[35–37] Mycobacterial infection must be excluded before a diagnosis of sarcoid is made. On the other hand, autoimmune symptoms have also been linked to HIV infection in the absence of immune reconstitution. Rheumatoid arthritis, reactive arthritis, diffuse interstitial lymphocytosis syndrome, subcorneal pustular dermatosis and pemphigus vulgaris have been reported in HIV disease.[38,39]

Therapy

Treatment of these disorders may require systemic immunosuppression. In pemphigus vulgaris, the role of cyclosporine has been explored, as it appears to have antiretroviral activity *in vitro*.[39]

OPPORTUNISTIC CUTANEOUS INFECTIONS IN HIV DISEASE

Bacterial Infections

S. aureus causes the majority of all pyodermas and soft-tissue infections (Fig. 64-5). Colonization of the anterior nares occurs in greater than 50% of HIV-infected individuals. From 1997 to 2000, it was the most common bacterial isolate in HIV-positive individuals, unlike HIV-negative individuals who are most frequently colonized by coagulase-negative *Staphylococci*. In addition, the number of isolates that are methicillin-resistant *S. aureus* (MRSA), as well as methicillin-resistant coagulase-negative *Staphylococci* is increasing in HIV-positive individuals over the rate noted in HIV-negative counterparts.[40] In a recent study of HIV-positive men who have sex with men, the frequency of community acquired MRSA was associated with high-risk sexual and drug-using behaviors but not with immune status.[41] Intravascular catheters and cutaneous infections are the most common sources of *S. aureus* bacteremia.

Rarely, as the result of trauma, *S. aureus* can infect the skin in the form of deep nodules, ulcers or verrucous plaques that discharge granules via sinuses. Lesions are usually found in the lower extremities and may be tender and pruritic.

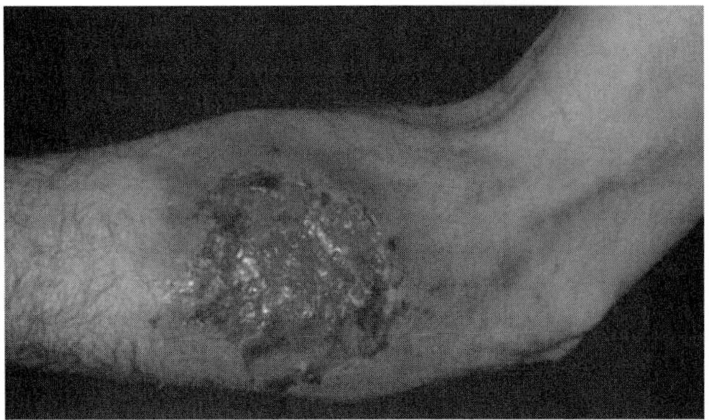

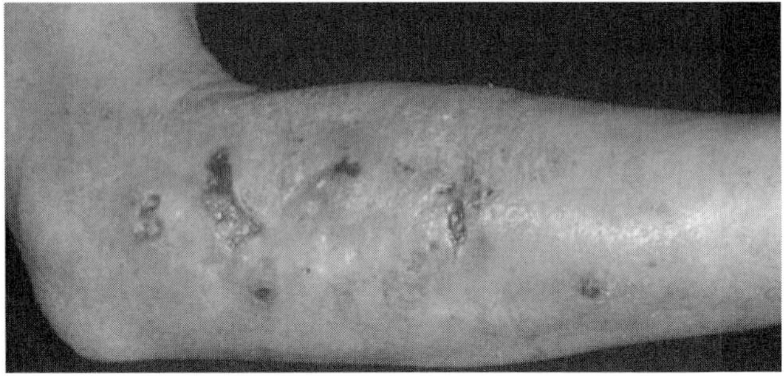

Figure 64-5 ■ MRSA infection: injection-site infections.

Botryomycosis in the HIV host is a chronic disease and diagnosis is made on histopathology and culture. Antibiotics are usually not sufficient to eradicate infection, and surgical excision is recommended. The disease is mostly cutaneous, though visceral botryomycosis has been reported.[42]

Therapy

Mupirocin ointment is effective in eradicating colonizing *S. aureus*. Benzoyl peroxide used as a wash is effective for treatment of colonized cutaneous sites or lesions. Alcohol-based hand gels, such as Purell and Cal Stat may also be of benefit. Oral antibiotic therapy with dicloxacillin or cephalexin is useful for those patients with methicillin-sensitive *S. aureus* (MSSA); in recent years, however, the incidence of MRSA is such that it should be assumed that most cutaneous *S. aureus* infections are due to MRSA and should be treated as such. In most cases, treatment with TMP-SMX, clindamycin, or doxycycline are effective. Vancomycin or linezolid is indicated only for more invasive or difficult to treat cutaneous infections.

Gram-negative folliculitis may be observed in HIV disease. Patients present with follicularly based papules and pustules, that may be occasionally tender or pruritic. Diagnosis is made by culture. Therapy, though initially empiric, should be guided by antibiotic sensitivities. Recently, *Acinetobacter baumanii* folliculits was reported in patients with AIDS. The patient cleared after treatment with intravenous ticarcillin/clavulanic acid (3 g/200 mg) four times daily.[43]

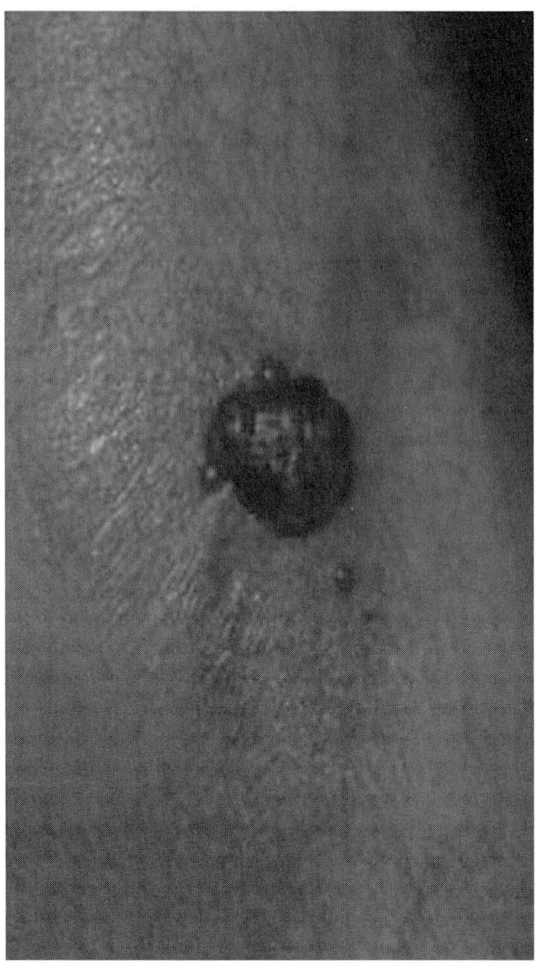

Figure 64-6 ■ Bacillary angiomatosis: arm, thigh, calf.

Bacillary Angiomatosis

Bacillary angiomatosis (BA) and bacillary peliosis (BAP), caused by the genus *Bartonella*, *B. henselae* and *B. quintana*, occur most commonly in the setting of HIV-induced immunodeficiency, characterized by angioproliferative lesions resembling cherry hemangiomas, pyogenic granulomas, or Kaposi sarcoma (KS) (*see* Chapter 42; Fig. 64-6).[44,45] Lesions may be multiple, varying in size from 1 mm to several centimeters, or may present as a single, painful, subcutaneous nodule. Currently, the prevalence of BA in North America and Western Europe is very low due to improved immune function with HAART and to prophylaxis given for infections such as *Mycobacterium avium* complex (MAC).[46] Diagnosis may be delayed because the organism is difficult to culture. Serological studies are plagued by cross-reactivity between organisms in the species. Histopathological examination with Warthin–Starry silver stain can help in diagnosis, but does not differentiate among species.

Therapy

Treatment should include either clarithromycin 500 mg twice daily, azithromycin 250 mg once daily, erythromycin 500 mg

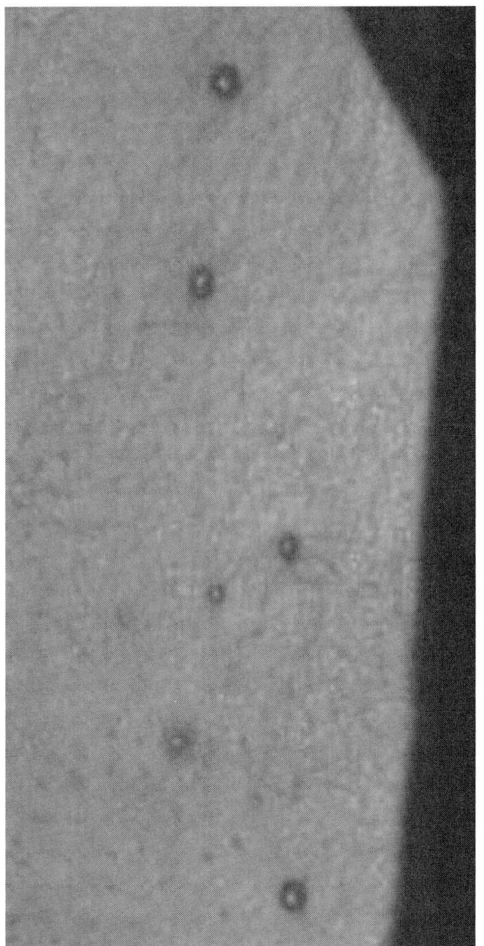
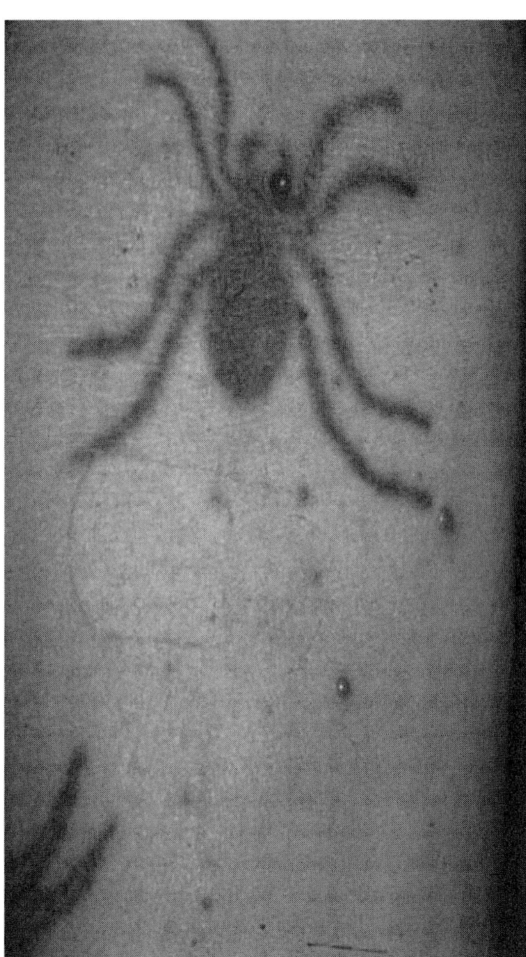

Figure 64-6 ■ Bacillary angiomatosis (*Continued*).

four times a day, or doxycycline 100 mg twice a day for a period of at least 4 weeks (*see* Chapter 42). Alternative therapies include rifampin, fluoroquinolones or TMP-SMX.[47]

In developing countries, tuberculosis is the most common OI in HIV disease; however, cutaneous tuberculosis is relatively uncommon. In non-HIV-infected persons with tuberculosis, the incidence of extrapulmonary tuberculosis is 15%; in HIV disease it is 20–40%. In advanced HIV disease, the incidence of extrapulmonary disease increases to 70% (*see* Chapter 40).

Tuberculosis

Tuberculids represent hypersensitivity reactions to hematogenous mycobacterial disease. Three morphological subtypes have been described. Papulonecrotic tuberculid (PNT) is the most common and presents as symmetrically distributed erythematous papules and pustules, primarily on the extensor surfaces of the extremities. Some lesions may develop central necrosis. PNT has a predilection for younger individuals and can be clinically misdiagnosed as PPE. Unlike PPE however, PNT is only mildly pruritic, if at all. It may heal spontaneously with only minimal scarring.

Lichen scrofulosorum is very rare and found in young individuals. It presents as very small erythematous papules with superficial scale that surround the hair follicles and heal without scarring. Erythema induratum of Bazin presents as an erythematous painful nodule, usually in the posterior, lower extremities. It is most common in women, and may ulcerate and heal with atrophic scars. In 2005, five cases of a "new" subtype were described and were termed 'nodular tuberculid'. Like erythema induratum, nodular disease also presents as erythematous nodules, but granulomatous vasculitis is observed additionally on histopathologic evaluation.[48] Treatment for tuberculids is geared at eradicating infection with multiple-agent antibiotic regimens. Supportive care for cutaneous hypersensitivity with topical steroids, emollients and antipuritics can be helpful.

Fungal Infections

Cutaneous fungal infections occur as superficial infections (dermatomycoses), invasive fungal infections, or hematogenous dissemination of systemic fungal infection to the skin. The two most common dermatomycoses are dermatophytoses and candidiasis; both of these infections occur with increased frequency in the setting of compromised local or systemic immunity.

Dermatophytoses

Dermatophytes, especially *Trichophyton rubrum*, can infect any keratinized epidermal structure, i.e., epidermis (tinea pedis, tinea cruris, tinea manuum, tinea corporis, tinea facialis, tinea incognito), nails (tinea unguium or onychomycosis) and hair (tinea capitis, tinea barbae, dermatophytic folliculitis).[49,50] Dermatophytes infect nonviable tissue in otherwise healthy individuals, however, in the compromised host, direct invasion of the dermis may occur. Up to 20% of HIV-positive patients with cell counts below 400 cells/μL will develop dermatophytic infections.[51] Dermatophytoses are of importance for three reasons: the morbidity and disfigurement caused by the dermatophyte infection itself, which can be quite extensive; the breakdown in the integrity of the skin that can occur, providing a portal of entry for other pathogens, particularly *S. aureus*; and also because such infections can cause clinical manifestations that mimic other dermatologic conditions.[52] For instance, widespread infection with *Trichophyton rubrum* can mimic KS.[53] Dermatophyte infections in the compromised host are more frequent, often widespread, atypical in appearance, or invasive.[54]

Trichophyton rubrum causes proximal subungual onychomycosis (PSO), an infection of the undersurface of the

Table 64-1 Agents Used in the Management of Dermatophyte Infections

Parameter	Comments
Prevention	Immune restitution with HAART markedly reduces the incidence of dermatophyte infections. Apply powder containing miconazole or tolnaftate to areas prone to fungal infection after bathing.
Topical antifungal preparations	These preparations may be effective for treatment of dermatophytoses of skin but not for those of hair or nails. Topical agents should be continued for at least 1 week after lesions have cleared. Apply at least 3 cm beyond advancing margin of lesion. These agents are comparable. Differentiated by cost, base, vehicle, and antifungal activity. Preparation is applied twice a day to involved area optimally for 4 weeks.
Imidazoles	Clotrimazole (Lotrimin, Mycelex) Miconazole (Micatin) Ketoconazole (Nizoral) Econazole (Spectazole) Oxiconazole (Oxistat) Sulconazole (Exelderm)
Allylamines	Naftifine (Naftin) Terbinafine (Lamisil)
Naphthiomates	Tolnaftate (Tinactin)
Substituted pyridone	Ciclopiroxolamine (Loprox)
Systemic antifungal agents	For infections of keratinized skin: use if lesions are extensive or if infection has failed to respond to topical preparations. Usually required for treatment of tinea capitis and tinea unguium. Also may be required for inflammatory tineas and hyperkeratotic moccasin-type tinea pedis.
Terbinafine	250 mg tablet. Allylamine.
Azole/imidazoles	Itraconazole and ketoconazole have potential clinically important interactions when administered with calcium-channel antagonists, warfarin, cyclosporin A, tacrolimus, oral hypoglycemic agents, phenytoin, protease inhibitors, terfenadine, theophylline, trimetrexate, and rifampin.
Itraconazole	Capsules (100 mg); oral solution (10 mg/mL); intravenous iriazole. Needs acid gastric pH for dissolution of capsule.
Fluconazole	Tablets (100, 150, 200 mg); oral suspension (10 or 40 mg/mL); 400 mg IV.
Ketoconazole	Tablets (200 mg) (little used currently).

proximal nail plate. PSO occurs most often in HIV-infected individuals; the diagnosis is an indication for HIV testing. Unless immunocompetence is restored, dermatophyte infections are chronic and recurrent.[55]

Therapy

Dermatophyte infections are managed with systemic as well as topical antifungal agents (Table 64-1). Infections of the epidermis (Table 64-1), nail apparatus (Table 64-2), and hair/hair follicle (Table 64-3) cannot be cured by topical agents alone, especially in the setting of immunocompromise. Though precautionary information abounds regarding combination of antiretroviral medications with antifungal agents, little data exists to support adverse effects, with the exception of combination therapy with indinavir and ketoconazole.[56] The HIV-infected patients who are taking oral imidazoles such as fluconazole or itraconazole for candidiasis or cryptococcosis, are also inadvertently treating dermatophytoses. Terbinafine, which is highly efficacious for dermatophytic infection, is not predictably effective for nondermatophytic fungal infections.

Cutaneous Candidiasis

Cutaneous *Candida* infections such as intertrigo, are common in adults with HIV disease (Table 64-4); concomitant diabetes mellitus associated with HAART may increase the prevalence. Candidiasis of moist, keratinized cutaneous sites such as the anogenital region occurs with some frequency in up to 90% of HIV-infected individuals (Fig. 64-7).[51] Candidal angular cheilitis occurs at the corners of the mouth as an intertrigo, unilaterally or bilaterally, and is more common in edentulous patients; it may occur in conjunction with oropharyngeal or esophageal disease or as the only manifestation of candidal infection. Children with HIV infection commonly experience

Table 64-2

Management of Dermatophytic Infections of the Nail Apparatus

Agent	Comments
Débridement	Dystrophic nails should be trimmed. In DLSO the nail and the hyperkeratotic nail bed should be removed with nail clippers. In SWO the abnormal nail can be debrided with a curette.
Topical agents	Available as lotions and lacquer. Usually not effective except for early DLSO and SWO after prolonged use (months). Amorolfine nail lacquer: reported to be effective when applied >12 months (available in Europe). Penlac: monthly professional nail debridement recommended.
Systemic agents	During systemic treatment of onychomycosis, nails usually do not appear normal after the treatment times recommended because of slow growth of nail. If cultures and KOH preparations are negative after these time periods, medication can nonetheless be stopped and the nail usually regrows normally.
Allylamines	Most effective against dermatophyte infections; also efficacious against select other fungi.
Terbinafine	Dose: 250 mg/day for 6 weeks for fingernails and 12 weeks for toenail.
Azoles	Drugs in this category are usually effective for treating nail infections caused by dermatophytes, yeasts, and molds.
Itraconazole[a]	Continuous therapy with 200 mg daily for 6 weeks (fingernails) or 12 weeks (toenails). Dose: 200 mg bid for first 7 days of each month for 2 months (fingernails) (pulse dosing). Although not approved for toenail onychomycosis, pulse dosing is used for 3–4 months.
Fluconazole[a]	Reported effective at dosing of 150–400 mg 1 day/week or 100–200 mg daily until the nails grow back normally. Effective against yeasts and less so for dermatophytes.
Secondary prophylaxis	Recommended for all patients. The entirety of both feet should be treated. Prophylaxis should be simple to use and inexpensive. Benzoyl peroxide bar for washing feet when bathing. Antifungal cream daily. Zeaborb (miconazole) AF lotion/powder on feet. Antifungal sprays or powders in shoes.

DLSO, distal and lateral subungual onychomycosis; SWO, superficial white onychomycosis; KOH, potassium hydroxide.
[a]Effective against dermatophytes and Candida.

Table 64-3 Management of Dermatophytic Infections of the Hair Shaft/Hair Follicle

Parameter	Comments
Prevention	Important to examine home and school contacts of affected children for asymptomatic carriers and mild cases of tinea capitis. Ketoconazole or selenium sulfide shampoo may be helpful for eradicating the asymptomatic carrier state.
Topical antifungal agents	Topical agents are ineffective for management of tinea capitis. Duration of treatment should be extended until symptoms have resolved and fungal cultures negative.
Oral antifungal agents	Of the systemic antifungals available, terbinafine and itraconazole are superior to ketoconazole, and all three are superior to griseofulvin. Side effects in increasing order: terbinafine, itraconazole, ketoconazole, griseofulvin.
Terbinafine	Dose: 250 mg qd. Reduce dosing according to weight in pediatric patients.
Itraconazole	Dose: 100 mg capsules or oral solution (10 mg/mL). Treatment duration: 4–8 weeks. Pediatric dose 5 mg kg^{-1} day^{-1}; adult dose 200 mg/day.
Fluconazole	Tablets (100, 150, 200 mg); oral solution (10 and 40 mg/mL). Dosage: 6–8 mg kg^{-1} day^{-1}. Treatment duration 3–4 weeks. Pediatric dose 6 mg kg^{-1} day^{-1} for 2 weeks; repeat at 4 weeks if indicated; adult dose 200 mg/day.
Ketoconazole	Tablets (200 mg). Treatment duration 4–6 weeks (little used currently). Pediatric dose 5 mg kg^{-1} day^{-1}; adult dose 200–400 mg/day.
Adjunctive therapy	
Prednisone	Dose: 1 mg kg^{-1} day^{-1} for 14 days for children with severe, painful kerion.
Systemic antibiotics	For secondary *S. aureus* or group A streptococcal infection: clindamycin, dicloxacillin, or cephalexin.
Surgery	Drain pus from kerion lesions.

Table 64-4 Classification of Candidiasis Involving Skin and Mucosa

Type	Site	Clinical Presentation
Occluded site (occurs where occlusion and maceration create warm, moist microecology)	Body folds	Axillae, inframammary, groins, intergluteal, abdominal panniculus
		Webspace: hands (erosio interdigitalis blastomycetica), feet
		Angular cheilitis; often associated with oropharyngeal candidiasis
	Genitalia	Balanitis, balanoposthitis
		Vulvitis
	Occluded skin	Under occlusive dressing, under cast, back in hospitalized patient
	Folliculitis	Back in hospitalized patient
	Area occluded under diaper	Diaper dermatitis
Nail apparatus	Paronychium	Chronic paronychia
	Nail plate	Onychia
	Hyponychium	Onycholysis
Chronic mucocutaneous	Extensive, multiple or 20 nails	In HIV-infected children, persistent or recurrent mucosal, cutaneous, and/or paronychial/nail infections
Genital	Vulva, vagina; preputial sac	Erythema, erosions, white plaques of candidal colonies
Mucosal	Oropharynx	Thrush; atrophic candidiasis; hyperplastic candidiasis
	Esophagus	Inflamed, eroded plaques
	Trachea, bronchi	Inflamed, eroded plaques
Candidemia	Skin, viscera	Skin: erythematous papules 6 hemorrhage

candidiasis in the diaper area, intertrigo in the axillae and neck fold. Fingernail chronic *Candida* paronychia with secondary nail dystrophy (onychia) is common in HIV-infected children.[57]

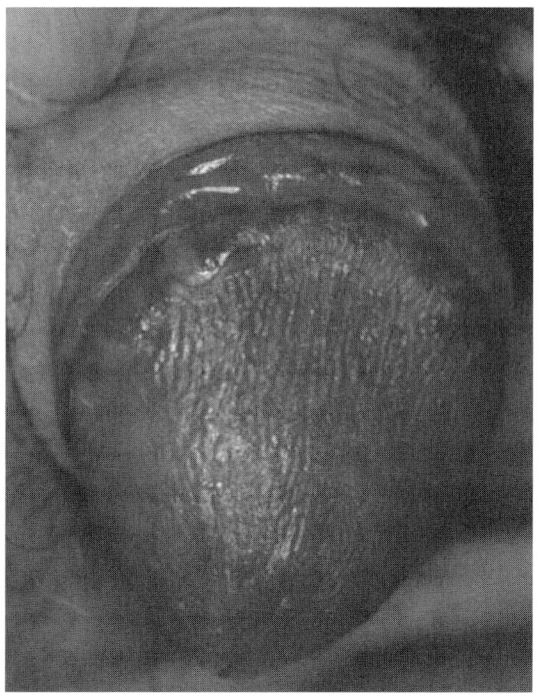

Figure 64-7 ■ Candidiasis: Balanoposthitis with HAART.

Therapy

Topical therapy is usually adequate, but systemic agents may be required in the setting of advanced immunocompromise (Tables 64-5 and 64-6). Chronic prophylaxis with fluconazole may lead to azole-resistance, and is currently not recommended unless CD4+ T-lymphocyte counts remain low or if recurrences are very frequent.[51]

Superficial Fungal Infections

Superficial fungal infections are confined to fully keratinized tissue, such as the stratum corneum, hair and nails. In advanced immunosuppression *Trichosporon beigelii*, the etiologic agent of white piedra, can disseminate and cause fever, pulmonary infiltrates, and disseminated erythematous macules and papules in skin. Diagnosis is made on biopsy and culture, as the organism may be mistaken for disseminated candidiasis. Treatment mandates systemic therapy but the disease is nearly always fatal.[47] In immunocompetent hosts, disease exhibits as white nodules on hair shafts on the head, often confused for lice nits. *Trichosporon beigelii* can manifest in the pubic area in HIV hosts. Clipping hair shafts is usually curative, but ketoconazole shampoos are also helpful.

Invasive Fungal Infections

Latent pulmonary fungal infections such as cryptococcosis, histoplasmosis, coccidioidomycosis, sporotrichosis, or penicillinosis can reactivate and disseminate to various organs including meninges and skin in persons with advanced HIV disease. The cutaneous findings, particularly those of

Management of Cutaneous Candidiasis

Table 64-5

Management	Comments
HAART	With immune restitution, candidiasis resolves and/or does not occur.
Prevention	Keep intertriginous areas dry (often difficult). Washing with benzoyl peroxide bar may reduce *Candida* colonization. Powder with miconazole applied daily.
Topical treatment Castellani's paint	Brings almost immediate relief of symptoms (i.e., candidal paronychia).
Corticosteroid preparation	Judicious short-term use speeds resolution of symptoms.
Topical antifungal agents	Antifungal preparation: nystatin, azole, or imidazole cream bid or more often with diaper dermatitis. Tolnaftate not effective for candidiasis. Terbinafine may be effective.
Nystatin cream	Effective for *Candida* only. Not effective for dermatophytosis.
Azole creams	Effective for candidiasis, dermatophytosis, and pityriasis versicolor.
Oral antifungal agents	Eliminate bowel colonization. Azoles treat cutaneous infection.
Nystatin (suspension, tablet, pastille)	Not absorbed from the bowel. Eradicates bowel colonization. May be effective for recurrent candidiasis of diaper area, genitalia, or intertrigo.
Systemic antifungal agents	See table 64.5.

HAART, highly active antiretroviral therapy.

Management of Oropharyngeal Candidiasis

Table 64-6

Management	Comments
HAART	With immune restitution, candidiasis resolves and/or does not occur.
Topical agents	Effective in most cases.
Nystatin	Vaginal tablets: 100 000 units qid dissolved slowly in the mouth. Oral suspension: 1–2 teaspoons held in mouth for 5 min and then swallowed.
Clotrimazole	Oral tablets (troche), 10 mg: one tablet 5 times daily.
Systemic therapy	Systemic therapy indicated if OPC fails to respond to topical agents.
Fluconazole	Oral: 200 mg PO once followed by 100 mg daily for 2–3, weeks, then discontinue. Increase the dose to 400–800 mg in resistant infection. IV also available.
Itraconazole	Capsules or oral solution: 100–200 mg PO 100 mg PO qd or bid for 2 weeks. Increase dose with resistant disease.
Ketoconazole	200 mg PO qd to bid for 1–2 weeks (little used currently).
Voriconazole	Investigational; may be useful for *Candida* species with relatively high MIC.
Fluconazole-resistant candidiasis	Defined as clinical persistence of infection following treatment with fluconazole 100 mg/day PO for 7 days. Occurs most commonly in HIV-infected individuals with CD4+ lymphocyte counts <50/mm^3 who have had prolonged fluconazole exposure. Chronic low-dose fluconazole treatment (50 mg/day) facilitates emergence of resistant strains.
Amphotericin B	For severe resistant disease. New liposomal preparations are effective and less toxic.

HAART, highly active antiretroviral therapy; MIC, minimal inhibitory concentration; OPC, oropharyngeal candidiasis.

cryptococcosis and coccidiodomycosis, most commonly resemble multiple molluscum contagiosum (MC)-like lesions that occur most often on the face and upper trunk.[58] Disseminated deep mycoses are much less common in the era of HAART (*see* Chapters 43–45).

Viral Infections

Viruses are major pathogens causing OIs in HIV disease, many of which are manifested at mucocutaneous sites, ranging from cosmetically disfiguring facial MC to extensive common or genital warts to life-threatening/invasive human papillomavirus (HPV) -induced squamous cell carcinoma. In the great majority of cases, viral OIs represent activation of subclinical infection (HPV, molluscum contagiosum virus (MCV)) or reactivation of latent infection (human herpesviruses: HSV-1, HSV-2, varicella-zoster virus (VZV), CMV, Epstein–Barr virus (EBV), and HHV-8 (KS-associated virus)).

HSV-1 and -2 Infections

With more advanced immunocompromise, lesions tend to be subacute or chronic, indolent, atypical, and respond less promptly to oral antiviral therapy. Chronic herpetic ulcers of greater than 1 months' duration are an AIDS-defining condition. Clinically, reactivated latent infections (ulcers) are larger and deeper. Ulcerated, crusted lesions at perioral, anogenital, or digital locations are usually HSV in etiology, in spite of atypical clinical appearances (Fig. 64-8). With increasing immunocompromise, recurrent HSV infection may become persistent and progressive (Fig. 64-9) (*see* Chapter 48). Erosions occurring at the typical sites (perioral, anogenital, and digital) enlarge and deepen into painful ulcers. In addition to ulceration, chronic HSV infections can also present as eroded tumors.

Therapy

Currently, three drugs are available for oral therapy of HSV infections; famciclovir and valacyclovir are absorbed with greater efficacy than acyclovir (Table 64-7; *see also* Chapter 48).[59] These agents can be prescribed to treat primary or reactivated infection or as suppressive therapy. In the management of chronic herpetic ulcers, immunocompromise should be corrected if possible. Though patients treated with HAART have similar rates of mucosal HSV shedding and HSV-2 reactivation than those who are not on therapy, treatment with HAART is associated with fewer days of symptomatic HSV lesions.[60] Chronic oral antiviral therapy has been

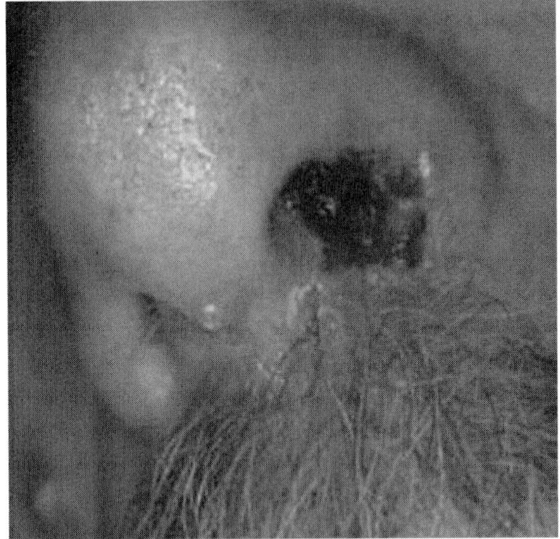

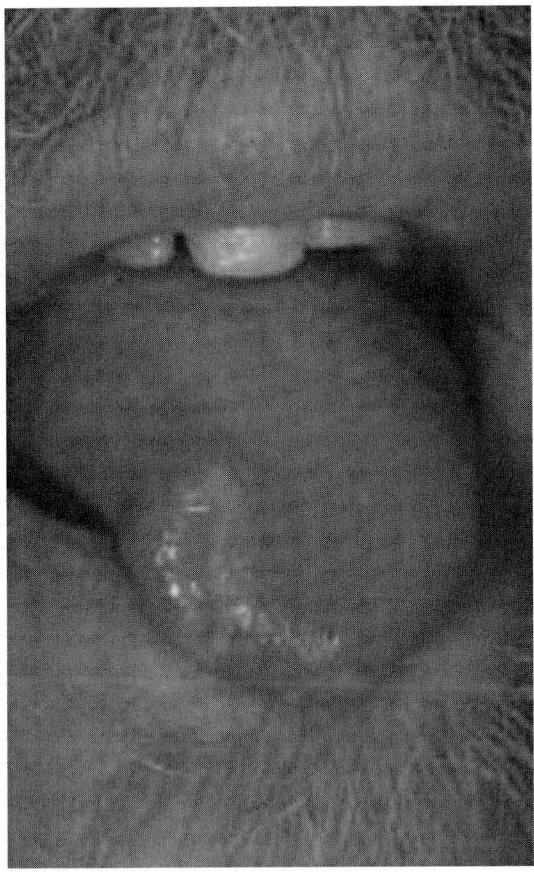

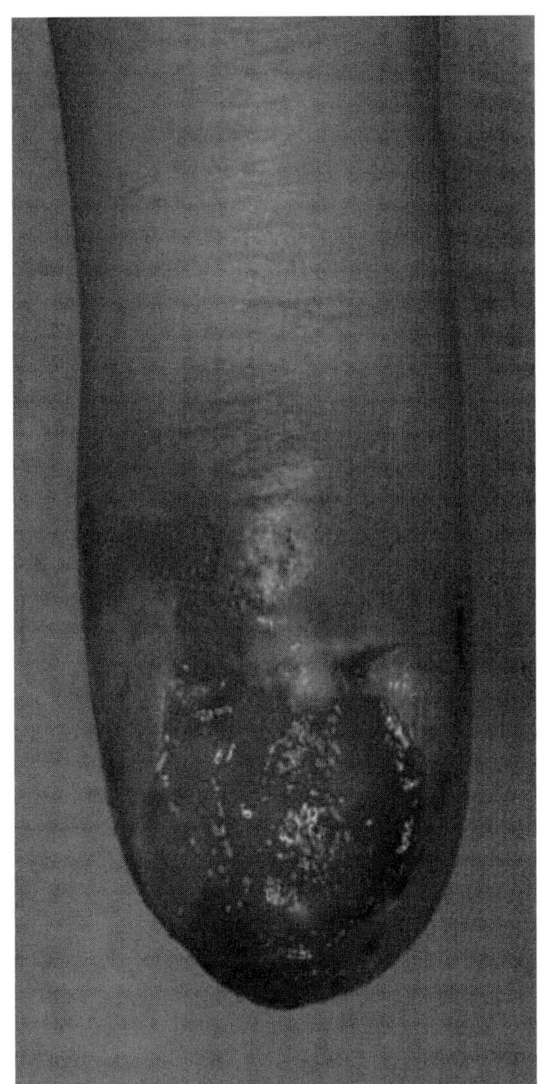

Figure 64-8 ■ HSV: chronic at multiple sites.

advocated for HSV infections in HIV disease, in that HIV viral loads have been reported to increase with reactivation of latent HSV infection.[61] Oral acyclovir is effective in suppressing recurrences of HSV in HIV-infected persons; a dosage of 600 mg/day is more efficacious than 400 mg/day.[62]

Improved blood levels of famciclovir and valacyclovir make oral therapy more effective than with oral acyclovir. Foscarnet and cidofovir are administered intravenously for infections caused by acyclovir-resistant HSV.[63] Cidofovir gel has been effective as a topical therapy of acyclovir-resistant HSV infections, although it is not available commercially and must be compounded by the pharmacist.[64] Imiquimod 5% cream is also an effective topical treatment for cutaneous herpetic infections, including those caused by acyclovir-resistant HSV strains. Imiquimod 5% cream is applied to the lesion(s) HS daily or qod if irritation occurs.[65]

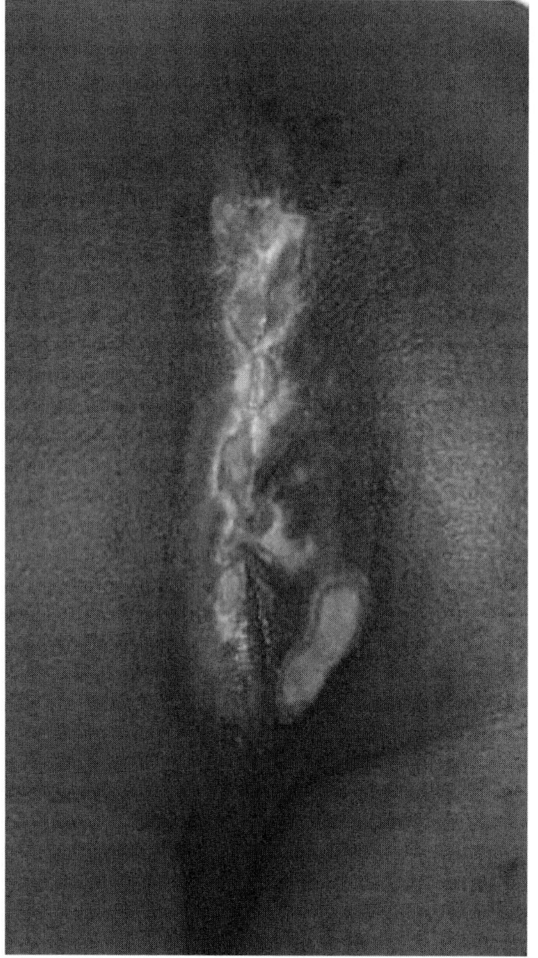

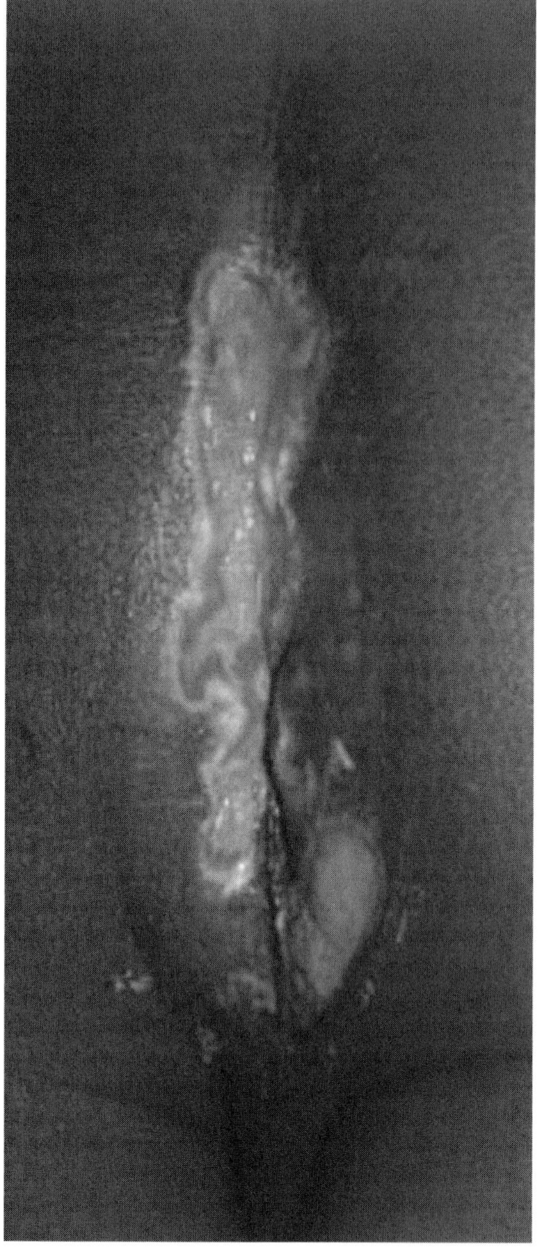

Figure 64-9 ■ HIV/HSV: chronic genital ulcers.

The management of recurrent HSV, particularly HSV-2 is important in HIV hosts and their sexual partners, as there is an increased risk of HIV-1 mucosal shedding in those who are HSV-2 seropositive and of infection in HIV-1-negative, but HSV-2 seropositive sexual partners.[66,67]

VZV Infections

Primary VZV infection manifests as varicella (chickenpox); reactivation of VZV from a dorsal-root ganglion or cranial-nerve ganglion manifests as herpes zoster (HZ; *see* Chapter 29). In the compromised host, VZV infection can present as severe varicella, persistent varicella, dermatomal HZ (Fig. 64-10), disseminated HZ (sometimes without dermatomal HZ), and chronic or recurrent HZ.[68] Disseminated HZ is defined as cutaneous involvement by greater than three contiguous dermatomes or more than 20 lesions scattered outside the initial dermatome (Fig. 64-11), or systemic infection (hepatitis, pneumonitis, encephalitis). Disseminated VZV infection in an individual harboring latent VZV can present with clinical pattern of scattered vesicles in the absence of dermatomal HZ. In immunocompetent individuals, the main complication of zoster is postherpetic neuralgia (defined as pain persisting more than 6 weeks after the development of cutaneous lesions).

HIV-infected individuals who are seronegative or have an indeterminate history of exposure to VZV, and hence are

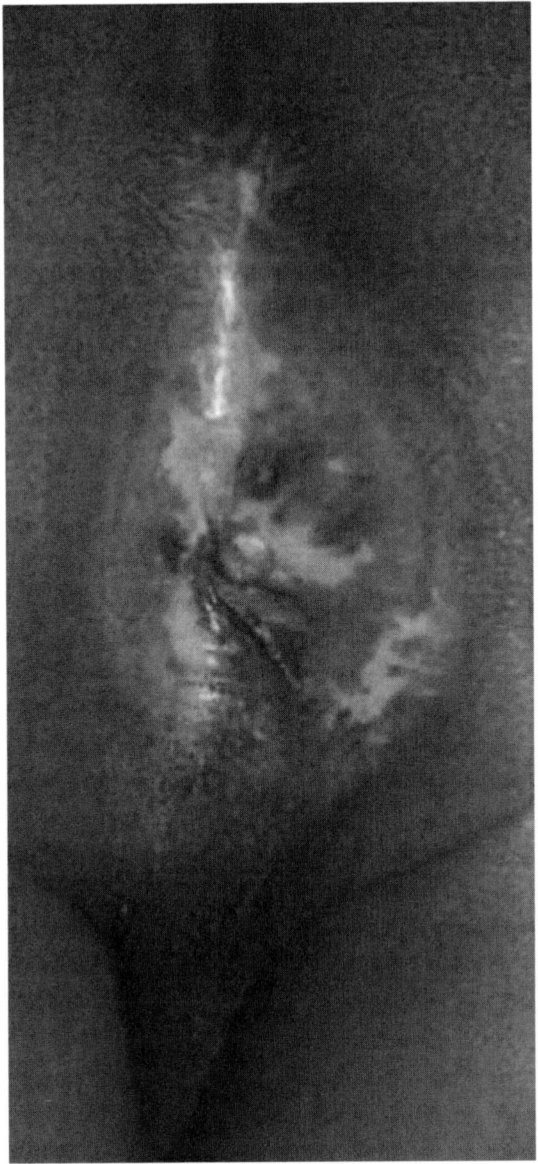

Figure 64-9 ■ Chronic ulcerative HSV (Continued)

at risk for primary infection, should promptly receive zoster immune globulin and immune plasma on exposure to the virus, and high-dose intravenous acyclovir (10 mg/kg every 8 h) instituted at the earliest signs of primary infection.

Therapy

Most persons with zoster occurring in early HIV disease do well without antiviral therapy. The same drugs approved for treatment of HSV are used for treatment of VZV infection: famciclovir, valacyclovir, and acyclovir (*see* Chapter 49). Intravenous acyclovir (10 mg/kg every 8 h) is given for severe infections. Because of the risk of visual impairment following ophthalmic zoster, intravenous acyclovir is usually given. As with HSV infections, acyclovir-resistant strains emerge following prolonged acyclovir treatment; most of these resistant strains respond to foscarnet therapy. Secondary prophylaxis is usually not indicated after VZV infection resolves. Administration of varicella vaccine in early HIV disease in children appears safe and beneficial. HIV-infected children exposed to VZV, whether varicella or zoster, may benefit from treatment with varicella-zoster immune globulin prophylactically, as well as acyclovir.

The management of reactivated VZV infections in patients with mild-to-moderate immunocompromise is identical to that in the immunocompetent host.[69] The cornerstone of treatment for severe VZV infection and/or VZV infection in the severely immunocompromised host is intravenous acyclovir (10 mg/kg IV q8h, until clinical resolution). Varicella in patients with AIDS carries a high mortality and initial therapy with intravenous acyclovir is recommended, though oral treatment may be started once the patient improves. As with HSV infection, acyclovir-resistant VZV has been reported following chronic acyclovir therapy for persistent or recurrent VZV infection.[70,71]

Oral Hairy Leukoplakia

EBV selectively infects certain types of squamous epithelium producing oral hairy leukoplakia (OHL) (*see* Chapter 51). OHL presents as a white plaque on the lateral aspects of the tongue, is nearly pathognomonic for HIV disease, and its occurrence correlates with moderate-to-advanced HIV-induced immunodeficiency.[72–76] OHL typically presents as hyperplastic, verrucous, whitish, epithelial plaques on the lateral aspects of the tongue, frequently extending onto the contiguous dorsal or ventral surfaces.[77] Usually, a single lesion or 3–6 discrete plaques separated by normal-appearing mucosa are observed. Although described as hairy, the most frequently noted appearance of the lesion occurring on the tongue is a corrugated appearance, with parallel white rows arranged nearly vertically.

Therapy

For the most part, OHL is asymptomatic, but its presence may be associated with some degree of anxiety. Patients should be reassured and advised that OHL is not thrush. With HAART, OHL often resolves without additional interventions.[78–80] In concerned patients with persistent lesions, topically applied podophyllin in benzoin is effective; recurrence within weeks to months is common. Topical tretinoin or imiquimod cream may also be effective. Acyclovir, valacyclovir, famciclovir, ganciclovir, or foscarnet, given for other indications, are often effective therapies for OHL.

Kaposi Sarcoma

Debate exists as to whether KS represents a malignant disease, a reactive process, or both. KS presents most commonly in the skin and the oral mucosa. Early lesions may be red, blue or purple, vascular-like, nonblanching patches that may progress to indurated papules and plaques (Fig. 64-12).

Management of Cutaneous HSV Infections

Table 64-7

Management	Comments
Scope	Lesions caused by HSV are relatively common among HIV-infected persons. For severe disease, IV acyclovir therapy may be required. If lesions persist among patients undergoing acyclovir treatment, resistance to acyclovir should be suspected.
HAART	With immune restitution, the incidence and severity of HSV infections are markedly reduced.
Oral antiviral therapy	Currently, anti-HSV agents are approved for use in genital herpes. Presumably, similar dosing regimens are effective for nongenital infections. Drugs for oral HSV therapy include acyclovir, valacyclovir, and famciclovir. Valacyclovir, the prodrug of acyclovir, has better bioavailability and is nearly 85% absorbed after oral administration. Famciclovir is equally effective for cutaneous HSV infections.
First episode	Primary infections are more severe and prolonged.
Acyclovir	Dose: 400 mg tid or 200 mg 5 times/day × 7–10 days.
Valacyclovir	Dose: 1 g bid × 7–10 days (not approved for first-episode disease).
Famciclovir	Dose: 250 mg tid × 5–10 days.
Recurrences	For severe recurrent disease, patients who start therapy at the beginning of the prodrome or within 2 days after onset of lesions may benefit from therapy by shortening and reducing severity of eruption. Recurrences cannot be prevented by intermittent therapy.
Acyclovir	Dose: 400 mg PO tid for 5 days or 800 mg PO bid for 5 days.
Valacyclovir	Dose: 500 mg bid × 5 days or 2 g bid for day 1, then 1 g bid on day 2.
Famciclovir	Dose: 125 mg bid for 5 days.
Chronic suppression	Decreases frequency of symptomatic recurrences and asymptomatic HSV shedding. After 1 year of continuous daily suppressive therapy, acyclovir should be discontinued to determine the recurrence rate.
Acyclovir	Dose: 400 mg bid.
Valacyclovir	Dose: 500–1000 mg qd.
Famciclovir	Dose: 250 mg bid.
Mucocutaneous HSV infections in advanced HIV disease	Neither the need for nor the proper increased dosage of acyclovir has been established conclusively. Patients with herpes simplex who do not respond to the recommended dose of acyclovir may require a higher oral dose of acyclovir, IV acyclovir, or be infected with an acyclovir-resistant HSV strain, requiring IV foscarnet. The roles of valacyclovir and famciclovir are not yet established.
Acyclovir	Dose: 5 mg/kg IV q8h for 7–14 days or 400 mg 5 times/day × 3 7–14 days.
Valacyclovir or famciclovir	Reduces the necessity for IV acyclovir therapy.
Acyclovir resistance	Usually occurs in individuals with long-standing HIV disease and chronic treatment with oral anti-HSV drugs. Chronic HSV infections are mucocutaneous, rarely invasive. Resistant HSV strains are thymidine-kinase deficient. Alternative drugs: foscarnet, cidofovir.
Foscarnet	For severe disease caused by proven or suspected acyclovir-resistant strains, hospitalization should be considered. Forscarnet, 40 mg/kg body weight until q8h clinical resolution is attained, appears to be the best available treatment.

HSV, herpes simplex virus; HAART, highly active antiretroviral therapy.

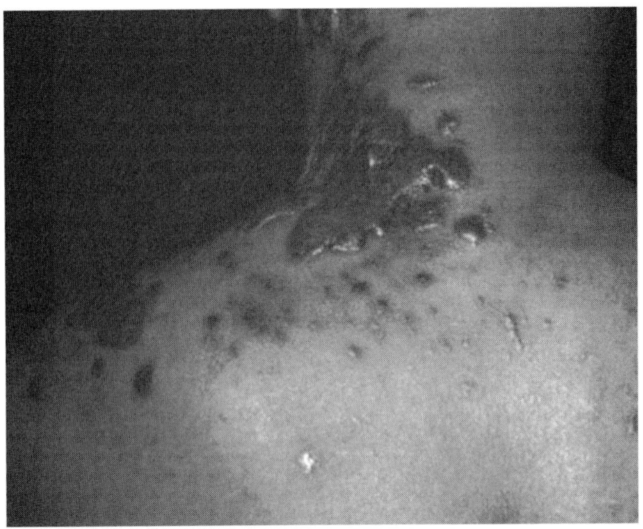

Figure 64-10 ■ VZV: post-HZ scarring.

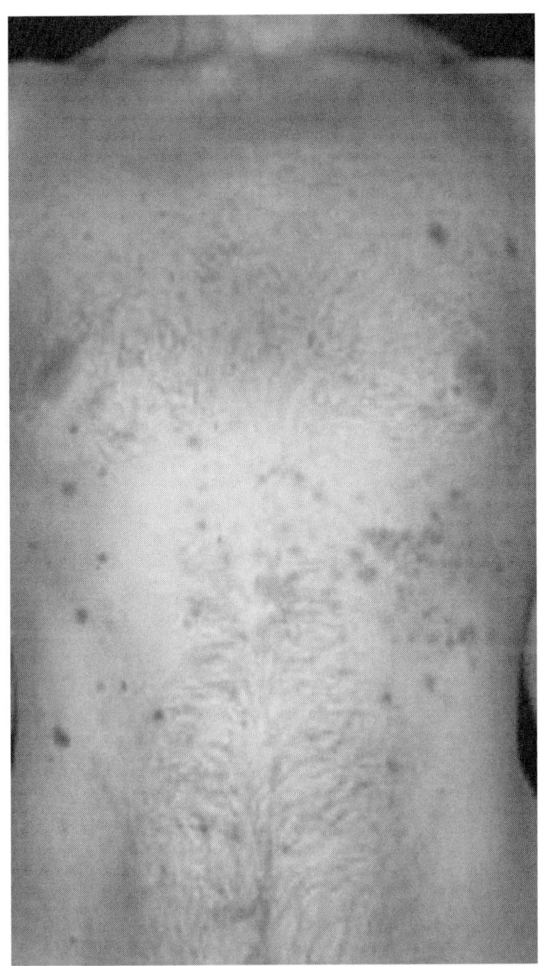

Figure 64-11 ■ VZV: Zoster with dissemination.

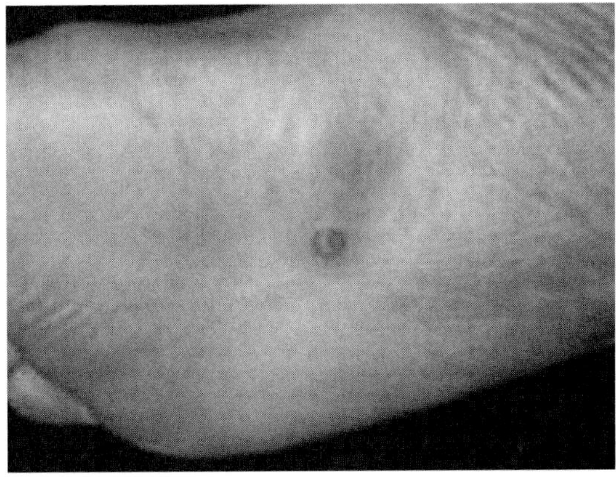

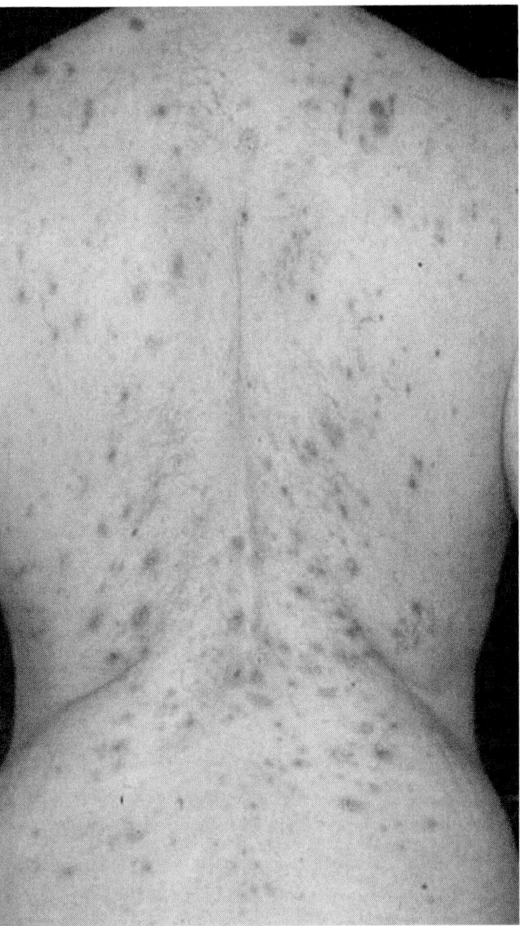

Figure 64-11 ■ VZV: Zoster with dissemination. (*Continued*)

More advanced lesions invade the subcutaneous tissue in nodular form. KS may regress, or can expand and coalesce into larger lesions and then ulcerate (Fig. 64-13). HIV infection promotes development of the most aggressive form, AIDS-defining KS, which occurs with CD4+ T-lymphocyte counts under 200 cells/μL. The role of the immune response in the development of this disease is further fortified by the realization that even local therapy with topical immunomodulators like tacrolimus ointment, may promote tumoral disease.[81]

Lesions can be noted anywhere, but preference for the upper trunk, face and distal extremities is observed. Clinical

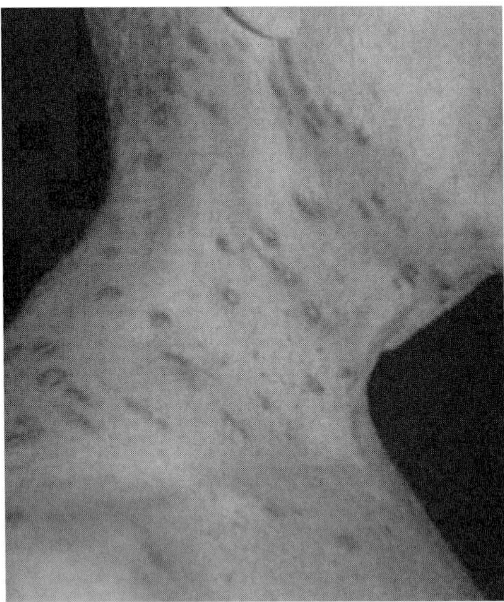

Figure 64-12 ■ KS: face, neck, ear, trunk.

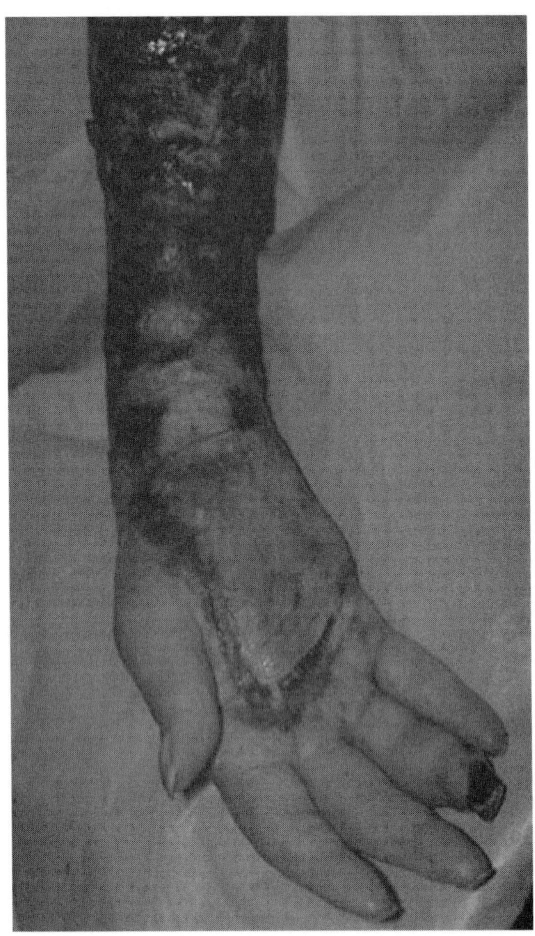

Figure 64-13 ■ KS: arm and hand.

presentation is varied and disease may present as a single lesion or as disseminated disease. About 20% of patients will have mucosal involvement, which is highly predictive of gastrointestinal disease.[82] In addition, the tumor can invade the lymph nodes and the lung; the latter carries a worse prognosis.

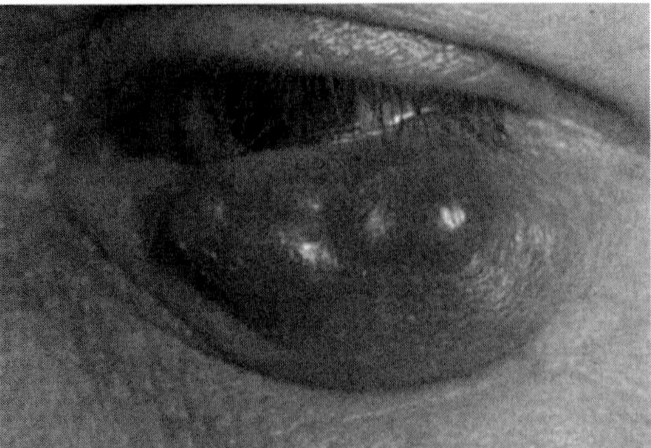

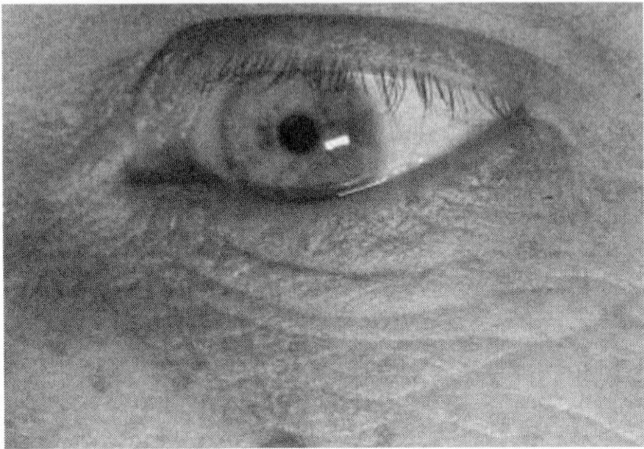

Figure 64-14 ■ KS management: before and after intralesional vinblastine.

Diagnosis is made by skin biopsy and immunohistochemistry, including the ability to stain for HHV-8. Interestingly, nodular lesions that are most aggressive have the highest amount of HHV-8 DNA.

Therapy

HAART is the most important therapy in early disease, and most people respond after restoration in CD4+ T-lymphocyte counts with clinical improvement and a decrease in HHV-8 DNA load in biopsied lesional skin. Individual lesions may be treated with destructive methods like cryotherapy, intralesional chemotherapy (Fig. 64-14), alitretinoin gel, radiotherapy, and interferon. In advanced cases, paclitaxel is used, though recurrent or recalcitrant cases have been successfully treated with docetaxel.[83] In addition, successful treatment of AIDS-related KS refractory to chemotherapy and HAART with imatinib mesylate has been documented (*see* Chapter 59).[84]

Molluscum Contagiosum

Molluscum congatiosum (MCV) commonly infects keratinized skin subclinically, can cause lesions at sites of minor trauma and in the infundibular portion of the hair follicle (Fig. 64-15).[85] The clinical course of MCV infection in HIV disease differs significantly from that in the normal host, and

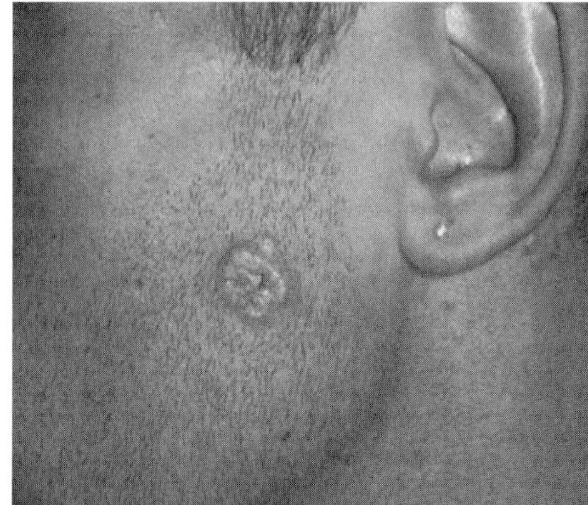

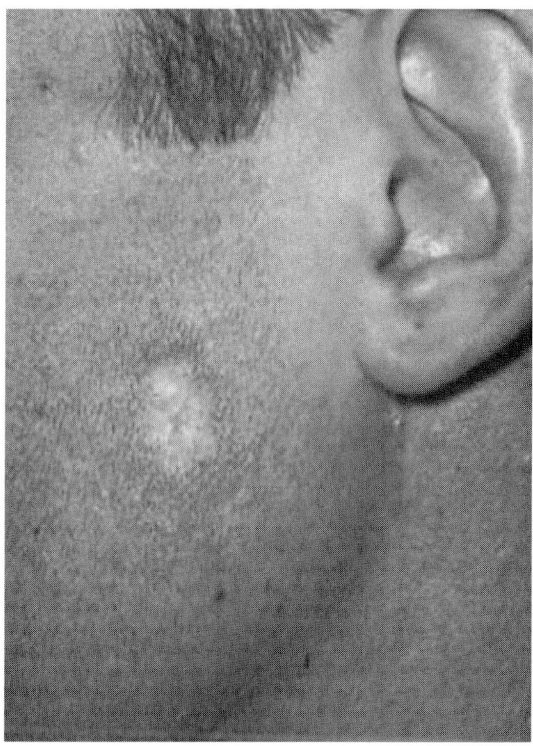

Figure 64-15 ■ Molluscum contagiosum: giant.

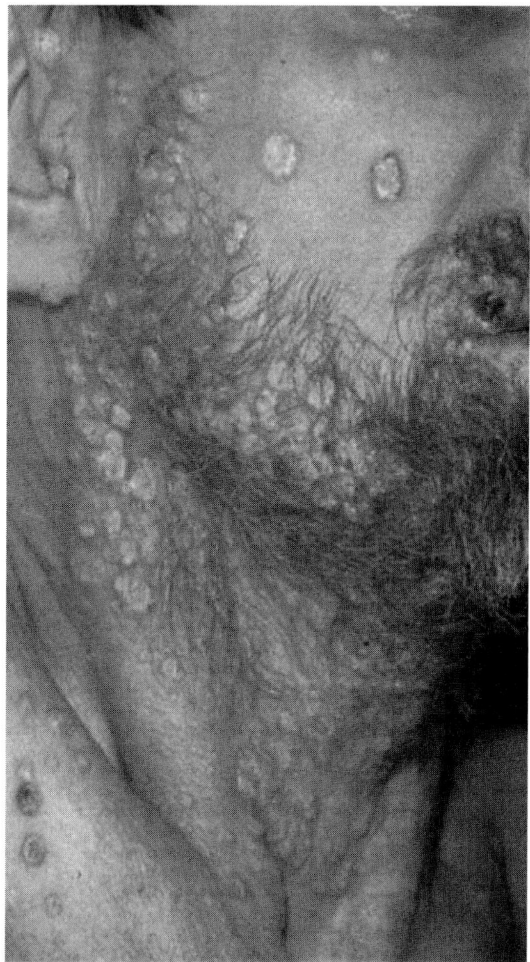

Figure 64-16 ■ Molluscum contagiosum: giant.

is an excellent clinical marker of the degree of immunodeficiency.[86] Large and confluent lesions cause significant morbidity and disfigurement (Fig. 64-16). Prior to HAART, MCV infections were detected in 10% of individuals with HIV disease, and in 30% of those with CD4+ T-lymphocyte cell counts under 100/μL, the number of lesions being inversely related to the CD4+ T-lymphocyte cell count.[87] In HIV-infected individuals, MCV infection tends to be progressive, and recurrent after the usual therapies. With response to HAART, MCV infections regress, resolve completely, or do not occur, associated with increased CD4+ T-lymphocyte cell counts and reduced viral load.[88]

Therapy

Therapeutically, the most efficacious approach toward MCV infection is correction of the underlying immunodeficiency; if this can be accomplished lesions regress. If correction of immunodeficiency is not possible, treatment is directed at controlling the numbers and bulk of cosmetically disturbing lesions rather than at eradication of all lesions (Table 64-8). Liquid nitrogen cryospray is the most convenient therapy, and usually must be repeated every 2–4 weeks. Simple curettage is effective for smaller lesions, but not practical for larger, more numerous lesions. Electrosurgery is more effective than cryosurgery; local anesthesia is required by most subjects with either injected lidocaine or EMLA cream. Imiquimod 5% cream applied three times a week is an effective patient administered therapy in children and adults.[89,90] Cidofovir, a nucleotide analog with activity against several DNA viruses, given either intravenously or topically as a cream, may be an effective therapy.[91–93] Combination therapy with cidofivir and cryotherapy has also been reported. Photodynamic therapy after application of 5-aminolevulinic acid has been used with success.[94,95]

Management of Molluscum Contagiosum

Table 64-8

Management	Comments
Prevention	Avoid skin-to-skin contact with individual having molluscum lesions. HIV-infected individuals with molluscum lesions in the beard area should be advised to minimize shaving facial hair or grow a beard.
HAART	With immune restitution, molluscum lesions resolve and/or do not occur.
Treatment of lesions	
Topical patient-directed therapy	Aldara cream (5% imiquimod) applied hs three times/week for up to 1–3 months.
Clinician-directed therapy (office)	These procedures are painful and traumatic, especially for young children. EMLA cream applied to lesions 1 h prior to therapy may reduce/eliminate pain.
Curettage	Small molluscum lesions can be removed with a small curette with little discomfort or pain.
Cryosurgery	Freezing lesions for 10–15 s is effective and minimally painful using either a cotton-tipped applicator or liquid nitrogen spray.
Electrodesiccation	For molluscum lesions refractory to cryosurgery, especially in HIV-infected individuals with numerous and/or large lesions, electrodesiccation or laser surgery is the treatment of choice. Large lesions usually require injected lidocaine anesthesia. Giant lesions may require several cycles of electrodesiccation and curettage to remove the large bulk of lesions; these lesions may extend through the dermis into the subcutaneous fat.

HAART, highly active antiretroviral therapy.

HTLV-1 and HIV

Dermatologic disease has been described in HTLV-1 infected individuals. Infective dermatitis is a chronic inflammatory dermatosis that resembles eczema. It is more common in children and adolescents from areas where HTLV-1 is endemic, including Brazil, the Caribbean and Africa. However, in Japan, where infection with HTLV-1 is also frequent, only a few cases have been reported. Lesions present as erythematous, scaly papules and plaques, primarily on the scalp, neck and retroauricular regions. Lichenoid papules and blepharoconjunctivitis are also seen frequently. Treatment is with TMP-SMX, antihistamines, emollients and topical steroids for at least 15 days.[96]

In a recent study of HTLV-1 endemic areas, up to 12% of patients with HIV were co-infected with HTLV-1, which in turn predisposes HIV-positive patients to additional inflammatory dermatoses. About 60% of co-infected patients may suffer from inflammatory dermatosis that include seborrheic dermatitis, prurigo, intertrigo, xeroderma and psoriasis. Some argue that in patients with HIV who present with inflammatory dermatoses, testing for HTLV-1 should be done, particularly in areas that are endemic for this virus.[97]

HPV Infections

Subclinical infection with HPV is nearly universal in humans. With immunocompromise, cutaneous and/or mucosal HPV infections (re)emerge from latency, presenting clinically on keratinized epithelium as verrucae, on non- or poorly keratinized mucosa as mucosal warts (condyloma acuminatum), squamous intraepithelial lesion (SIL), or invasive squamous cell carcinoma (SCC).[98]

Common Warts (Verruca Vulgaris, Verruca Plana, Verruca Plantaris), Squamous Cell Carcinoma In Situ (SCCIS), and Invasive SCC

In HIV-infected individuals, verrucae are not unusual in morphology, number, or response to treatment; however, with advancing disease, verrucae can enlarge, become confluent, and become unresponsive to therapy (Fig. 64-17).[99] HPV-5 can cause an unusual pattern of extensive verruca plana and pityriasis (tinea) versicolor-like warts, similar to the pattern seen in epidermodysplasia verruciformis. With moderate or advanced immunodeficiency, warts may become much more numerous, confluent, and refractory to usual treatment modalities (Fig. 64-18). Precancerous lesions identical to mucosal lesions, namely SIL and SCCIS, can occur periungually on the fingers. In some cases, invasive SCC can arise at one or multiple sites on the fingers and/or nail bed (Fig. 64-19). These tumors are aggressive and invade to the underlying periosteum and bone relatively early due the proximity of the underlying bony structures. In spite of immune restitution with HAART, HPV infections often persist and progress unlike other opportunistic viral infections.

Verrucae occurring in HIV-infected individuals are usually asymptomatic, with the most common complaint being a cosmetic one. Warts on the plantar aspect of the foot can become large and painful. Verruca vulgaris and verruca plantaris appear as well-demarcated keratotic papules or nodules,

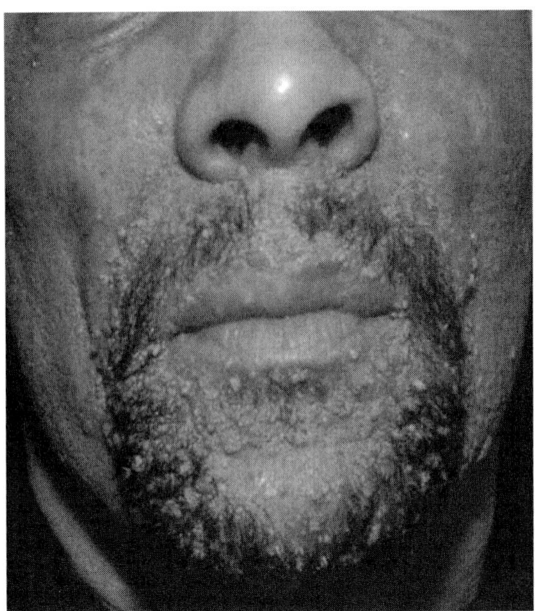

Figure 64-17 ■ HIV/HPV: flat wart.

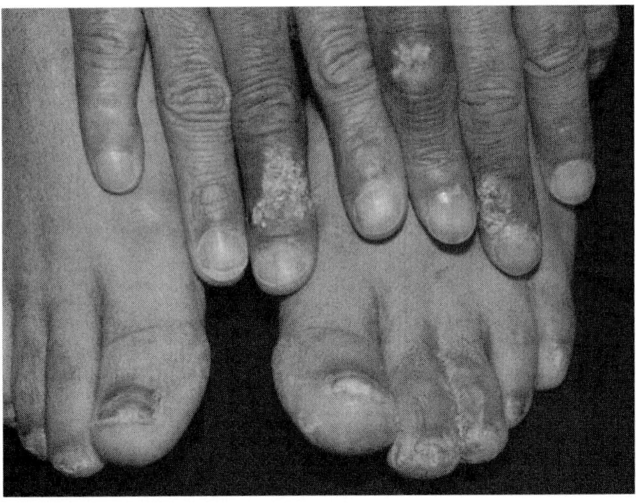

Figure 64-18 ■ HPV: verrucus vulgaris.

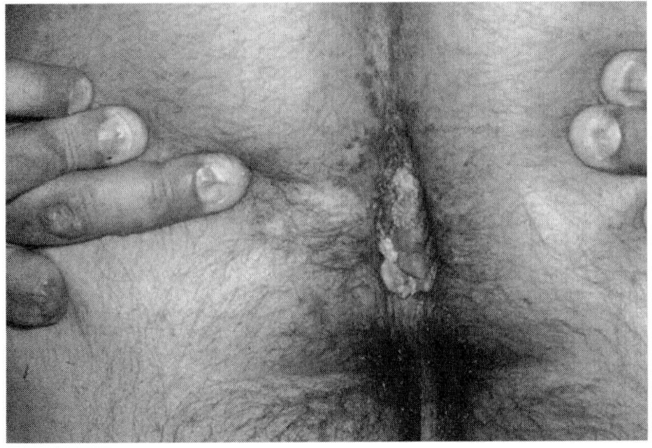

Figure 64-19 ■ HIV/HPV: invasive SCC of nail apparatus.

usually with multiple tiny red-brown dots representing thrombosed capillaries; palmar and plantar warts characteristically interrupt the normal dermatoglyphics. They may be very numerous and confluent, giving the appearance of a mosaic. Verruca plana appears as a well-demarcated, flat-topped papule, which lacks the dots seen in other types of verrucae.[100,101] When present in the beard area, hundreds of flat warts may be noted (Fig. 64-17). All types of verrucae may have a linear arrangement due to koebnerization or autoinoculation.

Therapy

Efficacy of treatment of verruca vulgaris (Table 64-9) and condyloma acuminatum in HIV disease varies with the degree of immunocompromise. In patients with early disease, these lesions should be managed as in the normal host. In patients with advanced HIV-induced immunodeficiency, complete eradication of benign HPV-induced lesions is often not possible, and aggressive treatment is contraindicated.[102] Intravenous cidofovir for refractory lesions of verruca vulgaris in HIV may be of benefit.[103] Cytologic smears and/or lesional biopsies should be obtained to monitor the evolution of benign neoplasia to dysplasia (SIL) to invasive SCC.

Mucosal HPV Infection

The greater majority of sexually active individuals are or have been subclinically infected with one or multiple HPV types. HPV-6 and -11 infect non- or scantily keratinized epithelium such as anogential sites and oropharynx and cause genital warts (condyloma acuminatum; Fig. 64-19); HPV-16 and -18 cause precancerous lesions low-grade SIL (LSIL), high-grade SIL (HSIL; Fig. 64-21), and invasive SCC (Fig. 64-22). Oropharyngeal HPV-induced lesions resemble anogenital condyloma, pink or white in color, but never the tan-to-brown color of some genital lesions. Extensive intraoral condyloma acuminatum (oral florid papillomatosis) presents as multiple large plaques, analogous to anogenital giant condylomata acuminata of Buschke–Löwenstein (64-20), and can also transform to verrucous carcinoma.

Therapy

Management of external genital warts can be office-based or patient initiated (Table 64-9). Similar therapies may be used for oral warts. Cidofovir 1–3% solution is beneficial in refractory oral warts in HIV.[104] Treatment of HIV with HAART, rather than the absolute level of immunosuppression, is predictive of HPV detection by PCR (*see* Chapter 56).[105]

LSIL, HSIL, SCCIS, Invasive SCC

The natural history of external anogenital HPV-induced dysplasia is not known. Prolonged, severe immunodeficiency provides the necessary milieu for the emergence of HPV-induced

Management of HPV Infections of Keratinized Skin: Cutaneous Warts (Verrucae)

Table 64-9

Management	Comments
HAART	Unlike other viral opportunistic infections, HPV infections may persist despite immune restitution.
Patient-initiated therapy	Minimal cost; no/minimal pain.
For small lesions	Salicylic acid (10–20%) and lactic acid in collodion.
For large lesions	Salicylic acid (40%) plaster for 1 week, then application of salicylic acid–lactic acid in collodion.
Aldara cream	At sites that are not thickly keratinized, apply with hs 3 times/week. Persistent warts may require occlusion. Hyperkeratotic lesions on palms/soles should be debrided frequently; Aldara used alternately with a topical retinoid such as tazarotene topical gel may be effective.
Clinician-initiated therapy	Costly, painful.
Cryosurgery	If patients have tried home therapies and liquid nitrogen is available, light cryosurgery using a cotton-tipped applicator or cryospray, freezing the wart and 1–2 mm of surrounding normal tissue for ~30 seconds, is quite effective. Freezing kills the infected tissue but not HPV. Cryosurgery is usually repeated about every 4 weeks until the warts have disappeared. Painful.
Electrosurgery	More effective than cryosurgery but also associated with a greater chance of scarring. EMLA cream can be used for anesthesia for flat warts. Lidocaine injection is usually required for thicker warts, especially palmar/plantar lesions.
CO_2 laser surgery	May be effective for recalcitrant warts but no better than cryosurgery or electrosurgery in the hands of experienced clinicians.
Surgery	Single, nonplantar verruca vulgaris: curettage after freon freezing; surgical excision of cutaneous HPV infections is not indicated in that these lesions are epidermal infections.
Intralesional bleomycin	Highly effective in the hands of experienced clinician.

HPV, human papillomavirus; HAART, highly active antiretroviral therapy.

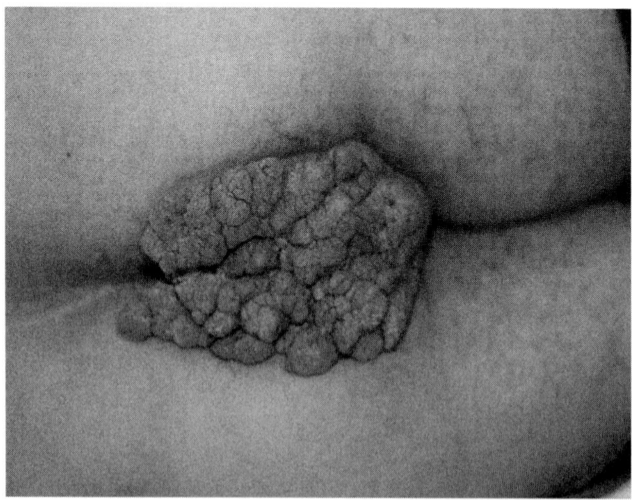

Figure 64-20 ■ HPV: giant condyloma perianal.

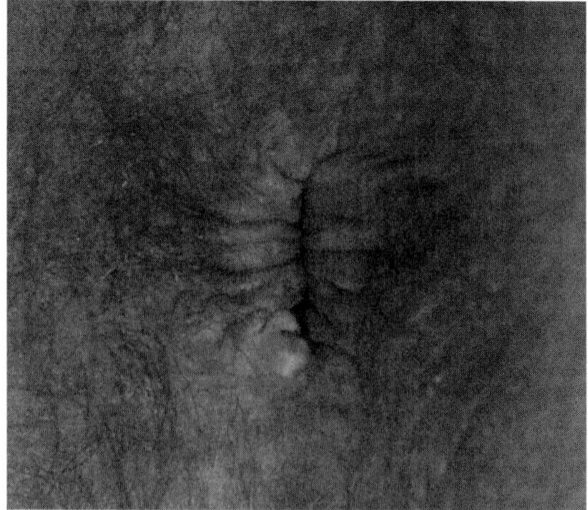

Figure 64-21 ■ HPV: SCCIS perianal.

anogenital neoplasia. The incidence of transformation of SCCIS to invasive SCC appears to be low. The relative risk for HPV-related anal invasive SCC is much higher in HIV-infected than in non-HIV-infected homosexual men, and is more likely in advanced HIV disease. The most common sites for HPV-induced SIL, SCCIS, and invasive SCC are cervix, anus, perineum, vulva, penis, oropharynx/tongue, conjunctivae, and nail apparatus.[106]

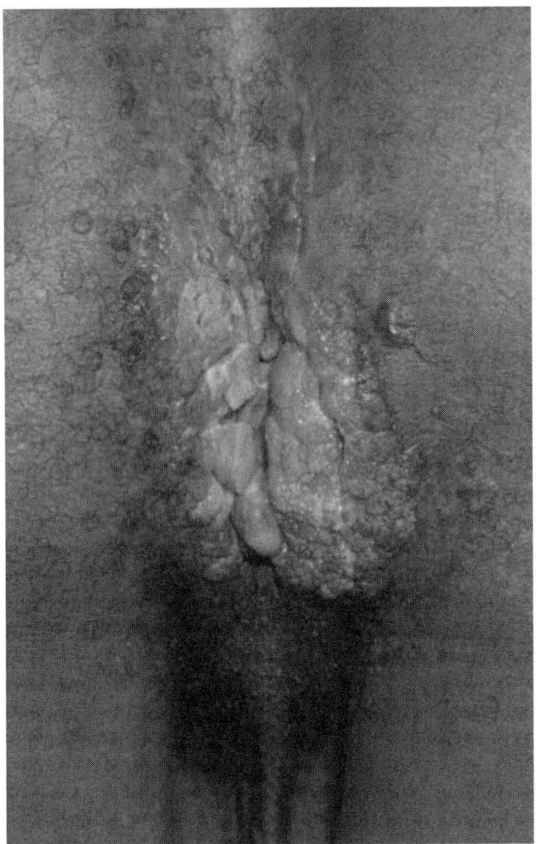

Figure 64-22 ■ HPV: verrucous carcinoma.

Anogenital neoplasias are likely to become more common manifestations of HIV disease as patients with profound immunodeficiency, who would previously have succumbed to OIs, are now surviving for extended periods because of HAART.[107] Cervical, anal, and external anogenital LSIL, HSIL, and invasive SCC have become more common in long-term survivors of HIV disease. In addition, the prevalence of anal intraepithelial neoplasia (AIN), the precursor for anal carcinoma, has not decreased since the introduction of HAART.[108] In a recent report, up to 86% of HIV-1-infected men who have sex with men and had a history of receptive anal intercourse, presented with evidence of anal HPV infection on their first visit. Twenty percent were diagnosed with AIN.[109] In addition, HIV infection and recurrent anal HPV co-infection are independent risk factors for high-grade dysplasia and anal cancer.[110] Invasive SCC arising on external anogenital (Fig. 64-21) sites is usually detected earlier and is less aggressive than that arising on the cervix or anal canal (Fig. 64-22).

Management of external anogenital HPV infection in HIV-infected individuals is directed at identifying HSIL before progression to invasive SCC has occurred. All HIV-infected individuals should be examined annually for evidence of HPV infection, especially those with prior HPV infections. In that HPV-induced neoplasia may extend to the cervix and/or anus, direct examination by speculum and anoscope should also be performed; samples for cytology should be obtained using a cervical brush and cytofix solution during the examination. High-resolution anoscopy and biopsy are done on individuals with HSIL.[110] Individuals with documented external anogenital SIL should be followed by periodic follow-up examinations (every 4–6 months), noting the appearance of new lesions at these sites or an enlarging nodule or ulcerated site; biopsy of these sites is recommended.

Therapy

LSIL and HSIL of the external anogenital epithelium can be treated by several methods: topical chemotherapy (imiquimod 5% cream or 80% trichloroacetic acid, especially for extensive multifocal lesions); surgical excision of single or several lesions; focal destruction of lesions by cryosurgery, electrosurgery, or laser surgery.[111] Unlike topical therapies like imiquimod, surgical modalities treat only clinically detectable lesions and not subclinical infection. For cervical intraepithelial neoplasia, referral to gynecology is indicated for loop electrosurgical excision (LEEP), cryosurgery, laser therapy or cold-knife conization. AIN may be treated similarly, with cryotherapy, fulguration, laser therapy and infrared coagulation.[112]

For minimally invasive SCC arising on the anal verge (nonkeratinized to keratinized epithelium) or on external anogenital sites (penis, vulva, perineum), surgical excision is recommended with adequate borders around the lesion. Invasive SCC of the anus (transformation zone) is treated with radiation therapy and chemotherapy. Prognosis for invasive anal SCC is better in those with higher CD4+ T-lymphocyte cell counts at the time of diagnosis.[113]

The potential role and development of preventive and therapeutic vaccination against HPV in both men and women with HIV-1 infection is currently under investigation.[109]

Sexually Transmitted Diseases

For discussion on sexually transmitted diseases (STDs) see Chapter 58.

Parasitic Infestations

Protozoan infections are among the most common OIs in HIV disease; mucocutaneous involvement, however, is uncommon, with the exception of leishmaniasis.[114]

Co-infection with leishmaniasis and HIV is becoming more frequent particularly in Mediterranean countries. Disease can present as limited cutaneous or mucocutaneous disease. Cutaneous disease results at the site of inoculation in the form of a papule or nodule that may ulcerate. Verrucous forms and atypical morphologies have also been described in HIV. Most lesions will resolve without scarring, though in some cases, scars remain. In the setting of severe immunosuppression, disseminated ulcerative disease may occur. After several years, mucocutaneous disease can develop, causing marked edema and infiltration of the nose and lips, deformation of the nasal cartilage and invasion of the vocal cords. When disease recurs at the site of inoculation, a yellow-brown, indurated plaque describes leishmania recidivans. Finally, a dermal reaction to treated visceral leishmaniasis has been described in the form of pedunculated fleshy papules and nodules that often resemble neurofibromas. Different species are responsible for cutaneous, mucocutaneous and visceral disease in the New and Old World (*see* Chapter 52). Diagnosis relies on identification of the parasite by touch preparations, culture or histopathologic evaluation. Serologic tests are not reliable.

Some species of *Leishmania* have been shown to upregulate HIV-replication and it is thought that they can facilitate HIV infection.[115] Interestingly, while mucocutaneous disease more currently recurs and is more difficult to treat in moderate-to-advanced HIV disease, reports have recently documented disseminated disease as well as exacerbation of previous lesions in the setting of immune reconstitution following HAART.[116,117]

Therapy

Treatment of leishmaniasis relies on pentavalent antimony, liposomal amphotericin, or pentamidine. Oral miltefosine has been used in recurrent cases.[118] Isolated cutaneous lesions have been treated successfully with 5% imiquimod cream.

Crusted (Norwegian) Scabies

Crusted or hyperkeratotic or Norwegian scabies occurs in compromised hosts. Currently in the United States, HIV disease is the most common associated immunocompromised state. In obtunded or compromised individuals, pruritus may be diminished or absent in crusted scabies. Scabetic infestation can be severe, with millions of mites infesting the skin, presenting as a hyperkeratotic dermatitis, but resembling atopic erythroderma, psoriasis vulgaris, keratoderma blennorrhagicum, keratosis follicularis (Darier's disease), or seborrheic dermatitis (in infants).[119] Thickly crusted plaques occur on the ears, buttocks, and extensor surfaces of the extremities, palms, and soles. Heavy infestation occurs around the nails with nail dystrophy and subungual and periungual scale-crust.[120,121] Scabetic infestation, which usually spares the head and neck in adults, can be generalized. *S. aureus* and gram-negative superinfection can occur, which has been complicated by septicemia and death.[122–124] Because of the high number of organisms in crusted scabies, recurrences are common, and hospital epidemics may occur. Use of potent topical corticosteroids for such previously diagnosed pruritic conditions may mask the presence of scabetic infestation.

Therapy

Eradication of the infestation is difficult because of the high number of organisms present. Topical treatment with gamma benzene hexachloride, permethrin lotion, or 10% sulfur ointment is effective; total-body application is required. Keratolytic agents are needed to debride hyperkeratotic areas, in conjunction with debridement of involved nails. Orally administered ivermectin 200 μg/kg given as a single dose has been reported to be very effective for common as well as crusted scabies.[125–127] Two to three doses separated by 1–2 weeks are usually required for heavy infestation or in those with advanced immunocompromised states.

OPPORTUNISTIC NEOPLASMAS (ON) IN HIV DISEASE

The prevalence of the ONs such as KS, HPV-induced neoplasia (SIL, SCCIS, invasive SCC of the cervix, external anogenitalia, and perineum), undifferentiated non-Hodgkin B-cell lymphoma (NHL), and primary central nervous system lymphoma is increased in HIV disease. The incidence of nonmelanoma skin cancers, melanoma and Hodgkin isease may also be increased, but in general, also have a more aggressive course in HIV-infected individuals.[128] Though less well-understood, the incidence of HPV-induced invasive SCC of the cervix and anus, T-cell lymphomas, and seminoma may also be increased. Many of these ONs (NHL, KS, and anogenital *in situ* SCC and invasive SCC) are associated with oncogenic human viruses (EBV, HHV-8, HPV) and diminished immune-mediated tumor surveillance.

Basal Cell Carcinoma and SCC

The prevalence of UVR-induced SCC appears to be increased in HIV disease as it is in immunosuppressed renal transplant recipients. As with transplant recipients, UVR-induced SCC in HIV disease may be more aggressive than in the immunocompetent host. In a report from San Francisco, thirty-three HIV-infected individuals with 97 SCCs were compared with 24 HIV-infected persons with 70 basal cell carcinomas (BCCs). Risk factors for the development of both types of carcinoma were fair skin and excessive sun exposure (more than 6 h/day during the previous 10 years). Those with SCCs tended to have outdoor occupations, were diagnosed at a younger age, had a higher risk of recurrence and metastasis as well as increased mortality.[129] SCCs occurred more often on the head and neck (Fig. 64-23); BCC, on the trunk. SCCs were diagnosed more commonly in individuals with advanced HIV disease than were BCCs. HPV was not an oncogenic factor in the development of these cutaneous tumors, however, p53 overexpression was hypothesized to play an etiologic role.

Response to therapy is in most cases the same as in the general population, however, aggressive SCCs, both UVL- and HPV-induced have been reported. Recently, more aggressive BCCs have also been noted in patients with advanced HIV.[130] Frequent follow-up examinations (every 4–6 months) for individuals with UVL-associated SCCs or BCCs is recommended, to detect recurrence of treated tumors or development of new lesions. Primary prevention with sunscreen use and sun avoidance is paramount. Whereas no data exists for more aggressive therapy in HIV-positive patients with BCC, some recommend aggressive therapy with margin control for the HIV-positive patient with biopsy-proven SCC.[131]

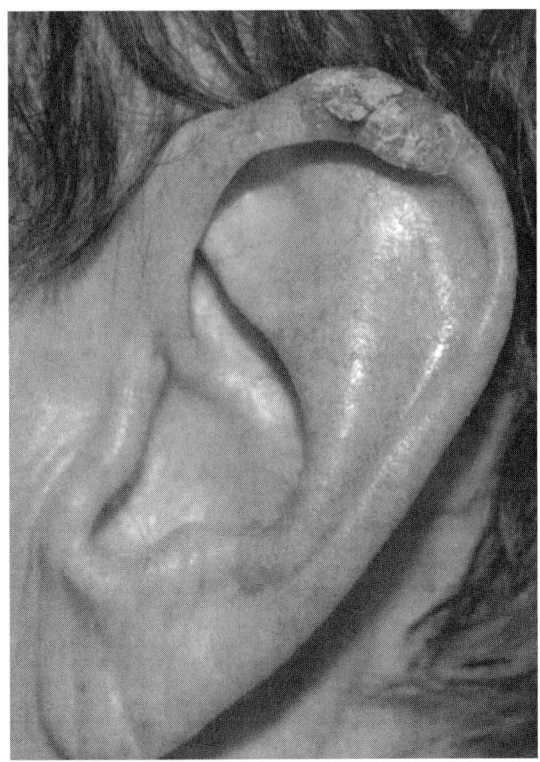

Figure 64-23 ■ Squamous cell carcinoma ear.

Merkel Cell Carcinoma

Merkel cell carcinoma (MCC) is a rare tumor of neuroendocrine cells that presents as an asymptomatic but firm, red, blue or purple papule in sun-exposed surfaces. Ulceration may occur in advanced stages. It originates in the dermis but is deeply invasive and readily metastasizes to lymph nodes and the lung. Biopsy is made on histopathologic evaluation. Main risk factors include sun exposure, immunosuppression after organ transplantation and HIV-disease. These risk factors may compound, as HIV patients with higher UVL exposure are at even greater risk. Treatment is controversial but in general, smaller tumors without positive lymph nodes are treated with wide surgical excision (2–3 cm margins) followed by radiation therapy with or without chemotherapy, whereas metastatic disease is often palliated with chemotherapy.[132] Interestingly, remission of metastatic MCC after therapy with HAART has been recently reported.[133]

HIV-Associated KS

For discussion on KS see Chapter 59.

ADVERSE CUTANEOUS DRUG REACTIONS

The incidence of adverse cutaneous drug eruptions adverse cutaneous drug reactions (ACDEs) to a variety of drugs is high in HIV disease (100 times more common than in the general population), and increases with advancing immunodeficiency.[134] Drug hypersensitivity complicated 3–20% of all prescriptions in one large series.[135]

The pathogenesis of the high rates of ACDE in HIV disease is unknown; pathogenetic factors include immune dysregulation with increased B-cell activity with IgE and IgA hyperimmunoglobulinemia and hypereosinophilia. The diagnosis can often be made on clinical findings; lesional skin biopsy is helpful in some cases, in order to differentiate an exanthematous reaction from drug-induced vasculitis.

In a report of 974 HIV-infected individuals followed for 46 months, 283 ACDEs occurred in 201 patients.[136] ACDE were noted more commonly in White than Black people. Acute or reactivated EBV or CMV infections were significantly more common in patients with ACDE. The onset of a majority of ACDEs was within 6–14 days of initiation therapy. TMP-SMX, other sulfonamide drugs, and penicillins were the causative agents in 75% of cases of ACDE. Exanthematous (morbilliform) eruptions were by far the most commonly occurring ACDE, occurring in 95% of cases; other ACDE observed were urticaria (four cases), erythema multiforme (EM, eight cases; EM major, two cases; EM minor, six cases), a lichenoid eruption (one case), and fixed-drug eruption (two cases). Systemic symptoms were reported in 20% of cases, including fever, headache, myalgia, and arthralgia.

The majority of ACDEs are mild, accompanied by pruritus, resolving promptly after the offending drug is discontinued. However, severe, life-threatening ACDRs do occur and are unpredictable. Drug eruptions can mimic virtually all the morphologic expressions in dermatology and must be first on the differential diagnosis in the sudden appearance of a symmetric eruption. Drug eruptions are caused by immunologic or nonimmunologic mechanisms and are provoked by systemic or topical administration of a drug. The majority are based on a hypersensitivity mechanism and may be of types I, II, III, or IV (see Table 64-10).

Nonimmunologic ACDE are classified in the following categories: (1) idiosyncrasy *sensu strictiori* (reactions due to hereditary enzyme deficiencies); (2) cumulation (dependent on the total amount of drug ingested: pigmentation, i.e., gold, amiodarone, or minocycline); (3) reactions due to the combination of a drug with ultraviolet irradiation, i.e., photosensitivity (either a toxic or immunologic (allergic) pathogenesis; (4) irritancy/toxicity of a topically applied drug (5-fluorouracil, imiquimod, podophyllotoxin); (5) individual idiosyncrasy to a topical or systemic drug; and/or (6) unknown mechanisms.

Guidelines for the assessment of possible ACDR include the following: (1) alternative causes should be excluded, especially infections, in that many infections (especially viral) are difficult to distinguish clinically from the adverse effects of drugs used to treat infections; (2) the interval between introduction of a drug and onset of the reaction should be examined; (3) any improvement after drug withdrawal should be noted; (4) the caregiver should determine whether similar reactions have been associated with the same

Table 64-10 Types of Allergic Cutaneous Drug Reactions

Reaction	Comments
Exanthematous (morbilliform) reactions	Most common type of ACDR. Can occur with nearly any drug. Onset: <14 days after drug therapy initiated. Same reaction recurs shortly after rechallenge with the sensitizing agent.
Urticaria/angioedema	Urticaria is the second most common type of ACDR after exanthematous reaction; in some cases, angioedema also occurs. Onset: usually within 36 h after initial exposure; within minutes after rechallenge. Agents: aspirin and NSAIDs are common causes; also codeine, penicillin, blood transfusion. Drugs that release mast cell mediator(s): opiates, codeine, amphetamine, polymyxin B, atropine, hydralazine, pentamidine, quinine, radiocontrast media. Drug that may cause urticaria/angioedema by pharmacologic mechanisms: cyclooxygenase inhibitors (aspirin, indomethacin).
Angioedema	Uncommon. Characterized by edema of deep dermis and subcutaneous and submucosal areas.
Anaphylaxis and anaphylactoid reactions	Most serious type of adverse drug reaction. Occurs within minutes or hours after administration of drug. May be systemic life-threatening reaction. Agents: radiographic contrast media, antibiotics, extracts of allergens. More common with parenteral than oral administration. Intermittent administration may predispose to anaphylaxis.
Serum sickness	Onset: 5–21 days after initial exposure. Minor form: fever, urticaria, arthralgia. Major (complete) form: fever, urticaria, angioedema, arthralgia, arthritis, lymphadenopathy, eosinophilia, ± nephritis, ± endocarditis. Agents: IV immunoglobulin G (IVIG), antibiotics, and bovine serum albumin (used oocyte retrieval during *in vitro* fertilization).
Erythema multiforme	Most cases considered to be associated with reactivated HSV infection.
Stevens–Johnson syndrome	Moderate mucocutaneous and systemic reaction. With more severe mucocutaneous and systemic involvement, clinical findings merge into toxic epidermal necrolysis.
Toxic epidermal necrolysis	Severe, life-threatening mucocutaneous and systemic reaction.
Fixed-drug eruptions	Appears 0.5–1.0 h after readministration in sensitized individuals. Lesions often solitary, recurring at same site; may be multiple. More numerous lesions occur after repeated administration; multiple bullous lesions can mimic those of TEN.
Lichenoid eruptions	Onset: weeks to months after initiation of drug therapy; may progress to exfoliative dermatitis. May be extensive. Adnexal involvement may result in alopecia, anhidrosis. Oral involvement occurs with some drugs. Resolution after discontinuation slow, 1–4 months; up to 24 months after gold. May be photodistributed or bullous.
Photosensitivity	Classified as phototoxic (occurring in all individuals if dosing high enough, only at sites of light exposure), photoallergic (may be eczematous or lichenoid), or photocontact reactions. Some drugs cause both phototoxic and photoallergic reactions.
Porphyria cutanea tarda (PCT), and photosensitivity	May be precipitated by drugs in sunexposed sites. Pseudo-PCT with bulla formation can also be a drug-induced reaction
Purpura (petechiae, ecchymoses)	Thrombocytopenia: allergic or cytotoxic; results in petechiae/ecchymoses if platelet counts are <30 000/mL.

(*Continued*)

(Continued)

Table 64-10

Reaction	Comments
	Hemorrhage into a morbilliform ACDR occurs not uncommonly on the legs. Oral, inhalation, and topical corticosteroid usage are associated with ecchymoses, usually on the extremities in areas of dermatoheliosis. Progressive pigmented purpura has also been reported to be associated with drug therapy.
Acneiform eruptions	Folliculocentric pustules, usually without comedones. Drugs: anabolic steroids/testosterone (replacement) corticosteroids (parenteral, topical), ACTH, anabolic steroids, oral contraceptives, halogens (iodides, bromides), isoniazid, danazol, lithium, azathioprine.
Pustular eruptions	Toxic pustuloderma, acute generalized exanthematous pustulosis. Must be differentiated from pustular psoriasis. Eosinophil in the infiltrate suggests ACDR. Drugs: ampicillin, amoxicillin, macrolides, tetracyclines.
Psoriasiform reactions	Drugs reported to exacerbate psoriasis: antimalarials; β-blockers; lithium salts; NSAIDs (ibuprofen, indomethacin); miscellaneous (captopril, cimetidine, clonidine, gemfibrozil, interferon, methyldopa, penicillamine, trazadone).
Eczematous eruptions	Systemic administration of a drug to an individual who has been previously sensitized to the drug by topical application can experience widespread eczematous dermatitis (systemic contact-type dermatitis medicamentosa) or urticaria. Systemically administered drugs that reactivate allergic contact dermatitis to related topical agents (systemic drug/topical agent): ethylenediamine antihistamines, aminophylline/aminophylline suppositories, ethylenediamine HCl; procaine/benzocaine; iodides, iodinated organic compounds, radiographic contrast media/iodine; streptomycin, kanamycin, paramomycin, gentamicin/neomycin sulfate; nitroglycerin tablets/nitroglycerin ointment; disulfuram/thiuram.
Exfoliative dermatitis and erythroderma	This widespread or generalized reaction may follow an exanthematous ACDR or begin with erythema and exudation in body folds and progress to become generalized. In individuals previously sensitized by topical administration of a drug, systemic administration of the sensitizing agent (or closely related compound) may cause a generalized eczematous dermatitis. The most commonly implicated drugs are sulfonamides, antimalarials, phenytoin, and penicillin.

ACDR, allergic cutaneous drug reaction; TEN, toxic epidermal necrolysis; NSAIDs, nonsteroidal antiinflammatory drugs.

compound; (5) any reaction on re-administration of the drug should be noted. Clinical patterns of ACDR vary tremendously and should be ruled out when a change in the clinical status of the patient is noted (see Table 64-10).

Skin findings indicating possible life-threatening ACDR include confluent skin pain, erythema, urticaria, facial edema or central facial involvement, palpable purpura (vasculitis), skin necrosis, blisters of epidermal detachment or a positive Nikolsky's sign (epidermis separates readily from dermis with lateral pressure). Mucosal findings correlating with a serious ACDR include mucous membrane erosions and swelling of the tongue. Systemic findings indicating possible serious adverse drug reactions include high fever (temperature >40ºC), hypotension, shortness of breath, wheezing, enlarged lymph nodes, arthralgias and/or arthritis.

In most cases, the implicated or suspected drug should be discontinued. In some cases, such as with morbilliform eruptions, the offending drug can be continued, and the eruption may resolve. In cases of urticaria/angioedema or early Stevens–Johnson syndrome/toxic epidermal necrolysis (TEN), the ACDR can be life-threatening, and the drug should be discontinued.

Antiretroviral Agents

Drug hypersensitivity commonly occurs with the non-nucleoside reverse transcriptase inhibitors (NNRTIs) nevirapine, delavirdine, and efavirenz; the NRTI abacavir; and the protease inhibitor amprenavir.[134] HIV-drug hypersensitivity is characterized principally by morbilliform/maculopapular/exanthematous rash, fever (often precedes rash), myalgias/fatigue, mucosal ulcerations, as well as the less common features (<5%) Stevens–Johnson syndrome, TEN, anicteric hepatitis, hypotension, acute interstitial nephritis, and acute interstitial pneumonitis. Nearly 20% of nevirapine-treated patients experience rash, most commonly an exanthematous eruption, which does not appear to be responsive to antihistamines like cetirizine, or to short courses of prednisone (40 mg/day for 2 weeks).[137,138] Less commonly Stevens–Johnson syndrome may develop requiring drug discontinuation.[134,139] About 18–50% of delavirdine-treated patients experience rash.

Approximately half the cases of antiretroviral hypersensitivity resolve despite continuation of therapy. Drug therapy should be discontinued if the following occur: mucosal involvement, blistering, exfoliation, clinically significant hepatic dysfunction, fever greater than 39°C, or intolerable fever or pruritus.[140] Rechallenge with abacavir has been associated with several deaths resulting from cardiovascular collapse.

Indinavir, which has a retinoid-like effect, caused cheilitis (57%), diffuse dryness and pruritus (41%), asteatotic dermatitis on the trunk, arms, and thighs (12%), and scalp defluvium (12%); pyogenic granulomas, single or multiple, have also been reported.[141] Symptoms resolve when indinavir is discontinued. Peripheral lipodystrophy syndrome occurs in 14% of subjects.

Longitudinal melanonychia, brown-black longitudinal streaks in the nail plate, occur in up to 40% of zidovudine (ZVD)-treated individuals, more commonly in Blacks than in Latinos or Whites. The pigmentary changes are usually noted in the finger- and/or toenails within 4–8 weeks after initiation of ZVD therapy but may occur as far as 1 year later. ZVD pigmented macules of mucous membranes is also common, occurring more commonly in more heavily melanized individuals. Diffuse hyperpigmentation mimicking primary adrenal insufficiency has been reported. Melanonychia and mucocutaneous pigmentation has also been reported with hydroxyrea in HIV disease.[142]

The newest class of antiretrovirals are the fusion inhibitors. Enfuvirtide/T-20 is the only member in this category, and its main dermatologic consequence is at injection sites in the form of erythema, induration, nodules and cyst formation.[143]

Amprenavir has been linked to development of acanthosis nigricans; eruptive xanthomas can follow treatment with ritonavir, and lichenoid drug eruptions have recently been reported with tenofovir.[144–146]

Trimethoprim–Sulfamethoxazole

Fifty to 60% of HIV-infected individuals treated with intravenous (IV) TMP-SMX develop an exanthematous eruption (often with fever) 1–2 weeks after starting therapy, at an incidence ten times greater than that in the general population.[147] Successful ‘desensitization’ has been accomplished in patients with prior exanthematous or urticarial reactions to TMP-SMX, sulfadiazine, and dapsone.[148–150] Desensitization in patients with prior Stevens–Johnson syndrome has also been reported.[151] Co-administration of corticosteriods with TMP-SMX reduced the incidence of adverse cutaneous reactions from 47% to 13%.[152] The occurrence of adverse reactions to TMP-SMX has also been associated with more rapid decline in CD4+ T-lymphocyte cell counts.[153]

Severe bullous eruptions appear to be more common in HIV disease. In a report of six cases of EM major and six of TEN, all adverse reactions were to sulfonamide: sulfadiazine (six cases), TMP-SMX (two cases), and sulfadoxine–pyrimethamine (Fansidar) (two cases). Of 14 cases of TEN over a 6-year period (1984–89), sulfa drugs were the most common causative agents.[154] The number of cases of TEN was 375 times that expected. TEN occurred in patients with advanced HIV disease, and had a 21% mortality rate.

Oral Corticosteroids

Oral corticosteroid therapy in HIV-infected individuals raises concerns regarding increased immunosuppression with exacerbations of OIs and ONs such as KS or HSV infections. A cohort of 44 asymptomatic HIV-infected individuals (200–799 CD4+ T-lymphocyte cells/μL) was treated with oral prednisolone (0.5 mg/kg for 6 months; 0.3 mg/kg thereafter).[155] After 1 year of prednisolone therapy, no major side effects or HIV disease-related events had occurred. Serum p24 antigen and HIV RNA load levels remained stable; CD4+ T-lymphocyte cell counts increased significantly at all time points (median increase at 1 year, 119 cells/μL). A more recent study concluded that short-term prednisone was well tolerated and reasonably safe.[156] The use of prednisone (0.5 mg kg^{-1} day^{-1}) in patients with ACDR, particularly in the setting of immune reconstitution when ACDRs are more common, while complicated by hyperglycemia and oral candidiasis has revealed no evidence of avascular necrosis or other untoward side effects.[157]

Short-term oral corticosteroid therapy appears to be safe in most HIV-infected individuals.

Foscarnet

Foscarnet (trisodium phosphonoformate) causes painful, penile erosions and/or ulcers in 30% of patients undergoing high-dose induction therapy for CMV retinitis, 7–24 days after starting treatment. The ulcers are caused by high urinary concentration of the urinary metabolites of foscarnet. Hyperhydration reduces the risk of ulceration; in some cases, the drug must be discontinued for the ulcers to heal.

LIPOATROPHY AND LIPODYSTROPHY

Treatment of lipoatrophy, lipodystrophy, and the metabolic syndrome are of increasing concern to patients, as characteristic features have made these entities increasingly recognized markers of HIV status even by those who are not in the medical profession (*see* Chapter 73). Discontinuation or replacement of protease inhibitor or NRTI therapy does not result in reversal of dysmorphic changes in most persons, and most changes are generally progressive.[158] Liposuction has been used to treat the buffalo hump, but the results are not very satisfactory.[159] Facial lipoatrophy has been treated with fat transfer from the abdominal panniculus or with injection of various inert agents (Fascian, Profill, Arteplast), again with limited cosmetic success.[160] Clinical effects achieved with Alloderm, produced from tissue bank donor dermal extracellular matrix, appear to be independent of the severity of lipoatrophy. Cosmetic results obtained with these agents, like those of most other fillers however, are short lasting and costly. Recently, the use of injectable poly-L-lactic acid has gained acceptance, showing improvement in cosmesis after 2 years and with limited side-effect profile.[161] In addition, permanent injectable silicone oil, though not currently FDA-approved for lipoatrophy, may become a cost-effective and safe therapy in the near future.[162] Treatment with metformin, thiazolidinediones, and recombinant human growth hormone, have limited effect on cutaneous disease, particularly on the face.

REFERENCES

1. Rico MJ, Myers SA, Sanchez MR. Guidelines of care for dermatologic conditions in patients infected with HIV: guidelines/outcomes committee. J Am Acad Dermatol 37:450, 1997.
2. Treating 3 million by 2005: making it happen. Geneva, Switzerland: WHO; 2003.
3. Krishnam Raju PV, Raghurama Rao G, Ramani TV, Vandana S. Skin disease: clinical indicator of immune status in human immunodeficiency virus (HIV) infection. Int J Dermatol 646, 2005.
4. Kahn JO, Walker BD. Acute human immunodeficiency virus type 1 infection. N Engl J Med 339:33, 1998.
5. Vanhems P, Dassa C, Lambert J, et al. Comprehensive classification of symptoms and signs reported among 218 patients with an acute HIV-1 infection. J Acquir Immune Defic Syndr 21:99, 1999.
6. Sardana K, Sehgal VN. Genital ulcer disease and human immunodeficiency virus: A focus [review]. Int J Dermatol 44:391, 2005.
7. Boonchai W, Laohasrisakul R, Manonukul J, Kulthanan K. Pruritic popular eruption in HIV seropositive patients: a cutaneous marker for immunosuppression. Int J Dermatol 38:348, 1999.
8. Rodwell GE, Berger TG. Pruritus and cutaneous inflammatory conditions in HIV disease. Clin Dermatol 18:479, 2000.
9. Gelfand JM, Rudikoff D. Evaluation and treatment of itching in HIV-infected patients. Mt Sinai J Med 68:298, 2001.
10. Bonacini M. Pruritus in patients with chronic human immunodeficiency virus, hepatitis B and C virus infections. Dig Liver Dis 32:621, 2000.
11. Maurer T, Poncelet A, Berger T. Thalidomide treatment for prurigo nodularis in human immunodeficiency virus-infected subjects. Arch Dermatol 140:845, 2005.
12. Rajendran PM, Dolev JC, Heaphy MR Jr, Maurer T. Eosinophilic folliculitis: before and after the introduction of antiretroviral therapy. Arch Dermatol 141:1227, 2005.
13. Milazzo F, Piconi S, Trabattoni D, et al. Intractable pruritus in HIV infection: immunologic characterization. Allergy 54:266, 1999.
14. Otley CC, Avram MR, Johnson RA. Isotretinoin treatment of human immunodeficiency virus-associated eosinophillic folliculitis: results of an open, pilot trial. Arch Dermatol 131:1047, 1995.
15. Lim HW, Vallurupalli S, Meola T, Sorter NA. UVB phototherapy in an effective treatment for pruritus in patients infected with HIV. J Am Acad Dermatol 37:414, 1997.
16. Toutous-Trellu L, Abraham S, Pechere M, et al. Topical Tacrolimus for effective treatment of eosinophilic folliculitis associated with human immunodeficiency virus infection. Arch Dermatol 141:1203, 2005.
17. Almagro M, Del Pozo J, Garcia-Silva J, et al. Acne is not a stigma of HIV infection: a review of 36 patients. Dermatology 211:114, 2005.
18. Resneck JS Jr, Van Beek M, Furmanski L, et al. Etiology of pruritic papular eruption with HIV infection in Uganda. JAMA 292:2614, 2004.
19. Singh F, Rudikoff D. HIV-associated pruritus: etiology and management. Am J Clin Dermatol 4:177, 2003.
20. Corominas M, Garcia JF, Mestre M, et al. Predictors of atopy in HIV-infected patients. Ann Allergy Asthma Immunol 84:607, 2000.
21. Bartke U, Venten I, Kreuter A, et al. Human immunodeficiency virus -associated psoriasis and psoriatic arthritis treated with infliximab [letter]. Br J Dermatol 150:784, 2004.
22. Yungmann MP, Ford MJ. Histoplasmosis presenting as erythroderma in a patient with acquired immunodeficiency syndrome. Int J Dermatol 42:636, 2003.
23. Schkenberg C, Lipsker D, Petiau P, et al. Photosensitivity as presenting sign of HIV infection. Control with triple antiretroviral therapy. Ann Dermatol Venereol 125:516, 1998.
24. Meola T, Sanchez, M, Lim HW, et al. Photosensitivity as presenting sign of HIV infection: control with triple antiretroviral therapy. Ann Dermatol Venereol 125:516, 1998.
25. Bilu D, Manelak AJ, Nguyen RH, et al. Clinical and epidemiological characterization of photosensitivity and HIV-positive individuals. Photoderm Photoimmunol Photomed 20:175, 2004.
26. Vin-Christian K, Epstein JH, Maurer TA, et al. Photosensitivity in HIV-infected individuals. J Dermatol 27:361, 2000.
27. Smith KJ, Skelton HG, Yeager J, et al. Pruritus in HIV-1 disease: therapy with drugs which may modulate the pattern of immune dysregulation. Dermatology 195:353, 1997.
28. Jacobson JM, Greenspan JS, Spritzler J, et al. Thalidomide in low intermittent doses does not prevent recurrence of human immunodeficiency virus-associated aphthous ulcers. J Infect Dis 183:343, 2001.
29. Cribier B, Rey D, Uhl G, et al. Abnormal urinary coproporphyrin levels in patients infected by hepatitis C virus with or without human immunodeficiency virus: a study of 177 patients. Arch Dermatol 132:1448, 1996.
30. Almehmi A, Deliri H, Szego GG, et al. Porphyria cutanea tarda in a patient with HIV-infection. West Virginia Med J 101:19, 2005.
31. O'Connor WJ, Murphy GM, Darby C, et al. Porphyria abnormalities in acquired immunodeficiency syndrome. Arch. Dermatol 132:1443, 1996.
32. Gisselbretcht M, Cohen P, Lortholary O, et al. Human immunodeficiency virus-related vasculitis: clinical presentation of and therapeutic approach to eight cases. Ann Med Interne (Paris) 149:398, 1998.
33. Calza L, Manfredi R, Colangelo V, et al. Systemic and discoid lupus erythematosus in HIV-Infected Patients treated with highly active antiretroviral therapy. Int J STD AIDS 14:356, 2003.
34. Chamberlain AJ, Hollowood K, Turner RJ, Byren I. Tumid lupus erythematosus occurring following highly active antiretroviral therapy for HIV infection: a manifestation of immune restoration. J Am Acad Dermatol 51:161, 2004.
35. Antony FC, Marsden RA. Vitiligo in association with human immunodeficiency virus infection. J Eur Acad Dermatol Venereol 17:456, 2003.
36. Pascual JC, Belinchon I, Silvestre JF, et al. Sarcoidosis after highly active antiretroviral therapy in patients with AIDS. Clin Exp Dermatol 29:156, 2004.

37. Tervenzoli M, Catekan AM, Marino F, et al. Sarcoidosis and HIV infection: a case report and review of the literature [review]. Postgrad Med J 79:535, 2003.
38. Calista D. Subcorneal pustular dermatosis in a patient with AIDS. J Eur Acad Dermatol Venereol 17:478, 2003.
39. Hodgson TA, Fidler SJ, Speight PM, et al. Oral pemphigus vulgaris associated with HIV infection. J Am Acad Dermatol 49:313, 2005.
40. Bar A, Hantschke D, Mirmohammadsadegh A, Hengge UR. Spectrum of bacterial isolates in HIV-positive patients with a skin and soft tissue infections: emergence of methicillin-resistant Staphylococci [letter]. AIDS 17:1253, 2003.
41. Lee NE, Talor MM, Bancroft E, et al. Risk factors for community-associated methicillin-resistant Staphylococcus aureus skin infections among HIV-positive men who have sex with men. CID 40:1529, 2005.
42. De Vries HJ, van Noesel CJ, Hoekzema R, Hulsebosch HJ. Botryomycosis in an HIV-positive subject [review]. J Eur Acad Dermatol Venereol 17:87, 2003.
43. Bachmeyer C, Landgraf N, Cordier F, et al. Acinetobacter baumanii folliculitis in a patient with AIDS. Clin Exp Dermatol 30:256, 2005.
44. Wong R, Tappero J, Cockrell CJ. Bacillary angiomatosis and other Bartonella species infections. Semin Cutan Med Surg 16:188, 1997.
45. Gazineo JL, Trope BM, Maceira JP, et al. Bacillary angiomatosis: description of 13 cases reported in five reference centers for AIDS treatment in Rio de Janeiro, Brazil. Rev Inst Med Trop Sao Paulo 43:1, 2001.
46. Plettenberg A, Lorenzen T, Burtsche BT, et al. Bacillary angiomatosis in HIV-infected patients-an epidemiological and clinical study. Dermatology 201:326, 2000.
47. Stevens DL, Bisno AL, Chambers HF, et al. Practice guidelines or the diagnosis and management of skin and soft tissue infections. CID 41:1373, 2005.
48. Friedman PC, Husain S, Grossman ME. Nodular tuberculid in a patient with HIV. J Am Acad Dermatol 53:s154, 2005.
49. Johnson RA. Dermatophyte infections in human deficiency virus (HIV) disease. J Am Acad Dermatol 43:135, 2000.
50. Korting HC, Blecher P, Stallman D, Hamm G. Dermatophyte on the feet of HIV infected patients: frequency, species distribution, localization and antimicrobial susceptibility. Mycoses 36:271, 1993.
51. Venkatesan P, Perfect JR, Myers SA. Evaluation and management of fungal infections in immunocompromised patients [review]. Dermatol ther 18:44, 2005.
52. Almeida L, Grossman M. Widespread dermatophyte infections that mimic collagen vascular disease. J Am Acad Dermatol 23:855, 1990.
53. Kwon KS, Jang HS, Son HS, et al. Widespread and invasive Trichophyton rubrum infection mimicking Kaposi's sarcoma in a patient with AIDS. J Dermatol 31:839, 2004.
54. Elewski BE, Sullivan J. Dermatophytes as opportunistic pathogens. J Am Acad Dermatol 30:1021, 1994.
55. Wright DC, Lennox JL, James WD. Generalized chronic dermatophytosis in patients with human immunodeficiency virus type I infection and CD4 depletion [letter]. Arch Dermatol 127:265, 1991.
56. Burkhart CN, Chang H, Gottwald L. Tinea corporis in human immunodeficiency virus-positive patients: case report and assessment of oral therapy [review]. Int J Dermatol 42:839, 2003.
57. Prose NS. HIV infection in children. J Am Acad Dermatol 22:1223, 1990.
58. Kantipong P, Walsh DS. Oral penicillinosis in a patient with human immunodeficiency virus in Northern Thailand. Int J Dermatol 39:926, 2000.
59. Schacker T, Hu HL, Koelle DM, et al. Famciclovir for the suppression of symptomatic and asymptomatic herpes simplex virus reactivation in HIV-infected persons: a double-blind placebo-controlled trial. Ann Intern Med 128:21, 1998.
60. Posavad CM, Wald A, Kuntz S, et al. Frequent reactivation of herpes simplex virus among HIV-1-infected patients treated with highly active antiretroviral therapy. J Infect Dis 109:693, 2004.
61. Conant M. Current clinical issues in the management of herpes simplex virus infections in patients with HIV. Dermatology 194:93, 1997.
62. Chang E, Absar N, Beall G. Prevention of recurrent herpes simplex virus (HSV) infections in HIV-infected persons. AIDS Patient Care 9:252, 1995.
63. Saint-Leger E, Fillet AM, Malvy D, et al. Efficacy of cidofivir in an HIV infected patient with an acyclovir and foscarnet resistant herpes simplex virus infection. Ann Dermatol Venereol 128:747, 2001.
64. Lalezari J, Schacter T, Feinberg J, et al. A randomized, double blind, placebo-controlled trail of cidofivir gel for the treatment of acyclovir-unresponsive mucocutaneous herpes simplex virus infection in patients with AIDS. J Infect D 176:892, 1997.
65. Gilbert J, Drehs M, Weinberg J, et al. Topical Imiquimod for acyclovir-unresponsive herpes simplex virus 2 infection. Arch Dermatol 127:1015, 2001.
66. Corey L, Wald A, Celum CL, Quinn TC. The effects of herpes simplex virus-2 on HIV-1 acquisition and transmission: a review of two overlapping epidemics [review]. J AIDS 35:435, 2004.
67. Freedman E, Mindel A. Epidemiology of herpes and HIV coinfection [review]. J HIV Ther 9:4, 2004.
68. Zampogna JC, Flowers FP. Persistent verrucous varicella as the initial manifestation of HIV infection. J Am Acad Dermatol 44:391, 2001.
69. Leautez S, Billaud E, Milipied B, Raffi F. Varicella zoster virus infection area in 39 HIV-infected patients: therapeutic management. Presse Med 28:473, 1999.
70. Safrin S, Berger TG, Gilson I, et al. Foscarnet therapy in five patients with AIDS and acyclovir-resistant varicella-zoster virus infection. Ann Intern Med 115:19–21, 1991.
71. Safrin S, Assaykeen T, Follansbee S, Mills J. Foscarnet therapy for acyclovir-resistant mucocutaneous herpes simplex virus infection in 26 AIDS patients: preliminary data. J Infect Dis 161:1078, 1990.
72. Patton LL, McKaig R, Strauss R, et al. Changing prevalence of oral manifestations of human immuno-deficiency virus in the era of protease inhibitor therapy. Oral Surg Oral Med Oral Pathol Oral Radiol Endod 89:299, 2000.
73. Patton LL. Sensitivity, specificity, and positive predictive value of oral opportunistic infections in adults with HIV/AIDS as markers of immune suppression and viral burden. Oral Surg Oral Med Oral Pathol Oral Radiol Endod 90:182, 2000.
74. Greenspan D, Komaroff E, Redford M, et al. Oral mucosal lesions and HIV viral load in women's interagency HIV study (WIHS). J Acquir Immune Defic Syndr 25:44, 2000.
75. Greenspan D, Greenspan JS, Hearst NG, et al. Relation of oral hairy leukoplakia to infection with human immunodeficiency virus and the risk of developing AIDS. J infect Dis 155:475, 1987.
76. Greenspan D, Greenspan JS. Oral manifestations of HIV infection. Dermatol Clin 9:517, 1991.
77. Alessi E, Berti E, Cusini M, et al. Oral hairy leukoplakia [see comments]. J Am Acad Dermatol 22:79, 1990.
78. Eyeson JD, Warnakulasuriya KA, Johnson NW. Prevalence and incidence of oral lesions-the changing scene. Oral Dis 6:267, 2000.

79. Logan RM, Coates EA, Pierce AM, Wilson SF. A retrospective analysis of oral hairy leukoplakia in South Australia. Aust Dent J 46:108, 2001.
80. Ceballos-Salobrena A, Gaitan-Cepeda LA, Ceballos-Garcia L, Lezama-Del Valle D. Oral lesions in HIV/AIDS patients undergoing highly active antiretroviral treatment including protease inhibitors: a new face of oral AIDS? AIDS patient care STDS 14:627, 2000.
81. Cho M, Puma I, Nguygen D, et al. Development of Kaposi's sarcoma in an AIDS patient after treatment with topical tacrolimus. J Am Acad Dermatol 50:149, 2004.
82. Sissolak G, Mayaud P. AIDS related Kaposi's sarcoma: epidemiological, diagnostic, treatment and control aspects in sub-Saharan Africa [review]. Trop Med Int Health 10:981, 2005.
83. Lim ST, Tupule A, Espina BM, Levine AM. Weekly docetaxel is safe and effective in the treatment of advanced-stage acquired immunodeficiency syndrome-related Kaposi sarcoma. Cancer 103:417, 2005.
84. Koon HB, Bubley GJ, Pantanowitz L, et al. Imatinib-induced regression of AIDS related Kaposi's sarcoma. J Clin Oncol 23:982, 2005.
85. Weinberg JM, Mysliwiec A, Turiansky GW, et al. Viral folliculitis. Atypical presentations of herpes simplex, herpes zoster, and molluscum contagiosum [see comments]. Arch Dermatol 133:983, 1997.
86. Myskowski PL. Molluscum contagiosum. New insights, new directions [editorial; comment]. Arch Dermatol 133:1039, 1997.
87. Koopman RJ, van Merrienboer FC, Vreden SG, Dolmas WM. Molluscum contagiosum; a marker for advanced HIV infection [letter]. Br J Dermatol 126:528, 1992.
88. Hicks CB, Myers SA, Giner J. Resolution of intractable molluscum contagiosum in a human immunodeficiency virus-infected patient after institution of antiviral therapy with ritonavir. Clin Infect Dis 24:1023, 1007.
89. Strauss RM, Doyle EL, Mohsen AH, Green ST. Successful treatment of molluscum contagiosum with topical imiquimod in a severely immunocompromised HIV-positive patient. Int J STD AIDS 12:264, 2001.
90. Liota E, Smith KJ, Bukley R, et al. Imiquimod therapy for molluscum contagiosum. J Cutan Med Surg 4:76, 2000.
91. Toro JR, Wood LV, Patel NK, Turner ML. Topical cidofovir: a novel treatment for recalcitrant molluscum contagiosum infections in children infected with human immunodeficiency virus 1. Arch Dermatol 136:983, 2000.
92. Calista D. Topical cidofovir for severe cutaneous human papillomavirus and molluscum contagiosum infections in patients with HIV/AIDS: a pilot study. J Eur Acad Dermatol Venereol 14:484, 2000.
93. Meadows KP, Tyring SK, Pavia AT, Rallis TM. Resolution of recalcitrant molluscum contagiosum virus lesions in human immunodeficiency virus-infected patients treated with cidofovir. Arch Dermatol 133:987, 1997.
94. Baxter KF, Highet AS. Tropical cidofovir and cryotherapy-combination treatment for recalcitrant molluscum contagiosum in a patient with HIV infection. J Eur Acad Dermatol Venerol 18:230, 2004.
95. Mollin A. Photodynamic therapy for molluscum contagiosum infection in HIV-coinfected patients: review of 6 patients. J Drugs Dermatol 2:637, 2003.
96. De Oliveira M, Brites C, Ferraz N, et al. Infective dermatitis associated with the human T cell lymphotropic virus type 1 in Salvador, Bahia, Brazil. Clin Inf Diseases 40:90, 2005.
97. Bonamigo RR, Borges K, Kietjen J, et al. Human T lymphotropic virus 1 and hepatitis C virus as risk factors for inflammatory dermatoses in HIV positive patients. Int J Dermatol 43:568, 2004.
98. Cohen LM, Tyring SK, Randy P, Callen JP. Human papillomavirus type II in multiple squamous cell carcinomas in a patient with subacute cutaneous lupus erythematosus. J Am Acad Dermatol 19:67, 1992.
99. Vaic J, Chardonnet Y, Euvard S, et al. Langerhans cells, inflammation markers and human papillomavirus infection in benign and malignant epithelial tumors from transplant recipients. J Dermatol 19:67, 1992.
100. Berger TG, Sawchuk WS, Leonardi C, et al. Epidermodysplasia verruciformis-associated papillomavirus infection complicating human immunodeficiency virus disease. Br J Dermatol 124:79, 1991.
101. Prose NS, von Knebel-Doeberitz, Miller S, et al. Widespread flat warts associated with human papillomavirus type 5: a cutaneous manifestation of human immunodeficiency virus infection. J Am Acad Dermatol 23:978, 1990.
102. Beck DE, Jaso RG, Zajac RA. Surgical management of anal condylomata in the HIV-positive patient. Dis Colon Rectum 33:180, 1990.
103. Hivnor C, Shepard JW, Shapiro MS, Vittorio CC. Intravenous cidofovir of recalcitrant verruca vulgaris in the setting of HIV. Arch Dermatol 140:13, 2004.
104. Husak R, Zouboulis CC, Sander-Bahr C, et al. Refractory human papillomavirus-associated oral warts treated topically with 1–3% cidofovir solutions in human immunodeficiency virus type 1-infected patients. Br J Dermatol 152:590, 2005.
105. Cameron JE, Maercante D, O'Brien M, et al. The impact of highly active retroviral therapy and immunodeficiency on human papillomavirus infection of the oral cavity of human immunodeficiency virus-seropositive adults. Sex Trans Dis 32:703, 2005.
106. Poblet E, Alfaro L, Fernander-Segoviano P, et al. Human papillomavirus-associated penile squamous cell carcinoma in HIV-positive patient. Dis Colon Rectum 33:180, 1990.
107. Goldstone SE, Winkler B, Ufford LJ, et al. High prevalence of anal squamous intraepithelial lesions and squamous cell carcinoma in men who have sex with men as seen in surgical practice. Dis Colon Rectum 44:690, 2001.
108. Palefsky JM, Holly EA, Efride JT, et al. Anal intraepithelial neoplasia in the highly active antiretroviral therapy era among HIV- positive men who have sex with men. AIDS 19:1407, 2005.
109. Kreuter A, Brockmeyer NH, Hochdorfer B, et al. Clinical spectrum and virologic characteristics of anal intraepithelial neoplasia in HIV infection. J Am Acad Dermatol 52:603, 2005.
110. Sobhani I, Walker F, Roudot-Thoraval F, et al. Anal Carcinoma: incidence and effect of cumulative infections. AIDS 18:1561, 2004.
111. Chin-Hong P, Palefsky J. Human papillomavirus anogenital disease in HIV-infected individuals. Dermatol Ther 18:67, 2005.
112. Pehoushek J, Smith KJ. Imiquimod and 5% fluorouracil therapy for anal and perianal squamous cell carcinoma in situ in an HIV-1-positive man. Arch Dermatol 137:14, 2001.
113. Place RJ, Gregoryck SG, Huber PJ, Simmang CL. Outcome analysis of HIV positive patients with anal squamous cell carcinoma. Dis Colon Rectum 44:506, 2001.
114. Piug L, Pradinaud R. Lesihmania and HIV-co-infection: dermatological manifestations. Ann Trop Med Parasit 97:107, 2003.
115. Olivier M, Badaro R, Medrano FJ, Moreno J. The pathogenesis of Leishmania/HIV co-infected: cellular and immunological mechanisms [review]. Ann trop med parasitol 97:79, 2003.
116. Coupie P, Clyti E, Sobesky M, et al. Comparative study of cutaneous leishmaniasis in human immunodeficiency virus (HIV)-infected patients and non-HIV-infected patients in French Guiana. Br J Dermatol 151:1165, 2004.

117. Posada-Vergara M, Lindoso J, Tolezano J, et al. Tegumentary Leishmaniasis as a manifestation of immune reconsitution inflammatory syndrome in 2 patients with AIDS. J Infect Dis 192:1819.
118. Sindermann H, Engel KR, Fischer C, Bommer W. Oral miltefosine for leishmaniasis in immunocompromised patients: compassionate use in 39 patients with HIV infection. Clin Infec Dis 39:1520, 2004.
119. Donabedian H, Khazan U. Norwegian scabies in a patient AIDS. Clin Infect Dis 14:162, 1992.
120. Portu JJ, Santamaria JM, Zubero Z, et al. Atypical scabies in HIV-positive patients. J Am Acad Dermatol 34:915, 1996.
121. Arico M, Noto J, La Rocca E, et al. Localized crusted scabies in the acquired immunodeficiency syndrome. Clin Exp Dermatol 17:339, 1992.
122. Hulbert TV, Larsen RA. Hyperkeratotic (Norwegian) scabies with gram-negative bacteremia as the initial presentation of AIDS [letter]. Clin Infec Dis 14:1164, 1992.
123. Glover A, Young L, Goltz AW. Norwegian scabies in acquired immunodeficiency syndrome: a report of a case resulting in death from associated sepsis [letter]. J Am Acad Dermatol 16:396, 1987.
124. Glover RA, Piaquiadio DJ, Kern S, Cockerell CJ. An unusual presentation of secondary syphilis in a patient with human immunodeficiency virus infection: a case report and review of the literature. Arch Dermatol 128:530, 1992.
125. Alberici F, Pagani L, Ratti G, Viale P. Ivermectin alone or in combination with benzyl benzoate in the treatment of human immunodeficiency virus-associated scabies. Br J Dermatol 142:969, 2000.
126. Meinking TL, Taplin D, Hermida JL, et al. The treatment of scabies with ivermectin. N Engl J Med 333:26, 1995.
127. Taplin D, Meinking TL. Treatment of HIV-related scabies with emphasis on the efficacy of ivermectin. Semin Cutan Med Surg 16:235, 1997.
128. Wilkins K, Turner B, Dolev J, et al. Cutaneous malignancy and human immunodeficiency virus disease. J Am Acad Dermatol 54:189, 2006.
129. Maurer TA, Christian KV, Kerschmann RL, et al. Cutaneous squamous cell carcinoma human immunodeficiency virus-infected patients: a study of epidemiologic risk factors, human papillomavirus and p53 expression. Arch Dermatol 133:577, 1997.
130. Oram Y, Orengo I, Griego RD, et al. Histologic patterns of basal cell carcinoma based upon patient immunostatus. Dermatol Surg 21:611, 1995.
131. Wilkins K, Dolev JC, Turner R, et al. Approach to the treatment of cutaneous malignancy in HIV-infected patients [review]. Dermatol Ther 18:77, 2005.
132. Colebunders R, Bottieau E, Van den Brande J, et al. Merkel cell carcinoma and multiple basal cell carcinoma in an African albino woman with HIV infection. HIV Med 5:452, 2004.
133. Burack J, Altschuler EL. Sustained remission of metastatic Merkel cell carcinoma with treatment of HIV infection. J Royal Soc Med 96:238, 2003.
134. Carr A, Copper DA. Adverse effects of antiviral therapy. Lancet 356:1423, 2000.
135. Coopman SA, Johnson RA, Platt R, Stren RS. Cutaneous disease and drug reactions in HIV infection. N Engl J Med 328:1670, 1993.
136. Smith KJ, Skelton HG, Yeager J, et al. Increased drug reactions in HIV-1 positive patients: a possible explanation based on patterns of immune dysregulation seen in HIV-1 disease. The Military Medical Consortium of the Advancement of Retroviral Research (MMCARR). Clin Exp Dermatol 22:118, 1997.
137. Knobel H, Miro JM, Mahillo B, et al. Failure of cetirizine to prevent nevirapine-associated rash: a double-blind placebo-controlled trial for the GESIDA 26/01 study. J AIDS 37:1276, 2004.
138. Montaner JS, Cahn P, Zala C, et al. Randomized, controlled study of the effects of a short course of prednisone on the incidence of rash associated with nevirapine in patients infected with HIV-1. J AIDS 33:41, 2003.
139. Metry DW, Lahart CJ, Farmer KL, Herbert AA. Stevens–Johnson syndrome caused by the antiretroviral drug nevirapine. J Am Achad Dermatol 22:354, 2001.
140. Max B, Sherer R. Management of the adverse effects of antiretroviral therapy medication adherence. Clin Infect Dis 30(Suppl 2):S96, 2000.
141. Calista D, Boschini A. Cutaneous side effects induced by indinavir. Eur J Dermatol 10:292, 2000.
142. Laughon SK, Shinn LL, Nunley JR. Melanonychia and mucocutaneous hyperpigmentation due to hydroxyurea use in an HIV-infected patient. In J Dermatol 39:928, 2000.
143. Kong H, Myers SA. Cutaneous effects of highly active antiretroviral therapy in HIV-infected patients [review]. Dermatol Ther 18:58, 2005.
144. Mur A, Seidel V, Lopez-Vilchez MA, et al. Acanthosis nigricans as an adverse effect of highly active antiretroviral therapy in an adolescent girl with human inmmunodeficiency virus infection. Ped Infect Disease J 24:742, 2005.
145. Geyer AS, MacGregor JL, Fox LP, et al. Eruptive xanthomas associated with protease inhibitortherapy [comment]. Arch Dermatol 140:617, 2004.
146. Wooley IJ, Veitch AJ, Harangozo CS, et al. Lichenoid drug eruption to tenofovir in an HIV/hepatitis B virus co-infected patient [letter]. AIDS 18:1857, 2004.
147. Roudier C, Caumes E, Rogeaux O, et al. Adverse cutaneous reactions to trimethoprim–sulfamethoxazole in patients with the acquired immunodeficiency syndrome and Pneumocystis carinii pneumonia. Arch Dermatol 130:1383, 1994.
148. Absar N, Daneshvar H, Beall G. Desensitization to trimethoprim/sulfamethoxazole in HIV infected patients. J Allergy Clin Immunol 93:1001, 1994.
149. Gluckstien D, Ruskin J. Rapid oral desensitization to trimethoprim–sulfamethoxazole (TMP-SMX): use in prophylaxis for Pneumocystis carinii pneumonia in patients with AIDS who were previously intolerant to TMP-SMX. Clin Infect Dis 20:849, 1995.
150. Yoshizawa S, Yashuoka A, Kikuchi Y, et al. A 5-day course of oral desensitization to trimethoprim/sulfamethoxazole (T/S) in patients with human immunodeficiency virus type-1 infection who were previously intolerant to T/S. Ann Allergy Asthma Immunol 85:241, 2000.
151. Douglas R, Spelman D, Czarny D, O'Hehir RE. Successful desensitization of two patients who previously developed Stevens–Johnson syndrome while receiving trimethoprim–sulfamethozazole. Clin Infect Dis 25:1480, 1997.
152. Caumes E, Roudier C, Rogeaux O, et al. Effect of corticosteroids on the incidence of adverse cutaneous reactions to trimethoprim–sulfamethoxazole during the treatment of AIDS-associated Pneumocystis carinii pneumonia. Clin Infect Dis 18:319, 1994.
153. Veenstra J, Veugelers PJ, Keet IP, et al. Rapid disease progression in human immunodeficiency virus type 1-infected individuals with adverse reactions to trimethoprim–sulfamethoxazole prophylaxis. Clin Infect Dis 24:936, 1997.
154. Roujeau JC, Chosidow O, Saiag P, Guillaume JC. Toxic epidermal necrolysis (Lyell syndrome). J Am Acad Dermatol 23:1039, 1990.
155. Andrieu JM, Lu W, Levy R. Sustained increases in CD4 cell counts in asymptomatic human immunodeficiency virus type 1-seropositive patients treated with prednisolone for 1 year. J Infect Dis 171:523, 1995.
156. McComsey GA, Whallen CC, Mawhorter SD, et al. Placebo-controlled trail of prednisone in advanced HIV-1 infection. AIDS 15:321, 2001.

157. Dolev J, Reyter I, Maurer T. Treatment of recurring cutaneous drug reactions in patients with human immunodeficiency virus 1 infection: a series of 3 cases. Arch Dermatol 140:1051, 2004.
158. Panse I, et al. Lipodystrophy associated with protease inhibitors. Br J Dermatol 142:496, 2000.
159. Wolfort FG, Cetrulo CL, Nevarre DR. Suction-assisted lipectmoy for lipodystrophy syndromes attributed to HIV-protease inhibitor use. Plast Reconstr Surg 104:1814, 1999
160. Fournier PF. Fat grafting: my technique. Dermatol Surg 26:1117, 2000.
161. Burgess CM, Quiroga RM. Assessment of the safety and efficacy of poly-L-lactic acid for the treatment of HIV-associated facial lipoatrophy. Am Acad Dermatol 52:233–239.
162. Jones DH, Carruthers A, Orentreich D, et al. Highly purified 1000-cSt Silicone oil for treatment of human immunodeficiency virus-associated facial lipoatrophy: an open pilot trial. Dermatol Surg 30:1279, 2004.

Chapter 65

Oropharyngeal Disease

Jeffrey D. Hill, DMD, David Reznik, DDS

Oral lesions are common throughout the course of HIV infection. They may represent the initial signs of infection in the undiagnosed individual or they may occur in patients with well-established disease. Severe pain and loss of dental function as a result of oral disease processes can significantly alter the patient's ability to sustain proper nutritional intake, to take oral medications, and to communicate effectively. Although the use of highly active antiretroviral therapy (HAART) has significantly reduced the incidence of opportunistic infections in general, oral lesions continue to occur and may be useful as clinical markers of disease progression.[1,2]

FUNGAL INFECTIONS

Superficial Diseases

Oropharyngeal candidiasis is the most common intraoral lesion among human immunodeficiency virus (HIV)-infected individuals (*see* Chapter 46). Reports indicate prevalence varying from less than 5% in adults living with HIV in developed countries to greater than 50% in those in the developing world.[3,4] Predominantly caused by *Candida albicans*,[5] this localized fungal infection is often a presenting sign of HIV infection. Closely associated with a low CD4+ T-lymphocyte count and high viral load,[6,7] it is a marker for progression of HIV disease.[8–10]

Four distinct clinical presentations of oral candidiasis can be seen: pseudomembranous candidiasis (Fig. 65-1), erythematous candidiasis (Fig. 65-2), hyperplastic candidiasis, and angular cheilitis (Fig. 65-3). Diagnosis is based on clinical appearance of the lesions, and may be confirmed by the presence of hyphae on a potassium hydroxide preparation.

Pseudomembranous oral candidiasis presents as a creamy-white plaque that can be scraped off mucous membranes with a tongue blade or cotton gauze, often leaving an erythematous surface beneath (Fig. 65-1A). Patients may complain of a mild burning sensation or a foul or metallic-like taste. The most common sites are the buccal mucosa, ventral tongue or floor of the mouth, and palate (Fig. 65-1A), but the lesions may appear anywhere in the oral cavity. Severe cases may lead to difficulty in eating or swallowing (Fig. 65-1B).

Erythematous oral candidiasis may be seen as a red macular lesion of the dorsal tongue, hard palate (Fig. 65-2A), or buccal mucosa. This form of oral candidiasis may appear as an erythematous, atrophic or 'bald' area of the middle of the dorsum of the tongue (Fig. 65-2B). This represents a loss of filiform papillae, which should regenerate with proper treatment. Patients

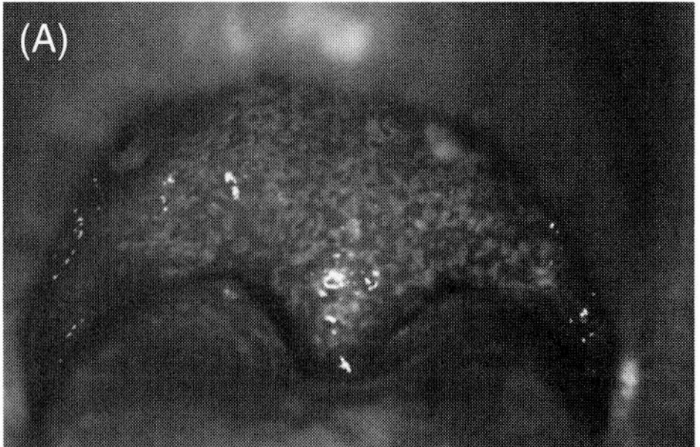

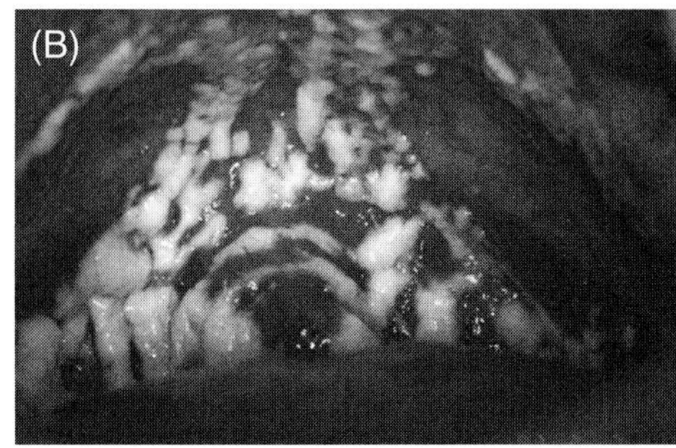

Figure 65-1 ■ (**A**) Moderate-severe pseudomembranous candidasis. (**B**) Azole-resistant, severe pseudomembranous candidasis.

Reprinted from the International AIDS Society-USA, From Reznik DA. Oral manifestations of HIV disease. TOP HIV Med 13:143, 2005.

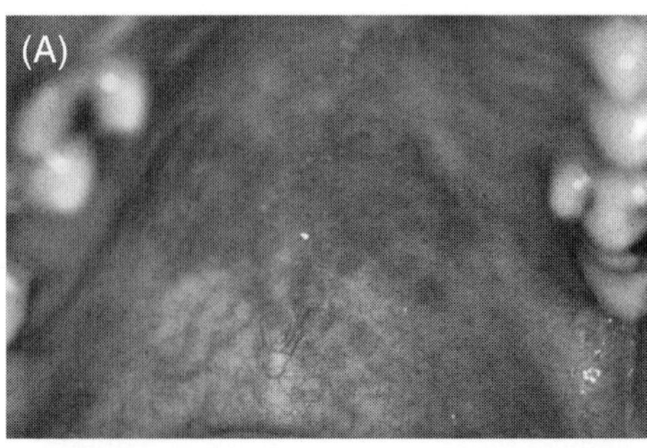

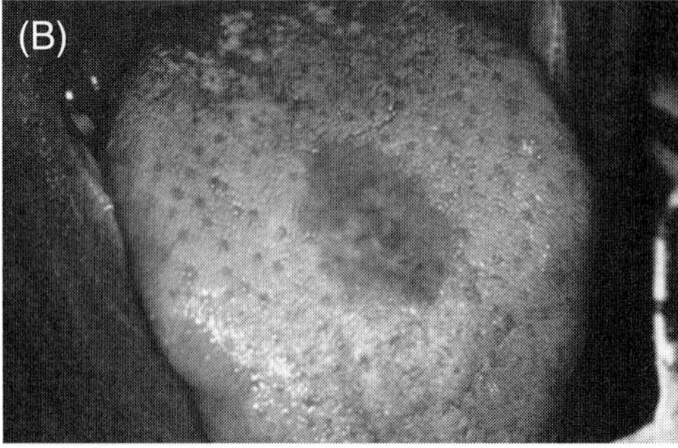

Figure 65-2 ■ (**A**) Erythematous candidasis on the roof of the mouth. (**B**) Erythematous candidiasis on the tongue.

Reprinted from the International AIDS Society-USA, from Reznik DA. Oral manifestations of HIV disease. TOP HIV Med 13:143, 2005.

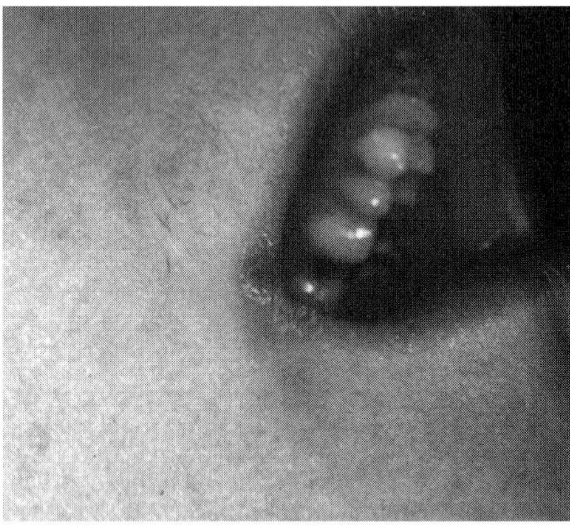

Figure 65-3 ■ Angular cheilitis at the corner of the mouth caused by *Candida* species.

Reprinted from the International AIDS Society-USA, from Reznik DA. Oral manifestations of HIV disease. TOP HIV Med 13:143, 2005.

may complain of a burning sensation when eating salty, spicy or acidic foods.

Chronic or hyperplastic oral candidiasis is a diffuse white or yellowish plaque which cannot be readily wiped off. These plaques cannot be easily removed because the long-standing infection has allowed the candidal hyphae to become anchored deep in the mucosa and therefore trapped in a layer of keratinized tissue. Chronic candidiasis may clinically resemble leukoplakia. This type of candidal infection is most often seen in patients with very low CD4+ T-lymphocyte counts.

Angular cheilitis presents as erythematous fissured, scaly patches at the angles of the mouth, with or without a pseudomembranous covering (Fig. 65-3). These sometimes painful lesions may appear unilaterally or bilaterally.

Therapy

Patients can be treated with topical, oral or intravenous regimens. Adherence, drug interactions, ability to take oral drugs, and likely fungal susceptibility results should influence the choice of agent. Topical therapy can be used for the treatment of mild to moderate episodes of pseudomembranous or erythematous candidiasis in which there is no esophageal involvement, although most clinicians choose systemic therapy.[13] Effective topical agents include clotrimazole (10 mg) oral troches, nystatin (200 000 U) oral pastilles, nystatin (100 000 U) vaginal troches, which have the advantage of not containing sugars, and nystatin swish and swallow (100 000 U/mL), which has a high sucrose content. The troches or pastilles are dissolved slowly in the mouth four to five times a day, for 14 days. Nystatin swish and swallow should be held in the mouth as long as possible four times a day for the 2 week treatment period. Topical preparations that contain high sugar content can exacerbate preexisting dental decay. The use of daily fluoride preparations should be employed to help reduce the risk of dental caries. Dentures should be removed during administration of the drug. The acrylic portion of dentures or partial dentures may also harbor fungus and should be thoroughly cleaned and disinfected, with either a 1–10 parts sodium hypochlorite and water solution, a 50% dilution of 0.12% chlorhexidine suspension and water, or nystatin suspension prior to re-insertion.

The following agents are effective in the management of angular cheilitis: ketoconazole cream (2%), clotrimazole cream (1%), or nystatin ointment (100 000 U). These agents are applied to the affected area three to four times a day, for at least 2 weeks. These topical creams and ointments can be used in conjunction with other therapies used in the treatment of intraoral candidiasis.

Systemic therapy should be reserved for moderate to severe cases of oropharyngeal candidiasis or in cases where patients cannot adhere to the multiple dosing involved with topical preparations. Systemic treatment is also warranted in cases where lesions are nonresponsive to topical therapy, following a review to verify proper regimen and patient compliance. Toxicities of oral azoles include headache, nausea, vomiting, diarrhea, abdominal pain, skin rash, and hepatotoxicity.[14] The recommended treatment duration is 14 days. Chronic suppressive therapy is indicated only if recurrences are frequent or severe.

Fluconazole is currently the preferred agent worldwide. Most clinicians use 200 mg PO as a loading dose to result in plasma concentrations close to steady state by the second day of therapy, followed by 100 mg PO/day for the remainder of the 14 day treatment period. Clinical evidence of oropharyngeal candidiasis generally resolves within several days, but treatment should be continued for at least 2 weeks to decrease the likelihood of recurrence. If the oral suspension (50 mg/5 mL or 200 mg/5 mL) is used, patients should swish and swallow 5 mL once a day. Fluconazole like the other azoles is metabolized by the cytochrome P450 system and can cause drug interactions, although much less frequently than other azoles used in the management of oral candidiasis. There have been increased reports of cases of oral infection with *Candida* species other than *C. albicans*, which are often inherently not susceptible to fluconazole (e.g., *C. glabrata*). Such cases may require alternative antifungal therapy (*see* Chapter 46).

Ketoconazole generally is no longer used in the United States. Other agents, such as itraconazole, are better absorbed, more active, and have fewer drug interactions. Itraconazole is available in tablet or suspension (two 100 mg tablets to be taken once daily with food or as the oral solution (10 mg/mL), 20 mL swished and swallowed once a day) .

Fluconazole-refractory oral candidiasis (FROC; Fig. 65-1B) is defined by failure to resolve within 14 days with treatment of 200 mg fluconazole per day, although this reflects dose-dependent resistance and can be temporarily overcome with doses of up to 800 mg/day. Factors associated with the development of FROC include CD4+ T-lymphocyte count <50 cells/μL, prior use of fluconazole, and frequent recurrences of candidiasis.[15,16] Voriconazole and posaconazole have good anticandidal activity and can be used as first-line therapy in FROC.[17,18] If oral agents are not effective in managing FROC, then the treatment of choice is an IV echinocandin class medication, such as caspofungin, or a liposomal amphotericin B.

Other Fungal Infections

Aspergillus species, *Mucor*, *Cryptococcus*, and *Histoplasma* occasionally can cause local invasion of oropharyngeal and nasal pharyngeal structures, and may be the initial presentation of these systemic fungal infections. Diagnosis is established by identification of characteristic organisms through biopsy and histologic examination. Cryptococcosis may present as a crater-like, nonhealing ulcer that is tender to palpation. Intraoral histoplasmosis may appear as a solitary, painful ulceration of several weeks duration with firm, rolled margins. Lesions present as white or erythematous areas with an irregular surface on the tongue, palate, and buccal mucosa.[21,22] All oral ulcerations that do not respond to traditional therapy should be biopsied.

Aspergillus, *Zygomyces*, and *Geotrichum candidum* can manifest as maxillary alveolar and/or palatal swelling.[21,23] A black, necrotic ulceration may be seen. Tissue damage to the maxillary sinus following tooth extraction or endodontic procedures, especially in the maxillary posterior region, can provide a portal of entry, but in most cases no predisposing anatomic factor can be found. These invasive fungal infections may initially present as localized pain and tenderness accompanied by nasal discharge.

VIRAL INFECTIONS

Herpes Simplex Virus

Recurrent herpes simplex virus (HSV) infections are one of the most common complications of HIV infection (*see* Chapter 48).[26,27] Most lesions are caused by HSV-1, although a few are caused by HSV-2. Oral mucosal involvement usually presents on keratinized mucosa. The lesions begin as an area of necrotic epithelium, then spread laterally to form a zone of erosion with a circinate, raised, yellow border. Multiple smaller lesions may coalesce forming an irregular pattern. Intraoral lesions usually appear in conjunction with herpes labialis.

A presumptive diagnosis of HSV infection can be made by clinical appearance (Fig. 65-4A,B). Viral culture can be performed if the diagnosis is in question, or if susceptibility testing is needed due to poor response to therapy. Biopsy or cytology is almost never necessary for the evaluation of herpetic lesions, although occasionally atypical lesions require biopsy.

Therapy

Treatment regimens for recurrent episodes include oral acyclovir, 400 mg three times per day for 7–10 days; valacyclovir, 500 mg orally twice daily for 7–10 days; or famciclovir, 500 mg twice daily for 7–10 days. Acyclovir is the least expensive oral option. Valacyclovir is the preferred choice for severe cases owing to higher drug levels and may require 14 days of therapy or more. Very severe cases may require IV acyclovir (5 mg/kg q8h × 10–14 days).

If recurrences are frequent or severe, chronic suppressive therapy with oral acyclovir, 800 mg/day, or valacyclovir 500 mg qd may be used. If the CD4+ T-lymphocyte count rises due to HAART, chronic therapy may be discontinued.

Patients with low CD4+ T-lymphocyte counts and frequent recurrences may develop acyclovir-resistant herpetic lesions (*see* Chapter 48). There is no effective oral regimen for such lesions. Depending on the mutation causing resistance, either intravenous cidofovir or intravenous foscarnet should be used. Interestingly, when such lesions recur, the isolate may be acyclovir-sensitive.

Epstein–Barr Virus

Oral hairy leukoplakia (OHL) is an Epstein–Barr virus (EBV)-associated lesion. OHL has been clearly linked to HIV disease progression.[29–32] OHL also been documented in patients with types of immunosuppression other than HIV infection.[33] Although the prevalence of OHL in the HIV-positive population has decreased dramatically with the widespread use of combination antiretroviral therapy (ART), it is still seen in ~12% of patients.[34]

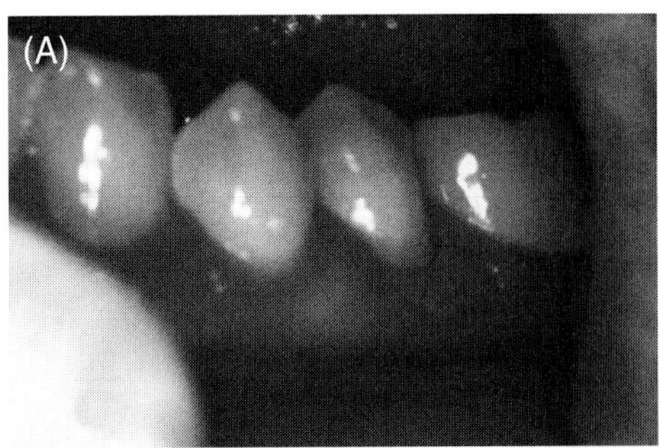

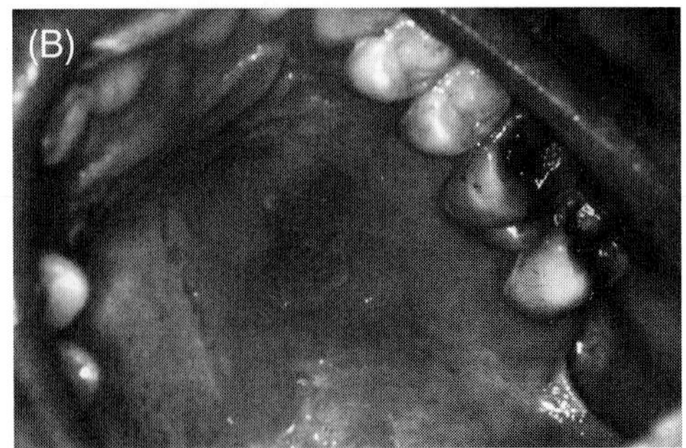

Figure 65-4 ■ Herpes simplex virus on gingiva (**A**) and palate (**B**).

Reprinted from the International AIDS Society-USA, from Reznik DA. Oral manifestations of HIV disease. TOP HIV Med 13:143, 2005.

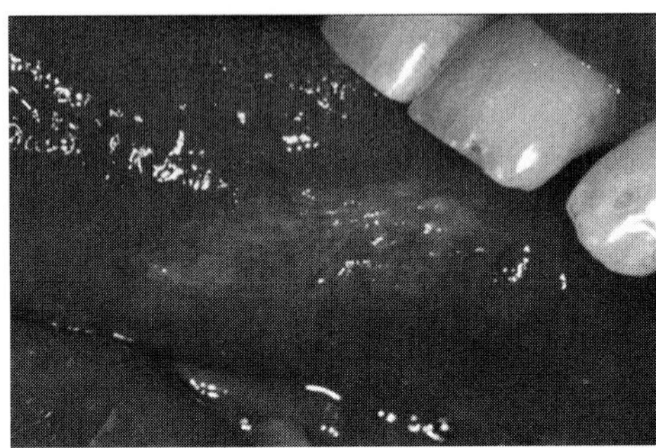

Figure 65-5 ■ Oral hairy leukoplakia on lateral border of tongue.

Reprinted from the International AIDS Society-USA, from Reznik DA. Oral manifestations of HIV disease. TOP HIV Med 13:143, 2005.

Diagnosis is established by clinical appearance (Fig. 65-5). OHL occurs most often on the lateral borders of the tongue, but can extend to the dorsal surface as well as other mucosal surfaces. The lesions range in appearance from faint white vertical streaks to thickened corrugated areas of leukoplakia, with a shaggy, or 'hairy', keratotic surface. These white plaques will not rub off helping to differentiate this clinical presentation from pseudomembranous candidiasis.

Therapy

Treatment of OHL is not necessary in most instances. In many cases, the lesions will spontaneously resolve once the patient is placed on active ART. If the patient is affected by the cosmetic appearance of the lesion and is not on ART, oral acyclovir 800 mg five times a day for 2 weeks is effective in temporarily reducing the clinical appearance of the lesion. Topical applications of podophyllin resin and tretinoin are also effective temporary therapies. The recurrence rate is high if patients do not respond to HAART.

Cytomegalovirus

Cytomegalovirus (CMV) disease can present as painful, nonhealing mucosal ulcerations.[35,36] The ulcers may appear anywhere in the oral cavity, with the gingiva, buccal mucosa, and palate being the most common sites. Oral ulcers that are nonresponsive to therapy should be biopsied, with histological verification, for a definitive diagnosis. If oral CMV lesions are documented, other sites of CMV disease such as the retina, should be sought. These oral lesions can be treated with oral valganciclovir or intravenous ganciclovir.

Varicella-Zoster Virus

Varicella-zoster virus can present with painful vesicles along the path of any of the branches of the trigeminal nerve, hence impacting the face and oral mucosa.[37,38] Diagnosis requires clinical suspicion and culture or biopsy.

Human Papillomavirus

The incidence of oral warts due to human papillomavirus (HPV) has dramatically increased in the HAART era. Certain "high-risk" types of HPV, such as HPV 16, 18, and 33, have been shown to be associated with the development of invasive oral carcinomas.[41–46] The potential for malignant transformation correlates with the presence of HPV DNA, the extent of the disease, and the degree of immunosuppression. Patients with a CD4+ T-lymphocyte count <200 cells/μL are at greatest risk.[47] HPV-associated oral lesions present as oral papillomas, condylomata, and focal epithelial hyperplasia. The lesions are usually multiple and may appear on any mucosal surface, most commonly the labial (Fig. 65-6A) and buccal mucosa (Fig. 65-6B), tongue, and gingiva. The vermilion border and labial commissures may also be involved. Lesions may be white, slightly erythematous, or normal in color. Clinical presentations vary from a pedunculated, exophytic lesion with numerous finger-like surface projections (papilloma), to multiple inconspicuous flat-topped papules or papillary areas (focal epithelial hyperplasia). Condylomata present as sessile, pink, exophytic masses with short, blunted surface projections. They are usually larger than papillomas and are typically multiple and clustered. Biopsy may be necessary to establish a diagnosis since the clinical appearance of some HPV-associated lesions may be nonspecific. Treatment should be directed at the removal of the associated

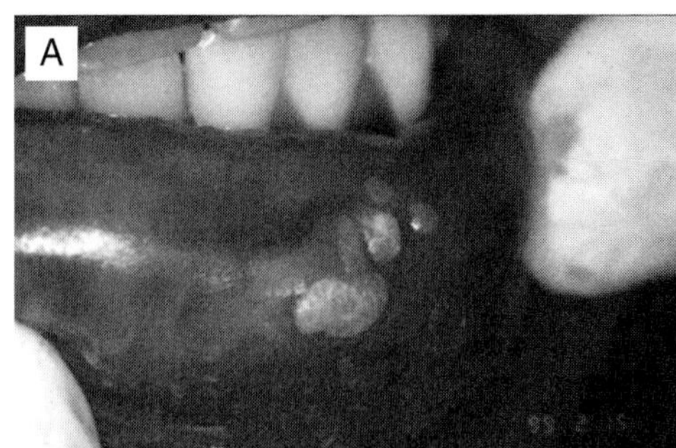

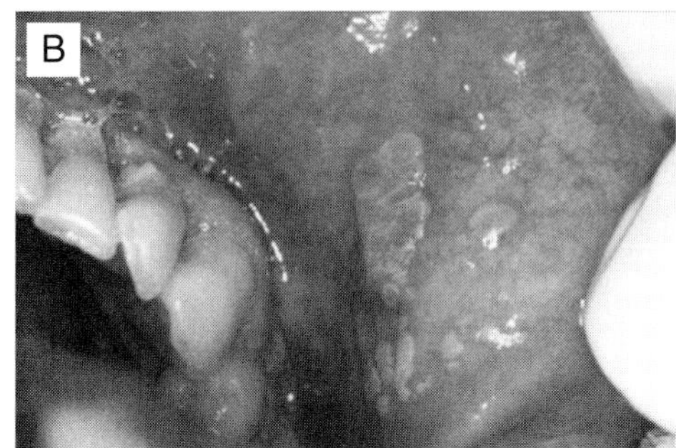

Figure 65-6 ■ Human papillomavirus warts on the lip (**A**) and buccal mucosa (**B**).

Reprinted from the International AIDS Society-USA, from Reznik DA. Oral manifestations of HIV disease. TOP HIV Med 13:143, 2005.

lesions by electrosurgery, cryotherapy, or scalpel excision. The recurrence rate is high, and repeated treatment is often necessary.

BACTERIAL INFECTIONS

Gingivitis and Periodontitis

There does not appear to be an increased incidence of conventional periodontal disease in patients with HIV infection.[48] Recent studies indicate there is no association between periodontal pocket depth or attachment loss (markers for periodontal disease) and CD4+ T-lymphocyte count.[51,52,57] However, severe forms of gingivitis and periodontitis can be seen in HIV-seropositive patients, especially those who are severely immunosuppressed.[49]

One manifestation of severe gingival disease is linear gingival erythema (LGE; Fig. 65-7). This presents as a distinctive linear band of erythema at the free gingival margin, extending 2–3 mm apically.[54] Petechial patches may be seen on the attached gingiva and adjacent alveolar mucosa. Mild pain and occasional bleeding have been reported but are not necessarily characteristic. LGE can be distinguished from conventional gingivitis by its failure to respond to routine plaque control measures and proper home care maintenance. Treatment of LGE should consist of a professional dental prophylaxis with thorough irrigation using a 0.12% chlorhexidine gluconate suspension or a 10% povidone-iodine solution, followed by 0.12% chlorhexidine gluconate rinse twice daily for 2 weeks. Frequent follow-ups and a maintenance dose of 0.12% chlorhexidine gluconate may be required.

Necrotizing ulcerative gingivitis (NUG) and necrotizing ulcerative periodontitis (NUP, Fig. 65-8) demonstrate a loss of gingival attachment and alveolar bone at affected sites respectively. Acute necrotizing ulcerative gingivitis (ANUG) is differentiated by interproximal gingival necrosis, bleeding, pain, and halitosis. The appearance of NUP is more closely associated with low CD4+ T-lymphocyte counts.[55,56] NUP is characterized by the presence of intense, deep-seated (non-gingival) pain, spontaneous bleeding, and the rapid destruction of soft tissue and supporting bone with minimal pocketing. This is often accompanied by loose teeth and fetid breath. The defects are usually localized and not in the diffuse pattern of routine periodontitis. NUP does not respond well to conventional periodontal therapy. Treatment consists of thorough debridement of necrotic tissues and scaling and root planing of affected teeth to remove all accumulated plaque, calculus, and debris. The area should be irrigated with either

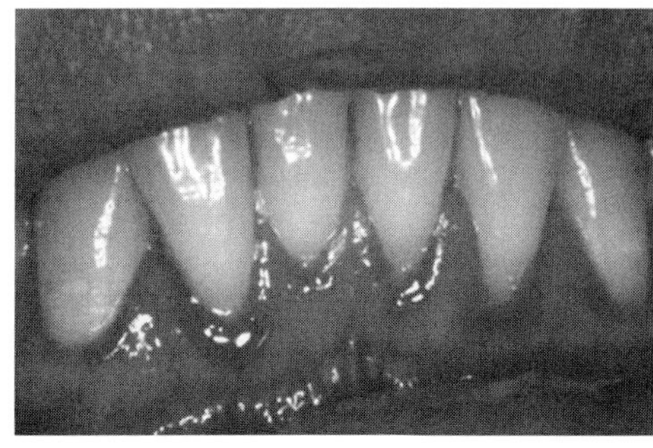

Figure 65-7 ■ Linear gingival erythema (LGE) presenting as red band along the free gingival margin.

Reprinted from the International AIDS Society-USA, from Reznik DA. Oral manifestations of HIV disease. TOP HIV Med. 13:143, 2005.

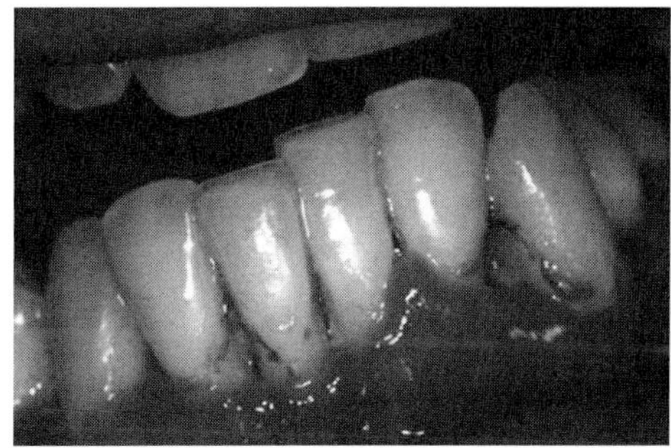

Figure 65-8 ■ Necrotizing ulcerative periodontitis (NUP).

Reprinted from the International AIDS Society-USA, from Reznik DA. Oral manifestations of HIV disease. TOP HIV Med 13:143, 2005.

a 0.12% chlorhexidine gluconate lavage or 10% povidone-iodine solution. Frequent follow-up appointments for the debridement of additional affected tissues may be necessary in the first 2–3 weeks. Diligent home care is very important and should include oral rinses with 0.12% chlorhexidine gluconate two times a day during the initial phase of therapy. Use of systemic antibiotics, such as metronidazole (500 mg tid), amoxicillin/clavulanic acid (875 mg bid), or clindamycin (300 mg tid), for 7 days, is necessary. Difficulty in chewing due to moderate to severe pain is a common complication, and pain medication is often required. Nutritional supplements should be considered as well. Frequent follow-up by a dental professional is necessary until the patient's overall periodontal condition has stabilized. Evaluations every 3 months thereafter are recommended.

Mycobacterium tuberculosis, *Mycobacterium avium-intracellulare*, *Klebsiella pneumoniae*, *Enterobacter cloacae*, *Actinomycosis*, *Escherichia coli*, *Neisseria gonorrhoeae*, and *Treponema pallidum* have each been associated with non-healing oral ulcerations.[57–64] Diagnosis requires direct microscopy, culture, and/or biopsy. Bacillary angiomatosis, caused by *Bartonella henselae* and *Bartonella quintana* also can present as oral lesions.[65]

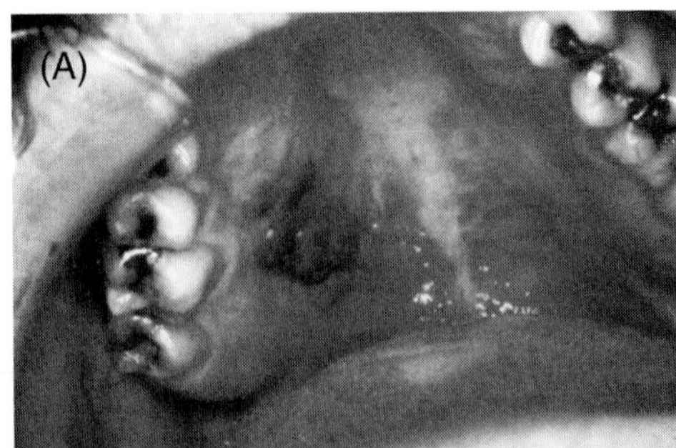

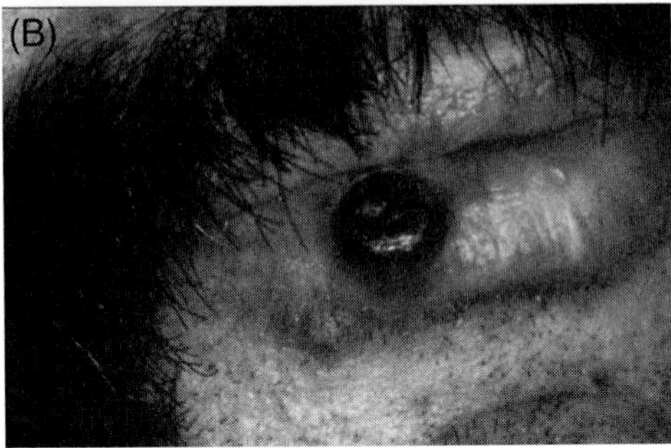

Figure 65-9 ■ Kaposi sarcoma (KS) on the hard palate (**A**) and lip (**B**).

Reprinted from the International AIDS Society-USA, from Reznik DA. Oral manifestations of HIV disease. TOP HIV Med 13:143, 2005.

NEOPLASMS

Kaposi Sarcoma

Kaposi sarcoma (KS) is the most common intraoral neoplasm seen in AIDS patients.[45,66–75] Intraoral KS is seen most often on the hard or soft palate (Fig. 65-9A), but may appear anywhere in the oral cavity (Fig. 65-9B). Initial lesions appear as painless diffuse, macular red-purplish, or dark patches which may resemble physiologic pigmentation. More advanced lesions become nodular with a darker purplish-brown appearance. Long-standing lesions may cover large areas, and develop painful ulcerations secondary to trauma which can become suprainfected by fungal or bacterial organisms. Multiple sites may be affected at once. Lesions involving the gingiva can be complicated by the accumulation of plaque and debris. Clinically, KS may resemble normal melanotic pigmentation or bacillary angiomatosis. Biopsy is necessary for a definitive diagnosis.

Therapy

Small intraoral lesions may be treated with intralesional injections of vinblastine sulfate (0.1 mg/cm^2) or the sclerosing solution sodium tetradecyl sulfate (up to 0.1 mL/cm^2) (*see* Chapter 59). Painful ulcerations and areas of necrosis may develop at the injection site. Surgical excision, cryotherapy, and removal with the carbon dioxide laser are also effective treatments. Larger, more bulky lesions require systemic chemotherapy or radiation therapy. Radiation therapy may be administered as a single, high-dose (800 cGy) regimen.[76] The use of fractionated therapy (2000 cGy in 10 fractions over 2 weeks) has been shown to be more successful in the complete resolution of palpable lesions.[77] Xerostomia, altered sense of taste, and severe mucositis are associated with radiation therapy to the oral cavity. These complications can be decreased by using 150-cGy fractions to a total of 1500 cGy.[76] For patients in whom systemic therapy is indicated, effective chemotherapeutic agents include paclitaxel[78] and the liposomal anthracyclines daunorubicin[79] and doxorubicin.[80] For moderate to advanced KS, simultaneous treatment with HAART and pegylated liposomal doxorubicin has been shown to be more effective than HAART alone.[81,82]

Non-Hodgkin's Lymphoma

Non-Hodgkin's lymphoma (NHL) presents with oral lesions in ~5% of cases.[87] Plasmablastic lymphoma is a novel subtype of AIDS-related NHL. This can be confused with non-lymphoid malignancies due to its unusual morphologic and immunophenotypic profile. Plasmablastic lymphomas are generally limited to the oral cavity at the time of diagnosis, and display a peculiar immunophenotypic pattern which is negative for the most common B-cell-associated surface antigens. These tumors consistently express high levels of plasma cell-associated markers, such as VS38c.[88] The risk of developing NHL following a plasmablastic lymphoma is related to the severity of immune suppression. This is a tumor associated with EBV[87–91] and human herpesvirus-8 (HHV-8).[92]

Intraoral NHL presents as a rapidly growing mass of the gingiva, posterior buccal vestibule, or retromolar area.

The lesions usually appear erythematous or purplish and may ulcerate. NHL may also be seen as a nontender, diffuse swelling of the posterior hard palate. Gingival lesions, which may be initially diagnosed as periodontal disease, can cause extensive necrosis of affected tissues and lead to severe mobility or loss of involved teeth. In some cases NHL originates in the jawbone, producing paresthesia and a vague pain or "toothache". The tumor may cause expansion of the bone, perforate the cortical plate and arise as a soft tissue swelling, usually without significant associated pain. This unusual presentation can be mistaken for a common dental abscess. The clinical appearance of intraoral NHL may often mimic other, more common lesions. Therefore, a biopsy should be obtained for a definitive diagnosis, especially if the lesion fails to clear with the appropriate standard therapy for the initial diagnosis. Treatment for NHL consists of chemotherapy and in some cases radiation therapy.

Squamous Cell Carcinoma

There is no compelling evidence suggesting an increased prevalence of oral squamous cell carcinoma (SCC) in HIV-infected patients. However, intraoral SCC can manifest at an earlier age in patients with HIV than that seen in individuals without HIV.[44–47] Intraoral SCC has a varied clinical presentation, including exophytic, ulcerating, leukoplakic, erythroplakic, or erythroleukoplakic forms. There is minimal pain during the early growth phase, which may allow the lesion to go unnoticed by the patient or delay the patient in seeking professional care.

OTHER LESIONS

Recurrent Aphthous Ulcers

Recurrent aphthous ulcers (RAU) are intensely painful lesions which in severe cases can be quite debilitating, interfering with the patient's ability to speak, eat, or take medications. RAU arise on nonkeratinized movable mucosa. The labial and buccal mucosa is affected most often, but lesions may occur on the ventral tongue, soft palate, floor of mouth, and oropharynx. Aphthous ulcers are covered by a yellowish-gray pseudomembrane, and surrounded by an erythematous halo (Fig. 65-10). This is in contrast to herpetic lesions which usually have a red center surrounded by a raised, yellow or white border.

Minor aphthae do not occur more often among HIV-positive patients,[95] but they are more severe and persistent. The lesions are usually round, measure 3–10 mm in diameter, and may occur singly or in groups of 1–5 each episode. Associated pain is often disproportionate for the size of the ulceration. Surface erosion is largely superficial, and healing occurs within 7–14 days without treatment and without scarring in immunocompetent patients. However, treatment with topical corticosteroids may be necessary for patients with advanced HIV disease. The greatest number of lesions with the most frequent recurrence can be seen in the herpetiform variant. The individual lesions are usually less than 3 mm in diameter, and as many as 100 can be present in a single recurrence. Smaller lesions may coalesce forming larger, irregular ulcerations. Recurrences tend to be closely spaced.

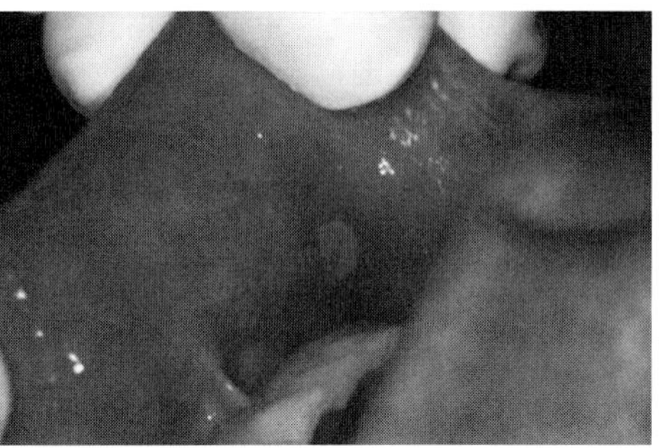

Figure 65-10 ■ Apthous ulcer on anterior buccal mucosa.

Reprinted from the International AIDS Society-USA, from Reznik DA. Oral manifestations of HIV disease. TOP HIV Med 13:143, 2005.

Major aphthous ulcerations most frequently occur in patients with CD4+ T-lymphocyte counts of less than 50 cells/μL.[93] Major aphthous ulcers can exceed 3 cm in diameter. They may extend onto keratinized mucosa, thus presenting in an irregular and atypical pattern for aphthae. Ulcerations are crater-like with a deeply eroded base, and are extremely painful, interfering with speech and swallowing. The lesions rarely undergo spontaneous healing, and may persist for 2–6 weeks or more. Multiple ulcers may be present simultaneously, and resolution of the lesions is often associated with scarring of the affected tissues. The patient's absolute granulocyte count (AGC) should be checked as large, fulminating ulcerations have been noted when the AGC drops below 800 cells/μL.

Therapy

Treatment for major aphthous ulcers involves the administration of topical or systemic glucocorticosteroids. Topical applications include fluocinocide ointment 0.05% or clobetasol ointment 0.05% mixed equally with Orabase and applied directly to the lesions four to six times a day. For multiple or hard to reach lesions, dexamethasone elixir (0.5 mg/5 mL), one tablespoon swished for at least 1 minute and expectorated, may be used four times a day. "Soothe-N-Seal" is an over-the-counter cyanoacrylate bioadhesive which provides a protective barrier against trauma and irritation from eating and speaking, thus reducing pain and promoting faster healing. The gel is applied directly to the lesion several times a day and lasts for up to 6 h. Systemic prednisone therapy is warranted for severe cases. Dosing of prednisone depends on the severity of the ulceration. Thalidomide may be used in an 8-week course, with an initial dosage of 400 mg/day for 1 week, followed by 200 mg/day for 7 weeks.[96] Until healing occurs, viscous lidocaine may be swished and expectorated several times a day to assist patients in taking their medications and to allow nutritional intake. "Gelclair", a rinse comprised of polyvinylpyrrolidone, hyaluronic acid, and glycyrrhetinic acid has been shown to be effective in managing oral pain due to mucositis and is effective in relieving pain due to large oral ulcerations.

Necrotizing Stomatitis

Necrotizing stomatitis (NS) is a localized acute, highly destructive ulceronecrotic lesion affecting mucosal tissue and underlying osseous structures.[98] NS begins as a mild to moderately painful gingival lesion and progresses rapidly to an intensely painful involvement of contiguous tissues. Without prompt treatment, necrotizing stomatitis may result in the exposure and sequestration of alveolar bone with subsequent spontaneous exfoliation of affected teeth. No specific causative pathogen has been identified. Necrotizing stomatitis is histopathologically similar to aphthous ulcers and may clinically resemble localized periodontal disease.

Therapy

Treatment should begin with a thorough debridement of necrotic tissues, plaque and calculus. A combination of topical and systemic antibacterial and corticosteroid therapy may be necessary to gain control of the lesion. Effective regimens have included the use of fluocinonide or clobetasol (0.05%) ointment, mixed in equal parts with Orabase and applied three to four times daily, and metronidazole (250 mg) taken four times a day. Treatment should continue for 5–7 days with appropriate follow-up appointments.

Xerostomia and Salivary Gland Disease

Xerostomia, or dry mouth, is a common complaint among HIV-positive individuals. This may be associated with salivary gland disease of the parotid or submandibular glands.[99] Salivary gland function is adversely affected early in HIV infection and HIV-seropositive individuals are at greater risk for xerostomia and salivary gland hypofunction.[40,100–102] Xerostomia is also a side-effect of a number of commonly prescribed medications, including antianxiolytics, anticholinergics, antidepressants, antihistamines, antihypertensives, decongestants, didanosine, foscarnet, meperidine, and zidovudine. Diuretics, including caffeinated beverages, may also cause dry mouth. Xerostomia may also be a consequence of tobacco, alcohol, or illicit drug abuse.

Decreased salivary flow contributes to the rampant development of caries, especially in the cervical region, and enhances the growth of fungal infections. Therefore, an oral healthcare referral for preventive care, including the use of topical fluorides, is encouraged. Oral dryness may be alleviated by the reduction or elimination of the causative factor, or can be managed with the use of sialagogs and artificial salivary substitutes. Salivary flow can be stimulated by chewing sugarless gum or sucking on sugarless candies. The mouth can be kept moist with frequent sips of water or by eating crushed ice. Sodas, diet sodas, juices, sports drinks, alcohol, tea and coffee should not be used in an effort to alleviate dryness. Due to the sugar and acid content, these products will only exacerbate the situation. Mouthwashes containing alcohol should also be avoided. Pilocarpine (2.5–7.5 mg three times a day) has been effective in increasing salivation.[103] Patients given this type of medication should be monitored for side-effects including nausea, excess sweating, and cardiovascular complications. Over-the-counter oral comfort products, such as Biotene (toothpaste, mouthwash, and chewing gum) and Oralbalance gel may also be of benefit to patients suffering from xerostomia.[104]

REFERENCES

1. Greenspan JS, Greenspan D. The epidemiology of oral lesions of HIV infection in the developed world. Oral Dis 8(Suppl 2):34, 2002.
2. Campo J, Del Romero J, Castilla J, et al. Oral candidiasis as a clinical marker related to viral load, CD4 lymphocyte count and CD4 lymphocyte percentage in HIV-infected patients. J Oral Pathol Med 31:5, 2002.
3. Eyeson JD, Tenant-Flowers M, Cooper DJ, et al. Oral manifestations of an HIV positive cohort in the era of highly active anti-retroviral therapy (HAART) in South London. L Oral Pathol Med 31:169, 2002.
4. Kerdon D, Pongsiriwet S, Pangsomboon K, et al. Oral manifestations of HIV infection in relation to clinical and CD4 immunological status in northern and southern Thai patients. Oral Dis 10:138, 2004.
5. Franker CK, Lucartorto FM, Johnson BS, et al. Characterization of the mycoflora from oral mucosal surfaces of some HIV-infected patients. Oral Surg Oral Med Oral Pathol 69:683, 1990.
6. Ramirez-Amador V, Ponce-de-Leon S, Sierra-Madero J, et al. Synchronous kinetics of CD4+ lymphocytes and viral load before the onset or oral candidiasis and hairy leukoplakia in a cohort of Mexican HIV-infected patients. AIDS Res Hum Retroviruses 21:981, 2005.
7. Coogan MM, Fidel PL, Komesu MC, et al. Candida and mycotic infections. Adv Dent Res 19:130, 2006.
8. Hilton JF. Functions of oral candidiasis episodes that are highly prognostic for AIDS. Stat Med 19:989, 2000.
9. Gaitan-Cepeda LA, Martinez-Gonzalez M, Ceballos-Salobrena A. Oral candidosis as a clinical marker of immune failure in patients with HIV/AIDS on HAART. AIDS Patient Care STDS 19:70, 2005.
10. Cassone A, Tacconelli E, De Bernardis F, et al. Antiretroviral therapy with protease inhibitors has an early, immune reconstitution-independent beneficial effect on Candida virulence and oral candidiasis in human immunodeficiency virus-infected subjects. J Infect Dis 15:188, 2002.
11. Martinez M, Lopez-Ribot JL, Kirkpatrick WR, et al. Replacement of Candida albicans with C. dubliniensis in human immunodeficiency virus-infected patients with oropharyngeal candidiasis treated with fluconazole. J Clin Microbiol 40:3135, 2002.
12. Messer SA, Diekema DJ, Boyken L, et al. Activities of micafungin against 315 invasive clinical isolates of fluconazole-resistant Candida spp. J Clin Microbiol 44:324, 2006.
13. Powderly WG, Gallant JE, Ghannoum MA, et al. Oropharyngeal candidiasis in patients with HIV: suggested

guidelines for therapy [review]. AIDS Res Hum Retroviruses 15:1619, 1999.
14. Munoz P, Moreno S, Berengeur J, et al. Fluconazole-related hepatotoxicity in patients with acquired immunodeficiency syndrome. Arch Intern Med 151:1020, 1991.
15. Goldman M, Cloud GA, Wade KD, et al. A randomized study of the use of fluconazole in continuous versus episodic therapy in patients with advanced HIV infection and a history of oropharyngeal candidiasis. AIDS Clinical Trails Group Study Team 323/Mycoses Study Group Study 40. Clin Infect Dis 41:1473, 2005.
16. Fichtenbaum CJ, Koletar S, Yiannoutsos C, et al. Refractory mucosal candidiasis in advanced human immunodeficiency virus infections. Clin Infect Dis 30:749, 2000.
17. Kofla G, Ruhnke M. Voriconazole: review of a broad spectrum triazole antifungal agent. Expert Opin Pharmacother 6: 1215, 2005.
18. Vazquez JA, Skiest DJ, Nieto L, et al. A multicenter randomized trial evaluating posaconazole versus fluconazole for the treatment of oropharyngeal candidiasis in subjects with HIV/AIDS. Clin Infect Dis 42:1187, 2006.
19. Saag MS, Fessel WJ, Kaufman CA, et al. Treatment of fluconazole-refractory oropharyngeal candidiasis with itraconazole oral solution in HIV-positive patients. AIDS Res Hum Retroviruses 15:1413, 1999.
20. Garbino J. Caspofungin – a new therapeutic option for oropharyngeal candidiasis. Clin Microbiol Infect 10:187, 2004.
21. Glick M, Cohen SG, Cheney RT, et al. Oral Manifestations of disseminated *Cryptococcus neoforans* in a patient with acquired immunodeficiency syndrome. Oral Surg Oral Med Oral Pathol 64:454, 1987.
22. Heinic GS, Greenspan D, MacPhail LA, et al. Oral Histoplasma capsulatum infection in association with HIV infection: a case report. J Oral Pathol Med 21:85, 1992.
23. Heinic GS, Greenspan D, MacPhail LA, et al. Oral Geotrichum candidus infection associated with HIV infection. Oral Surg Oral Med Oral Pathol 73:726, 1992.
24. Shannon MT, Sclaroff A, Cohen SJ. Invasive aspergillosis of the maxilla in an immunocompromised patient. Oral Surg Oral Med Oral Pathol 70:425, 1990.
25. Miller CS, Berger JR, Mootoor Y, et al. High prevalence of multiple human herpesviruses in saliva from human immunodeficiency virus-infected persons in the era of highly active antiretroviral therapy. J Clin Microbiol 44:2409, 2006.
26. Severson JL, Tyring SK. Relationship between herpes simplex viruses and human immunodeficiency virus infections. Arch Dermatol 135:1393, 1999.
27. Wutzler P, Doerr HW, Farber I, et al. Seroprevalence of herpes simplex virus type 1 and type 2 in selected German populations-relevance for the incidence of genital herpes. J Med Virol 61:201, 2000.
28. Hardy WD. Foscarnet treatment of acyclovir-resistant herpes simplex virus infection in patients with the acquired immunodeficiency syndrome: preliminary results of a controlled, randomized, regimen-comparative trial. Am J Med 92(Suppl 2A):305, 1992.
29. Moura MD, Grossmann S deM, Fonseca LM, et al. Risk factors for oral hairy leukoplakia in HIV-infected adults in Brazil. J Oral Pathol Med 35:321, 2006.
30. Greenspan D, Gange SJ, Phelan JA, et al. Incidence of oral lesions in HIV-1-infected women: reduction with HAART. J Dent Res 83:145, 2004.
31. Greenspan JS, Greenspan D, Lennette ET, et al. Replication of Epstein-Barr virus within the epithelial cells of oral "hairy" leukoplakia, on AIDS-associated lesion. N Engl J Med 313:1564, 1985.
32. Greenspan, D, Greenspan JS, Overby G, et al. Risk factors for rapid progression from hair leukoplakia to AIDS: a nested case-control study. J Acquir Immune Defic Syndr 4:652, 1991.
33. Syrjaren S, Laire P, Happoren R-P, et al. Oral hairy leukoplakia is not a specific sign of HIV-infection but related to immunosuppression in general. J Oral Pathol Med 18:28, 1989.
34. Patton LL, McKaig R, Strauss R, et al. Changing prevalence of oral manifestations of human immuno-deficiency virus in the era of protease inhibitor therapy. Oral Surg Oral Med Oral Pathol Oral Radiol Endod 89:299, 2000.
35. Jones AC, Freedman PD, Phelan JA, et al. Cytomegalovirus infections in the oral cavity. A report of six cases and review of the literature. Oral Surg Oral Med Oral Pathol 75:76, 1993.
36. Glick M, Muzyka BC, Lurie D, et al. Oral manifestations associated with HIV disease as markers for immune suppression and AIDS. Oral Surg Oral Med Oral Pathol 77:344, 1994.
37. Stewart JA, Reef SE, Pellet PE, et al. Herpesvirus infections in persons infected with human immunodeficiency virus. Clin Infect Dis 21(Suppl 1):5114, 1995.
38. Safrin S, Berger TG, Gilson I, et al. Foscarnet therapy in five patients with AIDS and acyclovir-resistant varicella-zoster virus infection. Ann Intern Med 115:19, 1991.
39. King MD, Reznik DA, O'Daniels CM, et al. Human papillomavirus-associated oral warts among human immunodeficiency virus-seropositive patients in the era of highly active antiretroviral therapy: an emerging infection. Clin Infect Dis 34:641, 2002.
40. Greenspan D, Canchola AL, MacPhail LA, et al. Effect of highly active antiretroviral therapy on frequency of oral warts. Lancet 357:1411, 2001.
41. Kreimer AR, Alberg AJ, Daniel R, et al. Oral human papillomavirus infection in adults is associated with sexual behavior and HIV serostatus. J Infect Dis 189:686, 2004.
42. Cameron JE, Mercante D, O'Brien M, et al. The impact of highly active antiretroviral therapy and immunodeficiency on human papillomavirus infection of the oral cavity of human immunodeficiency virus-seropositive adults. Sex Transm Dis 32:703, 2005.
43. Herrero R, Castellsague X, Pawlita M, et al. Human pailloma-virus and oral cancer. The International Agency for Research on Cancer Multicenter Study. J Natl Cancer Inst. 95:1772, 2003.
44. Sirera G, Videla S, Piaol M, et al. High prevalence of human papilloma virus infection in the anus, penis and mouth in HIV-positive men. AIDS 20:1201, 2006.
45. Womack SD, Chirenje ZM, Gaffikin L, et al. HPV-based cervical cancer screening in a population at high risk for HIV infection. Int J Cancer 85:206, 2000.
46. Bouda M, Gorgoulis VG, Kastrinakis NG, et al. "High risk" HPV types are more frequently detected in potentially malignant and malignant oral lesions, but not in normal oral mucosa. Mod Pathol 13:644, 2000.
47. Chopra KF, Tyring SK. The impact of human immunodeficiency virus on the human papillomavirus epidemic. Arch Dermatol 133:829, 1997.
48. Moore LVH, Moore WEC, Riley C, et al. Periodontal microflora of HIV positive subjects with gingivitis or adult periodontitis. J Periodontol 64:48, 1993.
49. Glick M, Muzyka BC, Salkin LM, et al. Necrotizing ulcerative periodontitis: a marker for immune deterioration and a predictor for the diagnosis of AIDS. J. Periodontol 65:393, 1994.
50. Yeung SCH, Stewart GJ, Cooper DA. Progression of periodontal disease in HIV seropositive patients. J Periodontol 64:651, 1993.
51. Alves M, Mulligan R, Passaro D, et al. Longitudinal evaluation of loss of attachment in HIV-infected women compared to HIV-uninfected women. J Periodontol 77:773, 2006.
52. Goncalves L deS, Ferreira SM, Silva A Jr, et al. Association of T CD4 lymphocyte levels and chronic periodontitis in

HIV-infected Brazilian patients undergoing highly active antiretroviral therapy: clinical results. J Periodontol 76:915, 2005.
53. Vastardis SA, Yukna RA, Fidel PL, et al. Periodontal disease in HIV-positive individuals: association of periodontal indices with stages of HIV disease. J Periodontol 74:1336, 2003.
54. Velegraki A, Nicolatou O, Theodoridou M, et al. Paediatric AIDS-related linear gingival erythema: a form of erythematous candidiasis? J Oral Pathol Med 28:178, 1999.
55. Winkler JR, Murray PA, Grassi M, et al. Diagnosis and management of HIV-associated periodontal lesions. J Am Dent Assoc 119(Suppl):25,1989.
56. Shangase L, Feller L, Blignaut E. Necrotising ulcerative gingivitis/periodontitis as indicators of HIV infection. SADJ 59:105, 2004.
57. Volpe F, Schwimmer A, Barr C. Oral manifestations of disseminated Mycobacterium avium-intracellulare in a patient with AIDS. Oral Surg Oral Med Oral Pathol 60:567, 1985.
58. Barone R, Ficarra G, Gaglioti D, et al. Prevalence of oral lesions among HIV-infected intravenous drug abusers and other risk groups. Oral Surg Oral Med Oral Pathol 69:169, 1990.
59. Greenspan D, Schiodt M, Greenspan JS, et al. AIDS and the Mouth. Copenhagen: Munksgaard; 1990.
60. Ficarra G, Shillitoe EJ. HIV-related infections of the oral cavity. Crit Rev Oral Biol Med 3:207, 1992.
61. Graden JD, Timpone JG. Emergence of unusual opportunistic pathogens in AIDS: a review. Clin Infect Dis 15:134, 1992.
62. Schmidt-Westhausen A, Fehrenbach FJ, Reichart PA. Oral enterobacteriaceae in patients with HIV infection. J Oral Pathol Med 19:229, 1990.
63. Ficarra G, Zaragoza AM, Stendardi L, et al. Early oral presentation of *lices maligna* in a patient with HIV infection. A case report. Oral Surg Oral Med Oral Pathol 75:728, 1993.
64. Yeager BA, Hoxie J, Weisman RA, et al. Actinomycosis in the acquired immunodeficiency syndrome-related complex. Arch Otolaryngol Head Neck Surg 112:1293, 1986.
65. Gasquet S, Maurin M, Brouqui P, et al. Bacillary angiomatosis in immunocompromised patients. AIDS 12:1793, 1998.
66. Glick M, Cleveland DB. Oral mucosal bacillary (epithelioid) angiomatosis in a patient with AIDS associated with rapid alveolar bone loss: report of a case. J Oral Pathol Med 22:235, 1993.
67. Engels EA, Pfeiffer RM, Goedert JJ, et al. Trends in cancer risk among people with AIDS in the United States 1980–2002. AIDS 20:1645, 2006.
68. Stebbing J, Sanitt A, Nelson M, et al. A prognostic index for AIDS-associated Kaposi's sarcoma in the era of highly active antiretroviral therapy. Lancet 367:1495, 2006.
69. Weinert M, Grimes RM, Lynch DP. Oral manifestations of HIV infection. Ann Intern Med 125:485, 1996.
70. Chang Y, Cesarman E, Pessin MS, et al. Identification of herpesvirus-like DNA sequences in AIDS-associated Kaposi's sarcoma. Science 266:1865, 1994.
71. Moore PS, Gao SJ, Dominguez G, et al. Primary characterization of a herpesvirus agent associated with Kaposi's sarcoma. J Virol 70:549, 1996.
72. Cannon MJ, Dolland SC, Black JB, et al. Risk factors for Kaposi's sarcoma in men seropositive for both human herpesvirus 8 and human immunodeficiency virus. AIDS 17:215, 2003.
73. Widmer IC, Erb P, Grob H, et al. Human herpesvirus 8 oral shedding in HIV-infected men with and without Kaposi's sarcoma. J Acquir Immune Defic Syndr 42:420, 2006.
74. Beral V, Peterman TA, Berkelmann RL, et al. Kaposi's sarcoma among persons with AIDS: a sexually transmitted infection? Lancet 335:123, 1990.
75. Dodd CL, Greenspan D, Greenspan JS. Oral Kaposi's sarcoma in a woman as a first indication of HIV infection. J Am Dent Assoc 122:61, 1991.
76. Berson AM, Quivey JM, Harris JW, et al. Radiation therapy for AIDS-related Kaposi's sarcoma. Int J Radiat Oncol Biol Phys 19:569, 1990.
77. Stelzer KJ, Griffin TW. A randomized prospective trial of radiation therapy for AIDS-associated Kaposi's sarcoma. Int J Radiat Oncol Biol Phys 27:1057, 1993.
78. Saville MW, Lietzau J, Pluda JM, et al. Treatment of HIV-associated Kaposi's sarcoma with paclitaxel. Lancet 346:26, 1995.
79. Presant CA, Scolaro M, Kennedy P, et al. Liposomal daunorubicin treatment of HIV-associated Kaposi's sarcoma. Lancet 341:1242, 1993.
80. Goebel F-D, Goldstein D, Goos M, et al. Efficacy and safety of stealth liposomal doxorubicin in AIDS-related Kaposi's sarcoma. Br J Cancer 73:989, 1996.
81. Lichterfeld M, Qurishi N, Hoffman C, et al. Treatment of HIV-1-associated Kaposi's Sarcoma with pegylated liposomal doxorubicin and HAART simultaneously induces effective tumor remission and CD4+ T cell recovery. Infection 33:140, 2005.
82. Martin-Carbonero L, Barrios A, Saballs P, et al. Pegylated liposomal doxorubicin plus highly active antiretroviral therapy versus highly active antiretroviral therapy alone in HIV patients with Kaposi's sarcoma. AIDS 18:1737, 2004.
83. Carbone A. AIDS-related non-Hodgkin's lymphomas: from pathology and molecular pathogenesis to treatment. Hum Pathol 33:392, 2002.
84. Matthews GV, Bower M, Mandalia S, et al. Changes in acquired immunodeficiency syndrome-related lymphoma since the introduction of highly active antiretroviral therapy. Blood 96:2730, 2000.
85. Grulich AE, Vajdic CM. The epidemiology of non-Hodgkin lymphoma. Pathology 37:409, 2005.
86. Singh B, Poluri A, Shaha AR, et al. Head and Neck manifestations of non-Hodgkin's lymphoma in human immunodeficiency virus-infected patients. Am J Otolaryngol 21:10, 2000.
87. Ziegler JL, Beckstead JA, Volberding PA, et al. Non-Hodgkin's lymphoma in 90 homosexual men: relation to generalized hymphadenopathy and the acquired immunodeficiency syndrome. N Eng J Med 311:565, 1984.
88. Carbone A, Gaidano G, Gloghini, A, et al. AIDS-related plasmablastic lymphomas of the oral cavity and jaws: a diagnostic dilemma. Ann Otol Rhinol Laryngol 108:95, 1999.
89. Shibata D, Weiss LM, Hernandez AM, et al. Epstein–Barr virus associated with non-Hodgkin's lymphoma in patients infected with the human immunodeficiency virus. Blood 81:2102, 1993.
90. Vilchez R, Shahab I, Kozinetz C, et al. The association of polyomavirus with AIDS-related systemic non-Hodgkin's lymphoma. In: Abstracts of the 8th Conference on Retroviruses and Opportunistic Infections, Chicago, IL, 2001, abstract No. 594.
91. Rabkin C, Gamache C, El-Omar E. Interleukin-6 (IL-6) promoter polymorphism associated with increased risk of AIDS-related non-Hodgkin's lymphoma. In: Abstracts of the 8th Conference on Retroviruses and Opportunistic Infections, Chicago, IL, 2001, Abstract No. 593.
92. Deloose ST, Smit LA, Pals FT, et al. High incidence of Kaposi's sarcoma-associated herpesvirus infection in HIV-related solid immunoblastic/plasmablastic diffuse large B-cell lymphoma. Leukemia 19:851, 2005.
93. Muzyka BC, Glick M. Major aphthous ulcers in patients with HIV disease. Oral Surg Oral Med Oral Pathol 77:116, 1994.
94. Pedersen A, Hougen HP, Kenrad B. T-lymphocyte subsets in oral mucosa of patients with recurrent aphthous ulceratus. J Oral Pathol Med 21:176, 1992.
95. Epstein JB, Silverman S Jr. Head and neck malignancies associated with HIV infection. Oral Surg Oral Med Oral Pathol 73:193, 1992.
96. Ramirez-Amador VA, Esquivel-Pedraza L, Ponce-de-Leon S, et al. Thalidomide as therapy for human immunodeficiency

virus-related oral ulcers: a double-blind placebo-controlled clinical trial. Clin Infect Dis 28:892, 1999.

97. Glick M, Muzyka BC. Alternate treatment for major aphthous ulcerations in patients with AIDS. J Am Dent Assoc 123:61, 1992.
98. Jones AC, Gulley ML, Freedman PD. Necrotizing ulcerative stomatitis in human immunodeficiency virus-seropositive individuals: a review of the histopathologic, immunohistochemical, and virologic characteristics of 18 cases. Oral Surg Oral Med Oral Pathol Oral R and Endo 89:323, 2000.
99. Schiodt M, Dodd CL, Greenspan D, et al. Natural history of HIV-associated salivary gland disease. Oral Surg Oral Med Oral Pathol 74:326, 1992.
100. Lin AL, Johnson DA, Stephan KT, et al. Alteration in salivary function in early HIV infection. J Dent Res 82:719, 2003.
101. Navazesh M, Mulligan R, Barron Y, et al. A 4-year longitudinal evaluation of xerostomia and salivary gland hypofunction in the Women's Interagency HIV Study participants. Oral Surg Oral Med Oral Pathol Oral Radiol Endod 95:693, 2003.
102. Patton LL, McKaig R, Strauss R, et al. Changing prevalence of oral manifestations of human immunodeficiency virus in the era of protease inhibitor therapy. Oral Surg Oral Med Oral Pathol Oral Radiol Endod 89:299, 2000.
103. Ferguson MM. Pilocarpine and other cholinergic drugs in the management of salivary gland dysfunction. Oral Surg Oral Med Oral Pathol 75:186, 1993.
104. Warde P, Kroll B, O'Sullivan B, et al. A phase II study of Biotene in the treatment of postradiation xerostomia in patients with head and neck cancer. Support Care Cancer 8:203, 2000.
105. Glick M. Dental Management of Patients with HIV. Chicago: Quintessence Publishing; 1994.
106. Brown JB, Rosenstein D, Mullooly J, et al. Impact of intensified dental care on outcomes in human immunodeficiency virus infection. AIDS Patient Care STDS 16:479, 2002.

Chapter 66

Ophthalmologic Disease

Douglas A. Jabs, MD, MBA, Jennifer E. Thorne, MD, PhD

Ocular manifestations are common in patients with AIDS, and in the era before highly active antiretroviral therapy (HAART), the majority of patients with AIDS developed some form of ocular involvement during the course of their disease (Table 66-1).[1] The most frequently encountered ocular manifestation was microangiopathy, most often recognized in the retina and often referred to as 'AIDS retinopathy', 'HIV retinopathy', or 'noninfectious HIV retinopathy'. Opportunistic ocular infections, particularly cytomegalovirus (CMV) retinitis, were common and a substantial cause of visual morbidity. Ocular structures also may be affected by those neoplasms seen in patients with AIDS, such as Kaposi sarcoma or lymphoma, by neuroophthalmic lesions, or by adverse drug side effects.

Most ocular symptoms are nonspecific, and any patient with visual symptoms should be referred to an ophthalmologist for evaluation. Most diagnoses can be made by an ophthalmologist on examination. Only occasionally will ancillary laboratory or imaging tests be necessary. For example, a review of the Johns Hopkins medical institutions' experience with CMV retinitis suggests that the diagnosis of CMV retinitis can be made accurately on the first evaluation by an experienced ophthalmologist using indirect ophthalmoscopy in over 95% of cases. With the exception of syphilis, serologic tests (e.g., for *Toxoplasma gondii*, CMV) are not needed. Occasionally, corneal cultures for keratitis and vitreous cultures or molecular diagnostic techniques (via vitreous aspirate or diagnostic vitrectomy) may be used for diagnosing bacterial endophthalmitis.

OCULAR MICROANGIOPATHY

Ocular microangiopathy is the most common ophthalmologic finding in patients with AIDS.[1–8] The most often recognized manifestation of this microangiopathy is retinopathy, consisting of

Table 66-1 Frequencies of Ocular Manifestations of AIDS in the Pre-HAART Era

Lesion	Frequency (%)
Microangiopathy	
Conjunctival	75
Retinal	50–67
Opportunistic ocular infections	
Cytomegalovirus retinitis	30
Varicella-zoster virus (VZV)	
Herpes zoster ophthalmicus	3–4
VZV retinitis	<1
Toxoplasmic retinitis	1–3
Pneumocystis choroidopathy	<1
Microsporidial keratitis	<1
Ocular syphilis	<1
Ocular neoplasms	
Kaposi sarcoma (lids, conjunctiva)	1–4
Lymphoma (orbital, intraocular)	<1
Neuroophthalmic lesions	5–10

cotton wool spots (Fig. 66-1) and less frequently intraretinal hemorrhages.[1–5] Cotton wool spots are microinfarcts of the nerve fiber layer of the retina and are due to occlusion of the retinal capillaries. In the pre-HAART era retinal microangiopathy was recognized clinically in about one-half of patients with AIDS but substantially less frequently in earlier stages of HIV infection.[1,5] Clinically evident HIV retinopathy is associated with low CD4+ T-lymphocyte counts, particularly <100 cells/μL.[6,7] Fluorescein angiographic studies and autopsy studies[3,4] have suggested that there was an even higher frequency of microangiopathic changes. Although conjunctival changes were reported less frequently, one study suggested that conjunctival vascular changes also were common in patients with AIDS.[8]

The pathogenesis of ocular microangiopathy is unknown; hypotheses have included (1) circulating immune complex disease,[2–4] (2) infection of the retinal vasculature by HIV,[9] and (3) hematological abnormalities.[10] Polyclonal B-cell activation is present in patients with AIDS,[11] circulating immune complexes have been reported,[2,12] and immunoglobulin deposition has been demonstrated within the retinal capillaries,[4] suggesting that immune complex deposition disease may account for the microangiopathy.[3] Alternatively, HIV infection of the retinal vascular endothelial cells has been demonstrated.[9] However, some authors have argued that the amount of HIV infection of the retinal vascular endothelial cells is inadequate to account for the retinal vasculopathy.[13]

HIV retinopathy generally is clinically silent.[1] Occasional patients will have larger vessel retinal disease, such as a branch vein occlusion or central retinal vein occlusion.[1,14] Patients with HIV infection and without infectious retinitis have been reported to have abnormalities in subjective measures such as visual acuity, visual field, and contrast sensitivity and in objective measures such as optical coherence tomography and electrophysiological testing.[15–20] Autopsy studies have reported loss of optic nerve fibers.[21] It has been speculated that this loss of optic nerve fibers may be due to either a cumulative insult from the microinfarcts of the nerve fiber or a direct HIV-related toxic effect on the optic nerve.

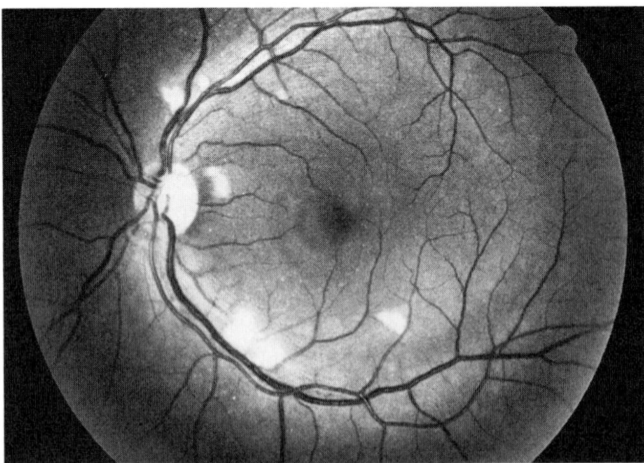

Figure 66-1 ■ Noninfectious retinal microangiopathy ('HIV retinopathy') in a patient with AIDS, manifested by cotton wool spots.

From Jabs DA. Ocular manifestations of HIV infection. Trans Am Ophthalmol Soc 93:623, 1995.

Although microangiopathy is the most common ocular involvement in patients with AIDS, opportunistic ocular infections, particularly CMV retinitis, account for most of the ocular morbidity.

CYTOMEGALOVIRUS RETINITIS

Epidemiology

Disease caused by CMV is among the most common opportunistic infections in patients with AIDS.[22,23] In the era before HAART, CMV disease affected an estimated 45% of patients.[23] Infection of the retina with CMV accounted for 75–85% of all CMV disease,[24,25] and it was estimated that 30% of patients with AIDS would develop CMV retinitis sometime between the diagnosis of AIDS and death.[25] CMV retinitis is a late-stage manifestation of AIDS, typically associated with CD4+ T-lymphocyte counts <50 cells/μL.[24–26] The incidence of CMV retinitis among patients with CD4+ T-lymphocyte counts <100 cells/μL was ~10% per year prior to the widespread use of HAART, and that among patients with a CD4+ T-lymphocyte count <50 cells/μL, it was ~20% per year.[24,26] HAART has resulted in a 55–95% decrease in the numbers of new cases of CMV retinitis at major urban medical centers throughout the United States since 1995.[27–29] This decline is due to a decrease in the cohort of patients with low CD4+ T-lymphocyte counts and low viral loads that is, those patients who are at risk for CMV retinitis and has occurred as a result of the improved immune function seen in patients treated with HAART. A similar, but much more modest and short-lived, drop in the incidence of CMV retinitis was seen when zidovudine was first introduced,[27] an observation consistent with this premise and the more modest effect of monotherapy with zidovudine on HIV. Recent data suggest that the incidence of CMV retinitis now has stabilized at ~20% of that in the era prior to HAART and that the majority of new cases are seen either in patients who are HAART-naive or who have failed at least one HAART regimen.[30–32]

Diagnosis and Natural History

CMV retinitis can be diagnosed reliably by an experienced ophthalmologist based on its clinical appearance (Fig. 66-2). CMV retinitis typically is described as a focal necrotizing retinitis, which may or may not be hemorrhagic. Unless there is immune reconstitution, untreated CMV retinitis spreads throughout the retina over a period of a few months, resulting in total retinal destruction and irreversible blindness.[32] The symptoms of CMV retinitis are nonspecific and include floaters, flashing lights, loss of visual field, or a vague sense of visual loss. CMV retinitis often is asymptomatic, and two studies estimated the prevalence of asymptomatic and undiagnosed CMV retinitis at 13–15% of patients with

CD4+ T-lymphocyte counts <50 cells/μL.[7,34] This fact led some experts to recommend routine evaluation of patients at high risk for CMV retinitis by an ophthalmologist using dilated indirect ophthalmoscopy in order to detect asymptomatic CMV retinitis. Although not universally accepted, and although no long-term outcome studies have been performed to validate this approach, a typical recommendation was that patients with CD4+ T-lymphocyte counts <50 cells/μL be seen every 3–4 months. Patients with CD4+ T-lymphocyte counts >100 cells/μL are at a low risk for the development of CMV retinitis and generally are seen annually. Patients with CD4+ T-lymphocyte counts between 50 and 100 cells/μL are often seen twice annually. Ophthalmoscopy using the direct ophthalmoscope through an undilated pupil evaluates only 10% of the retinal area and is inadequate for either the diagnosis or the routine evaluation of patients for CMV retinitis.

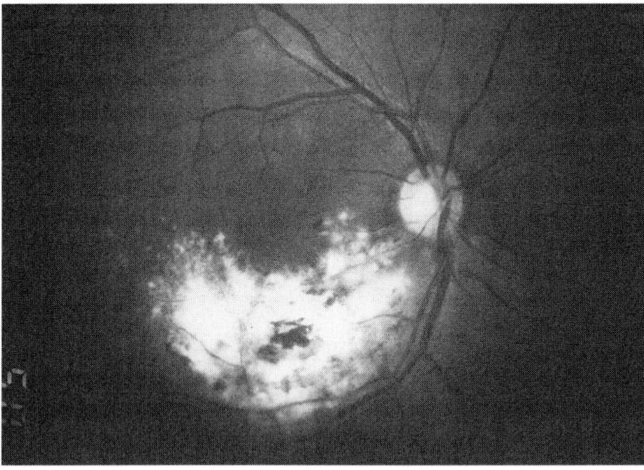

Figure 66-2 ■ CMV retinitis in a patient with AIDS.

From Jabs DA. Ocular manifestations of HIV infection. Trans Am Ophthalmol Soc 93:623, 1995.

The use of virologic assays of the peripheral blood (culture, antigen detection, or PCR) usually is unnecessary for establishing a diagnosis. In unusual cases, a diagnostic study of the peripheral blood, vitreous, or retina may be useful.

Treatment

The goal of treatment of CMV retinitis is to arrest progression of the disease, prevent further spread of infection in the retina, and preserve visual function. Treatment with anti-CMV agents suppresses viral replication in the eye but does not eliminate the virus.[35] Discontinuation of therapy in patients who remain immunocompromised is associated with prompt relapse of the retinitis.[36] Each relapse of retinitis is associated with retinal destruction and loss of visual field. Prior to the availability of HAART, the median time to bilateral visual acuity of 20/50 or worse ('visual impairment') was 16 months, and the median time to bilateral visual acuity of 20/200 or worse ('legal blindness') was 21 months.[1] Therefore, unless there is immune recovery from antiretroviral therapy (defined as an increase in CD4+ T-lymphocyte count to >100 cells/μL), long-term suppressive anti-CMV therapy is required.

Treatment options for CMV retinitis are outlined in Table 66-2. When systemically administered anti-CMV drugs are used, the treatment of CMV retinitis generally is performed in a two-step fashion. Initially a high dose of an anti-CMV drug is given to control the infection (induction), and subsequently a lower dose is given to prevent relapse (maintenance therapy or secondary prophylaxis). Four drugs have been approved by the US Food and Drug Administration (FDA) for the treatment of CMV retinitis: ganciclovir (Cytovene), foscarnet (Foscavir), cidofovir (Vistide), and fomivirsen (Vitravene). Ganciclovir is available both as an intravenous and oral formation and as a surgically placed slow-release implant (Vitrasert). A prodrug of ganciclovir, valganciclovir (Valcyte), has replaced the use of oral ganciclovir because its bioavailability is similar to

Table 66-2 **Treatment of CMV Retinitis**

Initial Therapy		Maintenance Therapy	Monitor
Ganciclovir implant plus valganciclovir 900 mg bid		Replace implant every 6–8 months plus valganciclovir 900 mg qd	CBC, creatinine
	OR		
Valganciclovir 900 mg bid for 14–21 days		Valganciclovir 900 mg qd	CBC, creatinine
	OR		
Intravenous ganciclovir 5 mg/kg bid for 14–21 days		Intravenous ganciclovir 5 mg/kg qd or valganciclovir 900 mg qd[a]	CBC, creatinine
	OR		
Intravenous cidofovir 5 mg/kg once weekly × 2		Intravenous cidofovir 5 mg/kg every other week	CBC, creatinine, urine analysis
	OR		
Intravenous foscarnet 60 mg/kg tid or 90 mg/kg bid for 14–21 days		Intravenous foscarnet 90–120 mg/kg qd	CBC, creatinine, electrolytes, calcium, magnesium

[a] Valganciclovir may be less effective than IV ganciclovir and is not as good a choice for zone 1 disease.

Note: In patients with immune recovery (CD4+ T cell count >100–150 cells/μL) due to HAART for greater than 3–6 months, maintenance therapy may be discontinued, but should be restarted for a drop in CD4+ T cell count to below 50 cells/μL.

that of IV ganciclovir.[37] Foscarnet and cidofovir are available only as intravenous formulations. Intravenous ganciclovir and intravenous foscarnet therapy require twice-daily intravenous infusions for induction therapy and once-daily intravenous infusion for maintenance therapy. Both require the placement of a permanent indwelling central venous catheter. Fomivirsen is available for intravitreous injection only, but currently is not being produced.[38] The intravenous formulation of ganciclovir, foscarnet, and cidofovir may be used for intravitreous injections as well. Intravenous ganciclovir and foscarnet therapy require twice-daily infusions for induction therapy and once-daily infusions for maintenance therapy. Both require the placement of a permanent indwelling central venous catheter. Because cidofovir is given once weekly for induction and once every other week for maintenance therapy, a permanent indwelling catheter is not required.

Despite the use of chronic maintenance therapy with systemically administered drugs, relapse of CMV retinitis in patients without immune recovery is typical and occurs in almost all such patients given sufficient time.[1] Therefore, the efficacy of an anti-CMV drug has been evaluated by its ability to prolong the time to relapse, typically defined as the time to progression. Progression is the movement of the border of a CMV lesion a specified distance, typically 750 μm, along a front of 750 μm, or the development of a new CMV lesion, one quarter of the size of the optic disc.[39,40] The comparative efficacy of two drugs is determined by their relative ability to prolong the time to progression.[40] The efficacy of a new anti-CMV drug is evaluated by comparing the ability of that drug to prolong the time to progression versus observation. This approach has been used to demonstrate the efficacy of intravenous ganciclovir, intravenous foscarnet, intravenous cidofovir, the ganciclovir implant, and intravitreous fomivirsen.[38,41–45]

The posterior pole of the retina (also referred to as the macula) contains the vital ocular structures, the optic nerve and fovea, responsible for good reading acuity. Lesions adjacent to the optic nerve or fovea are immediately vision threatening. For clinical trial purposes, the retina has been arbitrarily divided into three zones. Zone 1 encompasses a region within 3000 μm from the center of the fovea and 1500 μm from the edge of the optic nerve. Lesions in zone 1 are immediately vision threatening. Zone 2 goes from the edge of zone 1 to the equator of the eye, and zone 3 extends anteriorly from the equator to the pars plana of the retina. Lesions in zones 2 and 3 become vision threatening given sufficient time but are not immediately vision threatening. Therefore, patients with small 'peripheral' lesions located entirely in zone 2 or 3 may be observed for a short period of time without increased risk of loss of visual acuity.[43]

Ganciclovir

Ganciclovir was the first drug approved by the FDA for the treatment of CMV retinitis in immunocompromised patients.[1,33,39,41] It is a nucleoside analog, which is taken up by the virally infected cells, triphosphorylated, and inhibits viral replication through its effect on the viral DNA polymerase. The first phosphorylation step is performed by a virally encoded phosphotransferase, whereas the next two phosphorylation steps are performed by cellular enzymes. Ganciclovir induction is given for 2–3 weeks at a dose of 5 mg/kg every 12 h. Maintenance therapy is given at 5 mg/kg intravenously once daily. Ganciclovir has been demonstrated to be effective in the treatment of CMV retinitis in controlled studies.[33,41] The most frequently encountered side effect of ganciclovir is a reversible granulocytopenia. An absolute neutrophil count of <500 cells/μL occurs in approximately one-third of patients treated for 6 months with intravenous ganciclovir.[46] Granulocytopenia promptly reverses with discontinuation of the drug and typically is treated with hematologic growth factors, such as granulocyte colony-stimulating factor (filgrastim, Neupogen).[47] Clinically significant thrombocytopenia occurs in less than 10% of patients and is reversible with discontinuation of the drug. Maintenance therapy with IV ganciclovir requires the placement of a permanent indwelling catheter. The rate of complications from the indwelling catheter, including catheter-related infections, has been reported to be 0.44/person-years (PY) among patients with AIDS and CMV retinitis.[40,48]

An oral formulation of ganciclovir was used for maintenance therapy after induction with intravenous ganciclovir, but has lost favor due to its limited absorption from the gastrointestinal tract,[49] which makes it less effective than IV ganciclovir as maintenance therapy.[50] An oral ganciclovir prodrug, valganciclovir, appears to produce blood levels similar to that of IV ganciclovir.[37] The induction dose of valganciclovir is 900 mg twice daily, and the maintenance dose is 900 mg once daily.

Foscarnet

Foscarnet is a pyrophosphate analog that inhibits the CMV DNA polymerase. The induction dose of foscarnet is 90 mg/kg twice daily and the maintenance dose is 90 to 120 mg/kg once daily.[52] A randomized controlled clinical trial demonstrated that foscarnet is effective for controlling CMV retinitis,[42] and the Foscarnet–Ganciclovir Cytomegalovirus Retinitis Trial demonstrated that intravenous ganciclovir and intravenous foscarnet were equivalent for controlling CMV retinitis.[53] The most important side effect of foscarnet is reversible nephrotoxicity, which occurs in ~13% of patients treated for 6 months.[46] The serum creatinine and electrolytes (including potassium, calcium, and magnesium) must be monitored twice weekly during induction therapy and once weekly during maintenance therapy, and frequent dosage adjustments often are required. Other important side effects include metabolic abnormalities, and potassium, magnesium, and calcium supplementation often are required.[46] Much less common side effects include genital ulcers and infusion-related nausea.[46]

Cidofovir

Cidofovir is a nucleotide analog, and its intracellular activation requires two phosphorylation steps, which are mediated by cellular enzymes. Cidofovir has a prolonged duration of effect and can be given as an intermittent intravenous infusion. Cidofovir induction is given as 5 mg/kg once weekly for 2 weeks, and maintenance therapy is given once every 2 weeks at a 5 mg/kg dose. Because of its potential nephrotoxicity, cidofovir is given in conjunction with probenecid and saline hydration.[54] Two studies comparing cidofovir to observation in patients with small peripheral CMV lesions have demonstrated that cidofovir is effective for the treatment of CMV retinitis.[43,44] Cidofovir's major side effect is nephrotoxicity, which is not always reversible.[53] Because proteinuria appears to predate a rise in serum creatinine, all patients are monitored for proteinuria, as well as serum creatinine, prior to each cidofovir infusion. Persistent proteinuria of 3+ or greater that does not clear with hydration is an indication for discontinuation of cidofovir therapy. Proteinuria of 2+ or more occurs at a rate of 1.22/PY. Other indications for discontinuing cidofovir include a serum creatinine of 2.0 mg/dL or greater or a rise in the serum creatinine by 0.5 mg/dL or greater. Withdrawal of cidofovir resolves the proteinuria in 90% of cases.[55] Intravenous cidofovir also may cause uveitis and/or hypotony (low intraocular pressure), which may cause visual loss. A study of long-term follow-up of patients with CMV retinitis treated with cidofovir reported the incidence of cidofovir-related uveitis as 0.20/PY. Regular ophthalmologic monitoring for the development of cidofovir-related ocular side effects is necessary.

Despite the use of systemically administered anti-CMV drugs as maintenance therapy, relapse of CMV retinitis is a nearly universal phenomenon unless there is immune reconstitution. Although reinduction with the same drug may control the retinitis, the interval between the relapses successively declines, suggesting a decreasing ability of single-agent monotherapy to control CMV retinitis over time.[1,53] The primary reason for relapse appears to be the limited intraocular penetration of systemically administered anti-CMV drugs.[56–58] The efficacy of the ganciclovir implant, which delivers higher levels of ganciclovir to the eye and effectively suppresses retinitis in patients with newly diagnosed CMV until it runs out of drug,[45] supports this idea. The Cytomegalovirus Retinitis Retreatment Trial evaluated treatment strategies for patients who had relapsed.[59] In this trial, combination intravenous ganciclovir and foscarnet were substantially more effective than either monotherapy with ganciclovir alone or foscarnet alone in patients with relapsed retinitis. Although not more toxic and not associated with any greater impact on general health or mental health, combination therapy did have a greater negative treatment impact on quality of life because it required two intravenous infusions rather than one. In this trial, switching from one monotherapy to another was not more effective than staying on the same monotherapy for the treatment of relapsed retinitis.[59] Given the *in vitro* synergy of foscarnet and ganciclovir, the superiority of combination therapy perhaps is not surprising. Other approaches to combination therapy, including the use of the ganciclovir implant and intravenous foscarnet, oral ganciclovir and intravenous foscarnet, and intravitreous foscarnet combined with another mode of ganciclovir therapy, have been used and appear to have merit for the treatment of frequently relapsing retinitis.

Ganciclovir Implant

The ganciclovir implant contains a reservoir of ganciclovir that is surgically implanted into the eye. The implant slowly releases ganciclovir and obtains sustained intraocular levels of ganciclovir four to five times those achievable with systemically administered drugs. In patients with newly diagnosed retinitis, the implant suppresses retinitis for 6–8 months until it runs out of drug.[45,61,62] Scheduled replacement of the implant every 6–7 months appears to be able to effectively suppress the retinitis in patients with newly diagnosed disease and prevent its relapse. The implant appears to be less effective in patients with relapsed disease who have been previously treated with ganciclovir. Approximately 75–85% of relapsed patients will respond.[59–61] Because placement of the ganciclovir implant requires an intraocular surgical procedure, it is associated with the typical complications of ocular surgery, including bacterial endophthalmitis, and vitreous hemorrhage. Severe vision-threatening complications occur in less than 5% of patients. Although there were concerns that the implant could increase the retinal detachment rate in patients with CMV retinitis, studies have shown no increase in rate of retinal detachment between eyes with CMV retinitis treated with systemic therapy and those treated with the ganciclovir implant.[61–63] The surgical procedure is associated with a transient mild blurring of the patient's vision in the immediate postoperative period caused by a refractive change while the eye heals. However, the vision typically returns to normal within 1–2 weeks.[45] The primary disadvantage of the ganciclovir intraocular device is that it provides no systemic therapy for patients with CMV retinitis. Most patients with CMV retinitis have positive blood and/or urine cultures for CMV.[1,33] Prior to HAART, the use of the ganciclovir implant alone was associated with an incidence of contralateral ocular disease of 50% at 6 months and visceral disease of 31%,[45] rates which were higher than those seen in patients treated with systemically administered drugs.[53] As such, most patients treated with the ganciclovir implant also are given oral ganciclovir or valganciclovir in order to decrease the probability of involvement of the second eye and/or of the viscera. A clinical trial comparing implant with oral ganciclovir to the implant alone and to intravenous ganciclovir showed that the use of oral ganciclovir decreased the incidence of contralateral ocular and visceral disease when compared to the implant alone.[62] With the advent of HAART and immune recovery, oral ganciclovir or valganciclovir still is used as adjunctive therapy following placement of a ganciclovir implant in patients who are not taking HAART or have failed HAART and whose CD4+ T-lymphocyte counts remain below 100 cells/μL. In patients taking HAART who have immune recovery, oral ganciclovir or valganciclovir therapy typically is discontinued after 3–6 months of CD+ T cell counts >100–150 cells/μL.

The Ganciclovir Cidofovir Cytomegalovirus Retinitis Trial compared the regimen of the ganciclovir implant with oral ganciclovir to a regimen of intravenous cidofovir. This trial was performed in the HAART era and detected no difference between the two regimens in the rate of relapse of the retinitis.[64] In this trial, the rate of progression in the cidofovir group was substantially less than that seen in patients treated with systemic-only therapies in the era before HAART. These data suggest that HAART may have had an effect on retinitis progression, even though it did not have sufficient effect to prevent CMV retinitis.[64]

An alternative approach to the use of intraocular therapy for the treatment of CMV retinitis has been repetitive intravitreous injections.[65–69] Intravitreous ganciclovir typically is given 2 mg two to three times weekly as induction therapy, and once weekly as maintenance therapy.[65–67] Intravitreous foscarnet is given 2.4 mg two to three times weekly for 2–3 weeks as induction therapy and once weekly as maintenance therapy.[68] Intravitreous cidofovir is associated with uveitis and hypotony, and therefore it is not used in clinical practice.

Fomivirsen

Fomivirsen is a 21-nucleoside phosphorothiolate olignucleotide which hybridizes to complementary mRNA that encodes the proteins of the major immediate-early region (IE_2) of CMV.[38] The mechanism of action is an antisense mechanism in which the affected mRNA site shuts down the translation and production of specific proteins. Fomivirsen does not cross the blood-ocular barrier, and therefore, is given as an intravitreous injection only. The induction dose of fomivirsen is 330 μg in a single dose every 2 weeks for two cycles. The maintenance dose is one 330 μg intravitreal injection once every 4 weeks. Fomivirsen has been shown to be effective in the treatment of CMV retinitis in randomized, controlled, clinical trials.[38,70–72] No systemic side effects attributable to fomivirsen have been found in patients receiving the drug.[71] Ocular effects have included intraocular inflammation, cataract, and increased intraocular pressure.[38,70–73]

Intravitreous injections generally are used as an adjunct to therapy (e.g., intravitreous injections of foscarnet with the ganciclovir implant) in patients with relapsed disease, or as an initial induction therapy until the ganciclovir implant can be placed. They also are used in areas where the implant is not readily available. With the exception of fomivirsen, most of the data on intravitreous injection therapy comes from case series and not from controlled clinical trials.

Management Strategy

Management of the patient with CMV retinitis requires close cooperation between the ophthalmologist and the patient's primary care provider and/or infectious disease physician. Ophthalmologic examination, including dilated indirect ophthalmoscopy, should be performed at the time of diagnosis of the retinitis and monthly thereafter for patients who remain immunocompromised. For patients who are treated with the ganciclovir implant, typical postoperative follow-up (at 1 day, 1 week, and 1 month after the surgical procedure) also is required. Routine (monthly) fundus photographs using a standardized photographic technique that documents the entire photographic area of the retina provides the optimal method for following patients.[40,53] The ophthalmologist can then compare the patient's current appearance to the previous photographs and detect early relapse of the retinitis. The use of photographs is superior to ophthalmoscopy alone or ophthalmoscopy and retinal drawings.

Because of the toxicity of systemically administered drugs, routine long-term monitoring for toxicity is an important part of the management of these patients. For patients on intravenous ganciclovir or valganciclovir, weekly complete blood counts and monthly chemistries (for creatinine) should be performed. The complete blood count monitors for ganciclovir toxicity, and the serum creatinine evaluates renal function to adjust the ganciclovir dose appropriately. During foscarnet induction, patients should have serum chemistries, particularly creatinine, calcium, magnesium, and potassium, checked twice weekly, and during maintenance therapy once weekly. Because foscarnet is eliminated by the kidney and because its toxicity is primarily renal, frequent dose adjustments are necessary in order to avoid substantial nephrotoxicity. For patients being treated with cidofovir, because of its intermittent mode of administration, laboratory monitoring is done prior to each dose and typically consists of chemistries and a urinalysis. Persistent proteinuria that does not clear with hydration should result in discontinuation of cidofovir. In addition, patients receiving cidofovir therapy need regular ophthalmologic evaluation for the occurrence of cidofovir-associated uveitis. No systemic adverse events have been reported with intravitreous therapy and no laboratory abnormalities have been attributed to its use. Therefore, there are no specific recommendations for routine laboratory monitoring for patients treated only with intravitreous therapy.

Management of CMV retinitis is aimed at early, aggressive control of the retinitis with anti-CMV therapy in order to reduce the likelihood of complications related to CMV retinitis such as retinal detachment or immune recovery uveitis (IRU). Zone 1 CMV retinitis is typically treated with intravitreous injections or the ganciclovir implant in order to avoid involvement of the macula and loss of visual acuity. Use of systemic therapy, such as valganciclovir, in addition to local therapy is often employed in order to reduce the risk of extraocular CMV and of contralateral eye involvement in patients with unilateral CMV retinitis. Valganciclovir may be used as induction therapy for more peripheral CMV retinitis lesions (i.e., zone 3 disease) without increasing the risk of visual acuity loss. Among immunocompromised patients, anti-CMV therapy is continued after HAART is instituted until the CD4+ T-lymphocyte count is >100 cells/μL for 3–6 months before discontinuation of anti-CMV therapy is considered (*see section on* Withdrawal of Anti-CMV Therapy).

Resistance

Patients with CMV retinitis treated with long-term maintenance therapy may develop CMV which is resistant to ganciclovir, foscarnet, or cidofovir.[74–81] In the pre-HAART era, the rate of developing resistant CMV was ~0.25/PY for each drug.[77,80–82] The mechanism for low-level ganciclovir resistance is a mutation in the CMV *UL97* gene. This gene encodes for the phosphotransferase that catalyzes the first phosphorylation step of ganciclovir to ganciclovir triphosphate.[83–84] Eighty to ninety percent of all ganciclovir-resistant CMV isolates will have a mutation in the CMV *UL97* gene.[83,84,87] For high-level ganciclovir resistance, mutations in the CMV *UL97* gene and the *UL54* gene, the DNA polymerase gene, contribute to ganciclovir resistance.[87–90] Mutations in both the *UL97* and in the *UL54* genes appear to be responsible for cross-resistance to cidofovir as well.[87]

The detection of a ganciclovir-resistant isolate from either the blood or urine is associated with poorly controlled disease and an increased risk of adverse ocular outcomes.[79,80,91] Although a detectable CMV viral load in the blood correlates well with both genotypic and phenotypic resistance[92] as well as progression of CMV retinitis, the positive predictive value of CMV viral load for resistance is reported as 8%, making it of limited clinical utility as a marker for viral resistance.[93] In the past culture and susceptibility methods for detecting phenotypic antiviral resistance have been labor intensive and not used routinely in clinical practice. However, sequencing of the CMV *UL97* gene may be performed on PCR-amplified blood specimens, a procedure that can be performed in <48 h as opposed to >4 weeks for standard cultures, and this more rapid method for the detection of resistant CMV may prove to be clinically useful in the future.[94]

Retinal Detachments

In the era prior to HAART, retinal detachments were a common complication of CMV retinitis.[1,53,95–97] In long-term studies conducted prior to 1995, the incidence of a retinal detachment in either eye of a patient with CMV retinitis was ~25% at 6 months after diagnosis of retinitis and 50–60% at 1 year.[1,53,96] The detachment rate in an eye involved by CMV retinitis was 38% by 1 year,[98] and a patient with a CMV retinitis-related retinal detachment in one eye would have a 28–46% chance of developing a detachment in the other eye.[1,99] With the advent of HAART, CMV retinitis-related retinal detachment occurs less frequently. In a study of the incidence of retinal detachment in 773 eyes with CMV retinitis from 511 patients with AIDS from both the pre-HAART and HAART eras, patients treated with HAART had a 60% reduction in the retinal detachment rate when compared to patients not taking HAART.[63] A multicenter cohort study[100] found an overall incidence of CMV retinitis-related retinal detachment of 0.06/PY, which represents an approximate 80% reduction from the incidence of retinal detachment in the pre-HAART era. The rate of retinal detachment reported among patients with CD4+ T-lymphocyte counts <50 cells/μL (0.30/PY) was similar to the rate reported in the pre-HAART era (0.50/PY).[100]

Prior to HAART, repair of CMV retinitis-related retinal detachments typically consisted of a vitrectomy surgical technique with silicone oil injection, with 75–85% of patients achieving an ambulatory visual acuity in the repaired eye.[99,101] Surgical repair without the use of silicone oil was associated with unacceptably high failure rates for retinal reattachment.[96] Long-term retinal reattachment repair using silicone oil often is associated with cataract formation, necessitating cataract surgery in these patients. Delimiting laser photocoagulation has been used to check the spread of small peripheral retinal detachments.[102] Most, if not all, of these detachments will break through the laser barrier ultimately, but some patients may be spared vitreoretinal surgery, and the approach is useful in some patients. Overall however, because of improved control of CMV retinitis among patients treated with HAART, and because patients with immune recovery due to HAART are more apt to mount an inflammatory response and form scarring allowing for ease of reattachment of the retina, surgical repair without silicone oil as well as laser barrier therapy are being used more often and with greater success, although the published experience remains limited.[102–104]

Prophylaxis

Two published studies evaluated oral ganciclovir as prophylaxis to prevent the occurrence of CMV disease in patients at high risk for the development of CMV retinitis. Spector et al[105] reported that oral ganciclovir prophylaxis resulted in a 49% reduction in the incidence of CMV disease, primarily retinitis. In contrast, Brosgart et al[106] used a similar, but not identical study design, and reported that oral ganciclovir was ineffective as primary prophylaxis. Due to the expense of oral ganciclovir as CMV primary prophylaxis,[107] the conflicting results of the two studies, and the decreased incidence of CMV disease as a consequence of HAART, primary prophylaxis for CMV disease is not widely used, nor is it recommended in the US Public Health Service (USPHS)/Infectious Disease Society of America (IDSA) guidelines.

CMV Retinitis in the Era of HAART

The clinical course of CMV retinitis has been altered by the use of HAART. Immune reconstitution secondary to HAART typically restores specific CMV immunity, reduces the population of patients with AIDS at risk for CMV disease, and has led to the decline in the incidence of CMV retinitis to ~20% of that observed in the pre-HAART era.[32] Prior to the availability of HAART, recurrence of CMV retinitis in untreated patients occurred within 3 weeks.[1,27,32] Among patients treated with anti-CMV therapy, the progression rate in the pre-HAART era was ~3.0/PY.[1,59,108] In the Longitudinal Studies of Ocular Complications of AIDS (LSOCA), a cohort study taking place entirely within the era of HAART, the overall rate of progression of CMV retinitis was 0.10/PY and in patients with CD4+ T-lymphocyte counts <50 cells/μL, the progression rate was 0.58/PY.[108] In patients who had undergone immune recovery (defined as a rise in CD4+ T-lymphocyte count levels of >50 cells/μL to a level of >100 cells/μL at enrollment), the rate of CMV retinitis progression was substantially lower (0.06/PY), but was not zero.[108] Further, patients with newly diagnosed CMV retinitis who had lower CD4+ T-lymphocyte counts, higher HIV viral loads, and were less likely to have immune recovery at enrollment, still had lower rates of retinitis progression when compared to patients followed in the pre-HAART era.[108–110] Rates of contralateral eye involvement in patients with unilateral CMV retinitis also have declined in the era of HAART.[100] In the era prior to HAART the rate of developing CMV retinitis in the unaffected eye was 0.40/PY.[33,43,53,100] Overall, the rate of second eye involvement has declined by ~80% with use of HAART (rate of second eye involvement in the era of HAART = 0.07/PY). Decreasing incidence rates of retinitis progression[108] and involvement of the second eyes with CMV retinitis in patients with unilateral disease,[100] along with a 60–80% reduction in the occurrence of retinal detachment[63,100] may explain the reported decreased risk of visual acuity loss among patients taking HAART compared to those in the pre-HAART era in a single center retrospective study of the risk of visual acuity loss in patients with AIDS and CMV retinitis.[111] Use of HAART also has increased survival in patients with CMV retinitis and AIDS.[109,112–114] Although the overall mortality rate in patients with CMV retinitis has declined,[112–114] CMV remains an independent risk factor for mortality, primarily in patients with CD4+ T-lymphocyte counts <100 cells/μL.[112,113]

Withdrawal of Anti-CMV Therapy

With the restoration of specific CMV immunity as a consequence of HAART, it is possible to discontinue anti-CMV maintenance therapy. Several uncontrolled case series of successful discontinuation of anti-CMV therapy in patients with immune recovery have been published.[115–121] In these case series, the CD4+ T-lymphocyte count typically has increased to levels >100–150 cells/μL, and the increase has been sustained for 6 months or more. As long as the CD4+ T-lymphocyte count remains above 50 cells/μL, relapse of the retinitis has occurred only rarely.[120,122]

However, there is a lag between the restoration of specific CMV immunity and the rise in CD4+ T-lymphocyte count due to response to HAART. Patients have been reported to develop CMV retinitis within the first 2 months after initiation of HAART, despite a rise in CD4+ T-lymphocyte count,[123–125] and the risk of progression of existent CMV retinitis appears to be greatest during the first 6 months after initiating HAART.[123,126] Therefore, most experts recommend that the CD4+ T-lymphocyte count be >100 cells/μL, and that this increase be sustained for 3–6 months before discontinuation of anti-CMV therapy.[127,128] Although there have been occasional case reports of CMV retinitis entering remission during treatment with HAART without specific anti-CMV therapy,[129,130] many of the ocular complications of CMV retinitis are related to the size of the CMV retinitis lesion. Therefore, HAART-naive patients with CMV retinitis should be treated with specific anti-CMV therapy, as well as started on HAART, until there has been an immune recovery for 3–6 months before discontinuation of the anti-CMV therapy is considered. Relapse of CMV retinitis may occur in patients that stop HAART or have immunological failure of HAART.[122,126] However, in some cases CMV retinitis may recur despite CD4+ T-lymphocyte counts >100 cells/μL and with apparent immune recovery.[124,131–134] This paradoxical effect presumably occurs due to a lack of restoration of CMV-specific immunity[133,135] and supports the need for routine monitoring of patients with CMV retinitis despite immune recovery.[127,132] Therefore, the USPHS/IDSA guidelines recommend that if patients have inactive disease, have had a CD4+ T-lymphocyte count >100–150 cells/μL for greater than 6 months, and have regular ophthalmologic follow-up, then maintenance therapy can be stopped.[136]

Immune Recovery Uveitis

Prior to HAART, CMV retinitis rarely was associated with substantial intraocular inflammation. Since the introduction of HAART, a new ocular inflammatory disorder termed HAART-induced IRU has been described in patients with CMV retinitis and immune recovery.[137–143] IRU is also known as immune recovery vitritis and is characterized by intraocular inflammation in conjunction with immune recovery. IRU may occur soon after initiating HAART (<1 month), but also has been reported to occur as long as 3 years after starting HAART.[139–141] The most common complications of IRU are cystoid macular edema and epiretinal membrane formation. Other reported complications of IRU include optic disk edema, cataract, retinal neovascularization, and neovascular glaucoma.[142–145] The complications of IRU may result in substantial decrease in vision.[137–147] IRU typically has been treated with topical or periocular corticosteroids or short courses of oral corticosteroids, without recurrence of CMV retinitis.[138,141,142] Approximately 50% of patients treated will have a decrease in IRU and improvement in vision.[142,148,149] Treatment with valganciclovir also has been reported to improve visual acuity among patients with IRU-related macular edema in a single, small case series.[150]

A proposed pathogenesis for IRU is that immunologic improvement in response to HAART causes the restoration of specific anti-CMV immunity which leads to an inflammatory response directed at CMV antigen present in the eye.[138,140,151] The method of treatment of CMV retinitis may influence the rate of IRU.[138,146,151] Patients treated with the ganciclovir implant, which delivers intraocular levels of ganciclovir five times higher than that of IV ganciclovir, appear to be less likely to develop IRU although this finding has not been consistent from study to study.[138,151] The reported incidence of IRU has been as high as 0.83/PY,[139] although most estimates suggest a rate between 0.10/PY and 0.20/PY.[138] Use of cidofovir has been reported to increase the risk of IRU.[146,151] Large CMV lesion size has been reported to be associated with an increased prevalence[151] and incidence[143] of IRU, which suggests that a higher CMV antigen load in the retina may increase the likelihood of IRU. These results suggest that aggressive therapy of CMV retinitis to minimize the quantity of retinal virus may be a useful strategy to minimize the likelihood that IRU will occur.

OTHER OCULAR INFECTIONS

Use of HAART has decreased substantially the incidence of other opportunistic ocular infections in patients with AIDS, as well as that of CMV retinitis.

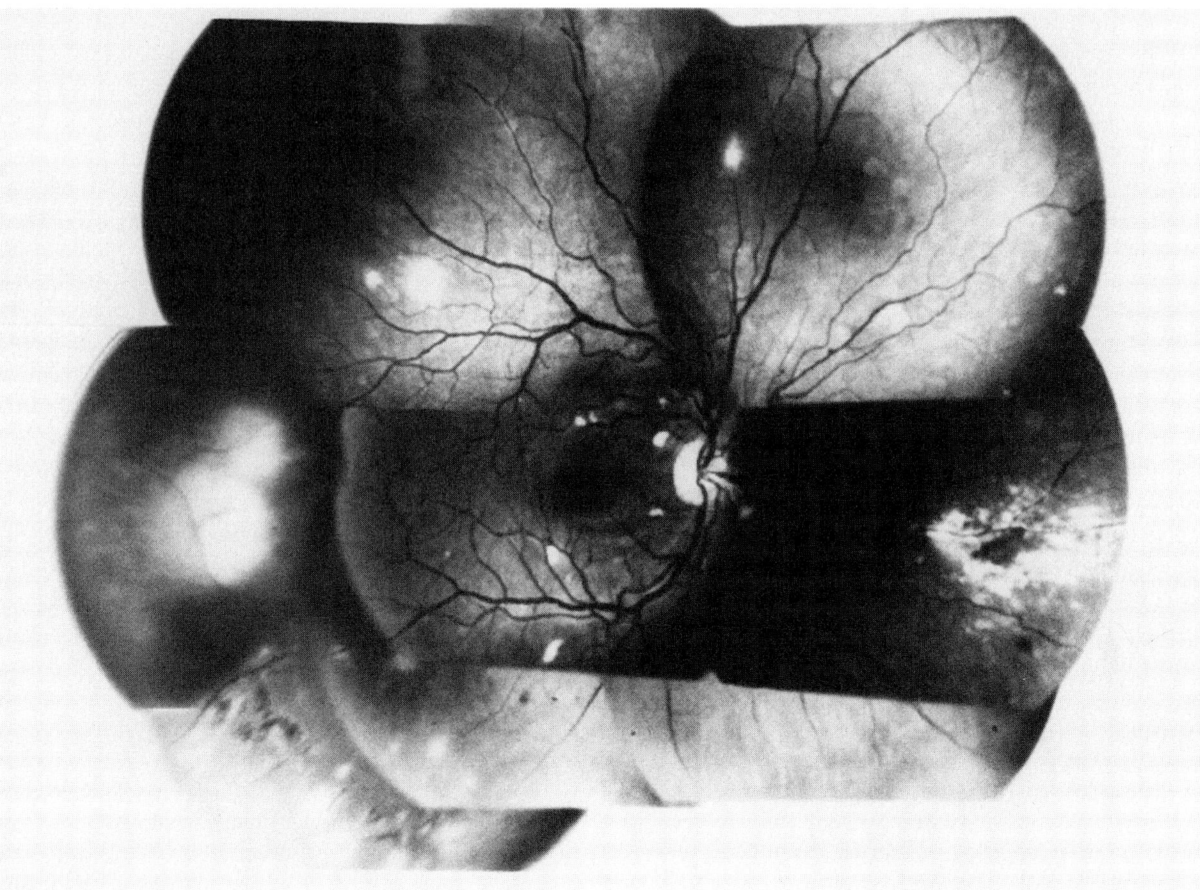

Figure 66-3 ■ Varicella-zoster retinitis in a patient with AIDS. The patient also had a small area of CMV retinitis nasally.
From Jabs DA. Ocular manifestations of HIV infection. Trans Am Ophthalmol Soc 93:623, 1995.

Varicella-Zoster Virus

Varicella-zoster virus is the second most common ocular pathogen in patients with HIV infection. Prior to HAART, herpes zoster ophthalmicus occurred in 3–4% of patients with HIV infection. Herpes zoster ophthalmicus can occur at all stages of HIV infection.[1,152,153] A diagnosis of herpes zoster ophthalmicus is suggested by the occurrence of typical zosteriform lesions over the distribution of the ophthalmic branch of the fifth cranial nerve. Disseminated cutaneous disease may be more common in immune-compromised patients. Diagnosis can be confirmed by obtaining a Tzank preparation of a lesion to demonstrate typical inclusion bodies, or by demonstrating virus by culture or immunofluorescence. Because of the high frequency of the occurrence of ocular complications in patients with herpes zoster ophthalmicus and the association of zoster retinitis, patients with herpes zoster ophthalmicus should have prompt ophthalmologic examination, including dilated indirect ophthalmoscopy. Ocular complications occur in 49% of HIV-infected patients with herpes zoster ophthalmicus. The most common ocular complications include keratitis, uveitis, and scleritis, occurring in 26%, 23%, and 6% of patients respectively. Other reported complications are less common and include sixth cranial nerve palsies, conjunctivitis, and ischemic neuropathy (an infarct of the optic nerve).[1] In HIV-infected patients with immunocompromise, herpes zoster ophthalmicus can cause a widespread necrotizing and destructive cutaneous lesion that damages the eyelids, resulting in long-term problems with corneal exposure.

Herpes zoster ophthalmicus in HIV-infected patients responds to standard treatments for varicella-zoster virus, including acyclovir, valacyclovir, and oral famciclovir. However, HIV-infected patients may require intravenous acyclovir as opposed to oral acyclovir for severe ocular involvement, and chronic suppressive therapy is required unless there is immune reconstitution.

Varicella-zoster virus retinitis was estimated to occur in 0.6% of patients with AIDS in the pre-HAART era.[1] In HIV-infected patients, varicella-zoster virus retinitis may occur in one of two clinical syndromes. The first is the acute retinal necrosis syndrome, which also may be seen in immunologically normal hosts.[154,155] Acute retinal necrosis can occur at any stage of HIV infection and is characterized by prominent anterior chamber reaction, vitritis, occlusive retinal vasculitis, and a full-thickness retinal necrosis (Fig. 66-3). Typically the retinal lesions begin peripherally and extend circumferentially. Retinal detachment occurs in 66–80% of patients. Affected patients may have a history of cutaneous herpes zoster occurring either proceeding or simultaneously with the retinitis. The acute retinal necrosis syndrome can be managed successfully with intravenous acyclovir at a dose of 500 mg/m^2 every 8 h for 10–14 days followed by long-term suppression with oral acyclovir, valacyclovir, or famciclovir.

The second clinical syndrome occurs in patients with low CD4+ T-lymphocyte counts, typically <50 cells/μL, and is sometimes known as the progressive outer retinal necrosis syndrome.[156–160] This variant is characterized by multifocal retinal opacification that progresses rapidly and is associated with little or no ocular inflammation. Approximately two-thirds of patients will develop bilateral disease and, as opposed to the acute retinal necrosis syndrome, the progressive outer retinal necrosis syndrome often begins in the posterior pole and can involve the optic nerve.[156–159] Medical therapy of the progressive outer retinal necrosis syndrome is problematic. This variant of varicella-zoster retinitis does not appear to respond to intravenous acyclovir or other forms of monotherapy.[1,158–160] Anecdotal reports have suggested that combination foscarnet and intravenous acyclovir may be effective in controlling the retinitis.[1] However, retinal detachments occur in ~70% of patients with this syndrome and often result in a poor visual outcome.[158,159]

Ocular Toxoplasmosis

In the United States, infection of the eye by *T. gondii* occurred in ~1% of patients with AIDS in the era prior to HAART.[1] In other countries, where the baseline seroprevalence of antibodies to *T. gondii* was higher, ocular toxoplasmosis was seen more often in patients with AIDS; in France, the frequency was 3%.[161] Although ocular toxoplasmosis may occur in immunologically normal hosts and at any stage of HIV infection, ocular toxoplasmosis most often is seen in patients with CD4+ T-lymphocyte counts <100 cells/μL.[161] Concurrent encephalitis occurs in 29–56% of patients with ocular toxoplasmosis and AIDS,[1,161] suggesting that patients with ocular toxoplasmosis and AIDS should be considered for neuroimaging. Unlike immunocompetent patients, who generally develop ocular toxoplasmosis as a result of reactivation of a congenitally acquired ocular infection, patients with AIDS may develop ocular toxoplasmosis due to primary infection or due to reactivation of latent disease.[161,162] In one large series of patients with ocular toxoplasmosis, only 4% of HIV-infected patients with toxoplasmic retinitis had retinal scars to suggest local reactivation.[161,162]

The clinical appearance of ocular toxoplasmosis in patients with AIDS (Fig. 66-4) is variable; although a focal white, full-thickness necrotizing retinitis similar to those lesions seen in immunocompetent patients may be seen, patients may also have a diffuse necrotizing retinitis, which could be mistaken for CMV infection, or a multifocal disease with a 'miliary' appearance.[162–165] Vitritis and anterior uveitis are common but are not required for the diagnosis. The disease is primarily unilateral, although it may be bilateral.

Diagnosis is generally established on the basis of the clinical appearance of the lesion. Patients with ocular toxoplasmosis should have a positive serum IgG test for toxoplasmosis, although many laboratories use relatively insensitive assays that may yield false-negative results if patients have low titers. Occasionally IgM tests are helpful, particularly for those with acquired disease (12% of ocular toxoplasmosis in patients with AIDS).[161]

Most cases of toxoplasmic retinitis in patients with AIDS respond to standard antitoxoplasmic treatment within 6 weeks. Regimens typically include pyrimethamine with sulfadiazine, and/or clindamycin. Double-strength trimethoprim–sulfamethoxazole (Bactrim) also has been effective. Atovaquone may have value in patients intolerant of other drugs. Prior to HAART, long-term maintenance therapy typically was required in order to prevent relapse of the disease.[161,162] There are few data currently to provide information about whether or not it is safe to stop maintenance therapy in patients who have responded immunologically to HAART. Oral corticosteroid therapy, often given to immunocompetent hosts with ocular toxoplasmosis to reduce the 'innocent bystander' damage to the retina, was not needed in patients with AIDS and ocular toxoplasmosis, because infection responded to antibiotics alone.

Pneumocystis carinii Choroidopathy

Choroidal infection with *P. carinii* is uncommon clinically, occurring in less than 1% patients with AIDS.[1] Choroidal pneumocystosis, however, accounted for 22% of infectious choroidopathies identified in one autopsy series in the pre-HAART era.[166–169] Most, but not all, patients with *P. carinii* choroiditis have a history of *P. carinii* pneumonia,[1,169] and, in an aggregate series from several centers,[169] 86% of patients with *P. carinii* choroidopathy had received aerosolized pentamidine as their *Pneumocystis* prophylaxis. *Pneumocystis carinii* choroidopathy typically was associated with other extrapulmonary lesions, but may be the initial and/or only sign of disseminated disease.

Clinically, the lesions are 1/3 to 2 disk diameters in size, creamy yellow to white, round or oval, and located at the level

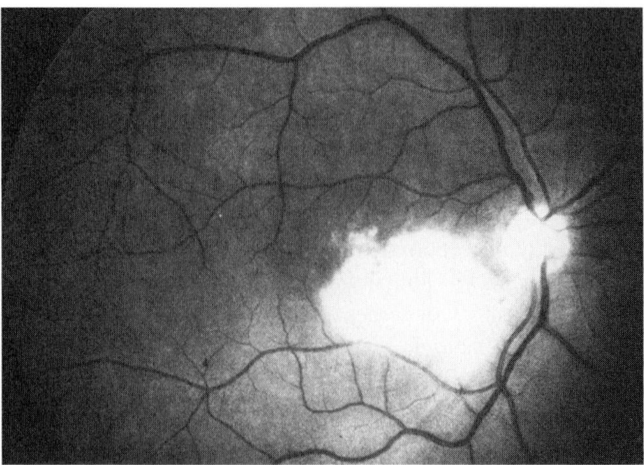

Figure 66-4 ■ Ocular toxoplasmosis in a patient with AIDS.
From Jabs DA. Ocular manifestations of HIV infection. Trans Am Ophthalmol Soc 93:623, 1995.

of the choroid (Fig. 66-5).[166,167] They usually are multifocal and bilateral,[168,169] and usually are found in the posterior pole or midperiphery of the retina.[169] Over time the lesions can become confluent and appear multilobulated.[136] There is no overlying vitritis.[166–169] The lesions generally are asymptomatic, although an occasional patient may complain of blurred vision.[166–169] Pathologically, an eosinophilic, amorphic, acellular, foamy infiltrate is identified in the inner choroid and choriocapillaris,[166–169] and organisms can be identified with electron microscopy. *Pneumocystis carinii* choroidopathy responds to systemic trimethoprim–sulfamethoxazole, pentamidine, or dapsone alone or in combination. In the pre-HAART era, lifelong maintenance was necessary to prevent recurrence.[166–169]

With the widespread use of trimethoprim–sulfamethoxazole as prophylaxis for *P. carinii* pneumonia, the frequency of *Pneumocystis* choroidopathy decreased, and HAART appears to have further reduced the incidence of *Pneumocystis* choroidopathy.

Bacterial Infections Including Mycobacterial Lesions

Before the advent of HAART, mycobacterial infection of the choroid with *Mycobacterium avium* complex or *Mycobacterium tuberculosis* were demonstrated at autopsy[5,166] but were uncommon clinically. Although there are case reports of choroidal granulomata caused by *M. tuberculosis* producing clinical disease,[170,171] one study estimated that only 5% of patients with active tuberculosis and HIV infection had clinical ocular lesions that produced signs or symptoms.[1]

The most common bacterial eye infection in HIV-infected patients is ocular syphilis, which may occur at any stage of HIV infection.[1] Ocular manifestations of syphilis include iridocyclitis, retinitis, neuroretinitis, panuveitis, papillitis, optic perineuritis, and retrobulbar optic neuritis.[172–176] However, 90% of HIV-infected patients presented with uveitis.[176] Patients with suspected syphilitic uveitis should have an FTA-abs performed regardless of the results of nonspecific testing (Rapid Plasma Reagin (RPR) or Venereal Disease Research Laboratory (VDRL) tests) as one-third of patients with syphilitic uveitis will have a negative nonspecific test.[177] Although many patients with ocular syphilis were staged clinically as secondary syphilis, approximately two-thirds of the patients had a positive cerebrospinal fluid VDRL test and neurologic disease.[172–176] Therefore, all patients with syphilitic uveitis should undergo a lumbar puncture and be treated with an antibiotic regimen for neurosyphilis (e.g., 12–24 million units penicillin/day intravenously for 10–14 days).

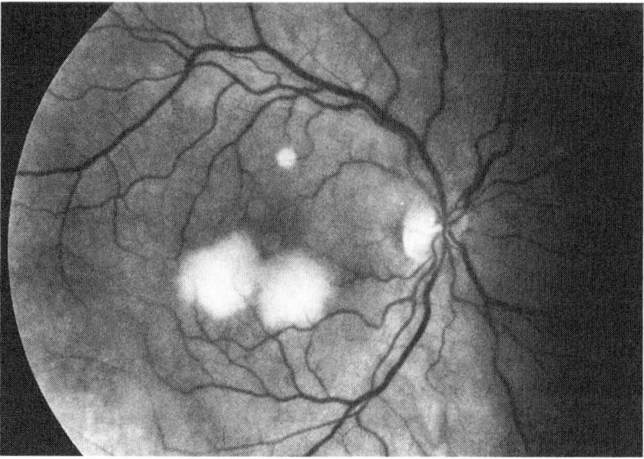

Figure 66-5 ■ *Pneumocystis* choroidopathy in a patient with AIDS. From Jabs DA. Ocular manifestations of HIV infection. Trans Am Ophthalmol Soc 93:623, 1995.

Fungal Infections

Intraocular infection with *Cryptococcus neoformans* is rare and occurred in less than 1% of patients with AIDS,[2] 2.5% of patients with systemic cryptococcosis, and 6% of patients with cryptococcal meningitis in the pre-HAART era.[1,178–180] Cryptococcal choroiditis nearly always is diagnosed in the presence of cryptococcal meningitis. The route of ocular infection is presumably hematogenous dissemination to the eye.[1,178] Cryptococcal lesions of the choroid clinically appear to be deep, hypopigmented or yellow-white, often multifocal spots and range from 1/5 to 1 disk diameter in size.[1,178,179] Treatment of cryptococcal infection typically is amphotericin B or fluconazole, and choroidal lesions have been reported to decrease in size and fade in coloration with adequate treatment.[5,178] Isolated cases of choroidal infection with *Histoplasma capsulatum* and *Aspergillus fumigatus* have been reported but are rare.[166,181,182] *Candida* retinitis and/or endophthalmitis also is uncommon in patients with AIDS and was reported to occur in less than 1% of patients with AIDS.[1] Most HIV-infected patients with *Candida* endophthalmitis were injection drug users, and the candidal infection was related to the injection drug use rather than the HIV infection.

Other Ocular Infections

Other ocular infections reported in patients with AIDS include corneal ulcers, molluscum contagiosum, and microsporidial keratoconjunctivitis.[1,183–186] Herpes simplex virus keratitis has not been shown to be more common in HIV-infected patients than in the general population; however, when it does occur, it may be atypical, more severe, and take longer to heal.[1] Microsporidial keratoconjunctivitis is caused by eukaryotic obligate intracellular protozoa of the *Encephalitozoon* species, usually *E. hellum* or *E. cuniculi*,[183–186] and occurs in less than 1% of patients with AIDS.[1] It is characterized by a fine to coarse corneal punctate epitheliopathy with associated conjunctival hyperemia with or without conjunctival staining with fluorescein. Agents with activity against these parasites include fumagillin, itraconazole, propamidine isethionate, and the benzimidazoles. Topical fumagillin (Fumadil B) 3 mg/mL instilled hourly for 1 week and then tapered over several weeks appears to be effective. The required duration of therapy remains undefined, but, given the persistence of spores with therapy, indefinite suppressive therapy may be needed.

OCULAR NEOPLASMS

Prior to the HAART era ocular involvement by Kaposi sarcoma was reported in 2% of patients with AIDS and in 15–22% of patients with AIDS and Kaposi sarcoma elsewhere.[1,187,188] Either the eyelids or the conjunctiva could be involved. Conjunctival Kaposi sarcoma may not require treatment. The lesions are slow growing, do not invade the eye, and often do not compromise vision. When removal is necessary, small, early lesions of the conjunctiva do well with surgical excision with a clear margin.[189] Larger lesions of the conjunctiva often recur with simple excision.[189] Eyelid involvement by Kaposi sarcoma may require therapy if it causes functional problems with the eyelid. Local excision, cryotherapy, radiation therapy, and local or systemic chemotherapy have all been reported to have a good response in some patients.[187–190]

In patients with HIV infection, high-grade lymphoma is an AIDS-defining disorder. Orbital and intraocular involvement by lymphoma have been reported[191–194] but occurs in less than 1% of patients with AIDS.[1] The clinical appearance of intraocular lymphoma is that of multifocal, yellow-white chorioretinal lesions associated with vitritis, retinal vascular disease, and disk edema. Intraocular lymphoma may be associated with central nervous system lymphoma.

NEUROOPHTHALMOLOGIC DISEASE

Before the advent of HAART neuroophthalmic lesions were reported in 5–10% of patients with AIDS.[1,5] Reported lesions included cranial nerve palsies, papilledema, optic neuropathy, hemianopsias, and cortical blindness.[1,195–203] The most common etiology for a neuroophthalmic lesion in a patient with AIDS was cryptococcal meningitis, accounting for up to 54% of these lesions.[1,178] Of patients with AIDS and cryptococcal meningitis, ~25% would have a neuroophthalmic lesion.[1] Papilledema is the most common finding in patients with cryptococcal meningitis; other findings include cranial nerve palsies and optic nerve damage.[1,178] Visual loss from cryptococcal meningitis was reported in 1–9% of patients, as a result of either direct invasion of the optic nerve by *C. neoformans*, elevated intracranial pressure, or adhesive arachnoiditis.[1,196–198] Other causes of neuroophthalmic lesions include herpes zoster ophthalmicus, syphilis, viral encephalitis, and central nervous system lymphoma.[1] Subtle ocular motility defects also can be detected in patients with AIDS by eye movement recordings using infrared oculography. These defects include slowed saccades, fixational instability, and abnormal pursuit. They appear to be related to HIV infection itself rather than to opportunistic ocular or neurologic infections, and they may correlate with the severity of the AIDS dementia complex.[199–201] Although lacking definitive proof, HIV may be responsible for some cases of optic neuritis or optic neuropathy. Case reports of optic neuropathies in the setting of HIV infection but without other identified cause have been described.[1,202,203]

DRUG-INDUCED OCULAR SIDE EFFECTS

Several drugs used to treat HIV and its complications have been associated with adverse ocular effects. Clofazamine, used to treat *M. avium* complex infections, has been associated with a bull's-eye maculopathy.[204] Didanosine, used to treat HIV, has been reported to cause well-circumscribed areas of retinal pigment epithelial atrophy in 7% of children treated with high-dose therapy.[205] However, no ocular toxicity has been reported in adults treated with didanosine. Rifabutin, an antimycobacterial agent, has been linked to the development of a fulminant anterior uveitis, which may mimic infectious endophthalmitis.[206–211] This uveitis may be seen in association with the rifabutin polyarthralgia/polyarthritis syndrome but may also develop on its own. The use of concurrent fluconazole and/or clarithromycin has been suggested as a cofactor for rifabutin-associated uveitis because of the pharmacokinetic effect of raising serum levels of rifabutin. Rifabutin uveitis responds well to topical steroids and discontinuing rifabutin or reducing the dose. Thirty-nine percent of 59 patients randomized to receive rifabutin 600 mg/day, clarithromycin, and ethambutol for the treatment of *M. avium* complex infections as part of one study developed iridocyclitis.[206] The incidence appears to be lower with lower doses, such as 300 mg/day. This uveitis may be unilateral or bilateral, and 55–100% of patients reported presented with a hypopyon.

Complications of cidofovir uveitis include hypotony (low intraocular pressure) and decreased vision.[43,55] Uveitis also has been described in patients with parenteral cidofovir, and the rate has been estimated at 0.20–0.24/PY.[43,55] As such, all patients receiving cidofovir therapy for CMV retinitis should undergo regular ocular examinations, even if the retinitis is well controlled, and such examinations should include measurement of the intraocular pressure. Fomivirsen also may cause uveitis, elevated intraocular pressure, cataract, and possibly a peripheral pigmentary retinopathy.[38,73] Drugs associated with ocular toxicity used in nonimmunosuppressed patients, such as ethambutol, are likely to have similar toxicity profiles in patients with HIV infection.

REFERENCES

1. Jabs DA. Ocular manifestations of HIV infection. Trans Am Ophthalmol Soc 93:623, 1995.
2. Holland GN, Pepose JS, Pettit TH, et al. Acquired immune deficiency syndrome: ocular manifestations. Ophthalmology 90:859, 1983.
3. Newsome DA, Green WR, Miller ED, et al. Microvascular aspects of acquired immune deficiency syndrome retinopathy. Am J Ophthalmol 98:590, 1984.
4. Pepose JS, Holland GN, Nestor MS, et al. Acquired immune deficiency syndrome: pathogenic mechanisms of ocular disease. Ophthalmology 92:472, 1985.
5. Jabs DA, Green WR, Fox R, et al. Ocular manifestations of acquired immune deficiency syndrome. Ophthalmology 96:1092, 1989.

6. Freeman WR, Chen A, Henderly DE, et al. Prevalence and significance of acquired immunodeficiency syndrome-related retinal microvasculopathy. Am J Ophthalmol 107:229, 1989.
7. Kuppermann BD, Petty JG, Richman DD, et al. Correlation between CD4+ counts and prevalence of cytomegalovirus retinitis and human immunodeficiency virus-related noninfectious retinal vasculopathy in patients with acquired immunodeficiency syndrome. Am J Ophthalmol 115:575, 1993.
8. Teich SA. Conjunctival vascular changes in AIDS and AIDS-related complex. Am J Ophthalmol 103:332, 1987.
9. Pomerantz RJ, Kuritzkes R, Monte M, et al. Infection of the retina by human immunodeficiency virus type I. N Engl J Med 317:1643, 1987.
10. Engstrom RE, Holland GN, Hardy WD, et al. Hemorheologic abnormalities in patients with human immunodeficiency virus infection and ophthalmic microvasculopathy. Am J Ophthalmol 109:153, 1990.
11. Lane HC, Masur H, Edgar LC, et al. Abnormalities of B-cell activation and immunoregulation in patients with the acquired immunodeficiency syndrome. N Engl J Med 309:453, 1983.
12. Gupta S, Licorish K. Circulating immune complexes in AIDS. N Engl J Med 310:1530, 1984.
13. Faber DW, Wiley CA, Lynn GB, et al. Role of HIV and CMV in the pathogenesis of retinitis and retinal vasculopathy in AIDS patients. Invest Ophthalmol Vis Sci 33:2345, 1992.
14. Dunn JP, Yamashita A, Kempen JH, Jabs DA. Retinal vascular occlusion in patients infected with human immunodeficiency virus. Retina 25:759, 2005.
15. Quiceno JI, Capparelli E, Sadun AA, et al. Visual dysfunction without retinitis in patients with acquired immunodeficiency syndrome. Am J Ophthalmol 113:8, 1992.
16. Geier SA, Hammel G, Bogner JR. HIV-related ocular microangiopathic syndrome and color contrast sensitivity. Invest Ophthalmol Vis Sci 35:3011, 1994.
17. Plummer DJ, Sample PA, Freeman WR. Visual dysfunction in HIV-positive patients without infectious retinopathy. AIDS Patient Care 1998;12:171–9.
18. Plummer DJ, Sample PA, Arevalo JF, et al. Visual field loss in HIV-positive patients without infectious retinopathy. Am J Ophthalmol 122:542–9, 1996.
19. Latkany PA, Holopigian K, Lorenzo-Latkany M, et al. Electroretinographic and psychophysical findings during early and late stages of human immunodeficiency virus infection and cytomegalovirus retinitis. Ophthalmology 104:445–53, 1997.
20. Kozak I, Bartsch D, Cheng L, et al. Objective analysis of retinal damage in HIV-positive patients in the HAART era using OCT. Am J Ophthalmol 139:295–301, 2005.
21. Tenhula WN, Xu S, Madigan MC, et al. Morphometric comparisons of optic nerve loss in acquired immunodeficiency syndrome. Am J Ophthalmol 113:14, 1992.
22. Moore RD, Chaisson RE. Natural history of opportunistic disease in an HIV-infected urban clinic cohort. Ann Intern Med 124:633, 1996.
23. Hoover DR, Saah J, Bacellar H, et al. Clinical manifestations of AIDS in the era of *Pneumocystis* prophylaxis. N Engl J Med 329:1922, 1993.
24. Gallant JE, Moore RD, Richman DD, et al. Incidence and natural history of cytomegalovirus disease in patients with advanced human immunodeficiency virus disease treated with zidovudine: The Zidovudine Epidemiology Group. J Infect Dis 166:1223, 1992.
25. Hoover DR, Peng Y, Saah A, et al. Occurrence of cytomegalovirus retinitis after human immunodeficiency virus immunosuppression. Arch Ophthalmol 114:821, 1996.
26. Pertel P, Hirschtick JP, Phair J, et al. Risk of developing cytomegalovirus retinitis in persons infected with the human immunodeficiency virus. J Acquir Immune Defic Syndr 5:1069, 1992.
27. Jabs DA, Bartlett JG. AIDS and ophthalmology: a period of transition. Am J Ophthalmol 124:227, 1997.
28. Palella FJ, Delaney KM, Moorman AC, et al. Declining morbidity and mortality among patients with advanced human immunodeficiency virus infection. N Engl J Med 338:853, 1998.
29. Holtzer DC, Jacobson MA, Hadley WK, et al. Decline in the rate of specific opportunistic infections at San Francisco General Hospital. AIDS 12:1931, 1998.
30. Jacobson MA, Stanley H, Holtzer C, et al. Natural history and outcome of new AIDS-related cytomegalovirus retinitis diagnosed in the era of highly active antiretroviral therapy. Clin Inf Dis 30:231, 2000.
31. Wohl DA, Pedersen S, van der Horst CM. Routine ophthalmologic screening for cytomegalovirus retinitis in patients with AIDS. J Acquir Immune Defic Syndr 23:438, 2000.
32. Jabs DA. Editorial. AIDS and ophthalmology in 2004. Arch Ophthalmol 122:1040, 2004.
33. Jabs DA, Enger C, Bartlett JG. Cytomegalovirus retinitis and acquired immunodeficiency syndrome. Arch Ophthalmol 107:75, 1989.
34. Baldassano V, Dunn JP, Feinberg J, et al. Cytomegalovirus retinitis and low CD4+ T-lymphocyte counts. N Engl J Med 333:670, 1995.
35. Pepose JS, Newman C, Bach MC, et al. Pathologic features of cytomegalovirus retinopathy after treatment with the antiviral agent ganciclovir. Ophthalmology 94:414, 1987.
36. Jacobson MA, O'Donnell JJ, Brodie HR, et al. Randomized prospective trial of ganciclovir maintenance therapy for cytomegalovirus retinitis. J Med Virol 25:339, 1988.
37. Hoffman VF, Skiest DJ. Therapeutic developments in cytomegalovirus retinitis. Expert Opinions Invest Drugs 9:207, 2000.
38. De Smet MD, Meenken C, van den Horn GJ. Fomivirsen – a phosphorothioate oligonucleotide for the treatment of CMV retinitis. Ocul Immunol Inflamm 7:189, 1999.
39. Holland GN, Buhles WC, Mastre B, et al. A controlled retrospective study of ganciclovir treatment for cytomegalovirus retinopathy: use of a standardized system for the assessment of disease outcome. Arch Ophthalmol 107:1759, 1989.
40. Studies of Ocular Complications of AIDS Research Group, in collaboration with the AIDS Clinical Trials Group. Studies of ocular complications of AIDS foscarnet–ganciclovir cytomegalovirus retinitis trial: rationale, design, and methods. Control Clin Trials 13:22, 1992.
41. Spector SA, Weingeist T, Pollard RB, et al. A randomized, controlled study of intravenous ganciclovir therapy for cytomegalovirus peripheral retinitis in patients with AIDS. J Infect Dis 168:557, 1993.
42. Palestine AG, Polis MA, DeSmet MD, et al. A randomized, controlled trial of foscarnet in the treatment of cytomegalovirus retinitis in patients with AIDS. Ann Intern Med 115:665, 1991.
43. Studies of Ocular Complications of AIDS Research Group in Collaboration with the AIDS Clinical Trial Group. Parenteral cidofovir for cytomegalovirus retinitis in patients with AIDS: the HPMPC peripheral cytomegalovirus retinitis trial. Ann Intern Med 126:264, 1997.
44. Lalezari JP, Stagg RJ, Kuppermann BD, et al. Intravenous cidofovir for peripheral cytomegalovirus retinitis in patients with AIDS: a randomized, controlled trial. Ann Intern Med 126:257, 1997.
45. Martin DF, Parks DJ, Mellow SD, et al. Treatment of cytomegalovirus retinitis with an intraocular sustained-release ganciclovir implant: a randomized controlled clinical trial. Arch Ophthalmol 112:1531, 1994.
46. Studies of Ocular Complications of AIDS Research Group, in collaboration with the AIDS Clinical Trials Group. Morbidity and toxic effects associated with ganciclovir and foscarnet therapy in a randomized cytomegalovirus retinitis trial. Arch Intern Med 155:65, 1995.

47. Davidson M, Min YI, Holbrook JT, et al. Use of filgrastim as adjuvant therapy in patients with AIDS-related cytomegalovirus retinitis. AIDS 16:757, 2002.
48. Thorne JE, Jabs DA, Vitale S, et al. Catheter complications in AIDS patients treated for cytomegalovirus retinitis. AIDS 12:2321, 2002.
49. Spector SA, Busch DF, Follansbee S, et al. Pharmacokinetic, safety and antiviral profiles of oral ganciclovir in persons infected with human immunodeficiency virus: a Phase I/II study. J Infect Dis 171:1431, 1995.
50. The Oral Ganciclovir European and Australian Cooperative Study Group. Intravenous versus oral ganciclovir: European/Australian comparative study of efficacy and safety in the prevention of cytomegalovirus retinitis recurrence in patients with AIDS. AIDS 9:471, 1995.
51. Lalezari J, Friedberg D, Bisset J, et al. A comparison of the safety and efficacy of 3 g, 4.5 g, and 6 g doses of oral ganciclovir vs IV ganciclovir for maintenance treatment of CMV retinitis. In: Abstracts of the XI International Conference on AIDS, Vancouver, 7–12 Jul 1996, p 225.
52. Katlama C, Dohin E, Caumes E, et al. Foscarnet induction therapy for cytomegalovirus retinitis in AIDS: comparison of twice-daily and three-times-daily regimens. J Acquir Immune Defic Synd 5(Suppl 5):S18, 1992.
53. Studies of Ocular Complications of AIDS Research Group, in collaboration with the AIDS Clinical Trials Group. Foscarnet–ganciclovir cytomegalovirus retinitis trial 4: visual outcomes. Ophthalmology 101:1250, 1994.
54. Lalezari JP, Drew WL, Glutzer E, et al. (S)-1-[3-hydroxy-2-(phosphonylmethoxy) propyl] cytosine (cidofovir): results of a phase I/II study of a novel antiviral nucleotide analogue. J Infect Dis 171:788, 1995.
55. Studies of Ocular Complications of AIDS Research Group, in collaboration with the AIDS Clinical Trials Group. Long-term follow-up of patients with AIDS treated with parenteral cidofovir for CMV retinitis: the HPMPC Peripheral CMV Retinitis Trial. AIDS 14:1571, 2000.
56. Jabs DA, Wingard JR, de Bustros S, et al. BW B759U for cytomegalovirus retinitis: intraocular drug penetration. Arch Ophthalmol 104:1436, 1986.
57. Kupperman BD, Quiceno JI, Flores-Aguilar M, et al. Intravitreal ganciclovir concentration after intravenous administration in AIDS patients with cytomegalovirus retinitis: implications for therapy. J Infect Dis 168:1506, 1993.
58. Arevalo JF, Gonzalez C, Capparelli EV, et al. Intravitreous and plasma concentrations of ganciclovir and foscarnet after intravenous therapy in patients with AIDS and cytomegalovirus retinitis. J Infect Dis 172:951, 1995.
59. Studies of the Ocular Complications of AIDS Research Group, in collaboration with the AIDS Clinical Trials Group. Combination foscarnet and ganciclovir therapy vs monotherapy for the treatment of relapsed cytomegalovirus retinitis in patients with AIDS: the cytomegalovirus retreatment trial. Arch Ophthalmol 114:23, 1996.
60. Marx JL, Kapusta MA, Patel SS, et al. Use of the ganciclovir implant in the treatment of recurrent cytomegalovirus retinitis. Arch Ophthalmol 114:815, 1996.
61. Hatton MR, Duker JS, Reichel E, et al. Treatment of relapsed cytomegalovirus retinitis with the sustained-release ganciclovir implant. Retina 18:50, 1998.
62. Martin DF, Kupperman BD, Wolitz RA, et al. Oral ganciclovir for patients with cytomegalovirus retinitis treated with a ganciclovir implant. N Engl J Med 340:1063, 1999.
63. Kempen JH, Jabs DA, Dunn JP, et al. Retinal detachment risk in cytomegalovirus retinitis related to the acquired immune deficiency syndrome. Arch Ophthalmol 119:33, 2001.
64. The Studies of Ocular Complications of AIDS Research Group, in collaboration with The AIDS Clinical Trials Group. The ganciclovir implant plus oral ganciclovir versus parenteral cidofovir for the treatment of cytomegalovirus retinitis in patients with AIDS: The Ganciclovir Cidofovir Retinitis Trial. Am J Ophthalmol 131:457, 2001.
65. Heinemann MH. Long-term intravitreal ganciclovir therapy for cytomegalovirus retinopathy. Arch Ophthalmol 107:1767, 1989.
66. Cochereau-Massin I, Lehoang P, Lautier-Frau M, et al. Efficacy and tolerance of intravitreal ganciclovir in cytomegalovirus retinitis in acquired immune deficiency syndrome. Ophthalmology 98:1348, 1992.
67. Young SH, Morlet N, Heery S, et al. High dose intravitreal ganciclovir in the treatment of cytomegalovirus retinitis. Med J Aust 157:370, 1992.
68. Diaz-Llopis M, Espana E, Munoz G, et al. High dose intravitreal foscarnet in the treatment of cytomegalovirus retinitis in AIDS. Br J Ophthalmol 78:120, 1994.
69. Kirsch LS, Arevalo JF, DeClercq E, et al. Phase I/II study of intravitreal cidofovir for the treatment of cytomegalovirus retinitis in patients with the acquired immunodeficiency syndrome. Am J Ophthalmol 119:466, 1995.
70. The Vitravene Study Group. A randomized controlled clinical trial of intravitreous fomivirsen for treatment of newly diagnosed peripheral cytomegalovirus retinitis in patients with AIDS. Am J Ophthalmol 133:467, 2002.
71. The Vitravene Study Group. Safety of intravitreous fomivirsen for treatment of cytomegalovirus retinitis in patients with AIDS. Am J Ophthalmol 133:484, 2002.
72. The Vitravene Study Group. Randomized dose-comparison studies of intravitreous fomivirsen for treatment of cytomegalovirus retinitis that has reactivated or is persistently active despite other therapies in patients with AIDS. Am J Ophthalmol 133:475, 2002.
73. Boyer DS, Muccioli C, Leiberman RM, et al. Phase 3 results of the efficacy and safety of fomivirsen in the treatment of CMV retinitis. Opthalmology 152S:167, 1998.
74. Drew WL, Miner RC, Busch DF. Prevalence of resistance in patients receiving ganciclovir for serious cytomegalovirus infection. J Infect Dis 163:716, 1991.
75. Drew WL, Miner RC, Saleh E. Antiviral susceptibility of cytomegalovirus: criteria for detecting resistance to antivirals. Clin Diagn Virol 1:179, 1993.
76. Jabs DA, Dunn JP, Enger C, et al. Cytomegalovirus retinitis and viral resistance: prevalence of resistance at diagnosis, 1994. Arch Ophthalmol 114:809, 1996.
77. Jabs DA, Enger C, Dunn JP, et al. Cytomegalovirus retinitis and viral resistance. 4. Ganciclovir resistance. J Infect Dis 177:770, 1998.
78. Jabs DA, Enger C, Dunn JP, et al. Cytomegalovirus retinitis and viral resistance: 3. culture results. Am J Ophthalmol 126:543, 1998.
79. Erice A, Chou S, Biron KK, et al. Progressive disease due to ganciclovir-resistant cytomegalovirus in immunocompromised patients. N Engl J Med 320:289, 1989.
80. Dunn JP, MacCumber MW, Forman MS, et al. Viral sensitivity testing in patients with cytomegalovirus retinitis clinically resistant to foscarnet or ganciclovir. Am J Ophthalmol 119:587, 1995.
81. Studies of Ocular Complications of AIDS (SOCA) in collaboration with the AIDS Clinical Trial Group. Cytomegalovirus (CMV) culture results, drug resistance, and clinical outcome in patients with AIDS and CMV retinitis treated with foscarnet or ganciclovir. J Infect Dis 176:50, 1997.
82. Jabs DA, Enger C, Forman M, et al. Incidence of foscarnet resistance and cidofovir resistance in patients treated for cytomegalovirus retinitis. Antimicrob Agents Chemother 42:2240, 1998.
83. Chou S, Erice A, Jordan MC, et al. Analysis of the UL97 phosphotransferase coding sequence in clinical cytomegalovirus

isolates and identification of mutations conferring ganciclovir resistance. J Infect Dis 171:576, 1995.
84. Chou S, Guentzel S, Michels KR, et al. Frequency of UL97 phosphotransferase mutations related to ganciclovir resistance in clinical cytomegalovirus isolates. J Infect Dis 172:239, 1995.
85. Hanson MN, Preheim LC, Chou S, et al. Novel mutation in the UL97 gene of a clinical cytomegalovirus strain conferring resistance to ganciclovir. Antimicrob Agents Chemother 39:1204, 1995.
86. Wolf DG, Smith IL, Lee DJ, et al. Mutations in human cytomegalovirus UL97 gene confer clinical resistance to ganciclovir and can be detected directly in patient plasma. J Clin Invest 95:257, 1995.
87. Smith IL, Cherrington JM, Jiles RE, et al. High-level resistance of cytomegalovirus to ganciclovir is associated with alterations in both the UL97 and DNA polymerase genes. J Infect Dis 176:69, 1997.
88. Lurain NS, Thompson KD, Holmes EW, et al. Point mutations in the DNA polymerase gene of human cytomegalovirus that result in resistance to antiviral agents. J Virol 66:7146, 1992.
89. Jabs DA, Martin BK, Forman MS, et al. Mutations conferring ganciclovir resistance in a cohort of patients with acquired immunodeficiency syndrome and cytomegalovirus retinitis. J Infect Dis 183:333, 2001.
90. Jabs DA, Martin BK, Forman MS, et al. Longitudinal observations on mutations conferring ganciclovir resistance in patients with acquired immunodeficiency syndrome and cytomegalovirus retinitis: The Cytomegalovirus and Viral Resistance Study Group Report Number 8. Am J Ophthalmol 132:700, 2001.
91. Jabs DA, Martin BK, Forman MS, et al. for the Cytomegalovirus Retinitis and Viral Resistance Study Group. Cytomegalovirus resistance to ganciclovir and clinical outcomes of patients with cytomegalovirus retinitis. Am J Ophthalmol 135:26, 2003.
92. Jabs DA, Forman M, Enger C, Jackson JB for the Cytomegalovirus Retinitis and Viral Resistance Study Group. Comparison of cytomegalovirus loads in plasma and leukocytes of patients with cytomegalovirus retinitis. J Clin Microbiol 37:1431, 1999.
93. Jabs DA, Martin BK, Forman MS, Ricks MO (for the Cytomegalovirus Retinitis and Viral Resistance Research Group). Cytomegalovirus (CMV) blood DNA load, CMV retinitis progression, and occurrence of resistant CMV in patients with CMV retinitis. J Infect Dis 192:640, 2005.
94. Jabs DA, Martin BK, Ricks MO, Forman MS (for the Cytomegalovirus Retinitis and Viral Resistance Study Group). Detection of ganciclovir resistance in patients with AIDS and cytomegalovirus retinitis: correlation of genotypic methods with viral phenotype and clinical outcome. J Infect Dis 193:1728, 2006.
95. Freeman WR, Henderly DE, Wan WL, et al. Prevalence, pathophysiology, and treatment of rhegmatogenous retinal detachment in treated cytomegalovirus retinitis. Am J Ophthalmol 103:527, 1987.
96. Jabs DA, Enger C, Haller J, et al. Retinal detachments in patients with cytomegalovirus retinitis. Arch Ophthalmol 109:794, 1991.
97. Freeman WR, Friedberg DN, Berry C, et al. Risk factors for development of rhegmatogenous retinal detachment in patients with cytomegalovirus retinitis. Am J Ophthalmol 116:713, 1993.
98. Studies of Ocular Complications of AIDS Research Group, in collaboration with the AIDS Clinical Trials Group. Rhegmatogenous retinal detachment in patients with cytomegalovirus retinitis: the foscarnet–ganciclovir CMV retinitis trial. Am J Ophthalmol 124:61, 1997.
99. Freeman WR, Quiceno JI, Crapotta JA, et al. Surgical repair of rhegmatogenous retinal detachment in immunosuppressed patients with cytomegalovirus retinitis. Ophthalmology 99:466, 1992.
100. Jabs DA, Van Natta ML, Thorne JE, et al (for the Studies of Ocular Complications of AIDS Research Group). Course of cytomegalovirus retinitis in the era of highly active antiretroviral therapy. 2. Second eye involvement and retinal detachment. Ophthalmology 111:2232, 2004.
101. Lim JI, Enger C, Haller JA, et al. Improved visual results after surgical repair of cytomegalovirus-related retinal detachments. Ophthalmology 101:264, 1994.
102. McCluskey P, Grigg J, Playfair TJ. Retinal detachments in patients with AIDS and CMV retinopathy: a role for laser photocoagulation. Br J Ophthalmol 79:153, 1995.
103. Canzano JC, Morse LS, Wendel RT. Surgical repair of cytomegalovirus-related retinal detachment without silicone oil in patients with AIDS. Retina 19: 274, 1999.
104. Freeman WR. Retinal detachment in cytomegalovirus retinitis: should our approach be changed? Retina 19:27, 1999.
105. Spector SA, McKinley GF, Lalezari JP, et al. Oral ganciclovir for the prevention of cytomegalovirus disease in persons with AIDS. N Engl J Med 334:1491, 1996.
106. Brosgart C, Louis TA, Hillman DW, et al. A randomized, placebo-controlled trial of the safety and efficacy of oral ganciclovir for prophylaxis of cytomegalovirus disease in HIV-infected individuals. Terry Beirn Community Programs for Clinical Research on AIDS. AIDS 12:269, 1998.
107. Moore RD, Chaisson RE. Cost-utility analysis of prophylactic treatment with oral ganciclovir for cytomegalovirus retinitis. J Acquir Immune Defic Syndr Hum Retroviral 16:15, 1997.
108. Jabs DA, Van Natta ML, Thorne JE, et al (for the Studies of Ocular Complications of AIDS Research Group). Course of cytomegalovirus retinitis in the era of highly active antiretroviral therapy. 1. Retinitis progression. Ophthalmology 111:2224, 2004.
109. Deayton JR, Wilson P, Sabin CA, et al. Changes in the natural history of cytomegalovirus retinitis following the introduction of highly active antiretroviral therapy. AIDS 14:1163, 2000.
110. Jabs DA, Van Natta ML, Kempen JH, et al. Characteristics of patients with cytomegalovirus retinitis in the era of highly active antiretroviral therapy. Am J Ophthalmol 133:48, 2002.
111. Kempen JH, Jabs DA, Wilson LA, et al. Risk of vision loss in patients with cytomegalovirus retinitis and the acquired immunodeficiency syndrome. Arch Ophthalmol 121:466, 2003.
112. Jabs DA, Holbrook JT, Van Natta ML, et al. Risk factors for mortality in patients with AIDS in the era of highly active antiretroviral therapy. Ophthalmology 112:771, 2005.
113. Kempen JH, Jabs DA, Wilson LA, et al. Mortality risk for patients with cytomegalovirus retinitis and the acquired immune deficiency syndrome. Clin Infect Dis 37:1365, 2003.
114. Walsh JC, Jones CD, Barnes EA, et al. Increasing survival in AIDS patients with cytomegalovirus retinitis treated with combination antiretroviral therapy including HIV protease inhibitors. AIDS 12:613, 1998.
115. Whitcup SM, Fortin E, Lindblad AS, et al. Discontinuation of anticytomegalovirus therapy in patients with HIV infection and cytomegalovirus retinitis. JAMA 282:1633, 1999.
116. Tural C, Romeu J, Sirera G, et al. Long-lasting remission of cytomegalovirus retinitis without maintenance therapy in human immunodeficiency virus-infected patients. J Infect Dis 177:1080, 1998.
117. Macdonald JC, Torriani FJ, Morse LS, et al. Lack of reactivation of cytomegalovirus (CMV) retinitis after stopping CMV maintenance therapy in AIDS patients with sustained elevations in CD4 T cells in response to highly active antiretroviral therapy. J Infect Dis 177:1182, 1998.
118. Jabs DA, Bolton SG, Dunn JP, et al. Discontinuing anticytomegalovirus therapy in patients with immune reconstitution after combination antiretroviral therapy. Am J Ophthalmol 126:817, 1998.

119. Vrabec TR, Baldassano VF, Whitcup SM. Discontinuation of maintenance therapy in patients with quiescent cytomegalovirus retinitis and elevated CD4+ counts. Ophthalmology 105:1259, 1998.
120. Macdonald JC, Karavellas MP, Torriani FJ, et al. Highly active antiretroviral therapy-related immune recovery in AIDS patients with cytomegalovirus retinitis. Ophthalmology 197:877, 2000.
121. Uthayakumar S, Birthistle J, Hay PE. Cytomegalovirus retinitis after initiation of highly active antiretroviral therapy (correspondence). Lancet 350:588, 1997.
122. Torriani FJ, Freeman WR, Macdonald JC, et al. CMV retinitis recurs after stopping treatment in virological and immunological failure of potent antiretroviral therapy. AIDS 14:173, 2000.
123. Jacobson MA, Zegans M, Pavan PR, et al. Cytomegalovirus retinitis after initiation of highly active antiretroviral therapy. Lancet 349:1443, 1997.
124. Gilquin J, Piketty C, Thomas V, et al. Acute cytomegalovirus infection in AIDS patients with CD4 counts above 100×10^6 cells/l following combination antiretroviral therapy including protease inhibitors [letter]. AIDS 111:1659, 1997.
125. van den Horn GJ, Meenken C, Danner SA, et al. Effects of protease inhibitors on the course of CMV retinitis in relation to CD4+ lymphocyte responses in HIV patients. Br J Ophthalmol 82:998, 1998.
126. Berenguer J, Gonzalez J, Pulido F, et al. Discontinuation of secondary prophylaxis in patients with cytomegalovirus retinitis who have responded to highly active antiretroviral therapy. Clin Infect Dis 34:394, 2002.
127. Jabs DA. Discontinuing anticytomegalovirus therapy in patients with cytomegalovirus retinitis and AIDS. Br J Ophthalmol 85:381, 2001.
128. Nussenblatt RB, Lane HC. Perspective – Human immunodeficiency virus disease: changing patterns of intraocular inflammation. Am J Ophthalmol 125:374, 1998.
129. Reed JB, Schwab IR, Gordon J, et al. Regression of cytomegalovirus retinitis associated with protease inhibitor treatment in patients with AIDS. Am J Ophthalmol 124:199, 1997.
130. Whitcup SM, Cunningham ET, Polis MA, et al. Spontaneous and sustained resolution of CMV retinitis in patients receiving highly active antiretroviral therapy [letter]. Br J Ophthalmol 82:845, 1998.
131. Johnson SC, Benson CA, Johnson DW, Weinberg A. Recurrences of cytomegalovirus retinitis in a human immunodeficiency virus-infected patient, despite potent antiretroviral therapy and apparent immune reconstitution. Clin Infect Dis 32:815, 2001.
132. Cassoux N, Bodaghi B, Fillet AM, et al. Relapses of CMV retinitis after 2 years of highly active antiretroviral therapy. Br J Ophthalmol 84:1203, 2000.
133. Lilleri D, Piccinini G, Baldanti F, et al. Multiple relapses of human cytomegalovirus retinitis during HAART in an AIDS patient with reconstitution of CD4+ T cell count in the absence of HCMV-specific CD4+ T cell response. J Clin Virol 26:95, 2003.
134. Song MK, Schrier RD, Smith IL, et al. Paradoxical activity of CMV retinitis in patients receiving highly active antiretroviral therapy. Retina 22:262, 2002.
135. Komanduri KV, Feinberg J, Hutchins RK, et al. Loss of cytomegalovirus-specific CD4+ T cell responses in human immunodeficiency virus type 1-infected patients with high CD41 T cell counts and recurrent retinitis. J Infect Dis 183:1285, 2001.
136. USPHS/IDSA Prevention of Opportunistic Infections Working Group. 1999 USPHS/IDSA guidelines for the prevention of opportunistic infections in persons infected with human immunodeficiency virus. MMWR Recomm Rep 48(RR-10):1, 1999.
137. Karavellas MP, Lowder CY, Macdonald C, et al. Immune recovery vitritis associated with inactive cytomegalovirus retinitis: a new syndrome. Arch Ophthalmol 116:169, 1998.
138. Nguyen QD, Kempen JH, Bolton SG, et al. Immune recovery uveitis in patients with AIDS and cytomegalovirus retinitis after highly active antiretroviral therapy. Am J Ophthalmol 129:634, 2000.
139. Karavellas MP, Plummer DJ, Macdonald JC, et al. Incidence of immune recovery vitritis in cytomegalovirus retinitis patients following institution of successful highly active antiretroviral therapy. J Infec Dis 179:697, 1999.
140. Zegans ME, Walton RC, Holland GN, et al. Transient vitreous inflammatory reactions associated with combination antiretroviral therapy in patients with AIDS and cytomegalovirus retinitis. Am J Ophthalmol 125:292, 1998.
141. Robinson MR, Reed G, Csaky KG, et al. Immune-recovery uveitis in patients with cytomegalovirus retinitis taking highly active antiretroviral therapy. Am J Ophthalmol 130:49, 2000.
142. Karavellas MP, Song M, Macdonald JC, et al. Long-term posterior and anterior segment complications of immune recovery uveitis associated with cytomegalovirus retinitis. Am J Ophthalmol 130:57, 2000.
143. Karavellas MP, Azen SP, MacDonald JC, et al. Immune recovery vitritis and uveitis in AIDS: clinical predictors, sequelae, and treatment outcomes. Retina 21:1, 2001.
144. Wright ME, Suzman DL, Csaky KG, et al. Extensive retinal neovascularization as a late finding in human immunodeficiency virus-infected patients with immune recovery uveitis. Clin Infect Dis 36:1063, 2003.
145. Goldberg DE, Freeman WR. Uveitic angle closure glaucoma with inactive cytomegalovirus retinitis and immune recovery uveitis. Ophthal Surg Lasers 33:421, 2002.
146. Song MK, Azen SP, Buley A, et al. Effect of anti-cytomegalovirus therapy on the incidence of immune recovery uveitis in AIDS patients with healed cytomegalovirus retinitis. Am J Ophthalmol 136:696, 2003.
147. Goldberg DE, Wang H, Azen SP, Freeman WR. Long-term visual outcome of patients with cytomegalovirus retinitis treated with highly active antiretroviral therapy. Br J Ophthalmol 87:853, 2003.
148. Henderson HW, Mitchell SM. Treatment of immune recovery vitritis with local steroids. Br J Ophthalmol 83:540, 1999.
149. Arevalo JF, Mendoza AJ, Ferretti Y. Immune recovery uveitis in AIDS patients with cytomegalovirus retinitis treated with highly active antiretroviral therapy in Venezuela. Retina 23:495, 2003.
150. Kosobucki BR, Goldberg DE, Bessho K, et al. Valganciclovir therapy for immune recovery uveitis complicated by macular edema. Am J Ophthalmol 137:636, 2004.
151. Kempen JH, Min YI, Freeman WR, et al. Risk of immune recovery uveitis with AIDS and cytomegalovirus retinitis. Ophthalmology 113:684, 2006.
152. Cole EL, Meisler DM, Calabrese LH, et al. Herpes zoster ophthalmicus and acquired immune deficiency syndrome. Arch Ophthalmol 102:1027, 1984.
153. Sandor EV, Millman A, Croxson S, et al. Herpes zoster ophthalmicus in patients at risk for the acquired immune deficiency syndrome (AIDS). Am J Ophthalmol 101:153, 1986.
154. Jabs DA, Schachat AP, Liss R, et al. Presumed varicella zoster retinitis in immunocompromised patients. Retina 7:9, 1987.
155. Sellitti TP, Huang AJW, Schiffman J, et al. Association of herpes zoster ophthalmicus with acquired immunodeficiency syndrome and acute retinal necrosis. Am J Ophthalmol 116:297, 1993.
156. Forster DJ, Dugel PU, Frangieh GT, et al. Rapidly progressive outer retinal necrosis in the acquired immunodeficiency syndrome. Am J Ophthalmol 110:341, 1990.
157. Johnston WH, Holland GN, Engstrom RE, et al. Recurrence of presumed varicella-zoster virus retinopathy in patients with

acquired immunodeficiency syndrome. Am J Ophthalmol 116:42, 1993.
158. Margolis TP, Lowder CY, Holland GN, et al. Varicella-zoster virus retinitis in patients with the acquired immunodeficiency syndrome. Am J Ophthalmol 112:119, 1991.
159. Engstrom RE Jr, Holland GN, Margolis TP, et al. The progressive outer retinal necrosis syndrome: a variant of necrotizing herpetic retinopathy in patients with AIDS. Ophthalmology 101:1488, 1994.
160. Morley MG, Duker JS, Zacks S. Successful treatment of rapidly progressive outer retinal necrosis in the acquired immunodeficiency syndrome. Am J Ophthalmol 117:264, 1994.
161. Cochereau-Massin I, Lehoang P, Lautier-Frau M, et al. Ocular toxoplasmosis in human immunodeficiency virus-infected patients. Am J Ophthalmol 114:130, 1992.
162. Holland GN, Engstrom RE, Glasgow BJ, et al. Ocular toxoplasmosis in patients with the acquired immunodeficiency syndrome. Am J Ophthalmol 106:653, 1988.
163. Parke DW, Font RL Diffuse toxoplasmic retinochoroiditis in a patient with AIDS. Arch Ophthalmol 104:571, 1986.
164. Weiss A, Margo CE, Ledford DK, et al. Toxoplasmic retinochoroiditis as an initial manifestation of the acquired immune deficiency syndrome. Am J Ophthalmol 101:248, 1987.
165. Berger BB, Egwuagu CE, Freeman WR, et al. Miliary toxoplasmic retinitis in acquired immunodeficiency syndrome. Arch Ophthalmol 111:373, 1993.
166. Morinelli EN, Dugel PU, Riffenburgh R, et al. Infectious multifocal choroiditis in patients with acquired immune deficiency syndrome. Ophthalmology 100:1014, 1993.
167. Rao NA, Zimmerman PL, Boyer D, et al. A clinical, histopathologic, and electron microscopic study of *Pneumocystis carinii* choroiditis. Am J Ophthalmol 107:218, 1989.
168. Dugel PU, Rao NA, Forster DJ, et al. *Pneumocysitis carinii* choroiditis after long-term aerosolized pentamidine therapy. Am J Ophthalmol 110:113, 1990.
169. Shami MJ, Freeman W, Friedberg D, et al. A multicenter study of *Pneumocystis* choroidopathy. Am J Ophthalmol 112:15, 1991.
170. Croxatto JO, Mestre C, Puente S, et al. Nonreactive tuberculosis in a patient with acquired immune deficiency syndrome. Am J Ophthalmol 105:659, 1986.
171. Blodi BA, Johnson MW, McLeish WM, et al. Presumed choroidal tuberculosis in a human immunodeficiency virus infected host. Am J Ophthalmol 108:605, 1989.
172. Passo MS, Rosenbaum JT. Ocular syphilis in patients with human immunodeficiency virus infection. Am J Ophthalmol 106:1, 1988.
173. Carter JB, Hamill RJ, Matoba AY. Bilateral syphilitic optic neuritis in a patient with a positive test for HIV. Arch Ophthalmol 105:1485, 1987.
174. Becerra LI, Ksiazek SM, Savino PJ, et al. Syphilitic uveitis in human immunodeficiency virus-infected and noninfected patients. Ophthalmology 96:1727, 1989.
175. McLeish WM, Pulido JS, Holland S, et al. The ocular manifestations of syphilis in the human immunodeficiency virus type 1-infected host. Ophthalmology 97:196, 1990.
176. Shalaby IA, Dunn JP, Semba RD, et al. Syphilitic uveitis in human immunodeficiency virus-infected patients. Arch Ophthalmol 115:469, 1997.
177. Tamesis RR, Foster CS. Ocular syphilis. Ophthalmology 97:1281, 1990.
178. Kestelyn P, Taelman H, Bogaerts J, et al. Ophthalmic manifestions of infections with *Cryptococcus neoformans* in patients with the acquired immunodeficiency syndrome. Am J Ophthalmol 116:721, 1993.
179. Carney MD, Coombs JL, Waschler W. Cryptococcal choroiditis. Retina 10:27, 1990.
180. Charles NC, Boxrud CA, Small EA. Cryptococcosis of the anterior segment in acquired immune deficiency syndrome. Ophthalmology 99:813, 1992.
181. Specht CS, Mitchell KT, Bauman AE, et al. Ocular histoplasmosis with retinitis in a patient with acquired immune deficiency syndrome. Ophthalmology 98:1356, 1991.
182. Macher A, Rodrigues MM, Kaplan W, et al. Disseminated bilateral chorioretinitis due to histoplasma capsulatum in a patient with the acquired immunodeficiency syndrome. Ophthalmology 92:1159, 1985.
183. Friedberg DN, Stenson SM, Orenstein JM, et al. Microsporidial keratoconjunctivitis in acquired immunodeficiency syndrome. Arch Ophthalmol 108:504, 1990.
184. Lowder CY, Meisler DM, McMahon JT, et al. Microsporidia infection of the cornea in a man seropositive for human immunodeficiency virus. Am J Ophthalmol 109:242, 1990.
185. Metcalfe TW, Doran RML, Rowlands PL, et al. Microsporidial keratoconjunctivitis in a patient with AIDS. Br J Ophthalmol 76:177, 1992.
186. Rastrelli PD, Didier E, Yee RW. Microsporidial keratitis. Ophthalmol Clin North Am 7:617, 1994.
187. Schuler JD, Holland GN, Miles SA, et al. Kaposi sarcoma of the conjunctiva and eyelids associated with the acquired immunodeficiency syndrome. Arch Ophthalmol 107:858, 1989.
188. Dugel PU, Gill PS, Frangieh GT, et al. Ocular adnexal Kaposi's sarcoma in acquired immunodeficiency syndrome. Am J Ophthalmol 119:500, 1990.
189. Dugel PU, Gill PS, Frangieh GT, et al. Treatment of ocular adnexal Kaposi's sarcoma in acquired immunodeficiency syndrome. Ophthalmology 99:1127, 1992.
190. Ghabrial R, Quivey JM, Dunn JP Jr, et al. Radiation therapy of acquired immunodeficiency syndrome-related Kaposi's sarcoma of the eyelids and conjunctiva. Arch Ophthalmol 110:1423, 1992.
191. Schanzer MC, Font RL, O'Malley RE. Primary ocular malignant lymphoma associated with the acquired immune deficiency syndrome. Ophthalmology 98:88, 1991.
192. Antle CM, White VA, Horsman DE, et al. Large cell orbital lymphoma in a patient with acquired immune deficiency syndrome: case report and review. Ophthalmology 97:1494, 1990.
193. Stanton CA, Sloan DB III, Slusher MM, et al. Acquired immunodeficiency syndrome-related primary intraocular lymphoma. Arch Ophthalmol 110:1614, 1992.
194. Matzkin DC, Slamovits TL, Rosenbaum PS. Simultaneous intraocular and orbital non-Hodgkin lymphoma in the acquired immune deficiency syndrome. Ophthalmology 101:850, 1994.
195. Keane JR. Neuro-ophthalmologic signs of AIDS: 50 patients. Neurology 41:841, 1991.
196. Lipson BK, Freeman WR, Beniz J, et al. Optic neuropathy associated with cryptococcal arachnoiditis in AIDS patients. Am J Med 107:523, 1989.
197. Rex JH, Larsen RA, Dismukes WE, et al. Catastrophic visual loss due to *Cryptococcus neoformans* meningitis. Medicine 72:207, 1993.
198. Cohen DB, Glasgow BJ. Bilateral optic nerve cryptococcosis in sudden blindness in patients with acquired immune deficiency syndrome. Ophthalmology 100:1689, 1993.
199. Hamed LM, Schatz NJ, Galetta SL. Brainstem ocular motility defects in AIDS. Am J Ophthalmol 106:437, 1988.
200. Nguyen N, Rimmer S, Katz B. Slowed saccades in the acquired immunodeficiency syndrome. Am J Ophthalmol 107:356, 1989.
201. Currie J, Benson E, Ramsden B, et al. Eye movement abnormalities as a predictor of the acquired immunodeficiency syndrome dementia complex. Arch Neurol 45:949, 1988.
202. Sweeney BJ, Manji H, Gilson RJC, et al. Optic neuritis and HIV-1 infection. J Neurol Neurosurg Psychiatry 567:705, 1993.

203. Newman NJ, Lessell S. Bilateral optic neuropathies with remission in two HIV-1 positive men. J Clin Neuroophthalmol 12:1, 1992.

204. Cunningham CA, Friedberg DN, Carr RE. Clofazimine-induced generalized retinal degeneration. Retina 10:131, 1990.

205. Whitcup SM, Butler KM, Caruso R, et al. Retinal toxicity in human immunodeficiency virus-infected children treated with 2,3-dideoxyinosine. Am J Ophthalmol 113:1, 1992.

206. Shafran SD, Deschenes J, Miller M, et al (The MAC Study Group of the Canadian HIV Trials Network). Uveitis and pseudojaundice during a regimen of clarithromycin, rifabutin and ethambutol. N Engl J Med 330:438, 1994.

207. Jacobs DS, Piliero PJ, Kuperwaser MG, et al. Acute uveitis associated with rifabutin use in patients with human immunodeficiency virus infection. Am J Ophthalmol 118:716, 1994.

208. Rifai A, Peyman GA, Daun M, et al. Rifabutin-associated uveitis during prophylaxis for *Mycobacterium avium* complex infection. Arch Ophthalmol 113:707, 1995.

209. Karbassi M, Nikou S. Acute uveitis in patients with acquired immunodeficiency syndrome receiving prophylactic rifabutin. Arch Ophthalmol 113:699, 1995.

210. Saran BR, Maguire AM, Nichols C, et al. Hypopyon uveitis in patients with acquired immunodeficiency syndrome treated for systemic *Mycobacterium avium* complex infection with rifabutin. Arch Ophthalmol 112:1159, 1994.

211. Siegal FP, Eilbott D, Burger H, et al. Dose-limiting toxicity of rifabutin in AIDS-related comples: syndrome of arthralgia/arthritis. AIDS 4:433, 1990.

Chapter 67

Hematologic Disease

Richard D. Moore, MD

Hematologic abnormalities are widely recognized and are of significant clinical importance in the management of patients with human immunodeficiency virus (HIV) infection. The etiology of these hematologic abnormalities is multiple. HIV infection of lymphocytes, monocytes, and macrophages is thought to induce abnormalities in cytokine production that in turn have marked effects on the regulation of both the hematopoietic and immune systems. Studies involving HIV infection of bone marrow progenitor cells have been conflicting.[1–3] Although some early data suggested that CD34+ bone marrow progenitor cells might be the targets of HIV infection,[4–7] other, more recent, findings have indicated that these cells are infrequently infected with HIV.[8,9] Similarly, HIV RNA in protein products have been found in committed myeloid and erythroid progenitor cells,[7] while another study failed to detect HIV in these cells.[10] The presence or absence of accessory cells in the bone marrow can also influence hematopoiesis through the local production of growth factors.[11] These accessory cells, such as T lymphocytes, monocytes, endothelial cells, and fibroblasts are targets for HIV and may serve as a reservoir for the virus in the bone marrow. HIV-infected accessory cells may be less able to produce local hematopoietic growth factors such as granulocyte colony-stimulating factor (G-CSF) and interleukin-3 (IL-3), which in turn may slow normal hematopoiesis or facilitate apoptosis.[12–13] These accessory cells may also produce inhibitors of hematopoiesis such as transforming growth factor beta, interferon gamma, and tumor necrosis factor alpha (TNF-alpha) or other suppressive cytokines.[11,14–18] HIV may also inhibit the hematopoietic process more directly, such as with antibodies to gp120 or through functioning of accessory genes.[19,20]

In addition to ineffective hematopoiesis, myelosuppression resulting from drugs, infections, and malignancies contribute to an increased incidence of cytopenia in patients with HIV. Correction of these defects involves inhibition of HIV replication, treatment of infections and tumors, discontinuation or reduction in dosages of myelosuppressive medications, correction of nutritional or other deficiencies, and augmentation with hematopoietic growth factors to facilitate the proliferation, maturation, and differentiation of mature blood cells.

CYTOPENIAS

Cytopenias were some of the first recognized signs of HIV infection. The untreated natural history of HIV infection is associated with a relatively high prevalence of anemia, neutropenia, and thrombocytopenia. The prevalence of each of these cytopenias tends to increase as HIV infection progresses from asymptomatic infection to advanced disease and acquired immunodeficiency syndrome (AIDS).[21–23] As will be discussed in subsequent sections, cytopenias also contribute to some of the morbidity associated with HIV and AIDS because they hinder therapy directed at HIV and the opportunistic infections and neoplasms of AIDS may increase the risk of bacterial infection, and affect quality of life.

Anemia

Anemia is the most common hematologic abnormality seen in patients with HIV infection (Fig. 67-1). Specific determination of the prevalence and incidence of anemia in HIV infection has been hampered by inconsistent definitions of anemia. Nevertheless, a number of studies have consistently demonstrated a prevalence of anemia of 10–20% in untreated asymptomatic HIV infection, and from 50% to 85% with overt AIDS.[1,24–26] A large study of over 32 800 HIV-infected persons in care in nine US cities, the multistate Adult and Adolescent Spectrum of HIV Disease Surveillance study (AASHD), assessed anemia as defined by a hemoglobin level <10 g/dL or a physician's diagnosis of anemia from 1990 to 1996, prior to the widespread

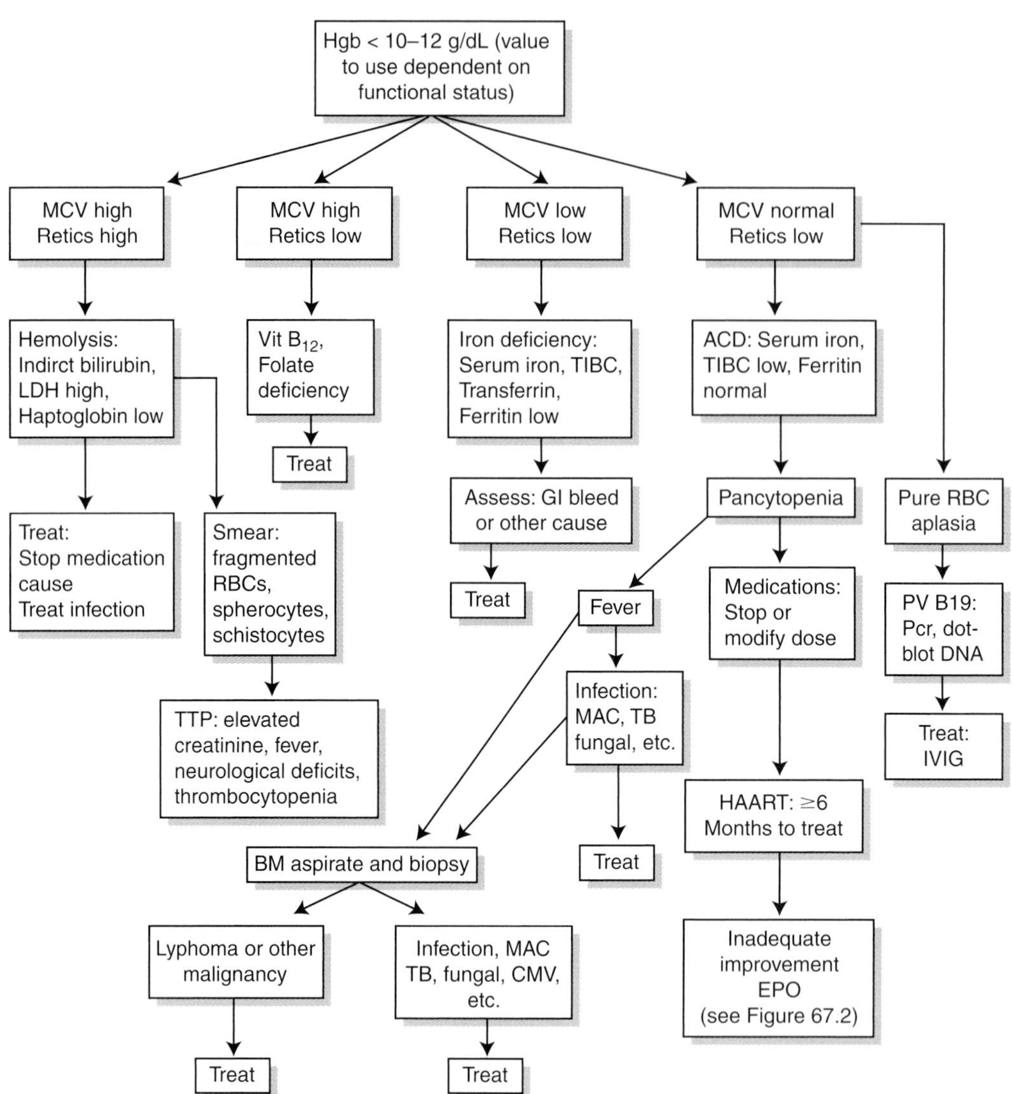

Figure 67-1 ■ Schema for evaluation of anemia in HIV infection.

availability of HAART. The annual incidence of anemia was 37% in those with clinical AIDS, 12% in immunologic AIDS (CD4+ T-cell count of >200 cells/μL) and 3% in HIV-infected individuals without AIDS.[27] In this cohort and others, HIV-infected women have been found to have a higher prevalence and incidence of anemia than men.[27–29] It has also been shown that HIV-infected African-Americans are more likely to have anemia than other racial/ethnic groups, and the HIV-infected persons with a history of injecting drug use are at higher risk for anemia than are other HIV transmission risk groups.[26,30–32]

There has been a consistent association between anemia and decreased survival in patients infected with HIV. This association has been demonstrated in observational studies and clinical trials since the mid-1980s.[33] The strongest association with a decreased survival is for a hemoglobin level of less than 10 g/dL. In the AASHD, the risk of dying was 48% greater in those with anemia compared to those who did not have anemia.[27] In another study using data from a clinical HIV cohort in Baltimore, the relative risk of dying for a patient with a hemoglobin level <9.5 g/dL was threefold that of those patients with higher hemoglobin levels.[34] Data for both of these analyses preceded HAART, but did control for other prognostic variables such as the CD4+ T-cell count. However, an analysis from the multicountry EuroSIDA cohort performed using data collected after 1996, when HAART was available, showed that the highest risk of dying (RR = 7.1) was for a hemoglobin level <8 g/dL, but that the risk remained elevated in the 8–14 g/dL range (RR = 2.2).[35] In the Human Immunodeficiency Virus Epidemiology Research Study (HERS), anemia was associated with a relative hazard of 1.64 for dying among HIV-infected women.[29] Similarly in the Women's Interagency HIV Study (WIHS), anemia was independently associated with decreased survival (relative hazard = 2.58).[36] These studies of anemia and mortality were all conducted in high socioeconomic countries. An association has also been found between anemia and survival in Haiti[37] and more recently, anemia was shown to be an independent predictor of mortality and immunologic progression of disease among HIV-infected women in Tanzania with a relative hazard of 2.06 for moderate anemia (hemoglobin <11 g/dL) and 3.19 for severe anemia (hemoglobin <8.5 g/dL).[38]

Anemia has also been shown to be associated with HIV progression to AIDS, and with the development of specific opportunistic illnesses. In data from the Multicenter AIDS Cohort Study (MACS), there was a 29% decrease in risk of progression to AIDS from HIV over 6 months for each one-point increase in the hemoglobin.[39] Anemia has been associated with development of early dementia[40] and the rapid progression of disseminated *Mycobacterium avium* complex.[41] The importance of anemia as a prognostic factor for AIDS progression and death has led it to be incorporated into a prognostic algorithm developed using data from EuroSIDA. In this study, a multivariate analysis identified four factors; CD4+ T-cell count, HIV RNA, a history of clinical AIDS, and the hemoglobin level as independent predictors of HIV disease progression and death.[42]

It is important to note that this consistent association may not be causal, but instead may be an epiphenomenon of impaired erythropoiesis which is secondary to rapidly advancing HIV disease. Notably, some studies have suggested that resolving anemia is associated with improved survival in patients infected with HIV.[17,34] Several studies have adjusted or otherwise controlled for a number of other prognostic factors such as CD4+ T-cell count, HIV RNA, AIDS diagnoses and antiretroviral and prophylaxis medications, yet found anemia to be an independent prognostic factor for survival. Nevertheless, short of a randomized clinical trial designed to assess treating versus not treating anemia in HIV infection, it will remain unknown whether anemia independently increases the risk of dying with HIV infection.

Anemia is also associated with a reduced quality of life, particularly as it relates to functional status. The association between anemia and a reduced functional status has been found in several studies of cancer treatment.[43–45] Until recently, there were few data examining the association between anemia and quality of life in HIV infection. An earlier observational study showed that an increase in the hematocrit from <30% to >38% was associated with significant improvement in several quality of life measures.[46] In a multicenter study of 221 patients receiving zidovudine who had a hemoglobin level <11 g/dL, a mean increase of 2.5 g/dL was associated with a significantly improved functional status.[47] In another multicenter, prospective cohort study of 1406 individuals, a higher hemoglobin level was associated with higher energy scores and physical functioning scores, after adjusting for CD4+ T-cell count, sex, age, race, and HIV transmission risk factor.[48] In a recent clinical trial of treatment of 650 patients who had anemia (hemoglobin <11 g/dL), there was a mean increase in hemoglobin of 2.5 g/dL, which corresponded to a 41% increase in the mean Linear Analog Scale Assessment (LASA) quality of life scale, and a 37% improvement in the (Medical Outcomes Study) MOS-HIV quality of life measure.[49] In both cancer and HIV infection, improvements in the quality of life appear to occur until the hemoglobin reaches the 12–13 g/dL range, suggesting the need to achieve and maintain hemoglobin >12 g/dL in an effort to preserve and maximize quality of life benefits.[50]

Etiology

Impaired Erythropoiesis

The major cause of anemia in HIV-infected patients is impaired erythropoiesis (Table 67-1), either as a direct consequence of HIV infection of erythrocyte precursors or, more likely, as a result of inappropriate release of inflammatory cytokines such as TNF-alpha, a potent inhibitor of erythroid maturation *in vitro*.[51,52] There is also a decreased production of erythropoietin, similar to that seen with other chronic inflammatory diseases.[53] The anemia of HIV infection is typically classified as an anemia of chronic disease and is usually normochromic and normocytic, although it may be mildly hypochromic and microcytic. There is usually a low serum iron level and iron-binding capacity, but a normal to elevated ferritin level and adequate iron stores in the bone marrow. The reticulocyte count is inappropriately low. Macrocytosis is unusual except in patients treated with zidovudine, and less so with stavudine.[54–56]

Table 67-1 Causes of Anemia in HIV Infection

Anemia – Impaired RBC Production
HIV infection – anemia of chronic disease

Other infection
- *M. avium* complex
- *M. tuberculosis*
- Cytomegalovirus
- Fungal
- Parvovirus B19

Malignancy infiltrating bone marrow
- Lymphoma
- Kaposi sarcoma
- Other

Drugs (see Table 67-2)
- Nutritional
- Iron-deficiency
- Vitamin B_{12} deficiency
- Folate deficiency

Anemia – Shortened RBC Life
Coomb's positive hemolytic anemia
TTP
DIC
G6PD deficiency and oxidant drug use (see Table 67-2)
Other drugs (see Table 67-2)

Neutropenia
HIV infection
Drugs (see Table 67-2)

Thrombocytopenia
HIV infection
ITP
TTP
DIC
Drugs (see Table 67-2)

Some other common causes of anemia in patients with HIV infection are infiltrative diseases of the bone marrow, such as that caused by *Mycobacterium avium* complex (MAC) in patients with advanced HIV disease.[57,58] Patients with MAC infections often have profound anemia with hematocrits as low as 15–20%. Fungal infections, cytomegalovirus, and neoplasms may also infiltrate bone marrow and cause profound anemia, often with associated neutropenia and thrombocytopenia.

Persistent infection with B19 parvovirus is also associated with intractable anemia in immunosuppressed patients.[59–61] Parvovirus B19 can selectively infect actively replicating erythroid progenitors, resulting in loss of red blood cells and erythroid hypoplasia. Parvovirus B19 is common in childhood (fifth disease), and as many as 80% of adults have antibodies to the virus. Control of this infection is mediated by an intact humoral immune response; therefore immunocompromised patients may fail to clear this infection because they are unable to maintain an adequate antibody response to this virus.[61–63] IgG and IgM antibodies are often absent, however, B19 parvovirus infection is reliably diagnosed by polymerase chain reaction (PCR) or by *in situ* hybridization using sequence-specific DNA probes for parvovirus B19. The presence of giant, abnormal pronormoblasts in the bone marrow is also pathognomonic for parvovirus B19 infection.

Nutritional deficiencies have been described in patients with HIV infection and may include disorders of iron metabolism or iron deficiency.[1,32,64] Iron deficiency may result from chronic blood loss, from Kaposi sarcoma, lymphoma of the gastrointestinal tract, or various infectious enterocolitides. Recent data suggest that HIV-infected injecting drug users may be at higher risk for iron deficiency anemia (adjusted RR = 6.65) than other HIV transmission risk groups.[31] The prevalence of HIV infection in women has increased over the past decade, and iron deficiency is a common nutritional disorder in premenopausal women. Although advanced HIV disease and AIDS may be associated with diminished menses, women with effectively treated and asymptomatic HIV infection may have normal menstruation and be at risk for iron deficiency. Alcohol abuse is not uncommon in HIV infection, and hemorrhagic gastritis can be a complication. The causes of iron deficiency are myriad, and it is important to ensure that the patient has had a sufficient evaluation to determine the specific cause.

Vitamin B_{12} deficiency occurs in up to 30% of HIV-infected patients.[1,32,64–66] Patients usually do not have other manifestations of vitamin B_{12} deficiency and often do not improve markedly with parenteral repletion.[67] The low vitamin B_{12} levels may result from abnormalities in vitamin B_{12}-binding proteins and decreased serum transport of vitamin B12,[68] however, abnormal absorption of vitamin B_{12} may also occur in patients with advanced HIV infection.[69–71] Folate deficiency is not prevalent in this patient population, and would most likely occur in advanced HIV infection associated with poor food intake. Both vitamin B_{12} and folate deficiency may occur in the setting of alcohol abuse.

Finally, several drugs used to treat HIV (e.g., zidovudine) and the complications of HIV can cause anemia. The most common of these are listed in Table 67-2.

Hemolysis

Hemolysis can occur in individuals with glucose 6-phosphate dehydrogenase (G6PD) deficiency who are exposed to antioxidant drugs (Table 67-1). In HIV infection, most commonly used antioxidant drugs are dapsone and primaquine, and less commonly, sulfonamides. Over 100 G6PD variants are inherited on the X-chromosome, but the most frequent are Gd^{A-} found in 10% of black men and in 1–2% of black women, and Gd^{med}, found predominantly in men from the Mediterranean area, India, and Southeast Asia. Rarer causes of hemoloysis include thrombotic thrombocytopenic purpura (TTP) a multisystem disease that is also associated with thrombocytopenia,

Table 67-2 Drugs Commonly Associated With Cytopenias in HIV Infection

Anemia	Neutropenia	Thrombocytopenia
Zidovudine	Cancer chemotherapy (various drugs)	Sulfonamides
Interferon-alpha	Zidovudine	Thiazides
Ribavirin	Ganciclovir	Heparin
Ganciclovir	Valganciclovir	Quinidine/quinine
Pyrimethamine	Foscarnet	Alcohol
Dapsone (G6PD deficiency)	Sulfonamides	Cocaine
Primaquine (G6PD deficiency)	Pyrimethamine	
Sulfonamides	Pentamidine	
Phenytoin	Interferon-alpha	
Cancer chemotherapy (various drugs)	Amphotericin	
Amphotericin	Flucytosine	
Alcohol	Alcohol	

renal impairment, fever and neurologic abnormalities, and disseminated intravascular coagulation (DIC).

Between 20% and 44% of asymptomatic HIV-infected patients are Coombs' test-positive, with the numbers increasing up to 85% in those with frank AIDS,[72,73] although it is usually nonspecific, and antibody-mediated hemolysis is rare in patients with HIV infection. Although these antibodies may be reactive with specific minor antigens on erythrocytes, in most cases nonspecific binding of antiphospholipid antibodies or deposition of immune complexes on erythrocytes are responsible for these positive Coombs' tests.[74]

Treatment of Anemia

The hemoglobin level for which anemia should be treated may vary somewhat. The World Health Organization (WHO) recommends treatment in women with a hemoglobin <12 g/dL and in men with a hemoglobin <13 g/dL. Studies that demonstrated improvement in the quality of life in anemic HIV-infected women and men, found such improvements with treatment of hemoglobin <10 g/dL or <11 g/dL, respectively. Many HIV-treating physicians now would consider treatment of anemia to maintain the hemoglobin level above 12 g/dL for men and above 11 g/dL for women.[75] The strongest association between anemia and adverse clinical outcomes appears to be for a hemoglobin level <10 g/dL, but it has not been shown whether treatment of anemia will actually alter the clinical prognosis of HIV infection. Finally, anemia may need to be treated if this allows for the use of antiretroviral drugs (e.g., zidovudine) or therapy for HIV complications that would otherwise be withheld or discontinued.

It is reasonable to assess the HIV-infected patient for possible treatment when the hemoglobin level meets the WHO thresholds. Simple assessments of functional status and other quality of life measures can be done with the LASA[44] or using questions from the MOS-HIV.[76] Although it may be difficult to determine when anemia is causing a decrease in quality of life in the setting of HIV infection and other complications, a decrease in functional status or other measures may clinically correlate with a decline in hemoglobin level.

When anemia occurs, it is important to determine the reason for the decline in hemoglobin level. As noted previously, there are myriad causes of anemia and it is important that a co-morbidity that should be treated not be overlooked. The MCV and reticulocyte count can be particularly helpful in categorizing the potential etiology of the anemia, with additional laboratory testing as needed (Table 67-3).

Prior to the introduction of highly active antiretroviral therapy (HAART), there was no evidence that antiretroviral treatment of HIV infection would also improve anemia. However, several studies have now demonstrated that HAART is effective in improving hemoglobin levels within 6 months to 1 year of initiating therapy in both men and women, and in whites and blacks.[35,36,77–81] These studies consistently showed improvements of 2–3 g/dL in the hemoglobin level over 1 year on HAART. However, the hemoglobin may not return completely to normal levels even when HAART results in HIV RNA suppression and there is effective immune restoration. Using zidovudine as part of an otherwise effective HAART regimen may decrease the likelihood that the hemoglobin level returns to normal.[82]

Administration of effective antiretroviral therapy may influence hematopoiesis by decreasing various inhibitory processes, and be critical to alleviating cytopenias in patients with HIV. In a study of the effects of antiretroviral therapy on cytokine and chemokine production by bone marrow and stromal cells in HIV-infected patients, there was decreased IL-2, elevated TNF-alpha, MIP-1 alpha, MIP-1 beta, and RANTES levels compared to uninfected controls. Antiretroviral therapy with protease inhibitors was associated with a restoration of stromal cell pattern and functions, and an increased IL-2 production and diminution of TNF-alpha levels. There was an increase in bone marrow colony growth in both HIV-infected patients and normal individuals in parallel with the normalization of functional and morphologic characteristics of stromal cells.[83] In another study, increases in hemoglobin levels in the first 6 months on HAART were shown to be strongly correlated with a decrease in sTNFR II and neopterin concentrations, immune activation markers of proinflammatory cytokine activity.[80]

Nutritional causes of anemia are treated by replacement of the specific nutrient. Mild to moderate iron deficiency may be treated with oral iron replacement such as ferrous sulfate at 300 mg three times daily. Parenteral iron is not typically necessary for most causes of nutritional iron loss. Because vitamin B_{12} may be malabsorbed in the GI tract, parenteral replacement with 100 μg IM is recommended. Replacement with oral folic acid (1–5 mg/day) is indicated should this deficiency occur, although GI malabsorption may interfere with folic acid replacement, particularly in advanced AIDS.

Treatment of parvovirus B19 infection involves a course of intravenous immunoglobulin (IVIG) over several days. Generally a dose of 400 mg kg^{-1} day^{-1} is given for 5 days and is effective in more than 75% of patients. Repeat administration of a course of IVIG may be necessary in patients with severe immune deficiencies who are unable to generate their own antibody response to B19 parvovirus infection. Some patients require maintenance IVIG of 400 mg kg^{-1} $month^{-1}$ to maintain red blood cell counts. Treatment with folate and other hematinics may also be necessary to sustain an erythropoietic response.

Studies of recombinant hematopoietic growth factors in patients with HIV disease have proven their overall effectiveness in increasing blood cell numbers and correcting cytopenias. Exogenous administration of growth factors offers the potential of ameliorating some of the adverse effects of HIV infection on normal hematopoiesis and may allow continued or heightened use of erythrosuppressive drugs necessary to manage HIV and its related complications.

The hematopoietic growth factor, erythropoietin is a glycoprotein that regulates the production of hematopoietic cells and the process of terminal differentiation and maturation. It also suppresses apoptosis,[84] and can enhance the function of terminally differentiated hematopoietic cells.[85] Most

Table 67-3 Diagnosing and Treating Causes of Cytopenia in HIV Infection

Diagnosis	Diagnosis	Treatment
Anemia		
Iron-deficiency anemia	Fe < 60 μg/dL, transferrin < 300 μg/dL, ferritin < 40 ng/mL, MCV < 80, reticulocytes > 2.0	Ferrous sulfate 300 mg po tid
HIV-induced anemia (chronic disease)	Fe < 60 μg/dL, transferrin < 300 μg/dL, ferritin >80 ng/mL, normal BM iron, low erythropoietin level, MCV low-normal, retics < 2.0	HAART (1–2 g/dL increase in hemoglobin over 6–12 months), epoetin-alpha
Vitamin B_{12} deficiency	MCV > 100, retics < 2.0, serum vitamin B_{12} (cyanocobalamin) < 125–175 pg/mL	Vitamin B_{12} 1 mg IM daily × 7 days, then monthly
Folate deficiency	MCV > 100, retics < 2.0, serum folate < 2–3 ng/mL	Folate 1–5 mg po daily × 1 month
Parvovirus B19	Severe pure RBC aplasia. Hemoglobin < 10, hematocrit < 24%, retics low-absent, positive IgG and IgM serology, positive PCR of dot-blot hybridization for PV B19	HAART IVIG 400 mg kg^{-1} day^{-1} × 5 days, repeat as necessary
Bone marrow infiltration by infection or tumor	MCV 80–100, retics < 2.0, possible pancytopenia, BM biopsy abnormal	Treat specific etiology
Drug induced	MCV > 100 (zidovudine and stavudine)	Discontinue drug, epoetin-alpha
G6PD deficiency and use of oxidant drugs, and other hemolysis	MCV 80–100, increased retics, indirect bilirubin > 1.2 mg/dL, LDH > 220 IU, haptoglobin <25 mg/dL, spherocytes and fragmented RBCs on smear	Discontinue drug, transfusion Severe methemoglobinemia (G6PD deficiency) can be treated with IV methylene blue (1 mg/kg)
Thrombocytopenia		
TTP	Hemolysis (see G6PD above), anemia, thrombocytopenia, increased creatinine, neurologic signs, fever	Plasma exchange with fresh frozen plasma (7–15 exchanges may be needed until normal platelets and LDH)
DIC	Hemolysis (see G6PD above), thrombocytopenia	Heparin
HIV-ITP	Platelets < 20 000, increased megakaryocytes in BM	Prednisone 30–60 mg daily, taper with response IVIG 1000 mg/kg × 2 days, then day 14, and every 2–4 weeks as needed Anti-Rh (anti-D) 25–50 μg/dk, repeat day 3–4, then 3–4 week intervals as needed in Rh-positive, non splenectomized Splenectomy (with prophylactic vaccination) RBC transfusion and platelet transfusion for active bleeding
Neutropenia		
HIV induced, drug induced, others	ANC < 250–500	G-CSF 5 μg/kg SQ daily, titrate as needed by adjusting dosing interval to qod, 3× −2× weekly, or reduce dose. Goal of ANC > 1000–2000 GM-CSF 250 μg/m^2 SQ daily, titrate by dosing interval or dose. Goal of ANC > 1000–2000 Pegylated G-CSF (Pegfilgrastim) 6 mg SQ weekly or less

HIV-infected patients with anemia have adequate erythropoietic capacity but are unable to augment it during periods of demand in large part because of relatively inadequate erythropoietin (EPO) levels.[53,86] Inappropriately low endogenous levels (<500 mU/mL) of serum EPO are seen in most AIDS patients with anemia.[86,87] In addition, cytokines that are produced in response to HIV infection, such as IL-1 and TNF-alpha, blunt the normal rise in hemoglobin with rising serum EPO levels. Circulating antierythropoietin antibodies have also been correlated with anemia in a subset of patients with HIV.[88–89]

Placebo-controlled trials have shown that small amounts of recombinant human erythropoietin (epoetin alpha) can increase hemoglobin and significantly reduce transfusion requirements of patients with HIV infection and anemia.[90] In these trials, epoetin alpha was well tolerated and significantly reduced transfusion requirements, increased the hematocrit, and improved the quality of life of patients with HIV infection and anemia. Patients whose EPO levels were less than 500 mU/mL had statistically significant reductions in red blood cell transfusions and increases in hematocrit compared to placebo-treated patients after 6–8 weeks of therapy. Patients with endogenous epoetin alpha levels of more than 500 mU/mL did not experience significant increases in hematocrit or reduction in transfusion requirements when compared to placebo-treated patients.[90]

A randomized controlled trial of epoetin alpha (100 to 300 IU/kg subcutaneously three times per week) in anemic HIV-infected patients in the community setting also showed significant increases in hemogloblin levels that were independent of the baseline CD4+ T-lymphocyte counts. The mean quality of life score, as measured by the Functional Assessment of HIV Infection (FAHI) scale, improved significantly, with increases in hemoglobin after epoetin alpha use.[91]

In a 16-week randomized trial of 285 HIV-infected adults with anemia (hemoglobin <12 g/dL) on stable antiretroviral therapy, once weekly epoetin alpha at 40 000 IU subcutaneously was as effective as three times weekly dosing in improving hemoglobin (2.9 g/dL for weekly vs 2.5 g/dL for thrice weekly).[92] In still another randomized trial of 650 patients with a hemoglobin <11 g/dL, there was a significant increase in hemoglobin level of 2.5 g/dL after 16 weeks with the weekly use of epoetin alpha at 40 000 IU with dose escalation to 60 000 IU weekly if the hemoglobin increase was <1 g/dL after 4 weeks.[49] Weekly use of epoetin alpha has also been shown to be effective for increasing the hemoglobin level in HIV-infected individuals in other studies, including in HIV/hepatitis C co-infected individuals being treated with interferon/ribavirin for the treatment of hepatitis C infection.[93]

The erythropoiesis stimulating protein, darbepoetin alpha, is a possible alternative to epoetin alpha for treating anemia. This drug has a longer half-life than epoetin alpha which may allow less frequent dosing. Currently, darbepoetin alpha has only been shown to effectively treat anemia associated with cancer chemotherapy and in renal failure, with limited data assessing its effectiveness in HIV infection.[94,95] Currently, epoetin alpha is only approved for use in patients with anemia as a result of zidovudine therapy, and the initial recommended dose is 100 IU/kg three times weekly. Failure to respond to this treatment after 6–8 weeks would warrant increasing the dose and possibly performing a bone marrow aspiration and biopsy to exclude other possible causes of myelosuppression. A serum erythropoietin level >500 IU/mL is associated with a significantly decreased rate of response. Though not an FDA-approved dose, many HIV-treating physicians would use once-a-week epoetin alpha for convenience. Recent evidence indicates that epoetin alpha is associated with an increased risk of serious cardiovascular events and death when administered to a target hemoglobin >12 g/dL.[96,97] Recommendations for the use of growth factors in HIV-infected patients are in Figure 67-2 and in Table 67-3.

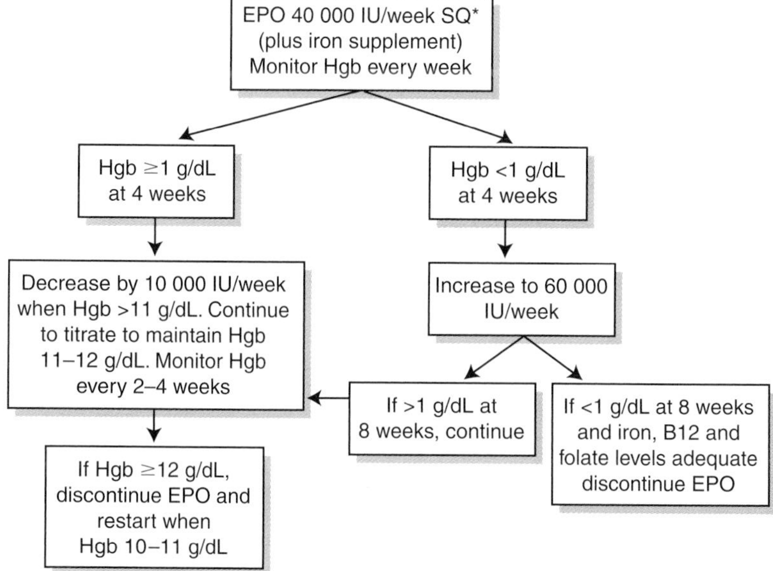

Figure 67-2 ■ Use of hematopoietic growth factor to treat anemia in HIV infection.

Administration of a hematopoietic growth factor offers an alternative to transfusions and their potential morbidity and mortality. Transfusions may be immunosuppressive,[96] and the time to progression to AIDS is shorter in those who are given transfusions.[97] Use of transfusion may also be associated with a higher mortality rate in HIV infection.[34,98] Data suggest an increase in HIV replication in those receiving red blood cell transfusions as well,[99] and a possible increased risk in opportunistic infection.[100] There is also a risk of exposure to new infectious agents with transfusions and a risk of transfusion reactions despite the immunodeficiency caused by HIV.[101] If one does need to transfuse red blood cells in an HIV-infected patient to treat severe hemorrhage or to maintain a hemoglobin level that is not otherwise treatable by other means, results from the Viral Activation Transfusion Study did not show any advantage to using leukocyte-reduced red blood cells in a large prospective randomized controlled study.[102]

The use of iron and hematinics is recommended for patients on long-term hematopoietic growth factor therapy as functional iron deficiency can rapidly ensue unless individuals are iron-overloaded from prior transfusions. Oral iron given as ferrous sulfate at 300 mg three times daily or an equivalent oral preparation may be adequate. However, moderate to severe iron deficiency can develop and the use of parenteral iron (iron gluconate or iron sucrose) should be considered.[103]

In an observational study of 200 HIV-infected patients, low testosterone levels were associated with anemia, and the use of supplemental androgens was associated with a decreased odds of anemia.[104] Supplemental testosterone or other androgens have not otherwise been assessed and cannot be recommended in the treatment of anemia.

Neutropenia

Infection with HIV affects lymphocytes, neutrophils, and macrophages/monocytes. The hallmark of HIV infection is progressive and profound depletion of CD4+ T-lymphocytes, presumably through direct viral invasion of these cells and enhanced cytolysis and apoptosis.[51,105] Infection of macrophages and monocytes also occurs and may result in significant perturbation of the complex network of growth factor and cytokine generation seen with HIV infection.

Among patients with early symptomatic HIV infection, 10–30% are neutropenic, and this may progress to 75% of those with frank AIDS.[21,22] Myelotoxic medications, including various antiretroviral drugs and drugs used to treat opportunistic infections and malignancies, are the major cause of neutropenia in patients with HIV infection. In addition, impaired myelopoiesis has been described in patients with leukopenia and HIV infection.[106,107] Deficiencies in G-CSF production in response to neutropenia have been described in patients with HIV infection, although the G-CSF response to infection and febrile episodes appears to be normal.[108] About one-third of patients have anti-neutrophil antibodies, but their presence does not appear to correlate with the incidence or severity of neutropenia.[1,109] Accelerated neutrophil apoptosis has also been described in patients with HIV.[110]

Defects in qualitative functions of neutrophils, such as chemotaxis, deficient degranulation responses, inhibition of leukocyte migration, ineffective killing of pathogens, and deficient superoxide generation, have been described in neutrophils from patients with HIV infection.[111,112] *In vitro*, decreased opsonization and intracellular killing of bacterial and fungal organisms by granulocytes have been seen.[113] The clinical importance of these functional neutrophil defects in terms of host defense among HIV-infected individuals is unclear, although an increasing incidence of bacterial infections such as sinusitis and pneumonia does occur in patients with advanced HIV disease. Finally, several medications used to treat HIV and its complications are also associated with the development of neutropenia (Table 67-2).

Neutropenia and Infection

Consistent evidence supports an increased risk of bacterial infection in patients receiving chemotherapy for the treatment of malignancy when the absolute neutrophil count (ANC) falls below 1000 cells/dL. Several studies have also assessed the risk of infection associated with neutropenia in HIV-infected persons, although at a similar degree of neutropenia, the risk appears to be lower than in cancer patients.[109–114] Another study showed that the risk of bacterial infection increased over twofold for an ANC <1000 cells/dL and over sevenfold for an ANC < 500 cells/dL. However, the absolute risk of bacterial infection remained low at 3–5 infections per 100 person-months even for an ANC <500 cells/dL.[115] In other studies, a nadir ANC of <500 cells/dL[116] and an ANC <250 cells/dL[117] were associated with an increased relative risk of bacterial infection.

Treatment of Neutropenia

As in the treatment of anemia, there is not an agreed upon threshold ANC level that mandates treatment of neutropenia (Fig. 67-3). The data presented above suggest that an ANC <250 cells/dL and possibly <500 cells/dL are indications for treatment. Similar to anemia, treatment of neutropenia may allow drugs necessary to manage HIV (e.g., zidovudine), important myelosuppressive antibiotics and antitumor drugs to be used in HIV-infected individuals.

Though not as dramatic as the effect of HAART on anemia, the use of HAART has been associated with a nonsignificant improvement in neutropenia.[118] Further data are needed to determine if HAART alone would be recommended for treatment of neutropenia.

In contrast, G-CSF, produced by activated, monocyte-stimulated endothelial cells and fibroblasts, has clearly been shown to increase neutrophil counts and reverse severe neutropenia in patients with HIV infection. Improvement in neutrophil function has also been demonstrated in patients receiving G-CSF. Improvements in chemotaxis, superoxide generation, and neutrophil killing of bacterial pathogens have been demonstrated with G-CSF.[119] Reduction in accelerated apoptosis of neutrophils with HIV was also seen with G-CSF.[120] Open-label

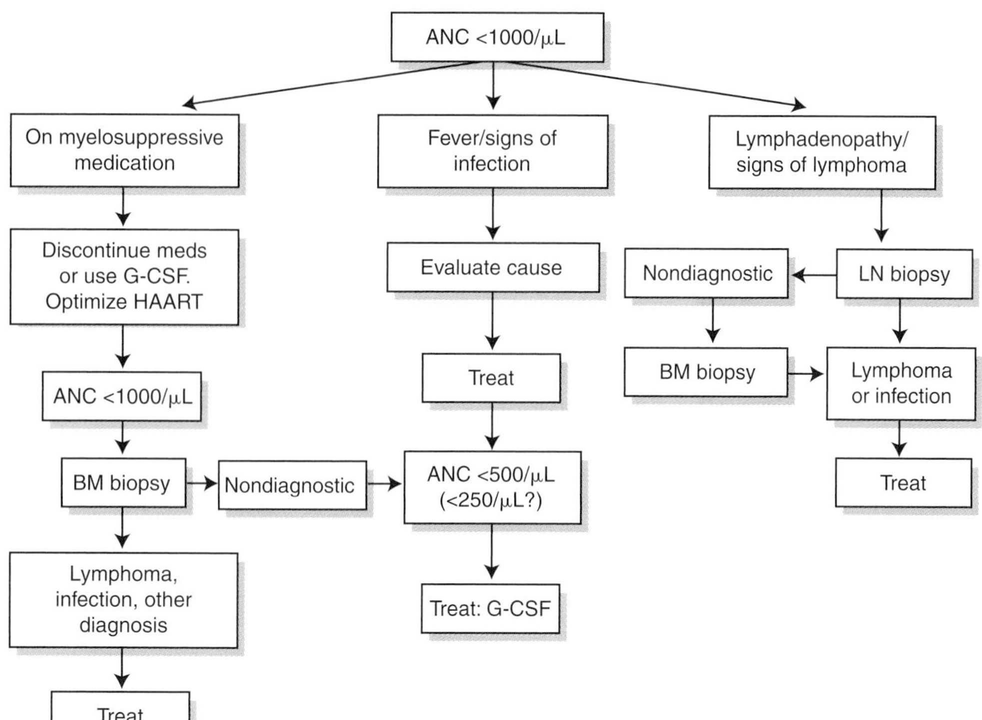

Figure 67-3 ■ Schema for evaluation of neutropenia in HIV infection.

studies of G-CSF for the treatment of neutropenia in patients with HIV infection have shown almost universal correction of neutropenia that is maintained for long periods of time with induction doses of 1–4 μg kg^{-1} day^{-1} followed by a maintenance dose of 300 μg one to seven times a week.[121] No significant changes in CD4+ or CD8+ T-cell counts or in HIV replication have been seen.[121,122]

Clinical studies have shown that G-CSF allows myelosuppressive medications to be given as scheduled and permits additional myelosuppressive drugs to be added when necessary.[121,123–125] In a large, multicenter trial that included more than 200 neutropenic HIV-infected patients, G-CSF reversed neutropenia in 98%, with a mean time of 2 days to reversal. G-CSF also allowed more than 84% of patients to increase or maintain doses of myelosuppressive medications or add them to their therapy.[121] Epoetin alpha may be combined with G-CSF in patients with both neutropenia and anemia with good multilineage effects.[126]

G-CSF may reduce infectious complications associated with neutropenia, including the need for hospitalization and the use of intravenous antibiotics. Improvements in survival have been seen in HIV-infected patients receiving G-CSF compared to those not receiving this agent in retrospective studies of patients with advanced HIV disease in general and in HIV patients with MAC infections.[125,127–130] In a large randomized study, the use of G-CSF to prevent severe neutropenia (ANC <500 cells/μL) was studied in 258 moderately neutropenic (ANC 750–1000 cells/μL) HIV-infected individuals with CD4+ T-lymphocyte counts of less than 200 cells/ μL.[129] Patients were randomized to receive subcutaneous G-CSF (either 1.0 μg kg^{-1} day^{-1} or 300 μg two to five times per week, titrated to maintain the ANC between 2000 and 10 000 cells/μL) or to an observational control group. The incidence of severe neutropenia was significantly lower during the 24-week study period in the groups of patients receiving G-CSF (1.7%) compared with controls, (22%) (P <0.001). The incidence of all bacterial infections was 31% lower in the G-CSF-treated group (2.93/1000 vs 4.24/1000 patient-days). G-CSF-treated patients also had 54% fewer severe bacterial infections and required less frequent use of intravenous antibiotics than control patients. No difference in plasma HIV-1 RNA levels was seen between the groups. This suggests that G-CSF is effective in preventing severe neutropenia and reducing the incidence of bacterial infections in HIV-infected individuals. A longer-acting pegylated form of G-CSF is now available that has the potential to simplify the management of neutropenia by allowing for less frequent dosing.[131]

The growth factor, granulocyte/macrophage colony-stimulating factor (GM-CSF), is produced primarily by stimulated fibroblasts and endothelial cells, and is also produced by T-cells. Administration of GM-CSF, as with G-CSF, results in a dose-dependent elevation in neutrophils. The kinetic basis of the elevation in neutrophils differs from that of G-CSF in that GM-CSF prolongs the circulating half-life of neutrophils rather than decreasing the production time.[132] Unlike G-CSF, GM-CSF results in a significant increase in eosinophils and monocytes.[132] Corrections of granulocyte and macrophage/ monocyte functional defects have been noted in patients receiving this drug where deficiencies have been observed.[133] Additionally, enhancement of antimicrobial function of leukocytes has been demonstrated in several *in vitro* studies.

Factors GM-CSF and G-CSF have different effects on HIV-infected cells.[126,132,134,135] Whereas G-CSF does not seem to alter HIV replication in cells that are targets for the growth factor, GM-CSF may stimulate HIV replication *in vitro* in infected monocytes.[135–137] However, other data indicate that GM-CSF inhibits HIV replication in monocytes and macrophages.[138] When GM-CSF is administered in conjunction with zidovudine, the result is enhanced antiviral effects seen *in vitro*, perhaps because of an increase in the concentration of the phosphorylated active form of the drug in monocytes.[135] However, in a randomized trial of GM-CSF in 105 HIV-infected patients receiving nucleoside reverse transcriptase inhibitor therapy, those who received GM-CSF had a greater reduction in HIV RNA than those patients who received antiretroviral therapy alone.[139] A study of GM-CSF in HIV-infected individuals refractory to antiretroviral therapy also demonstrated some enhancement of the antiretroviral effect of protease inhibitors.[140] In contrast, another randomized placebo-controlled clinical trial of 116 patients on stable antiretroviral therapy who received GM-CSF three times a week for 16 weeks, followed by open-label treatment for an additional 32 weeks demonstrated greater HIV RNA levels (+0.48 vs −0.13 log copies/mL, $P = 0.036$) in the GM-CSF group.[141]

Thrombocytopenia

Although granulocytopenia and anemia may occur concomitantly and their severity appears to parallel the course of HIV infection, thrombocytopenia (Fig. 67-4) can occur independently of other cytopenias and at all stages of HIV infection.[1,32,142–144] Thrombocytopenia to one degree or another occurs in 30–60% of HIV-infected patients.[145–147] Most patients with HIV-related immune thrombocytopenia have only minor submucosal bleeding, characterized by petechiae, ecchymosis, and occasional epistaxis. Rare patients have gastrointestinal blood loss. Splenomegaly occurs in some individuals with HIV-associated thrombocytopenia. Laboratory findings include isolated thrombocytopenia with typically normal peripheral blood smears and nonspecific bone marrow findings except for increased numbers of megakaryocytes. Sullivan found a 1-year incidence of thrombocytopenia (<50 000 /μL) in the AASHD of 8.7% in patient with clinical AIDS, 3.1% in immunologic AIDS and 1.7% in HIV-infected without AIDS,[47] however, thrombocytopenia has not been as directly correlated with the stage of HIV infection in all studies.[148] As with anemia and neutropenia, the use of certain drugs is associated with thrombocytopenia (Table 67-2).

Etiology

Idiopathic thrombocytopenic purpura (ITP) with immune destruction of platelets is the major cause of thrombocytopenia in HIV-infected patients. ITP can result in bruising

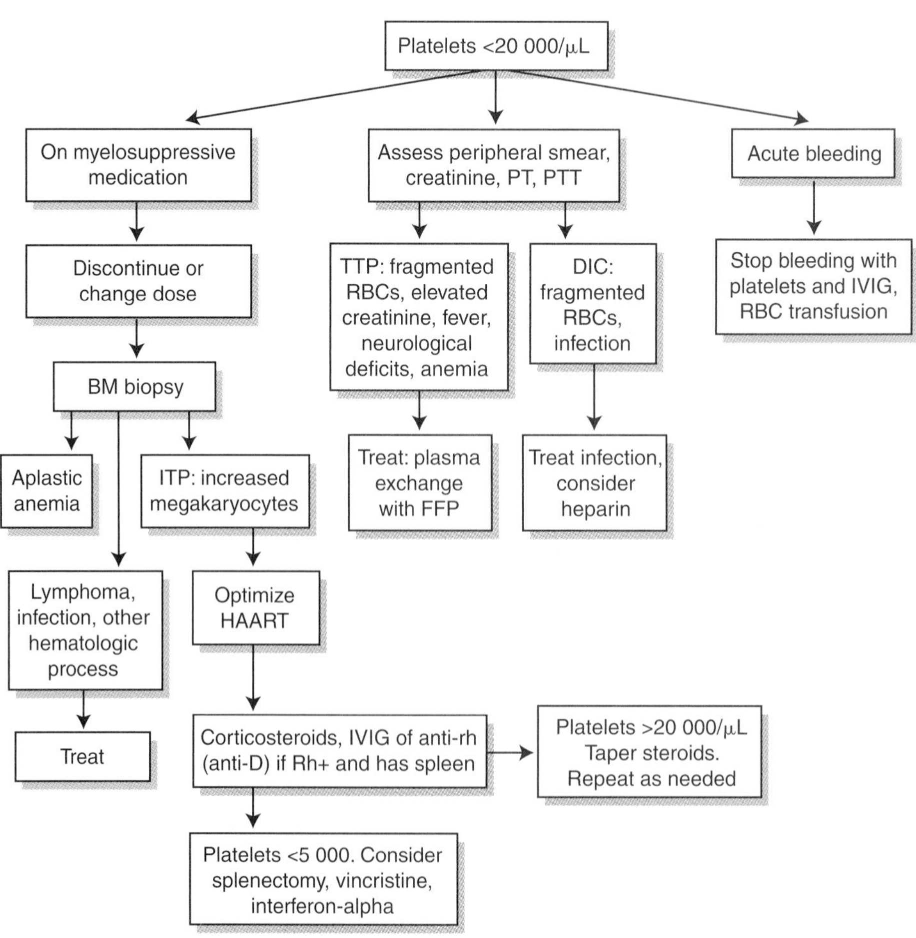

Figure 67-4 ■ Schema for evaluation of thrombocytopenia in HIV infection.

or bleeding from the mucous membranes and skin, yet ITP-related bleeding in HIV infection is less common than with *de novo* ITP, with a relatively low risk of bleeding until the platelet count is <10 000/μL.[149] In many patients with HIV infection antibodies coat the platelets.[149–157] Nonspecific binding of immune complexes to platelets and more specific molecular mimicry between gpl60/120 antigens of HIV and the gpIIb/IIIa of platelets lead to specific platelet-associated antibodies.[149–151,158] Another hypothesis holds that a specific IgG antiplatelet antibody binds to a 25 kDa antigen on the platelet membrane, resulting in platelet destruction.[141] Nonspecific binding of anti-HIV immune complexes to the platelet Fc receptor may make platelets more susceptible to phagocytosis by macrophages.[158,159] There is no direct correlation between the presence of platelet-associated antibodies and the platelet count because of additional defective reticuloendothelial clearance of platelets in HIV-infected patients.[153] In addition to immune destruction, peripheral destruction of platelets occurs as a result of infections and fevers that reduce the life span of circulating platelets, as well as other nonimmune destruction of circulating platelets such as occurs with TTP, which have been described in patients with HIV.[141,160–162]

A less common cause of thrombocytopenia is reduced bone marrow production. Reduction in the productive capacity of megakaryocytes may be due to direct suppression of platelet production by HIV because megakaryocytes are potential targets of infection for the virus.[163,164] Subpopulations of megakaryocytes express CD4[165,166] and CXCR-4.[167,168] It has also been shown that HIV can be internalized by megakaryocytes.[165] HIV may also indirectly suppress platelet production by exposing or altering antigen expression on the surface of megakaryocytes, which renders them targets of anti-platelet antibodies.[158] Alteration in cytokine and growth factor production during HIV infection may also modify platelet production.[163]

Treatment of Thrombocytopenia

Most evaluations of various treatments for HIV-associated thrombocytopenia are hampered by the relative lack of well-controlled, prospectively randomized trials of various treatment options for HIV-associated thrombocytopenia. Spontaneous remissions have been reported in 1–20% of patients.[154] In many with sustained decreases of platelet counts, therapy is not always necessary because the incidence of significant bleeding is low despite low platelet counts.[141,154] It is difficult to predict the risk of bleeding based solely on platelet counts.[154,155]

Thrombocytopenia associated with HIV infection may be corrected with the administration of zidovudine (Fig. 67-4). Zidovudine elevates the platelet count in at least 30% of treatment-naive patients within 12 weeks of initiating therapy.[156,157] Doses of 1000 mg/day are most effective.[169] The mechanism by which zidovudine increases platelet counts is unknown. Anecdotal responses and small case series have also indicated that other effective antiretroviral treatment will improve thrombocytopenia,[170–174] although there are no prospective, randomized controlled trials of the efficacy of HAART in treating thrombocytopenia. One small study suggested that dapsone may also elevate platelet counts.[175]

Corticosteroids and immunoglobulin therapy can be initiated for patients needing immediate restoration of platelet counts. Corticosteroids elevate platelet counts in 40–80% of patients with HIV-associated thrombocytopenia, although long-term remission occurs in only 10–20% of patients.[141,155] Although chronic low-dose corticosteroids may be effective in maintaining an acceptable platelet count,[155] side-effects of long-term corticosteroid use preclude their routine use. Infusion of gamma globulin (400 mg kg^{-1} day^{-1} for 4–5 days) may be used to increase the platelet count rapidly, although its effect is transient, lasting 2–3 weeks.[176] Acute response rates of 70–90% have been reported,[141,177] although sustained remission from a single course of such therapy occurs in fewer than 10% of patients.[141] A higher dose, 1000–2000 mg/kg over 2–5 days, resulted in responses in 20/22 HIV-infected individuals with the mean platelet count increasing from 22 000 to 182 000/μL. Repeat infusions of IVIG every 3 weeks were required in 75% of the patients.[178] The high cost and transient nature of immunoglobulin therapy limit its use to situations of acute bleeding or as a preoperative intervention for patients undergoing splenectomy, when rapid elevation of platelet count is necessary.

A similar response has been seen with anti-Rh antibody (anti-D), which produces a short-term response of 75% and a more sustained platelet response than with gamma globulin.[179] As with gamma globulin infusion, re-administration is effective in elevating the platelet count in patients who respond initially.[141,180] The mechanism of its effect is the binding of anti-Rh-coated Rh-positive red blood cells to the Fc receptor of macrophages in the spleen. The red blood cells compete with the antibody-coated platelets. As there is likely to be red blood cell hemolysis because of phagocytosis of the bound red blood cells in the spleen, the hemoglobin level should tolerate a 1–2 g/dL decrease, and anti-D is generally not effective with splenectomized patients or those who are Rh-negative. Fever and chills may occur in 5–10% of patients. Immunoglobulin infusion and anti-D may also work by increasing the production of thrombopoietic cytokines, such as IL-6, from cells of the reticuloendothelial system in addition to decreasing platelet destruction, anti-D has the advantage of requiring lesser amounts of antibody to be administered than gamma globulin.[181] Anti-D is only 5–10% the cost of gamma globulin.

Splenectomy is also a successful therapeutic intervention for patients who fail to respond to corticosteroid therapy and is generally not associated with greater morbidity or mortality than in patients with non-HIV-associated thrombocytopenia.[182,183] Splenectomy has a short-term response rate in 60–100%, with durable responses occurring in 40–60% of patients.[141] No demonstrated detrimental effects of splenectomy have been seen on progression.[184] This procedure can, however, result in artificial elevation of CD4+ T-lymphocyte counts because of peripheral lymphocytosis.[184] In a study of 68 patients who had splenectomy performed to treat HIV-ITP after an average of 13 months on medical therapies, 92% had a response with the mean platelet count increasing from 18000 to 223000/μL. There was no evidence of shortened survival or increased rate of AIDS progression compared to 117 patients with HIV-ITP who were not splenectomized.[182] Similar results were seen in a series of 22 patients with HIV-ITP.[185] There is an increased risk of infection with *Streptococcus pneumoniae* and *Haemophilus influenzae*,[182] emphasizing the need for prophylactic vaccination before surgery.

A small uncontrolled study of splenic irradiation as an alternative to splenectomy has also demonstrated a short-term response rate of 70% with a durable response occurring in 40% in small numbers of patients.[186,187] The total dose used was 900–1000 cGy administered over the course of a month.

For patients who do not require immediate increases in platelet count, the institution of or alteration in antiretroviral therapy is warranted to suppress HIV. Other modalities of treatment include vincristine and anabolic steroids, with an overall response rate of ~10%.[188,189] Interferon alpha has also been shown in controlled trials to have some efficacy in zidovudine-resistant HIV-associated thrombocytopenia.[190] One potential mechanism by which interferon alpha restores platelet production may be by increasing the levels of IL-6, a cytokine with trophic effects on megakaryocytes.[191] Partial responses to interferon alpha appear to be more common than complete normalization of the platelet count, and the drug is generally well tolerated at doses of 3 million units given subcutaneously three times a week.[192,193] The nonandrogenizing testosterone danazole was thought initially to reverse HIV-ITP, but has not proved efficacious in large-scale trials.[188]

The potential use of pegylated recombinant human megakaryocyte growth and development factor (PEG-rHuMGDF) and recombinant human thrombopoietin (rHu-TPO) in patients with HIV-induced thrombocytopenia has become of interest. PEG-rHuMGDF has been given twice weekly to HIV-positive-thrombocytopenic patients, and their platelet counts rose 10-fold within 14 days and were sustained for the 16 weeks of the study before falling to baseline levels within 14 days of discontinuing therapy.[194,195]

COAGULATION ABNORMALITIES ASSOCIATED WITH HIV INFECTION

Coagulation abnormalities are frequently encountered in patients with HIV infection. The most common is the lupus anticoagulant, which is one of several antibodies to acidic phospholipids that can occur as a result of the abnormal immune responses seen with HIV infection. An incidence of 20–66% has been reported for the lupus anticoagulant in patients with HIV infection.[196–199] The IgG or IgM antibody titer increases with active opportunistic infections. The presence of this anti-phospholipid antibody is established by the use of phospholipid-dependent coagulation assays such as the activated partial thromboplastin time (aPTT) or the Russell viper venom clotting time; or is confirmed on an enzyme-linked immunosorbent assay.[198,201] These antibodies may give false-positive test results for the Venereal Disease Research Laboratory (VDRL) and anticardiolipin antibody assays. The most commonly seen abnormality is an elevation in the aPTT that is not corrected with 1:1 mixing of normal and patient plasma. The prothrombin time may be prolonged to a mild degree in ~10% of patients who have the lupus anticoagulant. Also abnormal is the dilute thromboplastin inhibition assay and the Russell viper venom clotting time. There is also evidence of deficiency of heparin cofactor II[202] and anticardiolipin antibodies,[203] though the clinical significance of this in HIV infection is not known.

Once thought to be clinically insignificant, the lupus anticoagulant in HIV-infected patients may be associated with major thromboembolic events.[200,201] Thromboembolic events may also occur as a result of reduced production of active protein S. This peptide is a cofactor for protein C by localizing active protein C to the phospholipid surface. Free protein S levels are statistically lower in HIV-infected patients with or without thrombosis than in healthy controls.[204,205] The total protein S level does not correlate with the CD4+ T-lymphocyte count or the stage of the HIV infection. Protein S binds to C4b-binding protein. The chronic inflammatory state encountered with HIV infection results in increased C4b-binding protein and more binding of protein S by C4b-binding protein, so less is available to prevent abnormal thrombotic events.[204] In addition, higher levels of antiprotein S antibodies have been detected that may bind protein C.[206] Anticoagulant therapy is appropriate in patients with documented deficiencies of protein S.

Clinical data now indicate that the incidence of thrombotic disease is increased in HIV-infected individuals.[207] The AASHD found an incidence of thrombosis of 2.6/1000 person-years of time. Risk factors included older age, concomitant AIDS-defining and other infections, immobility, and use of Megace.[207] Other observational studies provide further supporting evidence of an increased incidence of thrombotic disease in HIV infection.[208–213] A recent systematic review of venous thromboembolic disease in HIV infection assessed ten relevant epidemiologic studies which showed a two- to 10-fold increase in the incidence compared to a healthy population of the same age. Since most of these studies were retrospective and confounding factors were not always addressed, the authors recommended further study to better establish this association.[214]

TTP results from deficiency of von Willebrand factor-cleaving protease activity (vWF-cp). Plasma exchange is the recommended therapy. In a case series of eight HIV-infected patients with TTP, all recovered with the use of plasma exchange and HAART. Normalization of vWF-cp activity was associated with recovery. Relapse occurred in two patients who discontinued HAART.[215] A case report from the University of Alabama supports the effectiveness of HAART for TTP even when plasma exchange is ineffective.[216]

The Collaborations in Human Immunodeficiency Virus Outcomes Research/US (CHORUS) cohort found a prevalence of 0.3% of thrombotic miroangiopathy (TMA) with incidences per 100 person-years of 0.079 for TMA, 0.009 for TTP, and 0.069 for hemolytic-uremic syndrome. Factors associated with TMA included more advanced immunosuppression and AIDS, a higher HIV RNA level, and infection with *M. avium* complex and hepatitis C.[217] TMA was also found in 7% of 350 consecutively hospitalized HIV-infected patients in a Baltimore cohort.[218]

Infection with CMV and herpes simplex virus types 1 and 2 may affect normal vascular endothelial cells and their procoagulant expression. Alterations of the surface phospholipid expression may activate the coagulation system locally and result in microangiopathies, such as TTP and other localized coagulation defects.[160,161,219]

OTHER BONE MARROW ABNORMALITIES

Bone marrow in most patients with HIV infection exhibits nonspecific morphologic abnormalities[2,24,220] that increase with progression of HIV infection.[1,101,221] Hypercellularity occurs in 50–60% of patients and does not seem to correlate with peripheral cell counts or with the stage of HIV infection.[2,220] The myeloid/erythroid cell ratio tends to be normal or to exhibit a mild myeloid predominance. Hypocellularity of the marrow is rare, and is usually a manifestation of advanced HIV disease. Atrophy or necrosis of the bone marrow may be seen in the late stages of HIV infection.[101]

Dysplasia of one or more cell lines occurs in 30–70% of HIV-infected patients.[222,223] This dysplasia may be indistinguishable from myelodysplastic syndrome.[25,222] Dysplasia of the granulocyte series is most common, with vacuolation of peripheral neutrophils and granulocyte precursors in the marrow often seen.[222] The degree of dysplastic changes in the bone marrow increases with progression of HIV infection and with concurrent opportunistic infections.

Other common abnormalities in the bone marrow include lymphoid aggregates, which are encountered in 20% of patients and may be seen in patients even with peripheral lymphopenia.[222] About 20% of patients with advanced HIV infection have focal or diffuse increases in reticulin deposits in the marrow. Other nonspecific morphologic changes seen in the bone marrow with HIV infection include eosinophilia, plasmacytosis, and histiocytic erythrophagocytosis.[1,220,222,224,225]

The bone marrow is also involved in about one-third of patients with AIDS-related lymphoma. The extent of bone marrow replacement by these malignant cells does not correlate well with peripheral blood counts.[226] Several opportunistic infections can also involve the bone marrow and contribute to bone marrow failure. Bone marrow may reveal disseminated mycobacterial or fungal infections long before other indications of the infection become apparent in the AIDS patient.[227,228] Small studies have shown that bone marrow examination or cultures are positive for mycobacteria or fungi in at least 75% of patients who are subsequently found to have these infections.[227–229] The most common manifestation of these infections is diffuse infiltration of bone marrow with the organisms, with loose aggregates and clusters of macrophages. These cells may organize into granulomas, which are less prominent in the presence of more advanced disease. Pseudo-Gaucher cells may also be a manifestation of these infections.[230] Marrow involvement with fungal or mycobacterial organisms may also result in marrow fibrosis.

Cytomegalovirus (CMV) can also infect bone marrow progenitor cells and render them less responsive to colony-stimulating factors.[231] CMV can affect the bone marrow stromal cells as well, interfering with their hematopoietic supporting function largely by decreasing local growth factor production by these cells.[231] CMV does not cause distinctive histologic changes of the bone marrow. It is best cultured from the buffy coat of blood and not from the bone marrow itself.

Human herpesvirus-6 (HHV-6) targets CD4+ T-lymphocytes and monocytes.[232,233] Immunosuppression as a result of HIV infection may result in loss of latency of this virus. Subsequent exposure of bone marrow precursor cells to this virus may inhibit their ability to respond to growth factors. Infection of T lymphocytes by this virus may also cause further suppression of T-cell function. Despite these laboratory observations, the clinical relevance of HHV-6 in this population is unclear.

REFERENCES

1. Scadden DT, Zon LI, Groopman GE. Pathophysiology and management of HIV-associated hematologic disorders. Blood 74:1455–63, 1989.
2. Calenda V, Chermann JC. The effects of HIV on hematopoiesis. Eur J Haematol 48:181–6, 1992.
3. Sugiura K, Oyaizu N, Pahwa R. Effect of human immunodeficiency virus-1 envelope glycoprotein on in vitro hematopoiesis of umbilical cord blood. Blood 80:1463–69, 1992.
4. Louache F, Debili N, Marandin A, et al. Expression of CD4 by human hematopoietic progenitors. Blood 84:3344–55, 1994.
5. Zauli G, Furlini G, Vitale M, et al. A subset of human CD34+ hematopoietic progenitors express low levels of CD4, the high-affinity receptor for human immunodeficiency virus-type 1. Blood 84:1896–905, 1994.
6. Deichmann M, Kronenwett R, Haas R. Expression of the human immunodeficiency virus type-1 coreceptors CXCR-4 (fusin, LESTR) and CKR-5 in CD34+ hematopoietic progenitor cells. Blood 89:3522–8, 1997.
7. Bagnara G, Zauli G, Gionvannini M, et al. Early loss of circulating hematopoietic progenitor in human immunodeficiency virus I infected cells. Exp Hematol 18:426–30, 1990.
8. Shen H, Cheng T, Preffer FI, et al. Intrinsic human immunodeficiency virus type 1 resistance of hematopoietic stem cells despite coreceptor expression. J Virol 73:728–37, 1999.
9. Koka PS, Jamieson BD, Brooks DG, Zack JA. Human immunodeficiency virus type 1 induced hematopoietic inhibition is independent of productive infection of progenitor cells in vivo. J Virol 73:9089–97, 1999.
10. Molina JM, Scadden DT, Sakaguchi M, et al. Lack of evidence for infection of or effect on growth of hematopoietic progenitor cells after in vivo or in vitro exposure to human immunodeficiency virus. Blood 76:2476–82, 1990.
11. Moses AU, Williams S, Henevild ML, et al. Human immunodeficiency virus infection of bone marrow endothelium reduces induction of stromal hematopoietic growth factors. Blood 87:919–25, 1996.
12. Re MC, Zauli G, Furlini G, et al. GM-CSF production by CD4+ T lymphocytes is selectively impaired during the course

of HIV-l infection: a possible indication of a preferential lesion of a specific subset of peripheral blood CD4+ T-lymphocytes. Microbiologica 15:265–70, 1992.
13. Re MC, Zauli G, Gibellini D, et al. Uninfected haematopoietic progenitor (CD34+) cells purified from the bone marrow of AIDS patients are committed to apoptotic cell death in culture. AIDS 7:1049–55, 1993.
14. Dubois CM, Ruscetti RW, Stankova J, et al. Transforming growth factor-beta regulates c-kit message stability and cell surface protein expression in hematopoietic progenitors. Blood 83:3138–45, 1994.
15. Scadden DT, Zeira M, Woon A, et al. Human immunodeficiency virus infection of human bone marrow stromal fibroblasts. Blood 76:317–22, 1990.
16. Maciejewski JP, Weichold FF, Young NS. HIV-1 suppression of hematopoiesis in vitro mediated by envelope glycoprotein and TNF-α. J Immunol 153:4304–10, 1994.
17. Berman MA, Zaldivar F Jr, Imfeld KL, et al. HIV-1 infection of macrophages promotes long-term survival and sustained release of interleukins 1-α and 6. AIDS Res Hum Retroviruses 10:529–39, 1994.
18. Schwartz BN, Kessler SW, Rothwell SW, et al. Inhibitory effects of HIV-1 infected stromal cell layers on the production of myeloid progenitor cells in human long term bone barrow cultures. Exp Hematol 22:1288–96, 1994.
19. Zauli G, Re MC, Furlini G, et al. Human immunodeficiency virus type 1 envelope glycoprotein gp120-mediated killing of human haematopoietic progenitors (CD34+ cells). J Gen Viral 73:417–21, 1992.
20. Kulkosky J, Laptev A, Shetty S, et al. Human immunodeficiency virus type 1 Vpr alters bone marrow cell function. Blood 93:1906–15, 1999.
21. Zon L, Arkin C, Groopman JE. Hematologic manifestations of the human immunodeficiency virus (HIV). Semin Hematol 25:208–19, 1988.
22. Mitsuyasu R. AIDS Clin Review 1993/4. Marcel Dekker, New York, NY 1993:189–210.
23. Moses A, Nelson J, Bagby GC Jr. The influence of human immunodeficiency virus-1 on hematopoiesis. Blood 91:1479–95, 1998.
24. Hambleton J. Hematologic complications of HIV infection. Oncology 10:671–80, 1996.
25. Ganser A. Abnormalities of hematopoiesis in the acquired immunodeficiency syndrome. Blut 56:49–53, 1988.
26. Belperio PS, Rhew DC. Prevalence and outcomes of anemia in individuals with human immunodeficiency virus: a systematic review of the literature. Am J Med 116(Suppl 7A):27S–43S, 2004.
27. Sullivan PS, Hanson DL, Chu SY, et al. Epidemiology of anemia in human immunodeficiency virus (HIV)-infected persons: results from the Multi-State Adult and Adolescent Spectrum of HIV Disease Surveillance Project. Blood 91: 301–8, 1998.
28. Levine AM, Berhane K, Masri-Lavine L, et al. Prevalence and correlates of anemia in a large cohort of HIV-infected women: women's interagency HIV study. J Acquir Immune Defic Syndr 26:28–35, 2001.
29. Semba RD, Shah N, Klein RS, et al. Prevalence and cumulative incidence of and risk factors for anemia in a multicenter cohort study of human immunodeficiency virus-infected and uninfected women. Clin Infect Dis 34:260–6, 2002.
30. Fangman JJ, Scadden DT. Anemia in HIV-infected adults: epidemiology, pathogenesis, and clinical management. Curr Hematol Rep 4:95–102, 2005.
31. Dancheck B, Tang AM, Thomas AM, et al. Injection drug use is an independent risk factor for iron deficiency and iron deficiency anemia among HIV-seropositive and HIV-seronegative women. J Acquir Immune Defic Syndr 40:198–201, 2005.
32. Evans RH, Scadden DT. Haematological aspects of HIV infection. Ballieres Clin Haematol 13:215–30, 2000.
33. Moore RD. Human immunodeficiency virus infection, anemia, and survival. Clin Infect Dis 29:44–9, 1999.
34. Moore RD, Keruly JC, Chaisson RE. Anemia and survival in HIV infection. J Acquir Immune Defic Syndr 19:29–33, 1998.
35. Mocroft A, Kirk O, Barton SE, et al. Anaemia is an independent predictive marker for clinical prognosis in HIV-infected patients from across Europe. AIDS 13:943–50, 1999.
36. Berhane K, Karim R, Cohen MH, et al. Impact of highly active antiretroviral therapy on anemia and relationship between anemia and survival in a large cohort of HIV-infected women: women's interagency HIV study. J Acquir Immune Defic Syndr 37:1245–52, 2004.
37. Deschamps MM, Fitzgerald DW, Pape JW, et al. HIV infection in Haiti: natural history and disease progression. AIDS 14:2515–21, 2000.
38. O'Brien ME, Kupka R, Msamanga GI, et al. Anemia is an independent predictor of mortality and immunologic progression of disease among women with HIV in Tanzania. J Acquir Immune Defic Syndr 40:219–25, 2005.
39. Graham N, Piantadosi S, Park LP, et al. CD4+ lymphocyte response to zidovudine as a predictor of AIDS-free time and survival time. J AIDS 6:1258–66, 1993.
40. McArthur J, Hoover DR, Bacellar H, et al. Dementia in AIDS patients: incidence and risk factors. Multicenter AIDS Cohort Study. Neurology 43:2245–52, 1993.
41. Sathe SS, Gascone P, Lo W, et al. Severe anemia is an important negative predictor for survival with disseminated *Mycobacterium avium-intracellulare* in acquired immunodeficiency syndrome. Am Rev Respir Dis 142:1306–12, 1990.
42. Lundgren JD, Mocroft A, Gatell JM, et al. A clinically prognostic scoring system for patients receiving highly active antiretroviral therapy: results from the EuroSIDA study. J Infect Dis 185:178–87, 2002.
43. Demetri G, Wade J, Cella D. Epoetin alfa improves quality of life in cancer patients receiving cytotoxic treatment independent of disease response: prospective clinical trial results. Blood 90:175a, 1997.
44. Glaspy J, Bukowski R, Steinberg D, et al. Impact of therapy with epoetin alfa on clinical outcomes in patients with nonmyeloid malignancies during cancer chemotherapy in community oncology practice. J Clin Oncol 15:1218–34, 1997.
45. Gabrilove JL, Cleeland CS, Livingston RB, et al. Clinical evaluation of once weekly dosing of epoetin alfa in chemotherapy patients: improvements in hemoglobin and quality of life are similar to three times weekly dosing. J Clin Oncol 19:2875–82, 2001.
46. Revick DA, Brown RE, Henry DH, et al. Recominant human erythropoietin and health-related quality of life of AIDS patients with anemia. J Acquir Immune Defic Syndr 7:474–84, 1994.
47. Abrams Di, Steinhart C, Frascio R. Epoetin alfa therapy for anemia in HIV infected patients: impact on quality of life. Int J STD AIDS 11:659–65, 1000.
48. Semba RD, Martin BK, Kempen JH, et al. The impact of anemia on energy and physical functioning in individuals with AIDS. Arch Int Med 165:2229–36, 2005.
49. Saag MS, Bowers P, Leitz GJ, et al. Once-weekly epoetin alfa improves quality of life and increases hemoglobin in anemic HIV+ patients. AIDS Res Hum Retroviruses 20:1037–45, 2004.
50. Levine AM. Anemia in the setting of cancer and human immunodeficiency virus. Clin Infect Dis 37(Suppl 4):S304–14, 2003.
51. Fauci A, Schnittman S, Poli G, et al. Immunopathogenic mechanisms in human immunodeficiency virus (HIV) infection. Ann Intern Med 114:678–93, 1991.
52. Zhang Y, Harada A, Bluethmann H, et al. Tumor necrosis factor (TNF) is a physiologic regulator of hematopoietic cells: increase

of early hematopoietic cells in TNF receptor p55-deficient mice in viva and potent inhibition of progenitor cell proliferation by TNF in vitro. Blood 86:2930–7, 1995.
53. Spivak JL, Barnes DC, Fuchs E, Quinn TC. Serum immunoreactive erythropoietin in HIV infected patients. JAMA 261:3104–7, 1989.
54. Geene D, Sudre P, Anwar D, et al. Causes of macrocytosis in HIV-infected patients not treated with zidovudine. Swiss HIV Cohort Study. J Infect 40:160–3, 2000.
55. Eyer-Silva WA, Arabe J, Pinto JF, Morais-De-SA CA. Macrocytosis in patients on stavudine. Scan J Infect Dis 33:239–40, 2001.
56. Richman DD, Fischl MA, Grieco MH, et al. The toxicity of azidothymidine (AZT) in the treatment of patients with AIDS and AIDS-related complex. N Engl J Med 317:192–7, 1987.
57. Gascon P, Sathe S, Rameshwar P. Impaired erythropoiesis in the acquired immunodeficiency syndrome with disseminated *Mycobacterium avium* complex. Am J Med 94:41–8, 1993.
58. Jacobson MA, Hopewell PC, Yajiko DM, et al. Natural history of disseminated *Mycobacterium avium* complex infection in AIDS. J Infect Dis 164:994–8, 1991.
59. Koduri PR. Parvovirus B19 anemia in HIV-infected patients. AIDS Patient Care STDS 14:7–11, 2000.
60. Gyllensten K, Sonnerborg A, Jorup-Ronstrom C, et al. Parvovirus B19 infection in HIV-1 infected patients with anemia. Infection 22:356–8, 1994.
61. Chernak E, Dubin G, Henry D, et al. Infection due to parvovirus B19 in patients infected with human immunodeficiency virus. Clin Infect Dis 20:170–3, 1995.
62. Naides S, Howard EJ, Swack NS, et al. Parvovirus B19 infection in HIV type 1-infected persons failing or intolerant to zidovudine therapy. J Infect Dis 168:101–5, 1993.
63. Bremner J, Beard B, Cohen A, et al. Secondary infection with parvovirus B19 in an HIV-positive patient. AIDS 7:1131–2, 1993.
64. Gupta S, Inman A, Licorish K. Serum ferritin in acquired immune deficiency syndrome. J Clin Lab Immunol 20:11–13, 1986.
65. Harriman GR, Smith PD, Horne MK, et al. Vitamin B_{12} malabsorption in patients with acquired immunodeficiency syndrome. Arch Intern Med 149:2039–41, 1989.
66. Herbert V, Fong W, Gulle V, Stopler T. Low holotranscobalamin: It is the earliest serum marker for subnormal vitamin B_{12} (Cobalamin) absorption in patients with AIDS. Am J Hematol 34:132–9, 1990.
67. Remacha AF, Riera A, Cadafalch J, et al. Vitamin B_{12} abnormalities in HIV-infected patients. Eur J Haematol 47:60–4, 1991.
68. Remacha AF, Cadafalch J. Cobalamin deficiency in patients infected with the human immunodeficiency virus. Semin Hematol 36:75–87, 1999.
69. Beach RS, Mantero-Atienza E, Shor-Posner G, et al. Specific nutrient abnormalities in asymptomatic HIV-1 infection. AIDS 6:701–8, 1991.
70. Ehrenpreis E, Carlson SJ, Boorstein HL, et al. Malabsorption and deficiency of vitamin B_{12} in HIV-infected patients with chronic diarrhea. Dig Dis Sci 39:2159–62, 1994.
71. Paltiel O, Falutz J, Veilleux M, et al. Clinical correlates of subnormal vitamin B_{12} levels in patients infected with the human immunodeficiency virus. Am J Hematol 49:318–22, 1995.
72. Saif MW. HIV-associated autoimmune hemolytic anemia: an update. AIDS Patient Care STDs 15:217–24, 2001.
73. Toy P, Reid M, Burns M. Positive direct antiglobulin test associated with hyperglobulinemia in acquired immunodeficiency syndrome. Am J Hematol 19:145–50, 1985.
74. McGinniss M, Macher A, Rook A, et al. Red cell autoantibodies in patients with acquired immune deficiency syndrome. Transfusion 26:405–9, 1986.
75. Volberding P. Consensus statement: anemia in HIV infection–current trends, treatment options, and practice strategies: anemia in HIV working group. Clin Ther 22:1004–20, 2000.
76. Wu AW, Rubin HR, Mathews WC, et al. A health status questionnaire using 30 items from the Medical Outcomes Study: preliminary validation in persons with early HIV infection. Med Care 29:786–98, 1991.
77. Semba RD, Shah N, Klein RS, et al. Highly active antiretroviral therapy associated with improved anemia among HIV-infected women. AIDS Patient Care STDS 15:473–80, 2001.
78. Semba RD, Shah N, Vlahov D. Improvement of anemia among HIV-infected injection drug users receiving highly active antiretroviral therapy. J Acquir Immune Defic Syndr 26: 315–19, 2001.
79. Moore RD, Forney D. Anemia in HIV infected patients receiving highly active antiretroviral therapy. J Acquir Immune Defic Syndr 29:54–7, 2002.
80. Sarcletti M, Quirchmair G, Weiss G, et al. Increase of haemoglobin levels by antiretroviral therapy is associated with a decrease in immune activation. Eur J Haematol 70:17–25, 2003.
81. Servais J, Nkoghe D, Schmit JC, et al. HIV-associated hematologic disorders are correlated with plasma viral load and improve under highly active antiretroviral therapy. J Acquir Immune Defic Syndr 28:221–5, 2001.
82. Moyle G, Sawyer W, Law M, et al. Changes in hematologic parameters and efficacy of thymidine analogue-based, highly active antiretroviral therapy: a meta-analysis of six prospective, randomized, comparative studies. Clin Ther 26:92–7, 2004.
83. Isgro A, Aiuti A, Leti W, et al. Immunodysregulation of HIV disease at bone marrow level. Autoimmun Rev 4:486–90, 2005.
84. Williams GT, Smith CA, Spooncer E, et al. Haematopoietic colony stimulating factors promote cell survival by suppressing apoptosis. Nature 343:76–9, 1990.
85. Groopman J, Feder D. Hematopoietic growth factors in AIDS. Semin Oncol 19:408–14, 1992.
86. Spivak J, Barnes DC, Fuchs E, et al. Serum immunoreactive erythropoietin in HIV-infected patients. JAMA 261:3104–7, 1989.
87. Fischl M, Galpin JE, Levine JD, et al. Recombinant human erythropoietin for patients with AIDS treated with zidovudine. N Engl J Med 322:1488–93, 1990.
88. Sipas NV, Kokori SI, loannidis JP, et al. Circulating autoantibodies to erythropoietin are associated with human immunodeficiency virus type 1-related anemia. J Infect Dis 180:2044–7, 1999.
89. Erslev A. Erythropoietin. N Engl J Med 324:1339–44, 1991.
90. Henry D, Beall G, Benson C, et al. Recombinant human erythropoietin in the therapy of anemia associated with HIV infection and zidovudine therapy: overview of four clinical trials. Ann Intern Med 117:739–48, 1992.
91. Abrams Dl, Steinhart C, Frascino R. Epoetin alfa therapy for anemia in HIV-infected patients: impact on quality of life. Int J STD AIDS 11:659–65, 2000.
92. Grossman HA, Goon B, Bowers P, et al. Once-weekly epoetin alfa dosing is as effective as three times-weekly dosing in increasing hemoglobin levels and is associated with improved quality of life in anemic HIV-infected patients. J Acquir Immune Defic Syndr 34:368–78, 2003.
93. Sulkowski MS, Dieterich DT, Bini EJ, et al. Epoetin alfa once weekly improves anemia in HIV/hepatitis C virus-coinfected patients treated with interferon/ribavirin: a randomized controlled trial. J Acquir Immune Defic Syndr 39:504–6, 2005.
94. Vansteenkiste J, Wouters I. The use of darbepoetin alfa for the treatment of chemotherapy-induced anaemia. Expert Opin Pharmacother 6:429–40, 2005.
95. Robinson DM, Easthope SE. Darbepoetin alfa: its use in anemia associated with chronic kidney disease. BioDrugs 19: 327–43, 2005.

95a. Singh AK, Szczech L, Tang KL, et al. Correction of anemia with epoetin alfa in chronic kidney diseasae. N Engl J Med 355:2085–98, 2006.
95b. Drueke TB, Locatelli F, Clyne N, et al. Normalization of hemoglobin level in patients with chronic kidney disease and anemia. N Engl J Med 355:2071–84, 2006.
96. Brunson ME, Alexander JW. Mechanisms of transfusion-induced immunosuppression. Transfusion 30:651–8, 1990.
97. Vamvakas E, Kaplan HS. Early transfusion and length of survival in acquired immune deficiency syndrome: experience with a population receiving medical care at a public hospital. Transfusion 33:111–18, 1993.
98. Buskin SE, Sullivan PS. Anemia and its treatment and outcomes in persons infected with human immunodeficiency virus. Transfusion 44:826–32, 2004.
99. Mudido PM, Georges D, Dorazio D, et al. Human immunodeficiency virus type 1 activation after blood transfusion. Transfusion 36:860–5, 1996.
100. Sloand E, Kuman P, Klein HJG, et al. Transfusion of blood components to persons infected with human immunodeficiency virus type 1: relationship to opportunistic infection. Transfusion 34:48–53, 1994.
101. Perkocha LA, Rodgers GM. Hematologic aspects of human immunodeficiency virus infection. Am J Hematol 29:94–105, 1992.
102. Collier AC, Kalish LA, Busch MP, et al. Leukocyte-reduced red blood cell transfusion in patients with anemia and human immunodeficiency virus infection: the Viral Activation Transfusion Study: a randomized controlled trial. JAMA 285:1592–601, 2001.
103. Eschbach JW. Iron requirements in erythropoietin therapy. Best Pract Res Clin Haematol 18:347–61, 2005.
104. Behler C, Shade S, Gregory K, et al. Anemia and HIV in the antiretroviral era: potential significance of testosterone. AIDS Res Hum Retroviruses 21:200–6, 2005.
105. Brizzi M, Porcu P, Porteri A, et al. Haematologic abnormalities in the acquired immunodeficiency syndrome. Haematologica 75:454–63, 1990.
106. Israel D, Plaisance K. Neutropenia in patients infected with human immunodeficiency virus. Clin Pharm 10:268–79, 1990.
107. Leiderman I, Greenberg M, Adlesberg B, et al. A glycoprotein inhibitor of in vitro granulopoiesis associated with AIDS. Blood 70:1267–72, 1987.
108. Mauss S, Steinmetz HT, Willers R, et al. Induction of granulocyte colony-stimulating factor by acute febrile infection but not by neutropenia in HIV-seropositive individuals. J Acquir Immune Defic Syndr 14:430–4, 1997.
109. Donahue R, Johnson M, Zon L. Suppression of in vitro hematopoiesis following human immunodeficiency virus infection. Nature 326:200–3, 1987.
110. Pitrak DL, Mullane KM, Bilek ML, et al. Impaired phagocyte oxidative capacity in patients with human immunodeficiency virus infection. J Lab Clin Med 132:284–93, 1998.
111. Murphy P, Lane C, Fauci A, et al. Impairment of neutrophil bactericidal capacity in patients with AIDS. J Infect Dis 158:627–30, 1998.
112. Valone F, Payan D, Abrams D, et al. Defective polymorphonuclear leukocyte chemotaxis in homosexual men with persistent lymph node syndrome. J Infect Dis 150:267–71, 1984.
113. Elis M, Gupta S, Galant S, et al. Impaired neutrophil function in patients with AIDS or AIDS-related complex: a comprehensive evaluation. J Infect Dis 158:1268–76, 1988.
114. Hermans P, Sommereijns B, Van Cutsen N, Clumeck N. Neutropenia in patients with HIV infection: a case control study in a cohort of 1403 patients between 1982 and 1993. J Hematother Stem Cell Res (Suppl 8):S23–S32, 1999.
115. Moore RD, Keruly J, Chaisson RE, et al. Neutropenia and bacterial infection in acquired immunodeficiency syndrome. Arch Intern Med 155:1965–70, 1995.
116. Moore DA, Benepal T, Portsmouth S, et al. Etiology and natural history of neutropenia in human immunodeficiency virus disease: a prospective study. Clin Infect Dis 32:469–75, 2001.
117. Meynard J-L, Guiguet M, Arsac S, et al. Frequency and risk factors of infectious complications in neutropenic patients infected with HIV. AIDS 11:995–8, 1997.
118. Huang SS, Barbour JD, Deeks SG, et al. Reversal of human immunodeficiency virus type 1 associated hematosuppression by effective antiretroviral therapy. Clin Infect Dis 30:504–10, 2000.
119. Pitrak DL, Bak P, DeMarais P, et al. Depressed neutrophil superoxide production in HIV infection. J Infect Dis 167: 1406–10, 1993.
120. Pitrak DL. Filgrastim treatment of HIV-infected patients improves neutrophil function. AIDS 13(Suppl 2):S25–S30, 1999.
121. Hermans P, Rozenbaum W, Jou A, et al. Filgrastim to treat neutropenia and support myelosuppressive medication dosing in HIV infection. G-CSF 92105 Study Group. AIDS 10: 1627–33, 1996.
122. Davidson M, Min YI, Holbrook JT, et al. Influence of filgrastim (granulocyte colony-stimulating factor) on human immunodeficiency virus type 1 RNA in patients with cytomegalovirus retinitis. J Infect Dis 186:1013–18, 2002.
123. Jacobson MA, Kramer F, Bassiakos Y, et al. Randomized phase I trial of two different combination foscarnet and ganciclovir chronic maintenance therapy regimens for AIDS patients with CMV retinitis: ACTG 151. J Infect Dis 170: 189–93, 1994.
124. Dubreuil-Lemaire ML, Gori A, Vittecoq D, et al. Lenograstim for the treatment of neutropenia in patients receiving ganciclovir for cytomegalovirus infection: a randomized placebo-controlled trial in AIDS patients: GCS3O9 European study group. Eur J Haematol 65:337–43, 2000.
125. Kuritzkes DR. Neutropenia, neutrophil dysfunction, and bacterial infection in patients with human immunodeficiency virus disease: the role of granulocyte colony-stimulating factor. Clin Infect Dis 30:256–60, 2000.
126. Miles SA, Mitsuyasu RT, Moreno J, et al. Combined therapy with recombinant granulocyte colony-stimulating factor and erythropoietin decreases hematologic toxicity from zidovudine. Blood 77:2109–17, 1991.
127. Keiser P, Higgs E, Scanton J. Neutropenia is associated with bacteremia in patients with HIV. Am J Med Sci 312:118–22, 1996.
128. Keiser P, Rademacher S, Smith JW. et al. Granulocyte colony-stimulating factor use is associated with decreased bacteremia and increased survival in neutropenic HIV-infected patients. Am J Med 104:48–55, 1998.
129. Kuritzkes DR, Parenti D, Ward DJ, et al. Filgrastim prevents severe neutropenia and reduces infective morbidity in patients with advanced HIV infection; results of a randomized, multicenter, controlled trial: G-CSF 930101 study group. AIDS 12:65–74, 1998.
130. Keiser P, Rademacher S, Smith J, Skiest D. G-CSF association with prolonged survival in HIV-infected patients with disseminated *Mycobacterium avium* complex infection. Int J STD AIDS 9:394–9, 1998.
131. Lyman GH. Pegfilgrastim: a granulocyte colony-stimulating factor with sustained duration of action. Expert Opin Biol Ther 5:1635–46, 2005.
132. Lieschke GJ, Burgess AW. Granulocyte colony-stimulating factor and granulocyte-macrophage colony-stimulating factor (first of two parts). N Engl J Med 327:28–35, 1992.
133. Baldwin C, Gasson J, Quan S. Granulocyte-macrophage colony-stimulating factor enhances neutrophil function in acquired immunodeficiency syndrome patients. Proc Natl Acad Sci USA 85:2763–6, 1988.

134. Pluda JM, Yarchoan R, Smith PH, et al. Subcutaneous recombinant granulocyte-macrophage colony-stimulating factor used as a single agent and in an alternating regimen with azidothymidine in leukopenic patients with severe human immunodeficiency virus infection. Blood 76:463–72, 1990.
135. Perno CF, Cooney DA, Gao W-Y, et al. Effects of bone marrow stimulatory cytokines on human immunodeficiency virus replication and the antiviral activity of dideoxynucleosides in cultures of monocyte/macrophages. Blood 80:995–1003, 1992.
136. Hammer SM, Gillis JM, Pinkston P, et al. Effect of zidovudine and granulocyte-macrophage colony-stimulating factor on human immunodeficiency virus replication in alveolar macrophages. Blood 75:1215–19, 1990.
137. Koyanagi Y, O'Brien WA, Zhao JQ, et al. Cytokines alter production of HIV-1 from primary mononuclear phagocytes. Science 241:1673–5, 1988.
138. Kedzierska K, Maerz A, Warby T, et al. Granulocyte-macrophage colony stimulating factor inhibits HIV-1 replication in monocyte-derived macrophages. AIDS 14:1739–48, 2000.
139. Jacobson JM, Lederman MM, Spritzler J, Valdez H, et al. Granulocyte-macrophage colony-stimulating factor induces modest increases in plasma human immunodeficiency virus (HIV) type 1 RNA levels and CD4+ lymphocyte counts in patients with uncontrolled HIV infection. J Infect Dis 18:1804–14, 2003.
140. Skowron G, Stein D, Drusano G, et al. The safety and efficacy of granulocyte-macrophage colony-stimulating factor (sargramostim) added to indinavir- or ritonavir-based antiretroviral therapy: a randomized double-blind, placebo controlled trial. J Infect Dis 180:1064–71, 1999.
141. Brites C, Gilbert MJ, Pedral-Sampaio D, et al. A randomized, placebo-controlled trial of granulocyte-macrophage colony stimulating factor and nucleoside analogue therapy in AIDS. J Infect Dis 182:1531–5, 2000.
142. Evatt BL. HIV infection and thrombocytopenia. Curr Hematol Rep 4:149–53, 2005.
143. Pechere M, Samii K, Hirschel B. HIV related thrombocytopenia. N Engl J Med 328:1785–6, 1993.
144. Miguez-Burbano MJ, Jackson J Jr, Hadrigan A. Thrombocytopenia in HIV disease: clinical relevance, physiopathology and management. Curr Med Chem Cardiovasc Hematol Agents 3:365–76, 2005.
145. Stricker RE. Hemostatic abnormalities in HIV disease. Hematol Oncol Clin North Am 5:249–65, 1991.
146. Perkocha LA, Rodgers GM. Hematologic aspects of human immunodeficiency virus infection: laboratory and clinical considerations. Am J Hematol 29:94–105, 1988.
147. Sullivan PS, Hanson DL, Chu SY, et al. Surveillance for thrombocytopenia in persons infected with HIV: results from the multistate Adult and Adolescent Spectrum of Disease Project. J Acquir Immune Defic Syndr 14:374–9, 1997.
148. Holzman RS, Walsh CM, Karpatkin S. Risk for the acquired immunodeficiency syndrome among thrombocytopenic and nonthrombocytopenic homosexual men seropositive for the human immunodeficiency virus. Ann Intern Med 106:383–6, 1987.
149. Bettaieb A, Fromont P, Louache F, et al. Presence of cross-reactive antibody between human immunodeficiency virus (HIV) and platelet glycoproteins in HIV-related immune thrombocytopenic purpura. Blood 80:162–9, 1992.
150. Stanworth DR, Solder B, Lewin IV, et al. Related epitopes in HIV viral coat protein and human IgG. Lancet 1:1458–9, 1989.
151. Gonzalez-Conejero R, Rivera J, Rosillo MC, et al. Association of antibodies against platelet glycoproteins Ib/IX and IIb/IIIa, and platelet reactive anti-HIV antibodies in thrombocytopenic narcotic addicts. Br J Hematol 93:464–71, 1996.
152. Nardi M, Karpatkin S. Anti-idiotype antibody against platelet anti-GPIIIa contributes to the regulation of thrombocytopenia in InV-1-ITP patients. Exp Med 191:2093–100, 2000.
153. Bender BS, Quinn TC, Spival JL. Homosexual men with thrombocytopenia have impaired reticuloendothelial system Fc receptor specific clearance. Blood 70:392–5, 1987.
154. Walsh C, Kriegel R, Lennette E, et al. Thrombocytopenia in homosexual patients. Ann Intern Med 103:542–5, 1985.
155. Karpatkin S. Immunologic thrombocytopenic purpura in HIV-seropositive homosexuals, narcotic addicts and hemophiliacs. Semin Hematol 25:219–29, 1988.
156. Oksenhendler E, Bierling P, Ferchal F. Zidovudine for thrombocytopenia purpura related to human immunodeficiency virus infection. Ann Intern Med 110:365–8, 1989.
157. Swiss Group for Clinical Studies on AIDS. Zidovudine for the treatment of thrombocytopenia associated with human immunodeficiency virus. Ann Intern Med 209:718–21, 1988.
158. Dominguez A, Gamallo G, Garcia R, et al. Pathophysiology of HIV related thrombocytopenia: an analysis of 41 patients. J Clin Pathol 47:999–1003, 1994.
159. Walsh C, Nardi MA, Karpatikin S. On the mechanism of thrombocytopenic purpura in sexually active homosexual men. N Engl J Med 311:635–9, 1984.
160. Leaf AN, Laubenstein LH, Raphael B, et al. Thrombotic thrombocytopenic purpura associated with human immunodeficiency virus type 1 (HIV-1) infection. Ann Intern Med 109:194–7, 1988.
161. Thompson CE, Damon LE, Ries CA, et al. Thrombotic microangiopathies in the 1980s: clinical features, response to treatment, and the impact of the human immunodeficiency virus epidemic. Blood 80:1890–5, 1992.
162. Badesha PS, Saklayen MG. Hemolytic uremic syndrome as a presenting form of HIV infection. Nephron 72:472–5, 1996.
163. Ballem PJ, Belzberg A, Devine DV, et al. Kinetic studies of the mechanisms of thrombocytopenia in patients with human immunodeficiency virus infection. N Engl J Med 327:1779–84, 1992.
164. Zucker-Franklin D, Cao Y. Megakaryocytes of human immunodeficiency virus-infected individuals express viral RNA. Proc Natl Acad Sci USA 86:5595–9, 1989.
165. Basch RS, Kouri YH, Karpatkin S. Expression of CD4 by human megakaryocytes. Proc Natl Acad Sci USA 87:8085–9, 1990.
166. Kouri YH, Borkowsky W, Nardi M, et al. Human megakaryocytes have a CD4 molecule capable of binding human immunodeficiency virus-1. Blood 81:2664–70, 1993.
167. Wang JF, Liu ZY, Groopman JE. The alpha-chemokine receptor CXCR4 is expressed on the megakaryocytic lineage from progenitor to platelets and modulates migration and adhesion. Blood 92:756–64, 1998.
168. Riviere C, Subra F, Cohen-Solal K, et al. Phenotypic and functional evidence for the expression of CXCR4 receptor during megakaryocytopoiesis. Blood 93:1511–23, 1999.
169. Landonio G, Cinque P, Nosari A, et al. Comparison of two dose regimens of zidovudine in an open, randomized, multicenter study for server HIV related throbocytopenia. AIDS 7:209–12, 1993.
170. Piketty C, Gilquin J, Kazatchkine M. Successful treatment of HIV-related thrombocytopenia with didanosine. J Acquir Immune Defic Syndr 7:521–2, 1994.
171. Maness LJ, Blair DC, Newman N, et al. Elevation of platelet counts associated with indinavir treatment in human immunodeficiency virus-infected patients. Clin Infect Dis 26:207–8, 1998.
172. Arranz Caso JA, Sanchez MC, Garcia TJ. Effect of highly active antiretroviral therapy on thrombocytopenia in patients with HIV infection. N Eng J Med 341:1239–40, 1999.
173. Tozzi V, Narcisco P, Sebastiani G, et al. Effects of indinavir treatment on platelet and neutrophil counts in patients with advanced HIV disease. AIDS 11:1067–8, 1997.
174. Caso JAA, Mingo CS, Tena JG. Effect of highly active antiretroviral therapy on thrombocytopenia in patients with HIV infection. N Engl J Med 16:1239–40, 1999.

175. Durand JM, Lefevre P, Hovette P, et al. Dapsone for thrombocytopenic purpura related to human immunodeficiency virus infection. Am J Med 90:675–7, 1991.
176. Yap PL, Todd AA, Williams PE, et al. Use of intravenous immunoglobulin in acquired immune deficiency syndrome. Cancer 68:1440–50, 1991.
177. Pollak AN, Janinis J, Green D. Successful intravenous immune globulin therapy for human immunodeficiency virus-associated thrombocytopenia. Arch Intern Med 148:695–7, 1988.
178. Bussel JB, Haimi JS. Isolated thrombocytopenia in patients infected with HIV: treatment with intravenous gammaglobulin. Am J Hematol 28:79–84, 1988.
179. Oskenhendler E, Bierling P, Brossard, et al. Anti-Rh immunoglobulin therapy for human immunodeficiency virus-related immune thrombocytopenia. Blood 71:1499–502, 1989.
180. Biniek R, Malessa R, Brochmeyer NH, et al. Anti-Rh(D) immunoglobulin for AIDS-related thrombocytopenia. Lancet 2:627, 1986.
181. Than S, Oyaizu N, Pahwa RN. Effect of human immunodeficiency virus type-1 envelope glycoprotein gp120 on cytokine production from cord-blood T cells. Blood 84:184–8, 1994.
182. Oksenhendler E, Bierling P, Chevret S, et al. Splenectomy is safe and effective in HIV-related immune thrombocytopenia. Blood 82:29–32, 1993.
183. Schneider P, Abrams D, Rayner A, et al. Immunodeficiency-associated thrombocytopenic purpura: response to splenectomy. Arch Surg 122:1175–8, 1987.
184. Zambello R, Trentin L, Agostini C, et al. Persistent polyclonal lymphocytosis in human immunodeficiency virus-1 infected patients. Blood 81:3015–21, 1993.
185. Kemeny MM, Cooke V, Melester TS, et al. Splenectomy in patients with AIDS and AIDS-related complex. AIDS 7:1063–7, 1993.
186. Calverley DC, Jones GW, Kelton JG. Splenic radiation for corticosteroid-resistant immune thrombocytopenia. Ann Intern Med 116:977–81, 1992.
187. Blauth J, Fisher S, Henry D, Nichini F. The role of splenic irradiation in treating HIV-associated immune thrombocytopenia. Int J Radiat Oncol Biol Phys 45:457–60, 1999.
188. Ahn YS. Efficacy of danazol in hematologic disorders. Acta Haematol 84:122–9, 1990.
189. Minter DM, Real FX, Jovino L, et al. Treatment of Kaposi's sarcoma and thrombocytopenia with vincristine in patients with the acquired immunodeficiency syndrome. Ann Intern Med 102:200–2, 1985.
190. Marroni M, Gresele P, Landonio G, et al. Interferon-alpha is effective in the treatment of HIV-1-related, severe, zidovudine-resistant thrombocytopenia: a prospective, placebo-controlled, double-blind trial. Ann Intern Med 121:423–9, 1994.
191. Zauli G, Re MC, Gugliotta L, et al. The elevation of circulating platelets after IFN-alpha therapy in HIV-seropositive thrombocytopenic patients correlates with increased plasma levels of 11–6. Microbiologica 16:27–34, 1993.
192. Stellini R, Rossi G, Paraninfo G. Interferon therapy in intravenous drug-users with HIV-associated idiopathic thrombocytopenic purpura. Haematologica 77:418–20, 1992.
193. Vianelli N, Cantani L, Gugliotta L. Recombinant alpha interferon 2b in the therapy of HIV-related thrombocytopenia. AIDS 7:823–7, 1993.
194. Harker LA. Physiology and clinical application of platelet growth factors. Curr Opin Hematol 6:127–34, 1999.
195. Harker LA, Carter RA, Marzec UM, et al. Correction of thrombocytopenia and ineffective platelet production in patients infected with human immunodeficiency virus by PEG-rHuMGDF therapy. Blood 92(Suppl 1):707a, 1998.
196. Cohen AJ, Phillips TM, Kessler CM. Circulating coagulation inhibitors in the acquired immunodeficiency syndrome. Ann Intern Med 104:175–80, 1986.
197. Gold JE, Haubenstock A, Zalusky R. Lupus anticoagulant and AIDS. N Engl J Med 314:1252–3, 1986.
198. Bloom EJ, Abrams DL Rodgers GM. Lupus anticoagulant in the acquired immunodeficiency syndrome. JAMA 256:491–3, 1986.
199. Cohen H, Mackie IJ, Anagnostopoulos N, et al. Lupus anticoagulant, anticardiolipin antibodies, and human immunodeficiency virus in haemophilia. Clin Pathol 42:629–33, 1989.
200. Cappell MS, Simon T, Tiku M. Splenic infarction associated with anticardiolipin antibodies in a patient with acquired immunodeficiency syndrome. Dig Dis Sci 38:1152–5, 1993.
201. Roubey RAS. Autoantibodies to phospholipid-binding plasma proteins: a new view of lupus anticoagulants and other 'antiphospholipid' autoantibodies. Blood 84:2854–67, 1994.
202. Toulon P, Lamine M, Ledjev I, et al. Heparin cofactor II deficiency in patients infected with the human immunodeficiency virus. Throm Haemost 70:730–5, 1993.
203. Stimmler MM, Quismorio FP, McGehee WG, et al. Anticardiolipin antibodies in acquired immunodeficiency syndrome. Arch Intern Med 149:1833–5, 1989.
204. Stahl CP, Sideman CS, Spira TJ, et al. Protein S deficiency in men with long-term human immunodeficiency virus infection. Blood 81:1801–7, 1993.
205. Bissuel F, Berruyer M, Causse X, et al. Acquired protein S deficiency: correlation with advanced disease in HIV-1 infected patients. J Acquir Immune Defic Syndr Hum Retrovirol 5: 484–9, 1992.
206. Lafeuillade A, Sorice M, Griggi T, et al. Role of autoimmunity in protein S deficiency during HIV-1 infection. Infection 22:201–3, 1994.
207. Sullivan PS, Dworkin MS, Jones JF, Hooper WC. Epidemiology of thrombosis in HIV-infected individuals. AIDS 14:321–4, 2000.
208. Fultz SL, McGinnis KA, Skanderson M, et al. Association of venous thromboembolism with human immunodeficiency virus and mortality in veterans. Am J Med 420–3, 2004.
209. Saber AA, Aboolian A, LaRaja RC, et al. HIV/AIDS and the risk of deep vein thrombosis: a study of 45 patients with lower extremity involvement. Ann Surg 67:645–7, 2001.
210. George SL, Swindells S, Knudson R, Stapleton JT. Unexplained thrombosis in HIV-infected patients receiving protease inhibitors: report of seven cases. Am J Med 107: 624–30, 1999.
211. Copur AS, Smith PR, Gomez V, et al. HIV infection is a risk factor for venous thromboembolism. AIDS Patient Care STDS 16:205–9, 2002.
212. Howling SJ, Shaw PJ, Miller RF. Acute pulmonary embolism in patients with HIV disease. Sex Trans Infect 75:25–9, 1999.
213. Saif MW, Bona R, Greenberg B. AIDS and thrombosis: retrospective study of 131 HIV-infected patients. AIDS Patient Care STDS 15:311–20, 2001.
214. Klein SK, Slim EJ, de Kruif MD, et al. Is chronic HIV infection associated with venous thrombotic disease? A systematic review. Neth J Med 63:129–36, 2005.
215. Miller RF, Scully M, Cohen H, et al. Thrombotic thrombocytopaenic purpura in HIV-infected patients. Int J STD AIDS 16:538–42, 2005.
216. Gruszecki AC, Wehrli G, Ragland BD, et al. Management of a patient with HIV infection-induced anemia and thrombocytopenia who presented with thrombotic thrombocytopenic purpura. Am J Hematol 69:228–31, 2002.
217. Becker S, Fusco G, Fusco J, et al. HIV-associated microangiopathy in the era of highly active antiretroviral therapy: an observational study. Clin Infect Dis 39(Suppl 5):S267–75, 2004.
218. Moore RD. Schistocytosis and a thrombotic microangiopathy-like syndrome in hospitalized HIV-infected patients. Am J Hematol 60:116–20, 1999.
219. Nair J, Bellevue R, Bertoni M, et al. Thrombotic thrombocytopenic purpura in patients with the acquired immunodeficiency syndrome-related complex. Ann Intern Med 109:209–12, 1988.

220. Harris C, Biggs, JC, Concannon AJ, et al. Peripheral blood and bone marrow findings in patients with acquired immune deficiency syndrome. Pathology 22:206–11, 1990.
221. Goasguen JE, Bennett JM. Classification and morphologic features of myelodysplastic syndromes. Semin Oncol 19:4–13, 1992.
222. Candido A, Rossi P, Menichella G, et al. Indicative morphological myelodysplastic alterations of bone marrow in overt AIDS. Haematologica 75:327–33, 1990.
223. Katsarou O, Terpos E, Patsouris E, et al. Myelodysplastic features in patients with long-term HIV infection and haemophilia. Haemophilia 7:47–52, 2001.
224. Abrams D, Chinn E, Lewis B. Hematologic manifestations in homosexual men with Kaposi's sarcoma. Am J Clin Pathol 81:13–8, 1984.
225. Sasadeusz J, Buchanan M, Speed B. Reactive haemophagocytic syndrome in human immunodeficiency virus infection. J Infect 20:65–8, 1990.
226. Seneviratne LS, Tulpule A, Mummaneni M, et al. Clinical, immunological and pathologic correlates of bone marrow involvement in 253 patients with AIDS-related lymphoma. Blood 92(Suppl 1):244A, 1998.
227. Poropatich CO, Labriola AM, Tuazon CU. Acid-fast smear and culture of respiratory secretions, bone marrow and stools as predictors of disseminated *Mycobacterium avium* complex infection. J Microbiol 25:929–30, 1987.
228. Neubauer MA, Bodensteiner DC. Disseminated histoplasmosis in patients with AIDS. South Med J 85:1166–70, 1992.
229. Cohen RJ, Samoszuk MK, Busch D, et al. Occult infections with *M. intracellulare* in bone marrow biopsy specimens from patients with AIDS. N Engl J Med 308;1475–6, 1983.
230. Solis OQ, Belmonte AH, Ramaswamy G. Pseudo-Gaucher cells in *Mycobacterium avium intracellulare* infection in the acquired immune deficiency syndrome (AIDS). Am J Clin Pathol 85;233–5, 1986.
231. Maciejewski JP, Bruening EE, Donahue RE, et al. Infection of hematopoietic progenitor cells by human cytomegalovirus. Blood 80:170–8, 1992.
232. Flamand L, Gosselin J, Stefanescu I, et al. Immunosuppressive effect of human herpesvirus 6 on T-cell functions: suppression of interleukin-2 synthesis and cell proliferation. Blood 85:1263–71, 1995.
233. Carrigan DR, Knox KK. Human herpes virus 6 (HHV-6) isolated from bone marrow: HHV-6 bone marrow suppression in bone marrow transplant patients. Blood 84:3307–10, 1994.

Chapter 68

Cardiovascular Disease in HIV

Jens D. Lundgren, MD, DMSc, Anette Sjøl, MD

Cardiovascular disease (CVD) has emerged as a looming problem for patients infected with HIV, because of two principal factors. First, combination antiretroviral therapy (ART) has led to a dramatic improvement in survival prognosis rendering patients susceptible to age-related morbidities including CVD.[1–3] Second, exposure to ART is associated with an accelerated risk of CVD[4–7] likely by accelerating the progression of atherosclerosis. In addition to atherosclerosis and its varied clinical presentation, this chapter also outlines other cardiac problems seen in HIV-infected persons.

ATHEROSCLEROSIS IN HIV

The Time Course of the Pathology

Atherosclerosis is a condition within the arterial wall.[8,9] The pathological evolution starts with the formation of fatty streaks, followed by lipid-rich plaque formation. LDL cholesterol exits the plasma and is engulfed in macrophages within the fatty streaks and plaques and inflammation develops.[10] Over time, a lipid core possibly mixed with crystallized calcium is formed within a fibrous cap.

In the normal population, fatty streaks can be observed in 30–50% of otherwise healthy persons in their second and third decades of life[11] and increase in number and extent thereafter. Fatty streaks and plaques are usually not associated with symptoms, but can become clinically detectable in either of two ways:

- Thrombosis: The plaque ruptures leading to thrombosis formation, which usually completely occludes the arterial lumen. In this case the symptoms are of acute onset.
- Stenosis: The plaque grows to such a size that it compromises a sufficient flow of blood through the artery required to cover the metabolic requirement of the tissue to which the artery supplies blood. Tissues only supplied by a single artery as opposed to tissues with collateral artery supply are at excess risk of suffering. Symptoms develop gradually, and are first seen in situations where the metabolic requirements of the tissue are enhanced (e.g., during exercise and postprandial).

The risk of CVD in the background population starts to emerge around age 45 for men and some 10 years later for women, increasing exponentially for both genders thereafter. Usually, thrombotic events precede stenotic events. The usual HIV-infected populations with median age of 35–40 years are hence relatively 'young' in CVD risk terms. Consequently, most of the emphasis of this chapter is focused on prevention of CVD. The specifics of the clinical presentation of atherosclerosis (ischemic heart disease (IHD), peripheral arterial atherosclerosis and stroke) are discussed in the subsequent sections.

Risk Factors Other Than HIV and ART

A multitude of factors influence the risk of atherosclerosis and its clinical manifestations in HIV (in Table 68-1 suspected and documented risk factors in HIV-infected populations are outlined). Most of these risk factors are well described in the general population (except of course those related to HIV and ART), and the contribution to risk of IHD is fairly comparable in HIV-infected populations and in the general population.

Table 68-1

Risk Factors Known or Suspected to Influence the Risk of Ischemic Heart Disease (IHD) in HIV-Infected Persons

Factor	Aggravates Traditional Risk Factors for IHD	Independent Predictor of IHD Risk in HIV?
Exposure to:		
Antiretroviral treatment	Yes	Yes
Protease inhibitors	Yes	Yes
NNRTIs	No	No
NRTIs	Yes (stavudine)	?
Age	–	Yes
Gender	–	Yes
Diabetes	–	Yes
History of CVD	–	Yes
Hypertension	–	Yes
Smoking	–	Yes
Family history of premature CVD	–	No
Total cholesterol	–	Yes
HDL cholesterol	–	Yes
Triglycerides	–	No
Replication of HIV	Yes	No
Level of immunodeficency	Yes	No
Development of lipoatrophy	Yes	No

CVD: cardiovascular disease; IHD: ischemic heart disease.

Source: The Data collection of Adverse effects of anti-HIV drugs (D:A:D) study [7] and updates from this study in 2005[45] and 2006.[43]

The current understanding of the risk factors depicted in Table 68.1 and their role in determining CVD/IHD risk in the general population and in HIV-infected populations is outlined below. Most of the knowledge cited below is derived from studies of the general population, and it appears reasonable to generally extrapolate most of this knowledge to the HIV-infected population. However, there are caveats surrounding certain aspects of doing such an extrapolation as noted below. Furthermore, the risk factors described in the table depict our current understanding of the situation in HIV, and this may be revised (expanded or reduced) as additional experience accumulates. Regardless, the success of preventive interventions is closely linked with intimate knowledge of this area.

Age and gender have already been mentioned.[12] Of key relevance, the atherosclerotic process takes decades to develop, and lack of clinical symptoms should not necessarily lead to complacency in managing the cardiovascular health of a person. Conversely, risk factors for normal health other than CVD may very well take priority in younger patients infected with HIV, and the expected benefit versus the potential risk from interventions to prevent CVD should be carefully considered in younger patients also.

A family history of premature CVD also adversely affects the risk of CVD.[13] The definition of 'prematurity' differs in various studies, but one operational definition is 'CVD before the age of 50 in a first-degree relative'. In part, this risk factor is related to dietary and genetic predisposition of well-known risk factors (e.g., congenital lipid disorders), and hence the clinical relevance of this risk factor is low in populations extensively screened for the risk factors described below.

Patients with a history of CVD have a six- to ninefold increased risk of having a reoccurrence of a CVD compared with patients without such a history.[14] Patients with diabetes mellitus have comparable excess risk.[14,15] Hence, diabetes can be considered a so-called 'CVD equivalent'. The reason why patients with diabetes have such a high risk of CVD is likely not linked to the abnormal glucose metabolism *per se*, whereas intense management of traditional CVD risk factors reduces the risk of CVD in patients with diabetes.[16]

Smoking, especially cigarettes, accelerates the risk of CVD.[17,18] Higher absolute consumption, longer duration of consumption, inhalation of the fumes, female gender, and younger age of the patient are all associated with relatively larger detrimental effects from smoking. Although the relative excess risk of CVD for smokers (vs nonsmokers) is greater for persons below 65 years of age, continued smoking also after this age is associated with excess risk.[19] Conversely, cessation of smoking is associated with a gradual reduction in risk of CVD over the first 5 years (~50% reduction in risk), whereas the detrimental influence on total mortality takes approximately twice as long to overcome (Fig. 68-1).[20]

LDL cholesterol is an integral part of the pathology of atherosclerosis and it is therefore not surprising that the risk of CVD is closely positively correlated with the plasma levels of this lipid. Importantly, there is a linear correlation between LDL cholesterol levels and the risk of CVD without any lower threshold (Fig. 68-2).[21] The level of LDL cholesterol

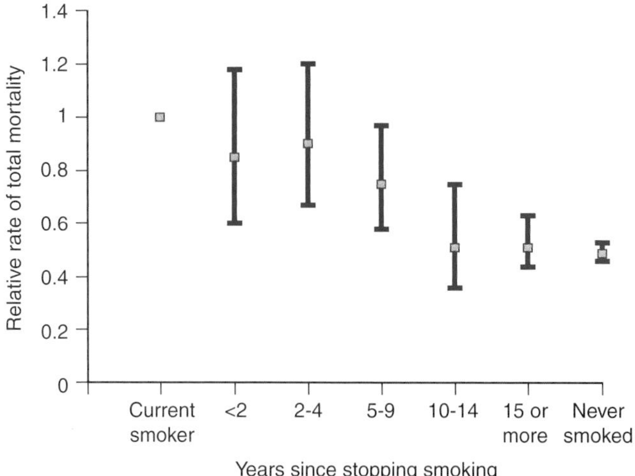

Figure 68-1 ■ Relative risk of total mortality from the time since quitting smoking. The relative risk of total mortality is comparable between ex-smokers 10 years after quitting smoking and persons who have never smoked. Note, the CVD protective effect of quitting smoking is more rapidly seen – the risk of CVD is comparable in persons from 5 years after quitting smoking compared with persons who have never smoked. Modified from Kawachi I, Colditz GA, Stampfer MJ et al. Smoking cessation in relation to total mortality rates in women. A prospective cohort study. Ann Intern Med 119:992, 1993.

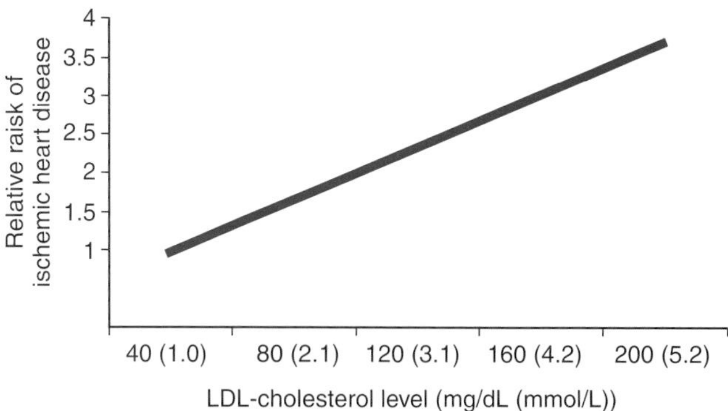

Figure 68-2 ■ The association between the relative risk of IHD (on a logarithmic scale) and plasma levels of LDL cholesterol. This relationship is consistent with a large body of epidemiological data and with data available from clinical trials of lipid-lowering therapy. These data suggest that for every 30 mg/dL (0.8 mmol/L) change in LDL cholesterol, the relative risk of IHD is changed in proportion by ~30%. The relative risk is set at 1.0 for LDL cholesterol = 40 mg/dL (1.0 mmol/L). Modified from Grundy SM, Cleeman JI, Merz CN et al. Implications of recent clinical trials for the National Cholesterol Education Program Adult Treatment Panel III guidelines. Circulation 110:227, 2004.

is linked to diet with persons consuming a Western-type diet having the highest levels. Interventions aimed at reducing the plasma levels of LDL cholesterol have conclusively demonstrated a reduction in the risk of CVD.[22]

Conversely, HDL cholesterol tends to transport LDL cholesterol away from the arterial plaques, reduce it in size and hence slow the progressive atherosclerotic process. The level of HDL cholesterol is inversely correlated with the risk of CVD.[22,23] Nonmedical interventions aimed at increasing HDL levels are associated with a reduced risk of CVD, whereas medical interventions principally designed to increase HDL cholesterol levels remain to be developed for routine clinical usage.

It is controversial whether fasting triglyceride plasma levels *per se* influence the risk of CVD. Elevated triglyceride levels are usually seen in conjunction with other CVD risk factors such as elevated LDL cholesterol, insulin resistance, and other manifestations of the metabolic syndrome (see discussion below), and it appears that once these other risk factors are controlled, the adverse association of high triglyceride and increased risk of IHD is removed.[24,25] The combination of high triglycerides and low HDL cholesterol may, however, constitute a situation where the risk of IHD remains increased.[26]

Beta-adrenoceptor blockers, thiazide diuretics, estrogens, androgens, thyroid hormone replacement preparations, and glucocorticoids may increase cholesterol and triglyceride levels.

Hypertension is a risk factor in many types of CVD, especially in stroke (see below).

Several versions of the definition of the metabolic syndrome exist.[27] The principal components are, however, the same, namely; insulin resistance, abdominal obesity, dyslipidemia (low HDL cholesterol and high triglyceride levels), and hypertension.[28] Much focus has been placed on this syndrome for two reasons. First, these factors are interlinked (perhaps causally) and coexist in many people, and second, it may be that patients with the metabolic syndrome have a risk of CVD that exceeds the contribution of the risk factors when present on their own. Whereas the first reason is definitively true, it remains to be clearly demonstrated whether the second reason is also true, especially in situations where drugs used in a population (e.g., ART, see below) are able to induce components of the syndrome. In the background population, the prevalence of the metabolic syndrome has increased markedly in recent times, predominantly because of an increasing prevalence of obesity. More studies are required in HIV-infected populations before the clinical relevance of assessing the metabolic syndrome in this population can be determined. However, as patients fulfilling the definition of the metabolic syndrome have several risk factors for CVD (as per definition), such patients should be targeted for interventions to modify each of these risk factors.

Physical inactivity is causally related with excess risk of CVD. There is a dose–response relation between baseline physical activity and health benefit. When sedentary, even a modest increase in physical activity is beneficial.[29] The mechanisms by which physical activity decreases the risk of CVD include improvement in HDL cholesterol level,[30] reduction in insulin resistance,[31] lowering of body weight,[32] and reduced blood pressure.[33] Among patients with a history of IHD, exercise training reduces the need for revasculation procedures.[34]

As already discussed above, diet affects LDL-cholesterol levels. Especially, saturated fat and cholesterol content are of influence.

Elevated C-reactive protein (CRP), determined by ultrasensitive (us) techniques, is associated with excess risk of

CVD.[35,36] However, the place for usCRP measurements in routine practice as a clinically useful determinant for assessing the risk of CVD remains to be defined, especially in HIV-infected populations where unrelated ongoing infection may increase usCRP levels as part of an acute inflammatory reaction.

Of key importance, the factors described above that contribute to the risk of CVD do so independently of each other. That is, when more than one factor is present in an individual patient, the CVD risk factors increase additively (Fig. 68-3).[37]

HIV Infection as a CVD Risk Factor

Advanced untreated and treated HIV infection is associated with reduced total, LDL-, and HDL-cholesterol levels and hypertriglyceridemia.[38–40] The risk of IHD in untreated HIV infection is low in absolute terms[7] and lower than what would be expected when assessing the expected IHD risk from risk equations used to assess risk of IHD in the background population.[41] It may be hypothesized that the metabolic alterations and the immunodeficiency may adversely affect the risk of CVD in untreated HIV infection, but the information available so far does not suggest that this is of major clinical importance.

ART as a CVD Risk Factor

Several studies have consistently shown that duration of exposure to ART is associated with a gradually increased risk of IHD in particular[4,6,7] (Fig. 68-4) and CVD in general.[5] This adverse effect of ART is at least partly driven via the effects that components of ART have on various metabolic factors, most prominently LDL-cholesterol elevation (*see* Chapters 71 and 72). In populations exposed to antiretrovirals, elevation of cholesterol is associated with suppressed viral replication and higher CD4+ T-lymphocyte counts[42] suggesting that ART reverses (and possibly exacerbates) the reductions in total cholesterol seen in advanced cases of untreated HIV.

Not all drug classes and not all drugs within a class are likely associated with comparable risk. Presently, it appears that an excess risk is carried from exposure to drugs within the protease inhibitor class.[43] Some (but not all)[44] of this effect is mediated by how these drugs affect cholesterol metabolism, in particular LDL levels. Whether all individual drugs within this class affect the risk of IHD equally remains

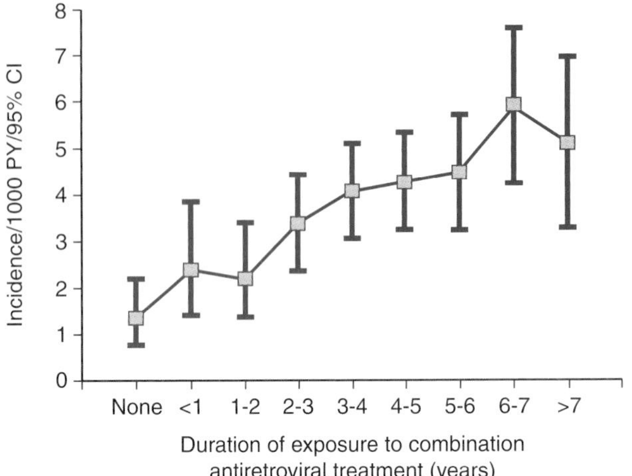

Figure 68-4 ■ Incidence of myocardial infarction according to exposure to combination antiretroviral treatment. Note the linear relationship between exposure to antiretroviral treatment and incidence of myocardial infarction. The risk of myocardial infarction is approximately doubled after 5 years of exposure to antiretroviral treatment.

From Writing committee: Friis-Møller N, Reiss P, El-Sadr W, et al., on behalf of the D:A:D study group. Class of Antiretroviral Drugs and the Risk of Myocardial Infarction. N Engl J Med 26;356: 1723–35, 2007

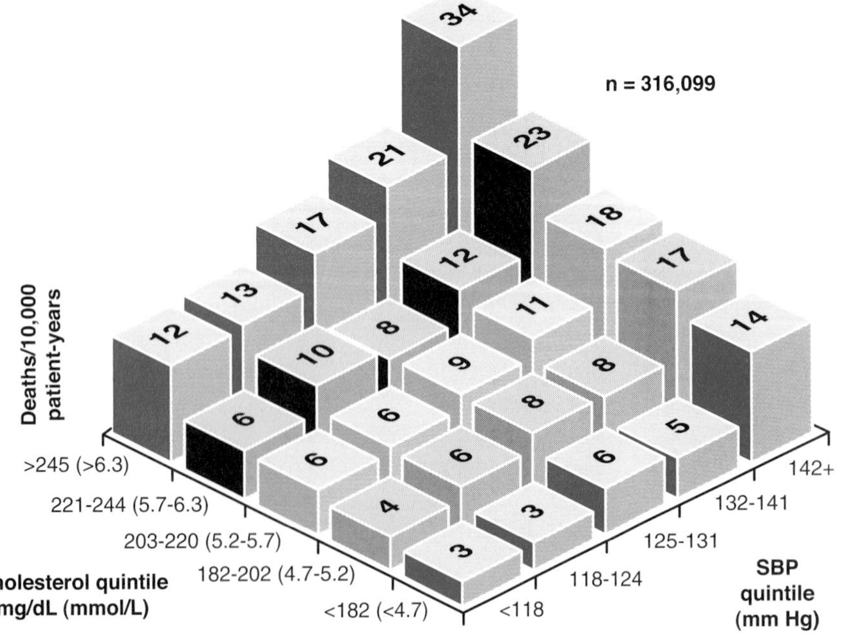

Figure 68-3 ■ Combined effects of systolic blood pressure and cholesterol level on coronary heart disease-related mortality. Note that the two factors add additively to the risk of coronary heart disease-related mortality.

Modified from Neaton JD, Wentworth D. Serum cholesterol, blood pressure, cigarette smoking, and death from coronary heart disease. Overall findings and differences by age for 316,099 white men. Multiple Risk Factor Intervention Trial Research Group. Arch Intern Med 152:56, 1992.

to be determined; some differences for example exist in how these drugs affect lipids (*see* Chapter 72).

The size of the added risk for IHD from being exposed to a drug from the protease inhibitor drug class has been expressed in the literature as the added risk per year of exposure.[43,45] This added risk amounts to 16% per year of exposure.[43] However, as this risk accumulates for each additional year of exposure, for example, 5 years of exposure is equal to 110% ($1.16^5 = 2.10$ (i.e., slightly more than a doubling of risk)). However, as mentioned, some of this added risk is mediated via how these drugs affect lipid levels. Once lipids are controlled for, the remaining added risk per year of exposure to the protease inhibitor class is 10% (60% per 5 years of exposure).[43] Additionally, these projections are based on the assumption that the added risk per year of exposure is comparable for each year of exposure. This assumption appears valid for up to 7 years of exposure (Fig. 68-4), whereas it remains unknown whether it is also true for even longer periods of exposure. Hence, extrapolations of these risk estimates for decades of exposure should not be done until additional experience has accumulated.

Conversely, exposure to the two main drugs within the non-nucleoside reverse transcriptase inhibitor drug class (efavirenz and nevirapine) appears not to be associated with an adverse risk of CVD,[43] although knowledge on effects from longer-term exposure is limited at present. Of note, both non-nucleoside reverse transcriptase inhibitors increase HDL, but not LDL-cholesterol levels.[46,47] Finally, whether one or more drugs within the nucleoside reverse transcriptase class also affects risk of CVD remains to be determined, although stavudine is linked to increase in cholesterol levels (Table 68-1).[48] Lipodystrophy is associated with dyslipidemia and insulin resistance (*see* Chapter 71–73), but IHD is not seen more frequently in patients with lipodystrophy.[7]

It is important to underline that the mechanism behind the excessive risk of CVD associated with exposure to ART remains to be fully clarified. This is indeed an area where knowledge expands quickly and many questions remain unanswered – primarily the clinical consequence of exposure to various combinations and how best to reduce the impact on CVD derived from exposure to ART. Furthermore, most of the evidence comes from observational studies, which have intrinsic methodological weaknesses rendering them susceptible to several types of bias (most notably confounding by indication and selection).

Clinical Evaluation and Interventions Aimed at Reducing Risk of CVD

HIV-infected persons are usually seen routinely every 3–4 months for their HIV care. These visits provide an opportunity to also assess CVD risk factors and appropriately intervene to reduce the risk as appropriate. However, no specific studies have documented the clinical benefit of cardiovascular preventive interventions in HIV. Such studies would be important, as extrapolations from the experience in the background population is problematic for two reasons: (1) components of ART accelerate the risk of CVD in HIV, a situation without resemblance in the general population for obvious reasons; (2) medical interventions are provided to HIV-infected patients already receiving treatment with the potential for drug–drug interaction and poorer compliance.

Until the time when such studies have been completed, the most reasonable approach nevertheless appears to be utilizing the strategies applied to the general population.[49]

The interventions consist of lifestyle changes and medical interventions. A large body of literature exists concerning the general population, documenting the benefits derived from four types of intervention: blood-pressure reduction in patients with hypertension, reduction of LDL cholesterol, use of acetylsalicylic acid (ASA) in patients with prior CVD, and smoking cessation. In Table 68-2 the relative benefit that can be expected from using each of these interventions, either alone or in combination, is depicted.

Smoking can be expected to be associated with the largest reduction in risk. Normalization of blood pressure reduces the risk of stroke more than the risk of IHD. Combination of the interventions results in added benefit (Table 68-2).[50,51] When all interventions are combined, the risk of CVD may be reduced by as much as 80%. For example, in a male smoker with a prior myocardial infarction, hypertension and dyslipidemia leading to a projected 30% risk of a new IHD in the next 10 years; this risk can be reduced to 6% by appropriate interventions. Of note, the net benefit (in absolute terms, in the example, 30−6% = 24% over a 10-year period) from these interventions obviously depends on the patient's *a priori* absolute CVD risk. For example, if the *a priori* risk was only 5% risk of IHD in the next 10 years, an 80% reduction constitutes a 1% risk of IHD (i.e., a 4% absolute risk reduction). Whereas lifestyle interventions have no apparent disadvantages (except impairment of quality-of-life which adversely affects adherence to the intervention), medical interventions are all associated with potential harm. Hence, a guiding principle in CVD prevention is to assess the individual person's absolute CVD risk, focusing the most aggressive interventions on those with the largest expected benefit in absolute terms.

A prediction of absolute risk is usually focused on the risk of IHD, as several so-called 'risk equations' exist that determine this risk. It is currently debated as to how to apply these risk equations in HIV, since none of them have been appropriately validated in this population and do not include the entirety of risk factors for CVD identified in HIV (most notably, none of them account for exposure to ART).[52] One study[40] has compared predicted and observed absolute risk of myocardial infarction in HIV infection, and found that the Framingham equation[53] fairly accurately predicted the observed incidence, whereas the 'Copenhagen risk equation'[54] under-predicted the observed risk by 40%. There is an ongoing effort to develop a risk equation specific for HIV infection. Until this work has been completed, use of the Framingham equation to predict the absolute risk of IHD in HIV (see: http://www.cphiv.dk/TOOLS/Framingham/tabid/302/Default.aspx) is recommended.

Table 68-2 The Expected Benefit From Interventions Aimed at Reducing Risk of Ischemic Heart Disease (IHD) and Stroke

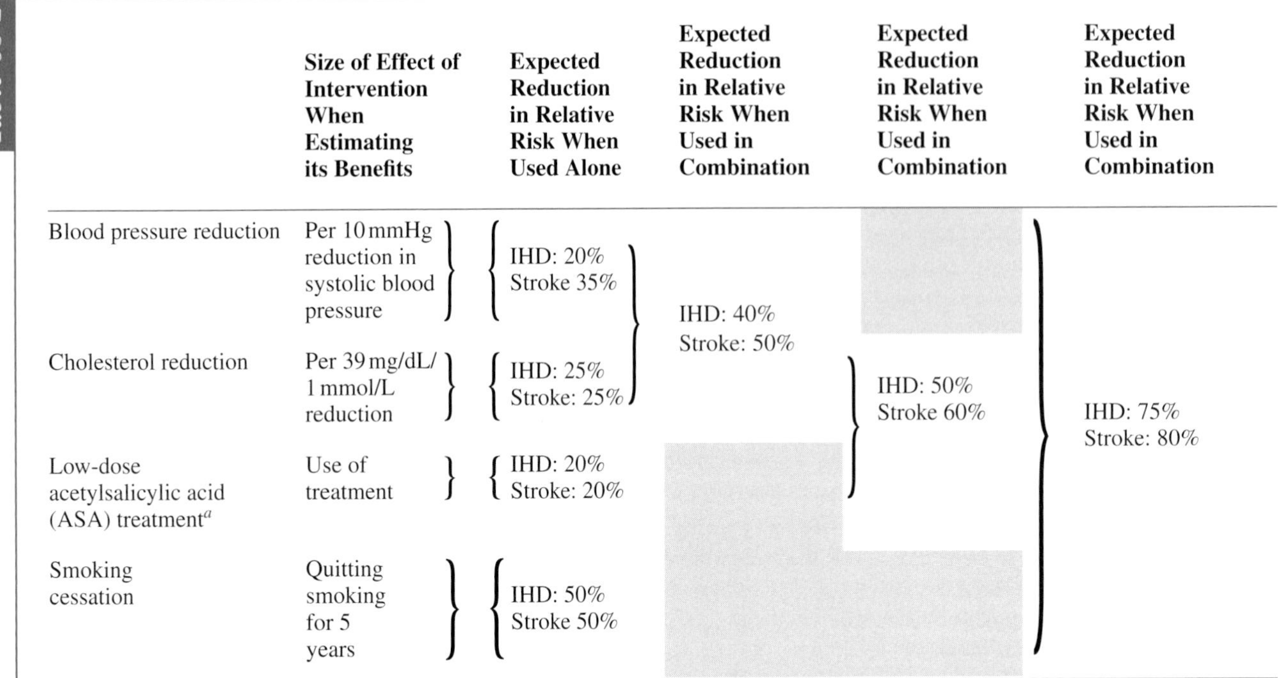

	Size of Effect of Intervention When Estimating its Benefits	Expected Reduction in Relative Risk When Used Alone	Expected Reduction in Relative Risk When Used in Combination	Expected Reduction in Relative Risk When Used in Combination	Expected Reduction in Relative Risk When Used in Combination
Blood pressure reduction	Per 10 mmHg reduction in systolic blood pressure	IHD: 20% Stroke 35%	IHD: 40% Stroke: 50%		IHD: 75% Stroke: 80%
Cholesterol reduction	Per 39 mg/dL/1 mmol/L reduction	IHD: 25% Stroke: 25%		IHD: 50% Stroke 60%	
Low-dose acetylsalicylic acid (ASA) treatment[a]	Use of treatment	IHD: 20% Stroke: 20%			
Smoking cessation	Quitting smoking for 5 years	IHD: 50% Stroke 50%			

Note, as interventions are used in combination, the reduction in the relative risk of IHD improves further.

The percentage reduction in absolute risk of IHD can be exemplified for individual patients by doing the following: (1) estimate the 10-year absolute risk of IHD using the size of risk factors for IHD determined prior to initiating the intervention(s) by use of a risk equation (e.g., www.nhlbi.nih.gov/guidelines/cholesterol); (2) then reduce this 10-year absolute risk with the percentage reduction in IHD indicated for the intervention(s) applied.

[a]Acetylsalicylic acid. Only for use in high-risk patients as risk of intracerebral bleeding increased by 25% and extracerebral bleeding by 50%, and hence the harm exceeds the benefit if risk of CHD is relatively low.[51a]

Source: Summary of the entirety of randomized controlled trials that have assessed these four interventions. Modified from MacMahon.[51]

Practicalities of Using the Interventions

In Figure 68-5 is outlined an algorithm for routine evaluation and interventions aimed at reducing LDL cholesterol in HIV infection, based on modification from the 'National Cholesterol Education Programme' (NCEP) III guidelines[55] and comparable guidelines in Europe.

First, the absolute risk of IHD is assessed and the population is stratified into three main categories of risk: low (<10% risk of IHD over the next 10 years), intermediate (10–20% risk), and high (>20% risk). The proportion of contemporarily followed HIV-infected patients with a 10-year risk of IHD exceeding 10% (intermediate to high risk) is 10–15% and this percentage is projected to be doubled by 2015, merely due to aging of the population.[41]

Lifestyle interventions are the first interventions to be considered (Fig. 68-5). The aggressiveness is intensified as the absolute risk increases, although all patients should be targeted. Exercise, quitting smoking, and diet modifications are the key components to consider.

Suggested key elements of the daily diet are:

- less than 7% of the total calorie intake should consist of saturated fat;
- less than 20% of the total calorie intake should consist of cholesterol (maximum 200–300 mg/day);
- 25–35% of the total calorie intake should consist of fat;
- the daily fiber intake should be at least 30 g/day.

Hence, the diet should preferably consist of five to six pieces of fruit daily, fish (not deep-fried) twice-weekly, and limited mammalian fat intake (including fat-containing milk).

All adults are recommended at least 30 min of moderately intensive physical activity daily.[29] Management of the addiction to nicotine[56] as well as the commitment of the patient to cease smoking are key determinants in successfully quitting this lifestyle. The diet modifications and the intensification of exercise may reduce LDL-cholesterol levels.

A dilemma for rational management of CVD in HIV infection is, how most appropriately to medically intervene in case of elevated LDL cholesterol that is not correctable by lifestyle interventions. The definition for an elevated LDL-cholesterol level requiring intervention depends on the absolute CVD risk of the individual patient (Fig. 68-5). There are two principal possibilities, namely switch in components of ART known to enhance LDL-cholesterol levels or providing lipid-lowering medication.[56,57]

Switch in ART is preferable if it is plausible that the new regimen will result in better metabolic control58,59 and if the

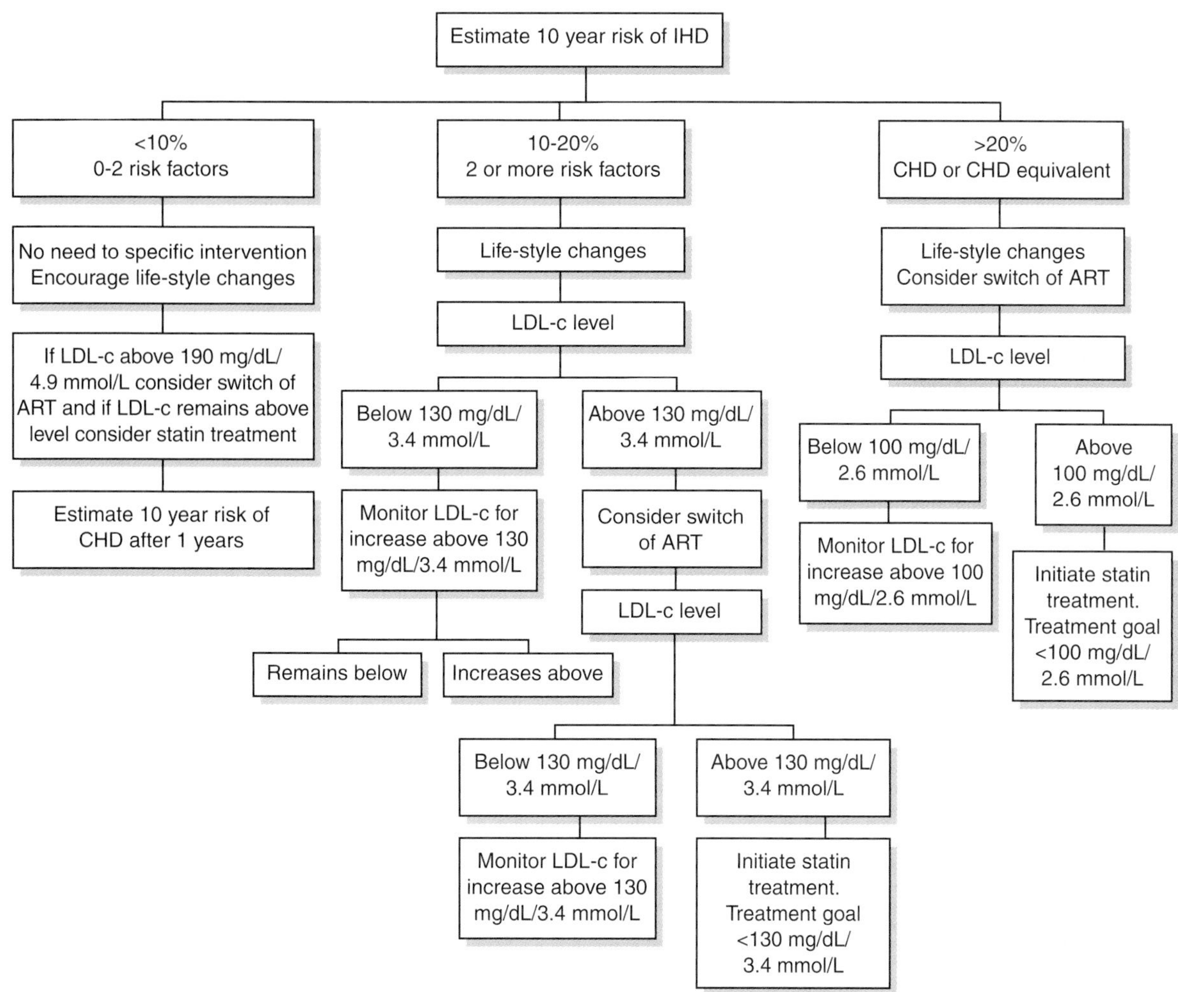

Figure 68-5 ■ Algorithm for the prevention of cardiovascular disease in HIV-infected patients. Estimation of 10-year risk of IHD – use http://www.cphiv.dk/TOOLS/Framingham/tabid/302/Default/aspx. Risk factors: smoking, age (>45 years for men; 55 years for women), hypertension (well controlled), HDL cholesterol <40 mg/dL, family history of premature CHD. Lifestyle changes: daily intake of saturated fats <7% of total calories, daily intake of cholesterol <200 mg, increase vegetables, and fiber intake, weight reduction and increased physical activity (30–60 minutes per day). Goals for treatment aimed at reducing LDL cholesterol: the LDL level above which the treatment is indicated (note, this level differs depending on the absolute CVD risk). In case the LDL cholesterol cannot be determined because of high triglyceride levels, the nonHDL cholesterol level is calculated (total cholesterol minus HDL cholesterol), and 30 mg/dL (0.8 mmol/L) is added to the levels indicated in the figure.

intended switch(es) do not render the patient more susceptible to virological failure due to archived viral resistance or inferior intrinsic antiviral activity of the new drug combination planned to be used. The treatment history and previously performed resistance tests can be used to assess the presence of archived resistance, whereas the reader is referred to the Chapters in section 3, Anti-retroviral therapy for information on differences in intrinsic antiviral activity of various combinations of anti-HIV drugs.

The lipid levels vary in the background population (as they do in patients infected with HIV receiving ART)[60] due to genetic and diet differences. Switch in components of ART can only be expected to reduce lipids in patients where ART increased the levels in the first place. In an attempt to separate preexisting from drug-induced dyslipidemia, screening patients for metabolic abnormalities prior to commencing ART is recommended. Switches are especially encouraged in case the patient is receiving a protease inhibitor. Of note, in the background population, there is a small increase in LDL and a decrease in HDL cholesterol associated with increasing age[61] which should be incorporated into considerations when changes are assessed in lipids in individual patients over many years.

Statins can be used in the case of elevated LDL cholesterol. Of note, drug–drug interactions may arise because certain statins and anti-HIV drugs are metabolized via the same pathway (see below), and the choice of statins is reduced (see below). The level of LDL cholesterol above which statin treatment is indicated varies according to the patient's absolute risk of IHD (Fig. 68-5). The aim of using the statin is to reduce the level of LDL cholesterol below this level. If statin monotherapy is not sufficient to reduce LDL-cholesterol levels sufficiently, combination therapy with bile acid resins (e.g., cholestipol, cholestyramin), ezetimibe, or nicotinic acid can be considered.[62] Ezetimibe adds additively to the LDL-reducing ability of statins,[63] but the potential for side effects and drug–drug interactions suggest that combination therapy should be reserved for high-risk patients only.

If the triglyceride levels are high, LDL-cholesterol levels cannot be calculated. In such situations, make sure that lipids are measured in fasting (at least 8 h without food) condition as food intake predominantly adversely affects triglyceride levels.[64] Cessation from long-term massive alcohol-intake, triglyceridemia-inducing drugs (discussed earlier), and certain antiretroviral drugs (most pronouncedly lopinavir, ritonavir,[65,66] and stavudine)[48] tend to reduce triglyceride levels. If the triglyceride level cannot be reduced sufficiently, non-HDL cholesterol levels can be used as a surrogate for LDL-cholesterol levels. The target non-HDL cholesterol level (total cholesterol minus HDL level) is 30 mg/dL (0.8 mmol/L) higher than the corresponding LDL cholesterol target (Fig. 68-5).

Fibrates can be considered in situations where triglyceride levels are high and constitute the major lipid abnormality and where alcohol cessation, diet restriction, other nonmedical interventions, and possible substitutions of drugs that may increase triglyceride levels are not able to improve the situation. One definition of 'high' triglyceride levels is when the plasma concentration of triglycerides exceeds 8 mmol/L (700 mg/dL), except for patients with a history of pancreatitis where interventions should be considered if plasma triglyceride levels exceed 5 mmol/L (440 mg/dL). The clinical benefit from using fibrates in HIV infection is however questionable. First, the level of triglycerides in plasma appears not to be a strong independent risk factor for CVD in HIV infection and in the general population (as discussed earlier). Second, the overall clinical benefit from fibrate treatment is not apparent from the review of three randomized intervention studies of non-HIV-infected populations.[67–70] Third, although more than 20% of HIV-infected patients have increased triglyceride plasma levels, the rate of pancreatitis is low and associated with traditional risk factors[71] (Lundgren, personal communication), and hence it is questionable whether the risk of pancreatitis is increased in HIV-infected persons with high triglyceride levels. Finally, triglyceride levels in HIV are often due to drugs or lipoatrophy, and only rarely associated with obesity and the metabolic syndrome, which is often the case in the background population. Only in very selected cases is it recommended to combine a statin and a fibrate because of risk of drug–drug interaction, and if this is done, fenofibrate appears most suitable.[72,73]

Both statins and fibrates have been demonstrated to reduce LDL cholesterol and triglycerides, respectively, in HIV-infected persons on ART.[74–77] These studies serve as proof-of-concept that ART-induced dyslipidemia is medically correctable, although they also point out that the desired optimal effect (reduction to below levels indicated in Table 68.5) is rarely met.

Many clinics have introduced screening for insulin resistance by use of a 2-h oral glucose tolerance test. Antiretroviral drugs can induce insulin resistance[78,79] and overt diabetes, and lipodystrophy is associated with insulin resistance.[80] Other than addressing these issues, the clinical implications from detecting an abnormal oral glucose tolerance test not fulfilling the criteria of diabetes are limited for CVD prevention. The insulin sensitizers (roziglitazone has been most extensively studied) improve determinants of insulin resistance but also aggravate dyslipidemia[81–84] and have other adverse effects and should not be used routinely. However, the oral glucose tolerance test is well suited to identify patients at excess risk of prestages of diabetes or overt diabetes.

The physician responsible for the management of the patient's HIV-infection should be responsible for the interventions discussed above being implemented appropriately. It is not advisable to merely refer patients to cardiologists or lipidologists not familiar with the special considerations required to manage HIV-infected persons. Conversely, many HIV specialists have limited experience and knowledge of issues related to CVD prevention. Hence, for patients at intermediate and especially at high risk of CVD, close consultation is required.

IHD: CORONARY ATHEROSCLEROSIS

IHD is one of the most prevalent diseases in the world. Almost all myocardial infarctions result from coronary atherosclerosis generally with superimposed coronary thrombosis. The acute coronary syndrome includes unstable angina, non-ST elevation-infarction, and ST elevation-infarction. The diagnosis is based on the combination of symptoms, changes in the electrocardiogram (ECG) and biochemical markers.

In patients with acute coronary syndrome the clinical examination and history of chest pain, possibly with radiation to the left arm, is important. An ECG identifies ST-segment changes that occur acutely after occlusion or severe hypoperfusion of a coronary culprit artery. Biochemical markers (troponin T (TNT), cardiac troponin I (TNI), creatine kinase isoenzyme MB (CK-MB), or myoglobin) should be measured to further establish the diagnosis.[85] TNT and TNI only exist within cardiomyocytes, and are not usually present in the peripheral circulating blood. As the assays to detect these proteins are extremely sensitive, this is the most sensitive and specific biomarker of myocardial necroses available. The proteins can be detected with a mean time to initial elevation of 3–12 h after the blood supply has been impaired. Conversely, the CK-MB also exists in other organ (including muscle) cells, and myocardial infarction should only be suspected if the 'CK-MB to total creatine kinase' ratio is larger than 5%. This ratio becomes abnormal at the same time as for the troponins. Conversely, within 1 h of occlusion of the coronary arteries, elevation of myoglobin can be detected. However, the elevation of myoglobin disappears within the first 24 h, whereas the other measurements discussed above remain abnormal for the first couple of days, expanding the diagnostic window. Additional information can be derived from serial determinations ensuring the return to normal levels.

IHD may also present with more subtle angina symptoms. Suspected cases should be referred to an exercise test. This test follows a protocol that requires the patient to exercise until symptoms of angina appear, ECG evidence of ischemia is seen, or a target of 80% of maximum workload has been reached. If this test is inconclusive, myocardial perfusion can be visualized by thallium-201 during exercise or pharmacological (dipyridamole, adenosin, or dobutamine) stress.

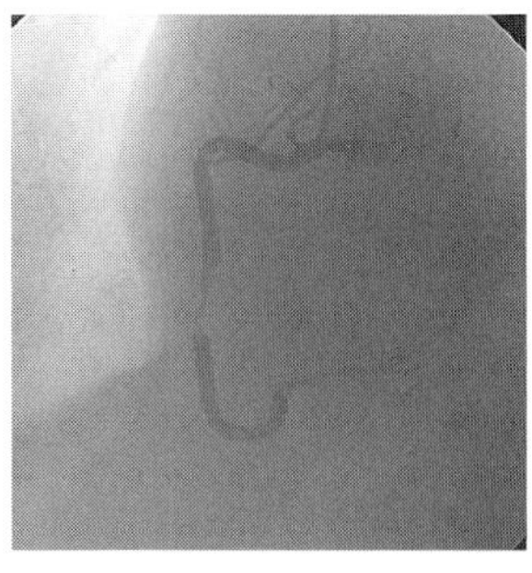
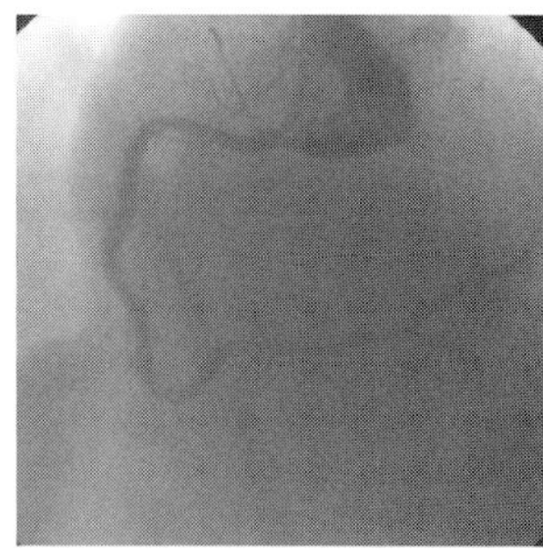

Figure 68-6 ■ Coronary arteriography of a patient with a coronary artery stenosis before (left) and after (right) angioplasty.

Coronary arteriography visualizes the coronary arteries (Fig. 68-6). It is not only used for primary investigation but also in conjunction with angioplasty for the diagnosis of coronary obstructions. This investigation does not provide information on the functional significance of coronary lesions; the exercise test is the best measure to evaluate myocardial oxygen demand. Several novel methodologies of assessing the extent of coronary atherosclerosis (e.g., coronary calcification by computer tomography) and myocardial oxygen demand (e.g., color flow echocardiography) might become routine in the future.

Treatment

A combination of nitrates, analgesics (morphine), oxygen and beta-adrenoceptor blockers is used to control the pain. Additional thrombosis formation is hindered by the administration of ASA along with clopidogrel and low molecular heparin. In the acute phase a statin drug is added. Acute coronary arteriography with percutaneous intravascular intervention (angioplasty)[86,87] has become standard-of-care in myocardial infarctions associated with ST elevation in the ECG (Fig. 68-6). In non-ST elevation myocardial infarctions, a coronary arteriography should be conducted within 1 week of onset of symptoms.

Angina pectoris is treated with angioplasty, nitroglycerin, aspirin, statin, beta-adrenoceptor blockers, and in addition eventually slow-release nitrates and calcium channel antagonists.

PERIPHERAL ARTERIAL ATHEROSCLEROSIS

Peripheral arterial disease compromises the mobility of the patient,[88] reduces quality of life, and is accompanied by enhanced cardiovascular morbidity and mortality. Intermittent claudication is due to functional insufficiency of the arterial function of the lower extremities and is clinically detected as pain in the legs while walking and relief from rest. The walking distance until pain emerges is associated with the severity of the disease; in severe cases this distance is less than 20–30 m.[89]

The most common etiology is atherosclerotic artery disease. Important risk factors are smoking, dyslipidemia, hypertension, and diabetes mellitus.

The clinical symptoms are suggestive. Assessment of peripheral perfusion pressure is a noninvasive technique that reliably informs of possible compromised arterial function. In suspected cases, angiography will establish the location of the occlusion.

Treatment

The key intervention is smoking cessation.[90] Additionally, exercise rehabilitation reduces the claudication pain. Other modifiable atherosclerotic risk factors should be managed as described above. Balloon treatment and bypass surgery is a possibility for severe peripheral artery disease confirmed by arteriography.

STROKE

Apoplexy cerebri is caused either by infarction (thrombosis or emboli) or hemorrhage (located intracerebrally, subarachnoidally, subdurally, or epidurally). Compromised flow of a cerebral artery leads to ischemia and infarction of the surrounding area and hence compromised neuronal function. Depending on the location and size of the neural tissue affected, patients complain of specific motor deficiencies or become unconscious. Transient cerebral ischemia is defined if symptoms persist for less than 24 h.

The background of an ischemic apoplexy is usually generalized atherosclerosis, especially in hypertensive patients.

In suspected cases computer tomography or magnetic resonance computer tomography of the brain is crucial to separate infarctions from hemorrhagic causes. Ultrasonic investigation of the carotid arteries and echocardiography of the heart should also be performed. In severely immunosuppressed HIV-infected patients, intracerebral opportunistic infections[91] and primary lymphomas[92] are important differential diagnoses of stroke-like symptoms.

Treatment

Antithrombolytic therapy is indicated in infarction along with risk factor modification as for other atherosclerotic diseases. Cerebral hemorrhage is treated conservatively or by surgery to evacuate the accumulated blood depending on the size and the localization. Rehabilitation is essential for all patients to enhance life quality.

HYPERTENSION

The prevalence of hypertension is related to the definition used by the WHO (Table 68-3).

Most patients with hypertension remain asymptomatic for extended periods of time, but the elevated blood pressure may lead to headache, sweating, palpitations, nervousness, and in the most severe cases nausea and vomiting. Hypertension should be actively investigated in patients presenting with IHD or stroke.

In HIV infection, hypertension is seen more frequently in men and is associated with obesity and older age.[65,93,94] The modifiable risk factors for hypertension in the background population include physical activity, over- and underweight, dyslipidemia, alcohol consumption, left ventricular hypertrophy, and microalbuminuria. There is no clear evidence to suggest that ART[93,95] or the underlying HIV infection affect the risk of hypertension. In most cases, no specific underlying cause can be identified. Only ~5% have secondary hypertension, often due to nephrotic illness, neurovascular hypertension, or hormonal disease.

The method of measuring blood pressure is essential in determining a correct diagnosis. The diagnosis must rely on repetitive measurements using a standardized procedure and after the patient has rested for at least 5 min. Of note, white-coat hypertension denotes artificially elevated blood pressure at the doctor's office but not at home[96] and should be suspected, especially in HIV-infected patients who are anxious about their underlying disease. Monitoring of blood pressure in the patient's usual surroundings can reliably be used to identify this problem. A validated upper arm monitor should be used for self-measurement of blood pressure.

Treatment

All patients diagnosed with hypertension should receive advice on lifestyle modifications, including enhancement of physical activity, reduction of body weight, if smoking, then cessation and modification of alcohol, fat, and salt consumption.

For grade 2 and 3 hypertension (Table 68-3), medical intervention is indicated. The goal is to reduce blood pressure to normal levels. The most frequent antihypertensive drugs used are thiazide diuretics, beta-adrenoceptor blockers, calcium channel antagonists, angiotensin 2 receptor antagonists, and angiotensin-converting enzyme inhibitors. The patient often needs two or three drugs combined in order to reach the desired goal.

LEFT AND RIGHT VENTRICULAR DYSFUNCTION

HIV has been isolated in myocardial cells[97,98] raising the possibility that HIV may induce myocarditis. However, it remains controversial whether these findings constitute a clinically significant pathological phenomenon. If significant, one would expect that the echocardiographically detectable consequence of this – dilated cardiomyopathy with left ventricular dysfunction – would be seen with higher frequency in HIV-infected persons. In the early years of the epidemic, some studies suggested such a high frequency. Of note, the study with the largest sample size was retracted by the editors of the publishing journal.[99] Furthermore, other studies did not support this among asymptomatic HIV-infected persons.[100] An emerging epidemic of heart failure due to left ventricular dysfunction among HIV-infected persons has not materialized (personal communication). In a recently reported carefully controlled study the prevalence was low (1%) and not apparently different from what can be expected to be observed in the general population.[101] However, several factors – other than HIV *per se* – may render HIV-infected persons at risk of ventricular dysfunction as reviewed below.

Left and Right Ventricular Dysfunction

Ventricular dysfunction can be expected to emerge as a growing problem as patients survive longer with chronic heart diseases. It is important to seek evidence of the underlying heart disease in both left and right ventricular dysfunction.

Previous IHD, hypertension, valvular disease/rheumatic fever, and palpitations are common causes of left ventricular dysfunction, whereas pulmonary arterial hypertension gives rise to cor pulmonale and thereby right ventricular dysfunction. Infectious disease can also give rise to ventricular dysfunction, as described below.

Table 68-3 Definition of Hypertension

	Systolic Blood Pressure (mmHg)		Diastolic Blood Pressure (mmHG)
Normal blood pressure	<140	and	<90
Grade 1 hypertension	140–159	and/or	90–99
Grade 2 hypertension	160–179	and/or	100–109
Grade 3 hypertension	⩾180	and/or	⩾110
Systolic hypertension	>140	and	<90
White coat hypertension	>140 (in office)	and/or	>90 (in office)
	<140 (at home)[a]	and	<90 (at home)[a]

The blood pressure should only be measured when the patient has rested (horizontally) for at least 5 minutes.

[a]Using an upper-arm certified blood pressure monitor.

Left Ventricular Dysfunction

Regional dyskinesia in the left ventricle due to IHD is the prominent cause of systolic left ventricular dysfunction in the Western world. It gives rise to a variety and degrees of chronic heart failure. It is critical to identify and manage the coronary artery disease (discussed earlier) and combine this with proper heart failure management (see below).

Cardiomyopathy

Cardiomyopathy constitutes a group of diseases where the pathology primarily involves the myocardium diffusively and is not due to ischemia. Three types of functional impairment have been described:

1. Dilated cardiomyopathy: this is the most common form, with either one or both right and left ventricular global dilation, systolic contractile dysfunction, and symptoms of congestive heart failure.
2. Hypertrophic cardiomyopathy with inappropriate left ventricular hypertrophy often with asymmetric involvement of the interventricular septum, usually with preserved or enhanced contractile function.
3. Restrictive cardiomyopathy marked by impaired diastolic filling, sometimes with endocardial scarring of the ventricle.

The distinction between these three functional categories is not always absolute, and overlapping is seen.

A complete understanding of the causes of dilated cardiomyopathy remains unclear although three basic mechanisms have been identified: genetic factors, viral myocarditis, and other cytotoxic insults and immunologic reactions.

Myocarditis

Myocarditis is defined as inflammation of the heart muscle. The inflammation may be caused by an infectious agent, is immune-mediated, or is the consequence of drug toxicity.[102] Myocarditis may be clinically asymptomatic, may lead to acute fully reversible dilated cardiomyopathy associated with congestive heart failure, or may persist as chronic dilated cardiomyopathy.[100,103–105]

The infectious etiology can be viral, bacterial, or fungal (Table 68-4).[106,107] The infectious agents cause myocardial damage by three mechanisms: (1) invasion of the myocardium; (2) production of a myocardial toxin; and (3) immunologically mediated myocardial damage. Once the infection has been cleared, fibrosis may persist.

The systemic illness should be characterized and treated. Treatment of heart failure is discussed below. Arrhythmias may develop. Note that patients with myocarditis may be more sensitive to digoxin.

Cor pulmonale

Acute cor pulmonale is defined as right heart strain or overload secondary to acute arterial pulmonary hypertension, often due to a large pulmonary embolism. Chronic cor pulmonale is characterized by hypertrophy and dilation of the right ventricle secondary to pulmonary hypertension. It can be due to diseases affecting the pulmonary vasculature (e.g., thrombo-embolic disorders), pressure due to tumors, diseases in the neuromuscular system and chest wall, or diseases affecting the air passage and alveoli (e.g., chronic obstructive pulmonary disease, infiltrative diseases).[108] A rare but real entity entitled 'HIV-associated pulmonary hypertension' has been described (occurring in 1 of 200 persons infected).[109,110]

Diuretics are used to treat right ventricular decompensation, possibly in combination with digoxin. Supplementary oxygen in hypoxemic patients with chronic cor pulmonale reduces right ventricular afterload and improves survival.

Heart Failure

Symptoms of suspected heart failure are dyspnea, fatigue, and edema.

It is critical to identify the cardiac origin of these nonspecific symptoms and at the same time seek the evidence of the possible underlying heart disease by clinical history, and examination, and investigation such as:

- ECG (sinus tachycardia, left ventricular hypertrophy, ST segment, T and Q wave abnormalities, ventricular and supraventricular arrhythmias),
- chest X-ray (dilated left ventricular and interstitial lung congestion), and
- echocardiogram (dilation of the ventricle, dyscontractility of the ventricle wall or increased left ventricular mass, depending on etiology of the underlying disease).

Treatment includes both nonmedical and medical interventions, depending on whether it is right or left ventricular dysfunction.[111]

Nonmedical: weight control, low-salt diet, fluid restriction, avoidance of alcohol and smoking, and use of regular physical exercise.

Medical: Diuretics (loop diuretics, thiazides, and spironolactone). Drugs blocking the neuroendocrine response (angiotensin-converting enzyme inhibitors and angiotensin 2 receptor antagonists) have become a cornerstone in the management of heart failure, as a large number of trials have documented improvement in survival rates in patients with left ventricular dysfunction. Beta-adrenoceptor blockers reduce mortality in left ventricular dysfunction. Antiarrythmic drugs are required in some patients, in others a biventricular pacemaker is required to synchronize the ventricular contractions.

Table 68-4

Infectious Complications of the Heart in HIV Seen More Frequently in Severely Immunodeficient Patients[a]

Section of Heart Infected	Pathogen – Bacteria, Virus, and Fungus	Associated with Immunodeficiency
Pericarditis	Tuberculosis, *Mycobacterium avium* complex, *Nocardia asteroides*	Yes
	Cytomegalovirus, herpes-simplex virus, Coxsackie virus, Adenovirus	Yes (for CMV)
	Cryptococcus neoformans, Aspergillus spp.	Yes
Myocarditis	Tuberculosis, *Mycobacterium avium* complex	Yes
	Cytomegalovirus, Coxsachie virus, Epstein–Barr virus-associated lymphomas, Human herpes virus 8-associated Kaposi sarcoma, HIV (?)	Yes
	Cryptococcus neoformans, Aspergillus spp., *Candida* spp., *Histoplasmosis capsulatum, Coccidioides immitis*	Yes
Endocarditis	*Staphylococcus aureus, Streptococcus viridans, Salmonella* spp.	No
	No viruses	–
	Aspergillus spp., *Cryptococcus neoformans, Candida* spp.	Yes

[a]Pericarditis is the most frequently observed condition in noninjecting drug users, whereas injecting drug users are at excessive increased risk of bacterial endocarditis regardless of level of immunodeficiency. All other infections are seen more frequently in patients with severe immunodeficiency and hence rarely seen in patients responding to antiretroviral therapy.

Source: Anderson et al,[106] Rerkpattanapipat et al,[107] Valencia and Miro,[112] and Heidenreich et al.[116]

ENDOCARDITIS

Infective endocarditis is the condition in which there is a microbial infection of the endothelial surface of the heart. There will be characteristic lesions in the form of vegetations which are variable in size and often situated at the heart valves. The infectious cause is usually bacteria such as *streptococci, staphylococci, enterococci*, and fastidious Gram-negative bacteria that reside in the oral cavity and upper respiratory tract. In patients with severe immunodeficiency, various fungal pathogens (Table 68-4) are an important differential diagnosis.

In HIV infection, most cases of endocarditis are seen in persons injecting illicit drugs intravenously and in patients requiring longer-term intravenous catheterization. The right side of the heart is usually affected, and the responsible bacteria is *Staphylococcus aureus*.[112–114] Available data suggest that the underlying HIV infection does not influence the clinical presentation, response to treatment, and outcome of bacterial endocarditis.

Treatment

Early recognition, precise identification of the infecting organism and prompt, aggressive antibiotic therapy, specifically directed at the offending organism, reduces complications.[115] The complications include valve destruction, infectious pulmonary emboli, congestive heart failure, proliferative glomerulonephritis, neurological manifestations such as embolic stroke, intracranial hemorrhage, and abscesses.

PERICARDIAL DISEASE

Acute pericarditis is a syndrome due to inflammation of the pericardium characterized by chest pain, a pericardial friction rub, and serial electrocardiographic abnormalities. Usually, ECHO viruses (coxsachie and adenoviruses) are responsible, although tuberculous pericarditis is a feared complication of tuberculosis in other organs (Table 68-4).[116] Tuberculosis should especially be suspected in patients originating from tuberculosis-endemic areas of the world.[117] Single cases of pericardial involvement of other HIV-related opportunistic infections have been reported.

Ballooning of the profile of the heart on a chest radiogram is usually seen in exudative pericarditis, and the pericardial effusion can be visualized by echocardiography. It is important to establish whether the pericarditis is related to an underlying disease that requires specific therapy or not. Examination of aspirated fluid may identify the causal agent. Of note, most cases of viral-induced acute pericarditis are nonexudative, and the diagnosis relies in these cases on the presence of retrosternal pain in the typical location and electrocardiographic abnormalities.

Table 68-5 Clinically Significant Drug Interactions Between Antiretroviral Drugs and Drugs Used to Prevent or Treat Cardiovascular Disease

Drugs Used to Treat Cardiovascular Disease	Non-Nucleoside Reverse Transcriptase Inhibitors	Protease Inhibitors
Acetylsalicylic acid	Use	Use
Anti-arrhythmics		
Digoxin	Use	$[\text{Anti-arrhythmics}]_p \uparrow$
Disopyramide, lidocaine, mexiletine,	$[\text{Anti-arrhythmics}]_p \downarrow$	$[\text{Anti-arrhythmics}]_p \uparrow$
Amiodarone, flecainide, propaferone,	$[\text{Anti-arrhythmics}]_p \downarrow$	Contraindicated
Beta-blockers		
Atenolol, bisoprolol, propranolol	Use	Use
Carvedilol	Unknown	Unknown
Calcium channel antagonists (Ca^{2+} ch. antag.)		
Amlodipine, diltiazem, nicardipine, nifedipine, nisoldipine, verapamil	$[Ca^{2+}\text{ ch. antag.}]_p \downarrow$	$[Ca^{2+}\text{ ch. antag.}]_p \uparrow$
Statins		
Fluvastatin, pravastatin, rosuvastatin	Use	Use
Atorvastatin	$[\text{Atorvastatin}]_p \downarrow$	$[\text{Atorvastatin}]_p \uparrow$
Lovastatin, simvastatin	Contraindicated	Contraindicated

If the plasma concentration of the first drug is reduced after co-administration with the HIV drug, higher than normal doses of the first drug may be required to accomplish the desired effect.

If the plasma concentration of the first drug is increased after co-administration with the HIV drug, lower than normal doses of the first drug may be required to accomplish the desired effect.
Source: www.hiv-druginteractions.org.

Treatment

The pain of the pericarditis responds normally to nonsteroidal anti-inflammatory agents. In some more severe cases it may be necessary to use corticosteroids for a short period of time. If the pericarditis becomes exudative, antibiotics are indicated and if ventricular function is compromised surgical drainage should be done.

Recurrent episodes of pericardial inflammation are a troublesome complication. Such cases are treated with high doses of nonsteroidal anti-inflammatory agents followed by gradual tapering over several months. Seldom intravenous methylprednisolone given as pulse therapy may be useful.

DRUG–DRUG INTERACTIONS OF DRUGS USED TO TREAT CARDIOVASCULAR DISEASE AND HIV INFECTION

Clinical relevant drug–drug interactions exist between non-nucleoside reverse transcriptase inhibitors and protease inhibitors on one side and anti-arrhythmics, beta-blockers, calcium channel antagonists, and statins on the other side (Table 68-5). In general non-nucleoside reverse transcriptase inhibitors tend to reduce plasma concentrations of some of these drugs, whereas protease inhibitors tend to have the opposite effect. One exception to this is that nelfinavir (a protease inhibitor) may reduce concentration of pravastatin.[118] Drugs used for the treatment of CVD do not affect the pharmacology of drugs used to treat HIV.

It is advisable to check for possible drug–drug interactions prior to commencing a combination of drugs used to treat CVD and HIV (e.g., www.hiv-druginteractions.org), and titrate the former drugs depending on the direction of the pharmacological interaction.

CARDIAC-RELATED ADVERSE EVENTS OF DRUGS COMMONLY USED IN HIV INFECTION

Cocaine and Methamfetamine

Excessive intake of cocaine can induce tachycardia, angina pectoris, and myocardial infarction,[119] and is frequently used by many HIV-infected patients, and hence is a relevant differential diagnosis to consider for cases suspected of IHD. Excessive intake of methamfetamine may induce similar symptoms.[120] It has been suggested that cocaine use may accelerate the atherosclerotic process in HIV infection.[121]

Arrythmias

Supraventricular arrythmias may develop in patients with congestive heart failure. If the antiarrythmic digoxin is used to manage such patients, a potential drug–drug interaction can occur with co-administration of ritonavir. Ritonavir slows the excretion of digoxin[122] maybe by inhibiting digoxin transport

Table 68-6

Drug Classes with Examples of Drugs and Cardiac Conditions with the Potential for QT-Prolongation and Torsades De Pointe[a]

Antihistamines	Cardiotherapy	Anti-Infectives
Astemizole[b]	Digoxin	Erythromycin and other macrolides
Terfenadine[b]	Calcium channel antagonists	Pentamidine
	Procainamide	Fluoroquinolones
Sedatives	Pimozide	Ketoconazole, itraconazol
Methadone		HIV-protease inhibitors
Antipsycotics	**Antidepressants**	**Cardiac Conditions**
Chlorpromazine	Amitryptiline	Ischemic heart disease
Haloperidol	Doxepine	Cardiomyopathy
Pimozide[b]	Desipramine	
Lithium	Imipramine	

[a]The risk of QT prolongation increased if drugs are combined – especially in situations where drug slow excretion of other drugs (e.g., calcium channels antagonists and HIV protease inhibitors (see Table 68-5)).

[b]Drugs where there is absolute contraindication for co-administration with HIV protease inhibitors due to excessive risk of QT-prolongation.

Source: www.torsades.org.

via P-glycoprotein (P-gp). This leads to increased serum digoxin and the potential for atrio-ventricular blockage.[123]

Of the possible ventricular arrythmias, in HIV infection, the primary focus should be on QT-prolongation. There is a growing body of evidence to suggest that protease inhibitors may prolong the QT interval of the contractile cycle of the heart in a few patients, rendering such patients at excess risk of developing torsades de pointes and other arrythmias.[124,125] The mechanism for this appears to be that protease inhibitors can block a potassium channel relevant to normal dissemination of the electrical current within the myocardium. Of note, a number of other drugs – many of which are used in HIV – are also able to prolong the QT interval (Table 68-6).[125,126] The QT prolongation is dose dependent, and special care should be observed when combining drugs that can affect the QT prolongation, especially as some of these drugs elevate the plasma concentrations of other drugs (Table 68-5). An example of this is the administration of the antihistamine terfenadine in patients receiving ritonavir, a combination absolutely contraindicated. Congestive heart failure is the cardinal symptom of torsades de pointes, and an ECG can confirm the diagnosis.

Chemotherapeutics and Cardiomyopathy

Anthracyclines inhibit the proliferation of rapidly growing Kaposi sarcoma, but prolonged exposure (more than 400–500 mg/m^2) may result in cardiomyopathy. Of note, anthracyclines are metabolized via the P450 enzyme system, rendering the patient at risk of higher than intended plasma concentrations if used together with inhibitors of this enzyme system, e.g., protease inhibitors.[127]

Perinatal Exposure to Antiretroviral Drugs

Concerns arising from preclinical studies of whether pre- and/or postnatal exposure to zidovudine leads to impairment of normal myocardiocyte development[128] are not supported by longitudinal studies of infants exposed to this drug.[129] Recent studies suggest that left ventricular function deteriorates in the first 3 years of life of HIV-infected infants.[130]

OPEN-HEART SURGERY

HIV-infected persons should be offered open-heart surgery and cardiac transplantation using comparable criteria to those applied for non-HIV-infected patients. The published case series of valve replacement shows reasonable outcome.[131,132] There is one case report of successful heart transplantation in an HIV-infected patient.[133]

REFERENCES

1. Mocroft A, Vella S, Benfield TL, et al. Changing patterns of mortality across Europe in patients infected with HIV-1. EuroSIDA Study Group. Lancet 352:1725, 1998.
2. Mocroft A, Ledergerber B, Katlama C, et al. Decline in the AIDS and death rates in the EuroSIDA study: an observational study. Lancet 362:22, 2003.
3. Palella FJ, Jr, Delaney KM, Moorman AC, et al. Declining morbidity and mortality among patients with advanced human immunodeficiency virus infection. HIV Outpatient Study Investigators. N Engl J Med 338:853, 1998.
4. Mary-Krause M, Cotte L, Simon A, et al. Increased risk of myocardial infarction with duration of protease inhibitor therapy in HIV-infected men. AIDS 17:2479, 2003.
5. d'Arminio A, Sabin CA, Phillips AN, et al. Cardio and cerebrovascular events in HIV-infected persons. AIDS 18:1811, 2004.
6. Iloeje UH, Yuan Y, L'italien G, et al. Protease inhibitor exposure and increased risk of cardiovascular disease in HIV-infected patients. HIV Med 6:37, 2005.
7. Friis-Moller N, Sabin CA, Weber R, et al. Combination antiretroviral therapy and the risk of myocardial infarction. N Engl J Med 349:1993, 2003.
8. Skalen K, Gustafsson M, Rydberg EK, et al. Subendothelial retention of atherogenic lipoproteins in early atherosclerosis. Nature 417:750, 2002.

9. Barter P. The inflammation: lipoprotein cycle. Atheroscler Suppl 6(2):15–20, 2005.
10. Ross R. Atherosclerosis – an inflammatory disease. N Engl J Med 340:115, 1999.
11. Berenson GS, Srinivasan SR, Bao W, et al. Association between multiple cardiovascular risk factors and atherosclerosis in children and young adults. The Bogalusa Heart Study. N Engl J Med 338:1650, 1998.
12. Tunstall-Pedoe H. Myth and paradox of coronary risk and the menopause. Lancet 351:1425, 1998.
13. Acton RT, Go RC, Roseman JM. Genetics and cardiovascular disease. Ethn Dis 14:S2, 2004.
14. Haffner SM, Lehto S, Ronnemaa T, et al. Mortality from coronary heart disease in subjects with type 2 diabetes and in nondiabetic subjects with and without prior myocardial infarction. N Engl J Med 339:229, 1998.
15. Huxley R, Barzi F, Woodward M. Excess risk of fatal coronary heart disease associated with diabetes in men and women: meta-analysis of 37 prospective cohort studies. BMJ 332:73, 2006.
16. Huang ES, Meigs JB, Singer DE. The effect of interventions to prevent cardiovascular disease in patients with type 2 diabetes mellitus. Am J Med 111:633, 2001.
17. Doll R, Peto R. Mortality in relation to smoking: 20 years' observations on male British doctors. BMJ 2:1525, 1976.
18. Parish S, Collins R, Peto R, et al. Cigarette smoking, tar yields, and non-fatal myocardial infarction: 14,000 cases and 32,000 controls in the United Kingdom. The International Studies of Infarct Survival (ISIS) Collaborators. BMJ 311:471, 1995.
19. Prescott E, Hippe M, Schnohr P, et al. Smoking and risk of myocardial infarction in women and men: longitudinal population study. BMJ 316:1043, 1998.
20. Kawachi I, Colditz GA, Stampfer MJ, et al. Smoking cessation in relation to total mortality rates in women. A prospective cohort study. Ann Intern Med 119:992, 1993.
21. Grundy SM, Cleeman JI, Merz CN, et al. Implications of recent clinical trials for the National Cholesterol Education Program Adult Treatment Panel III guidelines. Circulation 110:227, 2004.
22. Executive Summary of The Third Report of The National Cholesterol Education Program (NCEP) Expert Panel on Detection, Evaluation, and Treatment of High Blood Cholesterol In Adults (Adult Treatment Panel III). JAMA 285:2486, 2001.
23. Wood D, De Backer G, Faergeman O, et al. Prevention of coronary heart disease in clinical practice: recommendations of the Second Joint Task Force of European and other Societies on Coronary Prevention. Atherosclerosis 140:199, 1998.
24. Egger M, Smith GD, Pfluger D, et al. Triglyceride as a risk factor for ischaemic heart disease in British men: effect of adjusting for measurement error. Atherosclerosis 143:275, 1999.
25. Criqui MH, Heiss G, Cohn R, et al. Plasma triglyceride level and mortality from coronary heart disease. N Engl J Med 328:1220, 1993.
26. Jeppesen J, Hein HO, Suadicani P, et al. High triglycerides/low high-density lipoprotein cholesterol, ischemic electrocardiogram changes, and risk of ischemic heart disease. Am Heart J 145:103, 2003.
27. Eckel RH, Grundy SM, Zimmet PZ. The metabolic syndrome. Lancet 365:1415, 2005.
28. Dekker JM, Girman C, Rhodes T, et al. Metabolic syndrome and 10-year cardiovascular disease risk in the Hoorn Study. Circulation 112:666, 2005.
29. Pate RR, Pratt M, Blair SN, et al. Physical activity and public health. A recommendation from the Centers for Disease Control and Prevention and the American College of Sports Medicine. JAMA 273:402, 1995.
30. Blair SN, Cooper KH, Gibbons LW, et al. Changes in coronary heart disease risk factors associated with increased treadmill time in 753 men. Am J Epidemiol 118:352, 1983.
31. Helmrich SP, Ragland DR, Leung RW, et al. Physical activity and reduced occurrence of non-insulin-dependent diabetes mellitus. N Engl J Med 325:147, 1991.
32. Despres JP, Pouliot MC, Moorjani S, et al. Loss of abdominal fat and metabolic response to exercise training in obese women. Am J Physiol 261:E159–E167, 1991.
33. Arroll B, Beaglehole R. Does physical activity lower blood pressure: a critical review of the clinical trials. J Clin Epidemiol 45:439, 1992.
34. Hambrecht R, Walther C, Mobius-Winkler S, et al. Percutaneous coronary angioplasty compared with exercise training in patients with stable coronary artery disease: a randomized trial. Circulation 109:1371, 2004.
35. Danesh J, Whincup P, Walker M, et al. Low grade inflammation and coronary heart disease: prospective study and updated meta-analyses. BMJ 321:199, 2000.
36. Danesh J, Wheeler JG, Hirschfield GM, et al. C-reactive protein and other circulating markers of inflammation in the prediction of coronary heart disease. N Engl J Med 350:1387, 2004.
37. Neaton JD, Wentworth D. Serum cholesterol, blood pressure, cigarette smoking, and death from coronary heart disease. Overall findings and differences by age for 316,099 white men. Multiple Risk Factor Intervention Trial Research Group. Arch Intern Med 152:56, 1992.
38. Grunfeld C, Kotler DP, Hamadeh R, et al. Hypertriglyceridemia in the acquired immunodeficiency syndrome. Am J Med 86:27, 1989.
39. Grunfeld C, Pang M, Doerrler W, et al. Lipids, lipoproteins, triglyceride clearance, and cytokines in human immunodeficiency virus infection and the acquired immunodeficiency syndrome. J Clin Endocrinol Metab 74:1045, 1992.
40. Riddler SA, Smit E, Cole SR, et al. Impact of HIV infection and HAART on serum lipids in men. JAMA 289:2978, 2003.
41. Law MG, Friis-Moller N, El Sadr WM, et al. The use of the Framingham equation to predict myocardial infarctions in HIV-infected patients: comparison with observed events in the D:A:D study. HIV Med, 7:218–230, 2006.
42. Friis-Moller N, Weber R, Reiss P, et al. Cardiovascular disease risk factors in HIV patients – association with antiretroviral therapy. Results from the DAD study. AIDS 17:1179, 2003.
43. Writing committee: Friis-Moller N, Reiss P, El-Sadr W, et al, on behalf of the D:A:D study group. Class of Antiretroviral Drugs and the Risk of Myocardial Infarction. N Engl J Med 26;356:1723–35, 2007.
44. Zhou H, Pandak WM Jr, Lyall V, et al. HIV protease inhibitors activate the unfolded protein response in macrophages: implication for atherosclerosis and cardiovascular disease. Mol Pharmacol 68:690, 2005.
45. Lundgren JD, Sabin CA, Weber R, et al. Cardiovascular outcomes in HIV infection. 12th Conference on Retroviruses and Opportunistic Infections, Boston, USA #62: 2005.
46. van Leth F, Phanuphak P, Stroes E, et al. Nevirapine and efavirenz elicit different changes in lipid profiles in antiretroviral-therapy-naive patients infected with HIV-1. PLoS Med 1: e19, 2004.
47. van der Valk M, Kastelein JJ, Murphy RL, et al. Nevirapine-containing antiretroviral therapy in HIV-1 infected patients results in an anti-atherogenic lipid profile. AIDS 15:2407, 2001.
48. Gallant JE, Staszewski S, Pozniak AL, et al. Efficacy and safety of tenofovir DF vs stavudine in combination therapy in antiretroviral-naive patients: a 3-year randomized trial. JAMA 292:191, 2004.
49. Dube MP, Stein JH, Aberg JA, et al. Guidelines for the evaluation and management of dyslipidemia in human immunodeficiency virus (HIV)-infected adults receiving antiretroviral therapy: recommendations of the HIV Medical Association

of the Infectious Disease Society of America and the Adult AIDS Clinical Trials Group. Clin Infect Dis 37:613, 2003.

50. Neal B, MacMahon S, Chapman N. Effects of ACE inhibitors, calcium antagonists, and other blood-pressure-lowering drugs: results of prospectively designed overviews of randomised trials. Blood Pressure Lowering Treatment Trialists' Collaboration. Lancet 356:1955, 2000.
51. MacMahon S. Can a 'Polypill' Cut Heart Disease Risk in People With HIV? International Workshop on Adverse Drug Reactions and Lipodystrophy in HIV, Dublin, November, 2005.
51a. Collaborative meta-analysis of randomised trials of antiplatelet therapy for prevention of death, myocardial infarction, and stroke in high risk patients. BMJ 324:71, 2002.
52. Bergersen BM, Sandvik L, Bruun JN, et al. Elevated Framingham risk score in HIV-positive patients on highly active antiretroviral therapy: results from a Norwegian study of 721 subjects. Eur J Clin Microbiol Infect Dis 23:625, 2004.
53. Anderson KM, Odell PM, Wilson PW, et al. Cardiovascular disease risk profiles. Am Heart J 121:293, 1991.
54. Thomsen TF, Davidsen M, Ibsen H, et al. A new method for CHD prediction and prevention based on regional risk scores and randomized clinical trials; PRECARD and the Copenhagen Risk Score. J Cardiovasc Risk 8:291, 2001.
55. Ardern CI, Katzmarzyk PT, Janssen I, et al. Revised Adult Treatment Panel III guidelines and cardiovascular disease mortality in men attending a preventive medical clinic. Circulation 112:1478, 2005.
56. Silagy C, Lancaster T, Stead L, et al. Nicotine replacement therapy for smoking cessation. Cochrane Database Syst Rev CD000146, 2002.
57. Aberg JA. Cardiovascular risk among HIV-positive patients on antiretroviral therapy. J Int Assoc Physicians AIDS Care 2(Suppl 2):S24–S39, 2003.
58. Young J, Weber R, Rickenbach M, et al. Lipid profiles for antiretroviral-naive patients starting PI- and NNRTI-based therapy in the Swiss HIV cohort study. Antivir Ther 10:585, 2005.
59. Fontas E, van Leth F, Sabin CA, et al. Lipid profiles in HIV-infected patients receiving combination antiretroviral therapy: are different antiretroviral drugs associated with different lipid profiles? J Infect Dis 189:1056, 2004.
60. Tarr PE, Taffe P, Bleiber G, et al. Modeling the influence of APOC3, APOE, and TNF polymorphisms on the risk of antiretroviral therapy-associated lipid disorders. J Infect Dis 191:1419, 2005.
61. Johnson CL, Rifkind BM, Sempos CT, et al. Declining serum total cholesterol levels among US adults. The National Health and Nutrition Examination Surveys. JAMA 269:3002, 1993.
62. Vasudevan AR, Jones PH. Effective use of combination lipid therapy. Curr Atheroscler Rep 8:76, 2006.
63. Bays HE, Ose L, Fraser N, et al. A multicenter, randomized, double-blind, placebo-controlled, factorial design study to evaluate the lipid-altering efficacy and safety profile of the ezetimibe/simvastatin tablet compared with ezetimibe and simvastatin monotherapy in patients with primary hypercholesterolemia. Clin Ther 26:1758, 2004.
64. Roge BT, Katzenstein TL, Gerstoft J. Comparison of P-triglyceride levels among patients with human immunodeficiency virus on randomized treatment with ritonavir, indinavir or ritonavir/saquinavir. Scand J Infect Dis 33:306, 2001.
65. Dragsted UB, Gerstoft J, Youle M, et al. A randomized trial to evaluate lopinavir/ritonavir versus saquinavir/ritonavir in HIV-1-infected patients: the MaxCmin2 trial. Antivir Ther 10:735, 2005.
66. Walmsley S, Bernstein B, King M, et al. Lopinavir-ritonavir versus nelfinavir for the initial treatment of HIV infection. N Engl J Med 346:2039, 2002.
67. Radermacher J, Chavan A, Bleck J, et al. Use of Doppler ultrasonography to predict the outcome of therapy for renal-artery stenosis. N Engl J Med 344:410, 2001.
68. Behar S, Brunner D, Kaplinsky E, et al. Secondary prevention by raising HDL cholesterol and reducing triglycerides in patients with coronary artery disease: the Bezafibrate Infarction Prevention (BIP) study. Circulation 102:21, 2000.
69. Keech A, Simes RJ, Barter P, et al. Effects of long-term fenofibrate therapy on cardiovascular events in 9795 people with type 2 diabetes mellitus (the FIELD study): randomised controlled trial. Lancet 366:1849, 2005.
70. Rubins HB, Robins SJ, Collins D, et al. Gemfibrozil for the secondary prevention of coronary heart disease in men with low levels of high-density lipoprotein cholesterol. Veterans Affairs High-Density Lipoprotein Cholesterol Intervention Trial Study Group. N Engl J Med 341:410, 1999.
71. Guo JJ, Jang R, Louder A, et al. Acute pancreatitis associated with different combination therapies in patients infected with human immunodeficiency virus. Pharmacotherapy 25:1044, 2005.
72. Davidson MH. Statin/fibrate combination in patients with metabolic syndrome or diabetes: evaluating the risks of pharmacokinetic drug interactions. Expert Opin Drug Saf 5:145, 2006.
73. Chang JT, Staffa JA, Parks M, et al. Rhabdomyolysis with HMG-CoA reductase inhibitors and gemfibrozil combination therapy. Pharmacoepidemiol Drug Saf 13:417, 2004.
74. Moyle GJ, Lloyd M, Reynolds B, et al. Dietary advice with or without pravastatin for the management of hypercholesterolaemia associated with protease inhibitor therapy. AIDS 15:1503, 2001.
75. Aberg JA, Zackin RA, Brobst SW, et al. A randomized trial of the efficacy and safety of fenofibrate versus pravastatin in HIV-infected subjects with lipid abnormalities: AIDS Clinical Trials Group Study 5087. AIDS Res Hum Retroviruses 21:757, 2005.
76. Benesic A, Zilly M, Kluge F, et al. Lipid lowering therapy with fluvastatin and pravastatin in patients with HIV infection and antiretroviral therapy: comparison of efficacy and interaction with indinavir. Infection 32:229, 2004.
77. Penzak SR, Chuck SK, Stajich GV. Safety and efficacy of HMG-CoA reductase inhibitors for treatment of hyperlipidemia in patients with HIV infection. Pharmacotherapy 20:1066, 2000.
78. Murata H, Hruz PW, Mueckler M. Indinavir inhibits the glucose transporter isoform Glut4 at physiologic concentrations. AIDS 16:859, 2002.
79. Noor MA, Seneviratne T, Aweeka FT, et al. Indinavir acutely inhibits insulin-stimulated glucose disposal in humans: a randomized, placebo-controlled study. AIDS 16:F1-F8, 2002.
80. Hadigan C. Diabetes, insulin resistance, and HIV. Curr Infect Dis Rep 8:69, 2006.
81. Hadigan C, Yawetz S, Thomas A, et al. Metabolic effects of rosiglitazone in HIV lipodystrophy: a randomized, controlled trial. Ann Intern Med 140:786, 2004.
82. van Wijk JP, de Koning EJ, Cabezas MC, et al. Comparison of rosiglitazone and metformin for treating HIV lipodystrophy: a randomized trial. Ann Intern Med 143:337, 2005.
83. Sutinen J, Hakkinen AM, Westerbacka J, et al. Rosiglitazone in the treatment of HAART-associated lipodystrophy – a randomized double-blind placebo-controlled study. Antivir Ther 8:199, 2003.
84. Carr A, Workman C, Carey D, et al. No effect of rosiglitazone for treatment of HIV-1 lipoatrophy: randomised, double-blind, placebo-controlled trial. Lancet 363:429, 2004.
85. Rajappa M, Sharma A. Biomarkers of cardiac injury: an update. Angiology 56:677, 2005.

86. Smith SC Jr, Feldman TE, Hirshfeld JW Jr, et al. ACC/AHA/SCAI 2005 Guideline Update for Percutaneous Coronary Intervention – summary article: a report of the American College of Cardiology/American Heart Association Task Force on Practice Guidelines (ACC/AHA/SCAI Writing Committee to Update the 2001 Guidelines for Percutaneous Coronary Intervention). Circulation 113:156, 2006.
87. Serruys PW, Kutryk MJ, Ong AT. Coronary-artery stents. N Engl J Med 354:483, 2006.
88. McDermott MM, Liu K, Greenland P, et al. Functional decline in peripheral arterial disease: associations with the ankle brachial index and leg symptoms. JAMA 292:453, 2004.
89. Dormandy JA, Rutherford RB. Management of peripheral arterial disease (PAD). TASC Working Group. TransAtlantic Inter-Society Concensus (TASC). J Vasc Surg 31:S1–S296, 2000.
90. Hankey GJ, Norman PE, Eikelboom JW. Medical treatment of peripheral arterial disease. JAMA 295:547, 2006.
91. Kumwenda JJ, Mateyu G, Kampondeni S, et al. Differential diagnosis of stroke in a setting of high HIV prevalence in Blantyre, Malawi. Stroke 36:960, 2005.
92. d'Arminio MA, Cinque P, Mocroft A, et al. Changing incidence of central nervous system diseases in the EuroSIDA cohort. Ann Neurol 55:320, 2004.
93. Seaberg EC, Munoz A, Lu M, et al. Association between highly active antiretroviral therapy and hypertension in a large cohort of men followed from 1984 to 2003. AIDS 19:953, 2005.
94. Jerico C, Knobel H, Montero M, et al. Hypertension in HIV-infected patients: prevalence and related factors. Am J Hypertens 18:1396, 2005.
95. Thiebaut R, El Sadr WM, Friis-Moller N, et al. Predictors of hypertension and changes of blood pressure in HIV-infected patients. Antivir Ther 10:811, 2005.
96. Celis H, Den Hond E, Staessen JA. Self-measurement of blood pressure at home in the management of hypertension. Clin Med Res 3:19, 2005.
97. Grody WW, Cheng L, Lewis W. Infection of the heart by the human immunodeficiency virus. Am J Cardiol 66:203, 1990.
98. Calabrese LH, Proffitt MR, Yen-Lieberman B, et al. Congestive cardiomyopathy and illness related to the acquired immunodeficiency syndrome (AIDS) associated with isolation of retrovirus from myocardium. Ann Intern Med 107:691, 1987.
99. Drazen JM, Curfman GD. Barbaro G, et al. Incidence of dilated cardiomyopathy and detection of HIV in myocardial cells of HIV-positive patients. N Engl J Med 339: 1093, 1998.
100. Himelman RB, Chung WS, Chernoff DN et al. Cardiac manifestations of human immunodeficiency virus infection: a two-dimensional echocardiographic study. J Am Coll Cardiol 13:1030, 1989.
101. Lebech AM, Gerstoft J, Hesse B, et al. Right and left ventricular cardiac function in a developed world population with human immunodeficiency virus studied with radionuclide ventriculography. Am Heart J 147:482, 2004.
102. Feldman AM, McNamara D. Myocarditis. N Engl J Med 343:1388, 2000.
103. Jacob AJ, Sutherland GR, Bird AG, et al. Myocardial dysfunction in patients infected with HIV: prevalence and risk factors. Br Heart J 68:549, 1992.
104. Coudray N, de Zuttere D, Force G, et al. Left ventricular diastolic function in asymptomatic and symptomatic human immunodeficiency virus carriers: an echocardiographic study. Eur Heart J 16:61, 1995.
105. Cohen IS, Anderson DW, Virmani R, et al. Congestive cardiomyopathy in association with the acquired immunodeficiency syndrome. N Engl J Med 315:628, 1986.
106. Anderson DW, Virmani R, Reilly JM, et al. Prevalent myocarditis at necropsy in the acquired immunodeficiency syndrome. J Am Coll Cardiol 11:792, 1988.
107. Rerkpattanapipat P, Wongpraparut N, Jacobs LE, et al. Cardiac manifestations of acquired immunodeficiency syndrome. Arch Intern Med 160:602, 2000.
108. Farber HW, Loscalzo J. Pulmonary arterial hypertension. N Engl J Med 351:1655, 2004.
109. Speich R, Jenni R, Opravil M et al. Primary pulmonary hypertension in HIV infection. Chest 100:1268, 1991.
110. Mesa RA, Edell ES, Dunn WF, et al. Human immunodeficiency virus infection and pulmonary hypertension: two new cases and a review of 86 reported cases. Mayo Clin Proc 73:37, 1998.
111. Jessup M, Brozena S. Heart failure. N Engl J Med 348:2007, 2003.
112. Valencia E, Miro J. Endocarditis in the setting of HIV infection. AIDS Rev 6:97, 2004.
113. Manoff SB, Vlahov D, Herskowitz A, et al. Human immunodeficiency virus infection and infective endocarditis among injecting drug users. Epidemiology 7:566, 1996.
114. Nahass RG, Weinstein MP, Bartels J, et al. Infective endocarditis in intravenous drug users: a comparison of human immunodeficiency virus type 1-negative and -positive patients. J Infect Dis 162:967, 1990.
115. Mylonakis E, Calderwood SB. Infective endocarditis in adults. N Engl J Med 345:1318, 2001.
116. Heidenreich PA, Eisenberg MJ, Kee LL, et al. Pericardial effusion in AIDS. Incidence and survival. Circulation 92:3229, 1995.
117. Ntsekhe M, Hakim J. Impact of human immunodeficiency virus infection on cardiovascular disease in Africa. Circulation 112:3602, 2005.
118. Aberg JA, Rosenkranz SL, Fichtenbaum CJ, et al. Pharmacokinetic interaction between nelfinavir and pravastatin in HIV-seronegative volunteers: ACTG Study A5108. AIDS 20:725, 2006.
119. Lange RA, Hillis LD. Cardiovascular complications of cocaine use. N Engl J Med 345:351, 2001.
120. Yu Q, Larson DF, Watson RR. Heart disease, methamphetamine and AIDS. Life Sci 73:129, 2003.
121. Lai S, Lima JA, Lai H et al. Human immunodeficiency virus 1 infection, cocaine, and coronary calcification. Arch Intern Med 165:690, 2005.
122. Penzak SR, Shen JM, Alfaro RM, et al. Ritonavir decreases the nonrenal clearance of digoxin in healthy volunteers with known MDR1 genotypes. Ther Drug Monit 26:322, 2004.
123. Phillips EJ, Rachlis AR, Ito S. Digoxin toxicity and ritonavir: a drug interaction mediated through p-glycoprotein? AIDS 17:1577, 2003.
124. Kikuchi Y, Genka I, Ishizaki A, et al. Serious bradyarrhythmia that was possibly induced by lopinavir-ritonavir in 2 patients with acquired immunodeficiency syndrome. Clin Infect Dis 35:488, 2002.
125. Anson BD, Weaver JG, Ackerman MJ, et al. Blockade of HERG channels by HIV protease inhibitors. Lancet 365:682, 2005.
126. Gil M, Sala M, Anguera I, et al. QT prolongation and torsades de pointes in patients infected with human immunodeficiency virus and treated with methadone. Am J Cardiol 92:995, 2003.
127. Rosenthal E, Sala F, Chichmanian RM, et al. Ergotism related to concurrent administration of ergotamine tartrate and indinavir. JAMA 281:987, 1999.
128. Walker DM, Poirier MC, Campen MJ, et al. Persistence of mitochondrial toxicity in hearts of female B6C3F1 mice exposed in utero to 3′-azido-3′-deoxythymidine. Cardiovasc Toxicol 4:133, 2004.

129. Lipshultz SE, Easley KA, Orav EJ, et al. Absence of cardiac toxicity of zidovudine in infants. Pediatric Pulmonary and Cardiac Complications of Vertically Transmitted HIV Infection Study Group. N Engl J Med 343:759, 2000.
130. Fisher SD, Easley KA, Orav EJ, et al. Mild dilated cardiomyopathy and increased left ventricular mass predict mortality: the prospective P2C2 HIV Multicenter Study. Am Heart J 150:439, 2005.
131. Chong T, Alejo DE, Greene PS, et al. Cardiac valve replacement in human immunodeficiency virus-infected patients. Ann Thorac Surg 76:478, 2003.
132. Trachiotis GD, Alexander EP, Benator D, et al. Cardiac surgery in patients infected with the human immunodeficiency virus. Ann Thorac Surg 76:1114, 2003.
133. Calabrese LH, Albrecht M, Young J, et al. Successful cardiac transplantation in an HIV-1-infected patient with advanced disease. N Engl J Med 348:2323, 2003.

Chapter 69

Respiratory Disease

Laurence Huang, MD

Patients with human immunodeficiency virus (HIV) infection can develop respiratory dysfunction due to a wide variety of disorders. Although the immediate focus is often directed at opportunistic infection (OI), clinicians caring for HIV-infected patients presenting with dyspnea, cough, chest pain, with or without fever, must approach the differential diagnosis methodically. In addition to HIV-associated OIs, patients with HIV infection are also susceptible to community-acquired pathogens (e.g., influenza or *Mycoplasma*) and hospital-acquired organisms (e.g., methicillin-resistant *Staphylococcus aureus* or extended-spectrum β-Lactamase-producing enteric organisms). Risk factors for HIV infection, such as injection drug use, may contribute to pulmonary disease (e.g., endocarditis with septic pulmonary emboli, aspiration pneumonia secondary to altered mentation, noncardiogenic pulmonary edema, talc granulomatosis). Clinicians should also recognize that HIV-infected persons might have preexisting or concurrent chronic pulmonary disease (e.g., asthma or chronic obstructive pulmonary disease) unrelated to their HIV infection. Thus, a rational approach to respiratory dysfunction in patients with HIV infection should include the same considerations as any immunologically normal patient, as well as consideration for the processes that occur with special frequency or severity in patients with HIV infection (Table 69-1). This chapter presents an approach to lower respiratory tract and upper respiratory tract infections in this patient population.

EPIDEMIOLOGIC PERSPECTIVE

The clinical setting – outpatient, inpatient, or ICU – influences the relative frequency of respiratory diseases that are observed. The Pulmonary Complications of HIV Infection Study (PCHIS) was a prospective, observational cohort study that followed more than 1 150 HIV-infected subjects for ~5 years at six sites across the United States prior to the era of highly active antiretroviral therapy (HAART).[1,2] PCHIS documented that patients who presented to an outpatient clinic with respiratory illness more often had upper respiratory tract infections and acute bronchitis than pneumonias due to bacteria or *Pneumocystis*.[2] In contrast, bacterial pneumonia and *Pneumocystis* pneumonia (PCP) are the most frequent causes of pneumonia in hospital-based series. Pneumonias due to bacteria (*Streptococcus pneumoniae*: 21% of all pneumonias in HIV-infected subjects) and *Pneumocystis* (27%) greatly exceeded those due to viruses, mycobacteria, and fungi (each <5%) in a year-long hospital-based study of community-acquired pneumonia at Johns Hopkins Hospital.[3] PCP (35%) and bacterial pneumonia (27%) were also the most common etiologies reported in a hospital-based study of community-acquired pneumonia from Atlanta.[4] Finally, PCHIS showed that the most common pulmonary diseases observed among HIV-infected patients requiring critical care were PCP followed by bacterial pneumonia.[5] These results from the multicenter PCHIS are similar to those reported from single institutions such as San Francisco General Hospital [6–8] as well as cohorts in Europe.[9]

The geographic location of the clinic or hospital may also influence the frequency of the diagnoses. In specific populations or geographic regions, mycobacterial and endemic fungal pneumonias are important considerations. Worldwide, tuberculosis (TB) is a leading cause of death. In endemic areas, diseases caused by *Histoplasma capsulatum* or *Coccidioides immitis* are among the most frequent infections seen,[10] whereas at San Francisco General Hospital they are rarely encountered. Table 69-2 lists diagnostic clues to the causes of respiratory disease in patients with HIV infection.

LOWER RESPIRATORY TRACT DISEASE: PNEUMONIA

One of the first decisions that clinicians face is whether or not to place a patient in isolation. Suspicion of TB, influenza, or respiratory syncytial virus (RSV) infection based on history,

Table 69-1 Causes of Pulmonary Dysfunction Seen with Increased Frequency or Severity in Patients with HIV Infection

Opportunistic Infections

Bacteria
- *Streptococcus pneumoniae*
- *Haemophilus influenzae*
- *Staphylococcus aureus*
- *Pseudomonas aeruginosa*
- *Klebsiella pneumoniae*
- *Rhodococcus equi*
- *Mycobacterium tuberculosis*
- Atypical mycobacteria[a]

Fungi
- *Pneumocystis jirovecii* (formerly *P. carinii*)
- *Cryptococcus neoformans*
- *Histoplasma capsulatum*
- *Coccidioides immitis*
- *Aspergillus* species
- *Penicillium marneffei*

Viruses
- CMV[a]
- VZV

Protozoa
- *Toxoplasma gondii*
- *Strongyloides stercoralis*[b]

Neoplasms
- Lymphoma
- Kaposi sarcoma
- Bronchogenic carcinoma (?)

Other Disorders
- Lymphocytic interstitial pneumonitis
- Nonspecific interstitial pneumonitis
- Asthma (?)
- Chronic obstructive pulmonary disease (?)
- Pulmonary arterial hypertension
- Immune reconstitution syndrome
- Sarcoid (?)

Upper Respiratory Tract Infection
- Bronchitis

VZV, varicella-zoster virus.

[a]Cytomegalovirus (CMV) and *Mycobacterium avium* complex (MAC) are rarely the cause of pulmonary dysfunction in patients with HIV infection regardless of their CD4+ T-lymphocyte and neutrophil counts.

[b]Although disseminated Strongyloides is an AIDS-defining disease, it has rarely been documented in patients with HIV infection.

clinical presentation, chest radiograph, or initial laboratory tests are examples of situations that would mandate respiratory (e.g., TB or influenza) or contact (e.g., RSV) isolation. Clinicians must recognize the risk that transmissible respiratory pathogens pose to other patients, hospital staff, and visitors. It is far preferable to be liberal in the use of isolation precautions until the specific diagnosis is established than to risk the spread of transmissible pathogens. Respiratory isolation is especially important to consider during procedures likely to increase pathogen aerosolization such as sputum induction, bronchoscopy, or intubation.

HIV TRANSMISSION CATEGORY AND HABITS

A patient's HIV transmission category and habits influence the relative frequency of various HIV and nonHIV-associated pulmonary diseases (Table 69-2). Kaposi sarcoma is seen almost exclusively in men who report having sexual contact with other men (MSM). Approximately 95% of the cases of HIV-associated Kaposi sarcoma occur in MSM; and although described, the occurrence of Kaposi sarcoma in women is quite uncommon.[11] Bacterial pneumonia and TB are more common in HIV-infected patients who are injection drug users than in HIV-infected patients without a history of injection drug use.[12,13] The PCHIS found that the rate of bacterial pneumonia was 11.1 episodes per 100 person-years among injection drug users, compared with 4.1 and 3.8 episodes per 100 person-years among MSM ($P < 0.001$) and female heterosexuals ($P = 0.003$), respectively.[12] Furthermore, injection or other illicit drug use can cause a variety of acute nonHIV-related pulmonary diseases (e.g., aspiration pneumonia secondary to central nervous system depression, endocarditis-related septic pulmonary emboli and drug-induced pulmonary edema) and a variety of chronic diseases (e.g., talc granulomatosis and pulmonary hypertension).[14]

As in the general population, HIV-infected patients who are cigarette smokers are at an increased risk of several respiratory illnesses. Bacterial bronchitis and pneumonia are more common in HIV-infected cigarette smokers than in HIV-infected nonsmokers or former smokers. This is especially true for persons with a CD4+ T-lymphocyte count of less than 200 cells/μL.[12] In addition, HIV-infected patients who report a long history of cigarette use may present with manifestations of chronic obstructive pulmonary disease (COPD) as the cause of their symptoms.[15] In fact, HIV-infected cigarette smokers appear to be at greater risk for COPD than comparable HIV negative smokers.[16] Most cases of lung cancer reported in HIV-infected patients have developed in those persons with a history of cigarette smoking. One can speculate that the incidence of nonHIV-associated pulmonary conditions – many related to cigarette smoking – will increase among HIV-infected patients receiving antiretroviral therapy (ART) as they live longer and as the incidence of HIV-associated OIs and neoplasms and the resulting mortality declines among them. Studies have demonstrated that HIV-positive patients who currently smoke have increased mortality and decreased quality of life, as well as increased respiratory symptoms, compared to nonsmokers.[17] As such, increased focus on strategies to reduce cigarette smoking is warranted.

TRAVEL AND RESIDENCE

TB is especially common in certain geographic areas and in certain populations.[18,19] HIV-infected patients who were

Approach to Respiratory Disease: Diagnostic Clues

Table 69-2

Clinical Setting
Ambulatory care/outpatient clinic: upper respiratory tract infections > acute bronchitis > bacterial pneumonia + PCP[a]
Hospital: bacterial pneumonia > PCP > tuberculosis > pulmonary Kaposi sarcoma = cryptococcosis[b]
Intensive care unit: PCP > bacterial pneumonia[c]

Geographic Location
Mycobacterium tuberculosis
Endemic fungi (e.g., *Histoplasma capsulatum, Coccidioides immitis*)

CD4+ T-lymphocyte Count
see Table 69-4

Patient Background
HIV transmission category
  MSM: increased incidence of Kaposi sarcoma
  IDU: increased incidence of bacterial pneumonia, tuberculosis, and IDU-related pulmonary complications
Habits: cigarette smoking – increased incidence of bacterial bronchitis, bacterial pneumonia, COPD, bronchogenic carcinoma
Travel and residence: assess risk for tuberculosis, endemic fungal diseases

Medical Background and Use of Prophylaxis
Prior disease increases incidence of recurrence: bacterial pneumonia, PCP, fungal pneumonias
Prophylaxis decreases incidence of disease: PCP, tuberculosis (if PPD+)

Symptoms and Signs
Respiratory symptoms: especially cough (productive or nonproductive) and symptom duration
Symptoms suggesting extrapulmonary or disseminated disease
Physical examination of chest: focal or nonfocal
Signs suggesting extrapulmonary or disseminated disease

Laboratory Tests
Arterial blood gas: nonspecific but useful for prognosis, management decisions (e.g., whether to hospitalize and whether corticosteroids are indicated for PCP)
White blood cell count: elevated or, if normal, elevated relative to baseline: bacterial pneumonia
Serum lactate dehydrogenase: elevated: nonspecific but classically seen in PCP

Chest Radiography
see Table 69-5

COPD, chronic obstructive pulmonary disease; IDU, injection drug users; MSM, men who have sex with men; PCP, *Pneumocystis* pneumonia; PPD, purified protein derivative.

In HIV-infected persons, PPD is considered positive if ≥5 mm induration.

[a]Most frequent causes of respiratory illness among HIV-infected outpatients from the multicenter Pulmonary Complications of HIV Infection Study.
[b]Most frequent causes of pneumonia among HIV-infected persons hospitalized at San Francisco General Hospital 1996–98 (Huang, unpublished data). PCP and *Streptococcus pneumoniae* were the two most common causes of community-acquired pneumonia among HIV-infected persons hospitalized at Johns Hopkins Hospital, 11/90 to 11/91.
[c]Most frequent causes of pneumonia among HIV-infected persons admitted to intensive care from the multicenter Pulmonary Complications of HIV Infection Study.[5]

born in or have traveled to a country with a high prevalence of TB and patients who are homeless, unstably housed, or previously incarcerated are at higher risk for exposure to *Mycobacterium tuberculosis*. Injection drug users, especially if anergic, are another population at increased risk for TB.[20] Patients who have a positive tuberculin skin test (defined as a ≥5 mm induration in HIV-infected persons), especially if recent converters, are also at increased risk for developing TB.[18,21]

Travel to or residence in a geographic region that is endemic for fungi such as *H. capsulatum*, *C. immitis*, or *Penicillium marneffei* is a strong determinant of the risk of exposure, infection, and ultimately disease.

PRIOR ILLNESS AND USE OF PROPHYLAXIS

Many HIV-associated OIs are recurrent. Recognition that bacterial pneumonias are common in HIV-infected patients and frequently recur led to the inclusion of recurrent pneumonia (i.e., two or more episodes within a 12-month period) as an AIDS-defining condition in the 1993 Expanded Surveillance Case Definition for AIDS by the US Centers for Disease Control and Prevention (CDC).[22] Often patients with multiple, recurrent episodes of severe bacterial pneumonia develop airway damage or bronchiectasis, which in turn predisposes them to further bacterial infections.[15] Some such patients develop multidrug-resistant bacteria that are refractory to treatment.

Patients with prior PCP are at high risk for recurrence, and current recommendations advise secondary PCP prophylaxis unless ART has produced a sustained (e.g., >3 months) CD4+ T-lymphocyte count of more than 200 cells/μL.[23] Similarly, patients with a history of cryptococcosis, coccidioidomycosis, or histoplasmosis are at high-risk for relapse and should receive chronic maintenance therapy with fluconazole (cryptococcosis and coccidioidomycosis) or itraconazole (histoplasmosis).[23] Patients with a significant CD4+ T-lymphocyte count response to ART can discontinue maintenance therapy provided their cell count remains above the threshold associated with an increased risk of disease (e.g., >100–200 cells/μL sustained for >6 months for cryptococcosis).

Chronic antimicrobial use clearly influences the likelihood of the targeted pathogen recurring, but it also affects the likelihood and the drug susceptibility of other organisms causing respiratory disease. For example, at San Francisco General Hospital, the dramatic rise in bacteria resistant to trimethoprim-sulfamethoxazole has coincided with use of trimethoprim-sulfamethoxazole for PCP prophylaxis.[24]

In HIV-infected patients, failure to adhere to recommended maintenance with the prescribed regimens frequently results in recurrent or relapsed disease. The corollary also can be used. Adherence to the prescribed regimen lessens the probability of disease, although even complete adherence to these regimens cannot completely prevent subsequent recurrence. HIV-infected patients, especially at the lowest CD4+ T-lymphocyte counts, may develop recurrent disease despite prophylaxis.

Current guidelines recommend pneumococcal vaccine and annual influenza immunization.[23] Their efficacy is best established in patients with CD4+ T-lymphocyte counts of more than 200–500 cells/μL and is likely to be diminished in patients with low CD4+ T-lymphocyte cell counts. Pneumococcal immunization can be repeated every 5 years and consideration given to repeat immunization for patients who were immunized prior to a rise in CD4+ T-lymphocyte counts >200 cells/μL induced by ART.[23] There is also evidence that heptavalent pneumococcal vaccination for children in the household or in the community leads to a reduction in pneumococcal disease among HIV-infected adults. Moreover, community immunization programs lead to change in the serotype of strains infecting HIV-infected adults to nonvaccine strains.[25]

SYMPTOMS AND SIGNS

The approach to respiratory disease in an HIV-infected patient begins with a thorough history and physical examination. Although nonspecific, constellations of particular symptoms and signs can often point to a specific diagnosis (Table 69-2).

Respiratory symptoms are more common in HIV-infected persons compared to HIV-negative individuals.[26] The PCHIS demonstrated that respiratory symptoms are a frequent complaint in HIV-infected persons, and that symptoms increase in frequency as the CD4+ T-lymphocyte count decreases. In this study, subjects reported cough at 27% of more than 12 000 routine visits, dyspnea at 23%, and fever at 9% (Huang, unpublished data). These symptoms increased in frequency in the subset of subjects with a CD4+ T-lymphocyte count of less than 200 cells/μL.

All of the HIV-associated respiratory diseases may present with cough,[27] dyspnea, and less frequently pleuritic chest pain. Particular aspects of these symptoms may be especially useful for suggesting a specific diagnosis. Most patients with bacterial bronchitis or pneumonia present with a cough productive of purulent sputum, whereas most patients with PCP note a dry, nonproductive cough.[15] In addition to the specific symptoms themselves, the duration of symptoms may also be useful. Bacterial pneumonias due to *S. pneumoniae* and *Haemophilus* spp. characteristically present with an acute onset and a symptom duration of 3–5 days. In contrast, PCP usually presents with a subacute, more insidious onset and a typical symptom duration of 2–4 weeks. Kovacs and co-workers found a median symptom duration of 28 days among 49 HIV-infected patients with PCP.[28] Thus, in an HIV-infected patient with a CD4+ T-lymphocyte count of less than 200 cells/μL (and hence at risk for both bacterial pneumonia and PCP), the presence of cough productive of purulent sputum of a few days' duration favors the diagnosis of bacterial infection (Table 69-3). In contrast, a nonproductive cough of a few weeks' duration strongly favors the diagnosis of PCP.

Clinicians should be aware of one caveat: patients may have dual infections (e.g., bacterial infection and PCP). Afessa and colleagues reported that more than 10% of the 111 episodes of bacterial pneumonia reviewed were accompanied by PCP.[29] A similar proportion (10%) of patients with PCP present with findings consistent with bacterial co-infection (Fig. 69-1). Although HIV-infected patients can present with multiple concurrent illnesses, extrapulmonary symptoms, when present, are often useful for suggesting a specific, unifying diagnosis, as many of the HIV-associated pulmonary diseases have important extrapulmonary manifestations. For example, the presence of headache in a patient with a CD4+ T-lymphocyte cell count of less than 200 cells/μL and respiratory complaints suggest the possibility of *Cryptococcus neoformans* meningitis and pneumonia. In fact, although the lungs are the portals of entry for *Cryptococcus*, many patients present with asymptomatic or minimally symptomatic pulmonary disease, and the diagnosis is only suggested by the presence of extrapulmonary symptoms. In a series of 106 patients with *C. neoformans* infection, 89 patients (84%) presented with meningitis; cough or dyspnea was present in fewer than one-third of these patients (n = 28, 31%).[30] In the National Institute of Allergy and Infectious Diseases Mycoses Study Group and the AIDS Clinical Trials Group (ACTG) study of treatment regimens for cryptococcal meningitis, 31% of the patients randomized to amphotericin B and 35% of those randomized to amphotericin B and flucytosine reported cough; 90% and 89% of the subjects, respectively, reported headache.[31]

Table 69-3 Presentation of Bacterial and *Pneumocystis* Pneumonia

Parameter	Bacteria	*Pneumocystis*
CD4+ T-lymphocyte count	Any	≤200 cells/μL
Symptoms	Fever, chills or rigors Dyspnea Pleuritic chest pain Productive cough Purulent sputum	Fever Dyspnea Nonproductive cough
Symptom duration	Typically 3–5 days	Typically 2–4 weeks
Signs: lung examination	Focal findings	Often unremarkable Inspiratory crackles
Laboratory tests	WBC frequently elevated LDH varies ABG nonspecific[a]	WBC varies LDH frequently elevated ABG nonspecific[a]
Chest radiography		
Distribution	Patchy, focal > multifocal	Diffuse > focal
Location	Unilateral, segmental/lobar	Bilateral
Pattern	Consolidation	Reticular-granular
Associated findings		
Cysts	Rarely	15–20%
Pleural effusions	25–50%	Very rarely
Adenopathy	Rarely	Very rarely
Pneumothorax	Rarely	Occasionally
Normal radiograph	Never	Occasionally

ABG, arterial blood gases; LDH, lactate dehydrogenase; WBC, white blood cell count.

[a]Used to determine severity of disease and whether adjunctive corticosteroids are indicated.

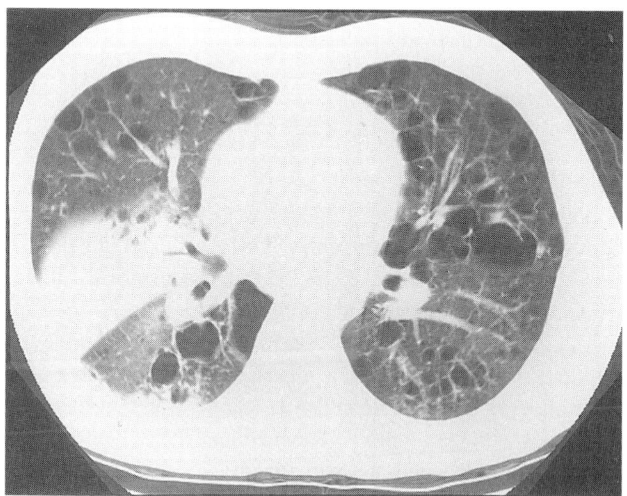

Figure 69-1 ■ Chest computed tomographic (CT) scan of an HIV-infected patient, CD4+ T-lymphocyte count less than 200 cells/μL with multiple bilateral cysts secondary to *Pneumocystis* and a focal alveolar consolidation secondary to *S. pneumoniae*.

Courtesy of Laurence Huang, MD.

Knowledge of extrapulmonary disease can also be used occasionally to infer the pulmonary diagnosis without specific microbiologic or pathologic confirmation. For example, patients diagnosed with non-Hodgkin lymphoma from a biopsy of a nonpulmonary site who also have findings suggestive of thoracic involvement might potentially receive initial therapy for non-Hodgkin lymphoma and might have specific pulmonary diagnostic procedures reserved for situations where the pulmonary disease progresses despite this therapy.

Patients with pneumonia who are HIV-positive are usually febrile, tachycardic, and tachypneic. Evidence of systemic hypotension suggests a fulminant disease process (e.g., bacterial septicemia, the sepsis-like syndrome seen with disseminated histoplasmosis, or rarely PCP). Pulse oximetry provides a helpful estimate of the severity of the disease. The presence of exercise-induced oxygen desaturation is reported to be a sensitive (but not specific) indicator of PCP. Importantly, this simple test is often useful when making decisions regarding the need for hospitalization. Patients whose oxygen saturation declines on exertion are usually unable to care for themselves at home and are more likely to need respiratory support and hospitalization.

Patients with bacterial pneumonia often have focal lung examinations suggestive of consolidation, pleural effusion, or both, whereas patients with PCP may have bilateral inspiratory crackles (Table 69-3). Wheezing in a patient with a history of asthma suggests an exacerbation of that condition, whereas diminished breath sounds in a longtime cigarette smoker may indicate emphysema. Absent breath sounds suggest pneumothorax in a patient complaining of pleuritic chest pain, dyspnea, or both. Occasionally, abnormal findings on lung examination are the result of nonpulmonary disease. For example, rales in association with an S3 cardiac gallop and an elevated jugular venous pressure suggest a cardiac etiology for the respiratory complaints.

The remainder of the physical examination may also suggest an etiology for the respiratory symptoms. For example, in a patient whose CD4+ T-lymphocyte count is less than 200 cells/μL, an altered mental status may be secondary to *C. neoformans* meningitis, whereas a focal neurologic examination may be secondary to *Toxoplasma gondii* encephalitis. Peripheral lymphadenopathy or hepatosplenomegaly suggests either disseminated mycobacterial or fungal disease or non-Hodgkin lymphoma. New cutaneous lesions may be manifestations of a disseminated fungal disease. The presence of mucocutaneous Kaposi sarcoma lesions may point toward pulmonary involvement with that disease. However, the absence of Kaposi sarcoma lesions on visual examination of the skin and mucous membranes does not preclude the possibility of significant visceral disease, including the lung. Huang and colleagues found that 15% of 168 patients with pulmonary Kaposi sarcoma diagnosed by bronchoscopy had no evidence of concurrent or preexisting mucocutaneous Kaposi sarcoma.[32]

LABORATORY TESTS

CD4+ T-Lymphocyte Counts

The CD4+ T-lymphocyte count is an excellent indicator of an HIV-infected patient's risk of developing a specific OI or neoplasm (Table 69-4). The CD4+ T-lymphocyte count is relevant to the occurrence of bacterial pneumonia as well as more traditional OIs. Hirschtick and colleagues in the PCHIS found that the risk of bacterial pneumonia among subjects with a CD4+ T-lymphocyte count of less than 200 cells/μL was more than five and a half times greater than that for subjects whose count was more than 500 cells/μL.[12] In addition, as the CD4+ T-lymphocyte count decreases, the incidence of bacterial pneumonia accompanied by bacteremia or septicemia and of *M. tuberculosis* infection accompanied by extrapulmonary or disseminated disease increase.[33,34] Nonspecific interstitial pneumonitis (NSIP), whose clinical presentation and chest radiographic features may be indistinguishable from PCP, differs from PCP in that NSIP may present at a CD4+ T-lymphocyte count of more than 200 cells/μL. In a series reported by Sattler and associates, the mean CD4+ T-lymphocyte count of 16 patients with NSIP was 492 cells/μL.[35]

At CD4+ T-lymphocyte counts of less than 200 cells/μL, PCP and *Cryptococcus neoformans* pneumonia become important diagnoses to consider, whereas neither is common in patients with counts that are significantly higher than 200 cells/μL. In a retrospective review of episodes of opportunistic pneumonia diagnosed at the Clinical Center of the National Institutes of Health, 46 of 49 patients (94%) diagnosed with PCP had a CD4+ T-lymphocyte count of less than 200 cells/μL.[36] The Multicenter AIDS Cohort Study demonstrated that subjects with a CD4+ T-lymphocyte count of less than 200 cells/μL had a nearly five-fold higher risk of developing PCP than subjects who had a count higher than 200 cells/μL at study entry.[37] Stansell and the PCHIS showed that 95% of 145 cases of PCP occurred in subjects whose CD4+ T-lymphocyte count was less than 200 cells/μL (median count 29 cells/μL).[38] Darras-Joly et al in a review of 76 patients with cryptococcal disease, found a mean CD4+ T-lymphocyte count of 46 cells/μL (range 2–220 cells/μL) in 65 patients with meningitis.[39] The median CD4+ T-lymphocyte counts among 381 patients with cryptococcal meningitis randomized to either amphotericin B alone or amphotericin B with flucytosine for initial treatment were 18 and 20 cells/μL, respectively.[31]

At CD4+ T-lymphocyte counts of less than 100 cells/μL, pulmonary diseases caused by *Pseudomonas aeruginosa*, *T. gondii*, and Kaposi sarcoma are increasingly common. A study of 64 patients with pulmonary toxoplasmosis diagnosed by bronchoalveolar lavage (BAL) reported a mean CD4+ T-lymphocyte count of 40 cells/μL; 82% had a count of less than 50 cells/μL; and only 4% had a count of more than 200 cells/μL.[40] One series of 168 consecutive patients with pulmonary Kaposi sarcoma diagnosed by bronchoscopy

Table 69-4 CD4+ T-Lymphocyte Count Ranges for Selected Respiratory Disease

Any CD4+ T-lymphocyte Count
Upper respiratory tract infection
Acute bronchitis/sinusitis
Asthma
Chronic obstructive pulmonary disease
Pulmonary arterial hypertension
Bacterial pneumonia (most often *Streptococcus pneumoniae*, *Haemophilus* spp.)
Mycobacterium tuberculosis pneumonia
Non-Hodgkin lymphoma
Bronchogenic carcinoma
Nonspecific interstitial pneumonitis
CD4+ T-lymphocyte Count <200 cells/μL
Pneumocystis pneumonia
Cryptococcus neoformans pneumonia
Bacterial pneumonia accompanied by bacteremia or septicemia
Extrapulmonary or disseminated *M. tuberculosis*
CD4+ T-lymphocyte Count <100 cells/μL
Bacterial pneumonia due to *Pseudomonas aeruginosa*
Toxoplasma gondii pneumonia
Pulmonary Kaposi sarcoma
CD4+ T-lymphocyte Count <50 cells/μL
Histoplasma capsulatum: usually associated with disseminated disease
Coccidioides immitis: usually associated with disseminated disease
Aspergillus species (most often *A. fumigatus*) pneumonia
Cytomegalovirus pneumonia: usually associated with disseminated disease
Mycobacterium avium complex: usually associated with disseminated disease

reported a median CD4+ T-lymphocyte count of 19 cells/μL; 68% had a count below 50 cells/μL, and only 4% had a count above 200 cells/μL.[32] Finally, at CD4+ T-lymphocyte counts of less than 50 cells/μL, diseases may be caused by endemic fungi (*H. capsulatum, C. immitis*) and nonendemic fungi (*Aspergillus* spp.). Cytomegalovirus (CMV) and nontuberculous mycobacteria (*Mycobacterium avium* complex) can also cause disease but such cases are quite unusual.

Numerous studies have indicated that the current CD4+ T-lymphocyte count is the best reflection of the risk for a specific OI.[23,41] For PCP, several studies have demonstrated that it is safe to discontinue primary or secondary PCP prophylaxis in HIV-infected subjects whose CD4+ T-lymphocyte count has risen from below to above 200 cells/μL.[42–49] However, as noted above, cases of PCP are well documented to occur occasionally at CD4+ T-lymphocyte cell counts above 200 cells/μL both in patients who have never received ART, and in patients whose CD4+ T-lymphocyte cell counts have risen from low levels to above 200 cells/μL.[50] For example, a patient previously had been able to discontinue treatment successfully for disseminated *M. avium* complex and disseminated fungal disease without relapse. Yet, despite a CD4+ T-lymphocyte count of 300 cells/μL just prior to the onset of PCP, PCP developed 4 months after secondary PCP prophylaxis was discontinued.[50] Thus, although important, the CD4+ T-lymphocyte count should be a guide as to which pulmonary diseases are most common in that population. Exceptions to such guidelines occurred before the era of ART, and exceptions continue to occur.

Arterial Blood Gases

Arterial blood gas (ABG) analysis is indicated for persons with clinical evidence of moderate to severe pulmonary disease (Table 69-2). ABG analysis is also useful for prognosis and for making clinical decisions regarding whether (and where) to admit the patient and whether adjunctive corticosteroids are indicated in patients with suspected or confirmed PCP. Laboratory tests that may be useful for suggesting a specific diagnosis include the white blood cell (WBC) count and differential count as part of the complete blood count and the serum lactate dehydrogenase (LDH) assay. Beyond their potential use as part of the diagnostic evaluation, these tests serve as prognostic markers and baseline values for subsequent measurements. Serial measurements are useful in any patient who fails to improve or who worsens despite apparent appropriate therapy.

WBC Count

Even for patients with HIV infection, the WBC count is frequently elevated in persons with bacterial infection. This elevation may be relative to the patient's baseline value; that is, an elevation from 2000 cells/μL to 6000 cells/μL suggests a bacterial process. Frequently, a left shift is also present in persons with bacterial infection. HIV-infected patients with neutropenia are at high-risk for bacterial infections and fungal infections such as those caused by *Aspergillus* spp. Pancytopenia suggests the presence of an infectious or neoplastic process in the bone marrow.

Serum LDH

Serum LDH is often (but not invariably) elevated in patients with PCP.[15] However, LDH may also be elevated in other pulmonary (including bacterial pneumonia and TB) and nonpulmonary conditions, making this test more useful for prognosis than diagnosis. Most of the studies reporting a high sensitivity of serum LDH for PCP consisted of hospitalized patients, some of whom had acute respiratory failure and were mechanically ventilated. The study that reported the lowest sensitivity examined outpatients presenting to a clinic.[51] This suggests that PCP severity and the patient population studied affect the diagnostic sensitivity of the test.

The degree to which the serum LDH is elevated has been shown to correlate with prognosis and response to therapy.[15] Patients with PCP and an initial markedly elevated serum LDH level or a rising serum LDH level despite PCP treatment have a poor prognosis. Patients with PCP that is responding to treatment have a decline in their LDH toward the normal range.[52]

IMAGING

Standard Chest Radiography

The characteristic chest radiographic findings for selected HIV-associated pulmonary diseases are presented in Table 69-5. For each disease, the findings from a large series (n >30 cases) are presented as an overview. When no large series has been reported, summary data from smaller series are provided. Differences in the description of radiographic findings and the absence of a standardized approach to interpreting and presenting radiographic data limit the ability to combine studies on a specific pulmonary disease into a single summary table.

Bacterial pneumonia is the most common pulmonary disease among HIV-infected persons in the United States. The chest radiographic presentation is similar to that of the overall population: focal, segmental, or lobar consolidation. One study reported that of 55 patients with bacterial pneumonia, 40% presented with focal, segmental, or lobar alveolar infiltrates, whereas 38% had diffuse reticulonodular infiltrates, 16% had focal reticulonodular infiltrates, and 5% had nodular or cavitary infiltrates on the chest radiograph.[53] Another study of 99 patients found that 54% of the patients with bacterial pneumonia had a lobar infiltrate, 17% had an interstitial infiltrate, 10% had a nodular infiltrate, and only 1% had a cavitary infiltrate on their radiograph. Pleural effusions were seen in 7% and intrathoracic adenopathy in 2%.[54] In this study, multivariate analysis demonstrated that the presence of a lobar infiltrate on chest radiograph was independently predictive of bacterial pneumonia. These studies, however, considered

Table 69-5 Characteristic Chest Radiographic Findings for Selected Pulmonary Diseases[a]

Pulmonary Disease	Author (year)	No. of patients	Distribution (%)	Pattern (%)	Associated Findings (%)
Bacteria[b]	Magnenat[53] (1991)	55		Alveolar (40%) Diffuse (38%) or focal (16%) reticulonodular Nodular/cavitary (5%)	
Bacteria[b]	Selwyn[54] (1998)	99	Focal (71%) Diffuse (29%)	Lobar (54%) Interstitial (17%) Nodular (10%)/Cavitary (1%)	Pleural effusion (7%) Adenopathy (2%)
Pneumocystis[c]	DeLorenzo[66] (1987)	104	Bilateral (95%), Diffuse (48%)	Interstitial or mixed (87.5%) Alveolar (12.5%)	Cysts (7%) Honeycomb lesions (4%)
M. tuberculosis, CD4+ T-lymphocyte <200 cells/μL	Abouya[71] (1995)	45	Miliary (9%)	Cavitary (29%) Noncavitary (58%)	Adenopathy (20%) Pleural effusion (11%)
M. tuberculosis, CD4+ T-lymphocyte 200–399 cells/μL	Abouya[71] (1995)	36	Miliary (6%)	Cavitary (44%) Noncavitary (44%)	Adenopathy (14%) Pleural effusion (11%)
M. tuberculosis, CD4+ T-lymphocyte ⩾400 cells/μL	Abouya[71] (1995)	30	Miliary (0%)	Cavitary (63%) Noncavitary (33%)	Adenopathy (0%) Pleural effusion (3%)
M. tuberculosis, CD4+ T-lymphocyte <200 cells/μL	Perlman[72] (1997)	98	Normal (9%)	Infiltrate (52%) Cavitary (7%) Interstitial (27%) Nodules(s) (18%)	Adenopathy (30%) Pleural effusion (7%)
M. tuberculosis, CD4+ T-lymphocyte ⩾200 cells/μL	Perlman[72] (1997)	30	Normal (3%)	Infiltrate (67%) Cavitary (20%) Interstitial (17%) Nodules(s) (20%)	Adenopathy (7%) Pleural effusion (10%)
C. neoformans	Batungwanayo[84] (1994)	37	Diffuse (76%)	Interstitial or mixed (76%) Alveolar (19%) Nodular/nodules (5%)	Cavitation (11%) Adenopathy (11%) Pleural effusion (5%)
C. neoformans	Meyohas[97] (1995) (plus review)	17	Normal (6%)	Interstitial (76%) Alveolar (35%) Nodular (6%)	Cavitation (12%) Adenopathy (18%) Pleural effusion (24%)
Cytomegalovirus	Salomon[99] (1997)	18	Normal (33%)	Reticular-granular (33%) Alveolar (22%) Nodular (11%)	Cavitation (11%) Cyst (6%) Pleural effusion (33%) Adenopathy (11%)
Cytomegalovirus	Rodriguez-Barradas[98] (1996)	17	Bilateral (71%), Unilateral (29%)	Interstitial (82%) Alveolar (18%)	Pleural effusion (12%)
T. gondii	Rabaud[40] (1996)	43	Normal (23%), Bilateral (58%)	Interstitial (53%) Nodular (16%)	Pleural effusion (7%) Pneumothorax (2%)

(Continued)

Table 69-5

Pulmonary Disease	Author (year)	No. of patients	Distribution (%)	Pattern (%)	Associated Findings (%)
Kaposi sarcoma	Gruden[73] (1995)	76	Normal (3%), Bilateral (96%), Diffuse or mid-lower lung zones (92%)	BWT+ coalescence (95%) Nodules (78%)	Kerley B lines (71%) Pleural effusion (53%) Adenopathy (16%)
Non-Hodgkin lymphoma	Eisner[101] (1996)	38	Normal (3%)	Nodules (40%) or mass (24%) Lobar (40%) Reticular (24%)	Cavitation (3%) Pleural effusion (44%) Adenopathy (21%)

BWT, bronchial wall thickening.

[a]Chest radiograph presentations can vary significantly depending on a number of factors, including severity of disease and use of prophylaxis.
[b]The characteristic chest radiograph presentation is influenced by the specific bacteria (see text).
[c]Although the largest chest radiographic series, this study predates the widespread use of PCP prophylaxis. Multiple studies have documented 'atypical' upper lung zone findings in patients receiving aerosolized pentamidine prophylaxis. At present, it is unclear what, if any, effect oral prophylaxis regimens (trimethoprim-sulfamethoxazole, dapsone, and atovaquone) have on the chest radiographic presentation.

all bacterial pathogens together. Numerous reports as well as clinical experience demonstrate that the frequency of specific radiographic findings is dependent on the specific bacteria.

Studies suggest that radiographic presentations may differ among *S. pneumoniae*, *Haemophilus* spp., and *P. aeruginosa*.[3,12,55] A review of English-language articles and abstracts from 1981 to 1990 on *S. pneumoniae* disease in HIV-infected persons found that three-fourths of bacterial pneumonias due to *S. pneumoniae* presented with segmental, lobar, or multilobar consolidation on chest radiography.[56] Garcia-Leoni et al reported that a classic lobar alveolar pattern was seen in 67% and a diffuse alveolar pattern in 10% of 21 patients with *S. pneumoniae* pneumonia.[57] Schlamm and Yancovitz found similar proportions in 34 patients with *H. influenzae* pneumonia; in this study, focal or diffuse lobar infiltrates were noted in 74%.[58] However, another series of 12 patients with *H. influenzae* pneumonia discovered that the presentation may be clinically and radiographically indistinguishable from that of PCP.[59] The patients complained of nonproductive cough and dyspnea with a median symptom duration of 4 weeks. All presented with bilateral interstitial or mixed interstitial-alveolar infiltrates similar to PCP. Cordero et al found that 35% of 26 patients with *H. influenzae* pneumonia presented with an interstitial pattern on chest radiograph.[60] A series of 16 patients with *P. aeruginosa* pneumonia showed that the pneumonia was community-acquired in 15 patients.[61] Chest radiographs revealed cavitary infiltrates on admission in 50%, and an additional 19% presented with pulmonary infiltrates that subsequently cavitated. The frequency of cavitary infiltrates in *P. aeruginosa* pneumonia was also noted in a study of 25 patients: 24% had cavitary pneumonia.[62] Thus the presence of a cavitary pneumonia may be more suggestive of *Pseudomonas* than either *Streptococcus* or *Haemophilus*. However, the differential diagnosis of a pulmonary cavitary lesion is extensive and includes TB, endemic fungal diseases, and *Rhodococcus equi*.

Pneumonia due to bacteria such as *Legionella* spp., *Mycoplasma pneumoniae*, and *Chlamydia* spp. occurs in HIV-infected patients.[63] The frequency of these pathogens as causes of community-acquired pneumonia in HIV-infected patients appears to parallel that of HIV-uninfected patients. A study in Baltimore performed extensive diagnostic testing on 180 HIV-infected patients: *Legionella pneumophila* (3%), *Chlamydia pneumoniae* (4%), and *M. pneumoniae* (<1%) were rarely detected.[3] The frequency of these pathogens matched these of the 205 HIV-uninfected patients (3%, 3%, and 1%, respectively) admitted during the same period.

Rhodococcus equi and *Nocardia* spp. (especially *N. asteroides*) have been described as causes of pneumonia in HIV-infected patients.[64,65] Neither is recognized often.

PCP remains a common AIDS-defining OI in the United States. The classic PCP presentation is bilateral interstitial-reticular or granular opacities that are often diffuse. One large study of 104 patients with PCP revealed that 87.5% presented with an interstitial pattern (75.0%) or a mixed interstitial-alveolar pattern (12.5%); the remaining patients had an alveolar pattern.[66] In addition, 7% of the radiographs had thin-walled cysts (i.e., pneumatoceles), and 4% had honeycomb lesions. Infiltrates were bilateral in 95% and unilateral in 5%; they involved the entire lung in 48%. This study remains the largest radiology series of patients with PCP, but it predates the widespread use of PCP prophylaxis. Since then, a number of reports have described the radiographic findings in patients receiving aerosolized pentamidine (AP) prophylaxis; these radiographs characteristically reveal an upper lung zone predominance that can mimic mycobacterial disease.[67] However, this upper lung zone predominance can also be seen in patients who have never received AP prophylaxis, and the pattern seen (i.e., reticular or granular) is more important than the distribution for suggesting the diagnosis of PCP. In the PCHIS, 467 subjects presenting for evaluation of new or worsening respiratory complaints underwent chest radiography.[68] In a multivariate analysis of the 174 subjects with an abnormal radiograph, the presence of interstitial infiltrates on the chest radiograph was an independent predictor of PCP.

TB can present with a variety of chest radiographic findings, including upper lung-zone infiltrates often with cavitation, middle or lower lung zone consolidation mimicking bacterial pneumonia, miliary disease, nodule(s), pleural effusions, and intrathoracic adenopathy. TB may also present with a normal chest radiograph. The frequency of these radiographic findings is influenced by the patient's CD4+ T-lymphocyte count.[69] Jones and colleagues reported that mediastinal adenopathy was found in 13% of the 30 patients with a CD4+ T-lymphocyte count higher than 200 cells/μL compared with 36% of the 58 patients with a count less than 200 cells/μL ($P = 0.02$).[70] Abouya and coworkers reviewed the chest radiographic presentation of 111 HIV-infected patients with TB. The proportion of patients with cavitary infiltrates decreased as the CD4+ T-lymphocyte count decreased from more than 400 cells/μL to 200 to 399 cells/μL, and then to less than 200 cells/μL ($P < 0.05$), whereas the proportions with noncavitary infiltrates and intrathoracic adenopathy increased as the count decreased (both $P < 0.05$).[71] Perlman and colleagues in the Terry Beirn Community Programs for Clinical Research on AIDS (CPCRA) and the ACTG pooled data from 128 patients with culture-positive TB.[72] When they combined their data with those from published studies, the authors found a significant association between the presence of infiltrates, cavitation (both more likely in patients with a CD4+ T-lymphocyte count of 200 cells/μL or more), and intrathoracic adenopathy (more likely in patients with a count of less than 200 cells/μL). Thus, the radiographic key to the diagnosis of pulmonary TB is knowledge of the patient's CD4+ T-lymphocyte count and an understanding of which patterns are more common at that count.

Pulmonary Kaposi sarcoma characteristically presents with bilateral opacities in a central or perihilar distribution and a middle/lower lung zone predominance. Linear densities, nodules, and pleural effusions are all common. In a study of 76 patients with pulmonary Kaposi sarcoma, 95% of the chest radiographs had peribronchial cuffing and tram track opacities or had extensive perihilar coalescent opacities.[73] Small nodules (50%) or nodular opacities (28%) were seen in 78%, Kerley B lines in 71%, and pleural effusions in 53% of the radiographs. No patient presented with either Kerley B lines or pleural effusions without concurrent parenchymal findings. Sixteen percent of these patients had hilar or mediastinal lymph node enlargement.

Chest Computed Tomography

For most evaluations of symptomatic HIV-infected patients, a computed tomography (CT) scan is unnecessary because the clinical and chest radiographic presentation suggests a single diagnosis or a few diagnoses to consider.[74,75] However, a chest high-resolution CT (HRCT) is extremely useful in cases of clinically suspected PCP in which the chest radiograph is normal or unchanged, a phenomenon that occurred in 39% of one reported series.[76] Most patients with respiratory symptoms suggestive of PCP whose radiograph is normal or unchanged do not have PCP. Subjecting these patients to diagnostic procedures such as bronchoscopy or to empiric PCP treatment with its associated toxicities is ill-advised. In these cases, a sensitive test is needed to select which patients require diagnostic procedures or empiric therapy and, just as important, which patients can be observed without either of the above. The chest HRCT scan is one of several such tests. Patients with PCP and a normal chest radiograph have patchy areas of ground-glass opacities (GGOs) on HRCT.[74,75] Although the presence of GGOs is nonspecific and may be seen with a number of pulmonary disorders, its absence strongly argues against the presence of PCP. In one study, none of the 40 HIV-infected patients with clinically suspected PCP, a normal or nonspecific chest radiograph, and an HRCT without GGOs had PCP diagnosed by BAL fluid examination or 60 days of clinical follow-up.[77] In fact, no patient with a normal chest radiograph and an HRCT without GGOs has been diagnosed with PCP at San Francisco General Hospital (Laurence Huang, personal observation).

Chest CT can also be useful for suggesting a diagnosis in cases in which the chest radiograph reveals multiple pulmonary nodules. A predominance of nodules smaller than 1 cm in diameter in a centrilobular distribution strongly suggests the presence of an OI, whereas a predominance of nodules larger than 1 cm in diameter is suggestive of a neoplasm.[78,79] In cases where the nodules are mostly smaller than 1 cm in diameter, the presence of intrathoracic adenopathy, especially if low attenuation (another potential use for CT) indicates that mycobacterial (or fungal) disease is probable.[80] In cases in which the nodules are mostly larger than 1 cm, the finding of associated peribronchovascular thickening inevitably results in a diagnosis of pulmonary Kaposi sarcoma. Finally, chest CT scans are useful for guiding diagnostic procedures such as bronchoscopy, CT-guided transthoracic needle aspiration, and surgical procedures.

Gallium 67 Scans

Gallium scans are sensitive but nonspecific indicators of PCP. The sensitivity and specificity for PCP depend in part on the criteria used to define a positive scan. When a positive test is defined as any gallium uptake (1+) over the lung parenchyma, the sensitivity and specificity of gallium for PCP have been reported to be 99% and 50%, respectively.[81] However, using more stringent criteria and defining a positive test as one with uptake equal to (3+) or greater than (4+) that of the liver, the sensitivity of gallium for PCP decreases to 60% (although the specificity increases to 80%). In either case, given the inherent time delays for obtaining results from gallium scans and the availability of HRCT and pulmonary function tests, gallium scans are rarely used at San Francisco General Hospital for evaluating AIDS-related pulmonary disease.

One situation where gallium scans can be extremely useful is for evaluation of a patient with suspected pulmonary Kaposi sarcoma in whom bronchoscopy fails to document endobronchial Kaposi sarcoma lesions. The reason for this is that pulmonary Kaposi sarcoma, unlike OIs, non-Hodgkin lymphoma, and lymphocytic interstitial pneumonitis, is gallium-negative. Thus, in an HIV-infected patient with mucocutaneous Kaposi sarcoma and a chest radiograph suggestive of pulmonary Kaposi sarcoma, a negative gallium scan is strongly suggestive of Kaposi sarcoma. In a patient with known pulmonary Kaposi sarcoma who develops progressive respiratory complaints and a worsening chest radiograph, a negative gallium scan indicates that progressive Kaposi sarcoma is the probable etiology rather than a superimposed OI.

Pulmonary Function Tests

In HIV-infected patients complaining of dry cough or dyspnea whose chest radiograph is normal, spirometry may diagnose airflow obstruction that may be responsive to bronchodilators.[82] The diffusing capacity for carbon monoxide (DL_{co}) is a sensitive but nonspecific indicator of PCP, and a normal DL_{co} makes the diagnosis of PCP unlikely.[68]

Although the DL_{co} can be useful for evaluating symptomatic patients, it has no role as a screening test to detect, for example, early PCP in asymptomatic individuals. In an evaluation of 64 patients who experienced more than a 20% decrease in their DL_{co} from a baseline value in the absence of new respiratory symptoms or new chest radiographic findings, none of the patients was found to have PCP or other OI on sputum induction, bronchoscopy, or clinical follow-up.[83] Care should be taken, especially with HIV-infected patients given their varied clinical and radiographic presentations, to exclude a diagnosis of TB before pulmonary function testing.

MICROBIOLOGIC TESTS

Blood Culture

Because *S. pneumoniae* is the most frequent cause of bacterial pneumonia and pneumococcal pneumonia is often accompanied by bacteremia (especially when the CD4+ T-lymphocyte count is less than 200 cells/μL), blood cultures should always be obtained in cases of suspected bacterial pneumonia (Table 69-6). When positive, blood cultures are specific for the diagnosis and, in an era of increasing antibiotic resistance, the utility of drug susceptibility testing cannot be overemphasized. Blood cultures should also be obtained for mycobacteria and fungi in the appropriate clinical settings.

Serology

The serum cryptococcal antigen (CRAG) is an extremely sensitive and specific test for the presence of cryptococcemia and cryptococcal meningitis. However, the serum CRAG assay may be negative in patients who have isolated cryptococcal pneumonia. In a study of 37 HIV-infected patients with cryptococcal pneumonia, the serum CRAG was positive in only eight of 26 patients (31%).[84] A serum CRAG assay should be performed on all patients with suspected cryptococcal disease; patients with a positive CRAG assay should have an evaluation to determine the extent of disease (i.e., lumbar puncture for possible meningitis), whereas those with a negative CRAG assay but respiratory complaints or chest radiograph findings should undergo further pulmonary evaluation (i.e., bronchoscopy with BAL) for possible isolated cryptococcal pneumonia.

The *H. capsulatum* polysaccharide antigen test is a sensitive and specific test for the presence of histoplasmosis. The antigen can be measured in blood and other fluids including BAL.[85] The *Toxoplasma* immunoglobulin G (IgG) is positive in most cases of toxoplasmosis. In a study of 64 patients with pulmonary toxoplasmosis, *Toxoplasma* IgG was positive in 55 of 60 cases (92%) for which prior serology results were available.[40] An additional three patients (5%) in this study seroconverted (IgA, IgM, and IgG all detected after previous negative results) at the time that toxoplasmosis was diagnosed, whereas the final two patients (3%) remained seronegative even after diagnosis. Thus, a negative *Toxoplasma* IgG assay makes the diagnosis of toxoplasmosis unlikely but not unprecedented. There is no test for *Toxoplasma* antigen or nucleic acid that is commercially available for use on blood or BAL fluid.

Sputum

Similar to HIV-uninfected persons, the diagnostic sensitivity of sputum culture for bacteria is low. Hirschtick and colleagues demonstrated that sputum culture identified a specific bacterial pathogen in ~40% of cases of bacterial pneumonia,[12] and Mundy and associates were unable to identify any pathogen in 26% of cases of community-acquired pneumonia.[3] Nevertheless, sputum Gram stain and culture should be examined for all hospitalized patients with suspected bacterial pneumonia.[86]

Most patients with PCP have a dry, nonproductive cough. In most cases, sputum cannot be produced unless it is induced. This can be accomplished by inhaling hypertonic saline via a hand-held nebulizer. Sputum induction should be performed in a properly engineered room to minimize transmission of infectious microorganisms. Sputum induction is a sensitive diagnostic test for PCP, with a reported sensitivity ranging from 55% in early studies to 95% when specimens are carefully obtained, concentrated by centrifugation, and stained with fluorescent antibody.[87,88] There is no difference in the sensitivity of induced sputum examination for PCP between patients on aerosolized pentamidine (AP) and those on no prophylaxis; nor is there a difference in the sensitivity of induced sputum examination whether the PCP episode was a first or second episode. At San Francisco General Hospital and at the National Institutes of Health (NIH), the use of sputum induction has permitted 80–95% of the PCP cases to be definitively diagnosed without resorting to bronchoscopy.[87,88] In a review of 992 episodes of PCP over

Table 69-6 Diagnostic Tests for Selected Pulmonary Diseases

Pulmonary Disease	Serology or Blood Cultures	Sputum	BAL ± TBBX	Pleural Fluid	Important Other Sites[a]	Suggestive Tests
Bacteria	**Blood cultures** (esp. *S. pneumoniae*)	**Gram stain and culture**	Rarely quantitative cultures	Consider (esp. if concern for empyema)		
M. tuberculosis	**Blood cultures**	**AFB smear and culture × 3**	Occasionally BAL and TBBX	Consider (with biopsy)	Lymph nodes, bone marrow	
Pneumocystis	No	**Induced sputum examination**	**BAL ± TBBX** (depends on respective sensitivities at institution)	Rarely		HRCT-GGO; PFTs-↓ DL_{co}. gallium ↑ uptake; O_2 sat. ↓ with exercise
C. neoformans	**Serum CRAG[b] Blood cultures**	Occasionally	**BAL**	Rarely	Cerebrospinal fluid, skin	
Cytomegalovirus	CMV-PCR	No	**TBBX**	No	Retina, GI tract	
T. gondii	***T. gondii* IgG, IgM**	Occasionally	**BAL**	Rarely	Central nervous system	Head CT/MRI with multiple lesions
Kaposi sarcoma	?HHV-8	No	**Visualization of lesions ± TBBX**	No	Mucocutaneous	Gallium-negative
Non-Hodgkin lymphoma	No	No	**TBBX, Wang needle**	Cytology, biopsy	Extranodal disease	

Tests in **boldface** are usual diagnostic tests of choice. Other tests should be considered if tests of choice are nondiagnostic.

AFB, acid-fast bacilli; BAL, bronchoalveolar lavage; CRAG, cryptococcal antigen; CT, computed tomography; DL_{co}, diffusing capacity for carbon monoxide; GGO, ground-glass opacities; GI, gastrointestinal; HHV-8, human herpes virus-8 (Kaposi sarcoma herpes virus, KS-HV); HRCT, chest high-resolution computed tomography; MRI, Magnetic resonance imaging; PFTs, pulmonary function tests; TBBX, transbronchial biopsies.

[a]Many of the pulmonary diseases present with important extrapulmonary sites of involvement that may dominate the clinical presentation. In such cases, pulmonary disease (if classic presentation) may be presumed in selected patients if the diagnosis is established from another site.

[b]The serum CRAG may be negative in isolated cryptococcal pneumonia.

a 4-year period, sputum induction accounted for 800 of the 992 (80%) diagnoses.[87] In addition, induced sputum aided in the diagnosis of TB and fungal pneumonias, bacterial bronchitis, and bronchopneumonia. Thus, sputum induction should be the initial diagnostic test for patients with pulmonary disease at institutions where it is available.

Sputum acid-fast bacilli (AFB) smear and culture are the foundations for the diagnosis of pulmonary TB. Sputum should be obtained on three consecutive days, ideally from the first morning specimen produced. Expectorated sputum is appropriate for patients with a productive cough, and sputum induction should be performed for those patients with a nonproductive or minimally productive cough. Several studies report that the sensitivity of sputum AFB smears and cultures in HIV-infected patients are similar to those seen in the overall population. The sensitivity of sputum AFB smears for *M. tuberculosis* ranged from 50% to 60% in two large series; the sensitivity of sputum AFB smears in persons presenting with disseminated disease was 90%.[89,90] Thus, patients with suspected TB, even if respiratory complaints are minimal and chest radiograph findings are absent, should have three sputum specimens submitted for AFB smears and culture.

One caveat regarding AFB smears and cultures: A positive sputum AFB smear can be due to a nontuberculous mycobacteria such as *M. kansasii* or *M. avium* complex (MAC).[91] The positive predictive value of a sputum AFB smear for *M. tuberculosis* depends in part on the relative frequencies of the other mycobacteria in that population. Nevertheless, any patient whose sputum smear reveals AFB must be approached as if it represents *M. tuberculosis*, and appropriate management (i.e., respiratory isolation if hospitalized, initiation of TB therapy) must be maintained until a definitive diagnosis is established. The use of molecular techniques such as nucleic-acid amplification (NAA) probes that are specific for *M. tuberculosis* can dramatically shorten the time until diagnosis. Sputum AFB specimens should be sent for culture, regardless of the results of the AFB smear, and all *M. tuberculosis* isolates should be sent for drug susceptibility testing.

Mycobacterium kansasii has been reported to present in a clinical and radiographic pattern indistinguishable from that of TB.[92] However, unlike *M. tuberculosis*, *M. kansasii* may be a nonpathogen in 8% to as many as 12% of cases.[93,94] The identification of MAC from a single sputum or BAL specimen cannot be presumed to indicate that MAC is the cause of the pulmonary pathology. In fact, one review of 200 HIV-infected patients with disseminated MAC found evidence for pulmonary disease in only five individuals.[95] Similarly, *Mycobacterium xenopi* rarely requires specific treatment.[96] *Mycobacterium gordonae* almost always represents a laboratory contaminant from a water source or from the laboratory.

Sputum examination, culture, or both can be used occasionally to diagnose fungal pneumonias, including those due to *C. neoformans*, *H. capsulatum*, and *C. immitis*, but not invasive *Aspergillus* spp. disease. It can be used to diagnose *T. gondii* and other parasitic pneumonias (e.g., *Strongyloides stercoralis*) as well.

Bronchoscopy

In general, bronchoscopy should be considered for any HIV-infected patient with pulmonary disease for which the severity warrants a prompt and accurate diagnosis, for patients with suspected pulmonary Kaposi sarcoma, for patients in whom the diagnosis is unclear despite less invasive diagnostic tests (e.g., sputum), and for those who are failing empiric therapy for a presumed pathogen.

Bronchoscopy with BAL is the gold standard diagnostic test for PCP and the initial test of choice at institutions where sputum induction is either unavailable or its sensitivity is low. Numerous studies have reported that the sensitivity of BAL for PCP is 95–98%. At San Francisco General Hospital, we perform bronchoscopy with BAL for patients with suspected PCP whose induced sputum examination is negative. From 992 cases of PCP diagnosed over a 4-year period, Huang and colleagues found that only two of the episodes (0.2%) were diagnosed by transbronchial biopsy (TBBX) alone; all of the remaining cases were diagnosed by sputum induction ($n = 800$) or BAL ($n = 190$).[87] This is not to imply that TBBX is an insensitive test for PCP; rather, it demonstrates that most cases of PCP can be diagnosed by other less invasive (e.g., sputum induction) or less risky (e.g., BAL) procedures. To estimate the sensitivity of BAL for PCP, the authors reviewed the medical records of 100 randomly selected patients who had both a negative induced sputum and a negative BAL fluid examination for *Pneumocystis* and had no other diagnosis established. The authors found that two patients were diagnosed with PCP during the 60 days after their negative BAL; one was diagnosed 46 days after the BAL and the other 51 days after. These results suggest that BAL alone is sufficient to diagnose most cases of PCP and that it is both sensitive and specific. It is important to note, however, that there are institutional differences in the sensitivity of the BAL examination. At institutions where the yields of BAL and TBBX are complementary and procedure-related complications are rare, both procedures are warranted.

Bronchoscopy is an important test for diagnosing cryptococcal pneumonia, especially if the disease is limited to the lungs. Batungwanayo and coworkers reported that BAL fluid culture was positive in 27 of 33 HIV-infected patients (82%) with cryptococcal pneumonia.[84] These results are similar to those reported by Meyohas and colleagues in which 23 of 27 HIV-infected patients (85%) with pulmonary cryptococcosis had a positive BAL fluid culture.[97] In this study, two of the patients with a negative BAL fluid culture had a positive BAL CRAG assay, and the remaining two had pleural cryptococcosis that was diagnosed by pleural fluid culture and pleural fluid CRAG assay.

Bronchoscopy with careful visual inspection of the airways is the procedure of choice for the diagnosis of pulmonary Kaposi sarcoma.[32] In these patients, neither endobronchial biopsy nor TBBX adds to the diagnostic yield when characteristic Kaposi sarcoma lesions are seen. However, the absence of visible Kaposi sarcoma lesions does not preclude their presence in more distal airways, nor does it preclude the possibility of parenchymal Kaposi sarcoma involvement. In these patients, TBBX can occasionally establish the diagnosis, but a diagnosis of Kaposi sarcoma may be difficult for the pathologist to establish with TBBX because of the small size of the sample and the crush artifact the procedure produces. In some cases, open lung biopsy is indicated.

TBBX can improve the diagnostic yield for mycobacterial and fungal pneumonias. In addition, TBBX or open lung biopsy is required to establish the diagnosis of CMV pneumonia.[98,99] Tissue from TBBX should reveal evidence of CMV inclusions and virologic changes. The isolation of CMV from BAL fluid or lung tissue cannot distinguish between asymptomatic viral shedding and pneumonia.[100] Similarly, biopsy is an important tool for diagnosing pulmonary non-Hodgkin lymphoma.[101]

Occasionally, endobronchial lesions are encountered on bronchoscopic visualization.[102] The clinical presentation and endobronchial appearance of these lesions may suggest the correct diagnosis. In these cases, establishing an appropriate differential diagnosis at the time of visualization is important, as certain lesions require specific biopsy techniques, and several etiologies require special stains.

Other Procedures

Diagnostic thoracentesis should be considered for any HIV-infected patient with evidence of pleural effusion in whom other tests are nondiagnostic and for whom infection is a concern. In most cases pleural fluid culture, antigen testing, molecular probes, or cytology can establish the diagnosis. However, for patients with pleural effusion and suspected pleural TB, the yield is improved with the addition of pleural biopsies.

Transthoracic needle aspiration with CT guidance is an important and useful diagnostic procedure for selected patients. HIV-infected patients with focal parenchymal lesions, most often peripheral nodules or masses that may be beyond the reach of a bronchoscope, are ideal candidates for CT-guided aspiration. In one study of 32 HIV-infected patients undergoing this procedure, a diagnosis was established in 27 patients.[103] Mediastinoscopy should be considered for patients with a mediastinal mass, intrathoracic lymphadenopathy, or both.

Occasionally, despite all of these efforts, HIV-infected patients with pulmonary disease may elude a definitive diagnosis. In such patients, consideration should be given to open lung biopsy, although such procedures have a low yield for diagnosing treatable disease and thereby favorably affecting the prognosis.

Interpretation of Radiologic, Microbiologic, and Other Diagnostic Information

Clinicians must exercise their clinical judgment to determine whether pneumonia is in fact present or organisms identified by the microbiology laboratory are the cause of the pulmonary dysfunction. As emphasized earlier, not all dyspnea, cough, hypoxia, or pulmonary infiltrates are due to pneumonia (i.e., pulmonary infection). Even if the constellation of symptoms, signs, and laboratory tests suggest that pneumonia is present, the microorganisms seen by direct microscopy or identified by culture or rapid tests may not be causative. Some organisms, such as *M. tuberculosis*, *Pneumocystis jirovecii*, and *H. capsulatum* should almost always be considered pathogens and be treated as such. If MAC, *Aspergillus*, or CMV is identified, it may represent a colonizer of the respiratory tract rather than the cause of the disease. Whether such organisms should be treated or other processes sought is an issue that requires considerable judgment and cannot be determined by a simple formula or algorithm.

PNEUMONIA: PRACTICAL CASE SCENARIOS

The following case scenarios illustrate how the CD4+ T-lymphocyte cell count and the chest radiograph interact to form a differential diagnosis that is further refined by information from the history, physical examination, and selected laboratory tests. Knowledge of the frequency of the various OIs and neoplasms in the demographic or regional setting assists the clinician in suggesting the most likely diagnosis. This, in turn, suggests a therapeutic approach.

Case Scenario 1: HIV-Infected Patient with CD4+ T-Lymphocyte Count Higher than 200 cells/μL

The differential diagnosis of pulmonary disease in an HIV-infected patient whose CD4+ T-lymphocyte count is higher than 200 cells/μL includes those HIV-associated pulmonary diseases that can present in persons without underlying immunodeficiency: bacterial pneumonia, viral or atypical pneumonias, TB, non-Hodgkin lymphoma, and occasionally fungal pneumonia (Fig. 69-2). In most clinical settings in the United States, bacterial pneumonia is the most common HIV-associated pulmonary disease. Rarely, PCP or fungi can present when the CD4+ T-lymphocyte cell count is higher than 200 cells/μL. Because each of these illnesses has a characteristic chest radiographic presentation, the specific radiographic findings influence the diagnostic tests and management.

If the chest radiograph reveals a focal, segmental, or lobar infiltrate in an alveolar pattern, bacterial pneumonia is the most likely diagnosis (Fig. 69-3). The suspicion for bacterial pneumonia is increased if the patient reports an acute onset of symptoms, typically fevers, chills or rigors, pleuritic chest pain, and a cough productive of purulent sputum. Other suggestive factors include the presence of focal findings on lung examination, an elevated WBC count with a left shift, a history of cigarette or injection drug use, and a history of prior bacterial pneumonia. In this case, the diagnostic approach typically includes sputum Gram stain, sputum and blood cultures for bacteria, and empiric therapy to cover the most common bacterial organisms, *S. pneumoniae* and *Haemophilus* spp. The presence of a pleural effusion should prompt consideration of thoracentesis.

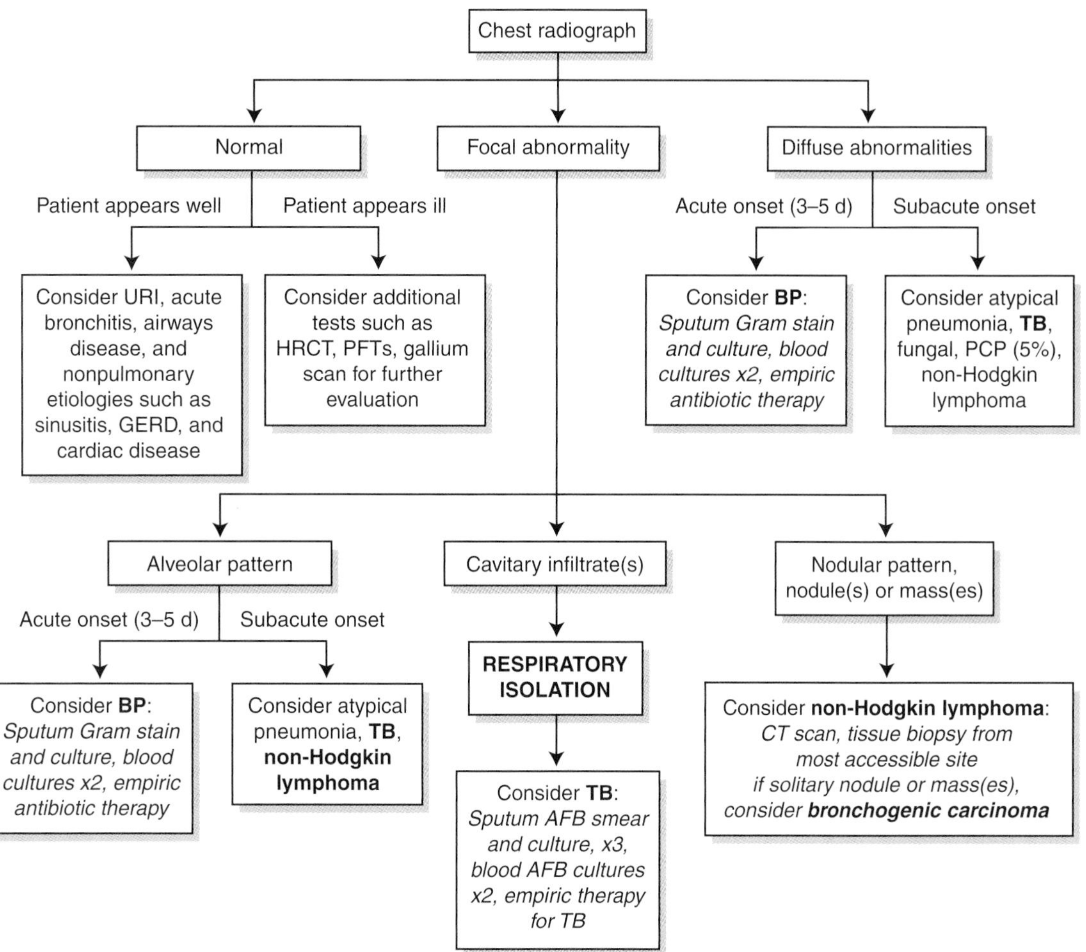

Figure 69-2 ■ Diagnostic approach to an HIV-infected patient, CD4+ T-lymphocyte count of more than 200 cells/μL. AFB, acid-fast bacilli; BP, bacterial pneumonia; CT, chest computed tomography; GERD, gastroesophageal reflux disease; HRCT, chest high-resolution computed tomography; PCP, *Pneumocystis* pneumonia; PFTs, pulmonary function tests; TB, tuberculosis; URI, upper respiratory tract infection.

If the chest radiograph reveals unilateral or bilateral upper lung zone infiltrates with cavitation, TB is the primary consideration (Fig. 69-4). The clinical suspicion for TB increases if the patient reports a subacute onset of fevers, cough, and constitutional complaints (night sweats, anorexia, weight loss), especially if the patient is at increased risk for exposure to *M. tuberculosis*. In this case, the diagnostic approach should include respiratory isolation (if the patient is hospitalized), examination of three morning sputum samples for AFB, sputum and blood cultures for mycobacteria, and empiric TB therapy with four drugs in addition to pyridoxine. For HIV-infected patients who are to receive concurrent therapy against HIV (with ART) and TB, special attention must be paid to interactions between the protease inhibitors and non-nucleoside reverse transcriptase inhibitors and the rifamycins. These interactions frequently require dose adjustments from the standard antiviral and antituberculous doses of these medications. In such cases, expert consultation is often warranted. Clinicians should also be aware that 'paradoxical reactions' to the initiation of therapy may occur; that is, the chest radiograph and pulmonary manifestations may worsen during the first few weeks despite effective antimycobacterial therapy. This phenomenon has been reported prior to the HIV era but has recently been noted when ART is initiated (*see* Chapter 5). This syndrome appears to be caused by an improved immunologic response to AFB, not to antimicrobial failure.

Case Scenario 2: HIV-Infected Patient with CD4+ T-Lymphocyte Count Less than 200 cells/μL

As the CD4+ T-lymphocyte count declines, the number of possible pulmonary diagnoses to consider increases. Still, the combination of the CD4+ T-lymphocyte count and the chest radiograph often suggests a probable diagnosis (Fig. 69-5).

A number of clinical possibilities and approaches exist if the chest radiograph is normal. In general, if the patient appears ill, additional tests are indicated to determine whether an occult pulmonary disease is present. As described, patients with PCP may have a normal chest radiograph; in these cases, chest HRCT scan may be useful. An HRCT with GGOs (Fig. 69-6) should prompt an evaluation for PCP (because this finding is not specific for PCP), whereas an HRCT without GGOs makes the diagnosis unlikely.

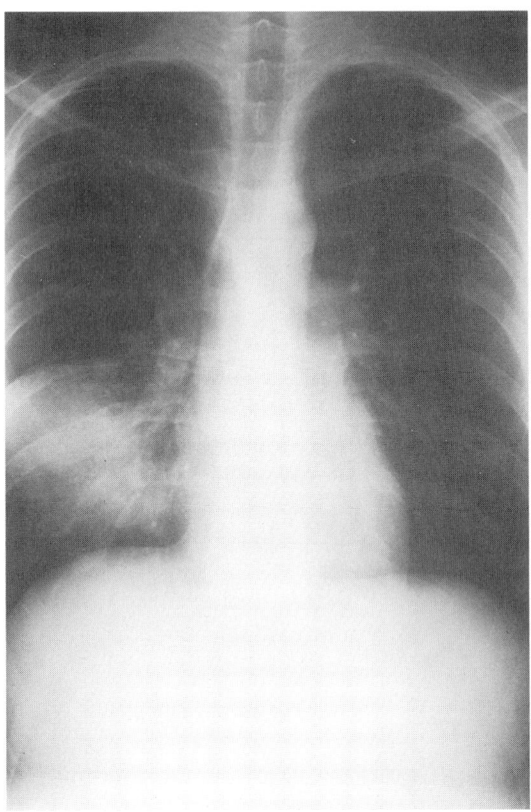

Figure 69-3 ■ Chest radiograph of an HIV-infected person, CD4+ T-lymphocyte count of more than 200 cells/μL, revealing right middle lobe consolidation. Sputum and blood cultures were positive for *S. pneumoniae*.

Courtesy of Laurence Huang, MD.

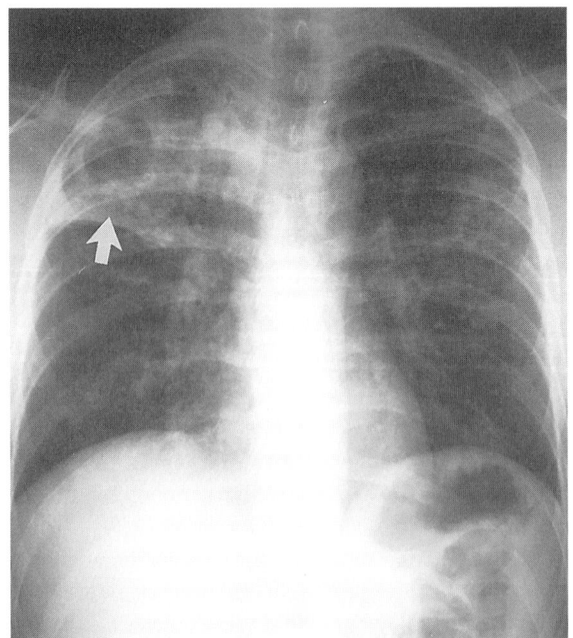

Figure 69-4 ■ Chest radiograph of an HIV-infected person, CD4+ T-lymphocyte count of more than 200 cells/μL, revealing right upper lobe infiltrate, with areas of cavitation. Sputum acid-fast bacillus stain was positive, and multiple sputum cultures grew *M. tuberculosis*.

Courtesy of Laurence Huang, MD.

If the chest radiograph reveals a focal infiltrate in an alveolar pattern (Figs 69-3 and 69-7), bacterial pneumonia is still the most likely diagnosis. However, if the patient presents with a subacute onset of symptoms and, especially if the patient has risk factors for exposure to *M. tuberculosis*, the possibility of TB must be strongly considered and three sputum AFB specimens must be examined. In Fig. 69-7, the key to the eventual diagnosis of TB was knowledge of the patient's CD4+ T-lymphocyte count (i.e., <200 cells/μL) and understanding that TB can present with middle or lower lung zone consolidation (or both) in these patients rather than the "classic" upper lung zone infiltrates with cavitation. Because of the higher incidence of mycobacteremia and disseminated or extrapulmonary disease, blood AFB cultures should be examined, and patients should have a careful physical examination for extrapulmonary sites of disease; for example, peripheral lymphadenopathy should prompt a lymph node aspirate or biopsy that may provide the diagnosis.

If the chest radiograph reveals bilateral symmetric interstitial-reticular or granular opacities (Fig. 69-8), PCP is the most likely diagnosis. Suspicion for PCP is increased if the patient reports a subacute onset of symptoms, typically fever, dyspnea, and a dry, nonproductive cough. Other suggestive factors include an elevated serum LDH. In this case, the diagnostic approach includes sputum induction and/or BAL and empiric PCP therapy. *C. neoformans* pneumonia also frequently presents below this CD4+ T-lymphocyte count range and with bilateral interstitial-reticular opacities. Cryptococcal infection is the leading diagnosis if the patient has evidence of concomitant neurologic dysfunction (e.g., headache, altered mental status). In this case, a serum CRAG assay is an excellent screening test and, if positive, should prompt analysis of cerebrospinal fluid. In addition, the diagnosis of cryptococcal disease can be made by fungal cultures of blood and respiratory specimens from sputum or bronchoscopy. The serum CRAG assay may be negative in cases of isolated cryptococcal pneumonia.

A patient with a CD4+ T-lymphocyte count less than 50 cells/μL whose chest radiograph or chest CT demonstrates a miliary pattern (Fig. 69-9) likely has either disseminated mycobacterial disease (e.g., miliary TB) or disseminated fungal disease. A history of risk factors for exposure to *M. tuberculosis* or residence in or travel to a geographic region that is endemic for certain fungal diseases may be useful when deciding which diagnosis is most likely and whether to begin empiric four-drug TB therapy or empiric antifungal therapy.

Finally, a patient with a CD4+ T-lymphocyte count less than 100 cells/μL whose chest radiograph reveals bilateral, diffuse coalescent opacities in a central distribution (usually with associated smaller nodules, Kerley B lines, pleural effusions, and occasionally intrathoracic adenopathy) likely has pulmonary Kaposi sarcoma (Fig. 69-10). This diagnosis is further supported by the presence of mucocutaneous Kaposi sarcoma lesions and can be confirmed by bronchoscopy and visualization of multiple characteristic Kaposi sarcoma lesions (Fig. 69-11).

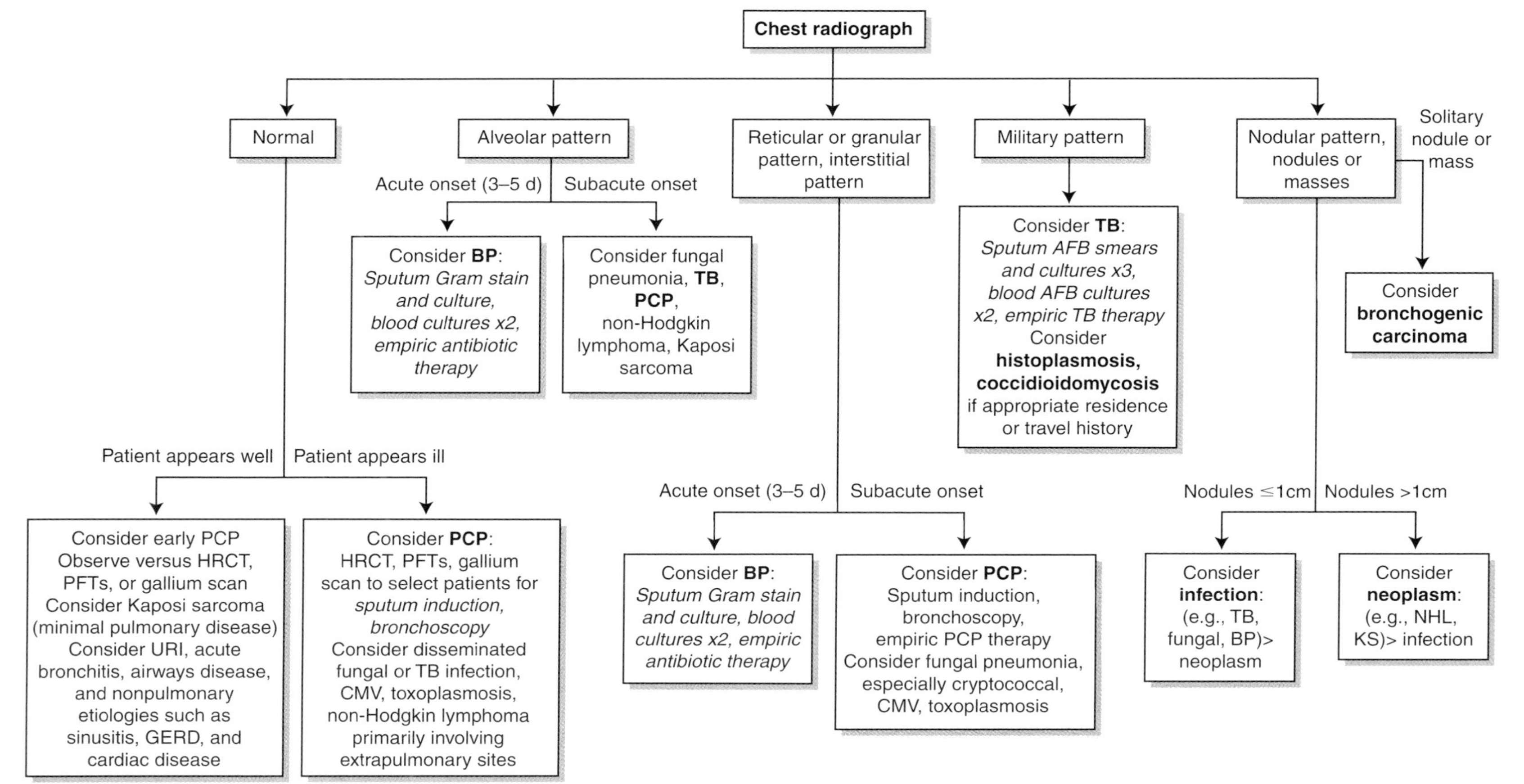

Figure 69-5 ■ Diagnostic approach to an HIV-infected patient, CD4+ T-lymphocyte count of less than 200 cells/μL. *Some of the diagnoses occur when the CD4+ T-lymphocyte count is less than 100 cells/μL or even less than 50 cells/μL. AFB, acid-fast bacilli; BP, bacterial pneumonia; CMV, Cytomegalovirus; GERD, gastroesophageal reflux disease; HRCT, chest high-resolution computed tomography; KS, Kaposi sarcoma; NHL, non-Hodgkin lymphoma; PCP, *Pneumocystis* pneumonia; PFTs, pulmonary function tests; TB, tuberculosis; URI, upper respiratory tract infection.

These case scenarios illustrate the most common HIV-related OIs and neoplasms. HIV-infected patients can develop a wide spectrum of pulmonary illnesses that include nonHIV-related conditions; HIV-related OIs due to bacterial, mycobacterial, fungal, viral, and parasitic pathogens; and HIV-related neoplasms. Usually, these diseases occur singly, but experience with HIV has reinforced the fact that occasionally diseases present simultaneously or develop rapidly one after another. Clinicians caring for HIV-infected patients must be vigilant for these situations and must have a low threshold for investigating any signs of clinical deterioration that may be due to a concurrent process that was missed initially.

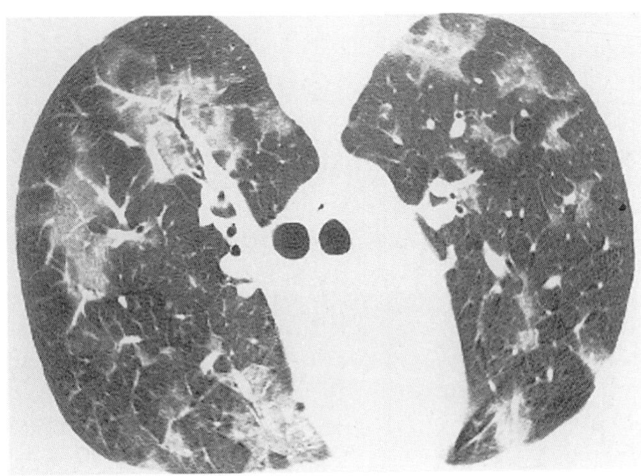

Figure 69-6 ■ Chest high-resolution computed tomographic (HRCT) scan of an HIV-infected person, CD4+ T-lymphocyte count of less than 200 cells/μL, whose chest radiograph was normal. Because of a clinical suspicion for *Pneumocystis* pneumonia (PCP), the patient underwent HRCT, which demonstrated the characteristic patchy ground-glass opacities of PCP. Induced sputum examination revealed *Pneumocystis* organisms.

Courtesy of Laurence Huang, MD.

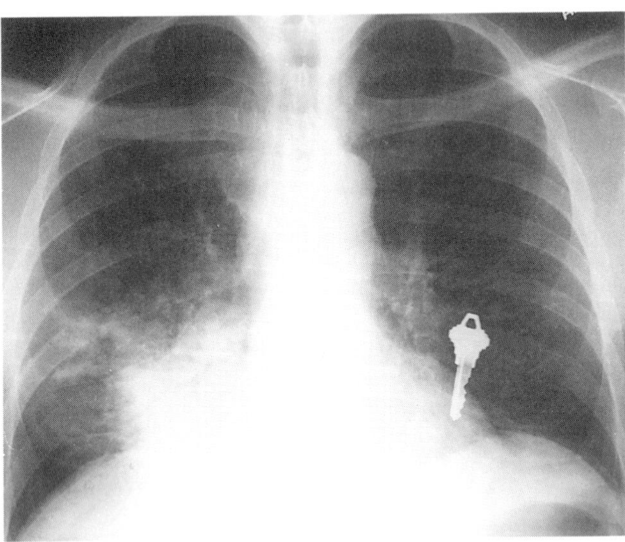

Figure 69-7 ■ Chest radiograph of an HIV-infected person, CD4+ T-lymphocyte count of less than 200 cells/μL, revealing right lower lung consolidation with air bronchograms. Sputum culture grew *M. tuberculosis* that was monorifampin-resistant. In this case the key to the diagnosis of tuberculosis was knowledge of the patient's CD4+ T-lymphocyte count and understanding that tuberculosis can present in this manner in such an individual.

Courtesy of Laurence Huang, MD.

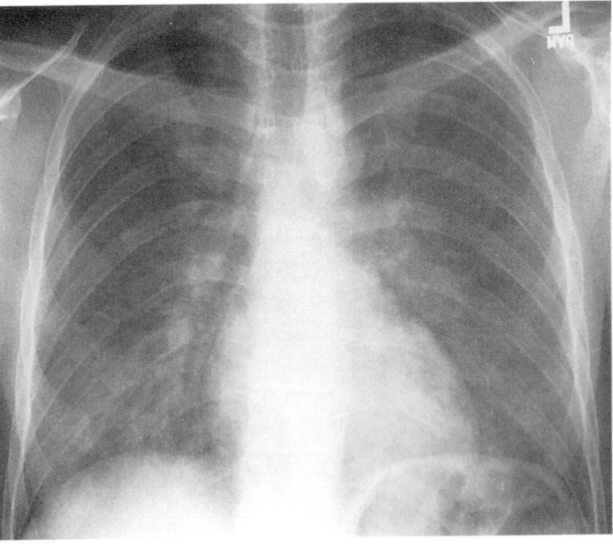

Figure 69-8 ■ Chest radiograph of an HIV-infected person, CD4+ T-lymphocyte count of less than 200 cells/μL demonstrating the characteristic bilateral, reticular-granular opacities of *Pneumocystis* pneumonia. Bronchoscopy with bronchoalveolar lavage fluid examination revealed *Pneumocystis* organisms.

Courtesy of Laurence Huang, MD.

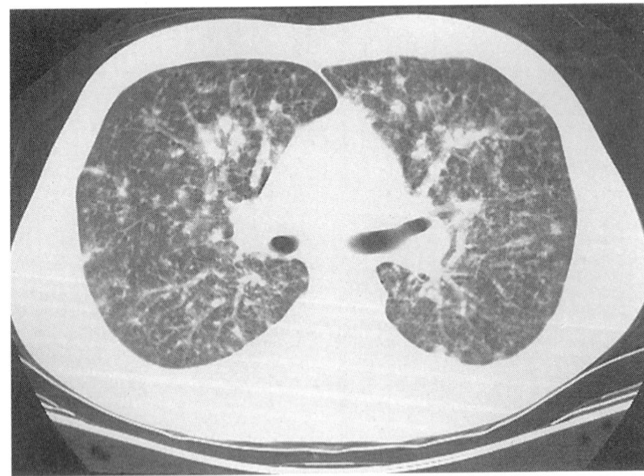

Figure 69-9 ■ Chest computed tomographic (CT) scan of an HIV-infected person, CD4+ T-lymphocyte count of less than 50 cells/μL with a miliary pattern. This radiographic pattern is nonspecific and may be seen in disseminated mycobacterial, fungal, and occasionally *Pneumocystis* infection. The diagnosis of *C. immitis* was suggested by a history of significant travel to the southwestern United States and was simultaneously confirmed by sputum, blood, and bronchoscopy cultures.

Courtesy of Laurence Huang, MD.

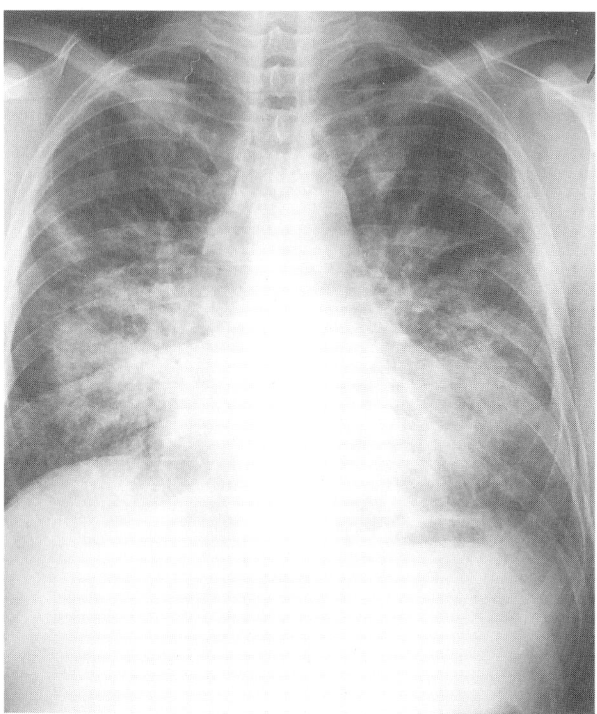

Figure 69-10 ■ Chest radiograph of an HIV-infected person, CD4+ T-lymphocyte count of less than 100 cells/μL with the characteristic bilateral, middle and lower lung zone, predominantly central distribution of abnormalities of pulmonary Kaposi sarcoma. The patient had no evidence of mucocutaneous Kaposi sarcoma, and the diagnosis of pulmonary disease was made by bronchoscopy with visualization of the characteristic erythematous-violaceous Kaposi lesions throughout the visible airway (see Fig. 69-11).

Courtesy of Laurence Huang, MD.

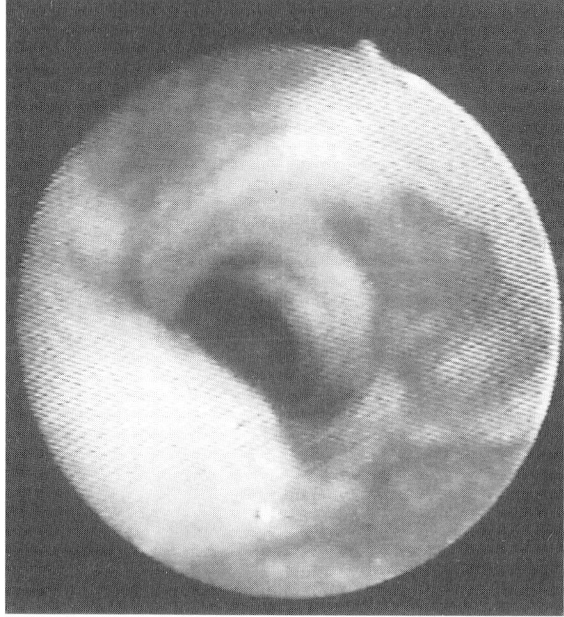

Figure 69-11 ■ Characteristic Kaposi sarcoma lesions located in the trachea in an HIV-infected person, CD4+ T-lymphocyte count of less than 100 cells/mL. Concurrent bronchoalveolar lavage also revealed *Pneumocystis* pneumonia.

Courtesy of Laurence Huang, MD.

APPROACH TO THERAPY

Without appropriate therapy, HIV-infected patients with certain types of pneumonia can progress rapidly to respiratory failure and death. Patients require a prompt evaluation and institution of treatment, especially those with low CD4+ T-lymphocyte counts, low neutrophil counts, or moderate, severe, or rapidly progressive disease. Unless disease is mild, or diagnostic facilities are unavailable, empiric therapy without any diagnostic evaluation is seldom justified. Specific antimicrobial therapy based on a well-established diagnosis can avoid unnecessary drug toxicity and drug interactions, reduce unnecessary ecologic pressure that can produce drug-resistant pathogens, and avoid expensive delays in instituting appropriate therapy, delays that can adversely affect outcome.

INITIAL THERAPY FOR SUSPECTED BACTERIAL PNEUMONIA

The principles of the treatment of patients with community-acquired bacterial pneumonia are the same in HIV-infected as in HIV-uninfected persons.[86,104] The choice of antimicrobial agent should be based on a number of factors, including the sputum Gram stain, the clinical and radiographic presentation, the severity of the pneumonia, and the patient's co-morbid conditions (e.g., COPD, alcohol use). Initial empiric therapy should include coverage against likely organisms (e.g., *S. pneumoniae*, *Haemophilus* spp.). Local or institutional drug-resistance patterns must be considered when selecting an antibiotic. For those patients with CD4+ T-lymphocyte counts of less than 100 cells/μL, especially if associated with recent hospitalization, neutropenia, broad-spectrum antimicrobial use, or a chest radiograph with evidence of cavitation, consideration should be given to including coverage against *P. aeruginosa*. Patients with underlying bronchiectasis and prior *P. aeruginosa* infection should receive antipseudomonal therapy based on prior sensitivity results. The duration of antibiotic therapy is similar in HIV-infected and nonHIV-infected persons, and the response rates appear to be comparable.[105]

Specific recommended regimens for non-ICU inpatients include either an extended spectrum cephalosporin (e.g., ceftriaxone or cefotaxime), often with a macrolide, or a fluoroquinolone with activity against *S. pneumoniae* (e.g., levofloxacin, moxifloxacin, or gemifloxacin).

Cordero and colleagues evaluated the prognosis and factors associated with mortality in 355 HIV-infected patients with community-acquired pneumonia.[106] They found that the mortality rate attributable to pneumonia was 9%. Patients meeting the American Thoracic Society criteria for severe pneumonia had a significantly higher mortality rate than those with nonsevere pneumonia (13% vs 3.5%; $P = 0.02$). Multivariate analysis revealed that patients with (1) a CD4+ T-lymphocyte count less than 100cells/μL, (2) septic shock, (3) cavities, (4) multilobar infiltrates, or (5) pleural effusions were at an increased risk of death. Importantly, when these five predictors were assessed as a group, patients without any of the five risk factors were at a low-risk for death (1.3%). This suggests that these criteria could be used to determine whether to admit an HIV-infected patient with community-acquired pneumonia or to treat the individual as an outpatient.

APPROACH TO THE PATIENT WHO IS FAILING PCP THERAPY

Regardless of which approach (definitive diagnosis or empiric therapy) has been selected, a percentage of patients fail to improve despite apparent appropriate therapy and there are several important factors to consider (Table 69-7). The case of a patient with PCP who is worsening despite treatment with trimethoprim-sulfamethoxazole is used to illustrate several of these considerations. First, how was the original diagnosis of PCP established? Strong consideration should be given to pursuing a definitive diagnosis, as several HIV-associated OIs can present in a fashion indistinguishable from that of PCP. Bronchoscopy is the procedure of choice, as it will provide the maximal diagnostic yield. Occasionally, patients require elective intubation and transfer to an intensive care unit for this procedure to be performed.

Next, careful consideration should be given to the possibility of a concurrent pulmonary process, either infectious or noninfectious (e.g., noncardiogenic pulmonary edema, pulmonary embolism). A review of the microbiology results may reveal a coexistent infection. A chest radiograph should be repeated to evaluate for a supervening process. At this stage, sputum and blood cultures against bacteria, fungi, and mycobacteria should be obtained or repeated. A serum CRAG assay should be undertaken, as cryptococcal pneumonia frequently presents with a clinical and radiographic picture that is indistinguishable from that of PCP.

For patients with a CD4+ T-lymphocyte count below 50 cells/μL, ophthalmology consultation should be sought for a dilated retinal examination for CMV. Patients with evidence of CMV retinitis require induction therapy, which also treats presumed CMV pneumonitis. Alternatively, a definitive diagnosis of CMV pneumonitis may be pursued with TBBX. The diagnosis depends on identifying multiple inclusion bodies. If the patient is known to have mucocutaneous Kaposi sarcoma, bronchoscopy may also provide a diagnosis of pulmonary Kaposi sarcoma by identifying endobronchial lesions.

Occasionally, a patient's "failure" to respond to PCP treatment is the result of noninfectious etiologies such as noncardiogenic edema, where a trial of diuresis may result in symptomatic and radiographic improvement. Concurrent with these considerations, a review of the patient's PCP therapy should consider whether the patient is receiving the "best" treatment option, whether adjuvant corticosteroids are warranted, and if the patient has nausea/vomiting or diarrhea whether a switch to an intravenous route is prudent.

Patients with PCP may have slow resolution of their disease, and it may be several days to a week or more until their clinical status improves. A general rule of thumb: the number of days a patient was symptomatic before treatment was begun is approximately the number of days it takes for resolution or near-resolution of the symptoms. Nevertheless, one expects a patient with PCP to manifest initial signs of improvement by day 7–10 of treatment. The chest radiograph tends to lag behind the clinical response.[107] If a patient fails to improve after this time or there is progressive deterioration, an evaluation for an alternate process is recommended and a switch in PCP therapy may be indicated.

Finally, the specter of drug-resistant *Pneumocystis* is often raised.[108–111] Unfortunately, the lack of a culture system for human *Pneumocystis* has limited our ability to confirm drug resistance in *Pneumocystis*. Several studies have reported that specific point mutations in the *Pneumocystis* dihydropteroate synthase gene – the enzymatic target of sulfamethoxazole and dapsone – are associated with an increased risk of trimethoprim-sulfamethoxazole PCP treatment failure and

Table 69-7 Diagnostic Approach to Clinical Failure of PCP Therapy

Review diagnosis

How was the initial diagnosis of PCP established?
- Empiric? Strongly consider diagnostic procedure.
- Induced sputum? Bronchoscopy?

Was there a concurrent process initially?
- Review microbiology results and cultures.
- Obtain or repeat sputum and blood cultures, serologies (e.g., serum CRAG).

Has another process supervened (consider infectious and noninfectious etiologies)?
- Repeat diagnostic tests (e.g., chest radiograph).
- Obtain or repeat sputum and blood cultures, serologies (e.g., serum CRAG).
- Strongly consider diagnostic procedure.

Review treatment

Is the patient receiving the best PCP treatment?
Is the dose of the medication correct?
Is the patient receiving adjuvant corticosteroids?
Does the patient have nausea/vomiting or diarrhea? Switch to intravenous therapy.
Allow adequate time for initial therapy to work (usually 5–8 days).

Consider further evaluation

Consider bronchoscopy.
- If initial diagnosis of PCP was empiric, bronchoscopy may confirm diagnosis or provide alternate diagnosis.
- If initial diagnosis of PCP was obtained from induced sputum examination, bronchoscopy may provide higher yield for other infections or may provide a diagnosis of pulmonary Kaposi sarcoma.
- If initial diagnosis of PCP was obtained from BAL examination, repeat bronchoscopy may provide evidence for new infection.

increased mortality.[112–116] These results have been interpreted to imply that the *Pneumocystis* in these patients has developed "resistance" to trimethoprim-sulfamethoxazole.

IMMUNE RECONSTITUTION SYNDROMES

The use of ART has resulted in dramatic declines in AIDS deaths and OI rates. Among patients who have experienced dramatic, sustained rises in their CD4+ T-lymphocyte counts, primary and secondary OI prophylaxis and chronic maintenance therapy have been successfully discontinued. However, the initiation of combinations of ART and the subsequent improvement in immune function has also resulted in several syndromes that have important clinical implications.[117] Interestingly, in some of the examples provided, the use of ART serves to exacerbate the disease transiently, whereas in others its use is seemingly solely responsible for the reported improvements. Finally, in some cases the use of ART has been associated with the development of pulmonary disease that is host-mediated.

The transient worsening of clinical symptoms, signs, and chest radiograph findings of TB after the initiation of appropriate antituberculous therapy have been well-recognized. These "paradoxical" reactions are thought to represent an enhanced antituberculous immune response and usually resolve without specific therapy.[118] HIV-infected patients who develop TB and receive concurrent antiretroviral and antituberculous therapies appear to have an increased incidence of paradoxical worsening. Narita and colleagues found that 36% of HIV-infected TB patients receiving these dual therapies developed a paradoxical reaction compared to 7% of HIV-infected TB patients who received TB therapy alone and 2% of TB patients without concomitant HIV infection.[119] Three-fourths of the patients who developed paradoxical reactions while on dual antiretroviral and antituberculous therapies developed hectic fevers, and three patients with severe paradoxical reactions required systemic corticosteroids for symptomatic relief. Fishman and colleagues noted transient worsening on serial chest radiographs in 45% of HIV-infected TB patients receiving dual HIV and TB therapies.[120] The radiographic worsening consisted of new or worsening parenchymal disease in 32%, new or worsening intrathoracic lymphadenopathy in 23%, and new or worsening pleural effusion in 19%. However, the diagnosis of paradoxical reaction must be one of exclusion. HIV-infected TB patients with suspected paradoxical reactions must also be thoroughly evaluated for progressive TB due to drug resistance or patient nonadherence and for the presence of a concurrent, superimposed OI. A similar syndrome has been described for patients with PCP who institute ART, during acute PCP therapy.[121]

The use of ART, often in the absence of specific chemotherapy, has resulted in clinical regression and occasionally complete resolution of Kaposi sarcoma (including pulmonary Kaposi sarcoma) lesions.[122] Several cases of clinically symptomatic pulmonary Kaposi sarcoma diagnosed by bronchoscopic visualization have been noted that responded to ART alone. In these cases, subsequent chest radiographs and, in one patient, subsequent bronchoscopy demonstrated complete resolution of disease. One question of major clinical importance that remains largely unanswered is whether the addition of ART to standard OI treatment is beneficial or potentially harmful if paradoxical reactions develop in patients with OIs. Given the still significant mortality associated with respiratory failure due to OIs, this question is particularly important to HIV-associated pneumonias.

Improved immune function may also play a role in the development of host-mediated pulmonary disease. There are several reports of sarcoidosis or a sarcoidosis-like disease developing after the initiation of ART.[123–128] In addition, subacute hypersensitivity pneumonitis to avian antigen that developed only when the patient's immune function improved on ART has also been described.[129] Diseases in which the host immune response plays an essential role in pathogenesis can be expected to become more prevalent as more HIV-infected patients receive ART.

LOWER RESPIRATORY TRACT DISEASE: NEOPLASMS AND NONINFECTIOUS INFLAMMATORY DISORDERS

The initial evaluation of respiratory disease usually focuses on the diagnosis of HIV-associated OIs. This stems from the frequency of infectious complications, the need for their prompt treatment, and in the case of TB the concern for transmission to other persons, both HIV-infected and nonHIV-infected. However, HIV-infected patients are also susceptible to a number of noninfectious respiratory complications, whose aspects are summarized briefly.

Two HIV-associated malignancies, Kaposi sarcoma and non-Hodgkin lymphoma, may include pulmonary involvement. With both neoplasms, intrathoracic disease is usually a manifestation of disease already recognized elsewhere, but occasionally Kaposi sarcoma and non-Hodgkin lymphoma present with isolated pulmonary disease.

Kaposi Sarcoma

The most common HIV-associated malignancy is Kaposi sarcoma. One of the phenomena of the AIDS epidemic during the early 1980s was the occurrence of this previously rare disease. Although the incidence of Kaposi sarcoma has decreased dramatically since then, significant advances have been made in our understanding of its pathogenesis, including its association with human herpesvirus 8 (HHV-8).

Almost all of the HIV-infected patients with Kaposi sarcoma are MSM. Pulmonary Kaposi sarcoma is detected clinically in approximately one-third of patients with known Kaposi sarcoma, with the proportion detected at autopsy approaching 50–75%.[130,131] Clinically symptomatic pulmonary Kaposi sarcoma presents at the lower range of CD4+

T-lymphocyte counts, but tracheobronchial lesions may be seen in patients with higher CD4+ T-lymphocyte counts who are undergoing bronchoscopy for other reasons. Most but not all patients with clinically diagnosed pulmonary Kaposi sarcoma have concomitant mucocutaneous disease.[32] Importantly, a significant proportion of patients with pulmonary Kaposi sarcoma also have concurrent OI. Huang and colleagues found that 45 of the 168 patients (27%) with pulmonary Kaposi sarcoma had an accompanying OI, most frequently PCP.[32] These observations underscore the critical need to evaluate each patient with suspected or known pulmonary Kaposi sarcoma for an OI. Patients with pulmonary Kaposi sarcoma who develop OI can also experience rapid progression of their Kaposi sarcoma.

Pulmonary Kaposi sarcoma characteristically presents with a nonproductive cough, slowly progressive dyspnea, and occasionally fever.[130,131] Chest pain and hemoptysis are noted less frequently. Rarely, Kaposi sarcoma lesions may involve the larynx or trachea to such an extent as to cause hoarseness or stridor. Symptoms are usually present for weeks or even months but may also progress rapidly in a manner that is indistinguishable from that of an OI.

As described previously, pulmonary Kaposi sarcoma characteristically presents with bilateral middle-lower lung zone opacities in a central or perihilar distribution on chest radiograph (Fig. 69-10). Typical chest radiographic findings include linear densities (bronchial wall thickening), nodules or nodular opacities of varying size, Kerley B lines, pleural effusions, and intrathoracic adenopathy.[132] The latter finding may be underappreciated on the chest radiograph given the perihilar distribution of parenchymal disease. Chest CT scans often demonstrate the characteristic peribronchovascular distribution with associated nodules.[74,75]

The diagnosis of pulmonary Kaposi sarcoma is usually established by bronchoscopy. Finding the characteristic endobronchial, reddish-purplish, flat or slightly raised lesions is sufficient to diagnose pulmonary disease in the proper clinical context (Fig. 69-11). Most patients with chest radiographic findings suggestive of pulmonary Kaposi sarcoma have multiple endobronchial Kaposi sarcoma lesions seen below the level of the carina. However, the presence of these lesions does not preclude a concurrent infection, nor does their absence in the observable airway preclude more distal airway disease or parenchymal, pleural, or nodal involvement. In cases where there is a strong clinical suspicion for pulmonary Kaposi sarcoma but no endobronchial lesions are seen, transbronchial biopsies should be considered to establish the diagnosis. However, accurately and reliably identifying Kaposi sarcoma in a small piece of crushed transbronchoscopically obtained tissue is difficult.

Patients with pleural effusions may be considered candidates for thoracentesis, primarily to exclude the presence of infection but also to provide symptomatic relief if the effusions are large. Although most Kaposi sarcoma effusions are exudative, pleural effusions may be transudate or exudate, serous, serosanguineous, or even frankly bloody.[131] Several chylous effusions due to lymphatic obstruction from Kaposi sarcoma have also been seen.

Non-Hodgkin Lymphoma

Intrathoracic involvement is more common in Kaposi sarcoma than in non-Hodgkin lymphoma. Most patients with non-Hodgkin lymphoma present with disseminated disease and extranodal involvement. Frequent extranodal sites include liver, spleen, bone marrow, meninges, and gastrointestinal tract. Intrathoracic involvement is seen in a smaller proportion. The reported incidence of intrathoracic disease varies from 0% to 31% of non-Hodgkin lymphoma patients at the time of clinical diagnosis and is usually higher at the time of autopsy.[131] Occasionally, the lung is the only site involved. Non-Hodgkin lymphoma can present at a wide range of CD4+ T-lymphocyte counts. The median CD4+ T-lymphocyte count is ~100 cells/μL, and 75% of patients have a count less than 50 cells/μL.

When the lungs are involved, the most common symptoms are cough and dyspnea, with pleuritic chest pain and hemoptysis occurring less frequently. One study found that these symptoms were present in 71%, 63%, 26%, and 11%, respectively, of the 38 patients reported.[101] The presence of B symptoms, such as fever, sweats, and weight loss, are also common features. Physical examination of the chest may reveal a variety of findings, including crackles, rhonchi, wheezes, decreased breath sounds, and egophony.

The most common chest radiographic parenchymal findings are multiple nodular opacities or masses, lobar infiltrates, and diffuse bilateral interstitial infiltrates.[101,131,133] Occasionally, a solitary nodule or mass is seen. More rarely, endobronchial lesions have been reported.[102] Pleural effusions are the most common radiographic abnormality, occurring in 40–70% of cases, and they may occur in the absence of parenchymal disease.[101,131] The effusions may be unilateral or bilateral and may vary in size. Hilar and mediastinal adenopathy can be found in up to 60% of these patients. Chest CT scans are useful for deciding on the optimal diagnostic procedure and for follow-up.

The diagnosis of non-Hodgkin lymphoma requires demonstration of malignant lymphocytes on cytology or biopsy specimens. Most often fine needle aspiration or biopsy of an extrathoracic site establishes the diagnosis. Persons presenting with isolated intrathoracic involvement should undergo bronchoscopy with biopsies or CT-guided fine-needle aspiration. Other options include mediastinoscopy, thoracoscopy, and open-lung biopsy. For patients with pleural effusions, pleural fluid cytology, biopsy, or both are often diagnostic.[131]

Bronchogenic Carcinoma

There is significant debate whether other malignancies that involve the lung (i.e., bronchogenic carcinoma) are also associated with HIV disease.[131] In contrast to Kaposi sarcoma and non-Hodgkin lymphoma, there is no increase in bronchogenic carcinoma seen in persons with other immunosuppressive disorders. Nevertheless, a number of reports have suggested that bronchogenic carcinoma is increased in frequency, occurs at a younger age, and has a more aggressive course in HIV-infected patients. One study that cross-matched the HIV/AIDS and cancer registries in Texas found a 6.5-fold increased incidence of bronchogenic carcinoma in HIV/AIDS patients compared to the rest of the US population.[134] Johnson and colleagues in the PCHIS found a bronchogenic carcinoma rate of ~180 cases per 100000 person-years in their HIV-infected cohort.[135] Other studies, however, found no significant increase. Nevertheless, one can expect the number of bronchogenic carcinomas in HIV-infected persons to increase as these individuals survive longer because of ART and OI prophylaxis and as they reach an age where lung cancer rates are increased.

Most HIV-infected patients who develop bronchogenic carcinoma are cigarette smokers.[131] Although all pathologic types are seen, adenocarcinoma has been the most frequent type reported, similar to that seen in nonHIV-infected patients younger than 40 years of age who develop bronchogenic carcinoma. Bronchogenic carcinoma can develop at a wide range of CD4+ T-lymphocyte counts. In the PCHIS, the range of CD4+ T-lymphocyte counts among the patients who developed lung cancer was 127–1026 cells/μL.[135] The characteristic presentation of bronchogenic carcinoma is familiar and includes respiratory symptoms such as cough occasionally with hemoptysis, dyspnea, and chest pain. Constitutional symptoms such as severe fatigue, anorexia, and weight loss may also be present. The chest radiographic presentation appears to include parenchymal nodules or masses, pleural effusion, and central parenchymal or hilar masses and mediastinal adenopathy.[73,136] Chest CT scans provide additional important details that are crucial for optimum diagnosis and management.

The diagnosis and treatment of bronchogenic carcinoma in HIV-infected patients is similar to that in nonHIV-infected individuals. HIV infection should be considered an important concurrent underlying medical problem, much the same as one would consider underlying cardiopulmonary disease. Surgical resection should be considered for any patient whose staging and medical condition supports such an approach.[137,138]

INTERSTITIAL PNEUMONITIS

Although OI and, to a lesser extent, neoplasia dominate the clinical spectrum of HIV-associated pulmonary disease, occasionally patients present with one of the interstitial pneumonitides: lymphocytic interstitial pneumonitis (LIP) or nonspecific interstitial pneumonitis (NSIP).[139]

Lymphocytic Interstitial Pneumonitis

The most striking feature of HIV-associated LIP is the effect of age on its incidence. Early in the AIDS epidemic, one-third to one-half of AIDS-defining diagnoses in children were due to LIP. In contrast, LIP is rare in adults, and there are only scattered case reports throughout the literature.[140]

The symptoms of LIP include slowly progressive dyspnea, nonproductive cough, and fever. Lung examination may be normal or may reveal inspiratory crackles. These clinical features are indistinguishable from an OI (e.g., PCP). In children, additional physical examination findings include clubbing, salivary gland enlargement, lymphadenopathy, and hepatosplenomegaly.

The chest radiograph presentation of LIP is nonspecific and characteristically shows bilateral reticulonodular "interstitial" infiltrates with a lower lung zone predominance.[141] Hilar or mediastinal adenopathy is occasionally seen and can potentially be used to distinguish LIP from PCP. Pulmonary function tests often reveal a restrictive ventilatory defect (decreased total lung capacity) and a decreased diffusing capacity. Chest CT scans may reveal small (2–4 mm) nodules often in a peribronchovascular distribution or diffuse areas of ground-glass opacification. Gallium scintigraphy may note diffuse pulmonary uptake, indistinguishable from that of PCP, although all patterns have been described. The diagnosis of LIP requires histologic confirmation by biopsy. Reports on treatment are limited, but ART has been used with success.[142,143]

Nonspecific Interstitial Pneumonitis

The symptoms of NSIP include dyspnea, nonproductive cough, and fever. Lung examination may be normal or may reveal inspiratory crackles. These clinical features are indistinguishable from those of PCP. However, NSIP may present at CD4+ T-lymphocyte counts of more than 200 cells/μL, whereas PCP rarely does.[35,139,144] In one large series of 67 HIV-infected patients with NSIP, the mean CD4+ T-lymphocyte count for patients with NSIP was 492 cells/μL compared to 57 cells/μL for matched controls with PCP.[35]

The chest radiographic presentation of NSIP is nonspecific and usually indistinguishable from that of PCP. As with PCP, NSIP can present with a normal radiograph. One study of patients with NSIP found that 16 of 36 patients (44%) with NSIP had a normal chest radiograph.[145] The most common radiographic abnormality seen was a diffuse interstitial pattern. Other abnormalities include pleural effusions, alveolar infiltrates, and nodules. Pulmonary function tests often reveal a mildly decreased diffusing capacity.[139] The diagnosis of NSIP requires histologic confirmation and exclusion of other etiologies.

OTHER DISORDERS

Pulmonary Hypertension

Numerous reports of pulmonary arterial hypertension (PAH) in HIV-infected patients are scattered throughout the literature.[146] One series compared 20 HIV-infected patients with PAH to 93 HIV-uninfected patients with PAH.[147] At the time of pulmonary hypertension being diagnosed, the HIV-infected patients were significantly younger, and the proportion with

New York Heart Association functional class III or IV was significantly lower (50% vs 75%; $P<0.01$). Pulmonary hypertension was thought to be the cause of death in 8 of the 10 HIV-infected patients who died within 1 year after the diagnosis of pulmonary hypertension. Pathologic findings resembled those of plexogenic pulmonary arteriopathy. Often, multiple potential factors (including injection drug use, cigarette use, history of underlying cardiac or pulmonary disease, and prior pulmonary OIs) complicate the clinical picture and the classification of these patients as having PAH.

The characteristic clinical presentation is one of progressive dyspnea, with a nonproductive cough, chest pain, and syncope or near-syncope seen in a small number.[146] Physical examination usually reveals evidence of right heart failure, with bipedal edema being the most consistent finding. Chest radiographic findings include cardiomegaly and prominence of the pulmonary arteries.

The chest radiograph or electrocardiogram with evidence of right ventricular hypertrophy often first suggests the diagnosis of pulmonary hypertension. Most commonly, the diagnosis is confirmed by echocardiogram. Patients diagnosed with pulmonary hypertension should undergo a thorough evaluation for secondary (potentially treatable) causes, including underlying cardiac disease (i.e., left ventricular failure, mitral or aortic valvular disease) and pulmonary disease (i.e., COPD, recurrent pulmonary emboli).

Treatment for HIV-infected patients with PAH should focus on oxygen supplementation (if the patient is hypoxemic); discontinuation of cigarette use, intravenous drug use, and other potential contributing factors; and aggressive treatment of underlying cardiopulmonary disease. More recently, HIV-infected patients with PAH have responded to standard PAH therapies, and there are a few reports of the possible beneficial effects of ART.[148-150]

Upper Respiratory Tract Disease

Sinusitis

Sinusitis is more common in HIV-infected persons than in immunocompetent ones.[151] Furthermore, the incidence of sinusitis appears to increase in frequency as the CD4+ T-lymphocyte count declines. These episodes often alternate with episodes of bronchitis.[152] This "ping-pong" effect results in a chronic, relapsing condition that is challenging to clinicians and frustrating to patients.

The clinical presentation of sinusitis in HIV-infected persons is similar to that in immunocompetent persons. Patients often report frontal headaches with sinus or nasal congestion, fever, and postnasal drip or purulent nasal discharge. Physical examination may reveal sinus tenderness and occasionally even facial swelling. The diagnosis of sinusitis is usually established on clinical grounds, especially in a patient with prior radiographic evidence of disease and a characteristic presentation. Sinus radiographs are used to diagnose maxillary involvement, but sinus CT scanning is a more sensitive diagnostic test for nonmaxillary disease. The treatment for sinusitis in HIV-infected persons is similar to that in immunocompetent persons and often includes a combination of decongestants, nasal vasoconstrictors, nasal corticosteroids, and antibiotics for selected patients. *S. pneumoniae* and *Haemophilus* spp. are the most common bacterial pathogens identified, so antibiotic therapy, if indicated, should target these pathogens. However, patients with apparent refractory sinusitis may have more ominous etiologies: *Aspergillus*, *Mucor*, or *Fusarium* infections and lymphoma have been reported.[153–155] Erosion of bone adjacent to the sinuses in particular should prompt an aggressive diagnostic evaluation. In these patients, ENT consultation for invasive diagnostic and therapeutic procedures may be warranted.

Bronchitis

Similar to sinusitis, bronchitis is more common in HIV-infected persons than in immunocompetent ones.[2] Bronchitis also appears to increase in frequency as the CD4+ T-lymphocyte count declines, and recurrent infections occasionally lead to more permanent airway damage and bronchiectasis.

The clinical presentation of bronchitis in HIV-infected persons is similar to that in immunocompetent persons. Patients often report a cough that is usually productive of purulent sputum and fever. Physical examination may reveal coarse rhonchi. The chest radiograph is without infiltrate, but the presence of bronchial wall thickening or peribronchial cuffing should alert the clinician to the presence of underlying airways disease. Chest HRCT can be useful for demonstrating bronchiectasis. The treatment for bronchitis in HIV-infected persons is similar to that in immunocompetent persons, and issues regarding whether the episode is bacterial or viral in etiology pertain. HIV-infected patients with recurrent bronchitis or bronchiectasis who are cigarette smokers should be strongly encouraged to quit smoking, and preventive measures such as pneumococcal vaccine and annual influenzae vaccine should be offered.

REFERENCES

1. Pulmonary Complications of HIV Infection Study Group. Design of a prospective study of the pulmonary complications of human immunodeficiency virus infection. J Clin Epidemiol 46:497, 1993.
2. Wallace JM, Hansen NI, Lavange L, et al. Respiratory disease trends in the pulmonary complications of HIV infection study cohort. Pulmonary Complications of HIV Infection Study Group. Am J Respir Crit Care Med 155:72, 1997.
3. Mundy LM, Auwaerter PG, Oldach D, et al. Community-acquired pneumonia: impact of immune status. Am J Respir Crit Care Med 152:1309, 1995.
4. Rimland D, Navin TR, Lennox JL, et al. Prospective study of etiologic agents of community-acquired pneumonia in patients with HIV infection. AIDS 16:85, 2002.
5. Rosen MJ, Clayton K, Schneider RF, et al. Intensive care of patients with HIV infection: utilization, critical illnesses, and outcomes. Pulmonary Complications of HIV Infection Study Group. Am J Respir Crit Care Med 155:67, 1997.

6. Nickas G, Wachter RM. Outcomes of intensive care for patients with human immunodeficiency virus infection. Arch Intern Med 160:541, 2000.
7. Morris A, Creasman J, Turner J, et al. Intensive care of human immunodeficiency virus-infected patients during the era of highly active antiretroviral therapy. Am J Respir Crit Care Med 166:262, 2002.
8. Morris A, Masur H, Huang L. Current issues in critical care of the human immunodeficiency virus-infected patient. Crit Care Med 34:42, 2006.
9. Casalino E, Wolff M, Ravaud P, et al. Impact of HAART advent on admission patterns and survival in HIV-infected patients admitted to an intensive care unit. AIDS 18:1429,2004.
10. Ampel NM. Coccidioidomycosis in persons infected with HIV type 1. Clin Infect Dis 41:1174,2005.
11. Haramati LB, Wong J. Intrathoracic Kaposi's sarcoma in women with AIDS. Chest 117:410, 2000.
12. Hirschtick RE, Glassroth J, Jordan MC, et al. Bacterial pneumonia in persons infected with the human immunodeficiency virus. Pulmonary Complications of HIV Infection Study Group. N Engl J Med 333:845, 1995.
13. Dworkin MS, Adams MR, Cohn DL, et al. Factors that complicate the treatment of tuberculosis in HIV-infected patients. J Acquir Immune Defic Syndr 39:464, 2005.
14. O'Donnell AE, Selig J, Aravamuthan M, et al. Pulmonary complications associated with illicit drug use: an update. Chest 108:460, 1995.
15. Huang L, Stansell JD. AIDS and the lung. Med Clin North Am 80:775, 1996.
16. Diaz PT, King MA, Pacht ER, et al. Increased susceptibility to pulmonary emphysema among HIV-seropositive smokers. Ann Intern Med 132:369, 2000.
17. Crothers K, Griffith TA, McGinnis KA, et al. The impact of cigarette smoking on mortality, quality of life, and comorbid illness among HIV-positive veterans. J Gen Intern Med 20:1142, 2005.
18. Markowitz N, Hansen NI, Hopewell PC, et al. Incidence of tuberculosis in the United States among HIV-infected persons. The Pulmonary Complications of HIV Infection Study Group. Ann Intern Med 126:123, 1997.
19. Munyati SS, Dhoba T, Makanza ED, et al. Chronic cough in primary health care attendees, Harare, Zimbabwe: diagnosis and impact of HIV infection. Clin Infect Dis 40:1818, 2005.
20. Selwyn PA, Sckell BM, Alcabes P, et al. High risk of active tuberculosis in HIV-infected drug users with cutaneous anergy. JAMA 268:504, 1992.
21. Markowitz N, Hansen NI, Wilcosky TC, et al. Tuberculin and anergy testing in HIV-seropositive and HIV-seronegative persons. Pulmonary Complications of HIV Infection Study Group. Ann Intern Med 119:185, 1993.
22. Centers for Disease Control and Prevention. From the Centers for Disease Control and Prevention: 1993 revised classification system for HIV infection and expanded surveillance case definition for AIDS among adolescents and adults. JAMA 269:729, 1993.
23. Kaplan JE, Masur H, Holmes KK. Guidelines for preventing opportunistic infections among HIV-infected persons – 2002. Recommendations of the U.S. Public Health Service and the Infectious Diseases Society of America. MMWR Recomm Rep 51:1, 2002.
24. Martin JN, Rose DA, Hadley WK, et al. Emergence of trimethoprim-sulfamethoxazole resistance in the AIDS era. J Infect Dis 180:1809, 1999.
25. Nuorti JP, Butler JC, Gelling L, et al. Epidemiologic relation between HIV and invasive pneumococcal disease in San Francisco Count, California. Ann Intern Med, 132:182–190, 2000.
26. Diaz PT, Wewers MD, Pacht E, et al. Respiratory symptoms among HIV-seropositive individuals. Chest 123:1977, 2003.
27. Rosen MJ. Cough in the immunocompromised host: ACCP evidence-based clinical practice guidelines. Chest 129:204S, 2006.
28. Kovacs JA, Hiemenz JW, Macher AM, et al. Pneumocystis carinii pneumonia: a comparison between patients with the acquired immunodeficiency syndrome and patients with other immunodeficiencies. Ann Intern Med 100:663, 1984.
29. Afessa B, Green B. Bacterial pneumonia in hospitalized patients with HIV infection. The Pulmonary Complications, ICU Support, and Prognostic Factors of Hospitalized Patients with HIV (PIP) study. Chest 117:1017, 2000.
30. Chuck SL, Sande MA. Infections with Cryptococcus neoformans in the acquired immunodeficiency syndrome. N Engl J Med 321:794, 1989.
31. van der Horst CM, Saag MS, Cloud GA, et al. Treatment of cryptococcal meningitis associated with the acquired immunodeficiency syndrome. National Institute of Allergy and Infectious Diseases Mycoses Study Group and AIDS Clinical Trials Group. New England J Med 337:15, 1997.
32. Huang L, Schnapp LM, Gruden JF, et al. Presentation of AIDS-related pulmonary Kaposi's sarcoma diagnosed by bronchoscopy. Am J Respir Crit Care Med 153:1385, 1996.
33. Ong A, Creasman J, Hopewell PC, et al. A molecular epidemiological assessment of extrapulmonary tuberculosis in San Francisco. Clin Infect Dis 38:25, 2004.
34. Yang Z, Kong Y, Wilson F, et al. Identification of risk factors for extrapulmonary tuberculosis. Clin Infect Dis 38:199, 2004.
35. Sattler F, Nichols L, Hirano L, et al. Nonspecific interstitial pneumonitis mimicking Pneumocystis carinii pneumonia. Am J Respir Crit Care Med 156:912, 1997.
36. Masur H, Ognibene FP, Yarchoan R, et al. CD4 counts as predictors of opportunistic pneumonias in human immunodeficiency virus (HIV) infection. Ann Intern Med 111:223, 1989.
37. Phair J, Munoz A, Detels R, et al. The risk of Pneumocystis carinii pneumonia among men infected with human immunodeficiency virus type 1: Multicenter AIDS Cohort Study Group. N Engl J Med 322:161, 1990.
38. Stansell JD, Osmond DH, Charlebois E, et al. Predictors of Pneumocystis carinii pneumonia in HIV-infected persons: Pulmonary Complications of HIV Infection Study Group. Am J Respir Crit Care Med 155:60, 1997.
39. Darras-Joly C, Chevret S, Wolff M, et al. Cryptococcus neoformans infection in France: epidemiologic features of and early prognostic parameters for 76 patients who were infected with human immunodeficiency virus. Clin Infect Dis 23:369, 1996.
40. Rabaud C, May T, Lucet JC, et al. Pulmonary toxoplasmosis in patients infected with human immunodeficiency virus: a French national survey. Clin Infect Dis 23:1249, 1996.
41. Kovacs JA, Masur H. Prophylaxis against opportunistic infections in patients with human immunodeficiency virus infection. N Engl J Med 342:1416, 2000.
42. Furrer H, Egger M, Opravil M, et al. Discontinuation of primary prophylaxis against Pneumocystis carinii pneumonia in HIV-1-infected adults treated with combination antiretroviral therapy. Swiss HIV Cohort Study. N Engl J Med 340:1301, 1999.
43. Schneider MM, Borleffs JC, Stolk RP, et al. Discontinuation of prophylaxis for Pneumocystis carinii pneumonia in HIV-1-infected patients treated with highly active antiretroviral therapy. Lancet 353:201, 1999.
44. Weverling GJ, Mocroft A, Ledergerber B, et al. Discontinuation of Pneumocystis carinii pneumonia prophylaxis after start of highly active antiretroviral therapy in HIV-1 infection: EuroSIDA study group. Lancet 353:1293, 1999.
45. Kirk O, Lundgren JD, Pedersen C, et al. Can chemoprophylaxis against opportunistic infections be discontinued after an increase in CD4 cells induced by highly active antiretroviral therapy? AIDS 13:1647, 1999.

46. Mussini C, Pezzotti P, Govoni A, et al. Discontinuation of primary prophylaxis for Pneumocystis carinii pneumonia and toxoplasmic encephalitis in human immunodeficiency virus type I-infected patients: the changes in opportunistic prophylaxis study. J Infect Dis 181:1635, 2000.
47. Furrer H, Opravil M, Rossi M. Discontinuation of primary prophylaxis in HIV-infected patients at high risk of Pneumocystis carinii pneumonia: prospective multicentre study. AIDS 15: 501, 2001.
48. Lopez Bernaldo de Quiros J, Miro J, Pena J. A randomized trial of the discontinuation of primary and secondary prophylaxis against Pneumocystis carinii pneumonia after highly active antiretroviral therapy in patients with HIV infection. N Engl J Med 344:159, 2001.
49. Ledergerber B, Mocroft A, Reiss P. Discontinuation of secondary prophylaxis against Pneumocystis carinii pneumonia in patients with HIV infection who have a response to antiretroviral therapy. N Engl J Med 344:168, 2001.
50. Crothers K, Huang L. Recurrence of Pneumocystis carinii pneumonia in an HIV-infected patient: apparent selective immune reconstitution after initiation of antiretroviral therapy. HIV Med 4:346, 2003.
51. Katz MH, Baron RB, Grady D. Risk stratification of ambulatory patients suspected of Pneumocystis pneumonia. Arch Intern Med 151:105, 1991.
52. Garay SM, Greene J. Prognostic indicators in the initial presentation of Pneumocystis carinii pneumonia. Chest 95:769, 1989.
53. Magnenat JL, Nicod LP, Auckenthaler R, et al. Mode of presentation and diagnosis of bacterial pneumonia in human immunodeficiency virus-infected patients. Am Rev Respir Dis 144: 917, 1991.
54. Selwyn PA, Pumerantz AS, Durante A, et al. Clinical predictors of Pneumocystis carinii pneumonia, bacterial pneumonia and tuberculosis in HIV-infected patients. AIDS 12: 885, 1998.
55. Burack JH, Hahn JA, Saint-Maurice D, et al. Microbiology of community-acquired bacterial pneumonia in persons with and at risk for human immunodeficiency virus type 1 infection: implications for rational empiric antibiotic therapy. Arch Intern Med 154:2589, 1994.
56. Janoff EN, Breiman RF, Daley CL, et al. Pneumococcal disease during HIV infection: epidemiologic, clinical, and immunologic perspectives. Ann Intern Med 117:314, 1992.
57. Garcia-Leoni ME, Moreno S, Rodeno P, et al. Pneumococcal pneumonia in adult hospitalized patients infected with the human immunodeficiency virus. Arch Intern Med 152:1808, 1992.
58. Schlamm HT, Yancovitz SR. Haemophilus influenzae pneumonia in young adults with AIDS, ARC, or risk of AIDS. Am J Med 86:11, 1989.
59. Moreno S, Martinez R, Barros C, et al. Latent Haemophilus influenzae pneumonia in patients infected with HIV. AIDS 5: 967, 1991.
60. Cordero E, Pach-n J, Rivero A, et al. Haemophilus influenzae pneumonia in human immunodeficiency virus-infected patients: the Grupo Andaluz para el Estudio de las Enfermedades Infecciosas. Clin Infect Dis 30: 461, 2000.
61. Schuster MG, Norris AH. Community-acquired Pseudomonas aeruginosa pneumonia in patients with HIV infection. AIDS 8:1437, 1994.
62. Dropulic LK, Leslie JM, Eldred LJ, et al. Clinical manifestations and risk factors of Pseudomonas aeruginosa infection in patients with AIDS. J Infect Dis 171: 930, 1995.
63. Pedro-Botet ML, Sabria M, Sopena N, et al. Legionnaires disease and HIV infection. Chest 124:543, 2003.
64. Weinstock DM, Brown AE. Rhodococcus equi: an emerging pathogen. Clin Infect Dis 34:1379, 2002.
65. Uttamchandani RB, Daikos GL, Reyes RR, et al. Nocardiosis in 30 patients with advanced human immunodeficiency virus infection: clinical features and outcome. Clin Infect Dis 18:348, 1994.
66. DeLorenzo LJ, Huang CT, Maguire GP, et al. Roentgenographic patterns of Pneumocystis carinii pneumonia in 104 patients with AIDS. Chest 91:323, 1987.
67. Kennedy CA, Goetz MB. Atypical roentgenographic manifestations of Pneumocystis carinii pneumonia. Arch Intern Med 152:1390, 1992.
68. Huang L, Stansell JD, Osmond D, et al. Performance of an algorithm to detect P. carinii pneumonia in HIV-infected patients. Chest 115:1025, 1999.
69. Geng E, Kreiswirth B, Burzynski J, et al. Clinical and radiographic correlates of primary and reactivation tuberculosis: a molecular epidemiology study. JAMA 293:2740, 2005.
70. Jones BE, Young SM, Antoniskis D, et al. Relationship of the manifestations of tuberculosis to CD4 cell counts in patients with human immunodeficiency virus infection. Am Rev Respir Dis 148:1292, 1993.
71. Abouya L, Coulibaly IM, Coulibaly D, et al. Radiologic manifestations of pulmonary tuberculosis in HIV-1 and HIV-2-infected patients in Abidjan, Cote d'Ivoire. Tuber Lung Dis 76:436, 1995.
72. Perlman DC, el-Sadr WM, Nelson ET, et al. Variation of chest radiographic patterns in pulmonary tuberculosis by degree of human immunodeficiency virus-related immunosuppression: the Terry Beirn Community Programs for Clinical Research on AIDS (CPCRA); The AIDS Clinical Trials Group (ACTG). Clin Infect Dis 25:242, 1997.
73. Gruden JF, Webb WR, Yao DC, et al. Bronchogenic carcinoma in 13 patients infected with the human immunodeficiency virus (HIV): clinical and radiographic findings. J Thorac Imaging 10:99, 1995.
74. Naidich DP, McGuinness G. Pulmonary manifestations of AIDS: CT and radiographic correlations. Radiol Clin North Am 29:999, 1991.
75. Hartman TE, Primack SL, Muller NL, et al. Diagnosis of thoracic complications in AIDS: accuracy of CT. AJR Am J Roentgenol 162: 547, 1994.
76. Opravil M, Marincek B, Fuchs WA, et al. Shortcomings of chest radiography in detecting Pneumocystis carinii pneumonia. J Acquir Immune Defic Syndr 7:39, 1994.
77. Gruden JF, Huang L, Turner J, et al. High-resolution CT in the evaluation of clinically suspected Pneumocystis carinii pneumonia in AIDS patients with normal, equivocal, or nonspecific radiographic findings. Am J Roentgenol 169: 967, 1997.
78. Edinburgh KJ, Jasmer RM, Huang L, et al. Multiple pulmonary nodules in AIDS: usefulness of CT in distinguishing among potential causes. Radiology 214:427, 2000.
79. Jasmer RM, Edinburgh KJ, Thompson A, et al. Clinical and radiographic predictors of the etiology of pulmonary nodules in HIV-infected patients. Chest 117:1023, 2000.
80. Jasmer RM, Gotway MB, Creasman JM, et al. Clinical and radiographic predictors of the etiology of computed tomography-diagnosed intrathoracic lymphadenopathy in HIV-infected patients. J Acquir Immune Defic Syndr 31: 291, 2002.
81. Woolfenden JM, Carrasquillo JA, Larson SM, et al. Acquired immunodeficiency syndrome: Ga-67 citrate imaging. Radiology 162:383, 1987.
82. Morris AM, Huang L, Bacchetti P, et al. Permanent declines in pulmonary function following pneumonia in human immunodeficiency virus-infected persons. The Pulmonary Complications of HIV Infection Study Group. Am J Respir Crit Care Med 162: 612, 2000.
83. Kvale PA, Rosen MJ, Hopewell PC, et al. A decline in the pulmonary diffusing capacity does not indicate opportunistic lung disease in asymptomatic persons infected with the human immunodeficiency virus: Pulmonary Complications of HIV Infection Study Group. Am Rev Respir Dis 148:390, 1993.

84. Batungwanayo J, Taelman H, Bogaerts J, et al. Pulmonary cryptococcosis associated with HIV-1 infection in Rwanda: a retrospective study of 37 cases. AIDS 8:1271, 1994.
85. Wheat LJ, Connolly-Stringfield P, Williams B, et al. Diagnosis of histoplasmosis in patients with the acquired immunodeficiency syndrome by detection of Histoplasma capsulatum polysaccharide antigen in bronchoalveolar lavage fluid. Am Rev Respir Dis 145:1421, 1992.
86. Benson CA, Kaplan JE, Masur H, et al. Treating opportunistic infections among HIV-infected adults and adolescents: recommendations from CDC, the National Institutes of Health, and the HIV Medicine Association/Infectious Diseases Society of America. MMWR Recomm Rep, 53:1,2004.
87. Huang L, Hecht FM, Stansell JD, et al. Suspected Pneumocystis carinii pneumonia with a negative induced sputum examination: is early bronchoscopy useful? Am J Respir Crit Care Med 151:1866, 1995.
88. Kovacs JA, Ng VL, Masur H, et al. Diagnosis of Pneumocystis carinii pneumonia: improved detection in sputum with use of monoclonal antibodies. N Engl J Med 318:589, 1988.
89. Greenberg SD, Frager D, Suster B, et al. Active pulmonary tuberculosis in patients with AIDS: spectrum of radiographic findings (including a normal appearance). Radiology 193:115, 1994.
90. Smith RL, Yew K, Berkowitz KA, et al. Factors affecting the yield of acid-fast sputum smears in patients with HIV and tuberculosis. Chest 106: 684, 1994.
91. Griffith DE, Aksamit T, Brown-Elliot BA, et al. An official ATS/IDSA statement: diagnosis, treatment, and prevention of nontuberculous mycobacterial diseases. Am J Respir Crit Care Med. 175(4) 367–416, 2007.
92. Witzig RS, Fazal BA, Mera RM, et al. Clinical manifestations and implications of coinfection with Mycobacterium kansasii and human immunodeficiency virus type 1. Clin Infect Dis 21:77, 1995.
93. Marras TK, Morris A, Gonzalez LC, et al. Mortality prediction in pulmonary Mycobacterium kansasii infection and human immunodeficiency virus. Am J Respir Crit Care Med 170:793, 2004.
94. Marras TK, Daley CL. A systematic review of the clinical significance of pulmonary Mycobacterium kansasii isolates in HIV infection. J Acquir Immune Defic Syndr 36:883, 2004.
95. Kalayjian RC, Toossi Z, Tomashefski JF Jr, et al. Pulmonary disease due to infection by Mycobacterium avium complex in patients with AIDS. Clin Infect Dis 20:1186, 1995.
96. Kerbiriou L, Ustianowski A, Johnson MA, et al. Human immunodeficiency virus type 1-related pulmonary Mycobacterium xenopi infection: a need to treat? Clin Infect Dis 37:1250, 2003.
97. Meyohas MC, Roux P, Bollens D, et al. Pulmonary cryptococcosis: localized and disseminated infections in 27 patients with AIDS. Clin Infect Dis 21:628, 1995.
98. Rodriguez-Barradas MC, Stool E, Musher DM, et al. Diagnosing and treating cytomegalovirus pneumonia in patients with AIDS. Clin Infect Dis 23:76, 1996.
99. Salomon N, Gomez T, Perlman DC, et al. Clinical features and outcomes of HIV-related cytomegalovirus pneumonia. AIDS 11:319, 1997.
100. Whitley RJ, Jacobson MA, Friedberg DN, et al. Guidelines for the treatment of cytomegalovirus diseases in patients with AIDS in the era of potent antiretroviral therapy. Recommendations of an international panel: International AIDS Society-USA. Arch Intern Med 158: 957, 1998.
101. Eisner MD, Kaplan LD, Herndier B, et al. The pulmonary manifestations of AIDS-related non-Hodgkin's lymphoma. Chest 110:729, 1996.
102. Judson MA, Sahn SA. Endobronchial lesions in HIV-infected individuals. Chest 105:1314, 1994.
103. Gruden JF, Klein JS, Webb WR. Percutaneous transthoracic needle biopsy in AIDS: analysis in 32 patients. Radiology 189:567, 1993.
104. Mandell LA, Bartlett JG, Dowell SF, et al. Update of practice guidelines for the management of community-acquired pneumonia in immunocompetent adults. Clin Infect Dis 37: 1405,2003.
105. Christensen D, Feldman C, Rossi P, et al. HIV infection does not influence clinical outcomes in hospitalized patients with bacterial community-acquired pneumonia: results from the CAPO international cohort study. Clin Infect Dis 41:554, 2005.
106. Cordero E, Pach-n J, Rivero A, et al. Community-acquired bacterial pneumonia in human immunodeficiency virus-infected patients: validation of severity criteria; the Grupo Andaluz para el Estudio de las Enfermedades Infecciosas. Am J Respir Crit Care Med 162:2063, 2000.
107. Datta D, Ali SA, Henken EM, et al. Pneumocystis carinii pneumonia: the time course of clinical and radiographic improvement. Chest 124:1820, 2003.
108. Morris A, Lundgren JD, Masur H, et al. Current epidemiology of Pneumocystis pneumonia. Emerg Infect Dis 10:1713, 2004.
109. Huang L, Crothers K, Atzori C, et al. Dihydropteroate synthase gene mutations in Pneumocystis and sulfa resistance. Emerg Infect Dis 10:1721, 2004.
110. Beard CB, Roux P, Nevez G, et al. Strain typing methods and molecular epidemiology of Pneumocystis pneumonia. Emerg Infect Dis 10:1729, 2004.
111. Stein CR, Poole C, Kazanjian P, et al. Sulfa use, dihydropteroate synthase mutations, and Pneumocystis jirovecii pneumonia. Emerg Infect Dis 10:1760, 2004.
112. Ma L, Borio L, Masur H, et al. Pneumocystis carinii dihydropteroate synthase but not dihydrofolate reductase gene mutations correlate with prior trimethoprim-sulfamethoxazole or dapsone use. J Infect Dis 180:1969, 1999.
113. Helweg-Larsen J, Benfield TL, Eugen-Olsen J, et al. Effects of mutations in Pneumocystis carinii dihydropteroate synthase gene on outcome of AIDS-associated P. carinii pneumonia. Lancet 354:1347, 1999.
114. Kazanjian P, Armstrong W, Hossler PA, et al. Pneumocystis carinii mutations are associated with duration of sulfa or sulfone prophylaxis exposure in AIDS patients. J Infect Dis 182:551, 2000.
115. Navin T, Beard CB, Huang L. Mutations in the Pneumocystis carinii dihydropteroate synthase gene do not affect outcome of P. carinii pneumonia in HIV-infected patients. Lancet 358:545, 2001.
116. Crothers K, Beard CB, Turner J, et al. Severity and outcome of HIV-associated Pneumocystis pneumonia containing Pneumocystis jirovecii dihydropteroate synthase gene mutations. AIDS 19: 801,2005.
117. Hirsch HH, Kaufmann G, Sendi P, et al. Immune reconstitution in HIV-infected patients. Clin Infect Dis 38:1159, 2004.
118. Lawn SD, Bekker LG, Miller RF. Immune reconstitution disease associated with mycobacterial infections in HIV-infected individuals receiving antiretrovirals. Lancet Infect Dis 5:361, 2005.
119. Narita M, Ashkin D, Hollender ES, et al. Paradoxical worsening of tuberculosis following antiretroviral therapy in patients with AIDS. Am J Respir Crit Care Med 158:157, 1998.
120. Fishman JE, Saraf-Lavi E, Narita M, et al. Pulmonary tuberculosis in AIDS patients: transient chest radiographic worsening after initiation of antiretroviral therapy. Am J Roentgenol 174:43, 2000.
121. Wislez M, Bergot E, Antoine M, et al. Acute respiratory failure following HAART introduction in patient's treated for Pneumocystis carinii pneumonia. Am J Respir Crit Care Med 164:847, 2001.

122. Aboulafia DM. Regression of acquired immunodeficiency syndrome-related pulmonary Kaposi's sarcoma after highly active antiretroviral therapy. Mayo Clin Proc 73:439, 1998.
123. Naccache JM, Antoine M, Wislez M, et al. Sarcoid-like pulmonary disorder in human immunodeficiency virus-infected patients receiving antiretroviral therapy. Am J Respir Crit Care Med 159:2009, 1999.
124. Mirmirani P, Maurer TA, Herndier B, et al. Sarcoidosis in a patient with AIDS: a manifestation of immune restoration syndrome. J Am Acad Dermatol 41:285, 1999.
125. Gomez V, Smith PR, Burack J, et al. Sarcoidosis after antiretroviral therapy in a patient with acquired immunodeficiency syndrome. Clin Infect Dis 31:1278, 2000.
126. Blanche P, Gombert B, Rollot F, et al. Sarcoidosis in a patient with acquired immunodeficiency syndrome treated with interleukin-2. Clin Infect Dis 31:1493, 2000.
127. Morris DG, Jasmer RM, Huang L, et al. Sarcoidosis following HIV infection: evidence for CD4+ lymphocyte dependence. Chest 124: 929,2003.
128. Foulon G, Wislez M, Naccache JM, et al. Sarcoidosis in HIV-infected patients in the era of highly active antiretroviral therapy. Clin Infect Dis, 38:418,2004.
129. Morris AM, Nishimura S, Huang L. Subacute hypersensitivity pneumonitis in an HIV infected patient receiving antiretroviral therapy. Thorax 55:625, 2000.
130. Aboulafia DM. The epidemiologic, pathologic, and clinical features of AIDS-associated pulmonary Kaposi's sarcoma. Chest 117:1128, 2000.
131. White DA. Pulmonary complications of HIV-associated malignancies. Clin Chest Med 17:755, 1996.
132. Gruden JF, Huang L, Webb WR, et al. AIDS-related Kaposi sarcoma of the lung: radiographic findings and staging system with bronchoscopic correlation. Radiology 195:545, 1995.
133. Bazot M, Cadranel J, Benayoun S, et al. Primary pulmonary AIDS-related lymphoma: radiographic and CT findings. Chest 116:1282, 1999.
134. Parker MS, Leveno DM, Campbell TJ, et al. AIDS-related bronchogenic carcinoma: fact or fiction? Chest 113:154, 1998.
135. Johnson CC, Wilcosky T, Kvale P, et al. Cancer incidence among an HIV-infected cohort. Pulmonary Complications of HIV Infection Study Group. Am J Epidemiol 146:470, 1997.
136. Bazot M, Cadranel J, Khalil A, et al. Computed tomographic diagnosis of bronchogenic carcinoma in HIV-infected patients. Lung Cancer 28:203, 2000.
137. Thurer RJ, Jacobs JP, Holland FW II, et al. Surgical treatment of lung cancer in patients with human immunodeficiency virus. Ann Thorac Surg 60:599, 1995.
138. Massera F, Rocco G, Rossi G, et al. Pulmonary resection for lung cancer in HIV-positive patients with low (<200 lymphocytes/mm×) CD4+ count. Lung Cancer 29:147, 2000.
139. Ognibene FP, Masur H, Rogers P, et al. Nonspecific interstitial pneumonitis without evidence of Pneumocystis carinii in asymptomatic patients infected with human immunodeficiency virus (HIV). Ann Intern Med 109:874, 1988.
140. Schneider RF. Lymphocytic interstitial pneumonitis and nonspecific interstitial pneumonitis. Clin Chest Med 17:763, 1996.
141. Oldham SA, Castillo M, Jacobson FL, et al. HIV-associated lymphocytic interstitial pneumonia: radiologic manifestations and pathologic correlation. Radiology 170:83, 1989.
142. Dufour V, Wislez M, Bergot E, et al. Improvement of symptomatic human immunodeficiency virus-related lymphoid interstitial pneumonia in patients receiving highly active antiretroviral therapy. Clin Infect Dis 36:e127, 2003.
143. Innes AL, Huang L, Nishimura SL. Resolution of lymphocytic interstitial pneumonitis in an HIV infected adult after treatment with HAART. Sex Transm Infect 80:417, 2004.
144. Griffiths MH, Miller RF, Semple SJ. Interstitial pneumonitis in patients infected with the human immunodeficiency virus. Thorax 50:1141, 1995.
145. Simmons JT, Suffredini AF, Lack EE, et al. Nonspecific interstitial pneumonitis in patients with AIDS: radiologic features. Am J Roentgenol 149:265, 1987.
146. Mehta NJ, Khan IA, Mehta RN, et al. HIV-related pulmonary hypertension: analytic review of 131 cases. Chest 118:1133, 2000.
147. Petitpretz P, Brenot F, Azarian R, et al. Pulmonary hypertension in patients with human immunodeficiency virus infection: comparison with primary pulmonary hypertension. Circulation 89:2722, 1994.
148. Opravil M, Pechére M, Speich R, et al. HIV-associated primary pulmonary hypertension: a case control study. Swiss HIV Cohort Study. Am J Respir Crit Care Med 155:990, 1997.
149. Nunes H, Humbert M, Sitbon O, et al. Prognostic factors for survival in human immunodeficiency virus-associated pulmonary arterial hypertension. Am J Respir Crit Care Med 167:1433, 2003.
150. Zuber JP, Calmy A, Evison JM, et al. Pulmonary arterial hypertension related to HIV infection: improved hemodynamics and survival associated with antiretroviral therapy. Clin Infect Dis 38:1178, 2004.
151. Porter JP, Patel AA, Dewey CM, et al. Prevalence of sinonasal symptoms in patients with HIV infection. Am J Rhinol 13:203, 1999.
152. Zurlo JJ, Feuerstein IM, Lebovics R, et al. Sinusitis in HIV-1 infection. Am J Med 93:157, 1992.
153. Upadhyay S, Marks SC, Arden RL, et al. Bacteriology of sinusitis in human immunodeficiency virus-positive patients: implications for management. Laryngoscope 105:1058, 1995.
154. Marks SC, Upadhyay S, Crane L. Cytomegalovirus sinusitis. a new manifestation of AIDS. Arch Otolaryngol Head Neck Surg 122:789, 1996.
155. Hunt SM, Miyamoto RC, Cornelius RS, et al. Invasive fungal sinusitis in the acquired immunodeficiency syndrome. Otolaryngol Clin North Am 33:335, 2000.

Chapter 70

HIV-Related Renal Disease

Jonathan A. Winston, MD, Paul E. Klotman, MD

Diseases of the kidney are generally classified into one of two broad clinical syndromes, acute renal failure (ARF) and chronic kidney disease (CKD), which are distinguished by the rate of change in glomerular filtration rate (GFR). This classification helps in the diagnosis, treatment and prognosis of the underlying disorder. However, these syndromes are not mutually exclusive, and some overlap exists. For example, HIV-associated nephropathy is the single most common cause of CKD in HIV-infected patients but it can present as an ARF syndrome. Similarly, although attention has focused on the potential for antiviral agents to cause ARF, recent reports suggest that some agents may be associated with subacute and/or chronic reductions in renal function. Also, appropriate use of antivirals in CKD is an area of growing importance. The distinction between acute and CKD can narrow the differential diagnosis, but accurate diagnosis can only be made with a detailed history and physical, relevant laboratory data including urinalysis, an assessment of kidney size and structure, knowledge of the nephrotoxic potential of concomitant medications, and often a kidney biopsy. This chapter will update the definitions of the important renal syndromes, review the disorders that commonly occur in HIV, and provide a clinical framework for diagnosis and treatment.

CHRONIC KIDNEY DISEASE

CKD is defined as kidney damage or reduced kidney function lasting longer than 3 months, regardless of diagnosis.[1] Abnormal renal pathology on biopsy or a surrogate marker, such as proteinuria or an abnormal imaging study, is the standard for defining kidney damage. Patients with a normal GFR (>90 mL/min per 1.73 m^2), or mild reductions in GFR (60–89 mL/min per 1.73 m^2) are classified as stage 1 and 2 CKD, respectively, when kidney damage (proteinuria or an abnormal imaging study) is also present. A GFR lower than 60 mL/min per 1.73 m^2 defines reduced kidney function. CKD stages 3–5 are classified according to the magnitude of the reduction in GFR, irrespective of the cause of kidney disease or whether proteinuria or an abnormal imaging study can be demonstrated (see Table 70-1(2)). The primary outcome of interest for patients with CKD is the risk of progressing to end-stage renal disease (ESRD) requiring dialysis. But CKD also places patients at risk for other co-morbid conditions, such as hypertension, cardiovascular disease, anemia, and hyperparathyroidism. Finally, impaired renal function places patients at risk for adverse events or drug toxicity caused by improper dosing of drugs that are excreted by the kidneys.

The prevalence of CKD in the United States is alarmingly high, estimated at 19–20 million people.[2] The rate of hospitalizations, cardiovascular events and all-cause mortality increases inversely with GFR, reaching three- to sixfold when GFR is reduced to moderate or severe levels.[3] Medicare patients with CKD are 5–10 times more likely to die from cardiovascular disease than to reach ESRD.[4] These striking epidemiologic data have stimulated several major public health initiatives aimed at increasing awareness of kidney disease so that patients can be identified early in the course of their disease when medical intervention could be more effective. The past several years have witnessed tremendous growth in our understanding of the epidemiology of early stages of CKD, including kidney diseases associated with HIV infection.

The Prevalence of CKD in HIV-Infected Patients

Several studies provide insight into the prevalence of CKD associated with HIV-infection. Fourteen percent of women in the WIHS cohort met criteria for CKD, as defined by two consecutive dipsticks for proteinuria of 1+ or greater (30–100 mg/dL).[5] Kidney disease was associated with older age, black race, a history of hypertension or diabetes, lower BMI, and a prior

Classification and prevalence of CKD in the United States

Table 70-1

Stage	Description	GFR (mL/min/1.73m^2)	Prevalence 1000s	Prevalence (%)
1	Kidney damage, normal GFR	≥90	5900	3.3
2	Kidney damage, mild decrease in GFR	60–89	5300	3
3	Moderately decreased GFR	30–59	7600	4.3
4	Severely decreased GFR	15–29	400	0.2
5	Kidney failure	<15 or dialysis	300	0.1

Adapted from Coresh, et al.[2]

AIDS-defining illness. In an analysis of the HERS cohort, kidney disease was defined as a serum creatinine >1.4 mg/dL or urine dipstick >2+ on any research visit between 1993–97.[6] Kidney disease was present in 7.2% of women at baseline, and was three-fold higher compared to controls (seronegative women selected because of high-risk behavior). Similar to associations described in the WIHS cohort, kidney disease in the HERS study was associated with black race and older age. HCV co-infection, injection drug use and HIV viral load were also independent risk factors. After a mean follow-up of 21 months, renal abnormalities were four times more frequent in seropositive women compared to controls (15.6% vs 4.3%). Gupta et al, studying patients in an urban hospital, defined CKD as a doubling of serum creatinine from the time of their initial examination through follow-up visits.[7] Two percent of the entire cohort and 9% of black patients met this definition. This is certainly an underestimate because, by today's standards, a doubling of serum creatinine is an insensitive marker for CKD. Twenty-nine percent of patients had dipstick proteinuria >1+. The prevalence of CKD was reviewed in a clinic, located in an urban medical center. Of 1200 patients, most of whom were black or Hispanics, 9% had an estimated GFR <60 mL/min per 1.73 M^2 as determined by the modification of diet in renal disease study (MDRD) formula.[8] A high prevalence of hypertension and diabetes was noted in the cohort. Jung et al. also reported a strong association between renal disease (proteinuria) and hypertension in HIV-infected patients. Proteinuria was present in 41% of their hypertensive patients.[9]

The prevalence of renal disease in HIV-infected patients from developing countries is even more alarming. Olson et al, reporting on the experience of Doctors without Borders, found that 19% of patients in Guatemala city, and, astonishingly, 43% of patients in Arua (Uganda) have estimated GFR values <50 mL/min, by Cockroft–Gault formula, when initiating antiretroviral therapy.[10] The high prevalence of kidney disease, particularly in Africa, could be spurious because of calibration differences in measuring serum creatinine. But, it is important to recognize the possibility that this represents the beginnings of a kidney disease epidemic in sub-Saharan Africa, based on the high prevalence of kidney disease in HIV infection and the kidney disease risk associated with black race.

A recent presentation of data from the CDC's Adult/Adolescent Spectrum of HIV Disease Project followed serum creatinine in ~10 000 outpatients.[11] Their findings were similarly dramatic. MDRD GFR was <60 mL/min per 1.73 m^2 in 9% of subjects. GFR was between 60–89 mL/min per 1.73 m^2 in 35%. While care must be taken in interpreting the significance of GFR levels between 60–89 mL/min per 1.73 m^2, it is reasonable to estimate that as many as 10% of HIV-infected patients of African descent have CKD based on a reduction in GFR. Futhermore, as many as 20–30% may have CKD using proteinuria as the criterion.

ASSESSING KIDNEY FUNCTION IN HIV

Glomerular Filtration Rate

GFR is the most important measure of kidney function, and serum creatinine is the most clinically useful estimate of GFR. Serum creatinine levels are not precise indicators of GFR, however, because serum levels reflect both renal clearance and creatinine generation in muscle. Creatinine generation reflects skeletal muscle mass, body habitus, and protein intake. Elderly patients, vegetarians, and patients with protein malnutrition have reduced muscle mass. Women also have lower muscle mass than men. Thus, based on the specific situation, serum creatinine concentration can be well within the normal range even in the face of a clinically significant reduction in GFR.

Several equations have been developed to predict GFR more reliably than serum creatinine alone, using best-fit or maximum likelihood mathematical models. These models equate variables associated with muscle mass and creatinine generation to a reference standard for GFR, either the renal clearance of an endogenous marker (a timed urine collection for calculated creatinine clearance) or an exogenous marker (infused iothalamate). The Cockroft–Gault formula and the MDRD equation, shown in Table 70-2, have been validated more than any others. The Cockroft–Gault formula was derived from a cohort of 290 patients and uses age, gender, and weight to predict endogenous creatinine clearance as the reference standard for GFR.[12] The MDRD equation was

Table 70-2 Comparison of Cockroft–Gault Formula and Modified MDRD Equation

	Cockroft–Gault Formula **140 − Age(yrs) × Weight (kg)** **(72 × Scr) × (0.85 if female)**	**MDRD Equation** **186 × (Scr)$^{-1.154}$ × (Age)$^{-0.203}$** **× (0.742 if female)** **(× 1.21 if African American)**
Publication	Nephron 1976; 16:31–41	Levey et al Ann Int Med 1999; 130:461–470
Prediction model	Best fit	Stepwise linear regression
Response variable	24 h urine creatinine clearance	^{125}I iothalamate clearance
Validation	200 hospitalized patients with wide range of clearance values	1600 patients with CKD and GFR 20–60 mL/min/1.73 m^2
Caveats	Assumes lean body mass; not validated in special populations, including HIV	Not validated for GFR > 60 mL/min/1.73m^2, and in special population, including HIV
Recommended uses	Dose adjustment for drugs excreted by kidneys	Reliable estimate of GFR

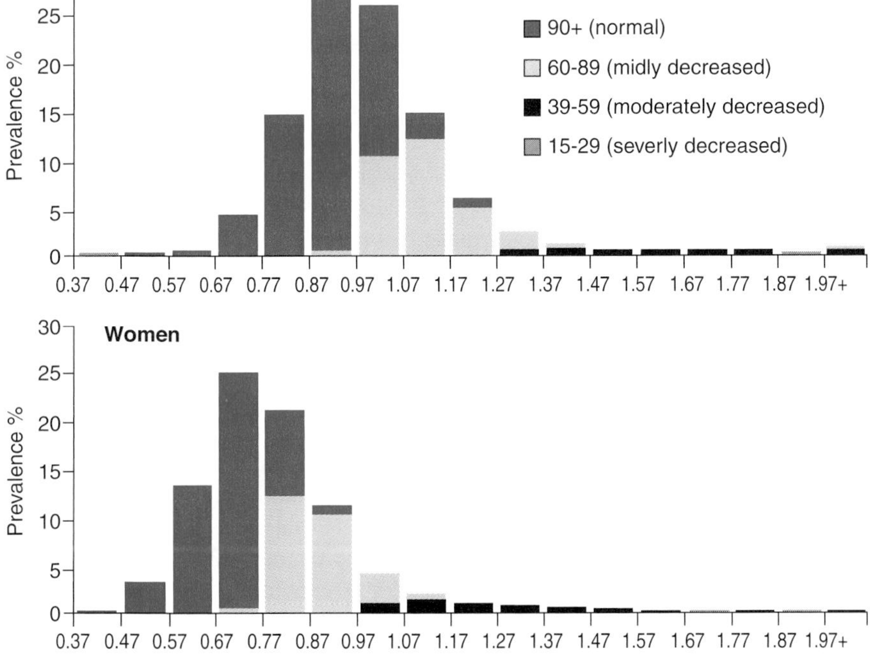

Figure 70-1 ■ Chronic Kidney Disease and Serum Creatinine values from *NHANES III*. Calculated GFR is superimposed on serum creatinine levels.

Adapted from Coresh J, et al. Prevalence of chronic kidney disease and decreased kidney function in the adult US population. Third National Health and Nutrition Examination Survey. Am J Kidney Dis **41**:1–12, 2003.

derived from ~1600 patients with CKD who participated in the NIH-sponsored, multicenter, MDRD study.[13] The full equation incorporates several predictor variables and GFR is measured by the clearance of infused iothalamate, the gold standard reference. Several variables have subsequently been dropped from the original equation, resulting in what is now termed the modified MDRD equation. This modification has increased clinical utility of this method without a loss of precision.[1]

Either equation is superior to serum creatinine alone when evaluating kidney function in clinical practice. The Cockroft–Gault formula has been used to estimate kidney function when studying drug clearance and it remains the standard to use when adjusting drug dose in kidney disease. The MDRD equation is a more accurate measure, especially in the range of 20–60 mL/min per 1.73 m^2. The importance of either equation in clinical practice cannot be overstated. As illustrated in Figure 70-1 and Table 70-3, these estimates

Table 70-3. Estimating GFR: Similar Serum Creatinine Levels do not Mean Similar GFR

P Creat	Age	Gender	Race	CG GFR	MDRD
1.4	45	M	C	71	58
1.4	45	M	B	71	68
1.4	45	F	C	52	44
1.4	45	F	B	52	52
1.4	70	M	C	52	54
1.4	70	M	B	52	63
1.4	70	F	C	38	41
1.4	70	F	B	38	48

Data from Levey et al.[13]

help identify patients with impaired kidney function when serum creatinine levels are within the upper limits of normal or only mildly elevated. In Figure 70-1, GFR, as measured by the MDRD equation, is superimposed on serum creatinine values obtained in the NHANES III survey.[2] A considerable proportion of people have mild to moderate reductions in GFR even when serum creatinine levels are well within the normal range. This is especially true for women. Table 70-3 depicts a wide range of GFRs, depending on age, gender, and race, for individual patients with a serum creatinine of 1.4 mg/dL.[13] While there are differences between the MDRD and Cockroft–Gault estimates, they remain more accurate than serum creatinine alone. Far greater differences exist across age, gender, and race, than which of the formulas is used to estimate GFR.

Most healthcare providers recognize the significance of high serum creatinine levels (>2 mg%). Unfortunately, many underestimate the importance of high normal or mildly elevated creatinine levels and fail to recognize that their patients have kidney disease when serum creatinine is between 1 and 2 mg%. The National Kidney Disease Education Program encourages clinical laboratories to include GFR estimates when they report serum creatinine.[14] This should increase awareness of CKD so we can identify more patients in the early stages and improve quality of care. These reports are now routine in many laboratories and may soon be mandated by several state health departments.

Estimates of GFR are not perfect, however. The MDRD equation was validated in a cohort with a GFR range from 20 to 60 mL/min per 1.73 m^2 and its precision in measuring GFR above 60 mL/min per 1.73 m^2 is uncertain. Current recommendations for clinical labs are to report unique GFR values below 60 mL/min per 1.73 m^2, while levels above this threshold should be reported as '>60 mL/min per 1.73 m^2.' From the perspective of clinical care or clinical research, patients with GFR in the range of 60–89 mL/min per 1.73 m^2 do not have CKD without evidence for kidney damage, such as proteinuria. Several clinical reports describe the prevalence of mild (stage II) CKD in HIV infection based on estimated GFR, but they do not accurately reflect the true prevalence unless they include patients with increased urinary protein excretion. Finally, the MDRD equation has not been validated in children, in individuals older than 70 years, in those with exceptional dietary intakes (vegetarians, creatine supplements) or in those patients with changing muscle mass (amputation, malnutrition, weight gain, or muscle wasting). The latter is especially relevant for patients with malnutrition or wasting associated with AIDS.

Proteinuria

Testing for proteinuria in adults is performed using a routine dipstick urinalysis.[1] Patients with a positive dipstick (1+ or greater) should undergo confirmation with an untimed, 'spot' urine tested for either albumin or protein and creatinine concentrations. Albumin is the more sensitive marker for CKD and is the recommended approach, particularly in diabetics. Medical therapy at the albuminuric stage of diabetic kidney disease improves long-term outcome. If albumin-specific dipsticks or albumin assays are unavailable, testing for total proteinuria is a reasonable alternative. The concentration of albumin or protein in the urine depends on whether the urine is concentrated or dilute, but the amount excreted can be readily interpreted when albumin or protein concentration are normalized for urine creatinine concentration. Usual creatinine excretion is ~1 g/day. Urinary albumin concentration should not exceed 30 mg/gram creatinine, and urinary total protein concentration should not exceed 200 mg per day. Thus, the urinary protein to creatinine ratio should not be greater than 1:5. A ratio of 1.0 estimates protein excretion at 1 g/day and a ratio of >2 g/day approaches nephrotic-range proteinuria. Because 24 h urine collections are cumbersome for the patient and require an additional office visit, the random urine sample for protein/creatinine ratio has largely supplanted timed collections in clinical practice.

Spectrum of Kidney Disease in HIV

A wide spectrum of kidney diseases has been described in association with HIV. Those commonly confirmed by kidney

BOX 70-1 Kidney Disease in HIV: Summary of Biopsy Reports

- HIV-Associated Nephropathy (Collapsing variant of FSGS, specific for Black race)
- Mesangial Glomerulonephritis (GN) with immune deposits (IgA, Henoch-Schonlein purpura)
- Lupus-like GN
- Minimal change disease, membranous nephropathy
- Membranoproliferative GN (associated with HCV)
- TTP/HUS
- Paraprotein nephropathies (Amyloid, light chain disease)
- ATN, allergic interstitial nephritis
- Crystal-induced nephropathy, Fanconi syndrome
- Lymphoma, infiltrative disease

Adapted from Balow JE. Nephropathy in the context of HIV infection. Kidney Int **67**:1632–3, 2005.

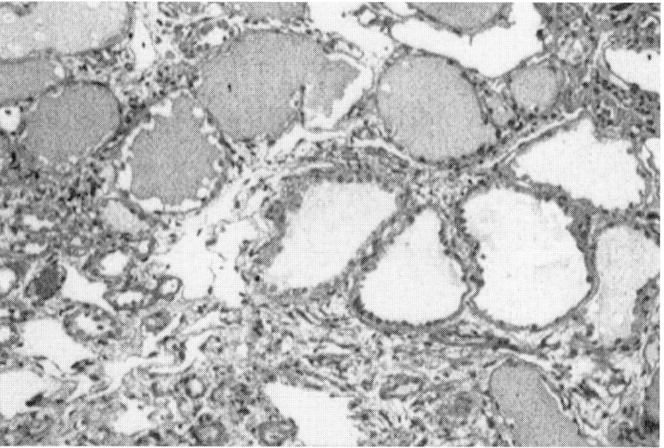

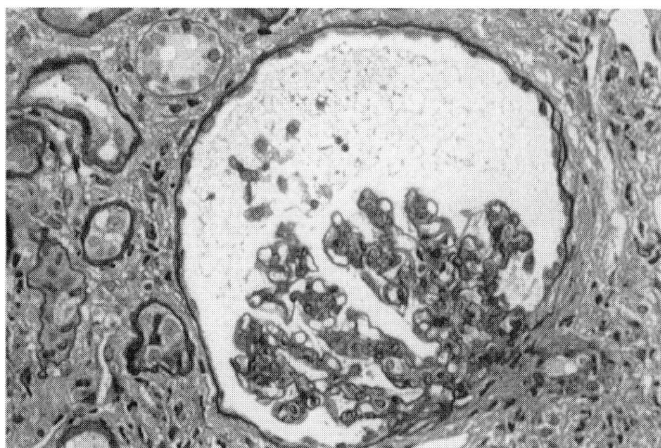

Figure 70-2 ■ Light microscopic findings in HIV-associated nephropathy. Top, Characteristic microcystic tubule disease. Tubule lumens are dilated and filled with proteinaceous casts. Tubules are surrounded by interstitial edema, fibrosis, and inflammatory cells. Bottom, Characteristic retraction of the glomerular tuft. Several proliferating visceral epithelial cells can be seen in the urinary space.

biopsy are listed in Box 70-1.[15] Biopsies are performed in a relatively small proportion of patients even though the prevalence of kidney disease in HIV is high. Therefore, patients undergoing a kidney biopsy represent a selected sampling group, usually with a more rapid progression. Their kidney disease is often unexplained or they have a remarkable clinical presentation, such as heavy proteinuria, an active urinary sediment (proteinuria, hematuria, and red blood cell casts), prolonged ARF or CKD that progresses to renal failure over a relatively short period of time. The frequency of fulminant renal failure in HIV infection has decreased over time, probably due to the widespread use of HAART.[16] As a result, many fewer biopsies are performed and kidney disease in these patients is often attributed to coexisting hypertension or diabetes, and a definitive diagnosis is not made.

HIV-associated nephropathy (HIVAN) is the single most common cause of CKD found by biopsy in patients with HIV infection.[17] It is defined morphologically by collapse of the glomerular capillary tuft, glomerulosclerosis, and microcystic tubulointerstitial disease[18] (Fig. 70-2). HIVAN's association with black race is striking. In biopsy reports throughout North America, Europe, and Asia[19,20] over 90% of affected patients are of African descent. This racial predilection accounts for differences in prevalence reported from individual centers. When reports of renal disease in HIV-1-infected subjects come from mainly Caucasian populations, such as reported in studies from San Francisco, Italy, Asia and northern Europe, HIVAN is not a frequent cause of CKD.[21–24] When blacks comprise a large proportion of the population under study, as in reports from New York, Washington, DC, Miami, and the African or Afro-Caribbean communities of Paris and London, HIVAN is by far the most common cause of renal disease. It is second only to sickle cell-associated renal disease in its racial clustering in blacks. HIVAN is now the third leading cause of ESRD in blacks between the age of 20 and 64 years, more common than lupus nephritis, polycystic disease, or primary glomerulonephritis.[25] A better understanding of the pathogenesis and genetic basis for HIVAN promises to uncover important information about renal susceptibility genes in patients of African descent.[26]

The characteristic clinical presentation of HIVAN is heavy proteinuria, often in the nephrotic range, with varying degrees of renal insufficiency in an HIV-infected patient of African descent. Renal ultrasound examination often shows normal to large kidney size. The predictive value of these clinical characteristics in distinguishing HIVAN from other forms of glomerulonephritis is limited, and numerous reports confirm that the clinical impression is not always borne out by the biopsy findings.[27,28] Prior to the HAART era, the clinical course was marked by progression to renal failure requiring dialysis within weeks to a month, but the natural history has changed dramatically. Now, patients who are receiving antiviral therapy have a more indolent course, with mild to moderate proteinuria and an impaired but stable GFR. In this clinical form, HIVAN may be contributing to more cases of

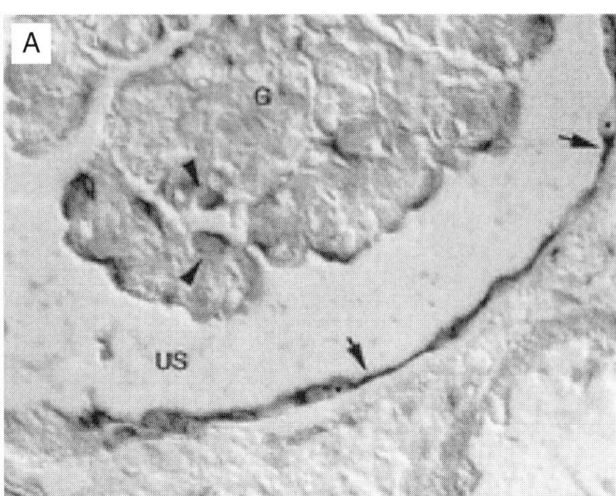

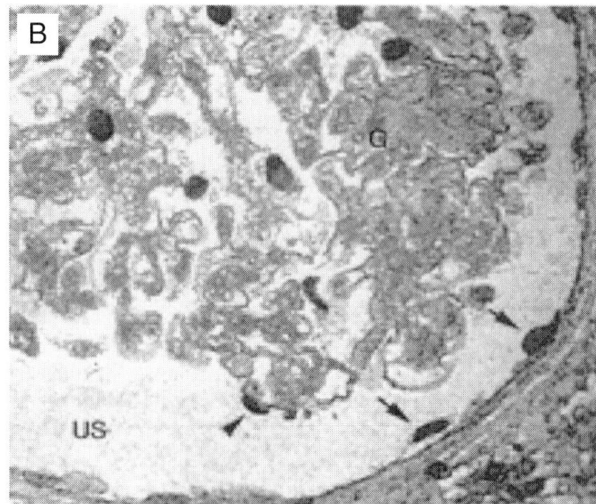

Figure 70-3 ■ Detection of infected glomerular epithelial cells by mRNA *in situ* hybridization and DNA *in situ* polymerase chain reaction (PCR). A, Viral mRNA expression in podocytes (arrowheads) and the cytoplasm of parietal epithelial cells (arrows). B, *In situ* PCR demonstrates the presence of viral DNA in the same cells.

From Bruggeman LA, Ross MD, Tanji N, et al. Renal epithelium is a previously unrecognized site of HIV-1 infection. J Am Soc Nephrol **11:**2079–2087, 2000.

CKD than has been appreciated but it remains undiagnosed in the absence of a definitive kidney biopsy.

Experiments in a murine model of disease support a direct role for HIV-1 in disease pathogenesis. Mice of the TG26 line contain copies of the HIV-1 proviral DNA pNL4-3d1443, generated by deletion of a 3-kb SphI/BalI fragment within pNL4-3 spanning the *gag* and *pol* genes. The construct, under the transcriptional control of the native promoter, the long terminal repeat (LTR), is noninfectious and nonreplicating.[29] Heterozygote mice develop kidney disease morphologically and functionally indistinguishable from HIVAN in man.[30] Cross-transplantation experiments prove that transgene expression is required for disease to develop. HIVAN appears in kidneys transplanted from transgenic mice to normal littermates, but does not develop when normal kidneys are transplanted into a transgenic mouse.[31] Renal transgene expression in glomerular epithelial (podocytes) and tubule epithelial cells precedes the development of nephropathy[31] (Fig. 70-3). Following transgene expression, cells undergo dedifferentiation and proliferation. Several viral genes, have been implicated in the pathogenesis, particularly the *Nef* and *Vpr* genes.[32–34]

Studies in man confirm the important role of renal epithelial cell infection in human disease. Viral mRNA is expressed in glomerular and tubule epithelial cells obtained from kidney biopsies of patients with HIVAN.[35] These cells are primary targets of disease pathogenesis in the murine model and in man. Infected mononuclear cells can also be detected in the interstitial compartment. They may be important in delivering virus to the kidney and contributing to disease pathogenesis through cytokine generation. Dysregulated cytokine expression and matrix accumulation does occur *in vivo*.[36] A recent microarray study demonstrates prominent upregulation of pro-inflammatory genes in HIV-infected renal tubule cells.[37] These data provide insight into the mechanism for tubulo-interstitial inflammation and progressive renal injury in HIVAN.

The effects of antiretroviral therapy on the natural history of HIVAN lend further support for the important role of the virus in HIVAN pathogenesis. Several small cohorts of patients with HIV infection and proteinuric kidney disease typical of HIVAN demonstrate a slower progression to ESRD in patients treated with HAART.[5,38] Fewer cases of fulminant renal failure have been observed in the HAART era.[16] Several well-described case reports provide unequivocal evidence that HAART can reverse the structural and functional abnormalities in HIVAN, particularly when therapy is initiated early in the course of disease before glomerulosclerosis has been established.[39,40] Antiretroviral therapy eliminates new rounds of renal cell infection, which interrupts the disease process. Viral mRNA is still detectable in renal cells in patients with HIVAN who have stable GFR and nondetectable circulating viral RNA. Thus, the kidney can be a reservoir for HIV-1 even during HAART.[40,41]

HIVAN accounts for ~800 incident cases of ESRD each year.[42,43] The number of new patients with HIV-ESRD has stabilized in the HAART era, but has not decreased in parallel to the decline in mortality and opportunistic infections (OIs). This is likely due to the increased pool of patients at risk for developing renal disease as the number of patients living with AIDS continues to rise steadily. A mathematical model has quantified the dynamics of new ESRD cases before and after the widespread use of effective antiretrovirals. HAART is responsible for at least a 30% reduction in new ESRD cases from HIVAN. Looking to the future, however, unless there is a dramatic decrease in cases of HIV infection in the black community, the beneficial effect of HAART to slow the progression of kidney disease will be offset by an ever-growing risk pool, and the number of new cases of ESRD will likely begin to increase again.

Two other classes of drugs have been advocated for the treatment of HIVAN; angiotensin converting enzyme inhibitors (ACE-I) and steroids. Evidence for their respective efficacy is limited by the absence of randomized controlled trials. Agents that block the renin-angiotensin system, either converting enzyme inhibitors or angiotensin receptor blocking (ARB) agents, have demonstrated efficacy in preventing progressive kidney failure of diverse etiologies. They have been tested in types 1 and 2 diabetes and in a cohort with advanced chronic renal insufficiency, irrespective of etiology.[44–47] Their mechanism(s) of action, although still unclear, are ascribed to reducing glomerular capillary hydrostatic pressure, altering glomerular basement membrane porosity and lowering transcapillary protein flux, or reducing the renal generation of cytokines, such as TGFβ. {ΣX}β{/ΣX}. Several studies suggest that converting enzyme inhibitor therapy delays the progression to renal failure in HIVAN.[48–51] The studies are limited by the use of nonrandomized controls, small numbers of patients, and are confounded by the beneficial effects of newer, more effective antiretrovirals. Nevertheless, ACE-Is and/or ARBs have become part of a standard regimen for CKD, especially when hypertension or proteinuria are conspicuous, and their use should be encouraged in patients with HIVAN or other kidney diseases associated with HIV infection.[52] Studies in HIV-infected transgenic mice seem to confirm the clinical impression that converting enzyme inhibitors may provide some benefit. Transgenic mice fed captopril in their drinking water survived longer than those fed vehicle although levels of blood urea nitrogen and urinary protein excretion rates were unchanged.[53] The mechanism(s) of action of captopril in this setting remain unresolved and deserve additional study.

Steroids have been tested in HIVAN because they can reduce urinary protein excretion and/or improve GFR in several forms of CKD. Several studies using steroids for HIVAN were performed before the introduction of HAART, based on case reports describing benefits.[54–58] In a nonrandomized trial, many patients responded with a brief improvement in GFR and/or urinary protein excretion, but by the end of the first year, only two had survived without ESRD. Another group has recently reported their experience with steroids prior to the widespread use of HAART.[59] Steroids were dosed at 60 mg of prednisone for 1 month, and gradually tapered over 2–4 months. Patients were not randomized, but selected for treatment according to individual physician standards and/or preferences. Kidney function did stabilize or improved more in the steroid-treated patients when compared to the untreated group and patients receiving prednisone did not have an increased risk of OI during the period of follow-up. The decision to use steroids in HIVAN must be individualized. Patients with prominent interstitial inflammation on biopsy could benefit, while those with predominant fibrosis would be less likely to benefit. The optimal dose and duration of therapy has not been studied adequately.

The pathogenesis, natural history, and therapy of other renal diseases commonly associated with HIV infection are less well defined because of the relatively small number of patients at any one center and the lack of joint collaborative studies or randomized controlled trials. The high prevalence of diabetes and hypertension has been discussed. Although treatment recommendations should be individualized, hypertensives with proteinuria should be treated with an ACE-I or ARB. Target blood pressure should be according to JNC guidelines.[60] Urinary albumin excretion should be tested in diabetics with kidney disease, and albuminuric patients should also be treated with an ACE-I or ARB.

Co-infection with hepatitis C virus (HCV) is associated with renal disease, at least in observational studies, but its exact role is unclear. HCV infection could be a marker for high-risk behavior such as intravenous drug use (IDU), it could directly affect kidney function, or its effects could be mediated through abnormal liver function. Antibodies to HCV can induce immune-complex glomerular disease. By histologic examination, these patients generally have membranoproliferative glomerulonephritis (MPGN), characterized by thickening of the glomerular basement membrane, proliferation of mesangial cells, and influx of mononuclear inflammatory cells. Electron microscopy reveals electron dense deposits of immune complexes in the glomerular basement membrane. The clinical presentation can be indistinguishable from HIVAN.[61] Clues to the diagnosis include an active urinary sediment with red cells and red blood cell casts and serologic tests that confirm the presence of circulating immune-complexes. Serum complement can be low, circulating cryoglobulins are often present, usually type 2 polyclonal IgG and monoclonal IgM kappa, and the latex-fixation test may be positive.

Antiviral therapy with interferon-alpha and ribavirin is the treatment of choice for HCV infection and MPGN. Improved kidney function has been reported in single cases and small cohorts. The decision to initiate treatment is often simplified by the fact that it is indicated for the liver disease *per se*, with or without cryoglobulinemia. It is realistic to anticipate that kidney function will improve if therapy effectively eradicates the virus. A more difficult decision arises when antiviral therapy is ineffective yet the kidney disease is active, as defined by heavy proteinuria or a progressive fall in GFR. Treatment options in this setting include steroids, plasma exchange, and, more recently, rituxamab, a human-mouse chimeric monoclonal antibody to CD20 that selectively targets B cells.[62] These approaches require careful monitoring and are especially risky in co-infected patients with low CD4+ T-lymphocyte count and/or high HIV viral loads.

Irrespective of the cause of the underlying kidney disease, patients with GFR $<60\,mL/min$ per $1.73\,m^2$ remain a special clinical challenge because of the high risk for co-morbid illness and progression to end-stage renal failure. Treatment must be initiated to control lipid abnormalities, Ca/PO_4 metabolism and anemia. Hypertension must also be treated, although several reports indicate that hypertension is conspicuously absent in patients with HIVAN.[63] As GFR falls, the therapeutic focus must shift to preparation for renal replacement therapy. Proper planning for hemodialysis, peritoneal dialysis or kidney transplantation should be made well in advance of uremic symptoms. Kidney transplantation is a viable option in selected patients. Its safety and efficacy is currently under study through a cooperative research program sponsored by the National Institute of Allergy and Infectious Diseases (NIAID).[64] Criteria for transplantation include undetectable viral RNA for at least 3 months, CD4+ T-lymphocyte count >200/μL and no history of an OI or neoplasm. Most or all of these issues are best managed with input from a nephrologist.

In those patients who are likely to start hemodialysis, an AV fistula should be created months before an anticipated start date. Although this can be especially difficult in the IDU patient because they often lack appropriate veins for fistula construction and medical follow-up is often inconsistent, venous mapping and close collaboration with vascular surgeons can increase the success rate of fistula creation. Fistulae are far superior to polytetrafluoroethylene (PTFE, Gore-Tex) grafts or percutaneous dialysis catheters because of reduced thrombosis and infection rates.[65] The long-term prognosis of patients with HIV infection on dialysis is determined by the stage of AIDS and these patients, too, must be aggressively treated with HAART. One- to two-year survival for ESRD patients has improved dramatically in the HAART era, with 1-year survival now approaching 80%. Survival on dialysis should continue to improve with newer antiviral drug therapies.[66] Antiretroviral drug pharmacokinetics and dose adjustments during hemodialysis are the subject of recent reviews.[52,67]

Asymptomatic Urinary Abnormalities

Microscopic hematuria and mild proteinuria are mostly asymptomatic. By themselves they have little clinical impact, but their presence may indicate an early form of a serious disease. In the general population, microscopic hematuria (>3 RBC/hpf) is a useful sign for a variety of genito-urinary (GU) disturbances, most important of which are occult neoplasms. As is true for the general population, the underlying causes of hematuria in HIV-1 infection is determined in part by the age of the population under study, their selection from either an inpatient service, a general medical clinic or a GU subspecialty clinic, and the presence of other GU symptoms. The prevalence of asymptomatic hematuria approaches 25% in a young, unselected cohort of HIV-1-infected individuals.[67a] In this setting, a workup for medically important illness has proved unrewarding, because most cases are mild and transient. An OI of the GU tract must be considered in the differential diagnosis, but this is unlikely in an otherwise asymptomatic patient. As in the general population, a selective diagnostic approach to hematuria is recommended in HIV-1-infected patients. The extent of evaluation should be based on the individual's age, stage of HIV-1 infection, general medical status and the presence of other symptoms. The risk of occult malignancy increases in patients approaching 50 years of age. In these older patients a complete evaluation for microscopic hematuria is warranted, including renal imaging by IVP or CT scan and cystoscopy. When hematuria is accompanied by proteinuria, underlying kidney disease is more likely.

Evaluating Kidney Disease in HIV Infection

The general approach to evaluating CKD in HIV infection has recently been published as Infectious Disease Society of America (IDSA) guidelines,[52] and includes baseline and periodic assessment. All patients should be screened for kidney disease at least once. Patients at risk for kidney disease, including family history, black race, diabetes, hypertension or HCV co-infection should be evaluated annually. Initial evaluation includes estimating GFR using Cockroft-Gault or MDRD formula, and performing a urinalysis to test for proteinuria. Patients with dipstick proteinuria (1+ or greater) or estimated GFR <60 mL/min per 1.73 m^2 require further testing. Urinary protein excretion should be quantified by a spot urine for protein and creatinine and, a renal ultrasound obtained to assess kidney size and structure. Further evaluation is often best performed with input from a nephrologist, and includes examination of urinary sediment, detailed history and physical, and maybe even a kidney biopsy. An overview of the clinical characteristics of the common kidney diseases in HIV infection is summarized in Table 70-4.

ACUTE RENAL FAILURE (ARF)

ARF is defined as an abrupt, detectable fall in GFR, usually recognized by either a 50% increase in serum creatinine or creatinine rising by at least 0.5 mg/dL. Depending on the clinical setting, this may occur in an otherwise asymptomatic patient or it may be associated with the clinical stigmata of underlying sepsis, dehydration, hypotension, or a systemic disease. The diagnostic approach is based on the context of the clinical setting, microscopic examination of the urine, and imaging studies that evaluate kidney structure and exclude urinary tract obstruction. Renal sonography is the preferred imaging study to exclude obstruction and should be obtained in virtually all cases of ARF.

The incidence, risk factors and outcomes for ARF in HIV infection have been studied recently. Franceschini et al reported 111 episodes in 71 subjects in an ambulatory clinic population of over 700 patients; the overall incidence rate was 5.9 per 100 person-years.[68] ARF was more likely to occur in patients with an AIDS-defining condition and HCV co-infection. Ischemia was the most common underlying cause, accounting for 65 events, 43 of which were diagnosed as prerenal azotemia and 22 events as ischemic injury attributable to acute tubular necrosis (ATN). Cirrhosis and/or hepatorenal syndrome, sepsis or infection, and adverse events from drugs were common contributors. Common drug-related syndromes include nephrotoxic ATN, interstitial nephritis, radiocontrast-induced ARF and crystalluria. Amphotericin was the drug most commonly associated with ARF. Wyatt et al, using an observational database, reported

Table 70-4

Brief Overview of Syndromes and Clinical Characteristics of Acute and Chronic Kidney Disease in HIV-Infected Persons

Type of Kidney Disorder	Underlying Causes	Clinical Characteristics
Acute Renal Failure		
Prerenal Azotemia	Dehydration, cirrhosis and hepatorenal syndrome, infection	Oliguria, urine specific gravity >1.015, Urine sodium concentration <20 meq/l bland urine sediment
Nephrotoxicity	Ace-inhibitors, nonsteroidals, aminoglycosides, tenofovir, radiocontrast, lithium, indinavir	Appropriate clinical context and temporal association (radiocontrast, NSAIDs), Fanconi syndrome (tenofovir), hematuria or crystalluria (indinavir)
ATN	Ischemic renal failure	Sepsis or hypotension. Oliguria or nonoliguria. Urine SG ~1.010, urine Na >20 mag/L, pigmented casts on urinalysis
Glomerular Disease	HIVAN, membranoproliferative GN, post-infectious GN	Heavy proteinuria, hematuria and red blood cell casts. (MPGN and post-infectious GN)
Tubulointerstitial disease	Drug-induced:abacavir, indinavir, penicillins, rifampin, NSAIDs, sulfonamides	Hematuria, pyuria, crystalluria
Obstructive uropathy		Characteristic hydronephrosis on renal ultrasound
Chronic Kidney Disease		
	Diabetes, hypertension, HIVAN, IgA Nephropathy, Amyloid, lupus-like	Heavy proteinuria, characteristic findings by sonogram, blood serology, kidney biopsy

a 6% incidence of ARF in hospitalized patients.[69] ARF was associated with traditional risk factors of older age, black race, diabetes and preexisting CKD. HCV infection, cirrhosis and acute hepatic failure commonly complicated these hospitalizations. Mortality rate was six-fold higher in patients with ARF.

Drug-induced crystalluria from indinavir was discussed in a previous edition, and has become relatively infrequent because the drug is used less commonly. Drug-induced crystalluria was observed in 20–40% of patients[70–72] and recognized by leukocyturia, hematuria, and characteristic crystals seen under light microscopy. These appear as needle-shaped crystals, grouped in forms of fans or rectangular-shaped. A hydration protocol of 1–2 L prior to drug ingestion is advocated to prevent high intratubule concentrations of the drug. Sulfadiazine also produces crystalluria.[73] The crystals are recognized as characteristic "shocks of wheat" under light microscopy. Treatment is with hydration and urinary alkalinization.

Rhabdomyolysis and myoglobin-induced ARF occurs as a direct result of HIV-1 infection, in association with zidovudine (ZDV), and complicating trauma, convulsions, cocaine use and from statins that are prescribed for protease inhibitor (PI)-induced dyslipidemia.[74] Statins and PI share a common metabolic pathway (CYP3A4) and the combination may result in high-tissue drug levels. Myoglobinuria-induced renal failure is relatively unusual when CPK levels are appreciably lower than 10 000 U/L. Treatment is aimed at reducing urinary myoglobin solubility through a combination of IV hydration and urinary alkalinization.

Commonly used agents with direct nephrotoxic potential include aminoglycosides, amphotericin, acyclovir, ganciclovir, pentamidine, foscarnet and trimethoprim-sulfamethoxazole. Rifampin and penicillins are relatively common causes of drug-induced interstitial nephritis.[75]

Tenofovir disoproxil fumarate (TDF) is an acyclic nucleotide analog reverse transcriptase inhibitor (NRTI) that has been approved for the treatment of HIV-1 infection since October 2001. Its efficacy has been demonstrated in several major trials, it is in widespread clinical use,[76,77] and it is currently recommended as part of the NRTI backbone in combination with efavirenz for initial treatment of HIV infection.[78] Tenofovir is structurally related to cidofovir and adefovir dipivoxil, compounds that are transported and concentrated in the renal proximal tubule and have been associated with proximal tubule dysfunction and ARF.[79] Approximately 25 case reports and small series describe patients with tenofovir-induced ARF.[80] The usual clinical presentation is a steady decrease in GFR (rise in serum creatinine) sometimes associated with signs of proximal tubule dysfunction, including hypophosphatemia, renal phosphate wasting, glycosuria and modest increases in urinary protein excretion (up to 1 g/day).[81–83] Abrupt changes in GFR have also been reported but less often. These case reports have attracted considerable attention, and at the 2006 Conference on Retroviruses and Opportunistic Infections (CROI), a poster session was devoted to understanding the incidence of renal dysfunction in the clinical setting.[84] Overall, tenofovir has been proven to be extremely safe and effective, as demonstrated in several major clinical trials.[76,77,85,86] Renal adverse events are rare, occurring in less than 1% of cases. Several cohort studies, most notably the Johns Hopkins cohort, have demonstrated a small but statistically significant decreases in GFR but within the normal range.[87] The clinical significance of these changes is unknown, and the fall in estimated GFR has not been associated with an increased rate of drug discontinuation. The small changes in estimated GFR associated with tenofovir in these cohort studies must be interpreted with caution. When first introduced, the drug was used as salvage therapy. In most series, therefore, treated patients tend to be older, have lower CD4+ T-lymphocyte counts and more frequently have a history of ADI.[88] These factors are all associated with increased risk of renal disease, regardless of the drugs used. Tenofovir can be used in all groups of patients, including African-Americans, diabetic and hypertensives. In treated patients, serum creatinine should be assessed at baseline and at routine clinic visits, every 3–4 months.[52,89] Dosing adjustments according to the manufacturer's instructions should be followed for patients with estimated GFR <50 mL/min.

In conclusion, physicians will encounter many forms of kidney disease in HIV-1 infection. The clinical course of disease is changing with the introduction of new antiretroviral therapies. As the population ages, the prevalence of CKD is likely to increase. The risk pool for HIVAN is increasing as patients with AIDS live longer, and HIV-1-infected patients are at risk for secondary causes of CKD more common in the aging population, such as type 2 diabetes, hypertension, and atherosclerotic vascular disease. The diagnostic approach is based on a careful history, physical examination, examination of the urine sediment and renal imaging. Kidney biopsies should be performed to establish the precise diagnosis when significant proteinuria is present. Physicians should be proactive, and screen for kidney disease in all HIV-infected patients. Careful attention to renal function is critical in high-risk patients. Multicenter clinical trials are necessary to better define the spectrum of kidney diseases in the HAART era, and to best define the optimal therapy.

REFERENCES

1. K/DOQI clinical practice guidelines for chronic kidney disease: evaluation, classification, and stratification. Am J Kidney Dis 39(2 Suppl 1):S1-266, 2002.
2. Coresh J, Astor BC, Greene T, et al. Prevalence of chronic kidney disease and decreased kidney function in the adult US population: Third National Health and Nutrition Examination Survey. Am J Kidney Dis 41:1–12, 2003.
3. Go AS, et al. Chronic kidney disease and the risks of death, cardiovascular events, and hospitalization. N Engl J Med 351:1296–305, 2004.
4. U.S. Renal Data System, USRDS 2005 Annual Data Report: Atlas of End-Stage Renal Disease in the United States. Bethesda, MD: National Institutes of Health, National Institute of Diabetes and Digestive and Kidney Diseases; 2005.
5. Szczech LA, et al. Association between renal disease and outcomes among HIV-infected women receiving or not receiving antiretroviral therapy. Clin Infect Dis 39:1199–206, 2004.
6. Gardner LI, et al. Development of proteinuria or elevated serum creatinine and mortality in HIV-infected women. J Acquir Immune Defic Syndr 32:203–9, 2003.
7. Gupta SK, et al. Prevalence of proteinuria and the development of chronic kidney disease in HIV-infected patients. Clin Nephrol 61:1–6, 2004.
8. Winston JA, et al. Chronic kidney disease in HIV infection. J Am Soc Nephrol 16:560A, 2005.
9. Jung O, et al. Hypertension in HIV-1-infected patients and its impact on renal and cardiovascular integrity. Nephrol Dial Transplant 19:2250–8, 2004.
10. Olson D, et al. Impaired renal function of patients initiating HAART in 2 developing countries. In: 13th Conference on Retroviruses and Opportunistic Infections, Denver, CO, 2006.
11. Heffelfinger J, et al. Renal impairment associated with the use of tenofovir. In 13th Conference on Retroviruses and Opportunistic Infections, Denver, CO, 2006.
12. Cockcroft DW, Gault MH. Prediction of creatinine clearance from serum creatinine. Nephron 16:31–41, 1976.
13. Levey AS, Bosch JP, Lewis JB, et al. A more accurate method to estimate glomerular filtration rate from serum creatinine: a new prediction equation. Modification of Diet in Renal Disease Study Group. Ann Intern Med 130:461–70, 1999.
14. http://www.nkdep.nih.gov/professionals/estimated_gfr.htm.
15. Balow JE. Nephropathy in the context of HIV infection. Kidney Int 67:1632–3, 2005.
16. Lucas GM, et al. Highly active antiretroviral therapy and the incidence of HIV-1-associated nephropathy: a 12-year cohort study. Aids 18:541–6, 2004.
17. Klotman PE. HIV-associated nephropathy (clinical conference). Kidney Int 1999. 56:1161–76.
18. D'Agati V, Appel GB. Renal pathology of human immunodeficiency virus infection. Semin Nephrol 18:406–21, 1998.
19. Laradi A, et al. HIV-associated nephropathy: outcome and prognosis factors. Groupe d' Etudes Nephrologiques d'Ile de France. J Am Soc Nephrol 9:2327–35, 1998.
20. Cantor ES, Kimmel PL, Bosch JP. Effect of race on expression of acquired immunodeficiency syndrome-associated nephropathy. Arch Intern Med 1991. 151:125–8.
21. Casanova S, et al. Pattern of glomerular involvement in human immunodeficiency virus- infected patients: an Italian study. Am J Kidney Dis 26:446–53, 1995.
22. Praditpornsilpa K, et al. Renal pathology and HIV infection in Thailand. Am J Kidney Dis 33:282–6, 1999.
23. Nochy D, et al. Renal disease associated with HIV infection: a multicentric study of 60 patients from Paris hospitals. Nephrol Dial Transplant 8:11–9, 1993.
24. Humphreys MH. Human immunodeficiency virus-associated glomerulosclerosis. Kidney Int 48:311–20, 1995.
25. Ross MJ, Klotman PE. HIV-associated nephropathy. Aids 18:1089–99, 2004.
26. Gharavi AG, et al. Mapping a locus for susceptibility to HIV-1-associated nephropathy to mouse chromosome 3. Proc Natl Acad Sci USA 101:2488–93, 2004.
27. Atta MG, et al. Nephrotic range proteinuria and CD4 count as noninvasive indicators of HIV-associated nephropathy. Am J Med 118:1288, 2005.
28. Winston JA, Klotman ME, Klotman PE. HIV-associated nephropathy is a late, not early, manifestation of HIV-1 infection [see comments]. Kidney Int 55:1036–40, 1999.
29. Lu TC, He JC, Klotman P. Animal models of HIV-associated nephropathy. Curr Opin Nephrol Hypertens 15:233–7, 2006.
30. Kopp JB, et al. Nephropathy in HIV-transgenic mice. Contrib Nephrol 107:194–204, 1994.

31. Bruggeman LA, et al. Nephropathy in human immunodeficiency virus-1 transgenic mice is due to renal transgene expression. J Clin Invest 100:84–92, 1997.
32. Husain M, et al. HIV-1 Nef induces dedifferentiation of podocytes in vivo: a characteristic feature of HIVAN. Aids 19:1975–80, 2005.
33. He JC, et al. Nef stimulates proliferation of glomerular podocytes through activation of Src-dependent Stat3 and MAPK1,2 pathways. J Clin Invest 114:643–51, 2004.
34. Dickie P, et al. Focal glomerulosclerosis in proviral and c-fms transgenic mice links Vpr expression to HIV-associated nephropathy. Virology 322:69–81, 2004.
35. Bruggeman LA, et al. Renal epithelium is a previously unrecognized site of HIV-1 infection. J Am Soc Nephrol 11: 2079–87, 2000.
36. Ray PE, et al. bFGF and its low affinity receptors in the pathogenesis of HIV-associated nephropathy in transgenic mice. Kidney Int 46:759–72, 1994.
37. Ross MJ, et al. HIV-1 infection initiates an inflammatory cascade in human renal tubular epithelial cells. J Acquir Immune Defic Syndr 42:1–11, 2006.
38. Cosgrove CJ, Abu-Alfa AK, Perazella MA. Observations on HIV-associated renal disease in the era of highly active antiretroviral therapy. Am J Med Sci 323:102–6, 2002.
39. Wali RK, et al. HIV-1-associated nephropathy and response to highly-active antiretroviral therapy (letter). Lancet 352:783–4, 1998.
40. Winston JA, et al. Nephropathy and establishment of a renal reservoir of HIV type 1 during primary infection. N Engl J Med 344:1979–84, 2001.
41. Marras D, et al. Replication and compartmentalization of HIV-1 in kidney epithelium of patients with HIV-associated nephropathy. Nat Med 8:522–6, 2002.
42. Schwartz EJ, et al. Highly active antiretroviral therapy and the epidemic of HIV+ end-stage renal disease. J Am Soc Nephrol 16:2412–20, 2005.
43. Eggers PW, Kimmel PL. Is there an epidemic of HIV Infection in the US ESRD program? J Am Soc Nephrol 15:2477–85, 2004.
44. Randomised placebo-controlled trial of effect of ramipril on decline in glomerular filtration rate and risk of terminal renal failure in proteinuric, non-diabetic nephropathy. The GISEN Group (Gruppo Italiano di Studi Epidemiologici in Nefrologia). Lancet 349:1857–63, 1997.
45. Brenner BM, et al. Effects of losartan on renal and cardiovascular outcomes in patients with type 2 diabetes and nephropathy. N Engl J Med 345:861–9, 2001.
46. Lewis EJ, et al. Renoprotective effect of the angiotensin-receptor antagonist irbesartan in patients with nephropathy due to type 2 diabetes. N Engl J Med 345:851–60, 2001.
47. Lewis EJ, et al. The effect of angiotensin-converting-enzyme inhibition on diabetic nephropathy. The Collaborative Study Group. N Engl J Med 329:1456–62, 1993.
48. Burns GC, et al. Effect of angiotensin-converting enzyme inhibition in HIV-associated nephropathy. J Am Soc Nephrol 8:1140–6, 1997.
49. Kimmel PL, Mishkin GJ, Umana WO. Captopril and renal survival in patients with human immunodeficiency virus nephropathy. Am J Kidney Dis 28:202–8, 1996.
50. Wei A, et al. Long-term renal survival in HIV-associated nephropathy with angiotensin-converting enzyme inhibition. Kidney Int 64:1462–71, 2003.
51. Szczech LA, et al. Protease inhibitors are associated with a slowed progression of HIV- related renal diseases. Clin Nephrol 57:336–41, 2002.
52. Gupta SK, et al. Guidelines for the management of chronic kidney disease in HIV-infected patients: recommendations of the HIV Medicine Association of the Infectious Diseases Society of America. Clin Infect Dis 40:1559–85, 2005.
53. Bird JE, et al. Captopril prevents nephropathy in HIV-transgenic mice. J Am Soc Nephrol 9:1441–7, 1998.
54. Appel RG, Neill J. A steroid-responsive nephrotic syndrome in a patient with human immunodeficiency virus (HIV) infection. Ann Intern Med 113:892–3, 1990.
55. Briggs WA, et al. Clinicopathologic correlates of prednisone treatment of human immunodeficiency virus-associated nephropathy. Am J Kidney Dis 28:618–21, 1996.
56. Watterson MK, Detwiler RK, Bolin P Jr. Clinical response to prolonged corticosteroids in a patient with human immunodeficiency virus-associated nephropathy. Am J Kidney Dis 29:624–6, 1997.
57. Smith MC, et al. Effect of corticosteroid therapy on human immunodeficiency virus-associated nephropathy. Am J Med 97:145–51, 1994.
58. Smith MC, et al. Prednisone improves renal function and proteinuria in human immunodeficiency virus-associated nephropathy. Am J Med 101:41–8, 1996.
59. Eustace JA, et al. Cohort study of the treatment of severe HIV-associated nephropathy with corticosteroids. Kidney Int 58:1253–60, 2000.
60. Chobanian AV, et al. The Seventh Report of the Joint National Committee on Prevention, Detection, Evaluation, and Treatment of High Blood Pressure: the JNC 7 report. JAMA 289:2560–72, 2003.
61. Cheng JT, et al. Hepatitis C virus-associated glomerular disease in patients with human immunodeficiency virus coinfection. J Am Soc Nephrol 10:1566–74, 1999.
62. Kamar N, Rostaing L, Alric L. Treatment of hepatitis C-virus-related glomerulonephritis. Kidney Int 2006. 69:436–9.
63. D'Agati V, Appel GB. HIV infection and the kidney. J Am Soc Nephrol 8:138–52, 1997.
64. http://spitfire.emmes.com/study/htr/index.html 2006.
65. Feldman HI, Kobrin S, Wasserstein A. Hemodialysis vascular access morbidity. J Am Soc Nephrol 7:523–35, 1996.
66. Ahuja TS, Grady J, Khan S. Changing trends in the survival of dialysis patients with human immunodeficiency virus in the United States. J Am Soc Nephrol 13:1889–93, 2002.
67. Izzedine H, et al. An appraisal of antiretroviral drugs in hemodialysis. Kidney Int 60:821–30, 2001.
67a. Cespedes RD, Peretsman SJ, Blatt SP. The significance of hematuria in patients infected with the human immunodeficiency virus. J Urol 154:1455–56, 1995.
68. Franceschini N, et al. Incidence and etiology of acute renal failure among ambulatory HIV-infected patients. Kidney Int 67:1526–31, 2005.
69. Wyatt CM, et al. Acute renal failure in hospitalized patients with HIV: risk factors and impact on in-hospital mortality. Aids 20:561–5, 2006.
70. Kopp JB, et al. Crystalluria and urinary tract abnormalities associated with indinavir [see comments]. Ann Intern Med 127:119–25, 1997.
71. Tashima KT, Horowitz JD, Rosen S. Indinavir nephropathy. N Engl J Med 336:138–40, 1997.
72. Wu DS, Stoller ML. Indinavir urolithiasis. Curr Opin Urol 10:557–61, 2000.
73. Becker K, Jablonowski H, Haussinger D. Sulfadiazine-associated nephrotoxicity in patients with the acquired immunodeficiency syndrome. Medicine (Baltimore) 75: 185–94, 1996.
74. Dube MP, et al. Preliminary guidelines for the evaluation and management of dyslipidemia in adults infected with human immunodeficiency virus and receiving antiretroviral therapy: Recommendations of the Adult AIDS Clinical Trial Group Cardiovascular Disease Focus Group. Clin Infect Dis 31:1216–24, 2000.
75. Rao TK. Acute renal failure syndromes in human immunodeficiency virus infection. Semin Nephrol 18:378–95, 1998.

76. Gallant JE, et al. Tenofovir DF, emtricitabine, and efavirenz vs. zidovudine, lamivudine, and efavirenz for HIV. N Engl J Med 354:251–60, 2006.
77. Gallant JE, et al. Efficacy and safety of tenofovir DF vs stavudine in combination therapy in antiretroviral-naive patients: a 3-year randomized trial. JAMA 292:191–201, 2004.
78. Guidelines for the use of antiretroviral agents in HIV-1-infected adults and adolescents. Washington, D.C.: Department of Health and Human Services. Available: http://AIDSinfo.nih.gov 2006.
79. Ho ES, et al. Cytotoxicity of antiviral nucleotides adefovir and cidofovir is induced by the expression of human renal organic anion transporter 1. J Am Soc Nephrol 11:383–93, 2000.
80. Winston JA. What do we know about tenofovir and renal function? Contagion 2:2–4, 2005.
81. Peyriere H, et al. Renal tubular dysfunction associated with tenofovir therapy: report of 7 cases. J Acquir Immune Defic Syndr 35:269–73, 2004.
82. Zimmermann AE, et al. Tenofovir-associated acute and chronic kidney disease: a case of multiple drug interactions. Clin Infect Dis 42:283–90, 2006.
83. Parsonage MJ, et al. The development of hypophosphataemic osteomalacia with myopathy in two patients with HIV infection receiving tenofovir therapy. HIV Med 6:341–6, 2005.
84. Tenofovir -Associated Renal Dysfunction. In: 13th Conference on Retroviruses and Opportunistic Infections. Denver, CO, 2006.
85. Schooley RT, et al. Tenofovir DF in antiretroviral-experienced patients: results from a 48-week, randomized, double-blind study. AIDS 16:1257–63, 2002.
86. Izzedine H, et al. Long-term renal safety of tenofovir disoproxil fumarate in antiretroviral-naive HIV-1-infected patients. Data from a double-blind randomized active-controlled multicentre study. Nephrol Dial Transplant 20:743–6, 2005.
87. Gallant JE, et al. Changes in renal function associated with tenofovir disoproxil fumarate treatment, compared with nucleoside reverse-transcriptase inhibitor treatment. Clin Infect Dis 40:1194–8, 2005.
88. Mauss S, Berger F, Schmutz G. Antiretroviral therapy with tenofovir is associated with mild renal dysfunction. AIDS 19: 93–5, 2005.
89. Winston JA, Shepp DH. The role of drug interactions and monitoring in the prevention of tenofovir-associated kidney disease. Clin Infect Dis 42:1657–8; author reply 1658, 2006.

Chapter 71

Diabetes and Insulin Resistance

Colleen Hadigan, MD, MPH, Steven Grinspoon, MD

INTRODUCTION

Insulin resistance and type 2 diabetes mellitus are increasingly recognized as common among individuals with HIV infection who are receiving antiretroviral therapy.[1–3] One important consequence of diabetes and insulin resistance is the associated increased risk of cardiovascular disease in HIV-infected patients.[4] In a large prospective cohort study, Friis-Moller and colleagues[4] demonstrated increased rates of acute myocardial infarction with increased duration of exposure to HAART, such that each year of HAART use was associated with a 1.26 (95% CI 1.12–1.41, $P < 0.001$) relative increase in risk for acute myocardial infarction (AMI). In addition to the risk of HAART, traditional independent risk factors for cardiovascular disease were identified and diabetes was associated with a 2.38-fold increased relative AMI risk (95% CI 1.38–4.10, $P = 0.002$). These findings suggest that insulin resistance and diabetes may contribute to cardiovascular disease among HIV-infected patients. This chapter summarizes new data on the prevalence of diabetes and insulin resistance in HIV-infected patients, summarizes our understanding to date of the mechanisms of insulin resistance and diabetes in the HIV-infected population and highlights a rational approach to the management of diabetes and insulin resistance in HIV-infected patients.

DEFINING DIABETES, IMPAIRED GLUCOSE TOLERANCE, AND INSULIN RESISTANCE IN THE HIV-INFECTED POPULATION

Diabetes is defined by the WHO as a fasting plasma glucose equal to 126 mg/dL or more, or a 2-h glucose 200 mg/dL or more during a 75 g oral glucose tolerance test (OGTT).[5] Impaired glucose tolerance (IGT) is defined as a 2-h plasma glucose 140 mg/dL or above during a 75 g OGTT,[5] and impaired fasting glucose (IFG) is defined more recently as a fasting plasma glucose 100 mg/dL or more.[6] Both diabetes and IGT are associated with increased cardiovascular risk.[7–10] In addition, patients with IGT have a substantial risk of going on to develop diabetes. In a prospective study of over 3000 individuals, the Diabetes Prevention Program found an estimated cumulative incidence of diabetes of 29% after 3 years of follow-up for subjects with IGT who did not receive any intervention.[11]

Insulin resistance is more difficult to define clinically, but is usually marked by hyperinsulinemia, and decreased insulin action (e.g., decreased insulin-mediated glucose transport into muscle and impaired insulin action to inhibit lipolysis). Numerous tests exist to determine abnormal glucose homeostasis, as listed in Table 71-1. A simple fasting blood glucose or 75 g OGTT are most useful clinically to diagnose diabetes or IGT. A fasting insulin level or index of fasting glucose and insulin (e.g., HOMA and QUICKI, see Table 71-1.) is relatively easy to obtain and can be useful for the evaluation of insulin resistance.[12] More sophisticated techniques such as the euglycemic hyperinsulinemic clamp are not practical clinically, but remain important research tools to quantify insulin resistance. While useful in the care and monitoring of patients with known diabetes, the hemoglobin A1c, an integrated measure of the average glucose over the prior few months, is not a useful measure in patients with significant insulin resistance but normal fasting glucose levels, which is common in HIV infection.

PREVALENCE OF DIABETES AND ABNORMAL GLUCOSE HOMEOSTASIS IN HIV-INFECTED PATIENTS

Early reports of hyperinsulinemia among HIV-infected men and women indicate that insulin resistance was prevalent even before the widespread introduction of HAART. For example,

Table 71-1 Summary of Tests to Determine Abnormal Glucose Homeostasis

Test	Utility	Standards	Benefits	Limitations
FPG[6]	Screening for DM, IFG	DM ≥126 mg/dL (7.0 mmol/L)[5,6] IFG 100−125 mg/dL (5.6−6.9 mmol/L)[6]	Requires single fasting blood sample	Diagnosis of DM[a] is provisional; should be confirmed by 2 h OGTT[5,6]
2 h OGTT (75 g oral glucose load)	Diagnoses DM, IGT	Postload glucose $_{DM}$ ≥200 mg/dL (11.1 mmol/L)[5,6] Postload glucose $_{IGT}$ 140–199 mg/dL (7.8–11.0 mmol/L)[5,6]	Distinguish DM from IGT for borderline FPG levels	Lacks insulin measures to identify IR[59]
Fasting insulin	Indicates insulin resistance	Normal range varies with assay[b]	Requires single fasting sample	Standardization for insulin values is assay-specific
QUICKI	Indicates insulin resistance	QUICKI[60] = 1/(log fasting insulin μIU/mL + log FPG mg/dL)	Correlates highly with SI_{clamp}.[61, 62] Requires single fasting sample	Standardization specific to insulin assay. No established normal range
HOMA-IR	Indicates insulin resistance	HOMA-IR[12] = (fasting insulin μIU/mL × FPG mmol/L)/22.5	Correlates highly with SI_{clamp}.[12, 63] Requires single fasting sample	Standardization specific to insulin assay. No established normal range
IVGTT	Whole-body glucose and Si; indicates pancreatic function	Minimal model analysis[64] calculates SI, Sg (glucose effectiveness), and AIRg (acute insulin response to glucose); no established normal ranges	Estimates whole-body insulin sensitivity with minimal complexity.[65] Correlates highly with SI_{clamp}[66]	Research only; multiple samples required and impractical for large, epidemiologic studies
Hyperinsulinemic clamp	Whole-body glucose disposal and insulin sensitivity (euglycemic clamp), and β-cell sensitivity to glucose (hyperglycemic clamp)	Calculations of M[67] (measure of glucose tolerance) and SI_{clamp} based on glucose infusion rate and insulin level; no established normal ranges	Provides most reliable, direct measure of insulin-stimulated glucose utilization[65]	Research only; impractical for large, epidemiologic studies; most technically complex method

Abbreviations: FPG = fasting plasma glucose; DM = diabetes mellitus; IFG = impaired fasting glucose (glycemia); OGTT = oral glucose tolerance test; IGT = impaired glucose tolerance; IR = insulin resistance; HOMA-IR = homeostasis model assessment of insulin resistance; SI = insulin sensitivity; QUICKI = quantitative insulin sensitivity check index; IVGTT = intravenous glucose tolerance test.

[a] If a fasting plasma glucose sample cannot be obtained, DM may also be diagnosed by the presence of classic symptoms of DM (polyuria, polydipsia, and unexplained weight loss) in addition to a casual (nonfasting) plasma glucose concentration ≥200 mg/dL.[1]

[b] Suggested reference range for normal fasting insulin: 6–20 μIU/mL (varies with insulin assay).

compared to weight-matched healthy controls, HIV-infected men and women with a history of wasting or prior weight loss demonstrated increased fasting insulin levels and markers of insulin resistance.[13,14] In both studies, there was no association between insulin levels and the use of protease inhibitors (PIs), the component of HAART most often associated with insulin resistance. Furthermore, more than 40% of the men[14] and 75% of the women[13] were not on HAART regimens in these studies. Increased relative truncal adiposity was demonstrated in relationship to hyperinsulinemia even among a population of nonobese HIV-infected patients with a history of weight loss.[13,14] Studies have also demonstrated insulin resistance among HIV-infected patients using HAART regimens containing a PI.[15,16]

More recently, Brown et al[2] investigated the prevalence and incidence of diabetes mellitus in a large cohort of HIV-infected men in the Multicenter AIDS Cohort Study. In this study of 710 HIV-seronegative men and 568 HIV-infected men, the prevalence of diabetes was significantly greater among HIV-infected men based on a fasting glucose above 126 mg/dL or self-reported diabetes mellitus (overall prevalence of diabetes: 12% HIV+ vs 5% HIV−). When subjects were further categorized according to current use of HAART, HIV-infected men not receiving HAART demonstrated a prevalence ratio of 2.21 (95% CI 1.12–4.38) compared to controls. In contrast, men receiving HAART demonstrated a prevalence ratio of 4.64 (95% CI 3.03–7.10) compared to controls, after adjusting for age and body mass index. Similarly, the incidence of diabetes between April 1999 and March 2003 was significantly increased among the HIV-infected men receiving HAART compared to HIV-seronegative controls (incidence rate: 4.7 per 100 person-years and the adjusted rate ratio was 4.11 (95% CI 1.85–9.16)). In a subanalysis to identify potential risk factors associated with diabetes mellitus and IGT, ritonavir was the only PI associated with increased risk (rate ratio 1.70 (95% CI 1.08–2.68)) of diabetes or IFG (i.e., fasting blood glucose between 100 and 125 mg/dL) when considered together. However, 94% of the participants using ritonavir were also receiving another PI in combination with ritonavir, which was used for its 'boosting effects' to improve the pharmacokinetic profile of other PIs, making it more difficult to interpret these results. Brown et al also demonstrated that men with a lower CD4 nadir had a greater risk of incident glucose abnormalities, suggesting that severity of HIV disease may be related to an increased risk of diabetes or insulin resistance. In a 4-year follow-up period, this study identified newly diagnosed diabetes mellitus in 10% of HIV-infected men on HAART. A fourfold increased incidence of diabetes compared to HIV-seronegative men was observed after adjusting for age and body mass index.

The risk and prevalence of diabetes and insulin resistance among women with HIV infection is less clear. Justman and colleagues[3] reported a threefold increase of incident diabetes mellitus among HIV-infected women receiving a PI compared to women receiving nonPI-based antiretroviral therapy in a cohort of 1785 women followed in the Women's Interagency HIV Study (WIHS) between 1994 and 1998. In addition to PI use, increasing age and body mass index were identified as significant independent risk factors for self-reported diabetes mellitus.[3] More recently, Howard et al[17] reported OGTT results from a large cohort of HIV-infected women ($n = 133$) and HIV-uninfected, age-matched controls ($n = 88$) without a history of diabetes. Here, 13.5% of HIV-infected women demonstrated IGT (i.e., 2-h postchallenge glucose level ≥140 mg/dL and <200 mg/dL) and 4.5% demonstrated previously unrecognized diabetes. Rates between the HIV-infected and HIV-uninfected groups did not differ significantly, but women in the control group had higher body mass index and waist circumference, and therefore may have had greater risk for abnormal glucose metabolism.

Danoff et al[18] published a subsequent study of women enrolled in the WIHS cohort, evaluating prospective oral glucose tolerance testing in 258 women. The study tested 88 HIV-seronegative, 74 HIV-infected women not receiving HAART, and 96 women with HIV infection receiving HAART. Fourteen percent of the HIV-infected participants had 'prediabetes' defined as a fasting blood sugar above 100 mg/dL or a 2-h postchallenge glucose level between 140 mg/dL and 200 mg/dL. The prevalence of diabetes was not increased in the HIV-infected women receiving HAART (4%) or the HIV-infected women not receiving HAART (8%) compared to the control women (10%), but this study also reported data from relatively overweight control subjects enrolled in the WIHS study. Indeed, in the study of Danoff et al, body mass index emerged as the single most important predictor of diabetes and prediabetes.[18] In summary, abnormalities in glucose metabolism may be seen in up to 14% of HIV-infected women, but the limited data currently available do not yet support an increased prevalence of diabetes mellitus in women living with HIV compared to a well-matched HIV-uninfected control group.

Although fewer data are available in children, preliminary studies indicate that insulin resistance may be increased, particularly among HIV-infected children on HAART. For example, in a small cross-sectional study of HIV-infected children on a PI-containing regimen ($n = 33$) compared to PI-naive children ($n = 15$), Bitnun and colleagues[19] identified lower insulin sensitivity in children after adjusting for potential confounders. In a larger, multicenter, 2-year prospective study of 130 HIV-infected children designed to assess lipodystrophy and associated metabolic complications, Beregszaszi et al found 13.2% of children to have hyperinsulinemia (defined as an insulin level greater than the 95th percentile from a normoglycemic healthy population matched for pubertal status).[20] After 2 years of follow-up, this percentage doubled to 25.6% ($P = 0.01$). Although children in the study were not found to have diabetes mellitus by fasting hyperglycemia, fasting hyperinsulinemia was common and could represent an early stage in the ultimate development of diabetes among HIV-infected children.

RISK FACTORS FOR INSULIN RESISTANCE AND DIABETES IN HIV

The use of PIs was one of the first factors identified with increased risk of insulin resistance and diabetes among HIV-infected patients. Recognition of lipodystrophy and metabolic complications associated with antiretroviral therapy occurred with the widespread introduction of PIs and HAART. However, increasing evidence suggests that, while antiretroviral medications can have direct effects on insulin sensitivity and glucose metabolism, e.g., via inhibition of glucose uptake into muscle by individual PIs,[21] indirect effects of antiretroviral medications on body fat distribution and lipids can contribute to impaired insulin sensitivity in HIV-infected patients. HIV infection itself may also contribute to chronic inflammation, and insulin resistance in this regard. Finally, changes in body composition, including truncal adiposity, may be associated with inflammatory cytokines and adipocytokines, such as tumor necrosis factor-α (TNF-α), interleukin-6 (IL-6), and adiponectin, which may further contribute to insulin resistance in HIV-infected patients.[22]

In an early cross-sectional study designed to compare HIV-infected patients with evidence of fat redistribution to age and BMI-matched subjects from the Framingham Offspring Cohort, 71 HIV-infected men and women complaining of changes in body fat distribution and 213 healthy age, sex, and weight-matched control subjects were studied.[1] HIV-infected patients with abnormal fat distribution had significantly increased rates of previously unrecognized diabetes (7% vs 0.5% in the control subjects) and increased rates of IGT (35.2% vs 5.2% in control subjects). In a subanalysis of 30 HIV-infected subjects without changes in body fat, there was no increase in diabetes or IGT compared to 90 age, sex, and weight-matched control subjects. These data suggest that fat distribution *per se* is an important factor in the development of insulin resistance among HIV-infected patients, who demonstrated increased central adiposity and waist-to-hip ratios compared to control subjects.

Lipoatrophy of the peripheral subcutaneous fat, as well as increased visceral fat, may contribute to insulin resistance in HIV. Mynarcik et al[23] identified an association between insulin sensitivity and peripheral limb fat in a study of HIV-infected subjects with and without lipodystrophy in comparison to healthy volunteers. Reduced limb fat was associated with increased insulin resistance, similar to the observation in HIV-uninfected patients with congenital lipodystrophy. Lipoatrophy is increasingly recognized as a direct effect of antiretroviral therapy, including nucleoside reverse transcriptase inhibitors (NRTIs).[24] Indeed, cumulative exposure to NRTIs and not PIs was identified as the strongest drug class association with markers of insulin resistance in the Multicenter AIDS Cohort Study of 755 HIV-infected men.[25] The putative mechanism for this observation is through lipoatrophy and mitochondrial toxicity to adipose tissue. In addition, mitochondrial toxicity to muscle may also contribute to insulin resistance, via increased intramyocellular lipid accumulation.

Several studies have also identified a strong positive relationship between visceral fat and insulin resistance in HIV disease.[13,19,26–28] For example, using positron emission tomography (PET) with administration of 2-Deoxy-2 [^{18}F] Fluoro-D-glucose, insulin stimulated glucose uptake in subcutaneous and visceral fat and skeletal muscle were assessed in patients with HIV-associated lipoatrophy and healthy controls.[28] Under insulin-stimulated conditions, visceral adipose depot size was correlated most significantly with whole-body glucose uptake (see Fig. 71-1), as well as regional muscle and fat glucose uptake. Therefore, as demonstrated in the general population with obesity and the metabolic syndrome, increased visceral adiposity may be an important determinant of insulin sensitivity in the HIV-infected population.

In order to separate the direct effects of antiretroviral medications on insulin resistance from potential long-term effects on body fat distribution and to distinguish such effects from the potential confounding effects of HIV, studies have been conducted in tissue culture and *in vivo* in healthy HIV seronegative volunteers. For example IL-6 and TNF-α, inflammatory cytokines associated with muscle and adipose tissue insulin resistance, are increased in adipocyte cultures after exposures to NRTIs and PIs.[29] In 3T3-L1 cultured adipocytes, Murata et al[21] demonstrated a direct effect of various PIs to inhibit insulin-mediated glucose uptake by adipocytes, via inhibition of glucose transporter GLUT4. Short-term (4 week) and single-dose administrations of a PI, indinavir, were associated with

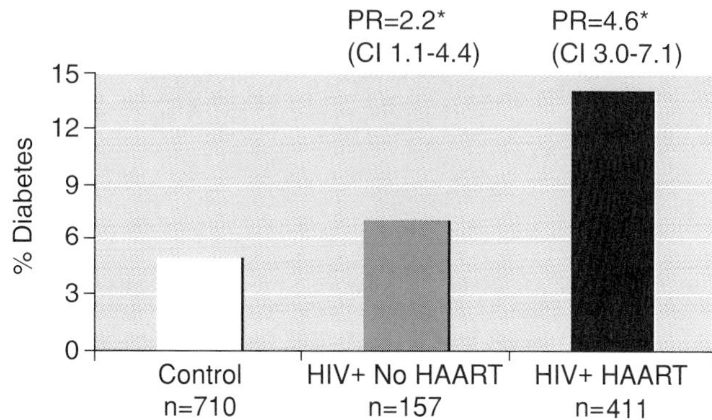

Figure 71-1 ■ Prevalence of diabetes mellitus among HIV-infected men on highly active antiretroviral therapy (HAART) compared to those not on HAART and HIV seronegative controls. PR= prevalence ratio relative to control. * indicates analyses are adjusted for age and body mass index.

Adapted from Brown TT, Cole SR, Li X, et al. Antiretroviral therapy and the prevalence and incidence of diabetes mellitus in the multicenter AIDS cohort study. Arch Intern Med 165:1179–1184, 2005.

reductions in whole-body glucose disposal of ~25%, as measured by hyperinsulinemic clamp techniques among HIV-seronegative volunteers in the absence of any significant changes in fat distribution.[30,31] A similar study of the short-term effects of lopinavir/ritonavir and atazanavir in healthy volunteers demonstrated decreased insulin sensitivity with lopinavir/ritonavir but not atazanavir.[32] Taken together, these data support a direct effect of specific HIV PIs to impair insulin-stimulated glucose disposal, independent of HIV infection and alterations in body composition. However, these data also argue against a class-specific effect of PI on insulin sensitivity.

Increased circulating fatty acids and inappropriate lipid accumulation in muscle and liver are known to be associated with insulin resistance in obesity and type 2 diabetes.[33] HIV-infected patients demonstrate increased lipids,[1] increased rates of lipolysis and circulating fatty acids,[34,35] and increased intramyocellular lipid content, which may contribute to decreased insulin sensitivity in the context of lipodystrophy and HAART.[36] In reports by Reeds et al[37] and Behrens et al,[38] HIV-infected men with dyslipidemia demonstrated impaired suppression of lipolysis as well as impaired glucose disposal in response to insulin stimulation. Conversely, acute suppression of lipolysis and reduction in circulating fatty acids have been shown to improve insulin sensitivity[39] and glucose disposal[40] in HIV-infected men with lipodystrophy (Fig. 71-2). Adipocytokines, in particular adiponectin, may play an important role in the relationship between adipocyte and lipid metabolism and insulin sensitivity.[28,37] Reduced adiponectin levels were identified among HIV-infected men in association with increased truncal adiposity, reduced extremity fat, and insulin resistance,[41] suggesting a potential therapeutic target in the HIV-infected population with lipodystrophy.

Hepatitis C infection is an important known risk factor for insulin resistance and diabetes. Hepatitis C was shown to be a risk factor for diabetes among non-HIV-infected patients[42]

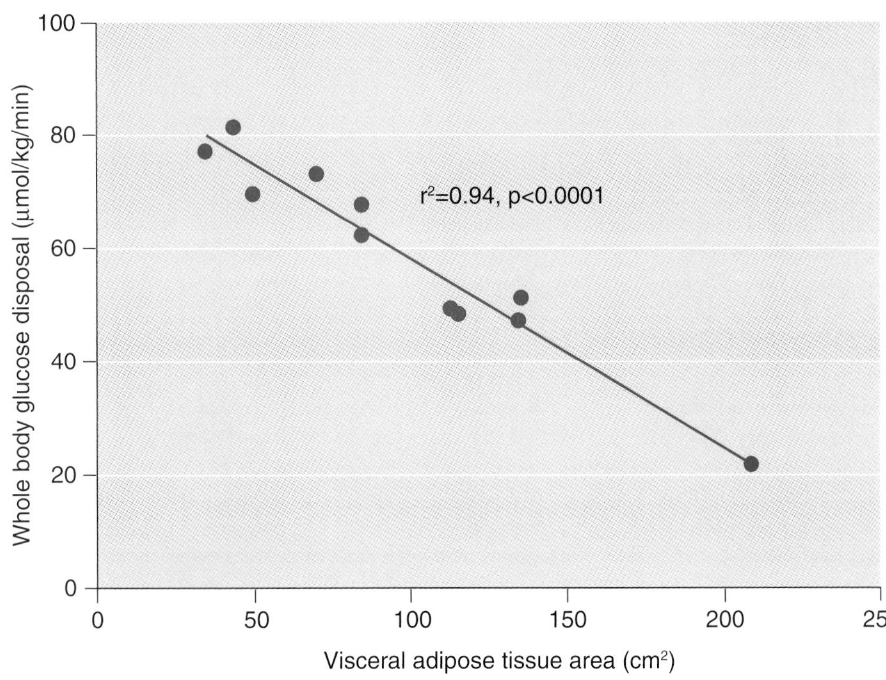

Figure 71-2 ■ Relationship between insulin-stimulated whole body glucose disposal and visceral adipose tissue area in HIV-infected men with lipodystrophy (n = 6) and healthy controls (n = 5).

Adapted from Hadigan C, Kamin D, Liebau J, et al. Depot specific regulation of glucose uptake and insulin sensitivity in HIV-lipodystrophy. Am J Physiol Endocrinol Metab, 2005.

and may also predispose co-infected patients with HIV disease to diabetes. In a cross-sectional analysis of 1389 antiretroviral-naive HIV-infected subjects with and without hepatitis C co-infection, Visnegarwala[43] reported that individuals with HIV and hepatitis C co-infection had a significantly increased prevalence of type 2 diabetes compared to patients with HIV monoinfection (5.9% vs 3.3%, respectively), controlling for differences in age and body weight. Thus, emerging data suggest that HIV-infected patients with hepatitis C may be at significantly increased risk for diabetes mellitus, and should be monitored accordingly.

STRATEGIES FOR THE TREATMENT OF INSULIN RESISTANCE AND DIABETES IN HIV INFECTION

Currently, there are no published reports evaluating the efficacy of treatment strategies for type 2 diabetes in HIV-infected patients, but insulin may be necessary when blood glucose levels increase significantly. Use of sulfonylureas is not recommended for HIV-infected patients with insulin resistance in the absence of increased fasting glucose levels, as these agents work by further stimulating pancreatic insulin secretion, without sensitizing to insulin action. In contrast, a number of randomized controlled trials have been completed to evaluate the benefits of insulin sensitizing agents, including metformin and rosiglitazone, in the treatment of HIV-infected patients (Table 71-2). Importantly, these studies differ with respect to treatments used, duration of therapy, and degree of baseline insulin resistance. The use of metformin has consistently been shown to improve insulin sensitivity and markers of insulin resistance, in addition to reducing triglyceride levels in some studies.[44,45] Clinically significant adverse effects on lactic acid levels have not been shown in studies of metformin in HIV infection. Administration of rosiglitazone also resulted in consistent improvements in insulin resistance among HIV-infected patients, but was also associated with modest but significant increases in lipid levels.[45–48]

Metformin and rosiglitazone result in differential effects on fat distribution.[49] Metformin tends to reduce weight and central adiposity,[44,49] whereas rosiglitazone has resulted in improved extremity and subcutaneous fat in some studies,[46,50,51] and with increased levels of adiponectin.[46–48,50] In contrast, Carr et al did not show an increase in subcutaneous fat in one large, randomized study, but the use of NRTI stavudine was more common in the treatment group, potentially affecting the study results.[47] Taken together, these studies demonstrate the potential utility and limitations of insulin-sensitizing agents in the treatment of insulin resistance in HIV-infected patients. A number of critical questions remain unanswered with respect to the use of insulin-sensitizing agents in patients with HIV lipodystrophy. Most important among these are whether the long-term use of these agents will reduce the risk of developing type 2 diabetes mellitus and the cardiovascular sequelae of chronic insulin resistance.

With the recognition that a number of antiretroviral classes and agents directly contribute to metabolic disturbances such as lipodystrophy, dyslipidemia, and insulin resistance, increased efforts are underway to develop HAART regimens that may have fewer metabolic effects. For example, use of the PI atazanavir has thus far not been associated with significant insulin resistance in limited clinical studies.[32,52] In addition, strategies are being developed to safely switch antiretroviral classes to avoid or improve metabolic toxicities while maintaining virological suppression. For example, several studies have demonstrated improvements in hyperlipidemia with institution of PI-sparing regimens, but few have been able to identify benefits in insulin sensitivity with changes in

Table 71-2

Summary of Randomized Trials Evaluating the Efficacy of Insulin Sensitizing Agents in HIV-Infected Patients

	Randomized PBO Controlled	IR Required	Duration	N	Effect on Insulin Resistance
Metformin					
Saint-Marc et al[44]	RZ	Yes	12 weeks	27	Improved
Hadigan et al[50]	RZ–PC	Yes	12 weeks	26	Improved
Martinez et al[68]	RZ–PC	No	48 weeks	108	Improved
Rosiglitazone					
Sutinen et al[48]	RZ–PC	No	24 weeks	30	Improved
Carr et al[47]	RZ–PC	No	48 weeks	108	Improved
Hadigan et al[46]	RZ–PC	Yes	12 weeks	28	Improved
Metformin vs Rosiglitazone					
Van Wijk et al[49]	RZ	No	24 weeks	39	Both arms improved
Tomazic et al[45]	RZ	Yes	48 weeks	90	Both arms improved

RZ = randomized treatment assignment, PC = placebo controlled, IR = insulin resistance, yes indicates a marker of insulin resistance was required for enrollment in the study.

HAART.[53] A large, randomized trial, designed to decrease the mitochondrial toxicity and potentially reverse lipoatrophy by replacement of stavudine or zidovudine with abacavir, showed increases in limb fat after 24 weeks, but did not identify any beneficial effects of the switch on insulin sensitivity.[54]

Diet and lifestyle modifications, including increased physical activity, remain the first-line recommendations for the management of insulin resistance and type 2 diabetes, but there are limited data available directly evaluating the potential benefits of lifestyle modification in HIV-infected patients. Regular physical activity appears to be protective against the development of insulin resistance and hyperlipidemia in HIV infection,[55] but prospective studies of exercise effects on metabolic parameters are limited and have demonstrated mixed results with regard to insulin sensitivity. Yarasheski and colleagues[56] showed that 16 weeks of resistance exercise training reduced triglyceride levels but did not reduce insulin concentrations in 18 HIV-infected men on antiretroviral therapy. Of note, the subjects studied by Yarasheski et al were not selected for specific metabolic abnormalities. In contrast, Driscoll et al[57] demonstrated significant added reductions in insulin resistance with aerobic and resistance training above and beyond the benefits of metformin therapy in HIV-infected patients with lipodystrophy and hyperinsulinemia. Additional studies are needed to fully assess the role of diet and exercise in the amelioration or prevention of insulin resistance and type 2 diabetes in HIV-infected patients receiving antiretroviral therapy.

CLINICAL RECOMMENDATION FOR GLUCOSE MONITORING

It is recommended that all HIV-infected patients undergo monitoring of fasting blood glucose yearly and after the initiation of new antiretroviral agents.[58] Testing with the 2-h 75 g OGTT may also be useful to diagnose IGT. Assessment of insulin levels is an excellent research tool, but clinical standards to define insulin resistance have not yet been developed. Patients with diabetes mellitus should be treated according to clinical guidelines, with the caveat that oral hypoglycemics have not been tested in this population and may be less effective if severe insulin resistance exists. Treatment of patients with IGT may be reasonable with metformin, especially in the context of severe visceral fat hypertrophy. Among patients with insulin resistance and severe lipoatrophy, use of a thiazolidinedione may be considered, but possible exacerbation of preexisting hyperlipidemia should be considered.

SUMMARY

Insulin resistance and diabetes are increasingly recognized as potential consequences of chronic HIV infection and long-term exposure to antiretroviral therapy. Insulin resistance may result from direct effects of HIV and inflammation, direct effects of specific antiretroviral agents, or via effects of fat redistribution. Insulin resistance in combination with hyperlipidemia may confer increased risk of cardiovascular disease and constitute important targets for risk modification. Prompt recognition and management of diabetes in this patient population is important, but studies are ongoing to determine whether insulin sensitizing strategies, among those with insulin resistance, but without clinical diabetes, may be useful to decrease cardiovascular risk.

REFERENCES

1. Hadigan C, Meigs JB, Corcoran C, et al. Metabolic abnormalities and cardiovascular disease risk factors in adults with human immunodeficiency virus infection and lipodystrophy. Clin Infect Dis 32:130–9, 2001.

2. Brown TT, Cole SR, Li X, et al. Antiretroviral therapy and the prevalence and incidence of diabetes mellitus in the multicenter AIDS cohort study. Arch Intern Med 165:1179–84, 2005.
3. Justman JE, Benning L, Danoff A, et al. Protease inhibitor use and the incidence of diabetes mellitus in a large cohort of HIV-infected women. J Acquir Immune Defic Syndr 32:298–302, 2003.
4. Friis-Moller N, Sabin CA, Weber R, et al. Combination antiretroviral therapy and the risk of myocardial infarction. N Engl J Med 349:1993–2003, 2003.
5. Part 1: Diagnosis and classification of diabetes mellitus. In: Definition, diagnosis and classification of diabetes mellitus and its complications. Geneva: World Health Organization; 1999, p 59.
6. American Diabetes Association. Diagnosis and classification of diabetes mellitus. Diabetes Care 28(Suppl 1):S37–S42, 2005.
7. Kannel WB, McGee DL. Diabetes and cardiovascular disease. The Framingham study. JAMA 241:2035–8, 1979.
8. Kannel WB, McGee DL. Diabetes and glucose tolerance as risk factors for cardiovascular disease: the Framingham study. Diabetes Care 2:120–6, 1979.
9. Coutinho M, Gerstein HC, Wang Y, et al. The relationship between glucose and incident cardiovascular events. A meta-regression analysis of published data from 20 studies of 95,783 individuals followed for 12.4 years. Diabetes Care 22:233–40, 1999.
10. Stamler J, Vaccaro O, Neaton JD, et al. Diabetes, other risk factors, and 12-yr cardiovascular mortality for men screened in the Multiple Risk Factor Intervention Trial. Diabetes Care 16:434–44, 1993.
11. Knowler WC, Barrett-Connor E, Fowler SE, et al. Reduction in the incidence of type 2 diabetes with lifestyle intervention or metformin. N Engl J Med 346:393–403, 2002.
12. Matthews DR, Hosker JP, Rudenski AS, et al. Homeostasis model assessment: insulin resistance and beta-cell function from fasting plasma glucose and insulin concentrations in man. Diabetologia 28:412–19, 1985.
13. Hadigan C, Miller K, Corcoran C, et al. Fasting hyperinsulinemia and changes in regional body composition in human immunodeficiency virus-infected women. J Clin Endocrinol Metab 84:1932–7, 1999.
14. Hadigan C, Corcoran C, Stanley T, et al. Fasting hyperinsulinemia in human immunodeficiency virus-infected men: relationship to body composition, gonadal function, and protease inhibitor use. J Clin Endocrinol Metab 85:35–41, 2000.
15. Walli R, Herfort O, Michl GM, et al. Treatment with protease inhibitors associated with peripheral insulin resistance and impaired oral glucose tolerance in HIV-1-infected patients. AIDS 12:F167–73, 1998.
16. Carr A, Samaras K, Thorisdottir A, et al. Diagnosis, prediction, and natural course of HIV-1 protease-inhibitor-associated lipodystrophy, hyperlipidaemia, and diabetes mellitus: a cohort study. Lancet 353:2093–9, 1999.
17. Howard AA, Floris-Moore M, Arnsten JH, et al. Disorders of glucose metabolism among HIV-infected women. Clin Infect Dis 40:1492–9, 2005.
18. Danoff A, Shi Q, Justman J, et al. Oral glucose tolerance and insulin sensitivity are unaffected by HIV infection or antiretroviral therapy in overweight women. J Acquir Immune Defic Syndr 39:55–62, 2005.
19. Bitnun A, Sochett E, Dick PT, et al. Insulin sensitivity and beta-cell function in protease inhibitor-treated and -naive human immunodeficiency virus-infected children. J Clin Endocrinol Metab 90:168–74, 2005.
20. Beregszaszi M, Dollfus C, Levine M, et al. Longitudinal evaluation and risk factors of lipodystrophy and associated metabolic changes in HIV-infected children. J Acquir Immune Defic Syndr 40:161–8, 2005.
21. Murata H, Hruz PW, Mueckler M. The mechanism of insulin resistance caused by HIV protease inhibitor therapy. J Biol Chem 275:20251–4, 2000.
22. Dolan SE, Hadigan C, Killilea KM, et al. Increased cardiovascular disease risk indices in HIV-infected women. J Acquir Immune Defic Syndr 39:44–54, 2005.
23. Mynarcik DC, McNurlan MA, Steigbigel RT, et al. Association of severe insulin resistance with both loss of limb fat and elevated serum tumor necrosis factor receptor levels in HIV lipodystrophy. J Acquir Immune Defic Syndr 25:312–21, 2000.
24. Mallal SA, John M, Moore CB, et al. Contribution of nucleoside analogue reverse transcriptase inhibitors to subcutaneous fat wasting in patients with HIV infection. AIDS 14:1309–16, 2000.
25. Brown TT, Li X, Cole SR, et al. Cumulative exposure to nucleoside analogue reverse transcriptase inhibitors is associated with insulin resistance markers in the Multicenter AIDS Cohort Study. AIDS 19:1375–83, 2005.
26. Meininger G, Hadigan C, Rietschel P, et al. Body-composition measurements as predictors of glucose and insulin abnormalities in HIV-positive men. Am J Clin Nutr 76:460–5, 2002.
27. Kosmiski LA, Kuritzkes DR, Lichtenstein KA, et al. Fat distribution and metabolic changes are strongly correlated and energy expenditure is increased in the HIV lipodystrophy syndrome. AIDS 15:1993–2000, 2001.
28. Hadigan C, Kamin D, Liebau J, et al. Depot specific regulation of glucose uptake and insulin sensitivity in HIV-lipodystrophy. Am J Physiol Endocrinol Metab 290:289–298, 2005.
29. Lagathu C, Bastard JP, Auclair M, et al. Antiretroviral drugs with adverse effects on adipocyte lipid metabolism and survival alter the expression and secretion of proinflammatory cytokines and adiponectin in vitro. Antivir Ther 9:911–20, 2004.
30. Noor MA, Lo JC, Mulligan K, et al. Metabolic effects of indinavir in healthy HIV-seronegative men. AIDS 15:F11–8, 2001.
31. Noor MA, Seneviratne T, Aweeka FT, et al. Indinavir acutely inhibits insulin-stimulated glucose disposal in humans: a randomized, placebo-controlled study. AIDS 16:F1–8, 2002.
32. Noor MA, Parker RA, O'Mara E, et al. The effects of HIV protease inhibitors atazanavir and lopinavir/ritonavir on insulin sensitivity in HIV-seronegative healthy adults. AIDS 18:2137–44, 2004.
33. Petersen KF, Dufour S, Befroy D, et al. Reversal of nonalcoholic hepatic steatosis, hepatic insulin resistance, and hyperglycemia by moderate weight reduction in patients with type 2 diabetes. Diabetes 54:603–8, 2005.
34. Hadigan C, Borgonha S, Rabe J, et al. Increased rates of lipolysis among HIV-infected men receiving highly active antiretroviral therapy. Metabolism 51:1143–7, 2002.
35. Sekhar RV, Jahoor F, White AC, et al. Metabolic basis of HIV-lipodystrophy syndrome. Am J Physiol Endocrinol Metab 283: E332–7, 2002.
36. Gan SK, Samaras K, Thompson CH, et al. Altered myocellular and abdominal fat partitioning predict disturbance in insulin action in HIV protease inhibitor-related lipodystrophy. Diabetes 51:3163–9, 2002.
37. Reeds DN, Yarasheski KE, Fontana L, et al. Alterations in liver, muscle, and adipose tissue insulin sensitivity in men with HIV infection and dyslipidemia. Am J Physiol Endocrinol Metab 290(1):E47–E53, 2005.
38. Behrens GM, Boerner AR, Weber K, et al. Impaired glucose phosphorylation and transport in skeletal muscle cause insulin resistance in HIV-1-infected patients with lipodystrophy. J Clin Invest 110:1319–27, 2002.
39. Hadigan C, Rabe J, Meininger G, et al. Inhibition of lipolysis improves insulin sensitivity in protease inhibitor-treated HIV-infected men with fat redistribution. Am J Clin Nutr 77:490–4, 2003.

40. Lindegaard B, Petersen AM, Plomgaard P, et al. Suppression of lipolysis decreases skeletal muscle insulin resistance in HIV-infected patients with lipodystrophy. Antivir Ther 10:L32, 2005.
41. Tong Q, Sankale JL, Hadigan CM, et al. Regulation of adiponectin in human immunodeficiency virus-infected patients: relationship to body composition and metabolic indices. J Clin Endocrinol Metab 88:1559–64, 2003.
42. Mehta SH, Brancati FL, Sulkowski MS, et al. Prevalence of type 2 diabetes mellitus among persons with hepatitis C virus infection in the United States. Ann Intern Med 133:592–9, 2000.
43. Visnegarwala F, Chen L, Raghavan S, et al. Prevalence of diabetes mellitus and dyslipidemia among antiretroviral naive patients co-infected with hepatitis C virus (HCV) and HIV-1 compared to patients without co-infection. J Infect 50:331–7, 2005.
44. Saint-Marc T, Touraine JL. Effects of metformin on insulin resistance and central adiposity in patients receiving effective protease inhibitor therapy. AIDS 13:1000–2, 1999.
45. Tomazic J, Karner P, Vidmar L, et al. Effect of metformin and rosiglitazone on lipid metabolism in HIV infected patients receiving protease inhibitor containing HAART. Acta Dermatovenerol Alp Panonica Adriat 14:99–105, 2005.
46. Hadigan C, Yawetz S, Thomas A, et al. Metabolic effects of rosiglitazone in HIV lipodystrophy: A randomized controlled trial. Ann Intern Med 140:786–94, 2004.
47. Carr A, Workman C, Carey D, et al. No effect of rosiglitazone for treatment of HIV-1 lipoatrophy: randomized, double-blind, placebo-controlled trial. Lancet 363:429–38, 2004.
48. Sutinen J, Hakkinen AM, Westerbacka J, et al. Rosiglitazone in the treatment of HAART-associated lipodystrophy – a randomized double-blind placebo-controlled study. Antivir Ther 8:199–207, 2003.
49. Hadigan C, Corcoran C, Basgoz N, et al. Metformin in the treatment of HIV lipodystrophy syndrome: A randomized controlled trial. JAMA 284:472–7, 2000.
50. van Wijk JP, de Koning EJ, Cabezas MC, et al. Comparison of rosiglitazone and metformin for treating HIV lipodystrophy: a randomized trial. Ann Intern Med 143:337–46, 2005.
51. Gelato MC, Mynarcik DC, Quick JL, et al. Improved insulin sensitivity and body fat distribution in HIV-infected patients treated with rosiglitazone: a pilot study. J Acquir Immune Defic Syndr 31:163–70, 2002.
52. Jemsek JG, Arathoon E, Arlotti M, et al. Body fat and other metabolic effects of atazanavir and efavirenz, each administered in combination with zidovudine plus lamivudine, in antiretroviral-naive HIV-infected patients. Clin Infect Dis 42:273–80, 2006.
53. Tebas P, Yarasheski K, Henry K, et al. Evaluation of the virological and metabolic effects of switching protease inhibitor combination antiretroviral therapy to nevirapine-based therapy for the treatment of HIV infection. AIDS Res Hum Retroviruses 20:589–94, 2004.
54. Carr A, Workman C, Smith DE, et al. Abacavir substitution for nucleoside analogs in patients with HIV lipoatrophy: a randomized trial. JAMA 288:207–15, 2002.
55. Gavrila A, Tsiodras S, Doweiko J, et al. Exercise and vitamin E intake are independently associated with metabolic abnormalities in human immunodeficiency virus-positive subjects: a cross-sectional study. Clin Infect Dis 36:1593–601, 2003.
56. Yarasheski KE, Tebas P, Stanerson B, et al. Resistance exercise training reduces hypertriglyceridemia in HIV-infected men treated with antiviral therapy. J Appl Physiol 90:133–8, 2001.
57. Driscoll SD, Meininger GE, Lareau MT, et al. Effects of exercise training and metformin on body composition and cardiovascular indices in HIV infected patients. AIDS 18:465–73, 2004.
58. Schambelan M, Benson CA, Carr A, et al. Management of metabolic complications associated with antiretroviral therapy for HIV-1 infection: recommendations of an International AIDS Society-USA panel. J Acquir Immune Defic Syndr 31:257–75, 2002.
59. Gelato MC. Insulin and carbohydrate dysregulation. Clin Infect Dis 36(Suppl 2):S91–5, 2003.
60. Katz A, Nambi SS, Mather K, et al. Quantitative insulin sensitivity check index: a simple, accurate method for assessing insulin sensitivity in humans. J Clin Endocrinol Metab 85:2402–10, 2000.
61. Yokoyama H, Emoto M, Fujiwara S, et al. Quantitative insulin sensitivity check index and the reciprocal index of homeostasis model assessment are useful indexes of insulin resistance in type 2 diabetic patients with wide range of fasting plasma glucose. J Clin Endocrinol Metab 89:1481–4, 2004.
62. Katsuki A, Urakawa H, Gabazza EC, et al. Quantitative insulin sensitivity check index is a useful indicator of insulin resistance in Japanese metabolically obese, normal-weight subjects with normal glucose tolerance. Endocr J 52:253–7, 2005.
63. Bonora E, Targher G, Alberiche M, et al. Homeostasis model assessment closely mirrors the glucose clamp technique in the assessment of insulin sensitivity: studies in subjects with various degrees of glucose tolerance and insulin sensitivity. Diabetes Care 23:57–63, 2000.
64. Boston RC, Stefanovski D, Moate PJ, et al. MINMOD Millennium: a computer program to calculate glucose effectiveness and insulin sensitivity from the frequently sampled intravenous glucose tolerance test. Diabetes Technol Ther 5:1003–15, 2003.
65. Radziuk J. Insulin sensitivity and its measurement: structural commonalities among the methods. J Clin Endocrinol Metab 85:4426–33, 2000.
66. Bergman RN, Prager R, Volund A, et al. Equivalence of the insulin sensitivity index in man derived by the minimal model method and the euglycemic glucose clamp. J Clin Invest 79:790–800, 1987.
67. DeFronzo RA, Tobin JD, Andres R. Glucose clamp technique: A method for quantifying insulin secretion and resistance. Am J Physiol 237:E214–23, 1979.
68. Martinez E, Domingo P, Ribera E, et al. Effects of metformin or gemfibrozil on the lipodystrophy of HIV-infected patients receiving protease inhibitors. Antivir Ther 8:403–10, 2003.

Chapter 72

Lipid Disorders

Peter Reiss, MD, PhD, Marc van der Valk, MD, PhD

INTRODUCTION

The use of highly active antiretroviral therapy (HAART)[1–3] is frequently associated with side effects. Among the most significant of these is lipodystrophy, manifested as an abnormal distribution of body fat. Characteristically fat is lost subcutaneously, particularly from the face, limbs, and buttocks, and visceral fat may be increased.[4–6] In addition to these changes in fat distribution, a large proportion of patients develop insulin resistance (*see* Chapter 70) and elevated plasma lipid concentrations. The combination of dyslipidemia, insulin resistance, and visceral fat accumulation closely resembles the abnormalities seen in 'the metabolic syndrome'[7] and has given rise to the concern that HIV-1-infected patients treated with potent combination antiretroviral therapy (ART) may be at increased risk of developing premature coronary artery disease (CAD). In this chapter we discuss the evidence so far with respect to this concern, discuss the differential effects of antiretroviral drugs on plasma lipid concentrations, review current hypotheses with respect to the pathogenesis of dyslipidemia, and address recommendations for its treatment and prevention. However, this cannot be discussed without first addressing the effects HIV infection itself has on plasma lipid concentrations and cardiovascular risk.

DYSLIPIDEMIA AND CAD DURING THE NATURAL COURSE OF HIV INFECTION

Early in the natural course of HIV infection, as seen in other infections and chronic inflammatory conditions, plasma total cholesterol (TC), high-density lipoprotein cholesterol (HDL-C) and low-density lipoprotein cholesterol (LDL-C) concentrations slightly decrease.[8,9] This decrease is followed by a decrease in the size of LDL particles leading to an increase in more atherogenic small dense LDL particles (LDL type B).[10] Late in the infection, when patients progress to a clinical diagnosis of AIDS, triglyceride concentrations may increase as well.[9] This latter increase is probably caused by both an increased production of triglyceride-rich VLDL particles and a decreased clearance of VLDL by the liver. This correlates closely with circulating concentrations of interferon-α which is strongly related with disease progression in untreated HIV-1-infected patients.[11] Consistent with this notion, both triglycerides and interferon-α levels were described to decrease in patients with advanced HIV disease using zidovudine monotherapy.[12] Recently, Riddler et al published a longitudinal study of investigated lipid profiles in HIV seroconverters (Table 72-1).[13] This study confirmed the previous findings from cross-sectional studies showing decreases in total, LDL, and HDL-C following seroconversion but prior to the initiation of HAART in asymptomatic HIV-infected individuals with a mean CD4-cell count of 307/μL at the time of second measurement.

Several cases and a single case-control study concerning CAD in patients with HIV infection have been published in the pre-HAART era. A small series of eight necropsies was described by Tabib in 1992 which demonstrated significant coronary lesions in deceased young HIV-infected patients (23–32 years old).[14] None of these patients had a known positive family history for coronary heart disease (CHD) or other known risk factors. All eight subjects showed fibrosis of their coronary arteries with foam cells, generally widely disseminated occluding 40–50% of the coronary arterial lumens similar to the lesions generally seen in older populations and quite distinct from the concentric pattern of the accelerated forms of (postgrafting) coronary disease. These results were confirmed in a relatively small case-control study using ultrasound showing an increased incidence of asymptomatic plaques in peripheral arteries in HIV-1-infected individuals compared to matched controls.[15]

Table 72-1 Plasma Lipid Changes After HIV-Seroconversion

	Pre Seroconversion	Post Seroconversion
Total-C (mg/dL)	201 (5.26 mmol/L)	−30 (−0.78 mmol/L)
HDL-C (mg/dL)	51 (1.35 mmol/L)	−12 (−0.31 mmol/L)
LDL-C (mg/dL)	122 (3.13 mmol/L)	−22 (−0.57 mmol/L)

Plasma lipid changes following HIV-1 seroconversion.

Mg/dL: milligram per deciliter.

mmol/L: millimol per liter.

Total-C: total cholesterol; HDL-C: high density lipoprotein cholesterol; LDL-C low density lipoprotein cholesterol.

DYSLIPIDEMIA AND CARDIOVASCULAR RISK DURING HAART

Soon after the introduction of HAART several case reports were published suggesting that patients receiving HAART were prone to the development of premature CAD.[5,16–18] This concern led to numerous studies addressing the question as to whether HAART is an independent risk factor for CAD. When addressing this question, it is very important to take into account the prevalence of known cardiovascular risk factors in the HIV-infected population being studied. For instance, the Data collection of Adverse effects of anti-HIV Drugs (D:A:D) study,[19] found that HIV-1-infected patients (both treated or therapy-naive; $n = 17\,852$ patients) showed an above average prevalence of various well-known risk factors for CAD. For instance, 50% of all HIV-infected individuals were current smokers compared to 30–40% in the general population. Furthermore, 8% of patients at the time of enrollment into this study had hypertension, 22% had elevated TC, 28% elevated triglyceride concentrations, and 25% were 45 years of age or older.

Retrospective Studies

The largest retrospective analysis of whether HAART results in an increased incidence of CAD is a study by Bozzette et al who extracted data from the Master Veteran Record National Database and VA National Patient Care databases in the United States (Table 72-2). These anonimized databases contain information on virtually all patients receiving care within the VA system.[20] In this study 36 766 HIV-1-infected patients (almost exclusively men) were followed for an average of 40 months from 1993 to 2001 (total patient-years of follow-up (PYFU) 121 936 years). The authors concluded that the overall incidence of cardiovascular and cerebrovascular events did not change over time. Furthermore, the authors did not find an increased incidence of CAD in the patients taking protease-inhibitor (PI)-based HAART compared to patients that did not. One important issue that might have biased the interpretation of the results is the fact that only patients admitted to a VA clinic were identified as cases. Since patients who receive ambulatory care within the VA system for acute coronary events are often admitted to hospitals outside of the system, this may have led to an underestimation of the true incidence of CAD. Furthermore, the duration of exposure to PI was relatively short (16 months). Another large study was published by Mary-Krause et al[21] utilizing the national French Hospital Database among 34 976 French HIV-1-infected men with a total of 88 029 PYFU. This study did find a relation between more prolonged use of PI and the occurrence of myocardial infarction (MI). Exposure to PI was associated with a relative hazard for MI of 2.56 (95%CI 1.03–6.34). The standardized morbidity ratio of men exposed to PI for >30 months compared to the general French male population, was 2.9 (range 1.5–5.0). The California Medicaid database consisting of 28 513 HIV-1-infected patients with 71 286 PYFU found that the overall incidence of CAD was increased for young men and women.[22] In 18–33-year-old men the relative risk was 2.16–6.76 ($P < 0.0001$), whereas in 18–44-year-old women this was 1.53–2.47 ($P < 0.011$) compared to matched healthy uninfected controls. The relatively small Kaiser Permanente registry study looked at discharge diagnoses in 4159 HIV-1-infected individuals with 14 823 PYFU.[23] They found an increased age-adjusted event rate of CAD (6.3 per 1000 patient-years) in HIV-1-infected individuals compared to HIV negative (3.7 per 1000 patient-years, $P < 0.01$). Of note is the fact that in those HIV-positive the prevalence of smoking was increased twofold in HIV-positive patients compared to the HIV-negative persons. In this latter study PI-usage was not identified as being an independent risk-factor for CAD.

Prospective Studies

Currently, there are two large prospectively designed cohort studies that have reported data regarding the incidence of coronary and cerebrovascular events in HIV-infected individuals (Table 72-2).

The largest cohort is the D:A:D.[24] This multicontinental study included cohorts from Europe, Australia, and the United States and consisted of 23 468 patients who had been included into the study between December 1999 and April 2001. During 36 199 PYFU, 126 MIs occurred. The incidence of MI increased with longer exposure to combination ART (adjusted relative rate per year of exposure, 1.26 (95% confidence interval (CI), 1.12–1.41); $P < 0.001$). This implies a 26% increase in the relative risk of having an MI per additional year of HAART usage. This effect was independent of a number of known CAD risk factors which were also significantly associated with MI, including older age (adjusted relative rate per additional 5 years, 1.38 (95% CI, 1.26–1.50); $P < 0.001$), history of current or former smoking (adjusted relative rate, 2.17 (95% CI, 1.30–3.62); $P = 0.007$), previous cardiovascular disease (adjusted relative rate, 5.84 (95% CI, 3.51–9.72); $P < 0.001$) and male gender (adjusted

Table 72-2

Cardiovascular Risk in Cohort Studies of HIV-Infected Individuals Using Art

	PYFU	Event Rate	Conclusions and Limitations
Retrospective Studies			
Veterans study[20]	1 21 936	N/A	No effect of HAART on CAD Ascertainment of events likely incomplete for patients receiving care for CAD outside of the VA system
French Hospital Database Cohort[21]	88 029	60 MI	Exposure to PI associated with increased risk of MI Degree of risk attributed to PI possibly overestimated as a result of insufficient information concerning known risk factors such as smoking and hypertension
California Medicaid[22]	71 286	410 MI	CAD risk increased with ART usage in young men and women compared to healthy age-matched controls
Kaiser Permanente[23]	14 823	47 MI	CAD risk increased compared to healthy matched controls Important limitation: smoking prevalence was twofold increased HIV vs non-HIV
Prospective Studies			
DAD[24]	36 199	126 MI	ART associated with increased risk of MI and cerebrovascular disease events
Updated analysis DAD[28]	76 577	277 MI	After adjustment for known risk factors including plasma lipids RR for MI 1.1 in HIV-infected individuals
HOPS[31]	17 712	21 MI	Greater risk of MI with PI usage

ART: antiretroviral therapy; PYFU: patient years of follow up; MI: myocardial infraction; RR: relative risk; PI: protease inhibitor; CAD: coronary artery disease.

relative rate, 1.99 (95% CI, 1.04–3.79; $P = 0.04$). A higher total serum cholesterol level, a higher triglyceride level, and the presence of diabetes were also associated with an increased incidence of MI. As noted before the prevalence of known cardiovascular risk factors was high in this population (56% of the total population were either current or former smokers). A substudy from D:A:D demonstrated differential effects of different types of regimens on plasma lipoprotein profiles in previously therapy-naive HIV-1-infected patients.[25] In the majority of patients first-line therapy consisted of a backbone of two nucleoside reverse transcriptase inhibitors (NRTIs) with the addition of either a PI, or a non-nucleoside reverse transcriptase inhibitor (NNRTI). The PI-based regimens resulted in a potentially more atherogenic lipid profile compared to both therapy-naive and NNRTI-based regimes. This differential effect is similar to the results previously found in a prospective randomized clinical trial comparing PI with NNRTI-based therapy.[26,27] A recent update from D:A:D showed that PI exposure was associated with an increased risk of MI which was markedly similar to that found in the initial analysis for exposure to combination ART as a whole (RR 1.16 (1.10–1.23), $P = 0.0001$).[28] This effect was not seen for NNRTI exposure. The effect of PI on the increased risk of MI could partly, but not fully, be explained by the dyslipidemia known to be induced by this drug class.

The original analysis within D:A:D with regard to MI has also been extended to cardiovascular and cerebrovascular disease events (CCVE).[29] The endpoint of this analysis was the occurrence of a first CCVE during prospective follow-up, defined as the first of any of the following events: acute MI, performance of an invasive cardiovascular procedure (specifically coronary artery angioplasty, bypass, or carotid artery endarterectomy), stroke, or death from other CCVE. A total of 268 events occurred in 207 patients over 36 145 PFYU. There were 134 MI among 126 patients (first event in 126 patients), 87 invasive cardiovascular procedures in 82 patients (first event in 39 patients), 41 strokes in 39 patients (first event in 38 patients), and six patients died from CCVE (first event in four patients). The multivariate analysis showed results similar to the original analysis which only looked at cases of first MI. Smoking, older age, a previous history of CCVE, a positive family history of CCVE or male gender were independently associated with an increased prevalence of CCVE. After controlling for these variables the incidence rate of CCVE increased by 26% per additional year of exposure to combination ART (RR per year of exposure, 1.26; 95% CI, 1.14–1.38; $P = 0.0001$). This analysis was not adjusted for current or previous antiretroviral agents used by patients. Additional analyses tested the association between CCVE and a number of possible metabolic and physiological causative factors. Factors independently associated with the risk of CCVE from these analyses were (time-updated): cholesterol (RR 1.11; 95% CI 1.03–1.19 per mmol higher; $P = 0.008$); triglycerides (RR 1.30; 95% CI 1.12–1.51 per $\log_2$ mmol higher; $P = 0.0006$); diabetes mellitus (RR 2.22; 95% CI 1.46–3.37; $P = 0.0002$); and hypertension (RR 1.79; 95% CI 1.25–2.56; $P = 0.001$). Adjustment for these factors in multivariable models that also included the risk factors for CCVE, led to a small reduction in the RR associated with exposure to ART, although this variable remained significantly associated with CCVE in all analyses (relative rates ranging from 1.21 to 1.25 in the individual analyses). A similar effect was recently reported within D:A:D for risk factors for a first MI, now including 277 cases of first MI during 76 577 PYFU.[30] The relative rate of MI per additional year of exposure to HAART, after adjusting for age, gender, history of smoking, prior CAD, and family history, was 1.17 (95% CI 1.08–1.26) in this updated analysis. After also adjusting for time-updated changes in total and HDL cholesterol as well as triglycerides, the relative rate was reduced to 1.10 (95% CI 1.01–1.19). This again suggests that the association between HAART use and risk of MI may partly, but not completely, be explained by the effect of treatment on lipids.

The second large prospective cohort study is the HIV Outpatient Study (HOPS) consisting of 5672 patients with 17712 PYFU.[31] The majority of patients were men (82%), and the incidence of MI rose over time. A total of 21 MIs occurred. Nineteen events were in patients on PI-containing regimens resulting in an odds ratio of 1.42 per 1000 person-years of observation, compared to only 2 in patients who did not use a PI (0.46 per 1000 person-years of observation). Controlling for known CAD risk factors showed similar results. These findings suggest the risk of CAD is increased in patients using PI-based therapy.

Surrogate Endpoints

In recent years several noninvasive imaging tools have been introduced for assessing atherosclerosis progression/regression in the general population, as potential surrogates for clinical endpoints (Table 72-3). A recent paper by Sankatsing et al provides an extensive overview of these different techniques.[32]

The technique most frequently utilized in HIV-infected individuals is the measurement of carotid intima-media thickness (IMT) by high-resolution B-mode ultrasonography. This noninvasive technique allows for real-time *in vivo* imaging of all stages of atherosclerosis and offers a good reproducibility under standardized conditions. Three large observational studies have shown that carotid IMT in the general population is an independent risk factor for CAD and can be used as a surrogate marker for cardiovascular disease.[33–35] In numerous intervention studies with statins conducted in the general population, carotid IMT has proven to be a reliable parameter to assess efficacy of lipid-lowering therapy.[36,37] Moreover carotid IMT is strongly correlated with other cardiovascular risk factors such as LDL-C and HDL-C and hypertension. However, a potential problem may lie in the great variability between available measurement protocols.

Following the report by Seminari et al in 2002 of a small cross-sectional study suggestive of increased carotid IMT values in patients with PI-induced hyperlipidemia,[38] several larger studies have been published with different results.

Table 72-3

Cardiovascular Surrogate Markers Studied in HIV-Infected Individuals

	n	Study Type	Conclusions and Limitations
Intima Media Thickness (IMT)			
Seminari et al[38]	28	Cross-sectional cohort	HIV-PI (n = 28) vs HIV-naive (n = 15) vs healthy (n = 16) IMT HIV PI > naive and HIV-negative difference explained by elevated plasma lipids. Small study
Martin[39]	154	Cross-sectional cohort	IMT increased with PI-usage Limitation: therapy not specified
Maggi[41]	293	Cross-sectional cohort	PI usage associated with increased IMT Limitation: risk factors not equal between groups
Hsue[42]	211	Prospective cohort	HIV (n = 148); healthy controls (n = 63) IMT increase associated with traditional risk factors Limitation: Smoking HIV 55% vs 25% in healthy group
Currier[40]	134	Prospective matched cohort	HIV-PI (n = 44) vs HIV-non-PI (n = 45) vs healthy (n = 45) IMT increase associated with traditional risk factors. No association with PI-usage or HIV-status
Mercie[43]	423	Prospective cohort	IMT increase associated with traditional risk factors
Thiebaut[44]	233	Prospective cohort	Initial IMT increase which decreased after 3 years of follow-up as a result of therapeutic interventions (statin/fibrate/HIV-therapy modification)
FMD of Brachial Artery			
Nolan[45]	48	Cross-sectional	HIV-PI (n = 24) vs healthy (n = 24) No difference in FMD between arms despite differences in plasma lipids
Stein[46]	37	Cross-sectional	HIV-PI (n = 22) vs HIV-naive (n = 15) FMD impaired in HIV-PI group associated with elevated plasma lipids

FMD: flow mediated dilation of the brachial artery; *n*: number of patients included; PI: protease inhibitor; healthy: healthy controls.

The key issues when interpreting the results of all of these studies are whether the effects seen on carotid IMT directly result from any of the individual antiretroviral agents being used, or are secondary to therapy-induced lipid changes, as well as to the influence of HIV itself, the immune system and other known CAD risk factors.

A recent single-center cross-sectional cohort study by Martin et al examined 154 patients and found that carotid IMT was significantly correlated with known cardiovascular risk factors including systolic blood pressure, plasma lipoprotein and glucose concentrations and age.[39] Before adjustment for such cardiovascular risk factors the cumulative exposure to PI but not NRTI or NNRTI was correlated with carotid IMT ($P = 0.02$). Unfortunately, the authors did not specify the exact number of patients in the different treatment groups making it very hard to interpret these results. After adjustment for known cardiovascular risk factors the cumulative exposure to lopinavir/ritonavir (RTV) remained correlated with carotid IMT ($P = 0.01$). Interestingly, in 35 patients without a history of prior cardiovascular events, who either had carotid IMT values greater than 0.75 mm and/or a Framingham risk score greater than 3, the authors performed myocardial perfusion scintigraphy during exercise and did not identify a single case who would qualify for a cardiovascular intervention.

A prospective matched cohort study by Currier et al compared HIV-infected individuals using PI-based therapy for more than 2 years ($n = 44$), with those who did not ($n = 45$) and with an HIV-uninfected control group ($n = 45$). All were matched for age, sex, ethnicity, smoking status, blood pressure, and menopausal status.[40] This study found an association between carotid IMT and traditional CAD risk factors but not with HIV infection or with the use of PI.

A cross-sectional cohort study of 293 patients by Maggi et al concluded that PI-treated patients ($n = 105$) had a higher prevalence of premature carotid lesions. However, patients were not matched for cigarette smoking and family history of cardiovascular disease which represents an important potential bias.[41] Hsue et al in a prospective study demonstrated that carotid IMT was increased in 148 HIV-infected individuals compared to healthy controls and was clearly related to traditional risk factors.[42] Again, there was a significant difference in the percentage of smoking between the groups (HIV-infected 55% vs 25% in non-HIV-infected, $P < 0.01$). In another large prospective cohort study with 1 year follow-up ($n = 346$) Mercie et al likewise concluded that traditional risk factors were associated with an increase in carotid IMT.[43] In light of the latter two studies Thiebaut et al published a prospective cohort study with 3 years of follow-up in 233 HIV-infected individuals (86% using HAART at baseline) that clearly showed that although carotid IMT initially increased at 12 months it normalized to baseline values at 36 months of follow-up.[44] This decrease seemed to be largely driven by increased prescribing of statins and/or fibrates and/or switching to more lipid-friendly antiretroviral regimens which resulted in a decrease in total and LDL cholesterol, which may have been the result of an increased awareness among physicians concerning CAD risk in patients with HIV.

A very early sign of atherogenesis which precedes the occurrence of atherosclerotic lesions is endothelial dysfunction which can be measured using flow-mediated dilatation (FMD) of the brachial artery and is associated with all known risk factors such as hypertension, smoking, hypercholesterolemia and diabetes mellitus. Two small studies showed contrary results with respect to the effect of PI on FMD.[45,46] Related to this, a study by Dressman et al in mice suggested that PI may not only affect endothelial atherosclerosis indirectly through effects on lipids, but also directly through other mechanisms.[47] Mice in this study were treated with the PI RTV, indinavir or amprenavir at both low and high doses for 8 weeks. At high doses plasma triglycerides and TC levels increased (RTV > indinavir > amprenavir), whereas at low doses no changes in plasma lipoproteins were observed in that study. When the ascending aortas from these mice were examined, extensive atherosclerotic lesions were observed in both groups, albeit more so at high rather than low doses of PI. Therefore, the development of atherosclerosis in these mice seemed at least in part independent of the induction of dyslipidemia. The direct effect of PI was mediated by an up-regulation of the scavenger receptor CD36 in macrophages. The administration of PI to CD36 knock-out mice did not result in atherosclerosis.

With respect to the possible direct effects of PI on endothelial function in humans, 4 weeks of treatment with indinavir in healthy HIV-negative men resulted in significantly impaired endothelial function in the absence of significant effects on plasma lipoprotein concentrations.[48] The authors speculate that this effect was induced by an impairment of nitric oxide production at the level of the endothelium which was previously demonstrated *in vitro*.[49] The administration of indinavir in these healthy men did result in statistically significant reduction in insulin sensitivity. Based on earlier studies, this probably results from a direct impairment of the activity of the glucose transporter GLUT-4 by indinavir.[50–55] However, since the observed changes in insulin concentrations were relatively small and not correlated with changes in endothelial function the authors suggested that an as yet unexplained direct effect of PI on endothelial function may exist. Several recent *in vitro* studies demonstrated that another PI RTV decreases endothelium-dependent vasorelaxation in cultured porcine carotid arteries.[56–59] This seemed to be mediated by an increase in superoxide anion production resulting in increased oxidative stress. Bonnet et al, in a cross-sectional case-control study of endothelial function and carotid IMT in HIV-infected children (including a large proportion of therapy-naive patients), reported endothelial function to be impaired in both treatment-naive and treated HIV-infected children compared to age- and sex-matched healthy children, whereas no changes in carotid IMT were found.[60] No differences were found between treated and therapy-naive children. Since most of the traditional risk factors for CAD are not present in children, this strongly suggests that HIV infection itself may contribute to the development of

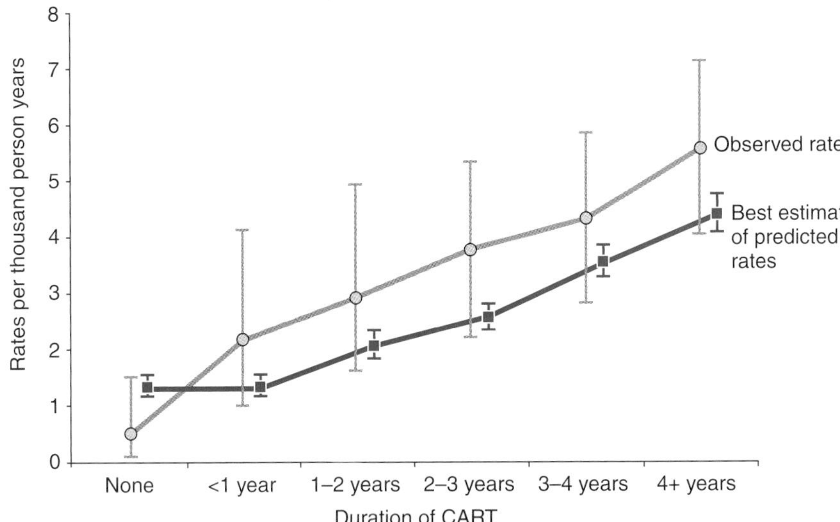

Figure 72-1 ■ Observed and predicted rates of myocardial infarction by duration of CART.

Reprinted with permission from Law et al. The Use of the Framingham Equation to Predict Myocardial Infarctions in HIV-infected Patients: Comparison with Observed Events in the D:A:D Study' HIV Medicine.[62]

endothelial dysfunction. Indirect evidence for this is also provided by the results of a recent AIDS Clinical Trials Group (ACTG) study A5152s.[61] In this large randomized clinical trial which compares PI-sparing (2 NRTIs + efavirenz) with NNRTI-sparing (2 NRTIs + lopinavir/RTV) and NRTI-sparing (efavirenz + lopinavir/RTV) therapy in previously antiretroviral-naive patients endothelial function was prospectively assessed in a subgroup of 82 patients. Although the investigators remain blinded to the actual treatment, significant improvements in endothelial function as measured by FMD of the brachial artery were seen following 24 weeks of therapy in each of the treatment arms. Interestingly, although significant differences were observed between treatments with respect to changes in plasma lipoproteins, no consistent correlation could be found between changes in FMD and changes in any lipoproteins. This again suggests that HIV infection *per se* may have an effect on endothelial function which may be reversed by suppressing HIV at least over the short term.

As indicated before, an updated analysis from the D:A:D study suggests that the association between HAART use and risk of MI may partly, but not completely, be explained by the effect of treatment on lipids.[30] This may also explain why the rate of MI which was observed in D:A:D was consistently higher than the one predicted when using the Framingham algorithm[62] (Fig. 72-1). Another potential explanation may be that the D:A:D population is younger than the one on which the Framingham algorithm has been based, and many of the same CVD risk factors are known to carry a higher risk in younger compared to older individuals. Importantly, both curves are parallel which suggests that algorithms such as Framingham can reasonably be used clinically for broadly assessing CAD risk in patients with HIV until an algorithm has been developed which is specific to HIV-infected populations. However, given that changes in plasma lipid profiles do explain at least some of the incremental risk of MI, differences between individual drugs and ART regimens on lipids are important to address.

Antiretroviral Drugs/Drug Classes: Effects on Plasma Lipids

Soon after the first indication that ART might be associated with hyperlipidemia the measurement of plasma lipid profiles was incorporated in many randomized clinical trials. As briefly mentioned before it became clear that different antiretroviral regimens differ with respect to their effects on plasma lipids. For instance, patients at time of entry into the D:A:D study who were on first-line regimens including PIs had higher TC and triglyceride concentrations as well as higher TC over HDL cholesterol ratios than did antiretroviral-naive patients.[25] In contrast, NNRTI-based therapy showed a potentially more cardio-protective plasma lipoprotein profile, by virtue of being associated with higher levels of HDL-C. Similar results were reported by Young et al from the Swiss HIV cohort study.[63]

NON-NUCLEOSIDE REVERSE TRANSCRIPTASE INHIBITORS

Treatment with a nevirapine-containing regimen in a trial conducted in antiretroviral-naive patients was associated with a 49% increase in HDL cholesterol and a decrease in the ratio of TC over HDL-cholesterol when compared to an indinavir-based regimen as well as a regimen consisting of three nucleosides, in the absence of significant differences in antiviral potency.[26] The study which has provided the best data comparing the effect of nevirapine and efavirenz is the 2NN study. In this trial, again conducted in previously ART-naive patients, both nevirapine- and efavirenz-containing regimens showed increases in HDL-C and a reduction in the ratio of total over HDL cholesterol, with these changes being most profound in the nevirapine-treated patients.[64] Both in the 2NN and D:A:D study, efavirenz-based therapy was associated with a higher plasma triglyceride concentration, whereas this was not the case for nevirapine-containing regimens.[25] Treatment with delavirdine resulted in a 13.2% increase in HDL-C after 8 weeks of treatment, whereas no changes were observed in PI-treated patients.[65]

Taken together, these data suggest that the pronounced effect on HDL-C may be a characteristic of NNRTI as a class. However, at this time data on HDL-C is not available for the new NNRTI etravirine (TMC-125).

PROTEASE INHIBITORS

In data from the D:A:D-study,[25] RTV-containing therapy, when used as a booster in combination with other PI or in its therapeutic dose, was associated with the most pronounced elevations in TC, ratio of total over HDL-C, and triglycerides. Saquinavir- and nelfinavir (NFV)-containing regimens were associated with a lesser likelihood of such changes. When all studies are put into perspective, of all the PIs RTV has the most pronounced effects on plasma lipids, and particularly on triglycerides. The effects of RTV are dose dependent. However, a recent study in healthy volunteers showed that even a dose as low as 100 mg bid of RTV monotherapy resulted in a 10% increase in TC, 16% in LDL-C, and a 26% increase in triglycerides.[66]

A large study compared NFV- versus RTV-boosted lopinavir (r/LPV)-containing regimens in previously ART-naive patients. Forty-eight weeks of treatment with r/LPV resulted in 9% grade 3 or 4 elevations in both triglyceride and TC concentrations in the lopinavir arm, compared to 5% for TC and 1% for triglycerides in NFV-treated patients.[67] The mean increase in triglycerides was significantly higher in patients randomized to lopinavir compared to NFV ($P < 0.001$). In a large observational cohort study of patients initiating lopinavir/RTV-based therapy, Martinez et al likewise reported significant increases in triglycerides in a substantial proportion of patients.[68]

Another trial compared RTV-boosted saquinavir (r/SQV 100 mg/1000 mg bid) with r/LPV-based regimens (100 mg/400 mg bid) in 324 patients.[69] This population was a mixture of antiretroviral treatment-naive, as well as PI-naive or PI-experienced patients with either virological failure or intolerance to PI. After 48 weeks of treatment regimens containing r/LPV resulted in significantly higher triglyceride concentrations. No significant differences were found in TC and HDL cholesterol between the two arms. Similarly, the comparison of r/SQV (100 mg/1000 mg bid) with RTV-boosted indinavir (r/IDV) (100 mg/800 mg bid) by the same investigators in a similar patient population also showed a more favorable lipoprotein profile in patients randomized to r/SQV.[70]

In contrast to what has been observed for most of the PIs which have been available for quite some time, the more recently licensed PI atazanavir (ATV) has not been associated with clinically relevant increases in TC, LDL-C, or fasting triglyceride concentrations. In two separate trials in previously ART-naive patients ATV (400 mg qd) was compared to treatment with NFV (1250 mg bid).[71,72] A summary of the results from these two randomized clinical trials has been provided by Cahn et al.[73] NFV-treated patients demonstrated mean percent increases from baseline in fasting lipid concentrations of 25–28% for TC, 27–31% for LDL-C, and 40–50% for triglycerides. Mean percent changes in the same parameters at week 48 in the ATV treatment groups ranged from +5% to +7% for TC, −6 to +6% for LDL-C, and +2% to +7% for triglycerides. Comparable mean percent increases in HDL-C were observed between the ATV- and NFV-treatment arms within the individual trials. In the ATV-treatment groups, the proportions of patients with TC within desirable levels defined by the NCEP ATP III criteria (<200 mg/dL) were consistent between baseline and 48 weeks in both trials. In contrast, the proportion of NFV-treated patients with desirable TC levels decreased from 83% at baseline to 40–49% in both trials.[73]

Tipranavir is the PI which has most recently been licensed in the US, and in Europe. It has primarily been developed for use in patients failing prior PI-containing regimens. Two pivotal phase III trials (RESIST-1 and RESIST-2) have been conducted in three drug class-experienced patients, failing a PI-containing regimen at entry into the trials. Based on a screening genotype, one of four best RTV-boosted PI regimens (boosted lopinavir, indinavir, saquinavir, or amprenavir) was selected plus an optimized background treatment. Patients were then randomized to optimized background along with either RTV-boosted tipranavir (200 mg/500 mg bid) or with the RTV-boosted control PI (cPI/r). A combined analysis of RESIST 1 and 2 after 48 weeks of treatment showed that grade 3 or 4 elevations of TC were observed in 2.1 versus 0.4%, and of triglycerides in 24.9 versus 13% of patients assigned to TPV/r and cPI/r, respectively).[74,75]

Another PI currently under investigation is darunavir (TMC-114). In a phase II trial that included triple class experienced patients currently failing (HIV-RNA > 1000 copies/mL), a stable PI-containing therapy, four different doses of darunavir/r with low-dose RTV added (400/100 mg qd, 800/100 mg qd, 400/100 bid, 600/100 mg bid) were compared to a PI that was selected by the investigator. The incidence of grade 2–4 elevation of TC and triglycerides was similar between the darunavir/r treated individuals (1.6–10.8 and 12.3–22.2 percent, respectively) and the control arm (1.6 and 28.6 percent, respectively) after 24 weeks of treatment. Lipid-lowering therapy was used concomitantly by 21% of all darunavir/r-treated patients and 29% of controls.[76]

Nucleoside Reverse Transcriptase Inhibitors

Apart from the clear effect PIs have on plasma lipids, there is considerable evidence that NRTIs also influence plasma lipid concentrations. In this light a large prospective randomized clinical trial ($n = 602$) compared two different potent regimens that both lack PI.[77] In this study stavudine (40 mg bid) was compared to tenofovir (300 mg qd), and both were combined with a backbone of efavirenz (600 mg qd) and lamivudine (150 mg bid) in 602 HIV therapy-naive individuals. Treatment with stavudine-containing therapy in ~160 patients after 144 weeks resulted in significantly greater changes in triglycerides (+134 mg/dL = 1.51 mmol/L), TC (+58 mg/dL = 1.5 mmol/L) and LDL-C (+26 mg/dL = 0.67 mmol/L), compared to +1 mg/dL (0.01 mmol/L) for triglycerides, +30 mg/dL (0.78 mmol/L) for TC and +11 mg/dL (0.28 mmol/L) for LDL-C in patients allocated to the tenofovir arm (n=170) (P<0.001 for all between group comparisons). It is likely that at least part of this difference in changes in lipids can be explained by the striking difference in the report of disturbances in fat distribution between both arms of the trial (3% in the tenofovir arm compared to 19% in the stavudine arm, P<0.001). The additional effect of thymidine analog NRTI on lipids is supported by the findings from another recently presented randomized clinical trial conducted in 509 antiretroviral-naive patients, which compared the combination of tenofovir (300 mg qd) and emtricitabine (200 mg qd) (Emtriva©) to zidovudine (300 mg bid) and lamivudine (150 mg bid) (ZDV/3TC) with a backbone of efavirenz (600 mg qd) in both arms.[78] Forty-eight weeks of treatment in individuals in the tenofovir/emtricitabine arm resulted in a 21 mg/dL increase in TC compared to 35 mg/dL in the ZDV/3TC arm (P<0.001). Changes in triglycerides were 3 mg/dL in the tenofovir/emtricitabine arm as compared to 31 mg/dL in the ZDV/3TC arm (P = 0.384). Whether thymidine analog NRTIs such as stavudine and zidovudine may also contribute to triglyceride elevation by adversely affecting mitochondrial function and thereby fatty acid oxidation in skeletal muscle remains to be determined.

Mechanisms of PI-Induced Hyperlipidemia

Several groups have looked at the effect of different PIs on plasma lipid profiles in healthy HIV-uninfected individuals. These studies convincingly show effects of certain PIs on plasma lipids which are independent of the presence of HIV infection and therefore are directly drug-related. The first study was performed by Purnell et al who demonstrated that 14 days of treatment with RTV 500 mg bid in a placebo-controlled trial resulted in significant elevations in TC [(4.4 mmol/L (170 mg/dL) 5.4 mmol/L (208 mg/dl); P<0.001)], triglycerides [from 1.2 mmol/L (106 mg/dL) to 3.1 mmol/L (273 mg/dl); P<0.01)] in 11 healthy controls compared to no changes in eight healthy individuals given placebo.[79,80] As a potential mechanism they suggested increased VLDL production.

Four weeks of treatment with indinavir in 10 healthy volunteers had no effect on plasma lipid concentrations. It did however result in insulin resistance as discussed before.[54]

The same experiment was repeated with 4 weeks of treatment with r/LPV again in 10 healthy volunteers.[81] This had no effect on TC, whereas triglyceride concentrations doubled from 0.89 mmol/L (79 mg/dL) at baseline to 1.63 mmol/L (144 mg/dL) after 4 weeks. When treatment for 5 days with r/LPV was compared with unboosted ATV in a randomized, double-blind, placebo-controlled trial in 30 healthy uninfected individuals similar results with respect to the effect of r/LPV on plasma triglyceride concentrations were demonstrated.[82] In contrast, unboosted ATV had no effects on plasma lipids. ATV is often used with a boosting dose of 100 mg qd of RTV. The effect of 10 days of treatment with RTV-boosted ATV (100/300 mg qd) on metabolic markers in 25 healthy volunteers was recently reported. Although treatment did not result in any significant changes in TC, triglycerides increased by ~30% (P < 0.01).[83] This suggests that a daily dose of RTV as low as 100 mg may still have an effect on lipids. Although the effect of RTV itself at a dose of 100 mg qd has not been studied in healthy volunteers, as mentioned before increases in lipids were clearly observed when given at 100 mg bid.[66]

A mechanism which was initially suggested to cause dyslipidemia was inhibition of the LDL-receptor-related protein (LRP) by PIs.[84] LRP is a receptor located on hepatocytes which plays an important role in the clearance of lipoproteins from the circulation. The catalytic site of HIV-1 protease was found to have 63% homology with the lipid-binding domain in LRP. A complex of LRP with lipoprotein lipase is also expressed on endothelial cells, and this complex facilitates the uptake of fatty acids from circulating triglycerides into adipocytes. Binding of both hepatic and endothelial LRP by PI could potentially lead to hypertriglyceridemia, but this hypothesis has not been further explored.

It has also been suggested that PI may induce hyperlipidemia by increasing hepatic VLDL production.[80] This hypothesis is supported by the demonstration that in HepG2 cells, several PIs (lopinavir, saquinavir, NFV, and RTV) increase triglyceride synthesis.[85] Furthermore, in fasting AKR/J mice treated with a detergent that inhibits triglyceride clearance, NFV and RTV more than doubled triglyceride levels.[85] Previously it was shown that PIs inhibit the proteosomal degradation of nascent apolipoprotein B, which is the principal protein component of triglyceride and cholesterol-rich plasma lipoproteins, which suggests a molecular basis for PI-induced hyperlipidemia.[86] A recent *in vitro* study by Parker et al shows that PIs induce endoplasmic reticulum stress that might dysregulate lipogenic pathways in hepatocytes and adipocytes by PI-induced inhibition of proteosome activity. In hepatocytes this resulted in an up-regulation of lipogenic and cholesterolgenic gene expression whereas in adipocytes the opposite occurred.[87]

In contrast, a recent study by den Boer et al tried to elucidate the mechanism of RTV-induced hypertriglyceridemia in a transgenic mouse model but yielded discrepant results.[88] APOE*3-Leiden transgenic mice were used as an experimental model, because these mice have a humanized lipoprotein profile and are susceptible to diet- and drug-induced hyperlipidemia, obesity, and atherosclerosis.[89–91] Similar to humans, APOE*3-Leiden transgenic mice have a much lower clearance rate of very low-density lipoproteins-triglyceride (VLDL-TG) than wild-type mice. As a consequence, APOE*3-Leiden mice were expected to represent a suitable animal model for studying RTV-associated hyperlipidemia. In this study RTV was not found to increase hepatic VLDL-TG production, but increased postprandial hypertriglyceridemia as a result of defective clearance of TG-rich lipoproteins. RTV decreased the plasma clearance of injected TG-rich VLDL-like emulsion particles and decreased post-heparin plasma total lipoprotein lipase (LPL) activity. In addition, the uptake of fatty acids derived from VLDL-TG, as well as albumin-bound fatty acids, was decreased selectively in adipose tissue where LPL is highly expressed in the postprandial state. Therefore, the authors conclude that RTV inhibits LPL-mediated triglyceride clearance in this mouse model.

LPL activity can be influenced by several cofactors, including apolipoprotein CII which is an essential cofactor for LPL and by apolipoprotein CIII which inhibits LPL. During HIV treatment, a strong association exists among PI therapy, patients who have certain apo C-III genetic variants, and dyslipidemia characterized by hypertriglyceridemia and low HDL-C.[92,93] It has been suggested that PIs interfere with normal regulation of the apo C-III leading to apo C-III overexpression and subsequent inhibition of LPL activity.

A reason why a single mechanism has not been identified to explain PI-induced hyperlipidemia might be that the initiation of ART, which consists of a combination of different classes of antiretrovirals, also induces other metabolic changes which are associated with hyperlipidemia in the general population. PIs acutely induce insulin resistance by the inhibition of GLUT-4,[54] whereas chronologically NRTIs and PIs are associated with the development of peripheral lipoatrophy and central fat accumulation, which are associated with insulin resistance.[94,95] In patients using PI-based therapy replacement of the PI by either abacavir or an NNRTI (nevirapine or efavirenz) resulted in a significant decrease in triglyceride concentrations.[96] This decrease of the same extent was not seen in patients with moderate to severe lipodystrophy as compared to those without lipodystrophy. This indicates that the changes in fat distribution *per se* may contribute to maintenance of hyperlipidemia. Van Wijk et al studied postprandial lipid metabolism and showed that in patients with clinical lipoatrophy, the clearance of free fatty acids and triglycerides was delayed compared to patients without lipoatrophy.[97] Furthermore, the lipoatrophic patients had a delayed and higher peak of hydroxybutyric acid (HBA) which is a product of FFA oxidation in the liver. HBA levels were significantly correlated with the severity of lipoatrophy.

Another factor which may be important in assessment of the effects of ART including PIs on lipids is co-infection with hepatitis C virus (HCV). A retrospective analysis of data from 881 participants of the Veterans Ageing Cohort 3 Site Study showed that a positive HCV antibody status was independently associated with lower TC and LDL-C levels, but not with lower HDL-C or triglyceride levels. After controlling for HIV medication use, glucose level, history of binge drinking, liver function, HIV viral load, current illegal drug use and CD4 cell count, HCV-seropositive patients had LDL levels 18.99 mg/dL (95% CI: −27.1 to −10.9) lower, and TC levels 13.65 mg/dL (95% CI: −21.6 to −5.7) lower than HCV-seronegative subjects.[98]

Guidelines for Evaluation of Dyslipidemia in HIV-Infected Individuals

Given the amount of evidence from both prospective studies and surrogate endpoint studies it seems very likely that HAART is associated with an increased risk of atherosclerotic vascular disease. It was against this background that the Infectious Disease Society of America (IDSA) and the ACTG have issued guidelines for the management of dyslipidemia in HIV-infected individuals[99] which were primarily based on those from the National Cholesterol Education Program Adult Treatment Panel III (NCEP ATP III).[100]

Evaluation of dyslipidemia in an individual patient starts with a measurement of serum lipids after an overnight fast, ideally prior to the initiation of ART. This should include TC, HDL-C, and triglyceride concentrations from which LDL-C and non-HDL-cholesterol can be calculated. This assessment should be repeated 3–6 months after the initiation of ART and yearly thereafter so that an intervention can be initiated as soon as lipid abnormalities occur. Target lipid levels to be achieved and the aggressiveness of instituting lipid-lowering strategies are based on a patient's individual estimated cardiovascular risk. Up until now no algorithm has been developed for specifically assessing this risk in HIV-infected individuals. Therefore, risk assessment currently employs algorithms developed for the general population such as the one derived from the Framingham study. The patients at high risk are those with prior CHD or those with a coronary risk equivalent. The latter category includes patients with cerebrovascular disease, peripheral vascular disease, diabetes mellitus or patients with multiple factors which jointly predict a 10-year risk of cardiovascular death or MI which exceeds 20% using the Framingham algorithm. A risk calculator based on the Framingham algorithm is available on the internet at http://www.nhlbi.nih.gov/guidelines/cholesterol. This site also includes the latest updates of the NCEP ATP guidelines. It is important to realize that the Framingham risk calculator has not been validated for the relatively young HIV-infected population, and does not take into account the duration of exposure to risk factors such as smoking. Most of the ART-induced changes in plasma lipids occur in a time frame of just months and therefore might importantly bias the calculation. Also other predisposing factors such as obesity, physical activity, and socioeconomic status are not included in the Framingham calculation. Finally, any effect that HIV infection *per se* and immune activation may have on the risk of atherogenesis, as well as the mitigating effects of ART on these parameters, are obviously also not incorporated. Nevertheless, the Framingham algorithm is a good starting point for the evaluation of cardiovascular risk and

Table 72-4

Risk Factors to be Assessed in Order to Determine LDL-C Target to be Achieved

Risk Factor	Definition
Cigarette smoking	
Hypertension	Systolic blood pressure >140 mmHg or antihypertensive therapy
Low HDL-C	<40 mg/dL (<1 mmol/L)
Family history of CHD	Male first-degree <55 OR Female first-degree <65 yrs old
Age	>45 years for men >55 years for women

An elevated HDL-C >60 mg/dL (>1.55 mmol/L) is considered a negative risk factor. If present subtract 1 factor from the above risk factor total.

management strategies in HIV-infected patients which is supported by the finding that in the D:A:D study the observed and Framingham-predicted rates of MI increased in a parallel fashion with increased duration of ART (Fig. 72-1).[62]

As mentioned before patients with established CHD or a CHD equivalent are those considered to be at high risk (10-year risk of cardiac death or MI > 20%) and should be treated most aggressively. The remaining patients are categorized by counting the number of risk factors present (Table 72-4). These include cigarette smoking, hypertension (>140/90 mmHg or use of antihypertensive treatment), low HDL-C (<40 mg/dL ~ <1 mmol/L), increased age (women >55 years; men >45 years), family history of premature CHD (in a male first-degree relative <55 years old or a first-degree female relative <65 years old). An elevated HDL-C (>60 mg/dL > 1.55 mmol/L) is a negative risk factor that neutralizes one other risk factor. If more than two of these risk factors are present, NCEP ATP III and IDSA/AACTG guidelines recommend calculating the 10-year risk of cardiac death or MI using the Framingham calculator. The LDL-C target to be achieved with lipid-lowering therapy is dependent on the total number of these risk factors present (see below).

Determining Target Lipids

The determination of target lipid levels should be determined once the 10-year coronary risk has been calculated. According to IDSA/AACTG guidelines in a patient with zero to 1 risk factor the target LDL-C for considering lipid lowering therapy is 190 mg/mL (4.9 mmol/L). For patients with two or more risk factors and an estimated 10-year coronary risk below 10% the target LDL-C is below 160 mg/dL (4.1 mmol/L). In patients with more than two risk factors and an estimated 10-year coronary risk between 10–20% the target LDL-C is 130 mg/dL (3.3 mmol/L) and for high-risk patients below 100 mg/dL (< 2.6 mmol/L). Following the publication of the IDSA/AACTG guidelines, NCEP updated their guidelines as a result of five large statin intervention trials.[101] The target level for LDL-C was adjusted downward to 70 mg/dL (0.79 mmol/L), particularly in high-risk patients with LDL-C concentrations less than 100 mg/dL (<2.6 mmol/L) and in those with a recent acute coronary syndrome, established cardiovascular disease or with multiple suboptimally treated lifestyle factors. In the moderate-risk group the LDL-C target level was adjusted to less than 100 mg/dL (<2.6 mmol/L) in those individuals with more than two risk factors and a 10-year risk of 10–20%. Furthermore, NCEP guidelines stress the fact that in high- or moderate-risk individuals LDL-C concentrations should decrease at least by 30–40%, regardless of the baseline LDL-C concentration. Moreover, any person at high or moderate risk who has lifestyle-related risk factors (obesity, physical inactivity, or metabolic syndrome) is a candidate to modify these risk factors.

When patients have triglycerides >200 mg/dL (2.2 mmol/L) the cholesterol content of triglyceride-rich lipoproteins is increased and the estimated LDL-C using the Friedewald calculation underestimates the total number of atherogenic particles. Non-HDL-C (calculated as TC minus HDL-C) or its mathematical equivalent (the TC/HDL-C ratio) can be used as an important secondary target of therapy in those cases. This is important in HIV-infected persons, given the fact that ART may frequently increase triglyceride concentrations in particular. The non-HDL-C target is simply the LDL-C target plus 30 mg/dL, since the latter represents the usual cholesterol concentration in VLDL particles.

Treatment of Dyslipidemia

Lifestyle changes and the initiation of lipid-lowering therapy are recommended if lipid levels are higher than their previously described targets. Another strategy to consider to achieve lower lipid levels is to replace individual antiretrovirals thought to exert particularly detrimental effects on lipids by more 'lipid-friendly' agents. Such a strategy however, should only be employed if it does not jeopardize maintenance of virus suppression. Switching from a PI to either nevirapine or abacavir or ATV may result in a significant improvement in TC and triglyceride concentrations (Fig. 72-2).[96,102,103]

The effects of switching ART versus the initiation of lipid-lowering therapy with a statin or fibrate has recently been studied in a randomized fashion. In a relatively small clinical trial 130 patients on their first PI-containing HAART regimen with fasting triglycerides >200 mg/dL (>2.2 mmol/L) and TC >250 mg/dL (>6.5 mmol/L) were randomized to switch their PI to either nevirapine (n = 29) or efavirenz (n = 34), or to treatment with pravastin (n = 36) or bezafibrate (n = 31).[104] Patients with severe hypertriglyceridemia (fasting plasma triglyceride levels >750 mg/dL (>8.5 mmol/L)) or severe hypercholesterolemia (fasting plasma TC levels > 350 mg/dL (> 9.1 mmol/L)) were excluded from the study. ART remained unchanged during follow-up in the patients receiving either a statin or a fibrate. In all groups a

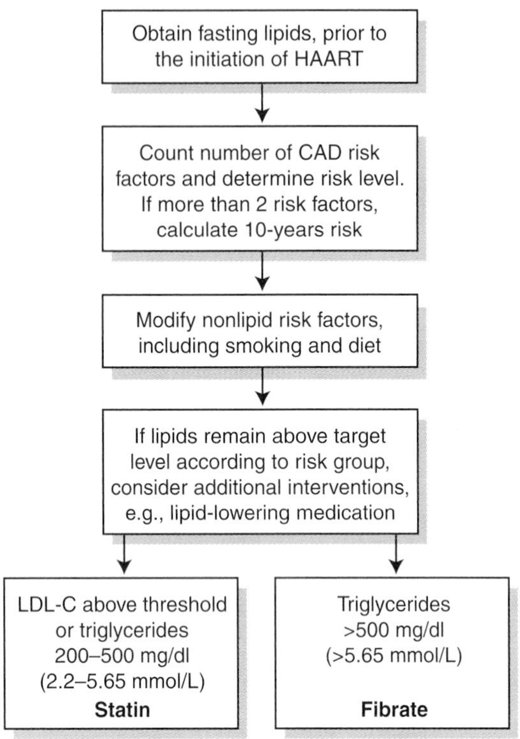

Figure 72-2 ■ General approach to lipid disorders and cardiovascular risk in HIV-infected patients receiving HAART. CAD, coronary artery disease; yr, year; LDL, low-density lipoprotein.

hypolipidemic diet and regular physical exercise were persistently and consistently recommended. This study concluded that treatment with a statin was superior to switching to nevirapine with respect to reduction of TC (46% vs 27%), LDL-C (40% vs 25%), and triglycerides (41% vs 25%). Switching to efavirenz was least successful and the effects on lipids were minor compared to switching to nevirapine. HDL-C increased 10% in the statin group versus 3% in the nevirapine arm. Fenofibrate was more or less equipotent compared to pravastatin. However, another recent ACTG randomized clinical trial showed that treatment with either pravastatin or fenofibrate did not result in achieving NCEP target lipid levels in the majority of participants.[105] In this study of the 83 individuals randomized to monotherapy with 40 mg of pravastatin for 12 weeks, only 36% reached LDL, 49% HDL, and 18% triglycerides target levels. Treatment with 200 mg of fenofibrate (n = 87) led to 9%, 66% and 48% of subjects who achieved their LDL, HDL, and TG goals, respectively. After 12 weeks of treatment in individuals who failed to achieve composite NCEP goals, pravastatin and fenofibrate were combined (n = 136). The remaining 38 patients either continued monotherapy or opted out of the study. Combination therapy resulted in only 21%, 65%, and 49% patients who met NCEP goals at week 28 for LDL, HDL, and triglycerides concentrations, respectively.

When pharmacologic therapy is needed following an insufficient effect of lifestyle modification, in patients with extremely high triglyceride concentrations (>500 mg/dL; >5.65 mmol/L)) a fibrate (gemfibrozil or fenofibrate) should be prescribed as first choice with niacin as an alternative. For patients with lower triglyceride concentrations reduction of LDL-C should be the primary target. A statin then is the first choice. Preferred statins in the IDSA/AACTG guidelines are pravastatin and atorvastatin, given their lesser propensity for drug–drug interactions with antiretrovirals. Nevertheless, since most statins are metabolized to some extent by CYP3A4, physicians should remain conscious of the potential for drug–drug interactions. Pravastatin and atorvastatin levels decrease in the presence of NNRTI in healthy volunteers whereas simvastatin levels significantly increase by 58%.[106] This increase could potentially result in an increased risk of clinically relevant toxicity, and therefore simvastatin should not be prescribed together with an NNRTI. No significant effects of statins on efavirenz concentrations have been described.

Another healthy volunteer study studied the combination of RTV/saquinavir (RTV/SQV) (400 mg/400 mg) with statins.[107] RTV/SQV increased simvastatin concentrations 30-fold. Atorvastatin concentrations increased threefold whereas no significant effect on pravastatin concentrations were described. No clinically significant effects on PI concentrations were described. Taken together, pravastatin seems to be the safest option in the HIV-infected patient population where polypharmacy is often the rule rather than the exception. Physicians also need to be aware of the fact that statins may cause elevations in hepatic transaminases. Therefore, the IDSA/AACTG guidelines recommend the monitoring of transaminases 6 weeks after commencing statin treatment. Routine monitoring of muscle enzymes is not recommended. Another interesting and relatively new statin is rosuvastatin. This drug seems to have no effect on the cytochrome P450 system which is crucial in the metabolism of both PIs and NNRTIs. In a small pilot study in 16 patients rosuvastatin seemed safe.[108] However, this result needs to be confirmed in larger studies before rosuvastatin can be safely recommended for use in patients on HAART.

The combination of a statin and a fibrate should be avoided as much as possible in view of an increased risk of both hepatic and muscle toxicity. However, when there is a need to combine these two drug classes in patients on HAART, fenofibrate seems the best option since almost no interactions between these two drugs occur in either healthy volunteers or HIV-infected individuals.[105,109]

CONCLUSIONS

Hyperlipidemia is an important side effect of HIV therapy and combination ART has been associated with an increased risk of CAD. However, it is important to realize that the major gain in health and survival provided by HAART far outweighs this risk. Therefore, concerns about CAD risk should never preclude the use of ART in any person with HIV. Nevertheless, because of the success of HAART, we shall be facing an increasingly aging HIV-infected population, and the incidence of CAD is expected to increase.

A systematic assessment and modification of known risk factors for CAD is thus warranted as part of the primary care of patients with HIV infection. Although the precise causes of the increased risk of CAD associated with ART remain to be further elucidated, it is clear that treatment-associated dyslipidemia importantly contributes to that risk. Because currently available antiretrovirals differ importantly in their effect on particular lipid fractions, choices among antiretroviral combination regimens to be prescribed should take into account the risk of CAD in the individual.

REFERENCES

1. Delta Coordinating Committee. Delta: a randomised double-blind controlled trial comparing combinations of zidovudine plus didanosine or zalcitabine with zidovudine alone in HIV-infected individuals. Lancet 348:283–91, 1996.
2. Palella FJ, Jr, Delaney KM, Moorman AC, et al. Declining morbidity and mortality among patients with advanced human immunodeficiency virus infection. HIV Outpatient Study Investigators. N Engl J Med 338:853–60, 1998.
3. Mocroft A, Vella S, Benfield TL, et al. Changing patterns of mortality across Europe in patients infected with HIV-1. EuroSIDA Study Group. Lancet 352:1725–30, 1998.
4. Carr A, Samaras K, Thorisdottir A, et al. Diagnosis, prediction, and natural course of HIV-1 protease-inhibitor-associated lipodystrophy, hyperlipidaemia, and diabetes mellitus: a cohort study. Lancet 353:2093–9, 1999.
5. Carr A, Samaras K, Burton S, et al. A syndrome of peripheral lipodystrophy, hyperlipidaemia and insulin resistance in patients receiving HIV protease inhibitors. AIDS 12:F51–8, 1998.
6. Lo JC, Mulligan K, Tai VW, et al. Body shape changes in HIV-infected patients. J Acquir Immune Defic Syndr Hum Retrovirol 19:307–8, 1998.
7. Reaven GM. Banting lecture 1988. Role of insulin resistance in human disease. Diabetes 37:1595–607, 1988.
8. Grunfeld C, Pang M, Doerrler W, et al. Lipids, lipoproteins, triglyceride clearance, and cytokines in human immunodeficiency virus infection and the acquired immunodeficiency syndrome. J Clin Endocrinol Metab 74:1045–52, 1992.
9. Grunfeld C, Kotler DP, Hamadeh R, et al. Hypertriglyceridemia in the acquired immunodeficiency syndrome. Am J Med 86:27–31, 1989.
10. Feingold KR, Krauss RM, Pang M, et al. The hypertriglyceridemia of acquired immunodeficiency syndrome is associated with an increased prevalence of low density lipoprotein subclass pattern B. J Clin Endocrinol Metab 76:1423–7, 1993.
11. Grunfeld C, Kotler DP, Shigenaga JK, et al. Circulating interferon-alpha levels and hypertriglyceridemia in the acquired immunodeficiency syndrome. Am J Med 90:154–62, 1991.
12. Mildvan D, Machado SG, Wilets I, Grossberg SE. Endogenous interferon and triglyceride concentrations to assess response to zidovudine in AIDS and advanced AIDS-related complex. Lancet 339:453–6, 1992.
13. Riddler SA, Smit E, Cole SR, et al. Impact of HIV infection and HAART on serum lipids in men. JAMA 289:2978–82, 2003.
14. Tabib A, Greenland T, Mercier I, et al. Coronary lesions in young HIV-positive subjects at necropsy. Lancet 340:730, 1992.
15. Constans J, Marchand JM, Conri C, et al. Asymptomatic atherosclerosis in HIV-positive patients: A case-control ultrasound study. Ann Med 27:683–5, 1995.
16. Behrens G, Schmidt H, Meyer D, et al. Vascular complications associated with use of HIV protease inhibitors. Lancet 351:1958, 1998.
17. Henry K, Melroe H, Huebsch J, et al. Severe premature coronary artery disease with protease inhibitors. Lancet 351:1328, 1998.
18. Gallet B, Pulik M, Genet P, et al. Vascular complications associated with use of HIV protease inhibitors. Lancet 351:1958–9, 1998.
19. Friis-Moller N, Weber R, Reiss P, et al. Cardiovascular disease risk factors in HIV patients association with antiretroviral therapy. Results from the DAD study. AIDS 17:1179–93, 2003.
20. Bozzette SA, Ake CF, Tam HK, et al. Cardiovascular and cerebrovascular events in patients treated for human immunodeficiency virus infection. N Engl J Med 348:702–10, 2003.
21. Mary-Krause M, Cotte L, Simon A, et al. Increased risk of myocardial infarction with duration of protease inhibitor therapy in HIV-infected men. AIDS 17:2479–86, 2003.
22. Currier JS, Taylor A, Boyd F, et al. Coronary heart disease in HIV-infected individuals. J Acquir Immune Defic Syndr 33:506–12, 2003.
23. Klein D, Hurley LB, Quesenberry CP Jr, Sidney S. Do protease inhibitors increase the risk for coronary heart disease in patients with HIV-1 infection? J Acquir Immune Defic Syndr 30:471–7, 2002.
24. Friis-Moller N, Sabin CA, Weber R, et al. Combination antiretroviral therapy and the risk of myocardial infarction. N Engl J Med 349:1993–2003, 2003.
25. Fontas E, van LF, Sabin CA, et al. Lipid profiles in HIV-infected patients receiving combination antiretroviral therapy: are different antiretroviral drugs associated with different lipid profiles? J Infect Dis 189:1056–74.
26. van der Valk M, Kastelein JJ, Murphy RL, et al. Nevirapine-containing antiretroviral therapy in HIV-1 infected patients results in an anti-atherogenic lipid profile. AIDS 15:2407–14, 2001.
27. van Leeuwen R, Katlama C, Murphy RL, et al. A randomized trial to study first-line combination therapy with or without a protease inhibitor in HIV-1-infected patients. AIDS 17:987–99, 2003.
28. Friis-Moller N, Reiss P, El-Sadr W, et al. Class of antiretroviral drugs and the risk of myocardial infarction. N Engl J Med 26(356): 1723–35, 2007.
29. d'Arminio A, Sabin CA, Phillips AN, et al. Cardio- and cerebrovascular events in HIV-infected persons. AIDS 18:1811–7, 2004.
30. El-Sadr W, Reiss P, De Wit S, et al. Relationship between prolonged exposure to combination ART and myocardial infarction: effect of sex, age, and lipid changes. 12th conference on retroviruses and opportunistic infections, February 22–25, Boston, MA; 2005.
31. Holmberg SD, Moorman AC, Williamson JM, et al. Protease inhibitors and cardiovascular outcomes in patients with HIV-1. Lancet 360:1747–8, 2002.
32. Sankatsing RR, de GE, Jukema JW, et al. Surrogate markers for atherosclerotic disease. Curr Opin Lipidol 16:434–41, 2005.
33. Chambless LE, Heiss G, Folsom AR, et al. Association of coronary heart disease incidence with carotid arterial wall thickness and major risk factors: the Atherosclerosis Risk in Communities (ARIC) Study, 1987–1993. Am J Epidemiol 146:483–94, 1997.
34. O'Leary DH, Polak JF, Kronmal RA, et al. Carotid-artery intima and media thickness as a risk factor for myocardial infarction and stroke in older adults. Cardiovascular Health Study Collaborative Research Group. N Engl J Med 340: 14–22, 1999.
35. Bots ML, Hoes AW, Koudstaal PJ, et al. Common carotid intima-media thickness and risk of stroke and myocardial infarction: the Rotterdam Study. Circulation 96:1432–37, 1997.
36. Smilde TJ, van WS, Wollersheim H, et al. Effect of aggressive versus conventional lipid lowering on atherosclerosis progression

in familial hypercholesterolaemia (ASAP): a prospective, randomised, double-blind trial. Lancet 357:577–81, 2001.

37. Jukema JW, Bruschke AV, van Boven AJ, et al. Effects of lipid lowering by pravastatin on progression and regression of coronary artery disease in symptomatic men with normal to moderately elevated serum cholesterol levels. The regression growth evaluation statin study (REGRESS). Circulation 91:2528–40, 1995.
38. Seminari E, Pan A, Voltini G, et al. Assessment of atherosclerosis using carotid ultrasonography in a cohort of HIV-positive patients treated with protease inhibitors. Atherosclerosis 162:433–8, 2002.
39. Martin LD, Vandhuick O, Guillo P, et al. Premature atherosclerosis in HIV positive patients and cumulated time of exposure to antiretroviral therapy (SHIVA study). Atherosclerosis 185(2):361–7, 2006.
40. Currier JS, Kendall MA, Zackin R, et al. Carotid artery intima-media thickness and HIV infection: traditional risk factors overshadow impact of protease inhibitor exposure. AIDS 19:927–33, 2005.
41. Maggi P, Lillo A, Perilli F, et al. Colour-Doppler ultrasonography of carotid vessels in patients treated with antiretroviral therapy: a comparative study. AIDS 18:1023–8, 2004.
42. Hsue PY, Lo JC, Franklin A, et al. Progression of atherosclerosis as assessed by carotid intima-media thickness in patients with HIV infection. Circulation 109:1603–8, 2004.
43. Mercie P, Thiebaut R, urillac-Lavignolle V, et al. Carotid intima-media thickness is slightly increased over time in HIV-1-infected patients. HIV Med 6:380–7, 2005.
44. Thiebaut R, urillac-Lavignolle V, Bonnet F, et al. Change in atherosclerosis progression in HIV-infected patients: ANRS Aquitaine Cohort, 1999–2004. AIDS 19:729–31, 2005.
45. Nolan D, Watts GF, Herrmann SE, et al. Endothelial function in HIV-infected patients receiving protease inhibitor therapy: does immune competence affect cardiovascular risk? QJM 96: 825–32, 2003.
46. Stein JH, Klein MA, Bellehumeur JL, et al. Use of human immunodeficiency virus-1 protease inhibitors is associated with atherogenic lipoprotein changes and endothelial dysfunction. Circulation 104:257–62, 2001.
47. Dressman J, Kincer J, Matveev SV, et al. HIV protease inhibitors promote atherosclerotic lesion formation independent of dyslipidemia by increasing CD36-dependent cholesteryl ester accumulation in macrophages. J Clin Invest 111:389–97, 2003.
48. Shankar SS, Dube MP, Gorski JC, et al. Indinavir impairs endothelial function in healthy HIV-negative men. Am Heart J 150:933, 2005.
49. Dressman J, Combs B, Greenberg RN, et al. HIV protease inhibitors impair endothelial nitric oxide synthase-mediated vasodilatation in response to acetylcholine and bradykinin. 11th Conference on retroviruses and Opportunistic Infections 2004, San Francisco 2004.
50. Murata H, Hruz PW, Mueckler M. Indinavir inhibits the glucose transporter isoform Glut4 at physiologic concentrations. AIDS 16:859–63, 2002.
51. Hruz PW, Murata H, Qiu H, Mueckler M. Indinavir induces acute and reversible peripheral insulin resistance in rats. Diabetes 51:937–42, 2002.
52. Murata H, Hruz PW, Mueckler M. The mechanism of insulin resistance caused by HIV protease inhibitor therapy. J Biol Chem 275:20251–4, 2000.
53. Schwarz JM, Lee GA, Park S, et al. Indinavir increases glucose production in healthy HIV-negative men. AIDS 18:1852–4.
54. Noor MA, Seneviratne T, Aweeka FT, et al. Indinavir acutely inhibits insulin-stimulated glucose disposal in humans: a randomized, placebo-controlled study. AIDS 16:F1–8, 2002.
55. Noor MA, Lo JC, Mulligan K, et al. Metabolic effects of indinavir in healthy HIV-seronegative men. AIDS 15:F11–18, 2001.
56. Fu W, Chai H, Yao Q, Chen C. Effects of HIV protease inhibitor ritonavir on vasomotor function and endothelial nitric oxide synthase expression. J Acquir Immune Defic Syndr 39:152–8, 2005.
57. Conklin BS, Fu W, Lin PH, et al. HIV protease inhibitor ritonavir decreases endothelium-dependent vasorelaxation and increases superoxide in porcine arteries. Cardiovasc Res 63:168–75, 2004.
58. Chai H, Yang H, Yan S, et al. Effects of 5 HIV protease inhibitors on vasomotor function and superoxide anion production in porcine coronary arteries. J Acquir Immune Defic Syndr 40:12–9, 2005.
59. Chen C, Lu XH, Yan S, et al. HIV protease inhibitor ritonavir increases endothelial monolayer permeability. Biochem Biophys Res Commun 335:874–82, 2005.
60. Bonnet D, Aggoun Y, Szezepanski I, et al. Arterial stiffness and endothelial dysfunction in HIV-infected children. AIDS 18:1037–41, 2004.
61. Torriani FJ, Parker RA, Murphy RL, et al. Antiretroviral therapy improves endothelial function in treatment-naïve HIV-infected subjects: A prospective, randomized multicenter trial (A5152s). Program and abstracts of the 10th European AIDS Conference; November 17–20, 2005, Dublin, Ireland 2005, abstract PS5–3.
62. Law M, Friis-Moller N, El-Sadr W, et al. The use of the framingham equation to predict myocardial infarctions in HIV-infected patients: comparison with observed events in the D:A:D Study. HIV Med 7(4):218–30, 2006.
63. Young J, Weber R, Rickenbach M, et al. Lipid profiles for antiretroviral-naive patients starting PI- and NNRTI-based therapy in the Swiss HIV cohort study. Antivir Ther 10:585–91, 2005.
64. van Leth F, Phanuphak P, Stroes E, et al. Nevirapine and efavirenz elicit different changes in lipid profiles in antiretroviral-therapy-naive patients infected with HIV-1. PLoS Med 1:e19, 2004.
65. Roberts AD, Liappis AP, Chinn C, et al. Effect of delavirdine on plasma lipids and lipoproteins in patients receiving antiretroviral therapy. AIDS 16:1829–30, 2002.
66. Shafran SD, Mashinter LD, Roberts SE. The effect of low-dose ritonavir monotherapy on fasting serum lipid concentrations. HIV Med 6:421–5, 2005.
67. Walmsley S, Bernstein B, King M, et al. Lopinavir-ritonavir versus nelfinavir for the initial treatment of HIV infection. N Engl J Med 346:2039–46, 2002.
68. Martinez E, Domingo P, Galindo MJ, et al. Risk of metabolic abnormalities in patients infected with HIV receiving antiretroviral therapy that contains lopinavir-ritonavir. Clin Infect Dis 38:1017–23, 2004.
69. Dragsted UB, Gerstoft J, Youle M, et al. A randomized trial to evaluate lopinavir/ritonavir versus saquinavir/ritonavir in HIV-1-infected patients: the MaxCmin2 trial. Antivir Ther 10:735–43, 2005.
70. Dragsted UB, Gerstoft J, Pedersen C, et al. Randomized trial to evaluate indinavir/ritonavir versus saquinavir/ritonavir in human immunodeficiency virus type 1-infected patients: the MaxCmin1 Trial. J Infect Dis 188:635–42, 2003.
71. Murphy RL, Sanne I, Cahn P, et al. Dose-ranging, randomized, clinical trial of atazanavir with lamivudine and stavudine in antiretroviral-naive subjects: 48-week results. AIDS 17:2603–14, 2003.
72. Sanne I, Piliero P, Squires K, et al. Results of a phase 2 clinical trial at 48 weeks (AI424-007): a dose-ranging, safety, and efficacy comparative trial of atazanavir at three doses in combination with didanosine and stavudine in antiretroviral-naive subjects. J Acquir Immune Defic Syndr 32:18–29, 2003.
73. Cahn PE, Gatell JM, Squires K, et al. Atazanavir – a once-daily HIV protease inhibitor that does not cause dyslipidemia in

newly treated patients: results from two randomized clinical trials. J Int Assoc Physicians AIDS Care (Chic Ill) 3:92–8, 2004.

74. FDA Tipranavir Review Team (HFD-530). 2005. Report No. 2005-4139b1-01-fda. Available: http://www.fda.gov/ohrms/dockets/ac/05/briefing/2005-4139b1-01-fda.pdf.
75. Cahn P, Hicks C. RESIST-1 (R-1) and RESIST-2 (R-2) 48 week meta-analyses demonstrate superiority or protease inhibitor (PI) tipranavir+ritonavir (TPV/r) over an optimized comparator PI (CPI/r) regimen in antiretroviral (ARV) experienced patients. Program and abstracts of the 10th European AIDS Conference; November 17–20, 2005, Dublin, Ireland 2005,abstract LBPS3–8.
76. Grinsztejn B, Arasteh K, Clotet B, et al. TMC114/r is well tolerated in 3-class-experienced patients: Week 24 primary safety analysis of POWER 1 (TMC114–C213). 3rd IAS Conference on HIV Pathogenesis and Treatment; July 24–27, 2005, Rio de Janeiro, Brazil 2005, abstract WePeLB6.201.
77. Gallant JE, Staszewski S, Pozniak AL, et al. Efficacy and safety of tenofovir DF vs stavudine in combination therapy in antiretroviral-naive patients: a 3-year randomized trial. JAMA 292:191–201, 2004.
78. Pozniak AL, Gallant JE, Dejesus E, et al. Superior outcome for tenofovir DF (TDF), emtricitabine (FTC) and efavirenz (EFV) compared to fixed dose zidovudine/lamivudine (CBV) and EFV in antiretroviral naive patients. 3rd IAS Conference on HIV Pathogenesis and Treatment; July 24–27, 2005, Rio de Janeiro, Brazil 2005, abstract WeOa0203.
79. Stein JH. Dyslipidemia in the era of HIV protease inhibitors. Prog Cardiovasc Dis 45:293–304, 2003.
80. Purnell JQ, Zambon A, Knopp RH, et al. Effect of ritonavir on lipids and post-heparin lipase activities in normal subjects. AIDS 14:51–7, 2000.
81. Lee GA, Seneviratne T, Noor MA, et al. The metabolic effects of lopinavir/ritonavir in HIV-negative men. AIDS 18:641–9, 2004.
82. Noor MA, Parker RA, O'Mara E, et al. The effects of HIV protease inhibitors atazanavir and lopinavir/ritonavir on insulin sensitivity in HIV-seronegative healthy adults. AIDS 18:2137–44, 2004.
83. Noor MA, Flint OP, Parker RA, et al. Evaluation of insulin sensitivity in healthy volunteers treated with low-dose ritonavir combined with atazanavir (ATV/RTV) or lopinavir (LPV/RTV): a prospective, randomized study using hyperinsulinaemic, euglycaemic clamp and oral glucose tolerance testing. Antivir Ther 10:L11, 2005.
84. Carr A, Samaras K, Chisholm DJ, Cooper DA. Pathogenesis of HIV-1-protease inhibitor-associated peripheral lipodystrophy, hyperlipidaemia, and insulin resistance. Lancet 351:1881–3, 1998.
85. Lenhard JM, Croom DK, Weiel JE, Winegar DA. HIV protease inhibitors stimulate hepatic triglyceride synthesis. Arterioscler Thromb Vasc Biol 20:2625–9, 2000.
86. Liang JS, Distler O, Cooper DA, et al. HIV protease inhibitors protect apolipoprotein B from degradation by the proteasome: a potential mechanism for protease inhibitor-induced hyperlipidemia. Nat Med 7:1327–31, 2001.
87. Parker RA, Flint OP, Mulvey R, et al. Endoplasmic reticulum stress links dyslipidemia to inhibition of proteasome activity and glucose transport by HIV protease inhibitors. Mol Pharmacol 67:1909–19, 2005.
88. den Boer MAM, Berbee JFP, Reiss P, et al. Ritonavir impairs LPL-mediated lipolysis and decreases uptake of fatty acids in adipose tissue. Arterioscler Thromb Vasc Biol 26(1):124–9, 2006.
89. van Vlijmen BJ, van den Maagdenberg AM, Gijbels MJ, et al. Diet-induced hyperlipoproteinemia and atherosclerosis in apolipoprotein E3-Leiden transgenic mice. J Clin Invest 93:1403–10, 1994.
90. van den Maagdenberg AM, Hofker MH, Krimpenfort PJ, et al. Transgenic mice carrying the apolipoprotein E3-Leiden gene exhibit hyperlipoproteinemia. J Biol Chem 268:10540–5, 1993.
91. van Vlijmen BJ, van't Hof HB, Mol MJ, et al. Modulation of very low density lipoprotein production and clearance contributes to age- and gender-dependent hyperlipoproteinemia in apolipoprotein E3-Leiden transgenic mice. J Clin Invest 97:1184–92, 1996.
92. Fauvel J, Bonnet E, Ruidavets JB, et al. An interaction between apo C-III variants and protease inhibitors contributes to high triglyceride/low HDL levels in treated HIV patients. AIDS 15:2397–406, 2001.
93. Tarr PE, Taffe P, Bleiber G, et al. Modeling the influence of APOC3, APOE, and TNF polymorphisms on the risk of antiretroviral therapy-associated lipid disorders. J Infect Dis 191:1419–26, 2005.
94. van der Valk M, Gisolf EH, Reiss P, et al. Increased risk of lipodystrophy when nucleoside analogue reverse transcriptase inhibitors are included with protease inhibitors in the treatment of HIV-1 infection. AIDS 15:847–55, 2001.
95. van der Valk M, Bisschop PH, Romijn JA, et al. Lipodystrophy in HIV-1-positive patients is associated with insulin resistance in multiple metabolic pathways. AIDS 15:2093–100, 2001.
96. Fisac C, Fumero E, Crespo M, et al. Metabolic benefits 24 months after replacing a protease inhibitor with abacavir, efavirenz or nevirapine. AIDS 19:917–25, 2005.
97. van Wijk JP, Cabezas MC, de Koning EJ, et al. *In vivo* evidence of impaired peripheral fatty acid trapping in patients with human immunodeficiency virus-associated lipodystrophy. J Clin Endocrinol Metab 90:3575–82, 2005.
98. Polgreen PM, Fultz SL, Justice AC, et al. Association of hypocholesterolaemia with hepatitis C virus infection in HIV-infected people. HIV Med 5:144–50, 2004.
99. Dube MP, Stein JH, Aberg JA, et al. Guidelines for the evaluation and management of dyslipidemia in human immunodeficiency virus (HIV)-infected adults receiving antiretroviral therapy: recommendations of the HIV Medical Association of the Infectious Disease Society of America and the Adult AIDS Clinical Trials Group. Clin Infect Dis 37:613–27, 2003.
100. Executive summary of the third report of the national cholesterol education program (NCEP) expert panel on detection, evaluation, and treatment of high blood cholesterol in adults (adult treatment panel III). JAMA 285:2486–97, 2001.
101. Grundy SM, Cleeman JI, Merz CN, et al. Implications of recent clinical trials for the national cholesterol education program adult treatment panel III guidelines. Circulation 110:227–39, 2004.
102. Gatell J, Salmon Ceron D, Lazzarin A. Efficacy and safety of atazanavir (ATV) based HAART in patients switching from a stable boosted/unboosted protease inhibitor (PI) treatment: the SWAN study. Program and abstracts of the 10th European AIDS Conference, November 17–20, 2005, Dublin, Ireland 2005, abstract PS1.
103. Mobius U, Lubach-Ruitman M, Castro-Frenzel B, et al. Switching to atazanavir improves metabolic disorders in antiretroviral-experienced patients with severe hyperlipidemia. J Acquir Immune Defic Syndr 39:174–80, 2005.
104. Calza L, Manfredi R, Colangeli V, et al. Substitution of nevirapine or efavirenz for protease inhibitor versus lipid-lowering therapy for the management of dyslipidaemia. AIDS 19:1051–8, 2005.
105. Aberg JA, Zackin RA, Brobst SW, et al. A randomized trial of the efficacy and safety of fenofibrate versus pravastatin in HIV-infected subjects with lipid abnormalities: AIDS clinical trials group study 5087. AIDS Res Hum Retroviruses 21: 757–67, 2005.

106. Gerber JG, Rosenkranz SL, Fichtenbaum CJ, et al. Effect of efavirenz on the pharmacokinetics of simvastatin, atorvastatin, and pravastatin: results of AIDS clinical trials group 5108 study. J Acquir Immune Defic Syndr 39:307–12, 2005.
107. Fichtenbaum CJ, Gerber JG, Rosenkranz SL, et al. Pharmacokinetic interactions between protease inhibitors and statins in HIV seronegative volunteers: ACTG Study A5047. AIDS16:569–77, 2002.
108. Calza L, Colangeli V, Manfredi R, et al. Rosuvastatin for the treatment of hyperlipidaemia in HIV-infected patients receiving protease inhibitors: a pilot study. AIDS 19:1103–5, 2005.
109. Pan WJ, Gustavson LE, Achari R, et al. Lack of a clinically significant pharmacokinetic interaction between fenofibrate and pravastatin in healthy volunteers. J Clin Pharmacol 40:316–23, 2000.

Chapter 73

Abnormalities of Fat Distribution in HIV Infection

Carl Grunfeld, MD, PhD

Shortly after the introduction of combination antiretroviral therapy with HIV protease inhibitors (PIs), changes in fat (Table 73-1) and serum metabolites were seen that were attributed to PI drugs. In 1997, three early case reports described phenomena such as hypertrophy of the breasts and upper chest fat accompanied by enlargement of the abdomen and thinning of the buttocks and legs,[1] benign symmetric lipomatosis,[2] and loss of subcutaneous fat.[3] At the same time, papers describing dyslipidemia,[4] hyperglycemia, and eventually insulin resistance[5,6] that were attributed to PI therapy were published. The next manifestation was the appearance of 'buffalo hump', a fat pad on the upper back, between the shoulders, often extending to the neck.[7–9] Increased abdominal size with increased visceral (intra-abdominal) fat was also reported.[10] Shortly thereafter, a flood of reports were published of fat loss in the periphery (face, legs, and arms) and gain of fat centrally.[11]

The striking loss of fat in the face became the new stigma of HIV. It 'outed' patients who were now healthy and no longer had wasting or Kaposi sarcoma to identify them as HIV-infected.[12] The presence of lipoatrophy greatly decreases quality of life at a time of restoration to health.[13–15] Indeed, some patients stopped antiretroviral therapy in the hope of reversing the changes.[16]

The combination of hyperlipidemia, insulin resistance, and abdominal obesity was evocative of the metabolic syndrome, which predicts increased risk of cardiovascular disease. The findings were rapidly synthesized into a single syndrome called HIV-lipodystrophy or fat redistribution syndrome which coupled peripheral fat loss to central fat gain, accompanied by insulin resistance and hyperlipdemia.[17,18] The syndrome was proposed to be due to PI drugs.

Table 73-1 Fat Distribution Changes Reported in HIV Infection in the Era of Combination Antiretroviral Therapy

Reported Finding	Description	Current Status
Buffalo hump	Increased fat in between the scapula, going up the neck	A result of lipoatrophy being more severe in the lower body. With weight gain, more fat is put on upper trunk and neck
Peripheral lipoatrophy	Loss of fat in legs and face	Now recognized to be subcutaneous lipoatrophy with legs more affected than upper trunk
Visceral obesity	Increased fat within the abdomen	Unrelated to lipoatrophy
Central lipohypertrophy	Increased fat in abdomen and trunk	Visceral obesity as above. In most patients central subcutaneous fat is reduced. With gain in fat, it is disproportionately placed in the upper trunk
Breast enlargement	Increased fat in breast	A result of subcutaneous lipoatrophy and weight gain, as above
Lipomatosis	Multiple fat tumors	A rare presentation. Relation to HIV unclear

The proposed syndrome neglected the abnormalities previously seen in patients with HIV infection, such as cachexia, low LDL and HDL, hypertriglyceridemia, and perhaps even increased sensitivity to insulin.[19,20] As will be delineated in this chapter, it is now clear that many of these changes are not linked in a single syndrome (e.g., peripheral fat wasting is not associated with central fat gain). Subcutaneous lipoatrophy at peripheral and central sites is the lesion most characteristic of HIV infection; the lower body is affected more than the upper body. There are multiple factors that may contribute to each change, rather than them all being due to PI therapy. The increase in visceral fat is not HIV-related. Finally, once lipoatrophy occurs, it is difficult to reverse.

ASSESSING CLINICAL SYNDROMES

A large number of reports on HIV lipodystrophy and its metabolic consequences relied on subjective criteria that differed among research groups.[11,21] Four different descriptions were used: (1) both peripheral lipoatrophy and central lipohypertrophy; (2) either peripheral lipoatrophy or central lipohypertrophy; (3) only peripheral lipoatrophy; and (4) only central lipohypertrophy. There were at least four ascertainment methods, which were not quantitative and also varied among the reports: (1) self-report of change in fat; (2) exam finding of fat abnormalities; (3) self-report of change in fat confirmed by exam finding of fat abnormalities; and (4) review of charts for report of HIV lipodystrophy. Perhaps as a consequence of these techniques, the prevalence of the 'HIV-lipodystrophy syndrome' was reported to vary between 2% and 84%.[11]

More important, there were major disagreements over the cause of the 'HIV-lipodystrophy syndrome'.[11,21] Some blamed PI drugs, while others blamed NRTI drugs. Other factors proposed to contribute included HIV itself, diagnosis of AIDS, history of CD4 counts, and age. The fact that differing definitions were used for HIV lipodystrophy led to disagreement over what were the potential causal factors.

However, the failure to begin by properly determining which findings were associated with each other likely diluted out the ability to assess potential factors. Research protocols often assumed that peripheral lipoatrophy and central lipohypertrophy were linked; as a consequence they only asked about loss of peripheral fat and gain of central fat. If a study preselected for either or both peripheral lipoatrophy and central lipohypertrophy, the study could not determine whether the contributing factors to these two changes were different.

Buffalo Hump

The reports of buffalo hump in HIV infection were accompanied by photographs (Figure 73-1) of large fat deposits in the upper back, often wrapping around the neck and cervical fat pads.[7–9,22] Many patients have difficulty sleeping on their backs due to the large fat deposits. Given that the majority of AIDS patients were wasted (cachectic) before the introduction of effective combination therapy, this change was striking. Furthermore buffalo hump appeared rapidly (over a few months) in some patients.

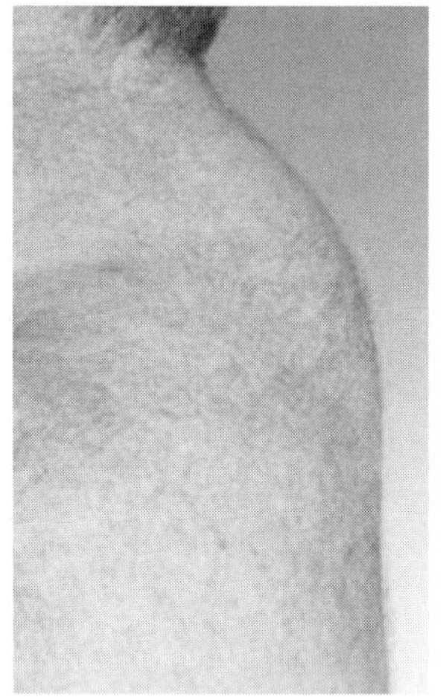
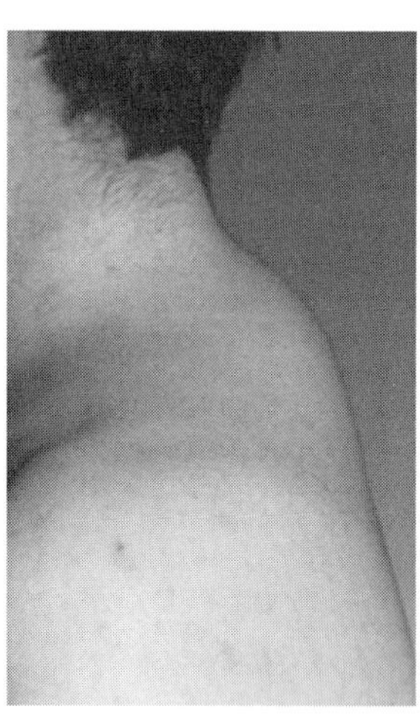

Figure 73-1 ■ A buffalo hump. A deposit of fat in the middle of the upper back, going up the neck.

Buffalo hump is found in patients with Cushing syndrome due to glucocorticoid excess. The first reports of buffalo hump ruled out circulating glucocorticoid excess as the cause of buffalo hump in HIV infection.[7,8] It is still possible that there is an indirect contribution of glucocorticoids to the appearance of buffalo hump, as upper body fat may convert more corticosterone to cortisol, the active glucocorticoid, leading to increased intracellular cortisol, promoting proliferation similar to that seen in Cushing syndrome.

In the earliest report of buffalo hump in HIV infection, half of the subjects were not on PI drugs.[7] These data were unfortunately ignored as others pursued PI drugs as the cause of a pooled syndrome or lipohypertrophy.

Increased Abdominal Fat

The finding of increases in abdominal fat also seemed striking after years of having cachectic patients with HIV infection.[10] This change was often called 'Crix belly', after Crixivan® (indinavir), one of the first effective PI drugs. It is not clear why this change was not initially linked to the use of ritonavir or saqunavir, but the gastrointestinal side effects of the early preparations and/or high doses of these drugs may have decreased weight gain.

CT and MRI imaging showed that many HIV-infected patients with large bellies had increased visceral adipose tissue (VAT),[10] which is associated with metabolic abnormalities and increased risk of cardiovascular disease. It should be noted that a high percentage of the non-HIV-infected population in the industrialized world has obesity; some studies find that one-third are obese and another one-third are overweight.[23] Several factors including age, race, and gender influence visceral obesity.[24] Obesity progresses with age and age is the major determinant of increased VAT even in the absence of obesity. Men have more VAT than women. Caucasians are more susceptible to increased VAT.

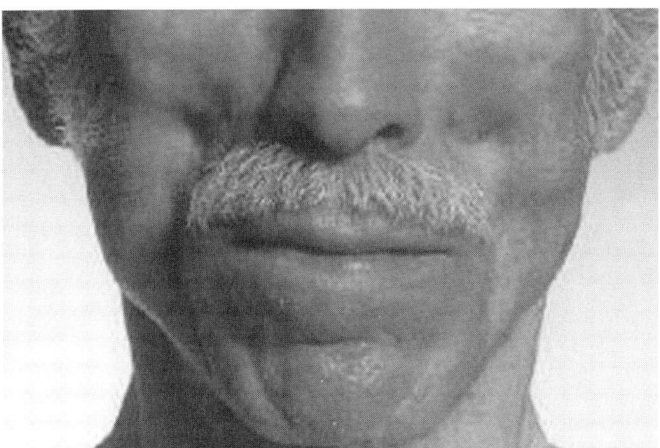

Figure 73-2 ■ Facial lipoatrophy. Loss of fat in the face, especially in Bichat's fat pad below the eyes and beside the nose.

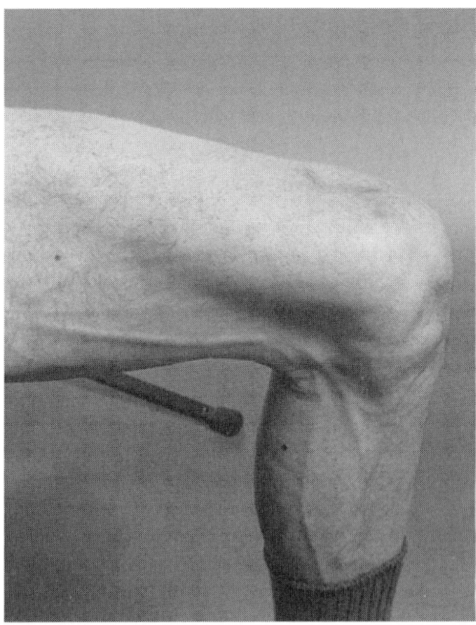

Figure 73-3 ■ Peripheral lipoatrophy. Prominence of the veins and muscles.

Increased Breast Size

The initial reports of changes in fat in HIV-infected women, emphasized central obesity and, in particular, increases in breast size.[1,25,26] In addition to pendulous breasts, large amounts of fat in the chest and upper back were reported. These findings paralleled the upper trunk fat seen in many patients with buffalo hump.

While the syndrome was described in women on PI, an early report found an association with lamivudine use.[26] Given the small size of the seminal studies, it is difficult to assess the role of any drug or class of drugs that were commonly used and in particular to distinguish that from therapy *per se*.

Peripheral Lipoatrophy

The most striking change reported was loss of subcutaneous fat in the peripheral sites of the face, legs, and arms.[27] Some patients had virtually no facial fat in Bichat's fat pad, the area of the cheeks below the eyes (see Figure 73-2). This change is not characteristic of other diseases with cachexia. Furthermore, the decrease in fat in the face, legs, and arms occurred when muscle mass was being restored due to effective therapy, a finding that is the antithesis of the cachexia seen for decades in patients with HIV infection. Veins and muscle appeared very prominent in affected arms and legs (see Figure 73-3). Careful examination of some of the photographs of HIV-infected patients with protuberant bellies revealed decreased subcutaneous fat in the abdomen.[27]

The first reports of peripheral lipoatrophy attributed it to PI drugs.[3,17] However, soon thereafter a role for NRTI emerged. Reports appeared of HIV-infected patients with peripheral lipoatrophy who were only on NRTI drugs and had never taken a PI.[28,29] Stavudine was more strongly linked to the presentation of peripheral lipoatrophy than any other NRTI. In the early days of PI therapy, not all patients were on NRTI combinations that are now deemed highly active; one analysis found that even among patients reported to have PI-associated fat distribution changes, those with lipoatrophy were twice as likely to be on stavudine and/or lamivudine (mostly on both in combination) than those with fat accumulation.[30]

WHAT IS THE HIV-ASSOCIATED SYNDROME OF LIPODYSTROPHY?

Peripheral Lipoatrophy Is Not Linked to Central Lipohypertrophy

In most early studies of HIV-lipodystrophy, entry was by clinical presentation, but measurement of fat was performed in some studies. Although many of the patients were clinically described as having increased abdominal fat (or girth), direct measurements of fat mass by dual-energy X-ray absorptiometry (DXA) revealed less truncal fat compared to those without the HIV-lipodystrophy syndrome.[11,17] These measurements were the first indication that the clinical presentations might not accurately represent the actual findings. They also raised the question of 'pseudo-truncal obesity', where loss of fat in arms and legs made the abdomen look prominent.[11]

As discussed above, many of the clinical instruments used assumed that the syndrome was peripheral fat loss and central fat gain. The instruments were unidirectional, i.e., the studies only measured peripheral fat loss or looked for peripheral lipoatrophy; they did not consider peripheral fat gain. More importantly, the instruments measured the central gain and looked for central lipohypertrophy; they did not look for central fat loss. As a consequence, these studies were never able to determine whether there was a statistical association of peripheral lipoatrophy and central lipohypertrophy or whether central depots had lipoatrophy.

The study of Fat Redistribution and Metabolic Change in HIV Infection (FRAM), a large (1183 HIV-infected subjects and 297 controls), multicenter study included clinical instruments similar to other studies, as well as direct measurements of fat.[31] However, the FRAM surveys of self-report of change in fat and examinations of fat were bidirectional. For example, subjects were asked about fat loss or fat gain in each body area. The FRAM study found that HIV-infected subjects reporting loss of fat in the periphery more often reported loss of or less gain of central fat than subjects not reporting peripheral fat loss.[32,33] Subjects with abnormally low peripheral fat on examination had less central fat than those who did not have peripheral fat loss. Thus, even in the 'clinical syndrome', there was no indication that loss of peripheral fat was linked to gain of central fat, providing evidence against using those two findings as part of a single syndrome.

Mimicking many early studies, FRAM defined lipoatrophy as self-report of loss of fat in an anatomical area confirmed by abnormally less fat in that area on examination. Likewise, lipohypertrophy was defined as gain of fat in an anatomical area confirmed by abnormally more fat in that area on examination. Because bidirectional scales were used, it was possible to study lipoatrophy and lipohypertrophy at both central and peripheral sites. Peripheral lipoatrophy was found in 38% of HIV-infected men and somewhat less frequently in HIV-infected women; the rates were less than 5% in controls.[32,33] Central lipoatrophy was less common, but occurred more often in HIV-infected subjects than controls. Central lipohypertrophy was found in 40% of HIV-infected men and slightly more often in HIV-infected women. However, central lipohypertrophy was actually less frequent in HIV-infected men than control men, while the rates in HIV-infected and control women were similar. Peripheral lipohypertrophy was uncommon in HIV-infected subjects.

FRAM then determined the association among the potential clinical syndrome.[32,33] Rather than finding a link between peripheral lipoatrophy and central lipohypertrophy, FRAM showed that the two findings were disassociated (for men the odds ratio of peripheral lipoatrophy occurring with central lipohypertrophy was OR = 0.7, CI = 0.47–1.1, P = 0.10; for women OR = 0.39, 95% C.I. = 0.20–0.75, P = 0.006). Thus, peripheral lipoatrophy and central lipohypertrophy could not be part of a single syndrome.

Measurements of Fat Prove Lipoatrophy and Lipohypertrophy Are Independent

The Women's Interagency HIV Study (WIHS) asked subjects at sequential visits about change in fat and estimated amounts of fat by anthropometric measurements.[34] They defined lipoatrophy as report of loss of fat accompanied by a decrease in fat measured by anthropometry. They defined lipohypertrophy as report of gain of fat accompanied by an increase by anthropometry. HIV-infected women in WIHS had more peripheral and central lipoatrophy than control women. HIV-infected women had less peripheral lipohypertrophy, than controls, but similar central lipohypertrophy. The authors concluded that lipoatrophy, in both peripheral and central sites, was the hallmark lesion in HIV infection; there was little evidence for excess central lipohypertrophy in HIV-infected women.[34]

In the Multi-center AIDS Cohort Study (MACS) anthropometric measurements were also performed in HIV-infected men and controls.[35] In MACS, HIV-infected subjects had less fat than controls as estimated by anthropometrics in both peripheral and central sites. They concluded that HIV-infected men receiving HAART were characterized by lipoatrophy, not lipohypertrophy.[35]

The control group from MACS is from the same at-risk cohort and the controls groups in WIHS were recruited to be similar. In both WIHS and MACS, the control groups had a tendency to be heavier than equivalent age subjects in the NHANES study that is representative of the US population.[34,35]

The FRAM study performed whole-body MRI for body composition.[31] Subcutaneous adipose tissue (SAT) volumes were measured in the peripheral sites of the leg and arm and the central sites of the abdomen/back and chest/back. VAT was also measured. There were no inverse relationships between peripheral adipose tissue depots and central adipose tissue depots.[32,33] HIV-infected subjects with the clinical syndrome of peripheral lipoatrophy had less adipose tissue in both peripheral and central sites than HIV-infected subjects without the clinical syndrome of peripheral lipoatrophy. Within the group with peripheral lipoatrophy, there was a positive correlation between all peripheral and central sites (not an inverse correlation), although the correlation between leg and VAT was not statistically significant. The HIV-infected group without clinical peripheral lipoatrophy had lower leg SAT than controls, but similar VAT in men and increased VAT in women. Thus, the clinical syndrome underestimates the prevalence and amount of lipoatrophy. For both HIV-infected groups, leg SAT showed the greatest decrease compared to controls, while upper trunk showed the least decrease. Indeed, in HIV-infected women without the clinical syndrome of peripheral lipoatrophy (a group that had a higher body mass index (BMI)), chest and upper back fat was higher than controls.

All HIV-infected groups had ranges of VAT that were similar to the controls.[32,33] Thus, there is a wide spectrum of HIV-infected patients with decreased leg SAT and some have increased VAT. However, there is no association of decreased leg SAT with increased VAT. The measurements of fat also demonstrate that there is no link between peripheral lipoatrophy and central lipohypertrophy. Rather, the abnormal syndrome in HIV infection is loss of subcutaneous fat in both peripheral and central depots, with lower sites affected more than upper sites. Increased VAT is not part of the syndrome.

WHAT FACTORS CONTRIBUTE TO LIPOATROPHY AND LIPOHYPERTROPHY?

Epidemiology Based on Clinical Syndromes

As discussed above, pooling two clinical syndromes that do not belong together (lipoatrophy and lipohypertrophy) dilutes the ability to look for causal factors. While one early study predominantly looking at lipoatrophy implicated PIs,[17] another early study of lipoatrophy found an association with stavudine use.[28] Subsequent studies of the clinical syndrome have been consistent with each of these findings.

In the HOPS study, moderate to severe lipoatrophy was associated with any use of stavudine, use of indinavir for longer than 2 years, increasing age, and measures of duration and severity of HIV disease.[36] They also concluded that if nondrug risk factors were absent, lipoatrophy was unusual regardless of the duration of drug use. Increasingly, the clinical studies of lipoatrophy implicated stavudine as having the strongest effect at inducing lipoatrophy, with a lesser effect of zidovudine. However, later in the epidemic, new cases of lipoatrophy were often not associated with the same factors. The HOPS study later found that white race, a low BMI, and a low CD4 count were major factors; the latter two could reflect the onset of HIV-associated cachexia which represents true wasting of both muscle and fat.[37]

Epidemiology Based on Fat Measurement

A key early study looked at DXA scans of patients on various antiretroviral regimens and found no difference in fat distribution of those on PI or not on PI.[38] A subsequent study followed patients for the onset of fat wasting using DXA.[39] They found that stavudine-containing regimens were associated with more and faster fat wasting than zidovudine-containing regimens. They also found that fat wasting was accelerated when NRTIs were used in combination with PIs.[39]

The FRAM study reviewed charts and interviewed subjects to obtain complete antiretroviral drug histories; it then determined which drugs or regimens were associated with leg SAT or VAT.[32,33] In both men and women, duration of stavudine use was strongly associated with less leg SAT. In men, indinavir use was also associated with less leg SAT, whereas in women, NNRTI use was associated with less leg SAT. In men no antiretroviral drug was associated with more VAT; rather nevirapine use was associated with less VAT. In women, any form of HAART was associated with more VAT, but no specific drug or class of drugs was found to be associated. Thus no drug or regimen was associated with lower leg SAT and more VAT. On the other hand, older age, being male, and being Caucasian was associated with lower leg SAT and more VAT. Physical activity and smoking were associated with lower fat in both depots.[32]

Table 73-2 Current Views of the Etiology of Fat Distribution Changes in HIV Infection

Finding	Associated Etiologic Factors
Subcutaneous lipoatrophy	Stavudine, zidovudine, didanosine ?, protease inhibitors (especially indinavir), NNRTI in women, age, Caucasian, male sex
Visceral obesity	Age, Caucasian, male sex, restoration to health, effective antiretroviral therapy

Antiretroviral Trials with Fat Measurements

Prospective data of body composition measurements with initiation of antiretroviral therapy was informative even before randomized trials were performed. In one study, the first changes that occurred were increases in fat in all areas over the first 24 weeks, followed by loss of predominantly limb fat later.[40] In multivariate analysis, the major factor associated with loss of limb fat was use of stavudine.[40]

In one study, antiretroviral-naive subjects were randomized to HAART with two different NRTI backbones.[41] Those on a stavudine with diadanosine backbone did worse than those on abacavir with lamivudine.

In another similar study, antiretroviral-naive patients were randomized to nelfinavir, efavirenz, or both on NRTI backbones of stavudine with diadanosine or zidovudine with lamivudine.[42] Again, subjects first gained fat, and then lost fat, especially in the limbs. More fat was lost in the stavudine with diadanosine backbone than the zidovudine with lamivudine backbone. More fat was lost with nelfinavir than with efavirenz.

The results of these etiology studies and switch studies described below are summarized in Table 73-2. In aggregate, these studies suggest that the major contributor to lipoatrophy is stavudine, with a lesser effect of zidovudine and possibly didanosine. PIs also contribute, perhaps aggravating the effect of thymidine analogs. Whether specific PIs have less effect of lipatrophy needs to be demonstrated by comparative trials.

THERAPY FOR FAT CHANGES IN HIV

Many of the trials of therapies for HIV-associated lipodystrophy were designed before the syndrome was defined or the etiology understood. Hence, some studies selected patients with both lipoatrophy and lipohypertrophy, while others only lipoatrophy. Some studies required that subjects have a particular metabolic change for entry. Some switch studies were negative, but they contribute to our understanding of the syndrome.

Switching Antiretroviral Drugs

While the etiology of the changes in fat distribution was being debated, switch studies were performed in which the proposed candidate drugs were stopped and others started. Many of these studies had direct measurements of fat. The results indicate that recovery from lipoatrophy is at best slow and perhaps never complete. The switch studies also implicated stavudine and to a lesser extent zidovudine as the most deleterious drugs.

Given the early focus on PIs as the cause of lipodystrophy, many studies switched patients off PI drugs, but little improvement was seen. Substitution of a PI with efavirenz caused no improvement in subcutaneous fat despite improvements in triglycerides and sensitivity to insulin.[43–45] Likewise, substitution of a PI with nevirapine had no effect on fat despite improvement in serum triglycerides.[45–47] Furthermore, substitution of abacavir for a PI had little effect on body fat although it improved lipids and reduced lipolysis.[45,48,49] Likewise, substitution of nevirapine, abacavir, adefovir, and hydroxyurea as an intensive alternative to PI drugs on an NRTI base led to no improvement in fat wasting.[50] These results imply that PIs are not the major contributors to lipoatrophy and also imply that abnormalities in triglyceride or glucose metabolism are not the cause of changes in fat distribution.

In contrast, switching from certain NRTI regimens consistently led to small improvements in limb and subcutaneous fat although subjects were not restored to normal. Switching from stavudine to abacavir led to small increases in limb fat.[48] Switching from either stavudine or zidovudine to abacavir led to small increases in limb fat (~1 kg), but lipoatrophy remained even after 2 years off thymidine analogs.[51–53] These data imply that thymidine analog-induced changes either take a very long time to reverse or that that thymidine analogs are not the only factors contributing to lipoatrophy.

Likewise, switching from a regimen containing both stavudine and a PI to zidovudine, lamivudine, and abacavir led to small increases in limb fat by DXA and subcutaneous fat by CT, but no change in VAT.[54] Small improvements in fat were also found when switching from stavudine to either abacavir or zidovudine.[55]

These switch data support the concept that stavudine-containing regimens induce more lipoatrophy than zidovudine containing regimens, but the sum of data indicates that avoidance of any thymidine analog leads to even less lipoatrophy.

Pharmacological Approaches

When the syndrome was viewed as a single entity of peripheral lipoatrophy combined with central lipohypertrophy and metabolic disturbances such as insulin resistance, certain pharmacological approaches were appealing. The studies described below had varying entry criteria. Some studies required insulin resistance for entry. Others selected for lipohypertrophy as well as lipoatrophy. Some of these approaches had not been previously tested in syndromes that were dominantly lipoatrophy.

Thiazolidinedione Drugs

Thiazolidinedione drugs were logical drugs to test as one drug of the class, troglitazone (which has been removed from the market), had been shown to increase subcutaneous fat and decrease visceral fat while improving insulin resistance and glucose control in mildly obese patients with type 2 diabetes in poor control.[56] Furthermore, troglitazone was shown to increase subcutaneous, but not visceral fat in patients with non-HIV-related lipoatrophy and lipodystrophy.[57]

Six randomized trials have been performed with thiazolidinedione drugs. Four found minimal increases in limb fat by DXA or subcutaneous fat by CT,[58–61] while two studies found no changes in these fat depots.[62,63] In one study VAT decreased,[60] but in the others there was no change in VAT.[58,59,62] One patient with severe lipoatrophy developed multiple symmetric lipomatosis with rosiglitazone treatment that improved on cessation of the drug.[64]

Thiazolidinediones improve insulin resistance[58,60,62] and decrease the clotting factor PAI-1[65] in patients with HIV-associated lipodystrophy of varying definitions. However, one drug in the class, rosiglitazone, may increase triglycerides and LDL cholesterol and decrease HDL cholesterol.[58,59,62,66] A well-known complication of all thiazolidinedione drugs is peripheral edema.

Metformin

Metformin is the oral hypoglycemic drug that is preferred as the first-line therapy in obese type 2 diabetics. It decreases fasting blood glucose by decreasing hepatic glucose production, improves insulin sensitivity, and decreases weight. Its use was logical when the syndrome was thought to be both lipoatrophy and lipohypertrophy. Two studies have shown that metformin decreased VAT in HIV-infected patients with lipodystrophy, many of whom had lipohypertrophy[58] but another found no change.[67] However, metformin also decreased SAT. Metformin improved insulin resistance in these patients and may lower triglyceride levels, but raised LDL cholesterol.[59]

Growth Hormone and Growth Hormone-Releasing Hormone (GHRH) Analogs

Growth hormone has been shown to decrease visceral fat in patients with growth hormone deficiency or obesity. In adult and adolescent patients with HIV-associated changes in fat who were selected for likely visceral obesity, growth hormone therapy decreases VAT, but also decreases SAT.[68–71] Many doses have been tried; in general the higher the dose, the greater the effect on VAT, but the more the complications.[71,72] Some trials of growth hormone excluded those with abnormalities on glucose tolerance testing. Growth hormone therapy, especially at higher doses, can cause worsening of glucose levels and insulin resistance, although with time insulin resistance returns toward normal.[71] Growth hormone improves LDL and non-HDL cholesterol, the atherogenic cholesterol.[68]

A GHRH analog has also been shown to induce small decreases in VAT in HIV-associated lipodystrophy, but with no change in SAT.[73,74] There were few changes in metabolic parameters. Whether higher doses of such compounds that induce more loss of VAT will reduce SAT and change metabolism remains to be seen.

Exercise

In patients with HIV infection and increased girth, exercise decreases abdominal and limb fat.[75–78] The combination of exercise plus metformin was more effective at reducing both VAT and SAT than metformin alone.[67]

CONCLUSION

The HIV-specific lipodystrophy syndrome is lipoatrophy. The major contributor is exposure to stavudine, which is worse in combination with a PI. Zidovudine and didanosine may also have effects. Once established, lipoatrophy is difficult to reverse. Therefore, prevention by avoiding or delaying suspect antiretroviral drugs is the best approach. Increased visceral adipose tissue is a product of restoration to health, but looks abnormal in HIV-infected subjects with loss of abdominal fat. The standard therapies for obesity and its metabolic complications should be used with the same indications in patients with HIV infection.

ACKNOWLEDGMENT

This study is supported by NIH grants RO1-DK57508 and HL74814.

REFERENCES

1. Herry I, Bernard L, de Truchis P, Perronne C. Hypertrophy of the breasts in a patient treated with indinavir. Clin Infect Dis 25:937–8, 1997.
2. Hengel RL, Watts NB, Lennox JL. Benign symmetric lipomatosis associated with protease inhibitors. Lancet 350:1596, 1997.
3. Massip P, Marchou B, Bonnet E, et al. Lipodystrophia with protease inhibitors in HIV patients. Therapie 52:615, 1997.
4. Sullivan AK, Nelson MR. Marked hyperlipidaemia on ritonavir therapy. AIDS 11:938–9, 1997.
5. Dube MP, Johnson DL, Currier JS, Leedom JM. Protease inhibitor-associated hyperglycaemia. Lancet 350:713–14, 1997.
6. Martinez E, Casamitjana R, Conget I, Gatell JM. Protease inhibitor-associated hyperinsulinaemia [letter]. AIDS 12:2077–9, 1998.
7. Lo JC, Mulligan K, Tai VW, Algren H, Schambelan M. 'Buffalo hump' in men with HIV-1 infection. Lancet 351:867–70, 1998.
8. Miller KK, Daly PA, Sentochnik D, Doweiko J, Samore M, Basgoz NO, Grinspoon SK. Pseudo-Cushing's syndrome in human immunodeficiency virus-infected patients. Clin Infect Dis 27:68–72, 1998.
9. Saint-Marc T, Touraine JL. 'Buffalo hump' in HIV-1 infection. Lancet 352:319–20, 1998.
10. Miller KD, Jones E, Yanovski JA, et al. Visceral abdominal-fat accumulation associated with use of indinavir. Lancet 351:871–5, 1998.
11. Safrin S, Grunfeld C. Fat distribution and metabolic changes in patients with HIV infection. AIDS 13:2493–505, 1999.
12. Oette M, Juretzko P, Kroidl A, et al. Lipodystrophy syndrome and self-assessment of well-being and physical appearance in HIV-positive patients. AIDS Patient Care STDS 16:413–17, 2002.
13. Collins E, Wagner C, Walmsley S. Psychosocial impact of the lipodystrophy syndrome in HIV infection. AIDS Read 10:546–50, 2000.
14. Blanch J, Rousaud A, Martinez E, et al. Impact of lipodystrophy on the quality of life of HIV-1-infected patients. J Acquir Immune Defic Syndr 31:404–7, 2002.
15. Nicholas PK, Kirksey KM, Corless IB, Kemppainen J. Lipodystrophy and quality of life in HIV: Symptom management issues. Appl Nurs Res 18:55–8, 2005.
16. Duran S, Saves M, Spire B, et al. Failure to maintain long-term adherence to highly active antiretroviral therapy: The role of lipodystrophy. AIDS 15:2441–4, 2001.
17. Carr A, Samaras K, Burton S, et al. A syndrome of peripheral lipodystrophy, hyperlipidaemia and insulin resistance in patients receiving HIV protease inhibitors. AIDS 12:F51–8, 1998.
18. Carr A, Samaras K, Thorisdottir A, et al. Diagnosis, prediction, and natural course of HIV-1 protease-inhibitor-associated lipodystrophy, hyperlipidaemia, and diabetes mellitus: a cohort study. Lancet 353:2093–9, 1999.
19. Hommes MJ, Romijn JA, Endert E, et al. Insulin sensitivity and insulin clearance in human immunodeficiency virus-infected men. Metabolism 40:651–6, 1991.
20. Grunfeld C, Pang M, Doerrler W, et al. Lipids, lipoproteins, triglyceride clearance, and cytokines in human immunodeficiency virus infection and the acquired immunodeficiency syndrome. J Clin Endocrinol Metab 74:1045–52, 1992.
21. Tien PC, Grunfeld C. What is HIV-associated lipodystrophy? Defining fat distribution changes in HIV infection. Curr Opin Infect Dis 17:27–32, 2004.
22. Roth VR, Kravcik S, Angel JB. Development of cervical fat pads following therapy with human immunodeficiency virus type 1 protease inhibitors. Clin Infect Dis 27:65–7, 1998.
23. Flegal KM, Carroll MD, Ogden CL, Johnson CL. Prevalence and trends in obesity among US adults, 1999–2000. JAMA 288:1723–7, 2002.
24. Stanforth PR, Jackson AS, Green JS, et al. Generalized abdominal visceral fat prediction models for black and white adults aged 17–65 y: the HERITAGE family study. Int J Obes Relat Metab Disord 28:925–32, 2004.
25. Dong KL, Bausserman LL, Flynn MM, et al. Changes in body habitus and serum lipid abnormalities in HIV-positive women on highly active antiretroviral therapy (HAART). J Acquir Immune Defic Syndr 21:107–13, 1999.
26. Gervasoni C, Ridolfo AL, Trifiro G, et al. Redistribution of body fat in HIV-infected women undergoing combined antiretroviral therapy. AIDS 13:465–71, 1999.
27. Carr A, Cooper DA. Images in clinical medicine. Lipodystrophy associated with an HIV-protease inhibitor. N Engl J Med 339:1296, 1998.
28. Saint-Marc T, Partisani M, Poizot-Martin I, et al. A syndrome of peripheral fat wasting (lipodystrophy) in patients receiving long-term nucleoside analogue therapy. AIDS 13:1659–67, 1999.
29. Madge S, Kinloch-de-Loes S, Mercey D, et al. Lipodystrophy in patients naive to HIV protease inhibitors. AIDS 13:735–7, 1999.
30. Benson JO, McGhee K, Coplan P, et al. Fat redistribution in indinavir-treated patients with HIV infection: A review of postmarketing cases. J Acquir Immune Defic Syndr 25:130–9, 2000.

31. Tien PC, Benson C, Zolopa AR, et al. The study of fat redistribution and metabolic change in HIV infection (FRAM): methods, design, and sample characteristics. Am J Epidemiol, 163:860–9. 2006.
32. Bacchetti P, Gripshover B, Grunfeld C, et al. Fat distribution in men with HIV infection. J Acquir Immune Defic Syndr 40:121–31, 2005.
33. Tien P, Bacchetti P, Cofrancesco J, Heymsfield S. The study of fat distribution and metabolic change in HIV infection (FRAM). Fat distribution in women with HIV infection. JAIDS 42:562–71, 2006.
34. Tien PC, Cole SR, Williams CM, et al. Incidence of lipoatrophy and lipohypertrophy in the women's interagency HIV study. J Acquir Immune Defic Syndr 34:461–6, 2003.
35. Palella FJ Jr, Cole SR, Chmiel JS, et al. Anthropometrics and examiner-reported body habitus abnormalities in the multicenter AIDS cohort study. Clin Infect Dis 38:903–7, 2004.
36. Lichtenstein KA, Ward DJ, Moorman AC, et al. Clinical assessment of HIV-associated lipodystrophy in an ambulatory population. AIDS 15:1389–98, 2001.
37. Lichtenstein KA, Delaney KM, Armon C, et al. Incidence of and risk factors for lipoatrophy (abnormal fat loss) in ambulatory HIV-1-infected patients. J Acquir Immune Defic Syndr 32:48–56, 2003.
38. Kotler DP, Rosenbaum K, Wang J, Pierson RN. Studies of body composition and fat distribution in HIV-infected and control subjects. J Acquir Immune Defic Syndr Hum Retrovirol 20:228–37, 1999.
39. Mallal SA, John M, Moore CB, et al. Contribution of nucleoside analogue reverse transcriptase inhibitors to subcutaneous fat wasting in patients with HIV infection. AIDS 14:1309–16, 2000.
40. Mallon PW, Miller J, Cooper DA, Carr A. Prospective evaluation of the effects of antiretroviral therapy on body composition in HIV-1-infected men starting therapy. AIDS 17:971–9, 2003.
41. Shlay JC, Visnegarwala F, Bartsch G, et al. Body composition and metabolic changes in antiretroviral-naive patients randomized to didanosine and stavudine vs. abacavir and lamivudine. J Acquir Immune Defic Syndr 38:147–55, 2005.
42. Dube MP, Parker RA, Tebas P, et al. Glucose metabolism, lipid, and body fat changes in antiretroviral-naive subjects randomized to nelfinavir or efavirenz plus dual nucleosides. AIDS 19:1807–18, 2005.
43. Martinez E, Garcia-Viejo MA, Blanco JL, et al. Impact of switching from human immunodeficiency virus type 1 protease inhibitors to efavirenz in successfully treated adults with lipodystrophy. Clin Infect Dis 31:1266–73, 2000.
44. Knechten H, Sturner KH, Hohn C, Braun P. Switch to efavirenz in a protease inhibitor-containing regimen. HIV Clin Trials 2:200–4, 2001.
45. Martinez E, Arnaiz JA, Podzamczer D, et al. Substitution of nevirapine, efavirenz, or abacavir for protease inhibitors in patients with human immunodeficiency virus infection. N Engl J Med 349:1036–46, 2003.
46. Ruiz L, Negredo E, Domingo P,et al. Antiretroviral treatment simplification with nevirapine in protease inhibitor-experienced patients with HIV-associated lipodystrophy: 1-year prospective follow-up of a multicenter, randomized, controlled study. J Acquir Immune Defic Syndr 27:229–36, 2001.
47. Martinez E, Conget I, Lozano L, et al. Reversion of metabolic abnormalities after switching from HIV-1 protease inhibitors to nevirapine. AIDS 13:805–10, 1999.
48. Moyle GJ, Baldwin C, Langroudi B, et al. A 48-week, randomized, open-label comparison of three abacavir-based substitution approaches in the management of dyslipidemia and peripheral lipoatrophy. J Acquir Immune Defic Syndr 33:22–8, 2003.
49. van der Valk M, Allick G, Weverling GJ, et al. Markedly diminished lipolysis and partial restoration of glucose metabolism, without changes in fat distribution after extended discontinuation of protease inhibitors in severe lipodystrophic human immunodeficient virus-1-infected patients. J Clin Endocrinol Metab 89:3554–60, 2004.
50. Carr A, Hudson J, Chuah J, et al. HIV protease inhibitor substitution in patients with lipodystrophy: a randomized, controlled, open-label, multicentre study. AIDS 15:1811–22, 2001.
51. Smith DE, Carr A, Law M, et al. Thymidine analogue withdrawal for lipoatrophic patients on protease-sparing therapy improves lipoatrophy but compromises antiviral control: the PIILR extension study. AIDS 16:2489–91, 2002.
52. Martin A, Smith DE, Carr A, et al. Reversibility of lipoatrophy in HIV-infected patients 2 years after switching from a thymidine analogue to abacavir: the MITOX Extension Study. AIDS 18:1029–36, 2004.
53. Carr A, Workman C, Smith DE, et al. Abacavir substitution for nucleoside analogs in patients with HIV lipoatrophy: a randomized trial. JAMA 288:207–15, 2002.
54. John M, McKinnon EJ, James IR, et al. Randomized, controlled, 48-week study of switching stavudine and/or protease inhibitors to combivir/abacavir to prevent or reverse lipoatrophy in HIV-infected patients. J Acquir Immune Defic Syndr 33:29–33, 2003.
55. McComsey GA, Ward DJ, Hessenthaler SM, et al. Improvement in lipoatrophy associated with highly active antiretroviral therapy in human immunodeficiency virus-infected patients switched from stavudine to abacavir or zidovudine: the results of the TARHEEL study. Clin Infect Dis 38:263–70, 2004.
56. Mori Y, Murakawa Y, Okada K, et al. Effect of troglitazone on body fat distribution in type 2 diabetic patients. Diabetes Care 22:908–12, 1999.
57. Arioglu E, Duncan-Morin J, Sebring N, et al. Efficacy and safety of troglitazone in the treatment of lipodystrophy syndromes. Ann Intern Med 133:263–74, 2000.
58. Hadigan C, Corcoran C, Basgoz N, et al. Metformin in the treatment of HIV lipodystrophy syndrome: A randomized controlled trial. JAMA 284:472–7, 2000.
59. van Wijk JP, de Koning EJ, Cabezas MC, et al. Comparison of rosiglitazone and metformin for treating HIV lipodystrophy: a randomized trial. Ann Intern Med 143:337–46, 2005.
60. Gelato MC, Mynarcik DC, Quick JL, et al. Improved insulin sensitivity and body fat distribution in HIV-infected patients treated with rosiglitazone: a pilot study. J Acquir Immune Defic Syndr 31:163–70, 2002.
61. Slama L, Lanoy E, Valentin MA, et al. Effect of Pioglitazone on HIV-1 Related Lipodystrophy: A Randomized Double-blind Placebo-controlled Trial (ANRS 113) with 130 Patients. In 13th Conference on Retroviruses and Opportunistic Infections, Denver, CO, 2006, p 102.
62. Sutinen J, Hakkinen AM, Westerbacka J, et al. Rosiglitazone in the treatment of HAART-associated lipodystrophy – a randomized double-blind placebo-controlled study. Antivir Ther 8:199–207, 2003.
63. Carr A, Workman C, Carey D, et al. No effect of rosiglitazone for treatment of HIV-1 lipoatrophy: randomised, double-blind, placebo-controlled trial. Lancet 363:429–38, 2004.
64. Mafong DD, Lee GA, Yu S, et al. Development of multiple lipomas during treatment with rosiglitazone in a patient with HIV-associated lipoatrophy. AIDS 18:1742–4, 2004.
65. Yki-Jarvinen H, Sutinen J, Silveira A, et al. Regulation of plasma PAI-1 concentrations in HAART-associated lipodystrophy during rosiglitazone therapy. Arterioscler Thromb Vasc Biol 23:688–94, 2003.
66. Moyle GJ, Daar E, Gertner J, et al. Growth hormone improves lean body mass, physical performance and quality of life in subjects with HIV-associated weight loss or wasting on highly active antiretroviral therapy. J Acquir Immune Defic Syndr 35:367–75, 2004.

67. Driscoll SD, Meininger GE, Lareau MT, et al. Effects of exercise training and metformin on body composition and cardiovascular indices in HIV-infected patients. AIDS 18:465–73, 2004.
68. Kotler DP, Muurahainen N, Grunfeld C, et al. Effects of growth hormone on abnormal visceral adipose tissue accumulation and dyslipidemia in HIV-infected patients. J Acquir Immune Defic Syndr 35:239–52, 2004.
69. Engelson ES, Glesby MJ, Mendez D, et al. Effect of recombinant human growth hormone in the treatment of visceral fat accumulation in HIV infection. J Acquir Immune Defic Syndr 30:379–91, 2002.
70. Vigano A, Mora S, Manzoni P, et al. Effects of recombinant growth hormone on visceral fat accumulation: pilot study in human immunodeficiency virus-infected adolescents. J Clin Endocrinol Metab 90:4075–80, 2005.
71. Lo JC, Mulligan K, Noor MA, et al. The effects of recombinant human growth hormone on body composition and glucose metabolism in HIV-infected patients with fat accumulation. J Clin Endocrinol Metab 86:3480–7, 2001.
72. Lo JC, Mulligan K, Noor MA, et al. The effects of low-dose growth hormone in HIV-infected men with fat accumulation: a pilot study. Clin Infect Dis 39:732–5, 2004.
73. Koutkia P, Canavan B, Breu J, et al. Growth hormone-releasing hormone in HIV-infected men with lipodystrophy: a randomized controlled trial. JAMA 292:210–18, 2004.
74. Falutz J, Allas S, Kotler D, et al. A placebo-controlled, dose-ranging study of a growth hormone releasing factor in HIV-infected patients with abdominal fat accumulation. AIDS 19:1279–87, 2005.
75. Jones SP, Doran DA, Leatt PB, et al. Short-term exercise training improves body composition and hyperlipidaemia in HIV-positive individuals with lipodystrophy. AIDS 15:2049–51, 2001.
76. Roubenoff R, Schmitz H, Bairos L, et al. Reduction of abdominal obesity in lipodystrophy associated with human immunodeficiency virus infection by means of diet and exercise: case report and proof of principle. Clin Infect Dis 34:390–3, 2002.
77. Roubenoff R, Weiss L, McDermott A, et al. A pilot study of exercise training to reduce trunk fat in adults with HIV-associated fat redistribution. AIDS 13:1373–5, 1999.
78. Smith BA, Neidig JL, Nickel JT, Mitchell GL, Para MF, Fass RJ. Aerobic exercise: effects on parameters related to fatigue, dyspnea, weight and body composition in HIV-infected adults. AIDS 15:693–701, 2001.

Chapter 74

Lactic Acidosis and Other Mitochondrial Disorders Associated with HIV Therapy

David Nolan, MD, Simon Mallal, MD

INTRODUCTION

Nucleoside analog reverse transcriptase inhibitors (NRTI) were the first class of drugs to demonstrate potent efficacy against HIV infection, being introduced into clinical practice in 1987 (with the advent of zidovudine monotherapy) within a short period of the widespread recognition of AIDS and of HIV as its underlying cause. However, the ongoing use of NRTI therapy into the second decade of HIV therapy highlights the need for a comprehensive understanding of NRTI-induced drug toxicities,[1–3] as HIV infection becomes a more manageable disease with greatly reduced morbidity and mortality.[4,5] This chapter will review current knowledge of the role of mitochondrial toxicity in the pathogenesis of clinical toxicity syndromes associated with NRTI drug therapy, including lactic acidosis as well as a number of tissue-specific treatment complications (e.g., lipoatrophy, neuropathy).

The NRTI-associated toxicities that are described in this chapter first came to light as clinical syndromes that (like AIDS) were denoted as either "present" or "absent". It is only with increased knowledge of the underlying pathogenic mechanisms (e.g., tissue-specific mitochondrial DNA depletion) and markers of disease progression over time (e.g., longitudinal body composition assessments for lipoatrophy) that we have come to appreciate how these disease processes can be assessed and monitored. This underlines one important treatment principle: as with the management of HIV, it is apparent that more advanced and clinically apparent disease represents less reversible disease. This appears to be particularly true where the toxic effect of drug therapy leads to tissue loss and damage – as seen most readily in the cases of lipoatrophy and neuropathy.

The risk of developing severe toxicities such as lactic acidosis appears to have declined significantly in recent years.[6] However, it is also apparent that certain long-term HIV drug toxicities provide an ongoing burden of disease, so that established clinical syndromes may not improve substantially even years after the removal of the causative NRTI drug. In this context, there is an ongoing need not only to prevent NRTI complications wherever possible, but also to develop effective treatment strategies for those affected by these treatment complications.

MODE OF ACTION OF NRTI DRUGS

The antiretroviral efficacy of NRTI drugs is conferred by their ability to inhibit HIV reverse transcriptase, the viral RNA-dependent DNA polymerase that allows the virus to create a DNA sequence based on its own RNA template (Fig. 74-1). Following intracellular phosphorylation, NRTI drugs compete with naturally occurring nucleotides for utilization by HIV reverse transcriptase. Incorporation of the "false" NRTI substrate then causes DNA chain termination, as these nucleotides lack a hydroxyl group that is critical for chain elongation. The effectiveness of NRTI drugs as inhibitors of HIV replication is therefore determined primarily by their ability to inhibit HIV reverse transcriptase. However, the efficiency with which NRTI drugs are delivered to the appropriate cell population and intracellular compartment – determined by factors such as oral bioavailability, cellular transport mechanisms, and the efficiency of cellular kinases responsible for activating NRTI drugs to their triphosphate form – is also an important factor in determining drug efficacy.

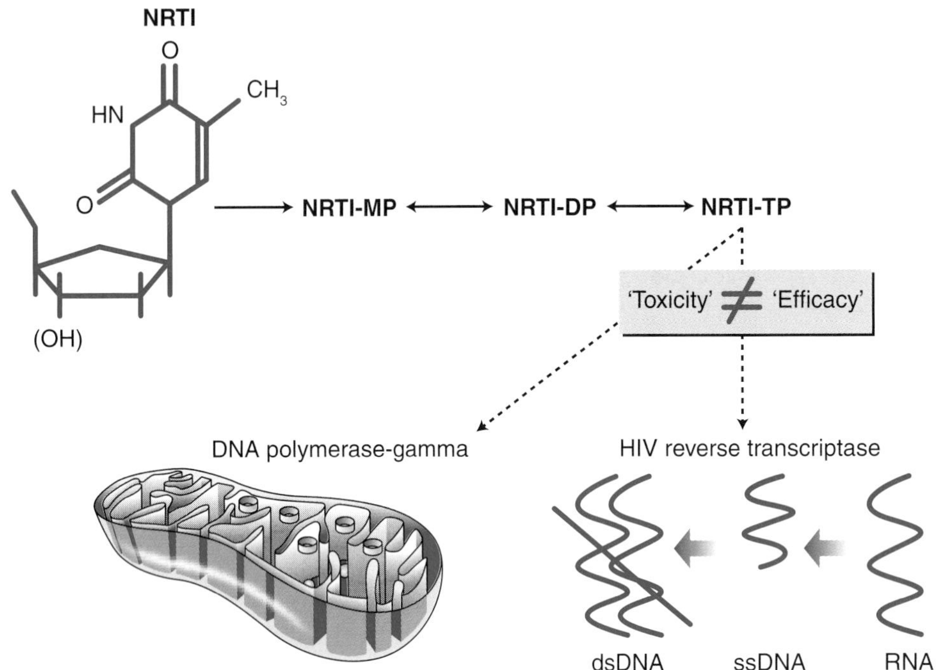

Figure 74-1 ■ The basis of NRTI-associated mitochondrial toxicity, according to the "pol-gamma" model. NRTI drugs differ from natural nucleoside compounds in that the 5′-hydroxyl group (blue) is modified or removed, so that incorporation into a nascent DNA chain leads to chain termination. Note that the affinity of a given NRTI drug for DNA polymerase-gamma (a determinant of its ability to cause mitochondrial DNA depletion) is not related to its affinity for HIV reverse transcriptase (a determinant of antiretroviral efficacy).

POTENTIAL MECHANISMS OF NRTI-MEDIATED MITOCHONDRIAL TOXICITY

The study of NRTI-associated toxicity syndromes has also been possible due to information available on the pharmacology of these drugs,[1–3] and particularly by their capacity to inhibit a specific host DNA polymerase (mitochondrial DNA polymerase-gamma) through a mechanism that is similar to its therapeutic activity as an HIV reverse transcriptase inhibitor. However, it is worth stating at the outset that the toxic and therapeutic profiles of individual NRTI drugs are not correlated, so that an increased efficacy is not necessarily accompanied by increased toxicity.[7] Indeed, over the past 15 years there has been an increasing trend toward using NRTI drugs that combine high levels of antiviral efficacy with benign toxicity profiles. This trend toward reduced toxicity may also reflect the avoidance of NRTI combinations that have synergistic toxicity profiles, as may be seen in the case of NRTI-associated neuropathy where stavudine and didanosine each contribute to increased risk. This will be discussed further.

Mitochondria are the energy powerhouses of the cell, and are unique among intracellular organelles in containing their own genome that is extrachromosomal and replicates independently of nuclear DNA. Hence, mitochondrial DNA can be synthesized in postmitotic and resting cells, utilizing a unique DNA polymerase (polymerase-gamma) whose evolutionary origins[8] and enzymatic activities[9] are distinct from the multiple DNA polymerases involved in nuclear DNA synthesis. Importantly, DNA polymerase-gamma is also unique among the human polymerases in that it is unable to discriminate between naturally occurring nucleotides and nucleoside analogue drugs.[8] Hence, NRTI drugs are capable of inhibiting cellular mitochondrial DNA synthesis via their effects on DNA polymerase-gamma (Fig. 74-1). The proposal that NRTI-induced polymerase-gamma inhibition represents a common pathway for tissue-specific adverse effects of this drug class has been reviewed extensively by Lewis and Dalakas,[10] Brinkman,[11] and more recently by Kakuda[4] and White.[5] The basic premise of the "pol-gamma" hypothesis is that NRTI-induced inhibition of this DNA polymerase leads to cellular mitochondrial DNA depletion (i.e., reduced numbers of mitochondrial DNA copies per cell). Cellular, and ultimately organ toxicity is the consequence of loss of mitochondrial bioenergetic function, when mitochondrial DNA levels have fallen beyond a critical level at which the production of the 13 mitochondrial DNA-encoded protein subunits of the mitochondrial respiratory chain is insufficient to meet energy requirements (see Fig. 74-2).

At the cellular level, there is an increasing understanding that while the ability of a specific NRTI to induce mitochondrial DNA depletion is primarily determined by its relative affinity for polymerase-gamma, the relevance of this effect to the development of tissue toxicity is modulated by other factors, such as that drug's ability to access the mitochondrial compartment within the cell cytosol in an activated form. This is highlighted by the recent discovery of a mitochondrial inner membrane transporter that is able to facilitate the entry of active NRTI diphosphate and triphosphate derivatives into mitochondria.[12]

In addition to the mechanism described above, zidovudine may exert at least some of its mitochondrial toxicity effects through "non-pol-gamma" mechanisms, with a body

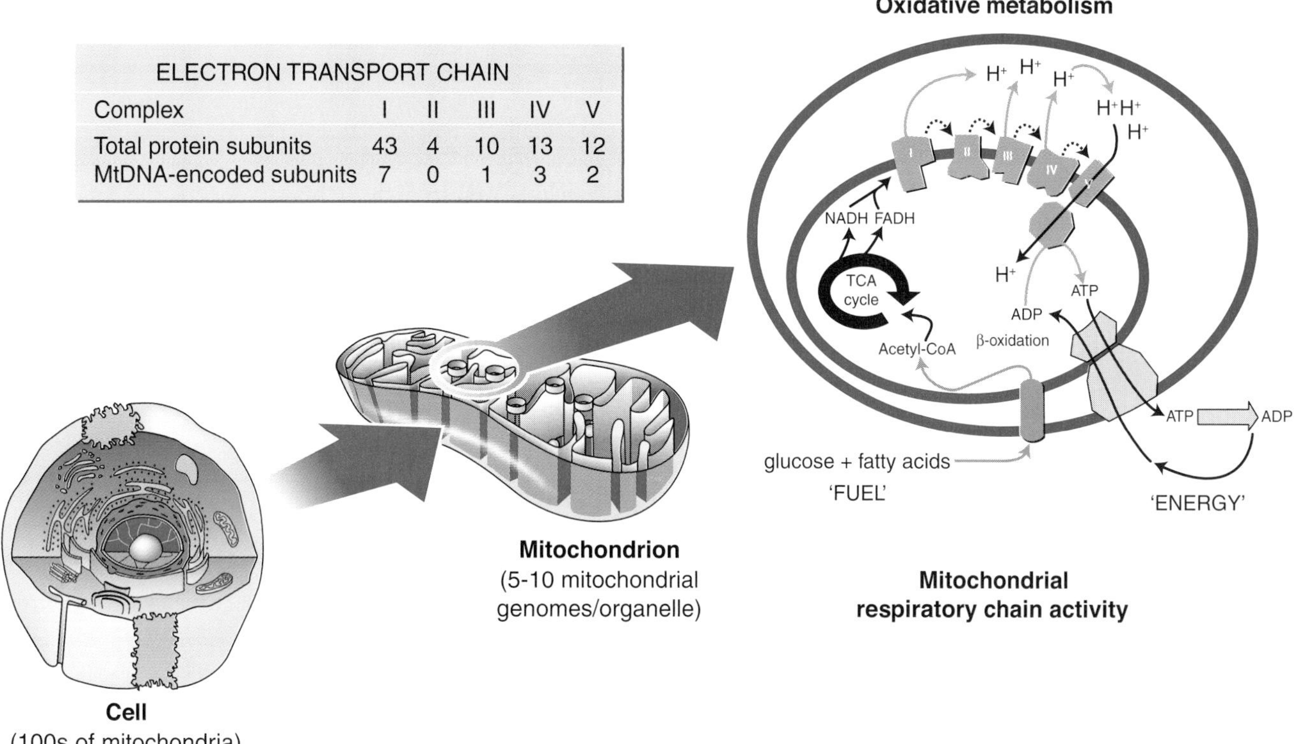

Figure 74-2 ■ The mitochondrial organelle and its role in oxidative phosphorylation. Mitochondria are ubiquitous organelles responsible for cellular energy production through oxidative phosporylation. This requires the concerted action of mitochondrial DNA-encoded subunits (13) and nuclear DNA-encoded subunits (~70) of the five respiratory chain complexes. Note also that all proteins involved in determining mitochondrial organellar number and structure, as well as in maintaining biochemical pathways within the mitochondrial matrix (e.g., beta-oxidation, Krebs' cycle) are nuclear DNA-encoded.

of research evidence indicating that zidovudine has direct effects on critical components of the mitochondrial membrane involved in cellular energy metabolism (e.g., the ADP/ATP transporter that exports mitochondrial-derived ATP to the cytosol).[13,14] In this context, it is also interesting to note that the mitochondrial ADP/ATP transporter also appears to be a target for selected HIV protease inhibitors (PIs) such as nelfinavir, which are thought to exert antiapoptotic effects through mitochondrial membrane stabilization.[15] However, this effect, now well-characterized in a number of *in vitro* and *in vivo* studies, is yet to find a widespread clinical application.

It is also important to recognize that inhibiting mitochondrial DNA polymerase-gamma may affect the fidelity of mitochondrial DNA synthesis – resulting in increased risk of mitochondrial DNA mutation – as well as causing mitochondrial DNA depletion.[16,17] The clinical importance of this effect has not been established, although neurologic syndromes attributable to mitochondrial DNA mutations have been seen in association with NRTI therapy, including five published cases of Leber's hereditary optic neuropathy (characterized by rapidly evolving bilateral optic atrophy and blindness).[18–21] It is likely that these individuals were genetically susceptible to this condition, in which the development of the clinical phenotype generally requires a very high proportion of mutated mitochondrial DNA, and that NRTI therapy may have "unmasked" the syndrome. However, the development of an unusual neurologic syndrome in an NRTI-treated individual should alert the clinician to the possibility of a "mitochondrial disease". Similarly, mitochondrial DNA mutation may be considered in rare cases in which mitochondrial dysfunction appears to be progressive despite cessation of NRTI therapy.

MITOCHONDRIAL TOXICITY AND PREGNANCY: FETAL AND MATERNAL CONSIDERATIONS

Before returning to more "typical" manifestations of mitochondrial toxicity associated with NRTI therapy, there has been concern that fetal exposure to NRTI therapy *in utero* may lead to the development of mitochondrial disease in infants, following the report of eight children with consistent clinical features.[22] A comprehensive US epidemiologic study examining this issue ($n = 1954$, including 188 deaths at age <5 years, with evidence of mitochondrial dysfunction rated from "unlikely" (class 1) to "highly likely/proven" (class 4)) has not identified increased mortality attributable to mitochondrial disease among NRTI-exposed infants,[23] and concluded that the benefits of perinatal zidovudine therapy are likely to outweigh the risks.[23,24] However, the French investigators who initially described this association have gone on to demonstrate an 18-month incidence of "established" mitochondrial dysfunction (i.e., clinical syndrome supported by histopathology and evidence of mitochondrial respiratory chain defects) among ~0.3% infants in a similarly large population-based study (7/2644 cases among NRTI-exposed infants, 0/1748 in unexposed controls).[25] "Possible" mitochondrial dysfunction was identified in a further 14 NRTI-exposed infants. This study also identified a relatively coherent clinical syndrome, consisting of (1) neurological symptoms (developmental delay, seizures, behavioral disturbances); (2) cerebral magnetic resonance imaging (MRI) abnormalities (white matter and brainstem lesions)[26]; and (3) hyperlactatemia. Risk factor analysis including both "possible" and "established" cases suggested increased risk associated with combined NRTI therapy (15/21 cases; zidovudine + lamivudine, $n = 14$) compared with zidovudine monotherapy (6/21 cases) (RR = 2.5, 95% CI 1–6.5). Intravenous zidovudine therapy was utilized in 20/21 cases. However, duration of NRTI therapy was not found to be different among cases and controls, and mitochondrial DNA depletion was not found in affected tissues despite the presence of histopathological and biochemical evidence of mitochondrial toxicity. The authors stressed that these findings do not argue against the usefulness of NRTI therapy in pregnancy.

With respect to the risks of maternal mitochondrial toxicity associated with NRTI use in pregnancy, however, there is increasing evidence that stavudine therapy, particularly when combined with didanosine, is associated with risk of lactic acidosis in late pregnancy.[27,28] This has prompted the manufacturers to issue product information in 2001 warning that the combination of stavudine and didanosine should be avoided during pregnancy "unless the potential benefit clearly outweighs the potential risks".[29]

IN VITRO STUDIES: ESTABLISHING TOXICITY PROFILE FOR NRTI DRUGS

In vitro studies have provided important information regarding the potential of specific NRTI drugs to cause DNA polymerase-gamma inhibition, mitochondrial DNA depletion, and mitochondrial dysfunction.[9,30–32] A consistent ranking of the potency of mitochondrial DNA synthesis inhibition has emerged from these studies, with decreasing potency associated with ddC (zalcitabine) ≫ ddI (didanosine) > d4T (stavudine) > AZT (zidovudine). These studies also suggest that no significant mitochondrial polymerase-gamma inhibition occurs at pharmacological concentrations of lamivudine, abacavir, and tenofovir. One caveat to these findings is that NRTI-associated mitochondrial toxicity is tissue-specific, so that *in vitro* studies should ideally utilize human cell cultures that are relevant to the clinical toxicity profile of the drug.

CLINICAL NRTI-INDUCED TOXICITY SYNDROMES

While the prototypic NRTI-associated toxicity syndrome is zidovudine myopathy, this syndrome is now rare in clinical practice,[33,34] possibly reflecting either the use of lower zidovudine doses in the HAART era, or the involvement of uncontrolled HIV infection *per se* in the pathogenesis of this syndrome. Currently, the most concerning adverse effects involving NRTI therapy are lactic acidosis and other less serious disorders of lactate metabolism; the progressive subcutaneous fat wasting syndrome that is viewed as part of the lipodystrophy syndrome; neuropathy; and pancreatitis (Fig. 74-3).

LACTIC ACIDOSIS AND HYPERLACTATEMIA

Lactic acidosis is probably the most recognizable feature of mitochondrial dysfunction in clinical disease, in which loss of mitochondrial oxidative function leads to increased reliance on "anaerobic" metabolism and the inevitable accumulation of lactate (and thus, of acid). In the setting of NRTI therapy, there is now an appreciation of a spectrum of clinical phenotypes associated with elevated systemic lactate levels.[35] At one end of this spectrum is a relatively common syndrome of mild, asymptomatic, nonprogressive hyperlactatemia (generally <2.5 mmol/L), which appears to represent a "compensated" homeostatic system in which elevated lactate production is balanced by effective mechanisms of lactate clearance. While the degree of hyperlactatemia appears to be greater in the presence of stavudine or didanosine therapy compared with zidovudine or abacavir, this syndrome appears to be benign irrespective of the choice of NRTI therapy.[36–40]

In contrast, lactic acidosis and hepatic steatosis represents a relatively uncommon (~1–2 per 1000 person-years) but life-threatening clinical syndrome in which lactate homeostasis is completely "decompensated", allowing the rapid, progressive accumulation of lactate and development of acidosis in affected patients. A critical aspect of lactic acidosis is its unpredictability, as it typically occurs in patients who have been on stable NRTI regimens for months or even years, and is not generally heralded by increased lactate levels before the development of the fulminant syndrome.[36,41] Host risk factors have been identified for NRTI-associated lactic acidosis, including concurrent liver disease, female gender[42] (reviewed in chapter 42), and obesity. The association between female gender and risk of NRTI-induced lactic acidosis is a striking one, with a United States Food and Drug Administration (FDA) report of 60 cases finding that 83% occurred in women, including 85% of fatal cases.[43] In relation to drug treatment, the majority of reported cases in recent years have involved stavudine-based HAART, although it is important to recognize that cases involving zidovudine therapy also occur (reviewed in Chapters 35 and 41). It is encouraging to note that a Swiss HIV cohort study has documented a declining

Non-tissue-specific mitochondrial toxicity syndromes

Lactic acidosis: NRTIs
- abdo. pain, lethargy, tachypnea
- neuromuscular weakness
- may be asymptomatic
- often unheralded, acute onset
- elevated lactate, ↓HCO_3
- ~0.1 case/100 patient years

Infantile NRTI toxicity syndrome:
- developmental delay, seizures
- MRI abnormalities
- hyperlactatemia
- rare: <0.3% 18-mth incidence
- prognosis uncertain

Adult "mitochondrial diseases":
- Leber neuropathy described
- bilateral optic neuritis
- likely in genetically-susceptible individuals, may have positive family history

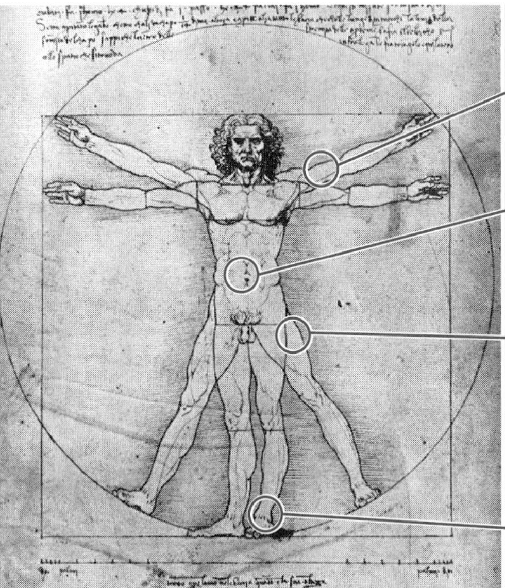

Tissue-specific mitochondrial toxicity syndromes

Myopathy: AZT
- myalgia, weakness
- elevated creatine kinase
- very rare in clinical practice

Pancreatitis: d4T and/or ddI
- central abdominal pain
- elevated amylase/lipase
- ~1 case/100 patient years

Lipoatrophy: d4T>AZT
- fat loss: esp legs, face>trunk
- measurable with DEXA scans
  -subclinical changes common
- no biological features
- common: d4T~40%, AZT~15%

Neuropathy: ddc>ddI, d4T
- painful sensory neuropathy
- abnormal electophysiology
  -subclinical changes common
- no biological features
- common: ddC/ddI/d4T≥40%

Figure 74-3 ■ Major clinical syndromes attributed to NRTI-associated mitochondrial toxicity.

incidence of both hyperlactatemia (lactate >2.4 mmol/L) and lactic acidosis (lactate >5 mmol/L) over time, with hyperlactatemia and lactic acidosis rates progressively falling by ~60% and 85%, respectively, in the interval between 1999 and 2003.[6] In this study, this pattern appeared to reflect reduced prescription of stavudine/didanosine dual NRTI therapy over the study period.

The cornerstone of management of this condition is early recognition of the clinical manifestations: abdominal symptoms including nausea, vomiting, anorexia, abdominal pain and distension, fatigue, with biochemical evidence of hepatocellular liver dysfunction and lactate level generally >5 mmol/L. These clinical and laboratory abnormalities should lead to prompt cessation of NRTI therapy. A more recently identified clinical syndrome accompanying lactic acidosis is progressive, severe neuromuscular weakness mimicking the Guillain–Barré syndrome.[44] Initial reports by the FDA identified 25 cases, including seven fatal cases (notably, NRTI therapy was continued after the diagnosis was made in all but one of these individuals). A more recent retrospective analysis has identified 55 cases (44 associated with stavudine therapy), with a 25% mortality rate among the 36 patients with documented follow-up.[45] Overall, the mortality associated with NRTI-associated lactic acidosis remains unacceptably high, at ~50%.[43]

Given the association between lactic acidosis and hepatic steatosis, it is worth noting that hepatic steatosis is not an infrequent finding in liver biopsy samples obtained from HIV-infected patients who develop abnormal liver function tests on long-term antiretroviral therapy, where it may represent a common element in a number of disparate disorders (e.g., alcoholic and nonalcoholic steatohepatitis, diabetes mellitus). Hence, this finding is not highly predictive of lactic acidosis, nor is it specific to this syndrome.

An "intermediate" hyperlactatemia syndrome has also been described, characterized by symptomatic hyperlactatemia or hepatic steatosis without systemic acidosis. This syndrome is almost uniformly associated with stavudine therapy, with an incidence of ~13 per 1000 person-years.[46,47] Of importance, there is evidence that lactate levels and symptoms can be controlled following modification of NRTI therapy to zidovudine or abacavir.[48]

With regard to the pathogenesis of hyperlactatemia syndromes, evidence has been provided from studies using exogenous lactate loading that increased lactate production is the fundamental defect in chronic asymptomatic hyperlactatemia, rather than decreased clearance of lactate (which primarily involves the liver).[49] Indeed, lactate clearance appears to be upregulated as a compensatory response to an elevated systemic lactate load.[49] The source of this excessive lactate production is unknown, although a carefully conducted exercise physiology study indicates that skeletal muscle is an unlikely candidate.[50] By contrast, lactic acidosis represents a complete failure of lactate homeostasis, in which lactic acid accumulation progresses inexorably while NRTI therapy is maintained. In this scenario, the prominent role of liver mitochondrial dysfunction (indicated by the presence of microvesicular hepatic steatosis)[37,43,46] leading to a shift from hepatic lactate consumption to lactate production would be predicted to have dramatic consequences for systemic lactate metabolism.

LIPOATROPHY

There is now strong evidence that the choice and duration of NRTI drugs represents the dominant risk factor for developing pathological loss of fat tissue, referred to as lipoatrophy. The importance of treatment choices in determining the risk of developing lipoatrophy is highlighted by the fact that this long-term complication is extremely rare in the general population as well as in treatment-naïve HIV-infected individuals.[51] Hence, there are no known modifiable risk factors for developing lipoatrophy that are present in the general population. This may be contrasted with other aspects of the broader clinical syndrome commonly referred to as "lipodystrophy", which also includes metabolic complications such as dyslipidemia and insulin resistance, and visceral/abdominal fat accumulation that often accompanies these metabolic changes[52] (*see* Chapters 70 and 72). These metabolic complications of therapy, which have a much stronger association with HIV PI therapy than with NRTI drugs, are also highly prevalent in the general population, suggesting that risk may be modified by "nondrug" factors such as diet and physical activity. This topic will not be addressed here.

Clinical studies have demonstrated that NRTI therapy alone provides sufficient conditions for the development of lipoatrophy[53–55] and that NRTI therapy is an independent risk factor for its occurrence in HAART-treated individuals.[56–58] Clinical trials data have now confirmed the findings of observational cohort studies [59] that stavudine therapy is associated with approximately twofold increased risk of lipoatrophy compared with zidovudine, so that the risk of clinically apparent lipoatrophy over 30 months is ~10–20% in zidovudine-treated individuals, and 40–50% among those treated with stavudine.[60–62] Significant differences in limb fat between stavudine and zidovudine treatment arms in the ACTG 384 trial have also been documented from 48 weeks onwards.[63] Finally, switching NRTI therapy from stavudine to abacavir in an observational study[64] and more recently in two randomized trials[65,66] has been associated with significant improvements in fat wasting. In contrast, over 30 trials investigating HIV PI discontinuation as a therapeutic strategy[67] have failed to demonstrate beneficial effects on fat wasting, although metabolic abnormalities such as dyslipidemia and insulin resistance did improve. It is notable, however, that improvement in fat wasting up to 96 weeks appear to be modest at best, with absolute increases in limb fat of ~1%.[65] Therefore, it would seem prudent to focus on identifying HAART regimens with a low risk of inducing fat wasting, since restoration of established fat wasting appears to be a slow, and possibly incomplete process.

The histopathological correlates of this syndrome also indicate that adipose tissue-specific mitochondrial toxicity is central to lipoatrophy pathogenesis. At the ultrastructural level, abnormal mitochondrial architecture and organellar proliferation are prominent features,[68–70] while increased adipocyte apoptosis associated with lipoatrophy has been shown to improve after discontinuing stavudine therapy in favor of abacavir,[71] but not after switching HIV PI therapy.[72] Mitochondrial DNA depletion in adipose tissue samples has also been documented using semiquantitative techniques,[70,73] and in studies of adipose tissue using precise real-time polymerase chain reaction quantitation methods which have demonstrated significant mitochondrial DNA depletion particularly associated with stavudine compared with zidovudine.[74,75] Stavudine treatment has also been associated with more severe adipocyte mitochondrial DNA depletion and fat wasting over time compared with zidovudine therapy,[76] as well as more severe effects on mitochondrial function.[77]

The role of NRTI drugs other than stavudine and zidovudine as risk factors for lipoatrophy has been more difficult to discern, particularly as lamivudine and didanosine are generally used in combination with these thymidine analog drugs. Thus far, no independent effect of these "second" NRTI drugs has emerged, with results from the available clinical trials completed to 30 months showing similar risk of lipoatrophy if stavudine is combined with didanosine or with lamivudine.[60–62] Data regarding the concurrent use of zidovudine and didanosine is more difficult to obtain, although an early study of dual NRTI therapy by Saint-Marc and colleagues included a number of patients on didanosine with stavudine (d4T/ddI = 13/27, 48%) and zidovudine treatment groups (AZT/ddI = 13/16, 81%) that were well-matched for NRTI therapy duration.[53] In this study, use of stavudine remained the most significant risk factor for lipoatrophy (relative risk 1.95 compared with zidovudine), while no significant didanosine effect could be demonstrated. Use of didanosine compared with lamivudine also had no significant effect on adipose tissue mitochondrial DNA depletion in a recent analysis of 232 biopsy samples, after adjustment for the effect of stavudine treatment.[75] In terms of the newer drugs abacavir (an NRTI) and tenofovir (a nucleotide reverse transcriptase inhibitor), which would be predicted to have reduced predisposition to cause mitochondrial toxicity,[30,31] clinical trials data show no evidence of an association with lipoatrophy. Indeed, 144-week data from the Gilead 903 study involving comparisons of tenofovir and stavudine therapy (combined with lamivudine and efavirenz in both arms), objectively measured limb fat was reduced by ~40% in the stavudine arm compared with those on tenofovir.[78]

NEUROPATHY

There are a number of issues to be considered in addressing the possible associations between NRTI therapy, mitochondrial toxicity, and neuropathy. First, neuropathic changes frequently do not come to the attention of clinicians as the symptoms are of gradual onset, and clinical signs of nerve damage are not generally sought in clinical practice. Hence, the prevalence and potential long-term impact of neuropathy is likely to be underestimated. Second, there is a definite contribution of HIV disease *per se* to the pathogenesis of a form of distal sensory neuropathy that is clinically and electrophysiologically indistinguishable from so-called "toxic neuropathy from antiretroviral drugs".[79] It is therefore difficult to dissect out the relative contribution of disease-associated and drug-associated factors in the syndrome, as these effects are likely to be synergistic. The clinical syndrome common to both HIV-associated and toxic sensory polyneuropathy is dominated by peripheral pain and dysesthesia, with rare motor involvement.

In general, the relative risk of toxic polyneuropathy associated with specific NRTI drugs correlates well with their ability to inhibit mitochondrial DNA polymerase-gamma *in vitro*. The greatest risk has been associated with zalcitabine, an NRTI with equivalent affinity for mitochondrial DNA polymerase-gamma and HIV reverse transcriptase, thus providing for a narrow therapeutic window.[9] Neuropathy was a consistent and dose-limiting toxicity in trials of zalcitabine, occurring in approximately one-third of patients receiving low-dose therapy (2.25 mg/day) for less than a year,[80,81] while higher doses were associated with almost universal development of neuropathy (100% with >0.04 mg kg^{-1} day^{-1}, 80% with 0.04 mg kg^{-1} day^{-1}).[80] Consistent with the "pol-gamma" hypothesis, Dalakas and colleagues[82] have provided *in vivo* evidence of significant mitochondrial DNA depletion in peripheral nerves associated with this complication of zalcitabine therapy.

Stavudine and didanosine have also been associated with increased risk of neuropathy in the large Johns Hopkins AIDS Service cohort study ($n = 1116$). Compared with a crude incidence rate of 6.8 cases per 100 person-years for didanosine, stavudine use was associated with a relative risk of 1.4, while concurrent use of these drugs further increased risk (3.5-fold relative risk for stavudine/didanosine compared with didanosine alone). Concurrent hydroxyurea therapy had an additional effect (7.8-fold relative risk of stavudine/didanosine/hydroxyurea compared with didanosine alone, giving a crude incidence of 28.6 cases per 100 person-years).[83]

As already mentioned, markers of progressive HIV disease also correlate with the development of sensory polyneuropathy, with evidence for associations between reduced CD4 T-cell counts and increased risk of neuropathy,[84] and increased pain scores in patients with higher HIV viral load.[85] However, in a cohort of 144 ambulatory patients with longer duration of exposure to stavudine and/or didanosine and average CD4 T-cell counts greater than 400/μL, the prevalence of sensory neuropathy was found to be 44%,[86] suggesting that among patients with prolonged survival and effective immunological and virological outcomes, choice and duration of NRTI therapy will ultimately become the dominant risk factor for neuropathy. In this analysis, use of a "d" drug (i.e., stavudine, didanosine and zalcitabine) was associated with an odds ratio of 26 developing clinical neuropathy, while disease-associated factors were not found to be significant in multivariate analysis.

Consistent with the lipoatrophy data, reversal of established neuropathy appears to be a slow process that is dependent on cessation of the offending NRTI drug. The identification of L-carnitine deficiency, and the use of L-acetyl-carnitine therapy, may also have beneficial effects on nerve regeneration.[87,88] Lamotrigine therapy has also been associated with improved pain symptoms in the context of NRTI-associated toxic polyneuropathy.[79] As with any clinical neuropathy, a search for contributing factors such as diabetes, excessive alcohol consumption, and vitamin deficiencies (e.g., thiamine, B_{12}, and folate) should be undertaken.[89] Ideally, these factors should also be considered prior to initiating NRTI therapy.

PANCREATITIS

There is a differential diagnosis for pancreatitis occurring in an HIV-infected individual that includes NRTI-associated disease, in which case pancreatitis may be an isolated event or may occur in the context of systemic lactic acidosis.[90] Other causes must also be considered including pancreatitis secondary to severe HIV PI-induced hypertriglyceridemia,[91,92] and the effects of other drugs such as pentamidine.[93] In this review, pancreatitis will be considered as a diagnosis that includes clinical symptoms of abdominal pain combined with elevated serum amylase levels. This excludes cases of isolated hyperamylasemia, which is increased in prevalence among HIV-infected patients with moderate to severe immune deficiency,[94] as the relationship between this biochemical abnormality and pancreatitis is uncertain.

The most comprehensive data concerning risk factors for NRTI-associated pancreatitis comes from the Johns Hopkins AIDS Service cohort ($n = 2613$, 33 cases).[90] In this analysis, didanosine and stavudine were associated with roughly equivalent risk of pancreatitis, with estimated incidence rates of 0.8 and 1.1 cases per 100 person-years, respectively. Zidovudine therapy was associated with an incidence of 0.1 per 100 person-years. Combining stavudine and didanosine increased risk approximately twofold, while the concurrent use of didanosine and hydroxyurea increased relative risk approximately eightfold.[90] Risk associated with didanasine and stavudine therapy was also highlighted in the ACTG 5025 study, which involved switching to a regimen of stavudine/didanosine/indinavir with or without hydroxyurea ($n = 6$ 8 in each arm) compared with ongoing zidovudine/lamivudine/indinavir ($n = 66$) in stable, aviremic patients with CD4+ T-cell counts greater than 200/μL. Stavudine and didanosine treatment was associated with a 4% incidence of pancreatitis (three in each arm), including three fatal cases in patients receiving hydroxyurea.[95]

HEMATOLOGICAL COMPLICATIONS OF NRTI THERAPY

These complications have assumed less importance in clinical management in the HAART era, reflecting the fact that HIV disease severity, and particularly the presence of one or more AIDS-defining illnesses, contributes significantly to the risk of anemia and other hematological events (e.g., thrombocytopenia, neutropenia) in untreated individuals.

Nevertheless, zidovudine therapy has been associated with increased risk of anemia in HAART recipients compared with other NRTI drugs (relative risk ~1.15),[96] suggesting that this drug should be used with caution when hemoglobin levels are low prior to treatment. This may be particularly relevant when initiating antiretroviral therapy in resource-poor countries where patients may be more prone to have reduced hemoglobin levels as a result of concomitant parasitic infection (malaria, hookworm), malnutrition, or genetically determined hemoglobinopathies.

Recent studies have also suggested that combined full-dose didanosine and tenofovir treatment may contribute to a targeted toxicity against lymphocytes, resulting in reduced CD4+ T-cell counts despite the presence of undetectable viral loads,[97] affecting >50% of patients receiving this drug combination in one clinical trial. Hence, drug toxicity should be considered as a potential explanation when there is significant discordance between virological suppression and CD4+ T-cell responses on HAART while employing this particular combination of antiretrovirals.

TENOFOVIR RENAL SAFETY

The renal safety of tenofovir is now a topic of considerable interest, following a number of reports (involving more than 30 cases) of significant renal toxicity with renal tubular damage and/or acute renal failure. In the large Gilead 903 study in which patients were selected for normal renal function at baseline, no evidence of significant renal toxicity could be identified over a 3-year treatment period using serum creatinine measures.[78] However, a recent study has observed reductions in glomerular filtration rate (~10%) along with ~20% increase in rate of proteinuria >130 mg/day.[98] Hence, simple measurements of serum creatinine may not be sufficient to capture the true effects of this drug on renal function. Further clinical data are awaited, but in the meantime it would be prudent to carefully consider more stringent assessments of glomerular filtration rate (as well as markers of renal tubular toxicity such as hypophosphatemia). Here, calculated methods such as the Cockcroft–Gault equation that adjust for body weight and gender may be useful for monitoring purposes. In addition, it would seem prudent to only use tenofovir with caution in patients with already compromised renal function. When doing so, proper dose adjustment needs to be employed.

The potential for nucleotide analog-associated renal toxicity is concerning given that this tissue-specific toxicity was observed with another drug of this class (adefovir,[99] and that tenofovir and adefovir can be transported across the renal tubular membrane by a specific protein (human renal organic anion transporter 1, hOAT1).[100] The manufacturers of tenofovir have carefully examined the effects of this drug in human proximal tubular cells, as well as other tissues *in vitro*,[31] finding no evidence of cellular or mitochondrial toxicity across a range of doses (3–300 μM). Whether these rare events represent mitochondrial toxicity is currently unknown.

PREVENTING NRTI-ASSOCIATED MITOCHONDRIAL TOXICITIES

From the data already presented it is apparent that NRTI drugs are associated with differential risks of mitochondrial toxicity, and that these toxicity syndromes are tissue-specific. The selection of NRTI drugs to minimize risk of toxicity is therefore of primary importance. However, in the clinical setting this is obviously not a straightforward decision when there are other factors at play such as drug resistance, and the potential risk of other adverse effects such as abacavir hypersensitivity. In this regard, there has been progress toward identifying a highly predictive genetic marker of the abacavir hypersensitivity syndrome within the human leukocyte antigen (HLA) region.[101]

A common feature of these mitochondrial toxicity syndromes, with the exception of lactic acidosis, is that risk is increased in patients with advanced immune deficiency at the commencement of antiretroviral therapy (i.e., with CD4 T-cell counts <200/μL). This is true for lipoatrophy[102] as it is for neuropathy,[84] pancreatitis[90] and anemia.[96] Hence, delaying the introduction of antiretroviral therapy does not seem supportable as a strategy for preventing NRTI-associated toxicity.

Otherwise, the recognition of other factors that may contribute independently to risk of toxicity syndromes is also important. This is most relevant to neuropathy and pancreatitis, where the risk factors in the general population are well known. In the case of lipoatrophy, no modifiable host risk factors have emerged, although risk of this complication is increased in those of white race and older age.[102] There have been reports that risk of mitochondrial toxicity is increased when NRTI therapy is combined with ribavirin and interferon-alpha for the treatment of hepatitis C co-infection.[103–105] This is certainly plausible, as ribavirin is a purine analogue[106,107] (like didanosine), while interferon-alpha may inhibit mitochondrial DNA transcription.[108]

MONITORING NRTI-ASSOCIATED MITOCHONDRIAL TOXICITIES

As a general principle, the identification and management of mitochondrial toxicities associated with NRTI therapy depends on clinical assessment rather than the use of laboratory markers. It is therefore important that clinicians are aware of the contribution of NRTI therapy to specific toxicity syndromes, as well as the relevant clinical manifestations of these syndromes. Perhaps even more importantly, the early recognition of these toxicities (by both clinician and patient) is critical if there is to be a realistic expectation that these adverse effects can be reversed.

Several research groups have developed highly precise assays for the measurement of mitochondrial DNA depletion in tissue samples and blood.[51,106,107,109,110] These assays are an attractive diagnostic tool, as the mitochondrial DNA level per cell is likely to reflect the direct consequences of NRTI therapy in affected tissue early in the treatment course, which may therefore predict the subsequent progression of tissue pathology to clinically apparent disease over time. This may be seen as analogous to the role of HIV viral load in determining the rate of disease progression. However, there is no widespread clinical application for these tools at present. A fundamental aspect of these syndromes is their tissue specificity, so that while important data can be obtained from the relevant target tissue (i.e., adipose tissue in lipodystrophy studies, and peripheral nerve tissue or neurites in neuropathy studies), these effects are not reflected in more readily obtained samples such as blood samples. For example, in a recent study involving 62 patients who had concurrent blood and adipose tissue samples collected at 6-monthly intervals (160 study visits in total),[75] mitochondrial DNA depletion in adipose tissue was strongly associated with stavudine use, but not didanosine, in adipose tissue ($P = 0.001$ and $P = 0.71$, respectively). In contrast, didanosine therapy was the dominant determinant of peripheral blood mitochondrial DNA depletion ($P = 0.07$), while stavudine therapy had no significant effect ($P = 0.80$). The specific association between peripheral blood mitochondrial DNA depletion and the use of didansoine and/or zalcitabine (but not zidovudine or stavudine) has also been documented in other studies.[111–113]

Similarly, routine measurement of systemic lactate levels does not appear to allow prediction of the more severe forms of lactic acidosis, or of tissue-specific NRTI toxicities,[6,114] although routine screening of lactate levels in pregnant women receiving NRTI therapy does seem warranted. Hence, even in hyperlactatemia syndromes (in which biochemical rather than clinical assessment would appear logical), the importance of clinical syndrome recognition cannot be overstated.

It is also important to recognize that the clinical manifestations of NRTI-associated toxicity, which form the basis of diagnostic classification systems, are likely to represent advanced and potentially irreversible tissue pathology. In this regard, active assessment for symptoms and signs according to the specific toxicity profile of a given NRTI drug is essential in order to identify reversible disease.

REFERENCES

1. Squires KE. An introduction to nucleoside and nucleotide analogues. Antiviral Ther 6(Suppl 3):1–14, 2001.
2. Kakuda TN. Pharmacology of nucleoside and nucleotide reverse transcriptase inhibitor-induced mitochondrial toxicity. Clin Ther 22:685–708, 2000.
3. White AJ. Mitochondrial toxicity and HIV therapy. Sex Transm Infect 77:158–73, 2001.
4. Palella FJ Jr, Delaney KM, Moorman AC, et al. The HIV Outpatient Study Investigators. Declining morbidity and mortality among patients with advanced human immunodeficiency virus infection. N Engl J Med 338:853–60, 1998.
5. Piot P, Bartos M, Ghys PD, et al. The global impact of HIV/AIDS. Nature 410:968–73, 2001.
6. Imhof A, Lederberger B, Gunthard HF, et al. Swiss HIV Cohort Study. Risk factors for and outcome of hyperlactatemia in HIV-infected persons: is there a need for lactate monitoring? Clin Infect Dis 41:721–8, 2005.
7. Martin JL, Brown CE, Matthews-Davis N, Reardon JE. Effects of antiviral nucleoside analogs on human DNA polymerases and mitochondrial DNA synthesis. Antimicrob Agents Chemother 38:2743–9, 1994.
8. Burgers PM, Koonin EV, Bruford E, et al. Eukaryotic DNA polymerases: proposal for a revised nomenclature. J Biol Chem 276:43487–90, 2001.
9. Longley MJ, Ropp PA, Lim SE, Copeland WC. Characterization of the native and recombinant catalytic subunit of human DNA polymerase-gamma Identification of residues critical for exonuclease activity and dideoxynucleotide sensitivity. Biochem 37:10529–39, 1998.
10. Lewis W, Dalakas MC. Mitochondrial toxicity of antiviral drugs. Nat Med 1:417–22, 1995.
11. Brinkman K, ter Hofstede HJ, Burger DM, et al. Adverse effects of reverse transcriptase inhibitors: mitochondrial toxicity as common pathway. AIDS 12:1735–44, 1998.
12. Dolce V, Fiermonte G, Runswick MJ, et al. The human mitochondrial deoxynucleotide carrier and its role in the toxicity of nucleoside antivirals. Proc Nalt Acad Sci USA 98:2284–8, 2001.
13. Barile M, Valenti D, Quagliarello E, Passarella S. Mitochondria as cell targets of AZT (zidovudine). Gen Pharmacol 31:531–8, 1998.
14. Masini A, Scotti C, Calligaro A, et al. Zidovudine-induced experimental myopathy: dual mechanism of mitochondrial damage. J Neurol Sci 166:131–40, 1999.
15. Weaver JGR, Tarze A, Moffat TC, et al. Inhibition of adenine nucleotide translocator pore function and proteaction against apoptosis in vivo by an HIV protease inhibitor. J Clin Invest 115:1828–38, 2005.
16. Lewis W, Copeland WC, Day BJ. Mitochondrial DNA depletion, oxidative stress, and mutation: mechanisms of dysfunction from nucleoside reverse transcriptase inhibitors. Lab Invest 81:777–90, 2001.
17. Martin AM, Hammond E, Nolan D, et al. Accumulation of mitochondrial DNA mutations in human immunodeficiency virus-infected patients treated with nucleoside-analogue reverse-transcriptase inhibitors. Am J Hum Genet 72:549–60, 2003.
18. Luzhansky JZ, Pierce AB, Hoy JF, Hall AJ. Leber's hereditary optic neuropathy in the setting of nucleoside analogue toxicity. AIDS 15:1588–9, 2001.
19. Shaikh S, Ta C, Basham AA, Mansour S. Leber hereditary optic neuropathy associated with antiretroviral therapy for human immunodeficiency virus infection. Am J Ophthalmol 131: 143–5, 2001
20. Warner JE, Ries KM. Optic neuropathy in a patient with AIDS. J Neuroophthalmol 21:92–4, 2001.
21. Mackey DA, Fingert JH, Luzhansky JZ, et al. Leber's hereditary optic neuropathy triggered by antiretroviral therapy for human immunodeficiency virus. Eye 17:312–7, 2003.
22. Blanche S, Tardieu M, Rustin P, et al. Persistent mitochondrial dysfunction and perinatal exposure to antiretroviral nucleoside analogues. Lancet 354:1084–9, 1999.
23. Bulterys M, Nesheim S, Abrams EJ, et al. Perinatal Safety Review Working Group. Lack of evidence of mitochondrial dysfunction in the offspring of HIV-infected women. Retrospective review of perinatal exposure to antiretroviral drugs in the Perinatal AIDS Collaborative Transmission Study. Ann N Y Acad Sci 918:212–21, 2000.
24. Tuomala RE, Shapiro DE, Mofenson LM, et al. Antiretroviral therapy during pregnancy and the risk of an adverse outcome. N Engl J Med 346:1863–70, 2002.
25. Barret B, Tardieu M, Rustin P, et al. Persistent mitochondrial dysfunction in HIV-1-exposed but uninfected infants: clinical screening in a large prospective cohort. AIDS 17:1769–85, 2003.

26. Tardieu M, Brunelle F, Raybaud C, et al. Cerebral MR imaging in uninfected children born to HIV-seropositive mothers and perinatally exposed to zidovudine. Am J Neuroradiol 26: 695–701, 2005.
27. Mandelbrot L, Kermarrec N, Marcollet A, et al. Case report: nucleoside analogue-induced lactic acidosis in the third trimester of pregnancy. AIDS 17:272–3, 2003.
28. Sarner L, Fakoya A. Case report: acute onset lactic acidosis and pancreatitis in the third trimester of pregnancy in HIV-1 positive women taking antiretroviral medication. Sex Transm Infect 78:58–9, 2002.
29. Bristol-Myers Squibb Company. Healthcare provider important warning letter. 5 January 2001.
30. Johnson AA, Ray AS, Hanes J, et al. Toxicity of antiviral nucleoside analogs and the human mitochondrial DNA polymerase. J Biol Chem 276:40847–57, 2001.
31. Birkus G, Hitchcock MJ, Cihlar T. Assessment of mitochondrial toxicity in human cells treated with tenofovir: comparison with other nucleoside reverse transcriptase inhibitors. Antimicrob Agents Chemother 46:716–23, 2002.
32. Walker UA, Setzer B, Venhoff N. Increased long-term mitochondrial toxicity in combinations of nucleoside analogue reverse-transcriptase inhibitors. AIDS 16:2165–73, 2002.
33. Manfredi R, Motta R, Patrono D, et al. A prospective case-control survey of laboratory markers of skeletal muscle damage during HIV disease and antiretroviral therapy. AIDS 16: 1969–71, 2002.
34. Simpson DM, Katzenstein DA, Hughes MD, et al. Neuromuscular function in HIV infection: analysis of a placebo-controlled combination antiretroviral trial. AIDS 12:2425–32, 1998.
35. John M, Mallal S. Hyperlactatemia syndromes in people with HIV infection. Curr Opin Infect Dis 15:23–9, 2002.
36. John M, Moore CB, James IR, et al. Chronic hyperlactatemia in HIV-infected patients taking antiretroviral therapy. AIDS 15:717–23, 2001.
37. Boubaker K, Flepp M, Sudre P, et al. Hyperlactatemia and antiretroviral therapy: the Swiss HIV Cohort Study. Clin Infect Dis 33:1931–7, 2001.
38. Moyle GJ, Datta D, Mandalia S, et al. Hyperlactataemia and lactic acidosis during antiretroviral therapy: relevance, reproducibility and possible risk factors. AIDS 16:1341–9, 2002.
39. Vrouenraets SM, Treskes M, Regez RM, et al. Hyperlactataemia in HIV-infected patients: the role of NRTI-treatment. Antivir Ther 7:239–44, 2002.
40. Hocqueloux L, Alberti C, Feugeas JP, et al. Prevalence, risk factors and outcome of hyperlactataemia in HIV-infected patients. HIV Med 4:18–23, 2003.
41. Falco V, Rodriguez D, Ribera E, et al. Severe nucleoside-associated lactic acidosis in human immunodeficiency virus-infected patients: report of 12 cases and review of the literature. Clin Infect Dis 34:838–46, 2002.
42. Clark R. Sex differences in antiretroviral therapy adverse events. Drug Saf 2005;28:1075–83.
43. Boxwell DE, Styrt BA. Lactic acidosis in patients receiving nucleoside reverse transcriptase inhibitors. 39th Interscience Conference on Antimicrobial Aents and Chemotherapy, 1999, San Francisco, CA, USA, abstract 1284.
44. Wooltorton E. HIV drug stavudine (Zerit, d4T) and symptoms mimicking Guillain–Barré syndrome. CMAJ 166:1067, 2002.
45. Simpson D, Estanislao L, Marcus K, et al. HIV-associated neuromuscular weakness syndrome. 10th Conference on Retroviruses and Opportunistic Infections, 2003, Boston, MA, USA, abstract 87.
46. Gerard Y, Maulin L, Yazdanpanah Y, et al. Symptomatic hyperlactataemia: an emerging complication of antiretroviral therapy. AIDS 14:2723–30, 2000.
47. Lonergan JT, Behling C, Pfander H, et al. Hyperlactatemia and hepatic abnormalities in 10 HIV-infected patients receiving nucleoside analogue combination regimens. Clin Infect Dis 31:162–6, 2000.
48. Lonergan T, McComsey G, Fisher R, et al. Improvements in symptomatic hyperlactatemia are observed after 12 weeks when stavudine is replaced by either abacavir or zidovudine. Antiviral Ther 6(Suppl 4):55–6. Abstract 81, 2001.
49. Leclercq P, Roth H, Bosseray A, Leverve X. Investigating lactate metabolism to estimate mitochondrial status. Antiviral Ther 6(Suppl 4):16. Abstract 21, 2001.
50. Roge BT, Calbet JA, Moller K, et al. Skeletal muscle mitochondrial function and exercise capacity in HIV-infected patients with lipodystrophy and elevated p-lactate levels. AIDS 16: 973–82, 2002.
51. Palella FJ Jr, Cole SR, Chmiel JS, et al. Anthropometrics and examiner-reported body habitus abnormalities in the multicenter AIDS cohort study. Clin Infect Dis 38:903–7, 2004.
52. Nolan D, John M, Mallal S. Antiretoviral therapy and the lipodystrophy syndrome, part 2: concepts in aetiopathogenesis. Antivir Ther 6:145–60, 2001.
53. Saint-Marc T, Partisani M, Poizot-Martin I, et al. A syndrome of peripheral fat wasting (lipodystrophy) in patients receiving long-term nucleoside analogue therapy. AIDS 13:1659–67, 1999.
54. Madge S, Kinloch-de-Loes S, Mercey D, et al. Lipodystrophy in patients naive to HIV protease inhibitors. AIDS 13:735–7, 1999.
55. Carr A, Miller J, Law M, Cooper DA. A syndrome of lipoatrophy, lactic acidemia and liver dysfunction associated with HIV nucleoside analogue therapy: contribution to protease inhibitor-related lipodystrophy syndrome. AIDS 14:F25–32, 2000.
56. Mallal SA, John M, Moore CB, et al. Contribution of nucleoside analogue reverse transcriptase inhibitors to subcutaneous fat wasting in patients with HIV infection. AIDS 14:1309–16, 2000.
57. Saint-Marc T, Partisani M, Poizot-Martin I, et al. Fat distribution evaluated by computed tomography and metabolic abnormalities in patients undergoing antiretroviral therapy: preliminary results of the LIPOCO study. AIDS 14:37–49, 2000.
58. van der Valk M, Gisolf EH, Reiss P, et al. Increased risk of lipodystrophy when nucleoside analogue reverse transcriptase inhibitors are included with protease inhibitors in the treatment of HIV-1 infection. AIDS 15:847–55, 2001.
59. John M, Nolan D, Mallal S. Antiretroviral therapy and the lipodystrophy syndrome. Antivir Ther 6:9–20, 2001.
60. Chene G, Angelini E, Cotte L, et al. Role of long-term nucleoside-analogue therapy in lipodystrophy and metabolic disorders in human immunodeficiency virus-infected patients. Clin Infect Dis 34:649–57, 2002.
61. Amin J, Moore A, Carr A, et al. Combined analysis of two-year follow-up from two open-label randomized trials comparing efficacy of three nucleoside reverse transcriptase inhibitor backbones for previously untreated HIV-1 infection: Ozcombo 1 and 2. HIV Clin Trials 4:252–61, 2003.
62. Joly V, Flandre P, Meiffredy V, et al. Increased risk of lipoatrophy under stavudine in HIV-1-infected patients: results of a substudy from a comparative trial. AIDS 16:2447–54, 2002.
63. Dube MP, Zackin R, Tebas P, et al. Prospective study of regional body composition in antiretroviral-naive subjects randomized to receive zidovudine + lamivudine or didanosine + stavudine combined with nelfinavir, efavirenz, or both: A5005s, a substudy of ACTG 384. 4th International Workshop on Adverse Drug Reactions and Lipodsystrophy. September 22–25, 2002, San Diego, California, USA, abstract 27.
64. Saint-Marc T, Touraine JL. The effects of discontinuing stavudine therapy on clinical and metabolic abnormalities in patients suffering from lipodystrophy. AIDS 13:2188–9, 1999.
65. Carr A, Workman C, Smith DE, et al. Abacavir substitution for nucleoside analogs in patients with HIV lipoatrophy: a randomized trial. JAMA 288:207–15, 2002.

66. Lafeuillade A, Clumeck N, Mallolas J, et al. Comparison of Metabolic Abnormalities and Clinical Lipodystrophy 48 Weeks After Switching from HAART to Trizivir trade mark Versus Continued HAART: The Trizal Study. HIV Clin Trials 2003 Jan-Feb;4:37–43.
67. Dreschler H, Powderly WG. Switching effective antiretroviral therapy: a review. Clin Infect Dis 35:1219–30, 2002.
68. Nolan D, Hammond E, Martin A, et al. Mitochondrial DNA depletion and morphologic changes in adipocytes associated with nucleoside reverse transcriptase inhibitor therapy. AIDS 17:1329–38, 2003.
69. Lloreta J, Domingo P, Pujol RM, et al. Ultrastructural features of highly active antiretroviral therapy-associated partial lipodystrophy. Virchows Arch 441:599–604, 2002.
70. Walker UA, Bickel M, Lutke Volksbeck SI, et al. Evidence of nucleoside analogue reverse transcriptase inhibitor-associated genetic and structural defects of mitochondria in adipose tissue of HIV-infected patients. J Acquir Immune Defic Syndr 29:117–21, 2002.
71. Thompson K, McComsey G, Paulsen D, et al. Improvements in body fat and mitochondrial DNA levels are accompanied by decreased adipose tissue apoptosis after replacement of stavudine therapy with either abacavir or stavudine. 10th Conference on Retroviruses and Opportunistic Infections. February 10–14, 2003, Boston, USA, abstract 728.
72. Domingo P, Matias-Guiu X, Pujol RM, et al. Switching to nevirapine decreases insulin levels but does not improve subcutaneous adipocyte apoptosis in patients with highly active antiretroviral therapy-associated lipodystrophy. J Infect Dis 184: 1197–201, 2001.
73. Shikuma CM, Hu N, Milne C, et al. Mitochondrial DNA decrease in subcutaneous adipose tissue of HIV-infected individuals with peripheral lipoatrophy. AIDS 15:1801–9, 2001.
74. Nolan D, Hammond E, James I, et al. Contribution of nucleoside-analogue reverse-transcriptase inhibitor therapy to lipoatrophy from the population to the cellular level. Antivir Ther 8:617–26, 2003.
75. Cherry C, Nolan D, James I, et al. Longitudinal associations between antiretroviral treatments and quantification of tissue mitochondrial DNA from ambulatory subjects with HIV infection. 10th Conference on Retroviruses and Opportunistic Infections. February 10–14, 2003, Boston, USA, abstract 133.
76. Nolan D, Hammond E, James I, et al. Contribution of nucleoside-analogue reverse-transcriptase inhibitor therapy to lipoatrophy from the population to the cellular level. Antivir Ther 8:617–26, 2003.
77. Hammond E, Nolan D, James I, et al. Reduction of mitochondrial DNA content and respiratory chain activity occurs in adipocytes within 6–12 months of commencing nucleoside reverse transcriptase inhibitor therapy. AIDS 18:563–5, 2004.
78. Gallant JE, Staszewski S, Pozniak AL, et al. Efficacy and safety of tenofovir DF vs stavudine in combination therapy in antiretroviral-naive patients: a 3-year randomized trial. JAMA 292:191–201, 2004.
79. Keswani SC, Pardo CA, Cherry CL, et al. HIV-associated sensory neuropathies. AIDS 16:2105–17, 2002.
80. Berger AR, Arezzo JC, Schaumburg HH, et al. 2′,3′-dideoxycytidine (ddC) toxic neuropathy: a study of 52 patients. Neurology 43:358–62, 1993.
81. Blum AS, Dal Pan GJ, Feinberg J, et al. Low-dose zalcitabine-related toxic neuropathy: frequency, natural history, and risk factors. Neurology 46:999–1003, 1996.
82. Dalakas MC, Semino-Mora C, Leon-Monzon M. Mitochondrial alterations with mitochondrial DNA depletion in the nerves of AIDS patients with peripheral neuropathy induced by 2′3′-dideoxycytidine (ddC). Lab Invest 81:1537–44, 2001.
83. Moore RD, Wong WM, Keruly JC, McArthur JC. Incidence of neuropathy in HIV-infected patients on monotherapy versus those on combination therapy with didanosine, stavudine and hydroxyurea. AIDS 14:273–8, 2000.
84. Simpson DM. Selected peripheral neuropathies associated with human immunodeficiency virus infection and antiretroviral therapy. J Neurovirol 8(Suppl 2):33–41, 2002.
85. Simpson DM, Haidich AB, Schifitto G, et al. Severity of HIV-associated neuropathy is associated with plasma HIV-1 RNA levels. AIDS 16:407–12, 2002.
86. Cherry C, McArthur J, Costello K, et al. Increasing prevalence of neuropathy in the era of highly active antiretroviral therapy (HAART). 9th Conference on Retroviruses and Opportunistic Infections. February 24–28, 2002, Seattle, WA, USA, abstract 69.
87. Famularo G, Moretti S, Marcellini S, et al. Acetyl-carnitine deficiency in AIDS patients with neurotoxicity on treatment with antiretroviral nucleoside analogues. AIDS 11:185–90, 1997.
88. Hart AM, Terenghi G, Johnson M, et al. Immunohistochemical quantification of cutaneous innervation in HIV-associated peripheral neuropathy: a study of L-acetyl-carnitine therapy. Antiviral Ther 5(Suppl 2):32, 2000.
89. Moyle GJ, Sadler M. Peripheral neuropathy with nucleoside antiretrovirals: risk factors, incidence and management. Drug Saf Dec;19(6):481–94, 1998.
90. Moore RD, Keruly JC, Chaisson RE. Incidence of pancreatitis in HIV-infected patients receiving nucleoside reverse transcriptase inhibitor drugs. AIDS 15:617–20, 2001.
91. Routy JP, Smith GH, Blank DW, Gilfix BM. Plasmapheresis in the treatment of an acute pancreatitis due to protease inhibitor-induced hypertriglyceridemia. J Clin Apheresis 16:157–59, 2001.
92. Perry RC, Cushing HE, Deeg MA, Prince MJ. Ritonavir, triglycerides, and pancreatitis. Clin Infect Dis 28:161–62, 1999.
93. Wilmink T, Frick TW. Drug-induced pancreatitis. Drug Saf 14:406–23, 1996.
94. Argiris A, Mathur-Wagh U, Wilets I, Mildvan D. Abnormalities of serum amylase and lipase in HIV-positive patients. Am J Gastroenterol 94:1248–52, 1999.
95. Havlir DV, Gilbert PB, Bennett K, et al. Effects of treatment intensification with hydroxyurea in HIV-infected patients with virologic suppression. AIDS 15:1379–88, 2001.
96. Belperio PS, Rhew DC. Prevalence and outcomes of anemia in individuals with human immunodeficiency virus: a systematic review of the literature. Am J Med 116:27S–43S, 2004.
97. Negredo E, Molto J, Burger D, et al. Unexpected CD4 cell count decline in patients receiving didanosine and tenofovir-based regimens despite undetectable viral load. AIDS 18:459–63, 2004.
98. Mauss S, Berger F, Schmutz G. Antiretroviral therapy with tenofovir is associated with mild renal dysfunction. AIDS 19:93–5, 2005.
99. Fisher EJ, Chaloner K, Cohn DL, et al. The safety and efficacy of adefovir dipivoxil in patients with advanced HIV disease: a randomized, placebo-controlled trial. AIDS 15:1695–700, 2001.
100. Cihlar T, Ho ES, Lin DC, Mulato AS. Human renal organic anion transporter 1 (hOAT1) and its role in the nephrotoxicity of antiviral nucleotide analogs. Nucleosides Nucleotides Nucleic Acids 20:641–8, 2001.
101. Mallal S, Nolan D, Witt C, et al. Association between presence of HLA-B*5701, HLA-DR7, and HLA-DQ3 and hypersensitivity to HIV-1 reverse-transcriptase inhibitor abacavir. Lancet 359:727–32, 2002.
102. Lichtenstein KA, Delaney KM, Armon C, et al. Incidence of and risk factors for lipoatrophy (abnormal fat loss) in ambulatory HIV-1-infected patients. J Acquir Immune Defic Syndr 32:48–56, 2003.

103. Nolan D, Mallal S. Effects of sex and race on lipodystrophy pathogenesis. J HIV Ther 6:32–6, 2001.
104. Lafeuillade A, Hittinger G, Chadapaud S. Increased mitochondrial toxicity with ribavirin in HIV/HCV coinfection. Lancet 357:280–1, 2001.
105. Kakuda TN, Brinkman K. Mitochondrial toxic effects and ribavirin. Lancet 357:1802–3, 2001.
106. Salmon-Ceron D, Chauvelot-Moachon L, Abad S, et al. Mitochondrial toxic effects and ribavirin. Lancet 357:1803–4, 2001.
107. Hong Z, Cameron CE. Pleiotropic mechanisms of ribavirin antiviral activities. Prog Drug Res 59:41–69, 2002.
108. Inagaki H, Matsushima Y, Ohshima M, Kitagawa Y. Interferons suppress mitochondrial gene transcription by depleting mitochondrial transcription factor A (mtTFA). J Interferon Cytokine Res 17:263–9, 1997.
109. Hammond EL, Sayer D, Nolan D, et al. Assessment of precision and concordance of quantitative mitochondrial DNA assays: a collaborative international quality assurance study. J Clin Virol 27:97–110, 2003.
110. Gahan ME, Miller F, Lewin SR, et al. Quantification of mitochondrial DNA in peripheral blood mononuclear cells and subcutaneous fat using real-time polymerase chain reaction. J Clin Virol 22:241–7, 2001.
111. Reiss P, Casula M, De Ronde A, et al. Greater and more rapid depletion of mitochondrial DNA in blood of patients treated with dual (zidovudine + didanosine or zidovudine + zalcitabine) vs. single (zidovudine) nucleoside reverse transcriptase inhibitors. HIV Med 5:11–4, 2004.
112. Petit C, Mathez D, Barthelemy C, et al. Quantitation of blood lymphocyte mitochondrial DNA for the monitoring of antiretroviral drug-induced mitochondrial DNA depletion. Acquir Immune Defic Syndr 33:461–9, 2003.
113. Miura T, Goto M, Hosoya N, et al. Depletion of mitochondrial DNA in HIV-1-infected patients and its amelioration by antiretroviral therapy. J Med Virol 70:497–505, 2003.
114. Brinkman K. Management of hyperlactatemia: no need for routine lactate measurements. AIDS 15:795–7, 2001.

Chapter 75

Bone Disorders

Val Amorosa, MD, Pablo Tebas, MD

OSTEOPOROSIS

Introduction

Osteoporosis is a disease characterized by low bone mass and microarchitectural deterioration of bone tissue, leading to enhanced bone fragility and an increase in fracture risk. Osteoporosis is a silent disease until its long-term consequences become apparent: fractures of the hip, vertebra and distal radius.[1] Osteoporosis and decreased bone mineral density (BMD) are extraordinarily common in the general population, and may become more so as populations live longer, having an increasingly significant impact on global health costs, morbidity and mortality. Long-term complications of osteoporosis are more common among women due to lower peak bone mass and the bone loss associated with menopause.

Because large epidemiologic studies have correlated BMD measured by dual energy X-ray absorptiometry (DXA) and increased fragility fracture risk, in 1994, the World Health Organization (WHO) adopted definitions of osteopenia and osteoporosis based on bone mass and the number of standard deviations of an individual BMD as measured by DXA compared to a young population average at the peak of bone mass (30 years of age), adjusted for gender and race (T-score). Table 75-1 summarizes the WHO diagnostic categories of osteopenia/osteoporosis based on bone densitometry.[2] Fragility fractures are fractures occurring as a result of force that would not ordinarily cause fracture and WHO defines this as equivalent to a fall from a standing height or less. Osteoporosis is defined as a BMD that is more than 2.5 SD below the young mean adult value (T-score less than −2.5). Osteopenia is defined as a T-score between −2.5 and −1 SDs. Severe or established osteoporosis requires in addition the presence of fragility fractures (Table 75-1). The use of T-scores to diagnose osteopenia or osteoporosis in children and adolescents is inappropriate since bone mass has not yet reached its peak until age 30. Z-scores are more appropriate in this group (matching for gender, race and age). Absolute BMD values should be compared to a normative database, such as that made available by the Body Composition Laboratory at the Children's Nutrition Research Center at Baylor University (http://www.bcm.edu/bodycomplab/mainbodycomp.htm).

Osteopenia and osteoporosis are found frequently in persons with HIV infection,[3–14] and although as yet no increased incidence of fractures has been reported,[15] one assumes that low BMD in the long term will be associated with the same adverse sequelae as is seen in the general population. With the improved survival of HIV-infected individuals thanks to highly active antiretroviral therapy (HAART) and the aging of HIV-infected populations, the detrimental consequences of osteoporosis and osteopenia are likely to increase in significance in the future.

Table 75-1 WHO Classification of Bone Mineral Density

Category	Definition
Normal	T-score above −1
Osteopenia (or low bone mass)	T-score between −1 and −2.5
Osteoporosis	T-score at or below −2.5
Severe osteoporosis (or established osteoporosis)	Osteoporosis and the presence of one or more fragility fractures

From World Health Organization. Assessment of Fracture Risk and Its Application to Screening for Postmenopausal Osteoporosis. Geneva, Switzerland: World Health Organization; 1994.

Epidemiology of Osteopenia and Osteoporosis in HIV-Infected Individuals

Although currently available epidemiological studies have methodological limitations, multiple cross-sectional studies have consistently observed an increased prevalence of osteopenia/osteoporosis in HIV-infected individuals. Twelve studies were included in a recent metanalysis[16] of cross-sectional studies published in English to determine the pooled odds ratios (OR) of reduced BMD and osteoporosis in HIV-infected patients compared with HIV seronegative controls.[3–6,8,9,13,17–20] Of the 884 HIV-infected patients, 67% had reduced BMD of whom 15% had osteoporosis, yielding a pooled OR of 6.4 (95% CI: 3.7, 11.3) and 3.7 (95% CI: 2.3, 5.9), respectively, compared to HIV-seronegative controls (n = 654) (Fig. 75-1). While the conclusions of these studies should be interpreted with caution because of the high likelihood of reporting bias and the fact that many of the included studies did not adjust for important covariates like HIV-disease severity, treatment duration, and cumulative antiretroviral (ARV) exposure, despite these limitations, the results demonstrate an extraordinarily high prevalence of osteopenia/osteoporosis among HIV-infected individuals.

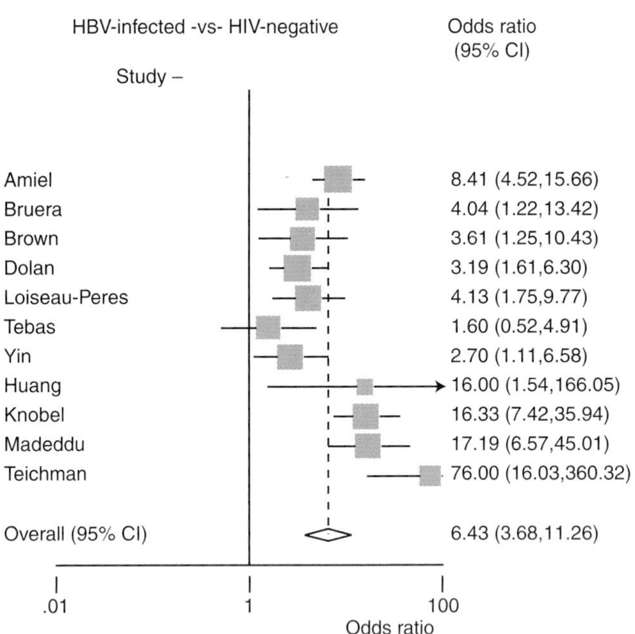

Figure 75-1 ■ Odds of reduced bone mineral density (osteopenia) in HIV-infected versus HIV-negative individuals. The size of the square is proportional to the weight of the study.

Redrawn from Brown TT, Qaqish RB. Antiretroviral therapy and the prevalence of osteopenia and osteoporosis: a meta-analysis. In: AIDS; 20:2165–2174, 2006. The studies listed correspond to references 3–5, 8, 9, 13, 17–20.

The prevalence of decreased bone density in HIV-infected women has also been directly examined. Huang et al noted that reduced BMD in HIV+ women with wasting was associated with reduced muscle mass.[21] The same group then looked at BMD in 84 HIV-infected women and 63 uninfected (average age 42 years) women of normal weight and noted reduced BMD in HIV-infected women versus age-matched controls at the L-spine and hip using DXA.[17] Osteopenia was present in 54% of the HIV-infected women versus 30% of controls and osteoporosis was present in 10% versus 5% of controls. Total body fat was significantly lower in the HIV-infected women than controls, but lean body mass was similar. Among the HIV-infected women, current body mass index (BMI), lowest adult weight, fat and lean body mass were all associated with BMD at the hip and spine. BMD was decreased in oligomenorrheic versus eumenorrheic women suggesting that this contributes to decreased BMD in a subset of women. Duration and class of antiretroviral therapy (ART) were not predictors of BMD.

Postmenopausal women with HIV infection are especially vulnerable to osteoporosis. Yin et al examined the prevalence of osteoporosis in 31 HIV+ African-American and Hispanic postmenopausal HIV+ women.[20] The women were compared to historic controls and were noted to have a 42% prevalence of osteoporosis at the spine, compared to 23% (P = .03) in controls. Of concern, at the hip the prevalence was 10% versus 1% in controls (P = .003). Rather than HIV-related risk factors such as CD4 T-lymphocyte count or ART, time since menopause and weight were the significant predictors of BMD.

Another potentially high-risk group for future fractures is HIV-infected children in whom several researchers have noted decreased BMD by DXA.[22–24] Several investigators have now studied HIV-infected children longitudinally for evidence of bone loss. Following-up on an earlier cross-sectional study noting decreased BMD in HIV+ children on HAART versus HAART-naive children and healthy children,[22] Mora et al studied a cohort of 32 HIV-infected children on HAART and healthy controls longitudinally over 1 year to assess gains in bone density in the two groups.[23] They found a decreased baseline BMD in the HIV+ children versus controls, a relatively similar 1 year increment in BMD at the L-spine and a smaller total body increment in BMD over the year. McComsey and Leonard followed 23 HIV+ children, 11 with baseline osteoporosis and six with baseline osteopenia over a median of 10 months and did not note a significant decrease in BMD at the spine or hip as measured by DXA over the course.[25] Ramos et al followed 35 HIV-infected children, 30 of whom were on HAART, over 13 months, noting 40% were osteopenic at baseline.[26] There was no significant increase in osteopenia prevalence or decrease in Z-score at follow-up.[26] It is important to remember that the use of T-scores in childhood and adolescence is not appropriate and that Z-scores are preferred with comparison to a normative database of individuals of the same gender, age, and size.

The increased incidence of osteopenia and osteoporosis among HIV positive individuals has not translated to an increased incidence of fragility fractures,[15] although follow-up has been too short and study sample sizes too small to detect an increased risk. One uncontrolled study suggests that

Table 75-2

Baseline Bone Mineral Density Characteristics of HIV Positive, Treatment-Naive Individuals Enrolled in Gilead 903

	TFV+3TC+EFV (n = 299)	D4T+3TC+EFV (n = 301)	Total (n = 600)
Normal	221 (74%)	206 (68%)	427 (71%)
Osteopenia	70 (23%)	83 (28%)	153 (26%)
Osteoporosis	8 (3%)	12 (4%)	20 (3%)

From Gallant JE, Staszewski S, Pozniak AL, et al. Efficacy and safety of tenofovir DF vs stavudine in combination therapy in antiretroviral-naive patients: a 3-year randomized trial. JAMA 292:191–201, 2004.

the incidence of fragility fractures in this population might be underreported.[27]

Etiology and Pathogenesis

Bone remodeling occurs in an orderly fashion, with bone resorption always followed by bone formation in a "coupled" process. If this balanced process is not matched (by increases in bone resorption or decreases in bone formation) then bone loss occurs. Several studies have suggested that this organized process can become unregulated during HIV infection.[10,13,28,29]

The Impact of HIV Infection on the Bone

Reports before the HAART era did not demonstrate a dramatically increased prevalence of osteoporosis and osteopenia in HIV-infected persons versus noninfected,[29–31] although the small sample size of those studies limit the strength of their conclusions.

The largest study to date examining the prevalence of osteopenia/osteoporosis among HIV-infected treatment-naive individuals is the Gilead study 903.[32] This was a randomized controlled trial of 600 ARV-naive patients who received either tenofovir/lamivudine (3TC)/efavirenz or stavudine (d4T)/3TC/efavirenz over 144 weeks. Because there were concerns about the potential bone toxicity of tenofovir, all 600 study participants underwent localized DXAs (hip and lumbar spine) every 24 weeks. The mean age at baseline was 36 years, participants were mostly white (64%) males (75%) with a mean HIV RNA viral load of 4.9 $\log_{10}$ copies/mL and a CD4 T-lymphocyte count of 280 cells/μL. The baseline data 33 clearly demonstrates that bone abnormalities are frequent among HIV-infected patients in the absence of ART. The prevalence of osteopenia of 26% for the whole group was higher than the expected 16% in the general population at this age. Osteoporosis was present in 3% of the individuals (Table 75-2). In a linear regression analysis of baseline demographic characteristics, male sex, lower weight and older age at enrollment correlated with lower spine T-scores at baseline.

The mechanism/s responsible for this low BMD in the absence of ART are not well understood. Traditional risk

Table 75-3

Risk Factors for Osteoporotic Fractures

Low bone mineral density	Consumption of >16 g of alcohol per day
Previous low-trauma fracture	Family history of hip fracture
Low body mass index	Falls and frailty
Current cigarette smoking	Increased age
Steroid exposure	Premature menopause of primary and secondary amenorrhea or hypogonadism
Rheumatoid arthritis	Low calcium or vitamin D intake

From Kanis JA, Borgstrom F, De Laet C, et al. Assessment of fracture risk. Osteoporos Int 16:581–9, 2005.

factors (Table 75-3) for osteopenia/osteoporosis and increased fracture risk are commonly present in HIV infected individuals and may play significant contributing roles. Smoking, wasting and nutritional deficits are frequent among HIV-infected individuals. It is also possible that HIV-induced alterations in cytotoxic T-cell numbers, circulating cytokines and T-cell turnover rates affect bone metabolism as is seen in other inflammatory diseases. Pro-inflammatory cytokines exert their regulatory effects on bone turnover by stimulating both the secretory and proliferative activities of mature cells. They also condition the differentiation of immature cells into phenotypes that favor osteoclastogenesis. Advanced AIDS is a state with high levels of T-cell activation and increased levels of tumor necrosis factor-alpha (TNF-alpha) and other cytokines, which may contribute to the significant bone loss seen in this population (*see* Chapter 27).

The Role of ARV Treatment

Initial descriptions of low BMD among HIV-infected patients suggested that ART, especially protease inhibitors (PIs) might be a significant contributor to the development of osteopenia and osteoporosis.[3]

Cross-sectional studies have shown that individuals receiving ART have a higher likelihood of osteoporosis. Brown's meta-analysis[16] of eight studies[4,6,7,9,11,18,34,35] determined the

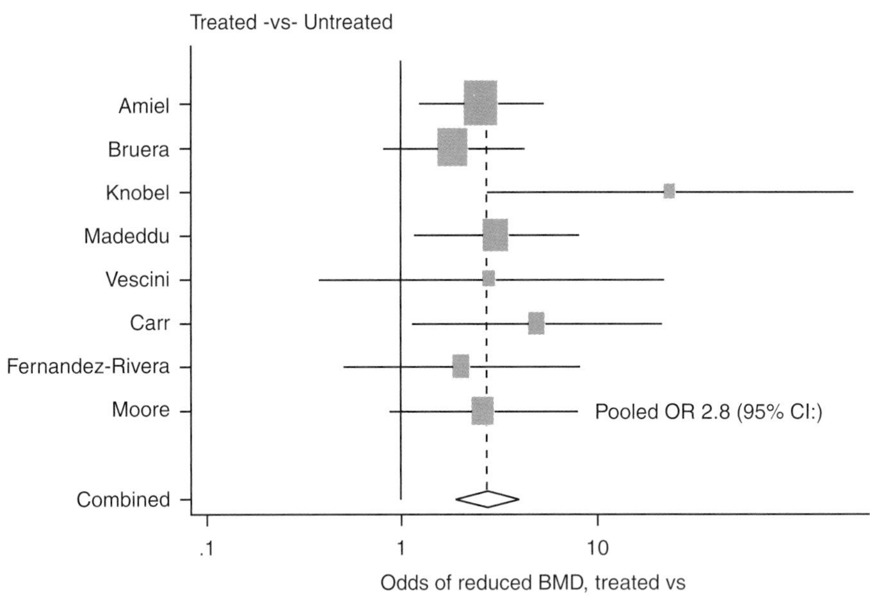

Figure 75-2 ■ Odds of reduced bone mineral density (osteopenia) in HIV-infected patients receiving treatment versus Treatment-naive. The size of the square is proportional to the weight of the study.

Redrawn from Brown TT, Qaqish RB. Antiretroviral therapy and the prevalence of osteopenia and osteoporosis: a meta-analysis. In: 7th International Workshop on Adverse Drug Reactions and Lipodystrophy in HIV. Antivir Ther 10:L52 (abstract 87), 2005. The studies listed correspond to references 4, 6, 7, 9, 11, 18, 34, 35.

odds of reduced BMD in ARV-treated patients (n = 802) compared to ARV-naive individuals (n = 189). HIV-infected individuals on therapy had a 2.8-(1.9-4.1) fold increase of reduced BMD and an OR of 2.6 of osteoporosis (Fig. 75-2). These findings suggest that ART might play a role in the development of osteopenia/osteoporosis in this population; however, because of the cross-sectional nature of the studies included and the risk of reporting bias, one must interpret the findings with caution.

Longitudinal studies avoid the biases of cross-sectional studies. Several longitudinal studies have now examined BMD over time in patients on HAART.[10,12,36] All these longitudinal studies included patients already receiving ART at the time of enrollment, so an early effect of medications on BMD could be missed. In a study of 54 patients over 54 weeks, pretreatment BMI was associated with lower baseline BMD.[12] Neither indinavir nor nelfinavir-based regimens was associated with decrease in BMD over time (0.31 increase Z-score/year on indinavir, no significant BMD change on nelfinavir). In a 72-week follow-up of 93 patients on HAART, Mondy et al noted that the most significant factors associated with low baseline bone density were BMI, body weight, duration of HIV infection and smoking history.[10] Over the study period overall BMD increased significantly at the spine and hip and was not associated with PI therapy. The main conclusion of these two longitudinal studies is that in patients on stable ART there seems to be a stable or slight improvement of BMD.

Nonetheless, the initiation of ART seems to be associated with some bone loss, seen to varying extent with different regimens. In the Gilead 903 study described above, over 144 weeks, BMD at the spine decreased by 2.2% in the tenofovir arms versus 1.0% in the d4T arm ($P < 0.001$) and at the hip it decreased 2.8% in the tenofovir arms versus 2.4% in the d4T arm ($P = 0.064$) 32 (Fig. 75-3). The overall prevalence of osteoporosis and osteopenia increased slightly over time with a 28% prevalence of osteopenia in the tenofovir group, a 27% prevalence in the d4T group (13% vs 8% increase) at study's end, and a 5% prevalence of osteoporosis in each group.[33] Twenty-eight percent of tenofovir-treated patients versus 21% of the stavudine-treated patients lost at least 5% of BMD at the spine or 7% of BMD at the hip. Clinically relevant fractures (excluding fingers and toes) were reported in four patients in the tenofovir group and eight patients in the stavudine group. In addition, there were significant increases in biochemical markers of bone metabolism (serum bone-specific alkaline, serum osteocalcin, serum C-telopeptide and urinary N-telopeptide) in the tenofovir group relative to the stavudine group, suggesting increased bone turnover. The initiation of ARV treatment has been associated with bone mineral loss in other studies without widely disseminated results (ACTG 384/5005[37] and BMS AI424-034[38]; M Dube and M Noor, personal communication), but not in others.[39] This initial modest bone loss after initiation of therapy tends to stabilize over time, analogous to the acute bone loss seen after transplantation and steroid initiation. Its clinical significance and implications for patients receiving intermittent ARV remains unclear.

The initial descriptions of bone loss among HIV-positive persons tended to focus on the potential contributory role of PIs to decreased BMD.[3] Subsequent publications tended to ameliorate the strength of the association.[3–6,9–12,17,18,21,34,35]

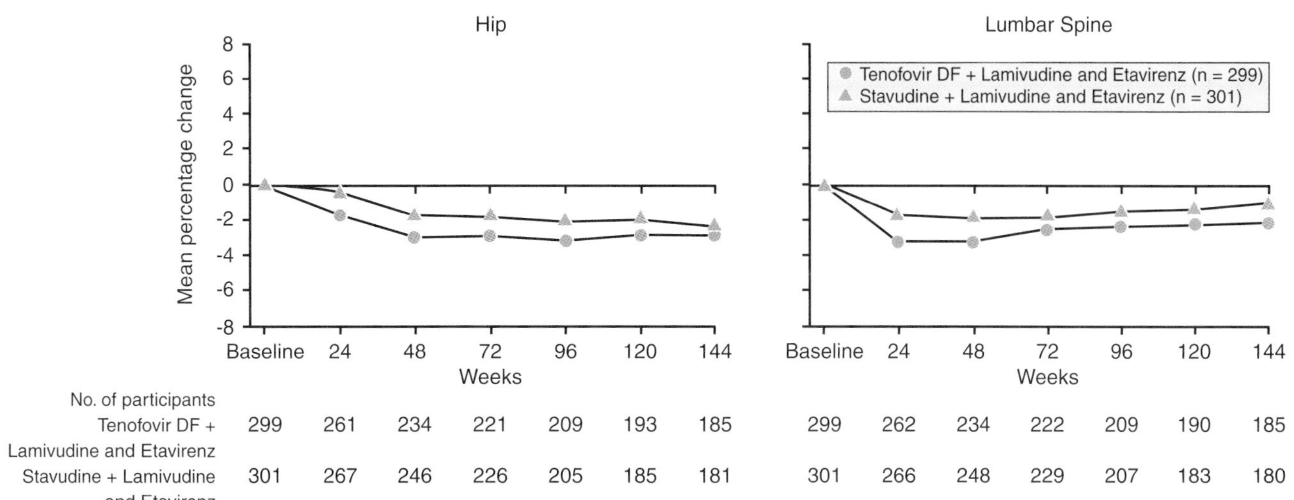

Figure 75-3 ■ Mean percentage change in hip and lumbar spine bone mineral density from baseline to week 144 in Gilead study 903. Redrawn from Gallant JE, Staszewski S, Pozniak AL, et al. Efficacy and safety of tenofovir DF vs stavudine in combination therapy in antiretroviral-naive patients: a 3-year randomized trial. JAMA 2004; 292:191–201.

In Brown's meta-analysis 16 of more than 10 published studies, PI-treated patients (n = 768) had increased odds of reduced BMD (OR 1.5; 95% CI: 1.1, 1.6) and osteoporosis (OR 1.6 95% CI: 1.08, 2.5) when compared to HIV-infected patients not treated with PIs (n = 402); however, the ORs are much lower than the association of low BMD and HIV infection or its treatment.

Contributing to the prevailing idea that PIs do not play a unique role in the development of osteopenia/osteoporosis, are studies in which switches to non-PI-based regimens do not seem to affect BMD. In ACTG 5125, 62 patients were randomized to switch a PI-based regimen to a non-nucleoside reverse transcriptase inhibitor (NNRTI)-based regimen or to switch to a nucleoside reverse transcriptase inhibitor (NRTI)-sparing regimen containing lopinavir/ritonavir and efavirenz.[40] At a median follow-up of 104 weeks there was no significant change in BMD within or between groups. Previously BMD longitudinal has also been evaluated over 48 weeks in 18 patients that switched from PI-based regimens to nevirapine-containing, PI-sparing regimens and no significant changes in BMD among the patients over the period were found.[41]

In Vitro and Animal Studies

In vitro studies have tried to evaluate the effects of HIV itself on bone metabolism and cytokine activation as well as direct drug effects on bone cells and metabolic pathways as potential contributors to bone demineralization among HIV-infected individuals. Unfortunately results have been confusing and occasionally difficult to correlate to clinical findings. A recent review summarizes the most recent *in vitro* data (Table 75-4).[42] The overall sense from these studies is that the alterations in bone mineralization observed in HIV-infected patients are probably multifactorial, and do not represent a "unique" pathogenic mechanism.

Chronic cytokine activation in persons with rheumatoid arthritis and other inflammatory diseases has been associated with osteoporosis. This has led to the hypothesis that chronic immune activation in patients with advanced AIDS could lead to increased bone resorption. Receptor of activated NF-κB ligand (RANKL) is a cytokine secreted from T cells and osteoblasts that stimulates osteoclast differentiation through activation of NF-κB and other pathways. TNF, which is characteristically elevated in patients with advanced HIV infection upregulates RANKL and osteoclastogenesis, probably via interleukin (IL)-1.[43] Because advanced HIV disease correlates with high levels of TNF[44] and because patients with advanced HIV infection (defined as a mean CD4 T-lymphocyte count cell count of 20 cells/μL) have markers of bone resorption that positively correlate with activation of TNF,[28] increased bone resorption in some patients may be due to increased cytokine activation and may contribute to decreased BMD. Fakruddin et al[45] demonstrated higher levels of RANKL in serum specimens from HIV-infected women than in serum specimens from HIV-uninfected women, regardless of ART use, suggesting a role for this cytokine pathway in HIV-associated bone loss.

In vitro effects of ARVs on bone resorption and formation pathways may eventually provide molecular explanations for the diverse effects on BMD of different ARVs, although as yet published *in vitro* studies present some discordant results. For example Wang et al found that indinavir inhibits osteoblast differentiation and leads to decreased BMD over time in a juvenile mouse model and that ritonavir inhibits osteoclast differentiation via blockade of RANKL-induced downstream signaling,[46] however, Fakruddin found that ritonavir (at lower concentrations than above) and saquinavir but not indinavir or nelfinavir lead to potentiation of osteoclastic activity.[47] Other authors have suggested that NRTIs like zidovudine (ZDV) increases osteoclast formation by upregulating NF-κB transcription factor activity in osteoclasts.[48]

Table 75-4

Summary of *In Vitro* Effects of HIV and ARVs on Bone Metabolism

Study	Finding	Reference
Viral factors		
Fakruddin et al	HIV GP120 led to upregulation of RANKL in PBMCs and increased osteoclastic activity.	47
Fakruddin et al	HIV Vpr increased RANKL expression in PBMCs in conjunction with endogenous and synergistically with exogenous glucocorticoids.	45
Wang et al	Indinavir inhibits osteoblast differentiation and leads to decreased BMD over time in a juvenile mouse model.	92, 93
Antiretroviral factors		
Wang et al	Ritonavir inhibits osteoclast differentiation via blockade of RANKL-induced downstream signaling.	46
Fakruddin and Laurence	Ritonavir (at lower concentrations than above) and saquinavir but not indinavir or nelfinavir lead to potentiation of osteoclastic activity.	47
Jain and Lenhard	In rat model, ritonavir, nelfinavir, indinavir, and saquinavir but not lopinavir or amprenavir were associated with increased osteoclast activity.	94
Pan et al	AZT increased osteoclast formation *in vitro* by upregulating NF-κβ downstream of RANKL. In mice, increased osteoclastogenesis led to decreased BMD.	48
Effect on vitamin D metabolism		
Cozzolino et al	*In vitro* ritonavir, indinavir, and nelfinavir decrease hepatic 25-hydroxylase, macrophage 1-alpha-hydroxylase activity and effects 1,25 dihydroxyvitamin D degradation, all with a final effect of decreased macrophage 1,25 dihydroxyvitamin D activity.	49

From Amorosa V, Tebas P. Bone disease and HIV infection. Clin Infect Dis 42:108–14, 2006.

The effects of ARVs on vitamin D metabolism present another mechanism by which ARVs may influence bone metabolism. Calcitriol, or 1,25 dihydroxyvitamin D, the steroid hormone that promotes intestinal calcium absorption and regulates osteoblast function, becomes activated by cytochrome enzymes, first in the liver, then in the kidney and in macrophages. In intact cells, HIV PIs markedly suppress the activities of 25- and 1alpha-hydroxylase, which are critical in 1,25(OH) vitamin D synthesis, while exerting mild inhibition of 24-hydroxylase, responsible for 1,25(OH) vitamin D catabolism. If PIs elicit a similar potency in inhibiting these critical steps for 1,25(OH) vitamin D homeostasis *in vivo*, defective 1,25(OH) vitamin D production could contribute to the bone demineralization in HIV patients.[49]

Cytochrome enzyme interactions could lead to osteoporosis via effects on exogenous hormone metabolism as well as illustrated by a case series in which osteoporosis and Cushing's syndrome developed in six patients on inhaled corticosteroids while taking a ritonavir-boosted PI.[50]

Recently much concern has been raised about decreased BMD on tenofovir. The large Gilead 903 study[32] and the observational study of Jacobson et al[36] both suggest that tenofovir may have more deleterious effects on bone than other studied ARVs, though this is of unclear clinical significance as yet. A longitudinal study of 18 HIV-infected children demonstrated significantly decreased BMD in five of them over 48 weeks on tenofovir.[51] Particularly at supra-therapeutic levels of prolonged duration as shown in macaque studies, tenofovir is capable of causing a Fanconi-like syndrome with renal phosphate wasting and concomitant osteomalacia.[52] While reports of Fanconi syndrome were more common with high-dose adefovir, reports for tenofovir have emerged as well.[53–56]

In vitro and animal studies provide fascinating insights into the mechanisms by which ARVs may directly lead to bone loss, but given the multiplicity of factors in a physiologic system, the *in vitro* studies do not correlate well with significant clinical effects. In addition, any negative *in vitro* role for ARVs in bone metabolism has to be balanced against their presumed positive impact in antagonizing the effects of HIV-associated wasting, chronic viremia and inflammation on bone.

Diagnosis

The frequency of osteopenia and osteoporosis is so high among HIV-infected individuals that the threshold to evaluate BMD in this population should be low. Current guidelines for HIV positive patients tend to be conservative and recommend evaluation only of individuals with other risk factors for osteoporosis or when a patient develops a fragility fracture.[57] Unfortunately, waiting for a fragility fracture is too late. At that time even antiresorptive treatment will not reduce the potential for future fractures to the risk seen in individuals without osteoporosis. Patients who develop fragility fracture are at very high risk for development of future fracture.[58] Yet even in HIV-infected individuals who have already developed fragility fractures, measurement of BMD was rarely performed.[27] A wider screen use of BMD measurements has been shown in prospective trials to decrease the risk for subsequent fragility fractures, as providers are more likely to treat if they are aware of the low BMD of the particular individual.[59]

The most widely used technique for determining BMD is DXA. DXA scanning measures bone mass and density in central regions of interest (hip and spine) as well as appendicular regions (wrist, forearm, heel). DXA scans are acquired quickly, accurately and safely. The ionizing radiation exposure is less than that received during a diagnostic chest radiograph (~40 mrem). Increased BMD measured by DXA scanning has correlated with reduced fracture risk in large-scale clinical trials of antiresorptive therapies, such as raloxifene, the selective estrogen receptor modulator[60] and is thus repeatedly shown to be an appropriate surrogate marker for fracture risk and for measurement of the therapeutic effectiveness of osteoporosis therapy. DXA has become the gold standard to which all other bone densitometry technologies are compared.

The International Society of Clinical Densitometry recommends that the diagnosis of osteoporosis be made by DXA using the lowest T-score of the lumbar spine (L1 to L4), total proximal femur, femoral neck, or trochanter, and that Ward's triangle area, a nonanatomical DXA-generated result should never be used for diagnosis.[61] A limitation in DXA's sensitivity in older patients is the presence of osteoarthritis and sclerosis in the lumbar spine that can artificially increase the BMD measurements.

DXA is also used to monitor the effectiveness of a therapeutic intervention on BMD. With most antiresorptive therapies, the spine will show BMD increases of several percent per year during the first year of therapy, whereas peripheral sites will remain stable (or in some cases, decline). Both for longitudinal evaluation of a population and for the evaluation of specific interventions to prevent or treat osteoporosis, it is important to allow an appropriate time interval to evaluate BMD changes. For most treatments and circumstances, at least a 2-year interval is recommended for assessing response at the spine. If possible the measurements should be made with the same device and in the same facility that was previously used.

Quantitative computed tomography (QCT)[62] and ultrasonography are alternative methods to directly measure or estimate bone density. QCT is rarely used outside research protocols, as it is more expensive, less reproducible, and requires a higher radiation dose than DXA. Quantitative ultrasound appears to be a good predictor of fractures in men and women, but its cost-effectiveness over screening using regular DXA is questionable.[63]

Biochemical markers of bone turnover measure the rate of bone formation and resorption. They are useful for the management of osteoporosis because they provide information that is different and complementary to BMD measurement. Baseline biochemical measures may reflect the current rate of bone loss and can predict future fracture risk,[64] although this is still controversial. The measurement of bone markers enhances the predictive value of bone mass measurement. High bone turnover independently predicts fracture risk in postmenopausal women.[65] Bone markers also provide the clinician critical information on the effectiveness of interventions, skeletal effects of treatment and potential long-term outcome of BMD measures. After an intervention, follow-up of bone markers is recommended at 3–6 months, by which time most of them have reached nadir levels.[64] The most frequent markers of bone resorption include N-telopeptide cross-linked collagen type 1 (NTx), deoxypyridinoline (Dpd), and C-telopeptide. Bone formation can be evaluated with osteocalcin, bone-specific alkaline phophatase and amino-terminal propeptide of type 1 collagen (P1NP). HIV-infected individuals in the absence of ARV treatment tend to have a state of low bone turnover. The initiation of ART is associated with a quick increase in markers of bone formation and resorption that tend to stay elevated while ARV treatment is maintained.[5,10,28]

At the time of the evaluation of patients with HIV infection and significant bone loss it is important to exclude causes of secondary osteoporosis, although it is unclear as yet how extensively and aggressively one should search for secondary causes. Secondary causes of osteoporosis include endocrine disorders like hyperthyroidism and hyperparathyroidism. Hypogonadism, which is frequent among patients with HIV infection (*see* Chapter 75) also leads to low BMD. Cushing syndrome, hyperprolactinemia, acromegaly, eating disorders associated with low BMI and diabetes are other diseases that can be associated with significant bone loss. Osteoporosis can also be a manifestation of gastrointestinal disorders associated with severe malabsortion such as celiac disease, severe liver disease and other diseases with massive infiltration of the bone marrow, including metastatic cancer and multiple myeloma, while renal disease can lead to renal osteodystrophy. The use of certain drugs is associated with low BMD, most notably corticosteroids, alcohol, and thyroid hormone replacement. A detailed discussion of all the secondary causes of osteoporosis is beyond the scope of this chapter. The prevalence of secondary osteoporosis in HIV infection is not known and has not been studied systematically. In postmenopausal women with osteoporosis up to 20% have some secondary cause of osteoporosis that might have contributed to the bone loss that is not identified readily by history.[66] A recent study of women with osteoporosis[66] showed that a workup including measurements of complete blood count, chemistry profile, 24 h urinary calcium, serum calcium, parathyroid hormone (PTH), thyroid-stimulating hormone (TSH), and vitamin D level determination would identify 98% of women with secondary osteoporosis. The most frequent secondary causes of osteoporosis in that study were hypercalciuria (10%), malabsorption (8%), primary or secondary hyperparathyroidsm (7%), and severe vitamin D deficiency (4%). In patients treated for hypothyrodism or thyroid cancer overdosing of thyroid hormones can be a common cause of osteopenia. In the absence of data in the HIV-infected population, such a workup should be reserved for the more severe cases (T-scores less than −2 or −2.5) or cases with other clinical clues suggestive of secondary diagnoses (see Fig. 75-4).

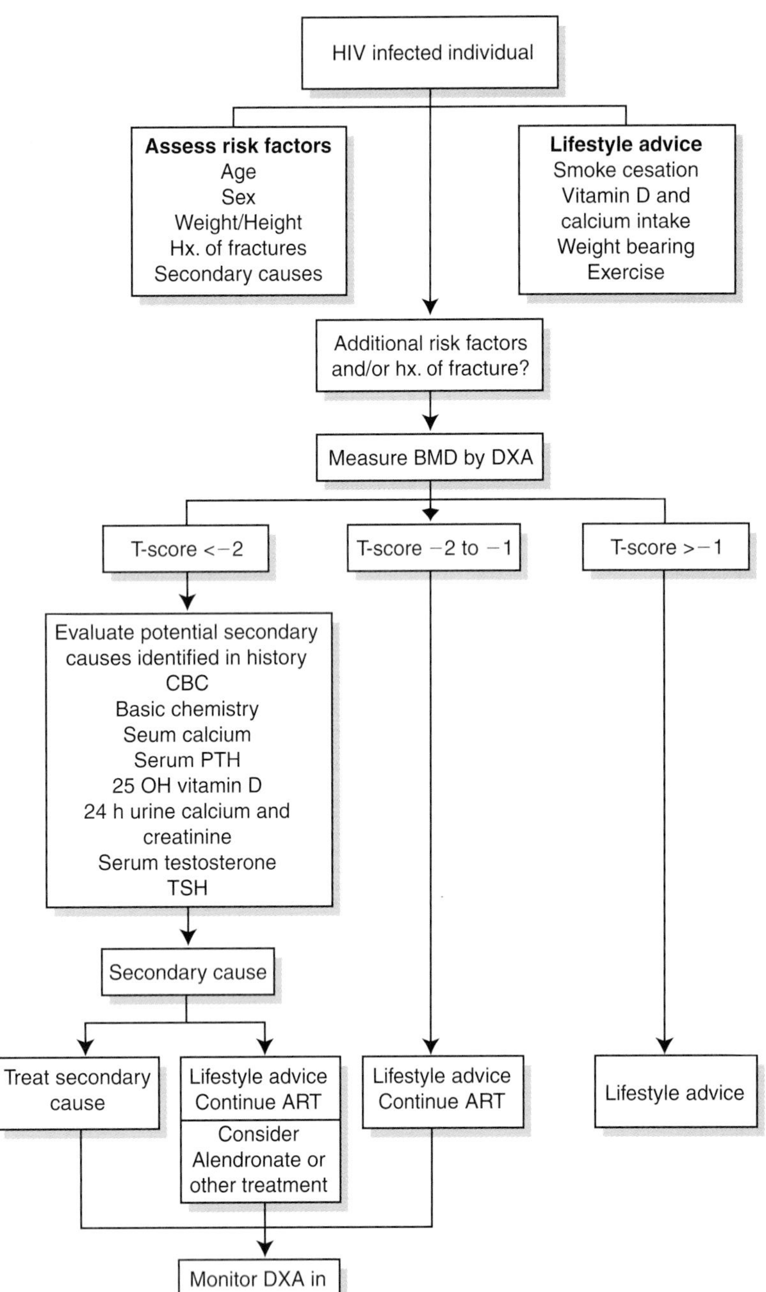

Figure 75-4 ■ General approach to the diagnosis and treatment of osteopenia and osteoporosis in HIV-infected individuals.

Bone biopsy is rarely needed, except when there is a strong suspicion of osteomalacia. Very few studies in HIV-infected individuals have been published that included the evaluation of bone biopsies.[10,29] Those studies showed that osteoporosis among HIV-infected individuals is a heterogeneous process with no uniform histological findings. Osteomalacia is uncommon in these studies, despite the potential for PIs to affect vitamin D metabolism.[49]

Treatment

The National Osteoporosis Foundation[67] recommends in its guidelines to initiate therapy to reduce fracture risk in women with; BMD T-scores below −2.0 by hip DXA with no risk factors or BMD T-scores below −1.5 by hip DXA with one or more risk factors and a prior vertebral or hip fracture. Although it is unclear whether these guidelines should be followed in HIV-infected men and premenopausal women, they seem to be a reasonable starting point. As HIV infection itself and its treatment are risks factors for bone loss, BMD T-scores less than −1.5 should be considered an indication for intervention. Patients with osteopenia should be followed with DXA every 1–2 years to evaluate the extent of change and those with a yearly decline >5% should be considered for therapy. The effects of treatment should be similarly evaluated. The management of osteopenia and osteoporosis is summarized in Figure 75-4.

General Measures

Once the diagnosis of osteopenia/osteoporosis has been made, and the need for treatment has been established some general measures are indicated. If the ostoepenia/osteoporosis is secondary to other pathology such as hypogonadism, hyperthyroidism or vitamin D deficiency, it should be treated appropriately. Any contributing risks such as steroids, alcohol and tobacco should be eliminated if possible. HIV-infected men or women with osteoporosis should receive adequate calcium (1000 mg/day) and vitamin D (400–800 IU/day) supplementation. However, it is important to remember that neither calcium nor vitamin D supplementation is effective for the treatment of established osteoporosis[68] nor do they decrease the risk of fracture in postmenopausal women.[69]

A weight-bearing exercise regimen also may be beneficial given the association of reduced physical activity with bone loss, especially in patients with advanced HIV infection and the known positive effect of exercise in women and men with osteoporosis.[70,71]

Androgen Therapy

Testosterone replacement increases BMD in men with hypogonadism. Hypogonadism is a frequently encountered problem among HIV-infected individuals, and when it is present it should be treated aggressively. However, the use of testosterone supplementation in eugonadal patients is more controversial. Farfield et al conducted a study to determine the effects of testosterone and progressive resistance training on BMD and bone turnover in 54 eugonadal men with AIDS wasting (weight $<90\%$ of ideal body weight or weight loss $>10\%$ from pre-illness baseline) who received either testosterone enanthate (200 mg/week, IM) or placebo and participated in progressive resistance training (3 times/week) or no training in a 2×2 factorial study design for 3 months. Lumbar spine BMD, as assessed on regional total-body DXA scan, increased over the 12-week treatment period in response to testosterone ($+2.4 \pm 1.3$ vs $-1.3 \pm 1.0\%$, testosterone vs placebo, respectively; $P = 0.02$), but not in response to training ($+0.8 \pm 1.0$ vs $+0.4 \pm 1.3\%$, training vs no training; $P = 0.70$).

In a much larger study of older men with low testosterone concentrations (<475 ng/dL) the administration of testosterone did not increase the lumbar spine BMD.[72] However, in a post-hoc analysis the individuals with a baseline concentration below 200 ng/dL obtained a benefit with testosterone supplementation.

Because of the myriad of potential side effects of androgen supplementation, the use of testosterone supplementation in eugonadal HIV-infected individuals for the treatment of osteopenia/osteoporosis is not recommended.

Bisphosphonates

Bisphosphonates are approved for the treatment of osteoporosis in both men and women. Mondy et al[73] conducted a small randomized trial comparing calcium and vitamin D supplementation with or without weekly alendronate for the treatment of HIV-infected individuals with evidence of osteopenia or osteoporosis. Thirty-one HIV-infected subjects with lumbar spine BMD T-scores less than -1.0 on ART for a minimum of 6 months, were randomized to receive (n = 15) or not (n = 16) 70 mg of alendronate weekly for 48 weeks in addition to calcium (1000 mg) and vitamin D supplementation (400 IU daily). At baseline, the median T-score in the lumbar spine was -1.52, and the median T-score in the hip was -1.02. Alendronate in combination with vitamin D and calcium increased lumbar spine BMD by 5.2% at 48 weeks compared with an increase of 1.3% in subjects receiving vitamin D and calcium alone. One subject discontinued treatment in each arm. There were no serious adverse events. Although small, the study established the safety of alendronate in HIV-infected individuals with decreased BMD. The improvements in this HIV-infected population were similar to that observed in a large randomized trial of daily alendronate in 241 men with osteoporosis, that demonstrated a significant reduction in the risk of new vertebral fractures.[74] Other smaller studies have demonstrated similar results using alendronate.[75,76] The AIDS Clinical Trials Group is conducting a larger randomized trial evaluating this compound for the treatment of osteoporosis associated with HIV infection with results available in mid-2006.

If alendronate is selected for the treatment of osteopenia/osteoporosis associated with HIV infection, the once weekly 70 mg formulation is the most convenient for the patients. No pharmacological interactions are expected between alendronate and ARV drugs. Patients should be instructed on proper administration and monitored for esophagitis, an infrequent complication.

There are no studies available evaluating the use of other biphosphonates like ibandronate[77] (Boniva, usual dose 150 mg PO once a month), risedronate[78] (Actonel) (5 mg q day or 35 mg q week), or intravenous zoledronic acid[79] (4 mg/year) in HIV-infected individuals.

Parathyroid Hormone

Teriparatide (Forteo®) was approved in 2001 for the treatment of osteoporosis in women and men at "high-risk" for fracture, individuals with a previous osteoporotic fracture, multiple risk factors for fracture, or previous therapeutic failure. The drug is effective in decreasing the number of fractures in women.[80] The largest trial in men included 437 men with spine or hip BMD more than 2 SD below the young adult male mean. Patients were randomized to placebo, SQ teriparatide 20 μg, or SQ teriparatide 40 μg in addition to supplemental calcium and vitamin D. By the end of treatment (11 months) spine BMD in individuals that received PTH was greater than in placebo subjects and greater than baseline by 5.9% (20 μg) and 9.0% (40 μg).[81] This drug should not be used in combination with alendronate as combinations studies have demonstrated that alendronate impair the ability of PTH to increase BMD.[82]

PTH is indicated of the treatment of osteoporosis with a decreased rate of bone formation. Patients with HIV infection appear to have a state of high bone turnover.[10] Because of this, in addition to the high cost, concerns about the development of osteosarcomas in animal models of teriparatide and the need of parenteral administration, the drug does not appear to have a role in the treatment of HIV-associated osteopenia/osteoporosis.

Raloxifene

Raloxifene, is a selective estrogen receptor modulator, effective in increasing BMD and reducing the risk of fracture in women[60] and maybe in men with prostate cancer.[83] There are no studies evaluating the use of raloxifene in HIV-infected individuals. This drug potentially could be useful on postmenopausal women with HIV infection who have a contraindication to bisphophonate therapy or cannot tolerate bisphosphonates.

Other Drugs

There is very limited or no data about the use of calcitonin, other estrogens, fluoride, isoflavones, calcitrol, statins, or thiazides in the management of osteoporosis in HIV-infected individuals. Because of the limited utility of these drugs in the noninfected population they are probably not indicated for first-line treatment in HIV-infected individuals.

OSTEONECROSIS

Osteonecrosis, also known as aseptic necrosis or avascular necrosis (AVN), is a pathological process that has been associated with HIV infection as well as with numerous other conditions and therapeutic interventions. The mechanisms by which this disorder develops are not fully understood. However, a compromise of the arterial blood supply to the bone appears to be the final common pathway. The process is progressive, resulting in joint destruction within three to 5 years if left untreated.

Epidemiology

Osteonecrosis seems to be more frequent among HIV-infected individuals than in HIV-negative controls. In a large published series, the National Institute of Health (NIH) screened 339 HIV positive asymptomatic patients along with 118 HIV-negative age and sex-matched controls.[84] Fifteen (4.4% (95% CI, 2.5% to 7.2%)) of 339 HIV-infected participants had osteonecrotic lesions of the hip on magnetic resonance imaging (MRI), while no lesions were found in HIV-negative participants. Among HIV-infected participants, osteonecrosis occurred more frequently in those who used systemic corticosteroids, lipid-lowering agents, or testosterone; those who exercised routinely by bodybuilding; and those who had detectable levels of anticardiolipin antibodies. Factors that did not seem to be associated with AVN were CD4 T-lymphocyte count cell count, HIV RNA level, or use of a PI. A follow-up of this cohort has subsequently been presented. 235 patients with no evidence of osteonecrosis on the first MRI underwent a second MRI scan a median of 23 months after the initial scan. Three patients (1.3%) were diagnosed with osteonecrosis of the femoral head (all bilateral), for an incidence rate of 0.7 cases/100 patient-years. This illustrates a significantly high incidence of osteonecrosis among HIV positive individuals.[85]

Other recent series confirm an increased incidence of AVN among HIV positive individuals, although these studies point to traditional risk factors rather than HIV or ARV as most responsible for AVN. In Spain, among the 23 cases reported by Gutiérrez et al,[86] 86% occurred in patients with non-HIV-specific risk factors including alcohol abuse, corticosteroid use, megestrol acetate use, hypertriglyceridemia, trauma and a hypercoagulable state. Hasse et al[87] examined risk factors for AVN within the Swiss cohort over the 11 years from 1991 to 2002. There were 26 patients with AVN (22 of them at the hip) and the investigators performed a case-control study comparing the patients to 260 HIV-infected controls. The risk factors found to be associated with AVN were lower CD4 T-lymphocyte count nadirs, prior opportunistic infections and higher BMI, whereas duration of diagnosed HIV and duration of ART use were not associated. Similar findings were reported by Lawson-Ayayi et al from the Aquitaine cohort in France.[88] They performed a case-control study and found that the factors associated with AVN in HIV-infected individuals using a multivariate regression model were heavy alcohol consumption and steroid use.

AVN can also affect children with HIV infection. In a large case-control study involving the Pediatric AIDS Clinical Trial Group, the prevalence of AVN in perinatally infected HIV-positive children was nine times the prevalence in uninfected controls, with six cases among 2014 infected patients.[89] There were no associations with the use of steroids, however, the number of cases was too small to find significant associations.

Clinical Manifestations

AVN is often first suspected when acute pain develops in a joint, typically a large joint such as the hip or shoulder. The femoral head is the most commonly affected region and patients usually present with severe hip pain and difficulty walking. Physical findings are largely nonspecific. Patients may have pain in the groin or the buttock area and eventually limitation on range of motion. Osteonecrosis in HIV-infected patients can also involve multiple sites.[90,91]

Diagnosis

The evaluation for suspected osteonecrosis of the femoral head should begin with anterior-posterior and frog-leg lateral films, but characteristic changes can be significantly delayed in regular X-rays. MRI of the joint is the most sensitive technique and should be used in cases in which there is a strong suspicion for AVN.

Treatment

The treatment of osteonecrosis remains a controversial area, and consultation with an orthopedic surgeon with experience in the management of AVN is recommended. Although the goal of therapy is to preserve the native joint for as long as possible, if the area of necrosis is greater than 15%, a surgical approach with joint replacement is often required. Some asymptomatic patients might not need specific interventions until symptoms appear, as was the case in several patients from the NIH cohort. Among the 15 patients with osteonecrosis diagnosed on the initial screening MRI, six had bilateral and nine had unilateral disease. At a median follow-up of 5.8 years, five patients remained asymptomatic, four reported mild pain symptoms, one underwent bilateral total hip replacement (THR), three patients died and one was lost to follow-up. Among 19 additional symptomatic patients referred to the study following diagnosis of osteonecrosis, 15 had bilateral involvement of the femoral heads, and seven had osteonecrosis involving other bones. Nine of the 19 required surgical intervention for pain control, with six patients undergoing THR.[85] Changing ART to a non-PI-containing regimen does not appear to help, but treating concomitant predisposing conditions that could cause further osteonecrosis is reasonable.

ACKNOWLEDGMENTS

This chapter is based in part on a review article recently published: Amorosa V, Tebas P. Bone disease and HIV infection. Clin Infect Dis 42:108–14, 2006. Supported in part by AI32783.

REFERENCES

1. Consensus development conference: diagnosis, prophylaxis, and treatment of osteoporosis. Am J Med 94:646–50, 1993.
2. World Health Organization. Assessment of Fracture risk and Its Application to Screening for Postmenopausal Osteoporosis. Geneva, Switzerland: World Health Organization; 1994.
3. Tebas P, Powderly WG, Claxton S, et al. Accelerated bone mineral loss in HIV-infected patients receiving potent antiretroviral therapy. AIDS 14:F63-7, 2000.
4. Amiel C, Ostertag A, Slama L, et al. BMD is reduced in HIV-infected men irrespective of treatment. J Bone Miner Res 19:402–9, 2004.
5. Brown TT, Ruppe MD, Kassner R, et al. Reduced bone mineral density in human immunodeficiency virus-infected patients and its association with increased central adiposity and postload hyperglycemia. J Clin Endocrinol Metab 89:1200–6, 2004.
6. Bruera D, Luna N, David DO, et al. Decreased bone mineral density in HIV-infected patients is independent of antiretroviral therapy. Aids 17:1917–23, 2003.
7. Carr A, Miller J, Eisman JA, Cooper DA. Osteopenia in HIV-infected men: association with asymptomatic lactic acidemia and lower weight pre-antiretroviral therapy. Aids 15:703–9, 2001.
8. Huang JS, Rietschel P, Hadigan CM, et al. Increased abdominal visceral fat is associated with reduced bone density in HIV-infected men with lipodystrophy. AIDS 15:975–82, 2001.
9. Madeddu G, Spanu A, Solinas P, et al. Bone mass loss and vitamin D metabolism impairment in HIV patients receiving highly active antiretroviral therapy. Q J Nucl Med Mol Imaging 48:39–48, 2004.
10. Mondy K, Yarasheski K, Powderly WG, et al. Longitudinal evolution of bone mineral density and bone markers in human immunodeficiency virus-infected individuals. Clin Infect Dis 36:482–90, 2003.
11. Moore AL, Vashisht A, Sabin CA, et al. Reduced bone mineral density in HIV-positive individuals. AIDS 15:1731–3, 2001.
12. Nolan D, Upton R, McKinnon E, et al. Stable or increasing bone mineral density in HIV-infected patients treated with nelfinavir or indinavir. AIDS 15:1275–80, 2001.
13. Teichmann J, Stephan E, Lange U, et al. Osteopenia in HIV-infected women prior to highly active antiretroviral therapy. J Infect 46:221–7, 2003.
14. Landonio S, Quirino T, Bonfanti P, et al. Osteopenia and osteoporosis in HIV+ patients, untreated or receiving HAART. Biomed Pharmacother 58:505–8, 2004.
15. Struble K, Murray J, Schneider B, Soon G. Bone fracture rates in HIV+ patients receiving PI vs non-PI containing regimens. In: 41st Interscience Conference on Antimicrobial and Antiviral Chemotherapy, Chicago, 2001, abstract I-1329.
16. Brown TT, Qaqish RB. Antiretroviral therapy and the prevalence of osteopenia and osteoporosis: a meta-analysis. In: 7th International Workshop on Adverse Drug Reactions and Lipodystrophy in HIV. Antivir Ther 10:L52 (abstract 87), 2005.
17. Dolan SE, Huang JS, Killilea KM, et al. Reduced bone density in HIV-infected women. AIDS 18:475–83, 2004.
18. Knobel H, Guelar A, Vallecillo G, et al. Osteopenia in HIV-infected patients: is it the disease or is it the treatment? AIDS 15:807–8, 2001.
19. Loiseau-Peres S, Delaunay C, Poupon S, et al. Osteopenia in patients infected by the human immunodeficiency virus. A case control study. Joint Bone Spine 69:482–5, 2002.
20. Yin M, Dobkin J, Brudney K, et al. Bone mass and mineral metabolism in HIV+ postmenopausal women. Osteoporos Int 16:1345–52, 2005.
21. Huang JS, Wilkie SJ, Sullivan MP, Grinspoon S. Reduced bone density in androgen-deficient women with acquired immune deficiency syndrome wasting. J Clin Endocrinol Metab 86:3533–9, 2001.
22. Mora S, Sala N, Bricalli D, et al. Bone mineral loss through increased bone turnover in HIV-infected children treated with highly active antiretroviral therapy. AIDS 15:1823–9, 2001.
23. Mora S, Zamproni I, Beccio S, et al. Longitudinal changes of bone mineral density and metabolism in antiretroviral-treated human immunodeficiency virus-infected children. J Clin Endocrinol Metab 89:24–8, 2004.
24. Rojo Conejo P, Ramos Amador JT, et al. Decreased bone mineral density in HIV-infected children receiving highly active antiretroviral therapy. An Pediatr (Barc) 60:249–53, 2004.
25. McComsey GA, Leonard E. Metabolic complications of HIV therapy in children. Aids 18:1753–68, 2004.
26. Ramon J, Rojo P, Ruano C, et al. Stability of osteopenia in HIV-infected children over time. In: Eleventh Conference on Retroviruses and Opportunistic Infections, San Francisco, Feb 2004, abstract 745.
27. McComsey GA, Huang JS, Woolley IJ, et al. Fragility fractures in HIV-infected patients: need for better understanding of diagnosis and management. J Int Assoc Physicians AIDS Care (Chic Ill) 3:86–91, 2004.
28. Aukrust P, Haug CJ, Ueland T, et al. Decreased bone formative and enhanced resorptive markers in human immunodeficiency virus infection: indication of normalization of the bone-remodeling process during highly active antiretroviral therapy. J Clin Endocrinol Metab 84:145–50, 1999.
29. Serrano S, Marinoso ML, Soriano JC, et al. Bone remodelling in human immunodeficiency virus-1-infected patients. A histomorphometric study. Bone 16:185–91, 1995.
30. Paton NI, Macallan DC, Griffin GE, Pazianas M. Bone mineral density in patients with human immunodeficiency virus infection. Calcif Tissue Int 61:30–2, 1997.

31. Hernandez Quero J, Ortego Centeno N, Munoz-Torres M, et al. Alterations in bone turnover in HIV-positive patients. Infection 21:220–2, 1993.
32. Gallant JE, Staszewski S, Pozniak AL, et al. Efficacy and safety of tenofovir DF vs stavudine in combination therapy in antiretroviral-naive patients: a 3-year randomized trial. JAMA 292:191–201, 2004.
33. Powderly WG, Cohen C, Gallant J, et al. Similar incidence of osteopenia and osteoporosis in antiretroviral-naïve patients treated with tenofovir DF or stavudine in combination with lamivudine and efavirenz over 144 weeks. In: 12th Conference on Retrovirus and Opportunistic Infections, Boston, MA, 2005, abstract 823.
34. Fernandez-Rivera J, Garcia R, Lozano F, et al. Relationship between low bone mineral density and highly active antiretroviral therapy including protease inhibitors in HIV-infected patients. HIV Clin Trials 4:337–46, 2003.
35. Vescini F, Borderi M, Buffa A, et al. Bone mass in HIV-infected patients: focus on the role of therapy and sex. J Acquir Immune Defic Syndr 33:405–7, 2003.
36. Jacobson D, Huang JS, Shevitz A, et al. Duration of ART and change in bone mineral density over time. In: Twelfth Conference on Retroviruses and Opportunistic Infections, Boston, 22–25 Feb 2005, abstract 825.
37. Dube MP, Parker RA, Tebas P, et al. Glucose metabolism, lipid, and body fat changes in antiretroviral-naive subjects randomized to nelfinavir or efavirenz plus dual nucleosides. AIDS 19:1807–18, 2005.
38. Jemsek JG, Arathoon E, Arlotti M, et al. Body fat and other metabolic effects of atazanavir and efavirenz, each administered in combination with zidovudine plus lamivudine, in antiretroviral-naive HIV-infected patients. Clin Infect Dis 42:273–80, 2006.
39. Dube MP, Qian D, Edmondson-Melancon H, et al. Prospective, intensive study of metabolic changes associated with 48 weeks of amprenavir-based antiretroviral therapy. Clin Infect Dis 35:475–81, 2002.
40. Tebas P, Zhang J, Yarasheski K, et al. Switch to a protease inhibitor-containing/nucleoside reverse transcriptase inhibitor-sparing regimen increases appendicular fat and serum lipid levels without affecting glucose metabolism or bone mineral density. The results of a prospective randomized trial, ACTG 5125s.. In: Twelfth Conference on Retroviruses and Opportunistic Infections, Boston, 22–25 Feb 2005, abstract 40.
41. Tebas P, Yarasheski K, Henry K, et al. Evaluation of the virological and metabolic effects of switching protease inhibitor combination antiretroviral therapy to nevirapine-based therapy for the treatment of HIV infection. AIDS Res Hum Retroviruses 20:589–94, 2004.
42. Amorosa V, Tebas P. Bone disease and HIV infection. Clin Infect Dis 42:108–14, 2006.
43. Wei S, Kitaura H, Zhou P, et al. IL-1 mediates TNF-induced osteoclastogenesis. J Clin Invest 115:282–90, 2005.
44. Aukrust P, Liabakk NB, Muller F, et al. Serum levels of tumor necrosis factor-alpha (TNF alpha) and soluble TNF receptors in human immunodeficiency virus type 1 infection – correlations to clinical, immunologic, and virologic parameters. J Infect Dis 169:420–4, 1994.
45. Fakruddin M, Yin M, Laurence J. Pathophysiologic correlates of RANKL deregulation in HIV infection and its therapy.. In: Twelfth Conference on Retroviruses and Opportunistic Infections, Boston, 22–25 Feb 2005, abstract 822.
46. Wang MW, Wei S, Faccio R, et al. The HIV protease inhibitor ritonavir blocks osteoclastogenesis and function by impairing RANKL-induced signaling. J Clin Invest 114:206–13, 2004.
47. Fakruddin JM, Laurence J. HIV envelope gp120-mediated regulation of osteoclastogenesis via receptor activator of nuclear factor kappa B ligand (RANKL) secretion and its modulation by certain HIV protease inhibitors through interferon-gamma/RANKL cross-talk. J Biol Chem 278:48251–8, 2003.
48. Pan G, Wu X, McKenna MA, et al. AZT enhances osteoclastogenesis and bone loss. AIDS Res Hum Retroviruses 20:608–20, 2004;.
49. Cozzolino M, Vidal M, Arcidiacono MV, et al. HIV-protease inhibitors impair vitamin D bioactivation to 1,25-dihydroxyvitamin D. AIDS 17:513–20, 2003.
50. Samaras K, Pett S, Gowers A, et al. Iatrogenic Cushing's syndrome with osteoporosis and secondary adrenal failure in human immunodeficiency virus-infected patients receiving inhaled corticosteroids and ritonavir-boosted protease inhibitors: six cases. J Clin Endocrinol Metab 90:4394–8, 2005.
51. Hazra R, Gafni RI, Maldarelli F, et al. Tenofovir disoproxil fumarate and an optimized background regimen of antiretroviral agents as salvage therapy for pediatric HIV infection. Pediatrics 116:e846–54, 2005.
52. Van Rompay KK, Brignolo LL, Meyer DJ, et al. Biological effects of short-term or prolonged administration of 9-[2-(phosphonomethoxy)propyl]adenine (tenofovir) to newborn and infant rhesus macaques. Antimicrob Agents Chemother 48:1469–87, 2004.
53. James CW, Steinhaus MC, Szabo S, Dressier RM. Tenofovir-related nephrotoxicity: case report and review of the literature. Pharmacotherapy 24:415–18, 2004.
54. Karras A, Lafaurie M, Furco A, et al. Tenofovir-related nephrotoxicity in human immunodeficiency virus-infected patients: three cases of renal failure, Fanconi syndrome, and nephrogenic diabetes insipidus. Clin Infect Dis 36:1070–3, 2003.
55. Rifkin BS, Perazella MA. Tenofovir-associated nephrotoxicity: Fanconi syndrome and renal failure. Am J Med 117:282–4, 2004.
56. Verhelst D, Monge M, Meynard JL, et al. Fanconi syndrome and renal failure induced by tenofovir: a first case report. Am J Kidney Dis 40:1331–3, 2002.
57. Schambelan M, Benson CA, Carr A, et al. Management of metabolic complications associated with antiretroviral therapy for HIV-1 infection: recommendations of an International AIDS Society-USA panel. J Acquir Immune Defic Syndr 31:257–75, 2002.
58. Ross PD, Davis JW, Epstein RS, Wasnich RD. Pre-existing fractures and bone mass predict vertebral fracture incidence in women. Ann Intern Med 114:919–23, 1991.
59. Kern LM, Powe NR, Levine MA, et al. Association between screening for osteoporosis and the incidence of hip fracture. Ann Intern Med 142:173–81, 2005.
60. Ettinger B, Black DM, Mitlak BH, et al. Reduction of vertebral fracture risk in postmenopausal women with osteoporosis treated with raloxifene: results from a 3-year randomized clinical trial. Multiple Outcomes of Raloxifene Evaluation (MORE) Investigators. JAMA 282:637–45, 1999.
61. Hamdy RC, Petak SM, Lenchik L. Which central dual X-ray absorptiometry skeletal sites and regions of interest should be used to determine the diagnosis of osteoporosis? J Clin Densitom 5(Suppl):S11–18, 2002.
62. Lang TF, Guglielmi G, van Kuijk C, et al. Measurement of bone mineral density at the spine and proximal femur by volumetric quantitative computed tomography and dual-energy X-ray absorptiometry in elderly women with and without vertebral fractures. Bone 30:247–50, 2002.
63. Marin F, Lopez-Bastida J, Diez-Perez A, Sacristan JA. Bone mineral density referral for dual-energy X-ray absorptiometry using quantitative ultrasound as a prescreening tool in postmenopausal women from the general population: a cost-effectiveness analysis. Calcif Tissue Int 74:277–83, 2004.
64. Garnero P, Hausherr E, Chapuy MC, et al. Markers of bone resorption predict hip fracture in elderly women: the EPIDOS Prospective Study. J Bone Miner Res 11:1531–8, 1996.

65. Miller PD, Baran DT, Bilezikian JP, et al. Practical clinical application of biochemical markers of bone turnover: consensus of an expert panel. J Clin Densitom 2:323–42, 1999.
66. Tannenbaum C, Clark J, Schwartzman K, et al. Yield of laboratory testing to identify secondary contributors to osteoporosis in otherwise healthy women. J Clin Endocrinol Metab 87:4431–7, 2002.
67. National Osteoporosis Foundation. Available: http://www.nof.org/_vti_bin/shtml.dll/physguide/index.htm 10 Feb 2005.
68. Ebeling PR, Wark JD, Yeung S, et al. Effects of calcitriol or calcium on bone mineral density, bone turnover, and fractures in men with primary osteoporosis: a two-year randomized, double blind, double placebo study. J Clin Endocrinol Metab 86:4098–103, 2001.
69. Jackson RD, LaCroix AZ, Gass M, et al. Calcium plus vitamin D supplementation and the risk of fractures. N Engl J Med 354:669–83, 2006.
70. Greendale GA, Barrett-Connor E, Edelstein S, et al. Lifetime leisure exercise and osteoporosis. The Rancho Bernardo study. Am J Epidemiol 141:951–9, 1995.
71. Wolff I, van Croonenborg JJ, Kemper HC, et al. The effect of exercise training programs on bone mass: a meta-analysis of published controlled trials in pre- and postmenopausal women. Osteoporos Int 9:1–12, 1999.
72. Snyder PJ, Peachey H, Hannoush P, et al. Effect of testosterone treatment on bone mineral density in men over 65 years of age. J Clin Endocrinol Metab 84:1966–1972, 1999.
73. Mondy K, Powderly WG, Claxton SA, et al. Alendronate, vitamin D, and calcium for the treatment of osteopenia/osteoporosis associated with HIV infection. J Acquir Immune Defic Syndr 38:426–31, 2005.
74. Orwoll E, Ettinger M, Weiss S, et al. Alendronate for the treatment of osteoporosis in men. N Engl J Med 343:604–10, 2000.
75. Negredo E, Martinez-Lopez E, Paredes R, et al. Reversal of HIV-1-associated osteoporosis with once-weekly alendronate. AIDS 19:343–5, 2005.
76. Guaraldi G, Orlando G, Madeddu G, et al. Alendronate reduces bone resorption in HIV-associated osteopenia/osteoporosis. HIV Clin Trials 5:269–77, 2004.
77. Reginster JY, Adami S, Lakatos P, et al. Efficacy and tolerability of once-monthly oral ibandronate in postmenopausal osteoporosis: 2-year results from the MOBILE study. Ann Rheum Dis 65:654–61, 2006.
78. Harris ST, Watts NB, Genant HK, et al. Effects of risedronate treatment on vertebral and nonvertebral fractures in women with postmenopausal osteoporosis: a randomized controlled trial. Vertebral Efficacy with Risedronate Therapy (VERT) Study Group. JAMA 282:1344–52, 1999.
79. Reid IR, Brown JP, Burckhardt P, et al. Intravenous zoledronic acid in postmenopausal women with low bone mineral density. N Engl J Med 346:653–61, 2002.
80. Neer RM, Arnaud CD, Zanchetta JR, et al. Effect of parathyroid hormone (1–34) on fractures and bone mineral density in postmenopausal women with osteoporosis. N Engl J Med 344:1434–41, 2001.
81. Orwoll ES, Scheele WH, Paul S, et al. The effect of teriparatide [human parathyroid hormone (1–34)] therapy on bone density in men with osteoporosis. J Bone Miner Res 18:9–17, 2003.
82. Finkelstein JS, Hayes A, Hunzelman JL, et al. The effects of parathyroid hormone, alendronate, or both in men with osteoporosis. N Engl J Med 349:1216–26, 2003.
83. Smith MR, Fallon MA, Lee H, Finkelstein JS. Raloxifene to prevent gonadotropin-releasing hormone agonist-induced bone loss in men with prostate cancer: a randomized controlled trial. J Clin Endocrinol Metab 89:3841–6, 2004.
84. Miller KD, Masur H, Jones EC, et al. High prevalence of osteonecrosis of the femoral head in HIV-infected adults. Ann Intern Med 137:17–25, 2002.
85. Morse CG, Kovacs JA. Metabolic and skeletal complications of HIV infection: the price of success. JAMA. 296:844–54, 2006. In: 7th International Workshop on Adverse Drug Reactions and Lipodystrophy in HIV, Dublin, Ireland, 13–16 Nov 2005, abstract 86.
86. Gutierrez F, Padilla S, Ortega E, et al. Avascular necrosis of the bone in HIV-infected patients: incidence and associated factors. AIDS 16:481–3, 2002.
87. Hasse B, Ledergerber B, Egger M, et al. Antiretroviral treatment and osteonecrosis in patients of the Swiss HIV Cohort Study: a nested case-control study. AIDS Res Hum Retroviruses 20:909–15, 2004.
88. Lawson-Ayayi S, Bonnet F, Bernardin E, et al. Avascular necrosis in HIV-infected patients: a case-control study from the Aquitaine Cohort, 1997–2002, France. Clin Infect Dis 40:1188–93, 2005.
89. Gaughan DM, Mofenson LM, Hughes MD, et al. Osteonecrosis of the hip (Legg–Calve–Perthes disease) in human immunodeficiency virus-infected children. Pediatrics 109:E74-4, 2002.
90. Gerster JC, Camus JP, Chave JP, et al. Multiple site avascular necrosis in HIV infected patients. J Rheumatol 18:300–2, 1991.
91. Monier P, McKown K, Bronze MS. Osteonecrosis complicating highly active antiretroviral therapy in patients infected with human immunodeficiency virus. Clin Infect Dis 31:1488–92, 2000.
92. Wang MW, Wei S, Teitelbaum SL, Ross FP. The HIV protease inhibitor indinavir uniquely inhibits bone formation [abstract]. J Bone Miner Res 16(Suppl):S372, 2001.
93. Wang MWH, Teitelbaum SL, Tebas P. Indinavir administration leads to bone loss in mice. In: Ninth Conference on Retroviruses and Opportunistic Infections, Seattle, Feb 2002.
94. Jain RG, Lenhard JM. Select HIV protease inhibitors alter bone and fat metabolism ex vivo. J Biol Chem 277:19247–50, 2002.

Chapter 76

Adrenal, Gonadal, and Thyroid Disorders

Joan C. Lo, MD, Morris Schambelan, MD

A variety of endocrine disorders have been reported in association with human immunodeficiency virus (HIV) infection and the acquired immunodeficiency syndrome (AIDS). Although direct viral infection may be responsible for organ dysfunction, most endocrine and metabolic perturbations are a consequence of systemic illness, opportunistic infections, neoplastic processes, weight loss, changes in body composition, pharmacologic therapy, or immune reconstitution. These abnormalities range from subclinical perturbations in hormone balance to overt glandular failure. While clinical presentations may bear some similarity to that in immunocompetent individuals, many aspects appear to be unique to HIV-infected patients. The goals of this chapter are to review the adrenal, gonadal, and thyroid abnormalities associated with HIV infection and AIDS and to provide a general approach to the diagnosis and management of these disorders.

ADRENAL GLAND

Adrenal Pathology

Pathologic involvement of the adrenal gland occurs frequently in AIDS, with abnormalities noted in up to two-thirds of patients during postmortem examination.[1,2] However, patients are typically asymptomatic, as clinical adrenal insufficiency generally does not manifest until more than 80–90% of the adrenal gland has been destroyed.[3,4] Cytomegalovirus adrenalitis appears to be the most frequent finding, although infection with *M. tuberculosis* and *avium* complex, *C. neoformans* and *T. gondii* have also been reported.[1,2,5] Other pathologic findings include hemorrhage, fibrosis, infarction, and focal necrosis.[5,6] Infiltration with Kaposi sarcoma or lymphoma occurs infrequently and is generally not associated with clinical adrenal insufficiency.[5,7]

Alterations in Adrenal Function

In normal individuals, corticotropin-releasing hormone (CRH) is secreted by the hypothalamus and stimulates production of adrenocorticotropic hormone (ACTH) by the anterior pituitary gland. ACTH, in turn, stimulates production of cortisol by the adrenal cortex, and both hormones manifest a diurnal circadian rhythm. Homeostatic regulation of the hypothalamic-pituitary-adrenal (HPA) axis is maintained by cortisol feedback at the level of the hypothalamus and pituitary. In response to acute illness, infection, or stress, increased hypothalamic activation leads to an increase in circulating cortisol levels. The adrenal gland also produces the mineralocorticoid hormone, aldosterone, which is primarily under regulation of the renin–angiotensin system.

Individuals infected with HIV commonly demonstrate an elevation in basal cortisol levels, frequently in association with lower levels of ACTH and the adrenal steroid dehydroepiandrosterone (DHEA).[8] Moreover, the adrenal reserve of the 17-deoxysteroids (corticosterone, deoxycorticosterone, 18-OH-deoxycorticosterone) appears to be impaired.[9] This shift in steroid metabolism may represent an adaptive response to systemic illness[10] or the effect of nonpituitary factors (e.g., cytokines) on adrenocortical function.[8] Reports of increased ACTH and cortisol levels in some HIV-infected patients have led others to speculate that hypothalamic activation may occur,[11] although individuals with advanced HIV illness often demonstrate blunted pituitary-adrenal responsiveness to CRH infusion.[12] Increased ACTH levels may also be compensatory, particularly in patients with subclinical defects in adrenocortical function.[13] In addition, glucocorticoid resistance should be considered in patients with AIDS who present with hypercortisolism, ACTH elevation, and paradoxical features of Addison's disease.[14]

Pituitary-adrenal function has also been studied in the setting of HIV-associated fat redistribution, particularly in patients who present with dorsocervical fat pad enlargement and visceral adiposity. Although these features are somewhat reminiscent of Cushing syndrome, overt hypercortisolism has not been found upon biochemical examination.[15–17] In addition, individuals with protease inhibitor (PI)-associated fat redistribution exhibit normal diurnal cortisol excretion as well as normal cortisol secretory dynamics after administration of ovine CRH.[17] Nevertheless, subtle changes in cortisol metabolism based on urinary steroid excretion profiles have been noted in these patients, although the significance of these findings is unclear.[17] An exception to the above observations has been the development of exogenous Cushing syndrome in patients treated with ritonavir in the setting of inhaled or nasal fluticasone (a glucocorticoid) where; ritonavir administration impairs the metabolism of fluticasone via effects on the cytochrome P450 3A4 enzyme system, resulting in high plasma levels of fluticasone and relative adrenal suppression.[18–20]

A number of drugs used to treat HIV-related disorders are known to affect adrenocortical function. For example, ketoconazole inhibits multiple steps in the pathway of cortisol biosynthesis and can cause clinical adrenal insufficiency, particularly in patients with limited adrenal reserve.[21] Rifampin increases the metabolic clearance of cortisol and may also lead to diminished cortisol levels in patients with limited adrenal reserve or those receiving glucocorticoid replacement therapy.[22] Megestrol acetate, a progestational agent with intrinsic glucocorticoid-like activity, has been shown to suppress the HPA axis and result in glucocorticoid deficiency when treatment is discontinued, particularly in patients who have had long-term therapy.[23,24] There have also been isolated reports of Cushing syndrome and diabetes mellitus in patients receiving megestrol acetate therapy.[24–26]

Diagnostic Approach and Therapy

Despite the abnormalities in adrenocortical function described above, most patients are asymptomatic and clinically significant adrenal impairment is uncommon with HIV infection. However, glucocorticoid insufficiency in patients with AIDS is clearly more prevalent than in the general population, so it is important to perform tests of adrenal function in patients who present with features suggestive of adrenal insufficiency (Fig. 76-1). The signs and symptoms of adrenal insufficiency include weakness, orthostasis, nausea, abdominal pain, weight loss, hyponatremia and hypoglycemia, as well as hyperkalemia and metabolic acidosis in patients with primary adrenal

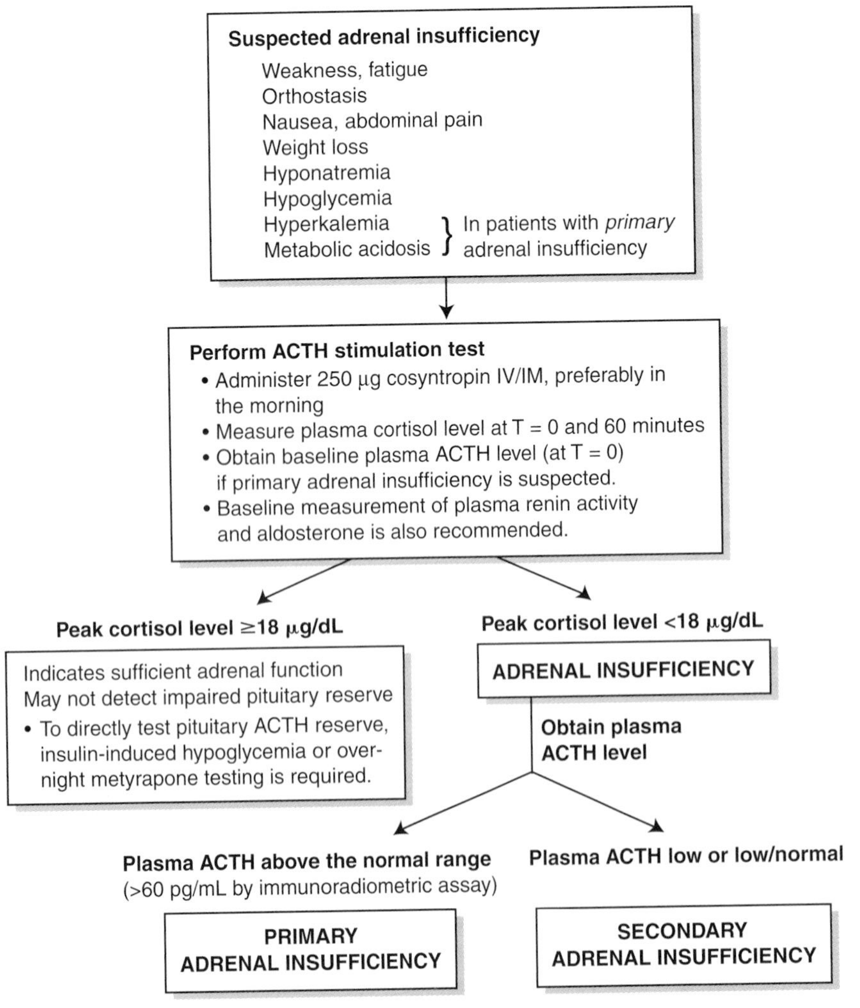

Figure 76-1 ■ Diagnostic approach to patients with suspected adrenal insufficiency.

failure. Hyperkalemia and renal sodium wasting have also been noted in patients receiving trimethoprim, an effect that is mediated through inhibition of the sodium channel in the distal nephron.[27]

The ACTH stimulation test provides the most direct means of assessing adrenal function. In patients with frank adrenal insufficiency, intravenous (or intramuscular) administration of cosyntropin (250 mcg) results in little or no increase in plasma cortisol, whereas normal individuals generally achieve peak cortisol levels above 20 mcg/dL (540 nmol/L). Basal glucocorticoid production is generally low in these patients, although the presence of low baseline cortisol levels alone should not be used for a definitive diagnosis. The ACTH stimulation test may not detect patients with impaired pituitary reserve, however, and in selected cases, insulin-induced hypoglycemia or the metyrapone test may ultimately be warranted to assess the HPA axis.[28]

Once the diagnosis of adrenal insufficiency has been established, it is important to distinguish between primary and secondary adrenal failure. Individuals with primary adrenal failure (Addison's disease) invariably have high ACTH levels, and biochemical findings (hyperkalemia, metabolic acidosis) are generally consistent with concomitant mineralocorticoid deficiency. Aldosterone levels are low despite increased plasma renin levels. Adrenal computed tomography (CT) imaging may yield information about the etiology of adrenal disease in some patients,[29] although in many cases the findings are nondiagnostic. Conversely, ACTH levels are low to low normal (<20 pg/mL by immunoradiometric assay) in patients with secondary hypoadrenalism due to pituitary ACTH deficiency. Such patients have normal levels of plasma renin and aldosterone.

Patients with documented adrenal insufficiency, based on failure to respond to stimulation with ACTH, should be treated with glucocorticoid replacement therapy. Hydrocortisone (20–30 mg/day) is generally administered in two divided doses, with higher doses in the morning to simulate normal circadian rhythmicity. In addition, fludrocortisone (0.05–0.10 mg/day) is usually added for mineralocorticoid replacement therapy in patients with primary adrenal insufficiency, although many patients with Addison's disease can be managed with cortisol and adequate dietary sodium intake alone. Larger doses of glucocorticoid are required for periods of stress, generally a two- to threefold increase for moderate stress and maximal stress doses (hydrocortisone 100 mg every 8 h) for severe illness or trauma. The role of glucocorticoid therapy in patients with elevated basal cortisol levels who show somewhat diminished responsiveness to ACTH is less clear, however, and each case should be evaluated individually. A number of these patients respond to prolonged (72 h) ACTH infusion,[9] suggesting that patients with a "borderline" response to acute ACTH stimulation may not require routine glucocorticoid maintenance therapy. However, some clinicians would give glucocorticoids to such patients at times of stress, provided the treatment is limited in duration, thereby avoiding the adverse consequences of prolonged steroid therapy. Routine glucocorticoid supplementation in patients with modest perturbations in the HPA axis is probably not warranted.

Special consideration should also be given to patients terminating pharmacologic glucocorticoid or megestrol acetate therapy because long-term treatment with these agents can lead to secondary adrenal insufficiency.[23,24] Although adrenal function generally recovers, the process can take months; and patients with subnormal ACTH stimulation test results may have to be maintained on low glucocorticoid replacement doses until a normal cortisol response is achieved.[30]

DHEA and HIV Infection

DHEA is a weak androgen produced by the adrenal gland. Although present in highest concentration during early adulthood, levels decline with advancing age and chronic illness, in contrast to cortisol levels, which remain relatively stable.[31,32] It has been postulated that the decline in DHEA levels may be responsible, in part, for the various immunologic, cognitive, and body composition changes associated with the aging process, leading to the widespread use of DHEA for its purported "fountain of youth" properties.[31] Furthermore, a number of preliminary studies support the role of DHEA as a potential immunomodulatory agent,[33–36] including pilot studies demonstrating inhibition of HIV replication *in vitro*,[37,38] and have led to renewed interest in DHEA therapy in the HIV community.[39] However, a recent small randomized trial did not show any benefit of DHEA on antiviral, immunomodulatory or hormonal effects.[40] Rather, nonsignificant increases in titers of infectious HIV culturable from blood were seen in the DHEA arm and thus it was recommended that DHEA be used with caution.[40] This same study did show an improvement in quality of life with DHEA administration. Higher dose DHEA supplementation has also been shown to improve mood in HIV-infected men with mild depression and significantly increase circulating sex steroid levels.[41,42]

TESTES AND OVARIES

Testicular Pathology

Examination of the testes at autopsy in men with AIDS have demonstrated a number of histopathologic changes, including hypospermatogenesis, basement membrane thickening, interstitial fibrosis, and tubular atrophy.[43–46] Multiple factors contribute to these findings, such as prolonged HIV illness, direct HIV cytopathic effects, chronic infection, fever, malnutrition, wasting, and the use of gonadotoxic and antiandrogenic drugs. Fewer than one-third of patients demonstrate specific testicular infection.[43,44] Direct testicular involvement by opportunistic infection has been seen most commonly with cytomegalovirus, *T. gondii*, and *Mycobacterium avium* complex.[43,44,46] Neoplastic processes affecting the testes occur infrequently, although Kaposi sarcoma and lymphoma of the testes have been observed in patients with disseminated disease.[7,46] Changes in semen quality have been reported in men with advanced HIV infection, including decreased sperm count and motility, reduced semen volume, increased abnormal sperm forms, and pyosemia.[47–49]

Alterations in Testicular Function

In normal individuals, gonadotropin-releasing hormone (GnRH) synthesized in the hypothalamus stimulates release of luteinizing hormone (LH) and follicle-stimulating hormone (FSH) from the anterior pituitary gland. LH, in turn, stimulates production of testosterone by testicular Leydig cells, and FSH promotes spermatogenesis in Sertoli cells. Both FSH and LH secretion are regulated by androgen concentrations; LH levels reflect testosterone feedback, and FSH levels are predominantly regulated by inhibin produced by the Sertoli cells. Early in the course of HIV infection, total and free testosterone levels may be normal or slightly elevated;[50,51] an exaggerated LH response to infusion of GnRH has been observed in a subset of patients.[51] However, testosterone levels tend to fall with advanced HIV illness, generally as a consequence of gonadal and extragonadal factors that lead to testicular dysfunction.[50,52,53] At that point, bioavailable or free testosterone levels may be the most sensitive indicator of hypogonadism, as sex hormone-binding globulin levels can be elevated in the setting of HIV infection[52,54,55] (Fig. 76-2).

With primary gonadal failure, FSH or LH levels (or both) are increased in the presence of decreased androgen production. Contributing factors include direct viral or opportunistic infection, prolonged fever, malignant infiltration, and administration of gonadotoxic agents, although the underlying cause is often not identified.[53,56] Ketoconazole inhibits steroidogenesis in the adrenal gland and testes, and prolonged treatment can lead to primary hypogonadism and gynecomastia, particularly at high doses.[21] The majority of HIV-infected patients with low circulating testosterone levels have secondary or central hypogonadism, which is established biochemically by detecting low or inappropriately normal serum FSH and LH concentrations in the presence of low testosterone levels. In most cases the etiology is not known but is likely multifactorial, as systemic illness, malnutrition, and wasting are common causes of central gonadotropin suppression.[7,53] A significant number of patients with the AIDS wasting syndrome have some degree of testosterone deficiency, and it has been suggested that the decline in circulating androgen levels may contribute to the critical loss of lean body mass.[54,57] In addition, systemic administration of glucocorticoids, megestrol acetate, and opiate drugs may also contribute to central hypogonadism,[58–60] as can previous treatment with anabolic androgenic steroids in cases in which recovery of the pituitary-gonadal axis is delayed. Direct pituitary destruction by opportunistic pathogens or malignant processes occurs rarely.[61,62]

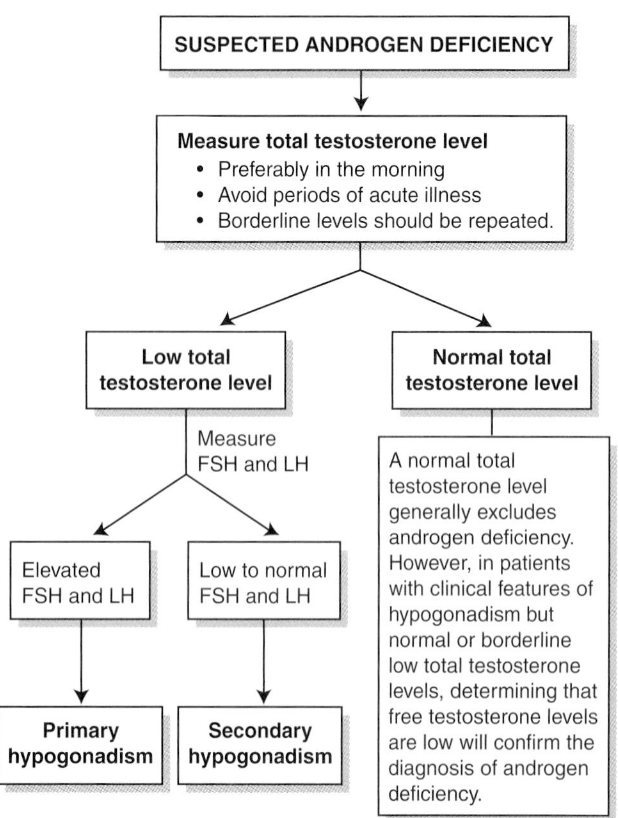

Figure 76-2 ■ Diagnostic approach to male patients with suspected androgen deficiency.

The emergence of gynecomastia in the setting of antiretroviral therapy (e.g., protease inhibitors (PIs), efavirenz or stavudine)[63–66] has additionally prompted consideration that HIV-specific treatment may alter the sex steroid bioavailability or action, since benign gynecomastia has traditionally been associated with a lower ratio of testosterone to estrogen. A number of these cases have been associated with the fat redistribution syndrome, suggesting a potential underlying metabolic component,[65] although it is important that pseudogynecomastia due to increased fatty tissue accumulation (lipomastia) in the breast be distinguished.[64] Other possible contributing factors to the development of gynecomastia in HIV-infected men include chronic alcoholism, marijuana or opiate drug use, liver disease, and use of medications known to cause gynecomastia. In the clinical setting, however, the most frequent cause of gynecomastia in an HIV-infected man will likely be hypogonadism.[67]

Diagnostic Approach and Therapy

Once the diagnosis of hypogonadism has been established, pituitary gonadotropins (FSH, LH) should be measured to distinguish between primary and secondary (central) hypogonadism. A careful history should also be obtained to exclude reversible etiologies prior to initiating testosterone replacement. For patients with secondary hypogonadism who manifest other pituitary deficiencies, visual field defects, or additional findings suggestive of a central mass lesion, magnetic resonance imaging (MRI) of the pituitary and hypothalamus is warranted. However, it should be noted that the incidence of direct pituitary involvement by infectious, inflammatory, or malignant processes is extremely low.

Androgen replacement therapy is indicated in patients with symptomatic hypogonadism. Although bioavailable testosterone levels are often subnormal and not extremely low, most individuals respond to replacement therapy with symptomatic improvement. Currently, there are three main routes of testosterone delivery. The testosterone esters enanthate and cypionate have traditionally provided a safe, effective, inexpensive approach to androgen replacement therapy. For men, starting doses range from 150 to 200 mg administered by intramuscular injection every 2 weeks[68] (or 300 mg every 3 weeks) although dosages may have to be adjusted for a clinical response. Because interval injections lead to large fluctuations in serum testosterone levels, some patients prefer treatment with smaller, more frequent doses (e.g., 100 mg/week). The transdermal testosterone delivery systems (patch or gel) provide a more stable, continuous mode of testosterone administration and may be preferred in patients who experience disturbing fluctuations in energy level and sexual function, although the disadvantage is that they require daily application. The testosterone patch can be associated with a local skin rash. Care should be taken with use of testosterone gel since vigorous skin contact in the applied area can lead to significant drug transfer, as residual testosterone remains on the skin after application.[68] It should also be noted that the transdermal testosterone formulations may not deliver an adequate testosterone concentration at the recommended doses in every individual, so measurements to assess whether therapeutic levels are achieved should be considered. Testosterone replacement is contraindicated in men with known breast or prostate malignancies; and prostate-specific antigen (PSA) levels should be measured in older patients before and at least 3 months after testosterone treatment.[68,69]

Sexual dysfunction is prevalent among men with HIV infection, particularly in the setting of advanced HIV disease.[70] However, not all HIV-infected men are hypogonadal, because diminished libido and erectile dysfunction may be related to a variety of other factors, such as neurologic disease, vascular causes, systemic illness, medications, substance abuse and psychosexual issues.[70–73] Erectile dysfunction remains prevalent in the current era of potent combination antiretroviral therapy,[73,74] potentially attributable to the aging male HIV population or, as suggested in some case series, the effect of PI therapy.[73,75–78]

In many patients, phosphodiesterase 5 (PDE5) inhibitors have been used successfully to improve erectile function (in the absence of other treatable causes such as hypogonadism). However, clinicians should be aware that the three available PDE5 inhibitors (sildenafil, vardenafil and tadalafil) are primarily metabolized by cytochrome P450 3A4, the hepatic microsomal enzyme involved in the metabolism of various PIs (e.g., saquinavir, ritonavir, indinavir, nelfinavir).[79,80] Hence, co-administration of PIs with PDE5 inhibitors should be done with caution at the recommended low doses to avoid substantial elevation in PDE5 inhibitor concentration, particularly with indinavir and ritonavir, and risk of PDE5 inhibitor-related adverse events.[79,80]

Hypogonadism with decreased testosterone levels has been reported in HIV-infected women as well, although the true incidence of this disorder in women is poorly characterized. The approach to diagnosis is the same as in men, however replacement doses of testosterone should be ~300 μg/day, preferably delivered via a transdermal patch.[81,82]

Ovarian Pathology and Function

Because the ovaries have not been systematically examined during autopsy studies in women with AIDS, little is known regarding ovarian pathology in the setting of HIV infection. Thus far there has been rare reports of cytomegalovirus (CMV) oophoritis in women with CMV infection.[83,84] HIV infectivity has also been demonstrated in tissues of the female reproductive tract,[85] and the presence of HIV RNA has also been detected in follicular fluids and cumulous oophorus cells in HIV-infected women undergoing *in vitro* fertilization.[86]

Changes in menstrual function among women with HIV infection have been more carefully evaluated since the early 1990s. It has been suggested that rates of menstrual disturbances are increased in HIV-infected women without AIDS-defining illnesses,[87] although other studies indicate that infection with HIV and related immunosuppression do not have clinically significant effects on either menstruation or vaginal bleeding.[88,89] Data from two large cohorts also demonstrated that HIV serostatus *per se* has little overall effect on menstrual cycle length, variability, and rates of amenorrhea; however, among HIV-infected women, low CD4+ T-lymphocyte counts and high HIV viral loads were associated with polymenorrhea and increased cycle length.[90] The prevalence of amenorrhea is increased in women with AIDS wasting compared to women with AIDS who are weight-stable or manifest only mild weight loss,[91] findings that are not unexpected for women with a severe catabolic illness complicating their HIV infection. In addition, the use of narcotics, marijuana, and chronic alcohol consumption may similarly affect menstrual status and ovulation.[59] Among HIV positive women who do report regular menstrual cycles, normal circulating levels of the ovarian hormones estradiol and progesterone have been observed during the follicular and luteal phases.[92]

During the era of highly active antiretroviral therapy (HAART), various body shape changes, including breast enlargement, abdominal obesity, and wasting of fat in the extremities and gluteal region, have been observed in women with HIV infection.[93–95] These alterations in fat distribution have generally occurred in the absence of overt endocrine perturbations, except for rare cases associated with polycystic ovary syndrome[96] or tumor-level serum testosterone concentration.[97] While a preliminary study found that women with HIV-associated fat redistribution have higher concentration of androgens, insulin and LH/FSH, compared to HIV-infected women without fat redistribution and seronegative controls[98] most HIV-infected women do not have features of polycystic ovary syndrome despite significant hyperinsulinemia and abdominal fat accumulation.[99]

Diagnostic Approach and Therapy

The approach to management of ovarian failure and associated symptomatology is similar to that for immunocompetent individuals. However, the pros and cons of estrogen replacement therapy need to be considered carefully, particularly given the increased cardiovascular risk profile of HIV-infected patients and two large clinical trials demonstrating no benefit and potential early adverse cardiovascular risk of combined estrogen and progestin treatment in seronegative postmenopausal women with and without established coronary heart disease.[100,101]

Androgen replacement therapy and treatment with androgenic anabolic steroids have also been considered as a possible therapeutic strategy in HIV-infected women, particularly since circulating total and free testosterone levels are lower in HIV-infected women (with and without HIV-associated weight loss) than in healthy seronegative controls.[102] Several studies have shown that low-dose twice-weekly transdermal administration of testosterone is generally well tolerated in women,[81,103,104] although efficacy of this treatment on weight gain and quality-of-life parameters in women with HIV-associated weight loss remains equivocal and may be dose-dependent.[81,82] In a multicenter study among HIV-infected women with weight loss, administration of nandrolone decanoate increased weight and lean body mass and appeared to have a tolerable safety profile.[105] For the postmenopausal woman, combination estrogen-androgen replacement has been used, but the methyltestosterone component may contribute to hepatic dysfunction, and concomitant progestin treatment would still be necessary for women with an intact uterus to prevent endometrial hyperplasia.[106]

THYROID

Thyroid Pathology

Opportunistic infections of the thyroid occur infrequently in patients with AIDS. Reported pathogens include *Pneumocystis carinii*, CMV, *C. neoformans*, *Aspergillus*, *Mycobacterium avium-intracellulare*, and *M. tuberculosis*.[107–109] *P. carinii* thyroiditis has historically been the most common pathogen, occurring primarily among patients receiving aerosolized pentamidine for *P. carinii* pneumonia (PCP) prophylaxis in an earlier HIV era.[108,110] Affected patients typically present with an enlarging neck mass (diffuse goiter or nodule) that is often tender on physical examination. Depending on the extent of follicular tissue destruction, *P. carinii* thyroiditis may be accompanied by hypothyroidism or transient hyperthyroidism.[110–112] Neoplastic infiltration of the thyroid seldom occurs in patients with AIDS. However, there have been a few isolated cases of Kaposi sarcoma involvement of the thyroid gland in patients with preexisting cutaneous manifestations, where clinical presentations have ranged from asymptomatic thyroid nodules to diffuse glandular infiltration.[108,113,114] Presumably, thyroid lymphoma may also occur (as either primary or metastatic disease) based on observations in seronegative individuals, but few cases have been reported in the setting of HIV infection.[115]

Alterations in Thyroid Function

In the normal individual, thyrotropin-releasing hormone (TRH) from the hypothalamus stimulates the synthesis and release of thyroid-stimulating hormone (TSH) from the anterior pituitary gland. TSH, in turn, stimulates the secretion of thyroxine (T4) and triiodothyronine (T3) from the thyroid, which exert negative feedback at the level of both the pituitary and hypothalamus to maintain homeostasis. Although circulating T4 concentrations are high relative to T3, peripheral conversion to T3 is required for activity. During the so-called sick euthyroid state, decreased conversion of T4 to T3 with enhanced deiodination of T4 to reverse T3 is seen, resulting in lower T3 and increased reverse T3 levels.[116,117] T3 reduction is thought to be adaptive during illness, as the body attempts to conserve protein stores and reduce energy expenditure during a time of stress.[117] With severe nonthyroidal illness, both T4 and T3 levels may be low.[116,117] TSH levels may also fall, although they tend to increase above the normal range during the recovery phase of acute illness.

Abnormal thyroid homeostasis occurs frequently in patients with AIDS, usually in the absence of direct thyroid pathology. In general, findings similar to those in the sick euthyroid state are observed,[118] although T3 levels are often higher and reverse T3 levels lower than expected for chronic illness.[119] Because similar changes in free (unbound) T3 levels are also seen, these findings cannot be attributed to the increased thyroid hormone-binding globulin levels observed with HIV infection.[120,121] This has led to the concern that inappropriate maintenance of "normal" T3 levels may contribute to weight loss and body wasting.[119] However, most patients with AIDS do develop lower T3 levels during secondary infection, anorexia, and weight loss.[119,120] Mild TSH elevations within the normal range have also been reported, with lower free T4 levels and enhanced TSH responsiveness to TRH; these hypothyroid-like findings may be adaptive to the hypermetabolic changes associated with HIV infection.[122]

Effect of Drugs on Thyroid Function

Thyroid function may also be affected by medications used to treat HIV infection and associated opportunistic infections (Table 76-1). Both rifampin and ketoconazole increase the metabolic clearance of thyroid hormone through induction of hepatic microsomal enzymes and can precipitate hypothyroidism in patients with diminished thyroid reserve. Thus higher doses of thyroxine may be required in patients receiving replacement therapy.[123] An increased maintenance dose requirement for levothyroxine has also been reported in a hypothyroid patient treated with ritonavir, a known inducer of hepatic glucuronosyl transferase activity, presumably due to increased metabolism of levothyroxine through the glucuronidation pathway.[124]

Table 76-1

Therapeutic Agents Used to Treat HIV-Related Disease and Their Effects on Adrenal, Gonadal, and Thyroid Function

Therapeutic Agent	Adrenal, Gonadal, and Thyroid Effects
Ketoconazole	Inhibits adrenal and gonadal steroid synthesis Adrenal insufficiency Hypogonadism Increases levothyroxine metabolism
Rifampin	Increases cortisol metabolism Increases levothyroxine metabolism
Megestrol acetate	Cushing syndrome Adrenal insufficiency (following withdrawal) Hypogonadism
Opiates	Hypogonadism
Marijuana	Hypogonadism
Androgenic steroids	Suppresses endogenous testicular function
Interferon-α	Autoimmune hyperthyroidism (Grave disease) Autoimmune hypothyroidism (Hashimoto's thyroiditis) Subacute or destructive thyroiditis
Protease inhibitors (PIs)	Immune restoration may unmask latent Graves' disease or other autoimmune thyroid disorders Ritonavir may increase levothyroxine metabolism Ritonavir impairs fluticasone metabolism and may induce Cushing syndrome

Among patients with hepatitis C infection, treatment with interferon (INF)-alpha, a cytokine with antiviral and immunomodulatory properties, has been associated with the development of thyroid dysfunction, including autoimmune hyper- and hypothyroidism (Graves' disease and Hashimoto's thyroiditis, respectively) as well as subacute or destructive thyroiditis.[125–132] Individuals with evidence of preexisting or development of thyroid autoantibodies during treatment are at higher risk for INF-alpha-induced autoimmune thyroid disease.[125,128,130,131] Thus, it has been suggested that thyroid function and thyroid autoantibodies (e.g., thyroid peroxidase antibody) be monitored prior to, during, and up to 6 months after INF-alpha treatment.[128,130] In many cases, thyroid function normalizes after discontinuation of INF-alpha, although sustained thyroid disease has been observed and longer-term follow-up may be necessary.[128,130] Treatment with interleukin-2, another cytokine currently being studied as an immunomodulatory agent in HIV care, has similarly been associated with the development of autoimmune thyroid disease.[133]

During the current treatment era, a number of patients have presented with activation of Graves' disease in the setting of immune restoration, typically 1–3 years after initiation of potent antiretroviral therapy resulting in effective virologic suppression.[134–136] Based on the timing of thyroid autoantibody appearance and the rise in CD4+ T-lymphocyte count from nadir levels (compatible with thymic production of naive CD4+ T-lymphocytes), it has been hypothesized that thyroid-specific autoimmunity results from abnormal reconstitution of a markedly altered T-lymphocyte repertoire;[135] thus disease manifestation is usually delayed after initiation of potent antiretroviral therapy. This is supported by additional evidence that autoimmune thyroid disease coincides with the second phase of T-cell repopulation by naive CD4+ T-lymphocyte subsets.[136] Presumably this phenomenon might also lead to the development of Hashimoto's thyroiditis and so-called hashitoxicosis in the setting of immune reconstitution has been reported.[136] However, the higher prevalence of clinical and subclinical hypothyroidism in patients with HIV may also be due to other antiretroviral and disease-related effects on thyroid hormone metabolism in addition to effects on autoimmunity.[137–140]

Diagnostic Approach and Therapy

Overall, patients with AIDS demonstrate subtle alterations in thyroid function which, in many ways, parallel the changes seen with the euthyroid sick syndrome. The significance of these findings is unclear, however, and thyroid function studies should be interpreted in their clinical context. In general, measurement of serum TSH provides the most sensitive indicator of overt thyroid dysfunction, and free T4 levels provide a more quantitative measure of hormone deficiency or excess. Symptoms and signs of hypothyroidism include cold intolerance, weight gain, fatigue, constipation, muscle cramps, dry skin, and myxedema. Often a goiter is present on physical examination, and thyroid indices are notable for increased TSH levels and subnormal free T4 levels. Replacement therapy should be approached gradually to avoid exacerbation of AIDS-related cachexia in select patients,[108] and lower doses of levothyroxine (25–50 μg/day) are advised initially with dose titration every 4–6 weeks to achieve normal TSH levels.

Patients with hyperthyroidism typically present with symptoms of heat intolerance, irritability, fatigue, weight loss, sweats, palpitations, and an increased frequency of bowel movements. The diagnosis is confirmed by documentation of a suppressed TSH level in the setting of elevated thyroid hormone levels. A radioactive iodine uptake scan is generally required to distinguish among the common causes of hyperthyroidism, such as Graves' disease, toxic nodule(s), and subacute thyroiditis. The clinical management for each of these processes in patients with HIV is similar to that for immunocompetent individuals. β-Adrenergic antagonists are prescribed initially to decrease symptoms related to tachycardia and, in the case of propanolol, decrease peripheral conversion of T4 to T3. Recommended therapeutic options for Graves' disease include antithyroid drugs (methimazole, propylthiouracil), thyroid ablation with radioactive iodine therapy, and rarely subtotal thyroidectomy. Patients with toxic nodules should receive radioactive iodine, as the antithyroid drugs are used only as a temporizing measure. Patients with subacute thyroiditis typically present with hyperthyroid symptoms, a tender enlarged thyroid gland, elevated erythrocyte sedimentation rate, and reduced radioactive iodine uptake. These individuals should be treated with supportive care alone, as spontaneous resolution is generally the rule. However, a tender thyroid gland in a patient with advanced HIV/AIDS should also prompt further investigation for an opportunistic infection of the thyroid.

As with immunocompetent individuals, solitary thyroid masses or nodules require evaluation by fine-needle aspiration biopsy to exclude the possibility of malignant disease. In addition, opportunistic infections and malignancies involving the thyroid gland should be considered in the differential diagnosis of any patient with AIDS who has an abnormal thyroid examination. For patients with *Pneumocystis carinii* thyroiditis, the diagnosis is established by Gomori methenamine silver staining of the fine-needle aspirate.[110,111,141] Kaposi sarcoma of the thyroid is also diagnosed by fine-needle aspiration biopsy and should be considered in patients with preexisting cutaneous lesions or disseminated disease.

CONCLUSIONS

A wide spectrum of adrenal, gonadal, and thyroid disorders are associated with HIV infection and AIDS, with presentations ranging from subtle biochemical aberrations to clinically manifest disease. Although these disorders may reflect cytopathic changes induced by HIV itself, they are more often a consequence of opportunistic infections, medications to prevent or treat these infections, malignancy, or therapies directed at slowing HIV-related disease progression. Furthermore, in the current era of potent antiretroviral therapy, there are additional endocrine manifestations that may be directly or indirectly related to specific antiretroviral drugs or a consequence of immune reconstitution. A clearer understanding of these disorders is crucial to the appropriate diagnostic and therapeutic management of these patients. Clinicians caring for HIV-infected patients should maintain a high suspicion for endocrine dysfunction; however, this vigilance should be balanced by the recognition that many subtle abnormalities do not require aggressive therapy.

ACKNOWLEDGMENTS

This work was supported in part by grants from the National Institute of Diabetes and Digestive and Kidney Diseases (DK45833, DK063640, DK069185) and the National Center for Research Resources (RR00083) of the National Institutes of Health.

REFERENCES

1. Bricaire F, Marche C, Zoubi D, et al. Adrenocortical lesions and AIDS. Lancet 1:881, 1988.
2. Welch K, Finkbeiner W, Alpers CE, et al. Autopsy findings in the acquired immune deficiency syndrome. JAMA 252:1152–9, 1984.
3. Barker NW. The pathologic anatomy in twenty-eight cases of Addison's disease. Arch Pathol 8:432, 1929.
4. Sellmeyer DE, Grunfeld C. Endocrine and metabolic disturbances in human immunodeficiency virus infection and the acquired immune deficiency syndrome. Endocr Rev 17:518–32, 1996.
5. Glasgow BJ, Steinsapir KD, Anders K, Layfield LJ. Adrenal pathology in the acquired immune deficiency syndrome. Am J Clin Pathol 84:594–7, 1985.
6. Reichert CM, O'Leary TJ, Levens DL, et al. Autopsy pathology in the acquired immune deficiency syndrome. Am J Pathol 112:357–82, 1983.
7. Dobs AS, Dempsey MA, Ladenson PW, Polk BF. Endocrine disorders in men infected with human immunodeficiency virus. Am J Med 84:611–6, 1988.
8. Villette JM, Bourin P, Doinel C, et al. Circadian variations in plasma levels of hypophyseal, adrenocortical and testicular hormones in men infected with human immunodeficiency virus. J Clin Endocrinol Metab 70:572–7, 1990.
9. Membreno L, Irony I, Dere W, et al. Adrenocortical function in acquired immunodeficiency syndrome. J Clin Endocrinol Metab 65:482–7, 1987.
10. Parker LN, Levin ER, Lifrak ET. Evidence for adrenocortical adaptation to severe illness. J Clin Endocrinol Metab 60:947–52, 1985.
11. Verges B, Chavanet P, Desgres J, et al. Adrenal function in HIV infected patients. Acta Endocrinol (Copenh) 121:633–7, 1989.
12. Lortholary O, Christeff N, Casassus P, et al. Hypothalamo-pituitary-adrenal function in human immunodeficiency virus-infected men. J Clin Endocrinol Metab 81:791–6, 1996.
13. Findling JW, Buggy BP, Gilson IH, et al. Longitudinal evaluation of adrenocortical function in patients infected with the human immunodeficiency virus. J Clin Endocrinol Metab 79:1091–6, 1994.
14. Norbiato G, Bevilacqua M, Vago T, et al. Cortisol resistance in acquired immunodeficiency syndrome. J Clin Endocrinol Metab 74:608–13, 1992.
15. Lo JC, Mulligan K, Tai VW, et al. 'Buffalo hump' in men with HIV-1 infection. Lancet 351:867–70, 1998.
16. Miller KK, Daly PA, Sentochnik D, et al. Pseudo-Cushing's syndrome in human immunodeficiency virus-infected patients. Clin Infect Dis 27:68–72, 1998.
17. Yanovski JA, Miller KD, Kino T, et al. Endocrine and metabolic evaluation of human immunodeficiency virus-infected

patients with evidence of protease inhibitor-associated lipodystrophy. J Clin Endocrinol Metab 84:1925–31, 1999.

18. Chen F, Kearney T, Robinson S, et al. Cushing's syndrome and severe adrenal suppression in patients treated with ritonavir and inhaled nasal fluticasone. Sex Transm Infect 75:274, 1999.
19. Johnson SR, Marion AA, Vrchoticky T, et al. Cushing syndrome with secondary adrenal insufficiency from concomitant therapy with ritonavir and fluticasone. J Pediatr 148:386–8, 2006.
20. Samaras K, Pett S, Gowers A, et al. Iatrogenic Cushing's syndrome with osteoporosis and secondary adrenal failure in human immunodeficiency virus-infected patients receiving inhaled corticosteroids and ritonavir-boosted protease inhibitors: six cases. J Clin Endocrinol Metab 90:4394–8, 2005.
21. Sonino N. The use of ketoconazole as an inhibitor of steroid production. N Engl J Med 317:812–8, 1987.
22. Kyriazopoulou V, Parparousi O, Vagenakis AG. Rifampicin-induced adrenal crisis in addisonian patients receiving corticosteroid replacement therapy. J Clin Endocrinol Metab 59:1204–6, 1984.
23. Leinung MC, Liporace R, Miller CH. Induction of adrenal suppression by megestrol acetate in patients with AIDS. Ann Intern Med 122:843–5, 1995.
24. Mann M, Koller E, Murgo A, et al. Glucocorticoidlike activity of megestrol. A summary of Food and Drug Administration experience and a review of the literature. Arch Intern Med 157:1651–6, 1997.
25. Henry K, Rathgaber S, Sullivan C, McCabe K. Diabetes mellitus induced by megestrol acetate in a patient with AIDS and cachexia. Ann Intern Med 116:53–4, 1992.
26. Steer KA, Kurtz AB, Honour JW. Megestrol-induced Cushing's syndrome. Clin Endocrinol (Oxf) 42:91–3, 1995.
27. Velazquez H, Perazella MA, Wright FS, Ellison DH. Renal mechanism of trimethoprim-induced hyperkalemia. Ann Intern Med 119:296–301, 1993.
28. Grinspoon SK, Biller BM. Clinical review 62: Laboratory assessment of adrenal insufficiency. J Clin Endocrinol Metab 79:923–31, 1994.
29. Freda PU, Wardlaw SL, Brudney K, Goland RS. Primary adrenal insufficiency in patients with the acquired immunodeficiency syndrome: a report of five cases. J Clin Endocrinol Metab 79:1540–5, 1994.
30. Stockheim JA, Daaboul JJ, Yogev R, et al. Adrenal suppression in children with the human immunodeficiency virus treated with megestrol acetate. J Pediatr 134:368–70, 1999.
31. Baulieu EE. Dehydroepiandrosterone (DHEA): a fountain of youth? J Clin Endocrinol Metab 81:3147–51, 1996.
32. Orentreich N, Brind JL, Vogelman JH, et al. Long-term longitudinal measurements of plasma dehydroepiandrosterone sulfate in normal men. J Clin Endocrinol Metab 75:1002–4, 1992.
33. Clerici M, Galli M, Bosis S, et al. Immunoendocrinologic abnormalities in human immunodeficiency virus infection. Ann N Y Acad Sci 917:956–61, 2000.
34. Jacobson MA, Fusaro RE, Galmarini M, Lang W. Decreased serum dehydroepiandrosterone is associated with an increased progression of human immunodeficiency virus infection in men with CD4 cell counts of 200–499. J Infect Dis 164:864–8, 1991.
35. Mulder JW, Frissen PH, Krijnen P, et al. Dehydroepiandrosterone as predictor for progression to AIDS in asymptomatic human immunodeficiency virus-infected men. J Infect Dis 165:413–8, 1992.
36. Khorram O, Vu L, Yen SS. Activation of immune function by dehydroepiandrosterone (DHEA) in age-advanced men. J Gerontol A Biol Sci Med Sci 52:M1-7, 1997.
37. Henderson E, Yang JY, Schwartz A. Dehydroepiandrosterone (DHEA) and synthetic DHEA analogs are modest inhibitors of HIV-1 IIIB replication. AIDS Res Hum Retroviruses 8:625–31, 1992.
38. Yang JY, Schwartz A, Henderson EE. Inhibition of HIV-1 latency reactivation by dehydroepiandrosterone (DHEA) and an analog of DHEA. AIDS Res Hum Retroviruses 9:747–54, 1993.
39. Centurelli MA, Abate MA. The role of dehydroepiandrosterone in AIDS. Ann Pharmacother 31:639–42, 1997.
40. Abrams DI, Shade SB, Couey P, et al. Dehydroepiandrosterone (DHEA) effects on HIV replication and host immunity: A randomized placebo-controlled study. AIDS Res Hum Retroviruses 23(1): 77–85, 2007.
41. Poretsky L, Brillon DJ, Ferrando S, et al. Endocrine effects of oral dehydroepiandrosterone in men with HIV infection: a prospective, randomized, double-blind, placebo-controlled trial. Metabolism 55:858–70, 2006.
42. Rabkin JG, McElhiney MC, Rabkin R, et al. Placebo-controlled trial of dehydroepiandrosterone (DHEA) for treatment of non-major depression in patients with HIV/AIDS. Am J Psychiatry 163:59–66, 2006.
43. Chabon AB, Stenger RJ, Grabstald H. Histopathology of testis in acquired immune deficiency syndrome. Urology 29:658–63, 1987.
44. De Paepe ME, Waxman M. Testicular atrophy in AIDS: a study of 57 autopsy cases. Hum Pathol 20:210–4, 1989.
45. Shevchuk MM, Nuovo GJ, Khalife G. HIV in testis: quantitative histology and HIV localization in germ cells. J Reprod Immunol 41:69–79, 1998.
46. Shevchuk MM, Pigato JB, Khalife G, et al. Changing testicular histology in AIDS: its implication for sexual transmission of HIV. Urology 53:203–8, 1999.
47. Crittenden JA, Handelsman DJ, Stewart GJ. Semen analysis in human immunodeficiency virus infection. Fertil Steril 57:1294–9, 1992.
48. Krieger JN, Coombs RW, Collier AC, et al. Fertility parameters in men infected with human immunodeficiency virus. J Infect Dis 164:464–9, 1991.
49. Politch JA, Mayer KH, Abbott AF, Anderson DJ. The effects of disease progression and zidovudine therapy on semen quality in human immunodeficiency virus type 1 seropositive men. Fertil Steril 61:922–8, 1994.
50. Christeff N, Gharakhanian S, Thobie N, et al. Evidence for changes in adrenal and testicular steroids during HIV infection. J Acquir Immune Defic Syndr 5:841–6, 1992.
51. Merenich JA, McDermott MT, Asp AA, et al. Evidence of endocrine involvement early in the course of human immunodeficiency virus infection. J Clin Endocrinol Metab 70:566–71, 1990.
52. Laudat A, Blum L, Guechot J, et al. Changes in systemic gonadal and adrenal steroids in asymptomatic human immunodeficiency virus-infected men: relationship with the CD4 cell counts. Eur J Endocrinol 133:418–24, 1995.
53. Poretsky L, Can S, Zumoff B. Testicular dysfunction in human immunodeficiency virus-infected men. Metabolism 44:946–53, 1995.
54. Grinspoon S, Corcoran C, Lee K, et al. Loss of lean body and muscle mass correlates with androgen levels in hypogonadal men with acquired immunodeficiency syndrome and wasting. J Clin Endocrinol Metab 81:4051–8, 1996.
55. Martin ME, Benassayag C, Amiel C, et al. Alterations in the concentrations and binding properties of sex steroid binding protein and corticosteroid-binding globulin in HIV+ patients. J Endocrinol Invest 15:597–603, 1992.
56. Croxson TS, Chapman WE, Miller LK, et al. Changes in the hypothalamic-pituitary-gonadal axis in human immunodeficiency virus-infected homosexual men. J Clin Endocrinol Metab 68: 317–21, 1989.
57. Dobs AS, Few WL 3rd, Blackman MR, et al. Serum hormones in men with human immunodeficiency virus-associated wasting. J Clin Endocrinol Metab 81:4108–12, 1996.

58. Engelson ES, Pi-Sunyer FX, Kotler DP. Effects of megestrol acetate therapy on body composition and circulating testosterone concentrations in patients with AIDS. AIDS 9:1107–8, 1995.
59. Smith CG, Asch RH. Drug abuse and reproduction. Fertil Steril 48:355–73, 1987.
60. Wagner GJ, Rabkin JG. Testosterone, illness progression, and megestrol use in HIV-positive men. J Acquir Immune Defic Syndr Hum Retrovirol 17:179–80, 1998.
61. Milligan SA, Katz MS, Craven PC, et al. Toxoplasmosis presenting as panhypopituitarism in a patient with the acquired immune deficiency syndrome. Am J Med 77:760–4, 1984.
62. Sullivan WM, Kelley GG, O'Connor PG, et al. Hypopituitarism associated with a hypothalamic CMV infection in a patient with AIDS. Am J Med 92:221–3, 1992.
63. Evans DL, Pantanowitz L, Dezube BJ, Aboulafia DM. Breast enlargement in 13 men who were seropositive for human immunodeficiency virus. Clin Infect Dis 35:1113–9, 2002.
64. Jover F, Cuadrado JM, Roig P, et al. Efavirenz-associated gynecomastia: report of five cases and review of the literature. Breast J 10:244–6, 2004.
65. Manfredi R, Calza L, Chiodo F. Gynecomastia, lipodystrophy syndrome, and dyslipidemia occurring or worsening during antiretroviral regimens other than protease inhibitor-based ones. J Acquir Immune Defic Syndr 35:99–102, 2004.
66. Strub C, Kaufmann GR, Flepp M, et al. Gynecomastia and potent antiretroviral therapy. AIDS 18:1347–9, 2004.
67. Biglia A, Blanco JL, Martinez E, et al. Gynecomastia among HIV-infected patients is associated with hypogonadism: a case-control study. Clin Infect Dis 39:1514–9, 2004.
68. Bhasin S, Cunningham GR, Hayes FJ, et al. Testosterone therapy in adult men with androgen deficiency syndromes: an endocrine society clinical practice guideline. J Clin Endocrinol Metab 91:1995–2010, 2006.
69. Cofrancesco J, Jr, Whalen JJ 3rd, Dobs AS. Testosterone replacement treatment options for HIV-infected men. J Acquir Immune Defic Syndr Hum Retrovirol 16:254–65, 1997.
70. Tindall B, Forde S, Goldstein D, et al. Sexual dysfunction in advanced HIV disease. AIDS Care 6:105–7, 1994.
71. Jones M, Klimes I, Catalan J. Psychosexual problems in people with HIV infection: controlled study of gay men and men with haemophilia. AIDS Care 6:587–93, 1994.
72. Newshan G, Taylor B, Gold R. Sexual functioning in ambulatory men with HIV/AIDS. Int J STD AIDS 9:672–6, 1998.
73. Crum NF, Furtek KJ, Olson PE, et al. A review of hypogonadism and erectile dysfunction among HIV-infected men during the pre- and post-HAART eras: diagnosis, pathogenesis, and management. AIDS Patient Care STDS 19:655–71, 2005.
74. Ende AR, Lo Re V 3rd, DiNubile MJ, Mounzer K. Erectile dysfunction in an urban HIV-positive population. AIDS Patient Care STDS 20:75–8, 2006.
75. Colebunders R, Smets E, Verdonck K, Dreezen C. Sexual dysfunction with protease inhibitors. Lancet 353:1802, 1999.
76. Martinez E, Collazos J, Mayo J, Blanco MS. Sexual dysfunction with protease inhibitors. Lancet 353:810–1, 1999.
77. Schrooten W, Colebunders R, Youle M, et al. Sexual dysfunction associated with protease inhibitor containing highly active antiretroviral treatment. AIDS 15:1019–23, 2001.
78. Sollima S, Osio M, Muscia F, et al. Protease inhibitors and erectile dysfunction. AIDS 15:2331–3, 2001.
79. Merry C, Barry MG, Ryan M, et al. Interaction of sildenafil and indinavir when co-administered to HIV-positive patients. AIDS 13:F101–7, 1999.
80. Setter SM, Iltz JL, Fincham JE, et al. Phosphodiesterase 5 inhibitors for erectile dysfunction. Ann Pharmacother 39:1286–95, 2005.
81. Miller K, Corcoran C, Armstrong C, et al. Transdermal testosterone administration in women with acquired immunodeficiency syndrome wasting: a pilot study. J Clin Endocrinol Metab 83:2717–25, 1998.
82. Choi HH, Gray PB, Storer TW, et al. Effects of testosterone replacement in human immunodeficiency virus-infected women with weight loss. J Clin Endocrinol Metab 90:1531–41, 2005.
83. Familiari U, Larocca LM, Tamburrini E, et al. Premenopausal cytomegalovirus oophoritis in a patient with AIDS. AIDS 5:458–9, 1991.
84. Manfredi R, Alampi G, Talo S, et al. Silent oophoritis due to cytomegalovirus in a patient with advanced HIV disease. Int J STD AIDS 11:410–2, 2000.
85. Howell AL, Edkins RD, Rier SE, et al. Human immunodeficiency virus type 1 infection of cells and tissues from the upper and lower human female reproductive tract. J Virol 71: 3498–506, 1997.
86. Bertrand E, Zissis G, Marissens D, et al. Presence of HIV-1 in follicular fluids, flushes and cumulus oophorus cells of HIV-1-seropositive women during assisted-reproduction technology. AIDS 18:823–5, 2004.
87. Chirgwin KD, Feldman J, Muneyyirci-Delale O, et al. Menstrual function in human immunodeficiency virus-infected women without acquired immunodeficiency syndrome. J Acquir Immune Defic Syndr Hum Retrovirol 12:489–94, 1996.
88. Ellerbrock TV, Wright TC, Bush TJ, et al. Characteristics of menstruation in women infected with human immunodeficiency virus. Obstet Gynecol 87:1030–4, 1996.
89. Shah PN, Smith JR, Wells C, et al. Menstrual symptoms in women infected by the human immunodeficiency virus. Obstet Gynecol 83:397–400, 1994.
90. Harlow SD, Schuman P, Cohen M, et al. Effect of HIV infection on menstrual cycle length. J Acquir Immune Defic Syndr 24:68–75, 2000.
91. Grinspoon S, Corcoran C, Miller K, et al. Body composition and endocrine function in women with acquired immunodeficiency syndrome wasting. J Clin Endocrinol Metab 82:1332–7, 1997.
92. Cu-Uvin S, Wright DJ, Anderson D, et al. Hormonal levels among HIV-1-seropositive women compared with high-risk HIV-seronegative women during the menstrual cycle. Women's Health Study (WHS) 001 and WHS 001a Study Team. J Womens Health Gend Based Med 9:857–63, 2000.
93. Dong KL, Bausserman LL, Flynn MM, et al. Changes in body habitus and serum lipid abnormalities in HIV-positive women on highly active antiretroviral therapy (HAART). J Acquir Immune Defic Syndr 21:107–13, 1999.
94. Gervasoni C, Ridolfo AL, Trifiro G, et al. Redistribution of body fat in HIV-infected women undergoing combined antiretroviral therapy. AIDS 13:465–71, 1999.
95. Herry I, Bernard L, de Truchis P, Perronne C. Hypertrophy of the breasts in a patient treated with indinavir. Clin Infect Dis 25:937–8, 1997.
96. Wilson JD, Dunham RJ, Balen AH. HIV protease inhibitors, the lipodystrophy syndrome and polycystic ovary syndrome–is there a link? Sex Transm Infect 75:268–9, 1999.
97. Dahan MH, Lyle LN, Wolfsen A, Chang RJ. Tumor-level serum testosterone associated with human immunodeficiency virus lipodystrophy syndrome. Obstet Gynecol 103(5 Pt 2):1094–6, 2004.
98. Hadigan C, Corcoran C, Piecuch S, et al. Hyperandrogenemia in human immunodeficiency virus-infected women with the lipodystrophy syndrome. J Clin Endocrinol Metab 85:3544–50, 2000.
99. Johnsen S, Dolan SE, Fitch KV, et al. Absence of polycystic ovary syndrome features in human immunodeficiency virus-infected women despite significant hyperinsulinemia and truncal adiposity. J Clin Endocrinol Metab 90:5596–604, 2005.

100. Hulley S, Grady D, Bush T, et al. Randomized trial of estrogen plus progestin for secondary prevention of coronary heart disease in postmenopausal women. Heart and Estrogen/progestin Replacement Study (HERS) Research Group. JAMA 280:605–13, 1998.
101. Rossouw JE, Anderson GL, Prentice RL, et al. Risks and benefits of estrogen plus progestin in healthy postmenopausal women: principal results from the Women's Health Initiative randomized controlled trial. JAMA 288:321–33, 2002.
102. Sinha-Hikim I, Arver S, Beall G, et al. The use of a sensitive equilibrium dialysis method for the measurement of free testosterone levels in healthy, cycling women and in human immunodeficiency virus-infected women. J Clin Endocrinol Metab 83:1312–8, 1998.
103. Herbst KL, Calof OM, Hsia SH, et al. Effects of transdermal testosterone administration on insulin sensitivity, fat mass and distribution, and markers of inflammation and thrombolysis in human immunodeficiency virus-infected women with mild to moderate weight loss. Fertil Steril 85:1794–802, 2006.
104. Javanbakht M, Singh AB, Mazer NA, et al. Pharmacokinetics of a novel testosterone matrix transdermal system in healthy, premenopausal women and women infected with the human immunodeficiency virus. J Clin Endocrinol Metab 85:2395–401, 2000.
105. Mulligan K, Zackin R, Clark RA, et al. Effect of nandrolone decanoate therapy on weight and lean body mass in HIV-infected women with weight loss: a randomized, double-blind, placebo-controlled, multicenter trial. Arch Intern Med 165: 578–85, 2005.
106. Lo JC, Schambelan M. Reproductive function in human immunodeficiency virus infection. J Clin Endocrinol Metab 86:2338–43, 2001.
107. Frank TS, LiVolsi VA, Connor AM. Cytomegalovirus infection of the thyroid in immunocompromised adults. Yale J Biol Med 60:1–8, 1987.
108. Heufelder AE, Hofbauer LC. Human immunodeficiency virus infection and the thyroid gland. Eur J Endocrinol 134:669–74, 1996.
109. Kaw YT, Brunnemer C. Initial diagnosis of disseminated cryptococcosis and acquired immunodeficiency syndrome by fine needle aspiration of the thyroid. A case report. Acta Cytol 38:427–30, 1994.
110. Guttler R, Singer PA, Axline SG, et al. Pneumocystis carinii thyroiditis. Report of three cases and review of the literature. Arch Intern Med 153:393–6, 1993.
111. Battan R, Mariuz P, Raviglione MC, et al. Pneumocystis carinii infection of the thyroid in a hypothyroid patient with AIDS: diagnosis by fine needle aspiration biopsy. J Clin Endocrinol Metab 72:724–6, 1991.
112. Drucker DJ, Bailey D, Rotstein L. Thyroiditis as the presenting manifestation of disseminated extrapulmonary Pneumocystis carinii infection. J Clin Endocrinol Metab 71:1663–5, 1990.
113. Krauth PH, Katz JF. Kaposi's sarcoma involving the thyroid in a patient with AIDS. Clin Nucl Med 12:848–9, 1987.
114. Mollison LC, Mijch A, McBride G, Dwyer B. Hypothyroidism due to destruction of the thyroid by Kaposi's sarcoma. Rev Infect Dis 13:826–7, 1991.
115. Samuels MH, Launder T. Hyperthyroidism due to lymphoma involving the thyroid gland in a patient with acquired immunodeficiency syndrome: case report and review of the literature. Thyroid 8:673–7, 1998.
116. Cavalieri RR. The effects of nonthyroid disease and drugs on thyroid function tests. Med Clin North Am 75:27–39, 1991.
117. Wartofsky L, Burman KD. Alterations in thyroid function in patients with systemic illness: the "euthyroid sick syndrome." Endocr Rev 3:164–217, 1982.
118. Raffi F, Brisseau JM, Planchon B, et al. Endocrine function in 98 HIV-infected patients: a prospective study. AIDS 5:729–33, 1991.
119. LoPresti JS, Fried JC, Spencer CA, Nicoloff JT. Unique alterations of thyroid hormone indices in the acquired immunodeficiency syndrome (AIDS). Ann Intern Med 110:970–5, 1989.
120. Grunfeld C, Pang M, Doerrler W, et al. Indices of thyroid function and weight loss in human immunodeficiency virus infection and the acquired immunodeficiency syndrome. Metabolism 42:1270–6, 1993.
121. Lambert M, Zech F, De Nayer P, et al. Elevation of serum thyroxine-binding globulin (but not of cortisol-binding globulin and sex hormone-binding globulin) associated with the progression of human immunodeficiency virus infection. Am J Med 89:748–51, 1990.
122. Hommes MJ, Romijn JA, Endert E, et al. Hypothyroid-like regulation of the pituitary-thyroid axis in stable human immunodeficiency virus infection. Metabolism 42:556–61, 1993.
123. Isley WL. Effect of rifampin therapy on thyroid function tests in a hypothyroid patient on replacement L-thyroxine. Ann Intern Med 107:517–8, 1987.
124. Tseng A, Fletcher D. Interaction between ritonavir and levothyroxine. AIDS 12:2235–6, 1998.
125. Bell TM, Bansal AS, Shorthouse C, et al. Low-titre auto-antibodies predict autoimmune disease during interferon-alpha treatment of chronic hepatitis C. J Gastroenterol Hepatol 14:419–22, 1999.
126. Carella C, Mazziotti G, Amato G, et al. Clinical review 169: Interferon-alpha-related thyroid disease: pathophysiological, epidemiological, and clinical aspects. J Clin Endocrinol Metab 89:3656–61, 2004.
127. Falaschi P, Martocchia A, D'Urso R, Proietti A. Subacute thyroiditis during interferon-alpha therapy for chronic hepatitis C. J Endocrinol Invest 20:24–8, 1997.
128. Fernandez-Soto L, Gonzalez A, Escobar-Jimenez F, et al. Increased risk of autoimmune thyroid disease in hepatitis C vs hepatitis B before, during, and after discontinuing interferon therapy. Arch Intern Med 158:1445–8, 1998.
129. Hsieh MC, Yu ML, Chuang WL, et al. Virologic factors related to interferon-alpha-induced thyroid dysfunction in patients with chronic hepatitis C. Eur J Endocrinol 142:431–7, 2000.
130. Koh LK, Greenspan FS, Yeo PP. Interferon-alpha induced thyroid dysfunction: three clinical presentations and a review of the literature. Thyroid 7:891–6, 1997.
131. Prummel MF, Laurberg P. Interferon-alpha and autoimmune thyroid disease. Thyroid 13:547–51, 2003.
132. Roti E, Minelli R, Giuberti T, et al. Multiple changes in thyroid function in patients with chronic active HCV hepatitis treated with recombinant interferon-alpha. Am J Med 101:482–7, 1996.
133. Jimenez C, Moran SA, Sereti I, et al. Graves' disease after interleukin-2 therapy in a patient with human immunodeficiency virus infection. Thyroid 14:1097–102, 2004.
134. Gilquin J, Viard JP, Jubault V, et al. Delayed occurrence of Graves' disease after immune restoration with HAART. Highly active antiretroviral therapy. Lancet 352:1907–8, 1998.
135. Jubault V, Penfornis A, Schillo F, et al. Sequential occurrence of thyroid autoantibodies and Graves' disease after immune restoration in severely immunocompromised human immunodeficiency virus-1-infected patients. J Clin Endocrinol Metab 85:4254–7, 2000.
136. Chen F, Day SL, Metcalfe RA, et al. Characteristics of autoimmune thyroid disease occurring as a late complication of immune reconstitution in patients with advanced human immunodeficiency virus (HIV) disease. Medicine (Baltimore) 84:98–106, 2005.
137. Beltran S, Lescure FX, Desailloud R, et al. Increased prevalence of hypothyroidism among human immunodeficiency virus-infected patients: a need for screening. Clin Infect Dis 37:579–83, 2003.

138. Beltran S, Lescure FX, El Esper I, et al. Subclinical hypothyroidism in HIV-infected patients is not an autoimmune disease. Horm Res 66:21–6, 2006.
139. Grappin M, Piroth L, Verges B, et al. Increased prevalence of subclinical hypothyroidism in HIV patients treated with highly active antiretroviral therapy. AIDS 14:1070–2, 2000.
140. Madeddu G, Spanu A, Chessa F, et al. Thyroid function in human immunodeficiency virus patients treated with highly active antiretroviral therapy (HAART): a longitudinal study. Clin Endocrinol (Oxf) 64:375–83, 2006.
141. Walts AE, Pitchon HE. Pneumocystis carinii in FNA of the thyroid. Diagn Cytopathol 7:615–7, 1991.

Chapter 77

Diseases of the Esophagus, Stomach, and Bowel

C. Mel Wilcox, MD

The early years of the acquired immunodeficiency syndrome (AIDS) epidemic highlighted the gastrointestinal (GI) tract as a target for a variety of opportunistic disorders. Because of the prevalence of gastrointestinal diseases in these patients, the spectrum of potential etiologies, approach to evaluation and therapy, and indications for prophylaxis have become well established. Although our therapeutic armamentarium has continued to expand, truly effective therapy for some opportunistic infections remains elusive. Fortunately, since the introduction of protease inhibitors (PIs) and highly active antiretroviral therapy (HAART), there has been a major decline of gastrointestinal opportunistic disorders in AIDS patients.[1,2] Nevertheless, for areas of the world with limited access to HAART, GI disease remains widely prevalent mirroring the early years of the epidemic in developed countries.[3] AIDS-related complications also remain prevalent for those who are noncompliant and recently infected patients.[4,5] The long-term prognosis for most GI disorders is dictated primarily by the degree of underlying immunodeficiency.

INFECTIONS OF THE ESOPHAGUS

In the pre-HAART era, esophageal infections were common in patients with AIDS with at least one-third of these patients experiencing esophageal symptoms at some point during their illness.[6] With HAART, these infections have been reduced in frequency especially those caused by *Candida*.[1,7] When evaluating a patient with esophageal complaints, a clear distinction must be drawn between dysphagia (sensation of food or pills "sticking" in the chest) and odynophagia (substernal pain after swallowing). Other esophageal signs and symptoms resulting from esophageal infections include esophagospasm (spontaneous substernal chest pain), singultus ("hiccups"), and hematemesis. In patients with esophageal infections the physical examination is often unrevealing, except for the presence of thrush, which suggests the presence of esophageal candidiasis. The absence of thrush, however, does not exclude *Candida* esophagitis.[8] Oropharyngeal candidiasis is readily diagnosed by the characteristic multiple white-yellow plaques, which can be focal or completely coat the buccal mucosa. Occasionally, candidiasis manifests as mucosal erythema in the absence of recognizable plaques or angular cheilitis. It is important to differentiate oral hairy leukoplakia (nonremovable white plaques on the lateral aspect of the tongue) from thrush given the different etiologies and therapy.[9] Another important fact is that the esophagus may be involved by multiple concurrent processes.[10] The main diagnostic tools employed to diagnose esophageal infections in HIV-infected patients are empiric therapy, barium esophagography, and endoscopy. Barium studies are often nonspecific. Endoscopy with biopsy is the gold standard for diagnosis, and in addition, upper endoscopy permits direct visualization of lesions and retrieval of tissue for analysis (Fig. 77-1).

Etiology

The most common infectious cause of esophagitis in patients with HIV infection is *Candida*. While *Candida albicans* is by far the most common cause of candidiasis, several other non-*albicans* species, including *C. krusei*, *C. tropicalis*, *C. parapsilosis*, *C. glabrata*, and *C. dublinensis*, have been associated with oral and esophageal candidiasis in HIV-infected individuals, particularly after prolonged antifungal drug therapy.[11] Generally, determining the specific *Candida* species is not required; however, certain species are more often azole resistant than others. For example, the identification of *C. krusei* suggests that azole therapy is unlikely to be successful.

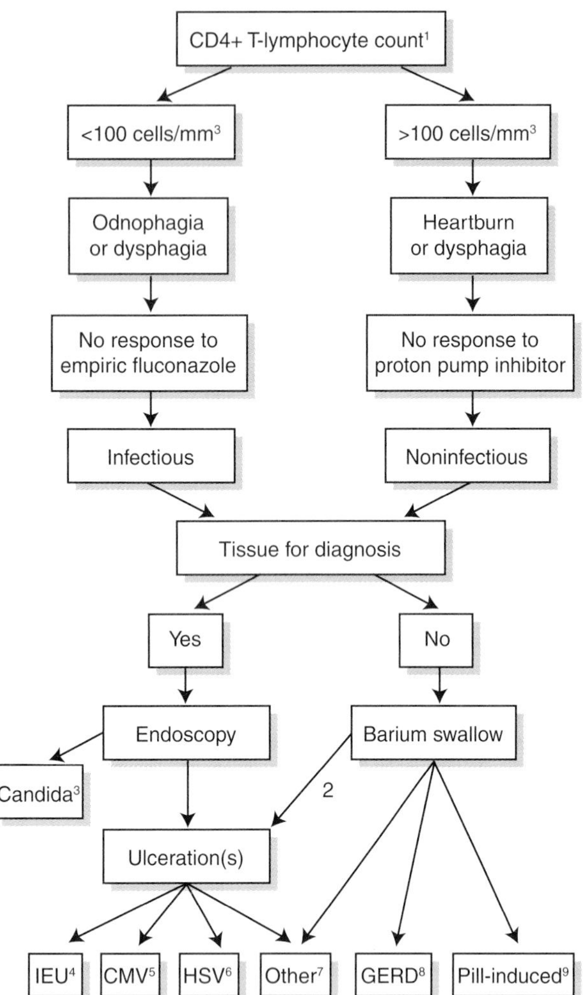

Figure 77-1 ■ Suggested approach to esophageal symptoms in patients with AIDS. 1, CD41 T-lymphocyte count is the major determining factor for the presence or absence of opportunistic infections. 2, Presence of ulcer on barium esophagogram requires endoscopy with biopsy. 3, *Candida albicans, C. krusei, C. tropicalis, C. parapsilosis, C. glabrata, C. guillermondi, C. dublinensis, C. inconspicua.* 4, Idiopatic esophageal ulcer. 5, Cytomegalovirus. 6, Herpes simplex virus (HSV) type 2. 7, Fungi: *Histoplasma capsulatum, Penicillium chrysogenum, Exophiala jeanselmani.* Viruses: Epstein–Barr virus, papovavirus, HSV-6. Bacteria: *Mycobacterium avium* complex, *M. tuberculosis, Rochalimae henselae, Nocardia asteroides, Actinomyces israelii.* Protozoa: *Pneumocystis carinii, Leishmania donovani.* 8, Gastroesophageal reflux disease. 9, Zalcitabine, zidovudine.

In general, *in vitro* azole resistance in patients with AIDS correlates with azole treatment failure for oropharyngeal candidiasis.[12] The major risk factor associated with the development of resistance was the prophylactic daily or intermittent use of fluconazole within the last 6 months. Fortunately, refractory mucosal candidiasis is now less common during the era of HAART.

Cytomegalovirus (CMV) is one of the most common opportunistic infections in patients with AIDS and typically occurs when the CD4+ T-lymphocyte count is less than 100 cells per cubic millimeter. In such patients who do not receive antiretroviral therapy, the incidence of disease may approach 21% at 2 years.[13,14] Although the retina is the most common target for CMV, CMV esophagitis and colitis remain significant causes of morbidity. Involvement of the stomach and small bowel is less common.

Herpes simplex virus (HSV) occasionally causes enteral disease. Because HSV infects primarily squamous mucosa, oropharyngeal, esophageal, and perianal involvement are the most common sites of disease. Oropharyngeal disease may be isolated or can occur in association with esophageal disease. In a large prospective study of 100 HIV-infected patients with ulcerative esophagitis, HSV esophagitis was identified in only 5%, compared to 50% for CMV.[15] Like CMV, the incidence of HSV disease rises as immunodeficiency worsens, with the greatest frequency occurring when the CD4+ T-lymphocyte count is less than 100 cells per cubic millimeter.[16]

An important cause of esophageal ulceration not clearly linked to a specific infection is HIV-associated idiopathic esophageal ulceration (IEU). These lesions can present at the time of seroconversion, although they typically occur when immunodeficiency is severe.[15] The median CD4+ T-lymphocyte count in these patients is less than 50 cells per cubic millimeter. Several studies have identified HIV-infected inflammatory cells in the ulcer base of these lesions, suggesting an etiologic role for HIV. However, HIV has not been identified in esophageal squamous mucosa but, rather, in inflammatory cells and has been found in HIV-infected patients with esophageal diseases other than IEU.[17] IEUs are almost as common as CMV esophagitis in patients with AIDS, comprising ~40% of esophageal ulcers in these patients.[15]

A variety of other infectious agents have been reported to involve the esophagus but are rare; they include protozoa (*Cryptosporidium, Pneumocystis carinii, Leishmania donovani, Trichomonas vaginalis*), bacteria (*Nocardia, Actinomyces*), mycobacteria (*Mycobacterium avium* complex, *M. tuberculosis*), fungi (*Histoplasma capsulatum, Penicillium chrysogenum, Exophiala jeanselmani*), and viruses (Epstein–Barr, human papillomavirus)[18] (Table 77-1). The numerous causes of esophageal disease in these patients underscore the importance of an accurate diagnosis.

Clinical Presentation

Esophageal candidiasis may be asymptomatic or may present as complete inability to swallow, with consequent dehydration, weight loss, and malnutrition. Dysphagia is the most frequent initial manifestation of esophageal candidiasis. Less commonly, odynophagia, heartburn, or retrosternal pain is reported. The presence of fever, nausea, vomiting, and epigastric pain suggests another etiology. As noted above, oropharyngeal candidiasis (thrush) is often present.

Patients with CMV esophagitis usually present with odynophagia which is characteristically severe.[15] In contrast to *Candida* esophagitis, dysphagia is distinctly uncommon. Heartburn is uncommon; nausea, vomiting, and low-grade fever may be reported. Concurrent oropharyngeal ulcerations are rare, whereas thrush is often present.

Etiology of Esophagitis in AIDS Patients

Table 77-1

Fungi	*Candida* species (*Penicillium chrysogenum*, *Pneumocystis carinii*, *Exophiala jeanselmani*, *Cryptococcus neoformans*, mucormycosis, *Aspergillus fumigatus*)
Viruses	Cytomegalovirus (CMV), herpes simplex virus type II (Epstein–Barr virus, papovavirus, human herpesvirus (HHV-6))
Idiopathic	idiopathic esophageal ulcer
Pill-induced	zalcitabine, zidovudine
Peptic	gastroesophageal disease
Bacteria	*Mycobacterium avium* complex (*Mycobacterium tuberculosis*, *Bartonella henselae*, *Nocardia asteroides*, *Actinomyces israelii*)
Protozoa	(*Cryptosporidium parvum*, *Leishmania donovani*, *Trichomonas vaginalis*)
Tumors	Non-Hodgkin lymphoma, Kaposi sarcoma (squamous cell carcinoma, adenocarcinoma, lymphomatoid granulomatosis)

Rare entities are shown in brackets.

Esophagitis due to HSV presents similarly to CMV esophagitis. The most common manifestations of esophageal HSV are odynophagia and dysphagia (82%), chest pain (68%), and fever (44%).[16] GI bleeding is rare. Ulcers of the oral mucosa, lips, and nares are often but not invariably present.

Patients with IEU present similarly to patients with ulcerative esophagitis from other causes. Severe odynophagia is almost uniformly present. Oral ulcers may be observed.

Diagnosis

Esophageal candidiasis is suspected clinically in the patient with moderately severe immunodeficiency (CD4+ T-lymphocyte count less than 100 cells per cubic millimeter) and esophageal symptoms, with or without thrush. Thrush is absent in one-third of patients with esophageal candidiasis.[8] Barium esophagography is relatively insensitive and nonspecific for detecting mild esophagitis and should not be performed for diagnostic purposes. The most common radiographic finding of *Candida* esophagitis is diffuse mucosal irregularity resulting in a "shaggy" appearance mimicking diffuse ulceration. Endoscopy is the most sensitive diagnostic method. Multiple yellow-white plaques with the appearance of "cottage cheese" are pathognomonic for esophageal candidiasis. A definitive diagnosis rests on the identification of typical yeast forms in endoscopic mucosal biopsies, esophageal brushings, or balloon cytology. The detection of *Candida* by these methods does not exclude other disorders, as *Candida* may coexist with additional esophageal processes in up to 25% of symptomatic patients.[6,10] Cultures of the esophagus may provide specimens for drug susceptibility testing but because *Candida* species can be cultured from patients without esophagitis; cultures are not as useful clinically.

On the barium esophagogram CMV may appear as one or multiple well circumscribed ulcers that may be shallow or deep. Endoscopically CMV results in large shallow or deep ulcerations that may be circumferential and may be multiple.[19] The diagnosis of CMV disease is best established by identifying a viral cytopathic effect (intranuclear inclusions) in GI mucosal biopsy specimens using routine hematoxylin and eosin (H & E) staining. The cytopathic effect of CMV is present in endothelial cells and mesenchymal cells; thus, it is imperative to obtain biopsy specimens from the ulcer base. Immunohistochemical stains of mucosal biopsies may be required to confirm the infection; viral culture of biopsy specimens is less sensitive and specific.[20] Blood cultures, serologic tests for CMV, as well as the presence of CMV antigenemia or viremia, are not useful for diagnosing CMV GI infection in HIV-infected patients, but have been linked to end-organ disease and higher mortality.[21,22]

A barium esophagram is seldom diagnostic of HSV esophagitis. The lesions endoscopically appear as superficial ulcers in most patients, where they tend to be small and discrete; they can have a characteristic volcano shape. The presence of small vesicles, as seen in normal hosts, is uncommon in HIV-infected patients. Mucosal biopsy is the most specific diagnostic method. The H & E stain reveals characteristic inclusion bodies; cytology, culture, and *in situ* hybridization of biopsy material provide alternative information that can be helpful for establishing a diagnosis. Because HSV infects squamous epithelium, it is essential to biopsy the ulcer edge to identify the viral cytopathic effect.

IEU appears endoscopically as one or multiple ulcers of variable depth with normal intervening mucosa. CMV esophagitis and IEU are indistinguishable clinically, radiographically, and endoscopically.[18] The diagnosis of IEU is one of exclusion; multiple biopsies (at least six) of the ulcer margins and ulcer base are necessary to exclude an infectious process.

Therapy

Given that esophageal candidiasis is the most common cause of esophageal infection in HIV-infected patients, it is common practice to administer an empirical trial of antifungal therapy in patients with esophageal complaints and thrush. A prospective study comparing empirical fluconazole to endoscopy for presumptive esophageal candidiasis in patients with AIDS showed that empirical fluconazole was a safe, cost-effective alternative to immediate endoscopy.[23] Fluconazole is administered with an oral or intravenous loading dose of 200 mg followed by 100 mg/day for 10–14 days. Failure to respond clinically in 3–7 days should prompt endoscopy to establish the etiology.

Although topical nystatin is effective for oropharyngeal candidiasis, clotrimazole troches have now largely replaced nystatin as the principal nonsystemic agent, given the ease of administration, palatability, negligible side effects, drug interactions, and effectiveness. Clinical cure is seen in 65–94% of patients following 14 days of clotrimazole therapy.[24] The use of systemic therapy with oral fluconazole for oropharyngeal candidiasis in HIV-infected patients achieves greater cure rates and lower relapse rates than clotrimazole troches[25] or nystatin.[26] Thus, neither nystatin nor clotrimazole is recommended. Single-dose therapy with fluconazole 150 mg is as efficacious as a 7-day treatment course for oral candidiasis.[27] Continuous and intermittent therapy are equivalent with refractory disease developing in ~4% at 42 months.[28] Unlike oropharyngeal disease, nonsystemic therapy (e.g., nystatin) is largely ineffective for esophageal candidiasis.

Three orally administered systemic azole antifungal agents have been investigated and used extensively to treat esophageal candidiasis: ketoconazole, fluconazole, and itraconazole. At most centers fluconazole has become the drug of choice for esophageal candidiasis associated with AIDS. Randomized trials have shown fluconazole to have efficacy superior to that of ketoconazole for both oropharyngeal and esophageal candidiasis.[25,29] The response rate of esophageal candidiasis to fluconazole tends to be rapid, with most patients experiencing significant clinical improvement within 5 days.[23,30] In the largest study reported to date, Barbaro et al[31] randomized 2213 HIV-infected patients with a first episode of *Candida* esophagitis to either fluconazole or itraconazole. Clinical cure was achieved in 81% of fluconazole-treated patients compared to 75% of itraconazole-treated patients ($P < 0.001$), although there was no difference in clinical and endoscopic cure at the end of the follow-up period (1 year). Approximately 25% of patients in both groups required an increase in dosage at 2 weeks.

Oral suspensions of both fluconazole and itraconazole have been developed, and their efficacy appears similar to that of pills. Results of comparative trials between fluconazole tablets and itraconazole suspension suggest equivalency in clinical response, mycologic eradication, and tolerability.[32]

Intravenous amphotericin B is highly effective against most *Candida* species. Because of its toxicity, this drug is used almost exclusively for candidiasis resistant to azole therapy. Lozenges containing amphotericin B and oral suspensions of amphotericin B have some efficacy and are available in Europe but not in the United States.[33] Low-dose amphotericin B (0.3–0.5 mg kg^{-1} day^{-1} for 7–14 days) is usually adequate therapy for oropharyngeal and esophageal candidiasis. Liposomal forms of amphotericin B are also effective and can be used if cost is not a factor and amphotericin B cannot be tolerated. Improved antiretroviral therapy, possibly by increasing the CD4+ T-lymphocyte count and thereby immune function, also leads to clearance of refractory thrush in some patients.

The newest agents available for candidal infection are the echinocandins.[34] These novel agents inhibit fungal cell wall synthesis through the inhibition of glucan synthase. Caspofungin, the first available agent in this class, has activity against both aspergillus and candida species including non-*albicans* strains. Prospective randomized trials have documented an efficacy and side effect profile similar to fluconazole for *Candida* esophagitis in AIDS,[35] and equal efficacy, better tolerability and comparable relapse rate than amphotericin B for azole resistant esophageal candidiasis.[36–38] Therefore, this drug has become the treatment of choice for resistant *Candida*. Other members of the echinocandin class have been less studied but are similarly effective.[39]

The incidence of azole-resistant mucosal candidiasis appears to be decreasing largely as a result of HAART. The risk factors, natural history, and outcome of fluconazole-resistant mucosal candidiasis have been examined.[40] The major risk factor associated with the development of resistance was the prophylactic daily or intermittent use of fluconazole within the last 6 months. The researchers also found that the prognosis of these patients was worse than that of patients with nonresistant *Candida*. In patients with fluconazole-resistant mucocutaneous candidiasis, treatment options include itraconazole (oral suspension or intravenous preparations), amphotericin, or more recently caspofungin.

Despite the frequency of oropharyngeal and esophageal candidiasis in HIV-infected patients, primary prophylaxis is not recommended. Although fluconazole prophylaxis decreases the occurrence of disease,[41] it is not recommended because these disorders are not life-threatening, acute therapy of individual episodes is highly effective, and there is concern that widespread use of primary prophylaxis will exacerbate the problem of drug resistance and drug-drug interactions. Therefore, we do not recommend primary prophylaxis for oropharyngeal or esophageal candidiasis. Whereas primary prophylaxis for *Candida* is rarely provided, secondary prophylaxis can be given if patients have multiple and frequent recurrences of oropharyngeal or esophageal candidiasis. Oral fluconazole 50–100 mg/day or 150 mg once-weekly is effective prophylaxis against recurrent oropharyngeal and esophageal candidiasis in patients with azole-sensitive disease.[25] Caspofungin has also been found effective in such cases but must be given intravenously.[38]

Treatment for GI CMV disease is limited to intravenous therapy with ganciclovir, foscarnet, and cidofovir. Valganciclovir has not been studied as primary therapy for enteric CMV disease.[42] A number of trials using intravenous ganciclovir in HIV-infected patients with GI CMV disease have demonstrated clinical improvement in ~75% of patients.[43,44] Open-label trials of foscarnet have yielded comparable results.[45] The only placebo-controlled trial of ganciclovir, which evaluated colitis, found no clinically significant differences between the treatment groups probably because the treatment period was only 2 weeks.[46] The only randomized controlled study comparing ganciclovir to foscarnet for therapy of CMV esophagitis found no difference between the agents regarding clinical activity, but there was more toxicity with foscarnet.[44] Marked endoscopic improvement was observed in 73% of the foscarnet-treated patients and 70% of the ganciclovir-treated patients. The symptomatic response was also similar for the two treatments: 82% of patients who received foscarnet and 80% of those treated with ganciclovir had a complete or at least a good clinical response. A randomized trial comparing ganciclovir to foscarnet in 48 AIDS patients with GI CMV disease found similar clinical efficacy (73%) regardless of the location of the disease (esophagus versus colon), with endoscopic improvement documented in more than 80%.[47] The time to progression of disease was similar (13–16 weeks) despite the use of maintenance therapy. Side effects occurred in half the patients in both groups. Mönkemüller and Wilcox described one case of CMV esophagitis that resolved after initiation of HAART without specific antiCMV therapy.[48] That report suggested that immune reconstitution with HAART can be associated with clearance of an opportunistic GI infection.

The decision to use either ganciclovir or foscarnet for GI CMV disease in AIDS should be based on the experience of the physician and the differing toxicities of each agent. The efficacy, tolerability, and cost of ganciclovir have established it as first-line therapy for GI CMV disease in AIDS. Our current policy for the therapy of GI CMV disease is to administer intravenous ganciclovir, assuming there are no major contraindications to this agent such as neutropenia or thrombocytopenia. The usual induction dose is 10–15 mg/kg administered twice a day for 3–4 weeks. In our experience, esophageal disease tends to respond more rapidly than does colonic disease. The response to therapy is judged by alleviation of symptoms and improved endoscopic findings. Ophthalmologic examination is mandatory at the time of diagnosis in all patients to exclude retinal disease. If retinal disease is absent and a complete symptomatic and endoscopic response is documented following induction therapy, we stop therapy and observe for recurrent symptoms. For patients with persistently low CD4+ T-lymphocyte counts, the relapse rate for esophageal and colonic disease is similar (30–50%).[43,44,47] Initiation of HAART therapy, or improving existing ART, plays an important role for prevention of recurrence. Endoscopic reexamination with biopsy of any mucosal abnormalities is important for patients with persistent symptoms following therapy. For those with frequent relapses of GI disease, long-term once-daily maintenance intravenous administration is appropriate. Although there are no reported data regarding the efficacy of oral valganciclovir for either maintenance therapy or treatment of acute GI disease, valganciclovir is likely to be effective in this setting and is a reasonable choice for treatment.[49] Failure to respond to ganciclovir may be the result of low serum levels[50] or drug resistance.[51]

For patients with major contraindications or failure to respond to ganciclovir, foscarnet is usually effective.[47,52] The recommended dosing schedule is 90 mg/kg IV bid daily for 14–21 days. Salzberger et al[53] demonstrated in an open-label, randomized trial that a frequency reduction of fosarnet from 7 to 5 days a week for 3 weeks was associated with equal response and fewer side effects than using the medication daily for 21 days. Combination therapy of foscarnet (90 mg/kg bid daily) and ganciclovir (5 mg/kg bid daily)[54] may be as effective for ganciclovir failures. A small study evaluated the safety of induction and maintenance therapy alternating ganciclovir (5 mg/kg every other day) and foscarnet (120 mg/kg every other day). There appears to be little benefit with their approach. The efficacy and incidence of side effects seemed to be equivalent to daily monotherapy or dual therapy.[54]

Although tested for retinitis, cidofovir has not been well studied for treatment of GI CMV disease but clinical experience suggests efficacy. The major side effect is renal toxicity. Since the drug can be given once-weekly, it may be an attractive option for selected patients.

Randomized placebo-controlled studies of oral ganciclovir for primary prophylaxis have demonstrated a reduction in the incidence of retinal involvement.[55] No definitive data exist on the effectiveness of primary prophylaxis for decreasing GI CMV disease in HIV-infected patients. Restoration of immune function with HAART is the primary strategy for prophylaxis.

For the patient with mild to moderate HSV esophagitis who is able to tolerate pills, oral administration of acyclovir 15–30 mg kg^{-1} day^{-1} is effective.[56] The drug is usually given in a dose of 400 mg PO five times a day for 2 weeks. Because absorption of oral acyclovir is inconsistent and may be as low as less than 30%,[57] valacyclovir 500–1000 mg bid PO has become the treatment of choice, especially for patients with more severe disease. Oral famciclovir is also highly effective against HSV. Intravenous administration of acyclovir should be applied when severe odynophagia limits oral intake or when the patient has not responded to high-dose oral therapy. Several studies have confirmed the safety and efficacy of intravenous foscarnet (40 mg/kg every 12 h) for treating HSV disease and supported the utility of this agent as maintenance therapy for delaying recurrences.[58] Primary prophylaxis is not currently recommended; secondary prophylaxis with valacyclovir (500 to 1000 mg/day) is usually provided to patients with frequent relapses of oropharyngeal or esophageal disease. Drug resistance is rare.[59]

Prospective studies of idiopathic esophageal ulcers have documented healing rates of more than 90% with oral corticosteroids.[60] The regimen most commonly employed is prednisone 40 mg/day tapering 10 mg/week for a 1-month treatment course.[60] Shorter courses of therapy may be effective for small ulcers. Although beneficial, intralesional injection of corticosteroids should be considered as second-line therapy. The side effects of corticosteroids are well recognized; patients with AIDS may be more likely to develop CMV disease while on therapy.[61] Because oropharyngeal and esophageal candidiasis may complicate steroid use and confuse the therapeutic response, we routinely use short courses of azole therapy while the patients are receiving prednisone.

The response to corticosteroids is rapid, with most patients experiencing significant pain relief within days. Although not as well studied, thalidomide appears to be highly effective for IEU.[62,63] In doses of 200–300 mg/day, thalidomide has been documented to result in a clinical response and endoscopic cure in more than 90% of treated patients.[63] Thalidomide is well tolerated, with the main side effect being somnolence; administration of the drug at bedtime tends to overcome this problem. Peripheral neuropathy and skin rash are infrequent side effects. The major fear with thalidomide is inadvertent use during the first trimester of pregnancy, which consistently results in severe birth defects. Therefore, most physicians do not prescribe this agent for women of childbearing age unless the patient is surgically sterile. Without improvement of immune function, the relapse rate of IEU is ~40–50% regardless of the initial therapy.[60,63]

INFECTIONS OF THE STOMACH

Symptomatic and clinically significant opportunistic gastric infections are uncommon in patients with HIV infection. While a number of opportunistic pathogens have been reported to infect the stomach in these patients, including cryptosporidia, *Toxoplasma gondii*, *Leishmania*, *Pneumocystis carinii*, *Treponema pallidium*, *Cryptococcus neoformans*, the most common is CMV.[64,65] All these infections may be asymptomatic or result in nausea and vomiting. Most present in the setting of disseminated disease and are associated with systemic symptoms (malaise, weakness, fever). Clues to the diagnosis may be found outside the GI tract. Epigastric pain or GI bleeding occur more frequently in the setting of ulcerative lesions such as peptic ulcer disease and CMV. The main diagnostic test for patients with these symptoms is upper endoscopy with biopsies.

Although earlier studies report that the prevalence of peptic ulcer disease and *Helicobacter pylori* infection were common in patients with HIV infection, subsequent studies performed since then have found that the prevalence of peptic ulcer disease and *H. pylori* is lower in HIV-infected patients, especially those with lower CD4 lymphocyte counts.[66,67] Possible explanations for this phenomenon include hypochlorhydria, antibiotic use, and inadequate mucosal inflammatory response.[68] Varsky et al studied 497 HIV-positive patients with upper digestive tract symptoms.[69] The investigators found that 5% of these patients had gastroduodenal ulcers (GDUs). *Helicobacter pylori* was detected in only 31% of patients with GDUs, whereas CMV was detected in 50% of these patients. In HIV-infected patients with chronic active gastritis without a GDU, other organisms such as *Cryptosporidium* and CMV were more prevalent than *H. pylori*. Based on their findings it is recommended that endoscopic biopsies be performed to search for opportunistic pathogens in AIDS patients with upper digestive symptoms. Most studies from Europe, Australia, and the United States have also found a low incidence of *H. pylori* in HIV-infected patients. In Italy, Cacciarelli et al found that the prevalence of *H. pylori* in HIV-positive patients with a CD4+ T-lymphocyte count of less than 200 cells per cubic millimeter was significantly less than that of HIV-negative patients.[66] The authors also found that the number of peptic ulcers was significantly less in HIV-infected patients. In New York, Marano et al found *H. pylori* in only 15.9% of symptomatic HIV-infected patients undergoing upper endoscopy, despite the presence of chronic active gastritis in 94.5% of them.[70] In Australia, Edwards et al found that the prevalence of *H. pylori* was 3% in patients with AIDS, compared to 22% in non-HIV-infected patients.[71] Mönkemüller et al reported that the incidence of opportunistic GI infections has declined, most likely secondary to the use of HAART.[1] During the same period they noted a rise in the number of nonopportunistic GI disorders in these patients, including peptic ulcer disease.[1]

ABDOMINAL PAIN

Abdominal pain is a common complaint among HIV-infected patients, with a reported incidence of 12%; there has been limited study of this symptom complex in the era of HAART. In the early stages of immunodeficiency, the causes of abdominal pain are similar to those of the nonimmunocompromised host. However with worsening immunodeficiency, opportunistic pathogens (CMV, protozoa, mycobacteria, fungi) and neoplasms become more prevalent etiologies either singularly or in combination of abdominal pain.

The diagnosis of abdominal pain can be a challenge given the broad spectrum of potential causes, including both opportunistic and nonopportunistic disorders.[72,73] In most cases a carefully performed history and physical examination in conjunction with the CD4+ T-lymphocyte count can help narrow the differential diagnosis. A thorough systematic evaluation is necessary to avoid overlooking potentially life-threatening conditions, such as hollow viscus perforation, appendicitis, intestinal obstruction, pancreatitis, and toxic megacolon. It is also important to remember that multiple conditions associated with ongoing, chronic abdominal pain such as CMV enteritis and non-Hodgkin lymphoma (NHL) can suddenly result in an acute abdomen due to intestinal perforation and obstruction.[73] Treatment of abdominal pain is directed by the underlying etiology.

Etiology

A cause of abdominal pain can be found in most HIV-infected patients, and treatment should be tailored accordingly. The most common causes of chronic abdominal pain in patients with advanced HIV disease (i.e., CD4+ T-lymphocyte count <100 cells per μL) are disseminated *Mycobacterium avium* complex (MAC), intestinal CMV disease, and neoplasms such as NHL and Kaposi sarcoma (KS) (Table 77-2).

Clinical Presentation

One of the largest studies evaluating the cause of abdominal pain in AIDS patients found that the predominant localization

Etiology of Abdominal Pain in Patients with HIV Infection

Table 77-2

Epigastric
Acute and chronic pancreatitis (CMV, drug-induced, TMP-SMX)
Peptic ulcer disease (gastric ulcer, duodenal ulcer)
Gastritis (*Helicobacter pylori*, CMV, *Cryptococcus neoformans*, *mucormycosis*, *cryptosporidia*, *Leishmania donovani*)
Duodenitis (CMV, *L. donovani*, *Cryptococcus neoformans*, *Cryptosporidium parvum*)
Nonulcer dyspepsia)

Periumbilical
Enteritis (viral: CMV, rotavirus, astrovirus, picorna virus, coronavirus; bacteria: *Salmonella*, MAC, *M. tuberculosis*; protozoa: *Isospora belli*, *cryptosporidia*, *microsporidia*, *Cyclospora cayetanensis*, *Giardia lamblia*; fungi: *Cryptococcus neoformans* (duodenum)
Lymphoma

Right Upper Quadrant
Cholecystitis (gallstones and acalculous). Acalculous most frequently secondary to infections: CMV, *Isospora belli*, *Candida*, *cryptosporidia*, *microsporidia*, *Salmonella* spp., *Campylobacter fetus*
AIDS-cholangiopathy (CMV, MAC, *Salmonella* spp., *Enterobacter* spp., *cryptosporidia*, *microsporidia*, *Cyclospora cayetanensis*)
Shingles (varicella zoster)
Hepatitis (A,B,C,D, CMV, EBV)
Perihepatitis (*Chlamydia trachomatis*, *Neisseria gonorrhoeae*), *Bartonella*

Left Upper Quadrant
Splenic abscess
Pancreatic abscess (TB)
Pancreatitis (ddI, ddC, pentamidine, TMP-SMX, *Cryptosporidium*, *Campylobacter*, CMV, HIV)
Shingles
Right Lower Quadrant
Lymphoma
Appendicitis
Inflammatory bowel disease
Pelvic inflammatory disease
Ectopic pregnancy

Left Lower Quadrant
Colitis (infectious: viral: CMV, rotavirus, astrovirus, picobirna virus, coronavirus, adenovirus, HSV; bacterial: Shigella, *Campylobacter*, *Salmonella*, *Clostridium difficile*, *Mycobacterium avium*, *Mycobacterium tuberculosis*, *Bartonella henselae*, *Aeromonas hydrophila*, protozoa: *Entamoeba histolytica*, *Isospora belli*, *Cryptosporidium*, *Toxoplasma gondii*, *Schistosoma mansonii*, *Dientamoeba fragilis*, *Blastocystis hominis*, *microsporidia*; fungi: *Histoplasma capsulatum*, *Candida albicans*, *Cryptococcus neoformans*, *Pneumocystis carinii* neoplastic: Kaposi sarcoma (Herpesvirus 8), non-Hodgkin lymphoma, idiopathic, drug-induced (acyclovir)
IBD (idiopathic, also can occur in association with KS)
Diverticulitis
IBS
Pelvic inflammatory disease
Ectopic pregnancy

Flanks
Kidney stones (drug-related: indinavir)
Pyelonephritis
Retroperitoneal lymphadenopathy (non-Hodgkin lymphoma, angioimmunoblastic lymphadenopathy, tuberculosis, MAC)

Suprapubic
Cervical cancer
Pelvic inflammatory disease
Ectopic pregnancy
Not localized to specific area:
- Toxic megacolon (CMV, *C. difficile*, *Cryptosporidium*, KS)
- Colonic perforation (CMV, histoplasmosis, idiopathic, diverticulum, neoplasm)
- Peritonitis
- Ileal perforation
- Neoplasm (lymphoma, Kaposi sarcoma)
- Adrenal failure

(*Continued*)

(Continued)

Table 77-2

Diffuse
Peritonitis (TB, CMV, *Toxoplasma gondii*, *Cryptococcus neoformans*, *Histoplasma capsulatum*)
Bowel perforation
Intraabdominal lymphadenopathy (lymphoma, KS, MAC, TB, angioimmunoblastic lymphadenopathy, bartonellosis)
Adrenal failure-adrenalitis
Mesenteric fibrosis
Omental fibrosis (*H. capsulatum*)
IBS

HIV-infected patients are at similar risk of suffering from diseases and abdominal pain due to the same etiologies as nonimmunocompromised patients. This list highlights some conditions seen frequently in HIV-infected patients.

Microsporidia: *Enterocytozoon bieneusi*, *Encephalocytozoon* (*Septata*) *intestinalis*, *Encephalocytozoon cuniculi*.

EBV, Epstein–Barr virus; IBD, inflammatory bowel disease; IBS, irritable bowel syndrome; KS, Kaposi sarcoma; MAC, *Mycobacterium avium* complex.

of abdominal pain had considerable value for establishing the final diagnosis.[72] In this study, upper abdominal pain most commonly resulted from gastric and duodenal involvement by nonopportunistic disorders such as pancreatitis and peptic ulcer disease and opportunistic processes such as CMV, KS, and NHL. Right upper quadrant pain most commonly resulted from cholangiopathy or hepatitis. It is important not to restrict the differential diagnosis to intraabdominal etiologies but to consider pulmonary, esophageal, and cardiac diseases as causes of upper abdominal pain (Table 77-2).

Accompanying symptoms such as nausea and vomiting or diarrhea are also helpful for determining the possible intra-abdominal organ involved. Vomiting is common with partial or complete bowel obstruction, kidney stones, and gallbladder diseases, whereas it is rarely reported with colitis. Isolated vomiting suggests the presence of central nervous system involvement. Patients with a retroperitoneal process, such as pancreatitis or lymphadenopathy, may find relief by leaning forward; ingestion of food aggravates the pain in patients with gastric ulcerations; an inability to find a comfortable body position is common in the presence of nephrolithiasis; and patients with peritonitis prefer to lie quietly. The presence of diarrhea suggests an intestinal source (colitis or enteritis). When abdominal pain is present in patients with enteritis, it is usually crampy and periumbilical in location. Symptoms such as nausea, vomiting, bloating, distension, and borborygmi are also commonly associated with small bowel diarrhea. In contrast, the pain in those with colitis tends to be localized to the lower abdominal quadrants, more commonly the left.[74]

Careful documentation of current medications is mandatory. Pancreatitis may occur as the result of the administration of pentamidine and trimethoprim-sulfamethoxazole (TMP-SMX) or the antiretroviral agents didanosine (ddI) and dideoxycytidine (ddC).[75] The presence of diarrhea and abdominal pain in a patient with recent use of antibiotics suggests the possibility of *Clostridium difficile* colitis. Flank pain in a patient receiving indinavir may be the result of nephrolithiasis. Persistent nausea and abdominal pain has been associated with nucleoside-related hepatic steatosis or lactic acidosis.

On physical examination careful attention should be given to any extra-abdominal findings, as conditions such as lower lobe pneumonia or pericarditis can result in upper abdominal pain. Fever, an important sign of infection in an immunocompetent person with abdominal pain, is an equally sensitive sign in AIDS patients. However, low-grade fever is a much less specific sign in AIDS patients because it may result from the HIV infection itself. Funduscopic examination is mandatory to exclude the presence of CMV retinitis; 20% with chronic diarrhea and abdominal pain from CMV have generalized CMV disease. The skin should be closely examined for KS lesions, as 40–50% of patients with skin or lymph node involvement by KS also have GI involvement. Jaundice suggests drug-induced liver disease, cholestatic hepatitis, or biliary tract obstruction secondary to infections or neoplasms (NHL, KS). Hepatomegaly is observed with infiltrative processes (MAC, neoplasm) and steatosis from the lactic acidosis syndrome caused by nucleoside agents. The presence of lymphadenopathy in the neck and inguinal regions suggests a systemic process such as MAC, tuberculosis (TB), or NHL. Decreased bowel sounds or high-pitched rushes is most often due to intestinal obstruction, whereas hyperactive bowel sounds are associated with diarrheal disorders. Tenderness on abdominal examination can be nonspecific, but localization to a specific quadrant can be helpful for pointing to the potentially affected organ (Table 77-2). Organomegaly can result from disseminated MAC, histoplasmosis, TB, bacillary angiomatosis, or tumors. Ascites may reflect underlying cirrhosis or represent a complication from TB, CMV enterocolitis, or toxoplasmosis. The anorectum should be examined carefully, as these patients can develop anal fissures and rectal ulcers.

Diagnostic Tests

Initial laboratory evaluation should include a white blood cell count and differential; assays for hemoglobin, liver and pancreatic enzymes, and albumin; coagulation studies; and urinalysis. Because of HIV-associated leukopenia, HIV-infected patients do not always exhibit leukocytosis as part of the systemic inflammatory response to intra-abdominal processes such as cholecystitis, colitis, and pancreatitis. Liver function tests are commonly abnormal and can be nonspecific, particularly when only minimally abnormal, or due to chronic viral hepatitis, drug-induced liver injury, or AIDS cholangiopathy.

Plain abdominal radiographs are not generally helpful for evaluating abdominal pain but are useful for detecting free subdiaphragmatic air in the presence of viscus perforation, air-fluid levels in the presence of bowel obstruction, or "thumbprinting" due to severe colitis.[74] Ultrasonography (US) is the test of choice for evaluating right upper quadrant pain. We employ US for the patient without jaundice in whom AIDS cholangiopathy or gallbladder disease is suspected, reserving computed tomography (CT) for those with marked hepatomegaly, jaundice, suspected mass lesions, or peritoneal diseases. In addition, CT scans of the abdomen and pelvis should be performed in the ill-appearing patient with unexplained abdominal pain, where it may demonstrate appendicitis, pancreatitis, intra-abdominal abscess, lymphadenopathy, or colitis.[76] Magnetic resonance imaging (MRI) is a reasonable alternative if reduced renal function prohibits the use of IV contrast. Hydroxyiminodiacetic acid (HIDA) scanning is often diagnostic for acalculous cholecystitis, demonstrating an absence of uptake into the gallbladder despite imaging of the common bile duct.

Endoscopy

Endoscopy is a valuable tool for evaluating chronic abdominal pain in AIDS, especially in the presence of specific symptoms such as epigastric pain, diarrhea, nausea, and vomiting. Endoscopic retrograde cholangiopancreatography is the most sensitive means of diagnosing AIDS cholangiopathy and should be strongly considered in the presence of biliary tract dilation.

Diagnostic Laparoscopy

Laparoscopy is useful for the evaluation of abdominal pain, hepatomegaly, fever of unknown origin, and ascites.[77] Diagnoses established using this technique include MAC, TB, KS, histoplasmosis, cryptosporidiosis, chronic active hepatitis, and cirrhosis. With the resolution of current CT scanning coupled with guided biopsy, laparoscopy is rarely required.

Therapy

Therapy should be directed by the cause of the abdominal pain. In most cases the treatment is medical; but when indicated, an aggressive surgical approach is warranted because the surgical morbidity and mortality rates are acceptable in these patients.[78]

Once a life-threatening condition has been excluded and a diagnosis is established, consideration should be given to adding antispasmodics and specific medications for appropriate pain control. In HIV-infected patients with abdominal pain, we suggest that during and following the initiation of definitive treatment mild to moderate pain may be treated with a nonsteroidal anti-inflammatory drug (NSAID) or acetaminophen on a fixed-dosage schedule. Narcotic agents should be given in more severe cases or when there is no response to scheduled NSAID or acetaminophen. Tricyclic antidepressants may be beneficial at low dosages especially for chronic pain syndromes. Narcotics and other anticholinergics should be avoided when there is a partial or evolving bowel obstruction.

DIARRHEA (ENTERITIS AND COLITIS)

Diarrhea is a frequent complaint among patients with HIV infection, and the frequency of opportunistic causes has fallen since the introduction of PIs and HAART in 1996.[1,2,79] A careful history may indicate the possible sites of involvement (i.e., enteritis or colitis). Small bowel diarrhea ("enteritis") is manifested as large-volume (>2 L/day), watery stools frequently associated with dehydration, electrolyte disturbances, and malabsorption. Abdominal pain, when present, is usually crampy and periumbilical. Low-grade fever and nausea are also common. In contrast, colitis is characterized by frequent, small-volume stools that contain mucus, pus, and blood and frequently accompanied by "proctitis symptoms" (tenesmus or a feeling of incomplete evacuation and dyskesia or pain on defecation). Abdominal pain tends to be localized to the lower quadrants, more commonly on the left. Nevertheless, in a number of patients, there is overlap among these symptoms and the location of disease may not be obvious. The physical examination is rarely diagnostic for the specific etiology of the diarrhea but is extremely important for assessing the patient's general condition and hydration status. In addition, if the patient has chronic malabsorptive diarrhea, physical findings associated with specific nutrient deficiencies may become evident (e.g., ecchymosis with vitamin K deficiency). The list of diagnostic tests available for evaluating acute and chronic infectious diarrhea in HIV-infected patients is exhaustive, but it is rarely necessary to use more than a few of these tests. The approach to the HIV-infected patient with diarrhea is generally "stepwise", beginning with simple tests and gradually progressing to more invasive tests (Table 77-3). A search for an etiology should always be attempted, as most causes of diarrhea are infectious and can be treated with specific antimicrobial agents.

When analyzing the stools, the first test should be a methylene blue stain to determine if fecal leukocytes are present. Their presence suggests an inflammatory (colonic) rather than a noninflammatory (small bowel) diarrhea. Stool cultures for *Salmonella*, *Shigella*, and *Campylobacter* should be done routinely, as well as a *Clostridium difficile* toxin screen. Routine stool stains should include a modified acid stain for cryptosporidia.[80]

Routine tests may be useful for evaluating the impact of the diarrhea on the host, such as malnutrition (hypoalbuminemia), hydration status, and electrolyte disturbances. The absolute CD4+ T-lymphocyte cell count is essential, as many organisms cause disease only in the presence of severe immunodeficiency.[81] Roentgenography is unimportant in the evaluation of HIV-associated diarrhea. Endoscopy (esophagogastroduodenoscopy, flexible sigmoidoscopy, colonoscopy) is important and may be an integral part of the workup of patients

Table 77-3 Diagnostic Evaluation for Diarrhea in HIV-Infected Patients

Acute Diarrhea (<14 days)

Step 1
- Stool methylene blue for leukocytes
- Stool culture for *Salmonella* spp.,[a] *Shigella* spp.,[a] and *Campylobacter jejunii*[a]; assay for *Clostridium difficile* toxin
- Stool microscopic examination for ova and parasites (*Giardia lamblia* and *Entamoeba histolytica*[b])
- Stool antibody testing (*Giardia lamblia*[c])

Step 2
- Flexible sigmoidoscopy
- Inspection and endoscopic characterization of colon
- Stool retrieval for cultures, ova and parasites, and *C. difficile* toxin (as above)

Chronic Diarrhea (>14 days)

Step 1
- Stool methylene blue for leukocytes
- Stool investigation for *Clostridium difficile* toxin
- Stool microscopic examination for ova and parasites (*microsporidia*,[d] *cryptosporidia*,[e] *Isospora belli*,[e] and *Cyclospora cayetanensis*)
- Blood cultures (*Mycobacterium avium* complex (MAC))

Step 2
- Endoscopy with biopsies
- Gastroduodenoscopy and duodenal biopsies (MAC, *microsporidia*)
- Flexible sigmoidoscopy or colonoscopy (cytomegalovirus (CMV), MAC, *microsporidia*, *Isospora belli*, *C. difficile*, inflammatory bowel disease)
- Biopsy specimens submitted for
  - Tissue stains[f]
  - Special tissue stains[g]
  - Culture of tissue[h]
  - Electron microscopy[i]

[a] Blood cultures (bacteremia with these bacteria is more common in HIV-infected patients).
[b] Hemophagocytosis needs to present to substantiate pathogenic *Entamoeba*.
[c] Electroimmunoassay (EIA) for *G. lamblia*.
[d] Gram stain, concentrated stool (zinc sulfate, Shether sucrose flotation).
[e] Modified Kinyoun acid-fast (*Cryptosporidium* and *Isospora belli*).
[f] Hematoxylin and eosin (CMV, herpes simplex virus (HSV), fungi), Giemsa or methenamine silver (*Candida*, *Histoplasma capsulatum*), Gram or methylene blue/azure II/basic fuchsin (microsporidia), Fite (*Mycobacteria*).
[g] *In situ* hybridization, immunoperoxide stains (CMV, HSV, adenovirus).
[h] Bacteria and fungi.
[i] *Microsporidia*, adenovirus.

suspected of having CMV or microsporidia and for patients with negative noninvasive studies.[82,83]

INFECTIONS OF THE SMALL INTESTINE (ENTERITIS)

Etiology

In most series before the era of HAART, *Cryptosporidium parvum* was the most common protozoal infection causing diarrhea, identified in up to 11% of symptomatic patients.[84] The prevalence of infection has been markedly reduced with the advent of potent antiretroviral therapy. Outbreaks of cryptosporidiosis are well described in both immunocompetent and immunodeficient hosts, and they result from contamination of public water sources. Microsporidia (*Enterocytozoon bieneusi* and *Encephalitozoon intestinalis*, formerly *Septata intestinalis*) involve a variety of organ systems causing either localized or disseminated disease[80] (Table 77-4). These parasites are common intestinal and biliary pathogens in patients with AIDS.[80,81,83,85] Kotler and Orenstein[86] found microsporidia in 39% of AIDS patients undergoing GI evaluation for diarrhea. *E. bieneusi* is the cause of most cases of GI disease. Co-infection with these two microsporidia or with other pathogens can occur. This high prevalence of intestinal microsporidiosis is probably not related to an increasing incidence of disease but, rather, to greater recognition and improved diagnostic testing. *Isospora belli* is a rare GI pathogen in HIV-infected patients in the United States, whereas it is endemic in many developing countries such as Haiti[80] and is an important cause of chronic diarrhea. As with other protozoa, it is primarily a small bowel pathogen. *Cyclospora*, another coccidial protozoon, has been recognized throughout the world as a GI pathogen in immunocompetent patients and in patients with AIDS.[87] The prevalence of *Cyclospora* in developed and developing countries is unknown. A number of similarities exist in the microbiology,

Enteric Pathogens in AIDS Patients

Table 77-4

Enteric Pathogens in AIDS Patients
Viruses
Cytomegalovirus
Astrovirus
Picornavirus
Coronavirus
Rotavirus
Herpesvirus
Adenovirus
Small round virus
HIV
Bacteria
Salmonella
Shigella
Campylobacter
Clostridium difficile
Mycobacterium avium complex
Mycobacterium tuberculosis
Treponema pallidum
Bartonella
Spirochaeta
Neisseria gonorrhoeae
Vibrio cholerae
Pseudomonas
Staphylococcus aureus
Parasites
Giardia lamblia
Entamoeba histolytica
Microsporidia
Enterocytozoon bieneusi
Septata intestinalis
Cyclospora
Cryptosporidium
Isospora belli
Blastocystis hominis
Fungi
Histoplasma
Candida albicans

epidemiology, and clinical expression of *Cyclospora* and cryptosporidia. *Cyclospora* spp. have a morphologic appearance similar to that of cryptosporidia, although they are larger (8–10 μm vs 4–6 μm). Giardiasis has no increased prevalence in HIV-infected patients, and the clinical presentation and diagnostic methods are similar to those for HIV seronegative patients. *Mycobacterium avium* complex (MAC), once common in AIDS, is now quite infrequent.[88] Small intestinal disease is the most common site of luminal GI involvement by MAC. It has been rarely reported to involve the esophagus, biliary tree, or colon.

Rotavirus has been linked to both acute and chronic diarrhea. Several unusual viruses have been identified in HIV-infected patients with chronic diarrhea, including astrovirus, picornavirus, and coronavirus.[89] Although the true incidence of these viruses as GI pathogens is unknown, it is probably low, and therapy is not currently available.

Clinical Presentation

In contrast to immunocompetent patients with cryptosporidiosis where spontaneous cure is uniform, in HIV-infected patients the natural history is much more variable.[90] This variability is related to the degree of immunodeficiency as patients with CD4+ T-lymphocyte counts higher than 180 cells per cubic millimeter usually have a self-limited illness.[90] In contrast, in patients with a CD4+ T-lymphocyte count of less than 50 cells per cubic millimeter the disease is often devastating, resulting in severe (voluminous) watery, nonbloody diarrhea with malabsorption, electrolyte disturbances, dehydration, and weight loss with a median survival of less than 12 weeks.[90] Abdominal cramps and weight loss are common. The parasite is distributed throughout the GI tract, although most commonly it infects the small bowel.

The most common clinical presentation of microsporidiosis is chronic, watery, nonbloody diarrhea of variable severity but infrequently voluminous. Substantial weight loss is uncommon. Abdominal pain and fever are not associated with intestinal involvement. In immunocompetent hosts the organism causes a self-limited illness characterized by crampy abdominal pain, flatulence, and diarrhea lasting 2–3 weeks.

Isosporiasis is typically a chronic illness characterized by profuse, nonbloody, watery diarrhea that may be indistinguishable from the diarrhea caused by microsporidia or cryptosporidia. Nausea and diffuse abdominal pain typically accompany the illness; fever and vomiting are uncommon. A malabsorption syndrome (steatorrhea and lactose intolerance) with weight loss of at least 10% often antedates the diagnosis.

The most frequent symptoms of giardiasis are flatulence, crampy abdominal pain, borborygmi, dyspepsia, and diarrhea. Fever and bloody stools are not associated with this infection.

Small bowel involvement by MAC is often diffuse. Massive infiltration of the small bowel mimicking Whipple's disease has been described and may account for the severe malabsorption observed in some patients.[91] The liver and spleen are the most common sites for dissemination. The most common manifestations of intestinal MAC infection are abdominal pain, fever, night sweats, wasting, and anemia.[92] Chronic watery diarrhea may result from small intestinal malabsorption.

Diagnosis

Cryptosporidiosis is diagnosed by stool analysis using a modified acid-fast stain. Although electron microscopy of small bowel biopsies is considered the gold standard for the diagnosis of microsporidiosis, studies have shown tissue stains (H & E, touch preparation with Giemsa, Brown-Brenn, Brown-Hopps, methylene blue azure II-basic fuchsin) of small bowel biopsies to have sensitivities of 77–83% with specificities approaching 100%.[93] When performing upper endoscopy, an attempt should be made to biopsy the most distal part of the small bowel, as microsporidia are mostly concentrated in the jejunum. The most commonly employed stool stain is a modified trichrome (chromotrope 2R) stain which is only modestly sensitive. The diagnosis of isosporiosis is best established using a modified Kinyoun acid-fast stool stain;[80] small bowel biopsy may also be diagnostic. *Cyclospora* are difficult to appreciate on routine microscopy of small bowel biopsies, although electron microscopy is often diagnostic. For the diagnosis of *Giardia*, it is well recognized that multiple stool tests (usually three) obtained on different days may be required, as intestinal shedding is sporadic;[94] moreover, only 40% of stools are positive in low excreters. Light microscopic detection of *Giardia* cysts (in semiformed stools) and trophozoites (in diarrheic stools) continues to be the mainstay of diagnosis. Fresh stool specimens should be examined or fixed with polyvinyl alcohol formalin and then stained with trichrome or iron hematoxylin. Cyst detection in stool can be increased by use of immunofluorescent antibody to cyst protein. Small bowel duodenal aspirate and biopsy may be diagnostic when stool testing is negative.

Positive blood cultures or bone marrow biopsy establish the diagnosis of disseminated MAC but do not establish the presence of active GI disease. The presence of a positive stool culture suggests, but does not prove, GI involvement; stool culture positivity is, however, a marker for subsequent disseminated disease.[95] Many laboratories, however, do not perform a MAC culture on stool.

Although many of these organisms (MAC, microsporidia, cryptosporidia) do not produce colitis *per se*, they may involve the colon. Thus, the diagnosis can be established based on colonic mucosal biopsies obtained during flexible sigmoidoscopy or colonoscopy. We present a simplified but focused algorithm for the evaluation of diarrhea in AIDS in Figure 77-2.

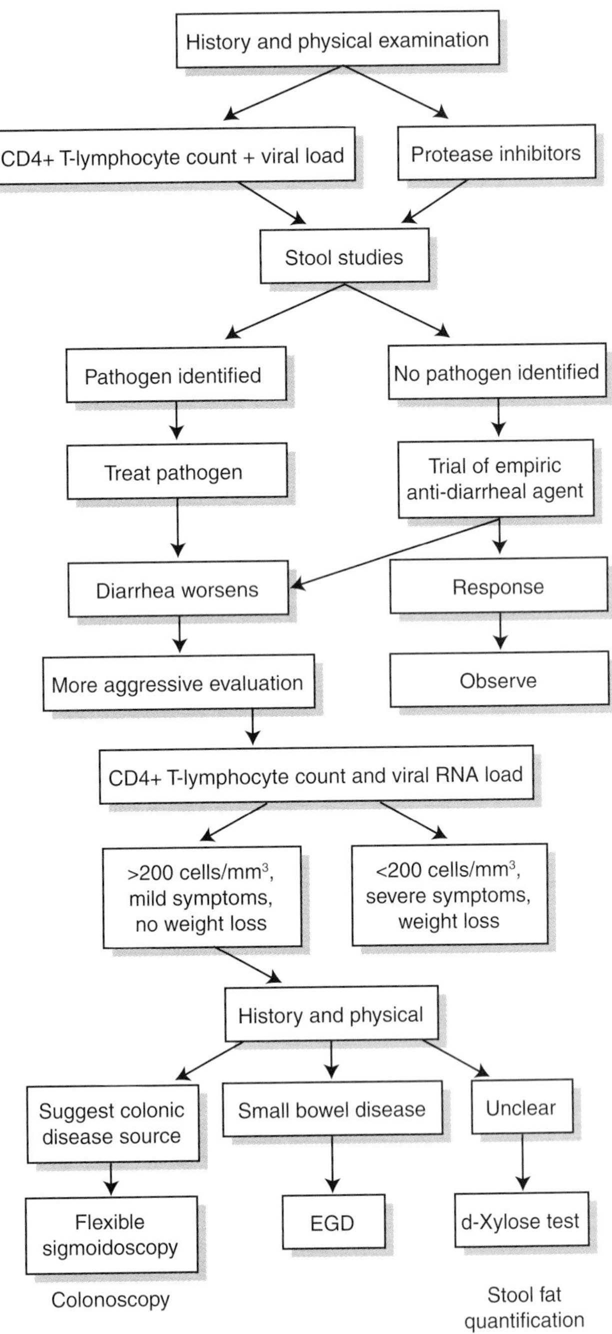

Figure 77-2 ■ Diagnostic algorithm for evaluating diarrhea in the HIV-infected patient.

Treatment

Numerous therapies have been used to treat intestinal cryptosporidiosis (*see* Chapter 38), most without success.[96] Immune reconstitution, through either potent antiretroviral therapy or improvements in nutritional status, may result in a clinical remission.[97]

The agent most commonly advanced as treatment of cryptosporidiosis is paromomycin.[96] In a study of 35 patients, a complete symptomatic response was seen in 20% of patients, with a partial response observed in an additional 43%;[98] responders had more preserved immune function as assessed by the CD4+ T-lymphocyte count. In a prospective open-label trial of 24 patients, 22 (92%) had a clinical response, with a complete remission observed in 18.[99] Among the 22 responders, clearance of the organisms was noted on follow-up stool studies, small bowel biopsy, or both. These results are in striking contrast to a randomized, double-blind placebo-controlled trial of 35 patients.[100] This study employed a 21-day placebo phase, but subsequently all patients then received an additional 21 days of active drug. A complete response was seen in 18% of the treated patients compared to 15% of the placebo patients. The findings from this study[100] are similar to our experience in that patients with the most severe disease (and most severe immunodeficiency) are the least likely to respond. For patients with a CD4+ T-lymphocyte count of less than 100 cells per microliter in whom therapy is clinically effective, long-term administration is required to prevent relapse, although relapse may still occur despite continued therapy. During the present era of HAART, it has been demonstrated that combination antiretroviral therapy that includes a PI can restore immunity to *C. parvum* in HIV-1-infected individuals, resulting in complete clinical, microbiologic, and histologic responses.[97] Therefore, the therapy for patients with AIDS and chronic diarrhea should focus on approaches to restore immune function (i.e., with HAART) rather than treating the opportunistic disorder itself.

Treatments for microsporidia are variably effective (*see* Chapter 39). Initial studies of metronidazole showed some efficacy,[101] although our experience has not been positive. Albendazole has shown promise in open-label trials,[102] with response rates of ~50% with a dose of 400 mg PO bid. Despite clinical improvement, the organisms persisted in the stool and small bowel biopsy specimens.[102] In contrast, studies of patients with *E. intestinalis* show response rates to albendazole of 66–100%, with some patients having clearance of the organism and no relapse.[103] With the recognition that two microsporidial species involve the bowel, it has become clear that albendazole is highly effective for *E. intestinalis* but largely ineffective for *E. bieneusi*. A recent study has shown that oral fumagillin is effective for *E. bieneusi*.[104] This response difference emphasizes the importance of a species-specific diagnosis of intestinal microsporidiosis. As with cryptosporidia, improvement in immune function with HAART can result in a clinical and histologic remission.[97]

In contrast to cryptosporidia and microsporidia, effective therapy is available for *Isospora belli* and *Cyclospora* (*see* Chapter 38). Cotrimoxazole or TMP-SMX results in cure in most patients. Because the relapse rate of isosporiasis is 50% once therapy is discontinued, lifelong suppressive therapy is required.[105] The widespread use of TMP-SMX for *Pneumocystis carinii* prophylaxis may be one explanation for the low incidence of these infections in developed countries. Therapy with metronidazole (500 mg bid × 5–7 days) is highly effective for treating giardiasis.

Table 77-5 Etiology of Colitis in HIV-Infected Patients

Bacteria
Shigella, Campylobacter, Salmonella
Clostridium difficile
Mycobacterium avium complex
Mycobacterium tuberculosis
Bartonella henselae
Aeromonas hydrophila
Viruses
Cytomegalovirus
Herpes simplex virus
Adenovirus
Protozoa
Entamoeba histolytica
Isospora belli
Blastocystis hominis
Cryptosporidium
Microsporidia
Toxoplasma gondii
Fungi
Histoplasma capsulatum
Candida albicans
Cryptococcus neoformans
Pneumocystis carinii
Other
Inflammatory bowel disease
Kaposi sarcoma (herpesvirus 8)

INFECTIONS OF THE COLON (COLITIS)

The spectrum of pathogens causing colitis is similar to that in the normal host, except for CMV (Table 77-5). In earlier studies of diarrhea in HIV-infected patients, bacteria were frequently identified. Unusual presentations of common bacterial diseases became apparent early in the AIDS epidemic where *Salmonella* sp. or *Campylobacter* sp. bacteremia. were reported as initial manifestations of AIDS.[74] The infection was characterized by frequent relapses despite appropriate antimicrobial therapy. Currently, the prevalence of these infections as causes of diarrhea is not well known, although it is probably lower than in the past given the widespread use of TMP-SMX for *Pneumocystis carinii* pneumonia (PCP) prophylaxis. *Clostridium difficile* is now one of the most common bacterial pathogens perhaps because of these patients' frequent exposure to antimicrobials and frequent hospitalizations-factors that have been linked to *C. difficile* disease.[106] CMV is the most common opportunistic cause of colonic disease. It usually presents as chronic diarrhea and is frequently associated with systemic disease (CMV retinitis). Adenovirus has been reported to cause diarrhea and colitis.[74] HIV-infected patients do not appear to have an increased susceptibility to *Entamoeba histolytica*. Amebic colitis is distinctly uncommon.[107]

Histoplasmosis infrequently involves the GI tract in patients with AIDS (*see* Chapter 44). GI tract involvement occurs in ~5% of patients with disseminated disease, may be the first site of disease, and the colon is the most common site of GI involvement (80%).[108] *Penicillium chrysogenum*, a fungal infection, has been described in the Far East.[109] Worms as symptomatic intestinal pathogens in AIDS patients are rare.[110]

Clinical Presentation and Diagnosis

Salmonella gastroenteritis presents with watery diarrhea, abdominal pain, nausea, and vomiting. Some patients present with classic "colitis" symptoms: dysentery (mucopurulent, bloody diarrhea) and fever. *Salmonella* bacteremia should be sought in the patient with diarrhea and fever, and when identified, prolonged antimicrobial therapy should be given. Shigellosis and campylobacteriosis present in a fashion similar to that of *Salmonella* gastroenteritis. Stool cultures are usually diagnostic; blood cultures are useful and occasionally are positive when stool cultures are negative. Colitis may be identified by flexible sigmoidoscopy; mucosal biopsies should be performed in severely immunocompromised patients, as CMV colitis may appear endoscopically similar.[74]

Colonic CMV infection typically presents with chronic watery diarrhea, abdominal pain, wasting, anorexia, and fever. When the distal colorectum is involved, symptoms of proctitis may be reported. GI bleeding without diarrhea may be the initial manifestation of CMV colitis. Perforation from small bowel ulcers or, less commonly, colonic ulcers are well recognized. Physical findings are nonspecific. CMV colitis almost always occurs when the CD4+ T-lymphocyte count is less than 100 cells per microliter. Serologic studies for CMV antibody are not specific. In the absence of a coinfection, stool tests are negative. White blood cells may be present with severe colitis. Abdominal radiographs are noncontributory unless the patient presents with toxic megacolon, where colonic dilation and "thumbprinting" of the mucosa may be observed. Barium enemas should not be used to evaluate colitis in HIV-infected patients. The main diagnostic tool is endoscopy with mucosal biopsies. In general, special histologic stains are not necessary for the diagnosis of CMV or other GI opportunistic disorders provided an experienced GI pathologist examines the biopsy specimens.[111] Sigmoidoscopy is generally sufficient; however, CMV disease may be isolated to the right colon, thereby requiring full colonoscopy for diagnosis.[83] Endoscopically, the most common appearance includes edema, submucosal hemorrhages, and multiple ulcerations. The viral cytopathic effect of CMV should be identified by histopathologic evaluation of multiple biopsy specimens to confirm the diagnosis.

The clinical presentation and response to therapy of *C. difficile* colitis are no different in HIV-infected or HIV-uninfected patients.[112] In the appropriate clinical setting, detection of *C. difficile* toxin is diagnostic. Fecal leukocytes are usually present (60%) and are an important clue to the diagnosis. Flexible sigmoidoscopy is warranted in the patient in whom the disease is suspected but stool toxin is negative.

Amebiasis presents classically as "dysentery" with mucopurulent, bloody diarrhea, tenesmus, crampy abdominal pain, and fever. Amebiasis can also present as fulminant colitis with toxic megacolon, ameboma, and liver abscess. These more virulent presentations are not increased in the HIV-infected patient. Ameba are frequently found on routine stool studies from both asymptomatic and symptomatic homosexual men. In these patients colonization with nonpathogenic ameba (nonpathogenic zymodemes), including *Entamoeba dispar*, *Entamoeba hartmanni*, and *Escherichia coli*, are likely, as they are indistinguishable by light microscopy from pathogenic ameba.[113] One might anticipate that colonization, even with nonpathogenic strains, would cause significant disease in immunocompromised patients. Instead, a benign clinical course has been found. A number of symptomatic patients in whom amebae were identified had other potential pathogens, suggesting that a search for other pathogens is always appropriate in a symptomatic HIV-infected patient with diarrhea and amebic cysts in the stool. In addition, despite clearance of these protozoa from the stool, treatment has not been shown to cure the diarrhea reliably, suggesting that in most patients they do not represent pathogens (i.e., *E. dispar*).

Amebiasis is generally diagnosed by microscopic examination of a rectal swab or a wet mount of fresh stool. As with *Giardia*, multiple stool samples (three to six) may be required because of the intermittent shedding of the cysts and trophozoites. Serologic tests (indirect hemagglutination), agar cell diffusion, counterimmunoelectrophoresis, and enzyme immunoassay techniques are sensitive and specific in patients with invasive *Entamoeba histolytica*.

The most frequent symptoms of GI histoplasmosis are fever, diarrhea, weight loss, and abdominal pain. The endoscopic appearance is that of a single segmental or constricting mass, but multiple ulcerations mimicking Crohn's disease have been described.[108] The diagnosis is made by identifying the fungus histologically and by culturing biopsy specimens.

Therapy

The antibiotic of choice for a presumed bacterial enterocolitis is a quinolone such as ciprofloxacin (500 mg PO bid). Potential drug-drug interactions must be carefully assessed. As with normal hosts infected with these organisms, the duration of therapy should be 7–10 days. Clinical experience with HIV-infected patients suggests that infections with *Shigella* sp. and *Campylobacter* sp. are occasionally recurrent after successful treatment and are more resistant to antimicrobial therapy. For the treatment of *C. difficile* diarrhea, two drugs are widely available and effective. Metronidazole (250–500 mg PO or IV tid for 7–10 days) represents first-line therapy. Vancomycin should be reserved for patients with a contraindication to or failure of metronidazole or when the disease is life-threatening; this agent is effective only when administered orally. Clinical cure can be obtained in essentially all patients. The relapse rate appears to be similar in HIV-infected and HIV-uninfected patients.

The treatment of CMV GI disease was discussed under infections of the esophagus.

Metronidazole (750 mg tid for 10–14 days) is highly effective for invasive *Entamoeba histolytica*, and relapse after curative therapy is rare. Because metronidazole is effective for cysts (which remain in the gut lumen), use of a luminally acting agent to eradicate intestinal colonization is recommended for those with invasive amebiasis or for the asymptomatic "cyst excretor" who has a positive serology. Three major luminally active agents are available: iodoquinol (650 mg PO tid for 20 days), diloxanide furoate (500 mg PO tid for 10 days), and paromomycin (25–30 mg kg^{-1} day^{-1} in three divided doses for 7 days). All have efficacy rates of 85–95% for the eradication of cyst passage. There is no convincing evidence of an increased incidence of either *Dientamoeba fragilis* or *Blastocystis hominis* in AIDS patients.

Therapy for MAC has improved substantially over the last decade. Previously used multidrug regimens were poorly tolerated, were associated with significant side effects, and had low efficacy.[114] It has now been clearly established that a macrolide (clarithromycin)-containing multidrug regimen is superior to a nonmacrolide-containing regimen for initial therapy of MAC disease.[115] Therapy and prophylaxis for GI MAC parallels that for disseminated infection.

Amphotericin B is the drug of choice for colonic histoplasmosis, and the recommended dosing is the same as for disseminated histoplasmosis. A liposomal preparation is required in some patients. Secondary prophylaxis should be provided with itraconazole, fluconazole, or weekly amphotericin B.

Symptomatic Therapies for Diarrhea

For patients in whom antimicrobial therapy is ineffective or no specific cause for diarrhea is found despite multiple stool analysis and endoscopy with biopsies, symptomatic therapy is necessary. When the diarrhea is mild, bulking agents (bismuth or Kaopectate) may provide relief. With more severe diarrhea, medications to reduce intestinal transit are required. We routinely use diphenoxylate (Lomotil) in doses up to 10 tablets/day. Larger doses may cause anticholinergic side effects, as diphenoxylate is combined with atropine in Lomotil.

Despite the potential for abuse, narcotic agents are also highly effective agents. In patients with severe diarrhea, tincture of opium (paregoric) is highly effective. It is usually provided with a dropper that provides a morphine concentration of 0.4 mg/mL. The normal dose is 5–10 mL/day in divided doses, and the dose can be titrated up to 20 mL/day. Some patients experience somnolence or abdominal cramps, which tend to dissipate over time.

Octreotide, a somatostatin analog, is an antisecretory agent with a variety of inhibitory functions throughout the GI tract. Initial studies in patients with AIDS found that this drug provides effective control of diarrhea in ~50% of patients. However, a large randomized placebo-controlled trial did not demonstrate efficacy of this agent in patients with and without identifiable pathogens.[116] The drug is given subcutaneously in doses of 50–500 μg tid. Side effects include decreased biliary motility (gallstones), diabetes, and steatorrhea, the latter of which can potentially exacerbate diarrhea. Although the drug has not been clearly proved to be effective, use in patients with severe diarrhea requiring hospitalization (e.g., *Cryptosporidia*) may be attempted. We define a clinical response as a reduction in stool frequency/volume of at least 50%.

REFERENCES

1. Mönkenmüller KE, Call SA, Lazenby AJ, Wilcox CM. Declining prevalence of opportunistic gastrointestinal disease in the era of combination antiretroviral therapy. Am J Gastroenterol 95:457–62, 2000.
2. San-Andres FJ, Rubio R, Castilla J, et al. Incidence of acquired immunodeficiency syndrome-associated opportunistic diseases and the effect of treatment on a cohort of 1115 patients infected with human immunodeficiency virus, 1989–1997. Clin Infect Dis 36:1177–85, 2003.
3. Chong VH, Lim CC. Human immunodeficiency virus and endoscopy: Experience of a general hospital in Singapore. J Gastroenterol Hepatol 2005;20:722–6.
4. Bonnet F, Lewden C, May T, et al. Opportunistic infections as causes of death in HIV-infected patients in the HAART era in France. Scand J Infect Dis 37:482–7, 2005.
5. Mönkenmüller KE, Lazenby AJ, Lee DH, et al. Occurrence of gastrointestinal opportunistic disorders in AIDS despite the use of highly active antiretroviral therapy. Dig Dis Sci 50:230–4, 2005.
6. Bonacini M, Young T, Laine L. The causes of esophageal symptoms in human immunodeficiency virus infection: a prospective study of 110 patients. Arch Intern Med 151:1567, 1991.
7. Mocroft A, Oancea C, van Lunzen J, et al. Decline in esophageal candidiasis and use of antimycotics in European patients with HIV. Am J Gastroenterol 100:1446–54, 2005.
8. Wilcox CM, Straub RF, Clark WS. Prospective evaluation of oropharyngeal findings in human immunodeficiency virus-infected patients with esophageal ulcer. Am J Gastroenterol 90:1938, 1995.
9. Weinert M, Grimes RM, Lynch DP. Oral manifestations of HIV infection. Ann Intern Med 125:485, 1996.
10. Wilcox CM. Evaluation of a technique to evaluate the underlying mucosa in patients with AIDS and severe *Candida* esophagitis. Gastrointest Endosc 42:360, 1995.
11. Sanglard D, Odds FC. Resistance of *Candida* species to antifungal agents: molecular mechanisms and clinical consequences. Lancet 2:73–85, 2002.
12. Troillet N, Durussel C, Bille J, et al. Correlation between in vitro susceptibility of *Candida albicans* and fluconazole-resistant oropharyngeal candidiasis in HIV-infected patients. Eur J Clin Microbiol Infect Dis 12:911, 1993.
13. Gallant JE, Moore RD, Richman DD, et al. Incidence and natural history of cytomegalovirus disease in patients with advanced human immunodeficiency virus disease treated with zidovudine. J Infect Dis 166:1223, 1992.
14. Salzberger B, Hartmann P, Hanses F, et al. Incidence and prognosis of CMV disease in HIV-infected patients before and after introduction of combination antiretroviral therapy. Infection 33:345–9, 2005.
15. Wilcox CM, Schwartz DA, Clark WS. Causes, response to therapy, and long-term outcome of esophageal ulcer in patients with human immunodeficiency virus infection. Ann Intern Med 122:143, 1995.
16. Genereau T, Lortholary O, Bouchaud O, et al. Herpes simplex esophagitis in patients with AIDS: report of 34 cases. Clin Infect Dis 22:926, 1996.
17. Wilcox CM, Zaki SR, Coffield LM, et al. Evaluation of idiopathic esophageal ulcer for human immunodeficiency virus. Mod Pathol 8:568, 1995.
18. Mönkemüller KE, Wilcox CM. Diagnosis and treatment of esophageal ulcers in AIDS. Semin Gastroeneterol 10:1, 1999.
19. Wilcox CM, Straub RA, Schwartz DA. Prospective endoscopic characterization of cytomegalovirus esophagitis in patients with AIDS. Gastrointest Endosc 40:481, 1994.
20. Wilcox CM, Rodgers W, Lazenby A. Prospective comparison of brush cytology, viral culture, and histology for the diagnosis of ulcerative esophagitis in AIDS. Clin Gastroenterol Hepatol 2:564–7, 2004.
21. Wohl DA, Zeng D, Stewart P, et al. Cytomegalovirus viremia, mortality, and end-organ disease among patients with AIDS receiving potent antiretroviral therapies. J Acquir Immune Defic Syndr 38:538–44, 2005.
22. Deayton JR, Prof Sabin CA, Johnson MA, et al. Importance of cytomegalovirus viraemia in risk of disease progression and death in HIV-infected patients receiving highly active antiretroviral therapy. Lancet 363:2116–21, 2004.
23. Wilcox CM, Alexander LN, Clark WS, Thompson SE. Fluconazole compared with endoscopy for human immunodeficiency virus-infected patients with esophageal symptoms. Gastroenterology 110:1803, 1996.
24. Pons V, Greenspan D, Derbruin M, et al. Therapy for oropharyngeal candidiasis in HIV-infected patients: a randomized, prospective multicenter study of oral fluconazole versus clotrimazole troches. J Acquir Immune Defic Syndr 6:1311, 1993.
25. Cha R, Sobel JD. Fluconazole for the treatment of candidiasis: 15 years experience. Expert Rev Anti Infect Ther 2:357–66, 2004.
26. Pons V, Greenspan D, Lozada-Nur F, et al. Oropharyngeal candidiasis in patients with AIDS: randomized comparison of fluconazole versus nystatin oral suspensions. Clin Infect Dis 24:1204, 1997.
27. DeWit S, Goosens H, Clumeck N. Single-dose versus 7 days of fluconazole treatment for oral candidiasis in human

immunodeficiency virus-infected patients: a prospective, random ized pilot study. J Infect Dis 168:1332, 1993.
28. Goldman M, Cloud GA, Wade KD, et al. A randomized study of the use of fluconazole in continuous versus episodic therapy in patients with advanced HIV infection and a history of oropharyngeal candidiasis: AIDS Clinical Trials Group Study 323/ Mycoses Study Group Study 40. Clin Infect Dis 41:1473, 2005.
29. Laine L, Dretler RH, Conteas CN, et al. Fluconazole compared with ketoconazole for the treatment of candida esophagitis in AIDS: a randomized trial. Ann Intern Med 117:655, 1992.
30. Wilcox CM. Time course of clinical response to fluconazole for *Candida* oesphagitis in AIDS. Aliment Pharmacol Ther 8:347, 1994.
31. Barbaro G, Barbarini G, Caladeron W, et al. Fluconazole versus itraconazole for *Candida* esophagitis in acquired immunodeficiency syndrome. Gastroenterology 111:1169, 1996.
32. Wilcox CM, Darouiche RO, Laine L, et al. A randomized, double-blind comparison of itraconazole oral solution and fluconazole tablets in the treatment of esophageal candidiasis. J Infect Dis 176:227, 1997.
33. Fichtenbaum CJ, Zackin R, Rajicic N, et al. Amphotericin B oral suspension for fluconazole-refractory oral candidiasis in persons with HIV infection. Adult AIDS Clinical Trials Group Study Team 295. AIDS 14:845, 2000.
34. Maschmeyer G, Glasmacher A. Pharmacological properties and clinical efficacy of a recently licensed systemic antifungal, caspofungin. Mycoses 48:227–34, 2005.
35. Villanueva A, Gotuzzo E, Arathoon EG, et al. A randomized double-blind study of caspofungin versus fluconazole for the treatment of esophageal candidiasis. Am J Med 113:294–9, 2002.
36. Arathoon EG, Gotuzzo E, Noriega LM, et al. Randomized, double-blind, multicenter study of caspofungin versus amphotericin B for treatment of oropharyngeal and esophageal candidiases. Antimicrob Agents Chemother 46:451–7, 2002.
37. Kartsonis N, DiNubile MJ, Bartizal K, et al. Efficacy of caspofungin in the treatment of esophageal candidiasis resistant to fluconazole. J Acquir Immune Defic Syndr 31:183–7, 2002.
38. Dinubile MJ, Lupinacci RJ, Berman RS, et al. Response and relapse rates of candidal esophagitis in HIV-infected patients treated with caspofungin. AIDS Res Hum Retroviruses 18:903, 2002.
39. de Wet N, Llanos-Cuentas A, Suleiman J, et al. A randomized, double-blind, parallel-group, dose-response study of micafungin compared with fluconazole for the treatment of esophageal candidiasis in HIV-positive patients. Clin Infect Dis 39:842–9, 2004.
40. Fichtenbaum CJ, Koletar S, Yiannotsos C, et al. Refractory mucosal candidiasis in advanced human immunodeficiency virus infection. Clin Infect Dis 30:749, 2000.
41. Willemot P, Klein MB. Prevention of HIV-associated opportunistic infections and diseases in the age of highly active antiretroviral therapy. Expert Rev Anti Infect Ther 2:521–32, 2004.
42. Cvetkovic RS, Wellington K. Valganciclovir: a review of its use in the management of CMV infection and disease in immunocompromised patients. Drugs 65:859–78, 2005.
43. Wilcox CM, Straub RF, Schwartz DA. Cytomegalovirus esophagitis in AIDS: a prospective study of clinical response to ganciclovir therapy, relapse rate, and long-term outcome. Am J Med 98:169, 1995.
44. Parente F, Bianchi Porro G. Treatment of cytomegalovirus esophagitis in patients with acquired immunodeficiency syndrome: a randomized controlled study of foscarnet versus ganciclovir; the Italian Cytomegalovirus Study Group. Am J Gastroenterol 93:317, 1998.
45. Blanshard C. Treatment of HIV-related cytomegalovirus disease of the gastrointestinal tract with foscarnet. J Acquir Immune Defic Syndr 5(Suppl 1):S25, 1992.
46. Dieterich DT, Kotler DP, Busch DF, et al. Ganciclovir treatment of cytomegalovirus colitis in AIDS: a randomized, double-blind, placebo-controlled multicenter study. J Infect Dis 167:278, 1993.
47. Blanshard C, Benhamou Y, Dohin E, et al. Treatment of AIDS-associated gastrointestinal cytomegalovirus infection with foscarnet and ganciclovir: a randomized comparison. J Infect Dis 172:622, 1995.
48. Mönkemüller KE, Wilcox CM. Esophageal ulcer caused by cytomegalovirus: resolution during combination antiretroviral therapy for acquired immunodeficiency syndrome. South Med J 93:818, 2000.
49. Freeman RB. Valganciclovir: oral prevention and treatment of cytomegalovirus in the immunocompromixed host. Expert Opin Pharmacother 5:2007–16, 2004.
50. Piketty C, Bardin C, Gilquin J, et al. Low plasma concentrations achieved with conventional schedules of administration of ganciclovir in patients with AIDS. J Infect Dis 174:188, 1996.
51. Chou SW. Cytomegalovirus drug resistance and clinical implications. Transpl Infect Dis 3 Suppl 2:20–4, 2001.
52. Dieterich DT, Poles MA, Dicker M, et al. Foscarnet treatment of cytomegalovirus gastrointestinal infections in acquired immunodeficiency syndrome patients who have failed ganciclovir induction. Am J Gastroenterol 88:542, 1993.
53. Salzberger B, Stoehr A, Jablonowski H, et al. Foscarnet 5 versus 7 days a week treatment for severe gastrointestinal CMV disease in HIV-infected patients. Infection 24:121–4, 1996.
54. Salzberger B, Stoehr A, Heise W, et al. Foscarnet and ganciclovir combination therapy for CMV disease in HIV-infected patients. Infection 22:197, 1994.
55. Spector SA, Mc Kinley, Lalezari JP, et al. Oral ganciclovir for the prevention of cytomegalovirus disease in persons with AIDS. N Engl J Med 334:1491, 1996.
56. Brady RC, Bernstein DI. Treatment of herpes simplex virus infections. Antiviral Res 61:73–81, 2004.
57. Laskin OL. Clinical pharmacokinetics of acyclovir. Clin Pharmacokinet 8:187, 1983.
58. Hardy WD. Foscarnet treatment of acyclovir-resistant herpes simplex virus infection in patients with acquired immunodeficiency syndrome: preliminary results of a controlled, randomized, regimen-comparative trial. Am J Med 92(2A):30S-5S, 1992.
59. Morfin F, Thouvenot D. Herpes simplex virus resistance to antiviral drugs. J Clin Virol 26:29–37, 2003.
60. Wilcox CM, Schwartz DA. Comparison of two corticosteroid regimens for the treatment of idiopathic esophageal ulcerations associated with HIV infection. Am J Gastroenterol 89:2163, 1994.
61. Nelson MR, Erskine D, Hawkins DA, Gazzard BG. Treatment with corticosteroids: a risk factor for the development of clinical cytomegalovirus disease in AIDS. AIDS 7:375, 1993.
62. Paterson DL, Georghiou PR, Allworth AM, Kemp RJ. Thalidomide as treatment of refractory aphthous ulceration related to human immunodeficiency virus infection. Clin Infect Dis 20:250, 1995.
63. Alexander LN, Wilcox CM. A prospective trial of thalidomide for the treatment of HIV-associated idiopathic esophageal ulcers. AIDS Res Hum Retroviruses 13:301, 1997.
64. Pensa E, Borum ML. Opportunistic infections. Gastric infections in HIV/AIDS. AIDS Read 10:347–9, 356–8, 2000.
65. Chiu HM, Wu MS, Hung CC, et al. Low prevalence of *Helicobacter pylori* but high prevalence of cytomegalovirus-associated peptic ulcer disease in AIDS patients: Comparative study of symptomatic subjects evaluated by endoscopy and CD4 counts. J Gastroenterol Hepatol 19:423–8, 2004.
66. Cacciarelli AG, Marano BJ Jr, Gualtieri NM, et al. Lower *Helicobacter pylori* infection and peptic ulcer disease prevalence

in patients with AIDS and suppressed CD4 counts. Am J Gastroenterol 91:1783, 1996.

67. AliMohamed F, Lule GN, Nyong'o A, et al. Prevalence of *Helicobacter pylori* and endoscopic findings in HIV seropositive patients with upper gastrointestinal tract symptoms at Kenyatta National Hospital, Nairobi. East Afr Med J 79: 226–31, 2002.
68. Olmos M, Araya V, Pskorz E, et al. Coinfection: *Helicobacter pylori*/ human immunodeficiency virus. Dig Dis Sci 49:1836–9, 2004.
69. Varsky CG, Correa MC, Sarmiento N, et al. Prevalence and etiology of gastroduodenal ulcer in HIV-positive patients: a comparative study of 497 symptomatic subjects evaluated by endoscopy. Am J Gastroenterol 93:935, 1998.
70. Marano BJ Jr, Smith F, Bonanno CA. *Helicobacter pylori* prevalence in acquired immunodeficiency syndrome. Am J Gastroenterol 88:687, 1993.
71. Edwards PD, Carrick J, Turner J, et al. *Helicobacter pylori*-associated gastritis is rare in AIDS: antibiotic effect or a consequence of immunodeficiency? Am J Gastroenterol 86:1761, 1991.
72. Thuluvath PJ, Connolly GM, Forbes A, et al. Abdominal pain in HIV infection. Q J Med 78:275, 1993.
73. Smith SJ, Du Toit RS. The acute AIDS abdomen – a prospective clinical and pathological study. S Afr J Surg 43:88, 2005.
74. Mönkemüller KE, Wilcox CM. Diagnosis and treatment of colonic disease in AIDS. Gastrointest Endosc Clin North Am 8:889, 1998.
75. Reisler RB, Murphy RL, Redfield RR, et al. Incidence of pancreatitis in HIV-1-infected individuals enrolled in 20 adult AIDS clinical trials group studies: lessons learned. JAIDS 39:159, 2005.
76. Jeffrey RB, Nyberg DA, Bottles K, et al. Abdominal CT in acquired immunodeficiency syndrome. AJR Am J Roentgenol 146:7, 1986.
77. Sauerland S, Agresta F, Bergamaschi R, et al. Laparoscopy for abdominal emergencies. Evidence-based guidelines of the European Association for Endoscopic Surgery. Surg Endosc 24, 2005 (Epub ahead of print).
78. Saltzman DJ, Williams RA, Gelfand DV, Wilson SE. The surgeon and AIDS: twenty years later. Arch Surg 140:961–7, 2005.
79. Call SA, Heudebert G, Saag M, Wilcox CM. The changing etiology of chronic diarrhea in HIV-infected patients with CD4 cell counts less than 200 cells/mm3. Am J Gastroenterol 95:3142–6, 2000.
80. Goodgame RW. Understanding intestinal spore-forming protozoa: *Cryptosporidia*, *Microsporidia*, *Isospora*, and *Cyclospora*. Ann Intern Med 124:429, 1996.
81. Sadraei J, Rizvi MA, Baveja UK. Diarrhea, CD4+ cell counts and opportunistic protozoa in Indian HIV-infected patients. Parasitol Res 97:270–3, 2005.
82. Blanshard C, Francis N, Gazzard BG. Investigation of chronic diarrhea in acquired immunodeficiency syndrome: a prospective study of 155 patients. Gut 39:824, 1996.
83. Wilcox CM, Rabeneck L, Friedman S. AGA technical review: malnutrition and cachexia, chronic diarrhea, and hepatobiliary disease in patients with human immunodeficiency virus infection. Gastroenterology 111:1724–52, 1996.
84. Connolly GM, Dryden MS, Shanson DC, Gazzard BG. Cryptosporidial diarrhea in AIDS and its treatment. Gut 29:593, 1988.
85. Bern C, Kawai V, Bargas D, et al. The epidemiology of intestinal microsporidiosis in patients with HIV/AIDS in Lima, Peru. J Infect Dis 191:1658–64, 2005.
86. Kotler DP, Orenstein JM. Prevalence of intestinal microsporidiosis in HIV-infected patients referred for gastroenterological evaluation. Am J Gastroenterol 89:1998, 1994.
87. Pape JW, Verdier R-I, Boncy M, et al. *Cyclospora* infection in adults infected with HIV: clinical manifestations, treatment, and prophylaxis. Ann Intern Med 121:654, 1994.
88. Kaplan JE, Hanson D, Dworkin MS, et al. Epidemiology of human immunodeficiency virus-associated opportunistic infections in the United States in the era of highly active antiretroviral therapy. Clin Infectious Dis 30-S5-14, 2000.
89. Grohmann GS, Glass RI, Pereira HG, et al. Enteric viruses and diarrhea in HIV-infected patients. N Engl Med 329:14, 1993.
90. Flanigan T, Whalen C, Turner J, et al. *Cryptosporidium* infection and CD4 counts. Ann Intern Med 116:840, 1992.
91. Benson C. Disseminated *Mycobacterium avium-intracellulare* complex in patients with AIDS. AIDS Res Hum Retroviruses 10:913, 1994.
92. Gordin FM, Cohn DL, Sullam PM, et al. Early manifestations of disseminated *Mycobacterium avium* complex disease; a prospective evaluation. J Infect Dis 176:126, 1997.
93. Orenstein JM. Diagnostic pathology of microsporidiosis. Ultrastruct Pathol 27:141–9, 2003.
94. Farthing MJ. Giardiasis. Gastroenterol Clin North Am 25: 493–515, 1996.
95. Chin DP, Hopewell PC, Yajko DM, et al. *Mycobacterium avium* complex in the respiratory or gastrointestinal tract and the risk of *M. avium* complex bacteremia in patients with human immunodeficiency virus infection. J Infect Dis 169:289, 1994.
96. Zardi EM, Picardi A, Afeltra A. Treatment of cyrptosporidiosis in immunocompromised hosts. Chemotherapy 51:193, 2005.
97. Carr A, Marriott D, Field A, et al. Treatment of HIV-1 associated microsporidiosis and cryptosporidiosis with combination antiretroviral therapy. Lancet 351:256, 1998.
98. White AC, Chappell CL, Hayat CS, et al. Paromomycin for cryptosporidiosis in AIDS: a prospective, double-blind trial. J Infect Dis 170:419, 1994.
99. Bissuel F, Cotte L, Rabodonirina M, et al. Paromomycin: an effective treatment for cryptosporidial diarrhea in patients with AIDS. Clin Infect Dis 18:447, 1994.
100. Hewitt RG, Yiannoutsos CT, Higgs ES, et al. Paromomycin: no more effective than placebo for treatment of cryptosporidiosis in patients with advanced human immunodeficiency virus infection. Clin Infect Dis 31:1084, 2000.
101. Eeftinck Schattenkerk JKM, van Gool T, van Ketel RJ, et al. Clinical significance of small-intestinal microsporidiosis in HIV-1-infected individuals. Lancet 337:895, 1991.
102. Dore GJ, Marriott DJ, Hing MC, et al. Disseminated microsporidiosis due to *Septata intestinalis* in nine patients infected with the human immunodeficiency virus: response to therapy with albendazole. Clin Infect Dis 21:70, 1995.
103. Molina JM, Oksenhendler E, Beauvais B, et al. Disseminated microsporidiosis due to *Septata intestinalis* in patients with AIDS: clinical features and response to albendazole therapy. J Infect Dis 171:245, 1995.
104. Molina JM, Tourneur M, Sarfati C, et al. Fumagillin treatment of intestinal microsporidiosis. N Engl J Med 346:1963, 2002.
105. DeHovitz JA, Pape JW, Boncy M, Johnson WD Jr. Clinical manifestations and treatment of *Isospora belli* infection in patients with acquired immunodeficiency syndrome. N Engl J Med 315:87, 1986.
106. Sanchez TH, Brooks JT, Sullivan PS, et al. Bacterial diarrhea in persons with HIV infection, United States, 1992–2002. Clin Inffect Dis 41:1621–27, 2005.
107. Wei SC, Hung CC, Chen MY, et al. Endoscopy in acquired immunodeficiency syndrome patients with diarrhea and negative stool studies. Gastrointest Endosc 51:427–32, 2000.
108. Kahi CJ, Wheat LJ, Allen SD, Sarosi GA. Gastrointestinal Histoplasmosis. Am J Gastroenterol 100:220–31, 2005.
109. Barcus AL, Burdette SD, Herchline TE. Intestinal invasion and disseminated disease associated with *Penicillium chrysogenum*. Ann Clin Microb Antibio 4:21, 2005 (Epub ahead of print).

110. Pinlaor S, Mootsikapun P, Pinlaor P, et al. Detection of opportunistic and non-opportunistic intestinal parasites and liver flukes in HIV-positive and HIV-negative subjects. Southeast Asian J Trop Med Public Health 36:841–5, 2005.
111. Mönkemüller KE, Bussian AH, Lazenby AJ, Wilcox CM. Special histologic stains are rarely beneficial for the evaluation of HIV-related gastrointestinal infections. Am J Clin Pathol 114:387, 2000.
112. Hutin Y, Molina JM, Casin I, et al. Risk factors for *Clostridium difficile*-associated diarrhoea in HIV-infected patients. AIDS 7:1441, 1993.
113. Kebede A, Verweij J, Dorigo-Zetsma W, et al. Overdiagnosis of amoebiasis in the absence of *Entamoeba histolytica* among patients presenting with diarrhoea in Wonji and Akaki, Ethopia. Trans R Soc Trop Med Hyg 97:305–07, 2003.
114. Kemper CA, Meng T-C, Nussbaum J, et al. Treatment of Mycobacterium avium complex bacteremia in AIDS with a four-drug oral regimen: rifampin, ethambutol, clofazimine, and ciprofloxacin. Ann Intern Med 116:466, 1992.
115. Karakousis PC, Moore RD, Chaisson RE. Mycobacterium avium complex in patients with HIV infection in the era of highly active antiretroviral therapy. Lancet Infect Dis 4: 557–65, 2004.
116. Simon DM, Cello JP, Valenzuela J, et al. Multicenter trial of octreotide in patients with refractory acquired immunodeficiency syndrome-associated diarrhea. Gastroenterology 108:1753, 1995.

Chapter 78

Hepatic and Hepatobiliary Diseases

Nicole M. Martin, MD, Raymond T. Chung, MD, Kenneth E. Sherman, MD, PhD

Diseases of the liver are a major source of morbidity and mortality in patients with human immunodeficiency virus (HIV) infection. Liver-related conditions accounted for 13% of HIV-related hospitalizations in the year 2000, having increased from 8% in 1996.[1] Although immune reconstitution and prevention of severe acquired immunodeficiency has decreased the prevalence of most opportunistic infections, the high prevalence of chronic hepatotropic viruses in this population has become increasingly troublesome.[2] Furthermore, the very medications that improve life expectancy in HIV-infected patients may alter hepatic metabolism and produce features of direct and indirect hepatotoxicity.[3] Finally, some of the more common metabolic disorders of the liver assume increased importance because of their contribution to chronic liver diseases. The evaluation and management of hepatic and hepatobiliary diseases has become a critical consideration for healthcare providers caring for patients with HIV infection.

CLINICAL EVALUATION

History

Obtaining a detailed history related to liver disease is perhaps the most crucial element of an evaluation of the patient with clinical or biochemical evidence of liver injury. Disease processes that must be considered include viral infections, medications, recreational drugs, toxic occupational exposures, vascular/thrombotic disorders, and inherited metabolic conditions. A detailed history of potential exposure to hepatotropic viruses is important for establishing a timeline for infection. This history should include the year of first exposure to intravenous drugs, nasal cocaine use, tattoos, body piercing, blood transfusion, and sexual exposures. Studies of injection drug users suggest that most of those with chronic hepatitis C virus (HCV) infection become infected during the first year of abuse. Risk of HCV was common in patients who received blood and blood products prior to 1991. Nearly all hemophilic men who required pooled factors prior to that time are HCV-infected. High-risk sexual behavior is a clear risk for hepatitis B infection and probably for HCV as well.[4] Recent analysis of clusters of acute HCV infection reveals that a history of unprotected receptive and insertive anal intercourse and fisting was highly associated with disease transmission.[5]

Medication history must be detailed and include all drugs started or stopped within a 3-month period. It is critical to include medications used transiently. For example, the use of common antibiotics such as amoxicillin-clavulinic acid (Augmentin) can cause severe cholestasis 2–12 weeks after a short drug course and is often missed by healthcare providers as a potential cause of liver injury.[6] Drug interactions must also be considered because some medications compete for active binding sites in hepatic mixed-function oxidase or cytochrome pathways, leading to toxic injury. Alcohol use should be estimated in terms of grams of ethanol ingested per day.

Family history is essential for establishing the possibility that the patient has an underlying inborn error of metabolism. A history of early cirrhosis (<45 years old) even in a relative should raise suspicion of a coexistent metabolic cause of injury. For instance, hereditary hemochromatosis and α_1-antitrypsin (AAT) deficiency are quite common in certain ethnic groups.[7]

A review of the medical history for a patient with HIV infection must also include a detailed assessment of immunologic status. Patients with very low CD4+ T-lymphocyte counts (<50 cells/μL) are more susceptible to hepatic injury from infiltrative processes (Kaposi sarcoma, non-Hodgkin lymphoma, granulomatous disease) and less susceptible to injury from hepatitis B than those with a CD4+ T-lymphocyte count higher than 500 cells/μL. Patients who have undergone immune reconstitution may represent a special risk in terms of injury from hepatitis B[8,9] and hepatitis C.[10] Because immune reconstitution is generally associated with use of highly active antiretroviral agents, which may independently cause liver toxicity, the healthcare provider must carefully document the timing of immunologic recovery as related to the onset of liver injury.

Physical Examination

The physical examination may provide valuable information related to chronicity and occasionally to etiology. The HEENT (head, ears, eyes, nose, throat) examination should focus on the presence or absence of scleral icterus. Mild jaundice may be observed by experienced clinicians when the serum bilirubin level is 2–3 mg/dL. The sclera are examined first, but the underside of the tongue may also yield evidence of mild yellowing. This feature may be particularly useful in dark-skinned patients with muddy sclerae. The eyelids may show xanthomatous changes, which can occur with chronic cholestasis.

The abdomen must be carefully evaluated in patients suspected of having liver disease. Hepatomegaly with palpation tenderness suggests an acute process, though several series have reported a high prevalence of hepatic enlargement in patients with HIV infection. Preferential hypertrophy of the left lobe is often seen with chronic liver disease. The triad of hepatomegaly, pain on liver palpation, and ascites suggest the possibility of a vascular thrombosis of the hepatic vein (Budd–Chiari syndrome). The presence of ascites mandates a workup for the etiology, but nonhepatic causes (including severe malnutrition and nephrotic syndrome) must be considered in addition to end-stage liver disease. The presence of a caput on the anterior surface of the abdomen suggests portal hypertension, as does splenomegaly.

The skin examination should include evaluation for spider angiomas on the chest and back and palmar erythema. The latter is not specific for liver disease, however, and in fact is seen in the absence of liver disease, particularly in women. The presence of excoriations raises the possibility of a severe cholestatic process associated with severe pruritus. Drug reactions may cause erythematous eruptions and urticaria.

Neurologic evaluation should include observation for asterixis (a "flap" of the extended hands), which is seen in patients with late-stage liver disease and reflects the presence of hepatic encephalopathy. A number connection tests to evaluate concentration is a valuable tool for clinical management of patients with encephalopathy.[11]

BIOCHEMICAL TESTS

Liver Injury and Synthetic Function

Biochemical screening tests for liver disease generally include a panel of tests that help identify and categorize the type of liver injury. Common tests of liver injury and function can be divided into three groups: (1) tests of hepatocellular injury; (2) tests of cholestatic injury; and (3) tests of liver function capacity.[12,13]

The serum transaminase assay provides an indication of the likelihood and severity of active liver injury. The most sensitive, specific test for hepatocellular injury is the serum alanine aminotransferase (ALT, SGPT) assay. ALT is found predominantly in the cytoplasm of hepatocytes, and death leads to release of ALT into the serum. Most laboratories utilize local ranges of normal derived from "healthy" controls combined with the determination of an arbitrary cutoff for the upper limit of normal determined by the distribution of the "normal" sample population. It is important to understand that the likelihood of liver disease is proportional to the increase in ALT but not absolutely so. Thus, not all patients with mildly increased ALT levels have discernible liver injury, and not all patients with ALT levels in the locally defined normal range lack liver injury. Women tend to have lower ALT levels than men, and standardization is often not gender-adjusted. Therefore the frequency of liver injury in women tends to be underestimated.

The other commonly reported serum transaminase is aspartate aminotransferase (AST, SGOT). This enzyme is present in hepatocytes but is found in high concentrations in muscle, erythrocytes, and other tissues as well. Therefore elevated AST levels are sometimes attributable to nonhepatic etiologies.

During the course of infection, up to 70% of patients with HIV infection have been reported to have abnormally high serum transaminase levels. This high prevalence has prompted a higher threshold for evaluating mild to moderately increased ALT/AST levels in HIV-infected patients. It is important to understand, though, that even mild chronic injury may result in fibrosis and eventual hepatic decompensation. An algorithm for evaluation of hepatocellular injury is shown in Figure 78-1.

Cholestatic injury is indicated by an elevated alkaline phosphatase level, an inducible enzyme produced by hepatocytes. Failure to excrete bile acids (as is seen with cholestasis) leads to induction of alkaline phosphatase, which is excreted into the serum. Bile acid concentration may be increased by a variety of mechanisms including drug-induced canalicular transport dysfunction (e.g., chlorpromazine), small bile duct injury (e.g., primary biliary cirrhosis), large bile duct narrowing (e.g., AIDS cholangiopathy, cholangiocarcinoma), or following acute hepatocellular injury (posthepatitic cholestasis). Because alkaline phosphatase levels can also be due to abnormalities in bone, intestine, and salivary glands, confirmation of a liver source generally requires a concomitant elevation of γ-glutamyl transpeptidase (GGT) or 5′-nucleotidase. These liver enzymes are also induced by bile acids, and the GGT is induced by a variety of drugs and alcohol as well. It is important to note that increased GGT merely suggests cholestasis; it is not a marker of hepatocellular injury, as is often mistakenly thought. The complete evaluation of patients with a cholestatic injury is described in Figure 78-2.

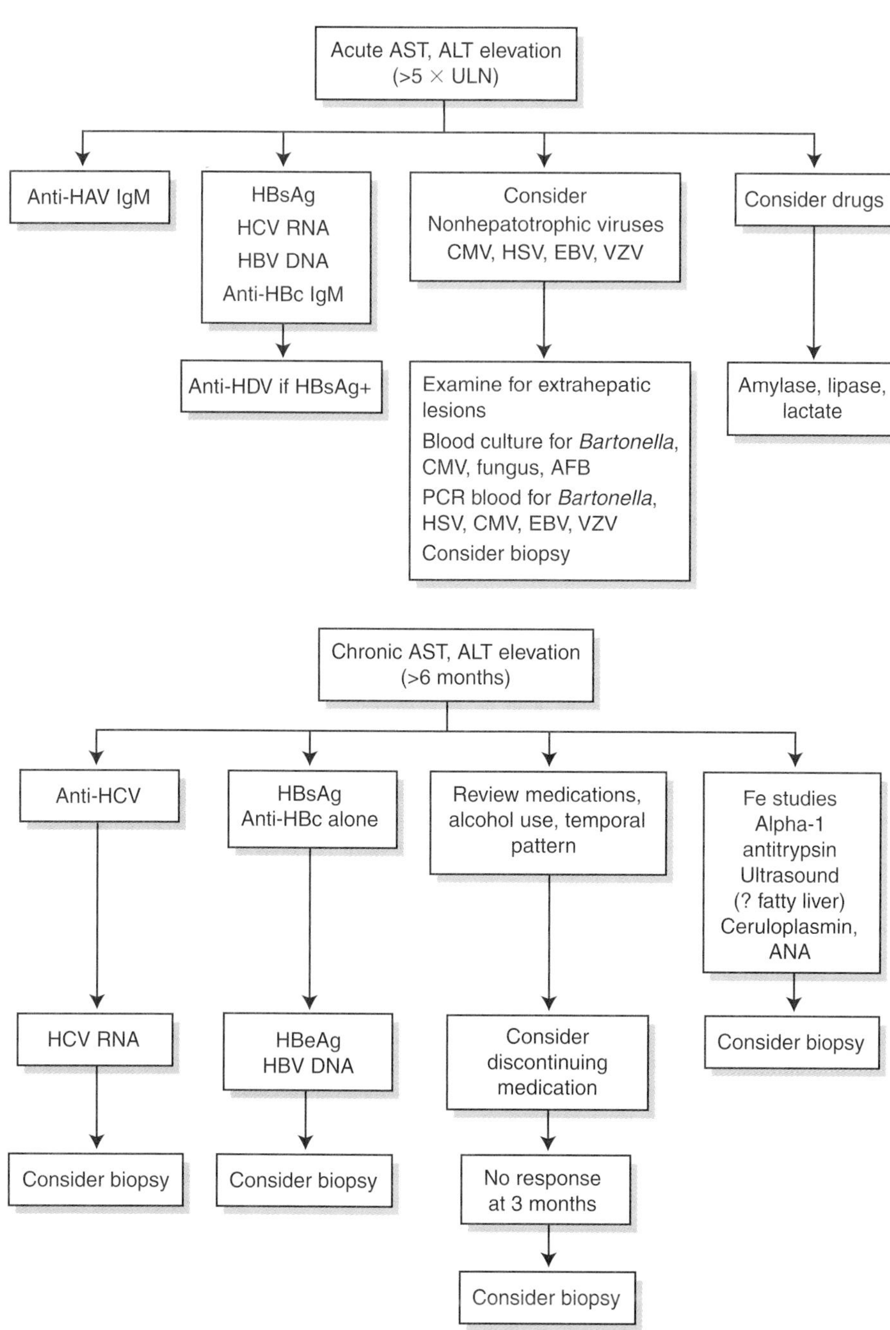

Figure 78-1 ■ Algorithm for evaluating HIV-infected patients with increased serum aminotransferases consistent with a hepatocellular injury pattern. The evaluation is divided between acute and chronic (lasting >6 months) elevations of AST and ALT. ALT, alanine aminotransferase; anti-HAV, hepatitis A antibody; anti-HDV, hepatitis D antibody; ART, antiretroviral therapy; AST, aspartate aminotransferase; HbeAg, hepatitis B "e" antigen; HbsAg, hepatitis B surface antigen; HBV DNA, hepatitis B DNA assay.

Frequently, the term "liver function tests (LFTs)" is used to describe basic biochemical tests of the liver; but this is a misrepresentation, as none of the above named tests measures liver function. Typical chemical profiles often include albumin, which is a measure of liver synthetic function. However, the serum albumin level may be abnormally low in patients with nephrotic-range proteinuria or in those with malnutrition. The prothrombin time (PT) is a more reliable measure of the liver's ability to manufacture clotting factors (II, VII, IX, X). Therefore, a prolonged PT is an indication of impaired synthetic function, although it may also be abnormal because of severe cholestasis and resultant malabsorption of fat-soluble vitamin K. Administration of parenteral vitamin K (10 mg SC or IV) corrects the PT within 3 days and therefore differentiates cholestasis from abnormal liver function due to a shortage of substrate. Specific measurements of liver function include studies of drug metabolism and clearance. Caffeine, bromsulphalein (BSP), and iodocyanine green clearance have all been utilized. Commercial test kits are available for evaluation of monoethylglycinexylidide (MEG-X), which is a metabolic by-product of liver metabolism of lidocaine. Recent studies by Shrestha et al have shown that calculation of a cholate shunt fraction may be a sensitive marker of liver function in patients with advanced liver disease.[14] These tests are generally used only in the research setting.

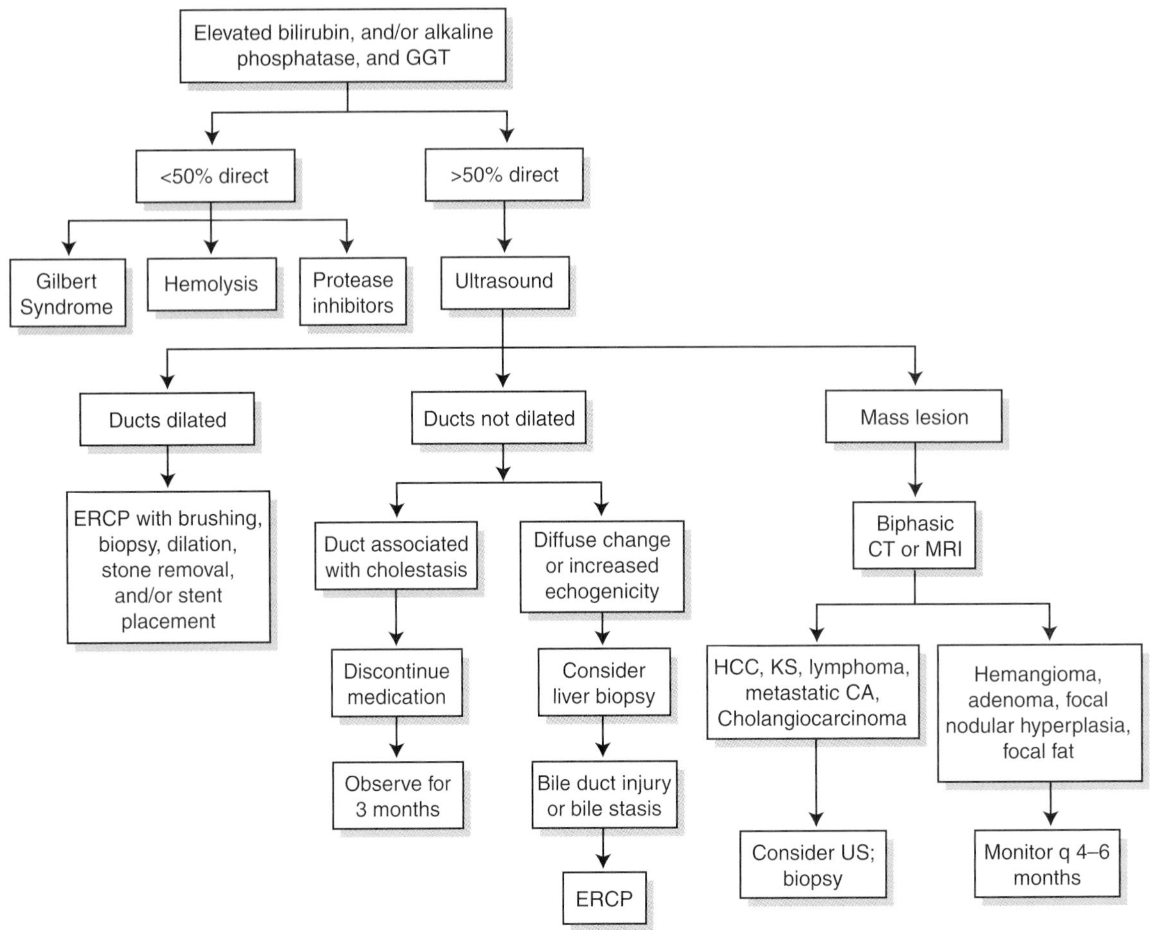

Figure 78-2 ■ Algorithm for evaluating HIV-infected patients with laboratory evidence of a cholestatic injury pattern (increased serum alkaline, phosphatase, GGT, with or without increased total bilirubin). ERCP, endoscopic retrograde cholangiopancreatography; FNH, focal nodular hyperplasia; GGT, γ-glutamyltranspeptidase; HCC, hepatocellular carcinoma; KS, Kaposi sarcoma; 5' NT, 5'-Nucleotidase.

Laboratory Evaluation for Disease Etiology

Although the tests described in the previous section define and classify liver injury, they do not necessarily identify specific etiologies. Some diagnoses are those of exclusion, combined with pertinent historical positives (e.g., drug injury), and others require specific biochemical or serologic tests to suggest or confirm the etiology. The range of diagnoses that must be considered is listed in Table 78-1.

The hepatotropic viruses represent the most important group of infectious agents. Their diagnoses are discussed in turn with specific reference to considerations in patients with HIV infection.

Acute hepatitis A virus (HAV) infection is identified by the appearance of immunoglobulin M (IgM) class antibodies against HAV. The assay turns positive shortly after infection and is considered diagnostic of acute hepatitis A. Many clinical laboratories utilize a test that detects a combination of IgM and IgG antibodies, requiring further testing of IgM class antibody alone to distinguish between acute infection and past exposure. Therefore, the clinician should request fractionation in cases of suspected acute hepatitis A. Prevention of hepatitis A is based on administration of a commercially available hepatitis A vaccine. A sometimes difficult decision for the clinician is whether to test for naturally acquired antibodies prior to vaccine administration. Prevaccination anti-HAV testing greatly enhances the cost-effectiveness of vaccination among the general public.[15] Although no formal analysis has demonstrated the cost-effectiveness of such testing in the HIV-infected population, many HIV-infected patients have a high pretest probability of prior hepatitis A exposure (low socioeconomic strata, homosexual men with multiple partners) and should therefore be tested for antibody prior to vaccine use.

Hepatitis B virus (HBV) infection is generally diagnosed by the presence of circulating hepatitis B surface antigen (HBsAg). The infection is classified as acute or chronic by distinguishing whether the antibodies directed against the virus core antigen (anti-HBc) are of the IgM or IgG class, respectively. Tests for IgG, IgM, and both (total) are available. As with HAV diagnosis, the clinician should select the

Table 78-1

Diseases Affecting the Liver and Biliary Tree in HIV Infection

Viral Hepatitis
Hepatotropic
- Hepatitis A virus
- Hepatitis B virus/hepatitis D virus
- Hepatitis C virus

Nonhepatotropic
- Cytomegalovirus
- Herpes simplex virus
- Epstein–Barr virus
- Varicella-zoster virus
- Human herpesvirus-6
- Adenovirus
- HIV

Fungal liver disease
- *Candida albicans*
- *Histoplasma capsulatum*

Parasitic liver disease
- *Leishmania donovani*
- *Pneumocystis carinii*
- *Microsporidia*

Bacterial liver disease
- *Bacillary angiomatosis*

Granulomatous liver disease
- *Mycobacterium* tuberculosis
- *Mycobacterium avium* complex

Toxic/metabolic liver disease
- Fatty liver, nonalcoholic steatohepatitis
- Nucleoside reverse transcriptase inhibitors (NRTIs)
- Protease inhibitors (PIs)
- Nonnucleoside reverse transcriptase inhibitors (NNRTIs)
- Alcohol
- Other medications

Neoplastic liver disease
- Kaposi sarcoma
- Non-Hodgkin lymphoma
- Hepatocellular carcinoma

AIDS cholangiopathy
- Sclerosing cholangitis
- Papillary stenosis
- Long extrahepatic bile duct strictures

Gallbladder disease
- Acalculous cholecystitis
- Hepatic and hepatobiliary diseases

correct test for the clinical setting. Patients with chronic hepatitis B should be evaluated for the degree of viral replication, which generally correlates with the degree of associated liver injury. In prior years, the replicative state has been determined by testing the level of HBV DNA in serum using a branched-chain-based assay (Quantiplex) or a hybridization-based assay. Whereas qualitative polymerase chain reaction (PCR) assays are not acceptable alternatives because their inordinate level of sensitivity fails to define the replicative state, quantitative PCR assays (Monitor) do provide useful information and have led to significant changes in prognostication and treatment paradigms. Hepatitis B "e" antigen (HBeAg) is generally associated with replicative levels of HBV DNA and may serve as a surrogate marker of replication. The presence of hepatitis B "e" antibody (HBeAb), conversely, is often a marker of a low or nonreplicative state. However, a large subset of persons will harbor HBeAg(–) replicative disease, a consequence of mutations in the HBV precore or core promoter region that results in failure to produce "e" antigen. These so-called precore mutants can be distinguished from nonreplicators by high levels of HBV DNA (>10 000 copies/mL). In patients with HIV infection, clinical scenarios uncommon in immunocompetent patients may occur. Some patients with IgG anti-HBc and without detectable HBsAg harbor active HBV replication with associated liver injury.[16,17] These cases can be definitively diagnosed only by using a sensitive PCR-based HBV DNA assay. With chronic HBV infection treated with lamivudine, a high rate of mutant virus breakthrough can be identified by the presence of HBV DNA by branched-chain or hybridization assays.[8] Testing for lamivudine-resistance mutations in an area called the YMDD motif is available in some clinical laboratories. Mutation is also observed with other HBV active agents including adefovir, tenofovir, and entecavir. A new generation of tests that permit evaluation of mutational patterns is now under development.

HCV infection can be detected by use of an enzyme-linked immunosorbent assay (ELISA or EIA). This test is highly sensitive, though false positives in patients with a low pretest probability of disease are common. False-negative reactions are sometimes observed in patients with HIV. The prevalence of this finding has been reported to range from 1.5% to ~10.0% in some series. Seroreversion associated with worsening immune function has also been described.[18] If HCV infection is strongly suspected and the HCV ELISA is negative, an HCV RNA test is indicated. Although HCV RNA detection represents the gold standard in terms of sensitivity and specificity, its accuracy and reliability have been low in some blind test panels of laboratories that routinely test for HCV RNA. Therefore, diagnosis and treatment decisions should not be based on a single HCV RNA assay alone. Recombinant immunoblot assays (RIBA) may also serve to confirm infection in patients with a low pretest probability of infection.

Hepatitis D virus (HDV) infection is uncommon in the United States but is much more prevalent in Mediterranean rim countries. Because it requires the presence of hepatitis B for its own replication, the diagnosis of HDV should be considered only in those patients who harbor HBsAg. The presence of HDV antibody or HDV RNA suggests active infection. HIV infection appears to increase the rates of hepatic decompensation and portal hypertension in patients with HDV.[19]

Hepatitis E virus (HEV) infection may be detected using commercial antibody assay kits. HEV infection is uncommon in the United States and Western Europe, but the prevalence of anti-HEV has been shown to be increased in HIV-infected patients in Argentina and Brazil. However, this association may result from common risk factors for the two infections, including low socioeconomic status.[20,21] HEV seropositivity does not bear a clear relationship to HIV infection in most other epidemiologic studies.

Other common liver diseases of adults that warrant investigation include AAT deficiency and hereditary hemochromatosis. The gene frequencies for defects in the AAT coding domain, which result in abnormal protein expression, exceed 5% in some populations. Initial testing makes use of a specific monoclonal antibody that binds serum AAT and can be used to determine the AAT level. Low levels are consistent with an AAT deficiency, which results from a conformational change in the protein. Confirmation of the diagnosis requires phenotyping on an isoelectric focusing gel. Wild-type AAT is classified as M, based on its migration to the midpoint of the gel; mutant proteins migrate differently. The "Z" phenotype (pi type) is considered an important factor in chronic liver disease.

Hereditary hemochromatosis results from a gene defect in duodenal transport of iron by the protein HFE, which leads to excess iron absorption and end-organ injury in the liver and other organs. This excess iron results in increases in the iron-storage protein ferritin, which suggests the presence of this disease. However, because ferritin is an acute-phase reactant, a more reliable index is the transferrin saturation (Fe/total iron-binding capacity(TIBC)). Saturations of more than 50% suggest the possible presence of hereditary hemochromatosis. Patients with hereditary hemochromatosis have substitution mutations in two loci in HFE, which can be tested by specific PCR amplification. Homozygosity for the C282Y mutation, seen in up to 90% of patients with hereditary hemochromatosis, and compound heterozygosity for C282Y and H63D, are associated with the disease. Tests for both of these mutations are available from specialized clinical laboratories. Ultimately, the extent of iron storage and severity of injury are determined by histologic evaluation of liver tissue. Quantitative evaluation of liver tissue permits calculation of an age-controlled index of hepatic iron content.

LIVER IMAGING

A number of modalities for liver imaging are available to clinicians. The strengths and weaknesses of liver imaging methods in the context of HIV-positive patients mirror the characteristics in subjects without HIV infection. However, some liver disease processes are more prevalent in HIV-infected patients, and the diagnosis may be enhanced by the correct choice of imaging study.

LIVER/SPLEEN SCAN AND SPECT

Use of radionuclides such as technetium-99m (^{99m}Tc)-labeled sulfur colloid relies on the functional capacity of liver phagocytes to take up the label, retain and concentrate it during the scanning process, and be quantitatively measured by a photon camera. The methodology assumes that there is uniform uptake of the radionuclide in the liver parenchyma. Thus, any disease process that alters the distribution or function of phagocytes alters the uptake pattern. Cysts, abscesses, and tumors fail to take up the sulfur colloid and appear as a "cold" spot on the subsequent image. Patients with portal hypertension demonstrate an altered pattern of uptake, with increased radionuclide in the spleen or bone marrow relative to the liver ("colloid shift"). Although ^{99m}Tc-labeled colloid studies are easily obtained in most centers, they have been largely supplanted by other imaging modalities in terms of accuracy, lesion discrimination, and resolution.

Traditional planar imaging efficacy may be improved by the use of single-photon emission computed tomography (SPECT), which permits three-dimensional evaluation of the radionuclide uptake. However, current computed tomography (CT) scanning and magnetic resonance imaging (MRI) permit resolution at levels much higher than with SPECT. The role of SPECT in evaluation of fibrosis in HIV-infected patients with hepatitis C is under clinical investigation; a pilot study has shown that SPECT is 86–90% sensitive and 62–83% specific for fibrosis and predicts the histological fibrosis score with 80–85% accuracy.[22]

Biliary Scintigraphy

Using ^{99m}Tc radiotracers attached to compounds that are taken up by hepatocytes and excreted into the biliary tract, biliary scintigraphy permits evaluation of bile excretion and creates images that define the biliary anatomy. A number of compounds have been studied, including *N;N*-(2,6-Dimethylp henyl)carbamoylmethyl iminodiacetic acid (HIDA) and other diacetic acid derivatives. Patients with severe liver disease lack the functional capacity for radiotracer uptake and fail to "light up" the liver during the early phases of scanning. Following uptake, scanning during the excretion phase might reveal blockage in the biliary tree evidenced by a discrete cutoff of photon emission in the areas distal to the obstruction. These studies may have some value for identifying biliary obstruction, but endoscopic retrograde cholangiopancreatography (ERCP) and MR cholangiography have largely supplanted reliance on these imaging studies. Small studies of hepatobiliary scintigraphy suggested a high correlation between biliary scintigraphy and ERCP in patients with AIDS-related cholangiopathy, but large clinical trials have not been reported.[23–25]

Ultrasonography and Doppler Ultrasonography

Sound pulses in the 2–5 MHz range are used to discern differences in soft tissues and fluids based on the "echo" return to a receiver probe. Transcutaneous ultrasonography has become an important noninvasive modality for assessing certain types of liver disease. Mass lesions can be discerned from normal liver tissue by the differences in the echogenicity of the lesion relative to its surroundings. A diffusely hyperechoic liver suggests the presence of an infiltrating process or a change in the water content of the hepatocytes. This finding may be observed in patients with diffuse fibrosis, fatty liver, or lymphoma. The bile ducts can be clearly visualized along with the gallbladder, and gallstones demonstrate a characteristic appearance with high echogenicity and shadowing. Ultrasonography is available in most clinical settings and is rapid and noninvasive – hence its popularity as a first-line choice for liver imaging, although the clinician must be aware of its limitations. It is extremely operator-dependent and is often performed by technicians, with only selected images reviewed by radiologists, and interpretation is highly subjective. Moreover, patients with truncal obesity may be too large to permit adequate penetration of the sound pulses to the liver below, and gas in the bowel may obscure the image. The limited resolution of ultrasound impedes detection of discrete lesions less than 1 cm in diameter. The bile ducts are well-visualized on ultrasound because of the interface between the liver parenchyma and each fluid-filled tube. Ultrasonography excels in defining the size and path of bile ducts as small as 3–5 mm and is the screening test of choice for patients with cholestatic patterns of liver disease. It is also excellent for identifying the presence or absence of ascites.

It is important to note that ultrasonography is not useful for defining the presence of fibrosis or cirrhosis, and it rarely helps define the etiology of noncholestatic disease processes. Beale et al found that 75% of 48 HIV-infected individuals had abnormal liver ultrasound scans. A diffusely hyperechoic liver was observed in 46% of patients, which was attributed mainly to steatosis. However, on biopsy, nearly half the patients had more than one histologic abnormality.[26] Albisetti et al reported that significant hepatic steatosis on liver biopsy was suspected in only 70% of the pediatric HIV-infected cases reviewed.[27] The portability and low cost of ultrasonography have resulted in its extensive use for evaluating HIV-infected patients in developing countries with a high prevalence of AIDS.[28]

Doppler ultrasonography allows for the detection of frequency shifts, which permits sophisticated software packages to define the presence and direction of blood flow. This modality permits evaluation of waveforms, which can suggest portal hypertension and portal and hepatic vein thrombosis as a cause of liver injury.

Computed Tomography

Along with ultrasonography, CT imaging of the liver is the most important modality for evaluating masses, abscesses, cystic lesions, and infiltrative processes. Biphasic CT scans of the liver should generally be performed because identification and differentiation of mass lesions requires rapid imaging through the arterial and venous phases of contrast administration. Meta-analysis has shown that baseline CT without contrast was significantly inferior to biphasic or triphasic studies for identifying small mass lesions.[29] Therefore, noncontrast CT scans are not recommended for hepatic imaging.

Knollmann et al described the results of abdominal imaging of 339 HIV-infected patients. This retrospective study reported that 82% of patients had abnormal imaging, including 11 patients with hepatic masses and seven with ascites. Both findings were associated with decreased survival relative to the studied cohort.[30] In another group of 259 HIV-infected patients, hepatomegaly was reported in ~39%, and focal hepatic lesions were seen in 19%.[31]

Magnetic Resonance Imaging

Most major medical centers now utilize MRI as a diagnostic modality. The underlying physical principle relies on changes in the spin of water and lipid nuclei in a strong magnetic field that release energy in the form of radio waves upon return to the baseline state. Therefore, differences between tissues of similar densities may be observed, even when CT and other modalities that rely on variable penetration of radiation fail to distinguish lesions or tissue planes. MRI is frequently used to help establish the presence and distribution of tumors and to evaluate vascular abnormalities. It is generally considered to be more sensitive than biphasic CT for detecting small hepatocellular carcinomas.

Magnetic resonance cholangiopancreatography (MRCP) is a variation of standard MRI that permits imaging of the biliary system. Studies comparing MRCP to ERCP, which is the gold standard for biliary duct imaging, demonstrate a high correlation.[32] Sensitivities for detecting primary sclerosing cholangitis (PSC) have ranged from 86.5% to 97%, with specificities of 64–99%.[33–35] There is no literature evaluating the efficacy of MRCP in HIV-infected patients with AIDS-related cholangiopathy, though it seems likely that a similar efficacy might be observed.

Endoscopic Retrograde Cholangiopancreatography

ERCP is regarded as the gold standard for evaluating the biliary duct system. Although somewhat invasive, the procedure is generally tolerable and, in the hands of experienced endoscopists, highly efficacious for diagnosing strictures, papillary stenosis and AIDS cholangiopathy, small stones, and masses in the biliary tree (Fig. 78-3). Somewhat better diagnostically than MRCP, it also offers the opportunity for immediate intervention, including stone removal, ductal dilation, sphincterotomy, and stent placement. Complications include pancreatitis in up to 5% of cases, though it is generally mild and self-limited. Some cases of severe pancreatitis occur, however.

Among patients with HIV infection, the literature supports use of ERCP for both diagnosis and intervention in patients with right upper quadrant pain and ultrasonographic evidence of ductal enlargement. Among 83 patients undergoing ERCP for abdominal pain or cholestatic liver enzyme abnormalities, 56 had AIDS-related cholangiopathy. Of the patients who underwent ampullary biopsy, 62.5% had evidence of opportunistic infection.[36] A review of this subject by Walden suggested that patients with a prominent component

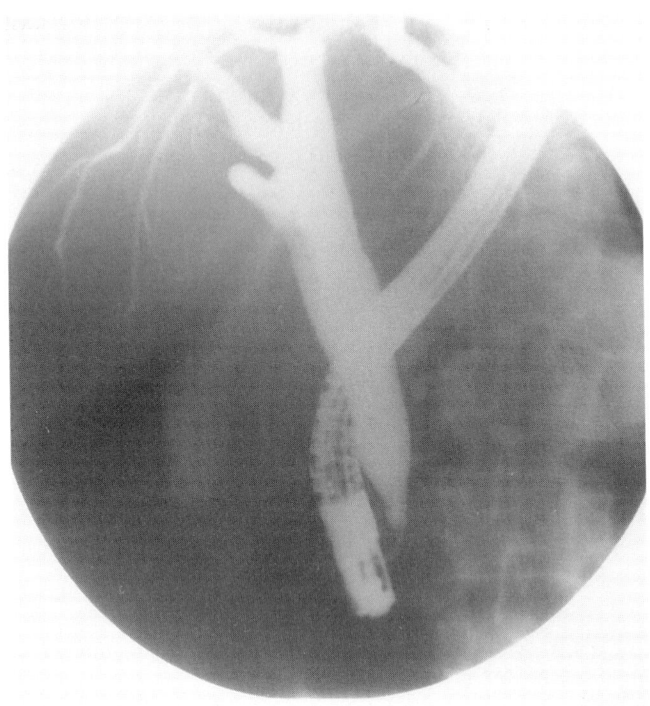

Figure 78-3 ■ HIV-related papillary stenosis. Endoscopic cholangiogram from a 47-year -old woman with HIV presenting with episodic severe right upper quadrant abdominal pain. The study reveals a diffusely dilated biliary tree and a smooth, stenotic distal common bile duct. There was no evidence of common bile duct stones. Endoscopic sphincterotomy produced immediate symptom relief. Multiple biopsies of the common duct and electron microscopy failed to reveal evidence of pathogens.

of pain may benefit from ERCP with sphincterotomy, but those with asymptomatic cholestatic enzyme elevations are much less likely to benefit from intervention.[37] Pancreatic ductal changes are common in patients diagnosed with AIDS cholangiopathy, and features suggestive of chronic pancreatitis may be observed in approximately half of these patients.[38]

Liver Biopsy

Histologic evaluation of liver tissue remains the definitive study for determination of liver disease activity and degree of fibrosis. It also helps confirm the presence of processes suspected during the biochemical and serologic workup phase. Occasionally, liver biopsy identifies previously unsuspected findings in terms of etiology or co-morbidity. Liver biopsies may also be obtained at the time of laparoscopy under direct liver visualization or via a transjugular route. One editorial suggested that radiologic guidance be restricted to patients with a suspected tumor or hepatic mass, obesity, or the rare case when physical examination fails to define the precise location of the liver. For cases of decompensated disease with coagulopathy, ascites, or significant thrombocytopenia, a transjugular approach is considered safer. All other cases may be performed by the percutaneous route, and physicians may or may not use ultrasound localization prior to biopsy.[39] While one pediatric study found that ultrasound did not change morbidity or mortality,[40] another showed that ultrasound improved the diagnostic yield and decreased the rate of minor complications.[41] Riley suggested that use of ultrasound prior to biopsy changed the management in 15.1% of cases[42]; moreover, an economic analysis supported the use of ultrasound prior to liver biopsy.[43]

The risk of complications from liver biopsy is highly variable based on the experience of the clinician, number of passes required, type of biopsy needle used, platelet count, prothrombin time, and type of lesion to be biopsied.[44] Serious complications are rare, although death has been reported to occur at a rate of nine per 100000 cases and hemorrhage, pneumothorax, and biliary peritonitis at rates of one per 1000 to three per 1000 cases.[45,46]

There is little in the literature on the safety of liver biopsy in patients with HIV. A retrospective review of 248 liver biopsies in HIV antibody-positive patients reported a hemorrhage rate of 2.0%, which is higher than might be expected. The exceptionally high mortality rate (1.6%) was attributed to a high prevalence of thrombocytopenia and coagulation abnormalities in the cohort.[47] The higher risk of bleeding and death may also be attributable to a high prevalence of disease etiologies that may increase the risk of postbiopsy bleeding, including malignancies such as Kaposi sarcoma and lymphoma and vascular abnormalities including peliosis due to bacillary angiomatosis. High-risk cases (e.g., patients with thrombocytopenia, coagulopathy, or liver lesions) with increased hemorrhage potential mandate screening and selection for safer biopsy approaches, such as transjugular liver biopsy.[48]

Deserving of special mention are patients with hemophilia who are frequently co-infected with HCV and HIV. There is often great reluctance to subject patients with heritable bleeding diatheses to liver biopsy, and the risk and cost of biopsy in hemophiliacs must be weighed against the value of the information obtained at liver biopsy. Current literature suggests that liver biopsy by the percutaneous or transjugular route can be performed safely in hemophiliacs following factor VIII replacement.[49–51] A consensus review of this subject confirms this opinion and provides guidance for clinicians managing patients with hemophilia and liver disease.[52]

The role of liver biopsy in patients with HIV infection has been controversial. Cappell et al described the outcomes of liver biopsy in 36 patients with HIV. The leading indication was unexplained fever (83%) and abnormal liver enzymes (89%). Previously unidentified etiologies were found most frequently in patients with increased alkaline phosphatase, suggesting the presence of a cholestatic process. Most of these patients had granulomas associated with *Mycobacterium* infection. The patients in whom biopsy was helpful were those with leukocytosis, those in whom full-blown AIDS was suspected, and those who were not known to have HIV infection prior to the biopsy.[53] Poles et al reported on the findings of liver biopsies from 501 HIV seropositive patients who underwent biopsy for indications similar to those described by Cappell et al. The most common diagnosis was mycobacterial infection (26.6% of the patients studied); 12% had chronic hepatitis. The study failed to determine if liver biopsy changed the treatment of the clinical diagnosis.[54] Similarly, a European study reported that among 24 patients with unexplained fever, liver biopsy provided a microbiologic diagnosis in 54%.[55] Among children with HIV infection, liver biopsy was found to be useful for determining a diagnosis when there was a strong suspicion of mycobacterial infection or the child was jaundiced (or both).[56] In HIV-infected patients with hepatitis B and C co-infection, liver biopsy is useful for staging disease and planning treatment.

Noninvasive Markers of Hepatic Fibrosis

Because liver biopsy can be attended by occasionally serious complications, development of validated noninvasive tests for hepatic fibrosis will continue to be important. While a composite index of serum markers have been validated in HIV-negative patients, only one index has been studied in HIV-infected persons with liver disease. The serum hyaluronic acid, albumin, and AST (SHASTA) index has been studied in an HIV–HCV co-infected cohort.[57] This index appeared to be sensitive for both moderate-to-severe fibrosis (Ishak fibrosis score = 3) and low fibrosis stages. Noninvasive measurement of liver stiffness by transient elastography (FibroScan) has also shown promise. In a small study among HIV–HCV co-infected patients, this method was found to be more accurate for the prediction of cirrhosis than the SHASTA index.[58] However, it remains unclear whether elastography will be less reliable among patients with hepatic steatosis or HIV-associated lipodystrophy/visceral adiposity. Elastography and biochemical testing may ultimately have complementary roles in the staging of hepatic fibrosis. These methods warrant further investigation in the HIV-infected population.

ETIOLOGIES OF LIVER DISEASE IN PATIENTS WITH HIV

Viral Liver Disease

Hepatotropic Viruses

In view of the markedly high rates of co-infection with hepatitis B and C viruses in HIV-infected persons, it has become increasingly clear that the enhanced survival during the era of HAART will make chronic liver disease with these pathogens important sources of morbidity and mortality. These infections are considered in more detail in Chapters 54 and 55.

Hepatitis A Virus

Seroepidemiologic surveys for HAV infection reveal an increased overall prevalence in the HIV-infected population; among risk groups, men who have sex with men and injection drug users are at increased risk for infection. Although most cases of acute hepatitis with this fecal-oral pathogen are self-limited episodes and are no more clinically severe in the HIV-infected host than in the general population,[59] HIV-infected patients treated for hepatitis A do exhibit prolonged viremia compared with HIV negative controls.[60] Individuals at particular risk for morbidity from hepatitis A are those who harbor chronic liver disease. Indeed, the risk of fatal acute hepatitis A is significantly increased in subjects with chronic HCV infection[61]; this has led to the recommendation that individuals with chronic HCV infection be actively immunized with an HAV vaccine.[62] HIV-infected individuals at continued risk for HAV infection should also be vaccinated. Vaccine response rates in HIV-infected adults range from 50–95%, and lower CD4+ T-lymphocyte counts appear to be associated with reduced efficacy.[63]

Hepatitis B Virus

Co-infection with HBV occurs frequently in view of its shared routes of transmission with HIV. Up to 95% of persons with AIDS have serologic markers of prior HBV infection (anti-HBs+ or anti-HBc+).[64,65] An estimated 7.6% of HIV-infected patients in the US are chronic HBV carriers (HBsAg+); co-infection rates may be higher than 20% in Asia, where HBV is endemic.[66] Although there is little evidence for a direct virologic interaction between HIV and HBV, the critical role of the immune system in mediating cell injury in chronic hepatitis B suggests that HIV alters its natural history. In support of this concept, the incidence of acute icteric hepatitis B is lower in the presence of HIV, and the risk of developing chronic HBV infection is increased substantially in patients with preexisting HIV infection.[67] Moreover, HIV appears to enhance and extend the period of HBV replication (HBeAg+, HBV DNA+) but without a concomitant increase in hepatic necroinflammatory activity. With advancing immunosuppression, markers of HBV replication appear to be reactivated. A 10-year cohort study of 5293 HIV positive men, including over 300 men with HBV–HIV co-infection, showed a 12.7-fold increase in mortality among HBsAg positive patients. Liver-related mortality was increased after 1996 (in the HAART era) and among those patients with low CD4 counts.[68,69] There is little evidence that HBV worsens the course of HIV disease. One large-scale retrospective analysis demonstrated no influence on the mortality of co-infected patients compared with HBsAg negative patients with HIV infection.[70]

Irrespective of whether HBV disease is hastened by HIV, alteration of the HIV treatment picture by introducing HAART increases the likelihood that HBV liver disease will become more problematic with control of HIV. Indeed, immune-mediated flares of HBV with successful pharmacologic reconstitution of the immune system have been described.[71,72] Furthermore, lamivudine withdrawal or YMDD-mutant breakthrough may precipitate acute liver injury in immunologically reconstituted patients who also have hepatitis B infection.[8,73]

The HIV–HBV co-infected patient should be treated for replicative HBV disease, defined by the following criteria: (1) presence of HBsAg, (2) abnormal serum ALT level,

(3) HBV DNA level >100000 copies/mL with HBeAg, or (4) HBV DNA level >10000 copies/mL without HBeAg (indicating infection with a precore or core promoter mutant strain of HBV). Goals of therapy include normalization of ALT, suppression of HBV replication, and seroconversion from HBeAg to anti-HBe when applicable. Improvement in liver histology can indicate a response to HBV therapy, but serologic indices are quite reliable and obviate the need for biopsy in most cases. However, liver biopsy remains advisable in HBV–HIV co-infected patients prior to initiation of HAART, since a flare of liver enzymes could precipitate hepatic failure in patients with cirrhosis.

The mainstays of HBV therapy in co-infected patients are nucleoside and nucleotide analogs. Interferon is less effective in co-infected patients than in HBV-monoinfected patients and is infrequently used in the former group.[74] Efficacy studies of pegylated interferon in co-infected subjects are underway, but no results have been published to date. Lamivudine, a nucleoside analog with activity against HIV reverse transcriptase and HBV DNA polymerase, lowers HBV DNA levels when used as a component of HAART in the short term but promotes emergence of YMDD mutants after years of treatment.[75,76] If a patient's HBV viral load increases during long-term HAART including lamivudine, a nucleotide analog should be added to the regimen. Lamivudine should not be stopped abruptly because a hepatic flare may occur.[77] A co-infected patient not on HAART should not receive lamivudine monotherapy for HBV, as lamivudine-resistant HIV mutants may emerge.[78] Other nucleoside analogs used to treat co-infected patients are emtricitabine, which, like lamivudine, has activity against both viruses but engenders YMDD resistance, and entecavir, which inhibits only HBV DNA polymerase and may be employed in the absence of HAART.[79]

Adefovir and tenofovir are nucleotide analogs that inhibit both HIV reverse transcriptase and HBV DNA polymerase. Unlike lamivudine, adefovir may be used as HBV monotherapy when HAART is not needed.[80,81] Adefovir-resistant HBV strains occur in 18% of monoinfected patients after 96 weeks of therapy.[82] However, an analysis of HIV–HBV co-infected patients treated with adefovir and lamivudine for up to 144 weeks did not reveal resistant HBV strains.[83,84] Furthermore, adefovir may be used to treat lamivudine-resistant HBV in co-infected patients; emergence of adefovir-resistant HIV has not been demonstrated in this context.[85] The major adverse effect of adefovir is nephrotoxicity, which is significantly less common in patients receiving the relatively low dose (10 mg/day) used to treat HBV than in those who receive higher doses for HIV.[86,87]

Tenofovir is a second-generation nucleotide analog that is effective against lamivudine-resistant HBV strains. This drug should therefore be included in HAART regimens for co-infected patients with lamivudine-resistant HBV. Tenofovir may reduce HBV viral load more rapidly than adefovir,[88] and no tenofovir-resistant HBV strains have yet been reported in co-infected patients. Promising treatment results were also described in a retrospective study by Benhamou et al.[89] This drug should not be co-administered with the antiretroviral didanosine (ddI) due to the increased risk of pancreatitis.[90]

Hepatitis C Virus

Among the 1 million persons infected with HIV in the United States, ~30%, or 300000, are co-infected with HCV.[91] Among drug users, co-infection rates of up to 92% have been cited.[92] When these rates are coupled with the known natural history of HCV (*see* Chapter 55), hepatic morbidity with this pathogen is a significant problem, as the life expectancy of the HIV cohort is increasing. Because of the important role of the immune system in containing HCV, it is not surprising that HCV viremia levels are ~10-fold higher with HIV co-infection than with HCV infection alone.[93] These findings mirror those found in other immunocompromised populations, such as those undergoing liver transplantation.[94] However, no clear correlation of HCV RNA with CD4+ T-lymphocyte counts or definite relationship between HCV and HIV levels has been established.

Influence of HIV on HCV-related liver disease

Retrospective analyses show that since the inception of HAART, mortality attributable to HCV-related end-stage liver disease has risen nearly fivefold, indicating that the prevalence of HCV-induced cirrhosis is increasing as co-infected patients live longer.[95] The most illuminating natural history studies have been performed in hemophiliacs, whose disease duration has been definable. Eyster et al[96] found that 9% of co-infected hemophiliacs developed liver failure within 10 to 20 years after HCV infection compared with none of the HIV-negative/HCV+ group. In this cohort, the risk of liver failure was more than half the risk of developing AIDS. Subsequently, at least three other studies confirmed accelerated liver failure in those with HCV-HIV co-infection.[97–99] A possible explanation for this finding may lie in the observation that HIV co-infection accelerates HCV fibrosis progression compared with single infection with HCV.[100] HAART seems to lessen the deleterious effects of HIV in HCV liver disease, decreasing the burden of cirrhosis by two-thirds over 25 years.[101]

The reciprocal relation is far less certain: does HCV influence HIV disease progression? An evaluation of the Swiss HIV cohort during the post-HAART era identified HCV as an important factor in increased progression to AIDS-defining complications and blunted immune recovery on HAART.[102] A recent meta-analysis showed that HIV-negative/HCV+ group co-infected patients have significantly smaller increases in CD4+ T-cells (mean 33.4 cells/μL lower) after HAART initiation than HIV-monoinfected patients.[103] However, two recent large studies failed to show adverse effects of HCV co-infection on progression to AIDS or requirement for HAART.[104,105]

Immune reconstitution and HCV

Initiation of HAART can cause an early rise in ALT and HCV RNA levels, followed by a return to baseline with continued treatment.[106] This pattern suggests a self-limited flare that is

Table 78-2 Sustained Virologic Response Rates (SVRs) with HCV Therapy in HCV/HIV Co-Infected patients[91]

	ACTG A5071		APRICOT			RIBAVIC	
Trial Response Rate	PEG/RBV	IFN/RBV	PEG/RBV	PEG	IFN/RBV	PEG/RBV	IFN/RBV
SVR	27%	12%	40%	20%	12%	27%	19%
genotype 1	14%	5%	29%	14%	7%	15%	5%
genotype 2/3	73%	33%	62%	36%	20%	43%	41%
SVR if >2 log drop at 12 weeks	51% (pooled for all)	51% (pooled for all)	56%	37%	30%	41%	35%

not readily attributable to drug hepatotoxicity. Among the protease inhibitors, nelfinavir is more commonly associated with immune reconstitution flares than a lopinavir-ritonavir combination.[10] Patients with increased aminotransferase levels early in HAART should be monitored vigilantly. If LFTs do not improve spontaneously, drug toxicity is much more likely than immune reconstitution.

Antiviral therapy for HCV in HIV Co-infected patients

The regimen of choice for treating HCV in HIV-co-infected patients consists of pegylated interferon-α(interferon complexed with inert polyethylene glycol, abbreviated PEG-IFN-α) and ribavirin (RBV). Interferon has both direct and indirect effects on HCV, including (1) possible prevention of viral binding, entry, and uncoating; (2) induction of antiviral host genes via the JAK-STAT kinase pathway; (3) upregulation of viral antigen presentation; and (4) induction of T and natural killer (NK) cell responses. PEG-IFN has a longer half-life than standard interferon, resulting in improved rates of sustained virologic response (SVR). Ribavirin is a synthetic analog of guanosine that is thought to decrease HCV infectivity by inducing RNA mutagenesis. It may also shift the profile of anti-HCV T-helper cell activity from Th2 to Th1. Although ribavirin itself does not affect HCV RNA levels, it significantly reduces postinterferon relapse rates and lowers serum ALT levels.[91]

The combination of PEG-IFN-α and RBV has been validated in three large clinical trials in HCV-HIV co-infected patients (Table 78-2).[91] The ACTG A5071 study, conducted in the United States, compared a PEG-IFN-α/RBV regimen with a standard IFN/RBV regimen.[107] Both regimens incorporated a dose escalation of RBV in order to minimize side effects; consequently, the dropout rate was only 12%. The overall SVRs were 27% for the PEG-IFN-α/RBV group and 12% for the IFN/RBV group. Among patients infected with HCV genotypes 2/3, the PEG-IFN-α/RBV regimen achieved SVR in 73%, compared with 33% in those receiving IFN/RBV. Genotype 1 patients did not respond as well, with SVR rates of only 14% and 5% on the two regimens, respectively. These low rates may have been due to the high prevalence of advanced fibrosis in the cohort, underdosing of ribavirin during the early stages of the trial, and the high proportion (33%) of African-American patients, who have lower rates of SVR in HCV monoinfection.

AIDS Pegasys Ribavirin International Coinfection Trial (APRICOT), the largest of the studies, included US and international patients and had three arms: PEG-IFN/RBV, standard IFN/RBV, and PEG-IFN alone.[108] The PEG-IFN/RBV regimen was most effective, inducing SVR in 40% overall (62% of genotype 2/3 patients, 29% of genotype 1 patients). The fact that only 16% of patients in this trial had bridging fibrosis and cirrhosis may have contributed to improved response rates in the genotype 1 group. Notably, genotype 1 patients with low viral loads (<800000 IU/mL) fared much better than those with high viral loads (SVR rates of 61% and 18%, respectively).

RIBAVIC was a French study that also compared PEG-IFN/RBV to standard IFN/RBV and had a large proportion (39%) of patients with advanced fibrosis.[109] For PEG-IFN/RBV, SVR was achieved in 27% (15% in genotype 1 and 43% of genotype 2/3 patients). Notably, this study had the highest dropout rate (31%). Fortunately, PEG-IFN/RBV treatment was not associated with progression of HIV disease in any of the trials.

While the results of these trials differ, they collectively establish PEG-IFN/RBV as standard treatment for HCV in HIV co-infection; unfortunately, the limited response rates in genotype 1 co-infection may limit the broad applicability of these regimens. A 48-week course of PEG-IFN/RBV is currently recommended for all genotypes. However, because the SVR rate in genotype 1 is low, the risks of treatment must be carefully weighed against potential benefits for each patient. Assessment of HCV RNA levels at week 12 provides useful prognostic information. If the viral load has not decreased by greater than 2 $\log_{10}$ from baseline, an early virologic response (EVR) is not achieved, and the odds of achieving SVR are effectively nil. However, even in the absence of EVR, the patient with advanced hepatic fibrosis may still benefit from extended treatment, as demonstrated by improved liver histology in some studies.[91] Figure 78-4 summarizes recommendations for HCV treatment in HIV co-infection.[110]

Despite their efficacy, both PEG-IFN-α and RBV are associated with problematic adverse effects in the HIV co-infected

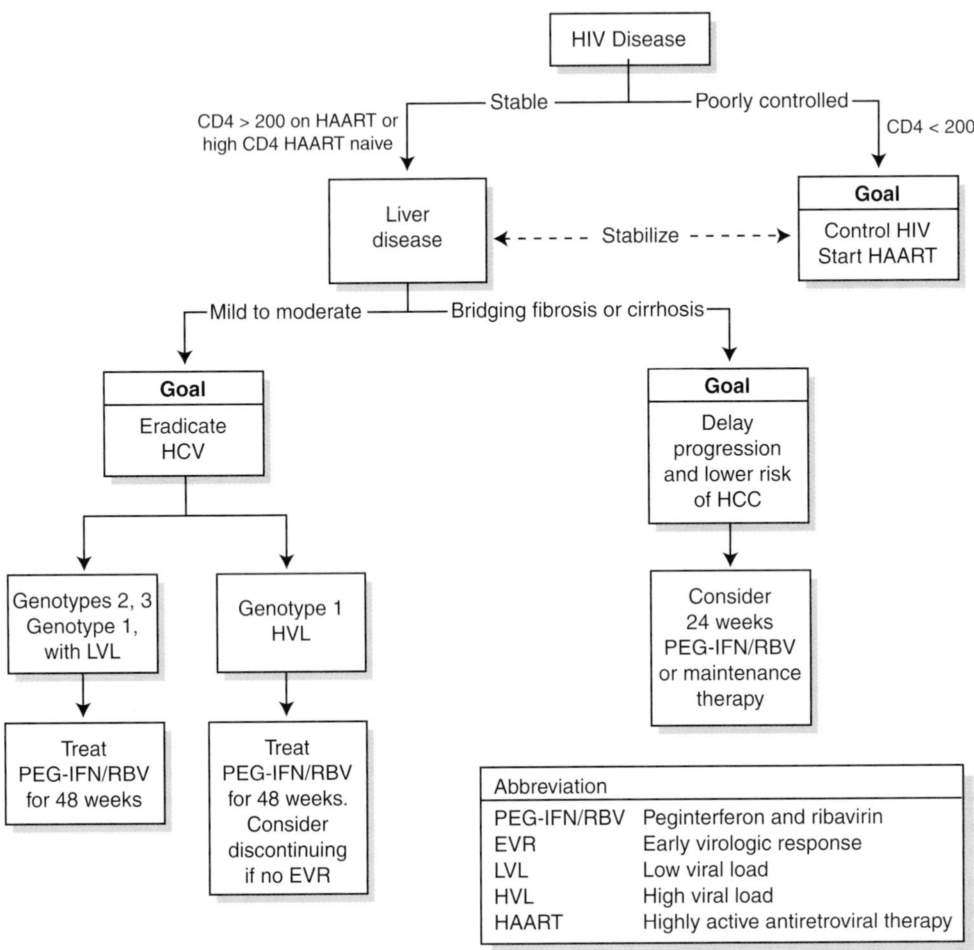

Figure 78-4 ■ Treatment of HCV in HIV co-infection.[110]

population. PEG-IFN-α may cause bone marrow suppression, flu-like symptoms, and neuropsychiatric disturbances.[111] RBV antagonizes the phosphorylation of the thymidine analogs zidovudine (AZT) and stavudine (d4T) *in vitro*, but this interaction has not been demonstrated *in vivo*.[112] RBV, a nucleoside analog, should not be used in combination with ddI or d4T because of the risk of mitochondrial toxicity (lactic acidosis and pancreatitis).[113,114] RBV also induces a dose-dependent hemolytic anemia, and AZT-associated anemia is often worsened by RBV.[115] Although this anemia can respond to supplemental erythropoietin, some consideration should be given to replacement of AZT with another antiretroviral agent prior to initiating RBV treatment.

Other Viral Etiologies

Cytomegalovirus

Cytomegalovirus (CMV) infection, common in patients with HIV, can produce a wide range of clinical outcomes, from asymptomatic seropositivity to a fulminant, disseminated illness. It is a frequent finding in the livers of patients with AIDS, usually in the setting of multiorgan CMV disease. CMV can produce both an acute hepatitis-like illness and biliary tract disease. Clinical illness correlates with more advanced states of immunocompromise. There is usually mild elevation of the serum aminotransferases and occasionally predominant elevation of the serum alkaline phosphatase level. Histological findings include a mild portal and periportal mononuclear infiltrate, sparse necrosis, and the presence of characteristic "owl's eye" intranuclear inclusions within hepatocytes, vascular endothelial cells, and biliary epithelium consistent with the broad cell tropism of this DNA virus. Less frequently, granulomatous reactions are seen. Imaging may show nonspecific findings such as hepatomegaly and increased parenchymal echogenicity. Serologic assays for diagnosis of active CMV disease are available but of limited utility. Amplification assays and antigenemia assays usually reveal positive tests for viremia once CMV hepatitis has developed.[116] Treatment with intravenous ganciclovir is indicated for CMV hepatitis.

Herpes Simplex Virus and Other Herpes Viruses

Herpes simplex virus (HSV) can cause significant acute hepatitis in HIV-infected hosts as part of a disseminated infection, with an occasional fulminant or subfulminant presentation. Aminotransferase elevations may be severe and accompanied by disseminated intravascular coagulation. Histologic examination reveals Cowdry type A intranuclear inclusions, but immunohistochemical staining may be required to distinguish HSV from CMV. Diffuse hepatocellular necrosis with sparse inflammatory reaction may be seen with severe hepatitis. Careful examination of the skin is therefore essential, as there is usually evidence of herpetic cutaneous lesions. Amplification assays for HSV DNA reveal high-titer viremia. Once the diagnosis is confirmed, prompt institution of intravenous acyclovir can be life-saving, particularly in patients with subfulminant or fulminant infection, among whom the case fatality rate is high.[117]

Other, less frequent herpes viruses implicated in liver disease in the HIV-infected person are varicella-zoster virus (VZV), Epstein-Barr virus, and human herpesvirus-6.[118] VZV hepatitis also presents in immunocompromised hosts as part of a disseminated syndrome with rash, fever, and pneumonitis. Treatment with intravenous acyclovir can shorten disease duration.[119]

Adenovirus

Disseminated adenovirus infection has been reported to cause acute hepatitis in HIV-infected persons.[120] Clinically, the picture can be severe, with high fever, respiratory symptoms, enteritis, rash, and hepatomegaly. The mortality rate is high in immunocompromised patients.[121] Histologically, hepatocyte necrosis with massive hemorrhagic foci has been reported. "Smoky" intranuclear inclusions adjacent to areas of necrosis can also be seen. The diagnosis, which can be supported serologically, is made by recovering virus from body fluids or tissues. Treatment is supportive. Adenovirus-associated cholangiohepatitis has occurred in immunocompromised children but has not been reported in adults.[122]

Human Immunodeficiency Virus

The p24 gag protein has been identified by immunohistochemistry in Kupffer cells and endothelial cells of the liver.[123] Furthermore, HIV replication has been demonstrated in Kupffer cell cultures. It has been speculated that this is due to the presence of CD4 receptors present in both cell types, and Kupffer cells (the macrophage-like cell type in the liver) may represent a reservoir for HIV. The clinical significance of these observations remains unclear but raises the possibility that HIV infection of the liver may serve as a portal of entry for other pathogens. Expression of p24 in hepatocytes has also been demonstrated and appears to be correlated with the severity of liver damage. This finding suggests that HIV infection may promote hepatocyte apoptosis.[124]

Fungal Liver Disease

Candidiasis

Candida species may cause invasive systemic infection with hepatic involvement in HIV-infected persons with advanced immunocompromise, especially in those who develop defects in neutrophil function.[125] The liver can become infected by *Candida albicans* in the setting of disseminated, multiorgan disease. HAART has reduced the incidence of nosocomial candidemia, but mortality from this condition remains high[126,127] With disseminated candidiasis involving the liver, clinical features include fever, abdominal pain and distension, nausea, vomiting, diarrhea, and tender hepatomegaly. The serum alkaline phosphatase level is almost invariably elevated, with variable elevations in serum aminotransferase and bilirubin levels. Although CT of the abdomen is highly sensitive for demonstrating hepatic and splenic candidal abscesses, which are often multicentric, MR may be superior.[128,129] In cases diagnosed antemortem, liver biopsy or laparoscopy reveals macroscopic nodules, necrosis with microabscess formation, and characteristic yeast or hyphal forms of *Candida*.[128,130] The results of cultures of biopsy material are negative in most cases. Treatment with intravenous amphotericin B is usually warranted for acute disseminated candidiasis, but response rates to therapy are limited.[131]

Histoplasmosis

Infection with *Histoplasma capsulatum* is acquired through the respiratory tract and, in most cases, is confined to the lungs. However, severely immunocompromised persons, such as those with AIDS, are predisposed to disseminated histoplasmosis. The liver can be invaded in both acute and chronic progressive disseminated histoplasmosis. Fever, oropharyngeal ulcers, hepatomegaly, and splenomegaly may be present in patients with chronic disease. Serum ALT and alkaline phosphatase levels are often elevated. Hepatosplenomegaly is present in ~30% of adults with acute disease, which is often the AIDS-defining illness. In AIDS patients with known disseminated histoplasmosis, an immune reconstitution inflammatory syndrome may occur after the initiation of HAART. Unusual manifestations of disseminated histoplasmosis, such as liver abscesses, compressive lymphadenitis, intestinal obstruction, uveitis, and arthritis, are seen in this syndrome.[132]

Yeast forms can be identified in sections of liver biopsies with standard hematoxylin and eosin staining. The most common hepatic histologic finding is portal lymphohistiocytic inflammation; discrete granulomas occur in less than 20% of involved livers.[133] The silver methenamine method is superior for detecting yeast forms in areas of caseating necrosis or granuloma formation (Fig. 78-5), but the organism is difficult to culture and almost never grows from biopsy specimens. Bone marrow biopsies produce a higher diagnostic yield than liver biopsy for stainable yeast.[134] Serologic testing for complement-fixing antibodies is therefore helpful for confirming the diagnosis. In immunocompromised persons who may not be capable of mounting an antibody response, detection of *H. capsulatum* antigens in urine and serum can be useful. Treatment with intravenous amphotericin, followed by a course of itraconazole, is warranted for disseminated disease[135] (*see* Chapter 44).

Parasitic Liver Disease

Leishmaniasis

Visceral leishmaniasis is caused by *Leishmania donovani*, *L. infantum*, and *L. chagasi* (now thought to be the same organism as *L. infantum*) and is endemic in the Mediterranean,

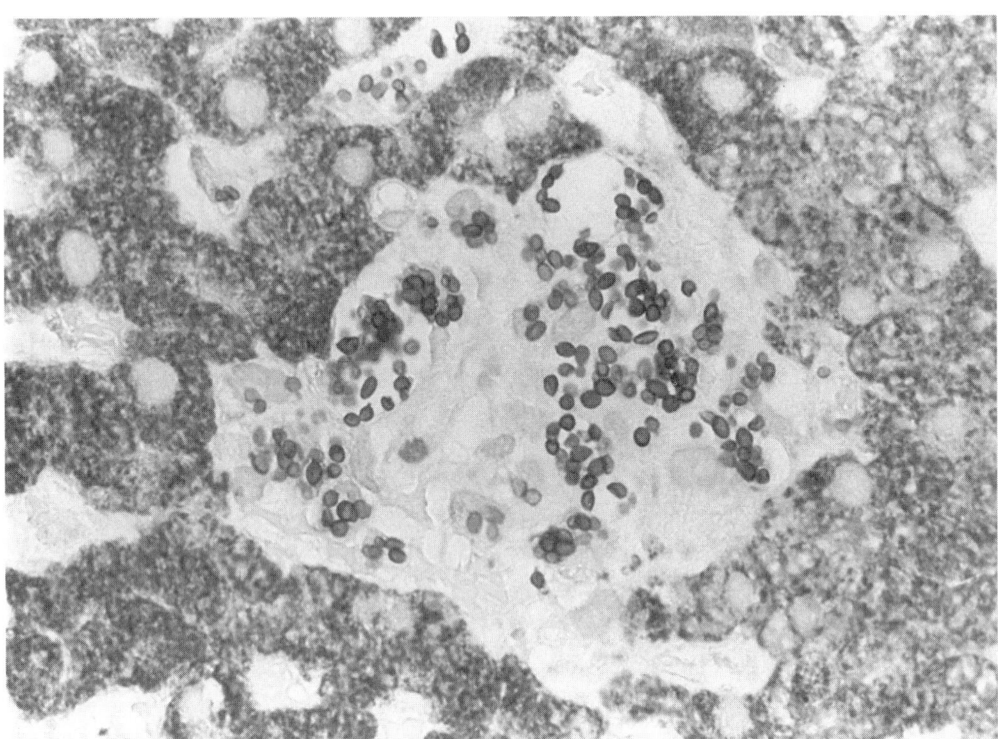

Figure 78-5 ■ Liver biopsy from an HIV-infected patient with recurrent fevers and cholestatic injury pattern of the liver. Grocott silver stain shows a granuloma containing *Histoplasma* yeast forms.

central Asia, the former Soviet Union, the Middle East, China, India, Pakistan, Bangladesh, Africa, Central America, and South America.[136] Amastigotes are ingested by the sandfly (*Lutzomyia* in the New World, *Phlebotomus* in the Old World) and become flagellated promastigotes. Following injection into the human host, the promastigotes are phagocytosed by macrophages in the reticuloendothelial system, where they multiply. Because cell-mediated immunity is needed to control leishmaniasis, AIDS patients are at increased risk for severe clinical manifestations.

Visceral leishmaniasis can usually be found in mononuclear phagocytes of the liver, spleen, bone marrow, and lymph nodes. Proliferation of Kupffer cells is often seen, and amastigotes can be detected in these cells.[137] Occasionally, parasite-bearing cells aggregate in noncaseating granulomas.[138] Hepatocyte necrosis is mild compared with the often severe necrosis seen in cutaneous leishmaniasis. Healing is accompanied by fibrous deposition, and occasionally the liver takes on a cirrhotic appearance. However, complications of chronic liver disease are rare.

Visceral infection caused by *L. donovani* begins with a papular or ulcerative skin lesion at the site of the sandfly bite. Following an incubation period of 2–6 months (sometimes years), intermittent fevers, weight loss, diarrhea (of bacillary, amebic, or leishmanial origin), and progressive painful hepatosplenomegaly develop, often accompanied by pancytopenia and a polyclonal hypergammaglobulinemia. Secondary bacterial infections resulting from suppression of reticuloendothelial cell function are important causes of mortality and include pneumonia, pneumococcal infection, and tuberculosis. Visceral leishmaniasis is almost uniformly fatal without treatment.

Physical findings include hepatomegaly; massive splenomegaly, jaundice, or ascites in severe disease; generalized lymphadenopathy; and muscle wasting. Cutaneous gray hyperpigmentation, which prompted the name kala-azar ("black fever"), is infrequent. Oral and nasopharyngeal nodules due to granuloma formation may also be seen.

The diagnosis is based on the history, physical examination, and microscopic demonstration of amastigotes in affected tissue samples. The highest yield (>95%) comes from aspiration of the spleen. The yield of a liver biopsy is almost as high and less risky. The yield of bone marrow aspiration is 55–97% and that of lymph node aspirates 60%.[139] Serologic testing (ELISA, immunofluorescence, immunochromatography, direct agglutination) can be used to support a presumptive diagnosis of visceral leishmaniasis. The newer methods of urinary antigen detection and blood and serum PCR are quite sensitive (>90% and >88%, respectively) and highly specific.[140–142] The leishmanin skin test (Montenegro test) is not helpful in the presence of acute visceral disease.

Pentavalent antimonial compounds are the drugs of choice for all forms of leishmaniasis. Parenteral sodium stibogluconate (Pentostam) is available through the Centers for Disease Control and Prevention (CDC) for treatment of infections in the United States. Alternative parenteral agents include liposomal amphotericin B, which is commonly used in India due to high rates of resistance to antimonials, aminosidine (parenteral paromomycin), and pentamidine.[139,143] Treatment with antimonials should be administered for at least 4 weeks. However, patients with AIDS and leishmaniasis often fail to respond to or relapse following treatment with conventional regimens.[139,144] Miltefosine, a phosphocholine analog administered orally, is highly efficacious against visceral leishmaniasis, with a reported cure rate of 97% in Phase 2 trials.[143,145] The oral agent sitamaquine is currently under study.[139,143]

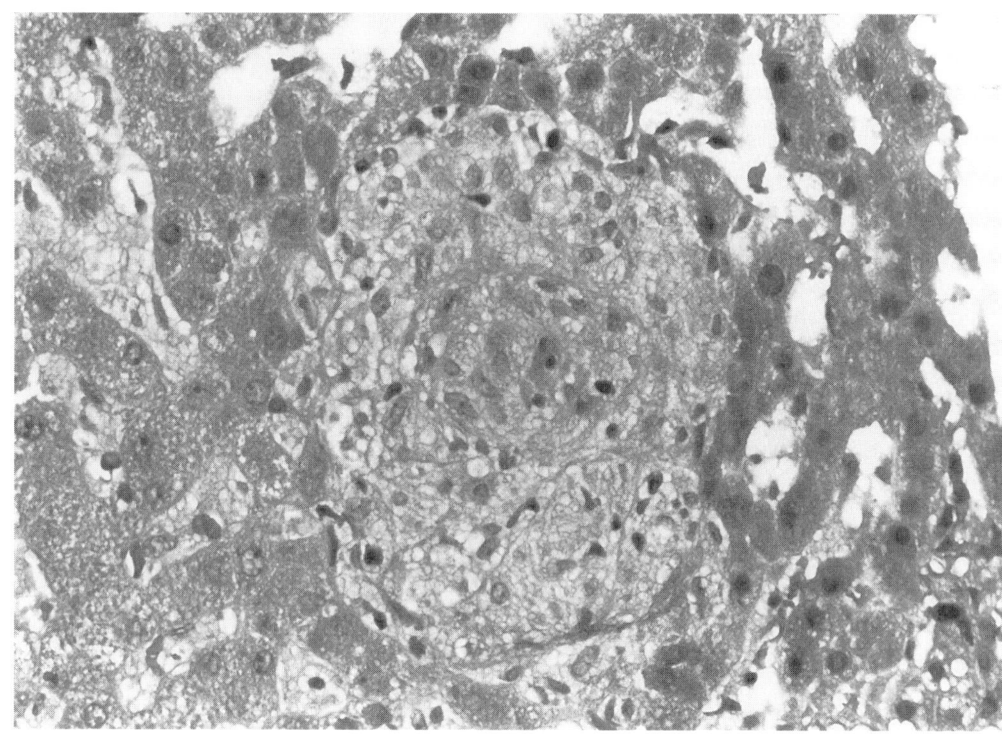

Figure 78-6 ■ Liver biopsy from an HIV-infected patient with recurrent fever shows a nonspecific granuloma on H&E staining. Silver stains for fungal elements and stains for acid-fast bacilli were negative for organisms.

Pneumocystis jiroveci

Hepatic involvement has been described frequently in patients with AIDS who present with disseminated extrapulmonary *Pneumocystis jiroveci* infection. In one study, *P. jiroveci* was found in 38% of cases.[146] It usually presents in persons who have received prophylactic aerosolized pentamidine or oral dapsone, which theoretically promotes emergence of extrapulmonary infection. Spread is also noted in lymph nodes, bone marrow, spleen, and liver, which is involved in 30–40% of extrapulmonary cases. Imaging studies may reveal low-attenuation lesions with rim-like calcifications. Biopsy discloses areas of granular necrosis without inflammation or nodules with foamy eosinophilic exudates. Methenamine silver stains reveal cystic forms in necrotic areas. Treatment with intravenous pentamidine or trimethoprim-sulfamethoxazole is successful in up to 45% of cases (*see* Chapter 36).

Microsporidia

In addition to biliary involvement, hepatic infection with protozoa of the order Microsporidia has been described. Histologically, focal granulomas can be seen in portal tracts, and parasites are seen in histiocytes by Giemsa staining. Albendazole is first-line therapy for pathogens other than *Enterocytozoon bieneusi*. No specific agent reliably eradicates *E. bieneusi*, but fumagillin and nitazoxanide have shown some benefit in intestinal microsporidiosis[147] (*see* Chapter 39).

Bacterial Liver Disease

Bacillary angiomatosis is an infectious disorder that primarily affects persons with AIDS or other immunodeficiency states. The causative agents have been identified as the Gram-negative bacilli *Bartonella henselae* and, in some cases, *Bartonella quintana*.[148] Infection with *B. henselae* is frequently associated with exposure to cats while *B. quintana* is associated with exposure to body lice.

Bacillary angiomatosis is characterized most commonly by multiple blood-red papular skin lesions, but disseminated infection with or without skin involvement has also been described.[149] The causative bacilli can infect liver, lymph nodes, pleura, bronchi, bones, brain, bone marrow, and spleen. Additional manifestations include persistent fever, bacteremia, and sepsis. Hepatic infection should be suspected when serum aminotransferase levels are elevated in the absence of other explanations.

Hepatic infection in persons with biliary angiomatosis may present as peliosis hepatis, or blood-filled cysts. Histologically, peliosis in patients with AIDS is characterized by an inflammatory myxoid stroma containing clumps of bacilli surrounding the blood-filled peliotic cysts. Culture and PCR-based methods are being used increasingly for diagnosis.[150]

Bacillary angiomatosis responds uniformly to therapy with erythromycin. For visceral infection, at least 16 weeks of treatment with erythromycin 2 g daily or doxycycline 100 mg every 12 h should be administered. Rifampin may be added for severely ill patients (*see* Chapter 42).

Granulomatous Liver Disease

Mycobacterium tuberculosis

Granulomas are commonly found in liver biopsy specimens (Fig. 78-6), and a wide variety of infectious, drug, and nonspecific etiologies have been implicated. Granulomas are identified in the liver in ~25% of persons with pulmonary tuberculosis and 80% of those with extrapulmonary tuberculosis. Tuberculous granulomas can be distinguished from sarcoid granulomas by central necrosis, acid-fast bacilli, and the presence of fewer granulomas with a tendency to coalesce.[151] Multiple granulomas in the liver may also be seen following vaccination with Bacillus Calmette-Guérin, especially in persons with an impaired immune response. Patients with multiple granulomas due to tuberculosis rarely have clinically significant liver disease.[152] Occasionally, tender hepatomegaly is found. Jaundice with elevated serum alkaline phosphatase levels may occur with miliary infections. The treatment of tuberculous granulomatous disease of the liver is the same as for active pulmonary tuberculosis, namely, four-drug therapy[135,151] (*see* Chapter 40).

Mycobacterium avium Complex

The most common pathogen producing granulomatous liver disease in HIV-infected individuals is *Mycobacterium avium* complex (MAC), which typically causes fatigue, malaise, low-grade fever, night sweats, elevated serum alkaline phosphatase levels, and less frequently hepatomegaly. MAC is found in the liver of up to 80% of autopsy studies in patients who die of AIDS. Liver biopsy reveals poorly formed, noncaseating granulomas with foamy macrophages and a paucity of lymphocytes. Special stains (Ziehl–Nielsen and periodic acid-Schiff) combined with tissue cultures can be used to establish the diagnosis, but histologic examination is more sensitive.

Treatment of MAC infection has markedly improved. Significant benefit has been reported with combinations of three or four drugs given for more than 3 months.[153] The most common regimens contain a macrolide (e.g., clarithromycin or azithromycin) and ethambutol, as well as rifabutin if the CD4+ T-lymphocyte count is less than 50 cells/μL, the mycobacterial load in the blood is greater than 2 $\log_{10}$ colony forming units/mL, or the patient is not on HAART. Alternatives to rifabutin include fluoroquinolones (ciprofloxacin or levofloxacin) and parenteral amikacin, although their benefits are less well-supported by existing data.[135] (*see* Chapter 41) Treatment can produce decreased mycobacterial load and symptomatic improvement as well as improved survival.[154,155]

Toxic and Metabolic Liver Disease

With the conversion of HIV infection to a chronic disease, liver disease has become an important source of morbidity and mortality in the HIV-infected population. In view of their shared routes of transmission, high co-infection rates with chronic viral hepatitis have been an important source of progressive liver disease and liver failure. Another major impediment to the successful initiation of HAART has been treatment-limiting hepatotoxicity. This may be a consequence of the antiretroviral therapies themselves or the effect of these drugs on livers already injured by viral hepatitis or metabolic liver disease, particularly fatty liver. Additionally, many medications used for the management and prevention of AIDS-related processes may cause liver toxicity. A list of commonly encountered drugs and the patterns of injury observed are shown in Table 78-3.

Fatty Liver (Hepatic Steatosis, Nonalcoholic Steatohepatitis)

Macrovesicular fatty infiltration of the liver is the most common specific histologic finding in patients with HIV infection who undergo liver biopsy. It is most commonly found in association with multiple metabolic derangements, including weight loss or gain, obesity, diabetes, hyperlipidemia, hyperalimentation, and alcohol use. Macrovesicular steatosis is randomly distributed throughout the liver lobule, generally unaccompanied by inflammation. Steatosis can lead to hepatomegaly and elevations of serum alkaline phosphatase and aminotransferases. Imaging studies may demonstrate increased density. Treatment is generally directed at the underlying predisposition, if identifiable. In addition, consideration should be given to holding antiretroviral medications, which have also been associated with steatosis (see ahead), particularly the nucleoside analogs AZT, d4T, ddC, ddI and to a lesser extent protease inhibitors (PIs). In general, withholding antiretroviral therapy is recommended once grade 3 elevations of the LFTs occur. However, with any chronic elevation of LFTs withholding of antiretroviral therapy should be considered, even when imaging studies suggest the presence of fatty liver. A significant subset of those persons with fatty liver also have fibrosis and are at increased risk for the subsequent progression to cirrhosis. These patients cannot be identified by imaging studies. It is unclear whether steatosis resolves with successful control of HIV infection.

Nucleoside Analog Reverse Transcriptase Inhibitors (NRTIs)-AZT, d4T, ddI, ddC, 3TC

The mode of action of NRTIs is competitive inhibition of the viral reverse transcriptase leading to premature viral chain termination. However, NRTIs have been associated with host mitochondrial toxicity. Mitochondria execute the key function of oxidative phosphorylation (OXPHOS) and generate ATP as energy for key cellular functions through the action of the electron transport chain. The mitochondrion is also the locus of fatty acid oxidation via medium-chain (MCAD) and long-chain (LCAD) acyl coenzyme A (coA) dehydrogenases. Mitochondrial proteins are encoded in large part by mitochondrial DNA (mtDNA), which is replicated separately by the mitochondrion-specific DNA polymerase γ. This is in contrast to nuclear DNA, which is replicated by DNA polymerases α, β, δ, and ϵ.

Because mtDNA has a high mutation rate, which is further accelerated by processes that enhance generation of reactive oxygen species, including chronic inflammation and aging, mitochondrial dysfunction related to drugs may occur at several levels. Toxicity would be expected to manifest as lactic acidosis (a result of enhanced pyruvate conversion to lactate) and microvesicular steatosis (a consequence of impaired fatty acid oxidation). Whereas phosphorylated

Hepatotoxicity of Drugs Commonly Used in Patients with HIV[190–193]

Table 78-3

	Pattern of Injury				
Type of Drug	**Hepatocellular**	**Microvesicular Steatosis**	**Cholestatic**	**Granulomas**	**Mixed**
Analgesics	Acetaminophen Ibuprofen Indomethacin Diclofenac Salicylates		Propoxyphene		Naproxen Piroxicam Sulindac
Anticonvulsants	Phenytoin	Valproate	Phenytoin	Phenytoin Carbamazepine	Carbamazepine Phenobarbital
Antidepressants	SSRIs Nefazodone Trazodone TCAs		Trazodone Tricyclic antidepressants		
	Venlafaxine				Venlafaxine
Antidiabetics	Pioglitazone Rosiglitazone			Rosiglitazone	Pioglitazone Metformin
	Glyburide		Glyburide		
Antipsychotics	Prochlorperazine Clozapine Risperidone Olanzapine		Haloperidol Chlorpromazine Prochlorperazine Clozapine Risperidone		
Antihypertensives	α-Methyldopa	Calcium channel blockers	Calcium channel blockers	α-Methyldopa	
	Labetalol Calcium channel blockers			Hydralazine	
	ACE inhibitors ARBs Hydralazine		ACE inhibitors ARBs		ACE inhibitors ARBs
Lipid-lowering agents	HMG-CoA reductase inhibitors		Lovastatin		Atorvastatin
	Gemfibrozil Fenofibrate Nicotinic acid		Simvastatin Nicotinic acid		Fluvastatin Pravastatin
Antimicrobials	Acyclovir Amphotericin B Ethionamide Isoniazid Ketoconazole Metronidazole Penicillins Pentamidine Pyrazinamide Quinacrine Rifampin Sulfonamides Dapsone Tetracycline Minocycline TMP-SMX 5-Flucytosine	Tetracycline (IV)	Albendazole Azithromycin Erythromycin Ketoconazole Penicillins Rifampin Thiabendazole TMP-SMX	TMP-SMX	TMP-SMX Terbinafine

(Continued)

(Continued)

Table 78-3

Type of Drug	Pattern of Injury: Hepatocellular	Microvesicular Steatosis	Cholestatic	Granulomas	Mixed
Antiretrovirals					
NRTIs		ddC d4T ddI AZT			
NNRTIs	Nevirapine Efavirenz				
PIs	Indinavir (increases in direct bilirubin) Saquinavir Nelfinavir Lopinavir Ritonavir (inhibits P_{450})				
Miscellaneous	Disulfiram Vitamin A		Anabolic steroids Contraceptive steroids		Chlordiazepoxide Diazepam

ACE, angiotensin converting enzyme; ARB, angiotensin receptor blocker; AZT, zidovudine; ddC, dideoxycytidine; ddI, didanosine; d4T, stavudine; HMG-CoA, 3-hydroxy-3-methylglutaryl-coenzyme A; TCA, tricyclic antidepressant; SSRI, selective serotonin reuptake inhibitor; TMP-SMX, trimethoprim-sulfamethoxazole.

nucleoside analogs have less affinity for cellular nuclear DNA polymerases, ddC, d4T, ddI, and to a lesser extent AZT are potent inhibitors of DNA polymerase, possibly leading to impairment of oxidative phosphorylation (OXPHOS), ATP production, and fatty acid oxidation. NRTIs may also promote generation of reactive oxygen species that, in turn, damage mtDNA.[156] Clinical manifestations of NRTI-induced oxidative stress include hepatic microvesicular steatosis, lactic acidosis, anemia, myopathy, neuropathy and pancreatitis. NRTI toxicity has been caused by fialuridine, or 1-(2-Deoxy-2-Fluoro-b-D-arabinofuranosyl)-5-Iodouracil (FIAU), an agent used to treat hepatitis B infection that produced irreversible lactic acidosis, liver failure, and death. An analogous effect has been reported with AZT (6/10 000 cases), with occasional severe toxicity (massive steatosis, enlarged irregular mitochondria).[157,158] Obese women were identified to be at particular risk for AZT hepatotoxicity,[159] raising the possibility that generating increased reactive oxygen species lowered the threshold for mitochondrial dysfunction. AZT appears to exert further toxicity by also directly inhibiting cytochrome C oxidase and citrate synthase, two key enzymes in OXPHOS.[160] Fulminant hepatitis due to NRTI therapy is rare (1.3–3.9/1000 person-years) but has a mortality of over 40%.[161,162] Grade 3 or 4 hepatotoxicity (ALT more than five times the upper limits of normal) is much more common, and occurred in ~5% of patients on dual nucleoside analog therapy in several studies.[3,163–165]

PIs (Indinavir, Ritonavir, Saquinavir, Nelfinavir)

Each PI is associated with its own spectrum of hepatotoxic potential, despite similar mechanisms of action. A distinct histologic pattern may be associated with PI therapy, including hepatocyte ballooning, Kupffer cell activation, and pericellular zone 3 fibrosis. This was seen in 26% of liver biopsies performed in a cohort of 110 patients.[166] In addition, PIs may be associated with the syndrome of peripheral lipodystrophy, central adiposity, hyperlipidemia, and insulin resistance, which may itself be associated with hepatic steatosis[71] (*see* Chapters 71–73). The precise basis for this finding is not known but may relate to inhibition of cytoplasmic retinoic acid-binding protein (CRABP-1) and LDL receptor-related protein (LRP), which bear 60% homology to HIV protease. Under such conditions PIs may impair triglyceride clearance by the endothelial LRP-lipoprotein lipase complex, leading to lipidemia, insulin resistance, and fatty liver.

A prospective study of the antiretroviral therapy in 298 patients found overall grade 3 or 4 hepatic toxicity in 10.4%, with no significant differences among patients treated with dual nucleoside analogs, saquinavir, indinavir, or nelfinavir. However, ritonavir hepatic toxicity, seen in 30% of patients exposed to the drug, was the single most important variable predicting grade 3 or higher toxicity.[3]

Among PIs, indinavir and atazanavir may cause asymptomatic indirect hyperbilirubinemia by inhibition of bilirubin UDP-glucuronosyltransferase (UGT).[167] There have been occasional reports of severe hepatitis associated with these medications. Histologic characterization of indinavir-induced hepatitis has suggested a hypersensitivity reaction, occurring in 6% of patients.[168] Saquinavir and nelfinavir may cause liver injury as direct hepatotoxins. However, a recent meta-analysis found that nelfinavir and indinavir were associated with hepatotoxicity in only 2.9% and 3.1% of patients, respectively.[169] Ritonavir is a potent inhibitor of the P450 system. Its use has been associated with a significantly increased risk of grade 3 toxicity when used alone or in combination (27–32%); the mechanism is unclear.[3] It is noteworthy that coexistent viral hepatitis was associated with only a slight quantitative increase in higher grades of hepatotoxicity, suggesting that ritonavir toxicity is a more important factor.[3] Amprenavir solution and capsules are contraindicated in hepatic failure.

Non-Nucleoside Reverse Transcriptase Inhibitors (NNRTIs)-Efavirenz, Nevirapine, Delavirdine

The NNRTIs efavirenz, nevirapine, and delavirdine, which inhibit HIV reverse transcriptase without blocking nucleotide chain incorporation, are theoretically at less risk of inhibiting mitochondrial DNA polymerase than nucleoside analogs. Studies suggest that the overall grade 3 to 4 hepatic toxicity rate is 2.4–3.6% for the NNRTIs, with the only grade 4 toxicities being associated with nevirapine.[170] Pregnant and underweight women, women with CD4+ T-lymphocyte counts over 250 cells/μL, and men with CD4+ T-lymphocyte counts over 400 cells/ μL appear to be at increased risk for nevirapine-induced hepatotoxicity.[171–173] Because of reports of severe hepatotoxicity, the US Food and Drug Administration (FDA) has issued an alert for nevirapine. Close monitoring is warranted, especially within the first 18 weeks of initiating therapy with this agent. Efavirenz is the NNRTI of choice for minimizing HAART hepatotoxicity.[91]

Alcohol and Liver Disease Progression

Alcohol abuse is common among HIV-infected patients, and afflicted over 30% of HIV-infected subjects in a Veterans' Administration study.[174] In a French cohort, excessive alcohol consumption was noted in 59% of patients who died from end-stage liver disease, as compared with 24% of patients who died from other causes.[175] Alcohol accelerates disease progression in HIV-HCV co-infected patients and appears to contribute as much to the rate of liver disease progression as does a low CD4 count. Consumption of more than 50 g of alcohol daily appears to produce the same compression of the time to development of cirrhosis as a CD4 count of less than 200/μL.[100] Alcohol abuse should be addressed and consumption minimized in persons with HIV infection, especially those with preexisting chronic liver disease.

Role of Viral Hepatitis in Drug Hepatotoxicity

It is reasonable to speculate that chronic viral hepatitis lowers the threshold for antiretroviral hepatotoxicity through a number of mechanisms, including (1) increasing the formation of reactive oxygen species; (2) directly inducing steatosis, as has been demonstrated in a transgenic mouse model overexpressing HCV core protein[176]; or (3) inducing direct mitochondrial alterations, as has been suggested in an ultrastructural study of HCV-infected hepatocytes.[177]

Notwithstanding these considerations, the data are mixed regarding relative risk posed by preexisting HCV for HAART hepatotoxicity. In one study, the relative risk for hepatotoxicity was 2.8 in HCV positive patients receiving three-drug HAART.[178] In the Johns Hopkins survey, the risk of hepatotoxicity was not increased by HCV in ritonavir users; however, the relative risk was increased by 3.7 in those receiving antiretroviral regimens not containing ritonavir. Overall, 88% of the patients with HBV or HCV infection did not develop hepatotoxicity.[3] A more recent study by the same group showed that 84% of HBV- and HCV-co-infected patients receiving NNRTIs were free from hepatotoxicity. However, HBV and HCV co-infection were risk factors for severe hepatotoxicity in this cohort, as were use of nevirapine, ritonavir, and PIs; baseline CD4+ T-lymphocyte count of less than 50 cells/μL; and increase in CD4+ T-lymphocyte count greater than 50 cells/mm^3 during therapy.[179] A biopsy series at Johns Hopkins showed steatosis in 40% of HIV–HCV co-infected patients with previous or ongoing HAART exposure, but in a multivariate analysis, only stavudine exposure was associated with an increased risk of steatosis.[180]

Several studies suggest that HAART can be continued safely in HCV-infected subjects despite a transient rise in aminotransferases and HCV RNA during the first 3 months of HAART,[106,181] implying that reactivation of HCV with immune reconstitution, not drug toxicity *per se*, explains these findings. In support of this idea, HCV-specific serologic and T-cell responses correlate with flares of liver tests in patients treated successfully with HAART.[182] However, the ability to noninvasively characterize HCV immune reconstitution remains limited. Although this phenomenon is usually self-limited, it may lead to hepatic decompensation in patients with underlying cirrhosis. Therefore, liver biopsy should be considered for all HIV–HCV and HIV-HBV co-infected patients before beginning HAART. For those co-infected patients who must discontinue HAART because of elevated transaminase levels, a course of therapy for HCV may facilitate successful reinitiation of HAART (Fig. 78-7).

Neoplastic Liver Disease

Kaposi Sarcoma

Kaposi sarcoma, although more frequently encountered in the luminal gastrointestinal tract, can also present as a mass lesion of the liver. Liver involvement is usually a manifestation of disseminated disease. Abdominal pain and hepatomegaly with disproportionate elevations of the serum alkaline phosphatase can be seen.

Non-Hodgkin Lymphoma

With advancing immunodeficiency, HIV-infected persons are at risk for developing non-Hodgkin lymphomas (NHLs),

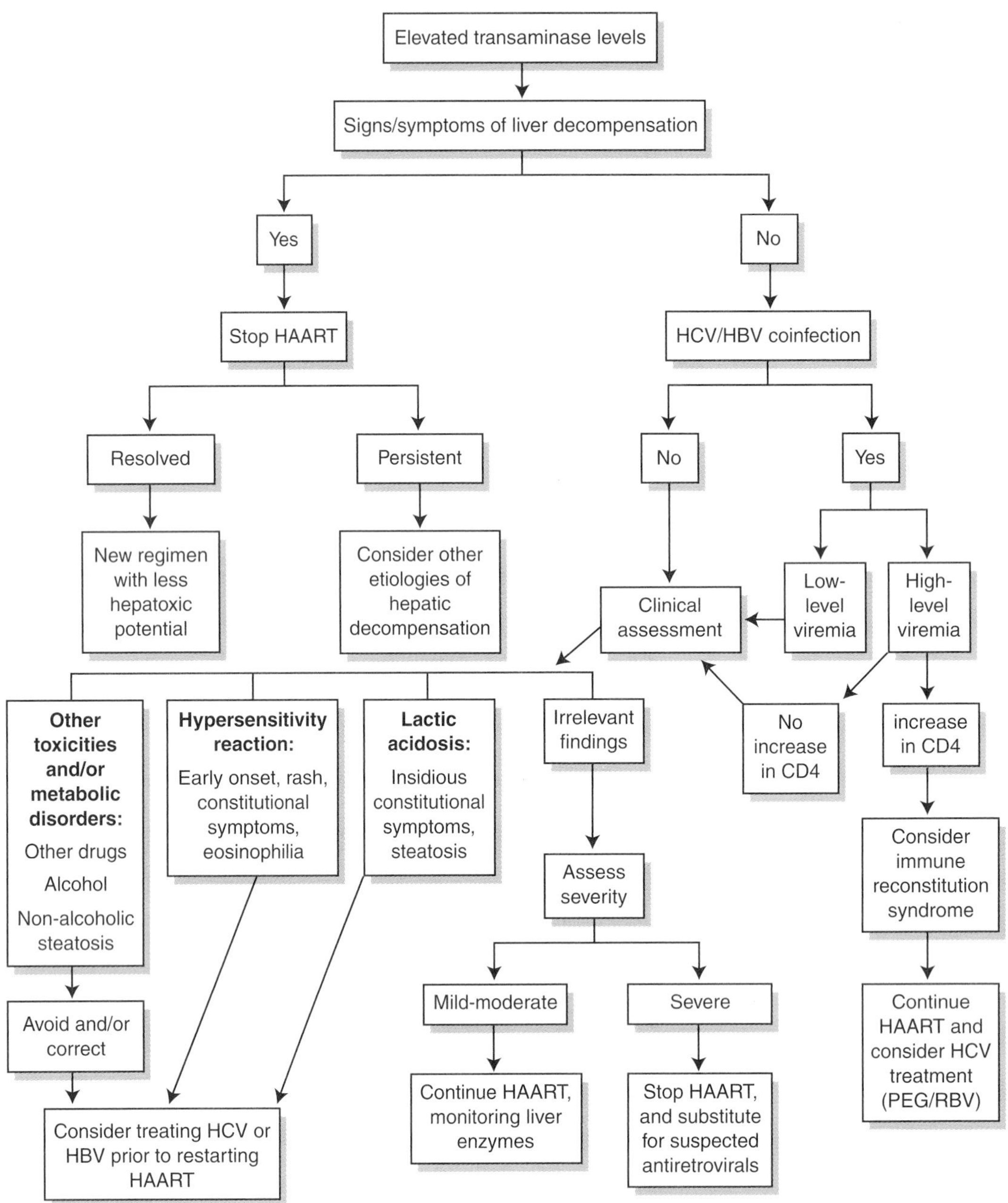

Figure 78-7 ■ Algorithm for evaluating liver test flares after initiation of HAART.[193]

predominantly of the B-cell type. These lymphomas present much more frequently extranodally in the HIV-infected population. About 10% of NHLs in the HIV-infected cohort involve the liver. Characteristic findings on ultrasound scans or CT scans (the preferred diagnostic modality) include the presence of mass lesion(s). The diagnosis is confirmed by an elevated serum alkaline phosphatase level. Jaundice may be seen as a manifestation of more advanced lymphoma or associated with biliary occlusion by portal adenopathy. When present, jaundice is usually associated with high short-term mortality, as lymphomas are usually of high biologic grade and respond poorly to treatment.

Hepatocellular Carcinoma

With an increasing prevalence of chronic liver disease and cirrhosis in the HIV-infected cohort, hepatocellular carcinoma (HCC), a frequent complication of HCV and HBV-related cirrhosis, is becoming more common as well. HCC should be suspected when a known cirrhotic individual experiences hepatic decompensation. Imaging studies disclose the presence of a mass lesion that exhibits arterial phase enhancement on CT or MRI. As compared with HIV negative patients, HIV positive patients are more likely to have multifocal, infiltrating, and metastatic disease upon first diagnosis with HCC.[183] Surveillance strategies for HCC include semiannual serum α_1-fetoprotein assays and ultrasonography. Hepatic resection and nonsurgical local-regional treatment (percutaneous ethanol injection, radiofrequency ablation, and transarterial embolization) improve survival in HIV positive patients.[184] Hepatic transplantation is a relatively new modality for management of HCC in those with HIV infection, and early results in selected centers appear promising.[185]

AIDS Cholangiopathy

Three overlapping clinical syndromes comprise AIDS cholangiopathy, which occurs late in HIV disease. Imaging studies suggest the diagnosis in most cases. Each syndrome can be diagnosed by ERCP. Signs and symptoms include fever, right upper quadrant abdominal pain, jaundice, and hepatomegaly. The predominant laboratory finding is an elevated serum alkaline phosphatase level. Aminotransferase elevations, when seen, are mild. The most commonly identified pathogens include *Cryptosporidium*, CMV, Microsporidia, and MAC. Causality is not proven, however, as therapeutic approaches directed at these pathogens do not produce meaningful responses in the outcome of cholangiopathy. HAART, on the other hand, is associated with reduced mortality from AIDS cholangiopathy.[186] The three syndromes are described below.

1. *Sclerosing cholangitis*. The clinical and cholangiographic picture of this syndrome is analogous to that seen with idiopathic primary sclerosing cholangitis. It is characterized by focal strictures alternating with dilations of the intrahepatic and extrahepatic biliary tree along with terminal pruning of the secondary or higher-order biliary radicals. The syndrome usually appears after AIDS is diagnosed. No medical therapy has been shown to be beneficial. In some cases, dominant focal strictures respond to biliary stenting.
2. *Papillary stenosis*. This discrete entity can occur alone or in conjunction with sclerosing cholangitis. ERCP reveals narrowing of the distal common bile duct that may extend into the intraduodenal segment (Fig. 78-5). A dilated proximal CBD is common. This entity can be responsive to sphincterotomy, resulting in significantly diminished abdominal pain. Repeat sphincterotomy may be required.
3. *Long extrahepatic bile duct strictures (with or without sclerosing cholangitis)*. This entity is likely a subset of sclerosing cholangitis and may respond to biliary stenting. Although stenting of large ducts may provide some decompression and pain relief, alkaline phosphatase levels may continue to rise as a result of progressive disease involving small intrahepatic bile ducts.

Acalculous Cholecystitis

Acalculous cholecystitis may be associated with a number of pathogens, including CMV, *Cryptosporidium, Isospora, Candida* sp., *Salmonella* sp., *Klebsiella, Campylobacter* sp., and *Serratia* sp. The presentation ranges from mild right upper quadrant pain to fulminant, gangrenous cholecystitis. Ultrasonography may reveal a thickened gallbladder wall, pericholecystic fluid, or ductal abnormalities. Technetium-HIDA scanning may be diagnostic, revealing an absence of gallbladder uptake. Both acute and chronic changes of cholecystitis can be seen pathologically. Under stable conditions, laparoscopic cholecystectomy can be performed with acceptable morbidity. More unstable patients may require open cholecystectomy or percutaneous cholecystectomy.

SUMMARY OF MANAGEMENT PRINCIPLES

Management of acute and chronic liver disease in patients with HIV infection is complex, partly because of the myriad linked etiologies that shade the decision process and partly because of the dearth of studies addressing this issue. The treatment algorithms provided herein describe a framework for the approach to patients. These are divided into acute (1a) and chronic (1b) hepatocellular injury patterns (Fig. 78-1) and cholestatic injury patterns (Fig. 78-2).

When a patient is first noted to have abnormal liver tests, it is often unclear whether the process is chronic or acute. However, serial enzyme profiles are available for some patients, and an acute process may be observed. As a general rule, acute elevations less than five times the upper limit of normal should be monitored to determine the trend. If the ALT/AST exceeds five times normal, it is reasonable to initiate a workup as shown in the acute AST/ALT elevation algorithm. A persistent transaminase abnormality lasting longer than 6 months should lead to initiation of a formal workup as shown in Figure 78-1. Key tests include evaluation for hepatitis B and C, medications and drugs associated with liver toxicity, and metabolic/autoimmune disorders. Liver biopsy is an important endpoint for all evaluations of chronic hepatitis.

Cholestatic processes that result in increased bilirubin, alkaline phosphatase, and GGT must be evaluated by a different process, as shown in Figure 78-2. As above, there are no absolute thresholds that determine whether to enter the diagnostic algorithm. However, bilirubin or alkaline phosphatase levels and GGT that are more than two times normal deserve further evaluation. Isolated GGT abnormalities are most commonly due to induction by medications and do not generally require an extensive workup. Hyperbilirubinemia due to PIs (particularly indinavir) may be troubling to the patient and clinician but does not generally require additional evaluation if the process is identified early. Visible jaundice may lead to a change of PI. For patients with jaundice, direct hyperbilirubinemia, and normal ducts, drug toxicity should be suspected. It is important to remember that cholestasis is slow to resolve, and months may pass before normalization after discontinuing the offending agent.

ROLE OF LIVER TRANSPLANTATION

The treatment of last resort for end-stage nonmalignant liver disease is liver transplantation. While HIV infection was once an absolute contraindication to transplantation, the HAART era has witnessed successful transplants in a number of HIV-infected patients at selected clinical centers.[187,188] One study has reported survival rates at 12, 24, and 36 months of 87.1%, 72.8%, and 72.8%, respectively, in HIV positive patients; these rates were not statistically different from those in HIV negative patients. However, survival was poorer among HIV-infected patients with HAART intolerance, post-transplant CD4+ T-cell counts less than 200 cells/μL, post-transplant HIV viral loads greater than 400 copies/mL, and HCV co-infection.[187] Of note, HIV positive patients have higher pre-transplant mortality than HIV negative patients with equivalent Model for End-stage Liver Disease (MELD) scores; most deaths on the waiting list are attributable to infection.[189] Therefore, HIV positive patients should be referred for transplant early and monitored closely for pre-transplant infection. The role of liver transplantation in the management of patients who develop end-stage liver disease requires further clarification in view of the disparity between the rapidly growing candidate list and the limited availability of donor organs. Active protocols for HIV positive and HCV-HIV co-infected individuals with end-stage liver disease whose HIV is effectively suppressed are ongoing in a limited number of US centers.

CONCLUSIONS

Prolongation of survival in HIV-infected patients has led to increased prominence of liver disease from a variety of viral, metabolic, and toxic etiologies. Healthcare workers caring for such patients must become conversant with common causes of liver injury, diagnostic modalities, and treatment interventions. Use of diagnostic algorithms included herein can aid in the management of such patients.

REFERENCES

1. Gebo KA, Fleishman JA, Moore RD. Hospitalizations for metabolic conditions, opportunistic infections, and injection drug use among HIV patients: trends between 1996 and 2000 in 12 states. J Acquir Immune Defic Syndr 40:609, 2005.
2. Sulkowski MS, Mast EE, Seeff LB, Thomas DL. Hepatitis C virus infection as an opportunistic disease in persons infected with human immunodeficiency virus. Clin Infect Dis 30 (Suppl 1):S77, 2000.
3. Sulkowski MS, Thomas DL, Chaisson RE, Moore RD. Hepatotoxicity associated with antiretroviral therapy in adults infected with human immunodeficiency virus and the role of hepatitis C or B virus infection. JAMA 283:74, 2000.
4. Alter MJ. Hepatitis C virus infection in the United States. J Hepatol 31:88, 1999.
5. Danta M et al. Evidence for sexual transmission of HCV in recent epidemic in HIV-infected men in the UK. CROI 2006, Abstract 86.
6. Reddy KR, Brillant P, Schiff ER. Amoxicillin-clavulanate potassium-associated cholestasis. Gastroenterology 96:1135, 1989.
7. Olynyk JK, Cullen DJ, Aquilia S, et al. A population-based study of the clinical expression of the hemochromatosis gene. N Engl J Med 341:718, 1999.
8. Bessesen M, Ives D, Condreay L, et al. Chronic active hepatitis B exacerbations in human immunodeficiency virus-infected patients following development of resistance to or withdrawal of lamivudine. Clin Infect Dis 28:1032, 1999.
9. Shire NJ, Sherman KE. Management of HBV/HIV-coinfected patients. Semin Liver Dis 25 (Suppl 1):48, 2005.
10. Sherman KE, Shire NJ, Cernohous P, et al. Liver injury and changes in hepatitis C virus (HCV) RNA load associated with protease inhibitor-based antiretroviral therapy for treatment-naive HCV-HIV-coinfected patients: lopinavir-ritonavir versus nelfinavir. Clin Infect Dis 41:1186, 2005.
11. Conn HO. Trailmaking and number-connection tests in the assessment of mental state in portal systemic encephalopathy. Am J Dig Dis 22:541, 1977.
12. Sherman KE. Alanine aminotransferase in clinical practice: a review. Arch Intern Med 51:260, 1991.
13. Aranda-Michel J, Sherman KE. Tests of the liver: use and misuse. Gastroenterologist 6:34, 1998.
14. Shrestha R, McKinley C, Showalter R, et al. Quantitative liver function tests define the functional severity of liver disease in early-stage cirrhosis. Liver Transpl Surg 3:166, 1997.
15. O'Connor JB, Imperiale TF, Singer ME. Cost-effectiveness analysis of hepatitis A vaccination strategies for adults. Hepatology 30:1077, 1999.
16. Hofer M, Joller-Jemelka HI, Grob PJ, et al. Frequent chronic hepatitis B virus infection in HIV-infected patients positive for antibody to hepatitis B core antigen only: Swiss HIV Cohort Study. Eur J Clin Microbiol Infect Dis 17:6, 1998.
17. Shire NJ, Rouster SD, Rajicic N, Sherman KE. Occult hepatitis B in HIV-infected patients. J Acquir Immune Defic Syndr 36:869, 2004.
18. Ragni MV, Ndimbie OK, Rice EO, et al. The presence of hepatitis C virus (HCV) antibody in human immunodeficiency virus-positive hemophilic men undergoing HCV "seroreversion." Blood 82:1010, 1993.
19. de Pouplana M, Soriano V, Samaniego JG, Enriquez A, et al. More severe course of delta hepatitis in HIV-infected patients. Genitourin Med 71:132, 1995.
20. Fainboim H, Gonzalez J, Fassio E, et al. Prevalence of hepatitis viruses in an anti-human immunodeficiency virus-positive population from Argentina. A multicentre study. J Viral Hepat 6:53, 1999.
21. Goncales NS, Pinho JR, Moreira RC, et al. Hepatitis E virus immunoglobulin G antibodies in different populations in Campinas, Brazil. Clin Diagn Lab Immunol 7:813, 2000.
22. Shiramizu B, Theodore D, Bassett R, et al. Adult AIDS Clinical Trials Group 5096 Team. Correlation of single photon emission computed tomography parameters as a noninvasive alternative to liver biopsies in assessing liver involvement in the setting of HIV and hepatitis C virus coinfection: a multicenter trial of the Adult AIDS Clinical Trials Group. J Acquir Immune Defic Syndr 33:329, 2003.
23. Bair HJ, Behr T, Rubbert A, et al. ^{99m}Tc-trimethyl-BrIDA scintigraphy in HIV-related cholangiopathy. Nuklearmedizin 34:252, 1995.
24. Buscombe JR, Miller RF, Ell PJ. Hepatobiliary scintigraphy in the diagnosis of AIDS-related sclerosing cholangitis. Nucl Med Commun 13:154, 1992.
25. Brunetti JC, Van Heertum RL, Kempf JS, et al. Tc-99m DISIDA hepatobiliary scintigraphy in AIDS cholangitis. Clin Nucl Med 19:36, 1994.
26. Beale TJ, Wetton CW, Crofton ME. A sonographic-pathological correlation of liver biopsies in patients with the acquired

immune deficiency syndrome (AIDS). Clin Radiol 50:761, 1995.
27. Albisetti M, Braegger CP, Stallmach T, et al. Hepatic steatosis: a frequent non-specific finding in HIV-infected children. Eur J Pediatr 158:971, 1999.
28. Tshibwabwa ET, Mwaba P, Bogle-Taylor J, Zumla A. Four-year study of abdominal ultrasound in 900 Central African adults with AIDS referred for diagnostic imaging. Abdom Imaging 25:290, 2000.
29. Catalano O, Cusati B, Sandomenico F, et al. Multiple-phase spiral computerized tomography of small hepatocellular carcinoma: technique optimization and diagnostic yield. Radiol Med (Torino) 98:53, 1999.
30. Knollmann FD, Maurer J, Grunewald T, et al. Abdominal CT features and survival in acquired immunodeficiency. Acta Radiol 38:970, 1997.
31. Radin R. HIV infection: analysis in 259 consecutive patients with abnormal abdominal CT findings. Radiology 197:712, 1995.
32. Macdonald GA, Peduto AJ. Magnetic resonance imaging and diseases of the liver and biliary tract. Part 2. Magnetic resonance cholangiography and angiography and conclusions. J Gastroenterol Hepatol 15:992, 2000.
33. Fulcher AS, Turner MA, Yelon JA, et al. Magnetic resonance cholangiopancreatography (MRCP) in the assessment of pancreatic duct trauma and its sequelae: preliminary findings. J Trauma 48:1001, 2000.
34. Weber C, Krupski G, Lorenzen J, et al. MRCP in primary sclerosing cholangitis. Rofo 175:203, 2003.
35. Textor HJ, Flacke S, Pauleit D, et al. Three-dimensional magnetic resonance cholangiopancreatography with respiratory triggering in the diagnosis of primary sclerosing cholangitis: comparison with endoscopic retrograde cholangiography. Endoscopy 34:984, 2002.
36. Teare JP, Daly CA, Rodgers C, et al. Pancreatic abnormalities and AIDS related sclerosing cholangitis. Genitourin Med 73:271, 1997.
37. Walden DT. Biliary problems in people with HIV disease. Curr Treat Options Gastroenterol 2:147, 1999.
38. Barthet M, Chauveau E, Bonnet E, et al. Pancreatic ductal changes in HIV-infected patients. Gastrointest Endosc 45:59, 1997.
39. Stotland BR, Lichtenstein GR. Liver biopsy complications and routine ultrasound. Am J Gastroenterol 91:1295, 1996.
40. Scheimann AO, Barrios JM, Al-Tawil YS, et al. Percutaneous liver biopsy in children: impact of ultrasonography and spring-loaded biopsy needles. J Pediatr Gastroenterol Nutr 31:536, 2000.
41. Nobili V, Comparcola D, Sartorelli MR, et al. Blind and ultrasound-guided percutaneous liver biopsy in children. Pediatr Radiol 33:772, 2003.
42. Riley TR. How often does ultrasound marking change the liver biopsy site? Am J Gastroenterol 94:3320, 1999.
43. Younossi ZM, Teran JC, Ganiats TG, Carey WD. Ultrasound-guided liver biopsy for parenchymal liver disease: an economic analysis. Dig Dis Sci 43:46, 1998.
44. Perrault J, McGill DB, Ott BJ, Taylor WF. Liver biopsy: complications in 1000 inpatients and outpatients. Gastroenterology 74:103, 1978.
45. Piccinino F, Sagnelli E, Pasquale G, Giusti G. Complications following percutaneous liver biopsy: a multicentre retrospective study on 68,376 biopsies. J Hepatol 2:1656, 1986.
46. McGill DB, Rakela J, Zinsmeister AR, Ott BJ. A 21-year experience with major hemorrhage after percutaneous liver biopsy. Gastroenterology 99:1396, 1990.
47. Churchill DR, Mann D, Coker RJ, et al. Fatal haemorrhage following liver biopsy in patients with HIV infection. Genitourin Med 72:62, 1996.
48. McAfee JH, Keeffe EB, Lee RG, Rosch J. Transjugular liver biopsy. Hepatology 15:726, 1992.
49. Ahmed MM, Mutimer DJ, Elias E, et al. A combined management protocol for patients with coagulation disorders infected with hepatitis C virus. Br J Haematol 95:383, 1996.
50. Fried MW. Management of hepatitis C in the hemophilia patient. Am J Med 107:85S, 1999.
51. Shin JL, Teitel J, Swain MG, et al. Virology and Immunology Committee of the Association of Hemophilia Clinic Directors of Canada. A Canadian multicenter retrospective study evaluating transjugular liver biopsy in patients with congenital bleeding disorders and hepatitis C: is it safe and useful? Am J Hematol 78:85, 2005.
52. Theodore D, Fried MW, Kleiner DE, et al. Liver biopsy in patients with inherited disorders of coagulation and chronic hepatitis C. Haemophilia 10:413, 2004.
53. Cappell MS, Schwartz MS, Biempica L. Clinical utility of liver biopsy in patients with serum antibodies to the human immunodeficiency virus. Am J Med 88:123, 1990.
54. Poles MA, Dieterich DT. Hepatitis C virus/human immunodeficiency virus coinfection: clinical management issues. Clin Infect Dis 31:154, 2000.
55. Cavicchi M, Pialoux G, Carnot F, et al. Value of liver biopsy for the rapid diagnosis of infection in human immunodeficiency virus-infected patients who have unexplained fever and elevated serum levels of alkaline phosphatase or gamma-glutamyl transferase. Clin Infect Dis 20:606, 1995.
56. Lacaille F, Fournet JC, Blanche S. Clinical utility of liver biopsy in children with acquired immunodeficiency syndrome. Pediatr Infect Dis J 18:143, 1999.
57. Kelleher TB, Mehta SH, Bhaskar R, et al. Prediction of hepatic fibrosis in HIV/HCV co-infected patients using serum fibrosis markers: the SHASTA index. J Hepatol 43:78, 2005.
58. de Ledinghen V, Douvin C, Kettaneh A, et al. Diagnosis of hepatic fibrosis and cirrhosis by transient elastography in HIV/Hepatitis C virus-coinfected patients. J Acquir Immune Defic Syndr 41:175, 2006.
59. Fonquernie L, Meynard JL, Charrois A, et al. Occurrence of acute hepatitis A in patients infected with human immunodeficiency virus. Clin Infect Dis 32:297, 2001.
60. Ida S, Tachikawa N, Nakajima A, et al. Influence of human immunodeficiency virus type 1 infection on acute hepatitis A virus infection. Clin Infect Dis 34:379, 2002.
61. Vento S, Garofano T, Renzini C, et al. Fulminant hepatitis associated with hepatitis A virus superinfection in patients with chronic hepatitis C. N Engl J Med 338:286, 1998.
62. CDC. Guidelines for Preventing Opportunistic Infections Among HIV-Infected Persons – 2002. Available: http://www.cdc.gov/mmwr/preview/mmwrhtml/rr5108a1.htm Dec 26, 2005.
63. Shire NJ, Welge JA, Sherman KE. Efficacy of inactivated hepatitis A vaccine in HIV-infected patients: a hierarchical bayesian meta-analysis. Vaccine 24:272, 2006.
64. Gordon SC, Reddy KR, Gould EE, et al. The spectrum of liver disease in the acquired immunodeficiency syndrome. J Hepatol 2:475, 1986.
65. Lebovics E, Dworkin BM, Heier SK, Rosenthal WS. The hepatobiliary manifestations of human immunodeficiency virus infection. Am J Gastroenterol 83:1, 1988.
66. Kellerman SE, Hanson DL, McNaghten AD, Fleming PL. Prevalence of chronic hepatitis B and incidence of acute hepatitis B infection in human immunodeficiency virus-infected subjects. J Infect Dis 188:571, 2003.
67. Bodsworth NJ, Cooper DA, Donovan B. The influence of human immunodeficiency virus type 1 infection on the development of the hepatitis B virus carrier state. J Infect Dis 163:1138, 1991.
68. Thio CL, Seaberg EC, Skolasky R Jr, et al. Multicenter AIDS Cohort Study. HIV-1, hepatitis B virus, and risk of liver-related mortality in the Multicenter Cohort Study (MACS). Lancet 360:1921, 2002.

69. Yachimski P, Chung RT. Update on Hepatitis B and C Coinfection in HIV. Curr Infect Dis Rep 7:299, 2005.
70. Scharschmidt BF, Held MJ, Hollander HH, et al. Hepatitis B in patients with HIV infection: relationship to AIDS and patients survival. Ann Intern Med 117:837, 1992.
71. Carr A, Samaras K, Chisholm DJ, Cooper DA. Pathogenesis of HIV-1-protease inhibitor-associated peripheral lipodystrophy, hyperlipidaemia, and insulin resistance. Lancet 351:1881, 1998.
72. Pol S, Lebray P, Vallet-Pichard A. HIV infection and hepatic enzyme abnormalities: intricacies of the pathogenic mechanisms. Clin Infect Dis 38 (Suppl 2):S65, 2004.
73. Wolters LM, Niesters HG, Hansen BE, et al. Development of hepatitis B virus resistance for lamivudine in chronic hepatitis B patients co-infected with the human immunodeficiency virus in a Dutch cohort. J Clin Virol 24:173, 2002.
74. Di Martino V, Thevenot T, Colin JF, et al. Influence of HIV infection on the response to interferon therapy and the long-term outcome of chronic hepatitis B. Gastroenterology 123:1812, 2002.
75. Benhamou Y, Bochet M, Thibault V, et al. Long-term incidence of hepatitis B virus resistance to lamivudine in human immunodeficiency virus-infected patients. Hepatology 30:1302, 1999.
76. Fang CT, Chen PJ, Chen MY, et al. Dynamics of plasma hepatitis B virus levels after highly active antiretroviral therapy in patients with HIV infection. J Hepatol 39:1028, 2003.
77. Lok AS, Heathcote EJ, Hoofnagle JH. Management of hepatitis B: 2000 – summary of a workshop. Gastroenterology 120:1828, 2001.
78. Ripamonti D, Maggiolo F, Suter F. HIV-1 and hepatitis B virus: time for a re-think? Lancet 363:1400, 2004.
79. Benhamou Y. Treatment algorithm for chronic hepatitis B in HIV-infected patients. J Hepatol 44 (Suppl 1):S90, 2006.
80. Brook M, Gilson R, Wilkins E. BHIVA Guidelines – HIV and Chronic Hepatitis: Co-Infection with HIV and Hepatitis B Virus Infection, updated October 2004. Available: http://www.bhiva.org/guidelines/2004/HBV/index.html Feb 5, 2006.
81. EASL Jury. EASL International Consensus Conference on Hepatitis B. 13–14 September, 2002: Geneva, Switzerland. Consensus statement (short version). J Hepatol 38:533, 2003.
82. Xiong S, Yang H, Westland CE, et al. Resistance surveillance of HbeAg-chronic hepatitis B (CHB) patients treated for two years with adefovir dipivoxil (ADV). J Hepatol 38 (Suppl 2):182, 2003.
83. Westland CE, Yang H, Delaney WE, et al. Resistance profile of adefovir dipivoxil (ADV) in immunocompetent and immunocompromised chronic hepatitis B patients after 48 weeks of adefovir dipivoxil therapy. J Hepatol 38 (Suppl 2):182, 2003.
84. Benhamou Y, Thibault V, Vig P, et al. Safety and efficacy of adefovir dipivoxil in patients infected with lamivudine-resistant hepatitis B and HIV-1. J Hepatol 44:62, 2006.
85. Delaugerre C, Marcelin AG, Thibault V, et al. Human immunodeficiency virus (HIV) Type 1 reverse transcriptase resistance mutations in hepatitis B virus (HBV)-HIV-coinfected patients treated for HBV chronic infection once daily with 10 milligrams of adefovir dipivoxil combined with lamivudine. Antimicrob Agents Chemother 46:1586, 2002.
86. Hannon H, Bagnis CI, Benhamou Y, et al. The renal tolerance of low-dose adefovir dipivoxil by lamivudine-resistant individuals co-infected with hepatitis B and HIV. Nephrol Dial Transplant 19:386, 2004.
87. Izzedine H, Hulot JS, Launay-Vacher V, et al. Adefovir Dipivoxil International 437 Study Group. Adefovir Dipivoxil International 438 Study Group. Renal safety of adefovir dipivoxil in patients with chronic hepatitis B: two double-blind, randomized, placebo-controlled studies. Kidney Int 66:1153, 2004.
88. van Bommel F, Wunsche T, Mauss S, et al. Comparison of adefovir and tenofovir in the treatment of lamivudine-resistant hepatitis B virus infection. Hepatology 40:1421, 2004.
89. Benhamou Y, Fleury H, Trimoulet P, et al. Anti-hepatitis B virus efficacy of tenofovir disoproxil fumarate in HIV-infected patients. Hepatology 43:548, 2006.
90. Martinez E, Milinkovic A, de Lazzari E, et al. Pancreatic toxic effects associated with co-administration of didanosine and tenofovir in HIV-infected adults. Lancet 364:65, 2004.
91. O'Leary JG and Chung RT. Management of HIV/HCV coinfected patients. AIDS Reader 16(6):313, 2006.
92. Kim AY, Chung RT, Polsky B. Human immunodeficiency virus and hepatitis B and C coinfection: pathogenic interactions, natural history, and therapy. AIDS Clin Rev 263, 2000–01.
93. Eyster ME, Fried MW, Di Bisceglie AM, Goedert JJ. Increasing hepatitis C virus RNA levels in hemophiliacs: relationship to human immunodeficiency virus infection and liver disease. Multicenter Hemophilia Cohort Study. Blood 84:1020, 1994.
94. Chazouilleres O, Kim M, Combs C, et al. Quantitation of hepatitis C virus RNA in liver transplant recipients. Gastroenterology 106:994, 1994.
95. Bica I, McGovern B, Dhar R, et al. Increasing mortality due to end-stage liver disease in patients with human immunodeficiency virus infection. Clin Infect Dis 32:492, 2001.
96. Eyster ME, Diamondstone LS, Lien JM, et al. Natural history of hepatitis C virus infection in multitransfused hemophiliacs: effect of coinfection with human immunodeficiency virus: the Multicenter Hemophilia Cohort Study. J Acquir Immune Defic Syndr 6:602, 1993.
97. Telfer P, Sabin C, Devereux H, et al. The progression of HCV-Associated liver disease in a cohort of haemophilic patients. Br J Haematol 87:555, 1994.
98. Makris M, Preston FE, Rosendaal FR, et al. The natural history of chronic hepatitis C in haemophiliacs. Br J Haematol 94:746, 1996.
99. Lesens O, Deschenes M, Steben M, et al. Hepatitis C virus is related to progressive liver disease in human immunodeficiency virus-positive hemophiliacs and should be treated as an opportunistic infection. J Infect Dis 179:1254, 1999.
100. Benhamou Y, Bochet M, Di Martino V, et al. Liver fibrosis progression in human immunodeficiency virus and hepatitis C virus coinfected patients: the Multivirc Group. Hepatology 30:1054, 1999.
101. Verma S, Wang CH, Govindarajan S, et al. Do type and duration of antiretroviral therapy attenuate liver fibrosis in HIV-hepatitis C virus-coinfected patients? Clin Infect Dis 42:262, 2006.
102. Greub G, Ledergerber B, Battegay M, et al. Clinical progression, survival, and immune recovery during antiretroviral therapy in patients with HIV-1 and hepatitis C virus coinfection: the Swiss HIV Cohort Study. Lancet 356:1800, 2000.
103. Miller MF, Haley C, Koziel MJ, Rowley CF. Impact of hepatitis C virus on immune restoration in HIV-infected patients who start highly active antiretroviral therapy: a meta-analysis. Clin Infect Dis 41:713, 2005.
104. Chung RT, Evans SR, Yang Y, et al. AIDS Clinical Trials Group 383 Study Team. Immune recovery is associated with persistent rise in hepatitis C virus RNA, infrequent liver test flares, and is not impaired by hepatitis C virus in co-infected subjects. AIDS 16:1915, 2002.
105. Sulkowski MS, Moore RD, Mehta SH, et al. Hepatitis C and progression of HIV disease. JAMA 288:199, 2000.
106. Rutschmann OT, Negro F, Hirschel B, et al. Impact of treatment with human immunodeficiency virus (HIV) protease inhibitors on hepatitis C viremia in patients coinfected with HIV. J Infect Dis 177:783, 1998.

107. Chung RT, Andersen J, Volberding P, et al. the AIDS Clinical Trials Group A5071 Study Team. Peginterferon alfa-2a plus Ribavirin versus Interferon alfa-2a plus Ribavirin for chronic Hepatitis C in HIV-coinfected persons. N Engl J Med 351:451, 2004.
108. Torriani FJ, Rodriguez-Torres M, Rockstroh JK, et al. APRICOT Study Group. Peginterferon alfa-2a plus ribavirin for chronic hepatitis C virus infection in HIV-infected patients. N Engl J Med 351:438, 2004.
109. Carrat F, Bani-Sadr F, Pol S, et al. ANRS HCO2 RIBAVIC Study Team. Pegylated interferon alfa-2b vs standard interferon alfa-2b, plus ribavirin, for chronic hepatitis C in HIV-infected patients: a randomized controlled trial. JAMA 292:2839, 2004.
110. Andersson K and Chung RT. Hepatitis C virus in the HIV-infected patient. Clin Liver Dis 2006; in press.
111. Mauss S. Treatment of viral hepatitis in HIV-coinfected patients-adverse events and their management. J Hepatol 44 (Suppl 1):S114, 2006.
112. Rodriguez-Torres M, Torriani FJ, Soriano V, et al. Effect of ribavirin on intracellular and plasma pharmacokinetics of nucleoside reverse transcriptase inhibitors in patients with human immunodeficiency virus-hepatitis C virus coinfection: results of a randomized clinical study. Antimicrob Agents Chemother 49:3997, 2005.
113. Moreno A, Quereda C, Moreno L, et al. High rate of didanosine-related mitochondrial toxicity in HIV/HCV-coinfected patients receiving ribavirin. Antivir Ther 9:133, 2004.
114. Uberti-Foppa C, De Bona A, Morsica G, et al. Recombinant interleukin-2 for treatment of HIV reduces hepatitis C viral load in coinfected patients. AIDS 13:140, 1999.
115. Brau N, Rodriguez-Torres M, Prokupek D, et al. Treatment of chronic hepatitis C in HIV/HCV-coinfection with interferon alpha-2b+ full-course vs. 16-week delayed ribavirin. Hepatology 39:989, 2004.
116. Griffiths PD, Emery VC. Cytomegalovirus. In: Richman DD, Whitley RJ, Hayden FG (eds). Clinical virology. New York: Churchill-Livingstone; 1997, p 445.
117. Kaufman B, Gandhi SA, Louie E, et al. Herpes simplex virus hepatitis: case report and review. Clin Infect Dis 24:334, 1997.
118. Knox KK, Carrigan DR. HHV-6 and CMV pneumonitis in immuno-compromised patients. Lancet 343:1647, 1994.
119. Schiff G. Hepatitis caused by other viruses. In: Schiff ER, Sorrell MF, Maddrey WC (eds). Disease of the Liver. Philadelphia: Lippincott-Raven; 1999, p 869.
120. Krilov LR, Rubin LG, Frogel M, et al. Disseminated adenovirus infection with hepatic necrosis in patients with human immunodeficiency virus infection and other immunodeficiency states. Rev Infect Dis 12:303, 1990.
121. Hierholzer JC. Adenoviruses in the immunocompromised host. Clin Microbiol Rev 5:262, 1992.
122. Brundler MA, Rodriguez-Baez N, Jaffe R, et al. Adenovirus ascending cholangiohepatitis. Pediatr Dev Pathol 6:156, 2003.
123. Housset C, Boucher O, Girard P. Immunohistochemical evidence for HIV-1 infection of liver Kupffer cells. Hum Pathol 21:404, 1990.
124. Jiang TJ, Zhao M, Zhao JM, et al. Immunohistochemical evidence for HIV-1 infection in the liver of HIV-infected patients. Zhonghua Shi Yan He Lin Chuang Bing Du Xue Za Zhi 19:152, 2005.
125. Schaffner F. The liver in HIV infection. Prog Liver Dis 9:505, 1990.
126. Myerowitz RL, Pazin GJ, Allen CM. Disseminated candidiasis: changes in incidence, underlying diseases, and pathology. Am J Clin Pathol 68:29, 1977.
127. Bertagnolio S, de Gaetano Donati K, Tacconelli E, et al. Hospital-acquired candidemia in HIV-infected patients. Incidence, risk factors and predictors of outcome. J Chemother 16:172, 2004.
128. Semelka RC, Shoenut JP, Greenberg HM, Bow EJ. Detection of acute and treated lesions of hepatosplenic candidiasis: comparison of dynamic contrast-enhanced CT and MR imaging. J Magn Reson Imaging 2:341, 1992.
129. Anttila VJ, Lamminen AE, Bondestam S, et al. Magnetic resonance imaging is superior to computed tomography and ultrasonography in imaging infectious liver foci in acute leukaemia. Eur J Haematol 56:82, 1996.
130. Phillips EH, Carroll BJ, Chandra M, et al. Laparoscopic-guided biopsy for diagnosis of hepatic candidiasis. J Laparoendosc Surg 2:33, 1992.
131. Rex JH, Walsh TJ, Sobel JD, et al. Practice guidelines for the treatment of candidiasis. Infectious Diseases Society of America. Clin Infect Dis 30:662, 2000.
132. Breton G, Adle-Biassette H, Therby A, et al. Immune reconstitution inflammatory syndrome in HIV-infected patients with disseminated histoplasmosis. AIDS 20:119, 2006.
133. Lamps LW, Molina CP, West AB, et al. The pathologic spectrum of gastrointestinal and hepatic histoplasmosis. Am J Clin Pathol 113:64, 2000.
134. Cappell MS. Hepatobiliary manifestations of the acquired immune deficiency syndrome. Am J Gastroenterol 86:1, 1991.
135. CDC. Treating Opportunistic Infections Among HIV-Infected Adults and Adolescents: Recommendations from CDC, the National Institutes of Health, and the HIV Medicine Association/Infectious Diseases Society of America. Available: http://www.cdc.gov/mmwr/ preview/mmwrhtml/rr5315a1.htm Dec 28, 2005.
136. Smith DH. Visceral leishmaniasis: human aspects. In: Giles HM (ed). Recent Advances in Tropical Medicine. Edinburgh: Churchill-Livingstone; 1984, p 79.
137. Gupta S. The liver in kala-azar. Ann Trop Med 50:252, 1956.
138. Moreno A, Marazuela M, Yebra M, et al. Hepatic fibrin-ring granulomas in visceral leishmaniasis. Gastroenterology 95:1123, 1988.
139. Murray HW, Berman JD, Davies CR, Saravia NG. Advances in leishmaniasis. Lancet 366:1561, 2005.
140. Murray HW, Pepin J, Nutman TB, et al. Tropical medicine. BMJ 320:490, 2000.
141. Islam MZ, Itoh M, Mirza R, et al. Direct agglutination test with urine samples for the diagnosis of visceral leishmaniasis. Am J Trop Med Hyg 70:78, 2004.
142. Gatti S, Gramegna M, Klersy C, et al. Diagnosis of visceral leishmaniasis: the sensitivities and specificities of traditional methods and a nested PCR assay. Ann Trop Med Parasitol 98:667, 2004.
143. Sundar S, Jha TK, Thakur CP, et al. Oral miltefosine for Indian visceral leishmaniasis. N Engl J Med 347:1739, 2002.
144. Dunn MA. Parasitic diseases. In: Schiff ER (ed). Disease of the Liver. Philadelphia: Lippincott; 1999, p 1533.
145. Jha TK, Sundar S, Thakur CP, et al. Miltefosine, an oral agent, for the treatment of Indian visceral leishmaniasis. N Engl J Med 341:1795, 1999.
146. Cohen O, Stoeckle M. *Pneumocystis carinii* infection in the acquired immunodeficiency syndrome. Arch Intern Med 151:1205, 1991.
147. Molina JM, Tourneur M, Sarfati C, et al. Agence Nationale de Recherches sur le SIDA 090 Study Group. Fumagillin treatment of intestinal microsporidiosis. N Engl J Med 346:1963, 2002.
148. Tompkins DC, Steigbigel RT. Rochalimaea's role in cat scratch disease and bacillary angiomatosis. Ann Intern Med 118:388, 1993.
149. Cotell SL, Noskin GA. Bacillary angiomatosis clinical and histologic features, diagnosis and treatment. Arch Intern Med 154:524, 1994.

150. Gasquet S, Maurin M, Brouqui P, et al. Bacillary angiomatosis in immunocompromised patients. AIDS 12:1793, 1998.
151. Alvarez SZ. Hepatobiliary tuberculosis. J Gastroenterol Hepatol 13:833, 1998.
152. Lizardi-Cervera J, Soto Ramirez LE, Poo JL, Uribe M. Hepatobiliary diseases in patients with human immunodeficiency virus (HIV) treated with non highly active antiretroviral therapy: frequency and clinical manifestations. Ann Hepatol 4:188, 2005.
153. Hoy J, Mijch A, Sandland M, et al. Quadruple-drug therapy for *Mycobacterium avium–intracellulare* bacteremia in AIDS patients. J Infect Dis 161:801, 1990.
154. Horsburgh CR, Metchock B, Gordon SM, et al. Predictors of survival in patients with AIDS and disseminated *Mycobacterium avium* complex disease. J Infect Dis 170:573, 1994.
155. Chin DP, Reingold AL, Stone EN, et al. The impact of *Mycobacterium avium* complex bacteremia and its treatment on survival of AIDS patients – a prospective study. J Infect Dis 170:578, 1994.
156. Ogedegbe AE, Thomas DL, Diehl AM. Hyperlactataemia syndromes associated with HIV therapy. Lancet Infect Dis 3:329, 2003.
157. Chariot P, Drogou I, de Lacroix-Szmania I, et al. Zidovudine-induced mitochondrial disorder with massive liver steatosis, myopathy, lactic acidosis, and mitochondrial DNA depletion. J Hepatol 30:156, 1999.
158. Sundar K, Suarez M, Banogon PE, Shapiro JM. Zidovudine-induced fatal lactic acidosis and hepatic failure in patients with acquired immunodeficiency syndrome: report of two patients and review of the literature. Crit Care Med 25:1425, 1997.
159. Freiman JP, Helfert KE, Hamrell MR, Stein DS. Hepatomegaly with severe steatosis in HIV-seropositive patients. AIDS 7:379, 1993.
160. Pan-Zhou XR, Cui L, Zou XJ, et al. Differential effects of antiretroviral nucleoside analogs on mitochondrial function in HepG2 cells. Antimicrob Agents Chemother 44:496, 2000.
161. Coghlan ME, Sommadossi JP, Jhala NC, et al. Symptomatic lactic acidosis in hospitalized antiretroviral-treated patients with human immunodeficiency virus infection: a report of 12 cases. Clin Infect Dis 33:1914, 2001.
162. Ristig M, Drechsler H, Powderly WG. Hepatic steatosis and HIV infection. AIDS Patient Care STDS 19:356, 2005.
163. Hammer SM, Katzenstein DA, Hughes MD, et al. A trial comparing nucleoside monotherapy with combination therapy in HIV-infected adults with CD4 cell counts from 200 to 500 per cubic millimeter: AIDS Clinical Trials Group Study 175 study team. N Engl J Med 335:1081, 1996.
164. Blackmore T, Gordon D. The Delta trial. Lancet 348:1238, 1996.
165. Randomised trial of addition of lamivudine or lamivudine plus loviride to zidovudine-containing regimens for patients with HIV-1 infection: the CAESAR trial. Lancet 349:1413, 1997.
166. Kemmer NM, Molina CP, Fuchs JE, et al. A distinctive histologic pattern of liver injury in HIV positive patients on HAART: a possible hepatotoxic effect of protease inhibitors. Hepatology 32:312A, 2000.
167. Zucker SD, Qin X, Rouster SD, et al. Mechanism of indinavir-induced hyperbilirubinemia. Proc Natl Acad Sci USA 98:12671, 2001.
168. Brau N, Leaf HL, Wieczorek RL, Margolis DM. Severe hepatitis in three AIDS patients treated with indinavir. Lancet 349:924, 1997.
169. Bruno R, Sacchi P, Maiocchi L, et al. Hepatotoxicity and nelfinavir: a meta-analysis. Clin Gastroenterol Hepatol 3:482, 2005.
170. Palmon R, Tirelli R, Braun JF, et al. Hepatotoxicity associated with non-nucleoside reverse transcriptase inhibitors for the treatment of HIV and the effect of HBV or HCV infection. Hepatology 32:312A, 2000.
171. Timmermans S, Tempelman C, Godfried MH, et al. Dutch HMF Study Group. Nelfinavir and nevirapine side effects during pregnancy. AIDS 19:795, 2005.
172. Sanne I, Mommeja-Marin H, Hinkle J, et al. Severe hepatotoxicity associated with nevirapine use in HIV-infected subjects. J Infect Dis 191:825, 2005.
173. Stern JO, Robinson PA, Love J, et al. A comprehensive hepatic safety analysis of nevirapine in different populations of HIV infected patients. J Acquir Immune Defic Syndr 34 (Suppl 1):S21, 2003.
174. Conigliaro J, Gordon AJ, McGinnis KA, et al. Veterans Aging Cohort 3-Site Study. How harmful is hazardous alcohol use and abuse in HIV infection: do health care providers know who is at risk? J Acquir Immune Defic Syndr 33:521, 2003.
175. Salmon-Ceron D, Lewden C, Morlat P, et al. The Mortality 2000 Study Group. Liver disease as a major cause of death among HIV infected patients: role of hepatitis C and B viruses and alcohol. J Hepatol 42:799, 2005.
176. Moriya K, Fujie H, Shintani Y, et al. The core protein of hepatitis C virus induces hepatocellular carcinoma in transgenic mice. Nat Med 4:1065, 1998.
177. Barbaro G, Di Lorenzo G, Asti A, et al. Hepatocellular mitochondrial alterations in patients with chronic hepatitis C: ultrastructural and biochemical findings. Am J Gastroenterol 94:2198, 1999.
178. Radriguez-Rosado R, Garcia-Samaniego J, Soriano V. Hepatotoxicity after introduction of highly active antiretroviral therapy. AIDS 12:1256, 1998.
179. Sulkowski MS, Thomas DL, Mehta SH, et al. Hepatotoxicity associated with nevirapine or efavirenz-containing antiretroviral therapy: role of hepatitis C and B infections. Hepatology 35:182, 2002.
180. Sulkowski MS, Mehta SH, Torbenson M, et al. Hepatic steatosis and antiretroviral drug use among adults coinfected with HIV and hepatitis C virus. AIDS 19:585, 2005.
181. Zylberberg H, Chaix ML, Rabian C, et al. Tritherapy for human immunodeficiency virus infection does not modify replication of hepatitis C virus in coinfected subjects. Clin Infect Dis 26:1104, 1998.
182. Stone SF, Lee S, Keane NM, et al. Association of increased hepatitis C virus (HCV)-specific IgG and soluble CD26 dipeptidyl peptidase IV enzyme activity with hepatotoxicity after highly active antiretroviral therapy in human immunodeficiency virus-HCV-coinfected patients. J Infect Dis 186:1498, 2002.
183. Puoti M, Bruno R, Soriano V, et al. HIV HCC Cooperative Italian-Spanish Group. Hepatocellular carcinoma in HIV-infected patients: epidemiological features, clinical presentation and outcome. AIDS 18:2285, 2004.
184. Bruno R, Puoti M, Sacchi P, et al. Management of hepatocellular carcinoma in human immunodeficiency virus-infected patients. J Hepatol 44 (Suppl 1):S146, 2006.
185. Neff GW, Sherman KE, Eghtesad B, Fung J. Review article: current status of liver transplantation in HIV-infected patients. Aliment Pharmacol Ther 20:993, 2004.
186. Ko WF, Cello JP, Rogers SJ, Lecours A. Prognostic factors for the survival of patients with AIDS cholangiopathy. Am J Gastroenterol 98:2176, 2003.
187. Ragni MV, Belle SH, Im K, et al. Survival of human immunodeficiency virus-infected liver transplant recipients. J Infect Dis 188:1412, 2003.
188. Neff GW, Bonham A, Tzakis AG, et al. Orthotopic liver transplantation in patients with human immunodeficiency virus and end-stage liver disease. Liver Transpl 9:239, 2003.

189. Ragni MV, Eghtesad B, Schlesinger KW, et al. Pretransplant survival is shorter in HIV-positive than HIV-negative subjects with end-stage liver disease. Liver Transpl 11:1425, 2005.
190. Chitturi S, George J. Hepatotoxicity of commonly used drugs: Nonsteroidal anti-inflammatory drugs, antihypertensives, antidiabetic agents, anticonvulsants, lipid-lowering agents, psychotropic drugs. Semin Liver Dis 22:169, 2002.
191. Ghali P, Lindor KD. Hepatotoxicity of drugs used for treatment of obesity and its comorbidities. Semin Liver Dis 24:389, 2004.
192. Maddrey WC. Drug-induced hepatotoxicity: 2005. J Clin Gastroenterol 39(Suppl 2):S83, 2005.
193. Nunez M, Soriano V. Hepatotoxicity of antiretrovirals: incidence, mechanisms and management. Drug Saf 28:53, 2005.

Chapter 79

Drug Interactions and Administration

Charles Flexner, MD, Paul A. Pham, PharmD

Pharmacology plays a critical role in the treatment of HIV infection affecting issues as diverse as adherence, efficacy, and tolerability. The era of HAART has been characterized by drug regimens that are potent but sometimes complicated, burdensome, and possessing a number of long-term toxicities. Most treated patients currently take at least three antiretrovirals, but may also take drugs for prophylaxis and treatment of opportunistic infections, and a variety of medications for supportive care of pain, depression, and other concomitant illnesses. Some patients are also receiving investigational agents and/or alternative medications from health food stores. While great strides have been made to improve formulations and reduce pill burden, the late-stage patient may still require in excess of 10 or more medications and administration of 30–40 pills each day.

Selecting appropriate medications and constructing an effective antiretroviral regimen can be difficult in this era of polypharmacy. In addition to contending with drug resistance, the clinician is faced with food effects, proper spacing of medications, drug–drug interactions, overlapping toxicities, and patient adherence with the regimen. These factors, combined with pharmacokinetic, formulation, and storage issues, further complicate the care of the HIV-infected patient.

FOOD EFFECTS

Food alters the absorption or bioavailability of several drugs commonly used in HIV-infected patients. Drug–food interactions can influence the scheduling of medications during the day, and can profoundly affect the quality of life of patients. Dosing of antiretrovirals can be very confusing for patients, who often have to schedule their meals around drug administration. For example, didanosine (ddI) tablets and sachets are formulated with a buffer that requires administration on an empty stomach because a low gastric pH leads to degradation of the drug.[1] Although not buffered, ddI enteric-coated capsules also must be given on an empty stomach since administration with food decreases the C_{max} and area under the concentration-time curve (AUC) by 46% and 19%, respectively.[2] Bioavailability of the other nucleosides is not significantly affected by food, although peak absorption may be delayed. For example, a high-fat[3] or high-protein[4] meal slows the rate of absorption of zidovudine, and may reduce the mean maximum concentration, but does not significantly alter the overall extent of absorption.

Several protease inhibitor (PI) regimens are particularly problematic in terms of food effects. When used alone, indinavir (IDV) must be given on an empty stomach or with a light meal containing less than 2 g of fat.[5] When combined with ritonavir (RTV), IDV can be administered without regard to food.[6] Conversely, nelfinavir requires administration with a meal that contains a minimum of 500 kcal with 20% fat for adequate absorption.[7] Tipranavir (TPV) and atazanavir (ATV) absorption are increased by 31% and 70%, respectively, and therefore should be administered with food.[8,9] On the other hand, lopinavir (LPV) and fosamprenavir (FPV) tablets are not significantly affected by food, and therefore may be taken without regard to meals.[10,11] While RTV capsule absorption is only increased by 15% in the presence of food, administration with a meal is recommended to decrease its gastrointestinal side effects.[12] A variety of HIV-related medications have specific food restrictions stemming from the possibility of increased or decreased absorption from the gastrointestinal tract; these restrictions are summarized in Table 79-1. A review of food restrictions should be an important part of patient counseling for a new or modified drug regimen.

Table 79-1

Food–Drug Interactions with HIV-Related Medications

Antiretrovirals	Food Effect	Recommendation
Atazanavir	AUC increased by 70% with light meal	Administer with food
Amprenavir	AUC decreased by 21% with high-fat meal	Take with or without food but high-fat meal should be avoided
Didanosine EC	AUC decreased by 18–27% with food	Administer 2 h before or 2 h after meals
Efavirenz	AUC increased by 22% and 50% with low-and high-fat meals	May be taken with or without meals but administer on an empty stomach during the first 2 weeks to minimize the risk of CNS side effects
Fosamprenavir	Not affected by food	May be taken with or without meals
Indinavir	High-fat caloric meal results in 77% decrease in AUC	May be taken with food when co-administered with ritonavir. Must be administered on empty stomach or with low-fat, light meal if not boosted with ritonavir
Lopinavir/r	Lopinavir tablets are not affected by food	Administer with or without food
Nelfinavir	AUC two- to fivefold higher when given with food	Administer with a minimum of 500 kcal with 20% fat meal
Saquinavir	Marked increase in AUC following high-fat meal	Administer within 2 h of a full meal. Food requirement is less of a factor with ritonavir co-administration
Tipranavir/r	AUC increased by 31% with high fat meal	Administer with food
Drugs for OIs		
Atovaquone	High-fat meal increases bioavailability up to threefold	Administer with food
Valganciclovir	AUC increased by 30% with food	Administer with food
Clarithromycin XL	AUC increased by 30% with food	Administer clarithromycin XL with food. Immediate-release clarithromycin can be taken with or without food
Isoniazid	Reduced absorption with food	Administer on an empty stomach
Itraconazole (caps)	Significant increase in bioavailability when taken with a full meal	Administer with food
Itraconazole (solution)	Maximal absorption when taken under fasting conditions	Administer without food
Ribavirin	Increased absorption with fatty food	Administer with food
Rifapentine	AUC increased by 43%	Administer with food
Voriconazole	AUC decreased by 24% with food	Administer 1 h before or 1 h after meals

AUC, area under the concentration–time curve.

SPACING OF MEDICATIONS

The specific administration times for some antiretrovirals, and how they are taken in relation to other medications, may affect their absorption and activity. For example, the antacids in ddI buffered sachets decrease the absorption of IDV and ATV by over 80% if they are administered concomitantly.[8,13] Thus, it is recommended to take ddI buffered powder 2h before the administration of ATV or IDV.[8,14] ddI enteric-coated (EC) tablets are preferred, since they do not alter IDV's or ATV's absorption and can be given concomitantly.[15,16]

Concentrations of some PIs in dual combination may differ depending on whether they are given concomitantly or in a staggered fashion. ACTG 378 was a study in healthy volunteers that evaluated single doses of dual combinations of PIs (saquinavir (SQV), RTV, or nelfinavir) given either simultaneously or when separated by 4h. The AUC of SQV was markedly lower when given 4h before RTV or nelfinavir; however, if RTV was given up to 48h before SQV, the levels of SQV were still significantly increased.[17] Dose separation of dual PI combinations is not recommended since this may increase the complexity of the antiretroviral regimen in addition to adversely affecting their pharmacokinetic profiles.

A number of dual PI combinations can be dosed once-daily (i.e., ATV/ritonavir (r), FPV/r, LPV/r) in antiretroviral-naive patients.[8,11,18] Such regimens would be particularly useful for selected populations such as prison inmates, methadone clinics, and those patients requiring directly observed therapy. Although these once-daily regimens would be more convenient, they might also require near-perfect adherence, since concentrations at the end of the 24-h dosing interval may be near the IC_{50} value. Therefore, a missed dose would result in suboptimal concentrations for a prolonged period, leading to increased risk of recurrent viral replication and drug resistance. Most PIs possess large interpatient and intrapatient pharmacokinetic variability, so that even with good adherence there may be a small proportion of patients with concentrations below the desired target at the end of a dosing interval. Although PK variability of PIs is minimized with the co-administration of RTV, it can still be quite large.[5]

DRUG INTERACTIONS

One of the greatest challenges for the HIV clinician is the recognition and management of drug interactions.[19] The HIV-infected patient often receives numerous medications and has a great potential for adverse drug interactions. Certain PI combinations may also be used to take advantage of beneficial pharmacokinetic interactions.

A number of medications used in HIV-infected patients can produce adverse drug interactions (Table 79-2).[19] In addition to over 300 drug interactions listed in the product labeling of antiretrovirals, there are potential interactions with other therapeutic classes not yet studied.[7–11,20–31] Although many of these interactions may be minor in nature, some are potentially serious, leading to severe toxicity or treatment failure. Fortunately, many interactions can be recognized, prevented, and corrected. Minor alterations in scheduling or selection of an appropriate alternative are usually all that is required to avoid a potential interaction. Other drug interactions may be beneficial by increasing plasma concentrations of co-administered PIs.

Drug interactions can generally be classified as pharmacokinetic, that is, affecting drug concentrations; or pharmacodynamic, that is, affecting drug activity. Pharmacokinetic interactions involve changes in absorption, distribution, metabolism, or excretion, whereas pharmacodynamic interactions may involve additive, synergistic, or antagonistic effects.

Pharmacokinetic Interactions

Altered Drug Absorption

Impairment of drug absorption can lead to a marked reduction in the bioavailability of certain agents. One of the most common interactions affecting drug absorption is chelation, the binding of drugs to metal ions or other substances in the gastrointestinal tract. The concomitant administration of a fluoroquinolone antibiotic with a di- or trivalent cation such as calcium, magnesium, aluminum, or iron results in a greater than 90% decrease in the AUC of the fluoroquinolone, possibly leading to therapeutic failure.[32–34] ddI formulations with a calcium and magnesium buffer (tablets) or citrate-phosphate buffer (sachet) can also alter fluoroquinolone disposition. Concomitant administration of ddI with ciprofloxacin has been shown to decrease the ciprofloxacin AUC from 15.5 to 0.26 $\mu g\ h^{-1}\ mL^{-1}$.[35] A similar interaction would be expected with other products such as antacids, sucralfate, or iron preparations. Administration of these agents should be separated from the fluoroquinolone by at least 2h, and the fluoroquinolone should be administered first, followed by the cation, to ensure adequate absorption. The newer EC formulation of ddI does not alter ciprofloxacin pharmacokinetics and can be given concomitantly.[2]

An increase in gastric pH significantly affects the absorption of azole antifungals (i.e., itraconazole) and ATV. An acidic environment is required for dissolution and absorption of ketoconazole, itraconazole, and ATV; thus concomitant administration with histamine-2 (H-2) antagonists, proton pump inhibitors (PPIs), and antacids should be avoided.[36–39] The ATV trough was decreased by 78% and 28% with omeprazole and famotidine co-administration, respectively. The interaction with PPIs cannot be overcome with higher ATV doses, dose separation, or "boosting" with RTV. If patients require acid suppression, H-2 blockers can be given 2h after or 10h before unboosted ATV administration; alternatively, "boosting" with RTV can minimize the decrease in ATV serum level observed with H-2 blockers.[38,39] Fluconazole or voriconazole are an appropriate alternative in patients requiring agents that raise gastric pH, or in those with achlorhydria, because their absorption is not dependent on gastric pH.[40,41] Alternatively, ketoconazole or itraconazole can be given with an acidic beverage such as Coca-Cola® to improve absorption, but this approach was not effective in reversing ATV-omeprazole interaction.[38,42]

Altered Drug Metabolism

Intestinal metabolism and P-glycoprotein

The cytochrome P450 (CYP) enzyme system consists of at least 12 families of enzymes common to all mammals, and represents the major enzyme system involved in drug metabolism.[43] In humans, the CYP1, CYP2, and CYP3 families are primarily responsible for drug metabolism, with the CYP3A subfamily involved in the metabolism of the largest number of drugs, including most available PIs and non-nucleoside reverse transcriptase inhibitors (NNRTIs). CYP-mediated metabolism largely takes place in the liver, although CYP enzymes are also present in other sites including enterocytes in the intestinal wall.[44] Thus, inhibitors of CYP3A4 may alter both drug absorption and hepatic metabolism. The 20-fold increase in plasma concentrations of SQV produced by RTV is likely caused by inhibition of CYP3A4 at both sites.[45] Grapefruit juice contains various substances that inhibit CYP3A4-mediated metabolism only in the gut wall, mainly by selective down regulation of CYP3A4 activity in

Clinically Significant Drug Interactions in HIV-Infected Patients

Table 79-2

Affected Drug	Interacting Drug	Effect	Comments
Midazolam, triazolam	All PIs, DLV, and potentially EFV	May significantly increase midazolam and triazolam serum levels	Co-administration is contraindicated. Alternative: Lorazepam or temazepam
Fentanyl	All PIs and DLV	May significantly increase fentanyl serum levels	Avoid co-administration. Alternative: Morphine
PIs and NNRTIs	Phenytoin, carbamazepine, phenobarbital	LPV AUC decreased by 33% and Phenytoin AUC decreased by 31%	Levels of all PIs and NNRTIs may be decreased. Alternative: valproic acid, Levetiracetam, and topiramate
All PIs (except NFV)	Efavirenz, nevirapine	Significant decrease PIs serum level when not co-administered with ritonavir	Co-administer protease inhibitor with ritonavir
Antiarrhythmics (amiodarone, disopyramide, dofetilide, flecainide, lidocaine, mexiletine, propafenone, and quinidine)	All PIs and DLV	May significantly increase antiarrhythmic serum levels	Avoid co-administration
Clarithromycin, erythromycin	All PIs and DLV	Clarithromycin AUC increased by 94% with ATV co-administration	QTc prolongation observed with ATV co-administration. Use 50% of clarithromycin dose with ATV co-administration. Use 50% of clarithromycin dose with boosted PIs in renal failure. Alternative: azithromycin
Ca Channel blocker	All PIs and DLV	Diltiazem AUC increased by 125%	Increase in PR interval observed. Start with 50% diltiazem dose and titrate slowly
ATV, DLV, itraconazole, ketoconazole	Proton pump inhibitor and antacid	ATV AUC decreased by 75%. DLV, itraconazole, and ketoconazole AUC may be significantly decreased	Co-administration contraindicated. ATV may be given 2 h before or 10 h after H-2 blockers
Rifampin	All PIs	Protease inhibitor AUC decreased by 70–92%	Co-administration contraindicated. Alternative: Dose adjusted rifabutin
Rifabutin	Ritonavir boosted PIs	Rifabutin AUC increased three- to fourfold	Decrease rifabutin to 150 mg 3x/week
Methadone	Nevirapine, efavirenz	Methadone AUC decreased by 46–57%	Monitor for withdrawal symptoms and titrate methadone dose to effect
Simvastatin, lovastatin	All PIs and DLV	Simvastatin AUC increased 32-fold with RTV-boosted PI	Co-administration contraindicated. Alternative: pravastatin and possibly atorvastatin and rosuvastatin
Erectile dysfunction agents (sildenafil, tadalafil, and vardenafil)	All PIs and DLV	Significant increase in AUC of erectile dysfunction agents	Do not exceed the following doses: Sildenafil 25 mg q48h; tadalafil 10 mg q72h; vardenafil 2.5 mg q72h
Ergot Alkaloid	All PIs, DLV, and EFV	May result in acute ergot toxicity	Co-administration contraindicated. Alternative: Sumatriptan

AUC, area under the concentration-time curve; PI, protease inhibitor; DLV, delavirdine; EFV, efavirenz; ATV, atazanavir, NFV, nelfinavir, LPV, lopinavir; NNRTI, non-nucleoside reverse transferase inhibitor.

the small intestine.[46] The AUC for SQV is increased by 1.5- to 2.5-fold during concomitant administration with grapefruit juice.[24] However, grapefruit juice should not be relied upon to increase the plasma concentrations of PIs because the amounts of inhibitors vary widely between brands and are affected by factors such as how much and how often the juice is consumed.[47]

P-glycoprotein (P-gp) is the product of the *mdr1* gene first described as a mediator of resistance to cancer chemotherapy. Enterocytes in the intestinal mucosa are a major site for expression of P-gp, one of several membrane-bound proteins that increase efflux of drugs from cells.[48] P-gp appears to contribute to the low bioavailability of some drugs, including certain PIs. P-gp in the brush border cells of the intestine can pump drug back into the gastrointestinal lumen, decreasing absorption. In the liver, P-gp pumps drug into bile; it is also present in the blood–brain barrier, where it can limit the uptake of drugs into the central nervous system. Several PIs are substrates for and inhibitors of P-gp. In theory, inhibition of P-gp could be used to increase PI concentrations in target sites such as the CNS.[49] However, P-gp expression has a profound negative impact on HIV replication. In two separate sets of experiments, cells expressing P-gp produced at least 40 to 70-fold less HIV than control cells. This was thought to be primarily due to inhibition of HIV entry and/or membrane fusion.[50,51] The clinical implications of these findings highlight a dilemma regarding how (or whether) P-gp should be altered in HIV-infected patients: the presence of P-gp may lead to decreased intracellular drug concentrations, but the fact that P-gp expression may make cells less susceptible to HIV infection might counteract these low drug concentrations. The clinical relevance of P-gp for antiretriovirals remains to be determined.

CYP enyzmes and P-gp in the intestine and liver can present a barrier to absorption of orally administered drugs, and have considerable impact on drug interactions. The overlap of tissue distribution and substrate specificity of CYP3A4 and P-gp complicates definition of the specific mechanisms of some drug interactions. Many drugs that are modulators of P-gp are also inhibitors of CYP3A4.[52] The effect of these two pathways on antiretroviral drug concentrations remains a fertile area for additional research.

Enzyme Induction

Inducers increase the rate of hepatic metabolism, usually through increased transcription of mRNA, and decrease serum concentrations of other drugs metabolized by the same hepatic isoenzyme. Rifampin and rifabutin are classic examples of enzyme inducers, and cause decreases in plasma concentrations of concomitant metabolized drugs. Both drugs can decrease concentrations of all HIV PIs. The Centers for Disease Control and Prevention (CDC) have issued guidelines for concomitant use of rifampin or rifabutin with HIV PIs in patients with tuberculosis.[53] Rifampin should be avoided with most PIs and NNRTIs but may be used with a higher efavirenz (EFV) dose (800 mg).[53] RTV with SQV should be avoided with rifampin co-administration due to a high incidence of hepatitis.[54] Although, the addition of extra RTV (300 mg bid) to LPV counteracted rifampin's enzyme induction, this strategy is limited due to a high incidence of undesirable side effect.[55] Patients receiving IDV or nelfinavir should receive a reduced dose of rifabutin and increased PI dose.[53,56]

Nevirapine is a mild to moderate hepatic enzyme inducer, and decreases the AUC of LPV, IDV, and SQV by 22–38%, but has a minimal effect on RTV and nelfinavir.[10,57,58] Boosting PIs with RTV or increasing the PI dose (i.e., LPV/r to 600/150 mg bid) can counteract the inducing effect of nevirapine.[10] EFV is a mixed inducer/inhibitor *in vitro*; however, *in vivo* a decrease in concentrations of FPV, ATV, LPV/r, SQV, and IDV is observed with co-administration. Increasing LPV/r dose to 600/150 mg twice-daily or the addition of RTV to ATV, FPV, and SQV is required with EFV co-administration.[59]

RTV and nelfinavir are also moderate enzyme inducers, and can increase hepatic glucuronidation as well as CYP activity. The AUC of the oral contraceptive ethinyl estradiol is decreased by ~40% with these agents, necessitating an alternative form of birth control.[7,60] Conversely, IDV and ATV are inhibitors of hepatic glucuronidation which resulted in a 24% and 48% increase in AUC of ethinyl estradiol, respectively.[26,61] RTV is also an inducer of CYP1A2 which is involved in the metabolism of theophylline and olanzapine.[62,63] Concomitant administration of RTV with theophylline or olanzapine has been reported to result in a decrease in the theophylline AUC of 43% and olanzapine AUC of 53%. Patients receiving these combinations should be monitored for reduced efficacy and the dose should be titrated to therapeutic effect.

TPV is a nonpeptidic HIV PI. In vivo, TPV is a substrate and potent inducer of the P-gp drug transporter (P-gp). In vitro metabolism studies with human liver microsomes also indicate that TPV is a substrate of CYP3A4.[64] RTV, a known inhibitor of CYP3A4 and P-gp, significantly decreases TPV clearance, resulting in a 29-fold increase in the TPV AUC.[64a] TPV is therefore dependent on RTV co-administration to achieve the desired pharmacokinetic parameters. TPV/r (500/200 mg BID) produces a net inhibition of CYP3A4, resulting in an increase in plasma concentrations of many CYP3A4 substrates (e.g., atorvastatin). However, for drugs that are dual substrates of CYP 3A4 and P-gp, a net induction results in a 45%, 49%, and 70% reduction in the amprenavir (APV), LPV (LPV/r), and SQV AUCs, respectively.[64b]

Enzyme Inhibition

There are a number of inhibitors of CYP that decrease the rate of hepatic metabolism and increase plasma concentrations of other drugs metabolized by the same isoenzyme. HIV PIs can be both CYP inhibitors and substrates, increasing concentrations of some metabolized drugs and having their own concentrations increased by other CYP inhibitors. With the exception of nelfinavir, all of the currently available PIs are primarily metabolized by CYP3A4.[5] These agents differ in the number and magnitude of potential drug interactions. RTV is associated with the greatest number of drug interactions, while SQV is the weakest enzyme inhibitor, and has less propensity to alter concentrations of other drugs. FPV, nelfinavir, and IDV inhibit CYP3A4 metabolism to a lesser extent than RTV. For example, all three drugs increase the rifabutin AUC approximately twofold, necessitating a 50% reduction in the rifabutin dose.[19] RTV increases the rifabutin AUC fourfold, which may lead to clinically significant adverse effects when clinicians did not reduce dose of rifabutin.[65,66] Since most PIs are co-administered with RTV, they have a similar drug interaction profile to that of RTV. However, there are some exceptions to this rule. For example, enzyme induction predominates when FPV and LPV/r are co-administered; this interaction resulted in a 64% and 48% decrease in amprenavir and LPV AUC, respectively.[67] Higher doses of both FPV and LPV only partially counteracted the observed interaction.[68] Similarly, when TPV is given with amprenavir/r, LPV/r, or SQV/r, a 45–70% decrease in AUC of the co-administered PI was observed.[69] Conversely, the clarithromycin AUC is increased 53% with IDV, 77% with RTV, and 94% with ATV. Clarithromycin dosage adjustment with most PIs is unnecessary in patients with normal renal function; however, a 50% dose reduction is recommended with ATV co-administration due to an observed QTc prolongation.[8,70] Azithromycin is primarily excreted by the biliary route and does not interact with inhibitors of CYP; therefore, it is a good alternative to clarithromycin.[71]

Life-Threatening Drug Interactions

The most serious potential interactions with CYP inhibitors involve concomitant administration with certain metabolized drugs such as terfenadine and cisapride (both removed from the US market), antiarrhythmics, and ergot alkaloids, which all have a low therapeutic index. In the case of cisapride and terfenadine, these combinations led to cardiotoxicity, with the potential for life-threatening arrhythmias.[72] Administration of PIs with some benzodiazepine sedative-hypnotics (i.e., midazolam and triazolam) and certain opiates (i.e., fentanyl) can result in exaggerated side effects such as oversedation and possible respiratory depression.[73,74]

Beneficial Drug Interactions

Drug interactions were initially viewed as a complication to be avoided in HIV-infected patients. The concept of using two PIs concomitantly to increase or "boost" plasma concentrations or improve convenience was first recognized with the combination of SQV and RTV. Simultaneous administration of two PIs takes advantage of beneficial pharmacokinetic interactions, and may circumvent many of the drugs' undesirable pharmacologic properties.[6] In addition, dual PIs decrease interpatient variability, making drug concentrations more predictable. Dual PI regimens have now been widely prescribed and are the standard of care in published treatment guidelines.[75] A number of potentially beneficial metabolic drug interactions exist for combinations of two HIV PIs. One drug, generally RTV, is used to inhibit the metabolism of the second agent, producing increased bioavailability, decreased clearance, or both. Two-, three-, and four-way interactions are no longer uncommon, in which case the pharmacokinetic profile of each drug can be benefited or adversely affected.

RTV-Boosted PI Combinations

Saquinavir-RITONAVIR

When SQV was first introduced, it possessed a number of disadvantages including poor bioavailability, three times daily dosing, and a pill burden of 18 capsules per day. However, when combined with even small doses of RTV, there is a marked increase in SQV bioavailability and a decrease in clearance, which allows twice-daily dosing with a lower pill burden (six per day). In a single-dose, crossover study in healthy volunteers, RTV increased the SQV AUC by 50- to 132-fold, and increased the SQV C_{max} by 23- to 35-fold.[45] Since RTV is a P450 inducer and undergoes autoinduction during the first 10–14 days of therapy,[76] steady-state concentrations of SQV should be lower when these two drugs are combined. Multiple-dose pharmacokinetic interaction studies found that the steady-state SQV AUC was increased only 20- to 30-fold.[77]

The effect of RTV on SQV plasma concentrations was evaluated in 120 patients receiving various SQV/r combinations.[78] Data from two dose-ranging trials of SQV/r given either twice daily or once daily were included in the analysis. A wide range of SQV doses (400–1800 mg) and RTV doses (100–400 mg) were evaluated. The investigators used multivariate linear and nonlinear regression to correlate steady-state SQV pharmacokinetic parameters (C_{min}, C_{max}, and half-life) with SQV and RTV doses. This model showed a strong effect of RTV on SQV C_{max} and C_{min}; however, these parameters were correlated only with SQV dosage, and the increase in SQV concentrations was similar for RTV dosages over the range of 100–400 mg twice daily. In this analysis there was no dose-dependent effect of RTV on SQV concentrations.

The poor oral bioavailability of SQV (1–12%, depending on formulation and conditions) likely reflects extensive first-pass metabolism rather than poor absorption. The increase in SQV concentrations with RTV is the result of improved bioavailability, perhaps to as much as 100%, with little effect on postabsorptive systemic clearance. In addition to effects on intestinal CYP 3A4, RTV is also an inhibitor of P-gp and its dual effects on both CYP3A4 and P-gp may account for the large magnitude of RTV's effect on SQV's oral bioavailability.[79]

Although the dose of 400 mg ritonavir/400 mg SQV twice daily was initially used, the high rate of GI intolerance, hepatitis, and hyperlipidemia led to "boosting" SQV with lower doses of RTV. In an open-label pharmacokinetic study, three SQV/r regimens (SQV/r 1600/100 mg once daily, 2000/100 mg once daily, and 1000/100 mg twice daily) were evaluated. SQV/r 2000/100 mg once daily resulted in a 71% higher AUC compared to SQV/r 1600/100 mg once daily. The AUC was comparable between SQV 1000/100 mg twice daily and SQV 2000/100 mg once daily, but the twice-daily arm achieved a significantly higher C_{min}.[45] Clinically, SQV/r 1000/100 mg bid was compared to LPV/r (400/100 mg bid), both with more than two NRTI/NNRTIs, in 324 HIV-infected patients. The population studied was heterogeneous and included 33% antiretroviral-naive, 48% PI-naive, and 32% who had experienced virologic failure with more than one PI. Risk of virologic failure was higher in the SQV/r arm than the LPV/r arm by intent-to-treat analysis.[80] In another trial, SQV/r 1600/100 mg qd also underperformed compared to EFV with NRTIs in 161 antiretroviral-naive patients. At 48 wks, viral suppression to below 50 copies/mL was 71% versus 51%, in the EFV and SQV/r arms, respectively.[81]

RTV-IDV

When used as a sole PI, IDV possesses a number of limitations including an every 8-h dosing regimen, food restrictions, hydration requirements, and large interindividual pharmacokinetic variability.[5] The combination of IDV with RTV alleviates many of these disadvantages.

In a steady-state pharmacokinetic interaction study in healthy volunteers involving 14 days of RTV treatment, the combination of 200 or 400 mg RTV with 400 or 600 mg IDV increased the IDV AUC by three- to sixfold compared to IDV 800 mg alone.[82] This mechanism primarily involves inhibition of hepatic CYP 3A4 with reduced first-pass metabolism making a minor contribution. RTV increased the IDV C_{max} up to twofold, and increased the IDV concentration 8 h after dosing by 11- to 33-fold.[82] Decreased RTV dose and increased IDV dose were examined in a separate study.[83] In healthy volunteers administered RTV for 14 days, the 24-h IDV AUC with a 800 mg bid IDV/100 mg bid RTV regimen was fourfold higher than with 800 mg q8h IDV alone. In the same study, the 24-h AUC of IDV with a 400/400 bid RTV-IDV regimen was 40% lower than with the 800/100 bid regimen and 55% lower than with a 800/200 bid regimen.[83] However, the mean 12-h trough concentrations of the 400/400 bid regimen and the 800/100 bid regimen were nearly the same. The 800/100 bid regimen is generally recommended due to the lower rate of GI intolerance, but if EFV or nevirapine is co-administered with IDV/RTV, the 800/200 mg bid regimen is recommended since EFV decreases the IDV AUC by 30%.[84]

In two studies, co-administration of RTV and IDV abolished the effect of food on IDV bioavailability. A high-fat meal reduced the bioavailability of unboosted IDV by up to 85%.[82] Doses of 100, 200, or 400 mg of RTV bid reversed the effect of a high- or low-fat meal on IDV pharmacokinetics, as compared to 800 mg IDV given in the fasted state.[83] RTV could enhance IDV oral bioavailability in the presence of food through inhibition of intestinal CYP or drug transporters such as P-gp. This finding suggests that the deleterious effects of food on IDV may be mediated by interaction with intestinal epithelial drug transporters or P450 complexes, processes potentially blocked by RTV.[6]

There is some concern that the high concentrations achieved with IDV/RTV may lead to an increased risk of nephrolithiasis. In patients taking IDV 800 mg q8h, a higher AUC and C_{max} were associated with increased risk of IDV nephrotoxicity in one study.[85] Increasing IDV C_{max} and C_{min} were associated with an increase in nephrolithiasis in patients taking IDV/RTV bid combinations of 400/100, 400/400, 600/100, or 800/100 mg; these regimens were associated with short-term nephrotoxicity risks of 0%, 2%, 6%, or 10%, respectively.[86] IDV/RTV regimens of 400/400 mg bid were not associated with an increased incidence of nephrolithiasis compared to IDV 800 mg q8h without RTV, although tolerability may be an issue with the higher RTV dose.[87]

Lopinavir-Ritonavir

LPV-RTV (Kaletra®) is the only co-formulated product designed to increase concentrations of a second PI by drug interaction. Each dose of Kaletra® contains 400 mg of LPV along with 100 mg of RTV (200/50 mg tablets × 2 tablets) which is given twice daily. LPV is a highly active PI but its bioavailability is low and its clearance rapid when given alone. However, in combination with low doses of RTV, the AUC is increased by greater than 100-fold,[88] due to inhibition of LPV's CYP3A4 metabolism in the liver and gastrointestinal tract. RTV's effect on the LPV AUC was several-fold greater than RTV's effect on the SQV AUC.[6]

In human volunteers mean trough concentrations of LPV were ~30-fold higher than the *in vitro* IC_{50} for HIV.[89] In 101 HIV-infected patients taking LPV 400 mg bid with RTV 100 mg bid with two nucleoside analogs for 48 weeks, HIV viral load (VL) was suppressed to less than 400 copies/mL in 93–100% of patients and to below 50 copies/mL in 83–86%.[90]

The addition of EFV to LPV-RTV results in a decrease of 40% in the LPV AUC.[91] Although concentrations are still relatively high despite this reduction, the manufacturer suggests the dose be increased to 600/150 mg (three tablets) bid when combined with EFV or nevirapine in order to offset the enzyme induction effects of the NNRTIs, especially if the patient is treatment-experienced and resistance is suspected.[10]

Fosamprenavir-Ritonavir

Administration of FPV with low-dose RTV increases the amprenavir AUC twofold and increases the trough concentration by approximately sixfold compared to FPV without RTV.[11] The current dosing recommendation is FPV/RTV 700/100 mg bid or 1400/200 mg once daily, but once-daily administration should be reserved for PI-naive patients due to lower amprenavir trough concentrations compared to twice-daily administration.[11]

In patients also receiving nevirapine or EFV, 100 mg bid of RTV does not appear to prevent a decrease in amprenavir concentrations (when given as the amprenavir capsule). In a small study, patients receiving 450 mg of amprenavir with 200 mg bid of RTV were switched to a 600/100 mg regimen and amprenavir trough values were decreased by 80%.[92] However, there was only a 17% decrease in amprenavir's trough when FPV/RTV 700/100 mg bid is co-administered with EFV.[11] EFV also decreased the IDV AUC by 30% when added to IDV/RTV 800/100 mg bid.[84] Thus, there appears to be a threshold dose of at least 200 mg of RTV that is required to prevent NNRTI-induced drug interactions for some PIs (i.e., amprenavir and IDV) but not others (i.e., ATV and FPV). The RTV dose should therefore be increased to 200 mg bid in IDV/RTV or amprenavir/RTV combinations with EFV or nevirapine.[10]

Clinically, FPV/RTV 700/100 mg bid, FPV/RTV 1400/200 mg qd, and LPV/RTV were compared in an open-label, randomized trial involving 315 PI-experienced patients. VL less than 50 through wk 48 was observed in 37%, 46%, and 50% receiving qd FPV, bid FPV, and LPV/RTV, respectively. The lower amprenavir trough may have contributed to the worse performance seen with the daily FPV regimen, and this regimen is not recommended for PI-experienced patients.[93]

RTV–Nelfinavir

Originally marketed as a thrice-daily drug, nelfinavir was studied in combination with RTV to reduce dosing frequency and evaluate the potential for once-a-day dosing. While RTV does increase nelfinavir concentrations modestly, overall, the AUC of nelfinavir was increased by only 30%. This combination is generally not widely used due to poor tolerability with only marginal pharmacokinetic benefit.[94] Dose limiting diarrhea or gastrointestinal adverse effects make this regimen less attractive than other dual PI combinations.[95]

Nelfinavir is the only HIV PI known to produce an active metabolite, the hydroxy-butylamide M8 (AG1402), which is the major metabolite of nelfinavir in humans and has equipotent anti-HIV activity *in vitro*.[96] RTV had a more significant beneficial impact on the pharmacokinetics of M8 than on nelfinavir itself. After 5 weeks of dosing, RTV use was associated with a 430% increase in the 500 mg M8 24-h AUC, and a 370% increase in the 750 mg M8 AUC, as compared to historical controls taking nelfinavir 750 mg tid alone.[6]

Atazanavir-Ritonavir

ATV is the first PI that is not dependent on RTV for once-daily dosing. However, in antiretroviral-experienced patients, unboosted ATV 400 mg qd is inferior to LPV/RTV (LPV/r 400/100 mg bid).[97] In an effort to improve the pharmacokinetic parameters of ATV, ATV 300 mg plus RTV 100 mg was evaluated. The ATV AUC and C_{min} increased twofold and 10-fold, respectively.[8] In a subsequent study involving antiretroviral-experienced patients, boosted ATV (ATV/r 300/100 mg qd) was compared to LPV/r 400/100 mg bid At 48 wks, 56% versus 58% achieved VL below 400 in ATV/r and LPV/r arm, respectively.[98] Thus, the beneficial pharmacokinetic interaction of boosted ATV resulted in improved clinical outcome in PI-experienced patients.

TPV-RTV

The pharmacokinetics of TPV, a nonpeptidic PI, are greatly improved by RTV. In an open-label, randomized, parallel-group trial involving 95 healthy subjects, RTV increased the TPV C_{min} 20-fold. This increase allows the TPV average steady-state C_{min} to be 20–57 times the protein-adjusted IC_{90} for PI-resistant HIV-1.[99] The potency of TPV/RTV (TPV/r) 500/200 mg bid in treatment-experienced patients with VL above 1000 copies/mL and more than one primary PI mutation was demonstrated in the RESIST I trial. At 24 wks, 34.7% in the TPV/r group and 16.5% of participants in the comparator PI group achieved a VL below 400 copies/mL.[100]

Dual-Boosted PI Combinations

Lopinavir/Ritonavir (LPV/r)-Atazanavir (ATV)

In a crossover pharmacokinetic study, the combination of ATV 300 mg qam with LPV/RTV (LPV/r) 400/100 mg bid resulted in a 45% higher ATV C_{min} compared to ATV/r 300/100 mg qd; however, ATV AUC_{0-24} and C_{min} were not significantly different. Additional boosting of ATV with RTV 100 mg qd when co-administered with LPV/r did not further increase the ATV C_{min} but did increase the LPV C_{min} by 28%. LPV PK parameters were comparable to historical data from volunteers receiving LPV/r 400/100 mg bid, at steady state, without ATV co-administration.[101] In several retrospective analyses involving both PI-experienced and naive patients, ATV with LPV/r combination as part of an antiretroviral regimen resulted in an undetectable VL in 77–97% of treated patients.[102–104] In a small pilot study in 12 patients who had failed at least two different PI-containing regimens, virologic suppression was reported in six of the 12 patients treated with ATV and LPV/r as part of their antiretroviral regimen.[105]

Lopinavir/ritonavir-Fosamprenavir

The combination of fosamprenavir (FPV) and lopinavir-ritonavir (LPV/r) may be a good option in treatment-experienced patients due to the nonoverlapping resistance mutations.[106] AIDS Clinical Trials Group (ACTG) Protocol 5143 was a randomized study that compared single-boosted PI regimens (LPV/r 400/100 mg bid or FPV/r 700/100 mg bid) to a dual-PI regimen (LPV/r 400/100 mg bid + FPV 700 mg bid) in combination with tenofovir DF and nucleosides in highly treatment-experienced patients.[107,108] Due to an adverse drug interaction in the dual-PI arm that resulted in a 55% and 60% decrease in the LPV and APV median AUC_{0-12}, respectively, study enrolment was stopped early after only 56 subjects out of a planned sample size of 216. Despite this interaction, at week 24, the dual-PI regimen had a comparable virologic response to the single-PI regimen, with 75% ($n = 28$) and 61% ($n = 28$) of patients having a greater than 1.0 log decline in VL from baseline with the dual-PI and single-PI regimens, respectively (intent-to-treat, $p = 0.17$). HIV-1 RNA was below 50 copies/mL in 54% and 46% of double and single PI subjects, respectively (intent-to-treat, $p = 0.37$).[107] The result of this study should be interpreted with caution, since the study was underpowered to detect a potential difference between the two groups.

Lopinavir/ritonavir-Saquinavir

The effect of lopinavir/ritonavir (LPV/r) on saquinavir (SQV) plasma concentrations was evaluated in 45 patients receiving LPV/r 400/100 mg bid and SQV 1000 mg bid. SQV exposure with LPV/r was not significantly lower compared to patients receiving SQV/r 1000/100 mg bid in the control arm, even though the RTV AUC was 55% lower. LPV concentrations were similar to historical control data.[109] The LPV with SQV combination was evaluated in a cohort study of 126 heavily pretreated patients who were experiencing treatment failure with nucleoside reverse transcriptase inhibitor (NRTI)-containing regimen. At week 48, a switch to LPV/r 400/100 mg with SQV 1000 mg bid without the addition of RTIs resulted in a VL decrease by a median 2.7 $\log_{10}$.[110]

RTV-Sparing Dual PI Combinations

A high incidence of hyperlipidemia and GI intolerance associated with RTV boosted PIs combination have led to the evaluation of dual PI combinations without RTV. Combining nelfinavir 750mg tid with 800mg tid of the soft-gel formulation of SQV produced an SQV AUC equivalent to 1200mg tid at steady state.[111] The substitution of SQV soft-gel capsule formulation with the commercially available formulation (SQV hard-gel capsules or tablets) will likely result in a similar pharmacokinetic profile, but this combination is less relevant to clinical practice due to the large pill burden and thrice-daily administration. IDV and SQV combinations, when dosed twice-daily at steady state had a disappointing pharmacokinetic enhancement profile, this led to only 45% of patients suppressing their plasma HIV RNA to less than 400 copies/mL after 72 weeks.[112] The IDV/SQV combination was reported to be antagonistic when used to inhibit HIV replication *in vitro*.[113] While the clinical relevance of this finding is unknown, this combination has not been evaluated in clinical studies and should be avoided.

The combination of FPV and ATV was evaluated in a prospective, randomized, open-label, three-way crossover pharmacokinetic study, in which 21 HIV-infected adults received FPV 1400mg, ATV 400mg, or both once-daily for 14 days. Although the AUC of FPV was increased by 78%, ATV AUC and C_{min} were decreased by 33% and 57%, respectively.[114] This combination is not recommended since ATV C_{trough} falls below the range of 150–850ng/mL which has been associated with the highest probability of virologic response.[115]

A small pilot study examined the pharmacokinetics of ATV 400mg qd when given alone compared to when given in combination with SQV 1200mg hard-gel capsules in 22 HIV-infected patients. Although the SQV AUC was increased threefold, the ATV pharmacokinetic profile was not enhanced by SQV co-administration.[8,116] The lack of a beneficial pharmacokinetic interaction between ATV 400mg qd and SQV 1200mg qd may partially explain the lower virologic response rate compared to ATV/r 300/100mg qd or LPV/r 400/100mg bid in treatment-experienced patients.[98] Numerous attempts to boost PI concentrations without RTV have fallen short in achieving the desired serum level needed to treat PI-experienced patients.

Other Antiretroviral Combinations

Other strategies for increasing concentrations of PIs through enzyme inhibition could include concomitant ketoconazole or delavirdine, both of which are CYP3A4 inhibitors. Delavirdine significantly increased the AUC of SQV by 520%, IDV by 72%, and nelfinavir by 92%.[117,118] However, due to the lack of clinical data and weak antiviral potency of delavirdine, these combinations are not recommended as initial therapy.[75]

Interactions with Herbal Therapies

Herbal remedies and nutritional supplements are widely used in HIV-infected patients although little attention has been paid to the pharmacokinetic effects of these compounds since they are considered benign. An increasing number of studies have shown that certain alternative therapies may cause drug interactions with agents used in the treatment of HIV infection. In healthy volunteers, St John's wort decreased the AUC of IDV by over 50%.[119] The mechanism of this interaction is complex and appears to be mediated by both induction of CYP3A4 and P-gp.[120,121] This herb should be avoided in patients taking PIs and NNRTIs, although there currently are no data on whether RTV can reverse this interaction.

Garlic supplements are sometimes used by HIV-infected patients because of their touted effects on lowering cholesterol. Raw garlic and garlic supplements inhibit the activity of CYP3A4 *in vitro* and in animals, and case reports have documented RTV-related gastrointestinal toxicity in two people after they ingested uncooked garlic preparations with RTV.[122] However, a study in healthy volunteers showed that garlic capsules taken bid for 3 weeks led to a mean decrease in SQV concentrations of ~50% probably as a consequence of reduced bioavailibility.[123] Even after a 10-day washout period, AUC values returned to only 60–70% of baseline suggesting a prolonged effect. Other herbs with reported *in vitro* effects on CYP450-mediated metabolism include silymarin (milk thistle), ginseng, and skullcap.[124] IDV C_{min} was decreased by 25% with milk thistle co-administration, but the AUC remained unchanged.[125] Clinicians need to include alternative medicines in their drug histories and consider them when adverse effects or treatment failure appear with no other cause.

Drug–Cytokine Interactions

Proinflammatory cytokines including interleukin (IL)-6, IL-1, and tumor necrosis factor (TNF)-α are released during periods of stress, trauma, or infection. A number of *in vitro* and clinical studies have shown that IL-6 and TNF-α inhibit CYP-mediated metabolism. This mechanism is not competitive but is a metabolic interaction at the level of transcription of CYP messenger RNA.[126]

Several immunodulating agents are being evaluated for the treatment of HIV-infection. One of the best studied is IL-2. Its exogenous administration has been shown to increase CD4+ T-lymphocyte cells, but results in a profound release of proinflammatory cytokines that are one likely cause of its problematic side effect profile. In HIV-infected patients receiving a 5-day continuous infusion of IL-2, IDV clearance significantly decreased and the AUC increased 75% as compared with baseline values before IL-2 administration.[127] The short-term administration (5 days) of IL-2 makes this interaction less clinically significant, although drug–cytokine interactions should be considered as additional investigational agents are used in a more chronic fashion.

Altered Excretion

Drug interactions may also be caused by alterations in renal elimination. This can be a consequence of either inhibition of tubular secretion or impairment of renal function. Probenecid and trimethoprim are inhibitors of renal tubular secretion, which may increase concentrations of some renally cleared drugs. The lamivudine AUC is increased by 44% with concomitant trimethoprim-sulfamethoxazole.[128] The acyclovir AUC is increased 40% with concomitant probenecid.[129] Inhibition of renal secretion with probenecid is a useful strategy to increase plasma concentrations of procaine penicillin, needed for the treatment of neurosyphilis.[130] tenofovir DF (TDF) clearance decreased by 16% with LPV/r co-administration The mechanism for this interaction is unknown. Although this interaction is not likely to be clinically significant, there have been several cases of nephrotoxicity when these two agents are co-administered.[131,132]

Intracellular Pharmacokinetic Interactions

The NRTIs are prodrugs that must undergo phosphorylation intracellularly to their active triphosphate forms. While these drugs are not generally affected by CYP450 interactions, there may be competition for intracellular activation pathways that result in clinically relevant drug interactions. Ribavirin decreases the phosphorylation of zidovudine and stavudine *in vitro*, resulting in decreased concentrations of the active triphosphate, but this interaction did not affect the antiviral effect of zidovudine or stavudine *in vivo*.[133–135] On the other hand, zidovudine may impair the intracellular phosphorylation of stavudine[134] and this combination is associated with unfavorable clinical outcomes as compared with other regimens containing two NRTIs.[136] Lamivudine inhibits zalcitabine phosphorylation and this combination should be avoided.[137]

ddI concentrations are increased when co-administered with TDF. The proposed mechanism of this interaction is an interference with ddI breakdown by direct inhibition of purine nucleoside phosphorylase (PNP) by tenofovir.[138] This interaction is not offset by taking both drugs together with food. However, when TDF is administered with a reduced dose of ddI (250 mg of the ECformulation in patients weighing 60 kg or 200 mg in patients weighing below 60 kg), the ddI AUC is comparable to that of ddI given at standard doses.[139]

In a longitudinal analysis, the combination of ddI and ribavirin resulted in acute pancreatitis and symptomatic hyperlactatemia in 28% and 17% patients, respectively. Two patients with pancreatitis and severe lactic acidosis died.[140–142] The proposed mechanism is inhibition of inosine monophosphate (IMP) dehydrogenase by ribavirin. This leads to an increase of the IMP pool, which acts as a phosphate donor for the transformation of ddI into deoxy IMP (dIMP). dIMP is then metabolised into ddATP, the triphosphorylated metabolite of ddI.[143] Increased intracellular ddATP may account for this increase in ddI-associated toxicities.

Recognizing and Circumventing Drug Interactions

Strategies for recognizing and avoiding drug interactions are shown in Box 79-1. A careful review of the patient's medication profile is essential to monitor for drug interactions. Patients should be asked to disclose all their medications, because they may often seek treatment from more than one healthcare provider. In addition, a medication history should include both prescription and nonprescription drugs, as well as any herbal, investigational, or alternative therapies. Clinicians should be familiar with those agents most commonly associated with drug interactions. Any patient receiving "red flag" drugs such as rifampin, RTV, or ketoconazole requires extra attention, and patients should be given a list of drugs that should not be administered concomitantly.

Finally, drug interactions can be avoided by simplifying drug regimens whenever possible. Selection of a therapeutically equivalent agent with fewer drug interactions may be wise. Azithromycin could be substituted for erythromycin or clarithromycin if appropriate for the clinical situation. Similarly, it may be advantageous to replace RTV with another PI for patients requiring medication with the potential for serious interactions. Care provider and patient need to work together to develop a tolerable regimen that meets therapeutic goals.

Strategies for Recognition and Avoidance of Drug Interactions

BOX 79-1

- Review of patient medication profiles
- Full medication profile, including over-the-counter and "alternative" medications
- Recognition of agents most commonly associated with interactions (i.e., protease inhibitors, ketoconazole, rifampin, etc)
- Recognition of agents with overlapping toxicities
- Proper staggering and scheduling of medications
- Knowledge of dietary restrictions with certain medications
- Selection of agents with fewer drug interactions if clinically appropriate.

OVERLAPPING TOXICITIES

Many of the drugs used in the HIV-infected patient share similar toxicity profiles. Some common examples are shown in Box 79-2. Although it would be ideal to prescribe drugs with nonoverlapping adverse effects, the limited choices for antiretroviral therapy and opportunistic infection treatment often preclude this. In the nucleoside analog class, stavudine, ddI, and zalcitabine are all associated with the development of peripheral neuropathy. Although a clinical study examining the combination of stavudine and ddI showed that only two patients developed peripheral neuropathy after 1 year of therapy,[144] other observational cohorts reported much higher incidence. The crude incidence rate of peripheral neuropathy observed in 1116 patients who received ddI, stavudine, ddI with stavudine, or ddI with stavudine and hydroxyurea were 6.8, 9.8, 17.5, and 28.6 per 100 person-years, respectively.[145]

BOX 79-2

Common Examples of Overlapping Toxicities of HIV-Related Medications

- **Bone marrow suppression**
  - Co-trimoxazole
  - Cytotoxic chemotherapy (i.e., doxorubicin, cyclophosphamide, vinblastine, etc)
  - Dapsone
  - Flucytosine
  - Ganciclovir
  - Interferon and peg-interferon
  - Pentamidine
  - Primaquine
  - Sulfadiazine/pyrimethamine
  - Trimetrexate
- **Peripheral neuropathy**
  - Didanosine
  - Ethambutol
  - Isoniazid
  - Stavudine
  - Zalcitabine
- **Renal dysfunction**
  - Aminoglycosides
  - Amphotericin B
  - Cidofovir
  - Foscarnet
  - Pentamidine (IV).

The same drug combinations are associated with an increased risk of severe pancreatitis. Since nucleoside-induced peripheral neuropathy may be irreversible if the implicating agents are not discontinued within 2 weeks of symptoms, clinicians should be vigilant about monitoring for these symptoms and, if present, should switch to an alternative NRTI (abacavir, tenofovir, zidovudine). Other examples of overlapping toxicities include pancreatitis with ddI and pentamidine, anemia with ribavirin and zidovudine, and nausea with high dose sulfadiazine and LPV/r. When the use of these combinations is unavoidable, supportive medications (i.e., erythropoietin, antiemetics, antidiarrheals) should be considered to lessen adverse effects.

A common dilemma is trying to identify which drug is actually causing an adverse effect. For example, LPV/r, zidovudine, and ddI are all associated with nausea and other gastrointestinal side effects. One strategy would involve stopping all medications until the side effects resolve and adding drugs back sequentially as tolerated. Note that this strategy is not an option for patients taking combination antiretroviral therapy, since it may induce resistance. Alternatively, single drugs could be removed and/or substituted in the regimen to see if the gastrointestinal symptoms resolve. This situation may be more difficult in the case of neutropenia, in which the adverse effect could be caused either by medications (Box 79-2) or by disease processes such as *M. avium* and CMV infections. For particularly toxic combinations such as zidovudine and ganciclovir, supportive care with granulocyte colony-stimulating factor may be a useful adjunctive therapy to allow continuation of the regimen.

MEDICATION ADHERENCE

Healthcare providers generally assume that patients take most or all of their prescribed medication. Numerous studies indicate that adherence to prescribed medication regimens varies greatly, and that few patients take all of their prescribed doses of drug. Imperfect adherence has probably been a medical fact of life since the dawn of civilization.

Using the most accurate means available to assess adherence, studies with single drugs suggest that fewer than 10% of patients take all prescribed doses of medication. Most patients are moderately compliant, taking between 70% and 90% of prescribed doses. About one-third of patients take less than 60% of prescribed doses.[146,147] These adherence estimates hold true in HIV-infected patients taking combination antiretroviral therapy[148] or treatment for opportunistic infections.[149] Adherence assessment of combination regimens is far more complicated because adherence behavior may be different for different agents prescribed at the same time.[150]

Even intelligent and highly motivated individuals with medical backgrounds have difficulty with adherence. A study in 36 medical students randomized to receive a twice-daily or thrice-daily placebo for 14 days found that the mean number of doses taken was only 71% of those prescribed,[151] a result similar to that seen in AIDS or epilepsy patients. Furthermore, less than 30% of dosing intervals were correct, regardless of assigned regimen. The two most common reasons cited for improper compliance in this study were "hectic schedule" and "irregular routine".

Healthcare providers cannot with great precision predict which patients will be adherent and which will not. Patient self-report and pill count also provide unreliable and inaccurate information.[147,152,153] Socioeconomic factors, racial and ethnic background, and disease state, which seem as if they ought to be related to degree of adherence, generally are not.[154] Therefore, care providers need to anticipate noncompliance and, whenever possible, avert any problems it may cause.

Studies suggest that poor adherence may be a major factor in the development of resistance to HIV PIs.[155] Overall adherence rates of less than 80% were associated with a significant increase in the risk of treatment failure.[156,157] The risk of treatment failure increased with decreasing adherence rate in patients taking PIs with two nucleoside analogs.[157] In one study, 78% of patients taking 95% or more of prescribed PI doses had undetectable VLs, while only 20% of those taking less than 80% of prescribed doses had undetectable VLs.[157] Viral suppression dropped off substantially with each decline in adherence rate.[157] It should be noted that most subjects evaluated in these studies were taking only a single PI without RTV enhancement, and therefore most were using a thrice-daily regimen. Such stringent adherence requirements may not be necessary with simpler NNRTI or PI-based regimens. Viral suppression to less than 400 copies was seen in greater than 62% of patient taking 54% or more of their prescribed NNRTI-based regimens.[158] This observation may in part be due to the long half-life of NNRTIs. Because NNRTIs have a low genetic barrier to resistance, this class is generally not considered ideal for patients with suboptimal adherence.

A number of interventions can promote better adherence.[148] Regimens involving fewer daily doses and fewer agents are easier to take. Once-a-day regimens promote adherence best; twice-daily regimens are only marginally better than thrice-daily regimens in recently published studies,[147,150,151] although these studies were conducted in patients taking only a single medication. An additional consideration is that the consequences of noncompliance may be more severe for agents dosed infrequently. For example, if a drug is dosed thrice-daily, then the daily therapeutic coverage is reduced by 33% if a single dose is missed; however, if a drug is dosed once-daily, then daily therapeutic coverage is reduced 100% if a single dose is missed. This may be less of an issue for drugs like EFV, with a steady-state half-life of more than 48 h, or tenofovir, with a reported intracellular diphosphate half-life of 60 h.

Effective pharmacotherapy for AIDS generally requires the incorporation into medical practice of means of improving adherence. Previous studies in patients with epilepsy and hypertension show that adherence can often be improved by modifying the drug regimen, physician practice, and patient behavior (Box 79-3). Steps include increasing recognition of the problem, counseling and educating the patient about the importance of good adherence and the dangers of poor adherence, providing environmental cues to habituate the taking of medicines, incorporating medication taking into established routines, monitoring outcomes and providing feedback to reinforce success, minimizing polypharmacy, and using twice-daily or once-daily regimens whenever possible.

Strategies for Improving Medication Adherence

BOX 79-3

- Recognize and anticipate the problem
- Educate the patient about the importance of good adherence
- Counsel the patient about the dangers of poor adherence
- Monitor the patient's adherence behavior
- Provide environmental cues for dosing
- Learn the patient's normal routine and incorporate dosing cues into that routine
- Provide positive feedback for clinical successes
- Emphasize patient self-reliance
- Provide realistic therapeutic goals and expectations for the patient
- Use bid or qd regimens whenever possible
- Minimize the number of agents prescribed.

THERAPEUTIC DRUG MONITORING

Therapeutic drug monitoring (TDM) refers to the adjustment of drug doses based on measured plasma concentrations to attain values within a "therapeutic window". Clinicians have used these principles for years to adjust doses of drugs including theophylline, aminoglycosides, digoxin, and anticonvulsants. There is growing evidence that TDM may be useful in some circumstances to ensure HIV-infected patients have adequate concentrations for efficacy without producing toxicity. Some antiretrovirals share many of the characteristics of drugs that require monitoring of plasma levels, including variable intersubject pharmacokinetics, serious consequences if there is a lack of effect or drug toxicity, documented relationships between concentration and effect or toxicity, and the availability of rapid and accurate assays. However, a number of inherent problems must be resolved before TDM becomes a standard practice.

The beneficial role of TDM in HIV clinical practice remains to be demonstrated. A number of studies have described relationships between antiretroviral drug concentrations and antiviral effect.[159–167] Results from three prospective, randomized trials of TDM in HIV-infected patients have been reported. In a pharmacokinetic sub-study of the ATHENA cohort, 147 treatment-naive patients who were prescribed nelfinavir, IDV, or IDV/r based regimen, were randomized to TDM or no TDM (control group). After 1 year of follow-up, 17.4% and 39.7% of patients discontinued therapy in the TDM group and control group, respectively. The significant differences in discontinuation rate were due to virologic failure in the nelfinavir-treated patients and toxicity in the IDV treated patients, but in a subanalysis of the study, patients who received RTV-boosted IDV did not benefit from TDM. In the intent-to-treat analysis (noncompleter equals failure), a higher proportion of patients randomized to TDM achieved a VL below 500 copies/mL after 12 month of treatment.[168] Conversely, PHARMADAPT, which used trough plasma PI concentrations to modify salvage therapy, did not show a significant improvement in virologic outcomes at 12 weeks with TDM.[169] Modification of PI therapy due to "subtherapeutic" troughs occurred for only 23.5 % of patients receiving PI TDM and dosage modifications did not occur until 8 weeks into therapy; this may have permitted the appearance of resistance mutations. In addition, wild type IC_{50}s were used as target trough concentrations in PHARMADAPT, and this target may be too low since the target for treatment-experienced patients may be higher. It was interesting to note that due to the wide inter- and intra-patient variability in concentrations, 14% of patients spontaneously changed from one "category" to the other between week 4 and 8 without any intervention.

GENOPHAR was another TDM study that randomized 134 patients to expert recommended therapy based on genotypic resistance only versus genotypic resistance with TDM. By intent-to-treat analysis, no difference in virologic response rate was observed between the two groups at 12 weeks; in the multivariate analysis, only prior exposure to at least two PIs predicted response.[170] GENOPHAR had similar trial design limitations as PHARMADAPT, in addition, both trials had a large proportion of patients on RTV-"boosted" PI regimens that may have made TDM intervention less critical, since concentrations of boosted-PIs are significantly higher.

TDM with the NNRTI class is limited to small observational studies. Adjusting EFV concentrations based on results obtained ~14 h after the last dose was associated with improved treatment response and central nervous system side effects.[171] On the other hand, in a small pharmacokinetic substudy of the ATHENA cohort, nevirapine TDM did not improve virologic success or adverse drug reaction rate.[172]

TDM with NRTIs is not recommended since there are only limited data showing a direct linear correlation between plasma concentrations of drugs like lamivudine, and ddI with their active intracellular triphosphate concentrations.[173,174] Technical challenges of measuring intracellular triphosphates of nucleoside analogs have limited these measurements to only a few research groups. In addition, validation across laboratories and variation in the source of the sample (cell cultures vs patient samples) have made standardization of intracellular triphosphate assays difficult.

Studies demonstrate that when the phenotype or "virtual" phenotype is used along with the plasma concentration, the ratio of the C_{min} (trough concentration) to the protein-adjusted IC_{50} is more predictive of virologic outcome in treatment experienced patients. This ratio is often called the Inhibitory Quotient or IQ.[175–180] Retrospective studies suggest that integration of pharmacokinetics and virus susceptibility to the drug provide more complete information than either measurement used alone. Ongoing prospective trials will evaluate if the IQ ratio will be a useful monitoring tool in HIV-infected patients.

A number of practical and logistical challenges limit the widespread use of TDM for antiretroviral therapy. A primary limitation of TDM is that it does not provide information on long-term adherence. A patient could have taken their drugs incorrectly for weeks but may improve adherence for the 2–3 days immediately before their clinic appointment if they know a TDM sample will be taken. The drug concentration in such a patient would appear to be adequate although the patient may be failing therapy due to nonadherence. Intrapatient variability also appears to be large for some antiretrovirals,[181] suggesting that clinical decisions should be made only after two or more trough samples are collected, and not based on a single determination. The definition of a true "therapeutic range" will also need to be determined for each drug, knowing that the target value may be very different for treatment-naïve and treatment-experienced patients. Finally, accurate sample collection, timely processing, storage and shipping of plasma, and rapid turnaround times for assay results must be assured.

Although current prospective studies do not support routine use, TDM can be considered in selected patient populations. Pregnant patients, pediatric patients, patients receiving nelfinavir, and patients receiving known enzyme inhibitors or inducers may be candidates for TDM.

PHARMACOKINETIC FACTORS

A number of pharmacokinetic factors, including oral and systemic bioavailability, distribution, and clearance, can be significant determinants of a patient's response to therapy. The importance of these factors as they apply to the administration of drugs for AIDS is emphasized below. The clinical pharmacokinetics of the available antiretroviral drugs are summarized in Chapter 61.

Drug Distribution and Protein Binding

Drug distribution and tissue penetration are a function of several factors, including the drug's size, lipophilicity, affinity for plasma binding proteins, and whether the drug is subject to active transport into or out of cells. For example, high-affinity binding to plasma proteins could affect a drug's ability to penetrate into cells, and this could affect a drug's antimicrobial activity.

Albumin, which accounts for ~50% of plasma protein, has a high capacity for drug binding but a generally low affinity. $Alpha_1$-acid glycoprotein (AAG) is a low-capacity but high-affinity drug-binding protein that may play a more important role in distribution. AAG is an inducible but minor component of plasma (<3% of total plasma protein). The addition of physiologic concentrations of AAG reduces the anti-HIV potency of a number of drugs *in vitro* by a factor of 10-fold or more.[182–185] This could contribute to reduced activity of such drugs under clinical circumstances.

For example, the HIV PI SC-52151 bound to AAG with particularly high affinity[183] failed to produce anti-HIV effects in phase II clinical studies[186] despite achieving total drug concentrations well in excess of its 90% inhibitory concentration.[187] The use of 2 mg/mL AAG (a slightly supraphysiologic concentration) prevented penetration of radiolabeled SC-52151 into cells[188]; this probably contributed to its lack of activity in clinical studies, because free drug concentrations were never high enough to exert a measurable anti-HIV effect.[187] High-affinity AAG binding can be overcome if total drug concentrations are high enough to saturate protein binding sites, as occurs with other highly AAG-bound drugs such as RTV.[189] This is of theoretical concern in HIV-infected patients because intercurrent infections and other illnesses may elevate AAG plasma concentrations and decrease free drug, although AAG concentrations remain in the normal range in asymptomatic patients with HIV infection.[187,190]

All of the available peptidomimetic HIV PIs are protein bound in plasma to varying degrees, although the protein binding of IDV is only ~60%, which has little or no effect on its disposition. Amprenavir, ATV, LPV, nelfinavir, RTV, and SQV are greater than 90% bound to protein in plasma.[5] Plasma protein binding is quite low for most of the nucleoside analogs[191] and plays no significant role in their disposition. Displacement of one drug by another from its plasma protein binding sites may lead to transient changes in free drug concentrations, potentially affecting activity or toxicity, but clinical relevance of such an interaction has never been demonstrated.

Central Nervous System Penetration

Penetration of drugs into the central nervous system (CNS) is essential for activity in CNS disease. The relationship between plasma concentrations and CNS concentrations of drugs is complex, and activity against CNS infections often does not require that cerebrospinal fluid (CSF) concentrations be as high as simultaneous plasma concentrations. Studies with PIs have shown that even agents with marginal CSF penetration, such as SQV and IDV, produce reductions in CSF VL comparable to those produced in the plasma.[192,193] The estimated fractional penetration of nelfinavir into CSF is less than 0.2%,[194] yet this drug is associated with remarkably good suppression of CSF VL.[195] Similarly, ATV concentrations in CSF are highly variable and 100-fold lower than plasma concentrations; these levels are not consistently higher than the wild type IC_{50}, but the clinical significance of this finding is unknown.[196] Only one of 17 subjects receiving amprenavir had a higher CSF VL than plasma VL in one study, and the magnitude of the difference in that single subject was small.[197] These findings suggest that the relatively low concentrations of free drug in the CSF are adequate to suppress HIV replication, or that CSF viral RNA may not adequately reflect virus replication in brain tissue.

Most nucleoside analogs penetrate the CNS to a limited extent, with CSF concentrations ranging from 10% to above 30% of simultaneous plasma concentrations.[191] Higher fractional penetration has been reported for zidovudine, but in most studies assessment is based on limited CSF sampling, with only a single CSF–plasma pair used to ascertain the ratio of drug concentrations. The relationship between CNS penetration and activity in HIV-associated encephalopathy has not been well characterized, although higher doses of zidovudine are associated with improved response in patients with CNS disease.[198]

Genital Tract Penetration

Genital secretions are a potential vector for sexual transmission of HIV, and drugs that penetrate into these fluids more extensively might better inhibit replication and transmission of the virus. Antiretroviral concentrations in seminal plasma are generally much higher than in the CSF, and some antiretrovirals, primarily NRTIs (i.e., zidovudine, lamivudine, tenofovir, and stavudine), appear to be concentrated in the semen as compared to the blood.[199–202] IDV concentrations in the semen equal plasma concentrations; RTV and SQV fractional penetration into seminal plasma is only 2–5%, perhaps reflecting the impact of plasma protein binding or drug transporters.[203] Similarly, fractional penetration in seminal plasma was poor with LPV, enfuvirtide, and EFV.[200,201,204,205]

Despite the differences in penetration into semen, IDV, RTV, and SQV use were associated with equivalent suppression of VL in the semen of treated patients.[203] Low concentrations of SQV or RTV are all that may be needed to suppress HIV in the genital tract. Alternatively, HIV measured in semen could originate in and reflect virus concentrations in the blood. Penetration of antiretrovirals into vaginal fluid is more difficult to quantify, and little information is available in the literature.

Drugs in the Pregnant Patient

Of increasing concern is administration of antiretroviral medication to pregnant patients. There are three situations in which this occurs: (1) an HIV-infected woman becomes pregnant while receiving standard pharmacotherapy; (2) a pregnant patient is newly diagnosed HIV positive and is placed on antiretroviral drugs to prevent maternal-fetal transmission; and (3) a pregnant healthcare worker suffers an occupational exposure to HIV and receives antiretroviral drugs to prevent infection. For each of these cases, the teratogenicity and the pharmacokinetics of antiretrovirals must be carefully considered. Teratogenicity data from clinical trials are available for certain antiretrovirals. Zidovudine, lamivudine, ddI, stavudine, nevirapine, nelfinavir, and SQV were not associated with an increased risk of teratogenicity.[206] Conversely, birth defects were observed with first trimester exposure to EFV; therefore, this drug is contraindicated in pregnancy. Clinicians should also counsel all women of child bearing potential receiving EFV about the importance of an adequate form of contraception.

Pregnant women may be at increased risk of lactic acidosis when prescribed stavudine and ddI in combination. Cases of lactic acidosis, in some cases fatal, have been reported, and therefore the combination of ddI and stavudine should be avoided.[207]

Unlike the CNS, the placenta does not, in general, act as a functional barrier to drug penetration. Most drugs, especially those with respectable oral bioavailability, cross the placenta to some degree. This is particularly true for lipophilic drugs; compounds that are large or highly ionized in plasma and therefore have limited penetration into extravascular compartments have reduced fetal penetration. Animal and human studies of placental drug penetration found that fetal concentrations of nucleoside analogs such as zidovudine were half as high that of concentrations in maternal plasma.[191] Although the placenta carries out some drug-metabolizing reactions, particularly glucuronidation, this is an inconsequential means of clearance for most drugs.

Penetration of drugs into breast milk is an important issue for women who are nursing. Like the placenta, mammary glands are no real barrier to drug penetration. Most orally available agents penetrate breast milk. Some lipophilic agents are actually concentrated in breast milk, and may reach concentrations higher than those in maternal plasma. For example, zidovudine concentrations in breast milk are ~50% higher, on average, than those in maternal plasma.[208]

Physiologic changes seen in pregnancy that may affect pharmacokinetics include: delayed gastric emptying, decreased intestinal motility, increase in volume of distribution by 30–50%, increased renal blood flow by 25–50% and increased glomerular filtration rate by 50%.[209–211] Drug concentrations may therefore fall during pregnancy. For example, SQV showed a substantial reduction in plasma concentrations during pregnancy, but concentrations were adequate when SQV was boosted with RTV.[212,213] Nefinavir concentrations fall on average by 24% in the third trimester of pregnancy with an even greater fall in concentrations of the metabolite M8.[214] Nelfinavir 750 mg tid achieved a target AUC of 10 mcg $h^{-1}mL^{-1}$ in only three of nine pregnant women; however, increasing the dose to 1200 mg bid resulted in improved pharmacokinetic parameters and undetectable VL in 82% of treated patients.[215] LPV concentrations are also decreased in pregnancy but this could be overcome by increasing the dose to 533/133 mg twice daily in the second and third trimester.[216] On the other hand, there is no difference in the pharmacokinetics of zidovudine, lamivudine, ddI, and nevirapine during pregnancy.[217–221]

Drugs in Other Special Populations

Genetics can play an important role in drug disposition and effect. Human genetic polymorphisms are well known for several drug-metabolizing enzymes, including *N*-acetyltransferases and the CYP isoforms 2C19 and CYP2D6. In recent years, an isoform CYP2B6 polymorphism has been identified as an important predictor of EFV pharmacokinetic parameters. The CYP2B6 T/T genotype at position 516 (GlnHis), which is more common in African-Americans (20%) than in European-Americans (3%), was associated with greater EFV plasma concentrations.[222]

On the other hand, most sex and racial effects in pharmacokinetics are of a minor magnitude. Formal pharmacokinetic evaluation showed no significant difference in the disposition of zidovudine, for example, as a function of sex or race.[223] However, nelfinavir and LPV concentrations are on average 30% higher in women than in men.

Pediatric pharmacokinetics are frequently different from those in adults, because renal and hepatic function change with age. This is especially true in neonates less than 1 month of age, in whom some drug-metabolizing enzymes, for example those involved in conjugation reactions, have not yet reached adult levels. For many drugs used in children greater than 12 months old, drug elimination as a function of body surface area is equivalent to that in adults. For example, surface area-adjusted zidovudine clearance in infants greater than 1 month of age is not significantly different from that in adults.[224] Nonetheless, pediatric drug dosing must be individualized and closely monitored, depending on age and size of the patient.

Liver disease can affect the clearance of all approved HIV PIs and NNRTIs, since elimination depends on hepatic CYP activity. In general, mild liver impairment does not warrant dose adjustment. Moderate cirrhosis increased the AUC of amprenavir by more than twofold as compared to that in healthy volunteers; severe cirrhosis increased the amprenavir AUC more than threefold.[30] Amprenavir oral solution contains propylene glycol. This formulation should be used with caution in patients with hepatic impairment and renal impairment, as these patients may be at increased risk of propylene glycol toxicity.[30]

Nelfinavir pharmacokinetics were highly variable in five patients with liver disease as compared to patients without liver disease. Calculated elimination half-life of nelfinavir was up to 20 h, compared to 3.5–5 h in patients without liver disease.[225] Formation of the nelfinavir M8 metabolite was reduced in these patients by ~10-fold as compared to patients without liver disease.[225] Doses were adjusted in these patients to achieve concentrations that were within the range of those seen in patients without liver disease. The AUC and half-life of IDV were modestly altered in patients with mild to moderate hepatic insufficiency and cirrhosis.[26] For some PIs (i.e., IDV, ATV, and FPV) doses need to be reduced in patients with moderate to severe hepatic impairment, as measured by Child–Pugh classification. TPV administration is not recommended for patients with liver disease.[9] Dose adjustment for other PIs should be based on published dosing guidelines.

Since most NRTI elimination depends on glomerular filtration and, to a lesser extent, tubular secretion, renal impairment can affect the clearance of all approved NRTIs with the exception of zidovudine and abacavir. On the other hand, the clearance of PIs and NNRTIs are not significantly affected, since they undergo hepatobiliary clearance. There are limited data on the pharmacokinetics of antiretrovirals in hemodialysis patients. Up to 25–46% of a stavudine, ddI, tenofovir, and nevirapine dose may be removed during a hemodialysis session.[226–229] In order to minimize an extended period of subtherapeutic antiretroviral exposure, timing of all antiretrovirals administration should be after the completion of the hemodialysis session.

Critically ill patients represent another special population with potential changes in pharmacokinetics. Altered distribution or clearance of many drugs, including aminoglycosides, phenytoin, and pentobarbital, have been reported in intensive care unit (ICU) patients.[230–232] It is important to note that absorption of oral medications is often poor in ICU patients, and some clinicians advocate the discontinuation of oral antiretrovirals because of the potential for suboptimal plasma concentrations. However, the consequence of viral rebound and development of resistance should be considered. Alternatively, antiretrovirals available as liquids may be given through feeding tubes. For some medications, the contents of a capsule or crushed tablet are mixed with a small amount of fluid or enteral nutrition formulas, and administered through the feeding tube. The absorption of antiretrovirals by this method of administration is unknown. Drug interactions may

Table 79-3

Number of Pills in Combination Regimens Using Standard Doses

Formulation Issues	Pill Burden
TDF, FTC, EFV	1
Epzicom, EFV	2
Combovir, EFV	3
Epzicom, ATV/r	3
Truvada, LPV/r	5
Trizivir, FPV/r	6
Truvada, AZT, LPV/r, SQV	11
LPV/r, ATV, Trizivir, T-20, TMP-SMX, fluconazole, clarithromycin, ethambutol, valganciclovir	16

TDF, tenofovir DF; FTC, emtricitabine; EFV, efavirenz; Epzicom, abacavir+lamivudine; Truvada, tenofovir DF+emtricitabine; Trizivir, zidovudine+lamivudine+abacavir; ATV/r, atazanavir+ritonavir; LPV/r, lopinavir+ritonavir; FPV/r, Fosamprenavir+ritonavir; SQV, saquinavir; TMP-SMX, co-trimoxazole.

also be a problem because of the large number of medications these patients receive.

FORMULATION ISSUES

Early HAART regimens often had complex dosing schedules and food restrictions, but adherence remains challenging even with the much simpler regimens commonly in use today. Table 79-3 lists the number of pills for some common anti-HIV regimens. In patients taking two or more PIs, the number of pills per day can be quite large. Some improvements in formulation include the combination of zidovudine with lamivudine (Combivir®), the combination of zidovudine, lamivudine and abacavir (Trizivir®), the combination of TDF and emtricitabine (Truvada®), and TDF, emtricitabine, and EFV (Atripla®). These products greatly simplify HAART regimen and require only one to two tablets per day.

ddI EC formulation is an enteric coated capsule that can be given once daily without many of the drug interactions seen with the buffered formulation. Pill burden with previous PI formulations has significantly improved with the introduction of LPV/r 200/50 mg tablets, FPV 700 mg tablets, and SQV 500 mg tablets. Two different combination products also exist for the treatment of tuberculosis. Rifamate® is a product containing 300 mg of rifampin and 150 mg of isoniazid, while Rifater® contains 120 mg of rifampin, 50 mg of isoniazid, and 300 mg of pyrazinamide. The use of these combination products provides a simple and convenient alternative if clinically warranted.

Many products are available in liquid formulations for use in pediatric patients or in adults with dysphagia. Antiretrovirals with liquid or reconstitutable formulations include ddI, stavudine, zidovudine, lamivudine, emtricitabine, LPV/r, RTV, amprenavir and nelfinavir. The taste of the RTV and amprenavir solutions is often described as unpleasant, and may cause adherence problems. RTV can be mixed with chocolate milk, Advera®, or Ensure® to mask the taste.[233] In addition, many of the medications for opportunistic infections, such as azithromycin, clarithromycin, atovaquone, and trimethoprim-sulfamethoxazole, are available as liquids.

STORAGE OF ANTIRETROVIRALS

Table 79-4 lists the storage requirements and stability of the Food and Drug Administration (FDA)-approved antiretrovirals. Clinicians should remind patients to follow general precautions regarding storage of all medications.[234] Clinicians must consider refrigeration requirement before prescribing certain antiretroviral formulations (i.e., RTV capsules, TPV capsules, and enfuvirtide injection) in resource-limited countries. In the absence of specific storage recommendations, medications should be kept in a cool, dry area, away from excessive heat, light, and moisture. They should not be stored in places that may be damp, such as the bathroom or near the kitchen sink.

SUMMARY

Polypharmacy of HIV infection has led to clinical success and a host of complicated drug delivery issues. Pill burden, adherence, overlapping side effects, and proper medication scheduling are just some of the problems that must be addressed. Although these complex treatment regimens require a certain amount of patient self-motivation, there are various strategies the HIV clinician can employ to simplify regimens and optimize patient care. Medication profiles need to be reviewed by the healthcare provider for duplication, drug interactions, and appropriateness of therapy. Patient counseling is critical to thoroughly explain how complicated regimens should be administered. Most importantly, each regimen should be individualized based on previous medication experience, genotype, history of side effects, willingness to understand and comply with the regimen, social factors, and the patient's overall quality of life. While this is a daunting task for the patient and clinician, antiretroviral drugs can achieve long-term viral suppression and prolong life when administered correctly.

TPV is a nonpeptidic HIV PI. *In vivo*, TPVis a substrate and potent inducer of the P-gp drug transporter (P-gp). *In vitro* metabolism studies with human liver microsomes also indicate that TPV is a substrate of CYP3A4.[64] RTV, a known inhibitor of CYP3A4 and P-gp, significantly decreases TPV clearance, resulting in a 29-fold increase in the TPV AUC.[64a] TPV is therefore dependent on RTV co-administration to achieve the desired pharmacokinetic parameters. TPV/r (500/200 mg bid) produces a net inhibition of CYP3A4, resulting in an increase in plasma concentrations of many CYP3A4 substrates (e.g., atorvastatin). However, for drugs

Storage and Stability of Antiretrovirals

Table 79-4

Generic	Brand	Dosage Form	Storage/Stability
Abacavir	Ziagen	Tablet, solution	Store both at room temperature 20–25°C (68–77°F). May refrigerate solution to improve palatability but do not freeze
Abacavir/lamivudine	Epzicom	Tablet	Store at room temperature 15–30°C (59–86°F)
Abacavir/lamivudine/zidovudine	Trizivir	Tablet	Store at room temperature 15–30°C (59–86°F)
Atazanavir	Reyataz	Capsule	Store at room temperature 15–30°C (59–86°F)
Delavirdine	Rescriptor	Tablet	Store at room temperature 20–25°C (68–77°F)
Didanosine	Videx EC	Delayed release capsules	Store at room temperature 15–30°C (59–86°F)
Efavirenz	Sustiva	Tablet, capsule	Store at room temperature 15–30°C (59–86°F)
Fosamprenavir	Lexiva	Tablet	Store at room temperature 15–30°C (59–86°F)
Emtricitabine	Emtriva	Capsule, Solution	Store capsules at room temperature 15–30°C (59–86°F). Refrigerate solution. Solution can be kept out at room temperature for 3 months only.
Emtricitabine/tenofovir	Truvada	Tablet	Store at room temperature 15–30°C (59–86°F). Keep in original factory container
Enfuvirtide	Fuzeon	Powder for injection	Store powder at room temperature at 15–30°C (59–86°F). Use immediately or store reconstituted solution under "refrigeration" at 2–8°C (36–46°F) for up to 24 h
Indinavir	Crixivan	Capsule	Store at room temperature 15–30°C (59–86°F). Capsules are very sensitive to moisture. Keep in a dry place and store in original factory bottle with desiccant inside
Lamivudine	Epivir	Tablet, solution	Store at room temperature 15–30°C (59–86°F)
Lamivudine/zidovudine	Combivir	Tablet	Store at 2–30°C (36–86°F)
Lopinavir/ritonavir	Kaletra	Tablet, capsule, solution	Store tablets at room temperature 20–25°C (68–77°F). Store tablets in original factory bottle. Keep tablets away from humidity. Can store tablets in other bottle or in humid areas for up to 2 weeks. Store capsules and solution in the refrigerator at 2–8°C (36–46°F) until expiration date or at room temperature for up to 2 months. Avoid exposing capsules and solution to excessive heat
Nelfinavir	Viracept	Caplets, tablets, powder	Store at room temperature 15–30°C (59–86°F). Store in original factory container. Store constituted powder in refrigerator for up to 6 h
Nevirapine	Viramune	Tablet, suspension	Store both at room temperature 15–30°C (59–86°F)
Ritonavir	Norvir	Capsule, solution	Store capsules in the "refrigerator" at 2–8°C (36–46°F). May store capsules out of refrigerator (at less than 25°C or 77°F) for up to 30 days. Protect from light and excessive heat. Store solution at room temperature 20–25°C (68–77°F) and do not refrigerate. Keep capsules and solution in original factory bottle
Saquinavir	Invirase	Tablet, Capsule	Store at room temperature 15–30°C (59–86°F)
Stavudine	Zerit	Capsule, Solution	Store capsule and solution powder at room temperature 15–30°C (59–86°F). After solution is constituted, store in the refrigerator at 2–8°C (36–46°F) for up to 30 days

(*Continued*)

(Continued)

Table 79-4

Generic	Brand	Dosage Form	Storage/Stability
Tenofovir	Viread	Tablet	Store at room temperature 15–30°C (59–86°F)
Tipranavir/ritonavir	Aptivus	Capsule	Store capsules in the "refrigerator" at 2–8°C (36–46°F). May store at room temperature at 15–30°C (59–86°F) for up to 60 days. Store in original factory container
Zalcitabine	Hivid	Tablet	Store at room temperature 15–30°C (59–86°F)
Zidovudine	Retrovir	Tablet, capsule, syrup, IV infusion	Store all at room temperature 15–25°C (59–77°F). Protect IV infusion vials from light

that are dual substrates of CYP 3A4 and P-gp, a net induction results in a 45%, 49%, and 70% reduction in the amprenavir (APV), LPV (LPV/r), and SQV AUCs, respectively.[64b]

REFERENCES

1. Knupp CA, Milbrath R, Barbhaiya RH. Effect of time of food administration on the bioavailability of didanosine from a chewable tablet formulation. J Clin Pharmacol 33:568, 1993.
2. Videx EC (didanosine) product monograph. Princeton, NJ: Bristol Myers-Squibb; 2001.
3. Unadkat JD, Collier AC, Crosby SS, et al. Pharmacokinetics of oral zidovudine (azidothymidine) in patients with AIDS when administered with and without a high-fat meal. AIDS 4:299, 1990.
4. Sahai J, Gallicano K, Garber G, et al. The effect of a protein meal on zidovudine pharmacokinetics in HIV-infected patients. Br J Clin Pharmacol 33:657, 1992.
5. Flexner C. HIV protease inhibitors. N Engl J Med 338:1281, 1998.
6. Flexner C. Dual protease inhibitor therapy in HIV-infected patients: pharmacologic rationale and clinical benefits. Annu Rev Pharmacol Toxicol 40:649–74, 2000.
7. Viracept (nelfinavir) product monograph. La Jolla, CA, Agouron Pharmaceuticals, 2004.
8. Reyataz (atazanavir) product monograph. Princeton, NJ: Bristol-Myers Squibb Company; 2005.
9. Aptivus (tipranavir) product monograph. Ridgefield, CT: Boehringer Ingelheim Pharmaceuticals, Inc.; 2005.
10. Kaletra (lopinavir/ritonavir) product monograph. North Chicago, Ill: Abbott Laboratories; 2003.
11. Lexiva (Fosamprenavir) product monograph. Research Triangle Park, NC: GlaxoSmithKline; 2004.
12. Lea AP, Faulds D. Ritonavir. Drugs 52:541, 1996.
13. Piscitelli SC, Gallicano KD. Interactions among drugs for HIV and opportunistic infections. N Engl J Med 344: 984–996, 2001.
14. Shelton MJ, et al. If taken 1 hour before indinavir (IDV), didanosine does not affect IDV exposure, despite persistent buffering effects. AAC 45: 298–300, 2001.
15. Damle BD, et al. Lack of effect of simultaneously administered didanosine encapsulated enteric bead formulation (Videx EC) on oral absorption of indinavir, ketoconazole, or ciprofloxacin. Antimicrob Agents Chemother 46: 385, 2002.
16. Kaul S, Bassi K, Damle B, et al. Pharmacokinetic evaluation of the combination of atazanavir, enteric coated didanosine, and tenofovir disoproxil fumarate for once-daily antiretroviral regimen. In: 43rd ICAAC, Chicago, IL, 2003, abstract A-1616.
17. Blaschke T, Flexner C, Sheiner L, et al. Effect of simultaneous or staggered dosing of saquinavir, ritonavir, and nelfinavir on pharmacokinetic interactions. In: Program and abstracts of the 7th Conference on Retroviruses and Opportunistic Infections, San Francisco, CA, Jan 30–Feb 4, 2000, abstract 76.
18. Johnson MA, Gathe JC Jr, Podzamczer D, et al. A once-daily lopinavir/ritonavir-based regimen provides noninferior antiviral activity compared with a twice-daily regimen. J Acquir Immune Defic Syndr 43:153–60, 2006.
19. Piscitelli SC, Gallicano KD. Interactions among drugs for HIV and opportunistic infections. N Engl J Med 344:984, 2001.
20. Retrovir (zidovudine) product monograph. Research Triangle Park, NC: GlaxoSmithKline; 2003.
21. Hivid (zalcitabine) product monograph. Nutley, NJ: Roche Laboratories; 2002.
22. Zerit (stavudine) product monograph. Princeton, NJ: Bristol Myers-Squibb; 2004.
23. Epivir (lamivudine) product monograph. Research Triangle Park, NC: Glaxo Smith Kline; 2004.
24. Invirase (saquinavir) product monograph. Nutley, NJ: Roche Laboratories; 2005.
25. Norvir (ritonavir) product monograph. Abbott Park, IL: Abbott Laboratories; 2005.
26. Crixivan (indinavir) product monograph. West Point, PA: Merck & Co; 2005.
27. Viramune (nevirapine) product monograph. Ridgefield, CT: Boehringer Ingelheim; 2005.
28. Rescriptor (delavirdine) product monograph. La Jolla, CA: Agouron Pharmaceuticals, Inc; 2001.
29. Sustiva (efavirenz) product monograph. Princeton, NJ: Bristol Myers-Squibb; 2005.
30. Agenerase (amprenavir) product monograph. Research Triangle Park, NC: Glaxo Smith Kline; 2004.
31. Abacavir (Ziagen) product monograph. Research Triangle Park, NC: Glaxo Smith Kline; 2004.
32. Polk RE. Drug–drug interactions with ciprofloxacin and other fluoroquinolones. Am J Med 87(Suppl 5A):8776S, 1989.
33. Noyes M, Polk RE. Norfloxacin and absorption of magnesium–aluminum. Ann Intern Med 109:168, 1988.
34. Lehto P, Kivisto KT. Effect of sucralfate on absorption of norflox acin and ofloxacin. Antimicrob Agents Chemother 38:248, 1994.
35. Sahai J, Gallicano K, Oliveras RT, et al. Cations in the didanosine tablet reduce ciprofloxacin bioavailability. Clin Pharmacol Ther 53:292, 1993.
36. Piscitelli SC, Goss TF, Wilton JH, et al. Effects of ranitidine and sucralfate on ketoconazole bioavailability. Antimicrob Agents Chemother 35:1765, 1991.

37. Lake-Bakaar G, Tom W, Lake-Bakaar D, et al. Gastropathy and ketoconazole malabsorption in the acquired immunodeficiency syndrome. Ann Intern Med 109:471, 1988.
38. Agarwala S, et al. Pharmacokinetic effect of Omeprazole and Atazanavir co-administration with RTV in healthy volunteers, In: Program and Abstracts of the 12th Conference on Retroviruses and Opportunistic Infections; abstract 658.
39. Agarwala S, Eley T, Child M, et al. Pharmacokinetic effect of famotidine on atazanavir with and without ritonavir in healthy subjects. In: Program and Abstracts of the 12th Conference on Retoviruses and Opportunistic Infections; abstract 658.
40. Blum RA, D'Andrea DT, Florentino BM, et al. Increased gastric pH and the bioavailability of fluconazole and ketoconazole. Ann Intern Med 114:755, 1991.
41. VFend package insert. New York, NY: Pfizer; 2003.
42. Lange D, Pavao JH, Wu J, et al. Effect of a cola beverage on the bioavailability of itraconazole in the presence of H2 blockers. J Clin Pharmacol 37:535, 1997.
43. Benet LZ, Kroetz DL, Sheiner LB. Pharmacokinetics: dynamics of drug absorption, distribution, and elimination. In Hardman JG, Limbird LE (eds). The Pharmacological Basis of Therapeutics, 9th edn. New York: McGraw-Hill; 1996.
44. Kolars JC, Lown KS, Schmiedlin-Ren P, et al. CYP3A gene expression in human gut epithelium. Pharmacogenetics 4:247–59, 1994.
45. Autar RS, Ananworanich J, Apateerapong W, et al. Pharmacokinetic study of saquinavir hard gel caps/ritonavir in HIV-1-infected patients: 1600/100 mg once-daily compared with 2000/100 mg once-daily and 1000/100 mg twice-daily. J Antimicrob Chemother 54:785–90, 2004.
46. Fuhr U. Drug interactions with grapefruit juice. Drug Safety 18:251–72, 1998.
47. Bailey DG, Arnold MJ, Spence JD. Grapefruit juice-drug interactions. Br J Clin Pharmacol 46:101–10, 1998.
48. Fojo AT, Ueda K, Slamon DJ, et al. Expression of multidrug-resistance gene in human tumors and tissues. Proc Natl Acad Sci USA 84:265–9, 1987.
49. Khaliq Y, Gallicano K, Venance S, et al. Effect of ketoconazole on ritonavir and saquinavir concentrations in plasma and cerebrospinal fluid from patients infected with human immunodeficiency virus. Clin Pharmacol Ther 68:637–46, 2000.
50. Lee CG, Ramachandra M, Jeang KT. Effect of ABC transporters on HIV-1 infection: inhibition of virus production by the MDR1 transporter. FASEB J 14:516–22, 2000.
51. Flexner C, Speck RR. Role of multidrug transporters in HIV pathogenesis. In: Eighth Conference on Retroviruses and Opportunistic Infections, Chicago, IL, Feb 2001, abstract S4.
52. Kim RB, Wandel C, Leake B, et al. Interrelationship between substrates and inhibitors of human CYP3A and P-glycoprotein. Pharm Res 16:408–14, 1999.
53. Centers for Disease Control and Prevention. Updated guidelines for the use of rifamycins for the treatment of tuberculosis among HIV-infected patients taking protease inhibitors or non-nucleoside reverse transcriptase inhibitors. MMWR Morb Mortal Wkly Rep 53: 37, 2004.
54. Dear Dr. Letter. Drug-Induced hepatitis with marked transaminase elevations has been observed in healthy volunteers receiving rifampin 600 mg once daily in combination with ritonavir 100 mg/ saquinavir 1000 mg twice daily. 2/07/2005. Roche Laboratories Inc.
55. La Porte C, et al. Pharmacokinetic of two adjusted dose regimen of LPV/RTV in combination with rifampin in healthy volunteers. 42nd International Conference on Antimicrobial Agents and Chemotherapy, San Diego, CA, 2002, abstract A-1823.
56. Hamzeh F, Benson C, Gerber J, et al. Steady-state pharmacokinetic interaction of modified-dose indinavir and rifabutin. In: Eighth Conference on Retroviruses and Opportunistic Infections, Chicago, IL, Feb 2001, abstract 742.
57. Murphy R, Gagnier P, Lamson M, et al. Effect of nevirapine on pharmacokinetics of indinavir and ritonavir in HIV-1 patients. In: Program and Abstracts of the 4th Conference on Retroviruses and Opportunistic Infections, Washington, DC. Alexandria, VA: Westover Management Group; 1997, p 374, Abstract No. 374.
58. Sahai J, Cameron W, Salgo M, et al. Drug interaction between saquinavir and nevirapine. In: Program and Abstracts of the 4th Conference on Retroviruses and Opportunistic Infections, Washington, DC. Alexandria, VA: Westover Management Group; 1997, abstract No. 614.
59. Barry M, Mulcahy F, Merry C. Pharmacokinetics and potential interactions amongst antiretroviral agents used to treat patients with HIV infection. Clin Pharmacokinet 36:289–304, 1999.
60. Ouellet D, Hsu A, Qian J, et al. Effect of ritonavir on the pharmacokinetics of ethinyl estradiol in healthy female volunteers. In: Program and Abstracts of the XIth International Conference on AIDS, Vancouver, 1996, abstract No. Mo.B.1198.
61. Tackett D, Child M, Agarwala S, et al. Atazanavir: a summary of two pharmacokinetic drug interaction studies in healthy subjects. 10th CROI, Boston, MA, 2003, abstract 543.
62. Hsu A, Granneman GR, Witt G, et al. Assessment of multiple doses of ritonavir on the pharmacokinetics of theophylline. In: Program and Abstracts of the XIth International Conference on AIDS, Vancouver, 1996, abstract No. Mo.B.1200.
63. Penzak SR, et al. Influence of ritonavir on olanzapine pharmacokinetics in healthy volunteers. J Clin Psychopharmacol 22: 366–70, 2002.
64. Flexner C, Bate G, Kirkpatrick P. Tipranavir: fresh from the pipeline. Nature Rev Drug Discov 4:955–6, 2005.
64a. MacGregor TR, Sabo JP, Norris SH, et al. Pharmacokinetic characterization of different dose combinations of coadministered tipranavir and ritonavir in healthy volunteers. HIV Clin Trials 5:371–82, 2004.
64b. Leith J et al. Pharmacokinetics and safety of TPV/r alone or in combination with SQV, APV, or LPV: Interim analysis of BI 182.51. In: 5th International Workshop on Clinical Pharmacology of HIV Therapy, Rome, Italy, 2004, abstract 5.1.
65. A, Cavanaugh JH, Shi H, et al. Assessment of multiple doses of ritonavir on the pharmacokinetics of rifabutin. In: Program and Abstracts of the XIth International Conference on AIDS, Vancouver, 1996, abstract No. Mo.B.175.
66. Sun E, Heath-Chiozzi M, Cameron DW, et al. Concurrent ritonavir and rifabutin increases the risk of rifabutin-associated adverse effects. In: Program and Abstracts of the XIth International Conference on AIDS, Vancouver, 1996, abstract No. Mo.B.171.
67. Kashuba AD, Tierney C, Downey GF, et al. Combining fosamprenavir with lopinavir/ritonavir substantially reduces amprenavir and lopinavir exposure: ACTG protocol A5143 results. AIDS 19:145–52, 2005.
68. Wire MB, Naderer OJ, Masterman AL, et al. The pharmacokinetic interaction between GW433908 and lopinavir/ritonavir (APV 10011 and APV 10012). In: 11th Conference on Retroviruses and Opportunistic Infections, San Francisco, CA, 2004, abstract 612.
69. Leith J, et al. Pharmacokinetic and safety of TPV/r alone or in combination with SQV, APV, LPV: Interim analysis of BI 1182.51. In: 5th International Workshop on Clinical Pharmacology of HIV Therapy, Noordwijk, the Netherlands, 2004, abstract 5.1.
70. Ouellet D, Hsu A, Granneman GR, et al. Assessment of the pharmacokinetic interaction between ritonavir and clarithromycin. Clin Pharmacol Ther 59:143, 1996.
71. Honig PK, Wortham DC, Zamani K, et al. Comparison of the effects of the macrolide antibiotics erythromycin, clarithromycin, and azithromycin on terfenadine steady-state pharmacokinetics and electrocardiographic parameters. Drug Invest 7:148, 1994.

72. Paris DG, Parente TF, Bruschetta HR, et al. Torsades de pointes induced by erythromycin and terfenadine. Am J Emerg Med 12:636, 1994.
73. Olkkola KT, Palkama VJ, Neuvonen PJ. Ritonavir's role in reducing fentanyl clearance and prolonging its half-life. Anesthesiology 91:681–685, 1999.
74. Merry C, Mulcahy F, Barry M, et al. Saquinavir interaction with midazolam: pharmacokinetic considerations when prescribing protease inhibitors for patients with HIV disease. AIDS 11:268–269, 1997.
75. Panel on Clinical Practices for Treatment of HIV Infection, Department of Health and Human Services. Guidelines for the use of antiretroviral agents in HIV-1-infected adults and adolescents, October 6, 2005. HIV/AIDS Treatment Information Service Web site: http://www.hivatis.org.
76. Hsu A, Granneman GR, Witt G, et al. Multiple-dose pharmacokinetics of ritonavir in human immunodeficiency virus-infected subjects. Antimicrob Agents Chemother 41:898–905, 1997.
77. Hsu A, Granneman GR, Bertz RJ. Ritonavir. Clinical pharmacokinetics and interactions with other anti-HIV agents. Clin Pharmacokinet 35:275, 1998.
78. Kilby M, Hill AM, Buss N. The effect of ritonavir on increases in saquinavir plasma concentration is independent of ritonavir dosage: combined analysis of 120 subjects. In: Program and abstracts of the 40th Interscience Conference on Antimicrobial Agents and Chemotherapy, Toronto, Canada, Sep 17–20, 2000, abstract1650.
79. Drewe J, Gutmann H, Fricker G, et al. HIV protease inhibitor ritonavir: a more potent inhibitor of P-glycoprotein than the cyclosporine analog SDZ PSC 833. Biochem Pharmacol 57:1147–52, 1999.
80. Youle M, Gerstoft J, Fox Z et al. The final week 48 analysis of a phase IV randomised open label multicentre trial to evaluate safety and efficacy of lopinavir/ritonavir (400/100 mg) vs saquinavir/ritonavir (1000/100 mg bid) in adult HIV-1 infection: the MaxCMin2 study. In: Second International AIDS Society Conference on HIV Pathogenesis and Treatment, Paris, 2003, abstract LB23.
81. Montaner JSG, Saag M, Barylski C, et al. FOCUS study: Saquinavir qd regimen versus efavirenz qd regimen 48 week analysis in HIV infected patients. In: 42nd Interscience Conference on Antimicrobial Agents and Chemotherapy, San Diego, 2002, abstract H-167.
82. Hsu A, Granneman GR, Cao G, et al. Pharmacokinetic interaction between ritonavir and indinavir in healthy volunteers. Antimicrob Agents Chemother 42:2784–91, 1998.
83. Saah AJ, Winchell G, Seniuk M, Deutsch P. Multiple-dose pharmacokinetics and tolerability of indinavir ritonavir combinations in healthy volunteers. In: Program and Abstracts of the 6th Conference on Retroviruses and Opportunistic Infections, Chicago, IL, Jan 31–Feb 4, 1999, abstract 136.
84. Aarnoutse RE, Burger DM, Hugen PWH, et al. A pharmacokinetic study to investigate the influence of efavirenz on a BID Indinavir/ritonavir regimen in healthy volunteers. In: 40th Interscience Conference on Antimicrobial Agents and Chemotherapy, Toronto, Canada, Sep 17–20, 2000, abstract 423.
85. Burger D, Felderhof M, Phanupak P, et al. Both short-term virological efficacy and drug-associated nephrotoxicity are related to indinavir (IDV) pharmacokinetics in HIV-1 infected Thai patients. In: Program and Abstracts of the 8th Conference on Retroviruses and Opportunistic Infections, Chicago, IL, 2001, Abstract 730.
86. Lamotte C, Peytavin G, Perre P, et al. Increasing adverse events (AE) with indinavir (IDV) dosages and plasma concentrations in four different ritonavir (RTV)-IDV containing regimens in HIV-infected patients. In: Program and abstracts of the 8th Conference on Retroviruses and Opportunistic Infections, Chicago, IL, 2001, Abstract 738.
87. Workman C, Whittaker W, Dyer W, Sullivan J. Combining ritonavir and indinavir decreases indinavir-associated nephrolithiasis. In: Program and Abstracts of the 6th Conference on Retroviruses and Opportunistic Infections, Chicago, IL, Jan 31–Feb 1 1999, Abstract 195.
88. Hurst M, Faulds D. Lopinavir. Drugs. 2000. 60:1371–9.
89. Bertz R, Lam W, Brun S, et al. Multiple-dose pharmacokinetics of ABT-378/ ritonavir in HIV+ subjects. In: 39th Interscience Conference on Antimicrobial Agents and Chemotherapy; San Francisco, CA, Sep 26–29, 1999, abstract 327.
90. Gulick R, King M, Brun S, et al. ABT-378/Ritonavir in antiretroviral naïve HIV+ patients: 72 weeks. In: 7th Conference on Retroviruses and Opportunistic Infections, San Francisco, CA, Jan 30–Feb 2, 2000, abstract 515.
91. Bertz R, Lam W, Hsu A, et al. Assessment of the pharmacokinetic interaction between ABT-378/ ritonavir and efavirenz in healthy volunteers and in HIV+ subjects. In: Program and Abstracts of the 40th Interscience Conference on Antimicrobial Agents and Chemotherapy, Toronto, Canada, Sep 17–20, 2000, abstract 424.
92. Degen O, Kurowski M, Van Lunzen J, et al. Amprenavir (APV) and ritonavir (RTV): intraindividual comparison of different doses and influence of concomitant NNRTI on steady-state pharmacokinetics in HIV-infected patients. In: Program and Abstracts of the 8th Conference on Retroviruses and Opportunistic Infections, Feb 4–8, 2001, Chicago, IL, abstract 739.
93. DeJesus E, LaMarca A, Sension M, et al. The context study: efficacy and safety of GW433908/RTV in PI-experienced subjects with virological failure (24 Week Results). In: 10th Conference on Retroviruses and Opportunistic Infections, Boston, MA, Feb 10–14, 2003, abstract 178.
94. Kurowski M, Kaeser B, Mroziekiewicz A, et al. The influence of low doses of ritonavir on the pharmacokinetics of nelfinavir 1250 mg twice daily. In: Program and abstracts of the 40th Interscience Conference on Antimicrobial Agents and Chemotherapy; Toronto, Canada, Sep 17–20, 2000, abstract 1639.
95. Flexner C, Hsu A, Kerr B, et al. Steady-state pharmacokinetic interactions between ritonavir (RTV), nelfinavir (NFV), and the nelfinavir active metabolite M8 (AG1402). Twelfth World AIDS Conference. Geneva, June 1998.
96. Zhang KE, Wu E, Patick AK, et al. Circulating metabolites of the human immunodeficiency virus protease inhibitor nelfinavir in humans: structural identification, levels in plasma, and antiviral activities. Antimicrob Agents Chemother 45:1086, 2001.
97. Nieto-Cisneros L, Zala C, Fessel WJ, et al. Antiviral efficacy, metabolic changes and safety of atazanavir (ATV) versus lopinavir/ritonavir (LPV/RTV) in combination with 2 NRTIs in patients who have experienced virologic failure with prior PI-containing regimen(s): 24-week results from BMS AI424-043. In: 2nd Conference on HIV Pathogenesis and Treatment, Paris, France, July 13–16, 2003, abstract 117.
98. DeJesus E, Grinsztejn B, Rodriguez C, et al. Efficacy and safety of atazanavir (ATV) with ritonavir (RTV) or saquinavir (SQV) vs lopinavir/ritonavir (LPV/RTV) in patients who have experienced virologic failure on multiple HAART regimens: 48-week results from BMS AI424-045; 11th CROI, San Francisco, California. 2004; Abstract 547.
99. Mac Gregor TR, Sabo JP, Norris SH, et al. Pharmacokinetic characterization of different dose combinations of coadministered tipranavir and ritonavir in healthy volunteers. HIV Clin Trials 5:371–82, 2004.
100. Hicks C, et al. RESIST-1: A phase 3, randomized, controlled, open-label, multicenter trial comparing tipranavir/ritonavir (TPV/r) to an optimized comparator protease inhibitor/r

(CPI/r) regimen in antiretroviral (ARV)-experienced patients: 24-week data. In: 44th ICAAC, Washington, DC, 2004, abstract LB H-1137.
101. Pham P, Flexner C, Parsons T, et al. Beneficial pharmacokinetic interaction between Atazanavir and Lopinavir/Ritonavir. J Acquir Immune Defic Syndr 45:201–205, 2007.
102. Duvivier C, Peytavin G, Ait-Mohand H, et al. Dual boosted atazanavir/lopinavir/ritonavir containing regimen in HIV-1 infected pretreated patients: plasma trough concentration and efficacy results [abstract WePe3.2C10]. Presented at: 3rd International AIDS Society (IAS) Conference on HIV Pathogenesis and Treatment, July 24–27, 2005.
103. Chan-Tack KM, Qaqish RB, Fantry LE, et al. Successful treatment with lopinavir/ritonavir (LPV/r) and atazanavir (ATV) combination therapy in protease inhibitor (PI)-naive and PI-experienced HIV-infected patients [abstract 796]. Presented at: 43rd Annual Meeting of the Infectious Disease Society of America (IDSA); 2005; San Francisco.
104. Ballinger J, Swaden L, Bhagani, et al. Double-boosted protease treatment using atazanavir and lopinavir/ritonavir. 11th Annual Conference of the British HIV Association.
105. Ribera E, Azuaje C, Lopez, RM, et al. Atazanavir and lopinavir/ritonavir: pharmacokinetics, safety and efficacy of a promising double-boosted protease inhibitor regimen. AIDS 20:1131–1139, 2006.
106. Paulsen D, Liao Q, Fusco G, et al. Genotypic and phenotypic cross-resistance patterns to lopinavir and amprenavir in protease inhibitor-experienced patients with HIV viremia. AIDS Res Hum Retroviruses. 18:1011–29, 2002.
107. Collier A, Tierney C, Downey G, et al. Randomized study of twice-daily lopinavir/ritonavir or fosamprenavir + ritonavir vs. lopinavir/ritonavir + fosamprenavir (with tenofovir DF and nucleosides) as rescue therapy. In: 12th Conference on Retroviruses and Opportunistic Infections, Boston, MA, Feb 22–25, 2005, abstract 577.
108. Kashuba AD, Tierney C, Downey GF, et al. Combining fosamprenavir with lopinavir/ritonavir substantially reduces amprenavir and lopinavir exposure: ACTG protocol A5143 results. AIDS. 19:145–52, 2005.
109. Stephan C, Hentig N, Kourbeti I, et al. SQV drug exposure is not impaired by the boosted double protease inhibitor combination of lopinavir/ritonavir. AIDS 18:503–8, 2004.
110. Staszewski S, Dauer B, Carlebach A, et al. The LOPSAQ salvage study: 48 week analysis of the full cohort treated with lopinavir (LPV/r) plus saquinavir (SQV) without any additional antiretroviral (ART) therapy. Presented at the XV International AIDS Conference, Bangkok, 2004, abstract B10840.
111. Kravcik S, Sahai J, Kerr B, et al. Nelfinavir mesylate increases saquinavir soft gel capsule exposure in HIV+ patients. In: Program and Abstracts of the 4th Conference on Retroviruses and Opportunistic Infections, Washington DC. Alexandria, VA: Westover Management Group; 1997, abstract No. 371.
112. Riddler S, Havlir DV, Squires K, et al. Coadministration of Indinavir and Nelfinavir in HIV-1 Infected Adults: Safety, Pharmacokinetics, and antiviral activity. Antimicrobial Agents and Chemotherapy 46: 3877–82, 2002.
113. Merrill DP, Manion DJ, Chou TC, Hirsch MS. Antagonism between human immunodeficiency virus type 1 protease inhibitors indinavir and saquinavir in vitro. J Infect Dis 176:265–8, 1997.
114. Clay P, Anderson P, Smith P, et al. Pharmacokinetics of Once-daily Fosamprenavir 1400 mg plus Atazanavir 400 mg without Ritonavir in HIV-negative Subjects. In: Conference on Retroviruses and Opportunistic Infections, Denver, CO, Feb 5–8, 2006, abstract 587.
115. Gonzalez de Requena D, Bonora S, Canta F, et al. Atazanavir Ctrough is associated with efficacy and safety: definition of therapeutic range. Conference on Retroviruses and Opportunistic Infections, Boston, MA, Feb 5–8, 2005, abstract 645.
116. Seminari E, Guffanti M, Villani P, et al. Steady-state pharmacokinetics of atazanavir given alone or in combination with saquinavir hard-gel capsules or amprenavir in HIV-1-infected patients. Eur J Clin Pharmacol 61:545–9, 2005.
117. Cox SR, Ferry JJ, Batts DH, et al. Delavirdine and marketed protease inhibitors: pharmacokinetic interaction studies in healthy volunteers. In: Program and Abstracts of the 4th Conference on Retroviruses and Opportunistic Infections, Washington, DC. Alexandria, VA: Westover Management Group; 1997, abstract No. 372.
118. Cox SR, Schneck BD, Herman BD, et al. Delavirdine and nelfinavir: a pharmacokinetic drug interaction study in healthy adult volunteers. In: Program and Abstracts of the 5th Conference on Retroviruses and Opportunistic Infections, Chicago. Alexandria, VA: Westover Management Group; 1998, abstract No. 345.
119. Piscitelli SC, Burstein AH, Chaitt D, et al. St. John's wort and indinavir concentrations. Lancet 355:547–8, 2000.
120. Roby CA, Anderson GD, Kantor E, et al. St John's Wort: effect on CYP3A4 activity. Clin Pharmacol Ther 67:451–7, 2000.
121. Johne A, Brockmoller J, Bauer S, et al. Pharmacokinetic interaction of digoxin with an herbal extract from St John's wort (Hypericum perforatum). Clin Pharmacol Ther 66:338–45, 1999.
122. Laroche M, Choudhri S, Gallicano K, Foster B. Severe gastrointestinal toxicity with concomitant ingestion of ritonavir and garlic. Can J Infect Dis9(Suppl A):471P, 1998.
123. Piscitelli SC, Burstein AH, Welden N, et al. Garlic supplements decrease plasma saquinavir concentrations. In: Program and Abstracts of the 8th Conference on Retroviruses and Opportunistic Infections, Chicago, IL, Feb 4–8, 2001, abstract 743.
124. Piscitelli SC. Use of Complementary Medicines by Patients With HIV Infection: Full Sail into Uncharted Waters. Available: www.medscape.com May 2000.
125. Piscitelli SC, Formentini E, Burstein AH, et al. The effect of milk thistle on the pharmacokinetics of indinavir in healthy volunteers. Pharmacother 22: 551–556, 2002.
126. Reiss WG, Piscitelli SC. Drug-cytokine interactions: mechanisms and clinical implications. BioDrugs 9:389–95, 1998.
127. Piscitelli SC, Vogel S, Figg WD, et al. Alteration in indinavir clearance during interleukin-2 infusions in HIV-infected patients. Pharmacotherapy 18:1212–6, 1998.
128. Moore KHP, Yuen GJ, Raasch RH, et al. Pharmacokinetics of lamivudine administered alone and with trimethoprimsulfamethoxazole. Clin Pharmacol Ther 59:550, 1996.
129. Laskin OL, De Miranda P, King DH, et al. Effects of probenecid on the pharmacokinetics and elimination of acyclovir in humans. Antimicrob Agents Chemother 21:804, 1982.
130. CDC Sexually transmitted diseases treatment guidelines MMWR 51: RR-6, 2002.
131. Kiser J, Carten M, Wolfe P, et al. Effect of Lopinavir/Ritonavir on the Renal Clearance of Tenofovir in HIV-infected Patients. In: Abstracts of the 13th Conference on Retroviruses and Opportunistic Infections. Denver, CO, 2005, poster No. 570.
132. Zimmermann A, Pizzoferrato T, Bedford J, et al. Tenofovir-associated acute and chronic kidney disease: a case of multiple drug interactions. Clin Infect Dis 42:283–90, 2006.
133. Sim SM, Hoggard PG, Sales SD, et al. Effect of ribavirin on zidovudine efficacy and toxicity in vitro: concentration-dependent interaction. AIDS Res Hum Retroviruses 14:1661–7, 1998.
134. Back D, Haworth S, Hoggard P, et al. Drug interactions with d4T phosphorylation in vitro. In: Program and Abstracts of the XI International Conference on AIDS, Vancouver, BC, Jul 1996, Abstract 88.

135. Rodriguez-Torres M, Torriani FJ, Soriano V, et al. Effect of Ribavirin on intracellular and plasma pharmacokinetics of nucleoside reverse transcriptase inhibitors in patients with human immunodeficiency virus-hepatitis C virus coinfection: results of a randomized clinical study. Antimicrob Agents Chemother 49: 3997–4008, 2005.
136. Havlir DV, Friedland G, Pollard R, et al. Combination zidovudine and stavudine therapy versus other nucleosides: report of two randomized trials (ACTG 290 and 298). In: 5th Conference on Retroviruses and Opportunistic Infections, Chicago, IL, Feb 1–5, 1998, abstract 79.
137. Veal GJ, Hoggard PG, Barry MG, et al. Interaction between lamivudine and other nucleoside analogs for intracellular phosphorylation. AIDS 10:546, 1996.
138. Ray AS, Olson L, Fridland A. Role of purine nucleoside phosphorylase in interactions between 2′,3′-dideoxyinosine and allopurinol, ganciclovir, or tenofovir. Antimicrob Agents Chemother 48:1089–95, 2004.
139. Bearney BP, Sayre JR, Flaherty, et al. Drug–drug and drug-food interactions between tenofovir disoproxil fumarate and didanosine. J Clin Pharmacol 45:1360–7, 2005.
140. Japour AJ, et al. A phase-I study of safety, pharmacokinetics, and antiviral activity of combination didanosine and ribavirin in patients with HIV-1 disease. J Acquir Immune Defic Syndr Hum Retroviral 13: 235–46, 1996.
141. US Food and Drug Administration. HIV/AIDS Historical Timeline. 2000–2003. Available: http://www.fda.gov/oashi/aids/miles20.html Nov 4, 2003.
142. Moreno A, Querada C, Moreno L, et al. High rate of didanosine-related mitochondrial toxicity in HIV-HCV co-infected patients receiving didanosine. Antiviral Ther 9: 133–8, 2004.
143. Balzarini J, Lee CK, Herdewijn P, et al. Mechanisms of the potentiating effect of ribavirin on the activity of 2′,3′-dideoxyinosine against human immunodeficiency virus, J Biol Chem 226: 21509–14, 1991.
144. Pollard RB, Peterson D, Hardy D, et al. Safety and antiretroviral effects of combined didanosine and stavudine therapy in HIV-infected individuals with CD4 counts of 200 to 500 cells/mm3. J Acquir Immune Defic Syndr 22:39, 1999.
145. Moore, RD., Wong, WE, Keruly J C, et al. Incidence of neuropathy in HIV-infected patients on monotherapy versus those on combination therapy with didanosine, stavudine and hydroxyurea. AIDS 14:273–8, 2000.
146. Evans L, Spelman M. The problem of noncompliance with drug therapy. Drugs 25:63, 1983.
147. Cramer JA, Mattson RH, Prevey ML, et al. How often is medication taken as prescribed? A novel assessment technique. JAMA 261:3723, 1989.
148. Chesney MA. Factors affecting adherence to antiretroviral therapy. Clin Infect Dis 30(Suppl 2):S171–6, 2000.
149. Flexner C, Noe D, Benson C, et al. ACTG 223 Study Team. Adherence patterns in patients with symptomatic Mycobacterium avium complex (MAC) infection taking a twice-daily clarithromycin regimen. Int Conf AIDS 12:585 (abstract no. 32324), 1998.
150. Kasstrisios H, Flowers NT, Suarez JR, et al. Assessment of differential compliance in ACTG Protocol 175. Clin Pharmacol Ther 55:191, 1994.
151. Kasstrisios H, Flowers NT, Blaschke TF. Introducing medical students to medication noncompliance. Clin Pharmacol Ther 59:577, 1996.
152. Rudd P, Byyny RL, Zachary V, et al. The natural history of medication compliance in a drug trial: limitations of pill counts. Clin Pharmacol Ther 46:169, 1989.
153. Waterhouse DM, Calzone KA, Mele C, et al. Adherence to oral tamoxifen: a comparison of patient self-report, pill counts, and microelectronic monitoring. J Clin Oncol 11:1189, 1993.
154. Cramer JA, Spilker B. Patient Compliance in Medical Practice and Clinical Trials. New York: Raven Press; 1991.
155. Vanhove GF, Schapiro JM, Winters MA, et al. Patient compliance and drug failure in protease inhibitor monotherapy. JAMA 276:1955, 1996.
156. Bangsberg DR, Hecht FM, Charlebois ED, et al. Adherence to protease inhibitors, HIV-1 viral load, and development of drug resistance in an indigent population. AIDS14:357–66, 2000.
157. Paterson DL, Swindells S, Mohr J, et al. Adherence to protease inhibitor therapy and outcomes in patients with HIV infection. Ann Intern Med 133:21–30, 2000.
158. Bangsberg D, Weiser S, Guzman D, et al. 95% Adherence is not necessary for viral suppression to less than 400 copies/mL in the majority of individuals on NNRTI Regimens. In: Program and abstracts of the 12th Conference on Retroviruses and Opportunistic Infections, Boston, MA, Feb 22–25, 2005, abstract 616.
159. Schapiro JM, Winters MA, Stewart F, et al. The effect of high-dose saquinavir on viral load and CD4+ T-cell counts in HIV-infected patients. Ann Intern Med 124:1039–50, 1996.
160. Molla A, Korneyeva M, Gao Q, et al. Ordered accumulation of mutations in HIV protease confers resistance to ritonavir. Nature Med 2:760–6, 1996.
161. Stein DS, Fish DG, Bilello JA, et al. A 24-week open-label phase I/II evaluation of the HIV protease inhibitor MK-639 (indinavir). AIDS 10:485–92, 1996.
162. Burger DM, Hoetelmans RMW, Mulder JW, et al. Low plasma levels of indinavir (IDV) are highly predictive of virological treatment failure in patients using IDV-containing triple therapy. In: 12th World AIDS Conference, Geneva, Switzerland, 1998, abstract 42275.
163. Pithavala Y, Zhang M, Knowles M, et al. Virologic response-plasma concentration relationship in phase III study of nelfinavir mesylate. In: 12th World AIDS Conference, Geneva, Switzerland, 1998, abstract 12304.
164. Lorenzi P, Yerly S, Abderrakim K, et al. Toxicity, efficacy, plasma drug concentrations and protease mutations in patients with advanced HIV infection treated with ritonavir and saquinavir. AIDS 11:F95–99, 1997.
165. Acosta EP, Henry K, Weller D, et al. Indinavir pharmacokinetics and relationships between exposure and antiviral effect. Pharmacotherapy 19:708–12, 1999.
166. Fletcher CV, Fenton T, Powell C, et al. Pharmacologic characteristics of efavirenz and nelfinavir associated with virologic response in HIV-infected children. In: Program and Abstracts of the 8th Conference on Retroviruses and Opportunistic Infections, Chicago, IL, Feb 4–8, 2001, abstract 259.
167. Durant J, Clevenbergh P, Garraffo R, et al. Importance of protease inhibitor plasma levels in HIV-infected patients treated with genotypic-guide therapy: pharmacologic data from the Viradapt Study. AIDS 14: 1333–9, 2000.
168. Burger DM, Hugen PWH, Reiss P, et al. Therapeutic drug monitoring of Nelfinavir and indinavir in treatment naïve HIV-1-infected individuals. AIDS 17: 1157–65, 2003.
169. Clevenbergh P, Garraffo R, Durant J, et al. PharmAdapt: a randomized prospective study to evaluate the benefit of therapeutic monitoring of protease inhibitors: 12 week results. AIDS 16: 2311–5, 2002.
170. Bossi B, Peytavin G, Ait-Mohand H, et al. GENOPHAR: a randomized study of plasma drug measurements in association with genotypic resistance testing and expert advice to optimize therapy in patients failing antiretroviral therapy. HIV Med 5:352–9, 2004.
171. Marzolini C, Amalio T, Decosterd LA, et al. Efavirenz plasma levels can predict treatment failure and central nervous system side effects in HIV-1 infected patients. AIDS 15: 71–5, 2001.

172. Crommentuyn K, Huitema AD, Brinkman K, et al. Therapeutic drug monitoring of efavirenz reduces pharmacokinetic variability bud does not affect toxicity or virologic success in the ATHENA study. Letters to the Editor. JAIDS 39: 249–50, 2005.
173. Anderson PL, Kakuda TN, Kawle S, et al. Antiviral dynamics and sex differences of zidovudine and lamivudine triphosphate concentrations in HIV-infected individuals. AIDS 17: 2159–68, 2003.
174. Stretcher BN, Pesce AJ, Frame PT, et al. Pharmacokinetics of zidovudine phosphorylation in peripheral blood mononuclear cells from patients infected with human immunodeficiency virus. Antimicrob Agents Chemother 38: 1541–7, 1994.
175. Kempf D, Hsu A, Jiang P, et al. Response to ritonavir intensification in indinavir recipients is highly correlated with inhibitory quotient. In: Program and abstracts of the 8th Conference on Retroviruses and Opportunistic Infections, Chicago, IL, Feb 4–8, 2001, abstract 523.
176. Fletcher CV, Anderson PL, Kakuda TN, et al. A novel approach to integrate pharmacologic and virologic characteristics: an in vivo potency index for antiretroviral agents. In: Program and Abstracts of the 8th Conference on Retroviruses and Opportunistic Infections, Chicago, IL, Feb 4–8, 2001, abstract 732.
177. Baxter JD, Merigan TC, Wentworth DN, et al. Both baseline HIV-1 drug resistance and antiretroviral drug levels are associated with short-term virologic responses to salvage therapy. AIDS 16:1131–8, 2002.
178. Hsu A, Issacson J, Brun S, et al. Pharmacokinetic-pharmacodynamic analysis of lopinavir-ritonavir in combination with efavirenz and two nucleoside reverse transcriptase inhibitors in extensively pretreated human immunodeficiency virus-infected patients. Antimicrob Agents Chemother 47:350–9, 2003.
179. Castagna A, Gianotti N, Galli L, et al. The NIQ of lopinavir is predictive of a 48-week virological response in highly treatment-experienced HIV-1-infected subjects treated with a lopinavir/ritonavir-containing regimen. Antivir Ther 9:537–43, 2004.
180. Kempf D, Hsu A, Isaacson J, et al. Evaluation of the inhibitory quotient as a pharmacodynamic predictor of the virologic response to protease inhibitor therapy. In: 2nd International Workshop on Clinical Pharmacology of HIV Therapy, Noordwijk, the Netherlands, Apr 2–4, 2001, abstract 7.3.
181. Nettles RE, Kieffer TL, Parsons T, et al. Marked intraindividual variability in antiretroviral concentrations may limit the utility of therapeutic drug monitoring. Clin Infect Dis 42:1189–1196, 2006.
182. Kageyama S, Anderson BD, Hoesterey BL, et al. Protein binding of human immunodeficiency virus protease inhibitor KNI-272 and alteration of its in vitro antiretroviral activity in the presence of high concentrations of protein. Antimicrob Agents Chemother 38:1107, 1994.
183. Zhang XQ, Schooley RT, Gerber JG. The effect of increasing alpha1-acid glycoprotein concentration on the antiviral efficacy of human immunodeficiency virus protease inhibitors J Infect Dis 180:1833–7, 1999.
184. Bilello JA, Bilello PA, Prichard M, et al. Reduction of the in vitro activity of A77003, an inhibitor of human immunodeficiency virus protease, by human serum α_1 acid glycoprotein. J Infect Dis 171:546, 1995.
185. Lazdins JK, Mestan J, Goutte G, et al. In vitro effect of a_1-acid glycoprotein on the anti-human immunodeficiency virus activity of the protease inhibitor CGP 61755: a comparative study with other relevant HIV protease inhibitors. J Infect Dis 175:1063, 1997.
186. Fischl MA, Richman DD, Flexner C, et al. Phase I study of the toxicity, pharmacokinetics, and activity of the HIV protease inhibitor SC-52151. J Acquir Immune Defic Syndr Hum Retrovirol 15:28, 1997.
187. Flexner C, Richman DD, Bryant M, et al. Effect of protein binding on the pharmacodynamics of an HIV protease inhibitor. Antiviral Res 26:A282, 1995.
188. Sommadossi J, Schinazi RD, McMillan A, et al. A human serum glycoprotein profoundly affects antiviral activity of the protease inhibitor SC-52151 by decreasing its cellular uptake. In: Program and Abstracts of the 2nd National Conference on Human Retroviruses and Related Infections. Washington, DC: American Society for Microbiology; 1995, abstract No. LB4.
189. Molla A, Vasavanonda S, Kumar G, et al. Human serum attenuates the activity of protease inhibitors toward wild-type and mutant human immunodeficiency virus. Virology 250:255, 1998.
190. Hendrix CW, Flexner C, Szebeni J, et al. Dipyridamole's effect on zidovudine pharmacokinetics and short-term tolerance in asymptomatic HIV-infected subjects. Antimicrob Agents Chemother 38:1036, 1994.
191. Flexner C, Hendrix C. Pharmacology of antiretroviral agents. In DeVita VT, Hellman S, Rosenberg SA (eds). AIDS Etiology, Diagnosis, Treatment, and Prevention. 4 edn. Philadelphia: Lippincott-Raven; 1997, p 479.
192. Moyle GJ, Sadler M, Hawkins D, et al. Pharmacokinetics of saquinavir at steady state in CSF and plasma: correlation between plasma and CSF viral load in patients on saquinavir containing regimens. In: Program and Abstracts of the 35th Annual Meeting of the Infectious Diseases Society of America, San Francisco. Alexandria, VA: Infectious Diseases Society of America; 1997, abstract No. 115.
193. Collier AC, Marra C, Coombs RW, et al. Cerebrospinal fluid indinavir and HIV RNA levels in patients on chronic indinavir therapy. In: Program and Abstracts of the 35th Annual Meeting of the Infectious Diseases Society of America, San Francisco. Alexandria, VA: Infectious Diseases Society of America; 1997, abstract No. 22.
194. Aweeka F, Jayewardene A, Staprans S, et al. Failure to detect nelfinavir in the cerebrospinal fluid of HIV-1-infected patients with and without AIDS dementia complex. J. Acquir. Immune Defic. Syndr 20:39–43, 1999.
195. Haas D, Clough L, Johnson B, et al. Quantification of nelfinavir and its active metabolite (M8) in CSF and Plasma, and correlation with CSF HIV-1 RNA response. In: Program and Abstracts of the 7th Conference on Retroviruses and Opportunistic Infections, San Francisco, CA, 2000, abstract 313.
196. Best B, Letendre S, Patel P, et al. Low atazanavir concentrations in cerebrospinal fluid. In: Program and Abstracts of the 13th Conference on Retroviruses and Opportunistic Infections, Denver, CO, 2000, Abstract 576.
197. Murphy R, Currier J, Gerber J, et al. Antiviral activity and pharmacokinetics of amprenavir with and without zidovudine/3TC in the cerebral spinal fluid of HIV-infected adults. In: Program and abstracts of the 7th Conference on Retroviruses and Opportunistic Infections, San Francisco, CA, 2000, abstract 314.
198. Sidtis JJ, Gatsonis C, Price RW, et al. Zidovudine treatment of the AIDS dementia complex: results of a placebo-controlled trial. AIDS Clinical Trials Group. Ann Neurol 33:343, 1993.
199. Kashuba AD, Dyer JR, Kramer LM, et al. Antiretroviral-drug concentrations in semen: implications for sexual transmission of human immunodeficiency virus type 1. Antimicrob. Agents Chemother 43:1817–26, 1999.
200. Taylor S, van Heeswijk R, Hoetelmans Richard M, et al. Concentrations of nevirapine, lamivudine and stavudine in semen of HIV-1-infected men. AIDS 14:1979–84, 2000.
201. Ghosn J, Chaix M, Peytavin G, et al. Penetration of enfuvirtide, tenofovir, efavirenz, and protease inhibitors in the genital tract of HIV-1-infected men. AIDS 18:1958–61, 2004.
202. Anderson PL, Noormohamed SE, Henry K, et al. Semen and serum pharmacokinetics of zidovudine and zidovudineglucuronide in men with HIV-1 infection. Pharmacotherapy 20: 917–22, 2000.

203. Taylor S, Back D, Drake S, et al. Antiretroviral drug concentrations in semen of HIV-infected men: differential penetration of indinavir (IDV), ritonavir (RTV), and saquinavir (SQV). J Antimicrob Chemother 48(3):351–4, 2001.
204. Isaac A, Taylor S, Cane P, et al. Lopinavir/ritonavir combined with twice-daily 400 mg indinavir: pharmacokinetics and pharmacodynamics in blood, CSF and semen. J Antimicrob Chemother 54:498–502, 2004.
205. Taylor S, Reynolds H, Sabin CA, et al. Penetration of efavirenz into the male genital tract: drug concentrations and antiviral activity in semen and blood of HIV-1-infected men. AIDS 15: 2051–3, 2001.
206. Perinatal HIV guidelines Working Group. Public Health Service Task Force Recommendations for Use of Antiretroviral Drugs in Pregnant HIV-1-infected Women for Maternal Health and Interventions to Reduce Perinatal HIV-1 Transmission in the United States. Safety and Toxicity of Individual Antiretroviral Agent in Pregnancy Supplement. Available: http://aidsinfo.nih.gov/ContentFiles/PerinatalGLSafetyTox_Sup.pdf Nov 2005.
207. Mandelbrot L, Kermarrec N, Marcollet A, et al. Case report: nucleoside analogue-induced lactic acidosis in the third trimester of pregnancy. AIDS 2003; 17: 272–3.
208. Ruff A, Hamzeh F, Lietman P, et al. Excretion of zidovudine (ZDV) in human breast milk. In: Program and Abstracts of the 34th Interscience Conference on Antimicrobial Agents and Chemotherapy, Orlando, FL. Washington, DC: American Society for Microbiology; 1994, abstract No. I-11.
209. Dunihoo DR. Maternal physiology. In: Dunihoo DR (ed). Fundamental of Gynecology and Obstetrics. Philadelphia: J.B. Lippincott Co; 1992, p 280.
210. Parry E, Shields R, Turnbull A. Transit time in the small intestine in pregnancy. J Obstet Gynaecol Br Commonw 77:900–1, 1970.
211. Davidson JM, Hytten FE. Glomerular filtration during and after pregnancy. J Obstet Gynaecol 81: 588–95, 1974.
212. Acosta EP, Zorrilla C, Van Dyke R, et al. Pharmacokinetics of saquinavir-SGC in HIV-infected pregnant women. HIV Clin Trials 2(6):460–5, 2001.
213. EP Acosta and others (Pediatric AIDS Clinical Trials Group 386 Protocol Team) Pharmacokinetics of saquinavir plus low-dose ritonavir in human immunodeficiency virus-infected pregnant women. Antimicrob Agents Chemother 48: 430–6, 2004.
214. van Heeswijk RP, Khaliq Y, Gallicano KD, et al. The pharmacokinetics of nelfinavir and M8 during pregnancy and post partum. Clin Pharmacol Ther 76: 588–97, 2004.
215. Bryson Y, Stek A, Mirochnick M, et al. Pharmacokinetics, Antiviral Activity, and Safety of Nelfinavir (NFV) with ZDV/3TC in Pregnant HIV-Infected Women and Their Infants: PACTG 353 Cohort 2. In: Program and Abstracts of the 9th Conference on Retroviruses and Opportunistic Infections, Seattle, WA,2002, abstract 795W.
216. Mirochnick M, Stek A, Capparelli E, et al. Adequate Lopinavir Exposure Achieved with a Higher Dose during the Third Trimester of Pregnancy. Program and abstracts of the 13th Conference on Retroviruses and Opportunistic Infections, San Francisco, CA,Feb 5–8, 2006, abstract 710.
217. Mirochnick M, Fenton T, Gagnier P, et al. Pharmacokinetics of nevirapine in human immunodeficiency virus type 1-infected pregnant women and their neonates. Pediatric AIDS Clinical Trials Group Protocol 250 Team. J Infect Dis 178:368–74, 1998.
218. Pharmacokinetic and antiretroviral acitivity of lamivudine alone or when coadministered with zidovudine in human immunodeficiency virus type 1-infected pregnant women and their offspring. J Infect Dis 178:1327–1333, 1998.
219. Schuman P, Kauffman R, Crane LR, et al. Pharmacokinetics of zidovudine during pregnancy. Int Conf AIDS 6: 94 (abstract no. F.B.17), 1990.
220. Wang Y, Liningston E, Patil S, et al. Pharmacokinetics of didanosine in antepartum and postpartum human immunodeficiency virus-infected pregnant women and their neonates: an AIDS clinical trial group study. JID 180: 1536–41, 1999.
221. Mirochnick M, Siminski S, Fenton T, et al. Nevirapine pharmacokinetics in pregnant women and in their infants after in utero exposure.Pediatr Infect Dis J 20:803–5, 2001.
222. Haas DW, Ribaudo, HJ, Kim RB, et al. Pharmacogenetics of efavirenz and central nervous system side effects: an Adult AIDS Clinical Trials Group study. AIDS 18:2391–400, 2004.
223. Fletcher CV, Acosta E, Strykowski JM. Gender differences in pharmacokinetics and pharmacodynamics. J Adolesc Health 15:619, 1994.
224. Mueller BU, Pizzo PA, Farley M, et al. Pharmacokinetic evaluation of the combination of zidovudine and didanosine in children with human immunodeficiency virus infection. J Pediatr 125:142, 1994.
225. Khaliq Y, Gallicano K, Seguin I, et al. Therapeutic drug monitoring of nelfinavir in HIV patients with liver disease. In: Program and Abstracts of the 6th Conference on Retroviruses and Opportunistic Infections, Chicago, IL, 1999, Abstract 369.
226. Knupp CA, Hak JL, Coakley DF, et al. Disposition of didanosine in HIV-seropositive patients with normal renal function or chronic renal failure: Influence of hemodialysis and continuous ambulatory peritoneal dialysis. Clin Pharmacol Ther 60: 535–42, 1996.
227. Grasela DM, Stoltz RR, Barry M, et al. Pharmacokinetics of Single-Dose Oral Stavudine in Subjects with Renal Impairment and in Subjects Requiring Hemodialysis. Antimicrob Agents Chemother 44:2149–53, 2000.
228. Viread package insert. Foster City, CA: Gilead Sciences, Inc; 2003.
229. Izzedine H, Launay-Vacher V, Aymard G, et al. Pharmacokinetic of nevirapine in haemodialysis. Nephrol Dial Transplant 16: 192–3, 2001.
230. Dasta JF, Armstrong DK. Variability in aminoglycoside pharmacokinetics in critically ill surgical patients. Crit Care Med 15:327, 1988.
231. Mlynarek ME, Peterson EL, Zarowitz BJ. Predicting unbound phenytoin concentrations in the critically ill neurosurgical patient. Ann Pharmacother 30:219, 1996.
232. Bayliff CD, Schwartz ML, Hardy GB. Pharmacokinetics of high dose pentobarbital in severe head trauma. Clin Pharmacol Ther 38:457, 1985.
233. Bertz R, Shi H, Cavanaugh J, et al. Effect of three vehicles, Advera, Ensure, and chocolate milk, on the bioavailability of an oral liquid formulation of Norvir. In: Abstracts of the 36th Interscience Conference on Antimicrobial Agents and Chemotherapy, New Orleans. Washington, DC: American Society for Microbiology; 1996, abstract No. A25.
234. USPDI Advice for the Patient. Drug Information in Lay Language. Rockville, MD: The United States Pharmacopoeia Convention, Inc; 1996.

Chapter 80

AIDS-Related Medications

Alice K. Pau, PharmD, Sarah Robertson, PharmD

INDEX OF MEDICATIONS

(Continued)

DEFINITIONS OF FDA PREGNANCY RISK FACTOR CATEGORIES

Category A: Controlled studies in women fail to show risk to fetus during first trimester (with no evidence of risk during later trimesters), and the possibility of fetal harm appears remote.

Category B: Either animal reproduction studies have not demonstrated a fetal risk (with no controlled studies in pregnant women) or animal reproduction studies have shown an adverse effect (other than a decrease in fertility) that was not confirmed in controlled studies of women during the first trimester (with no evidence of risk during later trimesters).

Category C: Either studies in animals have revealed adverse effects on the fetus (teratogenic, embryocidal, or other), with no controlled studies in pregnant women, or studies in women and animals are not available. Drugs should be given only if potential benefit justifies the potential risk to the fetus.

Category D: There is positive evidence of human fetal risk, but the benefits from use in pregnant women may be acceptable despite the risk (e.g., if the drug is needed in a life-threatening situation or for a serious disease for which safer drugs cannot be used or are ineffective).

Category X: Studies in animals or humans have demonstrated fetal abnormalities, there is evidence of fetal risk based on human experience, or both; and the risk of the use of the drug in pregnant women clearly outweighs any possible benefit. The drug is contraindicated in women who are or may become pregnant.

Abbreviations

AUC	Area under the concentration–time curve
C_{max}	Maximum concentration
CMV	Cytomegalovirus
CrCl	Creatinine clearance
CNS	Central nervous system
CSF	Cerebrospinal fluid
EC	enteric coated
GI	Gastrointestinal
HSV	Herpes simplex virus
IM	Intramuscular
IV	Intravenous
LFTs	Liver function tests
MAC	*Mycobacterium avium* complex
OTC	Over the counter
PCP	*Pneumocystis jiroveci (carinii)* pneumonia
SC	Subcutaneous
$t_{1/2}$	Half-life
T_{max}	Time to maximum concentration
Toxo	Toxoplasmosis
USPHS	US Public Health Service
VZV	Varicella-zoster virus

Prices listed are approximate and based on 2005 average wholesale price (AWP).

ANTIRETROVIRALS

Note: Please refer to the table at the end of this section for dosing recommendations of antiretroviral agents in patients with renal or hepatic dysfunction.

Abacavir (ABC)

Trade name: Ziagen (GlaxoSmithKline)

Available formulations:

300 mg tablets	$7.46
20 mg/mL oral solution, 240 mL	$117.71
Epzicom (abacavir 600 mg/lamivudine 300 mg)	$26.03
Trizivir (abacavir 300 mg/lamivudine 150 mg/zidovudine 300 mg)	$19.50

Class: Nucleoside reverse transcriptase inhibitor

Oral dose:

Adults:
As Ziagen: Abacavir 300 mg twice daily or 600 mg once daily
As Epzicom: One tablet once daily
As Trizivir: One tablet twice daily
Children (3 months): – 8 mg/kg (max 300 mg) twice daily

Storage and stability: Store at room temperature; oral solution may be refrigerated; do not freeze

Pharmacokinetics

T_{max}: 1 h

Bioavailability: 83%

Plasma half-life: 0.9–1.5 h (intracellular 12–26 h)

CSF penetration: Approximately 18% of plasma concentration

Plasma protein binding: Approximately 50%

Metabolism/elimination: Primarily metabolized by alcohol dehydrogenase and glucuronyl transferase

Food effects: Can be taken without regard to meals

Breast milk: Animal studies indicate that abacavir is excreted in breast milk. USPHS recommends that HIV+ mothers not breastfeed, to avoid transmission to infant

Side-effects: Systemic hypersensitivity reaction, associated with constitutional symptoms, fever, rash, gastrointestinal disturbances, and/or respiratory symptoms, reported in 2–9% of patients; reaction is strongly associated with carriage of the MHC class I allele *HLA-B*5701*. Abacavir should be discontinued and not rechallenged; rechallenge reactions can be severe, even fatal. This reaction has also been reported in patients who discontinue abacavir for reasons other than hypersensitivity. Other side-effects included asthenia, abdominal pain, diarrhea, nausea, vomiting, headache, hepatomegaly with steatosis, lactic acidosis

Pregnancy: Category C

Amprenavir (APV)

Trade name: Agenerase (GlaxoSmithKline)

Available formulations (150 mg capsule formulation is no longer available):

50 mg capsule	$0.54
15 mg/mL oral solution, 240 mL	$38.77

Note: Oral solution contains propylene glycol, not recommended in children less than 4-years old, pregnant women, patients with renal or liver failure, and patients on metronidazole or disulfiram.

Class: Protease inhibitor (PI)

Oral dose:

Adults:
Capsules: 1200 mg twice daily or (600 mg twice daily + ritonavir 100 mg twice daily) or (1200 mg once daily + ritonavir 200 mg once daily). Fosamprenavir should be considered for use in place of amprenavir in adults – as amprenavir 150 mg capsule is no longer available

Oral solution: 1400 mg (93.3 mL) twice daily

Children:
Capsules: <50 kg: 20 mg/kg twice daily or 15 mg/kg three times daily

Solution: <50 kg: 22.5 mg/kg twice daily or 17 mg/kg three times daily

Capsules and oral solution doses are not interchangeable on a milligram per milligram basis

Storage and stability: Store at room temperature

Pharmacokinetics

T_{max}: 1–2 h

Bioavailability: Not established

Half-life: 7–10 h

CSF penetration: Not established

Plasma protein binding: 91–95%

Metabolism/elimination: Extensive hepatic metabolism by CYP3A4; inhibitor and inducer of CYP3A4-mediated metabolism

Food effects: Can be taken without regard to meals, but not with a high-fat meal

Breast milk: Animal studies indicate that amprenavir is excreted in breast milk. USPHS recommends that HIV+ mothers not breastfeed, to avoid transmission to infant

Side-effects: Headache, nausea, vomiting, diarrhea, rash. PIs have been associated with metabolic effects including hyperglycemia, increased triglycerides and cholesterol, and fat redistribution

Pregnancy: Category C

Atazanavir (ATV)

Trade name: Reyataz (Bristol-Myers Squibb)

Available formulations:

100 mg	$14.29
150 mg	$14.29
200 mg	$14.29
300 mg	$28.57

Class: PI

Oral dose:

Adults: Treatment-naive patients: 400 mg once daily
Treatment-experienced patients and patients on efavirenz or tenofovir: 300 mg once daily + ritonavir 100 mg once daily
Children: Not approved for use in children

Storage and stability: Store at room temperature

Pharmacokinetics

T_{max}: 2.5 h

Bioavailability: Not established

Half-life: 7 h

CSF penetration: CSF to plasma ratio 0.0021–0.0226

Plasma protein binding: 86%

Metabolism/elimination: Substrate and inhibitor of CYP3A4 metabolism

Food effects: Bioavailability increases with food; administer with meals or snack. Avoid taking with antacids

Breast milk: Unknown. USPHS recommends that HIV+ mothers not breastfeed, to avoid transmission to infant

Side-effects: Nausea, headache, indirect hyperbilirubinemia, jaundice, prolonged PR interval (less common), asymptomatic first-degree AV block in some patients. Less hypertriglyceridemia than with other PIs

Pregnancy: Category B

Darunavir (Prezista™)

Class: Protease inhibitor

Oral dose:
Adults: 600 mg bid + ritonavir 100 mg bid (treatment-experienced)

Storage and stability: Tablets stable at room temperature.

Pharmacokinetics

T_{max}: 2.5 – 4 hours

Bioavailability: 37% (82% with ritonavir)

Half-life: approximately 10 hours (unboosted); 15 hours (with ritonavir)

CSF penetration: Unknown

Plasma protein binding: 95%

Metabolism/elimination: Darunavir is almost exclusively metabolized by CYP3A4. Both darunavir and ritonavir are inhibitors of CYP3A4.

Food effects: When administered with food, the C_{max} and AUC of darunavir, co-administered with ritonavir, increases 30% relative to the fasting state. Darunavir/ritonavir should be administered with meals.

Breast milk: Darunavir is secreted into the milk of lactating rats; extent of secretion in human milk is unknown. USPHS recommends that HIV+ mothers not breastfeed to avoid transmission to infant.

Dosage adjustment for organ failure: No dosage adjustment in the setting of renal impairment is necessary, as the renal clearance of darunavir is limited. No recommendations for patients with hepatic impairment; use with caution.

Side-effects: Diarrhea, headache, nausea, fatigue, nasopharyngitis, increased liver enzymes, increased pancreatic enzymes, and increased cholesterol and triglycerides.

Pregnancy: Category B

Delavirdine

Trade name: Rescriptor (Agouron)

Available formulations:

100 mg tablets	$0.88
200 mg tablets	$1.76

Class: Non-nucleoside reverse transcriptase inhibitor

Oral dose (adults): 400 mg three times daily

Storage and stability: Keep in tightly closed container at room temperature away from high humidity

Pharmacokinetics

T_{max}: 1 h

Bioavailability: 85%, increased when in slurry of water

Half-life: 5.8 h

CSF penetration: 0.4% of plasma concentration

Plasma protein binding: 98%

Metabolism/elimination: Extensively metabolized in liver by CYP3A4 and possibly CYP2D6. Inhibitor of CYP3A4-mediated metabolism

Food effects: Can be taken without regard to meals

Breast milk: Unknown. USPHS recommends that HIV+ mothers not breastfeed to avoid transmission to infant

Side-effects: Rash in 18% and severe in 3.6%, usually appears within 1–3 weeks of therapy initiation; nausea; increased serum transaminases

Pregnancy: Category C

Didanosine (ddI)

Trade name: Videx and Videx EC (Bristol-Myers Squibb); generic enteric-coated didanosine

Available formulations:

25 mg buffered tablets	$0.47
50 mg buffered tablets	$0.95
100 mg buffered tablets	$1.89
150 mg buffered tablets	$2.84
200 mg buffered tablets	$3.79
2 g/100 mL pediatric powder	$34.70

4 g/200 mL pediatric powder	$78.61
100 mg sachet	$1.89
167 mg sachet	$3.16
250 mg sachet	$4.74
125 mg EC capsules	$3.60
200 mg EC capsules	$4.96
250 mg EC capsules	$6.19
400 mg EC capsules	$9.91

Class: Nucleoside reverse transcriptase inhibitor

Oral doses:

EC capsules:
>60 kg: 400 mg once daily on an empty stomach
<60 kg: 250 mg once daily on an empty stomach

Buffered tablets:
>60 kg: 200 mg twice daily or 400 mg once daily on an empty stomach
<60 kg: 125 mg twice daily or 250 mg once daily on an empty stomach
Note: Two buffered tablets must be administered at each dose to ensure adequate buffering. Tablets should be chewed, crushed, or dispersed in water or clear apple juice

Sachet:
>60 kg: 250 mg twice daily on an empty stomach
<60 kg: 167 mg twice daily on an empty stomach
Mix with 4 ounces of water; stir until dissolved

Oral dose suspension (children):
Age 2 weeks to 8 months: 100 mg/m^2 twice daily
Age >8 months: 120 mg/m^2 twice daily
Suspension is dissolved in water and then mixed with equal amount of antacid

Storage and stability:
EC capsules: Store at room temperature
Tablets: Store at room temperature in tightly closed bottles. If dispersed in water or apple juice, stable for 1 h at room temperature
Sachet: Store at room temperature. If dissolved in water, stable for 4 h at room temperature
Suspension: Store bottles at room temperature. After reconstitution, store in refrigerator in tightly closed container for up to 30 days

Pharmacokinetics

T_{max}: 0.6–1.0 h

Bioavailability: Buffered tablet and EC capsule 40%; sachet 30%

Plasma half-life: 1.6 h (Intracellular >20 h)

CSF penetration: 21% of serum concentration (children 46%)

Plasma protein binding: Less than 5%

Metabolism/elimination: Primarily eliminated by renal excretion

Food effects: Requires administration on empty stomach, at least 30 min before or 2 h after a meal

Breast milk: Unknown. The USPHS recommends that HIV+ women not breastfeed to avoid transmission to infants

Side-effects: Nausea, diarrhea (mainly with buffered formulations), abdominal pain, peripheral neuropathy (12–34%, dose-related), pancreatitis (1–7%, dose-related), headache, rash, hepatomegaly with steatosis, lactic acidosis, retinal pigmentation

Pregnancy: Category B. Fatal lactic acidosis has been reported in pregnant women treated with a combination of ddI and stavudine

Efavirenz (EFV)

Trade name: Sustiva (Bristol-Meyers Squibb)

Available formulations:

50 mg capsules	$1.33
100 mg capsules	$2.66
200 mg capsules	$5.33
600 mg tablets	$15.98
Atripla (efavirenz 600 mg/ emtricitabine 200 mg/ tenofovir 300 mg)	$47.95

Class: Non-nucleoside reverse transcriptase inhibitor

Oral dose:
Adults: 600 mg once daily, recommended to be given at bedtime or before bedtime on an empty stomach.
As Atripla: One tablet at bedtime or before bedtime on an empty stomach
Children (3 years of age or older):

Weight (lbs)	Dose (mg)
22 to <33	200
33 to <44	250
44 to <55	300
55 to <71.5	350
71.5 to <88	400
≥88	600

Storage and stability: Store at room temperature

Pharmacokinetics

T_{max}: 3–5 h

Bioavailability: Not established

Half-life: 40–55 h with multiple dosing

CSF penetration: 0.65–1.20% of plasma concentration

Plasma protein binding: 99.5–99.75%

Metabolism/elimination: Primarily hepatic metabolism by CYP2B6 and CYP3A4; mixed inducer and inhibitor of CYP3A4

Food effects: Administer on an empty stomach; food increases EFV absorption and may result in increased toxicity

Breast milk: Animal studies indicate that EFV is excreted in breast milk. USPHS recommends that HIV+ women not breastfeed to avoid transmission to infants

Side-effects: Dizziness, paresthesias, headache, lightheadedness, confusion, vivid dreams (CNS-related symptoms may be minimized by administering drug at bedtime), nausea, rash (26% in adults, 40% in children), elevated LFTs, liver failure, elevated serum lipids

Pregnancy: Category D. EFV has been shown to cause major congenital anomalies in nonhuman primates following first trimester exposure; there are case reports of neural tube defects in humans following first trimester exposure

Emtricitabine (FTC)

Trade name: Emtriva (Gilead Sciences)

Available formulations:

200 mg capsule	$10.60
10 mg/mL oral solution 170 mL	$81.96
Truvada (FTC 200 mg/tenofovir 300 mg)	$26.03
Atripla (efavirenz 600 mg/ emtricitabine 200 mg/tenofovir 300 mg)	$47.95

Class: Nucleoside reverse transcriptase inhibitor active against HIV and hepatitis B

Oral dose:
Adults: 200 mg capsule once daily or 240 mg oral solution (24 mL) once daily
As Atripla: One tablet at bedtime or before bedtime on an empty stomach
Children (3 months to 17 years): 6 mg/kg (max 240 mg) oral solution once daily; capsules (for weight >33 kg): 200 mg once daily

Storage and stability: Store at room temperature

Pharmacokinetics

T_{max}: 1–2 h

Bioavailability: 93% capsules; 75% oral solution

Plasma half-life: 10 h (intracellular >20 h)

CSF penetration: Unknown

Plasma protein binding: <4%

Metabolism/elimination: Renal excretion by glomerular filtration and active tubular secretion

Food effects: Administer without regards to meals

Breast milk: Unknown. The USPHS recommends that HIV+ women not breastfeed to avoid transmission to infants

Side-effects: Minimal toxicity; nausea, headache, diarrhea, hyperpigmentation, lactic acidosis with hepatic steatosis (rare). Potential exacerbation of hepatitis B in co-infected patients following discontinuation of FTC change to alternative agent with activity against hepatitis B virus (HBV)

Pregnancy: Category B

Enfuvirtide (T20)

Trade name: Fuzeon (Hoffmann-LaRoche)

Available formulation:

Single-use vial of 108 mg enfuvirtide, to be reconstituted with 1.1 mL sterile water for delivery of 90 mg/1 mL	$35.29

Class: Fusion inhibitor

Dose:
Adults: 90 mg (1 mL) subcutaneous (SC) injection twice daily
Children: Not approved for children <6 years of age. In children 6 years of age: 2 mg/kg (max 90 mg) twice daily by subcutaneous injection

Storage and stability: Store vials at room temperature. Reconstituted solution should be stored under refrigeration and used within 24 h

Pharmacokinetics

T_{max}: 4 h

Bioavailability: 84.3%

Half-life: 3.8 h

CSF penetration: Unknown

Plasma protein binding: 92%

Metabolism/elimination: Catabolism to constituent amino acids

Food effects: Administer without regards to meals

Breast milk: Animal studies indicate that enfuvirtide is excreted in breast milk. The USPHS recommends that HIV+ women not breastfeed, to avoid transmission to infants

Side-effects: Local injection site reaction seen in almost all patients (pain, erythema, induration, nodules, pruritis); increased rate of bacterial pneumonia in patients receiving enfuvirtide was observed in clinical trials; hypersensitivity reaction (<1%)

Pregnancy: Category B

Fosamprenavir (f-APV)

Trade name: Lexiva (GlaxoSmithKline)

Available formulations:

700 mg tablet	$11.09
50 mg/mL oral suspension, 225 mL	

Class: PI

Oral dose:

Adult treatment-naive patients:
f-APV 1400 mg twice-daily OR
(f-APV1400 mg + ritonavir 200 mg) once-daily OR
(f-APV 700 mg + ritonavir 100 mg) twice daily
Adult treatment-experienced patients:
f-APV 700 mg twice daily + ritonavir 100 mg twice daily
Children:
Therapy-naive 2–5 years old:
30 mg/kg twice daily, not to exceed 1,400 mg twice daily

Therapy-naive ⩾ 6 years old:
30 mg/kg twice daily not to exceed 1,400 mg twice daily or 18 mg/kg plus ritonavir 3 mg/kg twice daily not to exceed 700 mg + ritonavir 100 mg twice daily

Therapy-experienced ⩾ 6 Years of Age:
18 mg/kg plus ritonavir 3 mg/kg administered twice daily not to exceed fosamprenavir 700 mg + ritonavir 100 mg twice daily

Storage and stability: Store at room temperature

Pharmacokinetics

T_{max}: 1.5–2.5 h

Bioavailability: Not established

Half-life: 7.7 h

CSF penetration: Unknown

Plasma protein binding: 90%

Metabolism/elimination: f-APV is rapidly and almost completely hydrolyzed to APV in the gut epithelium. The parent drug, APV, is extensively metabolism by CYP3A4, and is an inhibitor and inducer of CYP3A4-mediated metabolism

Food effects: Administer without regards to meals

Breast milk: Animal studies indicate that APV is excreted in breast milk. USPHS recommends that HIV+ mothers not breastfeed to avoid transmission to infant

Side-effects: Skin rash (19%), headache, nausea, vomiting, diarrhea. PIs have been associated with metabolic effects including hyperglycemia, increased triglycerides and cholesterol, and fat redistribution

Pregnancy: Category C

Indinavir (IDV)

Trade name: Crixivan (Merck)

Available formulations:

100 mg	$0.76
200 mg	$1.52
333 mg	$2.54
400 mg	$3.05

Class: PI

Oral doses:
800 mg every 8 h on an empty stomach, OR
IDV 800 mg + ritonavir (100 or 200 mg) twice daily with or without food

Storage and stability: Store at room temperature in original, tightly closed container with desiccant

Pharmacokinetics

T_{max}: 0.8 h

Bioavailability: 65%

Half-life: 1.5–2.0 h

CSF penetration: 2.2–76.0% in limited number of patients

Plasma protein binding: Approximately 60%

Metabolism/elimination: Hepatic metabolism by CYP3A4; less than 20% excreted unchanged in urine; inhibitor of CY3A4-mediated metabolism

Food effects: High-caloric, high-fat meal reduces bioavailability. Administer on empty stomach or with a low-fat, light meal. It can be administered with food when taken with ritonavir. Patients are advised to drink at least 1.5 L of fluid daily to avoid crystalluria and nephrolithiasis

Breast milk: Available data suggest distribution into milk. USPHS recommends that HIV+ mothers not breastfeed to avoid transmission to infant

Side-effects: Nephrolithiasis/urolithiasis, nausea, GI intolerance, indirect hyperbilirubinemia, headache, dizziness, rash, hemolytic anemia. PIs have been associated with metabolic effects, including hyperglycemia, increased triglycerides and cholesterol, and fat redistribution

Pregnancy: Category C

Lamivudine (3TC)

Trade name: Epivir (GlaxoSmithKline)

Available formulations:

150 mg tablet	$5.55
300 mg tablet	$11.11
10 mg/mL, 240 mL oral solution	$88.86
Combivir (3TC 150 mg + zidovudine 300 mg)	$12.04
Epzicom (3TC 300 mg + ABC 600 mg)	$26.03
Trizivir (3TC 150 mg + ABC 300 mg + zidovudine 300 mg)	$19.05

Class: Nucleoside reverse transcriptase inhibitor active against HIV and HBV

Oral dose:
Adults: 150 mg twice daily or 300 mg once daily
Children:
Neonatal/infants (<30 days): 2 mg/kg twice daily
Pediatric (<50 kg): 4 mg/kg twice daily (up to 150 mg twice daily)

Storage and stability: Store at room temperature in tightly closed containers

Pharmacokinetics

T_{max}: Approximately 1 h (fasting), 3.2 h (fed)

Bioavailability: 86% (66–68% in children)

Half-life: 5–7 h (intracellular 18–22 h)

CSF penetration: Unknown

Plasma protein binding: Less than 36%

Metabolism/elimination: Primarily eliminated unchanged in the urine

Food effects: Food delays absorption but not overall extent; give without regard to meals

Breast milk: Available data suggest that lamivudine is readily excreted in milk. USPHS recommends that HIV+ women not breastfeed to avoid transmission to infants

Side-effects: Nausea, headache, malaise, nasal congestion, pancreatitis in children (14%), hepatomegaly with steatosis, lactic acidosis. Potential exacerbation of hepatitis B in co-infected patients following discontinuation of 3TC– change to alternative agent with activity against HBV

Pregnancy: Category C

Lopinavir/Ritonavir (LPV/RTV)

Trade name: Kaletra (Abbott)

Available formulations:

Lopinavir 200 mg + ritonavir 50 mg tablet	$6.64
Lopinavir 80 mg/ritionavir 20 mg/mL oral solution, 180 mL	$351.75

Class: PI

Oral dose:
Adults, adolescents (>12 years): 400/100 mg twice daily or 800/200 mg once daily (treatment-naive patients only)
Children (6 months to 12 years):

7 to <15 kg	12/3 mg/kg twice daily
15 to 40 kg	10/2.5 mg/kg twice daily
>40 kg	Use adult dose

Storage and stability: Solution is stable in refrigerator until date on label; at room temperature, use within 2 months. Tablets are stored at room temperature

Pharmacokinetics

T_{max}: 4 h

Bioavailability: Not determined

Half-life: 5–6 h

CSF penetration: Negligible

Plasma protein binding: Approximately 98–99%

Metabolism/elimination: Substrate and inhibitor of CYP3A4 metabolism

Food effects: Food significantly increases plasma concentrations of the solution; administer with food. Tablets may be administered without regard to meals

Breast milk: Animal data suggest distribution into milk. USPHS recommends that HIV+ mothers not breastfeed to avoid transmission to infant

Side-effects: Nausea, diarrhea (higher incidence with once-daily dosing), abdominal pain, asthenia, headache, elevated LFTs. PIs have been associated with metabolic effects including hyperglycemia, increased triglycerides and cholesterol, and fat redistribution

Pregnancy: Category C

Maraviroc

Trade name: Selzentry (Pfizer)

Available formulation:
150 mg tablet
300 mg tablet

Class: Entry Inhibitor

Mechanism of Action: CCR5 Antagonist

Oral dose:
Adults:

When given with strong CYP3A inhibitors (with or without CYP3A inducers), including protease inhibitors (except tipranavir/ritonavir) and delavirdine	150 mg twice daily
With NRTIs, tipranavir/ritonavir, nevirapine and other drugs that are not strong CYP3A inhibitors or CYP3A inducers	300 mg twice daily
With CYP3A inducers including efavirenz (without a strong CYP3A inhibitor)	600 mg twice daily

Storage and stability: Room temperature

Pharmacokinetics

T_{max}: 0.5–4 h

Bioavailability: 33% (predicted, following a 300 mg dose)

Half-life: 14–18 h

CSF penetration: Unknown

Plasma protein binding: 76%

Metabolism/elimination: Maraviroc is principally metabolized by CYP3A, and is also a substrate for P-glycoprotein (P-gp). Renal clearance accounts for approximately 25% of maraviroc total clearance. When administered with CYP3A/P-gp inhibitors, maraviroc exposure is significantly increased, while CYP3A inducers rifampin and efavirenz significantly decrease maraviroc exposure. Tipranavir/ritonavir does not affect the PK of maraviroc

Food effects: Maraviroc may be taken with or without food

Breast milk: Maraviroc is extensively secreted into the milk of lactating rats; the extent of secretion into human milk is unknown. USPHS recommends that HIV+ mothers not breastfeed to avoid HIV transmission to infant

Dosage adjustment for organ failure: Maraviroc exposure may be increased in patients with renal impairment, especially when CYP3A inhibitors are coadministered. Patients with a CrCl < 50 mL/min should take maraviroc with a CYP3A inhibitor only if the potential benefit outweighs the risk of toxicity; monitor for side-effects. Maraviroc exposure is expected to be increased in patients with hepatic impairment; use with caution

Side-effects: The most common adverse events reported in clinical trials were cough, pyrexia, upper respiratory tract infection, rash, musculoskeletal symptoms, abdominal pain and dizziness. Laboratory abnormalities reported in clinical trials included increases in AST, ALT, total bilirubin, amylase and lipase, and decreased absolute neutrophil count

Pregnancy: Pregnancy Category B. Maraviroc has not been studied in pregnant women. Ensure adequate contraception in women of childbearing potential

Nelfinavir (NFV)

Trade name: Viracept (Agouron)

Available formulations:

250 mg tablet	$2.52
625 mg tablet	$6.05
50 mg/g oral powder, 144 g	$66.48

Class: PI

Oral dose:
Adults: 750 mg three times daily or 1250 mg twice daily with food
Children (≤2 years): 45–55 mg/kg twice daily with food or 25–35 mg/kg three times daily with food

Storage and stability: Oral powder may be mixed with water, milk/formula, soy milk/formula, and dietary supplements. Mixed powder may be stored in refrigerator up to 6 h. Store tablets at room temperature

Pharmacokinetics

T_{max}: 2–4 h

Bioavailability: 20–80%

Half-life: 3.5–5.0 h

CSF penetration: Negligible

Plasma protein binding: More than 98%

Metabolism/elimination: Extensive hepatic metabolism by CYP3A4 and CYP2C19, with metabolites excreted in feces. Inhibitor of CYP3A4-mediated metabolism

Food effects: Bioavailability increased with food. Administer with meals or snack

Breast milk: Animal data suggest that nelfinavir is distributed into breast milk USPHS recommends that HIV mothers do not breastfeed to avoid transmission to infant

Side-effects: Diarrhea, nausea, elevated serum transaminases, abdominal pain. PIs have been associated with metabolic effects including hyperglycemia, increased triglycerides and cholesterol, and fat redistribution

Pregnancy: Category B

Nevirapine (NVP)

Trade name: Viramune (Boeringer-Ingelheim)

Available formulations:

200 mg tablet	$12.97
10 mg/mL suspension, 240 mL	$91.98

Class: Non-nucleoside reverse transcriptase inhibitor

Oral dose:
Adults: 200 mg once daily for 14 days, then 200 mg twice daily
Children:
Neonatal/infant (through 2 months of age): 120 mg/m^2 once × 14 days, then 120 mg/m^2 twice a day × 14 days, then 200 mg/m^2 twice daily
2 months to <8 years: 4 mg/kg once daily × 14 days, then 7 mg/kg twice daily
≥ 8 years: 4 mg/kg once daily × 14 days, then 4 mg/kg once daily (max 200 mg twice a day)
Do not increase dosage if rash appears during escalation phase. If therapy is stopped for more than 7 days, reinitiate dose escalation

Storage and stability: Store at room temperature in tightly closed bottles

Pharmacokinetics

T_{max}: Within 4 h

Bioavailability: More than 90%

Half-life: 25–30 h

CSF penetration: 45% of concentration in plasma

Plasma protein binding: 60%

Metabolism/elimination: Substrate and inducer of CYP3A metabolism

Food effects: Not affected by food; administer without regard to meals

Breast milk: Detectable in breast milk. USPHS recommends that HIV+ mothers not breastfeed to avoid transmission to infant

Side-effects: Rash (17%) usually appears within the first 6 weeks of therapy; Stevens–Johnson syndrome has been reported. Nausea, fever, headache. Hepatotoxicity – can be severe, close monitoring of serum transaminases is recommended, particularly during first 18 weeks of therapy. Women have threefold greater risk of hepatotoxicity than men; contraindicated in women with CD4+ T-lymphocyte count >250 cells/mL and men with CD4+ T-lymphocyte count >400 cells/mL. Do not restart after severe hepatic, skin or hypersensitivity reaction

Pregnancy: Category C

Ritonavir (RTV)

Trade name: Norvir (Abbott)

Available formulations:

100 mg capsule	$10.29
80 mg/mL oral solution, 240 mL	$1728.24

Class: PI

Oral dose:
Adults: 600 mg twice daily (when used as sole PI); dose escalation required to reduce gastrointestinal side-effects
Doses of 100–400 mg/day (in 1–2 divided doses) are used as pharmacokinetic enhancer with other PIs. Solution may be mixed with Advera, Ensure, or chocolate milk to increase palatability
Children (>1 month): 350–400 mg/m^2; dose escalation required. Initiate with 250 mg/m^2 and increase in 50 mg/m^2 twice-daily increments every 2–3 days

Storage and stability: Store capsules in refrigerator; stable at room temperature for up to 30 days. Solution should not be refrigerated. Avoid exposure to extreme heat and protect from light

Pharmacokinetics

T_{max}: 2–4 h

Bioavailability: 60–80%

Half-life: 3–5 h

CSF penetration: Negligible

Plasma protein binding: 98–99%

Metabolism/elimination: Extensive hepatic metabolism by hepatic CYP3A4; potent inhibitor of CYP3A4-mediated metabolism

Food effects: Recommended to be administered with food: 15% increase in AUC with food

Breast milk: Unknown. USPHS recommends that HIV+ mothers not breastfeed to avoid transmission to infant

Side-effects: Predominantly GI side-effects (nausea and vomiting, diarrhea, abdominal pain) especially during first month of treatment, circumoral paresthesias, taste perversion, elevated serum transaminases, hypertriglyceridemia. PIs have been associated with metabolic effects including hyperglycemia, increased triglycerides and cholesterol, and fat redistribution

Pregnancy: Category B

Saquinavir (SQV)

Trade name: Invirase (Roche)

Available formulations:

200 mg hard gel capsule	$2.40
500 mg tablet	$5.99

Class: PI

Oral dose:
Adults: Unboosted SQV not recommended
Recommended RTV-boosted dose: (SQV 1000 mg + RTV 100 mg) twice daily
Not approved for use in children

Storage and stability: Store at room temperature

Pharmacokinetics

T_{max}: Approximately 3 h

Bioavailability: Approximately 4% with full meal (when sole PI)

Half-life: 1–2 h

CSF penetration: Negligible

Plasma protein binding: 98%

Metabolism/elimination: Metabolized primarily by CYP3A4; extensive first-pass metabolism. Inhibitor of CYP3A4

Food effects: Administer within 2 h of a full meal

Breast milk: Secreted in milk of laboratory animals; no data in humans. USPHS recommends that HIV+ mothers not breastfeed to avoid transmission to infant

Side-effects: Nausea and vomiting, abdominal pain, diarrhea, elevated serum transaminases, headache. PIs have been associated with metabolic effects including hyperglycemia, increased triglycerides and cholesterol, and fat redistribution

Pregnancy: Category B

Stavudine (d4T)

Trade name: Zerit (Bristol Myers Squibb)

Available formulations:

15 mg capsule	$5.49
20 mg capsule	$5.70
30 mg capsule	$6.06
40 mg capsule	$6.17
1 mg/mL, 200 mL	$69.64

Class: Nucleoside reverse transcriptase inhibitor

Oral dose:
Adults:
>60 kg: 40 mg twice daily; <60 kg: 30 mg twice daily
Children: <30 kg: 1 mg/kg per dose every 12 h. Weight ≤30 kg, follow adult recommendations

Storage and stability:
Capsules: store at room temperature in tightly closed bottles
Suspension: After reconstitution with water, store in refrigerator in tightly closed original container for up to 30 days

Pharmacokinetics

T_{max}: Within 1 h

Bioavailability: 86%

Half-life: 1.0–1.4 h (intracellular 7.5 h)

CSF penetration: 30% of serum levels

Plasma protein binding: Negligible

Metabolism/elimination: Primarily excreted renally (50%)

Food effects: AUC unchanged with food; give without regard to meals

Breast milk: Animal studies suggest d4T is excreted in breast milk. USPHS recommends that HIV+ women not breastfeed to avoid transmission to infants

Side-effects: Peripheral neuropathy (>20%), lipodystrophy, hypertriglyceridemia, rapidly progressive ascending neuromuscular weakness (rare), pancreatitis (especially if used with ddI), hepatomegaly with steatosis, lactic acidosis (can be severe, even fatal)

Pregnancy: Category C. Fatal lactic acidosis has been reported in pregnant women treated with a combination of d4T and ddI

Tenofovir Disoproxil Fumarate (TDF)

Trade name: Viread (Gilead)

Available formulations:

300 mg tablet	$16.75
Truvada (tenofovir 300 mg + emtricitabine 200 mg)	$26.03
Atripla (efavirenz 600 mg/emtricitabine 200 mg/tenofovir 300 mg)	$47.95

Class: Nucleotide reverse transcriptase inhibitor with activities against HIV and HBV

Oral dose (adults): 300 mg once daily
As Truvada: one tablet once daily
As Atripla: One tablet at bedtime or before bedtime on an empty stomach
Not approved for use in children

Storage and stability: Store at room temperature

Pharmacokinetics

T_{max}: 1 h under fasting condition, and 2 h when taken with food

Bioavailability: 25% in fasting state; 39% with high-fat meal

Half-life: 17 h (intracellular >60 h)

Metabolism/elimination: Primarily renal excretion by glomerular filtration and active tubular secretion

Food effects: Take without regard to meals

Breast milk: Animal studies suggest tenofovir is excreted in breast milk. USPHS recommends that HIV+ women not breastfeed, to avoid transmission to infants

Side-effects: Nausea, vomiting, headache, asthenia, increased serum creatinine, renal insufficiency, diabetes insipidus (rare), Fanconi-like syndrome

Pregnancy: Category C

Tipranavir (TPV)

Trade name: Aptivus (Boehringer Ingelheim Pharmaceuticals)

Available formulation:
250 mg capsules

Class: PI

Oral dose:
Adults: 500 mg twice daily + RTV 200 mg twice daily

Note: TPV should always be given with RTV. TPV is indicated in highly treatment-experienced patients or for patients with HIV-1 strains resistant to multiple PIs
Children: Not approved for use in children

Storage and stability: Capsules should be refrigerated. If stored at room temperature, must be used within 60 days

Pharmacokinetics

T_{max}: Approximately 3 h

Bioavailability: Not established

Half-life: 6 h when administered with RTV

CSF penetration: Unknown

Plasma protein binding: >99%

Metabolism/elimination: TPV is not appreciably metabolized when administered with RTV. TPV is a substrate and inducer of CYP3A and P-glycoprotein; when administered with RTV, the net effect is CYP3A4 inhibition and P-glycoprotein induction

Food effects: Bioavailability increases with a high fat meal; administer TPV and RTV with meals. Separate from antacid administration

Breast milk: Unknown. USPHS recommends that HIV+ mothers not breastfeed to avoid transmission to infant

Side-effects: Nausea, vomiting, diarrhea, fatigue, headache, mild to moderate rash (urticarial and maculopapular). TPV has a sulfonamide moiety; use with caution in patients with a sulfonamide allergy. Rare cases of intracranial hemorrhage have been reported. Hepatotoxicity – clinical hepatitis and hepatic decompensation, including some fatalities, have been associated with TPV/RTV; patients with chronic hepatitis B or C co-infection are at increased risk. Hyperglycemia and new-onset diabetes mellitus, increases in total cholesterol and triglycerides

Pregnancy: Category C

Zidovudine (AZT, ZDV)

Trade name: Retrovir (GlaxoSmithKline); generic ZDV tablets and syrup available

100 mg capsule	$2.16
300 mg tablet	$6.45
50 mg/5 mL, 240 mL oral solution	$51.91
10 mg/mL, 20 mL IV solution	$23.40
Combivir (ZDV 300 mg/3TC 150 mg)	$12.04
Trizivir (ZDV 300 mg/3TC 150 mg/ABC 300 mg)	$19.05

Class: Nucleoside reverse transcriptase inhibitor

Oral dose:
Adults: 300 mg twice daily or 200 mg three times daily
As Combivir: one tablet twice daily
As Trizivir: one tablet twice daily
Children (6 weeks to 12 years): 160 mg/m^2 PO every 8 h (maximum 200 mg q8h) or 120 mg/m^2 IV every 6 h
Neonates/Infants (<6 weeks): Starting within 12 h after birth: 2 mg/kg PO every 6 h × 6 weeks or 1.5 mg/kg IV over 30 min every 6 h

Storage and stability: Oral formulations are stable at room temperature; protect from moisture. Diluted IV solution is stable under refrigeration for 24 h

Pharmacokinetics

T_{max}: 0.5–1.5 h

Bioavailability: 60%

Half-life: 1.1 h (7 h intracellularly)

CSF penetration: 60% of serum level in adults; 68% in children

Plasma protein binding: 34–38%

Metabolism/elimination: Undergoes glucuronidation in liver; metabolite excreted in urine

Food effects: May be taken without regard to meals

Breast milk: Excreted in breast milk in similar concentration as serum. USPHS recommends that HIV+ women not breastfeed, to avoid transmission to infants

Side-effects: Subjective complaints (headache, nausea, vomiting, malaise, anorexia), bone marrow suppression: macrocytic anemia and neutropenia, myopathy, myositis, changes in nail and skin pigmentation, hepatomegaly with steatosis, lactic acidosis

Pregnancy: Category C. Indicated during pregnancy for reducing the risk of vertical transmission to fetus

HIV-related medications (*Note*: Only adult dosages are included in the following monographs. Please refer to product labeling for dosage recommendations in children)

Dosing of Antiretrovirals in the Presence of Renal or Hepatic Insufficiency in Adult HIV Patients

Antiretrovirals	Daily Dose	Dosing in Renal Insufficiency	Dosing in Hepatic Impairment
Nucleoside reverse transcriptase inhibitors[a]			
Abacavir (Ziagen)	300 mg PO bid	No need for dosage adjustment	No dosage recommendation
Didanosine (Videx EC)	>60 kg 400 mg PO qd <60 kg 250 mg qd	**CrCl (mL/min)** — Dose **>60 kg** / **<60 kg** 30–59: 200 mg / 125 mg 10–29: 125 mg / 100 mg <10: 125 mg / 75 mg *CAPD or HD patients:* use same dose as CrCl < 10 mL/min	No dosage recommendation
Emtricitabine (Emtriva)	200 mg oral capsule PO qd or 240 mg (24 mL) oral solution PO qd	**CrCl** — **Capsule** / **Solution** 30–49: 200 mg q48 h / 120 mg q24h 15–29: 200 mg q72h / 80 mg q24h <15: 200 mg q96h / 60 mg q24h or HD*	No dosage recommendation
Lamivudine (Epivir)	300 mg PO qd or 150 mg PO bid	**CrCl (mL/min)** — **Dose** 30–49: 150 mg qd 15–29: 150 mg × 1, then 100 mg qd 5–14: 150 mg × 1, then 50 mg qd <5: 50 mg × 1, then 25 mg qd or HD*	No dosage recommendation
Stavudine (Zerit)	>60 kg 40 mg PO bid <60 kg 30 mg PO bid	**CrCl (mL/min)** — Dose **>60 kg** / **<60 kg** 26–50: 20 mg q12h / 15 mg q12h 10–25: 20 mg q24h / 15 mg q24h or HD*	No dosage recommendation
Tenofovir (Viread)	300 mg PO qd	**CrCl (mL/min)** — **Dose** 30–49: 300 mg q48h 10–29: 300 mg twice weekly ESRD or HD: 300 mg q7d	No dosage recommendation
Tenofovir + Emtricitabine (Truvada)	1 tablet PO qd	**CrCl (mL/min)** — **Dose** 30–49: 1 tablet q48h <30 not recommended	No dosage recommendation
Zidovudine (Retrovir)	300 mg PO bid	'Severe' renal impairment or HD – 100 mg TID or 300 mg qd	No dosage recommendation
Non-Nucleoside Reverse Transcriptase Inhibitors			
Delavirdine (Rescriptor)	400 mg PO TID	No dosage adjustment necessary	No recommendation; use with caution in patients with hepatic impairment
Efavirenz (Sustiva)	600 mg PO qd	No dosage adjustment necessary	No recommendation; use with caution in patients with hepatic impairment
Nevirapine (Viramune)	200 mg PO bid	No dosage adjustment necessary	No data available; avoid use in patients with moderate to severe hepatic impairment

Antiretrovirals	Daily Dose	Dosing in Renal Insufficiency	Dosing in Hepatic Impairment
Protease Inhibitors			
Amprenavir (Agenerase)	1200 mg PO BID *Note*: oral solution not recommended in patients with renal or hepatic failure	No dosage adjustment necessary	**Child–Pugh Score** / **Dose** 5–8: 450 mg bid 9–12: 300 mg bid
Atazanavir (Reyataz)	400 mg PO qd	No dosage adjustment necessary	**Child–Pugh Class** / **Dose** 7–9: 300 mg qd >9: not recommended
Darunavir (Prezista, DRV)	DRV 600 mg + RTV 100 mg PO bid	No dosage adjustment necessary	No dosage recommendation; use with caution in patients with hepatic impairment
Fosamprenavir (Lexiva)	1400 mg PO bid	No dosage adjustment necessary	**Child–Pugh Score** / **Dose** 5–6: 700 mg bid ±RTV 100 mg qd 7–9: 700 mg bid or 450 mg bid + RTV 100 mg qd 10–12: 350 mg bid ritonavir boosting should not be used in patients with hepatic impairment
Indinavir (Crixivan)	800 mg PO q8h	No dosage adjustment necessary	Mild to moderate hepatic insufficiency due to cirrhosis: 600 mg q8h
Lopinavir/ ritonavir (Kaletra)	400 mg/100 mg PO bid or 800 mg/200 mg PO qd (qd dosing only for treatment-naive patients)	No dosage adjustment necessary	No dosage recommendation; use with caution in patients with hepatic impairment
Nelfinavir (Viracept)	1250 mg PO bid	No dosage adjustment necessary	No dosage recommendation; use with caution in patients with hepatic impairment
Ritonavir (Norvir)	600 mg PO bid	No dosage adjustment necessary	No dosage adjustment in mild hepatic impairment; no data for moderate to severe impairment, use with caution
Saquinavir (Invirase)	1000 mg bid + 100 mg ritonavir bid	No dosage adjustment necessary	No dosage recommendation; use with caution in patients with hepatic impairment
Tipranavir (Aptivus)	500 mg PO bid with ritonavir 200 mg PO bid	No dosage adjustment necessary	No dosage recommendation; use with caution in patients with hepatic impairment; TPV/RTV is contraindicated in pts with moderate to severe (Child–Pugh Class B & C) hepatic insufficiency
Fusion Inhibitors			
Enfuvirtide (Fuzeon)	90 mg SQ q12h	No dosage adjustment necessary	No dosage recommendation

Antiretrovirals	Daily Dose	Dosing in Renal Insufficiency	Dosing in Hepatic Impairment
CCR5			
Maravoric (Selzentry)	Daily dose differs based on concomitant medication, please refer to Ch 81 for dosing recommendation	No dosage recommendation; use with caution Patients with CrCL<50mL/min should receive MRV and CYP3A inhibitor only if potential benefit outweighs the risk	No dosage recommendations. Concentrations are likely increased in patients with hepatic impairment.
Integrase Inhibitors			
Raltegravir (Isentress)	400 mg twice daily	No dosage adjustment	No dosage adjustment

Child–Pugh Score

	Score Given		
Component	**1**	**2**	**3**
Encephalopathy*	None	Grade 1–2	Grade 3–4
Ascites	None	Mild or controlled by diuretics	Moderate or refractory despite diuretics
Albumin	>3.5 g/dl	2.8 to 3.5 g/dl	<2.8 g/dl
Total Bilirubin OR	<2 mg/dL	2 to 3 mg/dL	>3 mg/dL
Modified Total Bilirubin**	(<34 μmol/L)	(34 μmol/L to 50 μmol/L)	(>50 μmol/L)
	<4 mg/dL	4–7 mg/dL	>7 mg/dL
Prothrombin time	<4	4–6	>6
(sec prolonged) OR INR	<1.7	1.7–2.3	>2.3

* NB: Encephalopathy Grades –

Grade 1: Mild confusion, anxiety, restlessness, fine tremor, slowed coordination
Grade 2: Drowsiness, disorientation, asterixis
Grade 3: Somnolent but rousable, marked confusion, incomprehensible speech, incontinence, hyperventilation
Grade 4: Coma, decerebrate posturing, flaccidity

** Modified Total Bilirubin used to score patients who have Gilbert's syndrome or who are taking indinavir or atazanavir

Child–Pugh Classification – Child–Pugh Class A = score 5–6; Class B = score 7–9; Class C = score >9.

(Adapted from DHHS Guidelines for the Use of Antiretroviral Agents in Adults and Adolescents, October 10, 2006, http://www.aidsinfo.nih.gov.)

[a]Note: Use of combination formulations of: Combivir, Trizivir, Epzicom and Atripla – not recommended in patients with CrCl <50 mL/min; use of Truvada not – recommended in patients with CrCl <30 mL/min

qd, once daily; bid, twice daily; TID, three times daily; HD* = dose after hemodialysis on dialysis days; HD, hemodialysis; CAPD , chronic ambulatory peritoneal dialysis; ESRD, end stage renal disease.

Creatinine Clearance calculation:

Male: $\frac{(140\text{-age in yrs}) \times \text{weight (kg)}}{72 \times \text{S.Cr.}}$

Female: $\frac{(140\text{-age in yrs}) \times \text{weight (kg)} \times 0.85}{72 \times \text{S.Cr.}}$

ANTIMYCOBACTERIAL DRUGS

Amikacin

Trade name: Amikin (Bristol-Myers Squibb), generic (various manufacturers)

Available formulations: Various preparations and strengths in single and multiple doses

Generic 250 mg/mL–2 mL	\$6.00–\$7.80

Class: Aminoglycoside antibiotic

Mechanism of action: Binds to 30S ribosomal subunit, inhibiting protein synthesis

Dosage for treatment of MAC and other mycobacterial infections: 7.5–15.0 mg kg^{-1} day^{-1} as IV infusion. Administer each dose over 60 min

Storage and stability: Store vials at room temperature. After dilution, stable for 24 h at room temperature

Pharmacokinetics

Half-life: Approximately 2 h

CSF penetration: 10–20% of serum levels but may be higher with inflamed meninges

Plasma protein binding: 4–11%

Metabolism/elimination: Eliminated primarily by glomerular filtration

Breast milk: Unknown breastfeeding should be avoided

Dosage adjustment for organ failure: Dosage adjustment required for renal dysfunction. Creatinine clearance (CrCl) should be estimated and dosing interval adjusted to maintain peak and trough concentrations

Side-effects: Nephrotoxicity, ototoxicity, arthralgia, fever, rash, eosinophilia, neuromuscular blockade

Pregnancy: Category D. Aminoglycosides can freely cross placenta. Its use has been associated with bilateral, irreversible deafness in neonates exposed to the drug *in utero*. One must weigh the benefit to the mother against the potential risks to the fetus

Azithromycin

250 mg tablets	\$8.30
500 mg tablets	\$16.61
600 mg tablets	\$19.93
1 g powder	\$25.79
100 mg/5 mL suspension, 15 mL	\$35.16
200 mg/5 mL suspension, 15 mL	\$35.16
500 mg/vial for IV	\$29.46

Trade name: Zithromax (Pfizer)

Available formulations:

Class: Macrolide antibiotic

Mechanism of action: Binds to 50S ribosomal subunit, inhibiting protein synthesis

Oral doses (adults):
Treating MAC: 250–600 mg PO once daily
Treating gonococcal urethritis: 1 g PO, single dose
MAC prophylaxis: 1200 mg once weekly
IV dose: 250–500 mg given over at least 1 h for 1–2 days, then switch to PO when appropriate

Storage and stability:
Tablets: Store below 30ºC
Suspension: Store dry powder at below 30ºC; after reconstitution, store between 5ºC and 30ºC, administer within 10 days
IV: reconstituted solution stable for 24 h at room temperature

Pharmacokinetics

T_{max}: Within 2 h

Bioavailability: 34%

Half-life: Biphasic elimination half-life – in first 8–24 h, half-life ~11–14 h; after 24–72 h, half-life 35–40 h; after multiple doses, half-life can be up to 68 h

CSF penetration: Negligible; extensive tissue and intracellular uptake

Plasma protein binding: 7–50%; concentration-dependent

Metabolism/elimination: Biliary excretion primarily as unchanged drug

Food effects: Decreased absorption of tablets by 43%; suspension not affected by food

Breast milk: Secreted in breast milk

Dosage adjustment for organ failure: None

Side-effects: Gastrointestinal side-effects (loose stools, nausea, vomiting, abdominal pain), pruritus, rash, CNS disturbances (headache, dizziness, delirium, vertigo, agitation – have been reported), ototoxicity, elevation of serum transaminases

Pregnancy: Category B

Clarithromycin

Trade names: Biaxin (Abbott); Biaxin-XL (Abbott)

Available formulations:

Class: Macrolide antibiotic

Mechanism of action: Inhibits protein synthesis by binding to the 50S ribosomal subunit

Oral dose for treatment of MAC: 500 mg twice daily

Storage and stability: Store tablets and granules for suspension at 15–30ºC in a well closed container and protected from light. Store extended-release forumation at 20–25ºC. Reconstituted suspension stored at room temperature and used within 14 days. Do not refrigerate reconstituted suspension – lower temperature may result in bitter taste

Pharmacokinetics

T_{max}: 0.5–1.5 h

Bioavailability: 50%

Half-life: 250 mg dose, 3–4 h; 500 mg dose, 5–7 h

CSF penetration: Unknown; extensive distribution into tissues, phagocytic cells

Metabolism/elimination: 20% to 30% excreted unchanged in urine; extensive hepatic metabolism. Active metabolite 14-OH-clarithromycin accounts for 20%

Food effects: Food slightly delays absorption, but does not affect overall bioavailability

Breast milk: Unknown; caution should be exercised in nursing mothers

Dosage adjustment for organ failure: Dose should be reduced by half or the interval doubled in the presence of severe renal impairment (CrCl <30 mL/min) with or without hepatic disease

Side-effects: Gastrointestinal adverse effects (nausea, vomiting, abdominal pain, diarrhea (11%)), infrequent reports of metallic taste, elevated LFTs, ototoxicity

Pregnancy: Category C

Ethambutol

Trade name: Myambutol (Lederle)

Available formulations:

100 mg tablets	$0.62
400 mg tablets	$1.80

Class: Antimycobacterial

Mechanism of action: Appears to inhibit cell replication and metabolism by an unknown mechanism

Oral dose for MAC (adults): 15 mg kg^{-1} day^{-1}

	Weight (kg)		
	40–55	56–75	76–90
Daily, mg	800	1 200	1 600
Thrice weekly, mg	2 000	2 800	4 000

Suggested weight-based dosing in treatment of tuberculosis (MMWR 2003; Vol 52, RR-11)

Storage and stability: Store at room temperature. Protect from excessive moisture and heat

Pharmacokinetics

T_{max}: 2–4 h

Bioavailability: 75–80%

Half-life: 2.5–4 h

CSF penetration: considerable variation reported from 20% to 80%

Plasma protein binding: 10–30%

Metabolism/elimination: Primarily eliminated unchanged in the urine (50%); partial oxidative metabolism in the liver and 20% excreted in feces unchanged

Food effects: Absorption is not affected by food

Breast milk: Distributed into milk in concentrations similar to those in plasma

Dosage adjustment for organ failure: Dose every 24–36 h in patients with CrCl 10–50 mL/min; every 48 h if CrCl < 10 mL/min

Side-effects: Optic neuritis with decrease in visual acuity and fields, peripheral neuropathy, hyperuricemia, dermatitis, pruritus, hypersensitivity reaction, headache, malaise

Pregnancy: Category B

Isoniazid

Trade name: Nydrazid Injection (Apothecon); generic (various); Rifamate (in combination with rifampin); Rifater (in combination with pyrazinamide and rifampin)

Available formulations:

100 mg tablets	$0.05
300 mg tablets	$0.09
50 mg/ml syrup, 473 mL	$26.66
100 mg/mL, 10 mL vial for IM use	$249.00
Rifamate (isoniazid 150 mg + rifampin 300 mg) capsule	$2.65
Rifater (isoniazid 50 mg+pyrrzinamide 300 mg+ rifampin 120 mg) capsule	$1.96

Class: Antimycobacterial

Mechanism of action: Inhibition of mycolic acid synthesis; interference with metabolism of bacterial proteins, carbohydrates, and lipids. Isoniazid is bactericidal against both intracellular and extracellular organisms

Oral, IM, or IV dose: 5 mg/kg (max 300 mg) per day (plus pyridoxine 50 mg/day) or 15 mg/kg (max 900 mg) three times weekly (plus pyridoxine 100 mg three times weekly)

Storage and stability: Protect from light, air, and excessive heat. Keep in well-closed containers at room temperature

Pharmacokinetics

T_{max}: 1–2 h

Bioavailability: 90%

Half-life: 0.7–2 h in rapid acetylators; 2.3–3.5 h in rapid acetylators

CSF penetration: 90–100% of plasma concentrations at 3–6 h after oral dose

Plasma protein binding: 4–30%

Metabolism/elimination: Metabolized primarily in liver by acetylation. Acetylation status is determined genetically: persons may be rapid or slow acetylators

Food effects: Food may slightly reduce isoniazid concentrations

Breast milk: Distributed into breast milk

Dosage adjustment for organ failure: Administer 50% of normal dose in patients with CrCl<10 mL/min

Side-effects: Peripheral neuropathy, hepatitis, increased serum transaminases, gastrointestinal complaints, vitamin B_6 (pyridoxine) deficiency, pellagra, systemic lupus erythematosus, arthritis, ataxia, rash, fever

Pregnancy: Category C

Moxifloxacin

Trade name: Avelox

Available formulations:

Class: Fluoroquinolone

Mechanism of action: inhibits bacterial DNA topoisomerases required for bacterial DNA replication, transcription, repair, and recombination

Oral, or IV dose: 400 mg/day

Storage and stability:
Oral tablets: Store at 25°C, avoid humidity
IV solution: Store at 25°C, do not refrigerate. Refrigeration results in precipitation

Pharmacokinetics

T_{max}: 1–3 h after oral dose

Bioavailability: 90%

Half-life: 9–16 h

CSF penetration: good penetration in animal study, human data not available

Plasma protein binding: 50%

Metabolism/elimination: Metabolized via glucuronide and sulfate conjugation; not affected by the cytochrome P450 pathway. 15–20% excreted in the urine as unchanged drug

Food effects: Food may reduce the rate but not the extent of absorption

Breast milk: Distributed into breast milk

Dosage adjustment for organ failure: No dosage adjustment recommended in patients with renal or hepatic dysfunction

Side-effects: Nausea, headache, dizziness, nervousness, rash, QT prolongation, tendon rupture, interstitial nephritis

Pregnancy: Category C

Pyrazinamide

Trade name: Generic (Lederle); Rifater (combination with isoniazid and rifampin)

Available formulations:
Pyrazinamide 500 mg tablet $1.14
Rifater (pyrazinamide 300 mg + isoniazid 50 mg + rifampin 120 mg) $1.96

Class: Antimycobacterial

Mechanism of action: Bactericidal against intracellular *Mycobacterium tuberculosis* at acidic pH (<5.6)

Oral dose (adults):
Suggested weight-based dosing in treatment of tuberculosis (MMWR 2003; Vol 52, RR-11)

	Weight (kg)		
	40–55	56–75	76–90
Daily, mg	1000	1500	2000
Thrice weekly, mg	2000	3000	4000

Storage and stability: Store in well closed containers at room temperature

Pharmacokinetics

T_{max}: 1–4 h

Half-life: 9–10 h

CSF penetration: CSF and plasma concentration approximately equal

Plasma protein binding: 5–10%

Metabolism/elimination: Primarily renal excretion; 70% of dose excreted in urine within 24 h

Food effects: Can be given with or without food

Breast milk: Small amounts excreted in breast milk

Dosage adjustment for organ failure: Dosage reduction recommended in patients with renal dysfunction

Side-effects: Hyperuricemia, hepatotoxicity, arthralgia, myalgia, fever, gastrointestinal side-effects. May interfere with diabetic urine testing kits

Pregnancy: Category C

Rifabutin

Trade name: Mycobutin (Pharmacia & Upjohn)

Available formulations:
150 mg capsules $4.67

Class: Rifamycin antimycobacterial

Mechanism of action: Inhibits DNA-dependent RNA polymerase in certain bacteria; mechanism in MAC unknown

Oral dose (adults):
If not used with PIs or EFV: 300 mg/day
If used with EFV (without PIs): 450–600 mg/day
If used with PIs: 150 mg every other day or three times weekly

Storage and stability: Store at room temperature (15–30°C)

Pharmacokinetics

T_{max}: 2–4 h

Bioavailability: Approximately 53% in HIV-uninfected patients, but only 20% in HIV-infected patients

Half-life: 36–45 h

CSF penetration: Unknown

Plasma protein binding: 85%

Metabolism/elimination: Hepatic metabolism to multiple metabolites; 25-*O*-desacetyl metabolite has activity similar to parent drug. Metabolite excreted in feces and urine; substrate and inducer of CYP3A4-mediated metabolism

Food effects: Food may decrease the rate but not the extent of absorption

Breast milk: Unknown

Dosage adjustment for organ failure: Pharmacokinetics modified only slightly by renal and hepatic dysfunction

Side-effects: Discoloration of body fluids, rash, uveitis, neutropenia, thrombocytopenia, gastrointestinal disturbances

Pregnancy: Category B

Rifampin

Trade name: Rifadin (Hoechst Marion Roussel), Rimactane (Ciba Geneva); Rifamate (with isoniazid), Rifater (with isoniazid and pyrazinamide)

Available formulations:

150 mg capsules	$1.34
300 mg capsules	$1.91
600 mg IV vial	$74.40
Rifamate (isoniazid 150 mg + rifampin 300 mg) capsule	$2.65
Rifater (isoniazid 50 mg + pyrrzinamide 300 mg + rifampin 120 mg) capsule	$1.96

Class: Rifamycin antimycobacterial

Mechanism of action: Inhibition of DNA-dependent RNA synthesis in susceptible bacteria

Oral or IV dose: 10 mg/kg (up to 600 mg) once daily or three times weekly

Storage and stability:
Capsules: store in light-resistant container at room temperature
IV: Reconstitute with sterile water. Solution stable at room temperature for 24 h. Further dilution with D5W; use within 4 h

Pharmacokinetics

T_{max}: 1–4 h

Bioavailability: Approximately 90–95%

Half-life: 1.5–5 h

CSF penetration: Wide distribution to body tissues; CSF levels 10–20% of serum concentrations with inflamed meninges

Plasma protein binding: 60–90%

Metabolism/elimination: Metabolized in liver by cytochrome P450; excreted primarily in bile. Undergoes enterohepatic recirculation; potent inducer of CYP3A4-mediated metabolism

Food effects: Food may slightly reduce or delay absorption

Breast milk: Small amount may be distributed into breast milk

Dosage adjustment for organ failure: Hepatic disease: use with caution under frequent monitoring of liver function tests and clinical symptoms

Side-effects: Discoloration of body fluids, hepatotoxicity, nausea, abdominal cramps, heartburn, CNS disturbances such as headache, dizziness; flu-like symptoms, arthralgia, myalgia, thrombocytopenia, nephrotoxicity

Pregnancy: Category C

Streptomycin

Trade name: Generic (Pfizer)

Available formulations:

IM or IV preparation 1 g in 2.5 mL	$9.75

Class: Aminoglycoside antibiotic

Mechanism of action: Binds to 30S ribosomal subunit, inhibiting protein synthesis

IM or IV dose:
For patients $<$59 year old with normal renal function: 15 mg kg^{-1} day^{-1} (up to 1 g)
For patients $>$59 year old with normal renal function: 10 mg kg^{-1} day^{-1} (up to 750 mg)
Dose may be reduced to 2–3 times weekly after the first 2–4 months or after culture conversion

Storage and stability: Store ampoules in the refrigerator

Pharmacokinetics

T_{max}: 1 h

Half-life: 2.5 h (in patients with normal renal function)

CSF penetration: Low

Plasma protein binding: 35%

Metabolism/elimination: Eliminated primarily by glomerular filtration, with 80–95% of dose eliminated unchanged in urine

Breast milk: Small amounts excreted in breast milk

Dosage adjustment for organ failure: Requires adjustment in the presence of renal dysfunction. Significant removal by dialysis (25–50%)

Side-effects: Nephrotoxicity, ototoxicity (hearing loss, tinnitus, vertigo, dizziness), edema, rash, paresthesias, fever, neuromuscular blockade

Pregnancy: Category D. Aminoglycosides can freely cross placenta. Its use has been associated with bilateral, irreversible deafness in neonates exposed to the drug *in utero*. Must weigh the benefit to the mother against the potential risks to the fetus

AGENTS FOR TREATMENT OF *PNEUMOCYSTIS JIROVECI (CARINII)* PNEUMONIA (PCP) AND *TOXOPLASMA GONDII* INFECTIONS

Atovaquone

Trade name: Mepron (Glaxo Wellcome)

Available formulations:

Suspension (750 mg/5 mL), 210 mL	$778.79

Class: Antiprotozoal, anti-*Pneumocystis* agent

Mechanism of action: Inhibition of nuclear viral synthesis by inhibiting mitochondrial electron transport

Oral dose (adults):
For PCP treatment: 750 mg twice daily with food for 21 days
Prophylaxis: 1500 mg daily with food
For toxoplasmosis treatment: 1500 mg twice daily with food

Storage and stability: Store at 15–25°C; do not freeze

Pharmacokinetics

Bioavailability: 23–47%

Half-life: 30–84 h

CSF penetration: Less than 1% of plasma concentration

Plasma protein binding: More than 99%

Metabolism/elimination: Little or no excretion in urine; enterohepatic recycling with elimination in feces

Food effects: Absorption enhanced twofold with food; administer with meals

Breast milk: Animal data suggest distribution into breast milk

Dosage adjustment for organ failure: No dosage adjustment necessary

Side-effects: Rash, pruritus, nausea, diarrhea, headache, vomiting, fever, insomnia, asthenia, weakness, elevated serum transaminases, hyperglycemia, hyponatremia

Pregnancy: Category C

Clindamycin

Trade name: Cleocin (Pharmacia & Upjohn), generic (various)

Available formulations:

150 mg capsules	$ 1.19
300 mg capsules	$ 3.76
150 mg/mL, 4 mL IV	$ 4.31
150 mg/mL, 6 mL IV	$ 8.50

Class: Antibacterial with activities against *P. jiroveci* and *T. gondii*

Mechanism of action: Inhibits bacterial protein synthesis by attaching to the 50S subunit of bacterial ribosome

Dose:
IV: 600–900 mg every 6–8 h
PO: 300–450 mg every 6–8 h
For PCP: Use with primaquine × 14–21 days
For Toxoplasmosis: Use with pyrimethamine and leucovorin

Storage and stability:
Oral tablets: Store at 20–25°C
Parenteral preparations: Stable at room temperature

Pharmacokinetics

T_{max}: 45 min

Bioavailability: 90%

Half-life: 1.5–5.0 h

CSF penetration: Poor, even in the presence of inflamed meninges

Plasma protein binding: 60–95%

Metabolism/elimination: Extensively metabolized to clindamycin sulfoxide and *N*-dimethyl clindamycin

Breast milk: Detectable in human breast milk after oral and intravenous doses

Dosage adjustment for organ failure: Adjustment recommended in patients with active liver disease. No adjustment necessary in patients with renal impairment

Side-effects: Diarrhea, pseudomembranous colitis, rash, and ventricular arrhythmia reported after IV bolus of undiluted clindamycin solution

Pregnancy: Category B

Dapsone

Trade name: Generic (Jacobus)

Available formulations:

25 mg tablets	$0.20
100 mg tablets	$0.21

Class: Sulfone antimicrobial

Mechanism of action: Competitive antagonists of para-aminobenzoic acid (PABA) and prevent normal bacterial utilization of PABA for the synthesis of folic acid

Oral dose (adults):
For treatment of PCP (with trimethoprim): 100 mg daily × 14–21 days

For PCP prophylaxis alone: 100 mg daily or 50 mg twice daily
For PCP and toxoplasmosis prophylaxis: Dapsone 50 mg daily (+ pyrimethamine 50 mg/leucovorin 25 mg weekly); or (dapsone 200 mg + pyrimethamine 75 mg + leucovorin 25 mg) weekly

Storage and stability: Store in tight container at room temperature and protected from light

Pharmacokinetics

T_{max}: 4–8 h

Bioavailability: Near-complete absorption from GI tract

Half-life: 10–50 h

CSF penetration: Can penetrate into CSF

Plasma protein binding: 70–90%

Metabolism/elimination: Undergoes acetylation and hydroxylation in the liver (acetylation genetically determined); hydroxyalanine metabolite may be associated with hypersensitivity reactions

Food effects: Can be given without regard to meals

Breast milk: Excreted in high concentrations; neonatal hemolytic anemia has been reported. Weigh risk of neonatal exposure to benefits of treatment of maternal infection

Dosage adjustment for organ failure: None

Side-effects: Fever, rash, hepatitis, phototoxicity, gastrointestinal, peripheral neuropathy, glucose 6-phosphate dehydrogenase (G6PD) deficiency-associated hemolysis, methemoglobinemia, agranulocytosis, aplastic anemia

Pregnancy: Category C

Pentamidine

Trade name: Pentam 300, NebuPent (Fujisawa); generic (Abbott)

Available formulations:

Oral inhalation NebuPent 300 mg	$98.75
Pentamidine isethionate 300 mg injection	$53.44 (generic product)

Class: Antiprotozoal

Mechanism of action: Inhibition of dihydrofolate reductase and interference with aerobic glycolysis in protozoa

Dose
Inhaled dose (adults): PCP prophylaxis 300 mg once a month (using Respirgard II nebulizer)
IM/IV dose: 3–4 mg/kg once daily for 21 days; infuse IV over at least 1–2 h

Storage and stability: Oral inhalation reconstituted with 6 mL sterile water; stable for 48 h. IV preparation is reconstituted with sterile water and diluted with D5W 50 mg/250 mL; stable for 24 h at room temperature. Reconstituted solution in D5W should not be refrigerated, to avoid crystallization. Protect from light

Pharmacokinetics

Half-life: 6.4–9.4 h

CSF penetration: Minimal

Plasma protein binding: 69%

Metabolism/elimination: Extensive, prolonged uptake into tissues. Prolonged renal elimination over weeks appears to be the major route of elimination

Breast milk: Unknown

Dosage adjustment for organ failure: Half-life may be prolonged in patients with renal dysfunction, however, no dosage adjustment is recommended

Side-effects:
IV or IM: Nephrotoxicity, leukopenia, hypoglycemia, hyperglycemia, nausea, elevated serum transaminases, hypocalcemia, pancreatitis
IV: Hypotension and cardiac arrhythmia associated with rapid infusion
IM: Sterile abscess or pain at injection site
Aerosol: Cough, metallic taste, shortness of breath, dizziness, rash, nausea, congestion, bronchospasm

Pregnan cy: Category C

Primaquine Phosphate

Trade name: Generic (various)

Available formulations:

26.3 mg (15 mg base) tablet	$1.04

Class: Antimalarial

Oral dose: PCP treatment: 15–30 mg base daily with clindamycin for 14–21 days

Storage and stability: Store at room temperature

Pharmacokinetics

T_{max}: 1–2 h

Bioavailability: 96%

Half-life: 4–7 h

Metabolism/elimination: Extensively metabolized; 1% excreted renally

Breast milk: Unknown

Dosage adjustment for organ failure: No adjustment in renal failure. No recommendation for adjustment in hepatic failure, use with caution and monitor for toxicities

Side-effects: Acute hemolytic anemia in patients with G6PD deficiency, granulocytopenia, methemoglobinemia, abdominal pain, cramps

Pregnancy: Category C

Pyrimethamine

Trade name: Daraprim (GlaxoSmithKline)

Available formulations:
25 mg tablets $0.58

Class: Antitoxoplasmosis agent

Mechanism of action: Folic acid antagonist inhibition of dihydrofolate reductase

Oral dose (adults):
For toxoplasmosis treatment (use with sulfadiazine or clindamycin): Pyrimethamine 200 mg once, then 50–75 mg/day with sulfadiazine, then 25–50 mg/day
Note: use with leucovorin 5–25 mg/day to reduce bone marrow suppression
For PCP and toxoplasmosis prophylaxis (use with dapsone): Dapsone 50 mg daily (+ pyrimethamine 50 mg/leucovorin 25 mg weekly); or (dapsone 200 mg + pyrimethamine 75 mg + leucovorin 25 mg) weekly

Storage and stability: Store at 15–25ºC in a dry place and protect from light

Pharmacokinetics

T_{max}: 2–6 h

Bioavailability: Well absorbed

Half-life: 80–96 h

CSF penetration: 12–27%

Plasma protein binding: 7%

Metabolism/elimination: Metabolized hepatically to several metabolites, which are excreted in the urine

Food effects: Take with food or meals to minimize adverse GI effects

Breast milk: Approximately 5% of drug passed to infant in breast milk; discontinue nursing while on drug

Dosage adjustment for organ failure: Use with caution in the presence of hepatic disease

Side-effects: Nausea and vomiting, anorexia, megaloblastic anemia, leukopenia, thrombocytopenia, skin rash, hyperpigmentation

Pregnancy: Category C

Sulfadiazine

Trade name: Generic (various)

Available formulations:
500 mg tablets $1.44

Class: Sulfonamide antimicrobial

Mechanism of action: inhibits dihydropteroate synthase thus affecting synthesis of folic acid

Oral dose (use with pyrimethamine and leucovorin)
Toxoplasmosis treatment: 1000–1500 mg four times daily
Toxoplasmosis suppression: 500–1000 mg four times daily

Storage and stability: Store in well closed, light-resistant containers at 15–30ºC

Pharmacokinetics

T_{max}: 3–6 h

Bioavailability: More than 70%

Half-life: 7–17 h

CSF penetration: 40–60% of serum levels

Plasma protein binding: 38–48% bound to plasma proteins

Metabolism/elimination: Partially metabolized in liver by acetylation; metabolites and 43–60% unaltered parent drug in urine

Food effects: Food may delay but does not decrease absorption

Breast milk: Distributed into breast milk

Dosage adjustment for organ failure: Use with caution in the presence of renal failure to avoid crystalluria; alkalinizing the urine may reduce the incidence

Side-effects: Hypersensitivity reactions: fever, rash, myelosuppression, crystalluria, renal failure

Pregnancy: Category C

Trimethoprim/Sulfamethoxazole (TMP/SMX or Cotrimoxazole)

Trade name: Bactrim (Roche); Septra (GlaxoSmithKline); generics (various)

Available formulations

	Bactrim	Septra	Generic
400/80 mg tablet	$1.08	$1.17	$0.31
800/160 mg DS tablet	$1.95	$1.83	$0.36
Suspension (200 mg/40 mg/5 mL) 480 mL	$58.89		
IV (80 mg/mL and 16 mg/mL), 10 mL	$8.71		

Class: Antibacterial, ant i-*Pneumocystis* agent

Mechanism of action: Inhibition of sequential enzymes in pathway of folic acid synthesis

Oral dose (adults):
For PCP/Toxoplasma prophylaxis: One double-strength (DS) tablet once daily
Alternative dosing for PCP prophylaxis alone: one DS tablet three times a week or single-strength tablet once daily

For PCP treatment: 15–20 mg kg^{-1} day^{-1} (based on trimethoprim) in three or four divided doses
IV dose: PCP treatment: 15–20 mg kg^{-1} day^{-1} (based on trimethoprim) divided into three or four doses given every 6–8 h; infuse over 60–90 min; once stabilized, can switch to equivalent oral dose to complete a 21-day course

Storage and stability:
Tablets/suspension: store in well closed, light-protected containers at 15–25°C
IV: store vials at room temperature; admixtures with D5W stable for 2–6 h depending on concentration

Pharmacokinetics

T_{max}: 1–4 h; steady-state concentrations of TMP/SMX are ~1:20

Bioavailability: More than 90% for both agents

Half-life: TMP 6–17 h; SMX 8–11 h

CSF penetration: TMP 50% of plasma levels; SMX 40% of plasma levels

Plasma protein binding: TMP 44–62%; SMX 70%

Metabolism/elimination: 80% and 20% of TMP and SMX, respectively, are recovered unchanged in the urine. SMX metabolized by *N*-acetylation and conjugation

Food effects: Can be given without regard to meals

Breast milk: Both agents are distributed into breast milk

Dosage adjustment for organ failure: Recommended to reduce dose by 50% in patients with CrCl 15–30 mL/min

Side-effects: Nausea, vomiting, anorexia, rash, fever, hypersensitivity reactions, photosensitivity, bone marrow suppression, headache, crystalluria, hepatotoxicity, pancreatitis. IV: thrombophlebitis

Pregnancy: Category C

ANTIFUNGAL AGENTS

Amphotericin B (Various Formulations)

Trade name: Fungizone (amphotericin B deoxycholate: Bristol-Myers Squibb); Abelcet (amphotericin B lipid complex: Liposome); Amphotec (amphotericin B colloidal dispersion: Sequus); AmBisome (liposomal amphotericin B: Fujisawa)

Available formulations:

Fungizone	50 mg/vial	$20.45
Abelcet	100 mg/20 mL vial	$240.00
Amphotec	50 mg/vial	$93.33
	100 mg/vial	$160.00
AmBisome	50 mg/vial	$188.40

Class: Polyene antifungal

Mechanism of action: Binds to sterols in fungal cell membrane leading to change in permeability

IV dose:
Fungizone: 0.25–1.5 mg/kg once daily or qod by slow infusion over 2–6 h. Test dose of 1 mg over 20–30 min may be given
Abelcet: 5 mg kg^{-1} day^{-1} at rate of 2.5 mg kg^{-1} h^{-1}
Amphotec: 3–6 mg kg^{-1} day^{-1} over 2 h
AmBisome: 3–5 mg kg^{-1} day^{-1} over 1–2 h

Storage and stability:
Fungizone: Fungizone vials should be kept under refrigeration. If left at room temperature, stable for 2 weeks to 1 month
Abelcet: Abelcet vials should be kept under refrigeration, protected from light
Amphotec: Amphotec vials can be stored at room temperature (15–30°C)
AmBisome: AmBisome vials can be stored at room temperature (25°C)

Pharmacokinetics

Half-life: Terminal elimination half-life of 15 days

CSF penetration: Less than 2.5% of those in plasma

Plasma protein binding: More than 90%

Metabolism/elimination: Slow excretion by the kidneys over weeks to months; metabolism poorly understood. Extensive uptake by various tissues/organs including liver, spleen

Breast milk: Unknown

Dosage adjustment for organ failure: Dosage adjustment in the presence of renal failure suggested by decreasing dose or extending frequency. If renal failure occurs while on therapy, may suggest using alternative antifungal agents

Side-effects (lipid formulations appear to have less systemic as well as infusion-related side-effects than amphotericin B deoxycholate): Nephrotoxicity, infusion-related side-effects (chills, rigors, fever, hypotension), electrolyte abnormalities (especially hypokalemia and hypomagnesemia), nausea, vomiting, muscle and joint pain, anemia

Pregnancy: Category B

Anidulofungin

Trade name: Eraxis (Pfizer, Vicuron)

Available formulations:

50 mg vials	Not yet available

Class: echinocandin antifungal

Mechanism of action: Inhibition of the synthese of *b* (1,3)D-glucan, which is an integral component of fungal cell wall synthesis

Spectrum of Antifungal Activities: *Aspergillus* spp., *Candida* spp.

Dosage:

For Esophageal Candidiasis: 100 mg IV × 1 dose, then 50 mg once daily × at least 14 days or until 7 days after symptom resolution

For Candidemia or Other Serious Candidal Infections: 200 mg IV × 1, then 10 mg once daily – duration based on response to therapy

Storage and stability: Store at 25°C

Pharmacokinetics

Half-life: 25–30 hours

Plasma protein binding: 84% bound

CSF penetration: human data unknown; animal studies showed extensive tissue penetration, including brain tissues.

Metabolism/elimination: believed to be not metabolized in the liver nor excreted in the urine; anidulafungin undergoes slow chemical degradation in physiologic pH

Breast milk: human data unknown

Dosage adjustment in organ failure: No dosage adjustment in patients with renal or hepatic insufficiency

Side-effects: Histamine-related reactions such as skin rash, facial swelling or flushing, or pruritus occur infrequently, and can be prevented by infusing each dose at <1.1 mg per minute. Hepatotoxicity reported in patients with or without underlying hepatic dysfunction.

Pregnancy: Category C

Caspofungin

Trade name: Cancidas (Merck)

Available formulations:

70 mg vials	$509.33
50 mg vials	$395.36

Class: echinocandin antifungal

Mechanism of action: Inhibition of the synthese of β (1,3) D-glucan, which is an integral component of fungal cell wall synthesis

Spectrum of antifungal activities: *Aspergillus* spp., *Candida* spp.

Dosage for invasive Aspergillosis or *Candida* esophagitis:
Loading dose: 70 mg IV
Maintenance dose: 50 mg IV every 24 h

Storage and stability: Lyophilized vials should be refrigerated at 2–8°C

Pharmacokinetics

Half-lives: β-phase: 9–11 h; γ-phase: 40–50 h

Plasma protein binding: Approximately 97% bound to albumin

CSF penetration: Unknown

Metabolism/elimination: Metabolized by hydrolysis and *N*-acetylation

Breast milk: Unknown

Dosage adjustment in organ failure:
In moderate hepatic insufficiency (Child–Pugh score 7–9): maintenance dose at 35 mg every 24 h
In severe hepatic insufficiency (Child–Pugh score >9): no experience
No dosage adjustment is necessary in patients with renal insufficiency; hemodialysis does not appreciably remove caspofungin acetate

Side-effects: Histamine-related reactions such as skin rash, facial swelling or flushing, or pruritus. One case of anaphylaxis was reported in clinical trials. Other adverse effects: elevated serum transaminases (higher incidence when used with cyclosporine), thrombophlebitis, nausea, vomiting, headache

Pregnancy: Category C

Clotrimazole

Trade name: Mycelex (Bayer)

Available formulation for oral candidiasis:

10 mg troche	$1.82

Class: Azole antifungal agent

Mechanism of action: Alters cell membrane permeability by binding with phospholipids

Oral dose: One troche five times a day; dissolve slowly in the mouth

Storage and stability: Store at room temperature below 30°C; do not freeze

Pharmacokinetics

Duration of local effect: Clotrimazole present in saliva for 3 h after dissolving troche

Bioavailability: Minimal absorption systemically

Breast milk: Minimal absorption suggests clotrimazole not present in significant amounts in breast milk

Dosage adjustment for organ failure: None

Side-effects: Nausea, vomiting, diarrhea, anorexia, altered taste

Pregnancy: Category C

Fluconazole

Trade name: Diflucan (Pfizer)

Available formulations:

50 mg tablets	$6.72
100 mg tablets	$9.78
150 mg tablets	$18.71
200 mg tablets	$17.51

50 mg/5 mL oral suspension, 35 mL	$40.32
200 mg/5 mL oral suspension, 35 mL	$146.45
200 mg/100 mL IV	$116.52
400 mg/200 mL IV	$170.13

Class: Triazole antifungal agent

Mechanism of action: Inhibits ergosterol production, necessary for synthesis of cell membrane

Dosages:
Oroespohageal candidiasis: 50–200 mg (or up to 400 mg) oral or IV once daily
Cryptococcal meningitis: Induction therapy: 400–800 mg PO or IV once daily; maintenance therapy: 200–400 mg PO once daily
Coccidiodomycosis: Induction therapy: 400–800 mg PO or IV once daily; maintenance therapy: 400 mg PO once daily

Storage and stability:
Tablets and oral suspension: Tight container below 30ºC
IV: Keep prepacked IV solution between 5ºC and 25ºC. Protect from freezing

Pharmaockinetics

T_{max}: 1–2 h

Bioavailability: More than 90%

Half-life: 32–40 h for HIV-infected patients

CSF penetration: 50–94% of plasma concentrations

Plasma protein binding: 11–12%

Metabolism/elimination: Primarily renally excreted; 80% of dose excreted unchanged; inhibitor of CYP3A4-mediated metabolism

Food effects: Pharmacokinetics unaffected by food

Breast milk: Excreted in breast milk at concentrations similar to plasma; weigh the benefit of treating maternal infection to the risk of exposure to infant. Avoid breast feeding if possible

Dosage adjustment for organ failure: 50% of usual dose in patients with CrCl <50 mL/min

Side-effects: Nausea, headache, rash, vomiting, abdominal pain, diarrhea, elevated serum transaminases

Pregnancy: Category C. Craniofacial, cardiac, and limb defects reported in four infants born to mothers exposed to fluconazole during the first trimester of pregnancy

Flucytosine

Trade name: Ancobon (Roche)

Available formulations:

250 mg capsules	$4.89
500 mg capsules	$9.74

Class: Fluorinated pyrimidine antifungal

Mechanism of action: Deaminated to fluorouracil by cytosine deaminase; fluorouracil is an antimetabolite that interferes with RNA and protein synthesis

Oral dose: 100–200 mg kg^{-1} day^{-1} divided into four doses

Storage and stability: Store in tight, light-resistant container at room temperature

Pharmacokinetics

T_{max}: Within hours

Bioavailability: 78–89%

Half-life: 2.4–4.8 h

CSF penetration: Approximately 80% of serum concentration

Plasma protein binding: 2–4%

Metabolism/elimination: 75–90% of dose excreted unchanged in urine

Food effects: Food affects the rate but not the extent of absorption

Breast milk: Unknown

Dosage adjustment for organ failure:
Renal impairment: Requires dosage adjustment, maintain peak serum levels (2 h after oral dose) at less than 100 μg/mL
Hemodialysis: 20–50 mg/kg immediately after dialysis, q48–72 h

Side-effects: Nausea, vomiting, diarrhea, bone marrow suppression, elevated serum transaminases, urticaria, pruritus, photosensitivity

Pregnancy: Category C

Itraconazole

Trade name: Sporanox (Janssen)

Available formulations:

100 mg capsules	$9.96
10 mg/mL oral solution, 150 mL	$141.16
10 mg/mL IV preparation, 250 mg ampule	$213.41

Class: Triazole antifungal agent

Mechanism of action: Inhibits ergosterol production, necessary for synthesis of cell membrane

Oral dose (adults): 100–400 mg daily

Intravenous dose (adults): 200–400 mg daily

Storage and stability:
IV: Keep at <25ºC, protect from light, do not freeze
Capsule: Keep at 15–25ºC, protect from light and moisture
Oral solution: Keep at <25ºC, do not freeze

Pharmacokinetics

T_{max}: 3–5 h (capsules, under fed condition) or 2.5 h (oral solution, under fasting condition)

Bioavailability: 55% (capsules – absorption impaired in the presence of high stomach pH) – higher bioavailability for oral solution taken under fasting condition

Half-life: 35–64 h

CSF penetration: Negligible

Plasma protein binding: 99.8%

Metabolism/elimination: Extensive hepatic metabolism to multiple metabolites including major metabolite (hydroxyitraconazole). Less than 1% of dose excreted renally. Inhibits CYP3A4-mediated metabolism

Food effects: Capsules require administration with food or cola beverage; food impair absorption of oral solution

Breast milk: Excreted into breast milk; should be avoided in nursing mothers

Dosage adjustment for organ failure: No change for oral itraconazole is required in the presence of renal dysfunction. For IV preparation, not recommended in patients with CrCl <30 mL/min due to the potential accumulation of hydroxypropyl-(beta)-Cyclodextrin (a vehicle in this formulation). Use with caution in presence of hepatic disease

Side-effects: Nausea, vomiting, diarrhea, dyspepsia, flatulence, hepatotoxicity, rash, headache, dizziness, fatigue, congestive heart failure, peripheral edema, pulmonary edema, hypokalemia, sexual dysfunction

Pregnancy: Category C

Ketoconazole

Trade name: Nizoral (Janssen)

Available oral formulation:

200 mg tablets $4.55

Class: Imidazole antifungal

Mechanism of action: Impairs synthesis of ergosterol, leading to increased permeability of fungal cell membrane

Oral dose: 200–400 mg once daily

Storage and stability: Store at 15–30°C, protect from moisture

Pharmacokinetics

T_{max}: 1–2 h

Bioavailability: 75%, requires acidic pH for optimal absorption

Half-life: Biphasic elimination, with half-life of 2 h during the first 10 h, then 8 h thereafter

CSF penetration: Negligible

Plasma protein binding: 91–99%

Metabolism/elimination: Metabolized extensively in liver; 85–90% excreted in bile and feces. Inhibits CYP3A4-mediated metabolism

Food effects: Can be taken with food or without food

Breast milk: Can be excreted into breast milk; should be avoided or use alternative antifungal agent

Dosage adjustment for organ failure: Careful monitoring of LFTs required in patients with history of liver disease; not altered in renal failure; not dialyzable

Side-effects: Nausea, vomiting, abdominal pain, decrease in testosterone, hepatotoxicity, adrenal insufficiency with high doses, hypertension, alopecia, gynecomastia, rash, pruritus, myalgia, arthralgia

Pregnancy: Category C

Micafungin

Trade name: Mycamine (Fujisawa)

Available formulations:

50 mg vials $93.50

Class: Echinocandin antifungal

Mechanism of action: Inhibition of the synthesis of β (1,3) D-glucan, which is an integral component of fungal cell wall synthesis

Spectrum of antifungal activities: *Aspergillus* spp., *Candida* spp.

Dosage: 150 mg IV every 24 h

Storage and stability: Store powder at 25°C

Pharmacokinetics

Half-life: 14–15 h

Plasma protein binding: >99% bound to albumin

CSF penetration: Unknown

Metabolism/elimination: metabolized in the liver to three metabolites

Breast milk: presence in milk in lactating rat; human data unknown

Dosage adjustment in organ failure: No dosage adjustment in patients with renal insufficiency or with moderate liver impairment; no data in patients with severe liver damage

Side-effects: Histamine-related reactions such as skin rash, facial swelling or flushing, or pruritus. Other adverse effects: elevated serum transaminases, thrombophlebitis, nausea, vomiting, headache, hemolysis, hemolytic anemia

Pregnancy: Category C

Nystatin

Trade names: Mycostatin (Apothecon); Nilstat (Lederle); Nystex (Savage); generics (various)

Available formulations:

100 000 U/mL, 60 mL $16.94

Class: Polyene antifungal

Mechanism of action: Binds to sterols in cell membrane, resulting in changes in membrane permeability

Oral dose: 500 000 U (5 mL) swish and spit (or swallow) four times daily

Storage and stability: Store at room temperature

Pharmacokinetics:

Bioavailability: Negligible absorption

Metabolism/elimination: Eliminated unchanged in stool

Food effects: Topical agent, not affected by food

Breast milk: Not systemically absorbed

Dosage adjustment for organ failure: None

Side-effects: Nausea and vomiting, diarrhea, oral irritation or sensitization, taste perversion

Pregnancy: Category C

Voriconazole

Trade name: Vfend (Pfizer)

Available formulations:

50 mg tablets	$8.84
200 mg tablets	$35.37
45 g oral powder for suspension	$643.68
200 mg IV	$110.32

Class: Triazole antifungal

Mechanism of action: Inhibits fungal cytochrome P450-dependent ergosterol synthesis

IV dose: 6 mg/kg every 12 h × 24 h, then 4 mg/kg every 12 h

Oral maintenance dose: 200 mg orally every 12 h, may be increased to 300 mg every 12 h if therapeutic response is not achieved

Storage and stability:
IV: Unreconstituted powder should be stored at 15–30°C, protect from moisture
Oral tablets: Store at 15–30°C
Oral powder for suspension: Unreconstituted oral powder should be refrigerated at 2–8°C. Once reconstituted, the oral suspension should be kept in a tight container at 15–30°C, do not refrigerate or freeze. Unused portion should be discarded after 14 days

Pharmacokinetics (Large Interpatient Variability)

T_{max}: 1–2 h

Bioavailability: 96%, oral absorption reduced with food

Half-life: Approximately 6 h (large interpatient variability)

CSF penetration: CSF level detected in some reports

Plasma protein binding: 58%

Metabolism/elimination: Metabolized extensively in liver via CYP 2C19, 2C9, and 3A4. Voriconazole is a substrate and inhibitor of these enzymes

Food effects: Food significantly reduces voriconazole absorption – should be taken at least 1 h before or 1 h after meal

Breast milk: Unknown

Dosage adjustment for organ failure:
For renal insufficiency: Oral voriconazole can be used; IV therapy should be avoided if CrCl <50 mL/min unless benefit outweighs the risk of accumulation of sulfobutyl ether beta-Cyclodextrin sodium (SEBCD), a vehicle of the IV preparation
For hepatic insufficiency: In patients with mild to moderate hepatic insufficiency (Child–Pugh Class A and B): IV – loading dose of 6 mg/kg every 12 h ×2, then 2 mg/kg every 12 h; PO – dose at 100 mg every 12 h. Voriconazole is not recommended in patients with severe hepatic insufficiency unless benefit outweighs the risk

Side-effects: Nausea, vomiting, abdominal pain, photosensitivity, visual disturbances, neuropsychiatric disturbances, hepatotoxicity, infusion-related anaphylactoid reactions, QT prolongation, and rarely arrhythmia

Pregnancy: Category D – can cause fetal harm. Not recommended in pregnant women unless no other alternative and benefits to the mother outweigh the risks to the fetus

ANTICYTOMEGALOVIRUS, ANTIHERPES SIMPLEX VIRUS, AND ANTIVARICELLA-ZOSTER VIRUS AGENTS

Acyclovir

Trade name: Zovirax (GlaxoSmithKline); generic (various)

Available formulations:

Dosage, Formuations	Zovirax Cost	Generic Product
200 mg capsules	$1.78	$0.14
400 mg tablets	$3.45	$0.44
800 mg tablets	$6.70	$0.87
200 mg/5 mL oral suspension, 473 mL	$147.12	$137.77
500 mg IV preparation	$78.56	$56.51
5% ointment, 3 g	$26.51	
5% cream, 2 g	$37.04	

Class: Purine nucleoside analog antiviral

Mechanism of action: Converted intracellularly to triphosphate metabolite, which interferes with DNA polymerase and inhibits viral DNA synthesis; active against HSV and VZV

Oral dose:
HSV infections: 200 mg five times per day or 400 mg three times daily or 800 mg twice daily
Herpes zoster infections: 800 mg five times per day

IV dose:
HSV: 5 mg/kg every 8 h, administer each dose at least over 1 h
Herpes zoster infection: 10 mg/kg q8h administer at least over 1 h

Storage and stability:
Oral tablets, suspension, and topical products: store at 15–25°C
IV: Store powder for IV use and solution after reconstitution at 15–25°C. Solution should not be refrigerated as acyclovir precipitates at low temperature

Pharmacokinetics

T_{max}: 1.5–2.5 h

Bioavailability: 10–20%

Half-life: 2.5–3.3 h

CSF penetration: Approximately 50% of serum concentration

Plasma protein binding: 9–33%

Metabolism/elimination: Excreted primarily in urine; 30–90% of dose recovered in urine

Food effects: Absorption is unaffected by food; give without regard to meals

Breast milk: Distribution into breast milk in concentrations similar to maternal plasma concentration

Dosage adjustment for organ failure: Adjust in the presence of renal dysfunction in patients receiving IV therapy

Side-effects:
IV: phlebitis irritation at site, nausea and vomiting, pruritus, CNS changes, crystalluria, and renal failure associated with rapid IV infusion
Oral: nausea and vomiting, diarrhea, headache, dizziness, rash, asthenia

Pregnancy: Category B

Cidofovir

Trade name: Vistide (Gilead)

Available formulations:

IV: 75 mg/mL, 5 mL amp	$888.00

Class: Antiviral

Mechanism of action: Converted to cidofovir diphosphate, which inhibits CMV DNA polymerase

IV dose for CMV retinitis:
Induction: 5 mg/kg IV over 1 h per week for two consecutive weeks
Maintenance: 5 mg/kg IV over 1 h every other week
Note: Must be administered with probenecid: 2 g orally 3 h prior to dose, then 1 g orally 2 and 8 h after completion of the infusion (4 g total)
Hydration: Normal saline 1 L immediately before each infusion; if tolerated, another liter of normal saline is recommended during or immediately after cidofovir infusion

Storage and stability: Store vials at room temperature. Admixture in 100 mL normal saline stable in refrigerator for 24 h

Pharmacokinetics

Half-life: 2.6 h (intracellular half-life of metabolite 24–65 h)

CSF penetration: Undetectable concentrations in CSF in limited number of patients

Plasma protein binding: Less than 1%

Metabolism/elimination: Eliminated primarily by renal excretion

Breast milk: Unknown

Dosage adjustment for organ failure:
Reduce from 5 to 3 mg/kg for an increase in creatinine of 0.3–0.4 mg/dL above baseline. Discontinue for an increase in creatinine of 0.5 mg/dL or more above baseline or development of 3+ proteinuria. Not recommended for patients with baseline serum creatinine higher than 1.5 mg/dL, CrCl 55 mL/min or less, or 2+ proteinuria or more

Side-effects: Nephrotoxicity (rarely manifested as Fanconi syndrome), proteinuria, neutropenia, nausea and vomiting, diarrhea, hypotony, iritis, uveitis, abdominal pain, rash (most likely associated with probenecid), fever, anemia, headache, ototoxicity

Pregnancy: Category C

Famciclovir

Trade name: Famvir (SmithKline Beecham)

Available formulations:

125 mg tablets	$4.27
250 mg tablets	$4.65
500 mg tablets	$9.34

Class: Antiviral – guanosine nucleoside analog

Mechanism of action: Prodrug of penciclovir, hydrolyzed *in vivo* to penciclovir and phosphorylated to penciclovir triphosphate, which inhibits viral DNA synthesis

Oral doses:
Herpes zoster: 500 mg every 8 h
Recurrent genital herpes: 250–500 mg every 12 h
HSV suppression: 250 mg every 12 h

Storage and stability: Store at room temperature

Pharmacokinetics

T_{max}: 0.7–0.9 h; rapid conversion to penciclovir

Bioavailability: 77%

Half-life: 2–3 h (penciclovir)

CSF penetration: Unknown

Plasma protein binding: Less than 20%

Metabolism/elimination: Rapid conversion to penciclovir and 6-Deoxypenciclovir; 73% of penciclovir excreted through the kidneys

Food effects: Food does not affect bioavailability of penciclovir; give without regard to meals

Breast milk: It is not known if famciclovir or penciclovir is distributed into milk in humans

Dosage adjustment for organ failure: Adjust for renal dysfunction

Side-effects: Nausea, headache, vomiting, diarrhea, pruritus

Pregnancy: Category B

Foscarnet

Trade name: Foscavir (Astra)

Available formulations:

IV: 24 mg/mL, 250 mL	$83.24
IV: 24 mg/mL, 500 mL	$165.78

Class: Pyrophosphate analog antiviral

Mechanism of action: Inhibition of viral DNA polymerase (does not require activation by kinases)

Dosage:
CMV induction: 90 mg/kg IV every 12 h (1.5–2.0 h infusion) × 2–3 weeks or 60 mg/kg every 8 h (1 h or longer infusion) × 2–3 weeks
CMV maintenance: 90–120 mg/kg IV once daily over 2 h
HSV dose: 40 mg/kg every 8–12 h (at least 1 h infusion) × 2–3 weeks or until healing of herpetic lesions
Hydration: Each dose should be accompanied by 500–1000 mL IV hydration (preferably 0.9% sodium chloride) to reduce nephrotoxicity

Storage and stability: Store at 15–30°C, protect from excessive heat

Pharmacokinetics

Half-life: 3–6 h

CSF penetration: Variable, reported to be 13–103% of plasma concentration

Plasma protein binding: 14–17%

Metabolism/elimination: 80–90% excreted unchanged in the urine; eliminated by both tubular secretion and glomerular filtration

Breast milk: Animal data suggest foscarnet is secreted in breast milk at concentrations higher than those in plasma

Dosage adjustment for organ failure: Adjustment in renal impairment

Side-effects: Nephrotoxicity (may be reduced with 750–1000 mL hydration accompanying each dose), mineral and electrolyte imbalances (hypocalcemia, hypophosphatemia, hypomagnesemia, hypokalemia), seizures, granulocytopenia, anemia, nausea, vomiting, headache, penile ulceration, thrombophlebitis (if peripheral IV used)

Pregnancy: Category C

Ganciclovir

Trade name: Cytovene (Roche); Vitrasert (Chiron Vision)

Available formulations:

250 mg capsules	$4.80
500 mg capsules	$9.62
500 mg/10 mL IV vial	$44.81
4.5 mg ocular implant	$5000.00

Class: Guanine derivative nucleoside antiviral

Mechanism of action: Phosphorylated to triphosphate metabolite, which inhibits viral DNA synthesis

Oral dose: 1 g three times daily with food (as maintenance therapy) – if available, valganciclovir should be used in place of oral ganciclovir

IV dose:
Induction: 5 mg/kg IV every 12 h × 14–21 days
Maintenance: 5 mg/kg once daily IV or 6 mg/kg once daily IV × 5 days a week

Ocular Implant: 4.5 mg insert, should be replaced every 6–9 months if indicated

Storage and stability: Store capsules at 5–25°C, unreconstituted IV vials at <40°C, and ocular insert at 15–30°C, protect from freezing, excessive heat or light

Pharmacokinetics

T_{max}: Capsules: 4.5–15.6 h

Bioavailability: Capsules ~5% (fasting) to 9% (with food)

Half-life: 2.5–5.0 h

CSF penetration: 24–70% of serum concentrations

Plasma protein binding: 1–2%

Metabolism/elimination: Eliminated primarily by renal excretion with more than 90% of dose recovered in the urine unmetabolized

Food effects: Food increases overall bioavailability

Breast milk: Unknown

Dosage adjustment for organ failure: Adjustment in renal insufficiency

Side-effects:
Systemic therapy (IV > oral): Neutropenia, thrombocytopenia, anemia, CNS disturbances (headache, confusion, seizures), fever, nausea, vomiting, pruritus, thrombophlebitis (IV only). Ocular insert: retinal detachment, transient loss in visual acuity, vitreous hemorrhage, uveitis, cataracts, macular abnormalities

Pregnancy: Category C, teratogenic in animals, generally not recommended during pregnancy unless benefits to the mother outweigh the risks to the fetus

Valacyclovir

Trade name: Valtrex (GlaxoSmithKline)

Available formulations:

500 mg tablets	\$4.92
1 g tablets	\$8.97

Class: Antiviral (L-valyl ester of acyclovir)

Mechanism of action: Rapidly converted to acyclovir by intestinal and/or hepatic first-pass metabolism. Acyclovir undergoes phosphorylation in the presence of viral thymidine kinase to its active triphosphate form which inhibits viral DNA synthesis

Oral dose:
Herpes zoster: 1 g three times daily × 7 days
First episode genital herpes: 1 g twice daily × 10 days
Recurrent genital herpes: 500 mg twice daily × 3–5 days
Chronic HSV suppression: 500 mg twice daily or 1 g once daily

Storage and stability: Store at 15–25°C

Pharmacokinetics

T_{max}: Rapid conversion to acyclovir by first-pass metabolism; peak acyclovir concentration at 1–3 h

Bioavailability: 54%

Half-life: 2.5–3.3 h (acyclovir)

CSF penetration: 50% of serum concentration (acyclovir)

Plasma protein binding: 13.5–17.9%

Metabolism/elimination: Rapid conversion to acyclovir. Acyclovir primarily excreted in urine; 30–90% of dose recovered in urine

Food effects: Food does not affect absorption; give without regard to meals

Breast milk: Acyclovir is distributed to breast milk in concentrations similar to those in maternal plasma

Dosage adjustment for organ failure: Adjust for renal dysfunction

Side-effects: Nausea, headache, vomiting, diarrhea, abdominal pain, dizziness. Thrombotic thrombocytopenic purpura with hemolytic–uremic syndrome has been reported with doses of 8 g/day in immunocompromised patients, including advanced HIV-infected patients

Pregnancy: Category B

Valganciclovir

Trade name: Valcyte (Roche)

Available formulation:

450 mg tablet	\$31.73

Class: Pro-drug of ganciclovir (a guanine derivative nucleoside antiviral)

Mechanism of action: L-valyl ester (prodrug) of ganciclovir. After oral administration, valganciclovir is rapidly converted to ganciclovir. Ganciclovir is converted to ganciclovir triphosphate intracellularly which produces its virustatic effect by inhibition of viral DNA synthesis

Oral dose:
Induction therapy for CMV retinitis: 900 mg twice daily × 21 days with food
Maintenance therapy for CMV retinitis: 900 mg once daily with food

Storage and stability: Store at 25°C

Pharmacokinetics

T_{max}: 1.5 to 2 h (as ganciclovir)

Bioavailability: 60% (as ganciclovir)

Half-life: 4 h

Plasma protein binding: 1–2% (for ganciclovir)

Metabolism/elimination: Valganciclovir is rapidly hydrolyzed to ganciclovir. Major route of elimination is through renal excretion

Food effects: High-fat meal increases oral bioavailability of ganciclovir by 30%

Breast milk: No information available; because of the potential serious adverse events in infants, mothers should be instructed not to breastfeed if they are receiving valganciclovir tablet

Dosage adjustment in organ failure: Adjustment in patients with renal insufficiency

Side-effects: Anemia, neutropenia, thrombocytopenia, diarrhea, nausea, vomiting, abdominal pain, fever, headache, insomnia, sedation, seizure, confusion, retinal detachment

Pregnancy: Category C, teratogenic in animals. Valganciclovir is not recommended during pregnancy unless benefits to the mother outweigh risks to the fetus

HEPATITIS B AND HEPATITIS C TREATMENT

Adefovir Dipivoxil

Trade name: Hepsera (Gilead)

Available formulation:

10 mg tablet	\$1.54

Class: Diester prodrug of adefovir. Adefovir is an acyclic nucleotide analog

Mechanism of action: Adefovir is phosphorylated by cellular kinase to the active metabolite, adefovir diphosphate, which inhibits HBV DNA polymerase

Oral dose: 10 mg once daily

Storage and stability: Store at 25°C in the original container

Pharmacokinetics

T_{max}: 1.75 h

Bioavailability: 59%

Half-life: 4 h

Plasma protein binding: <4%

Metabolism/elimination: Adefovir is primarily renally excreted in the kidney by glomerular filtration and active tubular secretion

Food effects: No effect on bioavailability

Breast milk: No information available

Dosage adjustment in organ failure: Adjustment in patients with renal insufficiency

Side-effects: Inflammatory flare of hepatitis B infection may be seen soon after initiation of therapy; nephrotoxicity (rare but can occur), nausea, vomiting, headache

Pregnancy: Category C

Entecavir

Trade name: Baraclude (Bristol-Myers Squibb)

Available formulations:

0.5 mg tablet	$24.67
1.0 mg tablet	$24.67
0.05 mg/mL oral solution, 210 mL	$518.01

Class: Guanine nucleoside analog with selective activity against hepatitis B

Mechanism of action: Entacavir is phosphorylated to its triphosphate form which inhibits the activity of HBV polymerase

Oral dose:
For lamivudine-naive patients: 0.5 mg once daily on an empty stomach
For lamivudine-experienced patients: 1.0 mg once daily on an empty stomach

Storage and stability: Both oral tablet and oral solution can be stored at 25°C. Oral solution should be protected from light

Pharmacokinetics

T_{max}: 0.5–1.5 h

Bioavailability: 100% (oral tablet as compared to oral solution)

Half-life: Entecavir appears to be extensively distributed to different tissue compartments, with slow elimination rate. The terminal half-life is estimated to be between 128 and 149 h

Plasma protein binding: 13%

Metabolism/elimination: Entecavir is primarily renally excreted in the kidney by glomerular filtration and tubular secretion

Food effects: Food can reduce C_{max} by 44–46% and AUC by 18–20%. It should be taken at least 2 h before meal or 2 h after meal

Breast milk: Entecavir is excreted in milk in rats. No human experience at this point. Mothers should be discouraged from breastfeeding while taking entecavir

Dosage adjustment in organ failure: Adjustment in patients with renal insufficiency

Side-effects: Inflammatory flare of hepatitis B infection may be seen soon after initiation of therapy; headache, fatigue, diarrhea, dyspepsia

Pregnancy: Category C

Interferon-alfa 2b

Trade name: Roferon A (Roche), Intron A (Schering–Plough)

Available formulations: Various: 3–50 million units/vial. Approximately $35/3 million units

Class: Recombinant antitumor, antiviral, and immunomodulatory cytokine

Mechanism of action: Various intracellular mechanisms including induction of specific enzymes, suppression of cell proliferation, augmentation of cytotoxicity and phagocytosis, and inhibition of viral replication

Dose:
Kaposi sarcoma: 30 MIU/m^2 three times weekly IM or SC
Hepatitis B infection: 10 MIU three times weekly IM or SC or 5 MIU daily IM or SC
Hepatitis C infection: 3 MIU three times weekly IM or SC

Storage and stability: Store both powder and solution under refrigeration (2–8°C)

Pharmacokinetics

T_{max}: IM or SC 3–12 h

Bioavailability: IM: 80%; SC: 90%

Half-life: 2 h

Metabolism/elimination: Primarily metabolized by enzymes in the kidney

Breast milk: Animal studies suggest excretion into human milk

Dosage adjustment for organ failure: Use caution in patients with renal and liver diseases

Side-effects: Flu-like symptoms (fever, myalgia, arthralgia, malaise, fatigue), nausea, vomiting, diarrhea, neutropenia, thrombocytopenia, elevated LFTs, abnormal thyroid function, ophthalmic complications, alopecia, rash, dermatitis, pneumonitis, pancreatitis, may cause or aggravate neuropsychiatric, autoimmune, ischemic, or infectious disorders

Pregnancy: Category C

Peginterferon-alfa 2a

Trade names: Pegasys (peginterferon-Alfa 2a, Roche)

Available formulations:

Pegasys 180 μg/mL	$404.24

Class: Immunomodulatory cytokine, antiviral

Mechanism of action (for hepatitis C treatment): not yet established

Dosage (for hepatitis C treatment): 180 μg SC once weekly

Storage and stability: Store under refrigeration at 2–8°C, protect from light. Do not freeze or shake

Pharmacokinetics

T_{max}: 72–96 h

Bioavailability: 60%

Half-life: 80 h (50–140 h)

Metabolism/elimination: Extent of liver metabolism versus renal elimination unknown

Breast milk excretion: Not known

Dosage adjustment in organ failure: Adjust in patients with significant renal and hepatic insufficiency

Side-effects: Flu-like symptoms (fever, myalgia, arthralgia, malaise, fatigue), nausea, vomiting, diarrhea, neutropenia, thrombocytopenia, elevated LFTs, abnormal thyroid function, ophthalmic complications, alopecia, rash, dermatitis, pneumonitis, pancreatitis, may cause or aggravate neuropsychiatric, autoimmune, ischemic, or infectious disorders

Pregnancy: Category C

Peginterferon-alfa 2b

Trade name: PEG-Intron (peginterferon-alfa 2b, Schering)

Available formulations:

50 μg	$354.35
80 μg	$372.04
120 μg	$390.66
150 μg	$410.18

Class: Immunomodulatory cytokine, antiviral

Mechanism of action (for hepatitis C treatment): not yet established

Doses (weight based, use in combination with ribavirin):

<50 kg	50 μg SC once a week
40–50 kg	64 μg SC once a week
51–60 kg	80 μg SC once a week
61–75 kg	96 μg SC once a week
76–85 kg	120 μg SC once a week
>85 kg	150 μg SC once a week

Storage and Stability: Store at room temperature

Pharmacokinetics

T_{max}: 15–44 h

Bioavailability: 60%

Half-life: 40 h (22–60 h)

Metabolism/elimination: renal clearance ~30%

Breast milk excretion: Not known

Dosage adjustment in organ failure: should be used with caution in patients with CrCl < 50 mL/min, monitor for excessive toxicities. Ribavirin should not be used in these patients

Side-effects: Flu-like symptoms (fever, myalgia, arthralgia, malaise, fatigue), nausea, vomiting, diarrhea, neutropenia, thrombocytopenia, elevated LFTs, abnormal thyroid function, ophthalmic complications, alopecia, rash, dermatitis, pneumonitis, pancreatitis, may cause or aggravate neuropsychiatric, autoimmune, ischemic, or infectious disorders

Pregnancy: Category C

Ribavirin (Oral)

Trade name: Copegus (Roche), Rebetol (Schering), generic products

Available formulation:

200 mg capsules	$7.30 – $10.59 (depends on brand)
40 mg/mL oral solution, 100 mL	$232.80

Class: Synthetic nucleoside analog

Mechanism of action: Exact mechanism against hepatitis C virus – unknown

Dosages (should always use in combination with interferon-alfa or peginterferon-alfa):

= 75 kg	600 mg qam, 600 mg qpm
<75 kg	400 mg qam, 600 mg qpm

Storage and stability: Store capsules at 25°C. Oral solution may be refrigerated at 2–8°C or stored at 25°C

Pharmacokinetics

T_{max}: 1–1.6 h after single dose; 3 h after multiple dosing

Bioavailability: 64%

Half-life: 298 h after multiple dosing

Metabolism/elimination: metabolized via (1) a reversible phosphorylation pathway; and (2) a degradative pathway; then ribavirin and its metabolites are excreted renally

Food effects: High-fat meal increases AUC by 70%, clinical significance not known; recommended to be taken with or without food

Breast milk: Not known. Given the potential risks of ribavirin to the newborn, women should be advised not to breastfeed or to delay ribavirin therapy

Dosage adjustment in organ failure: monitor for toxicities in patients with renal insufficiency. Not recommended in patients with CrCl < 50 mL/min

Side-effects: hemolytic anemia, pulmonary symptoms such as dyspnea, fatal and nonfatal myocardial infarction have been reported in patients who developed anemia during ribavirin therapy

Pregnancy: Category X – ribavirin is teratogenic and embryotoxic for all animal species tested. Should never be used in pregnant women

BIOLOGICS MISCELLANEOUS

Darbepoietin

Trade name: Aranesp (Amgen)

Available formulations:

25 μg/mL	$128.16
40 μg/mL	$205.08
60 μg/mL	$307.56
100 μg/mL	$512.64

Class: Erythropoiesis-stimulating protein closely related to erythropoietin

Mechanism of action: Stimulation of erythropoiesis by interacting with progenitor stem cell to increase red blood cell production

SC/IV dose (dosing based on patients with chronic renal failure):
Initial dose to correct anemia – 0.45 μg/kg per week, dosage requirement varies from patient to patient. Maintenance dose should be titrated based on hemoglobin (Hgb) response. Hgb target should not exceed 12 g/dL

Storage and stability: Store under refrigeration at 2–8°C. Vials should not be frozen or shaken and should be protected from light

Pharmacokinetics

T_{max}: SC: absorption is slow and rate limiting. Peak concentration at 24–72 h in patients with chronic renal failure and 71–123 h in cancer patients

Bioavailability: SC: 37% compared to IV

Half-life: IV: 25 h in patients with renal failure; SC: 49 h

CSF penetration: Unknown

Metabolism/elimination: Metabolism and degradation not well defined; only small amounts recovered in urine

Breast milk: Not established

Dosage adjustment for organ failure: None

Side-effects: Hypertension, thrombotic events, iron deficiency, bone pain, peripheral edema, polycythemia, nausea, myalgia, arthralgia, headache, and rarely, pure red cell aplasia

Pregnancy: Category C

Erythropoietin

Trade name: Epogen (Amgen); Procrit (Ortho Biotech)

Available formulations:

2000 U/mL vial	$26.92
3000 U/mL vial	$40.38
4000 U/mL vial	$53.83
10 000 U/mL vial	$134.59
40 000 U/mL vial	$568.00

Class: Synthetic biological hematopoietic growth factor

Mechanism of action: Stimulation of erythropoiesis

SC/IV dose: 50–100 units/kg per dose three times weekly or 40 000 units once-weekly. Dose may be titrated based on Hgb response. Hgb target should not exceed 12 g/dL

Storage and stability: Store at 2–8°C. Do not freeze or shake

Pharmacokinetics

T_{max}: SC: 5–24 h

Bioavailability: SC: 22–31% compared to IV, although serum levels persist after SC administration for 3–4 days

Half-life: IV: 4–13 h in patients with renal failure; SC: ~27 h in patients with chronic renal failure; 40 h in cancer patients

CSF penetration: Negligible

Metabolism/elimination: Metabolism and degradation not well defined; only small amounts recovered in urine

Breast milk: Not established

Dosage adjustment for organ failure: None necessary

Side-effects: Hypertension, thrombotic events, iron deficiency, bone pain, peripheral edema, polycythemia, nausea, myalgia, arthralgia, headache, and rarely, pure red cell aplasia

Pregnancy: Category C

Filgrastim

Trade name: Neupogen (Amgen)

Available formulations:

300 μg/mL vial, 1 mL	$215.40
480 μg/mL vial, 1.6 mL	$343.20

Class: Granulocyte colony-stimulating factor

Mechanism of action: Promotion of proliferation and maturation of neutrophil precursors

IV/SC dose: Initiate at 5 μg kg^{-1} day^{-1} and titrate to response. For IV administration, give as a short infusion

(15–30 min). Many HIV-infected patients only require once- or twice-weekly dosing

Storage and stability: Refrigerate at 2–8°C. Do not freeze or shake. Discard if left at room temperature for more than 24 h

Pharmacokinetics

T_{max}: SC dosing 2–8 h

Bioavailability: SC: ~70%

Half-life: 3.5 h

Metabolism/elimination: Not well established, although neutrophil endocytosis and degradation is thought to be involved

Breast milk: Not established

Dosage adjustment for organ failure: None

Side-effects: Bone pain, nausea, injection site reaction, hypersensitivity reaction (including anaphylaxis), increased uric acid, increased alkaline phosphatase, myelodysplastic syndrome (rare, dose, and duration (years) related)

Pregnancy: Category C

MISCELLANEOUS – OTHER MEDICATIONS

Albendazole

Trade name: Albenza (GlaxoSmithKline)

Available formulations:
200 mg tablets $1.58

Class: Anthelminthic

Mechanism of action: Inhibition of tubulin polymerization resulting in loss of cytoplasmic microtubules

Oral dose:
For Giardiasis (dose based on HIV-uninfected patients): 400 mg once daily × 5 days
For Strongyloides infections: 400 mg once daily × 3 days
For Neurocysticercosis:
>60 kg: 400 mg twice daily
<60 kg: 15 mg kg^{-1} day^{-1} divided twice daily

Storage and stability: Store at 20–25°C

Pharmacokinetics

T_{max}: 2–2.5 h

Bioavailability: <5%, improve with food

Half-life: 8–12 h (sulfoxide)

CSF penetration: 20–50% of plasma

Plasma protein binding: 70%

Metabolism/elimination: Hepatic metabolism to the sulfoxide metabolite, then undergoes further metabolism to the sulfone and other metabolites; primarily excreted in bile

Food effects: Administration with a high-fat meal results in four- to sixfold higher concentrations; grapefruit juice increases concentration by 3.2-fold

Breast milk: Excreted into milk in animal studies; however, since albendazole is poorly absorbed orally, the extent of distribution in breast milk is probably negligible

Dosage adjustment for organ failure: Closely monitor patients with hepatic disease

Side-effects: Elevated serum transaminases, abdominal pain, nausea, vomiting, constipation, headache, dizziness, vertigo, rash, fever, granulocytopenia, pancytopenia, and eosinophilia

Pregnancy: Category C

Paromomycin

Trade name: Humatin (Monarch)

Available formulations:
250 mg capsules $3.37

Class: Aminoglycoside antibiotic

Mechanism of action: Not significantly absorbed; acts directly on intestinal lumen; binds to 30S ribosomal subunit inhibiting bacterial protein synthesis

Oral dose:
Intestinal amebiasis: 25–35 mg kg^{-1} day^{-1} in three divided doses × 5–10 days
Cryptosporidium: some success with 500 mg qid × 6 weeks

Storage and stability: Store at 15–30°C in airtight containers

Pharmacokinetics

Bioavailability: Minimal or negligible absorption from GI tract; ~100% of dose excreted unchanged in feces

Breast milk: Excretion into breast milk not expected owing to poor oral absorption

Dosage adjustment for organ failure: None

Side-effects: Abdominal cramps, nausea, diarrhea, superinfection, malabsorption; nephrotoxicity or ototoxicity may occur in patients with inadvertent absorption of paromomycin due to bowel ulceration

Pregnancy: Negligible absorption suggests low risk to fetus

Adult Antiretroviral Dosing Guidelines

Alice K. Pau, PharmD

Chapter 81

Anti-Retroviral Drugs	Adult Dosages	Renal Function Adjustment	Storage Instructions	Food Considerations
Nucleos(t)ide Reverse Transcriptase Inhibitors (NRTIs)				
Abacavir (ABC, Ziagen) *Yellow, capsule-shaped tablet*: 300 mg *Oral solution:* 20 mg/mL Also see Epzicom and Trizivir	300 mg bid (2 tab/day) or 600 mg qd (2 tabl/day) *Hypersensitivity Registry*: 1-800-270-0425	Not necessary	***Tablets***: Room temperature ***Oral solution***: Room temperature or refrigerate, DO NOT FREEZE	Can be taken with or without food
Didanosine (ddI, Videx, Videx-EC) *EC caps*: white, opaque cap: 125, 200, 250, 400 mg *Buffered tabs*: White, round tablets: 25, 50, 100, 150 mg; 200 mg tablets (for once daily dosing only) *Sachets*: 167 and 250 mg; *Pediatric suspension*: 2 and 4 Gm Powder, final solution: 10 mg/mL	**>60 kg** 1–400 mg EC cap qd, or 2–100 mg bid (4 tab/day)*, or 2–200 mg qd (2 tab/day), or Sachet: 250 mg bid *With tenofovir*: 250 mg qd (1 cap/d) **<60 kg** 1–250 mg EC cap qd, or 1–100 mg + 1–25 mg bid*, or 1–100 mg tab + 1–150 mg tab qd, or 1–200 mg tab + 1–50 mg tab), or Sachet: 167 mg bid *With tenofovir*: 200 mg qd (1 cap/d)	**>60 kg (if use with tenofovir, use dosing recommendation as <60 kg)** CrCl / Tablet / EC cap / Sachet 30–59: 100 mg bid or 200 mg qd / 200 mg qd / 100 mg bid 10–29: 150 mg qd / 125 mg qd / 167 mg qd <10: 100 mg qd / 125 mg qd / 100 mg qd **<60 kg** CrCl / Tablet / EC cap / Sachet 30–59: 150 mg qd or 75 mg bid / 125 mg qd / 100 mg bid 10–29: 100 mg qd / 125 mg qd / 100 mg qd <10: 75 mg qd / use tablet / 100 mg qd **CAPD or Hemodialysis Pt:** Use same dose as CrCl < 10 mL/min	Room temperature in tightly closed container ***Tablet***: stable for 1 h in room temperature after dispersed in apple juice or water ***Sachet***: stable for 4 h after dissolved in water ***Suspension***: Mix with antacid, *store in refrigerator* for up to 30 days	Empty stomach; ≥1/2 h before or ≥2 h after meals; space apart with all protease inhibitors (except for Videx EC, which can be taken with indinavir) Take with water or apple juice

* When buffered tablets are used, 2 tablets should be taken at the same time for adequate buffering effect.

(*Continued*)

Anti-Retroviral Drugs	Adult Dosages	Renal Function Adjustment	Storage Instructions	Food Considerations
Nucleos(t)ide Reverse Transcriptase Inhibitors (NRTIs) (Cont'd)				
Emtricitabine (FTC, Emtriva) *Blue and white capsule*: 200 mg *Oral solution*: 10 mg/mL Also see Truvada and Atripla	*Oral capsule*: 200 mg qd (1 cap/day) *Oral solution*: 240 mg (24 mL) qd	CrCl / Capsule / Solution 30–49 / 200 mg q48h / 120 mg (12 mL) q24h 15–29 / 200 mg q72h / 80 mg (8 mL) q24h <15 / 200 mg q96h / 60 mg (6 mL) q24h or HD (dose after dialysis if dose is due on dialysis day)	***Oral tablets***: Room temperature ***Oral solution***: Store in refrigerator until dispensing, if stored at room temperature (up to 25°C), use within 3 months	Take with or without food
Lamivudine (3TC, Epivir) White, diamond shape tab: 150 mg Gray, diamond shape tab: 300 mg *Oral solution*: 10 mg/mL Also see: Combivir, Epizicom, and Trizivir	150 mg bid (2 tab/day) or 300 mg qd (1 tab/day)	CrCl (ml/min) / Dose 30–49 / 150 mg qd 15–29 / 150 mg qd, then 100 qd 5–14 / 150 mg qd, then 50 qd < 5 / 50 qd, then 25 qd Not enough data on hemodialysis	Room temperature	Take with or without food
Stavudine (d4T, Zerit) 40 mg – dark orange cap; 30 mg – light and dark orange cap; 20 mg – light brown cap; 15 mg – light yellow and dark red cap *Oral solution*: 1 mg/mL	⩾60 kg 40 mg bid (2 tab/day) <60 kg 30 mg bid (2 tab/day)	CrCL / >60 kg dose / <60 kg dose 26–50 / 20 mg q12h / 15 mg q12h ⩽25 / 20 mg q24h / 15 mg q24h No data on hemodialysis	Room temperature *Oral suspension*: Store in refrigerator after reconstitution. Stable for up to 30 days	Take with or without food
Tenofovir DF (TDF, Viread) 300 mg – Almond-shaped light blue film-coated tablet Also see: Truvada and Atripla	300 mg qd (1 tab/day)	CrCl / Dose >50 / 300 mg qd 30–49 / 300 mg q48h 10–29 / 300 mg twice weekly ESRD / 300 mg once weekly	Room temperature	Take with or without food
Zidovudine (ZDV, AZT, Retrovir) Blue and white cap – 100 mg; White, round tab – 300 mg; *Oral syrup*: 50 mg/5mL Also see: Combivir and Trizivir	300 mg bid (2 tab/day); or 200 mg tid (6 cap/day) **IV** – 10 mg/mL	100 mg TID or 300 mg qd in pts with severe renal impairment or on hemodialysis	Room temperature	Take with or without food
Fixed Dosage Combination NRTI Products (listed in alphabetical order by trade names)				
Atripla™ – EFV 600 mg + FTC 200 mg + TDF 300 mg Pink, capsule-shaped film-coated tablet	One tablet qHS (1 tab/day)	Fixed dose combination product – *not recommended* in pts with CrCl < 50 mL/min – use individual products	Room temperature	Avoid high fat meal

Anti-Retroviral Drugs	Adult Dosages	Renal Function Adjustment	Storage Instructions	Food Considerations
Fixed Dosage Combination NRTI Products (listed in alphabetical order by trade names) (Cont'd)				
Combivir 3TC 150 mg + ZDV 300 mg White, oblong tablet	One tablet bid (2 tab/day)	Fixed dose combination product – *not recommended* in pts with CrCl <50 mL/min – use individual products	Room temperature	Take with or without food
Epzicom ABC 600 mg + 3TC 300 mg Orange, film-coated, modified capsule-shapted tablet	One table qd (1 tab/day)	Fixed dose combination product – *not recommended* in pts with CrCl <50 mL/min – use individual products	Room temperature	Take with or without food
Truvada FTC 200 mg + TDF 300 mg Blue, capsule-shaped, film-coated tablet	One tablet qd (1 tab/day)	CrCl / Dose >50: 1 tablet QD 30–49: 1 tablet q48h <30: Fixed dose combination not recommended	Room temperature	With or without food
Trizivir ABC 300 mg + ZDV 300 mg + 3TC 150 mg Pale blue oblong tablet	One tablet bid (2 tablets/day)	Fixed dose combination product – *not recommended* in pts with CrCl <50 mL/min – use individual products	Room temperature	With or without food
Non-Nucleoside Reverse Transcriptase Inhibitors (NNRTIs)				
Delavirdine (DLV, Rescriptor) White oblong tab – 100 and 200 mg	400 mg tid (12 tab/day)	Not necessary Hemodialysis: no effect	Room temperature	W/ or w/o food, avoid taking w/ antacids, ddI, or H_2-blockers; acidic beverages ↑ absorption; Can mix 4 tablets in 3 oz of water to make a dispersion (drink promptly)
Efavirenz (EFV, Sustiva) Yellow capsule shaped tab – 600 mg Gold cap – 200 mg White cap – 100 mg Gold and white cap – 50 mg Also see Atripla	600 mg qhs (1 tablet or 3 cap/day)	Not necessary	Room temperature	Take on an empty stomach for both capsule and tablet per labelling (Note: This is a change from previous recommendation of avoiding high fat meal)
Nevirapine (NVP, Viramune) White oval tab – 200 mg Oral suspension – 50 mg/5 mL	200 mg qd × 14 days, then 200 mg bid (2 tab/day)	Not necessary Hemodialysis – data not available	Room temperature	No specific consideration

(Continued)

Anti-Retroviral Drugs	Adult Dosages	Renal Function Adjustment	Storage Instructions	Food Considerations
Protease Inhibitors (PIs)				
Amprenavir (APV, Agenerase) *Oral Solution*: 15 mg/mL Agenerase oral capsule no longer in market, switch pts to fosamprenavir	1400 mg bid (93 mL bid)	Not necessary	Room temperature	No food restriction *Oral solution contains propylene glycol* – contraindicated in children <4 years pregnant women, pts w/ renal or hepatic failure, and pts treated w/ disulfiram w/ disulfiram or metronidazoles *Oral solution should not be used with ritonavir oral solution*
Atazanavir (ATV, Reyataz) Blue/white capsule – 100 mg Blue/powder blue cap – 150 mg Blue/blue capsule – 200 mg	ATV 400 mg qd (2 cap/day) *with EFV, TDF, or for PI-experienced salvage therapy:* (ATV 300 mg + RTV 100 mg) qd	Not necessary	Room temperature	Take with food – improve biovailability and reduce variability
Darunavir (DRV, Prezista™) Orange, oval shaped, film-coated tablet – 300 mg	(DRV 600 mg + RTV 100 mg) BID	Not necessary	Room temperature	Take with food
Fosamprenavir calcium (fAPV, Lexiva) Pink capsule-like tablet – 700 mg *Oral suspension*: 50 mg	***ARV-naive patients***: fAPV1,400 mg bid; or (fAPV1,400 mg + RTV 200 mg) qd; or (fAPV 700 mg + RTV 100 ng) bid ***PI-experience patients***: (fAPV 700 mg + RTV 100 mg) bid (once daily rtv-boosted regimen is not recommended in these patients) ***Co-adminstration w/ EFV***: If qd fAPV is used – additional 100 mg rtv should be added (total 300 mg RTV)	Not necessary	Room temperature	No food restriction

Anti-Retroviral Drugs	Adult Dosages	Renal Function Adjustment	Storage Instructions	Food Considerations
Protease Inhibitors (PIs) (Cont'd)				
Indinavir (IDV, Crixivan) Off white capsules – 200 mg, 333 mg and 400 mg	As sole PI-IDV 800 mg q8 h (6 cap/day); or *With EFV or NVP (w/o RTV)*: IDV 1000 mg q8h (IDV 800 mg + rtv 100 or 200 mg) bid	Not necessary No data on dialysis	Store in tightly closed original container *Do not discard dessicant*	Empty stomach or w/light, low fat meals *Drink 1–2 L of fluid per day No food restriction if taken with ritonavir*
Lopinavir/ritonavir (LPV/RTV, Kaletra) Yellow film-coated ovaloid tablets –200 mg LPV + 50 mg RTV per tab *Oral solution*: 400 mg LPV/ 100 mg RTV per 5 mL	***Tablet formulation***: 2 tabs (400 mg LPV + 100 mg RTV) bid; or 4 tabs (800 mg LPV + 200 mg RTV) qd *If used w/EFV or NVP*: Treatment-naive pts – 2 tabs bid Treatment-experienced pts – 3 tabs (600 mg LPV + 150 mg RTV) bid *Note:* qd dosing is not recommended for pts with PI-experience or in pts taking EFV or NVP	Not necessary	***Tablets:*** Room temperature ***Oral solution:*** Pharmacy store in refrigerator until dispense For pts, if stored at room temperature discard after 2 months	***For tablets:*** Take with or without food ***Oral solution:*** Take with food Take one h before or two h after ddI Oral solution contains 42.4% alcohol
Nelfinavir (NFV, Viracept) Light blue capsule-shaped tab – 250 mg White oral tablet – 625 mg tablet *Oral powder*: 50 mg of nelfinavir/ Gm (scoop)	750 mg tid (9 tab/day) or 1250 mg bid (4–10 tab/day)	Not necessary Hemodialysis – Not likely to affect clearance	Room temperature ***Oral powder:*** once mixed with liquid, use within 6 h	Take with food or light snack

(*Continued*)

Anti-Retroviral Drugs	Adult Dosages	Renal Function Adjustment	Storage Instructions	Food Considerations
Protease Inhibitors (PIs) (Cont'd)				
Ritonavir (RTV, Norvir) Off white soft gel cap – 100 mg *Oral solution*: 600 mg/7.5 mL	600 mg (7.5 cm^3) bid (titration from 300–400 mg bid to full dose in <2 weeks; total 12 cap/day); lower dose (100–400 mg/day) when used as PK enhancer	Not necessary Hemodialysis – not likely to affect clearance	***Oral capsules***: Refrigerate – discard if left at room temperature for >30 days ***Oral solution***: Do not refrigerate; Advise pt not to use pass expiration date on bottle	With meals if possible At least 2.5 h apart from ddI. Oral solution can be taken w/ Ensure, chocolate milk or Advera
Saquinavir (Invirase, INV) Light brown and green hard gel cap – 200 mg Oval cylindrical, biconvex light orange to grayish or brownish-orange film-coated tablet – 500 mg	Only to be used with RTV boosting FDA approved dose: (INV 1,000 mg + RTV 100 mg) bid	Not necessary Hemodialysis – not likely to affect clearance	Room temperature	Take with a meal or at up to 2 h after a meal
Tipranavir (Aptivus, TPV) Pink, oblong soft gel cap – 250 mg	**Tipranavir should not be used without ritonavir** (TPV 500 mg + RTV 200 mg) bid	Not necessary Hemodialysis – not likely to affect clearance	After opening the bottle: may be stored at up to 25°C for up to 60 days	Take with food
Fusion Inhibitor				
Enfuvirtide (T-20, Fuzeon) 108 mg lyophilized powder per vial + sterile water for injection	90 mg SQ q12h Reconstitute with 1.1 mL of sterile water for injection, inject 1.0 mL per dose Rotate injection sites	Not necessary	Room temperature Reconstituted solution can be kept in refrigerator and use within 24 h	Not applicable

Anti-Retroviral Drugs	Adult Dosages	Renal Function Adjustment	Storage Instructions	Food Considerations
CCR5 Antagonist				
Maraviroc (MRV, Selzentry) Blue, biconvex, oral film-coated tablets – 150 mg and 300 mg	With potent CYP3A inhibitors (w/ or w/o CYP3A inducers, except for TPV/r): 150 mg BID With NRTIs, TPV/r, NVP, & other drugs that are not potent CYP3A inhibitors or inducers: 300 mg BID With CYP3A inducers including EFV (w/o a potent CYP3A inhibitor): 600 mg BID	Not necessary	Room temperature	Take with or without food
Integrase Inhibitor				
Raltegravir (RAL, Isentress)	400 mg bid	Not necessary	Room temperature	Take with or without food

Chapter 82

HIV/AIDS-Related Internet Resources

Richard A. Colvin, MD, PhD

INTRODUCTION

The Internet and proliferation of the personal computer allowed information to be shared among scientists, clinicians, and patients at a speed and to an extent not easily imagined even 20 years ago. Together, the Internet and the World Wide Web have now become invaluable and ubiquitous tools for clinicians, scientists, and patients to communicate about research questions, patient care issues, and problems they may be facing with their disease or current therapies.

In this appendix, a framework is developed as a guide to AIDS-related resources on the Internet. Due to the difficulty in categorizing so many of the important web sites, anyone interested in AIDS will likely find interesting information in all of the categories listed below. The corollary to this is that the best way to get a sense of the resources available on the World Wide Web is to spend time on a computer looking at the various web pages then linking to other sites, many of which are not listed here. General searches are most easily performed using Google (http://www.google.com) or Google Scholar (http://scholar.google.com). All of the sites listed in this chapter have been found to be useful and with up to date and accurate information. The websites listed are predominantly sites based in the United States; however, there are a number of European and African websites listed as well. As of March 2006 the links, as listed, are functional.

INDEX AND COMPREHENSIVE SITES

Table 82-1 lists sites that are either HIV and AIDS specific, or general medical sites that give HIV and AIDS significant attention. The sites listed in Table 82-1 are good initial launching points for

Table 82-1

Index and Comprehensive Sites

Site	WWW Address	Source	Corporate Sponsors?
Johns Hopkins	http://hopkins-aids.edu	Johns Hopkins University	Yes
HIV Insite	http://hivinsite.ucsf.edu	University of California at San Francisco	Yes
AEGIS	http://www.aegis.com	AEGIS, non-profit site	Yes
International Association of Physicians in AIDS Care	http://www.iapac.org	International Association of Physicians in AIDS Care	Yes
Medscape	http://www.medscape.com	Medscape.com, commercial site	Yes
Infectious Diseases Society of America	http://www.idsociety.org/HIVMA_Template.cfm?Section=HIVMA	Infectious Diseases Society of America	No
The Body	http://www.thebody.com	The Body, commercial site	Yes
The Body Pro	http://www.thebodypro.com	The Body, commercial site	Yes

recent information about HIV and AIDS and frequently have links to more specific topics about HIV and AIDS.

PATIENT EDUCATION AND ADVOCACY SITES

Perhaps the most interesting change the Internet has brought to the world of medicine is the change that has occurred in the patient–doctor relationship due to the plethora of clinical information available to patients on the World Wide Web. Now patients have easy access to the primary literature as well as reviews and anecdotes from others living with the same condition. Table 82-2 lists websites with accurate and reliable information that may be useful for persons living with HIV, as well as clinicians treating HIV-infected patients. Several of the websites also specialize in patient advocacy.

WOMEN AND AIDS

It has now become clear that the global HIV pandemic significantly affects women in unequal ways. Many websites dedicated to the unique situation of HIV-infected women have been developed over the past several years. These websites provide general information about HIV and AIDS in women as well as topics such as child bearing and HIV, raising HIV-infected children, and the effects of medications on women (Table 82-3).

CLINICIAN AND PATIENT CARE SITES

As exists for HIV-infected persons, there is a plethora of information on the web devoted to the clinical practice of HIV and AIDS care. The websites in Table 82-4 provide general information about HIV-infected patient management. These sites also provide information or links to information on HIV/AIDS-related medications, side effects, and drug interactions.

Websites that specifically provide HIV-related treatment guidelines are listed in Table 82-5. These sites are updated regularly. Recently, a free web-based encyclopedia, the Wikipedia, has been developed. This website is updated as soon as information becomes available. The Wikipedia (http://www.wikipedia.org) is particularly interesting because it is collaboratively written by anyone and is also constantly updated and corrected. The Wikipedia has very useful information on HIV and AIDS as well as HIV treatment guidelines.

HIV drug therapy is often complicated by drug–drug interactions. Many websites have user-friendly tables or search functions that list important drug–drug interactions (Table 82-6).

CLINICAL TRIALS AND VACCINE DEVELOPMENT

The Internet has been used as an effective communication device to keep investigators informed of trial progress, for

Table 82-2 Patient Education and Advocacy Sites

Web Site	Web Address	Source	Corporate Sponsors?
AEGIS	http://www.aegis.com	AEGIS, non-profit site	Yes
The Body	http://www.thebody.com	The Body, commercial site	Yes
National AIDS Treatment Advocacy Program	http://www.natap.org	National AIDS Treatment Advocacy Project, non-profit organization	Yes
Gay Men's Health Crisis	http://www.gmhc.org	Gay Men's Health Crisis, non-profit organization	Yes
POZ	http://www.poz.com	POZ, magazine designed for HIV infected persons	Yes
Project Inform	http://www.projinf.org	Project Inform, non-profit organization	Yes
Treatment Action Group	http://www.aidsinfonyc.org/tag/	TAG, non-profit organization	Yes
AIDS Action	http://www.aidsaction.org/	AIDS Action, non-profit organization	Yes
Being Alive	http://www.beingalivela.org/	Being Alive, non-profit organization	No
Positive Nation	http://www.positivenation.co.uk/	Positive Nation, U.K.	Yes
Treatment Action Campaign	http://www.tac.org.za/	Treatment Action Campaign, South Africa	No
WebMD	http://www.webmd.com/diseases_and_conditions/hiv_aids.htm	WebMD, commercial site	Yes

Women and AIDS

Table 82-3

Web Site	Web Address	Source	Corporate Sponsors?
The Body – Women and AIDS	http://www.thebody.com/whatis/women.shtml	The Body, commercial site	Yes
UNAIDS	http://womenandaids.unaids.org/	United Nations	No
NIAID	http://www.niaid.nih.gov/factsheets/womenhiv.htm	NIAID	No
CDC	http://www.cdc.gov/hiv/pubs/facts/women.htm	CDC	No
The Well Project	http://www.thewellproject.org	The Well Project, non-profit corporation	Yes
WORLD	http://www.womenhiv.org/	WORLD, not for profit organization	No
GMHC	http://www.gmhc.org/health/women.html	Gay Men's Health Crisis, non-profit organization	Yes
Women, Children, and HIV	http://www.womenchildrenhiv.org/	UMDNJ and UCSF	No
Women's Health.gov	http://www.4woman.gov/hiv/	US Department of Health and Human Services	No
Black Women's Health	http://www.blackwomenshealth.com/HIV_AIDS.htm	Black Women's Health	Yes
Facts about Women and AIDS	http://www.cdc.gov/hiv/pubs/facts/women.htm	CDC	No

Clinician Sites/Patient Care Information

Table 82-4

Web Site	Web Address	Source	Corporate Sponsors?
Johns Hopkins AIDS Service	http://www.hopkins-adis.edu	Johns Hopkins University	Yes
Johns Hopkins HIV Guide	http://www.hopkins-hivguide.org/)	Johns Hopkins University	Yes
HIV Insite	http://hivinsite.ucsf.edu	University of California at San Francisco	Yes
International AIDS Society – USA	http://iasusa.org	International AIDS Society – USA	No
HIV Medicine.com	http://hivmedicine.com	HIV Medicine	No
IDSA	http://www.idsociety.org/	Infectious Diseases Society of America	No
Wikipedia	http://en.wikipedia.org/wiki/AIDS	Wikipedia	No

Treatment Guidelines

Table 82-5

Web Site	Web Address
NIH	http://aidsinfo.nih.gov/
IDSA – HIV MA	http://www.idsociety.org/HIVMA_Template.cfm?Section=HIVMA_HIV_AIDS_Practice_Guidelines
Johns Hopkins	http://www.hopkins-aids.edu/guidelines/guidelines.html
CDC	http://www.cdc.gov/hiv/topics/treatment/index.htm
UCSF	http://hivinsite.ucsf.edu/InSite?page=md-01-01
AEGIS	http://www.aegis.com/ni/topics/treatmnt.asp
Wikipedia	http://en.wikipedia.org/wiki/Talk:AIDS/treatment_guidelines

Drug Interactions

Table 82-6

Web Site	Web Address
US Food and Drug Administration	http://www.fda.gov/cder/index.html
University of Liverpool	http://www.hiv-druginteractions.org/
The Body	http://www.thebody.com/pinf/interact.html
Corey Nahman	http://www.coreynahman.com/antiHIVdrugdatabase61499.html
UCSF – HIV Insite	http://hivinsite.ucsf.edu/arvdb?page=ar-00-02
NY State Department of Health AIDS Institute	http://www.hivguidelines.org/public_html/a-drug/a-drug.htm
Project Inform	http://www.projectinform.org/fs/druginter.html
Toronto General Hospital	http://www.tthhivclinic.com/interact_tables.html

Clinical Trials and Vaccine Development

Table 82-7

Web Site	Web Address
AIDS Clinical Trial Information Service	http://www.actis.org
NIH Clinical Trials Site	http://clinicaltrials.gov
ACTG (AIDS Clinical Trial Group)	http://aactg.s-3.com/
Pediatric AIDS Clinical Trials Group	http://pactg.s-3.com/INDEX.HTM
AMFAR	http://www.amfar.org
Canadian HIV Trials Network	http://www.hivnet.ubc.ca/ctn.html
Initio	http://www.ctu.mrc.ac.uk/initio
ACRIA	http://www.acria.org
Forum for Collaborative HIV Research	http://www.hivforum.org
HIV Vaccine Trials Network	http://www.hivtn.org
MACS Study	http://www.statepi.jhsph.edu/macs/macs.html
Office of AIDS Research	http://www.nih.gov/od/oar/
HIV Vaccine Trials Network	http://www.hvtn.org/
NIH – HIV vaccine status	http://www.niaid.nih.gov/hivvaccines/statuslinks.htm
WHO vaccine initiative	http://www.who.int/vaccine_research/diseases/hiv/en/
International AIDS Vaccine Initiative	http://www.iavi.org/
HIV InSite status of HIV vaccine development	http://hivinsite.ucsf.edu/InSite?page=kb-02-01-06
South African HIV Vaccine Initiative	http://www.saavi.org.za/

reporting trial results to the public, and for recruiting patients to participate in trials. Table 82-7 lists websites that perform these functions for HIV therapies and for HIV vaccine-related trials.

RESEARCH SITES AND DATABASES

Biologists have been using resources on the World Wide Web for years to help them with ongoing research projects. These tools are very useful to AIDS researchers who have expanded and created specific tools to foster the understanding of HIV biology and therapy. The National Library of Medicine (NLM) provides access to MEDLINE, AIDSLINE, AIDSDRUGS, and AIDSTRIALS through PubMed (http://www.pubmed.gov). These databases allow access to the available scientific and clinical literature about HIV and AIDS. In addition to the general databases from the NLM, there are HIV specific databases (Table 82-8) available that are particularly useful to AIDS researchers. These include HIV sequence databases, HIV resistance databases, and websites that report statistics about HIV and AIDS. The AIDS Reagent Program (http://www.aidsreagent.org) provides a resource for researchers to obtain biological materials for use in HIV-related research.

Research and Database sites

Table 82-8

Web Site	Web Address
Medline	http://ncbi.nlm.nih.gov
HIV Sequence databank	http://hiv-web.lanl.gov
HIV ATIS	http://www.hivatis.org
HIV RT and Protease database	http://hivdb.stanford.edu/hiv/
HIV Protease database	http://www.ncifcrf.gov/HIVdb
AIDS Reagent program	http://www.aidsreagent.org
Anti-HIV compound list	http://www.niaid.gov/daids/dtpdb
CDC – HIV Statistics	http://www.cdc.gov/hiv/topics/surveillance/basic.htm
Avert – Global HIV Statistics	http://www.avert.org/
NAM – Global HIV Statistics	http://www.aidsmap.com/

United States Government AIDS-Related Information Sites

Table 82-9

Web Site	Web Address
NIAID	http://www.niaid.nih.gov/research/daids/htm
CDC HIV information	http://www.cdc.gov/hiv/
CDC National Prevention Information Network	http://www.cdcnpin.org
Food and Drug Administration	http://www.fda.gov/oashi/aids/hiv.html
AIDS Treatment Information Site	http://www.hivatis.org

Global Organizations

Table 82-10

Web Site	Web Address
UNAIDS	http://www.unaids.org
WHO	http://www.who.int/topics/hiv_infections/en/
ONE	http://www.one.org
DATA	http://www.data.org
Bill and Melinda Gates Foundation	http://gatesfoundation.org/GlobalHealth/Pri_Diseases/HIVAIDS/
Elizabeth Glaser Pediatric AIDS Foundation	http://www.pedaids.org/
Global AIDS Alliance	http://www.globalaidsalliance.org/
The Global Fund	http://www.theglobalfund.org/

UNITED STATES GOVERNMENT AND GLOBAL ORGANIZATION WEBSITES

Agencies within the US government report significant information on their websites. Table 82-9 lists the US government websites with the most useful information. Similarly, many websites are dedicated to fighting the global HIV pandemic. Some of the most significant organizations and their websites are listed in Table 82-10.

CONFERENCES AND MEETINGS

Many websites (Table 82-11) list upcoming scientific and clinical meetings as well as report on meetings as they occur.

Conference and Meeting Web Sites

Table 82-11

Web Site	Web Address
The IAPAC list of clinical meetings	http://www.iapac.org/
16th meeting on AIDS 2006	http://www.aids2006.com
Conference on Retroviruses and Opportunistic Infections	http://www.retroconference.org
ICAAC	http://www.asm.org
Meeting reviews at The Body	http://www.thebody.com/confs/confcov9798.html

Web Blogs

Table 82-12

Web Site	Web Address
TAG (Treatment Action Group)	http://tagbasicscienceproject.typepad.com/tags_basic_science_vaccin/
AIDS.about.com	http://aids.about.com/
Politics/HIV	http://blogs.law.harvard.edu/politicshiv/
AIDS Matters	http://www.aidsmatters.org/
Aetiology	http://scienceblogs.com/aetiology/

Journal Sites

Table 82-13

Web Site	Web Address
AIDS	http://www.aidsonline.com/
AIDS Patient Care and STDs	http://www.liebertpub.com/apc/default.htm
AIDS Research and Human Retroviruses	http://www.liebertpub.com/publication.aspx?pub_id=2
Annals of Internal Medicine	http://www.acponline.org/journals/annals/annaltoc.htm
Antimicrobial Agents and Chemotherapy	http://intl-aac.asm.org/
Antiviral Chemistry and Chemotherapy	http://www.intmedpress.com/IMPWeb/Journals/AVCC/avcchome.htm
Antiviral Therapy	http://www.intmedpress.com/IMPWeb/Journals/AVT/avthome.htm
British Medical Journal	http://www.bmj.com/
Cell	http://www.cell.com/
Clinical Infectious Diseases	http://www.journals.uchicago.edu/CID/home.htm
Emerging Infectious Diseases	http://www.cdc.gov/ncidod/eid/index.htm
HIV Clinical Trials	http://www.thomasland.com/_nonsearch/hctissues.htm
International Journal of STDs and AIDS	http://www.catchword.co.uk/titles/rsm/09564624/contp1-1.htm
Journal of Acquired Immune Deficiency Syndromes	http://www.jaids.com
Journal of the American Medical Association	http://jama.ama-assn.org
Journal of the Association of Nurses in AIDS Care	http://www.sagepub.com/Shopping/Journal.asp
Journal of Immunology	http://www.jimmunol.org/
Journal of Infectious Diseases	http://www.journals.uchicago.edu/JID/
Journal of Virology	http://jvi.asm.org
Lancet	http://www.thelancet.com/
Morbidity and Mortality Weekly Report	http://www.cdc.gov/mmwr
Nature	http://www.nature.com/
Nature Medicine	http://medicine.nature.com/
New England Journal of Medicine	http://www.nejm.org/content/index.asp
Pediatrics	http://www.pediatrics.org/
Public Library of Science	http://www.plos.org
Proceedings of the National Academy of Sciences	http://www.pnas.org/
Science	http://science-mag.aaas.org/

More recently, web blogs, or blogs for short (discussed next) report up to the minute news from major HIV clinical meetings.

WEB BLOGS (BLOGS)

A recent phenomenon on the World Wide Web has been the emergence of web blogs, or blogs for short. Blogs are websites that are regularly updated and usually are dedicated to a particular topic. They often publish news before other news outlets. Blogs also can provide a community to people who regularly post at these sites. Some blogs document the experience of persons living with HIV/AIDS (Table 82-12). Others, such as the Treatment Action Group Blog, focus on news about HIV-related research and therapies. The Conference on Retroviruses and Opportunistic Infections was "live-blogged" by a number of major HIV-related websites (e.g., Project Inform, http://www.projinf.org/conference/croi.html).

JOURNALS

Most peer-reviewed journals are now available online. Some of these are free of charge while others are free when accessed through a network with a site license. Many medical center libraries have thus accumulated electronic libraries containing many medical and scientific journals. Most of the journals allow the user to download copies of articles to their computer in the PDF format. The Acrobat Reader allowing display and printing of the article in its original published form can read the PDF format. Table 82-13 lists the web addresses of journals that are related to HIV and AIDS. Some require a subscription or site license for access to the full text of articles but all allow the viewing of the table contents and article abstracts and usually allows the user to search back-issues for topics of interest. In addition to the list below, the NLM, through PubMed, provides access to the full text of many other scientific journals.

CONCLUSION

The emergence and convergence of the AIDS epidemic and the World Wide Web have changed healthcare, the doctor–patient relationship, and the way science is conducted. Given the architecture of the World Wide Web, many important sites were left off from this list. The best way to get a feel for the amount of information available on the web is to start at one of the general sites like AEGIS and begin "surfing". One has to follow the links and see as to what can be got from the web. Finally, a word of caution: not all of the information available on the World Wide Web has been verified. Therefore, any information should be evaluated as to the source of the information and whether it has been confirmed by another source. The sources always need to be judged in the context of the funding and purpose of the website. The NIH has assembled a guideline on evaluating medical resources on the web (http://nccam.nih.gov/health/webresources/). The sites listed in this appendix have been found to be functional in July 2006 and been determined to provide useful information.

Index

Page numbers followed by the letter f refer to figures and those followed by t refer to tables. Those followed by b refer to boxes.

B

F

G

H

J

K

M

N

O

Q

R

U

W

X

Y

Z

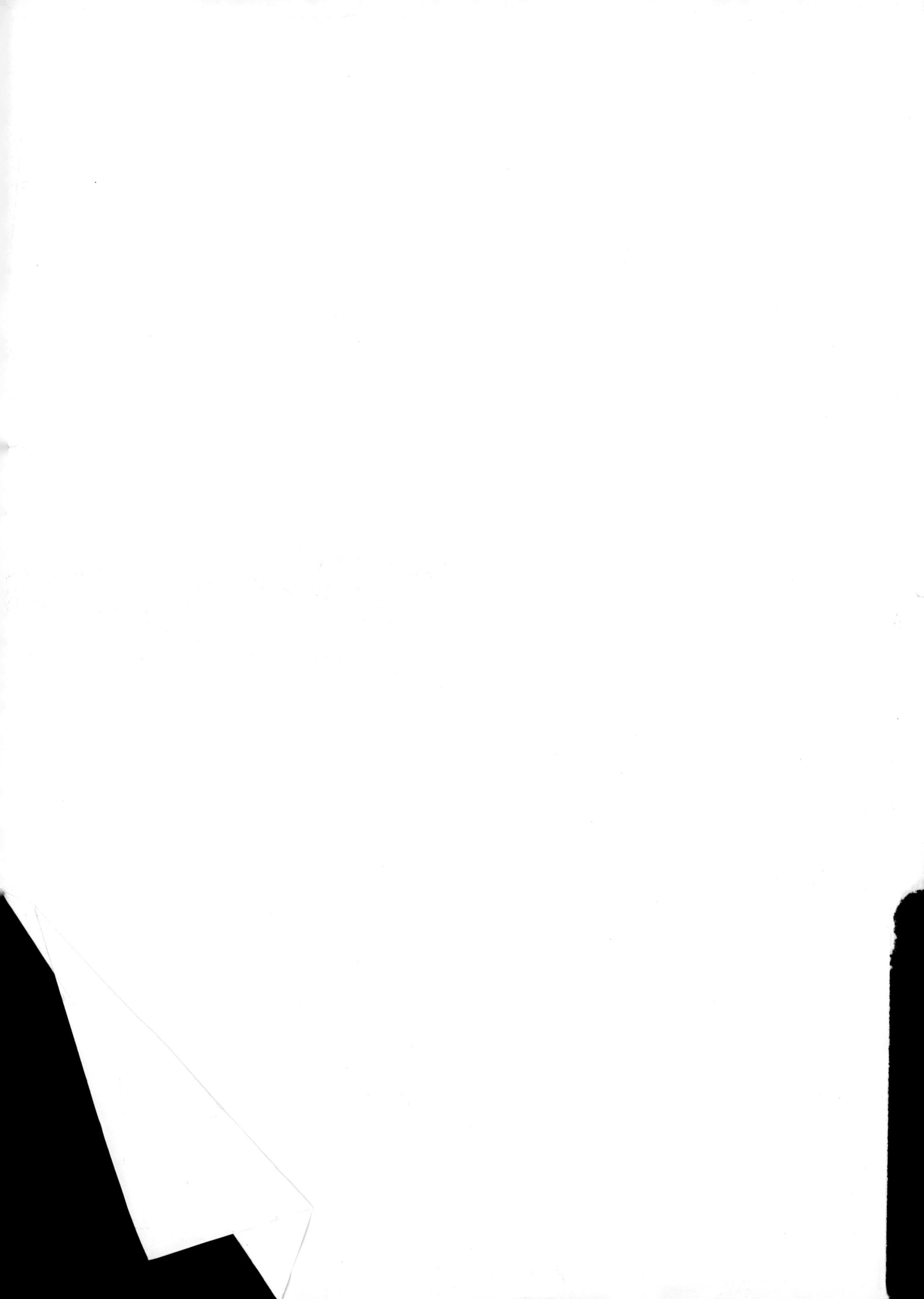